PEDIATRIC NEPHROLOGY

FIFTH EDITION

PEDIATRIC NEPHROLOGY

FIFTH EDITION

Edited By

ELLIS D. AVNER, M.D.

Gertrude Lee Chandler Tucker Professor and Chairman
Case Western Reserve University School of Medicine
Chief Medical Officer and Rainbow Chair for Excellence in Pediatrics
Rainbow Babies and Children's Hospital
Cleveland, Ohio

WILLIAM E. HARMON, M.D.

Associate Professor of Pediatrics
Harvard Medical School
Director, Division of Nephrology
Children's Hospital Boston
Boston, Massachusetts

PATRICK NIAUDET, M.D.

Professor of Pediatrics
Department of Pediatric Nephrology
Hôpital Necker Enfants Malades
Paris, France

with 132 contributing authors

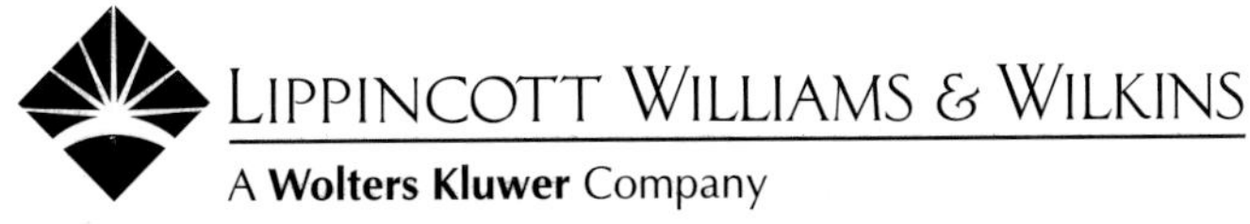

Philadelphia • Baltimore • New York • London
Buenos Aires • Hong Kong • Sydney • Tokyo

Acquisitions Editor: Timothy Y. Hiscock
Developmental Editor: Denise Martin
Supervising Editor: Mary Ann McLaughlin
Production Editor: Brooke Begin, Silverchair Science + Communications
Manufacturing Manager: Ben Rivera
Cover Designer: Christine Jenny
Compositor: Silverchair Science + Communications
Printer: Maple Press

530 Walnut Street
Philadelphia, PA 19106 USA
LWW.com

Printed in the USA

Library of Congress Cataloging-in-Publication Data

Pediatric nephrology / [edited by] Ellis D. Avner, William E. Harmon, Patrick Niaudet.-- 5th ed.
p. ; cm.
Includes bibliographical references and index.
ISBN 0-7817-3545-9
1. Pediatric nephrology. 2. Children--Diseases. I. Avner, Ellis D. II. Harmon, William, 1943- III. Niaudet, P.
[DNLM: 1. Kidney Diseases--Child. 2. Kidney Diseases--Infant. 3. Urinary Tract Infections--Child. 4. Urinary Tract Infections--Infant. WS 320 P371 2003]
RJ476.K5P4344 2003
618.92'61--dc22

2003060615

---

10 9 8 7 6 5 4 3 2 1

CONTENTS

SECTION X: ACUTE RENAL FAILURE 1221

SECTION XI: CHRONIC RENAL FAILURE 1267

SECTION XII: PEDIATRIC NEPHROLOGY AROUND THE WORLD 1479

CONTRIBUTING AUTHORS

Steven R. Alexander, M.D. Professor of Pediatrics, Stanford University School of Medicine; Chief of Pediatric Nephrology, Lucile Packard Children's Hospital at Stanford, Stanford, California

Carmelo A. Alfiler, M.D. Professor of Pediatrics, University of the Philippines Manila College of Medicine, Manila, Philippines

Uri S. Alon, M.D. Professor of Pediatrics, Department of Pediatric Nephrology, University of Missouri—Kansas City School of Medicine, Children's Mercy Hospital, Kansas City, Missouri

Alessandro Amore, M.D. Professor of Nephrology, Department of Nephrology, Dialysis, and Transplantation, Regina Margherita Children's Hospital, Torino, Italy

Sharon P. Andreoli, M.D. Professor of Pediatrics, Indiana University School of Medicine, James Whitcomb Riley Hospital for Children, Indianapolis, Indiana

Corinne Antignac, M.D., Ph.D. Professor of Medicine, Inserm U574 and Department of Genetics, Paris 5 University, Hôpital Necker Enfants Malades, Paris, France

Anthony Atala, M.D. Surgeon, Associate Professor of Surgery, Department of Urology, Children's Hospital, Boston, Massachusetts

Ellis D. Avner, M.D. Gertrude Lee Chandler Tucker Professor and Chairman, Case Western Reserve University School of Medicine; Chief Medical Officer and Rainbow Chair for Excellence in Pediatrics, Rainbow Babies and Children's Hospital, Cleveland, Ohio

Fred E. Avni, M.D., Ph.D. Professor of Radiology, Department of Medical Imaging, Erasme Hospital, Brussels, Belgium

T. Martin Barratt, M.B., F.R.C.P. Emeritus Professor of Paediatric Nephrology and Honorary Consulting Nephrologist, Institute of Child Health, Great Ormond Street Hospital for Children, London, England, United Kingdom

Stuart B. Bauer, M.D. Professor of Surgery, Department of Urology, Harvard Medical School; Senior Associate in Urology, Children's Hospital, Boston, Massachusetts

Jean U. Bender, M.D. Fellow in Nephrology and Pediatric Nephrology, Division of Pediatric Nephrology and Hypertension, University of Texas—Houston Medical School, Houston, Texas

Mark R. Benfield, M.D. Associate Professor of Pediatrics, University of Alabama School of Medicine, Birmingham, Alabama

Rajendra Bhimma, M.D., M.B.Ch.B., D.C.H., M.Med., F.C.P.P. Associate Professor of Pediatrics and Principal Specialist, Department of Pediatrics and Child Health, University of Natal, Durban, South Africa

Melvin A. Bonilla-Felix, M.D. Associate Professor of Pediatrics, University of Puerto Rico School of Medicine, San Juan, Puerto Rico

Ivy I. Boydstun, M.D. Assistant Professor, Department of Pediatrics, SUNY at Stony Brook School of Medicine Health Sciences Center, Stony Brook, New York

Matthias Brandis, M.D. Professor of Medicine, Department of Pediatrics and Adolescent Medicine, Freiburg University Hospital, Freiburg, Germany

Michael C. Braun, M.D. Assistant Professor of Pediatrics, The Institute of Molecular Medicine, University of Texas—Houston Medical School, Houston, Texas

Eileen D. Brewer, M.D. Professor of Pediatrics, Head, Renal Section, Department of Pediatrics, Baylor College of Medicine, Texas Children's Hospital, Houston, Texas

Michel J. C. Broyer, M.D. Professor Emeritus, Department of Pediatric Nephrology, Hôpital Necker Enfants Malades, Paris, France

Timothy E. Bunchman, M.D. Professor of Pediatrics, University of Alabama School of Medicine, Pediatric Nephrology and Transplantation, Children's Hospital of Alabama, Birmingham, Alabama

John R. Burke, M.B., F.R.A.C.P. Associate Professor of Medicine, Department of Nephrology, Royal Children's Hospital, Mater Children's Hospital, Princess Alexandra Hospital, Brisbane, Australia

Suzanne B. Cassidy, M.D. Professor of Pediatrics, University of California, Irvine, College of Medicine, Irvine, California

James C. M. Chan, M.D. Professor of Pediatrics, University of Vermont College of Medicine, Burlington, Vermont; Director of Research, Barbara Bush Children's Hospital, Maine Medical Center, Portland, Maine

Russell W. Chesney, M.D. Le Bonheur Professor and Chair, Department of Pediatrics, University of Tennessee, Memphis College of Medicine, Memphis, Tennessee

Robert L. Chevalier, M.D. Professor and Chair, Department of Pediatrics, University of Virginia Medical Center, Charlottesville, Virginia

Man-Chun Chiu, M.B.B.S., F.R.C.P., F.R.C.P.C.H., F.H.K.A.M. (Paed) Doctor, Department of Pediatrics and Adolescent Medicine, Princess Margaret Hospital, Hong Kong, China

Carol Clayberger, Ph.D. Professor of Pediatrics and Cardiothoracic Surgery, Stanford University School of Medicine, Stanford, California

Pierre Cochat, M.D. Professor of Pediatrics, Hôpital Edouard-Herriot, Lyon, France

Laure B. D. E. Collard, M.D. Department of Pediatrics, Division of Pediatric Nephrology, University of Liège—CHU, CHR, CHC, Liège, Belgium

Christopher S. Cooper, M.D. Chief of Pediatric Urology, Associate Professor of Urology, University of Iowa College of Medicine, Iowa City, Iowa

Rosanna Coppo, M.D. Professor of Pediatric Nephrology, Department of Nephrology, Department of Dialysis and Transplantation, Regina Margherita Hospital, Torino, Italy

Ira D. Davis, M.D. Associate Professor of Pediatrics, Case Western Reserve University School of Medicine; Director of Pediatric Nephrology, Rainbow Babies and Children's Hospital, Cleveland, Ohio

Katherine MacRae Dell, M.D. Assistant Professor of Pediatrics, Case Western Reserve University School of Medicine; Attending Pediatric Nephrologist, Rainbow Babies and Children's Hospital, Cleveland, Ohio

Prasad Devarajan, M.D. Louise M. Williams Endowed Professor of Pediatrics and Developmental Biology, Director of Nephrology and Hypertension, Cincinnati Children's Hospital Medical Center, Cincinnati, Ohio

David A. Diamond, M.D. Associate Professor of Surgery, Department of Urology, Harvard Medical School, Children's Hospital, Boston, Massachusetts

Michael J. Dillon, M.B.B.S., F.R.C.P., F.R.C.P.C.H., D.C.H. Professor of Pediatric Nephrology, Nephro-Urology Unit, Institute of Child Health, Great Ormond Street Hospital for Children, London, England, United Kingdom

Allison A. Eddy, M.D. Professor of Pediatrics, University of Washington School of Medicine, Children's Hospital and Regional Medical Center, Seattle, Washington

Jochen H. H. Ehrich, M.D., D.C.M.T. (London) Professor of Pediatrics, Hannover Medical School, Children's Hospital, Hannover, Germany

Felicia Eke, M.D. Professor of Pediatrics, University of Port Harcourt, Port Harcourt, Rivers, Nigeria

Jack S. Elder, M.D. Carter Kissell Professor of Urology, Case Western Reserve University School of Medicine, Director of Pediatric Nephrology, Rainbow Babies and Children's Hospital, Cleveland, Ohio

Anita Amina Elgendi, M.D. Department of Pediatric Nephrology, Children's Hospital, Hannover, Germany

Francesco Emma, M.D. Pediatric Nephrologist and Co-Director of the Pediatric Nephrology Laboratory, Department of Nephrology and Urology, Bambino Gesù Children's Hospital and Research Institute, Rome, Italy

Ramon Alfonso Exeni, M.D. Professor of Pediatrics, Department of Pediatric Nephrology, University of Buenos Aires, Hospital de Niños de San Justo, Beccar, Buenos Aires, Argentina

Jeffrey Fadrowski, M.D. Fellow, Department of Pediatrics, Johns Hopkins University School of Medicine, Baltimore, Maryland

Leonard G. Feld, M.D., Ph.D., M.M.M. Professor of Pediatrics, UMDNJ—New Jersey Medical School, Newark, New Jersey; Chairman of Pediatrics, Atlantic Health System, Morristown, New Jersey

Richard N. Fine, M.D. Professor and Chair, Department of Pediatrics, SUNY at Stony Brook School of Medicine Health Sciences Center, Stony Brook University Hospital, Stony Brook, New York

Joseph T. Flynn, M.D. Associate Professor of Clinical Pediatrics, Division of Pediatric Nephrology, Albert Einstein College of Medicine of Yeshiva University, Montefiore Medical Center, Bronx, New York

Agnes B. Fogo, M.D. Professor of Pathology, Medicine, and Pediatrics, Department of Pathology, Vanderbilt University Medical Center, Nashville, Tennessee

John W. Foreman, M.D. Professor of Pediatrics, Chief of Pediatric Nephrology, Duke University Medical Center, Durham, North Carolina

Susan L. Furth, M.D., Ph.D. Assistant Professor, Department of Pediatrics and Epidemiology, Johns Hopkins University School of Medicine, Baltimore, Maryland

Gian Marco Ghiggeri, M.D. Nephrology Unit, Researcher, Laboratory on Pathophysiology of Uremia, Department of Pediatrics and Basic Science, G. Gaslini Children's Hospital, Genoa, Italy

Stuart L. Goldstein, M.D. Assistant Professor, Department of Pediatrics, Baylor College of Medicine, Houston, Texas

Paul R. Goodyer, M.D. Professor of Pediatrics, McGill University Faculty of Medicine, Montreal, Quebec, Canada

Ira Greifer, M.D. Professor of Pediatrics, Albert Einstein College of Medicine of Yeshiva University Monte Fiore Medical Center, Bronx, New York

Lisa M. Guay-Woodford, M.D. Professor of Medicine and Pediatrics, University of Alabama School of Medicine, Birmingham, Alabama

Marie Claire Gubler, M.D. Directeur de Recherche, Hôpital Necker Enfants Malades, Paris, France

Jean-Pierre Guignard, M.D. Professor of Pediatrics, Centre Hospitalier Universitaire Vaudois, Lausanne, Switzerland

Michelle Hall, M.D. Professor of Pediatric Nephrology, Queen Fabiloa Brussels Free University; Pediatric Nephrologist, Dialysis and Transplantation, Children's Hospital, Brussels, Belgium

Sverker Hansson, M.D., Ph.D. Associate Professor of Pediatric Nephrology, Pediatric Uro-Nephrologic Center, Queen Silvia Children's Hospital, Göteborg, Sweden

William E. Harmon, M.D. Associate Professor of Pediatrics, Harvard Medical School; Director, Division of Nephrology, Children's Hospital Boston, Boston, Massachusetts

Laurence Heidet, M.D., Ph.D. Hôpital Necker Enfants Malades, Paris, France

John T. Herrin, M.B.B.S., F.R.A.C.P. Associate Clinical Professor of Pediatrics, Harvard Medical School; Director of Dialysis, Children's Hospital Boston, Boston, Massachusetts

Friedhelm Hildebrandt, M.D. Professor of Pediatrics and Human Genetics, Department of Pediatrics and Communicable Diseases and Human Genetics, University of Michigan Medical School, Ann Arbor, Michigan

Christer Holmberg, M.D., Ph.D. Professor of Pediatrics, University of Helsinki, Pediatric Nephrologist, Hospital for Children and Adolescents, Helsinki, Finland

Masataka Honda, M.D. Vice President, Department of Pediatrics, Division of Pediatric Nephrology, Tokyo Metropolitan Hachioji Children's Hospital, Hachioji, Tokyo

Iekuni Ichikawa, M.D., Ph.D. Professor of Pediatrics and Medicine, Department of Pediatric Nephrology, Vanderbilt University Medical Center, Nashville, Tennessee

Kathy Jabs, M.D. Associate Professor of Pediatrics, Director of Pediatric Nephrology, Vanderbilt University Medical Center, Nashville, Tennessee

Hannu J. Jalanko, M.D. Department of Pediatric Nephrology and Transplantation, University of Helsinki, Hospital for Children and Adolescents, Helsinki, Finland

Ulf Jodal, M.D., Ph.D. Professor of Pediatric Nephrology, Pediatric Uro-Nephrologic Center, Queen Silvia Children's Hospital, Göteborg, Sweden

Deborah P. Jones, M.D. Associate Professor of Pediatrics, Memphis College of Medicine, Memphis, Tennessee

Frederick J. Kaskel, M.D., Ph.D. Professor of Pediatrics, Albert Einstein College of Medicine of Yeshiva University; Chief, Section on Nephrology, Vice Chair, Affiliate and Network Affairs, Children's Hospital at Montefiore, Bronx, New York

Phyllis J. Kaskel, M.A., R.D., C.D.N. Director, Department of Clinical Nutrition, Mount Sinai Hospital of the Mount Sinai Medical Center, New York, New York

Marjo K. Kestilä, Ph.D. Senior Research Scientist, Department of Molecular Medicine, National Public Health Institute, Helsinki, Finland

Nine V. A. M. Knoers, M.D., Ph.D. Clinical Geneticist, Professor in Clinical Genetics, Department of Human Genetics, University Medical Centre Nymegen, Nymegen, The Netherlands

Valentina Kon, M.D. Associate Professor of Pediatric Nephrology, Vanderbilt University Medical Center, Nashville, Tennessee

Jordan A. Kreidberg, M.D., Ph.D. Assistant Professor of Pediatrics, Department of Medicine, Harvard Medical School, Children's Hospital, Boston, Massachusetts

Alan M. Krensky, M.D. Shelagh Galligan Professor, Department of Pediatrics, Stanford University School of Medicine, Stanford, California

Beatriz D. Kuizon, M.D. Department of Pediatrics, Kaiser Permanente Los Angeles Medical Center, Los Angelos, California

Craig B. Langman, M.D. Isaac A. Abt, M.D., Professor of Kidney Diseases, Department of Pediatrics, Northwestern University Medical School; Director of Nephrology, Children's Memorial Hospital, Chicago, Illinois

Michael Levin, Ph.D., M.B.B.C.H., F.R.C.P. Professor of Pediatrics, Imperial College London Faculty of Medicine, London, England, United Kingdom

Chanin Limwongse, M.D. Assistant Professor of Medicine, Mahidol University Faculty of Medicine, Siriraj Hospital, Bangkok, Thailand

Chantal Loirat, M.D. Professor of Pediatrics, Department of Pediatric Nephrology, Hôpital Robert Debré, Paris, France

Robert H. K. Mak, M.D., Ph.D. Professor and Chief, Division of Pediatric Nephrology, Oregon Health Sciences University School of Medicine, Portland, Oregon

Sudesh Paul Makker, M.D. Professor and Chief of Pediatric Nephrology, Department of Pediatrics, University of California, Davis, School of Medicine, Davis, California

Ruth A. McDonald, M.D. Associate Professor of Pediatrics, Department of Nephrology, University of Washington School of Medicine, Children's Hospital and Regional Medical Center, Seattle, Washington

Dawn L. McLellan, M.D., F.R.C.S.C. Fellow in Urology, Children's Hospital Boston, Boston, Massachusetts

Dawn S. Milliner, M.D. Professor of Pediatrics and Medicine, Division of Pediatric Nephrology, Mayo Clinic, Rochester, Minnesota

Leo A. H. Monnens, M.D., Ph.D. Professor, Department of Pediatric Nephrology, Nymegen University, Nymegen, The Netherlands

Bruce Z. Morgenstern, M.D. Associate Professor, Department of Pediatric and Adolescent Medicine, Division of Pediatric Nephrology, Mayo Clinic, Rochester, Minnesota

Bahia Hassan Moustafa, M.D. Professor of Pediatrics, Pediatric Nephrology Unit, Cairo University, Children's Hospital, Cairo, Egypt

Corina Nailescu, M.D. Fellow in Pediatric Nephrology, Department of Pediatrics, Albert Einstein College of Medicine of Yeshiva University, Children's Hospital at Montefiore, Bronx, New York

Koichi Nakanishi, M.D. Instructor of Pediatrics, Wakayama Medical University, Wakayama City, Japan

Patrick Niaudet, M.D. Professor of Pediatrics, Department of Pediatric Nephrology, Hôpital Necker Enfants Malades, Paris, France

Amitava Pahari, M.D.D.C.H., D.N.B., M.R.C.P., F.R.C.P.C.H. Senior Consultant, Department of Pediatric Nephrology, Apollo Gleneagles Hospital, Kolkatla, India

Craig A. Peters, M.D. Associate Professor of Surgery, Department of Urology, Harvard Medical School, Children's Hospital Boston, Boston, Massachusetts

Anthony A. Portale, M.D. Professor of Pediatrics, University of California, San Francisco, School of Medicine, San Francisco, California

Ronald J. Portman, M.D. Professor and Director, Division of Pediatric Nephrology and Hypertension, University of Texas—Houston Medical School, Houston, Texas

Gail E. Richards, M.D. Professor of Pediatrics, University of Washington School of Medicine, Children's Hospital and Regional Medical Center, Seattle, Washington

Juan Rodríguez-Soriano, M.D. Professor of Pediatrics, Basque University School of Medicine, Hospital de Cruces, Baracaldo, Spain

Jonathan A. Roth, M.D. Assistant Professor of Urology, University of Virginia School of Medicine, Charlottesville, Virginia

H. Gil Rushton, Jr., M.D., F.A.A.P. Professor of Urology and Pediatrics, George Washington University School of Medicine and Health Sciences, Chairman, Department of Pediatric Urology, Children's National Medical Center, Washington, D.C.

Rémi Salomon, M.D., Ph.D. Pediatric Nephrology, Hôpital Necker Enfants Malades, Paris, France

Isidro B. Salusky, M.D. Professor of Pediatrics, Department of Pediatric Nephrology, University of California, Los Angeles, UCLA School of Medicine, Los Angeles, California

Fernando Santos, M.D. Professor of Pediatrics, Hospital Universitario Central de Asturias and School of Medicine, Asturias, Spain

Franz Schaefer, M.D. Professor of Pediatrics, Pediatric Nephrology Division, University of Heidelberg, Children's Hospital, Heidelberg, Germany

Jon I. Scheinman, M.D. Professor of Pediatrics; Chief, Pediatric Nephrology, University of Kansas Medical Center, Kansas City, Kansas

George J. Schwartz, M.D. Professor of Pediatrics and Medicine, University of Rochester School of Medicine and Dentistry, Rochester, New York

Norman J. Siegel, M.D. Professor of Pediatrics and Medicine, Yale University School of Medicine, New Haven, Connecticut

William E. Smoyer, M.D. Robert C. Kelch Professor, Director, Pediatric Nephrology Division, University of Michigan Medical School, Ann Arbor, Michigan

Michael J. G. Somers, M.D. Assistant Professor of Pediatrics, Division of Nephrology, Harvard Medical School, Children's Hospital, Boston, Massachusetts

C. Frederic Strife, M.D. Professor of Medicine, Department of Nephrology and Hypertension, University of Cincinnati College of Medicine, Cincinnati Children's Hospital Medical Center, Cincinnati, Ohio

Endre Sulyok, M.D., Ph.D., D.Sci. Director and Professor of Pediatrics, County Children's Hospital, Pécs, Hungary

C. Mark Taylor, F.R.C.P. (London), F.R.C.P.C.H. Consultant Pediatric Nephrologist, Senior Clinical Lecturer, Department of Nephrology, Birmingham Children's Hospital, Birmingham, England, United Kingdom

Howard Trachtman, M.D. Professor of Pediatrics, Albert Einstein College of Medicine of Yeshiva University, Schneider Children's Hospital, Bronx, New York

Karl Tryggvason, M.D., Ph.D. Professor of Medical Chemistry, Department of Medical Biochemistry and Biophysics, Karolinska Institutet, Stockholm, Sweden

Rudolph P. Valentini, M.D. Assistant Professor, Director of Dialysis Services, Department of Pediatrics, Wayne State University School of Medicine, Children's Hospital of Michigan, Detroit, Michigan

Scott K. Van Why, M.D. Associate Professor, Department of Pediatrics, Medical College of Wisconsin, Milwaukee, Wisconsin

William G. van't Hoff, M.D., F.R.C.P., F.R.C.P.C.H. Consultant Pediatric Nephrologist, Great Ormond Street Hospital for Children, London, England, United Kingdom

Beth A. Vogt, M.D. Associate Professor of Pediatrics, Case Western Reserve University School of Medicine, Rainbow Babies and Children's Hospital, Cleveland, Ohio

Sam Walters, M.B., F.R.C.P. Senior Lecturer in Pediatric Infectious Diseases, Department of Pediatrics, Imperial College London, London, England, United Kingdom

Bradley A. Warady, M.D. Professor of Pediatrics; Chief, Section of Pediatric Nephrology, Director of Dialysis and Transplantation, Department of Pediatric Nephrology, University of Missouri—Kansas City School of Medicine, Kansas City, Missouri

Sandra L. Watkins, M.D. Professor of Pediatrics, University of Washington School of Medicine, Children's Hospital and Regional Medical Center, Seattle, Washington

Clark D. West, M.D. Emeritus Professor of Pediatrics, Department of Nephrology and Hypertension, University of Cincinnati College of Medicine, Cincinnati Children's Hospital Medical Center, Cincinnati, Ohio

Dilys A. Whyte, M.D. Assistant Professor of Pediatrics, Stony Brook University Hospital, Stony Brook, New York

Patricia D. Wilson, Ph.D. Professor, Department of Medicine, Mount Sinai School of Medicine of the City University of New York, New York, New York

William Wong, M.B.Ch.B., F.R.A.C.P. Pediatric Nephrologist, Starship Children's Hospital, Grafton, Auckland, New Zealand

Adrian S. Woolf, M.D., M.A., F.R.C.P.C.H. Professor of Nephrology, Nephro-Urology Unit, Institute of Child Health, London, United Kingdom

Robert P. Woroniecki, M.D. Assistant Professor of Pediatrics, Division of Pediatric Nephrology, Albert Einstein College of Medicine of Yeshiva University, Montefiore Medical Center, Bronx, New York

Hui-Kim Yap, M.D., M.B.B.S., M.Med. (Pediatrics), F.R.C.P.C.H., F.R.C.P. (Edin) Professor of Pediatrics, National University of Singapore, National University Hospital, Singapore, Chiña

Norishige Yoshikawa, M.D. Professor and Chair, Department of Pediatrics, Wakayama Medical University, Wakayama City, Japan

Israel Zelikovic, M.D. Associate Professor of Pediatrics, Technion—Faculty of Medicine, Director, Department of Pediatric Nephrology, Rambam Medical Center, Haifa, Israel

PREFACE AND DEDICATION

Through its past four editions, *Pediatric Nephrology* has become the standard medical reference for health care professionals treating children with kidney disease. This new edition is focused on providing critical information regarding the evaluation of children with symptoms of renal disease, the molecular and cellular pathophysiology of renal disorders, and the diagnosis and therapy of specific renal diseases in children. The text is particularly targeted to pediatricians, pediatric nephrologists, pediatric urologists, and physicians in training. It is also targeted to the increasing number of allied health professionals involved in the care of children with renal disease, including geneticists, genetic counselors, nurses, dialysis personnel, nutritionists, social workers, and mental health professionals. It is designed to serve the needs of primary care physicians (internists and family practitioners), as well as internist nephrologists who are increasingly involved in the initial evaluation and/or longitudinal care of children with renal disease under the managed care systems of health care delivery evolving throughout the world.

The fifth edition includes a total reorganization of content from previous editions and begins with an overview of the basic developmental anatomy, biology, and physiology of the kidney, which is critical to understanding the developmental nature of pediatric renal diseases. This is followed by a comprehensive presentation of the evaluation, diagnosis, and therapy of specific kidney diseases of childhood, including extensive clinical algorithms. Of particular note is the emphasis on how rapidly evolving research advances in molecular genetics and evidence-based medicine are being translated into new, effective clinical approaches to many children's kidney diseases. To keep pace with the dramatic evolution of pediatric renal medicine since the previous edition, the content of the fifth edition has been extensively revised, with approximately 40% of the chapters being entirely new and the remainder being revised by previous and/or new authors.

As has been the tradition of previous editions, the former senior editor of the text, Professor Martin Barratt, has stepped down, and Professor Ellis D. Avner serves as senior editor of the fifth edition. Professor William E. Harmon continues as second editor, and Professor Patrick Niaudet joins the editorial troika as junior editor for this edition. This rotation of editors continues to provide a dynamic mixture of continuity, new ideas, and new perspectives. The current editors are nationally and internationally recognized leaders in complementary areas of pediatric nephrology and reflect the international nature of the text and the subspecialty it serves. Professor Avner's focused interest is in developmental renal biology and congenital/genetic diseases of the kidney. He serves as Chairman of the Department of Pediatrics at Case Western Reserve University School of Medicine and Chief Medical Officer at Rainbow Babies and Children's Hospital in Cleveland, Ohio, and is the current President of the American Society of Pediatric Nephrology. Professor Harmon is a leading expert in the field of chronic renal failure and its therapy in children. He serves as the Director of Nephrology at Harvard Medical School and The Children's Hospital, Boston, Massachusetts, and is the current President of the American Society of Transplantation and Director of the North American Pediatric Renal Transplant Collaborative Study. Professor Niaudet is an internationally recognized educator and clinician-scientist in the evaluation and treatment of kidney disease in children, with a particular focus on childhood nephrosis. Professor Niaudet directs the Pediatric Nephrology Unit at The University of Paris and the Hôpital Necker Enfants Malades, is the former President of the European Society of Pediatric Nephrology, and currently directs the Continuing Medical Education Programs of the International Pediatric Nephrology Association.

The editors of *Pediatric Nephrology* take pleasure in dedicating the fifth edition of the text to the senior editor of the previous edition, Professor Martin Barratt, C.B.E., F.R.C.P., F.R.C.P.H. Over an extraordinarily productive career as one of the first pediatricians in the United Kingdom to specialize in nephrology, Professor Barratt has held leadership positions in the British Association for Pediatric Nephrology and the International Pediatric Nephrology Association and is internationally recognized for his scientific contributions in the fields of childhood nephrotic syndrome and hemolytic uremic syndrome. His distinguished career predominantly evolved at the Institute of Child Health and the Great Ormond Street Hospital for Children in London, where he served as Director of Clinical Services from 1989 to 1994. In 1992, he was awarded the coveted James Spence Medal of the Royal College of Pediatrics and Child Health. Professor Barratt has the reputation of being the "clinician's clinician" in recognition of his extraordinary clinical skills and acumen as a pediatrician and pediatric nephrologist. His work is distinguished for its clarity and logic—characteristics that he used well in reengineering and guiding *Pediatric Nephrology* through its second, third, and fourth editions. On a personal note, he has an extraordinary sense of humor and the ability to turn the most tedious of editorial tasks into an exciting adventure. He is a keen observer of human nature, finds pleasure in the extraordinary aspects of seemingly ordinary events, and takes great pride in mentoring trainees and junior colleagues. He has been an inspiration to all of the current editors of *Pediatric Nephrology*, as well as to countless trainees, colleagues, patients, and their families.

The editors also wish to acknowledge the outstanding editorial assistance of Shelly Parkhurst (Cleveland), Corinne Fleming (Boston), and Denise Martin, formerly of Lippincott Williams & Wilkins. Their dedicated efforts were essential in the publication of the fifth edition.

Ellis D. Avner, M.D.
William E. Harmon, M.D.
Patrick Niaudet, M.D.

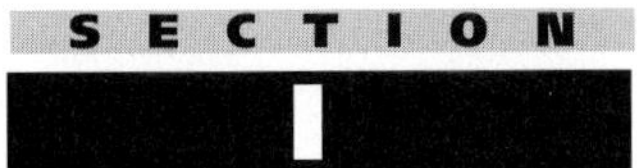

DEVELOPMENT

1

EMBRYOLOGY

ADRIAN S. WOOLF

In the last two decades, considerable advances have been made in understanding the mechanisms that control kidney development (1,2). In previous years, nephrogenesis was described in purely anatomic terms, but we can now interpret many of the key anatomic events as dynamic processes driven by the expression of specific genes. Although our long-term aim is to understand human kidney development, most functional studies have been performed in murine species; therefore, these animal experiments are described in some detail. As is obvious to any pediatric nephrologist, developmental disorders account for a wide spectrum of kidney diseases that cause considerable morbidity and mortality in the first years of life (3–5). Renal malformations, such as agenesis (absence of the kidney) and dysplasia (failure of normal renal differentiation), represent major defects of development, whereas enhanced proliferation, a characteristic of undifferentiated cells, occurs in Wilms' tumor and cystic kidney diseases. Although these diseases are described in detail elsewhere in this book, they are alluded to as illustrative examples of "nephrogenesis gone wrong": In some of these disorders, defined aberrations of cell biology and genetics shed light on normal human kidney development.

ANATOMY OF KIDNEY DEVELOPMENT

Overview

Potter has provided the most complete anatomic description of human kidney development (6). The reader is also referred to more recent reviews (1,2). Three sets of "kidneys" form in mammalian embryos: the pronephros, mesonephros, and metanephros. The metanephros is the direct precursor of the adult kidney, whereas the others essentially involute before birth. The anatomic events of human and mouse nephrogenesis are similar, but the timetable of development differs. Human gestation is 40 weeks, but mouse gestation is 20 days. The metanephros appears 5 to 6 weeks after fertilization in humans and on day 11 in mice. The first metanephric glomeruli form by 9 weeks in humans and day 14 in mice. The final layer of nephrons forms by 36 weeks' gestation in humans, whereas nephrogenesis continues for 1 to 2 postnatal weeks in mice. In addition, there are some anatomic differences. The human mesonephros contains glomeruli with capillary loops, but mouse mesonephric tubules have rudimentary glomerular tufts. Humans have approximately 0.9×10^6 glomeruli in each kidney (7), with a rather large normal range, from 0.7 to 1.0×10^6; mice and rats (8) have proportionately fewer glomeruli per kidney. Finally, whereas the human renal pelvis has multiple papillae, the murine kidney has one. An illustration of the early stages of human metanephric development is depicted in Figure 1.1, and a histologic analysis is shown in Figure 1.2. Figure 1.3 indicates the major cell lineages derived from the metanephros, and Figure 1.4 addresses the formation of blood vessels in the metanephros.

Pronephros and Mesonephros

The mesoderm forms during gastrulation, and embryonic kidneys subsequently develop from nephrogenic cords; masses of intermediate mesoderm, located behind the embryonic coelom between the dorsal somites; and the lateral plate mesoderm. At the height of their development, the pronephros and the mesonephros extend in series from the cervical to lumbar levels. They develop in a segmental manner as tubules that are induced to differentiate from mesoderm by the adjacent pronephric and mesonephric (or wolffian) duct. In humans, the pronephros develops from the third embryonic week and contains rudimentary tubules opening into the pronephric duct. The human mesonephros begins to develop in the fourth week of gestation and contains well-developed nephrons comprising vascularized glomeruli connected to proximal and distal-type tubules draining into the mesonephric duct, a continuation of the pronephric duct. The mesonephric duct extends to fuse with the cloaca, the urinary bladder precursor, at the end of the fourth week. The pronephros and mesonephros can be regarded as a single unit, and as the wave of differentiation spreads caudally, the cranial end of this organ complex begins to regress. By one-third of the way through human gestation, most cells in these organs have involuted. In the male, mesonephric tubules in the area of the gonad

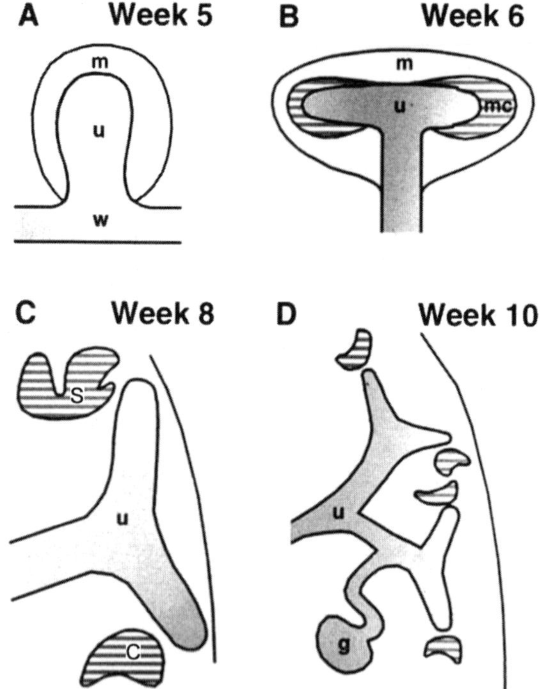

FIGURE 1.1. Early development of the metanephros. Cross-sectional diagrams of the human metanephros at approximately 5 weeks' **(A)**, 6 weeks' **(B)**, 8 weeks' **(C)**, and 10 weeks' gestation **(D)**. Note that the most primitive structures are located in the periphery of the maturing organ. c, comma-shaped body; g, glomerulus; m, mesenchyme; mc, mesenchymal condensate; s, S-shaped body; u, ureteric bud; w, wolffian duct.

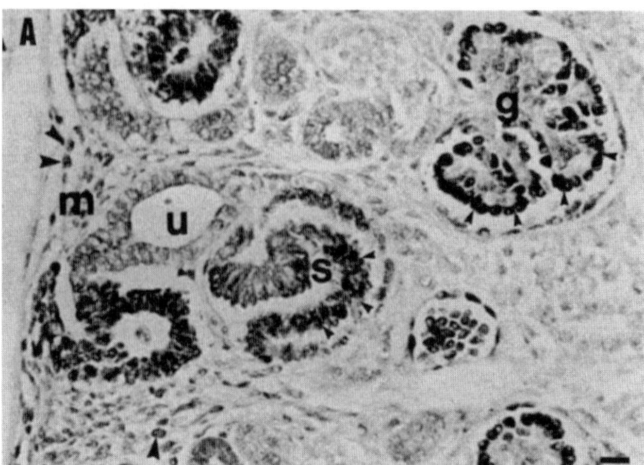

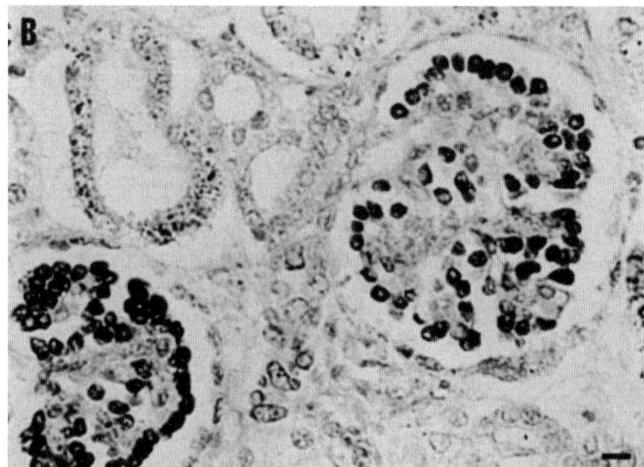

FIGURE 1.2. WT1 immunostaining in human fetal kidneys. **A:** Normal human fetal kidney shows a gradient of WT1 immunoreactivity (*black*) from nephrogenic cortex (*right*) to maturing nephrons (*left*). Cells in condensates and vesicles (*larger arrowheads*) are weakly positive for WT1. Expression increases in the mesenchymal (m) to epithelial transition, with high WT1 levels in the proximal limb of S-shaped bodies (s; *smaller arrowheads*) and the podocytes of fetal glomeruli (g). A ureteric bud branch tip (u) is negative. **B:** Intense WT1 expression is maintained in the podocytes of maturing glomeruli. Bars are 10 μm. (Courtesy of Dr. P. J. D. Winyard, Institute of Child Health, London.)

form the efferent ductules, and the mesonephric duct gives rise to the epididymis and ductus deferens. In the female, some mesonephric tubules persist as the epoophoron and para-oophoron.

Metanephros

The metanephros is the last embryonic kidney to develop and is identified in humans and consists of two components (2). These are the ureteric bud epithelium, which branches from the caudal part of the mesonephric duct at approximately 4 weeks of gestation, and the metanephric mesenchyme, which condenses from the intermediate mesoderm around the enlarging tip, or ampulla, of the bud. The human metanephric kidney can be first identified at approximately weeks 5 to 6 of gestation. The ureteric bud and its branches form epithelia of the collecting ducts, renal pelvis, ureter, and bladder trigone, whereas the metanephric mesenchyme differentiates into nephron tubules (glomerular, proximal tubule, loop of Henle, and distal tubular epithelia) and interstitial fibroblasts. These lineages may be more plastic than previously considered, as discussed later in this chapter. In humans, the renal pelvis and major calyces are apparent by the tenth to twelfth weeks of gestation. The pelvis forms from remodeling of the first six generations of ureteric bud branches, and the minor calyces arise from the next generation of branches. Each minor calyx is associated with 20 ampullae, which will form the papillary collecting ducts: These indent the calyx to form the familiar cup shape seen in intravenous urograms (2).

Up to 14 weeks' gestation, the formation of each new collecting duct is associated with the induction of a nephron from adjacent metanephric mesenchyme. The differentiation of each nephron starts with mesenchymal cell aggregation around ureteric bud branch tips. Each condensate subsequently forms a lumen (the vesicle stage) and elongates to form a tubule (the comma-shaped body), which then shows regional specialization into primitive glomerular and proximal tubular epithelia (the S-shaped body). The proximal end of each S-shape becomes the glo-

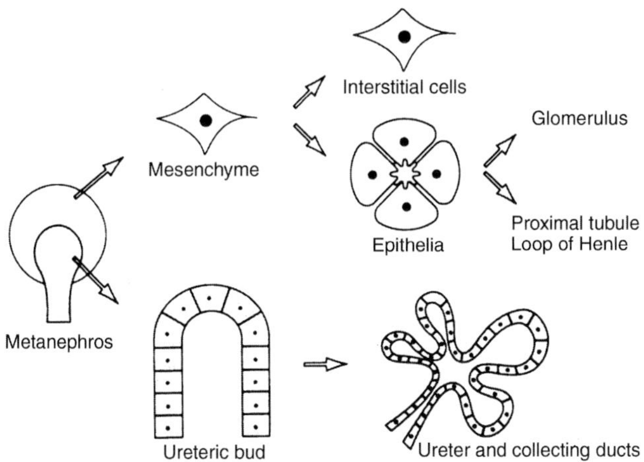

FIGURE 1.3. Main cell lineages arising in the metanephros. (Modified from Hardman P, Kolatsi M, Winyard PJD, et al. Branching out with the ureteric bud. *Exper Nephrol* 1994;2:211–219.)

merular epithelium, whereas the distal end of each tubule fuses with the adjacent branch of the ureteric bud. With each division of the ureteric bud, a new layer of nephrons is induced from stem cells in the periphery of the organ. Between 14 and 20 weeks, each ampulla induces three to six nephrons without dividing. During this process, the connecting tubule of the older, innermost nephron shifts the position of its point of attachment away from the ampulla to the connecting tubule of the next-formed nephron so they are joined together in arcades of four to seven nephrons. Up to 34 to 36 weeks' gestation, the ureteric bud branch tips advance further outward, and another four to seven nephrons form and attach separately just behind the ampullary tips. Thereafter, no new nephrons form, although each tubule continues to mature into the postnatal period. These changes include the elongation of the loops of Henle toward the medulla as well as convolution of the proximal tubule.

The adult kidney is highly vascular and receives approximately 20% of the cardiac output. However, at the inception of metanephric development, no mature vessels are present in the renal mesenchyme. The first patent capillaries are evident around the stalk of the ureteric bud, when it has branched once or twice, and capillaries later appear in the glomerular crevices of the S-shaped bodies (9). The primitive, multilayered, visceral glomerular epithelium subsequently forms a monolayer of podocytes, which abut glomerular capillary loops. At 9 to 10 weeks' human gestation, the most mature nephrons, located toward the center of the metanephros, are the first to acquire capillary loops and a patent Bowman's space. The forming glomerular basement membrane is believed to be synthesized by both the endothelium and epithelium (10). The fusion of the two embryonic membranes and its subsequent biochemical maturation correlate with the progressive restriction of filtration of macromolecules. At its inception, the human

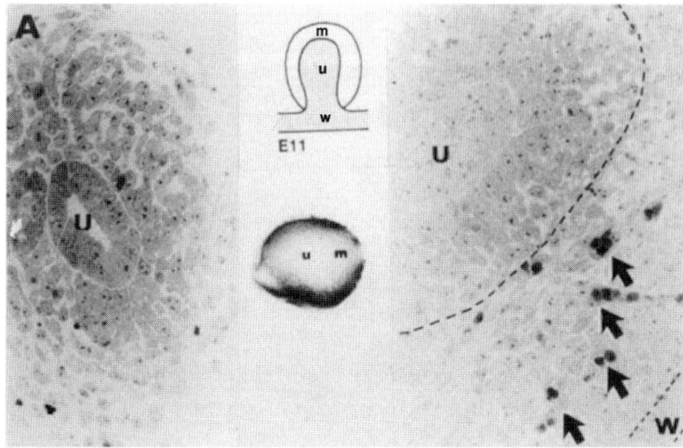

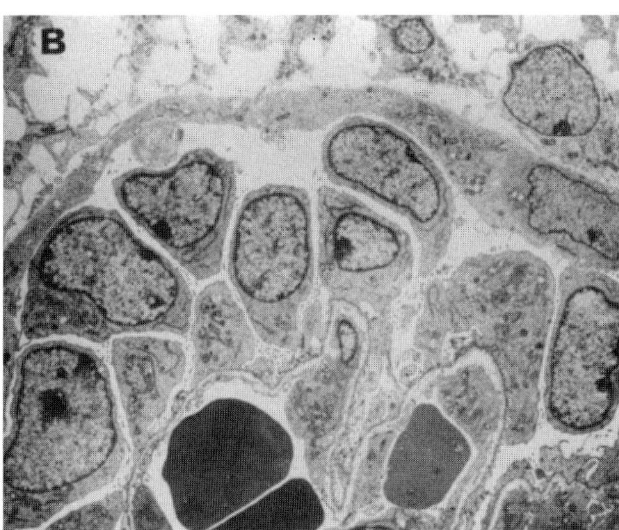

FIGURE 1.4. Capillary formation in the mouse metanephros. **A:** The mouse metanephros at the ureteric bud (u) stage contains no formed capillaries. Center panel shows diagram of the ureteric bud stage above a photograph of the intact organ. Flanking panels are histology sections of the organ in different planes: The right panel shows an area of loose connective tissue and capillaries (*arrows*; between the metanephros itself and the wolffian duct (w). Upper dashed line is lower limit of metanephros and lower dashed line marks upper limit of wolffian duct. **B:** Electron microscope image of a glomerulus that has formed in the metanephros. m, mesenchyme.

metanephros receives its blood supply from the lateral sacral branches of the aorta. As development proceeds, the organ is located at progressively higher levels and is supplied by higher branches of the aorta. By 8 weeks' gestation, the metanephros is located in the lumbar position, and ultimately, the definitive renal arteries arise from the aorta at the level of the second lumbar vertebra (2).

Ureter and Urinary Bladder

The lower urinary tract forms in synchrony with the metanephric kidney (1). The urogenital sinus is the urinary bladder rudiment, and it separates from the rectum by 4 weeks of human gestation. At this time, its epithelium fuses with that of the mesonephric duct, and the ureteric bud arises as a diverticulum from the posteromedial aspect of the mesonephric duct near where it enters the forming bladder. Between 4 and 5 weeks, the human ureter is patent, and it has been assumed because the cloaca is imperforate at that time, mesonephric urine maintains ureteral patency by increasing intraluminal pressure. The mesonephric duct above the ureteric bud becomes the vas deferens in males but involutes in females. At 5 weeks of gestation, the mesonephric duct below the ureteric bud, the "common excretory duct," is absorbed into the urogenital sinus to form the trigone; thereafter, ureteric orifices migrate cranially and laterally. Over the next few weeks, the ureter apparently becomes occluded and then recanalizes, the latter event perhaps coinciding with urine production from the first metanephric glomeruli. The embryonic "ascent" of the metanephros from the level of the sacral segments to the lumbar vertebrae is partly associated with ureteric elongation. The urinary bladder becomes a recognizable entity by approximately 6 weeks of gestation, and the urogenital membrane ruptures at approximately week 7, providing a connection between the bladder and outside of the body. The allantois, another potential outflow tract on the anterior of the developing bladder, involutes by 12 weeks. Toward the end of the first trimester, the ureteric urothelium assumes a pseudo-multilayered arrangement, and its walls become muscularized; by this time, the bladder wall has differentiated into circular and longitudinal smooth muscle fibers which continue to mature in the second trimester. The murine urinary bladder develops in a similar fashion, in synchrony with the metanephros (11).

METHODS USED TO STUDY THE BIOLOGY OF NEPHROGENESIS

Descriptive Studies of Gene Expression

Patterns of cell division, death, differentiation, and morphogenesis can be correlated with changes in spatial and temporal patterns of gene expression in terms of messenger RNA (mRNA) and protein by using *in situ* hybridization and immunohistochemistry (Figs. 1.2 and 1.5). Recently, "gene chip" technology has been used to study the spectrum of genes expressed during murine and human kidney development (12,13). These observations provide the essential data for the generation of hypotheses regarding the molecular control of nephrogenesis; the hypotheses can be tested by studying the effects of diverse interventions during normal development. These functional experiments can be performed in the intact animal, *in vivo*, or "in the test tube," *in vitro*.

Functional Studies *In Vitro*

Experiments performed by Grobstein several decades ago are classic examples of *in vitro* studies (14). Grobstein found that the mouse metanephros forms a small kidney in organ culture over days. Of note, other branching organs, such as the lung and the salivary gland, can also be grown in the same manner (Fig. 1.6). If either the renal mesenchyme or the ureteric bud were cultured in isolation, however, Grobstein noted that they failed to differentiate. This clearly demonstrated that embryonic tissue interactions are critical for kidney development, and we now know that growth factors are important signaling molecules involved in these inductive processes. Growth may be modulated in organ culture with antisense oligonucleotides that impair the transcription of metanephric mRNAs or with antibodies that block the bioactivity of secreted or cell surface proteins (15–17). Other technologic advances have made it feasible to transfer new genes into the metanephros *in vitro* (18–20). Qiao and Herzlinger used retroviral transduction to introduce a reporter gene into renal mesenchymal cells; they subsequently demonstrated that these precursors not only formed nephron tubules, as expected, but also differentiated into a minor proportion of cells within collecting duct epithelia (20). Finally, the generation of metanephric cell lines has made it feasible to study the expression of multiple genes in homogeneous populations of precursors (16) as well as in normal and abnormal differentiation of these cells in response to defined stimuli (21).

Functional Studies *In Vivo*

In vivo experiments on developing kidneys have used physical, teratogenic (e.g., chemical), and genetic strategies. For example, surgical interruption of the avian mesonephric duct prevents the conversion of intermediate mesoderm into mesonephric tubules and also prevents the formation of the metanephros (22). Complete obstruction of the sheep fetal ureter in midgestation generates hydronephrotic kidneys, with generation of cysts and disruption of nephrogenesis resembling human renal dysplasia (23,24). With regard to teratogenic studies, an example is the generation of urinary tract malformations after exposure to ethanol (25). Welham et al. (8) reported that the imposition of mild (9%) dietary protein restriction during rat pregnancy reduced numbers of glomeruli per kidney of offspring when measured postnatally. This was associated with enhanced apoptotic deletion of renal mesenchymal precursors at the start of metanephrogenesis (8). In humans, the equivalent developmental time frame is 5 to 7 weeks' gestation, and this might represent a critical window when fetal kidney morphogenesis is susceptible to maternal dietary influences.

The most powerful *in vivo* experiments, however, alter the expression of metanephric molecules by genetic engineering using transgenic animal technology. First, levels of a specific protein can be increased by inserting a coding DNA sequence, linked to a strong promoter, into the genome of early embryos. This is usually done by microin-

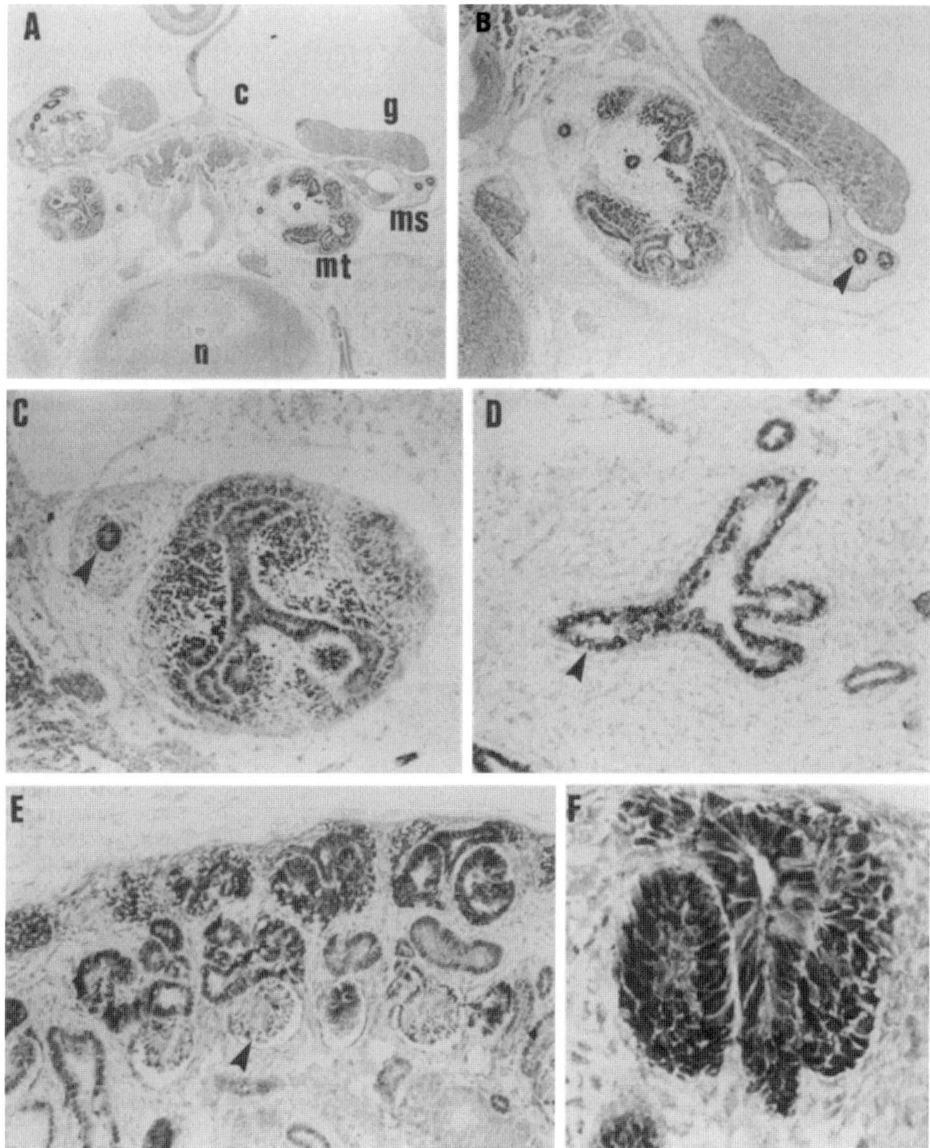

FIGURE 1.5. Early human metanephros (mt) and the mesonephros (ms). Sections are stained with antibody to PAX2 transcription factor: Positive nuclei appear black, whereas others are counterstained with methyl green and appear gray. **A:** Transverse section of a 5- to 6-week gestation of human embryo showing, on each side of the embryo, a mesonephros, a metanephros, and a gonadal ridge (g) (×5). Also shown is the central notochord (n) in a mass of cartilage that will form the vertebral body, and the coelom (c). **B:** Enlarged view of **A**. Note the mesonephros duct (*arrowhead*) stains for PAX2, as does the flanking paramesonephric duct (×10). **C:** High power of metanephros containing the first branches of the ureteric duct with adjacent mesenchymal condensates. The mesonephros duct (*arrowhead*) is nearby (×20). **D:** Medulla of an 11-week human kidney shows a major branch of the fetal ureter (*arrowhead*) branching to form collecting ducts: Most nuclei in these structures stain for PAX2 (×20). **E:** Cortex of an 11-week human fetal kidney shows presence of a nephrogenic outer cortex with increasingly mature nephrons and glomeruli (*arrowhead*) toward the center of the organ. Note that PAX2 is down-regulated in more mature elements (×20). **F:** High-powered image of **E**. Intense staining for PAX2 in the branch tip of a ureteric bud and the flanking renal mesenchymal condensates (×63). (Courtesy of Dr. P. J. D. Winyard, Institute of Child Health, London.)

jection into the male pronucleus of fertilized ova. The phenotype of such mice illustrates the effects of an excess of a molecule (26). Even more informative is the technique of homozygous recombination in which the function of a gene can be ablated. Here, mouse embryonic stem cells are genetically engineered *in vitro* and then incorporated into early embryos that develop into chimeric mice. If the altered cells contribute to the germline, animals with homozygous and heterozygous gene deletions can be generated by further breeding (27). The phenotypes of these null

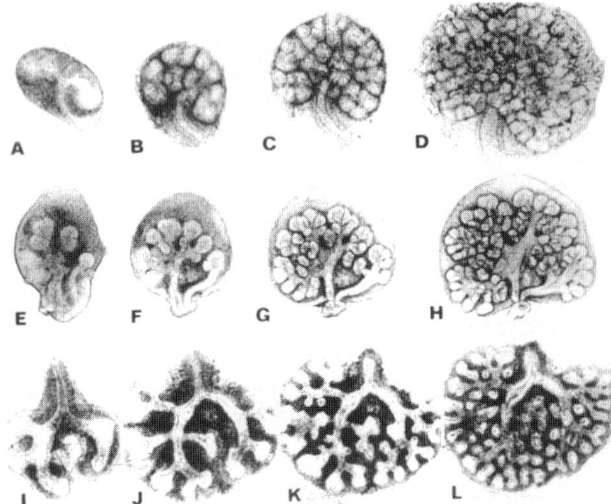

FIGURE 1.6. Growth of mouse embryonic tissues in organ culture. Note branching morphogenesis occurs over 1 week in organ culture. **A–D:** The metanephros. **E–H:** The salivary gland. **I–L:** The lung. (Modified from Hardman P, Kolatsi M, Winyard PJD, et al. Branching out with the ureteric bud. *Exp Nephrol* 1994;2:211–219.)

mutant or "knock-out" mice, which include the complete absence of metanephric development, have so far suggested that approximately 30 genes are essential for normal nephrogenesis *in vivo* (Table 1.1). Many of these animal models also have defects in nonrenal systems because the same genes are expressed in, and critical for, the normal development of organs other than the kidney.

Hundreds of molecules are known to be expressed during nephrogenesis (28), and tens of these have been considered to be functionally important based on organ culture studies. However, mice with null mutations of the same genes sometimes have normal kidney development *in vivo*. Hence, we can speculate that numerous metanephric molecules are of little functional significance or are redundant in the intact fetus. It also follows that organ culture must constitute a relatively stressful milieu in which it is comparatively easy to disrupt development by altering levels of a single molecule. Of note, the genetic background, or strain, of mice with defined mutations can affect the kidney phenotype, suggesting the presence of modifying genes (29). When two structurally similar molecules are expressed at identical locations in the metanephros, both loci may have to be ablated to generate a renal malformation *in vivo* (30,31).

TABLE 1.1. NULL MUTANT MICE WITH RENAL MALFORMATIONS

Transcription factor genes
BF2 (small, fused, and undifferentiated kidneys)
EYA1 (absent kidneys)
EMX2 (absent kidneys)
FOXC1/FOXC2[a] (duplex and hypoplastic kidneys)
HOXA11/HOXD11[a] (small or absent kidneys)
LIM1 (absent kidneys)
LMX1B (poorly formed glomeruli)
N-MYC (malformed mesonephric kidneys)
PAX2[b] (small or absent kidneys)
SALL1 (failure of ureteric bud outgrowth)
WT1[b] (absent kidneys)
Growth factors and receptor genes
Angiotensin II receptor 1 (poor papillary growth)
AT2 (diverse kidney and lower urinary tract malformations)
EGFR (cystic collecting ducts)
BMP4 (kidney and ureter malformations)
BMP7 (undifferentiated kidneys)
FGF7 (small kidneys with fewer glomeruli)
GDNF[b] and its receptor, *RET* (small or absent kidneys)
NOTCH2 (malformed glomeruli)
PDGFB chain and its receptor, *PDGFR*β (absent mesangial cells)
WNT4 (undifferentiated kidneys)
Adhesion molecules and receptor genes
α_3 *integrin* (decreased collecting duct branching)
α_8 *integrin* (impaired ureteric bud branching and nephron formation)
GPC3 (dysplastic kidneys)
s-laminin/laminin β_2 (nephrotic syndrome)
Other genes
BCL2 (small kidneys)
COX2 (small kidneys)
Formin (absent kidneys)
MPV17 (nephrotic syndrome)
Neuronal NOS (bladder outflow impairment)
RAR$\alpha\gamma/\alpha\beta_2$[a] (small or absent kidneys)
Uroplakin III (hydronephrosis and vesicoureteric reflux)

Note: Many mutants have aberrations of other organ systems: Please see references for details. Unless otherwise stated, the renal abnormalities are detected only in homozygous null mutant animals (i.e., both alleles of one gene are nonfunctional).
[a]Null mutations of two homologous but separate genes are required to produce the malformation.
[b]In these cases, heterozygous null mutations produce kidney malformations that are less severe than the homozygotes. In all other cases, heterozygotes appear to have normal nephrogenesis.

CELL BIOLOGY OF NEPHROGENESIS

Cell Proliferation and Cell Death

Proliferation is prominent in the tips of the ureteric bud branches and in the adjacent mesenchymal cells in the nephrogenic cortex of the metanephros (32). Renal mesenchymal stem cells are believed to reside within this area, and such cells are believed to divide to generate a copy of themselves and also another cell. These cells subsequently differentiate into nephron epithelia or interstitial cells (21). More recent evidence, discussed later in this chapter, suggests that cells in the renal mesenchymal compartment can also differentiate into glomerular capillaries and juxtaglomerular cells. Stem cells are generally considered to be absent from the mature kidney; although if they did exist, they might provide a source of cells for the regeneration of nephron epithelia after injury.

Not all cells born in the developing kidney are destined to survive the fetal period. In 1926, Kampmeier reported that the first layers of metanephric nephrons "disappeared" before birth (33), a process likely to be associated with the remodeling of the first divisions of the ureteric bud during formation of the pelvis. More recently, others have reported the normal occurrence of cell death in the mesenchyme adjacent to primitive nephrons, where it may regulate the number of cells in each tubule or the number of nephrons formed (8). These cells die by apoptosis, a process accompanied by nuclear condensation and fragmentation. These deaths are sometimes called *programmed* because they are part of the normal program of development, and each cell "commits suicide" by an active program of biochemical events, including digestion of genomic DNA into fragments of approximately 200 nucleotides by calcium-dependent endonucleases. Apoptosis also occurs in the developing medulla (Fig. 1.7) and it has been suggested that this process is implicated in the morphogenesis of the thin ascending limb of the loop of Henle (34) and also in deleting excess beta intercalated cells in the collecting duct (35).

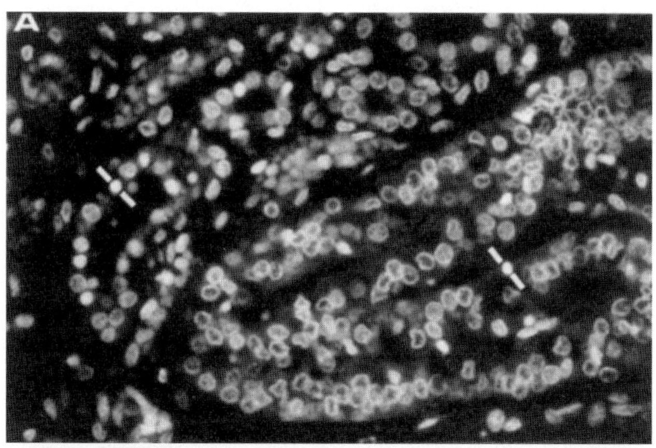

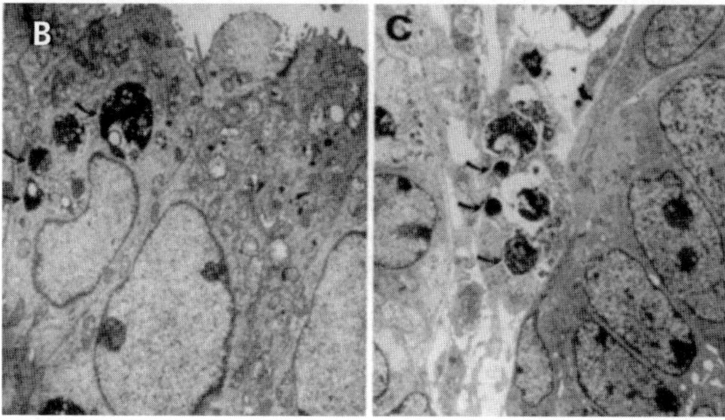

FIGURE 1.7. Cell death in normal nephrogenesis. **A:** Apoptotic cell death is detected in the outer medulla of the human metanephros, as assessed by bright, condensed, propidium-iodide–stained nuclei (between the *white bars*) in primitive loops of Henle and other tubules, probably collecting ducts (×63). (Courtesy of Dr. P. J. D. Winyard, Institute of Child Health, London.) **B,C:** Electron microscope images of the medulla of a mouse metanephros to show apoptotic nuclei (*curved arrows*) being engulfed by epithelial cells **(B)** and cells within the interstitium **(C)**.

Therefore, normal nephrogenesis involves a fine balance between cell proliferation and death. Excessive proliferation is associated with the generation of neoplasms (e.g., Wilms' tumor) and cysts (e.g., polycystic kidney diseases) (36). Conversely, excessive apoptosis would cause a reduction of kidney growth resulting in an organ with fewer nephrons than normal (e.g., a hypoplastic kidney) or even involution of a metanephric kidney (e.g., some dysplastic kidneys) (37,38).

Differentiation

As individual renal precursor cells become specialized, they undergo differentiation. For example, some renal mesenchymal cells differentiate into primitive nephron epithelia, whereas others differentiate into stromal cells or interstitial fibroblasts (39). Precursor cells later become "terminally differentiated" to enable them to perform specific functions of the adult organ. For example, cells within a nephron precursor form the glomerular parietal and visceral epithelia as well as the cells that comprise the proximal tubule and loop of Henle. The term *lineage* describes the series of phenotypes as a precursor differentiates into a mature cell.

Morphogenesis

Morphogenesis describes the developmental process by which groups of cells acquire complex three-dimensional shapes. Examples include the formation of nephron tubules from renal mesenchymal cells and the serial branching of the ureteric bud to form the collecting duct system. The process of morphogenesis also occurs during angiogenesis and vasculogenesis; modes of renal capillary formation is discussed later in this chapter (9). Angiogenesis also involves the fundamental cellular process of directional movement or migration.

MOLECULAR CONTROL OF NEPHROGENESIS

Overview

Three main classes of molecules are expressed during nephrogenesis: transcription factors, growth/survival factors, and adhesion molecules. Note that italics are used when referring to genomic sequences, whereas regular typescript is used for gene products (e.g., *PAX2* gene and PAX2 mRNA or protein). The following criteria should be satisfied for a molecule to be definitively involved in normal nephrogenesis: It must be expressed by the metanephros in an appropriate spatial or temporal manner; functional experiments should demonstrate that its absence perturbs kidney development in organ culture and *in vivo*; and the molecule should have appropriate bioactivity on isolated populations of precursor cells. At present, few molecules have been shown to fulfill all three criteria.

Transcription Factors

Transcription factor proteins bind to DNA and regulate expression of other genes. Because they can enhance or switch off the transcription of mRNAs, transcription factors have been likened to conductors of an orchestra during normal development. These molecules can be classified into families that share similar DNA-binding protein motifs and domains. One such motif is called the *zinc-finger*, which describes a projection of the molecule that intercalates with DNA. An example of a transcription factor with multiple zinc-fingers is the WT1 protein, which is expressed at the inception of the metanephros (32). Other examples of transcription factors expressed during nephrogenesis include members of the HOX family, which contain DNA-binding homeodomains, as well as the PAX family, which contain DNA-binding paired domains (40). At present, little is known about the specific targets of many of the transcription factors expressed in the developing kidney.

Growth Factors

The metanephros is rich in growth factors that modulate cell survival, proliferation, differentiation, and morphogenesis (41). Factors that have a positive effect on growth are epidermal growth factor (EGF), transforming growth factor (TGF) α, fibroblast growth factor (FGF)-2, glial cell line–derived neurotrophic factor (GDNF), hepatocyte growth factor (HGF), insulin-like growth factor (IGF)-1 and -2, keratinocyte growth factor (KGF; also called *FGF-7*), leukemia inhibitory factor, neurotrophin 3, pleiotrophin, and TGFβ. Factors that have been reported to have a negative effect on growth include activin, TGFβ, and tumor necrosis factor-α (TNF-α). In some cases, a single factor can have multiple effects by virtue of binding to more than one different receptor; for example, angiotensin (AT) II generally acts to promote growth through its type 1 receptor but also stimulates apoptosis through the AT 2 receptor (42).

When acting on the neighboring cell, growth factors are *paracrine* factors, but when acting on the producing cell, they are *autocrine* factors. Growth factors bind to cell-surface receptors, many of which are receptor tyrosine kinases that, after ligand binding, dimerize and become phosphorylated, thereafter transducing signals into the cell. Factors acting via receptor tyrosine kinases include angiopoietin, EGF, TGFα, FGFs, HGF, IGF-1 and -2, KGF, neurotrophin 3, nerve growth factor, platelet-derived growth factor A and B chains, and vascular endothelial growth factor (VEGF). Others, including bone morphogenetic proteins (BMP) types 4 and 7 and TGFβ, bind receptors with threonine and serine kinase activity. GDNF is a distant relative of TGFα but signals through a receptor tyrosine kinase after binding to an accessory receptor. Yet, other metanephric growth factors, including AT, leukemia inhibitory factor, and TNF-α, signal through different classes of receptors.

Adhesion Molecules

The third major class of molecules comprises the adhesion molecules (43). Some mediate the attachment of cells to one another, whereas a second group mediates attachment of cells to the surrounding matrix. Examples of the former include neural cell adhesion molecule, whose adhesive properties are independent of calcium, and E-cadherin, whose adhesive properties depend on calcium. Molecules in the second group include collagen, fibronectin, laminin, nidogen, and tenascin. Many bind to cell surfaces via integrin receptors to provide a physical framework for epithelial tubules and endothelia. Some of these interactions also modulate growth and differentiation in an analogous fashion to the binding of growth factors to their receptors. Proteoglycans, including syndecan and heparan sulfate, constitute another type of adhesion molecule. They also bind growth factors, such as FGFs and VEGF, hence sequestering and storing these molecules as well as modulating their binding to receptor tyrosine kinases.

CONVERSION OF METANEPHRIC MESENCHYME INTO NEPHRON EPITHELIA

Uninduced Metanephric Mesenchyme Is Preprogrammed to Form Nephrons

Isolated metanephric mesenchyme can be induced to form nephrons *in vitro* by recombination with the ureteric bud or by apposition to embryonic spinal cord. However, mesenchyme from other embryonic organs cannot be stimulated to produce nephrons by either the ureteric bud or heterologous inducers (14). Hence, by the time the metanephros can first be detected, the renal mesenchyme has already been programmed to form nephrons, but it requires additional, inductive signals from the ureteric bud to permit its differentiation. The molecules responsible for this preprogramming of the renal mesenchyme are currently undefined. The transcription factor LIM1 is expressed in the intermediate mesoderm before it forms the renal mesenchyme, and the metanephros fails to form in mice, which lack LIM1 (44). However, the embryonic expression of this gene is widespread, and diverse nonrenal organs are malformed in null mutants.

Uninduced Metanephric Mesenchyme Is Preprogrammed to Die

When cultured in isolation, murine renal mesenchyme fails to survive. In contrast, the recombination with either ureteric bud epithelium or embryonic spinal cord rescues mesenchymal cells from death and induces them to form nephrons.

Koseki et al. demonstrated that death of the isolated renal mesenchyme was mediated by apoptosis and that it was an active process, as assessed by a requirement for mRNA and protein synthesis (45). They also reported that isolated renal mesenchyme could be rescued from death by the addition of EGF (the adult homolog of TGFα) or by phorbol ester (a chemical that enhances the activity of protein kinase C). Perantoni et al. reported that FGF-2 could also facilitate survival of isolated renal mesenchyme (46)—an important observation considering that the ureteric bud secretes this factor (47). Barasch et al. (48) have reported that metalloproteinase-2 stimulates mesenchymal growth by preventing this cell population from dying.

The *WT1* gene produces multiple transcripts, some of which act as transcription factors, whereas others are likely to affect splicing of mRNA before export from the nucleus (49). WT1 is expressed at low levels in metanephric mesenchyme, and levels are upregulated during differentiation into nephron precursors (32) (Fig. 1.2). *In vivo*, absence of WT1 protein causes fulminant death of the intermediate mesoderm, which would normally form the metanephric mesenchyme, producing renal agenesis (50). A similar final phenotype can be generated in mice that are homozygous null mutants for *PAX2*, *formin,* or *GDNF/RET.* In these cases, the primary defect is a failure of outgrowth of the ureteric bud from the mesonephric duct: The defect in the renal mesenchyme is secondary to the loss of its normal inducing tissue *in vivo*. Nishinakamura et al. (51) have recently reported that mesenchymal expression of the SALL1 transcription factor is necessary for early inductive events in the murine kidney; the human homologue is mutated in the Townes-Brocks syndrome, a disorder associated with urinary tract malformations.

Condensation of Renal Mesenchyme

The first morphologic step in nephron formation is the aggregation of renal mesenchymal cells to form a condensate. At the same time, these nephrogenic precursor cells undergo a burst of proliferation and upregulate the expression of the transcription factors WT1 (32), PAX2 (Fig. 1.5) (32), and N-MYC. Other genes that are switched on or upregulated include MET (the HGF receptor) (Fig. 1.8) (52), $\alpha_8\beta_1$ integrin (53), and BCL2 (32). Inhibition of PAX2 by antisense oligonucleotides prevents condensation in metanephric organ culture (54), and mice lacking one copy of the *PAX2* gene are born with small kidneys (27,55). Mice with homozygous mutations of *N-MYC* have malformed mesonephric tubules but die before development of the metanephros (56). HGF induces epithelioid characteristics in MET-transfected 3T3 embryonic fibroblasts (57), a model for the conversion of mesenchymal into epithelial cells. This growth factor also induces the expression of epithelial markers in a murine renal mesenchymal cell line (58). Mice deficient in α_8 integrin have small, severely malformed kidneys,

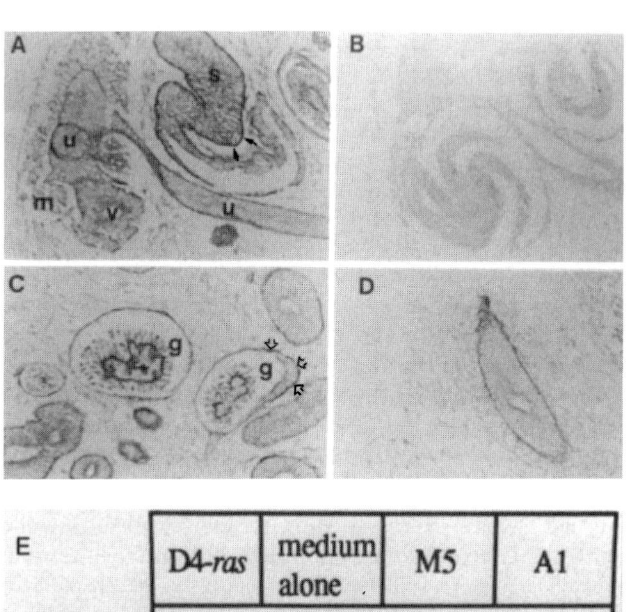

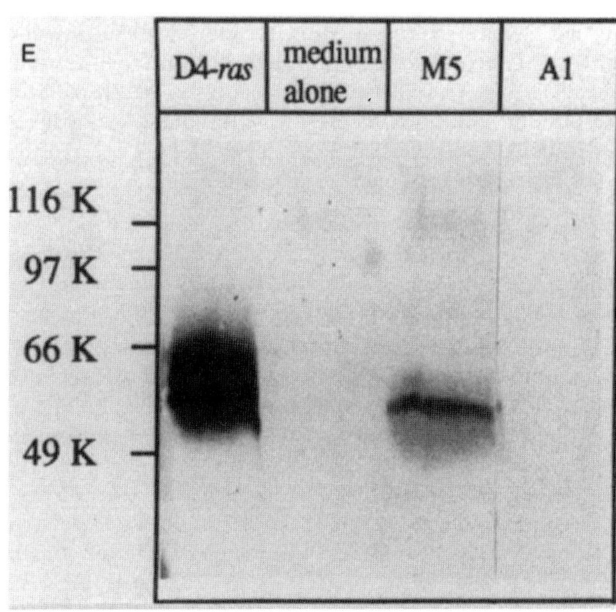

FIGURE 1.8. Hepatocyte growth factor and its receptor, MET, in the normal metanephros. **A–D:** Nine-week gestation of human metanephros. **A:** Positive MET staining in ureteric bud branches (u) and primitive nephrons, such as vesicles (v) and S-shaped bodies (s). Note marked staining on basal surface of primitive epithelia (*arrows*). Condensing renal mesenchyme (m) expresses a much lower level of MET in the cytoplasm. **B:** Similar field as **A**, after primary antibody was preabsorbed with MET peptide: no specific staining. **C:** MET staining in basal surface of epithelia of Bowman's capsule (*open arrows*) of fetal glomeruli (g). Mesangial and endothelial cells in the fetal glomeruli are MET-positive. **D:** The stalk of the ureteric bud shows positive MET immunostaining on the basal epithelial surface (immunostaining appears black). **E:** By Western blot, HGF protein is detected at 62 kDa in conditioned media from D4-*ras* NIH 3T3 cells (positive control) and from a mouse renal mesenchyme cell line (M5) but was not present in media from a more mature metanephric clone (A1) or in unconditioned medium. [Panels **A–D** from Kolatsi-Joannou M, Moore R, Winyard PJD, et al. Expression of hepatocyte growth factor/scatter factor and its receptor, MET, suggests roles in human embryonic organogenesis. *Pediatr Res* 1997;41:657–665; panel **E** from Woolf AS, Kolatsi-Joannou M, Hardman P, et al. Roles of hepatocyte growth factor/scatter factor and the MET receptor in early development of the metanephros. *J Cell Biol* 1995;128:171–184, with permission.]

with defective nephron formation and impaired ureteric bud branching (53). A ligand for $\alpha_8\beta_1$ integrin dimers is expressed on the surface of ureteric bud branches; therefore, these molecules most likely coordinate morphogenetic interactions between the mesenchymal condensate and the ureteric bud epithelium. BCL2 is located in the nuclear and mitochondrial membranes and prevents apoptosis, perhaps by interfering with lipid peroxidation. Homozygous null mutant mice have fulminant renal apoptosis during development and are born with small kidneys containing fewer nephrons than normal (renal hypoplasia) (37,59).

Putting the above experiments together, the following scenario can be envisaged: WT1 appears necessary for the induction and survival of renal mesenchymal cells; PAX2 and HGF/MET may drive the proliferation of nephron precursors; BCL2 may protect cells in the condensate stage from an untimely programmed death; and $\alpha_8\beta_1$ integrin plays a role in aggregation of nephron precursor cells around the ureteric bud branch tips. The application of either FGF-2 or lithium ions to uninduced renal mesenchyme *in vitro* appears to stimulate differentiation up to but not beyond this stage of mesenchymal condensation (46,60).

Morphogenesis into Nephron Tubules

Next, the mesenchymal condensate forms a lumen and differentiates into an increasingly mature nephron via the vesicle, comma shaped, and S-shaped stages. This process is associated with the replacement of the intermediate filament vimentin by cytokeratin in all segments apart from glomerular podocytes. In addition, there are profound changes of expression of adhesion molecules. The neural cell adhesion molecule becomes downregulated (61), whereas E-cadherin appears at sites of cell-cell contact (adherens junctions) in the primitive nephron (17). Numerous studies have implicated the latter molecule as playing a part in the genesis of epithelia (62,63). At the same time, the expression of the extracellular matrix molecules, collagen I and fibronectin, are downregulated, and primitive tubular epithelia begin to synthesize a basement membrane containing collagen IV, laminin, heparan sulfate, and nidogen (17,43). Evidence from organ culture experiments supports the concept that the interaction of laminin-1, a cruciform trimeric molecule, with a cell-surface receptor, $\alpha_6\beta_1$ integrin, is essential for lumen formation of the primitive nephron (17,64). Other interactions of laminin-1 with the α-dystroglycan complex (located on the cell surface) and with nidogen (a mesenchymal-derived matrix protein) are also critical for epithelial morphogenesis (65,66). As the nephron epithelia differentiate further into specific segments, other integrins are expressed: α_3 subunit is found in glomerular podocytes and binds laminin, and the α_2 subunit is expressed by distal tubules and collecting ducts and interacts with collagen IV and laminin (43). As the glomerular epithelium matures, the basement membrane becomes rich in s-laminin, the β_2 chain of laminin. Mice without the gene encoding this protein develop an infantile nephrotic syndrome, despite the presence of grossly normal-appearing glomeruli at birth (67).

Other types of molecules have been implicated in the growth of primitive nephrons. WNTs are glycoproteins, which are believed to be secreted signaling factors. WNT4, a member of this family, is upregulated in renal mesenchymal cells as they differentiate into nephrons and may have an autocrine role in this process. Mice with *WNT4* homozygous null mutations have metanephroi in which the renal mesenchyme is induced but "frozen" at the condensate stage (68). BMPs are members of the TGFβ superfamily and transduce growth signals through types 1 and 2 receptor serine/threonine kinases. BMP-7 is expressed by the branches of the ureteric bud and is also upregulated in primitive nephrons (69,70). Nephrogenesis is impaired in BMP-7 null mutant mice with formation of only a few nephrons and ureteric bud branches. Recent data suggest that leukemia inhibitory factor, a member of the interleukin-6 family, is secreted by the ureteric bud and can transform renal mesenchyme into epithelia, including proximal tubules and glomeruli, acting together with FGF-2 and TGFα (71). Indeed, several growth factors may have a permissive effect on epithelial growth at this stage, including HGF, FGF-2, IGF-1, IGF-2, and TGFα (16,71–73).

At present, little is known about the molecular controls of differentiation of primitive nephrons into the specialized cells in the mature mammalian nephron. However, this type of detailed analysis has been performed for cells in the Malpighian excretory tubule of embryonic *Drosophila* fruit flies (74). In mammals, there is evidence that expression of WT1 is essential for the maintenance of the mature podocyte (32), where it downregulates the transcription of PAX2 (75). In humans, mutation of a single *WT1* allele causes the Denys Drash syndrome in which nephrotic syndrome and structural glomerular abnormalities are key features (76), whereas the transgenic overexpression of PAX2 causes epithelial overgrowth and a congenital nephrotic syndrome in mice (26).

Negative Regulators of Nephrogenesis

The final form of the kidney is determined by not only growth but also negative processes, such as programmed cell death and as yet poorly defined mechanisms that terminate morphogenesis. In organ culture, TNF-α, a classical inflammatory cytokine, inhibits nephron differentiation and morphogenesis at the stage of mesenchymal condensation (77). This protein is localized at mesenchymal/epithelial interfaces and is expressed by renal mesenchymal cells and possibly also by macrophages that populate the metanephros from its inception. Rogers et al. reported that these *in vitro* actions of TGFβ are similar to those of TNF-α (78). Another factor that can inhibit nephrogenesis in organ culture is activin, a TGFβ-like molecule (79).

STROMAL CELL LINEAGE

Little is known about the mechanisms that control the differentiation of renal mesenchyme into stromal cells, or interstitial fibroblasts (80), but there is evidence that stromal cells are essential for epithelial development. For example, the G_{D3} ganglioside is expressed by stromal cells surrounding the stalk of the ureteric bud, and antibodies to this molecule prevent bud morphogenesis (81). Metanephric stromal cells also express the BF2 winged-helix transcription factor. Mice that were homozygous null mutants for this gene have impaired branching of the collecting ducts and also perturbed conversion of renal mesenchyme to nephrons (82). Other evidence emphasizes that metanephric stromal and epithelial cells are involved in complex reciprocal signaling loops, with expression of retinoic acid receptors in the stroma, playing important roles (83). A subset of metanephric stromal cells has neuronal characteristics, staining positively with neurofilament markers (84). The role of these cells is unknown, but their survival can be modulated by neurotrophin 3 (84). Although fibroblasts in the mature kidney are heterogeneous (e.g., only some make the hormone erythropoietin), it is not understood how this diversity is generated.

BRANCHING MORPHOGENESIS OF THE URETERIC BUD

Mesenchymal Factors and Ureteric Bud Growth

When the mouse ureteric bud is grown in organ culture with its adjacent renal mesenchyme, it undergoes branching morphogenesis; however, it fails to differentiate when cultured in isolation (14,85). It is established that the epithelia of the ureteric bud express various receptors, mostly tyrosine kinases that transduce differentiation signals by binding to mesenchyme-derived growth factors (85,86). The most important signaling system involves RET, a receptor tyrosine kinase expressed in mesonephric duct, ureteric bud, and its branching tips. GDNF causes tyrosine phosphorylation of RET after binding to a membrane-linked accessory receptor called GDNF receptor α (87). The ligand is expressed by condensing renal mesenchyme, whereas GDNF receptor α is expressed in the same cells as RET (85). Lower levels of the accessory receptor are found in renal mesenchyme, where it may concentrate the ligand and also prevent its diffusion with initiation of ectopic ureteric bud branches (85). Mice with homozygous null mutations of *RET* or *GDNF* do not develop kidneys because of deficient outgrowth of the ureteric bud (88–92). Experiments using culture of whole metanephric rudiments with blocking antibodies to GDNF demonstrate that this signaling system is critical for stimulation branching after initial outgrowth of the ureteric bud (85). Equally impressive, the addition of recombinant GDNF to cultured metanephroi induces ectopic ureters (85). When the ureteric bud is cultured as a monolayer, it dies by apoptosis over a few days, but GDNF can partially reverse this process (85). The factor also stimulates survival and morphogenesis of RET-transfected collecting duct cells (93). Hence, GDNF is a survival factor and morphogen for the ureteric bud epithelium.

Other metanephric growth factors affect ureteric bud growth. HGF induces branching morphogenesis of Madin-Darby canine kidney collecting duct cells grown in a collagen I matrix. This model system mimics ureteric bud morphogenesis (94). HGF is secreted by renal mesenchymal cells, whereas its receptor, tyrosine kinase MET, is located on the basal surface of ureteric bud epithelia (16,52) (Fig. 1.8). Functional studies demonstrate that HGF is required for growth and branching in metanephric organ culture (16,95,96) (Fig. 1.9). Transgenic mice overexpressing HGF commonly develop renal failure, although details of renal histopathology have not yet been reported (97). Mice with homozygous *HGF* or *MET* null mutations die at embryonic day 13 or 14 with placental, liver, and muscle pathologies, but early nephrogenesis is surprisingly normal (98,99). ROS is another receptor tyrosine kinase expressed in the ureteric bud lineage (100). Its ligand is unknown but is likely to be a mesenchymally derived factor, using the GDNF/RET and HGF/MET signaling systems as paradigms. Antisense oligonucleotides to ROS mRNA cause impaired growth in organ culture (100), but mice with homozygous *ROS* null mutations have normal nephrogenesis *in vivo* (101). Antisense experiments in metanephric organ culture have also implicated low-affinity nerve growth factor receptor in branching (15), but again, mice genetically engineered to lack this molecule have grossly normal nephrogenesis (102). Thus, it is easy to perturb branching morphogenesis in organ culture, but the process is more robust when the whole animal is challenged *in vivo*.

EGF and its embryonic homolog, TGFα, bind to the EGF receptor. EGF induces limited branching of isolated ureteric buds in collagen I gel (103), whereas blocking antisera to TGFα inhibit metanephric development in organ culture (73). Mice with homozygous null mutations of *EGFR* have collecting duct dilation and kidney failure, a strain-dependent phenotype, implicating the activity of modifying genes (29). An isoform of FGF receptor-2 with high affinity for KGF (FGF-7) is expressed in mesonephric duct and its derivatives (104). Furthermore, administration of KGF enhances proliferation of adult urothelial cells *in vivo* (105), whereas the factor modulates ureteric bud morphogenesis in organ culture (106). Finally, pleiotrophin, a heparin-binding protein, has recently been identified as a renal mesenchymal-secreted factor involved in ureteric bud branching (107).

Cell Adhesion Molecules and Ureteric Bud Growth

The stalk of the ureteric bud is surrounded by a basement membrane composed of laminin-1 and collagen IV, as well

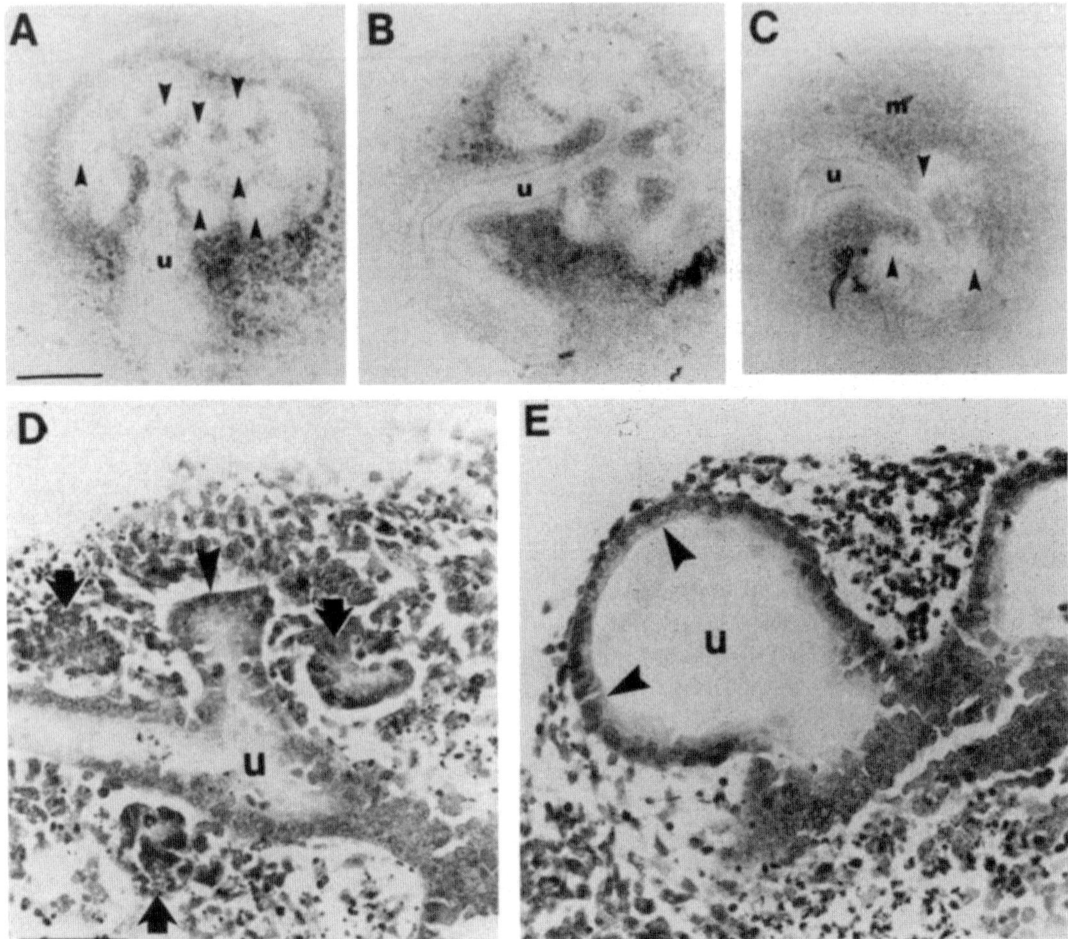

FIGURE 1.9. Blockade of hepatocyte growth factor in metanephric organ culture. **A–C:** Mouse rudiments after 3 days of culture in basal media **(A)**, nonimmune immunoglobulin G **(B)**, and anti-HGF immunoglobulin G **(C)**. Ureteric bud (u) branching and nephron formations are limited in organs treated with anti-HGF antibody. **D,E:** Photomicrographs of sections of a metanephros grown for 3 days in basal medium **(D)** or in the presence of anti-HGF antibody **(E)**. Note the condensations of mesenchyme (m) around the tips of the ureteric bud in **D** compared with the cystic dilation of the bud surrounded by loose mesenchyme with pyknotic nuclei in **E**. Arrowheads indicate the tips of the ureteric bud, and arrows indicate mesenchyme condensates **(D)**. Bars are 100 μm. Arrowheads in **A, C,** and **E** indicate ureteric bud branch tips. (Modified from Woolf AS, Kolatsi-Joannou M, Hardman P, et al. Roles of hepatocyte growth factor/scatter factor and the MET receptor in early development of the metanephros. *J Cell Biol* 1995;128:171–184.)

as nidogen/entactin and tenascin. As assessed by electron microscopy, the basement membrane is attenuated around the tips of the ureteric bud, and branching epithelia may be exposed to a renal mesenchymal matrix rich in collagen I and fibronectin. There is evidence that matrix molecules affect branching morphogenesis *in vitro*. In monolayer culture of ureteric bud epithelia, proliferation is enhanced by a fibronectin versus laminin substrate (85), consistent with the observation that cells at the branching tips have a high proliferation rate (32). Collagen I appears permissive for branching of Madin-Darby canine kidney cells, whereas some components of the basement membrane are inhibitory (108). Using the Madin-Darby canine kidney model, HGF-induced branching into collagen I is accompanied by an increase in matrix degrading molecules (e.g., collagenases, such as matrix metalloproteinases, and plasminogen activating proteases, such as urokinase) (109). TGFβ inhibits its branching and decreases the ratio of matrix-degrading molecules versus others that inhibit this process (e.g., tissue inhibitor of metalloprotease-1 and plasminogen activator inhibitor-1) (109). Further evidence that the basement membrane plays a critical role in collecting duct morphogenesis is provided by experiments that disrupt the signaling of extracellular matrix molecules to the cell surface. Mice genetically engineered to lack α_3 integrin, which forms functional dimers with β_1 subunits, have a reduced number of medullary collecting ducts (110). Finally, galectin-3 is a cell adhesion molecule expressed in the ureteric bud lineage, which may regulate the growth of collecting duct epithelia by interaction with laminin and other extracellular matrix molecules (111,112), whereas polycystin 1, the product of a gene mutated in autosomal-dominant polycystic kidney disease, is a putative cell adhesion molecule expressed in the ureteric bud lineage (113).

Transcription Factors and Ureteric Bud Growth

As yet, little is known about how the expression of transcription factors orchestrates the expression of growth factors and matrix molecules that directly affect the morphogenesis of the ureteric bud lineage. PAX2 appears to be particularly important because it is expressed in the mesonephric duct and in the ureteric bud branch tips (32,112). The expression of PAX2 in the human ureteric bud lineage correlates with proliferation, and both are downregulated as the ducts mature (32). In mice genetically engineered to lack PAX2, the ureteric bud fails to branch from the mesonephric duct, producing renal agenesis (27). Finally, mice lacking the expression of formin show no outgrowth of the ureteric bud from the mesonephric duct. The function(s) of this gene, which produces multiple transcripts, is unclear (114).

Further Differentiation of Collecting Ducts

As the bud branches, the stems mature into the collecting ducts, which contain three types of cells: the potassium-handling principal cells and the proton-handling α and β intercalated cells (115). Corticosteroids enhance collecting duct differentiation, and there is also some plasticity regarding the lineage of these cells based on *in vitro* studies (116,117). During this period of maturation, the Na^+-K^+–adenosine triphosphatase becomes relocated from the apical to basal plasma membrane, and this process is perturbed in some polycystic kidney diseases (118). Other cells that arise from the ureteric bud differentiate into the pseudostratified urothelium, which lines the renal calyces, pelvis, and ureter: The KGF receptor is expressed by these cells and the administration of KGF enhances urothelial proliferation *in vivo* (106). The human fetal ureter is not patent in early gestation, but the mechanisms of its canalization are unknown (119): a failure of this process is believed to occur in human multicystic dysplastic kidneys (3). AT II, acting through its AT 1 receptor, has recently been shown to be important for maturation of the ureter, partly by enhancing peristalsis and partly by a direct effect on morphogenesis (120).

FORMATION OF GLOMERULAR CAPILLARIES

Embryonic blood vessels arise by vasculogenesis or angiogenesis (9). In vasculogenesis, mesenchyme differentiates *in situ* to form capillaries. In contrast, angiogenesis involves ingrowth from existing capillaries. The first embryonic vessels of the yolk sac, endocardium, and dorsal aorta arise by vasculogenesis, but thereafter, descriptive studies alone cannot ascertain the origin of embryonic vessels. When avascular murine renal mesenchyme is induced to differentiate in organ culture, the glomeruli that develop lack capillaries as assessed by light and electron microscopy (121), a result used to argue against the possibility of glomerular vasculogenesis. When mouse metanephroi were transplanted onto avian chorioallantoic membranes, forming glomeruli acquired capillary loops but these were of host origin as assessed by a quail-specific nuclear marker and antisera to chick collagen IV, a component of endothelial basement membrane (10,122). These results were used to argue that glomerular vessels form by angiogenesis *in vivo*. However, neither organ culture nor chorioallantoic membrane is likely to provide a normal environment for growth of glomerular capillaries.

During endothelial differentiation, cells in the lineage express a defined sequence of receptor tyrosine kinases (9): VEGF receptor (VEGFR)-2, VEGFR-1, TIE2, and TIE1. VEGF is expressed at sites of embryonic vessel formation and is a ligand for VEGFR-1 and VEGFR-2, whereas angiopoietin 1 is a ligand for TIE2. VEGFR-1/-2 and TIE1 are expressed by uninduced metanephric mesenchyme, hence suggesting the presence of endothelial precursors (123). When a *TIE1/LACZ* transgenic mouse was used, in which a β-galactosidase reporter gene product can be detected histochemically, endothelial precursors were visualized in intermediate mesoderm condensing around the caudal end of the mesonephric duct, with a similar pattern noted in renal mesenchyme at the ureteric bud stage (123,124). Later in nephrogenesis, TIE1/LACZ was expressed by all endothelia, including glomerular endothelia. Loughna et al. (123) determined whether these precursors could differentiate into endothelia using a model in which metanephroi form filtering glomeruli after transplantation into the neonatal nephrogenic cortex (125). When transgenic avascular metanephroi were transplanted into wild-type hosts, differentiated donor tissue contained transgene-expressing glomerular arterioles and capillary loops (123) (Fig. 1.10). Other experiments support the conclusion that glomerular capillaries originate from endothelial precursors present at the inception of nephrogenesis. When wild-type mouse metanephroi were grafted into the anterior eye chamber of adult *ROSA26* transgenic mice, a strain in which the β-galactosidase reporter gene is expressed in all cells, glomerular endothelia were found to be of donor origin (126). Moreover, exposure of murine metanephroi to hypoxia increases endothelial growth in organ culture, whereas other experiments in mice and rats have demonstrated that addition of VEGF or angiopoietin-1 enhance the formation of metanephric capillaries in organ culture (127,128). One can speculate that capillary formation within the metanephros is at least in part driven by hypoxia and that low oxygen tension increases expression of diverse vascular growth factors and their receptors.

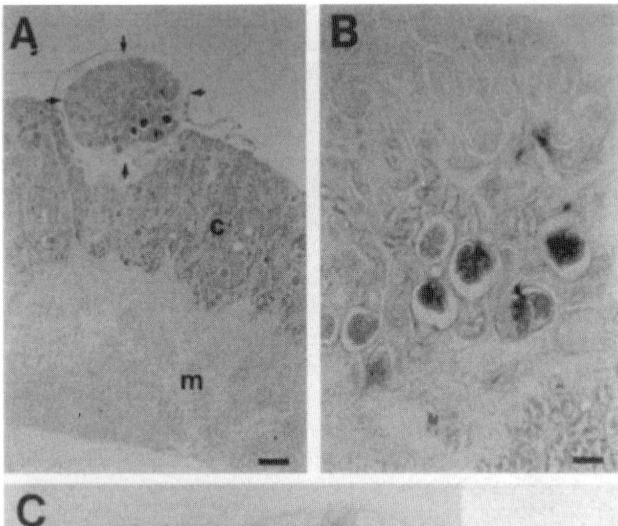

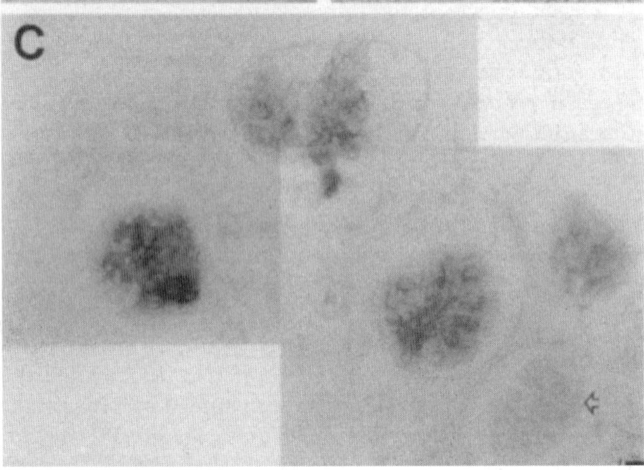

FIGURE 1.10. Transplantation of *TIE1/LACZ* metanephroi into wild-type neonates. **A:** After 1 week, the E11 transplant differentiated (*arrows*) in the host cortex (c). Transgene expression (black) was confined to the transplant. No staining was detected in host cortex or medulla (m). **B:** Donor glomeruli expressed the transgene intensely. **C:** Positive capillary loops in glomeruli are visible. Podocytes (*open arrow*) do not express the transgene. Bars: 120 μm in **A**; 30 μm in **B**; and 10 μm in **C**. (From Loughna S, Hardman P, Landels E, et al. A molecular and genetic analysis of renal glomerular capillary development. *Angiogenesis* 1997;1: 84–101, with permission.)

Other molecules are implicated in vascular growth within the metanephros. These include the Eph/ephrin family of membrane receptors, which appear to be critical in cell-cell recognition (129). Renin is widely expressed in perivascular cells in the arterial system of the metanephros but becomes restricted to juxtaglomerular cells during maturation. Recent evidence suggests that the metanephric mesenchyme contains renin-expressing precursor cells (130). In addition, other molecules required to generate bioactive AT are expressed in the metanephros, as are AT 1 and AT 2 receptors. In rats, there is evidence that AT II may enhance glomerular endothelial growth *in vivo* (131,132). This axis is also important in fetal glomerular hemodynamics, as discussed elsewhere in this text (see Chapter 2).

MESANGIAL CELL LINEAGE

It has been speculated that mesangial cells arise from the same lineage as glomerular capillaries because neither cell forms when the metanephros is cultured under standard organ culture conditions (121). It was assumed that mesangial cells were derived from cells outside the embryonic kidney. However, mesangial cells develop when metanephroi are grown *in oculo* (126), and thus, mesangial precursor cells may be present in renal mesenchyme. Whatever their origin, platelet-derived growth factor B and its receptor, tyrosine kinase platelet-derived growth factor receptor β, are crucial for the differentiation of mesangial cells *in vivo*. Mice with null mutations of either of these genes lack mesangial cells and develop bizarre, malformed glomeruli (133,134). Platelet-derived growth factor B is expressed by primitive nephron epithelia, and mesangial precursors express the receptor, suggesting a paracrine mode of action. As mesangial cells mature, both ligand and receptor are coexpressed, suggesting autocrine activity. Other growth factor–signaling systems may play roles in development of this lineage. For example, HGF and MET are coexpressed by immature mesangial cells (135).

NEURONS IN EARLY NEPHROGENESIS

Grobstein found that when an embryonic spinal cord was placed on the opposite side of a filter from metanephric mesenchyme, nephrons were induced to differentiate (14). Further investigations showed that neurons had penetrated the mesenchyme through the microscopic pores of the filter, and if the neurons in the spinal cord were destroyed, induction did not occur (136). As assessed by antibodies against neurofilaments and neural cell surface gangliosides, neuronal cell bodies can be observed around the ureteric bud *in vivo*, and their terminals surround mesenchymal condensates (137). These observations support the hypothesis that kidney development may partly depend on innervation. It is also interesting that embryonic neural tissues are capable of inducing the formation of mesonephric tubules from intermediate mesoderm (138).

HUMAN RENAL MALFORMATIONS: NEPHROGENESIS GONE WRONG

Overview

Renal malformations are the major causes of end-stage renal failure in children (3–5) (see Chapter 6). The term *renal malformation* encompasses a heterogeneous group of developmental aberrations. In the most extreme example, renal agenesis, the kidney is absent. *Renal dysplasia* describes an organ comprised of undifferentiated and metaplastic cells

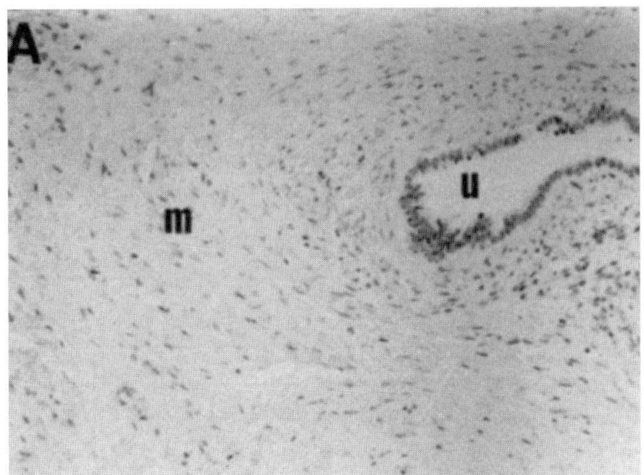

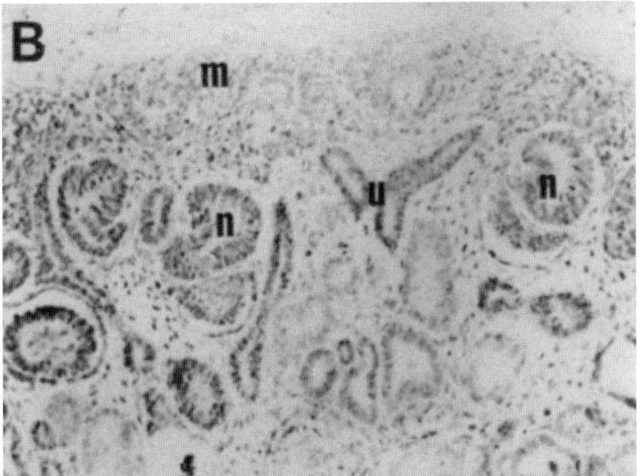

FIGURE 1.11. Histology of a human dysplastic kidney. **A:** Typical histology of a human dysplastic kidney. Primitive ducts, believed to be branches of the ureteric bud (u), are surrounded by undifferentiated tissue that superficially resembles normal renal mesenchyme (m). Note that no nephrons have differentiated from the mesenchyme compartment. **B:** For comparison, this plate shows a normal human metanephros or embryonic kidney at 10 weeks after fertilization. Note that there is a superficial similarity to the dysplastic kidney depicted in **A** because both structures contain primitive ureteric bud ducts and mesenchyme. In the normal embryonic kidney, however, there is evidence of conversion of mesenchyme to epithelial nephron precursors (n). (Courtesy of Dr. P. J. D. Winyard, Institute of Child Health, London.)

surrounding poorly branched ureteric bud derivatives (Fig. 1.11). These organs may be tiny (renal aplasia) or large enough to distend the abdomen (multicystic dysplastic kidneys). A hypoplastic kidney is small and has fewer nephrons than normal. These nephrons may be grossly enlarged in oligomeganephronia. Associated malformations of the urinary tract include agenesis, duplications, obstruction, and vesicoureteric reflux.

Renal Malformations as Dynamic Processes

The above classification of renal malformations is based on pathologic end points. Yet it is now known that normal kidney development is a highly dynamic process of proliferation, death, morphogenesis, and differentiation controlled by the temporal and spatial expression of specific genes (discussed above). It is interesting to reassess multicystic dysplastic kidneys with these perspectives in mind. Serial ultrasound scans performed both prenatally and postnatally have shown that some of these organs can increase to a massive size only to subsequently regress and even involute completely (139). Epithelia lining dysplastic cysts have a high rate of proliferation and overexpress both PAX2, a potentially oncogenic transcription factor, and BCL2, a survival molecule (32). Other evidence also suggests that mesenchymal-derived growth factors, such as TGFβ, HGF (Fig. 1.12), and IGFs, are involved in dysplastic epithelial growth (52,140,141). Conversely, undifferentiated tissues around cysts have a high rate of apoptosis associated with a lack of BCL2 expression, and these cells fail to form nephrons (38). Hence, phases of growth and involution correlate with cellular events and aberrant expression of nephrogenesis genes. An understanding of the dynamics that underlie these malformations now allows potential therapies, especially the administration of growth factors that prevent apoptosis and enhance normal differentiation into nephrons, to be envisaged (19). The deregulated expression of genes such as PAX2, BCL2, and TGFβ, although intriguing, is likely to be a secondary event. A major question remains: What are the primary causes of human malformation? To date, there are at least three answers: teratogens, physical obstruction of the urinary tract, and sporadic or inherited mutations of genes expressed in the developing kidney (2,142).

Teratogens

As discussed, animal experiments have implicated a wide variety of agents, including vitamin A and ethanol, as renal teratogens. In humans, both glucose (i.e., mothers with diabetes) (143) and AT-converting enzyme inhibitors (used to treat maternal hypertension) are associated with renal malformations. It is unusual, however, to elicit a history of exposure to known teratogens from the parents of children with renal malformations, but it remains possible that occult exposure is important. For example, a recent study suggested that the incidence of various malformations, including those of the genitourinary tract, was increased with a daily intake of vitamin A over 10,000 IU (144).

Physical Obstruction of the Developing Urinary Tract

It has long been recognized that a significant minority of kidney malformations in girls and perhaps half of all malformations in boys are associated with obstructed lower urinary tracts (3–5). Obstruction during the last third of gestation is associated with hydronephrosis, poor renal parenchymal growth, and subcortical cysts, whereas kid-

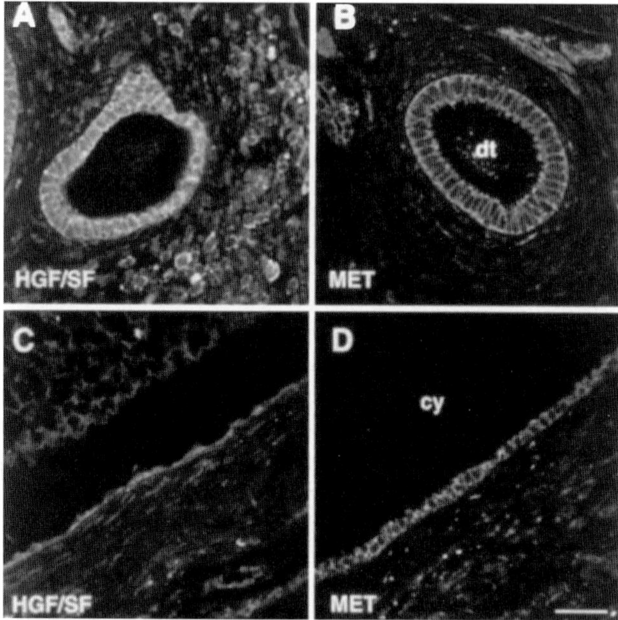

FIGURE 1.12. Hepatocyte growth factor (HGF) and MET immunohistochemistry in a dysplastic kidney. **A:** A dysplastic tubule within a postnatal human kidney malformation. HGF immunostaining is localized to the epithelium and also to scattered cells in the surrounding undifferentiated stromal/mesenchymal tissues. **B:** In a section adjacent to that depicted in **A**, MET immunostaining was confined to the epithelium. **C:** Other parts of the same organ contained large cysts. Faint HGF/SF immunoreactivity was noted in three locations: stromal; around the cyst, apparently coating the lining of the cyst; and in amorphous material inside the cyst. **D:** In a section adjacent to that depicted in **(C)**, MET immunostaining was prominent in epithelium, lining the cyst (cy). Bar is 50 μm. SF, scatter factor; dt, dysplastic tubule. (From Kolatsi-Joannou M, Moore R, Winyard PJD, et al. Expression of hepatocyte growth factor/scatter factor and its receptor, MET, suggests roles in human embryonic organogenesis. *Pediatr Res* 1997;41:657–665, with permission.)

neys associated with obstruction during early gestation are often dysplastic. Data suggest that experimental obstruction of murine kidneys in the neonatal period causes enhanced cell death by apoptosis, as well as aberrant expression of BCL2, TGF-β1, AT II, and EGF (145). Similar molecules are implicated in the pathogenesis of renal dysplasia, a phenotype that can be generated in animals, such as sheep, by ureteric obstruction much earlier during development (23,24). All of these molecules have been functionally implicated in metanephric growth in various other experiments using organ culture or transgenic mice.

Genetic Causes: Malformations Confined to the Urinary Tract

Primary vesicoureteric reflux (VUR) affects approximately 1% of white infants, and associated reflux nephropathy causes up to 15% of end-stage renal failure in children and adults (4,146). There is a 20- to 50-fold increased risk of VUR in immediate relatives of probands (147). Feather et al. (148) reported the first genome-wide search of VUR in seven families with dominant inheritance. Polymorphic markers were used, spaced at 10 centiMorgan (cM) through the genome, with affecteds-only parametric and nonparametric linkage analyses. The most positive locus spans 20 cM on chromosome 1p13, with a nonparametric lod score of 5.76 (p = .0002) and a parametric lod score of 3.16. Hence, VUR maps to chromosome 1, although the gene has yet to be defined. There was also evidence of genetic heterogeneity, and 12 additional loci were identified with $p < .05$. The results support the hypotheses that VUR is a genetic disorder and offers the future prospect of genetic screening to replace invasive cystograms for diagnosis. Other loci, yet to be defined, might be implicated in the rare families reported with inherited nonsyndromic kidney aplasia and dysplasia (149,150).

Genetic Causes: Multiorgan Malformation Syndromes

In some cases, congenital kidney or lower urinary tract disorders occur with a multiorgan malformation syndrome commonly affecting central nervous, cardiovascular, and skeletal systems. For a listing of such syndromes, see Chapter 6 and reference 151. Although individually rare, malformation syndromes collectively account for significant morbidity. Some are associated with gross chromosomal anomalies, such as monosomies, trisomies, 4p- syndrome, and dup (10p)/del (10q); however, gross cytogenetic defects are absent in most cases of children born with syndromic renal tract malformation. Many renal malformation syndromes are inherited in Mendelian patterns, and in some, specific mutations have been defined (Table 1.2) (151). Here, four such syndromes are highlighted.

The ablation of a single *PAX2* allele in mice causes impaired metanephric growth as well as megaureter, a finding consistent with gross VUR (27,55). These animals are blind because of maldevelopment of the retina, another site of embryonic PAX2 expression. There is a human syndrome that is strikingly similar to these mouse models, namely the renal-coloboma syndrome. This comprises blindness caused by optic nerve colobomas and renal failure and hypertension associated with vesicoureteric reflux and small, malformed kidneys. This resemblance was noted by a New Zealand–based laboratory that described heterozygous mutations of *PAX2* in individuals with this syndrome (152). These mutations most likely result in haploinsufficiency (a partial lack of functional protein), and they can arise *de novo* or be inherited in an autosomal-dominant manner. *PAX2* mutations have also been implicated in human inherited renal hypoplasia with a very mild ocular phenotype, emphasizing the utility of careful examination of the optic fundus in such cases (153).

X-linked Kallmann syndrome is caused by mutations of *KAL-1* (154,155). Anosmia and hypogonadotrophic hypogonadism occur in affected male patients because of defective prenatal elongation of axons of olfactory neurons and migration of gonadotrophin-releasing hormone–synthesizing neurons from the nasal placode into the forebrain.

TABLE 1.2. EXAMPLES OF HUMAN RENAL MALFORMATION SYNDROMES WITH A GENETIC BASIS

Associated with syndromes
- Apert syndrome (*FGFR2* mutation)
- Bardet Biedl syndrome (several loci and BBS genes defined)
- Beckwith-Wiedemann syndrome (*p57KIP2* mutations in a minority of patients)
- Branchio-oto-renal syndrome (*EYA1* mutation)
- Camptomelic dysplasia (*SOX9* mutation)
- Denys Drash syndrome (*WT1* mutation)
- Di George syndrome (locus on 22q11, possibly several genes mutated)
- Glutaric aciduria type II (*glutaryl–coenzyme A dehydrogenase* mutation)
- Fanconi anemia (*FAA* mutation)
- Kallmann syndrome (*KAL-1* mutation)[a]
- Meckel syndrome (locus on 17q21–q24)
- Nail-patella syndrome (*LMX1B* mutation)
- Oral-facial-digital syndrome type 1 (*OFD1* mutation)
- Renal-coloboma syndrome (*PAX2* mutation)[a]
- Renal cysts and diabetes syndrome (*HNF1β* mutation)[a]
- Simpson-Golabi-Behmel syndrome (*GPC3* mutation)[a]
- Townes-Brocks syndrome (*SALL1* mutation)
- Smith-Lemli-Opitz syndrome [*δ(7)-dehydrocholesterol reductase* mutation]
- WAGR syndrome (*WT1* and *PAX6* contiguous gene defects)
- Zellweger syndrome (peroxisomal protein mutation)

Nonsyndromic
- Congenital anomalies of the kidney and urinary tract (*AT2* polymorphism)
- Renal adysplasia (locus not defined)
- Primary vesicoureteric reflux (locus on 1p13 but condition is genetically heterogeneous)[a]

[a]Conditions discussed in more detail in the current text. For updated information on the genetics of these and other renal and urinary tract malformation syndromes, see reference 151.

Moreover, the olfactory bulb fails to grow and is hypoplastic. Approximately 30 to 40% of patients have a solitary functioning kidney, with presumed renal agenesis (156). Patients with urinary tract agenesis also lack the vas deferens, a structure derived from the mesonephric duct which also gives rise to the ureteric bud and its derivatives. Two children with X-linked Kallmann syndrome and unilateral multicystic dysplastic kidney have been reported (157): Perhaps the apparent "agenesis" phenotype seen in older individuals with the syndrome might be the result of spontaneous involution of multicystic organs, as is known to occur in non-Kallmann patients. *In vitro* studies demonstrate an adhesive role for the protein coded by *KAL-1. In vivo* KAL-1 is expressed in the embryonic human central nervous and excretory systems (Fig. 1.13) (155,157). The protein, called *anosmin-1*, immunolocalizes to the epithelial interstitial matrix and basement membranes of the mesonephric collecting tubules and mesonephric duct and to the first generations of metanephric collecting duct branches of the ureteric bud (158). It is possible that failure of growth of either the ureteric bud or its first branches, perhaps due

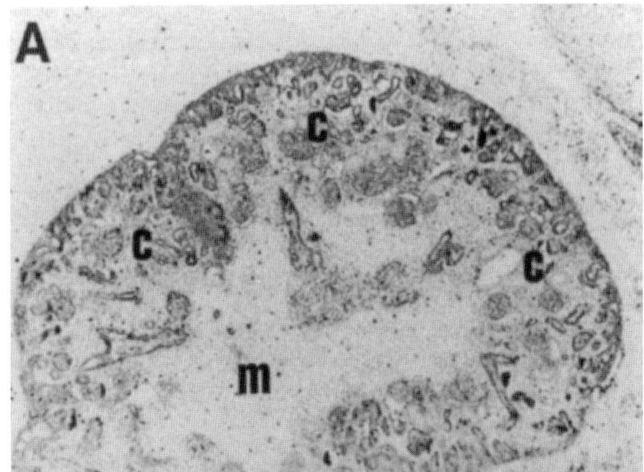

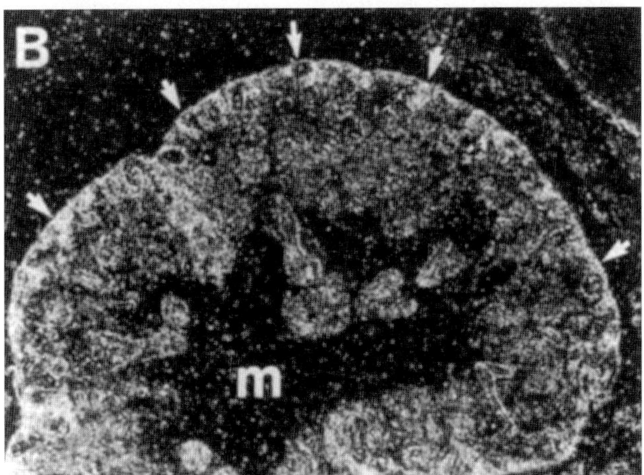

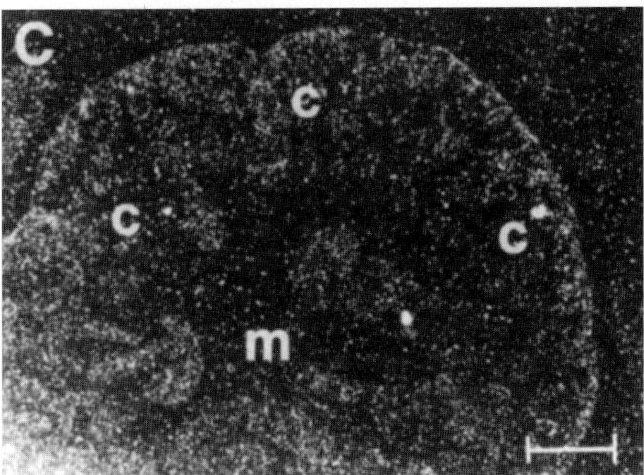

FIGURE 1.13. KAL expression in the developing human metanephros. **A:** Bright-field photomicrograph of section of the organ at 11 weeks' gestation counterstained with hematoxylin and eosin, showing the cortex (c) and medulla (m). **B:** *In situ* hybridization with dark field illumination: KAL antisense probe shows moderate signal over the nephrogenic cortex (*arrows*) with a weak signal from deeper tissues. **C:** Background signal from KAL sense probe. Bar is 40 μm. (From Duke V, Winyard PJD, Thorogood PV, et al. *KAL,* a gene mutated in Kallmann's syndrome, is expressed in the first trimester of human development. *Mol Cell Endocrinol* 1995;110:73–79, with permission.)

to alterations in cell adhesion, would lead to a failure of metanephric formation with consequent renal agenesis.

The Simpson-Golabi-Behmel syndrome is an X-linked condition characterized by prenatal and postnatal overgrowth with visceral and skeletal abnormalities. Affected males are often very tall with nephromegaly, renal cysts, hydronephrosis, double renal pelvis, dysplastic kidneys, and Wilms' tumor. The disease superficially resembles Beckwith-Wiedemann syndrome, an autosomal-dominant disorder linked to 11p, and the Perlman syndrome, which is inherited in an autosomal-recessive manner. Mutations of the *GPC3* gene (Xq26) have recently been reported in the Simpson-Golabi-Behmel syndrome (159). This gene encodes a putative extracellular proteoglycan, called *glypican 3*, that is expressed in the fetal kidney and other tissues that are derived from embryonic mesoderm. There is preliminary evidence that the protein product may bind to IGF-2 and modulate its action. This factor is made by the embryonic kidney and enhances metanephric growth in organ culture (72). It is overexpressed in some Wilms' tumors, perhaps because of loss of genetic imprinting of a normally silent *IGFII* allele or to derepression of transcription associated with *WT1* mutations. It has also been demonstrated that mice with *GPC3* null mutations have an overgrowth syndrome accompanied by deregulated metanephric cell turnover and malformed kidneys (160).

It has long been recognized that glucose is teratogenic for kidneys and other organs, with embryopathy associated with free radicals and vasculopathy (143,161). Recently, a genetic link was established between diabetes mellitus and renal cystic malformations, based on a spectrum of disorders associated with mutations of *hepatocyte nuclear factor 1β*; collectively, these have been called the renal cysts and diabetes syndrome (162–164). Human mutations were initially associated with maturity onset diabetes mellitus of the young; these individuals have a failure of pancreatic insulin secretion. Mutations in the DNA binding and transactivating domains of this transcription factor have been reported in patients with kidney malformations, including agenesis, dysplasia, hypoplasia, and glomerulocystic disease, a form of cystic kidney disease in which glomerular cysts predominate (see Chapter 38). The gene is expressed in human embryos: Hepatocyte nuclear factor 1β mRNA can be detected in normal human metanephroi, with the highest levels of transcripts localized to fetal medullary and cortical collecting ducts and low levels of expression in nephrogenic cortex mesenchyme, primitive nephron tubules, and immature glomeruli. The gene is also expressed in the embryonic pancreas, liver, gut, and lung. Most likely, this is an example of a gene involved in epithelial differentiation and branching in several organ systems.

REFERENCES

1. Woolf AS, Welham SJM, Hermann MM, Winyard PJD. Maldevelopment of the human kidney and lower urinary tract: an overview. In: Vize PD, Woolf AS, Bard JBL, eds. *The kidney: from normal development to congenital abnormalities.* New York: Elsevier Science Academic Press, 2003:377–393.
2. Risdon RA, Woolf AS. Development of the kidney. In: Jennette JC, Olson JL, Schwartz MM, Silva FG, eds. *Heptinstall's pathology of the kidney*, 5th ed. Philadelphia: Lippincott–Raven Publishers, 1998:67–84.
3. Risdon RA, Woolf AS. Developmental defects and cystic diseases of the kidney. In: Jennette JC, Olson JL, Schwartz MM, Silva FG, eds. *Heptinstall's pathology of the kidney*, 5th ed. Philadelphia: Lippincott–Raven Publishers, 1998:1149–1206.
4. Lewis M. Report of the paediatric renal registry. In: Ansell D, Feest T, eds. *The UK Renal Registry: the second annual report.* Bristol, UK: The Renal Association, 1999:175–187.
5. Woolf AS, Thiruchelvam N. Congenital obstructive uropathy—its origin and contribution to end-stage renal failure in children. *Adv Ren Replace Ther* 2001;8:157–163.
6. Potter EL. *Normal and abnormal development of the kidney.* Chicago: Year Book Medical Publishers, 1972.
7. Hinchliffe SA, Howard CV, Lynch MR, et al. Renal developmental arrest in sudden infant death syndrome. *Pediatr Pathol* 1993;13:333–343.
8. Welham SJM, Wade A, Woolf AS. Protein restriction in pregnancy is associated with increased apoptosis of mesenchymal cells at the start of rat metanephrogenesis. *Kidney Int* 2002;61:1231–1242.
9. Woolf AS, Yuan HT. The development of kidney blood vessels. In: Vize PD, Woolf AS, Bard JBL, eds. *The kidney: from normal development to congenital abnormalities.* New York: Elsevier Science Academic Press, 2003:251–266.
10. Sariola H, Timpl R, von der Mark K, et al. Dual origin of glomerular basement membrane. *Dev Biol* 1984;101:86–96.
11. Smeulders N, Woolf AS, Wilcox DT. Smooth muscle differentiation and cell turnover in mouse detrusor development. *J Urol* 2002;167:385–390.
12. Stuart RO, Bush KT, Nigam SK. Changes in global gene expression patterns during development and maturation of the rat kidney. *Proc Natl Acad Sci U S A* 2001;98:5649–5654.
13. Dekel B, Amariglio N, Kaminski N, et al. Engraftment and differentiation of human metanephroi into functional mature nephrons after transplantation into mice is accompanied by a profile of gene expression similar to normal kidney development. *J Am Soc Nephrol* 2002;13:977–990.
14. Grobstein C. Mechanisms of organogenetic tissue interaction. *Natl Cancer Inst Monogr* 1967;26:279–299.
15. Sariola H, Saarma M, Sainio K, et al. Dependence of kidney morphogenesis on the expression of nerve growth factor receptor. *Science* 1991;254:571–573.
16. Woolf AS, Kolatsi-Joannou M, Hardman P, et al. Roles of hepatocyte growth factor/scatter factor and the MET receptor in the early development of the metanephros. *J Cell Biol* 1995;128:171–184.
17. Klein G, Langegger M, Timpl R, et al. Role of laminin A chain in the development of epithelial cell polarity. *Cell* 1988;55:331–341.
18. Woolf AS, Bosch RJ, Fine LG. Gene transfer into the mammalian kidney: micro-transplantation of retrovirus-transduced metanephric tissue. *Exp Nephrol* 1993;1:41–48.

19. Woolf AS. Congenital kidney diseases: prospects for new therapies. In: Vize PD, Woolf AS, Bard JBL, eds. *The kidney: from normal development to congenital abnormalities.* New York: Elsevier Science Academic Press, 2003:487–492.
20. Qiao J, Herzlinger D. The metanephric blastema differentiates into collecting system and nephron epithelia in vitro. *Development* 1995;121:3207–3214.
21. Burrow C, Wilson PD. A putative Wilms tumor-secreted growth factor activity required for primary culture of human nephroblasts. *Proc Natl Acad Sci U S A* 1993;90:6066–6070.
22. Boyden EA. Experimental obstruction of the mesonephric ducts. *Proc Soc Exp Biol Med* 1927;24:572–576.
23. Attar R, Quinn F, Winyard PJD, et al. Short-term urinary flow impairment deregulates PAX2 and PCNA expression and cell survival in fetal sheep kidneys. *Am J Pathol* 1998;152:1225–1235.
24. Yang SP, Woolf AS, Quinn F, Winyard PJD. Deregulation of renal transforming growth factor-β1 after experimental short-term ureteric obstruction in fetal sheep. *Am J Pathol* 2001;159:109–117.
25. Gage JC, Sulik KK. Pathogenesis of ethanol-induced hydronephrosis and hydroureter as demonstrated following in vivo exposure of mouse embryos. *Teratology* 1991;44:299–312.
26. Dressler GR, Wilkinson JE, Rothenpieler UW, et al. Deregulation of Pax-2 expression in transgenic mice generates severe kidney abnormalities. *Nature* 1993;362:65–67.
27. Torres M, Gomez-Pardo E, Dressler GR, et al. Pax-2 controls multiple steps of urogenital development. *Development* 1995;121:4057–4065.
28. Davies J. *The kidney development database.* http://129.215.178.164/kidhome.html. Accessed April 2, 2003.
29. Threadgill DW, Dlugosz AA, Hansen LA, et al. Targeted disruption of mouse EGF receptor. Effect of genetic background on mutant phenotype. *Science* 1995;269:230–234.
30. Davis AP, Witte DP, Hsieh-Li HM, et al. Absence of radius and ulna in mice lacking hoxa-11 and hoxd-11. *Nature* 1995;375:791–795.
31. Mendelsohn C, Lohnes D, Decimo S, et al. Function of the retinoic acid receptors (RAR) during development. *Development* 1994;120:2749–2771.
32. Winyard PJD, Risdon RA, Sams VR, et al. The PAX2 transcription factor is expressed in cystic and hyperproliferative dysplastic epithelia in human kidney malformations. *J Clin Invest* 1996;98:451–459.
33. Kampmeier OF. The metanephros or so-called permanent kidney in part provisional and vestigial. *Anat Rec* 1926;33:115–120.
34. Kim J, Lee GS, Tisher CC, Madsen KM. Role of apoptosis in development of the ascending thin limb of the loop of Henle in rat kidney. *Am J Physiol* 1996;271:F831–F845.
35. Kim J, Cha JH, Tisher CC, Madsen KM. Role of apoptotic and nonapoptotic death in removal of intercalated cells from developing rat kidney. *Am J Physiol* 1996;270:F575–F592.
36. Nadasy T, Laszik Z, Lajoie G, et al. Proliferative activity of cyst epithelium in human renal cystic diseases. *J Am Soc Nephrol* 1995;5:1462–1468.
37. Veis DJ, Sorenson CM, Shutter JR, et al. Bcl-2-deficient mice demonstrate fulminant lymphoid apoptosis, polycystic kidneys and hypopigmented hair. *Cell* 1994;75:229–240.
38. Winyard PJD, Nauta J, Lirenman DS, et al. Deregulation of cell survival in cystic and dysplastic renal development. *Kidney Int* 1996;49:135–146.
39. Herzlinger D, Koseki C, Mikawa T, et al. Metanephric mesenchyme contains multipotent stem cells whose fate is restricted after induction. *Development* 1992;114:565–572.
40. Dressler GR, Woolf AS. PAX2 in development and renal disease. *Int J Dev Biol* 1999;43:463–468.
41. Woolf AS, Cale CM. Roles of growth factors in renal development. *Curr Opin Nephrol Hypertens* 1997;6:10–14.
42. Mikazaki Y, Ichikawa I. Role of the angiotensin receptor in the development of the mammalian kidney and urinary tract. *Comp Biochem Physiol A Mol Integr Physiol* 2001;128:89–97.
43. Ekblom P. Extracellular matrix and cell adhesion molecules in nephrogenesis. *Exp Nephrol* 1996;4:92–96.
44. Shawlot W, Behringer RR. Requirement for Lim1 in head-organizer function. *Nature* 1995;374:425–432.
45. Koseki C, Herzlinger D, Al-Awqati Q. Apoptosis in metanephric development. *J Cell Biol* 1992;119:1322–1333.
46. Perantoni AO, Dove LF, Karavanova I. Basic fibroblast growth factor can mediate the early inductive events in renal development. *Proc Natl Acad Sci U S A* 1995;92:4696–4700.
47. Barasch J, Pressler L, Connor J, et al. A ureteric bud cell line induces nephrogenesis in two steps by two distinct signals. *Am J Physiol* 1996;271:F50–F61.
48. Barasch J, Yang J, Qiao J, et al. Tissue inhibitor of metalloproteinase-2 stimulates mesenchymal growth and regulates epithelial branching during morphogenesis of the rat metanephros. *J Clin Invest* 1999;103:1299–1307.
49. Larsson SH, Charlieu J-P, Miyagawa K, et al. Subnuclear localization of WT1 in splicing of transcription factor domains is regulated by alternative splicing. *Cell* 1995;81:391–401.
50. Kreidberg JA, Sariola H, Loring JM, et al. WT-1 is required for early kidney development. *Cell* 1993;74:679–691.
51. Nishinakamura R, Matsumoto Y, Nakao K, et al. Murine homolog of *SALL1* is essential for ureteric bud invasion in kidney development. *Development* 2001;128:3105–3115.
52. Kolatsi-Joannou M, Moore R, Winyard PJD, et al. Expression of hepatocyte growth factor/scatter factor and its receptor, MET, suggests roles in human embryonic organogenesis. *Pediatr Res* 1997;41:657–665.
53. Muller U, Wang D, Denda S, et al. Integrin α8β1 is critically important for epithelial-mesenchymal interactions during kidney development. *Cell* 1997;88:603–613.
54. Rothenpieler UW, Dressler GR. Pax-2 is required for mesenchyme-to-epithelium conversion during kidney development. *Development* 1993;119:711–720.
55. Favor J, Sandulache R, Neuhauser-Klaus A, et al. The mouse Pax2[1Neu] mutation is identical to a human PAX2 mutation in a family with renal-coloboma syndrome and results in developmental defects of the brain, ear, eye and kidney. *Proc Natl Acad Sci U S A* 1996;93:13870–13875.
56. Stanton BR, Perkins AS, Tessarollo L, et al. Loss of N-MYC function results in embryonic lethality and failure of the epithelial component of the embryo to develop. *Genes Dev* 1992;6:2235–2247.
57. Tsarfaty I, Rong S, Resau JH, et al. The met proto-oncogene promotes mesenchymal to epithelial cell conversion. *Science* 1994;263:98–101.

58. Karp SL, Ortiz-Arduan A, Li S, et al. Epithelial differentiation of metanephric mesenchymal cells after stimulation with hepatocyte growth factor or embryonic spinal cord. *Proc Natl Acad Sci U S A* 1994;91:5286–5290.
59. Sorenson CM, Rogers SA, Korsmeyer SJ, et al. Fulminant metanephric apoptosis and abnormal kidney development in bcl-2-deficient mice. *Am J Physiol* 1995;268:F73–F81.
60. Davies JA, Garrod DR. Induction of early stages of kidney tubule differentiation by lithium ions. *Dev Biol* 1995;167:50–61.
61. Klein G, Langegger M, Garidis C, et al. Neural cell adhesion molecules during embryonic induction and development of the kidney. *Development* 1988;102:749–761.
62. Gumbiner B, Stevenson B, Grimalfi A. The role of the cell adhesion molecule uvomorulin in the formation and maintenance of the epithelial junctional complex. *J Cell Biol* 1988;107:1575–1587.
63. McNeil H, Ozawa M, Kemler R, et al. Novel function of the cell adhesion molecule uvomorulin as an inducer of cell surface polarity. *Cell* 1990;62:309–316.
64. Sorokin L, Sonnenberg A, Aumailley M, et al. Recognition of the laminin E8 cell-binding site by an integrin possessing the α6 subunit is essential for epithelial polarization in developing kidney tubules. *J Cell Biol* 1990;111:1265–1273.
65. Durbeej M, Larsson E, Ibraghimov-Beskrovnaya O, et al. Non-muscle α-dystroglycan is involved in epithelial development *J Cell Biol* 1995;130:79–91.
66. Ekblom P, Ekblom M, Fecker L, et al. Role of mesenchymal nidogen for epithelial morphogenesis in vitro. *Development* 1994;120:2004–2014.
67. Noakes PG, Miner JH, Gautam M, et al. The renal glomerulus of mice lacking s-laminin/laminin β_2: nephrosis despite molecular compensation by laminin β_1. *Nat Genet* 1995; 10:400–406.
68. Stark K, Vainio S, Vassileva G, et al. Epithelial transformation of metanephric mesenchyme in the developing kidney regulated by Wnt-4. *Nature* 1994;372:679–683.
69. Dudley AT, Lyons KM, Robertson EJ. A requirement for BMP-7 during development of the mammalian kidney and eye. *Genes Dev* 1995;9:2795–2807
70. Luo G, Hofmann C, Bronckers ALJJ, et al. BMP-7 is an inducer of nephrogenesis and is also required for eye development and skeletal patterning. *Genes Dev* 1995;9:2808–2820.
71. Barasch J, Yang J, Ware CB, et al. Mesenchymal to epithelial conversion in rat metanephros is induced by LIF. *Cell* 1999;99:377–386.
72. Rogers SA, Ryan G, Hammerman MR. Insulin-like growth factors I and II are produced in the metanephros and are required for growth and development in vitro. *J Cell Biol* 1991;113:1447–1453.
73. Rogers SA, Ryan G, Hammerman MR. Metanephric transforming growth factor-α is required for renal organogenesis in vitro. *Am J Physiol* 1992;262:F533–F539.
74. Skaer H. Cell proliferation and development of the Malpighian tubules in *Drosophila* melanogaster. *Exp Nephrol* 1996;4:116–119.
75. Ryan G, Steele-Perkins V, Morris JF, et al. Repression of Pax-2 by WT1 during normal kidney development. *Development* 1995;121:867–875.
76. Coppes MJ, Huff V, Pelletier J. Denys-Drash syndrome: relating a clinical disorder to alterations in the tumor suppressor gene WT1. *J Pediatr* 1993;123:673–678.
77. Cale CM, Klein NJ, Morgan G, Woolf AS. Tumour necrosis factor-α inhibits epithelial differentiation and morphogenesis in the mouse metanephric kidney in vitro. *Int J Dev Biol* 1998;42:663–674.
78. Rogers SA, Ryan G, Purchio AF, et al. Metanephric transforming growth factor β1 regulates nephrogenesis in vitro. *Am J Physiol* 1993;264:F996–F1002.
79. Rivtos O, Tuuri T, Eramaa M, et al. Activin disrupts epithelial branching morphogenesis in developing glandular organs of the mouse. *Mech Dev* 1995;50:229–245.
80. Ekblom P, Weller A. Ontogeny of tubulointerstitial cells. *Kidney Int* 1991;39:394–500.
81. Sariola H, Aufderheide E, Bernhard H, et al. Antibodies to cell surface ganglioside G_{D3} perturb inductive epithelial-mesenchymal interactions. *Cell* 1988;54:235–245.
82. Hatini V, Huh SO, Herzlinger D, et al. Essential role of stromal mesenchyme in kidney morphogenesis revealed by targeted disruption of Winged Helix transcription factor BF-2. *Genes Dev* 1996;10:1467–1478.
83. Batourina E, Gim S, Bello N, et al. Vitamin A controls epithelial/mesenchymal interactions through Ret expression. *Nat Genet* 2001;27:74–78.
84. Karavanov A, Sainio K, Palgi J, et al. Neurotrophin-3 rescues neuronal precursors from apoptosis and promotes neuronal differentiation in the embryonic metanephric kidney. *Proc Natl Acad Sci U S A* 1995;92:11279–11280.
85. Towers PR, Woolf AS, Hardman P. Glial cell line-derived neurotrophic factor stimulates ureteric bud outgrowth and enhances survival of ureteric bud cells in vitro. *Exp Nephrol* 1998;6:337–351.
86. Qiao J, Bush KT, Steer DL, et al. Multiple fibroblast growth factors support growth of the ureteric bud but have different effects on branching morphogenesis. *Mech Dev* 2001;109:123–135.
87. Jing S, Wun D, Yu Y, et al. GDNF-induced activation of the ret protein tyrosine kinase is mediated by GDNFR-α a novel receptor for GDNF. *Cell* 1996;85:1113–1124.
88. Schuchardt A, D'Agati V, Larsson-Blomberg L, et al. Defects in the kidney and nervous system of mice lacking the receptor tyrosine kinase receptor Ret. *Nature* 1994;367:380–383.
89. Schuchardt A, D'Agati V, Pachnis V, et al. Renal agenesis and hypodysplasia in *ret-k*⁻mutant mice result from defects in ureteric bud development. *Development* 1996;122:1919–1929.
90. Moore MW, Klein RD, Farinas I, et al. Renal and neuronal abnormalities in mice lacking GDNF. *Nature* 1996;382:76–79.
91. Pichel JG, Shen L, Sheng HZ, et al. Defects in enteric innervation and kidney development in mice lacking GDNF. *Nature* 1996;382:73–76.
92. Sanchez MP, Silos-Santiago I, Frisen J, et al. Renal agenesis and the absence of enteric neurones in mice lacking GDNF. *Nature* 1996;382:70–73.
93. O'Rourke DA, Sakurai H, Spokes K, et al. Expression of c-ret promotes morphogenesis and cell survival in mIMCD-3 cells. *Am J Physiol* 1999;276:F581–F588.
94. Montesano R, Matsumoto K, Nakamura T, et al. Identification of fibroblast-derived epithelial morphogen as hepatocyte growth factor. *Cell* 1991;67:901–908.

95. Santos OFP, Barros EJG, Yang X-M, et al. Involvement of hepatocyte growth factor in kidney development. *Dev Biol* 1994;163:525–529.
96. Davies J, Lyon M, Gallagher J, et al. Sulphated proteoglycan is required for collecting duct growth and branching but not nephron formation during kidney development. *Development* 1995;121:1507–1517.
97. Takayama H, La Rochelle WJ, Avner M, et al. Scatter factor/hepatocyte growth factor as a regulator of skeletal muscle and neural crest development. *Proc Natl Acad Sci U S A* 1996;93:5866–5871.
98. Schmidt C, Bladt F, Goedecke S, et al. SF/HGF is essential for liver development. *Nature* 1995;373:699–702.
99. Bladt F, Riethmacher D, Isenmann S, et al. Essential role for the c-met receptor in the migration of myogenic precursor cells into the limb bud. *Nature* 1995;376:768–771.
100. Kanwar YS, Liu ZZ, Kumar A, et al. Cloning of mouse c-ros renal cDNA, its role in development and relationship to extracellular matrix glycoproteins. *Kidney Int* 1995;48:1646–1659.
101. Sonnenberg-Riethmacher E, Walter B, Riethmacher D, et al. The c-ros tyrosine kinase receptor controls regionalization and differentiation of the epithelial cells of the epididymis. *Genes Dev* 1996;10:1184–1193.
102. Lee K-F, Li E, Huber J, et al. Targeted mutation of the gene encoding the low affinity NGF receptor p75 leads to deficits in the peripheral sensory nervous system. *Cell* 1992;69:737–749.
103. Perantoni AO, Williams CL, Lewellyn AL. Growth and branching morphogenesis of rat collecting duct anlagen in the absence of metanephrogenic mesenchyme. *Differentiation* 1991;48:107–113.
104. Orr-Urtreger A, Bedford MT, Bukarova T, et al. Developmental localisation of the splicing alternatives of fibroblast growth factor receptor-2 (FGFR2). *Dev Biol* 1993;158:475–486.
105. Yi ES, Shabaik AS, Lacey DL, et al. Keratinocyte growth factor causes proliferation of urothelium in vivo. *J Urol* 1995;154:1566–1570.
106. Qiao J, Uzzo R, Obara-Ishihara T, et al. FGF-7 modulates ureteric bud growth and nephron number in the developing kidney. *Development* 1999;126:547–554.
107. Sakurai H, Bush KT, Nigam SK. Identification of pleiotrophin as a mesenchymal factor involved in ureteric bud branching morphogenesis. *Development* 2001;128:3283–3293.
108. Santos OFP, Nigam SK. HGF-induced tubulogenesis and branching of epithelial cells is modulated by extracellular matrix and TGF-β. *Dev Biol* 1993;160:293–302.
109. Sakurai H, Nigam SK. Transforming growth factor-β selectively inhibits branching morphogenesis but not tubulogenesis. *Am J Physiol* 1997;410:F139–F146.
110. Kreidberg JA, Donovan MJ, Goldstein SL, et al. $\alpha_3\beta_1$ integrin has a crucial role in kidney and lung organogenesis. *Development* 1996;122:3537–3547.
111. Bullock SL, Johnson T, Bao Q, et al. Galectin-3 modulates ureteric bud branching in organ culture of the developing mouse kidney. *J Am Soc Nephrol* 2001;12:515–523.
112. Winyard PJD, Bao Q, Hughes RC, et al. Epithelial galectin-3 during human nephrogenesis and childhood cystic diseases. *J Am Soc Nephrol* 1997;8:1647–1657.
113. Geng L, Segay Y, Peissel B, et al. Identification and localisation of polycystin, the PKD1 gene product. *J Clin Invest* 1996;2674–2683.
114. Maas R, Elfering S, Glaser T, et al. Deficient outgrowth of the ureteric bud underlies the renal agenesis phenotype in mice manifesting the limb deformity (ld) mutation. *Dev Dyn* 1994;199:214–218.
115. Evan AP, Satlin LM, Gattone II VH, et al. Postnatal maturation of rabbit renal collecting duct. II. Morphological observations. *Am J Physiol* 1991;261:F91–F107.
116. Fejes-Toth G, Naray-Fejes-Toth A. Differentiation of renal α-intercalated cells to β-intercalated and principal cells in culture. *Proc Natl Acad Sci U S A* 1992;89:5487–5491.
117. Slotkin TA, Seidler FJ, Kavlock RJ, et al. Fetal dexamethasone exposure accelerates development of renal function: relationship to dose, cell differentiation and growth inhibition. *J Dev Physiol* 1992;17:55–61.
118. Avner ED, Sweeney WE, Nelson WJ. Abnormal sodium pump distribution during renal tubulogenesis in congenital murine polycystic kidney disease. *Proc Natl Acad Sci U S A* 1992;89:7447–7451.
119. Ruani-Gil D, Coca-Payeras A, Tejedo-Mateu A. Obstruction and normal recanalization of the ureter in the human embryo: its relation to congenital ureteric obstruction. *Eur Urol* 1975;1:287–293.
120. Funjinaka H, Mijazaki Y, Matsusaka T, et al. Salutary role for angiotensin in partial urinary tract obstruction. *Kidney Int* 2000;58:2018–2027.
121. Bernstein J, Cheng F, Roska J. Glomerular differentiation in metanephric culture. *Lab Invest* 1981;45:183–190.
122. Sariola H, Ekblom P, Lehtonen E, et al. Differentiation and vascularisation of the metanephric kidney grafted on the chorioallantoic membrane. *Dev Biol* 1983;96:427–435.
123. Loughna S, Hardman P, Landels E, et al. A molecular and genetic analysis of renal glomerular capillary development. *Angiogenesis* 1997;1:84–101.
124. Loughna S, Yuan HT, Woolf AS. Effects of oxygen on vascular patterning in *Tie1/LacZ* metanephric kidneys in vitro. *Biochem Biophys Res Commun* 1998;247:361–366.
125. Woolf AS, Palmer SJ, Snow ML, et al. Creation of a functioning chimeric mammalian kidney. *Kidney Int* 1990;38:991–997.
126. Hyink DP, Tucker DC, St. John PL, et al. Endogenous origin of glomerular endothelial and mesangial cells in grafts of embryonic kidneys. *Am J Physiol* 1996;270:F886–F899.
127. Tufro A, Norwood VF, Carey RM, Gomez RA. Vascular endothelial growth factor induced nephrogenesis and vasculogenesis. *J Am Soc Nephrol* 1999;10:2125–2134.
128. Kolatsi-Joannou M, Yuan HT, Li X, Suda T, Woolf AS. Expression and potential role of angiopoietins and Tie-2 in early development of the mouse metanephros. *Dev Dyn* 2001;222:120–126.
129. Takahashi T, Takahashi K, Gerety S, et al. Temporally compartmentalized expression of ephrin-B2 during renal glomerular development. *J Am Soc Nephrol* 2001;12:2673–2682.
130. Sequeira Lopez ML, Pentz ES, Robert B, et al. Embryonic origins and lineage of juxtaglomerular cells. *Am J Physiol Renal Physiol* 2001;281:F345–F356.
131. Bensoussan M, Heudes D, Nahmias C, et al. Organ culture of rat kidney: a model for angiotensin II receptor ontogenic studies. *Kidney Int* 1995;48:1635–1640.
132. Fogo A, Yoshida Y, Yared A, et al. Importance of angiogenic action of angiotensin II in the glomerular growth of maturing kidneys. *Kidney Int* 1990;38:1068–1074.

133. Leveen P, Pekny M, Gebre Medhin S, et al. Mice deficient for PDGFB show renal, cardiovascular, and hematological abnormalities. *Genes Dev* 1994;8:1875–1887.
134. Soriano P. Abnormal kidney development and hematological disorders in PDGFB receptor mutant mice. *Genes Dev* 1994;8:1888–1896.
135. Kolatsi-Joannou M, Woolf AS, Hardman P, et al. The hepatocyte growth factor/scatter factor (HGF/SF) receptor, MET, transduces a morphogenetic signal in renal glomerular fibromuscular mesangial cells. *J Cell Sci* 1995;108:3703–3714.
136. Sariola H, Ekblom P, Henke-Fahle S. Embryonic neurons as in vitro inducers of differentiation of nephrogenic mesenchyme. *Dev Biol* 1989;132:271–281.
137. Sariola H, Holm K, Henke-Fahle S. Early innervation of the metanephric kidney. *Development* 1988;104:563–589.
138. Gruenwald P. Stimulation of nephrogenic tissues by normal and abnormal inductors. *Anat Rec* 1943;86:321–335.
139. Mesrobian H-GJ, Rushton HG, Bulas D. Unilateral renal agenesis may result from in utero regression of multicystic dysplasia. *J Urol* 1993;150:793–794.
140. Mattsell DG, Bennett T, Armstrong RA, et al. Insulin-like growth factor (IGF) and IGF binding protein gene expression in multicystic renal dysplasia. *J Am Soc Nephrol* 1997;8:85–94.
141. Yang SP, Woolf AS, Yuan HT, et al. Potential biological role of transforming growth factor β1 in human congenital kidney malformations. *Am J Pathol* 2000;157:1633–1647.
142. Woolf AS, Winyard PJD. Molecular mechanisms of human embryogenesis: developmental pathogenesis of renal tract malformations. *Pediatr Dev Pathol* 2002;8:108–129.
143. Novak RW, Robinson HB. Coincident Di George anomaly and renal agenesis and its relation to maternal diabetes. *Am J Med Genet* 1994;50:311–312.
144. Rothman KJ, Moore LL, Singer MR, et al. Teratogenicity of high vitamin A intake. *N Engl J Med* 1995;333:1369–1373.
145. Chevalier RL. Growth factors and apoptosis in neonatal ureteral obstruction. *J Am Soc Nephrol* 1996;7:1098–1105.
146. Smellie J, Barratt TM, Chantler C, et al. Medical versus surgical treatment in children with severe bilateral vesicoureteric reflux and bilateral nephropathy: a randomised trial. *Lancet* 2001;357:1329–1333.
147. Feather S, Gordon I, Risdon RA, et al. Vesicoureteric reflux: is it all in the genes? *Lancet* 1996;348:725–728.
148. Feather SA, Malcolm S, Woolf AS, et al. Primary, non-syndromic vesicoureteric reflux and its nephropathy is genetically heterogeneous with a locus on chromosome 1. *Am J Hum Genet* 2000;66:1420–1425.
149. McPherson E, Carey J, Kramer A, et al. Dominantly inherited renal adysplasia. *Am J Med Genet* 1987;26:863–872.
150. Roodhooft AM, Birnholz JC, Holmes LB. Familial nature of congenital absence and severe dysgenesis of both kidneys. *N Engl J Med* 1984;310:1341–1345.
151. OMIM™ Mendelian Inheritance in Man. http://www4.ncbi.nlm.nih.gov/Omim/. Accessed April 2, 2003.
152. Sanyanusin P, Schimmentl LA, McNoe LA, et al. Mutations of the PAX2 gene in a family with optic nerve colobomas, renal anomalies and vesicoureteral reflux. *Nat Genet* 1995;9:358–364.
153. Nishimoto K, Iijima K, Shirakawa K, et al. PAX2 gene mutation in a family with isolated renal hypoplasia. *J Am Soc Nephrol* 2001;12:1769–1772.
154. MacColl G, Pouloux P, Quinton R. Kallmann syndrome: adhesion, afferents and anosmia. *Neuron* 2002;34:1–3.
155. Duke VM, Winyard PJD, Thorogood P, et al. *KAL*, a gene mutated in Kallmann's syndrome, is expressed in the first trimester of human development. *Mol Cell Endocrinol* 1995; 110:73–79.
156. Duke V, Quinton R, Gordon I, et al. Proteinuria, hypertension and chronic renal failure in X-linked Kallmann's syndrome, a defined genetic cause of solitary functioning kidney. *Nephrol Dial Transplant* 1998;13:1998–2003.
157. Deeb A, Robertson A, MacColl G, et al. Multicystic kidney and X-linked Kallmann's syndrome: a new association? *Nephrol Dial Transplant* 2001;16:1170–1175.
158. Hardelin JP, Julliard AK, Moniot B, et al. Anosmin-1 is a regionally restricted component of basement membranes and interstitial matrices during organogenesis: implications for the developmental anomalies of X chromosome-linked Kallman syndrome. *Dev Dyn* 1999;215:26–44.
159. Pilia G, Hughes-Benzie RM, MacKenzie A, et al. Mutations in GPC3, a glypican gene, cause the Simpson-Golabi-Behmel overgrowth syndrome. *Nat Genet* 1996;12: 241–247.
160. Cano-Gauci DF, Song HH, Yang H, et al. Glycipan-3-deficient mice exhibit developmental overgrowth and some of the abnormalities typical of Simpson-Golabi-Behmel syndrome. *J Cell Biol* 1999;146:255–264.
161. Woolf AS. Diabetes, genes and kidney development. *Kidney Int* 2000;57:1202–1203.
162. Bingham C, Bulman MP, Ellard S, et al. Mutations in the hepatocyte nuclear factor-1β gene are associated with familial hypoplastic glomerulocystic kidney disease. *Am J Hum Genet* 2001;68:219–224.
163. Kolatsi-Joannou M, Bingham C, Ellard S, et al. Hepatocyte nuclear factor 1β: a new kindred with renal cysts and diabetes, and gene expression in normal human development. *J Am Soc Nephrol* 2001;12:2175–2180.
164. Bingham C, Ellard S, Cole TRP, et al. Solitary functioning kidney and diverse genital tract malformations associated with hepatocyte nuclear factor-1β mutations. *Kidney Int* 2002;61:1243–1251.

2

GLOMERULAR CIRCULATION AND FUNCTION

VALENTINA KON
IEKUNI ICHIKAWA

The essential function of the kidney is to preserve constancy of body fluid and electrolytes by removing water and potentially harmful metabolic end-products (e.g., uric acids, sulfates, phosphates) while preserving blood pressure (BP) and essential solutes (e.g., sodium, chloride, bicarbonate, sugars, amino acids). The process begins in the renal glomerulus, where plasma is ultrafiltered under pressure through a semipermeable glomerular capillary wall. The ultrafiltration separates plasma water and crystalloids from blood cells and protein macromolecules, which remain in the glomerular circulation. The magnitude of this filtration process is enormous and requires a high rate of renal blood flow (RBF). Indeed, the entire plasma volume is cycled through the glomerular system 20 times per hour. The RBF and glomerular filtration rate (GFR) are interrelated such that maintenance of an adequate RBF is crucially important for optimal GFR while the glomerulus is an active participant in determining the RBF.

RENAL BLOOD FLOW

Blood flow to the kidneys comprises 20 to 30% of cardiac output (CO) and is determined by two factors: renal perfusion pressure (RPP), which is approximately equal to the systemic arterial BP, and renal vascular resistance (RVR), which is determined primarily by the afferent and efferent arterioles. The relationship can be expressed as RBF = BP/RVR. Although RBF is the parameter usually discussed, it is the renal plasma flow (RPF) that is clinically relevant. Thus, at a given level of RBF, RPF may vary with the volume of packed red cells. For example, RPF increases with anemia. Lambs bled to decrease their hematocrit from 33 to 14% double their RPF (1). Because RBF is partly determined by the need for oxygen delivery, RPF may be high with severe chronic anemia such as occurs with sickle cell disease. In such circumstances, both the RPF and the GFR are elevated because of decreased volume of red blood cells.

Like most organs, the kidneys possess intrinsic autoregulatory mechanisms that adjust local RVR when RPP changes. This autoregulation maintains RBF relatively constant in the face of changing BP and RPP under physiologic conditions (2). Many hormonal systems regulate RVR and, hence, RBF. The nature and magnitude of their effects are often age specific because anatomic factors (innervation), presence and distribution of receptor subtypes [angiotensin (AT) II receptors], and post–receptor signaling events change with development (3–6). In addition, autoregulatory efficiency is impaired in several conditions, including extracellular fluid depletion, diuretic exposure, congestive heart failure, and renal parenchymal damage (7–10). Each of these conditions makes the organism more susceptible to acute renal failure in the face of relatively minor changes in BP that cause substantial changes in RBF (see later).

Development of Renal Blood Flow

Prenatal Renal Blood Flow

Fetal RBF is low but increases with gestational age. Doppler ultrasound at 25 weeks of gestation shows the RBF to be 20 mL/min, whereas at 40 weeks, the RBF is 60 mL/min (11). Within the kidney, the relative perfusion varies with cortical depth, with deeper nephrons of the cortex receiving more blood flow than nephrons in the superficial layers (12). This distribution of blood flow parallels morphologic maturation because deeper nephrons are the first to form and mature; superficial nephrons are not completed until near term (13).

Although the kidneys in the human embryo produce urine by 12 weeks' gestation, the role of kidneys in fetal homeostasis is minor compared to the placenta. The percentage of CO perfusing the kidneys is low during intrauterine life. During late gestation, the kidneys of fetal lambs receive only approximately 2.5% of the CO whereas the placenta receives 40%. The kidneys of 10- to 20-week human fetuses receive only 3 to 7% of CO (14). Thus, the clinical relevance of intrauterine RBF and also glomerular filtration is less for the clearance of fetal plasma than for the formation of urine and, hence, amniotic fluid.

Fetal hemodynamics and urine formation are affected by maternal factors such as the maternal volume status, drugs, and vasoactive substances that cross the placenta. For example, acute oral hydration, which is sufficient to decrease plasma osmolality of healthy pregnant women, increases fetal urine production in near-term fetuses (15). Furosemide given to pregnant women induces diuresis in the fetus; likewise, maternally administered indomethacin lessens urine production and may lead to glomerular hypofiltration even after the baby is born (16,17). AT II has distinct effects on the maternal, ureteroplacental, and fetal hemodynamics. Maternal circulation appears to be most sensitive to the vasoconstrictive effects of AT II, which would tend to preserve ureteroplacental and fetal circulations (18,19). However, this fetoprotective effect disappears with long-term exposure to elevated levels of AT II. Thus, although the first 4 hours of AT II infusion into pregnant ewes did not compromise ureteroplacental/fetal perfusion, more than 20 hours of heightened AT II caused a dramatic decrease in the placental perfusion and compromised fetal gas exchange (20). These observations illustrate the important effect of AT II on the ureteroplacental circulation and, by extension, on fetal well-being. AT's actions to maintain BP *in utero* and at the same time maintain RVR at a high level can be compromised by inhibitors of its actions. AT-converting enzyme inhibitors (ACEIs) (e.g., captopril) lead to a decrease in fetal BP, RVR, and GFR in ewes, resulting in oligoanuria (21) and have been observed to cause anuria in the human fetus and newborn (22,23). These hemodynamic changes may result from decreased AT II synthesis or accumulation of bradykinin. AT II receptor antagonism did not affect BP or RVR in fetal piglets or puppies (24,25), whereas bradykinin receptor antagonism attenuated renal vasodilation after AT II receptor antagonism of neonatal rats (26). These findings indicate a role for vasodilatory role of kinins offsetting AT II–modulated vasoconstriction in the maturing kidney and complement the observations that the developing kidney expresses high levels of immunoreactive bradykinin and receptors (27,28). It is interesting that the kinin components localize to the deeper parts of the kidney (29), promoting preferential perfusion of the deeper rather than superficial nephrons characteristic of the fetal kidney.

Another vasodilator that likely plays an important role in fetal renal hemodynamics is nitric oxide (NO) (30). Basal production of NO in third-trimester fetal sheep maintains baseline RBF; its inhibition increased RVR by 50% and blocked the increase in GFR and the natriuresis that accompany volume loading. The NO effects may be direct or mediated by modulation of AT II actions. Overall, the low RBF *in utero* reflects incomplete renal mass that increases exponentially during fetal life, structural immaturity of resistance vessels (narrower vascular lumina), as well as unique modulation by vasoactive compounds (e.g., AT II, prostaglandins, kinins, and NO).

Postnatal Renal Blood Flow

RBF, measured as a clearance of paraamino hippurate (CPAH) and corrected for body size, is low in human neonates and correlates with gestational age. For example, CPAH is 10 mL/min/m^2 in babies born at 28 weeks and 35 mL/min/m^2 in those born at 35 weeks of gestation (31). After birth, RBF increases steadily, doubling by 2 weeks and reaching mature levels by 2 years of age (32). The postnatal change in RBF primarily reflects the considerable increase in the relative RBF to the outer cortex (33–35).

RBF is governed by two factors: CO and the ratio of renal to systemic vascular resistance. After birth, both an increase in CO and a decrease in RVR favor an increase in RBF. Furthermore, RVR decreases much more than systemic vascular resistance (12) allowing for a progressive increase in the renal fraction of CO. For example, RBF increases 18-fold in newborn pigs during the first 5 weeks of life, whereas CO (corrected for body surface area) increases only 7.2 times during the same period (Fig. 2.1). RVR is a function of the arteriolar resistance offered not only by the sum of the glomerular vessels, but also by the number of existing vascular channels. New nephron formation increases the number of channels and, hence, decreases RVR. New nephron formation contributes to the postnatal decrease in RVR and increase in RBF only in premature infants born before 36 weeks of gestation (13).

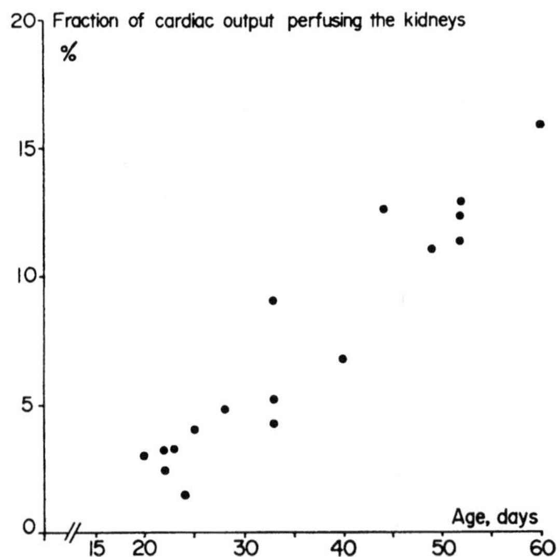

FIGURE 2.1. Renal blood flow as a percentage of cardiac output, plotted versus age, in growing rats between 17 and 60 days of age. (From Aperia A, Herin P. Development of glomerular perfusion rate and nephron filtration rate in rats 17 to 20 days old. *Am J Physiol* 1975;228:1319, with permission.)

Other factors that control the postnatal decrease in RVR largely affect the resistance of glomerular arterioles. In rats, both afferent and efferent arteriolar resistances decrease by a factor of three between 40 days of life and maturity (36). This decrease in RVR may be linked to a decrease in vasoconstrictors or activation of potent vasodilators. Catecholamines, but especially components of the renin-angiotensin system, are high in the early postnatal period of premature and term infants (37–41). The role of the renin-angiotensin system has been extensively studied. Angiotensinogen undergoes a dramatic postnatal increase in liver expression before decreasing and settling to adult levels (42). Renin production in neonates is robust and expands beyond the juxtaglomerular apparatus to include more proximal segments of the renal arterial tree (43). ACE is also abundant. Renal ACE increases postnatally such that within 2 weeks of birth the renal level surpasses the adult level as does the level of circulating ACE (44). Both the AT 1 and AT 2 receptor subtypes are expressed in the neonatal kidney (3,39–46). The AT 2 receptor is believed to play an important role in the apoptotic processes during organogenesis, which wanes postnatally (45,47). Expression of AT 1 receptors peaks postnatally at twice that of adult levels (46). Overall, the substrate, receptors, and the enzymes required for production and actions of AT II are abundantly expressed in the neonatal kidney and contribute to the vasoconstriction of the neonatal kidney. In addition, AT II has been shown to have an important role in the development and function of the renal outflow tract by inducing the development of the renal pelvis and by stimulating the proliferation and differentiation of smooth muscle cells around the ureters, thereby promoting ureteral peristalsis (48). Absence of these AT II–mediated effects promotes hydronephrosis.

Counteracting these vasoconstrictive effects are postnatal increases in the activities of prostaglandins, NO, and kinins, which contribute to the maturational increase in RBF. Indomethacin (which inhibits prostaglandin) lowers RBF in newborn rabbits (49) and decreases renal function in infants indicating an important role for vasodilator prostaglandins (49–52). Endothelium-derived NO release by the renal artery, as well as constitutive NO synthase activity in the renal microvasculature, increases with fetal and postnatal maturation of guinea pigs (53). This increase in NO production is paralleled by increased sensitivity of vascular smooth muscle to NO after birth, which contributes to NO's modulation of postnatal RBF. As *in utero,* vasodilators contribute to the maturational increase in RBF. However, as in the fetus, it may be linked to the renin-angiotensin system through the AT 2 receptor, a potent stimulator of prostaglandin, NO, and kinins (54).

Measurement of Renal Blood Flow

Concept of Clearance

Substances reaching the kidney through circulation may undergo glomerular filtration, tubular reabsorption, or tubular secretion. Most solutes are freely permeable across the glomerular capillary and undergo filtration, followed by tubular reabsorption or secretion along the various nephron segments. Renal clearance of a substance X (C_x) is the volume of plasma from which X is removed (or "cleared") by the kidney within a period of time. Glomerular filtration and tubular secretion facilitate clearance of a solute, whereas tubular reabsorption impedes it. Clearance is calculated as follows:

$$C_x = (U_x \times V)/P_x$$

where U_x and P_x are the concentrations of X in urine and plasma, respectively, and V is the urine flow. The units of clearance are volume per unit time, usually in milliliters per minute. For example, if P_x = 40 mg/mL, U_x = 80 mg/mL, and V = 100 mL/min, then C_x = 200 mL/min. Clearance is a more appropriate concept in describing the renal handling of a certain substance than is urinary excretion rate (i.e., $U_x \times V$) because clearance takes into account the plasma level of X.

If a plasma substance is totally excreted on a single passage through the kidneys, it can be used as a marker of RPF. However, in reality, only approximately 92% of the total RPF passes through the functioning excretory tissue, a fraction termed *effective RPF.* Effective RPF is commonly measured as a CPAH, a weak acid that is almost completely extracted by the renal tubule cells and eliminated in the urine (55). Measurement of effective RPF as CPAH requires a constant infusion of paraamino hippurate and multiple plasma and urine specimens. A simplified modification using a single injection technique, although less accurate, can be used. The use of CPAH as an estimate of RBF has a major limitation in young infants because the renal tubular extraction of paraamino hippurate is incomplete; it is 65% in infants younger than 3 months of age and reaches adult levels only by 5 months of age (56). Thus, CPAH underestimates RBF in infants younger than 5 months of age.

Indirect Assessment of Renal Blood Flow

Radionuclide markers and radiographic techniques can be used to assess RBF. Radiopharmaceuticals used in imaging of the kidneys can provide estimates of RBF or GFR. They have gained wide use in clinical studies of both children and adults because they do not require biochemical assays. The markers are usually labeled with radioactive iodine or technetium. Because of concern that radioactive iodine may accumulate in the thyroid, noniodine radioactive tags are preferred in children. A major value of nuclear methods is the ability to obtain "split" renal function (i.e., separate measurements for each kidney).

Radioactive hippuran is another agent used for assessing renal function. It is excreted by glomerular filtration (20%) and tubular secretion (80%), both governed by RPF. After intravenous injection, timed images are obtained and a computer-generated time activity curve is obtained for the region of interest drawn around each kidney. Split renal function is also calculated from the renogram by computer analysis. Other markers include iothalamate (57), ortho-iodohippurate (handled by the kidney in a manner similar to paraamino hippurate and, hence, a marker of RBF), pentaacetic acid, and dimercaptosuccinic acid (58,59). Although the risk of radiation injury from most radionuclide agents in use is minimal, they are usually reserved for selected cases when accurate estimation of renal function is necessary, such as in the evaluation of a child before urologic surgery (e.g., nephrectomy) or in the follow-up of renal transplantation.

Doppler ultrasonography is a radiologic method that assesses blood velocity in the renal vessels. Although limited in its sensitivity, this method can provide screening information regarding the patency and flow through the renal vessels and detect significant arterial stenosis (60). The resistive index is a crude index of the resistance of the kidneys to blood flow. It takes into account systolic and diastolic blood flow in the renal vessels, as measured by Doppler, and may be helpful in the diagnosis and follow-up of some forms of acute renal failure, such as transplant rejection.

GLOMERULAR FILTRATION

Whole kidney GFR represents filtration occurring in both kidneys and is the product of single-nephron glomerular filtration rate (SNGFR) and the number of filtering nephrons. Formation of new nephrons (nephrogenesis) occurs mainly during intrauterine life and proceeds at different rates in different species. In humans, it is complete by 36 weeks' gestation and proceeds at the same pace when infants are born prematurely (13). Nephronogenesis continues postnatally in rats until 1 week (33), in dogs until 3 weeks (61), and in guinea pigs until 6 weeks of age (62). However, regardless of the species, once nephrogenesis is complete, it is not reactivated even in the face of reduction in the functional renal mass (i.e., disease or surgical resection). Any increase in GFR after nephrogenesis reflects increased filtration of residual nephrons. The degree of this compensatory increase correlates with the magnitude of the initial loss and is more pronounced in the young (63–72). Apart from lack of new nephron formation after nephron loss, compensatory renal growth reflecting increased tubule length and interstitial expansion can start *in utero*. For example, in the model of unilateral obstruction in fetal lambs at 60 days and contralateral kidney, weight increased by 50%, together with an increase in indices of cell proliferation (hyperplasia); however, there is no increase in glomerular number (66,67). The increase in single nephron function that follows a loss of other nephrons early in life is greater in glomeruli in the outer cortex; however, when loss occurs later in life, the increase is more evenly distributed among all residual nephrons (73).

The number of glomeruli in healthy humans has been taken to be, on the average, approximately 1 million in each kidney. However, new observations indicate that there is considerable interindividual variability in the total number of nephron units. The final complement of nephrons has been shown to be affected by an assortment of prenatal factors. For example, low birth weight, especially fetal growth retardation; protein malnutrition; vitamin A deficiency; drugs, such as gentamicin, amino-penicillins, cyclosporine A, and glucocorticoids; as well as metabolic disorders, such as maternal hyperglycemia, have all been shown to cause a significant nephron deficit in the fetus (74–81). Due to the very large number of individual nephron units contributing to the filtration process and the capacity to increase filtration within a single glomerulus, it is unlikely that this interindividual variability in nephron number impacts whole kidney GFR, although no studies exist on this possibility. Instead, the relevance of these findings stems from observations that individuals who have even a modest decrease in the complement of number of nephrons are at an increased risk of developing hypertension and progressive chronic renal dysfunction (74,82,83).

Theoretic Considerations of Glomerular Filtration

As a filtering structure, the glomerulus is essentially a tuft of capillaries, and filtration is transudation of fluid across the capillary wall into Bowman's space (Fig. 2.2). Two characteristics distinguish glomerular ultrafiltration from transcapillary exchange in other organs: (a) The glomerular capillary wall exhibits an extraordinarily high net permeability to water and small solutes, with up to 33% of intraglomerular plasma being filtered; and (b) the glomerulus almost completely excludes plasma proteins the size of albumin and larger from its filtrate. The filtration rate is determined by the same Starling forces governing movement of fluid across other capillary walls (i.e., imbalance between transcapillary hydraulic and oncotic pressure differences). These can be summarized as follows:

1. Mean glomerular transcapillary hydraulic pressure difference [$\Delta P = (P_{GC} - P_{BS})$]
2. Systemic plasma colloid osmotic pressure (π_A)
3. Glomerular plasma flow rate (Q_A)
4. Glomerular capillary ultrafiltration coefficient ($K_f = k \times S$)

When the individual pressures are expressed as average values over the entire length of the capillary, SNGFR is given by the equation:

$$\text{SNGFR} = (k \times S) \times (\Delta P - \Delta\pi)$$

$$= K_f \times P_{UF}$$

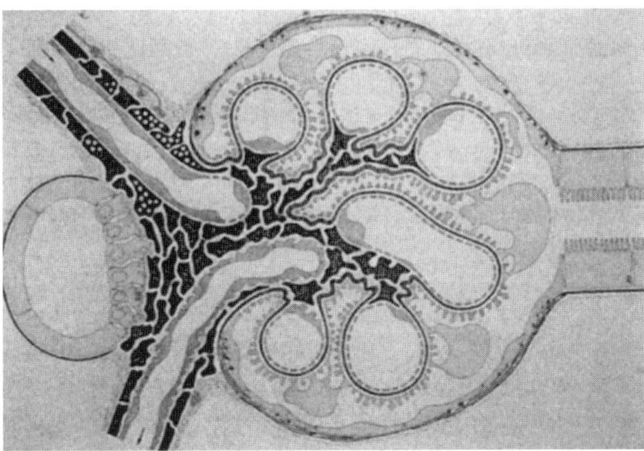

FIGURE 2.2. Schematic representation of a glomerulus. Blood enters the glomerular capillaries through the afferent arteriole, courses through the capillary tuft, and exits through the efferent arteriole. Filtration takes place across the capillary wall into Bowman's space. Mesangial cells are strategically located to control the filtration surface area. The juxtaglomerular apparatus, one of the sites of glomerulotubular feedback regulation, is depicted. Terminals from the renal nerve are also shown. (From the artist, Dr. W. Kriz, with permission.)

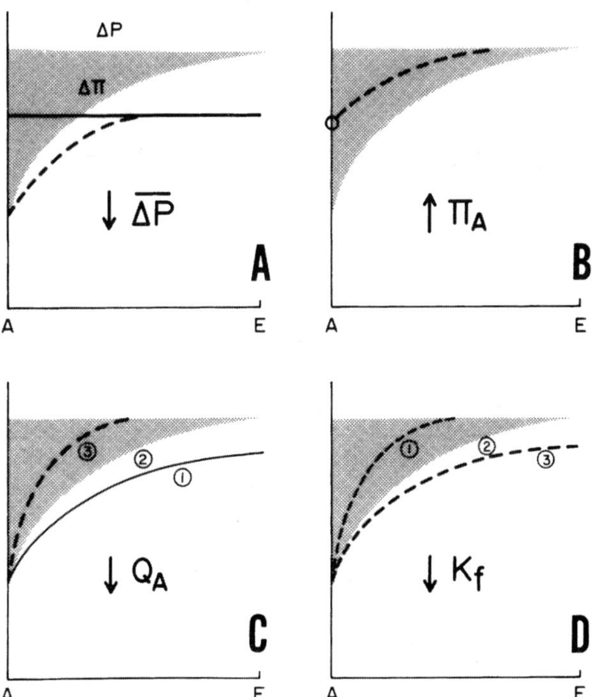

FIGURE 2.3. Schematic portrayals of the process of ultrafiltration as it proceeds from the afferent (*A*) to efferent (*E*) arteriole. **A:** Glomerulus with reduced mean transcapillary hydraulic pressure difference (ΔP). **B:** Increased systematic colloid osmotic pressure (π_A). **C:** Reduced glomerular plasma flow rate (Q_A). **D:** Reduced ultrafiltration coefficient (K_f). The shaded areas represent normal mean net ultrafiltration pressure (P_{UF}), determined by the normal profiles of hydraulic (ΔP) and oncotic (Δπ) pressure differences. The altered ΔP profile as a consequence of each of the above changes is given by an interrupted curve in each panel. Curve 1 in **C** and curve 3 in **D** represent conditions of filtration pressure disequilibrium, whereas curve 3 in **C** and curve 1 in **D** represent equilibrium. The Starling equation is also given and describes the determinants for single-nephron glomerular filtration rate (SNGFR).

where P_{GC} is the glomerular capillary hydraulic pressure and P_{BS} is the hydraulic pressure in the tubule; ΔP – Δπ are the mean glomerular transcapillary hydraulic and colloid osmotic pressure differences, respectively; k is the permeability of the glomerular capillary, and S is the total surface area available for filtration; and K_f, the glomerular ultrafiltration coefficient, is the product of k and S. In this equation, average values are used for ΔP – Δπ because ΔP decreases and Δπ increases as the plasma flows from the beginning to the end of the capillary within a given glomerulus.

Effect of Perturbation in Determinants of Single-Nephron Glomerular Filtration Rate

Mean Glomerular Transcapillary Hydraulic Pressure Difference

Changes in ΔP seldom play a significant role in altering SNGFR because the autoregulatory mechanism in the afferent arteriole sustains glomerular capillary pressure despite large changes in systemic BP (Fig. 2.3). For example, P_{GC} remained unchanged in Munich-Wistar rats despite a drop in RPP from 115 to 80 mm Hg induced by aortic constriction (8). Similarly, GFR in patients with mild to moderate hypertension is usually normal (84). As BP rises, spontaneously hypertensive rats maintain normal P_{GC} by increased afferent arteriolar resistance (85). However, when BP changes outside the autoregulatory range, both P_{GC} and GFR change accordingly. In circulatory collapse, GFR is severely reduced. Significant reductions in P_{GC} and SNGFR are noted in rats when BP falls below 80 mm Hg (8). As ΔP becomes equal to systemic plasma osmotic pressure (πA), filtration diminishes to zero. Conversely, when an increase in BP is extreme, P_{GC} and filtration increase despite a marked concurrent increase in preglomerular vascular resistance. During a decrease (or increase, respectively) in RPP, autoregulation of P_{GC} is largely determined by the ability of the afferent arteriole to constrict/dilate and of the efferent arteriole to respond conversely. It is important to note that the autoregulatory range is not fixed. For example, renal autoregulation is impaired by volume contraction. In volume-depleted animals, lowering BP leads to a reduction in P_{GC} and GFR at a relatively high RPP, whereas little or no change occurs in euvolemic animals (8). This effect and low circulating volume play significant roles in the reduction in GFR that accompanies hypovolemic shock. Renal autoregulation is also readjusted in severe chronic hypertension in which acute hypotensive treatment may lead to a decrease in GFR and a rise in serum creatinine (S_{Cr}). Such a phenomenon in the setting of chronic hypertension might reflect a structural (i.e., not readily reversible) rather than functional narrowing of arteriolar lumen as a consequence of long-standing elevation in RPP. Although this change may be beneficial in maintaining P_{GC} and GFR in the steady state, it leads to a loss of responsiveness of the renal vasculature and to an acute reduction in RPP.

Changes in ΔP can also occur because of changes in P_{BS}. These occur with acute urinary tract obstruction and some forms of acute renal failure. Early in acute ureteral obstruction, whether partial or complete, SNGFR is well maintained despite marked elevation in P_{BS} due to compensatory increases in both P_{GC} and Q_A. Twenty-four hours after complete ligation of a ureter, P_{BS} returns to near normal, yet GFR remains low as a result of a low Q_A secondary to vasoconstriction. In chronic, mild unilateral ureteral obstruction, total kidney GFR, SNGFR, P_{BS}, and Q_A are nearly the same as values in unobstructed control kidneys. This preservation of GFR is a result of the development of two opposing changes in SNGFR determinants: an increase in P_{GC} and a reduction in K_f.

Systemic Plasma Colloid Osmotic Pressure

Derived primarily from serum proteins, π_A is a function of the number of molecules of protein present per unit volume of solution. At the same concentration, a small protein (e.g., albumin) contributes more to oncotic pressure than does a large protein (e.g., globulin). An isolated change in systemic plasma protein concentration (C_A), and hence in π_A, would theoretically be expected to change SNGFR in an opposite direction (Fig. 2.3). However, this does not occur. Acute reductions in C_A from 5.5 g/dL to 3.5 g/dL, induced by infusion of colloid-free solutions into rats, did not increase SNGFR because the fall in π_A and, hence, the rise in P_{UF} elicited a decrease in K_f; the opposing influences of an increase in P_{UF} and a decrease in K_f maintained SNGFR nearly constant (34). Whether changes in π_A occurring chronically are also accompanied by changes in K_f is unknown. In the experimental rat model of nephrotic syndrome, K_f decreases significantly, accounting for a large decrease in SNFGR (86). This reduction of K_f observed in the nephrotic syndrome may account for the low or normal GFR rather than higher values that would be predicted when C_A is low and circulation volume is not appreciably affected (87).

Hypoproteinemia, in association with severe malnutrition, is often accompanied by a decrease in GFR (88,89). This decrease in GFR may be overlooked because S_{Cr} may not be elevated, consequent to a low muscle mass and creatinine production. GFR is reduced in protein malnutrition even when C_A is normal. The reduction in SNGFR is a result of reduced filtering surface area because glomerular size is smaller in protein-malnourished animals.

Glomerular Plasma Flow Rate

The impact of a change in Q_A on SNGFR depends on whether the other determinants of SNGFR have been concurrently modified (Fig. 2.3). For example, infusion of isooncotic plasma selectively increases Q_A, whereas constriction of the aorta or the renal artery decreases both Q_A and ΔP (8). Under certain circumstances, filtration does not occur along the entire length of the glomerular capillary but ceases at some point before its end. This is because plasma oncotic pressure increases progressively from the beginning to the end of the glomerular capillary. This progressive rise in oncotic pressure is accelerated when K_f is high or Q_A is low. Thus, a decrease in Q_A results in cessation of glomerular filtration at an earlier portion of the glomerular capillary tuft and, hence, a reduction in GFR. Experimental administration of renal vasodilators, such as prostaglandin E1, acetylcholine, bradykinin, or histamine causes substantial increase in RBF and RPF in humans or in animals, but GFR is unaffected. SNGFR remains constant because of the opposing influences of an increase in Q_A and a decrease in K_f that occur in response (90). The unexpected decrease in K_f could represent a direct action of these substances on the glomerular capillary, distinct from their known dilatory effects. Conversely, vasoconstrictors, such as AT II and norepinephrine, are capable of producing substantial reductions in RPF but little resultant change in GFR. Again, this is a result of a significant compensatory increase in P_{GC} as a consequence of the pressor-induced increase in efferent arteriolar resistance (91).

Glomerular Capillary Ultrafiltration Coefficient

Glomerular capillary ultrafiltration coefficient is the product of the glomerular capillary permeability to water (k) and the surface area available for filtration (s). Because changes in K_f inevitably lead to directionally similar changes in Dp (Fig. 2.3), changes in K_f, unless extreme, are not expected to cause major changes in SNGFR. Nevertheless, a profound fall in K_f can affect GFR as demonstrated in rats with various experimental conditions. Many of these are disease models, such as minimal change nephrotic syndrome, acute renal failure, acute and chronic extracellular fluid depletion, and congestive heart failure in which a reduction in K_f is the main factor in decreasing SNGFR (10,89,91). A variety of hormones and vasoactive substances, including antidiuretic hormone, adenosine, AT II, endothelin, catecholamines, prostaglandins, acetylcholine, and histamine, modulate SNGFR by reducing K_f (10,89,92). The mesangial cells are believed to be the main locus of their actions because they appear to have a capillary surface area–regulating function. They possess intracellular contractile myofilaments, bear receptors to vasoactive agents, and visibly contract in response to these agents (Fig. 2.4) (93). It is speculated that hormones and vasoactive substances regulate glomerular capillary filtering surface areas, and hence GFR, by affecting mesangial contractility.

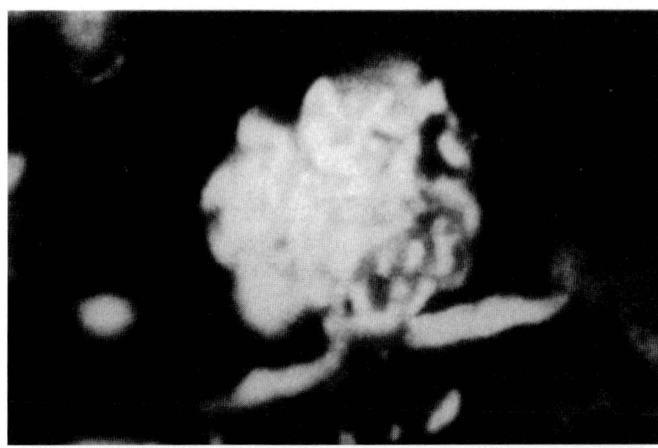

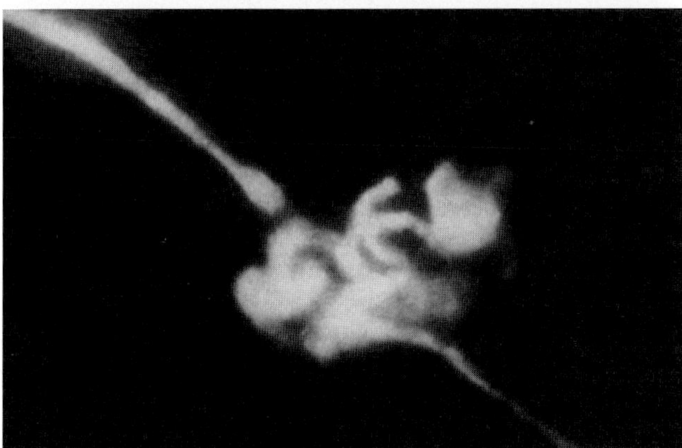

FIGURE 2.4. Structural expression of a reduction in the glomerular capillary ultrafiltration coefficient (K_f). The top panel represents the cast of a normal glomerulus; the bottom panel represents a glomerulus after a stimulus (renal nerve stimulation known to induce contraction of mesangial cells and a decrease in K_f) is applied. Mesangial cell contraction leads to obliteration of some of the glomerular capillaries (i.e., anatomic reduction in the surface area available for filtration), reflected as a decrease in the functional parameter K_f. (From Ichikawa I, Kon V. *Fed Proc* 1983;42:3078, with permission.)

Defense of Glomerular Filtration Rate

Nonmammalian vertebrates have effective homeostatic mechanisms to drastically alter GFR, which is critically important to maintain hydration in these species (94). They can afford to markedly alter GFR because toxic nitrogenous wastes are excreted through nonrenal organs such as gills, skin, and cloacae. In contrast, mammals, with their highly and variable fluid intake, have developed a greater capability to conserve and eliminate water from the body, largely through an expanded and highly regulated reabsorptive capacity of the renal tubules. However, because glomeruli are the only route for elimination of metabolic wastes and toxins, the GFR in mammals is remarkably constant and high relative to other species. Mammals have developed specific mechanisms that maintain GFR stable over a wide range of BP and extracellular fluid volume, which ensures an effective removal of large amounts of nitrogenous waste that are constantly produced. The mechanisms that maintain GFR stable depend on adjustments at the glomerular loci, namely the afferent and efferent arterioles, and likely also in the glomerular capillary bed itself (Fig. 2.5). Two mechanisms, namely the myogenic reflex and tubuloglomerular feedback, are important for the autoregulation of GFR during changes in BP. In the young, autoregulation of RBF is maintained through the same mechanisms but over a lower range of RPP that reflects the lower prevailing BP in the young (2,24).

Myogenic Reflex

The *myogenic reflex* describes the theory that an increase in transmural pressure increases vascular tone. In the renal circulation, this is particularly important in the afferent arteriole, which dilates in response to a decrease in RPP. This dilation also serves to preserve P_{GC}. At the same time, P_{GC} (and GFR) is also maintained in the adult animal through stimulation of renin release and the selective vasoconstrictor effect of AT II on the efferent renal arteriole (10). This reflex is independent of renal nerves or macula densa mechanisms and reflects the inherent characteristics of the vessel (24,95–97). This response has been demonstrated in isolated perfused renal vessels in which a change in vasomotor tone occurs in response to changes in the perfusion pressure in mature animals. However, a definitive role of the myogenic reflex during gestation and early life has not been defined.

Tubuloglomerular Feedback

Constancy of GFR is also determined by the tubuloglomerular feedback system, which describes the coupling of the distal nephron flow and SNGFR. In each nephron, the distal tubule returns to the parent glomerulus and contributes to the formation of the macula densa, which consists of specialized cells of the ascending loop of Henle located between the afferent and efferent arterioles and the glomerulus. In this system, the stimulus to adjust SNGFR is related to the rate of distal flow and also to the composition of the tubular fluid, particularly the chloride concentration and the tubule fluid osmolality (98–102). The signal is perceived in the macula densa and transmitted to the vascular structures of the nephron, particularly the afferent arteriole, but also to the efferent arteriole and the glomerular capillaries, which in concert adjust the rate of filtration. This feedback system is well suited to adjust the rate of filtration and maintain constancy of salt and water delivery to the distal nephron where tubular reabsorption is precisely regulated. Thus, an inverse relationship between filtration and tubular flow is established such that a decrease in tubular flow is anticipated to increase the rate of SNGFR and vice versa. The vascular response has been linked to several vasoactive substances, including adenosine, thromboxane A_2, endothelin, NO, and particularly AT II (103–106).

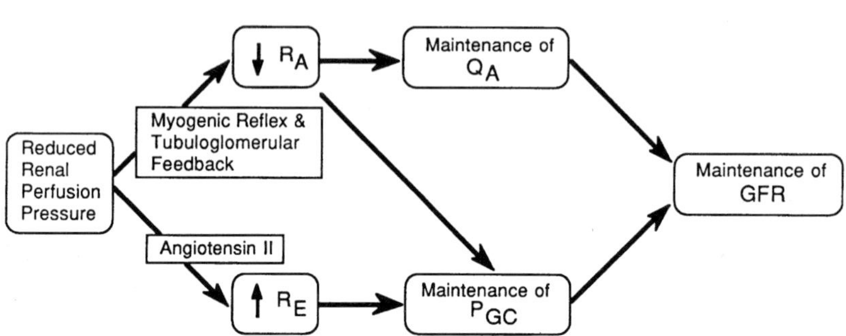

FIGURE 2.5. Mechanisms contributing to the autoregulatory maintenance of renal blood flow and glomerular filtration rates (GFR) in the face of a reduction in renal perfusion pressure. In the young animal, high baseline levels of angiotensin II, the inability to maximally activate the renin-angiotensin system on stimulation under certain circumstances, and low responsiveness of the vasculature to the constrictor action of angiotensin II may limit the ability to autoregulate GFR. P_{GC}, glomerular capillary hydraulic pressure; Q_A, glomerular plasma flow rate; R_A, afferent arteriolar resistance; R_E, efferent arteriolar resistance. (From Badr KF, Ichikawa I. Prerenal failure: a deleterious shift from renal compensation to decompensation. *N Engl J Med* 1988;319:623, with permission.)

The existence of a tubuloglomerular feedback mechanism has been established in the superficial nephrons of young (30-day-old) rats (107). Its sensitivity (i.e., the change of SNGFR induced by a given change in tubule flow rate) is maximal around the values of SNGFR and tubule flow rate prevailing under normal undisturbed conditions. As SNGFR and tubule flow rates increase with growth, adjustments in the tubuloglomerular feedback mechanism take place to maintain this relationship, and the relative sensitivity of the system remains unaltered.

As noted earlier, afferent arteriolar dilation and RBF adjust to decreasing RPP in both adults and immature animals. However, one study found that although decreasing the RPP by approximately 30% from baseline was accompanied by a minimal fall in the GFR in adult rats; in young rats, GFR plummeted by more than 80% (108). Micropuncture experiments revealed that the profound hypofiltration in the young rats reflected decreased glomerular capillary pressure. Because glomerular capillary pressure, in large part, reflects efferent arteriolar vasoconstriction maintained by AT II, the autoregulatory decompensation observed in the young animals likely reflects incompetence in the AT II–mediated vasoconstriction of the efferent vessels. In this connection, a similar degree of water deprivation causes a greater increase in the plasma renin activity in adult animals than in immature animals, and a higher dose of AT II is required in immature animals than in adult animals to effect a similar increase in glomerular capillary pressure (108). Taken together, it appears that the young have limited ability to activate AT II and that the immature efferent arteriole has a limited responsiveness to AT II. Thus, even in the face of afferent vasodilation after decreasing RPP, young animals develop hypofiltration. These observations provide a mechanism for dissociation between RBF and the GFR in that dilation in the afferent arteriole without sufficient vasoconstriction in the efferent arteriole is insufficient to maintain a transcapillary pressure that promotes glomerular hypofiltration in the young (Fig. 2.5).

As noted above, of the two currently recognized receptors for AT II, AT 1 and AT 2, the AT 1 is most abundantly expressed and transduces the bulk of the recognized actions of AT II including efferent arteriolar constriction (3,109). Glomerular AT II hyporesponsiveness in the neonatal kidney does not appear to reflect inadequate AT 1 receptor density, as kidney AT 1 expression peaks postnatally at twice the adult level (46). Further, as noted above, AT II availability is also maximized, reflecting an abundance of renal angiotensinogen, renin, and ACE (42–44). The observed hyporesponsiveness of the neonatal kidney, therefore, appears to reflect inadequate postnatal maturation of post-receptor processes. It is possible, however, that the blunted vasoconstriction of the neonatal efferent arteriole in response to AT II reflects the vasodilatory contribution of the AT 2 receptor, which is abundant during development but wanes with maturation. This may occur through a direct effect of the AT 2 receptor or through AT 2–mediated stimulation of NO and bradykinin (54).

Development of Glomerular Filtration Rate

Prenatal Glomerular Filtration Rate

GFR in the fetus correlates with gestational age and body weight and parallels the increase in renal mass (110,111). There remains controversy as to whether this increase continues throughout gestation (112) or plateaus between 28 and 35 weeks of gestation (113). However, even corrected for body weight, prenatal GFR at every stage of development is much lower than that in adults. For example, creatinine clearance (C_{Cr}) measured within 24 to 40 hours of birth in 30-week premature infants is less than 10 ml/min/1.73 m^2 body surface area (11); at 34 weeks, it is less than 15 mL/min/1.73 m^2, whereas at 40 weeks, it ranges between 10 and 40 mL/min/1.73 m^2 (Fig. 2.6) (114). Direct measurement of intrauterine glomerular function is obviously limited, and creatinine is not an ideal indicator of fetal renal function because it freely crosses the placenta such that the fetal level actually reflects maternal levels. Recently, endogenous low-molecular-weight proteins such as β_2-microglobulin and cystatin C have been shown to be useful in assessing renal function of adults, children, and infants and have been used to assess prenatal renal function (115–121). Cordocentesis measurements of β_2-

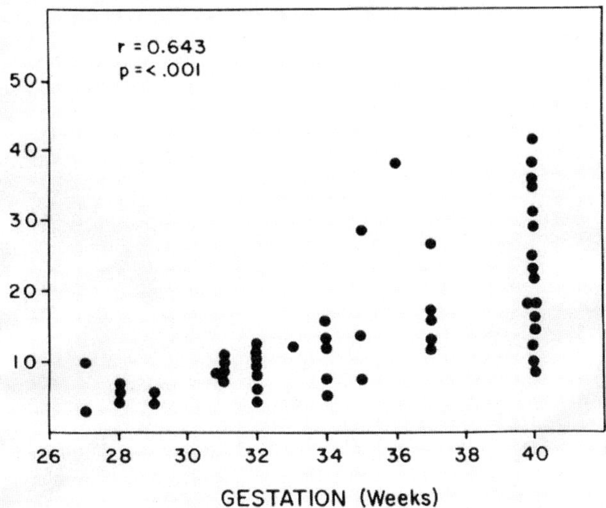

FIGURE 2.6. Creatinine clearance measured within 24 to 40 hours of birth in 30-week premature to 40-week full-term infants. [From Chevalier RL. Developmental renal physiology of the low birth weight preterm newborn. *J Urol* 1996;156(2 Pt 2):714–719, with permission.]

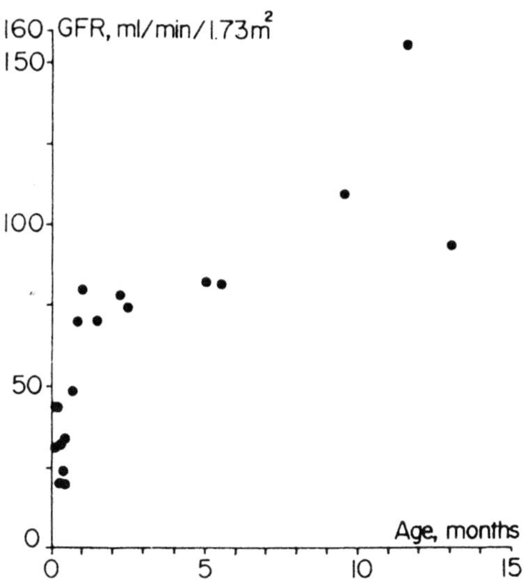

FIGURE 2.7. Glomerular filtration rate (GFR) during the first year of life. (From Aperia A, Broberger O, Thodenius K, et al. Development of renal control of salt and fluid homeostasis during the first year of life. *Acta Paediatr Scand* 1975;64:393.)

microglobulin and cystatin C have generated reference values in fetuses with normal amniotic fluid volume, normal chromosomes, and absence of sonographic evidence of renal/extrarenal abnormalities as well as fetuses with abnormalities in these parameters or postnatal evidence of renal dysfunction (115). The study found that β_2-microglobulin has higher sensitivity, and cystatin C has higher specificity of predicting impaired postnatal renal function, suggesting that these measurements may be a useful adjunct to the analysis of prenatal renal/urinary tract abnormalities.

Postnatal Glomerular Filtration Rate

At birth, the placental function of regulating fetal homeostasis becomes shifted to the kidneys. Compared to the adult, the GFR of a term newborn baby is less than 10% of the adult level whether expressed per gram of kidney weight, body weight, or surface area and correlates closely with the gestational age (Figs. 2.6 and 2.7) (122,123). However, during the first 2 weeks of life, the GFR doubles and continues to increase, reaching adult levels by 2 years of age (112,123). This increase lags in premature babies (124). As with RBF, development of GFR proceeds centrifugally, and the maturational increase in whole kidney GFR reflects primarily an increase in the SNGFR within superficial nephrons and less in the juxtamedullary nephrons (33,125,126).

All four determinants of SNGFR—ΔP, π_A, Q_A, and K_f—contribute to the maturational increase in GFR to varying degrees. In early stages, the systemic BP in humans averages 40 to 70 mm Hg, which is below the autoregulatory range (126,127) and likely contributes to a low P_{GC} and DP that has been shown in immature animals (36). Indeed, the BP in babies born at 28 to 43 weeks of gestation predicted their C_{Cr} (33,38). Plasma protein concentration, and therefore the resultant π_A, is lower in newborns than in older children (5 to 6 g/dL vs. 6 to 8 g/dL) and is a factor that increases ultrafiltration. However, the maturational increase in π_A that hinders ultrafiltration is offset by a more profound increase in P_{GC} having the net effect on P_{UF} to promote ultrafiltration. Experimental studies during later postnatal maturation indicate that π_A and P_{GC} are at adult levels and remain constant (36). The further increase in SNGFR is attributable to an increasing plasma flow rate, Q_A, that reflects an increasing caliber of afferent and efferent arterioles and decreasing resistances in these arterioles. Experimental and human observations support the parallel increase in plasma flow and GFR. Thus, increasing circulating blood volume by delayed clamping of the umbilical cord or intravenous fluid infusion increases inulin clearance (128,129). Finally, rising hydraulic conductivity as well as surface area of the glomerular capillaries likely contributes to maturational increase in the capillary ultrafiltration coefficient, K_f. Glomerular size, glomerular capillary basement membrane surface area, and capillary permeability to macromolecules all increase from neonatal period to adulthood (130–132). However, neither human nor animal data can provide the precise contribution of such changes to the increasing GFR.

CLINICAL ASSESSMENT OF GLOMERULAR FILTRATION RATE

Inulin Clearance

Assessment of GFR is the single most important measurement of renal function. Substances reaching the kidney may undergo one of several processes, including glomerular filtration, tubule reabsorption, tubule secretion, and intrarenal metabolism. These considerations necessitated the search for an "ideal GFR marker." Among various substances considered, inulin emerged and has remained the standard against which all other techniques of measuring GFR are compared to validate their accuracy (133). Inulin is a polymer of fructose, containing, on average, 32 fructose residues and has a molecular weight of approximately 5700 daltons. Natural inulin is derived from plant tubers such as dahlias, chicory, and Jerusalem artichokes. Although the molecular configuration of inulin varies depending on the source, the Stokes-Einstein radius that affects filtration is constant at approximately 5.0 nm. Inulin fulfills the following criteria:

1. It is freely and completely filterable at the glomerulus.
2. It is neither secreted nor reabsorbed by tubules.
3. It is neither metabolized nor synthesized by the kidney.
4. It is not bound to plasma proteins, or if it is, the free unbound as well as the bound components can be measured separately.
5. It is physiologically inert.

Because of these characteristics of inulin, the rate of inulin filtered into Bowman's space equals the urinary excretion of inulin. Moreover, inulin concentration in Bowman's space equals that of plasma. Thus, the flow rate of the fluid filtered into Bowman's space is

$$GFR = C_{In} = U_{In} \times V/P_{In}$$

where C_{In} is the clearance of inulin; U_{In} and P_{In} are the inulin concentrations in the urine and plasma, respectively; and V is the urinary flow rate. For example, if P_{In} = 0.5 mg/mL, U_{In} = 50 mg/mL, and V = 1.1 mL/min, then GFR = C_{In} = 110 mL/min. Although this is a straightforward relationship, there are several points worth emphasizing. It is plasma, not urine, that is being cleared of inulin. In the above example, all inulin is removed from 110 mL of plasma each minute. The inulin clearance is independent of the rate of urinary flow rate. Thus, the concentration of inulin in the urine increases as the volume decreases and vice versa at a given GFR. The inulin clearance is also independent of the concentration of inulin in the plasma; thus, as plasma inulin concentration increases, its appearance in the urine increases as more is filtered. Although inulin clearance remains the most accurate method of assessing GFR, it is cumbersome in routine clinical settings. The drawbacks include difficulty in obtaining the inulin, the preparation of the inulin, and requirement for continuous intravenous infusion to maintain constancy in its plasma concentration. Moreover, measurements of inulin levels are not routinely available in hospital clinical laboratories. These drawbacks have led to the development of other methods to estimate GFR.

Creatinine as a Marker of Glomerular Filtration Rate

In clinical practice, GFR is most often estimated from measurements of S_{Cr} concentrations and the clearance of endogenously produced creatinine. These require only collections of urine or blood samples. Most commonly, renal function is estimated simply by obtaining an S_{Cr} measurement as the initial screening assessment and in monitoring the increase as an estimate of the rate of deterioration of renal function. In the steady state, $U_{Cr} \times V$ (creatinine excretion rate) equals creatinine production rate, which is constant. GFR is inversely proportional to plasma creatinine concentration because GFR = $(U_{Cr} \times V)/P_{Cr}$. Thus, an increase in plasma creatinine from 1 to 2 mg/dL or from 4 to 8 mg/dL represents a functional loss of 50% of GFR between measurements, although the absolute decline in function is less in the latter as is the fractional residual function. The utility of S_{Cr} measurement stems from the relatively constant production of daily creatinine and is independent of diet, protein catabolism, and physical activity. Creatinine production is a function of muscle mass. Approximately 1 g creatinine is derived from 20 kg muscle mass in 1 day (i.e., 50 mg/kg muscle) (134). In individuals of average proportions, creatinine production is 15 to 20 mg/kg/day in boys and 10 to 15 mg/kg/day in girls and infants. This is the amount that is expected to be found in a complete 24-hour urine collection. Thus, if GFR completely ceases (e.g., acute renal failure), the plasma creatinine concentration is expected to increase by approximately 1.5 mg/mL/24 hr.

C_{Cr} is a well-accepted estimate of GFR (as measured by C_{In}) in patients who are older than 1 month of age (135) who have normal or have only moderately decreased renal function. However, in some settings, C_{Cr} is an unreliable estimate of GFR. C_{Cr} overestimates GFR with severely decreased renal function; when GFR falls below 20 mL/min/1.73 m^2, C_{Cr} overestimates C_{In} by approximately 20%. C_{Cr} has been shown to overestimate C_{In} in adults with nephrotic syndrome (136) and in kidney transplant donors and recipients (137,138). Both C_{Cr} and C_{In} underestimate GFR in some forms of acute renal failure in which the functional integrity of the renal tubule is disrupted. Under these conditions, filtered creatinine and inulin can be reabsorbed by passive back diffusion. In acute tubular necrosis after cardiac surgery, 50% of filtered inulin undergoes tubular back leak (139). Thus, measurements of GFR in the setting of acute renal failure with tubule injury are invalid. Notably, although the value of GFR is relatively preserved in this setting, the clearance of creatinine, inulin, and the toxic metabolic wastes represented by these markers is compromised. In practice, therefore, changes in GFR are reflected by changes in S_{Cr} with sufficient accuracy to follow the course of patients with acute renal failure.

Values for S_{Cr} in human newborns are somewhat higher than the maternal S_{Cr} level, reflecting a gradient that allows fetal creatinine to be cleared largely by the maternal kidneys. Over the first few days of life, S_{Cr} decreases and represents GFR maturation, which eliminates both the maternal creati-

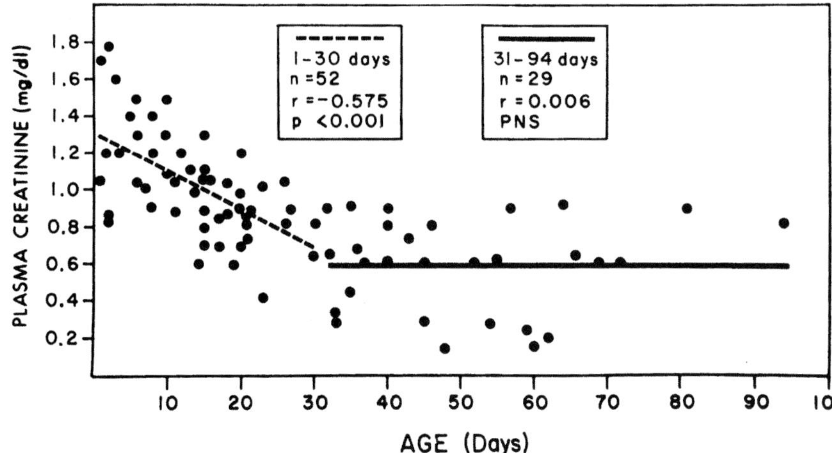

FIGURE 2.8. Plasma creatinine values during the first 3 months of life in low-birth-weight infants (less than 2000 g). (From Stonestreet BS, Oh W. Plasma creatinine levels in low-birth-weight infants during the first three months of life. Pediatrics 1978;61:788, with permission.)

nine and the newborn's endogenous creatinine production (Fig. 2.8). In normal premature infants, S_{Cr} values in the first 10 days of life range between 0.1 and 1.8 mg/dL with a mean of 1.3. During the first month of life, S_{Cr} declines gradually and becomes less than 1 mg/dL after 1 month of age (140). Low-birth-weight infants have daily urinary creatinine excretion rates during the first 2 weeks of life that correlate with birth weight, gestational age, and body length (141). S_{Cr} concentration in normal infants and children increases with age and is slightly higher at any age in male patients than in female patients (Fig. 2.9) (142). Estimation of GFR by C_{Cr} entails obtaining an accurately timed urine collection over a long period, ideally two 24-hour periods (see above). Investigators have attempted to derive formulas to estimate C_{Cr} from S_{Cr} level, in conjunction with anthropometric measurements such as height, weight, or body surface area. The following formula, derived by Schwartz and others, yields values of GFR that correlate with those obtained from C_{Cr} and C_{In} (143):

$$GFR = \delta L/S_{Cr}$$

where GFR is expressed in milliliters per minute per 1.73 m^2; L represents body length in centimeters; S_{Cr} is S_{Cr} in milligrams per deciliter; and δ, a constant of proportionality, is age and sex dependent. Although this formula is useful in day-to-day management, a more precise measurement of GFR (using C_{In} or iothalamate clearance) should be obtained whenever a high accuracy is desirable. New equations have been developed from the Modification of Diet in Renal Disease study that more accurately estimate GFR in adults than GFR measurements obtained by C_{Cr} (144). The equations take into account the individual's age, gender, race, and body size; however, the utility of these equations have not been tested in children.

Modifications of the Standard Clearance Method

Because of the difficulty in maintaining intravenous access and obtaining urine samples in newborn infants and young children, various modifications of the standard clearance tests have been used to yield indirect assessments of GFR. One modification uses an intravenous infusion of a GFR marker but does not require urine collection. Because at steady state the amount of marker infused per unit time (I)

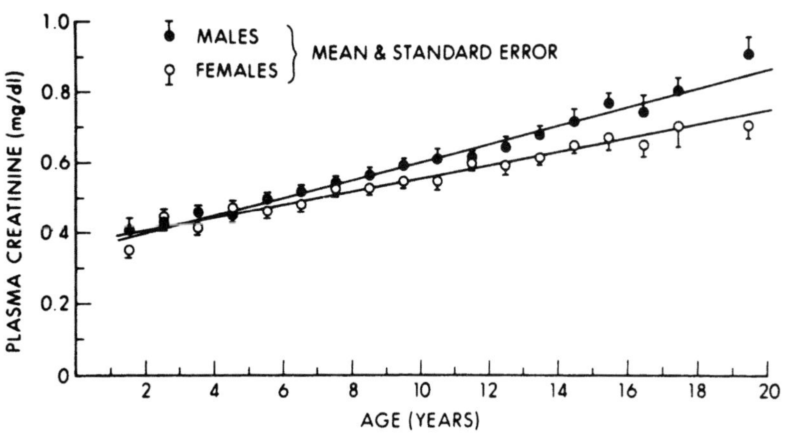

FIGURE 2.9. Mean plasma creatinine concentration (mg/dL) plotted against age for both sexes. The regression equations are for males: y = 0.35 + 0.025 × age, and for females: y = 0.37 + 0.018 × age. (From Schwartz GJ, et al. Plasma creatinine and urea concentration in children: normal values for age and sex. *J Pediatr* 1976;88:828, with permission.)

equals the amount excreted in the urine, as well as the amount filtered,

$$U_x \times V = I$$
$$= GFR \times P_x$$
$$\text{hence, } GFR = I/P_x$$

Thus, only blood sampling is required, together with accurate knowledge of infusion parameters (infusion rate and marker concentration) and certainty that a steady state has been attained. The method uses unlabeled iothalamate infused subcutaneously via a portable minipump (145). After steady state (8 to 24 hours), the marker clearance can be calculated, assisted by a computer program to correct for the child's age, gender, and body size. Some advantages of this method include its suitability for use in infants, in terms of its accuracy, simplicity, safety, and low cost.

Clearance of a marker has also been measured by a single injection of that marker, followed by analysis of its disappearance rate as assessed from repeated plasma samples. This method bypasses the necessity of continuous intravenous infusion and urine collection. A dose of inulin or polyfructosan (0.5 mL/kg of a 25% solution) is given intravenously, and seven or eight capillary blood samples are collected at 5, 10, 15, and 20 minutes, and then after 10- to 15-minute intervals; clearance of the marker is calculated using a mathematic model (146,147). Radiolabeled markers such as chromium-51–ethylene diameinetetraacetic acid (147) or iodine-125–iothalamate (57) have been used because they do not require biochemical assays. However, they remain costly and are still reserved for selected cases when accurate estimation of renal function is necessary.

Cystatin C as a Marker of Glomerular Filtration Rate

Although inulin clearance remains the gold standard and S_{Cr} concentration and C_{Cr} are currently most widely used to estimate GFR, a new endogenous marker has emerged that may obviate some of the limitations of the traditional methodologies. Cystatin C is a 13.6 kDa protease inhibitor constitutively synthesized by all nucleated cells that is freely filtered through the glomerulus and essentially completely reabsorbed and catabolized by tubular cells. Its measurement can now be performed by readily available immunoassay (118,148–151). Studies in adults and children, including premature babies, show that serum concentrations are not affected by gender, height, or muscle mass. It is important to note that the assay is also free from analytical interference from bilirubin and hemoglobin, which represent considerable confounders of S_{Cr} in newborns with jaundice or hemolysis from difficult blood draws.

A reference range has been established for adults (152–154). Recently, a pediatric reference range for cystatin C together with levels of S_{Cr} was published based on measurements in 291 children aged 1 day to 17 years, including infants with gestational age ranging from 24 to 36 weeks (154). The data are shown in Figure 2.10. The data obtained in this study reiterate the high creatinine values at birth and during the first week of life (see above) and the fall that occurs over the first month. Creatinine levels then remain constant until 2 years of age when they rise to adolescent values. The authors emphasize that, by contrast, cystatin C values more closely parallel functional clearance studies. Thus, premature babies have the highest levels of cystatin C (0.43 to 2.77 mg/L; mean, 1.56), followed by infants less than 1 year of age reflecting kidney immaturity (0.59 to 1.97 mg/L; mean, 1.20). By 1 year of age, the range 0.50 to 1.27 mg/L (mean, 0.82) approximates levels found in adults of 0.51 to 0.98 mg/L and indicates essentially constant cystatin C concentration beyond 1 year of age. Recent studies also find that cystatin C may be a more accurate serum marker than creatinine in individuals with impaired renal function (155–157). Finally, even fetal serum concentrations of cystatin C appear to be useful predictors of postnatal renal function suggesting that this may well become a more universal marker of glomerular function (115).

GLOMERULAR SIEVING OF MACROMOLECULES

The enormity in the quantity of filtration generated by the glomerulus underscores specific features of the glomerular capillary bed that allows high permeability to water and small molecules while at the same time providing efficient selectivity that bars cells, proteins larger than albumin, and charged molecules (158,159). This barrier function of the glomerular capillaries is influenced by the size, shape, and charge of the macromolecules. Micropuncture studies and urinary clearance analyses that compare concentration of a given macromolecule in Bowman's space/urine to plasma have been used to obtain the glomerular sieving coefficient for a variety of macromolecules. Sieving coefficients are inversely correlated with the effective radius of the macromolecules. Thus, clearance of the larger proteins, such as albumin and globulin, is markedly less than that of smaller proteins such as monomeric immunoglobulin light chains (160,161). Molecules without charge, including dextran and polyvinylpyrrolidone, that are neither reabsorbed nor secreted (unlike proteins), have been used extensively to study glomerular capillary size selectivity both in experimental settings and in human diseases (160–170). Greater restriction of anionic than of neutral or cationic molecules suggests an electrostatic barrier that is charge selective. The observation that for a given chromatographic radius and charge density, the protein sieving coefficient is smaller than that of neutral dextrans suggests that the glomerular capillary barrier is also shape selective. Thus, proteins are believed to behave as rigid spheres, whereas dextrans are more compliant so as to have a smaller effective radii (161).

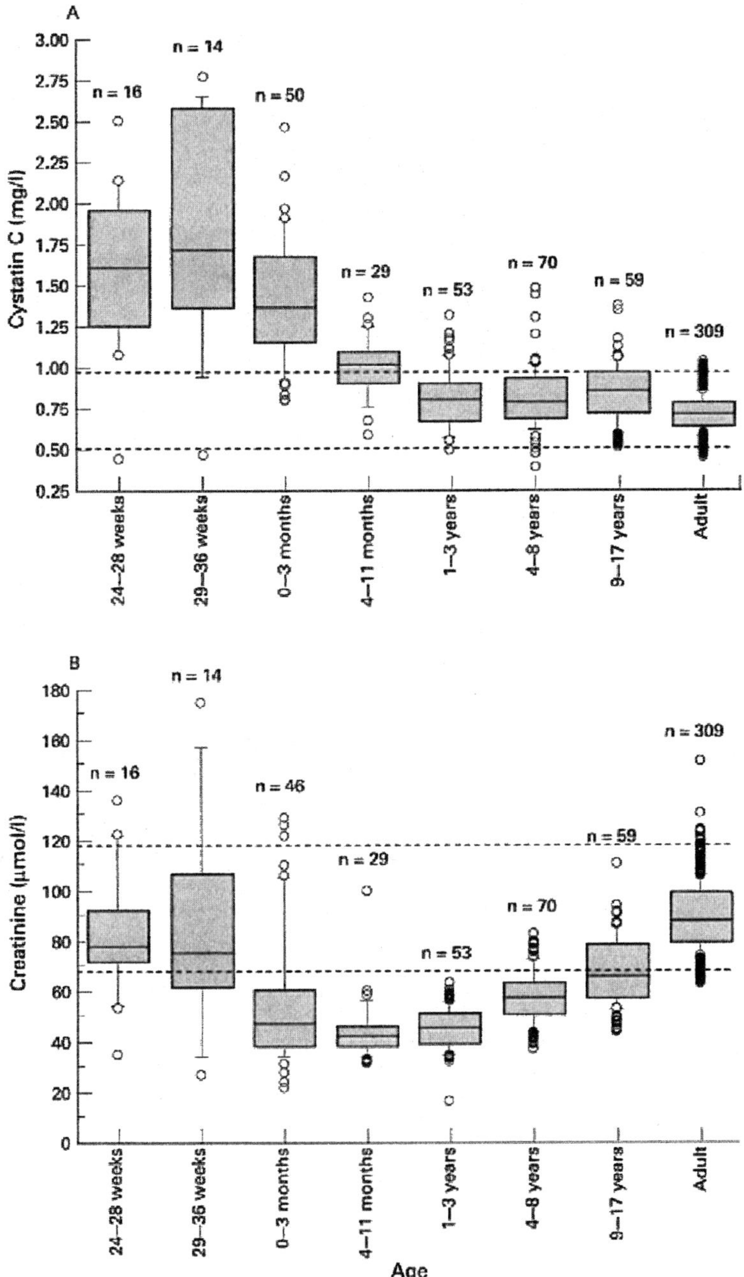

FIGURE 2.10. Range for cystatin C **(A)** and creatinine **(B)** measured in 291 children aged 1 day to 17 years. [From Finney H, Newman DJ, Thakkar H, et al. Reference ranges for plasma cystatin C and creatinine measurements in premature infants, neonates, and older children. *Arch Dis Child* 2000;82(1):71–75, with permission.]

It appears that each of the three major components of the glomerular capillary wall (endothelial cells, basement membrane, and epithelial cells with their podocytes and slit diaphragms) provide impedance to macromolecular filtration (Fig. 2.11). Both endothelial cells and epithelial cells are important in this barrier function as evidenced by the observation that permeability of the isolated glomerular basement membrane (GBM) is much higher than in the intact glomeruli (171). Indeed, native anionic ferritin particles accumulate in the endothelial fenestrae and in the lamina rara externa of the basement membrane. The GBM is increasingly being recognized as providing an important barrier to macromolecular passage. The composition of the GBM includes type IV collagen, laminin, and proteoglycans that provide size and charge-selective restriction to glomerular filtration. Type IV collagen is a trimeric basement membrane specific protein that represents six genetically distinct forms that assemble in specific combinations *in utero* and in different combinations postnatally (172). Defects in adult collagen IV lead to distortion of the GBM that characterizes Alport's syndrome (172). Laminin plays a role in basement membrane structure, cellular differentiation, and adhesion. Laminin also provides sieving impedance, as mice deficient in laminin-2 chain develop nephrotic syndrome (173). Perlecan and agrin are the major proteogly-

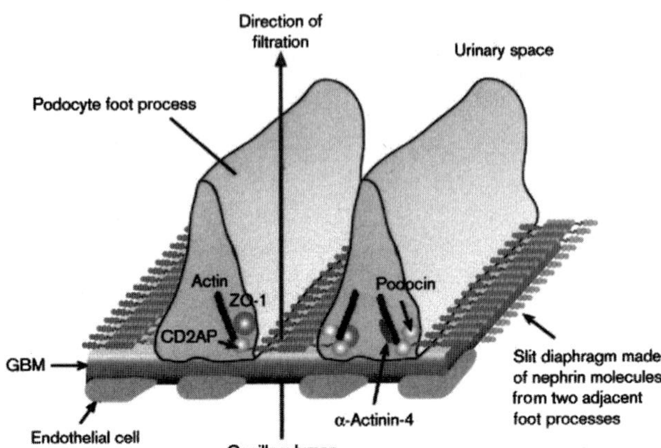

FIGURE 2.11. Molecular model of the glomerular filtration barrier. The three layers of the barrier are the fenestrated endothelial cells lining the inside of the glomerular capillary, the glomerular basement membrane (GBM), and the podocyte foot processes with their intervening slit diaphragm. CD2AP, CD2-associated protein; ZO-1, zonula occludens-1. (From Tryggvason K, Wartiovaara J. Molecular basis of glomerular permselectivity. *Curr Opin Nephrol Hypertens* 2001;10:543, with permission.)

cans in the GBM that contain high levels of negatively charged heparan sulfate moieties (174–176). Overall, it is currently believed that the endothelial cells together with the basement membrane components provide electrostatic impedance for negatively charged components of glomerular filtrate.

The epithelial cell layer of the glomerular capillary network is the site of restrictive size selection of macromolecular filtration. Indeed, the epithelial cells appear to provide the most significant element in glomerular permselectivity, and loss of epithelial podocytes has been shown to parallel the degree of proteinuria in patients with immunoglobulin A and diabetic nephropathies (177,178). Significant proteinuria is typically accompanied by dissolution of the normal interdigitation of epithelial podocytes. Notably, infusion of exogenous polycations, which cause proteinuria, also produce this podocyte lesion (179). Recent studies have clarified the molecular structure and functional implications of the epithelial podocyte slit diaphragms. Positional cloning has identified the gene mutated in congenital nephrotic syndrome of the Finnish type. The NPHS1 gene product, nephrin, is a transmembrane glycoprotein similar to immunoglobulin-like cell adhesion molecules, and nephrin is located in the podocyte slit diaphragms such that two adjacent molecules form the porous filter (180–184). Intracellularly, nephrin interacts with CD2-associated protein as well as other proteins such as podocin and zonula occludens-1 that connect with actin (185). Mice deficient in nephrin or CD2-associated protein have massive proteinuria and early death (173,181). These studies underscore the recent appreciation of the pivotal role of the podocyte and slit diaphragm in the glomerular filtration barrier function.

In addition to the structural characteristics of the capillary wall components that determine its permeability, individual determinants of SNGFR also impact filtration of macromolecules (Fig. 2.12). Glomerular capillary flow rate, but particularly the glomerular capillary pressure, modulates membrane pore structure such that an increase in glomerular pressure augments proteinuria. The mechanism for this effect has been attributed to AT II–induced proteinuria. Thus, infusion of AT II, or endogenous stimulation of AT II activity, increases the fractional excretion of protein, whereas decreasing the pressure has the opposite effect (186–188). These studies underscore that glomerular hemodynamic changes, through increasing the large nonselective pores in the glomerular membrane, can allow macromolecules to escape into the urinary space (Fig. 2.12). It is of interest that acute exercise-induced proteinuria, in which the sieving defect is believed to be linked to increased intraglomerular pressure, is lessened by pretreatment with ACEI (189). Conversely, antagonism of AT II actions by ACEI or AT II receptor antagonist acutely lessens proteinuria and is well documented to decrease protein excretion in many different chronic settings (190–196). The mechanism for this antiproteinuric effect is in part related to decreased efferent arteriolar resistance and there-

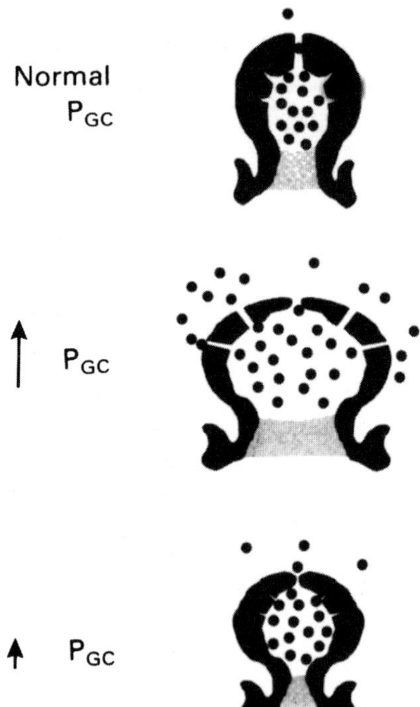

FIGURE 2.12. Schematic representation of the relationship between glomerular capillary pressure (P_{GC}), functional pores in the glomerular capillary wall, and glomerular macromolecular sieving. An increase in P_{GC}, as induced by angiotensin II, increases nonselective pores on the capillary wall allowing the bulk of macromolecules to escape into Bowman's space and then the urine. When the high P_{GC} is attenuated by saralasin, an angiotensin II antagonist, the abnormal presence of large nonselective pores and the sieving defect are largely corrected. (From Ichikawa I, Harris RC. Angiotensin actions in the kidney: renewed insight into the old hormone. *Kidney Int* 1991;40:586, with permission.)

fore glomerular capillary pressure (197). This effect occurs, at least in part, because of a decrease in AT II. However, it also occurs because of an increase in bradykinin, which is also elevated during ACE inhibition and can be abolished by bradykinin antagonism. It should be emphasized that although hemodynamic effects are important in modulating proteinuria, it is likely that more chronic antagonism of AT II activity by ACEI or AT II antagonists also therapeutically preserves glomerular structure and lessens proteinuria.

REFERENCES

1. Davis LE, Hohimer AR, Woods LL. Renal function during chronic anemia in the ovine fetus. *Am J Physiol* 1994;266(6 Pt 2):R1759–R1764.
2. Chevalier RL, Kaiser DL. Autoregulation of renal blood flow in the rat: effects of growth and uninephrectomy. *Am J Physiol* 1983;244(5):F483–F487.
3. Kakuchi J, Ichiki T, Kiyama S, et al. Developmental expression of renal angiotensin II receptor genes in the mouse. *Kidney Int* 1995;47(1):140–147.
4. Burrow C. Regulatory molecules in kidney development. *Pediatr Nephrol* 2000;14:240–253.
5. Miyazaki Y, Tsuchida S, Fogo A, Ichikawa I. The renal lesions that develop in neonatal mice during angiotensin inhibition mimic obstructive nephropathy. *Kidney Int* 1999; 55(5):1683–1695.
6. Pohl M, Bhatnagar V, Mendoza S, Nigam S. Toward an etiological classification of developmental disorders of the kidney and upper urinary tract. *Kidney Int* 2002;61:10–19.
7. Duchin KL, Peterson LN, Burke TJ. Effect of furosemide on renal autoregulation. *Kidney Int* 1977;12(6):379–386.
8. Robertson CR, Deen WM, Troy JL, Brenner BM. Dynamics of glomerular ultrafiltration in the rat. 3. Hemodynamics and autoregulation. *Am J Physiol* 1972;223(5):1191–1200.
9. Adams PL, Adams FF, Bell PD, Navar LG. Impaired renal blood flow autoregulation in ischemic acute renal failure. *Kidney Int* 1980;18(1):68–76.
10. Badr KF, Ichikawa I. Prerenal failure: a deleterious shift from renal compensation to decompensation. *N Engl J Med* 1988;8;319(10):623–629.
11. Veille JC, Hanson RA, Tatum K, Kelly K. Quantitative assessment of human fetal renal blood flow. *Am J Obset Gynecol* 1993;169:1399.
12. Gruskin AB, Edelmann CM Jr, Yuan S. Maturational changes in renal blood flow in piglets. *Pediatr Res* 1970;4(1):7–13.
13. Potter EL, Craig JM. Kidneys, ureters, urinary bladder and urethra. In: Potter EL, Craig JM, eds. *Pathology of the fetus and the infant*, 3rd ed. Chicago: Yearbook Medical Publishers, 1975;436.
14. Rudolph AM, Heymann MA, Teramo AW, et al. Studies on the circulation of the previable human fetus. *Pediatr Res* 1971;5:452–465.
15. Oosterhof H, Haak M, Aarnoudse J. Acute maternal rehydration increases the urine production rate in the near-term human fetus. *Am J Obstet Gynecol* 2000;183(1):226–229.
16. Hedriana H. Ultrasound measurement of fetal urine flow. *Clin Obstet Gynecol* 1997;40(2):337–351.
17. Gouyon JB, Petion AM, Sandre D, et al. Neonatal kidney insufficiency and intrauterine exposure to ketoprofen. *Arch Fr Pediatr* 1997;48:347–348.
18. Rosenfeld CR, Naden RP. Uterine and nonuterine vascular responses to angiotensin II in ovine pregnancy. *Am J Physiol* 1989;257:H17–H24.
19. Lumbers ER, Kingsford NM, Menzies RI, Stevens AD. Acute effects of captopril, an angiotensin-converting enzyme inhibitor, on the pregnant ewe and fetus. *Am J Physiol* 1992;262: R754–R760.
20. Stevens AD, Lumbers ER. The effects of long-term infusions of angiotensin II into the pregnant ewe on uterine blood flow and on the fetus. *J Cardiovasc Pharmacol* 1999; 34(6):824–830.
21. Lumbers ER, Burrell JH, Menzies RI, Stevens AD. The effects of a converting enzyme inhibitor (captopril) and angiotensin II on fetal renal function. *Br J Pharmacol* 1993; 110(2):821–827.
22. Shotan A, Widerhorn J, Hurst A, et al. Risks of angiotensin-converting enzyme inhibition during pregnancy: experimental and clinical evidence, potential mechanisms, and recommendations for use. *Am J Med* 1994;96:451–456.
23. Sedman AB, Kershaw DB, Bunchman TE. Recognition and management of angiotensin converting enzyme inhibitor fetopathy. *Ped Nephrol* 1995;9:382–385.
24. Jose PA, Slotkoff LM, Montgomery S, et al. Autoregulation of renal blood flow in the puppy. *Am J Physiol* 1975;229(4): 983–988.
25. Osborn JL, Hook JB, Bailie MD. Effect of saralasin and indomethacin on renal function in developing piglets. *Am J Physiol* 1980;238(5):R438–R442.
26. el-Dahr SS, Yosipiv IV, Lewis L, Mitchell KD. Role of bradykinin B2 receptors in the developmental changes of renal hemodynamics in the neonatal rat. *Am J Physiol* 1995; 269(6 Pt 2):F786–F792.
27. el-Dahr SS, Figueroa CD, Gonzalez CB, Muller-Esterl W. Ontogeny of bradykinin B2 receptors in the rat kidney: implications for segmental nephron maturation. *Kidney Int* 1997;51(3):739–749.
28. El-Dahr SS, Dipp S, Yosipiv IV, et al. The bradykinin/B2-receptor pair: an autocrine modulator of segmental nephron differentiation. *J Am Soc Nephrol* 1996;7:A1728(abst).
29. el-Dahr SS, Chao J. Spatial and temporal expression of kallikrein and its mRNA during nephron maturation. *Am J Physiol* 1992;262(5 Pt 2):F705–F711.
30. Bogaert GA, Kogan BA, Mevorach RA. Effects of endothelium-derived nitric oxide on renal hemodynamics and function in the sheep fetus. *Pediatr Res* 1993;34(6):755–761.
31. Fawer CL, Torrado A, Guignard JP. Maturation of renal function in full term and premature neonates. *Helv Paediatr Acta* 1979;34:11–21.
32. Rubin MI, Bruck E, Rapoport M. Maturation of renal function in childhood: clearance studies. *J Clin Invest* 1949; 28:114–1162.
33. Aperia A, Herin P. Development of glomerular perfusion rate and nephron filtration rate in rats 17–60 days old. *Am J Physiol* 1975;228(5):1319–1325.
34. Olbing H, Blaufox MD, Aschinberg LC, et al. Postnatal changes in renal glomerular blood flow distribution in puppies. *J Clin Invest* 1973;52(11):2885–2895.

35. Aperia A, Broberger O, Herin P. Maturational changes in glomerular perfusion rate and glomerular filtration rate in lambs. *Pediatr Res* 1974;8(8):758–765.
36. Ichikawa I, Maddox DA, Brenner BM. Maturational development of glomerular ultrafiltration in the rat. *Am J Physiol* 1979;236(5):F465–F471.
37. Eliot RJ, Lam R, Leake RD, et al. Plasma catecholamine concentrations in infants at birth and during the first 48 hours of life. *J Pediatr* 1980;96(2):311–315.
38. Sulyok E, Nemeth M, Tenyi I, et al. Postnatal development of renin-angiotensin-aldosterone system, RAAS, in relation to electrolyte balance in premature infants. *Pediatr Res* 1979; 13(7):817–820.
39. Kotchen TA, Strickland AL, Rice TW, Walters DR. A study of the renin-angiotensin system in newborn infants. *J Pediatr* 1972;80(6):938–946.
40. Harris JM, Gomez RA. Renin-angiotensin system genes in kidney development. *Microsc Res Tech* 1997;39:211–221.
41. Hohenfellner K, Fogo A, Kon V. Renin-angiotensin genes in renal development and the occurrence and progression of renal diseases. *Semin Nephrol* 1999;19:148–154.
42. Gomez RA, Cassis L, Lynch KR, et al. Fetal expression of the angiotensinogen gene. *Endocrinology* 1988;123:2298–2302.
43. Gomez RA, Lynch KR, Sturgill BC, et al. Distribution of renin mRNA and its protein in the developing kidney. *Am J Physiol* 1989;257(5 Pt 2):F850–F858.
44. Yosipiv IV, El-Dahr SS. Developmental biology of angiotensin-converting enzyme. *Pediatr Nephrol* 1998;12:72–79.
45. Maric C, Aldred GP, Harris PJ, Alcorn D. Angiotensin II inhibits growth of cultured embryonic renomedullary interstitial cells through the AT2 receptor. *Kidney Int* 1998; 53:92–99.
46. Tufro-McReddie A, Harrison JK, Everett AD, et al. Ontogeny of type 1 angiotensin II receptor gene expression in the rat. *J Clin Invest* 1993;91:530–537.
47. Nishimura H, Matsusaka T, Fogo A, et al. A novel in vivo mechanism for angiotensin type 1 receptor regulation. *Kidney Int* 1997;52:345–355.
48. Miyazaki Y, Tsuchida S, Nishimura H, et al. Angiotensin induces the urinary peristaltic machinery during the perinatal period. *J Clin Invest* 1998;102:1489–1497.
49. Chamaa, NS, Mosig D, Drukker A, Guignard J. The renal hemodynamic effects of ibuprofen in the newborn rabbit. *Pediatr Res* 2000;48(5):600–605.
50. Varvarigou A, Bardin CL, Beharry K, et al. Early ibuprofen administration to prevent patent ductus arteriosus in premature newborn infants. *JAMA* 1996;275:539–544.
51. Gersony WM, Peckham GJ, Ellison RC, et al. Effects of indomethacin in premature infants with patent ductus arteriosus: results of a national collaborative study. *J Pediatr* 1983;102:895–906.
52. Clyman RI. Recommendations for the postnatal use of indomethacin: an analysis of four separate treatment strategies. *J Pediatr* 1996;128:601–607.
53. Thompson LP, Weiner CP. Acetylcholine Relaxation of Renal Artery and Nitric Oxide Synthesis Activity of Renal Cortex Increase with Fetal and Postnatal Age. *Pediatr Res* 1996;40(2):192–197.
54. Carey R, Wang ZQ, Siragy HM. Role of the angiotensin type 2 receptor in the regulation of blood pressure and renal function. *Hypertension* 2000;35:155–163.
55. Warren JV, Brannon E, Merrill A. A method of obtaining renal venous blood in unanaesthetized persons, with observations on the extraction of O2 and sodium p-aminohippurate. *Science* 1944;100:108.
56. Calcagno PL, Rubin MI. Renal extraction of para aminohippurate in infants and children. *J Clin Invest* 1963;42: 1632–1639.
57. Brouhard BH, Travis LB, Cunningham RJ 3rd, et al. Simultaneous iothalamate, creatinine, and urea clearances in children with renal disease. *Pediatrics* 1977;59(2):219–223.
58. Chervu LR, Blaufox MD. Renal radiopharmaceuticals—an update. *Semin Nucl Med* 1982;12(3):224–245.
59. Bueschen AJ, Witten DM. Radionuclide evaluation of renal function. *Urol Clin North Am* 1979;6(2):307–320.
60. Pedersen EB. New tools in diagnosing renal artery stenosis. *Kidney Int* 2000;57(6):2657–2677.
61. Horster M, Valtin H. Postnatal development of renal function: micropuncture and clearance studies in the dog. *J Clin Invest* 1971;50(4):779–795.
62. Merlet-Benichou C, Pegorier M, Muffat-Joly M, Augeron C. Functional and morphologic patterns of renal maturation in the developing guinea pig. *Am J Physiol* 1981;241 (6):F618–F624.
63. Hayslett JP. Effect of age on compensatory renal growth. *Kidney Int* 1983;23(4):599–602.
64. Kaufman JM, Siegel NJ, Hayslett JP. Functional and hemodynamic adaptation to progressive renal ablation. *Circ Res* 1975;36:266–293.
65. Chevalier RL. Functional adaptation to reduced renal mass in early development. *Am J Physiol* 1982;242(2):F190–F196.
66. Northrup TE, Malvin RL. Cellular hypertrophy and renal function during compensatory renal growth. *Am J Physiol* 1976;231(4):1191–1195.
67. Peters CA, Gaertner RC, Carr MC, Mandell J. Fetal compensatory renal growth due to unilateral ureteral obstruction. *J Urol* 1993;150(2 Pt 2):597–600.
68. Celsi G, Larsson L, Seri I, et al. Glomerular adaptation in uninephrectomized young rats. *Pediatr Nephrol* 1989;3(3): 280–285.
69. Ogden DA. Donor and recipient function 2 to 4 years after renal homotransplantation. A paired study of 28 cases. *Ann Intern Med* 1967;67(5):998–1006.
70. Claesson I, Jacobsson B, Jodal U, Winberg J. Compensatory kidney growth in children with urinary tract infection and unilateral renal scarring: an epidemiologic study. *Kidney Int* 1981;20(6):759–764.
71. Wikstad I, Celsi G, Larsson L, et al. Kidney function in adults born with unilateral renal agenesis or nephrectomized in childhood. *Pediatr Nephrol* 1988;2(2):177–182.
72. Barrera M, Roy LP, Stevens M. Long-term follow-up after unilateral nephrectomy and radiotherapy for Wilms' tumour. *Pediatr Nephrol* 1989;3(4):430–432.
73. Carriere S, Gagnan-Brunette M. Compensatory renal hypertrophy in dogs: single nephron glomerular filtration rate. *Can J Physiol Pharmacol* 1976;55:105–110.
74. Merlet-Benichou C, Gilbert T, Vilar J, et al. Nephron number: variability is the rule. Causes and consequences. *Lab Invest* 1999;79:515–527.
75. Hinchliffe SA, Lynch MR, Sargent PH, et al. The effect of intrauterine growth retardation on the development of renal nephrons. *Br J Obstet Gynaecol* 1992;99:296–301.

76. Vilar J, Gilbert T, Moreau E, et al. Metanephros organogenesis is highly stimulated by vitamin A derivatives in organ culture. *Kidney Int* 1996;49:1478–1487.
77. Lelievre-Pegorier M, Vilar J, Ferrier ML, et al. Mild vitamin A deficiency leads to inborn nephron deficit in the rat. *Kidney Int* 1998;54:1455–1462.
78. Fernandez H, Bourget P, Delouis C. Fetal levels of tobramycin following maternal administration. *Obstet Gynecol* 1990;76:992–994.
79. Amri K, Freund N, Vilar J, et al. Adverse effects of hyperglycemia on kidney development in rats: in vivo and in vitro studies. *Diabetes* 1999;48:2240–2245.
80. Leroy B, Josset P, Morgan G, et al. Intrauterine growth retardation (IUGR) and nephron deficit: Preliminary study in man. *Pediatr Nephrol* 1992;6:3.
81. Merlet-Benichou C, Gilbert T, Vilar J, et al. Rat metanephric organ culture in terato-embryology. *Cell Biol Toxicol* 1996;12:305–311.
82. Brenner BM, Chertow GM. Congenital oligonephropathy: an inborn cause of adult hypertension and progressive renal injury? *Curr Opin Nephrol Hypertens* 1993;2:691–695.
83. Barker DJ, Osmond C, Golding J, et al. Growth in utero, blood pressure in childhood and adult life, and mortality from cardiovascular disease. *BMJ* 1989;298:564–567.
84. London GM, Safar ME, Levenson JA, et al. Renal filtration fraction, effective vascular compliance and partition of fluid volumes in sustained essential hypertension. *Kidney Int* 1981;20:99–103.
85. Arendshorst WJ. Autoregulation of renal blood flow in spontaneously hypertensive rats. *Circ Res* 1979;44:344–349.
86. Ichikawa I, Rennke HG, Hoyer JR, et al. Role for intrarenal mechanisms in the impaired salt excretion of experimental nephrotic syndrome. *J Clin Invest* 1983;71:91–103.
87. White RH, Glasgow EF, Mills RJ. Clinicopathological study of nephrotic syndrome in childhood. *Lancet* 1970;27;1(7661):1353–1359.
88. Ichikawa I, Purkerson ML, Klahr S, et al. Mechanism of reduced glomerular filtration rate in chronic malnutrition. *J Clin Invest* 1980;65(5):982–988.
89. Klahr S, Schreiner G, Ichikawa I. The progression of renal disease. *N Engl J Med* 1988;23;318(25):1657–1666.
90. Deen WM, Maddox DA, Robertson CR, Brenner BM. Dynamics of glomerular ultrafiltration in the rat. VII. Response to reduced renal mass. *Am J Physiol* 1974;227(3):556–562.
91. Deen WM, Robertson CR, Brenner BM. A model of glomerular ultrafiltration in the rat. *Am J Physiol* 1972;223(5):1178–1183.
92. Kon V, Ichikawa I. Hormonal regulation of glomerular filtration. *Annu Rev Med* 1985;36:515–531.
93. Schlondorff D. The glomerular mesangial cell: an expanding role for a specialized pericyte. *FASEB J* 1987;1(4):272–281.
94. Dantzler WH. Comparative physiology of the vertebrate kidney. In: Dantzler WH, ed. *Zoophysiology*, Vol. 22. Berlin: Springer-Verlag, 1989.
95. Martinez-Orgado J, Gonzalez R, Alonso MJ, et al. Endothelial factors and autoregulation during pressure changes in isolated newborn piglet cerebral arteries. *Pediatr Res* 1998;44:161–167.
96. Bayliss WM. On the local reaction of the arterial to changes of the internal pressure. *J Physiol Lond* 1902;28:220–231.
97. Harder DR, Kauser K, Roman RJ, Lomard JH. Mechanism of pressure-induced myogenic activation of cerebral and renal arteries: role of endothelium. *J Hypertens* 1989;7(Suppl):11–5.
98. Bell PD, McLean CB, Navar LG. Dissociation of tubuloglomerular feedback responses from distal tubular chloride concentration in the rat. *Am J Physiol* 1981;240(2):F111–F119.
99. Schnermann J, Persson AE, Agerup B. Tubuloglomerular feedback. Nonlinear relation between glomerular hydrostatic pressure and loop of Henle perfusion rate. *J Clin Invest* 1973;52(4):862–869.
100. Schnermann J, Ploth DW, Hermle M. Activation of tubuloglomerular feedback by chloride transport. *Pflugers Arch* 1976;6;362(3):229–240.
101. Bell PD, Reddington M. Intracellular calcium in the transmission of tubuloglomerular feedback signals. *Am J Physiol* 1983;245(3):F295–F302.
102. Bell PD, Reddington M, Ploth D, Navar LG. Tubuloglomerular feedback-mediated decreases in glomerular pressure in Munich-Wistar rats. *Am J Physiol* 1984;247(6 Pt 2):F877–F880.
103. Schnermann J, Briggs JP. Interaction between loop of Henle flow and arterial pressure as determinants of glomerular pressure. *Am J Physiol* 1989;256(3 Pt 2):F421–F429.
104. Welch WJ, Wilcox CS. Modulating role for thromboxane in the tubuloglomerular feedback response in the rat. *J Clin Invest* 1988;81(6):1843–1849.
105. Weihprecht H, Lorenz JN, Briggs JP, Schnermann J. Vasoconstrictor effect of angiotensin and vasopressin in isolated rabbit afferent arterioles. *Am J Physiol* 1991;261(2 Pt 2):F273–F282.
106. Mitchell KD, Navar LG. Enhanced tubuloglomerular feedback during peritubular infusions of angiotensins I and II. *Am J Physiol* 1988;255(3 Pt 2):F383–F390.
107. Briggs JP, Schubert G, Schnermann J. Quantitative characterization of the tubuloglomerular feedback response: effect of growth. *Am J Physiol* 1984;247(5 Pt 2):F808–F815.
108. Yared A, Yoshioka T. Uncoupling of the autoregulation of renal blood flow and glomerular filtration rate in immature rats: role of the renin-angiotensin system. *Kidney Int* 1988;33:414.
109. Okubo S, Ichikawa, I. Role of angiotensin: insight from gene targeting studies. *Kidney Int Suppl* 1997;63:S7–S9.
110. Robillard JE, Kulvinskas C, Sessions C, et al. Maturational changes in the fetal glomerular filtration rate. *Am J Obstet Gynecol* 1975;1;122(5):601–606.
111. Siegel SR, Oh W. Renal function as a marker of human fetal maturation. *Acta Paed Scand* 1976;65:481–485.
112. Bueva A, Guignard JP. Renal function in preterm neonates. *Pediatr Res* 1994;36(5):572–577.
113. van der Heijden AJ, Grose WF, Ambagtsheer JJ, et al. Glomerular filtration rate in the preterm infant: the relation to gestational and postnatal age. *Eur J Pediatr* 1988;148(1):24–28.
114. Chevalier RL. Developmental renal physiology of the low birth weight pre-term newborn. *J Urol* 1996;156(2 Pt 2):714–719.
115. Bökenkamp A, Dieterich C, Dressler F, et al. Fetal serum concentrations of cystatin C and beta2-microglobulin as predictors of postnatal kidney function. *Am J Obstet Gynecol* 2001;185(2):468–475.

116. Bökenkamp A, Domanetzki M, Zinck R, et al. Cystatin CA new marker of glomerular filtration rate in children independent of age and height. *Pediatrics* 1998;101:875–881.
117. Bokenkamp A, Domanetzki M, Zinck R, et al. Reference values for cystatin C serum concentrations in children. *Pediatr Nephrol* 1998;12(2):125–129.
118. Newman DJ, Thakkar H, Edwards RG, et al. Serum cystatin C measured by automated immunoassay: a more sensitive marker of changes in GFR than serum creatinine. *Kidney Int* 1995;47(1):312–318.
119. Berry SM, Lecolier B, Smith RS, et al. Predictive value of fetal serum beta 2-microglobulin for neonatal renal function. *Lancet* 1995;20;345(8960):1277–1278.
120. Randers E, Erlandsen EJ. Serum cystatin C as an endogenous marker of the renal function—a review. *Clin Chem Lab Med* 1999;37(4):389–395.
121. Nolte S, Mueller B, Pringsheim W. Serum alpha 1-microglobulin and beta 2-microglobulin for the estimation of fetal glomerular renal function. *Pediatr Nephrol* 1991;5(5):573–577.
122. Kleinman LI, Lubbe RJ. Factors affecting the maturation of glomerular filtration rate and renal plasma flow in the newborn dog. *J Physiol* 1972;223(2):395–409.
123. Guignard JP, Torrado A, Da Cunha O, Gautier E. Glomerular filtration rate in the first three weeks of life. *J Pediatr* 1975;87(2):268–272.
124. Vanpee M, Blennow M, Linne T, et al. Renal function in very low birth weight infants: normal maturity reached during early childhood. *J Pediatr* 1992;121(5 Pt 1):784–788.
125. Aperia A, Broberger O, Herin P, Joelsson I. Renal hemodynamics in the perinatal period. A study in lambs. *Acta Physiol Scand* 1977;99(3):261–269.
126. Spitzer A, Edelmann CM Jr. Maturational changes in pressure gradients for glomerular filtration. *Am J Physiol* 1971;221(5):1431–1435.
127. Allison ME, Lipham EM, Gottschalk CW. Hydrostatic pressure in the rat kidney. *Am J Physiol* 1972;223(4):975–983.
128. Oh W, Oh MA, Lind J. Renal function and blood volume in newborn infant related to placental transfusion. *Acta Paediatr Scand* 1966;55:197–210.
129. Leake RD, Zakauddin S, Trygstad CW, et al. The effects of large volume intravenous fluid infusion on neonatal renal function. *J Pediatr* 1976;89(6):968–972.
130. John E, Goldsmith DI, Spitzer A. Quantitative changes in the canine glomerular vasculature during development: physiologic implications. *Kidney Int* 1981;20(2):223–229.
131. Fetterman GH, Shuplock NA, Philipp FJ, et al. The growth and maturation of human glomeruli from term to adulthood. Studies by microdissection. *Pediatrics* 1965;35:601–619.
132. Spitzer A. Factors underlying the increase in glomerular filtration rate during postnatal development. In: Spitzer A, ed. *The kidney during development, morphology and function.* New York: Masson Publishing, 1982;127–113.
133. Gutman Y, Gottschalk CW, Lassiter WE. Micropuncture study of inulin absorption in the rat kidney. *Science* 1965;147:753–754.
134. Graystone JE. Creatinine excretion during growth. In: Cheek DB, ed. *Human growth.* Philadelphia: Lea & Febiger, 1968;182–197.
135. Arant BS Jr, Edelmann CM Jr, Spitzer A. The congruence of creatinine and inulin clearances in children: use of the Technicon AutoAnalyzer. *J Pediatr* 1972;81(3):559–561.
136. Carrie BJ, Golbetz HV, Michaels AS, Myers BD. Creatinine: an inadequate filtration marker in glomerular diseases. *Am J Med* 1980;69(2):177–182.
137. Rosenbaum RW, Hruska KA, Anderson C, et al. Inulin: an inadequate marker of glomerular filtration rate in kidney donors and transplant recipients? *Kidney Int* 1979;16(2):179–186.
138. Mak RH, Al Dahhan J, Azzopardi D, et al. Measurement of glomerular filtration rate in children after renal transplantation. *Kidney Int* 1983;23(2):410–413.
139. Myers BD, Chui F, Hilberman M, Michaels AS. Transtubular leakage of glomerular filtrate in human acute renal failure. *Am J Physiol* 1979;237(4):F319–F325.
140. Stonestreet BS, Oh W. Plasma creatinine levels in low-birth-weight infants during the first three months of life. *Pediatrics* 1978;61(5):788–789.
141. Sutphen JL. Anthropometric determinants of creatinine excretion in preterm infants. *Pediatrics* 1982;69(6):719–723.
142. Schwartz GJ, Haycock GB, Spitzer A. Plasma creatinine and urea concentration in children: normal values for age and sex. *J Pediatr* 1976;88(5):828–830.
143. Schwartz GJ, Brion LP, Spitzer A. The use of plasma creatinine concentration for estimating glomerular filtration rate in infants, children, and adolescents. *Pediatr Clin North Am* 1987;34(3):571–590.
144. Manjunath G, Sarnak MJ, Levey AS. Prediction equations to estimate glomerular filtration rate: an update. *Curr Opin Nephrol Hypertens* 2001;10:785–792.
145. Holliday M, Kogan B, Gambertoglio J. Measuring progression in patients with renal disease. *Curr Opin Urol* 1992;2.
146. Svenningsen NW. Single injection polyfructosan clearance in normal and asphyxiated neonates. *Acta Paediatr Scand* 1975;64(1):87–95.
147. Backlund L, Goransson M, Muller-Suur R, Olsen L. Evaluation of glomerular filtration rate in infants. *Acta Paediatr Scand Suppl* 1983;305:77–78.
148. Kyhse-Andersen J, Schmidt C, Nordin G, et al. Serum cystatin C, determined by a rapid, automated particle-enhanced turbidimetric method, is a better marker than serum creatinine for glomerular filtration rate. *Clin Chem* 1994;40:1921–1926.
149. Dworkin LD. Serum cystatin C as a marker of glomerular filtration rate. *Curr Opin Nephrol Hypertens* 2001;10:551–553.
150. Finney H, Newman DJ, Gruber W, et al. Initial evaluation of cystatin C measurement by particle-enhanced immunonephelometry on the Behring nephelometer systems (BNA, BN II). *Clin Chem* 1997;43:1016–1022.
151. Schwartz GJ, Brion LP, Spitzer A. The use of plasma creatinine concentration for estimating glomerular filtration rate in infants, children, and adolescents. *Pediatr Clin North Am* 1987;34(3):571–590.
152. Norlund L, Fex G, Lanke J, et al. Reference intervals for the glomerular filtration rate and cell-proliferation markers: serum cystatin C and serum β_2-microglobulin/cystatin C-ratio. *Scand J Clin Lab Invest* 1997;57:463–470.
153. Finney H, Newman DJ, Price CP. Adult reference ranges for serum cystatin C, creatinine and predicted creatinine clearance. *Ann Clin Biochem* 2000;37(Pt 1):49–59.

154. Finney H, Newman DJ, Thakkar H, et al. Reference ranges for plasma cystatin C and creatinine measurements in premature infants, neonates, and older children. *Arch Dis Child* 2000;82(1):71–75.
155. Mussap M, Vestra M, Fioretto P, et al. Cystatin C is a more sensitive marker than creatinine for the estimation of GFR in type 2 diabetic patients. *Kidney Int* 2002;61:1453.
156. Risch L, Huber AR. Serum cystatin C in transplantation. *Kidney Int* 2002;61(4):1548.
157. Leach TD, Kitiyakara C, Thakkar H, et al. Serum cystatin C concentrations in renal transplant recipients. *Kidney Int* 1999;55(6):2588.
158. Deen WM, Satvat B, Jamieson JM. Theoretical model for glomerular filtration of charged solutes. *Am J Physiol* 1980; 238(2):F126–F139.
159. Deen WM, Myers BD, Brenner BM. The glomerular barrier to macromolecules: theoretical and experimental considerations. In: Brenner BM, ed. *Contemporary issues in nephrology*, Vol. 9. New York: Churchill Livingstone, 1982; 1–29.
160. Deen WM, Bohrer MP, Brenner BM. Macromolecule transport across glomerular capillaries: application of pore theory. *Kidney Int* 1979;16(3):353–365.
161. Deen WM, Bridges CR, Brenner BM, Myers BD. Heteroporous model of glomerular size selectivity: application to normal and nephrotic humans. *Am J Physiol* 1985;249(3 Pt 2):F374–F389.
162. Alfino PA, Neugarten J, Schacht RG, et al. Glomerular size-selective barrier dysfunction in nephrotoxic serum nephritis. *Kidney Int* 1988;34(2):151–155.
163. Olson JL. Role of heparin as a protective agent following reduction of renal mass. *Kidney Int* 1984;25(2):376–382.
164. Myers BD, Winetz JA, Chui F, Michaels AS. Mechanisms of proteinuria in diabetic nephropathy: a study of glomerular barrier function. *Kidney Int* 1982;21(4):633–641.
165. Morelli E, Loon N, Meyer T, et al. Effects of converting-enzyme inhibition on barrier function in diabetic glomerulopathy. *Diabetes* 1990;39(1):76–82.
166. Remuzzi A, Perticucci E, Ruggenenti P, et al. Angiotensin converting enzyme inhibition improves glomerular size-selectivity in IgA nephropathy. *Kidney Int* 1991;39(6):1267–1273.
167. Guasch A, Deen WM, Myers BD. Charge selectivity of the glomerular filtration barrier in healthy and nephrotic humans. *J Clin Invest* 1993;92(5):2274–2282.
168. Guasch A, Myers BD. Determinants of glomerular hypofiltration in nephrotic patients with minimal change nephropathy. *J Am Soc Nephrol* 1994;4(8):1571–1581.
169. Ting RH, Kristal B, Myers BD. The biophysical basis of hypofiltration in nephrotic humans with membranous nephropathy. *Kidney Int* 1994;45(2):390–397.
170. Drumond MC, Kristal B, Myers BD, Deen WM. Structural basis for reduced glomerular filtration capacity in nephrotic humans. *J Clin Invest* 1994;94(3):1187–1195.
171. Daniels BS, Hauser EB, Deen WM, Hostetter TH. Glomerular basement membrane: in vitro studies of water and protein permeability. *Am J Physiol* 1992;262(6 Pt 2):F919–F926.
172. Hudson B, Reeders S, Tryggvason K. Type IV collagen: structure, gene organization, and role in human diseases: molecular basis of Goodpasture and Alport syndromes and diffuse leiomyomatosis. *J Biol Chem* 1993;268:26033–26036.
173. Shih N, Li J, Karpitskii V, et al. Congenital nephrotic syndrome in mice lacking CD2-associated protein. *Science* 1999;286:312–315.
174. Hassel J, Robey P, Barrach H, et al. Isolation of a heparan sulfate-containing proteoglycan from basement membrane. *Proc Natl Acad Sci U S A* 1980;77:4494–4498.
175. Groffen A, Ruegg M, Dijkman H, et al. Agrin is a major heparan sulfate proteoglycan in the human glomerular basement membrane. *J Histochem Cytochem* 1998;46:19–27.
176. Caulfield J, Farquhar M. Loss of anionic sites from the glomerular basement membrane in aminonucleoside nephrosis. *Lab Invest* 1978;39:505–512.
177. Lemley K, Lafayette R, Safai M, et al. Podocytopenia and disease severity in IgA nephropathy. *Kidney Int* 2002;61(4):1475–1485.
178. Lemley K, Blouch K, Abdullah I, et al. Glomerular permselectivity at the onset of nephropathy in type 2 diabetes mellitus. *J Am Soc Nephrol* 2000;11:2095–2105.
179. Hunsicker LG, Shearer TP, Shaffer SJ. Acute reversible proteinuria induced by infusion of the polycation hexadimethrine. *Kidney Int* 1981;20(1):7–17.
180. Putaala H, Sainio K, Sariola H, Tryggvason K. Primary structure of mouse and rat nephrin cDNA and structure and expression of the mouse gene. *J Am Soc Nephrol* 2000;11:991–1001.
181. Putaala H, Soininen R, Kilpeläinen P, et al. The murine nephrin gene is specifically expressed in kidney, brain and pancreas: inactivation of the gene leads to massive proteinuria and neonatal death. *Hum Mol Genet* 2001;10:1–8.
182. Ruotsalainen V, Ljungberg P, Wartiovaara J, et al. Nephrin is specifically located at the slit diaphragm of glomerular podocytes. *Proc Natl Acad Sci U S A* 1999;96:7962–7967.
183. Holthofer H, Ahola H, Solin M, et al. Nephrin localizes at the podocyte filtration slit area and is characteristically spliced in the human kidney. *Am J Pathol* 1999;155:1681–1687.
184. Holzman L, St. John P, Kovari I, et al. Nephrin localizes to the slit pore of the glomerular epithelial cell. *Kidney Int* 1999;56:1481–1491.
185. Tryggvason K, Wartiovaara J. Molecular basis of glomerular permselectivity. *Curr Opin Nephrol Hypertens* 2001;10(4):543–549.
186. Tencer J, Frick I, Oquist BW, et al. Size-selectivity of the glomerular barrier to high molecular weight proteins: upper size limitations of shunt pathways. *Kidney Int* 1998;53:709–715.
187. Yoshioka T, Mitarai T, Kon V, et al. Role for angiotensin II in an overt functional proteinuria. *Kidney Int* 1986;30(4):538–545.
188. Eisenbach GM, Liew JB, Boylan JW, et al. Effect of angiotensin on the filtration of protein in the rat kidney: a micropuncture study. *Kidney Int* 1975;8(2):80–87.
189. Cosenzi A, Carraro M, Sacerdote A, et al. Involvement of renin angiotensin system in the pathogenesis of postexercise proteinuria. *Scand J Urol* 1993;27:301–304.
190. Maschio G, Cagnoli L, Claroni F, et al. ACE inhibition reduces proteinuria in normotensive patients with IgA nephropathy: a multicentre, randomized, placebo-controlled study. *Nephrol Dial Transplant* 1994;9(3):265–269.

191. Ruilope LM, Alcazar JM, Hernandez E, et al. Long-term influences of antihypertensive therapy on microalbuminuria in essential hypertension. *Kidney Int Suppl* 1994;45:S171–S173.
192. Anderson S, Rennke HG, Brenner BM. Therapeutic advantage of converting enzyme inhibitors in arresting progressive renal disease associated with systemic hypertension in the rat. *J Clin Invest* 1986;77(6):1993–2000.
193. Tanaka R, Kon V, Yoshioka T, et al. Angiotensin converting enzyme inhibitor modulates glomerular function and structure by distinct mechanisms. *Kidney Int* 1994;45(2):537–543.
194. Taal MW, Brenner BM. Combination ACEI and ARB therapy: additional benefit in renoprotection? *Curr Opin Nephrol Hypertens* 2002;11(4):377–381.
195. Parving H. Diabetic nephropathy: prevention and treatment. *Kidney Int* 2001;60(5):2041–2055.
196. Lewis EJ, Hunsicker LG, Bain RP, Rohde RD. The effect of angiotensin-converting-enzyme inhibition on diabetic nephropathy. *N Engl J Med* 1993;329(20):1456–1462.
197. Kon V, Fogo A, Ichikawa I. Bradykinin causes selective efferent arteriolar dilation during angiotensin I converting enzyme inhibition. *Kidney Int* 1993;44(3):545–550.

3

TUBULAR FUNCTION

DEBORAH P. JONES
RUSSELL W. CHESNEY

ANATOMIC ORGANIZATION

The renal tubule forms an epithelial surface that, through the processes of reabsorption and secretion, adjusts glomerular filtrate so that excretion balances input and body composition is kept close to normal. In particular, this function maintains extracellular fluid (ECF) volume and electrolyte and acid-base homeostasis, maintains substrate levels, and excretes a wide variety of organic solutes, including drugs.

The renal tubule is divided into 12 segments; each has distinct morphologic and functional characteristics. The differences that set apart each segment result from the changes in distribution of transport systems on the apical and basolateral surface of the epithelial cells of each of these segments and to the anatomic arrangement in which cells from one segment influence the environment and function of another segment. The membrane properties of segments change as the tubule progresses from its proximal origin to its distal terminus. A series of at least 16 different tight junction proteins, termed *claudins*, are found in segment-specific expression patterns along the nephron in each of these 12 segments (1). Changes in the volume and composition of peritubular capillary fluid and of tubular luminal fluid also influence these transport processes.

Reabsorption is the net transfer of solutes from luminal fluid to pericapillary fluid; secretion is the reverse. The transfer may be transcellular across apical and basolateral membranes or paracellular across epithelial tight junctions into intercellular spaces. In many cases, it is bidirectional, and the net transfer may change from reabsorptive to secretory as conditions dictate.

Some solutes, particularly organic substrates and phosphates, are reabsorbed almost exclusively in the proximal convolution. Electrolytes, including hydrogen ions, are transferred by segments along the entire nephron, sometimes being reabsorbed and then secreted, or the reverse. Often, there are different transport systems for the same solute, such as glucose or organic acids. The proximal segments reabsorb the bulk of glomerular filtrate. The distal segments effect more precise adjustments of solutes, particularly electrolytes, and water. This fine-tuning preserves ECF and whole-body composition within the narrow margins we describe as normal and buffers change in ECF composition through disease.

Developmental Pattern

At birth, the infant is transformed from an organism dependent on the maternal placenta to an independent organism that relies largely on renal function to maintain homeostasis. From midgestation, the kidney develops rapidly so as to be able to fulfill its function at birth. Nephrogenesis is complete by 36 weeks' gestation; tubular maturation begins early in the second trimester, is very active during weeks 32 to 36 of gestation, and continues well into postnatal life (2,3). Factors that affect this maturation and transport capacity include the density, structure, and turnover of specific transporter proteins, in particular, the activity of Na^+-K^+-ATPase; the electrochemical gradient across the cell membrane; hormone responsiveness; membrane surface area, phospholipid content, and fluidity; and cell metabolic activity (3).

This chapter reviews the transport functions of the individual classes of solutes that are transferred, beginning with those specific to the proximal segments and proceeding to those transferred along the 12 segments of the nephron from origin to terminus. In each case, we consider overall tubular handling and the cellular mechanisms and regulatory systems involved in solute transfers. We also describe developmental features affecting each class of solutes.

Before describing the transport mechanisms for each class of solute, we note that three levels of active transport operate along the nephron. The *primary* active transport systems are those in which energy derived from adenosine triphosphate (ATP) hydrolysis is used. The major component of this primary system is Na^+-K^+-ATPase. Others include H^+-ATPase and Ca^{2+}-ATPase. *Secondary* active transporters are those in which sodium transport is coupled to the antiport or cotransport of another solute. These include Na^+-H^+ exchange; the Na^+-K^+-$2Cl^-$ cotransporter;

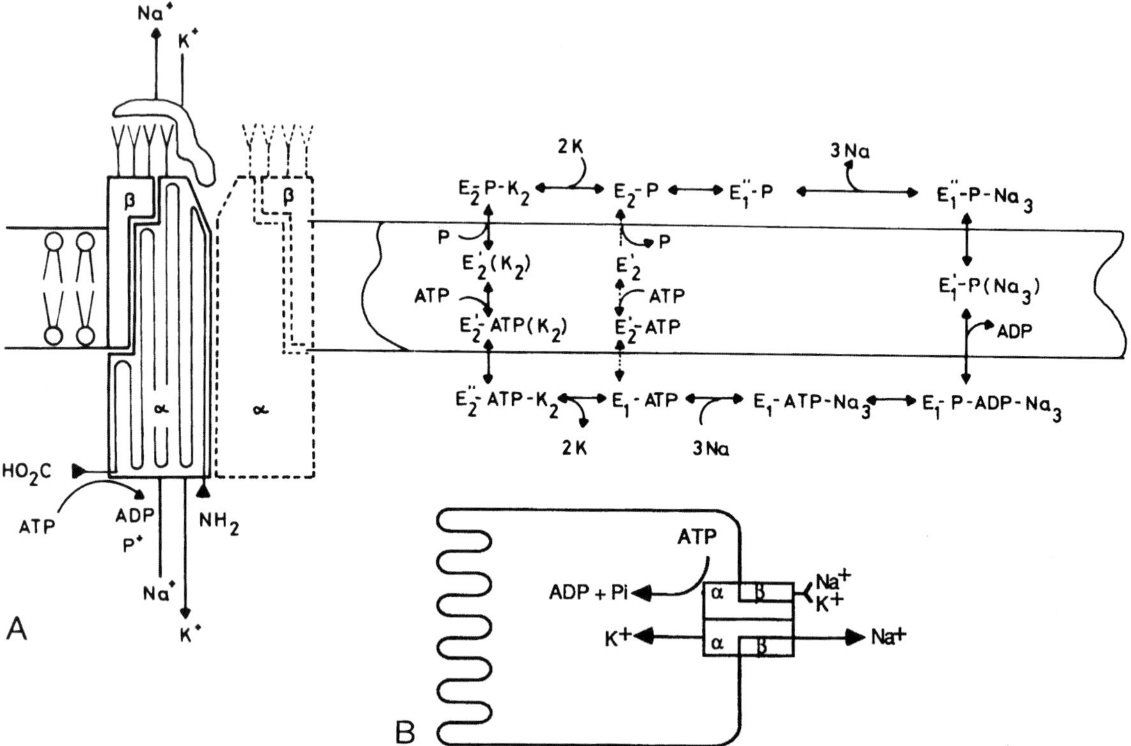

FIGURE 3.1. **A:** Model of Na^+-K^+–adenosine triphosphatase (ATPase) and biochemical reactions involved in the sodium-driven conformational changes of the α subunit. The 3 Na^+ bind to E_1-ATP to form phosphorylated E_1-P, which releases the 3 Na^+ at the outer surface and undergoes a conformational change to the E_1 form, then binds to 2 K^+ and is dephosphorylated at the inner surface, where it binds to ATP and releases the 2 K^+. The intermediate pathway represents reactions in the absence of extracellular K^+. **B:** Model of the cellular orientation of the Na^+-ATPase. ADP, adenosine diphosphate. (From Guder WG, Morel F. Biochemical characterization of individual nephron segments. In: Windhager EE, ed. *Handbook of physiology: renal physiology*. New York: Oxford University Press, 1992:2120–2164, with permission.)

and the amino acid, glucose, and phosphate cotransporters. These symport and antiport systems couple the downhill influx of sodium with the uphill flux of the other solute. *Tertiary* active transport systems are those that are coupled to secondary active transport processes. Examples are the Cl^--formate exchanger, which is coupled to Na^+-H^+ exchange, and the organic anion exchanger, which is coupled to ketoglutarate exchange. Selective ion channels enable ions to diffuse down their concentration gradients.

The use of human cell lines with extended *in vitro* growth potential, especially if they are fully differentiated, have permitted new insights into tubular transport function (4). Likewise, the use of tissue-engineered bioartificial renal tubules, in which porcine proximal tubule cells are seeded into the intraluminal space of a high-flux hollow-fiber hemofiltration cartridge, has permitted study of differentiated transport as well as the metabolic and endocrine functions of the kidney (5).

Na^+-K^+-ATPase

Na^+-K^+-ATPase transports sodium from cells in exchange for potassium uptake into cells. In the renal tubule, this activity is located on the basolateral cell membrane and is the energy-dependent step that regulates sodium chloride reabsorption. Sodium reabsorption begins with its passive transport from luminal fluid across the apical membrane into the intracellular space by secondary transporters (see earlier). It is actively transported out of the cell into peritubular fluid by Na^+-K^+-ATPase (Fig. 3.1). This step creates the favorable electrochemical gradient necessary for continued transport of solutes from luminal fluid into the cell and then into pericapillary fluid, which completes the reabsorptive process. The high level of renal Na^+-K^+-ATPase activity accounts for the high level of renal oxygen consumption and energy expenditure (6). With the hydrolysis of ATP, this pump exchanges three intracellular sodium ions for two extracellular potassium ions, thus maintaining a low intracellular sodium concentration and creating a sodium concentration gradient from lumen to cell. In addition, the high intracellular potassium concentration establishes a cell membrane potential difference (PD) of –60 mV inside the cell.

Na^+-K^+-ATPase is composed of two subunits, α and β, which link the hydrolysis of ATP to the translocation of Na^+ and K^+ (Fig. 3.1). The phosphorus from ATP phosphorylates an amino acid residue of the α subunit, which binds to potassium on the extracellular face. This binding site is the same as that for ouabain. Na^+ binds to the internal cell surface of the α subunit and is translocated to the extracellular face of the membrane along with adenosine diphosphate. The stoichiometry of the process is $3Na^+$ exchanged for $2K^+$ per ATP hydrolyzed. Three isoforms of the α subunit (α_1, α_2, and α_3) and two isoforms of the β subunit (β_1 and β_2) have been identified (7). The α_1 and β_1 forms are found in the mature kidney.

Regulation of Na^+-K^+-ATPase Activity

Agents with a natriuretic action, such as dopamine, atrial natriuretic factor (ANF), parathyroid hormone (PTH), endothelin, and prostaglandin E_2, inhibit Na^+-K^+-ATPase, whereas agents such as norepinephrine, α-adrenergic receptor agonists, insulin, and angiotensin (low dosages) stimulate Na^+-K^+-ATPase. In the dopaminergic system, CA1 receptors are coupled to adenylate cyclase such that dopaminergic agonists simultaneously increase cyclic adenosine monophosphate (cAMP) and phospholipase C_2 with activation of protein kinases, which phosphorylate a regulatory protein and potentially specific phosphorylation sites on the α subunit of Na^+-K^+-ATPase. Phosphorylation of the α subunit reduces ATP hydrolysis and changes the equilibrium between sodium binding E_1 and potassium binding E_2 forms (8).

Developmental Changes in Na^+-K^+-ATPase Activity

The activity of the Na^+-K^+-ATPase increases during development, as does the expression of the α and β subunits. Striking increases occur during weanling (9). The activity of the Na^+-K^+-ATPase in homogenized whole rabbit kidney and isolated tubules from rabbit is lower in neonatal kidney than in the adult kidney; however, the distribution and the affinity constants for Na^+ and K^+ are identical (10,11). The increase in Na^+-K^+-ATPase that occurs during development parallels the increase in sodium reabsorption. In developing rats, an increase in sodium reabsorption precedes an increase of Na^+-K^+-ATPase (12). Studies performed in guinea pig renal cortex demonstrate that pump activity increases fourfold to fivefold during transition from fetus to newborn. Most of the postnatal increase in basolateral pump activity was related to increased pump synthesis rather than redistribution of preformed pumps from internal stores. The increase in pump protein abundance was greater than the increase in mRNA for both α and β subunits, leading to the conclusion that posttranscriptional upregulation might account for the marked increase in pump abundance (13). Inhibition of the Na^+-H^+ pump, the major mechanism for active sodium entry into the cell, reduces the activity of the Na^+-K^+-ATPase in weanling rats, and manipulations that increase the Na^+-H^+ exchanger activity stimulate Na^+-K^+-ATPase (14). The rate of sodium entry into cells and intracellular sodium concentration regulate transcription of both subunits of Na^+-K^+-ATPase (15). Inhibition of Na^+-K^+-ATPase leads to an increased cell sodium concentration, which, within hours, stimulates synthesis of Na^+-K^+-ATPase (15). Glucocorticoid hormones increase transcription of both subunits of Na^+-K^+-ATPase in the newborn rat kidney (16). Na^+-K^+-ATPase activity is acutely affected by other hormones and intracellular second messenger systems. The immature kidney has a blunted response to dopamine and protein kinase C activation (17).

PROXIMAL TRANSPORT SYSTEMS

The proximal tubule has three nephron segments (S1, S2, and S3), which differ from each other morphologically. Cells of the early, or S1, segment have a greater density of microvilli and deeper basolateral membrane infoldings, as well as an abundance of mitochondria. Transport capacity for most solutes (NaCl, bicarbonate, glucose, amino acids, and phosphate) is greatest in the S1 and less in the S2 and S3 segments. This difference may result from the high permeability of the epithelium to solutes and water or to intrinsic differences in the density or kinetic properties of specific transport processes. Changes in the transport rate do not automatically imply a greater intrinsic transport capacity; for example, a decrease in transport rate may follow decreasing substrate concentration as luminal fluid moves distally along the proximal tubule (5,18). Later segments may be described as having less surface area and decreased capacity for transport, both transcellular and paracellular. However, these later segments are also less permeable to solutes and fluid because they have tighter junctional complexes; backleak is minimal in the region of these segments, and a higher concentration gradient is thereby achieved. This illustrates a common theme: The arrangement of transcellular transporters and intercellular permeability characteristics in series in the proximal tubule favors a higher flux in the proximal segment and creation of steeper concentration gradients in the later segments. This arrangement achieves almost complete absorption of nutrients and organic solutes as luminal fluid passes through the proximal tubule (5,18).

Functionally, the proximal tubule performs two major functions: the reabsorption of almost all of the filtered glucose, amino acids, phosphate, and bicarbonate and reabsorption of more than one-half of the sodium, chloride, and water. Figure 3.2 describes the relative reabsorption of various solutes along the length of the proximal tubule. The tubular fluid (TF):plasma (P) ratio of each solute relative to that of inulin is represented; a TF:P ratio less than 1 denotes a drop in TF concentration and indicates net reabsorption. The PD across the proximal tubular epithelium is lumen negative and that of the later (S3) is lumen positive (18).

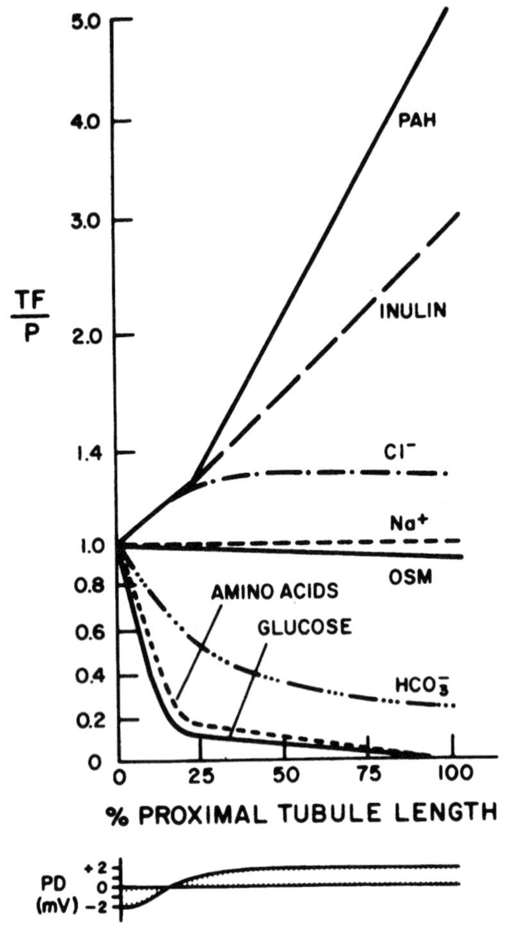

FIGURE 3.2. Reabsorption of solutes along the proximal tubule in relation to the TF:P ratios and potential difference (PD) across the tubular epithelium. TF/P represents the ratio of tubule fluid to plasma concentration. The area above the line denotes that the substance is secreted, and below the line that the solute is reabsorbed. OSM, osmolality; PAH, *p*-aminohippurate. (Adapted from Rector FC Jr. Sodium, bicarbonate, and chloride absorption by proximal tubule. *Am J Physiol* 1983;244:F461.)

Glucose

Glucose is almost completely reabsorbed by the proximal tubule; less than 0.05% of the filtered load appears in urine when the serum level is within the normal range. As the filtered load of glucose increases, the quantity of glucose reabsorbed also increases until the maximum rate of glucose reabsorption (Tm_G) is achieved. The plasma level of glucose at which glucose reabsorption is maximal is known as the *threshold for glucose.* The transport capacity (milligrams per minute) when the threshold is reached is called the Tm_G. The limited capacity for glucose transport is probably related to the number of carrier or transport molecules on the brush-border membrane surface and the basolateral membrane. These carrier systems work in series to transport glucose from the luminal fluid to the intracellular space and then into the pericapillary fluid. The transport maximum for glucose may be modified by factors other than the number of glucose transporters: ECF volume, glomerular filtration rate (GFR), intracellular sodium concentration, and the electrical potential across the tubular epithelium (19). A number of membrane-associated polypeptides are also found at the inner side of the plasma membrane. These influence incorporation and/or retrieval of transporters into the membrane, a process which alters membrane capacitance (20). The membrane protein, termed *RS1,* also influences the organic cation transporter (OCT2).

Heterogeneity of Glucose Transport Along the Tubule

The bulk of filtered glucose is reabsorbed by the first 3 mm of the proximal tubule (S1), with negligible reabsorption by S2 and S3 segments (Fig. 3.2). There are two components of glucose flux: nonsaturable, passive paracellular diffusion and saturable, active transport, which is transcellular. The rate-limiting step in glucose reabsorption is the activity of the glucose transporter, which is located on the brush-border membrane surface. The kinetic properties of the glucose transporter vary among the segments of the proximal tubule: in the S1 segment, there is a high-capacity (J_{max}), low-affinity (*Km*) system; in the S2 segment, a high-affinity, lower-capacity system; and in the S3 segment, an even higher-affinity, lower-capacity system (Table 3.1) (21). The permeability of the diffusion pathway decreases with increasing distance along the proximal tubule. Hence, the rate of glucose reabsorption decreases along the length of the proximal tubule as the character of the transport proteins change, the permeability of the diffusive pathway changes, and the concentration of glucose in luminal fluid declines. This diversity allows high glucose flux in the early proximal tubule and then a steep uphill reabsorption as the affinity for glucose increases along the late proximal tubule, where backleak is minimal. A question still remains: Do these heterogenous functions of the uphill glucose transporter (SGLT1) indicate two independent transporters or different transport modes through an oligomeric protein? The most likely explanation is that heteroassociation with regulatory subunit(s) contribute to this heterogeneity of glucose handling (22).

TABLE 3.1. COMPARISON OF KINETIC PARAMETERS FOR GLUCOSE TRANSPORT IN PROXIMAL TUBULE SEGMENTS

Segment	V_{max} (pmol/min/mm)	Km (mM)
Convoluted (S1)	83.2 ± 5.0	1.64 ± 0.19
Early straight (S2)	12.9 ± 1.1	0.70 ± 0.12
Late straight (S3)	7.9 ± 0.5	0.35 ± 0.05

V_{max}, maximum transport.
From Silverman M, Turner RJ. Glucose transport in the renal proximal tubule. In: Windhager EE, ed. *Handbook of physiology: renal physiology*. New York: Oxford University Press, 1992:2017–2038, with permission.

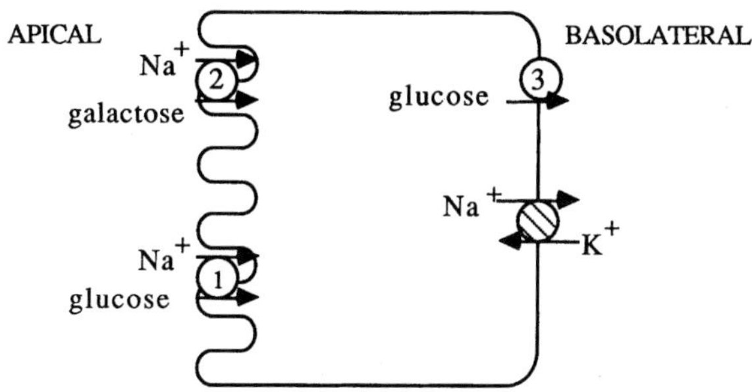

FIGURE 3.3. Model of glucose transport by the proximal tubular cell. (1) Glucose enters the proximal tubular cells by an apical brush-border cotransporter along with either one or two sodium ions, depending on the location of the transporter along the proximal tubule. (2) A transporter for other hexose sugars in addition to glucose is present on the apical surface. (3) Exit across the basolateral membrane of the cell occurs through a sodium-independent transporter. The Na^+-K^+-ATPase is also illustrated.

Cellular Processes Involved in Glucose Reabsorption

Three steps are involved in the reabsorption of glucose: uptake of glucose into the cell by a sodium-dependent glucose transporter in the apical membrane, diffusion of free glucose in the intracellular fluid, and exit from the cell via a specific sodium-independent transport process in the basolateral membrane (Fig. 3.3). The transport of glucose across the apical membrane is by secondary active transport dependent on the electrochemical sodium gradient that is produced by Na^+-K^+-ATPase. The transport is carried out by two structurally and kinetically distinct apical glucose transporter proteins (19,23): One has a high capacity and a low affinity (SGLT2) and the other a low capacity and high affinity (SGLT1) for glucose. The transporter-coupling ratios of sodium to glucose are 1:1 for the S1 segment and 2:1 for the S2 and S3 segments (24). The sensitivity of the two systems to phlorizin, a competitive inhibitor of the glucose transporter, also differs. Phlorizin binding appears to influence both the glucose- and Na^+-binding sites (25). The transitional steps involved in glucose uptake at the brush-border membrane have been elucidated. The initial binding of sodium at the luminal outside surface induces a conformational change that increases affinity of glucose binding. This is followed by presentation of sodium and glucose to the cytoplasmic side, in which the low sodium concentration favors disassociation of sodium, which reduces the affinity of the transporter for glucose that is then released into the cytosol. Then, the transporter orients sodium- and glucose-binding sites back toward the extracellular domain for repeated transport (26).

Molecular Studies of Sodium-Dependent and Sodium-Independent Systems

The distribution of the two apical sodium-dependent glucose transport systems may account for the kinetic differences mentioned earlier. There are two distinct sodium-dependent luminal sugar transporters in the proximal tubule. The SGLT2, which is localized to the early proximal segment, is specific for glucose, has a 1:1 stoichiometry with sodium, and accounts for approximately two-thirds of glucose absorption. The SGLT1 transporter accepts galactose as well as glucose, has a 2:1 stoichiometry (Na:sugar), and is found along the brush border of all proximal segments (22,26). The gene for the sodium-dependent glucose transporter has been localized to chromosome 16. The human transporter protein is 664 amino acids in length, with ten transmembrane helical domains and a molecular weight of approximately 73 kDa (26). The renal cortical, sodium-dependent glucose transporter is similar to that found in small intestine (27).

The basolateral glucose transport systems (GLUT) do not require Na^+ and are not inhibited by phlorizin. At least five distinct GLUT transporters are distributed among numerous tissues, with two predominantly expressed in renal tubule and intestine (28). One has higher affinity and lower capacity (GLUT 1), and the other has lower affinity and higher capacity (GLUT 2). These two systems are distributed differently along the renal tubule: GLUT 1 is present in the glomerulus and along the entire proximal tubule, whereas GLUT 2 is localized exclusively to the basolateral membrane of early proximal convoluted tubule (S1) (29). The specific locations of the two basolateral glucose transport systems parallel those of the apical, sodium-dependent systems. The basolateral glucose transporter system of renal cells is structurally similar to that of erythrocytes and hepatocytes (23,29).

Developmental Changes in Glucose Transport

The increase in glucose reabsorption during late fetal life through infancy and childhood parallels the increase in GFR. However, glucosuria is more common among neonates, and the levels of glucose in urine are highest in preterm infants (65 ± 78 mg/dL), lower in term infants (15 mg/dL), and even lower in adults (6 ± 2 mg/dL) (24). Tm_G, when adjusted to standard surface area and to GFR, tends to be lower in preterm and term infants (Table 3.2) than it is in adults (30).

Factors that increase the glucose absorptive capacity during growth from fetal life to maturity include development of new nephrons, increases in cell membrane surface area and in basolateral Na^+-K^+-ATPase, and changes in expression and density of transporter proteins (31–34). The maximal rate of glucose transport into brush-border vesicles is lower in preparations from fetal kidneys than in those from adult kidneys (Fig. 3.4); the density of transporter proteins is higher in adults (31). Age-related differences in glucose transport capacity correlate with differences in sodium conductance. Changes in membrane permeability to sodium affect membrane potential, a factor that modifies glucose reabsorption.

TABLE 3.2. NORMAL VALUES FOR TUBULAR MAXIMUM FOR GLUCOSE

	Tm_G[a] (mg/min/1.73 m²)	Tm_G/GFR[b] (mg/mL)
Adults	290–375	2.3-2.7
Children	250–400	1.8–2.9
Infants		
Term	35–290	0.9–2.9
Premature	25–190	2.3

[a]Maximum tubular reabsorption of glucose.
[b]Maximum tubular reabsorption of glucose per mL glomerular filtration rate (GFR).
Adapted from Brodehl J, Franken A, Gelissen K. Maximal tubular reabsorption of glucose in infants and children. *Acta Paediatr Scand* 1972;61:413–420.

Maturation of the glucose transport system parallels maturation of bicarbonate flux, fluid absorption, and basolateral surface area of the proximal tubule (Fig. 3.5). The reduced capacity for glucose absorption that characterizes the immature kidney is related to a less-developed basolateral membrane, in addition to the previously mentioned differences in membrane transporter density (35). In summary, the maturational increase in the capacity for tubular reabsorption of glucose is related to an increased number of apical symporter proteins, a more favorable electrochemical gradient, decreased turnover rate of transporter proteins, and decreased membrane fluidity (31). In addition, the membrane of the immature animal is leakier; nearly one-third of the glucose reabsorbed by the neonatal animal leaks back across the tubular membrane, compared with one-sixth of that in the adult (3,36).

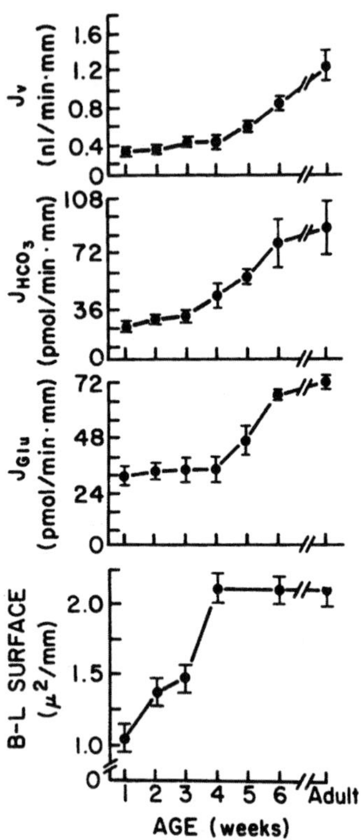

FIGURE 3.5. Absorption of fluid (J_v), bicarbonate (J_{HCO_3}), and glucose (J_{Glu}) and surface area of basolateral membrane (B-L surface) per millimeter of proximal convoluted tubule during development in the rat. (From Schwartz GJ, Evans AP. Development of solute transport in rabbit proximal tubule: I. HCO_3^- and glucose absorption. *Am J Physiol* 1983;245:F382–F390, with permission.)

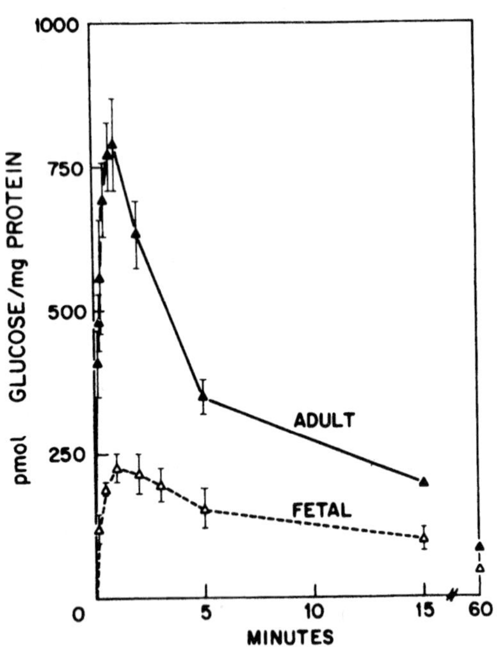

FIGURE 3.4. Maturation of glucose transport. Time course of glucose uptake into brush-border membrane vesicles from fetal and adult rabbits. (From Beck JC, Lipkowitz MS, Abramson RG. Characterization of the fetal glucose transporter in rabbit kidney. Comparison with the adult brush border electrogenic Na^+-glucose symporter. *J Clin Invest* 1988;82:379–387, with permission.)

AMINO ACIDS

The bulk of amino acid reabsorption occurs within the first 2 mm or the proximal one-third of the proximal tubule (S1 segment) (Fig. 3.2) (37). The luminal fluid concentration of amino acids drops as it passes this portion of the tubule and then remains fairly constant. This is indirect evidence for reabsorption of amino acids along the entire length of the proximal tubule. Under normal conditions, amino acids other than glycine, histidine, and taurine are completely reabsorbed. The capacity for amino acid reabsorption along the entire proximal tubule is high. The renal tubule has a mechanism to increase reabsorption in the event that the filtered load of any amino acid increases (38,39).

Although the loop of Henle is difficult to study, bidirectional amino acid transport for neutral amino acids and acidic amino acids has been reported (40,41). The physiologic role of loop amino acid transport has not been elucidated, and it seems unlikely that it would make a significant contribution to total tubular reabsorption because delivery of amino acids to the loop is minimal under normal conditions.

Cellular Mechanisms of Amino Acid Transport

The transepithelial transport of amino acids is an active, concentrative, sodium-requiring process that involves several specific steps (Fig. 3.6) (37). Luminal cell-surface transport is performed by specific amino acid transport systems that operate by secondary active transport, cotransporting amino acids uphill against their concentration gradient along with sodium. The electrochemical sodium gradient created by Na^+-K^+-ATPase enables amino acids to be accumulated. Once inside the cell, the amino acids may be used by the cell or may exit the cell by passive, downhill transport. Together, the apical and the basolateral amino acid transporters achieve the net reabsorption of amino acids from luminal to peritubular fluid. There is also bidirectional movement of amino acids. At the apical membrane, backleak occurs via a paracellular route, through the leaky "tight junctions" of the proximal tubule or via a transepithelial route, using the apical amino acid transporters. Studies in brush-border membrane vesicles (BBMVs) indicate that the transporters located on the brush border are stimulated by intravesicular, or cytoplasmic, amino acids (transstimulation). Therefore, the transport system on the apical membrane is probably bidirectional.

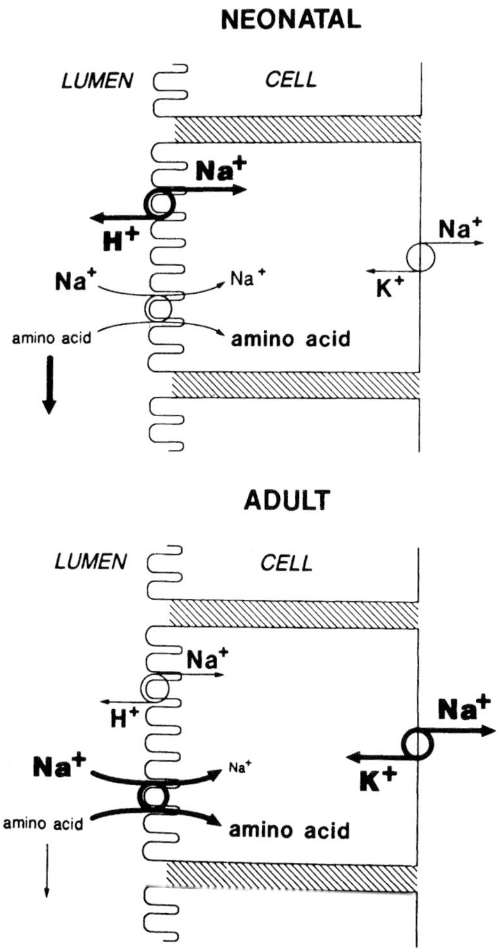

Amino acids may be coupled to sodium in a 1:1 or a 2:1 ratio, which allows the transport process to rely on the luminal to cellular transmembrane potential (Em) and the chemical potential for sodium. In addition to cellular accumulation of amino acids from the luminal membrane, amino acids may be taken up by cells from the basolateral surface to provide substrate, especially in the portions of the nephron that do not have high flux of amino acids via a luminal system (42).

The kinetics of glycine transport (43) in the convoluted tubule differ from those in the straight tubule. The transport maximum and the *Km* are lower in the straight portion. This allows the tubule to drastically reduce the intraluminal concentration of an amino acid by increasing the affinity of the transporter for substrate. In addition, the forces that favor backleak of amino acids are progressively reduced from convoluted to straight tubule.

FIGURE 3.6. Proposed factors responsible for the physiologic aminoaciduria of the immature animal. Factors include decreased activity of the amino acid-sodium cotransporter, increased Na^+-H^+ exchange at the luminal membrane, and decreased activity of the Na^+-K^+-ATPase at the basolateral membrane. (From Zelikovic I, Chesney RW. Development of renal amino acid transport systems. *Semin Nephrol* 1989;9:49–55, with permission.)

Amino Acid Transport Systems

Seven specific transport systems for amino acids have been identified (Table 3.3). Most of the amino acid transport processes are sodium dependent and have some degree of substrate specificity. The electrogenic properties of the sodium–amino acid transporter complex depend on the charge of the amino acid, the coupling ratio for sodium, the charge on the protein carrier complex, and the ionic dependence (Cl^- or K^+) (38). Acidic amino acids require potassium for transport (44). The anionic or acidic amino acids L-glutamate and L-aspartate are reabsorbed by a transporter that is stereospecific, requiring a primary two-amino group along with a positively charged two- to four-carbon chain for transport to occur (45,46). The glutamate transport system is unique in that it requires 2 Na^+ and a proton, which are exchanged for a potassium ion after the transporter undergoes a conformational change. The β-amino acid transport system requires chloride in addition to sodium (47). Protein kinase C activation may also modify taurine transporter activity by phosphorylation of a critical serine residue (48). Dibasic amino acids L-arginine and L-lysine and L-ornithine share at least one transport system (49,50); the luminal uptake step is sodium independent and passive. A sodium-dependent, electrogenic system on the basolateral membrane allows amino acid exit.

A large number of amino acid transport systems have now been cloned and characterized by structural homolo-

TABLE 3.3. AMINO ACID TRANSPORT SYSTEMS

Acidic	L-Glutamate
	L-Aspartate
Basic	L-Arginine
	L-Lysine
	L-Ornithine
Cystine	L-Cystine
	L-Cysteine
Glycine	Glycine
Imino acids	L-Proline
	L-Hydroxyproline
β-Amino acids	Taurine
	β-Alanine
	γ-Aminobutyric acid
Neutral	L-Phenylalanine
	L-Serine
	L-Alanine
	L-Leucine
	L-Phenylalanine
	L-Valine
	L-Asparagine
Glycine	L-Tryptophan
	L-Citrulline
	L-Methionine
	L-Tyrosine
	L-Glutamine

gies to be members of distinct gene families: the glycine transport system, the neutral amino acid transport system A, the basic amino acid transport system y+, and the acidic amino acid transport system X–.

A sodium-independent amino acid transport system (rBAT) for the dibasic amino acids, neutral amino acids, and cystine has been identified (51). As a member of the type II membrane glycoproteins, this transporter is found in the brush-border membrane of both the intestine and the kidney proximal tubule, in which it enables electrogenic exchange of neutral and dibasic amino acids. It shares sequence homology with a variety of amino acid transporters and α glucosidases as part of a family of transport regulators. The gene is located on human chromosome 2. Mutations of this protein have been identified in patients with cystinuria, a transport defect of ornithine, lysine, cystine, and lysine. This transport system is inhibited by heavy metals such as lead and mercury (52). These heteromeric amino acid transporters (HATs) have interesting biologic properties (53). If mutated, they form the molecular basis of the primary aminoacidurias cystinuria and lysinuric protein intolerance (54). They are composed of two polypeptides, a heavy and light subunit, which also may play a role in integrin activation. The genes encoding these transporters are SLC 3A1, SLC 7AG, and SLC 7A7 (54).

Developmental Changes in Amino Acid Transport

In general, urinary amino acid levels are higher in neonates than in mature animals, and the fractional excretion of all but a few amino acids is greater in immature animals. The increased excretion of amino acids results from reduced reabsorption. Factors that might account for the immaturity of the reabsorptive process include differences in the luminal transport system, decreased efflux of the amino acid from the contraluminal membrane, increased backleak through paracellular or transepithelial pathways, or nonspecific maturational differences in the cell membrane or cell metabolism (Fig. 3.6) (55). Altered renal amino acid handling is a highly sensitive marker for nephrotoxicity in immature rats (56).

The aminoaciduria that occurs in preterm and term neonates probably is not caused by a generalized abnormality, because not all of the filtered amino acids are wasted to the same degree (55). The excretion of glycine, imino acids (proline, hydroxyproline), dibasic amino acids, and taurine is preferentially higher than that of other amino acids (57–61). Acquisition of mature reabsorptive capacity of the amino acid system and the glycine transporter occurs at different developmental stages (57). When compared, the renal cortical accumulations of glycine, leucine, and glutamic acid are lower than those of lysine and alanine (55,62–64). Lysine uptake is similar in adult and neonatal animals, whereas cystine accumulation into cortical slices from neonatal kidney is lower than it is in adult kidneys until the age of 2 to 3 weeks (65). Urinary levels of proline are decreased by the postnatal age of 7 days, whereas those of glycine remain elevated until 3 weeks of age (66,67).

Most studies thus far have failed to demonstrate a change from one transporter protein isoform to another with maturation. Early studies of glycine and proline transport led investigators to conclude that the specific, high-affinity transporter was not present at birth but appeared at the time that amino acid reabsorption capacity reached mature levels. Later studies found that both a common glycine-proline transport system and individual transport systems were present from birth and that no new systems were acquired with maturation (55,66,67).

Intrinsic differences in the activity and transport capacity for certain individual transport systems exist. There is evidence of a decreased rate of efflux (66). Analysis of kinetic studies involving the uptake of proline by rat renal BBMVs reveals that the magnitude of proline uptake is reduced in neonates and that the characteristic uptake pattern is less pronounced in vesicles from young rats. This phenomenon is explained by differences in membrane permeability to sodium. The sodium gradient that is necessary for cellular or vesicular uptake of an amino acid is dissipated more rapidly in the vesicles from 7-day-old rats than in those from older rats (66).

Studies using isolated renal tubule preparations reveal that the initial transport rate of proline into neonatal rat tubules equals that of adults, yet the cellular amino acid levels are higher in the neonatal rats (60). This phenomenon is partially explained by metabolic studies. Metabolism of proline by tubules from adult rats is twice that of tubules from neonates. The maturational changes in the excretion of proline are related to metabolic changes within the cell as well as to changes in the transport system.

Two cystine transport systems have been detected in isolated proximal renal tubules from neonatal dogs. Both systems are present from birth, yet the activity of both systems, as judged by the transport maximum (J_{max}), is less in the tubules from puppies; these increase to adult levels by 3 weeks of age. The authors speculate that the postnatal increase in transport capacity is secondary to an increase in the number of transport sites for the sulfur amino acids (65).

Changes in the phospholipid composition of the membrane during maturation also affect the ionic and amino acid permeability characteristics. The change in composition of rat tubular brush-border membranes parallels change in membrane permeability to sodium (55). This may impair the ability of the immature renal tubular cell to maintain the electrochemical gradient necessary for reabsorption of amino acids.

The steady-state renal cell accumulation of the amino acids glycine, proline, and taurine is greater in young animals than it is in adults, probably because of slower egress of amino acids from immature animals (55). The intracellular concentration of amino acids is higher in younger animals. Although the luminal transport process is similar, the efflux step at the basolateral membrane is reduced. The net effect is decreased net transepithelial amino acid transport.

The kinetic characteristics of taurine accumulation by BBMVs have been extensively studied and are similar in adult and 28-day-old rats (68). The young rats responded to alterations in the supply of the substrate amino acids with changes in accumulation that were identical to responses in adults. Despite this, the urinary excretion of taurine is much greater in the immature animals. This probably is related to differences in the membrane permeability to taurine or reduced basolateral efflux in the immature rats. An age-related increase in the accumulation of the amino acid into BBMVs was found in younger rats (59). Taurine transport into vesicles isolated from nursing rats of three different ages (7, 14, and 21 days) was measured to examine the influence of dietary supply on uptake. Taurine uptake by the vesicles from 7-day-old rats was significantly lower than that of the older rats; there was little response to changes in dietary taurine intake (59). The efflux of taurine from cortical slices is decreased in the 7-day-old pups (69). Taurine accumulation increased as a function of age, being lower in the 14- and 21-day-old animals and increasing to adult levels by 28 days of age. These results suggest that age-related differences in taurine reabsorption and urinary excretion are related to reduced intrinsic apical transporter activity early in development and to differences in membrane permeability to taurine and Na^+ later in development, when the transporter capacity is at adult levels. The ability of the renal tubular cell to respond to dietary taurine is attained at 1 to 2 weeks of age in the rat. The maturational factors responsible for this capacity are unknown.

The urinary levels of taurine in low-birth-weight neonates are significantly elevated, with fractional excretion ranging from 38 to 68% (70). These infants were receiving parenteral nutrition devoid of taurine and had low plasma taurine levels. Therefore, immature animals cannot reabsorb as much filtered amino acids and are less able to adapt to deficiency, predisposing them to significantly reduced plasma taurine values. Because taurine is needed for normal retinal and CNS development, this may have deleterious consequences in the developing preterm infant.

PEPTIDE AND PROTEIN REABSORPTION

Peptides are reabsorbed in the proximal tubule by a variety of processes, including reabsorption by endocytosis, luminal hydrolysis with reabsorption as free amino acids, carrier-mediated reabsorption of small intact peptides, and peritubular uptake. Peptides reabsorbed by the proximal tubule include angiotensin II, bradykinin, and glucagon. These peptides are rapidly hydrolyzed by peptidases found along the brush-border membrane and are then reabsorbed as single amino acids. Certain properties confer resistance to peptidases, because peptides with disulfide bonds or β-amino acids may not undergo hydrolysis (37).

Dipeptides and tripeptides that are resistant to hydrolysis in the gastrointestinal tract are presented to the brush-border membrane, in which they are encountered by enzymes that may be reabsorbed by a Na^+-independent, electrogenic peptide transporter. The peptide transporter is located in cortex and medulla and shares similarities with the intestinal peptide transport system (71). Peptide transport is sodium independent and energized by an inwardly directed transmembrane proton gradient that depends on the inward negative membrane potential. This type of system is unique to the renal tubule, is more commonly found among prokaryotic cells, and remains the only example of uphill solute transport energized primarily by proton movement. Two distinct dipeptide transport systems have been characterized: a high-affinity system that is highly dependent on proton gradient and a lower-affinity system that may operate in the absence or presence of substrate concentration or inward proton gradient (71). A diverse group of dipeptides or tripeptides and xenobiotics with a peptide backbone are accepted by these systems, but free amino acids, or peptides with more than three amino acids, do not interact. Hydrophobicity seems to favor binding to transporter. Specific basolateral systems for peptide transport have not been demonstrated. However, many of these substances interact with basolateral systems for organic cations or anions. The *p*-aminohippurate (PAH) transporter reveals significant affinity for dipeptides and tripeptides and also seems to favor hydrophobic compounds. Peritubular uptake of peptides appears to be negligible.

Although not filtered freely like smaller peptides, proteins may reach the urinary space through glomerular filtration, in which they are reabsorbed by nonspecific adsorptive endocytosis or receptor-mediated endocytosis, or undergo hydrolysis by brush-border membrane enzymes such as peptidases (72). Handling of proteins by the brush-border membrane depends on size. The low-molecular-weight proteins are 10 to 44 kDa. Examples include growth hormone, PTH, many enzymes, immunoprotein fragments such as Bence Jones, and tissue-specific antigens such as β_2-microglobulin. These proteins are absorbed and then undergo hydrolysis.

Intermediate-molecular-weight proteins of 44 to 90 kDa (e.g., albumin) are normally filtered to a very small degree and are subsequently endocytosed and then hydrolyzed within lysosomes (72). Larger proteins, such as fibrinogen and immunoglobulins, normally do not reach the urinary space. If the normal barrier to filtration of high-molecular-weight proteins is disrupted, they may undergo endocytosis.

Examples of low-molecular-weight proteins that undergo hydrolysis by a nonspecific system are angiotensin II and bradykinin. Peptides such as insulin, PTH, and ANF are absorbed by specific receptor-mediated endocytosis hydrolysis. The nonspecific system is a high-capacity, low-affinity system, whereas the specific systems are usually low-capacity, high-affinity systems (72).

Phosphate

The fraction of plasma phosphate that is filtered depends on the plasma phosphate concentration and the distribution of ionized phosphate as determined by the Donnan equilibrium. In the rat, 92 to 98% of phosphate is present in the aqueous phase of plasma, and 90% of total plasma phosphate is filterable. The ultrafilterability of phosphate declines with increases in plasma calcium (73).

Phosphate reabsorption occurs primarily in the proximal tubule, in which approximately 76% of the filtered phosphate is reabsorbed (Table 3.4). Phosphate reabsorption occurs in both the convoluted and the straight portions of the proximal tubule (73). A small fraction of phosphate is reabsorbed in the distal tubule under conditions of sodium loading and in the absence of PTH. Phosphate reabsorption rates are three to four times greater in the early proximal tubule than in the S2 portion of the convoluted tubule and are lower still in the straight tubule (74). This axial heterogeneity in phosphate transport is postulated to be the result of TF acidification, which decreases the ratio of the divalent form (preferred substrate) to monovalent form (75) (see Peptide and Protein Reabsorption, Cellular Mechanisms). There are differences in the affinity and capacity for phosphate transport between the straight and convoluted portions of the proximal tubule (74,75). Affinity of the transporter for phosphate is low in the S1 and increases as one travels distally. This characteristic, which enables a large substrate flux proximally and more complete absorption distally, has been alluded to in the discussion of glucose transport. Higher affinity of the transporter for substrate allows more complete absorption by increasing the transporter efficiency in the face of lower tubular substrate concentrations.

TABLE 3.4. RENAL PHOSPHATE HANDLING IN NEWBORN AND ADULT GUINEA PIGS

	Newborn	Adult	*p* Value
GFR (mL/g kidney)	0.28 ± 0.06	0.55 ± 0.05	<.01
Plasma phosphate (mM)	2.18 ± 0.15	2.16 ± 0.14	>.90
Tubular reabsorption of P[a]			
% Filtered load	89.93 ± 2.55	78.25 ± 2.89	<.01
μmol/mL GFR	1.87 ± 0.14	1.53 ± 0.12	<.05
Fractional reabsorption of P[b] (% filtered load)			
Proximal	76.66 ± 2.75	67.21 ± 2.74	<.001
Distal	15.62 ± 2.11	10.51 ± 1.83	<.005

GFR, glomerular filtration rate.
[a]Whole kidney tubular reabsorption.
[b]Single nephron tubular reabsorption.
Adapted from Kaskel FJ, Kumar AM, Feld LG, et al. Renal reabsorption of phosphates during development: tubular events. *Pediatr Nephrol* 1988;2:129–134.

Cellular Mechanisms

Phosphate reabsorption is a unidirectional, transcellular movement of phosphate across the proximal tubule from luminal to peritubular fluid (Fig. 3.7A). Phosphate is reabsorbed by a sodium-dependent, cotransport system located on the apical, or brush-border, membrane. Uptake occurs against a small chemical gradient and a large electrical gradient (76). Phosphate uptake is driven by the electrochemical gradient for sodium, with a sodium-coupling ratio of 3:1 (77). The rate-limiting process for transepithelial phosphate reabsorption is the apical transport step (76,78). The transporter prefers the divalent form (HPO_4^{-2}) of inorganic phosphate to the monovalent form ($H_2PO_4^-$), although both are candidates for transport. Luminal fluid pH influences the activity of the Na^+-phosphate cotransporter; kinetically distinct transporter proteins also cause the rate of phosphate transport to vary.

Sodium is required for cotransport with phosphate and is postulated to activate the binding of phosphate to its transport site (78). The Na^+-phosphate cotransporter probably functions in a "glide symmetry" model, as illustrated in Figure 3.7C: Na^+ binds to the transporter protein first and then induces a conformational change to increase affinity of the protein for phosphate. The substrate-transporter complex is translocated to the interior of the cell, in which sodium and then phosphate dissociates (76).

Phosphate transport is stimulated by decreased intracellular pH (an outwardly directed proton gradient) (75). Two

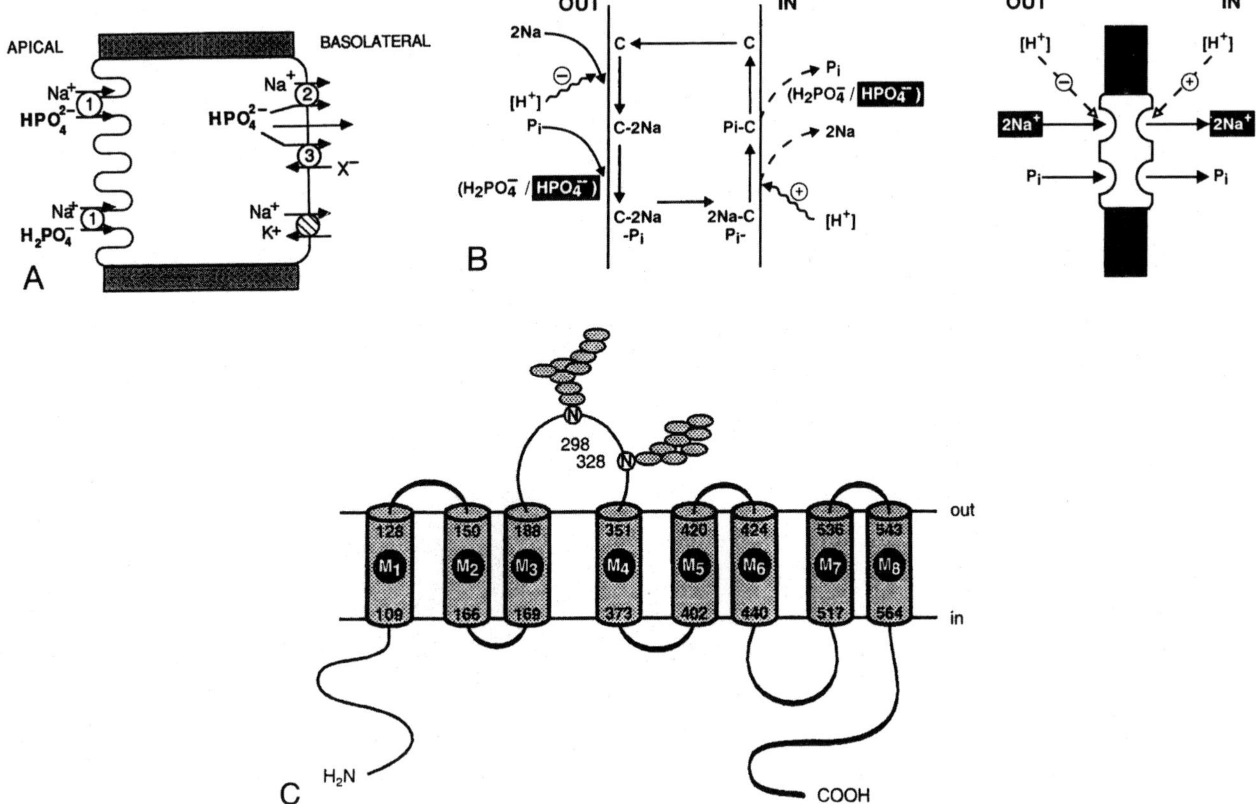

FIGURE 3.7. **A:** Model for sodium-phosphate cotransport by the proximal tubular cell (1). Both monovalent and divalent phosphates are cotransported with sodium at the brush-border membrane. Phosphate exits the basolateral membrane by a sodium cotransport process (2), or by anion exchange (3). **B:** Model for conformational changes and ionic interactions of the sodium-phosphate cotransporter. At high intratubular sodium concentrations, sodium binds to the transporter first and favors binding of phosphate to the transport site, followed by movement of the transporter-substrate complex to the cytoplasmic side of the cell where sodium dissociates first, decreasing protein affinity for phosphate, which then dissociates (glide symmetry model). **C:** Secondary structure prediction for the type II Na-P_1 cotransporter. Eight transmembrane-spanning regions are proposed. The transporter is *N*-glycosylated at the two positions indicated. (From Murer H. Cellular mechanisms in proximal tubular Pi reabsorption: some answers and more questions. *J Am Soc Nephrol* 1992;2:1649–1665, with permission.)

factors are responsible: Increasing the luminal fluid pH increases divalent phosphate, which is more readily transported; and there appears to be a direct effect of pH on the transporter protein, which alters its binding properties (79). Protons and sodium compete for binding sites of the transporter both inside and outside the cell. A decrease in the external pH reduces the affinity of the transporter and the rate of transport, whereas a decrease in intracellular pH increases the rate of transport (75,76,79).

Intracellular phosphate has many important functions in oxidative metabolism, protein synthesis, and enzyme action. The mechanism of phosphate exit has not been as clearly characterized; there is probably a passive component leading to phosphate transfer down its electrochemical gradient. Phosphate also exits the cell by the sodium-independent system, using a phosphate-OH^- antiport system (anion exchanger) (76,80). A basolateral, Na^+-phosphate cotransport system has been proposed that is based on the demonstration of sodium-coupled phosphate uptake into basolateral BBMVs; however, these findings may have resulted from contamination of the basolateral vesicles with vesicles from apical membranes (76).

Molecular Characterization

Structural characterization of at least two distinct Na-phosphate cotransport systems (NPT1 and NPT2) in the kidney indicates that the two classes are different, sharing only 20% homology. The NPT1 transporters are 465 amino acids in length, with a predicted seven to nine transmembrane domains. The NPT2 transporters have 635 amino acids and eight transmembrane domains (Fig. 3.7). Both transporters have been localized to the brush-border membrane of the proximal tubular cell, although the NPT1 is homogenously found throughout, whereas the NPT2 is most concentrated in the S1 segment (81). NPT1 transporter is less specific for phosphate and also accepts anions such as probenecid, chloride, and penicillin. The NPT2 is the PTH- and hormone-sensitive transporter that also responds to changes in dietary phosphate. The type II (NPT2) transporter forms the rate-limiting step in brush-border membrane transport (82). In addition to these two systems, Na-independent phosphate transporters have been identified that are also cell surface viral receptors Glvr-1 and Ram-1 and are widely expressed in mammalian tissues, in which they are proposed to serve a housekeeping function (81).

Hormonal Regulation

PTH is the principal hormone regulator of Na^+-phosphate transport. PTH reduces the transport maximum without changing the affinity of the transporter for substrate (76). PTH inhibits Na-dependent phosphate transport by mechanisms dependent on AMP protein kinase A and protein kinase C-phosphoinositide pathways. Other factors that stimulate cAMP production also inhibit phosphate transport (83). Apical and basolateral PTH receptors mediate the effect of PTH to reduce phosphate transport through an acute mechanism dependent on endocytosis or phosphorylation (81). Growth hormone, insulin-like growth factor-I, insulin, thyroid hormone, and 1,25-dihydroxyvitamin D_3 stimulate phosphate absorption, whereas PTH-related peptide, calcitonin, ANF, epidermal growth factor, transforming growth factor α, and glucocorticoids inhibit this process. Hormonal effects may be mediated through ligand-activated receptors that bind to response elements in the promotor region of the transporter gene.

Two major circulating factors also greatly influence phosphate reabsorption. The first, a membrane-bound endopeptidase encoded by the PHEX (protein with homology to endopeptidases on the X chromosome) gene, serves as an enzyme to degrade a protein, fibroblast growth factor 23, which in the absence of PHEX acts to massively reduce phosphate reabsorption (84). PHEX also appears to degrade PTH related peptide (85). Mutations of PHEX and fibroblast growth factor 23 have been associated with a number of hereditary or tumor-induced phosphaturic syndromes (84,86).

Developmental Changes in Phosphate Reabsorption

In contrast to most other transport processes, fractional reabsorption of phosphate is greater in the immature or neonatal animal than it is in the adult (Table 3.4) (87). Clearance studies performed in infants and children initially suggested that the increased plasma phosphate levels and reduced fractional excretion of phosphate during infancy are related, in part, to the lower GFR during the first year of life (88). However, subsequent studies per-

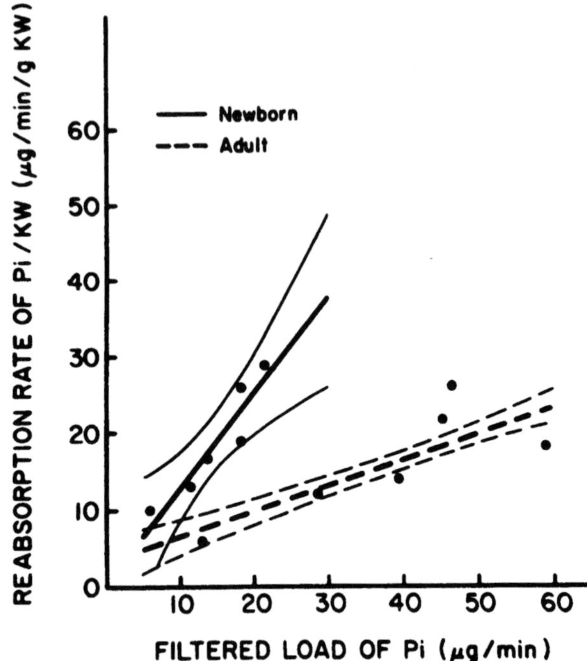

FIGURE 3.8. Relationship between the filtered load of phosphate and phosphate reabsorption in isolated perfused kidneys from mature and newborn guinea pigs. At a comparable filtered load, the reabsorption of phosphate is significantly greater in newborn animals than in adult animals. (From Johnson V, Spitzer A. Renal reabsorption of phosphate during development: whole-kidney events. *Am J Physiol* 1986;251:F251–F256, with permission.)

formed in the rat, guinea pig, and dog indicate that enhanced tubular reabsorption of phosphate is the primary contributing factor to the greater reabsorption and positive phosphate balance that characterize early extrauterine life (87). The tubular maximum for the reabsorption of phosphate is high in infants at a time when the accretion of phosphate is highest; it declines when the accretion of phosphate declines (89). The rate of phosphate reabsorption at any given filtered load of phosphate is greater in newborn guinea pigs than in adults (Fig. 3.8).

The mechanisms responsible for higher phosphate reabsorption by the neonatal kidney are intrinsic ones controlling the renal handling of phosphate and differences in hormonal regulation of phosphate transport. Investigators have used microperfusion techniques, the isolated perfused kidney, and BBMVs to assess whether the increased tubular reabsorption of phosphate is related to differences in the transport of phosphate at the brush-border surface of the proximal tubule. The fractional reabsorption of phosphate is higher in the newborn than it is in the adult guinea pig (Table 3.4) (90,91). The proximal tubular reabsorption is 77% of the filtered load in the newborn and 67% in the adult guinea pigs. The distal reabsorption of phosphate in newborns is 16% and in mature guinea pigs is 11%. Both proximal and distal tubular phosphate reabsorption are greater in newborns. This is remarkable in light of the relative structural immaturity of the newborn proximal tubule. Compared with adults, the maximum rate of phosphate reabsorption is greater in newborn guinea pigs (92). There is no significant difference in affinity (*Km*) of the transporter for phosphate. BBMVs from 2-month-old and 8- to 9-month-old rats demonstrate no difference in the activity of sodium phosphate cotransport (89). However, newborn rats have enhanced phosphate uptake due to changes in the affinity of the transporter (*Km*) for phosphate (90). Therefore, greater apical membrane density rather than conformational changes or structural isomers of the sodium phosphate cotransporter probably accounts for the greater phosphate absorption characteristic of the developing animal.

Increased phosphate reabsorption by the developing animal or child might be explained by relative insensitivity to the phosphaturic effect of PTH. The fractional excretion of phosphate after administration of PTH was lower in 6-week-old rats than in 20-week-old rats. However, studies indicate that the greater phosphate reabsorption characteristic of the newborn is intrinsic to the immature tubule and is independent of PTH. In parathyroidectomized rats, the capacity for phosphate reabsorption was greatest in the immature, or 3-week-old, animals and decreased with growth and development (91). Parathyroidectomy is accompanied by a greater increase in the maximal tubular reabsorption of phosphate in immature rats than in the mature rats (89). In the presence of parathyroid glands, the phosphate reabsorptive capacity was lower in all groups, but a decline in capacity was still noted as rats matured. Therefore, it appears that there is an enhanced intrinsic ability of the immature kidney to reabsorb phosphate, which is not simply related to noted maturational differences in PTH action on the renal tubule. PTH receptor–associated adenylate cyclase is less responsive to PTH stimulation in the immature renal tubule than in mature controls; however, hormone responsiveness in the rat increases threefold during the first several weeks of life (93).

The rate of phosphate transport is also regulated by the availability of phosphate. Dietary phosphate deprivation results in enhanced reabsorption of phosphate (92). A parallel has been drawn between the phosphate-replete state of the immature kidney and the adult kidney during phosphate depletion, because in both conditions phosphate reabsorptive capacity is enhanced independent of PTH (91,94). Factors observed to contribute to the enhanced reabsorption of phosphate during dietary deprivation include increased activity of the brush-border transport system, significant phosphate reabsorption in both distal and proximal tubules, and decreased responsiveness to PTH (90). As mentioned, these same factors contribute to the greater increase in phosphate reabsorption observed in the young kidney.

Conflicting results have been obtained from the study of the response of the newborn rat and guinea pig kidney to

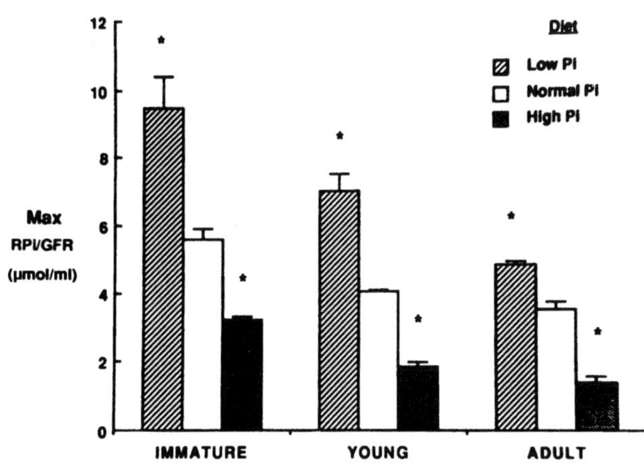

FIGURE 3.9. Age-related changes in the effect of dietary phosphate on maximal capacity for phosphate reabsorption in thyroparathyroidectomized rats given low-, normal-, and high-phosphate diets. GFR, glomerular filtration rate; Pi, inorganic phosphate; RPI, resting pressure index. (From Mulroney SE, Lumpkin MD, Haramati A. Antagonist to GH-releasing factor inhibits growth and renal Pi reabsorption in immature rats. *Am J Physiol* 1989;257:F29–F34, with permission.)

either low- or high-phosphate diets, depending on whether the whole organ or the proximal tubule is studied. Studies of whole-kidney phosphate reabsorption in the rat indicate that the immature kidney has enhanced capacity to respond to both decreases and increases in dietary phosphate and the filtered load of phosphate (Fig. 3.9) (89,91,95). Immature rats receiving low-phosphate diets had greater phosphate reabsorption than either immature animals receiving normal dietary phosphate or mature animals on low-phosphate diets. In contrast, a low-phosphate diet did not induce any changes in phosphate uptake by BBMVs from the newborn guinea pig, nor did a high-phosphate diet decrease phosphate uptake. The newborn animals experienced greater fluctuations in plasma phosphate (92). Proximal phosphate transport by immature rats, as assessed by BBMV studies, is greater than that of adults, yet there is diminished ability of the developing rat to sustain plasma phosphate as dietary phosphate is changed. These developmental changes in phosphate handling are analogous to those described for taurine (see earlier). Although immature animals have similar intrinsic transporter function with greater relative capacity, the ability of the renal proximal tubule to adapt to its environment is diminished.

The ability to respond to alterations in the filtered load of phosphate does not require PTH (91,95,96). The stimulation of phosphate reabsorption in the immature animal may be related to reduced intracellular levels of phosphate (97). Intracellular phosphate as measured by nuclear magnetic resonance is lower in 3-week-old rats than in 12-week-old rats (97). The investigators postulate that a low intracellular phosphate concentration in developing rats may stimulate synthesis and expression of phosphate transporter proteins.

Growth hormone also may regulate renal phosphate reabsorption during the neonatal period (96). Long-term administration of the growth hormone antagonist (GRF-AN) to immature and mature rats resulted in growth failure and increased urinary phosphate excretion in the immature rats only. Immature rats (4 weeks old) receiving GRF-AN exhibited decreased tubular capacity for phosphate reabsorption, whereas adult animals did not. These data indicate that the release of growth hormone during development may contribute to the elevated phosphate reabsorption characteristic of this period (95,98). Insulin-like growth factor-1 induces the increase in activity of the sodium phosphate transporter and prevents the decrease observed after GRF-AN administration (98,99). Preliminary studies suggest a role for tyrosine kinases in transduction of hormone-transporter events (99).

In summary, the renal retention of phosphate in the newborn is not an expression of an immature transport system; rather, it is an appropriate physiologic adaptation to the demands for phosphate during a period of rapid growth. The postnatal changes in phosphate reabsorption do not necessarily depend on GFR, PTH, or dietary phosphate. They may be regulated by growth hormone and insulin-like growth factor-1, as well as by intracellular phosphate concentration.

ORGANIC ANIONS

The proximal renal tubule is the primary site for the major organic anion transporters hOAT1 and hOAT3 (100). PAH is the prototypical substrate for the organic anion transport pathway. Organic anions may be filtered, reabsorbed, and secreted by the nephron. Excretion of a given anion is the sum of filtration and secretion less reabsorption. There is a great deal of variability in the renal handling of organic anions, depending on the species and organic anion studied (101). In humans, the major transporters are in the proximal tubule (100), whereas in mice, they are present in proximal tubule, Henle's loop, and cortical collecting duct (102). These anions may undergo bidirectional transport, with secretion being the predominant direction of flux. Many of the organic anions are highly protein bound and are not filtered to any extent at the glomerulus. Rather, these compounds may reach luminal fluid via transcellular transport movement across basolateral and apical membranes. PAH is secreted at a very high rate; as much as 90% is extracted from plasma by the proximal tubule in a single pass through the kidney. Because of this characteristic, PAH is used as a marker of renal blood flow. The urinary levels of PAH increase along the length of the proximal tubule (Fig. 3.2).

Tubular capacity for the secretion of organic anions increases as the plasma concentration increases, up to a maximum at which the transport system is saturated (101).

TABLE 3.5. ORGANIC ANIONS

p-Aminohippuric acid	Phenol red
Ascorbic acid	Phenylbutazone
Benzyl penicillin	Probenecid
Carbenicillin	Riboflavin
Folic acid	Salicylic acid
Methotrexate	Sulfisoxazole
Nicotinic acid	Taurocholic acid
Pantothenic acid	Uric acid
Phenobarbital	

A wide variety of organic anions are secreted by this transport system (Table 3.5). Although the secretion of all organic anions occurs in the proximal tubule, the rate of secretion by different proximal segments varies, depending on the compound and on the species studied (103). In the rat and the rabbit, PAH secretion is greatest in the straight tubule, specifically the S2 segment, whereas in the pig, it is greater in the convoluted portion of the proximal tubule (103). These differences in the secretory patterns probably are related to differences in transporter density on the basolateral membrane of the tubule (104).

Other factors that influence the excretion of organic anions include the degree of protein binding, the competition by other similar compounds for the same basolateral transport system, and the metabolic state of the animal, because many of these compounds are metabolic intermediates (103).

Cellular Mechanisms

Secretion of organic anions is accomplished by the cooperative interaction of several cotransport and countertransport systems located on the basolateral and apical membrane surfaces (Fig. 3.10A) (101,103). As the interior of the cell has a substantial net negative charge, the uptake of anions occurs against a steep electrochemical gradient. The basolateral transport of PAH is sodium- and energy-dependent but, as a tertiary active transport system, is not directly coupled to either sodium or energy expenditure. PAH enters the basolateral cell surface via an anion exchanger; ketoglutarate is thought to be the principal anion exchanged for PAH. This anion exchanger is coupled to a basolateral sodium-anion (ketoglutarate) cotransporter that allows the energy from ATP hydrolysis to be coupled to that of the anion exchanger through the recycling of ketoglutarate at the basolateral membrane. This process is similar to the apical C1-formate exchanger (see Sodium and Chloride: Whole Nephron). Once inside the cell, the organic anion diffuses through the cytoplasm and exits the apical side of the cell through another anion exchanger. The substrate specificity of the apical anion exchanger differs from that of the basolateral anion exchanger. Ketoglutarate is the preferred substrate for exchange with PAH on the basolateral surface, but many anions (lactate, pyruvate, hydroxybutyrate,

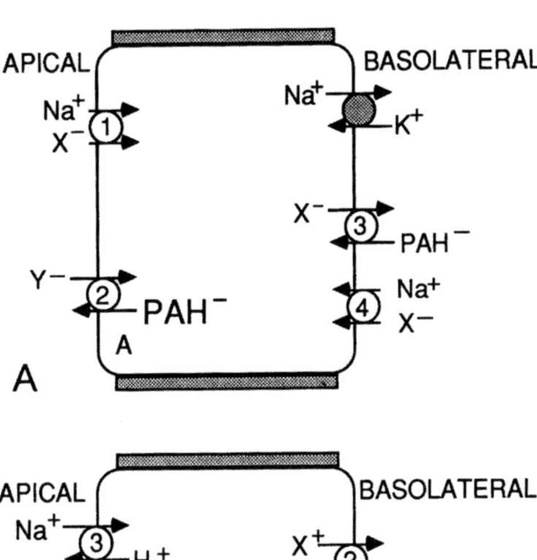

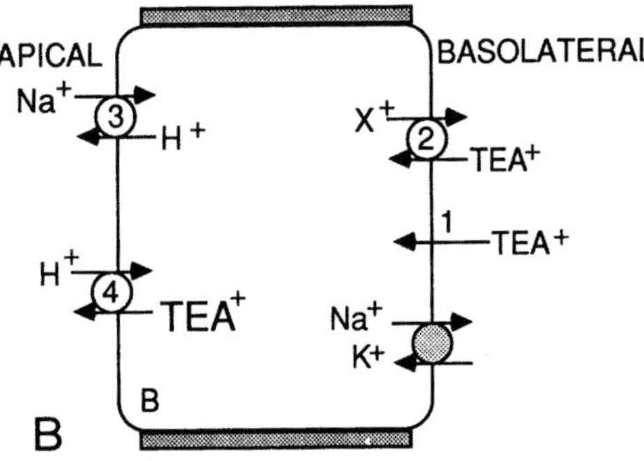

FIGURE 3.10. **A:** Organic anions [*p*-amino hippurate (PAH)] enter the proximal tubular cell on the basolateral surface by an anion exchanger (3) in association with a sodium anion cotransporter (4), which allows recycling of the anion across the basolateral membrane. PAH exits the cell by another anion exchanger (2) with different substrate specificity than the basolateral system. The apical anion exchanger is also associated with an anion sodium cotransport system (1). **B:** Organic cations [tetraethylammonium (TEA)] enter the proximal tubular cell on the basolateral surface by one of two mechanisms: cation exchange (2) or passive, facilitated diffusion (1). TEA exits the luminal membrane via a proton exchanger (4) that operates in association with a sodium-proton exchanger to allow recycling of a proton across the luminal membrane. (Adapted from Roch-Ramel F, Besseghir K, Murer H. Renal excretion and tubular transport of organic anions and cations. In: Windhager EE, ed. *Handbook of physiology: renal physiology*. New York: Oxford University Press, 1992:2179–2262.)

acetoacetate, succinate, ketoglutarate, urate, hydroxyl ions, bicarbonate, and chloride) may be exchanged for PAH by the apical exchanger. In addition to the anion exchanger on the apical surface, there is a sodium-coupled anion transporter that reabsorbs organic substances such as ketoglutarate for the reabsorption of metabolic substrates, as well as one specific for ketoglutarate that may be exchanged for PAH by the basolateral anion exchanger. Therefore, the net movement of PAH is from peritubular fluid to luminal fluid, and the net movement of the anion ketoglutarate is the reverse. Lithium inhibits the sodium-organic anion cotransporters, and probenecid inhibits the anion exchangers.

Molecular Characterization

The basolateral organic anion transporter system accomplishes organic anion-dicarboxylate exchange and is found on the basolateral membrane (100,102). The rat kidney transporter (OAT1) has 551 amino acid residues with 12 proposed transmembrane domains (105). OAT1 has wide substrate specificity, including cyclic nucleotides, prostaglandins, uric acid, and a variety of drugs. Expression is limited to an isolated basolateral segment of the proximal tubule (105). OAT1 shows approximately 38% structural homology to the organic cation transporter (OCT1). The human kidney transporter (hOAT3) has 543 amino acids and is localized to the basolateral membrane (106), with comparable structural homology.

Developmental Changes in Organic Anion Transport

The secretion of organic acids is low during the neonatal period; it increases gradually over the first few years of life (107,108). Limitations on the excretion of organic acids include low GFR, anatomic immaturity, reduced number of transporter sites, and incomplete metabolic capacity. In addition, the limited distribution of blood flow to the deep cortical structure reduces the concentration of organic acids available for secretion.

The kidney's ability to produce a concentration gradient of organic anions is present before birth and increases with maturation. Studies in newborn humans, dogs, and rats demonstrate a gradual increase in renal extraction of PAH with age (109–111). When PAH transport is examined using tissue slices, the slice:medium ratios (in rats) peak at approximately 1 month of age and then decline to adult values. The PAH extraction (GFR) of infants 3 months or younger is approximately 30% that of older children.

The increased secretory ability that occurs with maturation is the result of the intrinsic ability of the proximal tubule to transport organic acids without appreciable changes in the membrane permeability to PAH. When organic acid transporter activity is standardized for tubule length, an almost fivefold increase in transport capacity occurs with maturation (108). Both increased transporter density and tubular length contribute to the increased capacity for organic acid secretion that occurs with development.

In addition to age-related changes in transporter capacity, organic anion transport is regulated by substrate availability and hormones (112,113). The administration of organic acids induces the transport system (112,114). Administration of penicillin to 2- and 4-week-old rabbits resulted in enhanced basolateral uptake and excretion of PAH in the 2-week-old, but not in the 4-week-old, rabbits (112). Administration of the drugs to pregnant rabbits during the later part of pregnancy results in enhanced newborn PAH transport. The ability to induce transport activity depends on the species and the anion studied.

Premature infants have a reduced renal ability to excrete organic anion drugs because of the immaturity of the organic anion transport system. Thyroxin administration to

TABLE 3.6. ORGANIC CATIONS

Amiloride	Norepinephrine
Amphetamine	Procainamide
Atropine	Pseudoephedrine
Chloroquine	Quinine
Cimetidine	Tetraethylammonium
Histamine	Thiamine
Levamisole	Tolazoline
Methadone	Triamterene
Morphine	

young rats increases PAH uptake (115). This increased uptake is blocked by inhibitors of protein synthesis, suggesting that the thyroxin effect depends on synthesis of regulatory or transporter proteins.

ORGANIC CATIONS

Organic cations include endogenous primary, secondary, tertiary, and quaternary amines in addition to many drugs that are secreted by the proximal tubule (103). A partial list of organic cations is found in Table 3.6. Tetraethylammonium (TEA) is the model substrate for describing the organic cation system. The clearance of TEA is similar to that of PAH; there is nearly complete extraction with a single pass through the kidney. Secretory fluxes are greatest in the proximal convoluted (S1) segment and decrease in S2 and S3 (116). Changes in the activity of the organic cation transport system appear to be related to regional differences in luminal permeability to TEA along the proximal tubule and are not caused by changes in basolateral cation uptake (101).

Cellular Mechanisms

Organic cations move into the negatively charged cell interior by a saturable, electrogenic process that is located on the basolateral cell surface. Some organic cation uptake is through facilitated diffusion (Fig. 3.10B) (101,103). A luminal organic cation-proton antiporter that uses potential energy stored in a pH gradient to drive uphill movement of cations has been demonstrated in human, snake, dog, rat, and rabbit BBMVs. Cations diffuse through the cell cytosol and are either taken up into cell organelles or vesicles or exit through a luminal proton exchanger. At the luminal membrane, TEA is exchanged for a proton. This is another example of a tertiary transport process: The energy-requiring process is the Na^+-K^+-ATPase, which creates the major driving force for the apical Na^+-H^+ exchanger. In turn, the Na^+-H^+ exchanger provides protons for apical exchange with TEA. The luminal proton-TEA exchange is electroneutral. Therefore, the net movement of TEA is from the capillary fluid to the lumen; protons recycle across the apical membrane.

The fetal kidney is able to secrete organic cations; the ability to do so is probably less than that in adult animals (108,109,117,118). In general, the capacity to secrete organic cations precedes that of organic anions (101,103).

URIC ACID

Uric acid, a weak organic acid, is the biologic end-product of dietary and endogenous purine metabolism. Approximately 75% is excreted by the kidney. Urate is freely filtered at the glomerulus and is transported exclusively by the proximal tubule (119). In a number of species (human, monkey, rat, mongrel dog), the fractional excretion of urate is less than 100%, indicating net reabsorption. In other species (pig and rabbit), the fractional excretion of urate exceeds 100%, indicating net secretion. The degree to which there is secretion or reabsorption varies and depends on the species studied (119). Urate reabsorption is inhibited by probenecid, high luminal fluid flow rate, hexose, and anion exchange inhibitors. Urate secretion is inhibited by pyrazinoic acid, the active metabolite of the antituberculous drug pyrazinamide (120). The decrease in urinary excretion of urate after the administration of pyrazinamide or its metabolite pyrazinoate was initially thought to be related to a selective effect of the drug on the secretory component of urate excretion. However, recent work suggests that pyrazinoate may inhibit the reabsorptive component in addition to the secretory pathway. Thus, the pyrazinoate-suppressible excretion of urate is not totally caused by inhibition of the secretory component (120,121). Urate handling along the proximal tubule is theorized to proceed as follows: Initial reabsorption of urate occurs in the early proximal convoluted tubule (S1), and secretion occurs in the late convoluted, early straight tubule (S2) via a secretory pathway similar to that for PAH (121). Postsecretory reabsorption may occur but has not been well characterized. Clearance studies performed in human subjects demonstrated that blocking reabsorption prevented an increase in excretion that would be expected to follow probenecid administration (103).

Cellular Mechanisms

Because of the bidirectional nature, axial heterogeneity, and species-related variability of urate transport, any model describing urate transport is complex. Most likely, passive, paracellular, and active transcellular transport mechanisms affect urate secretion and reabsorption. A urate anion exchanger has been demonstrated in rat and dog BBMV (121–123). This system may use the hydroxyl, Cl^-, HCO_3^-, lactate, or succinate anion in exchange for urate. This system is specific for urate, but PAH is also accepted. Probenecid inhibits urate transport by this system (121–123). A sodium-urate cotransport system has been proposed, because the reabsorption of urate is closely coupled to sodium in studies involving intact animals and isolated perfused tubules. Such a system has not been demonstrated in isolated BBMVs. Most likely, urate transport is sodium dependent through the sodium-dependent cotransport of organic anions or dicarboxylates and is linked as a tertiary transport process to sodium flux.

An anion exchange system for urate has been described in basolateral membrane vesicles from the rat; this transport system is postulated to be distinct from the apical transport system because PAH and other organic anions do not interact with it (124).

The initial step for urate reabsorption is the anion exchanger at the apical membrane, with exit on the basolateral membrane by another anion exchanger or by a passive mechanism. Secretion of urate occurs by basolateral exchange of urate for chloride, with secretion by the apical anion exchanger. The differential distribution of these two systems along the proximal tubule probably determines the net flux of urate in a given segment. In the S1 segment, reabsorption predominates; in the S2 segment, secretion (pyrazinamide-sensitive) predominates. Both fluxes could be present in the S3 segment, with the net flux being in the direction of reabsorption in the human (119).

The human urate transporter (uHAT) has been cloned and it has two membrane-spanning domains. It acts as a highly selective urate ion channel. A second urate transporter (uHAT2) has also been cloned (125).

Developmental

The fractional excretion of urate is much higher in infants than in adults or older children. Plasma levels tend to be higher in premature and term newborns than in older children and adults (126). Urate fractional excretion is 70% at a gestational age of 29 to 31 weeks and 38% at term (127–129). The fractional excretion of urate decreases further during the early postnatal period, and this effect appears to be independent of gestational age (Fig. 3.11). Uptake of urate by neonatal kidney slices and by fetal and neonatal mouse kidney cortex slices is lower than uptake by slices from adult animals (128). This probably indicates decreased ability for urate secretion in the immature rodent (127,129). Therefore, the increased fractional excretion probably is not related to increased secretion. Instead, increased excretion of urate could be related to the relative volume-expanded state of the infant, as well as to the potential immaturity of reabsorptive pathways (130). Maturation of the superficial renal cortex, with its greater reabsorptive capacity, could also contribute to the postnatal decline in fractional urate excretion (127).

SULFATE

Sulfate and thiosulfate are freely filtered at the glomerulus. Both are reabsorbed by the proximal tubule; fractional excretion is approximately 10% (131). Sulfate is transported into the proximal tubular cell by a luminal, sodium-dependent process with a stoichiometry of 2 Na^+ to 1 SO_4^- (Fig. 3.12). The system is electroneutral and requires a proton. The proton acts as an allosteric activator of the transport system and modifies the stoichiometry of the transporter with respect to sodium. With an acidic internal pH, stoichiometry is 2:1; in an alkaline environment, it is 1:1 (132,133). On the basolateral cell surface, sulfate is transported by an anion exchanger that is sodium independent. Sulfate is exchanged for another anion (hydroxyl radical, bicarbonate, or thiosulfate). This anion exchanger does not accept Cl^-, phosphate, or other organic anions such as PAH or lactate, but it is inhibited by

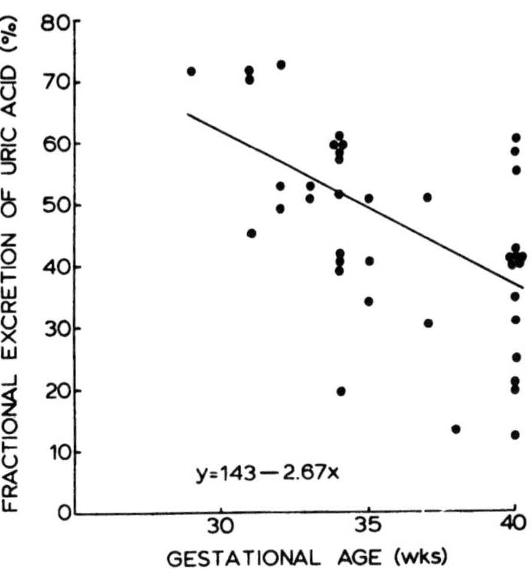

FIGURE 3.11. Fractional excretion of uric acid (clearance of uric acid/creatinine clearance ×100) during the first day of life. A significant inverse relationship was observed between the fractional excretion of urate and gestational age. (From Stapleton FB. Renal uric acid clearances in human neonates. *J Pediatr* 1983;103:290–294, with permission.)

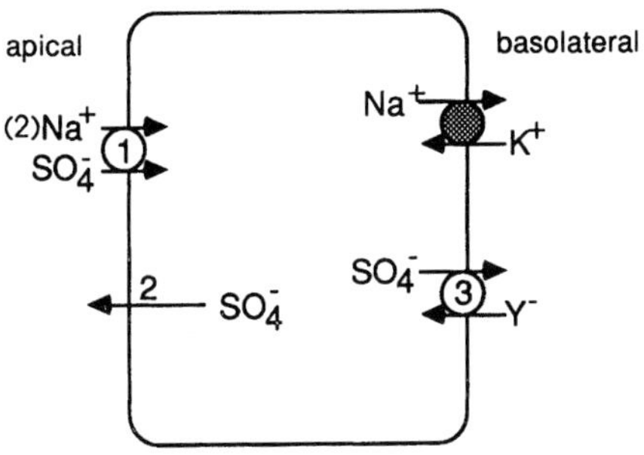

FIGURE 3.12. Model of sulfate transport by the proximal tubule. Sulfate is cotransported with two sodium ions at the brush-border membrane (1) and exits the cell by way of passive, facilitated diffusion on the apical membrane (backleak, 2) or by a sulfate-anion exchanger (3) on the basolateral surface of the cell. (From Murer H, Manganel M, Roch-Ramel F. Tubular transport of monocarboxylates, Krebs cycle intermediates and inorganic sulfate. In: Windhager EE, ed. *Handbook of physiology: renal physiology*. New York: Oxford University Press, 1992:2164–2188, with permission.)

typical anion transporter inhibitors, SITS and DIDS. Luminal sodium sulfate cotransport enables significant luminal chloride transport in the proximal tubule, through the coordinated luminal oxalate-sulfate exchanger and oxalate-chloride exchange systems.

CARBOXYLATES

The renal tubule has several specific transport systems for the reabsorption and absorption of monocarboxylates, dicarboxylates, and tricarboxylates (131). These substrates are divided into the monocarboxylates (lactate, pyruvate, acetoacetate, hydroxybutyrate, and fatty acids) and dicarboxylates/tricarboxylates (citrate, succinate, ketoglutarate, oxaloacetate, and fumarate) (131). Most of these compounds are metabolic intermediates or substrates that are important energy sources, hence the need for absorption and reabsorption, respectively.

Reabsorption of these compounds is predominantly in the proximal tubule. In general, tubular reabsorption is incomplete, which may be the combined result of incomplete absorption by the apical membrane surface or the efflux of these substrates from the cell back into the lumen when the intracellular concentrations are high (131).

Cellular Mechanisms

Monocarboxylates

There are both apical and basolateral transport processes for the monocarboxylates (Fig. 3.13A). Reabsorption from luminal fluid is by an apical-specific transporter that is sodium dependent and is not inhibited by other organic compounds such as PAH, urate, or dicarboxylates. The transporter requires a single carboxyl group, but it accepts both the D- and the L-isomer of the carboxylate. Studies using BBMVs indicate that there may be both a high-affinity/low-capacity system and a low-affinity/high-capacity system (131,134).

In addition to the sodium-monocarboxylate cotransport system, there is an apical anion exchange system. This system accepts a variety of anions (Cl^-, hydroxyl, bicarbonate, urate, PAH, and dicarboxylates). It is sensitive to SITS and DIDS, as well as furosemide and probenecid, indicating that this organic anion exchanger is nonspecific. This system probably functions to facilitate exit of metabolic intermediates and the shuttling of protons (formate-Cl exchanger), which are necessary for the electroneutral absorption of NaCl.

The basolateral system is sodium independent and specific for the D-isomer of lactate. The basolateral system is thought to be an anion exchanger that exchanges lactate for the hydroxyl ion or bicarbonate in a fashion similar to that described for sulfate (135–137). This system is bidirectional and allows the entry as well as the exit of monocarboxylates. This system can affect the net reabsorption of monocarboxylates from luminal fluid and release into pericapillary fluid, as well as effect basolateral uptake of these compounds as substrate for cell metabolism. The basolateral transport system is located in the S2 and S3 segments, which do not have an apical transport system for the monocarboxylates. In these segments, the transport system is crucial to the uptake of monocarboxylates as substrates needed for cell energy metabolism.

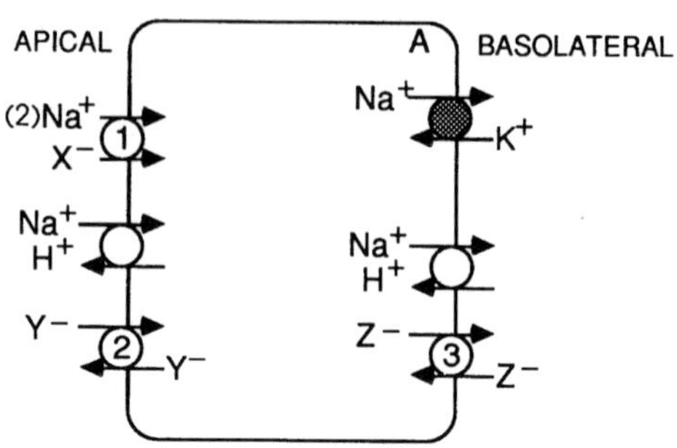

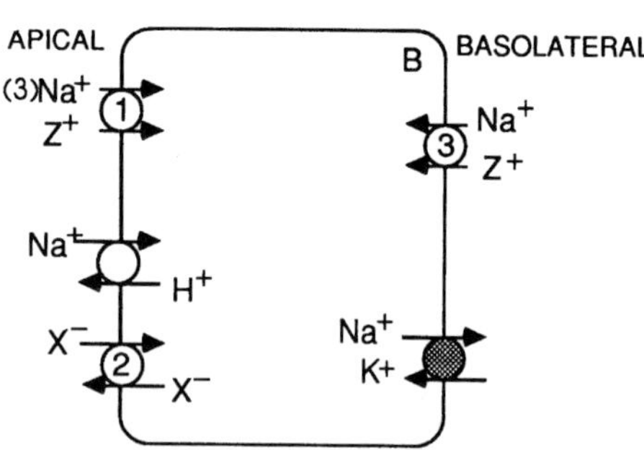

FIGURE 3.13. A: Model for monocarboxylate transport. Monocarboxylates enter the proximal tubular cell by one of two mechanisms: either a sodium cotransporter (1), where X = lactate, pyruvate, acetoacetate, or β hydroxybutyrate, or by an anion exchanger (2) with different substrate specificity (Y = OH^-, Cl^-, urate, bicarbonate, *p*-aminohippurate, ketoglutarate, lactate, pyruvate, acetoacetate, or β hydroxybutyrate). On the basolateral membrane, an anion exchanger enables the exit of these substances (3) (Z = lactate, pyruvate, OH^-, formate, Cl^-, sulfate, phosphate, or oxalate). **B:** Model for dicarboxylate/tricarboxylate transport. The substances enter the luminal membrane of the cell by a sodium cotransport system (1) (Z = pyruvate, succinate, citrate, malate, fumarate, or ketoglutarate) or an anion exchanger (2) (bicarbonate, lactate, pyruvate, acetoacetate, β hydroxybutyrate, malate, or succinate). In addition, a sodium cotransport system (3) similar to the apical system enables the basolateral transport of these substrates. (From Murer H, Manganel M, Roch-Ramel F. Tubular transport of monocarboxylates, Kreb's cycle intermediates and inorganic sulfate. In: Windhager EE, ed. *Handbook of physiology: renal physiology.* New York: Oxford University Press, 1992:2164–2188, with permission.)

Dicarboxylates/Tricarboxylates

The model substrate for the transport of dicarboxylates/tricarboxylates is α-ketoglutarate. Approximately 75% of the filtered load is reabsorbed by the proximal tubule, 20% of which is by the S3 segment. Secretion also has been demonstrated in the rat (138). Ketoglutarate reabsorption is effected by cotransport with sodium (stoichiometry 3:1) (Fig 3.13B) (139). This system accepts all the Krebs cycle intermediates as well as pyruvate, which is actually a monocarboxylate (140). Sodium must bind to the transporter protein to induce a conformational change that facilitates binding and transport of substrates. Lithium inhibits this process by binding in place of sodium (141,142). The same system is located on the basolateral surface of the cell to effect uptake of key substrates from peritubular fluid. The presence of arginine-349 and aspartate-373 of the Na^+/dicarboxylate cotransporter is important in the conformational states of the transport cycle (143). There is an additional anion exchanger that has affinity for many substrates and is probably the same transport system as that previously mentioned for the monocarboxylates.

Sodium and Chloride: Whole Nephron

Approximately 60% of the filtered sodium and 50% of filtered chloride is reabsorbed by the proximal tubule (144). The preferential reabsorption of amino acids, glucose, phosphate, and bicarbonate in the early proximal tubule creates a TF NaCl concentration greater than the plasma concentration. This augments the reabsorption of NaCl through both active and passive processes (144,145). The passive reabsorption of NaCl through a paracellular pathway accounts for two-thirds of the total NaCl flux in the S2 and S3 segments (144). In the early proximal tubule, a lumen-negative potential resulting from sodium-coupled absorption of substrates such as glucose and amino acids favors passive paracellular Cl transport. Sodium bicarbonate reabsorption via the luminal Na-H exchange is accompanied by fluid absorption so that the luminal Cl concentration increases in the late proximal tubule favoring Cl absorption, which creates a positive luminal charge that favors passive transcellular sodium absorption in the late proximal tubule (145). Additional Cl absorption is achieved via apical Cl exchange with formate or oxalate. This chloride-formate exchanger, expressed in the brush-border membrane, can also be found in the pancreas and heart (146).

Cellular Mechanisms: Proximal Tubule

Three apical transport systems operate in conjunction with the basolateral Na^+-K^+-ATPase transport system to effect sodium reabsorption (Fig. 3.14) (147): the Na^+-H^+ exchanger; the sodium-coupled transport with amino acids, phosphate, glucose, sulfate, and organic acids; and the sodium channels. The Na^+-H^+ exchanger accounts for the greatest fraction of reabsorbed sodium in the S1-3 segment. Sodium-coupled transport mechanisms are more important in the S1, and sodium channels are more important in the S2 and S3 segments (144). Active Na^+ transport occurs across the apical membrane by the coupling of Na^+-H^+ exchange and the Cl^--formate exchanger (147).

A significant amount of chloride reabsorption occurs in the proximal tubule by passive diffusion of Cl; the rate of reabsorption is lower in the early proximal tubule, in which sodium and bicarbonate reabsorption are favored. As TF moves distally, it becomes acidified, and the chloride concentration rises to a level greater than that of plasma (Fig. 3.2). The transtubular PD is negative in the early proximal tubule, but it becomes lumen positive later in the proximal tubule. In the early proximal tubule, the major driving force for passive Cl reabsorption is the lumen-negative PD and, in the later proximal tubule, an outwardly directed Cl^- concentration gradient. Active Cl reabsorption also occurs in the proximal tubule by tertiary active transport, because the driving force is generated by one of two secondary active transport systems: the Na^+-H^+ exchanger in parallel with Cl^- formate or the Na-sulfate exchanger in parallel with Cl^- oxalate. Cl^- transport is coupled indirectly to H^+ transport because the cell concentration of formate is affected by pH, and hydrogen ions are pumped out of the cell in exchange for sodium. In the case of Cl-oxalate exchange, oxalate is accumulated in exchange for sulfate, which is cotransported with sodium. Renal potassium-chloride cotransporters, which are electroneutral, are found in the proximal tubule and thick ascending limb (148).

Because Na-H exchange is vital in both $NaHCO_3$ and NaCl reabsorption, regulation of Na-H activity could be expected to affect both processes. In the setting of metabolic acidosis, a need for enhanced $NaHCO_3$ absorption results in upregulation of Na-H exchange via increased expression of NHE3 protein. NaCl transport would be expected to increase as well, but decreased formate-induced NaCl transport, decreased oxalate-induced NaCl transport, and Na-sulfate cotransport are observed during acidosis, thereby counteracting the increase in Na-H exchange activity on net Cl reabsorption (149). Phosphorylation of serine-982 in the Na^+ bicarbonate cotransporter shifts the HCO_3^-:Na^+ stoichiometry from 3:1 to 2:1 (150).

Na^+-H^+ Exchanger

The Na^+-H^+ exchanger is responsible for the bulk of $NaHCO_3$ and NaCl reabsorption in the proximal tubule (147). The Na^+-H^+ exchanger requires Na^+ and H^+ and is inhibited by amiloride in concentrations lower than those required for inhibition of the Na^+-K^+-ATPase but higher than those required for inhibition of sodium channels (149). The antiporter accepts NH_4^+, Li^+, Na^+, and H^+ but does not accept K^+, Rb^+, Cs^+, or choline (23). Na^+, Li^+, NH_4^+, and H^+ compete for the external binding site. There are two internal cation-binding sites; one is for transport and the other binds hydrogen ions as a means of regulating

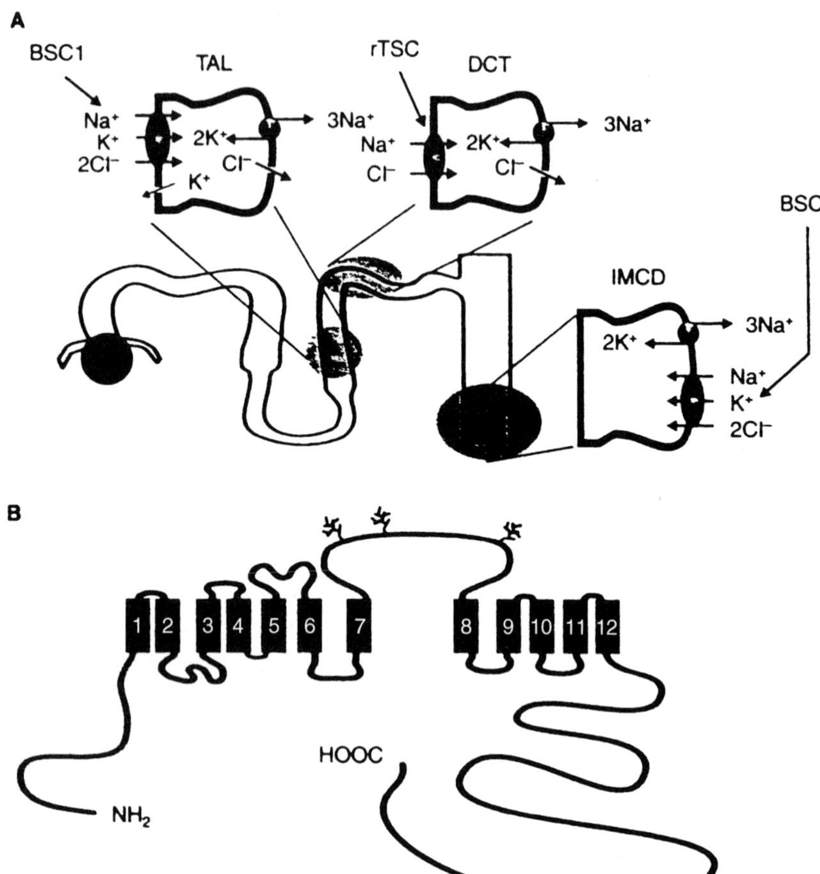

FIGURE 3.14. The Na-(K)-Cl cotransporters. **A:** Localization of cloned Na-(K)-Cl cotransporters along the mammalian nephron. **B:** Schematic model of the topology of the Na-(K)-Cl cotransporters. The proposed membrane-spanning helices are numbered 1 to 12. Putative *N*-glycosylation sites on the loop between membrane spans 7 and 8, and the amino-(NH_2) and carboxy-(COOH) termini are indicated. DCT, distal convoluted tubule; IMCD, inner medullary collecting duct; TAL, thick ascending limb. [From Hebert SC, Gamba G, Kaplan M. The electroneutral Na^+-(K^+)-Cl-cotransport family. *Kidney Int* 1996:1638–1641, with permission.]

the activity of the transporter (151). Increases in the hydrogen ion concentration induce protonation of the regulatory site and activation of the antiporter. Increasing intracellular pH inactivates the exchanger (23). Therefore, acidification of the cell cytosol activates the Na^+-H^+ exchanger by provision of protons and by allosteric activation.

The activity of the exchanger is regulated by acidosis, renal ablation, thyroxine, glucocorticoids, angiotensin II, catecholamines, and PTH (145,147). Activation of the Na^+-H^+ exchanger occurs either through the action of tyrosine-specific kinases or through activation of protein kinase C. Epidermal growth factor, platelet-derived growth factor, and insulin activate the Na^+-H^+ exchanger through the tyrosine-specific kinase. Thrombin, angiotensin II, vasopressin, and α-adrenergic agonists activate the Na^+-H^+ exchanger via protein kinase C (152–154). The Na^+-H^+ exchanger also maintains intracellular pH and the regulation of cell growth. The Na^+-H^+ exchanger is regulated in parallel with regulation of the basolateral system that is involved with bicarbonate reabsorption and the Na-3HCO_3 cotransporter. The latter also increases its transport capacity in response to chronic acidosis (155). The turnover of both transporters probably is regulated by the need for transepithelial bicarbonate transport or proton secretion.

Several isoforms of the Na^+-H^+ exchanger have been characterized. The eukaryotic housekeeping isoform gene, NHE1, encodes a protein that is composed of 10- to 12-membrane–spanning α helical segments and a large hydrophilic C-terminal domain with potential phosphorylation sites (145). The housekeeping form is expressed only on the basolateral membrane of proximal tubule segments. A total of five isoforms, NHE1-5, have been identified, with predicted proteins that have highly conserved sequences except for the C-terminal domains. All isoforms except NHE5 are found in the kidney and intestine. NHE3 is specifically expressed on the brush-border membrane of the proximal tubule, and expression is increased after acid loading (145). This isoform appears to be unique in that it is resistant to amiloride. In addition, apical membrane expression of NHE3 increases during maturation and after administration of glucocorticoids (156).

Chloride Formate Exchanger

The Cl^--formate exchanger is a tertiary transport system that recycles a base across the membrane and couples proton secretion and sodium reabsorption with chloride reabsorption. The base, which is usually formate, reenters the cell, dissociates, and is again available for exchange with Cl^-. The Cl^--formate exchanger has been studied in both BBMVs and intact proximal tubules (157–159). Addition of formate to luminal fluid increases NaCl reabsorption when the lumen pH is lower than the intracellular pH. The effect of pH is related to the H^+ gradient between luminal fluid and cell fluid and the recycling of the necessary base. Other bases have been considered as substrates for this exchanger, such as OH^-, bicarbonate, HCO_3^-, and oxalate (160). Oxalate has recently been noted to contribute to net Na reabsorption in a manner similar to formate, with anion exchange at the apical membrane of the proximal tubule. Oxalate is recycled via oxalate-sulfate exchange in parallel with oxalate-Cl exchange.

Basolateral

Several different pathways for Cl exit at the basolateral membrane include KCl cotransport, Na-dependent Cl-HCO_3 exchange, and Cl channels. Basolateral SITS—an anion exchange inhibitor—reduces NaCl reabsorption in rat proximal tubule by 50%; this suggests a role for a Cl^- base exchange in the basolateral Cl^- exit (147,161). The process is sodium dependent with a stoichiometry of Na:2 HCO_3^-:Cl^- and probably is responsible for most basolateral Cl^- exit (147). Recent evidence indicates that the largest component of Cl movement across the basolateral membrane is via Cl channels (sensitive to diphenylamine-2-carboxylate) (145).

Cellular Mechanisms: Thick Ascending Limb of the Loop of Henle

Sodium reabsorption in this segment proceeds via a luminal Na^+-K^+-Cl^- transporter that couples the reabsorption of 1 Na^+ and 1 K^+ with 2 Cl^- (Fig. 3.14) (128). Chloride leaves the cell via a basolateral Cl channel or KCl cotransporter (162,163). Potassium is recycled via K channels located on the apical membrane. These K channels are inhibited by choline, ammonium, ATP, and verapamil and are not regulated by Ca^{2+} (162). In addition, there is a mechanism for potassium exit from the basolateral membrane either by K^+ channels or by the previously mentioned KCl cotransport system (164). Polarization of most K^+ conductance on the apical membrane and most Cl channels on the basolateral membrane generates a lumen-positive charge that drives as much as 50% of total sodium reabsorption through passive paracellular pathways (162).

The Na^+-K^+-Cl^- cotransporter is an electroneutral transport system and is located on the apical surface of the thick ascending limb of the loop of Henle and the inner medullary collecting duct. In the presence of sodium and potassium, two Cl^- ions are transported with 1 Na^+ and 1 K^+. Lithium may be transported instead of sodium; however, other cations may not substitute for sodium (165). Rb^+, Cs^+, and $NH4^+$ may be transported instead of K^+. The high-affinity site is specific for Cl^- or Br^-. Once the high-affinity site is occupied, the remaining site is a low-affinity site that may accept Br^-, Cl^-, I^-, nitrate, or thiocyanate (166). This transport system provides the energy for countercurrent multiplication, which concentrates solutes in the renal medullary interstitium, allowing generation of a concentrated urine. Regulation of urinary-concentrating ability is, in part, a function of this system. The Na^+-K^+-Cl^- transporter is inhibited by furosemide and bumetanide. A separate secretory isoform of the Na-$^+$K$^+$-Cl^- cotransporter (NKCCl) (BSG-2) localizes to the basolateral membrane of the ∝ intercalated cell of the collecting duct. This form of the transporter serves to regulate cell volume, as well as to facilitate electrolyte and water transport (167).

The transporter gene (NKCC2) has recently been cloned (168). Homozygous mutations have been found to account for the Bartter's syndrome in numerous kindreds (168). As a member of the electroneutral cation-chloride cotransporter family, this transport system serves both an absorptive and a secretory function (cell volume regulation) (169). Sequence analyses show that these cotransporters are structurally similar, with 12 transmembrane-spanning helices and variable-length amino and carboxyterminal segments, which are cytosolic (Fig. 3.14). A long extracellular loop is proposed to be located between the seventh and eighth transmembrane domains with potential glycosylation sites. There is approximately 50% homology between the two Na^+-K^+-Cl^- cotransporters and the thiazide-sensitive Na-Cl cotransporter found in the distal tubule. Two isoforms of the Na^+-K^+-Cl^- cotransporter are found within the kidney. One is the absorptive form (BSC1), which is localized to the apical membrane of the cortical thick ascending limb of the loop of Henle. The more ubiquitous basolateral form, BSC2, is found in chloride secretory epithelia (169). In the kidney, BSC2 is localized to the basolateral membrane of the inner medullary collecting duct and to the extraglomerular mesangium (juxtaglomerular) and to a subpopulation of smooth muscle cells in the afferent arteriole (167,169). The function of the BSC2 cotransporter in the inner medullary collecting duct may be NaCl secretion through an ANF-inducible response. In addition, this transporter may enable H^+ and/or NH_3^+ secretion. The role of the BSC2 transporter in the afferent arteriole and juxtaglomerular region could be that of tubuloglomerular feedback. Increased Cl delivery to the cortical thick ascending limb has been postulated to be detected by a furosemide-inhibitable Na^+-K^+-Cl cotransporter, suggesting a direct role of chloride as the signal between cortical thick ascending loop chloride delivery and response from the macula densa to alter afferent arteriolar tone (170). Recent studies have indicated the precise distribution pattern of transport proteins in the human distal tubule (171).

The main regulating factors for the Na^+-K^+-Cl cotransporter are the cAMP/cyclic guanosine monophosphate system, the state of phosphorylation (phosphorylation stimulates), and cell shrinkage. Antidiuretic hormone stimulates the adenylate cyclase system, which increases the rate of NaCl reabsorption in the medullary thick ascending limb of the mouse. Enhanced luminal transport of NaCl occurs after insertion of additional transporter units into the plasma membrane (23). In addition, urea at high concentration inhibits the Na^+-K^+-Cl^- cotransporter independent of changes in cell volume (172). This is prevented by prior phosphorylation, which suggests that exposure to urea results in dephosphorylation of the cotransporter or a closely linked regulatory protein. Urea appears to alter cotransporter activity by decreasing the number of functional transporters. Long-term saline administration to rats increases the expression of the gene (BSC1) for the Na^+-K^+-Cl^- cotransporter. Long-term furosemide use also increases gene expression, as well as possibly inducing glycosylation of the cotransporter (173).

Cellular Mechanisms: Distal Convoluted Tubule

The thiazide-sensitive NaCl cotransporter of the distal collecting tubule is the primary source of active Na reabsorption distal to the loop of Henle. This transporter has structural homology with the Na^+-K^+-Cl^- cotransporter, as previously mentioned.

Also contributing to luminal sodium entry are the sodium channels. A ubiquitous class of transporters sensitive to amiloride, Na channels are regulated acutely by cAMP-dependent hormones such as vasopressin; G-proteins; and intracellular Na^+, Ca^+, and H^+, and chronically by aldosterone. There is a great deal of heterogeneity among amiloride-sensitive sodium channels. They may be characterized by their conductance, amiloride-binding affinity, and epithelial origin (174). Na channels are multimeric, with various combinations of subunits. Channel activity has been shown to be modified by phosphorylation (cAMP dependent). The guanosine triphosphate-binding protein, GαI-3, is associated with the channel protein complex and directly participates in channel activity. The G protein pathway is activated through phospholipase- and lipoxygenase-generated phospholipids. Nonphosphorylated channels are primarily closed. Exposure to protein kinase A in the presence of ATP shifts channel activity to a more open position (174). Other covalent modifications of the Na channel that affect its activity include pertussis toxin-induced ribosylation and aldosterone-mediated carboxyl methylation. All covalent modifications are induced by exposure of the channel complex from the internal surface and the opposite site of amiloride binding and depend on the state of phosphorylation (174).

Cellular Mechanisms: Collecting Tubule

In this segment, sodium is reabsorbed by transcellular pathways only (Fig. 3.14). The energy is provided by the basolaterally located Na^+-K^+-ATPase. Sodium enters the principal cell by way of highly selective, low-conductance Na^+ channels located on the apical membrane (147). Sodium reabsorption is regulated acutely by antidiuretic hormone (175) and chronically by aldosterone and dietary sodium intake (176). The reabsorption of sodium in this segment creates a lumen-negative charge. There is no chloride reabsorption by the principal cell; rather, chloride is reabsorbed by a paracellular route or via a transcellular pathway through intercalated cells. In addition, both arginine and lysine enhance cortical collecting duct Na^+ transport. Because lysine is not a nitrous oxide (NO) precursor, this is a cationic amino acid effect rather than a vasodilatory effect (177).

Comparison of the mechanisms of sodium reabsorption in the proximal tubule (S1-S3), loop of Henle, and the collecting duct reveals major differences. In the proximal tubule, a large amount of sodium is reabsorbed at low energy cost to the tubule because there is a substantial component of passive paracellular sodium flux; however, the ability of this segment to generate a concentration gradient is limited by the high sodium conductance (147). Therefore, a large fraction of sodium and chloride reabsorption takes place; however, because the luminal concentrations of Na^+ and Cl^- are similar to their plasma concentrations, a significant concentration gradient is not generated. In contrast, sodium reabsorption in the collecting duct occurs by a transcellular route that is expensive with respect to cellular energy. However, in the absence of a significant paracellular conductive pathway, the tubule can generate a large sodium concentration gradient. The thick ascending limb is a compromise between the proximal and collecting tubules; up to 50% of sodium reabsorption is passive.

Developmental Changes in Sodium and Fluid Transport

The reabsorptive capacity for fluid in the proximal tubule increases approximately twofold from 3 to 6 weeks of age in the rat (178) in parallel with increased luminal and basolateral membrane surface area. The postnatal increase in reabsorptive ability can be attributed to the increased activity of the Na^+-K^+-ATPase. The sodium-dependent proton flux in isolated, perfused tubules from rabbits is approximately one-third of adult levels at 2 weeks of age and increases to adult levels by 6 weeks of age (179). Studies in both proximal tubular cells in culture and BBMVs confirm that the Na^+-H^+ exchange system is less active in immature animals than it is in adults (180,181). This is related to differences in the abundance of the transport protein, because the Na^+-H^+ exchanger from newborn rats has characteristics identical with those of the adult rats except that the transport maximum (V_{max}) is one-fourth that obtained from adult rats (Fig. 3.15). Increases in V_{max} occur after the administration of glucocorticoids, indicating an increase in abundance of the transport protein (181).

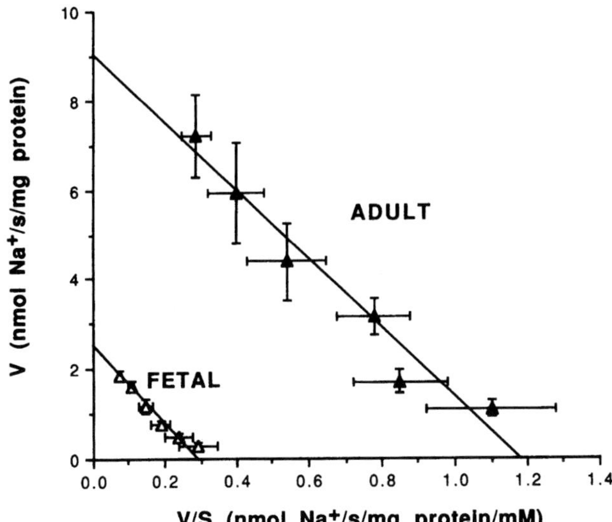

FIGURE 3.15. Developmental changes in Na^+-H^+ exchanger activity. Kinetic analysis of initial rate of amiloride-sensitive ^{22}Na uptake into brush-border membrane vesicles from adult and fetal rabbits. (From Ives HE, Chen PY, Verkman AS. Mechanism of coupling between C1 and OH transport in renal brush-border membranes. *Biochem Biophys Acta* 1986;863:91–100, with permission.)

This chapter has outlined various renal tubular transport processes that are vital to homeostasis. Subsequent chapters on water, acid-base, and potassium homeostasis detail those tubular transport systems. Transepithelial movement of solute and fluid tends to be massive in the early parts of the nephron with most of the renal tubular fine-tuning occurring in the more distal segments. Recent advances in the ability to characterize transporter proteins using molecular techniques has provided invaluable insights into the unique proteins that are arranged along the nephron in a polarized and highly segment-specific distribution. Distinct differences in protein structure allow kinetic variation along the proximal tubule so that an impressive concentration gradient from cell to lumen is maintained, allowing nearly complete reabsorption of a substrate.

Maturational changes in transporter protein abundance, metabolism, and regulational responses, in addition to less specific alterations in the cell membrane, explain the decreased functional capacity of the immature kidney. The exception to this generalized functional immaturity is phosphate transport, which is more active in the immature nephron than in the adult counterpart. The ability of both the adult and immature renal tubule to respond to changes in the external milieu through modification of gene transcription or protein trafficking and turnover at the plasma membrane serves as a means of adaptation to our external environment.

REFERENCES

1. Kiuchi-Saishin Y, Gotoh S, Furuse M, et al. Differential expression patterns of claudins, tight junction membrane proteins, in mouse nephron segments. *J Am Soc Nephrol* 2002;13:875–886.
2. Spitzer A, Schwartz GJ. The kidney during development. In: Windhager EE, ed. *Handbook of physiology: renal physiology*. New York: Oxford University Press, 1992:475–544.
3. Schwartz GJ, Evan AP. Development of solute transport in rabbit proximal tubule: I. HCO_3^- and glucose absorption. *Am J Physiol* 1983;245:F382–F390.
4. Racusen LC, Monteil C, Sgrignoli A, et al. Cell lines with extended in vitro growth potential from human renal proximal tubule: characterization, response to inducers, and comparison with established cell lines. *J Lab Clin Med* 1997;129:318–329.
5. Humes HD, MacKay SM, Funke AJ, et al. Tissue engineering of a bioartificial renal tubule assist device: in vitro transport and metabolic characteristics. *Kidney Int* 1999;55:2502–2514.
6. Guder WG, Morel F. Biochemical characterization of individual nephron segments. In: Windhager EE, ed. *Handbook of physiology: renal physiology*. New York: Oxford University Press, 1992:2120–2164.
7. Herrera VL, Emanuel JR, Ruiz-Opazo N, et al. Three differentially expressed Na, K-ATPase a subunit isoforms: structural and functional implications. *J Cell Biol* 1987;105:1855–1865.
8. Aperia A, Fryckstedt J, Holtback U, et al. Cellular mechanisms for bi-directional regulation of tubular sodium reabsorption. *Kidney Int* 1996;49:1743–1747.
9. Emanual JR, Garetz S, Stone L, et al. Differential expression of Na^+, K^+-ATPase alpha- and beta-subunit mRNAs in rat tissues and cell lines. *Proc Natl Acad Sci U S A* 1987;84:9030–9034.
10. Beyth Y, Gutman Y. Ontogenesis of microsomal ATPase in the rabbit kidney. *Biochim Biophys Acta* 1969;191:195–197.
11. Schmidt U, Horster M. Na-K-activated ATPase: activity maturation in rabbit nephron segments dissected in vitro. *Am J Physiol* 1977;233:F55–F60.
12. Larsson SH, Rane S, Fukuda Y, et al. Changes in Na influx precede post-natal increase in Na-K-ATPase activity in rat renal proximal tubule cells. A study of cells in short primary culture. *Acta Physiol Scand* 1990;138:243–244.
13. Guillery EN, Huss DJ, McDonough AA, et al. Posttranscriptional upregulation of Na-K-ATPase activity in newborn guinea pig renal cortex. *Am J Physiol* 1997;273:F254–F263.
14. Fukuda J, Aperia A. Differentiation of Na^+-K^+ pump in rat proximal tubule is modulated by Na^+-H^+ exchanger. *Am J Physiol* 1988;255:F552–F557.
15. Bowen JW, McDonough A. Pretranslational regulation of Na^+ K^+-ATPase in cultured canine kidney cells by low K^+. *Am J Physiol* 1987;252:C179–C189.
16. Celsi G, Nishi A, Akujarvi G, et al. Abundance of Na^+ K^+ ATPase mRNA is regulated by glucocorticoid hormones in infant rat kidneys. *Am J Physiol* 1991;260:F192–F197.
17. Fukuda Y, Bertorello A, Aperia A. Ontogeny of the regulation of Na^+-K^+ ATPase activity in the renal proximal tubule cell. *Pediatr Res* 1991;30:131–134.
18. Morel F, Doucet A. Functional segmentation of the nephron. In: Seldin DW, Giebisch G, eds. *The kidney: physiology and pathophysiology*. New York: Raven Press, 1992;1049–1086.

19. Silverman M, Turner RJ. Glucose transport in the renal proximal tubule. In: Windhager EE, ed. *Handbook of physiology: renal physiology*. New York: Oxford University Press, 1992:2017–2038.
20. Valentin M, Kuhlkamp T, Wagner K, et al. The transport modifier RS1 is localized at the inner side of the plasma membrane and changes membrane capacitance. *Biochim Biophys Acta* 2000;1468:367–380.
21. Barfuss DW, Schafer JA. Differences in active and passive glucose transport along the proximal nephron. *Am J Physiol* 1981;240:F332–F344.
22. Oulianova N, Berteloot A. Sugar transport heterogeneity in the kidney: two independent transporters or different transport modes through an oligomeric protein? *J Membr Biol* 1996;153:181–194.
23. Burchkhardt G, Kinne RKH. Cotransporters and countertransporters. In: Seldin DW, Giebisch G, eds. *The kidney: physiology and pathophysiology*. New York: Raven Press, 1992;537–586.
24. Turner RJ, Moran A. Heterogeneity of sodium-dependent D-glucose transporter. *J Membr Biol* 1982;67:73–80.
25. Oulianova N, Falk S, Berteloot A. Two-step mechanism of phlorizin binding to the SGLT1 protein in the kidney. *J Membr Biol* 2001;179:223–242.
26. Stevens BR, Fernandez A, Hirayama B, et al. Intestinal brush border membrane Na^+/glucose cotransporter functions in situ as a homotetramer. *Proc Natl Acad Sci U S A* 1990;87:1456–1460.
27. Kanai Y, Lee W, You G, et al. The human kidney low affinity Na/glucose cotransporter SGLT2. Delineation of the major renal reabsorptive mechanism for D-glucose. *J Clin Invest* 1994;93:397–404.
28. Debnam ES, Unwin RJ. Hyperglucemia and intestinal and renal glucose transport: Implications for diabetic renal injury. *Kidney Int* 1996;50:1101–1109.
29. Hediger MA, Rhoads DB. Molecular physiology of sodium-glucose cotransporters. *Physiol Rev* 1994;74:993–1026.
30. Brodehl J, Franken A, Gelissen K. Maximal tubular reabsorption of glucose in infants and children. *Acta Physiol Scand* 1972;61:413–420.
31. Beck JC, Lipkowitz MS, Abramson RG. Characterization of the fetal glucose transporter in rabbit kidney. Comparison with the adult brush border electrogenic Na^+-glucose symporter. *J Clin Invest* 1988;82:379–387.
32. Alexander DP, Nixon DA. Reabsorption of glucose, fructose and myoinositol by fetal and post-natal sheep kidney. *J Physiol* 1963;167:480–486.
33. Lelievre-Pegorier M, Geloso JP. Ontogeny of sugar transport in fetal rat kidney. *Biol Neonate* 1980;38:16–24.
34. Robillard JE, Sessions C, Kennedy RL, et al. Maturation of the glucose transport process by the fetal kidney. *Pediatr Res* 1978;12:680–684.
35. Foreman JW, Medow MS, Wald H, et al. Developmental aspects of sugar transport by isolated dog renal cortical tubules. *Pediatr Res* 1984;18:719–723.
36. Turner RJ, Silverman M. Sugar uptake into brush border vesicles from dog kidney. *Kinetics Biochem Acta* 1978;511: 470–486.
37. Silbernagl S. Tubular transport of amino acids and small peptides. In: Windhager EE, ed. *Handbook of physiology: renal physiology*. New York: Oxford University Press, 1992; 1937–1976.
38. Silbernagl S. The renal handling of amino acids and oligopeptides. *Physiol Rev* 1988;68:911–1007.
39. Silbernagl S. Tubular reabsorption of L-glutamine studies by free flow micropuncture and microperfusion of rat kidney. *Int J Biochem* 1980;12:9–16.
40. Silbernagl S, Ganapathy V, Leibch FH. H^+-gradient-driven dipeptide reabsorption in the proximal tubule of rat kidney. Studies in vivo and in vitro. *Am J Physiol* 1987;253:F448–F457.
41. Silbernagl S. Kinetics and localization of tubular reabsorption of "acidic" amino acids. A microperfusion and free flow micropuncture study in rat kidney. *Pflugers Arch* 1983;396: 218–224.
42. Samarzija I, Fromter E. Electrophysiological analysis of rat renal sugar and amino acid transport. Acidic amino acids. *Pflugers Arch* 1982;393:215–221.
43. Barfuss DW, Mays JM, Schafer JA. Peritubular uptake and transepithelial transport of glycine in isolated proximal tubules. *Am J Physiol* 1980;238:F324–F333.
44. Sacktor B. L-glutamate transport in renal plasma membrane vesicles. *Mol Cell Biochem* 1981;39:239–251.
45. Schneider EG, Sacktor B. Sodium gradient-dependent L-glutamate transport in renal brush border membrane vesicles. Evidence for an electroneutral mechanism. *J Biol Chem* 1980;255:7650–7656.
46. Silbernagl S, Volkl H. Molecular specificity of the tubular reabsorption of "acidic" amino acids. A continuous microperfusion study in rat kidney in vivo. *Pflugers Arch* 1983;396: 225–230.
47. Zelikovic I, Stejskal-Lorenz E, Lohstroh P, et al. Anion dependence of taurine transport by rat renal brush border membrane vesicles. *Am J Physiol* 1989;256:F646–F655.
48. Han X, Budreau AM, Chesney RW. Ser-322 is a critical site for PKC regulation of the MDCK cell taurine transporter (pNCT). *J Am Soc Nephrol* 1999;10:1874–1879.
49. Segal S, Smith I. Delineation of cystine and cysteine transport systems in rat kidney cortex by developmental patterns. *Proc Natl Acad Sci U S A* 1969;63:926–933.
50. Segal S, Smith I. Delineation of separate transport systems in rat kidney cortex for L-lysine and L-cystine by developmental patterns. *Biochem Biophys Res Commun* 1969;35: 771–777.
51. Lee WS, Wells RG, Sabbag RV, et al. Cloning and chromosomal location of a human kidney cDNA involved in cystine, dibasic, and neutral amino acid transport. *J Clin Invest* 1993;91:1959–1963.
52. Waldegger S, Schmidt F, Herzer T, et al. Heavy metal mediated inhibition of rBAT-induced amino acid transport. *Kidney Int* 1995;47:1677–1681.
53. Chillaron J, Roca R, Valencia A, et al. Heteromeric amino acid transporters: biochemistry, genetics and physiology. *Am J Physiol Renal Physiol* 2001;281:F995–F1018.
54. Zelikovic I. Molecular pathophysiology of tubular transport disorders. *Pediatr Nephrol* 2001;16:919–935.
55. Zelikovic I, Chesney RW. Development of renal amino acid transport systems. *Semin Nephrol* 1989;9:49–55.
56. Fleck C, Kretzschel I, Sperschneider T, et al. Renal amino acid transport in immature and adult rats during chromate

and cisplatinum-induced nephrotoxicity. *Amino Acids* 2001; 20:201–215.
57. Baerlocher KE, Scriver CR, Mohyuddin F. The ontogeny of amino acid transport in rat kidney 1: effect on distribution ratios and intracellular metabolism of proline and glycine. *Biochim Biophys Acta* 1971;249:353–363.
58. Brodehl J, Gelissen K. Endogenous renal transport of free amino acids in infancy and childhood. *Pediatrics* 1968;42:395–404.
59. Chesney RW, Jax DK. Developmental aspects of renal β-amino acid transport: I. Ontogeny of taurine reabsorption and accumulation in rat renal cortex. *Pediatr Res* 1979;13:854–860.
60. Hwang SM, Serahan MA, Toth KS, et al. L-proline transport by isolated renal tubules from newborn and adult rats. *Pediatr Res* 1983;17:42–46.
61. Medow MS, Foreman JW, Bovee KD, et al. Developmental changes of glycine transport in the dog. *Biochim Biophys Acta* 1982;693:85–92.
62. Webber WA. Amino acid excretion patterns in developing rats. *Can J Physiol Pharmacol* 1967;45:867–872.
63. Webber WA, Cairns JS. A comparison of the amino acid concentrating ability of the kidney cortex of newborn and mature rats. *Can J Physiol Pharmacol* 1968;46:165–169.
64. Webber WA. A comparison of the efflux rates of AIB from kidney cortex slices of mature and newborn rats. *Can J Physiol Pharmacol* 1968;46:765–769.
65. Foreman JW, Medow MS, Bovee KD, et al. Developmental aspects of cystine transport in the dog. *Pediatr Res* 1986;20: 593–597.
66. Goldman DR, Roth KS, Langfitt TW, et al. L-proline transport by newborn rat kidney brush border membrane vesicles. *Biochem J* 1979;178:253–256.
67. Medow MS, Roth KS, Goldman DR. Developmental aspects of proline transport in rat renal brush border membranes. *Proc Natl Acad Sci U S A* 1986;83:7561–7564.
68. Chesney RW, Gusowski N, Zelikovic I, et al. Developmental aspects of renal β-amino acid transport: V. Brush border membrane transport in nursing animals-effect of age and diet. *Pediatr Res* 1986;20:890–895.
69. Chesney RW, Jax DK. Developmental aspects of renal β-amino acid transport: II. Ontogeny of uptake and efflux processes and effect of anoxia. *Pediatr Res* 1979;13:861–867.
70. Zelikovic I, Chesney RW, Ahlfors EC. Very low birth weight (VLBW) infants receiving prolonged total parenteral nutrition (TPN) are taurine-depleted because of renal immaturity. *J Pediatr* 1990;116:301–306.
71. Daniel H, Herget M. Cellular and molecular mechanisms or renal peptide transport. *Am J Physiol* 1997;273: F1–F8.
72. Maack T. Renal handling of proteins and polypeptides. In: Windhager EE, ed. *Handbook of physiology: renal physiology*. New York: Oxford University Press, 1992:1937–1976.
73. Dennis VW. Phosphate homeostasis. In: Windhager EE, ed. *Handbook of physiology: renal physiology*. New York: Oxford University Press, 1992:1785–1815.
74. Brunette MG, Chan M, Maag U, et al. Phosphate uptake by superficial and deep nephron brush border membranes: effects of the dietary phosphate and parathyroid hormone. *Pflugers Arch* 1984;400:356–362.
75. Quamme GA, Wong NLM. Phosphate transport in the proximal convoluted tubule: effect of intraluminal pH. *Am J Physiol* 1984;246:F323–F333.
76. Murer H. Cellular mechanisms in proximal tubular Pi reabsorption: some answers and more questions. *J Am Soc Nephrol* 1992;2:1649–1665.
77. Murer H, Lotscher M, Kaissling B, et al. Renal brush border membrane Na/Pi-cotransport: Molecular aspects in PTH-dependent and dietary regulation. *Kidney Int* 1996;49:1769–1773.
78. Gmaj P, Murer H. Cellular mechanisms of inorganic phosphate transport in kidney. *Physiol Rev* 1986;66:36–70.
79. Amstutz M, Mohrmann M, Gmaj P, et al. Effect of pH on phosphate transport. *Am J Physiol* 1985;248:F705–F710.
80. Hoffman N, Thees M, Kinne R. Phosphate transport by isolated renal brush border vesicles. *Pflugers Arch* 1976;362:147–156.
81. Tenehouse HS. Cellular and molecular mechanisms of renal phosphate transport. *J Bone Miner Res* 1997;12:159–164.
82. Murer H, Hernando N, Forster I, et al. Molecular aspects in the regulation of renal inorganic phosphate reabsorption: the type IIa sodium/inorganic phosphate co-transporter as the key player. *Curr Opin Nephrol Hypertens* 2001;10:555–561.
83. Cai H, Puschett DB, Guan S, et al. Phosphate transport inhibition by KW-3902, an adenosine A1 receptor antagonist, is mediated by cyclic adenosine monophosphate. *Am J Kidney Dis* 1995;26:825–830.
84. Bowe AE, Finnegan R, Jan de Beur SM, et al. FGF-23 inhibits renal tubular phosphate transport and is a PHEX substrate. *Biochem Biophys Res Commun* 2001;284:977–981.
85. Boileau G, Tenenhouse HS, Desgroseillers L, et al. Characterization of PHEX endopeptidase catalytic activity: identification of parathyroid-hormone-related peptide 107-139 as a substrate and osteocalcin, PPi and phosphate as inhibitors. *Biochem J* 2001;355:707–713.
86. Shimada T, Mizutani S, Muto T, et al. Cloning and characterization of FGF23 as a causative factor of tumor-induced osteomalacia. *Proc Natl Acad Sci U S A* 2001;98:6500–6505.
87. Kaskel FJ, Kumar AM, Feld LG, et al. Renal reabsorption of phosphate during development: Tubular events. *Pediatr Nephrol* 1988;2:129–134.
88. Brodehl J, Gelissen K, Weber HP. Postnatal development of tubular phosphate reabsorption. *Clin Nephrol* 1982;17:163–171.
89. Caversasio J, Boujour JP, Flesch H. Tubular handling of Pi in young growing and adult rats. *Am J Physiol* 1982;242:F705–F710.
90. Haramati A. Phosphate handling by the kidney during development: immaturity or unique adaptations for growth? *News Physiol Sci* 1989;4:234–238.
91. Haramati A, Mulroney SE, Webster SK. Developmental changes in the tubular capacity for phosphate reabsorption in the rat. *Am J Physiol* 1988;255:F287–F291.
92. Neilberger RE, Barac-Nieto M, Spitzer A. Renal reabsorption of phosphate during development: transport kinetics in BBMV. *Am J Physiol* 1989;257:F268–F274.
93. Imbert-Teboul M, Chabardes D, Clique A, et al. Ontogenesis of hormone-dependent adenylate cyclase in isolated rat nephrol segments. *Am J Physiol* 1984;247:F316–F325.

94. Johnson V, Spitzer A. Renal reabsorption of phosphate during development: whole-kidney events. *Am J Physiol* 1986; 251:F251–F256.
95. Mulroney SE, Lumpkin MD, Haramati A. Antagonist to GH-releasing factor inhibits growth and renal Pi reabsorption in immature rats. *Am J Physiol* 1989;257:F29–F34.
96. Haramati A, Mulroney SE, Lumpkin MD. Regulation of renal phosphate reabsorption during development: implications from a new model of growth hormone deficiency. *Pediatr Nephrol* 1990;4:387–391.
97. Barac-Nieto M, Gupta RK, Spitzer A. NMR studies of phosphate metabolism in the isolated perfused kidney of developing rats. *Pediatr Nephrol* 1990;4:392–398.
98. Haramati A, Lumpkin MD, Winaver J, et al. Role of growth hormone/IGF-I axis in regulating renal phosphate homeostasis during growth. Proceedings of the Fifth International Workshop on Developmental Physiology, 1992.
99. Caverzasio J, Bonjour JP. Growth factors and renal regulation of phosphate transport. Proceedings of the Fifth International Workshop on Developmental Physiology, 1992.
100. Motohashi H, Sakurai Y, Saito H, et al. Gene expression levels and immunolocalization of organic ion transporters in the human kidney. *J Am Soc Nephrol* 2002;13:866–874.
101. Pritchard JB, Miller DS. Proximal tubular transport of organic anions and cations. In: Seldin DW, Giebisch G, eds. *The kidney: physiology and pathophysiology*. New York: Raven Press, 1992:2921–2945.
102. Kojima R, Sekine T, Kawachi M, et al. Immunolocalization of multispecific organic anion transporters, OAT1, OAT2, and OAT3, in rat kidney. *J Am Soc Nephrol* 2002;13:848–857.
103. Roch-Ramel F, Besseghir K, Murer H. Renal excretion and tubular transport of organic anions and cations. In: Windhager EE, ed. *Handbook of physiology: renal physiology*. New York: Oxford University Press, 1992:2179–2262.
104. Shumomura A, Chonko AM, Grantham JJ. Basis for heterogeneity of para-aminohippurate secretion in rabbit proximal tubules. *Am J Physiol* 1981;240:F430–F436.
105. Sekine T, Watanabe N, Hosoyamada M, et al. Expression cloning and characterization of a novel multispecific organic anion transporter. *J Biol Chem* 1997;272:18525–18529.
106. Cha SH, Sekine T, Fukushima JI, et al. Identification and characterization of human organic anion transporter 3 expressing predominantly in the kidney. *Mol Pharmacol* 2001;59:1277–1286.
107. Elbourne I, Lumbers ER, Hill KJ. The secretion of organic acids and bases by the ovine fetal kidney. *Exp Physiol* 1990;95:211–221.
108. Rennick B, Hamilton B, Evans R. Development of renal tubular transport of TEA and PAH in the puppy and piglet. *Am J Physiol* 1961;201:743–746.
109. Calcagno PL, Rubin MI. Renal extraction of para-aminohippurate in infants and children. *J Clin Invest* 1963;42: 1632–1639.
110. Horster M, Lewy JE. Filtration fraction and extraction of PAH during the neonatal period in the rat. *Am J Physiol* 1970;219:1061–1065.
111. Kleinman LI, Lubbe RJ. Factors affecting the maturation of renal PAH extraction in the newborn dog. *J Physiol* 1972; 223:411–418.
112. Stopp M, Braunlich H. Kinetics of p-aminohippurate (PAH) transport in renal cortical slices from neonatal and adult rats. *Biochem Pharmacol* 1977;26:1809–1812.
113. Stopp M, Braunlich H. In vitro analysis of drug-induced stimulation of renal tubular *p*-aminohippurate (PAH) transport in rats. *Biochem Pharmacol* 1980;29:983–986.
114. Hirsch GH, Hook JB. Maturation of renal organic acid transport: Substrate stimulation by penicillin. *Science* 1969; 165:909–910.
115. Braunlich H. Hormonal control of postnatal development of renal tubular transport of weak organic acids. *Pediatr Nephrol* 1988;2:151–155.
116. Montrose-Rafizadeh C, Roch-Ramel F, Sachall C. Axial heterogeneity of organic cation transport along the rabbit renal proximal tubule: Studies with brush border membrane vesicles. *Biochim Biophys Acta* 1987;904:175–177.
117. Michaly GW, Jones DB, Morgan DJ, et al. Placental transfer and renal elimination of cimetidine in maternal and fetal sheep. *J Pharmacol Exp Ther* 1983;227:441–445.
118. Szeto HH, Clapp III JF, Larrow RW, et al. Renal tubular secretion of meperidine by the fetal lamb. *J Pharmacol Exp Ther* 1980;213:346–349.
119. Kahn AM, Weinman EJ. Urate transport in the proximal tubule: in vivo and vesicle studies. *Am J Physiol* 1985;249: F789–F798.
120. Guggino SE, Aronson PS. Paradoxical effects of pyrazinoate and nicotinate on urate transport in dog renal microvillus membranes. *J Clin Invest* 1985;76:543–547.
121. Kahn AM, Aronson PS. Urate transport via anion exchange in dog renal microvillus membrane vesicles. *Am J Physiol* 1983;244:F56–F63.
122. Guggino SE, Martin GJ, Aronson PS. Specificity and modes of the anion exchanges in dog renal microvillus membranes. *Am J Physiol* 1983;244:F612–F621.
123. Kahn AM, Branhanm S, Weinman EJ. Mechanism of urate and *p*-aminohippurate transport in rat renal microvillus membrane vesicles. *Am J Physiol* 1983;245:F151–F158.
124. Kahn AM, Shelat H, Weinman EJ. Urate and p-aminohippurate in rat renal basolateral vesicles. *Am J Physiol* 1985; 249:F654–F661.
125. Lipkowitz MS, Leal-Pinto E, Rappoport JZ, et al. Functional reconstitution, membrane targeting, genomic structure, and chromosomal localization of a human urate transporter. *J Clin Invest* 2001;107:1103–1115.
126. Poulsen H. Uric acid in blood and urine of infants. *Acta Physiol Scand* 1955;33:372–377.
127. Passwell JH, Modan M, Brush M, et al. Fractional excretion of uric acid in infancy and childhood. Index of tubular maturation. *Arch Dis Child* 1974;49:878–882.
128. Stapleton FB. Renal uric acid clearances in human neonates. *J Pediatr* 1983;103:290–294.
129. Stapleton FB, Linshaw MA, Hassanein K, et al. Uric acid excretion in normal children. *J Pediatr* 1978;92:911–914.
130. Stapleton FB, Arant BS Jr. Ontogeny of uric acid excretion in the mongrel puppy. *Pediatr Res* 1981;15:1513–1516.
131. Murer H, Manganel M, Roch-Ramel F. Tubular transport of monocarboxylates, Krebs cycle intermediates and inorganic sulfate. In: Windhager EE, eds. *Handbook of physiology: renal physiology*. New York: Oxford University Press, 1992;2164–2188.

132. Schneider EG, Durham JC, Sacktor B. Sodium-dependent transport of inorganic sulfate by rabbit renal brush border membrane vesicles. *J Biol Chem* 1984;259: 14591–14599.
133. Turner RJ. Sodium-dependent sulfate transport in renal outer cortical brush border membrane vesicles. *Am J Physiol* 1984;247:F793–F798.
134. Jorgensen KE, Sheikh MI. Mechanisms of uptake of ketone bodies by luminal membrane vesicles. *Biochim Biophys Acta* 1985;814:23–34.
135. Fukuhara Y, Turner RJ. Sodium-dependent succinate transport in renal outer cortical brush border membrane vesicles. *Am J Physiol* 1983;245:F374–F381.
136. Hirayama B, Wright EM. Coupling between sodium and succinate transport across renal brush border membrane vesicles. *Pflugers Arch* 1986;407:S174–S179.
137. Wright SH, Hirayama B, Kippen I, et al. Effect of Na^+ and membrane potential on kinetics of succinate transport in renal brush border membranes, abstracted. *Fed Proc* 1982; 41:1264.
138. Ferrier B, Martin M, Baverel G. Reabsorption and secretion of a-ketoglutarate along the rat nephron: a micropuncture study. *Am J Physiol* 1985;248:F404–F412.
139. Samarzija I, Molnar V, Fromter E. The stoichiometry of Na^+-coupled anion absorption across the brush border membrane of rat renal proximal tubule. *Adv Physiol Sci* 1981;11:419–434.
140. Sheridan E, Rumrich G, Ullrich KJ. Reabsorption of dicarboxylic acids from the proximal convolution of rat kidney. *Pflugers Arch* 1983;399:18–28.
141. Wright SH, Hirayama B, Kaunitz JE, et al. Kinetics of sodium succinate cotransport across renal brush border membranes. *J Biol Chem* 1983;258:5456–5462.
142. Burchkhardt G. Sodium-dependent dicarboxylate transport in rat renal basolateral membrane vesicles. *Pflugers Arch* 1984;401:254–261.
143. Yao X, Pajor AM. Arginine-349 and aspartate-373 of the Na(+)/dicarboxylate cotransporter are conformationally sensitive residues. *Biochemistry* 2002;41:1083–1090.
144. Berry CA, Rector Jr. FC. Relative sodium to chloride permeability in the proximal convoluted tubule. *Am J Physiol* 1978;235:F592–F604.
145. Aronson PS. Role of ion exchangers in mediating NaCl transport in the proximal tubule. *Kidney Int* 1996;49:1665–1670.
146. Knauf F, Yang CL, Thomson RB, et al. Identification of a chloride-formate exchanger expressed on the brush border membrane of renal proximal tubule cells. *Proc Natl Acad Sci U S A* 2001;98:9425–9430.
147. Burchkhardt G, Gregor R. Principles of electrolyte transport across plasma membranes of renal tubular cells. In: Windhager EE, ed. *Handbook of physiology: renal physiology.* New York: Oxford University Press, 1992;639–657.
148. Mount DB, Gamba G. Renal potassium-chloride cotransporters. *Curr Opin Nephrol Hypertens* 2001;10:685–691.
149. Aronson PS, Giebisch G. Mechanisms of chloride transport in the proximal tubule. *Am J Physiol* 1997;273:F179–F192.
150. Gross E, Hawkins K, Pushkin A, et al. Phosphorylation of Ser(982) in the sodium bicarbonate cotransporter kNBC1 shifts the HCO(3)(–): Na(+) stoichiometry from 3:1 to 2:1 in murine proximal tubule cells. *J Physiol* 2001;537:659–665.
151. Aronson PS, Nee J, Suhm MA. Modifier role of internal H^+ in activating the Na^+-H^+ exchanger in renal microvillus membrane vesicles. *Nature* 1982;299:161–163.
152. Grinstein S, Rothstein A. Mechanisms of regulation of the Na^+/H^+ exchanger. *J Membr Biol* 1986;80:1–12.
153. Grinstein S, Rotin D, Mason MJ. Na^+/H^+ exchange and growth factor-induced cytosolic pH changes. Role in cellular proliferation. *Biochim Biophys Acta* 1989;988:73–97.
154. Sardet C, Counillon L, Franchi A, et al. Growth factors induce phosphorylation of the Na^+/H^+ antiporter, a glycoprotein of 110 kD. *Science* 1990;247:723–725.
155. Akiba T, Rocco VK, Warnock DG. Parallel adaptation of the rabbit renal cortical sodium/proton antiporter and sodium/bicarbonate cotransporter in metabolic acidosis and alkalosis. *J Clin Invest* 1987;80:308–315.
156. Baum M, Biemesderfer D, Gentry D, et al. Ontogeny of rabbit renal cortical NHE3 and NHE1: effect of glucocorticoids. *Am J Physiol* 1995;268:F815–F820.
157. Chen PY, Illsley NP, Verkman AS. Renal brush border chloride transport mechanisms characterized using a fluorescent indicator. *Am J Physiol* 1988;254:F114–F120.
158. Ives HE, Chen PY, Verkman AS. Mechanism of coupling between Cl and OH transport in renal brush border membranes. *Biochim Biophys Acta* 1986;863:91–100.
159. Karnishki LP, Aronson PS. Chloride/formate exchange with formic acid recycling: a mechanism for active chloride transport across epithelial membranes. *Proc Natl Acad Sci U S A* 1985;82:6362–6366.
160. Karnishki LP, Aronson PS. Anion exchange pathways for Cl transport in rabbit renal microvillus membranes. *Am J Physiol* 1987;253:F513–F521.
161. Ullrich KJ, Capasso G, Rumrich G, et al. Coupling between proximal tubular transport processes: studies with ouabain, SITS and HCO_3 free solutions. *Pflugers Arch* 1977;368:245–252.
162. Gregor R. Cl-transport mechanisms in the thick ascending limb of Henle's loop of the mammalian. *Nephron Physiol Rev* 1985;65:760–797.
163. Wangemann P, Wittner M, Di Stefano A, et al. Cl-channel blockers in the thick ascending limb of the loop of Henle. Structure activity relationships. *Pflugers Arch* 1986;407: S128–S141.
164. Gregor R, Schlatter E. Properties of the basolateral membrane of the cortical thick ascending limb of Henle's loop of rabbit kidney: a model for secondary active chloride transport. *Pflugers Arch* 1983;396:325–334.
165. Kinne R, Konig B, Hannafin J, et al. The use of membrane vesicle to study the NaCl/KCl cotransporter involved in active transepithelial chloride transport. *Pflugers Arch* 1985; 405:S101–S105.
166. Kinne R, Kinne-Saffran E, Scholermann B, et al. The anion specificity of the sodium-potassium-chloride cotransporter in rabbit kidney outer medulla: studies on medullary plasma membranes. *Pflugers Arch* 1986;407: S168–S173.
167. Wall SM, Fischer MP. Contribution of the Na^+-K^+-$2Cl^-$ Cotransporter (NKCCl) to transepithelial transport of H^+,

NH_4^+, K^+, and Na^+ in rat outer medullary collecting duct. *J Am Soc Nephrol* 2002;13:827–835.
168. Simon DB, Lifton RP. The molecular basis of inherited hypokalemic alkalosis: Bartter's and Gitelman's syndromes. *Am J Physiol* 1996;271:F961–F966.
169. Hebert SC, Gamba G, Kaplan M. The electroneutral Na^- $(K)^-$ Cl cotransport family. *Kidney Int* 1996;49:1638–1641.
170. Kaplan MR, Plotkin MD, Brown D, et al. Expression of the Mouse Na-K-2Cl cotransporter, mBSC2, in the terminal inner medullary collecting duct, the glomerular and extraglomerular mesangium and the glomerular afferent arteriole. *J Clin Invest* 1996;98:723–730.
171. Biner HL, Arpin-Bott MP, Loffing J, et al. Human cortical distal nephron: distribution of electrolyte and water transport pathways. *J Am Soc Nephrol* 2002;13:836–847.
172. Kaji DM, Diaz J, Parker JC. Urea inhibits Na-K-2Cl cotransport in medullary thick ascending limb cells. *Am J Physiol* 1997;272:C615–C621.
173. Ecelbarger CA, Terris J, Hoyer JR, et al. Localization and regulation of the rat renal Na-K-2Cl cotransporter, BSC-1. *Am J Physiol* 1996;271:F619–F628.
174. Benos DJ, Awayda MS, Berdiev BK, et al. Diversity and regulation of amiloride-sensitive Na^+ channels. *Kidney Int* 1996;49:1632–1637.
175. Schlatter E, Schafer JA. Electrophysiological studies in principal cells of rat cortical collecting tubules. *Pflugers Arch* 1983;396:210–217.
176. O'Neil RG, Helman SI. Transport characteristics of renal collecting tubules: influences of DOCA and diet. *Am J Physiol* 1977;233:F544–F558.
177. Howard DP, Cuffe JE, Boyd CA, et al. L-arginine effects on Na+ transport in M-1 mouse cortical collecting duct cells—a cationic amino acid absorbing epithelium. *J Membr Biol* 2001;180:111–121.
178. Aperia A, Larsson L. Correlation between fluid reabsorption and proximal tubule ultrastructure during development of the rat kidney. *Acta Physiol Scand* 1979;105:11–22.
179. Baum M. Neonatal rabbit juxtamedullary proximal convoluted tubule acidification. *J Clin Invest* 1990;85:499–506.
180. Ekblad H, Larsson SH, Aperia A. The capacity to recover from intracellular acidosis is lower in infant than in adolescent renal cells (Abstract). *Pediatr Nephrol* 1990;27: 327A.
181. Beck JC, Lipkowitz MS, Abramson RG. Ontogeny of Na/H antiporter activity in rabbit renal brush border membrane vesicles. *J Clin Invest* 1991;87:2067–2076.

4

PERINATAL UROLOGY

DAVID A. DIAMOND
CRAIG A. PETERS

The routine use of maternal-fetal ultrasound has introduced the field of perinatal urology. Fetal hydronephrosis, with an incidence of 1:100 to 1:500 maternal studies, is the most common abnormality detected. Other urologic abnormalities have been diagnosed prenatally as well, including renal cystic disease, renal agenesis, and even stones and tumors. For the pediatric urologist, these prenatal findings have opened a Pandora's box of questions that challenge our understanding of normal and abnormal renal embryology and physiology. In this chapter, we discuss the diagnosis of prenatal urologic abnormalities, the rationale behind prenatal intervention, and our clinical experience in managing children with prenatal urologic abnormalities.

DIAGNOSIS

In a large prospective Swedish study, the incidence of prenatally detected renal anomalies was 0.28% (1). Of these, two-thirds (0.18%) were hydronephrosis. A British study (2), in which 99% of the pregnant population in Stoke-on-Trent were scanned at 28 weeks' gestation, demonstrated hydronephrosis prenatally in 1.40% of cases, which was confirmed postnatally in 0.65% (2). These authors defined *prenatal hydronephrosis* as an anteroposterior (A-P) diameter of the renal pelvis greater than 5 mm but noted the lack of consensus on the definition of *antenatal hydronephrosis* (3–5).

When an abnormality of the urinary tract is determined by maternal-fetal ultrasound, several questions should be raised by the ultrasonographer and consulting urologist. Combinations of specific findings direct the differential diagnosis and permit more accurate prognosis and tailoring of postnatal evaluation. The principal findings and their implications are listed in Table 4.1.

Diagnostic Accuracy

The importance of accurate diagnosis is dependent on the context of the case. If intervention is to be considered, diagnostic accuracy needs to be high. In most cases, the detection of some degree of hydronephrosis permits appropriate postnatal evaluation, even if the responsible mechanism and precise level of obstruction are not discernible. Diagnostic accuracy of hydronephrosis in the fetus remains imperfect. An early report by Hobbins et al. suggested that the correct prenatal identification of the site of obstruction could be confirmed postnatally in 88% of cases (6). Subsequent studies reported fairly high false-positive rates ranging from 9 to 22% (3). The majority of false positives in these studies was nonobstructive causes of hydronephrosis, such as high-grade reflux or large, nonobstructed, extrarenal pelves or transient hydronephrosis.

Accurate diagnosis of posterior urethral valves (PUV), in which intervention might be considered, has proven difficult. In one series, the false-positive rate was as high as 58% (7), but the criteria for diagnosing valves were quite liberal and perhaps inappropriate. In another population-based series, the sensitivity in detecting valves was as low as 23% (3). Diagnosis of obstructive conditions based on the criteria of increased renal echogenicity and decreased amniotic fluid is very accurate (8). The distinction between mild and moderate degrees of obstruction and conditions such as reflux may be more challenging. The clinical impact of these distinctions depends on whether intervention should be considered for anything less than severe.

Ureteropelvic Junction Obstruction

The basic features of ureteropelvic junction obstruction (UPJO) in the fetus include dilation of the renal pelvis and collecting system with no evidence of ureteral dilation (Fig. 4.1). The best way to detect ureteral dilation is at the level of the bladder, preferably in transverse view. The degree of dilation becomes the critical issue determining postnatal recommendations. The threshold for recommending postnatal follow-up is largely arbitrary, yet most would agree that a unilateral A-P diameter over 7 or 8 mm in the third trimester (5 to 6 mm with bilateral dilation) mandates postnatal follow-up (9). In the case of unilateral UPJO, there is little

TABLE 4.1. MAJOR DIAGNOSTIC FINDINGS IN PRENATAL IMAGING

	Finding	Comment
Kidney	Hydronephrosis	Assess degree
	Unilateral vs. bilateral	May be different degrees
	Parenchymal echogenicity	Should be less than spleen or liver; if increased and organ enlarged, suggests autosomal recessive polycystic kidney disease
	Duplication	Often with dilation of upper pole; may be lower pole dilation
	Cysts	Small cysts associated with dysplasia; simple cyst of upper pole suggests duplication with ureterocele or ectopic ureter; genetic cystic disease
	Urinoma	Perinephric or subcapsular
Ureter	Dilation/tortuosity	Obstruction or reflux
Bladder	Distended	Variation with time
	Wall thickness	In relation to filling status
	Intravesical cystic structure	Ureterocele
	"Keyhole" pattern	Dilated posterior urethra; PUV
	Not visible	Exstrophy
Amniotic fluid	Absence; oligohydramnios	Impaired urine output
	Polyhydramnios	May be seen with mild-moderate hydronephrosis
Gender	Penis/scrotum/testes	Sex-associated conditions (e.g., PUV)
Spine	Meningocele	Neural tube defect

PUV, posterior urethral valves.

rationale for *in utero* intervention. In a few cases with massive dilation, therapeutic aspiration has been recommended for dystocia. In the case of bilateral UPJO, the efficacy of *in utero* intervention is difficult to assess.

Attempts to correlate prenatal ultrasound appearance with postnatal outcomes have been complicated by the long-standing controversy regarding postnatal evaluation and management of UPJO. Grignon et al. developed a system of grading hydronephrosis secondary to UPJO based on the diameter of the renal pelvis (RPD) and degree of calyceal dilatation (10). Mandell et al. attempted to correlate the degree of A-P RPD pelvic diameter relative to gestational age with subsequent need for postnatal surgical intervention (Fig. 4.2) (11). They found the "at risk" diameter to be greater than or equal to 5 mm at 15 to 20 weeks' gestation, greater than or equal to 8 mm at 20 to 30 weeks' gestation, and greater than 1 cm at over 30 weeks' gestation. An alternative system proposed by Kleiner et al. defined *hydronephrosis* as the ratio of A-P RPD to A-P diameter of kidney as being greater than 0.5 cm (12); caliectasis was later added as an additional indicator of significant hydronephrosis. Mild degrees of renal pelvic dilatation may resolve *in utero*. Mandell et al. noted this to occur in 23% of cases, with 66% remaining stable and 9% worsening over the course of the pregnancy (11). Severe forms of UPJO may be associated with urinary ascites or perinephric urinomas, which often precede nonfunction of the kidney (13).

Cystic Kidneys

The distinction between severe unilateral hydronephrosis and a multicystic dysplastic kidney may occasionally be unclear. The findings of multiple noncommunicating cysts, minimal or absent renal parenchyma, and the absence of a central large cyst are diagnostic of a multicystic dysplastic kidney. Bilaterally enlarged echogenic kidneys, particularly if associated with hepatobiliary dilatation or oligohydramnios, suggests autosomal recessive polycystic kidney disease (Fig. 4.3). A more challenging finding is normal-sized, diffusely echogenic kidneys that are not associated with other urologic lesions. Estroff et al. described 19 cases (14 bilateral), including 10 with normal function who survived and 4 with autosomal recessive polycystic kidneys who died (14).

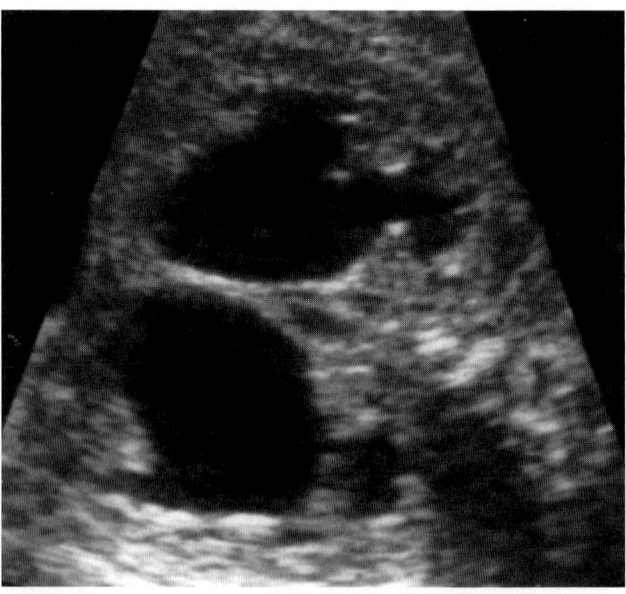

FIGURE 4.1. Bilateral ureteropelvic junction obstruction manifested as symmetric hydronephrosis with caliectasis and no ureteral dilation in a fetus.

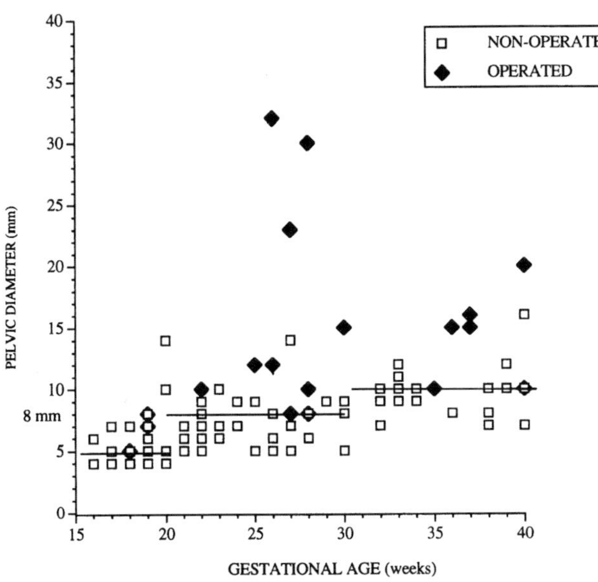

FIGURE 4.2. Prenatal renal pelvic diameter in operative and non-operative patients with hydronephrosis. [From Mandell J, Blyth BR, Peters CA, et al. Structural genitourinary defects detected in utero. *Radiology* 1991;178(1):193–196, with permission.]

Ureterovesical Junction Obstruction

Less common than UPJO, ureterovesical obstruction is characterized by ureteral dilation along with varying degrees of renal pelvic and calyceal dilation. More extreme cases may be confused with single system ectopic ureters, particularly in males. In general, the differentiation can be made postnatally.

Duplication Anomalies

Duplication anomalies, among the most interesting of prenatal urologic findings, are recognized on the basis of upper pole hydroureteronephrosis, associated with an obstructing ureterocele within the bladder or ectopic ureter, inserting outside of the bladder (15) (Fig. 4.4). Lower pole hydronephrosis may be present as a result of reflux or UPJO. Occasionally, lower pole dilation is due to upper and lower ureteral obstruction by a large ureterocele.

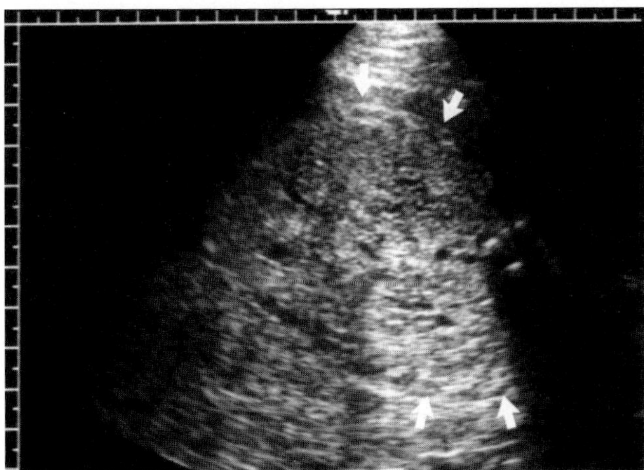

FIGURE 4.3. Markedly enlarged echogenic ("bright") kidneys (*arrows*) in a fetus with oligohydramnios, consistent with autosomal-recessive polycystic kidney disease.

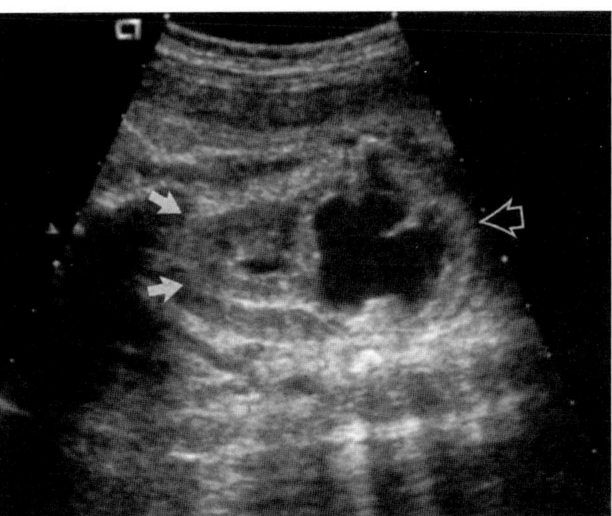

FIGURE 4.4. Fetal image of duplex kidney with marked upper pole hydronephrosis (*open arrow*) in contrast to a normal lower pole (*closed arrows*). This image is consistent with either ectopic ureter or ectopic ureterocele with duplication.

Vesicoureteral Reflux

One cannot make a firm diagnosis of vesicoureteral reflux based on prenatal ultrasound, although intermittent hydronephrosis or hydroureter is highly suggestive. Vesicoureteral reflux may be present in as many as 38% of children with prenatal hydronephrosis (16). Reflux occurred in 42% of children in whom postnatal imaging revealed persistent upper tract abnormalities and in 25% of those with normal findings on postnatal ultrasound but having a history of prenatal dilation. Tibballs and Debrun reported that in patients with prenatal dilation and postnatally normal renal units by ultrasound, 25% had grade III–V reflux (17). The incidence of high-grade reflux was greater in males than in females as noted in previous studies.

Posterior Urethral Valves

Perhaps the most important diagnosis to be made prenatally is that of PUV in the male fetus—a disorder that, at the very least, mandates prompt postnatal surgical correction. In some cases, prenatal intervention may be warranted. Fetal sonographic findings of PUV include bilateral hydroureteronephrosis, a thick-walled bladder with dilated posterior urethra, and, in more severe cases, dysplastic renal parenchymal changes with perinephric urinomas and urinary ascites (Figs. 4.5 and 4.6) (18). When characteristic

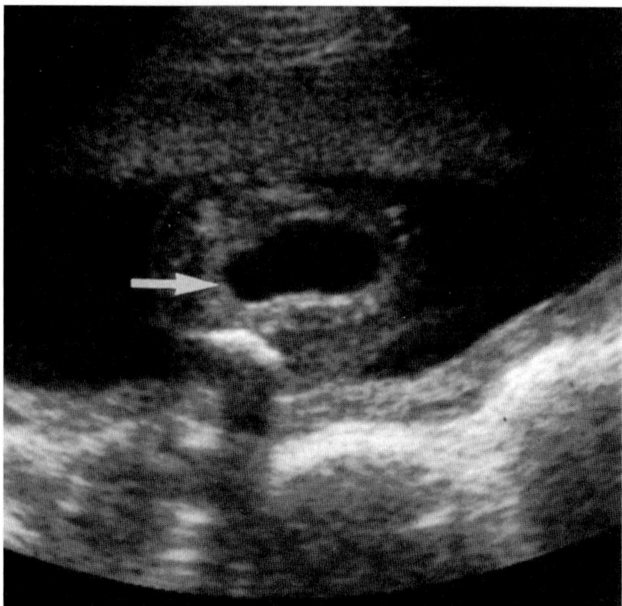

FIGURE 4.5. Image of fetal bladder associated with posterior urethral valves showing bladder wall thickening and a dilated posterior urethra (*arrow*), "keyhole sign."

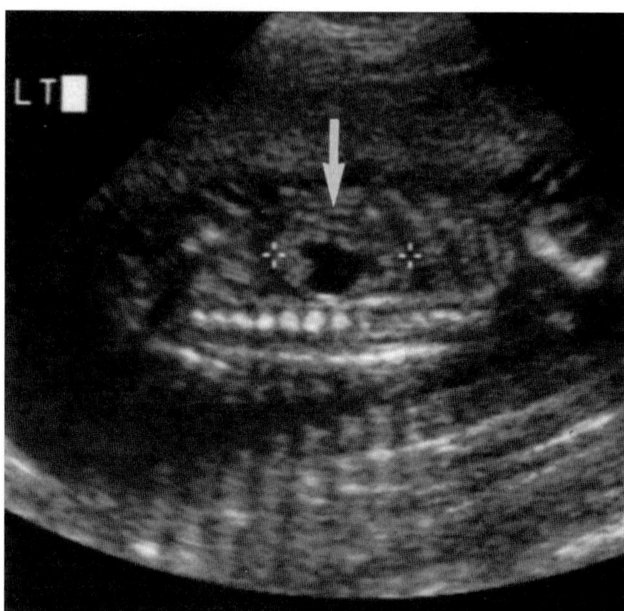

FIGURE 4.6. Echogenic hydronephrotic kidney (*arrow*) associated with posterior urethral valves in a 20-week fetus.

sonographic findings are present, the differential diagnosis includes prune belly syndrome (with or without urethral atresia), massive vesicoureteral reflux, and certain cloacal anomalies (in genetic females) (19,20). Prenatal diagnostic accuracy for PUV is far from perfect but is probably better than the 40% reported by Abbott et al. (7).

RATIONALE FOR PRENATAL INTERVENTION

The scientific rationale for prenatal treatment of hydronephrosis is to maximize normal development of renal and pulmonary function. These two aspects of fetal development are closely linked because urine comprises 90% of amniotic fluid volume, and oligohydramnios during the third trimester has been causally related to pulmonary hypoplasia.

Before prenatal surgical intervention for obstructive uropathy, it is critical to assess the risk-benefit ratio. The most widely accepted indicator of salvageable renal function is analysis of fetal urine. When the urinary sodium is less than 100 mg/dL and urine osmolarity less than 200 mOsm/dL, renal function appears to be salvageable with *in utero* intervention (Table 4.2) (21). The accuracy of these predictors has been challenged (22,23). More recently, serial aspirations of fetal urine have been reported to yield more valuable results (24). Guez et al. (25) reported ten fetuses who underwent multiple urine samplings and in whom severe obstruction reduced sodium and calcium reabsorption. They concluded that fetal urinary chemistries were reasonably predictive of severe but not moderate postnatal renal impairment. Other investigators have suggested the use of fetal urinary β_2-microglobulin as an indicator of tubular damage. Using this parameter, poor renal outcome has been predicted with a specificity of 83% and sensitivity of 80% (26).

The time of onset of oligohydramnios has been shown to be an important determinant of outcome by Mandell et al. (27). In fetuses in which adequate amniotic fluid was documented at up to 30 weeks' gestation in association with a urologic abnormality, pulmonary outcomes were satisfactory, and postnatal clinical problems were related to renal disease. It seems inappropriate to recommend late urinary tract decompression from a pulmonary or renal basis. It is unclear whether early delivery, to permit earlier postnatal urinary decompression, is beneficial.

CLINICAL EXPERIENCE WITH INTERVENTION FOR PRENATAL HYDRONEPHROSIS

The ability to diagnose severe prenatal hydronephrosis and knowledge of its outcomes has led to our desire to treat it. In 1982, Harrison et al. described the initial report of fetal surgery in a 21-week-old fetus with bilateral hydroureteronephrosis due to PUV (28). More interventions followed. After the 1986 report of the International Fetal Surgery Registry (29) in which outcomes did not seem to justify risk, a de facto moratorium on *in utero* urinary tract shunting evolved. More recently, with improved technology and renewed interest in fetal shunting, most cases have been referred to a small number of highly specialized centers actively engaged in prenatal surgery. The initial method of decompression with open surgery has largely been replaced by *in utero* shunt

TABLE 4.2. PRENATAL ASSESSMENT OF RENAL FUNCTIONAL PROGNOSIS

	Good		Poor	
Amniotic fluid	Normal to moderately decreased		Moderate to severely decreased	
Sonographic appearance of kidneys	Normal to echogenic		Echogenic to cystic	
Fetal urine	**Glick et al. (21)**	**Johnson et al. (24)**	**Glick et al. (21)**	**Johnson et al. (24)**
Sodium (mEq/L)	<100	<100	>100	>100
Chloride (mEq/L)	<90	—	>90	—
Osmolarity (mOsm/L)	<210	<200	>210	>200
Calcium (mg/dL)	—	<8	—	>8
β_2-Microglobulin (mg/L)	—	<4	—	>4
Total protein (mg/dL)	—	<20	—	>20
Output (mL/h)	>2	—	<2	—
Sequential improvement in urinary values	—	X	—	—

X, only in this series was the criterion used.

placement, although this has been complicated by technical problems of shunt dislodgement and, in the case of the double-J shunt, bowel herniation (30). Some investigators have explored the use of fetoscopic methods for direct intervention to provide prolonged bladder drainage (31–33), whereas others have attempted direct endoscopic valve ablation (34).

Harrison et al. have clearly outlined the indications and contraindications of intervention for prenatal obstructive uropathy (Table 4.3). (35) The principal reason for considering vesicoamniotic shunting is to prevent early neonatal pulmonary insufficiency and death. The risks that one accepts with intervention include induction of premature labor, perforation of fetal bowel and bladder, as well as hemorrhage and infection in the fetus and mother.

The need to consider *in utero* intervention for obstruction is rare. In a recent study, only 9 of 177 fetuses with a diagnosis of hydronephrosis were considered to have PUV, and only 3 warranted serious consideration of intervention (11).

The results of prenatal intervention for fetal hydronephrosis between 1982 and 1985 were reported by the International Fetal Surgery Registry (29). The largest group of fetuses that were treated had an indeterminate cause of their prenatal hydronephrosis (45%). Among those fetuses with a clear etiology of their hydronephrosis, PUV was the leading cause (29%). Surgical intervention in these cases led to a survival rate of 76%. Among the several reports of outcomes with fetal intervention for obstructive uropathy, true benefit is difficult to assess. This is due to variability in diagnosis, length of follow-up, and documentation of postnatal care. A compilation of these reports is shown in Figure 4.7. These data demonstrate improvement in survival and reduction in renal failure in patients with both good and poor prognostic features (36–38). Longer follow-up periods have demonstrated a high incidence of later renal failure and growth retardation (39). No direct, prospective trial of prenatal intervention for fetal hydronephrosis has been performed.

More recently, the ability to influence renal outcome in male patients with PUV but without oligohydramnios has been suggested as a possible indication for *in utero* intervention. The principal goal of intervention is not to prevent pulmonary hypoplasia and deaths but to prevent or delay end-stage renal failure. Although some reports have shown the ability to distinguish those fetuses with likely early renal failure from those with later-onset failure (40,41), the specificity and accuracy of methods using a combination of ultrasound and urinary chemistries (sodium, β_2-microglobulin, and calcium) has not been well defined. In summary, precise identification of those situations in which intervention may benefit the fetus with obstructive uropathy remains unclear.

POSTNATAL MANAGEMENT OF INFANT WITH PRENATALLY DIAGNOSED HYDRONEPHROSIS

A child with a prenatal diagnosis of hydronephrosis should be carefully evaluated and followed by a pediatric

TABLE 4.3. PRENATAL INTERVENTION FOR HYDRONEPHROSIS

Indications (prerequisites)	Contraindications
Presumed obstructive hydronephrosis, persistent or progressive, bilateral or in solitary unit	Unilateral hydronephrosis with an adequately functioning contralateral kidney
Otherwise healthy fetus	Chromosomal abnormalities or presence of associated severe anomalies
Oligohydramnios	Bilateral hydronephrosis without oligohydramnios
No overt renal dysplasia	Severely dysplastic kidneys
Adequate renal functional potential based on urinary indices (see text)	Evidence of urethral atresia
Informed consent	Presence of a normal twin

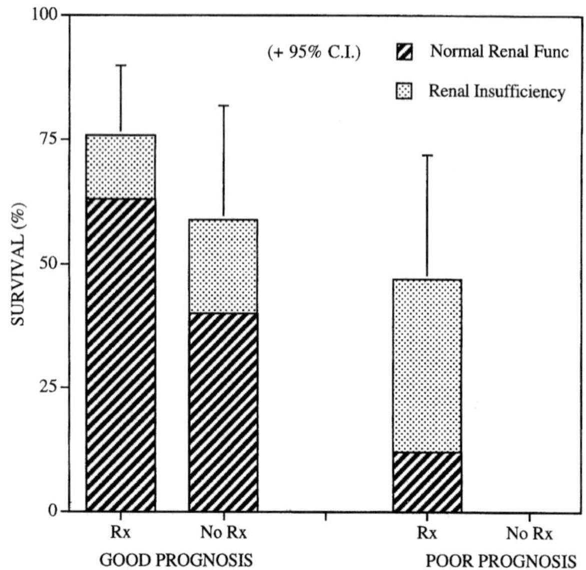

FIGURE 4.7. Survival and renal function in fetal interventions for bladder outlet obstruction comparing treated and untreated fetuses with good and poor prognostic indices. C.I., confidence interval; Rx, treatment. [Data from Crombleholme TM, Harrison MR, Golbus MS, et al. Fetal intervention in obstructive uropathy: prognostic indicators and efficacy of intervention. *Am J Obstet Gynecol* 1990;162:1239–1244; Johnson MP, Bukowski TP, Reitleman C, et al. In utero surgical treatment of fetal obstructive uropathy: a new comprehensive approach to identify appropriate candidates for vesicoamniotic shunt therapy. *Am J Obstet Gynecol* 1994;170(6):1770–1776; discussion 1776–1779; and Coplen DE, Hare JY, Zderic SA, et al. 10-year experience with prenatal intervention for hydronephrosis. *J Urol* 1996;156(3):1142–1145.]

urologist from birth. The vast majority of these children (with unilateral hydronephrosis and a contralateral normal kidney) appear entirely healthy and, in the absence of prenatal ultrasound findings, would not have any indications for regular urologic follow-up. Parental anxiety is common and should be addressed directly with prenatal counseling and education. The presence of unilateral dilation of the kidney warrants postnatal evaluation in a timely but nonurgent fashion (3 to 8 weeks of life) with an ultrasound (42). Early ultrasound is unlikely to miss a significant abnormality, but a normal result adds confusion as to the need for further evaluation (43). The precise indications for antibiotic prophylaxis (amoxicillin, 10 mg/kg/day or 50 mg/day) are unclear. A reasonable rule of thumb is that if a voiding cystourethrogram is requested, prophylactic antibiotics should be used. There are no outcomes-based assessments of follow-up protocols for children with mild to moderate dilation. An approach that seems reasonable and safe is to recommend functional imaging (diuretic renography or intravenous pyelography if there is calyceal dilation followed by serial ultrasonography. Serial ultrasonography with some plan for extending the interval between imaging studies seems reasonable but unproven.

For the child with bilateral hydroureteronephrosis suggestive of bladder outlet obstruction, an ultrasound and voiding cystourethrogram should be performed promptly. In boys, PUV is the most important diagnosis to be ruled out. In girls, an obstructing ectopic ureterocele would be the most likely cause for bladder outlet obstruction. In the event that an obstructive lesion is discovered, it should be corrected promptly. If high-grade reflux is noted, antibiotic prophylaxis with appropriate radiologic follow-up is indicated.

The timing of postnatal cystography in the setting of prenatally detected unilateral hydronephrosis remains controversial. Although some groups advocate postnatal cystography in any child with a history of prenatal hydronephrosis, others have questioned the value of this approach (44). A practical threshold for performing cystography used in many programs has been the presence of caliectasis, a dilated ureter, or variable hydronephrosis.

In a neonate with prenatally detected hydronephrosis, the importance of diagnosing vesicoureteral reflux remains controversial. Several studies have demonstrated that a high incidence of reflux is a major factor contributing to prenatally detected hydronephrosis, although its clinical significance is unclear. In several studies, the incidence of reflux is approximately 20 to 30% in all grades of hydronephrosis (45–50). The grade of hydronephrosis does not predict the likelihood or grade of reflux, and the absence of hydronephrosis does not rule out high-grade reflux. As with hydronephrosis in the neonatal period, reflux (and particularly high-grade reflux) occurs more commonly in boys. The natural history is less well defined, with some series demonstrating rapid resolution of higher grades of reflux (48,51). When neonates with grades 4 and 5 and higher reflux are studied with dimercaptosuccinic acid (scintigraphy) renal scanning, renal abnormalities are detected in up to 50% of children with no history of infection (49,52–54). This challenges current dogma that renal injury associated with reflux is only due to infection. It may be argued that the observed renal abnormalities are dysplastic and will not progress postnatally, yet this remains unproven. The relationship of bladder function to neonatal reflux is currently being defined and may be of critical importance, particularly in boys. Significant bladder instability has been documented in infants with high-grade reflux (55–57), and for this reason, managing bladder dysfunction is appropriate.

URETEROPELVIC JUNCTION OBSTRUCTION

Perhaps the most challenging aspect of managing prenatal hydronephrosis is determining when postnatal surgical correction for obstruction is appropriate. Despite the improved anatomic detail afforded by real-time ultrasound and the

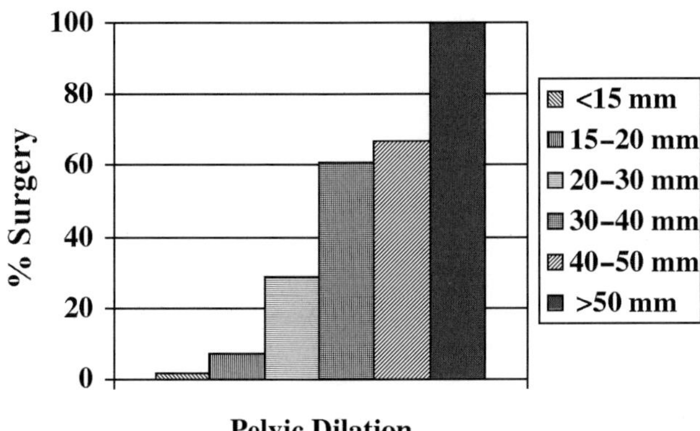

FIGURE 4.8. Renal pelvic dilation and occurrence of surgical intervention (based on declining function, increasing hydronephrosis, or symptoms). [Adapted from Dhillon HK. Prenatally diagnosed hydronephrosis: the Great Ormond Street experience. *Br J Urol* 1998;81(Suppl 2):39–44.]

increasing experience with functional nuclear medicine studies (mercaptotriglycylglycine) (see Chapter 25), no gold standard for physiologically significant obstruction exists. Over time, some kidneys have been seen to improve, whereas others appear to lose function. The natural history of prenatal hydronephrosis remains to be clearly defined.

The debate over the appropriate management of infants with prenatally detected unilateral hydronephrosis remains unsettled and will ultimately be determined by three key factors. It will be necessary to define the degree of hydronephrosis in a reproducible way to correlate initial presentation with outcome. Next, the natural history of various degrees of hydronephrosis must be defined in current clinical terms, as well as using novel means of marking the progression of renal function or response to the hydronephrotic condition. Finally, clinically useful indicators of the state of the developing kidney in the hydronephrotic state need to be defined to permit identification of "at risk" patients.

At present, it is commonly considered that a unilaterally hydronephrotic kidney with significantly reduced relative uptake on a renogram (i.e., less than 30%) should be considered for surgical repair. The group of kidneys with uptake from 30 to 40% are controversial: The London group recommends surgical repair based on a high incidence of later functional loss (58), whereas Koff and colleagues observe these patients with frequent diuretic renograms (59,60). Indeed, Koff has recommended scans as frequently as every 2 weeks for those with significantly reduced uptake. In kidneys with less than 10 to 15% uptake on renogram, it is questionable whether any attempt to salvage renal function is appropriate. The greatest difficulty lies in those patients with a unilateral kidney having severe dilation and normal uptake (i.e., greater than 45%). Some are found to have uptakes greater than 50%, which is as yet unexplained (61). The most predictive clinical parameter identified to date is the degree of renal pelvic dilation (A-P diameter). Dhillon et al. have shown that with increasing A-P diameter, there is a progressive risk of decrease in relative renal function or development of symptoms (Fig. 4.8) (62). These are minimal risks if the A-P diameter is less than 20 mm, whereas in those with dilation greater than 50 mm, it is almost 100%. It remains unknown if this relationship is time dependent and whether the risk of deterioration will increase at lesser degrees of dilation with increasing time. The few reports of prospective assessments of the risk of renal injury (functional deterioration, infection, or symptoms) are listed in Table 4.4 and indicate a 20 to 25% likelihood of patients with unilateral, significant UPJO warranting pyeloplasty by objective criteria. In most cases, functional loss was corrected by surgical intervention. A retrospective study by Chertin et al., however, observed that the functional status of comparable kidneys was better if the children had undergone earlier rather than delayed pyeloplasty (63).

Other indicators of potential deterioration have been proposed. Koff attempted using contralateral renal growth as an indirect indicator of ipsilateral obstructive injury, but this has not proved to be clinically useful (64). Urinary markers, including *N*-acetyl-β-D-glucosaminidase (65) and transforming growth factor-β1 (66), have been explored in limited series with suggestive but as yet clinically unproven predictive value. All of these markers have suggested that affected kidneys are not normal, but few data have been rigorously correlated with functional outcomes.

TABLE 4.4. REPORTS OF NONOPERATIVE MANAGEMENT OF UNILATERAL URETEROPELVIC JUNCTION OBSTRUCTION

Author (reference)	No. of patients	Study type	Crossover to pyeloplasty (%)
Ransley et al. (58)	100	Prospective, single arm	23
Cartwright et al. (68)	41	Prospective, single arm	15
Palmer et al. (69)	16	Prospective, double arm, randomized	25
Ulman et al. (60)	104	Prospective, single arm	22

From a practical standpoint, the clinician must balance possible spontaneous resolution of hydronephrosis without impairment of renal development with losing the opportunity to maximize potential renal function through surgical intervention. As in all of pediatric practice, the emphasis should remain on permitting maximal childhood growth and development while minimizing medical intrusion (67). Our current approach is to consider surgical repair in the setting of impaired relative renal function (i.e., less than 40%), marked or increasing dilation, decreasing function on serial radionuclide imaging, or the development of symptoms. Also critical is parental preference, with many parents remaining uncomfortable with a "watchful waiting" approach. Early counseling by all members of the pediatric healthcare delivery team can help avoid confusion and allay anxiety.

ACKNOWLEDGMENT

The authors acknowledge the assistance of Beryl Benacerraf, M.D., for providing many of the fetal ultrasound images.

REFERENCES

1. Helin I, Persson PH. Prenatal diagnosis of urinary tract abnormalities by ultrasound. *Pediatrics* 1986;78(5):879–883.
2. Livera LN, Brookfield DS, Egginton JA, et al. Antenatal ultrasonography to detect fetal renal abnormalities: a prospective screening programme. *BMJ* 1989;298(6685):1421–1423.
3. Scott JE, Renwick M. Urological anomalies in the Northern Region Fetal Abnormality Survey. *Arch Dis Child* 1993;68:22–26.
4. Scott JE, Wright B, Wilson G, et al. Measuring the fetal kidney with ultrasonography. *Br J Urol* 1995;76(6):769–774.
5. Scott JE, Renwick M. Screening for fetal urological abnormalities: how effective? *BJU Int* 1999;84(6):693–700.
6. Hobbins JC, Romero R, Grannum P, et al. Antenatal diagnosis of renal anomalies with ultrasound. I. Obstructive uropathy. *Am J Obstet Gynecol* 1984;148(7):868–877.
7. Abbott JF, Levine D, Wapner R. Posterior urethral valves: inaccuracy of prenatal diagnosis. *Fetal Diagn Ther* 1998;13(3):179–183.
8. Kaefer M, Peters CA, Retik AB, et al. Increased renal echogenicity: a sonographic sign for differentiating between obstructive and nonobstructive etiologies of in utero bladder distension. *J Urol* 1997;158(3 Pt 2):1026–1029.
9. Kent A, Cox D, Downey P, et al. A study of mild fetal pyelectasia—outcome and proposed strategy of management. *Prenat Diagn* 2000;20(3):206–209.
10. Grignon A, Filion R, Filiatrault D, et al. Urinary tract dilatation in utero: classification and clinical applications. *Radiology* 1986;160(3):645–647.
11. Mandell J, Blyth BR, Peters CA, et al. Structural genitourinary defects detected in utero. *Radiology* 1991;178(1):193–196.
12. Kleiner B, Callen PW, Filly RA. Sonographic analysis of the fetus with ureteropelvic junction obstruction. *AJR Am J Roentgenol* 1987;148(2):359–363.
13. Mandell J, Paltiel HJ, Peters CA, et al. Prenatal findings associated with a unilateral nonfunctioning or absent kidney. *J Urol* 1994;152:176–178.
14. Estroff JA, Mandell J, Benacerraf BR. Increased renal parenchymal echogenicity in the fetus: importance and clinical outcome. *Radiology* 1991;181(1):135–139.
15. Vergani P, Ceruti P, Locatelli A, et al. Accuracy of prenatal ultrasonographic diagnosis of duplex renal system. *J Ultrasound Med* 1999;18(7):463–467.
16. Zerin JM, Ritchey ML, Chang AC. Incidental vesicoureteral reflux in neonates with antenatally detected hydronephrosis and other renal abnormalities [see comments]. *Radiology* 1993;187(1):157–160.
17. Tibballs JM, DeBruyn R. Primary vesicoureteric reflux-how useful is postnatal ultrasound? *Arch Dis Child* 1996;75:444–447.
18. Peters CA. Lower urinary tract obstruction: clinical and experimental aspects. *Br J Urol* 1998;81(Suppl 2):22–32.
19. Kaefer M, Barnewolt C, Retik AB, et al. The sonographic diagnosis of infravesical obstruction in children: evaluation of bladder wall thickness indexed to bladder filling [see comments]. *J Urol* 1997;157(3):989–991.
20. Oliveira EA, Diniz JS, Cabral AC, et al. Predictive factors of fetal urethral obstruction: a multivariate analysis. *Fetal Diagn Ther* 2000;15(3):180–186.
21. Glick PL, Harrison MR, Golbus MS, et al. Management of the fetus with congenital hydronephrosis II: prognostic criteria and selection for treatment. *J Pediatr Surg* 1985;20(4):376–387.
22. Elder JS, OGrady JP, Ashmead G, et al. Evaluation of fetal renal function: unreliability of fetal urinary electrolytes. *J Urol* 1990;144:574.
23. Wilkins IA, Chitkara U, Lynch L, et al. The nonpredictive value of fetal urinary electrolytes: preliminary report of outcomes and correlations with pathologic diagnosis. *Am J Obstet Gynecol* 1987;157(3):694–698.
24. Johnson MP, Corsi P, Bradfield W, et al. Sequential urinalysis improves evaluation of fetal renal function in obstructive uropathy [see comments]. *Am J Obstet Gynecol* 1995;173(1):59–65.
25. Guez S, Assael BM, Melzi ML, et al. Shortcomings in predicting postnatal renal function using prenatal urine biochemistry in fetuses with congenital hydronephrosis. *J Pediatr Surg* 1996;31(10):1401–1404.
26. Tassis BMG, Trespidi L, Tirelli AS, et al. In fetuses with isolated hydronephrosis, urinary β_2-microglobulin and N-acetyl-β-D-glucosaminidase (NAG) have a limited role in prediction of postnatal renal function. *Prenat Diagn* 1996;16:1087–1093.
27. Mandell J, Peters CA, Estroff JA, et al. Late onset severe oligohydramnios associated with genitourinary abnormalities. *J Urol* 1992;148:515–518.
28. Harrison MR, Nakayama DK, Noall RA, et al. Correction of congenital hydronephrosis in utero II. Decompression reverses the effects of obstruction on the fetal lung and urinary tract. *J Pediatr Surg* 1982;17:965.
29. Manning FA, Harrison MR, Rodeck C. Catheter shunts for fetal hydronephrosis and hydrocephalus. Report of the Interna-

tional Fetal Surgery Registry. *N Engl J Med* 1986;315(5):336–340.
30. Robichaux AI, Mandell J, Greene M, et al. Fetal abdominal wall defect: a new complication of vesicoamniotic shunting. *Fetal Diagn Ther* 1991;6:11–13.
31. Estes JM, MacGillivray TE, Hedrick MH, et al. Fetoscopic surgery for the treatment of congenital anomalies. *J Pediatr Surg* 1992;27(8):950–954.
32. Luks FI, Deprest JA, Vandenberghe K, et al. A model for fetal surgery through intrauterine endoscopy. *J Pediatr Surg* 1994;29(8):1007–1009.
33. Kohl T, Szabo Z, Suda K, et al. Percutaneous fetal access and uterine closure for fetoscopic surgery. Lessons learned from 16 consecutive procedures in pregnant sheep. *Surg Endosc* 1997;11(8):819–824.
34. Quintero RA, Shukla AR, Homsy YL, et al. Successful in utero endoscopic ablation of posterior urethral valves: a new dimension in fetal urology. *Urology* 2000;55(5):774.
35. Harrison MR, Golbus MS, Filly RA, et al. Fetal hydronephrosis: selection and surgical repair. *J Pediatr Surg* 1987;22(6): 556–558.
36. Crombleholme TM, Harrison MR, Golbus MS, et al. Fetal intervention in obstructive uropathy: prognostic indicators and efficacy of intervention. *Am J Obstet Gynecol* 1990;162: 1239–1244.
37. Freedman AL, Bukowski TP, Smith CA, et al. Fetal therapy for obstructive uropathy: diagnosis specific outcomes. *J Urol* 1996;156(2 Pt 2):720–723; discussion 723–724.
38. Johnson MP, Bukowski TP, Reitleman C, et al. In utero surgical treatment of fetal obstructive uropathy: a new comprehensive approach to identify appropriate candidates for vesicoamniotic shunt therapy. *Am J Obstet Gynecol* 1994;170(6):1770–1776; discussion 1776–1779.
39. Holmes N, Harrison MR, Baskin LS. Fetal surgery for posterior urethral valves: long-term postnatal outcomes. *Pediatrics* 2001;108(1):E7.
40. Mandelbrot L, Dumez Y, Muller F, et al. Prenatal prediction of renal function in fetal obstructive uropathies. *J Perinat Med* 1991;1:283–287.
41. Muller F, Dommergues M, Mandelbrot L, et al. Fetal urinary biochemistry predicts postnatal renal function in children with bilateral obstructive uropathies. *Obstet Gynecol* 1993;82(5):813–820.
42. Clautice-Engle T, Anderson NG, Allan RB, et al. Diagnosis of obstructive hydronephrosis in infants: comparison sonograms performed 6 days and 6 weeks after birth. *AJR Am J Roentgenol* 1995;164:963–967.
43. Docimo SG, Silver RI. Renal ultrasonography in newborns with prenatally detected hydronephrosis: why wait? *J Urol* 1997;157(4):1387–1389.
44. Yerkes EB, Adams MC, Pope JCT, et al. Does every patient with prenatal hydronephrosis need voiding cystourethrography? *J Urol* 1999;162(3 Pt 2):1218–1220.
45. Scott JE. Fetal ureteric reflux. *Br J Urol* 1987;59(4):291–296.
46. Anderson PA, Rickwood AM. Features of primary vesicoureteric reflux detected by prenatal sonography. *Br J Urol* 1991;67(3):267–271.
47. Paltiel HJ, Lebowitz RL. Neonatal hydronephrosis due to primary vesicoureteral reflux: trends in diagnosis and treatment. *Radiology* 1989;170:787–789.
48. Elder JS. Commentary: importance of antenatal diagnosis of vesicoureteral reflux. *J Urol* 1992;148(5 Pt 2): 1750–1754.
49. Burge DM, Griffiths MD, Malone PS, et al. Fetal vesicoureteral reflux: outcome following conservative postnatal management. *J Urol* 1992;148(5 Pt 2):1743–1745.
50. Marra G, Barbieri G, Moioli C, et al. Mild fetal hydronephrosis indicating vesicoureteric reflux. *Arch Dis Child Fetal Neonatal Ed* 1994;70(2):F147–F149; discussion 149–150.
51. Farhat W, McLorie G, Geary D, et al. The natural history of neonatal vesicoureteral reflux associated with antenatal hydronephrosis. *J Urol* 2000;164(3 Pt 2): 1057–1060.
52. Marra G, Barbieri G, Dell'Agnola CA, et al. Congenital renal damage associated with primary vesicoureteral reflux detected prenatally in male infants. *J Pediatr* 1994;124: 726–730.
53. Bouachrine H, Lemelle F, Didier F, et al. A follow-up study of pre-natally detected primary vesicoureteric reflux: a review of 61 patients. *Br J Urol* 1996;78:936–939.
54. Nguyen HT, Bauer SB, Peters CA, et al. 99m technetium dimercapto-succinic acid renal scintigraphy abnormalities in infants with sterile high grade vesicoureteral reflux. *J Urol* 2000;164(5):1674–1679.
55. Sillen U, Hjalmas K, Aili M, et al. Pronounced detrusor hypercontractility in infants with gross bilateral reflux. *J Urol* 1992;148(2 Pt 2):598–599.
56. Sillen U, Bachelard M, Hermanson G, et al. Gross bilateral reflux in infants: gradual decrease of initial detrusor hypercontractility. *J Urol* 1996;155(2):668–672.
57. Yeung CK, Godley ML, Dhillon HK, et al. The characteristics of primary vesico-ureteric reflux in male and female infants with pre-natal hydronephrosis. *Br J Urol* 1997;80 (2):319–327.
58. Ransley PG, Dhillon HK, Gordon I, et al. The postnatal management of hydronephrosis diagnosed by prenatal ultrasound. *J Urol* 1990;144:584–587.
59. Koff SA, Campbell KD. The nonoperative management of unilateral neonatal hydronephrosis: natural history of poorly functioning kidneys. *J Urol* 1994;152(2 Pt 2): 593–595.
60. Ulman I, Jayanthi VR, Koff SA. The long-term followup of newborns with severe unilateral hydronephrosis initially treated nonoperatively. *J Urol* 2000;164(3 Pt 2): 1101–1105.
61. Oh SJ, Moon DH, Kang W, et al. Supranormal differential renal function is real but may be pathological: assessment by 99m technetium mercaptoacetyltriglycine renal scan of congenital unilateral hydronephrosis. *J Urol* 2001;165(6 Pt 2):2300–2304.
62. Dhillon HK. Prenatally diagnosed hydronephrosis: the Great Ormond Street experience. *Br J Urol* 1998;81(Suppl 2):39–44.
63. Chertin B, Fridmans A, Knizhnik M, et al. Does early detection of ureteropelvic junction obstruction improve surgical outcome in terms of renal function? *J Urol* 1999;162(3 Pt 2):1037–1040.
64. Koff SA, Peller PA, Young DC, et al. The assessment of obstruction in the newborn with unilateral hydronephrosis

by measuring the size of the opposite kidney. *J Urol* 1994; 152(2 Pt 2):596–599.
65. Carr MC, Peters CA, Retik AB, et al. Urinary levels of the renal tubular enzyme NAG in unilateral obstructive uropathy. *J Urol* 1993;151:442–445.
66. Furness PD 3rd, Maizels M, Han SW, et al. Elevated bladder urine concentration of transforming growth factor-beta1 correlates with upper urinary tract obstruction in children. *J Urol* 1999;162(3 Pt 2):1033–1036.
67. Peters CA. Urinary obstruction in children. *J Urol* 1995; 154:1874–1884.
68. Cartwright PC, Duckett JW, Keating MA, et al. Managing apparent ureteropelvic junction obstruction in the newborn. *J Urol* 1992;148(4):1224–1228.
69. Palmer LS, Maizels M, Cartwright PC, et al. Surgery versus observation for managing obstructive grade 3 to 4 unilateral hydronephrosis: a report from the Society for Fetal Urology. *J Urol* 1998;159(1):222–228.

5

RENAL DYSPLASIA/HYPOPLASIA

PAUL R. GOODYER

During normal kidney development, interactions between the branching ureteric bud and the metanephric mesenchyme generate the nephrons of each kidney. Nephrons eventually hang like apples, each on its own branch of the arborized collecting system. At birth, this crop of nephrons constitutes the individual's nephron endowment for life and ranges widely among normal humans from 0.3 to 1.1 million nephrons per kidney (1). "Normal" children at the low end of this nephron endowment spectrum are thought to be at increased risk for hypertension and renal insufficiency after an acquired renal insult later in life; suboptimal nephron number may also influence longevity of renal allografts (2–4). On occasion, renal hypoplasia may be more extreme. In one antenatal ultrasound screening study, it was estimated that approximately 1 in 400 neonates are born with at least one hypoplastic kidney (5). When renal hypoplasia is bilateral, nephron number may be insufficient for normal extrauterine life. As somatic growth outstrips nephron endowment, these children develop progressive renal insufficiency, generating approximately 20% of the pediatric end-stage renal disease population (6).

In this chapter, those clinical settings in which primary nephron number is suboptimal from birth are considered. In some, nephron number may be reduced even though the structure and function of nephrons is normal (pure renal hypoplasia). More often, renal hypoplasia is associated with histopathologic evidence of aberrant developmental fates of the metanephric mesenchyme and profound disturbances of the normal patterning of renal tissue (renal dysplasia). As suggested by Pohl et al., current approaches to classification of human kidney hypoplasia/dysplasia must integrate recent advances in the understanding of nephrogenesis with clinicopathologic observations (7). Because the former field is so rapidly evolving, any classification system should be considered a work in progress. In this chapter, primary renal agenesis and pure renal hypoplasia are considered in the context of key molecules that are either essential for initial steps in renal development or which optimize the rate of branching nephrogenesis. Then, renal dysplasia, which is often linked to aberrant outgrowth of the primary ureteric bud and/or disturbed interactions of bud with metanephric mesenchyme, is described. Although syndromes involving marked renal dysplasia are categorized in Chapter 6, examples of renal dysplasia and the evidence that obstruction of the fetal urinary tract can disturb mesenchymal cell fate during kidney development are considered in this chapter. Abnormalities of kidney position and macroscopic patterning, particularly multicystic/dysplastic kidneys (MCKDs), are reviewed in regard to failure of mechanisms normally involved in the terminal differentiation of renal epithelia.

RENAL AGENESIS

Bilateral Renal Agenesis

Bilateral failure of primary nephrogenesis during fetal life causes a characteristic pattern of facial compression and pulmonary hypoplasia (Potter syndrome) due to the absence of amniotic fluid. When severe, oligohydramnios is evident clinically or by ultrasonography in the second trimester (21 to 23 weeks), and should raise major concern about the postnatal viability of the infant (8). High-resolution color Doppler ultrasonography is helpful in detecting the fetal renal arteries and distinguishing renal hypoplasia from renal agenesis (9). Complete absence of renal parenchyma (renal agenesis) and amniotic fluid predicts severe pulmonary hypoplasia, often resulting in pneumothorax and/or inability to oxygenate in the newborn period. In those who initially survive, the decision about whether to embark on chronic peritoneal dialysis is usually based on whether: (a) lung development is sufficient to allow oxygenation without respiratory support beyond the perinatal period; (b) there is any functional renal parenchyma [identifiable by mercaptoacetyltriglycerine (MAG-3) imaging and/or ultrasonography]; (c) urine volume is sufficient to permit minimal long-term oral nutrition (100 kcal/kg/day); and (d) family and institutional resources can sustain dialytic therapy long enough to achieve growth and development sufficient to permit successful renal transplantation.

The causes of renal agenesis in humans are not well understood, but reports of absent renal arteries during the second trimester suggest arrest of kidney development at an early stage. Study of homozygous knock-out mice has identified a number of critical developmental genes causing experimental BRA. For example, inactivation of either glial cell line–derived neurotrophic factor (a growth factor expressed in the undifferentiated mesenchyme) or c-ret (the glial cell line–derived neurotrophic factor receptor, which is expressed at the surface of ureteric bud cells) results in failure of primary outgrowth of the ureteric bud (10,11). Knock-out mice lacking key transcription factor genes, such as PAX2 or WT1, are also anephric (12,13). Presumably, homozygous mutations for any one of these genes could account for occasional sporadic cases of complete renal agenesis in humans, but this has not yet been demonstrated. Most cases of Potter syndrome are associated with obstruction of the urinary tract or severe bilateral renal hypoplasia rather than complete BRA. Antenatal ultrasonography of 4000 normal Japanese pregnancies uncovered no examples of BRA, indicating its rarity (5).

Unilateral Renal Agenesis

In a recent study of American infants, the incidence of unilateral renal agenesis (URA) was 1 per 2900 births and was more common in infants of diabetic mothers and among black mothers than in others (adjusted odds ratio of 4.98 and 2.19, respectively) (14). In a screening study of normal Japanese newborns, 52 of 4000 newborns (1.3%) had evidence of unilateral hypoplastic/dysplastic kidneys (5). During follow-up of three of these cases, the abnormal renal tissue involuted in early postnatal life so that eventually no detectable kidney was evident (5). Thus, adults with congenital absence of one kidney may be born with at least some partial, though abortive, renal tissue that regresses at an early stage. In murine models, knock-out of both copies of the c-ret gene usually results in anephric fetuses. However, a small percentage manage to achieve outgrowth of the ureteric bud and generate a small, though suboptimal, kidney on one side (10). This suggests that some cases of URA may be caused by inherited mutant genes. Occasional cases of autosomal dominant URA have been reported (15).

At birth, nephron number is suboptimal in children with URA, and the contralateral kidney is stimulated to undergo postnatal compensatory hypertrophy. In most cases, plots of renal length or volume versus body length demonstrate gradual compensatory hypertrophy of the unaffected contralateral kidney over the first 3 to 4 months postnatally, crossing percentiles established for normal populations. Failure to undergo compensatory hypertrophy usually indicates contralateral renal dysplasia and may predict progressive renal insufficiency. In addition to monitoring contralateral growth, it is important to screen for residual functional renal tissue by nuclear dimercaptosuccinic acid (DMSA) or MAG-3 scanning. The presence of severely hypoplastic/dysplastic tissue is sometimes associated with hypertension, which might require excision of the dysplastic kidney.

URA has been associated with developmental abnormalities of other tissues, particularly the ear, genital tract, and axial skeleton. Among 40 girls with URA, 4 out of 40 (10%) had an ipsilateral mild-moderate sensorineural hearing deficit and 14 (35%) had mullerian duct abnormalities (16). In a retrospective study of patients with mullerian duct abnormalities, 30% had URA (17); this association was particularly strong for girls with uterus didelphys (13 of 16 cases), uterine agenesis (two of five cases), and unicornuate uterus (two of seven cases). URA was seen in all 11 cases of obstructed uterus didelphys, ipsilateral to the side of the obstructing transverse hemivaginal septum. The incidence of genital tract anomalies in boys with URA is not precisely known, but ipsilateral cystic dysplasia or seminal vesicle cysts and bilateral absence of the vas deferens (with ipsilateral syndactyly) have all been described (18–20). In a prospective study of 202 patients with congenital vertebral abnormalities, 54 (26.7%) had at least one genitourinary abnormality detected by intravenous pyelography or ultrasonography; the most frequent being URA (16). Although the pathogenetic mechanisms are not well understood, it is evident that defective developmental pathways or genes may disturb morphogenesis of mesenchyme in the ear, genital tract, and skeleton, and it is not unreasonable to screen children with URA for these associated anomalies.

PRIMARY RENAL HYPOPLASIA

Normal mature kidneys contain approximately 617,000 glomeruli with mean glomerular size of approximately 6 μm^3 (21). In the 1970s, pediatric nephrologists recognized a familial form of oligomeganephronia in which renal hypoplasia and progressive proteinuric renal failure in childhood were associated with unusually large but otherwise normal-appearing glomeruli (22). During the same period, an autosomal dominant syndrome of renal hypoplasia associated with colobomas of the optic nerve [renal-coloboma syndrome (RCS)] was also characterized (23). In 1995, Eccles showed that RCS was caused by heterozygous mutations of the PAX2 gene and drew attention to the high frequency of vesicoureteral reflux (VUR) in affected families (24–26). When patients with oligomeganephronia were subsequently reinvestigated, these patients also proved to have heterozygous PAX2 mutations, though the optic nerve abnormality was often barely detectable (27–29). Approximately 15 different inactivating mutations of the PAX2 gene have been described, and the most common (a single base-pair insertion in the second exon of PAX2) also causes RCS in the inbred *1Neu* mouse strain (30). Studies of fetal kidney development in *1Neu* mice have led to the hypothesis that a critical function of the PAX2 gene is to prevent apoptosis of cells in the branching ureteric bud during kidney development (31,32). Absence of one PAX2 gene is sufficient to permit increased ureteric bud cell apoptosis,

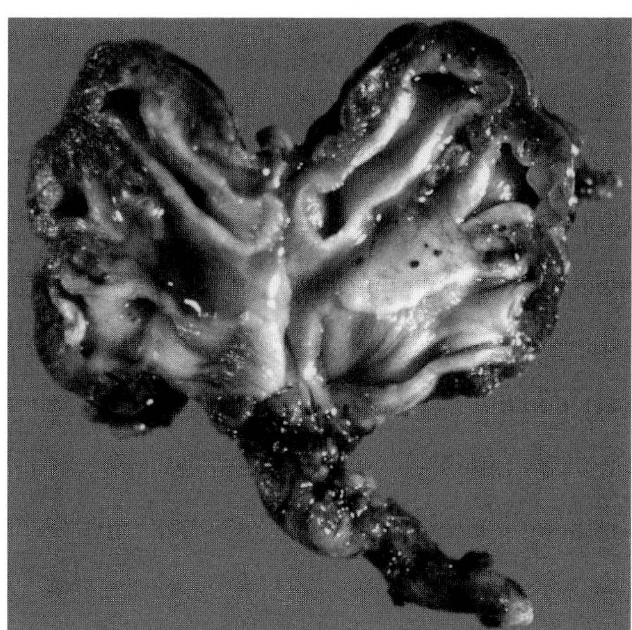

FIGURE 5.1. Hypoplastic kidney bisected to show presence of ureter and symmetric collecting system derived from initial branches of the ureteric bud. The thin outer rim of renal cortex has normal architecture, but nephron number is dramatically reduced.

compromising nephron number by slowing the rate of branching nephrogenesis. Presumably, PAX2 function also influences structure of the ureterovesical junction. In pure primary renal hypoplasia, there is little evidence of dysplasia, and glomerular hypertrophy is presumably the normal compensatory response to the deficit in nephron number (Fig. 5.1).

At least one other form of hereditary renal hypoplasia, branchiootorenal (BOR) syndrome (OMIM 113650), can be attributed to mutation of a single gene. The autosomal dominant BOR syndrome, involving variable degrees of renal hypoplasia, congenital lateral cervical fistulas or cysts, and ear abnormalities (preauricular tags or pits, a malformed auricle, atresia of the canal, anomalies of the middle ear, and hypoplasia of the cochlea or semicircular canals) is caused by mutations of the EYA1 gene (32,33). More than 20 different EYA1 mutations have been reported; end-stage renal failure may develop anywhere between 12 and 36 years of age. EYA1 is the human homolog (chromosome 18q13.3) of a small family of transcription factors originally identified in *Drosophila* because of their importance to eye development, but in humans the eye is unaffected. Within the same family, heterozygous mutations of EYA1 may cause renal defects ranging from BRA to mild unilateral hypoplasia (34). During normal renal development EYA1 is expressed in the metanephric mesenchyme, and homozygous EYA1 knock-out mice lack primary outgrowth of the ureteric bud with subsequent failure of nephron induction (35).

The otic defects in BOR syndrome can usually be delineated by computed axial tomography, but nuclear magnetic resonance imaging may be useful in diagnosis (36). It has been argued that renal defects are not common enough in children with external ear anomalies alone to warrant routine renal ultrasonography (37). On the other hand, several other syndromes involve renal anomalies and external ear deformities (38). Although renal hypoplasia can be quite variable in BOR, branchial arch defects with normal kidneys (BO syndrome) probably result from mutations of a different gene on chromosome 1q31 (39).

In the 1940s and 1950s, Wilson reported that severe vitamin A (retinol) deficiency caused renal agenesis (40,41). More recent observations indicate that even modest maternal retinol deficiency (50% reduction in circulating levels of retinol) can cause significant renal hypoplasia in rodents. In such studies, postnatal kidney weight is decreased by 24%, and nephron number is reduced by 20% (42). In these rodent studies, nephron number correlated with kidney size and varied directly with circulating retinol concentration. Normally, the fetus acquires retinol from the maternal circulation and converts it to an active metabolite, all-*trans*-retinoic acid, in the kidney and other peripheral tissues (43). In fetal rat kidneys cultured *ex vivo*, all-*trans*-retinoic acid (0.1 to 1.0 μmol) accelerates new nephron formation by two- to threefold (44,45). Vitamin A deficiency is widespread (15 to 25% of pregnant women) in many third world regions, and in North America a small but significant fraction (1%) of pregnant women have retinol levels in the low-normal range that could effect nephron number. As yet, however, it is unknown whether human maternal vitamin A deficiency limits nephrogenesis as it does in rats.

RENAL DYSPLASIA/HYPOPLASIA AND VESICOURETERAL REFLUX

During early fetal life, the two nephric (wolffian) ducts arise in the pronephric region of the intermediate mesoderm and migrate caudally. Just before arrival at the cloaca (approximately somite 25 in the mouse), ureteric buds emerge from the nephric ducts at a site corresponding to the future vesicoureteral junction and induce the metanephric kidneys from laterally adjacent metanephric mesenchyme. In 1975, Mackie and Stephens observed (by ureteroscopy) that many children born with duplex collecting systems and/or VUR also had malpositioned ureteric orifices (46). In Japanese perinatal screening studies, renal hypoplasia (approximately 1 in 400 normal births) was strongly correlated with VUR (5). Among neonates investigated for VUR, renal hypoplasia (reduced renal length by ultrasonography and reduced DMSA uptake by scintigraphy) was frequent, being symmetric in approximately one-third of cases and involving patchy scars of the renal parenchyma in others (47,48). Thus, disturbance of the

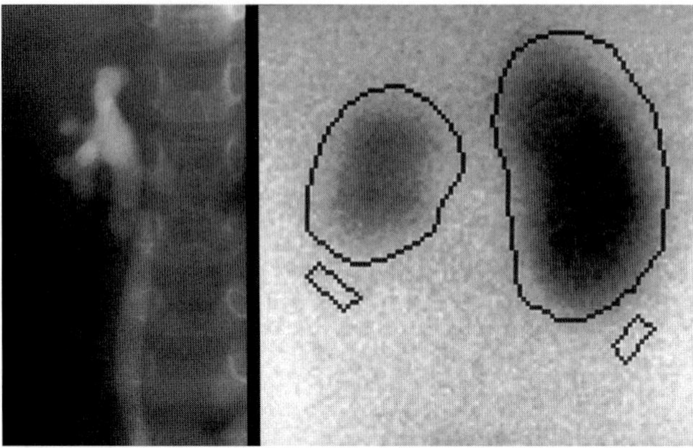

FIGURE 5.2. Renal hypoplasia associated with ipsilateral vesicoureteral reflux in a 2-year-old boy who presented with his first lower urinary tract infection. Dimercaptosuccinic acid scintigraphy demonstrates normal reniform appearance of the hypoplastic parenchyma, which contributes only approximately 10% of total renal function.

factors that regulate the proper timing or positioning of ureteric bud outgrowth appear to lead to ectopic ureteric orifices, abnormalities of ureter structure, and faulty induction of metanephric mesenchyme by the ectopic ureteric bud (Fig. 5.2). This hypothesis is supported by knock-out mouse experiments in which homozygous inactivation of a single transcription factor gene (*Foxc2*) may cause various anatomic abnormalities of the ureters associated with renal hypoplasia in approximately 60% of offspring (49). *Foxc2* is normally expressed in the metanephric mesenchyme and is thought to be involved in guiding outgrowth of the ureteric bud (49). The gross abnormalities were often unilateral (70 to 85% of offspring) and were highly dependent on the genetic background of the mice (49). To date, single gene mutations causing VUR and renal hypoplasia/dysplasia have not been identified in humans, but putative VUR loci have been reported (50).

RENAL HYPOPLASIA/DYSPLASIA AND FETAL URINARY TRACT OBSTRUCTION

Numerous observations indicate that antenatal obstruction of the urinary tract (UTO) may be associated with disturbances of normal nephrogenesis. Most commonly, renal hypoplasia/dysplasia is reported in males with posterior urethral valves but is also evident in other UTO settings such as prune-belly syndrome and urethral atresia (51–53) (Fig. 5.3). Dysplastic areas containing cysts, fibrotic interstitial zones, and even islands of cartilage may be scattered amid fairly normal-appearing renal tubules. In fetal monkeys, obstruction produced by injection of agaral beads into the collecting system at mid-gestation causes progressive diminution in renal size associated with evidence of apoptosis (particularly of collecting duct and glomerular cells), cysts with pericystic fibrotic collars, and a defect in branching of the ureteric bud (54). Thus, although the molecular mechanisms are not yet

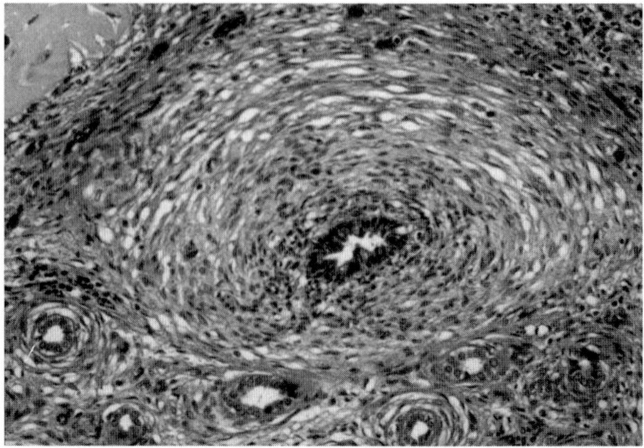

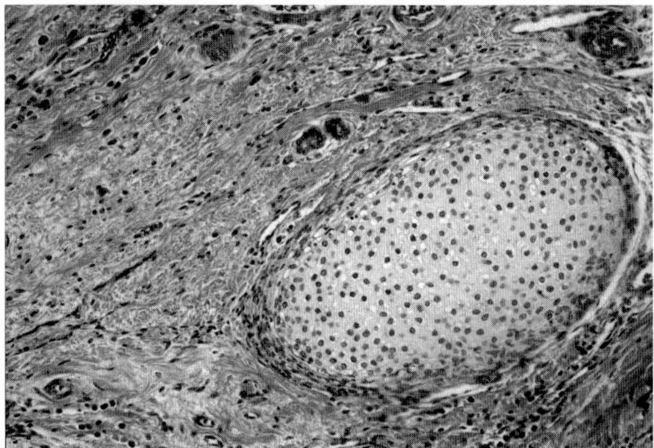

FIGURE 5.3. A: Renal dysplasia: peritubular fibrous cuff. **B:** Renal dysplasia: island of cartilage amid dysplastic tissue represents aberrant cell fate of metanephric mesenchyme.

well understood, fetal UTO appears to modify survival of selected cell lineages and affect signals regulating developmental cell fates. Timing of the fetal obstruction may be important; very early (50 days' gestation) obstruction of the urinary tract in lambs causes severe hypoplasia and interstitial fibrosis, whereas obstruction at 60 days results in a larger, cystic kidney with less fibrosis (55). In humans, striking obstruction has sometimes been reported in association with normal renal histology, prompting the speculation that UTO late in fetal life may have less effect on determinants of developmental cell fate (56).

As in other forms of renal hypoplasia/dysplasia, the risk of progressive renal insufficiency due to congenital UTO is highly influenced by the number of functioning nephrons at birth. The likelihood of developing end-stage renal disease ranges from 22 to 70% in various studies of boys with posterior urethral valves. A key predictor of long-term outcome is serum creatinine level 1 year after relief of obstruction (53,57). In 29 patients with prune-belly syndrome (deficient abdominal musculature, evidence of UTO, and cryptorchidism), approximately one-third die in the perinatal period from Potter syndrome, and most survivors develop end-stage renal disease (58,59).

SYNDROMIC RENAL HYPOPLASIA/DYSPLASIA

Renal dysplasia is associated with many different recognizable patterns of malformation, presumably involving genes or developmental pathways shared by multiple organs. Although a more complete list appears in Chapter 6, several syndromes of interest are mentioned briefly here. Mutations in the hepatocyte nuclear factor-1β gene (TCF2) are responsible for an autosomal dominant syndrome characterized by maturity-onset diabetes of the young, nondiabetic progressive nephropathy, genital malformations, and liver dysfunction (60). The hepatocyte nuclear factor-1β gene is normally expressed in the wolffian duct, metanephric tubules, and mullerian duct during fetal life; its absence results in a form of cystic renal dysplasia in which glomerular number is significantly reduced (61,62). Early-onset progressive nephropathy may be seen without evidence of diabetes mellitus in some cases, and renal dysplasia is quite variable, producing unilateral renal hypoplasia with cystic dysplasia in the contralateral kidney (62).

Renal dysplasia is also part of the autosomal dominant HDR syndrome (hypoparathyroidism, deafness, and renal anomalies) caused by mutations of another transcription factor gene, GATA3 (63) and is part of the Bardet-Biedl syndrome caused by mutations at six different loci, including the MKKS gene (64). Other monogenic syndromes with renal dysplasia include Townes-Brock syndrome (SALL1 gene) (65) and nail-patella syndrome (LMX1B gene) (66).

Variable degrees of renal dysplasia have been described in numerous syndromes for which the etiology is unknown. The causes of the VATER syndrome (*v*ertebral defects, *a*nal atresia, *t*rachio-*e*sophageal fistula, and *r*enal dysplasia) are thought to be heterogeneous but presumably identify a common developmental pathway in these tissues (67). In the VACTERL syndrome (with additional limb and cardiac defects), the majority of patients have renal dysplasia, which may be associated with vesicoureteral reflux (39%), unilateral aplasia (23%), or unilateral multicystic dysplasia (7%) (68). Similarly, renal dysplasia may be seen in association with developmental defects of the pancreas and liver (Ivemark syndrome) (69), jejunal atresia (70), and encephalocele (Meckel syndrome) (71), and with pancreatic fibrosis, liver dysgenesis, and *situs inversus* (72). In Perlman syndrome, renal dysplasia and Wilms' tumor are associated with fetal gigantism and multiple congenital anomalies (73,74).

MULTICYSTIC/DYSPLASTIC KIDNEY

Classically, MCKDs have been identified as unilateral multiloculated abdominal masses with thin-walled cysts that do not appear to connect (Fig. 5.4), distinguishing them from hydronephrotic kidneys. Nuclear scans often show no functional parenchyma, and ureters are usually atretic, indicating little or no urine formation from early fetal life. The cystic mass usually lacks a reniform shape; scanty tissue between cysts is hyperechoic, and there is usually no detectable renal artery by Doppler ultrasonography. Microscopic analysis reveals disorganized renal architecture with islands of undifferentiated mesenchymal cells, occasional bizarre differentiation (e.g., cartilage), and few if any normal-appearing nephrons. Cysts are often rimmed by collars of fibromuscular cells. The incidence of unilateral MCKD is approximately 1 in 4000 live births (75). Rarely, bilateral MCKD has been reported and is fatal in the newborn period (76).

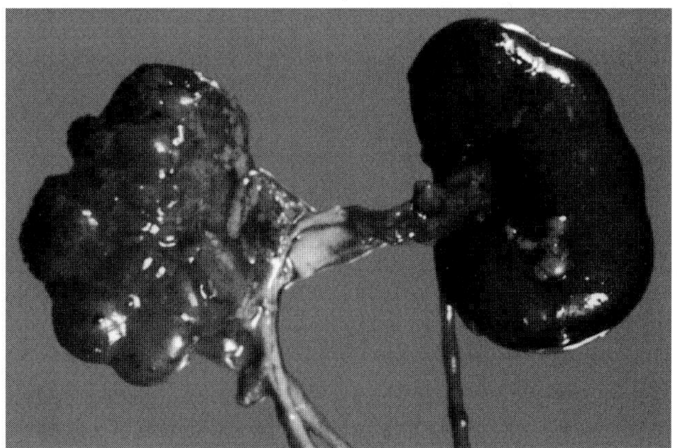

FIGURE 5.4. Nonfunctional multicystic/dysplastic right kidney and grossly normal-appearing left kidney from an infant who died in the perinatal period of nonrenal causes.

More recently, antenatal detection and long-term follow-up studies of unresected MCKDs have suggested that the pathogenesis and prognosis for this entity are more complex than was initially appreciated. In approximately 15% of unilateral cases, postnatal nuclear scans show some minimal functional renal tissue amid the dysplastic areas, so complete absence of renal function is no longer the *sine qua non* (77). Numerous cases of localized (restricted to one pole) cystic dysplasia have been reported (78,79). More important, the contralateral kidney often (20 to 30% of cases) exhibits some form of limited dysplasia (80–83). Approximately one-fourth of contralateral kidneys exhibit VUR, and this may be associated with recurrent urinary tract infections and progressive renal insufficiency (84). Careful evaluation of contralateral renal growth by serial postnatal ultrasonography, DMSA nuclear scans to detect foci of dysfunctional parenchyma, and voiding cystourethrography to identify contralateral VUR may be considered to identify cases with significant contralateral dysplasia (85).

Because experimental obstruction may produce cystic dysplasia, it has been proposed that first-trimester UTO might account for MCKD (75,86). However, the putative obstruction would have to be intrarenal as MCKD ureters are atretic, and lower tract obstruction could not explain cases of localized dysplasia. Furthermore, there are reports of autosomal dominant MCKD and chromosomal anomalies (87,88), suggesting that failure of key genes can lead to MCKD by perturbing the normal pattern of nephrogenesis. A high incidence of subtle genital and other nonrenal abnormalities suggests aberrations in shared developmental programs rather than UTO as the primary etiology (81,82).

On occasion, unilateral MCKD has been associated with hypertension; in some cases, hypertension resolves when the dysplastic tissue is resected (89). Ectopic renin gene expression has been documented in macrophage-like interstitial cells (90). Although hypertension is not commonly identified in children with unilateral MCKD (less than 5%), its prevalence may be underestimated. Subtle abnormalities of blood pressure were found in 5 of 25 such children when studied by ambulatory blood pressure monitoring (91).

It has long been appreciated that MCKDs may undergo complete or partial involution, but the significance of this observation is not yet clear (92). Involution of MCKD tissue has been observed during fetal life, and 20 to 25% of MCKDs involute completely in the first 1 to 2 years of postnatal life (93–95). When involution does not occur, the specter of rare malignant transformation is raised. Multiple cases of Wilms' tumor (approximately three- to tenfold increased incidence over the normal population) (96,97) and renal cell carcinoma (98–101) arising from within the cystic tissue have been reported. On the other hand, because Wilms' tumors grow rapidly, effective ultrasound screening would have to be done approximately every 3 months for 8 years (102); renal carcinomas may arise in adulthood. Several recent reports advise conservative management, and routine early excision of MCKDs has become much less common than in the past (102,103). However, the approach to MCKD tissue that does not involute is still made on an individual basis after discussion with the family.

ABNORMALITIES OF KIDNEY POSITION AND PATTERNING

Variations in the gross architecture of the kidney are fairly common. Nearly 1% of patients undergoing ultrasonography are found to have duplex kidneys; of these, 80% have ureteral duplication as well (104). However, there is no evidence that isolated duplication of the collecting system is associated with morbidity. Rarely, ectopic kidneys have been reported in the thorax, but these are usually nonfunctional and are identified when an unidentified chest mass is spotted incidentally (105).

Horseshoe kidneys represent the most common renal fusion abnormality and occur in every 400 to 800 individuals (106). They are unusually common (30%) in Turner syndrome (107). Horseshoe kidneys are usually detected by ultrasonography, but other imaging modalities are required to identify the anomaly in approximately one-third of cases. In one series, vesicoureteral reflux was noted in 32% and uretero-pelvic junction obstruction in 23% (108). The risk of Wilms' tumor is slightly increased in children with horseshoe kidney, and there are more than 40 reports of this association in the literature (109). However, regular screening for this complication is probably unwarranted. Although 0.5% of Wilms' tumors arise within a horseshoe kidney, this is only approximately three times the expected incidence. The arterial supply to the horseshoe kidney is highly variable, presenting a special technical challenge for transplantation. Nevertheless, horseshoe kidneys can be transplanted into recipients *en bloc* or after division of the isthmus, and the success rate is equivalent to normal cadaveric transplantation with either approach (106).

REFERENCES

1. Clark AT, Bertram JF. Molecular regulation of nephron endowment. *Am J Physiol* 1999;276:F485–F497.
2. Azuma H, Nadeau K, Mackenzie HS, et al. Nephron mass modulates the hemodynamic, cellular, and molecular response of the rat renal allograft. *Transplantation* 1997;63:519–528.
3. Mackenzie HS, Lawler EV, Brenner BM. Congenital oligonephropathy: the fetal flaw in essential hypertension? *Kidney Int* 1996;55[Suppl]:S30–S34.
4. Brenner BM, Chertow GM. Congenital oligonephropathy and the etiology of adult hypertension and progressive renal injury. *Am J Kidney Dis* 1994;23:171–175.
5. Hiraoka M, Tsukahara H, Ohshima Y, et al. Renal aplasia is the predominant cause of congenital solitary kidneys. *Kidney Int* 2002;6:1840–1844.
6. Lewy JE. Treatment of children in the U.S. with end-stage renal disease (ESRD). *Med Arh* 2001;55:201–202.
7. Pohl M, Bhatnagar V, Mendoza SA, Nigam SK. Toward an etiological classification of developmental disorder of the kidney and upper urinary tract. *Kidney Int* 2002;61:10–19.
8. Takeuchi H, Koyanagi T, Yoshizato T, et al. Fetal urine production at different ages: correlation to various compromised fetuses in utero. *Early Hum Develop* 1994;40:1–11.
9. Sepulveda W, Stagiannis KD, Flack NJ, Fisk NM. Accuracy of prenatal diagnosis of renal agenesis with color flow imaging in severe second-trimester oligohydramnios. *Am J Obstet Gynecol* 1995;173:1788–1792.
10. Schuchardt A, D'Agati V, Pachnis V, Costantini F. Renal agenesis and hypodysplasia in ret-k—mutant mice result from defects in ureteric bud development. *Development* 1996;122:1919–1929.
11. Sanchez MP, Silos-Santigo I, Frisen J, et al. Renal agenesis and the absence of enteric neurons in mice lacking GDNF. *Nature* 1996;382:70–73.
12. Torres M, Gomez-Pardo E, Dressler GR, Gruss P. PAX2 controls multiple steps of urogenital development. *Development* 1995;121:4057–4065.
13. Kreidberg JA, Sariola H, Loring JM, et al. WT1 is required for early kidney development. *Cell* 1993;74:679–691.
14. Parikh CR, McCall D, Engelman C, Schrier RW. Congenital renal agenesis: case control analysis of birth characteristics. *Am J Kidney Dis* 2002;39:689–694.

15. Doray B, Gasser B, Reinartz I, Stoll C. Hereditary renal adysplasia in a three generations family. *Genet Couns* 1999;10:251–257.
16. Rai AS, Taylor TK, Smith GH, et al. Congenital abnormalities of the urogenital tract in association with congenital vertebral malformations. *J Bone Joint Surg Br* 2002;84:891–895.
17. Li S, Qayyum A, Coakley FV, Hricak H. Association of renal agenesis and mullerian duct anomalies. *J Comput Assist Tomogr* 2000;24:829–834.
18. Cherullo EE, Meraney AM, Bernstein LH, et al. Laparoscopic management of congenital seminal vesicle cysts associated with ipsilateral renal agenesis. *J Urol* 2002;167:1263–1267.
19. Burns JA, Cooper CS, Austin JC. Cystic dysplasia of the testis associated with ipsilateral renal agenesis and contralateral crossed ectopia. *Urology* 2002;60:344.
20. McCallum T, Milunsky J, Munarriz R, et al. Unilateral renal agenesis associated with congenital bilateral absence of the vas deferens: phenotypic findings and genetic considerations. *Hum Reprod* 2001;16:282–288.
21. Nyengaard JR, Bendtsen TF. Glomerular number and size in relation to age, kidney weight, and body surface in normal man. *Anat Rec* 1992;232:194–201.
22. Carter JE, Lirenman DS. Bilateral renal hypoplasia with oligomeganephronia. Oligomeganephronic renal hypoplasia. *Am J Dis Child* 1970;120:537–542.
23. Weaver RG, Cashwell LF, Lorentz W, et al. Optic nerve coloboma associated with renal disease. *Am J Med Genet* 1988; 29:597–605.
24. Eccles MR, Schimmenti LA. Renal-coloboma syndrome: a multi-system developmental disorder caused by PAX2 mutations. *Clin Genet* 1999;56:1–9.
25. Schimmenti LA, Cunliffe HE, McNoe LA, et al. Further delineation of renal-coloboma syndrome in patients with extreme variability of phenotype and identical PAX2 mutations. *Am J Hum Genet* 1997;60:869–878.
26. Schimmenti LA, Pierpont ME, Carpenter BL, et al. Autosomal dominant optic nerve colobomas, vesicoureteral reflux, and renal anomalies. *Am J Med Genet* 1995;59:204–208.
27. Salomon R, Tellier AL, Attie-Bitach T, et al. PAX2 mutations in oligomeganephronia. *Kidney Int* 2001;59:457–462.
28. Nishimoto K, Iijima K, Shirakawa T, et al. PAX2 gene mutation in a family with isolated renal hypoplasia. *J Am Soc Nephrol* 2001;12:1769–1772.
29. Ford B, Rupps R, Lirenman D, et al. Renal-coloboma syndrome: prenatal detection and clinical spectrum in a large family. *Am J Med Genet* 2001;99:137–141.
30. Porteous S, Torban E, Cho NP, et al. Primary renal hypoplasia in humans and mice with PAX2 mutations: evidence of increased apoptosis in fetal kidneys of Pax2(1Neu) +/– mutant mice. *Hum Mol Genet* 2000;9:1–11.
31. Torban E, Eccles MR, Favor J, Goodyer PR. PAX2 suppresses apoptosis in renal collecting duct cells. *Am J Pathol* 2000;157:833–842.
32. Melnick M, Bixler D, Nance W, Silk K, Yune H. Familial branchio-oto-renal dysplasia: a new addition to the branchial arch syndromes. *Clin Genet* 1976;9:25–34.
33. Abdelhak S, Kalatzis V, Heilig R, et al. A human homologue of the *Drosophila* eyes absent gene underlies branchio-oto-renal (BOR) syndrome and identifies a novel gene family. *Nature Genet* 1997;15:157–164.
34. Frasier FC, Sproule JR, Hatal F. Frequency of the branchio-oto-renal syndrome in children with profound hearing loss. *Am J Med Genet* 1980;7:341–349.
35. Xu PX, Adams J, Peters H, et al. EYA1-deficient mice lack ears and kidneys and show abnormal apoptosis of organ primordia. *Nature Genet* 1999;23:113–117.
36. Ceruti S, Stinckens C, Cremers CW, Casselman JW. Temporal bone anomalies in the branchio-oto-renal syndrome: detailed computed tomographic and magnetic resonance imaging findings. *Otol Neurotol* 2002;23:200–207.
37. Kugelman A, Tubi A, Bader D, et al. Pre-auricular tags and pits in the newborn: the role of renal ultrasonography. *J Pediatr* 2002;141:388–391.
38. Wang RY, Earl DL, Ruder RO, Graham JM Jr. Syndromic ear anomalies and renal ultrasounds. *Pediatrics* 2001;108:E32.
39. Kumar S, Deffenbacher K, Marres HA, et al. Genomewide search and genetic localization of a second gene associated with autosomal dominant branchio-oto-renal syndrome: clinical and genetic implications. *Am J Hum Genet* 2000;66:1715–1720.
40. Wilson JG, et al. Malformations in the urinary tract induced by maternal vitamin A deficiency in the rat. *Am J Anat* 1948;83:357–407.
41. Wilson JG, et al. An analysis of the syndromes of malformations induced by maternal vitamin A deficiency. Effects of restoration of vitamin A at various times during gestation. *Am J Anat* 1953;92:189–217.
42. Lelievre-Pegorier M, Vilar J, Ferrier ML, et al. Mild vitamin A deficiency leads to inborn nephron deficit in the rat. *Kidney Int* 1998;54:1455–1462.
43. Ross SA, McCaffrey PJ, Drager UC, De Luca LM. Retinoids in embryonal development. *Physiol Rev* 2000;80:1021–1054.
44. Vilar J, Gilbert T, Moreau E, Merlet-Benichou C. Metanephros organogenesis is highly stimulated by vitamin A derivatives in organ culture. *Kidney Int* 1996;49:1478–1487.
45. Gilbert T, Merlet-Benichou C. Retinoids and nephron mass control. *Pediatr Nephrol* 2000;14:1137–1144.
46. Mackie GG, Stephens FD. Duplex kidneys: a correlation of renal dysplasia with position of the ureteral orifice. *J Urol* 1975;114:274–280.
47. Farhat W, McLorie G, Bagli D, Khoury A. Greater reliability of neonatal ultrasonography in defining renal hypoplasia with antenatal hydronephrosis and vesicoureteral reflux. *Can J Urol* 2002;9(Feb):1459–1463.
48. Stock JA, Wilson D, Hanna MK. Congenital reflux nephropathy and severe unilateral fetal reflux. *J Urol* 1998;160:1017–1018.
49. Kume T, Deng K, Hogan BLM. Murine forkhead/winged helix genes Foxc1(Mf1) and Foxc2 (Mhf1) are required for the early organogenesis of the kidney and urinary tract. *Development* 2000;127:1387–1395.
50. Feather SA, Malcolm S, Woolf AS, et al. Primary, nonsyndromic vesicoureteric reflux and its nephropathy is genetically heterogeneous, with a locus on chromosome 1. *Am J Hum Genet* 2000;66:1420–1425.
51. Haecker FM, Wehrmann M, Hacker HW, et al. Renal dysplasia in children with posterior urethral valves: a primary or secondary malformation? *Pediatr Surg Int* 2002;18:119–122.

52. Woolf AS, Thiruchelvam N. Congenital obstructive uropathy: its origin and contribution to end-stage renal disease in children. *Adv Ren Replace Ther* 2001;8:157–163.
53. Lal R, Bhatnagar V, Mitra DK. Long-term prognosis of renal function in boys treated for posterior urethral valves. *Eur J Pediatr Surg* 1999;9:307–311.
54. Matsell DG, Mok A, Tarantal AF. Altered primate glomerular development due to in utero urinary tract obstruction. *Kidney Int* 2002;61:1263–1269.
55. Kitagawa H, Pringle KC, Koike J, et al. Different phenotypes of dysplastic kidney in obstructive uropathy in fetal lambs. *J Pediatr Surg* 2001;36:1698–703.
56. Shigeta M, Nagata M, Shimoyamada H, et al. Prune-belly syndrome diagnosed at 14 weeks' gestation with severe urethral obstruction but normal kidneys. *Pediatr Nephrol* 1999; 13:135–137.
57. Roth KS, Carter WH Jr, Chan JC. Obstructive nephropathy in children: long-term progression after relief of posterior urethral valve. *Pediatrics* 2001;107:1004–1010.
58. Manivel JC, Pettinato G, Reinberg Y, et al. Prune belly syndrome: clinicopathologic study of 29 cases. *Pediatr Pathol* 1989;9:691–711.
59. Reinberg Y, Manivel JC, Pettinato G, Gonzalez R. Development of renal failure in children with the prune belly syndrome. *J Urol* 1991;145:1017–1019.
60. Lindner TH, Njolstad PR, Horikawa Y, et al. A novel syndrome of diabetes mellitus, renal dysfunction and genital malformation associated with a partial deletion of the pseudo-POU domain of hepatocyte nuclear factor-1beta. *Hum Mol Genet* 1999; 8:2001–2008.
61. Bingham C, Ellard S, Allen L, et al. Abnormal nephron development associated with a frameshift mutation in the transcription factor hepatocyte nuclear factor-1 beta. *Kidney Int* 2000;57:898–907.
62. Bingham C, Ellard S, Cole TR, et al. Solitary functioning kidney and diverse genital tract malformations associated with hepatocyte nuclear factor-1beta mutations. *Kidney Int* 2002;61:1243–1251.
63. Van Esch H, Groenen P, Nesbit MA, et al. GATA3 haplo-insufficiency causes human HDR syndrome. *Nature* 2000; 406:419–422.
64. Katsanis N, Beales PL, Woods MO, et al. Mutations in MKKS cause obesity, retinal dystrophy and renal malformations associated with Bardet-Biedl syndrome. *Nat Genet* 2000;26:67–70.
65. Kohlhase J. SALL1 mutations in Townes-Brocks syndrome and related disorders. *Hum Mutat* 2000;16(Dec):460–466.
66. Dreyer SD, Zhou G, Baldini A, et al. Mutations in LMX1B cause abnormal skeletal patterning and renal dysplasia in nail patella syndrome. *Nat Genet* 1998;19(May):47–50.
67. Quan L, Smith DW. The VATER association. Vertebral defects, anal atresia, T-E fistula with esophageal atresia, radial and renal dysplasia: a spectrum of associated defects. *J Pediatr* 1973;82:104–107.
68. Kolon TF, Gray CL, Sutherland RW, et al. Upper urinary tract manifestations of the VACTERL association. *J Urol* 2000;163:1949–1951.
69. Abbi R, Daum F, Kahn E. Ontogeny of renal dysplasia in Ivemark syndrome: light and immunohistochemical characterization. *Ann Clin Lab Sci* 1999;29(Jan-Mar):9–17.
70. Herman TE, McAlister WH. Familial type 1 jejunal atresias and renal dysplasia. *Pediatr Radiol* 1995;25:272–274.
71. Moerman P, Verbeken E, Fryns JP, et al. The Meckel Syndrome. Pathological and cytogenetic observations in eight cases. *Hum Genet* 1982;62:240–245.
72. Huang SC, Chen WJ. Renal dysplasia and situs inversus totalis: an autopsy case report and literature review. *Changgeng Yi Xue Za Zhi* 2000;23:43–47.
73. Neri G, Martini-Neri ME, Katz BE, Opitz JM. The Perlman syndrome: familial renal dysplasia with Wilms tumor, fetal gigantism and multiple congenital anomalies. *Am J Med Genet* 1984;19(Sept):195–207.
74. Schilke K, Schaefer F, Waldherr R, et al. A case of Perlman syndrome: fetal gigantism, renal dysplasia, and severe neurological deficits. *Am J Med Genet* 2000;91(Mar):29–33.
75. Winyard P, Chitty L. Dysplastic and polycystic kidneys: diagnosis, associations and management. *Prenat Diag* 2001;21: 924–925.
76. D'Alton M, Romero R, Grannum P, et al. Antenatal diagnosis of renal anomalies with ultrasound. IV. Bilateral multicystic kidney disease. *Am J Obstet Gynecol* 1986;154:532–537.
77. Roach PJ, Paltiel HJ, Perez-Atayde A, et al. Renal dysplasia in infants: appearance on 99mTc DMSA scintigraphy. *Pediatr Radiol* 1995;25:472–475.
78. Slywotzky CM, Bosniak MA. Localized cystic disease of the kidney. *AJR Am J Roentgenol* 2001;176(Apr):843–849.
79. Jeon A, Cramer BC, Walsh E, Pushpanathan C. A spectrum of segmental multicystic renal dysplasia. *Pediatr Radiol* 1999;29 (May):309–315.
80. Abidari JM, Park KH, Kennedy WA, Shortliffe LD. Serial followup of the contralateral renal size in children with multicystic dysplastic kidney. *J Urol* 2002;168:1821–1825.
81. Mathiot A, Liard A, Eurin D, Dacher JN. Prenatally detected multicystic renal dysplasia and associated anomalies of the genito-urinary tract. *J Radiol* 2002;83:731–735.
82. Feldenberg LR, Siegel NJ. Clinical course and outcome for children with multicystic dysplastic kidneys. *Pediatr Nephrol* 2000;14(Oct):1098–1101.
83. Lazebnik N, Bellinger MF, Ferguson JE 2nd, et al. Insights into the pathogenesis and natural history of fetuses with multicystic dysplastic kidney disease. *Prenat Diagn* 1999;19(May):418–423.
84. Fanos V, Sinaguglia G, Vino L, Pizzini C, Portuese A. Multicystic dysplastic kidney and contralateral vesicoureteral reflux. Renal growth. *Minerva Pediatr* 2001;53:95–98.
85. Rudnik-Schoneborn S, John U, Deget F, et al. Clinical features of unilateral multicystic renal dysplasia in children. *Eur J Pediatr* 1998;157(Aug):666–672.
86. Ranke A, Schmitt M, Didier F, Droulle P. Antenatal diagnosis of multicystic renal dysplasia. *Eur J Pediatr Surg* 2001;11:246–254.
87. Belk RA, Thomas DF, Mueller RF, et al. A family study and the natural history of prenatally detected unilateral multicystic dysplastic kidney. *J Urol* 2002;167:666–669.
88. Srivastava T, Garola RE, Hellerstein S. Autosomal dominant inheritance of multicystic dysplastic kidney. *Pediatr Nephrol* 1999;13:481–483.
89. Chen YH, Stapleton FB, Roy S 3rd, Noe HN. Neonatal hypertension from a unilateral multicystic dysplastic kidney. *J Urol* 1985;133:664–665.

90. Liapis H, Doshi RH, Watson MA, et al. Reduced renin expression and altered gene transcript profiles in multicystic dysplastic kidneys. *J Urol* 2002;168:1816–1820.
91. Seeman T, John U, Blahova K, et al. Ambulatory blood pressure monitoring in children with unilateral multicystic dysplastic kidney. *Eur J Pediatr* 2001;160:78–83.
92. Kessler OJ, Ziv N, Livne PM, Merlob P. Involution rate of multicystic renal dysplasia. *Pediatrics* 1998;102:E73.
93. Mesrobian HG, Rushton HG, Bulas D. Unilateral renal agenesis may result from in utero regression of multicystic renal dysplasia. *J Urol* 1993;150:793–794.
94. Kis E, Verebely T, Varkonyi I, Mattyus I. Multicystic dysplastic kidney: natural history of the affected and the contralateral kidney compared to the normal and solitary kidney. *Orv Hetil* 2002;143:19–23.
95. Aubertin G, Cripps S, Coleman G, et al. Prenatal diagnosis of apparently isolated unilateral multicystic kidney: implications for counselling and management. *Prenat Diagn* 2002;22:388–394.
96. Homsy YL, Anderson JH, Oudjhane K, Russo P. Wilms tumor and multicystic dysplastic kidney disease. *J Urol* 1997;158:2256–2259.
97. Minevich E, Wacksman J, Phipps L, et al. The importance of accurate diagnosis and early close followup in patients with suspected multicystic dysplastic kidney. *J Urol* 1997;158:1301–1304.
98. Nakada H, Ogawa M, Shirai M, Kitagawa T. A case of renal cell carcinoma developing from a dysplastic kidney. *Gan No Rinsho* 1985;31:1731–1736.
99. Rackley RR, Angermeier KW, Levin H, et al. Renal cell carcinoma arising in a regressed multicystic dysplastic kidney. *J Urol* 1994;152:1543–1545.
100. Birken G, King D, Vane D, Lloyd T. Renal cell carcinoma arising in a multicystic dysplastic kidney. *J Pediatr Surg* 1985;20:619–621.
101. Shirai M, Kitagawa T, Nakata H, Urano Y. Renal cell carcinoma originating from dysplastic kidney. *Acta Pathol Jpn* 1986;36:1263–1269.
102. Perez LM, Naidu SI, Joseph DB. Outcome and cost analysis of operative versus nonoperative management of neonatal multicystic dysplastic kidneys. *J Urol* 1998;160:1207–1211.
103. Rickwood AM, Anderson PA, Williams MP. Multicystic renal dysplasia detected by prenatal ultrasonography. Natural history and results of conservative management. *Br J Urol* 1992;69:538–540.
104. Lee CT, Hung KH, Fang JS, et al. Implications of sonographic identification of duplex kidney in adults. *Chang Gung Med J* 2001;24:779–85.
105. Stein JP, Kurzrock EA, Freeman JA, et al. Right intrathoracic renal ectopia: a case report and review of the literature. *Tech Urol* 1999;5:166–168.
106. Stroosma OB, Smits JM, Schurink GW, et al. Horseshoe kidney transplantation within the eurotransplant region: a case control study. *Transplantation* 2001;72:1930–1933.
107. Bilge I, Kayserili H, Emre S, et al. Frequency of renal malformations in Turner syndrome: analysis of 82 Turkish children. *Pediatr Nephrol* 2000;14:1111–1114.
108. Cascio S, Sweeney B, Granata C, et al. Vesicoureteral reflux and ureteropelvic junction obstruction in children with horseshoe kidney: treatment and outcome. *J Urol* 2002;167:2566–2568.
109. Neville H, Ritchey ML, Shamberger RC, et al. The occurrence of Wilms tumor in horseshoe kidneys: a report from the National Wilms Tumor Study Group (NWTSG). *J Pediatr Surg* 2002;37:1134–1137.

6

SYNDROMES AND MALFORMATIONS OF THE URINARY TRACT

CHANIN LIMWONGSE
SUZANNE B. CASSIDY

Birth defects involving the kidney and urinary system are common and often occur in association with other structural abnormalities. A congenital urinary tract anomaly may provide the first clue to the recognition of multiorgan developmental abnormalities. Nevertheless, many renal anomalies remain asymptomatic and undiagnosed.

Although the number of single malformations involving the kidney and urinary system is limited, combinations of such malformations with anomalies involving other organ systems are found in more than 500 syndromes. In addition, many well-known sequences and associations involve the kidney and urinary tract. This chapter discusses common malformations, sequences, and associations involving the kidney and urinary tract and provides a summary of conditions that have these anomalies as one of their features. In addition, Tables 6.1 through 6.3 summarize more detailed information about a large number of disorders associated with urinary tract anomalies. These tables can be used to (a) provide readily available information about potential urinary tract anomalies in patients with a diagnosed genetic syndrome and (b) develop a differential diagnosis when specific anomalies are identified. Readers interested in additional details about a specific syndrome are referred to standard reference textbooks and databases for further reading (4–7).

To understand the pathophysiologic basis of structural abnormalities, it is important to define certain terms used in describing malformations and syndromes.

Malformation refers to a single structural anomaly that arises from an error in organogenesis. Such an error may be due to the failure of cells or tissues to form, to regress (programmed cell death), or to induce others' anlagen. Examples include renal agenesis, horseshoe kidney, and bladder exstrophy.

Deformation refers to a single structural anomaly that arises from mechanical forces (e.g., intrauterine constraint). Examples include metatarsus adductus, torticollis, and congenital scoliosis. The underlying tissue may be normal or abnormal, and sometimes a malformation (e.g., renal agenesis) can predispose patients to a deformation (e.g., Potter's sequence from oligohydramnios).

Disruption refers to a single structural anomaly that results from a destructive event after normal morphogenesis. Such events can be caused by lack of vascular supply, infectious process, or mechanical factors. Examples include limb amputation from amniotic bands and abdominal wall defects from vascular insufficiency related to maternal cocaine use.

Sequence refers to a cascade of abnormalities that results from a single initiating anomaly. Sequences can be malformational, deformational, or disruptive, and they sometimes represent more than one of these categories. Obstruction of urine flow at the level of the ureter during early gestation, for example, can cause malformation of the kidneys, intestines, and abdominal wall—a malformation sequence. At the same time, decreased urine flow produces oligohydramnios, fetal compression, and multiple deformities of the face, limbs, and chest wall—a deformation sequence.

Syndrome refers to a consistently observed pattern of multiorgan anomalies consisting of malformations, deformations, or disruptions. Examples include Turner syndrome and fetal alcohol syndrome.

Association refers to a constellation of anomalies that occur together more often than expected by chance alone but cannot be explained by a single cause or sequence of events. Vertebral, anus, tracheoesophageal, radial, and renal (VATER) association, which is discussed later in this chapter, is a common example.

PREVALENCE OF URINARY TRACT ANOMALIES

The true incidence of urinary tract anomalies is difficult to ascertain because they are asymptomatic and, therefore, remain undetected. The reported incidence of many anoma-

TABLE 6.1. SYNDROMES AND DISORDERS THAT HAVE URINARY TRACT ANOMALIES AS A FREQUENT FEATURE

Syndromes	Urinary tract abnormalities											Other associated anomalies	Inheritance pattern	Reference
	Renal agenesis	Ectopia/horseshoe	Cystic/dysplasia	Duplication	Hypoplasia	Hydronephrosis/ureter	Diverticulae	Atresia/stenosis	Reflux	Nephritis/sclerosis	Tumor/nephromegaly			
Abruzzo-Erickson		H										Coloboma, cleft palate, hypospadias, deafness, short stature	Uncertain	44
Acrocephalopolydactylous dysplasia (Elejalde syndrome)			+		+	+						Acrodactyly, hand hexadactyly, overgrowth, visceromegaly, globular body, redundant neck skin	AR	45
Acrorenal (Dieker)	1	E		+	+	+	Ua					Ectrodactyly, oligodactyly, hypoplastic carpal/tarsal bones	Sporadic	46
Acrorenal (Johnson-Munson)	1, 2						U, Ua					Aphalangy, hemivertebrae, genital/intestinal/anal dysgenesis	AR	46
Acrorenal (Siegler)		E				+		U	+			Short stature, hypoplastic radii/ulnae/humeri, oligodactyly	Uncertain	46
Acro-renal-mandibular	1		+									Ectrodactyly, hypoplastic mandible	AR	47
Acro-renal-ocular	1	E			+		B					Hypoplastic thumb, optic coloboma, cleft lip/palate	AD	48
Adrenoleukodystrophy, neonatal												See Pseudo-Zellweger		
Aglossia-adactylia	1											Micrognathia, cranial nerve palsy	Sporadic	49
Agnathia-holoprosencephaly		H				+						Arrhinencephaly, situs inversus, midline defects	Sporadic	50
Alagille	1		+	+						+		Cholestasis, peripheral pulmonic stenosis, characteristic face	AD	51
Alport										+		Nephritis, proteinuria, deafness	AD, X-linked	52
Alsing										+		Nephritis, nephronophthisis, optic coloboma, hip dislocation	AR	53
Alstrom										+		Diabetes mellitus, retinopathy, short stature, deafness	AR	54
Amelogenesis imperfecta										+		Enamel hypoplasia, nephrolithiasis, enuresis	AR	55
Amyloidosis type 5										+		Nephropathy, proteinuria, cranial nerve palsy, cutis laxa	AD	56
Angiotensin converting enzyme inhibitor, maternal use										+		IUGR, oligohydramnios, patent ductus arteriosus, limb anomalies, renal artery stenosis, progressive renal failure	Sporadic	57
Aniridia-Wilms' tumor											+	Aniridia, ambiguous genitalia, hypospadia, short stature	AD	58

Axial mesoderma dysplasia	1											Bladder exstrophy, vertebral anomalies, Goldenhar-like	Uncertain	59
Baldellou	1											Hypoparathyroidism, ocular coloboma, MR, seizures	Uncertain	60
Baller-Gerold	+	E	+		+							Craniosynostosis, radial aplasia, malformed ear, anal atresia	AR	61
Barakat										+		Mesangial sclerosis, MR, optic atrophy, nystagmus	AR	62
Bardet-Biedl			+	+		+	+		+	+		Obesity, polysyndactyly, MR, retinopathy, hypogonadism	AR	63,64
Beckwith-Wiedemann		E	+	+		+					+	Overgrowth, macroglossia, omphalocele, embryonal tumors	Sporadic, AD	65–68
Berardinelli						+					+	Insulin resistance, lipodystrophy, acanthosis nigricans, MR	AR	69
Brachymesomelia-renal			+									Micrognathia, corneal opacity, craniofacial dysmorphism	Uncertain	70
Braddock-Carey			+									Robin sequence, thrombocytopenia, ACC	Uncertain	71
Branchio-oculo-facial	1											Philtrum hypertrophy, cleft lip/palate, branchial remnant	AD	72
Branchio-oto-renal	1, 2	E	+	+	+	+			+			Branchial remnant, preauricular pit/tag, microtia, deafness	AD	73
Branchio-oto-ureteral				+								Branchial remnant, preauricular pit/tag, microtia, deafness	AD	74
Braun-Bayer				+				U		+		Deafness, bifid uvula, digital anomalies	Uncertain	75
Cat eye												See Table 6.3	Chromosomal	
Caudal duplication	1, 2	E		+		+			+			Duplication of colon, sacrum, genitalia, vertebral defects	Sporadic	76
Caudal regression	1, 2	E, H			+	+	Ua		+			Atresia of colon, anus, genitalia, vertebral defects, transesophageal fistula	Sporadic, AR	77,78
Cerebro-hepato-renal (Passarge)			+									Hypotonia, abnormal ear, hepatomegaly, hypospadias	AR	79
Cerebro-oculo-hepato-renal			+									Cerebellar hypoplasia, hepatic fibrosis, Leber amaurosis	AR	80
Cerebro-osteo-nephro-dysplasia			+							+		Rhizomelic limb shortening, cerebral atrophy, MR, seizures	AR	81
CHARGE association	+	E	+		+	+	+	U	+			See text for details		30–33
Chondroectodermal dysplasia (Ellis van Creveld)	1		+			+				+		Acromelic dwarfism, polydactyly, nail dystrophy, tooth hypoplasia narrow thorax, CHD	AR	82,83
Cocaine, maternal use	1, 2				+	+	Ua		+			Vascular disruption anomalies affecting multiple organs	Sporadic	84
Cornelia de Lange	1		+		+	+					+	SS, microcephaly, limb defect, hirsutism, synophrys	Uncertain	87
Crossed renal ectopia-pelvic lipomatosis		E				+		U				Clubbing of fingers, gynecomastia	Uncertain	85
Czeizel						+		U				Ectrodactyly, spina bifida, megacystis	AD	86

continued

TABLE 6.1. *CONTINUED.*

Syndromes	Urinary tract abnormalities: Renal agenesis	Ectopia/horseshoe	Cystic/dysplasia	Duplication	Hypoplasia	Hydronephrosis/ureter	Diverticulae	Atresia/stenosis	Reflux	Nephritis/sclerosis	Tumor/nephromegaly	Other associated anomalies	Inheritance pattern	Reference
Diabetic mother, infant of	1, 2	E, H	+	+	+	+	Ua		+			Neural tube defect, cardiac/limb anomalies, sacral agenesis	Sporadic	88,89
DiGeorge/velocardiofacial	1, 3	E		+	+	+		+	+			See Table 6.3	Chromosomal	
Denys-Drash		E		+						+	+	Pseudohermaphroditism, Wilms' tumor, proteinuria	Sporadic	90
Down												See Table 6.3	Chromosomal	
Ectrodactyly-ectodermal dysplasia-clefting (EEC)	1		+	+		+			+			Ectrodactyly, hypohidrosis, sparse hair, cleft lip/palate	AD	91
Elejalde												See Acrocephalopolydactylous dysplasia		
Epstein									+			Thrombocytopenia, nerve deafness, cataract	AD	92
Facio-cardio-renal		H				+		U				Cardiomyopathy, conduction defect, MR, typical face	AR	93
Fanconi anemia	1	E, H	+	+	+	+						Pancytopenia, limb defects, leukemia, lymphoma	AR	94,95
Fetal alcohol	1	E, H	+	+	+	+						IUGR, DD, microcephaly, short palpebral fissure	Sporadic	96
Fibromatosis, infantile					+						+	Multiple myofibromatosis, myositis ossificans	AR	97
Fraser cryptophthalmos	1, 2		+					U				Fused eyelids, ear/genital anomalies, syndactyly	AR	98
Frasier					+					+		Male pseudohermaphrodite, amenorrhea, ovarian cysts	Uncertain	99
Goeminne			+							+		Congenital torticollis, keloids, cryptorchidism	X-linked	100
Goldenhar (oculo-auriculo-vertebral)	1	E	+	+	+	+			+			Hemifacial microsomia, ear anomalies, vertebral defects	Sporadic, AD	101
Goldston			+									Dandy-Walker malformation, cerebellar malformation	Uncertain	102
Graham			+								+	Cystic hamartoma of lung and kidney	Sporadic	103
Hemifacial microsomia (oculo-auriculo-vertebral)												See Goldenhar (oculo-auriculo-vertebral)		
Hemihyperplasia			+								+	Asymmetry, vascular malformation, embryonal tumors	Sporadic	104

Hepatic fibrosis			+								Congenital hepatic fibrosis	Sporadic	105
Holzgreve	2										Potter sequence, cardiac defect, polydactyly, cleft palate	Uncertain	106
Hypertelorism-microtia-clefting		E		+							Microcephaly, cleft lip/palate, MR	AR	107
Ivemark	1		+		+	+					Poly/asplenia, complex CHD, laterality defects	Sporadic, AR	108
Jeune			+								Narrow chest, short limbs, polydactyly, glomerulosclerosis	AR	82,83
Joubert			+								Vermis aplasia, apnea, jerky eyes, retinopathy, ataxia	AR	109
Juberg-Hayward		H			+						Microcephaly, cleft lip/palate, abnormal thumbs/toes	AR	110
Kabuki		H		+		+		U	+		MR, characteristic Kabuki-like face, large ears, cleft palate	Uncertain	111
Kallmann	1				+						Anosmia, cleft lip/palate, hypogonadotrophic hypogonadism	AD, AR, +R	112
Kaufman-McKusick		E	+	+		+		Ua			Hydrometrocolpos, polydactyly, anal/urogenital sinus defect	AR	113
Kivlin		E		+							Short stature, Peters' anomaly, MR, genital/cardiac defects	AR	114
Klippel-Feil	1	E		+							Short neck, cervical vertebral fusion, low posterior hairline	Sporadic, AD	115
Kousseff	1										Sacral meningocele, hydrocephalus, cardiac defects	AR	116
Leprechaunism (Donohue)			+							+	Insulin resistance, lipodystrophy, hirsutism	AR	117
Limb–body wall complex	1	E	+				U, Ua				Lateral body wall defect, limb reduction, CHD	Sporadic	118
Mammo-renal				+							Ipsilateral supernumerary breasts/nipples	Sporadic	119
Marden-Walker			+		+						Microcephaly, blepharophimosis, micrognathia, contractures	AR	120
Meckel-Gruber			+		+		U, Ua				Encephalocele, cardiac defects, cleft lip/palate, polydactyly	AR	121
Megacystis-microcolon						+		U			Large bladder, intestinal hypoperistalsis, oligohydramnios	AR	122
Melnick-Needles osteodysplasty							+	U			Bowing long bones, short upper limbs, micrognathia	X-linked	123
Mendelhall										+	Insulin resistance, acanthosis nigricans	AR	124
Microgastria–upper limb anomaly	1	E			+						Hypoplastic spleen, limb reduction defects	Uncertain	125
Miranda	+		+								Brain malformation, liver dysplasia	Uncertain	126
Moerman	1		+	+	+	+					Short limbs, brain malformation, cleft palate	Uncertain	127
MURCS association	1	E	+					U			See text for details	Sporadic	

continued

TABLE 6.1. *CONTINUED.*

Syndromes	Urinary tract abnormalities: Renal agenesis	Ectopia/horseshoe	Cystic/dysplasia	Duplication	Hypoplasia	Hydronephrosis/ureter	Diverticulae	Atresia/stenosis	Reflux	Nephritis/sclerosis	Tumor/nephromegaly	Other associated anomalies	Inheritance pattern	Reference
Nager acrofacial dysostosis	+			+		+			+			Facial bone hypoplasia, cleft eyelid, radial ray defect	AD	128
Nail-patella										+		Absent/hypoplastic nails and patellae	AD	129
Neu-Laxova	1											IUGR, lissencephaly, CHD, pterygia, ichthyosis	AR	130
Neuro-facio-digito-renal	1											Prominent forehead with vertical groove, MR, ear anomaly	Uncertain	131
Neurofibromatosis type I	1							Ua			+	Renal artery stenosis, hypernephroma, café-au-lait spots	AD	132
Nezelof			+							+		Arthrogryposis, hepatic impairment, hypotonia, club feet	AR	133
Noonan			+	+		+						Webbed neck, short stature, MR, pulmonic stenosis	AD	134
Occipital horn						+	B	Ua				Cranial exostosis, hyperextensibility, cutis laxa	X-linked	135
Ochoa				+		+		B, U, Ua +				Facial grimacing with lateral displacement of mouth	Uncertain	136
Oculo-auriculo-vertebral												See Goldenhar syndrome		
Oculo-hepato-encephalo-renal			+		+							Encephalocele, hepatic fibrosis, coloboma	AR	137
Oculorenal												See Pierson syndrome		139
Oculorenal (Karcher)	1				+					+		Optic nerve coloboma	AD	139
Oculo-renal-cerebellar										+		MR, spastic diplegia, choreoathetosis, retinopathy	AR	138
OEIS complex			+			+		Ua	+			Malrotation of colon, sacral defect, tethered spinal cord, pelvic bone abnormalities	Sporadic	
Otorenal			+			+	+	U				Renal pelvis diverticulae, nerve deafness	AD	140
Pallister-Hall	1, 2	E, H	+			+						Hypothalamic hamartoblastoma, polydactyly	AD	141,142
Pierson			+									Hypoplastic retina, cataract, anterior chamber anomalies	AR	143
Penoscrotal transposition		E	+		+	+	B	U				Abnormal placement of external genitalia	Sporadic	144

Perlman			+	+		+				+	+	Early overgrowth, typical face, nephroblastomatosis	AR	145
Polydactyly-obstructive uropathy						+	Ua		+			Postaxial polydactyly of hands and feet	Uncertain	146
Potter (oligohydramnios)	1, 2		+		+			Ua				See text for details	Uncertain	
Prune belly			+	+		+	Ua		+			See text for details	Sporadic	
Pseudo-Zellweger			+								+	Hypotonia, seizures, MR, typical face, FTT, hepatomegaly	AR	147–149
Pyloric stenosis		H	+	+	+	+						Cystic kidney	Sporadic	150
Rapadilino						+						Radial/patella hypoplasia, diarrhea, short stature, long nose	AR	152
Rass-Rothschild	+					+						Klippel-Feil anomaly, sacral agenesis, cryptorchidism	Uncertain	151
Renal dysplasia or adysplasia	1	E	+		+	+	Ua		+			Abnormal uterus in some patients	AD	154
Renal-hepatic-pancreatic dysplasia			+									Pancreatic cysts, extrahepatic biliary atresia, Caroli disease	AR	82,83
Renal/müllerian hypoplasia		H			+				+			Absent uterus, broad forehead, DD, large fontanel	AR	153
Retinoic acid, maternal use					+	+		U				Ear anomalies, CHD, cleft palate, neural tube defect	Sporadic	155,156
Roberts	1	H	+			+						Limb reduction, oligo/syndactyly, CHD, dysmorphic face	AR	157
Robson										+		MR, macrocephaly, deafness, proteinuria, Alport-like	X-linked	158
Rokitansky-Mayer-Kuster-Hauser	1	E	+	U	+							Absence of vagina, uterine anomalies, amenorrhea	Sporadic	159
Rubella, congenital	1		+	+								CHD, MR, deafness, cataract, growth retardation	Sporadic	160
Rubinstein-Taybi	1	E	+	+	+			Ua				SS, MR, broad thumbs and great toes, typical face	Sporadic	161,162
Russell-Silver						+		Ua				SS, triangular face, asymmetry, clinodactyly, hypoglycemia	Sporadic, AD	163
Santos	1											Hirschsprung's disease, hearing loss, postaxial polydactyly	AR	164
Say			+									SS, microcephaly, micrognathia, large ear, cleft palate	AD	165
Schimke										+		SS, spondyloepiphyseal dysplasia, immunodeficiency	AR	166
Schinzel-Giedion		E		U		+		U				CHD, distinctive face, figure 8 head shape, eyelid groove	AR	167
Senior-Loken			+							+		Nephronophthisis, tapeto retinal degeneration	AR	168
Setleis						+		U				Cutis aplasia with temporal scarring, abnormal eyelashes	AD, AR	169
Short rib, Beemer Langer			+		+	+		U				Hydrops, cleft lip, bowed long bones, atretic ear canal	AR	170
Short rib–polydactyly, types 1–3	1		+					Ua				Urethral fistula, CHD, cloacal/urogenital sinus anomalies	AR	170,171

continued

TABLE 6.1. *CONTINUED.*

Syndromes	Urinary tract abnormalities											Other associated anomalies	Inheritance pattern	Reference
	Renal agenesis	Ectopia/horseshoe	Cystic/dysplasia	Duplication	Hypoplasia	Hydronephrosis/ureter	Diverticulae	Atresia/stenosis	Reflux	Nephritis/sclerosis	Tumor/nephromegaly			
Silverman (dyssegmental dwarfism)						+		U				SS, flat face, cleft palate, generalized skeletal dysplasia	Uncertain	172
Simopoulos			+									Hydrocephalus, polydactyly	AR	173
Simpson-Golabi-Behmel			+			+					+	Overgrowth, polydactyly, typical face, arrhythmia	X-linked	174
Sirenomelia sequence	1, 2	E	+	+	+	+	+	+	+			See text for details	Sporadic	
Smith-Lemli-Opitz	1		+		+							SS, ambiguous genitalia, two to three toe syndactyly, brain anomalies	AR	175,176
Sommer	1											Iris aplasia, corneal opacity, glaucoma, prominent forehead	AD	177
Sorsby (coloboma-brachydactyly)	1											Ocular coloboma, brachydactyly type B, bifid thumbs	AD	178
Sotos								Ua			+	Overgrowth, MR, embryonal tumors, advanced bone age	Sporadic	179
Supernumerary nipples, renal anomalies		E	+	+	+	+						Familial polythelia	AD	180
Thalidomide, maternal use	1, 2	E, H	+		+	+	+		+			Limb reduction, phocomelia, neural tube defect	Sporadic	181,182
Thymic-renal-anal-lung	+		+					U				SS, absent thymus, parathyroid agenesis, urethral fistula	AR	183
Tolmie			+									Lethal multiple pterygia, long bone abnormalities	X-linked	184
Townes-Brocks	1		+		+			Ua	+			Triphalangeal thumb, imperforate anus, skin tag, deafness	AD	185
Trimethadione, maternal use	1							U				SS, CHD, omphalocele, distinctive face	Sporadic	186
Tuberous sclerosis			+								+	MR, seizures, cortical tuber, facial angiofibroma	AD	187
Turner												See Table 6.3	Chromosomal	
Ulnar-mammary	1											Oligodactyly, ulnar ray defect, nipple aplasia, genital defects	AD	188
Urogenital adysplasia	1, 2		+									Absent uterus, vaginal atresia, hydrometrocolpos	AD	189
VATER (VACTERL) association	1	E, H	+	+	+	+	+	+	+			See text for details		
Velocardiofacial	1, 2	E, H		+	+	+		+	+			See Table 6.3		

von Hippel–Lindau			+							+	Cerebello-retinal angiomatosis, pheochromocytoma	AD	190,191
Weinberg-Zumwalt			+							+	Multiple lung cysts, ascites, accessory spleen	Uncertain	192
Wenstrup	1		+		+	+		U			Female pseudohermaphrodite, imperforate anus	Uncertain	193
Weyers		H	+	+		+		U			Oligodactyly, pterygia, sternal defect, cleft palate	AR	194
Wiedemann-Beckwith											See Beckwith-Wiedemann syndrome		
Williams		E			+	+	B, U	U			See Table 6.3	Chromosomal	
Wilms' tumor–horseshoe kidney		H								+	Possible association	Sporadic	195
Wilms' tumor–hemihypertrophy										+	Ipsilateral vascular malformation, café-au-lait spots	Sporadic	104
Wilms' tumor–radial aplasia										+	Hypoplastic fibula/tibia, abnormal thumbs	Sporadic	196
Winter (oto-renal-genital)	1, 2		+								Middle ear anomalies, deafness, vaginal atresia	AR	197
Wolfram						+			+		Diabetes mellitus/insipidus, optic atrophy, nerve deafness	Mitochondrial	198
Zellweger	1		+			+					Hypotonia, seizures, hepatosplenomegaly, growth delay	AR	147–149

+, Feature present or reported; 1, unilateral renal agenesis; 2, bilateral renal agenesis; ACC, agenesis of corpus callosum; AD, autosomal-dominant; AR, autosomal-recessive; B, bladder; CHARGE, coloboma, heart disease, atresia choanae, retarded growth and development, genital hypoplasia, and ear anomalies; CHD, congenital heart disease; DD, developmental delay; E, ectopia; FTT, failure to thrive; H, horseshoe; IUGR, intrauterine growth retardation; MR, mental retardation; MURCS, müllerian, renal, cervicothoracic, somite abnormalities association; OEIS, omphalocele-cloacal exstrophy-imperforate anus-spinal dysraphism; SS, short stature; U, ureter; Ua, urethra; VACTERL, vertebral, anal, cardiac, tracheal, esophageal, renal, limb; VATER, vertebral, anus, tracheoesophageal, radial, and renal.

TABLE 6.2. WELL-KNOWN SYNDROMES ASSOCIATED WITH OCCASIONAL URINARY TRACT ANOMALIES

	Urinary tract abnormalities													
Syndromes	Renal agenesis	Ectopia/horseshoe	Cystic/dysplasia	Duplication	Hypoplasia	Hydronephrosis/ureter	Diverticulae	Atresia/stenosis	Reflux	Nephritis/sclerosis	Tumor/nephromegaly	Other associated anomalies	Inheritance pattern	Reference
Aase								Ua				Triphalangeal thumb, hypoplastic anemia	AD, AR	199
Achondrogenesis				+		+						Micromelic dwarfism, short trunk, fetal hydrops	AR	200
Acrocallosal	1		+									ACC, macrocephaly, polymicrogyria, polydactyly, CHD	AR	201
Acro-facial dysostosis		H										Abnormal thumb/toe, facial bone defect, ear anomalies	AR	202
Acromelic frontonasal dysplasia		E		+								Polydactyly, ACC, encephalocele, Dandy-Walker anomaly	Sporadic	203
Adrenal hypoplasia-MR						+		U	+			Aminoaciduria, MR, muscular dystrophy, visual abnormality	X-linked	205
Adrenogenital	1			+		+						Ambiguous genitalia, vomiting, salt losing, ureteropelvic junction obstruction	AR	204
Antley-Bixler		H		+								Craniosynostosis, radio-humeral synostosis, cardiac defects	AR	206
Apert (acrocephalosyndactyly)			+			+						Acrocephaly, craniosynostosis, syndactyly	AD	207
Bloom											+	Short stature, telangiectasias, leukemia, lymphoma	AR	208
Bowen-Conradi		H		+								Micrognathia, arthrogryposis, cloudy cornea, brain anomaly	AR	209
Brachydactyly type E	1				+							Vertebral anomalies, narrow auditory canal	Uncertain	210
3C (Ritscher-Schinzel)						+						SS, Dandy-Walker anomaly, typical face, CHD	AR	211
C-trigonocephaly	1											Polysyndactyly, abnormal ear, hypospadias, dislocated joints	AR	212
Campomelic dysplasia	1		+			+						Tibial bowing, pretibial dimples, ambiguous genitalia	AD	213
Carbohydrate deficient glycoprotein			+									FTT, abnormal fat pad, hepatosplenomegaly, neurodegeneration	AR	214
Carpenter										+		Aminoaciduria, polysyndactyly, craniosynostosis	AD	215
CHILD	1, 2					+						Unilateral erythroderma, ipsilateral limb defect	X-linked	216
Chondrodysplasia punctata, nonrhizomelic			+									Flat face, microcephaly, cataract, short femora/humeri, stippled epiphyses	AR	217
Coffin-Siris	1					+						MR, sparse scalp hair, hirsutism, coarse face, thick lips	AR	218
Cutis laxa type I							B					GI tract diverticulae, emphysema, diaphragmatic defect	AR	219
Disorganization-like	+											Polydactyly, duplication of lower limbs, skin appendages	Sporadic	220
Duane anomaly–radial defects	1											Limited ocular abduction, radial defects, blepharophimosis	AD	221

Ehlers-Danlos			+							Joint hypermobility, skin hyperextensibility, easy bruising	AD, AR	222
Epidermolysis bullosa						+	U			Skin blistering, pyloric stenosis, dystrophic nails, sparse hair	AR	223,224
Femoral hypoplasia-unusual facies	1									Various leg deformities, abnormal genitalia, typical face	Sporadic, AD	225
Floating-Harbor		E								SS, typical face, DD, delayed bone age	Uncertain	226
Focal dermal hypoplasia		H								Atrophy/linear skin pigmentation, hand/vertebral anomalies	X-linked	227
Freeman-Sheldon					+	+				Whistling face, ulnar deviation of hands, talipes equinovarus	AD	228
Fronto-metaphyseal dysplasia				+		+				Prominent supraorbital ridges, contractures, deafness	X-linked	229
Frontonasal dysplasia	+	E								Hypertelorism, broad nasal tip, median cleft nose	Sporadic	230
Fryns			+							Digital hypoplasia, diaphragmatic defect, cleft palate	AR	231
G (Opitz/BBB)				+			+	+		See Opitz (G/BBB)		
Glutaric aciduria, type II			+							Cerebral anomalies, pancreatic dysplasia, biliary dysgenesis	AR	232
Grieg cephalopolysyndactyly				+						Macrocephaly, polydactyly, hypertelorism	AD	233
Hajdu-Cheney			+							SS, Wormian bones, acro-osteolysis, osteoporosis	AD	234
Hydrolethalus						+	Ua			Hydrocephalus, polydactyly, polyhydramnios, cleft lip	AR	235
Jarcho-Levin						+				Spondylothoracic dysplasia, fused ribs, hemivertebrae	AR	236
Johanson-Blizzard						+				Pancreatic insufficiency, spiky hair, small alae nasi	AR	237
Killian-Pallister										See Table 6.3	Chromosomal	
Lacrimo-auriculo-dento-digital	1									Nasolacrimal duct stenosis, malformed ears/ enamel/digits	AD	238
Larsen	1					+				Multiple joint dislocations, flat face	AD, ?AR	239,240
Lenz microphthalmia	1		+			+				Ocular coloboma, ear/facial anomalies, syndactyly/ camptodactyly	X-linked	241
LEOPARD (multiple lentigines)	1									Hypertelorism, deafness, abnormal electrocardiogram, genital anomalies	AD	242
Marfan			+						+	Tall thin habitus, aortic root dilatation, lens subluxation, arachnodactyly	AD	243,244
Marshall-Smith						+				MR, FTT, accelerated bone maturation, broad phalanges	Sporadic	245
Miller-Dieker (lissencephaly)	1		+							See Table 6.3	Microdeletion	
Moebius-peripheral neuropathy				+						Peripheral neuropathy, anosmia, hypogonadism	Sporadic	246
Mohr-Majewski										See Orofaciodigital, type IV		
Multiple pterygium					+					Multiple soft tissue contractures, camptodactyly	AR	247
Myotonic dystrophy			+							Myotonia, muscle weakness, cataract, arrhythmia, diabetes	AD	248,249
Nijmegen breakage						+				MR, SS, microcephaly, immunodeficiency	AR	250
Opitz (G/BBB)										Hypertelorism, hypospadias, cleft lip/palate, dysphagia	AD, X-linked	251,252
Orofaciodigital, type I			+			+				Midline cleft lip, multiple frenulae, polydactyly, tongue nodules	X-linked	253

continued

TABLE 6.2. *CONTINUED.*

Syndromes	Urinary tract abnormalities: Renal agenesis	Ectopia/horseshoe	Cystic/dysplasia	Duplication	Hypoplasia	Hydronephrosis/ureter	Diverticulae	Atresia/stenosis	Reflux	Nephritis/sclerosis	Tumor/nephromegaly	Other associated anomalies	Inheritance pattern	Reference
Orofaciodigital, type IV	1		+									Cleft palate, multiple frenulae, polysyndactyly, lobed tongue	AR	253,254
Orofaciodigital, type VI	1		+									Midline cleft lip, multiple frenulae, polydactyly, tongue nodules	AR	253
Pallister-Killian												See Table 6.3	Chromo-somal	
Peutz-Jeghers			+									Hamartomatous intestinal polyposis, lip hyperpig-mentation	AD	255,256
Poland anomaly	1			+	+							Hypoplastic pectoralis, ipsilateral upper limb reduc-tion	Sporadic	257,258
Restrictive dermopathy				U								Aplasia cutis, rigid skin, contractures, typical face	AR	259
Robinow				+		+						Mesomelic dwarfism, typical face, abnormal genitalia	AD, ?AR	260
Rothmund-Thomson										+		Poikiloderma, alopecia, dysplastic nails, photosensi-tivity	AR	261
Serpentine fibula			+									Elongated curved fibulae, hirsutism, hypertelorism	Uncertain	262
Spondylocostal dysostosis	1		+									Sacral agenesis, anal atresia, bifid thumb, skin tags	Uncertain	263
Spondyloepimetaphyseal dysplasia						+		U				Joint laxity, kyphoscoliosis, talipes equinovarus, CHD	AR	264
Spondylometaphyseal dys-plasia										+		SS, platyspondyly, coxa vara, vertebral/long bone anomalies	AD	265
Syndactyly, type V		E			+							Bladder exstrophy, fusion of 4th and 5th metacar-pal bones	AD	266

+, Feature present or reported; 1, unilateral renal agenesis; 2, bilateral renal agenesis; ACC, agenesis of corpus callosum; AD, autosomal-dominant; AR, autosomal-recessive; B, bladder; CHD, congenital heart disease; CHILD, hemidysplasia with ichthyosiform erythroderma and limb defects; DD, developmental delay; E, ectopia; FTT, failure to thrive; H, horseshoe; LEOPARD, lentigines, electrocardiographic abnormality, ocular hypertelorism, pulmonic stenosis, abnormal genitalia, retardation of growth, and deafness; MR, mental retardation; SS, short stature; U, ureter; Ua; urethra.

TABLE 6.3. CHROMOSOMAL DISORDERS AND THEIR CONSISTENT ASSOCIATED URINARY TRACT ANOMALIES

Chromosomal disorders	Urinary tract abnormalities											Other associated anomalies	Reported familial cases	References
	Renal agenesis	Ectopia/horseshoe	Cystic/dysplasia	Duplication	Hypoplasia	Hydronephrosis/ureter	Diverticulae	Atresia/stenosis	Reflux	Nephritis/sclerosis	Tumor/nephromegaly			
3p deletion		E, H				+						MR, growth delay, ptosis, postaxial polydactyly, micrognathia	No	269
3q duplication		H		+	+	+						MR, SS, seizures, hirsutism, typical face, cardiac defects	No	270
Williams syndrome (7q deletion)		E			+	+	B, U	U				SS, typical face, supravalvar aortic stenosis, hypercalcemia	Yes	267
Trisomy 9 mosaicism			+			+	B					MR, joint contractures, cardiac defects, brain anomalies	No	268
10q duplication		H	+									MR, ptosis, short palpebral fissures, camptodactyly	Yes	269
Aniridia-Wilms' tumor (11p13 deletion)											+	Ambiguous genitalia, hypospadias, short stature	AD	270
Pallister-Killian syndrome (tetrasomy 12p)			+									SS, MR, hypogonadism, seizures, diaphragmatic defect	No	270
Patau syndrome (trisomy 13)	1, 2	H	+	+		+						Holoprosencephaly, midline anomalies, cleft lip/palate	No	268
Miller-Dieker syndrome (17p13 deletion)	1		+									MR, lissencephaly, microgyria, agyria, typical face, seizures	No	271
Edward syndrome (trisomy 18)	+	E, H	+	+		+						IUGR, CHD, clenched hands, rocker bottom feet	Yes	268
18q deletion		H										SS, MR, microcephaly, narrow external ear canals, long hands	Yes	272
Down syndrome (trisomy 21)		H	+	+								MR, hypotonia, CHD, typical face, clinodactyly	Yes	273
Cat eye syndrome (tetrasomy 22p)	1	H	+			+		U				MR, CHD, colobomas, anal/digital anomalies	Yes	274
Velocardiofacial syndrome (22q11 deletion)	1, 2	E, H	+	+	+	+		+	+			Conotruncal CHD, thymic aplasia, typical face, cleft palate	Yes	275,276
Turner syndrome (45,X or 46,X,i(Xq))	1	E, H	+	+	+	+			+			SS, amenorrhea, webbed neck, cubitus valgus, hypogonadism	No	277
Triploidy		H	+			+						Large molar placenta, IUGR, syndactyly of third and fourth digit, others	No	270

+, Feature present or reported; 1, Unilateral renal agenesis; 2, bilateral renal agenesis; AD, autosomal-dominant; B, bladder; CHD, congenital heart disease; E, ectopia; H, horseshoe; IUGR, intrauterine growth retardation; MR, mental retardation; SS, short stature; U, ureter.

TABLE 6.4. PREVALENCE OF URINARY TRACT ANOMALIES PER 1000 BIRTHS FROM METROPOLITAN ATLANTA CONGENITAL DEFECTS PROGRAM (MACDP), CALIFORNIA BIRTH DEFECTS MONITORING PROGRAM (CBDMP), AND WASHINGTON STATE BIRTH DEFECTS REGISTRY (WSBDR)

	Rates per 1000 liveborn infants		
Anomalies	MACDP 1983–1988	CBDMP 1983–1994	WSBDR 1987–1989
Renal agenesis/dysplasia	0.47	0.480	0.58
Horseshoe kidney	No data	0.040	0.16
Cystic kidney	No data	0.030	0.05
Obstruction of kidney/ureter	0.80	1.270	1.27
Double ureter	No data	0.004	0.05
Exstrophy of bladder	0.03	0.030	0.02
Obstruction of bladder/urethra	0.23	0.160	0.20
VATER, CHARGE, and MURCS associations	No data	0.210[a]	No data
Sirenomelia	No data	0.090[b]	No data

CHARGE, coloboma, heart disease, atresia choanae, retarded growth and development, genital hypoplasia, and ear anomalies; MURCS, müllerian, renal, cervicothoracic somite abnormalities; VATER, vertebral, anus, tracheoesophageal, radial, and renal.
[a]Rates include 39 other syndromes with related anomalies.
[b]Rates include 34 other syndromes with related anomalies.

lies reflects ascertainment bias because data are often derived from symptomatic individuals. Reliable data have been reported from several birth defects registries. In the United States, these include the Metropolitan Atlanta Congenital Defects Program, California Birth Defects Monitoring Program, and the Washington State Birth Defects Registry (1,2). Table 6.4 summarizes prevalence data for a number of distinct urinary anomalies reported from these registries.

When adjusted for race, sex, and maternal age, the prevalence of renal agenesis, cystic kidney, exstrophy of the bladder, and obstruction of the bladder or urethra do not show differences between geographic areas (1). In contrast, there appears to be a higher prevalence of obstruction of the kidney or ureter in California and Washington compared with Atlanta. It has been suggested that these differences are due to ascertainment bias; however, differences in prenatal teratogenic exposures (e.g., alcohol and cocaine) and differences in the genetic background of individuals in these geographic areas cannot be discounted. Overall, renal anomalies are found in approximately 3 to 6 per 1000 births (1,3). Genitourinary anomalies are responsible for approximately 6.8% of infant deaths in the United States (March of Dimes Perinatal Data Center 2002; http://www.marchofdimes.com/aboutus/1523.asp/).

APPROACH TO THE CHILD WITH A URINARY TRACT ANOMALY

The clinical approach to the child with a urinary tract anomaly is similar to that for other birth defects. The initial step is to establish a specific diagnosis if possible based on history, physical examination, and laboratory investigation. A thorough family history for both urinary tract anomalies and for any other type of congenital or developmental anomalies must be obtained. Many genetic disorders have variable expression even within the same family. A careful physical examination looking specifically for major and minor anomalies should be performed. Sometimes, a pattern of multiple anomalies can be recognized immediately as a well-described syndrome. Patterns of anomalies that cannot be recognized may require a literature or database search or referral to an expert in syndrome recognition. The search for a specific diagnosis is optimally accomplished by identifying the least common and most distinctive anomalies, thereby limiting the list of possible differential diagnoses. To aid in this effort, refer to Tables 6.1 through 6.3 in addition to tables listing the differential diagnosis that accompanies the description of each of the major urinary tract anomalies below (see Tables 6.5 through 6.15). For example, it is preferable to search for syndromes with urethral agenesis (22 syndromes) rather than renal dysplasia (more than 80 syndromes) when the two anomalies coexist. A search based on the more common anomalies can be performed if the first search does not reveal a match. Even after careful evaluation, a substantial number of children with multiple congenital anomalies remain undiagnosed.

A chromosome analysis is indicated in any child who has at least two major congenital anomalies or one isolated anomaly that is particularly associated with a defined chromosomal abnormality [e.g., aniridia (microdeletion 11p)]. Growth or developmental delay, dysmorphic features, or lack of familial resemblance should also prompt a chromosomal analysis. Chromosome abnormalities are found in approximately 10 to 12% of all renal anomalies (3,8). Table 6.3 lists common and distinct chromosomal disorders with their reported urinary tract anomalies.

For a child with no known urinary tract anomaly, findings that should prompt an evaluation of the urinary tract include oligohydramnios, undefined abdominal mass, abnormal genitalia, aniridia, hypertension, preauricular pits or tags, branchial cleft cyst or sinus, imperforate anus, symptoms indicative of renal dysfunction, urinary tract infection, or obstructive uropathy (3). For patients with known syndromes, the types of associated urinary tract anomalies are listed in Tables 6.1 and 6.2.

Ultrasonography is recommended in screening for urinary tract anomalies. It is noninvasive and provides excellent anatomic information. It is also the only method routinely used for the prenatal diagnosis of urinary tract anomalies. Additional radiographic studies and specialized genetic testing may then follow as part of a staged diagnostic evaluation. Corrective or reparative treatments are available for many anomalies (stenosis or atresia, bladder exstrophy, duplication, diverticula, and tumors).

Once a child with a urinary tract anomaly is identified, a search for related anomalies in first-degree relatives is indicated only when the proband has renal agenesis (9). Otherwise, the decision to investigate family members should be based on a thorough family history and whether the identified anomaly is part of a well-described inherited syndrome. Genetic counseling should be provided to the family, and reproductive options should be discussed in a nondirective fashion. For an isolated anomaly without a family history of similar or related anomalies, an empiric risk can be provided. Accurate risk figures can be determined for mendelian disorders, and estimated risks are available for associations.

All children with congenital anomalies need long-term follow-up. This is especially the case for children with undiagnosed multiple congenital anomalies, for whom follow-up examination may lead to a specific diagnosis. Additional relevant family information should be specifically sought for any newly affected member. Finally, for patients with a urinary tract anomaly who reach reproductive age, the recurrence risk for their offspring and reproductive options should be discussed.

DEVELOPMENT OF THE URINARY TRACT

Renal organogenesis is reviewed in Chapter 1. Embryogenesis of the lower urinary tract includes development of the mesonephric duct and urogenital sinus. The mesonephric duct inserts into the lower allantois, just above the terminal part of the hindgut, the cloaca. During the fourth to seventh weeks, mesoderm proliferates and forms the transverse mesodermal ridge, the urorectal septum. The urorectal septum divides the cloaca into the anterior portion (the primitive urogenital sinus) and the posterior portion (the cloacal sinus or anorectal canal). The mesonephric ducts open into the urogenital sinus and later become the ureters. The urorectal septum develops caudally and fuses with the cloacal membrane, dividing it into the urogenital membrane (anterior) and the anorectal membrane (posterior) by the end of the seventh week. The primitive perineal body forms at the site of fusion.

The primitive urogenital sinus develops primarily into the urinary bladder. The superior portion, originally continuous with the allantois, later becomes a solid fibrous cord (the urachus or median umbilical ligament), which connects the bladder to the umbilicus. The inferior portion of the urogenital sinus in the male divides into a pelvic portion, containing the prostatic and membranous urethra, and the long phallic portion, containing the penile urethra. The inferior portion in the female forms a small portion of the urethra and the vestibule. At the same time, the distal portion of the mesonephric ducts is incorporated into the endodermal vesicoureteral primordium, forming the trigone of the bladder. A part of the distal end of both mesonephric ducts just proximal to the trigone develops into the seminal vesicles and ductus deferens in the male. Finally, at the end of the twelfth week, the epithelium of the superior portion of the prostatic urethra proliferates to form buds that penetrate the surrounding mesenchyme. In the male, these buds form the prostate gland; in the female, they form the urethral and paraurethral glands.

URINARY TRACT ANOMALIES

Kidney Defects

Renal Agenesis

Renal agenesis refers to complete absence of one or both kidneys without identifiable rudimentary tissue. Renal agenesis is usually associated with agenesis of the ipsilateral ureter. The pathogenesis of renal agenesis is failure of formation of the metanephros. Causal heterogeneity has been shown, both by animal studies and by human observations (10–12), including failure of ureteric bud formation, failure of the bud to reach the metanephric blastema, or failure of the bud and the metanephric blastema, to create mutual inductive influence on one another (see Chapter 1). In addition, interruption in vascular supply and regression of a multicystic kidney can lead to renal agenesis in the fetal period (11).

Unilateral renal agenesis is usually asymptomatic and detected incidentally, whereas bilateral renal agenesis results in severe oligohydramnios and fetal or perinatal loss. Several studies have demonstrated that unilateral renal agenesis is associated with an increased frequency of anomalies in the contralateral kidney (9,13). Renal agenesis is often associated with anomalies of other organ systems. These anomalies can occur both in contiguous structures (e.g., vertebrae, genital organs, intestines, and anus) and in noncontiguous structures (e.g., limbs, heart, trachea, ear, and central nervous system). The diagnosis of renal agenesis is made by abdominal ultrasound. Care must be taken to

TABLE 6.5. SYNDROMES ASSOCIATED WITH UNILATERAL RENAL AGENESIS

Acrocallosal syndrome
Acrorenal syndrome, Dieker type
Acro-renal-mandibular syndrome
Acro-renal-ocular syndrome
Adrenogenital syndrome
Aglossia-adactylia syndrome
Alagille syndrome (arteriohepatic dysplasia)
Branchio-oto-renal syndrome
C-trigonocephaly syndrome
Campomelic dysplasia
Cat-eye syndrome
Chondroectodermal dysplasia
Coffin-Siris syndrome
Cornelia de Lange syndrome
Ectrodactyly-ectodermal dysplasia-clefting syndrome
Femoral hypoplasia–unusual facies syndrome
Fetal alcohol syndrome
Goldenhar syndrome
Ivemark syndrome
Kallmann syndrome
Klippel-Feil anomaly
Lacrimo-auriculo-dento-digital syndrome
Larsen syndrome
Lenz microphthalmia syndrome
LEOPARD syndrome (multiple lentigines)
Limb–body wall complex
Miller-Dieker syndrome
MURCS association
Neu-Laxova syndrome
Oro-facio-digital syndrome, types IV and VI
Pfeiffer syndrome
Poland anomaly
Renal dysplasia
Roberts syndrome
Rokitansky-Mayer-Kuster-Hauser syndrome
Rubella syndrome, congenital
Rubinstein-Taybi syndrome
Russell-Silver syndrome
Short rib polydactyly syndrome, types 1–3
Smith-Lemli-Opitz syndrome
Sorsby coloboma-brachydactyly syndrome
Spondylocostal dysostosis
Townes-Brocks syndrome
Trisomy 22
Turner syndrome
Ulnar-mammary syndrome
VATER (VACTERL) association
Zellweger syndrome

LEOPARD, lentigines, electrocardiographic abnormality, ocular hypertelorism, pulmonic stenosis, abnormal genitalia, retardation of growth, and deafness; VACTERL, vertebral, anal, cardiac, tracheal, esophageal, renal, limb; VATER, vertebral, anus, tracheoesophageal, radial, and renal.

exclude the possibility of ectopic kidney. Intravenous pyelography, computed tomography, and radionuclide studies can be helpful in equivocal cases.

The recurrence risk for renal agenesis can be estimated if the pattern of inheritance is known or if the proband has a recognizable syndrome. For nonsyndromic renal agenesis, an empiric risk of 3% can be used for families in which renal anomalies in first-degree relatives (siblings, parents) have been excluded (3). First-degree relatives of patients with nonsyndromic renal agenesis have an increased prevalence of related urogenital anomalies. In one study, 9.0% of first-degree relatives of infants with agenesis or dysgenesis of both kidneys had a related urogenital anomaly, and 4.4% had an asymptomatic renal malformation (13). Therefore, renal sonography is recommended for the first-degree relatives of the proband, unless renal agenesis in the proband is clearly sporadic or a specific cause without an increased recurrence risk is identified.

TABLE 6.6. SYNDROMES ASSOCIATED WITH UNILATERAL OR BILATERAL RENAL AGENESIS

Acrorenal, Johnson-Munson type
Alkylating agent, maternal use
Caudal duplication syndrome
Caudal regression syndrome
CHARGE association
Cocaine, maternal use
Diabetic mother, infant of
DiGeorge syndrome
Fraser (cryptophthalmos) syndrome
Holzgreve syndrome
Pallister-Hall syndrome
Potter (oligohydramnios) sequence
Sirenomelia sequence
Thalidomide embryopathy
Urogenital adysplasia
Velocardiofacial syndrome
Winter syndrome

CHARGE, coloboma, heart disease, atresia choanae, retarded growth and development, genital hypoplasia, and ear anomalies.

Tables 6.5 and 6.6 list the syndromes commonly associated with unilateral and bilateral renal agenesis, respectively. For more information about these disorders and other less common conditions with renal agenesis, see Tables 6.1 through 6.3.

Ectopic Kidney

Ectopic kidneys result from an error(s) of ascent. Most are pelvic kidneys that fail to ascend out of the pelvic cavity. Rare case reports of thoracic kidneys exist (14). Ectopic kidneys can be unilateral or bilateral. Bilateral pelvic kidneys often fuse into a midline mass of renal tissue, with two pelvises and a variable number of ureters, which is referred to as a *pancake* or *discoid kidney*. *Crossed renal ectopia* refers to an ectopic kidney whose ureter crosses the midline. Ectopic kidneys are usually hypoplastic and rotated and contain numerous small blood vessels and ureteric anomalies. Ectopic kidneys may be asymptomatic, but complications from ureteral obstruction, infection, and calculi are common. Table 6.7 provides a list of syndromes that include ectopic kidney, also described in Tables 6.1 through 6.3.

TABLE 6.7. SYNDROMES ASSOCIATED WITH ECTOPIC KIDNEY

Acromelic frontonasal dysplasia
Acrorenal syndrome, Dieker type
Acrorenal syndrome, Siegler type
Acro-renal-ocular syndrome
Baller-Gerold syndrome
Beckwith-Wiedemann syndrome
Branchio-oto-renal syndrome
Caudal regression syndrome
CHARGE association
Crossed ectopia–pelvic lipomatosis syndrome
DiGeorge syndrome
Drash (Denys-Drash) syndrome
Fanconi anemia syndrome
Fetal alcohol syndrome
Floating-Harbor syndrome
Frontonasal dysplasia
Goldenhar syndrome
Kaufman-McKusick syndrome
Klippel-Feil anomaly
Limb–body wall complex
MURCS association
Pallister-Hall syndrome
Penoscrotal transposition
Renal adysplasia
Rokitansky-Mayer-Kuster-Hauser syndrome
Rubinstein-Taybi syndrome
Schinzel-Giedion syndrome
Sirenomelia sequence
Turner syndrome
VATER (VACTERL) association
Velocardiofacial syndrome
Williams syndrome

CHARGE, coloboma, heart disease, atresia choanae, retarded growth and development, genital hypoplasia, and ear anomalies; MURCS, müllerian, renal, cervicothoracic somite abnormalities; VACTERL, vertebral, anal, cardiac, tracheal, esophageal, renal, limb; VATER, vertebral, anus, tracheoesophageal, radial, and renal.

Horseshoe Kidney

Horseshoe kidney refers to a condition in which the kidneys are fused at the lower poles with a renal parenchymal or, less commonly, fibrous isthmus. The embryopathogenesis of horseshoe kidney with parenchymal isthmus is believed to be abnormal migration of nephrogenic cells across the primitive streak before the fifth gestational week. Horseshoe kidney with fibrous isthmus is believed to originate from fusion after the fifth week, before renal ascent (15). Most horseshoe kidneys are located in the pelvis or at the lower lumbar vertebral level, as ascent is further prevented when the fused kidney reaches the junction of the aorta and inferior mesenteric artery.

Complications of horseshoe kidneys include obstructive uropathy, calculi, and urinary tract infection. Horseshoe kidneys are associated with other genitourinary anomalies as well as renal tumors (16). Wilms' tumor is the most common, but renal cell carcinoma, adenocarcinoma, transitional cell carcinoma, malignant teratoma, oncocytoma, angiomyolipoma, and carcinoid have all been reported.

TABLE 6.8. SYNDROMES ASSOCIATED WITH HORSESHOE KIDNEY

Acro-facial dysostosis syndrome
Agnathia-holoprosencephaly syndrome
Antley-Bixler syndrome
Bowen-Conradi syndrome
Caudal regression syndrome
Diabetic mother, infant of
Fanconi anemia syndrome
Fetal alcohol syndrome
Focal dermal hypoplasia
Juberg-Hayward syndrome
Kabuki syndrome
Pallister-Hall syndrome
Pyloric stenosis
Roberts syndrome
Thalidomide embryopathy
Trisomy 13, 18, 21, and 22
Turner syndrome
VATER (VACTERL) association
Weyers syndrome
Wilms' tumor

VACTERL, vertebral, anal, cardiac, tracheal, esophageal, renal, limb; VATER, vertebral, anus, tracheoesophageal, radial, and renal.

Table 6.8 lists syndromes associated with horseshoe kidney. For more details of these disorders, see Tables 6.1 and 6.2.

Dysplasia and Polycystic Kidney

Renal dysplasia (17–19) and polycystic kidney disease are extensively covered in Chapters 5 and 36, respectively. Table 6.9 summarizes well-known syndromes with renal dysplasia/cystic kidney. (See Tables 6.1 through 6.3.)

Obstruction and Hydronephrosis

Urinary obstruction is a complication of a primary anomaly, which can be stenosis or atresia of the ureteropelvic junction, ureter, or urethra; a poorly functional bladder causing stasis or reflux; a malformed dilated ureteral end (ureterocele); or extrinsic compression by other structures (e.g., anomalous blood vessels or tumors). Hydronephrosis and pelvocaliectasis are the most common urinary tract abnormalities detected by prenatal ultrasound examination (20). (See Chapter 4.)

Table 6.10 provides a list of syndromes commonly associated with obstruction and hydronephrosis. (See Tables 6.1 through 6.3.)

Ureter Defects

Duplication

Double ureters or collecting systems are caused by duplication of the ureteric bud. Early duplication results in a duplicated kidney, which is usually smaller and fused with

TABLE 6.9. SYNDROMES ASSOCIATED WITH RENAL DYSPLASIA/CYSTIC KIDNEY

Acro-renal-mandibular syndrome
Alagille syndrome (arteriohepatic dysplasia)
Baller-Gerold syndrome
Bardet-Biedl syndrome
Beckwith-Wiedemann syndrome
Branchio-oto-renal syndrome
Campomelic dysplasia
Carbohydrate deficient glycoprotein syndrome
CHARGE association
Chondrodysplasia punctata, nonrhizomelic
Cloacal exstrophy
Cornelia de Lange syndrome
Diabetic mother, infant of
Ectrodactyly-ectodermal dysplasia-clefting syndrome
Fanconi anemia syndrome
Fetal alcohol syndrome
Fraser (cryptophthalmos) syndrome
Fryns syndrome
Glutaric aciduria, type II
Goldenhar syndrome
Hajdu-Cheney syndrome
Ivemark syndrome
Jeune syndrome
Joubert syndrome
Kaufman-McKusick syndrome
Lenz microphthalmia syndrome
Leprechaunism (Donohue) syndrome
Limb–body wall complex
Marden-Walker syndrome
Marfan syndrome
Marshall-Smith syndrome
Meckel-Gruber syndrome
MURCS association
Noonan syndrome
OEIS complex
Oral-facial-digital syndrome, types I and VI
Pallister-Hall syndrome
Pallister-Killian syndrome
Potter (oligohydramnios) sequence
Prune-belly syndrome
Renal adysplasia
Roberts syndrome
Rokitansky-Mayer-Kuster-Hauser syndrome
Rubella syndrome, congenital
Short rib–polydactyly syndrome
Smith-Lemli-Opitz syndrome
Thalidomide embryopathy
Trisomy 8, 9, 13, 18, 21, and 22
Tuberous sclerosis
VATER (VACTERL) association
von Hippel–Lindau disease
Zellweger and pseudo-Zellweger syndromes

CHARGE, coloboma, heart disease, atresia choanae, retarded growth and development, genital hypoplasia, and ear anomalies; MURCS, müllerian, renal, cervicothoracic somite abnormalities; OEIS, omphalocele-cloacal exstrophy-imperforate anus-spinal dysraphism; VACTERL, vertebral, anal, cardiac, tracheal, esophageal, renal, limb; VATER, vertebral, anus, tracheoesophageal, radial, and renal.

TABLE 6.10. SYNDROMES ASSOCIATED WITH HYDRONEPHROSIS OR HYDROURETER

Acro-cephalo-polysyndactylous dysplasia
Acrorenal syndrome, Dieker and Johnson-Munson types
Barbet-Biedl syndrome
Branchio-oto-renal syndrome
Campomelic dysplasia
Caudal duplication and regression syndromes
CHARGE association
Cloacal exstrophy
Coffin-Siris syndrome
Cornelia de Lange syndrome
Crossed ectopia-pelvic lipomatosis syndrome
Diabetic mother, infant of
Ectrodactyly-ectodermal dysplasia-clefting syndrome
Fanconi anemia syndrome
Fetal alcohol syndrome
Goldenhar syndrome
Hydrolethalus syndrome
Kabuki syndrome
Kaufman-McKusick syndrome
Megacystis-microcolon syndrome
Noonan syndrome
Ochoa syndrome
OEIS complex
Pallister-Hall syndrome
Polydactyly–obstructive uropathy syndrome
Pyloric stenosis
Roberts syndrome
Schinzel-Giedion syndrome
Sirenomelia sequence
VATER (VACTERL) association

CHARGE, coloboma, heart disease, atresia choanae, retarded growth and development, genital hypoplasia, and ear anomalies; OEIS, omphalocele-cloacal exstrophy-imperforate anus-spinal dysraphism; VACTERL, vertebral, anal, cardiac, tracheal, esophageal, renal, limb; VATER, vertebral, anus, tracheoesophageal, radial, and renal.

the ipsilateral kidney and has ureters that enter into the bladder separately. Duplication that occurs later results in double ureters that may have separate openings into the bladder. On rare occasions, one of the ureters may have an ectopic opening into the vagina, vestibule, or urethra. Most double ureters are crossed, and the ureter from the higher pelvis enters the bladder more caudally. Duplication anomalies are common but usually asymptomatic; therefore, they often remain undetected. One autopsy study reported the prevalence of duplication anomalies to be as high as 1 in 25, with females approximately four times more likely to be affected than males (21). Unilateral duplication is five to six times more common than bilateral duplication (3). Double ureters are commonly associated with vesicoureteral reflux due to their ectopic opening into the urinary bladder or the ureterocele (22). In addition, ureteric obstruction can occur at the level of the vesicoureteric junction or that of the ureteropelvic junction.

Table 6.11 summarizes syndromes associated with duplication, and Tables 6.1 through 6.3 provide clinical information about these disorders.

TABLE 6.11. SYNDROMES ASSOCIATED WITH DUPLICATION OF URETERS OR COLLECTING SYSTEMS

Achondrogenesis
Acromelic frontonasal dysplasia
Adrenogenital syndrome
Antley-Bixler syndrome
Bardet-Biedl syndrome
Bowen-Conradi syndrome
Branchio-oto-ureteral syndrome
Braun-Bayer syndrome
Caudal duplication syndrome
Diabetic mother, infant of
Drash (Denys-Drash) syndrome
Ectrodactyly-ectodermal dysplasia-clefting syndrome
Fanconi anemia syndrome
Fetal alcohol syndrome
Frontometaphyseal dysplasia
G (Opitz-Frias) syndrome
Goldenhar syndrome
Kabuki syndrome
Kaufman-McKusick syndrome
Mammo-renal syndrome
Noonan syndrome
Ochoa syndrome
Perlman syndrome
Poland anomaly
Prune-belly syndrome
Robinow syndrome
Rubinstein-Taybi syndrome
Trisomy 8, 9, 13, 18, and 21
Turner syndrome
Weyers syndrome

Hydroureter

Hydroureter, or megaloureter, is caused by distal obstruction and is usually found with hydronephrosis, except in ureteropelvic junction obstruction. Hydroureter has the same etiology as hydronephrosis (see Obstruction and Hydronephrosis).

Bladder Defects

Anomalies of the bladder are rare. These include agenesis, hypoplasia, diverticulae, and dilatation or megacystis caused by distal obstruction or by nonobstructive causes. Agenesis of the bladder is usually associated with severe developmental anomalies of the urinary tract, such as in sirenomelia and caudal regression syndrome. Hypoplastic bladder can be found in conditions associated with bilateral renal agenesis because no urine is produced. Bladder diverticulae have heterogeneous causes. They may result from an intrinsic defect in the bladder wall (e.g., in cutis laxa or Ehlers-Danlos, Ochoa, occipital horn, and Williams syndromes). They can also be caused by increased intravesicular pressure from distal obstruction or by persistent urachus. For information about specific syndromes associated with bladder diverticulae, see Tables 6.1 through 6.3.

TABLE 6.12. SYNDROMES ASSOCIATED WITH BLADDER EXSTROPHY

Axial mesodermal dysplasia
Caudal duplication syndrome
Caudal regression syndrome
Cloacal exstrophy
Frontonasal dysplasia
OEIS complex
Sirenomelia sequence
Syndactyly, type V
Trisomy 18

OEIS, omphalocele-cloacal exstrophy-imperforate anus-spinal dysraphism.

Bladder exstrophy refers to a urinary bladder that is open anteriorly because of the lack of abdominal wall closure. It is usually associated with anomalies of the contiguous structures including epispadias and separation of the pubic rami. Exstrophy is believed to result from an overdeveloped cloacal membrane that interferes with inferolateral abdominal mesenchymal closure. Therefore, when the cloacal membrane ruptures, the inferior abdominal wall has not completely closed and the bladder cavity is exposed. It has been suggested that bladder exstrophy belongs to the spectrum of omphalocele-cloacal exstrophy-imperforate anus-spinal dysraphism complex (23,24). The extent of anomalies is determined by the timing of the cloacal membrane rupture. Rupture that occurs after the separation of cloaca by the urorectal septum results in bladder exstrophy, whereas one that occurs before the separation results in the more severe cloacal exstrophy and omphalocele-cloacal exstrophy-imperforate anus-spinal dysraphism complex. Bladder exstrophy is six times more common in males.

Table 6.12 lists syndromes associated with bladder exstrophy, and Tables 6.1 through 6.3 provide information about these disorders.

Urethral Defects

Agenesis and Atresia

Urethral agenesis is rare. It predominantly occurs in males, reflecting the complex embryogenesis of the male urethra. Urethral agenesis is often associated with the bladder obstruction sequence. Table 6.13 lists syndromes associated with urethral agenesis, and clinical information about these disorders is summarized in Tables 6.1 through 6.3.

Duplication

Duplication refers to complete or partial duplication of the urethra, which is a rare anomaly, found only in a few syn-

TABLE 6.13. SYNDROMES ASSOCIATED WITH URETHRAL AGENESIS

Aase syndrome
Acrorenal syndrome, Dieker and Johnson-Munson types
Adrenogenital syndrome
Caudal regression syndrome
Cocaine, maternal use
Hydrolethalus syndrome
Kaufman-McKusick syndrome
Limb–body wall complex
Meckel-Gruber syndrome
Occipital horn syndrome
Ochoa syndrome
OEIS complex
Potter (oligohydramnios) sequence
Prune-belly syndrome
Renal adysplasia
Russell-Silver syndrome
Short rib–polydactyly syndrome, types 1–3
Sirenomelia sequence
Sotos syndrome
Townes-Brocks syndrome
Trisomy 21

OEIS, omphalocele-cloacal exstrophy-imperforate anus-spinal dysraphism.

dromes. Those syndromes associated with urethral duplication are listed in Table 6.14, and their findings are provided in Tables 6.1 through 6.3.

Posterior Urethral Valves

Posterior urethral valves refer to abnormal mucosal folds that obstruct urine flow. Posterior urethral valves can be suspected prenatally when a dilated bladder is seen in association with obstructive uropathy. Recently, the "keyhole sign" has been demonstrated by prenatal ultrasonography in fetuses with subsequently confirmed posterior urethral valves (25). A voiding cystourethrogram or endoscopy is usually required for a definitive diagnosis. The embryogenesis of posterior urethral valves is unknown. Proposed hypotheses include an overdeveloped posterior urethral fold, a remnant of the mesonephric duct, and an anomalous opening of the ejaculatory duct. Table 6.15 lists syndromes in which posterior urethral valves can be seen, and the other findings in these disorders are provided in Tables 6.1 through 6.3.

TABLE 6.14. SYNDROMES ASSOCIATED WITH URETHRAL DUPLICATION

Amniotic band disruption sequence
Limb–body wall complex
OEIS complex
Prune-belly syndrome

OEIS, omphalocele-cloacal exstrophy-imperforate anus-spinal dysraphism.

TABLE 6.15. SYNDROMES ASSOCIATED WITH POSTERIOR URETHRAL VALVES

Acrorenal syndrome, Johnson-Munson type
Caudal regression syndrome
Diabetic mother, infant of
Kaufman-McKusick syndrome
Limb–body wall complex
Neurofibromatosis, type I
Ochoa syndrome
OEIS complex
Polydactyly–obstructive uropathy syndrome
Potter (oligohydramnios) sequence
Prune-belly syndrome
Renal adysplasia
Rubinstein-Taybi syndrome
Sirenomelia sequence
Townes-Brocks syndrome
VATER (VACTERL) association

OEIS, omphalocele-cloacal exstrophy-imperforate anus-spinal dysraphism; VACTERL, vertebral, anal, cardiac, tracheal, esophageal, renal, limb; VATER, vertebral, anus, tracheoesophageal, radial, and renal.

ASSOCIATIONS AND SEQUENCES INVOLVING THE URINARY TRACT

A number of associations and sequences involve anomalies of the urinary tract that are important for both diagnosis and clinical management. For this reason, such conditions are described in more detail in this section in addition to the information presented in Tables 6.1 and 6.2.

Association of Vertebral, Anus, Tracheoesophageal, Radial, and Renal Anomalies

VATER is an acronym used to designate a nonrandom occurrence of vertebral defects, imperforate anus, tracheoesophageal fistula, and radial and renal anomalies (26,27). *VACTERL* (vertebral, anal, cardiac, tracheal, esophageal, renal, limb), another acronym, has been proposed to broaden the spectrum of VATER to include cardiac defects and limb anomalies. The term *VATER* is not a diagnosis per se, but the designation provides clues for potentially associated anomalies and for recurrence risk counseling when no specific syndromic diagnosis can be made. Causes of VATER association include chromosomal disorders (e.g., trisomy 18), genetic syndromes (e.g., Goldenhar and Holt-Oram syndromes), and teratogenic exposures (e.g., infants of diabetic mothers and fetal alcohol syndrome). Recently, a family with a mitochondrial DNA mutation was identified in which the daughter was born with VACTERL association, and her mother and sister had classic mitochondrial cytopathy (28). Thus, all patients suspected to have VATER association should have a chromosome analysis, a careful family and prenatal exposure history, and a thorough examination for dysmorphic features. The spectrum of anomalies seen in VATER is broad. Associated renal anomalies are usually agenesis, ectopy, or obstruction (26,27).

Because there is apparent causal heterogeneity for VATER association, the inheritance pattern and recurrence risk vary with the cause. VATER association is usually sporadic, with an empirical recurrence risk of 1 to 3% when a specific cause cannot be identified (29). Autosomal recessive and X-linked inheritance have been reported for subsets of patients (e.g., for VATER with hydrocephalus), in which recurrence risk can be as high as 25% (28).

Association of Coloboma, Heart Disease, Atresia Choanae, Retarded Growth and Development, Genital Hypoplasia, and Ear Anomalies

CHARGE is an acronym used to designate an association of coloboma of iris, choroid or retina, heart defects, atresia choanae, retarded growth and development, genital anomalies or hypogonadism, and ear anomalies or deafness (30–33). In addition, unilateral facial palsy is a common finding. Renal anomalies found in CHARGE association include ectopy, dysplasia, renal agenesis, and ureteric anomalies. The presence of two or more anomalies associated with CHARGE association should prompt a search for the others. To prevent overuse of the term, it was suggested that at least three anomalies are required for the term *CHARGE* to be applied, and one of the anomalies should be either coloboma or choanal atresia (31). CHARGE association has phenotypic overlap with VATER association. Similar to VATER, a specific cause should be sought, although familial forms of CHARGE have been reported more often than for VATER, with recessive, dominant, and X-linked inheritance patterns identified. Conditions with anomalies in the spectrum of CHARGE include trisomy 13, trisomy 18, Wolf-Hirschhorn (deletion 4p), cat-eye, Treacher-Collins, velocardiofacial, Apert, Crouzon, and Saethre-Chotzen syndromes. Therefore, a careful physical examination for malformations and dysmorphic features should be conducted, and chromosome analysis including specific fluorescence *in situ* hybridization probes for velocardiofacial syndrome (deletion 22q) and 4p deletion should be performed. Because most cases of CHARGE association are sporadic, the empirical recurrence risk is low (30,33). In familial forms of CHARGE association, the recurrence risk is substantially higher and can be as much as 25%.

Association of Müllerian, Renal, Cervicothoracic Somite Abnormalities

MURCS refers to the rare association of müllerian duct aplasia, renal aplasia, and cervicothoracic somite dysplasia (34). Anomalies include absence of the proximal two-thirds of the vagina, uterine hypoplasia or aplasia, unilateral renal agenesis, ectopic kidney, renal dysplasia, C5-T1 vertebral anomalies (hypoplasia of vertebrae, fusion, hemivertebrae, and butterfly vertebrae), and short stature. Additional anomalies are common, including rib defects, facial asymmetry, limb anomalies, hearing loss, and brain anomalies (e.g., encephalocele and cerebellar cysts) (35).

The pathogenesis of MURCS association is unknown, but it is believed to be related to defects in the paraxial mesoderm, which gives rise to the cervicothoracic somites and the adjoining intermediate mesoderm. Most patients are diagnosed because of primary amenorrhea or infertility associated with normal secondary sexual characteristics, followed by recognition of reproductive organ atresia. MURCS association is usually sporadic. A report of vertebral and renal anomalies associated with azoospermia was proposed to represent the male version of MURCS association (36).

Oligohydramnios Sequence

Oligohydramnios of whatever cause leads to a recurrent pattern of abnormalities that has been called the *oligohydramnios sequence* (3,5). Oligohydramnios may be caused by decreased production of fetal urine from bilateral renal agenesis or dysplasia or by urinary obstruction, or it can result from amniotic fluid leakage. When oligohydramnios is prolonged and severe, the condition is lethal because of pulmonary hypoplasia. Moderate oligohydramnios from amniotic fluid leakage may result in a liveborn child with multiple congenital anomalies. These anomalies are both malformations and deformations. Intrauterine constraint leads to mechanical compression that leads to the characteristic flat facial profile (Potter's facies), limb deformities (e.g., talipes equinovarus), and intrauterine growth retardation. Decreased fetal movement as a result of intrauterine constraint causes multiple joint contractures (arthrogryposis). Breech presentation is common. Pulmonary hypoplasia can be the consequence of compression of the chest cavity coupled with decreased inspiration of amniotic fluid. Because the initial defect has many causes, recurrence risk is based on the underlying defect. When oligohydramnios is due to nonsyndromic bilateral renal agenesis or dysgenesis, related renal malformations occur at an increased frequency in first-degree relatives (13), and recurrence risk can be as high as 4 to 9%. The recurrence risk can be as high as 25% for an autosomal-recessive disorder causing bilateral renal agenesis or dysplasia.

Urethral Obstruction Sequence

The initial defect in this sequence is obstruction of the urethra leading to dilation of the proximal urinary tract, bladder distension, and hydroureter (3,5,37). Obstruction of urine flow interferes with normal nephrogenesis, resulting in renal dysplasia. Other potential anomalies related to bladder distension include cryptorchidism, malrotation of colon, persistent urachus, and limb deficiency caused by iliac vessel compression. In addition, oligohydramnios results from lack of urine and leads to the oligohydramnios sequence.

Prune-belly syndrome (37,38) is a rare entity referring to a constellation of anomalies that includes megacystis, abdominal wall muscle deficiency, hydroureter, renal dysplasia, and characteristic wrinkled abdominal skin. This condition, previously believed to be a form of urethral obstruction sequence, is, in fact, a nonobstructive cause of bladder distension that results from a malformation, thus now being properly designated a syndrome (25).

The most common cause of urethral obstruction is posterior urethral valves, but urethral agenesis/atresia or bladder neck obstruction can also be the cause. This anomaly occurs more often in males, with a male to female ratio of 20:1. Survival is rare in fetuses with complete obstruction, and severe urinary tract anomalies are always present in those who are liveborn. Prenatal diagnosis by ultrasound examination can detect the abnormally dilated bladder at the beginning of the second trimester (39), and intrauterine urinary decompression procedures, such as vesicoamniotic shunts, are options for treatment to decrease the occurrence of pulmonary hypoplasia, although their benefits have not been unequivocally shown (40,41). (See Chapter 4.)

Sirenomelia Sequence

Sirenomelia is a malformation characterized by the presence of a single lower extremity with posterior alignment of the knees and feet, sacral agenesis and other lower vertebral defects, imperforate anus and rectal agenesis, and absence of external and internal genitalia (42). The current view of the embryogenesis is that sirenomelia results from a vascular steal phenomenon (43). This is supported by the presence of abnormal vasculature in the caudal part of affected embryos. A single large vessel originating from the aorta, a derivative of the vitelline artery complex, connects the iliac arteries to the placenta rather than the two normal umbilical arteries. The area caudal to the origin of this vessel has minimal blood supply because of the lack of aortic branches. Therefore, a "vascular steal phenomenon" is generated, leading to a vascular disruption sequence.

Sirenomelia is a rare condition and has a broad spectrum of anomalies. Virtually any urinary tract anomaly can occur in sirenomelia sequence. Renal agenesis occurs in two-thirds of cases, and a variable degree of renal dysplasia is present in one-third of cases (3). Absence of the ureter and bladder are common. All cases of sirenomelia are sporadic and almost uniformly fatal because of pulmonary hypoplasia. Sirenomelia has been noted with an increased frequency among monozygotic twins in which only one of the twins is usually affected.

REFERENCES

1. Schulman J, Edmonds LD, McClearn AB, et al. Surveillance for and comparison of birth defect prevalences in two geographic areas—United States, 1983–88. *MMWR CDC Surveill Summ* 1993;42:1–7.
2. Metropolitan Atlanta Congenital Defects Program and Birth Defects Monitoring Program—congenital malformations surveillance. *Teratology* 1993;48:664–698.
3. Van Allen MI. Urinary tract. In: Stevenson RE, Hall JG, Goodman RM, eds. *Human malformations and related anomalies.* New York: Oxford University Press, 1993;11:501–550.
4. Gorlin RJ, Cohen MM Jr, Levin LS. *Syndromes of the head and neck,* 3rd ed. New York: Oxford University Press, 1990.
5. Jones KL. *Smith's recognizable patterns of human malformation,* 5th ed. Philadelphia: WB Saunders, 1997.
6. Winter RM, Baraitser M. *London dysmorphology database.* London: Oxford University Press, 1995.
7. Online Mendelian Inheritance in Man, OMIM™. National Center for Biotechnology Information. Available at: http://www.ncbi.nlm.nih.gov/omim/. Accessed April 2003.
8. Nicolaides KH, Cheng HH, Abbas A, et al. Fetal renal defects: associated malformations and chromosomal defects. *Fetal Diagn Ther* 1992;7:1–11.
9. Robson WLM, Leung AKC, Rogers RC. Unilateral renal agenesis. *Adv Pediatr* 1995;42:575–592.
10. Ekblom P. Genetics of kidney development. *Curr Opin Nephrol Hypertens* 1996;5:282–287.
11. Mesrobian HG, Rushton HG, Bulas D. Unilateral renal agenesis may result from in utero regression of multicystic renal dysplasia. *J Urol* 1993;150(2 Pt 2):793–794.
12. Atiyeh B, Husmann D, Baum M. Contralateral renal abnormalities in patients with renal agenesis and noncystic renal dysplasia. *Pediatrics* 1993;91:812–815.
13. Roodhooft AM, Birriholz JC, Holmes LB. Familial nature of congenital absence and severe dysgenesis of both kidneys. *N Engl J Med* 1984;310:1341–1345.
14. N'Guessen G, Stephens FD, Pick J. Congenital superior ectopic (thoracic) kidney. *Urology* 1984;24:219–228.
15. Domenech-Mateu JM, Gonzalez-Compta X. Horseshoe kidney: a new theory on its embryogenesis based on the study of a 16-mm human embryo. *Anat Rec* 1988;244:408–417.
16. Hohenfellner M, Schultz-Lampel D, Lampel A, et al. Tumor in the horseshoe kidney: clinical implications and review of embryogenesis. *J Urol* 1992;147:1098–1102.
17. Fisher C, Smith JF. Renal dysplasia in nephrectomy specimens from adolescents and adults. *J Clin Pathol* 1975;28:879–890.
18. Gotolt T, Koyanagi T, Tokunaka S. Pathology of ureterorenal units in various ureteral anomalies with particular reference to the genesis of renal dysplasia. *Int Urol Nephrol* 1987;19:231–243.
19. Winyard P, Chitty L. Dysplastic and polycystic kidneys: diagnosis, associations and management. *Prenat Diagn* 2001;21:924–935.
20. Hash F, Fontaine E, Muller F, et al. Antenatal diagnosis of obstructive uropathy: state of the art. *Prog Urol* 1994;4:398–407.
21. Campbell MF, Harrison JH. Anomalies of the ureter. In: Campbell MF, Harrison JH, eds. *Urology*, 3rd ed, vol. 2. Philadelphia: WB Saunders, 1970:1488, 1800.
22. Whitten SM, Wilcox DT. Duplex systems. *Prenat Diagn* 2001;21:952–957.

23. Pang D. Sacral agenesis and caudal spinal cord malformations. *Neurosurgery* 1993;32:755–778.
24. Carey JC, Greenbaum B, Hall BD. The OEIS complex (omphalocele, exstrophy, imperforate anus, spinal defects). *Birth Defects Orig Artic Ser* 1978;14(6B):253–263.
25. McHugo J, Whittle M. Enlarged fetal bladders: aetiology, management and outcome. *Prenat Diagn* 2001;21:958–963.
26. Ueliling DT, Gilbert E, Chesney R. Urologic implications of the VATER association. *J Urol* 1983;129:352–354.
27. Evans JA, Stranc LC, Kaplan P, et al. VACTERL with hydrocephalus: further delineation of the syndrome(s). *Am J Med Genet* 1989;34:177–182.
28. Damian MS, Seibel P, Schachenmayr W, et al. VACTERL with the mitochondrial np 3243 point mutation. *Am J Med Genet* 1996;62:398–403.
29. Harper PS. *Practical genetic counseling*, 3rd ed. London: Butterworths, 1988.
30. Pagon RA, Graham JM, Zonana J, et al. Coloboma, congenital heart disease and choanal atresia with multiple anomalies, CHARGE association. *J Pediatr* 1981;99:223–227.
31. Harris J, Robert E, Kallen B. Epidemiology of choanal atresia with special reference to the CHARGE association. *Pediatrics* 1997;99:363–367.
32. Davenport SLH, Hefner MA, Mitchell JA. The spectrum of clinical features in CHARGE syndrome. *Clin Genet* 1986; 29:298–310.
33. Toriello HV. CHARGE association. *J Am Acad Audiol* 1995;6:47–53.
34. Braun-Quentin C, Billes C, Bowing B. MURCS association: case report and review. *J Med Genet* 1996;33:618–620.
35. Lin HJ, Cornford ME, Hu B, et al. Occipital encephalocele and MURCS association: case report and review of central nervous system anomalies in MURCS patients. *Am J Med Genet* 1996;61:59–62.
36. Wellesley DG, Slaney SF. MURCS in a male? *J Med Genet* 1995;32:314–315.
37. Terada S, Suzuki N, Uchide K, et al. Etiology of prune belly syndrome: evidence of megalocystic origin in an early fetus. *Obstet Gynecol* 1994;83:865–868.
38. Sutherland RS, Mevorach RA, Kogan BA. The Prune belly syndrome: current insights. *Pediatr Nephrol* 1995;9:770–778.
39. Cazorla E, Ruiz F, Abad A, et al. Prune belly syndrome: early antenatal diagnosis. *Eur J Obstet Gynecol Reprod Biol* 1997;72:31–33.
40. Freedman AL, Bukowski TP, Smith CA. Fetal therapy for obstructive uropathy: diagnosis specific outcome. *J Urol* 1996;156:720–723.
41. Agarwal SK, Fisk NM. In utero therapy for lower urinary tract obstruction. *Prenat Diagn* 2001;21:970–976.
42. Langer B, Stoll C, Nicolau R, et al. Sirenomelia and situs inversus: case report and review of the literature. *Fetal Diagn Ther* 1996;11:79–84.
43. Stevenson RE, Jones KL, Phelan MC, et al. Vascular steal: the pathogenetic mechanism producing sirenomelia and associated defects of the viscera and soft tissues. *Pediatrics* 1986;78:451–457.
44. Abruzzo MA, Erickson RP. A new syndrome of cleft palate associated with coloboma, hypospadia, deafness, short stature, and radial synostosis. *J Med Genet* 1977;14:76–80.
45. Nevin NC, Herron B, Armstrong MJ. An 18 week fetus with Elejalde syndrome (acrocephalopolydactylous dysplasia). *Clin Dysmorphol* 1994;3:180–184.
46. Evans JA, Vitez M, Czeizel A. Pattern of acrorenal malformation associations. *Am J Med Genet* 1992;44:413–419.
47. Halal F, Desgranges MF, Leduc B, et al. Acro-renal-mandibular syndrome. *Am J Med Genet* 1980;5:277–284.
48. Halal F, Honisy M, Perreault G. Acrorenal-ocular syndrome: autosomal dominant thumb hypoplasia, renal ectopia, and eye defect. *Am J Med Genet* 1984;17:753–762.
49. Schuhl H. Aglossia-adactylia. A propos of a case. Review of the literature. *Ann Pediatr (Paris)* 1986;33:137–140.
50. Pauli RM, Pettersen JC, Arya S. Familial agnathia-holoprosencephaly. *Am J Med Genet* 1983;14:677–698.
51. Martin SR, Garel L, Alvarez F. Alagille's syndrome associated with cystic renal disease. *Arch Dis Child* 1996;74:232–235.
52. Kashtan CE. Clinical and molecular diagnosis of Alport syndrome. *Proc Assoc Am Phys* 1995;107:306–313.
53. Alsing A, Christensen C. A typical macular coloboma (dysplasia) associated with familial juvenile nephronophthisis and skeletal abnormality. *Ophthal Paed Genet* 1988;9:149–155.
54. Millay RH, Weleber RG, Heckenlively JR. Ophthalmologic and systemic manifestations of Alstrom's disease. *Am J Ophthalmol* 1986;102:482–490.
55. Lubinsky M, Angle C, Marsh PW, et al. Syndrome of amelogenesis imperfecta, nephrocalcinosis, impaired renal concentration, and possible abnormality of calcium metabolism. *Am J Med Genet* 1985;20:233–243.
56. Purcell JJ, Rodrigues M, Chishti MI, et al. Lattice corneal dystrophy associated with familial systemic amyloidosis (Meretoja's syndrome). *Ophthalmology* 1983;90:1512–1517.
57. Barr M Jr. Teratogen update: angiotensin-converting enzyme inhibitors. *Teratology* 1994;50:399–409.
58. Clericuzio CL. Clinical phenotypes and Wilms' tumor. *Med Pediatr Oncol* 1993;21:182–187.
59. Stewart FJ, Nevin NC, Brown S. Axial mesodermal dysplasia spectrum. *Am J Med Genet* 1993;45:426–429.
60. Baldellou A, Bone J, Tamparillas M, et al. Congenital hypoparathyroidism, ocular coloboma, unilateral renal agenesis and dysmorphic features. *Genet Couns* 1991;2:245–247.
61. Dallapiccola B, Zelante L, Mingarelli R, et al. Baller-Gerold syndrome: case report and clinical and radiological review. *Am J Med Genet* 1992;42:365–368.
62. Barakat AY, D'Albora JB, Martin MM, et al. Familial nephrosis, nerve deafness, and hypoparathyroidism. *J Pediatr* 1977;91:61–64.
63. Ozer G, Yuksel B, Suleymanova D, et al. Clinical features of Bardet-Biedl syndrome. *Acta Pediatr Jpn* 1995;37:233–236.
64. O'dea D, Parfrey PS, Harnett JD, et al. The importance of renal impairment in the natural history of Bardet-Biedl syndrome. *Am J Kidney Dis* 1996;27:776–783.
65. Elliot M, Bayly R, Cole T, et al. Clinical features and natural history of Beckwith-Wiedemann syndrome: presentation of 74 new cases. *Clin Genet* 1994;46:168–174.
66. Mulvihill DM, Mercado MG, Boineau FG. Beckwith-Wiedemann syndrome and its association with type 3 polycystic kidney disease. *Pediatr Nephrol* 1989;3:286–289.
67. Ponte P, Katz SM, Falkner B. Beckwith-Wiedemann syndrome. Renal pathology at 4 months of age. *Clin Pediatr* 1990;29:393–397.

68. Watanabe H, Yamanaka T. A possible relationship between Beckwith-Wiedemann syndrome, urinary tract anomaly and prune belly syndrome. *Clin Genet* 1990;38:410–415.
69. Moller DE, Flier JS. Insulin resistance-mechanisms, syndromes, and implications. *N Engl J Med* 1991;325:938–948.
70. Langer LO Jr, Nishino R, Yamaguchi A, et al. Brachymesomelia-renal syndrome. *Am J Med Genet* 1983;15:57–65.
71. Braddock SR, Carey JC. A new syndrome: congenital thrombocytopenia, Robin sequence, agenesis of the corpus callosum, distinctive facies and developmental delay. *Clin Dysmorphol* 1994;3:75–81.
72. Lin AE, Gorlin RJ, Lurie M et al. Further delineation of the branchio-oculo-facial syndrome. *Am J Med Genet* 1995;56:42–59.
73. Chitayat D, Hodgkinson KA, Chen MY, et al. Branchio-oto-renal syndrome: further delineation of an underdiagnosed syndrome. *Am J Med Genet* 1992;43:970–975.
74. Fraser FC, Ayme S, Halal F, et al. Autosomal dominant duplication of the renal collecting system, hearing loss, and external ear anomalies: a new syndrome? *Am J Med Genet* 1983;14:473–478.
75. Braun FC, Bayer JF. Familial nephrosis associated with deafness and congenital urinary tract anomalies in siblings. *J Pediatr* 1962;60:33–41.
76. Dominguez R, Rott J, Castillo M, et al. Caudal duplication syndrome. *Am J Dis Child* 1993;147:1048–1052.
77. Duncan PA, Shapiro LR, Mein RM. Sacrococcygeal dysgenesis association. *Am J Med Genet* 1991;41:153–161.
78. Adra A, Cordero D, Mejides A, et al. Caudal regression syndrome: etiopathogenesis, prenatal diagnosis, and perinatal management. *Obstet Gynecol Surv* 1994;49:508–516.
79. Passarge E, MeAdams AJ. Cerebro-hepato-renal syndrome. A newly recognized hereditary disorder of multiple congenital defects, including sudanophilic leukodystrophy, cirrhosis of the liver, and polycystic kidneys. *J Pediatr* 1967;71:691–702.
80. Matsuzaka T, Sakuragawa N, Nakayama H, et al. Cerebro-oculo-hepato-renal syndrome (Arima's syndrome), a distinct clinicopathological entity. *J Child Neurol* 1986;1:338–346.
81. Opitz JM, Lowry RE, Holmes TM, et al. Hutterite cerebro-osteo-nephrodysplasia; autosomal recessive trait in a Lehrerleut Hutterite family from Montana. *Am J Med Genet* 1985;22:521–529.
82. Caraballo A, Lopez Barrios A, Martin Govantes J, et al. Thoracic asphyxiant dystrophy and renal disease. *An Esp Pediatr* 1977;10:88–95.
83. Brueton LA, Dillon MJ, Winter RM. Ellis van Creveld syndrome, Jeune syndrome, and renal-hepatic-pancreatic dysplasia: separate entities or disease spectrum? *J Med Genet* 1990;27:252–255.
84. Chasnoff IJ, Chisum GM, Kaplan WE. Maternal cocaine use and genitourinary tract malformations. *Teratology* 1988;37:201–204.
85. Goswami RK, Rangnekar GV, Varshney S, et al. Crossed renal ectopia with pelvic lipomatosis: a new syndrome involving chromosome 1. *Hum Genet* 1992;89:666–670.
86. Czeizel A, Losonei A. Split hand, obstructive urinary anomalies and spina bifida or diaphragmatic defect syndrome with autosomal dominant inheritance. *Hum Genet* 1987; 77:203–204.
87. Jackson L, Kline AD, Barr MA, et al. de Lange syndrome: a clinical review of 310 individuals. *Am J Med Genet* 1993; 147:940–946.
88. Lynch SA, Wright C. Sirenomelia, limb reduction defects, cardiovascular malformation, renal agenesis in an infant born to a diabetic mother. *Clin Dysmorphol* 1997;6:75–80.
89. Grix A Jr, Curry C, Hall BD. Patterns of multiple malformations in infants of diabetic mothers. *Birth Defects Orig Artic Ser* 1982;18:55–77.
90. Mueller RF. Denys-Drash syndrome. *J Med Genet* 1994; 31:471–477.
91. London R, Heredia RM, Israel J. Urinary tract involvement in EEC syndrome. *Am J Dis Child* 1985;l39:1191–1193.
92. Turi S, Kobor J, Erdos A, et al. Hereditary nephritis, platelet disorders and deafness—Epstein's syndrome. *Pediatr Nephrol* 1992;6:38–43.
93. Nevin NC, Hill AE, Carson DJ. Facio-cardio-renal (Eastman-Bixler) syndrome. *Am J Med Genet* 1991;40:31–33.
94. Glaze A, Fraser FC. Spectrum of anomalies in Fanconi anemia. *J Med Genet* 1982;19:412–416.
95. Gordon-Smith EC, Rutherford TR. Fanconi anemia-constitutional aplastic anemia (Review). *Semin Hematol* 1991;28: 104–112.
96. Taylor CL, Jones KL, Jones MC, et al. Incidence of renal anomalies in children prenatally exposed to ethanol. *Pediatrics* 1994;94:209–212.
97. Davies RS, Carty H, Pierro A. Infantile myofibromatosis-a review. *Br J Radiol* 1994;67:619–623.
98. Gattuso J, Patton MA, Baraitser M. The clinical spectrum of the Fraser syndrome: report of three new cases and review. *J Med Genet* 1987;24:549–555.
99. Bailey WA, Zwingman TA, Reznik M et al. End-stage renal disease and primary hypogonadism associated with a 46,XX karyotype. *Am J Dis Child* 1992;146:1218–1223.
100. Goeminne L. A new probably X-linked inherited syndrome: congenital muscular torticollis, multiple keloids, cryptorchidism and renal dysplasia. *Acts Genet Med Gemel* 1968;17:439–467.
101. Ritchey NIL, Norbeck J, Huang C, et al, Urologic manifestations of Goldenhar syndrome. *Urology* 1994;43:88–91.
102. Goldston AS, Burke EC, DAgostino, A, et al. Neonatal polycystic kidney with brain defect. *Am J Dis Child* 1963; 106:484–488.
103. Graham J Jr, Boyle W, Troxell J, et al. Cystic harmartomata of lung and kidney: a spectrum of developmental abnormalities. *Am J Med Genet* 1987;27:45–59.
104. Hennessy WT, Cromie WJ, Duckett JW. Congenital hemihypertrophy and associated abdominal lesions. *Urology* 1981;18:576–579.
105. Lipschitz B, Berdon WE, Defelice AR, et al. Association of congenital hepatic fibrosis and autosomal dominant polycystic kidney disease. Report of a family with review of the literature. *Pediatr Radiol* 1993;23:131–133.
106. Thomas IT, Honore GM, Jewett T, et al. Holzgreve syndrome: recurrence in sibs. *Am J Med Genet* 1993;45:767–769.
107. Verloes A. Hypertelorism-microtia-clefting (HMC syndrome). *Genet Couns* 1994;5:283–287.
108. Larson RS, Rudloff MA, Liap H, et al. The Ivemark syndrome: prenatal diagnosis of an uncommon cystic renal

lesion with heterogeneous associations. *Pediatr Nephrol* 1995;9:594–598.
109. Cantani A, Lucenti P, Ronzani GA, et al. Joubert syndrome: review of the fifty-three cases so far published. *Ann Genet* 1990;33:96–98.
110. Verloes A, Le Mercer M, Davin JC, et al. The orocraniodigital syndrome of Juberg and Hayward. *J Med Genet* 1992; 29:262–265.
111. Niikawa N, Matsuura N, Fukushima Y, et al. The Kabuki-make up syndrome. *J Pediatr* 1981;99:565–569.
112. Honiball S, Sandler M. Kallmann's syndrome with unilateral renal agenesis. A case report. *S Afr Med J* 1986;70:489–491.
113. Schaap C, de Die-Smulder CEM, Kuijten RH, et al. McKusick-Kaufmann syndrome: the diagnostic challenge of abdominal distension in the neonatal period. *Eur J Pediatr* 1992;151: 583–585.
114. Hennekam RCM, Van Schooneveld MJ, Ardinger HH, et al. The Peters' plus syndrome: description of 16 patients and review of the literature. *Clin Dysmorphol* 1993;2:283–300.
115. Grise P, Lefort J, Dewald M, et al. Urinary malformations in synostoses of the cervical vertebrae (Klippel-Feil syndrome). Apropos of 35 cases. *Ann Urol* 1984;18:232–235.
116. Kousseff EG. Sacral meningocele and conotruncal heart defects: a possible autosomal recessive trait. *Pediatrics* 1984; 74:395–398.
117. Ellis EN, Kemp SF, Frindik JP, et al. Glomerulopathy in patients with Donohue syndrome (Leprechaunism). *Diabetes Care* 1991;14:413–414.
118. Russo R, D'Armiento M, Angrisami P, et al. Limb body wall complex: a critical review and a nosological proposal. *Am J Med Genet* 1993;47:893.
119. Goeminne L. Synopsis of mammo-renal syndrome. *Humangenetik* 1972;14:170–171.
120. Schrander-Stumpel C, de Die Schmulder C, de Krom M, et al. Marden-Walker syndrome: case report, literature review and nosologic discussion. *Clin Genet* 1993;43:303–308.
121. Blankenberg TA, Ruebner BH, Ellis WG, et al. Pathology of renal and hepatic anomalies in Meckel syndrome. *Am J Med Genet Suppl* 1987;3:395–410.
122. Penman DG, Lilford RJ. The megacystis-microcolon-intestinal hypoperistalsis syndrome: a fatal autosomal recessive condition. *J Med Genet* 1989;26:66.
123. LaMontagne AE. Urologic manifestations of Melnick-Needles syndrome: a case report and review of the literature. *J Urol* 1991;145:1020–1021.
124. Robinson S, Kessling A. Diabetes secondary to genetic disorders. *Baillieres Clin Endocrinol Metab* 1992;6:867–898.
125. Cunniff C, Williamson-Kruse L, Olney AH. Congenital microgastria and limb reduction defects. *Pediatrics* 1993;91: 1192–1194.
126. Miranda D, Schjnella RA, Finegold MJ. Familial renal dysplasia. *Arch Pathol* 1972;93:483–491.
127. Moerman P, Vandenberghe K, Fryns JP, et al. A new lethal chondrodysplasia with spondylocostal dysostosis, multiple internal anomalies and Dandy-Walker cyst. *Clin Genet* 1985;27:160–164.
128. McDonald MT, Gorski JL. Nager acrofacial dysostosis. *J Med Genet* 1993;30:779–782.
129. Rizzo R, Pavone L, Micali G, et al. Familial bilateral antecubital pterygia with severe renal involvement in nail-patella syndrome. *Clin Genet* 1993;44:1–7.
130. King JA, Gardner V, Chen S, et al. Neu-Laxova syndrome: pathological evaluation of a fetus and review of the literature. *Pediatr Pathol Lab Med* 1995;15:57–79.
131. Freire-Maia N, Pinheiro M, Opitz JM. The neurofaciodigitorenal (NFDR) syndrome. *Am J Med Genet* 1982;11:326–336.
132. Demierre MF, Gerstein W. Segmental neurofibromatosis with ipsilateral renal agenesis. *Int J Dermatol* 1996;35:445–447.
133. Saraiva JM, Lemos C, Goncalves I, et al. Arthrogryposis multiplex congenita with renal and hepatic abnormalities in a female infant. *J Pediatr* 1990;117:761–763.
134. George CD, Patton MA, el Sawi M, et al. Abdominal ultrasound in Noonan syndrome: a study in 44 patients. *Pediatr Radiol* 1993;23:316–318.
135. Tsukahara M, Imaizumi K, Kawai S, et al. Occipital horn syndrome: report of a patient and review of the literature. *Clin Genet* 1994;45:32–35.
136. Teebi AS, Hassoon MM. Urofacial syndrome associated with hydrocephalus due to aqueductal stenosis. *Am J Med Genet* 1991;40:199–200.
137. Hunter AGW, Rothman SJ, Hwang WS, et al. Hepatic fibrosis, polycystic kidney, colobomata and encephalopathy in siblings. *Clin Genet* 1974;6:82–89.
138. Hunter AGW, Jurenka S, Thompson D, et al. Absence of the cerebellar granular layer, mental retardation, tapetoretinal degeneration and progressive glomerulopathy: an autosomal recessive oculo-renal-cerebellar syndrome. *Am J Med Genet* 1982;11:383–395.
139. Weaver RG, Cashwell LP, Lorentz W, et al. Optic nerve coloboma associated with renal disease. *Am J Med Genet* 1988;29:597–605.
140. Morse MJ, Lirenman DS, Johnson HW. The association of renal pelviocaliceal dysmorphism with sensorineural deafness: a new syndrome. *J Urol* 1981;125:625–627.
141. Hall JG, Pallister M, Clarren SK, et al. Congenital hypothalamic hamartoblastoma, hypopituitarism, imperforate anus and postaxial polydactyly—a new syndrome. *Am J Med Genet* 1980;7:47–83.
142. Biesecker LG, Graham JM Jr. Pallister-Hall syndrome. *J Med Genet* 1996;33:585–589.
143. Winter RM, Baraitser M. *London dysmorphology database.* London: Oxford University Press, 1995.
144. MacKenzie J, Chitayat D, McLorie G, et al. Penoscrotal transposition: a case report and review. *Am J Med Genet* 1994;49:103–107.
145. Gorlin RJ, Cohen MM Jr, Levin LS. *Syndromes of the head and neck*, 3rd ed. New York: Oxford University Press, 1990.
146. Halal F. Distal obstructive uropathy with polydactyly: a new syndrome? *Am J Med Genet* 1986;24:753–757.
147. Singh I, Johnson GH, Brown FR 3rd. Peroxisomal disorders. Biochemical and clinical diagnostic considerations. *Am J Dis Child* 1988;142:1297–1301.
148. Moser AB, Rasmussen M, Naldu S, et al. Phenotype of patients with peroxisomal disorders subdivided into sixteen complementation groups. *J Pediatr* 1995;127:13–22.
149. Suzuki Y, Shimozawa N, Takahashi Y, et al. Peroxisomal disorders: clinical aspects. *Ann N Y Acad Sci* 1996;804:442–449.

150. Bidair M, Kalota SJ, Kaplan GW. Infantile hypertrophic pyloric stenosis and hydronephrosis: Is there an association? *J Urol* 1993;150:153–155.
151. Raas-Rothchild A, Goodman RM, Grunbaum M, et al. Klippel-Feil anomaly with sacral agenesis: an additional subtype, type IV. *J Cranio Genet Dev Biol* 1988;8:297–301.
152. Vargas FR, de Almeida JC, Llerena JC Jr, et al. RAPADILINO syndrome. *Am J Med Genet* 1992;44:716–719.
153. Davee MA, Moore CA, Bull MJ, et al. New syndrome? Familial occurrence of renal and Mullerian duct hypoplasia, craniofacial anomalies, severe growth and developmental delay. *Am J Med Genet* 1992;44:293–296.
154. Moerman P, Fryns J-P, Sastrowijoto HS, et al. Hereditary renal adysplasia: new observation and hypotheses. *Pediatr Pathol* 1994;14:405–410.
155. Rosa FW, Wilk AL, Ketsey FO. Teratogen update: vitamin A congeners. *Teratology* 1986;34:366.
156. Rothman M, Moore LL, Singer MR, et al. Teratogenicity of high vitamin A intake. *N Engl J Med* 1995;333:1369–1373.
157. Van Den Berg DJ, Francke U. Roberts syndrome: a review of 100 cases and a new rating system for severity. *Am J Med Genet* 1993;47:1104–1123.
158. Robson WLM, Lowry RB, Leung AM. X-linked recessive nephritis with mental retardation, sensorineural hearing loss and macrocephaly. *Clin Genet* 1994;45:314–317.
159. Strubbe EH, Cremers CWRJ, Willensen P, et al. The Mayer-Rokitansky-Kuster-Hauser syndrome without and with associated features: two separate entities. *Clin Dysmorphol* 1994;3:192–199.
160. Menser MA, Robertson SE, Dorman DC, et al. Renal lesions in congenital rubella. *Pediatrics* 1967;40:901–904.
161. Prosperi P, Ricotti Chessa G. Rubinstein-Taybi syndrome with renal malformations. *Minerva Pediatr* 1975;27:2230–2238.
162. Wallerstein R, Anderson CE, Hay B, et al. Submicroscopic deletions at 16p13.3 in Rubinstein-Taybi syndrome: frequency and clinical manifestations in a North American population. *J Med Genet* 1997;34:203–206.
163. Patton MA. Russell-silver syndrome. *J Med Genet* 1988;25: 557–560.
164. Santos H, Mateus J, Leal MJ. Hirschsprung disease associated with polydactyly, unilateral renal agenesis, hypertelorism and congenital deafness: a new autosomal recessive syndrome. *J Med Genet* 1988;25:204–208.
165. Abu-Libdeh B, Fujimoto A, Ehinger M. Syndrome of cleft palate, microcephaly, large ears and short stature (Say syndrome). *Am J Med Genet* 1993;45:358–360.
166. Ludman MD, Cole DEC, Crocker JFS, et al. Schimke immuno-osseous dysplasia: case report and review. *Am J Med Genet* 1993;47:793–796.
167. Okamoto N, Takeuchi M, Kitajinia H, et al. A patient with Schinzel-Giedion syndrome and a review of 20 patients. *Jpn J Hum Genet* 1995;40:189–193.
168. Cantani A, Bamonte G, Ceccoli D, et al. Familial juvenile nephronophthisis. A review and differential diagnosis. *Clin Pediatr* 1986;25:90–95.
169. Clark RD, Golabi M, Lacassie Y, et al. Expanded phenotype and ethnicity in Setleis syndrome. *Am J Med Genet* 1989; 34:354–357.
170. Tsai Y-C, ChangJ-M, Changchien CC, et al. Unusual short rib-polydactyly syndrome. *Am J Med Genet* 1992;44:31–36.
171. Silence D, Kozlowski K, Bar-Ziv J, et al. Perinatally lethal short rib-polydactyly syndromes 1. Variability in known syndromes. *Pediatr Radiol* 1987;17:474–480.
172. Aleck KA, Grix A, Clericuzio C, et al. Dyssegmental dysplasia: clinical, radiographic and morphologic evidence of heterogeneity. *Am J Med Genet* 1987;27:295–312.
173. Simoupoulos A, Brennan GC, Alivan A, et al. Polycystic kidneys, internal hydrocephalus, polydactylism in newborn siblings. *Pediatrics* 1967;39:931–934.
174. Verloes A, Massart B, Dehalleux I, et al. Clinical overlap of Beckwith-Wiedermann, Perlman and Simpson-Golabi-Behmel syndromes: a diagnostic pitfall. *Clin Genet* 1995;47:257–262.
175. Cunniff C, Kratz LE, Moser A, et al. Clinical and biochemical spectrum of patients with RSH/Smith-Lemli-Opitz syndrome and abnormal cholesterol metabolism. *Am J Med Genet* 1997;68:263–269.
176. Curry JCR, Carey JC, Holland JS, et al. Smith-Lemli-Opitz syndrome type II: multiple congenital anomalies with male pseudohermaphroditism and frequent early lethality. *Am J Med Genet* 1987;26:45–57.
177. Sommer A, Rathbun MA, Battles ML. A syndrome with partial aniridia, unilateral renal agenesis and mild psychomotor retardation. *J Pediatr* 1974;85:870–872.
178. Thompson EM, Baraitser M. Sorsby syndrome: a report on further generations of the original family. *J Med Genet* 1988;25:313–321.
179. Sotos JF. Syndromes and other disorders associated with overgrowth. *Clin Pediatr* 1997;36:89–103.
180. Jejart G, Seres E. Supernumerary nipples and renal anomalies. *Int Urol Nephrol* 1994;26:141–144.
181. McBride WG. Thalidomide embryopathy. *Teratology* 1977; 16:79–82.
182. Smithells BW, Newman CGH. Recognition of thalidomide defects. *J Med Genet* 1992;29:716–723.
183. Rudd NL, Curry C, Chen KTK, et al. Thymic-renal-anal-lung dysplasia in sibs: a new autosomal recessive error of early morphogenesis. *Am J Med Genet* 1990;37:401–405.
184. Tolmie JL, Patrick A, Yates JRW. A lethal multiple pterygium syndrome with apparent X-linked inheritance. *Am J Med Genet* 1987;27:913–919.
185. O'Callaghan M, Young ID. Townes-Brocks syndrome. *J Med Genet* 1990;27:457–461.
186. Kelly TE. Teratogenicity of anticonvulsant drugs. I: review of the literature. *Am J Med Genet* 1984;19:413–434.
187. Bernstein J, Robbins TO. Renal involvement in tuberous sclerosis. *Ann N Y Acad Sci* 1991;615:36–49.
188. Bamshad M, Root S, Carey JC. Clinical analysis of a large kindred with the Pallister ulnar-mammary syndrome. *Am J Med Genet* 1996;65:325–331.
189. Battin J, Lacombe B, Leng JJ. Familial occurrence of hereditary renal adysplasia with Mullerian anomalies. *Clin Genet* 1993;43:23–24.
190. Neumann HP, Zbar B. Renal cyst, renal cancer and von Hippel-Lindau disease. *Kidney Int* 1997;51:16–26.
191. Maher ER, Yates JRW, Harries R, et al. Clinical features and natural history of von Hippel-Lindau disease. *QJM* 1990; 77:1151–1163.
192. Weinberg AG, Zumwalt RE. Bilateral nephromegaly and multiple pulmonary cysts. *Am J Clin Pathol* 1976;67:284–288.

193. Wenstrup RJ, Pagon RA. Female pseudohermaphroditism with anorectal, Mullerian duct, and urinary tract malformations: report of four cases. *J Pediatr* 1985;107:751–754.
194. Turnpenny PD, Dean JCS, Dufty P, et al. Weyers' ulnar ray/oligodactyly and the association of midline malformations and ulnar ray defects. *J Med Genet* 1992;29:659–662.
195. Del Papa M, Attardo S, Mobilli M, et al. Critical considerations on a case of nephroblastoma in a horseshoe kidney. *G Chir* 1991;12:549–552.
196. Hewitt M, Lunt PW, Oalchill A. Wilms' tumor and a de novo (1;7) translocation in a child with bilateral radial aplasia. *J Med Genet* 1991;28:411–412.
197. King LA, Sanchez-Ramos L, Talledo OE, et al. Syndrome of genital, renal and middle ear anomalies: a third family and report of a pregnancy. *Obstet Gynecol* 1986;69:891–893.
198. Monller Gisberg J, Tano Pino F, Rodriguez Arteaga G, et al. Urologic manifestations in Wolfram syndrome. *Acta Urol Esp* 1996;20:474–477.
199. Hing AV, Dowton SB. Aase syndrome: novel radiographic feature. *Am J Med Genet* 1993;45:413–415.
200. Schulte JM, Lenz W, Vogel M. Lethale Achondrogenesis: eine Ubersicht uber 56 Falle. *Klin Padiatr* 1978;191:327–340.
201. Casamassima AC, Beneck D, Gewitz MH, et al. Acrocallosal syndrome: additional manifestations. *Am J Med Genet* 1989;32:311.
202. Petit P, Moerman P, Fryns J-P. Acrofacial dysostosis syndrome type Rodriguez: a new lethal MCA syndrome. *Am J Med Genet* 1992;42:343–345.
203. Toriello HV, Radecki LL, Sharda J, et al. Frontonasal "dysplasia," cerebral anomalies and polydactyly: report of a new syndrome and discussion from a developmental field perspective. *Am J Med Genet Suppl* 1986;2:89–96.
204. McMillan DD, McArthur RG. Williams JA, et al. Upper urinary tract anomalies in children with adrenogenital syndrome. *J Pediatr* 1976;89:953–955.
205. Petrykowski WV, Beckmann R, Bohm N, et al. Adrenal insufficiency, myotonic hypotonia, severe psychomotor retardation, failure to thrive, constipation, and bladder ectasia in 2 brothers: adrenomyodystrophy. *Helv Paediatr Acta* 1982;37:387–400.
206. Hassell S, Butler MG. Antley-Bixler syndrome: report of a patient and review of the literature. *Clin Genet* 1994;46:372–376.
207. Cohen MM Jr, Kreiborg S. Visceral anomalies in the Apert syndrome. *Am J Med Genet* 1993;45:758–760.
208. Cairney AEL, Andrews M. Wilms' tumor in three patients with Bloom syndrome. *J Pediatr* 1987;111:414–416.
209. Bowen P, Conradi GJ. Syndrome of skeletal and genitourinary anomalies with unusual facies and failure to thrive in Hutterite sibs. *Birth Defects Orig Artic Ser* 1976;12(6):101–108.
210. Temtamy SA, McKusick VA. The genetics of hand malformations. *Birth Defects Orig Artic Ser* 1978;14:261–262.
211. Kosaki K, Curry C, Roeder E, et al. Ritscher-Schinzel (3C) syndrome: delineation of the phenotype. *Am J Med Genet* 1997;68:421–427.
212. Antley RM, Hwang DS, Theopold W, et al. Further delineation of the C (trigonocephaly) syndrome. *J Med Genet* 1981;9:147–163.
213. Houston CS, Opitz JM, Spranger JW, et al. The campomelic syndrome. *J Med Genet* 1983;15:3–28.
214. Jaeken J, Carchon R. The carbohydrate deficient glycoprotein syndromes: an overview. *J Inherit Metab Dis* 1993;16:813–820.
215. Robinson LK, James HE, Mubarak SJ, et al. Carpenter syndrome: natural history and clinical spectrum. *Am J Med Genet* 1985;20:461–469.
216. Cullen SI, Harris DE, Carter CH, et al. Congenital unilateral ichthyosiform erythroderma. *Arch Dermatol* 1969;199:724–729.
217. Nuoffer JM, Pfammatter JP, Spahr A, et al. Chondrodysplasia punctata with a mild clinical course. *J Inherit Metab Dis* 1994;17:60–66.
218. Levy P, Baraitser M. Coffin-Siris syndrome. *J Med Genet* 1991;28:338–341.
219. Janik JS, Shandling B, Mancer K. Cutis laxa and hollow viscus diverticula. *J Pediatr Surg* 1982;17:318–320.
220. Woods CG, Treleaven S, Betheras FR, et al. Disorganization-like syndrome with 47,XXY and unilateral narrowing of the common iliac artery. *Clin Dysmorphol* 1995;4:82–86.
221. Cullen P, Rodgers CS, Callen CF, et al. Association of familial Duane anomaly and urogenital abnormalities with a bisatellited marker derived from chromosome 22. *Am J Med Genet* 1993;47:925–930.
222. Levard G, AigrainY, Ferkadji L, et al. Urinary bladder diverticula and the Ehlers-Danlos syndrome in children. *J Pediatr Surg* 1989;24:1184–1186.
223. Berger TG, Detlefs RL, Donatucci CF. Junctional epidermolysis bullosa, pyloric atresia, and genitourinary disease. *Pediatr Dermatol* 1986;3:130–134.
224. Eklof O, Parkkulainen K. Epidermolysis bullosa dystrophica with urinary involvement. *J Pediatr Surg* 1984;19:215–217.
225. Burn J, Winter RM, Baraitser M, et al. The femoral hypoplasia-unusual facies syndrome. *J Med Genet* 1984;21:331–340.
226. Patton MA, Hurst J, Donnai D, et al. Floating-Harbor syndrome. *J Med Genet* 1991;28:201–204.
227. Suskan E, Kurkcuoglu N, Uluoglu O. Focal dermal hypoplasia (Goltz syndrome) with horseshoe kidney abnormality. *Pediatr Dermatol* 1990;7:283–286,
228. Hashemi C, Mahloudji M. The whistling face syndrome: report of a case with a renal anomaly. *Birth Defects Orig Artic Ser* 1974;10:265–267.
229. Kanemura T, Orii T, Olitani M. Frontometaphyseal dysplasia with congenital urinary tract malformations. *Clin Genet* 1979;16:399–404.
230. Roizenblatt J, Wajntal A, Diament AJ. Median cleft face syndrome or frontonasal dysplasia: a case report with associated renal malformations. *J Pediatr Ophthalmol Strabismus* 1979;16:16–20.
231. Siebert JR, Benjamin DR, Jutil S, et al. Urinary tract anomalies associated with congenital diaphragmatic defects. *Am J Med Genet* 1990;37:1–5.
232. Hockey A, Knowles S, Davies D, et al. Glutaric aciduria type II, an unusual cause of prenatal polycystic kidneys: report of prenatal diagnosis and confirmation of autosomal recessive inheritance. *Birth Defects Orig Artic Ser* 1993;29:373–382.

233. Gallop TR, Fontes LR. The Grieg cephalopolysyndactyly syndrome: report of a family and review of the literature. *Am J Med Genet* 1985;22:59–68.
234. Kaplan P, Ramos F, Zackai EH, et al. Cystic kidney disease in Hajdu-Cheney syndrome. *Am J Med Genet* 1995;56:25–30.
235. Salonen R, Herva R. Hydrolethalus syndrome. *J Med Genet* 1990;27:756–759.
236. Devos EA, Leroy JG, Braeckman JJ, et al. Spondylocostal dysostosis and urinary tract anomaly: definition and review of the entity. *Eur J Pediatr* 1978;128:7–15.
237. Gershoni-Baruch R, Lemer A, Braun J, et al. Johanson-Blizzard syndrome: clinical spectrum and further delineation of the syndrome. *Am J Med Genet* 1990;35:546–551.
238. Horn D, Wakowski R. Phenotype and counseling in lacrimo-auriculodento-digital (LADD) syndrome. *Genet Couns* 1993; 4:305–309.
239. Raff ML, Byers PH. Joint hypermobility syndromes. *Curr Opin Rheumatol* 1996;8:459–466.
240. Silverman FN. Larsen syndrome: congenital dislocation of the knees and other joints, distinctive facies, and frequently, cleft palate. *Ann Radiol* 1972;15:297–328.
241. Traboulsi EI, Lenz W, GonzalesRamos M, et al. The Lenz microphthalmia syndrome. *Am J Ophthalmol* 1988;105:40–45.
242. Swanson SL, Santen RJ, Smith DW. Multiple lentigines syndrome: new findings of hypogonadotrophism, hyposmia, and unilateral renal agenesis. *J Pediatr* 1971;78:1037–1039.
243. Sbar GR Venkataseshan VS, Huang Z, et al. Renal disease in Marfan syndrome. *Am J Nephrol* 1996;16:320–326.
244. Biermann CW, Rutishauser G. Polycystic kidneys associated with Marfan syndrome in an adult. *Scand J Urol Nephrol* 1994;28:295–296.
245. Sharon A, Gillerot Y, Van Maldergem L, et al. The Marshall-Smith syndrome. *Eur J Pediatr* 1990;150:54–55.
246. Kawai M, Momoi T, Fujii T, et al. The syndrome of Moebius sequence, peripheral neuropathy and hypogonadotropic hypogonadism. *Am J Med Genet* 1990;37:578–582.
247. Willems PJ, Colpaert C, Vaerenbergh M, et al. Multiple pterygium syndrome with body asymmetry. *Am J Med Genet* 1993;47:106–111.
248. Roig M, Balliu PR, Navarro C, et al. Presentation, clinical course and outcome of the congenital form of myotonic dystrophy. *Pediatr Neurol* 1994;11:208–213.
249. Emery AEH, Oleesky S, Williams RT. Myotonic dystrophy and polycystic disease of the kidneys. *J Med Genet* 1967;4:26–28.
250. Taalman RDHM, Hustinx TWJ, Weemaes CM, et al. Further delineation of the Nijmegen breakage syndrome. *Am J Med Genet* 1989;32:425–431.
251. Robin NH, Opitz JM, Muenke M. Opitz/GBBB syndrome: clinical comparisons of families linked to Xp22 and 22q, and review of the literature. *Am J Med Genet* 1996;62:305–317.
252. Cappa M, Borrelli P, Marini R, et al. The Opitz syndrome: a new designation for clinically indistinguishable BBB and G syndromes. *Am J Med Genet* 1987;28:303–310.
253. Toriello HV. Review. Oral-facial-digital syndromes, 1992. *Clin Dysmorphol* 1993;2:95–105.
254. Meinecke P, Hayek H. Orofaciodigital syndrome type IV (Mohr-Majewski) with severe expression expanding the known spectrum of anomalies. *J Med Genet* 1990;27:200–202.
255. Kieselstein M, Herman G, Wahrman J, et al. Mucocutaneous pigmentation and intestinal polyposis (Peutz-Jeghers syndrome) in a family of Iraqi Jews with polycystic kidney disease, with a chromosome study. *Isr J Med Sci* 1969;5:81–90.
256. Kuwada SK, Burt RW. The clinical features of the hereditary and nonhereditary polyposis syndromes. *Surg Oncol Clin North Am* 1996;5:553–567.
257. Bouvet J, Maroteaux P, Briand-Guillemot M. Le syndrome de Poland: etudes clinique et genetique considerations physiopathologiques. *Nouv Presse Med* 1976;5:185–190.
258. Bamforth JS, Fabian C, Machin G, et al. Poland anomaly with a limb body wall disruption defect: case report and review. *Am J Med Genet* 1992;43:780–784.
259. Verloes A, Mulliez N, Gonzales M, et al. Restrictive dermopathy, a lethal form of arthrogryposis multiplex with skin and bone dysplasias: three new cases and review of the literature. *Am J Med Genet* 1992;43:539–547.
260. Butler MG, Wadlington WB. Robinow syndrome: report of two patients and review of the literature. *Clin Genet* 1987; 31:77.
261. Vennos EM, Collins M, James WD. Rothmund-Thomson syndrome: review of the world literature. *J Am Acad Dermatol* 1992;27:750–762.
262. Majewski F, Enders H, Ranke MB, et al. Serpentine fibula-polycystic kidney syndrome and Melnick-Needles syndrome are different disorders. *Eur J Pediatr* 1993;152:916–921.
263. Murr MM, Waziri MH, Schelper RL, et al. Case of multivertebral anomalies, cloacal dysgenesis, and other anomalies presenting prenatally as cystic kidneys. *Am J Med Genet* 1992;42:761–765.
264. Beighton P. Spondyloepimetaphyseal dysplasia with joint laxity (SEMWL). *J Med Genet* 1994;31:136–140.
265. Carter P, Burke JR, Searle J. Renal abnormalities and spondylometaphyseal dysplasia. *Austr Paediatr J* 1985;21: 115–117.
266. Robinow M, Johnson GF, Broock W. Syndactyly type V. *Am J Med Genet* 1982;11:475–482.
267. Pankau R, Partsch CJ, Winter M, et al. Incidence and spectrum of renal abnormalities in Williams-Beuren syndrome. *Am J Med Genet* 1996;63:301–304.
268. Sandoval R, Sepulveda W, Gutierrez J, Be C, Altieri E. Prenatal diagnosis of nonmosaic trisomy 9 in a fetus with severe renal disease. *Gynecol Obstet Invest* 1999;48:69–72.
269. Barakat AY, Butler MG. Renal and urinary tract abnormalities associated with chromosome aberrations. *Int J Pediatr Nephrol* 1987;8:215–226.
270. Jones KL. *Smith's recognizable patterns of human malformation,* 5th ed. Philadelphia: WB Saunders, 1997.
271. Van Zelderen-Bhola SL, Breslau-Siderius EJ, Beveratocks GC, et al. Prenatal and postnatal investigation in a case of Miller-Dieker syndrome due to a familial cryptic translocation t(17;20) (p13.3;q13.3) detected by prenatal fluorescence in situ hybridization. *Prenat Diagn* 1997;17:173–179.
272. Gorlin RJ, Cohen MM Jr, Levin LS. *Syndromes of the head and neck,* 3rd ed. New York: Oxford University Press, 1990.
273. Kupferman JC, Stewart CL, Kaskel FJ, et al. Posterior urethral valves in patients with Down syndrome. *Pediatr Nephrol* 1996;10:143–146.

274. Van Buggenhout GJ, Verbruggen J, Fryns JP. Renal agenesis and trisomy 22: case report and review. *Ann Genet* 1995; 38:44–48.
275. Goldberg R, Motzkin B, Scambler PJ, et al. Velo-cardio-facial syndrome: a review of 120 patients. *Am J Med Genet* 1993;45:313–319.
276. Greenberg F. DiGeorge syndrome: a historical review of clinical and cytogenetic features. *J Med Genet* 1993;30:803–806.
277. Flynn MT, Ekstrom L, De Arce M, et al. Prevalence of renal malformation in Turner syndrome. *Pediatr Nephrol* 1996; 10:498–500.

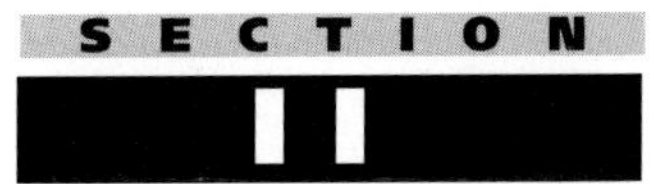

HOMEOSTASIS

7

SODIUM AND WATER

HOWARD TRACHTMAN

You may not discontinue the salt of your God's covenant from upon your meal offerings. . .

Leviticus 2:13

For the life of any creature—its blood represents its life. . .

Leviticus 17:14

This chapter reviews the physiologic mechanism involved in the control of sodium and water homeostasis. Using this knowledge as a basis, the common diseases that arise when these systems malfunction are analyzed, and a discussion of the optimal therapy for these conditions is presented.

BODY FLUID COMPARTMENTS AND THEIR COMPOSITION

Total Body Water and Its Compartments

On average, water comprises 60% of total body weight in adults. This proportion is higher in infants and even greater in babies born prematurely and very low birth weight neonates. Total body water (TBW) declines during early infancy and reaches the adult proportion by the end of the first year (1). The percentage of body weight that is water is higher in individuals who have lower adipose levels and higher muscle levels. In addition, TBW may be altered in disease states that are associated with altered salt handling, such as cystic fibrosis.

In general, the TBW is divided into two principal components: the intracellular water (ICW) and the extracellular water (ECW) spaces (2). These spaces are divided in a 2:1 ratio. In those states in which there is an increase in the TBW, the increase is manifested clinically by the increase in the ECW space. The ECW compartment is further divided into the interstitial and plasma spaces, which are separated in a 3:1 ratio. A component of the ECW, namely the interstitial fluid in skin and connective tissue, may serve as a reservoir that can mobilize water into the plasma volume to sustain circulation during conditions of hypovolemia (3). Finally, there are transcellular water compartments, such as the gastrointestinal lumen or cerebrospinal fluid, which need to be considered in a distinct category. They are not in direct contact with the rest of the fluid spaces and are separated by an epithelial membrane. Water and electrolytes enter these spaces via active transport processes.

Composition of Body Water Compartments

All of the major fluid compartments in the body are separated by semipermeable membranes (2,3). This type of barrier permits free passage of the solvent but may limit the movement of selective solutes across the membrane. Therefore, the solvent will always move down its concentration gradient to ensure that the osmolality of the solution is the same on both sides of the membrane. Despite marked differences in the makeup of the cationic and anionic solutes in the various body water compartments, under equilibrium conditions, osmolality or tonicity is always equal in all body fluids.

Because of the presence of active transporters and selective channels for various solutes within the cell membrane, there is an uneven distribution of solutes in the ICW and ECW compartments. The presence of the Na-K–adenosine triphosphatase (ATPase) pump in the cell membrane ensures that potassium is the principal cation in the intracellular compartment, and sodium is the primary ECW cation (4). Similar limitations in membrane permeability to chloride and bicarbonate result in these anions being found almost exclusively in the ECW space, whereas proteins and phosphate constitute the major intracellular anions. The differences in cell permeability and binding characteristics of specific ions are reflected in the coefficients that are used to determine the volume of distribution for individual solutes. For example, because of the permeability of cell membranes to water, the volume of distribution for sodium is equal to the TBW compartment, although sodium is confined to the ECW space. In contrast, the volume of distribution of bicarbonate is 0.3 × TBW. These considerations are important in formulating therapeutic regimens to treat specific disorders of sodium and water homeostasis (5).

Besides the presence of distinctive membrane permeability characteristics for specific solutes, the unequal distribution of ions across the membrane is, in part, due to the Gibbs-Donnan effect, which arises because of the presence of impermeant, negatively charged proteins, primarily albumin, in the intravascular space (3). Nonetheless, there is electroneutrality in all body fluids, and the osmolality, or the sum of all osmotically active particles, is equal in all body water compartments.

Under normal conditions, the serum osmolality is 286 ± 4 mOsm/kg water. Because sodium is the major cation in the ECW, osmolality can be estimated by the following formula:

$$\text{Serum osmolality} \approx 2 \times [\text{serum sodium concentration}]$$

A reflection coefficient of 1.0 indicates a totally non-permeant solute, whereas freely permeable molecules have a reflection coefficient of zero. The reflection coefficient for urea is approximately 0.4. Similarly, in the absence of insulin, the reflection coefficient for glucose is 0.5. Thus, in circumstances in which there is a pathologic elevation in the serum urea nitrogen (e.g., acute renal failure or glucose concentration) (diabetic ketoacidosis), these solutes will also contribute to osmolality, and the following formula should be used to calculate serum osmolality:

$$\text{Serum osmolality} = 2 \times [\text{serum sodium concentration}] + [\text{serum urea nitrogen}]/2.8 + [\text{serum glucose concentration}]/18$$

This formula is based on the molecular weights of urea nitrogen (28 d) and glucose (180 d) and the standard practice of reporting these serum concentrations as mg/100 mL. The calculated serum osmolality is normally within 1 to 2% of the value obtained by direct osmometry in clinical chemistry laboratories. However, there are circumstances in which the calculated serum osmolality is significantly lower than the value obtained by measurement with an osmometer. This "osmolal gap" reflects the accumulation of unmeasured osmoles such as organic solutes that are produced after an ingestion of ethanol or ethylene glycol (antifreeze) (6,7).

MAINTENANCE SODIUM AND WATER REQUIREMENTS

Sodium

It is established that sodium is an essential component of the diet. Not only is this cation necessary for the maintenance of the size of the extracellular fluid (ECF) space (see later), it is also required for normal growth. Wassner (8) has demonstrated that somatic growth of experimental animals is impaired if they are fed a sodium-deficient diet. This effect is independent of protein or calorie content of the diet.

Balance studies indicate that the daily sodium requirement is 2 to 3 mmol/kg body weight. This quantity is nearly two- to threefold higher in term and very low birth weight premature infants (9). This is a reflection of immaturity in renal tubular function coupled with the increased need for sodium to achieve the high rate of growth that is normally observed during the first few years of life. The sodium requirement is exaggerated by intrinsic (diarrhea, increased losses in children on chronic peritoneal dialysis, genetic defect in tubular sodium transport) or exogenous (administration of diuretics) factors that enhance losses of sodium. In most developed countries, the daily sodium intake is well in excess of the amount needed to promote growth or maintain body function. Under normal circumstances, the principal anion that accompanies sodium in the diet is chloride. In certain disease states, such as renal tubular acidosis, metabolic acidosis associated with chronic renal insufficiency, or urolithiasis, it may be advisable to provide a portion of the daily sodium requirement as the bicarbonate or the citrate salt.

Water

The daily requirement for water has traditionally been expressed as a quantity of mL per metabolic kg (10). However, in clinical practice, this is a very cumbersome and impractical method, and all calculations are based on body weight and size. Currently, three methods are used to estimate the daily fluid requirement. The first is a direct extension of the use of metabolic kg and uses the following formula:

Daily water requirement = 100 mL/kg for a child weighing less than 10 kg
+ 50 mL/kg for each additional kg up to 20 kg
+ 20 mL/kg for each kg in excess of 20 kg

The second method is based on body surface area and uses the following formula:

$$\text{Daily water requirement} = 1500\ \text{mL/m}^2\ \text{body surface area}$$

The last method is a refinement of the second and uses the following formula:

Daily water requirement = Urine output + insensible water losses

Based on clinical experience, under normal circumstances, urine output is approximately 1000 mL/m^2/day, and insensible losses amount to 500 mL/m^2/day.

Thus, consider a child weighing 30 kg and 123 cm in height with a body surface area of 1 m^2. According to the first method, the daily water requirement is 1700 mL, whereas the second method yields 1500 mL/day. This example illustrates the relative benefits of these two methods. Although the first is easier to apply, it tends to overestimate the water requirement as body weight increases. The third method is the most precise and should be applied in more unusual circumstances, such as when the patient has oliguria secondary to acute renal failure or increased insensible losses (e.g., diarrhea, increased ambient temperature, tachypnea, burns, or cystic fibrosis) (11). In addition to the daily energy requirement and insensible losses that are represented in the formulas, the amount of water excreted daily is dependent on the solute load. Because the urine has a minimum osmolality—approximately 50 mOsm/kg H_2O, even in the absence of arginine vasopressin (AVP)—increased dietary intake of solute will result in a larger obligatory urine volume to accommodate the larger solute load (12).

The daily sodium and water requirement are generally provided enterally. Intravenous administration of fluids and electrolytes should be used only under clinical circumstances that interfere with normal feeding, such as persistent vomiting or gastrointestinal tract surgery.

DISTINCT ROLES OF SODIUM AND WATER IN BODY FLUID HOMEOSTASIS

Sodium and water are inextricably linked in the determination of the serum sodium concentration. However, it is critical to recognize that sodium and water serve two distinct functions within the body. Sodium is instrumental in the maintenance of the size of the ECF space, whereas water is critical to the maintenance of the size of individual cells. The regulation of sodium and water homeostasis represents two distinct processes with discrete sensing and effector mechanisms. Although these systems may overlap from a physiologic and clinical perspective, a complete understanding of body fluids and electrolytes mandates separate evaluation of sodium and water.

As mentioned earlier, sodium is confined primarily to the ECW compartment as a consequence of active transport mechanisms in the cell membrane. Because sodium is the principal cation in this space, disturbances in total body sodium content are reflected by expansion or contraction in the ECW compartment. Adequacy of the ECW compartment is essential to maintain the intravascular space and sustain perfusion of vital organs. The primary step in the pathogenesis of disturbances in ECW compartment size is a perturbation in sodium balance. Under normal circumstances when TBW and sodium content are within the normal range, sodium balance is zero. This means that the daily intake of sodium is matched by the net losses in the urine, stool, and other insensible losses. Provided kidney function is normal, the dietary sodium intake can be as low as 0.1 mmol/kg or in excess of 10 mmol/kg without any derangement in ECF compartment size. If the alterations in diet are not abrupt, then sodium balance is maintained, even when kidney function is markedly impaired (13). In contrast, if the daily input of sodium exceeds the normal losses, then there is expansion of the ECF space that may manifest as edema. If the input does not match the daily losses, there will be symptoms and signs related to ECW space contraction. These disturbances are not associated with any obligatory changes in the serum sodium concentration.

Water homeostasis is a prerequisite for the normal distribution of fluid between the ICW and ECW compartments. Cell function is dependent on stabilization of cell volume to keep the cytosolic concentration of enzymes, cofactors, and ions at the appropriate level. Perturbations in water balance result in fluctuations in serum osmolality. Because cell membranes are semipermeable and generally permit free movement of water down an osmolal gradient, changes in osmolality will cause obligatory shifts in water between the cell and the ECW space. Any disorder that alters the 2:1 ratio of water volume in the ICW:ECW spaces will be reflected in changes in cell size and subsequent cellular dysfunction. Thus, under hypoosmolal conditions, water will move from the intravascular compartment into the cell, causing relative or absolute cell volume expansion. Conversely, if the serum osmolality is elevated, water will exit from the cell to the ECW space, resulting in absolute or relative cellular contraction (14).

Disturbances in cell function related to abnormalities in cell size occur throughout the body. However, this problem is especially prominent in cerebral cells. There are two reasons for this phenomenon. First, the blood-brain barrier, which is constituted by tight junctions between adjacent endothelial cells, limits the movement of solute between the ICW and ECW compartments, while permitting unrestricted flow of water down an osmolal gradient (15). Second, because the brain is contained within the skull, which is a closed, noncompliant space, and is tethered to the cranial vault by bridging blood vessels, it has limited tolerance of cell swelling or contraction. Thus, alterations in water balance and serum osmolality are dominated by clinical findings of central nervous system dysfunction, including lethargy, seizures, and coma (14).

Similar to the situation noted earlier in which disturbances in sodium balance do not necessarily imply specific abnormalities in serum sodium concentration, the presence of a disturbance in water balance and serum osmolality is not linked to a specific abnormality in the ECW compartment. The independent nature of disturbances in sodium and water balance is illustrated in Table 7.1. It is apparent that alterations in ECW size can occur in patients with hypoosmolality, isotonicity, or hypertonicity. Similarly, each alteration in serum osmolality can develop in patients with contraction or expansion of the ECW compartment.

Disturbances in sodium and water homeostasis need to be addressed separately in the clinical evaluation of patients with abnormalities in sodium and/or water. The clinical approach to these problems is outlined below.

SENSOR MECHANISMS: SODIUM AND WATER

For both sodium and water homeostasis, the sensor mechanisms that maintain the equilibrium state are primarily

TABLE 7.1. CLINICAL DISEASES OF SODIUM AND WATER HOMEOSTASIS: RELATIONSHIP BETWEEN EXTRACELLULAR WATER (ECW) SIZE AND TONICITY

	Tonicity		
ECW volume	Low	Normal	High
Low	Addison's disease *Salmonella* diarrhea Mannitol infusion	Isotonic dehydration	Hypertonic diarrheal dehydration Diabetes insipidus
Normal	SIADH	No disease	Acute sodium bicarbonate infusion
High	Acute renal failure Nephrotic syndrome Cirrhosis Congestive heart failure	Nephrotic syndrome	Salt intoxication Saltwater drowning

SIADH, syndrome of inappropriate secretion of antidiuretic hormone.

designed to be responsive to the secondary consequences of abnormalities in sodium or water balance (i.e., changes in ECW and cell size, respectively) rather than measuring the primary variable. They operate using negative feedback loops in which deviations from normal are detected, counterregulatory mechanisms are activated that antagonize the initiating event, and the system is restored to its original state.

Sodium

The detection of abnormalities in sodium balance is based on systems that sense the consequences of these changes. Thus, net sodium deficit is detected as a decrease in ECW space size, whereas net sodium excess is perceived as an obligatory expansion of the ECW space. These receptors, which are influenced by the filling pressure within the circulation, are called *baroreceptors* or *mechanoreceptors*. It is important to note that these signals are supplemented in certain instances by chemoreceptors that respond directly to changes in the serum sodium concentration and trigger adaptive modifications in renal sodium handling. These receptors may effect change by altering nervous system activity or by activating upstream promoter elements and stimulating the expression of relevant genes (16).

Atrial Receptors

There are ECW volume receptors on the venous (low pressure) and arterial (high pressure) sides of the circulation. Within the right atrium, there are sensors that possess the distensibility and compliance needed to detect alterations in intrathoracic blood volume by maneuvers such as negative intrathoracic pressure or head-out water immersion. Both of these maneuvers, which increase the central blood volume and raise central venous and right atrial pressures, are followed by a brisk natriuresis and diuresis (17). These changes are triggered even in the absence of concomitant change in the total ECW space size. Neural receptors that respond to mechanical stretch or changes in right or left atrial pressure convey the signal via the vagus nerve (17,18).

Hepatic Receptors

The enhanced effect on renal sodium excretion of saline infusions directly into the hepatic vein versus the systemic circulation suggests that there are also low-pressure sensors within the portal vein or hepatic vasculature. The hepatic responses to changes in sodium balance have been divided into two categories (19). The "hepatorenal reflex" involves direct activation of sodium chemoreceptors and mechanoreceptors in the hepatoportal region via the hepatic nerve and causes a reflex decrease in renal nerve activity. The "hepatointestinal reflex" uses chemoreceptors to respond to changes in sodium concentration and modulate intestinal absorption of sodium via signals conveyed along the vagus nerve. Activation of these hepatic volume sensors may contribute to the sodium retention and edema states that develop secondary to chronic liver disease and cirrhosis with their associated intrahepatic hypertension.

Pulmonary Receptors

There may also be pressure sensors within the pulmonary circulation that are activated by changes in pulmonary perfusion or mean airway pressure (20). The receptors in the lung may be located in the interstitial spaces and may influence the physical forces that modulate paracellular absorption of sodium and water. Similar receptors in the renal interstitium may also influence paracellular absorption of fluid and solutes along the nephron, especially in the proximal tubule segment (21).

Carotid Arch Receptors

There are also volume-dependent sensors on the high-pressure side of the circulation, including the carotid arch, the brain, and the renal circulation. Thus, occlusion of the carotid leads to increased sympathetic nervous system activity and alterations in renal sodium handling (18). The responsiveness of the carotid arch receptors may be modulated by chronic changes in ECF volume. For example, head-down bed rest and a high-salt diet blunt carotid baroreceptor activity and lead to natriuresis (22).

Cerebral Receptors

Alterations in the sodium concentration of the cerebrospinal fluid or brain arterial plasma lead to increased renal sodium excretion (23). Various lesions in discrete anatomic areas of the brain, such as the anteroventral third ventricle, alter renal sodium reabsorption and buttress the contention that there are central mechanisms of sensing changes in sodium balance and ECF volume. Derangements in the sensing system within the brain in patients with longstanding central nervous system diseases may contribute to the cerebral salt-wasting syndrome.

Of interest, if the arterial sensors perceive underfilling of the vascular space, this activates counterregulatory mechanisms to replete the ECW compartment size, even if the receptors in the venous system detect adequate or even overfilling of the venous tree. Despite normal or even excess total body sodium and net positive sodium balance, there are conditions in which the body perceives an inadequate circulating plasma volume. This has given rise to the notion of the "effective" intravascular volume, a concept that is applicable in the edema states such as congestive heart failure, cirrhosis, and nephrotic syndrome (24). For example, in patients with cardiac pump failure, the perceived underfilling of the arterial tree may occur despite significant venous distention and TBW overload (25). Similarly, women who develop edema during pregnancy may have primary peripheral vasodilatation and excess total body sodium (24).

In summarizing the sensor mechanisms that are involved in the regulation of sodium balance, there are those that are directly linked via mechanoreceptors to the status of the ECF volume. These sensor systems are activated by decreased size of the ECW compartment and respond to "underfilling" of the vasculature tree. However, there are other mechanisms that may be activated by chemoreceptors or localized intra-organ disturbances in perfusion that are dissociated from the ECF volume. These sensors can cause overfilling of the vascular compartment by stimulating renal sodium reabsorption. Correct interpretation of the balance between these two processes involved in sodium balance is critical to the proper diagnosis and management of the edema states (see later).

Water: Arginine Vasopressin

The receptors that are responsible for regulating water homeostasis are primarily osmoreceptors and are sensitive to alterations in cell size (26). These osmoresponsive cells are located in the anterolateral regions of the hypothalamus, adjacent to but distinct from the supraoptic nuclei. They shrink or swell in response to increases or decreases in plasma tonicity, and this change in cell size triggers the release of AVP and/or the sensation of thirst.

AVP is a peptide containing nine amino acids and has a molecular weight of 1099 d. It is synthesized by the cells in the hypothalamus, transported down the axon, and stored in the posterior pituitary in conjunction with larger proteins, called *neurophysins* (27). The gene for AVP is located on chromosome 20 and has a cyclic adenosine monophosphate response element in the promoter region. Prolonged stimulation of AVP release leads to upregulation of the AVP gene; however, synthesis does not keep up with the need for the peptide, because pituitary levels of AVP are usually depleted in states such as chronic salt loading and hypernatremia (28).

The principal solute that provokes the release of AVP is sodium. The infusion of sodium chloride to increase plasma osmolality results in increased secretion of AVP in the absence of parallel changes in ECW volume. This underscores the primary role of fluctuations in plasma osmolality per se in stimulating AVP release (26). Mannitol, an exogenous solute that is used in clinical practice to treat increased intracranial pressure, is nearly as effective as sodium in stimulating AVP release. Urea and glucose are less than 50% as effective as sodium in provoking AVP secretion, presumably because they are more permeable than sodium and cause less pronounced changes in osmoreceptor cell volume. However, in disease states such as acute renal failure or diabetic ketoacidosis in which urea or glucose act as osmotically active molecules or after the exogenous administration of mannitol, these solutes can also stimulate increases in AVP release. Likely there is coupling between mechanical changes in membrane structure and hormone release. However, the exact mechanism and the neurotransmitters that mediate the actions of the osmoreceptors on the cells of the posterior pituitary have not been identified.

There are a variety of nonosmotic stimuli to AVP release that may contribute to water handling in various disease states (26). Vomiting and acute hypoglycemia promote AVP release by neural-hormonal pathways that are not well defined. Stress associated with pain or emotional anxiety, physical exertion, high body temperature, acute hypoxia, and acute hypercapnia are other conditions that lead to increased secretion of AVP in the absence of a primary disturbance in water balance. There are numerous drugs that directly influence the hypothalamic release of AVP, including carbamazepine, cyclophosphamide, and vincristine. Finally, hemodynamic changes arising from primary alterations in sodium balance and the ECW space can trigger AVP release. If the ECW volume disturbance is mild, then the stimulation of AVP release is modest. However, in the face of severe ECW volume contraction, there is marked secretion of AVP. Under

TABLE 7.2. FACTORS THAT INCREASE ARGININE VASOPRESSIN RELEASE

↑ Plasma osmolality
Hemodynamic
↓ Blood volume
↓ Blood pressure
Emesis
Hypoglycemia
Stress
Elevated body temperature
Angiotensin II
Hypoxia
Hypercapnia
Drugs

↑, increased; ↓, decreased.

these circumstances, the imperative to protect the effective circulating blood volume takes precedence over the need to maintain plasma osmolality, and ECW volume is restored at the expense of hypoosmolality. This clinical observation indicates that despite rigorous intellectual attempts to separate sodium and water homeostatic mechanisms, these two factors are closely linked *in vivo*, and there can be significant overlap in sensor and effector mechanisms in the regulation of ECW and ICW compartment size. Table 7.2 lists the factors that modulate AVP release.

In addition to AVP release, the osmoreceptor cells also respond to the changes in serum osmolality in an independent manner to stimulate thirst and increase drinking (29). The stimuli for thirst are generally the same as those for AVP release, among which hypernatremia is the most potent trigger. The osmotic threshold for thirst in humans appears to be higher than for AVP secretion, namely 295 mOsm/kg. The sensing mechanism that leads to this increase in water intake is even more obscure than that for AVP release. It is likely that changes in ECW volume are also involved in this process, because angiotensin II, which rises in states of ECW volume contraction, is a potent dipsogen (30).

EFFERENT MECHANISMS: SODIUM AND WATER

The efferent mechanisms involved in maintaining sodium and water balance include a variety of neural and endocrine-humoral systems. There often is an overlap in the action of these effectors, with an individual effector having distinctive effects on sodium and water balance.

Sodium

Renin-Angiotensin-Aldosterone Axis

The major components of this system—renin, angiotensinogen, and angiotensin-converting enzyme—are found within the kidney and within the vasculature of most organs. Thus, these elements are linked in a large feedback loop involving the liver, kidney, and lung, as well as smaller loops within individual organs. This complex system accounts for the often-disparate data that have been accumulated about plasma renin activity and the expression of these components within the kidney during disturbances in ECW compartment size.

Angiotensin II is the major signal generated by this axis (3). The peptide interacts with two different receptors, and most of its biologic activity is mediated by the angiotensin type 1 (AT1) receptor. The AT2 receptor is expressed more prominently in the fetal kidney; however, interaction of angiotensin II with the AT2 receptor postnatally may stimulate the release of molecules, such as nitric oxide, that counteract the primary action of the peptide (31). The best-known effects of angiotensin II include peripheral vasoconstriction to preserve organ perfusion and stimulation of adrenal synthesis of aldosterone to enhance renal sodium reabsorption. These two actions serve to restore the ECW space to normal. However, angiotensin II also has direct actions on tubular function and stimulates both proximal and distal sodium reabsorption. The proximal tubule cells contain all of the elements needed to synthesize angiotensin II locally, and the peptide increases the activity of the sodium-hydrogen exchanger (32). In the distal tubule, angiotensin II modulates this exchanger as well as the amiloride-sensitive sodium channel (33). The effects of aldosterone on the renal tubule include both an immediate effect to increase apical membrane permeability to sodium and more extended effects that involve enhanced gene transcription and *de novo* synthesis of Na-K-ATPase. Aldosterone may also stimulate the synthesis of other enzymes involved in renal cell bioenergetics (e.g., citrate synthase) that are needed to sustain maximal tubular sodium transport (34).

Endothelin

This vasoactive molecule is part of a family of three peptides of which endothelin-1 is the most important in humans (35). It is converted in two steps from an inactive precursor to a biologically active 21–amino acid peptide. Endothelins react with two receptors, ETA and ETB, and cause vasoconstriction, which result in a decrease in renal blood flow (RBF) and glomerular filtration rate (GFR). With regard to sodium balance, the primary effect of endothelin is sodium retention mediated by the reduction in GFR. This would suggest that endothelin acts in concert with angiotensin II to protect ECW compartment size under conditions of sodium deficit. However, the situation may be more complicated, because direct exposure of proximal tubule and medullary collecting duct cells to endothelin *in vitro* inhibits sodium absorption.

Renal Nerves

There is abundant sympathetic nervous innervation of the renal vasculature and all tubular segments of the nephron

(36). The efferent autonomic fibers are postganglionic and originate in splanchnic nerves. The renal innervation is primarily adrenergic and involves α_1 adrenoreceptors in the blood vessels and both α_1 and α_2 receptors along the basolateral membrane of the proximal tubule. Renal sympathetic nervous system activity contributes to preservation of ECF volume by promoting renal vasoconstriction and lowering GFR and by increasing sodium reabsorption. Among the catecholamines involved in adrenergic transmission, norepinephrine exerts an antinatriuretic effect. The fact that dopamine, another sympathetic nervous system neurotransmitter, promotes a natriuresis suggests that there may be internal regulation of the effect of nerve activation on renal sodium handling (37).

Renal sympathetic nervous activity is inversely proportional to dietary salt intake (36). Drug-induced sodium retention and volume-dependent hypertension (e.g., with the use of cyclosporine) is mediated in part by activation of the sympathetic nervous system (38). In addition, increased adrenergic nervous signaling within the kidney is instrumental in the initiation of hypertension in experimental animals by causing a right-shift in the pressure-natriuresis curve (36). However, the observation that sodium balance is normal and ECF volume is maintained in the denervated transplanted kidney implies that the role of the sympathetic nervous system in maintaining sodium homeostasis is redundant and can be taken over by other regulatory mechanisms (36).

Atrial Natriuretic Peptide

Atrial natriuretic peptide (ANP) is a 28–amino acid peptide that is a member of a group of proteins that includes brain natriuretic peptide and C-type natriuretic peptide (39). It is synthesized as a prohormone that is stored in granules in the cardiac atria. Increases in right trial pressure provoke cleavage and release of the mature peptide. For each 1-mm Hg rise in central venous pressure, there is a corresponding 10- to 15-pmol/L increase in circulating ANP levels. Conversely, declines in atrial pressure secondary to sodium depletion or hemorrhage reduce ANP release. There are two receptors for ANP, and both are coupled to guanylate cyclase. The activation of this enzyme results in cytosolic accumulation of cyclic guanosine monophosphate, which, in turn, appears to diminish agonist-stimulated increases in intracellular calcium concentration. The principal effects of ANP are to promote an increase in GFR, diuresis, and, most important, natriuresis. The increased renal sodium excretion is, in part, mediated by an increase in filtered load secondary to the rise in GFR. However, ANP also exerts direct actions on renal tubular cells to diminish sodium reabsorption, including inhibition the Na-K-Cl cotransporter in the loop of Henle and the amiloride-sensitive sodium uptake in the medullary collecting duct. Finally, ANP antagonizes the action of several antinatriuretic signals in the kidney, including sympathetic nervous system activity, angiotensin II, and endothelin. The overall effects of ANP to counteract increases in ECW compartment have been demonstrated by short-term studies in which acute infusions of ANP improved cardiac status in patients with congestive heart failure and promoted a diuresis in patients with acute renal failure (40).

Prostaglandins

The kidney contains the enzymes required for constitutive (COX-1) and inducible (COX-2) cyclooxygenase that are necessary for the conversion of arachidonic acid to prostaglandins (PGs) (41). The major products of these pathways are PGE_2, $PGF_{2\alpha}$, PGD_2, prostacyclin (PGI_2), and thromboxane (TXA_2). In the cortical regions, PGE_2 and PGI_2 predominate, whereas PGE_2 is the major PG metabolite in the medulla. These two compounds increase GFR and promote increased urinary sodium excretion. In addition, they antagonize the action of AVP. These actions may mediate the adverse effects of hypercalcemia and hypokalemia on renal tubular function (41). The natriuretic effects of PGs in response to alterations in dietary sodium intake under normal circumstances are unclear. However, the role of PGs as efferent signals is more apparent in conditions associated with increased vasoconstrictor tone, such as congestive heart failure or reduced renal perfusion. In these conditions, PGs act to counteract the vasoconstrictor and sodium-retaining effects of angiotensin II and norepinephrine. Inhibition of PGs with cyclooxygenase inhibitors can be associated with dramatic declines in GFR and profound sodium retention and edema (42).

Kinins

Kinins are produced within the kidney and act via β_2 receptors. Their principal action is to promote renal vasodilatation and natriuresis. The kinins act in the distal tubule to reduce sodium reabsorption (43).

Nitric Oxide

The kidney contains all three isoforms of nitric oxide synthase (NOS) that are involved in NO synthase—neuronal NOS in the macula densa, inducible NOS in renal tubules and mesangial cells, and endothelial NOS in the renal vasculature. The neuronal and endothelial isoforms are calcium-dependent enzymes and produce small, transient increases in NO production. The inducible isoform is upregulated by various cytokines and inflammatory mediators, resulting in large, sustained elevations in NO release.

Activation of eNOS within the kidney increases the activity of soluble guanylate cyclase and causes vasodilatation and an increase in GFR. In addition to its effect on RBF and GFR, NO has direct effects to inhibit Na-K-

ATPase in cultured proximal tubule and collecting duct cells (44,45). The specific isoform of NOS that is responsible for modulating urinary sodium excretion is not as well known. Recent studies using inducible NOS, neuronal NOS, and endothelial NOS knock-out mice suggest that only the first two isoforms are involved in the regulation of sodium and water reabsorption in the proximal tubule (44). There is evidence to support a role of NO in maintaining sodium balance under normal conditions, because alterations in dietary salt intake are associated with parallel changes in urinary excretion of nitrite, the metabolic byproduct of NO release (46). In normotensive Wistar-Kyoto rats and spontaneously hypertensive rats, increased dietary sodium intake is associated with a modest increase in urinary nitrite excretion (47). This effect is less well documented in pediatric patients. Along with ANP and bradykinin, NO is part of the defense system against sodium excess and expansion of the ECW compartment. Derangements in renal NO synthesis and responsiveness to cyclic guanosine monophosphate may be instrumental in the pathogenesis of salt-dependent hypertension in experimental animals (47).

Adrenomedullin

Adrenomedullin is a 52–amino acid peptide that was isolated from human pheochromocytoma cells (48). It reacts with a G-protein cell receptor and causes vasodilatation, an effect that may be mediated by increased synthesis of NO. The resultant natriuresis secondary to the increase in GFR is accompanied by direct inhibition of tubular sodium reabsorption. Its role in sodium balance is under investigation.

Water

Arginine Vasopressin

The primary efferent mechanism in the maintenance of water homeostasis is AVP. This peptide fosters water retention by the kidney and stimulates thirst. The plasma AVP concentration is approximately 1 to 2 pg/mL under basal conditions (26). It is not known whether there is tonic release of AVP or whether there is pulsatile secretion in response to minute fluctuations in plasma osmolality. The set point, or osmotic threshold for AVP release, ranges from 275 to 290 mOsm/kg H_2O. The circulating hormone concentration rises approximately 1 pg/mL for each 1% increase in plasma osmolality. The sensitivity of the osmoreceptors in promoting AVP release varies from person to person, with some individuals capable of responding to as small as a 0.5 mOsm/kg H_2O increase in osmolality and others requiring greater than a 5 mOsm/kg H_2O increment to stimulate AVP release. Patients with essential hypernatremia possess osmoreceptors that have normal sensitivity, but the osmotic threshold for AVP release is shifted to the right. Because the relative distribution of water between the ECW and ICW compartments is undisturbed, these patients are clinically unaffected by their abnormally high-serum sodium concentration. Although there may be gender-related differences in AVP secretion in response to abnormal water homeostasis with increased sensitivity in women, this is not a relevant clinical concern in prepubertal children.

Angiotensin

Angiotensin II serves as an efferent system in water homeostasis primarily by stimulating drinking (30). Its role in water handling within the kidney is minor and may be related to modulation of the renal response to AVP.

Thirst

Thirst, or the consciously perceived desire to drink, is a major efferent system in water homeostasis (29). It is estimated that for each 1-pg/mL increase in the circulating plasma AVP level, there is a parallel rise of 100 mOsm/kg H_2O in urinary concentration. If the basal plasma osmolality and AVP concentration are approximately 280 mOsm/kg H_2O and 2 pg/mL, respectively, and the steady state urine osmolality is 200 mOsm/kg H_2O, then as soon as the plasma osmolality and AVP concentration reach 290 mOsm/kg H_2O and 12 pg/mL, respectively, the urine is maximally concentrated. Beyond this point, the only operational defense against further increases in plasma osmolality is increased free water intake. This underscores the essential role of thirst as an efferent mechanism in water homeostasis. Moreover, it highlights the increased risk of hyperosmolality developing in patients who do not have free access to water such as infants, those who are physically or mentally incapacitated, or the elderly (49).

Thirst is a very difficult biologic function to quantitate, because it is an expression of a drive rather than an actual behavior. At present, visual analog scales using colors or faces are the most useful tools for quantitating thirst under controlled condition. There can be dissociation between water intake and the sensation of thirst, as in patients with psychogenic polydipsia (e.g., schizophrenia, neurosis). It is not known whether specific drugs directly stimulate the dipsogenic response. The role of diet (e.g., high salt intake) in the regulation of thirst is unknown. The osmotic control of thirst may be suboptimal in both newborn infants and in the elderly (49).

Thirst and drinking behavior are stimulated by significant contraction of the ECF space or by hypotension. In addition, thirst and drinking behavior are modulated by signals that originate in the oropharynx and upper gastrointestinal behavior. Thus, in animals with hypernatremia, those that are given free access to water as the sole means of correcting the hyperosmolal state will stop drinking sooner than animals, which are corrected in part with supplemental intravenous fluid. This is most likely due to oropharyngeal stimuli that curtail drinking before complete normalization of the plasma osmolality (50).

EFFECTOR MECHANISMS: SODIUM AND WATER

The kidney is the principal organ that acts in response to sensory input, delivered via neural or humoral signals, to restore ECW volume size to normal after the full range of clinical problems. These are supplemented by specific anatomic features of the effector organ to achieve normal homeostasis. Although absorption of sodium and water across the intestinal epithelium may be modulated by chemoreceptors in the hepatic vasculature, the role of the gastrointestinal tract in the control of sodium balance is clearly secondary to the function of the kidney.

Sodium

Glomerular Filtration Rate

In children with normal kidney function, changes in GFR are generally associated with parallel alterations in sodium balance. This is accomplished by glomerular-tubular balance, in which proximal tubule sodium absorption and delivery of filtrate to the distal tubule is modulated in response to GFR (51). Thus, tubular sodium reabsorption increases in parallel with an increase in GFR. This, in part, reflects the load-dependent nature of sodium reabsorption in the proximal tubule. In addition, changes in GFR lead to changes in the oncotic pressure within the peritubular capillaries that also influence sodium reabsorption (52). Thus, an increased GFR is associated with higher hydrostatic pressures in the peritubular capillary network that retard fluid and solute reabsorption in the proximal tubule changes. Finally, tubuloglomerular feedback is activated by alterations in solute delivery to the distal nephron to bring GFR in line with alterations in tubular function. Many of the efferent signals, including renin, angiotensin, NO, and PGs, participate in this particular pathway. The release of these effector molecules is activated via myogenic stretch receptors and chemoreceptors located in the macula densa region of the distal nephron. Even in children with compromised renal function (GFR <20 to 30 mL/min/1.73 m^2) in whom there are adaptive changes in tubular function [e.g., increased fractional excretion of sodium (FE_{Na})], glomerulotubular balance is maintained in the face of gradual changes in GFR. However, patients with chronic renal failure are unable to respond to abrupt changes in sodium balance and ECF volume changes as rapidly as healthy children. Therefore, they are susceptible to volume contraction or hypervolemia if sodium intake is substantially reduced or increased over a short period of time (13).

Most of the neural and humoral factors described previously can modulate GFR. Agents that lower GFR may act predominantly on the vascular tone of the afferent arteriole and cause substantial reduction in RBF and the filtration fraction. Agents in this category include adrenergic nerve stimulation and endothelin. In contrast, angiotensin II acts primarily on efferent arteriolar tone and tends to preserve GFR more than RBF. Therefore, filtration fraction (GFR/RBF) is increased. This pattern is most evident in states of compromised effective perfusion such as congestive heart failure, cirrhosis, and nephrotic syndrome (24,25,53). The critical role of angiotensin II in maintaining GFR and sodium excretion in these conditions is manifest during the functional decline in GFR that occurs after the administration of angiotensin-converting enzyme inhibitors (54). This phenomenon also explains the reversible reduction in kidney function and sodium retention that are observed in patients with a critical renal artery stenosis in a kidney transplant after initiation of angiotensin-converting enzyme inhibitor therapy (54).

Proximal Tubule

Nearly 60 to 70% of the filtered sodium and water load are reabsorbed in the proximal tubule. Sodium and fluid reabsorption are isosmotic in this segment of the nephron. These processes are driven by Na-K-ATPase activity along the basolateral membrane surface with secondary active transport of solute across the apical membrane. The bulk of sodium reabsorption is driven by the sodium-hydrogen exchanger, with a lesser contribution by other cotransport systems for glucose, phosphate, organic anions, and amino acids. The linkage between disturbances in ECF volume and sodium reabsorption in the proximal tubule is created, in part, by changes in the physical forces that govern fluid and solute movement. These include changes in peritubular capillary hydrostatic pressure, peritubular capillary protein concentration and oncotic pressure, and changes in renal interstitial pressure that modulate water and solute movement across cells (transcellular) and along the paracellular pathway.

It is now evident that sympathetic nervous stimulation, norepinephrine release, and both filtered and locally synthesized angiotensin II stimulate the activity of the sodium-hydrogen antiporter and promote sodium reabsorption in conditions associated with decreased ECF volume. Conversely, ANP and the kinins act on proximal tubular cells to inhibit sodium reabsorption and limit expansion of the ECW space.

Distal Nephron Including Collecting Duct

This portion of the nephron is responsible for the reabsorption of approximately 10 to 25% of the filtered sodium and water load. Under most circumstances, it can adapt to changes in delivery arising from alterations in proximal tubule function. This segment of the nephron is responsive to virtually all of the humoral efferent signals and accomplishes the final renal homeostatic response to fluctuations in sodium balance. Sodium reabsorption in the distal tubule and connecting segment is responsive to circulating levels of aldosterone (34). In the collecting tubule, there are mineralocorticoid-responsive sodium reabsorptive pathways that are responsible for the final modulation of sodium excretion in response to alterations in sodium intake. The most prominent of these is the epithelial sodium channel (ENaC). This transepithelial protein is composed of three distinct chains—α, β, and γ—each of which is encoded by a separate gene (55). The complete protein has two membrane-spanning domains with an amino and carboxyl terminus within the cell. The α-chain appears to constitute the actual sodium-conducting pathway, whereas the β- and γ-chains may represent regulatory components that control the open/closed status of the channel. Genetic defects in each of the individual components have been described and linked to human disease. Thus, pseudohypoaldosteronism has been mapped to mutations in the α-, β-, and γ-chains, and Liddle's syndrome has been attributed to truncation in the β-chain (55).

Water

Arginine Vasopressin

AVP acts along several segments of the nephron. However, its primary site of AVP action for maintenance of water homeostasis is the collecting tubule (56). In the segment of the nephron, AVP reacts with a V2 receptor—a 371–amino acid protein that is coupled to a heterotrimeric G-protein—along the basolateral membrane of cells along the distal tubule and the collecting duct. The V2 receptor gene has been localized to region 28 of the X chromosome. This epithelial cell receptor is distinct from the V1 receptor in the vasculature that is linked to Ca-activation of the inositol triphosphate cascade, which mediates vasoconstrictor response to the hormone (56).

Binding of AVP to the V2 receptor activates basolateral adenylate cyclase and stimulates the formation of cyclic adenosine monophosphate within the cytosol. This intracellular second messenger then interacts with the cytoskeleton, specifically microtubules and actin filaments, and promotes fusion of intramembrane particles that contain preformed water channels with the apical membrane of principal cells in the collecting duct. The AVP-induced entry of preformed water channels involves clathrin-coated pits. Withdrawal of AVP is followed by endocytosis of the membrane segment containing the water channels into vesicles that can be localized to the submembrane domain of the cell. This results in termination of the hormone signal. The recycling of water channels from vesicles to the apical membrane and then back into vesicles has been demonstrated in freeze-fracture studies of cells exposed to AVP (56). The importance of the V2 receptor in water homeostasis has been confirmed by the documentation of numerous mutations in the gene and corresponding abnormalities in protein structure in children with X-linked congenital nephrogenic diabetes insipidus (57).

The water channels that mediate increased transmembrane movement of water across the collecting tubule in response to AVP have been identified and are called *aquaporins* (58). There are nine known members of this group of transmembrane water channels, all of which contain six membrane-spanning domains. The first member to be identified was aquaporin-1 (AQP-1; originally called channel-forming integral membrane protein of 28 kDa or CHIP-28). It is a transmembrane protein that mediates water movement across the erythrocyte membrane and along the proximal tubule. Mice that do not express AQP-1 have a normal phenotype and concentrate their urine normally. Aquaporin-2 (AQP-2) is the major AVP-sensitive water channel in the collecting tubule (59). Immunogold electron microscopy studies have confirmed that AQP-2 represents the water channel that is present within the cytosolic vesicles that fuse with the apical membrane after exposure of principal cells in the collecting duct to AVP. The contribution of AQP-3 and AQP-4 to the normal urinary-concentrating mechanism has been confirmed in mice that have been genetically manipulated and do not express these two proteins (60).

The importance of AQP-2 in mediating the normal response to AVP has been verified by the discovery of mutations in the AQP-2 gene in children with non–X-linked, autosomal recessive forms of nephrogenic diabetes insipidus (61). Moreover, alterations in AQP-2 protein expression have been documented in other states associated with a urinary-concentrating defect, such as lithium exposure, urinary tract obstruction, hypokalemia, and hypercalcemia (58).

It is important to acknowledge that water reabsorption in the collecting duct is not completely dependent on the presence of AVP. Thus, even in animals that are genetically deficient in AVP (Brattleboro rats) or in patients with central diabetes insipidus, the urinary osmolality does increase slightly above basal levels in the face of severe ECF volume contraction. This concentration may be the consequence of reduction in urinary flow rate along the collecting duct that enables some passive equilibration to occur between the luminal fluid and the hypertonic medullary interstitium.

Although the collecting duct is the primary site of regulation of net water reabsorption, the proximal tubule may contribute to water balance under circumstances of decreased ECW compartment size. Whereas the proximal tubule normally reabsorbs approximately 60% of the filtered water load, this proportion may exceed 70% when the ECF volume is diminished. Furthermore, by decreasing fluid delivery to the distal nephron, this may enhance the AVP-independent reabsorption of water along the collecting tubule. These combined effects may explain the beneficial effects that have been observed after administration of thiazide diuretics to patients with nephrogenic diabetes insipidus (62).

Countercurrent Mechanism

The primary locus of the urinary-concentrating mechanism is the medulla and involves the thin descending limb of Henle, the medullary thick ascending limb of Henle, the cortical thick ascending limb of Henle, and the collecting duct (63). Sodium and water reabsorption are isosmotic in all segments of the nephron proximal to the loop of Henle. To concentrate or dilute the urine, water and solute must be separated to enable excretion of free water or urine that is hyperosmolal relative to plasma. This process begins in the medullary and cortical thick ascending limb of Henle in which NaCl is reabsorbed independently of water, generating a hypotonic luminal fluid. This action is linked in series to the low water permeability of the distal tubule and the connecting segment, which together with continued sodium reabsorption enhances the hypotonicity of the urine in this segment. In a secondary step, the permeability to water along this segment of the nephron is much lower than in the descending limb of the loop of Henle. This enables water to move down its osmolal gradient from the tubule lumen into the interstitium as it enters the medulla in the descending limb. Finally, the third critical component of the countercurrent mechanism is the presence of vasa recta, which perfuse the inner medulla via vascular bundles that contain hairpin loop–shaped blood vessels. This facilitates the efficient removal of the water that exits in the descending limb of Henle from the medullary interstitium without washing out the solute gradient that passively drives water reabsorption in the collecting tubule. The final effector mechanism is the alteration in the water permeability of the collecting tubule in response to AVP and the generation of a concentrated urine or the excretion of solute free water in the absence of AVP (Table 7.3).

Osmoprotective Molecule (Compatible Osmolytes)

Besides the presence of effector mechanisms to maintain water balance, cells possess a wide range of adaptive mechanisms to counteract the undesirable movement of water between the cell and the ECW during hypotonic and hypertonic states and prevent neurologic dysfunction. These mechanisms include early response genes that result in the immediate accumulation of chaperone molecules that counteract the adverse effects of altered cell size on protein function (14). This immediate response is followed in short order by the uptake or extrusion of electrolytes as an acute response to the altered size cell. Because there are inherent limits on the ability to regulate cell volume exclusively with inorganic electrolytes, this is followed by a more extended response involving the membrane transport or synthesis/degradation of a variety of compatible solutes, called *osmolytes*, whose cytosolic concentration can be safely altered within the cell without perturbing cell function. These osmoprotective molecules include various carbohydrates (sorbitol, myo-inositol), amino acids (taurine, glutamate), and methylamines (betaine, glycerophosphorylcholine) (14). The osmolytes accumulate in the cytosol to preserve cell function during chronic osmolal disturbances. The cell volume regulatory response can be activated by electrolytes such as sodium or neutral molecules (e.g., urea and glucose) (14). The adequacy of the cell volume regulatory response and the accumulation of osmoprotective molecules in cerebral and renal cells may be dependent on the rate of rise in osmolality, as well as the magnitude of the absolute change (64).

Experimental data in animals and clinical experience in premenopausal women suggest that estrogens may impair the cell volume regulatory response to disturbances in plasma osmolality. This increases the risks associated with both the untreated abnormalities and therapy (65). Although there are some who assert that adaptive control of cell size is inadequate during development, it has been demonstrated that the accumulation of osmoprotective molecules during chronic hypernatremia is normal in preweanling rats and, in fact, there is a higher set-point to preserve the increased brain cell water content (66).

Failure to adequately account for the cell volume regulatory response to osmolal disorders contributes to some of the adverse effects associated with inappropriate correction of abnormalities in plasma osmolality. These effects include neurologic dysfunction, specifically seizures, during the treatment of hypernatremia; osmotic demyelinating syndrome during rapid reversal of hyponatremia; dialysis dysequilibrium syndrome that occurs during the initiation of dialysis in patients with acute or chronic renal failure; and cerebral edema and brain herniation in patients with diabetic ketoacidosis (67,68).

TABLE 7.3. FACTORS THAT CONTRIBUTE TO THE COUNTERCURRENT MECHANISM

Na-Cl-K–mediated solute absorption in the medullary thick ascending limb of Henle
Low water permeability of the distal tubule and connecting segment
High water permeability in the descending limb of Henle
Vasa recta and elimination of interstitial water volume
Arginine vasopressin responsiveness of the collecting tubule

LABORATORY ASSESSMENT OF SODIUM AND WATER BALANCE

There are no normal values for sodium and water intake or excretion, reflecting the wide range of normal daily intake for both sodium and water as a consequence of differences in dietary composition. Healthy individuals are in balance, and the excretion of sodium and water matches the daily intake. Therefore, laboratory assessment of sodium and water homeostasis is confined to disease states in which the clinicians must determine whether renal sodium and water handling are appropriate for the clinical circumstances, will maintain balance, and will prevent disturbances in ECF volume or water distribution between the ICW and ECW compartments.

Sodium

The urine sodium concentration is not a valid index of sodium balance, because the value may vary depending on the volume and concentration of the sample. Therefore, the renal handling of sodium is best evaluated using the FE_{Na}. After obtaining a random urine sample and a simultaneous blood sample and measuring the sodium and creatinine concentrations in both specimens, the FE_{Na} is calculated using the following formula:

$$FE_{Na} = \text{Excreted sodium/Filtered sodium}$$
$$= \text{Urinary sodium concentration} \times \text{urine flow rate/Plasma sodium concentration} \times \text{GFR}$$
$$= \frac{\text{Urine sodium concentration/Plasma sodium concentration}}{\text{Urine creatinine concentration/Plasma creatinine concentration}}$$

This formula is based on the insertion of the creatinine clearance as a measurement of GFR in the second equation and the cancellation of the urine flow rate term in the numerator and denominator. Therefore, the determination of the FE_{Na} is a particularly useful test in clinical practice, because the measurement does not require a timed urine collection. In healthy individuals, this value varies depending on the daily sodium intake. However, in patients with ECF volume contraction who are responding appropriately to retain sodium, the FE_{Na} is less than 1% (less than 3% in neonates). Conversely, in patients with expansion of the ECW compartment, the FE_{Na} typically will exceed 3% unless there is concomitant renal disease.

Water

Determination of the urine-specific gravity or osmolality in a random sample will vary depending on the water intake in the past 2 to 4 hours. Therefore, the assessment of water handling is best judged by determining these values under more controlled conditions such as in the water-deprived state or after administration of a water load (10 to 20 mL/kg body weight) to evaluate the urinary concentrating or diluting capacity, respectively.

The functional aspects of renal water handling are best assessed by determining the free water clearance. This represents the amount of solute-free water excreted by the kidney. It is calculated using the following formula:

$$\text{Free water clearance} = \text{Urine volume} - \text{osmolal clearance}$$
$$= \text{Urine volume} - [\text{Urine osmolality} \times \text{urine flow rate}]/\text{Plasma osmolality}$$

If the free water clearance is a positive number, then the urine/plasma osmolality ratio is less than 1, the urine is dilute, and the kidney is in a diuretic mode. When a water diuresis is maximal, the free water clearance measures the capacity of the kidney to excrete free water. In contrast, patients who are in an antidiuretic mode with urine:plasma osmolality ratio greater than 1 and who are able to concentrate their urine will have a negative free water clearance. As the solute excretion rate increases, both the maximum values for free water clearance and free water reabsorption increase. At any given solute excretion rate, the free water clearance greatly exceeds the free water reabsorption. This indicates that the renal water homeostatic mechanisms designed to protect against overhydration and dilution of the ECW are more robust than those used to defend against water deficit and dehydration.

OVERVIEW OF THE EVALUATION OF FLUID AND WATER ABNORMALITIES

In practice, the clinical information and laboratory data that are used to evaluate patients overlap with one another. However, in view of the different physiologic roles of sodium and water balance in body fluid homeostasis, the distinct regulatory mechanisms used to control these factors, and the varied therapeutic strategies that must be used to restore sodium and water balance to normal in disease states, it is essential that disturbances in sodium and water balance be evaluated separately. In realtime, these separate assessments are done in parallel, a reflection of the body's own method of operation.

When confronted with a child with a sodium and water disturbance, the first question that must be addressed is whether there is a life-threatening compromise in the size of the ECF volume. Thus, it is necessary to clarify whether the ECF volume is decreased or expanded. By implication, this is an assessment of sodium balance. Such patients have a life-threatening disease and may require emergency therapy such as volume resuscitation or acute ultrafiltration, reflecting the vital importance of a normal ECF volume to maintain intravascular volume within the normal range to sustain perfusion of vital organs.

After making this emergency determination and instituting appropriate therapy, it is important to grade the magnitude of the disturbance in ECF volume. Unfortunately, there are no laboratory tests that can reliably substitute for clinical judgment. Because acute changes in body weight always reflect alterations in sodium balance and ECW compartment size, serial measurements in body weight are the most reliable indicator of the presence and severity of disturbances in ECF volume. However, these measurements are often unavailable and, therefore, the evaluation of sodium balance is based on a wide range of clinical findings, including changes in mental status, level of alertness, irritability, presence of thirst, pulse rate, blood pressure, orthostatic changes, fullness of the anterior fontanelle in infants, the presence of tears, dryness of the mucus membranes, skin color, elasticity of the skin or tenting, capillary refill or turgor, peripheral edema, shortness of breath, and the presence of rales on auscultation of the chest. Some investigators have documented that capillary refill may be the most useful test to rapidly and accurately assess ECF volume and the response to treatment (69). Other findings on clinical examination include urinary-specific gravity and central venous pressure. Laboratory investigations include BUN, serum creatinine, and bicarbonate concentrations.

It is important to emphasize that assessment of ECF volume is a clinical determination. There is no laboratory test that is a valid surrogate marker. Moreover, despite the frequency of clinical disturbances in sodium balance, especially ECF volume contraction, no suitable scoring has been devised based on any combination of the previously mentioned elements that can be used to accurately and reliably distinguish different degrees of ECF volume contraction or expansion. This deficiency is in contrast to the Glasgow coma score or APACHE (acute physiology and chronic health evaluation) score that have been successfully applied to the initial assessment of patients with acute neurologic or multisystem illnesses.

The third step in the evaluation of a patient with a sodium and water disturbance is to evaluate the plasma osmolality. This evaluation indicates whether there will be an abnormal distribution of water between the ECW and ICW compartments. The most likely symptoms that will be present in affected patients will arise secondary to central nervous dysfunction. These include confusion, irritability, lethargy, obtundation, and seizures. These manifestations overlap significantly in patients with hyperosmolality or hypoosmolality. Moreover, there is no obligatory change in ECF volume. Therefore, unlike disorders of ECF volume, disturbances in water balance and distribution require a laboratory determination for confirmation and grading. The steps involved in the initial evaluation of a child with a disturbance in sodium and water balance are outlined in Table 7.4.

TABLE 7.4. STEPS IN THE INITIAL EVALUATION AND TREATMENT OF A CHILD WITH A DISTURBANCE IN SODIUM AND/OR WATER BALANCE

Step 1: Determine whether there is a life-threatening alteration in ECF volume.
  Volume resuscitation if there is ECF volume contraction.
  Consider ultrafiltration if there is ECF volume expansion.
Step 2: Grade severity of defect in sodium balance.
  Clinical determination of ECF volume.
Step 3: Determine whether there is a defect in water balance.
  Laboratory measurement of plasma osmolality.

ECF, extracellular fluid.

SODIUM BALANCE DISTURBANCES: DEFICIT AND EXCESS

Sodium Deficit

Diagnosis and Evaluation

In children with normal kidney function, consumption of a diet that is low or high in sodium does not generally cause a net negative or positive sodium balance, because the kidney can adaptively modify sodium reabsorption to parallel fluctuations in salt intake if the changes are not too abrupt or massive in nature.

Sodium deficits and ECF volume contraction are dangerous because decreased size of the intravascular fluid can lead to reduced perfusion and ischemia in organs such as the brain, heart, and kidneys. In children, the absence of concomitant atherosclerosis disease or endothelial dysfunction secondary to essential hypertension, smoking, hyperlipidemia, and diabetes decreases this risk. However, there are groups of pediatric patients who may be more susceptible to the adverse consequences of hypovolemia These include newborn babies in whom high circulating levels of vasoconstrictor hormones and impaired autoregulation render the glomerular microcirculation particularly sensitive to reduced perfusion (70). In addition, underlying diseases or medications may hinder the counterregulatory responses to ECF volume contraction and enhance the risks of hypovolemia.

Diseases that cause sodium deficiency can originate outside the kidney or within the kidney. It is unfortunate that the word *dehydration* is often used to describe these states because it deflects attention from the primary defect, namely a net negative sodium balance, and suggests that water deficit is the major pathophysiologic problem in these conditions (71,72). The critical role of the ECF space and sodium balance in the pathogenesis of states of volume contraction is highlighted by comparing them with diabetes insipidus. When sodium balance is perturbed, >60% of the fluid loss is derived from the ECW compartment, provoking the rapid onset of symptoms. In contrast, only 8% of the pure water loss that occurs in diabetes insipidus is derived from the ECF, accounting for the rare evidence of ECF volume contraction. Use of the term *denaturation* may provide a more accurate depiction of what is occurring in patients with primary deficits in sodium balance and contraction of the ECF volume (71).

Extrarenal causes can be attributed to losses of sodium in any body fluid or across any epithelial surface, including the cerebrospinal fluid, pleural fluid, biliary tree, gastrointestinal losses, or the skin. They can represent the result of a disease process, or they may be iatrogenic in nature. Renal diseases can cause sodium deficit as a result of limited homeostatic capacity caused by a compromise in GFR. Alternatively, there may be primary renal sodium loss that is not the consequence of a decrease in kidney function. Finally, renal sodium reabsorption may be diminished

TABLE 7.5. CAUSES OF NET SODIUM DEFICIT

- Renal causes
  - Compromised glomerular filtration rate
    - Acute decrease in sodium intake or increased losses
  - Tubular disorders
    - Osmotic diuresis
    - Diabetic ketoacidosis
    - Renal tubular acidosis
    - Pseudohypoaldosteronism
    - Obstructive uropathy
    - Bartter's syndrome
    - Renal dysplasia/hypoplasia
- Central nervous system
  - Cerebral salt wasting
  - Cerebrospinal fluid drainage procedures
- Hepatobiliary system
  - Biliary tract drainage
- Gastrointestinal tract
  - Infectious diarrhea
  - Chloride diarrhea
  - Laxative abuse
  - Malignancy (carcinoid, tumor-related)
- Adrenal diseases
  - Salt-losing congenital adrenal hyperplasia
  - Addison's disease
- Skin losses
  - Cystic fibrosis
  - Neuroectodermal diseases
  - Burns

because of reduced circulating levels of aldosterone or unresponsiveness to the hormone. The major causes of sodium deficiency are summarized in Table 7.5.

The diagnosis of the cause of a disturbance in sodium balance is made based on the history and physical examination. In most cases, this information is adequate to identify the source of the sodium losses. Previously, the degree of ECF volume contraction was categorized as mild, moderate, or severe if the changes in body weight were estimated to be less than 5%, 5 to 10%, or more than 10%, respectively. Life-threatening ECF volume contraction was thought to represent a more than 15% decrease in weight. Recent data, based on systematic body weights at the time of hospitalization and immediately after correction of the sodium deficit, suggest that these numbers overestimate the degree of sodium deficit and that the ECF volume contraction is better estimated to be less than 3%, 3 to 6%, and greater than 6% with a greater than 9% change in body weight representing an emergency (73).

If the losses are primarily extrarenal in nature, then renal sodium retentive mechanisms will be activated, and the specific gravity of the urine will be more than 1.015 and the FE_{Na} will be low, specifically less than 1%. Failure to increase the urine concentration and a high FE_{Na} in the face of clinical signs of ECF volume contraction points toward a renal or adrenal cause for the disorder. A renal ultrasound documenting the presence of small, misshaped kidneys or hydronephrosis may be indicative of congenital abnormalities of the kidney, such as dysplasia or obstructive uropathy.

Treatment

In the unusual circumstance in which the ECW is so severely contracted that vital organ perfusion is compromised, based on an altered mental status, orthostatic changes, and azotemia, then fluid resuscitation must be initiated on an emergent basis. This treatment is necessary to prevent the development of acute tubular necrosis, which may occur if there is hypotension and renal ischemia secondary to ECF volume contraction. The risk of acute renal failure is higher in children with preexisting renal disease, children who are receiving nephrotoxic medications, or children who have concomitant hemoglobinuria or myoglobinuria. If there is no evidence of cardiac or pulmonary disease, then the optimal therapy under these conditions is infusion of isotonic crystalloid (0.9% NaCl, Ringer's lactate), 20-mL/kg body weight. Although transfusions of whole blood are optimal for treatment of hemorrhagic shock, infusion of crystalloid solutions avoids difficulties caused by extravasation of the colloid into the interstitial compartment. Moreover, a systematic review of the literature does not support the use of colloid solutions for volume replacement in critically ill patients (74). This fluid is appropriate regardless of what the initial serum sodium or osmolality is, and concerns about the advisability of infusing Ringer's lactate are misplaced in view of the low potassium concentration (4 mmol/L) in this solution. A catheter should be placed in the bladder to facilitate monitoring of urine output. The infusion should be as rapid as possible, and the fluid dose should be repeated as often as necessary to achieve some evidence of clinical improvement, such as improved mental status, decrease in pulse, rise in blood pressure, or improved capillary refill.

After addressing and correcting the underlying disease, a fluid repletion plan should be initiated as soon as possible. Preference should be given to correcting sodium and electrolyte deficits with oral rehydration solutions (ORS). In general, patients can be repleted with a rapid (1 to 2 hour) intravenous infusion to restore ECF volume followed immediately by initiation of ORS (75). The only conditions that represent contraindications to the use of ORS are impaired neurologic status, persistent vomiting, or diseases associated with mucosal damage in the gastrointestinal lumen.

ORS fluids introduced by the World Health Organization contain sodium 90; potassium 20; bicarbonate 30; chloride; and glucose (20 g/L), 111 mmol/L. The sodium and glucose are present in a molar ratio that maximizes the secondary active uptake of these solutes via the sodium-glucose cotransporter across the gastrointestinal epithelium. Water is absorbed passively down its osmolal gradient. The presence of other solutes, such as potassium and bicarbonate, are not critical to the successful use of ORS. These fluids have been used for more than 30 years. They can be administered ad libitum in response to the child's own thirst, and they are effective and safe with minimal occurrence of hypernatremia or hyperkalemia. There is evidence that various alternatives to glucose, such as rice-syrup or amylase-resistant starch, may facilitate sodium and water reabsorption from ORS, decrease fecal fluid loss, and shorten recovery time after an episode of cholera (76,77). However, further clinical studies are needed to confirm the use of these additives because they may increase the cost and decrease the shelf life of ORS. These are important considerations in developing countries where there is a high incidence of infectious diarrhea in infants and children.

In specific circumstances when parenteral therapy is required to correct sodium and water deficits, the following guidelines can be applied when devising a therapeutic plan. First, in the absence of reliable data regarding the acute weight loss, it is easiest to calculate the maintenance and deficit therapy based on the clinical estimate of the percentage decrease in body weight. Second, it is advisable to discount any emergency fluid therapy, such as bolus infusions of isotonic saline, in computing the fluid prescription. Third, if the clinical problem has developed in less than 48 hours, then it should be considered an acute process, and the sodium and fluid losses are derived from the ICW and ECW in the ratio of 80 to 20%. If the patient has been ill for more than 48 hours and the process is chronic, then the sodium and fluid losses are derived from the ICW and ECW in the ratio of 60 to 40%. Under most conditions in which the sodium and water losses are isotonic, the ECW portion of the loss, in liters, can be multiplied by 140 mmol/L to determine the sodium loss. Similarly, the ICW portion of the loss, in liters, can be multiplied by 140 mmol/L to determine the potassium deficit. If the ECW and ICW fluid losses together with the respective sodium and potassium deficits are added to the maintenance requirements, then a total fluid volume can be determined. After selecting a fluid that most closely approximates the total sodium and water losses, the total fluid volume is divided by the time frame of the correction to determine the intravenous infusion rate.

As an example, if a 10-kg child is judged to have a 5% decrease in body weight over 36 hours, then the total fluid deficit of 500 mL can be divided into two components—400 mL ICW with 56 mmol potassium and 100 mL ECW containing 14 mmol sodium. The daily maintenance water and sodium requirements are 1000 mL and 30 mmol sodium. Adding these two quantities together results in a fluid that closely resembles 0.25% saline (37 mmol NaCl/L) containing 30 mmol KCl/L, and the infusion rate is approximately 60 mL/hr if the correction is designed to occur over 24 hours. In all cases, it is important to monitor and replace ongoing losses to insure that there is full resolution of the underlying clinical problem.

Sodium Excess

Diagnosis and Evaluation

These conditions, which generally are less common than sodium deficit, are evidenced by clinical signs of ECF volume expansion. The causes of net total body sodium excess are noted in Table 7.6. They can arise secondary to exogenous addition of sodium or abnormal retention of endogenous sodium. Because the normal kidney can rapidly excrete a sodium load, for the excess sodium to cause clinical symptoms and signs, there must be a concomitant factor that limits natriuresis.

Common causes of excess exogenous sodium are saltwater drowning, ingestion of a diet abnormally high in sodium, or therapeutic infusion of sodium-containing intravenous solutions, such as sodium bicarbonate during the resuscitation after a cardiopulmonary arrest. Examples of dietary excess of sodium include errors in the preparation of infant formulas. The widespread use of premixed baby formulas may decrease the incidence of these accidents.

The conditions associated with excessive endogenous sodium retention include acute renal failure and the edema states, namely nephrotic syndrome, cirrhosis, and congestive heart failure. In the first condition, which may occur owing to glomerulonephritis or tubular necrosis, the sodium retention is directly related to the decrease in GFR and diminished filtration of sodium. In the latter three states, renal sodium and water reabsorption are activated by a combination of mechanisms that are termed *underfill* and *overfill*. A critical review of available evidence in patients with nephrotic syndrome suggests that those diseases that are associated with an inflammatory infiltrate in the kidney develop primary sodium retention and overfilling of the ECF volume. This histopathologic feature is absent in most cases of minimal change nephrotic syndrome (78). Thus, in nephrotic syndrome, the total body sodium excess may be coupled with a diminished, normal, or expanded effective ECF volume, explaining the normal distribution of plasma renin activity values and the variability in measurements of plasma volume in these patients.

The clinical problems that accompany these conditions are mainly related to pulmonary venous congestion, impaired

TABLE 7.6. CAUSES OF NET SODIUM EXCESS

Exogenous sodium
- Saltwater drowning
- Errors in formula preparation
- Infusion of hypertonic sodium solutions (e.g., after cardiopulmonary arrest)

Endogenous sodium
- Acute renal failure (glomerulonephritis, acute tubular necrosis)
- Nephrotic syndrome
- Cirrhosis
- Congestive heart failure

gas exchange in the lung, and difficulty breathing. In idiopathic nephrotic syndrome, the intraalveolar pressure is often sufficient to prevent frank pulmonary edema. However, in other circumstances, there may be intrinsic capillary leak together with lowered plasma oncotic pressure, augmenting the development of pulmonary interstitial fluid. Peripheral edema may be associated with skin infection, peritonitis, or thromboembolic events.

All of the states associated with sodium excess should be evident on physical examination. The FE_{Na} is high if there is sodium loading and renal function is normal. In contrast, in the states associated with abnormal retention of endogenous sodium, the FE_{Na} is very low. The FE_{Na} is more useful than the urinary-specific gravity because it is likely to be elevated in all cases of sodium excess.

Therapy

The optimal therapy is targeted at correcting the underlying disease. This is most important in patients with cirrhosis or congestive heart failure. Ancillary therapies include administration of diuretics to facilitate urinary sodium excretion. Although thiazide diuretics may be adequate, a more potent loop diuretic may be required if the GFR is diminished. Supplemental oxygen may be necessary to alleviate shortness of breath and hypoxemia. In more severe cases, acute dialysis may be necessary to foster rapid clearance of the excess sodium. Patients with nephrotic syndrome may require combinations of diuretic agents that act in the proximal (e.g., metolazone) and distal (e.g., furosemide) segments of the nephron to promote an adequate natriuresis and diuresis. Infusions of albumin (1 g/kg body weight) may be necessary to promote and augment the medication-induced diuresis, especially in those with severe ECF volume contraction, reduced GFR, and azotemia (79). Finally, hemofiltration may be a safe and effective means to rapidly remove sodium and water in severely ECF-overloaded children with nephrotic syndrome (80).

WATER BALANCE DISTURBANCES: DEFICIT AND EXCESS

Hyponatremia

Diagnosis and Evaluation

Patients with hyponatremia have relative or absolute expansion of the ICW compartment. If renal function is normal, excess free water is eliminated within 2 to 4 hours. Therefore, for this problem to occur, two conditions must be satisfied—there must be continued AVP release that is inappropriate to the serum sodium concentration, and the patient must have continued access to free water. The symptoms and signs of hyponatremia, which generally involve central nervous system dysfunction, are vague and nonspecific. Therefore, laboratory confirmation is required to diagnose this abnormality. Moreover, the presence of hyponatremia has no predictive value about the status of the ECF volume. Therefore, this later issue must be assessed clinically to determine whether the child has hypovolemic hypotonicity, isovolemic hypotonicity, or hypervolemic hypotonicity.

It is important to recognize that the laboratory measurement of serum sodium concentration is no longer susceptible to technical errors. In the past, laboratory analyzers measured sodium concentration in the total supernatant phase obtained after centrifugation of blood samples, including lipids and proteins. Because these molecules are not water soluble, they displace sodium into a smaller aqueous phase, leading to a spurious reduction in the serum sodium concentration. All biochemical analyzers that are currently in use assay sodium concentration only in the aqueous phase and result in an accurate determination of the serum sodium level. Therefore, the entity called *pseudohyponatremia* is no longer clinically relevant. In contrast, the reduced serum sodium concentration noted in patients with increased circulating levels of an impermeant solute, such as mannitol, urea, contrast media, or glucose in patients with diabetic ketoacidosis, is valid and reflects osmotic redistribution of water from the ICW to the ECW space. The phenomenon is reflected in the following formula, which enables adjustment of the serum sodium in patients with severe hyperglycemia:

"Physiologic" sodium concentration =
measured serum sodium concentration + 1.6 ×
[Each 100 mg/dL increment in serum glucose >100 mg/dL]

The most common clinical causes of hyponatremia are classified by the concomitant ECF volume status in Table 7.7. In some diseases, such as congestive heart failure, the degree of hyponatremia may be a reflection of circulating AVP levels and sympathetic nervous system activation and provides a marker of disease severity. This relationship has not been demonstrated in patients with nephrotic syndrome or cirrhosis.

The syndrome of inappropriate AVP release causes hyponatremia with mild to modest ECF volume expansion. It can occur as a consequence of central neurologic lesions, pulmonary disease, or tumors. In addition, numerous drugs can result in abnormal secretion or action of AVP and lead to chronic hyponatremia. A list of these agents is provided in Table 7.8. The diagnosis of this problem requires confirmation that the urine is excessively concentrated relative to the plasma osmolality without any evidence of ECF volume contraction or adrenal or thyroid insufficiency. The two hormones are required to maintain the low water permeability of the collecting duct in the absence of AVP. Deficiencies of either hormone impair free water clearance, leading to euvolemic hyponatremia. In practice, this requires comparison of the urine-specific gravity or osmolality with the concurrent serum osmolality. The

TABLE 7.7. CAUSES OF HYPONATREMIA

Hypovolemic: ECF volume contraction
Renal
Mineralocorticoid deficiency
Mineralocorticoid resistance
Diuretics
Polyuric acute renal failure
Salt-wasting renal disease
Renal tubular acidosis
Metabolic alkalosis
Bartter's syndrome/Gitelman's syndrome
Gastrointestinal
Diarrheal dehydration
Gastrointestinal suction
Intestinal fistula
Laxative abuse
Transcutaneous
Cystic fibrosis
Heat exhaustion
"Third space" loss with inadequate fluid replacement
Burns
Major surgery, trauma
Septic shock
Euvolemic: Normal ECF volume
Glucocorticoid deficiency
Hypothyroidism
Mild hypervolemia: ECF volume expansion
Reduced renal water excretion
Antidiuretic drugs
Inappropriate secretion of ADH
Hypervolemic: ECF volume expansion
Acute renal failure (glomerulonephritis, ATN)
Chronic renal failure
Nephrotic syndrome
Cirrhosis
Congestive heart failure
Psychogenic polydipsia/compulsive drinking

ADH, antidiuretic hormone; ATN, acute tubular necrosis; ECF, extracellular fluid.

urine should normally be maximally dilute if the serum sodium concentration is <130 mmol/L or the plasma osmolality is <270 mOsm/kg H_2O. In addition, if the urinary sodium concentration is >40 mmol/L, there is adequate evidence against ECF volume contraction.

Treatment

In all cases, the first line of therapy should be directed at the underlying cause of the low serum sodium concentration. However, hyponatremia often warrants specific corrective treatment. Much ink has been spilled in detailing the appropriate therapy of this electrolyte abnormality. At times, this issue has been quite contentious, and the nephrology community has been divided into two supposedly distinct camps—those who advocate "rapid" versus "slow" correction of hyponatremia. The former group asserts that hyponatremia has direct adverse effects on central nervous system function, including impaired oxygenation that can lead to seizures or cardiopulmonary collapse before initiation of therapy (81). This risk may be especially prominent in premenopausal women. In contrast, there are others who emphasize the cerebral cell volume regulatory response to hyponatremia and highlight the risk of brain cell dehydration and osmotic demyelinating syndrome in patients who are corrected too quickly (82).

TABLE 7.8. DRUGS THAT CAUSE WATER RETENTION AND THE SYNDROME OF INAPPROPRIATE ARGININE VASOPRESSIN (AVP) RELEASE ACCORDING TO MODE OF ACTION

Increasing water permeability of the nephron
AVP (arginine or lysine vasopressin)
Vasopressin analogs (e.g., 1-deamino, 8-D-AVP)
Oxytocin
Promoting AVP release
Barbiturates
Carbamazepine
Clofibrate
Colchicine
Isoproterenol
Nicotine
Vincristine
Inhibition of prostaglandin synthesis
Salicylates
Indomethacin
Acetaminophen (paracetamol)
Other nonsteroidal antiinflammatory drugs
Potentiation of the action of AVP
Chlorpropamide
Cyclophosphamide

Taking into account the entire literature on the subject, current evidence suggests that the risk of hyponatremia is more closely related to the acuity of the change rather than the absolute size of the drop in serum sodium concentration (83). Thus, therapy should be guided by the clinical assessment of the time frame in which hyponatremia has developed. If the hyponatremia is acute—that is, less than 12 hours in duration—then the brain will behave as a perfect osmometer, leading to potentially life-threatening cerebral cell swelling. Under these circumstances, there is an urgent need to reverse the hyponatremia to counteract cell swelling. Clinical experience indicates that infusion of a 3% NaCl solution (513 mmol/L) in a volume designed to raise the sodium concentration by 3 to 5 mmol/L is sufficient to halt central nervous system dysfunction (84). The benefits and lack of adverse effects of acute correction have been confirmed in a series of 34 infants and children with acute water intoxication caused by the administration of dilute infant formula (85). After partial correction is achieved, the hyponatremia can be corrected more slowly. For example, if a 6-year-old child weighing 20 kg (TBW = 0.6 L/kg × 20 kg = 12 L) develops a seizure after a tonsillectomy and is noted to have a serum sodium concentration of 115 mmol/L, then 36 to 60 mmol of sodium are needed to raise the sodium concentration by 3 to 5 mmol/L.

This correction is accomplished by infusing 72 to 120 mL of the hypertonic saline.

If hyponatremia has developed over more than 12 hours or the duration of the problem is unclear, especially if the patient has no signs of neurologic dysfunction, then slow correction is the prudent course of action (82,83). The current definition of low correction includes two features:

1. The rate of rise in serum sodium concentration should be less than 0.6 mmol/L/hr throughout the correction phase.
2. The total increment and/or the final serum sodium concentration after 48 hours of treatment should not exceed 25 mmol/L or 130 mmol/L, respectively.

The more cautious criterion should be applied depending on the initial serum sodium level. If the child develops acute changes in mental status or new neurologic findings, during or shortly after the fluid treatment, then a serum sodium concentration should be checked. Imaging studies, specifically an MRI of the brain, may reveal the changes of osmotic demyelinating syndrome.

In patients with syndrome of inappropriate secretion of antidiuretic hormone, if the underlying cause cannot be corrected, then there are several therapeutic options. Restriction of free water intake to match insensible losses and urine output may be adequate to stabilize the serum sodium concentration. If this is not well tolerated, then administration of furosemide, 1 to 2 mg/kg/day, to promote a hypotonic diuresis together with oral administration of NaCl, 1 to 2 g/day, may correct the hyponatremia. If these measures fail, consideration can be given to treatment with lithium or demeclocycline, two drugs that interfere with AVP action in the collecting tubule to foster excretion of free water and raise the serum sodium concentration (86). Finally, orally active nonpeptide vasopressin antagonists have been developed that may be introduced into clinical practice for the treatment of chronic hyponatremia (87,88).

Hypernatremia

Diagnosis and Evaluation

The causes of hypernatremia are listed in Table 7.9. Hypernatremia may arise owing to excessive intake of sodium and ECF volume expansion. However, excessive water loss relative to the sodium deficit with hypovolemia is far more common. In a recent survey of hypernatremia in hospitalized children, the vast majority had significant underlying medical problems, and 76% of the cases were secondary to inadequate water intake (89). The prevalence of this electrolyte abnormality is much lower than hyponatremia. One of the common causes is diarrheal illness in infants; however, the reduction in the sodium concentration of most baby formulas to match the level in human breast milk has resulted in a dramatic decrease in the incidence of hypernatremic dehydration. Nonetheless, recent changes in medical practice with early discharge of newborn infants after delivery have resulted in a steady occurrence of hypernatremic dehydration in breast-fed babies (90). Patients with hypernatremia have relative or absolute contraction of the ICW compartment. Similar to the situation with hyponatremia, the clinical clues to the presence of hypernatremia are nonspecific. Therefore, laboratory confirmation is required to diagnose this abnormality. Moreover, the presence of hyponatremia must be evaluated in light of the status of the ECF volume.

Those patients with hypernatremia and ECF volume expansion are easy to diagnose. The children who represent a serious problem are those with hypovolemia. They may have some distinct features, including marked irritability, a high-pitched cry, and a doughy skin texture. Because the hyperosmolality of the ECW compartment provokes movement of water from the ICW down its osmolal gradient, these patients tend to preserve ECF volume until late in the disease course. Thus, their illness is usually chronic, and there is a greater contribution of the ICW to the water and electrolyte deficits. Assessment of the FE_{Na} is useful in assessing the ECF volume in these patients.

TABLE 7.9. CAUSES OF HYPERNATREMIA

Hypovolemic: ECF volume contraction
Gastrointestinal (diarrhea and vomiting)
Evaporative (high fever, high ambient temperature)
Hypothalamic diabetes insipidus (ADH deficiency)
Head trauma
Infarction (Sheehan's syndrome)
Tumors (e.g., craniopharyngioma)
Histiocytosis
Degenerative brain diseases
Infections
Hereditary central diabetes insipidus (usually dominant)
Idiopathic
Nephrogenic diabetes insipidus (ADH resistance)
Chronic renal failure
Hypokalemia
Hypercalcemia
Damage to renal medulla
Sickle cell disease
Nephronophthisis
Renal papillary necrosis
Chronic pyelonephritis (reflux nephropathy)
Euvolemic: normal ECF volume
Unconscious patients
Infants
Lack of access to water (lost in the desert)
Primary adipsia
Essential hypernatremia (osmoreceptor destruction or malfunction)
Hypervolemic: ECF volume expansion
Inappropriate IV fluid therapy
Salt poisoning
Mineralocorticoid excess

ADH, antidiuretic hormone; ECF, extracellular fluid.

Treatment

Because children with hypovolemic hypernatremia are usually very ill, they often require substantial infusions of isotonic saline to restore organ perfusion. Once adequate perfusion is accomplished, the fluid regimen should include the maintenance fluids, the estimated deficit with the assumption that 60% is derived from the ECW and 40% from the ICW. In addition, there is a free water deficit that can be calculated from the following formula:

$$\text{Water deficit (in L)} = 0.6 \times \text{Body weight} \times [(\text{Actual serum sodium concentration}/140) - 1]$$

There is some evidence that this formula may overestimate the water deficit, and it has been recommended that the following alternative equation (91) be used to estimate the change in serum sodium concentration that will be achieved after the infusion of 1 L of a given solution:

$$\text{Change in sodium concentration} = [\text{Infusate } Na^+ - \text{serum } Na^+]/(\text{TBW} + 1)$$

Finally, with regard to the rate of correction, it is standard practice to correct hypovolemic hypernatremia gradually over at least 48 hours. After the groundbreaking work of Finberg et al. (92), the risk of cerebral edema after rapid correction of chronic hypernatremia is now attributed to the inability of brain cells to extrude the osmoprotective solutes that accumulate during sustained hyperosmolal conditions in parallel with the decline in plasma osmolality during fluid therapy (93,94). Therefore, the osmolal gradient is reversed with plasma osmolality lower than cerebral cell osmolality, leading to ICW expansion and clinical signs of cerebral edema. This experimental observation was confirmed in a randomized trial, which demonstrated that the safest and most effective fluid therapy for hypovolemic hypernatremia is 0.18% NaCl given slowly over 48 hours, compared to 0.45% saline given slowly or rapidly over the same time period (95). Because hyperosmolality impairs insulin and parathyroid hormone release, patients should be monitored for hyperglycemia and hypocalcemia during the correction period.

REFERENCES

1. Shaffer SG, Bradt SK, Hall RT. Postnatal changes in total body water and extracellular volume in the preterm infant with respiratory distress syndrome. *J Pediatr* 1986;109:509–514.
2. Skorecki KL, Brenner BM. Body fluid homeostasis in man. *Am J Med* 1981;70:77–88.
3. Holliday MA. Extracellular fluid and its proteins: dehydration, shock, and recovery. *Pediatr Nephrol* 1999;13:989–995.
4. Kaplan JH. Biochemistry of Na,K-ATPase. *Ann Rev Biochem* 2002;71:511–535.
5. Trachtman H, Futterweit S, Tonidandel W, et al. The role of organic osmolytes in the cerebral cell volume regulatory response to acute and chronic renal failure. *J Am Soc Nephrol* 1993;12:1913–1919.
6. Glaser DS. Utility of the serum osmolal gap in the diagnosis of methanol or ethylene glycol ingestion. *Ann Emerg Med* 1996;27:343–346.
7. Schelling JR, Howard RL, Winter SD, et al. Increased osmolal gap in alcoholic ketoacidosis and lactic acidosis. *Ann Intern Med* 1990;113:580–582.
8. Wassner SJ. Altered growth and protein turnover in rats fed sodium-deficient diets. *Pediatr Res* 1989;26:608–613.
9. Sulyok E, Varga F, Nemeth M, et al. Furosemide-induced alterations in electrolyte status, the function of the renin-angiotensin-aldosterone system, and the urinary excretion of prostaglandins in newborn infants. *Pediatr Res* 1980; 14:765–768.
10. Holliday M. The evolution of therapy for dehydration: Should deficit therapy still be taught? *Pediatrics* 1996;98:171–177.
11. Bell EF, Neidich GA, Cashore WJ, et al. Combined effect of radiant warmer and phototherapy on insensible water loss in low-birth weight infants. *J Pediatr* 1979;94:810–813.
12. Schoorlemmer GH, Evered MD. Water and solute balance in rats during 10 h water deprivation and rehydration. *Can J Physiol Pharmacol* 1993;71:379–386.
13. Danovitch GM, Bourgoignie J, Bricker NS. Reversibility of the "salt losing" tendency of chronic renal failure. *N Engl J Med* 1976;296:14–19.
14. Trachtman H. Cell volume regulation: a review of cerebral adaptive mechanisms and implications for clinical treatment of osmolal disturbances. *Pediatr Nephrol* 1991;5:743–752 (Part I) and 1992;6:104–112.
15. Kleeman CR. Metabolic coma. *Kidney Int* 1989;36:1142–1158.
16. Morita H, Tanaka K, Hosomi H. Chemical inactivation of the nucleus tractus solitarius abolished hepatojejunal reflex in the rat. *J Autonom Nerv Syst* 1994;48:207–212.
17. Firth JD, Raine AEG, Ledingham JGG. Raised venous pressure: a direct cause of renal sodium retention in edema. *Lancet* 1988;331;1033–1035.
18. Fater D, Schultz HD, Sundet WD, et al. Effects of left atrial stretch in cardiac-denervated and intact conscious dogs. *Am J Physiol* 1982;242:H1056–H1064.
19. Levy M, Wexler MJ. Sodium excretion in dogs with low-grade caval constriction: role of hepatic nerves. *Am J Physiol* 1987;253:F672–F678.
20. Paintal AS. Vagal sensory receptors and their reflex effects. *Physiol Rev* 1973;53:159–227.
21. Kirchheim HR, Ehmke H, Hackenthal E, et al. Autoregulation of renal blood flow, glomerular filtration rate, and renin release in conscious dogs. *Pflugers Arch* 1987;410:441–449.
22. Quail AW, Woods RL, Korner PI. Cardiac and arterial baroreceptor influences in release of vasopressin and renin during hemorrhage. *Am J Physiol* 1987;252:H1120–H1126.
23. Harrigan MR. Cerebral salt wasting syndrome: a review. *Neurosurgery* 1996;38:152–160.
24. Schrier RW. Pathogenesis of sodium and water retention in high-output and low-output cardiac failure, nephrotic syndrome, cirrhosis, and pregnancy. *N Engl J Med* 1988; 319:1065–1072, 1127–1134.

25. Schrier RW. Hormones and hemodynamics in heart failure. *N Eng J Med* 1999;341:577–585.
26. Share L, Kimura T, Matsui K, et al. Metabolism of vasopressin. *Fed Proc* 1985;44:59–61.
27. Hays RM. Antidiuretic hormone. *N Engl J Med* 1976;295: 659–665.
28. Robinson AG, Roberts MM, Evron WA, et al. Hyponatremia in rats induces downregulation of vasopressin synthesis. *J Clin Invest* 1990;86:1023–1029.
29. Robertson GL. Abnormalities of thirst regulation. *Kidney Int* 1984;25:460–469.
30. Blair-West JR, Carey KD, Denton DA, et al. Evidence that brain angiotensin II is involved in both thirst and sodium appetite in baboons. *Am J Physiol* 1998;275:R1639–R1646.
31. Tsutsumi Y, Matsubara H, Masaki H, et al. Angiotensin II type 2 receptor overexpression activates the vascular kinin system and causes vasodilatation. *J Clin Invest* 1999;104:925–935.
32. Liu FY, Cogan MG. Role of angiotensin II in glomerulotubular balance. *Am J Physiol* 1990;259:F72–F79.
33. Ichikawa I, Harris RC. Angiotensin actions in the kidney: renewed insight into the old hormone. *Kidney Int* 1991;40: 583–589.
34. Verrey F. Early aldosterone action: toward filling the gap between transcription and transport. *Am J Physiol* 1999;277: F319–F327.
35. Hunley TE, Kon V. Update on endothelins: biology and clinical implications. *Pediatr Nephrol* 2001;16:752–762.
36. DiBona GF. Neural control of the kidney: functionally specific renal sympathetic nerve fibers. *Am J Physiol* 2000;279:R1517–R1524.
37. Jose PA, Eisner GM, Felder RA. Role of dopamine receptors in the kidney in the regulation of blood pressure. *Curr Opin Nephrol Hypertens* 2002;11;87–92.
38. Carvalho MJ, Van den Meiracker AH, Boomsma F, et al. Role of sympathetic nervous system in cyclosporine-induced rise in blood pressure. *Hypertension* 1999;34:102–106.
39. Levin ER, Gardner DG, Samson WK. Natriuretic peptides. *N Engl J Med* 1998;339:321–328.
40. Cody RJ, Atlas SA, Laragh JH. Atrial natriuretic factor in normal subjects and heart failure patients: plasma levels and renal, hormonal, and hemodynamic responses to peptide infusion. *J Clin Invest* 1986;78:1362–1374.
41. Smith WL, Garavito RM, DeWitt DL. Prostaglandin endoperoxide H synthases (cyclooxygenases)-1 and -2. *J Biol Chem* 1996;271:33157–33160.
42. Patrono C, Dunn MJ. The clinical significance of inhibition of renal prostaglandin synthesis. *Kidney Int* 1987;32:1–12.
43. Tonel J, Madrid MI, Garcia-Salom M, et al. Role of kinins in the control of renal papillary blood flow, pressure natriuresis, and arterial pressure. *Circ Res* 2000;86:589–595.
44. Wang T. Role of iNOS and eNOS in modulating proximal tubule transport an acid-base balance. *Am J Physiol* 2002;283: F658–F662.
45. Stoos BA, Carretero OA, Garvin JL. Endothelial-derived nitric oxide inhibits sodium transport by affecting apical membrane channels in cultured collecting duct cells. *J Am Soc Nephrol* 1994;4:1855–1860.
46. Schultz PJ, Tolins JP. Adaptation to increased dietary salt intake: role of endogenous nitric oxide. *J Clin Invest* 1992; 91:642–650.
47. Kagota S, Tamashiro A, Yamaguchi Y, et al. Downregulation of soluble guanylate cyclase induced by high salt intake in spontaneously hypertensive rats. *Br J Pharmacol* 2001;134:737–744.
48. Taylor MM, Samson WK. Adrenomedullin and the integrative physiology of fluid and electrolyte balance. *Microsci Res Tech* 2002;57:105–109.
49. Phillips PA, Rolls BJ, Ledingham JGG, et al. Reduced thirst after water deprivation in healthy elderly men. *N Engl J Med* 1984;311:753–759.
50. Thompson CJ, Burd JM, Baylis PH. Acute suppression of plasma vasopressin and thirst after drinking in hypernatremic humans. *Am J Physiol* 1987;252:R1138–R1142.
51. Dirks JH, Cirkensa WJ, Berliner RW. The effect of saline infusion on sodium reabsorption by the proximal tubule of the dog. *J Clin Invest* 1965;44:1875–1885.
52. Brenner BM, Troy JL, Daugharty TM. On the mechanism of inhibition of fluid reabsorption by the renal proximal tubule of the volume-expanded rat. *J Clin Invest* 1971;50:1596–1602.
53. Better OS, Schrier RW. Disturbed volume homeostasis in patients with cirrhosis of the liver. *Kidney Int* 1983;23:303–311.
54. Hricik D, Broning PJ, Kopelman R, et al. Captopril-induced functional renal insufficiency in patients with bilateral renal artery stenosis or renal artery stenosis in a solitary kidney. *N Engl J Med* 1983;308:373–376.
55. Stokes JB. Disorders of the epithelial sodium channel: insights into the regulation of extracellular volume and blood pressure. *Kidney Int* 1999;56:2318–2333.
56. Harris HW Jr, Strange K, Zeidel ML. Current understanding of the cellular biology and molecular structure of the antidiuretic hormone-stimulated water transport pathway. *J Clin Invest* 1991;88:1–8.
57. Knoers NV, Deen PM. Molecular and cellular defects in nephrogenic diabetes insipidus. *Pediatr Nephrol* 2001;16: 1146–1152.
58. Kozono D, Yasui M, King LS, et al. Aquaporin water channels: atomic structure and molecular dynamics meet clinical medicine. *J Clin Invert* 2002;109:1395–1399.
59. Deen PM, Verdijk MA, Knoers NV, et al. Requirement of human renal water channel aquaporin-2 for vasopressin-dependent concentration of urine. *Science* 1994;264:92–95.
60. Ma T, Song Y, Yang B, et al. Nephrogenic diabetes insipidus in mice lacking aquaporin-3 water channel. *Proc Natl Acad Sci U S A* 2000;97:4386–4391.
61. Morello JP, Bichet DG. Nephrogenic diabetes insipidus. *Ann Rev Physiol* 2001;63:603–630.
62. Kirchlechner V, Koller DY, Seidl R, et al. Treatment of nephrogenic diabetes insipidus with hydrochlorothiazide and amiloride. *Arch Dis Child* 1999;80:548–552.
63. Berliner RW. Mechanisms of urine concentration. *Kidney Int* 1982;22:202–211.
64. Cai Q, Michea L, Andrews P, et al. Rate of increase of osmolality determines osmotic tolerance of mouse inner medullary epithelial cell. *Am J Physiol* 2002;283:F792–F798.
65. Ayus JC, Arieff AI. Chronic hyponatremic encephalopathy in postmenopausal women: association of therapies with morbidity and mortality. *J Am Med Assoc* 1999;281:2299–2304.
66. Trachtman H, Yancey PH, Gullans SR. Cerebral cell volume regulation during hypernatremia in developing rats. *Brain Res* 1995;693:155–162.

67. Duck SC, Wyatt DT. Factors associated with brain herniation in the treatment of diabetic ketoacidosis. *J Pediatr* 1988; 113:10–14.
68. Harris GD, Fiordalisi I. Physiologic management of diabetic ketoacidemia: a 5-year prospective experience in 231 episodes. *Arch Pediatr Adol Med* 1994;148:1046–1052.
69. Saavedra JM, Harris GD, Finberg L. Capillary refill (skin turgor) in the assessment of dehydration. *Am J Dis Child* 1991;145:296–298.
70. Prevot A, Mosig D, Guignard JP. The effects of losartan on renal function in the newborn rabbit. *Pediatr Res* 2002;51: 728–732.
71. Trachtman H. Volume depletion state: dehydration or denatration? *Pediatr Nephrol* 1991;5:271–272.
72. Mange K, Matsuura D, Cizman B, et al. Language guiding therapy: the case of dehydration versus volume depletion. *Ann Intern Med* 1997;127:848–853.
73. Mackenzie A, Barnes , Shann F. Clinical signs of dehydration in children. *Lancet* 1989;334:605–607.
74. Schierhout G, Roberts I. Fluid resuscitation with colloid or crystalloid solutions in critically ill patients: a systematic review of randomized trials. *BMJ* 1998;316:961–964.
75. Holliday MA, Friedman AL, Wassner SJ. Extracellular fluid restoration in dehydration: a critique of rapid versus slow. *Pediatr Nephrol* 1999;13:292–297.
76. Pizarro D, Posada G, Sandi L, et al. Rice-based electrolyte solutions for the management of infantile diarrhea. *N Engl J Med* 1991;324:517–521.
77. Ramakrishna BS, Venkataraman S, Srinivasan P, et al. Amylase-resistant starch plus oral rehydration solution for cholera. *N Engl J Med* 2000;342:308–313.
78. Rodriguez-Iturbe B, Herrera-Acosta J, Johnson RJ. Interstitial inflammation, sodium retention, and the pathogenesis of nephrotic edema: a unifying hypothesis. *Kidney Int* 2002; 62:1379–1384.
79. Haws RM, Baum M. Efficacy of albumin and diuretic therapy in children with nephrotic syndrome. *Pediatrics* 1993;91: 1142–1146.
80. Forni LG, Hilton PJ. Continuous hemofiltration in the treatment of acute renal failure. *N Engl J Med* 1997;336:1303–1309.
81. Fraser CL, Arieff AI. Epidemiology, pathophysiology, and management of hyponatremic encephalopathy. *Am J Med* 1997;102:67–77.
82. Sterns RH. Severe hyponatremia: the case for conservative management. *Crit Care Med* 1992;20:534–539.
83. Berl T. Treating hyponatremia: damned if we do and damned if we don't. *Kidney Int* 1990;37:1006–1018.
84. Sarnaik AP, Meert K, Hackbarth R, et al. Management of hyponatremic seizures in children with hypertonic saline: a safe and effective strategy. *Crit Care Med* 1991;19:758–762.
85. Keating JP, Schears GJ, Dodge PR. Oral water intoxication in infants: an American epidemic. *Am J Dis Child* 1991;145:985–990.
86. Miller M. Inappropriate antidiuretic hormone secretion. *Curr Thera Endocrinol Metabol* 1994;5:186–189.
87. Fujisawa G, Ishikawa S, Tsuboi Y, et al. Therapeutic efficacy of non-peptide ADH antagonist OPC-31260 in SIADH rats. *Kidney Int* 1993;44:19–23.
88. Shimizu K. Aquaretic effect of the nonpeptide V2 antagonist OPC-31260 in hydropenic humans. *Kidney Int* 1995;48:220–226.
89. Moritz ML, Ayus JC. The changing pattern of hypernatremia in hospitalized children. *Pediatrics* 1999;104:435–439.
90. Cooper WO, Atherton HD, Kahana M, et al. Increased incidence of severe breastfeeding malnutrition and hypernatremia in a metropolitan area. *Pediatrics* 1995;96:957–960.
91. Adrogue HJ, Madias NE. Hypernatremia. *N Engl J Med* 2000;342:1493–1499.
92. Finberg L, Luttrell C, Redd H. Pathogenesis of lesion in the nervous system in hypernatremic states. II. Experimental studies of gross anatomic changes and alterations of chemical composition of the tissues. 1959;23:46–53.
93. Lee JH. Arcinue E, Ross BD. Organic osmolytes in the brain of an infant with hypernatremia. *N Engl J Med* 1994;334:439–442.
94. Lien YHH, Shapiro JI, Chan L. Study of brain electrolytes and organic osmolytes during correction of chronic hyponatremia: implications for the pathogenesis of central pontine myelinolysis. *J Clin Invest* 1991;88:303–309.
95. Banister A, Matin-Siddiqi SA, Hatcher G. Treatment of hypernatremic dehydration in infancy. *Arch Dis Child* 1975;50:179–186.

8

POTASSIUM

GEORGE J. SCHWARTZ

Potassium (K^+) is the most abundant intracellular cation. High concentrations of K^+ in the cytosol are required for many normal cellular functions, including metabolism and growth, cell division, optimal enzyme function, protein and DNA synthesis, volume regulation, and intracellular acid-base balance (1). In addition, a steep concentration gradient of K^+ across the cell membranes is required for nerve excitation and muscle contraction. These functions are achieved by maintaining high intracellular and low extracellular K^+ concentrations. The intracellular and extracellular fluids (ECFs) are separately controlled to maintain K^+ homeostasis. Whereas homeostasis in adults seeks to maintain zero K^+ balance, growing infants and children must accumulate K^+ for growth.

The intracellular K^+ concentration, 100 to 150 mEq/L, far exceeds its concentration in ECF, 3.5 to 5 mEq/L. This transcellular K^+ gradient is maintained by the action of the enzyme Na^+-K^+-adenosine triphosphatase (Na^+-K^+-ATPase) in the cell membrane, which pumps Na^+ out of and K^+ into the cell in a 3:2 ratio (2–4). Thus, serum potassium level provides only an indirect estimate of total body K^+ status because it represents only 2% of total body K^+.

BODY COMPOSITION AND INTAKE

Total body K^+ in adult men, estimated from total body counting of potassium-40, is approximately 50 mEq/kg, and 98% is within cells, mainly muscle (5–8). In proportion to muscle mass, total body K^+ is lower in females than in males (8), and the levels in all adults decline gradually after age 40. During growth, total body K^+ increases linearly with either height or weight without sex-related differences for height and weight below 135 cm and 30 kg, respectively (9,10) (Fig. 8.1). By the onset of puberty, gender-related differences in total body K^+ content develop, even when values are corrected for body weight or height. The rate of increase in body K^+ as a function of growth diminishes in girls (9,10). This change from the male pattern reflects the deposition of adipose tissue, which contains little K^+ (6). In boys postnatal growth is accompanied by an increase in total body K^+ from approximately 8 mEq/cm body height at birth to more than 14 mEq/cm body height by 18 years of age (9). In absolute terms, total body K^+ in infants (approximately 42 mEq/kg) is less than in older children (approximately 51 mEq/kg), and it increases more rapidly during the first 1.5 years of life than after age 3 (9–11) (Fig. 8.1).

The average intake of potassium in adults is quite variable, ranging from 50 to more than 500 mEq/day (12,13). In the healthy adult, K^+ output balances intake, so that constancy of body K^+ content is maintained. For a typical adult K^+ intake of 1.5 mEq/kg body weight, 90 to 95% is excreted in the urine and 5 to 10% in the stool (Fig. 8.2).

The process of growth requires that the growing organism be able to conserve K^+ and exist in a state of positive K^+ balance (14) to facilitate incorporation of K^+ into dividing cells. Infants fed human milk receive only 13 mEq of K^+/L (corresponding to 1.8 mEq/100 kcal or 1.8 mEq/kg/day), whereas other milk formulas may provide 1.5 to 3 times this amount (15). Under normal physiologic conditions the K^+ content of breast milk is sufficient, because there is little urinary excretion of K^+. In addition, the renal K^+ clearance (C_K), even corrected for the low absolute glomerular filtration rate of infants (that is, the fractional excretion of K^+, or FEK*), is less than in the older child (Table 8.1) (16). This tendency to retain K^+ early in postnatal life is observed in infants, who tend to have higher plasma K^+ concentrations than older children and adults. With maturation of renal K^+ excretion, however, adjustments of K^+ intake are essential. Maintenance K^+ intake in children is 2 to 3 mEq/100 kcal, approximately twice that in adults (17).

The 2% of total body K^+ that is located within the ECF is tightly regulated. Because of the dependence of so many vital processes on K^+ homeostasis and the ratio of intracellular to extracellular K^+, many mechanisms to regulate serum K^+ concentration and total body K^+ homeostasis

---

*Fractional excretion of K^+ is the percentage of filtered K^+ that appears in the urine:

$$FEK = \text{urinary } K^+ \text{ (mEq/L)}/\text{plasma } K^+ \text{ (mEq/L)} \times 100\%/[\text{urinary creatinine (mg/dL)}/\text{plasma creatinine (mg/dL)}]$$

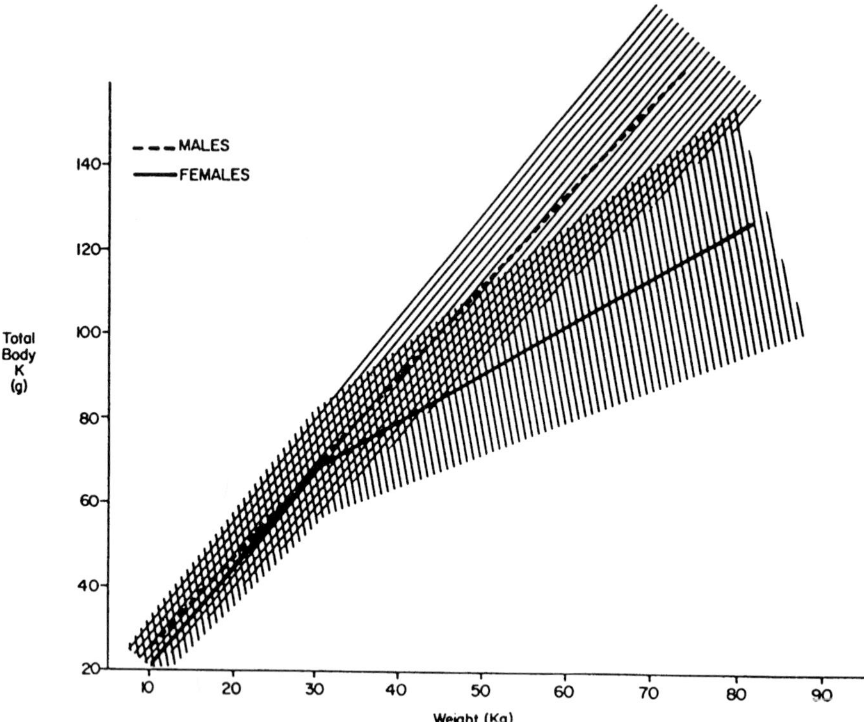

FIGURE 8.1. Total body potassium as a function of weight in males and females 3 to 18 years of age. The shaded regions represent the mean ± 1 standard deviation for 68% of the population of 432 children. (From Flynn MA, Woodruff C, Clark J, et al. Total body potassium in healthy children. *Pediatr Res* 1972;6:239, with permission.)

have evolved. The cellular volume of distribution for K^+ greatly exceeds that of the ECF volume, and the potential for intracellular redistribution provides protection against abrupt changes in serum K^+ concentrations.

Direct chemical analysis of various nonsecreting mature tissues (e.g., skeletal muscle) has provided estimates of intracellular fluid (ICF) K^+ concentration of 100 to 160 mEq/L (18–20). Comparable studies in the tissues of newborn humans and animals have revealed ICF K^+ concentrations that are 15 to 30% lower than those found in adults (19,21) (Fig. 8.3). The more rapid accretion of K^+ in infants probably reflects both a maturation of intracellular chemical composition and actual cellular growth.

DISTRIBUTION BETWEEN INTRACELLULAR AND EXTRACELLULAR FLUID

Potassium is readily absorbed from the gastrointestinal tract and enters the ECF. Relative constancy of plasma K^+ concentration during entry of K^+ into the ECF is maintained by hormonally mediated temporary shifts of this cation into cells, such as muscle, liver, red cells, and bone (Fig. 8.2) (22). To maintain zero K^+ balance, all of the dietary K^+ must be ultimately excreted, primarily by the kidney. However, the renal excretion of K^+ is rather slow, requiring several hours. Only approximately 50% of an oral load of K^+ is excreted during the first 4 to 6 hours after ingestion (23–25). Protection is achieved within minutes by hormonally mediated translocation of extracellular K^+ into cells (22–27).

Na^+-K^+-Adenosine Phosphatase Activity

The high ratio of intracellular to extracellular K^+ concentration is sustained primarily by the action of Na^+-K^+-ATPase, the sodium pump. This pump, generally present on the basolateral membranes of polarized epithelial cells, consumes energy (adenosine triphosphatase, or ATP) in the process of transporting three Na^+ ions out of and two K^+ ions into the cell, which generates a negative intracellular

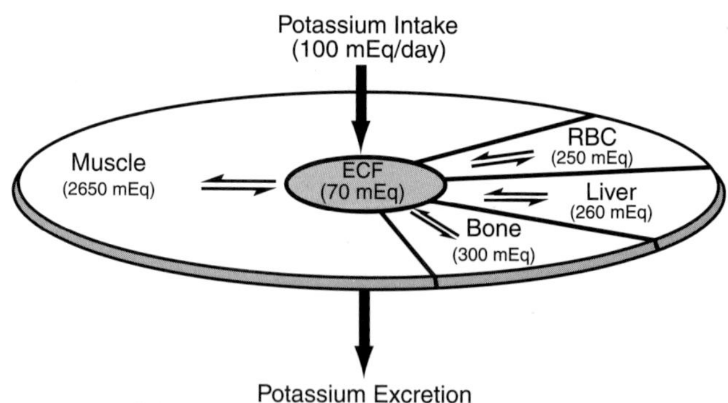

FIGURE 8.2. Potassium homeostasis depends on the maintenance of external and internal K^+ balance. External balance of K^+ in adults is determined by the rate of K^+ intake (approximately 100 mEq/day) and the rate of excretion in the urine (approximately 90 mEq/day) and feces (approximately 10 mEq/day). Internal K^+ balance depends on the distribution of K^+ between muscle, bone, liver, red blood cells (RBC), and extracellular fluid (ECF). (From Giebisch G. Renal potassium transport: mechanisms and regulation. *Am J Physiol* 1998;274:F817, with permission.)

TABLE 8.1. PLASMA K+ AND RENAL K+ CLEARANCES IN GROWING CHILDREN

Age (yr)	n	P_K	C_{Cr}	C_K	FEK	UNa/K
0.0–0.3	13	$5.2 \pm 0.8^{a,b}$	$62 \pm 26^{a,b,c}$	$5 \pm 3^{b,c}$	$8.5 \pm 3.8^{a,b}$	1.1 ± 1.1
0.4–1.0	10	$4.9 \pm 0.5^{a,b}$	$99 \pm 38^{a,b}$	14 ± 6^{a}	14.6 ± 5.0	0.8 ± 0.9
3–10	19	4.2 ± 0.5	141 ± 30	20 ± 11	14.5 ± 8.9	1.5 ± 1.1
11–20	17	4.3 ± 0.3	137 ± 21	21 ± 8	16.2 ± 8.2	1.4 ± 0.8

C_{Cr}, creatinine clearance in mL/min/1.73 m²; C_K, clearance of potassium in mL/min/1.73 m²; FEK, fractional excretion of potassium in percent; n, number of infants or children; P_K, plasma potassium in mEq/L; UNa/K, sodium to potassium ratio in urine.
Note: Mean plus/minus the standard deviation. Patients were on regular diets and were free of renal disease.
[a] $p < .05$ vs. 11–20 yr.
[b] $p < .05$ vs. 3–10 yr.
[c] $p < .05$ vs. 0.4–1.0 yr.
Data from Satlin LM, Schwartz GJ. Metabolism of potassium. In: Ichikawa I, ed. *Pediatric textbook of fluids and electrolytes.* Baltimore: Williams & Wilkins, 1990:90.

voltage. It is comprised of an α (catalytic) and a β (glycoprotein) heterodimer. The activity of Na^+-K^+-ATPase in red cells (28,29), kidney (30–33), and intestine (34) is low early in life, perhaps mediating lower cellular K^+ concentrations (19,21).

Na^+-K^+-ATPase activity is regulated by several hormones, namely, insulin, thyroid hormone, catecholamines, and aldosterone. Long-term stimulation of Na^+-K^+-ATPase by aldosterone and thyroid hormone is mediated by changes in gene expression, whereas short-term regulation may be mediated by altered phosphorylation of the pump (catecholamines) or by changes in the surface distribution of pumps (insulin, aldosterone) (35,36). A small rise in ECF K^+ (from dietary intake, exercise, or acute hyperosmolality) stimulates secretion of these hormones, activating Na^+-K^+-ATPase to transport more K^+ into cells.

Hormone Activity

Insulin is the most important hormonal regulator of internal K^+ balance. Insulin reduces serum K^+ by promoting the cellular uptake of K^+, probably by directly stimulating Na^+-K^+-ATPase activity (3,22,37,38). Basal insulin levels permissively facilitate K^+ entry into cells. An acute rise in plasma K^+ results in a two- to threefold increase in insulin levels (24,25,39–42).

Catecholamines influence K^+ distribution, with α receptors inhibiting and β_2 receptors stimulating cellular K^+ uptake. This results in a biphasic response manifested first by an initial increase followed by a prolonged decrease in plasma K^+ concentration to below baseline (22). The transient initial rise is due to α-adrenergic receptor stimulation, which causes release of K^+ from cells, whereas the β_2-receptor stimulation, via stimulation of adenylate cyclase and generation of cyclic adenosine monophosphate, activates Na^+-K^+-ATPase and mediates increased K^+ uptake by liver and muscle cells (22). Basal epinephrine levels are permissive in stimulating K^+ uptake by liver, skeletal muscle, adipose tissue, and cardiac muscle (22,23,43). Indeed, the increment in plasma K^+ concentration after a K^+ load or exercise is greater and more prolonged if the subject has been pretreated with the beta-blocker propranolol (23,44,45). The administration of a β_2-adrenergic agonist (albuterol) can reduce plasma K^+ concentration by stimulating K^+ uptake by cells and by stimulating insulin release, which independently stimulates K^+ uptake.

Blood levels of aldosterone are sensitively influenced by plasma K^+ concentration (46–48). The secretion of aldosterone protects against hyperkalemia primarily by increasing uri-

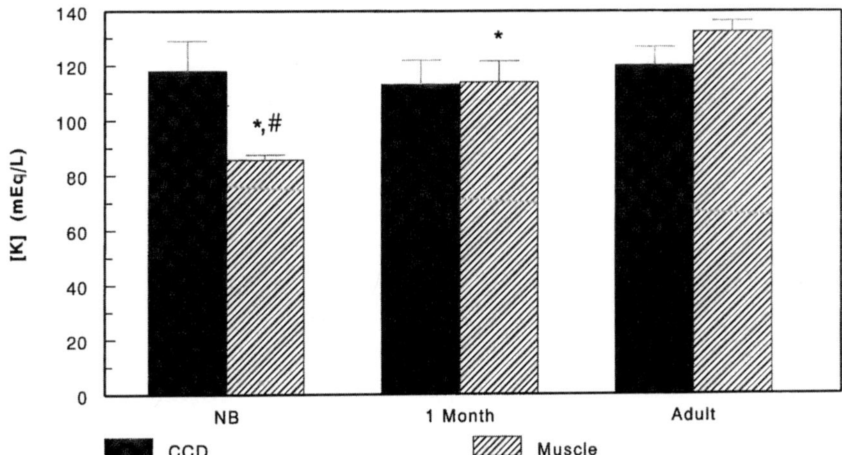

FIGURE 8.3. Comparison of cellular K^+ concentration (mEq/L) in the skeletal muscle (*slashed bars*) and cortical collecting duct (CCD, *solid bars*) of newborn (NB), 1-month-old, and adult rabbits. Mean values plus standard error are given for each age group. *, $p < .05$ versus adult; #, $p < .05$ versus 1-month-old. (Data from Satlin LM, Evan AP, Gattone VH III, et al. Postnatal maturation of the rabbit cortical collecting duct. *Pediatr Nephrol* 1988;2:135.)

nary and colonic K^+ excretion but also by promoting cellular K^+ uptake (13,25,49). Thyroid hormone, glucocorticoids, and growth hormone may also promote the cellular uptake of K^+ by chronically stimulating Na^+-K^+-ATPase (22,35,36).

Plasma K^+ Concentration

An increase in plasma K^+ concentration, independent of aldosterone and other factors, promotes K^+ entry into cells, probably by diminishing the K^+ concentration gradient against which the Na^+-K^+-ATPase–dependent sodium pump must function (24,25,50). Thus, plasma K^+ concentration generally varies directly with body K^+ stores (51). In those cells of the kidney and colon responsible for K^+ secretion, the resulting increase in cellular K^+ concentration enhances secretion by favoring increased K^+ diffusion into the tubular fluid down its concentration gradient.

Acid-Base Balance

Acute changes in acid-base balance may have important effects on K^+ distribution. During mineral-acid–induced acidosis, excessive protons are buffered in the cells and K^+ moves into the ECF, which results in an increase in plasma K^+ concentration; hyperkalemia may ensue (13,52,53). A common rule of thumb states that, for every 0.1-U decrease in blood pH, the plasma K^+ concentration increases by approximately 0.6 mEq/L (13,22,51,53).

Increases in plasma K^+ concentration are generally much smaller in acute organic acid acidosis, such as lactic acidosis and diabetic ketoacidosis (13,51,53–55). The concurrent entry into the cell of the anion with the proton may reduce the necessity for K^+ redistribution. Also, the hyperkalemia often observed in ketoacidosis reflects a larger flux of K^+ from cells to ECF due to insulin deficiency and hyperosmolality rather than to acidemia per se (13,26,51,53).

Acute metabolic alkalosis causes K^+ to shift into cells, with a resulting decrease in plasma K^+ concentration. The effect on serum K^+ concentration is generally smaller (0.2 to 0.4 mEq/L), probably due to the smaller degree of intracellular buffering and transcellular movement of protons (53,56). More prolonged alkalosis usually results in hypokalemia (13,51), due to a shift of K^+ into collecting duct cells that results in enhanced urinary excretion of K^+. Contributing to the variability of proton load and serum K^+ concentration, the concentration of plasma HCO_3^- itself can reciprocally affect plasma K^+ values, independent of a pH effect (13,53,57). Large changes in plasma K^+ concentration are rarely seen with respiratory acid-base disorders (13,52,53,56).

Exercise

Exercise can cause the release of K^+ from muscle, due in part to the discrepancy between the K^+ exit during depolarization and the reuptake of K^+ by the Na^+-K^+-ATPase sodium pump (58,59). With strenuous exercise, the reduction in ATP within muscle cells stimulates the opening of ATP-dependent K^+ channels, which further promotes an increase in K^+ release from cells (60). Finally, the release of K^+ from the myocyte takes place with H^+ exchange, and the exercise-induced hyperkalemia may result from a reduction in nondiffusible intracellular anions, which accompanies phosphocreatine hydrolysis (59).

Other Conditions

Any condition resulting in cell breakdown leads to the release of K^+ into the ECF and potentially to hyperkalemia (61,62). An acute increase in effective plasma hyperosmolality can also cause K^+ to leave cells, so that the plasma K^+ concentration may rise by 0.3 to 0.8 mEq/L for every 10 mOsm/kg elevation (63–67). Hyperglycemia is a common clinical example of this phenomenon, especially because the rise in ECF K^+ concentration may not be effectively modulated in a diabetic patient lacking insulin secretion (64). With permeant solutes, such as urea or ethanol, plasma hyperosmolality does not result in hyperkalemia, because there is no transcellular osmotic gradient.

RENAL POTASSIUM EXCRETION

Overview of the Renal Contribution to Potassium Homeostasis

Renal regulation of urinary K^+ excretion allows for adjustment of output to equal intake over a wide range. The kidney excretes 90 to 95% of the daily K^+ intake (7). Extreme adjustments cannot be achieved as rapidly as for sodium, nor are they as complete. Maximal rates of K^+ excretion may not be observed until several days after K^+ intake is increased (68). Whereas urinary Na^+ can be reduced to less than 1 mEq/day within 3 to 4 days of Na^+ restriction, a minimum urinary K^+ loss of 5 to 15 mEq/day persists in the adult on K^+ restriction (12,26,69–71).

There is a circadian rhythm of renal K^+ excretion in the adult that is independent of changes in serum aldosterone or K^+ concentration (72–74). The cause of this rhythmic K^+ excretion is unclear, but it may be due to hypothalamic oscillators characterized by maximum output during times of peak activity. In children, one study has shown no diurnal variation in urinary K^+ excretion (75).

Growing individuals maintain a state of positive K^+ balance (14,18). The relative conservation of K^+ early in life is generally associated with higher plasma K^+ values* than in

*Serum K^+ concentration runs approximately 0.5 mEq/L higher than in plasma, due to the release of K^+ from cells during clotting (78).

TABLE 8.2. FACTORS INFLUENCING K⁺ DISTRIBUTION BETWEEN CELLS AND EXTRACELLULAR FLUID

Factor	Effect on extracellular K^+ concentration
Physiologic	
Insulin	↓
Na-K–adenosine triphosphatase	↓
Catecholamines	
α receptor	↑
β receptor	↓
Mineralocorticoids	↓
↑ Plasma K^+ concentration	↑
Exercise	↑
Pathologic	
Metabolic acidosis	↑
Metabolic alkalosis	↓
Hyperosmolality	↑
Excessive cell breakdown	↑

the adult (14,76–78). Our own study of healthy human infants shows that plasma K^+ concentrations during the first 4 months of life average 1 mEq/L higher than in infants older than 1 year of age (Table 8.1).

FEK (Table 8.2) provides an additional assessment of renal K^+ handling under various physiologic and pathophysiologic states. Normally, FEK ranges from 10 to 30%, but FEK usually exceeds 40% and urinary Na^+/K^+ ratio is less than 1 with enhanced mineralocorticoid activity. During K^+ conservation FEK is less than 10% with urinary Na^+/K^+ ratios exceeding 2 or 3.

Children and adults ingesting a regular diet containing Na^+ in excess of K^+ excrete urine with an Na^+/K^+ ratio higher than 1 (Table 8.1) (76,77). Although the Na/K ratios of breast milk and commercial infant formulas are approximately 0.5 (15), the urinary Na/K ratio of the newborn also generally exceeds 1, due in part to a physiologic natriuresis, as well as preferential retention of K^+ as a function of growth. Premature infants may show urinary Na^+/K^+ ratios above 4, which reflects a relative hyporesponsiveness of the distal tubule and collecting duct to mineralocorticoid activity in addition to the substantial natriuresis that occurs during this period of gestation (14).

The renal adaptation to chronic K^+ loading is due primarily to an enhanced capacity for individual nephrons to secrete K^+. Infants can excrete K^+ at a rate that exceeds its filtration, which indicates the capacity for net tubular secretion (79); however, they cannot do this as rapidly or as efficiently as can adults (80–82).

Sites of Potassium Transport in the Kidney

The nephron sites of K^+ handling have been ascertained by micropuncture and *in vitro* microperfusion studies (Fig. 8.4). Filtered K^+ is reabsorbed mainly in proximal segments of the nephron, whereas the urinary K^+ is derived primarily from distal K^+ secretion. Although small amounts of K^+ are

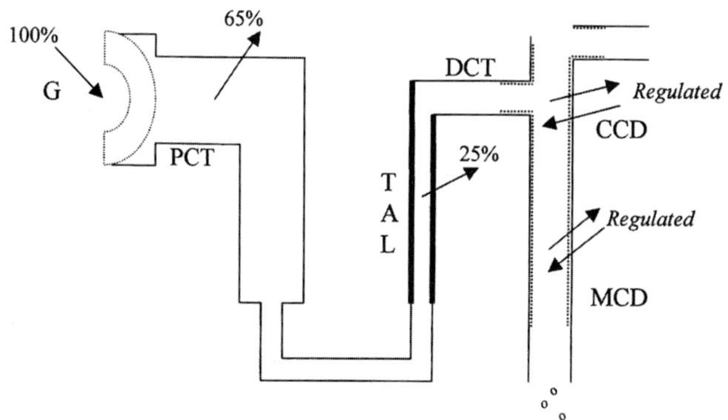

FIGURE 8.4. Schematic of K^+ transport along the nephron. Reabsorption occurs in the proximal tubule and thick ascending limb of the loop of Henle. The excretion of K^+ during varied K^+ intake is mainly regulated by the distal nephron (areas indicated by the *dotted lines* in the lumens). The handling of K^+ in the collecting duct during K^+ depletion is also influenced by reabsorptive processes mediated by H^+-K^+-ATPase in the collecting duct, a subject of active investigation. CCD, cortical collecting duct; DCT, distal convoluted tubule; G, glomerulus; MCD, medullary collecting duct; PCT, proximal convoluted tubule; TAL, thick ascending limb of loop of Henle.

lost each day in the stool (5 to 15 mEq) (83,84) and sweat (0 to 10 mEq) (26), K^+ homeostasis is regulated in large part by the rate of K^+ secretion in the distal nephron.

Segmental Potassium Transport

The renal handling of K^+ requires filtration at the glomerulus, reabsorption in the proximal nephron, and secretion by the distal tubule and cortical collecting duct (1,85). Micropuncture studies in adult rats by Malnic et al. (86) (Fig. 8.5) examined the clearance of K^+ factored by that of inulin. After being freely filtered at the glomerulus, K^+ is nearly completely reabsorbed in the proximal tubule and thick ascending limb of the loop of Henle, as seen by the progressive decrease in K/inulin (K/In) along the proximal nephron (Fig. 8.5). Proximal K^+ reabsorption is passive after that of Na^+ and water; 60 to 65% of the filtered K^+ load is reabsorbed in the proximal tubule of the adult rat (86) (Fig. 8.6A) (87), a fraction similar to that observed in the immature rat (88–91).

In the adult rat, only 5 to 15% of the filtered load of K^+ reaches the superficial distal tubule, which reflects further significant net reabsorption by the intervening nephron segments (86). Indeed, an additional 20 to 30% of the filtered load of K^+ is reabsorbed along the thick ascending limb of the loop of Henle, so that by the time the tubular fluid reaches the distal convoluted tubule, as little as 10% of the filtered K^+ load remains (K^+/In of <0.1; Fig. 8.5). The avid reabsorption of K^+ in the thick ascending limb is mediated by apical uptake through a secondary active electroneutral Na^+-K^+-$2Cl^-$ co-transporter driven by the electrochemical gradient for Na^+ that is generated by the basolateral Na^+-K^+-ATPase activity (Fig. 8.6B). There is passive K^+ exit across the

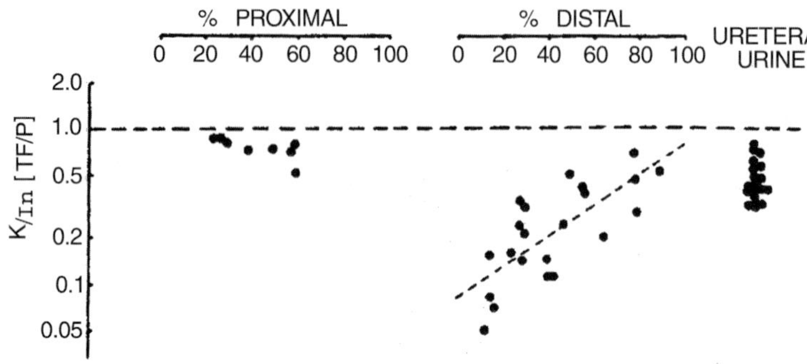

FIGURE 8.5. Determination of tubular fluid to plasma concentration ratios of potassium to inulin [K/In (TF/P)] as a function of tubular length along the nephron in rats undergoing hypertonic NaCl administration. (From Malnic G, Klose RM, Giebisch G. Micropuncture study of distal tubular potassium and sodium transport in rat nephron. *Am J Physiol* 1966;211:529, with permission.)

basolateral membrane by diffusion through K^+ channels or by co-transport with chloride or bicarbonate (85). There is also K^+ recycling back across the apical membrane through a K^+ channel, which assures adequate amounts of K^+ for the Na^+-K^+-$2Cl^-$ co-transporter and generates a positive potential in the lumen. The molecular identification of this apical channel is ROMK (*r*at *o*uter medullary *K*+ channel) (92–94). Mutations in ROMK have been identified in patients with

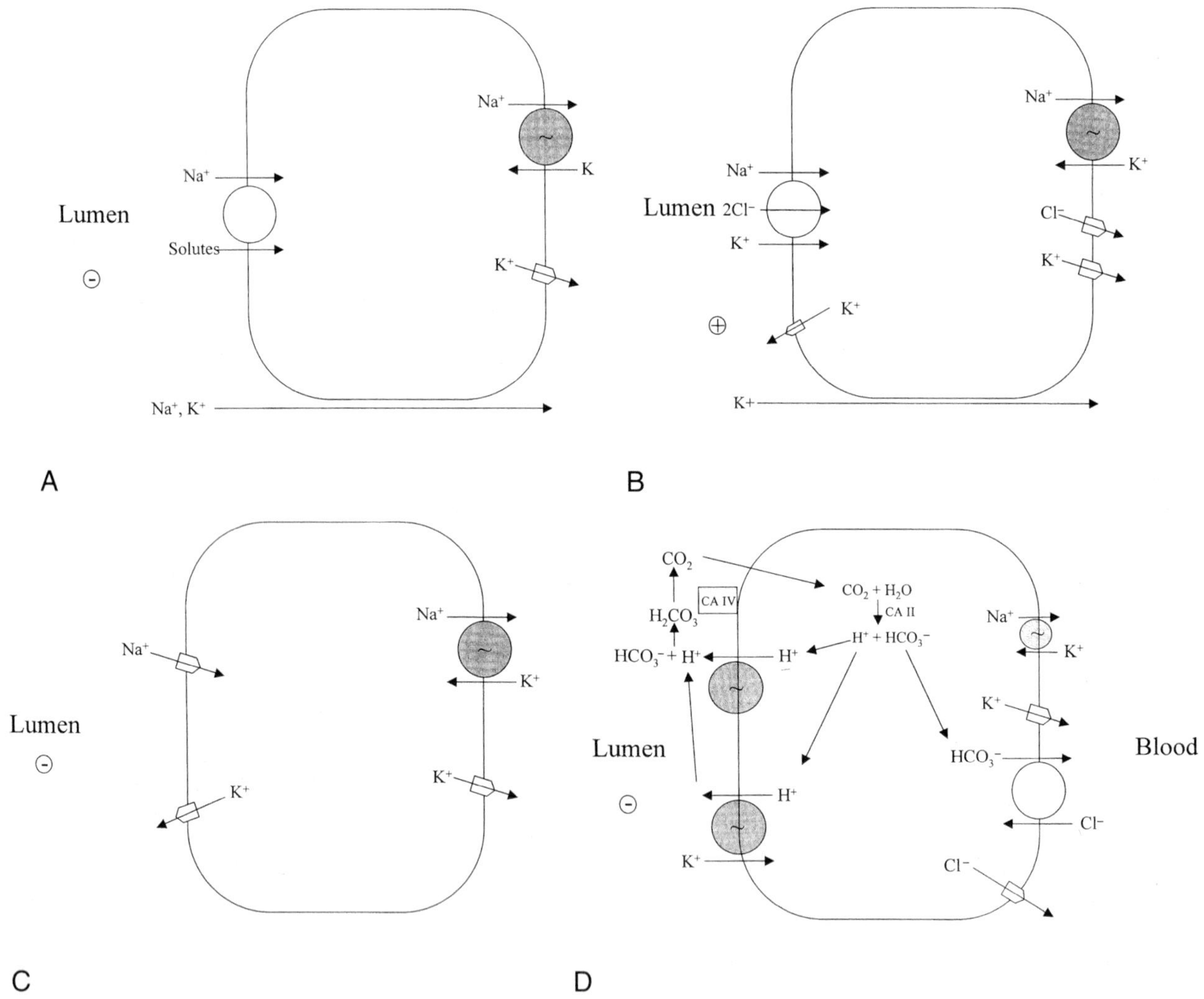

FIGURE 8.6. Cell models of K^+ transport pathways across apical and basolateral membranes and paracellularly through the tight junction. **A:** Proximal tubule. **B:** Thick ascending limb. **C:** Principal cell. **D:** Type A intercalated cell or outer medullary collecting duct cell. The circles enclosing the "~" indicate primary active transport; open circles represent exchangers. Channels are denoted by the pentagonal figures in the membranes. Transcellular transport is denoted by the long arrow. CA, carbonic anhydrase (isoform II or IV).

Bartter's syndrome, an inherited disease characterized by hyperreninemic hypokalemic metabolic alkalosis with secondary hyperaldosteronism and normal blood pressure (95). Significant amounts of K^+ are also reabsorbed via the paracellular pathway across the thick ascending limb, driven by the electropositive potential. The net reabsorption of K^+ in this segment can be changed to net K^+ secretion if the Na^+-K^+-$2Cl^-$ co-transporter is inhibited by loop diuretics.

The elevation of the K^+/In ratio along the distal tubule indicates that K^+ has been secreted into the tubular fluid. Potassium is secreted by the late distal tubule (initial collecting tubule), connecting segment, principal cells of the cortical and medullary collecting duct (Fig. 8.6C), and, under certain circumstances, the inner medullary collecting duct (7,86,96–100). Under conditions of excessive K^+ intake or depressed glomerular filtration rate, the rate of K^+ secretion may become so high that the net K^+ excretion rate exceeds the filtered load (86,101–103).

Secretion of K^+ in the distal nephron occurs in principal cells by Na^+-K^+-ATPase–mediated active uptake of K^+ across the basolateral membrane (4) and passive diffusion through secretory channels across the apical membrane into the luminal fluid (Fig. 8.6C). The magnitude of K^+ secretion depends on its electrochemical gradient and apical permeability. The electrochemical gradient is generated by the cell to lumen ratio of K^+ concentrations and the lumen-negative potential, which is driven by apical Na^+ entry through epithelial Na^+ channels (ENaCs) and transcellular Na^+ flux. The active cellular uptake of two K^+ ions in exchange for the extrusion of three Na^+ ions (via Na^+-K^+-ATPase at the basolateral membrane) generates a negative intracellular voltage with respect to the blood. Cell K^+ is then secreted passively down a favorable electrochemical gradient into the lumen through apical K^+-selective channels (104–106). The small conductance channel has a high open probability and is regulated by ATP. Its molecular identification is ROMK (93,94,107), and it is considered to mediate basal K^+ secretion (85,105,106). It has two potential membrane-spanning helices flanking a region that forms part of the channel pore in the voltage-gated K^+ channel (108). The channel has a unitary conductance of 30 to 40 picosiemens, high K^+/Na^+ selectivity, weak inward rectification, sensitivity to external Ba^{2+}, and marked inhibition to decreases in cytosolic pH within the physiologic range (108). The inward rectification permits significant outward K^+ current, as for K^+ secretion from principal cells. This same ROMK channel (105,106,108) is present in the apical membrane of thick ascending limb cells and therein allows the Na^+-K^+-$2Cl^-$ co-transporter to function optimally by providing readily available substrate, K^+ (109) (Fig. 8.6B). There is also a high-conductance, stretch- and calcium-activated maxi-K channel that is likely to mediate flow-stimulated K^+ secretion (110).

The lumen-negative potential in the cortical collecting duct, generated by apical Na^+ entry and electrogenic basolateral extrusion (via Na^+-K^+-ATPase), promotes both the secretion of K^+ and the paracellular reabsorption of Cl^-. Thus, the major determinants of passive K^+ secretion are the difference between cell and tubular fluid K^+ concentrations, the transepithelial negative voltage driven by Na^+ reabsorption through apical Na^+ channels, and the number of open K^+ channels in the luminal membrane.

Potassium reabsorption has been localized morphologically to collecting duct intercalated cells in the cortex and medulla (111–113). Distal K^+ secretion can be partially offset by this K^+ reabsorptive process in the cortical and medullary collecting ducts (112,114) and in the inner medullary collecting duct (96,115). This process is probably due to a luminal H^+-K^+-ATPase (Fig. 8.6D) in the collecting duct, an enzyme that exchanges a single K^+ ion for a proton while consuming ATP and thereby mediating both H^+ secretion and K^+ reabsorption (116–120). It is likely that both α and β intercalated cells express H^+-K^+-ATPase (1,112,121). Several isoforms of H^+-K^+-ATPases have been identified in the kidney, and they share some identity with the gastric and colonic ATPases (121–123). The activity of H^+-K^+-ATPase is increased by K^+ depletion and reduced by K^+ loading (111,119–121,124). The adaptation with severe K^+ depletion results in net K^+ reabsorption along the distal nephron (86,111,113).

Medullary K^+ recycling occurs when the K^+ reabsorbed in the thick ascending limb enters the medullary interstitium and is then secreted into the late proximal tubule or thin descending limb of the loop of Henle; this additional K^+ is reabsorbed when it enters the outer medullary collecting duct (125–128). This recycling of K^+ in the medulla results in a relatively high concentration of K^+ in the interstitium that tends to favor K^+ excretion by decreasing the gradients for passive K^+ efflux out of the collecting duct and thick ascending limb (7,129).

Factors Affecting K^+ Secretion in the Cortical Collecting Duct

Whereas 90% of filtered K^+ is reabsorbed in the proximal tubule and thick ascending limb, total body K^+ homeostasis is maintained by regulation of K^+ secretion along the distal nephron. The cortical collecting duct is the main regulatory site of K^+ secretion, capable of generating luminal K^+ concentrations in excess of 100 mmol/L in the adult (98). The principal cell of this cortical collecting duct secretes K^+ and absorbs Na^+. The major regulators of distal K^+ secretion are listed in Table 8.3.

Aldosterone

Aldosterone secretion rises after a K^+ load (130). Mineralocorticoids stimulate net sodium reabsorption and potassium secretion in the principal cells of the cortical collecting duct and adjacent cells of the connecting segment (97,131–134).

TABLE 8.3. FACTORS AFFECTING K^+ SECRETION IN THE CORTICAL COLLECTING DUCT

Factor
Aldosterone activity
Cell K^+ concentration
Tubular flow rate
Luminal Na^+ concentration
Luminal nonreabsorbable anion
Acid-base balance
Other hormones

Aldosterone binds to mineralocorticoid receptors of principal cells; the hormone-receptor complex is translocated to the nucleus, which results in activation of transcription and synthesis of physiologically active proteins (135). Cellular effects of aldosterone include an early enhancement in apical Na^+ permeability; this in turn increases the basolateral Na^+-K^+-ATPase turnover rate, which results in increased cell K^+ concentration (132,136–138). Later effects include increases in basolateral membrane infolding, insertion of additional Na^+-K^+-ATPase pumps into the membrane, and an increase in the apical K^+ conductance as K^+-channel density increases (105,134,136,137,139–142). Stimulation of Na^+ reabsorption leads to an increase in lumen negative transepithelial voltage, which further favors K^+ secretion (97,132,134,142). Mineralocorticoids stimulate both the electrochemical gradient and luminal membrane permeability across the principal cell, which results in increased K^+ secretion and Na^+ reabsorption (97,132,133,143,144). Prolonged administration of mineralocorticoids leads to a persistent kaliuresis but only a transient phase of Na^+ retention (143–145). After a significant extracellular volume expansion to a new steady state, there is a subsequent diuresis, which returns plasma volume toward normal (143,146). This "escape" phenomenon is probably due to decreased Na^+ reabsorption in some other nephron segment (147).

Plasma K^+ Concentration

The serum K^+ concentration directly affects renal K^+ excretion (130). An increase in dietary K^+ intake results in a transient rise in plasma K^+ concentration (50), which in turn stimulates renal potassium excretion and the adrenal release of aldosterone (68,99,130,148). The elevation in serum K^+ concentration favors the entry of K^+ into principal cells across the basolateral membrane and thereby drives K^+ secretion across the luminal membrane (149,150). Aldosterone enhances the electrochemical gradient, driving K^+ secretion in the distal tubule and collecting duct. In addition, plasma K^+ elevation, through unknown mechanisms, increases Na^+ reabsorption, luminal Na^+ permeability, and Na^+-K^+-ATPase activity independently of aldosterone (105,151–153). Also, a high-K^+ diet can induce increases in K^+ channel density in the apical membranes of principal cells (105,154).

In the first 4 hours after an exogenous K^+ load, approximately one-half is excreted by the kidneys, whereas the rest is distributed into cells (22). The rise in plasma K^+ concentration is transient, because only a small fraction of the K^+ load remains in the ECF. After the initial cell sequestration of K^+, the kidneys continue to excrete K^+ at an accelerated rate until the excess is eliminated and balance is restored (1,22,68). Most of the increase in urinary K^+ excretion is mediated by a rise in K^+ secretion by the distal tubule (99,155–158) and cortical collecting duct (159–163). An elevation of plasma K^+ concentration may also be modulated by K^+ uptake into cells of the proximal tubule, which results in decreased cellular H^+ concentration and thereby decreased HCO_3^- reabsorption. This proximal effect serves to increase tubular flow rate, which, in combination with increased cellular K^+ activity and aldosterone-induced effects, serves to increase urinary K^+ excretion (99).

Habitual ingestion of a high-K^+ diet leads to an acquired tolerance to K^+ in the distal nephron, an adaptation that augments the capacity of each individual nephron to secrete K^+ (164). In the principal cell, the cellular mechanisms underlying this adaptation include increases in basolateral surface area, Na^+-K^+-ATPase activity, and density of apical membrane K^+ and Na^+ channels; increased cellular K^+ concentration; and increased transepithelial voltage along the distal nephron (150,152,154,164,165–169)—events that together enhance K^+ movement from cell to lumen. The morphologic correlate of this adaptation is the major increase in basolateral membrane surface area, the site at which the Na^+-K^+-ATPase pumps are inserted (113). Distal K^+ secretion at comparable levels of serum K^+ concentration is approximately three times higher in K^+-adapted rats (99,113). A similar adaptive response seen in chronic renal insufficiency (170,171) allows K^+ balance to be relatively well maintained during the course of many forms of progressive renal disease. Finally, gastrointestinal excretion of K^+ can increase in response to K^+ loading or renal insufficiency to help maintain K^+ balance (172,173).

When there is chronic K^+ depletion, there is less K^+ secretion (86,113,174), due in part to decreased release of aldosterone and, later, diminished cellular K^+ concentrations (175). There is also an increase in active K^+ reabsorption by cortical and medullary intercalated cells expressing the luminal H^+-K^+-ATPase pump (111,113,124). This response is associated with morphologic alterations to increase luminal surface area in the intercalated cells (112).

Tubular Flow Rate

K^+ secretion is strongly influenced by the rate of tubular fluid flow and the concentration of K^+ in the tubular fluid (151,176–178). The higher the distal flow rate, the slower the rate of rise in tubular fluid K^+ concentration and the larger the driving force favoring additional K^+ secretion (149,177,178). Thus, volume expansion and diuretics, which increase distal delivery rates, enhance K^+ secretion in the distal nephron. By causing a concomitant reduction in extracellular volume, diuretics also stimulate aldosterone secretion, which further favors K^+ secretion.

Increased distal flow is usually associated with increased distal Na^+ delivery. The increased availability of Na^+ at distal sites results in two additional factors favoring K^+ secretion (177,179). First, the increase in Na^+ entry across the apical channels makes the luminal potential more negative, which creates a more favorable electrochemical gradient for K^+ secretion. Second, the increase in Na^+ transport makes more K^+ available to the cell via the basolateral Na^+-K^+-ATPase pump; the higher cell K^+ concentration stimulates distal K^+ secretion.

Relevant to flow dependence, the high-conductance maxi-K channel, which is not open at physiologic membrane potentials, can be activated by membrane depolarization, elevation of intracellular Ca^{2+} concentration, membrane stretch, or hypoosmotic stress (180). One study shows that high urinary flow rates and hydrostatic pressure alter intracellular Ca^{2+} or the membrane stretch to which renal epithelial cells are exposed, thereby stimulating apical stretch- and Ca^{2+}-activated maxi-K channels (110). Stimulation of these maxi-K channels is likely to mediate flow-dependent K^+ secretion in the cortical collecting duct, whereas baseline K^+ secretion occurs through the small-conductance ROMK channel.

Na^+ Concentration

The effect of luminal Na^+ concentration on the magnitude of K^+ secretion is determined by the entry of Na^+ into the cell across the apical membrane (149,178,181). In addition to increasing luminal electronegativity, enhanced Na^+ movement from the tubular fluid into the principal cell depolarizes the apical cell membrane, stimulates Na^+-K^+-ATPase activity, and accelerates basolateral K^+ uptake (149,181). The net effect of these events is creation of a more favorable electrochemical gradient driving passive diffusion of K^+ from cell to lumen. Maneuvers that decrease active Na^+ transport (e.g., blockers of Na^+ channels, such as the K^+-sparing diuretic amiloride) attenuate the lumen negative potential difference and thereby reduce K^+ secretion (177).

Once the luminal Na^+ concentration falls below 35 mEq/L, K^+ secretion declines and the transepithelial voltage becomes less negative (162,178,179). The decrease in Na^+ uptake into the principal cell hyperpolarizes the apical membrane and decreases the electrochemical gradient favoring K^+ secretion into the lumen. A reduction in cell Na^+ concentration also reduces the activity of the basolateral Na^+-K^+-ATPase pump, thereby further reducing K^+ secretion.

Prolonged increases in Na^+ delivery resulting from long-term diuretic treatment will augment the basolateral membrane area of distal convoluted tubule cells, connecting tubule cells, and principal cells (182–185). This structural adaptation is accompanied by increased Na^+ reabsorption and K^+ secretion, which results in a downstream attenuation of the diuretic-induced natriuresis and an increase in the kaliuresis.

Nonreabsorbable Anion

Anions are generally reabsorbed in the cortical collecting duct via the paracellular route, after the active transport of Na^+. The delay in the reabsorption of the anion creates the negative transepithelial difference (186). Distal delivery of Na^+ accompanied by an anion that is less reabsorbable than chloride, such as sulfate, bicarbonate, β-hydroxybutyrate, or carbenicillin, leads to an increase in luminal electronegativity in the cortical collecting duct; this further stimulates K^+ secretion (187–189), occasionally with clinical consequences (190).

Acid-Base Balance

Acute metabolic acidosis causes the urine pH and K^+ excretion to decrease, whereas both acute respiratory alkalosis and metabolic alkalosis result in increases in urine pH and K^+ excretion. Chronic metabolic acidosis has variable effects on urinary K^+ excretion. Metabolic changes in ECF pH produce reciprocal H^+ and K^+ shifts between cells. During acute acidemia, H^+ is taken up by cells while K^+ moves out of cells, and this tends to reduce K^+ secretion; in acute alkalemia, on the other hand, H^+ comes out of cells and K^+ moves into cells, and this tends to increase K^+ secretion (150,191–194). Moreover, a decrease in the pH of tubular fluid, as would be expected during metabolic acidosis, in itself inhibits K^+ secretion in the cortical collecting duct (192,195,196). Data indicate that cell acidification suppresses and cell alkalinization stimulates activity of the apical pH-sensitive K^+ secretory channels (176). Furthermore, low pH inhibits Na^+-K^+-ATPase activity (1), which reduces K^+ uptake and K^+ secretion in the distal nephron.

The effect of chronic acid-base disturbances on K^+ secretion is more complex and may be overridden by modifications of the glomerular filtrate (e.g., Cl^- and HCO_3^- concentration), tubular fluid flow rate, and circulating aldosterone levels (197–199). Indeed, chronic metabolic acidosis is a potent stimulus of renal K^+ excretion (192,193,200–203). Presumably, the acidosis causes hyperkalemia, which stimulates aldosterone secretion, and this results in the high rate of urinary K^+ excretion in this acid-base disorder. In addition, a reduction in plasma HCO_3^- inhibits fluid and Na^+ reabsorption in the proximal tubule, which leads to increased fluid and Na^+ distal delivery (192). The development of volume depletion that also results from this proximal inhibition stimulates the secretion of aldosterone, which further increases K^+ secretion. Thus, in contrast to acute metabolic acidosis in which K^+ secretion is reduced, chronic acidosis overrides this inhibition by inducing aldosterone- and flow-dependent K^+ secretion. The handling of K^+ in the organic acidurias (lactate, β-hydroxybutyrate) is dominated by the increased distal delivery of Na^+ with a poorly reabsorbable anion, plus volume depletion that stimulates aldosterone secretion—effects that offset those of acute acidosis and stimulate net distal K^+ secretion and ultimately K^+ depletion in the body (26).

Other Hormones

Glucocorticoids stimulate K^+ excretion through their action to enhance glomerular filtration, distal Na^+ delivery, and rate of urinary flow (133,204,205). The administration of vasopressin causes a small increase in urinary K^+ excretion despite a reduction in urinary flow rate, due in large part to an increase in the electrochemical driving force for K^+ secretion across the luminal membrane (206–208). Specifically, there is a vasopressin-induced initial increase in apical Na^+ permeability that leads to apical membrane depolarization, basolateral Na^+-K^+-ATPase activation with enhanced K^+ uptake, and increased K^+ secretion into the tubular fluid (155,209). In addition, the vasopressin-induced stimulation of K^+ secretion may also reflect an increase in density of apical K^+ secretory channels in the principal cell (210). Catecholamines decrease urinary K^+ excretion both directly and indirectly through catecholamine-induced alterations in renal hemodynamics and cell K^+ uptake in the liver and muscle (43,211). In addition, β-adrenergic agonists directly inhibit K^+ secretion in the cortical collecting duct via modifications in chloride transport and transepithelial voltage (212,213).

CONTRIBUTION OF THE GASTROINTESTINAL TRACT

In the adult under normal conditions, approximately 10% of daily K^+ intake is excreted in the stool (Fig. 8.2). The gastrointestinal tract normally absorbs approximately 85% of dietary K^+. This process is substantially more efficient in the neonate, probably related to a higher activity of K^+-absorptive pumps (214,215). The general pattern of K^+ handling by the intestine parallels that of the nephron, and the primary site of regulation of intestinal K^+ transport is the colon. Most dietary K^+ is absorbed along with water in the small intestine (84,214,216), so that a low volume of fluid with a high K^+ concentration is delivered to the colon. The direction of net K^+ transport in the colon, as in the distal nephron, is determined by the balance between K^+ secretion and K^+ absorption (172,217). In the colon, K^+ secretion requires basolateral uptake of K^+ via the Na^+-K^+-ATPase pump and Na^+-K^+-$2Cl^-$ co-transporter and its secretion across the apical membrane via K^+ channels (218). The absorption of K^+ is mediated by apical K^+-dependent ATPases, including a colonic H^+-K^+-ATPase (214,215).

Hormones (aldosterone, glucocorticoids, epinephrine, and prostaglandins) stimulate K^+ colonic secretion (22,219). A high-K^+ diet also stimulates colonic K^+ secretion (220). In addition, glucocorticoids stimulate maturation of neonatal colon K^+ secretion by opening up apical K^+ channels and increasing the activity of Na^+-K^+-ATPase (221,222). On the other hand, colonic K^+ secretion is inhibited by indomethacin and dietary K^+ restriction. Diarrheal illnesses are typically associated with hypokalemia, despite an adaptive reduction in renal K^+ excretion. Mucosal inflammation reduces K^+ absorption, whereas cyclic adenosine monophosphate–stimulated secretion during rotaviral enteritis may contribute to inappropriate colonic K^+ excretion (223).

Potassium adaptation in the colon is demonstrated by increased fecal K^+ excretion under conditions of K^+ loading (trauma, renal tubular K^+ secretory disorders, excessive K^+ intake), especially when exacerbated by renal insufficiency (164). Whereas stool K^+ content averages 5 to 10% of dietary intake in healthy adults, fecal K^+ excretion may triple in patients with severe renal insufficiency (22,172).

MATURATION OF RENAL K+ TRANSPORT

Newborns fed breast milk or formula with an Na^+/K^+ ratio of 0.5 to 0.6 demonstrate significant renal K^+ retention with an average urine Na^+/K^+ higher than 1 (Table 8.1). This relative conservation of K^+ in the newborn and immature animal is generally associated with a higher plasma K^+ concentration than in the adult and is a requirement for somatic growth (14,76,77,88,224). Clearance and micropuncture studies in the newborn consistently demonstrate low rates of urinary K^+ excretion under basal conditions (88,225,226) and an inability to excrete an exogenously administered potassium load as efficiently as the adult (14,79–82). Acute K^+ loading of experimental animals results in significantly lower rates of urinary K^+ excretion in weaning than in older rats (Fig. 8.7)

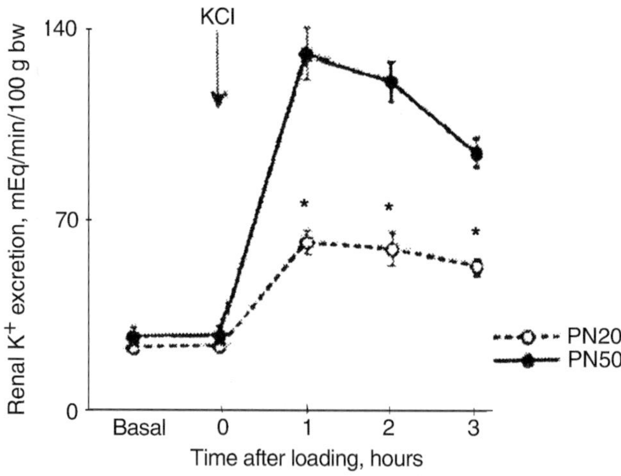

FIGURE 8.7. Renal K^+ excretion after intragastric KCl loading (0.7 mmol/100 g body weight) in unanesthetized infant (PN20) and adult (PN50) rats. Values are means ± the standard error of the mean; asterisks indicate statistically significant difference between infant and adult rats. bw, body weight.

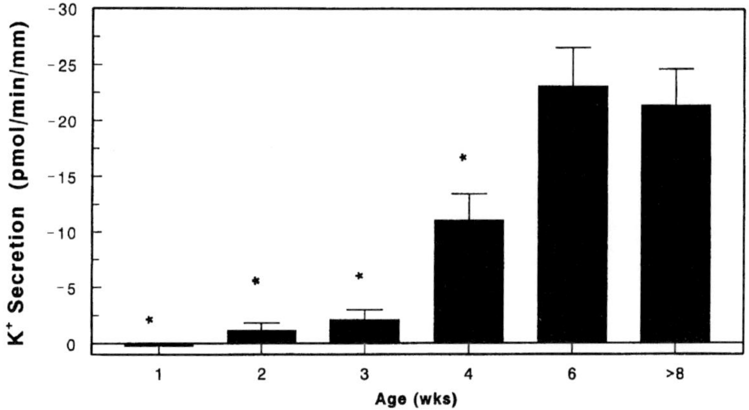

FIGURE 8.8. Maturation of net K^+ secretion in cortical collecting ducts obtained from 1-, 2-, 3-, 4-, 6-, and >8-week-old (adult) rabbits. Mean values plus standard error are given for each age group. *, $p < .05$ versus >8-week-old (adult). (Data from the Satlin LM. Postnatal maturation of potassium transport in rabbit cortical collecting duct. *Am J Physiol* 1994;266:F57.)

(215). Whereas infants, like adults, can excrete K^+ at a rate that exceeds its filtration (79), the rate of K^+ excretion expressed per unit of body or kidney weight is less than that observed in older subjects (80,82,214).

Micropuncture studies have shown that approximately 50% of the filtered load of K^+ is reabsorbed in the proximal tubule of both suckling and older rats (88,90). However, up to 35% of the filtered load of K^+ reaches the superficial distal tubule of the 13- to 15-day-old rat, which far exceeds the distal delivery measured in older animals and indicates functional immaturity of the loop of Henle (88,227). The fractional reabsorption of K^+ along the loop of Henle, expressed as a percentage of delivered load, increases from 57% at 13 to 15 days to 79% by 30 to 39 days of age (88).

Because the fractional excretion of K^+ in the immature rat is approximately the same as the percentage of the load delivered to the superficial distal tubule (88), it is likely that there is little net K^+ secretion along the immature distal nephron. Evidence indicates that the limitation in K^+ excretion is due, at least in part, to a greatly reduced K^+ secretory capacity of the cortical collecting duct early in life. Clearance experiments in saline-loaded puppies have provided indirect evidence for diminished capacity of the immature distal nephron to secrete K^+ (225). Comparison of early distal tubular fluid and final urine in the newborn suggests that the immature distal tubule and cortical collecting duct secrete less K^+ than do more mature segments (88).

Microperfusion experiments in rabbit cortical collecting ducts have conclusively shown that net K^+ secretion is absent at birth, first becomes evident at the fourth postnatal week, and increases sharply to reach adult levels by 6 weeks of age (Fig. 8.8) (228). These data indicate that the low rates of K^+ excretion characteristic of the newborn kidney are due, at least in part, to a low capacity for K^+ secretion by the immature cortical collecting duct. Whereas K^+ secretion in the mature cortical collecting duct is strongly stimulated by an increase in luminal flow rate, this is not observed in early life, at least until 6 weeks postnatally. Indeed, the developmental appearance of flow dependence 2 weeks after the appearance of basal K^+ secretion suggests that basal and flow-stimulated K^+ secretion are mediated by distinct channels with different developmental patterns of expression (229).

Ultrastructural comparison of principal cells from newborn and adult cortical collecting ducts lends support to the observation of relative functional immaturity of the K^+ secretory epithelium early in life (21,230). Whereas the principal cell of the neonatal cortical collecting duct possesses few organelles, smooth apical and basolateral surfaces, varying amounts of intracellular glycogen, and a low volume of mitochondria, the mature principal cell is devoid of glycogen and possesses twice the volume percentage of mitochondria, has more organelles and basolateral infoldings, and has a 35% larger apical perimeter (230).

Factors Limiting K^+ Secretion in the Cortical Collecting Duct

Several factors may limit urinary K^+ secretion in the neonatal principal cell, including an unfavorable electrochemical gradient (low cell K^+, low Na^+-K^+-ATPase activity, and/or low transepithelial voltage), high backleak of K^+ through paracellular routes, limited membrane permeability to K^+, low tubular fluid flow rates, and diminished principal cell sensitivity to mineralocorticoids. Alternatively, enhanced K^+ absorption by intercalated cell-rich distal nephron segments (e.g., inner cortical collecting duct, outer medullary collecting duct) may offset much of the distal K^+ secretion.

Na^+-K^+-ATPase

The high cellular potassium concentration is generated and maintained by the activity of Na^+-K^+-ATPase. Na^+-K^+-ATPase activity in the neonatal cortical collecting duct is only 50% of that measured in the mature segment, when expressed per unit of dry weight (32), in keeping with the smaller number of basolateral infoldings observed in neonatal principal cells (230). This lower level of Na^+-K^+-ATPase activity in the immature cortical collecting duct results in a reduced electrochemical K^+ gradient across the apical membrane. If one assumes that principal cell K^+

activity is similar in neonatal and mature collecting ducts (21), it is likely that the low rate of Na^+-K^+-ATPase activity observed early in life must be accompanied by a proportionally low rate of passive K^+ efflux from immature principal cells. The efflux of K^+ may be limited by an unfavorable electrochemical gradient opposing secretion, reduced apical membrane K^+ permeability, or low tubular flow rates prevailing in the neonate.

Flow Rate

The low distal flow rates characteristic of the newborn (88,231,232) could limit K^+ secretion early in life. To address the role of flow rate on K^+ secretion, Satlin measured the rates of K^+ transport in cortical collecting ducts. Flow-dependent stimulation of K^+ secretion was not observed until 6 weeks postnatally (228). These studies rule out a low *in vivo* tubular flow rate per se as a factor limiting K^+ secretion in the neonatal kidney.

Micropuncture studies in maturing rats show that the early distal tubular fluid concentration of K^+ decreases during maturation from 4.5 to 2.3 mmol/L (88,90). The higher K^+ concentration in the youngest rats reflects, in part, immaturity of K^+ reabsorption by the thick ascending limb of the loop of Henle. These data suggest that only a small increase in distal nephron K^+ secretion could be accounted for by this maturational decrement in chemical gradient along the collecting duct. Thus, the chemical driving force for K^+ secretion across the apical membrane of the principal cell appears to remain relatively constant after birth (228).

Electrical Gradient

The luminal electronegativity of the cortical collecting duct, driven by electrogenic Na^+ absorption (97,162), favors K^+ secretion from principal cell to lumen. Measurements of transepithelial voltage in cortical collecting ducts early in life have shown maturational increases from a few millivolts negative at birth to approximately 10 mV negative in the adult (228,233). These findings suggest that a smaller electrical gradient slightly limits K^+ secretion in the neonatal cortical collecting duct. Microperfused cortical collecting ducts isolated from 1-week-old rabbits show no significant Na^+ absorption (228). By 2 weeks of age the rate of net Na^+ absorption is approximately half that observed in cortical collecting ducts taken from mature animals. Concomitant with the postnatal increase in Na^+ absorption is a parallel increase in negativity of transepithelial voltage (228).

Finally, to secrete K^+, the principal cell requires functioning apical Na^+ channels to provide Na^+ for the Na^+ pump. The rate-limiting step for Na^+ absorption appears to be the expression of the apical Na^+ channel. Using patch-clamp analysis of the maturing rabbit principal cell, Satlin and Palmer (234) found that by 2 weeks of age the number of open Na^+ channels per patch reached a value similar to that observed in 5-week-old animals. The increase in the number of conducting channels is due to both an increase in the number of channels present per patch plus an increase in open probability (234). Thus, the presence of conducting Na^+ channels in the maturing cortical collecting duct approximately 1 week before net K^+ secretion is observed suggests that a low rate of Na^+ entry into the principal cell does not limit K^+ secretion early in life, unless little Na^+ is delivered to the distal nephron. *In vivo* measurements of distal tubular Na^+ concentrations in both adult and maturing rats generally exceed 30 mEq/L (86,88,179,232), which rules out the possibility that very low luminal Na^+ concentrations contribute to the reduced rate of distal K^+ secretion in the newborn.

Backleak

Paracellular K^+ conductance may be increased through leaky tight junctions in immature proximal tubules and cortical collecting ducts compared with mature segments (235,236). Thus, at the lower flow rates found in the immature kidney, enhanced tubular backleak of K^+ could severely limit net K^+ secretion. A cortical collecting duct microperfusion study showed that the difference between perfused and collected K^+ concentrations was less than 1.5 mol/L during the first 3 weeks of life (228). However, in the same age group, a lack of active secretion of K^+ over a wide range of flow rates suggests that backleak may not be a limiting factor early in life. Moreover, despite the absence of net K^+ secretion, active Na^+ absorption was evident as early as 2 weeks of age, at a rate that approached 50% of the mature level. Because the difference between perfused and collected Na^+ concentrations was nearly the same in immature and mature segments (228), it is not likely that postnatal development of the tight junctions comprising the paracellular pathway plays a major role in the maturation of K^+ secretion in the cortical collecting duct. On the other hand, data to suggest that backleak may be important in limiting K^+ transport come from the isotopic Na^+ studies performed by Vehaskari in maturing cortical collecting ducts (237), which showed high rates of passive Na^+ permeability during the first 2 weeks of postnatal life before a decrease to adult levels. Thus, a role for backleak in limiting K^+ secretion in the immature cortical collecting duct is still a significant possibility.

Aldosterone

Plasma aldosterone concentrations in the fetus and newborn are high compared with those in the adult (14,238–241). Yet, clearance studies demonstrate that young animals are less sensitive to mineralocorticoids than their mature counterparts (14,242). Both the density of aldosterone binding sites and receptor affinities are similar in mature and immature rats, which suggests that the early hyposensitivity to aldosterone is likely to be a postreceptor phenomenon (242). In addition, Vehaskari (237) showed that the administration of mineralocorticoid for 48 hours to 1- and 2-week-old rabbits had no effect on the sodium-22 absorptive flux in cortical collecting ducts isolated from these animals. Thus, the biological responsiveness to aldosterone is minimal early in life and increases with age; this development of aldosterone responsiveness may contribute to the maturation of K^+ secretion in the cortical collecting duct.

Apical K^+ Channels

The most likely explanation for both the low rate of K^+ secretion and the mature level of intracellular K^+ concentration despite the low activity of the Na^+-K^+-ATPase pump is a low apical permeability of the principal cell to K^+. The passage of K^+ across the apical membrane from the principal cell into the luminal fluid is likely mediated by a low conductance inwardly rectifying K^+-selective channel (105,106,108,154). Using patch-clamp technology, Satlin and Palmer (243) found a progressive increase with age in mean number of open K^+ channels per patch in rabbit principal cells (Fig. 8.9). This increase was due primarily to a developmental increase in the number of channels per patch, because the open probability remained constant after the second week of life. Because a major increase in net K^+ secretion occurs after the first 3 weeks of life and a major increment in mean number of open channels per patch occurs after the second week, it is likely that the increase in apical K^+ conductance of the principal cell substantially contributes to the maturational surge in the rate of K^+ secretion.

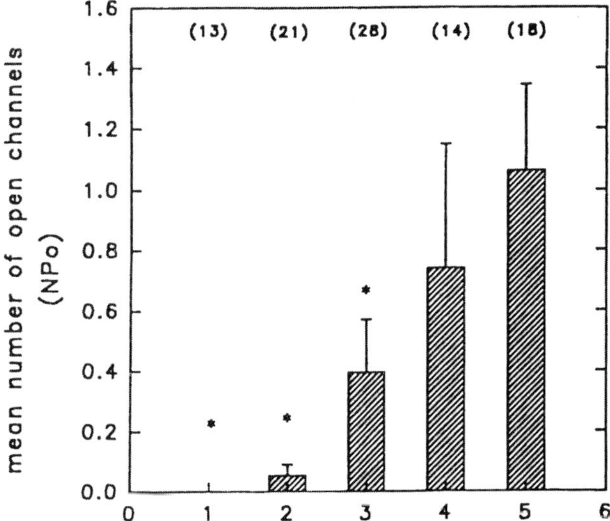

FIGURE 8.9. Maturation of K^+ conductance in split-open cortical collecting ducts obtained from 1-, 2-, 3-, 4-, and 5-week-old rabbits. Mean values of number of open channels per patch plus standard error are given for each age group. Segments from rabbits older than 5 weeks were not examined because the rate of successful patch-clamp experiments was too low. *, $p < .05$ versus 5-week-old. (From Satlin LM, Palmer LG. Apical K^+ conductance in maturing rabbit principal cell. *Am J Physiol* 1997;272:F397, with permission.)

The secretory K^+ channel characterized by Satlin and Palmer (243) is generally believed to have a major functional subunit called ROMK, based on similarities in biophysical properties (92,107,244,245). Using reverse transcriptase polymerase chain reaction, Benchimol et al. (246) showed that ROMK messenger RNA (mRNA) was regularly expressed by cortical collecting ducts isolated from animals 3 weeks of age and older. Only 30% of ducts from 2-week-old animals expressed ROMK mRNA and none expressed ROMK during the first week of life. Immunodetectable (247) and functional (243) apical low (ROMK) conductance channels, absent in neonatal principal cells, are present in principal cells from maturing rabbits, which indicates that the increase in ROMK mRNA contributes to the development of low-conductance secretory K^+ channels in the maturing cortical collecting duct.

K^+ Absorption by Intercalated Cells

Because net K^+ transport represents the sum of K^+ secretory and K^+ reabsorptive processes, it is possible that some K^+ absorption offsets the limited K^+ secretion in the neonatal cortical collecting duct. Clearance studies in saline-expanded dogs showed that newborn dogs reabsorbed 25% more of the distal K^+ load than did adult animals (80,225). Because micropuncture studies of immature rats indicated little K^+ reabsorption in the loop of Henle (88,90), the collecting duct was considered a likely segment for K^+ reabsorption. This K^+ reabsorption is probably mediated by an apical H^+-K^+-ATPase that couples K^+ reabsorption to H^+ secretion identified in collecting duct intercalated cells (117,118,121,248). Indeed, K^+ deficiency in adult animals is associated with selective hypertrophy of the apical membranes of medullary collecting duct intercalated cells (114). These anatomical changes are accompanied by functional data that show increased K^+ absorption (249) and H^+-K^+-ATPase protein and activity (124,250–252).

Functional studies indicate that neonatal cortical collecting duct intercalated cells possess an apical H^+-K^+-ATPase with activity comparable to that of mature intercalated cells (253). In addition, the higher tubular fluid K^+ concentration of the immature animal (88) should facilitate lumen to cell K^+ absorption mediated by the H^+-K^+-ATPase. Although direct studies of K^+ absorption by the immature collecting duct have not been performed, the preceding data suggest that parts of the neonatal collecting duct may absorb K^+ (233,253), which is essential for conserving some of the excessive K^+ presented to the immature distal nephron.

DISORDERS OF POTASSIUM METABOLISM

Hypokalemia

K^+ is predominantly an intracellular cation, yet clinical estimation of K^+ balance usually depends on the measurement of extracellular (serum or plasma) K^+ concentration. Accurate assessment of body potassium stores can be performed only by total-body counting methods, laborious measurements not readily available to the clinician. Hypokalemia, defined as a serum K^+ concentration below 3.5 mEq/L, usually indicates a deficit in total body potassium but may also represent a shift of K^+ from the extra- to the intracellular space in the setting of normal total body K^+ stores. To a first approximation, each 1 mEq/L decrease in serum K^+ concentration below 3 mEq/L corresponds to a 200- to 400-mEq (approximately 10%) deficit in total body potassium stores in the 70-kg adult. Total body K^+ depletion causing hypokalemia results from inadequate intake or from excessive loss of K^+ from the body via the kidney or gastrointestinal tract. A list of clinical disorders associated with K^+ redistribution and depletion is found in Table 8.4.

Clinical Disorders Associated with Hypokalemia

Insufficient K^+ Intake

Dietary Insufficiency. Potassium is virtually impossible to eliminate from the average diet except by limiting intake to foods containing a high percentage of carbohydrate or refined sugar or by administering K^+-free parenteral fluids for a prolonged period. The K^+ content of a variety of foods and beverages in the American diet are listed in Table 8.5.

In the adult a sharp reduction in dietary K^+ intake is followed within several days by a decrease in urinary K^+ excretion but only to a minimum rate of approximately 10 mEq/day, as the kidney is unable to produce a K^+-free urine (69). The combination of the limited ability to maximally conserve urinary K^+ and ongoing obligatory gastrointestinal losses may lead to significant K^+ depletion if dietary deprivation is prolonged.

Chloride Deficiency Syndrome. Dietary chloride deficiency syndrome, first recognized in infants fed chloride-deficient batches of commercial cow's milk formula, is characterized by hypochloremic metabolic alkalosis, hypochloruria, and hypokalemia (254,255). Clinically, these babies presented with failure to thrive, anorexia, muscular weakness, lethargy, vomiting, and dehydration. Renal K^+ excretion was lower in chloride-deficient patients than in age-matched controls offered formula of comparable K^+ content (254). The pathogenesis of the hypokalemia may be related to volume contraction due to lack of adequate chloride and resulting in secondary hyperaldosteronism, reduced intake of formula, pH-induced redistribution of extracellular K^+, and provision of nonreabsorbable anions.

Increased Entry of K^+ into Cells

Acute Alkalosis. Either metabolic or respiratory alkalosis can be associated with hypokalemia by promoting K^+ entry into cells in exchange for protons. The initial small transcellular shift of K^+ is exacerbated by volume contraction–induced hyperaldosteronism and the delivery of nonreabsorbable anions (bicarbonate) to potassium-secretory sites in the distal nephron.

TABLE 8.4. CLINICAL DISORDERS ASSOCIATED WITH HYPOKALEMIA

- Inadequate intake
  - Dietary insufficiency
  - Chloride deficiency syndrome
- Increased entry of K^+ into cells
  - Acute alkalosis (metabolic, respiratory)
  - Insulin administration
  - Elevated β-adrenergic activity
  - Hypokalemic periodic paralysis
  - Increased number of cells in plasma
  - Barium poisoning
  - Pseudohypokalemia
- Increased renal losses
  - Renal K^+ wasting disorders with low plasma renin activity
    - Disorders of excess mineralocorticoid activity
      - Primary hyperaldosteronism
        - Aldosterone-producing adenomas
        - Bilateral adrenal hyperplasia
      - Cushing syndrome
        - Primary adrenal disease
        - Effect of pharmacologic doses of corticosteroids
        - Secondary effect of nonendocrine tumor
        - Congenital adrenal hyperplasia
          - 11β-hydroxylase deficiency
          - 17α-hydroxylase deficiency
      - Excessive licorice ingestion
        - Inhibition of 11β-hydroxysteroid dehydrogenase
    - Liddle's syndrome (pseudoaldosteronism type 1)
    - Pseudoaldosteronism type 2 (mineralocorticoid receptor defect)
    - Glucocorticoid-remediable aldosteronism
    - Syndrome of apparent mineralocorticoid excess
  - Renal K^+-wasting disorders with high plasma renin activity
    - Excessive renin production
    - Bartter's syndrome
    - Gitelman's syndrome
    - Diuretic use
      - Thiazides and loop diuretics
      - Osmotic diuretics (mannitol, glucose)
      - Carbonic anhydrase inhibitors
    - Renal tubular acidosis
    - Other conditions associated with increased distal nephron flow
      - Renal diseases (interstitial nephritis, obstructive uropathy, dysplasia, hypercalcemia)
      - Antibiotic use (carbenicillin, nafcillin, penicillin, gentamicin, amphotericin B)
      - Leukemia
    - Miscellaneous
      - Hypomagnesemia
      - Vitamin D intoxication
      - Thyrotoxicosis
      - Primary polydipsia
      - Cardiopulmonary bypass
- Increased gastrointestinal loss
  - Gastric (vomiting, nasogastric suction, pyloric stenosis)
  - Large intestinal (diarrhea, VIPoma syndrome, villous adenoma, chronic laxative abuse, biliary drainage, ureterosigmoidostomy)
- Integumental loss
  - Excessive sweating
  - Full-thickness burns

VIPoma, vasoactive intestinal polypeptide tumor.

TABLE 8.5. POTASSIUM CONTENT OF VARIOUS FOODS

Food	K^+ (mg)	Food	K^+ (mg)
Beverages		Cookies/desserts	
Cola, 12 oz	4	Gingersnaps, 1 oz, 4 cookies	98
Pepsi, 12 oz	10	Doughnut, 1	60
Gingerale, 12 oz	4	Chocolate ice cream, 0.5 cup	164
Diet Coke, 12 oz	18	Vanilla ice cream, 0.5 cup	131
Coffee, 6 oz	96	Chocolate ice cream bar with chocolate coating, 1 bar	247
Cranberry-apple juice, 6 oz	50	Apple turnover, 1	33
Hawaiian punch, 8 oz	50	Orange sherbet, 0.5 cup	92
Orange juice, 6 oz	210	Jello, 0.5 cup	239
Black tea, brewed, 6 oz	66	Meals	
Citrus fruit juice drink, 8 oz (from frozen concentrate)	278	Scrambled egg (1) with milk	84
Apple juice, 8 oz	295	Macaroni and cheese, 1 cup	190
Grapefruit juice, 8 oz	378	Cheese pizza, 1 slice	85
Orange juice, 8 oz	436	Chicken pot pie, 1/3 of 9-in. pie	343
Tomato juice, 6 oz	400	Spaghetti with tomato sauce, 1 cup	408
Chocolate shake, 10 oz	566	Cheeseburger, 1 large	644
Candy		Hotdog, 1	143
Golden Almond Hershey's Chocolate 3.2-g bar	429	Mashed potatoes, 1/3 cup	235
Lollipop, 1	0	Fruit, fresh	
Marshmallow, 1	25	Apple, 1 medium	159
Milk chocolate, 1.55-oz bar	169	Banana, 1 medium	451
Snickers, 2.16-oz bar	206	Cantaloupe, 1 cup	494
Twizzlers, 2.5 oz	45	Grapefruit, one-half, medium	175
Cereals		Peach, 1 medium	171
Bran, 100%, 1 oz	277	Raisins, 2/3 cup	825
Cornflakes, 1.06 oz	35	Watermelon, 1 cup	186
Granola, Kellogg's lowfat, 1.7 oz	122	Bread	
Raisin bran, 2.08 oz	380	White, 1 slice	30
Special K, 1.09 oz	54	Whole wheat, 1 slice	71
Shredded Wheat, 1 oz	93	English muffin, with butter	69
Cheese		Vegetables	
American processed, 1 oz	46	Potato, with skin	903
Cream cheese, 1 oz	34	Tomato, 1	273
Chips		Green beans, 0.5 cup	185
Corn chips, 1 oz	40	Carrot, 1 medium	233
Potato chips, 1 oz	361	Lima beans, 1 cup boiled	955
Pretzels, 1 oz	41	Lentils, 1 cup boiled	731
		Broccoli, 0.5 cup raw	143

Data from Pennington JAP. *Bowes & Church's food values of portions commonly used*, 17th ed. Philadelphia: Lippincott–Raven, 1998.

Insulin Administration. Insulin promotes the entry of K^+ into skeletal muscle and liver cells (37,256), as observed most prominently in the treatment of diabetic ketoacidosis.

Elevated β-Adrenergic Activity. Nonselective β-adrenergic agonists (isoproterenol, epinephrine) and selective β_2-adrenergic agonists (albuterol, terbutaline) promote K^+ entry into cells (37). Thus, transient hypokalemia can be produced by stress-induced release of epinephrine, theophylline intoxication, treatment of asthma with albuterol (257), or treatment of premature labor with terbutaline (258). Arrhythmias may result from this hypokalemia when there is volume contraction induced by concomitant diuretic therapy (259) or by poor oral intake (260).

Hypokalemic Periodic Paralysis. Hypokalemic periodic paralysis is a rare disorder characterized by attacks of muscle weakness and episodes of flaccid paralysis of the limbs and thorax lasting 6 to 24 hours (261). Serum K^+ concentration is normal between attacks. In severe cases death from respiratory failure or cardiac arrhythmia may occur. Both sporadic and familial cases have been reported with a male to female preponderance of 3:1 and generally autosomal dominant inheritance. Familial forms are due to point mutations in the gene encoding the α-1 subunit of the L-type calcium channel, or voltage-gated dihydropyridine receptor (262,263). The dihydropyridine receptor functions as a voltage-gated calcium channel and is critical for excitation-contraction coupling in a voltage sensitive and calcium-independent manner (264). The defect in hypokalemic periodic paralysis is associated with a reduced sarcolemmal ATP-sensitive K^+ current (265).

The disorder usually becomes symptomatic during the first or second decade of life. Acute attacks generally occur at night, and the patient awakens paralyzed. Episodes are associated with sudden movement of K^+ into cells, which lowers plasma K^+ concentration by 1.5 to 2.5 mEq/L. Attacks are often precipitated by a carbohydrate meal, rest after exercise, or stressful events causing hypokalemia by a shift of K^+ into cells via the release of insulin or epinephrine. The paralysis is characterized by failure of propagation of the muscle action potential (266). After the attack, sequestered K^+ is released from cells and plasma K^+ concentration becomes normal.

Treatment with oral KCl usually aborts symptomatic attacks; intravenous K^+ may be required for severe attacks. Nonselective beta-blockers can reduce the number and severity of attacks, and limit the fall in plasma K^+ concentration (261). In most patients acetazolamide (20 to 40 mg/kg/day divided into four doses) may be more effective than K^+ supplementation or K^+-sparing diuretics in preventing severe attacks. The metabolic acidosis induced by acetazolamide may decrease the rate of K^+ entry into cells and thereby diminish the severity of the disease (267). Hyperthyroidism may be associated with hypokalemic periodic paralysis, probably because thyroid hormone stimulates Na^+-K^+-ATPase activity and sensitivity to catecholamines, and thereby drives K^+ into cells. Restoration of euthyroidism in thyrotoxic patients combined with beta-blockade generally prevents the hypokalemic attacks.

Barium Poisoning. Ingestion of soluble barium salts may result in a severe decrease in plasma K^+ concentration secondary to intracellular shifts of K^+ from the plasma (268). Barium acts on muscle cells to decrease K^+ conductance, thereby impairing outward diffusion of K^+ (269). Thus, the K^+ pumped into the cell via Na^+-K^+-ATPase cannot exit.

Increased Number of Cells in Plasma. A rapid increase in hematopoietic cell production associated with new cell K^+ uptake, such as resulting from the administration of folic acid or vitamin B_{12} to patients with megaloblastic anemia, can lead to hypokalemia and potentially to cardiac arrhythmias (270). Similarly, after the administration of granulocyte-macrophage colony-stimulating factor to correct neutropenia, a marked increase in white blood cell production may lead to hypokalemia (271).

Other Cellular Shifts. Hypothermia has been associated with hypokalemia as K^+ enters cells and is reversible on rewarming.

Pseudohypokalemia. Because metabolically active cells continue to take up K^+ after blood has been drawn, patients with very high white blood cell counts may become apparently hypokalemic if their blood has been allowed to stand for prolonged periods at room temperature (271,272).

Increased Renal Losses

Urinary K^+ excretion is determined primarily by K^+ secretion in the cortical collecting duct. Increased urinary losses usually result from increased flow of water and Na^+ to the cortical collecting duct and/or excessive mineralocorticoid. In the setting of adequate distal Na^+ delivery, the urine K^+ concentration is helpful in differentiating among the causes of hypokalemia.

Renal K^+ Wasting Disorders with Low Plasma Renin Activity

Disorders of Excess Mineralocorticoid Activity. Because mineralocorticoids stimulate K^+ secretion in the distal tubule and cortical collecting duct, conditions characterized by excessive mineralocorticoid activity are often associated with hypokalemia. The classic disorder of endogenous overproduction, *primary hyperaldosteronism,* may be associated with an adrenal adenoma or bilateral adrenal hyperplasia and is accompanied by hypertension, a variable degree of hypokalemia, and metabolic alkalosis (273,274).

Hypokalemia along with metabolic alkalosis may be observed in some patients with increased cortisol production (*Cushing syndrome*) or in those receiving *pharmacologic doses of corticosteroids,* presumably related to the mineralocorticoid effect of such hormones or to the fact that the rate of delivery of cortisol exceeds its rate of inactivation via 11β-hydroxysteroid dehydrogenase (11β-HSD) (275,276). Tumors of the lung, thymus, and pancreas that produce an adrenocorticotropic hormone (ACTH)–like substance are less prevalent in children than in adults but may lead to increased production of cortisol, desoxycorticosterone (DOC), and corticosterone, which results in severe hypokalemia (277).

Among the multiple forms of *congenital adrenal hyperplasia,* deficiencies of 11β-hydroxylase and 17α-hydroxylase are associated with hypertension and hypokalemic alkalosis. The 11β-hydroxylase deficiency leads to a block in synthesis of cortisol, enhanced secretion of ACTH, and subsequent stimulation of DOC and adrenal androgen production (278). The excess mineralocorticoid (DOC) activity results in hypokalemia and hypertension. The 17α-hydroxylase deficiency leads not only to a block in cortisol synthesis but also to defective production of adrenal androgens (278,279).

Ingestion of large quantities of European *licorice,* which contains glycyrrhetinic acid, a plant steroid with weak mineralocorticoid activity, can lead to a syndrome similar to primary hyperaldosteronism with sodium retention, edema, hypertension, and hypokalemia, except that plasma aldosterone levels are suppressed (280). Licorice and its analogues are also effective inhibitors of 11β-HSD, which converts cortisol to cortisone in the distal nephron (275,281). Cortisol binds to the mineralocorticoid receptors present in the cortical collecting duct with an avidity equal to that of aldosterone but circulates at much higher concentrations in plasma. However, cortisol is converted locally by 11β-HSD to inactive metabolites such as cortisone. This conversion is impaired with licorice-induced inhibition of 11β-HSD, which allows cortisol to activate the mineralocorticoid receptors and produce a clinical picture of primary hyperaldosteronism.

Liddle's Syndrome. Liddle's syndrome is a rare autosomal dominant disorder that presents a clinical picture similar to that of primary hyperaldosteronism with severe hypokalemic metabolic alkalosis and hypertension accompanied by Na^+ retention and substantial urinary K^+ excretion (282). Plasma renin and aldosterone levels are low, however, which gives rise to the clinical descriptor of pseudoaldosteronism (283).

This disease is caused by mutations in the carboxyterminal of the β or γ subunits of the ENaC (282,284). These gain-of-function mutations result in enhanced channel activity due to increased cell surface expression (and lack of downregulation) of functional Na^+ channels in the cortical collecting duct. The consequent increase in Na^+ reabsorption leads to severe hypertension. The hypokalemia reflects urinary K^+ wasting due to the secondary effects of increased apical Na^+ reabsorption, which results in an increased electrochemical driving force favoring K^+ secretion from the principal cell into the urinary space. The urinary Na^+ and K^+ abnormalities are not affected by spironolactone, a competitive aldosterone antagonist, but rather by the Na^+ channel blockers triamterene and amiloride (285).

Pseudoaldosteronism Type 2. This disorder results from a mutation in the hormone-binding domain of the mineralocorticoid receptor (286). The phenotype resembles that of Liddle's syndrome with autosomal dominant inheritance, hypertension, hypokalemia, suppressed plasma renin activity, and aldosterone secretion. However, a very severe presentation during pregnancy is also seen (284).

A serine to leucine mutation occurs at position 810 in the hormone-binding domain of the mineralocorticoid receptor that changes the affinity of the receptor for a variety of steroids. This mutation results in constitutive mineralocorticoid receptor activity and alters receptor specificity, so that progesterone and other steroids lacking 21-hydroxyl groups, normally mineralocorticoid receptor antagonists, become potent agonists (286).

Progesterone has a very high affinity for the mutated receptor, which accounts for the severe presentation during pregnancy. Because the receptor has constitutively stimulated basal activity and may respond to other endogenous steroids, the clinical phenotype can present in males and nonpregnant females as well. Spironolactone is an agonist for the mutated receptor, and its use is therefore contraindicated in this form of pseudoaldosteronism.

Glucocorticoid-Remediable Aldosteronism. In glucocorticoid-remediable aldosteronism, aldosterone and the weak mineralocorticoids 18-oxo-cortisol and 18-hydroxy-cortisol are produced in excess (287). This is a single-gene disorder that causes hypertension. It results from a relatively common autosomal dominant mutation that creates a chimeric gene comprised of 5' regulatory sequences of the 11β-hydroxylase gene fused to the 3' coding sequences of the gene encoding aldosterone synthase, the rate-limiting enzyme for aldosterone synthesis. This ectopic aldosterone synthesis in the zona fasciculata is under the control of ACTH, rather than the renin-angiotensin system, and results in salt and water retention, hypertension, and dramatic hypokalemia. The level of hypertension appears to correlate with the level of aldosterone secretion, and glucocorticoids suppress this hypertension (284). The mechanism for urinary K^+ wasting is similar to that observed in Liddle's syndrome.

Syndrome of Apparent Mineralocorticoid Excess. In the syndrome of apparent mineralocorticoid excess, inactivating mutations in the 11β-HSD type II gene allow cortisol to act as the major endogenous mineralocorticoid (284,288). This enzyme normally converts cortisol to cortisone, thereby preventing cortisol from activating the type I mineralocorticoid receptor in the kidney. In this rare autosomal recessive disorder characterized by pre- and postnatal growth failure, juvenile hypertension, hypokalemic metabolic alkalosis, and hyporeninemic hypoaldosteronism, reduced metabolism of cortisol to cortisone results in local cortisol excess and increased mineralocorticoid response, even in the absence of elevations in plasma cortisol level (289). The underlying mechanism for urinary K^+ wasting is similar to that in Liddle's syndrome. Treatment usually includes spironolactone (which competes for the mineralocorticoid receptor), K^+ supplements, and a low-salt diet.

Renal K^+ Wasting Disorders with High Plasma Renin Activity

Bartter's and Gitelman's Syndromes. Bartter's and Gitelman's syndromes are rare autosomal recessive disorders associated with urinary K^+ wasting, hypokalemia and metabolic alkalosis, hyperreninism, and hyperaldosteronism, but with normal blood pressure (282,290). Hypokalemia, chronic volume contraction, and high plasma concentrations of angiotensin, kallikrein, kinins, and vasopressin all stimulate the production of prostaglandin E_2. The absence of hypertension rules out primary mineralocorticoid excess, and the finding of high urinary chloride excretion rules out secondary hyperaldosteronism due to extrarenal fluid loss. Such findings occur only in Bartter's syndrome and with long-term diuretic therapy (282). The pathogenesis of Bartter's and Gitelman's syndromes is similar to that in long-term treatment with loop and thiazide diuretics, respectively. The genetic defect of Bartter's syndrome involves transporters in the thick ascending limb of the loop of Henle and collecting duct. Clinical disease is attributable to defective NaCl reabsorption in the thick ascending limb, where approximately 30% of the filtered salt is reabsorbed. Gitelman's syndrome presents with milder salt wasting due to abnormal salt transport in the distal convoluted tubule.

At least three phenotypically different subgroups of patients with Bartter's and Gitelman's syndromes can be identified. The neonatal variant, previously called hyperprostaglandin E syndrome, presents with dehydration, failure to thrive, dysmorphic facies, and a history of polyhydramnios and premature delivery (291,292). There is significant Na^+ wasting, polyuria, hypercalciuria, osteopenia, and nephrocalcinosis with normal serum magnesium levels. The pathophysiology is likely due to mutations in the gene encoding the bumetanide-sensitive Na-K-2Cl co-transporter in the thick ascending limb (293) or in the gene encoding the ATP-regulated K^+ channel (ROMK1) (291) in the thick ascending limb and cortical collecting duct.

The second type is classic Bartter's syndrome, which presents in childhood (younger than 5 years of age), often as failure to thrive with signs of severe intravascular volume depletion. Compared to the neonatal form, urine calcium is elevated less severely and nephrocalcinosis is generally absent (260). The pathogenesis is generally a loss-of-function mutation of the renal basolateral Cl^- channel (ClC-Kb).

The third type of hypokalemic metabolic alkalosis is known as Gitelman's syndrome, which presents in childhood or later and is not associated with salt craving or bouts of dehydration. The presentation is much milder than Bartter's from a clinical and biochemical viewpoint. Gitelman's syndrome is due to mutations in the thiazide-sensitive NaCl cotransporter (NCCT or TSC), which is localized in the distal convoluted tubule (294). This subgroup comprises the Bartter's-type patients with hypomagnesemia and hypocalciuria. Defective NaCl reabsorption in the distal convoluted tubule results in increased delivery to the cortical collecting duct, with consequent mild volume contraction and aldosterone-stimulated K^+ and H^+ secretion, which leads to a mild hypokalemic metabolic alkalosis. The extent of volume contraction and K^+ depletion appear to be less marked than in Bartter's syndrome and are not sufficient to raise prostaglandin E_2 production.

Treatment focuses on correcting the electrolyte abnormalities and preventing dehydration. Potassium chloride therapy is required to fully address the K^+ imbalance and NaCl helps manage the defect in Cl^- reabsorption. Spironolactone is often helpful. Indomethacin inhibits prostaglandin production and decreases renin and aldosterone production; this results in less renal K^+ wasting but can have adverse long-term effects on renal function. Despite treatment, patients with Bartter's syndrome often have persistent hypokalemia. Patients with Gitelman's syndrome need magnesium chloride supplements but rarely need volume resuscitation or prostaglandin synthase inhibition.

Renal Tubular Acidosis. The mechanisms responsible for hypokalemia and renal K^+ wasting differ for proximal (type II) and distal (type I) renal tubular acidosis (RTA). Despite the K^+ depletion, however, the plasma K^+ concentration may be normal because the acidemia promotes K^+ movement out of cells. Failure of intercalated cells in the distal nephron to secrete protons into the urinary fluid results in distal RTA. The defect in H^+ secretion increases tubular electronegativity, thereby enhancing K^+ secretion and limiting Na^+ reabsorption in the cortical collecting duct. Volume depletion and consequent secondary hyperaldosteronism further aggravate urinary K^+ losses. Hypokalemic variants of distal RTA may arise from abnormalities of the luminal H^+-K^+-ATPase, which mediates H^+ secretion and K^+ reabsorption in the distal nephron, or a defect in the membrane permeability of the distal nephron. Treatment with alkali to correct the acidosis and volume depletion may diminish urinary K^+ losses and normalize serum K^+ concentration when dietary intake of Na^+ and K^+ is adequate (295). However, flooding of the distal nephron segments with excessive bicarbonate ion will exacerbate urinary K^+ losses.

Proximal or type II RTA, characterized by a depression in the renal HCO_3^- threshold, may exist as an isolated proximal defect of HCO_3^- reabsorption or may be associated with other proximal tubular transport abnormalities as a Fanconi syndrome, in which patients excrete large amounts of HCO_3^-, phosphate, amino acids, and glucose. Distal deliveries of Na^+ and the poorly reabsorbed anion HCO_3^- are high, which results in excessive K^+ secretion. Secondary hyperaldosteronism due to Na^+ wasting and volume depletion further increases K^+ secretion, as does treatment with sodium bicarbonate. On the other hand, correction of the acidosis and hypokalemia can usually be accomplished by replacing some of the sodium bicarbonate with potassium citrate (296–298).

Diuretic Use. The most common cause of renal K^+ wasting is the administration of diuretics, particularly loop and thiazide diuretics. The major mechanisms for K^+ wasting include increased delivery of loop or distal tubular fluid to the cortical collecting duct, where K^+ secretion is flow dependent, and secondary hyperaldosteronism resulting both from the underlying disease and from the volume contraction induced by the diuretics (298–300). In addition, the metabolic alkalosis that accompanies the use of such diuretics is likely to promote additional K^+ secretion.

Diuretic-induced hypokalemia may be associated with an increased incidence of arrhythmias (301,302) and should be treated in patients with hypomagnesemia or cardiac disease, especially during digitalis therapy (303). Treatment is recommended with KCl supplements or K^+-sparing diuretics (such as spironolactone or triamterene); the latter will also partially correct diuretic-induced magnesium depletion by diminishing magnesium excretion (304).

Excessive Renin Production. Activation of the renin-angiotensin system provides a major stimulus for adrenal aldosterone synthesis with the development of hypertension and hypokalemia. Such findings may be observed in patients with poor oral intake, diuretic use, vomiting or diarrhea, renal vascular disease, malignant hypertension, and renin-producing tumors, including hemangiopericytomas and Wilms' tumor (298).

Secondary hyperaldosteronism in edema-producing states does not usually result in hypokalemia (305). Edematous patients do not experience increased urinary K^+ losses or become hypokalemic when administered Na^+ loads to ensure adequate distal delivery and flow (306). Thus, the development of significant K^+ depletion in the presence of Na^+ retention (nephrotic syndrome, cirrhosis, congestive heart failure) suggests that additional kaliuretic factors are involved; for example, the administration of potent diuretics or the presence of metabolic alkalosis.

Other Conditions Associated with Increased Distal Nephron Flow. Conditions associated with increased flow of water and salt to the distal nephron may result in hypokalemia. As described for diuretic use and Bartter's and Gitelman's syndromes, the initial renal Na^+ wasting leads to a secondary rise in aldosterone release, which further contributes to the tendency to hypokalemia. A variety of renal diseases, including *chronic interstitial nephritis, urinary tract obstruction*, and *dysplasia*, can cause hypokalemia by these mechanisms (271). Similarly, *hypercalcemia* is frequently associated with a urinary concentrating defect and high distal flow, because calcium-induced tubular damage may impair Na^+ reabsorption (307).

Hypokalemia and urinary K^+ wasting may follow administration of various antibiotics, including high-dose *penicillin and penicillin analogues*, such as carbenicillin and nafcillin. The penicillins behave as nonreabsorbable anions, enhancing transepithelial electronegativity in the distal nephron, and are often administered as sodium salts, so that they enhance distal Na^+ delivery and thus K^+ secretion (298). Hypokalemia associated with prolonged or high-dose administration of *aminoglycosides* (e.g., gentamicin) has been attributed to development of secondary hyperaldosteronism and drug-induced renal magnesium wasting (308,309). Polyene antibiotics, such as *amphotericin B*, frequently induce renal K^+ wasting by increasing K^+ permeability of the luminal membrane and by causing a distal acidification defect (310).

Renal K^+ wasting and hypokalemia can be seen in patients with various forms of *leukemia*. The elevated urinary excretion of lysozyme (a low-molecular-weight protein present in leukocytes), which is characteristic of these leukemias, may be toxic to the proximal tubule (311,312). The hypokalemia observed in childhood leukemia (acute lymphocytic leukemia, acute myelogenous leukemia) and other adult leukemias (chronic myelogenous leukemia, chronic lymphocytic leukemia) is probably multifactorial in origin and may be attributed to causes such as reduced K^+ intake, antibiotic-induced renal K^+ wasting, the mineralocorticoid effect of high-dose steroid therapy, increased K^+ entry into metabolically active leukemic cells, and the osmotic diuresis (and nephrotoxicity) encountered in the administration of some chemotherapeutic agents (e.g., cisplatinum) (271,298,313).

Miscellaneous Factors. Hypomagnesemia is a relatively common finding in hypokalemic patients (314,315). Hypomagnesemia can lead to K^+ depletion (314,316). The mechanism for the increased kaliuresis is not clear, but it may reflect decreased reabsorption of K^+ in the loop of Henle and possibly the cortical collecting duct. Magnesium deficiency may result in loss of cell K^+, either by impairment of Na^+-K^+-ATPase activity or alteration of cell membrane permeability to K^+. Magnesium depletion may enhance renin and thus aldosterone secretion, with the resulting hyperaldosteronism in turn promoting urinary K^+ excretion. Hypocalcemia is also commonly found in hypomagnesemic patients due to decreased secretion of parathyroid hormone and skeletal resistance to its effect. Indeed, the combination of hypokalemia plus hypocalcemia is highly suggestive of underlying magnesium depletion (316). Correction of the hypokalemia frequently requires the restoration of magnesium balance (314–316).

Other conditions have been associated with hypokalemia, including *vitamin D intoxication, thyrotoxicosis, lithium toxicity, primary polydipsia*, and *cardiopulmonary bypass* (298). Hypokalemia can also follow transfusion of previously frozen washed erythrocytes, which reflects avid uptake of K^+ by these K^+-depleted red cells (317).

Increased Gastrointestinal Losses

Gastric Loss. Vomiting and nasogastric suction often lead to hypokalemia despite the fact that gastric secretions contain only 10 to 20 mEq/L of K^+ (318). The major site of K^+ loss is, in fact, the kidney. Volume contraction after prolonged vomiting or nasogastric suction and consequent secondary hyperaldosteronism are primarily responsible for increased distal K^+ and H^+ losses. The metabolic alkalosis that accompanies significant vomiting causes an increase in both distal tubular cell K^+ concentration and distal delivery of HCO_3^-, a nonreabsorbable anion; these two factors, in addition to secondary hyperaldosteronism, stimulate urinary K^+ excretion.

Large Intestine Loss. Fecal excretion of K^+ usually amounts to between 5 and 15 mEq/day. Because gastrointestinal fluids (e.g., from stomach, ileum, cecum) contain approximately 10 mEq/L of K^+ and because colonic mucus is rich in K^+ (100 to 140 mEq/L) (319), diarrhea can induce significant K^+ loss. In cholera, daily stool losses may average 8 L of water, 1000 mEq of Na^+, and 130 mEq of K^+ (320). Comparable losses may occur in patients with *VIPoma syndrome*, a severe, watery diarrhea and histamine-fast achlorhydria that is usually but not always due to a vasoactive intestinal peptide–producing non–β-cell islet cell tumor (321). When volume contraction ensues, secondary hyperaldosteronism further stimulates renal and colonic K^+ secretion (322).

A similar picture may be seen early in the course of *congenital chloride diarrhea*, a rare autosomal recessive condition characterized by mutations in the downregulated adenoma gene (DRA) that codes for an intestinal Cl^--HCO_3^- exchanger in the terminal ileum and colon (323). Infants with the disorder have distended abdomens and absence of meconium, and fail to thrive. They develop metabolic alkalosis, dehydration, secondary hyperaldosteronism, and severe electrolyte disturbances, including hypochloremia, hyponatremia, and hypokalemia. Fecal Cl^- concentration always exceeds 90 mEq/L in patients with corrected electrolyte balance (324).

Severe diarrhea and dehydration (10 to 15%) in children can incur losses of between 7 and 14 mEq of K^+ per kilogram of body weight (325). Evaluation of such patients usually reveals a hyperchloremic metabolic acidosis, despite the secondary hyperaldosteronism, due to the marked bicarbonate and organic anion (potential alkali) losses in diarrheal fluid. The metabolic acidosis may induce K^+ to shift from the cells to the ECF, which thereby masks total body K^+ depletion.

Profound large intestine losses of K^+ are commonly observed in patients with villous adenomas of the colon and rectum (326). Ureterosigmoidostomies, surgical diversions performed to relieve chronic urinary tract obstruction, are typically associated with a hypokalemic hyperchloremic metabolic acidosis arising from colonic secretion of K^+ and HCO_3^- in exchange for Na^+ and Cl^-. This complication can be mitigated by implantation of the ureter into the ileum.

Those who habitually abuse laxatives frequently develop marked K^+ depletion (298). These patients, typically overly concerned with body image, may also abuse diuretics. With habitual use of either laxatives or diuretics, Na^+ depletion, volume contraction, secondary aldosteronism, and metabolic alkalosis may develop. Thus, these patients may present with a picture mimicking Bartter's syndrome. The habitual laxative abuser who has not recently taken diuretics usually shows a urinary Cl^- concentration below 25 mEq/L.

Excessive Integumental Losses

The concentration of K^+ in sweat is approximately 5 to 10 mEq/L (327). Vigorous exercise or heat stress usually results in a significant increase in the volume of sweat and its Na^+ concentration (though rarely exceeding 60 mEq/L), which leads to salt losses and volume contraction. The secondary hyperaldosteronism that ensues results in augmented K^+ secretion into both exocrine gland products (327) and urine, and thereby produces additional K^+ deficits. Excessive loss of sweat and its salts in patients with cystic fibrosis may lead to hypokalemia by similar mechanisms (328), with patients occasionally presenting with a picture resembling Bartter's syndrome.

Patients with full-thickness burns who develop volume contraction and consequent secondary hyperaldosteronism from massive integumental fluid losses often demonstrate an enhanced kaliuresis by 48 hours (298).

Clinical Manifestations of Hypokalemia

An acute fall in plasma K^+ concentration generally results in a more severe manifestation than does a chronic K^+ loss, which is often well tolerated.

Neuromuscular

Hypokalemia can induce skeletal muscle weakness and, in severe cases, paralysis (301). Excitable tissues require a specific transmembrane K^+ gradient for optimal function. Briefly, depolarization of excitable cells is characterized by the rapid entry of Na^+ ions and exit of K^+ ions. Repolarization of the membrane involves extrusion of the Na^+ ions in exchange for the lost K^+ ions. Hypokalemia results in a high intracellular to extracellular concentration ratio for K^+, which induces a state of electrical hyperpolarization and thereby slows nerve impulse conduction and muscle contraction. Neuromuscular dysfunction is most commonly manifest as skeletal muscle weakness. Usually the muscles of the lower extremities are affected first, followed by the quadriceps, then those of the trunk and upper extremities, and ultimately of respiration (271,301).

Potassium deficiency can also reduce skeletal muscle blood flow. During exercise and muscular contraction, muscle cells normally release K^+ to the interstitial fluid. The increasing concentration of interstitial K^+ is believed to act as a vasodilator (329). It has been suggested that severe K^+ depletion (plasma K^+ concentration lower than 2 mEq/L) leads to failure of the vasodilatory response to exercise, which results in muscle ischemia with subsequent muscle cramps, rhabdomyolysis, and myoglobinuria (330).

Hypokalemia-induced smooth muscle dysfunction is usually manifest as paralytic ileus with abdominal distention, anorexia, nausea, vomiting, and constipation. Impaired pressor responsiveness to angiotensin and catecholamines may lead to postural hypotension (331).

Cardiac

Hypokalemia contributes to cardiovascular morbidity and mortality by its effect on cardiac conduction and arterial blood pressure. The electrical disturbances of conduction and rhythm, manifest on the electrocardiogram as depression of the ST segment, diminished T-wave voltage, and appearance of U waves, are generally observed at plasma K^+ concentrations below 3 mEq/L (Fig. 8.10). Premature atrial and ventricular contractions and atrial arrhythmias may be seen. In patients who have congestive heart failure, cardiac ischemia, or left ventricular hypertrophy, or who are taking digoxin therapy, hypokalemia significantly increases the risk of cardiac arrhythmias (332).

A diet that is low in K^+, especially in the presence of high salt intake, has been implicated in the genesis of high blood pressure (333). The mechanism for hypokalemia-induced hypertension may relate to intravascular volume expansion as a result of renal Na^+ retention (334). The association between hypokalemia and hypertension is marked in African Americans, a population in whom a reduction in Na^+ intake and supplementation with K^+ may be particularly beneficial.

Metabolic

Potassium depletion interferes with both carbohydrate and protein metabolism. Potassium deficiency suppresses pancreatic insulin release, which results in increased glucose intolerance (335). However, a 10% reduction in body K^+ (corresponding roughly to a decrease in plasma K^+ concentration of 1 mEq/L) in healthy subjects results in only a mild impairment as measured by the glucose tolerance test, which

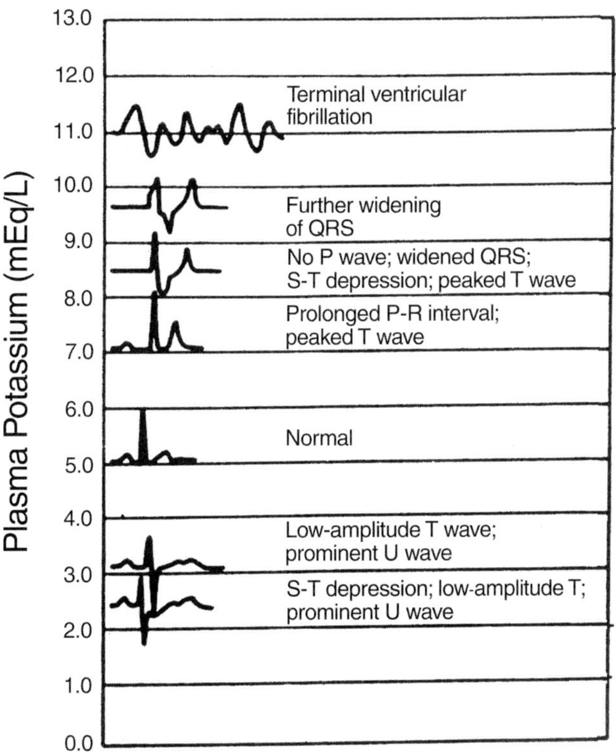

FIGURE 8.10. Relationship between plasma K^+ concentration and electrocardiographic changes. (From Winters RW. *The body fluids in pediatrics*. Boston: Little, Brown, 1973:134, with permission.)

suggests that more severe glucose intolerance in the presence of hypokalemia is associated with an underlying disorder, for example, subclinical diabetes. In diabetic patients hypokalemia impairs both insulin release and end-organ sensitivity to insulin, which aggravates the hyperglycemia.

Growth failure is commonly observed with chronic K^+ depletion (298). Although the mechanism is unclear, it may be due in part to a disturbance in protein metabolism. Because K^+ is the predominant intracellular cation, body K^+ depletion results in enhanced cellular uptake of other positively charged cations, specifically Na^+, H^+, and cationic amino acids (301). Thus, K^+ depletion results in an increase in the ratio of ECF volume to total body water volume, a decrease in the ratio of total body K^+ to body water, and a decrease in body noncollagen protein (8).

Renal

Potassium depletion, regardless of cause, produces a characteristic picture of structural and functional abnormalities in the kidney, known collectively as potassium-depletion nephropathy (301). One function that is preserved is the ability to conserve K^+ (336), mediated by decreased K^+ secretion as well as increased K^+ absorption via the H^+-K^+-ATPase in the collecting duct (111,124). A specific reversible vacuolar lesion of proximal tubular cells has been described in humans (336,337). Interstitial fibrosis, tubular atrophy, and cyst formation in the medulla also may be seen (338).

The most common renal functional abnormality associated with K^+ depletion is impaired urinary concentration, a deficit arising from a reduced osmolar gradient in the medullary interstitium (339). This concentrating defect is resistant to the administration of exogenous vasopressin and prolonged water deprivation (337). Hypokalemia inhibits activation of renal adenylate cyclase, which prevents vasopressin-stimulated urinary concentration in the inner medullary collecting duct. In addition to this direct tubular effect, K^+ depletion stimulates the central thirst center via increased production of angiotensin II (340). Enhanced proximal tubular Na^+ reabsorption (341) in the face of K^+ depletion leads to Na^+ retention, expansion of the ECF, and even frank edema (301).

Potassium depletion would be expected to result in increased net acid excretion because of enhanced cellular uptake of H^+ as a substitute for K^+; this leads to intracellular acidosis (and alkalemia) and stimulation of both H^+ secretion and renal ammonia production by renal tubular cells (342). Indeed, moderate K^+ depletion induced by restriction of dietary K^+ (substituting with Na^+ without changing dietary anion content) results in a mild systemic metabolic alkalosis unaccompanied by chloride depletion or hyperaldosteronism (343). The metabolic alkalosis is likely due to enhanced proximal reabsorption of HCO_3^-, mediated by an increase in the activity of the luminal Na^+-H^+ exchanger and basolateral Na^+-HCO_3^- co-transporter. This is manifest by an elevated plasma HCO_3^- concentration and is associated with the paradoxical excretion of an acid urine, possibly via the stimulation of H^+-K^+-ATPase isoforms.

Approach to the Patient with Hypokalemia

Diagnosis

The evaluation of a patient with hypokalemia should begin with taking a detailed history that includes the pattern of childhood growth, occurrence of chronic illness, family history of similar disease, use of medications and special diets, and symptoms associated with the present electrolyte disturbance. Physical examination must include measurement of growth indices and blood pressure and assessment of any evidence of edema and altered neuromuscular function.

The initial laboratory evaluation should include measurement of serum electrolytes and acid-base status and a complete blood count. These routine laboratory studies will identify whether or not the hypokalemia is due to K^+ uptake by abnormal leukocytes or is associated with the redistribution of K^+ from the extra- to the intracellular space. If the laboratory data do not support either of these two possibilities, the hypokalemia likely represents total body K^+ depletion due to K^+ losses via the gastrointestinal tract, skin, or kidney.

To evaluate these possibilities, a urine collection (preferably timed) on a controlled Na^+ and K^+ intake of 2 to 3 mEq/kg/day for each cation should be obtained to yield information on renal function and renal K^+ handling (urinary Na^+/K^+ ratio, absolute and fractional urinary K^+ excretion). A low urinary K^+ concentration (less than 15 mEq/L) in the absence of recent diuretic use implies near-maximal urinary K^+ conservation, which suggests that the K^+ deficit is secondary to extrarenal losses (gastrointestinal system, skin) or inadequate intake. The measurement of total body K^+ is not readily available to the clinician. Gastrointestinal K^+ losses occur from either vomiting, diarrhea, fistulas, nasogastric suction, or a villous adenoma. Laxative abuse should be considered in patients overly concerned with body image.

A child with a high rate of urinary K^+ excretion (greater than 15 mEq/L or exceeding intake by 0.5 to 1.0 mEq/kg/day, a fractional urinary K^+ excretion exceeding 30%, or a urinary Na^+/K^+ ratio consistently less than 1 in the absence of renal failure) has renal K^+ wasting. Inappropriate urinary K^+ wasting is often associated with hypertension and/or abnormalities of acid-base status. Hypokalemia associated with hypertension and metabolic alkalosis is classically found in hyperreninemic states, such as renal vascular stenosis, and primary hyperaldosteronism. The finding of hypokalemia and metabolic acidosis in a normotensive patient should suggest RTA or diabetic ketoacidosis. Bartter's and Gitelman's syndromes should be considered in patients with hypokalemic metabolic alkalosis, chronic salt wasting with volume depletion, and hyperreninemia and hyperaldosteronism.

TABLE 8.6. ORAL POTASSIUM PREPARATIONS

Potassium chloride (40 mEq K = 3 g KCl)			
Solution	10% (6.7 mEq/5 mL)		
	15% (10 mEq/5 mL)		
	20% (13.3 mEq/5 mL)		
Powder	15, 20, 25 mEq/packet		
Sustained-release tabs	6, 7, 8, 10, 20 mEq/tablet		
Sustained-release capsules	8, 10 mEq/capsule		
Potassium gluconate (40 mEq K = 9.4 g K gluconate)			
Elixir	20 mEq/15 mL		
Tablets	500 mg (2.15 mEq)		
	595 mg (2.56 mEq)		
Potassium citrate			
Liquid	Na^+	K^+	Citrate (HCO_3^-) each given as mEq/mL
Polycitra	1	1	2
Polycitra-K	0	2	2
Bicitra	1	0	1
Oracit	1	0	1
Extended-release tablets	5 mEq/tablet		Urocit-K (wax matrix)
	10 mEq/tablet		Urocit-K (wax matrix)

Data from Gunn VL, Nechyba C. *The Harriet Lane handbook: a manual for pediatric house officers*, 16th ed. Philadelphia: Mosby, 2002.

Therapy

The choice of K^+ replacement therapy depends primarily on the magnitude of the K^+ deficit. Treatment of the deficit, particularly in the presence of complicating factors that affect the transcellular distribution of K^+, must be performed cautiously, especially in patients with renal or cardiac disease.

Mild hypokalemia will often respond simply to dietary supplementation with foods having a high K^+ content (Table 8.5). Oral K^+ supplementation is necessary for moderate K^+ depletion (Table 8.6). Among the oral preparations available in liquid, powder, and slow-release preparations are potassium chloride, potassium citrate, and potassium gluconate. Potassium chloride is most commonly used; the citrate and gluconate formulations are ideal for patients with concomitant acidosis in whom the organic anion provides potential alkali. The adverse effects associated with oral therapy, especially after administration of KCl, include gastrointestinal irritation, ranging from vomiting to ulceration, and K^+ intoxication.

Intravenous K^+ supplementation therapy should be reserved for patients with severe hypokalemia, including those patients demonstrating neuromuscular or cardiac disturbances, those receiving amphotericin B, and diabetic patients in ketoacidosis. Administration of K^+ in dextrose-containing solutions may worsen the hypokalemia, because the sugar stimulates insulin secretion, which results in movement of K^+ into cells. Conventionally, parenteral K^+ should be infused in a solution containing no more than 40 mEq/L and infused at a rate not to exceed 0.5 to 1.0 mEq/kg of body weight per hour in children (298,344) or 10 to 20 mEq/hr in adults (334,345). When life-threatening paralysis or ventricular arrhythmias are present, or there are excessive ongoing losses such as with diabetic ketoacidosis, more aggressive K^+ replacement may be appropriate. Under these circumstances, adults have been shown to tolerate K^+ administered in concentrations of 40 to 100 mEq/L and infused at a rate not to exceed 40 mEq/hr, while serial electrocardiograms and frequent measurements of plasma K^+ concentration are monitored (334,346).

In patients with diuretic-induced hypokalemia who require continued use of their diuretic, addition of a potassium-sparing diuretic such as amiloride, triamterene, or spironolactone should be considered. Hypomagnesemia can lead to renal K^+ wasting and refractoriness to K^+ replacement. Magnesium repletion facilitates correction of the coexisting K^+ deficit.

Hyperkalemia

Hyperkalemia is defined as a serum K^+ concentration higher than 6.0 mEq/L in the newborn and 5.5 mEq/L in the older child and adult. Hyperkalemia is an uncommon finding in healthy subjects, because cellular and renal adaptations prevent significant accumulation of K^+ in the ECF. Because the kidney provides the primary means of eliminating excess K^+, hyperkalemia is frequently observed with major disturbances of renal excretory function. A classification of disorders associated with hyperkalemia is presented in Table 8.7.

Clinical Disorders Associated with Hyperkalemia

Pseudohyperkalemia

Pseudohyperkalemia represents an *in vitro* elevation of serum K^+ concentration in the absence of any clinical evidence of hyperkalemia and is attributable to K^+ movement out of cells during or after the drawing of the blood specimen. The serum K^+ concentration is normally up to 0.5 mEq/L higher than the plasma value due to release of K^+ by platelets and leukocytes during the *in vitro* clotting process. Potassium leakage by red blood cells, coincident with *in vitro* hemolysis, is readily demonstrable because of simultaneous release of hemoglobin into the plasma or serum. Hematologic disease associated with marked leukocytosis, thrombocytosis [especially with Kawasaki disease (347)], or familial disorders of erythrocyte membrane permeability (348,349) can lead to increases in serum, but not plasma, K^+ concentration. Inappropriate blood drawing can raise the apparent blood or plasma K^+ concentration by more than 2 mEq/L (350,351).

Transcellular Shift of K^+ from Cells to the Extracellular Fluid

Metabolic Acidosis. The relationship between acid-base balance and transcellular distribution of K^+ predicts that acute metabolic acidosis will often be accompanied by an increase in plasma K^+ concentration as excess protons enter the cell to be buffered intracellularly. Metabolic acidosis due to mineral acids such as hydrochloric acid or ammonium chloride is generally accompanied by an increase in plasma K^+ concentration of up to 1.5 mEq/L for every 0.1 unit reduction in arterial blood pH (53). In contrast, organic acids such as lactic acid, β-hydroxybutyric acid, and methylmalonic acid and respiratory acidosis usually provoke a lesser rise in the plasma K^+ concentration (352).

Hormones. Cellular uptake of K^+ is influenced by several hormones, including insulin, catecholamines, and mineralocorticoids. Impairment of hormonally mediated uptake processes may result in hyperkalemia. Thus, hyperkalemia may complicate insulin deficiency (353), exercise during treatment with beta-blockers such as propranolol and metoprolol (354), and hypoaldosteronism, either hyporeninemic or that which follows administration of angiotensin-converting enzyme (ACE) inhibitors (355) or angiotensin receptor antagonists.

Severe Exercise. Potassium is normally released from muscle cells during exercise (51), and this local release of K^+ plays a vasodilatory role to maintain enhanced blood flow to the exercising muscle (60,356). With more severe exercise and reduction of ATP levels in the cells, the ATP-dependent K^+ channels open, so that K^+ is released from muscle cells.

TABLE 8.7. CLINICAL DISORDERS ASSOCIATED WITH HYPERKALEMIA

- Pseudohyperkalemia
  - Hematologic disorders: leukocytosis, thrombocytosis, test tube hemolysis
  - Improper collection of blood
- Transcellular shift of K^+ from cells to the extracellular fluid
  - Metabolic acidosis
  - Impaired hormone activity
    - Insulin deficiency
    - Exercise (beta blockade)
  - Severe exercise
  - Hyperosmolality
  - Increased tissue catabolism
  - Drug effects
    - Succinylcholine
    - Digoxin (overdose)
    - β-adrenergic blockers and α-adrenergic agonists
    - Arginine hydrochloride
  - Familial hyperkalemic periodic paralysis
- Increased potassium load
  - Exogenous
    - Oral or parenteral potassium supplements
    - Salt substitutes
    - Potassium penicillin in high doses
    - Blood transfusion
    - Addition of KCl to parenteral fluid bags with poor mixing
  - Endogenous
    - Intravascular hemolysis
    - Rhabdomyolysis
    - Exercise
    - Infection
    - Trauma
    - Burns
    - Tumor lysis
    - Severe starvation
- Decreased renal excretory capacity
  - Renal failure
    - Acute
    - Chronic
    - Effective circulating volume depletion
  - Hypoaldosteronism
    - Hyporeninemia
    - Congenital adrenal enzymatic defects
      - 21-hydroxylase defects
      - Aldosterone synthase defects
      - Primary adrenal insufficiency
  - Impaired renal tubular secretion without abnormalities in mineralocorticoid production
    - Pseudohypoaldosteronism type I
    - Mutations in mineralocorticoid receptor (consider new pseudohypoaldosteronism type II)
    - Familial hyperkalemia with hypertension (originally pseudohypoaldosteronism type II)
      - Includes Spitzer-Weinstein and Gordon's syndromes
    - Acquired forms with normal mineralocorticoid production
      - Sickle cell disease
      - Renal transplantation
      - Systemic lupus erythematosus
      - Lead nephropathy
      - Papillary necrosis
      - Obstructive and reflux uropathy
    - Distal renal tubular acidosis (voltage-dependent defect)
  - Drug effects
    - Potassium-sparing diuretics
    - Prostaglandin synthesis inhibitors
    - Angiotensin-converting enzyme inhibitors
    - Miscellaneous (trimethoprim-sulfamethoxazole, pentamidine, heparin, cyclosporine A, tacrolimus)

Hyperosmolality. Hyperosmotic infusion of mannitol or saline, or acute hyperglycemia may lead to an acute increase in plasma K^+ concentration, as K^+ leaks from cells (63,65,67). With the rise in osmolality, there is a fluid shift from intracellular to extracellular space and a resulting increase in intracellular K^+ concentration. K^+ accompanies the fluid shift out of the cells via solvent drag. The higher cellular K^+ gradient stimulates K^+ efflux via K^+ channels in the membrane.

Increased Tissue Catabolism. When an increased rate of tissue breakdown occurs, large amounts of K^+ may be released into the ECF to cause hyperkalemia. Clinical examples of hypercatabolism include the use of cytotoxic drugs causing tumor lysis syndrome (61), extensive trauma (357), and massive hemolysis (358).

Drug Effects. Certain drugs alter the normal distribution of K^+ in the body. Depolarizing muscle relaxants used in general anesthesia such as *succinylcholine* cause release of K^+ from muscle during cellular depolarization (359). In healthy subjects the increment in plasma K^+ concentration is small, but in patients with neuromuscular disease, trauma, burns, tetanus, or renal insufficiency succinylcholine can induce an increase in plasma K^+ concentration of as much as 6 mEq/L (360–362). Patients who have taken an overdose of *digoxin*, a drug that inhibits cellular Na^+-K^+-ATPase so that intracellular K^+ leaks from cells, can also acutely develop marked hyperkalemia (363–365).

Nonspecific *β-adrenergic blockade* and *α-adrenergic stimulation* impair extrarenal disposal of K^+. Although beta-blockers normally produce only a small increment in plasma K^+ concentration, they should be used with caution in patients with renal insufficiency (366). Commonly used α-adrenergic agonists such as phenylephrine can also contribute to hyperkalemia. A relatively pure β_1-selective adrenergic blocker (metoprolol, atenolol) is safer in these settings (367).

Arginine hydrochloride may cause hyperkalemia as the cationic amino acid enters cells and displaces intracellular K^+ (368). Severe hyperkalemia has been reported in patients with renal and hepatic failure; patients in the latter group are unable to metabolize the arginine (352).

Hyperkalemic Periodic Paralysis. Hyperkalemic periodic paralysis is a rare familial disorder with autosomal dominant inheritance characterized by recurrent episodes of muscle weakness that occur in association with hyperkalemia (369). Episodes are precipitated by rest after strenuous exercise, exposure to cold or glucocorticoids, or ingestion of small amounts (0.5 to 1 mEq/kg) of exogenous K^+ (266), and are often aborted by carbohydrate feeding. Several characteristics of this disorder, aside from the association of hyperkalemia with the attacks, differ from those of the entity hypokalemic periodic paralysis. Attacks begin at a younger age (first or second decade of life) and are more frequent and of shorter duration (usually less than 2 hours) than those of the hypokalemic disorder.

The disease is associated with a point mutation of the gene encoding the α subunit of the voltage-gated Na^+ channel of human skeletal muscle (SkM1), which results in a single amino acid substitution of a highly conserved residue (369,370). The mutation leads to increased activity of the Na^+ channel (371) or disruption of fast inactivation of these channels after the action potential; this allows Na^+ entry into the cells, which depolarizes the membrane and favors K^+ diffusion out of the cells with the development of hyperkalemia.

Attacks can be aborted by treatment with β-adrenergic agonists such as albuterol, which drive K^+ back into cells (372). Other long-term treatment modalities include limiting exercise, consuming a low-K^+, high-carbohydrate diet, inducing mild K^+ depletion with a thiazide diuretic or mineralocorticoid, and adding a carbonic anhydrase inhibitor (373).

Increased K^+ Load

Exogenous K^+ Load. The healthy individual is easily able to tolerate an acute K^+ load due to both early cellular uptake, the predominant means of short-term disposal of K^+, and, later, renal excretion (22). However, oral K^+ loads exceeding 160 mEq in adults can cause fatal increases in plasma K^+ concentrations to above 8 mEq/L, even in patients with normal renal function (374). Severe hyperkalemia is more likely to occur with a rapid intravenous infusion or in infants, because of their small size (373). Infants, as well as adults, have become hyperkalemic after the administration of potassium penicillin in an intravenous bolus (1.7 mEq K^+ per 1 million U) (375,376) or after the use of stored blood (more than 5 days old) in exchange transfusions (377).

Most salt substitutes contain significant amounts of K^+ (10 to 13 mEq/g or 50 to 65 mEq per level teaspoon) (378) and can cause severe hyperkalemia in infants (379) or those who concurrently use ACE inhibitors. Many enteral nutrition products, including Boost and Ultracal (Mead Johnson), Ensure Plus (Nestle), Promote (Ross) and Scandishake (Scandipharm) contain K^+ in concentrations exceeding 40 mEq/L. Intravenous KCl preparations added to parenteral fluid bags without adequate mixing may layer out at the injection port, so that the initial solution administered to the patient has a markedly elevated K^+ concentration (380,381).

Endogenous K^+ Load. Massive cellular breakdown with endogenous K^+ release after intravascular coagulation, sickle cell hemolytic crisis, rhabdomyolysis, trama, burns, massive gastrointestinal bleeding, tumor lysis syndromes associated with chemotherapeutic destruction of lymphoproliferative malignancies (e.g., lymphoma), and, less frequently, solid tumors (e.g., neuroblastoma), as well as severe starvation, can rapidly induce hyperkalemia (62,353).

Decreased Renal Excretory Capacity

Potassium excretion is normally so efficient that even a massive long-term increase in K^+ intake will not produce hyperkalemia in healthy subjects (382). Thus, for hyperkalemia to persist, urinary K^+ excretory capacity must be reduced. Three major causes of reduced urinary K^+ excretion include renal failure, decreased effective circulating volume, and hypoaldosteronism.

Renal Failure. Hyperkalemia is a routine complication of acute renal failure. Not only does an acute decrease in glomerular filtration rate limit net urinary K^+ losses, but also the diminished urinary flow rate in the distal nephron, where K^+ secretion is flow dependent, markedly impairs further K^+ excretion (383,384). Hyperkalemia may develop in nonoliguric patients because of an acute increase in K^+ load requiring excretion, resulting from enhanced tissue breakdown, increased K^+ intake (see Table 8.5 for K^+ content of various foods), hypoaldosteronism, or therapeutic maneuvers such as blood transfusion. Although the rate at which endogenous hyperkalemia develops is variable, patients with uncomplicated abrupt cessation of renal function are expected to demonstrate a rise in plasma K^+ concentration at a rate of approximately 0.5 mEq/L/day (357,385).

In addition to decreased kaliuresis, K^+ uptake by cells is impaired in chronic renal failure (386,387). Cells have reduced K^+ concentrations in the basal state as well as after K^+ loading (22,388). Total body K^+ stores are normal or slightly reduced in stable chronic renal insufficiency (389–391). The reduction in K^+ content in leukocytes and muscle cells in uremic patients can be normalized by hemodialysis, which suggests that accumulation of a uremic toxin inhibits cellular Na^+-K^+-ATPase activity and results in impaired K^+ uptake into cells (392–394).

Plasma K^+ concentration in chronic renal failure may be maintained within normal limits by both renal and extrarenal adaptive mechanisms (170,395,396). Despite a marked decrease in glomerular filtration rate, renal adaptation provides for a rapid increase in K^+ excretion per surviving nephron to the extent that K^+ excretion may exceed filtered load in patients with a significant reduction in functional renal mass (101,170,391). However, the capacity of the surviving nephrons to excrete an additional acute K^+ load is generally impaired (391). Extrarenal adaptive mechanisms include increased excretion of K^+ by the colonic mucosa and increased cellular uptake due to high circulating levels of insulin and catecholamines. The finding of hyperkalemia in a stable patient with chronic renal failure suggests the presence of an increased excretory burden, possibly due to ingestion of K^+-rich foods and medications.

Acute renal failure is often accompanied by metabolic acidosis secondary to accumulation of organic acids, concomitant lactic acidosis, or ketoacidosis, factors that reduce cellular uptake of K^+ and exacerbate hyperkalemia (53,397). Although most patients with nonoliguric renal failure who maintain a reasonable urine output do not develop hyperkalemia, plasma K^+ concentrations exceeding 7 mEq/L have been observed in very-low-birth-weight neonates with nonoliguric renal failure (398). The hyperkalemia that develops in these infants, provided no exogenous K^+ source exists, likely reflects a shift of K^+ from the intracellular to the extracellular space during the transition from fetal to postnatal life, as well as a limited urinary K^+ excretory capacity (399).

Effective Circulating Volume Depletion. The ability to handle an acute K^+ load is diminished in hypovolemia, in which there is usually a low glomerular filtration rate and increased proximal Na^+ and fluid reabsorption; this results in decreased distal fluid delivery and impaired K^+ secretion, despite secondary hyperaldosteronism (86,400). Volume depletion from salt-losing nephropathy can also result in poor renal K^+ excretion and hyperkalemia (401).

Hypoaldosteronism. Mineralocorticoids stimulate K^+ secretion in both the colon and the kidney and so are of primary importance in maintaining K^+ homeostasis. Deficiencies in mineralocorticoid production or end-organ responsiveness can thus result in hyperkalemia. The most common causes are hyporeninemic hypoaldosteronism and the use of K^+-sparing diuretics in adults and adrenal enzyme deficiencies in children (298,373). In addition to hyperkalemia, varying degrees of Na^+ wasting and metabolic acidosis are present in hypoaldosteronism (because aldosterone normally stimulates Na^+ reabsorption and H^+ and K^+ secretion; see earlier). The metabolic acidosis is a type IV RTA.

Hyporeninemic hypoaldosteronism may account for more than half the cases of initially unexplained hyperkalemia in adults (402,403), after elimination of obvious causes. Most patients are adults who have a mild to moderate impairment of renal function that complicates diabetic glomerulosclerosis, or other chronic renal disease such as obstructive uropathy, sickle cell disease, tubulointerstitial nephritis, or even glomerulonephritis (298,404). Typically, the hyperkalemia and hyperchloremic metabolic acidosis found in these patients is disproportionate to the degree of renal insufficiency (353,402). A similar clinical picture has been observed in hyporeninemic children, who often have primary renal interstitial disease (405). Because angiotensin II and K^+ are the main physiologic stimuli to aldosterone secretion, hyporeninemia is clearly an important cause of the hyperkalemia. The mechanisms responsible may include a primary renal defect leading to decreased renin secretion, a primary adrenal defect in aldosterone biosynthesis or release, or a mixed disturbance (402,404).

Congenital adrenal enzymatic defects in mineralocorticoid production lead to depressed aldosterone synthesis. Whereas certain of these disorders are accompanied by an increased synthesis of other compounds with mineralocorticoid-like properties, such as DOC, other enzyme deficiencies may not allow production of alternate mineralocorticoid-like hormones. The most common of the latter disorders is *21-hydroxylase* deficiency, characterized by diminished mineralocorticoid and glucocorticoid production with consequent salt wasting, hyperkalemia, virilization, and failure to thrive (278, 406,407). Children with a defect in *aldosterone synthase* have isolated hypoaldosteronism (408–410). Infants affected by this rare autosomal recessive disorder have salt wasting, recurrent dehydration, hyperkalemia and failure to thrive (278,411).

Treatment varies with the type of enzyme deficiency. Mineralocorticoid replacement with fludrocortisone is sufficient in patients with isolated hypoaldosteronism, whereas those with 21-hydroxylase deficiency require replacement of both mineralocorticoid and glucocorticoid (as hydrocortisone or dexamethasone) (373).

In *primary adrenal insufficiency* there is diminished glucocorticoid as well as mineralocorticoid secretion, but the clinical picture is dominated by the complications of salt wasting, even though there may also be symptoms and signs of hyperkalemia (412). Severe hyperkalemia is more likely to occur in patients receiving inadequate mineralocorticoid replacement or in those with significant intravascular volume depletion and reduced glomerular filtration rate in whom low distal urinary flows further limit renal K^+ excretion (413).

Impaired Tubular Secretion without Abnormalities in Mineralocorticoid Production. *Pseudohypoaldosteronism type I* is an autosomal recessive disorder of end-organ resistance to aldosterone associated with renal salt wasting; elevated NaCl concentrations in sweat, stool, and saliva; hyperkalemia; and markedly elevated plasma renin activity and aldosterone concentrations (414,415). These findings resemble the aldosterone resistance caused by K^+-sparing diuretics, except that all aldosterone target organs are involved, including colon and sweat and salivary glands. The disorder is especially marked in the neonatal period, with vomiting, hyponatremia, failure to thrive, and occasionally respiratory distress syndrome. These infants do not respond to exogenous mineralocorticoids, but with vigorous salt replacement and control of hyperkalemia, they can survive. The severity of the disorder appears to lessen with maturation, and most patients ultimately outgrow the need for therapy (414–417). The defect appears to be a mutation in any one of the three ENaC subunits leading to a loss of function (418,419). Although many patients outgrow the need for therapy by age 4 years (298), the disorder has been reported in children as old as 7 years of age (420).

Low-birth-weight infants may demonstrate a similar transient disorder with salt wasting and hyperkalemia, abnormalities that usually resolve spontaneously by approximately 6 weeks of age (421,422). The underlying disorder appears to be a hyporesponsiveness of the immature distal tubule and cortical collecting duct to aldosterone (421). Unlike those with the ENaC mutations, these affected patients do not have pulmonary or other organ system involvement. In keeping with the hyporesponsiveness to aldosterone, studies have identified in affected patients and kindreds mutations in the mineralocorticoid receptor gene (MLR) (423).

Carbenoxolone, which inhibits 11β-HSD type II (the enzyme that converts cortisol to cortisone), can partially correct the apparent mineralocorticoid resistance in these patients (424). By slowing the conversion of cortisol to cortisone, carbenoxolone raises the intracellular cortisol concentration sufficiently to maintain high activation of the wild-type mineralocorticoid receptor and thus overcome the functional defect in the mutant receptor in this autosomal dominant disorder (284).

All index cases had presented with neonatal salt wasting with hyperkalemic acidosis despite high aldosterone levels, and all improved with age, so that none was symptomatic by 10 years of age. This mild disease contrasts with the more severe form of pseudohypoaldosteronism type I, which is mediated by mutations in ENaC genes, and might be considered as a new class of *pseudohypoaldosteronism type II* (284). A suggested nomenclature for these genetic disorders in which blood pressure and aldosterone secretion are inversely related is shown in Table 8.8. Similar improvement with age is seen in patients with congenital hypoaldosteronism due to aldosterone synthase deficiency, which probably reflects a reduced dependence on aldosterone action with increasing age (425). Therapy with Na^+ supplementation has been shown usually to correct the biochemical and clinical abnormalities, although plasma aldosterone levels remain elevated. High-dose fludrocortisone may be beneficial if a high-salt diet is ineffective or not tolerated (426).

Patients with sickle cell disease, renal transplants, systemic lupus erythematosus, lead nephropathy, papillary necrosis, or reflux or obstructive uropathy may present with a similar clinical picture that resembles hyporeninemic hypoaldosteronism but is characterized by normal levels of aldosterone in the plasma (435,437,438).

Familial hyperkalemia with hypertension (formerly pseudohypoaldosteronism type II) is manifest by a primary defect in renal distal nephron K^+ secretion. Rather

TABLE 8.8. SUGGESTED NOMENCLATURE FOR DISORDERS OF POTASSIUM HOMEOSTASIS IN WHICH BLOOD PRESSURE IS INVERSELY PROPORTIONAL TO ALDOSTERONE SECRETION

Descriptor	Inheritance	Mutations	Phenotype	OMIM
Pseudoaldosteronism				
PA1	AD	γ and β ENaC subunits	↑ BP, ↓ K, ↓ pH	177200
PA2	AD	S801L MR	↑ BP, ↓ K, ↓ pH	605115
Pseudohypoaldosteronism				
PHA1	AR	α, β, γ ENaC subunits	↑ K, ↑ pH, ↓ BP (neonatal)	264350
PHA2	AD	MR	↑ K, ↑ pH, ↓ BP (mild)	177735

↑, increased; ↓, decreased; AD, autosomal dominant; AR, autosomal recessive; BP, blood pressure; ENaC, epithelial sodium channel; K, plasma potassium concentration; MR, mineralocorticoid receptor; OMIM, Online Mendelian Inheritance in Man; PA, pseudoaldosteronism; pH, plasma pH; PHA, pseudohypoaldosteronism; S801L, serine to leucine mutation at position 801 of the MR.
From Warnock DG. Renal genetic disorders related to K^+ and Mg^{2+}. *Annu Rev Physiol* 2002;64:845, with permission.

than being volume depleted due to salt wasting, these patients present with hyperkalemia, volume expansion–mediated hypertension, normal glomerular filtration rate, low or low-normal plasma renin activity and aldosterone concentrations, metabolic acidosis, and short stature; all have normal dietary K^+ intake and Na^+ handling (Spitzer-Weinstein syndrome) (427–430). This syndrome is probably similar to Gordon's syndrome and the chloride shunt syndrome (431,432).

Despite the hyperkalemia, the fractional excretion of K^+ (2.8%) is an order of magnitude less than in controls studied similarly (427). Low-renin hypertension appears to become more severe with aging in this autosomal dominant disorder (433). The lack of Na^+ wasting and a normal antinatriuretic response to exogenous mineralocorticoids indicate that the underlying abnormality is not simply resistance to aldosterone. Enhanced NaCl reabsorption by the distal tubule leads to both volume expansion and decreased distal Na^+ and fluid delivery to the K^+-secreting cells of the cortical collecting duct, which thereby reduces K^+ secretion and causes hyperkalemia. Administration of a mineralocorticoid leads to an appropriate reduction in Na^+ excretion but does not appreciably affect that of K^+. On the other hand, urinary K^+ excretion increases dramatically after the infusion of Na^+ with a nonchloride anion, such as sulfate or bicarbonate (431).

Therapy consists of a high-Na^+, *low-K^+* diet and usually a thiazide diuretic; the latter suggests that the primary defect in this disorder may be increased activity of the thiazide-sensitive NaCl co-transporter in the luminal membrane of cells of the distal tubule and adjacent connecting segment (432,434,435).

Genetic studies of patients with this disorder (Online Mendelian Inheritance in Man No. 145260) have identified probable gain-of-function missense mutations in members of the WNK family of serine-threonine kinases that are expressed in the distal nephron (436). These kinases may serve to increase transcellular or paracellular Cl^- conductance in the collecting duct, thereby increasing salt reabsorption and intravascular volume, while concomitantly dissipating the electrical gradient and dissipating K^+ secretion. Another possibility is that the mutant kinases stimulate constitutive activity of the Na-Cl co-transporter in the cortical collecting duct or a marked increase in the activity of this transporter in the distal tubule (436).

Distal Renal Tubular Acidosis—Hyperkalemic Form. Hypokalemia is generally observed with distal RTA, in part because the decrease in H^+ secretion requires that Na^+ reabsorption occur in exchange for K^+ secretion. However, hyperkalemia may result when the underlying mechanism is a decrease in distal Na^+ reabsorption (439); this is the voltage-dependent defect. Hyperkalemic RTA most often occurs in patients with obstructive uropathy (440) and sickle cell disease (441). Unlike in hyporeninemic hypoaldosteronism, which is also observed in these disorders, in RTA the plasma aldosterone level is normal.

Drug Effects. Distal nephron K^+ secretion is inhibited by the *K^+-sparing diuretics*, which are used primarily to mitigate diuretic-induced K^+ depletion but are also administered to patients with cirrhosis. Spironolactone acts as a competitive inhibitor of aldosterone. Triamterene and amiloride diminish K^+ secretion independently of mineralocorticoids by directly closing the luminal Na^+ channel in cells of the distal nephron and thereby decreasing the negative luminal voltage. Severe hyperkalemia can develop in patients with compromised renal function and occasionally in patients with diabetes in whom cellular K^+ uptake is impaired in the absence of insulin (442).

Inhibitors of prostaglandin synthesis such as nonsteroidal antiinflammatory drugs also cause hyperkalemia. Inhibition of prostaglandin synthesis produces iatrogenic hyporeninemic hypoaldosteronism (443). Prostaglandins also inhibit NaCl reabsorption in the loop of Henle, thereby augmenting distal tubular delivery of Na^+.

ACE inhibitors such as captopril or enalapril increase plasma K^+ levels by blocking the conversion of angiotensin I to angiotensin II, the latter of which is a potent vasoconstrictor and stimulator of aldosterone release. Patients on long-term ACE inhibitor therapy do not routinely develop clinically significant hyperkalemia unless their course is complicated by renal or adrenal insufficiency, congestive heart failure with decreased renal perfusion, or administration of nonsteroidal antiinflammatory drugs.

Other drugs that are associated with hyperkalemia include trimethoprim-sulfamethoxazole, pentamidine, heparin, and calcineurin inhibitors (cyclosporin A, tacrolimus). High-dose trimethoprim therapy, commonly used for the treatment of *Pneumocystis carinii* infection, frequently causes a significant increase in plasma K^+ levels (by approximately 1 mEq/L). Like amiloride, trimethoprim and pentamidine cause hyperkalemia by blocking the luminal Na^+ channel, which decreases luminal electronegativity and thereby reduces K^+ secretion (444–446). Heparin reversibly suppresses adrenal aldosterone production and can thus be associated with a natriuresis and reduced urinary excretion of K^+ (447). Therefore, plasma K^+ concentration should be monitored in patients taking heparin for 3 or more days, particularly if these patients are at risk for development of hyperkalemia due to complicating renal insufficiency, diabetes, or use of other K^+-retaining drugs. Cyclosporine A (448) and tacrolimus (449), immunosuppressive drugs routinely used by transplant recipients, have been associated with hyperkalemia, even in patients with normal renal function and no evidence of transplant rejection.

Clinical Manifestations of Hyperkalemia

The clinical consequences of hyperkalemia are related to the adverse electrophysiologic effects of an altered transmembrane K^+ gradient on excitable tissues. Specifically, an increased extracellular K^+ concentration reduces the resting membrane potential, initially enhancing but ultimately suppressing tissue excitability ("depolarizing block").

Cardiac

Cardiac toxicity generally develops when the plasma K^+ concentration rises above 7 mEq/L, a concentration that should immediately signal the need for initiation of specific treatment for hyperkalemia (450,451). Regardless of the degree of hyperkalemia, however, treatment should be initiated in any patient with suspected hyperkalemia if electrocardiographic abnormalities characteristic of hyperkalemia are noted. It is important to remember that the extracellular K^+ concentration demonstrates at best a rough correlation with the onset and degree of cardiotoxicity. For example, adverse effects may be seen with a plasma K^+ concentration of less than 7 mEq/L if hyperkalemia has developed acutely or is accompanied by other metabolic derangements such as acidosis or hypocalcemia (373). The characteristic electrocardiographic changes accompanying hyperkalemia are depicted in Figure 8.10. The first and most specific abnormality seen is development of tall, peaked T waves, which usually become apparent with plasma K^+ levels above 6 mEq/L. The PR interval lengthens and the QRS complex then widens. At K^+ concentrations above 8 mEq/L, the P-wave amplitude decreases and may in fact disappear with atrial standstill. As ventricular conduction time continues to lengthen, the QRS complex merges with the peaked T wave, producing a "sine-wave" pattern. Finally, ventricular fibrillation or asystole may occur with K^+ levels above 10 mEq/L.

Neuromuscular

Hyperkalemia is clinically associated with changes in neuromuscular conduction. Persistent depolarization inactivates Na^+ channels in the cell membrane, thereby producing a net decrease in membrane excitability (373). This is manifested clinically by skeletal muscle weakness, paresthesias, and ascending flaccid paralysis. Such muscle weakness does not usually develop until the plasma K^+ concentration exceeds 8 mEq/L (452). Generally, the trunk and head muscles as well as muscles of respiration are spared.

Approach to the Patient with Hyperkalemia

Diagnosis

The diagnostic workup of a patient with hyperkalemia should begin with a complete history taking similar to that described earlier for hypokalemia. The physical examination must include measurement of growth indices and blood pressure, assessment of volume status, and evaluation for signs of chronic illness.

An electrocardiogram must be obtained promptly for any patient with hyperkalemia. Because renal failure is a common cause of hyperkalemia, additional laboratory evaluation should include a repeat set of plasma, not serum, electrolyte levels including glucose, calcium, blood urea nitrogen, and creatinine. Note that sequential measurements of plasma K^+ concentrations are expected to vary little from day to day. Increased K^+ load due to increased tissue breakdown can be assessed from the complete blood count and levels of uric acid, lactate dehydrogenase, and creatine phosphokinase enzymes. Renal function can be further assessed with a urinalysis. An abnormal urinary specific gravity or pH may suggest a renal tubular defect, such as obstructive uropathy or RTA, whereas the presence of casts or large amounts of protein or red blood cells is consistent with glomerular disease. Information regarding renal K^+ conservation can be obtained from a timed collection on a constant Na^+ and K^+ intake (2 to 3 mEq/kg/day), which will allow the calculation of creatinine clearance, absolute K^+ excretion

TABLE 8.9. PHARMACOLOGIC TREATMENT OF ACUTE HYPERKALEMIA[a]

Mechanism of action	Drug	Dosage	Route of administration	Onset of action	Duration of action
Antagonism	Calcium gluconate (10%)	100 mg/kg/dose (= 1 mL/kg/dose)	i.v. over 3–5 min	1–3 min	30 min
Redistribution	Glucose (25%) (insulin)	0.5 g/kg (= 2 mL/kg) (regular insulin, 0.1 U/kg)	i.v. over 15–30 min	30 min	2–4 h
	Albuterol (0.5%)	0.1–0.3 mg/kg for <12 yr 2.5–5.0 mg for >12 yr	Nebulized over 10 min	Within 30 min	4–6 h
	Sodium bicarbonate	1–2 mEq/kg	i.v. over 5–10 min	10–30 min	2 h
Removal	Furosemide	1–2 mg/kg	i.v. or i.m.	15–30 min	4–6 h
	Sodium polystyrene sulfonate resin	0.5–1.0 g/kg	Orally or rectally	60–120 min	4–6 h

[a]In the setting of acute or chronic renal failure or failure to remove adequate amount of potassium, dialytic removal may be necessary.

rate, fractional excretion of K^+, urinary Na^+/K^+ ratio, and transtubular K^+ gradient (TTKG) (see later).

Hyperkalemia is frequently due to a condition that causes impairment of urinary K^+ excretion. The most common conditions are advanced renal failure, severely reduced effective volume depletion, and hypoaldosteronism (because aldosterone is the primary hormone mediating urinary K^+ excretion). If renal function is normal or only modestly impaired and no other causes are obvious, the patient should be evaluated for hypoaldosteronism. In infants and children, enzyme deficiencies and type I pseudohypoaldosteronism are most common. Salt wasting may be very severe in infants with hypoaldosteronism, who typically present with volume depletion, hyperkalemia, hyponatremia, metabolic acidosis, and an elevated urinary Na^+ concentration. Ultimately, measurement of morning plasma renin activity and aldosterone and cortisol levels should be performed. The patient should be given 0.5 to 1 mg/kg of furosemide the night before the blood specimens are obtained. This regimen enhances aldosterone secretion (via stimulation of renin) in healthy subjects, but not in patients with hypoaldosteronism (402).

In addition to measuring plasma aldosterone level, one can estimate the degree of aldosterone activity by measuring the tubular fluid K^+ concentration at the end of the cortical collecting duct. In humans, this determination can be estimated clinically from the calculation of the TTKG, on the assumption that (a) urine osmolality at the end of the cortical collecting duct is comparable to that in plasma and (b) little or no K^+ is transported in the medullary collecting duct. The calculation is relatively accurate as long as the urine is not dilute and urine $[Na^+]$ is above 25 mEq/L (453,454). Thus,

$$\text{TTKG} = \{\text{urine } [K^+]/(\text{urine osmolality}/\text{plasma osmolality})\}/\text{plasma } [K^+]$$

Normally, TTKG is 8 to 9 on a regular diet and rises to above 11 with a K^+ load, which indicates increased K^+ secretion by the cortical collecting duct (454). Hypokalemia with a TTKG higher than 4 suggests renal K^+ loss due to increased distal K^+ secretion. A value below 7, and particularly below 5, in a hyperkalemic patient is highly suggestive of hypoaldosteronism. Limited urine flow (and distal Na^+ delivery), rather than a limitation in the secretion of K^+, may be seen in advanced congestive heart failure resulting in insufficient urinary K^+ excretion.

The TTKG is normally higher in infants (median 7.8) than in children (median 6.3) and correlates directly with the fractional excretion of K^+ and urine K^+/Na^+ ratios (455). In patients with hypoaldosteronism and pseudohypoaldosteronism, TTKG values varied between 1.6 and 4.1, and all were below the third percentile established for the age of the subject (455). The TTKG level is lower in preterm neonates than in term infants (456), which probably reflects the immaturity of renal tubular K^+ secretion or hyporesponsiveness to aldosterone.

Therapy

The presence of severe hyperkalemia (plasma K^+ concentration above 8 mEq/L) with electrocardiographic abnormalities or severe muscle weakness is a potentially life-threatening event that requires immediate therapeutic intervention with almost all of the measures listed in Table 8.9. Such treatment can prevent fatal cardiac arrhythmias. Treatment measures used in this medical emergency can be divided into three general categories: (a) those that rapidly antagonize the membrane effects of hyperkalemia, (b) those that rapidly enhance the transfer of extracellular K^+ into cells, and (c) those that remove K^+ from the body. Because the onset and duration of action of each of these maneuvers differ, and because the first two measures are only temporizing, several treatment methods, including at least one for inducing K^+ removal from the body, should be instituted simultaneously for symptomatic hyperkalemia (373). For asymptomatic hyperkalemia, treatment can be solely with a cation exchange resin, because rapid therapy is not necessary.

The effect of hyperkalemia on the cardiac cell membrane can be rapidly reversed with calcium. A rise in ionized calcium makes less negative the threshold potential at which excitation occurs and thereby mitigates the depolarizing blockade resulting from hyperkalemia. Calcium gluconate (10%) is the preparation most often used; it is infused slowly intravenously with continuous electrocardiographic monitoring. The duration of action is transient, and cardiotoxicity will reappear once the infused calcium is sequestered in bone or is excreted.

Somewhat more long-lasting effects (several hours) can be obtained by transferring extracellular K^+ into cells and thereby reestablishing a more physiologic transmembrane potential gradient. This can be well accomplished by inducing endogenous insulin release through infusion of glucose. It has been customary to give insulin as well, although this may not be necessary in the absence of diabetes. The dose of glucose with or without insulin may be repeated as needed, with monitoring for the complications of hyperglycemia or hypoglycemia.

Administration via nebulizer of β_2-agonists (albuterol, salbutamol), which promote K^+ uptake by cells, has been widely used in adults for the treatment of hyperkalemia in chronic renal failure (457) and has been shown to be safe and efficacious in children as well (458). A single dose of nebulized albuterol can lower plasma K^+ concentration by as much as 0.5 mEq/L (457,458); the more potent parenteral preparation is not available in the United States. Transient side effects associated with this class of drug include elevation of heart rate, tremor, and mild vasomotor flushing.

Although alkalinization of the ECF with sodium bicarbonate to promote the rapid cellular uptake of K^+ was formerly recommended as a mainstay of therapy, it is no longer considered to be useful. However, this maneuver remains valuable if metabolic acidosis is at all responsible for the hyperkalemia.

The treatment options discussed thus far are only temporizing. To remove K^+ from the body, renal K^+ excretion must be enhanced, for example, by stimulating flow-dependent K^+ secretion in the distal nephron through administration of loop or thiazide diuretics, a response that requires the presence of good renal function. Diuretics are useful in chronic hyperkalemia due to hypoaldosteronism, heart failure, or a selective K^+ secretory defect (373).

In patients with renal insufficiency, a cation exchange resin may be administered to promote gastrointestinal elimination. Sodium polystyrene sulfonate (Kayexalate) is the resin used most commonly. Within the intestinal lumen the resin binds 1 mEq of K^+ in exchange for 1 mEq of Na^+; 1 g/kg of resin is expected to reduce plasma K^+ concentration by 1 mEq/L. When given orally, each gram of resin is suspended in 3 to 4 mL water and mixed with 70% sorbitol or a 10% aqueous dextrose solution to reduce constipation. The resin is most often provided as a retention enema in sorbitol, to be retained for at least 15 to 30 minutes. Because the efficacy of K^+ removal by the resin is variable and the cation exchange is not entirely specific for K^+, plasma concentrations of K^+, Ca^{2+}, and Mg^{2+} as well as the electrocardiogram must be monitored frequently. Administration can be repeated at least six times in 24 hours.

Addition of sodium polystyrene sulfonate directly to infant formulas and nutritional supplements (1 g/mEq K^+ in the formula) effectively lowers the K^+ content by approximately 50% (459). However, caution should be exercised in routinely prescribing this mode of therapy, because pretreatment of the formulas is associated with a 200% increase in Na^+ concentration, a problem that may be avoided by using calcium polystyrene sulfonate (459). Failure of the resin to control hyperkalemia should prompt the clinician to evaluate whether K^+ is being continuously delivered to the ECF, possibly from extensive ongoing tissue damage or continued absorption of K^+-containing gastrointestinal contents.

If the amount of K^+ to be removed is of such magnitude that the administration of cation exchange resins does not suffice, dialysis may be necessary. Hemodialysis can remove up to 1 mEq/kg of body weight per hour in children and adults (460). Plasma K^+ concentration can be lowered by using a low dialysate K^+ concentration. Dialysis against a low-K^+ bath must be performed cautiously, however, because rapid fluctuations in plasma K^+ concentration can induce cardiac rhythm disturbances (461). One approach that is especially useful if frequent measurements of plasma K^+ concentration are not possible is to lower the K^+ concentration of the dialysate in gradual decrements over the course of the dialysis treatment (461). Continuous venovenous hemofiltration is also effective in removing total body K^+ from hemodynamically compromised patients. Peritoneal dialysis is less efficient in removing K^+ (462).

Patients with disease characterized by chronic hyperkalemia, such as chronic renal insufficiency (glomerular filtration rate less than 10% of normal), require indefinite dietary K^+ restriction and frequent monitoring of the plasma K^+ concentration. Because patients differ in their dietary intake, extrarenal handling of K^+, and rates of glomerular filtration and urinary flow, the regimen for K^+ restriction must be tailored to the individual. Occasionally, these patients require the use of supplemental oral cation exchange resins (0.1 g/kg three times a day) to maintain normokalemia.

Children with hypoaldosteronism often respond to the oral mineralocorticoid fludrocortisone acetate (0.1 to 1 mg/day). Fludrocortisone may exacerbate preexisting hypertension or edema, however, so that better control of the hyperkalemia is achieved using a low-K^+ diet and a loop or thiazide-type diuretic. Persistent hyperkalemia associated with K^+ secretory abnormalities in the absence of diminished renal function or hypoaldosteronism often improves with a thiazide diuretic.

ACKNOWLEDGMENTS

The studies in the author's laboratory have been supported by National Institutes of Health grants HD13232 and DK50603 and grants-in-aid from the New York Heart Association and American Heart Association. The author was an Established Investigator of the American Heart Association (1984–1989). Thanks to Ms. W. Lepsch for assistance in preparing the manuscript.

REFERENCES

1. Stanton BA, Giebisch GH. Renal potassium transport. In: Windhager EE, ed. *Handbook of physiology*. New York: Oxford University Press, 1992:813–874.
2. Doucet A. Function and control of Na-K-ATPase in single nephron segments of the mammalian kidney. *Kidney Int* 1988; 34:749–760.
3. Clausen T, Everts ME. Regulation of the Na,K-pump in skeletal muscle. *Kidney Int* 1989;35:1–13.
4. Katz AI. Renal Na-K-ATPase: its role in tubular sodium and potassium transport. *Am J Physiol* 1982;242:F207–F219.
5. Edelman IS, Leibman J. Anatomy of body water and electrolytes. *Am J Med* 1959;27:256–277.
6. Pierson RN Jr, Lin DHY, Phillips RA. Total-body potassium in health: effects of age, sex, height, and fat. *Am J Physiol* 1974;226:206–212.
7. Giebisch G, Malnic G, Berliner RW. Control of renal potassium excretion. In: Brenner BM, Rector FC Jr, eds. *The kidney*. Philadelphia: WB Saunders, 1996:371–407.
8. Forbes GB. *Human body composition. Growth, aging, nutrition, and activity*. New York: Springer-Verlag, 1987.
9. Flynn MA, Woodruff C, Clark J, et al. Total body potassium in normal children. *Pediatr Res* 1972;6:239–245.
10. Flynn MA, Clark J, Reid JC, et al. A longitudinal study of total body potassium in normal children. *Pediatr Res* 1975; 9:834–836.
11. Rutledge MM, Clark J, Woodruff C, et al. A longitudinal study of total body potassium in normal breastfed and bottle-fed infants. *Pediatr Res* 1976;10:114–117.
12. Schwartz WB. Potassium and the kidney. *N Engl J Med* 1955;253:601–608.
13. Kurtzman NA, Gonzalez J, DeFronzo R, et al. A patient with hyperkalemia and metabolic acidosis. *Am J Kid Dis* 1990;15:333–356.
14. Sulyok E, Nemeth M, Tenyi I, et al. Relationship between maturity, electrolyte balance and the function of the renin-angiotensin-aldosterone system in newborn infants. *Biol Neonate* 1979;35:60–65.
15. Winters RW, Heird WC. Special problems of the pediatric surgical patient. In: Winters RW, ed. *The body fluids in pediatrics. Medical, surgical, and neonatal disorders of acid-base status, hydration, and oxygenation*. Boston: Little, Brown, 1973:612–640.
16. Satlin LM, Schwartz GJ. Metabolism of potassium. In: Ichikawa I, ed. *Pediatric textbook of fluids and electrolytes*. Baltimore: Williams & Wilkins, 1990:89–98.
17. Winters RW. Maintenance fluid therapy. In: Winters RW, ed. *The body fluids in pediatrics. Medical, surgical, and neonatal disorders of acid-base status, hydration, and oxygenation*. Boston: Little, Brown, 1973:113–133.
18. Wilde WS. Potassium. In: Comar CL, Bronner F, eds. *Mineral metabolism*. New York: Academic Press, 1962:73–107.
19. Dickerson JWT, Widdowson EM. Chemical changes in skeletal muscle during development. *Biochem J* 1960;74: 247–257.
20. Vernadakis A, Woodbury DM. Electrolyte and nitrogen changes in skeletal muscle of developing rats. *Am J Physiol* 1964;206:1365–1368.
21. Satlin LM, Evan AP, Gattone VHI, et al. Postnatal maturation of the rabbit cortical collecting duct. *Pediatr Nephrol* 1988;2:135–145.
22. Bia MJ, DeFronzo RA. Extrarenal potassium homeostasis. *Am J Physiol* 1981;240:F257–F268.
23. Rosa RM, Silva P, Young JB, et al. Adrenergic modulation of extrarenal potassium disposal. *N Engl J Med* 1980;302:431–434.
24. DeFronzo RA, Sherwin RS, Dillingham M, et al. Influence of basal insulin and glucagon secretion on potassium and sodium metabolism. Studies with somatostatin in normal dogs and in normal and diabetic human beings. *J Clin Invest* 1978;61:472–479.
25. DeFronzo RA, Lee R, Jones A, et al. Effect of insulinopenia and adrenal hormone deficiency on acute potassium tolerance. *Kidney Int* 1980;17:586–594.
26. Rose BD. *Clinical physiology of acid-base and electrolyte disorders*. New York: McGraw-Hill, 1994:346–376.
27. Winkler AW, Hoff HE, Smith PK. The toxicity of orally administered potassium salts in renal insufficiency. *J Clin Invest* 1941;20:119–126.
28. Sigstrom L, Waldenstrom J, Karlberg P. Characteristics of active sodium and potassium transport in erythrocytes of healthy infants and children. *Acta Paediatr Scand* 1981;70: 347–352.
29. Whaun JM, Oski FA. Red cell stromal adenosine triphosphatase (ATPase) of newborn infants. *Pediatr Res* 1969;3: 105–112.
30. Schwartz GJ, Evan P. Development of solute transport in rabbit proximal tubule. III. Na-K-ATPase activity. *Am J Physiol* 1984;246:F845–F852.
31. Davis PW, Dixon RL. Selective postnatal development of Na,K-activated-adenosinetriphosphatase in rabbit kidneys. *Proc Soc Exp Biol Med* 1971;136:95–97.
32. Schmidt U, Horster M. Na-K-activated ATPase: activity maturation in rabbit nephron segments dissected in vitro. *Am J Physiol* 1977;233:F55–F60.
33. Mitchell W, Kim CS, O'Tuama LA, et al. Choroid plexus, brain and kidney Na^+,K^+-ATPase: comparative activities in fetal, newborn and young adult rabbits. *Neurosci Lett* 1982; 31:37–40.
34. Marin L, Aperia A. Colonic water and electrolyte transport in young and adult rats. *J Pediatr Gastroenterol Nutr* 1984;3: 471–474.
35. Ewart HS, Klip A. Hormonal regulation of the Na(+)-K(+)-ATPase: mechanisms underlying rapid and sustained changes in pump activity. *Am J Physiol* 1995;269:C295–C311.

36. Therien AG, Blostein R. Mechanisms of sodium pump regulation. *Am J Physiol* 2000;279:C541–C566.
37. Clausen T, Flatman JA. Effects of insulin and epinephrine on Na+-K+ and glucose transport in soleus muscle. *Am J Physiol* 1987;252:E492–E499.
38. Lytton J, Lin JC, Guidotti G. Identification of two molecular forms of (Na^+,K^+)-ATPase in rat adipocytes. Relation to insulin stimulation of the enzyme. *J Biol Chem* 1985;260: 1177–1184.
39. Pettit GW, Vick RL. Contribution of pancreatic insulin to extrarenal potassium homeostasis: a two-compartment model. *Am J Physiol* 1974;226:319–324.
40. DeFronzo RA, Felig P, Ferrannini E, et al. Effect of graded doses of insulin on splanchnic and peripheral potassium metabolism in man. *Am J Physiol* 1980;238: E421–E427.
41. Santeusanio F, Faloona GR, Knochel JP, et al. Evidence for a role of endogenous insulin and glucagon in the regulation of potassium homeostasis. *J Lab Clin Med* 1973;81:809–817.
42. Dluhy RG, Alexrod L, Williams GH. Serum immunoreactive insulin and growth hormone response to potassium infusion in normal man. *J Appl Physiol* 1972;33: 22–26.
43. DeFronzo RA, Bia M, Birkhead G. Epinephrine and potassium homeostasis. *Kidney Int* 1981;20:83–91.
44. Carlsson E, Fellenius E, Lundborg P, et al. β-adrenoceptor blockers, plasma-potassium, and exercise [Letter]. *Lancet* 1978;2:424–425.
45. Williams ME, Gervino EV, Rosa RM, et al. Catecholamine modulation of rapid potassium shifts during exercise. *N Engl J Med* 1985;312:823–827.
46. Young DB, Smith MJ Jr, Jackson TE, et al. Multiplicative interaction between angiotensin II and K concentration in stimulation of aldosterone. *Am J Physiol* 1984;247:E328–E335.
47. Himathongkam T, Dluhy RH, Williams GH. Potassium–aldosterone–renin interrelationships. *J Clin Endocrinol Metab* 1975;41:153–159.
48. Funder JW, Blair-West JR, Coghlan JP, et al. Effect of plasma $[K^+]$ on the secretion of aldosterone. *Endocrinology* 1969;85:381–384.
49. Bia MJ, Tyler KA, DeFronzo RA. Regulation of extrarenal potassium homeostasis by adrenal hormones in rats. *Am J Physiol* 1982;242:F641–F644.
50. Laragh JH, Capeci NE. Effect of administration of potassium chloride on serum sodium and potassium concentration. *Am J Physiol* 1955;180:539–544.
51. Sterns RH, Cox M, Feig PU, et al. Internal potassium balance and the control of the plasma potassium concentration. *Medicine* 1981;60:339–354.
52. Adler S, Fraley DS. Potassium and intracellular pH. *Kidney Int* 1977;11:433–442.
53. Adrogue HJ, Madias NE. Changes in plasma potassium concentration during acute acid-base disturbances. *Am J Med* 1981;71:456–467.
54. Oster JR, Perez GO, Vaamonde CA. Relationship between blood pH and potassium and phosphorus during acute metabolic acidosis. *Am J Physiol* 1978;235: F345–F351.
55. Fulop M. Serum potassium in lactic acidosis and ketoacidosis. *N Engl J Med* 1979;300:1087–1089.
56. Pitts RF. *Physiology of the kidney and body fluids*. Chicago: Year Book, 1974:178–241.
57. Fraley DS, Adler S. Correction of hyperkalemia by bicarbonate despite constant blood pH. *Kidney Int* 1977;12: 354–360.
58. Rose BD, Post TW. Potassium homeostasis. In: Wonsiewicz M, McCullough K, Davis K, eds. Clinical physiology of acid-base and electrolyte disorders. New York: McGraw-Hill, 2001:372–402.
59. Wasserman K, Stringer WW, Casaburi R, et al. Mechanism of the exercise hyperkalemia: an alternate hypothesis. *J Appl Physiol* 1997;83:631–643.
60. Daut J, Maier-Rudolph W, von Beckerath N, et al. Hypoxic dilation of coronary arteries is mediated by ATP-sensitive potassium channels. *Science* 1990;247: 1341–1344.
61. Arseneau JC, Bagley CM, Anderson T, et al. Hyperkalaemia, a sequel to chemotherapy of Burkitt's lymphoma. *Lancet* 1973;1:10–4.
62. Jones DP, Mahmoud H, Chesney RW. Tumor lysis syndrome: pathogenesis and management. *Pediatr Nephrol* 1995;9:206–212.
63. Conte G, Dal Canton A, Imperatore P, et al. Acute increase in plasma osmolality as a cause of hyperkalemia in patients with renal failure. *Kidney Int* 1990;38:301–307.
64. Viberti GC. Glucose-induced hyperkalaemia: a hazard for diabetics? *Lancet* 1978;1:690–691.
65. Moreno M, Murphy C, Goldsmith C. Increase in serum potassium resulting from the administration of hypertonic mannitol and other solutions. *J Lab Clin Med* 1969;73: 291–298.
66. Makoff DL, Da Silva JA, Rosenbaum BJ. On the mechanism of hyperkalaemia due to hyperosmotic expansion with saline or mannitol. *Clin Sci* 1971;41:383–393.
67. Makoff DL, Da Silva JA, Rosenbaum BJ, et al. Hypertonic expansion: acid-base and electrolyte changes. *Am J Physiol* 1970;218:1201–1207.
68. Rabinowitz L, Sarason RL, Yamauchi H, et al. Time course of adaptation to altered K intake in rats and sheep. *Am J Physiol* 1984;247:F607–F617.
69. Squires RD, Huth EJ. Experimental potassium depletion in normal human subjects. I. Relation of ionic intakes to the renal conservation of potassium. *J Clin Invest* 1959;38: 1134–1148.
70. Pak CYC, Ohata M, Lawrence EC, et al. The hypercalciurias: causes, parathyroid functions, and diagnostic criteria. *J Clin Invest* 1974;54:387–400.
71. Womersley RA, Darragh JH. Potassium and sodium restriction in the normal human. *J Clin Invest* 1955;34: 456–461.
72. Dyer AR, Martin GJ, Burton WN, et al. Blood pressure and diurnal variation in sodium, potassium, and water excretion. *J Hum Hypertens* 1998;12:363–371.
73. Rabinowitz L. Aldosterone and potassium homeostasis. *Kidney Int* 1996;49:1738–1742.
74. Rabinowitz L, Aizman RI. Circadian variation in the natriuresis produced by potassium intake in the rat. *Clin Exp Hypertens* 1997;19:1193–1203.

75. Vurgun N, Yiditodlu MR, Ypcan A, et al. Hypernatriuria and kaliuresis in enuretic children and the diurnal variation. *J Urol* 1998;159:1333–1337.
76. Widdowson EM, McCance RA. The effect of development on the composition of the serum and extracellular fluids. *Clin Sci* 1956;15:361–365.
77. Rodriguez-Soriano J, Vallo A, Castillo G, et al. Renal handling of water and sodium in infancy and childhood: a study using clearance methods during hypotonic saline diuresis. *Kidney Int* 1981;20:700–704.
78. Narins RG, Jones ER, Stom MC, et al. Diagnostic strategies in disorders of fluid, electrolyte and acid-base homeostasis. *Am J Med* 1982;72:496–520.
79. Tudvad F, McNamara H, Barnett HL. Renal response of premature infants to administration of bicarbonate and potassium. *Pediatrics* 1954;13:4–16.
80. Lorenz JM, Kleinman LI, Disney TA. Renal response of newborn dog to potassium loading. *Am J Physiol* 1986;251:F513–F519.
81. Kersten L, Mohr C, Braunlich H. Der mechanismus der renalen ausscheidung von natrium und kalium und seine altersabhangige entwicklung bei ratten vom 5. bis 240. lebenstag. *Acta Biol Med Ger* 1971;27:327–340.
82. McCance RA, Widdowson EM. The response of the newborn piglet to an excess of potassium. *J Physiol* 1958;141:88–96.
83. Phillips SF. Absorption and secretion by the colon. *Gastroenterology* 1969;56:966–971.
84. Turnberg LA. Electrolyte absorption from the colon. *Gut* 1970;11:1049–1054.
85. Giebisch G. Renal potassium transport: mechanisms and regulation. *Am J Physiol* 1998;274:F817–F833.
86. Malnic G, Klose RM, Giebisch G. Micropuncture study of distal tubular potassium and sodium transport in rat nephron. *Am J Physiol* 1966;211:529–547.
87. Kaufman JS, Hamburger RJ. Passive potassium transport in the proximal convoluted tubule. *Am J Physiol* 1985;248:F228–F232.
88. Lelievre-Pegorier M, Merlet-Benichou C, Roinel N, et al. Developmental pattern of water and electrolyte transport in rat superficial nephrons. *Am J Physiol* 1983;245:F15–F21.
89. Solomon S. Absolute rates of sodium and potassium reabsorption by proximal tubule of immature rats. *Biol Neonate* 1974;25:340–351.
90. Dlouha H. A micropuncture study of the development of renal function in the young rat. *Biol Neonate* 1976;29:117–128.
91. Solomon S. Maximal gradients of Na and K across proximal tubules of kidneys of immature rats. *Biol Neonate* 1974;25:327–339.
92. Boim MA, Ho K, Shuck ME, et al. ROMK inwardly rectifying ATP-sensitive K^+ channel. II. Cloning and distribution of alternative forms. *Am J Physiol* 1995;268:F1132–F1140.
93. Lee W-S, Hebert SC. ROMK inwardly rectifying ATP-sensitive K^+ channel. I. Expression in rat distal nephron segments. *Am J Physiol* 1995;268:F1124–F1131.
94. Hebert SC. An ATP-regulated, inwardly rectifying potassium channel from rat kidney (ROMK). *Kidney Int* 1995;48:1010–1016.
95. Simon DB, Karet FE, Rodriguez-Soriano J, et al. Genetic heterogeneity of Bartter's syndrome revealed by mutations in the K^+ channel, ROMK. *Nat Genet* 1996;14:152–156.
96. Diezi J, Michoud P, Aceves J, et al. Micropuncture study of electrolyte transport across papillary collecting duct of the rat. *Am J Physiol* 1973;224:623–634.
97. Schwartz GJ, Burg MB. Mineralocorticoid effects on cation transport by cortical collecting tubules in vitro. *Am J Physiol* 1978;235:F576–F585.
98. Grantham JJ, Burg MB, Orloff J. The nature of transtubular Na and K transport in isolated rabbit renal collecting tubules. *J Clin Invest* 1970;49:1815–1826.
99. Stanton BA, Giebisch GH. Potassium transport by the renal distal tubule: effects of potassium loading. *Am J Physiol* 1982;243:F487–F493.
100. Velazquez H, Ellison DH, Wright FS. Chloride-dependent potassium secretion in early and late renal distal tubules. *Am J Physiol* 1987;253:F555–F562.
101. Leaf A, Camara AA, Albertson B. Renal tubular secretion of potassium in man. *J Clin Invest* 1949;28:1526–1533.
102. Mudge GH, Foulks J, Gilman A. The renal excretion of potassium. *Proc Soc Exp Biol Med* 1948;67:545–547.
103. Berliner RW, Kennedy TJ Jr, Hilton JG. Renal mechanisms for excretion of potassium. *Am J Physiol* 1950;162:348–367.
104. O'Neil RG, Sansom SC. Characterization of apical cell membrane Na^+ and K^+ conductances of cortical collecting duct using microelectrode techniques. *Am J Physiol* 1984;247:F14–F24.
105. Wang W, Schwab A, Giebisch G. Regulation of small-conductance K^+ channel in apical membrane of rat cortical collecting tubule. *Am J Physiol* 1990;259:F494–F502.
106. Frindt G, Palmer LG. Low-conductance K channels in apical membrane of rat cortical collecting tubule. *Am J Physiol* 1989;256:F143–F151.
107. Ho K, Nichols CG, Lederer WJ, et al. Cloning and expression of an inwardly rectifying ATP-regulated potassium channel. *Nature* 1993;362:31–37.
108. Wang W, Hebert SC, Giebisch G. Renal K^+ channels: structure and function. *Annu Rev Physiol* 1997;59:413–436.
109. Greger R, Gogelein H. Role of K^+ conductive pathways in the nephron. *Kidney Int* 1987;31:1055–1064.
110. Woda CB, Bragin A, Kleyman TR, et al. Flow-dependent K^+ secretion in the cortical collecting duct is mediated by a maxi-K channel. *Am J Physiol* 2001;49:F786–F793.
111. Okusa MD, Unwin RJ, Velazquez H, et al. Active potassium absorption by the renal distal tubule. *Am J Physiol* 1992;262:F488–F493.
112. Stetson DL, Wade JB, Giebisch G. Morphological alterations in the rat medullary collecting duct following potassium depletion. *Kidney Int* 1980;17:45–56.
113. Stanton BA, Biemesderfer D, Wade JB, et al. Structural and functional study of the rat distal nephron: effects of potassium adaptation and depletion. *Kidney Int* 1981;19:36–48.
114. Hansen GP, Tisher CC, Robinson RR. Response of the collecting duct to disturbances of acid-base and potassium balance. *Kidney Int* 1980;17:326–337.
115. Jamison RL, Work J, Schafer JA. New pathways for potassium transport in the kidney. *Am J Physiol* 1982;242:F297–F312.

116. Wingo CS. Active proton secretion and potassium absorption in the rabbit outer medullary collecting duct. Functional evidence for proton-potassium-activated adenosine triphosphatase. *J Clin Invest* 1989;84:361–365.
117. Wingo CS, Madsen KM, Smolka A, et al. H-K-ATPase immunoreactivity in cortical and outer medullary collecting duct. *Kidney Int* 1990;38:985–990.
118. Wingo CS, Armitage FE. Rubidium absorption and proton secretion by rabbit outer medullary collecting duct via H-K-ATPase. *Am J Physiol* 1992;263:F849–F857.
119. Cheval L, Barlet-Bas C, Khadouri C, et al. K^+-ATPase-mediated Rb^+ transport in rat collecting tubule: modulation during K^+ deprivation. *Am J Physiol* 1991;260:F800–F805.
120. Garg LC, Narang N. Ouabain-insensitive K-adenosine triphosphatase in distal nephron segments of the rabbit. *J Clin Invest* 1988;81:1204–1208.
121. Wingo CS, Cain BD. The renal H-K-ATPase: physiological significance and role in potassium homeostasis. *Annu Rev Physiol* 1993;55:323–347.
122. DuBose TD Jr, Codina J, Burges A, et al. Regulation of H^+-K^+-ATPase expression in kidney. *Am J Physiol* 1995;269:F500–F507.
123. Wingo CS, Smolka AJ. Function and structure of H-K-ATPase in the kidney. *Am J Physiol* 1995;269:F1–F16.
124. Kraut JA, Hiura J, Besancon M, et al. Effect of hypokalemia on the abundance of HK alpha 1 and HK alpha 2 protein in the rat kidney. *Am J Physiol* 1997;272:F744–F750.
125. Jamison RL. Potassium recycling. *Kidney Int* 1987;31:695–703.
126. Jamison RL, Lacy FB, Pennell JP, et al. Potassium secretion by the descending limb or pars recta of the juxtamedullary nephron in vivo. *Kidney Int* 1976;9:323–332.
127. Arrascue JF, Dobyan DC, Jamison RL. Potassium recycling in the renal medulla: effects of acute potassium chloride administration to rats fed a potassium-free diet. *Kidney Int* 1981;20:348–352.
128. Dobyan DC, Lacy FB, Jamison RL. Suppression of potassium-recycling in the renal medulla by short-term potassium deprivation. *Kidney Int* 1979;16:704–709.
129. Milanes CL, Jamison RL. Effect of acute potassium load on reabsorption in Henle's loop in chronic renal failure in the rat. *Kidney Int* 1985;27:919–927.
130. Young DB, Paulsen AW. Interrelated effects of aldosterone and plasma potassium on potassium excretion. *Am J Physiol* 1983;244:F28–F34.
131. Kaufman JS, Hamburger RJ. Potassium transport in the connecting tubule. *Miner Electrolyte Metab* 1996;22:242–247.
132. Field MJ, Giebisch GJ. Hormonal control of renal potassium excretion. *Kidney Int* 1985;27:379–387.
133. Field MJ, Stanton BA, Giebisch GH. Differential acute effects of aldosterone, dexamethasone, and hyperkalemia on distal tubular potassium secretion in the rat kidney. *J Clin Invest* 1984;74:1792–1802.
134. Stokes JB. Mineralocorticoid effect on K^+ permeability of the rabbit cortical collecting tubule. *Kidney Int* 1985;28:640–645.
135. Marver D, Kokko JP. Renal target sites and the mechanism of action of aldosterone. *Miner Electrolyte Metab* 1983;9:1–18.
136. Sansom SC, O'Neil RG. Effects of mineralocorticoids on transport properties of cortical collecting duct basolateral membrane. *Am J Physiol* 1986;251:F743–F757.
137. Sansom SC, O'Neil RG. Mineralocorticoid regulation of apical cell membrane Na^+ and K^+ transport of the cortical collecting duct. *Am J Physiol* 1985;248:F858–F868.
138. Sansom S, Muto S, Giebisch G. Na-dependent effects of DOCA on cellular transport properties of CCDs from ADX rabbits. *Am J Physiol* 1987;253:F753–F759.
139. Garg LC, Knepper MA, Burg MB. Mineralocorticoid effects of Na-K-ATPase in individual nephron segments. *Am J Physiol* 1981;240:F536–F544.
140. Wade JB, O'Neil RG, Pryor JL, et al. Modulation of cell membrane area in renal collecting tubules by corticosteroid hormones. *J Cell Biol* 1979;81:439–445.
141. Petty KJ, Kokko JP, Marver D. Secondary effect of aldosterone on Na-K ATPase activity in the rabbit cortical collecting tubule. *J Clin Invest* 1981;68:1514–1521.
142. Stokes JB. Sodium and potassium transport by the collecting duct. *Kidney Int* 1990;38:679–686.
143. August JT, Nelson DH, Thorn GW. Response of normal subjects to large amounts of aldosterone. *J Clin Invest* 1958;37:1549–1555.
144. Mohring J, Mohring B. Reevaluation of DOCA escape phenomenon. *Am J Physiol* 1972;223:1237–1245.
145. Haas JA, Berndt TJ, Youngberg SP. Collecting duct sodium reabsorption in deoxycorticosterone-treated rats. *J Clin Invest* 1979;63:211–214.
146. Wright FS, Knox FG, Howards SS, et al. Reduced sodium reabsorption by the proximal tubule of Doca-escaped dogs. *Am J Physiol* 1969;216:869–875.
147. Ballermann BJ, Bloch KD, Seidman JG, et al. Atrial natriuretic peptide transcription, secretion, and glomerular receptor activity during mineralocorticoid escape in the rat. *J Clin Invest* 1986;78:840–843.
148. Young DB. Relationship between plasma potassium concentration and renal potassium excretion. *Am J Physiol* 1982;242:F599–F603.
149. Khuri RN, Wiederholt M, Strieder N, et al. Effects of flow rate and potassium intake on distal tubular potassium transfer. *Am J Physiol* 1975;228:1249–1261.
150. Khuri RN, Agulian SK, Kalloghlian A. Intracellular potassium in cells of the distal tubule. *Pflugers Arch* 1972;335:297–308.
151. Muto S, Giebisch G, Sansom S. An acute increase of peritubular K stimulates K transport through cell pathways of CCT. *Am J Physiol* 1988;255:F108–F114.
152. Stanton B, Pan L, Deetjen H, et al. Independent effects of aldosterone and potassium on induction of potassium adaptation in rat kidney. *J Clin Invest* 1987;79:198–206.
153. Garg LC, Narang N. Renal adaptation to potassium in the adrenalectomized rabbit. Role of distal tubular sodium-potassium adenosine triphosphatase. *J Clin Invest* 1985;76:1065–1070.
154. Palmer LG, Antonian L, Frindt G. Regulation of apical K and Na channels and Na/K pumps in rat cortical collecting tubule by dietary K. *J Gen Physiol* 1994;104:693–710.
155. Field MJ, Stanton BA, Giebisch GH. Influence of ADH on renal potassium handling: a micropuncture and microperfusion study. *Kidney Int* 1984;25:502–511.

156. Malnic G, Klose RM, Giebisch G. Microperfusion study of distal tubular potassium and sodium transfer in rat kidney. *Am J Physiol* 1966;211:548–559.
157. Malnic G, Klose RM, Giebisch G. Micropuncture study of renal potassium excretion in the rat. *Am J Physiol* 1964;206: 674–686.
158. Wright FS, Strieder N, Fowler NB, et al. Potassium secretion by distal tubule after potassium adaptation. *Am J Physiol* 1971;221:437–448.
159. Bengele HH, Evan A, McNamara ER, et al. Tubular sites of potassium regulation in the normal and uninephrectomized rat. *Am J Physiol* 1978;234:F146–F153.
160. O'Neil RG, Helman SI. Transport characteristics of renal collecting tubules: influences of DOCA and diet. *Am J Physiol* 1977;233:F544–F558.
161. Wingo CS, Seldin DW, Kokko JP, et al. Dietary modulation of active potassium secretion in the cortical collecting tubule of adrenalectomized rabbits. *J Clin Invest* 1982;70: 579–586.
162. Stokes JB. Potassium secretion by cortical collecting tubule: relation to sodium absorption, luminal sodium concentration, and transepithelial voltage. *Am J Physiol* 1981;241: F395–F402.
163. Wallmark B, Briving C, Fryklund J, et al. Inhibition of gastric H^+,K^+-ATPase and acid secretion by SCH 28080, a substituted pyridyl(1,2a)imidazole. *J Biol Chem* 1987;262: 2077–2084.
164. Hayslett JP, Binder HJ. Mechanism of potassium adaptation. *Am J Physiol* 1982;243:F103–F112.
165. Fujii Y, Mujais SK, Katz AI. Renal potassium adaptation: role of the Na^+-K^+ pump in rat cortical collecting tubules. *Am J Physiol* 1989;256:F279–F284.
166. Mujais SK, Chekal MA, Hayslett JP, et al. Regulation of renal Na^+-K^+-ATPase in the rat: role of increased potassium transport. *Am J Physiol* 1986;251:F199–F207.
167. Oberleithner H, Guggino W, Giebisch G. The effect of furosemide on luminal sodium, chloride and potassium transport in the early distal tubule of Amphiuma kidney. Effects of potassium adaptation. *Pflugers Arch* 1983;396:27–33.
168. Silva P, Brown RS, Epstein FH. Adaptation to potassium. *Kidney Int* 1977;11:466–475.
169. Doucet A, Katz AI. Renal potassium adaptation: Na-K-ATPase activity along the nephron after chronic potassium loading. *Am J Physiol* 1980;238:F380–F386.
170. Schultze RG, Taggart DD, Shapiro H, et al. On the adaptation in potassium excretion associated with nephron reduction in the dog. *J Clin Invest* 1971;50:1061–1068.
171. Schon DA, Silva P, Hayslett JP. Mechanism of potassium excretion in renal insufficiency. *Am J Physiol* 1974;227: 1323–1330.
172. Bastl C, Hayslett JP, Binder HJ. Increased large intestinal secretion of potassium in renal insufficiency. *Kidney Int* 1977; 12:9–16.
173. Fisher KA, Binder HJ, Hayslett JP. Potassium secretion by colonic mucosal cells after potassium adaptation. *Am J Physiol* 1976;231:987–994.
174. Linas SL, Peterson LN, Anderson RJ, et al. Mechanism of renal potassium conservation in the rat. *Kidney Int* 1979;15: 601–611.
175. Khalifah RG. Carbon dioxide hydration activity of carbonic anhydrase: paradoxical consequences of the unusually rapid catalysis. *Proc Natl Acad Sci U S A* 1973;70:1986–1989.
176. Engbretson BG, Stoner LC. Flow-dependent potassium secretion by rabbit cortical collecting tubule in vitro. *Am J Physiol* 1987;253:F896–F903.
177. Malnic G, Berliner RW, Giebisch G. Flow dependence of K^+ secretion in cortical distal tubules of the rat. *Am J Physiol* 1989;256:F932–F941.
178. Good DW, Wright FS. Luminal influences on potassium secretion: sodium concentration and fluid flow rate. *Am J Physiol* 1979;236:F192–F205.
179. Good DW, Velazquez H, Wright FS. Luminal influences on potassium secretion: low sodium concentration. *Am J Physiol* 1984;246:F609–F619.
180. Frindt G, Palmer LG. Ca-activated K channels in apical membrane or mammalian CCT, and their role in K secretion. *Am J Physiol* 1987;252:F458–F467.
181. Khuri RN, Wiederholt M, Strieder N, et al. Effects of graded solute diuresis on renal tubular sodium transport in the rat. *Am J Physiol* 1975;228:1262–1268.
182. Kaissling B. Structural aspects of adaptive changes in renal electrolyte excretion. *Am J Physiol* 1982;243:F211–F226.
183. Kaissling B, Stanton BA. Adaptation of distal tubule and collecting duct to increased sodium delivery. I. Ultrastructure. *Am J Physiol* 1988;255:F1256–F1268.
184. Stanton BA, Kaissling B. Adaptation of distal tubule and collecting duct to increased Na delivery. II. Na+ and K+ transport. *Am J Physiol* 1988;255:1269–1275.
185. Kaissling B, Le Hir M. Distal tubular segments of the rabbit kidney after adaptation to altered Na^- and K^- intake. I. Structural changes. *Cell Tissue Res* 1982;224:469–492.
186. Giebisch G, Malnic G, Klose RM, et al. Effect of ionic substitutions on distal potential differences in rat kidney. *Am J Physiol* 1966;211:560–568.
187. Bank N, Schwartz WB. The influence of anion penetrating ability on urinary acidification and the excretion of titratable acid. *J Clin Invest* 1960;39:1516–1525.
188. Velazquez H, Wright FS, Good DW. Luminal influences on potassium secretion: chloride replacement with sulfate. *Am J Physiol* 1982;242:F46–F55.
189. Carlisle EJF, Donnelly SM, Ethier JH, et al. Modulation of the secretion of potassium by accompanying anions in humans. *Kidney Int* 1991;39:1206–1212.
190. Lipner HI, Ruzany F, Dasgupta M, et al. The behavior of carbenicillin as a nonreabsorbable anion. *J Lab Clin Med* 1975;86:183–194.
191. Kubota T, Biagi BA, Giebisch G. Effects of acid base disturbances on basolateral membrane potential and intracellular potassium activity in the proximal tubule of Necturus. *J Membr Biol* 1983;73:61–68.
192. Stanton BA, Giebisch G. Effects of pH on potassium transport by renal distal tubule. *Am J Physiol* 1982;242:F544–F551.
193. Malnic G, de Mello Aires M, Giebisch G. Potassium transport across renal distal tubules during acid-base disturbances. *Am J Physiol* 1971;221:1192–1208.
194. Barker ES, Singer RB, Elkinton JR, et al. The renal response in man to acute experimental respiratory alkalosis and acidosis. *J Clin Invest* 1957;36:515–529.

195. Boudry JF, Stoner LC, Burg MB. Effect of acid lumen pH on potassium transport in renal cortical collecting tubules. *Am J Physiol* 1976;230:239–244.
196. Toussaint C, Vereerstraeten P. Effects of blood pH changes on potassium excretion in the dog. *Am J Physiol* 1962;202:768–772.
197. Scandling JD, Ornt DB. Mechanism of potassium depletion during chronic metabolic acidosis in the rat. *Am J Physiol* 1987;252:F122–F130.
198. Green R, Giebisch G. Ionic requirements of proximal tubular sodium transport. I. Bicarbonate and chloride. *Am J Physiol* 1975;229:1205–1215.
199. Brandis M, Keyes J, Windhager EE. Potassium-induced inhibition of proximal tubular fluid reabsorption in rats. *Am J Physiol* 1972;222:421–427.
200. Lemann J Jr, Lennon EJ, Goodman AD, et al. The net balance of acid in subjects given large loads of acid or alkali. *J Clin Invest* 1965;44:507–517.
201. Sartorius OW, Roemmelt JC, Pitts RF. The renal regulation of acid-base balance in man. IV. The nature of the renal compensations in ammonium chloride acidosis. *J Clin Invest* 1949;28:423–439.
202. Lowance DC, Garfinkel HB, Mattern WD, et al. The effect of chronic hypotonic volume expansion on the renal regulation of acid-base equilibrium. *J Clin Invest* 1972;51:2928–2940.
203. DeSousa RC, Harrington JT, Ricanati ES, et al. Renal regulation of acid-base equilibrium during chronic administration of mineral acid. *J Clin Invest* 1974;53:465–476.
204. Uete T, Venning EH. Interplay between various adrenal cortical steroids with respect to electrolyte excretion. *Endocrinology* 1962;71:768–778.
205. Bia MJ, Tyler K, DeFronzo RA. The effect of dexamethasone on renal electrolyte excretion in the adrenalectomized rat. *Endocrinology* 1982;111:882–888.
206. Barraclough MA, Jones NF. The effect of vasopressin on the reabsorption of sodium, potassium and urea by the renal tubules in man. *Clin Sci* 1970;39:517–527.
207. Johnson MD, Kinter LB, Beeuwkes R III. Effects of AVP and DDAVP on plasma renin activity and electrolyte excretion in conscious dogs. *Am J Physiol* 1979;236:F66–F70.
208. Sonnenberg H, Honrath U, Wilson DR. Effect of vasopressin analogue (dDAVP) on potassium transport in medullary collecting duct. *Am J Physiol* 1987;252:F986–F991.
209. Schlatter E, Schafer JA. Electrophysiological studies in principal cells of rat cortical collecting tubules. ADH increases the apical membrane Na^+-conductance. *Pflugers Arch* 1987;409:81–92.
210. Cassola AC, Giebisch G, Wang W. Vasopressin increases density of apical low-conductance K^+ channels in rat CCD. *Am J Physiol* 1993;264:F502–F509.
211. Johnson MD, Barger AC. Circulating catecholamines in control of renal electrolyte and water excretion. *Am J Physiol* 1981;240:F192–F199.
212. Kimmel PL, Goldfarb S. Effects of isoproterenol on potassium secretion by the cortical collecting tubule. *Am J Physiol* 1984;246:F804–F810.
213. Iino Y, Troy JL, Brenner BM. Effects of catecholamines on electrolyte transport in cortical collecting tubule. *J Membr Biol* 1981;61:67–73.
214. Aizman R, Grahnquist L, Celsi G. Potassium homeostasis: ontogenic aspects. *Acta Paediatr* 1998;87:609–617.
215. Aizman RI, Celsi G, Grahnquist L, et al. Ontogeny of K^+ transport in rat distal colon. *Am J Physiol* 1996;271:G268–G274.
216. Turnberg LA. Potassium transport in the human small bowel. *Gut* 1971;12:811–818.
217. Petrovic S, Cemerikic D. Intracellular pH in proximal tubular cells of doubly perfused frog kidney. *Period Biol* 1991;93:311–312.
218. Pacha J, Popp M, Capek K. Potassium secretion by neonatal rat distal colon. *Pflugers Arch* 1987;410:362–368.
219. Rechkemmer G, Frizzell RA, Halm DR. Active potassium transport across guinea-pig distal colon: action of secretagogues. *J Physiol* 1996;493:485–502.
220. Del Castillo JR, Sulbaran-Carrasco MC, Burguillos L. K+ transport in isolated guinea pig colonocytes: evidence for Na(+)-independent ouabain-sensitive K+ pump. *Am J Physiol* 1994;266:G1083–G1089.
221. Pacha J, Popp M, Capek K. Corticosteroid regulation of Na+ and K+ transport in the rat distal colon during postnatal development. *J Dev Physiol* 1988;10:531–540.
222. Wang Z-M, Yasui M, Celsi G. Differential effects of glucocorticoids and mineralocorticoids on the mRNA expression of colon ion transporters in infant rats. *Pediatr Res* 1995;38:164–168.
223. Woodard JP, Chen W, Keku EO, et al. Altered jejunal potassium (Rb+) transport in piglet rotavirus enteritis. *Am J Physiol* 1993;265:G388–G393.
224. Kersten L, Weisse H, Hafner E, et al. Natrium- und kalium-konzentrationen im serum sowie im Nieren- und muskelgewebe bei ratten verschiedenen alters und deren veranderungen nach belastung mit 0,9%iger NaCl-losung und nach gleichzeitiger applikation von diuretika. *Acta Biol Med Ger* 1972;29:707–721.
225. Kleinman LI, Banks RO. Segmental nephron sodium and potassium reabsorption in newborn and adult dogs during saline expansion (41637). *Proc Soc Exp Biol Med* 1983;173:231–237.
226. Satlin LM, Schwartz GJ. Renal regulation of potassium homeostasis. In: Edelmann CM Jr, ed. *Pediatric kidney disease.* Boston: Little, Brown, 1992:127–146.
227. Zink H, Horster M. Maturation of diluting capacity in loop of Henle of rat superficial nephrons. *Am J Physiol* 1977;233:F519–F524.
228. Satlin LM. Postnatal maturation of potassium transport in rabbit cortical collecting duct. *Am J Physiol* 1994;266:F57–F65.
229. Satlin LM. Regulation of potassium transport in the maturing kidney. *Semin Nephrol* 1999;19:155–165.
230. Evan AP, Satlin LM, Gattone VH II, et al. Postnatal maturation of rabbit renal collecting duct. II. Morphological observations. *Am J Physiol* 1991;261:F91–F107.
231. Spitzer A, Brandis M. Functional and morphologic maturation of the superficial nephrons: relationship to total kidney function. *J Clin Invest* 1974;53:279–287.
232. Aperia A, Elinder G. Distal tubular sodium reabsorption in the developing rat kidney. *Am J Physiol* 1981;240:F487–F491.

233. Mehrgut FM, Satlin LM, Schwartz GJ. Maturation of HCO_3^- transport in rabbit collecting duct. *Am J Physiol* 1990;259:F801–F808.
234. Satlin LM, Palmer LG. Apical Na^+ conductance in maturing rabbit principal cell. *Am J Physiol* 1996;270:F391–F397.
235. Horster M. Expression of ontogeny in individual nephron segments. *Kidney Int* 1982;22:550–559.
236. Horster M, Larsson L. Mechanisms of fluid absorption during proximal tubule development. *Kidney Int* 1976;10:348–363.
237. Vehaskari VM. Ontogeny of cortical collecting duct sodium transport. *Am J Physiol* 1994;267:F49–F54.
238. Sulyok E, Nemeth M, Tenyi I, et al. Postnatal development of renin-angiotensin-aldosterone system, RAAS, in relation to electrolyte balance in premature infants. *Pediatr Res* 1979;13:817–820.
239. Robillard JE, Nakamura KT. Neurohormonal regulation of renal function during development. *Am J Physiol* 1988;254:F771–F779.
240. Siegel SR, Fisher DA. Ontogeny of the renin-angiotensin-aldosterone system in the fetal and newborn lamb. *Pediatr Res* 1980;14:99–102.
241. Kowarski A, Katz H, Migeon CJ. Plasma aldosterone concentration in normal subjects from infancy to adulthood. *J Clin Endocrinol Metab* 1974;38:489–491.
242. Stephenson G, Hammet M, Hadaway G, et al. Ontogeny of renal mineralocorticoid receptors and urinary electrolyte responses in the rat. *Am J Physiol* 1984;247:F665–F671.
243. Satlin LM, Palmer LG. Apical K^+ conductance in maturing rabbit principal cell. *Am J Physiol* 1997;272:F397–F404.
244. Palmer LG, Choe H, Frindt G. Is the secretory K channel in the rat CCT ROMK? *Am J Physiol* 1997;273:F404–F410.
245. Zhou H, Tate SS, Palmer LG. Primary structure and functional properties of an epithelial K channel. *Am J Physiol* 1994;266:C809–C824.
246. Benchimol C, Zavilowitz B, Satlin LM. Developmental expression of ROMK mRNA in rabbit cortical collecting duct. *Pediatr Res* 2000;47:46–52.
247. Zolotnitskaya A, Satlin LM. Developmental expression of ROMK in rat kidney. *Am J Physiol* 1999;276:F825–F836.
248. Silver RB, Frindt G. Functional identification of H-K-ATPase in intercalated cells of cortical collecting tubule. *Am J Physiol* 1993;264:F259–F266.
249. Wingo CS. Potassium transport by medullary collecting tubule of rabbit: effects of variation in K intake. *Am J Physiol* 1987;253:F1136–F1141.
250. Codina J, Delmas-Mata JT, DuBose TD Jr. Expression of $HK\alpha_2$ protein is increased selectively in renal medulla by chronic hypokalemia. *Am J Physiol* 1998;275:F433–F440.
251. Kuwahara M, Fu W-J, Marumo F. Functional activity of H-K-ATPase in individual cells of OMCD: localization and effect of K^+ depletion. *Am J Physiol* 1996;270:F116–F122.
252. Buffin-Meyer B, Younes-Ibrahim M, Barlet-Bas C, et al. K depletion modifies the properties of Sch-28080–sensitive K-ATPase in rat collecting duct. *Am J Physiol* 1997;272:F124–F131.
253. Constantinescu A, Silver RB, Satlin LM. H-K-ATPase activity in PNA-binding intercalated cells of newborn rabbit cortical collecting duct. *Am J Physiol* 1997;272:F167–F177.
254. Rodriguez-Soriano J, Vallo A, Castillo G, et al. Biochemical features of dietary chloride deficiency syndrome: a comparative study of 30 cases. *J Pediatr* 1983;103:209–214.
255. Roy S III, Arant BS Jr. Alkalosis from chloride-deficient Neo-Mull-Soy. *N Engl J Med* 1979;301:615.
256. Cox M, Sterns RH, Singer I. The defense against hyperkalemia: the roles of insulin and aldosterone. *N Engl J Med* 1978; 299:525–532.
257. Wong CS, Pavord ID, Williams J, et al. Bronchodilator, cardiovascular, and hypokalaemic effects of fenoterol, salbutamol, and terbutaline in asthma. *Lancet* 1990;336:1396–1399.
258. Braden GL, vonOeyen PT, Germain MJ, et al. Ritodrine- and terbutaline-induced hypokalemia in preterm labor: mechanisms and consequences. *Kidney Int* 1997;51:1867–1875.
259. Lipworth BJ, McDevitt DG, Struthers AD. Prior treatment with diuretic augments the hypokalemic and electrocardiographic effects of inhaled albuterol. *Am J Med* 1989;86: 653–657.
260. Simon DB, Bindra RS, Mansfield TA, et al. Mutations in the chloride channel gene, *CLCNKB*, cause Bartter's syndrome type III. *Nat Genet* 1997;17:171–178.
261. Stedwell RE, Allen KM, Binder LS. Hypokalemic paralyses: a review of the etiologies, pathophysiology, presentation, and therapy. *Am J Emerg Med* 1992;10:143–148.
262. Ptacek LJ, Tawil R, Griggs RC, et al. Dihydropyridine receptor mutations cause hypokalemic periodic paralysis. *Cell* 1994;77:863–868.
263. Sillen A, Sorensen T, Kantola I, et al. Identification of mutations in the CACNL1A3 gene in 13 families of Scandinavian origin having hypokalemic periodic paralysis and evidence of a founder effect in Danish families. *Am J Med Genet* 1998;69:102–106.
264. Tanabe T, Beam KG, Powell JA, et al. Restoration of excitation-contraction coupling and slow calcium current in dysgenic muscle by dihydropyridine receptor complementary DNA. *Nature* 1988;336:134–139.
265. Tricarico D, Servidei S, Tonali P, et al. Impairment of skeletal muscle adenosine triphosphate-sensitive K+ channels in patients with hypokalemic periodic paralysis. *J Clin Invest* 1999;103:675–682.
266. Fontaine B, Lapie P, Plassart E, et al. Periodic paralysis and voltage-gated ion channels. *Kidney Int* 1996;49:9–18.
267. Resnick JS, Engel WK, Griggs RC, et al. Acetazolamide prophylaxis in hypokalemic periodic paralysis. *N Engl J Med* 1968;278:582–586.
268. Roza O, Berman LB. The pathophysiology of barium: hypokalemic and cardiovascular effects. *J Pharmacol Exp Ther* 1971;177:433–439.
269. Hermsmeyer K, Sperelakis N. Decrease in K+ conductance and depolarization of frog cardiac muscle produced by Ba^{++}. *Am J Physiol* 1970;219:1108–1114.
270. Lawson DH, Murray RM, Parker JLW. Early mortality in the megaloblastic anaemias. *Q J M* 1972;41:1–14.
271. Rose BD, Post TW. Hypokalemia. In: Wonsiewicz M, McCullough K, Davis K, eds. *Clinical physiology of acid-base*

and electrolyte disorders. New York: McGraw-Hill, 2001:836–887.
272. Adams PC, Woodhouse KW, Adela M, et al. Exaggerated hypokalaemia in acute myeloid leukaemia. *BMJ* 1981;282:1034–1035.
273. Biglieri EG. Spectrum of mineralocorticoid hypertension. *Hypertension* 1991;17:251–261.
274. Stewart PM. Mineralocorticoid hypertension. *Lancet* 1999;353:1341–1347.
275. Kenouch S, Coutry N, Farman N, et al. Multiple patterns of 11 β-hydroxysteroid dehydrogenase catalytic activity along the mammalian nephron. *Kidney Int* 1992;42:56–60.
276. Morris DJ, Souness GW. Protective and specificity-conferring mechanisms of mineralocorticoid action. *Am J Physiol* 1992;263:F759–F768.
277. Biglieri EG, Stockigt JR, Schambelan M. Adrenal mineralocorticoids causing hypertension. *Am J Med* 1972;52:623–632.
278. White PC. Mechanisms of disease: disorders of aldosterone biosynthesis and action. *N Engl J Med* 1994;331:250–258.
279. Biglieri EG, Herron MA, Brust N. 17-hydroxylation deficiency in man. *J Clin Invest* 1966;45:1946–1954.
280. Conn JW, Rovner DR, Cohen EL. Licorice-induced pseudoaldosteronism. Hypertension, hypokalemia, aldosteronopenia, and suppressed plasma renin activity. *JAMA* 1968;205:492–496.
281. Farese RV Jr, Biglieri EG, Shackleton CH, et al. Licorice-induced hypermineralocorticoidism. *N Engl J Med* 1991;325:1223–1227.
282. Scheinman SJ, Guay-Woodford LM, Thakker RV, et al. Genetic disorders of renal electrolyte transport. *N Engl J Med* 1999;340:1177–1187.
283. Liddle GW, Bledsoe T, Coppage WS Jr. A familial renal disorder simulating primary aldosteronism but with negligible aldosterone secretion. *Trans Assoc Am Physicians* 1963;76:199–211.
284. Warnock DG. Renal genetic disorders related to K^+ and Mg^{2+}. *Annu Rev Physiol* 2002;64:845–876.
285. Botero-Velez M, Curtis JJ, Warnock DG. Brief report: Liddle's syndrome revisited—a disorder of sodium reabsorption in the distal tubule. *N Engl J Med* 1994;330:178–181.
286. Geller DS, Farhi A, Pinkerton N, et al. Activating mineralocorticoid receptor mutation in hypertension exacerbated by pregnancy. *Science* 2000;289:119.
287. Lifton RP. Genetic determinants of human hypertension. *Proc Natl Acad Sci U S A* 1995;92:8545–8551.
288. Mune T, Rogerson FM, Nikkila H, et al. Human hypertension caused by mutations in the kidney isozyme of 11 beta-hydroxysteroid dehydrogenase. *Nat Genet* 1995;10:394–399.
289. van Uum SHM, Hermus ARMM, Smits P, et al. The role of 11β-hydroxysteroid dehydrogenase in the pathogenesis of hypertension. *Cardiovasc Res* 1998;38:16–24.
290. Gregory MJ, Schwartz GJ. Diagnosis and treatment of renal tubular disorders. *Semin Nephrol* 1998;18:317–329.
291. Karolyi L, Konrad M, Kockerling A, et al. Mutations in the gene encoding the inwardly-rectifying renal potassium channel, ROMK, cause the antenatal variant of Bartter syndrome: evidence for genetic heterogeneity. *Hum Mol Genet* 1997;6:17–26.
292. Proesmans W. Bartter syndrome and its neonatal variant. *Eur J Pediatr* 1997;156:669–679.
293. Simon DB, Karet FE, Hamdan JM, et al. Bartter's syndrome, hypokalaemic alkalosis with hypercalciuria, is caused by mutations in the Na-K-2Cl cotransporter *NKCC2*. *Nat Genet* 1996;13:183–188.
294. Simon DB, Nelson-Williams C, Bia MJ, et al. Gitelman's variant of Bartter's syndrome, inherited hypokalaemic alkalosis, is caused by mutations in the thiazide-sensitive Na-Cl cotransporter. *Nat Genet* 1996;12:24–30.
295. Sebastian A, McSherry E, Morris RC Jr. Renal potassium wasting in renal tubular acidosis (RTA). Its occurrence in types 1 and 2 RTA despite sustained correction of systemic acidosis. *J Clin Invest* 1971;50:667–678.
296. Schwartz GJ. Acid-base disorders. In: Burg FD, Ingelfinger JR, Polin RA, et al, eds. *Gellis and Kagan's current pediatric therapy*. Philadelphia: WB Saunders, 2002:24–29.
297. Schwartz GJ. General principles of acid-base physiology. In: Holliday MA, Barratt TM, Avner ED, eds. *Pediatric nephrology*. Baltimore: Williams & Wilkins, 1993:222–246.
298. Satlin LM, Schwartz GJ. Disorders of potassium metabolism. In: Ichikawa I, ed. *Pediatric textbook of fluids and electrolytes*. Baltimore: Williams & Wilkins, 1990:218–236.
299. Duarte CG, Chomety F, Giebisch G. Effect of amiloride, ouabain, and furosemide on distal tubular function in the rat. *Am J Physiol* 1971;221:632–639.
300. Wright FS. Flow-dependent transport processes: filtration, absorption, secretion. *Am J Physiol* 1982;243:F1–F11.
301. Welt LG, Hollander W Jr, Blythe WB. The consequences of potassium depletion. *J Chronic Dis* 1960;11:213–254.
302. Kuller LH, Hulley SB, Cohen JD, et al. Unexpected effects of treating hypertension in men with electrocardiographic abnormalities: a critical analysis. *Circulation* 1986;73:114–123.
303. Seelig M. Cardiovascular consequences of magnesium deficiency and loss: pathogenesis, prevalence and manifestations—magnesium and chloride loss in refractory potassium repletion. *Am J Cardiol* 1989;63:4G-21G.
304. Schnaper HW, Freis ED, Friedman RG, et al. Potassium restoration in hypertensive patients made hypokalemic by hydrochlorothiazide. *Arch Intern Med* 1989;149:2677–2681.
305. Levy M. Effects of acute volume expansion and altered hemodynamics on renal tubular function in chronic caval dogs. *J Clin Invest* 1972;51:922–938.
306. Chonko AM, Bay WH, Stein JH, et al. The role of renin and aldosterone in the salt retention of edema. *Am J Med* 1977;63:881–889.
307. Aldinger KA, Samaan NA. Hypokalemia with hypercalcemia. Prevalence and significance in treatment. *Ann Intern Med* 1977;87:571–573.
308. Cronin RE, Bulger RE, Southern P, et al. Natural history of aminoglycoside nephrotoxicity in the dog. *J Lab Clin Med* 1980;95:463–474.
309. Brinker KR, Bulger RE, Dobyan DC, et al. Effect of potassium depletion on gentamicin nephrotoxicity. *J Lab Clin Med* 1981;98:292–301.

310. Douglas JB, Healy JK. Nephrotoxic effects of amphotericin B, including renal tubular acidosis. *Am J Med* 1969;46:154–162.
311. Muggia FM, Heinemann HO, Farhangi M, et al. Lysozymuria and renal tubular dysfunction in monocytic and myelomonocytic leukemia. *Am J Med* 1969;47:351–366.
312. Evans JJ, Bozdech MJ. Hypokalemia in nonblastic chronic myelogenous leukemia. *Arch Intern Med* 1981;141:786–787.
313. Mir MA, Brabin B, Tang OT, et al. Hypokalemia in acute myeloid leukaemia. *Ann Intern Med* 1975;82:54–57.
314. Whang R, Oei TO, Aikawa JK, et al. Magnesium and potassium interrelationships experimental and clinical. *Acta Med Scand* 1981;647:139–144.
315. Whang R, Whang DD, Ryan MP. Refractory potassium repletion. A consequence of magnesium deficiency. *Arch Intern Med* 1992;152:40–45.
316. Shils ME. Experimental human magnesium depletion. *Medicine* 1969;48:61–86.
317. Gennari FJ. Hypokalemia. *N Engl J Med* 1998;339:451–458.
318. Witten TA, Bickel JG. Potassium in gastric juice. *Gastroenterology* 1970;59:330–332.
319. Crane CW. Observations on the sodium and potassium content of mucus from the large intestine. *Gut* 1965;6:439–443.
320. Watten RH, Morgan FM, Songkhla YN, et al. Water and electrolyte studies in cholera. *J Clin Invest* 1959;38:1879–1889.
321. Grier JF. WDHA (watery diarrhea, hypokalemia, achlorhydria) syndrome: clinical features, diagnosis, and treatment. *South Med J* 1995;88:22–24.
322. Richards P. Clinical investigation of the effects of adrenal corticosteroid excess on the colon. *Lancet* 1969;1:437–442.
323. Hoglund P, Haila S, Socha J, et al. Mutations of the Down-regulated in adenoma (DRA) gene cause congenital chloride diarrhoea. *Nat Genet* 1996;14:316–319.
324. Kere J, Lohi H, Hoglund P. Genetic disorders of membrane transport. III. Congenital chloride diarrhea. *Am J Physiol* 1999;276:G7–G13.
325. Dell RB. Pathophysiology of dehydration. In: Winters RW, ed. *The body fluids in pediatrics.* Boston: Little, Brown, 1973:134–154.
326. Agarwal R, Afzalpurkar R, Fordtran JS. Pathophysiology of potassium absorption and secretion by the human intestine. *Gastroenterology* 1994;107:548–571.
327. Grand RJ, diSant'Agnese PA, Talamo RC, et al. The effects of exogenous aldosterone on sweat electrolytes. *J Pediatr* 1967;70:346–356.
328. Gottlieb RP. Metabolic alkalosis in cystic fibrosis. *J Pediatr* 1971;79:930–936.
329. Dawes GS. The vaso-dilator action of potassium. *J Physiol* 1941;99:224–238.
330. Knochel JP, Dotin LN, Hamburger RJ. Pathophysiology of intense physical conditioning in a hot climate. I. Mechanisms of potassium depletion. *J Clin Invest* 1972;51:242–255.
331. Biglieri EG, McIlroy MB. Abnormalities of renal function and circulatory reflexes in primary aldosteronism. *Circulation* 1966;33:78–86.
332. Fisch C. Relation of electrolyte disturbances to cardiac arrhythmias. *Circulation* 1973;47:408–419.
333. Whelton PK, He J, Cutler JA, et al. Effects of oral potassium on blood pressure. Meta-analysis of randomized controlled clinical trials. *JAMA* 1997;277:1624–1632.
334. Weiner ID, Wingo CS. Hypokalemia—consequences, causes, and correction. *J Am Soc Nephrol* 1997;8:1179–1188.
335. Conn JW. Hypertension, the potassium ion and impaired carbohydrate tolerance. *N Engl J Med* 1965;273:1135–1143.
336. Relman AS, Schwartz WB. The nephropathy of potassium depletion. A clinical and pathological entity. *N Engl J Med* 1956;255:195–203.
337. Schwartz WB, Relman AS. Effects of electrolyte disorders on renal structure and function. *N Engl J Med* 1967;276:383–389.
338. Torres VE, Young WF Jr, Offord KP, et al. Association of hypokalemia, aldosteronism, and renal cysts. *N Engl J Med* 1990;322:345–351.
339. Manitius A, Levitin H, Beck D, et al. On the mechanism of impairment of renal concentrating ability in potassium deficiency. *J Clin Invest* 1960;39:684–692.
340. Berl T, Linas SL, Aisenbrey GA, et al. On the mechanism of polyuria in potassium depletion. The role of polydipsia. *J Clin Invest* 1977;60:620–625.
341. Bank N, Aynedjian HS. A micropuncture study of the renal concentrating defect of potassium depletion. *Am J Physiol* 1964;206:1347–1354.
342. Tannen RL. Relationship of renal ammonia production and potassium homeostasis. *Kidney Int* 1977;11:453–465.
343. Jones JW, Sebastian A, Hulter HN, et al. Systemic and renal acid-base effects of chronic dietary potassium depletion in humans. *Kidney Int* 1982;21:402–410.
344. Rodriguez-Soriano J. Potassium homeostasis and its disturbances in children. *Pediatr Nephrol* 1995;9:364–374.
345. Kruse JA, Clark VL, Carlson RW, et al. Concentrated potassium chloride infusions in critically ill patients with hypokalemia. *J Clin Pharmacol* 1994;34:1077–1082.
346. Pullen H, Doig A, Lambie AT. Intensive intravenous potassium replacement therapy. *Lancet* 1967;2:809–811.
347. Shimizu T, Yamashiro Y, Yabuta K. Pseudohyperkalaemia in Kawasaki disease. *Eur J Pediatr* 1992;151:497–498.
348. Stewart GW, Corrall RJ, Fyffe JA, et al. Familial pseudohyperkalaemia. A new syndrome. *Lancet* 1979;2:175–177.
349. Iolascon A, Stewart GW, Ajetunmobi JF, et al. Familial pseudohyperkalemia maps to the same locus as dehydrated hereditary stomatocytosis (hereditary xerocytosis). *Blood* 1999;93:3120–3123.
350. Don BR, Sebastian A, Cheitlin M, et al. Pseudohyperkalemia caused by fist clenching during phlebotomy. *N Engl J Med* 1990;322:1290–1292.
351. Weiner ID, Wingo CS. Hyperkalemia: a potential silent killer. *J Am Soc Nephrol* 1998;9:1535–1543.
352. Bushinsky DA, Gennari FJ. Life-threatening hyperkalemia induced by arginine. *Ann Intern Med* 1978;89:632–634.
353. DeFronzo RA, Bia M, Smith D. Clinical disorders of hyperkalemia. *Annu Rev Med* 1982;33:521–554.
354. Carlsson E, Fellenius E, Lundborg P, et al. Beta-adrenoceptor blockers, plasma-potassium, and exercise. *Lancet* 1978;2:424–425.

355. Textor SC, Bravo EL, Fouad FM, et al. Hyperkalemia in azotemic patients during angiotensin-converting enzyme inhibition and aldosterone reduction with captopril. *Am J Med* 1982;73:719–725.
356. Knochel JP, Schlein EM. On the mechanism of rhabdomyolysis in potassium depletion. *J Clin Invest* 1972;51:1750–1758.
357. Lordon RE, Burton JR. Post-traumatic renal failure in military personnel in Southeast Asia. Experience at Clark USAF hospital, Republic of the Philippines. *Am J Med* 1972;53:137–147.
358. Fortner RW, Nowakowski A, Carter CB, et al. Death due to overheated dialysate during dialysis. *Ann Intern Med* 1970;73:443–444.
359. Gronert GA, Theye RA. Pathophysiology of hyperkalemia induced by succinylcholine. *Anesthesiology* 1975;43: 89–99.
360. Cooperman LH. Succinylcholine-induced hyperkalemia in neuromuscular disease. *JAMA* 1970;213:1867–1871.
361. Walton JD, Farman JV. Suxamethonium hyperkalaemia in uraemic neuropathy. *Anaesthesia* 1973;28:666–668.
362. Birch AA Jr, Mitchell GD, Playford GA, et al. Changes in serum potassium response to succinylcholine following trauma. *JAMA* 1969;210:490–493.
363. Asplund J, Edhag O, Mogensen L, et al. Four cases of massive digitalis poisoning. *Acta Med Scand* 1971;189:293–297.
364. Smith TW, Willerson JT. Suicidal and accidental digoxin ingestion. Report of five cases with serum digoxin level correlations. *Circulation* 1971;44:29–36.
365. Reza MJ, Kovick RB, Shine KI, et al. Massive intravenous digoxin overdosage. *N Engl J Med* 1974;291:777–778.
366. Arthur S, Greenberg A. Hyperkalemia associated with intravenous labetalol therapy for acute hypertension in renal transplant recipients. *Clin Nephrol* 1990;33:269–271.
367. Castellino P, Bia MJ, DeFronzo RA. Adrenergic modulation of potassium metabolism in uremia. *Kidney Int* 1990;37:793–798.
368. Hertz P, Richardson JA. Arginine-induced hyperkalemia in renal failure patients. *Arch Intern Med* 1972;130:778–780.
369. Cannon SC. From mutation to myotonia in sodium channel disorders. *Neuromuscul Disord* 1997;7:241–249.
370. Rojas CV, Wang JZ, Schwartz LS, et al. A Met-to-Val mutation in the skeletal muscle Na+ channel alpha-subunit in hyperkalaemic periodic paralysis. *Nature* 1991;354:387–389.
371. Fontaine B, Khurana TS, Hoffman EP, et al. Hyperkalemic periodic paralysis and the adult muscle sodium channel alpha-subunit gene. *Science* 1990;250:1000–1002.
372. Wang P, Clausen T. Treatment of attacks in hyperkalaemic familial periodic paralysis by inhalation of salbutamol. *Lancet* 1976;1:221–223.
373. Rose BD, Post TW. Hyperkalemia. In: Wonsiewicz M, McCullough K, Davis K, eds. *Clinical physiology of acid-base and electrolyte disorders*. New York: Mc-Graw Hill, 2001: 888–930.
374. Illingworth RN, Proudfoot AT. Rapid poisoning with slow-release potassium. *BMJ* 1980;281:485–486.
375. Moss MH, Rausen AR. Potassium toxicity due to intravenous penicillin therapy [Letter]. *Pediatrics* 1962;29:1032–1034.
376. Bostic O, Duvernoy WF. Hyperkalemic cardiac arrest during transfusion of stored blood. *J Electrocardiol* 1972;5:407–409.
377. Scanlon JW, Krakaur R. Hyperkalemia following exchange transfusion. *J Pediatr* 1980;96:108–110.
378. Sopko JA, Freeman RM. Salt substitutes as a source of potassium. *JAMA* 1977;238:608–610.
379. Kallen RJ, Rieger CH, Cohen HS, et al. Near-fatal hyperkalemia due to ingestion of salt substitute by an infant. *JAMA* 1976;235:2125–2126.
380. Lankton JW, Siler JN, Neigh JL. Hyperkalemia after administration of potassium from nonrigid parenteral-fluid containers [Letter]. *Anesthesiology* 1973;39:660–661.
381. Williams RH. Potassium overdosage: a potential hazard of non-rigid parenteral fluid containers. *BMJ* 1973;1:714–715.
382. Rabelink TJ, Koomans HA, Hene RJ, et al. Early and late adjustment to potassium loading in humans. *Kidney Int* 1990;38:942–947.
383. Elkinton JR, Tarail R, Peters JP. Transfers of potassium in renal insufficiency. *J Clin Invest* 1948;28:378–388.
384. Gonick HC, Kleeman CR, Rubini ME, et al. Functional impairment in chronic renal disease. 3. Studies of potassium excretion. *Am J Med Sci* 1971;261:281–290.
385. Strauss MB. Acute renal insufficiency due to lower nephron nephrosis. *N Engl J Med* 1948;239:693–700.
386. Allon M, Takeshian A, Shanklin N. Effect of insulin-plus-glucose infusion with or without epinephrine on fasting hyperkalemia. *Kidney Int* 1993;43:212–217.
387. Salem MM, Rosa RM, Batlle DC. Extrarenal potassium tolerance in chronic renal failure: implications for the treatment of acute hyperkalemia. *Am J Kid Dis* 1991;18:421–440.
388. Bilbrey GL, Carter NW, White MG, et al. Potassium deficiency in chronic renal failure. *Kidney Int* 1973;4:423–430.
389. van Ypersele de Strihou C. Potassium homeostasis in renal failure. *Kidney Int* 1977;11:491–504.
390. Letteri JM, Asad SN, Caselnova R, et al. Creatinine excretion and total body potassium in renal failure. *Clin Nephrol* 1975;4:58–61.
391. Keith NM, King HE, Osterberg AE. Serum concentration and renal clearance of potassium in severe renal insufficiency. *Arch Intern Med* 1943;71:675–701.
392. Cole CH. Decreased ouabain-sensitive adenosine triphosphatase activity in the erythrocyte membrane of patients with chronic disease. *Clin Sci Mol Med* 1973;45:775–784.
393. Patrick J, Jones NF. Cell sodium, potassium and water in uraemia and the effects of regular dialysis as studied in the leucocyte. *Clin Sci Mol Med* 1974;46:583–590.
394. Bonilla S, Goecke IA, Bozzo S, et al. Effect of chronic renal failure on Na,K-ATPase alpha 1 and alpha 2 mRNA transcription in rat skeletal muscle. *J Clin Invest* 1991;88:2137–2141.
395. Mitch WE, Wilcox CS. Disorders of body fluids, sodium and potassium in chronic renal failure. *Am J Med* 1982;72: 536–550.
396. Bank N, Aynedjian HS. A micropuncture study of potassium excretion by the remnant kidney. *J Clin Invest* 1973; 52:1480–1490.
397. Magner PO, Robinson L, Halperin RM, et al. The plasma potassium concentration in metabolic acidosis: a re-evaluation. *Am J Kid Dis* 1988;11:220–224.

398. Brion LP, Schwartz GJ, Campbell D, et al. Early hyperkalaemia in very low birthweight infants in the absence of oliguria. *Arch Dis Child* 1989;64:270–272.
399. Lorenz JM, Kleinman LI, Markarian K. Potassium metabolism in extremely low birth weight infants in the first week of life. *J Pediatr* 1997;131:81–86.
400. Anderson HM, Laragh JH, Hall CW, et al. Renal excretion of potassium in normal and sodium depleted dogs. *J Clin Invest* 1958;37:323–331.
401. Popovtzer MM, Katz FH, Pinggera WF, et al. Hyperkalemia in salt-wasting nephropathy. Study of the mechanism. *Arch Intern Med* 1973;132:203–208.
402. DeFronzo RA. Hyperkalemia and hyporeninemic hypoaldosteronism. *Kidney Int* 1980;17:118–134.
403. Schambelan M, Sebastian A, Biglieri EG. Prevalence, pathogenesis, and functional significance of aldosterone deficiency in hyperkalemic patients with chronic renal insufficiency. *Kidney Int* 1980;17:89–101.
404. Kokko JP. Primary acquired hypoaldosteronism. *Kidney Int* 1985;27:690–702.
405. McSherry E. Renal tubular acidosis in childhood. *Kidney Int* 1981;20:799–809.
406. Iversen T. Congenital adrenocortical hyperplasia with disturbed electrolyte regulation. *Pediatrics* 1955;16:875–901.
407. Oetliker OH, Zurbrugg RR. Renal tubular acidosis in salt-losing syndromes of congenital adrenal hyperplasia (CAH). *J Clin Endocrinol Metab* 1970;31:447–450.
408. Veldhuis JD, Melby JC. Isolated aldosterone deficiency in man: acquired and inborn errors in the biosynthesis or action of aldosterone. *Endocr Rev* 1981;2:495–517.
409. Ulick S, Wang JZ, Morton DH. The biochemical phenotypes of two inborn errors in the biosynthesis of aldosterone. *J Clin Endocrinol Metab* 1992;74:1415–1420.
410. David R, Golan S, Drucker W. Familial aldosterone deficiency: enzyme defect, diagnosis, and clinical course. *Pediatrics* 1968;41:403–412.
411. Shizuta Y, Kawamoto T, Mitsuuchi Y, et al. Inborn errors of aldosterone biosynthesis in humans. *Steroids* 1995;60:15–21.
412. Daughaday WH, Rendleman D. Severe symptomatic hyperkalemia in an adrenalectomized woman due to enhanced mineralocorticoid requirement. *Ann Intern Med* 1967;66:1197–1203.
413. Pollen RH, Williams RH. Hyperkalemic neuromyopathy in Addison's disease. *N Engl J Med* 1960;263:273–278.
414. Oberfield SE, Levine LS, Carey RM, et al. Pseudohypoaldosteronism: multiple target organ unresponsiveness to mineralocorticoid hormones. *J Clin Endocrinol Metab* 1979;48:228–234.
415. Cheek DB, Perry JW. A salt wasting syndrome in infancy. *Arch Dis Child* 1958;33:252–256.
416. Petersen S, Giese J, Kappelgaard AM, et al. Pseudohypoaldosteronism. Clinical, biochemical and morphological studies in a long-term follow-up. *Acta Paediatr Scand* 1978;67:255–261.
417. Proesmans W, Geussens H, Corbeel L, et al. Pseudohypoaldosteronism. *Am J Dis Child* 1973;126:510–516.
418. Chang SS, Grunder S, Hanukoglu A, et al. Mutations in subunits of the epithelial sodium channel cause salt wasting with hyperkalaemic acidosis, pseudohypoaldosteronism type 1. *Nat Genet* 1996;12:248–253.
419. Strautnieks SS, Thompson RJ, Gardiner RM, et al. A novel splice-site mutation in the gamma subunit of the epithelial sodium channel gene in three pseudohypoaldosteronism type 1 families. *Nat Genet* 1996;13:248–250.
420. Satayaviboon S, Dawgert F, Monteleone PL, et al. Persistent pseudohypoaldosteronism in a 7-year-old boy. *Pediatrics* 1982;69:458–462.
421. Sulyok E. The relationship between electrolyte and acid-base balance in the premature infant during early postnatal life. *Biol Neonate* 1971;17:227–237.
422. Day GM, Radde IC, Balfe JW, et al. Electrolyte abnormalities in very low birthweight infants. *Pediatr Res* 1976;10:522–526.
423. Geller DS, Rodriguez-Soriano J, Boado AV, et al. Mutations in the mineralocorticoid receptor gene cause autosomal dominant pseudohypoaldosteronism type 1. *Nat Genet* 1998;19:279–281.
424. Hanukoglu A, Bistritzer T, Rakover Y, et al. Pseudohypoaldosteronism with increased sweat and saliva electrolyte values and frequent lower respiratory tract infections mimicking cystic fibrosis. *J Pediatr* 1994;125:752–725.
425. Pascoe L, Curnow KM, Slutsker L, et al. Mutations in the human CYP11B2 (aldosterone synthase) gene causing corticosterone methyloxidase II deficiency. *Proc Natl Acad Sci U S A* 1992;89:4996–5000.
426. Arai K, Tsigos C, Suzuki Y, et al. Physiological and molecular aspects of mineralocorticoid receptor action in pseudohypoaldosteronism: a responsiveness test and therapy. *J Clin Endocrinol Metab* 1994;79:1019–1023.
427. Spitzer A, Edelmann CM Jr, Goldberg LD, et al. Short stature, hyperkalemia and acidosis: a defect in renal transport of potassium. *Kidney Int* 1973;3:251–257.
428. Weinstein SF, Allan DM, Mendoza SA. Hyperkalemia, acidosis, and short stature associated with a defect in renal potassium excretion. *J Pediatr* 1974;85:355–358.
429. Paver WKA, Pauline GJ. Hypertension and hyperpotassaemia without renal disease in a young male. *Med J Aust* 1964;2:305–307.
430. Arnold JE, Healy JK. Hyperkalemia, hypertension and systemic acidosis without renal failure associated with a tubular defect in potassium excretion. *Am J Med* 1969;47:461–472.
431. Schambelan M, Sebastian A, Rector FC Jr. Mineralocorticoid-resistant renal hyperkalemia without salt wasting (type II pseudohypoaldosteronism): role of increased renal chloride reabsorption. *Kidney Int* 1981;19:716–727.
432. Gordon RD. Syndrome of hypertension and hyperkalemia with normal glomerular filtration rate. *Hypertension* 1986;8:93–102.
433. Disse-Nicodeme S, Achard JM, Desitter I, et al. A new locus on chromosome 12p13.3 for pseudohypoaldosteronism type II, an autosomal dominant form of hypertension. *Am J Hum Genet* 2000;67:302–310.
434. Take C, Ikeda K, Kurasawa T, et al. Increased chloride reabsorption as an inherited renal tubular defect in familial type II pseudohypoaldosteronism. *N Engl J Med* 1991;324:472–476.

435. DeFronzo RA, Goldberg M, Cooke CR, et al. Investigations into the mechanisms of hyperkalemia following renal transplantation. *Kidney Int* 1977;11:357–365.
436. Wilson FH, Disse-Nicodeme S, Choate KA, et al. Human hypertension caused by mutations in WNK kinases. *Science* 2001;293:1107–1112.
437. DeFronzo RA, Taufield PA, Black H, et al. Impaired renal tubular potassium secretion in sickle cell disease. *Ann Intern Med* 1979;90:310–316.
438. DeFronzo RA, Cooke CR, Goldberg M, et al. Impaired renal tubular potassium secretion in systemic lupus erythematosus. *Ann Intern Med* 1977;86:268–271.
439. Batlle DC. Segmental characterization of defects in collecting tubule acidification. *Kidney Int* 1986;30:546–554.
440. Batlle DC, Arruda JA, Kurtzman NA. Hyperkalemic distal renal tubular acidosis associated with obstructive uropathy. *N Engl J Med* 1981;304:373–380.
441. Batlle D, Itsarayoungyuen K, Arruda JA, et al. Hyperkalemic hyperchloremic metabolic acidosis in sickle cell hemoglobinopathies. *Am J Med* 1982;72:188–192.
442. Greenblatt DJ, Koch-Weser J. Adverse reactions to spironolactone. A report from the Boston Collaborative Drug Surveillance Program. *JAMA* 1973;225:40–43.
443. Bennett WM, Henrich WL, Stoff JS. The renal effects of nonsteroidal anti-inflammatory drugs: summary and recommendations. *Am J Kid Dis* 1996;28:S56–S62.
444. Ellison DH. Hyperkalemia and trimethoprim-sulfamethoxazole. *Am J Kid Dis* 1997;29:959–962.
445. Greenberg S, Reiser IW, Chou SY, et al. Trimethoprim-sulfamethoxazole induces reversible hyperkalemia. *Ann Intern Med* 1993;119:291–295.
446. Kleyman TR, Roberts C, Ling BN. A mechanism for pentamidine-induced hyperkalemia: inhibition of distal nephron sodium transport. *Ann Intern Med* 1995;122:103–106.
447. Oster JR, Singer I, Fishman LM. Heparin-induced aldosterone suppression and hyperkalemia. *Am J Med* 1995;98: 575–586.
448. Petersen KC, Silberman H, Berne TV. Hyperkalaemia after cyclosporin therapy. *Lancet* 1984;1:1470.
449. Katari SR, Magnone M, Shapiro R, et al. Clinical features of acute reversible tacrolimus (FK 506) nephrotoxicity in kidney transplant recipients. *Clin Transplant* 1997;11:237–242.
450. Winters RW. Acute renal failure in pediatrics. In: Williams GS, Klenk EL, Winters RW, eds. *The body fluids in pediatrics: medical, surgical, and neonatal disorders of acid-base status, hydration, and oxygenation.* Boston: Little, Brown, 1973:523–557.
451. Dobrin RS, Larsen CD, Holliday MA. The critically ill child: acute renal failure. *Pediatrics* 1971;48:286–293.
452. Finch CA, Sawyer CG, Flynn JM. Clinical syndrome of potassium intoxication. *Am J Med* 1946;1:337–352.
453. West ML, Marsden PA, Richardson RM, et al. New clinical approach to evaluate disorders of potassium excretion. *Miner Electrolyte Metab* 1986;12:234–238.
454. Ethier JH, Kamel KS, Magner PO, et al. The transtubular potassium concentration in patients with hypokalemia and hyperkalemia. *Am J Kid Dis* 1990;15:309–315.
455. Rodriguez-Soriano J, Ubetagoyena M, Vallo A. Transtubular potassium concentration gradient: a useful test to estimate renal aldosterone bioactivity in infants and children. *Pediatr Nephrol* 1990;4:105–110.
456. Nako Y, Ohki Y, Harigaya A, et al. Transtubular potassium concentration gradient in preterm neonates. *Pediatr Nephrol* 1999;13:880–885.
457. Allon M. Hyperkalemia in end-stage renal disease: mechanisms and management. *J Am Soc Nephrol* 1995;6:1134–1142.
458. McClure RJ, Prasad VK, Brocklebank JT. Treatment of hyperkalaemia using intravenous and nebulised salbutamol. *Arch Dis Child* 1994;70:126–128.
459. Bunchman TE, Wood EG, Schenck MH, et al. Pretreatment of formula with sodium polystyrene sulfonate to reduce dietary potassium intake. *Pediatr Nephrol* 1991;5:29–32.
460. Rodriguez-Soriano J. Potassium homeostasis and its disturbances in children. *Pediatr Nephrol* 1995;9:364–374.
461. Karnik JA, Young BS, Lew NL, et al. Cardiac arrest and sudden death in dialysis units. *Kidney Int* 2001;60:350–357.
462. Nolph KD, Popovich RP, Ghods AJ, et al. Determinants of low clearances of small solutes during peritoneal dialysis. *Kidney Int* 1978;13:117–123.

9

ACID-BASE HOMEOSTASIS

JAMES C. M. CHAN
ROBERT H. K. MAK

The importance of acid-base homeostasis is underscored by Hastings (1):

> To Faraday, we are indebted for naming the products of dissociation, ions—and thus we came by hydrogen ion, a term now synonymous with proton. . . . Tiny though it is, I suppose no constituent of living matter has so much power to influence biological behavior . . .

Endogenous cellular metabolism produces two kinds of hydrogen ion or acid (2). The first class of acid is the volatile, metabolizable acid that on complete oxidation is converted to carbon dioxide (CO_2) and water, with the CO_2 rapidly excreted by the lungs (3). The second category of acid is the nonvolatile, nonmetabolizable net acid, with the kidneys as its sole route of elimination (4). With the lungs and kidneys working in concert to maintain acid-base homeostasis, the normal blood pH can be maintained close to 7.40 despite challenges to acid-base homeostasis. This complex subject may seem difficult. A historical prospective on how the field developed may assist in this understanding (5).

HISTORICAL PERSPECTIVE

The first clinical account of severe disturbances in acid-base homeostasis was O'Shaughnessy's delineation of the massive loss of carbonate of soda in the watery diarrhea of cholera victims during the 1831 epidemic in London (6). No distinction was made between carbonate and bicarbonate at the time. Physiologic acid-base disturbances were next noted in 1877 when Walter (7) found that administration of hydrochloric acid by stomach tube to rabbits caused a virtual depletion of the CO_2 in blood. In 1909, Henderson's renowned monograph illustrated the interrelationships between the metabolic and respiratory components of acid-base equilibrium by an equation that subsequently became known as the *Henderson-Hasselbalch equation* (8). In the same year, Sorensen (9) perfected the first electrode to measure hydrogen ion concentration in the blood and coined the term *pH* to stand for the negative logarithm of the hydrogen ion concentration. In 1923, Bronsted and Lowry (10) set forth the modern definition of an *acid* as a substance that donates hydrogen ion and a *base* as a substance that accepts hydrogen ion. At the same time, Van Slyke (11), in collaboration with Wu and McLean in the Beijing Union Medical College and Hastings in the Rockefeller University, perfected the acid-base measuring equipment that has since come to be known as the *Van Slyke apparatus*. In the preinsulin era, these advances had major clinical implications in the early detection and treatment of diabetic ketoacidosis by averting diabetic coma and markedly improving the survival rate of patients (12,13).

PHYSICAL CHEMISTRY OF ACIDS AND BASES

In accordance with the universally accepted Bronsted and Lowry definition (10), an *acid* is a donor of proton or hydrogen ion, and a *base* is an acceptor of proton or hydrogen ion.

$$HA \rightleftharpoons H^+ + A^-$$

As visualized in the above equation, HA is an acid able to donate a hydrogen ion, and A^- is a base able to accept a hydrogen ion. The acid-base pair is intimately linked, with HA being the conjugate acid of A^-, and A^- being the conjugate base of HA. Acids and bases differ in "strength" contingent on their readiness to donate or accept a hydrogen ion. A strong acid yields its hydrogen ion promptly; a weak acid tends not to (e.g., hydrochloric acid is a strong acid because it dissociates almost completely into its hydrogen ion and chloride ion; in contrast, a weak organic acid does not readily dissociate into hydrogen ion and its conjugate base).

The blood pH of 7.40 is normally maintained within the range of 7.35 to 7.45, despite continuous dietary metabolic and endogenous production of acids and bases. Prevention of excess fluctuations of blood pH beyond these ranges is necessary for optimal cellular enzyme activity and membrane integrity. Substantial pH fluctuations can precipitate severe glycolysis and brain dysfunction (14,15).

In view of the fact that the term *pH* stands for the negative logarithm of hydrogen ion concentration, it is inappropriate to present calculated mean values of pH or to take percentage changes in pH values. The change in pH and the corresponding hydrogen ion concentration are shown below:

pH	H^+ (nEq/L)
7.35	44.7
7.40	39.8
7.45	35.5

BICARBONATE AND NONBICARBONATE BUFFERING SYSTEMS

The first line of defense against acid-base disturbances resides in the blood bicarbonate and nonbicarbonate buffering systems. In the plasma, the buffers consist of bicarbonate, inorganic phosphate, and protein. In the erythrocytes, the buffers consist of hemoglobin, oxyhemoglobin, inorganic and organic phosphate, and bicarbonate. At a normal blood pH of 7.40, 40% of the total buffering capacity of the blood resides in the plasma and erythrocyte bicarbonate buffering system. As metabolic acidosis develops and the blood pH falls to, for example, 7.30, more and more bicarbonate is used up. Thus, determination of the total blood bicarbonate concentration is a reliable indicator of the degree of metabolic acidosis.

In addition to the blood buffering system, two additional systems defend the acid-base homeostasis: the respiratory system and the renal system.

The respiratory compensation to any acid-base disturbance is prompt. In contrast, the renal response to acid-base disturbance is gradual, with stepwise increments of net acid excretion to a hydrogen ion load over 3 or 4 days until maximum renal acidification occurs and the excretion of hydrogen ion reaches a plateau (Fig. 9.1). Closer examinations of the normal responses show that the titratable acidity component of the renal net acid excretion rises abruptly, primarily with the phosphate buffering of the hydrogen ion in the urine. The ammonium component of the net acid excretion rises more gradually in a stepwise fashion until glutaminase-dependent ammonium formation reaches a plateau.

INTERRELATIONSHIP BETWEEN METABOLIC AND RESPIRATORY COMPONENTS

Changes of serum bicarbonate concentration correlate closely with changes in blood pH. Carbonic acid (H_2CO_3) concentration stays in balance with the CO_2 content of the blood because the lungs provide an open system of exchange. These relationships between the metabolic component (as represented by the plasma bicarbonate in mEq/L) and the respiratory component [as represented by the plasma partial pressure of CO_2 (P_{CO_2}) in mm Hg] are governed by the Henderson-Hasselbalch equation:

$$pH = pK + \log \frac{HCO_3^-}{S \times P_{CO_2}}$$

where HCO_3^- is the bicarbonate concentration (24.0 mEq/L); S is the solubility constant of H_2CO_3 (S = 0.03 at 37°C); P_{CO_2} is the partial pressure of CO_2 in blood (P_{CO_2} = 40 mm Hg); and pK is the dissociation constant for both CO_2 and H_2CO_3. With pK of 6.1 and the log of

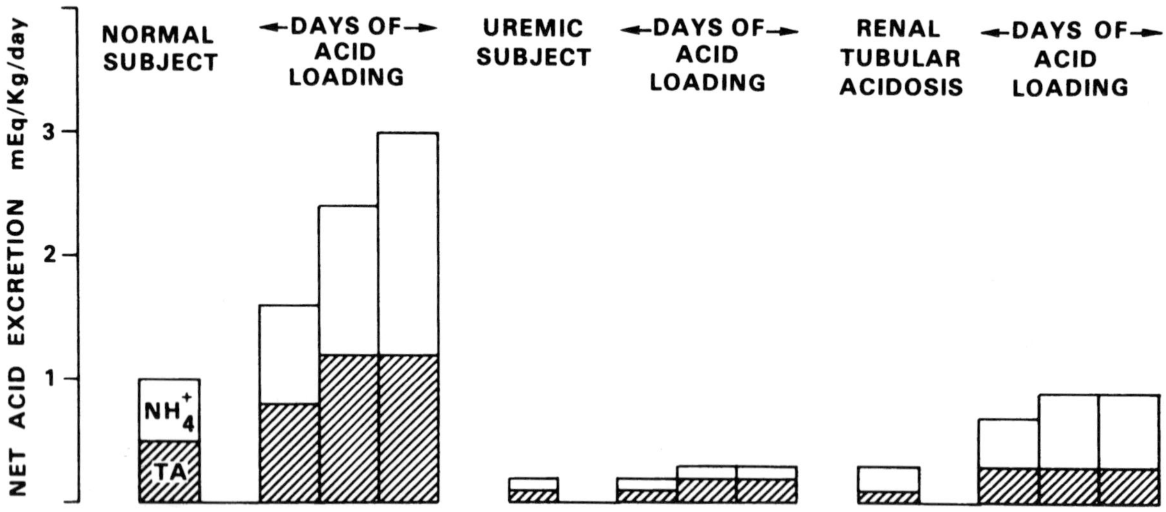

FIGURE 9.1. Net acid excretion of urinary titratable acid (TA) and ammonium (NH_4^+). With any acid load, the renal acidification rises in stepwise fashion until a maximum level is achieved in 3 or 4 days, after which a plateau is reached. In chronic renal failure, the urinary acidification is inadequate.

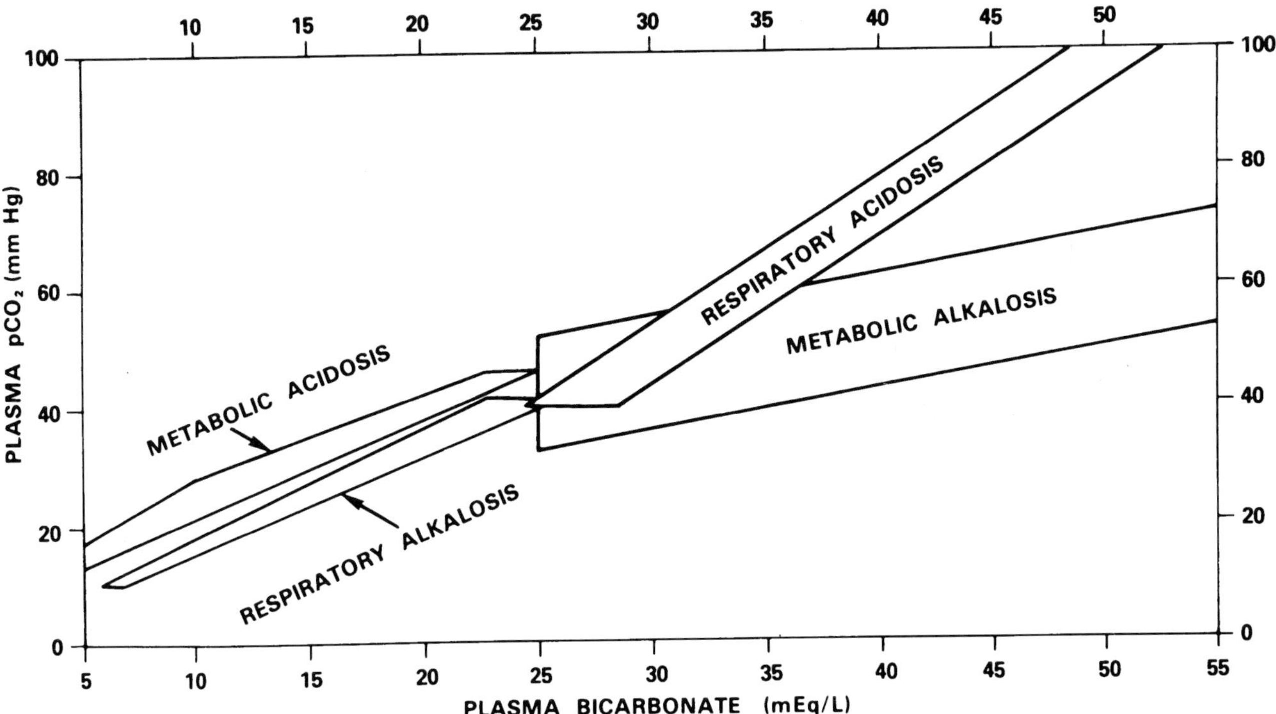

FIGURE 9.2. Relationship between the metabolic component (plasma bicarbonate) and the respiratory component [plasma partial pressure of carbon dioxide (PCO_2)] in clinical acid-base disturbances. The diagrams represent 95% confidence limits between changes in plasma bicarbonate (mEq/L) in relationship with a predictable increase or fall in PCO_2.

$HCO_3^-/S \times PCO_2 = 1.3$, the normal pH is 7.4.

In the clinical setting, the pH of blood is determined by the interrelationship between the metabolic component and the respiratory component. The metabolic component in blood and the respiratory component are shown in Figure 9.2 (2,16–18). There is a narrow confidence limit for the respiratory compensation to acid-base disturbance. The ninety-fifth percentile confidence limits for respiratory acidosis and metabolic acidosis are wide and are less useful clinically (Fig. 9.2).

Let us use the example of a child with severe metabolic acidosis secondary to diarrhea dehydration to illustrate the respiratory compensation to metabolic acidosis. The plasma bicarbonate has fallen to 10 mEq/L due to bicarbonate loss in the diarrhea. In this case, in the absence of any secondary process, the respiratory response (hyperventilation) brings the PCO_2 down to approximately 20 mm Hg, within the ninety-fifth percentile confidence limits for metabolic acidosis (Fig. 9.2). However, if the plasma PCO_2 should stay above the ninety-fifth percentile confidence limits, an independent secondary process interfering with CO_2 exchange (e.g., a pneumonitis or airway obstruction) would have to be considered. On the other hand, if the PCO_2 were to fall below the fifth percentile confidence limits, an independent secondary process stimulating the respiratory center (e.g., salicylate intoxication) would have to be postulated. Thus, any PCO_2 value outside of the ninety-fifth percentile confidence limits for metabolic acidosis would indicate a secondary process other than a normal respiratory compensation.

NUTRITION AND ACID-BASE HOMEOSTASIS

Hydrogen ion production from metabolism of dietary intake or endogenous production is eliminated by excretion in the urine. The impact of dietary intakes on the urinary acidity was first described by Claude Bernard (19):

> One day, rabbits from the market were brought into my laboratory. . . . I happened to observe that their urine was clear and acid. This fact struck me because rabbits, which are herbivore, generally have turbid and alkaline urine; while on the other hand carnivore, as we know, have clear and acid urine. . . . So I had rabbits fed on cold, boiled beef (which they eat very nicely when given nothing else). My expectation was again verified, and as long as the animal diet was continued, the rabbits kept their clear and acid urine.

As a result of Bernard's observation, the acidity of a carnivorous diet influencing the urinary pH and net acid excretion has become widely accepted (13,20). The urine of vegetarians has an average pH of 6.6 (21). However, some confusion remains because of the ambiguity of what consti-

TABLE 9.1. INFLUENCE OF DIETARY ALKALINE ASH AND METABOLISM OF SULFUR-CONTAINING AMINO ACIDS ON RENAL ACID EXCRETION

Diet	N	Alkaline ash (mEq/d)	Urinary sulfate (mEq/d)	Net acid excretion (mEq/d)	Urine pH
Milk	4	131.3	71.4	66.7	<7.00
Lettuces	2	40.1	56.7	60.4	<7.00
Vegan	2	58.8	23.5	29.2	>7.10
DL-methionine	1	—	92.1	92.9	5.10
Beef fillet	1	—	124.5	137.5	5.60

N, number of subjects studied.
Note: Calculated mean values from the original data of Hunt (21) in normal medical students and in vegan subjects.

tutes a typical vegetarian diet. In some cases, a vegetarian may simply eschew red meat while continuing to consume eggs, dairy products, and fish as well as vegetables and fruit. Those whose alkaline ash diets do have a small effect on urine pH are the vegans who consume only food of vegetable origin and exclude dairy products, eggs, and fish.

ALKALINE ASH IN FOOD

The acidity-alkalinity of dietary ash has been calculated by McCance and Widdowson (22) to be the cation content of sodium, potassium, calcium, and magnesium, minus the anion content of chloride and phosphorus. If the cations are in excess, as is the case in most vegetables, the foodstuff is considered to provide an alkaline ash.

Such excess of cation implies that the foods with an alkaline residue must contain a surplus of organic anions (e.g., citrate and bicarbonate). Therefore, it has been assumed that the ingestion of a high alkaline ash diet should result in an alkaline urine. Consistent with that assumption is the fact that ingestion of large amounts of sodium bicarbonate indeed alkalinizes the urine, the bicarbonate being recovered more or less quantitatively from the urine. The reasonableness of such an assumption may account for the scarcity of published experiments testing it. Until recently, the dietary and metabolic sources of acid in the urine do not appear to have been thoroughly investigated since the work of Sherman and Gettler (23). Subsequently, Sherman (24) came to the conclusion that most of the acid in the urine had its origin in the oxidation of sulfur from dietary sulfur-containing amino acids. However, confirmatory data were not available until the work of Hunt (21). To test the relationship between an alkaline ash diet and urinary output of acid, Hunt placed four students on a diet limited to 3 to 5 liters of milk per day for 4 days, supplying a caloric intake of 2100 to 3400 calories a day. Milk was chosen both because it is a "highly standardized food" with an alkaline ash and because it is a "complete food for infants" and, therefore, cannot be criticized as being "unnatural." The pH of the daily outputs of urine showed no increase, although the diet certainly had an alkaline ash. The total net acid excretion was confirmed to be more closely correlated with the urinary sulfate excretion (Table 9.1).

However, interpretation of Hunt's experimental results was clouded by the fact that the protein content of the diet was high and protein metabolism was known to promote acid urine. Therefore, another source of alkaline ash was used in a second experiment. Hunt (21) persuaded two volunteers to eat 4 kg of lettuce each day for 4 days, supplying an alkaline ash content of approximately 40 mEq/day. However, even such large amounts of alkaline ash did not neutralize the acid excreted through the kidney, whereas the sulfate output approximately matched the output of acid. Hunt (21) also collected data on two subjects who had lived on a vegan diet for several years, showing that their urinary output of acid was lower but well balanced by the urinary output of sulfate. Their urinary pH was greater than 7.

CONCEPT OF HYDROGEN ION BALANCE

To determine the influence of diets with a high content of sulfur, Hunt (21) supplemented the diet of one subject with 583 mEq of sulfur as DL-methionine. The mean urinary output of acid immediately increased to 92.9 mEq/day, and the urinary output of sulfur rose to 92.1 mEq/day—results clearly demonstrating that the sulfur of methionine is oxidized in the body to sulfate, which is then excreted in the urine together with a corresponding amount of net acid. In further studies, Hunt (21) provided another volunteer with 7 pounds of beef fillet only, most of which he ate in 2 days. His urinary net acid excretion, however, did not match his urinary sulfate excretion.

To reconcile these discrepancies, Lemann and Relman (25) conducted additional studies that confirmed Hunt's work by showing that sulfur-containing amino acids are oxidized to urea plus CO_2, water, sulfate, and hydrogen ion. From the amount of urinary sulfate excreted, the amount of hydrogen ion produced in this step of intermediary metabolism could be extrapolated. In view of the fact that the total net acid excretion was not fully accounted for, Relman et al. (26) searched for a second component of endogenous acid production, discovering that incompletely oxidized organic acid dissociates in the renal tubule to organic anion and hydrogen ion. By measurement of organic anions, the obligatory renal excretion of fixed, "nonmetabolizable" hydrogen ion produced by dissociation of organic acid could be extrapolated. Furthermore, because the hydrogen ion produced by dissociation of organic acid could be extrapolated from the two metabolic sources combined and approximated the net acid excretion measured, Relman et al. (26) proposed that endogenous acid production from intermediary metabolism can be estimated by summing urinary sulfate and organic anion. A typical daily acid production of 70 mEq was thus established.

In a later study (27), Lennon, Lemann, and Litzow found that the correlation between net acid excretion and endogenous acid production as computed by the sum of the sulfate and organic anions could be improved by subtracting the quantity of "undetermined anion" in the diet. As defined by McCance and Widdowson (22), the "undetermined anion" in foodstuff is the difference between the cations and the predominant anions, calculated as the sum of sodium, potassium, calcium, and magnesium minus the sum of chloride and phosphorus. Lennon et al. (27) further refined the correlation by taking the undetermined anion in the stool into consideration. The difference between undetermined dietary anion and undetermined stool anion constitutes the amount of undetermined anion absorbed.

Despite these refinements, the endogenous acid production continues to be estimated as the sum of sulfate and organic anions (27–29). Finally, in view of the fact that phosphorus is present in food as phosphates, phosphorus oxidation is negligible (21), and phosphoric acid production, once proposed as a third component of endogenous acid production (30), is consequently ignored in the computation of endogenous acid production (27–29). Rather, phosphate intake is accounted for in the dietary undetermined anion computations (27–29).

ACID-BASE BALANCES IN INFANTS AND CHILDREN

Chan (31) carried out metabolic balance studies in ten healthy, normal, 1-week-old infants receiving the milk formula Similac as their sole dietary intake. The sum of cations minus the sum of anions in the milk left a value of 8 mEq/kg body weight per day as the undetermined dietary anion fraction. Similarly computed, the undetermined stool anion fraction was 5 mEq/kg body weight per day. Thus, the undetermined anion fraction absorbed was an insignificant portion of the total dietary anions. Similar studies in ten adult volunteers who agreed to consume only milk for 14 days also revealed insignificant undetermined anion absorption (31).

Goodman, Lemann, and Lennon (32) demonstrated that, despite minor daily fluctuations, the cumulative acid balance in normal individuals is approximately zero. Typical acid production in adults is estimated at 70 mEq/day by extrapolating from urinary sulfate and organic anion. The urinary acid output is also estimated to be 70 mEq/day (32). Goodman et al. (32) demonstrated that with chronic renal insufficiency, serum CO_2 content reaches the acidotic level over a period of 6 days after withdrawal of bicarbonate therapy. The patient's net acid production is not matched by the compromised net acid excretion; therefore, a positive balance of 21 to 30 mEq of acid per day can be demonstrated (32). In other words, withdrawing the alkaline therapy of a patient with chronic renal disease led to a metabolic acidosis resulting primarily from hydrogen ion retention.

In view of the fact that acid retention may continue for months or years in patients with chronic renal acidosis, the base-donating tissue must have a large alkaline pool that can be expended very slowly. Evidence points toward bone as the source of the endogenous base.

The acidosis of chronic renal failure is accompanied by retention of such metabolic wastes as urea and creatinine. Moreover, in renal insufficiency, vitamin D metabolism is defective (33–35). Thus, the effects of metabolic acidosis on calcium metabolism are more appropriately examined in the "pure" state, namely in children with renal tubular acidosis (RTA) but normal renal function. Most adults with RTA have some renal impairment resulting from nephrocalcinosis and nephrolithiasis; for example, of adult patients with RTA studied by Goodman et al. (32), few had a normal glomerular filtration rate.

The acid balance data of two young brothers with distal type I RTA, studied by Chan, are shown in Figure 9.3A,B. Over a 6-day period, the patient in Figure 9.3B maintained a mean net acid balance of 22 $mEq/M^2/day$ and manifested persistent metabolic acidosis. In contrast, with the alkaline therapy increased to over 100 $mEq/M^2/day$, the patient in Figure 9.3A regained a normal serum CO_2 concentration and a zero acid balance by the end of the study period (41).

The major effects of alkaline therapy on mean daily calcium balances are shown in Figure 9.4. During the patient's acidotic period, his mean calcium intake was 44 mEq/day, and the stool and urinary calcium outputs were 25 and 8 mEq/day, respectively, leaving a mean calcium balance of 11 mEq/day. The dramatic threefold increase in his mean calcium balance to 32 mEq/day (p <.05) on correction of acidosis by alkaline therapy is clearly shown. Most of the improvement occurred through reduction of calcium losses in the stool; a lesser

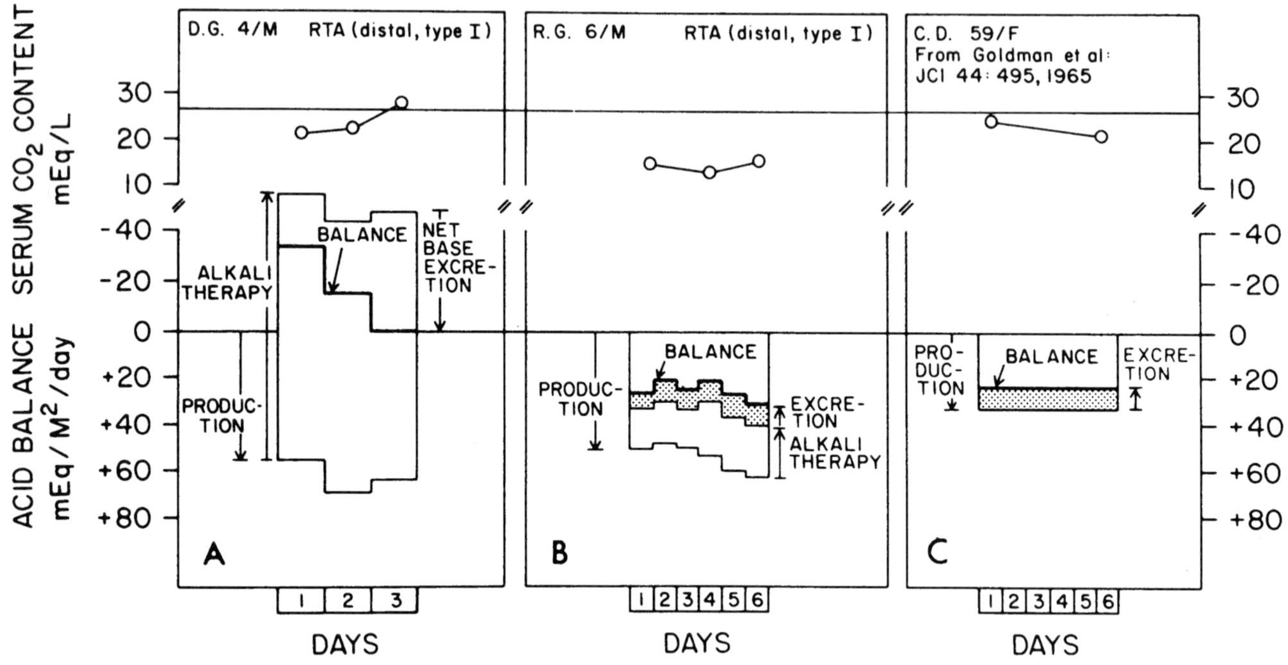

FIGURE 9.3. **A:** Serum CO_2 content and acid balance in a 4-year-old boy with type I renal tubular acidosis (RTA) who received alkaline therapy that increased to more than 100 mEg/M^2/day. **B:** Serum CO_2 content and acid-base balance in a 6-year-old boy with RTA-I. **C:** Fifty-nine-year-old woman with distal RTA and normal kidney functions.

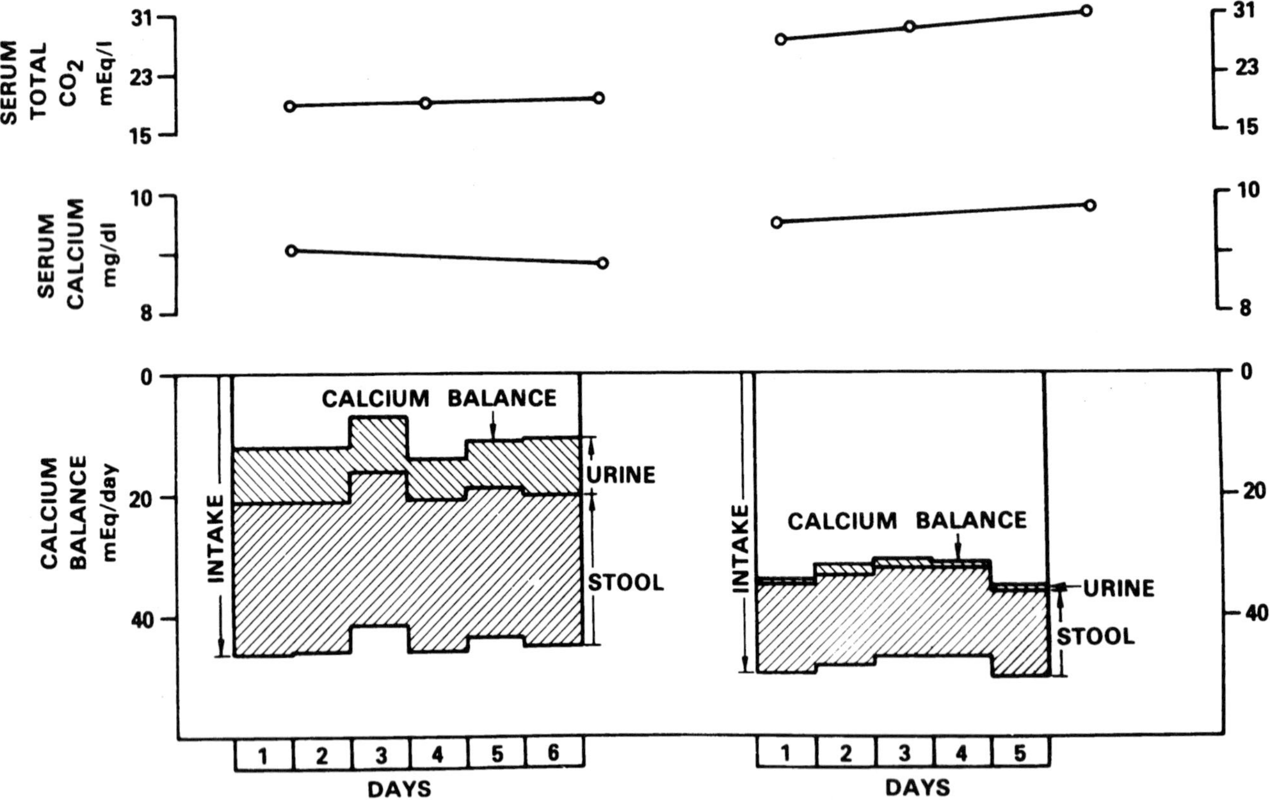

FIGURE 9.4. Serum CO_2 content and calcium balances in a 10-year-old girl with type I renal tubular acidosis. Redrawn from data of Chan (28).

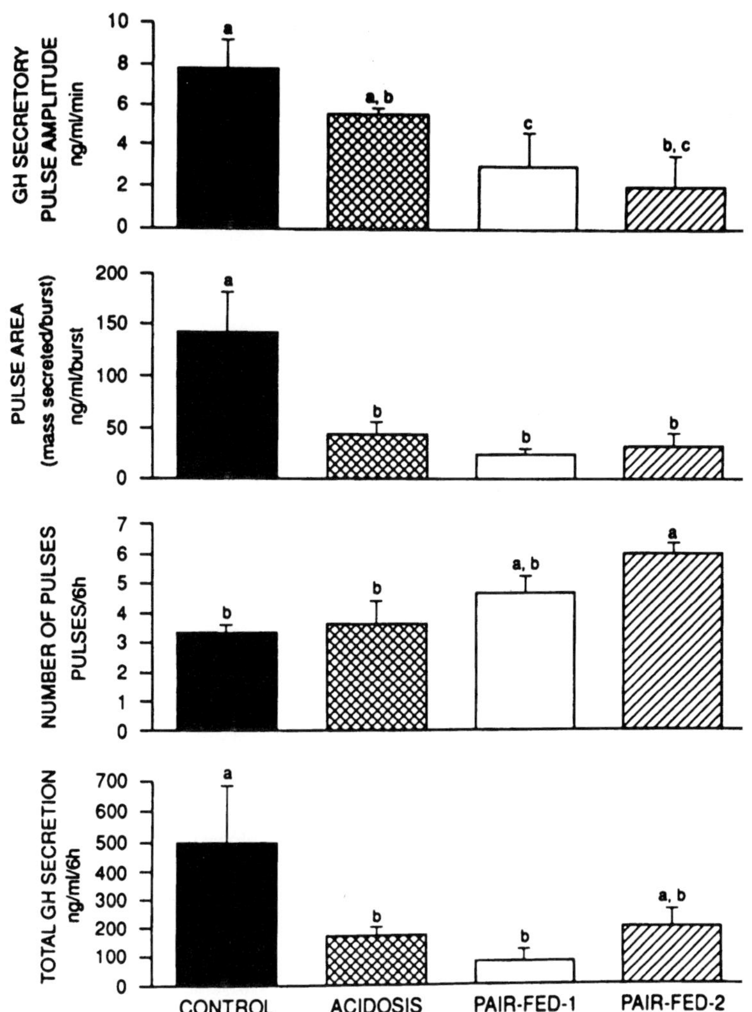

FIGURE 9.5. Data from deconvolution analysis of pulsatile growth hormone (GH) secretion in control (N = 9), acidotic (N = 9), pair-fed-1 (N = 8), and pair-fed-2 (N = 6) groups. Values for mean GH secretory pulse amplitude (height), pulse area (mass), pulse number, and total GH secreted as pulses are shown. Data are expressed as means ± standard error of means. *Pair-fed-1* indicates animals pair-fed in the morning, and *pair-fed-2* indicates pair-fed in the afternoon. In each panel, values with *a*, *b*, or *c* are significantly different (p = .05). (From Challa A, Krieg RJ, Thabet MA, et al. Metabolic acidosis inhibits growth hormone secretion in rats: mechanism of growth retardation. *Am J Physiol* 1993;265:E547–E553, with permission.)

effect was attributable to reduction of urinary calcium losses.

The data of Greenberg et al. (36,37) and of Cooke et al. (38) for children with RTA also show that their patients' calcium balances underwent improvement with correction of metabolic acidosis.

The underlying mechanism of the growth failure of children with RTA has remained unclear. It is commonly assumed that because negative calcium balances have been found to accompany positive acid balances and hypercalciuria in adults with renal acidosis secondary to renal parenchymal diseases, then negative calcium balances must also occur in children with RTA. The foregoing calcium balance data therefore contain some interesting information. First, in contrast to the persistent negative calcium in adults with stable metabolic acidosis secondary to parenchymal renal diseases, the children studied clearly maintained positive calcium balances in both the acidotic and the corrected states. The manifold augmentation of their calcium balances through reduction of fecal and urinary calcium losses as a consequence of acidosis correction amply demonstrates that metabolic acidosis diminishes intestinal calcium absorption in children with classic type I RTA.

In a recent study, Lee et al. (39) showed that the enzymatic hydroxylation of 25-hydroxyvitamin-D to 1,25-dihydroxyvitamin-D was impaired in rats made acutely acidotic by ammonium chloride ingestion. Despite some contrary evidence (40), the data of Lee et al. (39) reinforce the hypothesis, based on observations of children with classic RTA (12), that interference with vitamin D metabolism is the mechanism by which systemic metabolic acidosis provokes malabsorption of calcium through the intestinal tract.

MECHANISMS OF GROWTH RETARDATION IN CHRONIC ACIDOSIS

Growth retardation is a frequent, long-recognized complication of chronic metabolic acidosis (41). Preliminary studies in acidotic children with classic RTA have shown a blunted release of growth hormone (GH) in response to provocative stimuli (42). The growth retardation associated with acidosis can be reversed by systemic bicarbonate therapy (43). The release of GH under acidotic conditions has recently been revisited (44). Exploration in rats with normal anion gap acidosis from ingestion of ammonium chloride demonstrated aberrant GH secretion. Significant inhibition of pulsatile GH secretion was present in the acidotic rats such that both the amplitude of the GH secretory pulse and the area under the curve were significantly smaller than in controls (Fig. 9.5). These reductions in pulse amplitude and area were correlated to decreased growth (weight) in the acidotic rats (44). Using *in situ* hybridization histochemistry in combination with immunocytochemistry, the expression of GH/insulin-like growth factor (IGF)-1 in the tibial epiphyseal growth plate has been examined (45). Evaluation of tibial epiphyseal growth plate (IGF-1) gene expression in acidotic and control rats revealed that IGF-1 messenger RNA abundance was lower in the acidotic growth plates (45). IGF-1 peptide was predominantly localized to the hypertrophic zone of chondrocytes and was weakly detectable in the proliferative zone in both the acidotic and control rats' growth plates (45). Anthropomorphic measurements demonstrated that acidotic rats grew less than did control rats in both length and weight, and these physical measurements were reflected in the size of the tibial epiphyseal growth plates being significantly smaller in the acidotic rats compared with the control group. Taken together, these observations suggest that metabolic acidosis reduces IGF-1 message abundance and induces resistance to IGF-1 peptide action within the tibial epiphyseal growth plate. As demonstrated in two independent laboratories (46,47), the use of GH to stimulate growth in normal anion gap acidosis has been ineffective, despite enhancement of IGF-1 and IGF binding protein immunoreactivity within the stem-cell chondrocyte zone of the tibial epiphyseal growth plate.

CONCEPT OF UNDETERMINED ANION GAP

The serum undetermined anion gap is usually approximated by the difference between the measured cation, sodium (140 mEq/L), minus the measured anions, chloride (105 mEq/L), and bicarbonate (25 mEq/L). This typically gives a normal anion gap of 10 mEq/L. This anion gap is made up of the undetermined variables consisting of sulfate, phosphates, and others. In view of the variability in measurements of serum sodium, chloride, and bicarbonate, the normal anion gap varies between 8 and 15 mEq/L.

Significantly elevated anion gap, not related to laboratory errors in measurements of the cation and anions, can be found when there is accumulation of endogenous lactic acid and keto acids or in uremic acidosis related to accumulation of sulfate and phosphates. Intoxications with salicylate, paraldehyde, methanol, or ethylene glycol ("antifreeze") may give rise to acidosis with large anion gaps. Elevated anion gaps, in the absence of intoxication or uremia, are usually encountered in alcoholic ketoacidosis and diabetic ketoacidosis, with lactic acid, β-hydroxybutyric acid, and acetoacetic acid accumulation. The differential diagnosis of normal anion gap associated with acidosis, especially in the neonate, is presented in Table 9.2.

TABLE 9.2. DIFFERENTIAL DIAGNOSIS OF NEONATAL FAILURE TO THRIVE AND NORMAL ANION GAP METABOLIC ACIDOSIS

Distal renal tubular acidosis
Congenital hypothyroidism
Obstructive uropathy
Early uremic acidosis
Bicarbonate loss
Proximal renal tubular acidosis
Diarrhea
Intestinal fistula
Ureterosigmoidostomy
Medications: cholestyramine, magnesium sulfate, calcium chloride
Acid loading
Ammonium chloride
Arginine hydrochloride

Modified from Chan JCM, Scheinman JI, Roth KS. Renal tubular acidosis. *Pediatr Rev* 2001;22:277–286.

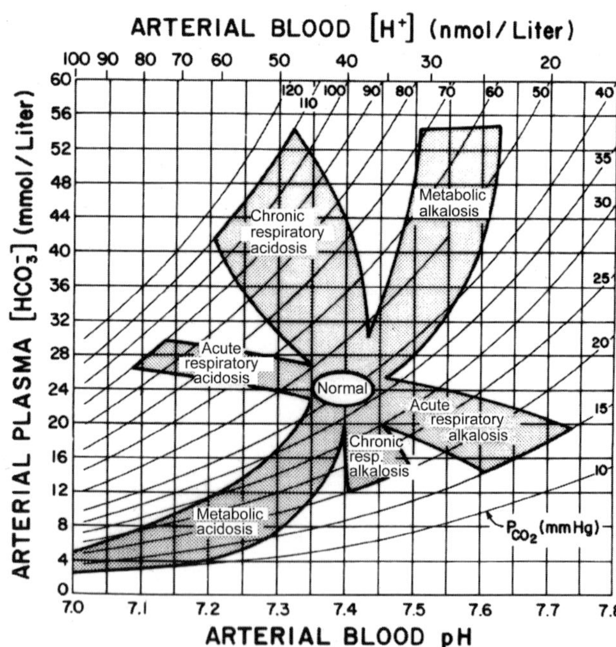

FIGURE 9.6. Acid-base nomogram. Shown are the 95% confidence limits of the normal respiratory (RESP) and metabolic compensations for primary acid-base disturbances. (From Dubose TD Jr, Cogan MG, Rector FC. Acid-base disorder. In: Brenner BM, Rector FC, ed. *Brenner and Rector's the kidney*, 5th ed. Philadelphia: WB Saunders, 1996:929–998, with permission.)

Abnormally depressed anion gap may be related to a reduction in serum albumin or secondary to overhydration. In addition, intoxications (e.g., lithium or polymyxin B) may give rise to significantly reduced anion gap due to increased undetermined cations. Increased serum cationic proteins in multiple myeloma should be in the differential diagnosis of a decreased anion gap.

RENAL REGULATION

The average American diet generates 1 to 3 mEq/kg/day of net acid in healthy infants and children (48,49) and 50 to 80 mEq/day in healthy adults (50). In addition, HCO_3^- may be lost in urine or stool. The kidney maintains acid-base homeostasis by reabsorption of HCO_3^- from the glomerular filtrate as well as hydrogen ion secretion into the urine. The balance of HCO_3^-, pH, and PCO_2 in acute and chronic abnormal acid-base states is shown in Figure 9.6. Most of the known transporters and exchangers involved have now been cloned and characterized. Mutations in the genes encoding these proteins form the molecular basis of the known inherited disorders of acid-base balance.

Proximal Mechanisms

The proximal tubule reabsorbs 80 to 90% of the filtered HCO_3^- and lowers luminal pH by only 0.5 to 0.7 pH units (50). HCO_3^- reabsorption in the proximal tubule is mediated primarily by H^+ ion secretion by a Na^+-H^+ exchanger (NHE)-3 at the luminal membrane (51,52) and HCO_3^- transport via a Na^+-HCO_3^- cotransporter (NBC)-1 (53). H_2CO_3 is formed within proximal tubular cells by hydration of CO_2, a reaction catalyzed by cytoplasmic carbonic anhydrase (CA) II (54). H_2CO_3 ionizes and H^+ ion is secreted in exchange for luminal Na^+. This mechanism is electron neutral and is driven by the lumen-to-cell Na^+ gradient, which is generated by the basolateral membrane Na^+-K^+–adenosine triphosphatase (ATPase). HCO_3^- exits across the basolateral membrane by mass action as well as by carrier-mediated cotransport by the Na^+-HCO_3^- exchanger (NBC-1). The secreted H^+ combines with filtered HCO_3^- to form luminal H_2CO_3, which is dehydrated by luminal CA IV to form H_2O and CO_2. Luminal CO_2 can freely diffuse back into the cell to complete the reabsorption cycle. These processes are described in Figure 9.7 (49). Approximately 20% of the filtered HCO_3^- is reabsorbed by passive back-diffusion along the paracellular pathway. Major factors that regulate the proximal acid-base processes include the filtered load, peritubular HCO_3^-, pH, PCO_2, and angiotensin (AT) II. Other less important or less well-defined factors include extracellular volume, peritubular protein concentration, NaCl reabsorption, K^+ depletion, parathyroid hormone (PTH), Ca^{2+}, and adrenergic nerve activity (49,50).

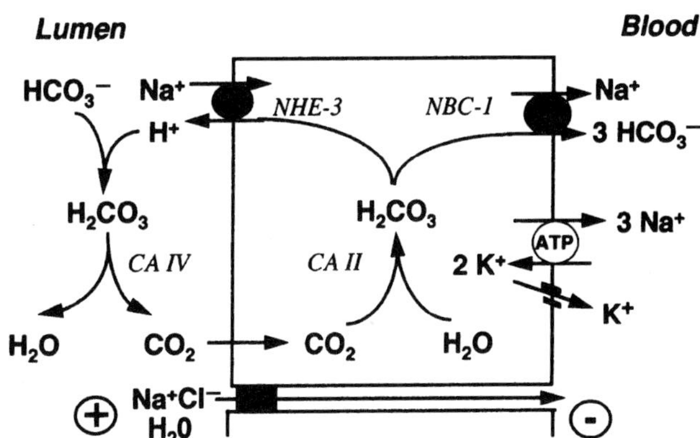

FIGURE 9.7. Schematic model of HCO_3^- reabsorption in proximal convoluted tubule. The processes occurring are H^+ secretion at the luminal membrane via a specific Na^+-H^+ exchanger (NHE) and HCO_3^- transport at the basolateral membrane via a 1 Na^+–3 HCO_3^- cotransporter. Cytoplasmic carbonic anhydrase (CA II) and membrane-bound carbonic anhydrase IV (CA IV) are necessary to reabsorb HCO_3^-. ATP, adenosine triphosphate. (From Rodriguez-Soriano J. Renal tubular acidosis: the clinical entity. *J Am Soc Nephrol* 2002;13:2160–2170, with permission.)

NHEs extrude protons from cells and take up sodium ions into cells. Six isoforms (NHE-1 to NHE-6) have been cloned. The housekeeping NHE-1 is located at the basolateral membrane of most renal tubular cells. NHE-2 is located apically in selected nephron segments. Both isoforms have minor roles in renal salt and water handling. NHE-3 is the predominant apical isoform in the proximal tubule and loop of Henle, whereas NHE-2 is the predominant isoform in the distal tubule (51,52). Fourteen isoforms of CA have been identified. Cytosolic CA II comprises approximately 95% of renal CA. CA II is expressed in the proximal convoluted and straight tubules, thin ascending and thick ascending limbs of the loop of Henle, and intercalated cells of the cortical and medullary cortical collecting duct; it is weakly expressed in principal cells and the inner medullary collecting duct. Membrane-associated CA is mostly CA IV, which is linked to the apical membrane via a glycosylphosphatidylinositol anchor. CA IV is also localized on the basolateral membranes of proximal tubules (54). There are four NBC isoforms and two NBC-related proteins. NBC-1 is expressed on the basolateral membrane of the proximal tubule, is electrogenic, and is directly stimulated by CA II, which binds to the carboxy terminal of NBC-1. NBC-2 has two variants—NBCn1 and mNBC3—both of which are electroneutral transporters. NBCn1 is expressed on the basolateral membrane of the thick ascending limb of Henle, whereas mNBC3 is expressed on the apical membrane of intercalated cells (53). Furthermore, an apical proton-translocating vacuolar ATPase (H^+-ATPase) is also present and contributes significantly to proximal HCO_3^- reabsorption. This is a multisubunit enzyme with a membrane-bound component (V_0 domain) and an intracellular catalytic component (V_1 domain) (55).

Distal Mechanisms

Urine acidification occurs in the distal tubule by three processes: (a) reabsorption of the remainder of the filtered HCO_3^-, which is left over from the proximal tubule (approximately 20%); (b) titration of divalent basic phosphate (HPO_4^-), which is converted to the monovalent acid form ($H_2PO_4^-$) or titratable acid; and (c) accumulation of ammonia intraluminally, which buffers H^+ to form nondiffusible ammonium (NH_4^+). These processes are described in Figure 9.8.

The thick ascending limb of the loop of Henle reabsorbs approximately 15% of the filtered HCO_3^- load through the apical NHE-3. It also participates in NH_3 transport. NH_4^+ absorption occurs in the apical membrane of the loop of Henle by both the Na^+K^+–2 Cl^- cotransport as well as K^+-H^+ antiport systems. The medullary thick ascending limb has low permeability to NH_3, which limits back-diffusion. A medullary NH_4^+ concentration gradient is generated and amplified by countercurrent multiplication through NH_4^+ secretion into the proximal tubule and possibly into the thin descending limb of the loop of Henle. The accumulation of NH_3 in the medullary interstitium increases the driving force for diffusion of NH_3 into the collecting tubule.

Distal urinary acidification occurs mainly in the collecting duct. In the cortical collecting tubule, the principal cells are in charge of Na^+ reabsorption and K^+ secretion, whereas the intercalated cells are involved in HCO_3^- absorption and H^+ secretion. There are two types of intercalated cells. The α cell is responsible for H^+ secretion, and the β cell is responsible for HCO_3^- absorption. There is a lack of consensus as to whether α and β intercalated cells are molecular images of each other or separate cell types. The cellular

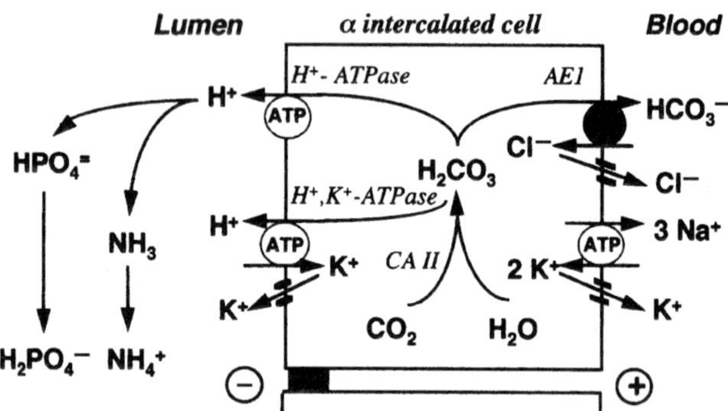

FIGURE 9.8. Schematic model of H^+ secretion in cortical collecting tubule. The main pump for luminal H^+ secretion in the α-type intercalated cell is a vacuolar H^+-adenosine triphosphatase (ATPase). An H^+,K^+-ATPase is also involved in H^+ secretion. Intracellularly formed HCO_3^- leaves the cell via Cl-HCO_3^- exchange, facilitated by an anion exchanger (AE1). Cytoplasmic carbonic anhydrase II (CA II) is necessary to secrete H^+. ATP, adenosine triphosphate. (From Rodriguez-Soriano J. Renal tubular acidosis: the clinical entity. *J Am Soc Nephrol* 2002;13:2160–2170, with permission.)

processes involved in distal acidification are described in Figure 9.8. H^+ is secreted by vacuolar H^+-ATPase on the luminal surface of α intercalated cells in the cortical collecting tubule and outer medullary collecting duct. The secreted H^+ is generated by intracellular CA on H_2CO_3. Basolateral Cl^--HCO_3^- exchanger facilitates exchange of Cl^- for HCO_3^-. A gastric-type H^+,K^+-ATPase is also present on the luminal surface of intercalated cells in the same regions and contributes to H^+ secretion and K^+ absorption. Buffer systems are present to prevent extreme luminal acidity. NH_3 is produced from glutamine and enters the lumen by nonionic diffusion. NH_3 captures H^+ to form NH_4^+. Filtered phosphate provides another buffer (Fig. 9.8). These acid salts comprise titratable acidity and enable urine acidification. NH_3 also stimulates the cortical collecting duct net HCO_3^- reabsorption by activating an apical H^+,K^+-ATPase independent of NH_3's known effects on intracellular pH. This mechanism is dependent on intracellular calcium and a zinc endopeptidase specific for vesicle-associated SNARE protein and appears to involve insertion of cytoplasmic vesicles into the apical plasma membrane of cortical collecting duct intercalated cells (56).

Mineralocorticoids, Na transport, buffer delivery, changes in systemic pH and PCO_2, luminal pH, and potassium status are important factors in the regulation of distal acidification. Aldosterone stimulates H^+-ATPase in the intercalated cells and sodium resorption by the principal cells. Distal acidification is subject to different regulatory factors along different segments. Acidification in the cortical collecting tubule is regulated by Na^+ transport–dependent changes in potential difference as well as chronic systemic acid-base status. The outer medullary cortical tubule has a high capacity for H^+ secretion but is not affected by systemic acid-base status or by sodium transport. The inner medullary duct is regulated by systemic acid-base status and K^+ balance (49,50).

H^+,K^+-ATPases belong to the X^+K^+-ATPase subfamily of P-type cation-transporting ATPase. H^+,K^+-ATPases are composed of at least 13 different subunits, organized into a membrane-anchored V_0 (stalk) domain through which protons are moved and a V_1 head that hydrolyzes ATP. At least two of the α intercalated cell apical pump's subunits, the β subunit in the V_1 domain and the α subunit in the V_0 domain, have been found to be different tissue-specific isoforms. Several isoforms of H^+,K^+-ATPase have been identified in the kidney. Renal tubular apical pumps contain β_1 rather than β_2 subunits and α_4 instead of α_1 subunits. Being ubiquitously expressed, β_2 and α_1 are regarded as the housekeeping isoforms. The colonic isoform, $H^+,K^+\alpha_2$, has been localized to the outer and inner renal medulla and appears to be site-specifically upregulated in response to chronic hypokalemia. $H^+,K^+\alpha_2$ assembles stably with β_1-Na^+K^+-ATPase in the renal medulla and in the distal colon (57–59). Apical tubular H^+,K^+-ATPase is functionally coupled to basolateral HCO_3^- exit (in exchange for Cl^-) via the anion exchanger (AE) AE1. Na^+-independent AEs—AE1, AE2, and AE3—are expressed in the kidney. The AE1 gene encodes erythrocyte eAE1 (band 3), the major intrinsic protein of the erythrocyte as well as kidney kAE1, the basolateral Cl^--HCO_3^- exchanger of the acid-secreting type A intercalated cell. Mutations in AE1 are responsible for distal tubular acidosis. The widely expressed AE2 participates in recovery from alkaline load and in regulatory cell volume increase after shrinkage. AE2 is regulated by NH_4^+. These properties are not shared by AE1. Less is known about AE3 in the kidney (60). Two other potential Cl^--HCO_3^- exchangers, pendrin and AE4, have been reported and may reside apically in the β intercalated cell (61–63).

RESPIRATORY REGULATION

The CO_2-HCO_3^- system in the respiratory tract provides the most important open buffer system for acid-base homeostasis in the body. Its significance can be appreciated if one considers the rate of development of acidosis during an acute respiratory tract obstruction versus that during an acute urinary tract obstruction. H^+ ions from the addition of acid combine with HCO_3^- to form H_2CO_3, which dissociates in the presence of CA into H_2O and CO_2. CO_2 is freely diffusible across alveolar barriers and cell membranes. The efficacy and potency of this system are due to the large buffer capacity in an open system, as CO_2 can rapidly escape from the fluid and be excreted in the lung. A constant PCO_2 is maintained by rapid adjustments in alveolar ventilation (50).

GASTROINTESTINAL REGULATION

Gastrointestinal disorders are common causes of acid-base imbalance in the pediatric age group. Diarrhea is the most common cause of metabolic acidosis in children and results from loss of large quantities of HCO_3^-. Compared with plasma, diarrheal stools contain a higher concentration of HCO_3^- as well as higher amounts of HCO_3^- decomposed by reactions with organic acids. Large quantities of K^+ are also lost in the stools and from the urine as high levels of renin and aldosterone result from hypovolemia. Urine pH may not be less than 5.5 because metabolic acidosis and hypokalemia enhance renal NH_4^+ synthesis and excretion. Thus, high urinary NH_4^+ may be the differentiating clinical feature for diarrhea-associated metabolic acidosis from RTA, which typically presents with low urinary NH_4^+. The urinary anion gap is a useful clinical tool for estimation of urinary NH_4^+. Gastrointestinal HCO_3^- loss can also result from external loss of pancreatic and biliary secretions. Coexistent lactic acidosis is also common in severe diarrheal diseases. On the other hand, H^+ loss through gastric secretions can be caused by vomiting, gastric aspiration, or presence of a gastric fistula and result in HCO_3^- retention and metabolic alkalosis. Hypovolemia from extracellular volume contraction also results in increased levels of renin and aldosterone, which enhance renal HCO_3^- reabsorption in exchange for Cl^-, which further potentiates the metabolic alkalosis (50).

MINERALOCORTICOID AND OTHER HORMONAL ACID-BASE REGULATION

Mineralocorticoids increase net acid excretion and result in hypokalemic metabolic alkalosis which is only sustained by sufficient distal Na^+ delivery and, therefore, dependent on adequate salt intake. The normal feedback is extracellular volume expansion and hypertension. There are several congenital forms of metabolic alkalosis with low-renin hypertension from conditions of mineralocorticoid excess or pseudoaldosteronism: Liddle's syndrome, glucocorticoid remediable alkalosis, and apparent mineralocorticoid excess. Congenital hyperkalemic metabolic acidosis may be caused by different forms of pseudohypoaldosteronism. These congenital disorders are now known to result from genetic mutations, and the underlying molecular pathophysiology is now well understood (see the section Molecular Genetics of Acid-Base Homeostasis). Renin generates AT II, which stimulates aldosterone. Renin is increased by diminished effective circulating volume, which is sensed by the kidney. AT stimulates H^+ transport by both Na^+-H^+ exchange and vacuolar H^+-ATPase in the late distal tubule and only in the early distal segments. This mechanism is mediated through the AT1 receptor (64). AT II, on the other hand, plays an important role in the adaptive enhancement of NH_4^+ secretion in the proximal tubule (65). Deficiency of 11α- or 17α-hydroxylase gives rise to hypokalemic metabolic alkalosis related to excess mineralocorticoids (e.g., deoxycorticosterone and corticosterone). Glucocorticoids stimulate renal tubule acidification both in proximal and distal nephrons by enhancing NH_4 production and net acid secretion. Excess glucocorticoids cause metabolic alkalosis.

Hypercalcemia and vitamin D excess may increase renal HCO_3^- reabsorption. Vitamin D poisoning and excessive ingestion of milk and antacids as in the milk alkali syndrome lead to metabolic alkalosis, nephrocalcinosis, and renal insufficiency (50). The effects of PTH on acid-base homeostasis is controversial. Hyperchloremic metabolic acidosis has been reported in both primary and secondary hyperparathyroid states, and PTH inhibits tubular reabsorption of HCO_3^- in rats under conditions of chronic hyperparathyroidism (66). PTH infusion in normal human subjects causes a biphasic response. An initial transient renal acidosis develops on the first day of PTH infusion, followed by a prompt increase in net acid excretion and an increase in plasma HCO_3^- to result in a steady state of mild metabolic alkalosis for up to 13 days (67). PTH is a potent inhibitor of renal proximal tubular NHE-3 (68). GH and IGF-I increase plasma HCO_3^- concentration by increasing renal NH_3 production and NH_4^+ net acid excretion (69).

PHYSIOLOGIC RESPONSES TO METABOLIC ACIDOSIS AND ALKALOSIS

An acute, nonvolatile acid load is distributed rapidly and attenuated by extracellular buffers within 20 to 30 minutes. A second phase of buffering by intracellular processes then occurs. Approximately two-thirds of this intracellular buffering is through Na^+-H^+ exchange and one-third through either K^+-H^+ or Cl^--HCO_3^- exchanges (70). Intracellular processes function as H^+ storage and restore normal arterial pH within 24 hours of an acute acid load. Renal mechanisms then increase net acid excretion by efficiently retaining all filtered HCO_3^- and increasing both titratable acid and NH_4^+ excretion. With chronic metabolic acidosis, renal acid excretion increases over the course of 3 to 5 days. Proximal conservation of

TABLE 9.3. CAUSES OF METABOLIC ACIDOSIS

Mechanism	Class of agents	Clinical conditions
↑ Production of acid	β-Hydroxybutyric acid and acetoacetic acid	Fasting or starvation
		Insulin deficiency
		Ethanol intoxication
		Ketotic hypoglycemia with hypoalaninemia
	Lactic acid	Hypoxia
		Muscular exercise
		Ethanol ingestion
		Type 1 glycogen storage disease
		Fructose-6-diphosphate deficiency
		Leukemia
		Diabetes mellitus
		Pancreatitis
		Cirrhosis
	Incompletely identified organic acids	Ethylene glycol ingestion
		Paraldehyde intoxication
		Salicylate intoxication
		Methanol intoxication
		Methylmalonic aciduria
		Propionyl coenzyme A carboxylase deficiency
	Acidifying salts	Arginine hydrochloride
		Ammonium chloride
		Lysine hydrochloride
		Hyperalimentation
	Sulfuric acid	Methionine
		Nutramigen
		High-protein milk formula
↑ Extra renal losses of base	Bicarbonate (or combustible base)	Diarrhea
		Ureterosigmoidostomy
		Drainage of pancreatic, biliary, or small bowel secretion
		Ingestion of calcium chloride, cholestyramine, and magnesium sulfate
Dilutional acidosis	Infusion of bicarbonate—free isotonic or hypertonic solutions	Impaired renal acidification
		Oliguria or salt-retaining states
		Renal tubular acidosis
Impaired renal acidification	Accumulation of fixed, nonmetabolizable acids	Polycystic kidney disease
		Hyperparathyroidism
		Adr enal insufficiency
		Pseudohypoaldosteronism
		Leigh's syndrome

↑, increased.

TABLE 9.4. CAUSES OF METABOLIC ALKALOSIS

Mechanism	Class of agents	Clinical conditions
Excessive loss of acid with volume contraction	Chloride deficiency syndromes	Normal blood pressure, high renin and aldosterone, low potassium: vomiting of gastric juices, gastric drainage fistula; diuretic and laxative abuse; Bartter's syndrome; chloride-deficient infant formula Cystic fibrosis; villous adenoma of the colon; congenital alkalosis with chloride diarrhea (Darrow)
Excessive gain of base	Base overload	Iatrogenic, especially in the context of renal insufficiency; milk alkali syndrome
	Conversion of lactate, acetate to base	Iatrogenic; dialysis excess
	Nonmetabolizable acid into cells	Glucose-induced alkalosis in fasting
	Excess proximal tubular bicarbonate reabsorption	Posthypercapnic state Phosphate excess Hypoparathyroidism
Increased (distal) bicarbonate reabsorption	Volume expansion, mineralocorticoid excess	Hypertension, high renin and aldosterone: secondary nonedematous aldosteronism (e.g., renal artery stenosis, intrarenal vascular disease, accelerated hypertension) Renin-secreting tumors Hypertension, low renin, high aldosterone: primary hyperaldosteronism; dexamethasone-suppressible hyperaldosteronism; adrenal carcinoma Hypertension, low renin, low aldosterone: adrenocorticosteroid excess; deficiency of 11-hydroxylation/17-hydroxylation; adrenal carcinoma; Liddle syndrome; licorice (glycyrrhizic acid) excess

HCO_3^- is achieved by low filtered load of HCO_3^- and enhanced proximal acid excretion. However, the secondary hypocapnia induced by metabolic acidosis may counteract proximal HCO_3^- conservation. The greatly reduced HCO_3^- delivery to the distal tubule plus stimulation of collecting duct H^+ secretion and NH_4^+ excretion result in urine with low pH, almost no HCO_3^-, and high levels of titratable acid and NH_4^+. Acidosis increases NH_4^+ production through stimulation of glutaminase and phosphoenolpyruvate carboxykinase in the proximal tubule. The increased distal delivery enhances NH_4^+ reabsorption by the thick ascending limb of the loop of Henle, thus increasing the inner medullary NH_3 concentration. This, in turn, increases NH_4^+ excretion in the medullary collecting duct. The net effect is an increase in both renal NH_4^+ production and excretion. Urinary NH_4^+ can increase up to approximately fivefold. The nature of the anion accompanying H^+ affects renal acid excretion. The nonreabsorbable anions enhance the ability to generate a distal tubule potential difference and augment H^+ excretion. Titratable acid excretion can increase by two- or threefold with an absorbable anion but by five- to tenfold with a nonabsorbable anion (e.g., organic anions during ketoacidosis). In severe cases, renal mechanisms may not account for total acid excretion. Bone may represent a major site of acute and chronic intracellular acid buffering. Calcium, phosphorus, and hydroxyproline excretion are increased during metabolic acidosis (50). Conditions that cause metabolic acidosis are described in Table 9.3, and conditions that cause metabolic alkalosis are described in Table 9.4.

An acute base load is rapidly distributed in the extracellular fluid within 25 minutes (71) followed by cellular buffering of the HCO_3^- load with a half-life of 3 hours. Only one-third of the base load is buffered cellularly, principally by H^+-Na^+ exchange and to a lesser extent by Cl^--HCO_3^- exchange. Modest hypokalemia also results. There is poorer stabilization of intracellular pH in the alkaline range than in the acid range. Neutralization of HCO_3^- by buffers results in an increase in PCO_2, which stimulates ventilation acutely. However, if the respiratory system is compromised, dangerous hypercapnia may ensue. The increase in PCO_2 is approximately 0.75 mm Hg/mEq/L in plasma HCO_3^-. The kidney excretes HCO_3^- more rapidly than acid. The proximal tubule is principally responsible for HCO_3^- excretion. Glomerular ultrafiltrate HCO_3^- rises in conjunction with plasma HCO_3^-, but absolute proximal HCO_3^- reabsorption does not increase because of suppression of proximal acidification processes by alkalemia. The most sensitive response to alkali input is a decline in the excretion of NH_4^+. The next level of response is to increase the excretion of unmeasured anions. This latter rise is quantitatively the most important process in eliminating alkali. The maximum excretion of citrate is approximately 70% of its filtered load. An even higher alkali load augments the excretion of 2-oxoglutarate to more than 400% of its filtered load. Only with the largest alkali load does bicarbonaturia become quantitatively important. Thus, renal mechanisms eliminate alkali while minimizing bicarbonaturia. This process of limiting changes in urine pH without sacrificing acid-base balance lessens the risk of kidney stone formation (72).

The physiologic adaptation to metabolic acidosis and alkalosis has also been studied at the molecular level. Chronic acid loading (7-day) is associated with an increase in apical NHE-3 in the renal proximal tubule. Because NHE-3 mediates both proton secretion and Na reabsorption, compensatory changes in Na handling develop, involving decreases in the abundance of the thiazide-sensitive Na^+-Cl^- cotransporter of the distal convoluted tubule and both the β and γ subunits of the amiloride-sensitive epithelial Na channel of the collecting duct. In addition, the renal cortical abundance of the proximal type 2 Na-dependent phosphate transporter was markedly decreased. In contrast, abundance of the bumetanide-sensitive Na-K–2 Cl cotransporter of the thick ascending limb and the α subunit of the epithelial Na channels were unchanged. A similar profile of changes is seen with short-term (16-hour) acid loading. Long-term (7-day) base loading with $NaHCO_3$ results in the opposite pattern of response, with marked increases in the abundance of the β and γ subunits of epithelial Na channel and type 2 Na-dependent phosphate. These adaptations may play critical roles in the maintenance of Na balance when changes in acid-base balance occur (73). Several targets have also been identified at the gene expression level to account for the adaptation of renal NH_4^+ synthesis and transport in response to an acid load. These are key enzymes of ammoniagenesis (mitochondrial glutaminase and glutamine dehydrogenase) and gluconeogenesis (phosphoenolpyruvate carboxykinase) in the proximal tubule, the apical Na^+-$K^+(NH_4^+)$–2 Cl^- cotransporter of medullary collecting ducts. Two major factors control the expression of these genes during metabolic acidosis, an acid pH and glucocorticoids, which appear to act in concert to coordinate the adaptation of various tubular cell types (74).

PHYSIOLOGIC RESPONSES TO RESPIRATORY ACIDOSIS AND ALKALOSIS

Respiratory acidosis (Tables 9.5 and 9.6), which follows hypercapnia, is initiated by an increase in arterial partial pressure of CO_2 ($PaCO_2$) and elicits acidification of body fluids. An acute increase in plasma HCO_3^- occurs and is complete within 5 to 10 minutes. This results from acidic titration of nonbicarbonate buffers, such as phosphates, hemoglobin, and intracellular proteins. When respiratory acidosis is chronic, renal adjustments worsen the acidemia by a further increase in plasma HCO_3^-. This chronic adjustment phase takes 3 to 5 days to complete and involves upregulation of the renal acidification mechanisms. Ninety-five percent confidence limits for graded degrees of acute and chronic respiratory acidosis are shown in Figure 9.6.

TABLE 9.5. CAUSES OF ACUTE RESPIRATORY ACIDOSIS

Mechanism	Conditions
Airway obstruction	Aspiration of vomitus or foreign body Laryngospasm and edema Bronchospasm Obstructive sleep apnea
Neuromuscular impairment	Injury of brain stem and high cord Botulism Tetanus Guillain-Barré syndrome Myasthenia gravis crisis Overdose of narcotic, sedatives Toxic agents (curare, succinylcholine) Aminoglycoids, organophosphate Hypokalemic myopathy Familial hypokalemic periodic paralysis
Thorax or pulmonary disorders	Respiratory distress syndrome Pneumothorax Hemothorax Smoke inhalation Severe pneumonitis
Inadequate ventilation	Large dead space mechanical ventilation Erroneous settings for tidal volume
Vascular accidents	Massive pulmonary embolism and edema Cardiac arrests
Central nervous system depression	General anesthesia Tranquilizer overdose Cerebral trauma or infarction Central sleep apnea

Respiratory alkalosis is initiated by a decrease in $PaCO_2$ from different causes (Table 9.7). Respiratory alkalosis causes alkalinization of body fluids. The acute response consists of a decrease in plasma and is complete within 5 to 10 minutes from the onset of hypocapnia. It occurs by alkaline titration of nonbicarbonate buffers of the body as well as increased production of organic acids. When respiratory alkalosis is chronic, renal adjustments worsen the alkalemia by an additional decrease in plasma HCO_3^-. This adaptation takes 2 to 3 days to complete and involves downregulation of renal acidification mechanisms. Ninety-five percent confidence limits for graded degrees of acute and chronic respiratory alkalosis are also shown in Figure 9.6. For the same $PaCO_2$, the degree of alkalemia is lower in chronic than in acute respiratory alkalosis (75). Conditions that cause respiratory acidosis are described in Tables 9.5 and 9.6, and conditions that cause respiratory alkalosis are described in Table 9.7.

Chronic but not acute respiratory acidosis stimulates activity of H^+-ATPase and H^+,K^+-ATPase in the proximal tubule, medullary thick ascending limb, and collecting tubule. By contrast, both acute and chronic respiratory alkalosis decrease both renal proton pumps. The stimulatory effect of respiratory acidosis and inhibitory effect of

TABLE 9.6. CAUSES OF CHRONIC RESPIRATORY ACIDOSIS

Mechanism	Conditions
Airway obstruction	Chronic obstructive airway disease: bronchitis, emphysema
	End-stage interstitial lung disease
Respiratory center depression	Chronic narcotic or tranquilizer overdose
	Primary hypoventilation (Ondine's curse)
	Brain tumor
Restrictive lesions	Kyphoscoliosis, spinal arthritis
	Diaphragmatic paralysis
	Hydrothorax
	Fibrothorax
	Interstitial fibrosis
	Prolonged pneumonitis
	Obesity hypoventilation syndrome (Pickwickian syndrome)
Neuromuscular defects	Poliomyelitis
	Multiple sclerosis
	Muscular dystrophy
	Amyotrophic lateral sclerosis
	Myxedema
	Myopathic polymyositis
	Acid maltase deficiency

respiratory alkalosis appear to be potassium and aldosterone independent. Although the precise mechanisms are not known, direct effects of P_{CO_2}, pH, or HCO_3^- delivery may be involved (76).

TABLE 9.7. CAUSES OF RESPIRATORY ALKALOSIS

Mechanism	Conditions
Reflex excitation of respiratory center via pulmonary stretch receptors	Pulmonary edema, cardiopulmonary disease
	Embolus
	Interstitial pulmonary disease
Primary excitation of central respiratory center	Anxiety
	Hyperventilation (voluntary or mechanical)
	Encephalitis, meningitis
	Cerebrovascular incidents, head trauma, brain tumor or vascular accidents
	Medications: salicylate, nicotine, xanthine, pressor agents, progesterone
	Heat exposure, fever, pain
	Pregnancy
Reflex excitation of respiratory center via peripheral chemoreceptor	Low inspirational oxygen (e.g., high altitude)
	Hypotension
	Tissue hypoxia (e.g., anemia, congestive heart failure, asthma)
	Arterial hypoxemia
Multiple mechanisms	Hepatic failure
	Gram negative sepsis
	Shock

PHYSIOLOGIC RESPONSES TO MIXED ACID-BASE DISORDERS

Metabolic acidosis and alkalosis primarily involve plasma HCO_3^- disturbances, whereas respiratory acidosis and alkalosis primarily involve P_{CO_2} disturbances. Figure 9.2 shows the 95% confidence limits of these simple acid-base disorders. Values that fall outside these limits imply that a mixed disorder may exist. Table 9.8 shows the possible combinations of mixed acid-base disturbances. Primary metabolic disturbances invoke secondary respiratory responses, whereas primary respiratory disturbances invoke secondary metabolic responses. Metabolic acidosis resulting from the addition of nonvolatile acids lowers the extracellular fluid HCO_3^- concentration and, hence, extracellular pH. Medullary chemoreceptors are stimulated by the low pH and invoke an increase in ventilation. The ratio of HCO_3^- to P_{CO_2} and subsequent pH are returned toward but not entirely to normal. Compensation is a physiologic consequence of the primary disturbance and does not represent a secondary alkalosis or acidosis. However, by definition, mixed acid-base disturbances exceed physiologic limits of compensation.

MOLECULAR GENETICS OF ACID-BASE HOMEOSTASIS

The advent of molecular biology and molecular genetics has advanced our understanding of the *in vivo* functions of acid-base transport proteins and the clinical syndromes caused by their genetic mutations. A gene family of Na^+-H^+ exchanger has been identified. One of its members, NHE-3, is identified as the Na^+-H^+ exchanger isoform responsible for transepithelial electroneutral Na^+ absorption in intestine and renal epithelial cells. The NHE-3 gene has been localized to 5p15.3 (77). The transient neonatal form of distal RTA may be caused by immaturity of the NHE-3 Na^+-H^+ exchanger isoform, which is known to undergo postnatal development (78). No human mutations of the NHE-3 exchange have been identified as yet. The human gene for NBC-1 has been cloned and maps to 4p-21. A nonsense mutation in the kidney NBC-1 gene (SLC4A4) has been identified. It predicts a truncated NBC-1 protein with loss of function, compatible with the phenotype of isolated proximal RTA. Other features of the syndrome include ocular abnormalities, mental retardation, and short stature (79).

Inherited defects in two of the key acid-base transporters involved in distal acidification, as well as mutations in cytosolic CA gene, can cause distal RTA. Both autosomal-dominant and autosomal-recessive patterns have been described. Recessive distal RTA present with either acute

TABLE 9.8. MIXED ACID-BASE DISORDERS

Mechanism	Disorders	Adaptation	Blood pH
Inadequate response	Mixed metabolic acidosis and respiratory acidosis	$Paco_2$ ↑↑ HCO_3 ↓↓	Depressed
	Mixed metabolic alkalosis and respiratory alkalosis	$Paco_2$ ↓↓ HCO_3 ↑↑	Elevated
Excessive response	Mixed metabolic acidosis and respiratory alkalosis	$Paco_2$ ↓↓ HCO_3 ↓↓	Normal or decreased or increased
	Mixed metabolic alkalosis and respiratory acidosis	$Paco_2$ ↑↑ HCO_3 ↑↑	Normal or increased or decreased
Triple acid-base disorders	Mixed metabolic alkalosis (diuretics or Cl-deficient intake), metabolic acidosis (lactic acids of sepsis to hypoxemia, hypotension), and respiratory acidosis or alkalosis	$Paco_2$ inappropriate HCO_3 inappropriate Anion gap exceeds 20 mEq/L	Variable
	Chronic respiratory acidosis, obstructive lung disease, superimposed acute respiratory acidosis from pneumonitis or congestive heart failure, acute respiratory alkalosis (intubation) mechanical ventilation	$Paco_2$ inappropriate HCO_3 inappropriate	Variable

↑↑, increased; ↓↓, decreased; $Paco_2$, partial pressure of CO_2.

illness or growth failure at a young age, sometimes accompanied by deafness, whereas dominant distal RTA is usually a milder disease and involves no hearing loss (80). The AE1 gene encodes band 3 Cl^--HCO_3^- exchangers that are expressed in the basolateral membranes of the intercalated cells in the distal tubule as well as erythrocytes. Several mutations of the AE1 gene cosegregate with dominant nonsyndromal distal RTA (81). However, the modest degree of loss of function exhibited *in vitro* by these mutations does not explain the abnormal distal acidification phenotype. Other AE1 mutations have been linked to the recessive syndrome of distal RTA without hemolytic anemia, in which loss of function can be demonstrated by *in vitro* studies of the mutations (82). Several mutations in the CA II gene are associated with the autosomal-recessive syndrome of RTA, osteopetrosis, and cerebral dysfunction (83). Mutations in ATP6B1, encoding the B subtype unit of the apical H^+-ATPase, are responsible for a group of patients with autosomal-recessive distal RTA associated with sensorineural deafness (84). Another gene, ATP6N1B, which encodes a noncatalytic accessory of the proton pump, is exclusively expressed on the luminal surface of the intercalated cells in the collecting duct and maps to chromosome 7. Nonsense, deletion, and splice-site mutations of this gene truncate the protein and result in the phenotype of distal tubular acidosis with preserved hearing (85).

Syndromes of aldosterone resistance [pseudohypoaldosteronism (PHA)] leading to hyperkalemic or type 4 RTA have also been characterized at the molecular level. PHA type I has a characteristic phenotype of neonatal salt wasting with dehydration, metabolic acidosis, hyperkalemia, and hypotension. Two forms of PHA-I exist. An autosomal-recessive form features severe disease with manifestations persisting into adulthood. This form is caused by loss-of-function mutations in genes encoding subunits of the amiloride-sensitive epithelial sodium channels (86–88). Autosomal-dominant or sporadic PHA-I is a milder disease that remits with age. Mineralocorticoid receptor gene mutations, including frameshifts, premature terminations codons, and splice donor mutations, have been identified with the autosomal-dominant or sporadic form of PHA-I (89). PHA type II, otherwise known as *Gordon's syndrome*, is an autosomal-dominant disorder with a phenotype of hyperkalemic hyperchloremic acidosis with normal renal function and volume-dependent, low-renin hypertension, which is responsive to thiazide diuretics. Recently, two genes causing PHA-II have been identified. Both genes encode members of the WNK (with no kinase) family of serine-threonine kinases and are on chromosomes 1 and 17. Disease-causing mutations in WNK1 are large intronic deletions that increase WNK1 expression. The mutations in WNK4 are missense, which cluster in a short, highly conserved segment of the encoded protein. Both proteins localize to the distal nephron. WNK1 is cytoplasmic, whereas WNK4 localizes to tight junctions (90).

Bartter's syndrome is an autosomal-recessive disease characterized by diverse abnormalities in electrolyte homeostasis including hypokalemic metabolic alkalosis. Mutations in the Na-K–2 Cl cotransporter (NKCC2) cause Bartter's syndrome with the phenotype of hypokalemic alkalosis, salt-wasting, hypercalciuria, and low blood pressure (91). NKCC2 mutations can be excluded in some Bartter's syndrome kindreds, prompting examinations of regulators of cotransporter activity. One such regulator is ROMK, an ATP-sensitive K^+ channel that recycles reabsorbed K^+ back to the tubule lumen. Examination of the ROMK gene reveals mutations that cosegregate with the disease and disrupt ROMK function in Bartter's kindreds. These findings establish the genetic heterogeneity of Bartter's syndrome and demonstrate the physiologic role of ROMK *in vivo* (92). The antenatal variant of Bartter's syndrome is also caused by mutations in ROMK (93). Bartter's syndrome type III phenotype is characterized by hypokalemic alkalosis with salt-wasting, low blood pressure, normal magnesium, and hyper- or normocalciuria with notable absence of nephrocalcinosis. Linkage of this phenotype has also been demonstrated to a segment of chromosome 1 containing the gene encoding the chloride channel CLCNKB. Loss-of-function mutations, including large deletions and nonsense and missense mutations of this gene, impair chloride reabsorption in the thick ascending limb of the loop of Henle (94). A variant of Bartter's syndrome, associated with sensorineural deafness and renal failure, has recently been mapped to chromosome 1 (95). A novel gene that encodes Bartin is expressed in the thin limb and the thick ascending limb of the loop of Henle in the kidney and in the dark cells of the inner ear (96). Bartin acts as an essential β subunit for basolateral CLC chloride channels, with which it colocalizes in basolateral membranes of renal tubules and of potassium-secreting epithelia of the inner ear (96). Gitelman's syndrome represents the predominant subset of Bartter's patients having hypomagnesemia and hypocalciuria. Complete linkage of Gitelman's syndrome has been demonstrated to the locus encoding the renal thiazide-sensitive Na-Cl cotransporter. A wide variety of nonconservative mutations has been identified, consistent with loss of function alleles, in affected subjects (97).

Mutations have also been identified in a number of mendelian disorders resulting in hypokalemic metabolic alkalosis as well as low-renin hypertension from conditions of mineralocorticoid excess or pseudoaldosteronism. Premature termination, frameshift (98), or missense (99) mutations in the gene encoding the β subunit of the amiloride-sensitive epithelial sodium channel cause constitutive activation of this channel leading to pseudoaldosteronism or Liddle's syndrome. Furthermore, mutations truncating the carboxy-terminus of the γ subunit of this channel also cause Liddle's syndrome (100). Chimeric gene duplications causing ectopic expression of aldosterone synthase enzymatic activity result in glucocorticoid-remediable aldosteronism (101). Point mutations in the HSD11B2 gene cause deficiency of 11β-hydroxysteroid dehydrogenase type 2, which is responsible for the conversion of cortisol to inactive metabolites, and result in the phenotype of apparent mineralocorticoid excess (102).

ACID-BASE CHANGES RELATED TO GROWTH AND DEVELOPMENT

Children with chronic metabolic alkalosis (e.g., Bartter's syndrome) do not grow well. However, the mechanism of this growth failure has not been well studied. Preliminary data have suggested the growth failure of Bartter's syndrome may be related to a primary effect of metabolic alkalosis or suppressing the IGF-GH axis (41). The effects of chronic hypokalemia in Bartter's syndrome on the growth axis have not been examined.

Children with chronic metabolic acidosis from RTA also suffer from failure to thrive and growth retardation (20). In an abstract presented in 1979, McSherry et al. (42) reported the blunting of GH release in children who have RTA. To determine how metabolic acidosis affects GH secretion and expression, Challa et al. (44) demonstrated that acidosis inhibits the GH pulse amplitude, pulse area, and total GH secretion in acidotic animals compared with that of control and pair-fed animals. They also demonstrated that serum IGF, hepatic IGF-1 mRNA, hepatic GH receptor mRNA, and gene expression of IGF at the growth plate of the long bone all are suppressed in the presence of metabolic acidosis (45,47,103). Thus, it appears that acidosis interferes with major aspects of the IGF-GH axis, although reduced nutrition from acidosis may contribute to decreased GH secretion. However, metabolic acidosis inhibits IGF-1 mRNA expression in the growth plate of the long bone and in the hepatic GH receptor mRNA specifically. These animal experiments showed that metabolic acidosis directly inhibited GH secretion and gene expression at target sites—anomalies that contribute to the growth failure of metabolic acidosis.

REFERENCES

1. Hastings AB. Part I: Acid base measurements in vitro: introductory remarks. *Ann N Y Acad Sci* 1966;133:15–24.
2. Kildeberg P. *Clinical acid-base physiology: studies in neonates, infants and young children.* Baltimore: Williams & Wilkins, 1968;228.
3. Kildeberg P, Engel K, Winters RW. Balance of net acid in growing infants: endogenous and transintestinal aspects. *Acta Paediatr Scand* 1969;58:321–329.
4. Relman AS, Lennon EJ, Lemann J Jr. Endogenous production of fixed acid and the measurements of the net balance of acid in normal subjects. *J Clin Invest* 1961;40:1621–1630.
5. Klahr S, Weiner ID. Disorders of acid-base metabolism. In: Chan JCM, Gill JR Jr, eds. *Kidney electrolyte disorders.* New York: Churchill Livingstone, 1990;1–58.

6. O'Shaughnessy WR. Experiments in blood in cholera. *Lancet* 1831;1:490.
7. Walter F. Untersuchungen uber die wirkung der sauren auf der thierischen organism. *Arch Exp Pathol Pharmacol* 1877; 7:148–178.
8. Henderson LJ. Das gleichgewicht zwischen basen und ssauren in tierschen organizmus. *Ergeb Physiol* 1909;8:254–325.
9. Sorensen SPL. Enzymstudiem: I. Uber die quantitative messung proteolytische spaltungen. *Biochem Z* 1908;7:45–101.
10. Bronsted JN. Einige bemerkungen uber der begriff der sauren und basen. *Rec Trav Chim Pays-Bas* 1923;42:718–728.
11. Van Slyke DD, Wu H, McLean FC. Studies of gas and electrolyte equilibrium in the blood: V. Factors controlling the electrolyte and water distribution in the blood. *J Biol Chem* 1923;56:765–849.
12. Santos F, Chan JCM. Renal tubular acidosis in children: diagnosis, treatment and prognosis. *Am J Nephr* 1986;6: 289–295.
13. Klahr SD. Disorders of acid-base metabolism. In: Chan JCM, Gill JR Jr, eds. *Disorders of mineral, water and acid-base metabolism.* New York: John Wiley & Sons, 1982.
14. Adrogue HJ, Madias NE. Management of life-threatening acid-base disorders, first of two parts. *N Engl J Med* 1998;338:26–34.
15. Adrogue HJ, Madias NE. Management of life-threatening acid-base disorders, second of two parts. *N Engl J Med* 1998;338:107–111.
16. Peters JP, Van Slyke DD. Hemoglobin and oxygen, carbonic acid and acid-base balance. Baltimore: Williams & Wilkins, 1932.
17. Chan JCM, Asch MJ, Lin S, Hays DM. Hyperalimentation with amino acid and casein hydrolysate solutions: mechanisms of acidosis. *JAMA* 1972;220:1700–1705.
18. Weil WB. A unified guide to parenteral fluid therapy. *J Pediatr* 1969;75:1–12.
19. Bernard C. *An introduction to the study of experimental medicine translated by Henry Copley Greene.* New York: Abelard-Schulman Inc., 1950.
20. Chan JCM, Scheinman JI, Roth KS. Renal tubular acidosis. *Pediatr Rev* 2001;22:277–286.
21. Hunt JN. The influence of dietary sulfur on the urinary output of acid in man. *Clin Sci* 1956;15:119–134.
22. McCance RA, Widdowson EM. *The chemical composition of foods.* London: HM Stationery Office, 1942.
23. Sherman HC, Gettler AO. The balance of acid-forming and base-forming elements in foods and its relation to ammonia metabolism. *J Biol Chem* 1912;11:323–338.
24. Sherman HC. *Chemistry of food and nutrition*, 6th ed. New York: Macmillan, 1941.
25. Lemann JJ, Relman AS. The relationship of sulfur metabolism to acid-base balance and electrolyte excretion: the effects of DL-methionine in normal man. *J Clin Invest* 1959;38:2215–2223.
26. Relman AS, Lennon EJ, Lemann J Jr. Endogenous production of fixed acid and the measurements of the net balance of acid in normal subjects. *J Clin Invest* 1961;40:1621–1630.
27. Lennon EJ, Lemann J Jr, Litzow JR. The effects of diet and stool composition on the net external acid balance of normal subjects. *J Clin Invest* 1966;45:1601–1607.
28. Chan JCM. Renal acidosis. In: Duarte CG, ed. *Renal function tests.* Boston: Little, Brown and Company, 1980;239–268.
29. Lemann J Jr, Litzow JR, Lennon EJ. The effects of chronic acid loads in normal man: further evidence for the participation of bone mineral in the defense against chronic metabolic acidosis. *J Clin Invest* 1966;45:1608–1614.
30. Lennon EJ, Lemann J Jr, Relman AS. The effects of phosphoprotein on acid balance in normal subjects. *J Clin Invest* 1962;41:637–645.
31. Chan JCM. Nutrition and acid-base metabolism. *Federation Proc* 1981;40:2423–2428.
32. Goodman AD, Lemann J Jr, Lennon EJ. Production, excretion and net balance of fixed acid in patients with renal acidosis. *J Clin Invest* 1965;44:495–506.
33. Chan JCM, Oldham SB, DeLuca HF. Effectiveness of 1-alpha-hydroxyvitamin D_3 in children with renal osteodystrophy associated with hemolysis. *J Pediatr* 1977;90:820–824.
34. Chan JCM, DeLuca HF. Calcium and parathyroid disorders in children: Chronic renal failure and treatment with calcitriol. *JAMA* 1979;241:1242–1244.
35. Chan JCM, Kodroff MB, Landwehr DM. Effects of 1,25-dihydroxyvitamin D_3 on renal function, mineral metabolism and growth in children with severe chronic renal failure. *Pediatrics* 1981;68:559–571.
36. Chan JCM, McEnery PT, Chinchilli VM, et al. A prospective, double-blind study of growth failure in children with chronic renal insufficiency and the effectiveness of treatment with calcitriol versus dihydrotachysterol. *J Pediatr* 1994;124:520–528.
37. Greenbreg AJ, McNamara H, McCrory WW. Metabolic balance studies in primary renal tubular acidosis: effects of acidosis on external calcium balances. *J Pediatr* 1966;69: 610–618.
38. Cooke RE, Kleeman CR. Distal tubular dysfunction with renal calcification. *Yale J Biol Med* 1950;23:199–206.
39. Lee SW, Russell J, Avioli LV. 25-Hydroxy-cholecalciferol to 1,25-dihydroxycholecalciferol: conversion impaired by systemic metabolic acidosis. *Science* 1977;195:994–996.
40. Weber HP, Gray RW, Dominguez JH, Lemann J Jr. The lack of effect of chronic metabolic acidosis on 25-OH-vitamin D metabolism and serum parathyroid hormone in humans. *J Clin Endocrinol Metab* 1976;43:1047–1055.
41. Chan JCM Acid-base disorders and the kidney. *Adv Pediatr* 1983;30:401–471.
42. McSherry E, Weberman J, Grumbach M. The effect of acidosis on human growth hormone (hGH) release in children with nonzotemic RTA. *Clin Res* 1980;28:535A(abst).
43. McSherry E, Morris RC Jr. Attainment and maintenance of normal stature with alkali therapy in infants and children with classic renal tubular acidosis. *J Clin Invest* 1978;61: 509.
44. Challa A, Krieg RJ, Thabet MA, et al. Metabolic acidosis inhibits growth hormone secretion in rats: mechanism of growth retardation. *Am J Physiol* 1993;265:E547–E553.
45. Hanna JD, Challa A, Chan JCM, Han VKM. Insulin-like growth factor-1 gene expression in the tibial epiphyseal growth plate of the acidotic and with nutritional limited rats. *Pediatr Res* 1995;37:363A(abst).

46. Chobanian MC, Friedman AL, Allen DB. Discordant effect of recombinant human growth hormone (rhGH) on bone, kidney, and linear growth in acidotic adult (A) and weanling (W) rats. *Pediatr Res* 1993;33:354A(abst).
47. Hanna JD, Lei CM, Han VKM. Tibial epiphyseal growth plate (TEGP) morphometrics, insulin-like growth factor-I (IGF-I) and insulin-like growth factor binding protein (IGFBP) immunoreactivity (IR) in acidotic growth hormone treated rats. *Pediatr Res* 1995;37:363A(abst).
48. Chan JCM. Calcium and hydrogen ion metabolism in children with classic (type 1/distal) renal tubular acidosis. *Ann Nutr Metab* 1981;25:65–78.
49. Rodriguez-Soriano J. Renal tubular acidosis: the clinical entity. *J Amer Soc Nephrol* 2002;13:2160–2170.
50. Dubose TD Jr, Cogan MG, Rector FC. Acid-base disorder. In: Brenner BM, Rector FC, ed. *Brenner and Rector's the kidney*, 5th ed. Philadelphia: WB Saunders, 1996;929–998.
51. Burckhardt G, Di Sole F, Helmle-Kolb C. The Na+/H+ exchanger gene family. *J Nephrol* 2002;15(Suppl 5):S3–S21.
52. Wang T, Hropot M, Aronson PS, Giebisch G. Role of NHE isoforms in mediating bicarbonate reabsorption along the nephron. *Amer J Physiol* 2001;281:F1117–F1122.
53. Soleimani M. Na+HCO3- cotransporter (NBC): expression and regulation in the kidney. *J Nephrol* 2002;(Suppl 5): S32–S40.
54. Schwartz GJ. Physiology and molecular biology of renal carbonic anhydrase. *J Nephrol* 2002;15(Suppl 5):S61–S74.
55. Nakhoul NL, Hamm LL. Vacuolar H+-ATPase in the kidney. *J Nephrol* 2002;(Suppl 5):S22–S31.
56. Frank AE, Wingo CS, Andrews PM, et al. Mechanisms through which ammonia regulates cortical collecting duct net proton secretion. *Amer J Physiol* 2002;282:F1120–F1128.
57. Doucet A. H+,K+-ATPase in the kidney: localization and function in the nephron. *Exper Nephrol* 1997;5:271–276
58. Codina, Wall SM, DuBose TD Jr. Contrasting functional and regulatory profiles of the renal H^+,K^+-ATPases. *Sem Nephrol* 1999;19:399–404.
59. Zies DL, Wingo CS, Cain BD. Molecular regulation of the HKalpha2 subunit of the H+, K+-ATPases. *J Nephrol* 2002;(Suppl 5):S54–S60.
60. Alper SL, Darman RB, Chernova MN, Dahl NK. The AE gene family of Cl/HCO3- exchangers. *J Nephrol* 2002;(Suppl 5):S41–S53.
61. Karet F. Inherited distal renal tubular acidosis. *J Amer Soc Nephrol* 2002;13:2178–2184.
62. Royaux IE, Wall SM, Karniski LP, et al. Pendrin, encoded by the Pendred syndrome gene, resides in the apical region of renal intercalated cells and mediates bicarbonate secretion. *Proc Natl Acad Sci U S A* 2001;4221–4226.
63. Parker MD, Ourmozdi EP, Tanner MJ. Human BTR1, a new bicarbonate transporter superfamily member and human AE4 from kidney. *Biochem Biophys Res Commun* 2001;282:1103–1109.
64. Malnic G, Fernandez R, Cassola AC et al. Mechanisms and regulation of H^+ transport in distal tubule epithelial cells. *Wien Klin Wochenschr* 1997;109:429–434.
65. Nagami GT. Enhanced ammonia secretion by proximal tubules from mice receiving NH4Cl: role of angiotensin II. *Amer J Physiol* 2002;282:F472–F477.
66. Hulter HN, Peterson JC. Acid-base homeostasis during chronic PTH excess in humans. *Kidney Int* 1985;28:187–192.
67. Jaeger P, Jones W, Kashgarian M, et al. Parathyroid hormone directly inhibits tubular reabsorption of bicarbonate in normocalcemic rats with chronic hyperparathyroidism. *Eur J Clin Invest* 1987;17:415–420.
68. Fan L, Wiederkehr MR, Collazo R, et al. Dual mechanisms of regulation of Na/H exchanger NHE-3 by parathyroid hormone in rat kidney. *J Biol Chem* 1999;274:11289–11295.
69. Sicuro A, Mahlbacher K, Hulter HN, et al. Effect of growth hormone on renal and systemic acid-base homeostasis in humans. *Amer J Physiol* 1998;274:F650–F657.
70. Swan JC, Pitts RF. Neutralization of infused acid by nephrectomized dogs. *J Clin Invest* 1955;34:205.
71. Singer RB, Clark JK, Barker ES, et al. The acute effects in man of rapid intravenous infusion of hypertonic sodium bicarbonate solution. *Medicine (Baltimore)* 1955;35:51.
72. Cheema-Dhadli S, Lin SH, Halperin SL. Mechanisms used to dispose of progressively increasing alkali load in rats. *Amer J Physiol* 2002;282:F1049–F1055.
73. Kim GH, Martin SW, Fernandez-Llama P, et al. Long-term regulation of Na-dependent cotransporters and EnaC: response to altered acid-base intake. *Amer J Physiol* 2000;279:F459–F467.
74. Karim Z, Attmane-Elakeb A, Bichara M. Renal handling of NH4+ in relation to the control of acid-base balance by the kidney. *J Nephrol* 2002;(Suppl 5):S128–S134.
75. Madias NE, Adrogue HJ. Acid base disturbances in pulmonary medicine. In: Arieff AI, DeFronzo RA, eds. *Fluid, electrolyte and acid-base disorders.* New York: Churchill Livingstone, 1995;223–253.
76. Eiam-ong S, Laski ME, Kurtzman NA, Sabatini S. Effect of respiratory acidosis and respiratory alkalosis on renal transport enzymes. *Amer J Physiol* 1994;267:F390–F399.
77. Brant SR, Bernstein M, Wasmuth JJ, et al. Physical and genetic mapping of a human apical epithelial Na^+/H^+ exchanger (NHE-3) isoform to chromosome 5p15.3. *Genomics* 1993;15: 668–672.
78. Guillery EN, Karniski LP, Matthews MS, Robillard JE. Maturation of proximal tubule Na^+/H^+ antiporter activity in sheep from fetus to newborn. *Amer J Physiol* 1994;267:E337–E345.
79. Igarashi T, Inatomi J, Sekine T, et al. Mutations in SLC4A4 cause permanent isolated proximal renal tubular acidosis with ocular abnormalities. *Nat Genet* 1999;23:264–266.
80. Batlle D, Ghanekar H, Jain S, Mitra A. Hereditary distal renal tubular acidosis, new understandings. *Ann Rev Medicine* 2001;52:471–484.
81. Bruce LJ, Cope Dl, Jones GK, et al. Familial distal renal tubular acidosis is associated with mutations in the red cell anion exchanger (band 3, AE1) gene. *J Clin Invest* 1997; 100:1693–1707.
82. Tanphaichitr VS, Sumboonnanonda A, Ideguchi H, et al. Novel AE1 mutations in recessive distal renal tubular acidosis. Loss-of-function is rescued by glycophorin A. *J Clin Invest* 1998;102:2173–2179.
83. Roth DE, Venta PJ, Tashian RE, Sly WS. Molecular basis of human carbonic anhydrase II deficiency. *Pro Nalt Acad Sci U S A* 1992;89:1804–1808.

84. Karet FE, Finberg KE, Nelson RD, et al. Mutations in the gene encoding B1 subunit of H⁺ATPase cause renal tubular acidosis with sensorineural deafness. *Nat Genet* 1999;21: 67–68.
85. Smith AN, Skaung J, Choate KA, et al. Mutations in ATP6N1B, encoding a new kidney vacuolar proton pump 116-kD subunit, cause recessive distal renal tubular acidosis with preserved hearing. *Nat Genet* 2000;26:71–75.
86. Strautniekds SS, Thompson RJ, Gardiner RM, Chung E. A novel splice-site mutation in the gamma subunit of the epithelial sodium channel gene in three pseudohypoaldosteronism type 1 families. *Nat Genet* 1996;13:248–253.
87. Chang SS, Grunder S, Hanukoglu A, et al. Mutations in subunits of the epithelial sodium channel cause salt wasting with hyperkalemic acidosis, pseudohypoaldosteronism type 1. *Nat Genet* 1996;12:248–253.
88. Grunder S, Firsov D, Chang SS, et al. A mutation causing pseudohypoaldosteronism type 1 identifies a conserved glycine that is involved in the gating of the epithelial sodium channel. *EMBO J* 1997;16:899–907.
89. Geller DS, Rodriguez-Soriano J, Ballor Boadao A, et al. Mutations in the mineralocorticoid receptor gene cause autosomal dominant pseudohypoaldosteronism type I. *Nat Genet* 1998;19:279–281.
90. Wilson FH, Disse-Nicodeme S, Choate KA, et al. Human hypertension caused by WNK kinases. *Science* 2001;293: 1107–1112.
91. Simon DB, Karet FE, Hamdan JM, et al. Bartter's syndrome, hypokalemic alkalosis with hypercalciuria, is caused by mutations in the Na-K-2Cl cotransporter NKCC2. *Nat Genet* 1996;13:183–188.
92. Simon DB, Karet FE, Rodriquez-Soriano J, et al. Genetic heterogeneity of Bartter's syndrome revealed by mutations in the K+ channel ROMK. *Nat Genet* 1996;14:152–156.
93. International Collaborative Study Group for Bartter-like Syndromes. Mutations in the gene encoding the inwardly-rectifying renal potassium channel, ROMK, cause the antenatal variant of Bartter syndrome: evidence for genetic heterogeneity. *Hum Mol Genet* 1997;6:17–26.
94. Simon KB, Bindra RS, Mansfield TA, et al. Mutations in the chloride channel gene, CLCNKB, cause Bartter's syndrome type III. *Nat Genet* 1997;17:171–178.
95. Birkenhager R, Otto E, Schurmann MJ, et al Mutations of BSND causes Bartter syndrome with sensorineural deafness and kidney failure. *Nat Genet* 2001;29:310–314.
96. Estevez R, Boettger T, Stein V, et al. Bartin is a Cl- channel beta-subunit crucial for renal Cl- reabsorption and inner ear K+ secretion. *Nature* 2001;414:558–561.
97. Simon DB, Nelson-Williams C, Bia MJ, et al. Gitelman's variant of Bartter's syndrome, inherited hypokalemic alkalosis, is caused by mutations in the thiazide-sensitive Na-Cl cotransporter. *Nat Genet* 1996;12:24–30.
98. Hansson JH, Schild L, Lu Y, et al. A *de novo* missense mutation of the beta subunit of the epithelial sodium channel causes hypertension and Liddle syndrome, identifying a proline-rich segment critical for regulation of channel activity. *Proc Natl Acad Sci U S A* 1995;92:11495–11499.
99. Shimkets RA, Warnock DG, Bositis CM, et al. Liddle's syndrome: heritable human hypertension caused by mutations in the beta subunit of the epithelial sodium channel. *Cell* 1994;79:407–414.
100. Hansson JH, Nelson-Williams C, Suzuki H, et al. Hypertension caused by a truncated epithelial sodium channel gamma subunit: genetic heterogeneity of Liddle syndrome. *Nat Genet* 1995;11:76–82.
101. Lifton RP, Dluhy RG, Powers M, et al. Hereditary hypertension caused by chimaeric gene duplications and ectopic expression of aldosterone synthase. *Nat Genet* 1992;2:66–74.
102. Wilson RC, Dave-Sharma S, Wei JQ, et al. A genetic defect resulting in mild low-renin hypertension. *Proc Nalt Acad Sci U S A* 1998;95:10200–10205.
103. Challa A, Chan W, Krieg RJ Jr, et al. Effect of metabolic acidosis on the expression of insulin-like growth factor and growth hormone receptor. *Kidney Int* 1993;44:1224–1227.

10

CALCIUM AND PHOSPHORUS

ANTHONY A. PORTALE

CALCIUM

Body Composition

Calcium is the most abundant electrolyte in the human body, and in healthy adults, accounts for approximately 2%, or 1300 g, of body weight. Approximately 99% of body calcium is in the skeleton, mainly in the form of hydroxyapatite crystals ($[Ca_{10}(PO_4)_6(OH)_2]$); the remainder is in teeth, soft tissue, and extracellular fluid. By contrast, at birth, calcium accounts for only approximately 0.9% of body weight (1). From birth to approximately 20 years of age, when the skeleton reaches its full size and density, calcium content increases by some 40-fold (2). During this period, the increase in skeletal weight and calcium content requires the net retention of 150 to 200 mg of calcium per day. Thus, in growing individuals, calcium balance must be positive to meet the needs of skeletal growth and consolidation. In adults, calcium balance is zero after peak bone mass is attained and becomes slightly negative as bone is slowly lost with aging.

Extracellular Metabolism of Calcium

Calcium in plasma exists in three fractions: protein-bound calcium (40%), which is not filtered by the renal glomerulus, and ionized calcium (48%) and complexed calcium (12%), which are filtered (3). Complexed calcium is that bound to various anions such as phosphate, citrate, and bicarbonate. Albumin accounts for 90% of the protein binding of calcium in plasma, and globulins for the remainder. Conditions that affect the concentration of albumin in plasma, such as nephrotic syndrome or hepatic cirrhosis, affect the measurement of total serum calcium concentration. A decrease in albumin concentration of 1 g/dL results in a decrease in protein-bound and hence total calcium concentration of approximately 0.8 mg/dL. Binding of calcium to albumin is strongly pH dependent between pH 7 and pH 8; an acute increase or decrease in pH of 0.1 pH units will increase or decrease protein-bound calcium, respectively, by approximately 0.12 mg/dL. Thus, in hypocalcemic patients with metabolic acidosis, rapid correction of acidemia with sodium bicarbonate can precipitate tetany, due to increased binding of calcium to albumin and a consequent decrease in the ionized calcium concentration.

The total serum calcium concentration exhibits a circadian rhythm characterized by a nadir at 1 to 3 a.m. and a peak at 12 to 1 p.m., with amplitude (nadir to peak) of approximately 0.5 mg/dL (4–6). This rhythm is thought to reflect hemodynamic changes in serum albumin concentration that result from changes in body posture (7). Prolonged upright posture or venostasis can cause hemoconcentration and thus increases of approximately 0.5 mg/dL in serum calcium concentration. There is little difference between values taken in fasting and nonfasting states.

Normal values of serum total calcium concentration differ among clinical laboratories and in general range from 9.0 to 10.6 mg/dL. The calcium concentration is higher in children than in adult subjects. It is highest at 6 to 24 months of age (mean of approximately 10.2 mg/dL), decreases to a plateau of approximately 9.8 mg/dL at 6 to 8 years, and decreases further to adult values at 16 to 20 years (8). In men, the calcium concentration decreases from a mean of approximately 9.6 mg/dL at age 20 to approximately 9.2 mg/dL at age 80 years; the decrease can be accounted for by a decrease in serum albumin concentration (9). In women, no change is observed with age.

Ionized calcium is the fraction of plasma calcium that is important for physiologic processes such as muscle contraction, blood coagulation, nerve conduction, hormone secretion and action (parathyroid hormone [PTH] and 1,25-dihydroxyvitamin D [$1,25(OH)_2D$]), ion transport, and bone mineralization. Measurement of the blood ionized calcium concentration is most useful in critically ill patients, particularly those in whom serum protein levels are decreased or acid-base disturbances are present, or to whom large amounts of citrated blood products are given, such as with cardiac surgery or hepatic transplantation. A decrease in the blood ionized calcium concentration can occur not only due to increased binding of calcium to albumin, such as in metabolic alkalosis, but also due to increased complexing with other anions. For example, in severe uremia, the ionized fraction of calcium can decrease due to increased complexing with phosphate, sulfate, and citrate (10). Based on *in vitro* studies of human serum (11), an increase in serum phosphorus concentration of 3.7 mg/dL was required to induce a decrease in ionized calcium of 0.1 mg/dL, the smallest decrease thought necessary to stimulate release of PTH (12,13).

Determinations of the concentration of ionized calcium in healthy individuals vary somewhat among laboratories depending on which technique is used and whether the measurement is made on serum, plasma, or heparinized whole blood. In healthy infants, ionized calcium levels decrease from approximately 5.8 mg/dL (1.4 mmol/L) at birth to a nadir of 4.9 mg/dL (1.2 mmol/L) at 24 hours of life (14), and increase slightly during the first week of life (15). Values in young children are slightly higher (by approximately 0.2 mg/dL) than those in adults until after puberty. In adult men and women, normal serum ionized calcium concentrations range from 4.6 to 5.3 mg/dL (1.0 to 1.3 mmol/L); there are no significant sex differences (16,17). The blood ionized calcium concentration exhibits a circadian rhythm characterized by a peak at 10 a.m. and a nadir at 6 to 8 p.m., with an amplitude of 0.3 mg/dL (4). Specimens must be obtained anaerobically to avoid spurious results due to *ex vivo* changes in pH.

Extracellular Calcium Homeostasis

Calcium homeostasis is maintained by the interaction between three major organ systems, bone, intestine, and kidney. It is regulated principally by PTH and 1,25(OH)$_2$D and, to a lesser extent, by calcitonin. In healthy adults, net intestinal absorption of calcium is 20 to 25% of dietary intake. To meet the demands of rapid skeletal growth, fractional calcium absorption in infants is higher, 40 to 45%, reaching values as high as 80% in low-birth-weight, breast-fed infants (18,19). The efficiency of calcium absorption also is increased during adolescence, during pregnancy, and with administration of vitamin D metabolites, and is decreased in vitamin D deficiency and in the elderly. Calcium is absorbed principally in the duodenum and proximal jejunum, both by a saturable, active transport mechanism that requires stimulation by 1,25(OH)$_2$D and by a nonsaturable, passive diffusion mechanism. A small amount of calcium is secreted into the intestinal lumen, presumably by paracellular diffusion. An overall schema of calcium metabolism is depicted in Figure 10.1.

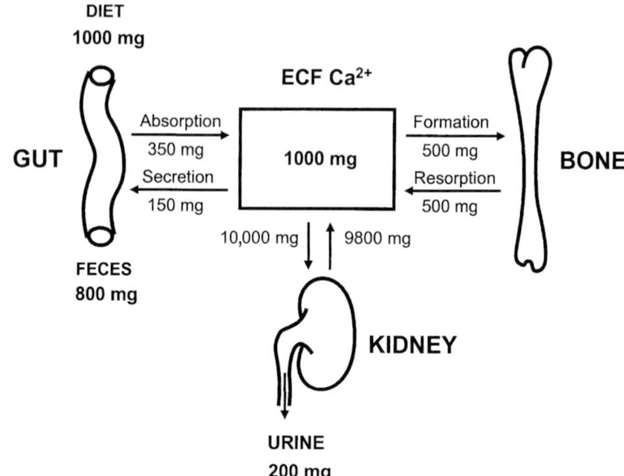

FIGURE 10.1. Calcium fluxes between body pools in the normal adult human in zero calcium balance. ECF, extracellular fluid.

Absorbed calcium enters the extracellular calcium pool, which is in equilibrium with the bone calcium pool; the latter includes a rapidly exchangeable pool, which plays an important role in maintaining extracellular calcium concentration, and a more stable bone mineral pool. Calcium is filtered by the renal glomerulus and is nearly completely reabsorbed by the renal tubule. In individuals in zero calcium balance, the amount of calcium excreted by the kidney is equal to the net amount absorbed by the intestine, and in growing children is less than the net amount absorbed due to deposition of calcium in bone. In response to a decrease in extracellular concentration of ionized calcium, secretion of PTH from the parathyroid gland is increased (Fig. 10.2). PTH acts on the kidney to decrease excretion of calcium, to increase excretion of phosphorus, and to stimulate the production of 1,25(OH)$_2$D. The 1,25(OH)$_2$D acts on the intestine to stimulate active absorption of calcium and phosphorus, and, together with PTH, acts on bone to stimulate release of calcium and phosphorus into the extracellular fluid. PTH action on bone is thought to occur in two phases: an initial rapid mobilization of bone mineral that occurs within hours, is associated with increased metabolic activity of osteoclasts, and does not require protein synthesis, and a later phase that occurs after 12 to 24 hours of exposure to PTH, is associated with an increase in both the activity and num-

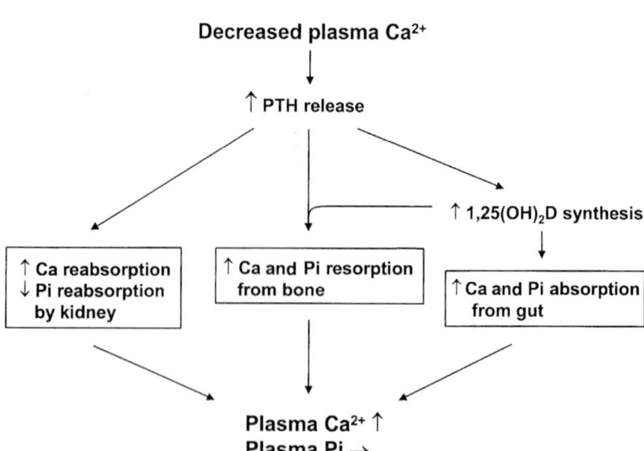

FIGURE 10.2. The homeostatic response to hypocalcemia. 1,25(OH)$_2$D, 1,25-dihydroxyvitamin D; Pi, inorganic phosphate; PTH, parathyroid hormone.

bers of osteoclasts, and does require protein synthesis (20). The combined effects of PTH and 1,25$(OH)_2$D on their target tissues results in an increase in extracellular calcium concentration toward normal values, with the serum phosphorus concentration being little changed.

Conversely, in response to an increase in blood ionized calcium concentration, secretion of PTH and production of 1,25$(OH)_2$D are decreased, and release of calcitonin is stimulated. The combined effects of these hormonal changes on bone, kidney, and intestine are opposite to those occurring with hypocalcemia and result in a decrease in calcium concentration toward normal values.

Calcium Receptor

Changes in the extracellular calcium concentration are detected by the extracellular calcium-sensing receptor (CaR) located on the plasma membrane of parathyroid cells. The CaR has been cloned from bovine, human, and rat parathyroid tissue (21–23) and from rat kidney (24). The receptor has a predicted molecular weight of approximately 120 kDa and is a member of the superfamily of receptors that couple with guanine-nucleotide-regulatory (G) proteins. Activation of the CaR results in increased activity of the enzyme phospholipase-C, which catalyzes the hydrolysis of the membrane-bound phospholipid inositol 4,5-bisphosphate to two second messengers, inositol 1,4,5-triphosphate (IP3) and diacylglycerol. Intracellular accumulation of IP3 induces release of calcium from storage pools and thereby a rapid increase in cytosolic calcium concentration, and possibly an increase in movement of calcium from the extracellular to the cellular compartment. In parathyroid cells, the increase in cytosolic calcium concentration is associated with a decrease in secretion of PTH.

Vitamin D

Vitamin D exists as either ergocalciferol (vitamin D_2) produced by plants, or cholecalciferol (vitamin D_3) produced by animal tissues and by the action of near-ultraviolet radiation (290 to 320 nm) on 7-dehydrocholesterol in human skin. Both forms of vitamin D are biologically inactive prohormones that must undergo successive hydroxylations at carbons 25 and 1 before they can bind to and activate the vitamin D receptor. The 25-hydroxylation of vitamin D occurs in the liver, catalyzed by one or more enzymes, including the mitochondrial enzyme vitamin D 25-hydroxylase. The activity of hepatic 25-hydroxylation is not under tight physiologic regulation, and thus circulating concentrations of 25OHD are determined primarily by dietary intake of vitamin D and exposure to sunlight. Although 25OHD is the most abundant form of vitamin D in the blood, it has minimal capacity to bind to the vitamin D receptor and elicit a biologic response.

The active form of vitamin D, 1,25$(OH)_2$D, is produced by the 1α-hydroxylation of 25OHD by the mitochondrial enzyme 25-hydroxyvitamin D-1α-hydroxylase (1α-hydroxylase or P450c1α). The circulating concentration of 1,25$(OH)_2$D primarily reflects its synthesis in the kidney; however, 1α-hydroxylase activity also is found in keratinocytes, macrophages, and osteoblasts (25–27). The 1α-hydroxylation is the rate-limiting step in the bioactivation of vitamin D, and enzyme activity in the kidney is tightly regulated. The steroid 1,25$(OH)_2$D is one of the principal hormonal regulators of calcium and phosphorus metabolism and thus is critically important for normal growth and mineralization of bone. The classical actions of 1,25$(OH)_2$D are to stimulate calcium and phosphorus absorption from the intestine and thereby maintain plasma concentrations of these ions at levels sufficient for normal growth and mineralization of bone. The hormone 1,25$(OH)_2$D also has direct actions on bone, kidney, parathyroid gland, and many other tissues unrelated to mineral metabolism (reviewed in 28).

The other important vitamin D–metabolizing enzyme, 25-hydroxyvitamin D-24-hydroxylase (24-hydroxylase), is found in kidney, intestine, lymphocytes, fibroblasts, bone, skin, macrophages, and possibly other tissues (29). The enzyme can catalyze the 24-hydroxylation of 25OHD to 24,25$(OH)_2$D and of 1,25$(OH)_2$D to 1,24,25$(OH)_3$D; both reactions are thought to initiate the metabolic inactivation of vitamin D via the C24-oxidation pathway. The kidney and intestine are major sites of hormonal inactivation of vitamin D by virtue of their abundant 24-hydroxylase activity.

The synthesis of 1,25$(OH)_2$D in the kidney is subject to complex regulation by PTH, calcium, phosphorus, and 1,25$(OH)_2$D (28,30,31). Synthesis of 1,25$(OH)_2$D can be stimulated by PTH, insulin-like growth factor-1, and phosphorus deficiency, and can be suppressed by plasma ionized calcium and 1,25$(OH)_2$D itself. The renal 1α-hydroxylase enzyme is a mitochondrial cytochrome P450 mixed-function oxidase that requires the presence of two electron transport intermediates for catalytic activity, a flavoprotein termed *ferredoxin reductase* and an iron-sulfur protein termed ferredoxin (32). These two proteins mediate the transfer of electrons from the reduced form of nicotinamide adenine dinucleotide phosphate to the 1α-hydroxylase. The complementary DNA (cDNA) for the 1α-hydroxylase, designated P450c1α, has been cloned from human, rat, mouse, and pig (33–38). The human P450c1α cDNA is 2.4 kilobases (kb) in length and encodes a protein of 508 amino acids with a predicted molecular mass of 56 kDa (33). The human gene for 1α-hydroxylase (officially termed CYP27B1) is single copy, comprises nine exons and eight introns, and is located on chromosome 12 (Fig. 10.3) (34,39). Although, at 5 kb, it is a substantially smaller gene than those for other mitochondrial P450 enzymes (39), its intron-exon organization is very similar, especially to that of P450scc (39,40). This strongly suggests that, although the mitochondrial P450 enzymes retain only 30 to 40% amino acid sequence identity with each other, they all belong to a single evolutionary lineage. The mouse P450c1α gene also has been cloned (41,42).

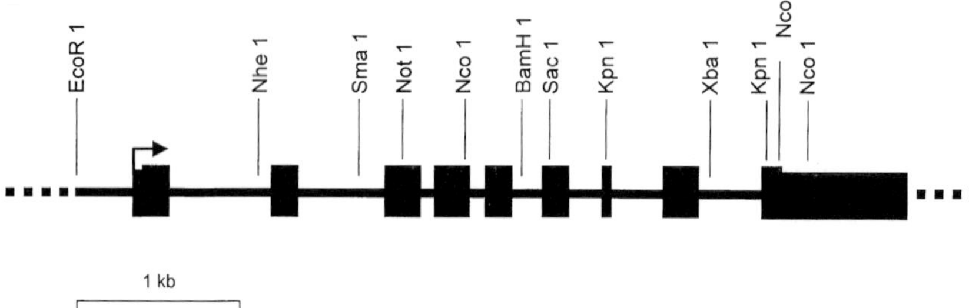

FIGURE 10.3. Scale diagram of the human P450c1α gene showing the intron-exon organization and principal restriction endonuclease cleavage sites. The lesser-thickness bars at the beginning and end of the first and last exons represent the 5' and 3' untranslated regions, respectively. (From Fu GK, Portale AA, Miller WL. Complete structure of the human gene for the vitamin D 1α-hydroxylase, P450c1α. *DNA Cell Biol* 1997;16:1499–1507, with permission.)

Loss-of-function mutations in the human P450c1α gene result in the autosomal recessive disease vitamin D 1α-hydroxylase deficiency (33,43–49), also known as *hereditary pseudo–vitamin D deficiency rickets* (50), *vitamin D dependency* (51), or *vitamin D–dependent rickets type I.* As of mid-2003 a total of 31 different mutations have been found on 88 distinct chromosomes since the first description of gene mutations in 1997 (33,48).

Cellular Metabolism of Calcium

A detailed discussion of intracellular calcium metabolism is found in comprehensive reviews (52–54). Most of the total amount of calcium in the cell, estimated at approximately 10^{-3} mol/L, is sequestered in intracellular storage compartments, principally the endoplasmic reticulum and mitochondria, or bound to specific cytoplasmic proteins such as calmodulin and calbindin-D. The cytosolic concentration of free ionized calcium is approximately 10^{-7} mol/L, 10,000-fold lower than that in extracellular fluid. Thus, a steep gradient exists that favors movement of calcium into the cell. Cytosolic calcium serves as an intracellular second messenger and plays a critical role in regulating physiologic functions, including muscle contraction, neurosecretion, hormone secretion and action, cell division and aggregation, membrane permeability, enzyme activity, and gene transcription. The cytosolic calcium concentration is tightly regulated by interplay between specific mechanisms of calcium entry into and exit from the cell, movement of calcium into and from intracellular storage compartments, and reversible complexing of calcium by high-affinity cytosolic calcium-binding proteins. Binding of calcium to such proteins provides for rapid and precise buffering of cytosolic calcium concentration. Long-term maintenance of the calcium gradient between the cytosol and extracellular environment is provided by calcium pumps and exchangers, which are intrinsic to the plasma membrane and the membranes of intracellular organelles. Mitochondria can buffer large amounts of ionized calcium when its cytosolic concentration increases to levels sufficient to activate the low-affinity mitochondrial transport systems.

Transepithelial Transport of Calcium

Transport of calcium across the plasma membrane of calcium-absorbing epithelia such as the intestine and renal tubule occurs via either the paracellular (between cells) or the transcellular (across cells) pathway, or via both pathways (Fig. 10.4). Paracellular transport is passive, linked to the net paracellular absorption (lumen-to-interstitium) of water, a process termed *solvent drag* or *convection.* Paracellular transport of calcium also can occur by passive diffusion driven by a chemical gradient, as occurs in the proximal convoluted tubule (PCT), or a lumen-positive transepithelial potential difference that results from sodium chloride reabsorption, as occurs in the thick ascending limb of the loop of Henle (TALH).

Transcellular transport of calcium is a three-step process consisting of passive entry across the apical membrane, diffusion through the cytosol facilitated by $1,25(OH)_2D$-dependent calcium-binding proteins (calbindins), and active extrusion across the basolateral membrane mediated by a high-affinity Ca^{2+}–adenosine triphosphatase (ATPase) and Na^+-Ca^{2+} exchanger (55).

Calcium Entry

Although calcium entry across the luminal membrane is favored by both electrical and chemical gradients (56,57), the physical and chemical properties of lipid bilayer membranes prevent passive diffusion of the positively charged Ca^{2+} ion across cell membranes. Thus, calcium entry across the luminal membranes of the kidney and intestine is thought to occur through Ca^{2+} channels. Studies using a variety of approaches, including Ca^{2+} channel agonists and antagonists, patch-clamp analysis, and cell-attached electrophysiologic techniques, have shown the presence of calcium channels in proximal and distal nephron segments and in cultured distal renal tubule cells (58). Using an expression cloning strategy, Hoenderop et al. (59) cloned and characterized the cDNA encoding a new epithelial Ca^{2+} influx channel, which is named ECaC by analogy with the amiloride-sensitive, aldosterone-dependent epithelial sodium channel, ENaC (60,61). ECaC is expressed exclusively in the distal renal tubule, proximal small intestine, and placenta. The rabbit ECaC cDNA encodes a protein of 730 amino acids with a predicted molecular mass of 83 kDa (59). In rabbit kidney, ECaC is present along the apical membranes of the distal convoluted tubule (DCT), connecting tubule (CNT), and cor-

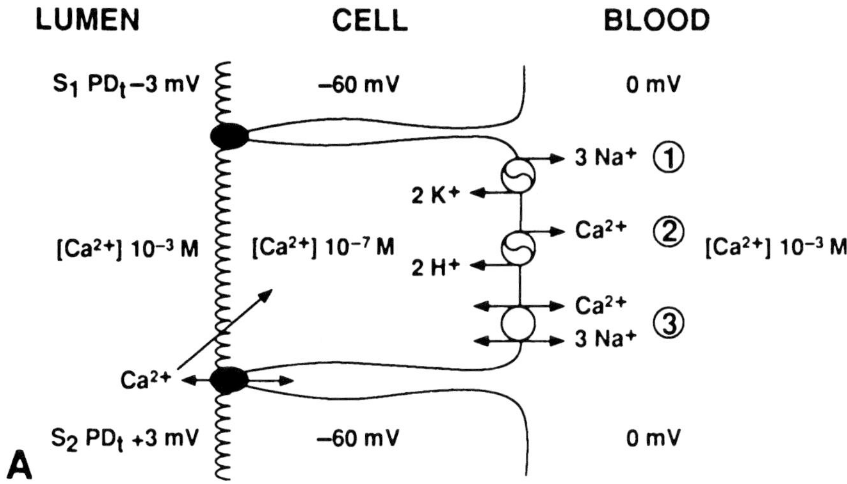

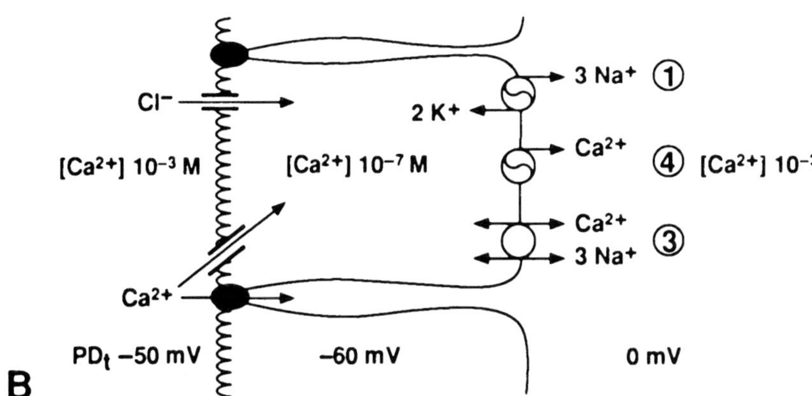

FIGURE 10.4. Possible cellular mechanisms involved in calcium transport in the proximal S1 and S2 tubule segments **(A)** and the distal convoluted tubule **(B)**. Major transport systems are (a) Na^+-K^+-adenosine triphosphatase; (b) adenosine triphosphate–dependent Ca^{2+}-H^+ exchanger; (c) Na^+-Ca^{2+} exchanger; and (d) Mg^{2+}-dependent Ca^{2+}-adenosine triphosphatase. For the distal tubule, calcium and chloride channels are depicted by "=." (From Suki WN, Rouse D. Renal transport of calcium, magnesium, and phosphate. In: Suki WN, Rouse D, eds. *Brenner and Rector's the kidney*. Philadelphia: WB Saunders, 1996:472–509, with permission.)

tical collecting duct, where it co-localizes with calbindin-D_{28K} (59,62). This part of the nephron is the major site of regulation of Ca^{2+} reabsorption by PTH and $1,25(OH)_2D$, and ECaC is thought to play a major role in such regulation. ECaC has been identified in several species, including rabbit, rat, mouse, and human (58,63).

Transcytoplasmic Calcium Movement

It is proposed that calcium diffusion through the cytoplasm is facilitated by the calcium-binding protein calbindin-D, whose synthesis is dependent on $1,25(OH)_2D$. Calbindins also are proposed to act as an intracellular Ca^{2+} buffer to keep the otherwise tightly regulated cytosolic calcium concentration within physiologic levels during periods of stimulated transcellular Ca^{2+} transport (64–68). Two forms of calbindin-D have been described: a 28-kDa protein (calbindin-D_{28K}) found in highest concentration in avian intestine and avian and mammalian kidney, brain, and pancreas, and a 9-kDa protein (calbindin-D_{9K}) found in highest concentration in mammalian intestine, placenta, and uterus but also present in kidney, lung, and bone (69,70). Much is now known about the amino acid sequence, x-ray crystal structure, and biophysical and calcium-binding properties of the calbindins. Calbindin-D_{28K} is highly conserved in evolution, with a high degree of sequence homology observed among the various mammalian and avian D_{28K} calbindins (71). By contrast, calbindin-D_{9K} is not highly conserved, and there is no amino acid sequence similarity between calbindin-D_{28K} and calbindin-D_{9K}. The genes for both rat calbindin species and chicken calbindin-D_{28K} have been cloned and sequenced, and their transcriptional regulation by $1,25(OH)_2D$, glucocorticoids, and other factors has been investigated (reviewed in 69 and 70).

The calbindins belong to the superfamily of EF-hand helix-loop-helix, high-affinity calcium-binding proteins (dissociation constant of 10^{-8} to 10^{-6} mol/L), which contains more than 250 proteins. Calbindin-D_{28K} binds 4 mol of calcium per mole of protein and calbindin-D_{9K} binds 2 mol of calcium per mole of protein. In the intestine, $1,25(OH)_2D$ stimulates both the synthesis of calbindin and the transfer of calcium across the luminal brush-border membrane (BBM). The rate and time course of active calcium absorption correlate well with the amount of calbindin-D over a wide variety of physiologic conditions (72,73), which provides strong support for the role of calbindin-D_{28K} and calbindin-D_{9K} in vitamin D–dependent active calcium transport. Calbindin-D may play a similar role in mediating active renal tubular reabsorption of calcium (74,75). In several mammalian species, both calbindin-D_{28K} and ECaC have been localized in the DCT and CNT (59,62,76,77), which are the major sites of active calcium reabsorption. Calbindin-D_{9K} also has been localized to the distal nephron in the rat and mouse (78,79).

Calcium Exit

At the basolateral membrane, calcium is actively extruded from the cell against its electrochemical gradient, a process mediated via a high-affinity, magnesium-dependent Ca^{2+}-ATPase or an electrogenic $3Na^{+}$-$1Ca^{2+}$ exchanger.

Ca^{2+}–Adenosine Triphosphatase

The plasma membrane Ca^{2+}-ATPase (Ca^{2+} pump) is an obligatory component of eukaryotic plasma membranes that mediates efflux of calcium from the cell. It is thought to play the most important role in maintaining the cytosolic calcium concentration within the normal range. The Ca^{2+} pump belongs to the family of P-type ATPases in that it forms a phosphorylated intermediate (an aspartylphosphate) during the reaction cycle. The pump has a high affinity for calcium, with an estimated Michaelis-Menton constant of 0.2 mmol/L and an apparent molecular weight of 120 to 140 kDa (reviewed in 80–84). The pump is activated by direct interaction with calmodulin, a specific calcium receptor protein present in the cytosol, which results in an increase in both the pump's affinity for calcium and its maximum transport velocity (V_{max}). The pump also is activated by cyclic adenosine monophosphate (cAMP)–dependent and protein kinase C–dependent phosphorylation of the pump protein, by limited proteolysis, and by exposure to acidic phospholipids. Transport of calcium from the cell is balanced by countertransport of hydrogen ion (H^{+}), and thus the activity of the Ca^{2+} pump can be either electroneutral (Ca^{2+}-$2H^{+}$) or electrogenic (Ca^{2+}-H^{+}).

The Ca^{2+} pump is located exclusively in the basolateral portion of the plasma membrane of renal tubule cells (85,86). In earlier studies, activity of the Ca^{2+} pump was found along the entire length of the rabbit nephron, with the activity highest in the distal tubule where the majority of active calcium reabsorption occurs (87). In later studies using monoclonal antibodies against the erythrocyte plasma membrane Ca^{2+} pump, an epitope of this enzyme was identified in human and rat kidneys in the basolateral portion of only the DCT (85,88). The purified Ca^{2+} pump protein co-localizes with calbindin-D_{28K} in this nephron segment (85,88). Analysis of different nephron segments of rat kidney using reverse transcription polymerase chain reaction revealed that the Ca^{2+} pump is expressed in both the distal and proximal nephron (89). In the intestine, the Ca^{2+} pump is stimulated by calmodulin and by $1,25(OH)_2D$, which acts to increase pump activity by increasing its V_{max} (90).

Four isoforms of the plasma membrane Ca^{2+} pump have been identified and their cDNAs cloned (91–95). In humans and rats, the isoforms are encoded by a family of four genes that have been mapped to chromosomes 12, 1, 3, and X. Additional isoforms of the enzyme are created by alternative RNA splicing of the primary gene transcript. The isoforms exhibit 81 to 85% amino acid homology among themselves, and a single isoform exhibits approximately 99% homology among different species (96,97). The deduced amino acid sequences of rat and human isoforms of the plasma membrane Ca^{2+} pump predict a secondary structure that contains 10 transmembrane domains, with four main units accounting for most of the pump mass protruding into the cytoplasm (80,81,97). The predicted secondary structure of the human plasma membrane Ca^{2+} pump is depicted in Figure 10.5.

Na^{+}-Ca^{2+} Exchanger

The Na^{+}-Ca^{2+} exchanger is an integral membrane protein that normally exports calcium from the cell, although under some circumstances it mediates calcium influx. The exchanger is a low-affinity, high-capacity transport system for calcium, which is driven by the inwardly directed transcellular electrochemical Na^{+} gradient that is normally maintained by the basolateral Na^{+}-K^{+}-ATPase. In excitable tissue such as heart and neurons, the exchanger is electrogenic, mediating the export of one intracellular calcium ion for the import of three extracellular sodium ions. Activity of the exchanger is regulated by intracellular calcium, by changes in the transmembrane voltage; it is inhibited by sodium ionophores and ouabain, which reduce the transmembrane sodium gradient, and is increased by ATP (reviewed in 98–100).

Complementary DNAs encoding functional Na^{+}-Ca^{2+} exchangers have been isolated from heart, kidney, and brain in a variety of species (101–107), which suggests that the protein plays an important role in different physiologic processes in various cell types. Three mammalian isoforms of the Na^{+}-Ca^{2+} exchanger (NCX), designated NCX1, NCX2, and NCX3, have been cloned and are the products of separate genes (108–111). NCX1 is expressed most abundantly in heart but is found in most tissues, including kidney, whereas expression of NCX2 and NCX3 is restricted to brain and skeletal muscle (111,112). A number of alternative splicing variants of NCX1 are expressed in a tissue-specific fashion, which is a common feature of a variety of transmembrane proteins (112). The three NCX proteins share 68 to 75% amino acid sequence identity, and all are predicted to share the same topology of 11 membrane-spanning segments with

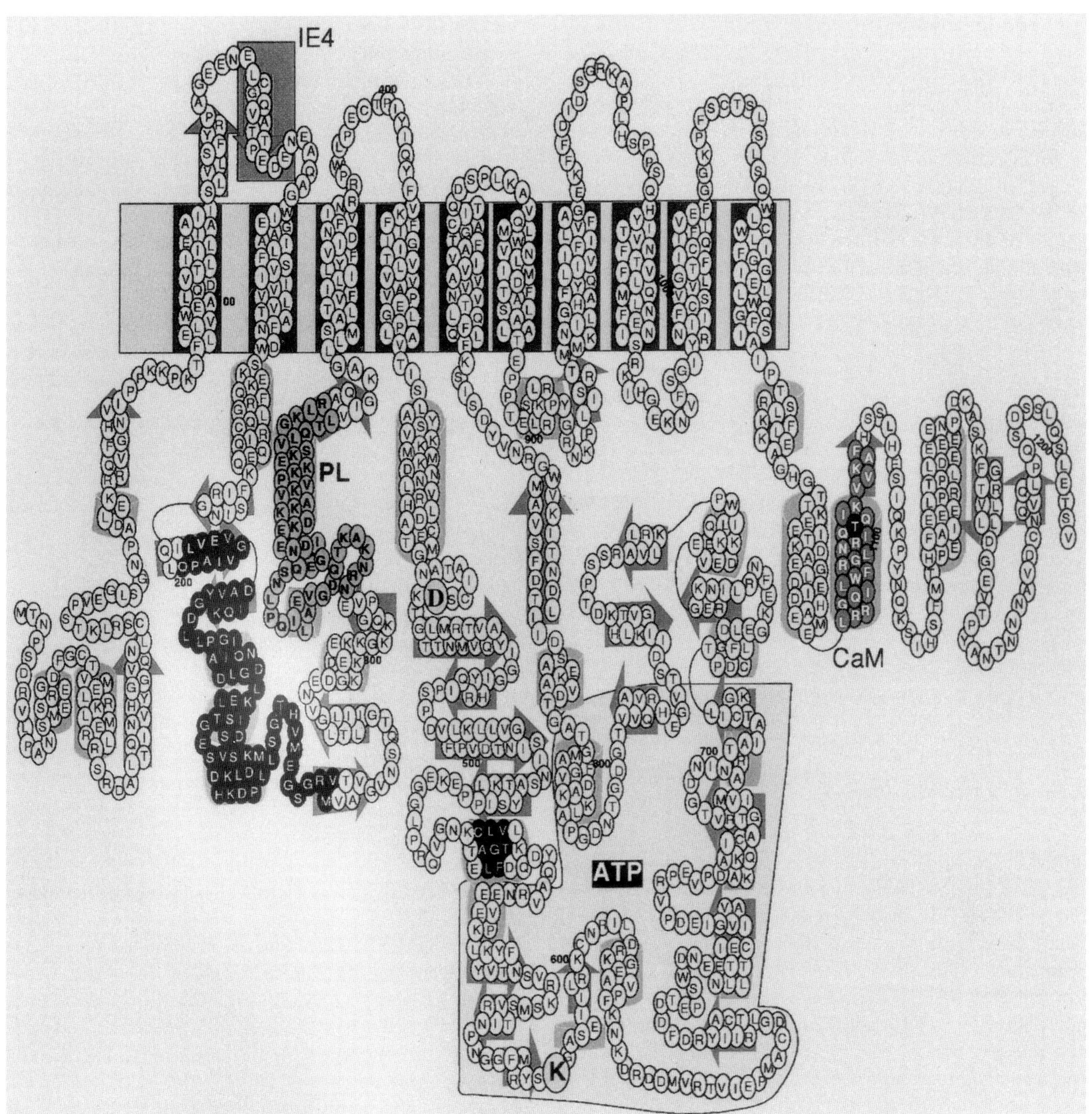

FIGURE 10.5. Sequence, predicted secondary structure, and topology of the plasma membrane Ca^{2+} pump showing ten membrane-spanning domains and four large cytoplasmic regions. CaM is the calmodulin-binding domain. PL is a sequence that interacts with acidic phospholipids. The shaded region (ATP) is the domain where adenosine triphosphate becomes bound. (From Carafoli E, Garcia-Martin E, Guerini D. The plasma membrane calcium pump: recent developments and future perspectives. *Experientia* 1996;52:1091–1100, with permission.)

a large hydrophilic cytoplasmic loop located between membrane-spanning segments 5 and 6. In NCX1, the cytoplasmic loop is thought to be a regulatory region and contains the binding site for Ca^{2+} and the location of the exchanger inhibitory peptide (XIP) sequence (Fig. 10.6).

Activity of the Na^{+}-Ca^{2+} exchanger is found only in basolateral membrane preparations of renal tubules (113) and is localized exclusively to the distal tubule in the rabbit and rat (114). Using antibodies that recognize the Na^{+}-Ca^{2+} exchanger in rabbit kidney, immunolocalization was detected predominately along the basolateral plasma membrane of cortical CNTs, with weak staining of principal cells of the collecting duct; no staining was detected in other cell types in either the cortex or medulla (115). When polymerase chain

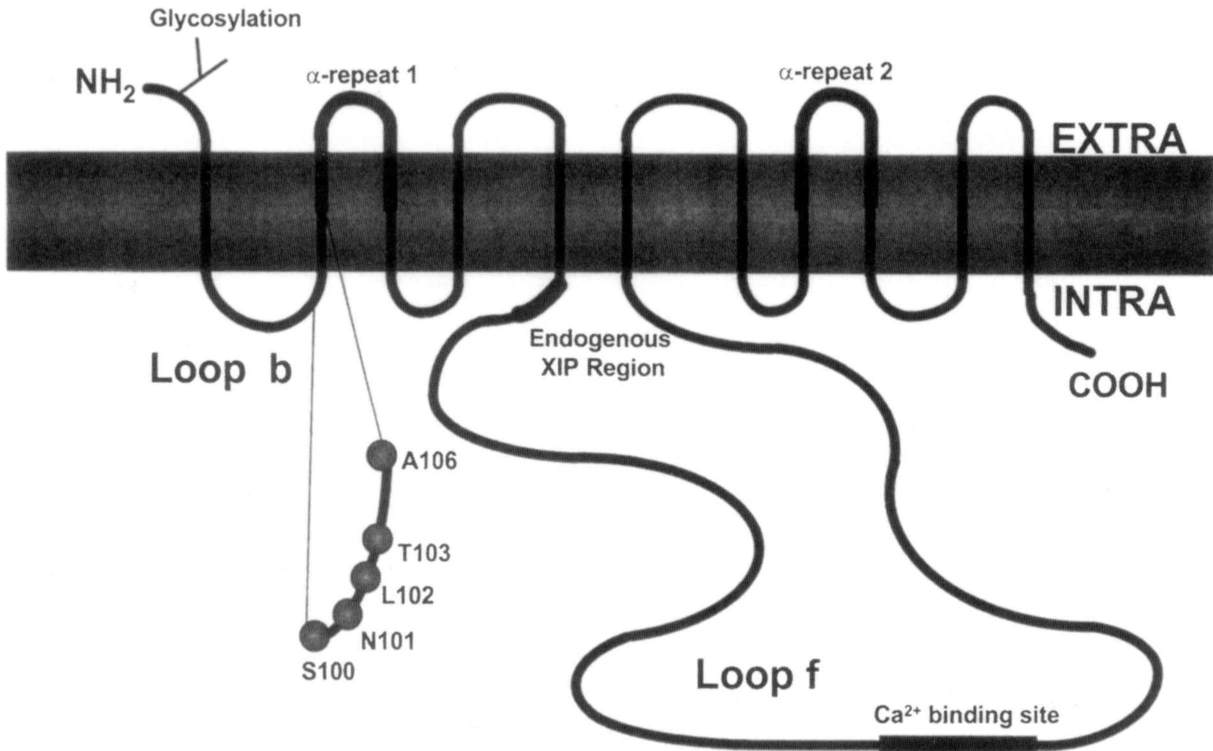

FIGURE 10.6. Topology of the Na^+-Ca^{2+} exchanger isoform NCX1 showing putative transmembrane-spanning domains 1 to 11 and a long intracellular loop, f. Loop f contains regions important in calcium regulation of exchanger activity (Ca^{2+} binding site) and in sodium-dependent inactivation (endogenous XIP region). The α-repeats in the transmembrane domains appear to be important in ion translocation. XIP, exchanger inhibitory peptide. (From Doering AE, Nicoll DA, Lu Y, et al. Topology of a functionally important region of the cardiac Na^+/Ca^{2+} exchanger. *J Biol Chem* 1998;273:778–783, with permission.)

reaction was used to localize the exchanger in microdissected segments of rat nephron, NCX1 expression was observed in the DCT but little or no expression was seen in other segments (116). Thus, the distal nephron exhibits Ca^{2+} pump and Na^+-Ca^{2+} exchanger activity, messenger RNA (mRNA) expression, and protein expression, which is consistent with the important role of this nephron segment in hormone-regulated calcium reabsorption.

Calcium Transport by the Nephron

Approximately 60% of plasma calcium is freely filtered by the glomerulus, as shown by a glomerular filtrate to plasma ratio for calcium that ranges between 0.63 and 0.70 (117,118). The fraction of plasma calcium that is filterable represents ionized calcium and complexed calcium. To maintain zero calcium balance, 98 to 99% of the filtered load of calcium, estimated at approximately 8 g/day in the adult, must be reabsorbed by the renal tubules. Clearance studies in humans and experimental animals show that an increase in the filtered load of calcium, as occurs with calcium infusion, results in an increase in both urine excretion and absolute tubular reabsorption of calcium (119–123). Thus it is thought that no maximum tubular reabsorptive rate exists for calcium within the normal physiologic range (124).

Approximately 70% of filtered calcium is reabsorbed in the proximal tubule; approximately 20% is reabsorbed between the late proximal and early distal tubule, primarily in the TALH; 5 to 10% is reabsorbed in the distal tubule; and less than 5% is reabsorbed in the collecting duct (Fig. 10.7) (117,125–127). Thus, 1 to 3% of filtered calcium is excreted in the urine. As discussed later, physiologic regulation of renal calcium reabsorption occurs in the distal nephron.

Proximal Nephron

The majority of filtered calcium is reabsorbed in the proximal tubule, with approximately 60% being reabsorbed by the end of the accessible portion of the superficial proximal tubule and an additional 10% reabsorbed in the proximal straight tubule. In the early PCT (S1 and S2 segments), calcium is reabsorbed passively in parallel with the reabsorption of sodium and water principally via the paracellular pathway, mediated by convection (solvent drag) across the tight junctions. Evidence for passive reabsorption of calcium is the finding that, in several species studied by micropuncture, the ratio of calcium concentration in tubular

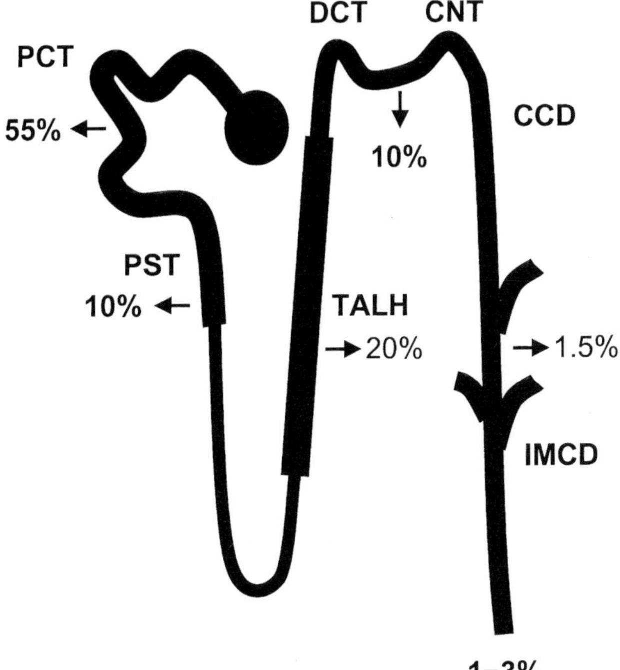

FIGURE 10.7. Profile of calcium reabsorption along the nephron, as derived from micropuncture data. CCD, cortical collecting duct; CNT, connecting tubule; DCT, distal convoluted tubule; IMCD, inner medullary collecting duct; PCT, proximal convoluted tubule; PST, proximal straight tubule; TALH, thick ascending limb of the loop of Henle. (From Friedman PA, Gesek FA. Calcium transport in renal epithelial cells. *Am J Physiol* 1993;264:F181–F198, with permission.)

fluid to that in glomerular ultrafiltrate is approximately 1.0 in the early PCT (127). In the late S1 segment, reabsorption of calcium lags slightly behind that of sodium, which thus creates a favorable chemical gradient for reabsorption downstream. In the S2 segment of the PCT, the transepithelial voltage is lumen positive; thus, the electrical gradient is favorable for passive calcium reabsorption. In rabbit early S2 segments, net flux of calcium was zero in the absence of both water transport and an electrochemical gradient (128), which provides further evidence for passive calcium reabsorption. There also is evidence that calcium reabsorption is active in the proximal nephron, particularly in the earliest segments of the PCT where the transepithelial voltage is lumen negative (127). Calcium reabsorption also appears to be active in the S3 segment of the proximal tubule, because it is not dependent on sodium, occurs against an electrochemical gradient, and is not inhibited by ouabain (129).

Loop of Henle

In the thin descending and ascending limbs of the loop of Henle, calcium transport is negligible (129,130). In the TALH, however, approximately 20% of the filtered calcium load is reabsorbed (127). In isolated, perfused segments of TALH, calcium reabsorption is passive, driven by the large lumen-positive transepithelial voltage difference in this segment (131–133) that results from the secondary active transport of sodium chloride out of tubular fluid. Inhibition of sodium chloride transport with furosemide reduces the transepithelial voltage and thus increases calcium excretion. In some studies, however, calcium transport in the TALH is found to be active (130,134,135). It has been proposed that axial heterogeneity may account for some of the differences observed in the studies reported (136). Calcium transport in the cortical TALH can be increased by addition of PTH to the bath (137) and, in medullary segments, by addition of calcitonin or cAMP (138).

Distal Convoluted Tubule and Connecting Tubule

Physiologic regulation of calcium excretion occurs in the DCT, which reabsorbs up to 10% of the filtered calcium load. The capacity for calcium transport in this segment appears to be high and to be limited mainly by the availability of transportable ions. Although calcium transport in the DCT normally occurs in parallel with that of sodium, it is not dependent on either sodium or the transepithelial voltage and occurs against an electrochemical gradient; thus, it is active and presumably transcellular. Reabsorption of calcium in the DCT can be dissociated from that of sodium by administration of thiazide diuretics, which increase reabsorption of calcium and decrease that of sodium. As discussed earlier, luminal calcium entry is thought to be mediated via the apical ECaC. Both vitamin D–dependent calbindin-D and the Ca^{2+}-ATPase co-localize in the DCT and are thought to facilitate transcellular movement and basolateral extrusion of calcium, respectively. The Na^+-Ca^{2+} exchanger also is localized, perhaps exclusively, to the basolateral membrane of the DCT and CNT (79,114–116), although its physiologic role in these segments remains to be defined.

Collecting Tubule

Net reabsorption in the collecting tubule accounts for less than 5% of filtered calcium (127). In the cortical collecting tubule, calcium transport probably is active, because both calbindin-D (77,79) and Ca^{2+}-ATPase activity (87) are found in this nephron segment. In the medullary collecting tubule, approximately 1% of the filtered load may be reabsorbed (139).

Determinants of Renal Handling of Calcium

Diet

A number of factors can influence renal tubular reabsorption and urine excretion of calcium (Table 10.1) (124,127). Expansion and contraction of the extracellular fluid volume induce an increase and decrease, respectively, in excretion of both calcium and sodium. Acute infusion of sodium chloride increases urine calcium excretion, an effect attributed to inhibition of calcium reabsorption in both the proximal and late distal tubule

TABLE 10.1. FACTORS AFFECTING RENAL CALCIUM EXCRETION

Factor	Ca excretion	Mechanism/nephron site
Diet		
Volume expansion	↑	↓ Distal reabsorption
Sodium chloride	↑	Undefined
Protein	↑	↑ Net acid and sulfate excretion
Phosphorus	↓	↓ Production of $1,25(OH)_2D$ ↓ Intestinal absorption of Ca ↑ Reabsorption distal nephron
Metabolism		
Acidosis	↑	↓ Proximal and distal reabsorption
Alkalosis	↓	↑ Proximal and distal reabsorption
Hypercalcemia	↑	↑ Filtered load of Ca ↓ Proximal and distal reabsorption (PTH)
Hormones		
PTH	↓	↑ Reabsorption TALH, DCT, and CNT
Vitamin D	↓	↑ Distal reabsorption, ? other sites
Insulin	↑	↓ Proximal and distal reabsorption
Glucagon	↑	? ↑ RBF and GFR
Growth hormone	↑	Undefined
Thyroid hormone	↑	↑ Filtered load of Ca, ↓ PTH
Calcitonin	↓	↑ Reabsorption TALH
Diuretics		
Mannitol	↑	↓ Proximal reabsorption
Furosemide	↑	↓ Reabsorption TALH
Thiazides, amiloride	↓	↑ Reabsorption DCT
Other		
Glucose	↑	↓ Proximal and distal reabsorption
Glucocorticoids	↑	? ↓ Bone resorption, volume expansion
Estrogens	↓	? ↓ Bone resorption

↑, increased; ↓, decreased; $1,25(OH)_2D$, 1,25 dihydroxyvitamin D; CNT, connecting tubule; DCT, distal convoluted tubule; GFR, glomerular filtration rate; PTH, parathyroid hormone; RBF, renal blood flow; TALH; thick ascending limb of loop of Henle.

(140). An increase in dietary sodium chloride induces an increase in urine calcium, although the intrarenal mechanisms responsible have not been defined.

Changes in dietary calcium within the normal range have only a modest effect on urine calcium excretion. A linear relationship exists between dietary protein intake and urine calcium excretion (141), an effect that is exaggerated in patients with recurrent nephrolithiasis. An increase in either oral or parenteral intake of phosphorus is associated with a decrease in urine calcium excretion, an effect mediated in part by increased calcium reabsorption in the distal nephron (142). Phosphorus loading can reduce intestinal calcium absorption and stimulate PTH secretion, both in part by decreasing the renal production and serum concentration of $1,25(OH)_2D$ (6,143). Conversely, phosphorus restriction increases urine calcium excretion (124,127). This effect is independent of vitamin D and is attributed to a reduction in tubular calcium reabsorption, principally in distal nephron segments, that is independent of PTH.

Hormones

PTH stimulates renal calcium reabsorption and is thought to be the principal hormonal determinant of urine calcium excretion. PTH acts to reduce calcium excretion in part by decreasing glomerular filtration rate (GFR) via a reduction in the glomerular capillary ultrafiltration coefficient K_f (144), and thus decreasing the filtered load of calcium. PTH also increases tubular calcium reabsorption in the cortical TALH, DCT, and CNT of the rabbit, with the principal effect being on the DCT (131,138,145–149). PTH action is attributed to activation of both the cAMP–protein kinase A and phospholipase-C–protein kinase C signaling pathways (126). The PTH-induced increase in calcium reabsorption is associated with an increase in the cytosolic calcium concentrations in cortical TALH, DCT, and CNT, which is mediated by an increase in the rate of calcium entry through dihydropyridine-sensitive channels (149–151). The role of ECaC in PTH-mediated stimulation of calcium reabsorption remains to be determined.

The effect of vitamin D on renal calcium reabsorption is variable, depending on vitamin D status, the activity of PTH, and the species studied (55). Although vitamin D has no detectable effect on calcium transport by the proximal tubule (152), $1,25(OH)_2D$ stimulates Ca^{2+} transport in distal nephron segments, including DCT of the dog and CNT and cortical collecting duct of the rabbit (55,153). The effect of $1,25(OH)_2D$ on expression of ECaC was studied in vitamin D–deficient rats. Administration of $1,25(OH)_2D$ induced an increase in the abundance of ECaC mRNA and protein in the distal part of the DCT and in CNT (154). The human ECaC promoter contains several putative vitamin D–responsive elements, which suggests that $1,25(OH)_2D$ stimulates ECaC expression at least in part at the transcriptional level (154). Thus, it is thought that $1,25(OH)_2D$ acts on the distal nephron to increase calcium reabsorption by increasing the expression of ECaC in this nephron segment.

Urine calcium excretion is increased by exposure to the following: insulin, glucose, glucagon, growth hormone, thyroid hormone, and corticosteroids; urine calcium is decreased by calcitonin and estrogens (127).

Metabolism

Both acute and chronic metabolic acidosis, as induced by ammonium chloride loading in humans and experimental animals, is attended by an increase in urine calcium excretion (155–157). This increase is irrespective of a change in filtered load of calcium or in circulating PTH and is attributed to a decrease in calcium reabsorption in the distal nephron (155). Hypercalciuria is reversed when the acidosis is corrected with administration of alkali (155,158,159). Conversely, metabolic alkalosis is associated with a decrease in calcium excretion (160,161). The effects of respiratory acid-base changes are similar to those of metabolically induced changes (162,163). Hypercalcemia, by increasing the filtered load of calcium, is associated with an increase in its excretion. This effect is mitigated to some extent by hypercalcemia-induced reduction in the ultrafilterability of calcium and phosphorus (164) and in GFR (165); the reduction in GFR is attributed to a PTH-dependent decrease in K_f. Hypercalcemia can decrease calcium reabsorption in the PCT, TALH, and distal nephron (124); the effect on this latter segment requires the presence of parathyroid glands (166).

Diuretics

Diuretic agents such as mannitol, which act on the proximal nephron, and furosemide or ethacrynic acid, which act on the TALH, induce an increase in both calcium and sodium excretion, because calcium reabsorption is passive and linked to that of sodium in these nephron segments. By contrast, thiazide diuretics and amiloride, which act on the DCT, decrease the excretion of calcium but increase that of sodium (127). The hypocalciuric effect of thiazide diuretics is due in part to increased calcium reabsorption by the DCT; the blockade of sodium chloride entry may reduce the cell sodium concentration sufficiently to enhance basolateral Na^+-Ca^{2+} exchange (167). The hypocalciuria induced by chronic administration of thiazide diuretics is thought to reflect enhanced calcium reabsorption by the proximal tubule (127); this effect can be reversed by increased salt intake.

PHOSPHORUS

Body Composition

In the adult, phosphorus accounts for approximately 1% of body weight, or 600 to 700 g (1). Approximately 85% of body phosphorus is in the skeleton and teeth, approximately 15% is in soft tissue, and the remainder is in extracellular fluid. At birth, phosphorus accounts for only approximately 0.6% of body weight (1). In growing individuals, the balance of phosphorus must be positive to meet the needs of skeletal growth and consolidation; in the adult, phosphorus balance is zero. Phosphorus not only is an important constituent of bone mineral but also plays a critical role in many metabolic processes within the cell, including those involved in energy metabolism, protein phosphorylation, nucleotide metabolism, and phospholipid metabolism.

Extracellular Metabolism of Phosphorus

Phosphorus exists in plasma in two forms, an organic form consisting principally of phospholipids and phosphate esters, and an inorganic form (168). Of the total plasma phosphorus concentration of approximately 14 mg/dL, approximately 4 mg/dL is in the inorganic form. In clinical settings, only the inorganic orthophosphate form is routinely measured. Approximately 10 to 15% of total plasma inorganic phosphorus is protein bound; the remainder, which is filtered by the renal glomerulus, exists principally either as the undissociated or "free" phosphate ions HPO_4^{2-} and $H_2PO_4^-$, which are present in serum in a ratio of 4:1 at pH 7.4, or as phosphate complexed with sodium, calcium, or magnesium.

The terms *phosphorus concentration* and *phosphate concentration* are often used interchangeably, and for clinical purposes the choice matters little. Phosphorus in the form of the phosphate ion circulates in blood, is filtered by the renal glomerulus, and is transported across plasma membranes. The content of "phosphate" in plasma, urine, tissue, or foodstuffs, however, is measured and expressed in terms of the amount of elemental phosphorus contained in the specimen, hence use of the term *phosphorus concentration.*

In healthy subjects ingesting typical diets, the serum phosphorus concentration exhibits a circadian rhythm, characterized by a rapid decrease in early morning to a nadir shortly before noon, a subsequent increase to a plateau in late afternoon, and a small further increase to a peak shortly after midnight (Fig. 10.8) (4,6). The normal circadian rhythm in serum phosphorus concentration can be described as the sum of sinusoidal functions with periodicities of 24 and 12 hours (6). The amplitude of the rhythm (nadir to peak) is approximately 1.2 mg/dL, or 30% of the 24-hour mean level. Restriction or supplementation of dietary phosphorus induces a substantial decrease or increase, respectively, in serum concentrations of phosphorus during the late morning, afternoon, and evening, but induces less or no change in the morning fasting phosphorus concentration (Fig. 10.8) (6). To minimize the impact of changes in dietary phosphorus on the serum phosphorus concentration, one should obtain specimens for analysis in the morning fasting state. Specimens obtained in the afternoon are more likely to be affected by diet and thus may be more useful to monitor the effect of dietary phosphorus on serum phosphorus concentrations, as in patients with renal insufficiency receiving phosphorus-binding agents to treat hyperphosphatemia.

Factors other than time of day and diet can affect the serum phosphorus concentration. Presumably because of movement of phosphorus into cells, the serum phosphorus concentration can be decreased acutely by intravenous infusion of glucose or insulin, ingestion of carbohydrate-rich meals, acute respiratory alkalosis, or infusion or endogenous release of epinephrine. The decrease in phosphorus concentration induced by acute respiratory alkalosis can be

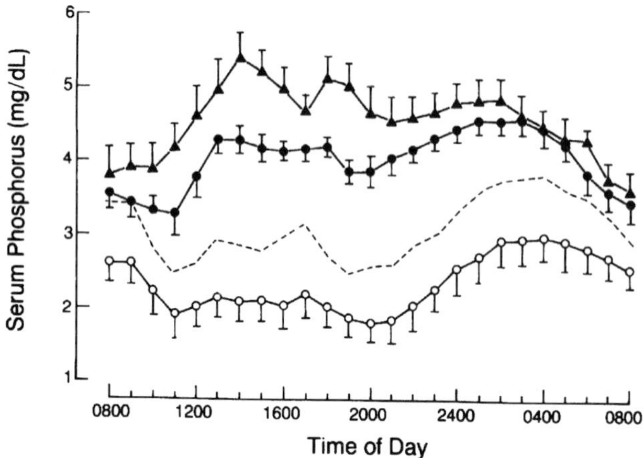

FIGURE 10.8. Effect of dietary phosphorus on the circadian rhythm of serum phosphorus concentration in healthy men. Blood was drawn from an indwelling venous needle at hourly intervals for 24 hours after subjects had received a normal intake (•) (1500 mg/day) of phosphorus for 9 days and after phosphorus was restricted for 1 day (- - -) and 10 days (o) (<500 mg/day), and then supplemented (▲) (3000 mg/day) for 10 days. Spectral analysis of the variations in serum phosphorus concentration over time (time series) revealed significant periodicities of 24 hours, 12 hours, or both in each of the subject studies. Depicted are mean values plus and/or minus the standard error of the mean. (From Portale AA, Halloran BP, Morris RC Jr. Dietary intake of phosphorus modulates the circadian rhythm in serum concentration of phosphorus: implications for the renal production of 1,25-dihydroxyvitamin D. *J Clin Invest* 1987;80:1147–1154, with permission.)

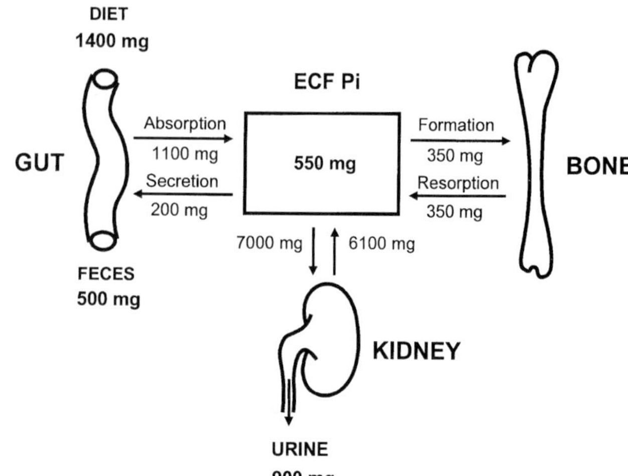

FIGURE 10.9. Phosphorus fluxes between body pools in the normal human adult in zero phosphorus balance. ECF, extracellular fluid; Pi, inorganic phosphate.

as much as 2.0 mg/dL (169). Serum phosphorus concentration can be increased acutely by metabolic acidosis and by intravenous infusion of calcium (127).

There are substantial effects of age on the fasting serum phosphorus concentration. Phosphorus levels are highest in infants, ranging from 4.8 to 7.4 mg/dL (mean, 6.2 mg/dL) in the first 3 months of life and decreasing to 4.5 to 5.8 mg/dL (mean, 5.0 mg/dL) at age 1 to 2 years (170). In mid-childhood, values range from 3.5 to 5.5 mg/dL (mean, 4.4 mg/dL) and decrease to adult values by late adolescence (8,171). In adult men, serum phosphorus levels decrease with age from approximately 3.5 mg/dL at age 20 years to 3.0 mg/dL at age 70 (9,171). In women, the values are similar to those of men until after menopause, when they increase slightly from approximately 3.4 mg/dL at age 50 years to 3.7 mg/dL at age 70. Because plasma phosphate is composed of divalent (HPO_4^{2-}) and monovalent ($H_2PO_4^-$) ions in a ratio of 4:1, the composite valence of phosphorus in serum (or intravenous solutions) at pH 7.4 is 1.8. At this pH, 1 mmol phosphorus is equal to 1.8 mEq.

Extracellular Phosphorus Homeostasis

In the adult in zero phosphorus balance, net intestinal absorption of phosphate (dietary phosphorus minus fecal phosphorus) is 60 to 65% of dietary intake. To satisfy the demands of rapid growth of bone and soft tissue, net intestinal absorption of phosphate is higher in infants than in adults and can exceed 90% of dietary intake (172,173). Metabolic balance studies in normal adult humans reveal that over the customary range of dietary phosphorus, net absorption is a linear function of intake (174). Phosphate is absorbed primarily in the duodenum and jejunum and to a lesser extent in the ileum and colon. Intestinal phosphate absorption occurs via two mechanisms: an active, sodium-dependent transcellular process that has been localized to the mucosal surface, and passive diffusion through the paracellular pathway. Under usual dietary circumstances, the bulk of phosphate absorption is thought to occur via passive diffusion, with active transport playing an important role when luminal phosphorus concentration is low, as when dietary phosphorus is restricted (175,176). The active absorption of phosphate across the luminal membrane involves a sodium-dependent high-affinity transport system that is simulated by $1,25(OH)_2D$ (177–180). This process is mediated by the now cloned intestinal sodium-phosphate cotransporter (type IIb), which is expressed in small intestine and other epithelial cells but not in kidney and plays a role in the physiologic regulation of intestinal phosphate absorption (181,182). A small amount of phosphate is secreted into the intestinal lumen in digestive fluids. An overall schema of phosphorus metabolism is depicted in Figure 10.9.

Absorbed phosphate enters the extracellular phosphate pool, which is in equilibrium with the bone and soft tissue phosphate pools. Phosphate is filtered at the glomerulus and is reabsorbed to a large extent by the renal tubule. In adults in neutral phosphorus balance, the amount of phosphorus excreted by the kidney is equal to the net amount absorbed by the intestine; in growing children it is less than the net amount absorbed due to deposition of phosphorus in bone.

The tubular reabsorption of phosphate plays a central role in the regulation of plasma phosphorus concentration and phosphate homeostasis. In response to a decrease in the extracellular phosphorus concentration, urine excretion of phos-

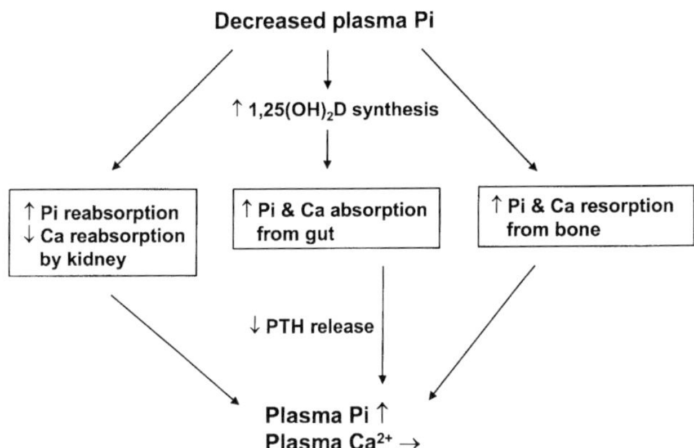

FIGURE 10.10. The homeostatic response to hypophosphatemia. 1,25(OH)$_2$D, 1,25-dihydroxyvitamin D; Pi, inorganic phosphate; PTH, parathyroid hormone.

phorus decreases promptly due to an increase in phosphate reabsorption by the proximal tubule (Fig. 10.10). This acute response reflects both a decrease in the filtered load of phosphate and an adaptive response of the nephron to increase phosphate reabsorption in response to a decrease in plasma concentration and dietary intake of phosphorus (see later). Hypophosphatemia is a potent stimulus for the renal production of 1,25(OH)$_2$D (183–185). In normal humans, moderate as well as severe restriction of dietary phosphorus can induce within 48 hours a substantial increase in the serum concentration of 1,25(OH)$_2$D (143,186,187); the increase is mediated by an increase in renal production of this hormone (143). In healthy humans in whom dietary phosphorus was manipulated throughout its normal range and beyond, the 24-hour mean serum phosphorus concentration varied inversely and significantly with the serum concentration of 1,25(OH)$_2$D (187). The increased serum 1,25(OH)$_2$D induced by hypophosphatemia acts to stimulate absorption of phosphorus and calcium by the intestine and mobilization of these minerals from bone. Hypophosphatemia also can directly promote mobilization of bone phosphate and calcium. The resulting increase in plasma calcium concentration induces suppression of PTH release, which leads to a further decrease in urine phosphorus excretion and an increase in calcium excretion. These homeostatic adjustments result in an increase in extracellular phosphorus concentration toward normal values, with little change in the serum calcium concentration. Conversely, in response to an increase in plasma phosphorus concentration, production of 1,25(OH)$_2$D is decreased and release of PTH is increased. The net effects of hyperphosphatemia on bone, kidney, and intestine are opposite to those occurring with hypophosphatemia, the net result being a decrease in phosphorus concentration toward normal values.

Renal Tubular Transport of Phosphate

In the proximal renal tubule, phosphate is transported across the luminal membrane against its electrochemical gradient by a unidirectional, transcellular, secondary active process, driven by the inwardly directed electrochemical sodium gradient that is maintained by the basolateral Na^+-K^+-ATPase. The transport of phosphate is dependent on the presence of luminal sodium and is coupled to that of sodium. Based on electrophysiologic and tracer studies of phosphate transport, it is proposed that three sodium ions and one phosphate ion are transported together via a transporter protein that spans the lipid bilayer of the BBM; both monovalent and divalent phosphate can interact with the transporter (188).

Factors Affecting Sodium-Phosphate Co-Transport by the Renal Tubule

The rate of phosphate reabsorption by the proximal tubule can be modulated by several factors, and this modulation reflects changes in sodium–inorganic phosphate (Na-Pi) co-transport by the BBM (124,189,190). Indeed, the BBM entry step is thought to be the final target of physiologic and pathophysiologic regulation of proximal tubular phosphate reabsorption (190–193). The rate of phosphate reabsorption by the proximal tubule decreases with decreasing pH of tubular fluid (194). In BBM vesicles isolated from rat kidney cortex, the rate of phosphate uptake decreased severalfold when extravesicular (luminal) pH was decreased from 8.0 to 6.0 or when extravesicular sodium was decreased from 175 to 10 mmol/L (195). The effect of luminal pH on phosphate reabsorption is sodium dependent; it is greater at lower luminal sodium concentrations. The decrease in phosphate reabsorption observed with acidic luminal pH is thought to be due to competition between protons and sodium ions for a common binding site on the phosphate transporter, which results in decreased affinity of the transporter for luminal sodium and thereby for luminal phosphate (196). Phosphate uptake by BBM vesicles is increased when intravesicular (cytosolic) pH is lowered (197,198); this finding is also consistent with an effect of hydrogen ion to decrease the transporter's affinity for sodium and hence for phosphate at the cytosolic side of the plasma membrane, which thus accelerates the transport cycle.

Changes in the lipid composition or fluidity state of the BBM are associated with changes in BBM Na-Pi co-transport (199–201). However, short-term (hours-long) restriction of dietary phosphorus induces an increase in phosphate uptake before changes in either BBM fluidity or cholesterol content are detectable, which suggests that neither fluidity nor cholesterol content is critical to the early adaptive response of the BBM to phosphorus restriction (202).

Cellular and Molecular Mechanisms

Attention has focused on the molecular events involved in regulation of renal tubular phosphate reabsorption. Using an expression cloning strategy, the laboratory of Murer cloned two different Na-Pi co-transporters, designated type I and

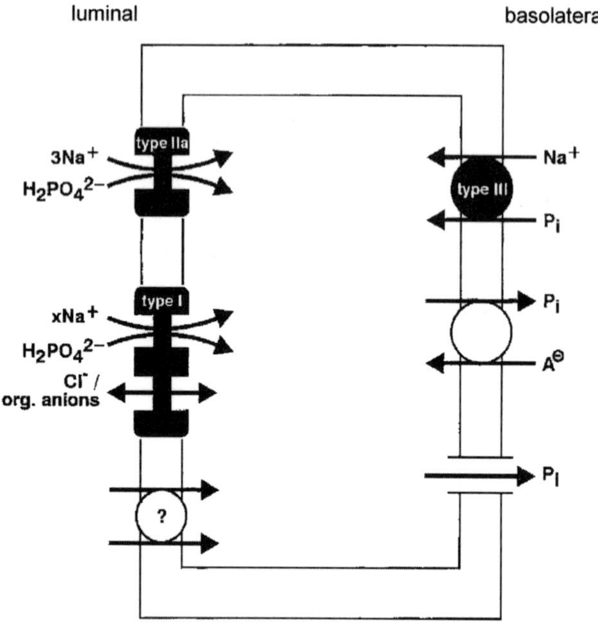

FIGURE 10.11. Location of identified and postulated Na-dependent and Na-independent phosphate transporters in the proximal tubule cell. Available data indicate that most proximal phosphate reabsorption occurs via the type IIa co-transporter, which is the major target of physiologic regulation of renal phosphate reabsorption. Org., organic; Pi, inorganic phosphate. (From Murer H, Forster I, Hernando N, et al. Posttranscriptional regulation of the proximal tubule NaPi-II transporter in response to PTH and dietary P_i. *Am J Physiol* 1999;277:F676–F684, with permission.)

type II (203,204). Currently, three types of Na-Pi co-transporters that mediate transport of phosphate from the extracellular to the intracellular compartment are identified: type I, type II, and type III (Fig. 10.11) (reviewed in 205).

The type I Na-Pi co-transporter is expressed primarily in apical BBMs of the proximal renal tubule, as determined by immunohistochemical analysis in rabbits and mice (206). Conditions that physiologically regulate proximal tubule phosphate transport such as dietary phosphorus or PTH do not alter type I Na-Pi co-transporter protein or mRNA expression. Thus, the type I co-transporter is not thought to be a major determinant of proximal tubule phosphate handling. The cDNA for the type I Na-Pi co-transporter was initially cloned from rabbit kidney, and its phosphate transport activity was expressed in *Xenopus laevis* oocytes (203); homologous cDNA has now been isolated from human, mouse, and rat kidney cortex and human brain (207–215). The rabbit cDNA encodes a protein of 465 amino acids with a predicted molecular mass of approximately 52 kDa and a secondary structure that contains six to eight transmembrane regions. The human gene encoding the type I Na-Pi co-transporter (*NPT1*) is located on chromosome 6 p21.3-p23.

The type IIa transporter is highly expressed in the apical region of the proximal tubule BBM and in subapical vesicular structures. The type IIa Na-Pi transporter is the principal determinant of overall Na-dependent phosphate reabsorption by the proximal tubule under physiologic and pathologic conditions, and the rate of transport is principally regulated by altering the abundance of type IIa protein in the BBM (188,193,205,216,217). Genetic disruption of the *NPT2* gene, which encodes the type IIa transporter, results in hypophosphatemia due to severe renal phosphate wasting (218). A related Na-Pi transporter, type IIb, is expressed in the BBM of the small intestine but not in kidney, and plays a role in the physiologic regulation of intestinal reabsorption of phosphate (181,182). A type IIa transporter appears to be expressed also in osteoclasts and may play a role in bone resorption (219). The type IIa Na-Pi co-transporter cDNA, initially cloned from rat and human kidney cortex libraries (204), encodes a protein of 637 amino acids with a predicted secondary structure containing eight transmembrane regions. Type II–related transporters have now been identified in renal cortex from rabbit (220), mouse (211,221), flounder (222), and opossum kidney cells (OK cells) (223), and from bovine renal NBL-1 cells (224). The human *NPT2* gene is located on chromosome region 5q35, and the corresponding mouse gene is located on chromosome region 13B (225–227). The structures of the *NPT2* genes are similar in both species; they are approximately 16 kb in length and consist of 13 exons and 12 introns. A high degree of homology is found within the promoter regions of the human, mouse, rat, and opossum genes. A model of the secondary structure of the rat type IIa Na-Pi co-transporter is depicted in Figure 10.12.

The viral receptors for gibbon ape leukemia virus (Glvr-1) and for mouse amphotropic retrovirus (Ram-1) exhibit Na-Pi co-transport activity when expressed in *X. laevis* oocytes (228–230). These receptors have been named PiT-1 and PiT-2, respectively, and are classified as type III Na-Pi co-transporters. Type III transporter mRNA is expressed in many tissues, including kidney, parathyroid glands, bone, liver, lung, striated muscle, heart, and brain (205); in mouse kidney, mRNA abundance of the type III transporter is two orders of magnitude less than that of the type IIa transporter (231). Type III transporter protein is localized to the basolateral region of the proximal tubule. The role of the type III transporter is thought to be that of "housekeeping" Na-Pi transport; that is, mediating phosphate flux into cells if luminal phosphate entry is not sufficient for metabolic processes

The mechanisms of phosphate efflux at the basolateral membrane are not well defined. Current evidence suggests that phosphate can exit the cell down its electrochemical gradient via (a) a low-capacity Na-Pi co-transport system that couples flux of one sodium ion with that of one divalent phosphate ion, and (b) a high-capacity phosphate-anion exchange mechanism (124).

Overall Phosphate Transport by the Nephron

Under normal physiologic conditions, 80 to 97% of the filtered load of phosphate is reabsorbed by the renal tubule

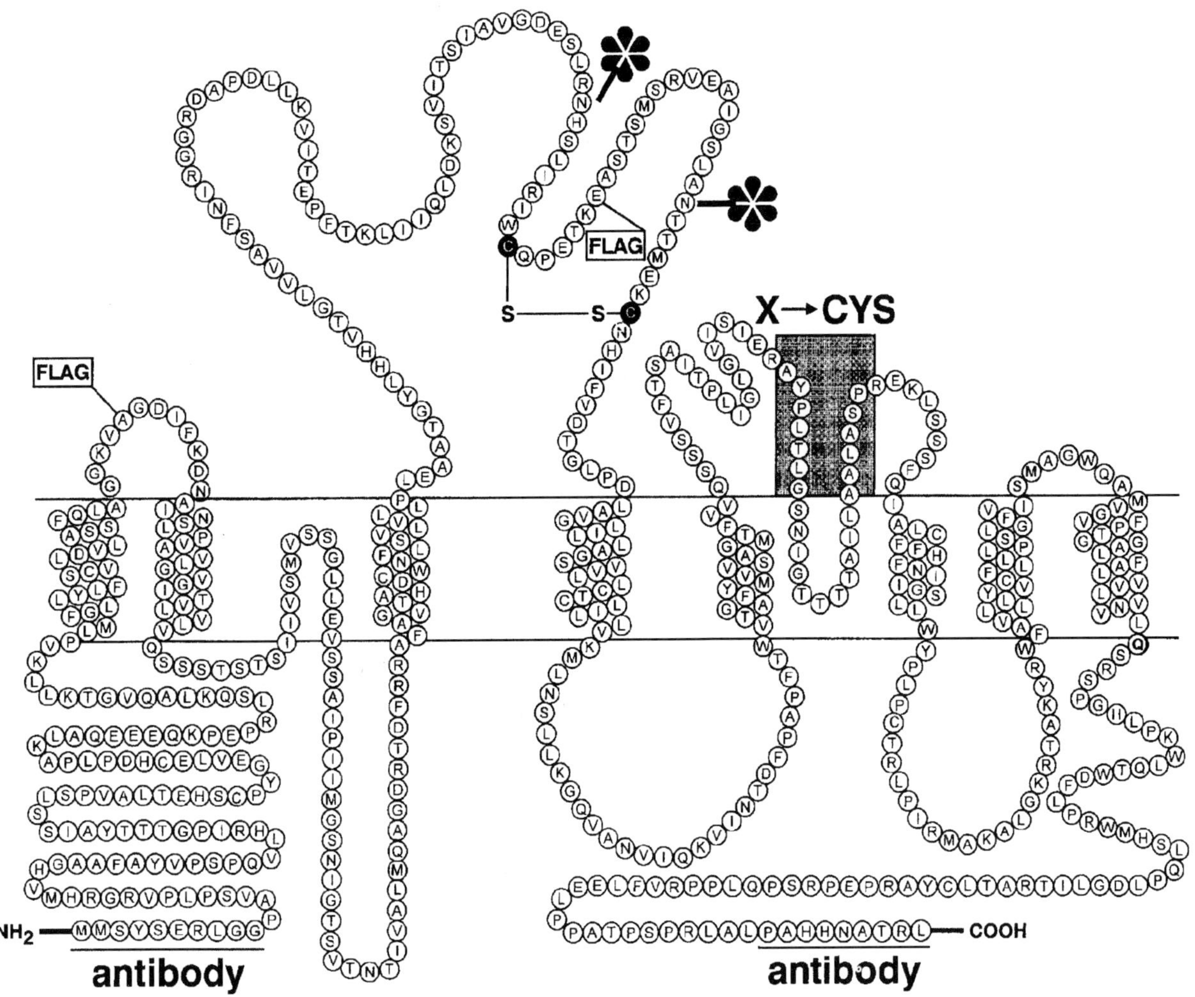

FIGURE 10.12. Model of the secondary structure of the rat type IIa Na-Pi co-transporter, derived from hydropathy predictions and experimentally supported (see reference 205). The two *N*-glycosylation sites in the secondary extracellular loop are indicated by asterisks. Cysteine residues likely to form a disulfide bridge and possibly important for function are shown in black. (From Murer H, Hernando N, Forster I, et al. Proximal tubular phosphate reabsorption: molecular mechanisms. *Physiol Rev* 2000;80:1373–1409, with permission.)

(124,127). Clearance studies in humans and experimental animals show that, when the filtered load of phosphate is progressively increased, phosphate reabsorption rises until a maximum tubular reabsorptive rate for phosphate, or TmP, is reached, after which phosphorus excretion increases in proportion to its filtered load. The measurement of TmP varies among individuals and within the same individual, due in part to variation in GFR. Thus, the ratio TmP/GFR, or the maximum tubular reabsorption of phosphate per unit volume of GFR, is the most reliable quantitative estimate of the overall tubular phosphate reabsorptive capacity and can be considered to reflect the quantity of Na-Pi co-transporters available per unit of kidney mass (175). The serum phosphorus concentration at which phosphate reabsorption is maximal is called the *theoretical renal phosphate threshold;* this value is equal to the ratio TmP/GFR and closely approximates the normal fasting serum phosphorus concentration. Thus, the renal reabsorptive capacity for phosphate is the principal determinant of the serum phosphorus concentration. Approximately 80% of filtered phosphate is reabsorbed in the proximal tubule, 5 to 10% is reabsorbed in the distal tubule, and 2 to 3% is reabsorbed in the collecting tubules (Fig. 10.13).

Proximal Tubule

Approximately 70% of the filtered load of phosphate is reabsorbed by the PCT. Under normal physiologic conditions, reabsorption rates in early convolutions (S1 segment) are as much as four times higher than those in late convolutions (S2 segment) and the pars recta (S3 segment) (232–234). Due to this axial heterogeneity in phosphate transport, most of the phosphate reabsorption in the PCT occurs within the first 25% of PCT length. Internephron heterogeneity is also seen in phosphate reabsorption in the proximal tubule; proximal

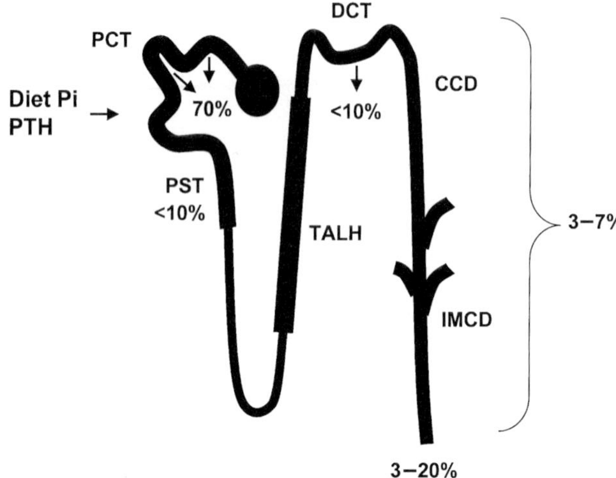

FIGURE 10.13. Profile of phosphate reabsorption along the mammalian nephron, as derived from micropuncture data. CCD, cortical collecting duct; DCT, distal convoluted tubule; IMCD, inner medullary collecting duct; PCT, proximal convoluted tubule; Pi, inorganic phosphate; PST, proximal straight tubule; PTH, parathyroid hormone; TALH, thick ascending limb of the loop of Henle. (Data from Suki WN, Rouse D. Renal transport of calcium, magnesium, and phosphate. In: Suki WN, Rouse D, eds. *Brenner and Rector's the kidney*. Philadelphia: WB Saunders, 1996:472–509.)

tubules of juxtamedullary nephrons have a greater capacity both to reabsorb phosphate (235–238) and to adapt to changes in its filtered load (239,240) than do proximal tubules of superficial nephrons. In the absence of PTH, up to an additional 10% of filtered phosphate can be reabsorbed in the proximal straight tubule.

Loop of Henle, Distal Convoluted Tubule, and Connecting Tubule

Little or no transport of phosphate is thought to occur in the loop of Henle except for the proximal straight tubule segment (127). Up to 10% of the filtered load of phosphate is reabsorbed by the DCT in the absence of PTH; an additional 3 to 7% may be reabsorbed beyond the accessible late DCT, presumably by the CNT (127).

Collecting Tubule

Although some investigators have failed to demonstrate phosphate reabsorption in isolated perfused cortical collecting tubules (241), others have shown a small but significant net efflux of phosphate in this portion of the nephron (242,243).

Physiologic Regulation of Renal Phosphate Transport

Dietary Phosphorus and Plasma Phosphorus

Dietary intake of phosphorus is one of the most important physiologic regulators of renal Na-Pi co-transport. An increase or decrease in dietary phosphorus predictably induces an increase or decrease, respectively, in urine excretion of phosphorus; with severe phosphorus restriction, urine phosphorus excretion is negligible. This adaptation is independent of changes in the filtered load of phosphate; does not depend on changes in extracellular fluid volume, plasma calcium level, growth hormone level, vitamin D status, or parathyroid activity; and appears to reflect changes in the rate of phosphate reabsorption by the proximal tubule, specifically, an increase or decrease in the V_{max} of Na-Pi co-transport activity. In addition, phosphorus restriction in animals can severely blunt the phosphaturic response to administration of PTH (196). The adaptation can be demonstrated both *in vivo* and in isolated perfused PCT segments and BBM vesicles taken from animals maintained on differing dietary intakes of phosphorus (244–249).

Renal tubule adaptation to changes in either dietary intake or plasma concentration of phosphorus can occur rapidly; an increase in BBM vesicle Na-Pi co-transport was observed after 2 to 4 hours of phosphorus restriction in the rat (250–252); conversely, a decrease in phosphate transport was induced after 1 hour of phosphorus infusion (253). The adaptation induced by short-term (hours-long) phosphorus restriction was preceded by a decrease in serum phosphorus concentration and was not inhibited by cycloheximide or actinomycin D, which suggests that protein synthesis is not required for the adaptation to occur (251). By contrast, the adaptation induced after long-term (3 days) phosphorus restriction was inhibited by cycloheximide and actinomycin D, which suggests that new protein synthesis is required (254). Similarly, exposure of cultured renal epithelial cells (LLC-PK1) to a low-medium phosphorus concentration induced both short-term (minutes-long) and long-term (hours-long) adaptations in Na-Pi co-transport (255–257). Thus, adaptation to changes in both dietary intake and plasma concentration of phosphorus involves two phases with different time courses: a rapid phase that is independent of protein synthesis and appears to involve activation or recruitment of preexisting transporter units, and a long-term phase that requires protein synthesis and permits a large increase (>100%) in phosphate transport rate (190,196,256).

Physiologic and pathologic changes in the renal handling of phosphate can be accounted for by changes in the abundance of type IIa Na-Pi co-transporter protein in the renal BBM. Short-term (hours-long) exposure of rats to a low-phosphorus diet induced an increase in both BBM Na-Pi co-transport activity and protein abundance but no change in Na-Pi–specific mRNA (258). The changes in transporter activity and protein abundance were blocked by prior treatment of the animals with colchicine, a microtubule-disrupting agent, but were not blocked by treatment with actinomycin D or cycloheximide (258). In opossum kidney (OK) cells, exposure to a low-phosphate medium induced within hours an increase in type IIa protein abundance in parallel with an increase in Na-Pi cotransport activity but no change in type II co-transporter mRNA abundance (259,260). Thus, acute regulation of Na-Pi co-transport activity appears to be independent of transcription and translation and is thought to result from retrieval (decrease) or insertion (increase) of preexisting transporters from or into the BBM (reviewed in 182, 193, 205, 261, and 262). An intact microtubular network is required for the acute adaptation to phosphorus restriction (258). In contrast, long-term (days-long) restriction of dietary phosphorus in mice, rats, and rabbits leads to an adaptive increase in BBM Na-Pi co-transport and in the abundance of type II Na-Pi co-transporter protein and mRNA (220,263–268); no change was observed in the abundance of type I transporter mRNA or protein (220). The increase in *Npt2* gene expression induced by a long-term (4 days) low-phosphorus diet was attributed to transcriptional mechanisms (269).

Hormones

Parathyroid Hormone

PTH is the principal hormonal regulator of renal phosphate reabsorption (124,270). PTH inhibits renal phosphate reabsorption in the convoluted and straight segments of the proximal tubule, where the majority of filtered phosphate is reabsorbed. Although PTH also inhibits proximal tubule reabsorption of bicarbonate, sodium, and fluid, the suppressive effect of PTH on phosphate reabsorption can be dissociated from that of sodium and fluid and thus is specific for phosphate (270). As further evidence of such specificity, in renal BBM vesicles isolated from animals treated with PTH *in vivo*, Na-Pi co-transport was reduced, whereas sodium-dependent transport of D-glucose and other solutes was unchanged (271,272). PTH-sensitive phosphate transport also is observed in the DCT and in the cortical collecting duct (135,243,273); however, the localization of PTH action along the nephron differs greatly in the various species studied (270).

PTH binds to its specific receptors on the apical and basolateral membranes of proximal tubule cells and activates adenylate cyclase, which results in an increase in intracellular cAMP and subsequent activation of protein kinase A. The phosphaturic effect of PTH can be mimicked by exogenous cAMP in intact animals, isolated perfused tubules, and BBM vesicles. PTH binding also activates the phosphoinositide-cytosolic calcium-dependent signaling pathway. In proximal tubule cells, PTH activates phospholipase C, which stimulates the production of diacylglycerol and IP3 (274); the latter induces an increase in the cytosolic calcium concentration (275,276). The formation of diacylglycerol and increase in cytosolic calcium result in activation of protein kinase C. In OK cells, exposure to PTH activates phospholipase C, stimulates production of IP3, and inhibits Na-Pi co-transport (274,277); activation of protein kinase C by phorbol esters also is associated with inhibition of phosphate transport (278,279). Based on findings in isolated perfused mouse tubules, binding of PTH to its receptor located on the apical surface primarily activates the phospholipase C–protein kinase C pathway, whereas binding to the receptor on the basolateral surface primarily activates the adenylate cyclase–protein kinase A pathway (280). Studies indicate that activation of the extracellular signal-related peptide/mitogen-activated protein kinase (ERK/MAPK) pathway also plays a central role in the regulation by PTH of renal phosphate transport (281).

The phosphaturic action of PTH is attributed to inhibition of phosphate transport by the BBM (205) and is associated with a reduction in the abundance of type IIa Na-Pi co-transporter protein, as determined by Western blot analysis of isolated proximal tubule BBMs and Na-Pi-IIa–specific immunofluorescence in convoluted and straight segments of proximal tubules (280,282). A prolonged increase in PTH also can induce a decrease in type II Na-Pi co-transporter mRNA abundance (282). The reduced abundance of type IIa Na-Pi co-transporter protein, induced acutely by infusion of PTH or feeding of a high-phosphorus diet, is attributed to endocytic internalization of phosphate transporters from the plasma membrane (205). The type IIa Na-Pi co-transporters are thought to be internalized via the same endocytic pathway as are soluble proteins (205,283) and, after internalization, are directed to the lysosomes for degradation. Studies in OK cells suggest that Na-Pi co-transporters, once internalized, are not immediately available for recycling back to the plasma membrane (284,285).

Vitamin D

Chronic administration of vitamin D or its metabolites is associated with a decrease in renal phosphate reabsorption. This effect is thought to be mediated by a vitamin D–induced increase in intestinal phosphate absorption and thus in phosphate balance, which induces an adaptive decrease in phosphate reabsorption by the proximal tubule (124,127). The effects of acute administration of vitamin D on phosphate transport appear to depend on the experimental conditions of study, including the dose of vitamin D administered and the prior vitamin D, PTH, and phosphorus status of the organism. In the rat, vitamin D depletion is associated with a decrease in renal phosphate reabsorption, which is rapidly corrected by physiologic amounts of 1,25-dihydroxyvitamin D_3. This effect is mediated by an increase in BBM Na-Pi co-transport (286) and is associated with a change in the lipid composition of the membrane (287,288). Vitamin D metabolites also stimulate renal phosphate reabsorption in hypophosphatemic or phosphorus-deprived states, or when basal phosphorus excretion is increased, as occurs with volume expansion or administration of PTH. By contrast, vitamin D induces phosphaturia in hyperphosphatemic or phosphorus-replete states (124).

Growth Hormone

Growth hormone acts to increase renal phosphate reabsorption, independently of PTH (191,289). In growth hormone–deficient subjects, the serum phosphorus concentration and the TmP/GFR ratio are reduced; both increase with administration of growth hormone (290,291). In patients with acromegaly, serum phosphorus concentrations are increased (292). Growth hormone also increases GFR, renal plasma flow, and renal gluconeogenesis (289). Growth hormone stimulates proximal tubular Na-Pi co-transport (293–296) and is mediated, at least in part, by increased production and release of insulin-like growth factor-1 (289,297). Receptors for growth hormone have been identified on the basolateral membrane of proximal tubule cells and appear to activate the phospholipase C pathway. Receptors for insulin-like growth factor-I also have been identified in proximal tubule membranes, and their effects may involve tyrosine kinase activity (289).

Phosphatonin

Attention has focused on the role of a circulating humoral factor(s), originally named phosphatonin (298), in the regulation of serum concentration and renal handling of phosphorus. Three disorders, autosomal dominant hypophosphatemic rickets (ADHR) (299–301), oncogenic hypophosphatemic osteomalacia (OHO) (also known as *tumor-induced osteomalacia*) (302–304), and X-linked hypophosphatemia (XLH) (305), each are characterized by hypophosphatemia due to renal phosphate wasting, inappropriately low or normal serum concentrations of $1,25(OH)_2D$, and rickets or osteomalacia (305). ADHR is caused by mutations in the *FGF23* gene, which encodes a novel secreted peptide that is processed to aminoterminal and carboxyterminal peptides. Affected individuals harbor mutations in the peptide's furin cleavage site, which prevent the processing of mutant fibroblast growth factor-23 (FGF-23) (306), presumably resulting in its accumulation in the plasma. FGF-23 is abundantly expressed in tumors that cause OHO (307,308), and serum concentrations of FGF-23 are greatly increased in patients with this disorder and also in patients with XLH (309,310). With surgical removal of the tumor, FGF-23 concentrations can decrease to normal values and the disorder resolves. Because extracts from these tumors inhibit phosphate transport in renal proximal tubule cells *in vitro* (298,311), it has been suggested that FGF-23 is responsible for this inhibition. In support of this hypothesis are the findings that recombinant FGF-23 inhibits phosphate transport in renal proximal tubule cells *in vitro* (312) and that administration of recombinant FGF-23 to mice induces hypophosphatemia and increased renal phosphate clearance (308). FGF-23–treated mice also exhibit decreased serum concentrations of $1,25(OH)_2D$ (308,313,314) due to reduced renal 1α-hydroxylase mRNA expression (308,314) and increased 24-hydroxylase mRNA expression (314). Taken together, these findings suggest that a common circulating factor, perhaps FGF-23, plays a central pathogenetic role in ADHR, OHO, and XLH. Further study is required, however, to determine the mechanisms by which FGF-23 or other peptide factor(s) regulates renal phosphate handling or vitamin D metabolism, and whether such factors play a role in the physiologic regulation of phosphorus or vitamin D metabolism.

Urine phosphorus excretion can be increased by exposure to the following: calcitonin, atrial natriuretic peptide, glucose, glucagon, and glucocorticoids; urine phosphorus excretion can be decreased by thyroid hormone and insulin (reviewed in 127, 205, and 315). The mechanism of action of such lipophilic substances as thyroid hormone, vitamin D, and glucocorticoids is unclear, although it is assumed that genomic mechanisms are involved (316).

Volume Status

Expansion of the extracellular fluid volume results in an increase, and volume contraction in a decrease, in urine excretion of phosphorus (Table 10.2) (124,127). The effect can be attributed in part to changes in the filtered load of phosphate and rate of phosphate reabsorption by the proximal tubule as well as to changes in plasma ionized calcium, the latter affecting secretion of PTH. A direct effect of volume expansion on tubular phosphate reabsorption also has been reported.

TABLE 10.2. FACTORS AFFECTING RENAL PHOSPHORUS EXCRETION

Factor	Pi excretion	Mechanism/ nephron site
Diet		
Volume expansion	↑	↑ Filtered load of Pi, ↓ proximal and distal reabsorption
Phosphorus restriction	↓	↑ Proximal reabsorption
Metabolism		
Acidosis	↑	↓ Tubular reabsorption
Alkalosis	↓	↑ Tubular reabsorption
Hormones		
PTH	↑	↓ Proximal and distal reabsorption
Vitamin D (long term)	↑	↓ Proximal reabsorption
Growth hormone	↓	↑ Proximal reabsorption, ↑ GFR
Calcitonin	↑	↓ Tubular reabsorption
Thyroid hormone	↓	↑ Tubular reabsorption
Insulin	↓	↑ Proximal reabsorption
Phosphatonin	↑	↓ Proximal reabsorption
Diuretics		
Mannitol, loop diuretics, thiazides	↑	↑ Tubular reabsorption, site varies
Other		
Growth and development	↓	↓ Proximal and distal reabsorption
Glucose	↑	Osmotic diuresis, ↓ reabsorption PCT
Glucocorticoids	↑	↓ Proximal reabsorption

↑, increased; ↓, decreased; GFR, glomerular filtration rate; PCT, proximal convoluted tubule; Pi, inorganic phosphate.

Acid-Base Status

Changes in acid-base status can significantly effect the renal handling of phosphate (124,270). Acute respiratory acidosis results in a decrease in renal phosphate reabsorption; this effect may depend on an increase in pCO_2 tension, but it does not depend on an increase in filtered load of phosphate, expansion of the extracellular fluid volume, or change in PTH or blood bicarbonate concentration (317). Conversely, acute respiratory alkalosis induces an increase in renal phosphate reabsorption and resistance to the phosphaturic action of both PTH and cAMP; these effects may depend on changes in pCO_2 tension but are independent of changes in plasma phosphorus concentration (318).

Although acute metabolic acidosis has minimal effects on urine phosphorus excretion (319), chronic metabolic acidosis can impair renal phosphate reabsorption independently of PTH and even when dietary phosphorus is severely restricted (320,321). The suppressive effect of metabolic acidosis on Na-Pi co-transport is demonstrable in BBM vesicles and is attributed to a decrease in the V_{max} of the transporter (321). The suppression of phosphate reabsorption might be mediated, in part, by changes in luminal and intracellular pH. Acute metabolic alkalosis induced by infusion of sodium bicarbonate reduces phosphate reabsorption when the prior dietary intake of phosphorus is high, but increases phosphate reabsorption when dietary phosphorus is normal (124,322–325). Chronic metabolic alkalosis predictably increases renal phosphate reabsorption (270).

Changes in the pH of luminal fluid can affect tubular reabsorption of phosphate. In rat proximal tubules, phosphate reabsorption was stimulated by increasing luminal pH when luminal phosphorus concentration was low (326). However, the effect of luminal pH on phosphate reabsorption was reduced or abolished when luminal phosphorus concentration was high (326), as occurs with intravenous infusion of phosphorus (327) or high dietary phosphorus (328). These findings suggest that the sensitivity of phosphate reabsorption to luminal pH depends on both luminal and peritubular and/or intracellular phosphorus concentration (196). The effects of luminal pH on phosphate transport observed *in vivo* are in good agreement with those observed in isolated BBM vesicles.

Growth and Development

As noted earlier, the serum phosphorus concentration is considerably higher in newborn infants and young children than in older children and adults. This finding is not due to a limitation of the immature kidney's ability to excrete phosphorus but rather reflects a higher rate of tubular phosphate reabsorption in infants and immature animals, as demonstrated by their higher values for the TmP/GFR ratio compared with values in adults (329). In newborn animals, as compared with adult animals, reabsorption of phosphate is greater, both in the early PCT and in more distal nephron segments, presumably the pars recta and segments beyond the DCT. In BBM vesicles, the V_{max} for Na-Pi co-transport is higher in newborn than in adult guinea pigs, a finding that cannot be accounted for by differences in plasma concentrations of phosphorus, ionized calcium, PTH, thyroxine, or calcitonin. The higher capacity for phosphate reabsorption by the immature kidney also may reflect its relatively greater number of juxtamedullary nephrons, which have a higher capacity to reabsorb phosphate. Newborn animals demonstrate a blunted phosphaturic response both to phosphorus loading and to administration of PTH, the latter despite a normal increase in urine cAMP. In phosphorus-restricted rats, the adaptive increase in phosphate reabsorption is much greater in immature animals than in adults. Growth hormone may play an important role in mediating the increased renal reabsorption of phosphate during development. The intracellular free phosphate concentration, as determined by phosphorus-31 nuclear magnetic resonance spectroscopy, is lower in the kidneys of growing rats than in those of adult rats; it has been suggested that this finding is due to age-related differences in cellular phosphate metabolism and results in part in an adaptive increase in tubular phosphate transport (330,331). It has also been suggested that most of the age-related changes in phosphate reabsorption can be explained by differences in BBM expression of the type II Na-Pi co-transporter (188). Thus, through a variety of mechanisms (329), phosphate handling by the immature kidney is regulated so that phosphate retention is promoted, presumably to meet the increased needs for phosphorus of the growing organism (329,332).

Diuretics

Although their mechanisms and sites of action differ, the following diuretic agents predictably induce phosphaturia: mannitol, acetazolamide, thiazide diuretics, and loop diuretics. Urine phosphorus excretion is little affected by amiloride, spironolactone, and triamterene (127).

REFERENCES

1. Nordin BEC. Nutritional considerations. In: Nordin BEC, ed. *Calcium, phosphate and magnesium metabolism.* New York: Churchill Livingstone, 1976:1–35.
2. Widdowson EM, Dickerson JWT. Chemical composition of the body. In: Comar CL, Bronner F, eds. *Mineral metabolism: an advanced treatise.* New York: Academic Press, 1964:1–247.
3. Moore EW. Ionized calcium in normal serum, ultrafiltrates, and whole blood determined by ion-exchange electrodes. *J Clin Invest* 1970;49:318–334.
4. Markowitz M, Rotkin L, Rosen JF. Circadian rhythms of blood minerals in humans. *Science* 1981;213:672–674.

5. Halloran BP, Portale AA, Castro M, et al. Serum concentration of 1,25–dihydroxyvitamin D in the human: diurnal variation. *J Clin Endocrinol Metab* 1985;60:1104–1110.
6. Portale AA, Halloran BP, Morris RC Jr. Dietary intake of phosphorus modulates the circadian rhythm in serum concentration of phosphorus: implications for the renal production of 1,25–dihydroxyvitamin D. *J Clin Invest* 1987;80:1147–1154.
7. Jubiz W, Canterbury JM, Reiss E, et al. Circadian rhythm in serum parathyroid hormone concentration in human subjects: correlation with serum calcium, phosphate, albumin, and growth hormone levels. *J Clin Invest* 1972;51:2040–2046.
8. Arnaud SB, Goldsmith RS, Stickler GB, et al. Serum parathyroid hormone and blood minerals: interrelationships in normal children. *Pediatr Res* 1973;7:485–493.
9. Keating FR Jr, Jones JD, Elveback LR, et al. The relation of age and sex to distribution of values in healthy adults of serum, calcium inorganic phosphorus, magnesium, alkaline phosphatase, total proteins, albumin, and blood urea. *J Lab Clin Med* 1969;73:825–834.
10. Walser M. The separate effects of hyperparathyroidism, hypercalcemia of malignancy, renal failure and acidosis on the state of calcium, phosphate, and other ions in plasma. *J Clin Invest* 1962;41:1454–1471.
11. Adler AJ, Ferran N, Berlyne GM. Effect of inorganic phosphate on serum ionized calcium concentration in vitro: a reassessment of the "trade-off hypothesis." *Kidney Int* 1985; 28:932–935.
12. Brent GA, LeBoff MS, Seely EW, et al. Relationship between the concentration and rate of change of calcium and serum intact parathyroid hormone levels in normal humans. *J Clin Endocrinol Metab* 1988;67:944–950.
13. Brown EM. Extracellular Ca^{2+} sensing, regulation of parathyroid cell function, and role of Ca^{2+} and other ions as extracellular (first) messengers. *Physiol Rev* 1991;71:371–411.
14. Loughead JL, Mimouni F, Tsang RC. Serum ionized calcium concentrations in normal neonates. *Am J Dis Child* 1988;142:516–518.
15. David L, Anast CS. Calcium metabolism in newborn infants: the interrelationship of parathyroid function and calcium, magnesium, and phosphorus metabolism in normal, "sick," and hypocalcemic newborns. *J Clin Invest* 1974;54:287–296.
16. Pesce AJ, Kaplan LA. *Methods in clinical chemistry.* St. Louis: CV Mosby, 1987.
17. Bowers GN, Brassard C, Sena S. Measurement of ionized calcium in serum with ion-selective electrodes: a mature technology that can meet the daily service needs. *Clin Chem* 1986;32:1437–1447.
18. Matkovic V, Heaney RP. Calcium balance during human growth: evidence for threshold behavior. *Am J Clin Nutr* 1992;55:992–996.
19. Liu Y-M, Neal P, Ernst J, et al. Absorption of calcium and magnesium from fortified human milk by very low birth weight infants. *Pediatr Res* 1989;25:496–502.
20. Fitzpatrick LA, Coleman DT, Bilezikian JP. The target tissue actions of parathyroid hormone. In: Coe FL, Favus MJ, eds. *Disorders of bone and mineral metabolism.* New York: Raven Press, 1992:123–148.
21. Brown EM, Gamba G, Riccardi D, et al. Cloning and characterization of an extracellular Ca^{2+}-sensing receptor from bovine parathyroid. *Nature* 1993;366:575–580.
22. Garrett JE, Capuano IV, Hammerland LG, et al. Molecular cloning and functional expression of human parathyroid calcium receptor cDNAs. *J Biol Chem* 1995;270(21):12919–12925.
23. Ruat M, Molliver ME, Snowman AM, et al. Calcium sensing receptor: molecular cloning in rat and localization to nerve terminals. *Proc Natl Acad Sci U S A* 1995;92(8):3161–3165.
24. Riccardi D, Park J, Lee WS, et al. Cloning and functional expression of a rat kidney extracellular calcium/polyvalent cation-sensing receptor. *Proc Natl Acad Sci U S A* 1995;92: 131–135.
25. Bikle DD, Nemanic MK, Gee E, et al. 1,25–dihydroxyvitamin D_3 production by human keratinocytes. *J Clin Invest* 1986;78:557–566.
26. Adams JS, Sharma OP, Gacad MA, et al. Metabolism of 25–hydroxyvitamin D_3 by cultured pulmonary alveolar macrophages in sarcoidosis. *J Clin Invest* 1983;72:1856–1860.
27. Howard GA, Turner RT, Sherrard DJ, et al. Human bone cells in culture metabolize 25–hydroxyvitamin D_3 to 1,25–dihydroxyvitamin D_3 and 24,25–dihydroxyvitamin D_3. *J Biol Chem* 1981;256:7738–7740.
28. Feldman D, Malloy PJ, Gross C. Vitamin D: metabolism and action. In: Marcus R, Feldman D, Kelsey J, eds. *Osteoporosis.* San Diego: Academic Press, 1996:205–235.
29. Armbrecht HJ, Okuda K, Wongsurawat N, et al. Characterization and regulation of the vitamin D hydroxylases. *J Steroid Biochem Mol Biol* 1992;43:1073–1081.
30. Fraser DR. Regulation of the metabolism of vitamin D. *Physiol Rev* 1980;60:551–613.
31. Reichel H, Koeffler HP, Norman AW. The role of the vitamin D endocrine system in health and disease. *N Engl J Med* 1989;320:980–991.
32. Miller WL. Molecular biology of steroid hormone synthesis. *Endocr Rev* 1988;9:295–318.
33. Fu GK, Lin D, Zhang MYH, et al. Cloning of human 25–hydroxyvitamin D-1α-hydroxylase and mutations causing vitamin D-dependent rickets type 1. *Mol Endocrinol* 1997;11: 1961–1970.
34. Monkawa T, Yoshida T, Wakino S, et al. Molecular cloning of cDNA and genomic DNA for human 25–hydroxyvitamin D_3 1α-hydroxylase. *Biochem Biophys Res Commun* 1997;239:527–533.
35. St-Arnaud R, Messerlian S, Moir JM, et al. The 25–hydroxyvitamin D 1–alpha-hydroxylase gene maps to the pseudovitamin D-deficiency rickets (PDDR) disease locus. *J Bone Miner Res* 1997;12:1552–1559.
36. Shinki T, Shimada H, Wakino S, et al. Cloning and expression of rat 25–hydroxyvitamin D_3–1α-hydroxylase cDNA. *Proc Natl Acad Sci U S A* 1997;94:12920–12925.
37. Takeyama K, Kitanaka S, Sato T, et al. 25–hydroxyvitamin D_3 1α-hydroxylase and vitamin D synthesis. *Science* 1997; 277(19):1827–1830.
38. Yoshida T, Yoshida N, Nakamura A, et al. Cloning of porcine 25–hydroxyvitamin D_3 1α-hydroxylase and its regulation by cAMP in LLC-PK_1 cells. *J Am Soc Nephrol* 1999;10(5):963–970.
39. Fu GK, Portale AA, Miller WL. Complete structure of the human gene for the vitamin D 1α-hydroxylase, P450c1α. *DNA Cell Biol* 1997;16:1499–1507.

40. Morohashi K, Sogawa K, Omura T, et al. Gene structure of human cytochrome P-450(SCC), cholesterol desmolase. *J Biochem (Tokyo)* 1987;101:879–887.
41. Kimmel-Jehan C, DeLuca HF. Cloning of the mouse 25–hydroxyvitamin D_3–1α-hydroxylase (CYP1α) gene. *Biochim Biophys Acta* 2000;1475(2):109–113.
42. Panda DK, Al Kawas S, Seldin MF, et al. 25–hydroxyvitamin D 1alpha-hydroxylase: structure of the mouse gene, chromosomal assignment, and developmental expression. *J Bone Miner Res* 2001;16(1):46–56.
43. Yoshida T, Monkawa T, Tenenhouse HS, et al. Two novel 1α-hydroxylase mutations in French-Canadians with vitamin D dependency rickets type I. *Kidney Int* 1998;54:1437–1443.
44. Kitanaka S, Takeyama K, Murayama A, et al. Inactivating mutations in the 25–hydroxyvitamin D_3 1α-hydroxylase gene in patients with pseudovitamin D-deficiency rickets. *N Engl J Med* 1998;338:653–661.
45. Wang JT, Lin CJ, Burridge SM, et al. Genetics of vitamin D 1α-hydroxylase deficiency in 17 families. *Am J Hum Genet* 1998;63:1694–1702.
46. Smith SJ, Rucka AK, Berry JL, et al. Novel mutations in the 1α-hydroxylase (P450c1) gene in three families with pseudovitamin D-deficiency rickets resulting in loss of functional enzyme activity in blood-derived macrophages. *J Bone Miner Res* 1999;14:730–739.
47. Kitanaka S, Murayama A, Sakaki T, et al. No enzyme activity of 25–hydroxyvitamin D_3 1α-hydroxylase gene product in pseudovitamin D deficiency rickets, including that with mild clinical manifestation. *J Clin Endocrinol Metab* 1999;84:4111–4117.
48. Wang X, Zhang MYH, Miller WL, et al. Novel gene mutations in patients with 1α-hydroxylase deficiency that confer partial enzyme activity *in vitro*. *J Clin Endocrinol Metab* 2002;87:2424–2430.
49. Portale AA, Miller WL. Rickets due to hereditary abnormalities of vitamin D synthesis or action. In: Glorieux FH, Pettifor JM, Juppner H, eds. *Pediatric bone*. San Diego: Academic Press, 2003:583–598.
50. Prader A, Illig R, Heierli E. Eine besondere form des primare vitamin-D-resistenten rachitis mit hypocalcamie und autosomal-dominanten erbgang: die hereditare pseudomangelrachitis. *Helv Paediatr Acta* 1961;16:452–468.
51. Scriver CR. Vitamin D dependency. *Pediatrics* 1970;45:361–363.
52. Carafoli E. The intracellular homeostasis of calcium: an overview. *Ann N Y Acad Sci* 1988;551:147–158.
53. Berridge MJ, Irvine RF. Inositol phosphates and cell signalling. *Nature* 1989;341:197–204.
54. Rasmussen H, Rasmussen JE. Calcium as intracellular messenger: from simplicity to complexity. In: Horecker BL, Chock PB, Stadtman ER, et al., eds. *Current topics in cellular regulation*. New York: Harcourt Brace Jovanovich, 1990:1–109.
55. Friedman PA, Gesek FA. Cellular calcium transport in renal epithelia: measurement, mechanisms, and regulation. *Physiol Rev* 1995;75:429–471.
56. Gmaj P, Murer H, Kinne R. Calcium ion transport across plasma membranes isolated from rat kidney cortex. *Biochem J* 1979;178:549–557.
57. Somermeyer MG, Knauss TC, Weinberg JM, et al. Characterization of Ca^{2+} transport in rat renal brush-border membranes and its modulation by phosphatidic acid. *Biochem J* 1983;214:37–46.
58. Hoenderop JG, Nilius B, Bindels RJ. Molecular mechanism of active Ca^{2+} reabsorption in the distal nephron. *Annu Rev Physiol* 2002;64:529–549.
59. Hoenderop JG, van der Kemp AW, Hartog A, et al. Molecular identification of the apical Ca^{2+} channel in 1, 25–dihydroxyvitamin D_3–responsive epithelia. *J Biol Chem* 1999;274(13):8375–8378.
60. Canessa CM, Horisberger JD, Schild L, et al. Expression cloning of the epithelial sodium channel. *Kidney Int* 1995;48(4):950–955.
61. Canessa CM, Schild L, Buell G, et al. Amiloride-sensitive epithelial Na^+ channel is made of three homologous subunits. *Nature* 1994;367(6462):463–467.
62. Hoenderop JG, Hartog A, Stuiver M, et al. Localization of the epithelial Ca^{2+} channel in rabbit kidney and intestine. *J Am Soc Nephrol* 2000;11:1171–1178.
63. Hoenderop JG, Muller D, Suzuki M, et al. Epithelial calcium channel: gate-keeper of active calcium reabsorption. *Curr Opin Nephrol Hypertens* 2000;9:335–340.
64. Kretsinger RH, Mann JE, Simmonds JG. Model of facilitated diffusion of calcium by the intestinal calcium binding protein. In: Norman AW, Schaefer K, Herrath DV, et al., eds. *Vitamin D: chemical, biochemical and clinical endocrinology of calcium metabolism*. New York: Walter de Gruyter, 1982:233–248.
65. Feher JJ, Fullmer CS, Fritzsch GK. Comparison of the enhanced steady-state diffusion of calcium by calbindin-D_{9k} and calmodulin: possible importance in intestinal absorption. *Cell Calcium* 1989;10:189–203.
66. Feher JJ. Facilitated calcium diffusion by intestinal calcium-binding protein. *Am J Physiol* 1983;244:C303–C307.
67. Bronner F, Pansu D, Stein WD. Analysis of calcium transport in rat intestine. *Adv Exp Med Biol* 1986;208:227–234.
68. Feher JJ, Fullmer CS, Wasserman RH. Role of facilitated diffusion of calcium by calbindin in intestinal calcium absorption. *Am J Physiol* 1992;262(2 Pt 1):C517–C526.
69. Christakos S, Beck JD, Hyllner SJ. Calbindin-D_{28K}. In: Feldman D, Glorieux FH, Pike JW, eds. *Vitamin D*. San Diego: Academic Press, 1997:209–221.
70. Thomasset M. Calbindin-D_{9K}. In: Feldman D, Glorieux FH, Pike JW, eds. *Vitamin D*. San Diego: Academic Press, 1997:223–232.
71. Kumar R, Wieben E, Beecher SJ. The molecular cloning of the complementary deoxyribonucleic acid for bovine vitamin D–dependent calcium-binding protein: structure of the full-length protein and evidence for homologies with other calcium-binding proteins of the troponin-C superfamily of proteins. *Mol Endocrinol* 1989;3:427–432.
72. Bronner F, Pansu D, Stein WD. An analysis of intestinal calcium transport across the intestine. *Am J Physiol* 1986;250:G561–G569.
73. Feher JJ. Facilitated diffusion by intestinal calcium-binding protein. *Am J Physiol* 1983;244:C303–C307.
74. Bronner F. Renal calcium transport: mechanisms and regulation—an overview. *Am J Physiol* 1989;257:F707–F711.
75. Johnson JA, Kumar R. Renal and intestinal calcium transport: roles of vitamin D and vitamin D-dependent calcium binding proteins. *Semin Nephrol* 1994;14:119–128.

76. Roth J, Brown D, Norman AW, et al. Localization of the vitamin D–dependent calcium-binding protein in mammalian kidney. *Am J Physiol* 1982;243:F243–F252.
77. Taylor AN, McIntosh JE, Bourdeau JE. Immunocytochemical localization of vitamin D–dependent calcium-binding protein in renal tubules of rabbit, rat and chick. *Kidney Int* 1982;21:765–773.
78. Li H, Christakos S. Differential regulation of 1,25 dihydroxyvitamin D_3 of calbindin-D_{9k} and calbindin-D_{28k} gene expression in mouse kidney. *Endocrinology* 1991;128:2844–2852.
79. Bindels RJM, Timmermans JAH, Hartog A, et al. Calbindin-D_{9k} and parvalbumin are exclusively located along basolateral membranes in rat distal nephron. *J Am Soc Nephrol* 1991;2:1122–1129.
80. Carafoli E. Calcium pump of the plasma membrane. *Physiol Rev* 1991;71:129–153.
81. Carafoli E, Chiesi M. Calcium pumps in the plasma and intracellular membranes. *Curr Top Cell Regul* 1992;32:209–241.
82. Carafoli E. The Ca^{2+} pump of the plasma membrane. *J Biol Chem* 1992;267:2115–2118.
83. Carafoli E. Biogenesis: plasma membrane calcium ATPase: 15 years of work on the purified enzyme. *FASEB J* 1994;8:993–1002.
84. Penniston JT, Enyedi A, Verma AK, et al. Plasma membrane Ca^{2+} pumps. *Ann N Y Acad Sci* 1997;834:56–64.
85. Borke JL, Minami J, Verman A, et al. Monoclonal antibodies to human erythrocyte membrane Ca^{++}-Mg^{++} adenosine triphosphatase pump recognize an epitope in the basolateral membrane of human kidney distal tubule cells. *J Clin Invest* 1987;80:1225–1231.
86. Brunette MG, Blouin S, Chan M. High affinity Ca^{2+} -Mg^{2+} ATPase in the distal tubule of the mouse kidney. *Can J Physiol Pharmacol* 1987;65:2093–2098.
87. Doucet A, Katz AI. High-affinity Ca^{++}-Mg^{++}-ATPase along the rabbit nephron. *Am J Physiol* 1982;242:F346–F352.
88. Borke JL, Minami J, Verma AK, et al. Co-localization of erythrocyte Ca^{++}-Mg^{++} ATPase and vitamin D–dependent 28–kDa-calcium binding protein. *Kidney Int* 1988;34:262–267.
89. Magosci M, Yamaki M, Penniston JT, et al. Localization of mRNAs coding for isozymes of plasma membrane Ca^{2+}-ATPase pump in rat kidney. *Am J Physiol* 1992;263:F7–F14.
90. Ghijsen WEJM, Van Os CH. 1α,25–dihydroxyvitamin D_3 regulates ATP-dependent calcium transport in basolateral plasma membranes of rat enterocytes. *Biochim Biophys Acta* 1982;689:170–172.
91. Shull GE, Greeb J. Molecular cloning of two isoforms of the plasma membrane Ca^{2+}-transporting ATPase from rat brain. Structural and functional domains exhibit similarity to Na^+,K^+- and other cation transport ATPases. *J Biol Chem* 1988;263:8646–8657.
92. Verma AK, Filoteo AG, Stanford DR, et al. Complete primary structure of a human plasma membrane Ca^{2+} pump. *J Biol Chem* 1988;263:14152–14159.
93. Greeb J, Shull GE. Molecular cloning of a third isoform of the calmodulin-sensitive plasma membrane Ca^{2+}-transporting ATPase that is expressed predominantly in brain and skeletal muscle. *J Biol Chem* 1989;264:18569–18576.
94. De Jaegere S, Wuytack F, Eggermont JA, et al. Molecular cloning and sequencing of the plasma-membrane Ca^{2+} pump of pig smooth muscle. *Biochem J* 1990;271:655–660.
95. Strehler EE, James P, Fischer R, et al. Peptide sequence analysis and molecular cloning reveal two calcium pump isoforms in the human erythrocyte membrane. *J Biol Chem* 1990;265:2835–2842.
96. Strehler EE. Recent advances in the molecular characterization of plasma membrane Ca^{2+} pumps. *J Membr Biol* 1991; 120:1–15.
97. Carafoli E, Garcia-Martin E, Guerini D. The plasma membrane calcium pump: recent developments and future perspectives. *Experientia* 1996;52:1091–1100.
98. Lytton J, Lee SL, Lee WS, et al. The kidney sodium-calcium exchanger. *Ann N Y Acad Sci* 1996;779:58–72.
99. Philipson KD, Nicoll DA, Matsuoka S, et al. Molecular regulation of the $Na(^+)$-Ca^{2+} exchanger. *Ann N Y Acad Sci* 1996;779:20–28.
100. Hryshko LV, Philipson KD. Sodium-calcium exchange: recent advances. *Basic Res Cardiol* 1997;92[Suppl 1]:45–51.
101. Nicoll DA, Longoni S, Philipson KD. Molecular cloning and functional expression of the cardiac sarcolemmal Na^+-Ca^{2+} exchanger. *Science* 1990;250:562–565.
102. Aceto JF, Condrescu M, Kroupis C, et al. Cloning and expression of the bovine cardiac sodium-calcium exchanger. *Arch Biochem Biophys* 1992;298:553–560.
103. Komuro I, Wenninger KE, Philipson KD, et al. Molecular cloning and characterization of the human cardiac Na^+/Ca^{2+} exchanger cDNA. *Proc Natl Acad Sci U S A* 1992;89:4769–4773.
104. Reilly RF, Shugrue CA. cDNA cloning of a renal Na^+-Ca^{2+} exchanger. *Am J Physiol* 1992;262:F1105–F1109.
105. Furman I, Cook O, Kasir J, et al. Cloning of two isoforms of the rat brain $Na(^+)$-Ca^{2+} exchanger gene and their functional expression in HeLa cells. *FEBS Lett* 1993;319:105–109.
106. Low W, Kasir J, Rahamimoff H. Cloning of the rat heart $Na(^+)$-Ca^{2+} exchanger and its functional expression in HeLa cells. *FEBS Lett* 1993;316:63–67.
107. Nakasaki Y, Iwamoto T, Hanada H, et al. Cloning of the rat aortic smooth muscle Na^+/Ca^{2+} exchanger and tissue-specific expression of isoforms. *J Biochem (Tokyo)* 1993;114:528–534.
108. Shieh BH, Xia Y, Sparkes RS, et al. Mapping of the gene for the cardiac sarcolemmal $Na(^+)$-Ca^{2+} exchanger to human chromosome 2p21–p23. *Genomics* 1992;12:616–617.
109. Li Z, Matsuoka S, Hryshko LV, et al. Cloning of the NCX2 isoform of the plasma membrane $Na(^+)$-Ca^{2+} exchanger. *J Biol Chem* 1994;269:17434–17439.
110. Kraev A, Chumakov I, Carafoli E. The organization of the human gene NCX1 encoding the sodium-calcium exchanger. *Genomics* 1996;37:105–112.
111. Nicoll DA, Quednau BD, Qui Z, et al. Cloning of a third mammalian Na^+-Ca^{2+} exchanger, NCX3. *J Biol Chem* 1996; 271:24914–24921.
112. Quednau BD, Nicoll DA, Philipson KD. Tissue specificity and alternative splicing of the Na^+/Ca^{2+} exchanger isoforms NCX1, NCX2, and NCX3 in rat. *Am J Physiol* 1997;272:C1250–C1261.
113. Borke JL, Penniston JT, Kumar R. Recent advances in calcium transport by the kidney. *Semin Nephrol* 1990;10:15–23.

114. Ramachandran C, Brunette MG. The renal Na^+/Ca^{2+} exchange system is located exclusively in the distal tubule. *Biochem J* 1989;257:259–264.
115. Reilly RF, Shugrue CA, Lattanzi D, et al. Immunolocalization of the Na^+/Ca^{2+} exchanger in rabbit kidney. *Am J Physiol* 1993;265:F327–F332.
116. Yu AS, Hebert SC, Lee SL, et al. Identification and localization of renal $Na(^+)$-Ca^{2+} exchanger by polymerase chain reaction. *Am J Physiol* 1992;263:F680–F685.
117. Lassiter WE, Gottschalk CW, Mylle M. Micropuncture study of tubular reabsorption of calcium in normal rodents. *Am J Physiol* 1963;204:771–775.
118. Harris CA, Baer PG, Chirito E, et al. Composition of mammalian glomerular filtrate. *Am J Physiol* 1974;227:972–976.
119. Chen PS Jr, Neuman WF. Renal excretion of calcium by the dog. *Am J Physiol* 1955;180:623–631.
120. Poulos PP. The renal tubular reabsorption and urinary excretion of calcium by the dog. *J Lab Clin Med* 1957;49:253–257.
121. Copp DH, McPherson GD, McIntosh HW. Renal excretion of calcium in man. *Metabolism* 1960;9:680–685.
122. Peacock M, Nordin BEC. Tubular reabsorption of calcium in normal and hypercalciuric subjects. *J Clin Pathol* 1968; 21:353–358.
123. Peacock M, Robertson WG, Nordin BEC. Relation between serum and urinary calcium with particular reference to parathyroid activity. *Lancet* 1969;1:384.
124. Yanagawa N, Lee DBN. Renal handling of calcium and phosphorus. In: Coe FL, Favus MJ, eds. *Disorders of bone and mineral metabolism.* New York: Raven Press, 1992:3–40.
125. Sutton RA, Dirks JH. The renal excretion of calcium: a review of micropuncture data. *Can J Physiol Pharmacol* 1975; 53:979–988.
126. Friedman PA, Gesek FA. Calcium transport in renal epithelial cells. *Am J Physiol* 1993;264:F181–F198.
127. Suki WN, Rouse D. Renal transport of calcium, magnesium, and phosphate. In: Suki WN, Rouse D, eds. *Brenner and Rector's the kidney.* Philadelphia: WB Saunders, 1996:472–509.
128. Ng RCK, Rouse D, Suki WN. Calcium transport in the rabbit superficial proximal convoluted tubule. *J Clin Invest* 1984;74:834–842.
129. Rouse D, Ng RCK, Suki WN. Calcium transport in the pars recta and thin descending limb of Henle of the rabbit, perfused in vitro. *J Clin Invest* 1980;65:37–42.
130. Rocha AS, Migaldi JB, Kokko JP. Calcium and phosphate transport in isolated segments of rabbit Henle's loop. *J Clin Invest* 1977;59:975–983.
131. Shareghi GR, Stoner LC. Calcium transport across segments of the rabbit distal nephron in vitro. *Am J Physiol* 1978;235:F367–F375.
132. Bourdeau JE, Burg MB. Voltage dependence of calcium transport in the thick ascending limb of Henle's loop. *Am J Physiol* 1979;236:F357–F364.
133. Shareghi GR, Agus ZS. Magnesium transport in the cortical thick ascending limb of Henle's loop of the rabbit. *J Clin Invest* 1982;69:759–769.
134. Imai M. Calcium transport across the rabbit thick ascending limb of Henle's loop perfused in vitro. *Pflugers Arch* 1978;374:255–263.
135. Suki WN, Rouse D, Ng RCK, et al. Calcium transport in the thick ascending limb of Henle. Heterogeneity of function in the medullary and cortical segments. *J Clin Invest* 1980;66:1004–1009.
136. Rouse D, Suki WN. Renal control of extracellular calcium. *Kidney Int* 1990;38:700–708.
137. Bourdeau JE, Burg MB. Effect of PTH on calcium transport across the cortical thick ascending limb of Henle's loop. *Am J Physiol* 1980;239:F121–F126.
138. Suki WN, Rouse D. Hormonal regulation of calcium transport in thick ascending limb renal tubules. *Am J Physiol* 1981;241:F171–F174.
139. Bengele HH, Alexander EA, Lechene CP. Calcium and magnesium transport along the inner medullary collecting duct of the rat. *Am J Physiol* 1980;239:F24–F29.
140. Agus ZS, Chiu PJS, Goldbeerg M. Regulation of urinary calcium excretion in the rat. *Am J Physiol* 1977;232:F545–F549.
141. Wasserstein AG, Stolley PD, Soper KA, et al. Case-control study of risk factors for idiopathic calcium nephrolithiasis. *Miner Electrolyte Metab* 1987;13:85–95.
142. Wong NLM, Quamme GA, Sutton RAL, et al. Effect of phosphate infusion on renal phosphate and calcium transport. *Renal Physiol* 1985;8:30–37.
143. Portale AA, Halloran BP, Murphy MM, et al. Oral intake of phosphorus can determine the serum concentration of 1,25–dihydroxyvitamin D by determining its production rate in humans. *J Clin Invest* 1986;77:7–12.
144. Ichikawa I, Humes HD, Dousa TP, et al. Influence of parathyroid hormone on glomerular ultrafiltration in the rat. *Am J Physiol* 1978;234:F393–F401.
145. Greger R, Lang F, Oberleither H. Distal site of calcium reabsorption in the rat nephron. *Pflugers Arch* 1978;374: 153–157.
146. Bourdeau JE, Burg MB. Effect of PTH on calcium transport across the cortical thick ascending limb of Henle's loop. *Am J Physiol* 1980;239:F121–F126.
147. Imai M. Effects of parathyroid hormone and N^6,O^{2-}dibutyryl cyclic AMP on Ca transport across the rabbit distal nephron segments perfused in vitro. *Pflugers Arch* 1981; 390:145–151.
148. Shimizu T, Yoshitomi K, Nakamura M, et al. Effects of PTH, calcitonin, and cAMP on calcium transport in rabbit distal nephron segments. *Am J Physiol* 1990;259:F408–F414.
149. Gesek FA, Friedman PA. On the mechanism of parathyroid hormone stimulation of calcium uptake by mouse distal convoluted tubule cells. *J Clin Invest* 1992;90:749–758.
150. Bourdeau JE, Lau K. Effects of parathyroid hormone on cytosolic free calcium concentration in individual rabbit connecting tubules. *J Clin Invest* 1989;83:373–379.
151. Bacskai GJ, Friedman PA. Activation of latent Ca^{2+} channels in renal epithelial cells by parathyroid hormone. *Nature* 1990;347:388–391.
152. Bouhtiauy I, Lajeunesse D, Brunette MG. Effect of vitamin D depletion on calcium transport by the luminal and basolateral membranes of the proximal and distal nephrons. *Endocrinology* 1993;132:115–120.
153. Bindels RJ, Hartog A, Timmermans J, et al. Active Ca^{2+} transport in primary cultures of rabbit kidney CCD: stimulation by 1,25–dihydroxyvitamin D_3 and PTH. *Am J Physiol* 1991;261(5 Pt 2):F799–F807.

154. Hoenderop JG, Muller D, van der Kemp AW, et al. Calcitriol controls the epithelial calcium channel in kidney. *J Am Soc Nephrol* 2001;12:1342–1349.
155. Sutton RAL, Wong NLM, Dirks JH. Effects of metabolic acidosis and alkalosis on sodium and calcium transport in the dog kidney. *Kidney Int* 1979;15:520–533.
156. Lemann J Jr, Litzow JR, Lennon EJ. Studies of the mechanism by which chronic metabolic acidosis augments urinary calcium excretion in man. *J Clin Invest* 1967;46:1318–1328.
157. Stacy BD, Wilson BW. Acidosis and hypercalciuria: renal mechanism affecting calcium, magnesium, and sodium excretion in the sheep. *Physiology* 1970;210:549–564.
158. Lemann J, Gray RW, Pleuss JA. Potassium bicarbonate, but not sodium bicarbonate, reduces urinary calcium excretion and improves calcium balance in healthy men. *Kidney Int* 1989;35:688–695.
159. Sakhaee K, Nicar M, Hill K, et al. Contrasting effects of potassium citrate and sodium citrate therapies and crystallization of stone-forming salts. *Kidney Int* 1983;24:348–352.
160. Parfitt AM, Higgins BA, Nassim JR, et al. Metabolic studies in patients with hypercalcemia. *Clin Sci* 1964;27:463–482.
161. Edwards NA, Hodgkinson A. Metabolic studies in patients with idiopathic hypercalciuria. *Clin Sci* 1965;29:143–157.
162. Anderson OS. Acute experimental acid-base disturbances in dogs. *Scand J Clin Lab Invest* 1962;66[Suppl]:1–20.
163. Gray SP, Morris JEW, Brooks CJ. Renal handling of calcium, magnesium, inorganic phosphate and hydrogen ions during prolonged exposure to elevated carbon dioxide concentration. *Clin Sci Mol Med* 1973;45:751–764.
164. Harris CA, Sutton RAL, Dirks JH. Effects of hypercalcemia on calcium and phosphate ultrafilterability and tubular reabsorption in the rat. *Am J Physiol* 1977;233:F201–F206.
165. Humes HD, Ichikawa I, Troy JL, et al. Evidence for a parathyroid hormone–dependent influence of calcium on the glomerular filtration. *J Clin Invest* 1978;62:32–40.
166. Edwards BR, Sutton RAL, Dirks JH. Effect of calcium infusion on renal tubular reabsorption in the dog. *Am J Physiol* 1974;227:13–18.
167. Costanzo LS, Windhager EE. Calcium and sodium transport by the distal convoluted tubule of the rat. *Am J Physiol* 1978;235:F492–F506.
168. Marshall RW. Plasma fractions. In: Nordin BEC, ed. *Calcium, phosphate and magnesium metabolism.* London: Churchill Livingstone, 1976:162–185.
169. Mostellar ME, Tuttle EP. Effects of alkalosis on plasma concentration and urinary excretion of inorganic phosphate in man. *J Clin Invest* 1964;43:138–149.
170. Brodehl J, Gellissen K, Weber HP. Postnatal development of tubular phosphate reabsorption. *Clin Nephrol* 1982;17:163–171.
171. Greenberg BG, Winters RW, Graham JB. The normal range of serum inorganic phosphorus and its utility as discriminant in the diagnosis of congenital hypophosphatemia. *J Clin Endocrinol* 1960;20:364–379.
172. Rowe J, Rowe D, Horak E, et al. Hypophosphatemia and hypercalciuria in small premature infants fed human milk: evidence for inadequate dietary phosphorus. *J Pediatr* 1984;104:112–117.
173. Giles MM, Fenton MH, Shaw B, et al. Sequential calcium and phosphorus balance studies in preterm infants. *J Pediatr* 1987;110:591–598.
174. Wilkinson R. Absorption of calcium, phosphorus and magnesium. In: Nordin BEC, ed. *Calcium, phosphate and magnesium metabolism.* New York: Churchill Livingstone, 1976:36–112.
175. Lee DBN, Kurokawa K. Physiology of phosphorus metabolism. In: Maxwell MH, Kleeman CR, Narins RG, eds. *Clinical disorders of fluid and electrolyte metabolism.* New York: McGraw-Hill, 1987:245–295.
176. Favus MJ. Intestinal absorption of calcium, magnesium, and phosphorus. In: Coe FL, Favus MJ, eds. *Disorders of bone and mineral metabolism.* New York: Raven Press, 1992:57–81.
177. Berner W, Kinne R, Murer H. Phosphate transport into brush-border membrane vesicles isolated from rat small intestine. *Biochem J* 1976;160:467–474.
178. Peterlik M, Wasserman RH. Effect of vitamin D on transepithelial phosphate transport in chick intestine. *Am J Physiol* 1978;234(4):E379–E388.
179. Danisi G, Bonjour J-P, Straub RW. Regulation of Na-dependent phosphate influx across the mucosal border of duodenum by 1,25–dihydroxycholecalciferol. *Pflugers Arch* 1980;388:227–232.
180. Lee DB, Walling MW, Corry DB. Phosphate transport across rat jejunum: influence of sodium, pH, and 1,25–dihydroxyvitamin D_3. *Am J Physiol* 1986;251(1 Pt 1):G90–G95.
181. Hilfiker H, Hattenhauer O, Traebert M, et al. Characterization of a murine type II sodium-phosphate co-transporter expressed in mammalian small intestine. *Proc Natl Acad Sci U S A* 1998;95:14564–14569.
182. Hattenhauer O, Traebert M, Murer H, et al. Regulation of small intestinal Na-P(i) type IIb cotransporter by dietary phosphate intake. *Am J Physiol* 1999;277(4 Pt 1):G756–G762.
183. Tanaka Y, DeLuca HF. The control of 25–hydroxyvitamin D metabolism by inorganic phosphorus. *Arch Biochem Biophys* 1973;154:566–574.
184. Baxter LA, DeLuca HF. Stimulation of 25–hydroxyvitamin D_3–1α-hydroxylase by phosphate depletion. *J Biol Chem* 1976;251:3158–3161.
185. Gray RW, Napoli JL. Dietary phosphate deprivation increases 1,25–dihydroxyvitamin D_3 synthesis in rat kidney in vitro. *J Biol Chem* 1983;258:1152–1155.
186. Maierhofer WJ, Gray RW, Lemann J Jr. Phosphate deprivation increases serum 1,25$(OH)_2$–vitamin D concentrations in healthy men. *Kidney Int* 1984;25:571–575.
187. Portale AA, Halloran BP, Morris RC Jr. Physiologic regulation of the serum concentration of 1,25–dihydroxyvitamin D by phosphorus in normal men. *J Clin Invest* 1989;83:1494–1499.
188. Murer H, Biber J. A molecular view of proximal tubular inorganic phosphate (Pi) reabsorption and of its regulation. *Pflugers Arch* 1997;433:379–389.
189. Biber J. Cellular aspects of proximal tubular phosphate reabsorption. *Kidney Int* 1989;36:360–369.
190. Murer H. Cellular mechanisms in proximal tubular P_i reabsorption: some answers and more questions. *J Am Soc Nephrol* 1992;2:1649–1665.

191. Murer H, Werner A, Reshkin S, et al. Cellular mechanisms in proximal tubular reabsorption of inorganic phosphate. *Am J Physiol* 1991;260:C885–C899.
192. Murer H, Biber J. Renal tubular phosphate transport. In: Seldin DW, Giebisch G, eds. *The kidney: physiology and pathophysiology*. New York: Raven Press, 1992:2481–2509.
193. Murer H, Biber J. Molecular mechanisms of renal apical Na/phosphate cotransport. *Annu Rev Physiol* 1996;58:607–618.
194. Murer H, Burckhardt G. Membrane transport of anions across epithelia of mammalian small intestine and kidney proximal tubule. *Rev Physiol Biochem Pharmacol* 1983;96:1–53.
195. Amstutz M, Mohrmann M, Gmaj P, et al. Effect of pH on phosphate transport in rat renal brush border membrane vesicles. *Am J Physiol* 1985;248:F705–F710.
196. Gmaj P, Murer H. Cellular mechanisms of inorganic phosphate transport in kidney. *Physiol Rev* 1986;66:36–70.
197. Kinoshita Y, Fukase M, Nakada M, et al. Defective adaptation to a low phosphate environment by cultured renal tubular cells from X-linked hypophosphatemic (*Hyp*) mice. *Biochem Biophys Res Commun* 1987;144:763–769.
198. Sacktor B, Cheng L. Sodium gradient-dependent phosphate transport in renal brush border membrane vesicles. *J Biol Chem* 1981;256:8080–8084.
199. Molitoris BA, Alfrey AC, Harris RA, et al. Renal apical membrane cholesterol and fluidity in regulation of phosphate transport. *Am J Physiol* 1985;249:F12–F19.
200. Levi M, Baird BM, Wilson PV. Cholesterol modulates rat renal brush border membrane phosphate transport. *J Clin Invest* 1990;85:231–237.
201. Levi M, Jameson DM, Wieb Van Der Meer B. Role of BBM lipid composition and fluidity in impaired renal Pi transport in aged rat. *Am J Physiol* 1989;256:F85–F94.
202. Levine BS, Knibloe KA, Golchini K, et al. Renal adaptation to dietary phosphate deprivation: role of proximal tubule brush-border membrane fluidity. *Am J Physiol* 1991;260: F613–F618.
203. Werner A, Moore ML, Mantei N, et al. Cloning and expression of cDNA for a Na/P_i cotransport system of kidney cortex. *Proc Natl Acad Sci U S A* 1991;88:9608–9612.
204. Magagnin S, Werner A, Markovich D, et al. Expression cloning of human and rat renal cortex Na/Pi cotransport. *Proc Natl Acad Sci U S A* 1993;90:5979–5983.
205. Murer H, Hernando N, Forster I, et al. Proximal tubular phosphate reabsorption: molecular mechanisms. *Physiol Rev* 2000;80:1373–1409.
206. Biber J, Custer M, Werner A, et al. Localization of NaPi-1, a Na/Pi cotransporter, in rabbit kidney proximal tubules. II. Localization by immunohistochemistry. *Pflugers Arch* 1993; 424:210–215.
207. Chong SS, Kristjansson K, Zoghbi HY, et al. Molecular cloning of the cDNA encoding a human renal sodium phosphate transport protein and its assignment to chromosome 6p21.3–p23. *Genomics* 1993;18:355–359.
208. Miyamoto K, Tatsumi S, Sonoda T, et al. Cloning and functional expression of a Na(+)-dependent phosphate co-transporter from human kidney: cDNA cloning and functional expression. *Biochem J* 1995;305(Pt 1):81–85.
209. Miyamoto K, Tatsumi S, Yamamoto H, et al. Chromosome assignments of genes for human Na(+)-dependent phosphate co-transporters NaPi-3 and NPT-1. *Tokushima J Exp Med* 1995;42(1–2):5–9.
210. Chong SS, Kozak CA, Liu L, et al. Cloning, genetic mapping, and expression analysis of a mouse renal sodium-dependent phosphate cotransporter. *Am J Physiol* 1995;268:F1038–F1045.
211. Collins JF, Ghishan FK. Molecular cloning, functional expression, tissue distribution, and in situ hybridization of the renal sodium phosphate (Na^+/P(i)) transporter in the control and hypophosphatemic mouse. *FASEB J* 1994;8:862–868.
212. Li H, Ren P, Onwochei M, et al. Regulation of rat Na+/Pi cotransporter-1 gene expression: the roles of glucose and insulin. *Am J Physiol* 1996;271(6 Pt 1):E1021–E1028.
213. Li H, Xie Z. Molecular cloning of two rat Na^+/Pi cotransporters: evidence for differential tissue expression of transcripts. *Cell Mol Biol Res* 1995;41(5):451–460.
214. Ni B, Du Y, Wu X, et al. Molecular cloning, expression, and chromosomal localization of a human brain-specific Na(+)-dependent inorganic phosphate cotransporter. *J Neurochem* 1996;66(6):2227–2238.
215. Ni B, Rosteck PR Jr, Nadi NS, et al. Cloning and expression of a cDNA encoding a brain-specific Na(+)-dependent inorganic phosphate cotransporter. *Proc Natl Acad Sci U S A* 1994;91(12):5607–5611.
216. Levi M, Kempson SA, Lotscher M, et al. Molecular regulation of renal phosphate transport. *J Membr Biol* 1996;154: 1–9.
217. Murer H, Hernando N, Forster I, et al. Regulation of Na/Pi transporter in the proximal tubule. *Annu Rev Physiol* 2003;65: 531–542.
218. Beck L, Karaplis AC, Amizuka N, et al. Targeted inactivation of Npt2 in mice leads to severe renal phosphate wasting, hypercalciuria, and skeletal abnormalities. *Proc Natl Acad Sci U S A* 1998;95(9):5372–5377.
219. Gupta A, Guo XL, Alvarez UM, et al. Regulation of sodium-dependent phosphate transport in osteoclasts. *J Clin Invest* 1997;100(3):538–549.
220. Verri T, Markovich D, Perego C, et al. Cloning of a rabbit renal Na-Pi cotransporter, which is regulated by dietary phosphate. *Am J Physiol* 1995;268:F626–F633.
221. Hartmann CM, Wagner CA, Busch AE, et al. Transport characteristics of a murine renal Na/Pi-cotransporter. *Pflugers Arch* 1995;430:830–836.
222. Werner A, Murer H, Kinne RK. Cloning and expression of a renal Na-Pi cotransport system from flounder. *Am J Physiol* 1994;267:F311–F317.
223. Sorribas V, Markovich D, Hayes G, et al. Cloning of a Na/Pi cotransporter from opossum kidney cells. *J Biol Chem* 1994;269:6615–6621.
224. Helps C, Murer H, McGivan J. Cloning, sequence analysis and expression of the cDNA encoding a sodium-dependent phosphate transporter from the bovine renal epithelial cell line NBL-1. *Eur J Biochem* 1995;228:927–930.
225. Kos CH, Tihy F, Econs MJ, et al. Localization of a renal sodium-phosphate cotransporter gene to human chromosome 5q35. *Genomics* 1994;19:176–177.
226. Hartmann CM, Hewson AS, Kos CH, et al. Structure of murine and human renal type II Na^+-phosphate cotransporter genes (Npt2 and NPT2). *Proc Natl Acad Sci U S A* 1996;93:7409–7414.

227. Kos CH, Tihy F, Murer H, et al. Comparative mapping of Na+-phosphate cotransporter genes, NPT1 and NPT2, in human and rabbit. *Cytogenet Cell Genet* 1996;75(1):22–24.
228. Kavanaugh MP, Kabat D. Identification and characterization of a widely expressed phosphate transporter/retrovirus receptor family. *Kidney Int* 1996;49:959–963.
229. Kavanaugh MP, Miller DG, Zhang W, et al. Cell-surface receptors for gibbon ape leukemia virus and amphotropic murine retrovirus are inducible sodium-dependent phosphate symporters. *Proc Natl Acad Sci U S A* 1994;91:7071–7075.
230. Olah Z, Lehel C, Anderson WB, et al. The cellular receptor for gibbon ape leukemia virus is a novel high affinity sodium-dependent phosphate transporter. *J Biol Chem* 1994;269: 25426–25431.
231. Tenenhouse HS, Roy S, Martel J, et al. Differential expression, abundance, and regulation of Na+-phosphate cotransporter genes in murine kidney. *Am J Physiol* 1998;275(4 Pt 2):F527–F534.
232. Baumann K, deRouffignac C, Roinel N, et al. Renal phosphate transport: inhomogeneity of local proximal transport rates and sodium dependence. *Pflugers Arch* 1975;356:287–298.
233. Ullrich KJ, Rumrich G, Kloss S. Phosphate transport in the proximal convolution of the rat kidney. *Pflugers Arch* 1977;372: 269–274.
234. McKeown JW, Brazy PC, Dennis VW. Intrarenal heterogeneity for fluid, phosphate and glucose absorption in the rabbit. *Am J Physiol* 1979;237:F312–F318.
235. Haas JA, Berndt T, Knox FG. Nephron heterogeneity of phosphate reabsorption. *Am J Physiol* 1978;234:F287–F290.
236. Haramati A, Haas JA, Knox FG. Nephron heterogeneity of phosphate reabsorption: effect of parathyroid hormone. *Am J Physiol* 1984;246:F155–F158.
237. Goldfarb S. Jextamedullary and superficial nephron phosphate reabsorption in the cat. *Am J Physiol* 1980;239:F336–F342.
238. deRouffignac C, Morel F, Moss N, et al. Micropuncture study of water and electrolyte movements along the loop of Henle in psammomys with special reference to magnesium, calcium, and phosphorus. *Pflugers Arch* 1973;344:309–326.
239. Knox FG, Haas JA, Berndt T, et al. Phosphate transport in superficial and deep nephrons in phosphate-loaded rats. *Am J Physiol* 1977;233:F150–F153.
240. Muhlbauer RC, Bonjour JP, Fleisch H. Tubular localization of adaptation to dietary phosphate in rats. *Am J Physiol* 1977;233:F342–F348.
241. Dennis VW, Bello-Reuss E, Robinson RR. Response of phosphate transport to parathyroid hormone in segments of rabbit nephron. *Am J Physiol* 1977;233:F29–F38.
242. Shareghi GA, Agus ZS. Phosphate transport in the light segment of the rabbit cortical collecting tubule. *Am J Physiol* 1982;242:F379–F384.
243. Peraino RA, Suki WN. Phosphate transport by isolated rabbit cortical collecting tubule. *Am J Physiol* 1980;238:F358–F362.
244. Stoll R, Kinne R, Murer H. Effect of dietary phosphate intake on phosphate transport by isolated rat renal brush border vesicles. *Biochem J* 1979;180:465–470.
245. Kempson SA, Dousa TP. Phosphate transport across renal cortical brush border membrane vesicles from rats stabilized on a normal, high or low phosphate diet. *Life Sci* 1979; 24:881–888.
246. Tenenhouse HS, Scriver CR. Renal brush border membrane adaptation to phosphorus deprivation in the Hyp/Y mouse. *Nature* 1979;281:225–227.
247. Brazy PC, McKeown JW, Harris RH, et al. Comparative effects of dietary phosphate, unilateral nephrectomy, and parathyroid hormone on phosphate transport by the rabbit proximal tubule. *Kidney Int* 1980;17:788–800.
248. Barrett PQ, Gertner JM, Rasmussen H. Effect of dietary phosphate on transport properties of pig renal microvillus vesicles. *Am J Physiol* 1980;239:F352–F359.
249. Cheng L, Liang CT, Sacktor B. Phosphate uptake by renal membrane vesicles of rabbits adapted to high and low phosphorus diets. *Am J Physiol* 1983;245:F175–F180.
250. Levine BS, Ho K, Hodsman A, et al. Early renal brush border membrane adaptation to dietary phosphorus. *Miner Electrolyte Metab* 1984;10:222–227.
251. Levine BS, Ho LD, Pasiecznik K, et al. Renal adaptation to phosphorus deprivation: characterization of early events. *J Bone Miner Res* 1986;1:33–40.
252. Caverzasio J, Bonjour JP. Mechanism of rapid phosphate (Pi) transport adaptation to a single low Pi meal in rat renal brush border membrane. *Pflugers Arch* 1985;404:227–231.
253. Cheng L, Dersch C, Kraus E, et al. Renal adaptation to phosphate load in the acutely thyroparathyroidectomized rat: rapid alteration in brush border membrane phosphate transport. *Am J Physiol* 1984;246:F488–F494.
254. Kempson SA, Shah SV, Werness PG, et al. Renal brush border membrane adaptation to phosphorus deprivation: effects of fasting versus low-phosphorus diet. *Kidney Int* 1980;18:36–47.
255. Biber J, Murer H. Na-Pi cotransport in LLC-PK cells: fast adaptive response to Pi deprivation. *Am J Physiol* 1985;249: C430–C434.
256. Caverzasio J, Brown CDA, Biber J, et al. Adaptation of phosphate transport in phosphate-deprived LLC-PK cells. *Am J Physiol* 1985;248:F122–F127.
257. Escoubet B, Djabali K, Amiel C. Adaptation to P_i deprivation of cell Na-dependent P_i uptake: a widespread process. *Am J Physiol* 1989;256:C322–C328.
258. Lotscher M, Kaissling B, Biber J, et al. Role of microtubules in the rapid regulation of renal phosphate transport in response to acute alterations in dietary phosphate content. *J Clin Invest* 1997;99:1302–1312.
259. Markovich D, Verri T, Sorribas V, et al. Regulation of opossum kidney (OK) cell Na/Pi cotransport by Pi deprivation involves mRNA stability. *Pflugers Arch* 1995;430:459–463.
260. Pfister MF, Hilfiker H, Forgo J, et al. Cellular mechanisms involved in the acute adaptation of OK cell Na/Pi-cotransport to high- or low-Pi medium. *Pflugers Arch* 1998;435(5):713–719.
261. Murer H, Biber J. Membrane permeability. Epithelial transport proteins: physiology and pathophysiology. *Curr Opin Cell Biol* 1998;10:429–434.
262. Murer H, Hernando N, Forster I, et al. Molecular aspects in the regulation of renal inorganic phosphate reabsorption: the type IIa sodium/inorganic phosphate co-transporter as the key player. *Curr Opin Nephrol Hypertens* 2001;10:555–561.
263. Werner A, Kempson SA, Biber J, et al. Increase of Na/Pi-cotransport encoding mRNA in response to low Pi diet in rat kidney cortex. *J Biol Chem* 1994;269:6637–6639.

264. Levi M, Lotscher M, Sorribas V, et al. Cellular mechanisms of acute and chronic adaptation of rat renal P(i) transporter to alterations in dietary P(i). *Am J Physiol* 1994;267:F900–F908.
265. Tenenhouse HS, Martel J, Biber J, et al. Effect of P(i) restriction on renal Na(+)-P(i) cotransporter mRNA and immunoreactive protein in X-linked Hyp mice. *Am J Physiol* 1995;268:F1062–F1069.
266. Beck L, Tenenhouse HS, Meyer RA Jr, et al. Renal expression of Na^+-phosphate cotransporter mRNA and protein: effect of the Gy mutation and low phosphate diet. *Pflugers Arch* 1996;431:936–941.
267. Katai K, Segawa H, Haga H, et al. Acute regulation by dietary phosphate of the sodium-dependent phosphate transporter (NaP(i)-2) in rat kidney. *J Biochem (Tokyo)* 1997;121(1):50–55.
268. Takahashi F, Morita K, Katai K, et al. Effects of dietary Pi on the renal Na^+-dependent Pi transporter NaPi-2 in thyroparathyroidectomized rats. *Biochem J* 1998;333[Pt 1]:175–181.
269. Kido S, Miyamoto K, Mizobuchi H, et al. Identification of regulatory sequences and binding proteins in the type II sodium/phosphate cotransporter NPT2 gene responsive to dietary phosphate. *J Biol Chem* 1999;274:28256–28263.
270. Mizgala CL, Quamme GA. Renal handling of phosphate. *Physiol Rev* 1985;65:431–466.
271. Evers J, Murer H, Kinne R. Effect of parathyrin on the transport properties of isolated renal brush-border vesicles. *Biochem J* 1978;172:49–56.
272. Hammerman MR, Karl IE, Hruska KA. Regulation of canine renal vesicle P_i transport by growth hormone and parathyroid hormone. *J Biol Chem* 1982;257:992–999.
273. Pastoriza-Munoz E, Colindres RE, Lassiter WE, et al. Effect of parathyroid hormone on phosphate reabsorption in rat distal convolution. *Am J Physiol* 235;1978:F321–F330.
274. Hruska KA, Moskowitz D, Esbrit P, et al. Stimulation of inositol triphosphate and diacylglycerol production in renal tubular cells by parathyroid hormone. *J Clin Invest* 1987;79:230–239.
275. Goligorsky MS, Loftus D, Hruska KA. Cytoplasmic Ca^{2+} in individual proximal tubular cells in culture: effects of parathyroid hormone. *Am J Physiol* 1986;251:F938–F944.
276. Hruska KA, Goligorsky M, Scoble J, et al. Effects of parathyroid hormone on cytosolic calcium in renal proximal tubular primary cultures. *Am J Physiol* 1986;251:F188–F198.
277. Cole JA, Eber SL, Poelling RE, et al. A dual mechanism for regulation of kidney phosphate transport by parathyroid hormone. *Am J Physiol* 1987;253:E221–E227.
278. Nakai M, Kinoshita Y, Fukase M, et al. Phorbol esters inhibit phosphate uptake in opossum kidney cells: a model of proximal renal tubular cells. *Biochem Biophys Res Commun* 1987;145:303–308.
279. Malstrom K, Stange G, Murer H. Intracellular cascades in the parathyroid hormone dependent regulation of Na^+/phosphate cotransport in OK cells. *Biochem J* 1988;251:207–213.
280. Traebert M, Volkl H, Biber J, et al. Luminal and contraluminal action of 1–34 and 3–34 PTH peptides on renal type IIa Na-P(i) cotransporter. *Am J Physiol Renal Physiol* 2000;278(5): F792–F798.
281. Bacic D, Schulz N, Biber J, et al. Involvement of the MAPK-kinase pathway in the PTH-mediated regulation of the proximal tubule type IIa Na^+/Pi cotransporter in mouse kidney. *Pflugers Arch* 2003;446:52–60.
282. Kempson SA, Lotscher M, Kaissling B, et al. Parathyroid hormone action on phosphate transporter mRNA and protein in rat renal proximal tubules. *Am J Physiol* 1995;268:F784–F791.
283. Traebert M, Roth J, Biber J, et al. Internalization of proximal tubular type II Na-P(i) cotransporter by PTH: immunogold electron microscopy. *Am J Physiol Renal Physiol* 2000;278: F148–F154.
284. Malmstrom K, Murer H. Parathyroid hormone regulates phosphate transport in OK cells via an irreversible inactivation of a membrane protein. *FEBS Lett* 1987;216:257–260.
285. Pfister MF, Ruf I, Stange G, et al. Parathyroid hormone leads to the lysosomal degradation of the renal type II Na/Pi cotransporter. *Proc Natl Acad Sci U S A* 1998;95:1909–1914.
286. Kurnik BRC, Hruska KA. Effects of 1,25-dihydroxycholecalciferol on phosphate transport in vitamin D–deprived rats. *Am J Physiol* 1984;247:F177–F182.
287. Kurnik BRC, Hruska KA. Mechanism of stimulation of renal phosphate transport by 1,25-dihydroxycholecalciferol. *Biochim Biophys Acta* 1985;817:42–50.
288. Kurnik BRC, Huskey M, Hruska KA. 1,25-dihydroxycholecalciferol stimulates renal phosphate transport by directly altering membrane phosphatidylcholine composition. *Biochim Biophys Acta* 1987;917:81–85.
289. Hammerman MR. The growth hormone–insulin-like growth factor axis in kidney. *Am J Physiol* 1989;257:F503–F514.
290. Gertner JM, Horst RL, Broadus AE, et al. Parathyroid function and vitamin D metabolism during human growth hormone replacement. *J Clin Endocrinol Metab* 1979;49:185–188.
291. Gertner JM, Tamborlane WV, Hintz RL, et al. The effects on mineral metabolism of overnight growth hormone infusion in growth hormone deficiency. *J Clin Endocrinol Metab* 1981;53:818–822.
292. McMillan DE, Deller JJ, Grodsky GM, et al. Evaluation of clinical activity of acromegaly by observation of the diurnal variation of serum inorganic phosphate. *Metabolism* 1968;17: 966–976.
293. Hammerman MR, Karl IE, Hruska KA. Regulation of canine renal vesicle P_i transport by growth hormone and parathyroid hormone. *Biochim Biophys Acta* 1980;603:322–335.
294. Mulroney SE, Lumpkin MD, Haramati A. Antagonist to GH-releasing factor inhibits growth and renal Pi reabsorption in immature rats. *Am J Physiol* 1989;257:F29–F34.
295. Caverzasio J, Montessuit C, Bonjour JP. Stimulatory effect of insulin-like growth factor-1 on renal Pi transport and plasma 1,25–dihydroxyvitamin D_3. *Endocrinology* 1990;127:453–459.
296. Quigley R, Baum M. Effects of growth hormone and insulin-like growth factor I on rabbit proximal convoluted tubule transport. *J Clin Invest* 1991;88(2):368–374.
297. Caverzasio J, Bonjour JP. Insulin-like growth factor I stimulates Na-dependent Pi transport in cultured kidney cells. *Am J Physiol* 1989;257:F712–F717.
298. Cai Q, Hodgson SF, Kao PC, et al. Brief report: inhibition of renal phosphate transport by a tumor product in a patient with oncogenic osteomalacia. *N Engl J Med* 1994;330:1645–1649.
299. Bianchine JW, Stambler AA, Harrison HE. Familial hypophosphatemic rickets showing autosomal dominant inheritance. *Birth Defects Orig Artic Ser* 1971;7:287–295.

300. Econs MJ, McEnery PT. Autosomal dominant hypophosphatemic rickets/osteomalacia: clinical characterization of a novel renal phosphate-wasting disorder. *J Clin Endocrinol Metab* 1997;82:674–681.
301. The ADHR Consortium. Autosomal dominant hypophosphataemic rickets is associated with mutations in FGF23. *Nat Genet* 2000;26:345–348.
302. Sweet RA, Males JL, Hamstra AJ, et al. Vitamin D metabolite levels in oncogenic osteomalacia. *Ann Intern Med* 1980;93:279–280.
303. Econs MJ, Drezner MK. Tumor-induced osteomalacia—unveiling a new hormone. *N Engl J Med* 1994;330:1679–1681.
304. Rasmussen H, Tenenhouse HS. Mendelian hypophosphatemias. In: Scriver CR, Beaudet AL, Sly WS, et al., eds. *The metabolic basis of inherited disease.* New York: McGraw Hill, 1998.
305. Tenenhouse HS, Econs MJ. Mendelian hypophosphatemias. In: Scriver CR, Beaudet AL, Sly WS, et al., eds. *The metabolic and molecular basis of inherited disease.* New York: McGraw Hill, 2001:5039–5068.
306. White KE, Carn G, Lorenz-Depiereux B, et al. Autosomal-dominant hypophosphatemic rickets (ADHR) mutations stabilize FGF-23. *Kidney Int* 2001;60:2079–2086.
307. White KE, Jonsson KB, Carn G, et al. The autosomal dominant hypophosphatemic rickets (ADHR) gene is a secreted polypeptide overexpressed by tumors that cause phosphate wasting. *J Clin Endocrinol Metab* 2001;86:497–500.
308. Shimada T, Mizutani S, Muto T, et al. Cloning and characterization of FGF23 as a causative factor of tumor-induced osteomalacia. *Proc Natl Acad Sci U S A* 2001;98(11):6500–6505.
309. Yamazaki Y, Okazaki R, Shibata M, et al. Increased circulatory level of biologically active full-length FGF-23 in patients with hypophosphatemic rickets/osteomalacia. *J Clin Endocrinol Metab* 2002;87:4957–4960.
310. Jonsson KB, Zahradnik R, Larsson T, et al. Fibroblast growth factor 23 in oncogenic osteomalacia and X-linked hypophosphatemia. *N Engl J Med* 2003;348:1656–1663.
311. Jonsson KB, Mannstadt M, Miyauchi A, et al. Extracts from tumors causing oncogenic osteomalacia inhibit phosphate uptake in opossum kidney cells. *J Endocrinol* 2001;169: 613–620.
312. Bowe AE, Finnegan R, Jan de Beur SM, et al. FGF-23 inhibits renal tubular phosphate transport and is a PHEX substrate. *Biochem Biophys Res Commun* 2001;284:977–981.
313. Saito H, Kusano K, Kinosaki M, et al. Human fibroblast growth factor-23 mutants suppress Na^+-dependent phosphate co-transport activity and 1α,25–dihydroxyvitamin D_3 production. *J Biol Chem* 2003;278:2206–2211.
314. Bai XY, Miao D, Goltzman D, et al. The autosomal dominant hypophosphatemic rickets R176Q mutation in FGF23 resists proteolytic cleavage and enhances in vivo biological potency. *J Biol Chem* 2003;278:9843–9849.
315. Kempson SA. Peptide hormone action on renal phosphate handling. *Kidney Int* 1996;49:1005–1009.
316. Dousa TP. Modulation of renal Na-Pi cotransport by hormones acting via genomic mechanism and by metabolic factors. *Kidney Int* 1996;49:997–1004.
317. Webb RK, Woodhall PB, Tisher CC, et al. Relationship between phosphaturia and acute hypercapnia in the rat. *J Clin Invest* 1977;60:829–837.
318. Hoppe A, Metler M, Berndt TJ, et al. Effect of respiratory alkalosis on renal phosphate excretion. *Am J Physiol* 1982;243:F471–F475.
319. Beck N. Effect of metabolic acidosis on renal action of parathyroid hormone. *Am J Physiol* 1975;228:1483–1488.
320. Beck N. Effect of metabolic acidosis on renal response to parathyroid hormone in phosphorus deprived rats. *Am J Physiol* 1981;241:F23–F27.
321. Kempson SA. Effect of metabolic acidosis on renal brush-border membrane adaptation to low phosphorus diet. *Kidney Int* 1982;22:225–233.
322. Kuntziger H, Amiel C, Couette S, et al. Localization of parathyroid hormone independent sodium bicarbonate inhibition of tubular phosphate reabsorption. *Kidney Int* 1980;17: 749–755.
323. Zilenovski AM, Kuroda S, Bhat S, et al. Effect of sodium bicarbonate on phosphate excretion in acute and chronic PTX rats. *Am J Physiol* 1979;236:F184–F191.
324. Quamme GA. Effects of metabolic acidosis, alkalosis, and dietary hydrogen ion intake on phosphate transport in the proximal convoluted tubule. *Am J Physiol* 1985;249:F769–F779.
325. Steele TH. Bicarbonate induced phosphaturia dependence upon the magnitude of phosphate reabsorption. *Pflugers Arch* 1977;370:291–294.
326. Lang F, Greger R, Knox FG, et al. Factors modulating the renal handling of phosphate. *Renal Physiol* 1981;4:1–16.
327. Quamme GA, Wong NLM. Phosphate transport in the proximal convoluted tubule: effect of intraluminal pH. *Am J Physiol* 1984;246:F323–F333.
328. Kumar R, DeLuca HF. Side chain oxidation of 1,25–dihydroxyvitamin D_3 in the rat: effect of removal of the intestine. *Biochem Biophys Res Commun* 1977;76:253–258.
329. Stewart CL, Devarajan P, Mulroney SE, et al. Transport of calcium and phosphorus. In: Polin R, Fox WW, eds. *Fetal and neonatal physiology.* Philadelphia: WB Saunders, 1992: 1223–1231.
330. Barac-Nieto M, Gupta RK, Spitzer A. NMR studies of phosphate metabolism in the isolated perfused kidney of developing rats. *Pediatr Nephrol* 1990;4:392–398.
331. Barac-Nieto M, Dowd TL, Gupta RK, et al. Changes in NMR-visible kidney cell phosphate with age and diet: relationship to phosphate transport. *Am J Physiol* 1991;261: F153–F162.
332. Spitzer A, Kaskel FJ, Feld LG, et al. Renal regulation of phosphate homeostasis during growth. *Semin Nephrol* 1983; 3:87–93.

11

DISORDERS OF PHOSPHORUS, CALCIUM, AND VITAMIN D

CRAIG B. LANGMAN

Patients who have disturbances in mineral homeostasis exhibit several different clinical pictures: a predominance of bone disease (rickets or hyperparathyroidism), the metabolic effects of disturbances in calcium (neurologic, musculoskeletal disorders) or phosphorus (cardiovascular, hematologic disorders), or evidence of phenotypic syndromes. Many of these disturbances result from or produce abnormalities in renal tubular divalent mineral handling.

In the evaluation of such patients, the clinician is expected to perform serum and urine biochemical analyses that involve phosphorus, calcium, and vitamin D. Such blood measurements include levels of ionized calcium, serum total calcium, serum phosphorus, intact parathyroid hormone (PTH), and 25-hydroxyvitamin D and 1,25-dihydroxyvitamin D [1,25 $(OH)_2D$]. Urinary studies may include quantitative determinations of excretion of calcium, phosphorus, and other ions of interest (oxalate, citrate). The results of such biochemical evaluations lend themselves to diagnostic schemes that involve the kidney in a primary or secondary manner. In what follows, these diagnostic schemes are arranged by primary abnormality in serum calcium or phosphorus and are then further organized by pattern of urinary biochemical findings. Because the changes in one component of mineral homeostasis often produce abnormalities in the other components of the system, the biochemical findings of any given disorder can be approached in a number of different ways that are discussed later.

The reader is referred to Chapter 10 for a discussion of the normal physiology and renal handling of calcium and phosphorus and to a published review of the physiology of vitamin D (1).

DISORDERS OF PHOSPHORUS HOMEOSTASIS

Hyperphosphatemia Associated with Reduced Urine Phosphorus Excretion

Tumoral Calcinosis

Tumoral calcinosis (2–10) is a rare but disabling disorder of mineral metabolism in which two pathophysiologic abnormalities occur: (a) an inability to excrete phosphorus and (b) the resultant hyperphosphatemia. Furthermore, the consequent hyperphosphatemia does not lead to an appropriate suppression of the production of $1,25(OH)_2D$, the active vitamin D metabolite, and thus normal serum levels of the hormone are present. The pathophysiologic basis of this disorder is unknown but presumably involves abnormalities of tubular phosphorus handling as well as of vitamin D metabolism. Thus, affected patients have hyperphosphatemia, a normal blood calcium level, and a reduction in urinary phosphorus excretion. This is the mirror image of the serum and urine profile of a patient with hypophosphatemic rickets. In tumoral calcinosis, serum levels of intact PTH are suppressed to low normal or frankly low values, as is nephrogenous cyclic adenosine monophosphate (cAMP) excretion. The physical-chemical product of calcium × phosphorus is greater than 70, and soft tissue calcifications occur. Of importance, a systemic osteopenia is seen in such patients, despite the elevation of the product of blood phosphorus × calcium.

The calcifications are commonly located along the extensor surfaces of major joints. Relief of symptoms often requires surgical removal of the calcifications. Without adequate control of the underlying disease, recurrence is universal. Neural compression is common. The tumors can ulcerate the overlying skin, leading to draining sinus tracts and chronic infections. Associated findings include anemia, splenomegaly, low-grade fevers, and regional lymphadenopathy. In some patients, a characteristic dental abnormality may occur. Although the disease is worldwide in distribution, in North America there is an ethnic bias toward African Americans; there is no gender bias.

The treatment of patients with tumoral calcinosis has been uniformly unrewarding. Simple surgical removal of calcifications provides temporary relief of painful symptoms. Radiation therapy and corticosteroid therapy have not been successful. The use of phosphate-binding antacids and a low dietary intake of phosphate and calcium has met with some success, but this regimen is generally difficult for patients to follow.

In an effort directly to promote phosphaturia and indirectly to increase suppressed levels of PTH with consequent phosphaturia, we have used long-term calcitonin administration (5 U/kg subcutaneously initially, and then repetitively but with increasing intervals between administrations) in these patients. Using calcitonin therapy in this manner, combined with dietary phosphate restriction and/or administration of oral phosphate binders, we have prevented the recurrence of the tumors in six such patients over the past several years. In addition, we have seen an increased bone density in nonaffected skeletal sites of such individuals.

Hypoparathyroidism

Absence of PTH biologic action is associated with significant hyperphosphatemia, hypocalcemia, and inappropriate renal tubular retention of phosphorus. It may occur as an inherited abnormality or be acquired through surgical removal of parathyroid gland tissue (for a general review, see reference 11).

Idiopathic hypoparathyroidism begins in early childhood and is part of the differential diagnosis of prolonged neonatal hypocalcemia. In the neonate, hypoparathyroidism is associated with aplasia of the glands, but beyond the neonatal age range, glandular hypoplasia is found instead. Idiopathic hypoparathyroidism may be X-linked, especially when it occurs in the neonate. The DiGeorge anomaly, a migrational disturbance in neural crest cells that results in abnormal development of the structures arising from the third and fourth branchial pouches, including anatomic cardiac defects and thymic dysplasia or absence, also is associated with a spectrum of abnormalities of the parathyroid gland ranging from frank hypoparathyroidism to a normocalcemic disorder termed *latent hypoparathyroidism.* Both normocalcemic children and adults with the DiGeorge anomaly may be unable to secrete PTH when faced with a hypocalcemic stimulus such as an infusion of ethylenediaminetetra-acetic acid (EDTA), which suggests that maximal secretion of serum PTH is occurring from hypoplastic parathyroid tissue (12). Furthermore, children with isolated conotruncal cardiac defects have a high frequency of latent hypoparathyroidism (13) associated with a 22q11 gene deletion commonly seen in DiGeorge anomaly (see reference 14 for general review). Evolution of the latent hypoparathyroidism associated with the 22q11 deletion into frank hypoparathyroidism (hypocalcemia, hyperphosphatemia) has been demonstrated across generations and over time within a generation (15).

Hypoparathyroidism (autosomal dominant, occasionally sporadic) may result from heterozygous mutations (16) in now-cloned extracellular calcium receptor, which sets a stable level of hypocalcemia (for a general review, see reference 17). Such patients appear to be uniquely sensitive to therapy with calcium and vitamin D analogues and must be closely monitored for the complications of nephrocalcinosis, nephrolithiasis, and renal insufficiency.

Hypoparathyroidism diagnosed in the latter part of the first decade of life may be associated with *autoimmune polyglandular disease* (Table 11.1). The disease is inherited in an autosomal recessive manner, and the other organ dysfunctions may occur years after the diagnosis of one component of the syndrome. PTH antibodies occur in 30 to 40% of cases. Associated clinical findings include the development of cataracts, basal ganglion calcifications, and steatorrhea in more than 25% of cases. Repetitive diagnostic testing for the diseases associated with this syndrome is suggested once the diagnosis of autoimmune hypoparathyroidism is made.

TABLE 11.1. FEATURES OF THE AUTOIMMUNE POLYGLANDULAR SYNDROME ASSOCIATED WITH HYPOPARATHYROIDISM

Feature	Frequency (%)
Addison disease (adrenal failure)	—
Chronic mucocutaneous candidiasis	—
Alopecia totalis	38
Steatorrhea	30
Primary hypogonadism	20
Pernicious anemia	15
Primary hypothyroidism	15
Chronic active hepatitis	12
Vitiligo	—

Other rare causes of isolated hypoparathyroidism in children and adults may also be inherited, with patterns varying from autosomal recessive to autosomal dominant (see earlier), with incomplete penetrances. Hypoparathyroidism is a commonly encountered component of mitochondrial myopathies and associated renal (tubular and glomerular) dysfunction, which are now understood to result from either deletions or mutations of mitochondrial, maternally inherited genes related to electron transport (18,19). Such diseases include complete or partial absence of *cytochrome c oxidase, Kearns-Sayre syndrome* (ophthalmoplegia, retinitis pigmentosa, and heart block), *MELAS* (mitochondrial encephalopathy, lactic acidosis, and stroke), and *MERRF* (mitochondrial encephalopathy with ragged red fiber myopathy). Hypoparathyroidism, transient or permanent, is also an integral part of *Kenny-Caffey syndrome,* which is marked by both growth retardation and tubular long bones with medullary stenosis (some children with this disorder have been noted to have pseudohypoparathyroidism; see below).

Pseudohypoparathyroidism

Pseudohypoparathyroidism is characterized by peripheral resistance to endogenously secreted PTH (for a general review, see reference 11). It may be inherited in an autosomal recessive, autosomal dominant, or X-linked manner. In addition to the lack of appropriate phosphaturia to endogenously secreted PTH, patients have hypercalciuria, reduced bony mobilization of calcium, and reduced renal production and subsequent serum levels of $1,25(OH)_2D$. Systemic osteopenia is present, and despite the lack of classic renal responses to endogenous PTH levels, excess bony resorption does occur.

Patients with pseudohypoparathyroidism may be classified by their response to exogenous administration of synthetic PTH. Most have an absence of urinary excretion of cAMP *(type I pseudohypoparathyroidism)* with administration of PTH; a few (fewer than 10%) have an intact generation of cAMP *(type II pseudohypoparathyroidism).*

Type I pseudohypoparathyroidism is associated with a characteristic clinical phenotype called *Albright hereditary osteodystrophy*, composed of facial dysmorphism, shortened metacarpals and metatarsals, short stature, mild mental retardation, thickened cranium, and abnormal carrying angles at the elbow, knee, and hip. Subcutaneous ossification may occur (and is seen with higher frequency in a disorder that resembles Albright osteodystrophy phenotypically but has normal serum phosphorus, calcium, and PTH levels and is termed *pseudopseudohypoparathyroidism;* frank hypoparathyroidism may develop later in life in this rare disorder). The disturbance in Albright osteodystrophy is a generalized decrease in the function of the stimulatory guanine nucleotide–binding protein (G_s) present in all cells (20,21). The decrease in function may be secondary to a point mutation in the α subunit of G_s (22). Because the G-protein signaling system mediates the response of other hormones, it is not unexpected that associated hormonal disturbances are seen in patients with Albright osteodystrophy, including hypergonadotropic hypogonadism and hypothyroidism (23).

Acute Tubular Necrosis

The abrupt cessation of effective glomerular filtration is associated with many pathophysiologic changes, including hyperphosphatemia and, usually, hypocalcemia. Levels of $1,25(OH)_2D$ are often reduced and, with the relief of oliguria, may increase above normal (24). Nonoliguric acute tubular necrosis is also associated with hyperphosphatemia from insufficient urinary phosphorus excretion.

Chronic Renal Insufficiency

Hyperphosphatemia occurs late in the course of chronic renal insufficiency, usually when the glomerular filtration rate (GFR) is less than 20% of normal. Functional nephrons filter more of the filtered phosphorus load, and thus phosphaturia is common in early chronic renal insufficiency. However, as the GFR declines to less than 20%, despite a low fractional reabsorption of filtered phosphorus, quantitative phosphorus excretion falls dramatically.

Hyperostosis

Closely linked but pathogenetically distinct from tumoral calcinosis is endosteal hyperostosis (25), which has also been associated with hyperphosphatemia. The disorder is inherited as either an autosomal recessive or autosomal dominant trait and has its onset in late childhood, often with asymmetric mandibular enlargement. Nasal bridge enlargement and mild frontal bossing are common accompanying signs; facial nerve palsies or neural deafness are seen occasionally from nerve entrapment.

Hyperphosphatemia Associated with Increased Urine Phosphorus Excretion

Disorders of Phosphorus Distribution and Systemic pH

Hyperphosphatemia with resultant phosphaturia may occur because phosphorus is released from intracellular stores into the extracellular fluid (ECF). This occurs commonly during *acute respiratory acidosis.* Aggressive treatment of the elevation in serum phosphorus is best approached by recognition of the systemic acid-base disturbance.

During the generation of *acute metabolic acidosis*, phosphorus is released into the ECF from intracellular stores, and phosphaturia results. However, during the maintenance phase of metabolic acidosis, ECF phosphorus levels are often reduced, but phosphaturia continues.

Disorders of Phosphorus Distribution

Cell Breakdown

Hyperphosphatemia and phosphaturia occur commonly in clinical diseases in which there is rapid cell lysis or turnover, including *tumor lysis syndrome* (most commonly seen with hematologic malignancies, Burkitt lymphoma, and metastatic breast or small cell lung carcinomas), *rhabdomyolysis* (of traumatic and nontraumatic causes, Table 11.2), and severe *hemolytic anemias.* The pathophysiology of the resultant abnormality in these diverse groups of diseases is the same: excessive egress of intracellular phosphate stores into the ECF compartment from cellular destruction exceeds the kidney's ability to excrete the released phosphorus load. Commonly associated findings with either tumor lysis or rhabdomyolysis are severe hypocalcemia and hyperkalemia. The latter results from the fact that potassium is the major intracellular cation released with cell breakdown.

The increased cell metabolic and turnover rates that occur in *thyrotoxicosis* or *Addison disease* are rare causes of hyperphosphatemia.

Increased Phosphorus Absorption

Long-term use of the *bisphosphonate* etidronate for the treatment of osteopenias of varying causes has been associated with mild hyperphosphatemia and phosphaturia. This first-generational bisphosphonate can now be replaced with more potent ones (amino-bisphosphonates) that have not been associated with such biochemical findings.

TABLE 11.2. CAUSES OF RHABDOMYOLYSIS ASSOCIATED WITH HYPERPHOSPHATEMIA AND PHOSPHATURIA

Hereditary	Exertional	Metabolic	Toxic
Phosphorylase deficiency	Anterior tibial syndrome	Carbon monoxide poisoning	Haff disease
Phosphofructokinase deficiency	Status epilepticus	Barbiturate, narcotic use	Chronic alcoholism
Muscle carnitine palmitoyltransferase deficiency	High-voltage electrical shock	Hypothermia	Heroin use
Malignant hyperthermia	Agitated delirium	Diabetic ketoacidosis, nonketotic hyperglycemic coma	Malayan snakebite poison
Defect unknown, familial distribution	Overexercise, often in excessively hot environment Crush injury Coma (crush by own body mass)	Systemic infection with fever Idiopathic paroxysmal paralytic myoglobinuria (Mayer-Batz disease)	K^+ loss: glycyrrhizate, carbenoxolone, amphotericin B associated

Infusion of inappropriate amounts of *sodium or potassium phosphate salts* during parenteral alimentation or intravenous fluid therapies may result in hyperphosphatemia and phosphaturia. More common is the severe hyperphosphatemia and phosphaturia caused by the use of sodium phosphate enema preparations (26). Tremendous quantities of phosphate can be absorbed by the dilated colon, and the use of such enemas in small children has been associated with renal failure and death.

As part of the syndrome of *vitamin D intoxication*, whether from the use of the parent compound or one of the available vitamin D metabolites, hyperphosphatemia and phosphaturia result. Such disturbances commonly have associated hypercalcemia. The disturbance in phosphate appears to result in part from increased vitamin D–driven dietary phosphate absorption.

Hypophosphatemia Associated with Reduced Urine Phosphorus Excretion

Phosphorus Deprivation

Dietary restriction of phosphorus, if severe, can lead to phosphorus deprivation and elimination of urine phosphorus excretion. Severe decreases in phosphorus intake may be simulated by the excessive use of *phosphate-binding antacids* or by the rare occurrence of an *enteroenteric fistula* that leads to excessive stool phosphorus losses. The clinical picture may be dominated by the accompanying caloric or protein deprivations. An elevated serum calcium level is common, and PTH levels are suppressed as a result. Acutely, increased serum $1,25(OH)_2D$ levels are present, but levels subside to subnormal after 10 to 14 days of dietary deprivation.

Disorders of Phosphorus Distribution and Systemic pH

Disorders associated with *respiratory alkalosis* cause an acute shift of extracellular phosphorus into the intracellular space because alkalosis stimulates production of the enzyme phosphofructokinase and increases formation of sugar phosphate moieties. Such disorders include acute hyperventilation (such as with temper tantrums), sepsis, heat stroke, or salicylate intoxication. In addition, patients with chronic bronchospastic pulmonary disorders can demonstrate hypophosphatemia and reduced urine phosphorus excretion during acute exacerbations.

Disorders of Phosphorus Distribution: Hormonal and Food-Fuel Effect

The following hormones promote a primary transport of phosphorus from the ECF into the intracellular fluid compartment: insulin, glucagon, androgens of adrenal or testicular origin, and β-adrenergic agonists. Endogenous physiologic overproduction or pharmacologic administration may produce the hypophosphatemia and associated reduction in urine phosphorus excretion. Insulin augments renal tubular reabsorption of phosphorus in addition to directing extracellular phosphorus to move to the intracellular compartment.

In addition, infusions of specific food-fuel nutrients promote the same translocation of phosphorus into the intracellular compartment. Such agents include glucose, fructose, lactate, and amino acid salts. Two other agents closely related to the food-fuels, glycerol and xylitol, also promote such phosphorus movement.

Increased Phosphorus Uptake into Bone

Two additional situations are associated with the production of hypophosphatemia and a reduced urine phosphorus excretion. After long-standing primary or secondary hyperparathyroidism is relieved, increased avidity of bone for calcium and phosphorus accumulation is seen. This has been termed the *hungry bone syndrome* and is commonly manifest with both hypophosphatemia and hypocalcemia, which may be symptomatic. Circumstances in which the hungry bone syndrome occurs include the immediately postoperative period after parathyroidectomy or after successful renal transplantation in cases of previous long-standing secondary hyperparathyroidism. However, the latter condition may also be associated with a phosphorus-losing tubulopathy as noted later.

The hungry bone syndrome has been observed also with vitamin D treatment of long-standing vitamin D deficiency. In this setting, long-standing secondary hyperparathyroidism produces hypophosphatemia with phosphaturia. Over a short time after reintroduction of vitamin D, the biochemical picture worsens with respect to the serum level of phosphorus, whereas the excessive urine phosphorus excretion ceases.

Miscellaneous Conditions

Chronic myelogenous leukemia in a proliferative *blast crisis* has been associated with hypophosphatemia and decreased phosphorus excretion. In this condition, the increased anabolic state of white blood cells necessitates a large amount of intracellular phosphorus transport.

Refeeding of a starved infant or child may promote increased phosphate transport into the intracellular compartment and a reduction in phosphaturia. The hypophosphatemia is rarely severe, unlike in the disorders mentioned earlier.

Hypophosphatemia Associated with Increased Urine Phosphorus Excretion

Fanconi Syndrome

For information regarding hypophosphatemia and Fanconi syndrome, see Chapter 41.

X-linked Hypophosphatemic (Vitamin D–Resistant) Rickets

Disorders of vitamin D metabolism and resultant rickets occur commonly in children and are most often related to a simple deficiency of the parent vitamin. Lack of subsequent hepatic production of the 25-hydroxyvitamin D substrate leads to insufficient amounts of the active, renally produced vitamin D metabolite $1,25(OH)_2D$. This results in profound hypocalcemia, secondary hyperparathyroidism, hypophosphatemia, and rachitic bone disease. Provision of modest amounts of the parent compound, vitamin D, cures the disorder.

The most commonly inherited form of rickets is X-linked hypophosphatemic rickets. Hypophosphatemic rickets in children is a systemic disorder in which renal phosphate wasting produces hypophosphatemia (27). Normocalcemia and normal levels of PTH are demonstrated. The circulating levels of the active vitamin D metabolite $1,25(OH)_2D$ also are often normal (28,29). The "defect" in vitamin D metabolism in this disorder is the inappropriately normal levels of $1,25(OH)_2D$, because reduced serum phosphorus levels represent a potent stimulus for increased renal production of the active metabolite of the vitamin D endocrine system (1,30,31). The gene for X-linked hypophosphatemic rickets has been cloned and is termed the *PHEX* gene for phosphate-regulating with homology to endopeptidase on the X chromosome (32). The disorder is now viewed as involving an abnormality of the phosphaturic factor fibroblast growth factor-23 (FGF-23). If PHEX is mutated, its natural substrate, FGF-23, is not inactivated by proteolysis and can exert its phosphaturic action (33). A study has documented the excessive levels of FGF-23 in this, and several other, rachitic hypophosphatemic disorders discussed later (34). It is not yet understood why there is a lack of appropriately increased synthetic ability of the renal 1α-hydroxylase enzyme that produces $1,25(OH)_2D$ in the face of such profound hypophosphatemia. Phenotypically normal family members of affected children with rickets have normal serum phosphorus levels, but serum levels of $1,25(OH)_2D$ have not been systematically studied.

The untreated disorder in children results in generalized rickets and often linear growth failure (35); other features appear in adults (36,37). Although there is controversy surrounding the efficacy of treatment, most clinicians believe that frequent phosphate supplementation and pharmacologic dosing with $1,25(OH)_2D$ are indicated (38). Despite the large doses of phosphate used, hypophosphatemia remains, and secondary hyperparathyroidism may be induced with long-term phosphate salt administration (39,40). Thus, a better understanding of the need for phosphate is required. The addition of $1,25(OH)_2D$ has improved the healing of the rickets (41,42). Recommendations for both phosphate therapy and $1,25(OH)_2D$ therapy are based on clinical experience. Neither the initial dosing nor subsequent modifications are based solely on measured serum levels of either phosphorus or the hormone, but rather on the clinical course of the child with respect to rickets, linear growth, or both. A recommendation for the starting dosage for toddler-aged children is elemental phosphorus 1 to 3 g/day in four to five divided doses and calcitriol 30 to 70 ng/kg/day in two or three divided doses (43).

Two different murine models of the human disease exist. In the affected *Hyp* mouse (44), the renal 25-hydroxyvitamin D–1α-hydroxylase defect is pervasive; it does not respond to PTH or phosphorus by increasing the production of $1,25(OH)_2D$. Calcitonin does stimulate hormonal synthesis, which suggests that the enzyme is capable of being upregulated in this animal model (45). Hormone catabolism also is increased in the *Hyp* mouse (46,47). In the *Gy* mouse, however, only the PTH-independent arm, the response to hypophosphatemia, is blunted (48). Thus, in response to dietary calcium restriction and subsequent secondary hyperparathyroidism, the renal production of $1,25(OH)_2D$ increases in the affected *Gy* mouse (49). Which murine model most resembles children with hypophosphatemic rickets with respect to renal 1α-hydroxylase is untested. Evidence from experimental animals suggests that the renal 1α-hydroxylase is regulated inversely by phosphorus during chronic metabolic acidosis, a disorder characterized by phosphaturia, mild hypophosphatemia, "normal" basal levels of 1,25(OH)$_2$D, and insufficient synthetic capacity in response to PTH-stimulation but intact response to phosphate restriction (50). Increasing the phosphate concentration of the bathing medium increases the *in vitro* production of 1,25(OH)$_2$D in kidney tubules from rats with chronic metabolic acidosis; tubules from nonacidemic controls show the expected decline in production. Similarly, tubules from control animals increase production of 1,25(OH)$_2$D during depletion of extracellular phosphorus, whereas tubules from the acidotic rats show only basal production. The data for humans with metabolic acidosis are controversial (51,52). Interestingly, administration of phosphate to the *Hyp* mouse increases peripheral receptors for 1,25(OH)$_2$D (53) and stimulates uptake of the hormone by target cells in the intestine (54).

Other Causes of Hypophosphatemic Rickets

Several other disorders of renal tubular phosphorus transport are associated with rickets similar to X-linked hypophosphatemic rickets. *Hereditary hypophosphatemic rickets with hypercalciuria* (55,56) is a rare disorder in which the hypophosphatemia is associated with increased levels of 1,25(OH)$_2$D. In turn, PTH secretion is suppressed, both from an increase in calcium consequent to the elevated levels of 1,25(OH)$_2$D and from direct inhibition of prepro-parathyroid hormone gene transcription by 1,25(OH)$_2$D. It is presumed that the inhibition of PTH leads to the hypercalciuria. The genetic transmission of the disorder remains unknown at present. In the few reports of this disease, children first manifest rickets from the first year of life through the end of the first decade of life (55). There are also unaffected relatives, children or adults, who manifest only the hypercalciuria portion of the disorder (56). Although clinically well, these unaffected relatives may have some or all of the biochemical abnormalities of their affected relatives, but with values closer to the normal values for age. Treatment consists of a high intake of phosphorus supplements alone. Unlike the disturbances in X-linked hypophosphatemic rickets, the rickets in this disorder is often healed by 6 to 9 months of therapy. Serum phosphorus levels increase and 1,25(OH)$_2$D levels decrease to normal. A study has documented that the kidney proximal tubular sodium–inorganic phosphate co-transporter is not mutated in this condition (57).

Some adolescents and young adults develop hypophosphatemic rickets at an advanced age, compared with the classic X-linked disturbance. There do not appear to be any specific differences in the pathophysiology or clinical consequences of this disease, termed *adolescent hypophosphatemic osteomalacia*, and the X-linked disorder discussed earlier. The treatment is the same and includes both phosphorus supplementation and administration of calcitriol. There is, in addition, an *autosomal dominant* variety of hypophosphatemic rickets. In general, final height is not as severely affected nor are levels of 1,25(OH)$_2$D as low as in patients with X-linked hypophosphatemic rickets. FGF-23 abnormalities have been implicated in each.

Frymoyer and Hodgkin described a large kindred with X-linked renal phosphate wasting in whom bone disease did not manifest as rickets but as osteomalacia (58). Adults showed progressive lower extremity bowing but were otherwise indistinguishable biochemically and clinically from patients with X-linked hypophosphatemic rickets. Scriver et al. described autosomal dominant transmission of a similar disorder in a different kindred (59,60). Both disorders have been called *nonrachitic hypophosphatemic osteomalacia.*

Phosphaturia, hypophosphatemia, and rickets or osteomalacia have been described in a handful of patients with *fibrous dysplasia* (monostotic or polyostotic, the latter in McCune-Albright syndrome), *epidermal nevus syndrome*, or other soft tissue *tumors of mesenchymal origin* (61) and has been termed *tumor-induced osteomalacia.* This is likely a heterogeneous disorder at the level of renal 1α-hydroxylase, because levels of 1,25(OH)$_2$D have been reported to be normal, elevated, or reduced; a minority of patients also have elevated serum PTH levels. Therapy with 1,25(OH)$_2$D may heal or worsen the underlying bone disease, but it generally improves the hypophosphatemia. Excision of the offending tumor, if possible, is curative. Again, FGF-23 has been implicated in the pathogenesis (53,54).

Vitamin D–Dependent Rickets

Children with the rare autosomal recessive disorder *vitamin D–dependent rickets, type 1* present with classic vitamin D–deficiency rickets but do not respond to replacement dosages of the parent vitamin D compound that are used to treat the deficient state. Rather, such children remain hypophosphatemic and severely hypocalcemic. The disease arises from a primary deficiency in the renal 1α-hydroxylase enzyme that produces the active vitamin D metabolite 1,25(OH)$_2$D (62). This is borne out by the lack of change of serum 1,25(OH)$_2$D levels when vitamin D or PTH is administered to such patients (63). Children with the disorder have elevated levels of the substrate of that reaction, 25-hydroxyvitamin D; children with deprivational rickets have reduced levels of 25-hydroxyvitamin D, or it is absent. Lifelong administration of the active hormone calcitriol is curative for the disorder. The gene for renal 25-hydroxyvitamin D–1α-hydroxylase has been cloned (64,65) and localized to 12q13.3. In patients with this disorder, inactivating mutations have been described in the gene, which lead to absence of enzyme activity in experimental systems (64,66) and explain the virtual absence of circulating 1,25(OH)$_2$D.

Since the original description in 1978 by Brooks et al. (67), fewer than four dozen patients have been reported with the classic clinical and radiographic findings of deprivational rickets but significantly increased serum levels of 1,25(OH)$_2$D and an associated resistance to the healing effect of 1,25(OH)$_2$D. Some patients also have alopecia (areata or universalis) or other ectodermal defects (oligodontia, milia, or epidermal cysts). This disease, *vitamin D–dependent rickets, type 2,* represents a disorder in which some aspect of the function of the vitamin D receptor is abnormal. The pathogenesis of the disturbance has been shown to involve one of a number of identified point mutations in the vitamin D receptor gene (68). Treatment consists of maintaining suprapharmacologic levels of 1,25(OH)$_2$D for prolonged periods (6 to 12 months minimum), which often requires parenteral therapy with the hormone and administration of oral or parenteral calcium. The response of the rachitic disorder to therapy probably depends on the exact defect in vitamin D receptor function (69).

Idiopathic (Genetic) Hypercalciuria

A minority of children with idiopathic (genetic) hypercalciuria (see later) have a primary renal phosphorus leak that leads to hypophosphatemia and phosphaturia in association with a frank elevation in serum 1,25(OH)$_2$D levels. In such children the response to phosphorus supplementation is reduced hypercalciuria, normalized serum phosphorus levels, and further exaggeration of urine phosphorus excretion.

Renal Transplantation

Several disturbances in phosphorus homeostasis may result after renal allograft transplantation (70–83). Hypophosphatemia and phosphaturia occur in 70% of all patients with successful renal allografts within the first year after transplantation, sometimes without distinct elevation in serum PTH levels. A distinct phosphorus-losing tubulopathy is less common and leads to a more pronounced hypophosphatemia indistinguishable from that of Fanconi syndrome. It is not associated with an elevation of serum 1,25(OH)$_2$D levels. Most often, the serum PTH level is in the upper range of normal to frankly elevated levels in this situation. Phosphorus supplementation may exaggerate the mild hyperparathyroidism, if present; if hyperparathyroidism is absent, it is the treatment of choice.

Primary Hyperparathyroidism

Primary hyperparathyroidism (see reference 84 and later in this chapter) is uncommon in the first decade of life but increases in incidence thereafter. It may occur as an isolated finding and most commonly presents with nephrolithiasis in the first several decades of life. Primary hyperparathyroidism may be associated with polyglandular endocrinopathy type II, which is characterized by medullary carcinoma of the thyroid, hypercalcitoninemia, and hypercalcemia. There is an adenomatous transformation of one of the four primary glands in more than 85% of children and young adults with primary hyperparathyroidism; infants and toddlers with primary hyperparathyroidism show diffuse glandular hyperplasia.

Severe neonatal hyperparathyroidism may result from homozygous inactivating mutations of the extracellular calcium receptor (85,86) or even from the presence of only one abnormal allele of the gene (87). In both cases, severe hypophosphatemia and phosphaturia are present. Total surgical parathyroidectomy is curative, and, interestingly, patients are often normocalcemic thereafter. (See Familial Hypocalciuric Hypocalcemia.)

Miscellaneous Disorders

Many clinical situations have been associated with hypophosphatemia and phosphaturia, although the exact relationship between the agents implicated and the biochemical findings is less certain than in the disorders described earlier. These situations include chronic *corticosteroid usage,* the *diuretic phase of acute tubular necrosis* or a *"postobstructive" diuresis,* chronic *glycosuria* (but not the entities of renal glycosuria), *hypokalemic disturbances* with a normal GFR, and chronic *alcohol abuse.*

DISORDERS OF CALCIUM HOMEOSTASIS

Hypercalcemia Associated with Hypocalciuria: Familial Hypocalciuric Hypercalcemia

The autosomal dominant condition familial hypocalciuric hypercalcemia (85,86,88,89), best characterized as an abnormality in the physiologic set point for serum calcium concentration, may begin in infancy or childhood with the development of hypercalcemia. The infant or child is generally asymptomatic, and the elevated blood calcium level is unexpected for the clinical disease being evaluated. The exception is the homozygous infant in whom life-threatening hypercalcemia and hyperparathyroidism have been reported (see reference 90 and earlier discussion).

The disease results most often from an inherited abnormality of the extracellular calcium receptor, an inactivating mutation of one of the two alleles of the gene (see earlier and reference 91). The gene defect changes the relationship between PTH release and serum calcium level; the sigmoid curve describing that relationship is shifted to the right. Thus, the calcium set point (i.e., the serum calcium level that suppresses maximal PTH release by 50%) is increased. Apparently, a similar set point for renal tubular calcium reabsorption is increased as well, which accounts for the relative hypocalciuria in the face of an elevated serum calcium level. However, there may be additional abnormalities in the disorder. PTH levels remain inappropriately normal despite the elevated serum calcium levels, and histopathologic abnormalities in the gland itself have been seen in up to 20% of patients who have frank hyperparathyroidism (92).

The treatment of the disorder is one of recognition and no specific therapy. Subtotal parathyroidectomies produce persistent hypercalcemia, and the production of hypoparathyroidism by total parathyroidectomy is of no benefit to the patient who is largely asymptomatic. Diagnostic clues include a family history, absence of the autoimmune polyglandular syndromes, a ratio of urinary calcium to creatinine (both values in milligrams) of 0.03 or less with elevated serum calcium levels and serum magnesium levels elevated between 3 and 4 mg/dL.

Hypercalcemia Associated with Hypercalciuria

Primary Hyperparathyroidism

Although primary hyperparathyroidism (84) is common in adult patients with *de novo* hypercalcemia, it is unusual in the first decade of life and occurs most commonly in neonates. In neonates and infants in the first 6 months of life, primary hyperparathyroidism has been reported approximately 100 times, always associated with extreme elevations in serum calcium levels (often greater than 14 mg/dL) and marked symptoms related to that elevation (93). The pathology in neonatal hyperparathyroidism is diffuse glandular hyperplasia in more than 90% of reported cases; adenomatous changes in one or more glands are responsible for the additional 10% of cases.

When primary hyperparathyroidism occurs in children younger than 10 years of age, a search for an associated endocrinopathy syndrome should be made (see later). In the second decade of life, the incidence of primary hyperparathyroidism increases dramatically (compared with younger ages) and may approach 1 in 1000 population. There does not seem to be a gender predilection among children and adolescents with primary hyperparathyroidism, which contrasts sharply with the female predominance of the disease in adults.

In addition to hypercalcemia and hypophosphatemia, the disease has other major features that result from the effects of elevated PTH levels on the skeleton and the kidney. The skeleton shows classically subperiosteal resorption in the distal phalanges, a "salt-and-pepper" appearance of the cranium, resorption and tapering of the clavicles, brown tumor formation in the long bones, and bone cysts as a result of chronic stimulation from PTH excess. In addition, severe osteopenia, especially in cortical bone, is demonstrated by determination of bone mineral density.

In the kidney, primary hyperparathyroidism is associated with calcium nephrolithiasis in up to 25% of patients in several series, a reduction in GFR, polyuria from an antidiuretic hormone–resistant concentrating defect, nephrocalcinosis, and systemic hypertension, especially with an acute onset of the disease. Other systemic manifestations may include a myopathy, now shown to be due to type II muscle fiber atrophy; peptic ulcer disease; pancreatitis; anemia; alteration in consciousness from lethargy through coma; nausea and vomiting; constipation; and clinical depression.

Primary hyperparathyroidism may occur as part of the multiple endocrine syndromes. In type 1 disease (hyperfunction of the parathyroid, pancreatic, and anterior hypophysis cells), 95% of patients develop hyperparathyroidism, whereas fewer than 30% develop the associated prolactinoma or gastrinoma. In type 2A disease (hyperfunction of the cells of the adrenal glands, parathyroid glands, and C cells of the thyroid glands), hyperparathyroidism occurs in only one-third of cases, whereas the development of C-cell cancer of the thyroid is more common. In the latter group of patients, the occurrence of a pheochromocytoma is associated with hypercalcemia in 15 to 20% of patients, independent of parathyroid gland pathology.

In addition to the isolated disease and the disease associated with multiple endocrine syndromes 1 and 2, another variant of primary hyperparathyroidism has been described, termed *cystic parathyroid adenomatosis*, which also indicates its pathology (94). The disorder is one of recurrent adenomatous change over time, but usually only in one gland at the time of hypercalcemia. To date, there have been no reports of children with the disorder. Associated fibrous tumors of the cheekbones are present in the patients described.

Diagnostically, primary hyperparathyroidism is characterized by an elevation in the level of circulating intact PTH in almost all patients, and an inappropriately high level of PTH for the degree of hypercalcemia in all patients. Corroborative findings include elevated nephrogenous cAMP levels, mildly elevated $1,25(OH)_2D$ levels, hypophosphatemia with phosphaturia, and mild renal tubular acidosis.

The treatment of symptomatic primary hyperparathyroidism in children is surgical with exploration of all four neck glands strongly recommended. Although "asymptomatic" primary hyperparathyroidism exists as an entity in adults, it is not clear that this occurs in children. Therefore, medical treatment of that disorder (phosphorus supplementation, the use of bisphosphonates, and provision of sex steroids) is probably inappropriate for most children with primary hyperparathyroidism.

A new class of drugs, called calcimimetics (95), has been designed to interact within the transmembrane-spanning domains of the extracellular calcium receptor and act allosterically to reduce the activation of the receptor by calcium levels in the ECF. Such agents may have great promise in the treatment of primary hyperparathyroidism, hyperparathyroidism that occurs in the course of chronic renal insufficiency and end-stage renal disease or after renal transplantation, and, perhaps, in severe neonatal hyperparathyroidism. Treatment with calcimimetic agents is also without study in children.

Syndromic Hypercalcemia

Two important syndromes in infants and children produce hypercalcemia: Williams syndrome and idiopathic infantile hypercalcemia. Williams described infants with supravalvular aortic stenosis, peculiar facies ("elfinlike"), and hypercalcemia during the first year of life (96,97). Currently, it is thought that the disorder represents a spectrum of abnormalities from the facial dysmorphism alone through all of the described abnormalities. A scoring system has been developed to categorize the suspected disease in infants as lying within or outside the syndrome itself (98). Two-thirds of infants with the disorder have been small for gestational age and many are born past their expected date of birth. Facial abnormalities include structural asymmetry, temporal depression, flat malae with full cheeks, microcephaly, epicanthal folds, lacy or stellate irises, a short nose with a long philtrum, an arched upper lip with a fuller lower lip, and small, maloccluded teeth. The vocal tone is hoarse. The children are affable and have been described as "cocktail party–like" with unusual friendliness to strangers. Additional cardiovascular abnormalities include other congenital heart defects and peripheral organ arterial stenoses of the renal, mesenteric, and celiac vessels. Hypercalcemia, if initially present, rarely remains by the end of the first year of life, but hypercalciuria persists throughout childhood and adolescence.

Several reports (99,100) have emphasized the renal abnormalities demonstrated by patients with Williams syndrome, including urinary frequency, daytime urinary incontinence, and some structural abnormalities, including hypoplasia or dysplasia.

The genetic defect for Williams syndrome is a heterozygous microdeletion of 7q11.23 and encompasses the elastin gene (101). Rarely, it may involve a defect of chromosome 11 [del(11)(q13.5q14.2)] or even chromosome 22 [r(22)(p11→q13)] (102).

The pathogenesis of the disturbance in calcium is unknown. Studies have largely focused on abnormalities of vitamin D metabolism (103–106). Previous studies of affected children have demonstrated increased circulating levels of 25-hydroxyvitamin D after vitamin D administration, increased levels of $1,25(OH)_2D$ during periods of hypercalcemia but not normocalcemia, and diminished levels of calcitonin during calcium infusions (107).

The treatment is directed toward the associated abnormalities, especially hypertension and cardiovascular anomalies. There are no data on the clinical effect of normalizing mildly elevated serum calcium levels, but the author has anecdotal evidence that normalization of persistent, mild hypercalcemia may improve the final neurologic outcome of children with Williams syndrome.

Idiopathic infantile hypercalcemia was reported by Lightwood (108) in the early 1950s in England and was ascribed to vitamin D intoxication. Other cases have been described subsequently in which maternal exposure to vitamin D was not an issue, which thus led to the designation of the disorder as "idiopathic" (109,110). Affected infants generally have much higher serum calcium levels than those with Williams syndrome, increased thirst, and the associated problems of symptomatic hypercalcemia. The distinction between this disorder and Williams syndrome remains a bit problematic because some infants have cardiovascular anomalies similar to those seen in the Williams disorder. Other clinical manifestations of idiopathic infantile hypercalcemia include hypertension, strabismus, inguinal hernias, disordered posture, kyphosis, radioulnar synostosis, and dislocated patellae. Hyperacusis is seen commonly, may be persistent, and is problematic.

We have identified (111) more than a dozen infants and young children with this disorder in whom an elevated level of N-terminal PTH-related protein (PTH-rp) was demonstrated at the time of hypercalcemia. Furthermore, in seven of those children who achieved normocalcemia, the levels of PTH-rp were normal or unmeasurably low, and in two children with persistent hypercalcemia, the levels of PTH-rp remained elevated. No other nonmalignant, hypercalcemic disorder that we have investigated, including Williams syndrome, includes elevated levels of the peptide.

The therapy for this disorder is normalization of the extremely high serum calcium level. We have not seen a recurrence of the disorder once the calcium level is normalized, although the systemic manifestations noted earlier are not changed.

Hypercalcemia with Malignancy

There are three general mechanisms whereby patients with malignancy develop hypercalcemia: lytic bone metastases, the ectopic production of PTH-rp, and the ectopic production of $1,25(OH)_2D$. Because most children with cancer develop hematologic malignancies, few of which metastasize to bone with enough tumor burden to produce hypercalcemia, and few children develop the solid organ malignancies associated with tumoral production of PTH-rp, the ectopic production of $1,25(OH)_2D$ is most often responsible for the hypercalcemia seen with leukemias and lymphomas in infants and children. Occasionally, primordial mesenchymal tumors produce an osteoclast-activating factor that may lead to local, osteolytic hypercalcemia. Such factors include interleukin-1 and tumor necrosis factor-α, which are potent promoters of bone resorption. Treatment of the malignancies eliminates the hypercalcemia from the ectopic production of hormones and cytokines (112).

Miscellaneous Disorders

Subcutaneous Fat Necrosis

Michael et al. (113) reported on the association of significant birth trauma with fat necrosis in two infants who were small for gestational age and who subsequently developed severe, symptomatic hypercalcemia. Histologic examinations of the violaceous pressure sites that developed revealed an inflammatory, mononuclear cell infiltrate and calcium-containing crystals. The author has noted such hypercalcemia in patients with subcutaneous fat necrosis associated with major trauma or disseminated varicella. The mechanism of the disorder is unknown but may be related to minimally elevated levels of 1,25$(OH)_2$D or excessive prostaglandin production from the tissue trauma site.

Granulomatous Disorders

Of children with sarcoidosis, an autoimmune disorder, 30 to 50% manifest hypercalcemia, and an additional 20 to 30% demonstrate isolated hypercalciuria (114). Some of the presenting signs and symptoms of children with sarcoid are related to hypercalcemia. Twins with cat-scratch disease were reported to develop symptomatic hypercalcemia associated with that granulomatous disorder (115). In such disorders, it is believed that expression of 25-hydroxyvitamin D–1α-hydroxylase, or another mixed-function microsomal oxidase capable of transforming 25-hydroxyvitamin D, is expressed and leads to unregulated production of 1,25$(OH)_2$D and consequent hypercalcemia. Treatment of the underlying disorder abolishes the supraphysiologic levels of 1,25$(OH)_2$D and the associated hypercalcemia.

Limb Fracture

Isolated fracture of a weight-bearing limb that requires immobilization for even a few days may be associated with hypercalcemia and hypercalciuria in young children or adolescents (116). Their occurrence probably reflects the more rapid skeletal turnover in this age group than in adults.

Vitamin D Metabolite Therapy

Children with renal osteodystrophy are commonly treated with calcitriol and develop hypercalcemia as a result once every 12 to 15 treatment-months per patient. Newer therapies of pulse oral or intravenous 1,25$(OH)_2$D may produce hypercalcemia every 6 to 9 treatment-months per patient. The use of calcitriol to treat other mineral disorders is associated with hypercalcemia only one-third as often as is the use of calcitriol or any other vitamin D metabolite to treat renal osteodystrophy. Treatment with the parent compound, vitamin D, may produce long-lasting hypercalcemia if used in excess, because of lipid storage (117).

Jansen Syndrome

Jansen syndrome presents in neonates with rickets and hypercalcemia and is a form of metaphyseal dysplasia. After infancy, the radiographic picture becomes one of mottled calcifications in the long bones, which represent partially calcified cartilage protruding into the diaphysis. The skull and spine may be affected in the neonate as well (118).

The biochemical picture of the affected infant or child with this disorder resembles that of those with primary hyperparathyroidism, but with some important exceptions: hypercalcemia, hypophosphatemia, and hypercalciuria are present but in the virtual absence of calciotropic hormones, including PTH, PTH-related peptide, and calcitriol. However, reports of patients with Jansen syndrome have demonstrated that, secondary to one of several point mutations in the structure of the PTH/PTH-rp receptor, ligand-independent activation of the receptor and consequent biologic action occur in such individuals (119–121).

Hypophosphatasia

Infantile hypophosphatasia, a disorder in which serum alkaline phosphatase activity is absent or significantly diminished, is associated with hypercalcemia, hypercalciuria, and radiological signs of rickets. The diagnosis is confirmed with demonstration of an increase in urinary phosphoethanolamine excretion. See Whyte (122) for a comprehensive review of this disorder.

Other Causes of Hypercalcemia

Additional causes of hypercalcemia are uncommon in infants and children. For the sake of completeness, one can list the following: thyrotoxicosis, adrenal insufficiency, VIPoma, leprosy, use of thiazide diuretics, lithium therapy, vitamin A toxicity, and milk-alkali syndrome. Aggressive treatment with calcitonin, and later with thiazide diuretics, has been shown to ameliorate the hypercalcemia often seen in the infantile forms (123).

Normocalcemic Hypercalciuria

Normal Levels of Calcium Excretion

Studies of several populations of children of diverse ethnicity have revealed a rather uniform degree of calcium excretion. On a daily basis, calcium excretion above 3.5 mg/kg is considered excessive (hypercalciuria) (124–127), although some normative data showing higher excretion rates may reflect the effect of a high dietary intake of sodium on calcium excretion dynamics (128). Data from multiple studies of adults and children with hypercalciuria have demonstrated that hypercalciuria is likely present when a randomly voided urine sample shows a calcium to creatinine ratio (both values in milligrams) exceeding 0.2 (or exceeding 0.5 for values in millimoles). Values of the ratio for randomly collected specimens of 0.15 to 0.2 (for measurements in milligrams) are highly suspicious for frank hypercalciuria and, in the author's experience, signal quantitative hypercalciuria in more than 65% of children. However, the clinician is encouraged to perform complete 24-hour urine collections to determine if hypercalciuria is indeed present, because there is a significant incidence of false-positive results when ratios are used (129).

Urinary calcium to creatinine ratios in neonates and infants younger than 3 months of age should be interpreted with caution, because such ratios have been shown to depend on both gestational age and source of milk protein (commercial formula vs. human milk) (130,131). In practice, the author does not use ratios for screening for hyper-

TABLE 11.3. DIFFERENTIAL DIAGNOSIS OF NORMOCALCEMIC HYPERCALCIURIA

Genetic (idiopathic) hypercalciuria
Furosemide therapy
Corticosteroid therapy
Sarcoidosis
Immobilization
Hereditary hypercalciuria with hypophosphatemic rickets
CLCN5 chloride-channel mutation
Bartter's syndrome
Seyberth syndrome
Prostaglandin E infusion
Vitamin D toxicity (early)
Limb fracture
Thyrotoxicosis
Distal renal tubular acidosis

calciuria in this population but proceeds to a formal collection. On formal collection, daily calcium excretion of more than 5 mg/kg is viewed as hypercalciuria.

Genetic Hypercalciurias

Hypercalciuria may result from an X-linked, recessively inherited disorder associated with one of several mutational defects in a renal chloride channel (132) or may be familial without a gene abnormality that has yet been described. The latter entity has been called idiopathic hypercalciuria. Chloride-channel defects in the kidney have a wide phenotypic expression, ranging from complete Fanconi syndrome with rickets, termed Dent's disease (133), to a disorder that is mild in childhood and is characterized by nephrolithiasis or nephrocalcinosis but that in adulthood appears to be progressive to chronic renal failure (134,135).

The differential diagnosis of normocalcemic hypercalciuria is shown in Table 11.3. Normocalcemic hypercalciuria that has been termed *idiopathic* is more prevalent than the chloride-channel defect (for a general review, see references 136–138). It may occur in 7 to 10% of all children. The inheritance of this disorder appears to be autosomal dominant with incomplete penetrance (139). The disorder is associated with nephrolithiasis, recurrent gross and microscopic hematuria, or otherwise unexplained pyuria, or solely with recurrent abdominal pain, and has been implicated in the frequency-dysuria syndrome (140–142).

Hypercalciuria may be seen in patients who ingest an excessive amount of dietary sodium, and the physician is encouraged to define the level of salt excretion in the assessment of urine calcium excretion. Especially in the small group of children with genetic hypercalciuria who form kidney stones (perhaps 2 to 3% of this group), other urine abnormalities may occur, including hypocitraturia in 25%, dietary hyperoxaluria in 30 to 40%, and hyperuricosuria in 20%.

The mechanisms of genetic hypercalciuria have been debated intensely in the literature, with evidence for primary overabsorption of calcium from intestinal sources vying with

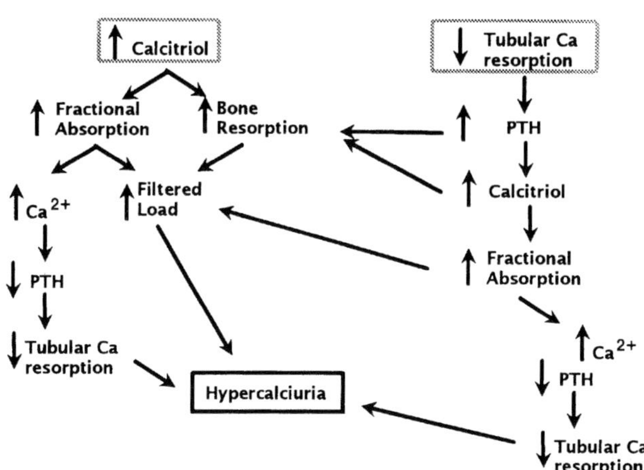

FIGURE 11.1. Pathophysiologic schemes for the production of normocalcemic hypercalciuria. The postulated "primary" defects in genetic hypercalciuria are depicted in the lightly shaded boxes. It can be seen that the two defects merge in the production of hypercalciuria (*solid box*). Up-pointing arrows represent increases in the associated physiologic process, and down-pointing arrows represent decreases in the associated physiologic process. Ca^{2+}, blood ionized calcium level; Ca, calcium; PTH, parathyroid hormone.

a primary renal calcium leak as a single pathophysiologic mechanism for the disorder. The current view is that both of these disease mechanisms occur in a child with genetic hypercalciuria. The pathophysiologic mechanism that dominates the clinical picture is wholly dependent on the dietary intake of calcium during the time diagnostic studies are performed. On a calcium-rich or calcium-sufficient diet, the gastrointestinal disorder manifests easily, whereas at very low levels of dietary calcium intake, "renal" hypercalciuria pertains. Alternatively, gastrointestinal absorption of calcium may contribute little to the final urinary calcium levels (143). Habitual dietary calcium intake determines the level of $1,25(OH)_2D$ found: normal with elevated calcium intake and elevated during dietary calcium restriction (144). Similarly, secondary hyperparathyroidism may be seen during dietary calcium restriction when the renal excretion of calcium is manifest (145) but may be absent during dietary calcium sufficiency (146). The two predominant mechanisms of genetic hypercalciuria are summarized Figure 11.1.

Thus, it remains unknown whether the primary disturbance in genetic hypercalciuria is at the level of the intestine or the kidney. Experimentally, the intestine may have an abnormal sensitivity to $1,25(OH)_2D$, perhaps because of the presence of a vitamin D receptor with a higher maximum transport velocity than that in normocalciuric experimental animals (147). Alternatively, the renal 1α-hydroxylase may produce more of $1,25(OH)_2D$ than is needed for systemic calcium homeostasis. Lastly, perhaps the abnormality in genetic hypercalciuria results from a disorder in the metabolic clearance of $1,25(OH)_2D$.

Until recently, it was not thought that bone calcium contributed to the urinary excess of calcium in patients with genetic hypercalciuria. Studies in adults with the disease and in children with genetic hypercalciuria have now convincingly shown that excessive bone resorption occurs (148–153). The bone loss is from both cortical and trabecular bone and is associated with serum markers that indicate increased bone resorption (C. B. Langman, *unpublished data*, 2002). Frank osteoporosis with fracturing bone disease has been seen in adults and children, especially when the latter group is placed on a calcium-restricted diet.

Treatment of genetic hypercalciuria is directed toward normalization of calcium excretion. In view of the tendency for bone disease to be part of the disorder, dietary calcium restriction seems contraindicated for most infants, children, and adolescents. Whether treatment of any sort need be given is dictated by the clinical picture and local customs. In the author's view, indications for therapy include stone formation, documentation of severe osteopenia without other cause, and symptomatic urinary findings. Treatment for gross hematuria alone in the absence of stone formation does not seem warranted, although in follow-up studies, it appears that children with gross hematuria from hypercalciuria had associated nephrolithiasis more often than did a control population of hypercalciuric children without gross hematuria (154).

If dietary sodium restriction does not ameliorate the hypercalciuria, an increase in dietary potassium may be initiated (155) in the absence of stone disease. If stone disease is present, the next therapy to institute is administration of thiazide diuretics in dosages used to treat mild primary hypertension. Such agents directly inhibit tubular calcium secretion in the cortical thick ascending limb (156,157) and promote whole-body calcium retention as well (158). Thiazides may have direct effects on bone mineralization, and these effects are currently being studied in children and adults in several centers. Some concern has been raised about long-term use because thiazides alter lipid metabolism in a proatherogenic manner (159).

Other treatments for hypercalciuria unresponsive to thiazide therapy alone may include the administration of supplemental alkali, usually in the form of citrate salts, and/or the provision of neutral phosphate salts to limit dietary calcium absorption. Careful attention to all components of the urine related to nephrolithiasis is mandatory when multiple therapies for genetic hypercalciuria are undertaken.

Bartter's Syndrome

See Chapter 38 for a discussion of Bartter's syndrome, a metabolic disorder. The overwhelming majority of infants and children with Bartter's syndrome are hypercalciuric (160), and occasionally hypercalciuria is the presenting sign of the disease. Hypercalciuria may be associated with the development of nephrolithiasis, but it is commonly associated with nephrocalcinosis.

Hyperprostaglandin Syndromes

Several disorders of prostaglandin metabolism in infants and children are associated with hypercalciuria, although the urinary finding rarely dominates the clinical picture. These include Seyberth (hyper–prostaglandin E) syndrome (161,162) and the use of prostaglandin infusions in neonates with congenital heart disease. Some data implicate excess urinary prostaglandin excretion in genetic (idiopathic) hypercalciuria (163,164).

Distal Renal Tubular Acidosis

An important feature of distal renal tubular acidosis is the attendant hypercalciuria that arises in part from an acquired defect in citrate metabolism secondary to the acidosis (165,166). Correction of the hypercalciuria with adequate alkali supplementation is critical to achieve normal growth in children with the disorder (167).

Juvenile Rheumatoid Arthritis

Children with clinically active juvenile rheumatoid arthritis have hypercalciuria and osteopenia (168,169). A reduction in disease activity improves both the osteopenia and the hypercalciuria (170).

Normocalcemic Hypocalciuria

Magnesium-Losing Tubulopathy (Gitelman's Syndrome)

Gitelman's syndrome may result in a frank hypokalemic metabolic alkalosis or have a more limited clinical expression in which renal magnesium wasting with hypomagnesemia occurs as an isolated entity (171) (see Chapter 38). Urine calcium excretion is generally under 0.5 mg/kg body mass per day. The lack of even normal levels of urine calcium excretion is unexpected, because severe hypomagnesemia inhibits the release or action of PTH. The disorder has an autosomal dominant inheritance, although incomplete phenotypic expression occurs commonly. Children manifest severe hypokalemia but grow and develop normally, unlike children affected with Bartter's syndrome

TABLE 11.4. CLINICAL FEATURES OF HYPOPHOSPHATEMIA

Acute hypophosphatemia	Chronic hypophosphatemia
Muscle weakness	Musculoskeletal complaints
Paresthesias	Paresthesias
Hyporeflexia	Depressed reflexes
Cranial nerve palsies	Tremor
Tremor	Seizures
Confusion → coma	Cardiac failure
	Respiratory failure
	Hemolytic anemia
	Rhabdomyolysis

TABLE 11.5. CLINICAL FEATURES OF HYPERCALCEMIA

Lethargy → confusion → coma	Hyporeflexia
Depression, paranoia	Abnormal electroencephalographic pattern
Muscle weakness	Nausea with or without emesis
Constipation	Bradycardia
Reduced QT_c interval on electrocardiogram	Polyuria with concentrating and diluting defects
Systemic hypertension	Nephrolithiasis
Nephrocalcinosis	Malignant venous thrombosis
Extraosseous calcifications	
Headache	

(172–174). Nephrocalcinosis is uncommon, and nephrolithiasis is slightly more common than in the general population; stones formed are composed of oxalate. When the disorder presents in infancy or early childhood, it may be associated with symptomatic hypocalcemia. In late adolescence and adulthood, chondrocalcinosis may develop whether the biochemical abnormalities have been effectively treated or not.

Cisplatinum Nephrotoxicity

Chronic cisplatinum nephrotoxicity is associated with a magnesium-losing tubulopathy that has a pronounced hypocalciuric component. Calcium excretion is often below 0.5 mg/kg body mass per day. The low urinary calcium excretion is unexpected, and its mechanism is unknown.

CLINICAL FEATURES OF MINERAL DISORDERS

Tables 11.4 to 11.6 list the most common manifestations of the disturbances discussed in this chapter. Whether or not an isolated blood mineral disturbance produces clinical features depends on the acuteness of the change and on the depth and chronicity of the directional changes.

TABLE 11.6. CLINICAL FEATURES OF HYPOCALCEMIA

Paresthesias	Muscle cramps
Seizures	Laryngospasm
Carpal pedal spasms	Tetany
Electroencephalographic changes	Irritability, depression, psychosis
Papilledema	Increased cerebrospinal fluid pressure
Intracranial calcification	Cataracts (hypoparathyroidism and pseudohypoparathyroidism)
Prolonged QT_c interval on electrocardiogram	Dental abnormalities

REFERENCES

1. Langman CB. Vitamin D physiology: normal and abnormal. In: Strauss J, ed. *Pediatric nephrology.* Coral Gables, FL: University of Miami Press, 1989:81–105.
2. Whyte MP. Tumoral calcinosis. In: Favus MJ, ed. *Primer on the metabolic bone diseases and disorders of mineral metabolism.* New York: American Society for Bone and Mineral Research, 1990:264–265.
3. Whyte MP. Metabolic and dysplastic diseases. In: Favus MJ, Coe FL, eds. *Disorders of bone and mineral metabolism.* New York: Raven Press, 1992:1019–1021.
4. Lyles KW, Burkes EJ, Ellis GJ, et al. Genetic transmission of tumoral calcinosis: autosomal dominant with variable clinical expressivity. *J Clin Endocrinol Metab* 1985;60:1093–1096.
5. Mozaffarian G, Lafferty FW, Pearson OH. Treatment of tumoral calcinosis with phosphate deprivation. *Ann Intern Med* 1972;77:741–745.
6. Prince MJ, Schaefer PC, Goldsmith RS, et al. Hyperphosphatemic tumoral calcinosis: association with elevation of serum 1,25-dihydroxyvitamin D concentrations. *Ann Intern Med* 1982;96:586–591.
7. Lyles KW, Halsey DL, Friedman NE, et al. Association of 1,25-dihydroxyvitamin D, phosphorus, and parathyroid hormone in tumoral calcinosis: potential pathogenetic mechanisms for the disease. *J Clin Endocrinol Metab* 1988;68:88–92.
8. Boskey AL, Vigorita VJ, Sencer O, et al. Chemical, microscopic, and ultrastructural characterization of mineral deposits in tumoral calcinosis. *Clin Orthop* 1983;178:258–270.
9. Davies M, Clements MR, Mawer EB, et al. Tumoral calcinosis: clinical and metabolic response to phosphorus deprivation. *J Med* 1987;242:493–503.
10. Salvi A, Cerudelli B, Cimino A, et al. Phosphaturic action of calcitonin in pseudotumoral calcinosis [Letter]. *Horm Metab Res* 1983;15:260.
11. Nagant de Deuxchasisnes C, Krane SM. Hypoparathyroidism. In: Avioli LV, Krane SM, eds. *Metabolic bone disease.* New York: Academic Press, 1978;2:218–415.
12. Gidding SS, Minciotti AM, Langman CB. Unmasking of hypoparathyroidism in familial partial DiGeorge syndrome by EDTA challenge. *N Engl J Med* 1988;319:1589–1591.
13. Cuneo BF, Langman CB, Hoo J, et al. Children with isolated conotruncal cardiac defects manifest reduced parathyroid hormone reserve. An expanded definition of latent hypoparathyroidism. *Circulation* 1996;93:1702–1708.
14. Gong W, Emanuel BS, Collins J, et al. A transcription map of the DiGeorge and velo-cardiofacial syndrome minimal critical region on 22q11. *Hum Mol Genet* 1996;5(6):789–800.
15. Cuneo BF, Driscoll DA, Gidding SS, et al. Evolution of latent hypoparathyroidism in familial 22q11 deletion syndrome. *Am J Med Genet* 1997;69:50–55.
16. Baron J, Winter KK, Yanovski JA, et al. Mutations in the Ca2+-sensing receptor gene cause autosomal dominant and sporadic hypoparathyroidism. *Nat Genet* 1995;11:389–394.
17. Brown EM, Pollak M. The extracellular calcium-sensing receptor: its role in health and disease. In: Coggins CH, Hancock EW, Levitt LJ, eds. *Annual review of medicine: selected topics in the clinical sciences.* Palo Alto, CA: Annual Reviews, 1998;49:15–30.

18. Lobes A, Bonilla E, DiMauro S. Mitochondrial encephalomyopathies. *Rev Neurol (Paris)* 1989;145:671–689.
19. Zupanc ML, Moraes CT, Shanske S, et al. Deletion of mitochondrial DNA in patients with combined features of Kearns-Sayre and MELAS syndromes. *Ann Neurol* 1991;29:680–683.
20. Levine MA, Downs RW Jr, Singer M. Deficient activity of guanine nucleotide regulatory protein in erythrocytes from patients with pseudohypoparathyroidism. *Biochem Biophys Res Commun* 1980;94:1319–1324.
21. Farfel Z, Brickman AS, Kaslow HR. Defect of receptor-cyclase coupling protein in pseudohypoparathyroidism. *N Engl J Med* 1980;303:237–242.
22. Patten JL, Johns DR, Valle D, et al. Mutation in the gene encoding the stimulatory G protein of adenylate cyclase in the Albright's hereditary osteodystrophy. *N Engl J Med* 1990;322:1412–1419.
23. Levine MA, Jap TS, Hung W. Infantile hypothyroidism in two sibs: an unusual presentation of pseudohypoparathyroidism type Ia. *J Pediatr* 1985;107:919–922.
24. Llach F, Felsenfeld AJ, Haussler MR. The pathophysiology of altered calcium metabolism in rhabdomyolysis-induced acute renal failure. Interactions of parathyroid hormone, 25-hydroxycholecalciferol, and 1,25-dihydroxycholecalciferol. *N Engl J Med* 1981;305:117–123.
25. Frame B, Honasoge M, Kottamasu S. *Osteosclerosis, hyperostosis, and related disorders*. New York: Elsevier, 1987.
26. Davis RF, Eichner JM, Bleyer WA, et al. Hypocalcemia, hyperphosphatemia, and dehydration following a single hypertonic phosphate enema. *J Pediatr* 1977;90:484–485.
27. Winters RW, Graham JB, Williams TF, et al. A genetic study of familial hypophosphatemia and vitamin D resistant rickets with a review of the literature. *Medicine* 1958;37:97–142.
28. Delvin EE, Glorieux FH. Serum 1,25-dihydroxyvitamin D concentration in hypophosphatemic vitamin D resistant rickets. *Calcif Tissue Int* 1981;33:77–79.
29. Lyles KW, Clark AG, Drezner MK. Serum 1,25-dihydroxyvitamin D levels in subjects with X-linked hypophosphatemic rickets and osteomalacia. *Calcif Tissue Int* 1982;34:125–130.
30. Baxter LA, DeLuca HF. Stimulation of 25-hydroxyvitamin D3-1alpha-hydroxylase by phosphate depletion. *J Biol Chem* 1976;251:3158–3161.
31. Gray RW, Wilz DR, Caldas AE, et al. The importance of phosphate in regulating plasma 1,25-dihydroxyvitamin D synthesis in rat kidney in vitro. *J Biol Chem* 1983;258:1151–1155.
32. The Hyp Consortium. A gene (PEX) with homologies to endopeptidases is mutated in patients with X-linked hypophosphatemic rickets. *Nat Genet* 1995;11:130–136.
33. Kumar R. New insights into phosphate homeostasis: fibroblast growth factor 23 and frizzled-related protein-4 are phosphaturic factors derived from tumors associated with osteomalacia. *Curr Opin Nephrol Hypertens* 2002;11:547–553.
34. Jonsson KB, Zahradnik R, Larsson T, et al. Fibroblast growth factor 23 in oncogenic osteomalacia and X-linked hypophosphatemia. *N Engl J Med* 2003;348:1656–1663.
35. Harrison HE. Primary hypophosphatemic rickets and growth retardation. *Growth Genet Horm* 1986;2:1–4.
36. Reid IR, Hardy DC, Murphy WA, et al. X-linked hypophosphatemia: a clinical, biochemical, and histopathologic assessment of morbidity in adults. *Medicine* 1989;68:336–352.
37. Reid IR, Hardy DC, Murphy WA, et al. X-linked hypophosphatemia: skeletal mass in adults assessed by histomorphometry, computed tomography, and absorptiometry. *Am J Med* 1991;90:63–69.
38. X-linked hypophosphatemia: an appreciation of a classic paper and a survey of progress since 1958 [editorial]. *Medicine* 1991;70:218–228.
39. Krohn KP, Offermann G, Brandis M, et al. Occurrence of hyperparathyroidism in children with X-linked hypophosphatemia under treatment with vitamin D and phosphate. *Adv Exp Med Biol* 1977;81:223–250.
40. Rith RG, Grant CS, Riggs BL. Development of hypercalcemic hyperparathyroidism after long-term phosphate supplementation in hypophosphatemic osteomalacia. Report of two cases. *Am J Med* 1985;78:669–673.
41. Costa T, Marie PJ, Scriver CR, et al. X-linked hypophosphatemia: effect of calcitriol on renal handling of phosphate, serum phosphate, and bone mineralization. *J Clin Endocrinol Metab* 1981;52:463–472.
42. Chesney RW, Mazess RB, Rose P, et al. Influence of calcitriol and supplemental phosphate in X-linked hypophosphatemic rickets. *Pediatrics* 1983;71:559–567.
43. Glorieux FH. Hypophosphatemic vitamin D-resistant rickets. In: Favus MJ, ed. *Primer on the metabolic bone diseases and disorders of mineral metabolism*, 3rd ed. New York: Lippincott-Raven, 1994:316–319.
44. Lobaugh B, Drezner MK. Abnormal regulation of renal 25-hydroxyvitamin D-1-alpha-hydroxylase activity in the X-linked hypophosphatemic mouse. *J Clin Invest* 1983;71:400–403.
45. Nesbitt T, Lobaugh B, Drezner MK. Calcitonin stimulation of renal 25-hydroxyvitamin D-1-alpha-hydroxylase activity in hypophosphatemic mice. Evidence that the regulation of calcitriol production is not universally abnormal in X-linked hypophosphatemia. *J Clin Invest* 1987;79:15–19.
46. Tenenhouse HS, Yip A, Jones G. Increased renal catabolism of 1,25-dihydroxyvitamin D_3 in murine X-linked hypophosphatemic rickets. *J Clin Invest* 1988;81:461–465.
47. Tenenhouse HS, Jones G. Abnormal regulation of renal vitamin D catabolism by dietary phosphate in murine X-linked hypophosphatemic rickets. *J Clin Invest* 1990;85:1450–1455.
48. Lyon MF, Scriver CR, Baker LRI, et al. The *Gy* mutation: another cause of X-linked hypophosphatemia in mouse. *Proc Natl Acad Sci U S A* 1986;83:4899–4903.
49. Davidai GA, Nesbitt T, Drezner MK. Normal regulation of calcitriol metabolism in *Gy* mice. Evidence for biochemical heterogeneity in the X-linked hypophosphatemic diseases. *J Clin Invest* 1990;85:334–339.
50. Bushinsky DA, Nalbantian-Brandt C, Favus MJ. Elevated Ca2+ does not inhibit the 1,25(OH)2D3 response to phosphorus restriction. *Am J Physiol (Renal Fluid Electrolyte Physiol)* 1989;256:F285–F289.
51. Portale AA, Halloran BP, Harris ST, et al. Metabolic acidosis reverses the increase in serum 1,25(OH)2D in phosphorus-restricted normal men. *Am J Physiol* 1992;263:E1164–E1170.
52. Krapf R, Vetsch R, Vetsch W, et al. Chronic metabolic acidosis increases the serum concentration of 1,25-dihydroxyvitamin D in humans by stimulating its production rate. Critical role of acidosis-induced renal hypophosphatemia. *J Clin Invest* 1992;90:2456–2463.

53. Nakajima S, Yamaoka K, Yamamoto T, et al. Decreased concentration of 1,25-dihydroxyvitamin D3 receptors in peripheral mononuclear cells of patients with X-linked hypophosphatemic rickets: effect of phosphate supplementation. *Bone* 1990;10:201–209.
54. Yamamoto T, Seino Y, Tanaka H, et al. Effects of the administration of phosphate on nuclear 1,25-dihydroxyvitamin D uptake by duodenal mucosal cells of Hyp mice. *Endocrinology* 1988;122:576–580.
55. Tieder M, Modai D, Samuel R, et al. Hereditary hypophosphatemic rickets with hypercalciuria. *N Engl J Med* 1985;312: 611–617.
56. Tieder M, Modai D, Shaked U, et al. "Idiopathic hypercalciuria" and hereditary hypophosphatemic rickets: two phenotypical expressions of a common genetic defect. *N Engl J Med* 1987;316:125–129.
57. Jones A, Tzenova J, Frappier D, et al. Hereditary hypophosphatemic rickets with hypercalciuria is not caused by mutations in the Na/Pi cotransporter NPT2 gene. *J Am Soc Nephrol* 2001;12:507–514.
58. Frymoyer JW, Hodgkin W. Adult-onset vitamin D-resistant hypophosphatemic osteomalacia. *J Bone Joint Surg* 1977;59: 101–106.
59. Scriver CR, MacDonald W, Reade T, et al. Hypophosphatemic nonrachitic bone disease: an entity distinct from X–linked hypophosphatemia in the renal defect, bone involvement, and inheritance. *Am J Med Genet* 1977;1: 101–117.
60. Scriver CR, Reade T, Halal F, et al. Autosomal hypophosphatemic bone disease responds to 1,25(OH)2D3. *Arch Dis Child* 1981;56:203–207.
61. Chesney RW. Phosphaturic syndromes. In: Gonick HC, Buckalew VM Jr, eds. *Renal tubular disorders: pathophysiology, diagnosis and management.* New York: Marcel Dekker, 1985:201–238.
62. Fraser D, Kooh SW, Kind HO, et al. Pathogenesis of hereditary vitamin D-dependent rickets: an inborn error of vitamin D metabolism involving defective conversion of 25–hydroxyvitamin D to 1,25–dihydroxyvitamin D. *N Engl J Med* 1973;289:817–822.
63. Rosen JF, Finberg L. Vitamin D-dependent rickets: action of parathyroid hormone and 25–hydroxycholecalciferol. *Pediatr Res* 1972;552–562.
64. Takeyama K, Kitanaka S, Sato T, et al. 25-Hydroxyvitamin D3 1a-hydroxylase and vitamin D synthesis. *Science* 1997;277: 1827–1830.
65. Fu GK, Lin D, Zhang MYH, et al. Cloning of human 25-hydroxyvitamin D-1a-hydroxylase and mutations causing vitamin D-dependent rickets type I. *Mol Endocrinol* 1997;11:1961–1970.
66. Kitanaka S, Takeyama KI, Murayama A, et al. Inactivating mutations in the 25-hydroxyvitamin D3 1a-hydroxylase gene in patients with pseudovitamin D-deficiency rickets. *N Engl J Med* 1998;338:653–661.
67. Brooks MH, Bell NH, Love L, et al. Vitamin D-dependent rickets, type II: resistance of target organs to 1,25-dihydroxyvitamin D. *N Engl J Med* 1978;293:996–999.
68. Hughes MR, Malloy PJ, Kieback DG, et al. Point mutations in the human vitamin D receptor gene associated with hypocalcemic rickets. *Science* 1988;242:1702–1705.
69. Lieberman UA, Eil C, Marx SJ. Resistance to 1,25-dihydroxyvitamin D3: association with heterogeneous defects in cultured skin fibroblasts. *J Clin Invest* 1983;71:192–200.
70. Moorehead JF, Ahmed KY, Varghese Z. Hypophosphataemic osteomalacia after cadaveric renal transplantation. *Lancet* 1974;20:694–697.
71. Ward HN, Pabico RC, McKenna BA, et al. The renal handling of phosphate by renal transplant patients: correlation with serum parathyroid hormone, cyclic 3',5'-adenosine monophosphate urinary excretion, and allograft function. *Adv Exp Med Biol* 1977;81:173–181.
72. Nielsen HE, Christensen MS, Melsen F, et al. Bone disease, hypophosphatemia and hyperparathyroidism after renal transplantation. *Adv Exp Med Biol* 1977;81:603–610.
73. Farrington K, Varghese Z, Newman SP, et al. Dissociation of absorption of calcium and phosphate after successful cadaveric renal transplantation. *BMJ* 1979;1:712–714.
74. Nielsen HE, Christensen MS, Melsen F. Spontaneous fractures following renal transplantation. Clinical and biochemical aspects, bone mineral content, and bone morphometry. *Miner Electrolyte Metab* 1979;2:323–330.
75. Walker GS, Peacock M, Marshall DH. Factors influencing the intestinal absorption of calcium and phosphorus following renal transplantation. *Nephron* 1986;26:225–229.
76. Kovarik J, Graf H, Stummvoll HK, et al. Tubular phosphate handling after successful kidney transplantation. *Klin Wochenschr* 1980;58:863–869.
77. Friedman A, Chesney RW. Fanconi's syndrome in renal transplantation. *Am J Nephrol* 1981;1:45–47.
78. Rosenbaum RW, Hruska KA, Korkor A, et al. Decreased phosphate reabsorption after renal transplantation: evidence for a mechanism independent of calcium and parathyroid hormone. *Kidney Int* 1981;19:568–578.
79. Lucas PA, Brown RC, Bloodworth L, et al. Vitamin D3 metabolites in hypercalcemic adults after kidney transplantation. *Proc Eur Dial Transplant Assoc* 1983;20:213–219.
80. Bonomini V, Feletti C, DeFelice A, et al. Bone remodeling after renal transplantation. *Adv Exp Med Biol* 1984;178:207–216.
81. Sakhaee K, Brinker K, Helderman JH, et al. Disturbances in mineral metabolism after successful renal transplantation. *Miner Electrolyte Metab* 1985;11:167–172.
82. Felsenfeld AJ, Gutman RA, Drezner M, et al. Hypophosphatemia in long–term renal transplant recipients: effects on bone histology and 1,25-dihydroxycholecalciferol. *Miner Electrolyte Metab* 1986;12:333–341.
83. Julian BJ, Benfield M, Quarles LD. Bone loss after organ transplantation. *Transplant Rev* 1993;7:82–95.
84. Bilezikian JP. Hypercalcemic states. Their differential diagnosis and acute management. In: Coe FL, Favus MJ, eds. *Disorders of bone and mineral metabolism.* New York: Raven Press, 1992;493–521.
85. Chattopadahyay N, Mithal A, Brown E. The calcium receptor: a new handle on the diagnosis and treatment of parathyroid disorders. *Endocr Rev* 1996;17:289–307.
86. Pollak M, Brown E, Chou Y. Mutations in the human Ca2+-sensing receptor gene cause familial hypocalciuric hypercalcemia and neonatal severe hyperparathyroidism. *Cell* 1993;75:1297–1303.
87. Pearce S, Trump D, Wooding C. Calcium-sensing receptor

mutations in familial benign hypercalcemia and neonatal hyperparathyroidism. *J Clin Invest* 1995;96:2683–2692.
88. Marx SJ, Attie MF, Levine MA, et al. The hypocalciuric or benign variant of familial hypercalcemia: clinical and biochemical features in fifteen kindreds. *Medicine* 1981;60:397–412.
89. Law WM Jr, Heath H III. Familial benign hypercalcemia (hypocalciuric hypercalcemia): clinical and pathogenetic studies in 21 families. *Ann Intern Med* 1985;102:511–519.
90. Marx SJ, Attie MF, Spiegel AM, et al. An association between neonatal severe primary hyperparathyroidism and familial hypocalciuric hypercalcemia. *N Engl J Med* 1982;306:257–264.
91. Heath H III, Odelberg S, Jackson C. Clustered inactivating mutations and benign polymorphisms of the calcium receptor gene in familial benign hypocalciuric hypercalcemia suggest receptor functional domains. *J Clin Endocrinol Metab* 1996;81:1312–1317.
92. Heath H III. Familial benign (hypocalciuric) hypercalcemia. A troublesome mimic of mild primary hyperparathyroidism. *Endocrinol Metab Clin North Am* 1989;18:723–740.
93. Bjernulf A, Hall K, Sjogren L, et al. Primary hyperparathyroidism in children. Brief review of the literature and a case report. *Acta Paediatr Scand* 1970;59:249–258.
94. Mallette LE, Malini S, Rappaport M, et al. Familial cystic parathyroid adenomatosis. *Ann Intern Med* 1987;107:49–54.
95. Nemeth E. Ca2+-receptor-dependent regulation of cellular function. *New Physiol Sci* 1995;10:1–5.
96. Williams JCP, Barratt-Boyes BG, Lowe JB. Supravalvular aortic stenosis. *Circulation* 1961;24:1311–1316.
97. Black JA, Bonham Carter RE. Association between aortic stenosis and facies of severe infantile hypercalcemia. *Lancet* 1963;2:745–748.
98. Preus M. The Williams syndrome: objective definition and diagnosis. *Clin Genet* 1984;25:422–428.
99. Pankau R, Partsch CJ, Winter M, et al. Incidence and spectrum of renal abnormalities in Williams-Beuren syndrome. *Am J Med Genet* 1996;63:301–304.
100. Schulman SL, Zderic S, Kaplan P. Increased prevalence of urinary symptoms and voiding dysfunction in Williams syndrome. *J Pediatr* 1996;129(3):466–469.
101. Perez Jurado LA, Peoples R, Kaplan P, et al. Molecular definition of the chromosome 7 deletion in Williams syndrome and parent-of-origin effects on growth. *Am J Hum Genet* 1996;59(4):781–792.
102. Joyce CA, Zorich B, Pike SJ, et al. Williams-Beuren syndrome: phenotypic variability and deletions of chromosomes 7, 11, and 22 in a series of 52 patients. *J Med Genet* 1996;33(12):986–992.
103. Taylor AB, Stern PH, Bell NH. Abnormal regulation of circulating 25OHD in the Williams' syndrome. *N Engl J Med* 1982;306:972–975.
104. Garabedian M, Jacqz E, Guillozo H, et al. Increased plasma 1,25(OH)2D3 concentrations in infants with hypercalcemia and an elfin facies. *N Engl J Med* 1985;312:948–952.
105. Martin ND, Snodgrass GJ, Makin HL, et al. Letter to the editor. *N Engl J Med* 1986;313:888–889.
106. Chesney RW, DeLuca HF, Gertner JM, et al. Letter to the editor. *N Engl J Med* 1986;313:889–890.
107. Culler FL, Jones KL, Deftos LJ. Impaired calcitonin secretion in patients with Williams' syndrome. *J Pediatr* 1985;107:720–723.
108. Lightwood RL. Idiopathic hypercalcemia with failure to thrive. *Arch Dis Child* 1952;27:302–303.
109. Martin ND, Snodgrass GJ, Cohen RD. Idiopathic infantile hypercalcemia—a continuing enigma. *Arch Dis Child* 1984; 59:605–613.
110. Aarskog D, Asknes L, Markstead T. Vitamin D metabolism in idiopathic infantile hypercalcemia. *Am J Dis Child* 1981;135:1021–1025.
111. Langman CB, Budayr AA, Sailer DE, et al. Nonmalignant expression of parathyroid hormone-related protein is responsible for idiopathic infantile hypercalcemia. *Bone Miner Res* 1992;7:593.
112. Orloff JJ, Stewart AF. Disorders of serum minerals caused by cancer. In: Coe FL, Favus MJ, eds. *Disorders of bone and mineral metabolism.* New York: Raven Press, 1992:539–562.
113. Michael AF, Hong R, West CD. Hypercalcemia in infancy. *Am J Dis Child* 1962;104:235–244.
114. Jasper PL, Denny FW. Sarcoidosis in children. *J Pediatr* 1968;73:499–512.
115. Bosch XB. Hypercalcemia due to endogenous overproduction of active vitamin D in identical twins with cat-scratch disease. *JAMA* 1998;279(7):532–534.
116. Rosen JF, Wolin DA, Finberg L. Immobilization hypercalcemia after single limb fractures in children and adolescents. *Am J Dis Child* 1978;132:560–564.
117. Chan JCM, Young RB, Alon U, et al. Hypercalcemia in children with disorders of calcium and phosphate metabolism during long-term treatment with 1,25(OH)2D3. *Pediatrics* 1983;72:225–233.
118. Frame B, Poznanski AK. Conditions that may be confused with rickets. In: Deluca HF, Anast CN, eds. *Pediatric diseases related to calcium.* New York: Elsevier, 1980: 269–289.
119. Schipani E, Kruse E, Juppner H. A constitutively active mutant PTH-PTHrP receptor in Jansen-type metaphyseal chondrodysplasia. *Science* 1995;268:98–100.
120. Schipani E, Langman CB, Parfitt AM, et al. Constitutively activated receptors for parathyroid hormone and parathyroid hormone-related peptide in Jansen's metaphyseal chondrodysplasia. *N Engl J Med* 1996;335:708–714.
121. Schipani E, Langman C, Hunzelman J, et al. A novel parathyroid hormone (PTH)/PTH-related peptide receptor mutation in Jansen's metaphyseal chondrodysplasia. *J Clin Endocrinol Metab* 1999;84:3052–3057.
122. Whyte MP. Hereditary metabolic and dysplastic skeletal disorders. In: Coe FL, Favus MJ, eds. *Disorders of bone and mineral metabolism.* New York: Raven Press, 1992:977–986.
123. Barcia JP, Strife CF, Langman CB. Infantile hypophosphatasia: treatment options to control hypercalcemia, hypercalciuria, and chronic bone demineralization. *J Pediatr* 1997;130(5): 825–828.
124. Moore ES, Coe FL, McMann BJ, et al. Idiopathic hypercalciuria in children: prevalence and metabolic characteristics. *J Pediatr* 1978;92:906–910.
125. Kruse K, Kracht U, Kruse U. Reference values for urinary calcium excretion and screening for hypercalciuria in children and adolescents. *Eur J Pediatr* 1984;143:25–31.
126. Paunier L, Borgeaud M, Wyss M. Urinary excretion of magnesium and calcium in normal children. *Helv Paediatr Acta* 1970;25:577–584.

127. De Santo NG, Di Iorio B, Capasso G, et al. Population based data on urinary excretion of calcium, magnesium, oxalate, phosphate and uric acid in children from Cimitile (southern Italy). *Pediatr Nephrol* 1992;6:149–157.
128. Chen YH, Lee AJ, Lin CS, et al. Oral calcium loading test and response to diuretics in normal Taiwanese school children. *Pediatr Nephrol* 1996;10(2):175–179.
129. Alconcher LF, Castro C, Quintana D, et al. Urinary calcium excretion in healthy school children. *Pediatr Nephrol* 1997; 11(2):186–188.
130. Reusz GS, Dobos M, Byrd D, et al. Urinary calcium and oxalate excretion in children. *Pediatr Nephrol* 1995;9(1):39–44.
131. Hoppe B, Hesse A, Neuhaus T, et al. Influence of nutrition on urinary oxalate and calcium in preterm and term infants. *Pediatr Nephrol* 1997;11:687–690.
132. Lloyd SE, Pearce SH, Fisher SE, et al. A common molecular basis for three inherited kidney stone diseases. *Nature* 1996;379(6564):445–449.
133. Fisher SE, van Bakel I, Lloyd SE, et al. Cloning and characterization of CLCN5, the human kidney chloride channel gene implicated in Dent disease (an X-linked hereditary nephrolithiasis). *Genomics* 1995;29(3):598–606.
134. Scheinman SJ, Pook MA, Wooding C, et al. Mapping the gene causing X-linked recessive nephrolithiasis to Xp11.22 by linkage studies. *J Clin Invest* 1993;91(6):2351–2357.
135. Frymoyer PA, Scheinman SJ, Dunham PB, et al. X-linked recessive nephrolithiasis with renal failure. *N Engl J Med* 1991;325(10):681–686.
136. Coe FL, Parks JH. Familial (idiopathic) hypercalciuria. In: Coe FL, Parks JH, eds. *Nephrolithiasis: pathogenesis and treatment.* Chicago: Year Book Medical Publishers, 1988:108–138.
137. Coe FL, Favus MJ. Nephrolithiasis. In: Brenner BM, Rector FC Jr, eds. *The kidney.* Philadelphia: WB Saunders, 1991; 1740–1747.
138. Pak CYC. Kidney stones. In: Wilson JD, Foster DW, eds. *Williams textbook of endocrinology.* Philadelphia: WB Saunders, 1992;1522–1526.
139. Coe FL, Parks JH, Moore ES. Familial idiopathic hypercalciuria. *N Engl J Med* 1979;300:337–341.
140. Langman CB, Moores ES. Hypercalciuria in clinical pediatrics. *Clin Pediatr* 1984;23:135–140.
141. Stapleton FB, Noe HN, Roy S, et al. Hypercalciuria in children with urolithiasis. *Am J Dis Child* 1982;136:675–678.
142. Alon U, Warady B, Hellerstein S. Hypercalciuria in the frequency-dysuria syndrome of childhood. *J Pediatr* 1990;116: 103–105.
143. Welch TR, Abrams SA, Shoemaker L, et al. Precise determination of the absorptive component of urinary calcium excretion using stable isotopes. *Pediatr Nephrol* 1995;9(3):295–297.
144. Stapleton FB, Langman CB, Bittle J, et al. Increased serum concentrations of 1,25(OH)2 vitamin D in children with fasting hypercalciuria. *J Pediatr* 1987;110:234–237.
145. Moore ES, Langman CB, Favus MJ, et al. Secondary hyperparathyroidism in children with idiopathic hypercalciuria. *J Pediatr* 1983;103:932–935.
146. Stapleton FB, McKay CP, Noe HN. Urolithiasis in children: the role of hypercalciuria. *Pediatr Ann* 1987;16:980–992.
147. Favus MJ, Coe FL. Evidence for spontaneous hypercalciuria in the rat. *Miner Electrolyte Metab* 1979;2:150–155.
148. Bataille P, Archard JM, Fournier A, et al. Diet, vitamin D and vertebral mineral density in hypercalciuric stone formers. *Kidney Int* 1991;93:1193–1205.
149. Malluche HH, Tschoepe W, Ritz E, et al. Abnormal bone histology in idiopathic hypercalciuria. *J Clin Endocrinol Metab* 1980;50:654–658.
150. Barkin J, Wilson DR, Manuel MA, et al. Bone mineral content in idiopathic calcium nephrolithiasis. *Miner Electrolyte Metab* 1985;11:19–24.
151. Peitschmann F, Breslau NA, Pak CYC. Reduced vertebral bone density in hypercalciuric nephrolithiasis. *J Bone Miner Res* 1992;7:1383–1388.
152. Perrone HC, Lewin S, Langman CB, et al. Bone effects of the treatment of children with absorptive hypercalciuria. Ninth Congress of the International Pediatric Nephrology Association. Jerusalem, Israel, 1992 (abst).
153. Garcia-Nieto V, Ferrandez C, Monge M, et al. Bone mineral density in pediatric patients with idiopathic hypercalciuria. *Pediatr Nephrol* 1997;11:578–583.
154. A report of the Southwest Pediatric Nephrology Study Group. Idiopathic hypercalciuria: association with isolated hematuria and risk for urolithiasis in children. *Kidney Int* 1990;37:807–811.
155. Osorio AV, Alon US. The relationship between urinary calcium, sodium, and potassium excretion and the role of potassium in treating idiopathic hypercalciuria. *Pediatrics* 1997;100:675–681.
156. Costanzo LS, Windhager EE. Calcium and sodium transport by the distal convoluted tubule of the rat. *Am J Physiol* 1978;235:F492–F499.
157. Edwards BR, Bael PG, Sutton RAL, et al. Micropuncture study of diuretic effects on sodium and calcium absorption in the dog nephron. *J Clin Invest* 1973;52:2418–2426.
158. Coe FL, Parks JH, Bushinsky DA, et al. Chlorthalidone promotes mineral retention in patients with idiopathic hypercalciuria. *Kidney Int* 1988;33:1140–1145.
159. Reusz GS, Dobos M, Tulassay T, et al. Hydrochlorothiazide treatment of children with hypercalciuria: effects and side effects. *Pediatr Nephrol* 1993;76(6):699–702.
160. Restreppo de Rovetto C, Welch TR, Hug G, et al. Hypercalciuria with Bartter syndrome: evidence for an abnormality of vitamin D metabolism. *J Pediatr* 1989;115:397–404.
161. Seyberth HW, Rascher W, Schweer H, et al. Congenital hypokalemia with hypercalciuria in preterm infants: a hyperprostaglandinuric syndrome different from Bartter syndrome. *J Pediatr* 1985;107:694–701.
162. Leonhardt A, Timmermanns G, Roth B, et al. Calcium homeostasis and hypercalciuria in hyperprostaglandin E syndrome. *J Pediatr* 1992;120:546–554.
163. Henriquez-La Roche C, Rodriguez-Iturbe B, Herrera J, et al. Increased excretion of prostaglandin E in patients with idiopathic hypercalciuria. *Clin Sci* 1988;75:581–587.
164. House M, Zimmerman B, Smith C, et al. Idiopathic hypercalciuria associated with hyperreninemia and high urinary prostaglandin E. *Kidney Int* 1984;26:176–182.
165. Norman ME, Feldman NI, Cohn RM, et al. Urinary citrate excretion in the diagnosis of distal renal tubular acidosis. *J Pediatr* 1978;92:394–398.
166. Restaino I, Kaplan BS, Stanley C, et al. Nephrolithiasis,

hypocitraturia, and a distal renal tubular acidification defect in type I glycogen storage disease. *J Pediatr* 1993;122:392–396.
167. McSherry E, Morris RC Jr. On the attainment and maintenance of normal stature with alkali therapy in infants and children with classical renal tubular acidosis. *J Clin Invest* 1978;61:509–527.
168. Stapleton FB, Hanissian AS, Miller LA. Hypercalciuria in children with juvenile rheumatic arthritis: association with hematuria. *J Pediatr* 1985;107:235–239.
169. Reed AM, Haugen M, Pachman LM, et al. Abnormalities in serum osteocalcin values in children with chronic rheumatic diseases. *J Pediatr* 1990;116:574–580.
170. Reed AM, Haugen M, Pachman LM, et al. The repair of osteopenia in children with juvenile rheumatoid arthritis. *J Pediatr* 1993;122:693–696.
171. Gitelman HJ, Graham JB, Welt LG. A new familial disorder characterised by hypokalemia and hypomagnesemia. *Trans Assoc Am Phys* 1966;79:221–224.
172. McCredie DA, Blair-West JR, Scoggins BA, et al. Potassium-losing nephropathy of childhood. *Med J Aust* 1971; 1:129–135.
173. Booth BE, Johanson A. Hypomagnesemia due to a renal tubular defect in reabsorption of magnesium. *J Pediatr* 1974;84:350–355.
174. Evans RA, Carter JN, George CRP, et al. The congenital "magnesium-losing kidney." Report of two patients. *J Med* 1981;50:197–209.

12

NUTRITION AND METABOLISM

CORINA NAILESCU
PHYLLIS J. KASKEL
FREDERICK J. KASKEL

NUTRITION AND METABOLISM IN CHRONIC KIDNEY DISEASE

Influences of Chronic Kidney Disease on Nutrition and Metabolism

Poor nutrition adversely affects weight gain, growth, and, likely, development of children with chronic kidney disease (CKD). The etiology of poor weight gain in CKD is thought to be multifactorial. There is evidence that most infants and young children with CKD have subnormal caloric intake (1). Foreman et al. found that mean caloric intake was 80 ± 23% [mean ± standard deviation (SD)], of the recommended dietary allowance (RDA) for age in these children (1). There was no correlation between caloric intake and height velocity. Calcium, vitamin B_6, zinc, and folate intakes were also low. The mean protein intake in these children was 153 ± 53% of the RDA. The same study suggested that the amount of energy per unit body weight (kcal/kg/day) consumed by children with CKD is comparable to that of age-matched healthy children, but because of their small size, children with CKD consume fewer total calories and have a lower %RDA. Despite the general use of supplemental feedings in children with CKD, it is still not known whether these supplements consistently improve height or weight gain (2). This review suggests that additional mechanisms may be responsible for the growth deficits in CKD.

CKD creates a state of glucose intolerance (3). The anabolic effect of insulin is blunted, including the glucose metabolism, as are amino acid uptake into cells and the lipoprotein lipase (LPL) activity. Clinically, this state usually consists of fasting euglycemia but abnormal glucose tolerance with a delayed decrease in blood glucose in response to insulin and hyperinsulinemia. The mechanisms responsible seem to be multiple, but the most prominent metabolic disturbance in uremic patients is insulin resistance, mainly due to a postreceptor defect (4,5). Chronic metabolic acidosis (CMA), frequently associated with CKD, contributes to insulin resistance, and its treatment increases insulin sensitivity (6). In addition to the insulin resistance, there is abnormal insulin release attributable to reduced adenosine triphosphate content in the pancreatic islets, induced partially by high intracellular calcium, secondary to augmented parathyroid hormone (PTH)–induced calcium entry into cells (4,5).

Regarding protein metabolism, abundant evidence from cross-sectional analyses indicates that low values of serum proteins and loss of muscle mass are commonly found in patients with CKD (7). In addition to an inadequate diet, CMA, inflammation, and resistance to anabolic hormones, especially to insulin, contribute to abnormalities in protein turnover and ultimately result in low-serum proteins (8). Each of these factors stimulates protein breakdown in muscle and activates a common proteolytic pathway, the *ubiquitin-proteasome pathway* (9–12). CMA stimulates amino acid and protein catabolism in children with CKD by either a primary effect of acidification or secondary effects due to changes in hormonal responses induced by acidification (13). For example, CMA causes resistance to insulin and impaired function of growth hormone (GH), thyroid hormone, and the conversion of vitamin D to its most active form, 1,25$(OH)_2$-cholecalciferol (14–16). Inflammatory proteins, such as acute-phase reactant proteins, tumor necrosis factor, and interleukins (IL), have been found in excess in serum from adult hemodialysis (HD) patients (17,18). These inflammatory factors could cause excessive protein catabolism and suppression of hepatic synthesis of albumin. Insulin deficiency causes loss of muscle mass and activates the ubiquitin-proteasome pathway to degrade muscle protein (19). Further characterization of the biochemical mechanisms that regulate the ubiquitin-proteasome and other catabolic pathways will be necessary to identify new strategies for preventing protein deficits in CKD.

Dyslipidemia increases the risk of cardiovascular events among individuals with CKD and contributes to the progression of renal disease itself (20). The characteristics of dyslipidemia are different in non-nephrotic patients compared with the nephrotic ones. Hyperlipidemias can occur in as many as 70% of the non-nephrotic patients with

CKD, as opposed to 100% in the nephrotics (21). The characteristic abnormality in plasma lipids in non-nephrotic patients with CKD includes elevated triglycerides (TG) accompanied by an increased concentration of very-low-density lipoproteins (VLDL), decreased high-density lipoproteins (HDL), and normal to below normal levels of low-density lipoproteins (LDL), which represents a type IV hyperlipoproteinemic pattern. In the nephrotic patients, serum lipoprotein patterns are nearly equally distributed among types IIa, IIb, and V. The finding of low total cholesterol (TC) level should not necessarily be reassuring, because it could be a marker of malnutrition associated with increased mortality risk in HD patients (22). The mechanism of this low cholesterol involves a defective catabolism of TG-rich lipoproteins and decreased activity of both LPL and hepatic TG-lipase (23). In addition, CMA and hyperinsulinemia depress LPL activity (24). Disordered lipoprotein metabolism results from complex interactions among many factors, including the primary disease process, use of medications such as corticosteroids, the presence of malnutrition or obesity, and diet.

The most recent data regarding growth in children with CKD is provided by the North American Pediatric Renal Transplant Cooperative Study (NAPRTCS, 2001). Patients with CKD are 1.4 SD below age- and gender-adjusted norms for height. Adolescents (older than 12 years) have less severe height deficits (−1.01 ± 0.04) at baseline, relative to infants (−1.81 ± 0.07; younger than 24 months) and toddlers (−1.77 ± 0.05; age, 2 to 5 years). The height deficit for females is marginally worse than for males, and patients with baseline glomerular filtration rate (GFR) less than the median of 36.5mL/min/1.73 m^2 have more severe growth retardation than the patients with higher GFR. Children with end-stage renal disease (ESRD) are, overall, approximately 1.6 SD below the appropriate age- and gender-adjusted height levels at the time of dialysis initiation, and younger patients, in particular, have more severe growth retardation. Although the weight deficits of dialysis patients are not as severe as height, patients are, on average, more than 1 SD below normal for weight.

The GH/insulin-like growth factor-1 (IGF-1) axis plays a fundamental role in the growth process during childhood. Although serum GH and IGF-1 levels are usually normal or high in growth-retarded CKD children (25), it was recognized long ago that uremic serum has a high IGF-1 binding capacity, resulting in low IGF-1 bioactivity (26,27). The mechanisms for this increased IGF-1 binding capacity seem to be related to decreased renal clearance of IGFBP (IGF binding proteins), because serum levels of IGFBP-1, -2, -4, and -6 were shown to correlate inversely with GFR (28,29). In addition, uremia raises hepatic mRNA levels for IGFBP-1 and -2 by an unknown mechanism (30).

Secondary hyperparathyroidism has significant effects on longitudinal growth. High PTH levels are associated with mobilization of calcium from bone. PTH also causes proliferation of the fetal growth plate chondrocytes, inhibits the differentiation of these cells into hypertrophic chondrocytes, and stimulates accumulation of cartilage-specific proteoglycans that are thought to act as inhibitors of mineralization (31). However, despite the high serum PTH levels, there is "PTH resistance" at the level of growth plates, owing to intertwined factors affecting the PTH/PTH-related peptide receptors. This receptor's mRNA expression was found to be downregulated in the kidney and growth plate of uremic rats, in the osteoblasts of patients with ESRD (32), and as a result of high-dose intermittent calcitriol therapy (33,34). On the other hand, PTH/PTH-related peptide expression is upregulated by GH and physiologic doses of calcitriol (33).

CMA may affect growth independently of uremia, because diseases such as renal tubular acidosis are associated with growth defects, and catch-up growth can be achieved when patients are given alkali therapy. When the blood pH is less than 7.25, length gain is diminished earlier than weight gain. A reduction of weight gain is observed only for more severe acidosis with pH less than 7.20 (35). This finding suggests that the longitudinal growth of bone is more sensitive to acidosis than are such factors as protein synthesis, which influences body weight. The mechanisms appear to be a profound *in vitro*–negative effect of CMA on the GH/IGF-1 axis, mainly through a downregulation of the receptors for both hormones (36) plus a stimulation of osteoclastic and a suppression of osteoblastic activity (37).

Nutritional Support for the Predialysis Child

Nutritional guidelines for children with chronic renal insufficiency (CRI) before dialysis are not as well established as those for children on dialysis. However, recent studies show that disturbances in nutritional intakes, bone biochemistry, and growth occur early in CRI and suggest the need for joint medical and dietary intervention in children even with mild and moderate CRI (38).

Children who are not yet on dialysis need nutritional intake to provide calories for both maintenance and catch-up growth. The protein requirements are slightly greater than for the normal healthy controls (39) (Table 12.1).

Vitamin and trace element supplementation may be indicated during the predialysis period if their estimated intake is considerably less than the RDA. Iron supplementation is usually required in the predialysis period when depletion of iron stores is documented by laboratory studies. Patients receiving erythropoietin generally require iron supplementation owing to increased turnover of red blood cells, and require regular checking of serum iron levels. Zinc supplementation is not routinely administered to children during the predialysis phase, but because foods rich in zinc are often limited owing to poor appetite, supplementation by pharmacologic means on the basis of RDA stan-

TABLE 12.1. PREDIALYSIS: FLUID AND NUTRIENT RECOMMENDATIONS FOR CHILDREN

	Infant (0–1 yr)	Toddler (1–3 yr)	Child (4–10 yr)	Adolescent (11–18 yr)
Energy	0–0.5 yr: ≥108 kcal/kg 0.5–1 yr: ≥98 kcal/kg	102 kcal/kg	4–6 yr: 90 kcal/kg 7–10 yr: 70 kcal/kg	Girls 11–14 yr: 47 kcal/kg Girls 15–18 yr: 40 kcal/kg Boys 11–14 yr: 55 kcal/kg Boys 15–18 yr: 45 kcal/kg
Protein	0–0.5 yr: 2.2 g/kg 0.5–1.0 yr: 1.6 g/kg	1.2 g/kg	4–6 yr: 1.2 g/kg 7–10 yr: 1 g/kg	11–14 yr: 1.0 g/kg 15–18 yr: 0.9 g/kg
Sodium	Generally unrestricted; 1–3 mEq/kg if edema or HTN present	Generally unrestricted; 1–3 mEq/kg if edema or HTN present	Generally unrestricted; 1–3 mEq/kg if edema or HTN present	Generally unrestricted; 1–3 mEq/kg if edema or HTN present
Calcium	0–0.05 yr: 400 mg/d 0.5–1.0 yr: 600 mg/day (provided hypercalcemia does not occur and calcium-phosphorus product does not exceed 70)	800 mg/d (provided hypercalcemia does not occur and calcium-phosphorus product does not exceed 70)	800 mg/d (provided hypercalcemia does not occur and calcium-phosphorus product does not exceed 70)	1200 mg/d (provided hypercalcemia does not occur and calcium-phosphorus product does not exceed 70)
Potassium	1–3 mEq/kg, if needed (usually not until GFR is <10% normal)	1–3 mEq/kg, if needed (usually not until GFR is <10% normal)	1–3 mEq/kg, if needed (usually not until GFR is <10% normal)	1–3 mEq/kg, if needed (usually not until GFR is <10% normal)
Phosphorus	Use low-content formula if serum levels of phosphate are elevated; restrict high-content foods	Usually 600–800 mg/d when serum levels are elevated	Usually 600–800 mg/d when serum levels are elevated	Usually 600–800 mg/d when serum levels are elevated
Vitamins	1 mL multivitamin drops; vitamin D metabolites if needed, based on serum calcium, PTH, and alkaline phosphatase levels	Multivitamin, if needed; vitamin D metabolites, if needed, based on serum calcium, PTH, and alkaline phosphatase levels	Multivitamin, if needed; vitamin D metabolite, if needed, based on serum calcium, PTH, and alkaline phosphatase levels	Multivitamin if needed; vitamin D metabolite if needed, based on serum calcium, PTH, and alkaline phosphatase levels
Trace minerals	Supplement zinc, iron, or copper, if needed	Supplement zinc, iron, or copper, if needed	Supplement zinc, iron, or copper, if needed	Supplement zinc, iron, or copper, if needed
Fluid	Unrestricted unless needed; then replace insensible + urinary output	Unrestricted unless needed; then replace insensible + urinary output	Unrestricted unless needed; then replace insensible + urinary output	Unrestricted unless needed; then replace insensible + urinary output

GFR, glomerular filtration rate; HTN, hypertension; PTH, parathyroid gland.
Adapted from Nelson P, Stover J. Nutrition recommendations for infants, children and adolescents with end-stage renal disease. In: Gillit D, Stover J, eds. *A clinical guide to nutrition care in end-stage renal disease*, 2nd ed. Chicago, IL: American Dietetic Association, 1994:79–97.

dards may be recommended if there is reason to suspect zinc deficiency. Fluoride supplementation is provided only when the water supply is not satisfactory (40).

Monitoring Energy and Protein Intake for the Child on Dialysis

The outcome measures chosen for adult studies, mainly mortality rates, are not appropriate for children, who generally have low mortality rates while being treated for ESRD. Alternatively, complications unique to younger patients, such as impaired growth, puberty, or school performance, are better end points for evaluation of treatment strategies in these children (41). An initial evaluation and ongoing monitoring of nutritional and growth status is a major component of providing optimal care to children with ESRD. For children on chronic renal replacement therapy, it is essential that the evaluations are done by experienced pediatric renal nutritionists with skills in age-appropriate data collection, interpretation, and counseling.

A thorough nutritional assessment should include observation of physical signs and symptoms, dietary intake assessment using the 24-hour or 3-day dietary history, biochemical values, anthropometric measurements, body composition data, and assessments of protein catabolic rate if available. The physical exam may lead to clues suggestive of deficiencies of proteins and vitamins (42).

The protein-caloric status in children with CKD is usually indirectly assessed by measuring albumin and transferrin, both of which are affected by inflammation, infection, malnutrition, acidosis, hormonal influences, liver disease, dialysis, and blood loss. More sophisticated measurements of protein stores involve protein turnover studies and biochemical analysis of skeletal muscle and the nitrogen balance (43).

Growth parameters in a pediatric patient on dialysis must be measured according to standardized protocols with consistent equipment and preferably performed by the same person. The most used parameters are weight, height, head circumference (in those less than 3 years of age), body mass index (BMI), mid-arm circumference, and skinfold thickness, for which nomograms are available depending on age and gender. Anthropometric measurements in relation to nutritional status can be thought of predominantly as methods of assessment of protein-calorie malnutrition (44).

Body composition data are generally used for research purposes only, owing to the difficulty of standardization (45). For determination of fat-free mass, the following methods can be used: total body water, total body potassium, total body nitrogen and calcium, bioelectrical impedance, and electromagnetic scanning. Determination of body fatness can be done by densitometry, inert gas absorption, or near-infrared interactance. Neutron activation or dual-energy x-ray absorptiometry can be used to determine the bone mineral content (46).

Nutrition evaluation and counseling are recommended at the initiation of dialysis, ideally within the first week, and after that, on an ongoing basis because of the dynamic nature of the child's medical condition and food preferences. The maximum time between such updates should be 3 to 4 months. Conditions that could dictate a more frequent evaluation of the nutrition plan of care include decreasing dry weight, ongoing decrease in oral intake, change in gastrointestinal function, significant change in SD scores (SDS), elevated or suboptimal laboratory values related to nutrients, ongoing excess interdialytic weight gain, concern for appropriate compliance with recommendations, change in psychosocial situation, or when placement of a tube for feeding is under consideration (42).

Compliance with the nutrition prescription and recommendations from other team members are important at any age, especially in adolescents. Integrating the treatment goals of the dietitian, social worker, child development specialist, nurse, and physician helps to maximize patient and family adherence to the overall plan of care.

Nutritional Support for the Child on Maintenance Hemodialysis

Chronic HD results in dialysate loss of amino acids and water-soluble vitamins. In addition, the HD procedure itself has catabolic effects (47). In adult studies, up to 8 g of free amino acids lost per HD session have been reported. This loss is further influenced by the choice of membrane: Newer synthetic polyacrylonitrile membranes have decreased losses relative to cellulose membranes (48).

In adults, multiple studies have reported that a good nutritional status predicts a better outcome in terms of mortality, morbidity, and rehabilitation (49,50). In pediatrics, similar studies have not been done owing to the small number of patients treated and the relatively short period of treatment before transplantation. Recently, data from the United States Renal Data System (USRDS) were used to identify all patients under the age of 18 years who initiated dialysis between 1995 and 1998. This multivariate analysis performed on almost 2000 pediatric patients demonstrated that each decrease in serum albumin of ~1 g/dL was associated with a 54% higher risk of death. This finding was independent of glomerular causes of their CKD and other potential confounding variables (51).

Good dialysis adequacy is a prerequisite for good nutritional status in adult dialysis patients. Observations made on pediatric patients undergoing dialysis in 13 units throughout the six-state New England region over a period of 18 months showed that vigorous dialysis, evidenced by a high Kt/V (urea amount cleared from plasma divided by distribution volume), did not appear to improve serum albumin concentrations in younger HD patients (52). However, most of these patients were well dialyzed, and thus this finding is likely consistent with the adult studies. Thus, there appears to be little additional benefit in nutritional status once a given level of clearance is attained. In a recent report of a combination of enhanced HD clearance and nutritional supplementation, this regimen was associated with improved growth in prepubertal to early-pubertal HD children monitored for more than 2 years while receiving an average of 90.6% and 155.9% of their recommended energy and protein intake, respectively. Average weekly treatment time was 14.8 hours, with a urea reduction ratio of 85% and Kt/V of 2.0 per treatment, all well above current guidelines (53). On this regimen, the patients gained, on average, more than 0.3 SD in height without GH and normal pubertal development was also described (53).

Children on maintenance HD require an adequate caloric intake not only for weight gain and growth, but also to avoid the use of proteins as an energy source. Current recommendations are that children treated with maintenance HD should receive caloric intake according to the RDA for chronologic age at the time of the initial evaluation. Furthermore, ongoing adjustments should be made, depending on the child's clinical and biochemical response (42).

Current recommendations regarding the dietary protein intake (DPI) in patients on maintenance HD are that, initially, DPI should be based on the RDA for chronologic age plus an additional increment of 0.4 g/kg/day to achieve a positive nitrogen balance (42) (Table 12.2).

Children on maintenance HD often have an insufficient intake of oral nutrients because of anorexia and dietary

TABLE 12.2. HEMODIALYSIS: FLUID AND NUTRIENT RECOMMENDATIONS FOR CHILDREN

	Infant (0–1 yr)	Toddler (1–3 yr)	Child (4–10 yr)	Adolescent (11–18 yr)
Energy	0–0.5 yr: ≥108 kcal/kg 0.5–1 yr: ≥98 kcal/kg	102 kcal/kg	4–6 yr: 90 kcal/kg 7–10 yr: 70 kcal/kg	Girls 11–14 yr: 47 kcal/kg Girls 15–18 yr: 40 kcal/kg Boys 11–14 yr: 55 kcal/kg Boys 15–18 yr: 45 kcal/kg
Protein	0–0.5 yr: 2.6 g/kg 0.6–1.0 yr: 2.0 g/kg	1.6 g/kg	4–6 yr: 1.6 g/kg 7–10 yr: 0.25 g/kg	11–14 yr: 1.4 g/kg 15–18 yr: 1.3 g/kg (males) 1.2 g/kg (females)
Sodium	1–3 mEq/kg, if needed	Same as for predialysis	Same as for predialysis	Same as for predialysis
Calcium	Same as for predialysis	Same as for predialysis	Same as for predialysis	Same as for predialysis
Potassium	Same as for predialysis	Same as for predialysis	Same as for predialysis	Same as for predialysis
Phosphorus	Use low-content formula if serum levels of phosphate are elevated; restrict high-content foods	600–800 mg/d	600–800 mg/d	600–800 mg/d
Vitamins	1 mL multivitamin drops, 1 mg folic acid, and vitamin D metabolites (in most cases)	Multivitamin, 1 mg folic acid, and vitamin D metabolites, as needed	B-complex vitamin containing 1 mg folic acid, 10 mg pyridoxine, 60 mg ascorbic acid, 5 mg pantothenic acid, 1.0 mg thiamin, 1.2 mg riboflavin, 3 μg vitamin B_{12}, 300 μg biotin; 15 mg niacin; active form of vitamin D, as needed	B-complex vitamin containing 1 mg folic acid, 10 mg pyridoxine, 60 mg ascorbic acid, 10 mg pantothenic acid, 1.5 mg thiamin, 1.7 mg riboflavin, 6 μg vitamin B_{12}; 300 μg biotin; 20 mg niacin; active form of vitamin D, as needed
Trace minerals	Supplement zinc, iron, or copper, if needed. Iron is usually needed with recombinant erythropoietin.	Supplement zinc, iron, or copper, if needed. Iron is usually needed with recombinant erythropoietin.	Supplement zinc, iron, or copper, if needed. Iron is usually needed with recombinant erythropoietin.	Supplement zinc, iron, or copper, if needed. Iron is usually needed with recombinant erythropoietin.
Fluid	Provide insensible + urinary output + ultrafiltration capacity (if possible)	Provide insensible + urinary output	Provide insensible + urinary output	Provide insensible + urinary output

Data from Nelson P, Stover J. Nutrition recommendations for infants, children and adolescents with end-stage renal disease. In: Gillit D, Stover J, eds. *A clinical guide to nutrition care in end-stage renal disease*, 2nd ed. Chicago, IL: American Dietetic Association, 1994:79–97; and K/DOQI Nutrition in chronic renal failure. *Am J Kidney Dis* 2000;35:S112–S115.

restrictions. The first step to provide nutritional support is by oral supplementation (54) (Table 12.3). This issue is most important during periods of very high-energy requirements during the first 2 years of life and the adolescent years (55). When oral supplementation fails, enteral feeding through a nasogastric or gastrostomy tube is commonly used and is successful in opposing growth retardation and achieving catchup growth in infants and young children (56,57).

Intradialytic parenteral nutrition (IDPN) can be initiated if enteral feeding has failed (58). Morbidity and mortality were lower in adult HD patients who received IDPN (59,60), and criteria exist for IDPN in this population (61). However, one study failed to demonstrate a beneficial effect of IDPN (62). One study evaluating the use of IDPN in the pediatric population demonstrated a dramatic increase in oral caloric intake and eventual weight gain after 3 months, secondary to the improved dietary status (63).

Possible side effects of IDPN are hyperglycemia associated with glucose infusion or rebound hypoglycemia when the infusion is suddenly terminated. A frequent complaint in patients receiving IDPN is painful cramps in the arm containing the fistula, an effect thought to be due to the rapid infusion of the hyperosmolar solution causing rapid fluid shifts from muscle cell to interstitium. A long-term complication of IDPN is the possible development of abnormal liver function tests due to fatty deposition in the liver and cholestasis. Therefore, the patients on IDPN require close monitoring in terms of glucose control, hepatic function, and lipid profile (58).

Pediatric IDPN indications and appropriate compositions are not well defined but involve the infusion of 5 to 6 mg/kg/min of glucose, 1.2 to 1.4 g/kg/day of protein, and possibly the addition of intralipids (63).

IDPN provides minimal supplementation, usually between 500 and 1500 kcal and is administered only three times per week. In addition, only approximately 70% of the infused amino acids are retained owing to rapid clearance by HD (58). Thus, in patients who are severely malnourished, IDPN could not provide sufficient nutrients, and total parenteral nutrition (TPN) is indicated. However, in patients with moderate malnutrition who are intolerant to further oral supplementation secondary to anorexia, a short course of IDPN may improve nutritional status sufficient to permit more physiologic oral supplementation (63).

TABLE 12.3. FORMULAS FOR CHILDREN WITH RENAL DISEASE

	Manufacturer	kcal/mL	Protein [g/L (sources)]	Fat [g/L (sources)]	Carbohydrate [g/L (sources)]	Na/K (mEq/L)	Ca/P (mg/L)	mOsm/kg water
Similac PM 60/40	Ross Products	0.67	16 (whey, caseinate)	38 (soy, coconut)	69 (lactose)	7/15	380/190	250
Amin-aid	R & D Laboratories	2	19 (free amino acids)	46 (partially hydrogenated soybean oil, soy lecithin, mono- and diglycerides)	365 (maltodextrin, sucrose)	<15/<15	–/–	700
Suplena	Ross Products	2	30 (caseinates)	96 (high oleic safflower and soy oil, soy lecithin)	255 (maltodextrin, sucrose, cornstarch)	34/29	1430/730	600
Renalcal Diet	Nestle Clinical Nutrition	2	34 (essential L-amino acids, select nonessential amino acids, whey protein concentrate)	82 (MCT oil, canola oil, corn oil, soy lecithin)	290 (maltodextrin, modified cornstarch)	–/–	–/–	600
Nepro	Ross Products	2	70 (caseinates)	69 (high oleic safflower and soy oil)	213 (corn syrup, sucrose, FOS)	37/27	1370/685	665

–/–, none; FOS, fructo-oligosaccharides.
Adapted from Winter HS, Madden J. Nutritional support of the chronically ill child. In: Lifschitz CH, ed. *Pediatric gastroenterology and nutrition in clinical practice*. New York: Marcel Dekker, 2002:405.

In conclusion, short-term IDPN is a promising safe and effective nutritional intervention in children on HD who are not receiving sufficient nutrition from enteral feedings. However, IDPN is quite expensive, and generally restrictive criteria prevent reimbursement. As soon as the patient can tolerate an increase in oral intake or becomes a candidate for tube feedings, enteral supplementation should be undertaken.

The practice of prescribing water-soluble vitamins for HD patients has not been rigorously tested but probably does little harm. There are losses of water-soluble vitamins in the dialysate fluid, particularly ascorbic acid (64). Vitamin B_6 and folate are important supplements, especially because they are useful in reducing the homocysteine levels (65). In view of the reports of peripheral neuropathy and hyperoxalemia with high-dose vitamin B_6 and vitamin C supplementation, megavitamin therapy with water-soluble vitamins should be avoided (66). Fat-soluble vitamins should be given only when there is a clear indication because of the risk of toxicity. Vitamin A levels are invariably increased in the plasma of CRI patients, because retinol-binding protein is increased in uremia (67).

Trace elements are indispensable components of many enzymes, and abnormalities are primarily the result of uremia and the dialysis procedure. Plasma trace element concentrations in adult HD patients are distinctly different compared to those of healthy controls. Elements such as cesium, magnesium, molybdenum, and rubidium are reduced, and cadmium, cobalt, and lead are accumulated in HD patients (68). Adequate water treatment, including reverse osmosis, prevents the accumulation of the majority of trace elements in HD patients. Zinc supplementation may be recommended for patients with proven zinc deficiency, but its use in all HD patients is questionable (69,70). Selenium deficiency is to be suspected in dialyzed patients, and supplementation may be beneficial by increasing glutathione peroxidase activity, cardioprotective effect, and immunostimulatory properties (71).

Nutritional Support for the Child on Chronic Peritoneal Dialysis

Malnutrition in children receiving chronic peritoneal dialysis (PD) has specific etiologies and treatments (72). Benefits of this modality, such as a more constant control of uremia, a liberalization of dietary restrictions, and an additional source of calories from the dialysate glucose absorption, are counter balanced by losses of proteins, amino acids, vitamins and trace elements in the dialysate, anorexia possibly related to the pressure effect of dialysate in the abdomen, and to the hyperglycemia effects of absorption of glucose from dialysate (73). Finally, there is a catabolic effect induced by episodes of peritonitis (74,75).

As with HD, good nutritional status in PD is associated with a better clinical outcome. Studies done in adults showed that markers of nutritional status, mainly albumin, correlate well with morbidity and mortality in patients on PD (76). In children, it was shown that better nutrition correlates with a reduced rate of infections, particularly peritonitis (77). Inter-

TABLE 12.4. PERITONEAL DIALYSIS: FLUID AND NUTRIENT RECOMMENDATIONS FOR CHILDREN

	Infant (0–1 yr)	Toddler (1–3 yr)	Child (4–10 yr)	Adolescent (11–18 yr)
Energy	0–0.5 yr: ≥108 kcal/kg 0.5–1 yr: ≥98 kcal/kg	102 kcal/kg	4–6 yr: 90 kcal/kg 7–10 yr: 70 gm/kg	Girls 11–14 yr: 47 kcal/kg Girls 15–18 yr: 40 kcal/kg Boys 11–14 yr: 55 kcal/kg Boys 15–18 yr: 45 kcal/kg
Protein	0–0.5 yr: 2.9–3.0 g/kg 0.5–1.0 yr: 2.3–2.4 g/kg	1.9–2.0 g/kg	4–6 yr: 1.9–2.0 g/kg 7–10 yr: 1.7–1.8 g/kg	11–14 yr: 1.7–1.8 g/kg 15–18 yr: 1.4–1.5 g/kg
Sodium	Same as for predialysis	Same as for predialysis	Same as for predialysis	Same as for predialysis
Calcium	Same as for predialysis	Same as for predialysis	Same as for predialysis	Same as for predialysis
Potassium	1–3 mEq/kg, if needed (usually not until GFR is <10% normal)	1–3 mEq/kg, if needed (usually not until GFR is <10% normal)	1–3 mEq/kg, if needed (usually not until GFR is <10% normal)	1–3 mEq/kg, if needed (usually not until GFR is <10% normal)
Phosphorus	Use low-content formula if serum levels of phosphate are elevated; restrict high-content foods	Usually 600–800 mg/d when serum levels are elevated	Usually 600–800 mg/d when serum levels are elevated	Usually 600–800 mg/d when serum levels are elevated
Vitamins	1 mL multivitamin drops, 1 mg folic acid, and vitamin D metabolites (in most cases)	Multivitamin, 1 mg folic acid, and vitamin D metabolites as needed	B-complex vitamin containing 1 mg folic acid, 10 mg pyridoxine, 60 mg ascorbic acid, 5 mg pantothenic acid, 1.0 mg thiamin, 1.2 mg riboflavin, 3 μg vitamin B_{12}, 300 μg biotin; 15 mg niacin; active form of vitamin D, as needed	B-complex vitamin containing 1 mg folic acid, 10 mg pyridoxine, 60 mg ascorbic acid, 10 mg pantothenic acid, 1.5 mg thiamin, 1.7 mg riboflavin; 6 μg vitamin B_{12}, 300 μg biotin; 20 mg niacin; active form of vitamin D, as needed
Trace minerals	Supplement zinc, iron, or copper, if needed. Iron is usually needed with recombinant ethropoietin.	Supplement zinc, iron, or copper, if needed. Iron is usually needed with recombinant ethropoietin.	Supplement zinc, iron, or copper, if needed. Iron is usually needed with recombinant ethropoietin.	Supplement zinc, iron, or copper, if needed. Iron is usually needed with recombinant ethropoietin.
Fluid	Provide insensible + urinary output + ultrafiltration capacity (if possible)	Unrestricted unless needed	Unrestricted unless needed	Unrestricted unless needed

Data from Nelson P, Stover J. Nutrition recommendations for infants, children and adolescents with end-stage renal disease. In: Gillit D, Stover J, eds. *A clinical guide to nutrition care in end-stage renal disease*, 2nd ed. Chicago, IL: American Dietetic Association, 1994:79–97; and K/DOQI Nutrition in chronic renal failure. *Am J Kidney Dis* 2000;35:S112–S115.

estingly, cardiovascular disease is also a surprisingly common cause of death in children on PD, and low serum albumin levels in children on dialysis have recently been shown to be associated with an increased risk of patient death (51,78).

Adequate dialysis may be an important factor for obtaining and maintaining adequate nutritional status and growth (79,80). The delta height velocity of children with a mean age at initiation of dialysis of 28.5 months was found to be significantly correlated with total creatinine clearance, residual GFR, and residual Kt/V_{urea} (81). On the other hand, on a cautionary note, Schaefer et al. have also described an important inverse correlation between growth rates and creatinine clearance in children on PD, perhaps attributable to dialytic losses of an essential factor (82). The change in height SDS over 18 months in children on PD revealed that high-transporter state and total dialysate volume had a negative effect, whereas higher dialytic creatinine clearance had a positive effect (83). Alternatively, Kt/V greater than 2.75 in PD patients had no effect on nutrition but resulted in increased albumin losses (52).

Malnutrition in PD patients is multifactorial. Increased losses of amino acids, water-soluble vitamins and trace elements occur, whereas protein losses are inversely related to the patient's weight and peritoneal membrane total area (73). During peritonitis, the permeability of the peritoneum for proteins and amino acids increases significantly by 50 to 100%. Between 100 and 300 mg of proteins/kg/day are lost in the drained peritoneal dialysate, which translates to up to 10% of the total protein intake (73,75). The main protein lost is albumin, but there are also losses of immunoglobulins, transferrin, opsonins (84), and water-soluble vitamins, such as vitamin B_6, vitamin C, and folic acid (84,85).

In addition to the nonspecific factors contributing to decreased caloric intake in CKD, there are specific factors related to PD, such as the abdominal fullness from the dialysate and the absorption of the glucose from dialysate. Whereas the glucose absorbed from the dialysate provides calories, it also contributes to the anorexia seen in PD patients (54,86). The number of calories provided by dialysate glucose absorption may be predicted by an equation applied in adults (87). Pediatric studies reported dialysate glucose absorption ranging from 9 to 18 kcal/kg/day, representing 7 to 15% of the total daily caloric intake, respectively (39).

Current recommendations for energy intake in children treated on PD should follow the RDA for chronologic age, including calories derived from the dialysate glucose, and adjusted accordingly (42). Malnourished children, however, will require "catchup" energy supplementation detailed by the American Academy of Pediatrics (88). Supplemental g-tube feeding facilitates weight gain in infants and older children receiving PD and arrests the decline in height SDS traditionally observed in infants with CRI total protein and albumin (89,90). Gastrostomy feedings via a button in children on PD significantly improved BMI (91).

Current recommendations regarding DPI in patients on PD are also based on the RDA for chronologic age, to which a supplement based on anticipated peritoneal losses should be added (42,73) (Table 12.4). Dietary recommendations for children on PD could be further defined using a series of nitrogen balance studies. The correlation between estimated DPI and nitrogen balance indicates that a DPI of more than 140% RDA and a total energy intake of more than 85% RDA are required to obtain an estimated nitrogen balance of at least 50 mg/kg/day, which is considered adequate for metabolic needs in children (92). High biologic value protein (e.g., meat, milk, eggs) should constitute 60 to 70% of the DPI (39).

The use of special amino acid–based dialysis solutions in children on PD may compensate for losses into the dialysate (93). Furthermore, the potential complications related to the dialysate glucose load, such as hyperlipidemia, excessive weight gain, and glucose intolerance, could be ameliorated (94,95). Usually, one exchange per day is replaced with the amino acid solution consisting of both essential and nonessential amino acids with electrolyte composition similar to that of standard dialysis solutions (96) (Table 12.5).

TABLE 12.5. COMPOSITION OF AMINO ACID 1.1% DIALYSIS SOLUTION (NUTRINEAL, BAXTER)

Essential amino acids (g/L)	
Valine	1.39
Leucine	1.02
Isoleucine	0.85
Methionine	0.85
Lysine	0.76
Threonine	0.65
Phenylalanine	0.57
Tryptophan	0.27
Histidine	0.71
Nonessential amino acids (g/L)	
Arginine	1.07
Alanine	0.95
Proline	0.60
Glycine	0.51
Serine	0.51
Tyrosine	0.30
Electrolytes (mmol/L)	
Sodium	132
Calcium	1.25
Magnesium	0.25
Chloride	105
Lactate (mmol/L)	40
Osmolarity (mOsm/L)	365
pH	6.7

Adapted from Schroder CH. The choice of dialysis solutions in pediatric chronic peritoneal dialysis: guidelines by an ad hoc European committee. *Perit Dial Int* 2001;21(6):568–574.

Between 50 and 90% of the amino acids are absorbed without any changes in ultrafiltration compared with standard dialysate (97). Side effects include a rise in blood urea nitrogen, metabolic acidosis, anorexia, and nausea (98,99). This promising nutritional intervention is still rather expensive and should be reserved for malnourished patients who fail more conservative nutritional support.

Dietary intake of water-soluble vitamins is lower than the RDA in the majority of children on PD and supplementation results in intakes that exceed the RDA (44,100,101). *Hyperhomocysteinemia*, an independent risk factor for cardiovascular disease in adults (102), is associated with deficiencies of folate, vitamin B_6, and vitamin B_{12} (103). Elevated plasma homocysteine levels in pediatric patients on PD were significantly reduced after administration of 2.5-mg folic acid daily for 4 weeks (104). Supplementation of trace elements is reserved for specific deficiencies such as zinc (72,105).

NUTRITION AND METABOLISM OF THE ACUTELY ILL CHILD

There is no conclusive evidence that acute renal failure (ARF) per se increases energy expenditure (EE). However, ARF is often associated with other organ system failures that increase energy demands (106). Metabolic changes occurring in such situations are different from the mechanisms associated with starvation alone. The optimal intake of nutrients in children with ARF is therefore influenced more by the nature of the disease causing ARF, the extent of catabolism, and the modality and frequency of renal replacement therapy, rather than by renal dysfunction itself.

The stress response is characterized by increased catabolism with subsequent release of large amounts of glucose, amino acids, and fatty acids from the body's stores. These metabolic changes are mediated by proinflammatory cytokines such as tumor necrosis factor-α and the ILs IL-1α, IL-1β, and IL-6. These changes have consistently been viewed as adaptive or beneficial, as they may reduce and redirect energy consumption, postpone anabolism, and at the same time activate the immunologic reaction (107). However, a prolonged stress response can trigger a sustained and irreversible catabolic state mediated by release of cytokines and by activation of the hypothalamic-pituitary axis (108,109).

The mortality rate remains very high in patients with ARF, reaching between 40 and 80% in adults (110,111) and between 30 and 80% in children (112,113). In adult populations, a correlation between energy balance and survival has been established (114). Although studies suggesting that nutrition improves outcome of ARF in children have not been documented, it is reasonable to suggest that the complication rate is reduced, and recovery is enhanced by adequate nutrition.

Assessment of the general nutritional status before the acute episode becomes very important. Studies performed in adults report that a poor prior nutritional status places the patient at risk in terms of morbidity and mortality: Malnourished patients have longer hospitalizations and increased morbidity and mortality (115). Unfortunately, surveys of hospitalized pediatric patients indicate a 20 to 40% prevalence of protein-energy malnutrition (116).

There are four primary goals in managing the nutritional needs of children in ARF: maintaining adequate caloric intake, avoiding excessive protein intake to control the rise in blood urea nitrogen, minimizing potassium and phosphate intake, and reducing fluid intake (117). Enteral nutrition should be considered first, whenever possible, because it also supports maintenance of the gut barrier and may prevent bacterial invasion (106). If the patient is not able to ingest adequate intake, tube feeding can be introduced. When this is not possible, TPN becomes necessary. If the child is oligo-anuric and sufficient calories cannot be achieved while maintaining appropriate fluid balance, an earlier initiation of dialysis should be instituted.

A hypermetabolic state occurs during critical illness in adults, characterized by an EE significantly greater than that in the normal resting state (118,119). Recent studies suggest the same EE state exists in pediatric patients with critical illnesses (120). In an effort to estimate the EE in stress situations, including ARF, one needs to determine the resting EE (REE) and the 24-hour EE (24h EE) for healthy children first. There are traditionally several methods for estimating REE in children, the most commonly used being the World Health Organization and the Schofield weight and weight-height equations (121,122). Recently, a study using the enhanced metabolic testing activity chamber, a new indirect calorimetry technology, was able to propose new equations to estimate the REE and 24h EE in infants 0 to 7 months of age (123). According to this study, both the World Health Organization and the Schofield equations underestimated REE by greater than 15 kcal/kg/day. The new proposed equations were within 4% of the REE obtained by using the enhanced metabolic testing activity chamber.

Extrapolating from adult studies, the energy requirements in critically ill children might be estimated by adding a stress-related correction to the REE (124,125). A recent prospective study using indirect calorimetry on children admitted to an intensive care unit (postcardiac surgery, sepsis, systemic inflammatory response syndrome) showed that EE predicted by the specific formulas grossly overestimates the actual EE, which means that 24h EE was closer

TABLE 12.6. EQUATIONS FOR PREDICTING BASAL METABOLIC RATE AND ENERGY REQUIREMENTS

Age range (yr)	Basal metabolic rate (kcal/d)
Males	
0–3	60.9 • weight – 54
3–10	22.7 • weight + 495
10–18	17.5 • weight + 651
Females	
0–3	61.0 • weight – 51
3–10	22.5 • weight + 499
10–18	12.2 • weight + 746
Level of activity	**Activity factor**
Confined to bed	1.2
Sedentary	1.5
Normal	1.7
Athlete	2.0

Note: Energy requirement = basal metabolic rate × activity factor. Adapted from WHO. Energy and protein requirements: report of a joint FAO/WHO/UNU expert consultation. WHO Technical Report Series No. 724. Geneva: World Health Organization, 1985.

to REE than predicted by the formulas (126). Therefore, direct measurement of EE is the only means currently available for accurate determination of caloric requirements.

For practical purposes, where indirect calorimetry is not available, one must rely on one of numerous methods that attempt to predict EE and, therefore, nutritional requirements, based on age, weight, and/or height. Caloric requirements are a summation of basal metabolic needs, activity, and growth (Table 12.6). In healthy children, REE accounts for approximately 50% of total EE, whereas activity and growth account for the remaining 50% of total EE (127). To predict energy requirements for critically ill children, one must first determine basal energy requirements and adjust for hypermetabolism (128) (Table 12.7).

Patients with ARF have high protein catabolic rates. Several studies done in adult populations reported between 1.4 and 1.8 g/kg/day protein catabolic rates (129,114). Another parameter that is used to measure the protein catabolic state, urea nitrogen appearance (UNA), has been found to be significantly elevated in children with ARF, with levels more than 180 mg/kg/day (130). A recent study of critically ill children demonstrated that protein turnover but not lipolysis correlated with the severity of the critically ill condition (131).

In addition to the catabolic effect of the illness, there are amino acid losses through dialysate solutions. Although the amino acid losses in conventional HD and PD were discussed earlier, it is worthwhile discussing the case of continuous renal replacement therapy–related amino acid losses. Amino acid clearances and calculated losses in adults on continuous venovenous hemofiltration have been reported between 2 and 11% of the dietary intake, whereas studies done for continuous venovenous HD found 8 to 22% dietary loss (132,133). The ultrafiltrate volumes, as well as blood flow rates, have varied widely between these individ-

TABLE 12.7. METHOD TO PREDICT METABOLIC RATES DURING CRITICAL ILLNESS

Average hospital energy requirements		Increases in energy with stress	
Body weight (kg)	kcal/kg/day		
0–10	100	Fever	12% per degree Celsius >37°C
10–20	1000 + 50/kg	Cardiac failure	15–25%
>20	1500 + 20/kg	Major surgery	20–30%
		Burns	Up to 100%
		Severe sepsis	40–50%

Adapted from Holliday MA, Segar WE. The maintenance need for water in parenteral fluid therapy. *Pediatrics* 1957;19:823–832; and Wesley JR, et al., eds. *Parenteral and enteral nutrition manual.* Chicago: Abbot Laboratories, 1980:17.

ual studies, making direct comparison among the treatments difficult. The only study performed in children reported amino acid losses of 11 to 12% of dietary intake. The patients had similar blood and dialysate/prefiltered replacement fluid flow rates, and there were equivalent amino acid losses and urea clearances with no significant difference in regard to modality, continuous venovenous hemofiltration, or continuous venovenous HD (134). A negative nitrogen balance occurred in those children despite the delivery of standard TPN containing 1.5 g/kg/day of proteins and caloric intake of 20 to 30% above REE.

It is possible to estimate the protein requirements by measuring the protein equivalent of total nitrogen appearance (PNA), which is an estimate of the protein losses (135). When the patient is in nitrogen balance, PNA should be equal to the protein intake. The PNA can be derived from the UNA by using the Bergström formula:

$$\text{PNA [g/day]} = 20.1 + 7.5 \text{ UNA [g/day]}$$

The UNA results from measuring the urea nitrogen content of all measurable outputs (urine, dialysate or ultrafiltrate, fistula drainage) plus the change in body urea nitrogen:

$$\text{UNA [g/day]} = \text{output urea nitrogen} + \text{change in body urea nitrogen}$$

Where change in body urea nitrogen [g/day] is given by:

$$(\text{SUN}_f - \text{SUN}_i)[\text{g/L/day}] \times \text{BW}_i[\text{kg}] \times 0.6[\text{L/kg}] + (\text{BW}_f - \text{BW}_i)[\text{kg/day}] \times \text{SUN}_f[\text{g/L}] \times (1 \text{ L/kg})$$

where i and f are the pre- and postdialysis moments in time, SUN is serum urea nitrogen, BW is the body weight, 0.6 is an estimate of the total body water and 1 L/kg is the volume of distribution of urea in the weight that is gained or lost.

The PNA is normalized to body weight to obtain the nPNA, which is expressed as g/kg/day.

In addition to the previously described particularities of ARF in regard to the energy intake and protein metabolism, such children also need daily intake of lipids, minerals, and vitamins, according to the normal daily requirements for age.

NUTRITIONAL AND METABOLIC CHANGES AFTER RENAL TRANSPLANTATION

Metabolic disorders post–renal transplantation result from a complex interaction of factors such as genetic susceptibility; medications; and physiologic changes related to ischemic, immunologic, vascular, and mechanical injury. Although other chapters discuss the electrolyte imbalances that frequently occur after renal transplantation, this subchapter focuses on common derangements pertinent to lipid and carbohydrate metabolism.

Posttransplant Hyperlipidemia

Hyperlipidemia is a risk factor for cardiovascular disease in adult transplant patients (136–139) and may also cause chronic allograft nephropathy (140), whereas no data exist in the pediatric transplant population.

The prevalence of hyperlipidemia is highest immediately posttransplant, declining to 30% after 5 years (139). A longitudinal evaluation of pediatric renal transplant recipients showed that the prevalence of elevated TC and TG declined from 70 to 35% and 46 to 15%, respectively, between 1 and 10 years posttransplant, most likely as the doses of immunosuppressive agents were decreased (141).

Causes of post–renal transplant hyperlipidemia include preexisting hyperlipidemia, especially with a familial history; medications (immunosuppressives, diuretics, and beta blockers); graft dysfunction; older age; male gender; obesity; and hypoalbuminemia secondary to nephrotic syndrome (142). Risk factors for high TC in transplanted children on cyclosporine A (CsA) include preexisting hyperlipidemia plus a family history and, unlike the adult studies, worsen with time (143). In the same study, elevated TG was associated with reduced GFR.

The specific lipid profile abnormalities posttransplant include increased TC, LDL, VLDL, and apolipoprotein B levels. HDL levels can be low, normal, or slightly elevated.

The chronic use of immunosuppressive medications is an important determinant of hyperlipidemia in posttransplant children. The most commonly used medications, corticosteroids and CsA, were clearly reported to produce hyperlipidemia. Tacrolimus seems to have a less prominent effect, whereas sirolimus has a more pronounced effect.

Corticosteroids were shown to be associated with increased TC and TG levels (144). They enhance lipogenesis by increasing the activity of acetyl–coenzyme A carboxylase and free fatty acid synthetase, thus increasing hepatic synthesis of VLDL, downregulating LDL receptor activity, and increasing the activity of 3-hydroxy-3-methylglutaryl coenzyme A reductase. Concurrently, they induce insulin resistance resulting in decreased activity of LPL, thus raising TG. Finally, the corticosteroid-induced decrease in adrenocorticotropic hormone release may contribute to the lipid abnormalities, because adrenocorticotropic hormone upregulates LDL receptor activity (142). Withdrawal of steroids posttransplantation significantly reduces TC and LDL levels (145). However, there is a simultaneous decrease in HDL levels, which may decrease the HDL:cholesterol ratio. Replacement of low-dose oral methylprednisone with deflazacort resulted in decreased TC and LDL and increased HDL in pediatric patients (146).

CsA is associated with increased TC and increased LDL, whereas HDL and TGs are not strongly affected (147). CsA is highly lipophilic, and up to 80% is transported in the blood mostly in the core of LDL particles (148). Its hyperlipidemic effect is due to several known mechanisms. It binds to the LDL receptor and raises LDL levels (149). In addition, CsA increases hepatic lipase activity and decreases LPL activity, resulting in impaired clearance of VLDL and LDL (142). On the other hand, like the corticosteroids, part of the hyperlipidemic effect seems to be secondary to the insulin resistance. Tacrolimus has an effect on lipid metabolism similar to that of CsA, but it seems to be less prominent (150,151). Sirolimus is associated mainly with high TG and, to a lesser extent, elevated TC. The mechanisms of sirolimus-induced hyperlipidemia have not been completely elucidated, and the effect is dose dependent and reversible (152).

Lipid-lowering agents, such as fluvastatin, are effective in adult transplant recipients (153–155). A prospective 12-week intensive dietary intervention study (American Heart Association step 2 diet) was effective in reducing hyperlipidemia in postrenal transplant children (156). Among pediatric cardiac transplant recipients, pravastatin was effective and well tolerated (157), whereas atorvastatin also effectively lowered lipids but was associated with rhabdomyolysis and asymptomatic creatine kinase elevation (158).

Posttransplant Glucose Intolerance

Hyperglycemia and posttransplant diabetes mellitus (PTDM) are well-known complications of organ transplantation, which worsen graft outcome and increase patient mortality. PTDM in adult liver transplant recipients results in an increase in the number of rejection episodes in the first posttransplant year and an increase in mortality in the second year (159). PTDM in adult post–renal transplant patients worsened mortality (160).

The incidence of PTDM in adult kidney transplant recipients ranges from 4 to 41% (161,162). The very wide range may be due to the lack of a standard definition of PTDM, as some patients have transient hyperglycemia after transplant, and other patients have persistent DM. In pediatric populations, the prevalence of PTDM parallels that of type 2 DM (163,164). A comprehensive study of pediatric renal transplant recipients reported a 7% prevalence of PTDM (serum glucose >200 mg/dL) (165).

In adults with PTDM, risk factors include the type of immunosuppressive regimen, ethnicity, age, BMI, family history of DM, episodes of rejection, and HLA type (166,167). PTDM in pediatric renal recipients occurred within 1.2 years posttransplant (range, 1 day to 6.2 years), especially with a family history of type 2 DM, tacrolimus use versus CsA (odds ratio, 9.1), and hyperglycemia in the immediate posttransplant period (165).

Corticosteroids increase insulin resistance in peripheral tissues by decreasing insulin receptor number and function, increasing hepatic glucose output, decreasing glucose uptake in muscle, and increasing lipolysis and free fatty acid release from adipose tissue (161). In addition, corticosteroids may inhibit insulin secretion by the pancreatic beta cells (168).

Tacrolimus has been clearly associated with PTDM in children (169). It may affect beta-cell function and peripheral insulin resistance and diminishes insulin secretion (170,171). Tacrolimus reversibly suppressed insulin gene transcription in normal rats (172). Furthermore, tacrolimus damages beta cells directly and possibly irreversibly (173). Beta-cell antibodies were transiently found in the setting of PTDM during tacrolimus use (174). Thus, in patients with a strong family history of type 2 DM or hyperglycemia in the immediate posttransplantation period, tacrolimus should be used cautiously (165). CsA also inhibits insulin secretion from beta cells and decreases glucose disposal by similar mechanisms.

INFLUENCES OF NUTRITION DISORDERS ON RENAL FUNCTION

Influences of Obesity on Renal Function

Obesity was found to be an important risk factor for a certain number of diseases, including cardiovascular diseases, hypertension, lipid and lipoprotein abnormalities, type 2 DM, nonalcoholic steato-hepatitis, pseudotumor cerebri, obstructive sleep apnea, and orthopedic problems such as Blount disease (175–177).

It is a problem of major concern that the prevalence and severity of obesity is increasing in the pediatric population. As a consequence, the prevalence of the sequelae of obesity is expected to be increasing as well. The last large investigation done by the National Health and Nutrition Examination Survey (NHANES III) reported a prevalence of childhood obesity of 25% in the United States, defined by a BMI of more than 95% for age and gender (178). This prevalence represented a 30% increase comparative to a previous similar investigation, NHANES II. The same trend has been observed in Western Europe in the past 30 years.

The association of obesity with proteinuria has been well described in adults (179–181). Despite the prevalence of childhood obesity, an association between obesity and renal abnormalities such as proteinuria has not been clearly reported until very recently (182). Obesity-associated proteinuria in adults is associated with focal segmental glomerulosclerosis (FSGS). However, the FSGS diagnosed in these patients shares clinical features distinctive from those usually seen with primary FSGS: Albumin levels tend to be higher, often above 3 g/dL; TC levels are only mildly elevated, often <300 mg/dL; proteinuria is moderate; blood pressure tends to be normal or only mildly elevated; and edema may be minimal to absent (183). Patients who lost weight successfully showed marked decreases in proteinuria. Histologic features of obesity-associated proteinuria in adults include focal segmental sclerotic changes often in a hilar location, mesangial proliferation and hypertrophy, foci of hyalinosis, and glomerulomegaly (184,185). In obesity-associated FSGS, on electron microscopy, the foot process fusion is often minimal and focal rather than diffuse, as opposed to idiopathic FSGS.

FSGS is the histologic expression of a variety of conditions that differ in cause, pathogenesis, clinical course, and response to therapy (186–189). Although the pathophysiology of obesity-related FSGS is unclear, potential etiologic factors seem to be hyperfiltration, hyperlipidemia, renal venous hypertension, and glomerular hypertrophy.

Based on the above clinical and pathologic characteristics, the patients with obesity-related FSGS seem to share features with a very diverse group of patients whose initiating factor is a reduction in renal mass. The reduction in renal mass can be due to reflux nephropathy (190), nephrectomy for Wilms' tumor (191), unilateral renal agenesis (192), or unilateral nephrectomy (193). These reduced numbers of glomeruli may be subjected to hemodynamic stress by taking on the filtration of a constant volume of plasma. This sets up a cascade of proteinuria, mesangial cell gene expression, and focal scarring. Similarly, in case of obesity, there is increased plasma volume and cardiac output that translates into a relative deficit in the number of glomeruli (194). In addition, obesity is associated with hypertension. Significant weight gain is accompanied by excess renal sodium resorption, leading to increased systemic arterial pressure and glomerular hyperfiltration (195). These changes result in glomerular capillary wall stress, leading to glomerular cell proliferation, matrix accumulation, and glomerular sclerosis.

Hyperlipidemia is another potential contributing factor, because the Zucker obese rat, a model in which FSGS develops, is hyperlipidemic, and reduction in serum lipids appears to decrease or prevent development of FSGS (196). A study of autopsies in obese adults noted that those with FSGS had higher lipid levels and showed lipid deposits in renal tubular epithelial cells (185).

Renal venous hypertension has been incriminated as another contributing factor to obesity-related FSGS. One study demonstrated that adult obese patients had increased plasma volume and increased right atrial pressure, which decreased with weight reduction along with parallel decreases in urinary protein losses (179). Other conditions also associated with increased right atrial pressure and presumed renal venous hypertension, such as tricuspid atresia, constrictive pericarditis, and pulmonary hypertension, have been associated with proteinuria and nephrotic syndrome (197,198).

The glomerular hypertrophy theory postulated a sequence of changes that may occur in the genesis of obesity-related FSGS from glomerular hypertrophy, stimulated in part by angiotensin II and other growth factors, leading to production of excess amounts of extracellular matrix in mesangial areas and the development of obesity-related FSGS (199).

Very recent studies showed the connection between adipose tissue and kidney at molecular level mediated by leptin, a small peptide mainly produced in adipose tissue, therefore directly reflecting the amount of body fat. In glomerular endothelial cells, leptin stimulates cellular proliferation, transforming growth factor β_1 (TGF-β_1) synthesis, and type IV collagen production. Conversely, in mesangial cells, leptin upregulates synthesis of the TGFβ type II receptor but not TGF-β_1 and stimulates glucose transport and type I collagen production through signal transduction pathways involving phosphatidylinositol-3-kinase. These data suggest that leptin triggers a paracrine interaction in which glomerular endothelial cells secrete TGF-β, to which sensitized mesangial cells may respond. Both cell types increase their expression of extracellular matrix in response to leptin. Infusion of leptin into normal rats produces the development of FSGS and proteinuria (200).

An association between obesity and renal abnormalities, such as proteinuria, has not been reported until very recently. In one study, seven obese black adolescent patients had FSGS and significant proteinuria but no edema; serum albumin levels were slightly low and TC was normal or mildly elevated. The histologic features included glomerular hypertrophy, FSGS, increased mesangial matrix and cellularity, relative preservation of foot process morphology, and absence of evidence of inflammatory or immune-mediated processes (182). These clinical and histologic characteristics resemble the descriptions of obesity-related FSGS found in the adult studies. Obesity-related FSGS may lead to ESRD (182). Children with FSGS in hilar areas, as commonly seen in obesity-associated FSGS, have a much higher likelihood of developing CKD than patients with peripherally located focal segmental lesions (201).

There is clearly a predisposition of the black children to develop obesity-related FSGS (182). Idiopathic primary FSGS is also much more common in adult black individuals (202). Epidemiologic data also suggest that there is a racial genetic component to susceptibility to renal injury as a complication of both type 2 DM and chronic hypertension in blacks compared with whites (203,204).

The treatment of obesity-related FSGS should include weight reduction. Obese Zucker rats showed a reduction in FSGS lesions with reduced dietary intake and subsequent reduced weight (196). Several studies reported that extensive reduction of body weight without use of any therapy markedly reduced or eliminated proteinuria in obese adult patients (205). In the pediatric study, one patient showed a dramatic reduction in proteinuria in response to weight reduction (182). The other treatment modality is the use of angiotensin-converting enzyme inhibitors. One study done in obese adults reported that patients with proteinuria who were given captopril had reductions in proteinuria similar to those seen with weight reduction alone. It is not clear whether the action of angiotensin-converting enzyme inhibitors in such cases is related to hemodynamic changes in efferent arteriolar resistance or to nonhemodynamic factors (205). In the pediatric study, three out of seven patients with obesity-related FSGS who were given angiotensin-converting enzyme inhibitors had significant reduction of proteinuria (182).

Influences of Malnutrition on Renal Function

Extensive data already showed in the sixties and seventies that renal development is influenced by many factors, including nutrition. Maternal diet may influence nephrogenesis, with the result that individuals whose mothers have low protein intake during gestation may have a relatively lower total number of nephrons at birth (206,207). After birth, the nutritional intake of an infant is a major stimulus to both renal growth and functional maturation. In early infancy, protein and amino acid intake can influence renal growth. GFR increases more rapidly in premature infants receiving a relatively high-protein diet than in those who do not (208). However, a high-protein diet has been reported to be associated with metabolic acidosis, failure to thrive, and even evidence of renal injury (209).

Later in life, renal function alterations are similar with diverse forms of malnutrition such as primary protein-calorie malnutrition, iatrogenic malnutrition, or anorexia nervosa. These changes include decrease in GFR, decrease in renal plasma flow, poor urinary concentrating ability, decreased ability to excrete sodium, and impaired acid excretion. In cases of malnutrition, GFR can be as low as 50%. A low-calorie diet and also a low-protein diet can independently produce a fall in GFR or renal plasma flow (210). These changes are usually reversible, not associated by renal structural damage, and are not explained by hypoproteinemia or edema, which can occur in these states (211).

REFERENCES

1. Foreman JW, et al. Nutritional intake in children with renal insufficiency: a report of the growth failure in children with renal diseases study. *J Am Coll Nutr* 1996;15(6):579–585.
2. Ellis EN, et al. The impact of supplemental feeding in young children on dialysis: a report of the North American Pediatric Renal Transplant Cooperative Study. *Pediatr Nephrol* 2001;16(5):404–408.
3. Alvestrand A. Carbohydrate and insulin metabolism in renal failure. *Kidney Int* 1997;62(Suppl):S48–S52.
4. Rasic-Milutinovic Z, Perunicic-Pekovic G. [Clinical importance and pathogenic mechanisms of insulin resistance in chronic renal insufficiency (part I): insulin resistance in patients with chronic renal insufficiency]. *Med Pregl* 2000; 53(1–2):45–50.
5. Rasic-Milutinovic Z, Perunicic-Pekovic G, Pljesa S. [Clinical significance and pathogenic mechanisms of insulin resistance in chronic renal insufficiency (part II): pathogenic factors of insulin resistance in chronic renal insufficiency]. *Med Pregl* 2000;53(3–4):159–163.
6. Mak RH. Effect of metabolic acidosis on insulin action and secretion in uremia. *Kidney Int* 1998;54(2):603–607.
7. Lim VS, Kopple J. Protein metabolism in patients with chronic renal failure: role of uremia and dialysis. *Kidney Int* 2000;58:1–10.
8. Mitch WE. Insights into the abnormalities of chronic renal disease attributed to malnutrition. *J Am Soc Nephrol* 2002; 13(Suppl 1):S22–S27.
9. Mitch WE, Goldberg A. Mechanisms of muscle wasting: the role of the ubiquitin-proteasome system. *N Engl J Med* 1996;335:1897–1905.
10. Mitch WE, Bailey J, Wang X, et al. Evaluation of signals activating ubiquitin-proteasome proteolysis in a model of muscle wasting. *Am J Physiol* 1999;276:C1132–C1138.
11. Bailey JL, Wang X, England BK, et al. The acidosis of chronic renal failure activates muscle proteolysis in rats by augmenting transcription of genes encoding proteins of the ATP-dependent, ubiquitin-proteasome pathway. *J Clin Invest* 1996;97:1447–1453.
12. Kaysen G. Biological basis of hypoalbuminemia in ESRD. *J Am Soc Nephrol* 1998;9:2368–2376.
13. Boirie Y, Broyer M, Gagnadoux MF, et al. Alterations of protein metabolism by metabolic acidosis in children with chronic renal failure. *Kidney Int* 2000;58:236–241.
14. Brungger M, Hulter H, Krapf R. Effect of chronic metabolic acidosis on the growth hormone/IGF-1 endocrine axis: new cause of growth hormone insensitivity in humans. *Kidney Int* 1997;51:216–221.
15. Brungger M, Hulter H. Krapf R. Effect of chronic metabolic acidosis on thyroid hormone homeostasis in humans. *Am J Physiol* 1997;272:F648–F653.

16. Krapf R, Vetsch R, Vetsch W, et al. Chronic metabolic acidosis increases the serum concentration of 1,25-dihydroxyvitamin D in humans by stimulating its production rate. *J Clin Invest* 1992;90:2456–2463.
17. Bergstrom J, Lindholm B, Lacson E Jr, et al. What are the causes and consequences of the chronic inflammation in chronic hemodialysis patients? *Semin Dialysis* 2000;13:163–176.
18. Qureshi AR, Alvestrand A, Danielsson A, et al. Factors predicting malnutrition in hemodialysis patients: a cross-sectional study. *Kidney Int* 1998;53:773–782.
19. Price SR, Bailey J, Wang X, et al. Muscle wasting in insulinopenic rats results from activation of the ATP-dependent, ubiquitin-proteasome pathway by a mechanism including gene transcription. *J Clin Invest* 1996;98:1703–1708.
20. Fried LF, Orchard TJ, Kasiske BL. Effect of lipid reduction on the progression of renal disease: a meta-analysis. *Kidney Int* 2001;59(1):260–269.
21. Attman PO, Alaupovic P. Lipid abnormalities in chronic renal insufficiency. *Kidney Int* 1991;31(Suppl):S16–S23.
22. Nishizawa Y, Shoji T, Ishimura E, et al. Paradox of risk factors for cardiovascular mortality in uremia: is a higher cholesterol level better for atherosclerosis in uremia? *Am J Kidney Dis* 2001;38(4 Suppl 1):S4–S7.
23. Oi K, et al. Role of hepatic lipase in intermediate-density lipoprotein and small, dense low-density lipoprotein formation in hemodialysis patients. *Kidney Int* 1999;71(Suppl):S227–S228.
24. Howard BV. Insulin resistance and lipid metabolism. *Am J Cardiol* 1999;84(1A):28J–32J.
25. Powell DR, et al. Insulin-like growth factor binding proteins as growth inhibitors in children with chronic renal failure. *Pediatr Nephrol* 1996;10(3):343–347.
26. Tonshoff B, et al. Serum insulin-like growth factors (IGFs) and IGF binding proteins 1, 2, and 3 in children with chronic renal failure: relationship to height and glomerular filtration rate. The European Study Group for Nutritional Treatment of Chronic Renal Failure in Childhood. *J Clin Endocrinol Metab* 1995;80(9):2684–2691.
27. Tonshoff B, Blum WF, Mehls O. Serum insulin-like growth factors and their binding proteins in children with end-stage renal disease. *Pediatr Nephrol* 1996;10(3):269–274.
28. Powell DR, et al. Insulin-like growth factor-binding protein-6 levels are elevated in serum of children with chronic renal failure: a report of the Southwest Pediatric Nephrology Study Group. *J Clin Endocrinol Metab* 1997;82(9):2978–2984.
29. Ulinski T, et al. Serum insulin-like growth factor binding protein (IGFBP)-4 and IGFBP-5 in children with chronic renal failure: relationship to growth and glomerular filtration rate. The European Study Group for Nutritional Treatment of Chronic Renal Failure in Childhood. German Study Group for Growth Hormone Treatment in Chronic Renal Failure. *Pediatr Nephrol* 2000;14(7):589–597.
30. Tonshoff B, et al. Decreased hepatic insulin-like growth factor (IGF)-I and increased IGF binding protein-1 and -2 gene expression in experimental uremia. *Endocrinology* 1997;138 (3):938–946.
31. Jikko A, et al. Effects of cyclic adenosine 3',5'-monophosphate on chondrocyte terminal differentiation and cartilage-matrix calcification. *Endocrinology* 1996;137(1):122–128.
32. Urena P, et al. PTH/PTHrP receptor mRNA is down-regulated in epiphyseal cartilage growth plate of uraemic rats. *Nephrol Dial Transplant* 1996;11(10):2008–2016.
33. Sanchez CP, Salusky I, Kuizon BD, et al. Growth of long bones in renal failure: Roles of hyperparathyroidism, growth hormone and calcitriol. *Kidney Int* 1998;54:1879–1887.
34. Kuizon BD, Goodman W, Juppner H, et al. Diminished linear growth during intermittent calcitriol therapy in children undergoing CCPD. *Kidney Int* 1998;53:205–211.
35. Maniar S, Caldas A, Laouari D, et al. Severity of chronic metabolic acidosis and growth of rats with chronic uremia. *Miner Electrolyte Metab* 1992;18:241–244.
36. Green J, Maor G. Effect of metabolic acidosis on the growth hormone/IGF-I endocrine axis in skeletal growth centers. *Kidney Int* 2000;57(6):2258–2267.
37. Bushinsky DA. Stimulated osteoclastic and suppressed osteoblastic activity in metabolic but not respiratory acidosis. *Am J Physiol* 1995;268(1 Pt 1):C80–C88.
38. Norman LJ, et al. Nutrition and growth in relation to severity of renal disease in children. *Pediatr Nephrol* 2000;15(3–4):259–265.
39. Nelson P, Stover J. Nutrition recommendations for infants, children and adolescents with end-stage renal disease. In: Gillit D, Stover J, eds. *A clinical guide to nutrition care in end-stage renal disease*. Chicago, IL: American Dietetic Association, 1994:79–97.
40. Borradori Tolsa C, Kuizon BD, Salusky IB. [Children with chronic renal failure: evaluation of the nutritional status and management]. *Arch Pediatr* 1999;6(10):1092–1100.
41. Warady BA, et al. Optimal care of the pediatric end-stage renal disease patient on dialysis. *Am J Kidney Dis* 1999;33 (3):567–583.
42. National Kidney Foundation. Clinical practice guidelines for nutrition in chronic renal failure. II. Pediatric guidelines. *Am J Kidney Dis* 2000;35(Suppl 2):S105–S136.
43. Goldstein-Fuchs D. Assessment of nutritional status in renal diseases. In: Mitch WE, Klahr S, eds. *Handbook of nutrition and the kidney*, 4th ed. Philadelphia: Lippincott Williams & Wilkins, 2002:42–92.
44. Filler G. The DOQI pediatric nutritional guidelines—critical remarks. *Perit Dial Int* 2001;21(Suppl 3):S192–S194.
45. Schaefer F, et al. Assessment of body composition in children with chronic renal failure. *Pediatr Nephrol* 2000;14(7):673–678.
46. Johnson VL, et al. Changes in body composition of children with chronic renal failure on growth hormone. *Pediatr Nephrol* 2000;14(7):695–700.
47. Swinford RD, Ingelfinger JR. Persistent renal disease. In: Walker WA, Watkins J, eds. *Nutrition in pediatrics*. Hamilton, Ontario: B.C. Decker 1997:504.
48. Hakim RM, Levin N. Malnutrition in hemodialysis patients. *Am J Kidney Dis* 1993;21(2):125–137.
49. Stefanovic V, Stojanovic M, Djordjevic V. Effect of adequacy of dialysis and nutrition on morbidity and working rehabilitation of patients treated by maintenance hemodialysis. *Int J Artif Organs* 2000;23(2):83–89.
50. Goldstein DJ, Callahan C. Strategies for nutritional intervention in patients with renal failure. *Miner Electrolyte Metab* 1998;24(1):82–91.

51. Wong CS, et al. Hypoalbuminemia and risk of death in pediatric patients with end-stage renal disease. *Kidney Int* 2002;61(2):630–637.
52. Brem AS, et al. Outcome data on pediatric dialysis patients from the end-stage renal disease clinical indicators project. *Am J Kidney Dis* 2000;36(2):310–317.
53. Tom A, et al. Growth during maintenance hemodialysis: impact of enhanced nutrition and clearance. *J Pediatr* 1999; 134(4):464–471.
53a. K-DOQI. Nutrition in chronic renal failure. *Am J Kidney Dis* 2000;35:S112–115.
54. Ikizler TA, Hakim RM. Nutrition in end-stage renal disease. *Kidney Int* 1996;50(2):343–357.
55. Brewer ED. Pediatric experience with intradialytic parenteral nutrition and supplemental tube feeding. *Am J Kidney Dis* 1999;33(1):205–207.
56. Claris-Appiani A, Ardissino GL, Dacco V, et al. Catch-up growth in children with chronic renal failure treated with long-term enteral nutrition. *JPEN J Parenter Enteral Nutr* 1995;19(3):175–178.
57. Reed EE, et al. Nutritional intervention and growth in children with chronic renal failure. *J Ren Nutr* 1998;8(3):122–126.
58. Shuler CL. Malnutrition and intradialytic parenteral nutrition in end-stage renal disease patients. In: Heinrich WL, ed. *Principles and practice of dialysis*, 2nd ed. Philadelphia: Lippincott Williams & Wilkins, 1999:381–382.
59. Chertow GM, et al. The association of intradialytic parenteral nutrition administration with survival in hemodialysis patients. *Am J Kidney Dis* 1994;24(6):912–920.
60. Capelli JP, et al. Effect of intradialytic parenteral nutrition on mortality rates in end-stage renal disease care. *Am J Kidney Dis* 1994;23(6):808–816.
61. Lazarus JM. Recommended criteria for initiating and discontinuing intradialytic parenteral nutrition therapy. *Am J Kidney Dis* 1999;33(1):211–216.
62. Siskind MS, Lien YH. Effect of intradialytic parenteral nutrition on quality of life in hemodialysis patients. *Int J Artif Organs* 1993;16(8):599–603.
63. Krause I, et al. Intradialytic parenteral nutrition in malnourished children treated with hemodialysis. *J Ren Nutr* 2002;12(1):55–59.
64. Bakaev VV, Efremov AV. [The excretion of ascorbic acid and its metabolites in uremia and hemodialysis]. *Patol Fiziol Eksp Ter* 2000;(2):22–24.
65. Malinow MR, NF, Kruger WD, et al. The effects of folic acid supplementation on plasma total homocysteine are modulated by multivitamin use and methylenetetrahydrofolate reductase genotypes. *Arterioscler Thromb Vasc Biol* 1997;17:1157–1162.
66. Maroni BJ, Mitch WE. Nutritional therapy in renal failure. In: Giebisch G. Seldin DW, eds. *The kidney: physiology and pathophysiology*, vol. 2, 3rd ed. Philadelphia: Lippincott Williams & Wilkins, 2000:2759–2788.
67. Gilmour ER, Hartley GH, Goodship THJ. Trace elements and vitamins in renal disease. In: Klahr S, Mitch WE, eds. *Nutrition and the kidney*. Philadelphia: Lippincott–Raven, 1998:107–122.
68. Krachler M, Wirnsberger GH. Long-term changes of plasma trace element concentrations in chronic hemodialysis patients. *Blood Purif* 2000;18(2):138–143.
69. Zima T, et al. Trace elements in end-stage renal disease. 1. Methodological aspects and the influence of water treatment and dialysis equipment. *Blood Purif* 1999;17(4):182–186.
70. Zima T, et al. Trace elements in end-stage renal disease. 2. Clinical implication of trace elements. *Blood Purif* 1999;17(4):187–198.
71. Gallieni M, et al. Trace elements in renal failure: are they clinically important? *Nephrol Dial Transplant* 1996;11(7):1232–1235.
72. Secker D, Pencharz P. Nutritional therapy for children on CAPD/CCPD: theory and practice. In: Fine RN, Alexander S, Warady BA, eds. *CAPD/CCPD in children*. Boston: Kluwer Academic, 1998:567–603.
73. Quan A, Baum M. Protein losses in children on continuous cycler peritoneal dialysis. *Pediatr Nephrol* 1996;10(6):728–731.
74. Canepa A, et al. Nutritional status in children receiving chronic peritoneal dialysis. *Perit Dial Int* 1996;16(Suppl 1):S526–S531.
75. Canepa A, et al. Protein and calorie intake, nitrogen losses, and nitrogen balance in children undergoing chronic peritoneal dialysis. *Adv Perit Dial* 1996;12:326–329.
76. Adequacy of dialysis and nutrition in continuous peritoneal dialysis: association with clinical outcomes. Canada-USA (CANUSA) Peritoneal Dialysis Study Group. *J Am Soc Nephrol* 1996;7(2):198–207.
77. Dabbagh S, et al. The effect of aggressive nutrition on infection rates in patients maintained on peritoneal dialysis. *Adv Perit Dial* 1991;7:161–164.
78. NIDDK/DKUHD, NIH. Excerpts from the United States Renal Data System's 2000 Annual Report: atlas of end-stage renal disease in the United States. *Am J Kidney Dis* 2000;36 (Suppl 2):S97–S114.
79. Katz A, Bock GH, Mauer M. Improved growth velocity with intensive dialysis. Consequence or coincidence? *Pediatr Nephrol* 2000;14(8–9):710–712.
80. Holtta T, et al. Clinical outcome of pediatric patients on peritoneal dialysis under adequacy control. *Pediatr Nephrol* 2000;14(10–11):889–897.
81. Chadha V, Blowey DL, Warady BA. Is growth a valid outcome measure of dialysis clearance in children undergoing peritoneal dialysis? *Perit Dial Int* 2001;21(Suppl 3):S179–S184.
82. Schaefer F, et al. Higher KT/V urea associated with greater protein catabolic rate and dietary protein intake in children treated with CCPD compared to CAPD. Mid-European Pediatric CPD Study Group (MPCS). *Adv Perit Dial* 1994;10:310–314.
83. Schaefer F, Klaus G, Mehls O. Peritoneal transport properties and dialysis dose affect growth and nutritional status in children on chronic peritoneal dialysis. Mid-European Pediatric Peritoneal Dialysis Study Group. *J Am Soc Nephrol* 1999;10(8):1786–1792.
84. Harty J, Gokal R. Nutritional status in peritoneal dialysis. *J Ren Nutr* 1995;5(1):2–10.
85. Wolk R. Micronutrition in dialysis. *Nutr Clin Pract* 1993; 8(6):267–276.
86. Wolfson M. Nutritional management of the continuous ambulatory peritoneal dialysis patient. *Am J Kidney Dis* 1996;27(5):744–749.
87. Grodstein GP, et al. Glucose absorption during continuous ambulatory peritoneal dialysis. *Kidney Int* 1981;19(4):564–567.
88. Kleinman R, Committee on Nutrition. *Pediatric nutrition handbook*, 4th ed. Elk Grove Village, IL: American Academy of Pediatrics, 1998:489.

89. Ramage IJ, et al. Efficacy of gastrostomy feeding in infants and older children receiving chronic peritoneal dialysis. *Perit Dial Int* 1999;19(3):231–236.
90. Warady BA, Weis L, Johnson L. Nasogastric tube feeding in infants on peritoneal dialysis. *Perit Dial Int* 1996;16(Suppl 1):S521–525.
91. Coleman JE, Norman LJ, Watson AR. Provision of dietetic care in children on chronic peritoneal dialysis. *J Ren Nutr* 1999;9(3):145–148.
92. Edefonti A, et al. Dietary prescription based on estimated nitrogen balance during peritoneal dialysis. *Pediatr Nephrol* 1999;13(3):253–258.
93. Kopple JD, et al. Treatment of malnourished CAPD patients with an amino acid based dialysate. *Kidney Int* 1995;47(4):1148–1157.
94. Qamar IU, et al. Effects of 3-month amino acid dialysis compared to dextrose dialysis in children on continuous ambulatory peritoneal dialysis. *Perit Dial Int* 1994;14(1): 34–41.
95. Qamar IU, et al. Effects of amino acid dialysis compared to dextrose dialysis in children on continuous cycling peritoneal dialysis. *Perit Dial Int* 1999;19(3):237–247.
96. Schroder CH. The choice of dialysis solutions in pediatric chronic peritoneal dialysis: guidelines by an ad hoc European committee. *Perit Dial Int* 2001;21(6):568–574.
97. Balfe JW. Intraperitoneal amino acids in children receiving chronic peritoneal dialysis. *Perit Dial Int* 1996;16(Suppl 1):S515–S516.
98. Canepa A, et al. Value of intraperitoneal amino acids in children treated with chronic peritoneal dialysis. *Perit Dial Int* 1999;19(Suppl 2):S435–S440.
99. Canepa A, et al. Acute effects of simultaneous intraperitoneal infusion of glucose and amino acids. *Kidney Int* 2001;59(5):1967–1973.
100. Pereira AM, et al. Oral vitamin intake in children receiving long-term dialysis. *J Ren Nutr* 2000;10(1):24–29.
101. Warady BA, et al. Vitamin status of infants receiving long-term peritoneal dialysis. *Pediatr Nephrol* 1994;8(3):354–356.
102. Dennis VW, Robinson K. Homocysteinemia and vascular disease in end-stage renal disease. *Kidney Int Suppl* 1996;57: S11–S17.
103. Dierkes J, et al. Homocysteine lowering effect of different multivitamin preparations in patients with end-stage renal disease. *J Ren Nutr* 2001;11(2):67–72.
104. Schroder CH, et al. Treatment of hyperhomocysteinemia in children on dialysis by folic acid. *Pediatr Nephrol* 1999;13 (7):583–585.
105. Coleman JE, Watson AR. Micronutrient supplementation in children on continuous cycling peritoneal dialysis (CCPD). *Adv Perit Dial* 1992;8:396–401.
106. Rosenblum ND, Balfe JW. Nutrition and metabolism. In: Barratt TM, Avner ED, Harmon WE, eds. *Pediatric nephrology*, 4th ed. Baltimore: Lippincott Williams & Wilkins, 1999:117–132.
107. Baumann H, Gauldie J. The acute phase response. *Immunol Today* 1994;15(2):74–80.
108. Chrousos GP. The hypothalamic-pituitary-adrenal axis and immune-mediated inflammation. *N Engl J Med* 1995;332 (20):1351–1362.
109. Van den Berghe G, de Zegher F, Bouillon R. Acute and prolonged critical illness as different neuroendocrine paradigms. *Crit Care Med* 1998;83:1827–1834.
110. Himmelfarb J. Dialytic therapy in acute renal failure: no reason for nihilism. *Semin Dial* 1996;9:230–234.
111. Kopple JD. The nutrition management of the patient with acute renal failure. *JPEN J Parenter Enteral Nutr* 1996;20 (1):3–12.
112. Maxvold NJ, et al. Management of acute renal failure in the pediatric patient: hemofiltration versus hemodialysis. *Am J Kidney Dis* 1997;30(5 Suppl 4):S84–S88.
113. Ronco C, Parenzan L. Acute renal failure in infancy: treatment by continuous renal replacement therapy. *Intensive Care Med* 1995;21(6):490–499.
114. Fiaccadori E, Lombardi M, Leonardi S, et al, Outcome of malnutrition in acute renal failure (ARF). *J Am Soc Nephrol* 1996;7:1372.
115. Galanos AN, et al. Relationship of body mass index to subsequent mortality among seriously ill hospitalized patients. SUPPORT Investigators. The Study to Understand Prognoses and Preferences for Outcome and Risks of Treatments. *Crit Care Med* 1997;25(12):1962–1968.
116. Hendricks KM, et al. Malnutrition in hospitalized pediatric patients. Current prevalence. *Arch Pediatr Adolesc Med* 1995; 149(10):1118–1122.
117. Haber BA, Deutschman CS. Nutrition and metabolism in the critically ill child. In: Rogers MC, Nichols DG, Ackerman AD, eds. *Textbook of pediatric intensive care*, 3rd ed. Baltimore: Williams & Wilkins, 1996:1141–1162.
118. Kinney JM. Metabolic responses of the critically ill patient. *Crit Care Clin* 1995;11(3):569–585.
119. Sugimoto H. [Energy substrate metabolism during stress]. *Nippon Geka Gakkai Zasshi* 1996;97(9):726–732.
120. Agus MS, Jaksic T. Nutritional support of the critically ill child. *Curr Opin Pediatr* 2002;14(4):470–481.
121. WHO. Energy and protein requirements: report of a joint FAO/WHO/UNU expert consultation. WHO Technical Report Series No. 724. Geneva: World Health Organization, 1985.
122. Schofield W. Predicting basal metabolic rate, new standards and review of previous work. *Hum Nutr Clin Nutr* 1985; 39(Suppl 1):5–41.
123. Duro D, et al. New equations for calculating the components of energy expenditure in infants. *J Pediatr* 2002;140 (5):534–539.
124. Reed M. Principles of total parenteral nutrition. In: Blumer JL, ed. *A practical guide to pediatric intensive care*, 3rd ed. St. Louis: Mosby Year Book 1990:582–591.
125. Cox JH, Cooning SW. Parenteral nutrition. In: Lang C, Queen PM, eds. *Handbook of pediatric nutrition*. Gaithersburg, MD: Aspen Publishers, 1993:279–314.
126. Briassoulis G, Venkataraman S, Thompson AE. Energy expenditure in critically ill children. *Crit Care Med* 2000;28 (4):1166–1172.
127. Holliday MA. Body composition, metabolism and growth. In: Holliday MA, ed. *Pediatric nephrology*, 3rd ed. Baltimore: Williams & Wilkins, 1994:152–163.
128. Kerner JJ. Parenteral nutrition. In: Walker WA, ed. *Pediatric gastrointestinal disease: pathophysiology, diagnosis, management*. Philadelphia: BC Decker, 1991:1647–1675.

129. Ikizler TA, Greene J, Wingard RL. Nitrogen balance in acute renal failure (ARF) patients. *J Am Soc Nephrol* 1995;6: 466.
130. Kuttnig M, et al. Nitrogen and amino acid balance during total parenteral nutrition and continuous arteriovenous hemofiltration in critically ill anuric children. *Child Nephrol Urol* 1991;11(2):74–78.
131. Cogo PE, et al. Protein turnover, lipolysis, and endogenous hormonal secretion in critically ill children. *Crit Care Med* 2002;30(1):65–70.
132. Mokrzycki MH, Kaplan AA. Protein losses in continuous renal replacement therapies. *J Am Soc Nephrol* 1996;7(10):2259–2263.
133. Novak I, et al. Glutamine and other amino acid losses during continuous venovenous hemodiafiltration. *Artif Organs* 1997;21(5):359–363.
134. Maxvold NJ, et al. Amino acid loss and nitrogen balance in critically ill children with acute renal failure: a prospective comparison between classic hemofiltration and hemofiltration with dialysis. *Crit Care Med* 2000;28(4):1161–1165.
135. Rocco MV, Blumenkrantz MJ. Nutrition. In: Daugirdas JT, Blake PG, Ing TS, eds. *Handbook of dialysis*, 3rd ed. Philadelphia: Lippincott Williams & Wilkins, 2001:420–445.
136. Kasiske BL, Guijarro C, Massy ZA, et al. Cardiovascular disease after renal transplantation. *J Am Soc Nephrol* 1996;7:158–165.
137. Kasiske BL, Chakkera HA, Roel J. Explained and unexplained ischemic heart disease risk after renal transplantation. *J Am Soc Nephrol* 2000;11:1735–1743.
138. Foley RN, Parfrey P, Sarnak MJ. Clinical epidemiology of cardiovascular disease in chronic renal disease. *Am J Kidney Dis* 1998;32:S112–S119.
139. Saland JM, Ginsberg H, Fisher EA. Dyslipidemia in pediatric renal disease: epidemiology, pathophysiology, and management. *Curr Opin Pediatr* 2002;14(2):197–204.
140. Massy ZA, Guijarro C, Weiderkehr MR, et al. Chronic renal allograft rejection: immunologic and nonimmunologic risk factors. *Kidney Int* 1996;49:518–524.
141. Milliner DS, et al. Lipid levels following renal transplantation in pediatric recipients. *Transplant Proc* 1994;26(1):112–114.
142. Shihab F. Metabolic complications. In: Turka LA, Norman DJ, eds. *Primer on transplantation*, 2nd ed. Thorofare, NJ: American Society of Transplantation 2001:247–256.
143. Silverstein DM, et al. Risk factors for hyperlipidemia in long-term pediatric renal transplant recipients. *Pediatr Nephrol* 2000;14(2):105–110.
144. Henkin Y, Como JA, Oberman A. Secondary dyslipidemia. Inadvertent effects of drugs in clinical practice. *JAMA* 1992;267:961–968.
145. Ingulli E, et al. Steroid withdrawal, rejection and the mixed lymphocyte reaction in children after renal transplantation. *Kidney Int Suppl* 1993;43:S36–S39.
146. Ferraris JR, et al. Effect of therapy with deflazacort on dyslipoproteinemia after pediatric renal transplantation. *J Pediatr* 1998;133(4):533–536.
147. Ballantyne CM, Podet E, Patsch WP, et al. Effects of cyclosporine therapy on plasma lipoprotein levels. *JAMA* 1989;262:53–56.
148. Gurecki J, Warty V, Sanghvi A. The transport of cyclosporine in association with plasma lipoproteins in heart and liver transplant patients. *Transplant Proc* 1985;17(4):1997–2002.
149. Raine A. Cardiovascular complications after renal transplantation. In: Morris P, ed. *Kidney transplantation: principles and practice*, 4th ed. Philadelphia: WB Saunders, 1994:339–355.
150. Henry M. Cyclosporine and tacrolimus (FK506): a comparison of efficacy and safety profiles. *Clin Transplant* 1999; 13:209–220.
151. McCune Thacker R, Thacker L, Peters TG, et al. Effects of tacrolimus on hyperlipidemia after successful renal transplantation: a Southeastern Organ Procurement Foundation multicenter clinical study. *Transplantation* 1998;65:87–92.
152. Ponticelli C, et al. Phase III trial of Rapamune versus placebo in primary renal allograft recipients. *Transplant Proc* 2001;33(3):2271–2272.
153. Akiyama T, Ishii T, Imanishi M, et al. Efficacy and safety of treatment with low-dose fluvastatin in hypercholesterolemic renal transplant recipients. *Transplant Proc* 2001;33:2115–2118.
154. Jardine A, Holdaas H. Fluvastatin in combination with cyclosporine in renal transplant recipients: a review of clinical and safety experience. *J Clin Pharm Ther* 1999;24:397–408.
155. Melchor JL, Gracida C. Treatment of hypercholesterolemia with fluvastatin in kidney transplant patients. *Transplant Proc* 1998;30:2054.
156. Delucchi A, et al. Dyslipidemia and dietary modification in Chilean renal pediatric transplantation. *Transplant Proc* 2001;33(1–2):1297–1301.
157. Penson MG, Fricker F, Thompson JR, et al. Safety and efficacy of pravastatin therapy for the prevention of hyperlipidemia in pediatric and adolescent cardiac transplant recipients. *J Heart Lung Transplant* 2001;20:611–618.
158. Chin C, Gamberg P, Miller J, et al. Efficacy and safety of atorvastatin after pediatric cardiac transplantation. *J Heart Lung Transplant* 2001;20:230.
159. Navasa M, Bustamante J, Marroni C, et al. Diabetes mellitus after liver transplantation: prevalence and predictive factors. *J Hepatol* 1996;25:64–71.
160. Lanerolle RD, de Abrew K, Fernando DJ, et al. Post-renal transplant diabetes in Sri Lanka. *Transplant Proc* 1996; 28:1945–1947.
161. Jindal RM, Sidner R, Milgrom ML. Post-transplant diabetes mellitus. The role of immunosuppression. *Drug Safety* 1997;16:242–257.
162. Onwubalili JK, Obineche E. High incidence of post-transplant diabetes mellitus in a single-centre study. *Nephrol Dial Transplant* 1992;7:346–349.
163. Rosenbloom AL, Joe J, Young RS, et al. Emerging epidemic of type 2 diabetes in youth. *Diabetes Care* 1999;22:345–354.
164. Pinhas-Hamiel O, Dolan L, Daniels SR, et al. Increased incidence of non-insulin-dependent diabetes mellitus among adolescents. *J Pediatr* 1996;128:608–615.
165. Greenspan LC, et al. Increased incidence in post-transplant diabetes mellitus in children: a case-control analysis. *Pediatr Nephrol* 2002;17(1):1–5.
166. Rao M, Jacob C, Shastry JC. Post-renal transplant diabetes mellitus—a retrospective study. *Nephrol Dial Transplant* 1992;7:1039–1042.
167. von Kiparski A, Frei D, Uhlschmid G, et al. Post-transplant diabetes mellitus in renal allograft recipients: a matched-pair control study. *Nephrol Dial Transplant* 1990;5:220–225.

168. Delaunay F, Khan A, Cintra A, et al. Pancreatic beta cells are important targets for the diabetogenic effects of glucocorticoids. *J Clin Invest* 1997;100:2094–2098.
169. Furth S, Neu A, Colombani P, et al. Diabetes as a complication of tacrolimus (FK-506) in pediatric renal transplant patients. *Pediatr Nephrol* 1996;10(1):64–66.
170. Filler G, Neuschulz I, Vollmer I, et al. Tacrolimus reversibly reduces insulin secretion in paediatric renal transplant recipients. *Nephrol Dial Transplant* 2000;15:867–871.
171. Strumph P, Kirsch D, Gooding W, et al. The effect of FK506 on glycemic response as assessed by the hyperglycemic clamp technique. *Transplantation* 1995;60:147–151.
172. Tamura K, Fujimura T, Tsutsumi T, et al. Transcriptional inhibition of insulin by FK506 and possible involvement of FK506 binding protein-12 in pancreatic beta-cell. *Transplantation* 1995;59:1606–1613.
173. Hirano Y, Mitamura T, Tamura T, et al. Mechanism of FK506-induced glucose intolerance in rats. *J Toxicol Sci* 1994;19:61–65.
174. Yoshioka K, Sato T, Okada N, et al. Post-transplant diabetes with anti-glutamic acid decarboxylase antibody during tacrolimus therapy. *Diab Res Clin Pract* 1998;42:85–89.
175. Sokol R. The chronic disease of childhood obesity: the sleeping giant has awakened. *J Pediatr* 2000;136:711–713.
176. Dietz W. Health consequences of obesity in youth: childhood predictors of adult disease. *Pediatrics* 1998;101:518–525.
177. Eckel RH, Krauss R. American Heart Association call to action: obesity as a major risk factor for coronary heart disease. AHA Nutrition Committee. *Circulation* 1998;97:2099–2100.
178. Curran JS, Barness LA. Nutrition. Obesity. In: Kliegman RM, Behrman RE, Jenson HB, eds. *Nelson textbook of pediatrics*, 16th ed. Philadelphia: W.B. Saunders Company, 2000:172–176.
179. Weisinger JR, Kempson RL, Eldridge FL, et al. The nephrotic syndrome: a complication of massive obesity. *Ann Intern Med* 1974;81:440–447.
180. Warnke RA, Kempson RL. The nephrotic syndrome in massive obesity: a study by light, immunofluorescence and electron microscopy. *Arch Pathol Lab Med* 1978;102:431–438.
181. Kasiske BL, Crosson JT. Renal disease in patients with massive obesity. *Arch Intern Med* 1986;146:1105–1109.
182. Adelman RD, et al. Proteinuria and focal segmental glomerulosclerosis in severely obese adolescents. *J Pediatr* 2001;138(4):481–485.
183. Praga M, Morales E, Herrero JC, et al. Absence of hypoalbuminemia despite massive proteinuria in focal segmental glomerulosclerosis secondary to hyperfiltration. *Am J Kidney Dis* 1999;33:52–58.
184. Kambham N, et al. Obesity-related glomerulopathy: an emerging epidemic. *Kidney Int* 2001;59(4):1498–509.
185. Verani R. Obesity-associated focal segmental glomerulosclerosis: pathological feature of the lesion and relationship with cardiomegaly and hyperlipidemia. *Am J Kidney Dis* 1992;20:629–634.
186. Devarajan P, Spitzer A. Towards a biological characterization of focal segmental glomerulosclerosis. *Am J Kidney Dis* 2002;39(3):625–636.
187. Ichikawa I, Fogo A. Focal segmental glomerulosclerosis. *Pediatr Nephrol* 1996;10:374–391.
188. Sharma M, Sharma R, McCarthy ET, et al. The FSGS factor: enrichment and in vivo effect of activity from focal segmental glomerulosclerosis plasma. *J Am Soc Nephrol* 1999;10:552–561.
189. Savin VJ, Sharma R, Sharma M, et al. Circulating factor associated with increased glomerular permeability to albumin in recurrent focal segmental glomerulosclerosis. *N Engl J Med* 1996;334:878–883.
190. Hinchliffe SA, Kreczy A, Ciftci AO, et al. Focal and segmental glomerulosclerosis in children with reflux nephropathy. *Pediatr Pathol* 1994;14:327–338.
191. Welch TR, McAdams A. Focal glomerulosclerosis as a late sequela of Wilms tumor. *J Pediatr* 1986;108:105–109.
192. Arfeen S, Rosborough D, Luger AM, et al. Familial unilateral renal agenesis and focal and segmental glomerulosclerosis. *Am J Kidney Dis* 1993;21:663–668.
193. Zucchelli P, Cagnoli L, Casanova S, et al. Focal glomerulosclerosis in patients with unilateral nephrectomy. *Kidney Int* 1983;24:649–655.
194. Welch T. Yet another target organ of obesity. *J Pediatr* 2001;138:455–456.
195. Hall JE, Brands M, Henegar JR. Mechanisms of hypertension and kidney disease in obesity. *Ann N Y Acad Sci* 1999;892:91–107.
196. Shimamura R. Focal glomerulosclerosis in obese Zucker rats and prevention of its development. *Kidney Int* 1983;24(S16):S259–S262.
197. Faustinella F, Uzoh C, Sheikh-Hamad, et al. Glomerulomegaly and proteinuria in a patient with idiopathic pulmonary hypertension. *J Am Soc Nephrol* 1997;8:1966–1970.
198. Jennette JC, Charles L, Grubb W. Glomerulomegaly and focal segmental glomerulosclerosis associated with obesity and sleep-apnea syndrome. *Am J Kidney Dis* 1987;10:470–472.
199. Fogo A, Ichikawa I. Evidence for a pathogenic linkage between glomerular hypertrophy and sclerosis. *Am J Kidney Dis* 1991;17:666–669.
200. Wolf G, et al. Leptin and renal disease. *Am J Kidney Dis* 2002;39(1):1–11.
201. Yoshikawa N, Ito H, Akamatsu R, et al. Focal segmental glomerulosclerosis with and without nephrotic syndrome in children. *J Pediatr* 1986;109:65–70.
202. McAdams AJ, Valentini RP, Welch TR. The nonspecificity of focal segmental glomerulosclerosis. The defining characteristics of primary focal glomerulosclerosis, mesangial proliferation and minimal change. *Medicine* 1997;76:42–52.
203. Freedman BI, Tuttle A, Spray BJ. Familial predisposition to nephropathy in African-Americans with non-insulin-dependent diabetes mellitus. *Am J Kidney Dis* 1995;25:710–713.
204. Bergman S, Key B, Kirk KA, et al. Kidney disease in the first-degree relatives of African-Americans with hypertensive end-stage renal disease. *Am J Kidney Dis* 1996;27:341–346.
205. Praga M, Hernandez E, Andres A, et al. Effects of body-weight loss and captopril treatment on proteinuria associated with obesity. *Nephron* 1995;70:35–41.

206. Ando A, Kawata T, Hara Y, et al. Effects of dietary protein intake on renal function in humans. *Kidney Int* 1989;27:S64–S67.
207. Goldstein RS, Hook JB, Bond JT. The effects of maternal protein deprivation on renal development and function in neonatal rats. *J Nutr* 1979;109(6):949–957.
208. Edelmann CM Jr, Wolfish NM. Dietary influence on renal maturation in premature infants. *Pediatr Res* 1968;2:421–422.
209. McCann ML, Schwartz R. The effects of milk solutes on urinary cast excretion in premature infants. *Pediatrics* 1966;38:555.
210. Ichikawa I, Purkerson M, Klahr S, et al. Mechanism of reduced glomerular filtration rate in chronic malnutrition. *J Clin Invest* 1980;65:982–988.
211. Klahr S, Alleyne G. Effects of chronic protein-calorie malnutrition on the kidney. *Kidney Int* 1973;3:129–141.

13

FLUID AND ELECTROLYTE THERAPY IN CHILDREN

MICHAEL J. G. SOMERS

The importance of fluid and electrolyte therapy in clinical pediatrics cannot be underestimated. In ambulatory practice, given the frequency with which children develop dehydrating illnesses, the clinician is often called on to formulate approaches to rehydration. In hospitalized children, myriad clinical and practice parameters impact fluid and electrolyte therapy and frequently go beyond merely providing adequate water and electrolytes to replace losses.

Over the last several years, the role of fluid and electrolyte therapy in clinical medicine has been subject to reinterpretation as a better understanding of the physiologic principles of fluid and electrolyte homeostasis has evolved and as common clinical practices have been critically reevaluated. Historically, it was two centuries ago that the first attempts to replace enteral losses from cholera led to an initial understanding of the profound morbidity and mortality that can accompany significant losses of salt and water (1). The recognition that affected patients improved simply by providing repeated intravenous infusions of a saline solution served as an impetus to define and develop parameters for fluid and electrolyte therapy. This understanding was later generalized to other illnesses in which there was an element of dehydration and ultimately helped to define the threshold for the minimum daily provision of fluid and electrolytes—so-called maintenance requirements—as well as a threshold of maximal tolerance.

In the first decades of the twentieth century, the work of Gamble and colleagues was especially significant to the development of fluid therapy in pediatrics (2). The concepts of extracellular and intracellular fluid compartments in the body helped to underscore the important role that renal mechanisms play in maintaining normal fluid and electrolyte balance. In turn, this enhanced knowledge of body fluid physiology spawned a tradition of clinical therapy grounded on rather elaborate guidelines for intravenous fluid and electrolyte replacement in the ill child based on continuing (maintenance) needs and past and current losses (deficits).

This so-called deficit therapy approach to fluid therapy in children, cogently outlined by Holliday and Segar in 1957 (3), has subsequently been taught as the gold standard to minimize complications and improve clinical outcomes. Recent reassessment of this traditional approach, again spawned in large measure by Holliday's work, has come to appreciate that such elaborate maneuvers are often unnecessary and may be counter-therapeutic (4). Rather, the use of standard oral rehydration and maintenance hydration fluids is a simple, safe, and efficacious alternative for most children in need of fluid and electrolyte therapy to restore intravascular volume in the setting of a dehydrating gastroenteritis (5).

Nonetheless, there continues to be a place for the more precise traditional assessment and prescription of fluid and electrolyte therapy, especially in children with nondiarrheal illness (6). In more complex disorders of fluid and electrolyte pathophysiology (e.g., frequently seen postoperatively or in critically ill children with sepsis, burns, or trauma), an understanding of the distribution of body fluids, usual fluid and electrolyte requirements, and the effect of perturbations in normal homeostatic balance remains vital to the correct prescription of initial therapy and the proper assessment of clinical response.

Such an understanding becomes more crucial when approaching the care of a child with renal disease. Frequently, the presence of a preexisting renal condition or the development of an acute renal dysfunction can complicate the fluid and electrolyte management of the child. Standard approaches to such therapy assume that normal renal homeostatic mechanisms come into play with the provision of adequate fluid and electrolytes. These approaches are ill advised for the child with renal disease in whom volume and electrolyte regulation may be deranged. Similarly, these approaches may have limited value with the critically ill child in whom normal fluid and electrolyte homeostasis may also be altered. In these circumstances, the clinician needs to approach fluid and electrolyte therapy systematically and with attention to individual clinical circumstance. Otherwise, in the absence of such a customized fluid and electrolyte prescription, the possibility arises that a therapeutic intervention may be deleterious, given preexisting reduced tolerance to alterations in body fluid volume, composition, or distribution.

DISTRIBUTION OF BODY FLUIDS

Total Body Water: Extracellular and Intracellular Fluid Compartments

Water makes up a large proportion of body weight, varying with age, body size, and body composition. In early gestation, 90% of the weight of the developing fetus may be water. In premature infants born early in the third trimester, total body water (TBW) approximates 80% of body weight. This falls to 70 to 75% in term infants, 65 to 70% in toddlers and young children, and eventually to 60% in older children and adolescents. Lean individuals have more body water than obese individuals, and pubertal adolescent boys with increasing muscle mass tend to have more TBW than adolescent girls. Although 60% is often the benchmark for estimating TBW in older children and adults, the actual percentage may be lower, especially in less well-conditioned individuals or the elderly (7).

Body water is distributed into intracellular and extracellular compartments. The intracellular compartment consists of water found within the cells of the body and comprises approximately two-thirds of TBW or 40% of body weight. The extracellular compartment comprises one-third of TBW or 20% of body weight and is divided into the interstitial fluid that bathes all cells and the plasma water that is carried intravascularly. The increased TBW seen in young children is due to an increased extracellular compartment, the result of a relatively increased surface area as compared to body weight (8).

The boundary between the intracellular and extracellular compartments is the cell membrane. Input or output from the body generally proceeds via some interface with the extracellular compartment. For instance, provision of intravenous fluid and electrolyte therapy is into the intravascular space, and subsequent delivery intracellularly depends on a host of factors.

Because most cell membranes are readily permeable to water, the distribution of water between the intracellular and extracellular spaces largely reflects osmotic forces. Each body space has a solute that is primarily sequestered within that compartment and that maintains its osmotic gradient (9,10). For instance, activity of the sodium-potassium pump found in cell membranes leads to an increased concentration of potassium intracellularly and an increased concentration of sodium in the interstitium. Thus, sodium serves as the effective osmole interstitially and potassium intracellularly. Similarly, plasma proteins, most notably albumin, exert an osmotic force to maintain water intravascularly. Osmotic force is counterbalanced by hydrostatic pressure pushing water across the capillary from the lumen to the interstitium. Perturbations in the distribution of effective osmoles can result in redistribution of water between the intracellular and extracellular spaces.

There is an ongoing dynamic equilibrium between the intracellular and extracellular spaces. Diffusional gradients, osmotic forces, and the activity of cellular pumps or transporters all combine to establish the differences in the composition of the body compartments. The intracellular space cannot be directly accessed. As a result, access to the intracellular space is achieved via its communication with the extracellular space. Thus, any intake by ingestion or infusion into the extracellular space results in a new equilibrium being established with the intracellular space as solute and fluid come to be exchanged. Ultimately, the final equilibrium is a result of complex biochemical, electrical, and physical interactions.

The communication between the cellular spaces can be bidirectional. In other words, there can be exchange from the intracellular space to the extracellular space allowing, for instance, for transfer or release of cell metabolites. In addition, because the extracellular space can communicate with the external milieu, any output from the extracellular space to the external milieu results in effective excretion from the body. There is, however, no direct communication between the intracellular space and the external milieu, and any output from the cells themselves is mediated via the cell's direct ability to interface with the interstitial fluid or the plasma water.

For the clinician, it is always important to remember that any impairment in the patient's normal homeostatic mechanisms regulating fluid and electrolyte balance has a striking impact on the patient's TBW and its extracellular and intracellular constituents. Clinically, a common example of this disruption of normal balance is the hypertension frequently exhibited by the renal patient with progressive renal dysfunction. As renal function declines, the ability of the kidney to excrete free water (CH_2O) also declines. Frequently, this is in the setting of decreased effective nephron number with concomitant impairment of overall tubular solute excretion, most notably salt. Often superimposed on this baseline tendency for dysregulation of solute and water balance are clinical factors (e.g., circulatory failure and decreased effective arterial volume) leading to further renal salt and water retention. This salt and water overload can lead to chronic expansion of the TBW and resulting systemic hypertension with expansion of the extracellular volume compartment. Appropriate therapy in this instance includes the judicious use of diuretics to reduce the total body burden of salt and water and to restore the TBW to a more physiologic state. In this instance, a clinician's failure to appreciate the preexisting expansion of the TBW because of chronic salt and water overload could prove deleterious to the patient if management did not include some measure to reduce the salt and water overload. This example also underscores the concept that fluid and electrolyte therapy may involve the removal of solute and water as well as the more usual notion that it is solely concerned with the correction of deficits of electrolytes and volume.

Effective Circulating Volume

The concept of effective circulating volume is somewhat more abstract than the division of body water into intracellular and extracellular fluid compartments. Through the circulation of the vascular volume, oxygen and nutrients are delivered to the intracellular space, and cellular metabolites are cleared from the intracellular space. The *effective circulating volume* refers to that portion of the extracellular vascular space that is actually perfusing the tissues and accomplishing such an exchange.

Any compromise in this exchange can prove deleterious to usual cell homeostasis; as a result, the body constantly senses and regulates effective perfusion of fluid through the intravascular space. Homeostatic feedback mechanisms include baroreceptors that respond to the stretch of specialized areas of the carotid arteries and the atrium. Hypoperfusion of these areas results in decreased stimulation of these stretch receptors, triggering the secretion of vasopressin and eventually leading to increased water reabsorption in the most distal nephron and expansion of the vascular volume. Similarly, in response to glomerular hypoperfusion, there is not only decreased afferent arteriolar stretch but also decreased glomerular filtration and delivery of sodium to the macula densa. Both of these stimuli can lead to the secretion of renin from the juxtaglomerular cells of the afferent arteriole. Renin release initiates a cascade of events resulting ultimately in increased aldosterone-mediated sodium reabsorption from the kidney as well as increased angiotensin-mediated vasoconstriction and sodium and water uptake.

Thus, the effective circulating volume is a product of multiple factors, not the least of which includes the size of the vascular space and the influence of various regulatory hormones. As a component of the extracellular body water, the size of the vascular space often parallels the size of the extracellular space. However, the size of the vascular space and the adequacy of the effective circulating volume do not necessarily vary coordinately. It is possible for the extracellular space to be replete or expanded and the actual effective circulating volume to be decreased. For instance, children with significant liver disease are often edematous, a sign of sodium retention and expansion of the interstitial component of the extracellular space. The intravascular component of their extracellular space may also be expanded due to factors resulting in avid salt and water reabsorption by the kidney. However, because of portal hypertension, splanchnic vessel congestion, and multiple arteriovenous spider angiomas generally seen with this condition, much of the expanded intravascular volume is ineffective—it does not serve to perfuse the tissues and accomplish effective cellular exchange. Thus, these children act as if they are volume depleted: They excrete little sodium in their urine, and they vigorously continue to expand their already overexpanded extracellular space by reabsorbing even more salt and water in response to the effects of aldosterone and antidiuretic hormone (ADH). Similarly, this paradoxic state of sodium avidity and ADH-mediated water reabsorption can be seen frequently in children with nephrotic syndrome or with cardiac failure despite their preexisting expansion of the extracellular space.

In managing all aspects of a patient's fluid and electrolyte therapy, the clinician must accurately assess both the patient's current extracellular volume status and effective circulating volume and reconcile these with potential causes of volume loss. At all times, it is most important to maintain an effective circulating volume and to make therapeutic decisions based on each patient's unique clinical circumstances at that time. This may require rather disparate therapeutic interventions. For instance, expansion of the extracellular volume with vigorous rehydration therapy may be called for in a child with poor perfusion secondary to gastroenteritis-induced dehydration, whereas another child with equally poor perfusion due to cardiodynamic compromise may be intravascularly replete and require the initiation of pressor therapy, and another child with edema from relapsed nephrotic syndrome may actually require fluid restriction. These examples underscore that loss of effective circulating volume generally arises as a result of one or more broad perturbations in the extracellular fluid compartment that impacts effective perfusion (Table 13.1).

Clinical signs and symptoms of effective circulating volume loss may be subtle. At times, there may be preservation of effective circulating volume in the face of an overall depleted extracellular fluid compartment. Failure to initiate appropriate fluid and electrolyte therapy in such a circumstance may result in eventual compromise of the effective circulating volume. Important initial clinical signs to assess in any patient being evaluated for fluid therapy include pulse rate and capillary refill. Tachycardia and sluggish refill generally precede more obvious signs of ineffective circula-

TABLE 13.1. ALTERATIONS IN EFFECTIVE CIRCULATING VOLUME

Cause	Mechanism
Contracted extracellular fluid space	Water or sodium chloride deficit
Massive vasodilatation	Loss of vascular tone sustaining perfusion pressure
Loss of intravascular osmotic pressure	Osmotic fluid losses into interstitium
Overfill of the intravascular space	Hydrostatic fluid losses into interstitium
Hemorrhage	Direct loss of blood and plasma water

tion (e.g., hypotension and oliguria). Clinical symptoms may also be nonspecific and include fatigue and lethargy that are often attributed to an underlying illness rather than to volume depletion. Proper restoration of effective circulating volume or extracellular fluid compartment depletion requires an understanding of baseline fluid and electrolyte needs as well as consideration of any extenuating clinical circumstances unique to the patient in question.

FLUID AND ELECTROLYTE REQUIREMENTS

Maintenance Water Therapy

The fluid and electrolytes required to replace daily losses and to maintain an overall net balance of zero fluid or electrolytes gained or lost are often termed *maintenance needs*. Such needs are a function of individual homeostatic and environmental factors and, thus, vary from day to day and from individual to individual. In the average child with adequate access to sources of fluid and nutrition, these maintenance needs are generally readily met (3,11). In the ill or hospitalized child who requires therapeutic intervention, these needs must be considered in the choice of fluid therapy provided.

To assist in estimating these needs, fluid and electrolyte requirements are generally calculated on the basis of weight or surface area, but individual clinical circumstance must be considered when making such calculations (12). For instance, the 20-kg child who is well requires a far different maintenance quantity of fluid and electrolytes than the 20-kg child who is tachypneic and febrile or the 20-kg child who is anuric and on a ventilator in the intensive care unit. Careful repeated assessment of the patient's volume status and close attention to a balance of overall daily input and output proves more useful at arriving at a correct estimate of daily fluid and electrolyte needs than reliance on mathematic formulas alone. With these caveats in mind, it is nonetheless a common clinical practice to make certain empirical assumptions regarding daily needs for water and the major electrolytes.

Historically, daily maintenance water needs have been estimated based on energy expenditure (Fig. 13.1) (3,11). Thus, for every kilocalorie (kcal) of energy used per day, 1 mL of water must be provided. Based on the computed energy expenditure of the average hospitalized patient, for the first 10 kg of body weight, 100 mL of water per kg is provided daily. For the next 10 kg of body weight, 50 mL of water per kg is provided daily, and for every kilogram of body weight in excess of 20 kg, 20 mL of water per kg is provided daily. In addition, in the process of oxidation of carbohydrate and fat, approximately 15 mL of water is generated for every 100 kcal of energy produced. This water of oxidation contributes significantly to overall water balance.

Maintenance water losses occur from insensible sources (almost exclusively evaporative and respiratory losses) and from urine output. In the child with average metabolic demands, for every 100 kcal of energy expended, 100 mL of water must be taken in. Of this 100 mL of water, 40 mL is lost insensibly, and 75 mL is lost as urine output. There is, however, 15 mL of water generated from the water of oxidation rendering net water balance equilibrated.

Clinical factors can have a striking impact on water losses (Table 13.2). Fever increases insensible losses by

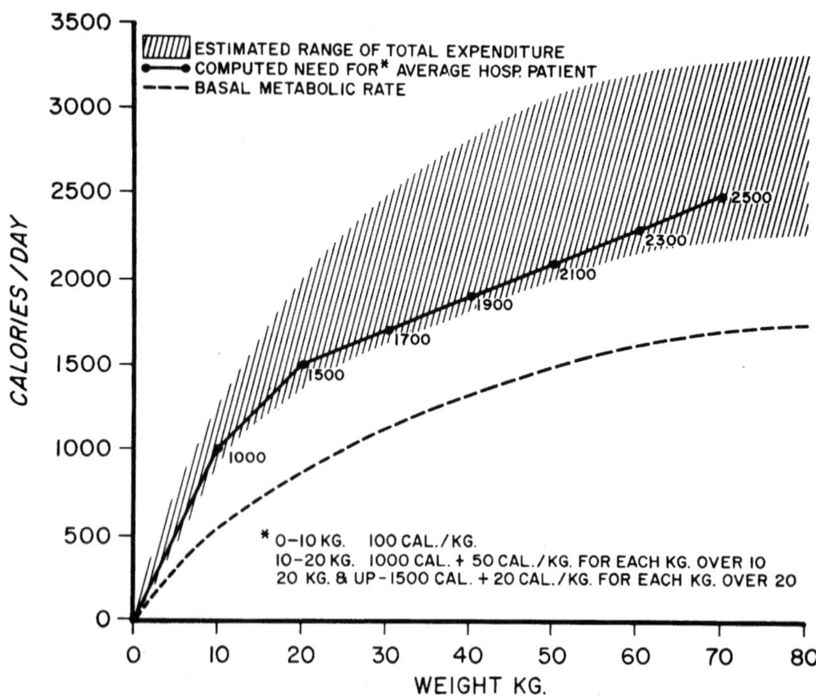

FIGURE 13.1. A comparison of the relation of estimated energy expenditure to weights over the range of 3 to 70 kg. (Courtesy of Malcolm Holliday.)

TABLE 13.2. FACTORS AFFECTING INSENSIBLE WATER LOSSES

Increased losses	Change (%)	Decreased losses	Change (%)
Prematurity	100–300	Enclosed incubator	25–50
Radiant warmer	50–100	Humidified air	15–30
Phototherapy	25–50	Sedation	5–25
Hyperventilation	20–30	Decreased activity	5–25
Increased activity	5–25	Hypothermia	5–15
Hyperthermia	12°C		

nearly 10% per degree Celsius. Premature infants with relatively increased surface areas for size can have insensible losses two- to threefold higher than baseline, especially if they are on open warmers or under phototherapy. On the other hand, children on ventilators being provided humidified oxygen may have only half of the insensible losses of a nonventilated child. Similarly, urinary output can vary tremendously. A child with a concentrating defect or ADH unresponsiveness may have urinary water losses of several liters per day, whereas an anuric child has no urinary losses. In any child with normal renal function, even in the setting of maximal ADH stimulation, there is a minimal volume of urinary water losses that is obligatory to excrete the osmotic load ingested by the diet and generated by basal metabolism. Thus, even the child concentrating urine at 1200 to 1400 mOsm/L loses approximately 25 mL of water as urine for every 100 kcal of energy expended (3).

Water Homeostasis and Serum Osmolality

Water homeostasis is crucial to maintaining a stable serum osmolality. The major factors contributing to serum osmolality are the serum concentrations of sodium, glucose, and blood urea nitrogen (BUN) (13). Serum osmolality is estimated by the following equation:

$$(2 \times \text{serum Na}) + (\text{serum glucose}/18) + (\text{BUN}/2.8)$$

where the serum sodium is measured in mEq/L and the glucose and BUN in mg/dL. Normally, the contributions of glucose and BUN to the effective osmolality are small, and the serum osmolality can be estimated by doubling the serum sodium concentration (14,15). Thus, most children have a serum osmolality between 270 and 290 mOsm/L, corresponding to serum sodium values of 135 to 145 mEq/L. Chemoreceptors in the hypothalamus constantly sense serum osmolality and respond to even small variations toward either limit of normal by adjusting ADH release from the posterior pituitary. Changes in osmolality in the setting of hypovolemia augment ADH release further. ADH effect on water permeability of the collecting tubule is a principal influence on the regulation of water balance.

Alterations in water intake or excretion result in the development of hypo- or hyperosmolality as the usual ratio of extracellular solute to water is perturbed. Because sodium is the largest component of extracellular osmolality, its concentration can be influenced profoundly by changes in water metabolism. An understanding of this link between water regulation and serum sodium values is crucial when prescribing fluid and electrolyte therapy. Most important, the clinician must recognize that hypo- or hypernatremia is usually a manifestation of impaired water regulation and that therapy must address regulation of water balance rather than alterations in body sodium stores.

Factors Contributing to Altered Water Homeostasis in Ill Children

In children with acute illness, vasoactive hormone levels appear to be increased, predisposing them to altered water homeostasis and changes in measured serum sodium levels. In one study of 103 acutely ill children, plasma vasopressin and renin levels were significantly elevated when compared to 31 control children awaiting elective surgery (16). These elevations were independent of the child's underlying illness and resulted in the ill children as a group having a lower measured serum osmolality than the control group.

In ill children, there are multiple causes of both physiologic and aberrant vasopressin effect (Table 13.3). As a result, in such at-risk children who receive hypotonic intravenous fluids for prolonged periods of time or in volumes exceeding those generally recommended, there is the risk of acute hyponatremia. After volume resuscitation with isotonic fluids, most hospitalized children are provided hypo-

TABLE 13.3. COMMON CAUSES OF VASOPRESSIN EFFECT IN HOSPITALIZED CHILDREN

Category	Specific etiology
Physiologic	Hyperosmolar state, hypovolemia
Pulmonary	Pneumonitis, pneumothorax, asthma, bronchiolitis, cystic fibrosis
Drug effect	Narcotics, barbiturates, carbamazepine, vincristine, cyclophosphamide
Metabolic	Hypothyroidism, hypoadrenalism, porphyria
Central nervous system	Infection (meningitis or encephalitis), tumor, trauma, hypoxia, shunt malfunction, nausea, pain, anxiety

tonic fluids for their maintenance therapy. Given the tendency for ill children to have vasopressin effect independent of the usual osmotic and volume-related stimuli, some investigators have suggested that isotonic fluids may be safer alternatives and should be continued as the source of maintenance fluid even after acute volume repletion (17).

Maintenance Electrolyte Therapy

Estimates for the maintenance requirements of the major electrolytes sodium, potassium, and chloride can also be made based on metabolic demands or, by extension, on daily water needs (3). For sodium and chloride, approximately 2 to 3 mEq/100 mL of water per day is required. For potassium, 1 to 2 mEq/100 mL of water per day is needed. Again, these estimates may require adjustment based on clinical circumstance, but the daily intake of most healthy individuals contains more than adequate electrolytes for maintenance needs. Although there can be significant electrolyte losses at times through the skin or the gastrointestinal tract, most electrolyte losses are urinary (12,18). Thus, in the setting of anuric renal failure, in the absence of concomitant electrolyte losses from other sources, a much lower level of maintenance electrolyte supplementation is needed, and often patients maintain adequate electrolyte balance with water supplementation alone to provide insensible fluid losses.

As with provision of water, it is vital in children who require electrolyte therapy to tailor their electrolyte prescription to their individual needs. For the provision of sodium and chloride, this requires careful assessment of the extracellular fluid space, especially the effective circulating volume. Providing too little sodium chloride results in volume contraction and circulatory compromise; providing too much causes volume overload and sequelae (e.g., hypertension and edema). Similarly, inappropriate potassium supplementation may have significant clinical ramifications. In children with diminished renal function or who are at risk of hyperkalemia for other reasons, it is usually appropriate to forego any maintenance potassium supplementation. When supplementation is given acutely, it is important to monitor serum potassium values closely. When chronic potassium supplementation is needed, there should continue to be periodic assessments. A course of supplemental potassium administered orally is safer than a bolus intravenous injection; intravenous potassium supplements rarely need to exceed 0.5 mEq/kg/hr (13).

PERTURBATIONS IN FLUID AND ELECTROLYTE HOMEOSTASIS

Alterations in Water Balance, Serum Sodium, and Cell Volume

As discussed earlier, the regulation of osmolality is achieved by alterations in water intake and excretion. Serum sodium levels often vary with these alterations in water balance. Generally, serum sodium is kept regulated at levels between 135 and 145 mEq/L. Serum sodium below 130 mEq/L or above 150 mEq/L is out of the range of normal homeostasis and is often indicative of some problem with water balance.

Because sodium is the major extracellular osmole, alterations in serum sodium can result in water flux between the intracellular and extracellular spaces. Because significant water flux into or out of cells could prove deleterious to cell function, cell volume is closely regulated to minimize such shifts (19). For instance, with hyponatremia, there is decreased effective osmolality in the extracellular space. As a result, water can shift from the plasma into the intracellular space, and cell swelling occurs acutely. To counterbalance such swelling, the cell acutely attempts to regulate its volume by transporting electrolytes, especially potassium, from the intracellular space into the extracellular space, thereby decreasing the osmotic gradient for water transfer. Over several days, when faced with chronic hyponatremia or chronic hypo-osmolality, the cells also achieve effective volume regulation by losing organic osmolytes (e.g., as taurine and inositol), thereby further diminishing the osmotic gradient for water transfer into the cell (20).

With hypernatremia, the osmotic gradient favors water flux out of the cells into the extracellular space. Without protective mechanisms, cell volume shrinks. Again, there are both acute and chronic mechanisms that attempt to minimize changes in cell volume. Acutely, there is transport of electrolytes intracellularly. Over time, there is stimulation of the production of organic idiogenic osmoles (20,21). Together, these act to ameliorate the loss of intracellular volume that would otherwise occur.

Thus, alterations in serum sodium values that arise slowly or are more chronic in nature tend to be better tolerated clinically than acute alterations. Chronic or slow changes allow for maximal counterregulation and fewer clinical sequelae. On the other hand, profound sudden alterations—serum sodium values falling to approximately 120 mEq or below or 160 mEq or above—are often accompanied by dramatic neurologic complications directly related to the acute changes in cell volume in the central nervous system (CNS).

These regulatory mechanisms must also be kept in mind when formulating specific therapeutic intervention. Acute perturbations can be corrected more rapidly than chronic conditions because the full gamut of responses to the imbalance has yet to come into play.

Hyponatremia: Initial Approach

Hyponatremia is usually defined as a serum sodium value less than 130 mEq/L. As noted earlier, low serum sodium values are less likely to arise secondary to depleted salt stores and more likely to be the result of persistent ADH effect and a relative surfeit of water for solute in the extracellular space.

TABLE 13.4. ETIOLOGY OF HYPONATREMIA

	Urinary Na (mEq/L)	
Circulating volume	**<20**	**>20**
Decreased	Burns Cystic fibrosis Diuretics—late Gastroenteritis	Adrenal insufficiency Diuretics—early Salt wasting
Normal or increased	Cardiac failure Hepatic cirrhosis Nephrotic syndrome	Renal failure Syndrome of inappropriate secretion of antidiuretic hormone Water intoxication

Infrequently, pseudohyponatremia may be seen. This is a result not of depletion of sodium stores but of an alteration in the usual makeup of the extracellular space such that the relative concentration of sodium is now depressed. Common etiologies of pseudohyponatremia include hyperglycemia, hyperlipidemia, and hyperproteinemia. In these clinical conditions, it is not uncommon for serum sodium values to be only modestly depressed. Because there is no underlying true anomaly in sodium or water stores in these conditions, the serum sodium need not be addressed with any therapeutic maneuvers. With the introduction of ion-sensitive electrodes for the measurement of plasma sodium concentration, pseudohyponatremia related to the presence of confounding factors in the laboratory assay is much less commonly encountered.

In attempting to clarify the etiology of the hyponatremia, it is often useful initially to assess the patient's extracellular volume status and determine if it is decreased, normal, or increased. Then, by quantitating urine sodium excretion and determining the renal response to the hyponatremia, it becomes easier to determine if the patient should receive sodium and water or if a sodium and water restriction is the appropriate therapy (Table 13.4).

Hyponatremia: Decreased Volume Status and Urine Sodium Less Than 20 mEq/L

Decreased circulating volume is usually seen with states of significant sodium loss. The most common site of this loss is the gastrointestinal tract as a result of vomiting, diarrhea, or tube drainage. The renal response to the decreased effective circulating volume includes increased activity of the renin-angiotensin axis and relatively high levels of aldosterone and angiotensin. As a result, urine sodium values are generally low (less than 20 mEq/L), and water reabsorption in the distal nephron is augmented by high levels of ADH. In the face of continuing sodium losses exceeding intake, this state of vigorous ADH effect leads to a relative excess of water and concomitant hyponatremia.

Such findings can also be seen in cystic fibrosis in which there are increased skin losses of sodium and chloride, with bleeding, with burns, with certain losses of fluid from the intravascular space of the extracellular fluid into the interstitial space ("third-spacing") as can occur postoperatively in conditions of vascular leak, or with peritonitis. Such hyponatremia can also be seen after a period of diuretic therapy. In response to chronic diuretic-mediated volume contraction, the mechanisms outlined above come into play. Thiazide diuretics, especially in combination with a loop diuretic (e.g., furosemide), are particularly prone to inducing such hyponatremia.

The appropriate therapeutic response to these conditions is the provision of sodium and water either by use of intravenous saline solutions or oral electrolyte solutions. This results in restoration of sodium balance and volume expansion.

Hyponatremia: Decreased Volume Status and Urine Sodium Greater Than 20 mEq/L

Decreased circulating volume and urinary sodium excretion greater than 20 mEq/L are indicative of renal salt wasting, either from an intrinsic tubulopathy or from early diuretic effect. Less commonly, adrenal insufficiency can cause sodium wasting from the principal cell of the distal nephron. Such cortisol deficiency can arise from an intrinsic endocrine defect (e.g., congenital adrenal hyperplasia related to 21-hydroxylase deficiency); from some secondary impairment of adrenal function caused by infection, bleeding, or malignancy; or from pharmacologic adrenal suppression without adequate replacement therapy. In the setting of adrenal insufficiency, replacement of appropriate adrenal hormones and provision of adequate sodium and water prove therapeutic. With renal salt wasting, supplementation with sodium and any other electrolytes exhibiting impaired renal reabsorption is useful.

Hyponatremia: Normal or Expanded Volume and Urine Sodium Less Than 20 mEq/L

Normal or increased circulating volume and urine sodium excretion less than 20 mEq/L can be seen in conditions in which there is an excess of both TBW and total body sodium. The three major disorders that cause this type of hyponatremia are the nephrotic syndrome, hepatic failure related to cirrhosis, and cardiac failure. In all these conditions, there is a state of sodium and water avidity related to high levels of ADH and aldosterone. Most commonly, this is in the setting of preexisting total body sodium overload as evidenced by edema. In all of these conditions, despite the increased extracellular or circulating volume, the effective circulating volume is often depressed. As a result of this ineffective perfusion of the tissues, sodium and water avidity is only heightened by stimulation of the renin-aldosterone-angiotensin axis, further exacerbating the total body excess of salt and water. Appropriate therapy includes striking a balance between interventions promoting the maintenance of effective circulating volume and restricting the provision of excess water and sodium that only contributes to further TBW and sodium overload.

Hyponatremia: Normal or Expanded Volume and Urine Sodium Greater Than 20 mEq/L

Hyponatremia in the setting of normal or increased effective circulating volume is always related to persistent ADH effect (10). If the urine sodium value is greater than 20 mEq/L, the most common clinical scenario is the syndrome of inappropriate secretion of ADH (SIADH). SIADH can arise from disparate clinical conditions, including in the postoperative child, the child with significant pain, or the child with pulmonary disease; as alluded to earlier, ill children are at risk for both SIADH and inappropriate ADH effect (22). In SIADH, despite a state of hypo-osmolality, the urine is inappropriately concentrated as a result of an inability to suppress ADH secretion and block ADH-mediated water reabsorption from the distal nephron. Appropriate therapy for SIADH includes restricting water intake and attending to any underlying clinical factors predisposing to this syndrome.

Normal or increased extracellular volume and high urine sodium concentration can also be seen in the setting of renal failure as glomerular filtration and water clearance fall and the fractional excretion of sodium rises. A more unusual cause of this form of hyponatremia is polydipsia, usually psychogenic in nature. Such water intoxication is rare in children but can occasionally be seen in emotionally disturbed older children or infants inappropriately provided large volumes of water or very hypotonic fluid. In both of these circumstances, restriction of the volume of CH_2O ingested on a daily basis may be beneficial.

Hypernatremia

Hypernatremia is defined as a serum sodium value greater than 150 mEq/L. Generally, higher serum sodium values can be tolerated, and significant clinical and neurologic effects of hypernatremia do not occur until sodium values exceed 160 mEq/L. As with hyponatremia, hypernatremia is more commonly a reflection of a problem with water balance rather than a sodium imbalance (23). In most instances, the patient has a relative deficiency of water for normal extracellular solute content.

Because sodium is the major determinant of plasma osmolality, as serum sodium levels rise, serum osmolality concomitantly increases. Increases in serum osmolality are sensed by hypothalamic osmoreceptors, triggering ADH release from the posterior pituitary once serum osmolality begins to increase over 280 mOsm (24). Increased serum osmolality also causes a sensation of thirst. Thus, in the normal state, as serum osmolality increases, there is increased fluid intake in the setting of high ADH levels. This results in increased reabsorption of CH_2O from the cortical collecting and reequilibration of serum sodium levels and serum osmolality before clinically significant hypernatremia or hyperosmolality occurs.

Outside infancy, hypernatremia as a result of sodium excess or salt poisoning is infrequently seen in pediatrics. Its major cause is improper preparation of powdered or liquid concentrated formula resulting in a hypertonic, hypernatremic solution. Because infants do not have free access to water, they cannot respond to their increasing sense of thirst as they develop hypernatremia. Exacerbating the whole situation are the facts that, most typically, caregivers continue to provide the same incorrectly prepared formula for further feedings and that young infants are unable to excrete sodium loads as efficiently as older children. Iatrogenic sodium loading can also be seen in children who have received large doses of sodium bicarbonate because of persistent acidosis or during a resuscitation or in children who have been given inappropriate amounts of sodium in peripheral nutrition. Iatrogenic sodium loading can also be seen in the child who has received repeated large volumes of blood products, generally isotonic or sodium-rich solutions.

Children who have hypernatremia from sodium excess should exhibit physical signs and symptoms compatible with extracellular space expansion. Thus, they frequently have peripheral edema and may have hypertension or symptoms of pulmonary edema. These children can respond to therapy aimed at augmenting the elimination of excess sodium. The use of diuretics and the provision of adequate CH_2O serve to decrease the total body sodium burden. Rarely, dialysis may need to be considered in cases in which it is clinically indicated to ameliorate the hypernatremia rapidly (25,26).

More commonly, hypernatremia is the result of a CH_2O deficit or a combined water and sodium deficit in which the water losses exceed the sodium losses. Hypernatremia secondary to a water deficit arises in the setting of inadequate access to water or an impairment in ADH release or response. It is uncommon to see hypernatremia secondary to poor water intake except in infants or young children who cannot get water for themselves in response to their sense of thirst (27). As for ADH-related anomalies, there are many causes of central or nephrogenic diabetes insipidus (28). Again, given normal access to water, it is rare for the older child to develop hypernatremia even with an impairment in the ADH axis because of the strong drive to drink in response to thirst (29). In very young children with diabetes insipidus, however, the issue of access to water arises, and hypernatremia may be a concern.

The most common etiology of hypernatremia in children is the loss of hypotonic fluid (i.e., fluid with a relative excess of water for its sodium content). In these situations, the TBW is decreased more than the total body sodium. The usual clinical scenario leading to such a condition is viral diarrheal illness in the setting of poor water intake or persistent vomiting. In this condition, there is loss of stool with a sodium content generally less than 60 mEq/L. These children tend to excrete small volumes of concentrated urine with urine sodium content less than 20 mEq/L, underscoring the fact that they are conserving both water and sodium. Their hypernatremia is not a manifestation of a total body excess of sodium but a depletion of sodium that is overshadowed by a larger relative depletion of body water. Therapy is aimed at restoring water and sodium balance by providing back the hypotonic fluid that was initially lost either by the use of intravenous saline solutions or with oral electrolyte therapy.

FLUID REPLACEMENT THERAPY

Most commonly, the importance of fluid replacement therapy lies with restoration of an adequate effective circulating volume. In its absence, significant metabolic derangements can occur, which only serve to exacerbate perturbations in fluid and electrolyte homeostasis. The volume of fluid replacement required varies with the extent and etiology of the compromised circulation. Children with mild dehydration, manifesting with less than 5% weight loss, usually respond to 30 to 50 mL/kg of fluid. In the setting of more significant dehydration or loss of vascular tone, more than 200 mL/kg may be needed. The clinician can approach such fluid resuscitation with either intravenous or oral rehydration therapy.

Clinical and Laboratory Assessment of Volume Depletion

In estimating the severity of dehydration, the most objective measure is usually the change in weight from baseline (30). As rehydration proceeds, following weights on a serial basis becomes an important adjunct in assessing the efficacy of fluid repletion. Frequently, the clinician is faced with the situation in which no baseline weight is known, and various parameters based on history and physical examination need to be used to judge the severity of dehydration (Table 13.5). Children with mild dehydration have minimal clinical signs and only a modest decline in urine output. As dehydration becomes more significant, more classical findings (e.g., dry mucous membranes, tenting skin, sunken eyes, and lethargy) become prominent. With profound dehydration, there is anuria, marked alterations in consciousness, and hemodynamic instability.

A capillary refill time greater than 2 seconds is a useful physical finding in effective volume depletion (31). However, delayed capillary refill is neither a sensitive nor specific marker of dehydration (32,33) and may be most useful if normal, as this does seem to exclude reliably severe dehydration. In a prospective cohort study of dehydrated Egyptian children between 3 and 18 months of age, the best correlation between clinical assessment of degree of dehydration and actual volume depletion came in children who had such clinical parameters of significant dehydration as prolonged skinfold tenting, a dry mouth, sunken eyes, and altered sensorium—findings generally associated with more substantial

TABLE 13.5. CLINICAL ASSESSMENT OF DEHYDRATION

	Degree of dehydration		
Physical sign	Mild	Moderate	Severe
Vital sounds			
Pulse	Normal	Rapid	Rapid and weak
Blood pressure	Normal	Normal to slightly low	Shock
Weight loss			
Infant	<5%	10%	>15%
Older child	<3%	6%	>9%
Mucous membranes	Tacky	Dry	Parched
Skin turgor	Slightly decreased	Decreased	Tenting
Eye appearance	Normal tears	Decreased tears ± sunken	No tears + very sunken
Capillary refill	Normal	Delayed (>3 s)	Very delayed (>5 s)
Urine output	Decreased	Minimal	Anuric

dehydration (34). Similarly, in a review of preschool children with dehydration, the best clinical indicators of volume depletion—decreased skin turgor, poor peripheral perfusion, and Kussmaul breathing—accompanied more significant dehydration (35), underscoring the difficulty with which more subtle degrees of dehydration may be estimated by the clinician without access to prior weights.

A study of 97 American children who needed intravenous fluids in an emergency department for rehydration underscored the difficulty in assessing accurately even severe dehydration by standard clinical estimates (36). Physicians' initial estimate of dehydration compared to the actual percent loss of body weight varied dramatically, with a sensitivity of 70% for severe dehydration (greater than 10% loss) but only 33% for moderate dehydration (6 to 10% loss). This study suggested that adding a serum bicarbonate level to the assessment may be useful, increasing the sensitivity of the clinical scales to 100% in severe dehydration and 90% in moderate dehydration if standard clinical features and a serum bicarbonate less than 17 mEq/L were found.

Other studies have found that laboratory studies by themselves are poor indicators of the degree of dehydration. In 40 children receiving intravenous fluids for dehydration, prehydration assessment of serum BUN, creatinine, uric acid, anion gap, venous pH, and venous base deficit were made, as well as assessment of urinary specific gravity, urinary anion gap, and fractional excretion of sodium. Only the serum BUN/creatinine ratio and serum uric acid significantly correlated with increasing levels of dehydration, but both lacked sensitivity or specificity for detecting more than 5% dehydration (37). Similarly, in a retrospective review of 168 dehydrated children, elevated serum urea levels and depressed serum bicarbonate levels were found to be useful adjuncts to clinical evaluation in accurately assessing the degree of dehydration but were not by themselves predictive (38).

In fact, with the most common clinical scenario (i.e., viral gastroenteritis) leading to dehydration in children, there rarely is a significant laboratory anomaly despite clinical volume depletion. In a cohort of children from the United Kingdom admitted for rehydration due to viral gastroenteritis, only 1% of admitted children had an electrolyte derangement (39–41).

In children with volume depletion accompanying trauma, sepsis, surgery, or underlying renal dysfunction, it is more likely to find perturbations in electrolyte and acid-base status. Thus, in the absence of a straightforward case of mild to moderate diarrheal dehydration, the general consensus is that blood should be obtained for assessments of electrolytes, bicarbonate, and renal function to help guide fluid and electrolyte therapy (42,43).

As the child is volume resuscitated, it is important to assess the child's response. Initial estimates as to the degree of dehydration may need to be adjusted if the child is not showing progressive improvement. Clinical parameters to follow include monitoring the child's general appearance and sensorium, the change in weight from initiation of rehydration, as well as urine output and urine osmolality. In children with some types of underlying renal dysfunction, there may often be a chronic urinary concentrating defect. In these children, relatively dilute urine flow may be maintained even in the face of clinical dehydration. In these children, markers other than urine output and osmolality should be followed.

Oral Rehydration Therapy

Parenteral fluid and electrolyte therapy have been the mainstays of medical treatment for most children presenting with fluid and electrolyte imbalances even though oral rehydration with electrolyte solutions is actually a safe, efficacious, and convenient alternative that can treat mild to severe volume depletion (44–47). Although this approach has been especially underused in North America, oral therapy has proved successful in clinical settings worldwide in resuscitating children of all ages with profound fluid and electrolyte anomalies; short of significant circulatory compromise, it can be used as first-line therapy in all fluid and electrolyte aberrations (48,49). An example of a situation in which oral hydration therapy is indicated is presented in the following case study:

> A healthy 5-year-old boy with no significant medical history presents to his pediatrician's office after 2 days of a febrile illness. For most of this time, his appetite has been severely depressed, and his parents estimate that he has only had a few cups of fluid in the last 8 to 12 hours. Today, he vomited once, prompting the office visit. He has continued to urinate, although urine volume is less than usual. On physical examination, the boy is nontoxic and alert. Initially, his pulse is 120 beats per minute; however, after acclimation to the examination, it has decreased to 100 beats per minute. His sitting blood pressure is 90/50 mm Hg, and he is not compliant with attempts at orthostatic vital signs. His mucous membranes are dry, and his weight today is 20 kg, exactly the same as his weight at a well-child examination 6 months previously. His parents are concerned that he is becoming dehydrated.

Pediatricians, family practitioners, and emergency room physicians face such clinical scenarios regularly. The otherwise well child with an apparent viral illness causing mild to moderate dehydration is frequently treated by intravenous therapy under the oftentimes misguided assumption that oral rehydration rarely succeeds, is too labor intensive, or takes too much time. In fact, such children are excellent candidates for oral rehydration. In most developed countries where a viral disease is believed to be

TABLE 13.6. ORAL REHYDRATION THERAPY (ORT) FOR PREVIOUSLY HEALTHY, WELL-NOURISHED CHILDREN

Type of dehydration	Rehydration prescription	Rehydration duration
Mild (<5%)	30–50 mL/kg ORT	3–4 h
Moderate (5–10%)	50–100 mL/kg ORT	3–4 h
Severe (>10%)	100–150 mL/kg ORT	3–4 h
Evidence of shock	20 mL/kg 0.9% NaCl IV	Repetitive infusions until perfusion restored then transition to ORT[a]
Accompanying hypernatremia	Per type of dehydration	≥12 h for ORT Monitor fall in serum Na

[a]With fluid containing 45 to 90 mmol/L Na, 90 mmol/L glucose, 20 mmol/L K, and 10 to 30 mmol/L citrate.

the etiology of the dehydration and there is little concern about a cholera-like enteritis, oral rehydration solutions with sodium contents from 30 to 90 mEq/L (54,55,57,59) can be chosen as oral therapy with expectation of success.

With this child, given his history and physical examination, it is unlikely that any electrolyte perturbations would be found; hence, there is little indication for assaying electrolytes or renal function before starting oral rehydration (39–41). The family is given a commercially available oral rehydration solution containing 75 mEq/L sodium, 20 mEq/L potassium, 30 mEq/L citrate, and 2.5% glucose. They are asked to provide 1 L of fluid (50 mL/kg) to the child over the next 4 hours. The child should be offered small aliquots of fluid very often—5 mL every 1 to 2 minutes at initiation. If this regimen is tolerated with no vomiting, the aliquots may be gradually increased in volume and the frequency reduced, aiming to deliver at least the prescribed total volume over approximately 4 hours.

A common cause of failure with oral rehydration is not recognizing that the initial provision of fluid given "little and often" is far more likely to be well tolerated than larger aliquots. If families are unwilling to provide the fluid in this manner, a nasogastric tube may be placed for continuous infusion.

Although some children may not respond to this approach and require intravenous rehydration, most children with mild to moderate rehydration can be rehydrated orally without a great deal of trouble. A guide for the volumes of fluid to provide and the duration of rehydration can be found in Table 13.6.

The first oral rehydration solutions were developed in the 1940s at academic medical centers. Within 10 years, a commercial preparation was available, but its use was associated with an increased incidence of hypernatremia (50). Several factors contributed to the development of this problem: The preparation was a powder meant to be reconstituted with water and was sometimes incorrectly administered as the powder itself or improperly diluted with too little water. When correctly reconstituted, the solution had a final carbohydrate concentration of 8% leading to an osmotic diarrhea in some children; it was a common practice at that time for parents to use high-solute fluids (e.g., boiled skim milk) as an adjunctive home remedy. Taken together, these early experiences contributed to a reluctance by many clinicians to use oral rehydration solutions.

Over time, there came to be a better understanding of the physiology of water and solute absorption from the gut. Of prime importance was the recognition that many substances actively transported across intestinal epithelium had an absolute or partial dependence on sodium for absorption and that sodium itself was actually better absorbed in their presence (51–53). This led to the routine introduction of glucose into oral rehydration solutions in a fixed molar ratio of no more than 2:1 with sodium. Moreover, it became clear that the sodium/glucose cotransporter remained intact not only in the face of enterotoxic gastroenteritis (e.g., as seen with cholera or *Escherichia coli*) but also in more common viral and bacterial enteritides (48,49).

The World Health Organization (WHO) and the United Nations Children's Fund have championed the use of a rehydrating solution that includes Na 90, Cl 80, K 20, base 30, and glucose 111 (2%) mmol/L. This WHO solution has proved useful in many clinical trials in children with dehydration from various causes, including secretory and nonsecretory diarrhea, and has been shown to reduce the morbidity and mortality associated with diarrheal illness regardless of its etiology (54,55). Most commercially available oral rehydration solutions differ from WHO solution in that they have a somewhat higher carbohydrate content, a lower sodium content, and a higher carbohydrate to sodium ratio (Table 13.7).

These formulation changes arose from concerns that using an oral rehydrating solution with a sodium content greater than 60 mmol/L may prove problematic in developed countries where most gastroenteritis is viral in nature and has a lower sodium content than the secretory diarrheas commonly seen in less developed areas. It was feared that if minimally dehydrated children losing small amounts of sodium in their stools were exclusively provided WHO solution without provision of some excess CH_2O, hyper-

TABLE 13.7. ORAL REHYDRATION SOLUTIONS

	Concentration (mmol/L)				
Product	Na	Glucose	K	Cl	Citrate
WHO ORS[a]	90	111	20	80	30
Rehydralyte (Ross)	75	140	20	65	30
Pedialyte (Ross)	45	140	20	35	30
Ricelyte (Mead Johnson)	50	170[b]	25	45	34

[a]Oral rehydrating solution provided as powder. Needs to be reconstituted with water.
[b]Rice-syrup solids substituted for glucose.

natremia might ensue. A few studies did indeed document iatrogenic hypernatremia related to such rehydration techniques (56). In cases of mild dehydration stemming from causes other than secretory diarrhea, solutions with lower sodium contents may be useful; in fact, solutions with sodium content ranging from 30 to 90 mmol have proved quite effective in this setting (57–59). A more recent metaanalysis of studies focused on the safety and efficacy of oral rehydration solution in well-nourished children living in developed countries documented little evidence that WHO solution was more likely to cause aberrations in serum sodium than oral rehydration solutions with lower sodium content.

Oral Rehydration with Fluids Other Than Oral Rehydration Solution

Despite the proven efficacy and fairly widespread availability of commercial oral rehydration solutions and the ease with which other electrolyte solutions can be mixed at home with recipes requiring few ingredients other than water, sugar, and salt, there are, nonetheless, many children who are given common household beverages in attempts at oral rehydration. In children with dehydration accompanied by electrolyte losses from vomiting or diarrhea, most common household beverages do not contain adequate sodium or potassium supplementation. Moreover, the base composition and the carbohydrate source are often suboptimal for the dehydrated child, especially in the setting of diarrheal illness (Table 13.8). Similarly, most beverages marketed as sports drinks for "rehydration" after exercise are also deplete of sufficient electrolytes given that the electrolyte composition of sweat is many times lower than the composition of gastrointestinal fluid. In prescribing oral rehydration to children in an ambulatory setting, the clinician should clarify for the family the appropriate fluid and volume for the child to ingest, emphasizing the need to use a fluid with appropriate electrolyte content if there is concern about evolving imbalances in sodium, potassium, or bicarbonate homeostasis.

Oral Rehydration and Significant Sodium Alterations

Although oral rehydration is often associated with the child with modest dehydration and no presumed electrolyte anomalies, it has also been used in cases of dehydration accompanied by hyponatremia or hypernatremia (60,61). It has met with overall success when a WHO-like solution has been used. In children with severe hypernatremia (greater than 160 mEq/L), although most can be successfully rehydrated orally, there have been reports of seizures, generally as a result of too rapid correction of serum sodium stemming from the provision of supplemental water in addition to the glucose-electrolyte solution (60–62). In those cases, the average serum sodium fell by 10 to 15 mEq/L over 6 hours rather than over 24 hours as advised. In follow-up studies, no seizure activity was seen in a similar cohort of hypernatremic children who received 90 mmol Na rehydration solution alone at a rate calculated to replace the infant's deficit over 24 hours (60). It is important for the practitioner to remember that once peripheral perfusion has been stabilized with initial volume expansion, there is no benefit to correcting any deficit rapidly, and tak-

TABLE 13.8. COMPOSITION OF COMMON ORAL FLUIDS

Fluid	Na (mEq/L)	K (mEq/L)	Source of base	Carbohydrate (g/100 mL)
Apple juice	<1	25	Citrate	12
Orange juice	<1	55	Citrate	12
Milk	20	40	Lactate	5
Cola	2	<1	Bicarbonate	10
Ginger ale	4	<1	Bicarbonate	8
Kool-Aid	<1	<1	Citrate	10
Gatorade	20	2.5	Citrate	4
Jell-O	25	<1	Citrate	14
Coffee	<1	15	Citrate	<0.5
Tea	2	5	Citrate	10

Adapted from Feld LG, Kaskel FJ, Schoeneman MJ. The approach to fluid and electrolyte therapy in pediatrics. *Adv Pediatr* 1988;35:497–536.

ing 24 to 48 hours may be a more prudent course in the face of significant electrolyte anomalies.

Oral Rehydration Schemes

Several oral rehydration schemes have been shown to be quite effective and well tolerated. In one approach used extensively in developing countries, the patient's volume deficit is calculated on the basis of weight loss and clinical appearance (63). The volume deficit is doubled; this is the target rehydration volume to be given over 6 to 12 hours. Two-thirds of this volume is given as a glucose-electrolyte solution containing 90 mmol Na over 4 to 8 hours; once this has been ingested, the remaining volume is provided as water alone over 2 to 4 hours. In cases of suspected or confirmed hypernatremia with serum sodium exceeding 160 mEq/L, the volume deficit is not doubled and is administered as 90 mmol Na glucose-electrolyte solution alone over 12 to 24 hours. Patients who refuse to take fluids by mouth have nasogastric tubes placed. With this approach, successful oral rehydration is the rule; 95% of children are fully rehydrated without the need for intravenous therapy.

An alternative approach has been to have the child begin by taking 15 mL/kg/hr of a 60- to 90-mmol Na rehydration solution by mouth or nasogastric tube (64). The solution is given in small, frequent quantities and increased up to 25 mL/kg/hr until hydration has improved, at which point solid feedings are reintroduced and volumes of 5 to 15 mL/kg of rehydration solution offered after feeds until the volume deficit has been delivered.

The American Academy of Pediatrics has issued guidelines for the treatment of fluid and electrolyte deficits with oral rehydration solutions (48). Children with acute dehydration and extracellular volume contraction should be provided 40 to 50 mL/kg of a glucose-electrolyte solution containing 75 to 90 mmol/L Na, 110 to 140 mmol/L glucose (2.0 to 2.5%), 20 mmol/L potassium, and 20 to 30 mmol/L base. This volume should be administered over 3 to 4 hours; once there has been amelioration of the extracellular volume contraction, the patient should be changed to a maintenance solution with 40 to 60 mmol Na at half the rate. If the child is still thirsty on this regimen, there should be free access to supplemental water or low-solute fluid (e.g., breast milk).

In a recent evidence-based guideline for treating dehydration in children from industrialized European countries, oral rehydrating solution containing 60 mmol/L of sodium, 90 mmol/L of glucose, 20 mmol/L of potassium, and 10 mmol/L of citrate was recommended, with rehydration occurring over 3 to 12 hours using from 30 to 150 mL/kg of fluid depending on the degree and type of dehydration (30). This rehydration scheme is summarized in Table 13.6.

Limited Use of Oral Rehydration Solutions

Despite the promulgation of guidelines for oral rehydration in a variety of clinical situations, less than 30% of a mixed group of American academic pediatricians, private practitioners, and pediatric house staff actually acknowledged using such therapy (57). Oral rehydration schemes have been shown to be used significantly more frequently by emergency room physicians who were familiar with the American Academy of Pediatrics' oral rehydration recommendations (65). Yet, even in these more knowledgeable emergency physicians, oral therapy was underused in children with all degrees of dehydration. Worldwide, WHO estimates that less than 25% of patients who could benefit from oral rehydration are actually treated with an appropriate oral therapy (66). Moreover, even in areas of the world, such as Bangladesh, where oral rehydration has been championed by both local and international medical agencies for decades, its use is still suboptimal (67,68).

When used, oral rehydration has been demonstrated to be quite successful, with more than 95% of children in a meta-analysis of oral rehydration studies achieving some degree of volume repletion (69). Other advantages to oral therapy include its ability to be administered readily anywhere by the child's usual caretaker, the safety and stability of the product despite its lengthy shelf-life, and avoidance of the discomfort and potential complications associated with intravenous catheter placement (70). In developed countries, there has been concern that the WHO solution may not be looked on by parents as a convenient hydration solution because it involves preparation from a powdered packet. In fact, in a randomized controlled trial of an urban pediatric clinic and a suburban medical practice in the United States, parents were equally as satisfied with the ease of administration and effectiveness of the WHO solution as compared to a commercially prepared oral rehydration solution (71).

Oral rehydration is somewhat less successful in hospitalized children than in children treated in an ambulatory setting (69). This difference may be directly related to the degree of dehydration or other complicating clinical issues leading to hospital admission. Moreover, the relatively labor-intensive, slower approach to oral rehydration may be problematic in medical facilities with time constraints or space limitations (70,72).

There are recent reports that frozen flavored oral rehydration solution may be more readily accepted than conventional oral solution. Its use resulted in higher rates of successful rehydration in children with mild to moderate dehydration, even if these children initially did not respond to conventional oral rehydration (70). Frozen flavored rehydration solution is now commercially available in some parts of the world, as is a variety of flavored rehydration solutions.

Another potential issue with oral rehydration is that its use does not alter the natural course of the child's illness. Thus, in gastroenteritis with dehydration, by far the most common illness requiring rehydration in children, oral rehydration does not lower stool output or change the duration of diarrheal illness (73). As a result, caretakers may abandon oral rehydration because the child is not getting

TABLE 13.9. COMPOSITION OF COMMON INTRAVENOUS FLUIDS

Fluid	Osmolarity (mOsm/L)	Na (mEq/L)	K (mEq/L)	Cl (mEq/L)	Buffer (source) (mEq/L)	Mg (mEq/L)	Ca (mEq/L)	Dextrose (g/L)
Crystalloids								
0.9% Saline	308	154	0	154	0	0	0	0
Lactated Ringer's solution	275	130	4	109	28 (lactate)	0	3	0
5% Dextrose water	252	0	0	0	0	0	0	50
Normosol	295	140	5	98	27 (acetate) 23 (gluconate)	3	0	0
Plasma-Lyte	294	140	5	98	27 (acetate) 23 (gluconate)	3	0	0
Colloids								
5% Albumin	309	130–160	<1	130–160	0	0	0	0
25% Albumin	312	130–160	<1	130–160	0	0	0	0
Fresh frozen plasma	300	140	4	110	25 (bicarbonate)	0	0	0
3.5% Haemaccel	301	145	5	145	0	0	6	0
6% Hetastarch	310	154	0	154	0	0	0	0
Dextran 40 or 70	310	154	0	154	0	0	0	0

better and is not appreciating the benefits of ongoing hydration. Oral rehydrating solutions have been formulated with lower electrolyte composition and different carbohydrate moieties with the goal to reduce the osmolarity of solutions and theoretically augment fluid absorption from the small intestine (74). The rice-based oral solutions have been studied most extensively. In these solutions, glucose is substituted with 50 to 80 g/L of rice powder. In a metaanalysis of 22 randomized clinical trials comparing rice-based solutions to conventional glucose-containing solutions, stool output dramatically decreased in children with cholera given rice-based hydration but did not change in children with other bacterial or viral enteritides (75).

There are some reports that suggest that providing children with noncholera enteritis with reduced osmolarity rehydration solution may be beneficial. In one study, 447 boys younger than 2 years of age admitted for oral rehydration were assigned to receive either the WHO solution (osmolarity, 311 mmol/L) or a solution containing less sodium and chloride (osmolarity, 224 mmol/L). Children who received the lower-osmolarity solution had reduced stool output, reduced duration of diarrhea, reduced rehydration needs, and reduced risk of requiring intravenous fluid infusion after completion of oral hydration (76). A metaanalysis of nine trials comparing WHO solution to reduced-osmolarity rehydration solution concluded that children admitted for dehydration had reduced needs for intravenous fluid infusion, lower stool volumes, and less vomiting when receiving the reduced-osmolarity solution (77).

Intravenous Therapy

Although absolute indications for parenteral intravenous therapy are limited, they do include any condition of impaired peripheral circulation or overt shock. In addition, there are occasional children who are truly unable to sustain an adequate rate of oral fluid intake despite concerted efforts or have such persistent losses that parenteral therapy comes to be necessary. The mainstays of fluid therapy in children are saline or buffered saline crystalloid solutions. Isotonic versions of these crystalloids are used for volume resuscitation, and hypotonic saline solutions may be used in addition to provide supplemental maintenance hydration. In addition to crystalloid solutions, there are several colloid fluids that are used by many clinicians. Table 13.9 lists the electrolyte content of some of the more common intravenous solutions used for pediatric fluid therapy.

Choice and Volume of Parenteral Fluid

Children with significant extracellular volume contraction (greater than 10% acute weight loss in an infant or 6% weight loss in an older child) should receive an isotonic crystalloid solution [e.g., 0.9% saline (154 mEq/L NaCl) or Ringer's lactate (130 mEq/L NaCl)] at a rate of 20 mL/kg over 30 to 60 minutes. Children with a more moderate degree of dehydration may not exhibit signs or symptoms of volume contraction. In certain situations, however, it may be clinically warranted to provide them with an initial rapid intravenous bolus to initiate rehydration therapy.

Concomitant with the placement of intravenous access, blood should be obtained for determination of serum electrolytes, osmolality, and renal function. Given that dehydrated children often have high levels of vasoactive hormones and high vasopressin levels, it is most circumspect to establish baseline electrolyte levels, as it is possible to alter electrolyte balance rapidly with intravenous therapy. In the face of inadequate tissue perfusion, a parenteral fluid infusion should begin immediately before the return of any pertinent laboratory results. If hemorrhagic shock is suspected, resuscitation with packed red blood cells is optimal. In cases of severe volume depletion, if the child does not improve with the initial 20-mL/kg crystalloid bolus, this should be repeated up to two additional times. In children who have not improved despite administration of 60 mL/kg of total volume over 1 hour or in children in whom underlying cardiac, pulmonary, or renal disease may make empiric aggressive rehydration more problematic, consideration should be given to placement of a central monitoring catheter to more accurately assess intravascular volume and cardiac dynamics (78). In some instances of profound ineffective circulating volume (e.g., those that might accompany certain cases of sepsis), initial volume resuscitation may require sequential infusions of fluid ultimately exceeding 100 mL/kg.

Within minutes of infusion of a crystalloid fluid, it becomes distributed throughout the extracellular space. Because this involves equilibration of the fluid between the two components of the extracellular space—the intravascular and interstitial spaces—actually only one-third to one-fourth of infused crystalloid stays in the blood vessels (78). This accounts for the need to give large volumes of crystalloid in the setting of circulatory collapse and leads some to suggest that colloid solutions (e.g., 5 or 10% albumin) should play a role in resuscitation (79,80).

Colloid Solutions for Volume Resuscitation

The use of colloid solutions for volume resuscitation is controversial. In the 1990s, colloids were included in a number of widely promulgated guidelines for the care of patients in emergency facilities and intensive care units both for hemorrhagic shock before the availability of blood and for nonhemorrhagic shock as an adjunct to crystalloid use (81). Types of colloids used included 5% albumin, fresh frozen plasma, modified starches, dextrans, and gelatins. These guidelines, generally aimed toward the fluid resuscitation of adults, were composed despite the prior publication of a systematic review of randomized controlled trials that demonstrated no effect on mortality rates when colloids were used in preference to crystalloids (82). Moreover, there is a distinct cost disadvantage to using colloid solutions.

Two subsequent systematic reviews have looked at this issue anew. In one meta-analysis of 38 trials comparing colloid to crystalloid for volume expansion, there was no decrease in the risk of death for patients receiving colloid (81). In the other review, albumin administration was actually shown to increase mortality by 6% compared to crystalloid (83). Proposed mechanisms contributing to this worse outcome include anticoagulant properties of albumin (84) and accelerated capillary leak (85).

A drawback of all these systematic reviews, however, has been the limited number of studies that included children other than ill premature neonates. As a result, generalization of these results from ill adults may not be germane to all critically ill, volume-depleted children. For instance, a report of 410 children with meningococcal disease suggests that albumin infusion in this population may not have been harmful, as case fatality rates were lower than predicted (86). Overall, however, there seem to be no substantive data to support the routine use of colloid to complement or replace crystalloid in fluid resuscitation. Rather, repetitive infusions of large volumes of crystalloid seem to be well tolerated in volume-depleted children; do not seem to predispose to excessive rates of acute respiratory distress syndrome or cerebral edema; and in some conditions (e.g., sepsis), play an important role in improved survival (87). A recent survey of pediatric anesthesiologists in western Europe reported that colloid solutions are being used less frequently in infants and older children and suggested that familiarity with some of the issues raised in these systematic reviews is affecting practice patterns (88).

Repetitive infusions of crystalloid may also prove problematic in some children. Most notably, if very large volumes of 0.9% saline are used acutely for volume resuscitation, it is not unusual for children to develop a hyperchloremic metabolic acidosis. This occurs as acidotic peripheral tissues begin to reperfuse and already depleted extracellular bicarbonate stores are diluted by a solution with an isotonic concentration of chloride (78,89). This acidosis can be ameliorated by supplemental doses of bicarbonate as well as the addition of supplemental potassium as needed. There is sometimes a tendency for clinicians to react to the hyperchloremic metabolic acidosis with further saline bolus infusions. In the face of corrected hypoxia or hypovolemia, however, such maneuvers may only exacerbate the chloride-driven acidosis (90). This hyperchloremic acidosis is seen less frequently when Ringer's lactate solution is used as the resuscitation fluid because of the metabolic conversion of lactate to bicarbonate. In the setting of significant preexisting acidosis or underlying hepatic dysfunction preventing the metabolism of lactate, infusion of Ringer's lactate solution may, however, exacerbate an acidosis.

Large-volume infusion of blood may predispose to electrolyte anomalies as well as manifestations of citrate toxicity. If aged whole blood is infused, there is the possibility that a large potassium load is delivered to the patient, as potassium, over time, migrates down its concentration gradient from less viable erythrocytes into plasma. Because most patients receive packed red blood cells instead of whole blood, this potential problem is minimized, as little plasma is infused; thus, the relatively small amount of infused potassium can be accommodated by movement intracellularly.

Citrate is used as the anticoagulant in stored blood. Because citrate complexes with calcium, there can be a fall in ionized calcium levels if large volumes of blood are infused rapidly or if there are concomitant perturbations in calcium homeostasis. Similarly, citrate may complex with magnesium, and magnesium depletion may occur. The liver usually metabolizes infused citrate into bicarbonate. Alkalosis may, therefore, occur if large volumes of citrate are metabolized. In the setting of hepatic dysfunction, however, citrate is not metabolized, serves as an acid load, and helps to create an acidosis or exacerbate any underlying acidosis.

Regardless of the initial infusion with either colloid or crystalloid, once sufficient volume to restore circulatory integrity has been infused, less rapid volume expansion is necessary. During this phase, the rapidity of fluid repletion is most probably not a concern unless there are severe underlying aberrations in the serum sodium or serum osmolality. In the absence of these derangements or profound volume deficit, if the child has improved significantly with the initial parenteral volume expansion, attempts should be made to reinstate oral rehydration. Prolonged intravenous therapy should rarely be needed.

Rapid Rehydration

Over the last decade, a scheme of rapid intravenous resuscitation and follow-up oral rehydration has been adopted by many pediatric emergency departments to successfully treat children with up to 10% dehydration secondary to vomiting and gastroenteritis (91). After infusion of 20 to 30 mL/kg on intravenous crystalloid, the child is allowed to take up to several ounces of a standard oral rehydration fluid; if this intake is tolerated without vomiting for 30 to 60 minutes, then the child is discharged home to continue rehydration, initially with a prescribed volume of standard rehydration solution.

If the child does not tolerate oral rehydration or if there are such significant electrolyte anomalies that there are concerns regarding potential adverse CNS sequelae of too rapid rehydration, then intravenous rehydration may be the best route for continued hydration. It is rare for children to become symptomatic from serum sodium aberrations until levels less than 120 mEq/L or greater than 160 mEq/L are reached. Children who have had very sudden fluxes in electrolytes may become symptomatic earlier. On the other hand, children whose severe sodium abnormalities are believed to be more chronic in nature must be treated in a more controlled fashion, as they are at higher risk for developing CNS symptoms during treatment.

The vast majority of children treated in emergency facilities for volume repletion do well with such rapid rehydration. These children are generally healthy with normal cardiac and renal function and have developed extracellular volume depletion relatively rapidly. As a result, they experience no ill effects from rapid rehydration. In fact, the clinical success of this aggressive restoration of extracellular volume underlies the calls to reexamine the traditional deficit therapy approach to rehydration with its tedious calculations of fluid and electrolytes losses and requirements (4,92).

Symptomatic Hyponatremia

In the setting of symptomatic hyponatremia, especially if the child has seizures, it is important to raise the serum sodium approximately 5 mEq/L acutely. Generally, this results in stabilization of the clinical situation and allows for further evaluation and treatment of the child to proceed in a nonurgent fashion. This is one of the few situations in which hypertonic saline (3% saline) should be used.

To calculate the proper volume of 3% saline to infuse, the child's TBW must be multiplied by the 5-mEq/L desired increase in serum sodium to determine the amount of sodium (in milliequivalents) to infuse. Because every milliliter of 3% saline contains 0.5 mEq of sodium, doubling the number of milliequivalents of sodium needed results in the proper volume in milliliters of 3% saline to infuse. Thus, in the 20-kg child, the TBW is approximately 12 L (0.6 L/kg × 20 kg), and the desired sodium dose is 60 mEq (12 L × 5 mEq/L). If 120 mL of 3% saline were infused, the serum sodium would be expected to rise by approximately 5 mEq/L. The infusion should be given at a rate to increase the serum sodium by no more than 3 mEq/L/hr and is often given more slowly over the course of 3 to 4 hours (93). If the child continues to be symptomatic from hyponatremia after this infusion, additional 3% saline may be given until the symptoms improve or the serum sodium is in the 120 to 125 mEq/L range. At that point, further correction of the hyponatremia should consist of a slower infusion of more dilute saline to cover the sodium deficit, the sodium maintenance needs, and any volume deficit.

Asymptomatic Hyponatremia

If a child has severe hyponatremia but is not symptomatic, there is no need to administer hypertonic saline based solely on a laboratory anomaly. With or without symptoms, in cases of severe hyponatremia, the child should be carefully evaluated as to the etiology of the hyponatremia, keeping in mind that hyponatremia may be the result of an imbalance of water regulation. If this is the case, CH_2O should be restricted and appropriate supplementation with intravenous saline solutions begun to provide maintenance sodium requirements of approximately 2 to 3 mEq/kg/day and any ongoing losses of sodium.

Besides these maintenance sodium needs, if the child has an element of dehydration, every kilogram of body weight lost from baseline represents a 1-L deficit of normal saline from the TBW as well. These losses are often referred to as *isotonic losses*. These account for a sodium deficit of 154 mEq/L that also must be included in the calculations for sodium replacement.

In the setting of hyponatremic dehydration, there have been additional sodium losses as well. Generally, this sodium deficit occurs because stool losses are replaced with fluids with a sodium content less than 60 mEq/L. To estimate these sodium losses, the difference between the child's desired serum sodium and current serum sodium is multiplied by the child's estimated TBW. This product represents the hyponatremic sodium losses that must be added to the maintenance sodium needs, any ongoing losses, and the sodium losses that accompanied weight loss. An example of the calculations and therapeutic maneuvers that need to be considered with significant hyponatremia is presented in the following case study:

A girl who normally weighs 10 kg presents having generalized seizures. She has had 1 week of gastroenteritis with intermittent fever and has been drinking water only, refusing any other feeds for several days. Emergency intravenous access is obtained. Lorazepam is administered, and the seizure activity stops. Blood work is obtained, and the child is weighed and found to be 8.8 kg. A bolus infusion of 200 mL of 0.9% NaCl is administered, after which the girl appears adequately perfused but still lethargic. She no longer has diarrhea but vomits any small volumes of oral rehydration solution offered. The serum sodium is then reported to be 112 mEq/L. While further evaluation of the child's overall status is ongoing, it is important to begin correcting the apparent symptomatic hyponatremia.

The child has actually already received approximately 30 mEq of sodium in the 0.9% NaCl bolus given because of her dehydration and poor perfusion. Given her TBW of roughly 5.4 L (weight in kg × 0.6 L/kg), this should result in her serum sodium having already increased by approximately 5 mEq/L. Because the child has had hyponatremic seizures and is still exhibiting some CNS effect with her lethargy, it is probably prudent to raise the serum sodium by approximately 5 mEq/L so that it is in the 120- to 125-mEq/L range. Because she is hemodynamically stable, it is probably best not to provide an excess of further volume until the child's brain is imaged to assess for cerebral edema, especially given the history of seizures, lethargy, and hyponatremia. By using a small volume of hypertonic saline, the serum sodium could begin to be raised in a controlled manner while further evaluation of the child continues. It would take approximately 22 mEq of sodium (TBW × desired increase in serum sodium = 5.4 L × 5 mEq/L) to accomplish the desired elevation. Because each milliliter of 3% saline contains approximately 0.5 mEq of sodium, a total of 44 mL of 3% saline could be infused over approximately 3 to 4 hours.

In addition to this acute management to restore circulation and perfusion and to raise the serum sodium to a safer level, plans must be formulated to attend to the patient's overall volume and sodium deficit. To prescribe the proper follow-up intravenous fluid, the patient's initial water and electrolyte deficits must be reconciled with her therapy thus far.

The child's water deficit is 1.2 L, reflecting the 1.2-kg weight loss. She has normal maintenance water needs of an additional 1 L/day based on her normal weight of 10 kg. She is having no other ongoing water losses and has already received nearly 250 mL in intravenous fluid in the form of 0.9% NaCl and 3% NaCl. Thus, her current water needs are 1950 mL.

The child's normal maintenance sodium needs are 30 mEq/day (3 mEq/kg/day). She has lost 1.2 kg in body weight that represents 185 mEq of sodium. In addition, she has hyponatremic sodium losses that have arisen as her diarrheal stool was replaced with water alone. To calculate these needs, her normal TBW needs to be multiplied by the difference in her serum sodium from a normal value of 135 mEq/L. Her TBW is 6 L (TBW = 0.6 L/kg × 10 kg), and the difference in serum sodium is 23 mEq/L (135 mEq/L to 112 mEq/L); her hyponatremic losses are, therefore, 138 mEq (6 L × 23 mEq/L). Thus, total sodium needs are 30 mEq of maintenance, 185 mEq of isotonic losses, and 138 mEq of hyponatremic losses, or a total of 353 mEq. She has already received 52 mEq of sodium from the 400 mL of 0.9% NaCl given in the emergency department. Her current sodium needs are, thus, approximately 300 mEq.

To choose the proper solution for this child, the deficit of 1950 mL of water should contain 300 mEq of sodium. This is best approximated by 0.9% NaCl with its NaCl content of 154 mEq/L NaCl. In the past, it has been suggested that half of the fluid and sodium deficit be replaced over 8 hours and the remainder over the ensuing 16 hours. Although such a plan can be followed, there is little evidence that more rapid correction of the hyponatremia is harmful except if the patient has been symptomatic with hyponatremia or has profound asymptomatic hyponatremia of chronic duration. In these cases, it is safest to plan to correct the serum sodium by no more than 12 to 15 mEq/L over 24 hours. More rapid correction has resulted in osmotic demyelination injury to the brain with devastating long-term neurologic outcomes (93,96,97).

Severe Hypernatremia

With hypernatremia, intravenous therapy is again guided by the clinical situation and is usually reserved for those children with very elevated serum sodium values. In cases of hypernatremia due to salt poisoning, there should be signs of overhydration and volume expansion. Excretion of sodium should be enhanced by using a loop diuretic to augment urine sodium losses and by replacing urine output with CH_2O. If the patient has significant renal or cardiac compromise because of the electrolyte imbalance, dialysis and ultrafiltration may be necessary (25,26). With hypernatremia and volume expansion, however, it is detrimental to provide further intravenous saline.

In hypernatremia accompanied by volume loss, any significant alterations in effective circulation should be addressed with 20-mL/kg bolus infusions of an isotonic crystalloid solution until effective peripheral perfusion is restored. Then, further provision of water and sodium should be provided based on calculated water and sodium needs. In the majority of cases, however, with mild elevations in serum sodium and minimal degrees of dehydration, the actual calculation of deficits is probably unnecessary, as the child is hemodynamically stable initially and a candidate for exclusive oral rehydration. In situations in which there is profound hypernatremia or circulatory compromise, it remains necessary, however, to be able to calculate a CH_2O deficit to tailor intravenous rehydration therapy. An example of such a situation is outlined in the following case study:

> After 2 days of refusing any fluid intake, a 5-kg infant with a viral syndrome presents in shock and is 15% dehydrated with a weight of 4.25 kg and a serum sodium of 170 mEq/L. She receives 300 mL of 0.9% NaCl in the emergency department and is now admitted for further therapy.
>
> The child has lost 750 g of weight. Because this is hypernatremic dehydration, there has been loss of water in excess to salt. Thus, part of the weight loss represents isotonic losses, but a larger proportion represents CH_2O loss. The child's CH_2O deficit can be calculated by the following equation:
>
> $$[(\text{serum Na actual})/(\text{serum Na desired}) \times \text{TBW}] - \text{TBW}$$
>
> Substituting the appropriate data for this baby:
>
> $$[(170/145) \times (0.6 \times 4.25)] - (0.6 \times 4.25) =$$
> $$(1.2 \times 2.55) - 2.55 = 0.51 \text{ L}$$
>
> Therefore, of this baby's 750-mL fluid deficit due to dehydration, 510 mL is CH_2O and 240 mL is normal saline.
>
> Too rapid correction of the child's serum sodium with CH_2O could result in cerebral edema as the water infused into the extracellular space follows osmotic forces and moves into the intracellular space. In cases of hypernatremia in which the serum sodium exceeds 160 mEq/L, it is considered safest to correct the serum sodium by no more than 15 mEq/day. In this baby's case, this means that correction to a serum sodium in the normal range would take approximately 2 days.
>
> If the fluid and electrolyte therapy must be given intravenously, the appropriate prescription again depends on calculation of water and sodium requirements and deficits. Her original fluid deficit was 750 mL, and her maintenance water needs are estimated at 500 mL/day. Thus, over the next 2 days, the fluid needs to replace her deficit and to provide maintenance are 1750 mL. Of this, she has already received 300 mL of fluid in the emergency department, so she has a net deficit of 1450 mL.
>
> The baby has maintenance sodium needs of 15 mEq/day (3 mEq/kg/day). Her sodium deficit reflects only her isotonic fluid losses that have been estimated above at 240 mL of normal saline or 37 mEq of sodium. Thus, over the next 2 days, her sodium needs are 67 mEq, of which she has already received the vast majority in the emergency department due to her need for initial volume expansion.
>
> Initiating an infusion of 30 mL/hr of CH_2O should result in the slow and steady correction of the hypernatremia over 2 days. The serum sodium should be monitored every 4 hours initially; if it is falling faster than desired (approximately 0.5 mEq/hr), then sodium should be added to the rehydration fluid.

FLUID AND ELECTROLYTE THERAPY WITH RENAL DYSFUNCTION

Impact of Renal Disease on Fluid and Electrolyte Therapy

Compromised renal function reduces the tolerance for changes in TBW as well as changes in the composition or distribution of volume between the intracellular and extracellular body spaces. Similarly, alterations in electrolyte balance are less readily tolerated because the normal homeostatic mechanisms are frequently perturbed. Thus, in the child with certain renal disorders (e.g., marked nephrosis or significant impairment in renal clearance), it becomes vital to approach the provision of fluids and electrolytes with great care.

As far as fluid therapy is concerned, it is important to recognize that any scheme to provide maintenance fluids or electrolytes presupposes normal renal function. Roughly two-thirds of any daily maintenance fluid prescription is to replace urinary water losses. Similarly, urinary electrolyte losses figure prominently in daily electrolyte balance. In the setting of oliguria or anuria, provision of maintenance fluids could contribute to and potentially exacerbate volume overload, and maintenance electrolyte therapy could result in electrolyte anomalies.

It is better to approach the fluid and electrolyte needs of the child with renal dysfunction in the context of his or her current volume status and electrolyte needs. The patient who is symptomatic due to volume depletion benefits from volume expansion regardless of urine output. Once volume is replete, the child's needs can be reassessed along with his or her current renal function. The child who is volume overloaded is best managed by volume restriction and provision of only insensible fluid losses of approximately 300 mL/m^2. Insensible fluid losses should be considered essentially CH_2O. The child who is volume replete should be kept volume replete. This is most readily accomplished by providing a combination of insensible losses as CH_2O and any other volume losses (urine output, diarrheal stool, surgical drain output, vomitus) on an additional milliliter-for-milliliter basis. If there are significant ongoing losses from a single source, the electrolyte composition of this fluid can be assayed so that the replacement fluid may more accurately reflect the electrolyte losses. Otherwise, a solution of 0.45% NaCl can be used initially and altered as the clinical situation continues to develop and further electrolyte determinations are made.

If the child's volume status or the adequacy of renal function is difficult to discern initially, it is probably best to provide the child with replacement of both insensible and ongoing losses. This should maintain the child's current volume status and allow for further determination of the appropriateness of more vigorous hydration or, conversely, fluid restriction as the clinical situation clarifies. Monitoring the child's weight on at least a daily basis and documenting the child's total fluid intake and output also assists in arriving at a proper hydration regimen.

Assessing the child's current electrolyte status and monitoring the loss of electrolytes in the urine or in any other source of significant electrolyte losses assist in tailoring the daily electrolyte prescription. An understanding of the pathophysiology underlying the child's renal dysfunction is also useful. The child who has profound tubular electrolyte losses requires more sodium on a daily basis than the child who is edematous and has total body salt overloaded from his or her nephrotic syndrome. The child with chronic renal insufficiency and hypertension mediated by long-standing salt and water overload may actually benefit from diuretic therapy to remove salt and water rather than any further volume expansion with saline.

Certainly, the provision of supplemental potassium to the child with renal dysfunction must be done judiciously. The oliguric or anuric child should receive no potassium until it is well documented that serum potassium levels are low or that there are extrarenal potassium losses (e.g., gut losses from diarrheal stool). The child with marginal renal function should receive small amounts of potassium (approximately 1 mEq/kg/day) with at least daily assessment of electrolyte balance to reassess the adequacy and appropriateness of continued potassium supplementation.

Fluid and Electrolyte Therapy in the Intensive Care Unit

Many children who are critically ill present a challenge to the clinician attempting to prescribe appropriate fluid and electrolyte therapy. Oftentimes, there may be renal dysfunction, and frequently there may be multiorgan failure complicating management decisions. What frequently creates significant fluid and electrolyte anomalies is rather rote reliance on standard formulas to prescribe fluid and electrolyte therapy. Rather than relying exclusively on a set maintenance requirement of fluid or electrolytes, it is almost always best to assess the patient's individual fluid and electrolyte needs in the context of the underlying pathophysiology, volume status, the efficacy of tissue perfusion, current ventilatory requirements, and current renal function. Whenever there is concern about incipient or exacerbating volume overload, it is important to review the volume and types of fluids being provided. Increasing the concentration of continuous medication drips and assessing medication compatibility for simultaneous infusion are important steps in limiting total daily fluid input. Initially, it is often appropriate in these critically ill children to ascertain that their intravascular space is replete to help maintain hemodynamic stability. Once the patient is believed to be intravascularly replete, maintaining euvolemia by providing insensible water losses as well as replacing any ongoing fluid and electrolyte losses should maintain the patient in fluid and electrolyte balance.

Oftentimes, despite a desire to limit fluids in the critically ill child, medication requirements, nutritional needs, and hemodynamic insufficiency may result in the development of significant volume overload. There may also be situations in which due to the "vascular leak" phenomenon, the critically ill child becomes massively volume overloaded but has a decreased effective circulating volume. In other words, renal and tissue perfusion may be a sluggish because fluid has leaked from the intravascular space into the interstitial space. In this setting, there may be a need to continue to administer large volumes of fluid to maintain circulatory integrity with the knowledge that such infusions only exacerbate the total body fluid overload. Aggressive diuretic therapy may prove useful especially if renal function is not compromised. Combination diuretic therapy using agents that work at separate sites along the renal tubule may be necessary. Ultimately, the use of either periodic or continuous ultrafiltration may be beneficial to these patients by allowing ongoing fluid administration but limiting the daily imbalance between fluid intake and output. Ultrafiltration may be accomplished via peritoneal dialysis, by intermittent hemodialysis with ultrafiltration, or by using one of the slow continuous ultrafiltration techniques now known as *continuous renal replacement therapy*.

If ultrafiltration is initiated, extreme vigilance is necessary to prevent exacerbation of intravascular depletion and the development of prerenal azotemia or frank renal failure. Special care must be taken with the continuous modalities to insure that ultrafiltration rates are periodically reassessed and readjusted. Furthermore, because the electrolyte losses that accompany the ultrafiltration of fluid are isotonic, the electrolyte content of infused fluids must be adjusted to match the composition of the ultrafiltrate. Serum electrolyte values need to be followed in a serial fashion with periodic review and readjustment of the composition of supplemental intravenous fluids.

Alterations in Serum Sodium Complicated by Renal Failure

Because of the important contribution of serum sodium to serum osmolality, alterations in serum sodium, especially coupled with alterations in BUN related to renal failure, can complicate the usual approach to a child with fluid and electrolyte anomalies. Generally, there are greater concerns with hypernatremia and renal failure, as the need to correct the sodium in a slow fashion can be problematic when renal replacement therapy needs to be initiated for clearance of urea. Balancing the correction of sodium and the hyperosmolar state with the clearance of urea requires a carefully considered plan that is grounded in a firm understanding of fluid and electrolyte homeostasis.

In most cases of hypernatremia related to severe dehydration, some degree of acute renal insufficiency is present. This renal failure is usually prerenal in nature, a result of a decreased effective circulating volume rather than an intrinsic glomerular or tubular disorder. Most often, in the course of rapid restoration of perfusion and early rehydration, the urine output increases, and the azotemia begins to resolve.

Alternatively, there are occasional cases in which, due to intrinsic renal dysfunction or acute tubular necrosis, the renal insufficiency does not respond to volume infusion; in fact, the provision of excess volume may contribute to significant volume overload. In these cases, there may be need to consider some form of renal replacement therapy to assist in the controlled correction of fluid and electrolyte derangements, especially if the renal failure is oliguric or anuric in nature. Such an example is detailed in the following case study:

> A 15-year-old boy presents with a several-week history of polyuria, severe weight loss, fatigue, and poor oral intake. He is diagnosed by his pediatrician as having diabetes mellitus with ketoacidosis and is referred to an emergency department for management. At this point, his serum sodium is 154 mEq/L, his creatinine is 3.0 mg/dL, and his BUN is 30 mg/dL. In the emergency department, the child receives several bolus infusions of normal saline supplemented with sodium bicarbonate and is started on an insulin drip. He is admitted and continues to receive brisk intravenous hydration with normal saline with bicarbonate supplementation. He is noted to be oliguric, and this does not improve with several more hours of hydration with normal saline. The next morning, laboratory values reveal a serum sodium of 165 mEq/L, a creatinine of 4.5 mg/dL, and a BUN of 50 mg/dL. He has made only 75 mL of urine in the last 8 hours and is developing some mild peripheral edema.
>
> In this case, the renal insufficiency and poor urine output have complicated the usual management of diabetic ketoacidosis and have exacerbated an underlying hypernatremia. Given the patient's evolving renal failure, it is not feasible to provide the necessary volume of CH_2O to correct the hypernatremia without contributing to further volume overload. Because of the apparent progressive renal failure, it is also useful to correct the hypernatremia in case dialysis becomes necessary for urea clearance. By performing controlled ultrafiltration on the patient and replacing back with CH_2O the volume ultrafiltered, the serum sodium could be corrected without exacerbating the volume status.

With a serum sodium of 165 mEq/L and an estimated TBW of 42 L (70 kg × 0.6 L/kg), this patient has CH_2O needs of 7.5 L to lower his serum sodium to the 140-mEq/L range [(165/140 × 42) – 42]. Because the patient is now significantly hypernatremic and has been subject to various fluid and electrolyte shifts as his diabetic ketoacidosis has been treated, it is prudent to correct his serum sodium by no more than 10 to 12 mEq/day over the course of 3 days. Thus, if the patient is ultrafiltered for 2.5 L/day, and the ultrafiltration volume each day is replaced back as CH_2O, the serum sodium should be in the normal range in 3 days' time. The ultrafiltration goal could be achieved over the course of a few hours each day if the patient were hemodynamically stable or over a more prolonged period of time each day if there were concerns regarding hypotension. Thus, a conventional hemodialysis setup could be used for relatively rapid ultrafiltration only or a continuous filtration circuit for either rapid or slow filtration.

Because the fluid removed in ultrafiltration is isonatremic to the serum sodium, the sodium concentration of each liter of ultrafiltrate should mirror the serum sodium concentration at the time of ultrafiltration. Thus, on the initial day of ultrafiltration, each liter of ultrafiltrate should contain a sodium content of 165 mEq/L. By providing back the volume ultrafiltered each day as CH_2O, the serum sodium content is expected to fall, in this case, by approximately 8 to 10 mEq/L/day.

It is important to recognize that CH_2O must be provided back to the patient to make up for the ultrafiltration losses. Otherwise, because the ultrafiltrate is isotonic, there is no change in the serum sodium concentration, and the ultrafiltration may potentially exacerbate the renal failure by depleting the intravascular space and the effective circulating volume.

Moreover, it is also important to recognize that the patient's overall daily fluid needs are greater than the daily ultrafiltration volume alone, as maintenance fluid requirements and any ongoing fluid losses must also be considered. Because the patient is in renal failure, his maintenance fluid needs are scaled back to insensible losses of 300 $mL/M^2/day$; in this case, there are no ongoing losses. Thus, each day for the next 3 days, this 70-kg patient needs to receive approximately 500 mL/day of insensible losses and 2500 mL/day of ultrafiltration replacement, or a total of 3000 mL/day. His maintenance sodium requirements are 3 mEq/kg/day. Although it may seem counterintuitive to provide a hypernatremic patient with maintenance sodium, disregarding these requirements results in a more rapid correction of the hypernatremia than desired. If the child were to receive a saline infusion of 0.45% NaCl at a rate of 125 mL/hr, this would provide just over 3 mEq/kg/day of sodium in a total volume of 3 L/day.

If the child with hypernatremia has profound renal failure and requires dialysis for urea clearance, the dialysis prescription must take into account the need to slowly correct the serum sodium. Normally, regardless of the modality of renal replacement therapy, most dialysate contains sodium isotonic to the normal serum sodium range. It may prove detrimental, however, to dialyze a patient who is very hypernatremic against a dialysate with a sodium concentration at least 30 mEq/L less than the patient's serum sodium concentration. The diffusional gradient during dialysis leads to more rapid correction of the serum sodium than the desired drop of approximately 1 mEq every 2 hours.

Although most hemodialysis machines can be readjusted so that the dialysate produced has a sodium content as high as the low to mid-150s, this still may not reduce the gradient sufficiently in cases of severe hypernatremia. In those situations, by maximizing the sodium concentration of the dialysate and by performing dialysis for limited amounts of time, one can minimize the drop in serum sodium. Still, there need to be frequent assessments of the serum sodium concentration, and overall clearance may need to be sacrificed to prevent too rapid correction of the serum sodium and a rapid concomitant decrease in the serum urea that may increase the chances for dialysis dysequilibrium.

Alternatively, a continuous hemodiafiltration technique such as continuous venovenous hemodiafiltration can be performed. By asking the hospital pharmacy to increase the sodium content of the dialysate fluid to within 10 to 12 mEq/L of the serum sodium concentration, the diffusional gradient for sodium clearance can be minimized. Then, by making appropriate adjustments in the sodium content of the dialysate as the serum sodium falls, the serum sodium levels can be reduced gradually by 10 to 12 mEq/L/day while adequate urea clearance and ultrafiltration for most situations are achieved.

Peritoneal dialysis has also been used in cases of severe hypernatremia (94,95). Again, the concentration of sodium in the dialysate may need to be adjusted upward in severe hypernatremia to prevent too rapid clearance of sodium. In addition, because the degree of clearance and ultrafiltration may not be as precisely controlled as with hemodialysis or hemodiafiltration, frequent assessment of electrolyte values is necessary. Manipulation of dwell volumes and dwell times also influences overall clearance, and the use of smaller dwell volumes for longer periods of time helps to minimize sodium clearance.

In contradistinction to hypernatremia, because hyperosmolality is less common with hyponatremia, in some ways it is easier to use renal replacement therapy in the setting of severe hyponatremia and concomitant renal insufficiency. Again, the focus needs to be on the rapidity of the correction of the serum sodium. In conditions of chronic severe but asymptomatic hyponatremia, the rate of correction of serum sodium should parallel the rate of correction recommended in hypernatremia—approximately 10 to 12 mEq/L/day. Correction of chronic hyponatremia at a more rapid rate has been associated with the development of central pontine demyelinosis.

All of the manipulations described above for hypernatremia and renal failure can be used with hyponatremia and renal failure with the understanding that the dialysate sodium concentration should now not exceed the serum sodium value by 10 to 12 mEq/L. Conventional hemodialysis machines can be adjusted to produce dialysate with a sodium concentration as low as the mid-120s. In the very rare situation in which a child with profound hypernatremia (less than 110 mEq/L) was being hemodialyzed, brief hemodialysis runs may be necessary initially to prevent too rapid correction of the serum sodium level and the attendant risk of central pontine demyelinosis. If dialysate is being custom prepared for peritoneal dialysis or hemodiafiltration, precise alterations in the electrolyte content can be made more readily to reduce the sodium gradient.

The local resources, the training of ancillary staff, the unique circumstances of each patient, and the comfort of the clinician with different modalities of renal replacement therapy guide the choice of therapy when faced with renal failure and significant serum sodium anomalies. The actual modality of renal replacement therapy used is less important than careful attention to the rate of correction of the electrolyte anomaly, to the rate of urea clearance being achieved, and to the clinical response of the patient to ongoing therapy.

REFERENCES

1. Cosnett JE. The origins of intravenous therapy. *Lancet* 1989;1:768–771.
2. Gamble JL. Early history of fluid replacement therapy. *Pediatrics* 1953;11:554–567.
3. Holliday MA, Segar WE. The maintenance need for water in parenteral fluid therapy. *Pediatrics* 1957;19:823–832.
4. Holliday M. The evolution of therapy for dehydration: should deficit therapy still be taught? *Pediatrics* 1996;98: 171–177.
5. Mahalanabis D, Snyder JD. Fluid and dietary therapy of diarrhoea. In: Walker WA, Durie PR, Hamilton JR, et al., eds. *Pediatric gastrointestinal disease: pathophysiology, diagnosis, management.* Philadelphia: Decker BC, 1996:1843–1850.
6. Schwartz R. Comments from another student of Gamble and Darrow on fluids. *Pediatrics* 1996;98:314.
7. Haas RE. Ions and IVs: Are we still using the Henry Ford model? *CRNA* 1996;7:71–80.

8. Yoshioka T, Iitaka K, Ichikawa I. Body fluid compartments. In: Ichikawa I, ed. *Pediatric textbook of fluids and electrolytes.* Baltimore: Williams & Wilkins, 1990:14–20.
9. Finberg L. Severe dehydration secondary to diarrhea. In: Dickerman JD, Lucey JF, eds. *The critically ill child: diagnosis and medical management,* 3rd ed. Philadelphia: WB Saunders, 1985:65–77.
10. Rose BD, Rennke HG. Regulation of salt and water balance. In: Rose BD, Rennke HG, eds. *Renal pathophysiology—the essentials.* Baltimore: Williams & Wilkins, 1994:29–66.
11. Talbot NB, Crawford JD, Butler AM. Homeostatic limits to safe parenteral fluid therapy. *N Engl J Med* 1953;248:1100–1108.
12. Clemmons MR. Fluid and electrolyte disorders. In: Merenstein GB, Kaplan DW, Rosenberg AA, eds. *Handbook of pediatrics,* 16th ed. Norwalk, CT: Appleton & Lange, 1991:107–117.
13. Besunder JB. Abnormalities in fluids, minerals, and glucose. In: Blumer JL, ed. *A practical guide to pediatric intensive care,* 3rd ed. St. Louis: Mosby–Year Book, 1990:545–563.
14. Trachtman H. Sodium and water homeostasis. *Pediatr Clin North Am* 1995;42:1343–1363.
15. Rose BD, Rennke HG. Disorders of water balance: hyponatremia, hypernatremia, and polyuria. In: Rose BD, Rennke HG, eds. *Renal pathophysiology—the essentials.* Baltimore: Williams & Wilkins, 1994:67–96.
16. Gerigk M, Gnehm HE, Rascher W. Arginine vasopressin and renin in acutely ill children: implication for fluid therapy. *Acta Paediatr* 1996;85:550–553.
17. Halberthal M, Halperin ML, Bohn D. Lesson of the week: acute hyponatraemia in children admitted to hospital: retrospective analysis of factors contributing to its development and resolution. *BMJ* 2001;322:780–782.
18. Choi M, Szerlip HM. Sodium and volume homeostasis. In: Szerlip HM, Goldfarb S, eds. *Workshops in fluid and electrolyte disorders.* New York: Churchill Livingstone, 1993:1–24.
19. Badr K, Ichikawa I. Physical and biological properties of body fluids and electrolytes. In: Ichikawa I, ed. *Pediatric textbook of fluids and electrolytes.* Baltimore: Williams & Wilkins, 1990:3–13.
20. Strange K. Regulation of solute and water balance and cell volume in the central nervous system. *J Am Soc Nephrol* 1992;3:12–27.
21. Morrison G. Hypernatremia. In: Szerlip HM, Goldfarb S, eds. *Workshops in fluid and electrolyte disorders.* New York: Churchill Livingstone, 1993:49–69.
22. Rose BD. Hypoosmolal states—hyponatremia. In: Rose BD, ed. *Clinical physiology of acid-base and electrolyte disorders.* New York: McGraw-Hill, 1989:601–638.
23. Conley SB. Hypernatremia. *Pediatr Clin North Am* 1990; 37:365–372.
24. Robertson GL. Physiology of ADH secretion. *Kidney Int* 1987;32:S20–S26.
25. Yang CW, Kim YS, Park IS, et al. Treatment of severe acute hypernatremia and renal failure by hemodialysis. *Nephron* 1995;70:372–373.
26. Pazmino PA, Pazmino BP. Treatment of acute hypernatremia with hemodialysis. *Am J Nephrol* 1993;13:260–265.
27. Molteni KH. Initial management of hypernatremic dehydration in the breastfed infant. *Clin Pediatr* 1994;33:731–740.
28. Baylis PH, Cheetham T. Diabetes insipidus. *Arch Dis Child* 1998;79:84–89.
29. Robertson GL. Abnormalities of thirst regulation. *Kidney Int* 1984;25:460–469.
30. Murphy MS. Guidelines for managing acute gastroenteritis based on a systematic review of published research. *Arch Dis Child* 1998;79:279–284.
31. Saavedra JM, Harris GD, Li S, et al. Capillary refilling (skin turgor) in the assessment of dehydration. *Am J Dis Child* 1991;145:296–298.
32. Gorelick MS, Shaw KN, Baker MD. Effects of ambient temperature on capillary refill in children. *Pediatrics* 1993; 92:699–702.
33. Baraff LJ. Capillary refill: Is it a useful clinical sign? *Pediatrics* 1993;92:723–724.
34. Duggan C, Refat M, Hashem M, et al. How valid are clinical signs of dehydration in infants? *J Pediatr Gastroenterol Nutr* 1996;22:56–61.
35. Mackenzie A, Barnes G, Shann F. Clinical signs of dehydration in children. *Lancet* 1989;2:605–607.
36. Vega RM, Avner JR. A prospective study of the usefulness of clinical and laboratory parameters for predicting percentage of dehydration in children. *Pediatr Emerg Care* 1997;13: 179–182.
37. Teach SJ, Yates EW, Feld LG. Laboratory predictors of fluid deficit in acutely dehydrated children. *Clin Pediatr (Phila)* 1997;36:395–400.
38. Yilmaz K, Karabocuoglu M, Citak A, et al. Evaluation of laboratory tests in dehydrated children with acute gastroenteritis. *J Paediatr Child Health* 2002;38:226–228.
39. Conway SP, Phillips RR, Panday S. Admission to hospital with gastroenteritis. *Arch Dis Child* 1990;65:579–584.
40. Jenkins HR, Ansari BM. Management of gastroenteritis. *Arch Dis Child* 1990;65:939–941.
41. Ellis ME, Watson B, Mandal BK, et al. Contemporary gastroenteritis of infancy: clinical features and prehospital management. *BMJ* 1984;288:521–523.
42. Armon K, Stephenson T, McFaul R, et al. An evidence and consensus based guideline for acute diarrhoea management. *Arch Dis Child* 2001;85:132–141.
43. American Academy of Pediatrics, Provisional Committee on Quality Improvement Subcommittee on Acute Gastroenteritis. Practice parameter: the management of acute gastroenteritis in young children. *Pediatrics* 1996;97:424–436.
44. Duggan C, Santosham M, Glass RI. The management of acute diarrhea in children: oral rehydration, maintenance, and nutritional therapy. Centers for Disease Control and Prevention. *MMWR Recomm Rep* 1992;41:1–20.
45. Pierce NF, Sack RB, Mitra R, et al. Replacement of electrolyte and water losses in cholera by an oral glucose-electrolyte solution. *Ann Intern Med* 1969;70:1173–1181.
46. Mahalanbais D, Wallace CK, Kallen RJ, et al. Water and electrolyte losses due to cholera in small children and infants: a recovery balance study. *Pediatrics* 1970;45:374–385.
47. Pizzaro D, Posada G, Mata L, et al. Oral rehydration of neonates with dehydrating diarrhoea. *Lancet* 1979;2:1209–1210.
48. Mauer AM, Dweck HS, Finberg L, et al. American Academy of Pediatrics Committee on Nutrition: use of oral fluid

therapy and posttreatment feeding following enteritis in children in a developed country. *Pediatrics* 1985;75:358–361.
49. Santosham M, Greenough WB. Oral rehydration therapy: a global perspective. *J Pediatr* 1991;118:S44–S51.
50. Finberg L. The role of oral electrolyte-glucose solutions in hydration for children—international and domestic aspects. *Pediatrics* 1980;96:51–54.
51. Nalin DR, Cash RA, Islam R, et al. Oral maintenance therapy for cholera in adults. *Lancet* 1968;2:370–372.
52. Hirschhorn N, Kinzie JL, Sachar D, et al. Decrease in net stool output in cholera during intestinal perfusion with glucose containing solutions. *N Engl J Med* 1968;279:176–181.
53. Phillips RA. Water and electrolyte losses in cholera. *Fed Proc* 1964;23:705–712.
54. World Health Organization. *Treatment and prevention of dehydration in diarrheal disease. A guide for use at the primary level.* Geneva: WHO, 1976.
55. World Health Organization. Cholera: can rehydration therapy be improved? *WHO Drug Information* 2000;14:88.
56. Nalin DR, Harland E, Ramlal A, et al. Comparison of low and high sodium and potassium content in oral rehydration solutions. *J Pediatr* 1980;97:848–853.
57. Snyder JD. Use and misuse of oral therapy for diarrhea: comparisons of US practices with American Academy of Pediatrics recommendations. *Pediatrics* 1991;87:28–33.
58. Leung AKC, Taylor PG, Geoffroy L, et al. Efficacy and safety of two oral solutions as maintenance therapy for acute diarrhea. *Clin Pediatr* 1988;27:359–364.
59. Santosham M, Daum RS, Dillman L, et al. Oral rehydration therapy of infantile diarrhea: a controlled study of well nourished children hospitalized in the United States and Panama. *N Engl J Med* 1986;306:1070–1076.
60. Pizarro D, Posada G, Levine MM. Hypernatremic diarrheal dehydration treated with "slow" (12-hour) oral rehydration therapy: a preliminary report. *J Pediatr* 1984;104:316–319.
61. Pizarro D, Posada G, Villavicencio N, et al. Oral rehydration in hypernatremic and hyponatremic diarrheal dehydration. *Am J Dis Child* 1983;137:730–734.
62. Pizarro D, Posada G, Villavicencio N, et al. Oral rehydration in hyper- and hyponatremic diarrheal dehydration. *Am J Dis Child* 1983;137:730–734.
63. Pizarro D, Posada G, Levine MM, et al. Oral rehydration of infants with acute diarrhoeal dehydration: a practical method. *J Trop Med Hyg* 1980;83:241–245.
64. Wittenberg DF, Ramji S. Paediatric diarrhoea—rehydration therapy revisited. *S Afr Med J* 1995;85:655–658.
65. Ozuah PO, Avner JR, Stein RE. Oral rehydration, emergency physicians, and practice parameters: a national survey. *Pediatrics* 2002;109:259–261.
66. Avery ME, Snyder JD. Oral therapy for acute diarrhea: the underused simple solution. *N Engl J Med* 1990;323:891–894.
67. Tanzi VL. An econometric study of the adoption of oral rehydration solution in Bangladesh. *Dissertation Abstracts International* 1999;60:1563.
68. Chowdhury AM, Karim F, Sarkar SK, et al. The status of ORT (oral rehydration therapy) in Bangladesh: how widely is it used? *Health Policy Plan* 1997;12:58–66.
69. Gavin N, Merrick N, Davidson B. Efficacy of glucose-based oral rehydration therapy. *Pediatrics* 1996;98:45–51.
70. Santucci KA, Anderson AC, Lewander WJ, et al. Frozen oral hydration as an alternative to conventional enteral fluids. *Arch Pediatr Adolesc Med* 1998;152:142–146.
71. Ladinsky M, Duggan A, Santosham M, et al. The World Health Organization oral rehydration solution in US pediatric practice: a randomized trial to evaluate parent satisfaction. *Arch Pediatr Adolesc Med* 2000;154:700–705.
72. American Academy of Pediatrics, Provisional Committee on Quality Improvement, Subcommittee on Acute Gastroenteritis. Practice parameter: the management of acute gastroenteritis in young children. *Pediatrics* 1996;97:424–435.
73. Rabbani GH. The search for a better oral rehydration solution for cholera. New *Engl J Med* 2000;342:345–347.
74. Hahn S, Kim S, Garner P. Reduced osmolarity oral rehydration solution for treating dehydration caused by acute diarrhoea in children. *Cochrane Database Syst Rev* 2002;1:CD002847.
75. Fontaine O, Gore SM, Pierce NF. Rice-based oral rehydration solution for treating diarrhoea. *Cochrane Database Syst Rev* 2000;2:CD000567.
76. International Study Group on reduced-osmolarity ORS solutions. Multicentre evaluation of reduced-osmolarity oral rehydration salts solution. *Lancet* 1995;345:282–285.
77. Hahn S, Kim Y, Garner P. Reduced osmolarity oral rehydration solution for treating dehydration due to diarrhoea in children: systematic review. *BMJ* 2001;323:81–85.
78. DeBruin WJ, Greenwald BM, Notterman DA. Fluid resuscitation in pediatrics. *Crit Care Clin* 1992;8:423–438.
79. Awazu M, Devarajan P, Stewart CL, et al. "Maintenance" therapy and treatment of dehydration and overhydration. In: Ichikawa I, ed. *Pediatric textbook of fluids and electrolytes.* Baltimore: Williams & Wilkins, 1990:417–428.
80. Tullis JL. Albumin. 2. Guidelines for clinical uses. *JAMA* 1977;237:460–463.
81. Alderson P, Schierhout G, Roberts I, et al. Colloids versus crystalloids for fluid resuscitation in critically ill patients. *Cochrane Database Syst Rev* 2000;2:CD000567.
82. Bisonni RS, Holtgrave DR, Lawler F, et al. Colloid versus crystalloids in fluid resuscitation: an analysis of randomized controlled trials. *J Fam Pract* 1991;32:387–390.
83. The Cochrane Injuries Group Albumin Reviewers. Human albumin administration in critically ill patients. *Cochrane Database Syst Rev* 2000;2.
84. Soni N. Wonderful albumin? *BMJ* 1995;310:887–888.
85. Fleck A, Raines G, Hawker F, et al. Increased vascular permeability: a major cause of hypoalbuminaemia in disease and injury. *Lancet* 1985;1:781–784.
86. Nichani S. Albumin: saint or sinner? *Arch Dis Child* 1999;81:189.
87. Carcillo JA, Fields AI. Clinical practice parameters for hemodynamic support of pediatric and neonatal patients in septic shock. *Crit Care Med* 2002;30:1365–1378.
88. Soderlind M, Salvignol G, Izard P, et al. Use of albumin, blood transfusion and intraoperative glucose by APA and ADARPEF members: a postal study. *Paediatr Anaesth* 2001;11:685–689.

89. Hirschhorn N. The treatment of acute diarrhea in children: an historical and physiological perspective. *Am J Clin Nutr* 1980;33:637–663.
90. Skellett S, Mayer A, Durward A, et al. Chasing the base deficit: hyperchloraemic acidosis following 0.9% saline fluid resuscitation. *Arch Dis Child* 2000;83:514–516.
91. Reid SR, Bonadio WA. Outpatient rapid intravenous rehydration to correct dehydration and resolve vomiting in children with acute gastroenteritis. *Ann Emerg Med* 1996;28:318–323.
92. Holliday MA, Friedman AL, Wassner SJ. Extracellular fluid restoration in dehydration: a critique of rapid versus slow. *Pediatr Nephrol* 1999;13:292–297.
93. Oh MS, Kim H-J, Carroll HJ. Recommendations for treatment of symptomatic hyponatremia. *Nephron* 1995;70:143–150.
94. Miller NI, Finberg L. Peritoneal dialysis for salt poisoning. *N Engl J Med* 1960;263:1347–1350.
95. Finberg L, Kiley J, Luttrell CN. Mass accidental salt poisoning in infancy. *JAMA* 1963;184:187–190.
96. Pradhan S, Jha R, Singh MN, et al. Central pontine myelinolysis following "slow" correction of hyponatremia. *Clin Neurol Neurosurg* 1995;97:340–343.
97. Faber MD, Kupin WL, Heilig CW, et al. Common fluid-electrolyte and acid-base problems in the intensive care unit: selected issues. *Semin Nephrol* 1994;14:8–22.

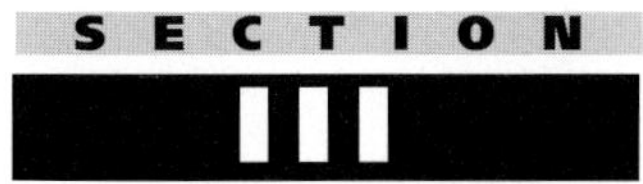

RESEARCH METHODS

14

MOLECULAR BIOLOGY

FRANCESCO EMMA
GIAN MARCO GHIGGERI

OVERVIEW OF MOLECULAR CELL BIOLOGY

The discipline of molecular biology began in the mid-1940s through an effort by scientists to discover the universal laws that govern the process of self-replication in living organisms (1). Earlier efforts by Mendel, Wilson, Morgan, and Garrod to study genetic inheritance used organisms with complex genomes. These studies were based entirely on the natural breeding systems of the organisms that were analyzed. As a result, a factor that determined a phenotypic future (i.e., a gene) could be shown to reside at a specific location, or locus. Until the advent of molecular biology, the concept of genes and loci remained intangible. Chromosomal loci were merely the sites determining differences, usually between "normal" and "mutant," and genes remained detectable only if mutated (2).

From the 1940s through the 1960s, these concepts were revolutionized. After Beadle and Tatum had established for the first time a link between genes and proteins, Griffith and Avery proposed that DNA was the molecule containing genetic information. Soon after, work by Wilkins, Franklin, Watson, and Crick described the structure of DNA as a double helix. The discovery of the genetic code and the establishment of the role of RNA in the synthesis of proteins laid the foundations for the development of modern-day molecular biology (3).

Efforts by many scientists have provided key technological innovations since the 1960s, allowing recombinant DNA technology to be applied to a wide variety of biologic problems. Major milestones include the discovery of restriction nucleases and DNA ligases; the development of DNA libraries (4), DNA cloning procedures, nucleic acid hybridization techniques, rapid sequencing techniques (5), and the polymerase chain reaction (PCR) (6); and the production of transgenic animals (7). These advances permit detection, amplification, and engineering of DNA sequences and delineation of the role of genes in cellular physiology and pathophysiology (2).

The molecular revolution has affected all of the sciences, including medical and clinical research, and has culminated in the completion of the human genome project (8). It has provided new insight into the complexity of living organisms that can only be partially studied with commonly available techniques.

The complexity of biologic systems presents new challenges for molecular biology in the post-genomic era. Recent progress in microengineering, computer technology, and bioinformatics has led to the development of nanotechnologies and to the emergence of new fields of investigation, including functional genomics and proteomics.

Basic Concepts

Central Dogma

The research efforts described led to the formulation of the so-called central dogma of molecular biology soon after the discovery of DNA structure in 1953. According to the central dogma, DNA sequences are transcribed into RNA molecules that carry the flow of genetic information out of the nucleus to be translated into proteins (1,3). These processes have been well defined and are detailed in most introductory cell biology texts (3,9). The simple concept of a one-way flow of information from DNA to RNA to protein has been thoroughly revised. Genetic information is conveyed in both directions through a complex series of feedback loops.

Proteins and Nucleic Acids: Different Molecules with Common Features Linked by a Genetic Code

Both DNA and proteins are composed of a limited number of units that are assembled sequentially in a step-by-step process that always proceeds in one unique direction (9). The link between nucleic acids and proteins is provided by the genetic code. To translate four nucleotides into 20 different amino acids, groups of at least three nucleotides (codons) yielding 64 possibilities are required. Of these, 61 correspond to specific amino acids, whereas three correspond to termination codons. The code is said to be degenerate, as it contains redundancies. Codons corresponding to the same amino acid generally differ by the nucleotide in the third position (3,9).

As a consequence of the degeneracy of the genetic code, nucleotide substitutions (point mutations) in the third nucleotide of a given codon may not change the primary sequence of a protein and are frequently found in nature, as they are not subject to natural selection. Point mutations in the first and second position result in an amino acid substitution or in a termination codon, either of which can dramatically alter protein structure and function.

In principle, each messenger RNA (mRNA) can be translated in any of the three possible reading frames determined by overlapping triplet codes. With few exceptions, only one reading frame produces a functional protein because stop codons encountered in the other two reading frames terminate translation. As the only punctuation signal is located at the start codon (ATG), the reading frame is set at the beginning of the translation and proceeds until a termination codon is reached. Thus, finding the correct reading frame and locating the start codon are essential steps in the process of cloning genes and defining their protein products. Mutations causing the deletion or insertion of one or two nucleotides result in a shift of the reading frame (frame-shift mutations) and cause the production of aberrant protein products.

Gene Structure

The complementary strands of chromosomal DNA are arranged in an antiparallel fashion as dictated by hydrogen bond pairing of nucleotide bases. It is estimated that the human genome is composed of approximately 3 billion base pairs of DNA containing 30,000 to 100,000 genes arrayed on 23 pairs of chromosomes (10). Overall, the amount of DNA containing genes comprises a minority of nuclear DNA.

Traditionally, a gene is depicted as a "transcriptional unit" as illustrated in Figure 14.1. The DNA double helix is represented as a line interrupted by rectangular boxes corresponding to exons, with its 5' end on the left and its 3' end on the right. Each gene is divided into two major regions, namely the promoter and the coding regions.

Typically, the promoter region is located upstream near the 5' boundary of the coding region and contains clusters of short sequences (fewer than ten base pairs) spread over a few hundred bases that bind transcription factors. These regulatory proteins mediate the attachment and activation of type II RNA polymerase, which mediates the transcription along the DNA while unwinding the duplex and adding nucleotides to the growing RNA molecule. DNA sequences in the promoter region that bind to transcription factors are referred as cis-*acting* elements. In some cases, transcription factors also interact with other *cis*-acting elements (termed *enhancers*) that are located at a greater distance (up to a few thousand bases) from the promoter.

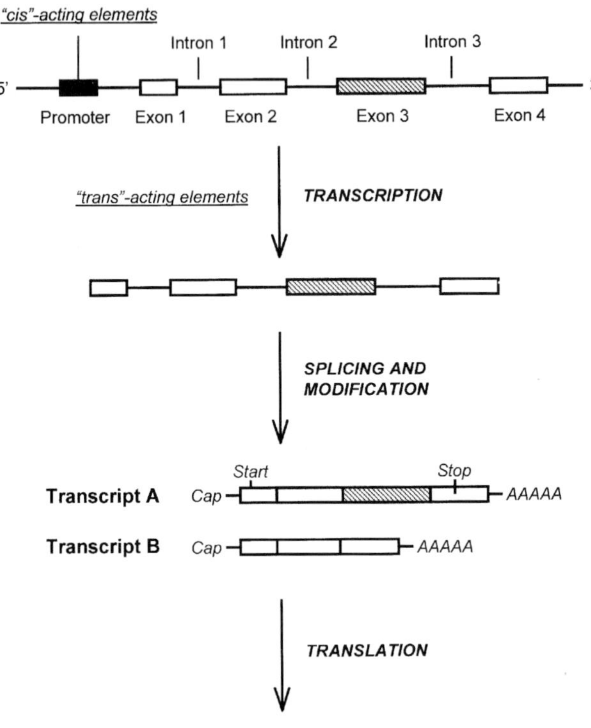

FIGURE 14.1. General organization and processing of a eukaryotic gene. A gene consisting of four exons and three introns is shown. The promoter region (*black box*) is located near the 5' end of the gene. Transcription of the gene yields a primary messenger RNA (mRNA) transcript that contains both exon and intron sequences. Differential splicing of this mRNA transcript yields two mature mRNA species by inclusion or exclusion of exon 3 (*hashed box*). To be exported into the cytosol and translated, mRNAs need to be modified by polyadenylation of their 3' end and capping of their 5' end with methylated guanosines. Differential splicing results in two different protein isoforms that are encoded by a single gene.

The physical gap between the enhancer and the promoter explains the need for accessory factors that convey transcriptional signals to the RNA-polymerase through protein-protein interactions (Fig. 14.2). All molecules, generally proteins, which are physically involved in the regulation of transcription are referred to as trans-*acting* elements, because their DNA sequence resides in a different location of the genome (3,9).

The coding region contains the information for protein synthesis. In this region, most genes are composed of a succession of exons and introns. Exons are coding sequences that ultimately transfer into mature mRNA, whereas introns are edited out of the newly synthesized transcript by a process called *splicing*.

Control of Gene Expression

As only a fraction of the available genes are expressed in a given cell at a given developmental stage, differential trans-

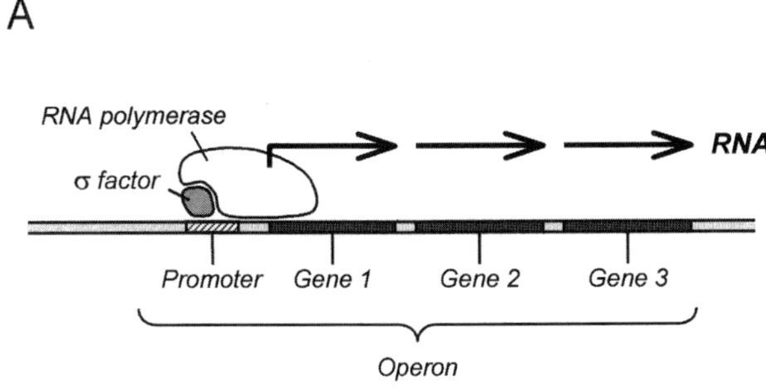

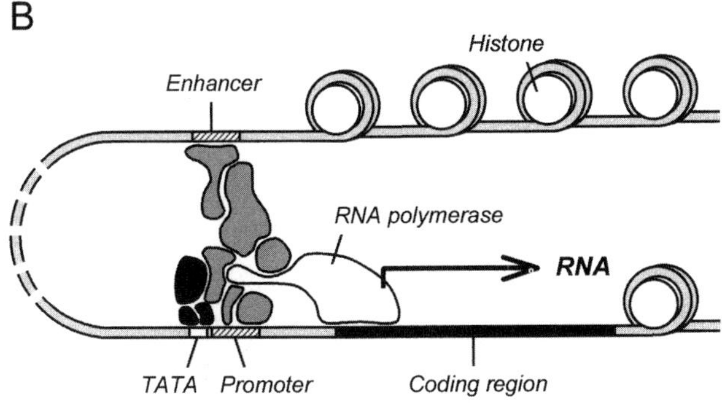

FIGURE 14.2. Transcriptional regulation in prokaryotes and eukaryotes. **A:** In prokaryotes, genes are organized in a cluster of related genes under the control of a single promoter, forming an operon. The RNA polymerase complex is constituted by a core enzyme that is activated on binding of a σ factor. **B:** This modular system is much more complex and sophisticated in eukaryotes. Different transcription factors bind to the promoter and enhancer regions and position type II RNA polymerase at the starting point of transcription. General transcription factors shown in black interact with the TATA box and hold together the enhancer-promoter-RNA polymerase complex. When not activated, eukaryotic genes are hidden in nucleosomes that are composed of a central core formed by histones. Activation of eukaryotic genes requires remodeling of the chromatin to allow the transcriptional apparatus to interact with the regulatory sequences.

cription and processing of genes provides for enormous diversity between cells within the same organism. Although gene expression can be controlled at different levels, transcriptional regulation generally predominates.

The information that governs transcription is located in DNA sequences that correspond to *cis*-acting elements or that encode for transcription factors. These sequences occupy a minimal portion of the entire genome but are the key determinants of cell organization by ensuring a balanced expression of different genes that preserves phenotypic stability. They also provide for differences among cell types within the same organisms and are at the core of the evolutionary process.

Gene Expression in Prokaryotes: A Simple Model of Regulation

The prokaryotic RNA polymerase has a simple structure formed by a core enzyme that mediates RNA transcription and a factor σ that recognizes the promoter region located 10 to 35 bases upstream to a transcription starting point (11) (Fig. 14.2). Thus, σ factors are the simplest examples of *trans*-acting elements. Once transcription begins, σ factors separate from the core enzyme. Sequential expression of different σ factors promotes the activation of different genes in a cascade of events that modifies the phenotype. During sporulation, for example, σ factor 43 promotes the transcription of specific genes involved in sporulation and the transcription of σ factors E and K that regulate and terminate this process (12). Conversely, intrinsic palindromic regions forming DNA hairpins or other *trans*-acting elements termed *p factors* that bind to the core enzyme can terminate transcription by the RNA polymerase. In addition, natural σ factor competitors, such as pN, NusH, or NuH6, can maintain RNA polymerase in an inactive state (13).

Therefore, gene expression in prokaryotes is controlled by balanced initiation and termination of transcriptional signals and by the specificity of different σ factors. However, this simple organization cannot provide for highly coordinated profiles of gene expression. This is achieved by physical alignment of clusters of genes termed *operons* behind the same promoter that enables sequential synthesis of proteins that are functionally related (14). The *lac*ZYA, for example, is a classic operon that codes for proteins involved in the β-galactose metabolism (breaking, transport, and acetylation of galactose) and is under the negative control of the *lac*I gene that encodes for the *lac* repressor (15). The repressor maintains the operon in the inactive state until it is inactivated by end-products of galactose metabolism (16). In this way, transcription of enzymes responsible for galactose metabolism is activated only in the presence of galactose in a highly efficient and ergometric manner. The *lacZ* gene is frequently inserted in recombinant bacterial plasmids, allowing colorimetric detection of colonies containing exogenous DNA material (Fig. 14.3).

Transcriptional Regulation in Eukaryotes

Three general principles govern the control of gene transcription in eukaryotes:

1. Unlike prokaryotes, genes operating within the same metabolic pathway are not usually physically aligned along genomic DNA and are often located on different chromosomes.
2. Recurrent structural motifs in DNA-binding domains (enhancers and promoters) indicate that the expression of functionally related genes is achieved by the activation of shared classes of transcription factors rather then by unique, gene-specific regulatory proteins.
3. Transcription factors are often involved in developmental regulation.

The eukaryotic type II RNA polymerase differs from its prokaryotic ancestor by the complexity of transcription fac-

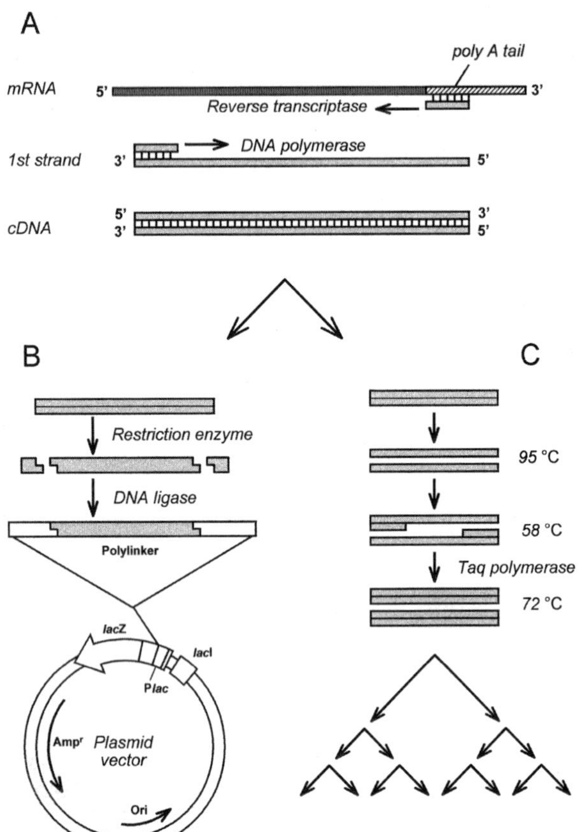

FIGURE 14.3. Basic enzymes and techniques in recombinant DNA technology. The figure summarizes basic procedures used in routine laboratory experiments. **A:** Messenger RNA (mRNA) molecules are reverse-transcribed into complementary DNA (cDNA) using the enzyme reverse transcriptase to synthesize the first cDNA strand, which is then used to generate double-stranded cDNA using a DNA polymerase. Both enzymes require priming with complementary oligonucleotides. **B:** cDNA and other DNA molecules can be amplified in bacteria after insertion into plasmids using restriction enzymes and DNA ligase. Recombinant plasmids generally contain a polylinker that offers different restriction sites to facilitate the insertion of exogenous DNA. In addition, they are engineered to contain antibiotic resistance genes (Amp^r) for selection of transformed bacteria and often contain other useful genes, such as the *lacZ* in this example, which allows color detection of colonies transformed with "empty" plasmids. **C:** Alternatively, DNA can be amplified by polymerase chain reaction (PCR) with the *Taq* polymerase. Repeated cycles of DNA denaturation (95°C), primer annealing (58°C in this example), and DNA synthesis (72°C) allow for exponential replication of DNA strands encompassed by the two primers. When reverse-transcription and PCR are combined, the procedure is referred to as *RT-PCR*.

tors that are required for its activation (17) (Fig. 14.2). This elaborate modular system allows for flexible and highly coordinated regulation of gene transcription.

On transcription, DNA rearranges to allow interaction between transcription factors located at the promoter and at the enhancer site. The TATA box, which contains consensus sequences recognized by general transcription factors (TFIID, TBP, and TAF), is usually located approximately 24 bases upstream from the promoter and acts as a bridge that holds together the enhancer-promoter-RNA polymerase complex and positions the enzyme at the starting point of transcription (18). Although enhancers are not essential, they increase promoter efficiency.

A second major characteristic of transcription in eukaryotic cells is related to the association of nuclear DNA with histones, forming nucleosomes. This particular organization prevents interaction between regulatory sequences and transcription factors unless conformational changes of the chromatin permit gene activation (Fig. 14.2).

It is suggested that chromatin remodeling is achieved by specific energy-dependent reactions that displace nucleosomes along the DNA strand. Alternatively, histone acetylation is thought to inactivate the natural binding of histones to DNA, allowing nucleosome remodeling, binding of transcription factors, and functional interactions between enhancers and promoters (18,19). This view is supported by the fact that histone acetylation correlates with the state of activation of gene expression.

Finally, gene transcription can also be chemically blocked in eukaryotic cells by methylation of specific DNA regions located near the promoter. Experimentally, the state of DNA methylation can be determined by inhibition of the nuclease activity of restriction enzymes, such as HpaII, that recognize non-methylated GC doublets.

Transcription Factors

The major characteristic of transcription factors is to contain specialized domains that allow for DNA interaction. Zinc-fingers, helix-turn-helix (HTH) domains, helix-loop-helix domains, and leucine zippers are examples of DNA-binding domains that are encountered in more than 80% of transcriptional factors (20).

Zinc-finger motifs are composed of a Zn ion holding together a peptide loop (the finger) through interaction with two histidines and two or four cysteines. The functional DNA binding domain is located in the amino acid residues at the base of the finger and recognizes specific consensus sequences that are generally located in the enhancer region. Steroid receptors are the most popular examples of this class of transcription factor, including glucocorticoid, mineralocorticoid, androgen, progesterone, thyroid hormone, and vitamin D receptors (21). Increasing evidence implicates the involvement of steroid receptors, such as the proto-oncogene bcl-6 or WT1, in cancer (22).

Similar DNA binding activity characterizes other classes of transcription factors. HTH domains are often found in proteins that have key roles during morphogenesis such as the homeobox group of transcription factors (23). Members of the helix-loop-helix class include proteins that control myogenesis, such as MyoD, that have been implicated in the *trans*-differentiation of myofibroblasts, which promote renal fibrosis (24). Leucine-zipper motifs are used by the Jun and Fos proteins. Both are members of the AP-1 heteromeric transcription complex that is involved in cell proliferation and regulation of cell matrix during fibrogenesis (25). An important transcription factor that is often implicated in renal diseases is nuclear factor-κB, which regulates many proinflammatory pathways and is itself under the control of other proteins, such as angiotensin II, known to promote inflammatory reactions in the renal parenchyma (26).

Transcriptional Control during Development

As discussed above, transcriptional regulation plays a central role during development by governing complex sequences of events that transform undifferentiated embryonic cells into highly specialized mature cells (3,9).

Three major classes of developmental regulatory genes have been identified. These include maternal genes, segmentation genes, and homeotic (Hox) genes. Each is expressed at different stages of cell maturation following complex sequences of activation in which gene products that are expressed at a given stage activate genes at a following stage. This highly sophisticated sequence of events creates a hierarchy according to which maternal, segmentation, and homeotic genes are expressed sequentially.

Four maternal systems activate the expression of specific transcription factors, termed *morphogens*, that are responsible for the initial patterning of the embryo. Segmentation genes are zinc-finger proteins that control the boundaries of compartments, whereas Hox genes control the differentiation steps of each segment. Hox genes are characterized by a common HTH-type DNA-binding motif at their carboxy-terminus termed *homeobox* and are organized in the human genome in four different clusters (A,B,C,D) containing up to ten genes each.

As the number of identified developmental transcription factors is rapidly increasing, their impact on renal development and involvement in congenital renal anomalies is a field of active research, as detailed in Chapter 1. Moreover, during the recovery phase of renal cell injury, cells reactivate several developmental genes in repair and restoration of function (27). Strategies to stimulate these patterns of expression are being investigated to promote early recovery from acute injury (28,29).

Messenger RNA Modification and Splicing

During cleavage and processing of primary RNA transcripts, the RNA molecules are capped at their 5' origin by the addition of methylated G nucleotides, and a segment of poly-A residues is attached near their 3' end (Fig. 14.1). These modifications are necessary to allow the export of the transcript from the nucleus, to stabilize mRNA molecules, and to allow interaction with ribosomes. The presence of a poly-A tail is a major characteristic of mRNAs and constitutes a key tool to isolate mRNAs from other RNA molecules, mostly ribosomal, using complementary oligo-dT primers.

Before RNA is exported into the cytosol, splicing of intron segments should be performed. The exact function of introns remains unclear. Because they facilitate recombination events, they have played a major role in the evolution of species and are often targeted in the process of generating knockout animals. Their physical structure may be more important than their actual nucleotide sequence, as these diverge more rapidly between species than exons (30).

Introns can range in size from 80 to several thousand nucleotides. They contain specific sequences at their extremities referred to as the *5' splice site* (always ending with 5'-GU-3') and the *3' splice site* (always ending with 5'-AG-3') that come together in the process of splicing. During splicing, a large catalytic heteromeric complex, termed *spliceosome*, is formed by the assembly of different ribonucleoproteins (31). After RNA binding, spliceosomes bridge together two exons and excise their intron segment.

In the majority of genes, each 5' splice site pairs with the closest 3' splice site in the spliceosome, producing only one form of mRNA. In some cases, however, splicing of RNA enables a single gene to produce different mRNA transcripts by jumping from a given 5' splice site to a more distant 3' splice site (Fig. 14.1). Each of these mRNAs yields different isoforms of the same protein that can be alternatively produced in different types of cells.

Recent genome-wide analysis of alternative splicing indicates that 40 to 60% of human genes have alternative splice isoforms (32), including molecules involved in kidney diseases such as angiotensin-converting enzyme and nephrin. Splicing of mRNA is an important regulatory step in the production of cell proteins that requires a high degree of accuracy. One pressing and still inadequately answered question is the functional meaning of these alternative transcripts. In general, DNA mutations that involve splice sites (splice site mutations) do not prevent splicing but instead cause the normal partner to seek alternative splice sites, producing the synthesis of various abnormal proteins lacking one or more exons, as, for example, in Frasier syndrome (33).

Translation of Messenger RNA into Proteins

Mammalian ribosomes are the site of mRNA translation and are composed of two asymmetric subunits, the 40S that binds mRNAs and the 60s that interacts with transfer RNAs. The genetic code is housed in the transfer RNA molecules that associate specific codons with the corresponding amino acid.

Eukaryotic cells can decrease their rate of protein synthesis in various conditions such as infections or heat shock. One important mechanism that mediates these types of nonselective responses involves phosphorylation of a repressor protein termed *elF-2* that interacts with target regions containing the AUG start codon preventing ribosomal binding.

A second gene-specific mechanism of translational regulation is termed *attenuation* and involves the formation of mRNA hairpins that block the translation. Similar mechanisms also regulate mRNA stability and degradation by RNases. Given the fact that each molecule of mRNA can serve as a template for multiple copies of proteins, the rate of mRNA degradation is a major determinant of protein abundance and is often the site of complex regulatory processes. In general, these processes operate primarily on unstable mRNAs (such as cytokines) that are stabilized under specific conditions by their interaction with *trans*-acting elements (34). The stability of transferrin mRNA, for example, increases during iron deprivation, triggering the synthesis of more transferrin molecules (35).

Protein Sorting and Degradation

Newly synthesized polypeptides are processed by a complex network of cellular enzymes and other binding proteins that are arranged in a highly organized fashion in various organelles in the cell. Information resident in the primary amino acid sequence as well as the folded structure of the proteins allow each to be recognized and targeted to its ultimate destination (3,9). Proteins that are synthesized in free cytosolic ribosomes are normally directed to the nucleus or to the mitochondria, whereas membranous ribosomes are the site of synthesis for proteins that enter the reticuloendothelial system (cotranslational transport) to be redirected to their final destination after being processed in the Golgi apparatus. An excellent example of this process is highly polarized epithelial cells in renal tubules. In these cells, transport proteins are located specifically on the apical or basolateral plasma membranes. This arrangement enables epithelial cells to perform net transport of solutes and water to either secrete or reabsorb fluid.

Some proteins are able to self-assemble by spontaneous interaction among reactive amino acid groups, whereas other proteins require the assistance of chaperon molecules such as the Hsp70 system and chaperonins. These molecules control the accessibility of reactive groups and maintain the peptide in a relatively flexible state until it reaches its final conformation.

The final fate of most cell proteins is degradation into proteosomes. A process called *ubiquitination* that involves covalent linkage of small peptides called *ubiquitins* to target proteins precedes this step. Ubiquitination is also involved in important signal-transduction pathways, such as the nuclear factor-κB pathway, in which inhibitory subunits are degraded after stimulatory signals and activate various signaling cascades (36).

RECOMBINANT DNA TECHNOLOGIES AND PROTEIN ANALYSIS

When reduced to its basics, molecular biology has until recently addressed two major objectives; namely, to identify genes and to analyze their function. With the completion of the human genome project, focus is gradually shifting from the first to the second goal and the more complex task of delineating complex patterns of gene expression. In the following sections, several recombinant DNA technologies are described to illustrate common experimental procedures that are routinely used in molecular diagnostics as well as basic research. A few examples of new, promising approaches are also provided.

Basic Recombinant DNA Technology

Hybridization and Detection of Nucleic Acids

The pairing of nucleotide bases in DNA and RNA allows a wide variety of specific recognition processes both *in vivo* and *in vitro*. These not only form the basis of many critical cellular functions but also provide the molecular biologist with tools to detect and study single genes. Based on specific hydrogen bonding arrangements, G pairs with C and A with T or U.

The extraordinary specificity of nucleic acid-base recognition has been exploited in the process of hybridization of complementary DNA or RNA *in vitro*. Under appropriate conditions, a unique nucleotide sequence present within a complex mixture of nucleic acids can be identified with a resolution of greater than one part per million (37). Using standard techniques, DNA or RNA is isolated from cells or tissues, stripped of proteins, and denatured into single strands. When incubated under conditions favoring renaturation, complementary sequences again reassociate. The experimental conditions (commonly temperature and salt concentration) can be altered to allow for only perfect or nearly perfect sequence matches. This is called *stringency*. Lowering stringency conditions is sometimes desirable to identify close relatives of particular nucleotide sequences. Thus, one can search for a gene or mRNA in kidney that is a close relative of a transcript expressed in other tissues as well as species (38,39).

Nucleic acids are commonly fractionated by agarose gel electrophoresis. Under these conditions, the agarose acts as a molecular sieve, retarding larger strands while allowing smaller strands to migrate in the electric field placed across the gel. Fractionated DNA or RNA is then eluted from the gel or transferred to a filter and exposed to a labeled DNA probe. When the filter contains DNA, this process is called a Southern blot (40), whereas it is called Northern blot if it contains RNA (41).

This same procedure has also been adapted to tissue sections to localize the expression of mRNA transcripts by specific cell types within a complex organ such as the kidney. This technique is called *in situ hybridization* (42).

Binding of specific DNA sequences to DNA or RNA species can also occur in solution. One example is protection of specific mRNA transcripts from digestion by S1 nuclease via hybridization (43). This technique, referred to as *S1 nuclease protection assay*, is more sensitive than standard Northern blotting.

Restriction Endonucleases

In eukaryotic chromosomes, strings of DNA are several million bases long. The discovery by Arber in 1962 of bacterial nucleases that cut DNA molecules at specific locations constitutes one of the cornerstone steps in the development of recombinant DNA techniques (44).

Most restriction enzymes recognize palindromic DNA sequences, meaning that the 5' to 3' sequence in the upper strand is identical to the 5' to 3' sequence in the lower strand. To date, nearly 1000 different restriction enzymes have been purified. Each enzyme can produce defined DNA restriction fragments possessing specific nucleotide sequences at each end from any given DNA sample.

With these enzymes, strings of DNA can be isolated, ligated into plasmid or phage genomes, and amplified (Fig. 14.3). Restriction nucleases have also allowed construction of the first detailed maps of various genomes (restriction maps) and are used for allelic discrimination by restriction fragment length polymorphism. In this technique, DNA mutations that modify the recognition sequence for specific restriction enzymes can be identified by the length of the restriction reaction product.

DNA Amplification Using Prokaryotic Systems

The possibility of replicating specific strings of DNA to obtain quantities sufficient for analysis and further manipulation is central to all recombinant DNA technologies. In the early 1970s, work by Boyer and by Cohen provided the first fundamental tools for DNA cloning with the discovery of DNA ligases and the characterization of bacterial plasmids. Plasmids are circular molecules of DNA that replicate in the cytoplasm of bacterial cells (Fig. 14.3).

Specific regions of plasmids not vital for vegetative growth under laboratory conditions can be engineered using restriction nucleases for the insertion of exogenous DNA fragments. When inserted into *Escherichia coli* cells, plasmid genes encoding for antibiotic resistance are expressed, allowing selection of bacteria that have been transformed. During this process, the inserted DNA is replicated along with the rest of the bacterial genome. This technology enables the amplification and characterization of virtually any DNA string of appropriate size. Because bacteria have a mean generation time of approximately 20 minutes during exponential growth and contain often as many as 500 copies of plasmids per bacterium, virtually limitless amounts of DNA can be grown and harvested routinely. Most available plasmids are engineered to incorporate a polylinker corresponding to a portion of DNA that contains multiple restriction sites that facilitate cloning of DNA fragments generated by various restriction enzymes.

Because of their simplicity, DNA is generally cloned into plasmids. The relatively low efficiency of bacteria transformation with plasmids limits their use, however, when generating DNA libraries. In this case, bacterial viruses, such as the *bacteriophage* λ, are more advantageously used. The λ phages are composed of a head that contains the viral genome and a tail that infects bacterial cells with high efficiency. Phages can be packaged *in vitro* after insertion of exogenous DNA and are replicated in bacteria.

Both λ phages and plasmids can amplify DNA fragments up to 20 kilobases (kb). They are ideal for cDNA and other relatively small DNA molecules, but are insufficient for large strings of genomic DNA. In these cases, other vectors can be used. These include cosmid vectors, containing elements of both plasmids and λ phages that can accommodate up to 45-kb fragments or bacteriophage P1 housing up to 100 kb of exogenous DNA. If even larger fragments need to be replicated, bacterial artificial chromosomes or yeast artificial chromosomes can incorporate up to 300 or 1000 kb of DNA, respectively (9).

DNA Amplification with Polymerase Chain Reaction

The second breakthrough in DNA amplification was achieved in 1985 by Mullis and coworkers who developed PCR (6). PCR relies on the binding of two priming oligonucleotides that flank a region of DNA to amplify the region located in between (Fig. 14.3). These two oligonucleotides are complementary to the opposite DNA strands. Addition of DNA polymerase results in the synthesis of new DNA. Repeated cycles of denaturation, annealing, and DNA synthesis are performed in a chain reaction such that the newly synthesized strands become templates for further DNA synthesis. This process exponentially increases the number of DNA copies containing the sequence of interest. Modern PCR uses thermostable DNA polymerase species derived from the thermophilic bacterium *Thermus aquaticus* (*Taq* polymerase), which retain activity after being heated to 95°C and obviate the need for addition of fresh enzyme after each round of DNA synthesis and denaturation (45). Several modified enzymes that guarantee more reliable DNA duplication or allow for the amplification of longer strings are also available.

PCR permits selective amplification of minute quantities of DNA, facilitating every aspect of molecular biology research and diagnostics (including forensic pathology), including site-directed mutagenesis, labeling, and sequencing of DNA. Even fixed tissues on slides or small tissue fragments, such as renal biopsy specimens, can provide sufficient material for PCR amplification.

Amplification of Messenger RNA with Reverse Transcription

Many experimental circumstances require direct amplification of mRNAs. Indeed, mRNA transcripts reflect the actual genes that are activated in a cell system and contain nucleotide sequences that can be directly translated into proteins, obviating the tedious task of sorting exon segments from introns when working with genomic DNA. This process is achieved with a reverse transcriptase derived from retroviruses, which are one major exception to the central dogma, as they harbor their genetic information in RNA molecules that are copied into DNA on infection of host cells. The DNA obtained by reverse-transcription is called *cDNA*, as it reflects the nucleotide sequences of mRNAs (Fig. 14.3). Similar to DNA polymerases, reverse transcriptase requires complementary oligonucleotide priming to begin transcription. Oligo-dT hybridizing to poly-A tails can be used to reverse-transcribe in a nonselective manner mRNA molecules (3,9). In other circumstances, gene-specific primers are designed to amplify selected mRNA molecules. Once converted into cDNA, nucleic acids are often ligated into plasmids or phages or directly amplified by the PCR reaction, a process that is referred as reverse transcription polymerase chain reaction (RT-PCR) (Fig. 14.3).

Sequencing Nucleic Acids

The highly specific binding of small oligonucleotides to DNA also lies at the heart of the dideoxy chain termination sequencing of DNA. DNA sequences are obtained from a uniform population of DNA, generally synthesized in large amounts by expansion in a bacterial plasmid or by PCR. After DNA is denatured, a complementary primer is added. In the traditional manual sequencing, synthesis of complementary radioactive DNA strands is initiated by DNA polymerase after addition of all four deoxynucleotides (dATP labeled with 35S, dGTP, dCTP, and dTTP) in four different reaction tubes containing one of the four dideoxynucleotide analogs of G, A, T, or C. In each reaction, chain termination can occur whenever a dideoxy analog is inserted in the newly formed DNA strand, preventing further extension. After resolution of each mixture of nested DNA fragments by gel electrophoresis, the nucleotide sequence is determined by reading the order of bands in the four lanes of the corresponding autoradiogram. Practically, 300 to 400 nucleotides can be determined with a single manual gel run. This sequence can be extended by construction of other oligonucleotides complementary to a short portion of the nucleotide sequence determined previously (46).

These procedures have been improved and automated. The basic principles behind automated sequencing remain similar to the manual technique. The major difference resides in the fluorescence labeling of one deoxynucleotide in each reaction tube using different dyes. The reaction mixtures are then pooled and separated in a single lane on a sequencing gel or electrophoresis capillary. As the bands advance along the electric gradient, they pass under a laser beam that excites their fluorescence, which is read and analyzed by a computer. Reliable DNA sequences can often be obtained for more than 500 nucleotides per run, and multiple lanes can be read simultaneously by the machine (46).

Analysis of Gene Expression

A critical issue in normal physiology and renal pathophysiology is the determination of the expression of given genes under different cellular and environmental conditions. Classically, gene expression analysis is performed by protein detection with specific antibodies in Western blotting or, when antibodies are not available, by measuring the amount of mRNA transcripts by Northern blotting or with the more sensitive S1 nuclease assay. Densitometric methods have been developed to compare the amount of expressed protein or mRNA with respect to a control preparation. These semiquantitative techniques, however, have severe limitations. They require relatively large amounts of starting material, can only study a limited numbers of genes simultaneously, and require development of specific probes such as antisera. To overcome some of these limitations, other techniques have recently been developed and are briefly reviewed.

Quantitative Reverse Transcription Polymerase Chain Reaction

RT-PCR is more sensitive than traditional Northern blot analysis and requires less RNA. The major difficulty in quantifying mRNA by RT-PCR is related to the exponential nature of the method.

In competitive RT-PCR, an internal standard sharing the same priming sequences as the transcript of interest is added to the mixture and acts as a competitor during the reaction (47,48). The abundance of mRNA is determined by comparing the signal obtained from the target signal with the internal standard. As this method is time consuming and often difficult to set up, it is increasingly replaced by real-time RT-PCR.

Real-time RT-PCR allows detection of products of the PCR reaction as they are being formed (Fig. 14.4). In the modern version of this technique, quenched fluorescent dyes linked to the 5' end of one primer are released by the 5' nuclease activity of the *Taq* DNA polymerase and become fluorescent (49). The emitted light is measured in real time during the PCR reaction and is proportional to the amount of PCR product. The number of cycles required to cross a given fluorescence threshold is inversely proportional to the amount of mRNA present in the original reaction mixture.

Multiplex real-time RT-PCR represents an extension of this technique and is based on differential fluorescent labeling of primers that amplify for different genes. This permits comparison within the same PCR reaction of the relative amount of different transcripts (50). By this method, housekeeping genes that are presumed to be stably expressed serve as internal controls, allowing correction of the results for the amount of RNA that was loaded in the initial sample reaction. Multiplex real-time RT-PCR allows

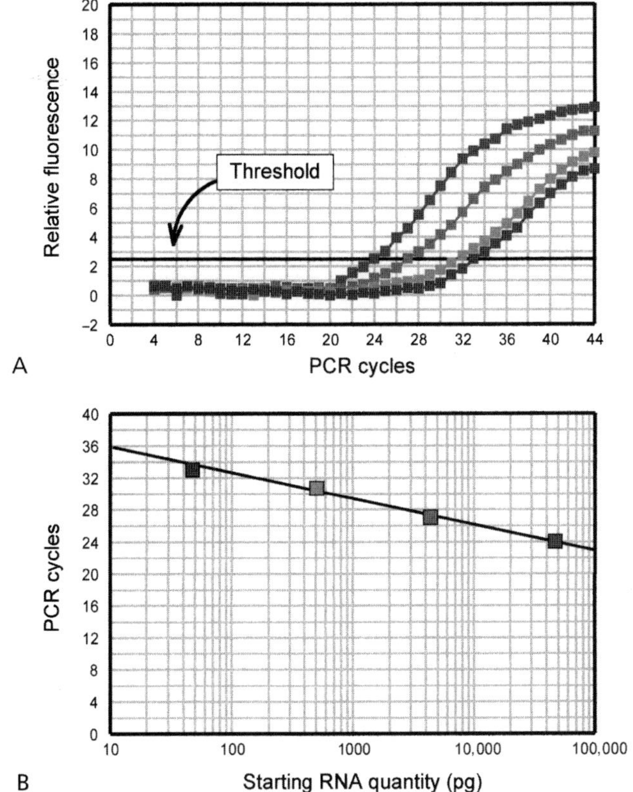

FIGURE 14.4. Real-time reverse transcription polymerase chain reaction (PCR). The figure illustrates an actin calibration curve. Total RNA was extracted from HK2 cells and loaded in increasing concentrations in the sample reaction. Fluorescence was measured in real time as primers were incorporated in newly synthesized PCR fragments with an ABI Prism 7700. The number of cycles required to cross a given fluorescence threshold **(A)** is proportional to the initial amount of loaded messenger RNA **(B)**. (See Color Plate 14.4.)

determination of gene expression even from extremely small samples, such as renal biopsies, and has been developed, for example, to detect gene expression in human renal specimens (51).

Differential Messenger RNA Display Using DNA Microarrays

With the identification of increasing numbers of genes, DNA microarray technology has rapidly developed as a valuable technique for comparative gene expression analysis.

DNA chips are composed of thousands of known expressed sequence tags (see Gene Cloning and Analysis of Cloned Sequences) or synthetic oligonucleotides that are deposited in gridded arrays by a robotic spotting device on a solid support such as a glass microscope slide or a membrane matrix. Oligonucleotide sequences are usually directly selected from databases such as GenBank, dbEST, or UniGene (52). As many as 10,000 genes can be spotted on a single microscope slide.

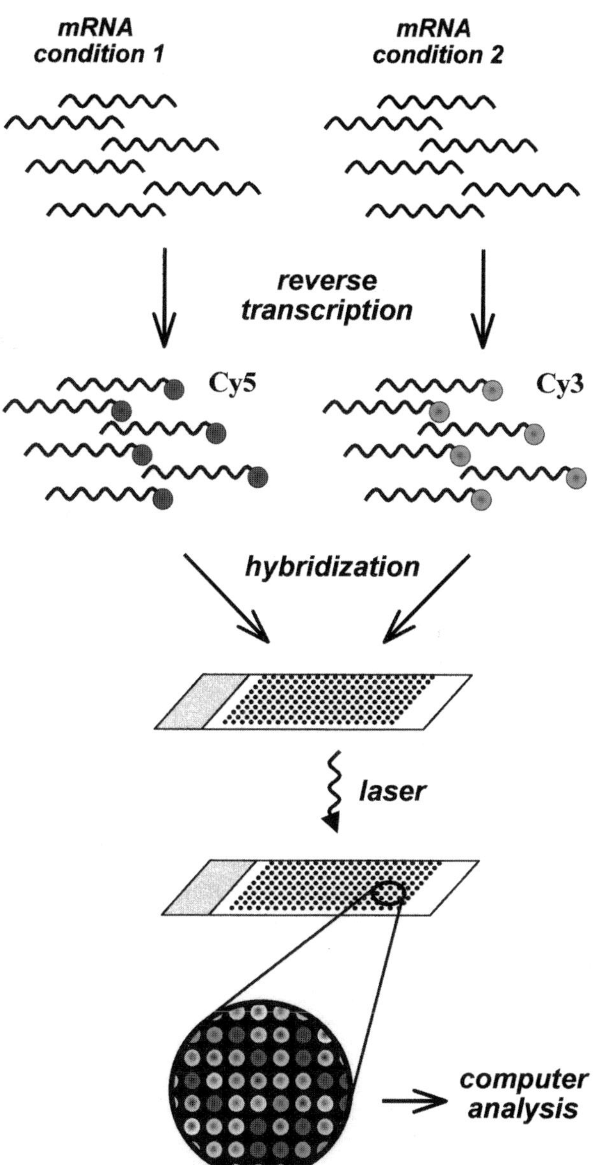

FIGURE 14.5. Differential display on DNA microarrays. Messenger RNA (mRNA) obtained from two different samples are labeled with two fluorescent cyanine dyes with one round of reverse transcription. The fluorescent targets are then pooled and hybridized under stringent conditions to the clones on the microarray chip. The emission light is measured with a scanning confocal laser microscope at two different wavelengths that are specific for each dye. Monochrome images are then pseudocolored, combined, and analyzed with suitable computer software. (See Color Plate 14.5.)

For differential display, two populations of mRNA are labeled with different fluorophores, hybridized to the chip and analyzed with a laser scanning device (Fig. 14.5). The intensity of fluorescence emitted by each dye is proportional to the amount of RNA that has hybridized at a given location, reflecting the level of a gene expression represented by that spot. The enormous quantity of information generated by expression data from thousands of genes requires sophisticated computer analysis to generate meaningful results (53).

Currently, DNA microarray technology is rapidly evolving. Despite increasing miniaturization and the development of more flexible techniques to generate "custom made" chips, it still has technical limitations, particularly in terms of chip reproducibility and variability in the efficiency of labeling and hybridization. New protocols and technical improvements are solving many of these limitations (52).

The major challenge of this technology is the development of computer-based inferential analysis strategies that recognize patterns of gene expression within complex genetic networks such as the human genome. The so-called cluster analysis is emerging as a powerful statistical tool, permitting the grouping of genes in hierarchical clusters that follow similar patterns of expression. This information can then be used as a molecular fingerprint in diagnosis or in monitoring response to therapy.

Gene Cloning and Analysis of Cloned Sequences

Cloning of genes responsible for genetic disorders can be achieved without prior knowledge of the molecular nature of the disease by a strategy termed *positional cloning*, which is based on the genomic localization of the locus of interest using genetic markers present at a known chromosomal location (54). (See Chapter 19.)

Alternatively, gene cloning is performed by screening tissue-specific collections of recombinant vectors containing sequences of foreign cDNA, called *cDNA libraries* (4). This basic approach can also be refined. Subtractive libraries, for example, are obtained by subtracting unwanted mRNA species from the library before screening (55).

Altogether, the success of any cDNA cloning strategy is related to the quality of the library to be screened and to the efficiency of the probing system that is used.

Since the 1990s, the process of cloning genes has been revolutionized by the creation of electronic databases. More than 53,000 partial sequences of cDNA called *expressed sequence tags* that cover most human genes have been collected (56). In addition, computer programs have been developed to identify putative genes within genomic databases by sorting out and mending together potential exon regions. All of these sequences and sequences from already cloned genes have been collected in databases that can be accessed online (www.ensembl.org and www.celera.com). Taken together, these databases constitute virtual DNA libraries that can be screened electronically using partial DNA or protein sequences. By this method, entire genes can sometimes be identified.

Screening Libraries by Nucleic Acid Hybridization

The object of screening a DNA library is to identify single plasmids or phages containing the nucleotide sequences of interest. Routinely, 50,000 phages (each containing a unique inserted DNA sequence) are plated on a lawn of bacteria in an agar plate. Phage DNA can be transferred in replicate fashion to a nylon filter and probed with a labeled DNA of interest to identify clones that hybridize with the probe. Individual plaques are picked from the plate, and the cloned DNA insert is characterized. When partial transcripts are obtained, these can be used to further screen libraries in search of overlapping sequences. Alternative procedures, termed *rapid amplification of cDNA ends*, allow the amplification of the missing 5' or 3' ends by RT-PCR (57).

This approach has tremendous flexibility and power. Knowledge of only a partial mRNA or protein sequence allows synthesis of oligonucleotides that can be used as probes. Because of the degeneracy of the genetic code (3,9), it is impossible to specify the exact nucleotide sequence corresponding to a specific peptide fragment. In these cases, mixtures of degenerate oligonucleotides containing several possible sequence combinations are used (58). Cloning strategies can also aim at identifying genes based on their homology with other proteins expressed in other tissues or species. By computer alignment of related sequences, constant regions that have been preserved throughout evolution within the same family of proteins can be identified and used to design degenerate oligonucleotides. By a similar approach, cDNA clones from related genes can serve directly as probes. By lowering the stringency of the hybridization conditions, homologous clones that contain high percentages of sequence identity with the probing DNA can be identified.

Library Screening with Antibodies, with Functional Assays, or by Protein-Protein Interaction

In addition to the use of DNA fragments or oligonucleotides as probes, phage plaques can be screened with antisera raised against purified proteins. Using expression plasmids, peptides encoded by exogenous cDNAs can be directly translated in the bacterial lawn and identified with specific antisera (59).

With a similar approach, phage epitope libraries expressing randomly generated oligopeptides can be screened to find domains recognized by antibodies or by other proteins (60). The recognized epitope sequence generally corresponds to a partial amino acid sequence contained in the natural antigen or binding protein. From this sequence, the protein can be identified or cloned. This technique is particularly powerful for identifying autoantibodies or to clone proteins by their reciprocal interactions such as in receptor-ligand association. The two-hybrid system is an alternative strategy that permits investigators to fish for clones that code for peptide that interact with other proteins offered as bait in the screening process (see Protein-Protein Interaction) (48).

Another powerful approach relies on screening cDNA clones that produce functionally active proteins when expressed in a suitable system. *Xenopus* oocytes have emerged as a favorite system to clone membrane transport proteins. Assays using oocytes have used electrode impalements, patch clamping, and optical or isotope flux techniques. Large quantities of RNA (cRNA) can be synthesized *in vitro* from cDNA libraries, fractionated, and used for injection into oocytes. When the oocyte demonstrates the expected physiologic response, smaller fractions of the original cRNA pool are injected until the process is narrowed down to a single clone (61).

Initial Analysis of Cloned Complementary DNAs

DNA sequences are generally read and entered into a suitable computer program for analysis and storage. Computer programs provide important clues as to the nature of newly cloned proteins, such as structural aspects, including membrane-spanning domains, antigenicity, and the presence of specialized amino acid sequences coding for phosphorylation or glycosylation. Sequence alignment in databases helps define the relationships with other genes and identify functional motifs, such as DNA-binding and protein-binding domains, that can give important clues to the biologic function of the newly cloned sequence (62).

Expression of Specific Genes in Various Experimental Systems

An important aspect of recombinant DNA technology is the demonstration that a clone selected from a library codes for a gene of interest. In cases in which structural analysis of the clone demonstrates a high degree of conservation with another homologous gene or cDNA, expression studies can compare these structural and functional differences. Site-directed mutagenesis studies can further refine knowledge of the function of various portions of a single protein (63).

Bacteria infected with recombinant phage can express polypeptides coded by cDNAs as fusion proteins. These fusion proteins can be purified in large quantities and used for functional studies or as immunogens to raise antisera.

Mammalian proteins expressed in bacteria, however, are not posttranslationally modified. This limitation has been circumvented by use of the baculovirus expression system, in which recombinant proteins are produced by viral infection of cultured insect cells (64). These proteins are then properly processed, glycosylated, and phosphorylated. Yeast has also been used extensively as an expression system (65). Detailed knowledge of yeast physiology and genetics coupled with the ability to mutagenize this organism has enabled detailed dissection of genomic control mechanisms as well as identification of proteins that regulate endocytosis and membrane fusion (66).

A variety of mammalian cells in culture, including green monkey kidney or COS cells, have been used to express various cDNAs using retroviral vectors. In these systems, viral promoters initiate and produce high levels of expression of the desired protein. However, such studies are often hampered by the transient nature of the expression of transfected genes. Using the same system, regulatory regions of genes may be transfected into cells and their effects on a neighboring gene determined using a gene product that is easily assayed, such as chloramphenicol acetyltransferase (67).

Sorting and trafficking of proteins within highly polarized epithelial cells of the kidney has been addressed using recombinant DNA technology and cultured epithelial cells such as the MDCK cell line. These cells maintain a polarized morphology and possess distinct apical and basolateral plasma membrane domains. Selective budding of viruses, such as vesicular stomatitis virus exclusively from the apical or basolateral membranes of MDCK cells, has permitted detailed study of the fundamental determinants of epithelial cell polarity (68).

Xenopus oocytes are a popular system to express membrane transport proteins. The cystic fibrosis gene was among the first gene to be isolated without knowledge of its actual function. Oocytes were used to demonstrate its function as an epithelial cell chloride channel (69). Other fundamental membrane transport proteins cloned using *Xenopus* oocytes include Na-H exchangers (70), bumetanide-sensitive Na-K-2Cl and thiazide-sensitive NaCl cotransporters (71), the renal outer medullary adenosine triphosphate–regulated potassium channel (72), multiple aquaphorin water channels (73), and the amiloride-inhibitable epithelial Na^+ channel, or ENaC (74). These data provide molecular links between epithelial cell transport data and the expression of specific genes within individual kidney epithelial cells. In turn, detailed knowledge of these transporter proteins has allowed the identification of specific gene abnormalities in humans that cause inherited disorders of renal tubular function, including nephrogenic diabetes insipidus (75) and Bartter's (76,77), Gitelman's (78), and Liddle's (79) syndromes.

Expression and Suppression of Specific Genes in Animal Models

Single cell expression systems cannot be used to study expression in multicellular organisms in which a gene's expression or lack thereof has complex effects on an animal's development and physiology. For these studies, the introduction and disruption of specific genes into amphibian, insect, and mammalian embryos have permitted studies of gene expression in the resultant offspring.

Xenopus and *Drosophila* embryos have been used to characterize various developmentally specific transcripts governing tissue-specific differentiation (3,9). This research is greatly facilitated by the ability to manipulate various cells of the earliest embryo stages, then transplant them to other embryos and allow them to develop. This research has produced a fundamental understanding of pattern formation in these animals. Homologs of these pattern genes have been characterized in mammals.

In a similar fashion, transgenic mice have been used extensively to produce a stable transfer of new or altered genes into the germ line of rodents (7). Both the homozygous and heterozygous offspring of transgenic animals can then be studied extensively. Production of transgenic animals involves injection of a new gene (transgene) into the pronucleus of a one-cell stage embryo so that it can integrate into the genome. This embryo is then implanted into a foster mother and allowed to develop. Transgenes are usually passed from parent to offspring. This permits propagation of the new trait. Inclusion of the appropriate regulatory elements of a gene allows study of gene expression in its various target tissues at precise times during the life span of the transgenic animal. This technology has been used on a large scale to determine not only gene functions that are critical to embryo development and survival but also genes that produce specific phenotypes that mimic human abnormalities (80).

Moreover, this technology has been carried one step further through development of gene targeting. Instead of introducing genes into cells, special vectors are designed to disrupt or knock out specific genes in mice. The offspring of these mice possess various copy numbers of the disrupted gene and can be examined using a wide array of anatomic, physiologic, and cellular methods (81).

Protein Analysis and Proteomics

Protein analysis involves protein detection, protein separation and purification, characterization of peptide sequences, and identification of interactive partners. Direct recognition of proteins is usually achieved with specific antibodies after protein separation in polyacrylamide gels (Western blotting) or can be directly performed *in situ* on biologic samples by immunocytochemistry. Antibodies can also be used to pull down or blot specific proteins from solutions, which are then used for further manipulations or are quantified (i.e., by enzyme-linked immunoassays).

Protein-Protein Interaction

One important question in protein analysis is to identify interactions between proteins, which regulate most intracellular signaling and are critical to the assembly of functional peptides. Protein-protein interaction assays have been developed in which labeled proteins are extracted from a crude mixture as they bind to target proteins linked to solid supports. These approaches can be further refined with recombinant DNA techniques, allowing for bacterial synthesis of partial protein fragments that are used as targets to identify specific domains that mediate protein-protein interaction.

The yeast two-hybrid system is also an attractive method based on the modular structure of gene activation, which complements or is used as an alternative to pull-down experiments. In the yeast two-hybrid system, the GAL4 transcriptional activator is often exploited (59). This transcription factor has a DNA-binding domain and an activation domain, both of which must be in close association to activate transcription. By DNA recombinant techniques, two protein sequences acting as bait and target are fused with sequences encoding with one of the GAL4 domains. When expressed in yeast cells, the activation domain and the DNA-binding domain are bridged together if the two proteins interact, thus promoting transcription of a reporter gene. These systems can be used to study interactions between known molecules or to clone new proteins using cDNAs libraries, as mentioned before.

Similar prokaryotic systems have been developed based on the modular structure of bacterial RNA polymerases, in which target and bait cDNAs are fused to either the core enzyme or a σ factor.

Protein-DNA Interaction

Techniques for protein separation also offer an important tool to study protein-DNA interactions. This permits analysis of regulation of DNA expression by transcriptional factors. Such experiments are essential to identify DNA binding sites and have been successfully used to purify and identify a number of regulatory proteins.

The basic principles behind these studies rely on the fact that protein-DNA interaction forms high molecular weight complexes that are retarded during polyacrylamide gel electrophoresis or protected from digestion with DNAse (82). In the example shown in Figure 14.6, a nuclear protein extract from cells stimulated with angiotensin II was coincubated with DNA strings containing the promotor sequences of collagen III. As shown, angiotensin II promotes the synthesis of a protein that binds to the ^{32}P-labeled DNA target, forming a macromolecular complex that is retarded in the gel (83).

Protein Separation and Purification

Separation of proteins is another important aspect of protein analysis required as a preliminary step for peptide sequencing or to perform other tasks such as functional assays. These complex sets of experimental procedures need high levels of expertise in protein biochemistry and are generally based on prior knowledge of the physical characteristics of the protein of interest, including size, isoelectric point, and hydrophobicity. The availability of antibodies or specific ligands greatly simplifies the experimental procedures by allowing detection of the final products or the use of alternative strategies such as the above-mentioned pull-down assay.

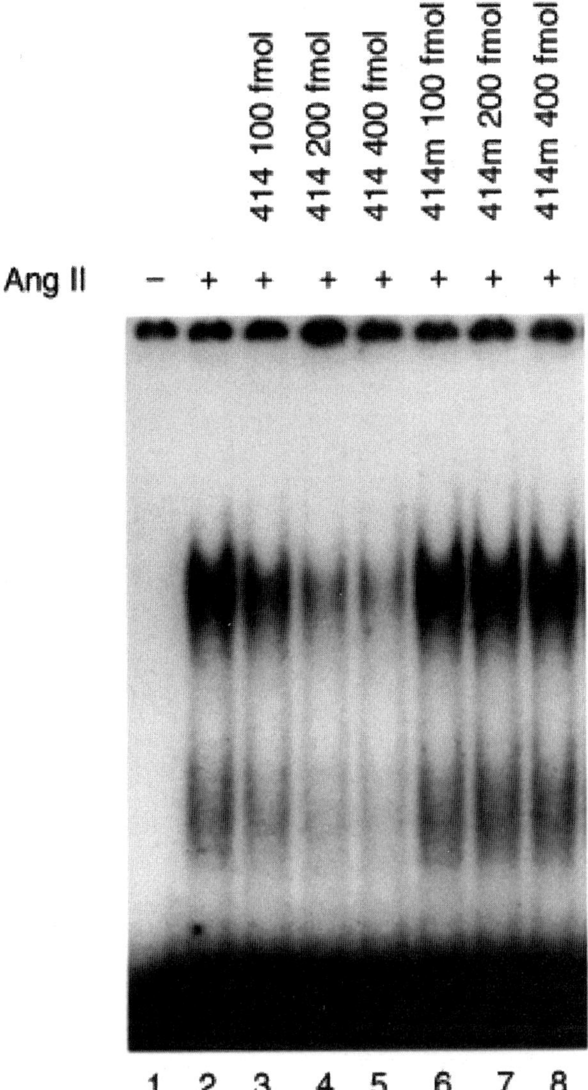

FIGURE 14.6. Gel retardation assay. The figure demonstrates binding of regulatory nuclear proteins to *cis*-elements in the COL3A1 promoter after angiotensin II (Ang II) stimulation. Nuclear extracts were obtained from Ang II–stimulated cells (Ang II+) and incubated with a ^{32}P-labelled oligonucleotide (414) that contains sequences +3 to +20 of the COL3A1 promoter. Ang II stimulates the synthesis of a peptide that binds to the target DNA and retards its migration in the gel (lane 2). This reaction can be competed with increasing amounts of nonlabeled, wild-type oligonucleotide (lanes 3 to 5) but not with a cold mutated analogue sequence (414m) (lanes 6 to 8). In the absence of Ang II stimulation (Ang II–), no DNA-protein complex generating gel retardation is observed (lane 1).

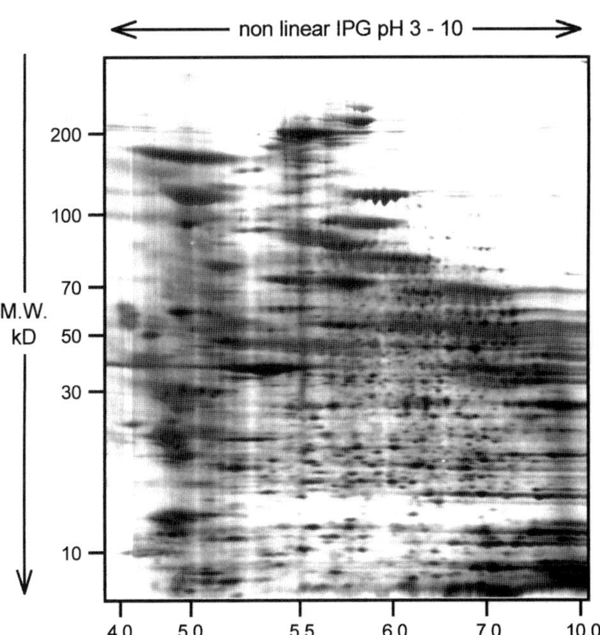

FIGURE 14.7. Two-dimensional electrophoresis analysis. The figure shows platelet proteins resolved in a low polyacrylamide–concentration, macroporous, two-dimensional gel. The initial protein mixture was solubilized with a tri-n-butyl phosphate:acetone:methanol solution according to an optimization protocol for high molecular weight proteins (85). Proteins were separated according to their isoelectric points using an immobilized pH gradient (IPG) in the first dimension (*horizontal*) and by their molecular weight (M.W.) in the second dimension (*vertical*). Single spots on the gel represent individual protein species.

In general, protein separation involves prepurification chromatographic steps that are performed with ion exchange, size exclusion, hydrophobic interaction, or affinity chromatography, followed by gel electrophoresis. Since the 1990s, two-dimensional electrophoresis has gained considerable favor. This powerful technique has been the object of major developments and permits fine resolution of proteins. Recent advances based on the use of new solvents and macroporous gels also allow for the detection of poorly soluble high molecular weight peptides (more than 150,000 kDa) that cannot be resolved by traditional gels (Fig. 14.7) (84). Moreover, new staining procedures based on silver stains or negative dyes offer increased sensitivity, with detection limits in the nanograms range (85).

Proteomics

One of the challenges of the post-genomic area is the characterization of global patterns of gene expression directly at the protein level. This new field of investigation has come to light in recent years with the combined developments of mass spectrometry techniques, nanotechnologies, and bioinformatics, and is generally referred to as *proteomics* (86). With a similar approach to differential transcription analysis, techniques permitting analysis of patterns of protein expression have been developed.

Although antibodies can only measure the expression of few proteins simultaneously, two-dimensional gels combined with chromatography techniques considerably increase the number of gene products that can be studied simultaneously. The complexity of peptide expression patterns represents, however, a major obstacle in proteomics. In general, the abundance of proteins in biologic samples is in the range of 10^6 whereas no more than 10^3 different proteins can be visualized even with high-quality two-dimensional gels. For these reasons, the initial step of any proteomic approach requires reduction of sample complexity by preliminary removal of uninteresting components using various affinity strategies.

In two-dimension differential protein display, proteins from different sources are labeled with different fluorescent cyanine dyes and run contemporaneously in the same gel. Similarly to differential display with DNA microarray techniques, the gel is analyzed with a laser beam scanner that measures the emitted fluorescence from each dye after excitation at different wavelengths. Computer analysis determines the relative contribution of the original protein mixtures to every spot on the gel, which correspond to unique protein species. These can then be recognized by their gel migration profile or with antibodies. If unknown, they can be analyzed by mass spectrometry (87).

Alternative new tools for protein expression analysis are also in the process of being developed, based on nanotechnologies. Similarly to DNA chips, recombinant proteins or small peptides containing protein binding domains or specific antibodies can be arrayed on miniaturized protein chips and used as probes to bind other proteins. At the moment, however, a number of technical problems still need to be resolved before protein chips become a reality in biomedical research.

Unlike DNA, peptide sequencing requires highly sophisticated techniques. Currently, mass spectrometry has replaced the classic Edman degradation technique. Fentomoles of proteins extracted from two-dimensional gel or protein chips can be analyzed by mass spectrometry, and different peptides can be detected within the same sample. Protein identification with mass spectrometry is performed with two possible strategies. In the first approach, matrix-assisted laser desorpition/ionization (MALDI) provides a peptide mass fingerprint of the eluted peptide mixture under study. The protein composition of the mixture is then derived from the analysis of the mass spectrum. In the second approach, referred to as *tandem mass spectrometry*, the MALDI step is followed by fragmentation of individual peptides into amino acids with a tandem mass spectrometer. Despite being more complex and time consuming, if coupled with electronic databases this approach permits identification of peptides directly from amino acid sequences, which produces more reliable results than peptide mass analysis (86).

REFERENCES

1. Micklos DA, Freyer GA. *DNA science.* Cold Spring Harbor, NY: Laboratory Press, 1990.
2. Fincham JRS. *Genetic analysis.* Oxford, UK: Blackwell Science Ltd, 1994.
3. Alberts B, Bray D, Lewis J, et al. *Molecular biology of the cell*, 3rd ed. New York: Garland Publishing Inc, 1994.
4. Huynh TV, Young RA, Davis RW. Constructing and screening cDNA libraries in lgt10 and lgt11. In: Glover DM, ed. *DNA cloning techniques: a practical approach.* Oxford, UK: IRL Press, 1984.
5. Sanger F. Determination of nucleotide sequences in DNA. *Science* 1981;214:1205–1210.
6. Mullis KB, Faloona FA. Specific synthesis of DNA in vitro via a polymerase chain reaction. *Methods Enzymol* 1987;155:335–350.
7. Hanahan D. Transgenic mice as probes into complex systems. *Science* 1989;246:1265–1274.
8. Lander ES, Linton LM, Birren B, et al. Initial sequencing and analysis of the human genome. *Nature* 2001;409:860–921.
9. Lodish H, Berk A, Zipursky SL, et al. *Molecular cell biology*, 4th ed. New York: W H Freeman & Co, 1999.
10. Risch NJ. Searching for genetic determinants in the new millenium. *Nature* 2000;405:847–856.
11. Grossman AD, Erickson JW, Gross CA. The htpR gene product of *E. coli* is a sigma factor for heat-shock promoters. *Cell* 1984;38:383–390.
12. Stragier P, Losick R. Molecular genetics of sporulation in *Bacillus subtilis. Annu Rev Genet* 1996;30:297–341.
13. Greenblatt J, Li J. Interaction of the sigma factor and the nusA gene protein of *E. coli* with RNA polymerase in the initiation-termination cycle of transcription. *Cell* 1981;24:421–428.
14. Jacob F, Monod J. Genetic regulatory mechanisms in the synthesis of proteins. *J Mol Biol* 1961;3:318–356.
15. Hu MC, Davidson N. The inducible lac operator-repressor system is functional in mammalian cells. *Cell* 1987;48:555–566.
16. Oehler S, Eismann ER, Kramer H, et al. The three operators of the lac operon cooperate in repression. *Embo J* 1990;9:973–979.
17. Nikolov DB, Burley SK. RNA polymerase II transcription initiation: a structural view. *Proc Natl Acad Sci U S A* 1967; 94:15–22.
18. Chen H, Lin RJ, Schiltz RL, et al. Nuclear receptor coactivator ACTR is a novel histone acetyltransferase and forms a multimeric activation complex with P/CAF and CBP/p300. *Cell* 1997;90:569–580.
19. Grant PA, Schieltz D, Pray-Grant MG, et al. A subset of TAF(II)s are integral components of the SAGA complex required for nucleosome acetylation and transcriptional stimulation. *Cell* 1998;94:45–53.
20. Pabo CO, Sauer RT. Transcription factors: structural families and principles of DNA recognition. *Annu Rev Biochem* 1992;61:1053–1095.
21. Tsai MJ, O'Malley BW. Molecular mechanisms of action of steroid/thyroid receptor superfamily members. *Annu Rev Biochem* 1994;63:451–486.
22. Coppes MJ, Campbell CE, Williams BR. The role of WT1 in Wilms tumorigenesis. *FASEB J* 1993;7:886–895.
23. Gehring WJ, Affolter M, Burglin T. Homeodomain proteins. *Annu Rev Biochem* 1994;63:487–526.
24. Weintraub H, Davis R, Tapscott S, et al. The myoD gene family: nodal point during specification of the muscle cell lineage. *Science* 1991;251:761–766.
25. Smart DE, Vincent KJ, Arthur MJ, et al. JunD regulates transcription of the tissue inhibitor of metalloproteinases-1

and interleukin-6 genes in activated hepatic stellate cells. *J Biol Chem* 2001;276:24414–24421.
26. Muller DN, Heissmeyer V, Dechend R, et al. Aspirin inhibits NF-kappaB and protects from angiotensin II–induced organ damage. *FASEB J* 2001;15:1822–1824.
27. Imgrund M, Grone E, Grone HJ, et al. Re-expression of the developmental gene Pax-2 during experimental acute tubular necrosis in mice 1. *Kidney Int* 1999;56:1423–1431.
28. Bohe J, Ding H, Qing DP, et al. IGF-I binding proteins, IGF-I binding protein mRNA and IGF-I receptor mRNA in rats with acute renal failure given IGF-I. *Kidney Int* 1998;54:1070–1082.
29. Hirschberg R, Kopple J, Lipsett P, et al. Multicenter clinical trial of recombinant human insulin-like growth factor I in patients with acute renal failure. *Kidney Int* 1999;55:2423–2432.
30. Sharp PA. Split genes and RNA splicing. *Cell* 1994;77:805–815.
31. Kramer A. The structure and function of proteins involved in mammalian pre-mRNA splicing. *Annu Rev Biochem* 1996;65:367–409.
32. Modrek B, Lee C. A genomic view of alternative splicing. *Nat Genet* 2002;30:13–19.
33. Klamt B, Koziell A, Poulat F, et al. Frasier syndrome is caused by defective alternative splicing of WT1 leading to an altered ratio of WT1 +/–KTS splice isoforms. *Hum Mol Genet* 1998;7:709–714.
34. Merrick WC. Mechanism and regulation of eukaryotic protein synthesis. *Microbiol Rev* 1992;56:291–315.
35. Cleveland DW. Gene regulation through messenger RNA stability. *Curr Opin Cell Biol* 1989;1:1148–1153.
36. Ben-Neriah Y. Regulatory functions of ubiquitination in the immune system. *Nat Immunol* 2002;3:20–26.
37. Hames BD, Higgins SJ. Nucleic acid hybridization: a practical approach. Oxford, UK: IRL Press, 1985.
38. Soleimani M, Burnham CE. Physiologic and molecular aspects of the Na+:HCO3– cotransporter in health and disease processes. *Kidney Int* 2000;57:371–384.
39. Gamba G, Saltzberg SN, Lombardi M, et al. Primary structure and functional expression of a cDNA encoding the thiazide-sensitive, electroneutral sodium-chloride cotransporter. *Proc Natl Acad Sci U S A* 1993;90:2749–2753.
40. Southern EM. Detection of specific sequences among DNA fragments separated by gel electrophoresis. *J Mol Biol* 1975;98:503–517.
41. Wahl GM, Meinloth JL, Kimmel AR. Northern and Southern blots. *Methods Enzymol* 1987;152:572–581.
42. Pardue ML. In situ hybridization. In: Hames BD, Higgins SJ, eds. *Nucleic acid hybridization: a practical approach.* Oxford, UK: IRL Press, 1985;179–202.
43. Ausubel FM, Brent R, Kingston RE, et al. *Short protocols in molecular biology*, 2nd ed. New York: Wiley, 1992.
44. Nathans D, Smith HO. Restriction endonucleases in the analysis and restructuring of DNA molecules. *Annu Rev Biochem* 1975;44:273–293.
45. Eisenstein BI. The polymerase chain reaction: a new method of using molecular genetics for medical diagnosis. *N Engl J Med* 1990;322:178–183.
46. Rosenthal N. Fine structure of a gene—DNA sequencing. *N Engl J Med* 1995;332:589–591.
47. Prediger EA. Quantitating mRNAs with relative and competitive RT-PCR. *Methods Mol Biol* 2001;160:49–63.
48. Freeman WM, Walker SJ, Vrana KE. Quantitative RT-PCR: pitfalls and potential. *Biotechniques* 1999;26:112–125.
49. Lie YS, Petropoulos CJ. Advances in quantitative PCR technology: 5' nuclease assays. *Curr Opin Biotechnol* 1998;9:43–48.
50. Wittwer CT, Herrmann MG, Gundry CN, et al. Real-time multiplex PCR assays. *Methods* 2001;25:430–442.
51. Von Schnakenburg C, Strehlau J, Ehrich JH, et al. Quantitative gene expression of TGF-beta1, IL-10, TNF-alpha and Fas Ligand in renal cortex and medulla. *Nephrol Dial Transplant* 2002;17:573–579.
52. Duggan DJ, Bittner M, Chen Y, et al. Expression profiling using cDNA microarrays. *Nat Genet* 1999; 21[Suppl]:10–14.
53. Lockhart DJ, Winzeler EA. Genomics, gene expression and DNA arrays. *Nature* 2000;405:827–836.
54. Caskey CT. Disease diagnosis by recombinant DNA methods. *Science* 1987;236:1229.
55. Donadel G, Marinos N, DeSilva MG, et al. Molecular cloning and characterization of a highly basic protein, IA-4, expressed in pancreatic islets and brain. *Neuroendocrinology* 1998;67:190–196.
56. Schuler GD, Boguski MS, Stewart EA, et al. A gene map of the human genome. *Science* 1996;274:540–546.
57. Schaefer BC. Revolutions in rapid amplification of cDNA ends: new strategies for polymerase chain reaction cloning of full-length cDNA ends. *Anal Biochem* 1995;227:255–273.
58. Wallace RB, Miyada CG. Oligonucleotide probes for the screening of recombinant DNA libraries. *Methods Enzymol* 1987;152:432–442.
59. Koenen M, Griesser H-W, Muller-Hill B. Immunological detection of chimeric β-galactosidases expressed by plasmid vectors. In: Glover DM, ed. *DNA cloning techniques: a practical approach*. Oxford, UK: IRL Press, 1984;89–100.
60. Yayon A, Aviezer D, Saran M, et al. Isolation of peptides that inhibit binding of basic fibroblast growth factor to its receptor from a random phage epitope library. *Proc Natl Acad Sci U S A* 1993;90:10643–10647.
61. Brown EM, Gamba G, Riccardi D, et al. Cloning and characterization of an extracellular Ca(2+)-sensing receptor from bovine parathyroid. *Nature* 1993;366:575–580.
62. Henikoff S, Greene EA, Pietrokovski S, et al. Gene families: the taxonomy of protein paralogs and chimeras. *Science* 1997;278:609–614.
63. Bai M, Quinn S, Trivedi S, et al. Expression and characterization of inactivating and activating mutations in the human Ca2+–sensing receptor. *J Biol Chem* 1996;271:19537–19545.
64. Miller LK. Baculoviruses as gene expression vectors. *Annu Rev Microbiol* 1988;42:177–199.
65. Geitz RD, Triggs-Raine B, Robbins A, et al. Identification of proteins that interact with a protein of interest: applications of the yeast two hybrid system. *Mol Cell Biochem* 1997;172:67–79.
66. Hopkins CR. Selective membrane protein trafficking: vectorial flow and filter. *Trends Biol Sci* 1992;17:27–32.
67. Southern PJ, Berg P. Transformation of mammalian cells to antibiotic resistance with a bacterial gene under control of

the SV40 early region promoter. *J Mol Appl Genet* 1982;1: 327–341.

68. Lisanti MP, Rodriguez-Boulan R. Glycophospholipid membrane anchoring provides clues to the mechanism of protein sorting in polarized epithelial cells. *Trends Biochem Sci* 1990; 15:113–118.
69. Anderson MP, Gregory RJ, Thompson S, et al. Demonstration that CFTR is a chloride channel by alteration of its anion selectivity. *Science* 1991;253:202–207.
70. Orlowski J, Grinstein S. Na+/H+ exchangers of mammalian cells. *J Biol Chem* 1997;272:22373–22376.
71. Gamba G, Miyanoshita A, Lombardi M, et al. Molecular cloning, primary structure and characterization of two members of the mammalian electroneutral sodium-(potassium)-chloride cotransporter family expressed in kidney. *J Biol Chem* 1994;269:17713–17722.
72. Ho K, Nichols CG, Lederer WJ, et al. Cloning and expression of an inwardly rectifying ATP-regulated potassium channel. *Nature* 1993;362:31–38.
73. Chrispeels MJ, Agre P. Aquaporins: water channel proteins of plant and animal cells. *Trends Biochem Sci* 1994;19:421–425.
74. Canessa CM, Schild L, Buell G, et al. Amiloride-sensitive epithelial Na+ channel is made of three homologous subunits. *Nature (Lond)* 1994;367:463–467.
75. Deen PMT, Verdijk MAJ, Knoers NVAM, et al. Requirement of human renal water channel aquaporin-2 for vasopressin-dependent concentration of urine. *Science* 1994; 264:92–95.
76. Simon RP, Lifton RP. The molecular basis of inherited hypokalemic alkalosis: Bartter's and Gitelman's syndromes. *Am J Physiol* 1996;271:F961–F969.
77. Karolyil L, Konrad M, Kockerling A, et al. Mutations in the gene encoding the inwardly-rectifying renal potassium channel, ROMK, cause the antenatal variant of Bartter syndrome: evidence for genetic heterogeneity. *Hum Mol Genet* 1997;6:17–26.
78. Lemmink HH, van den Heuvell LPWJ, van Dijk HA, et al. Linkage of Gitelman syndrome to the human thiazide-sensitive sodium-chloride cotransporter gene with identification of mutations in three Dutch families. *Pediatr Nephrol* 1996;10:403–407.
79. Hannson JH, Schild L, Lu Y, et al. A de novo missense mutation of the beta subunit of the epithelial sodium channel causes hypertension and Liddle's syndrome, identifying a proline-rich segment critical for regulation of channel activity. *Proc Natl Acad Sci U S A* 1995;92:11495–11499.
80. Musaro A, Rosenthal N. Transgenic mouse models of muscle aging. *Exp Gerontol* 1999;34:147–156.
81. Jentsch TJ, Stein V, Weinreich F, et al. Molecular structure and physiological function of chloride channels. *Physiol Rev* 2002;82:503–568.
82. Rosenthal N. Recognizing DNA. *N Engl J Med* 1995;333: 925–927.
83. Ghiggeri GM, Oleggini R, Musante L, et al. A DNA element in the alpha1 type III collagen promoter mediates a stimulatory response by angiotensin II. *Kidney Int* 2000; 58:537–548.
84. Righetti PG, Gelfi C. Electrophoresis gel media: the state of the art. *J Chromatogr B Biomed Sci Appl* 1997;699:63–75.
85. Candiano G, Musante L, Bruschi, et al. Two-dimensional maps in soft immobilized pH gradient gels: a new approach to the proteome of the Third Millennium. *Electrophoresis* 2002;23:292–297.
86. Pandey A, Mann M. Proteomics to study genes and genomes. *Nature* 2000;405:837–846.
87. Leimgruber RM, Malone JP, Radabaugh MR, et al. Development of improved cell lysis, solubilization and imaging approaches for proteomic analyses. *Proteomics* 2002;2:135–144.

15

IN VITRO METHODS IN RENAL RESEARCH

PATRICIA D. WILSON

Significant advances in the understanding of renal cell function, epithelial cell biology, and morphogenesis have been made in recent years by the application of *in vitro* techniques. The researcher today is presented with a wide choice of *in vitro* models, and the aim of this chapter is to provide not only an overview of techniques available but also sufficient information to allow insight into the advantages and limitations of each system. This provides the experimental pediatric nephrologist with an appreciation of the range of renal *in vitro* methods currently available and allows selection of the most appropriate *in vitro* system to adequately answer the questions posed. For a more complete methodologic review of isolation and culture techniques, the reader is referred to standard tissue culture texts (1–3).

RENAL CELL TYPES AND ISOLATION TECHNIQUES

The kidneys are extremely heterogeneous, predominantly epithelial organs, each containing 1 million nephrons that are highly segmented and composed of many different cell types (Fig. 15.1). Detailed studies of the properties of these individual cell types are needed for the fundamental understanding of normal function and development of the kidney, and progress toward achievement of this goal has accelerated dramatically since 1990.

The initial requirement for the establishment of renal cell culture was the development of reproducible and reliable isolation techniques for individual cell types. The most successful of these are summarized in Table 15.1 and include physical microdissection, size discrimination by graded sieving or centrifugation over a Percoll or other similar gradients, and removal of specific components by immunoabsorption (4–11). Certain fundamental differences between these starting isolates should be stressed. Most of these techniques use an initial period of tissue disaggregation by incubation in collagenase, pronase, or other dissociative enzyme solutions. The length of time and conditions of this incubation determine whether tubule fragments or single cells are obtained. However, enzyme pretreatment is now considered undesirable because of the resultant damage to cell membrane proteins, such as receptors, and the deleterious effects on cell adhesion properties, which limit viability. For these reasons, physical microdissection of tubules without enzyme pretreatment is often the preferred choice. Many segments of the nephron can be isolated with precision by microdissection, and the ease of dissection is increased by using pathogen-free animals or salt solution–perfused human kidneys. Although physical microdissection of tubules provides the most accuracy, only relatively small numbers of tubules can be obtained from a single isolate because of the limited period of tissue viability. This limitation can be alleviated to some extent by freezing tissue slices in 5% dimethyl sulfoxide–containing medium for subsequent use, but the technique remains time consuming and labor intensive.

If purity is less important than large quantities of cells, the isolation technique of choice is gentle enzymatic digestion and/or calcium chelation (by ethylenediaminetetraacetic acid) of thin tissue slices followed by differential sieving or Percoll centrifugation. These techniques are widely used for the derivation of highly enriched proximal tubule preparations from cortical slices, but no discrimination between S1, S2, and S3 segments is possible in these types of isolates. Similar techniques have been applied to isolate thick ascending limbs of Henle and collecting tubules using cortical, outer, or inner medullary slices. The limitation of compromised cell type purity of this technique can be addressed by the application of a subsequent immunoabsorption step using cell type–specific antibodies. In this case, the quality of the preparation is a function of the specificity of the antibodies used. In addition to tubule epithelial cells, it is also possible to isolate glomerular epithelia by trypsinization and two rounds of sieving to produce pure podocytes (12–14).

There are many obvious advantages to long-term study of defined cell populations *in vitro*. The ability to adapt conditions to allow the proliferation of isolated renal cells *in vitro* has led to a dramatic increase in our understanding of renal cell biology and provides a powerful tool for study of renal tubule function, development, and disease. Most

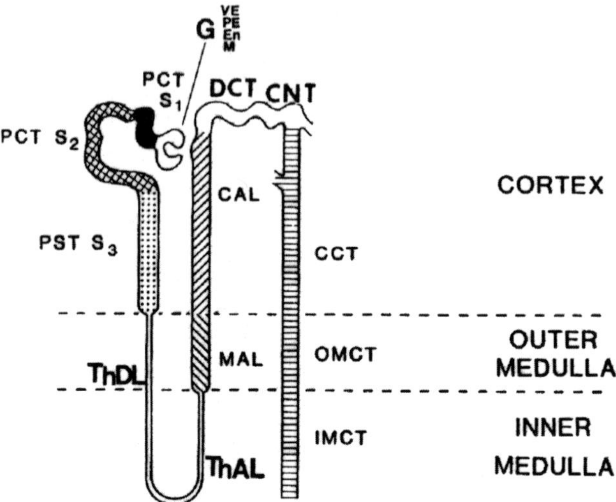

FIGURE 15.1. Schematic representation of distribution of cell types in the mammalian nephron. All tubule cell types can be isolated by microdissection techniques, and those shaded can be grown as primary culture monolayers in serum-free defined media. Glomeruli can be isolated by sieving and individual cell types grown in culture. Additional cells (not shown) include juxtaglomerular, vascular endothelia and smooth muscle cells, and interstitial fibroblasts of the cortical and medullary zones. CAL, cortical thick ascending limb of Henle's loop; CCT, cortical collecting tubule; CNT, connecting piece; DCT, distal convoluted tubule; En, endothelial cells; G, glomerulus; IMCT, inner medullary collecting tubule; M, mesangial cells; MAL, medullary thick ascending limb of Henle's loop; OMCT, outer medullary collecting tubule; PCT, proximal convoluted tubule; PE, parietal epithelial cells; PST, proximal straight tubule; ThDL, thin descending limb of Henle's loop; ThAL, thin ascending limb of Henle's loop; VE, visceral epithelial cells.

TABLE 15.1. ISOLATION TECHNIQUES

Technique	Tubule	Species	Collagenase	References
Microdissection	PCT S1, S2	Human, rabbit	–	19,21
	PST	Rabbit, human	–	20,21
	mTAL, cTAL	Rat, rabbit, human	+	—
	Tdl, DCT, CNT	Mouse	+	19–21
	CCT	Human, rabbit	–	19–21
	OMCT, IMCT	Human, rabbit	–	—
Sieve	Glomeruli	Human, rat	+	12–14
		Bovine	+	—
	PT, IMCT	Rabbit, mouse	+	4,7
Percoll	PT, CT	Dog, rabbit	+	8,9
Immunoabsorption	PT, CCT	Dog	+	6
	cTAL, mTAL	Rabbit, rat	+	10,11

CCT, cortical collecting tubule; CNT, connecting piece; cTAL, cortical thick ascending limb of Henle; DCT, distal convoluted tubule; IMCT, inner medullary collecting tubule; mTAL, medullary thick ascending limb of Henle; OMCT, outer medullary collecting tubule; PCT, proximal convoluted tubule; PST, proximal straight tubule; PT, proximal tubule; Tdl, thin descending limb of Henle.

tubule isolation techniques have used adult kidneys as starting material, but it has been easy to adapt these basic techniques to the isolation and proliferation of fetal tubules (2).

CELL AND TISSUE CULTURE

Cell and tissue culture techniques have been developed for the *in vitro* proliferation of many of the defined cell types in the kidney. These are summarized in Table 15.2, but for a more detailed survey, the reader is referred to several reviews (3,13,15).

Primary Cell Cultures

Traditional explant techniques, in which small pieces of the whole kidney (separated into cortex or medulla) are chopped and placed into tissue culture media containing serum and cell monolayer outgrowths studied in primary culture, are of little use in kidney research because of the extreme heterogeneity of cell types and the nonselective nature of serum stimulation of growth. These problems stimulated the development of cell type–specific isolation techniques. Significant advances in renal cell biology have been made by the application of these pure or highly enriched cell populations to defined culture media conditions. This has allowed the production of primary cultures of homogeneous populations of several renal cell types (Table 15.2).

Glomeruli can be readily isolated from mammalian kidney cortex by graded sieving (14), and the differential supplementation of culture media and extracellular matrix to the collagenase digests favors the primary outgrowth of epithelial, endothelial, or mesangial cells. Mesangial cells are the easiest to obtain because they grow on uncoated plastic in Roswell Park Medical Institute (RPMI) medium containing high levels (20%) of serum (16). Endothelial cells require gelatin for attachment and endothelial cell growth factor supplementation in the medium (17), whereas epithelial cells require collagen as matrix and supplementation of the medium with transferrin, insulin, dexamethasone, triiodothyronine, and prostaglandin E2 (18). These cells undergo few passages, and cloning is recommended for purity. Epithelial cells are usually considered to be visceral (podocyte) in origin because Bowman's capsules containing parietal epithelia are removed by the collagenase treatment. However, definitive marker analysis is required to substantiate this assertion (Table 15.3).

Primary cultures of defined renal tubule epithelia have been derived from several species, using a wide variety of techniques. As discussed earlier, microdissected tubules pro-

TABLE 15.2. MAMMALIAN RENAL CELL AND TISSUE CULTURES

Cell type	Species	References
Primary cultures		
Glomerular epithelia	Human, rat	13,18
Glomerular endothelia	Human, bovine, rat	15,17,23
Glomerular mesangial cells	Human, bovine, rat	16
Proximal convoluted tubule S1	Human, rabbit, mouse	3,19–21
Proximal convoluted tubule S2	Human, rabbit, mouse	3,19–21
Proximal straight tubule S3	Human (adult, fetal), rabbit, mouse	3,19–21
Mixed proximal tubules	Dog, rabbit, rat, mouse	7,8,10
Medullary thick ascending limb	Human, rabbit	19,20,24,25
Cortical thick ascending limb	Human, rabbit, mouse	19,20,24,26
Distal convoluted tubule	Rabbit, rat, mouse	26–28
Cortical collecting tubule	Human (adult, fetal), bovine, dog, rabbit	11,19,20,29
Intercalated cells	Rabbit	30
Principal cells	Rabbit	31
Outer medullary collecting tubule	Human, rabbit	19,20
Inner medullary collecting tubule	Human, rabbit, rat	19,20,32,33
Juxtaglomerular cells	Rat	34
Cortical interstitial fibroblasts	Human, rabbit, rat	22,35,36
Medullary interstitial fibroblasts	Rabbit, rat	36–38
Renal vascular smooth muscle cells	Rabbit	39
Spontaneous permanent cell lines		
Proximal-like: JTC-12, BSC-1, OK, LLC-PK1, PT	Monkey, opossum, pig, mouse	40–43
Distal-like: MDBK, MDCK, GRB-MAL, MmTAL-1C	Bovine, dog, rabbit, mouse	44–46
Fetal kidney	Human	44
Immortalized/transfected cell lines		
Glomerular epithelia	Human, mouse	47,48
Proximal tubule	Human, rabbit, rat	49–52
Distal convoluted tubule	Mouse	52,53
Cortical collecting tubule	Rabbit, human	54,55
Inner medullary collecting tubule	Mouse	56
Fetal kidney	Human	44

LLC-PK1, pig kidney; MDBK, Madin-Darby bovine kidney; MDCK, Madin-Darby canine kidney; MmTAL-1C, mouse medullary thick ascending limb; OK, opossum kidney; PT, proximal tubule.

vide maximum purity and allow discrimination between the S1, S2, and S3 portions of the proximal tubule (19–21). Commonly used and reliable techniques are available for the culture of proximal tubules, thick ascending limbs of Henle's loop, and collecting tubules of cortical and medullary origin, and these are used for the primary monolayer culture of cells of adult and fetal origin. In addition to epithelial cells, renal interstitial fibroblasts can also be cultured with ease from the cortical or medullary explants (22). These are fairly easy to generate because fibroblasts proliferate rapidly in response to 10% serum stimulation, whereas renal epithelial proliferation is inhibited under these conditions. This means that the renal fibroblasts initially present in mixed cell populations from explants eventually overgrow the cultures because of their selective growth in response to 10% serum in simple Dulbecco modified Eagle medium. Subculture with trypsin results in the acquisition of pure preparations of fibroblasts by the third passage, because renal epithelia are more sensitive to the destructive effects of trypsin than fibroblasts (22). Additional cell types, including juxtaglomerular and renal vascular smooth muscle cells, have also been grown in primary culture (34,39).

To assess the validity of any primary culture technique, marker analysis (Table 15.3) is essential because each cell type contains some specific protein(s) *in vivo*. This allows the analysis of both the purity of preparation and the maintenance of the differentiated state *in vitro*. If these criteria are fulfilled, primary cultures are particularly useful for the study of normal cell function. Most cell cultures derived from isolated glomerular or tubule preparations survive a few (three to five) passages but then die out. This is consistent with normal cell properties and is thought to represent the maximal repair capacity of renal cells *in vivo*. This contrasts with neoplastically transformed cells, which possess unlimited proliferative potential and produce tumors *in vivo* and immortal cell lines *in vitro*.

Permanent Cell Lines of Renal Origin

Several permanently growing cell lines of renal epithelia are in current use and can provide a convenient supply of large numbers of cells for the study of polarity, ion transport, and hormone receptor interactions. However, their limitations should be appreciated. Although LLC-PK1, OK, and JTC-

TABLE 15.3. MARKERS OF DIFFERENTIATED CELL TYPES: ADULT

Glomerulus	
Visceral epithelium	Podocalyxin, synaptopodin, podocin, laminin α_5, integrin α_3, C3B receptor, angiopoietin, VEGF
Parietal epithelium	Cytokeratin, VCAM1
Endothelial cells	Factor VIII, angiotensin-converting enzyme, Weibel-Palade bodies, acetylated low-density lipoprotein uptake, PDGFB, Tie 2
Mesangial cells	Actomyosin, contractility, angiotensin receptors, kinin receptors, protein kinase C, desmin, PDGFRβ
Tubules	
Proximal	Abundant brush border, alkaline phosphatase, γ-glutamyl transpeptidase, isomaltase, leucine aminopeptidase, meprin, aminopeptidase N, dipeptidylpeptidase Na-glucose transporter, Na-amino acid transporter, Na-amino acid transporter, parathyroid hormone receptors, aquaporin-1, midkine, NHE3; ClC5, rBAT, PEX, NBC, hUAT, GLUT-2, villin, 1,25-hydroxy $2D_3$
Thin descending limb of Henle	Aquaporin 1
Thick ascending limb of Henle	No brush border, abundant mitochondria, highest Na-K-ATPase activity, preproepidermal growth factor, ROMK channel, CaSR, Tamm-Horsfall protein, glucocorticoid receptor, osteopontin, NKCC2 (BSC1)
Juxtaglomerular apparatus	Renin
Distal convoluted tubule	Epidermal growth factor, osteopontin, Ca-ATPase, NCCT, claudin 16
Connecting tubule	Kallikrein, calbindin
Collecting tubule:	
Principal cells	Light cytoplasm, few organelles, calcium-binding protein, vasopressin, receptor V2 aquaporin 2, ENaC 11-hydroxysteroid dehydrogenase, mineralocorticoid receptor, AE1, aquaporin 4
Intercalated cells	Dense cytoplasm, many organelles, band 3, carbonic anhydrase II, H^+ATPase, mineralocorticoid receptor
Fibroblasts	
Cortical	Vimentin I; CAM-1; α_1, α_4, $\alpha_5\beta$, integrins
Medullary	Vimentin, tenascin

CaSR, calcium sensing receptor; ClC5, chloride channel; ENaC, epithelial sodium channel; GLUT-2, Na^+/glucose cotransporter; hUAT, urate transporter; PDGF, platelet-derived growth factor; PEX, Na/phosphate transporter; NBC, Na^+/HCO_3^- transporter; NCCT, Na^+/Cl^- transporter; NHE3, Na^+/H^+ exchanger; NKCC2 (BSC1), $Na^+K^+Cl^-$ transporter; rBAT, cystine and dibasic amino acid transporter; ROMK, renal outer medullary potassium clearance; VCAM1, V-cell adhesion molecule 1; VEGF, vascular endothelial growth factor.

12 cells have properties suggesting proximal tubule origin, and Madin-Darby canine kidney (MDCK) cells have some properties of distal tubules, the precise cells of origin of these spontaneously immortal lines is unknown. In addition, like all immortal cell lines, they have undergone genetic drift because of numerous passages, which has led to the loss of some properties and acquisition of other anomalous properties. Therefore, spontaneously immortal renal cell lines (40–46) may not be the system of choice for the study of normal epithelial function, although they have proved invaluable for the study of certain specific proteins, notably transporters, and for analysis of mechanisms controlling epithelial cell polarity. However, their value for studies of renal development is limited.

Immortalized Cell Lines

An important advance in the generation of cell lines for renal research has been the successful application of immortalization techniques using recombinant viral vectors introduced into cells by infection or transfection. Initial studies used oncogenic viruses such as adenovirus or papilloma virus to generate cell lines (47–57) (Table 15.2) such as HEK 293, HKC-8, mIMCD, and HK-2, which have proved to be very useful for several types of studies, not least because they are permissive to transfection. However, these types of cells also suffer from the limitation that they are permanently transformed with an abnormal proliferative phenotype conferred by the expression of the introduced oncogene.

Conditionally Immortalized Cell Lines

By far the most successful advance made toward the goal of production of large numbers of permanently proliferating but normally differentiated renal cell cultures has been the introduction of a temperature-ensitive (tsA58) allele-containing Simian virus (SV-40) T antigen into defined renal cell types (50,55,57–60). This has allowed for the immortalization by virtue of expression of the integrated SV-40 T antigen at the permissive temperature of 33°C but the differentiation and loss of T antigen expression after 7 to 10 days at nonpermissive, normal temperature (37°C). This technique has been successfully applied either by making cultures from renal tissues from the SV-40tsA58 transgenic mouse (58,61) or by transfection of human renal epithelial cells in culture (50). The latter technique has proved to have a wide use and has been used to conditionally immortalize renal epithelial cells of normal and diseased origin, including human normal fetal and normal adult proximal tubules, thick ascending limbs and collecting tubules, and epithelia from patients with cystinosis and

TABLE 15.4. CHARACTERIZATION OF CONDITIONALLY IMMORTALIZED CLONAL EPITHELIAL CELL LINES

	HFPT	HFCT	NHPT	NHTAL	NHCT	ADPKD	ARPKD
Keratin	+	+	+	+	+	+	+
Vimentin	–/+	–	–	–	–	+	+
Alkaline phosphatase	+	–	+	–	–	+(–)	–
Leucine aminopeptidase	–	–	+	–	–	+(–)	–
Multidrug resistance P-glycoprotein	+	–	+	–	–	+	–
Aquaporin 1	+	–	+	–	–	+(–)	–
NHE3	–	–	+	–	–	+	±
Epidermal growth factor receptor	+/–	+(A)	+(B)	–	–	+(A)	+(A)
Erb-B2	–	+(A)	–	–	–	+(A)	+(A)
α_2 Integrin	+/–	+	+	+/–	+/–	+	+
α_6 Integrin	–	–/+	+	+	+	+	+
β_1 Integrin	+	+	+	+	+	+	+
Tamm-Horsfall protein	–	–	–	+	–	–(+)	–
Aquaporin 2	–	+(–)	–	–	+(–)	+(–)	+
H^+ATPase	–	–(+)	+	–	+(–)	–(+)	–
Carbonic anhydrase II	–	–	–	–	+(–)	–(+)	–
ENaC	–	+	–	–	+	+	+
NaK-ATPase α_1	–	+(A)	+(B)	+(B)	+(B)	+(A)	+(A)
NaK-ATPase β_1	–	–	+(B)	+(B)	+(B)	+(C)	–
NaK-ATPase β_2	+(A)	+(A)	–	–	–	+(A)	+(A)
Polycystin 1	–	+	–	–	+	+(C)	+
Protein kinase	–	+	–	–	–	+	+
Sprouty-1	–	+	+	–	–	+	–(+)
WT1	–	–	–	–	–	+	–
Oct-1	–	+	–	–	–	+	+
Pax-2	–	+	–	–	–	+	+
Midkine	–	–	+	–	–	+	+/–

–/+, weak signal; +/–, most clones positive, few clones negative; (A), apical; ADPKD, autosomal dominant polycystic kidney disease; ARPKD, autosomal recessive polycystic kidney disease; (B), basal; (C), cytoplasmic; HFCT, human fetal collecting tubule; HFPT, human fetal proximal tubule; NHCT, normal human adult collecting tubule; NHPT, normal adult human proximal tubule; NHTAL, normal human adult thick ascending limb.

autosomal dominant and autosomal recessive polycystic kidney disease. By using actively proliferating microdissected renal tubule segments as starting material—6 weeks of neomycin selection and dilution analysis—clones have been isolated with the marker characteristics of their normal renal epithelia of origin (Table 15.4).

Role of Matrix

Studies in several in vitro systems have elucidated a major role for the extracellular matrix in the regulation of epithelial proliferation, differentiation, and gene expression (62). *In vivo*, the renal extracellular matrix is made up of the mesenchymal layer of interstitial fibroblasts that secrete types I and III collagen and the thin basement membrane on which epithelial cells rest, composed of type IV collagen, laminin, fibronectin, entactin, and heparan sulfate proteoglycans. Confluent renal tubule epithelial cells *in vitro* also secrete a basement membrane with normal structural and biochemical characteristics (19,63,64). Several of the techniques for primary cultures of renal tubule epithelia include precoating tissue culture dishes with type I (rat-tail) collagen or growth on collagen gels, EHS sarcoma matrix (matrigel), or amnion. This not only provides adhesion but also produces epithelial cultures with more differentiated characteristics. In addition, cultures of microdissected tubules and glomerular epithelia have an absolute requirement for extracellular matrix. By contrast, cells of mesenchymal origin in the adult kidney (i.e., mesangial and interstitial cells) have no matrix requirement and grow on uncoated plastic.

Role of Growth Factors

Soluble growth factors have long been known to play a major role in the control of cell proliferation. *In vitro*, serum was first used to induce cell growth. However, serum is a complex mixture of proteins, and detailed composition has not been fully elucidated. The value of serum in renal cell culture is that it favors the growth of fibroblasts at the expense of epithelia. In mixed epithelial and fibroblast cell populations, this enables the differential survival of fibroblasts because *in vitro*, after approximately three passages, the epithelial cells have disappeared and fibroblasts continue to proliferate. A significant advance for renal epithelial cell culture was the definition of serum-free growth factor–supplemented culture media that support the proliferation of renal epithelial cells (65). Modifications of the original formulation have led to the ability to culture most renal tubule epithelia in serum-free media. All epithelia have an absolute requirement for transferrin and proximal tubules are stimulated to proliferate by combinations of dexamethasone (or hydrocortisone) and insulin, although this requirement can be substituted by epidermal growth factor (EGF). Optimal proliferation of thick ascending limb epithelia requires additional supplementation with triiodothyronine, whereas collecting tubules require only dexamethasone and transferrin (19–21). Although it is not surprising that different renal epithelial cell segments with their individual complements of membrane proteins, including receptors, should require distinct hormone supplementation, the precise mechanisms regulating renal cell–type specific proliferation are not fully understood. Because normal renal epithelial cell division is complete before birth in humans, it is thought that the limited ability to proliferate *in vitro* represents a repair response.

ORGAN CULTURE TECHNIQUES

It is often desirable to study tissue and cell interactions, and although this can be accomplished by co-cultures of primary monolayers or cell lines, an alternative is to use an organ culture technique. Such techniques maintain the three-dimensional organization of the tissue of origin, including interactions with endogenous matrix proteins and intercalated growth factors. The emphasis in such systems is to retain viability of tissues rather than to encourage monolayer outgrowth of new cells.

These techniques have proved particularly useful for the study of renal development, because the embryonic organ can be removed and placed in organ culture in which the influence of a variety of inductive factors can be studied in detail. Most studies of this type have used mouse metanephric blastema (66–68), although rat and human renal organ culture have been reported (69,70). Small pieces of tissue or whole embryonic kidneys are dissected and placed on a stainless steel raft or membrane filter apparatus that has been placed in a tissue culture dish. Sufficient tissue culture medium is added to the dish to bathe the tissue from below and form a thin film of media above but not to submerge it. Organ culture techniques have also been used to study mechanisms of cyst formation and regression in normal mouse kidneys and in those cultured from mice with congenital recessive polycystic kidney disease (71,72). This technique is also now being used to microinject recombinant viral reporter-DNA constructs into either the blastema or the ureteric bud to analyze lineage tracing of progenitor cells or the effects of specific gene expression in the developing ureteric bud, respectively.

MORPHOGENESIS AND DIFFERENTIATION: APPLICATION OF *IN VITRO* TECHNIQUES TO RENAL DEVELOPMENT

Mammalian renal development is a complex process that involves the induction of undifferentiated mesoderm to form epithelia (73,74). As described in detail in Chapter 1, the ureteric bud (a branch of the mesonephric duct) invades and is induced to branch by the mesenchyme of the metanephric blastema and in return the ureteric bud induces the undifferentiated blastemal cells to proliferate, condense, and differentiate into primitive renal vesicles, comma bodies, and S-shaped bodies. The exquisite regulation of gene expression necessary to complete this elaborate set of reciprocal interactions is beginning to be understood (75).

Transfilter Techniques

For studies of renal development and nephrogenesis, the most important modification of organ culture, the *transfilter technique*, was first introduced by Grobstein (67) and continues to be used extensively. Metanephric blastemas are attached to a filter suspended above a tissue culture dish or well. To induce nephrogenesis, tissue fragments of ureter or spinal cord can be applied to the undersurface of the filter. Alternatively, the natural inducer, the ureteric bud is left in the blastema of a day 11 to 12 embryonic kidney, and culture on the membrane is carried out in optimized serum-free, supplemented media that can support the normal three-dimensional development of organogenesis in culture for up to 2 weeks.

Progressively refined analysis of the transfilter organ culture system has provided the basis for much of our present understanding of the cellular and molecular events associated with nephrogenesis and has led to an understanding of the complex temporally and spatially coordinated interactions involved. These include cell-cell contact and cell-matrix attachment, allowing regulated migration and cell shape changes as well as appropriate growth factor–receptor interactions regulating proliferation and apoptosis as well as epithelial polarization events associated with renal tubule maturation.

Proliferation and Differentiation of Primary Cultures

Cell culture techniques have been used to study renal development and epithelial differentiation and have included the isolation and culture of S-shaped bodies from newborn rabbit kidneys that give rise to the outgrowth of collecting duct principal cell monolayers (31). More recently, several primary and conditionally immortalized cell lines of normal human fetal proximal and collecting tubule epithelia have been generated from microdissected nephron segments providing a readily manipulatable system for the analysis of epi-

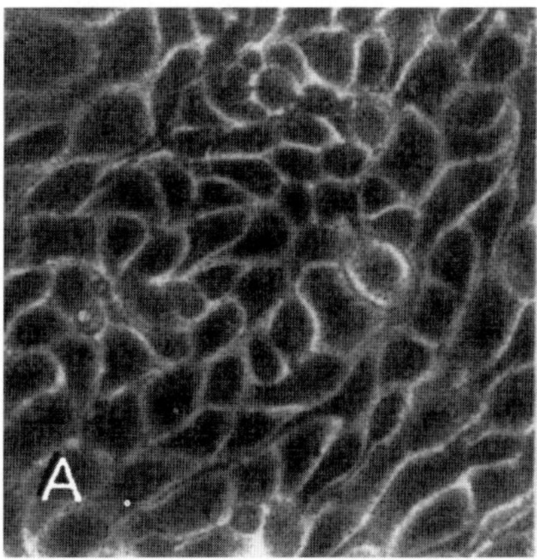

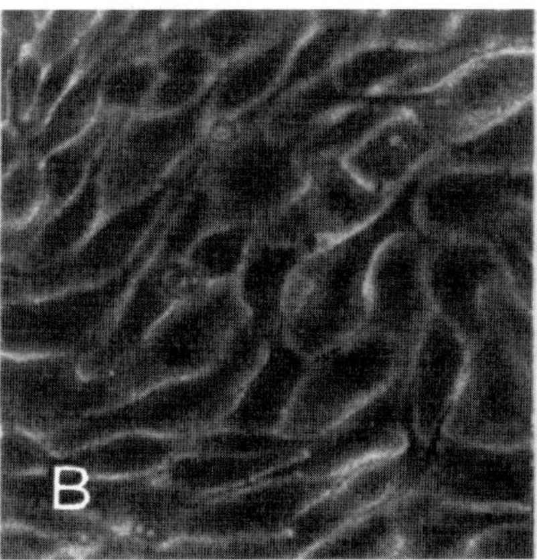

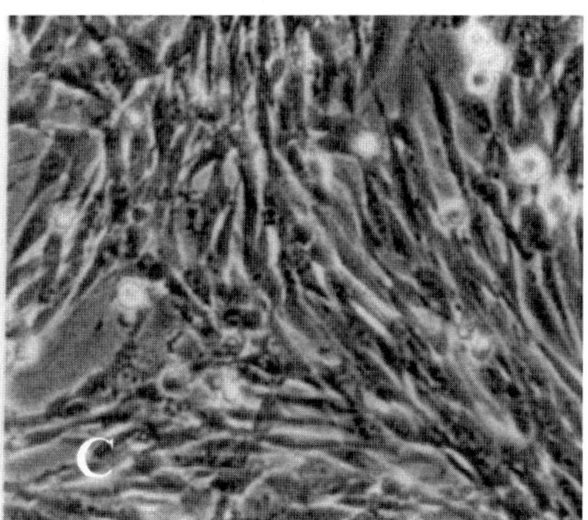

FIGURE 15.2. Phase-contrast light micrographs of confluent primary cultures. **A:** Epithelial monolayer grown from individually microdissected human fetal proximal tubule explanted onto type I collagen-coated plastic plates in Click–Roswell Park Medical Institute medium supplemented with human transferrin, dexamethasone, insulin, and fetal bovine serum (1%). Note polygonal morphology. **B:** Epithelial monolayer grown from individually microdissected human fetal collecting tubule explanted onto type I collagen-coated plastic plates in Click–Roswell Park Medical Institute medium supplemented with transferrin, dexamethasone, and fetal bovine serum (1%). Note polygonal morphology. **C:** Renal fibroblasts derived from cortical explants plated onto uncoated tissue culture plastic in Dulbecco modified Eagle medium supplemented with 10% fetal bovine serum. Note elongated spindle morphology.

thelial differentiation, polarization, and transport events (Fig. 15.2). These processes can be particularly well studied when cells are grown on filters suspended in a tissue culture well because there is individual access to the separate culture medium compartments bathing the apical and basal surfaces of the cell monolayer. For instance, the polarized fate of a radioactive tracer added to one compartment can easily be traced by scintillation techniques (Fig. 15.3). These types of studies have been widely applied in functional analysis of normal fetal, adult, and diseased (e.g., polycystic kidney disease) epithelia (76–78). An additional advantage of these membrane-grown cultures is that the differentiated and polarized characteristics of the cells are maximized under these conditions of nutrient access to both basal and apical cell surfaces.

Although much has been learned about induction and differentiation associated with nephrogenesis using the transfilter organ culture system, recent important technical advances provide the potential for more detailed molecular analyses of the underlying processes of induction and differentiation. Major advances have been made in the development of renal progenitor and ureteric bud cell culture systems. The isolation of normal human renal progenitor cells from 12- to 16-week human fetal kidneys and their dependence on conditioned media from a Wilms' tumor cell line (WT-CM) has led to the identification of a new soluble growth factor activity (midkine) involved in the control of renal progenitor proliferation (79–81). Human renal progenitor cells *in vitro* not only retain the distinctive morphology of renal cortical progenitors but also retain the capability to convert into epithelial phenotypes with appropriate switches in gene transcription and protein expression after withdrawal of WT-CM and addition of serum and/or collagen matrix (82) (Fig. 15.4). Most recently, similar studies have resulted in the isolation and characterization of renal progenitor cells from mouse kidneys and progress is being made in isolating subpopulations of epithelial, and stromal/fibroblast progenitors (D. Hyink, *personal communication*, 2002).

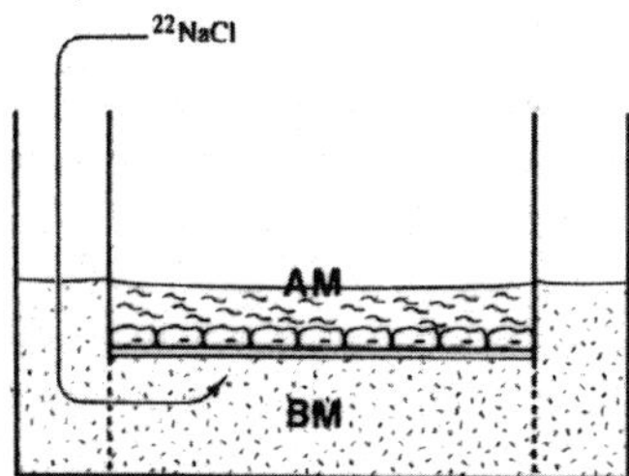

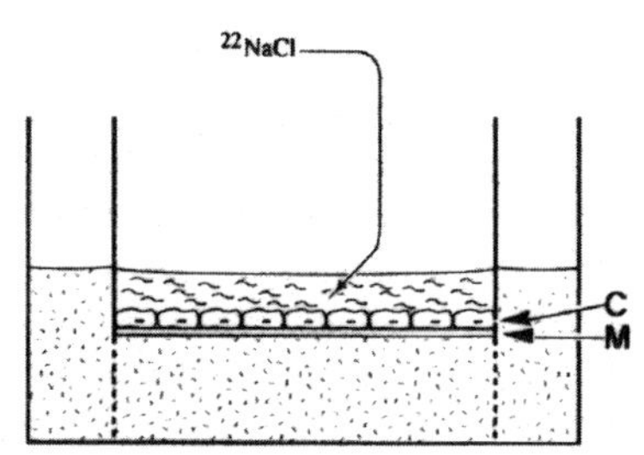

FIGURE 15.3. Schematic representation of *in vitro* system for study of transport and differentiation properties of epithelial monolayers. Cells (C) are seeded at high density on permeable, translucent membranes (M) mounted on a plastic ring and suspended in a tissue culture well. In this way, the medium overlying the apical surface of the cell monolayer (AM) is in a separate compartment from the medium bathing the basal surface of the cell monolayer (BM), which allows addition of radioactive tracer to either the basal or the apical compartment. Loss from that compartment or appearance in the contralateral compartment can be measured by scintillation counting of media aliquots.

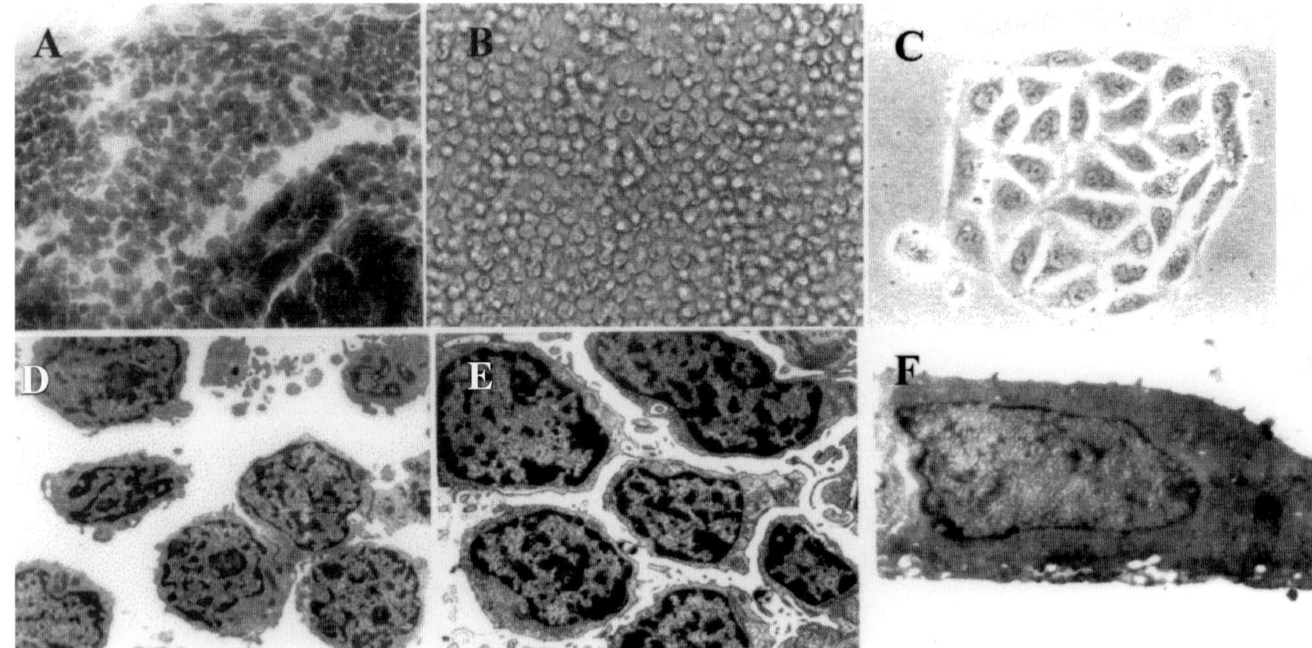

FIGURE 15.4. **A:** Outer cortical region of human fetal kidney of 14 weeks' gestation showing small, round undifferentiated mesenchymal blastemal cells. **B:** Phase-contrast light micrograph of human fetal nephroblasts *in vitro*, plated on gelatin and grown in serum-free medium containing Midkine from G401 conditioned media (CM). Cells show small round morphology, small overall diameter (4 μm), large nuclei, and thin rim of cytoplasm with few organelles. **C:** Light micrograph of differentiated focus of cultured renal epithelial progenitor cells after removal of G401 CM and addition of 10% fetal bovine serum. Note polygonal cells with large overall diameter and extensive cytoplasm. **D:** Electron micrograph of outer cortical region of kidney in **A**. **E:** Electron micrograph of cultured nephroblasts in **B**. **F:** Electron micrograph of epithelial focus in **C**.

TABLE 15.5. MARKERS OF RENAL DEVELOPMENT

Cell type or structure	Markers
Metanephric blastema (undifferentiated mesenchyme)	Vimentin; syndecan; integrins α_1, α_9; collagen I, III; laminin β_1, γ_1; fibronectin; N-CAM; IGF-II; GDNF HGF; c-Met; NGFR; midkine; CRABP; BF2; tenascin; WT1 cadherin-11; Hox AII; Hox DII; Six-2; Sca-1; P75NGFR; FGF2; BMP4; PNA+; apoptosis
Condensates	Vimentin, syndecan, α_8 integrin, N-CAM, N-myc, WT1, IGF-II, HGF, c-Met, NGFR, midkine, pax-2, wnt4, cadherin 6, E-cadherin
S-shaped bodies	Laminin α_1 integrin, E-cadherin, syndecan, tenascin, N-myc, NGFR, wnt4, Notch-1
Glomerular pole	Vimentin, WT1, α_3 integrin, podocalyxin, C3b receptor, IGF-II, nephrin B_2
Tubular pole	γGT, MDR, α_6 integrin, α_1-dystroglycan
Fetal tubule epithelia	Cytokeratin, laminin α_1, collagen IV, α_6 integrin, E-cadherin, desmoplakin, HGF, c-Met, LIM-1, α_1-dystroglycan
Proximal	Alkaline phosphatase, leucine aminopeptidase, renal peptidase, meprin, MDR, midkine, aquaporin 1, CFTR, cadherin 6
Thin descending limb	Aquaporin 1
Thick ascending limb	Na-K-ATPase $\alpha_1\beta_2$, Tamm-Horsfall protein, osteopontin, L-myc, integrin β_4, integrin α_2, calcium-binding protein, E-cadherin, Brn 4/1
Collecting tubule/ureteric bud	Midkine, Wnt7b, PKD-1, polycystin-1, CFTR, Pax-2, carbonic anhydrase, H-ATPase, aquaporin 2, Hox B7, c-ret, calbindin, Pax-2, E-cadherin and DBA+
Fetal glomeruli	Vimentin; integrin α_3, β_1; podocalyxin; C3bR; WT1; ACE
Fetal interstitium/stroma	Vimentin, tenascin, GD-3, ganglioside, IGF-II, FGFa, NGFR, RARα, RARβ, BF-2

ACE, angiotensin-converting enzyme; ATPase, adenosine triphosphatase; BMP, bone morphogenetic protein; CAM, cell adhesion molecule; CFTR, cystic fibrosis transmembrane regulator; FGF, fibroblast growth factor; GDNF, glial derived factor; γGT, γ-glutamyl transpeptidase; HGF, hepatocyte growth factor; IGF, insulin-like growth factor; MDR, multidrug resistance; NGFR, nerve growth factor receptor; RAR, retinoic acid receptor; WT1, Wilms' tumor 1.

Differentiation of Immortalized Cell Lines

Mouse metanephric renal progenitor cells have also been transfected with SV-40 T antigen (83,84) and provide a useful system for the analysis of growth factor interactions. Together with immortalized cells derived from the ureteric bud (85), these cellular approaches promise to increase our molecular understanding of proliferation, induction, and differentiation in nephrogenesis.

Marker Analysis

The differentiation process involved in conversion of undifferentiated, nonadhesive, nonpolarized mesenchymal cells into polarized, adhesive, highly specialized renal tubule (and glomerular) epithelia involves several stages of modification under strict temporal control. These include specific matrix (laminin) and receptor (integrin) expression, intercellular tight-junction formation and E-cadherin expression, and segregation of membrane proteins to apical and basolateral domains. This is followed by elaboration of specialized membrane and cytoplasmic proteins, including enzymes, transporters, receptors, and structural components of the brush border and cytoskeleton (86–89). To study such a complex array of events in cell or organ cultures, a series of developmental cell- and stage-specific markers are necessary. Known markers derived from tissue localization studies are summarized in Table 15.5. These markers can be used to characterize a culture system and evaluate its relevance for further study. For instance, in cultures of undifferentiated human and mouse renal progenitors, vimentin and syndecan expression is strong. After differentiation into cells with epithelial characteristics, however, the former are lost, and E-cadherin, alkaline phosphatase, and cytokeratin are highly expressed (79,82), whereas Pax-2 and N-CAM are appropriately, transiently expressed. The use of the renal progenitor cell system for study rests on the fidelity of expression of these markers before and after induction *in vitro*.

Regulation of Differentiation by Matrix and Soluble Factors

The interactions of extracellular matrix (e.g., collagens I, III, IV, and V; laminin; and proteoglycans) with specific matrix receptors such as syndecan and integrins are critically important in nephrogenesis (74,86,87,90). These interactions appear to be of particular importance in establishing cell polarity, a prerequisite for epithelial differentiation, in which laminin α_1-chain expression and interaction with an epithelial integrin α_6 subunit is required (86,87). An important role for the adhesion protein E-cadherin (uvomorulin) has also been proposed (88). *In vitro* techniques allow the analysis of the influence of matrix proteins on proliferation (64), but few studies have been carried out in fetal cells. An absolute requirement for collagen has been demonstrated for the attachment and growth of human fetal proximal and collecting tubules, whereas undifferentiated renal progenitor cells not only grow in suspension in the absence of matrix but also require its absence to retain their undifferentiated state.

The action of soluble factors via specific receptors plays an important role in proliferation and nephrogenesis, but studies in transfilter organ cultures were unable to identify a role for many candidate growth factors (90). More recently, however, the combination of embryonic kidney organ culture and cell culture studies has begun to identify important roles for a variety of growth factor ligands, including midkine, neuregulin, fibroblast growth factor, and leukemia inhibitory factor (81,85,91,92).

Establishment of Epithelial Cell Polarity

Reabsorption and secretion in the kidney are the byproducts of vectorial transport—the physiologic hallmark of renal epithelia. This is possible because renal tubule epithelial cells are polarized with asymmetric distributions of membrane proteins on their apical and basolateral membranes. This polar distribution of transporters, channels, and other proteins is a characteristic of fully differentiated functionally competent adult renal epithelia. Polarity is not only a functional characteristic but also reflects structural differences of apical and basolateral membranes. Typically, the apical (luminal) membrane is elaborated into a brush border, although the degree of specialization of microvilli depends on the tubule cell type. The basal membrane is characterized by its close proximity to the secreted basement membrane, which is composed of a thin electron-dense layer and separated from the epithelial cell by a thin electron-lucent zone. Proteins of the apical and basolateral domains are prevented from intermixing by the occluding tight junctional complexes that form a continuous belt between epithelial cells at the apical pole of the cell and serve to prevent intercellular leakage. When renal tubule epithelia are grown in culture, they also establish polarity characterized by formation of tight junctions and segregation of membrane proteins to appropriate apical or basolateral domains. This results in the vectorial transport of ions characteristic of those epithelia *in vivo*. The degree of polarization achieved *in vitro* is dependent on the cell type and the culture conditions. Polarization begins when cells attach to a substrate, which can be glass or plastic but is induced by collagen. Maximal polarization of epithelia is seen when cells are grown to confluence on collagen-coated filter membrane (transwell) inserts in which feeding is from the basal as well as the apical surface.

During renal development, a key feature of nephrogenesis is the conversion of undifferentiated, nonpolarized mesenchymal cells of the metanephric blastema through several stages into polarized, highly specialized tubule and glomerular epithelia. After induction by reciprocal interaction with the ureteric bud, mesenchymal cells first adhere to one

TABLE 15.6. MARKERS OF POLARITY: NORMAL ADULT

Apical	Basal and lateral
Influenza hemagglutinin	VSV G
Alkaline phosphatase	Na-K-ATPase
γ-Glutamyl transpeptidase	Ankyrin
5'-Nucleotidase	Fodrin
Meprin	E-cadherin
Diaminopeptidase IV, meprin	V_2 receptors
Aminopeptidases M, N, P	Epidermal growth factor receptors
Maltase	Insulin-like growth factor-1 receptors
H^+-ATPase	Laminin receptors
Trehalase	Type IV collagen receptors
Carcinoembryonic antigen	HSPG receptors
Na-glucose transporter GLUT2	Integrin α_6
Na-amino acid transporter	Integrin α_2
Na-H exchanger NHE3	Integrin β_1
Aquaporin 2	Integrin β_4
$Na^+K^+2Cl^-$ symporter	Cl/HCO_3 transporter, AEI
Urate transporter	AQP 4

AQP, aquaporin; ATPase, adenosine triphosphatase; HSPF, heparin sulfate proteoglycan.

another in the condensate stage and then begin to establish polarity in the vesicle and S-body stages. An important role for the adhesion protein E-cadherin has been suggested (88), and inhibitory antibody studies suggest a critical role for laminin α_1 chain and its receptor $\alpha_6\beta_1$ integrin because these are expressed concomitantly with onset of epithelial polarization (86,87). The formation of occluding tight junctions between cells has also been correlated with the expression of adherens junction and desmosomal plaque proteins, including ZO-1, catenins, and desmoglein (93, 94). Subsequent differentiation into tubule cell types is a result of further insertion of polarized tubule cell–specific membrane proteins. This is particularly marked on the apical surface, which is elaborated into a brush border to provide increased surface area to accommodate an array of enzymes, transporters, and receptors. Table 15.6 shows some typical markers of apical and basolateral membranes in renal tubular epithelia, which might be used to analyze differentiation processes. The analysis of cell polarization events in monolayer primary cultures derived from differentiated renal progenitors will in the future provide a temporal and spatial map of sequential events involved in tubule maturation during nephrogenesis.

EPITHELIAL-MESENCHYMAL INTERACTIONS

The regulation of ordered growth in the developing kidney and the subsequent maintenance of differentiation is a function of reciprocal interactions between the epithelial and mesenchymal components of the organ (95,96). In the embryonic kidney, the mesenchyme provides a pool of progenitor cells that differentiate along epithelial (glomerular and tubule), vascular, and fibroblast lineages, and morphogenesis can be studied by embryonic organ culture techniques. Co-culture techniques of epithelial and fibroblast components have also shown the importance of these interactions in the adult kidney (97).

Morphogenesis Assays

Three-Dimensional Gels

Experimental confirmation of the role of mesenchymal and extracellular matrix induction on normal renal epithelia has also been shown by the ability of collagen or reconstituted basement membrane gels to promote the development of three-dimensional tubule-like structures from mouse (inner medullary collecting duct) and bovine (MDCK) collecting tubules (98,99) as well as human, dog, and rabbit proximal tubules (3). When initially seeded into type I collagen gels, MDCK and LLC-PK1 cells form cysts (100,101), the specific polarity of which is a reflection of the responsiveness of the epithelium to inductive signals from the collagen matrix (95,96). Landmark studies showed that co-cultures of MDCK cysts in type I collagen gels with fibroblasts or the addition of fibroblast-conditioned media elicits a tubulogenic effect on MDCK cells in collagen gels that is mediated by hepatocyte growth factor (102,103). These studies have led to the wide use of this technique to further dissect the mechanisms of hepatocyte growth factor regulation (104,105) as well as to elucidate the role of cyclic adenosine monophosphate, protein kinase A, and protein kinase X (106,107). The use of this system is that it provides a robust three-dimensional assay system to analyze the roles of cell-cell, cell-matrix, and cell-soluble factor interactions. The concentration on MDCK cells will most likely in the future give way to the use of more normal cell lines derived from conditionally immortalized mouse and human nephron segments from adult and fetal kidneys.

Embryonic Organ Culture

An increased level of three-dimensional organization and normal cell-cell, cell-matrix, and cell-soluble factor interactions can be achieved by organ culture. Because fetal mouse kidneys can now be encouraged to grow and differentiate relatively normally for periods up to and exceeding 14 days, this system can be used very successfully for analysis by adding growth factors, antibodies, or even antisense to the media or by introducing genes into the organ rudiments. Studies of this type have been instrumental in identifying important matrix and growth factors in the regulation of ureteric bud branching and progenitor cell production including laminin, $\alpha_6\beta_1$-integrin, sulfated proteoglycans, galectin-3, ganglioside D3, retinoic acid, midkine, EGF, and neuregulin (75,91,108–113).

TABLE 15.7. *IN VITRO* TECHNIQUES FOR THE STUDY OF CELL INJURY AND DISEASES

Insult or abnormality	Cell type	Species	References
Ischemia (anoxia)	PT, PCT, PST	Human, rat	117
	cTAL, mTAL, CCT	Rabbit	118
Gentamicin	LLC-PK1, PT PCT, PST, CCT	Human, dog, rabbit	119–122
Cyclosporine	LLC-PK1, PCT, PST, TAL, CCT, mesangial, endothelia, vascular smooth muscle	Human, dog, rabbit	123–126
Nephropathic cystinosis	T	Human	50
ADPKD	Primary monolayer: epithelia fibroblasts	Human	22,63
	Conditionally immortalized: epithelia	Human	50,55
ARPKD	Primary monolayer epithelia	Human, mouse	127–130
	Conditionally immortalized epithelia	Human, mouse	50,55,131
	Organ culture	Mouse	72
Nephronophthisis	Primary monolayer	Human	132
Wilms' tumor	G401, SK-NEP, WIT 13, GOS-4	Human	44,133
Renal adenocarcinoma	A704, AHCN RAG	Human, mouse	44
Renal carcinoma	CAKI-1, 2: A-498; RC-1; RCC; CCF-RC1, -2	Human	44,123, 134–136

ADPKD, autosomal dominant polycystic kidney disease; ARPKD, autosomal recessive polycystic kidney disease; CCT, cortical collecting tubule; cTAL, cortical thick ascending limb of Henle; mTAL, medullary thick ascending limb of Henle; PCT, proximal convoluted tubule; PST, proximal straight tubule; PT, proximal tubule.

IN VITRO TECHNIQUES FOR ANALYSIS OF RENAL CELL INJURY AND DISEASE

Renal tubule cell injury *in vivo* can be induced by ischemia, nephrotoxins, genetic abnormalities, or cancer. An understanding of some of the cellular and molecular mechanisms involved is beginning to emerge, in large part because of the use of *in vitro* techniques, as summarized in Table 15.7.

Glomerular Disease

The availability of pure glomerular cell types *in vitro* has led to their use in elucidating cellular mechanisms of disease. For example, glomerular epithelial cells in culture have been exposed to Heymann nephritis antigen and provided experimental evidence for binding in coated pits, patching, capping, and final shedding from the cell surface (114). More recently, the advent of well-differentiated, conditionally immortalized podocyte cell systems from normal mice and their genetically manipulated diseased counterparts has significantly contributed to the understanding of the roles of collagen 4α4 in Alport's syndrome, nephrin in Finnish-type nephropathy, and podocin in immunoglobulin A nephropathies (61,115). Glomerular epithelial cell cultures have also been used to demonstrate a role for loss of negative charge and adhesive properties in puromycin aminonucleoside nephrosis. Mesangial cell cultures have also been used as a model system to study diabetes by their isolation from diabetic kidneys and/or by addition of glucose, transforming growth factor β, interleukin-1β, or galectin-3 to their tissue culture media *in vitro* (110,116).

Ischemic Injury

Isolated tubules were the first preparations used to study anoxic and ischemic injury *in vitro*. These studies identified a role for increased calcium in postischemic cell death (117). Subsequent studies also showed protective effects of extracellular acidosis and glycine. Molecular mechanisms of cell injury can be studied easily in long-term cultures, but permanent cell lines including MDCK and LLC-PK1 are not well suited for the study of ischemic damage because they have adapted to the relatively hypoxic conditions of tissue culture and are abnormally resistant to ischemic damage. However, primary cultures of rat, rabbit, and human renal tubule epithelial cells retain their sensitivity to hypoxic and postischemic reperfusion injury. They have been used successfully to demonstrate differential tubule cell sensitivity and attenuation of cell death by polyethylene glycol, extracellular calcium restriction, calcium channel blockers, and inhibitors of calmodulin and cysteine protease activities (117,118).

Nephrotoxic Injury

LLC-PK1 and primary cultures of rabbit and human proximal tubules and conditionally immortalized human proximal, thick ascending limb, and collecting tubules have been used to reproduce the characteristics of gentamicin and aminoglycoside antibiotic toxicity *in vivo*. They have demonstrated a major role for lipid changes, including decreased turnover and degradation caused by reductions in sphingomyelinase activity in cellular injury primarily in the proximal tubule (50,119–122).

Cyclosporine toxicity can also be studied in LLC-PK1 rabbit proximal tubule and human proximal, thick ascending limb, and collecting tubule cultures and has been shown to exert differential toxic effects on proximal tubule cells. These toxic effects can be attenuated by extracellular calcium restriction, calcium channel blockers, and cysteine protease inhibition. The mechanism of action may be through intracellular binding to cyclophilin and increased intracellular calcium-dependent protease activity (123,124). Renal vascular effects have also been demonstrated by observation of increased proliferation of endothelial and vascular smooth muscle cells in culture as well as increases in intracellular free calcium in mesangial cells (125,126) that are inhibited by cyclosporine.

Genetic Renal Tubular and Cystic Diseases

The first cell culture system devised for the study of genetic cystic disease was for human autosomal dominant polycystic kidney disease (ADPKD) in which individual cysts were microdissected and grown in primary culture (63). Subsequently, several primary, immortalized, and conditionally immortalized monolayer systems for human ADPKD, human and mouse autosomal recessive polycystic kidney diseases (ARPKD), and nephronophthisis (132) have been established (Table 15.7). Monolayer primary cultures were particularly instrumental in delineating the excessive tubule epithelial cell proliferation, matrix adhesion, and polarity and fluid secretion defects in cystic epithelia (137) (Chapter 35). The advantages of these *in vitro* monolayer culture techniques are the capacity to carry out strict comparisons of normal and abnormal cells, which have allowed structural and functional characterization of the modified phenotype in ADPKD epithelia, compared with similarly cultured normal tubule epithelia of proximal, thick ascending limb or collecting tubule origin. Use of these techniques in combination with *in vivo* studies has identified several abnormalities and determined their functional consequences. Mislocalization of Na-K-ATPase to the apical membranes of ADPKD epithelia is associated with similarly mislocated ankyrin, fodrin, and E-cadherin and a basal-to-apical vectorial transport of sodium, suggesting a mechanism for the secretion of ions and fluids into cysts (138). A mechanism for increased proliferation in ADPKD cyst epithelia is suggested by detection of hypersensitivity of ADPKD epithelia *in vitro* to the mitogenic effects of EGF, apical secretion of EGF into cyst fluids, and mislocalization of EGF receptors to apical cell membranes of ADPKD epithelia. Similar abnormalities in Na-K-ATPase and EGF receptor proteins have been found in human ARPKD, in cpk/cpk, and PKD1 and PKD2 knock-out mice, which is consistent with their fundamental roles in cyst formation in genetically determined polycystic kidney disease. However, ADPKD differs from ARPKD in that cysts are derived from all segments of the nephron, and there are additional interstitial abnormalities, including increased extracellular matrix (heparan sulfate proteoglycan) turnover and overproliferation of fibroblasts (22,64). The identification of the PKD-1–encoded protein polycystin-1 and its localization to cell membranes of normal fetal collecting duct and ADPKD epithelia *in vivo* and *in vitro* correlates with demonstrated abnormal fetal patterns of gene transcription in adult epithelia from ADPKD kidneys. Primary and conditionally immortalized cell lines derived from these cell types provide an essential tool to analyze the precise function of polycystin-1 and to determine the primary effects of PKD-1 mutations (Table 15.4).

In addition to monolayer cultures, organ cultures of embryonic and postembryonic kidneys from cystic and other disease states have provided invaluable information (72). As more mouse models of genetic disease become available and developmental defects suspected, these types of techniques are likely to be used increasingly. Not only will the results from the mutant phenotype be analyzed but also the effects of addition of exogenous compounds or introduction of DNA constructs will allow for *in vitro* testing of potential therapeutic agents.

Culture techniques are also being used increasingly to study mechanisms of disease from genetically engineered mice such as the *orpk* model of ARPKD and the *gy* model of X-linked hypophosphatemia (139). It is to be anticipated that further crosses with the immortomouse (58) will lead to isolation of cells from a variety of mouse models of disease. To advance the study of human disease, the same temperature-sensitive conditionally immortalizing construct was first used to generate a unique model for analysis of nephropathic cystinosis (50), as well as human ADPKD and ARPKD (55). The success of generating immortal cell lines from these human disease states that retain their unique characteristics suggests the general use of this approach for the future. In addition, the ability to generate identical clonal cells will facilitate the detailed analysis of the functional effects of mutations.

Cancer: Wilms' Tumor

Although it has been surprisingly difficult to culture cells from primary Wilms' tumors, some permanently growing cell lines are available for study, the most widely used of which are G401 and SK-NEP. The Wilms' tumor suppressor gene, WT1, localized on chromosome 11p13, is a zinc-finger DNA-binding protein involved in normal renal development, and the deletion of this gene *in vivo* results in

Wilms' tumor formation, and, therefore, cell lines that fail to express WT1 should provide a suitable model system for the study of Wilms' tumor. Four candidates have been described: WIT 13, GOS-4, G401, and SKNEP (Table 15.7). Each has limitations, however. WIT 13 has two different 11p13 deletions (both lacking the WT1 locus), grows slowly, and has fibroblast morphology because it was derived from the stromal component of a Wilms' tumor. GOS-4 and G401 have intact 11p13 regions but fail to transcribe WT1 mRNA, suggesting that the primary disturbance in growth control is related to a mutation in an unlinked gene. It is a consistent finding that primary cultures of Wilms' tumors rarely produce immortal cell lines. Typically, they have been subcultured but could be maintained only for 15 to 25 passages, did not produce tumors in nude mice, and did not demonstrate WT1 deletions.

Renal Cell Carcinoma

Renal cell carcinoma is associated with deletions on chromosome 3p at 14.2. Several permanent cell lines have been derived (Table 15.7), representing adenocarcinoma and clear cell carcinoma with metastatic and nonmetastatic phenotypes. Surprisingly, few studies of cellular abnormalities have been carried out using these lines, which therefore provide an underused source of material for experimental analysis of the tumorigenic renal epithelial cell phenotype.

Interstitial Fibrosis

Interstitial fibrosis is an important manifestation of renal disease and cause of renal functional decline. Experimental analyses of rat cortical fibroblasts implicate increases in α_5, β_1, and α_v integrins, as well as nonintegrin matrix receptors and discoidin domain receptors in fibrotic responses (35,140). Using renal biopsy specimens, fibroblasts cultured from interstitial fibrosis and from ADPKD end-stage kidneys have been used to analyze matrix protein synthesis and growth characteristics, providing a new tool for the analysis of inappropriate fibroblast proliferation in response to disease (22).

CONCLUSION AND PERSPECTIVES

The ability to culture pure populations of renal cells has increased dramatically in the last decade, which has led to a concomitant increase in our understanding of renal cell biology. Recent additional progress in conditional immortalization by transfection techniques, the sequencing of the human genome, the generation of genetically engineered mouse models, and improvements in embryonic organ culture technology sets the stage for a new explosion in the application of renal *in vitro* analysis.

ACKNOWLEDGMENTS

I am indebted to Drs. Christopher Burrow, Deborah Hyink, Katalin Polgar, and Jill Norman for continued stimulating discussion concerning the application of renal *in vitro* techniques for studies of normal and abnormal renal development.

REFERENCES

1. Freshney RI. *Culture of animal cells*, 2nd ed. New York: AR Liss, 1987.
2. Potter EL. *Normal and abnormal development of the kidney.* Chicago: Year Book Medical Publishers, 1972.
3. Kreisberg JI, Wilson PD. Renal cell culture. *J Electron Microsc Tech* 1988;9:235–263.
4. Chung SD, Alavi N, Livingston D, et al. Characterization of primary rabbit kidney cultures that express proximal tubule functions in a hormonally defined medium. *J Cell Biol* 1982;85:118–126.
5. Vinay P, Gougoux A, Lemieux G. Isolation of pure suspension of rat proximal tubules. *Am J Physiol* 1981;240:F403–F411.
6. Smith WL, Garcia-Perez A. Immunodissection: use of monoclonal antibodies to isolate specific types of renal cells. *Am J Physiol* 1985;248:F1–F7.
7. Blumenthal SS, Lewand DL, Buday MA, et al. Effect of pH on growth of mouse renal cortical tubule cells in primary culture. *Am J Physiol* 1989;257:C419–C426.
8. Goligorsky MS, Menton DN, Hruska KA. Parathyroid hormone-induced changes of the brush border topography and cytoskeleton in cultured renal proximal tubule cells. *J Membr Biol* 1986;92:151–162.
9. Bello-Reuss E, Weber MR. Electrophysiologic characterization of primary cultures of kidney cells. *Am J Physiol* 1987;252:F899–F909.
10. Stanton RC, Mendrick DL, Rennke HG, et al. Use of monoclonal antibodies to culture rat proximal tubule cells. *Am J Physiol* 1986;251:C780–C786.
11. Fejes-Toth G, Fejes-Toth AN. Differentiated transport functions in primary cultures of rabbit collecting ducts. *Am J Physiol* 1987;253:F1302–F1307.
12. Mundell P, Reiser J, Kriz W. Induction of differentiation in cultured rat and human Podocytes. *J Am Soc Nephrol* 1997; 8:697–705.
13. Striker GE, Striker LJ. Biology of disease: glomerular cell culture. *Lab Invest* 1985;53:122–131.
14. Misra RP. Isolation of glomeruli from mammalian kidneys by graded sieving. *Am J Clin Pathol* 1972;58:135–139.
15. Striker LJ, Tannen RL, Lange MA, et al. The contribution of cell culture to the study of renal diseases. *Int Rev Exp Pathol* 1988;30:55–105.
16. Kreisberg JI, Karnovsky MJ. Glomerular cells in culture. *Kidney Int* 1983;23:439–447.
17. Ballerman BJ. Regulation of bovine glomerular endothelial cell growth in vitro. *Am J Physiol* 1989;256:C182–C189.
18. Harper PA, Robinson JM, Hoover RL, et al. Improved methods for culturing rat glomerular cells. *Kidney Int* 1984;26:875–880.

19. Wilson PD, Dillingham MA, Breckon R, et al. Defined human renal tubular epithelia in culture: growth, characterization and hormonal response. *Am J Physiol* 1985;248:F436–F443.
20. Wilson PD, Anderson RJ, Breckon RD, et al. Retention of differentiated characteristics by cultures of defined rabbit kidney epithelia. *J Cell Physiol* 1987;130:245–254.
21. Wilson PD. Monolayer cultures of microdissected renal tubule epithelial segments. *J Tissue Cult Meth* 1991;13:137–142.
22. Kuo N, Norman JT, Wilson PD. Acidic FGF regulation of hyperproliferation of fibroblasts in human autosomal dominant polycystic kidney disease. *Biochem Mol Med* 1997;61: 178–191.
23. Castellot JR, Hoover RL, Karnovsky MJ. Glomerular endothelial cells secrete a heparin-like inhibitor and a peptide stimulator of mesangial cell proliferation. *Am J Pathol* 1987;125:493–500.
24. Allen LM, Nakao A, Sonnenburg WS, et al. Immunodissection of cortical and medullary thick ascending limb cells from rabbit kidney. *Am J Physiol* 1988;255:F704-F710.
25. Drugge ED, Carroll MA, McGiff JC. Cells in culture from rabbit medullary thick ascending limb of Henle's loop. *Am J Physiol* 1989;256:C1070–C1081.
26. Pizzonia JH, Gesk FA, Kennedy SM, et al. Immunomagnetic separation, primary culture and characterization of cortical thick ascending limb plus distal convoluted tubule cells from mouse kidney. *In Vitro Cell Dev Biol* 1991;27A:409–416
27. Merot J, Bidet M, Gachot B, et al. Electrical properties of rabbit early distal convoluted tubule in primary culture. *Am J Physiol* 1989;257:F288–F299.
28. Caviedes R, Croxatto HR, Corthorn J, et al. Identification of kallikrein in cultures of adult renal cells. *Cell Biol Int Rep* 1987;11:735–743.
29. Garcia-Perez A, Smith WL. Use of monoclonal antibodies to isolate cortical collecting tubule cells: AVP induces PGE release. *Am J Physiol* 1983;244:C211–C220.
30. Van Adelsberg J, Edwards JC, Herzlinger D, et al. Isolation and culture of HCO_3-secreting intercalated cells. *Am J Physiol* 1989;256:1004–1011.
31. Minuth W. Induction and inhibition of outgrowth and development of renal collecting duct epithelium. *Lab Invest* 1983;48:543–548.
32. Grenier FC, Rollins TE, Smith WL. Kinin-induced prostaglandin synthesis by renal papillary collecting tubule cells in culture. *Am J Physiol* 1981;241:F94–F104.
33. Sato M, Dunn MJ. Interaction of vasopressin, prostaglandins and cAMP in rat renal papillary collecting tubules in culture. *Am J Physiol* 1984;247:F423–F433.
34. Rightsel WA, Okamura T, Inagami T, et al. Juxtaglomerular cells grown as monolayer culture contain renin, angiotensin I-converting enzyme and angiotensins I and II/III. *Circ Res* 1982;50:822–829.
35. Lewis MP, Norman JT. Differential response of activated versus non-activated renal fibroblasts to tubular epithelial cells: a model of initiation and progression of fibrosis. *Exp Nephrol* 1998;6:132–143.
36. Rodemann HP, Muller GA, Knecht A, et al. Fibroblasts of rabbit kidney in culture. Characterization and identification of cell-specific markers. *Am J Physiol* 1991;261:F283–F291.
37. Knecht A, Fine LG, Kleinman KS, et al. Fibroblasts of rabbit kidney in culture. II. Paracrine stimulation of papillary fibroblasts by PDGF. *Am J Physiol* 1991;261:F292–F299.
38. Fontoura BM, Nussenzvieg DR, Pelton KM, et al. Atrial natriuretic factor receptors in cultured renomedullary interstitial cells. *Am J Physiol* 1990;258:C692–C699
39. Dussaule JC, Bea ML, Baud L, et al. Effects of bradykinin on prostaglandin synthesis and cytosolic calcium in rabbit subcultured renal cortical smooth muscle cells. *Biochim Biophys Acta* 1989;1005:34–44.
40. Takaoka T, Katsuta H, Endo M, et al. Establishment of a cell strain, JTC-12, from cynomolgus monkey kidney tissue. *Jpn J Exp Med* 1962;32:351–365.
41. Walsh-Reitz MM, Toback FG. Vasopressin stimulates growth of renal epithelial cells in culture. *Am J Physiol* 1983;245: C365–C370.
42. Koyama H, Goodpasture C, Miller MM, et al. Establishment and characterization of a cell line from the American opossum (*Didelphys virginiana*). *In Vitro* 1978;14:239–246.
43. Hull RN, Cherry WR, Weaver GW. The origin and characteristics of a pig kidney cell strain LLC-PK1. *In Vitro* 1976;12:670–677.
44. American Type Culture Collection. *Catalogue of cell lines and hybridomas*, 7th ed. Rockville, MD: The Collection, 1992.
45. Green N, Algren A, Hoyer J, et al. Differentiated lines of cells from rabbit renal medullary thick ascending limbs grown on amnion. *Am J Physiol* 1985;249:C97–C104.
46. Valentich JD, Stokols MF. An established cell line from mouse kidney medullary thick ascending limb. I. Cell culture techniques, morphology and antigenic expression. *Am J Physiol* 1986;251:C299–C311.
47. Delarue F, Virone A, Hagege J, et al. Stable cell line of T-SV40 immortalized human glomerular visceral epithelial cells. *Kidney Int* 1991;40:906–912.
48. Mackay K, Striker LJ, Elliot S, et al. Glomerular epithelial, mesangial, and endothelial cell lines from transgenic mice. *Kidney Int* 1988;33:677–684.
49. Ryan MJ, Johnson G, Kirk J, et al. HK-2: an immortalized proximal tubule epithelial cell line from normal adult human kidney. *Kidney Int* 1994;45:48–57.
50. Racusen LC, Wilson PD, Hartz PA, et al. Renal proximal tubular epithelium from patients with nephropathic cystinosis: immortalized cell lines as in vitro model systems. *Kidney Int* 1995;48:536–543.
51. Tang SS, Jung F, Diamant D, et al. Temperature-sensitive SV40 immortalized rat proximal tubule cell line has a functional rennin-angiotensin system. *Am J Physiol* 1995;268:F435–F436.
52. Bland RE, Walker A, Hughes SV, et al. Constitutive expression of 25-hydroxyvitamin D3-1 alpha-hydroxylase in a transformed human proximal tubule cell l line: evidence for direct regulation of vitamin D metabolism by calcium. *Endocrinology* 1999;140:2027–2034.
53. Friedman PA, Coutermarsh BA, Rhim JS, et al. Characterization of immortalized mouse distal convoluted tubule cells. *J Am Soc Nephrol* 1991;2:737.
54. Brandsch M, Brandsch C, Prasad PD, et al. Identification of a renal cell line that constitutively expresses the kidney-specific high-affinity H^+/peptide cotransporter. *FASEB J* 1995; 9:1489–1496.

55. Geng L, Burrow CR, Li H, et al. Modification of the composition of polycystin-1 multiprotein complexes by calcium and tyrosine phosphorylation. *Biochim Biophys Acta* 2000;1535:21–35.
56. Barasch J, Pressler L, Connor J, et al. A ureteric bud cell line induces nephrogenesis in two steps by two distinct signals. *Am J Physiol* 1996;271:F50–F61.
57. Wilson, PD Geng L, Li X, et al. The PKD1 gene product, "polycystin-1," is a tyrosine phosphorylated protein that colocalizes with alpha2beta1 integrin in focal clusters in adherent renal epithelia. *Lab Invest* 2000;79:1311–1323.
58. Jat P, Noble M, Ataliotis N, et al. Direct derivation of conditionally immortal cell lines from an H-$2K_b$-tsA58 transgenic mouse. *Proc Natl Acad Sci U S A* 1991;88:5096–5100.
59. Danos O, Mulligan RC. Safe and efficient generation of recombinant retroviruses with amphotropic and ecotropic host ranges. *Proc Natl Acad Sci U S A* 1988;85:6460–6464.
60. Frederiksen K, Jat PS, Valtz, et al. Immortalization of precursor cells from the mammalian CNS. *Neuron* 1988;1:439–448.
61. Mundel P, Reiser J, Borja AZ, et al. Rearrangements of the cytoskeleton and cell contacts induce process formation during differentiation of conditionally immortalized mouse podocyte cell line. *Exp Cell Res* 1997;236:248–258.
62. Bissell MJ, Hall HG, Parry G. How does the extracellular matrix direct gene expression? *J Theor Biol* 1982;99:31–68.
63. Wilson PD, Schrier RW, Breckon RD, et al. A new method for studying human polycystic kidney disease epithelia in culture. *Kidney Int* 1986;30:371–378.
64. Wilson PD, Hreniuk D, Gabow PA. Abnormal extracellular matrix and excessive growth of human adult polycystic kidney disease epithelia. *J Cell Physiol* 1992;150:360–369.
65. Taub M, Sato G. Growth of functional primary cultures of kidney epithelial cells in defined medium. *J Cell Physiol* 1980;105:369–378.
66. Grobstein C. Inductive epithelio mesenchymal interaction in cultured organ rudiments of the mouse. *Science* 1953;118:52–55.
67. Grobstein C. Trans-filter induction of tubules in mouse metanephrogenic mesenchyme. *Exp Cell Res* 1956;10:424–440.
68. Saxen L, Lehtonen E. Embryonic kidney in organ culture. *Differentiation* 1987;36:2–11.
69. Davis H, Gascho C, Kiernan JA. Effects of aprotinin on organ cultures of the rat's kidney. *In Vitro* 1976;12:192–197.
70. Crocker JFS. Human embryonic kidneys in organ culture: abnormalities of development induced by decreased potassium. *Science* 1973;181:1178–1179.
71. Avner ED, Sweeney W, Piesco NP, et al. Growth factor requirements of organogenesis in serum-free metanephric organ culture. *In Vitro Cell Dev Biol* 1985;21:297–304.
72. Avner E, Sweeney W, Ellis D. In vitro modulation of tubular cyst regression in murine polycystic kidney disease. *Kidney Int* 1989;36:960–968.
73. Ekblom P. Determination and differentiation of the nephron. *Med Biol* 1981;59:139–160.
74. Ekblom P. Developmentally regulated conversion of mesenchyme to epithelium. *FASEB J* 1989;3:2141–2150.
75. Burrow CR. Regulatory molecules in kidney development. *Pediatr Nephrol* 2000;14:240–253.
76. Wilson PD, Sherwood AC, Palla K, et al. Reversed polarity of Na^+K^+-ATPase: mislocation to apical plasma membranes in polycystic kidney disease. *Am J Physiol* 1991;260:F420–F430.
77. Wilson PD, Burrow CR. Autosomal dominant polycystic kidney disease: cellular and molecular mechanisms of cyst formation. *Adv Nephrol* 1992;21:125–142.
78 Rohatgi R, Greenberg A, Burrow CR, et al. Na transport in ARPKD cyst lining epithelial cells. *J Am Soc Nephrol* 2003;14:827–836.
79. Burrow CR, Wilson PD. A putative Wilms' tumor-secreted growth factor activity required for primary culture of human nephroblasts. *Proc Natl Acad Sci U S A* 1993;90:6066–6070.
80. Ratovitsky EA, Kotzbauer PT, Milbrandt J, et al. Midkine induces tumor cell proliferation and binds to a high affinity signaling receptor associated with JAK tyrosine kinases. *J Biol Chem* 1998;273:3654–3660.
81. Qiu L, Escalante C, Aggarwal, et al. Monomeric midkine induces tumor cell proliferation in the absence of cell-surface proteoglycan binding. *Biocehemistry* 2000;39:5977–5987.
82. Burrow CR, Wilson PD. Renal progenitor cells: problems of definition, isolation and characterization. *Exp Nephrol* 1994;2:1–12.
83. Woolf AS, Kolatsi-Joannou M, Hardmann P, et al. Roles of hepatocyte growth factor/scatter factor and the Met receptor in the early development of the metanephros. *J Cell Biol* 1995;128:171–184.
84. Karp SL, Ortiz-Arduan A, Li S, et al. Epithelial differentiation of metanephric mesenchymal cells after stimulation with hepatocyte growth factor or embryonic spinal cord. *Proc Natl Acad Sci U S A* 1994;91:5286–5290.
85. Barasch J, Qiao J, et al. Ureteric bud cells secrete multiple factors, including bFGF, which rescue renal progenitors from apoptosis *Am J Physiol* 1997;273:F757–F767.
86. Klein G, Langegger M, Timpl R, et al. Role of laminin A chain in the development of epithelial cell polarity. *Cell* 1988;55:331–314.
87. Sorokin L, Sonnenberg A, Aumailley M, et al. Recognition of the laminin E8 cell-binding site by an integrin possessing alpha 6 subunit is essential for epithelial polarization in developing kidney tubules. *J Cell Biol* 1990;111:1265–1273.
88. McNeill J, Ozawa M, Kemler R, et al. Novel function of the cell adhesion molecule uvomorulin as an inducer of cell surface polarity. *Cell* 1990;62:309–316.
89. Rodriquez-Boulan E, Nelson WJ. Morphogenesis of the polarized epithelial cell type. *Science* 1989;245:718–725.
90. Weller A, Sorokin L, Illgen E, et al. Development and growth of mouse embryonic kidney in organ culture and modulation of development by soluble growth factors. *Dev Biol* 1991;144:248–261.
91. Amsler K, Burrow CR, Hyink DP, et al. Heregulin induces renal blastemal cell proliferation and aberrant ureteric bud branching. *J Am Soc Nephrol* 2000;11:373A.
92. Yang J, Blum A, Novak T, et al. An epithelial precursor is regulated by the ureteric bud and by the renal stroma. *Dev Biol* 2002;246:296–310.
93. Pasdar M, Krzeminski K, Nelson WJ. Regulation of desmosome assembly in MDCK epithelial cells: coordination of

membrane core and cytoplasmic plaque domain assembly at the plasma membrane. *J Cell Biol* 1991;113:645–655.
94. Schnabel E, Anderson JM, Farquhar MG. The tight junction protein ZO-1 is concentrated along slit diaphragms of the glomerular epithelium. *J Cell Biol* 1990;111:1255–1263.
95. Hodges GM. Tumour formation: the concept of tissue (stroma-epithelium) regulatory disfunction. *Br Soc Cell Biol Symp* 1982;5:333–356.
96. Cunha GR, Bigsby RM, Cooke PS, et al. Stromal-epithelial interactions in adult organs. *Cell Differ* 1985;17:137–148.
97. Bard JB. Epithelial-fibroblastic organization in cultures grown from human embryonic kidney: its significance for morphogenesis in vivo. *J Cell Sci* 1979;39:291–298.
98. Taub M, Wang Y, Szczesny M, et al. Epidermal growth factor or transforming growth factor alpha is required for kidney tubulogenesis in matrigel cultures in serum-free medium. *Proc Natl Acad Sci U S A* 1990;87:4002–4006.
99. Gospodarowicz D, Lepine J, Massoglia S, et al. Comparison of the ability of basement membranes produced by corneal endothelial and mouse-derived endodermal PF-HR-9 cells to support the proliferation and differentiation of bovine kidney tubule epithelial cells in vitro. *J Cell Biol* 1984;99:947–961.
100. Hall HG, Farson DA, Bissell MJ. Lumen formation by epithelial cell lines in response to collagen overlay: a morphogenetic model in culture. *Proc Natl Acad Sci U S A* 1982; 79:4672–4676.
101. Wohlwend A, Montesano R, Vassalli J, et al. LLC-PK1 cysts: a model for the study of epithelial polarity. *J Cell Physiol* 1985;125:533–539.
102. Montesano R, Schaller G, Orci L. Induction of epithelial tubular morphogenesis in vitro by fibroblast-derived soluble factors. *Cell* 1991;66:697–711.
103. Montesano R, Matsumoto K, Nakamura T, et al. Identification of a fibroblast-derived epithelial morphogen as hepatocyte growth factor. *Cell* 1991;67:901–908.
104. Sakurai H, Tsukamoto T, Kjelsberg CA, et al. EGF receptor ligands are a large fraction of in vitro branching morphogens secreted by the embryonic kidney. *Am J Physiol* 1997;273: F463–F472
105. Balkovetz DF. Hepatocyte growth factor and Madin-Darby canine kidney cells: in vitro models of epithelial cell movement and morphogenesis. *Microsc Res Tech* 1998;43:456–463.
106. Gupta JR, Piscionne TD, Grisaru S, et al. Protein kinase A is a negative regulator of renal branching morphogenesis and modulates inhibitory and stimulatory bone morphogenetic proteins. *J Biol Chem* 1999;274:26305–26314.
107. Li X, Li H, Amsler K, et al. PRKX, a phylogenetically and functionally distinct cAMP-dependent protein kinase, activates renal epithelial cell migration and morphogenesis. *Proc Natl Acad Sci U S A* 2002;99:9260–9265.
108. Ekblom M, Klein G, Mugrauer G, et al. Transient and locally restricted expression of laminin A chain mRNA by developing epithelial cells during kidney organogenesis. *Cell* 1990;60:337–346.
109. Falk M, Salmivirta K, Durbeej M, et al. Integrin alpha 6B beta 1 is involved in kidney tubulogenesis in vitro. *J Cell Sci* 1996;109:2801–2810.
110. Bullock SL, Johnson TM. Galectin-3 modulates ureteric bud branching in organ culture of the developing mouse kidney. *J Am Soc Nephrol* 2001;12:515–523.
111. Davies J, Lyon M. Sulphated proteoglycan is required for collecting duct growth and branching but not nephron formation during kidney development. *Development* 1995;121:1507–1517.
112. Qiu L, Gans WH, Hyink D, et al. Midkine promotes selective expansion of the nephrogenic mesenchyme during kidney organogenesis. *Development* 2003: (*in press*).
113. Sariola H, Aufderheide E, Bernhard H, et al. Antibodies to cell surface ganglioside GD3 perturb inductive epithelial-mesenchymal interactions. *Cell* 1988;54:235–245.
114. Couser WG, Abrass CK. Pathogenesis of membranous nephropathy. *Annu Rev Med* 1988;39:517–527.
115. Mundel P, Schwarz K, Reiser J. Podocyte biology: a footstep further. *Adv Nephrol Necker Hosp* 2001;31:235–241.
116. Sasaki S, Bao Q, Hughes RC. Galectin-3 modulates rat mesangial cell proliferation and matrix synthesis during experimental glomerulonephritis induced by anti-Thy 1.1 antibodies. *J Pathol* 1999;187:481–489.
117. Wilson PD, Schrier RW. Nephron segment and calcium as determinants of anoxic cell death in renal cultures. *Kidney Int* 1986;29:1172–1179.
118. Wilson PD. Use of cultured renal tubular cells in the study of cell injury. *Miner Electrolyte Metab* 1986;12:71–84.
119. Hori R, Yamamoto K, Saito H, et al. Effect of aminoglycoside antibiotics on cellular functions of kidney epithelial cell line (LLC-PK1): a model system for aminoglycoside nephrotoxicity. *J Pharmacol Exp Ther* 1984;230:742–748.
120. Schwertz DW, Kreisberg JI, Venkatachalam MA. Gentamicin-induced alterations in pig kidney epithelial (LLC-PK1) cells in culture. *J Pharmacol Exp Ther* 1986;236: 254–262.
121. Ramsammy LS, Josepovitz C, Lane B, et al. Effect of gentamicin on phospholipid metabolism in cultured rabbit proximal tubular cells. *Am J Physiol* 1989;256:C204–C213.
122. Ghosh P, Chatterjee S. Effects of gentamicin on sphingomyelinase activity in cultured human renal proximal tubular cells. *J Biol Chem* 1987;262:12550–12556.
123. Wilson PD, Hreniuk D. Nephrotoxicity of cyclosporine in renal tubule cultures and attenuation by calcium restriction. *Transplant Proc* 1988;20:709–711.
124. Wilson PD, Hartz PA. Mechanisms of cyclosporine A toxicity in defined cultures of renal tubule epithelia: a role for cysteine proteases. *Cell Biol Int Rep* 1991;15: 1243–1258.
125. Lau DCW, Wong K, Hwang WS. Cyclosporine toxicity on cultured rat microvascular endothelial cells. *Kidney Int* 1989;35:604–613.
126. Jonasson L, Holm J, Hansson GK. Cyclosporine A inhibits smooth muscle proliferation in the vascular response to injury. *Proc Natl Acad Sci U S A* 1988;85:2303–2306.
127. Hjelle JT, Waters DC, Golinska BT, et al. Autosomal recessive polycystic kidney disease: characterization of human peritoneal and cystic kidney cells in vitro. *Am J Kidney Dis* 1990;2:123–136.
128. Wilson PD, Falkenstein DF. The pathology of human renal cystic disease. In: Dodd SM, ed. *Current topics in pathology*. Berlin, Heidelberg: Springer-Verlag, 1995;88: 1–50.

129. Van Adelsberg J. Murine polycystic kidney cells have increased integrin-mediated adhesion to collagen. *Am J Physiol* 1994;267:F1082–F1093.
130. Yoder B, Tousson A. Polaris, a protein disrupted in orpk mutant mice, is required for assembly of renal cilium. *Am J Physiol* 2002;282:F541–F552.
131. Sweeney WE, Kusner L, Carlin CR, et al. Phenotypic analysis of conditionally immortalized cells isolated from the BPK model of ARPKD. *Am J Physiol* 2001;281:C1695–C1705.
132. Berteelli R, Ginevri F, Candiano G, et al. Tubular epithelium culture from nephronophthisis-affected kidneys: a new approach to molecular disorders of tubular cells. *Am J Nephrol* 1990;10:463–469.
133. Haber DA, Park S, Maheswaren S, et al. WT1-mediated growth suppression of Wilms tumor cells expressing a WT1 splicing variant. *Science* 1993;262:2057–2059.
134. Sherwood JB, Shouval D. Continuous production of erythropoietin by an established human renal carcinoma cell line: development of the cell line. *Proc Natl Acad Sci U S A* 1986;83:165–169.
135. Moon TD, Morley J, Vessella J, et al. The role of calmodulin in human renal cell carcinoma. *Biochem Biophys Res Commun* 1983;114:843–849.
136. Hashimura T, Tubbs RR, Connelly R, et al. Characterization of two cell lines with distinct phenotypes and genotypes established from a patient with renal cell carcinoma. *Cancer Res* 1989;49:7064–7071.
137. Wilson PD. Pathogenesis of polycystic kidney disease: altered cellular function. In: Watson ML, Torres VE, eds. *Polycystic kidney disease.* Oxford: Oxford University Press, 1996:125–163.
138. Wilson PD. Epithelia cell polarity and disease. *Am J Physiol* 1997;272:F434–F442.
139. Nesbitt T, Drezner MK. Phosphate transport in renal cell cultures by gy mice: evidence of a single defect in X-linked hypophosphatemia. *Am J Physiol* 1997;273:F113–F119.
140. Norman JT, Fine LG. Progressive renal disease: fibroblasts, extracellular matrix and integrins. *Exp Nephrol* 1999;7:167–177.

16

ANIMAL MODELS

JORDAN A. KREIDBERG

The use of animal models has been an essential aspect of nearly all areas of nephrologic research since its earliest days. Research on kidney formation and malformation, physiology and pathophysiology, immunologic injury, and tolerance or transplant rejection all depend on the use of animal experimentation. This chapter emphasizes genetic approaches that use animals, as this area has shown the most progress in the development of novel technologies since the previous edition of this book.

INSTITUTIONAL OVERSIGHT

There is increasing public awareness of the use of animals in research and with this comes increasing concern about the appropriateness of the use of animals and whether much of the research that does involve animal models could be accomplished using nonanimal models. Therefore, it is important to note that all animal research in the United States must be evaluated by institutional committees before any experimentation may commence. Furthermore, the U. S. Department of Agriculture provides constant oversight through the use of frequent and usually unannounced visits to animal facilities of research institutions. These regulatory committees and agencies are charged with evaluating animal protocols to make certain that animals are used in an ethical manner, with proper use of anesthetics or analgesics to minimize or eliminate any source of pain during experimentation. They are also charged with verifying that animals are indeed required for the specific research in question, that large animals are not used when smaller ones would suffice, and that the investigators are trained and knowledgeable about proper use of animals. Despite these several layers of oversight, in the end, it is up to the principal investigator to be thoughtful about whether the intended experimental approach will yield sufficiently important and worthwhile results to justify the use of laboratory animals.

GENETIC MODELS

The early 1990s to the present have witnessed an explosion in the use of genetic approaches to understand development and physiology, and, thus, they receive appropriate emphasis in this chapter. Several genetic approaches are available for use with animal model systems. There are *reverse* genetic systems, in which a gene of interest is mutated using gene targeting or expressed in transgenic mice in such a way to interfere with its normal function. Using *forward* genetic approaches, one starts with a phenotype of interest, which could either be obtained as a spontaneous mutation or from mice treated with a mutagen, and an effort is made to identify the mutated gene responsible for the phenotype. Reverse genetic approaches using gene-targeted or transgenic mice are useful for a wide variety of developmental and physiologic studies in which there is a need to study the function of a known gene. Forward genetic approaches, on the other hand, are mainly used in projects in which the goal is the identification of novel genes.

Gene Targeting

Gene targeting was originally used to introduce a deletion or interruption into a gene of interest, using the scheme shown in Figure 16.1, such that it could be determined whether mice would be able to develop in the absence of that gene's function. In cases in which a gene was shown not to be essential for development, the homozygous mutant mouse might serve as a useful model in which to study the role of a specific gene in a physiologic or disease process. For example, targeted deletions of the Wt1 (1), Pax2 (2), GDNF (3–5), Wnt4 (6), and BMP7 (7,8), among others, showed these genes to be essential for various aspects of early kidney development. On the other hand, the absence of many immunology-related genes does not result in any developmental impairment, but these mice have served as useful models to study the role of the immune system in transplant rejection.

The advent of gene targeting was made possible through the use of two technologies developed mainly in the 1980s. The first was the development of tissue culture conditions that allowed embryonic stem (ES) cell lines to be grown indefinitely in culture while retaining their totipotency (9). ES cells grown in culture could then be introduced into mouse preimplantation embryos or blastocysts and become fully integrated into those embryos such that their descendant cells would give

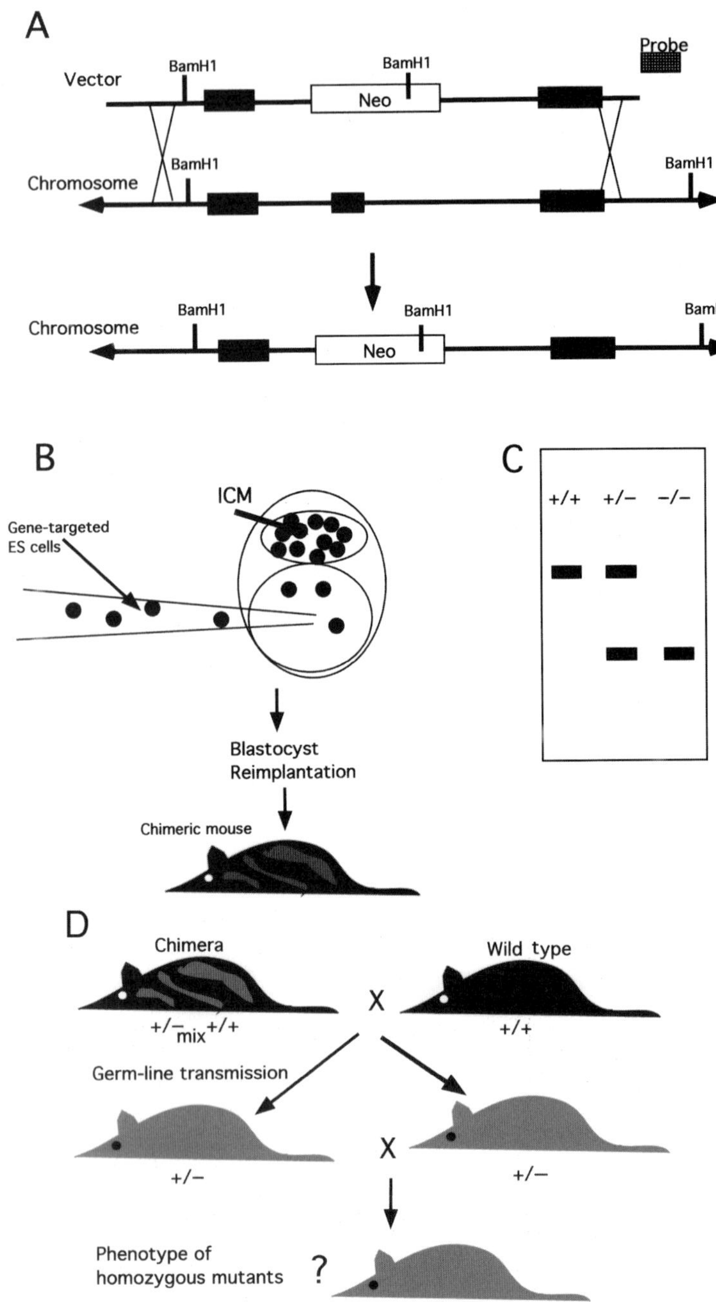

FIGURE 16.1. Gene targeting in mice. **A:** The scheme for targeting a deletion of an exon in embryonic stem (ES) cells. Exons are shown as black boxes along a chromosome. Restriction sites for restriction enzyme BamH1A are shown. The replacement vector is constructed such that the neomycin resistance gene (neo) is shown as an open box, in place of one of the exons. An external probe specifically does not overlap with the replacement vector. A double homologous recombination results in the integration of the vector into the chromosome, thus replacing the exon with the Neo gene. The BamH1 site within the neo gene results in a shorter BamH1 restriction fragment detected by probe after homologous recombination. **B:** ES cells can be injected through a micropipette into a blastocyst, in which they become part of the inner cell mass. The injected blastocyst is introduced into the uterus of a hormonally primed mouse and gives rise to a chimeric mouse, partially derived from the ES cells and partially from the original inner cell mass (ICM) cells. If the ES cells and blastocysts are derived from strains with different coat colors, then the chimeric mouse will have a variegated coat color pattern on its fur, providing an indication of its overall extent of chimerism. In the best cases, the resultant mouse is nearly entirely derived from ES cells. **C:** Shows a possible pattern obtained in a Southern blot, based on the scheme shown in **A**, using the external probe. A wild-type mouse shows only the longer band. A heterozygous mouse shows both the wild-type and gene-targeted band, and the homozygous mutant shows only the shorter band, due to the presence of the BamH1 site in the neo gene. **D:** The mating involved in obtaining germ-line transmission of the mutation and subsequently obtaining homozygous mutant mice.

rise to all developmental lineages that are found in adult mice (10). The second technology involved is the use of homologous recombination to introduce mutations into mammalian genes (11–13). As shown in Figure 16.1, when long stretches of genomic DNA in recombinant DNA constructs are introduced into cells in culture, this DNA will, at variable and often quite low frequency, recombine into the locus from which the genomic DNA was originally derived. Therefore, homologous recombination of the correctly designed genomic fragment can be used to introduce a deletion or insertion into a genomic locus that renders the gene unable to be expressed. This ES cell would in essence be heterozygous for a mutation in the targeted gene, and heterozygous ES cells can be isolated and expanded to provide a population for injection into blastocysts. Therefore, by combining the ES cell technology and homologous recombination, it became possible to target mutations into genes in ES cells and then introduce ES cells carrying these mutations into blastocysts, finally obtaining a mutant adult mouse.

In a typical experiment, gene-targeted ES cells would contain one mutated allele and one normal or wild-type allele for the gene under study. The targeted ES cells would be injected into preimplantation blastocysts, and groups of these blastocysts would be introduced into female mice that were previously hormonally primed to allow implantation of the injected blastocysts into their uteri to begin a pregnancy. The resultant mice from these injections are termed *chimeras*, because any specific cell is either derived from an ES cell or the original injected embryo (i.e., the chimeric mouse essentially has four parents, the male and female that provided the blastocyst and the male and female that provided the embryo from which the ES cell line in use was originally derived). In the best cases, a chimera might be nearly entirely derived from the ES cells. Among the tissues that ES cells contribute to are the germ cells: spermatocytes or oocytes. When ES cells heterozygous for a mutation are used to make a chimera, germ cells derived from the ES cells have a 50% chance of carrying the mutant rather than the wild-type allele. Therefore, mating a chimeric and wild-type mice can result in some of the offspring being true heterozygotes for the mutated gene. After obtaining both male and female heterozygotes, they can be mated to obtain homozygous mutant embryos or mice, depending on whether or not the gene is essential for development.

Conditional Gene Targeting

The process described in the preceding section results in the inactivation of a target gene from the beginning of embryogenesis. In this situation, an embryo will become nonviable at the first point at which expression of the inactivated gene becomes essential for survival. However, it may be highly desirable to study the function of a gene product in many later events during development or adult life. Conditional gene targeting allows the inactivation of a gene in particular tissues or at particular times during development or adult life (14–16). This technology has been developed more recently, and has proved more difficult to use on a widespread basis thus far, for reasons that are discussed next.

The general approach to conditional gene targeting is shown in Figure 16.2. This is a variation on traditional gene targeting, in that it also relies on homologous recombination to introduce a segment of recombinant DNA into the locus of a gene in ES cells. However, whereas traditional gene targeting inactivates the gene, conditional gene targeting must modify the gene such that it can be expressed until such time as its inactivation is desired. The most commonly used approach involved the insertion of LOX sites, which are 34 base pair sites involved in site-specific recombination by Cre recombinase, an enzyme originally derived from a bacteriophage (15). Because LOX sites are rather small, it is usually possible to insert them in introns in which they have no effect on gene expression. By placing two LOX sites in a gene to flank an exon, Cre can be used to inactivate a gene by recombining out the DNA seg-

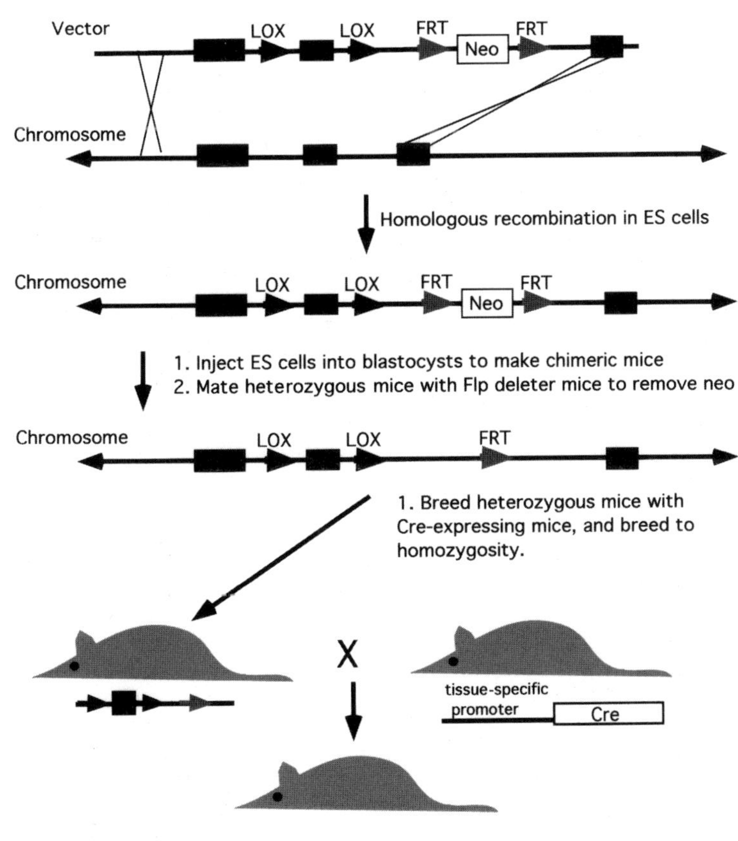

FIGURE 16.2. Conditional gene targeting. The targeting vector is different from the previous figure in that LOX sites flank the exon that will eventually be deleted, and the Neo gene is flanked by FRT sites. The vector is incorporated into the chromosome through homologous recombination, and embryonic stem (ES) cells with this knock-in are used to make chimeric mice, and germline transmission is obtained. Although the LOX sites should not interfere with expression of the gene, the Neo gene is likely to interfere with normal gene expression. However, in most cases, mice will tolerate one inactive gene, as long as the other allele is functional. After obtaining heterozygous mice, they are mated with Flp –deleter mice, that express Flp recombinase in germ cells. Flp will recombine the FRT sites and eliminate the neo gene. Mice without the neo gene, but still containing the exon flanked by LOX sites, are mated with mice expressing Cre in a particular tissue or cell type, or expressing an inducible Cre, to obtain the conditional knock-out. The breeding scheme shown in the figure is oversimplified. In the actual experiment, a more complicated breeding scheme is required to obtain a mouse that is homozygous for alleles with LOX sites and that also has the Cre-expressing transgene. An alternative is to breed mice with the conditional allele with mice carrying a traditional knock-out. This has the advantage that to obtain the conditional knock-out, Cre must only recombine one, and not two, pairs of LOX sites in each cell.

ment containing the exon that was situated between the two LOX sites, thus inactivating the gene. There are experimental approaches for expressing Cre in temporally or spatially specific manners or both. Spatial- or lineage-specific expression of Cre is most often obtained by placing the Cre cDNA downstream of a known tissue-specific promoter. Sometimes this is achieved by using homologous recombination to insert the Cre gene into the genomic locus of a gene with known tissue-specific expression, such that Cre replaces the first exon of that gene. Temporally, specific expression of Cre has proved more difficult to obtain. One approach is to regulate Cre using the tetracycline system for inducible gene expression (17). The other approach makes use of a fusion protein consisting of Cre and a portion of the estrogen receptor that confers steroid-mediated nuclear localization (18,19). The latter is modified to bind tamoxifen or tamoxifen derivatives instead of estrogen. The Cre-modified estrogen receptor fusion protein will remain in the cytoplasm and therefore not be able to mediate site-specific recombination of LOX sites until tamoxifen is administered to the mouse to induce nuclear translocation of the Cre fusion protein. This system can be used to induce recombination in embryos when tamoxifen is administered to pregnant mice. The major obstacle to using conditional gene targeting on a widespread basis is the availability of promoter/enhancer elements that are able to confer robust tissue or cell-lineage–specific expression of Cre recombinase. For example, in the kidney, there are not promoters available that are able to direct expression of a transgene in every distinct cell lineage or groups of lineages. However, this situation is gradually improving. For example, the nephrin and podocin promoters have recently been shown to confer podocyte-specific expression (20–22), and the upstream region of the aquaporin-2 promoter confers expression in collecting ducts (23).

As more tissue-promoter elements become available, conditional gene targeting promises to have a large impact on genetic approaches to kidney disease. As noted earlier, there are many genes expressed both in the developing and adult kidney, in which the knock-out of the gene results in embryonic lethality. This precludes study of how the product of that gene might function in postnatal kidneys or why a mutation in that gene leads to kidney disease in humans. It also raises the question of why humans carrying such mutations are able survive, albeit with a genetic disease, when mice carrying mutations in the same gene do not survive embryogenesis. Sometimes this is simply because mice and humans differ in their respective requirements for specific genes, but more often, it is because humans with genetic disease often have point mutations that lead to partial loss of function, whereas mouse knock-outs often involve complete loss of function mutations. Conditional gene targeting can sometimes offer a solution to this problem by allowing normal gene expression during embryogenesis and then inactivating a gene in adult mice. Alternatively, there are variations on the Cre-LOX approach that allow the introduction of point mutations into mice. The introduction of point mutations into mice has been greatly facilitated by recent advancements that facilitate homologous recombination into BACs (bacterial artificial chromosomes) in *Escherichia coli* (Fig. 16.3). BACs are used because they contain large amounts of genomic DNA and, thus, are ideal for use as gene-

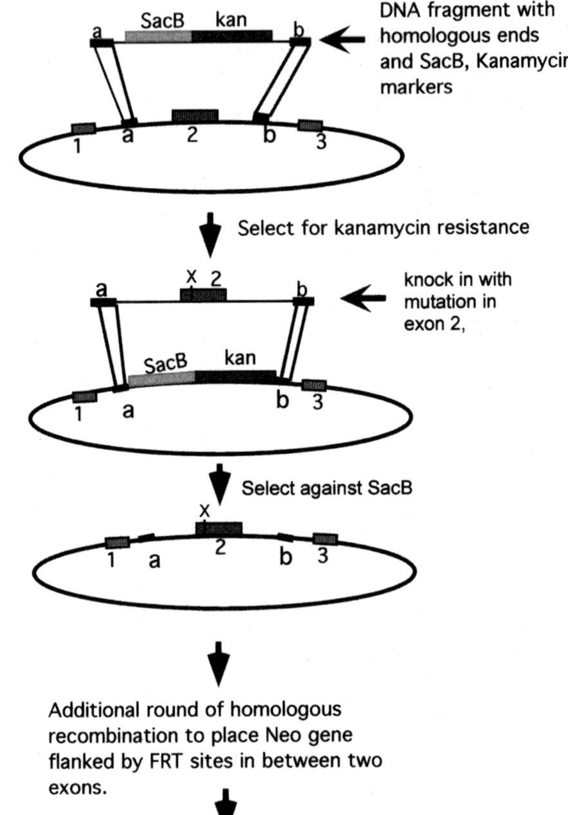

FIGURE 16.3. Gene targeting using bacterial artificial chromosome (BAC) clones. Homologous recombination is done in *Escherichia coli* instead of in embryonic stem (ES) cells. In the first step, a DNA fragment is prepared that contains the kanamycin resistance–positive selectable marker, and the SacB-negative selectable marker, which also contains homologous ends (a and b, each approximately 50–60 bp), is introduced into *E. coli*. This fragment can usually be prepared by polymerase chain reaction, using primers that contain the homologies to the genomic region and also to a vector containing the selectable markers. Usually, a strain of *E. coli* is used that allows transient activation of the enzymes required for homologous recombination. Selection for kanamycin resistance obtains BAC clones where the selectable markers have recombined into the BAC. In a second round of homologous recombination, a DNA fragment with the same homologous ends but containing a mutated exon 2, denoted by the "X," is introduced into the *E. coli* containing the BAC. Selection against SacB obtains BACs in which the mutated exon 2 has replaced the selectable markers. A third round of homologous recombination is used to insert the Neo gene, flanked by FRT sites, so that the BAC can be used for homologous recombination in ES cells. As shown, this scheme is used to introduce point mutations or small deletions into a gene. It can also be used to construct conditional knock-out vectors, similar to those shown in Figure 16.2. An additional use is to knock-in a green fluorescent protein or β-galactosidase (LacZ) reporter gene into a locus to obtain information about patterns of gene expression.

targeting vectors. The longer length of BACs compared with shorter genomic clones should improve the frequency of homologous recombination in ES cells.

TRANSGENIC MICE

As mentioned earlier, many mutations that result in human disease are point mutations that result in *hypomorphic*, or partial, loss of function alleles of a gene. In this case, a disease state may result from decreased activity of a gene product. In other cases, a point mutation or deletion mutation may produce a protein that interferes with the function of the normal gene; this is referred to as a dominant negative effect. This could occur in instances in which a protein requires homodimerization for activity, and dimerization of a wild-type and a mutant form of a protein leads to an inactive complex. Dominant-negative effects can also be found in cases in which two proteins heterodimerize, and an inactive mutant protein is able to complex with its partner protein, but the complex is inactive. Dominant-negative effects can be studied in animal models using transgenic mice. Although gene-targeted mice discussed in the previous sections can also be considered to be transgenic because foreign DNA is used to disrupt the endogenous gene, here the term *transgenic* is reserved for those mice in which foreign DNA has been inserted into the murine genome through pronuclear injection. In contrast to gene-targeting schemes in which genes are modified in ES cells and ES cells are then used to derive chimeric mice, in transgenic strategies, DNA is directly microinjected into the pronucleus of a fertilized egg or zygote, and the injected zygotes are then reimplanted into the oviduct of a hormonally primed female mouse. The injected DNA is able to recombine by nonhomologous or illegitimate recombination into random locations within the genome and in variable amounts from zygote to zygote. Once mice are derived from the injected zygotes, they are tested to determine whether they carry the injected DNA within their genomes as a transgene, and if they do, whether the transgene is expressed. By injecting DNA constructs that contain a tissue-specific promoter and a mutated gene of interest, it is possible to study whether expression of the mutant gene leads to an observable phenotype. In other instances, the gene to be expressed is not mutated, and the experiment is designed to determine whether overexpression or *de novo* expression of the gene results in an observable phenotype or disease model.

FORWARD AND REVERSE GENETICS

Forward genetic approaches begin with a phenotype and attempt to identify the gene. These phenotypes may be obtained through mutagenesis screens or from spontaneous mutations identified within a population. In contrast, reverse genetic approaches start with a known gene and attempt to characterize the phenotype resulting from mutation of that gene. Knock-out mice described earlier are one type of reverse genetic approach; ENU mutagenesis described later is an example of a forward genetic approach. This approach would also be used with spontaneous mutations that affect renal function. In either case, whether or not a mutagen is applied, these projects are designed to lead to the identification of the gene whose mutation is causing the phenotype. Now that the human and mouse genomes have been sequenced, forward genetic approaches may tend more often to assign diseases to previously identified genes than identify the gene outright.

Animal models of disease that have a genetic basis may either result from spontaneous or induced mutations. Spontaneous mutations or phenotypes are those noticed either by chance or through the directed observation of large numbers of mice that were not otherwise treated to induce a mutation. In contrast, induced mutations are those resulting from the treatment of mice with irradiation or mutagenic agents known to introduce point mutations or deletions into the genome. At present, several major efforts in several countries involve the use of *N*-ethyl-*N*-nitrosourea (ENU) to introduce small mutations throughout the mouse genome (24–31). These large genome-scale approaches, which can involve very large mouse colonies, are justified by the following arguments:

1. Most disease-related human mutations are caused by point mutations; therefore, an ENU-mutagenic approach may have a greater chance of producing a phenotype resembling a human disease than will gene-targeted mutations that usually completely inactivate a gene.
2. An ENU-based approach does not rely on previous identification or cloning of the gene (i.e., any gene is a theoretical target and can be studied) to the extent that some degree of compromise in the gene product's activity will result in an observable phenotype. The obvious disadvantage in comparison with gene targeting is that a large amount of work lies between the observation of a phenotype and the final identification of the mutated gene.
3. Given a large enough effort, it should be possible to eventually "saturate" the genome with mutations—that is, examination of several hundred thousand mutagen-treated mice is likely to provide the opportunity to observe the effects of placing a mutation in every gene capable of causing an observable phenotype.

However, one important point remains to be mentioned that dramatically increases the labor and expense of an ENU-based effort. Most observable phenotypes tend to be genetically recessive instead of dominant, meaning that they are not apparent in the first-generation offspring of mutagen-treated mice. Instead, it is necessary to breed a

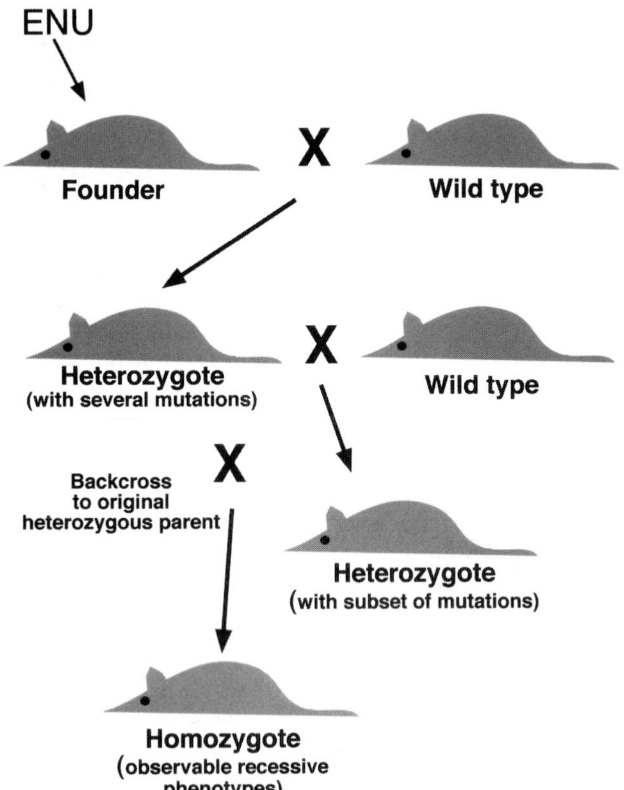

FIGURE 16.4. *N*-ethyl-*N*-nitrosourea (ENU) mutagenesis. A scheme is depicted for finding recessive phenotypes through ENU mutagenesis. Dominant phenotypes require a less complicated approach, as phenotypes will be apparent in the first generation derived from crossing founders with wild-type mice. In this scheme, a mutagenized male founder that probably carries many mutations after mutagenesis is mated with a wild-type mouse to produce heterozygote offspring that carry a subset of these mutations. These heterozygotes are mated with wild-type mice to produce a second generation, which will carry a smaller subset of the original mutations. These are then mated to the original heterozygous offspring of the founders, and 25% of the offspring of this cross will be homozygous for any particular mutation that was present in the second heterozygous generation.

second generation and then backcross it to the first-generation mice, resulting in a third generation (Figure 16.4). Doing this on a large scale will result in many third-generation mice that are now homozygous for mutations resulting from the original mutagenic treatment, and some will have observable phenotypes that can be studied for biologic interest and to map the responsible gene.

Mapping sites of induced or spontaneous mutations in mice has been greatly aided by the development of sets of microsatellite repeat markers. Microsatellite repeats used in mapping are stretches of CA dinucleotide repeats that are found interspersed throughout mammalian genomes (32,33). Typically, these CA repeats contain 10 to 20 CA dinucleotides. These CA repeats are flanked by unique sequences, and thus it is possible to design pairs of polymerase chain reaction primers that correspond to these flanking sequences that will amplify the $(CA)_n$ sequence between the two primers. Within a genetically inbred strain of mice, each individual mouse will contain the same number of CA dinucleotides at each repeat. However, similar to the variation observed between human individuals, different inbred strains may differ in the number of CA dinucleotides at any particular repeat. In addition, there are species of mice closely related to *Mus musculus*, such as *Mus spretus*, that provide even greater differences in the number of CA dinucleotides at many repeats than are found between the inbred strains of *M. musculus*. As depicted in Figure 16.5, genetic mapping using microsatellite markers takes the following approach: A mouse (or mice) with a phenotype produced by induced or spontaneous mutagenesis is mated with a mouse from a different inbred strain or from a different species, such as *M. spretus*, to produce F1 mice that are now heterozygous at all loci, containing one allele from each of the two parental strains and one mutant allele. In the case of a recessive phenotype, these F1 mouse are now either backcrossed to the original mutant strain or intercrossed among themselves to produce approximately 100 progeny mice, approximately 25% of which can be expected to show the mutant phenotype. For dominant phenotypes, the backcross can be to a wild-type mouse of either parental strain, and 50% will display the phenotype. Importantly, during this back- or intercross, there is independent segregation of chromosomes, such that each individual of the 100 mice is genetically unique, in that at any given locus it may be homozygous for alleles from a parental strain or heterozygous, containing an allele from each strain. A set of polymerase chain reaction primers corresponding to approximately 40 to 50 microsatellite repeats (about two to three per mouse chromosome) are used in the first round of analysis. These are chosen such that the two parental strains are known to differ in the length of the CA repeat between each primer pair. DNA samples are now obtained from all the progeny and are tested for the length of the CA sequence at each of the microsatellites, and these results are correlated with the observed phenotypes (in practice, a computational result, called a lod score is produced). Most of the microsatellites will not be genetically linked to the locus containing the mutation, and there will be no observable correlation between the strain genotype at a particular microsatellite and the presence or absence of the phenotype. In contrast, if a microsatellite marker is sufficiently closely linked to the site of a mutation causing a recessive phenotype, both alleles of the microsatellite marker are more likely to be derived from the parental strain originally containing the mutation. Thus, the goal of the first round of screening is to identify at least one marker that is linked to the mutation. Thereafter, subsequent rounds will use sets of markers linked to the original positive marker, with the expectation that it will be possible to identify a marker or pair of markers very closely linked to the mutation that will delimit the region of a single chromosome on which the mutation is

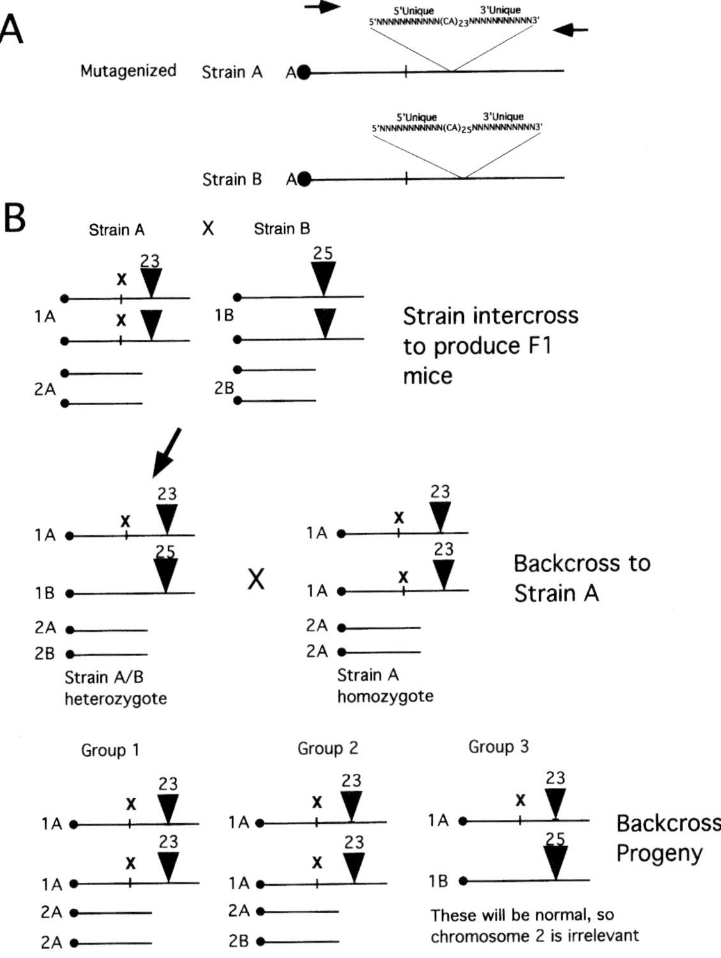

FIGURE 16.5. A scheme for mapping a mutation to a genetic locus. **A:** Depicts the use of microsatellite CA repeats. Strains A and B are two inbred strains of mice that differ in the length of many CA repeats, including the one shown here. Strain A has 23 CA dinucleotide repeats, whereas strain B has 25. They have the same unique 5' and 3' sequences flanking the CA repeats; thus, the same polymerase chain reaction primers can be used for both strains, but amplification will yield a longer product from strain B than A. **B:** The mating scheme to begin mapping the mutation. Only chromosomes 1 and 2 are shown. Strain A has a homozygous mutation on chromosome 1, marked as an "X" that is linked to the CA repeat, here designated by the black inverted triangle. This recessive mutation yields an observable phenotype. Strains A and B are mated to produce an F1 progeny, which will be heterozygous at all loci, including the one mutated in strain A. They will also be heterozygous for all CA repeats, including those on chromosome 2. Thus, any CA repeats that differ between the two strains will yield two bands on a polymerase chain reaction using the flanking unique primers for that CA repeat. F1 mice are backcrossed to strain A homozygotes, and many offspring are examined. Fifty percent of these offspring should be homozygous for X and have the observable phenotype. When these mice are analyzed for the CA repeat close to the locus for X, most mice with the phenotype will show only the strain A amplification product, whereas most of those without the phenotype will show both the strain A and strain B bands. In contrast, amplification of any CA repeats from chromosome 2 or any other chromosome will not show any correlation of strain A homozygosity with the observed phenotype.

located. This can then be used to initiate either a candidate gene approach or a chromosome walking approach to eventually identify the mutated gene. Newer sets of markers include single nucleotide repeats and improved radiation hybrid maps that will also aid in the mapping and identification of mutated genes (34,35).

These forward genetic approaches are not only suited to study developmental anomalies. Some of the large-scale efforts on mouse mutagenesis ongoing around the world involve performing basic blood work, urinalyses, and renal structural studies on each mouse from the group being screened for new phenotypes. Thus, this approach has the potential to identify genes involved in disease progression, as well as those responsible for morphogenetic processes.

GENETIC MODELS IN OTHER SPECIES

The previous discussion focuses on mice as the obvious model for genetic approaches to kidney development or disease. Mice are the most popular model system for genetic approaches, given their long history of study, the availability of many inbred lines, and that they are the most inexpensively maintained mammal. However, it should be mentioned that other animals may provide advantages that suggest them as an alternative to mice. Zebrafish are much less expensive to maintain than mice, and genetic tools to map zebrafish mutations will soon equal those available for mice (36–38). The zebrafish excretory system involves a pronephric duct and glomus that bears important similarity to mammalian nephrons and has already been the subject of many research studies (39–46). Alternatively, there is often a desire to use genetic approaches in animals that allow more complex physiologic studies than are usually done with mice. Rats provide an alternative, although the availability of genetic markers has not progressed as far as for murine systems (33,47), and they are more expensive than mice to maintain.

ANIMAL MODELS OF KIDNEY DISEASE

The selection of an animal model for some aspect or type of kidney disease takes several factors into consideration. Most important, the similarity to human disease that can be observed in a particular model is taken into account. Other important factors include the cost of the animals involved: The cost of maintaining animals larger than rodents increases dramatically with size, and the numbers of animals that can be studied consequently decreases. For this reason, some studies may begin with a rodent model, and then progress to a larger model once the rodent model establishes the feasibility of the hypothesis under study. The size of an animal may be important to the extent that it affects the ability to perform surgical manipulations or physiologic measurements. However, because it has become increasingly desirable to obtain physiologic measurements on various strains of knock-out mice, the equipment available to perform these measurements has improved and become commercially available.

MODELS OF RENAL FAILURE

Approaches to the study of renal failure include acute and chronic models. Acute renal failure has been induced using pharmacologic agents, antisera against kidney tissue or other antigens in which immune complex formation leads to glomerular disease (48–54). Ischemia-reperfusion models of acute renal failure, achieved by temporarily ligating a renal artery, allow study of the pathologic processes involved in tubular damage, as well as the effect of various pharmacologic treatments on the pathologic process (55–75).

There is often considerable variability in the response to a treatment among animals of a particular species. For example, different species of rats or mice may respond differently to different treatments. This difference in response is presumably due in a large part to genetic differences between different strains of rats or mice. The identification of so-called modifier genes that are responsible for these interstrain differences may contribute importantly to the understanding of human disease (76–82). Differences among humans in the sensitivity to nephrotoxic agents or differences in the severity of a disease process among different individuals may be due to polymorphisms in these same modifier genes.

MODELS OF IMMUNOLOGIC INJURY

There are many models of autoimmune injury to the kidney. The traditional model for a lupus-like autoimmune disease is the New Zealand black mouse, which has been studied for many years (83–87). These mice develop autoantibodies similar to those observed in humans with systemic lupus erythematosus and other related autoimmune disorders. More recently, many strains of mice carrying mutations in genes involved in the regulation of the immune response have been used to increase our understanding of the role the immune system plays in the onset and progression of kidney disease (88–98). These knock-out strains have allowed investigators to begin a genetic dissection of genes involved in autoimmune and other disorders.

TRANSPLANT MODELS

Animal models have been used extensively to study transplant rejection and in efforts to understand how tolerance to transplanted tissue may be improved. Over the past 20 years, there has been an extraordinary advancement in our mechanistic understanding of the immune function, and this has been brought to bear on the study of transplant rejection and tolerance (99–105). Important models under study include skin and heart transplants in mice and kidney transplants in rats (106–113). In addition, it is possible to produce "humanized" mice by transplanting human tissue into immunodeficient or irradiated mice whose immune system has been reconstituted with human lymphocytes, thus allowing the study of human immune function in an animal model (114–117). One area of research that remains controversial is involving xenografts (118,119). Because the supply of human kidneys and other organs for transplants continues to fall far short of the demand, there is a desirability of determining whether nonhuman animals provide an alternative source of organs for transplantation. The major concerns here include the strong immunologic rejection to a xenograft that must be overcome and the danger that xenografts might serve as vectors for the introduction of novel infectious agents into the human population.

ANIMAL MODELS FOR THE STUDY OF RENAL PHYSIOLOGY

Historically, several animal models have been used to study renal physiology, including swine, sheep, guinea pigs, rabbits, rats, and mice. Fetal lambs have been a particularly important model in which developmental aspects of physiology have been studied, particularly relating to obstructive uropathy (120–132). As alluded to earlier, when genes encoding proteins involved in the regulation of physiologic processes are knocked out, there is a desirability to perform physiologic studies in murine systems to determine how physiologic responses are altered in the absence of a particular protein (133–140). Although gene knock-outs are not yet done in rats, the availability of genetic models and gene mapping of physiologic traits has yielded important information (141–145). The ability to perform sophisticated physiologic experiments in mice has improved dramatically over the past several years, as new equipment has become available (139). As in other situations, there is a constant need to balance the advantages of a large animal model with the lower costs of smaller animal models.

SUMMARY

Animal models are of increasing importance in the study of kidney disease. An important shift since the early 1990s is the use of rodent models and the use of genetic models.

Large animal use remains an important aspect of these studies. The use of large versus small animals must take into account cost and ethical considerations.

REFERENCES

1. Kreidberg JA, et al. WT-1 is required for early kidney development. *Cell* 1993;74(4):679–691.
2. Torres M, et al. Pax-2 controls multiple steps of urogenital development. *Development* 1995;121(12):4057–4065.
3. Moore MW, et al. Renal and neuronal abnormalities in mice lacking GDNF. *Nature* 1996;382:76–79.
4. Pichel JG, et al. Defects in enteric innervation and kidney development in mice lacking GDNF. *Nature* 1996;382:73–76.
5. Sanchez MP, et al. Renal agenesis and absence of enteric ganglions in mice lacking GDNF. *Nature* 1996;382:70–74.
6. Kispert A, Vainio S, McMahon AP. Wnt-4 is a mesenchymal signal for epithelial transformation of metanephric mesenchyme in the developing kidney. *Development* 1998;125 (21):4225–4234.
7. Dudley AT, Lyons KM, Robertson EJ. A requirement for bone morphogenetic protein-7 during development of the mammalian kidney and eye. *Genes Dev* 1995;9(22):2795–2807.
8. Luo G, et al. BMP-7 is an inducer of nephrogenesis, and is also required for eye development and skeletal patterning. *Genes Dev* 1995;9(22):2808–2820.
9. Robertson EJ, ed. *Isolation of embryonic stem cells, in teratocarcinomas and embryonic stem cells: a practical approach.* Oxford: IRL Press, 1987.
10. Bradley A. Production and analysis of chimeric mice. In: Robertson EJ, ed. *Teratocarcinomas and embryonic stem cells: a practical approach.* Oxford: IRL Press, 1987:113–151.
11. Thomas KR, Capecchi MR. Targeting of genes to specific sites in the mammalian genome. *Cold Spring Harb Symp Quant Biol* 1986;51(1):1101–1113.
12. Thomas KR, Deng C, Capecchi MR. High-fidelity gene targeting in embryonic stem cells by using sequence replacement vectors. *Mol Cell Biol* 1992;12(7):2919–2923.
13. Capecchi MR. The new mouse genetics: altering the genome by gene targeting. *Trends Genet* 1989;5(3):70–76.
14. Orban PC, Chui D, Marth JD. Tissue- and site-specific DNA recombination in transgenic mice. *Proc Natl Acad Sci U S A* 1992;89(15):6861–6865.
15. Sauer B. Inducible gene targeting in mice using the Cre/lox system. *Methods* 1998;14(4):381–392.
16. Stricklett PK, Nelson RD, Kohan DE. The Cre/loxP system and gene targeting in the kidney. *Am J Physiol* 1999;276(5 Pt 2):F651–F657.
17. Furth PA, et al. Temporal control of gene expression in transgenic mice by a tetracycline responsive promoter. *Proc Natl Acad Sci U S A* 1994;91:9302–9306.
18. Sohal DS, et al. Temporally regulated and tissue-specific gene manipulations in the adult and embryonic heart using a tamoxifen-inducible Cre protein. *Circ Res* 2001;89(1):20–25.
19. Verrou C, et al. Comparison of the tamoxifen regulated chimeric Cre recombinases MerCreMer and CreMer. *Biol Chem* 1999;380(12):1435–1438.
20. Moeller MJ, et al. Two gene fragments that direct podocyte-specific expression in transgenic mice. *J Am Soc Nephrol* 2002;13(6):1561–1567.
21. Wong MA, Cui S, Quaggin SE. Identification and characterization of a glomerular-specific promoter from the human nephrin gene. *Am J Physiol Renal Physiol* 2000;279:F1027–F1032.
22. Eremina V, et al. Glomerular-specific gene excision in vivo. *J Am Soc Nephrol* 2002;13:788–793.
23. Stricklett PK, Nelson RD, Kohan DE. Targeting collecting tubules using the aquaporin-2 promoter. *Exp Nephrol* 1999;7 (1):67–74.
24. Hrabe de Angelis M, Strivens M. Large-scale production of mouse phenotypes: the search for animal models for inherited diseases in humans. *Brief Bioinform* 2001;2(2):170–180.
25. Beier DR. Sequence-based analysis of mutagenized mice. *Mamm Genome* 2000;11(7):594–597.
26. Nolan PM, et al. Implementation of a large-scale ENU mutagenesis program: towards increasing the mouse mutant resource. *Mamm Genome* 2000;11(7):500–506.
27. Chen Y, et al. Genotype-based screen for ENU-induced mutations in mouse embryonic stem cells. *Nat Genet* 2000; 24(3):314–317.
28. Anderson KV. Finding the genes that direct mammalian development: ENU mutagenesis in the mouse. *Trends Genet* 2000;16(3):99–102.
29. Justice MJ, et al. Mouse ENU mutagenesis. *Hum Mol Genet* 1999;8(10):1955–1963.
30. Hrabe de Angelis M, Balling R. Large scale ENU screens in the mouse: genetics meets genomics. *Mutat Res* 1998;400(1–2): 25–32.
31. Shelby MD, Tindall KR. Mammalian germ cell mutagenicity of ENU, IPMS and MMS, chemicals selected for a transgenic mouse collaborative study. *Mutat Res* 1997;388(2–3):99–109.
32. Dietrich WF, et al. Mapping the mouse genome: current status and future prospects. *Proc Natl Acad Sci U S A* 1995; 92(24):10849–10853.
33. Brown DM, et al. An integrated genetic linkage map of the laboratory rat. *Mamm Genome* 1998;9(7):521–530.
34. Lindblad-Toh K, et al. Large-scale discovery and genotyping of single-nucleotide polymorphisms in the mouse. *Nat Genet* 2000;24(4):381–386.
35. Van Etten WJ, et al. Radiation hybrid map of the mouse genome. *Nat Genet* 1999;22(4):384–387.
36. Fishman MC. Zebrafish genetics: the enigma of arrival. *Proc Natl Acad Sci U S A* 1999;96(19):10554–10556.
37. Shimoda N, et al. Zebrafish genetic map with 2000 microsatellite markers. *Genomics* 1999;58(3):219–232.
38. Knapik EW, et al. A microsatellite genetic linkage map for zebrafish (Danio rerio). *Nat Genet* 1998;18(4):338–343.
39. Drummond IA, et al. Early development of the zebrafish pronephros and analysis of mutations affecting pronephric function. *Development* 1998;125(23):4655–4667.
40. Liu S, et al. A defect in a novel Nek-family kinase causes cystic kidney disease in the mouse and in zebrafish. *Development* 2002;129(24):5839–5846.
41. Briggs JP. The zebrafish: a new model organism for integrative physiology. *Am J Physiol Regul Integr Comp Physiol* 2002;282(1):R3–9.

42. Serluca FC, Fishman MC. Pre-pattern in the pronephric kidney field of zebrafish. *Development* 2001;128(12):2233–2241.
43. Majumdar A, Drummond IA. The zebrafish floating head mutant demonstrates podocytes play an important role in directing glomerular differentiation. *Dev Biol* 2000;222(1):147–157.
44. Drummond IA. The zebrafish pronephros: a genetic system for studies of kidney development. *Pediatr Nephrol* 2000;14(5):428–435.
45. Majumdar A, et al. Zebrafish no isthmus reveals a role for pax2.1 in tubule differentiation and patterning events in the pronephric primordia. *Development* 2000;127(10):2089–2098.
46. Majumdar A, Drummond IA. Podocyte differentiation in the absence of endothelial cells as revealed in the zebrafish avascular mutant, cloche. *Dev Genet* 1999;24(3–4):220–229.
47. Twigger S, et al. Rat genome database (RGD): mapping disease onto the genome. *Nucleic Acids Res* 2002;30(1):125–128.
48. Chugh S, et al. Aminopeptidase A: a nephritogenic target antigen of nephrotoxic serum. *Kidney Int* 2001;59(2):601–613.
49. Cook HT, et al. Treatment with an antibody to VLA-1 integrin reduces glomerular and tubulointerstitial scarring in a rat model of crescentic glomerulonephritis. *Am J Pathol* 2002; 161(4):1265–1272.
50. Hiromura K, et al. Podocyte expression of the CDK-inhibitor p57 during development and disease. *Kidney Int* 2001; 60(6):2235–2246.
51. Lin F, et al. Decay-accelerating factor confers protection against complement-mediated podocyte injury in acute nephrotoxic nephritis. *Lab Invest* 2002;82(5):563–569.
52. Topham PS, et al. Lack of chemokine receptor CCR1 enhances Th1 responses and glomerular injury during nephrotoxic nephritis. *J Clin Invest* 1999;104(11):1549–1557.
53. Xu Y, et al. Induction of urokinase receptor expression in nephrotoxic nephritis. *Exp Nephrol* 2001;9(6):397–404.
54. Yanagita M, et al. Essential role of Gas6 for glomerular injury in nephrotoxic nephritis. *J Clin Invest* 2002;110(2):239–246.
55. Carmago S, Shah SV, Walker PD. Meprin, a brush-border enzyme, plays an important role in hypoxic/ischemic acute renal tubular injury in rats. *Kidney Int* 2002;61(3):959–966.
56. Chatterjee PK, et al. Calpain inhibitor-1 reduces renal ischemia/reperfusion injury in the rat. *Kidney Int* 2001;59 (6):2073–2083.
57. Fernandez M, et al. Exacerbated inflammatory response induced by insulin-like growth factor I treatment in rats with ischemic acute renal failure. *J Am Soc Nephrol* 2001;12(9):1900–1907.
58. Gimelreich D, et al. Regulation of ROMK and channel-inducing factor (CHIF) in acute renal failure due to ischemic reperfusion injury. *Kidney Int* 2001;59(5):1812–1820.
59. Gretz N. The development of hypertension in the remnant kidney model after either pole resection or partial infarction of the kidney. *J Am Soc Nephrol* 1995;5(10):1839–1840.
60. Jia ZQ, et al. The effects of artery occlusion on temperature homogeneity during hyperthermia in rabbit kidneys in vivo. *Int J Hyperthermia* 1997;13(1):21–37.
61. Kakoki M, et al. Effects of vasodilatory antihypertensive agents on endothelial dysfunction in rats with ischemic acute renal failure. *Hypertens Res* 2000;23(5):527–533.
62. Knoll T, et al. Therapeutic administration of an endothelin-A receptor antagonist after acute ischemic renal failure dose-dependently improves recovery of renal function. *J Cardiovasc Pharmacol* 2001;37(4):483–488.
63. Kren S, Hostetter TH. The course of the remnant kidney model in mice. *Kidney Int* 1999;56(1):333–337.
64. Kwon O, Phillips CL, Molitoris BA. Ischemia induces alterations in actin filaments in renal vascular smooth muscle cells. *Am J Physiol Renal Physiol* 2002;282(6):F1012–F1019.
65. Lieberthal W, et al. Rapamycin impairs recovery from acute renal failure: role of cell-cycle arrest and apoptosis of tubular cells. *Am J Physiol Renal Physiol* 2001;281(4):F693–F706.
66. Lloberas N, et al. Postischemic renal oxidative stress induces inflammatory response through PAF and oxidized phospholipids. Prevention by antioxidant treatment. *FASEB J* 2002; 16(8):908–910.
67. Megyesi J, et al. Positive effect of the induction of p21WAF1/CIP1 on the course of ischemic acute renal failure. *Kidney Int* 2001;60(6):2164–2172.
68. Meldrum KK, et al. Simulated ischemia induces renal tubular cell apoptosis through a nuclear factor-kappaB dependent mechanism. *J Urol* 2002;168(1):248–252.
69. Modolo NS, et al. Acute renal ischemia model in dogs: effects of metoprolol. *Ren Fail* 2001;23(1):1–10.
70. Mister M, et al. Propionyl-L-carnitine prevents renal function deterioration due to ischemia/reperfusion. *Kidney Int* 2002;61(3):1064–1078.
71. Okusa MD. The inflammatory cascade in acute ischemic renal failure. *Nephron* 2002;90(2):133–138.
72. Power JM, Tonkin AM. Large animal models of heart failure. *Aust N Z J Med* 1999;29(3):395–402.
73. Textor SC. Pathophysiology of renal failure in renovascular disease. *Am J Kidney Dis* 1994;24(4):642–651.
74. Vaneerdeweg W, et al. A standardized surgical technique to obtain a stable and reproducible chronic renal failure model in dogs. *Eur Surg Res* 1992;24(5):273–282.
75. Yoshida T, et al. Global analysis of gene expression in renal ischemia-reperfusion in the mouse. *Biochem Biophys Res Commun* 2002;291(4):787–794.
76. Andrews KL, et al. Quantitative trait loci influence renal disease progression in a mouse model of Alport syndrome. *Am J Pathol* 2002;160(2):721–730.
77. Woo DD, et al. Genetic identification of two major modifier loci of polycystic kidney disease progression in pcy mice. *J Clin Invest* 1997;100(8):1934–1940.
78. Sommardahl C, et al. Phenotypic variations of orpk mutation and chromosomal localization of modifiers influencing kidney phenotype. *Physiol Genomics* 2001;7(2):127–134.
79. Yeung RS, et al. Genetic identification of a locus, Mot1, that affects renal tumor size in the rat. *Genomics* 2001;78(3):108–112.
80. Kamba T, et al. Failure of ureteric bud invasion: a new model of renal agenesis in mice. *Am J Pathol* 2001;159(6):2347–2353.
81. Montagutelli X. Effect of the genetic background on the phenotype of mouse mutations. *J Am Soc Nephrol* 2000;11(Suppl 16):S101–S105.

82. Upadhya P, et al. Genetic modifiers of polycystic kidney disease in intersubspecific KAT2J mutants. *Genomics* 1999;58 (2):129–137.
83. Foster MH. Relevance of systemic lupus erythematosus nephritis animal models to human disease. *Semin Nephrol* 1999;19(1):12–24.
84. Morel L, Wakeland EK. Susceptibility to lupus nephritis in the NZB/W model system. *Curr Opin Immunol* 1998;10 (6):718–725.
85. Walport MJ, Davies KA, Botto M. C1q and systemic lupus erythematosus. *Immunobiology* 1998;199(2):265–285.
86. Gavalchin J, Staines NA. T and B cell recognition of idiotypes of anti-DNA autoantibodies. *Lupus* 1997;6(3):337–343.
87. Isenberg DA, et al. The role of antibodies to DNA in systemic lupus erythematosus—a review and introduction to an international workshop on DNA antibodies held in London, May 1996. *Lupus* 1997;6(3):290–304.
88. Pickering MC, et al. Uncontrolled C3 activation causes membranoproliferative glomerulonephritis in mice deficient in complement factor H. *Nat Genet* 2002;31(4):424–428.
89. Salvador JM, et al. Mice lacking the p53-effector gene Gadd45a develop a lupus-like syndrome. *Immunity* 2002; 16(4):499–508.
90. Tabata N, et al. Establishment of monoclonal anti-retroviral gp70 autoantibodies from MRL/lpr lupus mice and induction of glomerular gp70 deposition and pathology by transfer into non-autoimmune mice. *J Virol* 2000;74(9):4116–4126.
91. Cruse JM, Lewis RE, Dilioglou S. Fate of immune complexes, glomerulonephritis, and cell-mediated vasculitis in lupus-prone MRL/Mp lpr/lpr mice. *Exp Mol Pathol* 2000; 69(3):211–222.
92. Ophascharoensuk V, et al. The cyclin-dependent kinase inhibitor p27Kip1 safeguards against inflammatory injury. *Nat Med* 1998;4(5):575–580.
93. Cattell V, et al. Anti-GBM glomerulonephritis in mice lacking nitric oxide synthase type 2. *Kidney Int* 1998;53(4): 932–936.
94. Quigg RJ, et al. Immune complex glomerulonephritis in C4- and C3-deficient mice. *Kidney Int* 1998;53(2):320–330.
95. Tang T, et al. A role for Mac-1 (CDIIb/CD18) in immune complex-stimulated neutrophil function in vivo: Mac-1 deficiency abrogates sustained Fcgamma receptor-dependent neutrophil adhesion and complement-dependent proteinuria in acute glomerulonephritis. *J Exp Med* 1997;186 (11):1853–1863.
96. Ito MR, et al. Rheumatic diseases in an MRL strain of mice with a deficit in the functional Fas ligand. *Arthritis Rheum* 1997;40(6):1054–1063.
97. Haas C, Ryffel B, Le Hir M. IFN-gamma is essential for the development of autoimmune glomerulonephritis in MRL/ Ipr mice. *J Immunol* 1997;158(11):5484–5491.
98. Hibbs ML, et al. Multiple defects in the immune system of Lyn-deficient mice, culminating in autoimmune disease. *Cell* 1995;83(2):301–311.
99. Gudmundsdottir H, Turka LA. T cell costimulatory blockade: new therapies for transplant rejection. *J Am Soc Nephrol* 1999;10(6):1356–1365.
100. Dong VM, Womer KL, Sayegh MH. Transplantation tolerance: the concept and its applicability. *Pediatr Transplant* 1999;3(3):181–192.
101. Bromberg JS, Murphy B. Routes to allograft survival. *J Clin Invest* 2001;107(7):797–798.
102. Light J, et al. Bone marrow transfusions in cadaver renal allografts: pilot trials with concurrent controls. *Clin Transplant* 2002;16(5):317–324.
103. Knechtle SJ, et al. Tolerance and near-tolerance strategies in monkeys and their application to human renal transplantation. *Immunol Rev* 2001;183:205–213.
104. Inverardi L, Ricordi C. Tolerance and pancreatic islet transplantation. *Philos Trans R Soc Lond B Biol Sci* 2001;356 (1409):759–765.
105. Field EH, Strober S. Tolerance, mixed chimerism and protection against graft-versus-host disease after total lymphoid irradiation. *Philos Trans R Soc Lond B Biol Sci* 2001;356 (1409):739–748.
106. Decker CJ, et al. The novel IMPDH inhibitor VX-497 prolongs skin graft survival and improves graft versus host disease in mice. *Drugs Exp Clin Res* 2001;27(3):89–95.
107. Yoshimura R, et al. Induction of hyperacute rejection of skin allografts by CD8+ lymphocytes. *Transplantation* 2000; 69(7):1452–1457.
108. Gardner CR. The pharmacology of immunosuppressant drugs in skin transplant rejection in mice and other rodents. *Gen Pharmacol* 1995;26(2):245–271.
109. Tepper MA, et al. Tolerance induction by soluble CTLA4 in a mouse skin transplant model. *Transplant Proc* 1994;26 (6):3151–3154.
110. Sho M, et al. New insights into the interactions between T-cell costimulatory blockade and conventional immunosuppressive drugs. *Ann Surg* 2002;236(5):667–675.
111. Rolls HK, et al. T-cell response to cardiac myosin persists in the absence of an alloimmune response in recipients with chronic cardiac allograft rejection. *Transplantation* 2002;74 (7):1053–1057.
112. Zhai Y, et al. Allograft rejection by primed/memory CD8+ T cells is CD154 blockade resistant: therapeutic implications for sensitized transplant recipients. *J Immunol* 2002; 169(8):4667–4673.
113. Fedoseyeva EV, et al. Modulation of tissue-specific immune response to cardiac myosin can prolong survival of allogeneic heart transplants. *J Immunol* 2002;169(3):1168–1174.
114. Coates PT, et al. Human myeloid dendritic cells transduced with an adenoviral interleukin-10 gene construct inhibit human skin graft rejection in humanized NOD-scid chimeric mice. *Gene Ther* 2001;8(16):1224–1233.
115. Fahy O, et al. Chemokine-induced cutaneous inflammatory cell infiltration in a model of Hu-PBMC-SCID mice grafted with human skin. *Am J Pathol* 2001;158(3):1053–1063.
116. Moulton KS, et al. Angiogenesis in the huPBL-SCID model of human transplant rejection. *Transplantation* 1999;67(12): 1626–1631.
117. Briscoe DM, et al. The allogeneic response to cultured human skin equivalent in the hu-PBL-SCID mouse model of skin rejection. *Transplantation* 1999;67(12):1590–1599.
118. Hammerman MR. Xenotransplantation of renal primordia. *Curr Opin Nephrol Hypertens* 2002;11(1):11–16.

119. Palmer DB, Lechler R. Can the thymus be a useful tool to induce specific tolerance to xenoantigens? *Transplantation* 1999;68(11):1628–1630.
120. Edouga D, et al. Recovery after relief of fetal urinary obstruction: morphological, functional and molecular aspects. *Am J Physiol Renal Physiol* 2001;281(1):F26–F37.
121. Kitagawa H, et al. Glomerular size in renal dysplasia secondary to obstructive uropathy: a further exploration of the fetal lamb model. *J Pediatr Surg* 2000;35(11):1651–1655.
122. Kitagawa H, et al. Early fetal obstructive uropathy produces Potter's syndrome in the lamb. *J Pediatr Surg* 2000;35(11): 1549–1553.
123. Smith LM, et al. Antenatal glucocorticoids alter postnatal preterm lamb renal and cardiovascular responses to intravascular volume expansion. *Pediatr Res* 2000;47(5):622–627.
124. Kitagawa H, et al. The pathogenesis of dysplastic kidney in a urinary tract obstruction in the female fetal lamb. *J Pediatr Surg* 1999;34(11):1678–1683.
125. Wang J, Rose JC. Developmental changes in renal renin mRNA half-life and responses to stimulation in fetal lambs. *Am J Physiol* 1999;277(4 Pt 2):R1130–R1135.
126. Gimonet V, et al. Nephrogenesis and angiotensin II receptor subtypes gene expression in the fetal lamb. *Am J Physiol* 1998;274(6 Pt 2):F1062–F1069.
127. Nguyen HT, Kogan BA. Renal hemodynamic changes after complete and partial unilateral ureteral obstruction in the fetal lamb. *J Urol* 1998;160(3 Pt 2):1063–1069.
128. Wang J, Perez FM, Rose JC. Developmental changes in renin-containing cells from the ovine fetal kidney. *J Soc Gynecol Investig* 1997;4(4):191–196.
129. Berry LM, et al. Preterm newborn lamb renal and cardiovascular responses after fetal or maternal antenatal betamethasone. *Am J Physiol* 1997;272(6 Pt 2):R1972–R1979.
130. Matsell DG, Bennett T, Bocking AD. Characterization of fetal ovine renal dysplasia after mid-gestation ureteral obstruction. *Clin Invest Med* 1996;19(6):444–452.
131. Peters CA, et al. Fetal compensatory renal growth due to unilateral ureteral obstruction. *J Urol* 1993;150(2 Pt 2): 597–600.
132. Peters CA, et al. Effect of in utero vesicostomy on pulmonary hypoplasia in the fetal lamb with bladder outlet obstruction and oligohydramnios: a morphometric analysis. *J Urol* 1991;146(4):1178–1183.
133. Ma X, Abboud FM, Chapleau MW. Analysis of afferent, central, and efferent components of the baroreceptor reflex in mice. *Am J Physiol Regul Integr Comp Physiol* 2002;283(5): R1033–R1040.
134. Ishii T, et al. Postnatal development of blood pressure and baroreflex in mice. *Auton Neurosci* 2001;94(1–2):34–41.
135. Gross V, et al. Heart rate variability and baroreflex function in AT2 receptor-disrupted mice. *Hypertension* 2002;40(2):207–213.
136. Rokosh DG, Simpson PC. Knockout of the alpha 1A/C-adrenergic receptor subtype: the alpha 1A/C is expressed in resistance arteries and is required to maintain arterial blood pressure. *Proc Natl Acad Sci U S A* 2002;99(14):9474–9479.
137. Besnard S, et al. Smooth muscle dysfunction in resistance arteries of the staggerer mouse, a mutant of the nuclear receptor RORalpha. *Circ Res* 2002;90(7):820–825.
138. Vecchione C, et al. Cardiovascular influences of alpha1b-adrenergic receptor defect in mice. *Circulation* 2002;105(14): 1700–1707.
139. Gross V, Luft FC. Adapting renal and cardiovascular physiology to the genetically hypertensive mouse. *Semin Nephrol* 2002;22(2):172–179.
140. Holschneider DP, et al. Increased baroreceptor response in mice deficient in monoamine oxidase A and B. *Am J Physiol Heart Circ Physiol* 2002;282(3):H964–H972.
141. Shiozawa M, et al. Evidence of gene-gene interactions in the genetic susceptibility to renal impairment after unilateral nephrectomy. *J Am Soc Nephrol* 2000;11(11):2068–2078.
142. Kwitek-Black AE, Jacob HJ. The use of designer rats in the genetic dissection of hypertension. *Curr Hypertens Rep* 2001;3 (1):12–18.
143. Stoll M, Jacob HJ. Genetic rat models of hypertension: relationship to human hypertension. *Curr Hypertens Rep* 2001; 3(2):157–164.
144. Stoll M, et al. A genomic-systems biology map for cardiovascular function. *Science* 2001;294(5547):1723–1726.
145. Jacob HJ, Kwitek AE. Rat genetics: attaching physiology and pharmacology to the genome. *Nat Rev Genet* 2002;3(1):33–42.

17

CLINICAL INVESTIGATION

SUSAN L. FURTH
JEFFREY FADROWSKI

CLINICAL RESEARCH QUESTION

How can we best evaluate, treat, and assess long-term risks for children with kidney disease? Who is at risk of developing end-stage renal disease (ESRD) in childhood or young adulthood? Clinicians are often faced with questions such as these with uncertain answers in the practice of pediatric nephrology. Parents ask, "Why did my child get this disease?" "What is the most effective method to treat this condition?" "What's the prognosis of this condition in my child?" Frequently, these answers are not known, and these questions are the inspiration for high-quality clinical research. The first step in developing a valuable clinical study is determining whether the initial query can be translated into a good research question.

Hallmarks of a Good Research Question

A good research question gives *useful* information, is interesting to the researcher, builds on what is known, and can be answered with available resources. Research is a labor of love, demanding attention to detail, perseverance, honesty, and imagination. Developing a good research question is an iterative process. One needs input from knowledgeable colleagues and collaborators. The researcher must become thoroughly familiar with what is already known about the topic by reviewing the literature and consulting with experts in the area. Investigating what is already known has several benefits. First, it can reveal that the candidate research question has already been answered adequately. Second, learning what is already known provides insight into potentially useful methods for addressing a research question. For example, previous studies may demonstrate good ways to measure a variable of interest or provide background information for determining sample size. Third, a literature review may suggest ways to frame the research question at hand. For example, a literature review may reveal that particular modifiable risk factors are consistently associated with a disease process, and an intervention to modify these risk factors may form a sound basis for a clinical trial.

Finally, a good research question needs to be answerable with available resources. These include subjects available for study, technical expertise of the research staff, and the time and money that can be devoted to the project. Once a question is framed, the researcher needs to outline the study protocol or methods, which include specifying the recruitment method, number of subjects and how they will be recruited, how each variable will be operationally defined, and the plan for data analysis. A poorly designed study is worse than no study at all because, like imprecise measurements and an improper analytic plan, it can also lead to false conclusions.

Steps in Refining a Good Research Question

A good research question usually begins with a broadly stated concept. The initial question is then made more specific by identifying independent and dependent variables. Often, research questions are concerned with causal relationships. *Independent variables* are those conceptualized to be causes; *dependent variables* are those conceptualized to be effects. The research question can be modified to ask about the role of multiple potential causes in leading to the specific outcome. A simple research question asks whether *x* (independent variable) causes *y* (dependent variable). More complex research questions could assess the relative importance of *x* and other variables (e.g., a and b) as causes of *y*. A different research question might ask how strongly *x* predicts *y* in one population versus another.

The next step is to translate a research question into a hypothesis. In our simple example, the researcher may hypothesize that *x* causes *y*. In the actual research project, the information collected is examined to determine whether it is reasonable to conclude that *x* does cause *y*. In examining the data, the investigator tests the *null hypothesis* that *x* does not cause *y* versus the *alternative hypothesis* that it does.

SCIENTIFIC METHOD

A study's potential value is determined by the relevance of the research question. Its ultimate worth is determined by the study methods. Methodologic issues concern the **study**

design, subject selection, data collection techniques, and the **analytic plan.** Subsequent sections in this chapter discuss each of these aspects. As a foundation, this section describes the concepts of inference, generalizability, and validity.

Inference

As Figure 17.1 shows, scientific research begins with the research question. It then moves (clockwise in the figure) to the controlled arena of the study design and then through the implementation of the actual study and findings. Inferences from the findings in the study approximate the "truth in the study." From these "truths" we attempt to infer the applicability of the findings to general clinical practice. Researchers describe and explain reality by sampling a portion of it, measuring characteristics of the sample, analyzing the measurements, and interpreting the results. Researchers make inferences from the sample measures of operationally defined variables to the hypothesized relationships of the theoretical constructs in the larger population of interest. Errors in the design or implementation of the study can lead to false conclusions. The strength of inference depends largely on the research methods used in the recruitment of study subjects (sampling) and in the choice and integrity of the study design.

Statistical inference depends on the methods used to define and sample the population. The researcher uses inferential statistics to *extrapolate* the sample findings to the larger population of children from which the sample was drawn. Inferential statistics assume that the studied sample is drawn by probability methods and can be used to make inferences about the larger population. The size of a probability sample determines the certainty of inferences from it. All other things being equal, the larger the sample size, the greater the certainty of inferences to the population.

The researcher's ability to make a *causal inference* from study results depends largely on issues of study design. Study designs are *observational* when the investigator does not manipulate the risk factor but merely selects children with and without disease and compares them in terms of the risk factor(s). Study designs are experimental when the investigator not only observes but actually manipulates the relationship between two variables. Observational designs provide somewhat weaker evidence of causation, because they fail to rule out explanations other than association between the variables studied. Experimental designs can provide much stronger evidence for causation. In an experimental study, the investigator controls the independent variable, which is the factor hypothesized to produce change in a dependent variable. In an experimental study, subjects are randomized to receive or not receive the independent variable. The goal of the process of randomization is to produce study groups that are "balanced" in terms of other factors that could influence the dependent variable. Unfortunately, experimental designs often are not feasible, ethical, or desirable. Epidemiologic studies of disease preclude manipulation of risk factors in humans. Health services researchers studying the public health impact of changes in health policy rarely can control these changes.

Within the broad categories of observational and experimental designs, there are many variations. These variations, distinguishing characteristics, primary uses, strengths, and weaknesses are discussed in the section Study Design. Study design also influences the validity of study results.

Validity

Validity is the extent to which study findings correctly reflect and explain reality. The concepts of internal and external validity are illustrated in Figure 17.2. As a research question's relevance increases, so does the need for validity. To some extent, every research question worth answering is controversial because of its implications for policy and practice and because it addresses areas in which existing evidence is scant or contradictory. If a question is not contro-

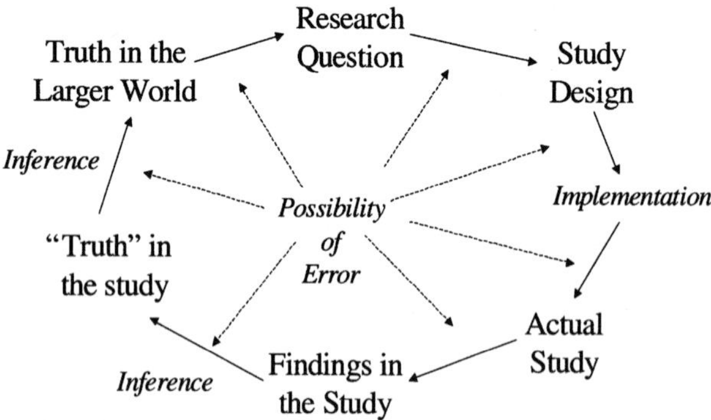

FIGURE 17.1. The role of inference in drawing conclusions from clinical research studies.

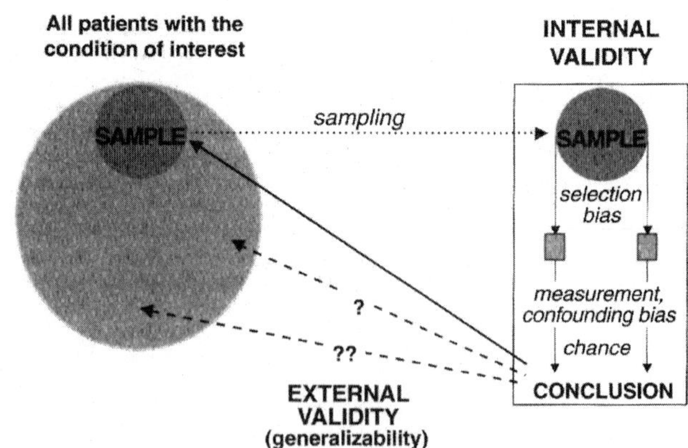

FIGURE 17.2. External and internal validity in experimental designs. (From Fletcher RH, Fletcher SW, Wagner EH. *Clinical epidemiology: the essentials*, 3rd ed. Baltimore: Williams & Wilkins, 1996:12, with permission.)

versial, there is little need for a scientifically rigorous search for its answer. The clarity and rigor of study design as well as the careful implementation of the research plan increase the likelihood that inferences from the study are valid.

Cook and Campbell (1) define several aspects of validity. *Statistical validity* is the correctness of study conclusions regarding the existence of a relationship between two variables. A study lacks statistical validity when it concludes there is no relationship between variables when in fact there is one or when it concludes there is a relationship when in fact there is none. Statistical validity is jeopardized most often by inadequate sample size and by improper use of statistical tests.

If there is a relationship between two variables, *internal validity* (Fig. 17.2) is the correctness of conclusions about whether the relationship between the operationally defined independent and dependent variables is causal. Internal validity is jeopardized when a study design fails to control for factors that could confound the hypothesized causal relationship.

Finally, given a causal relationship between the independent and dependent variables, *external validity* (Fig. 17.2) is the correctness of generalizing to other persons, settings, and times. Poor choice of a study population and inadequate research procedures are common challenges to external validity.

In summary, the scientific method involves extrapolating inferences from a study situation to the larger world. The value of research depends on the validity of such inferences, which in turn is determined by the researcher's choice of methods. The following sections explain the strengths and weaknesses of the methodologic choices available.

STUDY DESIGN

Observational Studies

There are four major types of observational studies: case series, cross-sectional, case-control, and cohort. Observational designs are weaker than interventional designs in establishing causation, but they are useful when it is not feasible to manipulate the independent variable. Studies of disease etiology usually are observational. In these types of observational studies, risk factors or exposures are the independent variables, and disease is the dependent variable.

Case Series

In a *case series* study, a sample of cases is chosen, and the presence of the risk factor is measured. A case series study is easy to conduct and is useful as a preliminary study to reinforce anecdotal evidence, to generate hypotheses, or to establish variable distributions in planning future research. Case series can sometimes identify previously unrecognized constellations of symptoms or morbidities attributed to exposures to drugs or toxins. An example of a case series is the report by Furth et al. on diabetes associated with the use of tacrolimus in pediatric renal transplant recipients (2). The authors identified a number of pediatric transplant recipients treated with tacrolimus who developed diabetes. The authors summarized the case histories and reviewed existing literature regarding diabetes associated with immunosuppressive therapy in adult transplant recipients. A case series such as this can provide useful information for the clinician. However, as a method to determine the risk associated with a particular factor, this design is extremely weak because there is no means of comparison. Even if a risk factor is highly prevalent among the cases (in this example, all the cases of diabetes posttransplant had been treated with tacrolimus), there is no way of knowing whether the risk of the disease is greater with exposure to tacrolimus than with exposure to other immunosuppressive medications—for example, cyclosporine or steroids. The case series design cannot provide an estimate of risk.

Cross-Sectional Design

A *cross-sectional study* is one in which the disease and risk factors are measured at the same time in a sample of subjects. Subjects can be categorized as either having or not having the risk factor. Within each group, the presence of the disease can be determined. Analytically, the association between a particular risk factor and the disease is measured as the relative prevalence of the disease among those with, versus those without, the risk factor.

The cross-sectional study design is superior to the case series in that it provides a means for comparison. Cross-sectional studies are relatively economic, easy to conduct, and allow simultaneous examination of multiple risk factors. An example of a cross-sectional study is the analysis of demographic factors associated with rates of hospital admissions for infection in pediatric ESRD patients in the U.S. Renal Data System (USRDS). In this analysis, presented in Figure 17.3, admissions for infection from 1997–1999 for incident and prevalent pediatric ESRD patients were described according to age, race, gender, and ESRD treatment modality (3). In this analysis, the youngest patients were at highest risk for hospital admission because of infection, and dialysis patients were at greater risk than transplant patients.

Cross-sectional studies have a number of limitations. For example, in the analysis of risk factors for hospitalization for infection in the USRDS, patients studied are those with hospitalization data in the USRDS database. These are patients that have survived ESRD long enough to be counted in the database. If they died early after developing ESRD, they may not be included. In addition, because of varying Medicare eligibility criteria (which influences the data available in this particular database), patients who have gone on to have long-term successful kidney transplants may not be included. Therefore, the characteristics increasing risk for hospitalizations for infection in this study may not be generalized to all pediatric

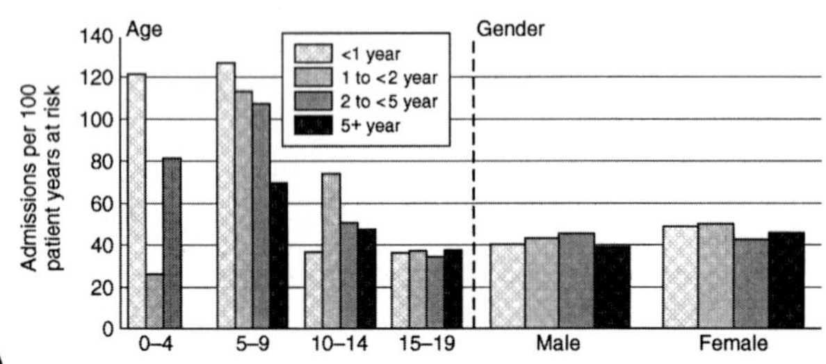

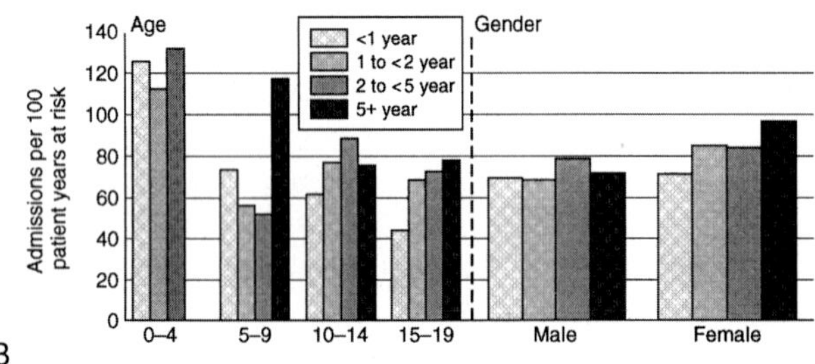

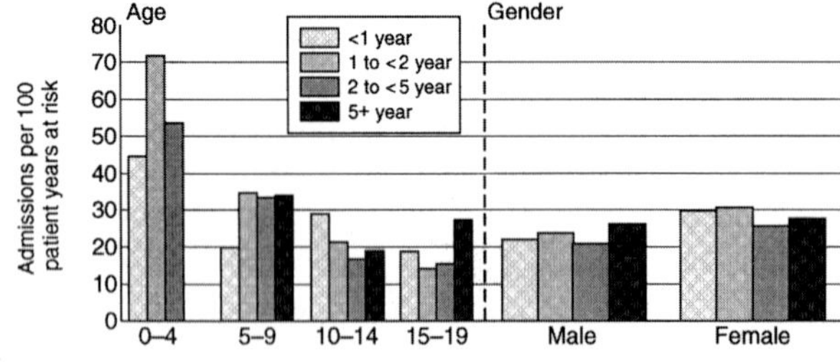

FIGURE 17.3. Cross-sectional study of risk factors for infection in pediatric end-stage renal disease (ESRD). HD, hemodialysis; PD, peritoneal dialysis. (From U.S. Renal Data System. USRDS 2001 Annual Data Report: atlas of end-stage renal disease in the United States. Bethesda, MD: National Institute of Health, National Institute of Diabetes and Digestive and Kidney Diseases, 2001:114, with permission.)

patients with ESRD. Studying prevalent patients runs the risk of missing those patients who were "cured" or who died soon after developing the disease. Also, because in cross-sectional analyses the presence or absence of two factors is assessed at the same time, it is not possible to attribute causality.

Case-Control Studies

Case-control studies are also known as case-referent, compeer, retrospective, case history, and cohort studies. A case-

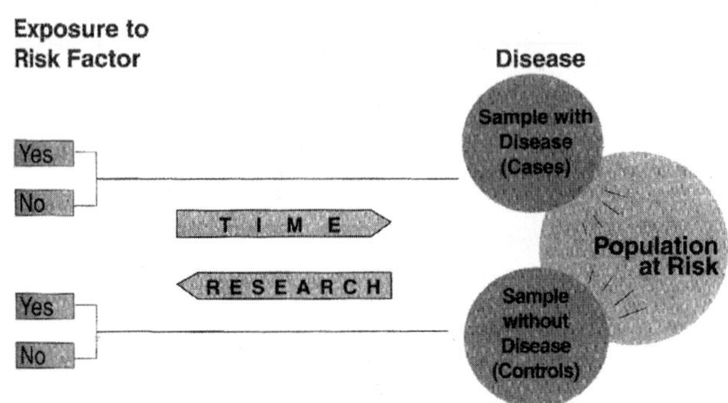

FIGURE 17.4. Design of a case-control study. (From Fletcher RH, Fletcher SW, Wagner EH. *Clinical epidemiology: the essentials*, 3rd ed. Baltimore: Williams & Wilkins, 1996:213, with permission.)

control study starts with the identification of persons with the disease or other outcome variables of interest in the population at risk (Fig. 17.4). A suitable control group of persons without the disease or outcome is also selected from the population at risk. This is pictured on the right side of Figure 17.4. To examine the possible relation of one or more exposures to the given disease or outcome, the researcher then looks back in time to compare the proportions of the cases and controls exposed and not exposed to the risk factor in question.

The case-control design has several advantages. It provides stronger evidence of causation than the cross-sectional design. In a cross-sectional study, outcomes and exposures are assessed simultaneously, and the investigator must infer cause and effect relationships because the temporal sequence cannot be established. In a case-control design, an attempt to establish a temporal relationship between the outcome and exposure is made by starting with a population of persons with and without the outcome and then working backwards to examine suspected exposures. Thus, compared to the cross-sectional design, the investigator is more confident that the exposure of interest came before the outcome, not as a result of the outcome. As compared to other study designs, case-control studies are efficient in the study of rare diseases or those with long latent periods between exposure and outcome. Whereas cross-sectional or cohort designs would require a large number of subjects and time to identify risk factors for a rare disease, a well-designed case-control study can identify similar risk factors with comparatively fewer subjects and much less time and expense. Also adding to the efficiency of the case-control design, several potential risk factors for a disease or outcome can be examined simultaneously.

A recent case-control study by Fored et al. confirmed the association of acetaminophen and aspirin with chronic renal failure (4). Adult Swedish patients with early-stage chronic renal failure were identified as cases (N = 918) from monthly reports of serum creatinine measurements from medical laboratories. Controls were randomly selected throughout the ascertainment period from the Swedish Population Register (N = 980). Aspirin and acetaminophen were used regularly by 37 and 25%, respectively, of the patients with renal failure and by 19 and 12%, respectively, of the controls. Regular use of either drug in the absence of the other was associated with an increase by a factor of 2.5 (odds ratio via logistic regression) in the risk of chronic renal failure from any cause.

Case-control studies yield an odds ratio as an estimate of relative risk. This measure is calculated by dividing the odds that a patient was exposed to a given risk factor by the odds that a control was exposed to the risk factor. It can also be obtained from logistic regression analysis. Logistic regression allows the investigator to obtain the odds ratio for a given risk factor independent of other potential risk factors or confounders using the technique of adjustment. Odds ratios are generally a good approximation of relative risk if the outcome is rare.

As with any study design, the case-control method has limitations. Case-control studies allow for the study of only one disease at a time, as opposed to cross-sectional or cohort studies. This design does not allow for the measurement of incidence, prevalence, or excess risk. Case-control studies are also subject to error, or bias, which can threaten the validity of the study. Selection and information biases, the two major categories of bias, are possible in the case-control design. Selection bias arises if the manner in which cases and controls were selected yields an apparent association when, in reality, exposure and disease are not associated. For example, cases, by definition, include only individuals who have been identified as having the disease and who are available for study. Those who have not been diagnosed, have been misdiagnosed, or have died are excluded. If diagnosis or availability is related to the exposure being studied, the sample of cases will be biased.

Avoiding selection bias can be even more challenging in the selection of controls. The control group must be comparable to the cases. They should not be chosen in such a way that important differences between cases and controls exist that might influence exposure history and thus limit the inferences derived from the study. A number of strategies exist to select a control group that is at risk for the disease and otherwise representative of the same population as the cases. These include sampling cases and controls in the same way (e.g., from the same clinical setting), matching controls to cases on key variables related to the disease (e.g., age), using multiple control groups, and using population-based samples of both cases and controls (e.g., using disease registries).

Information bias occurs when the case and control groups differ in terms of the quality of the data collected to measure risk factors. The retrospective approach to measuring an exposure in the case-control design introduces the possibility of differential recall between the cases and controls. Cases may have been asked more often about the presence of a given exposure and/or may be more circumspect in their recall of such exposures. This introduces *recall bias*, a form of information bias because of better, and sometimes exaggerated, recollection of exposures by cases as compared to controls.

It can be difficult for an investigator to remain objective in collecting exposure information. In interviewing subjects and in reviewing records, there may be a tendency to look more carefully or evaluate evidence differently for cases than for controls. Strategies for dealing with this problem include the use of objective measures and to ensure that the individuals collecting data are unaware of the subject's group status (*blinding/masking*). The more subjective the method for measuring the exposure, the more important it is to mask the observer. Blinding as to the specific exposure being studied or study hypothesis is useful and also can be used to attempt to control recall bias.

Nested case-control studies and nested case-cohort studies are alternative case-based hybrid designs that have many advantages. A nested case-control study involves selecting all cases and control subjects from a known cohort. In this design, the controls are free of the outcome or disease. Nested case-control studies eliminate the problem of recall bias, because the exposure information is obtained before the outcome has developed (cohort design). Also, the temporal sequence between exposure and outcome is defined. This design is also much more economical and efficient; the entire cohort need not be analyzed for a given exposure (e.g., via a laboratory specimen). Nested case-cohort studies also use the selection of cases and controls from a known cohort. However, in this design, controls are randomly selected from the initial cohort irrespective of outcome. This design permits the delineation of *relative risk* for an exposure.

Cohort Design

Various names, including prospective, follow-up, and longitudinal, have been used to label cohort studies in the past, reflecting the temporal sequence of exposure and disease in this category of observational studies (Fig. 17.5). The word *cohort* originated from the Latin word *cohors*, describing a group of warriors that marched together. Clinical investigators have adapted this term to a

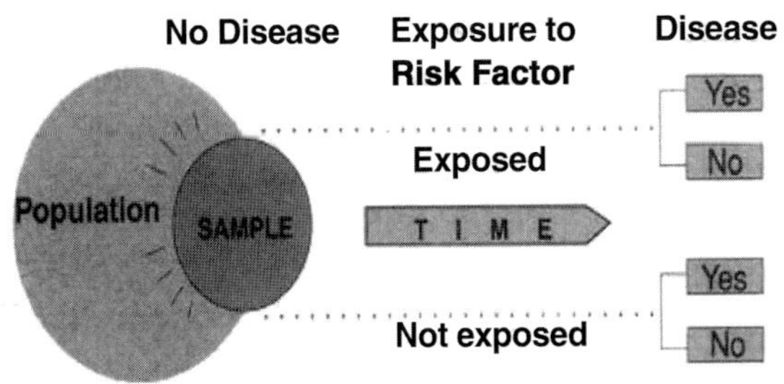

FIGURE 17.5. Design of a cohort study. (From Fletcher RH, Fletcher SW, Wagner EH. *Clinical epidemiology: the essentials*, 3rd ed. Baltimore: Williams & Wilkins, 1996:102, with permission.)

specific type of research study: a group of individuals free of the disease(s) of interest is assembled, their risk status is determined, and the group is followed over time to measure the incidence of disease. Comparison of the incidence of disease (or rate of death from disease) between those with and without the exposure of interest permits measurement of the association between the risk factor and the disease.

The significance of the cohort design has been emphasized by the wealth of scientific data obtained from famous cohorts such as the Framingham Study or the Physicians Health Study. Pediatric nephrology has also benefited from studies using the cohort design. For example, Wong et al. used the cohort design to demonstrate a 17-fold increase in the risk of hemolytic uremic syndrome (HUS) associated with antibiotic use in children with *Escherichia coli* O:157 diarrheal infections (5). In this study, children with *E. coli* O:157 were followed to assess risk factors for the development of HUS.

The cohort design has an obvious niche in clinical research. Ethical and practical considerations often do not allow for randomization of individuals to an exposure of interest. Cohort designs allow for the examination of exposure and disease associations under such circumstances.

Cohort studies can be classified as concurrent or nonconcurrent. In a concurrent cohort study (also referred to as a prospective or longitudinal study), the clinical investigator identifies the population and collects extant exposure information and then follows the cohort to a designated point in the future. Nonconcurrent cohort studies (i.e., retrospective, historical, and nonconcurrent prospective) require the investigator to identify a cohort that has been delineated in the past, along with information regarding the exposure(s) of interest. This population can then be followed for the development of a given disease in the more recent past, the present, or into the future.

Traditionally, the outcome of interest in cohort studies is the ratio of the incidence of disease in those with the exposure divided by the incidence of disease in those without the exposure. This can be interpreted as the *relative risk* for disease in many cases. When calculating and interpreting risks in the cohort design, the absence of randomization must be taken into account. Because the investigator is merely observing the exposure and not controlling for it via randomization, subjects with and without the risk factor might differ in terms of other characteristics that are related to the disease. If the characteristic is related to both the exposure being evaluated and the disease, it can lead to a misleading association between the exposure and the disease. Such a characteristic would be a *confounder*.

To avoid misinterpreting such an association, the investigator must measure potential confounders and adjust for them in the analysis. Multivariable analyses are examples of statistical tools used to adjust for confounders. However, unsuspected confounders might still jeopardize the validity of conclusions.

For example, Wong et al. (5) used a multivariate logistic-regression analysis to account for potential confounders in the association of antibiotic use for *E. coli* O:157–associated diarrhea and HUS. Adjustments were made for the initial white blood cell count and the day of illness on which the initial stool culture was obtained for analysis. These factors had been previously associated with increased risk of HUS. A higher initial white blood cell count could be a potential confounder, for example, because it is associated with an increased risk of HUS (the outcome) and might make the physician more likely to prescribe antibiotics (the exposure), thus potentially falsely linking antibiotic usage with HUS. After adjustment for these factors, the multivariate analysis revealed a persistent association, reassuring the discerning reader.

Cohort studies have several advantages. Because risk factors are measured before disease, the temporal sequence of risk and disease is established, and the potential for biased risk measurement is avoided. Several diseases or outcomes can be measured, and disease occurrence can be measured in terms of incidence, not just prevalence. Cohort studies often require large sample sizes and are unsuitable for studying rare diseases. Large sample size and long follow-up periods can make cohort studies costly. A nonconcurrent cohort design can reduce cost, but it decreases the investigator's control over subject selection and risk factor measurement.

Experimental Design

In an experimental design, the investigator controls the independent variable or intervention and uses randomization to determine which subjects will receive the intervention (the intervention, study, or experimental group) and which subjects will not (the control or placebo group) (Fig. 17.6).

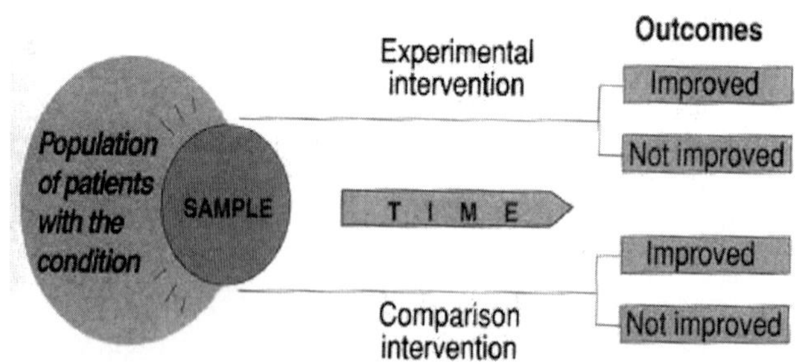

FIGURE 17.6. Design of a randomized trial. (From Fletcher RH, Fletcher SW, Wagner EH. *Clinical epidemiology: the essentials*, 3rd ed. Baltimore: Williams & Wilkins, 1996:139, with permission.)

The North American IgA Nephropathy Study is an example of a randomized controlled clinical trial. In this study, eligible patients younger than 40 years with immunoglobulin A (IgA) nephropathy on kidney biopsy, glomerular filtration rate >50 mL/min/1.73 m^2, and evidence of proteinuria are randomly assigned to receive alternate day prednisone, fish oil, or placebo (6). The goal of this study is to determine the relative benefits of fish oil or alternate day prednisone on the progression of IgA nephropathy. In this and other controlled clinical trials, randomization is the key feature of its experimental nature. Through randomization, all potential confounders, both those recognized by the investigator and those that are not suspected, are likely to be balanced between the study groups. In other words, the three groups in this study are considered to be the same except for the treatment they receive. Differences in rates of progression of kidney disease in the three groups are attributable to the intervention, because the effect of confounders has been ruled out by the balance achieved by randomization. Therefore, experimental designs offer stronger evidence of causality than do observational designs.

In an experimental study, it is important to ensure that subject assignment is truly random. This can be achieved by using random numbers, either through computer-assisted assignment or manually, with a table of random numbers. Sometimes *blocking* is used in conjunction with random assignment. A block of subjects is simply a set number of consecutive study enrollees. Within each block, a predetermined number of subjects is randomly assigned to each study group. For example, if the block size is set at six and two study groups of equal size are desired, then three subjects in each block of six are randomly assigned to one group and three to the other. Blocking is useful when study enrollment is expected to be prolonged. Over extended periods, both study procedures and outside conditions can change. Blocking ensures that the study groups will be balanced with regard to such changes.

Experimental studies, like observational studies, are subject to measurement bias. Research staff should be masked or blinded to the subject's group assignment during data collection, especially if any outcome measures are not strictly objective. In the IgA study, for example, both the research staff and the study subjects are unaware of which treatment they receive. In one arm of the study, placebo capsules are made to look exactly like fish oil capsules. In another arm, placebo tablets are distributed that are identical to prednisone. If outcomes are measured without subject or staff knowledge of the subject's group status, they are less likely to be influenced by expectations about potential differences between treatment and control group outcomes.

Quasi-Experimental Designs

In a quasi-experimental study, the investigator maintains control over the intervention but cannot use randomization to assign subjects to study groups. Such designs are useful in evaluating programs that are targeted to groups of individuals (e.g., a community-based health education program). In this case, the investigator might control the program's design but cannot randomly assign community residents to be exposed to it.

Quasi-experimental designs fall into two broad categories: nonequivalent control group designs and time series designs. In the former, two or more study groups are compared. The investigator tries to assemble groups that are comparable but cannot be assured of their comparability. In time series designs, the investigator measures the outcome of interest at several points in time before and after the intervention. Agreement between hypothesized and observed patterns of outcome measures supports a causal relationship between intervention and outcome. There are many variations on these two broad types of quasi-experimental designs. Some variations incorporate both types. For example, studies of community health programs often involve time series analysis of two or more communities, some with the health program and some without.

In summary, many research designs are available to the investigator. No single design is best for all research questions. Although experimental designs are superior to observational designs in addressing threats to internal validity, they are not always feasible or ethical. The most appropriate design for a given research question is the design that maximizes internal validity within the constraints of the research environment.

IMPORTANT ISSUES IN CARRYING OUT A RESEARCH PLAN

Selection of Subjects

In any research study, one would like to extrapolate the findings to all patients with the condition of interest (Fig. 17.2). The study population is the group that is meant to represent the target population from which a sample is drawn. Sampling decisions involve defining the study population and sample.

Defining the Target Population

Although there is no one single ideal target population, the investigator needs to consider the ramifications of one definition versus another. If the investigator were interested in studying risk factors for a specific disease, the target population could be defined as all children with this disease or a subset of them (e.g., children of a certain age). The broader the target population, the greater the generalizability of the study findings. On the other hand, the increased heterogeneity of a broadly defined target population could introduce variability among subgroups in terms of the importance of risk factors. For example, a particular characteristic could be a major risk factor in some population subgroups but not in others. Assessing the importance of risk factors within subgroups requires a larger study sample and perhaps a more complex sampling design.

Defining the Study Population

A practical consideration in defining the target population is availability of the population for study. The investigator could have all children available seen in a particular clinical setting. Insofar as children seen in this setting are representative of the target population, the clinical site would be a good choice for study; the experience of its enrollees could be considered *generalizable* to the target population. If children enrolled in the clinical setting differ systematically from the target population, *sampling bias* is introduced. For example, tertiary care pediatric nephrology centers might be more likely to serve children with advanced stages of the kidney disease or more severe or complicated cases. Studying only these cases may introduce bias toward only studying the most complex forms of a particular disease. Sampling bias impairs the generalizability of study findings. Representativeness, therefore, is a prime consideration in defining a study population. Investigators should evaluate the representativeness of candidate settings and the likely implications of potential biases. One possible approach to this in studies of patients with kidney disease is to compare the characteristics of participants in a study to known characteristics of the larger population to whom one would like to generalize the results.

Defining the Sampling Scheme

Just as we generalize from the study population to the target population, we generalize from the study sample to the study population. *Sample statistics* are measures that pertain to the samples that are studied. A sample mean, for example, is the sample's average score on a particular measure, and a sample standard deviation expresses the variability of the sample scores. The sample statistics are the investigator's best estimates of the *population parameters.* The sample mean is the best estimate of the population mean; the sample standard deviation is the best estimate of the population standard deviation.

Extending beyond inference to hypothesis testing, sample statistics of the association between variables are the best estimates of these associations in the target population. The association between a hypothesized risk factor and the occurrence of disease in the study sample (perhaps measured by odds ratios or relative risks) is the investigator's best estimate of the association between the risk factor and disease in the target population.

Probability theory is the rationale for extrapolating inferences from a study sample to the reference population. A *probability sample* is one in which every subject, or element, in the study population has a known probability of being selected. A *nonprobability sample* is one in which the probabilities of selection are unknown. It is legitimate to extrapolate from a sample to its population only if probability sampling has been used.

There are several types of probability sampling. In *simple random sampling*, each element has an equal chance of being selected. In *systematic sampling*, each element in the population is assigned a consecutive number, and every *nth* element is sampled. Systematic sampling is easy to use, but it will generate a biased sample if the sampling fraction (e.g., every tenth case) is the same as some periodicity in the ordering of cases in the population. For example, if every tenth patient is sampled in a clinic where ten patients are seen each session and the most complex cases are scheduled first, then the sample will contain either all complex cases or no complex cases, depending on the first element drawn. *Stratified random sampling* is useful when one believes that population subgroups differ in important ways. The population is divided into the subgroups, or *strata*, of interest. Simple or systematic random samples are then drawn from each stratum. *Cluster sampling* is useful when it is difficult or costly to sample elements in a population individually. Instead of elements, groups of elements are sampled. For example, in a study of school children, the investigator could take a probability sample of classrooms and then study all the students within each selected classroom. The selected classrooms, in combination, must be representative of the overall population. As with stratified sampling, formulas for calculating variance must be modified, and consultation with a statistician is recommended.

Nonprobability sampling techniques include *convenience sampling, quota sampling,* and *purposive sampling.* A convenience sample is one that is most readily obtained without the use of random sampling. A quota sample is a convenience sample drawn to assure specified numbers of subjects in specified strata, without the use of random sampling. A purposive

TABLE 17.1. EXAMPLE ILLUSTRATING HOW α, β, AND EFFECT SIZE AFFECT SAMPLE SIZE

Confidence $1-\alpha$ (%)	Power $1-\beta$ (%)	Effect size (%)	Total sample No.
95	80	$10 \rightarrow 40$	76
95	90	$10 \rightarrow 40$	96
95	90	$10 \rightarrow 20$	572
95	99	$10 \rightarrow 40$	156

Adapted from Sample size calculator (Statcalc) in Epi-info Stat Calc. Available at: http://www.cdc.gov/epiinfo/. Accessed April 11, 2003.

sample is one in which subjects are selected because they are judged to be representative of the population of interest.

Probability sampling is preferred but not always possible. In clinical research, the investigator is often limited to a particular clinic population. If a clinic population is believed to be representative and if it is larger than the number of subjects needed for study, the investigator should use a probability sampling technique to draw the study sample.

An example of probability sampling using stratified sampling techniques can be seen in a recent survey study of adult and pediatric nephrologists (7). The authors created a survey containing ten case vignettes to assess whether increased experience with pediatric patients influenced nephrologists' recommendations for peritoneal or hemodialysis in otherwise identical patients with ESRD described in the vignettes. Because the authors wanted the survey respondents to represent the population of U.S. adult and pediatric nephrologists, they randomly selected a representative sample of nephrologists in five geographic regions of the United States. Each randomly selected nephrologist was mailed a survey containing ten case vignettes to assess what factors affected the nephrologists' dialysis recommendations.

Determining Sample Size

In any study, several factors determine the required sample size. This section describes those that come into play in several common types of investigations. Detailed sample-size formulas and tables are beyond the scope of this chapter, but several excellent references are listed in Suggested Reading. Briefly, to estimate sample size, the researcher needs to set the acceptable level of α (probability of type I error), β (probability of type II error), and determine the effect size that one is likely to see. In determining sample size, the probability of making a type I error, α, is usually set at 0.05. This is the probability of concluding that an association between two variables exists when it does not. β error is the probability of concluding that no association exists, when in fact it does. The reader will be more familiar with β error in terms of its relationship to "power." The power of a study is equal to 1-β. In many studies, β is customarily set at 0.2 for a power of 80%. If β is set to 0.1, the power of the study is 90%.

In addition to specifying α and β, the researcher must also determine an estimate of the response to treatment in one of the groups (in a clinical trial) or the rate of occurrence of disease (in a cohort study). The effect size is an estimate of how much better than the comparison group you expect a treatment group to be in a clinical trial or how increased the risk of a particular disease is in the setting of a particular risk factor (in a cohort study). An illustration of estimated sample sizes for given α, β, and effect sizes is shown in Table 17.1 for a study comparing differences in proportions in two groups (8).

Table 17.1 illustrates how varying the acceptable levels of α, β, and effect size influences sample size. For example, if we designed a study to determine whether a new drug could "cure" 40% of patients compared to an old drug that "cured" 10% of patients, we would have 90% power to see such an effect with 95% confidence in a total sample of 96 patients (see row 2 in Table 17.1). In contrast, to obtain a significant result documenting a smaller effect size from the old drug cure rate of 10% to a new drug cure rate of 20% with the same α = 0.05 and 90% power, we would need to study 572 patients.

Attrition of Study Subjects

Sample size calculations determine the number of subjects needed at the study's conclusion. In determining the number of subjects to enroll, the investigator must estimate attrition rates and enroll a sufficiently large sample to compensate for study dropout.

Even if probability sampling is used to define the study, subject attrition could produce a biased sample at the study's conclusion. An attrition rate of more than 25% is cause for concern. In data analysis, subjects completing the study should be compared with those who drop out to determine whether the two groups differ in a clinically significant way. Such differences must be considered in interpreting the study findings.

DATA COLLECTION: MEASUREMENT

Decisions on what data to collect and how to do so begin with specifying the variables that need to be measured and operationally defining each. The investigator will need to evaluate the suitability of existing measures and determine whether to use an existing measure or develop a new one. The data sources for each variable must also be identified. Finally, the investigator should specify the level of measurement of each variable. An efficient way to document the data collection plan is to make a table with columns listing the variables to be measured, their operational definitions, the data source(s) for each variable, and level of measurement for each. This section describes issues pertaining to each of these tasks.

Identifying the Variables to Be Measured

Researchers are often tempted to collect as much information as possible. This can be costly, in terms of time, money, and data quality. The investigator should be able to justify each variable to be measured. Most important are the hypothesized independent and dependent variables. In addition, identified potential confounders should be measured. Finally, data characterizing the study population and sample will be needed to describe the study's generalizability.

Sources of Data

Study data can be collected from existing sources or can be generated specifically for the specific research hypothesis being tested, using surveys, interviews, or observations. Most studies combine both strategies.

An enormous variety of existing data sources is available, including medical records, vital records, national and local health surveys, and census data. Health programs often keep records of services provided, and billing records can be especially helpful. Examples of existing data sources in pediatric kidney disease include the USRDS (3) and data collected by the North American Pediatric Renal Transplant Case Study (NAPRTCS) (9). Existing sources can provide data for time periods and individuals otherwise unavailable to the investigator. The number of studies published by the NAPRTCS and their tremendous contribution to our understanding of clinical outcomes in pediatric kidney transplantation and dialysis illustrate this point. The chief disadvantage of existing sources gleaned from registry data is that the data are often not collected as systematically as in a prospective research study. Important data elements are sometimes missing. Incomplete data and inaccuracies are also possible with registry data.

Primary data collection is expensive and is limited to subjects available to the investigator. On the other hand, the investigator's control over data collection makes data quality more certain. Many primary data collection strategies are available, including mail surveys, mass-administered questionnaires, telephone and in-person structured and unstructured interviews, direct observation, and videotaping and audiotaping. Choosing a strategy should be based on the research question, the sensitivity of the data to be collected, the literacy of the population to be studied, and the resources available for the study. The key factor should be data quality—that is, which method will provide the most complete and accurate information within budgetary constraints.

Assessing Data Quality

One strategy to enhance data quality is to train research staff thoroughly. Often, data-collection staff work independently. To ensure that they follow study procedures, the protocol for data collection should be detailed in a study manual. Training sessions should be held to explain the study's aim to staff, as well as how each one's role fits into the big picture. Staff should be given ample time to practice their data-collection skills. Once the fieldwork of the main study begins, staff should be encouraged to bring problems to the attention of supervisory staff. Such problems should be resolved in a timely fashion, and the resolution should be documented and added to the study manual. In this way, research staff are kept apprised of changes in the study protocol and are impressed with the importance of adhering to it.

After the instrument pretesting and staff training, the investigator should pilot test the data-collection activities. A pilot test is a dress rehearsal of the activities for selecting study subjects, contacting them, securing informed consent, and collecting and processing data. Activities that do not work as planned should be modified and the pilot testing continued until the fieldwork procedures run smoothly.

Data quality should be monitored during the main study. Interviews and questionnaires should be reviewed as they are completed to allow recontacting subjects to correct errors. The reliability of subjective measures and those requiring special technical skill should be assessed. For studies with unsupervised interviewing of subjects, it is wise to validate a portion of the completed interviews handed in by fieldworkers. This can be done by recontacting a random sample of subjects and then asking them to verify their responses to a sub-sample of the interview questions.

ANALYTIC PLAN

Data Analysis

Investigators often defer considering data analysis until the data have been collected. This is a serious mistake. Study planning should include an analytic plan of the steps needed to answer the study questions once the fieldwork is completed.

Use of Statistical Tests

As noted earlier, statistical validity is the correctness of study conclusions regarding group differences and variable relationships. A key threat to statistical validity is the use of inappropriate statistical tests. *Parametric statistical tests* are based on assumptions about parameters of the population and are the most powerful tests available in situations in which these assumptions are met. *Nonparametric statistical tests* are based on fewer assumptions about the population, so they are appropriate in situations in which the assumptions underlying parametric statistics are not met.

Assumptions vary by statistical test. If a test is used in a situation that violates its assumptions, it will be inaccurate, leading to a misleading measure of statistical significance. This, in turn, will lead to an incorrect estimate of the likelihood of a type I error.

In developing the analytic plan, the investigator should consider the assumptions of candidate tests in determining which ones to use. A discussion of specific statistical tests is beyond the scope of this chapter, but a framework for deciding which tests to use can be given. In this framework, three factors determine the type of test to use: the major analytic question to be answered, the levels of measurement used, and the number and independence of comparison groups.

In preparing the analytic plan, the investigator needs to translate the research question into analytic terms. Three major analytic approaches are to describe characteristics of the sampled population, to compare groups of subjects,

TABLE 17.2. BIVARIATE STATISTICAL TESTS

	Two groups		Three or more groups	
Level of measurement	Independent (unpaired groups)	Paired groups	Independent (unmatched groups)	Matched groups
Nominal dichotomy	Chi-square or Fisher's exact test	McNemar's test	Chi-square	Cochran's test
More than two categories	Chi-square	McNemar's test	Chi-square	Cochran's test
Ordinal	Mann-Whitney test	Sign test	Kruskal-Wallis one-way analysis of variance (ANOVA)	Friedman two-way ANOVA
		Wilcoxon matched-pairs signed-ranks test		
Interval	*t* Test for groups	*t* Test for pairs	One-way ANOVA	ANOVA for repeated measures

and to measure associations among variables. In addition, the appropriate analytic test is determined by the level of measurement of the variables of interest. Measurements can be normal, ordinal, or interval.

Where group comparisons are to be made, the appropriate statistical test is also determined by the number of groups to be compared (two vs. three or more) and by whether comparison groups are independent or matched. Thus, in a study of cases matched with sibling controls, it would be inappropriate to use a statistical test for independent groups.

As decisions about level of measurement and the selection of study groups are part of study planning, it is easy to see how these decisions are better informed if their ramifications for data analysis are considered. Level of measurement, study group formation, and data analysis are all interrelated, and all should be considered part of study planning.

When the study's purpose is to describe a population, the investigator makes inferences from sample statistics to population parameters. Sample proportions and measures of central tendency (mean, median, and mode) and dispersion (standard deviation, range) are used to estimate these parameters in the population. Confidence intervals can be constructed around proportions and means to express the certainty of the sample-based population estimates. When the study's objective is to compare two or more groups, sample group differences in proportions and means are used to estimate such differences in the population. Statistical tests of significance can be used to assess the certainty of sample-based inferences about group differences in the population. The appropriate statistical test depends on the number of groups compared, whether subjects in the groups are matched, and the level of measurement of the variable on which the groups are being compared. Table 17.2 displays bivariate statistical tests commonly used in assessing the significance of group differences.

When the research aim is to measure the association between variables, sample statistics again are used to estimate population parameters. The variables' levels of measurement determine the appropriate statistical measure of the strength of their association, the appropriate test of the statistical significance of the association, and the certainty of estimates of its strength. For dichotomous variables, the odds ratio and relative risk are measures of the degree of association. For continuous data, Pearson's correlation coefficient is used to measure association.

Studies of the combined and relative impacts of multiple independent variables, or the effect of an independent variable after controlling for other factors, will require multivariable analytic tests. The appropriateness of a multivariable technique is determined by the levels of measurement of the independent and dependent variables. The references cited at the end of this chapter describe the applicability and interpretation of the most commonly used multivariable statistical tests.

Statistical Significance and Confidence Intervals

Most readers of the medical literature will be familiar with the term *statistical significance*, which is most often referred to in clinical reports as a "p value <.05." This highly sought after result of a statistical test refers to the probability of α, or a type I error. A p value of .05 in a study means that there is a 5% chance that the results seen in the study could have occurred by chance. However, the authors have concluded that this probability is low enough for them to accept the alternative hypothesis (that there is a real difference between groups) and to reject the null hypothesis (there is no difference between groups). It is important to note that the p value in a study result depends on the size of the observed difference between the groups in question and the size of the sample of patients studied. Standing alone, the p value does not convey any sense of the magnitude of the treatment effect seen in the study or the precision of the estimate of the size of the treatment effect. Confidence intervals, in contrast to p values, can convey this information in a more meaningful way.

For any estimated value, it is useful to have an idea of the uncertainty of the estimate in relation to the true value it is trying to approximate. For example, if we designed a study to estimate the beneficial effect of a new lipid-lowering medication in chronic renal failure in adolescents, we would try to recruit a large representative sample of hyperlipidemic adolescents and randomize them to treatment with a new lipid-lowering medication. From our study, we might want to estimate the magnitude of lipid level reduction associated with the new medicine. We might also want to use this estimate as an approximation for the "true" reduction in lipid levels that would be seen in the "universe" of pediatric patients with hyperlipidemia and chronic renal failure. To estimate the "true" reduction in lipid levels (which can never be directly measured), we can generate a confidence interval around our estimate.

In any study, construction of a *confidence interval* around the point estimate gives us a range of values in which we can be confident that the true value resides. A confidence interval gives a sense of the estimate's precision; it extends evenly on either side of the estimate by a multiple of the standard error (SE) of the estimate. In our example, our study might yield an estimate of the drop in serum low-density lipoprotein cholesterol levels of the treatment group of 30% with a standard deviation of that estimate of 20%. One could then use this estimate to generate a confidence interval around this estimate. In the medical literature, one will most often see references to 95% confidence intervals. The general equation for a 95% confidence interval is equal to the estimate ±1.96 times the SE of the estimate. The factor 1.96 comes from the standard normal distribution, in which 95% of estimates would fall within ±1.96 SEs of the mean. If one wanted to increase the probability of including the true estimate in the confidence interval, one could generate a 99% confidence interval, which would equal the estimate ±2.56 times the SE of the estimate. Because the SE of an estimate is equal to the standard deviation of the population divided by the square root of the sample size, N, one can see that a larger sample size is needed in a study to generate a precise estimate of a treatment's effect. Given the same standard deviation, the SE in our study would be smaller if we studied 100 children compared to 20 children. The larger study would generate a narrower 95% confidence interval. The strict interpretation of a 95% confidence interval is that this is the range of values for the true population estimate that is consistent with the data observed in the study. In our hypothetical example, the smaller study might give us the opportunity to conclude that the new lipid lowering is associated with a 30% reduction in low-density lipoprotein cholesterol with a relatively broad 95% confidence interval of 21 to 39%, whereas the larger study yields a more precise estimate. The 95% confidence interval around the same point estimate of a 30% reduction is 26 to 34% in the study with the larger sample size.

EVALUATING THE LITERATURE: RATING THE STRENGTH OF SCIENTIFIC EVIDENCE

Health care decisions should be based on research-based evidence. Whether the individual nephrologist is making a clinical decision or a national organization is developing clinical practice guidelines, efforts should be made to systematically assess the strengths of scientific evidence related to a particular clinical diagnostic or treatment plan. Guidelines first developed more than 20 years ago at the Department of Clinical Epidemiology and Biostatistics at McMaster University first introduced tools to allow clinicians to critically review original articles on etiology, diagnosis, prognosis, and therapy (10). In the following decade, the series was widely read and cited, was modified for use by the general public, and was published in clinical epidemiology texts (11). At the same time, clinicians at McMaster University and across North America continued to expand and improve the guidelines. Their focus has expanded to include clinicians' ability to access, summarize, and apply information from the literature to everyday clinical problems, transforming the Readers' Guides to Users' Guides (12–35).

Such systematic approaches have also been adapted to assess entire bodies of research on particular subjects. In 1999, the U.S. Congress directed the Agency for Health Care Policy Research and Quality to identify methods to assess health care research results. The results of that effort were published in a report entitled "Systems to rate the strength of scientific evidence" (36). Key features of this report and the users' guides are summarized in Randomized Controlled Trials.

Randomized Controlled Trials

If a clinician or researcher is interested in evaluating the evidence that a cause-effect relationship exists between a treatment and a result, a randomized experiment is the design of choice. In evaluating the quality of the randomized clinical trial, one must assess whether a number of important elements are addressed in the clinical trial. These are outlined in Table 17.3. The study population should be clearly defined. Randomization should have resulted in study groups that are balanced at the start of the study in terms of potential confounders. The reader should be wary of two threats to this balance. The first is differential group attrition during the course of the study, resulting in groups that are no longer balanced with respect to confounders by the study's end. To guard against this, the investigator should provide evidence of low attrition rates or should analyze treatment effectiveness on the basis of "intent to treat," including in the analysis of all study subjects both those who completed the study and those dropping out. An intent-to-treat analysis maintains individuals and their outcomes in the treatment group to which they were assigned. This maintains the balance achieved by randomization and is the most conservative analysis plan. The second threat to validity is biased outcome measurement. The reader should look for evidence that outcome measurement was objective and not biased by observer knowledge of subject group status. Finally, in determining treatment impact, the investigator should provide evidence that both statistical and clinical

TABLE 17.3. IMPORTANT DOMAINS AND ELEMENTS FOR ASSESSING STRENGTH OF EVIDENCE IN RANDOMIZED CONTROLLED TRIALS

Domain	Element
Study question	Clearly focused and appropriate question
Study population	Description of study population Specific inclusion and exclusion criteria Sample size justification
Randomization	Adequate approach to sequence generation Adequate concealment method used Similarity of groups at baseline
Blinding	Double-blinding (e.g., of investigators, caregivers, subjects, assessors, and other key study personnel as appropriate) to treatment allocation
Interventions	Intervention(s) clearly detailed for all study groups (e.g., dose, route, and timing for drugs and details sufficient for assessment and reproducibility for other types of interventions) Compliance with intervention Equal treatment of groups except for intervention
Outcomes	Primary and secondary outcome measures specified Assessment method standard, valid, and reliable
Statistical analysis	Appropriate analytic techniques that address study withdrawals, loss to follow-up, missing data, and intention to treat Power calculation Assessment of confounding Assessment of heterogeneity, if applicable
Results	Measure of effect for outcomes and appropriate measure of precision Proportion of eligible subjects recruited into study and followed up at each assessment
Discussion	Conclusions supported by results with possible biases and limitations taken into consideration
Funding or sponsorship	Type and sources of support for study

From Agency for Healthcare Research and Quality. Systems to rate the strength of scientific evidence. AHRQ Publication No. 02-E016, April 2002. Rockville, MD: Agency for Healthcare Research and Quality. Available at: http://www.ahrq.gov/clinic/strevinv.htm. Accessed May 2003, with permission.

relevance were considered in establishing sample size and in drawing conclusions.

Observational Studies

In a study of disease etiology, a randomized experiment is seldom possible. When a randomized trial is not feasible, the reader should determine whether the investigator has used the strongest alternative observational design possible. Important domains and elements to assess for the quality of observational

TABLE 17.4. IMPORTANT DOMAINS AND ELEMENTS FOR ASSESSING STRENGTH OF EVIDENCE IN OBSERVATIONAL STUDIES

Domain	Element
Study question	Clearly focused and appropriate question
Study population	Description of study populations Sample size justification For all observational studies Specific inclusion/exclusion criteria for all groups Criteria applied equally to all groups Comparability of groups at baseline with regard to disease status and prognostic factors Study groups comparable to nonparticipants with regard to confounding factors Use of concurrent controls Comparability of follow-up among groups at each assessment Additional criteria for case-control studies Explicit case definition Case ascertainment not influenced by exposure status Controls similar to cases except without condition of interest and with equal opportunity for exposure
Exposure or intervention	Clear definition of exposure Measurement method standard valid and reliable Exposure measured equally in all study groups
Outcome measurement	Primary/secondary outcomes clearly defined Outcomes assess blind exposure or intervention status Method of outcome assessment standard valid and reliable Length of follow-up adequate for question
Statistical analysis	Statistical tests appropriate Multiple comparisons taken into consideration Modeling and multivariate techniques appropriate Power calculation provided Assessment of confounding Dose-response assessment, if appropriate
Results	Measure of effect for outcomes and appropriate measure of precision Adequacy of follow-up for each study group
Discussion	Conclusions supported by results with biases and limitations taken into consideration
Funding or sponsorship	Type and sources of support for study

From Agency for Healthcare Research and Quality. Systems to rate the strength of scientific evidence. AHRQ Publication No. 02-E016, April 2002. Rockville, MD: Agency for Healthcare Research and Quality. Available at: http://www.ahrq.gov/clinic/strevinv.htm. Accessed May 2003, with permission.

studies are outlined in Table 17.4. The reader should look for additional evidence of a causal relationship as well, such as the consistency of findings across studies, confirmation that the cause preceded the effect temporally, and the presence of a dose-response effect. As with an experimental study, measurements of cause and outcome should be objective and unbiased, and both clinical and statistical relevance should be considered in the analysis. Finally, because available designs do not achieve balance between study groups with respect to confounders, it is important that the investigators identify and control for potential confounders in the analysis.

In evaluating an observational study of the prognosis of disease, the reader should focus on subject selection, measurement, and analysis. The primary purpose of this type of study is to describe the clinical course of patients with a particular disease. As in studies of etiology, the investigator might also seek to identify factors influencing outcome. It is essential that those studied be representative of such patients, including both those who will eventually recover and those who will die. The reader's first task, therefore, is to seek evidence that the study sample was selected early in their disease. The next task is to determine the adequacy of subject follow-up. As the number of subjects lost to follow-up increases, the representativeness of the sample becomes suspect. Assuming a representative sample and adequate follow-up, the reader should then determine whether patient outcomes were measured reliably in ways that can be related to the reader's own practice. Finally, the reader should determine whether the investigator controlled for potential confounders in assessing the role of prognostic factors. As in studies of etiology, it is impossible to randomly assign patients to groups with and without a prognostic factor. Therefore, it is essential that potential confounders be controlled for in the analysis.

TABLE 17.5. IMPORTANT DOMAINS AND ELEMENTS FOR ASSESSING STRENGTH OF EVIDENCE IN DIAGNOSTIC STUDIES

Domain	Element
Study population	Subjects similar to populations in which the test would be used and with a similar spectrum of disease
Adequate description of test	Details of test and its administration sufficient to allow for replication of study
Appropriate reference standard	Appropriate reference standard ("gold standard") used for comparison
	Reference standard reproducible
Blinded comparison of test and reference	Evaluation of test without knowledge of disease status, if possible
	Independent, blind interpretation of test and reference
Avoidance of verification bias	Decision to perform reference standard not dependent on results of test under study

From Agency for Healthcare Research and Quality. Systems to rate the strength of scientific evidence. AHRQ Publication No. 02-E016, April 2002. Rockville, MD: Agency for Healthcare Research and Quality. Available at: http://www.ahrq.gov/clinic/strevinv.htm. Accessed May 2003, with permission.

Studies Evaluating Diagnostic Tests

In reviewing a study evaluating a diagnostic test, the reader's chief concerns are subject selection and measurement (Table 17.5). The study sample should be representative of the population of interest in terms of spectrum of disease. Regarding measurement, it is essential that the can-

TABLE 17.6. IMPORTANT DOMAINS AND ELEMENTS FOR ASSESSING STRENGTH OF EVIDENCE IN SYSTEMATIC REVIEWS

Domain	Element
Study questions	Question clearly specified and appropriate
Search strategy	Sufficiently comprehensive and rigorous with attention to possible publication biases
	Search restrictions justified (e.g., language or county of origin)
	Documentation of search terms and databases used
	Sufficiently detailed to reproduce study
Inclusion and exclusion criteria	Selection methods specified and appropriate, with a priori criteria specified if possible
Interventions	Intervention(s) clearly detailed for all study groups
Outcomes	All potentially important harms and benefits considered
Data extraction	Rigor and consistency of process
	Number and types of reviewers
	Blinding of reviewers
	Measure of agreement of reproducibility
	Extraction of clearly defined interventions/exposures and outcomes for all relevant subjects and subgroups
Study quality and validity	Assessment method specified and appropriate
	Method of incorporation specified and appropriate
Data synthesis and analysis	Appropriate use of qualitative and/or quantitative synthesis, with consideration of the robustness of results and heterogeneity issues
Results	Narrative summary and/or quantitative summary statistic and measure of precision, as appropriate
Discussion	Conclusion supported by results with possible biases and limitations taken into consideration
Funding or sponsorship	Types and sources of support for study

From Agency for Healthcare Research and Quality. Systems to rate the strength of scientific evidence. AHRQ Publication No. 02-E016, April 2002. Rockville, MD: Agency for Healthcare Research and Quality. Available at: http://www.ahrq.gov/clinic/strevinv.htm. Accessed May 2003, with permission.

didate test be compared with a "gold standard," that the comparison is unbiased, and that the reliability of the test is established. From a practical standpoint, it is important that the diagnostic test procedures, as evaluated in the research, can be used in clinical practice.

Systematic Reviews

As opposed to a traditional invited review, a systematic review is an organized method of locating, assembling, and evaluating a body of literature on a particular topic using a set of specific predefined criteria. If the systematic review includes a quantitative pooling of data, then it is referred to as a metaanalysis. As systematic reviews have been more frequently used in recent years as part of the development of practice guidelines, criteria for evaluating the quality of systematic reviews have also been developed (Table 17.6). An example of a systematic review in pediatric nephrology is the evidence-based assessment of treatment options for children with IgA nephropathy by Hogg and Wyatt (37).

In summary, the busy clinician can afford to be selective in reviewing the literature. In rating the strength of scientific evidence in evaluating a specific clinical problem or treatment, one needs to be selective. The simplest criteria for choosing which studies to read in detail or which to weigh heavily in evidence are clinical relevance and methodologic soundness. This chapter has introduced a simple framework for evaluating such features in the context of sound clinical research methodology and has outlined the most recent guidelines for assessing the strength of scientific evidence for making decisions in clinical care. These tools for systematic assessment of existing research can also guide the clinical investigator toward areas that require further study in which current evidence for treatment or outcomes is scant.

SUGGESTED READING

DeAngelis C. *Introduction to clinical research.* New York: Oxford University Press, 1990.

Hulley SB, Cummings SR. *Designing clinical research,* 2nd ed. Philadelphia: Lippincott Williams & Wilkins, 2001.

Clinical Epidemiology

Gordis L. *Epidemiology,* 2nd ed. Philadelphia: Saunders, 2000.

Fletcher RH, Fletcher SW, Wagner EH. *Clinical epidemiology: the essentials,* 3rd ed. Baltimore: Williams & Wilkins, 1996.

Lilienfeld AM, Lilienfeld DE. *Foundations of epidemiology,* 2nd ed. New York: Oxford University Press, 1980.

Sackett DL, Haynes RB, Guyatt GH, et al. *Clinical epidemiology: a basic science for clinical medicine,* 2nd ed. Boston: Little, Brown, 1991.

Study Design

Cook TD, Campbell DT. *Quasi-experimentation: design and analysis issues for field settings.* Boston: Houghton-Mifflin, 1979.

Meinert CL. *Clinical trials: design, conduct and analysis.* New York: Oxford University Press, 1986.

Schiesselman JJ. *Case-control studies: design, conduct, analysis.* New York: Oxford University Press, 1982.

General Statistic References

Dawson-Saunders B, Trapp RG. *Basic and clinical biostatistics,* 3rd ed. New York: Lange Medical Books–McGraw-Hill, 2001.

Fleiss JL. *Statistical methods for rates and proportions.* New York: John Wiley & Sons, 1981.

Glaser AN. *High yield biostatistics.* Pennsylvania: Williams & Wilkins, 2001.

Hollander M, Wolfe DA. *Nonparametric statistical methods,* 2nd ed. New York: John Wiley & Sons, 1999.

Kleinbaum DG, Kupper LL. *Applied regression analysis and other multivariate methods,* 3rd ed. Pacific Grove: Duxbury Press, 1998.

Tabachnick BG, Fidell LS. *Using multivariate statistics.* 4th ed. Boston: Allyn and Bacon, 2001.

Zar JH. *Biostatistical analysis,* 4th ed. Upper Saddle River, NJ: Prentice-Hall, 1999.

REFERENCES

1. Cook TD, Campbell DT. *Quasi-experimentation: design and analysis issues for field settings.* Boston: Houghton Mifflin, 1979.
2. Furth SL, Neu AM, Colombani P, et al. Diabetes as a complication of FK506 in pediatric renal transplant patients. *Pediatr Nephrol* 1996;10:64–66.
3. U.S. Renal Data System. USRDS 2001 Annual Data Report: atlas of end-stage renal disease in the United States. Bethesda, MD: National Institutes of Diabetes and Digestive and Kidney Disease, 2001.
4. Fored CM, Ejerblad E, Lindblad P, et al. Acetaminophen, aspirin, and chronic renal failure. *N Engl J Med* 2001;345:1801–1808.
5. Wong CS, Jelacic S, Habeeb RL, et al. The risk of the hemolytic-uremic syndrome after antibiotic treatment of *Escherichia coli* 0157:H7 infections. *N Engl J Med* 2000; 342:1930–1936.
6. Hogg RJ for the SPNSG. A randomized, placebo-controlled, multicenter trial evaluating a) alternate day prednisone; b) fish oil supplements in young patients with IgA nephropathy. *Am J Kidney Dis* 1995;26:792–796.
7. Furth SL, Hwang W, Yang C, et al. Relation between pediatric experience and treatment recommendations for children and adolescents with kidney failure. *JAMA* 2001;258:1027–1033.
8. What is Epi info? Available at: http://www.cdc.gov.epiinfo/. Accessed July 8, 2002.
9. North American Pediatric Renal Transplant Cooperative Study. NAPRTCS 2001 annual report. Available at: http://spitfire.emmes.com/study/ped/annlrept/. Accessed July 8, 2002.
10. Department of Clinical Epidemiology and Biostatistics. McMaster University. How to read clinical journals. I. Why to read them and how to start reading them critically. *Can Med Assoc J* 1981;124:555–558.
11. Sackett DL, Haynes RB, Guyatt GH, et al. *Clinical epidemiology: a basic science for clinical medicine,* 2nd ed. Boston: Little, Brown, 1991.

12. Guyatt GH, Rennie D. Users' guides to the medical literature (editorial). *JAMA* 1993;270:2096–2097.
13. Oxman AD, Sackett DL, Guyatt GH. Users' guide to the medical literature: I. How to get started. *JAMA* 1993;270: 2093–2095.
14. Guyatt GH, Sackett DL, Cook DJ. Users' guides to the medical literature: II. How to use an article about therapy or prevention A. Are the results of the study valid? *JAMA* 1993;270:2598–2601.
15. Guyatt GH, Sackett DL, Cook DJ. Users' guides to the medical literature: II. How to use an article about therapy or prevention B. What were the results and will they help me in caring for my patients? *JAMA* 1994;271:59–63.
16. Jaeschke R, Guyatt G, Sackett DL. Users' guide to the medical literature: III. How to use an article about a diagnostic test A. Are the results of the study valid? *JAMA* 1994;271:389–391.
17. Jaeschke R, Guyatt G, Sackett DL. Users' guide to the medical literature: III. How to use an article about a diagnostic test B. What are the results and will they help me in caring for my patients? *JAMA* 1994;271:703–707.
18. Levine M, Walter S, Lee H, et al. Users' guide to the medical literature: IV. How to use an article about harm. *JAMA* 1994;271:1615–1619.
19. Laupacis A, Wells G, Richardson WS, et al. Users' guide to the medical literature: V. How to use an article about prognosis. *JAMA* 1994;272:234–237.
20. Oxman AD, Cook DJ, Guyatt GH. Users' guide to the medical literature: VI. How to use an overview. *JAMA* 1994;272:1367–1371.
21. Richardson WS, Detsky AS. Users' guide to the medical literature: VII. How to use a clinical decision analysis. A. Are the results valid? *JAMA* 1995;273:1292–1295.
22. Richardson WS, Detsky AS. Users' guide to the medical literature: VII. How to use a clinical decision analysis. B. What are the results and how will they help me in caring for my patients? *JAMA* 1995;273:1610–1613.
23. Hayward RSA, Wilson MC, Tunis SR, et al. Users' guide to the medical literature: VIII. How to use clinical practice guidelines. A. Are the guidelines valid? *JAMA* 1995;274:570–574.
24. Hayward RSA, Wilson MC, Tunis SR, et al. Users' guide to the medical literature: VIII. How to use clinical practice guidelines. B. What are the recommendations and how will they help you in caring for your patients? *JAMA* 1995;274:1630–1632.
25. Guyatt GH, Sackett DL, Sinclair JC, et al. Users' guide to the medical literature: IX. A method for grading health care recommendations. *JAMA* 1995;274:1800–1804.
26. Naylor CD, Guyatt GH. Users' guide to the medical literature: X. How to use an article reporting variations in the outcomes of health services. *JAMA* 1996;275:554–558.
27. Dans AL, Dans LF, Guyatt GH, et al. Users' guides to the medical literature: XIV. How to decide on the applicability of clinical trial results to your patient. Evidence-Based Medicine Working Group. *JAMA* 1998;279(7):545–549.
28. Richardson WS, Wilson MC, Guyatt GH, et al. Users' guides to the medical literature: XV. How to use an article about disease probability for differential diagnosis. Evidence-Based Medicine Working Group. *JAMA* 1999;281(13):1214–1219.
29. Berlin JA, Rennie D. Measuring the quality of trials: the quality of quality scales. *JAMA* 1999;282(11):1083–1085.
30. McGinn TG, Guyatt GH, Wyer PC, et al. Users' guides to the medical literature: XXII: how to use articles about clinical decision rules. Evidence-Based Medicine Working Group. *JAMA* 2000;284(1):79–84.
31. Giacomini MK, Cook DJ. Users' guides to the medical literature: XXIII. Qualitative research in health care B. What are the results and how do they help me care for my patients? Evidence-Based Medicine Working Group. *JAMA* 2000;284(4):478–482
32. Richardson WS, Wilson MC, Williams JW Jr, et al. Users' guides to the medical literature: XXIV. How to use an article on the clinical manifestations of disease. Evidence-Based Medicine Working Group. *JAMA* 2000;284(7):869–875.
33. Shah NR. What is the best evidence for making clinical decisions? *JAMA* 2000;284(24):3127–3128.
34. Altman DG. Poor-quality medical research: what can journals do? *JAMA* 2002;287(21):2765–2767.
35. Guyatt. *Users' guides to the medical literature: essentials of evidence-based clinical practice*. Chicago: AMA Press, 2002.
36. Agency for Healthcare Research and Quality. Systems to rate the strength of scientific evidence. AHRQ Publication No. 02-E016, April 2002. Rockville, MD: Agency for Healthcare Research and Quality. Available at: http://www.ahrq.gov/clinic/strevinv.htm. Accessed May 2003.
37. Hogg RJ, Wyatt RJ. Evidence-based assessment of treatment options for children with IgA nephropathies. *Pediatr Nephrol* 2001:16:156–167.

18

GENETICS

LISA M. GUAY-WOODFORD

The principles of classic genetics were established by Gregor Mendel in 1865. Based on controlled breeding experiments with the garden pea, Mendel determined that physical characteristics (phenotypes) were transmitted by "hereditary units" from one generation to the next in a predictable fashion. These hereditary units (genes) exist in alternate forms (alleles) that determine the expression of a particular phenotype. Mendel's first law of heredity describes the segregation of alleles: *Alleles have no permanent effect on one another when present in the same organism, but they segregate unchanged by passing into different gametes.* An organism is homozygous if both alleles of a given gene are identical, and it is heterozygous if the alleles are different. Alleles typically have dominance properties. For example, one dominant allele determines the phenotype regardless of the dominance characteristics of the other allele. The recessive phenotype only appears when the organism is homozygous for the recessive allele. Mendel also determined that alleles of one gene and alleles of another gene are transmitted independently to gametes; thus he formulated his second law of heredity: *The assortment (transmission) of one gene does not influence the assortment of another* (1).

Mendel's laws were first applied to human disease by Sir Archibald Garrod in 1909. Based on his clinical observations, Garrod reasoned that alkaptonuria, albinism, cystinuria, and pentosuria were transmitted as mendelian recessive traits. With alkaptonuria, he postulated that an essential enzyme was defective, a so-called inborn error of metabolism (2). The one gene–one enzyme concept later postulated by George Beadle and Edward Tatum had immediate implications for the inborn errors of metabolism described by Garrod. Indeed, shortly thereafter, the era of biochemical genetics began with the identification of specific enzyme defects as the genetic basis of recessive methemoglobinemia, von Gierke disease, and phenylketonuria (2). Subsequent studies in the 1940s and early 1950s determined that the genetic information in each cell is encoded in double-stranded DNA molecules. These findings set the stage for the modern era of molecular genetics.

PATTERNS OF INHERITANCE

Pedigree Analysis

The family history is a critical tool for assessing inherited disorders and determining inheritance patterns. The key issues to investigate are (a) whether anyone in the family has had a condition similar to the patient and, if so, whether this condition "runs in the family"; and (b) whether the family has suffered fetal losses late in gestation or whether there have been unexplained infant deaths. In the case of rare disorders, the possibility of consanguinity should be explored by inquiring whether the parents are related, whether their grandparents or great-grandparents may have intermarried, or whether the parental families originate from the same village or small community.

With the details obtained from a careful family history, the disease distribution within the family or kindred can be evaluated. The pattern of inheritance is documented by constructing a pedigree (Fig. 18.1) in which the first identified patient is designated as the proband or index case. Pedigree analysis indicates whether the disease behaves as a single mendelian trait (i.e., whether it is transmitted according to Mendel's principles of segregation and independent assortment). Alternatively, if the inheritance pattern does not conform to mendelian principles, the genetic trait may arise from (a) polygenic inheritance, (b) genomic imprinting, (c) uniparental disomy, or (d) mitochondrial inheritance.

Mendelian Inheritance

Single-gene disorders that follow a mendelian pattern of inheritance are manifested as (a) autosomal-dominant traits, (b) autosomal-recessive traits, (c) X-linked dominant traits, or (d) X-linked recessive traits. Genes involved in human autosomal disorders are carried on any one of the 22 pairs of nonsex chromosomes (autosomes). The terms *X-linked dominant* and *X-linked recessive* refer to trait expression in females. In comparison, males carry only one X chromosome and, therefore, are hemizygous for X-linked traits.

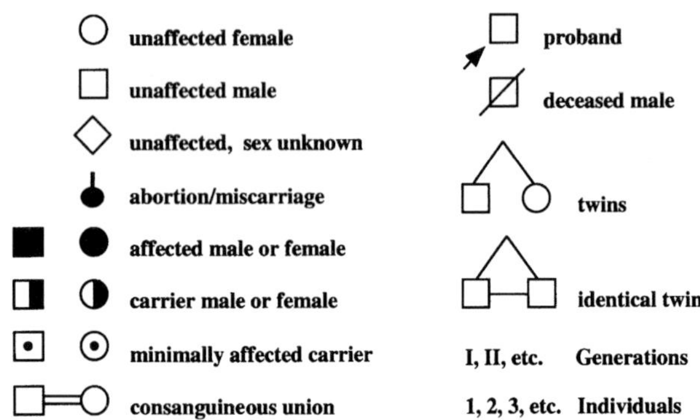

FIGURE 18.1. Standard pedigree symbols.

Dominant disorders are expressed in heterozygotes, hemizygotes, as well as homozygotes, whereas recessive disorders are only expressed in homozygotes and hemizygotes. It is important to note that the terms *dominant* and *recessive* refer to the inheritance of the disease phenotype rather than to the expression of the mutant gene. For example, in the case of autosomal-dominant polycystic kidney disease (ADPKD), the disease phenotype is inherited as an autosomal-dominant trait. However, in cystic epithelia of *PKD1* and *PKD2* patients, there appears to be a "second hit," which results in the somatic cell loss of the normal allele. These data therefore suggest that *PKD1*- and *PKD2*-associated diseases behave in a recessive fashion at the molecular level (3).

Autosomal-Dominant Traits

Dominant traits are expressed when only one mutant allele is inherited. The characteristic pattern of autosomal-dominant inheritance is shown in Figure 18.2. When large numbers of patients are evaluated, an equal number of males and females are affected. An affected child typically has an affected parent, and vertical transmission of the trait occurs through successive generations. Each child of an affected individual has a 50% risk of inheriting the mutant allele. The *sine qua non* of autosomal-dominant inheritance is father-to-son transmission.

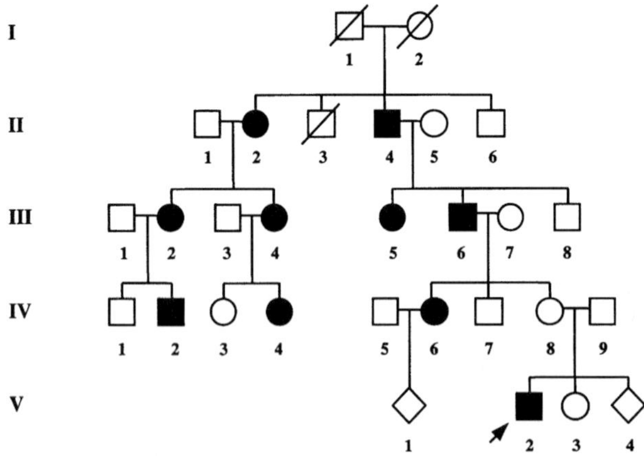

FIGURE 18.2. Pedigree illustrating an autosomal-dominant pattern of inheritance. Note the male-to-male transmission (individual II:4 to individual III:6) and nonpenetrance (individual IV:8).

Many autosomal-dominant disorders are characterized by delayed clinical onset as well as variability in the disease phenotype between families and even within families. These issues are important (e.g., when evaluating fetuses and neonates with presumed polycystic kidney disease). In ADPKD, clinical disease is typically manifested after the third decade of life. Given this delayed clinical presentation, individuals who carry a mutant ADPKD allele may be clinically asymptomatic throughout their child-bearing years. However, ADPKD can be diagnosed *in utero*; for approximately 30% of these fetuses, parental sonographs can identify the previously unaware, transmitting parent (4).

Occasionally, the expression of the dominant trait is so minimal that clinical disease appears to have "skipped" a generation. Individuals who carry a mutant allele for an autosomal-dominant trait but who have little evidence of clinical disease are said to demonstrate decreased or incomplete penetrance (Fig. 18.2). In contrast, when an individual inherits a mutant allele for an autosomal-dominant trait from each parent, the clinical phenotype can be very severe. For example, clinical disease in individuals with the dominant disorder familial hypocalciuric hypercalcemia may proceed undetected. However, the union of two such heterozygotes can produce a child with two mutant alleles who then manifests the often fatal disorder neonatal severe hyperparathyroidism (5).

Although each child of an individual with a specific autosomal-dominant disorder has a 50% risk of inheriting the disease trait, not every affected child necessarily has an affected parent. This is because in every autosomal-dominant disorder, affected individuals can develop the disease phenotype as the result of a new (spontaneous) mutation rather than through inheritance of a mutant allele. A reasonable estimate of the frequency of mutation is on the order of 10^{-6} mutations per allele per generation (1). Many new mendelian mutations occur in the gametes of fathers who are of relatively advanced age, the so-called paternal age effect (2). Most of these mutations either do not impair the function of the gene product or behave as recessive alleles. However, others cause a defective gene product that gives rise to a dominant trait. In these situations, the parent in whose gametes the mutation arose remains clinically unaffected. Similarly, the siblings of the affected individual are also clinically unaffected because spontaneous mutations typically affect only one or a few germ cells.

Before concluding that a dominant trait in a given individual is the result of a spontaneous mutation, two other possibilities must be considered. First, the disease gene may be carried by one parent in whom the disease phenotype is either nonpenetrant or incompletely penetrant. Second, the father may be someone other than the designated man.

Studies in various cultures around the world have detected nonpaternity in approximately 3 to 5% of children (2).

A number of different molecular mechanisms may cause the disease phenotype associated with dominant traits. One mechanism involves haploinsufficiency, in which 50% of the normal gene product is insufficient to maintain a normal phenotype. This mechanism may be operative in disorders involving cellular receptors (e.g., familial hypercholesterolemia) and key regulatory enzymes (e.g., porphyrias). A second mechanism involves a dominant-negative effect in which the incorporation of an abnormal subunit disrupts the function of a multimeric protein (e.g., enzyme pumps, transport proteins, and complex ion channels). This mechanism may be operative in autosomal-dominant forms of nephrogenic diabetes insipidus (6). A third mutational mechanism involves a gain of function in which the mutation causes overexpression of the protein product or results in a new, aberrant function of the protein. This mechanism may be responsible for one form of autosomal-dominant hypocalcemia, in which a mutation in the gene encoding the calcium-sensing receptor causes expression of an overactivated receptor (7). A fourth mechanism for a dominant phenotypic effect results when a heterozygous mutation becomes homozygous at the cellular level due to a second somatic mutation or a "second hit." This mechanism appears to underlie the molecular pathogenesis of ADPKD (3) and tuberous sclerosis (8).

Autosomal-Recessive Disorders

Autosomal-recessive conditions are clinically apparent only in the homozygous state (i.e., when both alleles of a particular gene carry mutations). In most autosomal-recessive disorders, the clinical presentation tends to be more uniform than in dominant diseases, and the onset is often early in life. In recessive pedigrees, the parents are clinically unaffected; on average, one-fourth (25%) of the children are affected, with an equal gender distribution. Given the small family sizes typical in many societies, pediatricians usually see isolated or sporadic cases of a recessive disorder. A typical simplex pedigree is shown in Figure 18.3A. In these situations, a high index of suspicion is required to make the correct genetic diagnosis.

Multiply affected families do occur, particularly in the context of parental consanguinity (Fig. 18.3B). In general, the less frequent the disease phenotype, the more likely it is that an affected child resulted from a consanguineous union. On the other hand, certain recessive disorders have a relatively high carrier frequency in specific populations (e.g., cystic fibrosis in whites and hemoglobin S in blacks). In these populations, recessive diseases usually do not involve consanguinity in the parents.

New mutations for recessive diseases occur, but because they generate an asymptomatic heterozygote, these mutations are not clinically detectable. In the homozygous state,

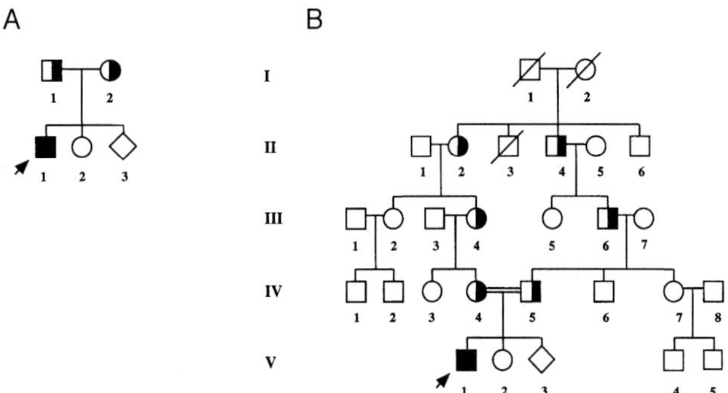

FIGURE 18.3. Pedigrees illustrating autosomal-recessive patterns of inheritance. **A:** A simplex family. **B:** A consanguineous family.

recessive alleles generally cause a complete or nearly complete loss of protein function. For example, a specific monomeric enzyme is rendered nonfunctional in the majority of inborn errors of metabolism. Affected individuals may be homozygous for the same mutant allele, as in the case of parental consanguinity, or they may have inherited a different mutant allele from each parent. In the latter case, the affected individual is referred to as a *compound heterozygote.*

X-Linked Inheritance

Diseases or traits that result from genes located on the X chromosome are termed *X-linked.* Because the female has two X chromosomes, the terms *X-linked dominant* and *X-linked recessive* refer only to expression of the trait in females. Affected males transmit their X chromosome to all of their daughters, rendering them all obligate carriers of an X-linked disease trait. Affected males do not transmit an X chromosome to their sons. Thus, an important feature of X-linked inheritance is the absence of father-to-son transmission.

The female carries two X chromosomes in each cell, but only one is expressed per cell. Both X chromosomes are apparently active early in development. However, through the process of lyonization, one of the X chromosomes is randomly inactivated in each cell during differentiation (9). Once inactivated, the cell's X chromosome is permanently nonfunctional such that all of its daughter cells inherit the same inactivated X chromosome. Therefore, depending on the proportion of mutant and normal X chromosomes in key tissues, a genetically heterozygous female may be clinically normal, may have mild disease, or, in rare cases, may have even severe disease manifestations.

Recognizing new mutations can be more complicated in X-linked disorders than in autosomal disorders. A new mutation may arise in one of the mother's two X chromosomes, and a single affected male may be born to a woman who is not a known carrier. Alternatively, the new mutation may arise in the maternal grandfather's X chromosome. In this scenario, a woman without a known family history of an X-linked disease may have one or more affected sons.

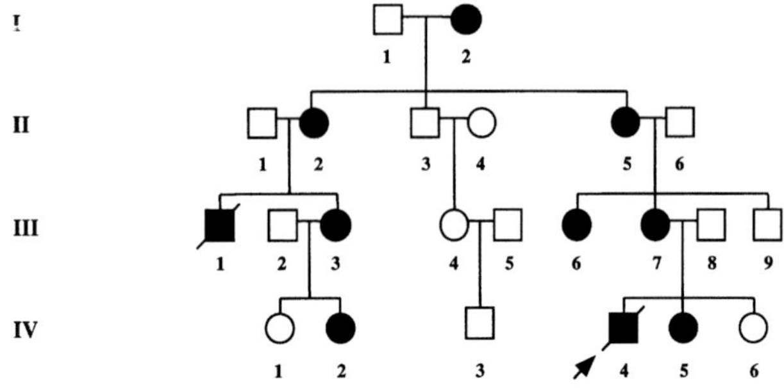

FIGURE 18.4. Pedigree illustrating an X-linked dominant pattern of inheritance. Note lethality in hemizygous males.

X-Linked Dominant Traits

The X-linked dominant pattern is a rare mode of inheritance characterized by a disease frequency in females that is often twice that evident in males. Vitamin D–resistant rickets is an example of an X-linked dominant trait (10). Heterozygous females transmit the trait to offspring of both genders, whereas hemizygous males transmit the trait to all of their daughters and none of their sons. The disease expression is more variable and generally less severe in heterozygous females than in hemizygous males. In other rarer X-linked dominant disorders (e.g., oral-facial-digital syndrome type I) (11), the phenotype may be expressed only in the heterozygous female because the condition is lethal in the hemizygous male (Fig. 18.4).

X-Linked Recessive Traits

In comparison to X-linked dominant inheritance, X-linked recessive inheritance is relatively common. These disorders are fully expressed in the hemizygous affected male. The pedigree pattern tends to be oblique in that affected males have affected uncles and nephews (Fig. 18.5). This oblique pattern is readily distinguished from the vertical transmission in autosomal-dominant inheritance and the horizontal pattern of autosomal-recessive inheritance. Heterozygous females are usually phenotypically normal. Depending on the pattern of lyonization in key tissues, these females may occasionally exhibit mild features of the disease and may rarely be severely affected.

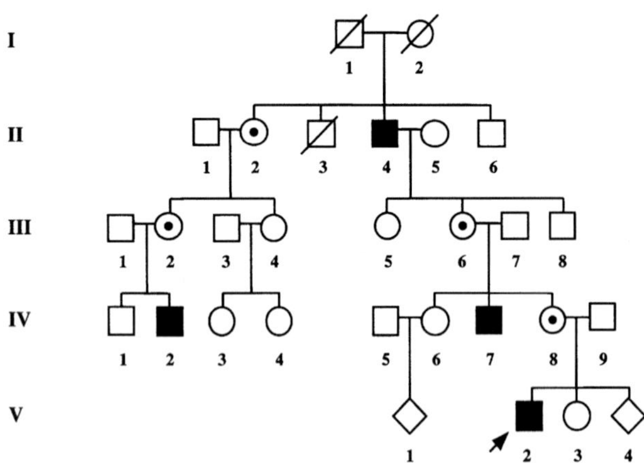

FIGURE 18.5. Pedigree illustrating an X-linked recessive pattern of inheritance.

Nonmendelian Inheritance

Polygenic Inheritance

In general, most phenotypic traits are determined by the interaction of several genes rather than by single gene effects. In terms of genetic disease, polygenic inheritance provides the basis for understanding many diseases that have a genetic component but lack a clear-cut pattern of mendelian inheritance. These disorders include congenital malformations (e.g., most forms of congenital heart disease), meningomyelocele and other neural tube defects, and vesicoureteral reflux, as well as many familial adult-onset diseases (e.g., essential hypertension, type II diabetes, and coronary artery disease) (2).

In multifactorial genetic diseases, multiple different genes interact with one another and with certain environmental factors to cause disease. An individual who inherits a particular combination of interacting genes has a relative risk of developing disease. When this genetic component interacts with a set of environmental factors, a biologic threshold is crossed and disease expression occurs (2). For example, maternal folate deficiency is an important environmental contributor to defective neural tube development in the fetus. Population studies have demonstrated that folic acid treatment in women before and during pregnancy reduces the incidence of neural tube defects by nearly half. These observations prompted efforts to identify variations in genes encoding enzymes of the folic acid metabolic pathway. Recent studies have determined that women carrying specific variants in several of these genes have an increased risk of bearing a child with neural tube defects (12).

Genomic Imprinting

Genomic imprinting refers to the phenomenon in which the phenotypic abnormalities of a given disorder differ depending on the sex of the transmitting parent. Genomic imprinting reflects a functional modification in which there is a temporary change in the function or expression of a gene depending on whether it is maternally or paternally derived (9).

Strong evidence for genomic imprinting in humans has resulted from molecular studies of two chromosomal deletion syndromes, Prader-Willi syndrome and Angelman syndrome. Although clinically quite distinct, both syndromes share similar cytogenetic deletions involving chromosome

15q11-13. The key factor that determines the specific phenotype is not the size of the deletion but the parental origin of the deleted chromosome. Prader-Willi syndrome occurs when the deletion is on the paternally derived chromosome 15, and Angelman syndrome occurs when the deletion is on the maternally derived chromosome 15. These parent-of-origin differences are believed to occur through methylation or other modifications of DNA, which differentially modify the expression of a small number of genes. Therefore, instead of the typical situation in which both maternal and paternal alleles of a gene are expressed, genomic imprinting acts by silencing the expression of one of the parental alleles. This differential expression of certain genes depending on the parent of origin appears to be effaced and reestablished during gametogenesis at each generation (13).

Uniparental Disomy

Uniparental disomy refers to the phenomenon in which both chromosomes of a given pair are inherited from only one parent. This phenomenon appears to result from errors in chromosome segregation during gamete formation. Uniparental isodisomy occurs when both chromosomes in the pair are completely identical, and uniparental heterodisomy results when the two chromosomes come from one parent but are different (14). Uniparental disomy can cause genetic disease either by rendering a mutant allele from the transmitting parent homozygous in the child or by unmasking an imprinted gene.

Mitochondrial Inheritance

The inheritance of nuclear chromosomes forms the basis for mendelian inheritance. In contrast, mitochondrial genes are inherited only from the mother. Mitochondria are passed from generation to generation via the cytoplasm of the oocyte. Because sperm do not contribute mitochondria to the zygote, mitochondrial genes have a strictly maternal pattern of inheritance (15). In theory, if penetrance were complete, then all of the sons and daughters of an affected female would be affected. In reality, penetrance is rarely complete; thus, confusing inheritance patterns can result.

Most cells contain hundreds or thousands of mitochondria, and each mitochondrion contains two to ten mitochondrial DNA (mtDNA) molecules (15). The mitochondrial genome is a small, circular, 16.6-kilobase, double-stranded DNA molecule that contains no introns. In the normal situation, each mtDNA molecule in a given individual is identical. However, the mutation rate in mtDNA is five to ten times greater than in nuclear DNA (16). Cells that contain a mixture of wild-type and mutant mtDNA are termed *heteroplasmic*, whereas cells with a single identical mtDNA are termed *homoplasmic*. Because mitochondria partition to daughter cells in an entirely random fashion, the cellular phenotype depends on the relative proportions of mutant and wild-type mtDNAs within a given cell and the degree to which that cell depends on oxidative phosphorylation. The central nervous system is most dependent on mitochondrial energy, followed by the heart, skeletal muscle, liver, and kidney. Therefore, defects in the mitochondrial genome and the associated impairment of oxidative phosphorylation typically manifest as neuromuscular disease but may also cause renal tubular dysfunction or glomerular disease (16).

MEDICAL GENETICS

Genomic Organization and the Transmission of Genetic Information

The genetic complement of each individual is arrayed in 23 pairs of chromosomes (the diploid genome). One-half of each individual's chromosomes, or one haploid genome, is maternally derived, and the other half is of paternal origin. Each diploid genome is composed of 22 pairs of autosomes, numbered in order of descending size, and one pair of sex chromosomes (females, XX; males, XY). Chromosomes are stored in the cell nucleus and distributed to daughter cells by either mitotic or meiotic cell division. In both processes, the chromosomes are unwound and the two DNA strands are copied. The replicated strands, called *chromatids*, remain joined at the centromere. The chromatids, which can be visualized at this stage by light microscopy, are composed of two asymmetric arms. The shorter of the two is termed the *p arm*, whereas the longer of the two is called the *q arm*. When chromosomes are arranged systematically in pairs 1 to 23, they comprise the karyotype.

During somatic cell division, the process of mitosis distributes one chromatid of each chromosome pair to the daughter cells; thus, the full diploid complement of 23 chromosome pairs is transmitted. In contrast, germ cells undergo a reduction division called *meiosis*, in which only one chromatid is transmitted to each gamete. The diploid germ cell therefore generates haploid oocytes or sperm that contain 23 individual chromosomes. During fertilization, the union of the oocyte and sperm constitutes a diploid zygote with 23 pairs of chromosomes.

Recombination and Genetic Mapping

Meiosis is the process by which the chromosome number of diploid germ cells (N = 46) is reduced to the haploid number (N = 23) in the gametes. The independent assortment of chromosomes into gametes during meiosis produces a remarkable variety of possible genotypes in the progeny. For a given set of parents, there are 2^{23} different chromosome combinations possible in their offspring; thus, the likelihood that this set of parents will produce two independent offspring with an identical complement of chromosomes is 1 in 84 million (1 in 2^{23}) (2). The phenomenon of genetic recombination during meiosis adds further to the enormous genetic diversity in humans and provides the basis for genetic mapping.

During the first meiotic division, chromatids pair with their homologues (e.g., the maternally derived chromosome 1 chromatids pair with the paternally derived chromosome 1 chromatids). This close proximity allows the exchange of segments between maternal and paternal homologues, a process termed *crossing over*. These exchanges, which result in genetic recombination, occur on average approximately 50 times during meiosis, with a slightly higher frequency in female germ cells than male germ cells. With the completion of this first meiotic division, each daughter cell has 46 chromosomes but only one copy of each chromatid pair. This separation of maternal and paternal chromosome homologues is referred to as a *reduction division*. The second meiotic division proceeds without further chromosome replication. The resulting gametes have a haploid chromosome complement.

Due to genetic recombination, two genes that are located on opposite ends of a given chromosome typically behave as if they are on different chromosomes (i.e., they segregate in an entirely random fashion). In comparison, recombination events are less likely between genes that are located close to one another. The distance between two such genes can be quantitated either in terms of genetic distance (i.e., the probability of recombination events per generation) or physical distance [i.e., millions of base pairs (megabases)]. Genetic distance is measured in centimorgans (cM). For two genes that are 1 cM apart, there is a 1% chance of a recombination event occurring between them in a given meiotic division. Although on average in the human genome, 1 cM corresponds to approximately 1 megabase of DNA, the frequency of recombination may vary in specific chromosomal regions and between female and male germ cells (2).

Mutations

A *mutation* is a stable alteration of the DNA sequence that can be passed from a parent cell to daughter cells. Alterations of DNA sequences in cells other than germ cells are termed *somatic mutations*. Although these alterations are not transmitted to the next generation, the mutations are passed on to the progeny of those mutated cells. When a somatic mutation occurs early in development, the resulting individual may be a mosaic or a combination of normal cells and mutant cells. Once development is complete, somatic mutations can be silent (i.e., they may not be associated with a specific phenotype). Alternatively, somatic mutations (e.g., those involved in ADPKD) play a central role in disease pathogenesis.

In comparison, germ-line mutations are transmitted from one generation to the next. On average, the rate of mutation is approximately 10^{-6} per locus per generation (1). Most of these mutations occur in noncoding sequences and typically are detected as variations or polymorphisms in the population. In comparison, mutations in coding sequences often cause disease. From an evolutionary perspective, these coding sequence mutations appear to play an important role in generating genetic diversity and thereby permit environmental adaptation of the species through the process of natural selection.

Single base changes that occur in coding regions cause three types of mutations: (a) a silent mutation, in which the base change results in a different three-base code (codon) for the same amino acid; (b) a missense mutation, in which the base change results in a new codon (i.e., the wild-type amino acid is replaced by a new amino acid); and (c) a nonsense mutation, in which the base substitution changes the amino acid codon to a termination (stop) codon. The deletion or insertion of a single base or a few bases within the coding region can cause a frame shift mutation in which the reading frame of the genetic code is altered. Frame shift mutations alter the amino acid sequence and often lead to premature truncation of the peptide by generating a new stop codon.

Germ-line mutations can also involve millions of base pairs and cause gross chromosomal alterations, including duplications, insertions, deletions, or translocations. Such alterations may disrupt the coding sequence and cause either an absence of the protein product, as in juvenile nephronophthisis (NPH1) (17), or the fusion of two closely related protein products, as in glucocorticoid-remediable aldosteronism (18). Finally, sequence alterations in the DNA flanking the coding regions may lead to changes in RNA splicing, transcriptional efficiency, or regulated tissue expression.

STRATEGIES FOR GENE IDENTIFICATION

After the seminal report by Watson and Crick in 1953 describing the structure of DNA, identification of disease-causing genes was predicated on first identifying the defective protein (functional cloning). Perhaps the best known successes of the functional cloning approach involve disease gene identification in phenylketonuria and sickle cell disease. However, for most human diseases, our level of insight into the fundamental pathogenic mechanisms remains rather limited; thus, functional cloning has not been a broadly applicable approach.

To a certain extent, the candidate gene approach also depends on functional insight into disease pathogenesis. By itself, this knowledge is not sufficient to precisely pinpoint the gene; rather, it provides a framework to form a series of educated guesses. For example, clinical studies of Bartter syndrome patients indicated a primary defect in transepithelial sodium chloride transport in the thick ascending limb of the loop of Henle. With the cloning of genes encoding the key transport proteins in the thick ascending limb [e.g., the bumetanide-sensitive sodium-potassium-chloride cotransporter (*NKCC2*), the apical adenosine triphosphate–regulated potassium channel (*ROMK*), and the kidney-specific basolateral chloride channel (*ClC-Kb*)], direct molecular studies became possible. Loss-of-function mutations in the genes for each of these transport proteins have been demonstrated in patients with either antenatal Bartter syndrome or the more classic phenotype (19).

Beginning in 1986, positional cloning or map-based gene discovery became the leading method for identifying disease susceptibility genes in inherited disorders. With the availability of the human genome sequence, the positional candidate approach has rapidly emerged as the preferred method for elucidating the molecular basis of genetic disease. This strategy combines genetic mapping, usually by linkage analysis, with information from databases that catalogue the human genomic sequence and its transcripts [e.g., those maintained by the National Center for Biotechnology Information (http://www.ncbi.nlm.nih.gov)]. Once a candidate disease-susceptibility gene is mapped to a chromosomal subregion, the databases can then be surveyed to identify attractive candidate genes within the interval.

To date, the successes in gene discovery have primarily involved single-gene disorders. Investigators have determined that the phenotypic expression of these disorders is due to different mutations within the disease-susceptibility gene. In addition, disease expression appears to be influenced by the modifying effects of other genes (modifying genes) that are involved in the same molecular pathway(s) (20). In comparison to single-gene disorders, multifactorial genetic diseases involve genetic susceptibility and environmental factors. In these disorders, the expression of the disease phenotype depends on the complement of risk genes that is inherited and the interaction of these risk genes with certain environmental factors. The major challenge facing molecular geneticists is to elucidate and characterize the molecular components involved in both single-gene and multifactorial disorders and to determine how these molecular factors influence the disease phenotype.

GENETIC TESTING

The immediate clinical impact of gene mapping and identification is the potential for gene-based diagnostic testing. DNA-based diagnosis of single-gene disorders is well established in prenatal, pretransplant, and presymptomatic contexts. For mendelian traits, such genetic testing can be performed in one of two ways: (a) indirect testing, which usually involves linkage analysis, or (b) direct gene-based testing.

Before genetic testing can be offered, the molecular "specifics" for a given disorder must be evaluated. The practicality of genetic testing depends on a number of factors, including (a) the number of genes/loci involved; (b) the genetic map for those disease genes that have yet to be cloned; (c) the size and the complexity of the disease genes; and (d) the number and distribution of different mutations within the disease genes. In addition to the technical challenges of genetic testing, issues such as phenotype-genotype correlation, sensitivity and specificity, proper informed consent, and access to genetic counseling must be addressed before a test is ready for clinical use (21).

It is important to stress that genetic tests differ from other medical tests. They have direct implications for family members and for reproductive decision making. They often raise issues of privacy, independence, insurability, and discrimination, and the test results may have dire emotional consequences (21). Therefore, genetic counseling should precede genetic testing to allow informed decision making.

Linkage Analysis

Linkage analysis is an indirect method for diagnostic genetic testing. It is useful in mendelian disorders in several contexts: (a) when the disease gene has not yet been identified; (b) when the disease gene is very large or complex; and (c) or when the mutations are too heterogeneous to be readily identified. In linkage-based testing, the disease gene is not directly analyzed. Rather, its presence is inferred by family studies that track the cosegregation of flanking polymorphic markers and a specific disease phenotype.

The principal advantage of linkage-based testing is that it can be applied to any mapped mendelian trait. The disadvantages of linkage analysis include (a) the absolute dependence of the test on correct phenotypic diagnosis; (b) the requirement for DNA typing of an affected proband as well as other affected and unaffected family members; and (c) the limitation of the maximum confidence level to 95 to 99%. Such confidence limits are inherent to linkage analyses because of the possibility that recombination events could occur between the marker and the mutant gene, with the probability directly related to the genetic distance between them. The risk of possible error can be minimized when intragenic and multiple flanking markers are used for testing. Although linkage-based testing is a powerful diagnostic tool in many disorders, diagnoses based on such an indirect methodology are estimates and should be treated as such.

Direct Mutation Analysis

Once a disease gene is cloned, direct mutation detection strategies can be designed to identify the genetic defect that is causally responsible for the disease phenotype. Direct mutation analysis can be performed by several methods. The details of these testing modalities are beyond the scope of this chapter and the reader is referred to several excellent reviews (22–25). In general, the choice of method depends on the types and numbers of mutations that cause the disorder.

TABLE 18.1. GLOSSARY OF TERMS

Term	Definition
Allele	An alternative form of a gene. Humans carry two sets of alleles for every gene or genetic marker, one from each parent.
Alternative splicing	A regulatory mechanism by which exons are variably incorporated into the mRNA, leading to the production of more than one related protein or isoform.
Autosomes	All of the chromosomes except for the sex chromosomes and the mitochondrial chromosome.
cDNA	A DNA sequence made from an mRNA molecule. cDNAs contain only exonic sequences.
Cloning	The process of generating multiple copies of a particular piece of DNA.
Codon	A three-base sequence of DNA or RNA that specifies a single amino acid.
Conservation	Sequence similarity for genes that are present in two distinct organisms. Conservation can be detected by measuring the sequence similarity at the nucleotide (DNA or RNA) or the amino acid level.
Epigenetic	A term describing nonmutational phenomena (e.g., methylation and histone modification) that modify the expression of a gene.
Euchromatin	The gene-rich regions of the genome.
Exon	A region of a gene that encodes a portion of its protein product.
Genomics	The study of the functions and interactions of all the genes in the genome, including their interactions with environmental factors.
Genotype	The set of genes that an individual carries; usually refers to the particular pairs of alleles that the individual has at a given region of the genome.
Haplotype	A group of nearby alleles that are closely linked (i.e., likely to be inherited together).
Heterochromatin	Compact gene-poor regions of the genome that are difficult to clone and thus are usually ignored in genome sequencing.
Intron	A region of a gene that does not code for a protein.
mRNA	The template for protein synthesis. A precursor RNA is constructed from the gene sequence and then processed with removal of the introns by splicing. Spliced RNAs contain only exonic sequences from which proteins are synthesized.
Microarray	High-dimensional tool that allows expression analysis of thousands of genes (or proteins) in a single hybridization experiment.
Monogenic disease	Caused by mutations in a single gene.
Multifactorial disease	Caused by the interaction of multiple genetic and environmental factors.
Mutation	An alteration in an individual's genomic sequence compared to a reference sequence. These sequence variants can have harmful effects (pathogenic mutations) or no harmful effects (silent mutations or polymorphisms).
Penetrance	The likelihood that a person carrying a particular mutant gene will have an altered phenotype.
Phenotype	The observable properties and physical characteristics of an individual.
Polymorphism	A region of the genomic sequence that varies between individual members of a population.
Proteomics	The study of the functions and interactions of all the proteins encoded in the genome.
SNP	A polymorphism caused by the change of a single nucleotide. The human genome is estimated to contain approximately 10 million SNPs.
Transcription	The process of copying a gene into RNA.
Transcriptosome	The complete set of RNAs transcribed from the genome.
Translation	The process of using an mRNA sequence to build a protein.

cDNA, complimentary DNA; mRNA, messenger DNA; SNP, single-nucleotide polymorphism.
Modified from Venter J, Adams M, Myers E, et al. The sequence of the human genome. *Science* 2001;291:1304–1351; and Guttmacher A, Collins F. Genomic medicine—a primer. *N Engl J Med* 2002;347:1512–1520.

When compared with linkage-based testing, direct mutation analysis has several advantages. Most notable among these are (a) a previously affected sibling is not essential, and (b) studies on other family members are not typically required. The pitfalls can include (a) locus heterogeneity, in which the same phenotype can be caused by mutations in more than one gene; (b) no *a priori* knowledge of the specific mutation segregating in a family or present in a given individual; and (c) the inability of a given technique to detect all mutations.

With current technologies, detection of mutations can be time-consuming and expensive. In the postgenomic era, the search for clinically useful assays will emphasize the use of newer DNA sequencing technologies as well as the development of microarray-based genomic and proteomic screening.

INSIGHTS FROM THE HUMAN GENOME PROJECT

In February 2001, the draft sequence of the human genome was published by two groups, the International Human Genome Sequencing Consortium (26) and Celera Genomics (27). The estimated size of the human genome is 3.2×10^9 base pairs or gigabases. The sequence is approximately 90% complete for the 2.95 gigabases of euchro-

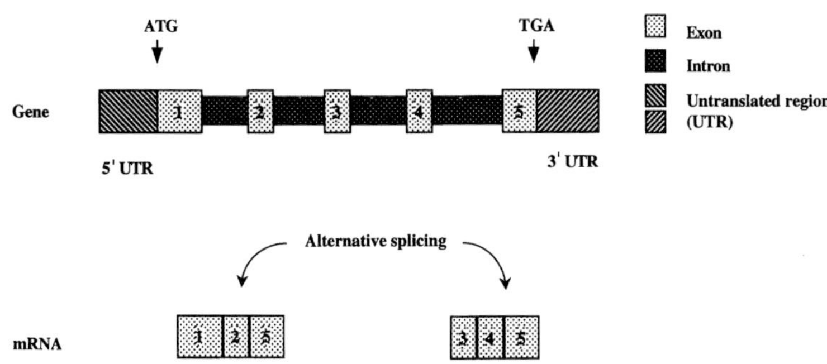

FIGURE 18.6. Schema of a typical eukaryotic gene and RNA splicing. The nontranslated portion of the gene contains DNA control regions that specify the RNA transcription start site and define the specificity of tissue expression. The sequences that encode the polypeptide product are organized into discrete units (exons) and specific sequences within the exons determine the translation start site (ATG) and stop site (TGA). The exons are interrupted by noncoding sequences (introns). The DNA sequence is transcribed in the nucleus into an RNA product, and the intervening introns are removed or "spliced out." By alternative splicing, a single gene can produce multiple related proteins. mRNA, messenger RNA. 1–5, exons.

matic or weakly staining gene-rich regions of the human genome (Table 18.1). Based on initial analyses, investigators predict that the human genome contains 30,000 to 35,000 protein-encoding genes (Fig. 18.6), which comprise 1.1 to 1.4% of the total sequence (28). The number of coding genes in the human sequence compares with 6000 for the yeast *Saccharomyces cerevisiae*; 13,000 for *Drosophila*; 18,000 for the roundworm *Caenorhabditis elegans*; and 26,000 for the mustard weed *Arabadopsis* (29). Therefore, our complexity as a species derives from more than just our complement of genes. Factors such as variations in gene regulation, gene expression, the splicing of gene transcripts, and modifications of proteins after translation probably all contribute to our complexity.

The human genome sequence is providing new tools and new challenges for genetic investigators (29). This information has already begun to revolutionize biologic investigation by allowing researchers to examine global gene expression in different cells, tissues, and disease states using high dimensional tools, such as microarrays. The power of these genomic tools will be enhanced as the genomic sequence is annotated so that the full complement of genes as well as their regulatory regions is defined. By extension, the genomic sequence will inform our understanding of the full complement of human proteins, the proteome. Ultimately, this information will permit detailed characterization of the cellular pathways and networks in which these proteins interact.

In addition, the human genome sequencing effort has demonstrated that individual humans differ from one another by approximately one base pair per thousand. By examining the patterns of these single-nucleotide polymorphisms in patients and controls, researchers can evaluate the contribution of individual genes to relative susceptibility or resistance to disease. This genetic variation may also provide insights into individual responses to pharmaceutical treatment (30).

FUTURE CONSIDERATIONS

To date, genetic discoveries have largely focused on identifying the genes involved in rare mendelian disorders. In the postgenomic era, methods for automated mutation detection, array-based systems for gene and protein expression, and polymorphism profiles of disease susceptibility will all become feasible. These advances will facilitate both the diagnosis of mendelian disorders (e.g., autosomal-recessive polycystic kidney disease) and the evaluation of genetic susceptibility to more common, multifactorial disorders (e.g., vesicoureteral reflux).

Detailed understanding of the molecular pathophysiology of human disease will provide new opportunities for diagnosis and treatment of both rare and common disorders (Fig. 18.7). Some of these treatments may entail

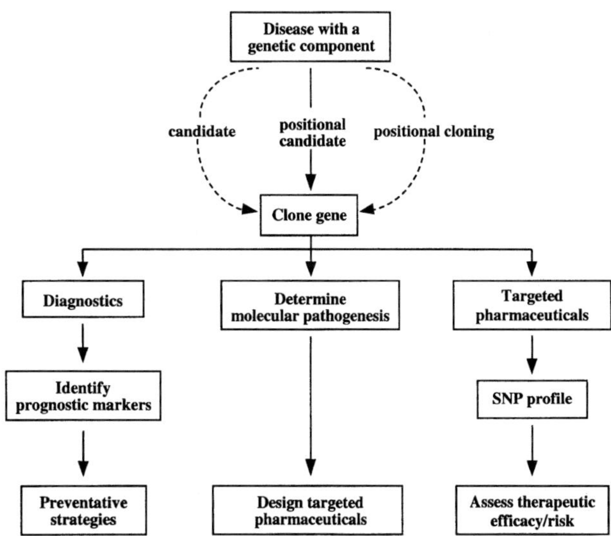

FIGURE 18.7. Advances in molecular genetics and the clinical implications. In the postgenomic era, positional candidate approaches can be applied to identify disease-susceptibility genes for mendelian and, eventually, polygenic disorders. Gene discovery can be translated into DNA-based diagnostic tests. In a growing number of instances, improved diagnostic specificity can lead to the identification of specific genetic risk factors and ultimately facilitate the development of preventative medicine strategies. In addition, gene discovery will open up new treatment options involving pharmaceuticals that target specific aspects of the molecular pathogenesis. Increasingly, the efficacy and risk of these new pharmaceuticals for a given individual will be assayed using single-nucleotide polymorphism (SNP)-based profiles. (Modified from Collins F. Positional cloning moves from perditional to traditional. *Nat Genet* 1995;9:347–350.)

sophisticated gene therapy techniques, but others will involve the development of targeted pharmaceuticals based on more precise understanding of molecular physiology. Single-nucleotide polymorphism profiling will afford risk assessment for an individual's genetic susceptibility to certain illnesses (e.g., type II diabetes), and specific preventative medicine programs will be developed to target this risk. In addition, it will become standard practice to use single-nucleotide polymorphism-based profiles to predict drug responses in individual patients (31). Pediatricians and pediatric subspecialists must become familiar with the advances in the postgenomic era to incorporate these changes into their practices.

REFERENCES

1. Lewin B. *Genes VI.* New York: Oxford University Press, 1997.
2. Beaudet A, Scriver C, Sly W, Valle D. Genetics, biochemistry, and molecular basis of variant human phenotypes. In: Beaudet A, Scriver C, Sly W, Valle D, eds. *The metabolic and molecular bases of inherited disease,* 6th ed. New York: McGraw-Hill, 1995:53–118.
3. Igarashi P, Somlo S. Genetics and pathogenesis of polycystic kidney disease. *J Am Soc Nephrol* 2002;13:2384–2398.
4. Fick G, Johnson A, Strain J, et al. Characteristics of very early onset autosomal dominant polycystic kidney disease. *J Am Soc Nephrol* 1993;3:1863–1870.
5. Pollak M, Brown E, Chou Y-H, et al. Mutations in the human Ca2+-sensing receptor gene cause familial hypocalciuric hypercalcemia and neonatal severe hyperparathyroidism. *Cell* 1993;75:1297–1303.
6. Knoers N, Deen P. Molecular and cellular defects in nephrogenic diabetes insipidus. *Pediatr Nephrol* 2001;16:1146–1152.
7. Pollak M, Brown E, Estep H, et al. Autosomal dominant hypocalcemia caused by a Ca2+-sensing receptor gene mutation. *Nat Genet* 1994;8:303–307.
8. Cheadle J, Reeve M, Sampson J, Kwiatkowski D. Molecular genetic advances in tuberous sclerosis. *Hum Genet* 2000; 107:97–114.
9. Langlois S, Lopez-Rangel E, Hall J. New mechanisms for genetic disease and non-traditional modes of inheritance. *Adv Pediatr* 1995;42:91–111.
10. Beur SJd, Levine M. Molecular pathogenesis of hypophosphatemic rickets. *J Clin Endocrinol Metab* 2002;87:2467–2473.
11. Ferrante M, Giorgio G, Feather S, et al. Identification of the gene for oral-facial-digital type I syndrome. *Am J Hum Genet* 2001;68:569–576.
12. Brody L, Conley M, Cox C, et al. A polymorphism, R653Q, in the trifunctional enzyme methylenetetrahydrofolate dehydrogenase/methenyltetrahydrofolate cyclohydrolase/formyltetrahydrofolate synthetase is a maternal genetic risk factor for neural tube defects: report of the Birth Defects Research Group. *Am J Hum Genet* 2002;71:1207–1215.
13. Paulsen M, Ferguson-Smith A. DNA methylation in genomic imprinting, development, and disease. *J Pathol* 2001;195:97–110.
14. Robinson W. Uniparental disomy and their clinical consequences. *Bioessays* 2000;22:452–459.
15. Grossman L, Shoubridge E. Mitochondrial genetics and human disease. *Bioessays* 1996;18:983–991.
16. Niaudet P. Mitochondrial disorders and the kidney. *Arch Dis Child* 1998;78:387–390.
17. Hildebrandt F, Omram H. New insights: nephronophthisis-medullary cystic kidney disease. *Pediatr Nephrol* 2001;16: 168–176.
18. Lifton RP, Dluhy RG, Powers M, et al. A chimaeric 11-B-hydroxylase aldosterone synthase gene causes glucocorticoid-remediable aldosteronism and human hypertension. *Nature* 1992;355:262–265.
19. Scheinman S, Guay-Woodford L, Thakker R, Warnock D. Genetic disorders of renal electrolyte transport. *N Engl J Med* 1999;340:1177–1187.
20. Dipple K, McCabe E. Phenotypes of patients with "simple" Mendelian disorders are complex traits: thresholds, modifiers, and systems dynamics. *Am J Hum Genet* 2000;66: 1729–1735.
21. Korf B. Genetic testing for patients with renal disease: procedures, pitfalls, and ethical considerations. *Semin Nephrol* 1999;19:319–326.
22. Korf B. Genetic testing and medical practice. *Curr Opin Pediatr* 2001;13:547–549.
23. Yan H, Kinzler K, Vogelstein B. Genetic testing—present and future. *Science* 2000;289:1890–1892.
24. Kiechle F, Zhang X. The postgenomic era: implications for the clinical laboratory. *Arch Pathol Lab Med* 2002;126:255–262.
25. Amos J, Patnaik M. Commercial molecular diagnostics in the U.S.: the human genome project to the clinical laboratory. *Hum Mutat* 2002;19:324–333.
26. International Human Genome Sequencing Consortium. Initial sequencing and analysis of the human genome. *Nature* 2001;409:860–921.
27. Venter J, Adams M, Myers E, et al. The sequence of the human genome. *Science* 2001;291:1304–1351.
28. Guttmacher A, Collins F. Genomic medicine—a primer. *N Engl J Med* 2002;347:1512–1520.
29. Baltimore D. Our genome unveiled. *Nature* 2001;409:814–816.
30. Chakravati A. Single nucleotide polymorphisms: to a future of genetic medicine. *Nature* 2001;409:822–823.
31. Roses A. Pharmacogenetics. *Hum Mol Genet* 2001;10: 2261–2267.

19

TISSUE ENGINEERING

ANTHONY ATALA

Regenerative medicine, a recently defined field, involves the diverse areas of tissue engineering, stem cells, and cloning toward the common goal of developing biologic substitutes that would restore and maintain normal tissue and organ function.

Tissue engineering follows the principles of cell transplantation, materials science, and engineering toward the development of biologic substitutes that restore and maintain normal function. Tissue engineering may involve matrices alone, wherein the body's natural ability to regenerate is used to orient or direct new tissue growth, or the use of matrices with cells.

When cells are used for tissue engineering, donor tissue is dissociated into individual cells that are either implanted directly into the host or expanded in culture, attached to a support matrix, and reimplanted after expansion. The implanted tissue can be heterologous, allogeneic, or autologous. Ideally, this approach might allow lost tissue function to be restored or replaced *in toto* and with limited complications (2). The use of autologous cells avoids rejection, wherein a biopsy of tissue is obtained from the host, the cells are dissociated and expanded *in vitro*, reattached to a matrix, and implanted into the same host.

One of the initial limitations of applying cell-based tissue-engineering techniques to urologic organs had been the previously encountered inherent difficulty of growing genitourinary-associated cells in large quantities. In the past, it was believed that urothelial cells had a natural senescence that was hard to overcome. Normal urothelial cells could be grown in the laboratory setting but with limited expansion. Several protocols were developed over the last two decades that improved urothelial growth and expansion (3–6). Using these methods of cell culture, it is possible to expand a urothelial strain from a single specimen that initially covers a surface area of 1 cm^2 to one covering a surface area of 4202 m^2 (the equivalent area of one football field) within 8 weeks (3).

Biomaterials in genitourinary tissue engineering may function as an artificial extracellular matrix and elicit biologic and mechanical functions of native extracellular matrix found in tissues in the body. The design and selection of the biomaterial is critical in the development of engineered genitourinary tissues. The biomaterial must be capable of controlling the structure and function of the engineered tissue in a predesigned manner by interacting with transplanted cells and/or the host cells. Generally, the ideal biomaterial should be biocompatible, promote cellular interaction and tissue development, and possess proper mechanical and physical properties.

In general, three classes of biomaterials have been used for engineering genitourinary tissues: naturally derived materials (e.g., collagen and alginate), acellular tissue matrices (e.g., bladder submucosa and small intestinal submucosa), and synthetic polymers [e.g., polyglycolic acid (PGA), polylactic acid, and poly(lactic-co-glycolic acid)]. These classes of biomaterials have been tested in respect to their biocompatibility with primary human urothelial and bladder muscle cells (7,8). Naturally derived materials and acellular tissue matrices have the potential advantage of biologic recognition. Synthetic polymers can be produced reproducibly on a large scale with controlled properties of their strength, degradation rate, and microstructure.

TISSUE ENGINEERING OF GENITOURINARY STRUCTURES

Urethra

Various strategies have been proposed over the years for the regeneration of urethral tissue. Woven meshes of PGA have been used to reconstruct urethras in animals (9,10). PGA has been also used as a cell transplantation vehicle to engineer tubular urothelium *in vivo* (11). When using cells for transplantation, it has been shown that cells from an abnormal environment, if genetically stable, are able to be engineered into normal tissues (12). A homologous free graft of acellular urethral matrix was used in a rabbit model (13). All tissue components were seen in the grafted matrix after 3 months, with further improvement over time; however, the smooth muscle in the matrix was less than in normal rabbit urethra and was not well oriented.

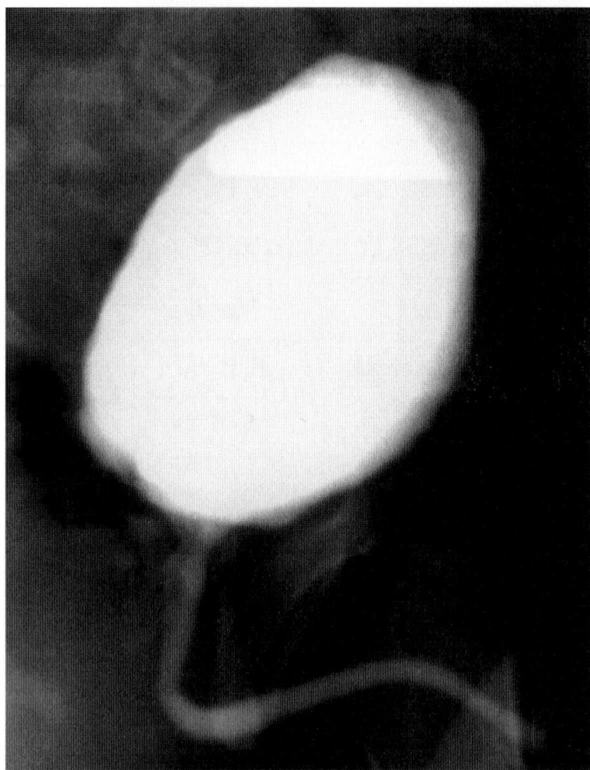

FIGURE 19.1. Urethrogram 6 months postoperatively of a patient who had a portion of his urethra replaced using tissue-engineering techniques.

Acellular collagen matrices obtained from donor bladder submucosa have proven to be suitable grafts for repairing urethral defects both experimentally and clinically at our institution. Rabbit neourethras reconstructed with acellular matrices demonstrated a normal urothelial luminal lining and organized muscle bundles without any signs of strictures or complications (14). These results were confirmed clinically in a series of patients with a history of failed hypospadias reconstruction, wherein the urethral defects were repaired with human bladder acellular collagen matrices in an onlay fashion, with the size of the created neourethras ranging from 5 to 15 cm (Fig. 19.1) (15). The same technique was used to repair urethral strictures on more than 40 adult patients (16). One of the advantages over nongenital tissue grafts used for urethroplasty is that the collagen-based acellular material is "off the shelf." This eliminates the necessity of additional surgical procedures for graft harvesting, which may decrease operative time as well as the potential morbidity due to the harvest procedure.

It has also been noted that although acellular collagen-based grafts may be suitable for partial onlay urethral replacement, they are not effective for the replacement of tubularized segments, as this results in the collapse of the grafts, with subsequent stricture formation (17). Tubularized urethral repairs require the application of collagen-based grafts seeded with both urothelial and muscle cells (17). Total urethral replacement is possible with the use of tissue-engineered constructs composed of urothelial and muscle cell seeded matrices.

Bladder

Currently, gastrointestinal segments are commonly used as tissues for bladder replacement or repair. However, gastrointestinal tissues are designed to absorb specific solutes, whereas bladder tissue is designed for the excretion of solutes. When gastrointestinal tissue is in contact with the urinary tract, multiple complications may ensue, such as infection, metabolic disturbances, urolithiasis, perforation, increased mucous production, and malignancy (18). Owing to the problems encountered with the use of gastrointestinal segments, numerous investigators have attempted alternative methods, materials, and tissues for bladder replacement or repair.

Seromuscular grafts and deepithelialized bowel segments, either alone or over a native urothelium, have been attempted (19–26). The concept of demucosalizing organs is not new to urologists. More than four decades ago, in 1961, Blandy proposed the removal of submucosa from intestinal segments used for augmentation cystoplasty to insure that mucosal regrowth would not occur (19). Hypothetically, this would avoid the complications associated with using bowel in continuity with the urinary tract (20,21). Since Blandy's initial report, 25 years transpired before there was a renewed interest in demucosalizing intestinal segments for urinary reconstruction (22). Since 1988, several other investigators have pursued this line of research (23–26). These investigative efforts have emphasized the complexity of both the anatomic and cellular interactions present when combining tissues with different functional parameters. The complexity of these interactions is emphasized by the observation that the use of demucosalized intestinal segments for augmentation cystoplasty is limited by either mucosal regrowth or contraction of the intestinal patch (23,24). It has been noted that removal of only the mucosa may lead to mucosal regrowth, whereas removal of the mucosa and submucosa may lead to retraction of the intestinal patch (27,28).

Some researchers have combined the techniques of autoaugmentation with enterocystoplasty. An autoaugmentation is performed, and the diverticulum is covered with a demucosalized gastric or intestinal segment. In a series of autoaugmentation (25) enterocystoplasty, patients with a neurogenic bladder had either incorporation of stomach or colon. In both groups of patients, the mucosa of the enteric segment was dissected away from the underlying muscle, and the resulting mucosa-free graft was used to cover a newly created bladder diverticulum. A satisfactory increase in bladder capacity and compliance was achieved in most patients. In another series of patients who underwent seromuscular colocystoplasty,

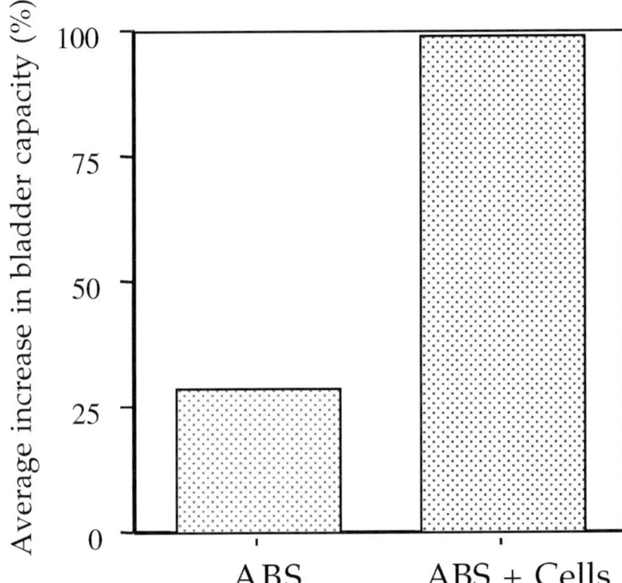

FIGURE 19.2. Bladders augmented with a collagen matrix derived from bladder submucosa seeded with urothelial and smooth muscle cells [allogenic bladder submucosa (ABS) + cells] showed a 100% increase in capacity compared to bladders augmented with the cell-free ABS, which showed only a 30% increase in capacity within 3 months after implantation. (See Color Plate 19.2.)

the bladder capacity increased an average of 2.4-fold in 14 patients (26). Ten patients had a postoperative bladder biopsy. Seven patients demonstrated urothelium covering the augmented portion of the bladder, two had regrowth of colonic mucosa, and one showed a mixture of colonic mucosa and urothelium. Although colonic mucosal regrowth is seen, there is a subset of patients who may benefit from these procedures, wherein mucous secretion may be reduced or eliminated (26).

Bladder grafts, initially used experimentally in 1961, have been used recently by various investigators (29–32). The allogenic acellular bladder matrix has served as a scaffold for the ingrowth of host bladder wall components. The matrix is prepared by mechanically and/or chemically removing the cellular components.

Allogenic bladder submucosa was used as a biomaterial for bladder augmentation in dogs (31). Biomaterials preloaded with cells before their implantation showed better tissue regeneration compared to biomaterials implanted with no cells in which the tissue regeneration depended on the ingrowth of the surrounding tissue. The bladders showed a significant increase in capacity of 100% when augmented with scaffolds seeded with cells, compared to a capacity of 30% for scaffolds without cells (Fig. 19.2).

Small-intestinal submucosa derived from pig small intestine has been used for augmentation cystoplasty in dogs (33). Preoperative mean bladder capacity was 51 mL compared to a postoperative mean capacity of 55 mL. Histologically, the muscle layer was not fully developed. A large amount of collagen was interspersed between a smaller number of muscle bundles. A computerized assisted image analysis demonstrated a decreased muscle-to-collagen ratio with a loss of the normal architecture in the small-intestinal submucosa–regenerated bladders. *In vitro* contractility studies performed on the small-intestinal submucosa–regenerated dog bladders showed a decrease in maximal contractile response by 50% from those of normal bladder tissues. Cholinergic and purinergic innervation was present (34).

In multiple studies using different materials as an acellular graft for cystoplasty, the urothelial layer was able to regenerate normally, but the muscle layer, although present, was not fully developed (30–33). Engineering tissue using selective cell transplantation may provide a means to create functional new bladder segments (11). The success of using cell transplantation strategies for bladder reconstruction depends on the ability to use donor tissue efficiently and to provide the right conditions for long-term survival, differentiation, and growth.

Urothelial and muscle cells can be expanded *in vitro*, seeded onto the polymer scaffold, and allowed to attach and form sheets of cells. The cell-polymer scaffold can then be implanted *in vivo*. A series of *in vivo* urologic-associated cell-polymer experiments were performed in mice, rabbits, and dogs (3,11,31,35).

To better address the functional parameters of tissue-engineered bladders, an animal model was designed that required a subtotal cystectomy with subsequent replacement with a tissue-engineered organ (36). Dogs underwent a trigone-sparing cystectomy. The animals were randomly assigned to one of three groups. Animals underwent closure of the trigone without a reconstructive procedure, underwent reconstruction with a cell-free bladder-shaped biodegradable matrix, or underwent reconstruction using a bladder-shaped biodegradable matrix that delivered autologous urothelial and smooth muscle cells. The cell populations had been separately expanded from a previously harvested autologous bladder biopsy. Preoperative and postoperative urodynamic, radiographic, gross, histologic, and immunocytochemical analyses were performed serially, at 1, 2, 3, 4, 6, and 11 months postoperatively (36).

The cystectomy only controls and polymer-only grafts maintained average capacities of 22% and 46% of preoperative values, respectively. An average bladder capacity of 95% of the original precystectomy volume was achieved in the tissue-engineered bladder replacements. These findings were confirmed radiographically. The subtotal cystectomy reservoirs, which were not reconstructed, and polymer-only reconstructed bladders showed a marked decrease in bladder compliance (10% and 42%). The compliance of the tissue-engineered bladders showed almost no difference from preoperative values that were measured when the native

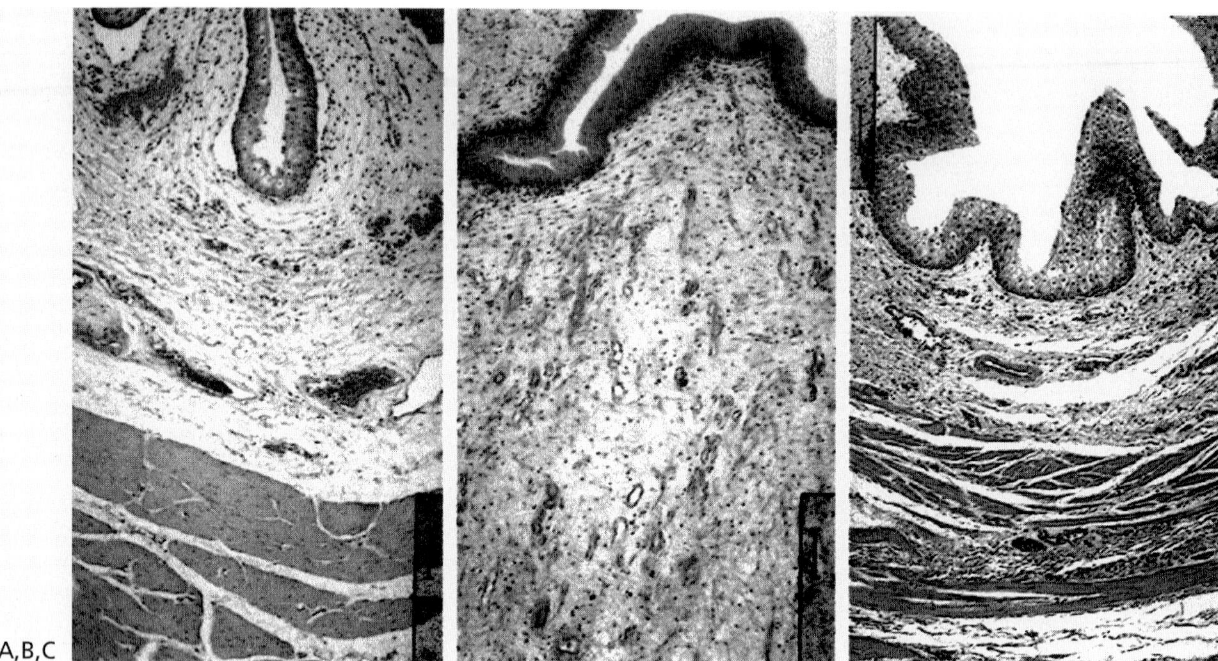

FIGURE 19.3. Hematoxylin and eosin histologic results 6 months after surgery (original magnification: ×250). **A:** Normal canine bladder. **B:** The bladder dome of the cell-free polymer reconstructed bladder consists of normal urothelium over a thickened layer of collagen and fibrotic tissue. Only scarce muscle fibers are apparent. **C:** The tissue-engineered neo-organ shows a histomorphologically normal appearance. A tri-layered architecture consisting of urothelium, submucosa, and smooth muscle is evident.

bladder was present (106%). Histologically, the polymer-only bladders presented a pattern of normal urothelial cells with a thickened fibrotic submucosa and a thin layer of muscle fibers. The retrieved tissue-engineered bladders showed a normal cellular organization, consisting of a trilayer of urothelium, submucosa, and muscle (Fig. 19.3). Immunocytochemical analyses for desmin, α-actin, cytokeratin 7, pancytokeratins AE1/AE3, and uroplakin III confirmed the muscle and urothelial phenotype. S-100 staining indicated the presence of neural structures. The results from this study showed that it is possible to tissue engineer bladders that are anatomically and functionally normal (36). Human bladders have been created using the same techniques.

Clinically, cells used for tissue engineering may be harvested from abnormal bladders. We investigated the contractility of tissue-engineered bladder smooth muscle derived from patients with functionally normal bladders and functionally abnormal neuropathic and exstrophic bladders (12). The tissue-engineered cells showed similar expression of smooth muscle marker proteins (α-actin and myosin) regardless of their origin. All scaffolds showed similar muscle formation and were α-actin positive. At retrieval, the muscle cell–seeded scaffolds exhibited contractile activity to electrical field stimulation and carbachol. There was no statistical difference between the three different types of muscle cells seeded (normal, neurogenic, exstrophic). The results of this study were also consistent with prior findings that, in diseased bladders, a large portion of the pathologic effects seen are due to increased fibrosis, whereas the cells retain their genetic stability.

Genital Tissues

Reconstructive surgery is required for a wide variety of pathologic penile conditions, such as penile carcinoma, trauma, severe erectile dysfunction, and congenital conditions like ambiguous genitalia, hypospadias, and epispadias. The creation of autologous functional and structural corporal tissue *de novo* would be beneficial clinically. Studies conducted in our laboratory showed that cultured human corporal smooth muscle cells may be used in conjunction with biodegradable polymers to create corpus cavernosum tissue *de novo*. The formation of normal corporal cavernosa tissue is enhanced with the addition of corporal endothelial cells (37,38).

Further studies show that it is possible to replace entire cross-sectional segments of both corporal bodies in the protruding penis *in vivo* by interposing autologous engineered tissue (39). Rabbits had a small corporal biopsy. Cavernosal smooth muscle and endothelial cells were harvested and expanded. Matrices were obtained using cell lysis techniques from donor penile tissues. Cavernosal smooth muscle and endothelial cells were seeded on the matrices. The entire cross section of the protruding rabbit phallus was excised, leaving the urethra intact. The experimental corporal bodies demonstrated intact structural integrity by cavernosography and only a slight decrease in pressure by cavernosometry when compared to the controls. Mating activity in the animals with the engineered corpora normalized by 3 months. Mating activity in the animals with the matrix alone was low throughout the study. The presence of sperm was confirmed during mating, and was present in all the rabbits with the engineered corpora but in only two with the matrix alone. Gross examination of the corporal implants with cells showed continuous integration of the graft into native tissue. The acellular matrices demonstrated the presence of fibrosis. Histologically, sinusoidal spaces and walls lined with endothelium and smooth muscle were observed in the engineered grafts. However, grafts without cells contained fibrotic tissue and calcifications with sparse corporal elements. Each cell type was identified immunocytochemically using antibodies to smooth muscle and endothelium. These studies demonstrate the possibility of engineering autologous penile corpora cavernosa tissue. The engineered tissue is able to achieve adequate structural and functional parameters. This technology may be potentially applicable to patients who require additional tissues for phallic reconstruction; however, additional studies involving larger phallic structures need to be completed. These studies are currently being performed in our laboratory.

Other alternative tissues are also being studied as possible replacements for silicone penile prostheses. Although silicone is an accepted biomaterial for penile prostheses, biocompatibility is a concern (40). The use of a natural prosthesis composed of autologous cells may be advantageous. A feasibility study for creating natural penile prostheses made of cartilage was performed (41). Cartilage, harvested from the articular surface of calf shoulders, was isolated, grown, and expanded in culture. The cells were seeded onto preformed cylindrical PGA polymer rods. The cell-polymer scaffolds were implanted in the subcutaneous space of athymic mice and retrieved up to 6 months postimplantation. At retrieval, the polymer scaffolds seeded with cells formed milky-white, rod-shaped, solid cartilaginous structures, maintaining their preimplantation size and shape. Biomechanical analyses showed that the engineered cartilage rods possessed the mechanical properties required to maintain penile rigidity. Histologic examination showed the presence of mature and well-formed cartilage.

In a subsequent study using an autologous system, the feasibility of applying the engineered cartilage rods *in situ* was investigated (42). Autologous chondrocytes harvested from rabbit ears were grown, expanded in culture, and seeded onto biodegradable polymer rods. The cell-polymer rods were implanted into the corporal spaces of rabbits. All animals tolerated the implants for the duration of the study (6 months) without any complications. Gross examination at retrieval showed the presence of well-formed milky-white cartilage structures within the corpora at 1 month. All polymers were fully degraded by 2 months. There was no evidence of erosion or infection in any of the implant sites. The animals could copulate and impregnate their female partners without problems.

We further investigated the feasibility of engineering biomechanically adequate large autologous human cartilage rods that could be used clinically as penile prostheses (43). Chondrocytes were isolated from human auricular cartilage and expanded *in vitro*. The chondrocytes were seeded onto preformed rod-shaped biodegradable polymer scaffolds (1.2 cm in diameter, 6.0 cm in length) and maintained in a cell culture bioreactor for 1 month. Subsequently, the cell-seeded scaffolds were implanted into the subcutaneous space of athymic rats. The cell-seeded scaffolds formed milky-white cartilaginous rods that maintained the same size and shape as the initial implants. Histologic analyses using hematoxylin and eosin, toluidine blue, and Alcian blue demonstrated mature and well-formed chondrocytes. Tensile tests showed that the engineered cartilaginous rods were readily elastic and could withstand high degrees of tensile force (1.78 ± 0.29 kg), which was not significantly different from the Jonas (2.64 ± 0.24 kg) or AMS 700 inflatable prostheses (2.35 ± 0.21 kg). Dynamic bending tests demonstrated that the cartilaginous rods were flexible and durable. None of the cartilage rods ruptured during the continuous strenuous mechanical tests. The results from the above studies demonstrate that autologous human auricular cartilage tissue can serve as a cell source for engineering cartilaginous penile prostheses. Clinically, a cartilage biopsy would be obtained from the patient's ear, and the cells would be expanded and seeded onto biodegradable rod-shaped scaffolds sized for the patient. One month after being in a bioreactor, the engineered cartilage rods could be implanted surgically into the patient. Further long-term functional studies are currently being performed to apply this technology to the clinical setting.

Kidney

Although the kidney was the first organ to be substituted by an artificial device and was the first successfully transplanted organ (1), current modalities of treatment are far from satisfactory. In addition to the inherent shortage of transplant organs, complications associated with renal transplantation are yet to be resolved. The kidney is probably the most challenging organ to reconstruct using tissue-engineering techniques in the genitourinary system owing to its complex structure and function. Extracorporeal assist devices may be improved by implanting isolated renal cell lines on bioartificial hemofilters (44). This may aid in the replacement of specific aspects of renal function, such as improved selected metabolic and endocrinologic parameters. Eventually, reconstruction of a tissue-engineered kidney by renal cell expansion *in vitro* and subsequent transplantation *in vivo* may be possible. To achieve this prospect, there are still many technical challenges to be solved.

The feasibility of achieving renal cell growth, expansion, and *in vivo* reconstitution using tissue-engineering techniques was explored in our laboratory. In one set of experiments, distal tubules, glomeruli, and proximal tubules from donor rabbit kidneys were plated separately *in vitro*, seeded onto biodegradable PGA polymer scaffolds, and implanted subcutaneously into host athymic mice. At retrieval, the scaffolds histologically showed progressive formation and organization of the nephron segments within the polymer fibers over time (45). To examine the tubular reconstitution process, nephron elements from animal kidneys were harvested and the cells were expanded *in vitro*, seeded on biodegradable polymers with a single-cell suspension, and reimplanted into syngeneic hosts (46). Sequential retrieval of the seeded polymers over time revealed that the renal epithelial cells first organized into a cord-like structure with a solid center. Subsequent canalization into a hollow tube could be seen by 2 weeks. Histologic examination with nephron segment–specific lectins showed successful reconstitution of proximal tubules, distal tubules, loops of Henle, collecting tubules, and collecting ducts.

In a third set of experiments, an attempt was made to harness the reconstitution of renal epithelial cells for the generation of functional nephron units. Renal cells were harvested and expanded in culture. The cells were seeded onto a tubular device constructed from a polycarbonate membrane, connected at one end with a silastic catheter, which terminated into a reservoir. The device was implanted in the subcutaneous space of athymic mice (47). Histologic examination of the implanted device revealed extensive vascularization, formation of glomeruli, and highly organized tubule-like structures. Immunocytochemical staining with anti-osteopontin antibody, which is secreted by proximal and distal tubular cells and the cells of the thin ascending loop of Henle, stained the tubular sections. Immunohistochemical staining for alkaline phosphatase stained proximal tubule-like structures. Uniform staining for fibronectin in the extracellular matrix of newly formed tubes was observed. Yellow fluid was collected from inside the implant, and uric acid and creatinine levels were determined. The fluid collected from the reservoir contained 66 mg/dL uric acid (as compared to 2 mg/dL in plasma). The creatinine assay performed on the collected fluid showed an 8.2-fold increase in concentration (27.91 ± 7.56 mg/dL), as compared to serum (4.49 ± 0.08 mg/dL). These results suggested that the reconstituted tubules are capable of unidirectional secretion and concentration of solutes. The fluid retrieved was consistent with the make-up of dilute urine, as evidenced by its creatinine and uric acid concentrations. Similar studies were performed with renal cells obtained through nuclear transfer (48). The renal cells were expanded, seeded onto polycarbonate membrane devices, and implanted into steers. The seeded constructs were able to form well-defined renal structures that secreted dilute urine. The retrieved structures demonstrated the presence of nephron units (Fig. 19.4).

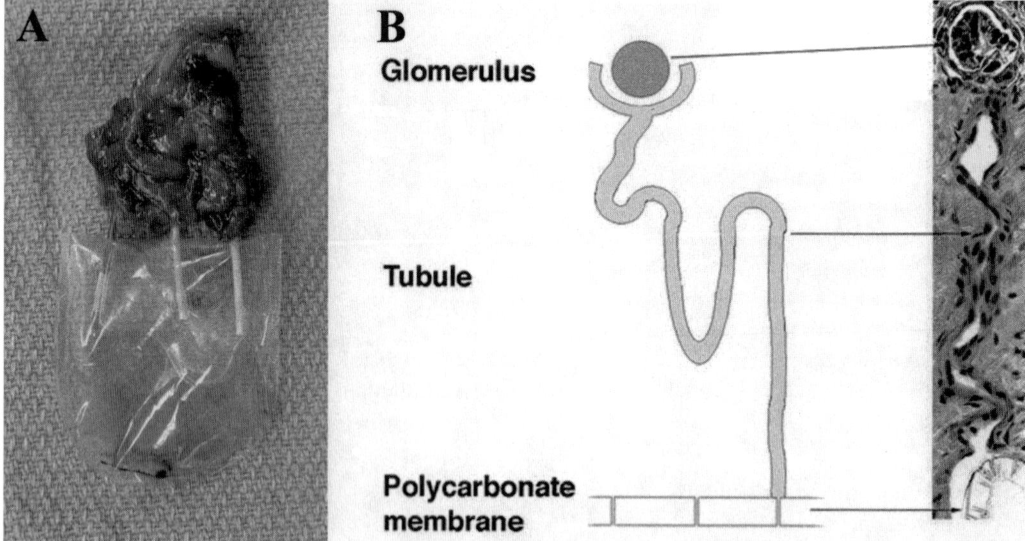

FIGURE 19.4. Tissue-engineered renal units. **A:** Retrieved tissue-engineered renal unit shows the excretion of yellow fluid in the reservoir. **B:** The engineered tissue showed a clear unidirectional continuity between the mature glomeruli, their tubules, and the reservoir. (See Color Plate 19.4.)

The results of these studies demonstrate that renal cells can be successfully harvested, expanded in culture, and implanted *in vivo*. The single cells form multicellular structures and become organized into functional renal units that are able to excrete high levels of solutes through a urine-like fluid. Further challenges await this technology, including the expansion of this system to larger three-dimensional structures.

Fetal Tissue Engineering

There are several strategies that may be pursued using today's technologic and scientific advances that may facilitate the future prenatal management of patients with urologic disease. Having a ready supply of urologic-associated tissue for surgical reconstruction at birth may be advantageous. Theoretically, once the diagnosis of the pathologic condition is confirmed prenatally, a small tissue biopsy could be obtained via ultrasound guidance. These biopsy materials could then be processed and the different cell types expanded *in vitro*. Using tissue-engineering techniques, reconstituted structures *in vitro* could then be readily available at the time of birth for reconstruction. Toward this end, a series of experiments were conducted using fetal lambs. Bladder exstrophy was created surgically in 90- to 95-day gestation fetal lambs. A small fetal bladder specimen was harvested via fetoscopy. The bladder specimen was separated, and muscle and urothelial cells were harvested and expanded separately. Seven to 10 days before delivery, the expanded bladder muscle cells were seeded on one side and the urothelial cells on the opposite side of a biodegradable polymer scaffold. After delivery, one-half of the lambs had surgical closure of their bladder using the tissue-engineered bladder tissue. No fetal bladder harvest was performed in the other lambs, and bladder exstrophy closure was performed using only the native bladder. Cystograms were performed 3 and 8 weeks after surgery. The engineered bladders were more compliant ($p = .01$) and had a higher capacity ($p = .02$) than the native bladder closure group (49). Similar prenatal studies were performed in lambs, engineering skin for reconstruction at birth. In addition to being able to manage the bladder exstrophy complex in utero with tissue-engineering techniques, one could also manage patients after birth in a similar manner whenever a prenatal diagnosis is not assured. In these instances, bladder tissue biopsies could be obtained at the time of the initial surgery. Different tissues could be harvested and stored for future reconstruction, if necessary.

Injectable Therapies

Both urinary incontinence and vesicoureteral reflux are common conditions affecting the genitourinary system, wherein injectable bulking agents can be used for treatment. The goal of several investigators has been to find alternate implant materials that would be safe for human use (50). Long-term studies were conducted to determine the effect of injectable chondrocytes *in vivo* (51). It was initially determined that alginate, a liquid solution of gluronic and mannuronic acid, embedded with chondrocytes, could serve as a synthetic substrate for the injectable delivery and maintenance of cartilage architecture *in vivo*. A biopsy of the ear could be easily and quickly performed, followed by chondrocyte processing and endoscopic injection of the autologous chondrocyte suspension for therapy.

Chondrocytes can be readily grown and expanded in culture. Neocartilage formation can be achieved *in vitro* and *in vivo* using chondrocytes cultured on synthetic biodegradable polymers (51). This system was adapted for the treatment of vesicoureteral reflux in a porcine model (52). Chondrocytes were harvested from the left auricular surface of surgically created refluxing mini-swine and expanded. The animals underwent endoscopic repair of reflux with the injectable autologous chondrocyte solution on the right side only. Serial cystograms showed no evidence of reflux on the treated side and persistent reflux in the uncorrected control ureter in all animals. The harvested ears had evidence of cartilage regrowth within 1 month of chondrocyte retrieval.

At the time of sacrifice, gross examination of the bladder injection site showed a well-defined rubbery to hard cartilage structure in the subureteral region. Histologic examination of these specimens showed evidence of normal cartilage formation. The polymer gels were progressively replaced by cartilage with increasing time. Aldehyde fuchsin–Alcian blue staining suggested the presence of chondroitin sulfate.

Using the same line of reasoning as with the chondrocyte technology, the possibility of using autologous muscle cells was also investigated (53). *In vivo* experiments were conducted in mini-pigs, and reflux was successfully corrected. In addition to its use for the endoscopic treatment of reflux and urinary incontinence, the system of injectable autologous cells may also be applicable for the treatment of other medical conditions, such as rectal incontinence, dysphonia, plastic reconstruction, and wherever an injectable permanent biocompatible material is needed.

Recently, the first human application of cell-based tissue-engineering technology for urologic applications has occurred with the injection of chondrocytes for the correction of vesicoureteral reflux in children (Fig. 19.5) and for urinary incontinence in adults. The clinical trials are currently ongoing (50,54–56).

The potential use of injectable, cultured myoblasts for the treatment of stress urinary incontinence has recently been investigated in preliminary experiments (57). Primary myoblasts obtained from mouse skeletal muscle were transduced *in vitro* to carry the β-galactosidase reporter gene and were then incubated with fluorescent microspheres that serve as markers for the original cell population. Cells were then directly injected into the proximal urethra and lateral bladder walls of nude mice with a microsyringe in an open

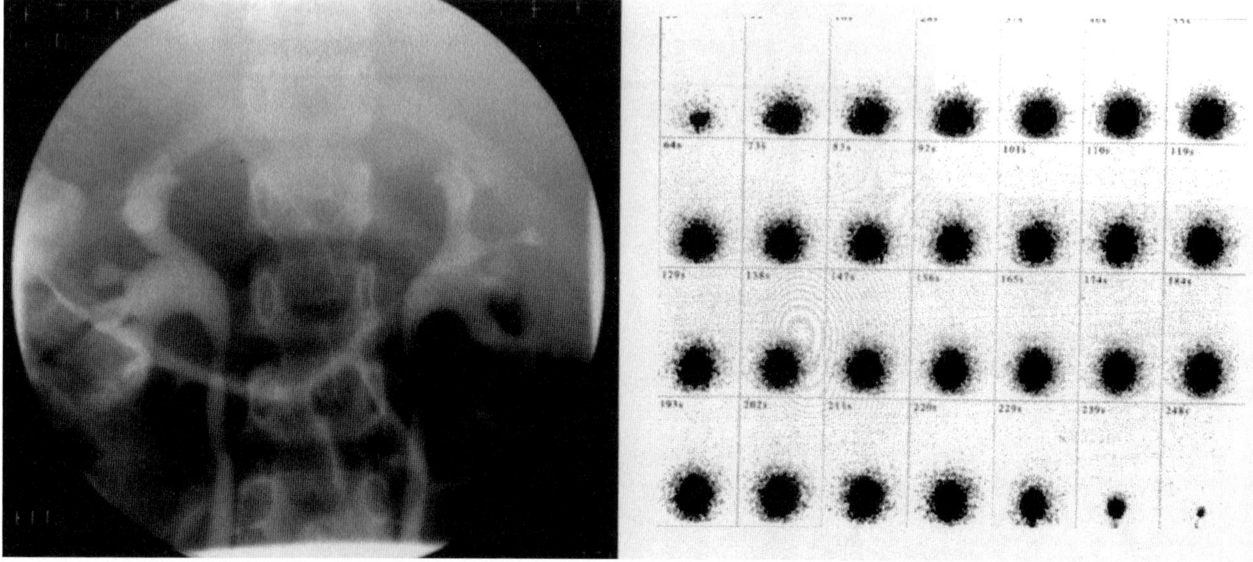

A,B

FIGURE 19.5. **A:** Preoperative voiding cystourethrogram of a patient showing bilateral reflux. **B:** Postoperative radionuclide cystogram of the same patient 6 months after the injection of autologous chondrocytes.

surgical procedure. Tissue was harvested up to 35 days postinjection, analyzed histologically, and assayed for β-galactosidase expression. Myoblasts expressing β-galactosidase and containing fluorescent microspheres were found at each of the retrieved time points. In addition, regenerative myofibers expressing β-galactosidase were identified within the bladder wall. By 35 days postinjection, some of the injected cells expressed the contractile filament a–smooth muscle actin, suggesting the possibility of myoblastic differentiation into smooth muscle. The authors reported that a significant portion of the injected myoblast population persisted *in vivo*. The fact that myoblasts can be transfected, survive after injection, and begin the process of myogenic differentiation further supports the feasibility of using cultured cells of muscular origin as an injectable bioimplant.

Testicular Hormonal Replacement

Leydig cells are the major source of testosterone production in males. Patients with testicular dysfunction require androgen replacement for somatic development. Conventional treatment for testicular dysfunction consists of periodic intramuscular injections of chemically modified testosterone or, more recently, of skin patch applications. However, long-term nonpulsatile testosterone therapy is not optimal and can cause multiple problems, including erythropoiesis and bone density changes.

A system was designed wherein Leydig cells were microencapsulated for controlled testosterone replacement. Microencapsulated Leydig cells offer several advantages, such as serving as a semipermeable barrier between the transplanted cells and the host's immune system, as well as allowing for the long-term physiologic release of testosterone.

Purified Leydig cells were isolated, characterized, suspended in an alginate solution, and extruded through an air jet nozzle into a 1.5% $CaCl_2$ solution in which they gelled and were further coated with 0.1% poly-L-lysine. The encapsulated cells were pulsed with human chorionic gonadotropin every 24 hours. The medium was sampled at different time points after human chorionic gonadotropin stimulation and analyzed for testosterone production. Cell viability was confirmed daily. The encapsulated Leydig cells were injected into castrated animals, and serum testosterone was measured serially. The castrated animals receiving the microencapsulated cells were able to maintain testosterone levels long term (58). These studies suggest that microencapsulated Leydig cells may be able to replace or supplement testosterone into situations in which anorchia or testicular failure is present. A similar system is currently being applied for estrogen.

Gene Therapy and Tissue Engineering

Genetically Engineered Cells

Cells can be engineered to secrete growth factors for various applications, such as for promoting angiogenesis for tissue regeneration. *Angiogenesis*, the process of new blood vessel formation, is regulated by different growth factors. These growth factors stimulate endothelial cells that are already present in the patient's body to migrate to the implanted area of need, where they proliferate and differentiate into blood vessels (59). One of the major molecules that promote and regulate angiogenesis is vascular endothelial growth factor (VEGF) (60). Several methods have been used experimentally to deliver VEGF *in vivo*. The growth factor protein can be directly injected into tissues (61); however, the rapid clearance of VEGF proteins from the vascular system limits its effect to only minutes. The VEGF gene could be delivered to tissues using various techniques; however, the transfection efficiency is low, the onset of action is delayed for up to 48 to 72 hours after the VEGF cDNA is incorporated, and the effect is transient, lasting only several days (61,62).

An approach that has been pursued in our laboratory to increase and stimulate rapid vascularization *in vivo* was to engineer a cell line to secrete high levels of VEGF proteins by gene transfecting the cells with the VEGF cDNA. The VEGF-secreting cells were encapsulated in polymeric microspheres. The microspheres would allow nutrients to reach the cells, while the VEGF proteins secreted from the cells diffused into the surrounding tissues. The microspheres protect the coated cells from the host immune environment. This novel system of neovascularization was tested *in vitro* and *in vivo* in an animal model. The degree of VEGF secretion and the period of delivery can be regulated by modulating the number of engineered cells that are encapsulated per microsphere, as well as the number of microspheres injected. A similar strategy has also been pursued for the genetic engineering of antiangiogenic factor–secreting cells (63). These strategies could be useful for antitumor therapy in urology.

Gene Therapy for Tissue-Engineered Constructs

Based on the feasibility of tissue-engineering techniques in which cells seeded on biodegradable polymer scaffolds form tissue when implanted *in vivo*, the possibility was explored of developing a neo-organ system for *in vivo* gene therapy (64). In a series of studies conducted in our laboratory, human urothelial cells were harvested, expanded *in vitro*, and seeded on biodegradable polymer scaffolds. The cell-polymer complex was then transfected with PGL3-luc, pCMV-luc, and pCMVβ-gal promoter-reporter gene constructs. The transfected cell-polymer scaffolds were then implanted *in vivo*, and the engineered tissues were retrieved at different time points after implantation. Results indicate that successful gene transfer may be achieved using biodegradable polymer scaffolds as a urothelial cell delivery vehicle. The transfected cell/polymer scaffold formed organ-like structures with functional expression of the transfected genes (64). This technology is applicable throughout the spectrum of diseases, which may be manageable with tissue engineering. For example, one can envision the use of effecting *in vivo* gene delivery through the *ex vivo* transfection of tissue-engineered cell/polymer scaffolds for the genetic modification of diseased corporal smooth muscle cells harvested from impotent patients. Theoretically, the *in vitro* genetic modification of corporal smooth muscle cells harvested from an impotent patient, resulting in either a reduction in the expression of the transforming growth factor-1 gene or the overexpression of genes responsible for prostaglandin E1 production, could lead to the resumption of erectile functionality once these cells were used to repopulate the diseased corporal bodies.

Stem Cells for Tissue Engineering

Most current strategies for engineering urologic tissues involve harvesting of autologous cells from the host diseased organ. However, in situations in which extensive end-stage organ failure is present, a tissue biopsy may not yield enough normal cells for expansion. Under these circumstances, the availability of pluripotent stem cells may be beneficial. Pluripotent embryonic stem cells are known to form teratomas *in vivo*, which are composed of a variety of differentiated cells. However, these cells may be immunocompetent and may require immunosuppression if used clinically.

The possibility of deriving pluripotent cells from postnatal mesenchymal tissue from the same host and inducing their differentiation *in vitro* and *in vivo* was investigated. Pluripotent cells were isolated from human foreskin-derived fibroblasts. Adipogenic, myogenic, and osteoblastic lineages were obtained from these progenitor cells. The cells were grown, expanded, seeded onto biodegradable scaffolds, and implanted *in vivo*, where they formed mature tissue structures. This was the first demonstration that stem cells can be derived from postnatal connective tissue and can be used for engineering tissues *in vivo ex situ* (65).

Therapeutic Cloning for Tissue Engineering

Recent advances with the cloning of embryos and newborn animals have expanded the possibilities of this technology for tissue engineering and organ transplantation. There are many ethical concerns with cloning in terms of creating humans for the sole purpose of obtaining organs. However, the potential for retrieving cells from early-stage cloned embryos for subsequent regeneration is being proposed as an ethically viable benefit of therapeutic cloning (Fig. 19.6). The feasibility of engineering syngeneic tissues *in vivo* using cloned cells was investigated.

Unfertilized donor bovine eggs were retrieved, and the nuclear material was removed. Bovine fibroblasts from the skin of a steer were obtained. The nuclear material was removed from the fibroblast and microinjected into the donor eggshell (nuclear transfer). A short burst of energy was delivered, initiating neo-embryogenesis. These techniques replicate what was performed to clone the first mammal—Dolly the sheep. However, instead of implanting the embryo into a uterus, the goal would be to harvest stem cells from the embryo, which was created not from the union of a sperm and an egg but rather

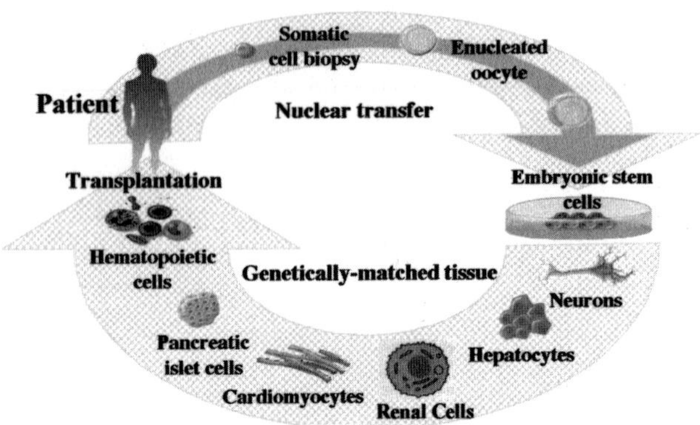

FIGURE 19.6. Schematic diagram of therapeutic cloning approach for the isolation of genetically matched tissues. (See Color Plate 19.6.)

from a skin cell and an eggshell, devoid of any genetic material. To achieve a proof of principle, bypassing the *in vitro* differentiation, the embryos were placed in the same steer uterus from which the fibroblasts had been obtained. The cloned embryo, with identical genetic material as the steer, was retrieved for tissue harvest. Various cell types were harvested, expanded *in vitro*, and seeded on biodegradable scaffolds. The cell-polymer scaffolds were implanted into the back of the same steer from which the cells were cloned. The implants were retrieved at various time points for analyses. Renal tissue, cardiac, and skeletal muscle were engineered successfully using therapeutic cloning.

These studies demonstrated that cells obtained through nuclear transfer can be successfully harvested, expanded in culture, and transplanted *in vivo* with biodegradable scaffolds in which the single suspended cells form and organize into tissue structures, which are the same genetically as the host. These studies were the first demonstration of the use of therapeutic cloning for the regeneration of tissues *in vivo* (48). One could envision taking one skin cell from a patient and having the ability to generate most types of tissues for replacement or transplantation, which would be genetically identical and fully biocompatible. Thus, each patient could conceivably have a ready-made supply of his or her own tissues available on demand.

CONCLUSION

Tissue-engineering efforts are currently being undertaken for every type of tissue and organ within the urinary system. Primary autologous cells, stem cells, and therapeutic cloning are being applied for the creation of tissues and organs. Tissue-engineering techniques require expertise in growth factor biology, a cell culture facility designed for human application, and personnel who have mastered the techniques of cell harvest, culture, and expansion. Polymer scaffold design and manufacturing resources are essential for the successful application of this technology.

The first human application of cell-based tissue engineering for urologic applications occurred at our institution with the injection of autologous cells for the correction of vesicoureteral reflux in children. The same technology has been recently expanded to treat adult patients with urinary incontinence. Trials involving urethral tissue replacement using processed collagen matrices are in progress at our center for both hypospadias and stricture repair. Bladder replacement using tissue-engineering techniques is being explored. Recent progress suggests that engineered urologic tissues may have a wider clinical applicability in regenerative medicine.

REFERENCES

1. Murray JE, Merrill JP, Harrison JH. Renal homotransplantation in identical twins. *Surg Form* 1955;6:432–436.
2. Atala A. Tissue engineering in the genitourinary system. In: Atala A, Mooney D, eds. *Tissue engineering.* Boston: Birkhauser Press, 1997:149.
3. Cilento BG, Freeman MR, Schneck FX, et al. Phenotypic and cytogenetic characterization of human bladder urothelia expanded in vitro. *J Urol* 1994;152:655.
4. Scriven SD, Booth C, Thomas DF, et al. Reconstitution of human urothelium from monolayer cultures. *J Urol* 1997;158 (3 Pt 2):1147–1152.
5. Liebert M, Wedemeyer G, Abruzzo LV, et al. Stimulated urothelial cells produce cytokines and express an activated cell surface antigenic phenotype. *Semin Urol* 1991;9(2):124–130.
6. Puthenveettil JA, Burger MS, Reznikoff CA. Replicative senescence in human uroepithelial cells. *Adv Exp Med Biol* 1999;462:83–91.
7. Pariente JL, Kim BS, Atala A. In vitro biocompatibility assessment of naturally-derived and synthetic biomaterials using normal human urothelial cells. *J Biomed Mat Res* 2001; 55:33–39.
8. Pariente JL, Kim BS, Atala A. In vitro biocompatibility evaluation of naturally derived and synthetic biomaterials using normal human bladder smooth muscle cells. *J Urol* 2002; 167:1867–1871.
9. Bazeed MA, Thüroff JW, Schmidt RA, et al. New treatment for urethral strictures. *Urology* 1983;21:53–57.
10. Olsen L, Bowald S, Busch C, et al. Urethral reconstruction with a new synthetic absorbable device. *Scand J Urol Nephrol* 1992;26:323–326.
11. Atala A, Vacanti JP, Peters CA, et al. Formation of urothelial structures in vivo from dissociated cells attached to biodegradable polymer scaffolds in vitro. *J Urol* 1992;148:658.
12. Lai JY, Yoon CY, Yoo JJ, et al. Phenotypic and functional characterization of in vivo tissue engineered smooth muscle from normal and pathological bladders. *J Urol* 2002;168: 1853–1858.
13. Sievert KD, Bakircioglu ME, Nunes L, et al. Homologous acellular matrix graft for urethral reconstruction in the rab-

bit: histological and functional evaluation. *J Urol* 2000; 163(6):1958–1965.

14. Chen F, Yoo JJ, Atala A. Acellular collagen matrix as a possible "off the shelf" biomaterial for urethral repair. *Urology* 1999;54:407–410.
15. Atala A, Guzman L, Retik A. A novel inert collagen matrix for hypospadias repair. *J Urol* 1999;162:1148–1151.
16. El-Kassaby EA, Retik A, Yoo J, et al. Urethral stricture repair with an off-the-shelf collagen matrix. *J Urol* 2003; 169:170–173.
17. DeFilippo RE, Yoo JY, Chen F, et al. Urethral replacement using cell-seeded tubularized collagen matrices. *J Urol* 2002; 168:1789–1793.
18. McDougal WS. Metabolic complications of urinary intestinal diversion. *J Urol* 1992;147:1199.
19. Blandy JP. Neal pouch with transitional epithelium and anal sphincter as a continent urinary reservoir. *J Urol* 1961; 86:749.
20. Blandy JP. The feasibility of preparing an ideal substitute for the urinary bladder. *Ann Royal Coll Surg* 1964;35:287.
21. Harada N, Yano H, Ohkawa T, et al. New surgical treatment of bladder tumors: mucosal denudation of the bladder. *Br J Urol* 1965;37:545.
22. Oesch I. Neourothelium in bladder augmentation. An experimental study in rats. *Eur Urol* 1988;14:328.
23. Salle J, Fraga C, Lucib A, et al. Seromuscular enterocystoplasty in dogs. *J Urol* 1990;144:454.
24. Cheng E, Rento R, Grayhack TJ, et al. Reversed seromuscular flaps in the urinary tract in dogs. *J Urol* 1994;152:2252.
25. Dewan PA. Autoaugmentation demucosalized enterocystoplasty. *World J Urol* 1998;16:255–261.
26. Gonzalez R, Buson H, Reid C, et al. Seromuscular colocystoplasty lined with urothelium (SCLU). Experimental in 16 patients. *Urology* 1995;45:124.
27. Atala A. Commentary on the replacement of urologic associated mucosa. *J Urol* 1995;156:338.
28. Atala A. Autologous cell transplantation for urologic reconstruction. *J Urol* 1998;159:2.
29. Tsuji I, Ishida H, Fujieda J. Experimental cystoplasty using preserved bladder graft. *J Urol* 1961;85:42.
30. Probst M, Dahiya R, Carrier S, et al. Reproduction of functional smooth muscle tissue and partial bladder replacement. *Br J Urol* 1997;79:505–515.
31. Yoo JJ, Meng, J, Oberpenning F, et al. Bladder augmentation using allogenic bladder submucosa seeded with cells. *Urology* 1998;51:221.
32. Sutherland RS, Baskin LS, Hayward SW, et al. Regeneration of bladder urothelium, smooth muscle, blood vessels, and nerves into an acellular tissue matrix. *J Urol* 1996; 156:571–577.
33. Kropp BP, Rippy MK, Badylak SF, et al. Small intestinal submucosa: urodynamic and histopathologic evaluation in long term canine bladder augmentations. *J Urol* 1996; 155:2098–2104.
34. Vaught JD, Kroop BP, Sawyer BD, et al. Detrusor regeneration in the rat using porcine small intestine submucosal grafts: functional innervation and receptor expression. *J Urol* 1996;155:374–378.
35. Atala A, Freeman MR, Vacanti JP, et al. Implantation in vivo and retrieval of artificial structures consisting of rabbit and human urothelium and human bladder muscle. *J Urol* 1993;150:608.
36. Oberpenning FO, Meng J, Yoo J, et al. De novo reconstitution of a functional urinary bladder by tissue engineering. *Nat Biotechnol* 1999;17:2.
37. Park HJ, Kershen R, Yoo J, et al. Reconstitution of human corporal smooth muscle and endothelial cells in vivo. *J Urol* 1999;162:1106–1109.
38. Kershen RT, Yoo JJ, Moreland RB, et al. Reconstitution of human corpus cavernosum smooth muscle in vitro and in vivo. *Tiss Eng* 2002;8:529–538.
39. Kwon TG, Yoo JJ, Atala A. Autologous penile corpora cavernosa replacement using tissue engineering techniques. *J Urol* 2002;168:1754–1758.
40. Thomalla JV, Thompson ST, Rowland RG, et al. Infectious complications of penile prosthetic implants. *J Urol* 1987; 138(1):65–67.
41. Yoo JJ, Lee I, Atala A. Cartilage rods as a potential material for penile reconstruction. *J Urol* 1998;160:1164.
42. Yoo J, Park H, Lee I, et al. Autologous engineered cartilage rods for penile reconstruction. *J Urol* 1999;162:1119–1121.
43. Kim BS, Yoo JJ, Atala A. Engineering of human cartilage rods: potential application for penile prostheses. *J Urol* 2002; 168:1794–1797.
44. Humes DH, Ceileski DA, Funke AJ. Cell therapy for erythropoietin (EPO) deficient anemias. *J Am Soc Nephrol* 1995; 6:535.
45. Atala A, Schlussel RN, Retik AB. Renal cell growth in vivo after attachment to biodegradable polymer scaffolds. *J Urol* 1995;153:4.
46. Fung LCT, Elenius K, Freeman M, et al. Reconstitution of EGFr-poor renal epithelial cells into tubular structures on biodegradable polymer scaffold. *Pediatrics* 1996;98(Suppl): S631.
47. Yoo JJ, Ashkar S, Atala A. Creation of functional kidney structures with excretion of urine-like fluid in vivo. *Pediatrics* 1996;98(Suppl):605.
48. Lanza RP, Chung HY, Yoo JJ, et al. Generation of histocompatible tissues using nuclear transplantation. *Nat Biotechnol* 2002;20:689–696.
49. Fauza DO, Fishman S, Mehegan K, et al. Videofetoscopically assisted fetal tissue engineering: bladder augmentation. *J Pediatr Surg* 1998;33:7.
50. Kershen RT, Atala A. Advances in injectable therapies for the treatment of incontinence and vesicoureteral reflux. *Urol Clin* 1999;26:81–94.
51. Atala A, Cima LG, Kim W, et al. Injectable alginate seeded with chondrocytes as a potential treatment for vesicoureteral reflux. *J Urol* 1993;150:745.
52. Atala A, Kim W, Paige KT, et al. Endoscopic treatment of vesicoureteral reflux with chondrocyte-alginate suspension. *J Urol* 1994;152:641.
53. Cilento BG, Atala A. Treatment of reflux and incontinence with autologous chondrocytes and bladder muscle cells. *Dial Pediatr Urol* 1995;18:11.
54. Diamond DA, Caldamone AA. Endoscopic correction of vesicoureteral reflux in children using autologous chondrocytes: preliminary results. *J Urol* 1999;162:1185.
55. Caldamone AA, Diamond DA. Long-term results of the endoscopic correction of vesicoureteral reflux in children

using autologous chondrocytes. *J Urol* 2001;165(6 Pt 2): 2224–2227.
56. Bent AE, Tutrone RT, McLennan MT, et al. Treatment of intrinsic sphincter deficiency using autologous ear chondrocytes as a bulking agent. *Neurourol Urodyn* 2001;20(2):157–165.
57. Yokoyama T, Chancellor MB, Watanabe T, et al. Primary myoblasts injection into the urethra and bladder as a potential treatment of stress urinary incontinence and impaired detrusor contractility; long term survival without significant cytotoxicity. *J Urol* 1999;161:307.
58. Machlouf M, Orsola A, Atala A. Controlled release of therapeutic agents: slow delivery and cell encapsulation. *World J Urol* 2000;18:80–83.
59. Polverini PJ. The pathophysiology of angiogenesis. *Crit Rev Oral Biol Med* 1996;6:230.
60. Klagsbrun M, D'Amore PA. Regulation of angiogenesis. *Ann Rev Physiol* 1991;53:217.
61. Bauters C, Asahara T, Zheng LP, et al. Physiological assessment of augmented vascularity induced by VEGF in ischemic rabbit hindlimb. *Am J Physiol* 1994;267:263.
62. Takeshita S, Tsurumi Y, Couffinahl T, et al. Gene transfer of naked DNA encoding for three isoforms of vascular endothelial growth factor stimulates collateral development in vivo. *Lab Invest* 1996;75:487.
63. Joki T, Machluf M, Atala A, et al. Continuous release of endostatin from microencapsulated engineered cells for tumor therapy. *Nat Biotechnol* 2001;19(1):35–39.
64. Yoo JJ, Atala A. A novel gene delivery system using urothelial tissue engineered neo-organs. *J Urol* 1997;158:1066–1070.
65. Bartsch GC, Yoo JJ, De Coppi P, et al. Dermal stem cells for pelvic and bladder reconstruction. *J Urol* 2002;167:59a.

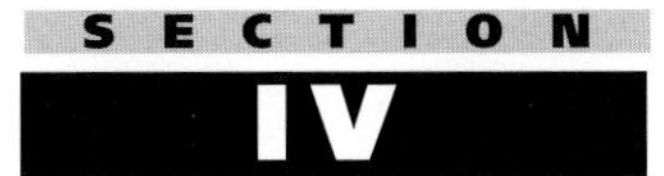

CLINICAL METHODS

20

CLINICAL EVALUATION

T. MARTIN BARRATT
PATRICK NIAUDET

Section IV is concerned with methods for evaluating children with kidney disease. This chapter addresses their presentation, the relevant features in their clinical history, and the findings to be sought on physical examination. This wide canvas is illustrated by didactic algorithms and frequent reference to other chapters in the book rather than by conventional citations of the medical literature, and we have drawn on our personal experience in the selection of material presented.

The clinical evaluation should follow the classic path of history, physical examination, and urinalysis, leading to a problem list with differential diagnoses, plan of investigation, and proposals for immediate management. It must, however, be modified to take into account the age of the child, the socioeconomic circumstances and medical resources available, the local epidemiology of renal disease, and the mode of presentation of the problem.

The proper recording of the clinical findings in the medical notes is essential for the management of the case, audit, retrospective review, and medicolegal purposes. It is the duty of the medical staff to maintain accurate records and of the clinical director of the service to ensure that this is done.

AGE AND RENAL DISEASE

The span of pediatric nephrology runs from conception to adolescence. At one end there is an overlap of responsibility with the geneticist and obstetrician, at the other with the "adult" nephrologist, and throughout with the pediatric urologist.

Fetus

The risk of inherited renal disease in the child may be evident from the family history, and several techniques are available for confirming the diagnosis in early pregnancy (see Chapter 21).

Structural malformations of the fetal kidneys or urinary tract are frequently revealed by the midtrimester maternal ultrasound scan that is part of routine obstetric care and is now the most common route for infants to reach pediatric urologic services (see Chapter 4). Some abnormalities such as unilateral hydronephrosis are relatively minor; others like renal agenesis or severe bladder outflow obstruction are accompanied by oligohydramnios, a consequence of intrauterine renal failure, and pulmonary hypoplasia (the Potter sequence) (see Chapter 5).

Neonates

Congenital renal abnormalities and inherited disorders are present at birth but may not be immediately apparent, in part because the placenta is an efficient excretory organ masking renal failure and in part because the low glomerular filtration rate of the neonatal kidney may conceal genetically determined disorders of renal tubular function. The congenital nephrotic syndrome is present *in utero*: Affected infants are edematous at birth and have a high placenta/body weight ratio (see Chapter 25). Polycystic kidneys, particularly the autosomal recessive variety, are easily palpable (see Chapter 36).

Congenital abnormalities such a posterior urethral valve may be missed in a midtrimester scan and present in the neonatal period with urinary retention and overflow. Urologic malformations may be associated with absent abdominal wall muscles and undescended testicles. Congenital abnormalities in other systems may suggest a syndrome with renal involvement (see Chapter 6).

The immaturity of glomerular and tubular function in the neonate is exaggerated in the premature infant, predisposing them to acidosis and hyponatremia. Perinatal crises may be associated with renal venous thrombosis, characterized by hematuria, firm enlarged kidneys, and renal failure (see Chapter 64). A urinary tract infection (UTI) may be a pointer to an underlying urologic abnormality.

Children

The clinical evaluation of young children requires special pediatric skills. They cannot articulate their symptoms: A

UTI may present as fever or vomiting (see Chapter 53) and chronic renal failure (CRF) as failure to thrive. The presentation of renal disease in older children is similar to adults, but it must be remembered that growth failure may be a pointer to occult renal disease (see Chapter 22). The psychosocial problems of chronic renal disease may be particularly troublesome in adolescents, and the possibility of noncompliance with therapy must be borne in mind.

SOCIAL AND ECONOMIC CIRCUMSTANCES

The clinical practice of pediatric nephrology described in this book is largely derived from and in reality only applicable to the 10% of the World's children who inhabit the industrialized countries of what might be called (without entering the political debate) the *Developed World* (see Chapter 75A). Three patterns can be discerned on the basis of the development of the specialty itself and the availability of renal replacement therapy for children. In the *Developed World* there are approximately one to two pediatric nephrologists per million total population, and renal transplantation is available for all children for whom it is clinically appropriate; in the *Developing World*, such services are patchy, and in the *Underdeveloped World* they are inappropriate in relation to the other medical needs of children.
The sick in poor countries are doubly disadvantaged: The gross national product is low, and a smaller proportion of it is made available for health care. Medical equipment and drugs are expensive, access to medical centers for children in rural communities is difficult, and civil war may disrupt services.

Children fare badly in the competition with adults for limited resources. Those with renal disease may be lost among the many who die from malnutrition and diarrhea: They tolerate salt and water depletion poorly. Protein-calorie malnutrition predisposes to postinfectious glomerulonephritis, aggravates the edema of the nephrotic syndrome, and is a major factor in the growth failure of CRF (see Chapter 68).

EPIDEMIOLOGY

There are considerable differences in the pattern of renal disease in children around the world. A major distinction exists between tropical and temperate regions, arising from racial variations in the susceptibility to renal disease, compounded by the socioeconomic factors described earlier. Thus, sickle cell nephropathy is restricted to Afro-Caribbean children, whereas vesicoureteric reflux (VUR) and associated UTI are more common in white children. The high incidence of glomerulonephritis in children in tropical countries is related to frequent bacterial and viral infections, and human immunodeficiency virus nephropathy is emerging as a major problem (see Chapter 51).

PRESENTATION

A renal or urologic disorder may present with symptoms such as hematuria or dysuria, obviously pointing to the urinary tract, or the kidneys may be involved as part of a more widespread syndrome (e.g., systemic lupus erythematosus). Similarly, a disordered pattern of micturition or change in urine volume or composition may indicate renal pathology. However, serious renal disease may be present without any symptoms at all or be associated with symptoms and signs that do not point directly to the urinary tract.

Abnormalities of Urine Appearance

Hematuria

The addition of even small amounts of blood to urine results in obvious macroscopic hematuria (Fig. 20.1). However, apparently clear urine may contain an abnormal number of red blood cells (RBCs), referred to as *microscopic hematuria*. If the bleeding is brisk, the urine will be red and may even contain clots, but usually the pigment changes to the more brown color of acid hematin. The presence of blood in the urine should be confirmed by dipstick testing with Hemastix (Bayer Diagnostics, Pittsburgh) (see Hemastix). Microscopy will distinguish hematuria from hemoglobinuria and myoglobinuria, which are also characterized by dark brown Hemastix-positive urine but without RBCs.

Bleeding may originate from the glomeruli or from the urinary tract: A distinction may be made by careful microscopy of the urine, with "glomerular hematuria" being characterized by deformed, misshapen RBCs. Red cell casts and proteinuria also point to a glomerular origin, but a urologic disorder, particularly tumor, hydronephrosis, or stone, must always be ruled out by careful ultrasound examination, even if there is obvious evidence of glomerular disease (see Chapters 57 and 58). Hematuria may be associated with hypercalciuria even without evident calculi. Blood in the initial part of the urinary stream suggests a urethral origin of the bleeding; terminal hematuria, particularly if associated with suprapubic pain or a disturbance of micturition, points to a bladder cause requiring investigation by cystourethroscopy. However, in most affected children, hematuria has its origin in the upper urinary tract, and endoscopy is not necessary as a routine investigation unless other features suggestive of lower tract pathology accompany the bleeding.

If the hematuria is persistent and accompanied by heavy proteinuria or reduced renal function, it is usually necessary to proceed to renal biopsy to determine the glomerular lesion. Recurrent episodes of isolated macroscopic hematuria with normal urine in between are usually benign and suggestive of immunoglobulin A nephropathy (see Chapter 31). Persistent microscopic hematuria, particularly with a suggestive family history, should prompt

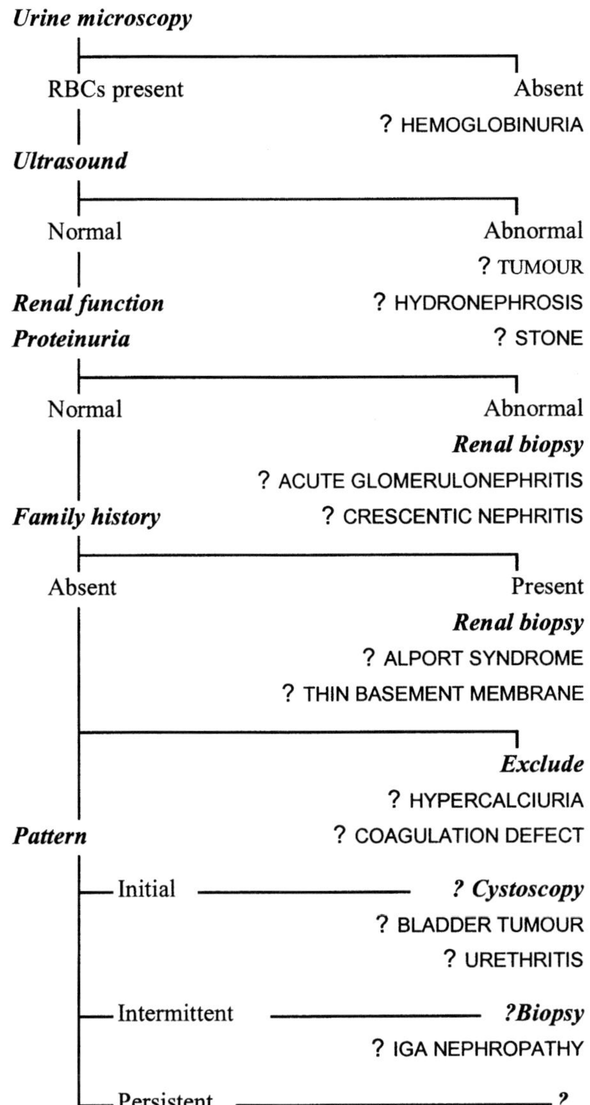

FIGURE 20.1. Hematuria. (Hemastix + ve.) RBC, red blood cell.

urine screening of all first-degree relatives and is best evaluated by renal biopsy, provided full facilities for its evaluation (including electron microscopy) are available (see Chapters 24 and 26).

Cloudy, Offensive Urine

Cloudy, offensive urine suggests a UTI, particularly if associated with local symptoms of dysuria and frequency or systemic symptoms of fever and loin pain, although significant bacteriuria may be asymptomatic (see Chapter 53) (Fig. 20.2). However, normal concentrated urine, when cooled, will form a precipitate of calcium phosphate; conversely, significant bacteriuria may be present without obvious macroscopic abnormality of the urine. Microscopy and culture of a properly collected and processed urine sample are essential in making the diagnosis of UTI, and screening tests are unreliable. Children with a proven UTI should have a careful abdominal ultrasound examination to exclude a urologic abnormality; boys and younger girls or those with recurrent UTI may require a cystogram to exclude VUR or other lower urinary tract abnormality. If VUR is present, a technetium-99m dimercaptosuccinic acid is the most sensitive method for determining the extent of associated renal scarring, but there is currently debate about protocols for the investigation of children with UTI (see Chapters 23, 53, and 54).

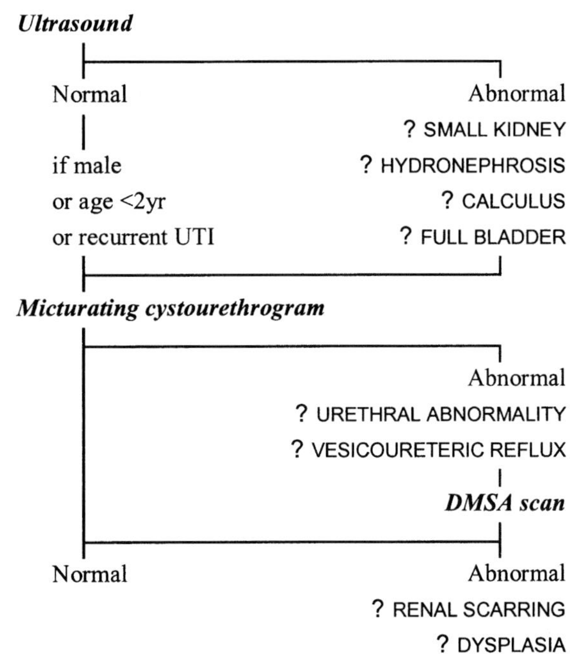

FIGURE 20.2. Urinary tract infection (UTI). (Hemastix + ve.) DMSA, dimercaptosuccinic acid.

Stone

The passage of a stone is an unusual event in childhood (see Chapter 57) (Fig. 20.3). Renal calculi may cause hematuria or UTI and, if obstructive, renal colic. They may consist of calcium salts (phosphates or oxalates), struvite (the triple salt of magnesium, ammonium, and phosphate with organic matrix), cystine, uric acid, or rarely one of the other purines (xanthine or dihydroxyadenine). In the United Kingdom, the most common variety is struvite, typically found in the upper urinary tract of young boys with a UTI caused by *Proteus*. In the United States, the most common variety is calcium-containing stones in older children living in the "stone belt." Children with renal calculi, especially if associated with nephrocalcinosis, require full investigation to rule out an underlying metabolic cause, particularly distal

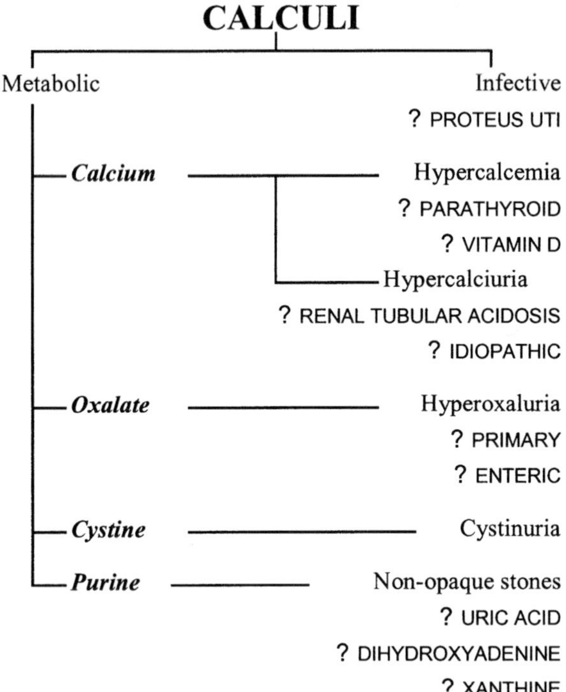

FIGURE 20.3. Calculi. UTI, urinary tract infection.

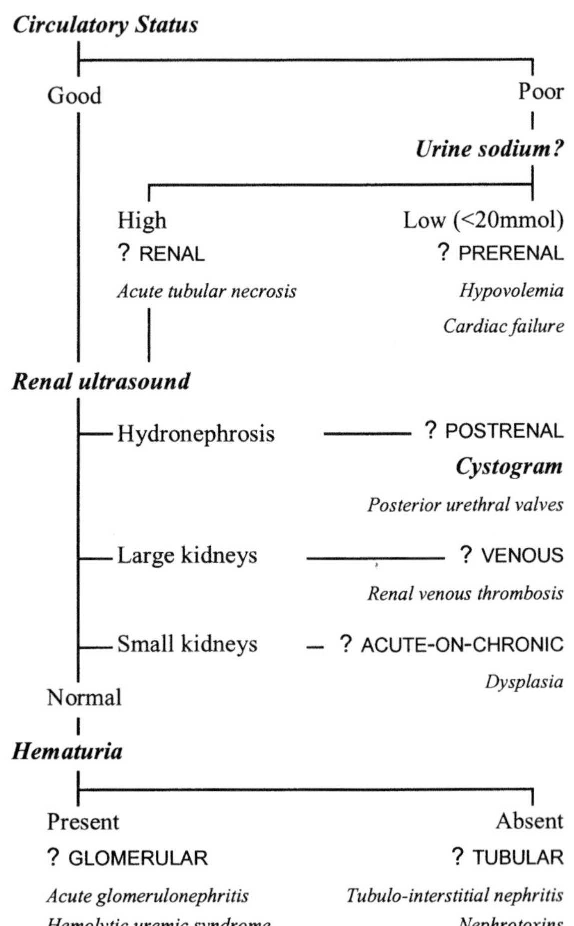

FIGURE 20.4. Acute renal failure. Oliguria <500 mL/1.73 m^2 SA/24 hr.

renal tubular acidosis (see Chapter 39) and primary hyperoxaluria (see Chapter 42). By comparison with adults, primary hyperparathyroidism is rare.

Abnormalities of Urine Volume

Oligoanuria

Anuria is the complete suppression of urine; oliguria is the passage of an insufficient volume to maintain homeostasis, usually taken to be less than 500 mL/24 hr/1.73 m^2 surface area, which in infants approximates 1.0 mL/hr/kg body weight. Urine volume in breast-fed, full-term babies averages 20 mL/24 hr in the first 2 days of life, rising to 200 mL by the tenth day. In newborn infants, 92% pass urine in the first 24 hours, and 98% do so within the first 48 hours of birth (see Chapter 56). Oliguria with acute renal failure may represent the physiologic response of a healthy kidney to inadequate perfusion ("prerenal"), parenchymal renal disease ("renal"), or obstruction of the urinary tract ("postrenal") (Fig. 20.4) (see Chapter 64).

Polyuria

Polyuria results from an excessive intake of fluid, a failure of release of antidiuretic hormone, osmotic diuresis, or renal resistance to the action of antidiuretic hormone (see Chapter 40) (Fig. 20.5). The distinction between primary polydipsia and primary polyuria may be inferred from the relative osmolality of plasma and urine and the response to controlled water deprivation. The distinction between pituitary and renal causes of polyuria may be made by the plasma arginine–vasopressin concentration and the urinary response to des-D-amino-arginine vasopressin.

A defect of urine concentration should be suspected in any infant with unexplained irritability, failure to thrive, fever, dehydration, or hypernatremia. Older children are more likely to have nocturnal enuresis accompanied by a clear history of polyuria and polydipsia. However, it is difficult to define the threshold of polyuria with accuracy, but it is usually not apparent as an isolated clinical symptom unless the urine is persistently hypotonic to plasma. Under these circumstances there is increased thirst, and infants in particular are at risk of dehydration. The principal renal diseases that result in antidiuretic hormone–resistant polyuria of this severity are nephrogenic diabetes insipidus (see Chapter 40), cystinosis (see Chapter 41), Bartter's syndrome (see Chap-

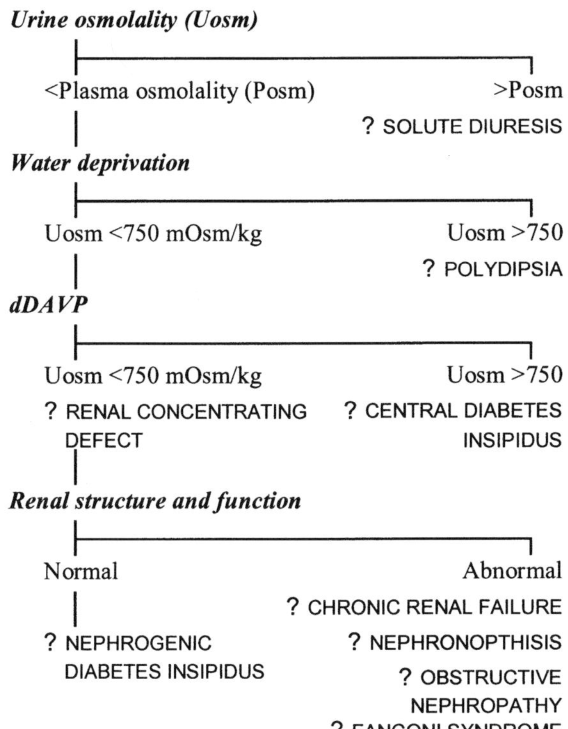

FIGURE 20.5. Polyuria (>200 mL/1.73 m^2 SA/24 hrs). dDAVP, des-D-amino-arginine vasopressin.

ter 38), obstructive nephropathy (see Chapter 55), and juvenile nephronophthisis (see Chapter 35).

Abnormalities of Micturition

Incontinence and Enuresis

Daytime urinary continence usually is achieved by 3 years of age (see Chapter 56). At the age of 5 years, approximately 15% of children wet the bed at night, falling to approximately 7% at 10 years. Nocturnal enuresis on its own is usually a benign self-limiting condition, whereas incontinence by day is commonly a behavioral problem. The development of incontinence in a child who has previously been dry raises the possibility of either organic disease or a psychological disturbance. Diurnal incontinence requires careful evaluation for the possibility of a neuropathic bladder, especially if associated with chronic constipation. Persistent dribbling incontinence associated with otherwise apparently normal micturition suggests an ectopic ureter opening below the bladder neck.

Giggle incontinence is usually a complaint of girls and younger women and is often associated with urgency. The definition is implicit in the name and is often a pointer to an unstable bladder with inappropriate detrusor contractions during filling. Younger girls with this complaint may squat on their heels to prevent voiding, a trick known as Saint Vincent's curtsy.

Poor Urinary Stream

Infrequent or difficult micturition may indicate inadequate bladder contraction or a functional failure of coordination between detrusor contraction and sphincter relaxation, suggesting a neuropathic bladder. A poor urinary stream in a male infant, particularly if associated with a full bladder, strongly suggests an obstructive pathology such as a posterior urethral valve. Observation of the urinary stream is an essential part of the physical examination of a child suspected of having a disorder of the urinary tract. Urinary retention is an uncommon problem in childhood and demands urgent and expert urologic attention to exclude a congenital anomaly, neuropathic bladder, tumor, or stone.

Frequency and Dysuria

Children of both genders between 5 and 14 years of age pass urine approximately four to eight times per day. Increased urinary frequency is seldom a primary complaint and is usually associated with other symptoms, such as urgency. An increased frequency of micturition may be due to polyuria, a reduced bladder capacity, or, most commonly, bladder irritability as with a UTI. Painful passage of urine (dysuria) usually indicates urethritis or cystitis secondary to UTI, but dysuria may also be a consequence of vulvovaginitis in girls and balanitis in boys.

Abnormalities of Hydration

Dehydration

Pure water depletion, resulting, for example, from defects in urine concentration, is associated, particularly in infants, with feeding difficulties and fever. If there is no concomitant salt depletion, there will be hypernatremia. The extracellular fluid (ECF) volume may be relatively well maintained, with the brunt of the fluid depletion being borne by the intracellular fluid (ICF) compartment, in which case the principal symptom is thirst. With salt depletion as well, ECF volume is depleted, resulting in hypotension and sensations of faintness and fatigue. Chronic salt-wasting is often associated with an increased salt appetite and a preference for savory rather than sweet foods (see Chapter 7).

Edema

ECF expansion results in edema, often first evident as swelling of the eyelids and sometimes mistaken for an allergic phenomenon; more generalized edema is characterized by pitting of the legs and abdominal swelling caused by ascites (Fig. 20.6). There are two distinct renal mechanisms of edema formation. In the first, characteristic of the acute nephritic syndrome and renal failure, a primary failure to excrete salt and water results in edema accompanied by expansion of the intravascular volume, hypertension, and

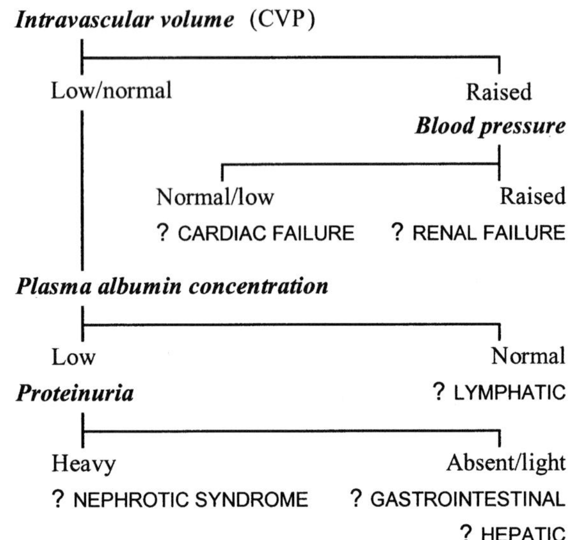

FIGURE 20.6. Edema. CVP, central venous pressure.

pulmonary congestion (see Chapter 30). In the second, as in the nephrotic syndrome, edema results from hypoproteinemia, the diminished colloid osmotic pressure of plasma leading to seepage of fluid from the intravascular into the interstitial compartment, with contraction of the plasma volume secondarily causing salt and water retention. In the nephrotic syndrome, there is also evidence for a primary increase in distal tubular sodium reabsorption. Hypoproteinemic edema is more gravity dependent than the edema of renal failure and may be accompanied by the symptoms of faintness and abdominal pain attributable to hypovolemia (see Chapter 27). The distinction between the edema of the acute nephritic syndrome, with its accompanying hematuria and hypertension, and the nephrotic syndrome is usually straightforward, but intermediate cases occur.

General Symptoms

Malaise

The symptoms associated with uremia are vague ill health, lassitude, anorexia, and vomiting. It is now rare for a child to reach such a condition without having come to medical attention, but an occasional case presenting as acute renal failure will in fact be found to have CRF. Anemia may contribute to the symptomatology, as attested by the improvement in general well-being with erythropoietin therapy.

Growth Failure

Children with CRF and some renal tubular disorders grow poorly and may indeed present with this problem. The causes are numerous and their interaction complex: poor calorie intake, acidosis, uncontrolled osteodystrophy, anemia, chronic salt and water depletion, and uremia per se, as well as (in some cases) a disordered pattern of growth hormone release (see Chapters 67 and 68). CRF may be overlooked as a cause of growth failure in young children because the plasma creatinine concentration may not be significantly elevated if muscle bulk is poor.

Gastrointestinal Problems

Feeding difficulties, vomiting, and anorexia dominate the clinical picture of CRF in young children. Again, the situation is complex: There is a disturbance of foregut motor function, often with gastroesophageal reflux; taste sensation is disturbed, leading to anorexia because of chronic salt and water depletion; and there may well have been a seriously disturbed weaning period. These factors combine to produce a situation in which inadequate caloric intake becomes a major factor in the failure to grow.

Asymptomatic Presentation

Renal disease is often asymptomatic, only coming to light as a consequence of routine examination or screening programs. This has led to various proposals for population screening. However, the issue is complicated because it can be assumed neither that the natural history of a disorder detected in this way is necessarily the same as one that presented symptomatically nor that it requires the same protocol of investigation and treatment.

Antenatal Ultrasound

The routine use of diagnostic ultrasound in pregnancy has led to the detection of urologic abnormality in many fetuses (see Chapter 4). The most common abnormality detected is simple hydronephrosis caused by presumed pelviureteric junction obstruction, followed by multicystic dysplastic kidney. Bilateral renal dysplasia or agenesis associated with oligohydramnios may be detected, and severe infravesical obstruction has led to attempts of uncertain benefit to drain the urinary tract *in utero*. However, the antenatal diagnosis of posterior urethral valves may be missed unless a scan is undertaken late in pregnancy. There is still much to be learned about the natural history and implications for postnatal investigation and management of urologic disorders diagnosed antenatally.

Routine Neonatal Examination

The routine examination of the neonate should include abdominal palpation, which may reveal evidence of renal disease (e.g., a palpable bladder or renal masses caused by hydronephrosis, cystic disease, venous thrombosis, or tumor). Renal agenesis or severe dysplasia should be suspected if there is a history of oligohydramnios associated with compression deformities [e.g., crumpled ears, Potter's facies, talipes, dislocated hips, or pulmonary hypoplasia (sometimes with pneumothorax)] (see Chapter 5). An absence of abdominal wall muscles (prune belly syndrome) is associated with bilateral cryptorchidism and a wide range of urologic abnormalities. There is an increased incidence of renal anomalies in association with other congenital defects, particularly those of the cardiovascular system, gastrointestinal tract (especially imperforate anus), and genitalia (see Chapter 6).

Urine Screening Programs

Because of the association between UTI, VUR, and renal scarring, a large number of studies have been directed at the role of screening for bacteriuria to prevent renal damage. Because some 5% of schoolgirls will at some stage develop bacteriuria, the yield of such surveys is large. However, it is by no means established that the widespread application of screening will reduce the incidence of end-stage renal failure. Regular urinalysis of school children is practiced in Japan (see Chapter 75C).

Family Studies

The diagnosis of an inherited disorder in a child, particularly if dominant or X-linked, should lead to a review of the extended family, which may identify several individuals previously unaware of having a renal abnormality. This raises ethical problems (see Chapter 18).

Routine Biochemical Evaluation

The kidney is involved in a wide variety of multisystem disorders, and, with the modern generation of multichannel biochemical analyzers, the serendipitous discovery of renal disease in a sick child is now not an uncommon occurrence.

HISTORY

Family History

A detailed family history is an essential part of the clinical evaluation because it may well provide an important clue to the diagnosis. Genetic factors are relevant in a wide variety of renal diseases such as inherited disorders of renal tubular function, familial glomerulonephritis, and cystic disease of the kidneys. The relevance may not be immediately obvious. Knowledge of the genetic abnormality carries implications for counseling the family. It is good practice to obtain the family tree for the case records.

A clue to dominantly inherited conditions may sometimes come from minor abnormalities in a parent: the diagnosis of autosomal dominant polycystic kidney disease may only become clear when the parents have had an ultrasound, and a family history of diabetes in a child with cystic kidneys may be a pointer to a hepatocyte nuclear factor-1β mutation (see Chapter 36).

Disorders transmitted as autosomal recessive traits are usually readily apparent and should be considered if there is parental consanguinity. They may have escaped notice if the expression of the disease is mild, as in some cases of recessive polycystic kidney disease, or in the early stages (e.g., in younger siblings of patients with juvenile nephronophthisis or familial idiopathic nephrotic syndrome).

Clues to X-linked recessive disorders may sometimes only be revealed on inquiry into the history of previous generations, such as the loss of the male infant relative of a mother of a child with nephrogenic diabetes insipidus or a male relative with deafness and renal failure in an Alport kindred (see Chapter 26).

Polygenic inheritance, genetic heterogeneity, or incomplete penetrance of a dominant gene may be operative in the etiology of VUR, with at least 10% of first-degree relatives being affected (see Chapter 54).

Obstetric and Neonatal History

The role of antenatal ultrasonography in the detection of urologic abnormalities and oligohydramnios is described earlier. An edematous or hypertrophied placenta, more than 25% of the child's birth weight, is a feature of the congenital nephrotic syndrome (see Chapter 25). Perinatal asphyxia, particularly if associated with macroscopic hematuria, may have been responsible for renal venous thrombosis and should be considered in the differential diagnosis of an older child with renal scarring, particularly if there is no suggestion of VUR.

General Medical History

Because the kidney or urinary tract is commonly involved in syndromes of congenital malformation or multisystem disorders, attention must be paid to all aspects of the child's medical history. Consultation with the department of otolaryngology for a deaf child may point to Alport's or the branchiootorenal syndromes; at the ophthalmology department, a diagnosis of retinitis pigmentosa may suggest Laurence-Moon-Biedl syndrome or juvenile nephronophthisis. The orthopedic department may be involved because of bony deformity as a result of osteodystrophy; slipped femoral capital epiphysis; or Perthes' disease, which is more common with renal abnormalities even without renal failure. Renal involvement may be part of a multisystem disorder, such as systemic lupus erythematosus, juvenile rheumatoid arthritis, or other vasculitic disorders (see Chapter 46). Drug nephrotoxicity may arise in many different groups of patients, particularly from antimicrobials, diuretics, and anticancer drugs (see Chapter 52). In a major children's hospital, the nephrologist may be as much involved with internal as with external referrals and must be familiar with the renal complications of systemic disorders and iatrogenic problems.

Urine and Micturition

A micturition history with specific detail about urinary stream is essential. The ages at which daytime and nocturnal urinary continence were achieved should be documented. A history of hematuria or features suggesting UTI may be relevant to the current renal problem.

Dietary History

A review of nutrition and feeding problems, beginning with the neonatal period, should be undertaken: whether the child was breast- or bottle-fed, episodes of vomiting or anorexia, thirst, or dietary preferences. Chronic salt-wasting, a feature of CRF, is commonly associated with an increased salt appetite and a preference for savory rather than sweet foods. For children with growth retardation or renal failure, a formal assessment of protein, energy, and other nutrient intake should be undertaken by a dietitian skilled in the management of problems of renal disease in childhood (see Chapter 67).

Gastrointestinal Symptoms

A prodrome of diarrhea strongly suggests infection with a verotoxin-producing *Escherichia coli* as the cause of hemolytic uremic syndrome (see Chapter 47).

Psychosocial Review

Many children with renal disease come from families with severe social problems. Some disorders (e.g., nephritis secondary to skin sepsis) are more common in deprived social classes. However, more important is the effect that social circumstances have on the ability of the family to cope with such minor symptoms as enuresis or to participate in the major upheaval of a renal replacement program. The involvement of a skilled social worker is essential in all cases. The commitment of the family to the child must be assessed. If the disease is congenital, particularly if prolonged hospitalization has been required or an inappropriately pessimistic prognosis has been given, problems may arise from inadequate mother-child bonding, and the opinion of a family-oriented child psychiatrist is often helpful.

The impact of the disease on the child's intellectual, emotional, and social progress must be assessed. In general, renal disease does not retard cognitive development, although there may be some delay if renal failure is severe in early life. A more common feature is emotional immaturity amounting to infantilism as a consequence of growth retardation, eliciting a response from society more appropriate to the child's size than chronologic age. Later, toward puberty, there will always be concern as to whether or when dialysis and transplantation will be necessary. A detailed educational history should be obtained and communication with the school authorities established. A children's renal unit should have a dedicated teacher whose opinion should be sought in individual cases, and an appropriate educational program should be worked out for each child.

Expertise in this area, as much as experience in organic renal disease in childhood, distinguishes skilled pediatric nephrologists from their colleagues in internal medicine.

PHYSICAL EXAMINATION

General Assessment

A preliminary rapid assessment should be made of how sick the child is, whether there is circulatory failure or shock, if ventilation is adequate, what the level of consciousness is, and whether the child is in pain. The child's mood and demeanor should be noted (e.g., whether happy or fractious, alert and lucid, or somnolent and obtunded). The child's state of care should be assessed (i.e., does the child appear to be kempt or disheveled?). Inspection of the mucous membranes, conjunctivae, and nailbeds may provide evidence of anemia. Other features suggesting long-standing CRF are growth retardation and skeletal deformity caused by uremic osteodystrophy.

Growth and Nutrition

Proper assessment of the child's growth necessitates accurate measurement of height with a stadiometer and weight with scales, both accurate to 0.1%, together with charts of height and weight percentiles appropriate for the child's age, race, and gender (see Chapter 22). Pubertal development must be formally assessed. An impression should be formed of muscle bulk and body fat, but nutritional status is difficult to assess. The relationship between weight and height may underestimate the degree of loss of muscle tissue because there is often subclinical expansion of ECF.

State of Hydration

Assessment of the state of hydration is a skilled matter. Consideration should first be given to total body water and its partition between ECF and ICF, then to ECF and its partition between intravascular and interstitial compartments, and finally to intravascular volume and circulatory status (see Chapters 7 and 13). There is, unfortunately, no simple clinical way to estimate total body water, although some clues may be obtained from a review of recent changes in body weight, which largely reflect changes in total body water. In isotonic states (i.e., with normal plasma sodium concentration), dehydration of moderate severity implies a deficit of total body water of some 5% of body weight and severe dehydration, a deficit of 10%. The partition of fluid between ICF and ECF is determined by osmotic forces, in effect by sodium; changes in body water alone without changes in body sodium principally affect ICF volume and are difficult to detect clinically. Both ICF contraction and expansion (water intoxication) principally affect the brain because of the volume constraints imposed by the skull.

Changes in ECF volume are easier to detect clinically than changes in ICF volume, although edema is not usually evident until the ECF has been expanded by some 10%. The partition of fluid between the intravascular and interstitial compartments is determined by colloid osmotic forces, in effect the plasma albumin concentration; and the integrity of the capillary wall. Expansion of the interstitial compartment results in peripheral edema, most easily detected by pretibial pitting; expansion of the intravascular compartment results in hypertension, raised central venous pressure (CVP), and pulmonary edema. Conversely, contraction of the interstitial compartment causes diminished skin turgor, and a reduction of the intravascular compartment (hypovolemia) results in hypotension and circulatory failure with a low CVP. Occult hypovolemia may be revealed by an exaggerated fall in blood pressure on standing.

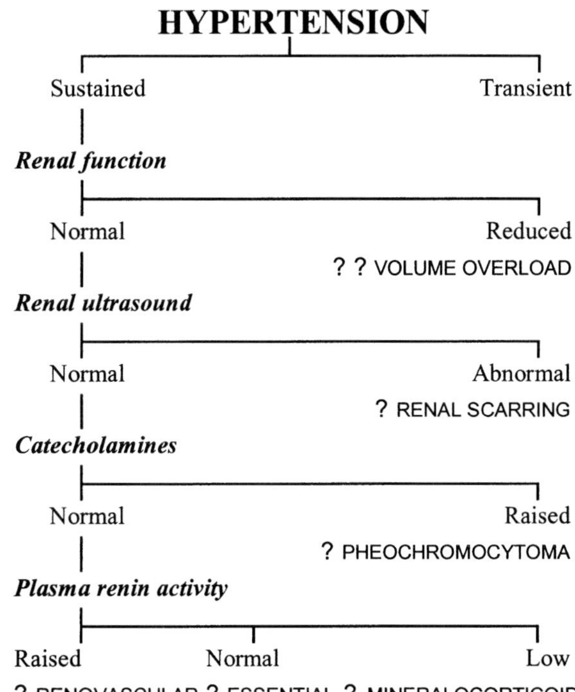

FIGURE 20.7. Hypertension.

System Review

Circulatory Status

Hypotension and poor peripheral perfusion, characterized by cold extremities and a peripheral-to-central temperature gap greater than 2°C indicate poor cardiac output. If the CVP is low, hypovolemia is the cause; if the CVP is raised, the problem is cardiac. Assessment of the CVP is an important observation. In the older child, inspection of the jugular venous pressure in the semirecumbent position may be helpful, but it is often impossible to be confident of the situation in a younger child. Cardiac size as shown on chest radiograph may be helpful, but the sick child under intensive care usually requires formal CVP monitoring.

Cardiorespiratory System

Pulse

The pulses should be examined and the rate, rhythm, and volume recorded. The femoral pulses should always be palpated; coarctation of the aorta may present with renal failure and/or hypertension. Auscultation for bruits over major arteries (e.g., carotid and renal) may indicate extensive vascular disease or renal artery stenosis.

Blood Pressure

Frequent observation of the blood pressure is an integral part of the management of the child with renal disease. It is one of the most difficult aspects of the physical examination and should not be delegated to the most junior doctor or nurse. Technical aspects of measuring the blood pressure are important, along with standards of blood pressure for age and height (see Chapter 61). Twenty-four-hour monitoring gives a more accurate assessment of the situation. Sustained hypertension in children requires full investigation (Fig. 20.7).

Precordium

Cardiomegaly may reflect volume overload or long-standing hypertension. Murmurs may indicate a congenital cardiac anomaly that might be the seat of subacute bacterial endocarditis or may simply reflect a high-output state arising from anemia. Pericarditis with rub is a feature of a severe uremic state.

Lungs

Adequacy of ventilation should be assessed clinically by cyanosis, but the anemia that accompanies uremia may mask desaturation. If there is any doubt, particularly with incipient or actual pulmonary edema, pulse oximetry or formal blood gas analysis is essential. Hyperventilation suggests metabolic acidosis (Kussmaul respiration). The lungs should be examined in the conventional manner, the most important physical sign being the diffuse fine crepitations at both lung bases, which indicate pulmonary edema.

Skin

Examination of the skin may reveal the maculopapular rash of Henoch-Schönlein syndrome typically most severe on the buttocks, the painful purple lesions involving the fingers or toes of a vasculitis, or the butterfly rash across the nose and cheeks characteristic of systemic lupus erythematosus (see Chapters 45 and 46). Multiple café-au-lait spots point to neurofibromatosis, which may be associated with renal artery stenosis and hypertension; adenoma sebaceum and shagreen patches point to tuberous sclerosis; and angiokeratoma to Fabry's disease. Dystrophic nails suggest the possibility of the nail-patella syndrome. Ichthyosis is associated with a lethal variant of Fanconi syndrome.

Inspection of the mouth is an important part of the physical examination. Poor or mixed primary and secondary dentition is a feature of CRF; gingival hypertrophy may be a consequence of cyclosporin toxicity, a tongue too large for the mouth may point to Beckwith-Wiedemann syndrome (associated with renal medullary dysplasia), and lumps on the tongue suggest the orofaciodigital syndrome (associated with polycystic kidneys).

Abdomen

Abdominal Distention

Abdominal distention in relation to renal disease may be a consequence of ascites, renal enlargement because of hydronephrosis or tumor, or retention of urine in the bladder. Absent abdominal wall musculature, characteristic of the prune belly syndrome and a consequence of intrauterine abdominal distension, is obvious in infancy but is sometimes less evident in older children or in cases of partial absence, and it may be revealed only by asking the recumbent child to put his arms across the chest and raise his shoulders off the bed. In affected cases, upward movement of the umbilicus will be observed.

Renal Enlargement

Detection of renal enlargement by palpation is a skilled physical maneuver. The kidneys can often be palpated in a healthy neonate but not in an older child. Palpable enlargement of the kidneys has the following characteristics: the mass can be lifted from the loin, and in contrast to the spleen, it is possible to get above it; there is not much movement of the mass with respiration; and it is resonant to percussion anteriorly because the bowel intervenes. Some inferences can be drawn from the nature of the mass, although it is difficult to distinguish clinically between the firm enlargement of polycystic disease and tumor or, in an infant, between the soft enlargement of hydronephrosis and a multicystic kidney.

Hepatosplenomegaly

The causes of hepatic enlargement are legion, among which glycogen storage disease should be noted for its association with glomerulosclerosis (see Chapters 50). Hepatosplenomegaly in association with renal disease has a more restricted differential diagnosis, suggesting a multisystem disorder, such as systemic lupus erythematosus or juvenile rheumatoid arthritis; an infection, such as bacterial endocarditis or shunt nephritis; a neoplastic process, perhaps complicated by uric acid nephropathy; or hypersplenism as a consequence of the hepatic fibrosis associated with the autosomal recessive form of polycystic kidney disease.

Bladder

Enlargement of the bladder should be sought by palpation and percussion. If detected, the child should be asked to pass urine and then be reexamined. It is sometimes difficult to detect bladder enlargement in the neonate when the umbilical cord is still *in situ*; an ultrasound scan easily resolves the issue.

Genitalia

There is a natural but inexcusable tendency to omit examination of the genitalia. The presence of the foreskin in a male and the position of the urethral meatus must be ascertained in both genders because anomalies are common. However, hypospadias is only rarely associated with upper tract abnormalities. Bilateral cryptorchidism is a feature of prune belly syndrome. Male pseudohermaphroditism with cryptorchidism is associated with nephroblastoma and glomerular disease in the Denys-Drash syndrome. Female pseudohermaphroditism suggests the possibility of adrenal hyperplasia with salt-wasting.

Anus

In the neonate, an imperforate or abnormally positioned anal opening may represent only one feature of complex congenital abnormalities, including those affecting the renal tract.

Nervous System

Neurologic Examination

A careful examination of the central nervous system is always appropriate, particularly in children who have severe hypertension, multisystem disorders, or are in intensive care. Convulsions may be due to uremia, hypertension, hyponatremia or hypernatremia, hypocalcemia, hypomagnesemia, or disorders such as hemolytic uremic syndrome or a systemic vasculitis, which affects both the kidney and the brain. Tetany may be due to hypocalcemia or alkalosis.

Severe hypertension may present with a facial palsy, may cause a cerebral hemorrhage, and, if the blood pressure is controlled too vigorously, may be associated with anterior visual pathway infarction, blindness, and abnormal pupillary responses.

Eyes

The eyes offer many clues in the evaluation of renal disease, and the assistance of an experienced pediatric ophthalmologist is helpful. Scleral calcification may be a consequence of hypercalcemia or uncontrolled hyperphosphatemia. The crystal deposits in the cornea characteristic of cystinosis are best detected by slit lamp examination, but the earliest manifestation in this disorder is a peripheral retinal pigmentary disorder. Alport's syndrome may be associated with keratoconus or, more commonly, with a macular abnormality. Buphthalmos is a feature of Lowe's syndrome. Aniridia is accompanied by an increased incidence of nephroblastoma. Iridocyclitis may complicate juvenile rheumatoid arthritis and associated amyloid nephropathy or may be found in association with idiopathic interstitial nephritis (see Chapter 43). Cataracts occur in many disorders, among which galactosemia may be noted for its association with renal tubular dysfunction. Posterior lenticular opacities may be a consequence of long-term corticosteroid therapy and with careful examination are commonly found, but they rarely give rise to visual handicap.

The examination of the fundus may reveal the ravages of hypertension with arterial narrowing, hemorrhages, exudates, and papilledema. Papilledema is also the major sign of raised intracranial pressure, as, for example, with cerebral edema in acutely ill children or after corticosteroid withdrawal. Diabetic retinopathy tends to parallel nephropathy and is rarely observed in childhood. Tapetoretinal degeneration is found in some cases of juvenile nephronophthisis (see Chapter 35), and retinitis pigmentosa is characteristic of Laurence-Moon-Biedl syndrome in which renal failure caused by medullary dysplasia is the principal cause of early death. The retinal changes in infantile oxalosis are striking (see Chapter 42).

Ears

Deformities of the external ear may result from oligohydramnios and even in its absence may be associated with renal anomalies. Preauricular tags and branchial fistulae are features of the branchiootorenal syndrome. High-tone sensorineural deafness is characteristic of Alport's syndrome and may be insidious in its onset, detectable at first only by audiography. Nerve deafness is also associated with some cases of distal renal tubular acidosis (see Chapter 39). Deafness may be a consequence of the previous administration of aminoglycoside antimicrobials, particularly in the neonatal period, or of high dosages of furosemide.

Skeletal System

Bones

The classic features of rickets may be a consequence of the early osteomalacic phase of renal osteodystrophy or of renal tubular disease. Hypophosphatemic vitamin D–resistant rickets is a feature of several genetically determined renal tubular disorders (see Chapter 11). Genu valgum is common with renal osteodystrophy and should be quantified by measuring the intermalleolar distance. Congenital dislocation of the hips is common in infants with renal disease and should be sought with great care. Slipped femoral capital epiphysis is a feature of uremic osteodystrophy, and avascular necrosis of the head of the femur may complicate corticosteroid therapy, particularly in transplanted patients (see Chapter 69). Polydactyly is found in many syndromes with a renal component (see Chapter 6) and may be missed because the accessory digit was removed in infancy.

Deformities of the spine, such as meningomyelocele, are obvious, but subtle signs, such as a patch of pigmentation or a tuft of hair, may point to an underlying spinal dysraphism responsible for a neuropathic bladder. Sacral agenesis, in particular, is easily overlooked. Unequal leg growth may be a consequence of spinal abnormalities. Hemihypertrophy is occasionally associated with nephroblastoma, with or without Beckwith-Wiedemann syndrome, or with medullary sponge kidney.

Joints

Arthropathy is a classic feature of systemic lupus erythematosus and the Henoch-Schönlein syndrome. It is occasionally observed in children with idiopathic membranous nephropathy. Juvenile rheumatoid arthritis may be complicated by amyloid or interstitial nephritis or associated with drug nephrotoxicity. The Lesch-Nyhan syndrome may present as a renal disorder, either as calculi or renal failure in infancy, and may be associated with a gouty arthropathy affecting the interphalangeal joints.

ROUTINE URINALYSIS

Examination of the urine is an integral part of the clinical evaluation and is the responsibility of the clinician. In today's increasingly busy clinical practice, dipstick testing of the urine is frequently delegated to the clinic nurse and microscopy to the microbiology laboratory. Nonetheless, the clinician must be conversant with the methods of urinalysis, their interpretation, and their sources of error and ensure that the correct procedures are followed.

Dipstick Tests

Urine samples should be inspected and routinely tested for blood, protein, and glucose, using commercially available dipsticks.

Hemastix

Hemastix rely on the peroxidase-like activity of hemoglobin to catalyze the reaction of a hydroperoxide with tetramethylbenzidine to give a green-blue color; myoglobin also gives a positive reaction. The test is capable of detecting as little as

150 μg/L of free hemoglobin and is so sensitive that a negative test excludes significant hematuria.

Albustix

Protein in urine is most conveniently detected by the so-called protein error of indicators principle with Albustix (Ames Company). These reagent strips are impregnated with tetrabromphenol blue buffered with citrate. Protein binds with the dye and causes a color change from yellow to green by displacement of the transformation range of the indicator. Free light chains (Bence-Jones protein) and other low-molecular-weight "tubular proteins" are not readily detected by Albustix. A dilute urine specimen may give a false-negative result. False-positive results occur with very alkaline urine, with concentrated samples, and with those contaminated with quaternary ammonium salts such as chlorhexidine. If the stick is left to soak in the urine or if there is a delay in reading the strip, false-positive readings can also occur.

Occasionally, protein is excreted in the urine in the upright posture but not when recumbent. Such postural proteinuria does not indicate renal disease and should be ascertained by examination of an overnight specimen of urine. Sustained proteinuria requires full investigation (Fig. 20.8) (see Chapter 21).

Clinistix

Clinistix (Ames Company) detect glucose in urine by a glucose oxidase-peroxidase linked reaction. The system is sensitive to a glucose concentration of approximately 0.5 mmol/L, but it is inhibited to some degree by glutathione and other substances in the urine, so the trace amounts of glucose in normal urine are below the threshold of the test.

Multistix

Multistix (Ames Company) combine the above with tests for pH (based on a double-indicator principle), osmolality (based on the change of pKa of certain polyelectrolytes in relation to ionic concentration), ketones, bilirubin, urobilinogen, and nitrite. The pH and osmolality are not sufficiently accurate for diagnostic purposes; pH should be measured in the laboratory by a pH meter and osmolality with an osmometer (see Chapter 21).

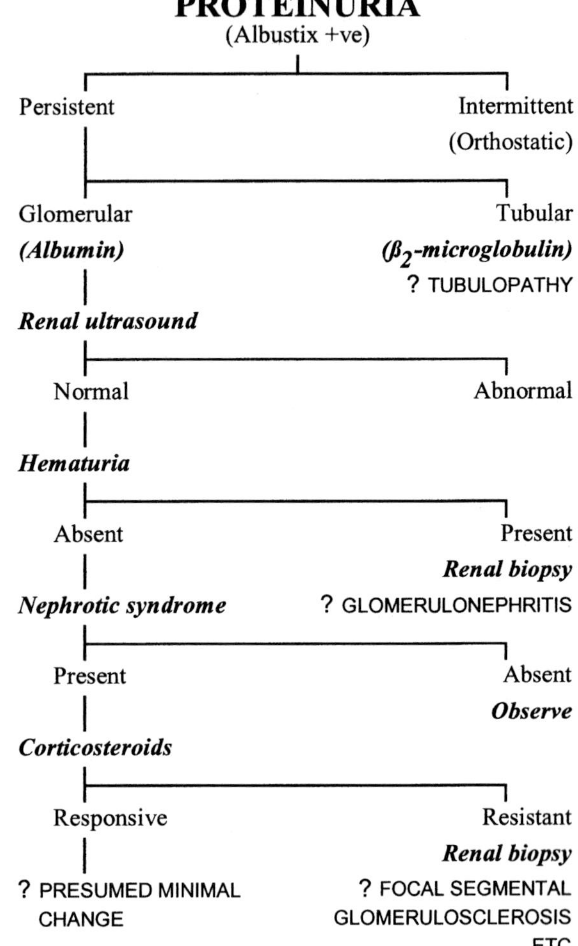

FIGURE 20.8. Proteinuria.

Microscopy and Culture

Urine microscopy in wards or clinics used to be part of the repertoire of every clinical nephrologist. Now, the availability of dipsticks for routine urinalysis and the sophistication of equipment have tended to transfer urine microscopy to the laboratory. There are some disadvantages in this: The immediate relevance of the findings to the clinical situation is lost, and it is difficult to ensure that the sample is fresh.

Midstream urine specimens should be collected and dispatched to the laboratory for microscopy and culture without delay (see Chapter 53).

21

LABORATORY INVESTIGATIONS

JEAN-PIERRE GUIGNARD
FERNANDO SANTOS

The validity of the recommendation by the American Academy of Pediatrics that all asymptomatic children have screening urinalyses at four intervals from infancy through adolescence has been questioned recently (1). The usefulness of routine multidipstick has, on the contrary, been emphasized by experienced pediatric nephrologists (2). Routine dipstick urinalysis is discussed in Chapter 20. The child with positive dipstick screening should be investigated to exclude or confirm the presence of renal disease.

PROTEINURIA

Pathophysiology of Proteinuria

The normal glomerulus restricts the filtration of proteins on both size and electrical charge. The size selectivity of the glomerular capillary is largely determined by the cellular layers rather than by the glomerular basement membrane (GBM) (3). With a molecular weight (MW) of 69 kDa, albumin passes the filter in small quantities, so that the ultrafiltration in Bauman's capule contains 10 mg/L or less of albumin. The permeability of the glomerular capillary to large protiens also depends on the electrical change. The glomerular capillary wall is indeed charged negatively due to its rich heparan sulfate content (4). Because of the electrostatic interaction with the filtration barrier, negatively charged macromolecules are more restricted than are neutral or positively charged molecules of similar MW. The electrical charge does not influence the filtration of small molecules of ions. The combined impairment of both barrier charge selectivity and size selectivity is required to account for the massive proteinuria observed in nephrotic patients.

Almost all of the filtered proteins are reabsorbed in the proximal tubule by endocytosis at the luminal membrane. Significant proteinuria occurs when this energy-requiring mechanism is saturated. In the tubular cells, the proteins are degraded by lysosomal enzymes to low-molecular-weight (LMW) fragments and amino acids. By this mechanism, the kidney plays a major role in the catabolism of many polypeptide hormones such as insulin and parathormone. Smaller peptides, such as angiotensin and vasopressin, are directly catabolized by peptidases located in the proximal luminal plasma membranes.

Types of Proteinuria

In normal individuals, the major constituent of nonplasma proteins is the Tamm-Horsfall protein (Uromodulin) (5). It is a glycoprotein (MW, 95 kDa) actively secreted by the tubular cells in the ascending thick limb. The Tamm-Horsfall protein has no clinical significance. Significant proteinuria can be classified into (a) glomerular proteinuria, (b) tubular proteinuria, and (c) overflow proteinuria.

Glomerular Proteinuria

Altered permselectivity of the glomerular barrier results in the abnormal passage of an increased fraction of the glomerular ultrafiltrate through the large nonselective pores (3). The altered permselectivity may be the consequence of physical damage to the filtering membranes or may be transient and hemodynamically or hormonally mediated (6). Glomerular proteinuria may be selective or nonselective. Selective proteinuria is characterized by the predominance of albumin as compared to other proteins of higher MW.

Albumin, immunoglobulin G (IgG), and transferrin are proteins used to characterize the selectivity of glomerular proteinuria. A permeability index based on the IgG/albumin or the IgG/transferrin clearance ratios can be used. An index below 0.1 is indicative of highly selective proteinuria (7). The clinical usefulness of this index is questionable. A high selectivity index is usually found in the steroid-sensitive minimal changes nephrotic syndrome as well as in the Finnish-type congenital nephrotic syndrome. The selectivity is low in orthostatic proteinuria (8). The excretion rate of urinary proteins and/or albumin is probably the best independent predictor of end-stage renal disease in nondiabetic proteinuric chronic nephropathies (9).

TABLE 21.1. MARKERS USED FOR THE CLASSIFICATION OF PROTEINURIA

Diagnosis	Marker	MW (d)	Excretion/creatinine	
			g/mol creatinine	mg/mol creatinine
Glomerular proteinuria	Proteins	—	<20	<180
Glomerular selectivity	Albumin	67'000	<1.17	<0.21
	Transferrin	80'000	—	—
	Immunoglobulin G	150'000	<5.8	<50
Tubular proteinuria	β_2-microglobulin	11'800	<0.040	<0.35
	α_1-microglobulin	30'000	<2.2	<19
	Retinol-binding protein	21'400	<0.024	<0.21
Tubular injury	Lysozyme	14'400	<0.065	<0.6

The loss of charge selectivity of the GBM can be assessed by the clearance of two proteins of similar MW but with different electric charges. Two pairs of molecules can be used: (a) the nonglycated and the negatively glycated albumin and (b) the neutral IgG and the negatively charged IgG_4 subclass. The ratio of their clearances is modified when the GBM has lost its charge selectivity (3). Loss of glomerular anionic charges may be the first step in the development of some nephropathies, as, for instance, type 1 diabetic nephropathy.

Tubular Proteinuria

Most LMW proteins (MW below 40 kDa) are filtered and reabsorbed in the proximal tubule. Impaired proximal tubular reabsorption of LMW proteins results in tubular proteinuria. This is observed in tubulopathies such as the Fanconi syndrome. Drug (aminoglycosides) or heavy-metal intoxication may induce tubular proteinuria.

The exclusive presence of LMW proteins in the urine characterizes the tubular proteinuria. Three markers are commonly used (Table 21.1) (10).

1. β_2-microglobulin, which is not bound to proteins, is easy to measure, but is unstable in acid urine.
2. α_1-microglobulin is stabler than β_2-microglobulin but has a higher MW and thus a more variable filterability.
3. Retinol-binding protein is stable at low urine pH, but it strongly binds to plasma proteins.

Overflow Proteinuria

An unusual increase in the protein filtered load results in significant proteinuria. Overflow proteinuria may be seen in multiple myeloma (Bence-Jones proteins), hemoglobinuria, and myoglobinuria.

Markers of Acute Tubular Necrosis

Two enzymes synthesized in the proximal tubular cells, the lysosomal enzyme *N*-acetyl-glucosaminidase and alanine-aminopeptidase, present in the brush border are urinary markers of tubular necrosis. The urinary excretion of these two enzymes is increased in various conditions associated with acute tubular necrosis. *N*-acetyl-glucosaminidase is stabler than alanine-aminopeptidase. Other enzymes may detect an injury of the proximal tubular cells (α-glutathione transferase) or the distal tubular cells (π-glutathione transferase). Lysozyme (MW, 14.4 kDa) is a marker of tubular proteinuria and of acute tubular necrosis (11) but is less sensitive than other markers.

Quantification of Urinary Proteins

Reagent Test Strips

Positive dipstick screening for proteinuria warrants quantification of the proteinuria.

Protein/Creatinine Ratio

The protein/creatinine (prot/creat) ratio is measured in a random urine sample. The second morning urine specimen is most suitable. The urine prot/creat ratio correlates well with the 24-hour urine protein excretion (13,14). Comparison of the ratio measured in the first morning urine specimen with that of urine collected during the day is used for the diagnosis of orthostatic proteinuria. Normal values of the urine prot/creat ratio observed at different ages are given in Table 21.2. By definition, nephrotic range proteinuria is superior to 400 g/mol creatinine. The albuminuria can also be expressed as an albumin/creatinine ratio. The upper-normal value is 1.17 g/mol creatinine.

Quantitative Proteinuria

Quantitative urine protein excretion can be made using a 24-hour urine collection, an overnight collection, or a shorter urine collection over a few hours. The 24-hour collection in children is cumbersome for the patient and subject to errors. Normal values are defined as less than 4 $mg/m^2/hr$ or 100 $mg/m^2/day$. Values above 40 $mg/m^2/hr$ define the nephrotic range proteinuria. *Microalbuminuria* is defined as an albumin excretion between 0.7 and 7.0 $mg/m^2/hr$ or 170 $mg/m^2/day$.

TABLE 21.2. NORMAL VALUES OF PROTEIN EXCRETION AS A FUNCTION OF AGE

	Proteinuria	
Age (yr)	g/mol creatinine	g/g creatinine
0.1–0.5	80	0.70
0.5–1.0	60	0.55
1–2	45	0.40
2–3	30	0.30
3–5	20	0.20
5–7	19	0.15
7–17	18	0.15

Analytic Procedures

The urinary proteins are usually measured by an autoanalyzer-adapted turbidimetry micromethod that uses benzethonium chloride to precipitate the urinary proteins at an alkaline pH. The quantification of albuminuria is achieved by enzyme-linked immunoabsorbent assays, immunoturbidimetry, or laser nephelometry (12).

Electrophoretic separation of urinary proteins by means of polyacrylamide or agarose gel electrophoresis is used to distinguish glomerular, tubular, and mixed proteinuria. Different markers are used to differentiate glomerular from tubular proteinuria (Table 21.1).

Etiology of Proteinuria

Orthostatic Proteinuria

Orthostatic proteinuria is only present when the patient is upright. The proteinuria is usually mild and not selective (8). Orthostatic proteinuria is often seen in slender adolescent patients. The prognosis of orthostatic proteinuria is excellent. No treatment is needed.

Transient Proteinuria

Transient proteinuria is usually associated with exercise, stress, fever, and dehydration. It does not reflect renal disease.

Persistent Proteinuria

Persistent proteinuria indicates renal disease. Proteinuria may *per se* also lead to renal injury (15) and should be thoroughly investigated (16).

URINE SOLUTE EXCRETION

Quantification

The renal elimination of a given solute is highly dependent on a number of factors such as diet content, water intake, intestinal absorption, extrarenal losses, and internal distribution of the solute in the body. Solute excretion varies with age.

Urine solute excretion can be expressed in mg or mmol/day/kg or per m^2, by the solute/creatinine concentration ratio, and/or by calculating the solute fractional excretion (FE). Solute/creatinine concentration ratios and FE can be calculated in random urine samples without the need for timed urine collection. Calculation of FE requires drawing a blood sample at the time of urine collection. The FE is calculated as follows: $FE_S = (U_S/P_S) \times (P_{Cr}/U_{Cr}) \times 100$, where U_S and P_S represent the urine and plasma concentrations of a solute (S) and P_{Cr} and U_{Cr} represent the plasma and urinary concentrations of creatinine, respectively. FE_S expresses the percent of filtered solute that is excreted in the urine. This concept is equivalent to the fractional clearance of S (FC_S), which is calculated with the same formula but expressed as mL/dL of glomerular filtrate. Calculation of glomerular filtration rate (GFR) by means of the creatinine clearance is $GFR = (U_{Cr} / P_{Cr}) \times V$, where V represents the mL of urine eliminated by minute and GFR is expressed in mL/min. For a GFR = 100 mL/min, $V = 100 \times (P_{Cr} / U_{Cr})$ and represents the mL of urine eliminated by 100 mL of GF. Thus, FC_S may be calculated by the formula $FC_S = U_S / P_S \times (P_{Cr} / U_{Cr}) \times 100$, which is identical to that used to calculate FE_S. FC_S represents the mL of each 100 mL of GF that have been cleared of S and is expressed in mL per 100 mL GFR. As noted in the above formula, its calculation is independent of the volume of urine and, therefore, does not require timed urine collection.

For those solutes not undergoing tubular secretion, the difference $100 - FE_S$ represents the percentage of solute that is reabsorbed. Thus, the tubular reabsorption of phosphate (TRP) equals $100 - FE_P$ and represents the percentage of filtered phosphate that is reabsorbed in the convoluted proximal tubule. The TRP is frequently expressed as TmP/GFR. TmP, representing the maximum tubular phosphate reabsorption, may be calculated by using phosphate infusions (see Glucose Titration Test and Fig. 21.1). However, TmP can also be deduced using a more practical approach. TRP is the difference between filtered phosphate and excreted phosphate. Individuals on a normal Western diet ingest a large amount of phosphate. Therefore, in the presence of normal GFR, the rate of phosphate reabsorption approaches the maximal capacity of proximal tubules to reabsorb phosphate. Thus, $TmP = GFR \times S_P - U_P \times V$, where S_P and U_P are the phosphate concentrations in serum and urine. In this equation, S_P represents the renal threshold for phosphate (as explained in the section Glucose Titration Test) when $U_P \times V$ is equal to 0. Therefore, TmP/GFR value equals the threshold concentration for serum phosphate and is considered as the best indicator of the renal tubular handling of phosphate (17).

According to Bijvoet et al., TmP/GFR can be calculated as follows: $TmP/GFR = TRP \times S_P$, or $TmP/GFR = [1 - (U_P \times S_{Cr} / S_P \times U_{Cr})]\ S_P$, or $TmP/GFR = S_P - (U_P \times S_{Cr} / U_{Cr})$ (18).

A nomogram for the determination of TmP/GFR based on the plasma phosphate concentration and TRP has been

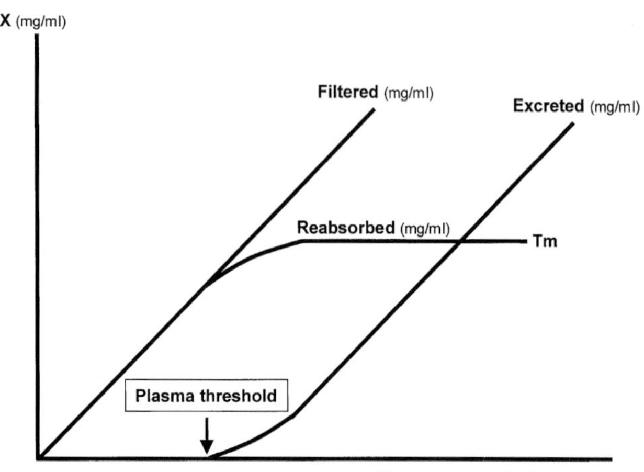

FIGURE 21.1. Representative renal titration curve for a substance (X) with an active and saturable mechanism of proximal tubular reabsorption, like that of glucose or phosphate.

developed by Walton and Bijvoet (19). The usefulness of this nomogram in children has been questioned, the use of TmP/GFR or the simple use of TP/GFR in well-nourished children appearing more relevant (20–23).

Sodium, Chloride, and Potassium

The daily urinary excretion of sodium varies widely in response to change in dietary salt intakes. On a normal Western diet, children excrete approximately 3 to 4 mmol/kg/day of sodium. Body fluid composition requires independent regulation of sodium and water balances as intake of water and sodium may vary separately. Thus, concentration of sodium in the final urine is highly related to the degree of urinary concentration or dilution. The extracellular fluid volume is regulated by changes in sodium excretion and when the extracellular fluid volume is contracted (i.e., dehydration, nephrotic syndrome), sodium can be virtually undetectable in the urine. Although there is no predictable relationship between the plasma sodium concentration and urinary sodium excretion, mild hypernatremia has recently been shown to induce natriuresis in humans (24). Normal urinary sodium/creatinine ratios in children are shown in Table 21.3.

Urinary chloride excretion is closely associated with that of sodium. Chloride excretion is dependent on the salt content of diet, and it is also retained during volume depletion. The measurement of urinary chloride concentration may be particularly useful in the diagnostic approach to metabolic alkalosis, because urine sodium and chloride concentrations may be dissociated. A urinary chloride concentration above 10 mmol/L is indicative of metabolic alkalosis of renal origin, whereas lower concentrations of urinary chloride or a reduced chloride/creatinine concentration ratio (25) suggests volume contraction as the cause of the metabolic alkalosis. However, even in the presence of volume contraction and active renal reabsorption, urinary sodium may be high because it is eliminated in the urine with the bicarbonate anion to keep electroneutrality. Normal urinary chloride/creatinine values are given in Table 21.3.

Urinary potassium excretion ranges from 1 to 2 mmol/kg/day in a child on a normal diet. The kidney regulates potassium balance by changing the secretion rate of potassium in the distal nephron. This regulation is mostly dependent on aldosterone and the amount of sodium and water delivered to the distal nephron. The renal ability to retain potassium is not as efficient as that of sodium, and, in the face of potassium depletion, urinary potassium does not decrease to less than 15 mmol/L. Normal urinary potassium/creatinine ratios are shown in Table 21.3.

The excretion of sodium, chloride, and potassium is frequently expressed as FE rates. In European children older

TABLE 21.3. URINARY SOLUTE/CREATININE (CREAT) RATIOS (FIFTH AND NINETY-FIFTH PERCENTILES) AS A FUNCTION OF AGE

Solute/creat	Age (yr)															
	1/12–1		1–2		2–3		3–5		5–7		7–10		10–14		14–17	
mol/mol	P5	P95	P5	P95	P5	P95	P5	P95	P5	P95	P5	P95	P5	P95	P5	P95
Sodium/creat	2.5	54	4.8	58	5.9	56	6.6	57	7.5	51	7.5	42	6	34	—	28
Potassium/creat	11	74	9	68	8	63	6.8	48	5.4	33	4.5	22	3.4	15	—	13
Calcium/creat	0.09	2.2	0.07	1.5	0.06	1.4	0.05	1.1	0.04	0.8	0.04	0.7	0.04	0.7	0.04	0.7
Magnesium/creat	0.4	2.2	0.4	1.7	0.3	1.6	0.3	1.3	0.3	1	0.3	0.9	0.2	0.7	0.2	0.6
Phosphate/creat	1.2	19	1.2	14	1.2	12	1.2	18	1.2	5	1.2	3.6	0.8	3.2	0.8	2.7
Oxalate/creat	0.06	0.17	0.05	0.13	0.04	0.1	0.03	0.08	0.03	0.07	0.02	0.06	0.02	0.06	0.02	0.06
Urate/creat	0.7	1.5	0.5	1.4	0.47	1.3	0.4	1.1	0.3	0.8	0.26	0.56	0.2	0.44	0.2	0.4

Adapted from Matos V, Melle G van, Boulat O, et al. Urinary phosphate/creatinine, calcium/creatinine, and magnesium/creatinine ratios in a healthy pediatric population. *J Pediatr* 1997;131:252–257; and Matos V, Melle G van, Werner D, et al. Urinary oxalate and urate to creatinine ratios in a healthy pediatric population. *Am J Kidney Dis* 1999;34:1–6.

than 1 year of age, not fasted, and on a normal diet, FE_{Na} has been shown to range from 0.3 to 1.6%, this variation being the result of the different dietary salt intakes (26). Calculation of FE_{Na} is widely used to explore whether the kidney responds adequately to extracellular volume depletion. In this situation, FE_{Na} is expected to fall as a result of compensatory avid sodium reabsorption. Thus, in patients with prerenal acute renal failure, FE_{Na} is expected to fall below 1%, whereas it is generally above 3% in acute tubular necrosis. In normal conditions, FE_K approximates 10 to 15%. Values of FE_K above 100% can be found in renal failure patients as a compensatory mechanism to maintain potassium balance.

Calcium

Urinary elimination of calcium is highly dependent not only on the diet but also on the child's age. Although the range of normal urinary calcium elimination may vary in different geographical regions, *hypercalciuria* is usually defined as urinary calcium excretion rates above 4 to 5 mg/kg/day (0.100 to 0.125 mmol/kg/day) and is suspected when the calcium/creatinine ratio is above 0.20 mg/mg (0.60 mol/mol) (27–29). The upper-normal limit of the urinary calcium/creatinine ratio is much higher in infants (30). Recent reference values for urinary calcium to creatinine concentration ratios in spot urines of children of different ages have been provided by Matos et al. and are shown in Table 21.3 (31). Under identical dietary conditions, urine calcium has been shown to be lower in black than in white children (32).

Phosphate

Similarly to calcium, phosphaturia expressed per unit of weight, as well as phosphatemia, markedly decreases with age. In adults, normal urinary phosphate excretion equals 10 to 15 mg/kg/day (0.3 to 0.5 mmol/kg/day), whereas values up to 20 to 25 mg/kg/day (0.6 to 0.8 mmol/kg/day) are found in young children. Recent reference values for urinary phosphate to creatinine concentration ratios in children are shown in Table 21.3 (31). Values of TP/GFR vary from 6.9 in neonates to 4.4 at 5 years of age and 3.2 mg/dL GFR at 6 years of age (21).

Magnesium

Daily elimination of urinary magnesium has been reported to decrease from a mean value of 2.44 ± 0.69 (SD) mg/kg/day (0.10 ± 0.03 mmol/kg/day) in Italian children 3 to 5 years of age to 1.77 ± 0.65 (SD) mg/kg/day (0.07 ± 0.03 mmol/kg/day) in children 15 to 16 years old (33). These values are quite similar to those obtained in other European studies and markedly higher than those found in children from Oriental origin (34–37). Reference values for urinary magnesium to creatinine concentration ratios in a pediatric population are shown in Table 21.3 (31). Calculation of FE_{Mg} allows an assessment of magnesuria in relation to the level of plasma magnesium. Under normal conditions, approximately 5% of filtered magnesium is excreted in urine, but in the face of magnesium deprivation, FE_{Mg} quickly falls below 1% (38). Thus, an FE_{Mg} equal to or greater than 5% with simultaneous hypomagnesemia indicates inappropriate loss of magnesium in the urine.

Uric Acid and Oxalate

Elevated urinary concentrations of uric acid and oxalate and decreased levels of urinary citrate are significant risk factors for the development of urolithiasis and/or nephrocalcinosis. It has been shown that the urinary excretion of uric acid corrected to 1.73 m^2 is independent of age in children aged 2 to 15 years, mean values being 520 ± 147 (SD) mg/1.73 m^2/day (3093 ± 874 μmol/1.73 m^2/day) (39). Calculation of urine uric acid concentration corrected for creatinine clearance in single fasting morning urine and blood specimens (urine uric acid × plasma creatinine/urine creatinine) has been used as a diagnostic criterion of hyperuricosuria, defined by a value above 0.53 mg/dL of GFR (32 μmol/L of GFR) in children between 2 and 12 years of age (40,41). Mean values of urinary oxalate have been reported to be 36.9 ± 13.7 (SD) mg/1.73 m^2/day (0.42 ± 0.16 mmol/1.73 m^2/day) and 1.0 ± 0.6 (SD) mg/kg/day (0.01 ± 0.06 mmol/kg/day) in Spanish and Italian children older than 3 years, respectively (33,42). Reference values for urinary oxalate and urate to creatinine ratios in infants, children, and adolescents are shown in Table 21.3 (43). There is a high positive correlation (R = 0.75) between oxalate excretion measured in 24-hour urine and the oxalate/creatinine ratio measured in the first morning urine sample (44).

Citrate

Values of citrate excretion in healthy children aged 3 to 14 years followed a normal distribution and were equal to 9.62 ± 4.05 (SD) mg/kg/day (45.78 ± 19.28 μmol/kg/day) (45). A moderate correlation (R = 0.49) was found between citruria determined in 24-hour urine specimens and citrate/creatinine concentration ratios in the second morning urine samples. A citrate to creatinine concentration ratio measured in 24-hour urine below 300 mg/g (0.176 mol/mol) in girls and 125 mg/g (0.074 mol/mol) in boys has been proposed as indicative of hypocitruria (41,46). Blau et al. have recently reported the simultaneous determination of oxalate, glycolate, citrate, and sulfate in spot urine samples dried on filter papers (47). This procedure may facilitate the study of these anions in large series of children.

Anion Gap

Metabolic acidosis may be classified according to whether it is associated with elevated or normal serum anion gap

(AG). To keep the electroneutrality of the extracellular fluid, the sum of the cation concentrations must equal that of the anions. This can be expressed by the equation: Na^+ + UC = Cl^- + HCO_3^- + UA, where UC and UA represent unmeasured cations and unmeasured anions, respectively. UC includes K^+, Ca^{2+}, and Mg^{2+}, whereas PO_4^{3-}, SO_4^{2-}, proteins, and organic anions form the UA. The serum AG is defined by the formula AG = $Na^+ - (HCO_3^- + Cl^-)$ = UA – UC. The normal values range from 8 to 16 mmol/L.

A related concept is that of the urine AG, which can be calculated by the formula: Urine AG = $(Na^+ + K^+) - Cl^-$, where Na^+, K^+, and Cl^- represent the urinary concentrations of these solutes in mmol/L (48–50). During metabolic acidosis, urine AG is a rough and inverse estimate of the ammonium (NH_4^+) eliminated in the urine. If large amounts of NH_4^+ are present in urine, the urinary chloride concentration is greater than the sum of sodium and potassium concentrations, and urinary AG becomes negative. Thus, in subjects with type II proximal renal tubular acidosis (RTA) or in patients with metabolic acidosis associated with diarrhea, urine AG is negative. In acidotic patients with impaired NH_4^+ excretion, such as those with type I RTA, type IV RTA, or chronic renal failure, urine AG remains positive.

Transtubular Potassium Concentration Gradient

The transtubular potassium concentration gradient (TTKG) provides an estimation of the regulatory mechanisms of distal potassium secretion, thus facilitating the clinical approach to disorders of potassium excretion. The measurement of the final concentration of potassium in urine gives limited information because this concentration depends not only on the distal secretion of potassium induced by aldosterone but also on the degree of water reabsorption along the medullary collecting duct.

The TTKG index attempts to evaluate the gradient between luminal and peritubular potassium concentrations in the late distal tubule and the cortical collecting duct as a reflection of aldosterone bioactivity. The test assumes that the systemic venous plasma potassium equals the peritubular potassium concentration in the renal cortex and that the luminal potassium concentration in the distal tubule and the cortical collecting duct can be deduced by dividing the urine potassium concentration by the urine to plasma osmolality ratio—that is, adjusting the urinary potassium concentration for medullary water reabsorption. These assumptions require that sufficient sodium be delivered to the distal nephron for exchange with potassium and that urine be hypertonic (51,52).

Based on the preceding rationale, TTKG can be calculated as follows:

$$TTKG = U_K/(U_{OSM}/P_{OSM})/P_K \text{, or}$$

$$TTKG = (U_K \times P_{OSM})/(P_K \times U_{OSM})$$

In adults, a TTKG value greater than 5 indicates that aldosterone is acting, whereas a value at or below 3 indicates lack of mineralocorticoid activity (52). In the face of hyperkalemia, a TTKG below 4.1 in children or below 4.9 in infants should be taken as indicative of a state of relative hypo- or pseudohypoaldosteronism. A TKKG higher than 2 in a hypokalemic child should be taken as indicative of lack of aldosterone suppression (53).

GLOMERULAR FILTRATION RATE

GFR is the best estimate of the functional renal mass. It is the most widely used indicator of kidney function in patients with renal disease. The severity and the prognosis of the disease are predicted on this parameter. The assessment of GFR is thus invaluable in the follow-up of patients with progressive renal failure. It is also of great value in a variety of clinical conditions, as an estimate of GFR may be required to rationally prescribe fluids, electrolytes, or drugs excreted by the kidney.

Physiology of Glomerular Filtration

Ultrafiltration occurs through the permselective capillary wall. Ultrafiltration is driven by Starling forces across the glomerular capillaries. Changes in renal perfusion and in the Starling forces alter GFR. Both renal blood flow (RBF) and GFR are held within narrow limits by the phenomenon of autoregulation. Autoregulation is an intrarenal mechanism with two components: (a) the "myogenic mechanism" and (b) the "tubuloglomerular feedback mechanism." Both mechanisms represent an effective means for uncoupling renal perfusion and GFR from abrupt changes in blood pressure.

The glomerular barrier filters molecules on the basis of size and electric charges. It behaves as if it were a filtering membrane containing aqueous pores with a diameter of 7.5 to 10.0 nm. Molecules with a diameter smaller than 3.6 nm are filtered freely. Molecules with a diameter larger than 7.2 nm are not filtered. Albumin, with an effective diameter of 7.1 nm, is filtered in minute amounts. The electrical charges of the molecules play an important role in their filterability. Filtration of large anionic molecules is restricted by the presence of negatively charged glycoproteins on the surface of all components of the glomerular membrane barrier. In the glomerulus, the MW cut-off for the filter is approximately 70 kDa. With an MW of 69 kDa, albumin passes through the filter in minute quantities. The glomerular filter is freely permeable to those molecules with an MW less than 7 kDa. Filtration of proteins, with consequent proteinuria, is increased in a number of glomerular diseases associated with the loss of negative charges on the glomerular filtration barrier.

The GFR is proportional to the sum of the Starling forces across the glomerular capillaries ($\Delta P - \Delta\pi$) times the ultrafiltration coefficient (K_f): GFR = $K_f \times (\Delta P - \Delta\pi)$, where ΔP and $\Delta\pi$ represent the capillary transglomerular hydrostatic and oncotic pressure difference, respectively.

K_f is the product of the intrinsic permeability of the glomerular capillary and the glomerular surface area available for filtration. The permeability of the glomerular capillaries is 100 times higher than that of the capillaries elsewhere in the body.

Concept of Clearance

The most common measurement of GFR is based on the concept of clearance, which relates to the volume of plasma that in a given unit of time would be completely "cleared" of a substance. The clearance of substance (x) is expressed by the formula $C_x = U_x \times V/P_x$, where V represents the urine flow rate and U_x and P_x the urine and plasma concentration of substance x, respectively.

For its plasma clearance to be equal to the rate of glomerular filtration, a marker must have the following properties: (a) it must be freely filterable through the glomerular capillary membranes—that is, not bound to the plasma proteins or sieved in the process of ultrafiltration; (b) it must be biologically inert and neither reabsorbed nor secreted by the renal tubules; (c) it must not be toxic; and (d) it must not alter renal function when infused in quantities that permit adequate quantification in plasma and urine. Several substances, endogenous or exogenous, have been claimed to have the preceding properties: creatinine, inulin, iohexol, and three compounds labeled with radioisotopes: diethylenetriamine-penta-acetic acid (DTPA), ethylenediaminetetra-acetic acid (EDTA), and sodium iothalamate. The experimental evidence that this is true has only been produced for inulin. Although inulin is the most accurate marker, creatinine is the most commonly used in children.

Methods Available for Assessing Glomerular Filtration Rate

A variety of markers (Table 21.4) can be used to assess GFR using different methods, the principles of which are described in the following sections.

Standard Urinary Clearance

Endogenous Markers

The urinary excretion of the endogenous marker is measured over a few hours, and its excretion rate is divided by the plasma concentration present during the urine collection period. When urine flow rate is expressed in mL/min/1.73 m^2, the standard urinary clearance (UV/P) formula also expresses GFR in mL/min/1.73 m^2. Duration of the collection may last from 3 to 24 hours. Short periods are best in children to avoid inaccuracies in urine collection. Creatinine is the endogenous marker that is used for assessing GFR.

Exogenous Markers

The exogenous marker is infused at a constant rate over 3 to 4 hours to achieve constant plasma concentrations. To shorten the time of equilibration, a priming dose of the marker is administered at the onset of the clearance study. When stable plasma concentrations are attained, urine and blood samples are collected at regular intervals, and the UV:P ratio is calculated. The ideal exogenous marker is inulin. Other markers include iohexol and unlabeled iothalamate.

Constant Infusion Technique without Urine Collection

The constant infusion technique assumes that the rate of infusion (IR) of a marker (x) needed to maintain constant its plasma concentration is equal to the rate of its excretion (54,55). After equilibration of the marker in its distribution space, the excretion rate must thus be equal to the IR, hence the formula:

$$C_x = U_x \times V/P_x = IR_x/P_x$$

The flow rate of the test solution containing the marker is expressed in mL/min/1.73 m^2 and so is the clearance C_x.

To accelerate the achievement of a steady concentration of the marker, a loading dose precedes the constant intravenous (i.v.) infusion. The constant infusion method may overestimate GFR if steady concentration of the marker is not achieved when the plasma concentration is measured. Depending on the conditions, the equilibration of the

TABLE 21.4. CHARACTERISTICS OF THE GLOMERULAR MARKERS

	Inulin	Creatinine	Iohexol	DTPA	EDTA	Iothalamate
Molecular weight	5200	113	811	393	292	637
Elimination half-life (min)	70	200	90	110	120	120
Plasma protein binding (%)	0	0	<2	5	0	<5
Space of distribution	EC	TBW	EC	EC	EC	EC

DTPA, diethylenetriaminepenta-acetic acid; EC, extracellular space; EDTA, ethylenediaminetetra-acetic acid; TBW, total body water.

marker within its distribution space may only be achieved after several hours of constant infusion. In newborn infants, the proportionally greater extracellular space and the low GFR require a much longer period for steady plasma concentrations to be attained. Inulin is the marker of choice for this technique, which is used when urine collection is not possible.

Plasma Disappearance Curve (Single Injection Technique)

The mathematical model for the plasma disappearance curve (single injection technique) is an open, two-compartment system (56). The glomerular marker is injected in the first compartment, equilibrates with the second compartment, and is excreted from the first compartment by glomerular filtration. The plasma disappearance curve of the marker follows two consecutive patterns. In the first, the plasma concentration falls rapidly but at a progressively diminishing rate. This reflects the diffusion of the marker in its distribution volume as well as its renal excretion. In the second, the slope of the decline of the plasma concentration reflects its renal excretion rate only. During this phase, the marker concentration decreases at the same exponential rate in all the compartments where it is distributed.

To obtain a well-defined plasma disappearance curve, and therefore an accurate calculation of the plasma clearance, numerous blood samples are required. Extension of the sampling period to 4 to 5 hours improves the precision of the results. Simplified techniques have been proposed that are based on a single-compartment model. They obviate the need for frequent blood sampling but result in greater accuracy.

The plasma disappearance curve is most often used when assessing GFR with radionuclides. Infusion of radionuclides for several hours is indeed undesirable, and they are best reserved for single injection studies in which the radioisotope is more rapidly eliminated from the kidney. Commonly used markers include technetium 99m (^{99m}Tc)-DTPA, chromium 51 (^{51}Cr)-EDTA, and iodine 125 (^{125}I)-iothalamate, and, more recently, cold iohexol. Clearance values derived from the plasma disappearance curve should be analyzed critically, particularly in patients with reduced GFR and those with edema and circulatory disturbances.

Plasma Concentration

The concentration of endogenous markers, such as creatinine, increases when GFR decreases. The increase in plasma creatinine is not linear, however. Several attempts have thus been made to develop reliable methods that will allow a correct estimate of creatinine clearance from its plasma concentration (P_{creat}) alone, without urine collection. The following formula has been developed that allows an estimate of GFR derived from the child's creatinine plasma concentration and height.

$$GFR = k \times Height/P_{creat}$$

where k is a constant, Height represents the body height, and P_{creat} the plasma creatinine concentration. This formula is based on the assumption that creatinine excretion is proportional to body height and inversely proportional to plasma creatinine (57). The value of factor k can be obtained from the formula $k = GFR \times Height/P_{creat}$. Under steady state conditions, k should be directly proportional to the muscle component of body weight, which corresponds reasonably well to the daily urinary creatinine excretion rate.

The serum concentration of cystatin C has been proposed to assess GFR. Although the serum concentration of cystatin C may be superior to P_{creat} in distinguishing normal from abnormal GFR, a rational numerical estimate of GFR cannot be derived from its plasma concentration (58).

Estimation of Glomerular Filtration Rate in Clinical Practice with Different Markers

Inulin

The Marker

Inulin, a fructose polysaccharide derived from dahlia roots and Jerusalem artichokes, has an Einstein-Stokes radius of 1.5 nm and an MW of approximately 5.2 kDa. It diffuses as would a spherical body of such radius. Inulin is inert, not metabolized, and can be recovered quantitatively in the urine after parenteral administration. Evidence that inulin in neither reabsorbed nor secreted by the renal tubules has been well demonstrated in experimental micropuncture studies (59,60).

The rate of excretion of inulin is directly proportional to the plasma concentration of inulin. Its clearance (UV/P) is consequently independent of its plasma concentration. Because the renal excretion of inulin occurs exclusively by glomerular filtration, its clearance is the most accurate index of GFR. Estimates of inulin clearance provide the basis for a standard reference against which the route or mechanism of excretion of other substances can be ascertained.

Sinistrin is a readily soluble preparation of polyfructose with side branching (extracted from the bulb of *Urginea maritima*), which is more suitable for clinical use and readily available in Europe. This compound is identical to inulin.

Measurement of Inulin

In the classical anthrone method, inulin is hydrolyzed to fructose by sulfuric acid, and the fructose is then measured by colorimetry (61). Carbohydrates present in the plasma and urine also react in the assay (62). The method has a variation coefficient close to 6%. A specific, highly sensitive, enzymatic method has been described by Kuehnle et al. (63).

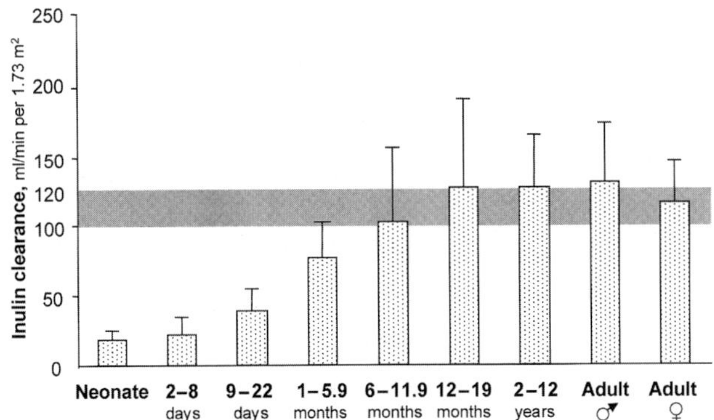

FIGURE 21.2. Inulin clearance as a function of age X ± SD.

In this method, inulin is hydrolyzed by insulinase, with simultaneous oxidation of the native glucose using glucose oxidase and H_2O_2. The fructose generated by inulinase is then converted to glucose-6-phosphate. This method has a variation coefficient below 5% in serum and urine samples. A fully automated enzymatic inulin assay, with minimal sample prehandling and capable of complete sinistrin hydrolysis, has been described (64). The coefficient of variation was reported at 4.4%.

Inulin Urinary Clearance

Inulin or sinistrin urinary clearance (UV/P) is the gold standard for the assessment of GFR. In the classical method, inulin is administered as a priming dose to achieve plasma concentrations close to 200 to 400 mg/L. It is then constantly infused to maintain constant levels over the 3-hour clearance study. After an equilibration period of 90 minutes, urine and blood samples are collected at intervals of 30 minutes. The mean value of three to four clearance periods is considered as representing the child's GFR. In small children, the urine samples are collected through an indwelling bladder catheter. In preschool and school children, urine is collected by spontaneous voiding. Generous oral water loading (~300 mL/m²/hr) is given to maintain high urine flow rates. Sugar (e.g., glucose, fructose, and saccharose)-containing drinks must be avoided, as these glucosides interfere with the measurement of inulin in both the plasma and urine.

The use of sinistrin has been associated with anaphylactic reaction (65) in a 45-year-old white patient, whereas anaphylaxis from inulin in vegetables has been reported in a 39-year-old man (66).

The rise in GFR from birth to adulthood is illustrated in Figure 21.2 and given in Table 21.5. Mature values of GFR range from 100 to 120 mL/min/1.73 m². In a study by Koopman et al. in adult volunteers, GFR, as assessed by inulin clearance, had a circadian rhythm (67). It started to decrease during late afternoon or evening and rose again at the end of the night. The mean amplitude of the rhythm was 36 mL/min.

Constant Infusion Technique of Inulin without Urine Collection

The constant infusion technique of inulin without urine collection yields reproducible results, as long as sufficient time is given for steady concentrations to be reached (54,55,68). This may take as long as 12 hours in adults and even longer in infants (68,69). During the equilibration period, inulin is excreted by filtration, while at the same time diffusing into the extracellular space. Calculations of the infusion (IR/P) clearance before equilibration overestimate clearance values up to 30% above the urinary clearance. The shorter the time of infusion, the larger is the overestimation. The constant infusion method is useful when timed urine collections are difficult or unreliable, such as in small babies, children with hydronephrosis, or those with neurogenic bladder.

The result of the study comparing the "3-hour constant infusion" with the urinary clearance of inulin in 60 children older than 1 year showed a significant correlation, but the calculated regression line differed significantly from the line of identity, and the scatter of points was considerable (70). These results did not confirm an earlier report by Cole et al. demonstrating virtual superposition of inulin clearance values generated with and without urine collection (55). The constant infusion technique should be reserved for studies when the precise collection of urine cannot be performed and its result interpreted with caution.

Plasma Disappearance Curve of Inulin

The total body clearance of inulin can be estimated from the plasma disappearance curve after a bolus i.v. short infu-

TABLE 21.5. NORMAL VALUES OF THE GLOMERULAR FILTRATION RATE (GFR) AS MEASURED BY CREATININE CLEARANCE AND RENAL PLASMA FLOW (RPF) AS MEASURED BY *P*-AMINOHIPPURIC ACID AND REFERENCE VALUES OF MAXIMAL URINE OSMOLALITY

	Neonate	1–2 wk	6–12 mo	1–3 yr	Adult
GFR[a] mL/min × 1.73 m²	26 ± 2	54 ± 8	77 ± 14	96 ± 22	118 ± 18
RBF[a] mL/min × 1.73 m²	88 ± 4	154 ± 34	352 ± 73	537 ± 122	612 ± 92
Maximal urine osmolality[a] mOsm/kg H_2O	543 ± 50	619 ± 81	864 ± 148	750 ± 1330	825 ± 1285

[a]Mean values ± SEM.
Adapted from García-Nieto V, Santos F. Pruebas funcionales renales. In: Garcia-Nieto V, Santos F, eds. *Nefrología pediátrica*. Madrid: Aula Médica, 2000; and García-Nieto V, Santos F, eds. *Grupo aula medica*. Madrid: Aula Médica, 2000;15–26.

sion (<5 minutes) of inulin at a dose of 100 mg/kg. The amount of inulin injected is such as to acutely increase the plasma concentration to 0.5 to 1.0 g/L (71). The concentration of inulin is ideally followed for at least 4 hours after the injection. Studies comparing the single injection with the urinary clearance of inulin have reported significant correlations between the two methods (72,73), but the single injection significantly overestimated the urinary clearance in a study by Florijn et al. (72). Pharmacokinetic adaptation of the standard technique can probably reduce the overestimation, but the procedure implies the collection of a blood sample for as long as 10 hours after the bolus injection in patients with impaired renal function (74).

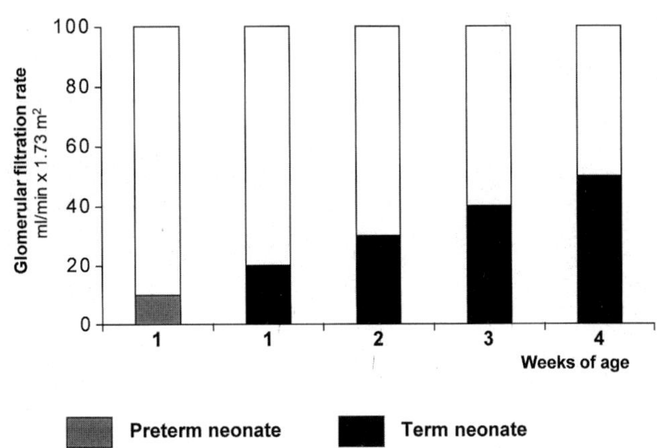

FIGURE 21.3. Postnatal increase in glomerular filtration rate in term and preterm infants. Open part in columns represents mature levels of glomerular filtration rates. (Adapted from Guignard JP, Torrado A, Da Cunha O, et al. Glomerular filtration rate in the first three weeks of life. *J Pediatr* 1975;87:268–272.)

Inulin as a Marker of Glomerular Filtration Rate in the Neonate

Studies comparing the clearance of inulin with that of other glomerular markers have led to the hypothesis that glomerular pore size could be related to body size and that inulin may not be freely filtered by the immature glomerulus (75). This hypothesis has not been confirmed by studies of inulin handling in rats or fetal lambs, both failing to demonstrate any restriction to the filtration of inulin (76,77). The same conclusion was reached from clinical studies in preterm infants showing that high-molecular-weight inulin or polysaccharides did not accumulate in the plasma of very immature babies infused with these glomerular markers for several days, thus excluding any retention of the larger molecules (78,79).

Studies on standard urinary inulin clearance in neonates are scarce. Those performed during the first 2 days of life of preterm and term neonates have shown that GFR at birth approximates 20 mL/min/1.73 m^2 in term neonates and 12 to 13 mL/min/1.73 m^2 in preemies of 28 to 30 weeks of gestation (80). The GFR matures rapidly in the early postnatal period, doubling during the first 2 weeks of life (80) (Fig. 21.3). The velocity of the maturation is somewhat slower in the most premature infants.

Conflicting results have been observed in neonates studied by the inulin constant infusion technique over a few hours. Although Cole et al. and Leake et al. found an excellent correlation between the constant infusion clearance and the urinary clearance of inulin (R = 0.999), Alinei and Guignard found the constant infusion technique to greatly overestimate (~30%) the urinary clearance of inulin in infants (55,81,82). The overestimation declined with time but remained substantial after 3 hours of infusion. The same conclusion was reached by Coulthard, who also observed an overestimation of GFR by the constant infusion technique in spite of the fact that the plasma inulin concentration was apparently stable (69). Reliable estimates of GFR could, however, be obtained when inulin was constantly infused for 24 hours, with or without a bolus injection at the start of the test. The main disadvantage of the method is that of requiring a constant infusion of long duration, as well as careful supervision of the test. Using the 24-hour constant infusion method in preterm infants, Van der Heijden et al. confirmed that GFR increases rapidly after birth (83).

Results comparing data obtained by the single injection technique with those obtained with the urinary clearance of inulin are conflicting. Early optimistic results have not been confirmed (84). A 30% overestimation of the true GFR was described by Fawer et al. in neonates 1 to 3 days old (85). These results were confirmed by Coulthard in preterm babies, who also described a large coefficient of variation for the single injection technique (69).

Creatinine

The Marker

Creatinine is the anhydrase of creatine, a compound present in skeletal muscle as creatine phosphate. It has an MW of 113 d. The serum creatinine levels reflect total body supplies of creatinine and correlate with muscle mass. After initial decrease during the first month of life (Table 21.6), it increases steadily with age (Table 21.7). The excretion rate varies according to body weight and age, both reflecting muscle mass. The renal excretion pattern of endogenous creatinine is similar to that of inulin in humans and several animal species. However, in addition to being filtered through the glomerulus, creatinine is secreted in part by the renal tubular cells.

The validity of creatinine as a marker of GFR has been questioned because creatinine is not only secreted by the renal tubular cells, but could also be reabsorbed under certain conditions. Such reabsorption has been shown to occur in rats and dogs at low urine flow rates (86,87). Substantial tubular secretion and reabsorption of creatinine has been suggested in humans in relation to the degree of hydration (88,89).

TABLE 21.6. MEAN VALUES OF PLASMA CREATININE DURING THE FIRST WEEKS OF LIFE OF TERM AND VERY LOW BIRTH WEIGHT NEONATES

	Plasma creatinine (μmol/L)[a]			
	Postnatal period (d)			
Birth weight (g)	1–2	8–9	15–16	22–23
1001–1500	95 ± 5	64 ± 5	49 ± 4	35 ± 3
1501–2000	90 ± 5	58 ± 7	50 ± 8	30 ± 2
2001–2500	83 ± 5	47 ± 8	38 ± 8	30 ± 10
Term	66 ± 3	40 ± 4	30 ± 8	27 ± 7

[a]Mean values ± SEM.

Overestimation of GFR by creatinine clearance is more pronounced at low GFR. Indeed, as GFR falls progressively during the course of renal diseases, the renal tubular secretion of creatinine contributes to an increasing fraction of urinary excretion, so that creatinine clearance may substantially exceed the actual GFR. Diffusion of creatinine into the gut may also interfere with the accuracy of its clearance in uremic patients. At a normal plasma concentration, the amount of creatinine entering the gut is negligible. It may become significant during renal failure when the plasma creatinine concentration increases (90). This phenomenon explains in part why creatinine clearance overestimates true GFR in patients with renal failure.

Measurement of Creatinine

Creatinine concentration in plasma and urine is usually based on the Jaffe reaction, characterized by the production of an orange-red color when creatinine reacts with alkaline sodium picrate. The method is not very specific, noncreatinine chromogens generating sufficient color to account for 0.2 to 0.3 mg/dL (~30 μmol/L) of "false creatinine." The interference of noncreatinine chromogen obviously is highest at the lowest values of creatinine, as present in newborn infants (91). Negative interference by conjugated and unconjugated bilirubin makes the use of the Jaffe reaction questionable in neonates. Other interference substances include acetoacetate, pyruvate, uric acid, the cephalosporins, and cotrimoxazole (91). The noncreatinine chromogens do not interfere significantly in the urine.

TABLE 21.7. PLASMA CREATININE IN CHILDREN

	Plasma creatinine		Creatininuria	
Age (yr)	μmol/L	mg/dL	μmol/kg/d	mg/kg/d
<2	35–40	0.4–0.5	62–88	7.1–9.9
2–8	40–60	0.5–0.7	108–188	12.2–21.2
9–18	50–80	0.6–0.9	132–212	14.9–23.9

Adapted from García-Nieto V, Santos F. Pruebas funcionales renales. In: Garcia-Nieto V, Santos F, eds. *Nefrología pediátrica*. Madrid: Aula Médica, 2000; and García-Nieto V, Santos F, eds. *Grupo aula medica*. Madrid: Aula Médica, 2000;15–26.

Modified kinetic Jaffe techniques have improved the specificity of creatinine measurement. Enzymatic methods have subsequently been developed that are more specific than the Jaffe reaction. Their cost and questionable precision have limited their widespread use.

Determination of serum creatinine by isotope dilution mass spectrometry has been described as the potential "definitive" method (92). High-performance liquid chromatography (HPLC) will undoubtedly become the reference method for creatinine determination (93,94), even if its routine use is still not possible in most clinical laboratories.

Creatinine Urinary Clearance

The urinary clearance of creatinine (UV/P) is the most commonly used method for assessing GFR in children. The urine is collected over 4 to 24 hours, with the plasma sample collected at the middle of the urine collection period. The plasma creatinine concentration can be significantly increased by cooked-meat feeding (95). Drugs, such as trimethoprim and cimetidine, increase the plasma creatinine by interfering with the renal tubular secretion, presumably by competition for the organic cation secretory passageway (96,97).

Estimation of GFR by measuring the urinary clearance of creatinine yields values that have been shown to correlate variably with inulin clearance. The best correlation is seen when GFR is normal. This results from the balance between two artifacts: (a) the excretion rate of creatinine is higher than the filtered rate because of the tubular secretion of creatinine and (b) the measured plasma creatinine is higher than the true creatinine because of the presence of noncreatinine chromogens that interfere with a standard colorimetric analysis of creatinine in the Jaffe reaction.

Overestimation of GFR by the urinary creatinine clearance is usually maximal at low levels of GFR (98). The ratio of the urinary creatinine clearance to urinary inulin clearance has been shown to vary between 1.14 and 2.27 in adult subjects. Dodge et al. and Kim et al. have long ago suggested that creatinine clearance should not be used for the estimation of GFR, as this clearance varies with tubular secretion of creatinine, which follows no apparent pattern (99,100). In the latter study, 42% of patients with decreased renal function would have been diagnosed as normal using urinary creatinine clearance. Like those of Rosenbaum, data obtained by Guignard et al. in 72 children older than 1 year showed a substantial overestimation of GFR by creatinine clearance at all levels of GF (70,101).

Assessment of Glomerular Filtration Rate by the Formula $(2\,C_{creat} + C_{urea})/3$

In children undergoing simultaneous inulin and creatinine urinary clearance studies, the overestimation of GFR by creatinine clearance was "corrected" when the clearance of urea was also taken into account (70). When using the for-

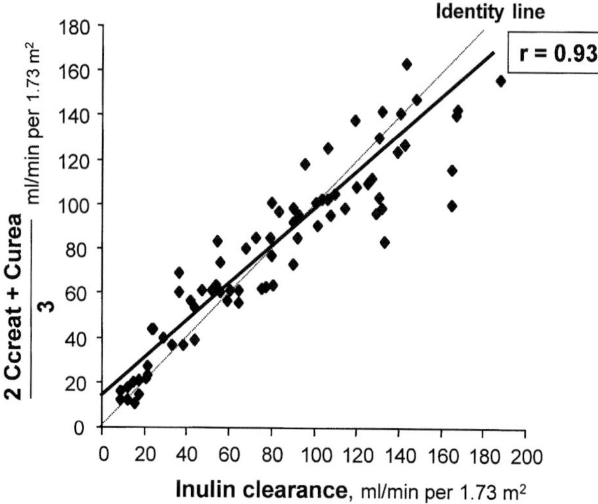

FIGURE 21.4. Relationship between standard urinary clearance of inulin and the (2 C_{creat} + C_{urea}) / 3 formula. (Adapted from Guignard JP, Torrado A, Feldmann H, et al. Assessment of glomerular filtration rate in children. *Helv Pediatr Acta* 1980;35:437–447.)

mula (2 C_{creat} + C_{urea})/3, the regression line correlating this formula to inulin clearance was indistinguishable from the line of identity (Fig. 21.4). The scatter of points around the regression line was, however, not negligible.

Clearly, creatinine clearance alone is not a good alternative to inulin clearance when a precise measurement of GFR is needed. The use of the formula (2 C_{creat} + C_{urea})/3, calculated over 3 to 4 hours in well-hydrated children, is recommended when the clinical situation does not warrant the cumbersome measurement of inulin clearance or when the technique is not available.

The GFR = k × Height/P_{creat} Formula

Numerous studies have used the GFR = k × Height/P_{creat} formula, first described in 1976 by Counahan et al. and Schwarz et al. (102,103). A critical review of the use of this formula has been published by Haycock (104). The formula provides useful data when used cautiously. It cannot be used in obese or malnourished children in whom body height does not accurately reflect muscle mass. Ideally, the exact value of k should be derived from the laboratory where the plasma creatinine is measured and from inulin clearance as the reference method for estimating GFR. The values of k, as derived from creatinine clearance in different age groups by Schwarz et al., are given in Table 21.8 (57). In a study involving 200 patients aged 1 month to 23 years, Haenggi et al. compared the values of k derived from the urinary inulin clearance to that derived from simultaneous urinary creatinine clearance (89). The value of k derived from creatinine or inulin clearance differed significantly, being lower when calculated from C_{inulin}. The effect of the state of hydration was assessed in 18 children in a "hydropenic state" (urine flow rate, 3.5 ± 0.6 mL/min/1.73 m²; mean urine osmolality, 407 ± 61 mOsm/kg H_2O) or undergoing water diuresis (urine flow rate, 8.5 mL/min/1.73 m²; mean urine osmolality, 163g ± 20 mOsm/kg H_2O). In hydropenic children, the values of k were identical when derived from C_{inulin} or C_{creat} (49 ± 2 and 50 ± 3, respectively). They differed significantly when k was derived from urinary creatinine clearance in children undergoing water diuresis (50 ± 3 vs. 64 ± 4; p <.001). Increased secretory rates of creatinine at high urine flow rates probably account for the elevated value of k calculated from C_{creat} in well-hydrated children. Extensive tubular secretion and reabsorption of creatinine in relation to the degree of hydration has been well described in humans (86). In spite of its relative inaccuracy, the k × height/P_{creat} formula has proved valuable as a rapid rough estimate of GFR in clinical practice.

TABLE 21.8. VALUES OF K FOR VARIOUS AGE GROUPS

	k values when P_{creat} expressed in:	
	µmol/L	mg/dL
Low-birth-weight infants <2.5 kg	29	0.33
Normal infants 0–18 mo	40	0.45
Girls 2–16 yr	49	0.55
Boys 2–13 yr	49	0.55
Boys 13–16 yr	62	0.70

Note: Values of k for estimating creatinine clearance by the k × height/P_{creat} formula.
Adapted from Schwartz GJ, Brion LP, Spitzer A. The use of plasma creatinine concentration for estimating glomerular filtration rate in infants, children, and adolescents. *Pediatr Clin North Am* 1987;34:571–590.

Creatinine as a Marker of Glomerular Filtration Rate in the Neonate

In tiny premature neonates, the clearance of creatinine underestimates inulin clearance (105,106). Studies in piglets and newborn rabbits suggest that the filtered creatinine is significantly reabsorbed by the immature tubule (107,108). Creatinine reabsorption by the immature kidney probably occurs by passive back-diffusion of filtered creatinine across leaky tubules. Significant reabsorption of filtered creatinine supposedly accounts for the transient increase in plasma creatinine in the first 3 days of life of very low birth weight infants (Fig. 21.5) (109–111). After the neonatal period, P_{creat} rises steadily throughout infancy and childhood toward adult levels (Table 21.7).

In spite of these drawbacks in the assessment of GFR by creatinine clearance in newborn infants, the latter method has been used commonly in this age group. Studying very low birth weight infants, Stonestreet et al. have reported a correlation coefficient of 0.78 when values of creatinine clearance were compared to those of inulin clearance (106). In recent studies in premature and term neonates, creatinine clearance has been shown to be low at birth and to rise

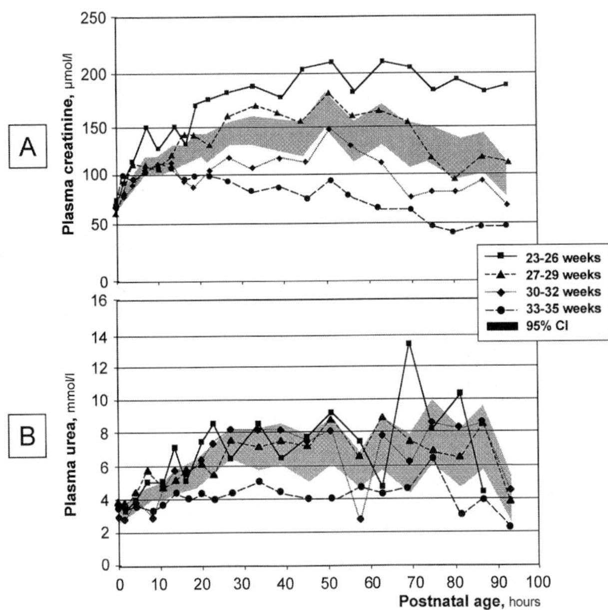

FIGURE 21.5. Changes in plasma creatinine **(A)** and urea **(B)** concentrations during the first 100 hours of life of premature neonates of variable gestational age. The shaded area represents 95% Cis for the mean plasma creatinine or urea of all infants. (Adapted from Miall LS, Henderson MJ, Turner AJ, et al. Plasma creatinine rises dramatically in the first 48 hours of life in preterm infants. *Pediatrics* 1999;104:e76.)

rapidly after birth (111,112). The slope of maturation was steeper in the most mature infants (112). The increase in creatinine clearance correlated with the postnatal increase in systemic blood pressure as well as with gestational and postnatal age (111–113). Creatinine clearance close to 42 mL/min/1.73 m^2 in term neonates and 27 mL/min/1.73 m^2 in premies younger than 27 weeks of gestation were recorded on the fifty-second day of life (111). Mature levels close to 100 mL/min/1.73 m^2 are reached at the end of the first year of life.

Iohexol

Iohexol is a nonionic contrast agent with an MW of 821 d. It does (almost) not bind to plasma proteins, diffuses into the extracellular space (114), and is eliminated exclusively via the kidneys (115). Iohexol has an elimination half-life of approximately 90 minutes. Total urine recovery of iohexol after i.v. injection occurs within 12 hours (114). Iohexol can be measured by x-ray fluorescence and HPLC methods (74). More recently, iohexol has been successfully measured by the capillary electrophoresis technique, with results similar to those obtained by the HPLC method (74). The capillary electrophoresis technique is less expensive, more rapid, and more sensitive than both the HPLC and x-ray fluorescence methods. Good correlations have been reported between plasma iohexol clearance and that of ^{51}Cr-EDTA (116). Clinical studies have, however, suggested that the diffusion of iohexol in its distribution volume is slow, and that it may take more than 4 to 6 hours to reach equilibrium after an i.v. injection of the agent (117). This may limit the usefulness of iohexol as a marker of GFR, even if significant correlations have been demonstrated between standard inulin clearance and values generated by the plasma disappearance curve of iohexol (74).

Cystatin C

Cystatin C, a nonglycosated, 13-d basic protein, is a proteinase inhibitor involved in the intracellular catabolism of proteins (118). It is produced by all nucleated cells at a constant rate apparently independent from inflammatory conditions, muscle mass, and gender (119). It is freely filtered across the glomerular capillaries, almost completely reabsorbed, and catabolized in the proximal tubular cells (120). Being reabsorbed, cystatin is not a classical glomerular marker as strictly defined (121). Fully automated assays using particle-enhanced turbidimetry or particle-enhanced nephelometry are available for the measurement of cystatin in plasma and serum (122,123). The assays are precise, rapid, and usable in clinical routine practice.

Cystatin C does not cross the placenta, and there is no correlation between maternal and neonatal serum cystatin C levels (124). Cystatin C concentrations are high at birth and then decrease to stabilize after 12 months of age (119) (Fig. 21.6). Whether cystatin C is significantly higher in premature infants as compared to term infants is not yet clear (119,125). Bökenkamp et al. found serum cystatin levels between 0.70 and 1.38 mg/L in children older than 1 year (126).

Serum cystatin C concentrations are closely related to GFR as are serum creatinine levels. Serum cystatin C increases when GFR decreases. The reciprocal values of cystatin C correlate linearly with GFR, and cystatin C has been claimed to be at least as good as serum creatinine for the evaluation of GFR in adults (127). In children aged 1.8 to 18.8 years with various levels of GFR, serum cystatin C has been found to be broadly equivalent or even superior to serum creatinine as an estimate of GFR (58,126). The fact that cystatin C is independent of age, gender, height, and body composition has been considered an advantage (126).

The major drawbacks in using cystatin C are that it is not a true glomerular marker and its clearance cannot be calculated. A recent study by Martini et al. compared the reliability of different estimates of GFR to distinguish impaired from normal GFR, with a cut-off at 100 mL/min/1.73 m^2 (128). Although plasma cystatin was slightly superior to plasma creatinine in diagnosing renal insufficiency, it was significantly less sensitive than both urinary creatinine clearance and the estimated k × Height / P_{creat}. The authors concluded that simply measuring the child's height in addition to the plasma creatinine was a simpler, cheaper, and better means of rapidly assessing GFR in children than measuring the plasma cystatin C. The recent observation that the urine cystatin C/

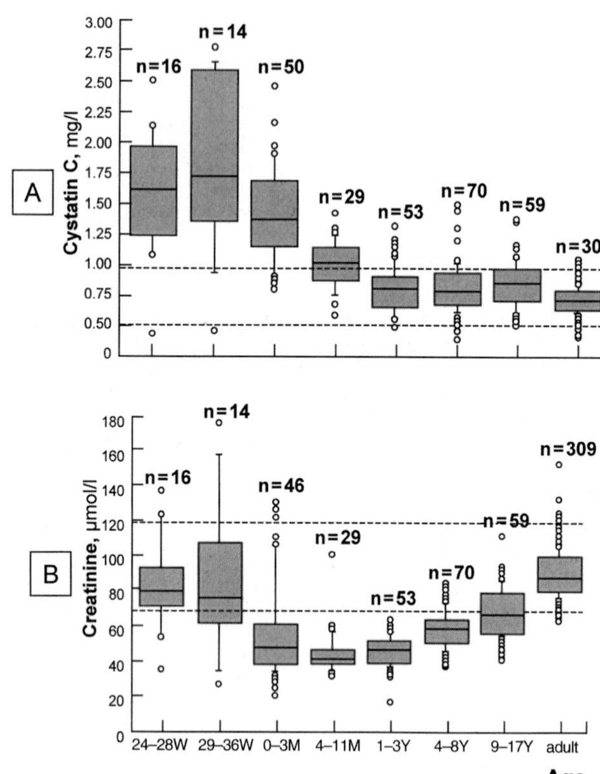

FIGURE 21.6. Box plot distributions showing **(A)** cystatin C and **(B)** creatinine values (tenth, twenty-fifth, fiftieth, and ninetieth percentiles) across the age groups. The categories of 24 to 36 and 29 to 36 weeks refer to gestational ages of preterm babies. Dotted lines indicate 95% confidence interval of adult range. Preterm babies born between 24 to 36 weeks' gestation were 1 day old. (Adapted from Finney H, Newman DJ, Thakkar H, et al. Reference ranges for plasma cystatin C and creatinine measurements in premature infants, neonates and older children. *Arch Dis Child* 2000;82:71–75.)

creatinine ratio could provide information on both glomerular function and tubular injury casts doubts on the real value of cystatin C as the best estimate of GFR (129).

Radionuclides

Radionuclides, such as ^{51}Cr-EDTA, ^{99m}Tc-DTPA, and ^{125}I-iothalamate, have been used as alternative filtration markers (Table 21.4). They permit accurate detection of minute concentrations of the markers in plasma and urine samples. Their urinary clearance, as calculated after a constant infusion of the marker, was initially reported as fairly similar to that of inulin (130). Prolonged radioactive exposure during the infusion of radiolabeled markers has limited the use of these compounds to single injection studies only. Even in these conditions, radioactive markers are best avoided in pregnant women and small children.

^{99m}Tc-DTPA

DTPA has an MW of 393 d. It appears to be excreted mainly by glomerular filtration (131). Protein binding of DTPA is minimal. Its clearance approximates that of inulin (132). The occurrence of extrarenal elimination of DTPA is, however, suggested by the observation that the plasma clearance of ^{99m}Tc-DTPA exceeds the urinary clearance of the compound by a variable but significant amount (130,132). A significant drawback in using ^{99m}Tc-DTPA as a glomerular marker is the fact that the ^{99m}Tc-DTPA can significantly dissociate from DTPA during a clearance study (133). In the neonate, ^{99m}Tc-DTPA scans are characterized by poor visualization of the kidneys and a relatively flat renal curve. Better-quality dynamic isotope scans are generally only achieved at the end of the neonatal period, when GFR has reached higher values.

^{51}Cr-EDTA

EDTA is a glomerular marker similar to DTPA. EDTA has an MW of 292 d and is used as a chelate of ^{51}Cr. Its plasma disappearance curve measured after a bolus i.v. injection exceeds its urinary clearance by an average of 6 mL/min, thus suggesting an extrarenal route of elimination (134). This phenomenon is particularly evident at low filtration rates.

Iothalamate

Iothalamate sodium has an MW of 637 d. Iothalamate has been used as ^{125}I-radiolabeled or without radioactive label, its plasma concentration being then assessed by x-ray fluorescence or by HPLC, or, more recently, by capillary electrophoresis (135). A recent study showed an excellent correlation between the clearance of ^{125}I-iothalamate and cold iothalamate, as assessed by capillary electrophoresis (136). Critical studies have, however, unequivocally demonstrated that iothalamate is actively secreted by renal tubular cells, and perhaps also undergoes tubular reabsorption in human and animal species (137). The urinary clearance of iothalamate significantly exceeds that of inulin in patients with normal renal function (138). When present, the agreement of iothalamate clearance with inulin clearance appears to be a fortuitous cancellation of errors between tubular excretion and protein binding (139). The use of iothalamate as a glomerular marker is presently not recommended.

Renal Functional Reserve

It has been considered for a long time that GFR in healthy individuals is remarkably stable from day to day over a period of years (121). This concept has been challenged by the observation that GFR in normal subjects could vary with their diet protein content (140). Alterations in protein intake thus result in variations in GFR that are independent of changes in renal mass. Patients with renal disease on a low-protein diet may thus have a reduction of GFR unrelated to the progression of renal disease (140). Variations in GFR also occur during the circadian rhythm, and upsurges in GFR are observed in patients with burns, women during pregnancy, and patients infused with amino acids (67).

The baseline or "resting" GFR theoretically depends on the working level of the intact nephrons and is the consequence, in part, of the amount of proteins ingested per day. The renal functional reserve represents the potential of the kidney to increase GFR from a baseline or resting value to a maximal one (the so-called maximal filtration capacity) in response to increased physiologic demands. Depending on the daily protein intake, GFR may vary from 30 to 143 mL/min/1.73 m^2 in normal individuals (140).

The maximal filtration capacity can be measured in patients undergoing inulin clearance studies before and after an oral load of proteins, during the infusion of amino acids, or during the combined administration of amino acids and dopamine (see section Protocol for Measuring the Functional Reserve Capacity). The maximal filtration capacity in young adults has been shown to reach values close to 160 mL/min/min (140,141).

The renal functional reserve represents the difference between the resting GFR and the maximal GFR. The magnitude of the renal functional reserve obviously depends on the resting GFR (142). Normal individuals with the lowest protein intake have the highest renal reserve. In patients with renal disease, the maximal filtration capacity decreases as the disease progresses. The resting GFR is insensitive as an indicator of renal damage. On the contrary, the filtration capacity is a good indicator of renal damage as it decreases proportionally to the extent of injury to the kidney. In patients with GFR below 40 mL/min/1.73 m^2, the renal functional reserve is usually negligible or absent, indicating that at this level of function, all nephrons are working maximally at all times. In most conditions, the increase in GFR observed after protein loading or i.v. amino acid infusion is associated with a parallel increase in RBF. The increase in RBF is probably the consequence of decreased intrarenal vascular resistance, mainly at the level of the afferent and efferent arterioles.

Several mechanisms may play a role in mediating the renal response to protein loading or amino acid infusion, including a number of circulating or locally acting hormonal factors and intrinsic intrarenal mechanisms (143).

Experimental data suggest that growth hormone and atrial natriuretic peptide are not involved in the response to protein or amino acid administration, but that prostaglandins, nitric oxide, and the kallikrein-kinin system could play key roles (143). Intrinsic renal mechanisms, namely, tubular transport and tubuloglomerular feedback mechanisms, could also play key roles in mediating the amino acid or the protein-stimulated renal vasodilatation and hyperfiltration. Amino acids could cause a primary stimulation of proximal tubular sodium reabsorption and in turn cause renal vasodilatation and hyperfiltration (144). The finding that the response to a meat meal is inhibited by acetazolamide, an inhibitor of sodium transport in the proximal tubule, but not by amiloride provided strong support for the hypothesis that normal proximal tubular sodium reabsorption capacity is required for protein-stimulated renal vasodilatation and hyperfiltration (145).

Protocol for Measuring the Functional Reserve Capacity

The functional reserve is assessed during a standard clearance test, using inulin and *p*-aminohippuric acid (PAH) as markers of GFR and effective renal plasma flow (ERPF), respectively. After a priming dose of inulin 25% [64 mg/kg body weight (BW)] and PAH 20% (9 mg/kg BW), a continuous infusion of 1 to 2 mg/kg/min inulin and 0.15 to 0.30 mg/kg/min PAH is given intravenously. Water diuresis is induced by an oral ingestion of 20 mL/kg BW (maximum, 1200 mL) during the first hour, and then 5 mL/kg BW (maximum, 300 ml) every 30 minutes. Urine samples are collected by spontaneous micturition at 30-minute intervals and blood samples drawn midway through each urine collection period. After an equilibration period of 60 minutes and 3-minute baseline periods, an oral protein load of 1.5 mg/kg BW (mixed meal containing meat with milk protein as a supplement) is given within 30 minutes. After the meal, the creatinine test is continued for an additional 3-hour period (6 periods of 30 minutes each).

The baseline GFR and ERPF corresponds to the mean values of the three periods before the protein-rich meal. The *maximal filtration capacity* is defined as the peak values observed after the protein-rich meal. The functional reserve is calculated by subtracting the baseline GFR and ERPF from their maximal values observed after the protein-rich meal. The renal function reserve is also expressed as fractional increase (%) from the baseline values. Another method for assessing the functional reserve consists of an i.v. infusion of a 7.5% solution of amino acids at a rate of 0.08 mL/min/kg. Dopamine (2 μg/kg BW/min) can be infused concomitantly to the infusion of amino acids.

RENAL BLOOD FLOW

Physiology

RBF approximates 20% of resting cardiac output—that is, 1200 mL/min/1.73 m^2. Most of this flow supplies the metabolic active renal cortex, whereas 10% of RBF is directed toward the outer medulla and only 1 to 2% into the capillary tissue. A small part goes to the capsule and perirenal fat. Several factors, such as a high-protein diet, can increase RBF both acutely and chronically. RBF also increases during pregnancy under the influence of gestational hormones.

RBF is proportional to the pressure gradient across the renal vasculature (renal artery pressure minus renal vein pressure) and inversely proportional to the total renal vascular resistance. Most of the resistance resides in three major segments: (a) the intralobular arteries, (b) the afferent arterioles, and (c) the efferent arterioles. The renal vascular tone is affected by neural impulses and by circulating intrarenal vasoactive compounds such as angiotensin II, prostaglandins, nitric oxide, endothelin, bradykinin, and adenosine.

RBF is autoregulated by an intrinsic myogenic mechanism. The vessels have the capacity to constrict when blood pressure rises and to vasodilate when it decreases. RBF is thus independent of the perfusion pressure over the range of autoregulation (~80 to 180 mm Hg).

The major role of blood supply to the kidney is to provide blood for filtration. The fraction of plasma that is filtered through the glomeruli, the so-called filtration fraction, approximates 20% in normal conditions. When RBF is reduced, GFR is usually maintained by angiotensin II–induced efferent arteriolar vasoconstriction. This is evidenced by an increase in the filtration fraction.

Measurement of Renal Blood Flow

Measurement of RBF is based on the Fick principle. According to this principle, any substance completely extracted from the blood during a single pass through the kidney would allow the measurement of true RBF. In addition to being completely extracted from the blood, the substance should not be metabolized by the kidney, not bound to proteins, and accurately measurable in blood and urine. PAH is the only known compound that meets the required properties. It has an MW of 194 d, is filtered through the glomerular capillaries, and is secreted by the proximal tubular cells (146). It is almost completely removed from the plasma by a single pass. At low arterial plasma concentrations (~20 mg/L) the concentration in the renal vein is negligible. The plasma perfusing the kidney being completely cleared of PAH and the extracted PAH quantitatively excreted in the urine, the clearance of PAH can be used to estimate renal plasma flow (RPF). By measuring the hematocrit, RBF can be derived from RPF by the formula RBF = RPF/1-hematocrit.

The clearance of PAH underestimates slightly the true RPF, as PAH extraction is only approximately 90% complete because part of the blood delivered to the kidney goes to sites not available for secretion in the proximal tubule (medulla, capsule, perinatal fat). The PAH clearance thus assesses cortical plasma flow more than true total RPF. The term *effective renal plasma flow* is often used to described the value derived from PAH clearances. The extraction ratio can vary in disease states or under the influence of certain drugs, thus making the measurement of renal vein concentration necessary for accurate determination of RPF.

Because PAH undergoes acetylation by the liver, its clearance estimated by the constant infusion technique without urine collection or by the plasma disappearance curve significantly overestimates the urinary clearance. The clearance of PAH can be affected by drugs, such as penicillin, salicylates, or sulfinpyrazone, that compete for the same secretory passageway. The extraction efficiency of PAH may also be depressed by drugs commonly used in renal patients (i.e., angiotensin-converting enzyme inhibitors and cyclosporine) (147,148).

Measurement of *p*-Aminohippuric Acid Clearance

The clearance of PAH is usually measured concomitantly with that of inulin. A priming dose of PAH is given at a dose of 9 mg/kg BW, followed by a continuous infusion of 0.15 to 0.30 mg/kg/min to maintain plasma concentration between 10 and 20 mg/L. Water intake is administered as for the inulin clearance test (20 mL/kg BW during the first hour, and then 5 mL/kg BW every 30 minutes). Urine and blood samples are collected as described for the inulin clearance test.

Determination of p*-Aminohippuric Acid*

PAH in plasma and urine can be measured by the classical colorimetric reaction of Bratton and Marshall (149). Several compounds interfere with the reaction, in particular those with a para-amino ring, including acebutolol, sotalol, procaine, cotrimoxazole, and furosemide (62). PAH can be measured more accurately by HPLC (150).

Adverse Effects of p*-Aminohippuric Acid*

The administration of PAH is usually well tolerated but may be associated with nausea, vomiting, vasomotor disturbances, flushing, tingling, cramps, and a feeling of warmth, and sometimes the urge to urinate or defecate.

Drawbacks in the Interpretation of C_{PAH}

The main drawbacks in the use of PAH clearance to assess RPF resides in the fact that the extraction of PAH is not complete and that it can vary under the influence of disease states, drug administration, and age. Newborn infants have low extraction ratios that limit the usefulness of PAH in the first month of life (151).

Other Cold Markers of Renal Plasma Flow

5-Hydroxyindoleacetic acid (5-HIAA) is the major metabolite of serotonin. Its renal elimination, analogous to that of PAH and other weak organic acids, is achieved by glomerular filtration and by probenecid-sensitive active secretion in the proximal tubule (152). A renal extraction ratio of 78% has been measured in hypertensive adult patients with normal renal function (153). This ratio is lower than the PAH extraction ratio measured in human subjects at plasma PAH concentrations below the maximum transport. The efficient renal tubular secretion of 5-HIAA is further illustrated by the 5-HIAA to inulin ratio as high as 6.3 ± 0.66

(SEM) in healthy subjects and in patients with reduced GFR (153). Plasma levels of 5-HIAA have been shown to correlate inversely (R = 0.85) with the PAH clearance.

The extraction of 5-HIAA in newborn animals, like that of PAH, is well below its level in mature subjects. The low extraction of PAH in neonates has been ascribed to the shunting of blood to the nonextracting renal tissues, to the relative decrease in tubular mass, and to the immaturity of the renal tubular secretory passageways (154). This endogenous marker, easily assayed in plasma by using liquid chromatography and electrochemical detection (155), may prove useful for a quick orientation on RPF in clinical practice (153).

Radionuclides as Markers of Renal Plasma Flow

Orthoiodohippurate (Hippuran)

Hippuran is eliminated by the kidney in a way similar to PAH. Its extraction ratio is, however, significantly lower than that of PAH (70 to 85% as compared to 90%) (156). Protein binding of Hippuran is not negligible. The urinary clearance of Hippuran underestimates RPF more than does that of PAH (157). Hippuran can easily be labeled by a simple iodine exchange reaction; most often it is labeled with either ^{131}I or ^{123}I. ^{123}I-Hippuran can be used in children in larger doses than ^{131}I-Hippuran, while still imparting a lower radiation burden to the patient. Its short half-life and greater cost limit its widespread use.

^{99m}Tc-Mercaptoacetyltriglycerine

In spite of early claims, mercaptoacetyltriglycerine (MAG-3) is not a marker of RPF. In normal volunteers, ^{99m}Tc-MAG-3 and ^{123}I-Hippuran showed comparable image quality, renal extraction, blood clearance, and time to peak height of the renogram curve. Overall, the clearance of ^{99m}Tc-MAG-3 is, however, approximately only 80% of the simultaneous clearance of ^{131}I-Hippuran (158).

Newer Imaging Techniques for the Assessment of Renal Perfusion

Newer promising imaging techniques have been developed in the last years, both in animals and humans (159). None can be a substitute to the clearance of PAH to precisely assess RPF. These techniques may, however, provide reliable estimates of total renal or regional renal blood perfusion.

Contrast-Enhanced Ultrasound

An excellent correlation has been found in dogs between cortical nutrient blood flow using microbubbles and ultrasonic flow probe–derived RBF values (R = 0.82; p <.001) over a wide range of flows (160). A similar correlation (R = 0.84) has been found in dogs when blood flow calculated from contrast ultrasonography was compared with direct measurement obtained with an electromagnetic flow probe (161).

Quantification with Color Flow and Pulsed Doppler Ultrasound

Estimates of total RBF have been produced in neonates by estimating the vessel diameter from color flow diameter and flow velocity from pulse Doppler ultrasound measurements (162).

Electron-Beam Computed Tomography

From studies in anesthetized dogs, comparing data from electron-beam computed tomography with those of electromagnetic flow probe, Lerman et al. (163) concluded that electron-beam computed tomography could provide credible quantification of RBF.

Dynamic Magnetic Resonance Imaging and Gadolinium-DTPA

By the use of a T1-weighted fast gradient sequence after an i.v. bolus injection of gadolinium-DTPA, dynamic images of the kidney have been obtained in patients presenting with well-functioning native or transplanted kidneys, patients with significant artery stenosis, or patients with renal failure (164). The authors concluded that realistic quantitative data on renal perfusion could be obtained by standard magnetic resonance imaging sequence after injection of a contrast medium. This method awaits confirmation.

TESTS TO ASSESS TUBULAR FUNCTION

Functional tests explore specific aspects of renal function under conditions in which the tubule must develop an adaptive response aimed at preserving body homeostasis. The use of functional tests often allows nephron disorders not apparent or hardly recognizable under basal conditions to be disclosed. Some tests are cumbersome, thus limiting their use in the clinical setting.

Description of the tests includes (165) (a) the function that is tested, (b) the rationale of the test, (c) the method and normal results, and (d) the indications for and limitations of the test.

Glucose Titration Test

Function tested: Characteristics of glucose tubular reabsorption.

Rationale: The amount of glucose filtered per minute is a linear function of its plasma concentration provided that GFR remains steady (Fig. 21.1). Below a threshold level, all filtered glucose is reabsorbed, and no glucose is detected in the urine. When the load of filtered glucose saturates the mechanism of transport in all nephrons, the maximum tubular reabsorption is achieved. From then on, the urinary elimination of glucose runs parallel to the filtered glucose. The same rationale may be applied to other substances with an active and saturable mechanism of proximal tubular reabsorption (Fig. 21.1).

Method and normal results: Starting from a plasma concentration below the threshold—that is, when glucosuria is negative—3 mL/min/1.73 m^2 of i.v. 5% dextrose is infused. Dextrose solution concentration is increased by 5% each 30 minutes until glycemia reaches 350 to 400 mg/dL (19 to 22 mmol/L). The maximal concentration of dextrose that can be infused in a peripheral vein is 35%. Urine samples collected during the last 15 minutes of each 30-minute period and plasma samples drawn in the midpoint of each urine collection period are used for calculation. Normal plasma threshold is approximately 180 mg/dL (9.9 mmol/L). Mean reference values of the maximum tubular reabsorption are 375 and 303 mg/min/1.73 m^2 (2.1 and 1.7 mmol/min/1.73 m^2) for males and females, respectively.

Indications and limitations: The test may be used for diagnostic classification of renal glucosurias. In some cases, the renal threshold for glucose is so low that it cannot be achieved without risk to the patient. Accurate collection of frequent and timed urine samples may require bladder catheterization in young children.

Bicarbonate Loading Test

Function tested: Characteristics of tubular reabsorption of bicarbonate (HCO_3^-) and hydrogen ion (H^+) distal secretory capacity in the face of a favorable chemical gradient.

Rationale: The test assesses the tubular reabsorption of HCO_3^- on the basis of a theoretical background similar to that described above for glucose. The difference between filtered and excreted HCO_3^- accounts for the HCO_3^- reabsorbed along the renal tubule, mostly in the proximal tubule. In addition, HCO_3^- loading will give rise to alkaline urine with pH higher than that of blood. This stimulates H^+ secretion by alpha-intercalated cells of the collecting duct. Hydrogen ions so secreted combine with HCO_3^- anions to form carbonic acid. As at this level of the nephron, there is no carbonic anhydrase in the luminal side of the tubule; carbonic acid dehydrates very slowly into carbon dioxide (CO_2) and water. The medullary trapping of CO_2 and the unfavorable surface-to-volume relationship in the lower urinary tract limit the diffusion of CO_2 out of the tubular lumen. As a result, the measurement of the partial pressure of CO_2 (PCO_2) in alkaline urine can be used as a reliable index of distal H^+ secretion (166).

Method and normal results: An i.v. solution of 0.3 to 0.5 mol/L of $NaHCO_3^-$ is infused at a rate calculated to increase bicarbonatemia by 2 to 3 mmol/L/hr in a subject with spontaneous or induced metabolic acidosis. For diagnostic purposes, the calculation of the plasma threshold for HCO_3^- is seldom required. It is usually sufficient to calculate $FE_{HCO_3^-}$ in the presence of normal bicarbonatemia—that is, 20 to 22 mmol/L in infants and 22 to 24 mmol/L in older children—and to measure the PCO_2 in alkaline urines (pH above 7.45 to 7.60 and bicarbonaturia higher than 80 mmol/L) induced by a single oral dose of 3 to 4 mmol/kg of $NaHCO_3^-$ (1 g = 12 mmol). Normal values are $FE_{HCO_3^-}$ less than 5% and urinary PCO_2 above 70 mm Hg, which is equivalent to a urine minus blood PCO_2 difference (Δ PCO_2) greater than 20 to 30 mm Hg. Urine HCO_3^- can be calculated by the Henderson-Hasselbalch equation:

$$pH = pK + \log (HCO_3^-/H_2CO_3)$$

Knowing that

1. $H_2CO_3 = CO_2 + H_2O = 0.03\ PCO_2$, where PCO_2 is the partial pressure of CO_2 measured in mm Hg, as determined by a pH/blood gas analyzer in urine collected and processed in anaerobic conditions, and 0.03 is the solubility constant of CO_2 in aqueous solutions.
2. The pK of the $NaHCO_3^-$ buffer system in urine is 6.33 – 0.5 multiplied by the square root of the sum of the urine sodium and potassium concentrations expressed in mol/L.

Indications and limitations: The test may be used in the differential diagnosis of the types of RTA. $FE_{HCO_3^-}$ is below 5% in type I distal RTA, above 15% in type II proximal RTA, and between 5% and 15% in type IV RTA. ΔPCO_2 is well below 20 mm Hg in children with primary forms of type I RTA. Calculation of $FE_{HCO_3^-}$ in the face of normal bicarbonatemia may give a clue to the dose of alkali to be recommended in recently diagnosed RTA children. The measurement of PCO_2 in alkaline urine has been proposed as a sensitive method to detect subtle defects of distal acidification (167,168). An accurate assessment of $FE_{HCO_3^-}$ requires a nonexpanded extracellular fluid volume. Otherwise, proximal tubular reabsorption is inhibited, giving rise to high values of $NaHCO_3^-$ excretion. Because of the massive bicarbonaturia, normal bicarbonatemia is hard to achieve and maintain in children with proximal RTA.

Phosphate Loading Test

Function tested: Secretory capacity of H^+ by the distal nephron in the face of large availability of intraluminal buffer. The use of phosphate infusions to assess phosphate tubular reabsorption has largely been replaced by the indices described above.

Rationale: A high luminal concentration of phosphate stimulates H^+ secretion. When urine pH is close to the urinary pK of the phosphate buffer system, disodium phosphate combines with the secreted H^+ to form acid phosphate that, in turn, reacts with $NaHCO_3^-$ to form H_2CO_3 and to increase PCO_2 in the final urine. Measurement of urinary PCO_2 reflects distal H^+ secretion.

Method and normal results: Concentrations of urinary phosphate greater than 20 mmol/L can usually be induced by oral administration of 50 mg/kg/day of elemental phosphorus given as a mixture of monosodium and disodium phosphate salts over a 3-day period. Alternatively, 0.6 mmol/kg of neutral sodium phosphate diluted in 180 mL of normal saline may be infused at 1 mL/min for 3 hours. Urinary PCO_2 measured in urine samples with pH of approximately 6.80 should normally exceed blood PCO_2 by 20 to 25 mm Hg (169).

Indications and limitations: The test may be used to explore the mechanism of defective acidification in patients with distal type I RTA. A normal Δ PCO_2 in individuals with distal RTA suggests that the acidification defect is due to back-leak of secreted acid.

Acidification Test

Minimal Urinary pH and Net Acid Excretion

Function tested: Secretory capacity of H^+ by the distal nephron in the face of metabolic acidosis.

Rationale: Metabolic acidosis stimulates distal secretion of H^+. The secreted H^+ will be found in the urine in free form, estimated by the urinary pH, and will be bound to the two major urinary buffers, phosphate, and, mainly, ammonia generated by the proximal tubule. Net acid excretion is equal to the sum of titratable acid plus NH_4^+ minus bicarbonate. *Titratable acid* refers to the amount of alkali needed to bring the pH of an acid urine back to a value of 7.4.

Method and normal results: The measurements are done in situations of spontaneous or exogenously induced metabolic acidosis. Ammonium chloride is the agent of choice for inducing metabolic acidosis. It is given at a dose of 75 to 100 mmol/m^2 (1 g = 18.7 mmol) either intravenously over 4 to 6 hours in a 0.9% solution, or by oral route in enteric coated capsules given over 1 hour. Ammonium chloride is an irritating agent and may produce vomiting. To avoid this effect, 1.9 mmol/kg/day of ammonium chloride may be given in a 3- to 5-day period, which, in addition, represents a much more potent stimulus of ammonia production than the short test. A state of moderate metabolic acidosis (blood pH less than 7.33 and bicarbonatemia below 16 to 18 mmol/L) is usually sufficient to assess urine acidification. Normal individuals lower urine pH below 5.5 and increase net acid excretion above 70 µmol/min/1.73 m^2.

Indications and limitations: The test is useful in the differential diagnosis of RTA. Patients with type I distal RTA are unable to both maximally decrease urinary pH and increase net acid excretion up to normal values. In type II proximal RTA, minimal urinary pH and normal net acid excretion are achieved once plasma bicarbonate falls below the renal threshold. Subjects with type IV RTA show normal ability to decrease urinary pH and defective excretion of ammonium. A urine pH equal to or below 6.0 in the second morning urine in fasting conditions has been proposed as a reliable screening tool to exclude incomplete or minor forms of distal RTA. However, the range of urine pH determined in the early morning urine in normal children ranges from 5.16 to 7.07 (170). As pH is a measurement of free H^+ concentration, patients unable to properly concentrate urine may in turn be unable to decrease urine pH to normal minimal values. Similarly, in subjects with contracted extracellular volume, the urinary acidification defect may be a result of the lack of sodium at the lumen of the distal nephron. Accordingly, a proper evaluation of urinary acidification requires the measurement of urinary sodium and urine osmolality as well as the simultaneous determination of urine pH and NH_4^+ because a low pH associated with reduced ammoniuria does not exclude a defective distal acidification, and, on the contrary, a high ammoniuria may be responsible for the fact that pH does not decrease below 5.5.

Furosemide Test

Function tested: Secretory capacity of H^+ by the distal nephron in the presence of large amounts of sodium delivered to the distal nephron and a favorable electronegative lumen potential.

Rationale: Furosemide inhibits reabsorption of sodium chloride in the thick ascending limb of the loop of Henle. Early distal reabsorption of sodium cation leaves behind the chloride anion, enhancing the electronegativity of tubular lumen, which stimulates H^+ secretion.

Method and normal results: Furosemide is given at a dose of 1 mg/kg, orally or intravenously. In normal subjects, a minimal urine pH below 5.5, associated with a kaliuretic response, is usually found within 3 to 4 hours after furosemide administration. Mean (SD) values of minimal urinary pH and maximal FE_K reported in 20 normal children, aged 2 to 14 years, given 1 mg/kg of i.v. furosemide are 4.96 (0.32) and 34.4% (8.9%), respectively (171). The H^+ secretion stimulated by furosemide also increases ammoniuria above 30 µmol/min/1.73 m^2 (172).

Indications and limitations: The test is used in the differential diagnosis of RTA. Type 1 distal RTA patients with an intrinsic defect in the proton pump cannot maximally decrease urine pH in response to furosemide. Subjects with type IV RTA and those with subnormal distal H^+ secretion secondary to low distal delivery of sodium (i.e., nephrotic syndrome) or reversible impairment of sodium distal reabsorption (i.e., sickle cell anemia or lithium administration) respond normally.

Acetazolamide Test

Function tested: Ability of distal nephron to secrete H^+ in the face of a favorable chemical gradient.

Rationale: By inhibiting carbonic anhydrase, acetazolamide reduces proximal tubular reabsorption of bicarbonate and causes bicarbonaturia and alkaline urine. Measurement of PCO_2 in urine samples with pH above that of blood reflects the ability of the distal nephron to secrete H^+.

Method and normal results: Oral acetazolamide is given at a dose of 0.5 to 1.0 g/1.73 m^2. A normal response is characterized by urinary PCO_2 above 70 mm Hg or Δ PCO_2 above 20 to 30 mm Hg.

Indications and limitations: The test is used to explore the mechanism of defective acidification in distal type I RTA. Children with primary defects of the distal proton pump do not increase urine PCO_2. Alon et al. found similar response to oral bicarbonate (2.5 mmol/kg) or acetazolamide (17 ± 2 mg/kg) in terms of urine bicarbonate concentration and PCO_2 (173).

Concentrating Ability

Urinary Concentration during Hydropenia

Function tested: Ability to concentrate urine in response to fluid suppression.

Rationale: Fluid restriction increases blood tonicity, thus stimulating vasopressin secretion. As a result, free water is reabsorbed, and the urine becomes concentrated.

Method and normal results: Urinary osmolality is measured at the end of a 12- to 16-hour period of fluid deprivation. During this period, children are allowed to eat solid foods except those having a high content in salt and water. In healthy children older than 2 years of age, mean (SD) values of urinary osmolality in the second and third urine voided in the morning during fluid suppression since noon have been reported to be equal to 1035 and 1127 (128) mOsm/kg H_2O (174,175). When fluid intake is suppressed since 5 or 6 p.m., the urinary osmolality measured in the second urine of the following morning is normally higher than 725 mOsm/kg H_2O. If the determination of osmolality is not available, urinary density values above 1025 are usually indicative of normal renal concentration capacity.

Indications and limitations: The test is used to investigate the origin of polyuric states as well as to disclose subclinical defects of urine concentrating ability. Prolonged fluid restriction may be harmful in infants and poorly tolerated in subjects with chronic primary polydipsia. In addition, these patients have a hypotonic medullary interstitium and may require much longer periods of hydropenia to maximally concentrate the urine. In these cases, a progressive reduction in fluid intake over days or weeks is necessary before exposing the child to a thirst test.

Vasopressin Administration

Function tested: Ability to concentrate urine in response to vasopressin administration.

Rationale: As urinary osmolality is strongly influenced by plasma concentrations of vasopressin, administration of pharmacologic amounts of a vasopressin analogue results in maximally concentrated urine even in the absence of fluid restriction.

Method and normal results: The compound most often used is the 1-desamino-8-D-arginine vasopressin (DDAVP). It can be given intranasally at doses of 10 μg in infants and 20 μg in children (175). In infants, usual fluid intake must be restricted to 50% in the 12 hours after DDAVP administration because of the risk of overhydration and hyponatremia. Osmolality is measured in individual urine samples collected over a 6- to 8-hour period after DDAVP administration. Normal values of maximal urine osmolality are shown in Table 21.5 (172,176). Recently, it has been proposed that assessment of renal concentrating capacity by administration of DDAVP at bedtime and measurement of osmolality in one urine sample taken the following morning may be reliable and easy to perform in children (177).

Indications and limitations: The DDAVP test represents a good alternative to thirst stimulus in infants and polyuric subjects in whom, as stated above, fluid suppression is hardly feasible. The test may also be used in moderately polyuric subjects sequentially after a period of fluid restriction when maximal urine osmolality obtained by hydropenia has not achieved normal values. In these cases, a DDAVP-induced increment of urine osmolality below 10% suggests tubular resistance to antidiuretic hormone, whereas a 40 to 60% increment in urinary osmolality indicates defective vasopressin release or primary polydipsia. In these sequential tests, a correct interpretation of the results requires that after DDAVP administration the child be allowed to drink an amount of fluid similar to that of urine voided. Thus, the degree of plasma hypertonicity induced by hydropenia remains unchanged.

Dilution Ability (Free Water Clearance)

Hypotonic Saline Loading

Function tested: Chloride, sodium, and potassium handling along the nephron under conditions of maximal urinary dilution and in the absence of hormonal influences.

Rationale: Maximal urine dilution and suppression of aldosterone and antidiuretic hormone are induced by extracellular volume expansion with hypo-osmolar fluid loading. Under these conditions, maximal excretion of electrolyte-free water is generated in the diluting segments of the tubule. An indirect estimate of solute reabsorption in the different segments of the nephron may be obtained by calculation of several urinary indices, as shown in Table 21.9.

Method and normal results: After oral administration of 20 mL/kg of water, a constant i.v. infusion of 2000 mL/ 1.73 m^2 of 0.45% saline is administered over 2 hours. Cal-

TABLE 21.9. NORMAL VALUES OF MAXIMAL FREE WATER CLEARANCE INDICES DURING HYPOTONIC SALINE DIURESIS

	Infants (n = 22)	Children (n = 17)
Urine osmolality (mOsm/kg)	51.8 ± 12.8	54.1 ± 13.3
Urine volume (mL/dL GF)	22.8 ± 3.6	17.2 ± 2.7[a]
Osmolar clearance (C_{osm}) (mL/dL GF)	4.3 ± 1.3	3.2 ± 0.7[a]
Free water clearance (C_{H_2O}) (mL/dL GF)	18.5 ± 2.9	14.0 ± 2.6[a]
Sodium clearance (C_{Na}) (mL/dL GF)	1.9 ± 0.8	1.4 ± 0.4[a]
Potassium clearance (C_K) (mL/dL GF)	19.9 ± 12.0	12.9 ± 5.2[a]
Chloride clearance (C_{Cl}) (mL/dL GF)	2.7 ± 1.1	2.1 ± 0.7a
Percentage of distal sodium reabsorption: $100 \times C_{H_2O} / (C_{H_2O} + C_{Na})$ (%)	90.8 ± 4.5	90.9 ± 3.3
Percentage of distal chloride reabsorption: $100 \times C_{H_2O} / (C_{H_2O} + C_{Cl})$ (%)	87.2 ± 5.3	86.7 ± 4.1
Creatinine clearance (mL/min/1.73 m²)	88.5 ± 27.1	124.8 ± 25.2[a]

GF, glomerular filtration (values are × ± SD).
[a]Significantly different from infants.
$C_{H_2O} + C_{Na}$: Sodium delivery to the distal nephron. $C_{H_2O} + C_{Cl}$: Chloride delivery to the distal nephron. C_{H_2O}: Reabsorption of sodium chloride in the distal nephron. $C_{H_2O} / (C_{H_2O} + C_{Na})$: Fraction of sodium reabsorbed in the distal nephron. $C_{H_2O} / (C_{H_2O} + C_{Cl})$: Fraction of chloride reabsorbed in the distal nephron.
Adapted from Rodríguez-Soriano J, Vallo A, Castillo G, Oliveros R. Renal handling of water and sodium in infancy and childhood: a study using clearance methods during hypotonic saline diuresis. *Kidney Int* 1981;20:700–704.

culations are made in maximally diluted urine samples, those with urinary osmolality below 70 mOsm/kg and the highest free-water clearance. Normal results of the test are given in Table 21.9. Sodium and chloride FC are calculated as explained above. C_{H_2O} is calculated as follows: $C_{H_2O} = V - C_{osm}$, where V is the volume of urine eliminated per 100 mL of GFR and C_{osm} is the osmolar fractional clearance.

$$V = (P_{Cr}/U_{Cr}) \times 100 \text{ and } C_{osm} = (\text{Urine osmolality/Plasma osmolality}) \times V$$

Indications and limitations: The test is used to localize the site of defective reabsorption in tubular disorders, such as Bartter syndrome, with exaggerated loss of chloride, sodium, or potassium. The various indices, based on theoretical assumptions, should be interpreted with caution, but can provide valuable information in conditions associated with tubular reabsorption defects.

REFERENCES

1. Kaplan RE, Springate JE, Feld LG. Screening dipstick urinalysis: a time to change. *Pediatrics* 1997;100:919–921.
2. Linshaw MA, Gruskin AB. The routine urinalysis: to keep or not to keep; that is the question. *Pediatrics* 1997;100: 1031–1032.
3. Deen WM, Lazzare MJ, Myers BD. Structureal determinants of glomerular permeability. *Am J Physiol Renal Physiol* 2001:281:F579–F596.
4. Kanwar YS. Biophysiology of glomerular filtration and proteinuria. *Lab Invest* 1984;51:7–21.
5. Kumar S, Muchmore A. Tann-Horsfall protein-uromodulin (1950–1990). *Kidney Int* 1990;37:1395–1401.
6. Yoshioka T, Mitarai T, Kon V, et al. Role for angiotensin II in an overt functional proteinuria. *Kidney Int* 1986;30:538–545.
7. Houser M. Assessment of proteinuria using random urine samples. *J Pediatr* 1984;104:845–848.
8. Ginsberg JM, Chang BS, Matarese RM, et al. Use of single voided urine samples to estimate quantitative proteinuria. *N Engl J Med* 1983;309:1543–1546.
9. Sawick PT, Heinemann L, Berger M. Comparison of methods for determination of microalbuminuria in diabetic patients. *Diabetic Med* 1989;6:412–415.
10. Bergon E, Granados R, Fernandez-Segoviano P, et al. Classification of renal proteinuria: a simple algorithm. *Clin Chem Lab Med* 2002;40:1143–1150.
11. Vehaskari VM. Mechanism of orthostatic proteinuria. *Pediatr Nephrol* 1990;4:328–330.
12. Ruggenenti P, Perna A, Mosconi L, et al. Urinary protein excretion rate is the best independent predictor of ESRF in non-diabetic proteinuric chronic nephropathies. *Kidney Int* 1998;53:1209–1216.
13. Tomlinson PA, Dalton RN, Hartley B, et al. Low molecular weight protein excretion in glomerular disease: a common analysis. *Pediatr Nephrol* 1997;11:285–290.
14. Barratt TM, Crawford R. Lysozyme excretion as a measure of renal tubular dysfunction in children. *Clin Sci* 1970;39: 457–465.
15. Remuzzi G. A unifying hypothesis for renal scarring linking protein trafficking to the different mediators of injury. *Nephrol Dial Transplant* 2000;15:58–60.
16. Hogg RJ, Portman RJ, Milliner D, et al. Evaluation and management of proteinuria and nephrotic syndrome in children: recommendations from a pediatric nephrology panel established at the National Kidney Foundation Conference on proteinuria, albuminuria, risk, assessment, detection, and elimination (Parade). *Pediatrics* 2000;105:1242–1249.

17. Alon U. Clinical assessment of plasma phosphate and renal tubular threshold for phosphate. In: Alon U, Chan JCM, eds. *Phosphate in pediatric health and disease.* Boca Raton, FL: CRC Press 1993;104–114.
18. Bijvoet OLM. Relation of plasma phosphate concentration to renal tubular reabsorption of phosphate. *Clin Sci* 1969;37:23–36.
19. Walton RJ, Bijvoet OLM. Nomogram for derivation of renal threshold phosphate concentration. *Lancet* 1975;II:309–310.
20. Kruse K, Kracht U, Gopfert G. Renal threshold phosphate concentration ($TmPO_4$/GFR). *Arch Dis Child* 1982;57:217–223.
21. Stark H, Eisenstein B, Tieder M, et al. Direct measurement of TP/GFR: a simple and reliable parameter of renal phosphate handling. *Nephron* 1986;44:125–128.
22. Brodehl J, Krause A, Hoyer PF. Assessment of maximal tubular phosphate reabsorption: comparison of direct measurement with the nomogram of Bijvoet. *Pediatr Nephrol* 1988;2:183–189.
23. Alon U, Hellerstein S. Assessment and interpretation of the tubular threshold for phosphate in infants and children. *Pediatr Nephrol* 1994;8:250–251.
24. Andersen LJ, Andersen JL, Pump B, et al. Natriuresis induced by mild hypernatremia in humans. *Am J Physiol Regul Integr Comp Physiol* 2002;282:R1754–R1761.
25. Mersin SS, Ramelli GP, Laux-End R, et al. Urinary chloride excretion distinguishes between renal and extrarenal metabolic alkalosis. *Eur J Pediatr* 1995;154:979–982.
26. Rossi R, Danzebrink S, Linnenbürger K, et al. Assessment of tubular reabsorption of sodium, glucose, phosphate and amino acids based on spot urine samples. *Acta Paediatr* 1994;83:1282–1286.
27. Ubalde E, García de Jalón A, et al. Excreción urinaria de calcio en niños sanos. Estudio colaborativo y multicéntrico. *Nefrología* 1988;8:224–230.
28. Sweid HA, Bagga A, Vaswani M, et al. Urinary excretion of minerals, oxalate, and uric acid in north Indian children. *Pediatr Nephrol* 1997;11:189–192.
29. Alconcher LF, Castro C, Quintana D, et al. Urinary calcium excretion in healthy school children. *Pediatr Nephrol* 1997;11:186–188.
30. Sargent JD, Stukel TA, Kresel J, et al. Normal values for random urinary calcium to creatinine ratios in infancy. *J Pediatr* 1993;123:393–397.
31. Matos V, Melle G van, Boulat O, et al. Urinary phosphate/creatinine, calcium/creatinine, and magnesium/creatinine ratios in a healthy pediatric population. *J Pediatr* 1997;131:252–257.
32. Bell NH, Yergey AL, Vieira NE, et al. Demonstration of a difference in urinary calcium, not calcium absorption, in black and white adolescents. *J Bone Miner Res* 1993;8:1111–1115.
33. De Santo NG, Di Iorio B, Capasso G, et al. Population based data on urinary excretion of calcium, magnesium, oxalate, phosphate and uric acid in children from Cimitile (southern Italy). *Pediatr Nephrol* 1992;6:149–157.
34. Paunier L, Borgeaud M, Wyss M. Urinary excretion of magnesium and calcium in normal children. *Helv Paediatr Acta* 1970;25:577–584.
35. Ghazali S, Barratt TM. Urinary excretion of calcium and magnesium in children. *Arch Dis Child* 1974;49:97–101.
36. Hernández MR, Nuñez GF, Martínez C. Excreción urinaria de calcio, magnesio, ácido úrico y ácido oxálico en niños normales. *An Esp Pediatr* 1988;29:99–104.
37. Chen YH, Lee AJ, Chen CH, et al. Urinary mineral excretion among normal Taiwanese children. *Pediatr Nephrol* 1994;8:36–39.
38. Sutton RAL, Domrongkitchaiborn S. Abnormal renal magnesium handling. *Miner Electrolyte Metab* 1993;19:232–240.
39. Stapleton FB, Linshaw MA, Hassanein K, et al. Uric acid excretion in normal children. *J Pediatr* 1978;92:911–914.
40. Stapleton FB, Nash DA. A screening test for hyperuricosuria. *J Pediatr* 1983;102:88–90.
41. La Manna A, Polito C, Marte A, et al. Hyperuricosuria in children: clinical presentation and natural history. *Pediatrics* 2001;107:86–90.
42. Martul MV, Baeza JF, Vila S, et al. Eliminación urinaria de citrato, magnesio y oxalato en niños normales. Indices urinarios litogénicos. *Nefrología* 1995;15:550–558.
43. Matos V, Melle G van, Werner D, et al. Urinary oxalate and urate to creatinine ratios in a healthy pediatric population. *Am J Kidney Dis* 1999;34:1–6.
44. Reusz GS, Dobos M, Byrd D, et al. Urinary calcium and oxalate excretion in children. *Pediatr Nephrol* 1995;9:39–44.
45. Areses R, Arruebarrena D, Arriola M, et al. Estudio Haurtxo. Valores de referencia del citrato en plasma y orina en la edad pediátrica. *Nefrología* 1994;14:302–307.
46. Norman ME, Feldman NI, Cohn RM, et al. Urinary citrate excretion in the diagnosis of distal tubular acidosis. *J Pediatr* 1978;82:394–400.
47. Blau N, Matasovic A, Lukasiewicz-Wedlechowicz A, et al. Simultaneous determination of oxalate, glycolate, citrate, and sulfate from dried urine filter paper spots in pediatric population. *Clin Chem* 1998;44:1554–1556.
48. Sulyok E, Guignard JP. Relationship of urinary anion gap to urinary ammonium excretion in the neonate. *Biol Neonate* 1990;57:98–106.
49. Abelow B. Urinary anion gap. In: Abelow B. *Understanding acid-base.* Baltimore: Williams & Wilkins, 1998;A57–A59.
50. Kirschbaum B, Sica D, Anderson FP. Urine electrolytes and the urine anion and osmolar gaps. *J Lab Clin Med* 1999; 133:597–604.
51. West ML, Bendz O, Chen CB, et al. Development of a test to evaluate the transtubular potassium concentration gradient in the cortical collecting duct in vivo. *Mineral Electrolyte Metab* 1986;12:226–233.
52. West ML, Marsden PA, Richardson RMA, et al. New clinical approach to evaluate disorders of potassium excretion. *Mineral Electrolyte Metab* 1986;12:234–238.
53. Rodríguez-Soriano J, Ubetagoyena M, Vallo A. Transtubular potassium concentration gradient: a useful test to estimate renal aldosterone bio-activity in infants and children. *Pediatr Nephrol* 1990;4:105–110.
54. Earle DP, Berliner RW. A simplified clinical procedure for measurement of glomerular filtration rate and renal blood flow. *Proc Soc Exp Biol Med* 1946;62:262–264.
55. Cole BR, Giangiacomo J, Ingelfinger JR, et al. Measurement of renal function without urine collection. A critical evaluation of the constant-infusion technique for determi-

nation of inulin and para-aminohippurate. *N Engl J Med* 1972;287:1109–1114.

56. Sapirstein LA, Vidt DG, Mandel MJ, et al. Volumes of distribution and clearances of intravenously injected creatinine in the dog. *Am J Physiol* 1955;181:330–335.
57. Schwartz GJ, Brion LP, Spitzer A. The use of plasma creatinine concentration for estimating glomerular filtration rate in infants, children, and adolescents. *Pediatr Clin North Am* 1987;34:571–590.
58. Stickle D, Cole B, Hock K, et al. Correlation of plasma concentration of cystatin C and creatinine to inulin clearance in a pediatric population. *Clin Chem* 1998;44:1334–1338.
59. Marsh D, Frasier C. Reliability of inulin for determining volume flow in rat renal cortical tubules. *Am J Physiol* 1965;209:283–286.
60. Tanner GA, Klose RM. Micropuncture study of inulin reabsorption in *Necturus* kidney. *Am J Physiol* 1966;211:1036–1038.
61. Wright HK, Gann DS. An automatic anthrone method for the determination of inulin in plasma and urine. *J Lab Clin Med* 1966;67:689–693.
62. Brenna S, Grigoras O, Drukker A, et al. Pitfalls in measuring inulin and para-amino-hippuric acid clearance. *Pediatr Nephrol* 1998;12:489–491.
63. Kuehnle HF, Dahl VK, Schmidt FH. Fully enzymatic inulin determination in small volume samples without deproteinization. *Nephron* 1992;62:104–107.
64. Soper CPR, Bending MR, Barron JL. An automated enzymatic inulin assay, capable of full sinistrin hydrolysis. *Eur J Chem Clin Biochem* 1995;33:497–501.
65. Chandra R, Barron JL. Anaphylactic reaction to intravenous sinistrin (Inutest). *Ann Clin Biochem* 2002;39:76.
66. Gay-Crosier F, Schreiber G, Hauser C. Anaphylaxis from inulin in vegetables and processed food. *N Engl J Med* 2000;342:1372.
67. Koopman MG, Koomen GCM, Krediet RT, et al. Circadian rhythm of glomerular filtration rate in normal individuals. *Clin Sci* 1989;77:105–111.
68. Hellerstein S, Barenbom M, Alon U, et al. The renal clearance and infusion clearance of inulin are similar, but not identical. *Kidney Int* 1993;44:1058–1061.
69. Coulthard MG. Comparison of methods of measuring renal function in preterm babies using inulin. *J Pediatr* 1983;102:923–930.
70. Guignard JP, Torrado A, Feldmann H, et al. Assessment of glomerular filtration rate in children. *Helv Pediatr Acta* 1980;35:437–447.
71. Rahn KH, Heidenreich S, Brückner D. How to assess glomerular filtration rate in humans? *J Hypertens* 1999;17:309–317.
72. Florijn KW, Barendregt JN, Lentjes EG, et al. Glomerular filtration rate measurement by "single-shot" injection of inulin. *Kidney Int* 1994;46:252–259.
73. Müller-Suur R, Göransson M, Olsen L, et al. Inulin single injection clearance. Microsamples technique useful in children for determination of glomerular filtration rate. *Clin Physiol* 1983;3:19–27.
74. Gaspari F, Noberto P, Remuzzi G. Application of newer clearance techniques for the determination of glomerular filtration rate. *Curr Opin Nephrol Hypertens* 1998;7:675–680.
75. Arturson G, Groth T, Grotte G. Human glomerular membrane porosity and filtration pressure: dextran clearance data analysed by theoretical models. *Clin Sci* 1971;40:137–158.
76. Harris CA, Baer PG, Chirito E, et al. Composition of mammalian glomerular filtrate. *Am J Physiol* 1974;227:972–976.
77. Rankin JH, Gresham EL, Battaglia FC, et al. Measurement of fetal renal inulin clearance in a chronic sheep preparation. *J Appl Physiol* 1972;32:129–133.
78. Coulthard MG, Ruddock V. Validation of inulin as a marker for glomerular filtration in preterm babies. *Kidney Int* 1983;23:407–409.
79. Wilkins BH. The glomerular filterability of polyfructosan-S in immature infants. *Pediatr Nephrol* 1992;6:319–322.
80. Guignard JP, Torrado A, Da Cunha O, et al. Glomerular filtration rate in the first three weeks of life. *J Pediatr* 1975;87:268–272.
81. Leake RD, Trygstad CW, Oh W. Inulin clearance in the newborn infant: relationship to gestational and postnatal age. *Pediatr Res* 1976;10:759–762.
82. Alinei P, Guignard JP. Assessment of glomerular filtration rate in infants. *Helv Pediatr Acta* 1987;42:253–262.
83. Van der Heijden AJ, Grose WF, Ambagtsheer JJ, et al. Glomerular filtration rate in the preterm infant: the relation to gestational and postnatal age. *Eur J Pediatr* 1988;148:24–28.
84. Svenningsen NW. Single injection polyfructosan clearance in normal and asphyxiated neonates. *Acta Paediatr Scand* 1975;64:87–95.
85. Fawer CL, Torrado A, Guignard JP. Single injection clearance in the neonate. *Biol Neonate* 1979;35:321–324.
86. Namnum P, Insogna K, Baggish D, et al. Evidence for bidirectional net movement of creatinine in the rat kidney. *Am J Physiol* 1983;244:F719–F723.
87. Lee KE, Behrendt U, Kaczmarczyk G, et al. Estimation of glomérulaire filtration rate in conscious dogs following a bolus of creatinine. *Pflügers Arch* 1983;396:176–178.
88. Sjöstrom PA, Odlind BG, Wolgast M. Extensive tubular secretion and reabsorption of creatinine in humans. *Scand J Urol Nephrol* 1988;22:129–131.
89. Haenggi MH, Pelet J, Guignard JP. Estimation du débit de filtration glomérulaire per la formula DFG = $k \times T/P_{creat}$. *Arch Pediatr* 1999;6:165–172.
90. Jones JD, Burnett PC. Implication of creatinine and gut flora in the uremic syndrome: induction of "creatininase" in colon contents of the rat by dietary creatinine. *Clin Chem* 1972;18:280–284.
91. Rossano TG, Ambrose RT, Wu AHB, et al. Candidate reference method for determining creatinine in serum: method development and interlaboratory validation. *Clin Chem* 1990;36:1951–1955.
92. Welch MJ, Cohen A, Hertz HS, et al. Determination of serum creatinine by isotope dilution mass spectrometry as a candidate definitive method. *Anal Chem* 1986;58:1681–1685.
93. Chiou WL, Gadalla MA, Peng GW. Simple, rapid and micro high-pressure liquid determination of endogenous "true" creatinine in plasma, serum, and urine. *J Pharm Sci* 1978;67:182–187.
94. Ambrose RT, Ketchum DF, Smith JW. Creatinine determined by "high-performance" liquid chromatography. *Clin Chem* 1983;29:256–259.

95. Meyersohn M, Conrad KA, Achari R. The influence of a cooked meat meal on creatinine plasma concentration and creatinine clearance. *Br J Clin Pharmacol* 1983;15:227–230.
96. Guignard JP, Tabin R, Vienny H, et al. Effect of trimethoprim-sulfamethoxazole on renal function. *Curr Ther Res* 1983;34:801–806.
97. Dubb JW, Stole RM, Familiar RG. Effect of cimetidine on renal function in normal man. *Clin Pharmacol Ther* 1978; 24:76–83.
98. Arant BS, Edelmann CM, Spitzer A. The congruence of creatinine and inulin clearance in children: use of the Technicon Auto-Analyser. *J Pediatr* 1972;81:559–561.
99. Dodge WF, Travis LB, Daeschner CW. Comparison of endogenous creatinine clearance with inulin clearance. *Am J Dis Child* 1967;113:683–692.
100. Kim KE, Onesti G, Ramirez O, et al. Creatinine clearance in renal disease: a reappraisal. *BMJ* 1969;4:11–14.
101. Rosenbaum JL. Evaluation of clearance studies in chronic kidney disease. *J Chronic Dis* 1970;22:507–514.
102. Counahan R, Chantler C, Ghazali S, et al. Estimation of glomerular filtration rate from plasma creatinine concentration in children. *Arch Dis Child* 1976;51:875–878.
103. Schwartz GJ, Haycock GB, Edelmann CM Jr, et al. A simple estimate of glomerular filtration rate in children derived from body length and plasma creatinine. *Pediatrics* 1976; 58:259–263.
104. Haycock GB. Creatinine, body size and renal function. *Pediatr Nephrol* 1989;3:22–24.
105. Coulthard MG, Hey EN, Ruddock V. Creatinine and urea clearances compared to inulin clearance in preterm and mature babies. *Early Hum Dev* 1985;11:11–19.
106. Stonestreet BS, Bell EF, Oh W. Validity of endogenous creatinine clearance in low birthweight infants. *Pediatr Res* 1979;13:1012–1014.
107. Alt JM, Colenbrander B, Forsling ML, et al. Perinatal development of tubular function in the pig. *Q J Exp Physiol* 1984; 69:693–702.
108. Matos P, Duarte-Silva M, Drukker A, et al. Creatinine reabsorption by the newborn rabbit kidney. *Pediatr Res* 1998;44: 639–641.
109. Guignard JP, Drukker A. Why do newborn infants have a high plasma creatinine? *Pediatrics* 1999;103:e49.
110. Miall LS, Henderson MJ, Turner AJ, et al. Plasma creatinine rises dramatically in the first 48 hours of life in preterm infants. *Pediatrics* 1999;104:e76.
111. Gallini F, Maggio L, Romagnoli C, et al. Progression of renal function in preterm neonates with gestational age ≤ 32 weeks. *Pediatr Nephrol* 2000;15:119–124.
112. Bueva A, Guignard JP. Renal function in preterm neonates. *Pediatr Res* 1994;36:572–577.
113. Fawer CL, Torrado A, Guignard JP. Maturation of renal function in full-term and premature neonates. *Helv Paediat Acta* 1979;34:11–21.
114. Krutzen E, Back SE, Nilsson-Ehle, et al. Plasma clearance of a new contrast agent, iohexol: a method for the assessment of glomerular filtration rate. *J Lab Clin Med* 1984;104:955–961.
115. Gaspari F, Perico N, Ruggenenti P, et al. Plasma clearance of nonradioactive iohexol as a measure of glomerular filtration rate. *J Am Soc Nephrol* 1995;6:257–263.
116. Frennby B, Sterner G, Almen T, et al. Clearance of iohexol, ^{51}Cr-EDTA and endogenous creatinine for determination of glomerular filtration rate in pigs with reduced renal function: a comparison between different clearance techniques. *Scand J Clin Lab Invest* 1997;57:241–252.
117. Back SE, Masson P, Nilsson-Ehle P. A simple chemical method for the quantification of the contrast agent iohexol, applicable to glomerular filtration rate measurements. *Scand J Clin Lab Invest* 1998;48:825–829.
118. Olafsson I. The human cystatin C gene promoter: functional analysis and identification of heterogenous mRNA. *Scand J Clin Lab Invest* 1995;55:597–607.
119. Finney H, Newman DJ, Thakkar H, et al. Reference ranges for plasma cystatin C and creatinine measurements in premature infants, neonates and older children. *Arch Dis Child* 2000;82:71–75.
120. Tenstad O, Roald AB, Grubb A, et al. Renal handling of radiolabelled human cystatin C in the rat. *Scand J Clin Lab Invest* 1996;56:409–414.
121. Pitts RF, ed. *Physiology of the kidney and body fluids*, 2nd ed. Chicago: Yearbook Medical Publishers Inc, 1978.
122. Kyhse-Andersen J, Schmidt C, Nordin G, et al. Serum cystatin C, determined by a rapid automated particle-enhanced turbimetric method, is a better marker than serum creatinine for glomerular filtration rate. *Clin Chem* 1994;40: 1921–1926.
123. Finney H, Newman DJ, Grubb W, et al. Initial evaluation of cystatin C measurement by particle-enhanced immunonephelometry on the Behring nephelometer systems (BNA, BNII). *Clin Chem* 1997;4:1016–1022.
124. Cataldi L, Mussap M, Bertelli L, et al. Cystatin C in healthy women at term pregnancy and in their infant newborns: relationship between maternal and neonatal serum levels and reference values. *Am J Perinatol* 1999;16:287–295.
125. Harmoinen A, Ylinen E, Ala-Houhala M, et al. Reference intervals for cystatin C in pre- and full-term infants and children. *Pediatr Nephrol* 2000;15:105–108.
126. Bökenkamp A, Domanetzki M, Zinck R, et al. Reference values for cystatin C serum concentration in children. *Pediatr Nephrol* 1998;12:125–129.
127. Randers E, Erlandsen EJ. Serum cystatin C as an endogenous marker of the renal function—a review. *Clin Chem Lab Med* 1999;37:389–395.
128. Martini S, Prévot A, Masig D, et al. Glomerular filtration rate: measure creatinine and height rather than cystatin C! *Acta Paediatr* 2003;(*in press*).
129. Uchida K, Gotoh A. Measurement of Cystatin C and creatinine in urine. *Clin Chem Acta* 2002;323:121–128.
130. Rehling M, Møller ML, Thamdrup B, et al. Simultaneous measurement of renal clearance and plasma clearance of ^{99m}Tc-labelled diethylenetriaminepenta-acetate, ^{51}Cr-labelled ethylenediaminetetra-acetate and inulin in man. *Clin Sci* 1984;66: 613–619.
131. Piepsz A, Denis R, Ham HR, et al. A simple method for measuring separate glomerular filtration rate using a single injection of ^{99m}Tc-DTPA and the scintillation camera. *J Pediatr* 1978;93:769–774.
132. LaFrance ND, Drew HH, Walser D. Radioisotopic measurement of glomerular filtration rate in severe chronic renal failure. *J Nucl Med* 1988;29:1927–1930.

133. Carlsen JE, Møller ML, Lund JO, et al. Comparison of four commercial Tc[99m] (Sn) DTPA preparations used for the measurement of glomerular filtration rate: concise communications. *J Nucl Med* 1980;2:126–129.
134. Piepsz A, Pintelon H, Ham HR. Estimation of normal chromium-51 EDTA clearance in children. *Eur J Nucl Med* 1994;21:12–16.
135. Boschi S, Marchesini B. High-performance liquid chromatographic method for the simultaneous determination of iothalamate and o-iodohippurate. *J Chromatogr* 1981;224:139–143.
136. Wilson DM, Bergert JH, Larson TS, et al. GFR determined by nonradiolabelled iothalamate using capillary electrophoresis. *Am J Kidney Dis* 1997;30:646–652.
137. Odlind B, Hallgren R, Sohtell M, et al. Is ^{125}I iothalamate an ideal marker of glomerular filtration? *Kidney Int* 1985;27:9–16.
138. Perrone RD, Steinman TI, Beck GJ, et al. Utility of radioisotopic filtration markers in chronic renal insufficiency: simultaneous comparison of ^{125}I-iothalamate, [169]Yb-DTPA, ^{99m}Tc-DTPA, and inulin. The Modification of Diet in Renal Disease Study. *Am J Kidney Dis* 1990;16:224–235.
139. Russell CD. Radiopharmaceuticals used to assess kidney function and structure. In: Tauxe WN, Dubowski EV, eds. *Nuclear medicine in clinical urology and nephrology*. Norwalk, CT: Appleton-Century-Crofts 1985;5–31.
140. Bosch JP. Renal reserve: a functional view of glomerular filtration rate. *Semin Nephrol* 1995;15:381–385.
141. Regazzoni B, Genton N, Pelet J, et al. Long-term follow-up of renal functional reserve capacity after unilateral nephrectomy in childhood. *J Urol* 1998;160:844–848.
142. Molina E, Herrera J, Rodriguez-Iturbe B. The renal functional reserve in health and renal disease in school age children. *Kidney Int* 1988;34:809–816.
143. Woods LL. Intrarenal mechanisms of renal reserve. *Semin Nephrol* 1995;15:386–395.
144. Claris-Appiani A, Assael BM, Tirelli AS, et al. Proximal tubular function and hyperfiltration during amino acid infusion in man. *Am J Nephrol* 1988;8:96–101.
145. Woods LL, Smith BE, De Young DR. Regulation of renal hemodynamics after protein feeding: effects of proximal and distal diuretics. *Am J Physiol* 1993;264:R337–R344.
146. Elbourne I, Lumbers ER, Hill KJ, et al. The secretion of organic acids and bases by the ovin fetal kidney. *Exp Physiol* 1990;75:211–221.
147. Wenling GJ, Derkx FH, Tan-Tjiong LH, et al. Risks of angiotensin converting enzyme inhibitors in renal artery stenosis. *Kidney Int* 1987;31:S180–S183.
148. Myers BD, Ross J, Newton L, et al. Cyclosporine-associated chronic nephropathy. *N Engl J Med* 1984;311:699–705.
149. Bratton AC, Marshall EK Jr. A new coupling component for sulfanilamide determination. *J Biol Chem* 1939;128:537–550.
150. Prueksaritanont T, Chen ML, Chiou WL. Simple and micro high-performance liquid chromatographic method for the simultaneous determination of *p*-aminohippuric acid and iothalamate in biological fluids. *J Chromatogr* 1984; 306:89–97.
151. Calgagno PL, Rubin MI. Renal extraction of para-aminohippurate in infants and children. *J Clin Invest* 1963;42: 1632–1639.
152. Hakim R, Watrous WM, Fujimoto JM. The renal tubular transport and metabolism of serotonine (5-HT) and 5-hydroxyindol-acetic acid (5-HIAA) in the chicken. *J Pharmacol Exp Ther* 1970;175:749–762.
153. Hannedouche T, Laude D, Deschaux M, et al. Plasma 5-hydroxyindoleacetic acid as an endogenous index of renal plasma flow. *Kidney Int* 1989;35:95–98.
154. Sulyok E, Nagy L, Baranyai Z, et al. Comparison of 5-hydroxyindol-acetic acid and para-amino hippurate clearances in newborn rabbits. *Clin Chim Acta* 1995;240:155–161.
155. Le Quan-Bui KH, Elghosi JL, Devynck MA, et al. Rapid liquid chromatographic determination of 5-hydroxyindoles and dihydroxyphenyllacetic acid in cerebrospinal fluid of the rat. *Eur J Pharmacol* 1982;81:315–320.
156. Maher FT, Strong CG, Elveback LR. Renal extraction ratios and plasma binding studies of radio-iodinated o-iodo hippurate and iodopyracet and of *p*-amino-hippurate in man. *Mayo Clin Proc* 1971;46:189–192.
157. Visscher CA, De Zeeuw D, Navis G, et al. Renal ^{131}I-hippurate clearance overestimates true renal blood flow in the instrumented conscious dog. *Am J Physiol* 1996;271:F269–F274.
158. Durand E, Prigent A. The basics of renal imaging and function studies. *Q J Nucl Med* 2002;46:249–267.
159. Young LS, Regan MC, Barry MK, et al. Methods of renal blood flow measurement. *Urol Res* 1996;24:149–160.
160. Wei K, Le E, Bin JP, et al. Quantification of renal blood flow with contrast-enhanced ultrasound. *J Am Coll Cardiol* 2001;37:1135–1140.
161. Aronson S, Wiencek JG, Feinstein SB, et al. Assessment of renal blood flow with contrast ultrasonography. *Anesth Analg* 1993;76:964–970.
162. Visser MO, Leighton JO, Van de Bohr, et al. Renal blood flow in neonates: quantification with color flow and pulsed Doppler US. *Radiology* 1992;183:441–444.
163. Lerman LO, Bell MR, Lahera V, et al. Quantification of global and regional renal blood flow with electron beam computed tomography. *Am J Hypertens* 1994;7:829–837.
164. Vallee JP, Lazeyras F, Khan HG, et al. Absolute renal blood flow quantification by dynamic MRI and Gd-DTPA. *Eur Radiol* 2000;10:1245–1252.
165. Santos F, Orejas G, Foreman JW, Chan JCM. Diagnostic workup of renal disorders. *Curr Probl Pediatr* 1991;21:48–74.
166. DuBose TD Jr. Hydrogen ion secretion by the collecting duct as a determinant of the urine to blood PCO_2 gradient in alkaline urine. *J Clin Invest* 1982;69:145–156.
167. Batlle DC, Grupp M, Gaviria M, Kurtzman NA. Distal renal tubular acidosis with intact capacity to lower urinary pH. *Am J Med* 1982;72:751–758.
168. Strife CF, Clardy CW, Varade WS, et al. Urine-to-blood carbon dioxide tension gradient and maximal depression of urinary pH to distinguish rate-dependent from classic distal renal tubular acidosis in children. *J Pediatr* 1993;122:60–65.
169. Batlle DC, Sehy JT, Roseman MK, et al. Clinical and pathophysiologic spectrum of acquired distal renal tubular acidosis. *Kidney Int* 1981;20:389–396.
170. Skinner R, Cole M, Pearson ADJ, et al. Specificity of pH and osmolality of early morning urine sample in assessing distal renal tubular function in children. *BMJ* 1996;312:1337–338.
171. Rodríguez-Soriano J, Vallo A. Renal tubular hyperkalemia in childhood. *Pediatr Nephrol* 1988;2:498–509.

172. García-Nieto V, Santos F. Pruebas funcionales renales. In: García-Nieto V, Santos F, eds. *Nefrología pediátrica*. Madrid: Grupo Aula Médica, 2000;15–26.
173. Alon U, Hellerstein S, Warady BA. Oral acetazolamide in the assessment of (urine-blood) PCO_2. *Pediatr Nephrol* 1991;5: 307–311.
174. Edelmann CM Jr, Barnett HL, Stark H, et al. A standardized test of renal concentrating capacity in children. *Am J Dis Child* 1967;114:639–644.
175. Aronson AS, Svenningsen NW. DDAVP tests for estimation of renal concentrating capacity in infants and children. *Arch Dis Child* 1974;49:654–659.
176. Marild S, Jodal U, Jonasson G, et al. Reference values for renal concentrating capacity in children by the desmopressin test. *Pediatr Nephrol* 1992;6:254–257.
177. Marild S, Rembratt A, Jodal U, Norgaard JP. Renal concentrating capacity test using desmopressin at bedtime. *Pediatr Nephrol* 2001;16:439–442.

22

EVALUATION OF GROWTH AND DEVELOPMENT

SANDRA L. WATKINS
GAIL E. RICHARDS

NORMAL GROWTH

Growth is such a valuable biologic indicator of health during childhood that careful assessment of growth should be a routine part of initial and ongoing care of children with documented or suspected renal disease. To appreciate the implications of growth perturbation caused by renal disease, it is necessary to understand normal growth and the uses and limitations of methods of growth evaluation.

MEASUREMENT OF GROWTH

Linear Growth

The growth charts that are commonly used in clinical settings are derived from cross-sectional data and are useful to determine how the growth of an individual compares to age- and gender-matched peers (Fig. 22.1). To see the impact over time of both normal physiology and superimposed growth abnormalities, it is crucial to have accurate longitudinal data. The importance of accurate measurements cannot be overemphasized. Accurate measuring equipment and accurate measuring technique are crucial. Inaccurate positioning of a child on an infant-measuring board or stadiometer can lead to significant misinterpretation of growth trends. Figure 22.2 demonstrates proper positioning of an infant (Fig. 22.2A) and an older child (Fig. 22.2B). Special attention should be paid to positioning of the feet and head. Feet must be flat and positioned against the same board as the head. Usually an assistant should hold the feet in position to assure that the patient does not rise as the measurement is being taken. Buttocks and shoulder blades should be touching the back board. For infants, it is usually necessary for an assistant to hold the knees down and hold the feet flat against the end board. The head should be in the Frankfurt plane, with the outer canthus of the eye and the external auditory meatus describing a line that is perpendicular to the back board of the stadiometer of the infant-measuring board. For standing measurements, the neck should be gently stretched while being sure that feet remain flat on the ground. Socks and shoes should be removed so that any lifting of the feet can be seen and corrected. Balance beam scales should not be used for the assessment of height, as the measurements are not accurate owing to the flexibility of the measurement arm.

Inaccurate plotting of measurements can lead to significant misinterpretations of growth data. It is crucial to plot the height as close to the fractional age as possible rather than plotting on the nearest year or half-year. Use of a growth chart appropriate to the measurement technique is also important. Standard charts for infants that often extend to 36 months are meant to be used with supine measurements taken on an infant-measuring board. Use of standing heights on these charts can lead to an erroneous conclusion that growth has slowed, because standing heights are shorter than recumbent lengths. Similarly, growth charts that include 2 years to 18 years or more are meant to be used for standing heights only and should not be used to plot recumbent lengths.

Most growth charts are expressed in terms of percentiles for a reference population. This is useful if a child's measurement lies within the percentiles. If, however, height is below the percentiles, an alternative method of height quantitation is needed. The SD score (SDS or Z score) is the number of SDs below or above the age- and gender-appropriate mean for a given height measurement. The concept of SDS is useful for most biologic variables and can be used for weight and body mass index (BMI) as well as for height and height velocity to compare individuals to the reference population and to follow change accurately. To use SDS accurately, a computer program is required that will convert height, weight, birth date, and measurement date to SDS scores. These programs are readily available and should be part of the standard armamentarium of pediatric nephrologists.

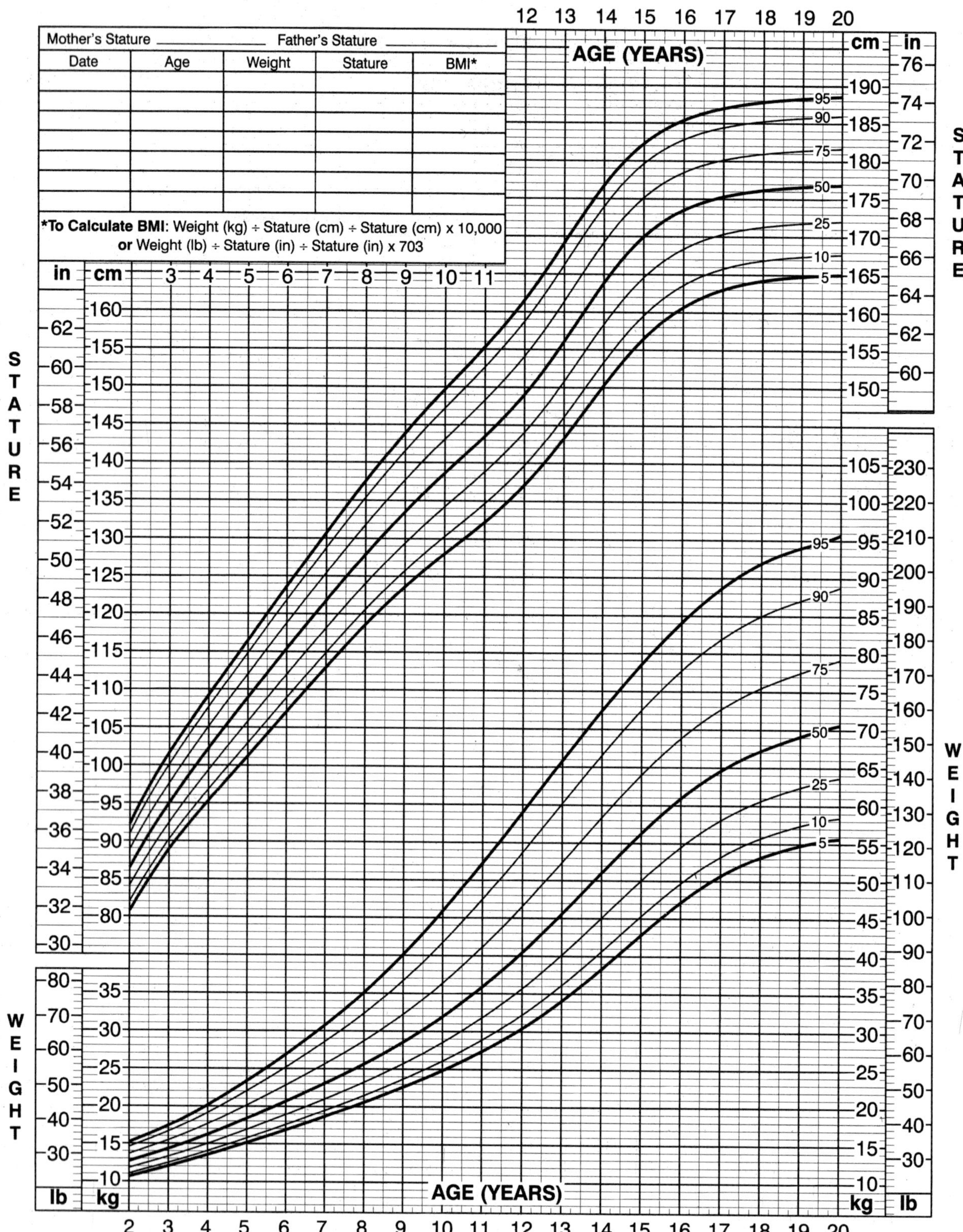

A

FIGURE 22.1. A: Height percentiles in boys 2 to 20 years of age. (*continued*)

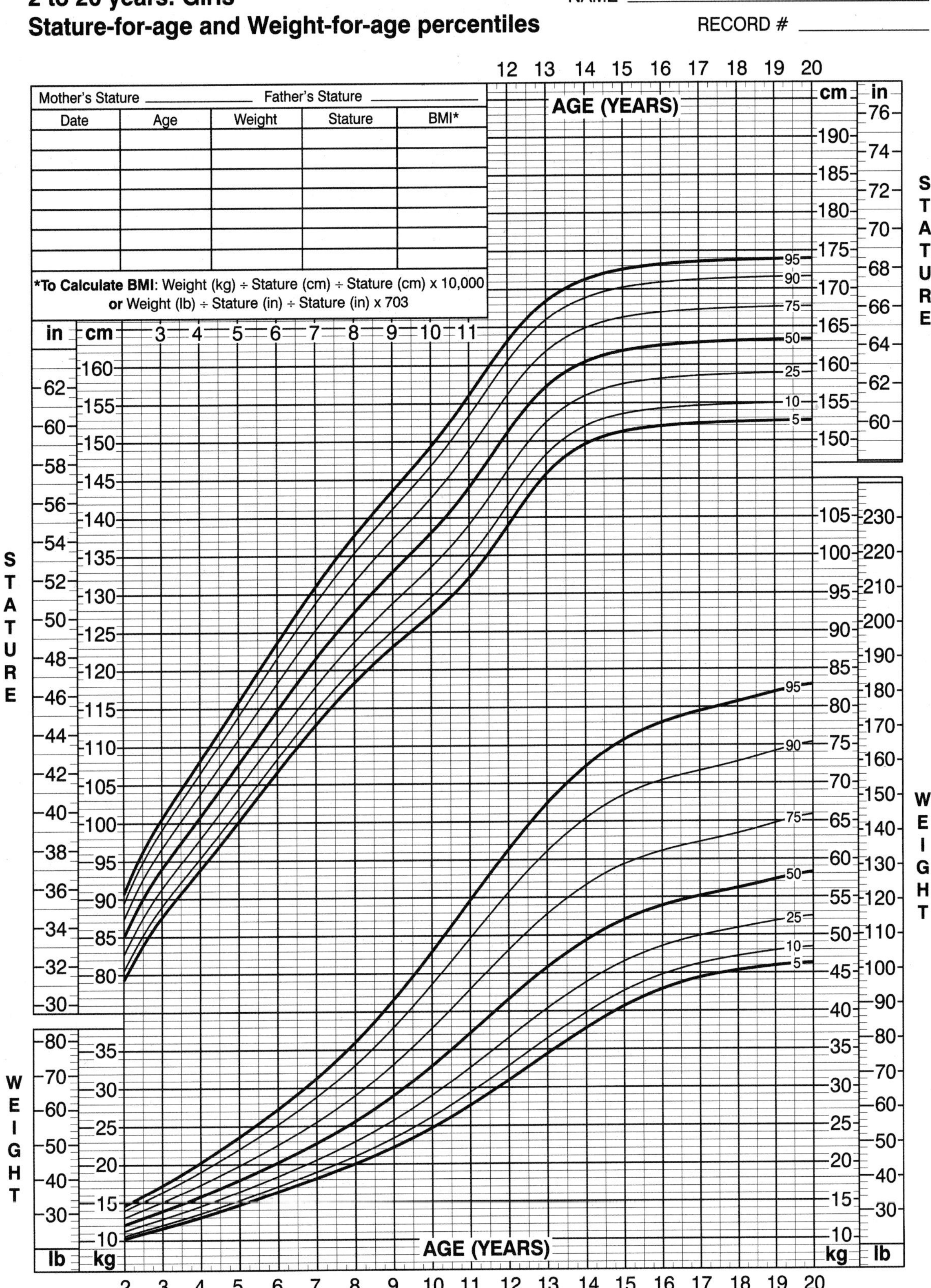

B

FIGURE 22.1. (*continued*) **B:** Height percentiles in girls 2 to 20 years of age.

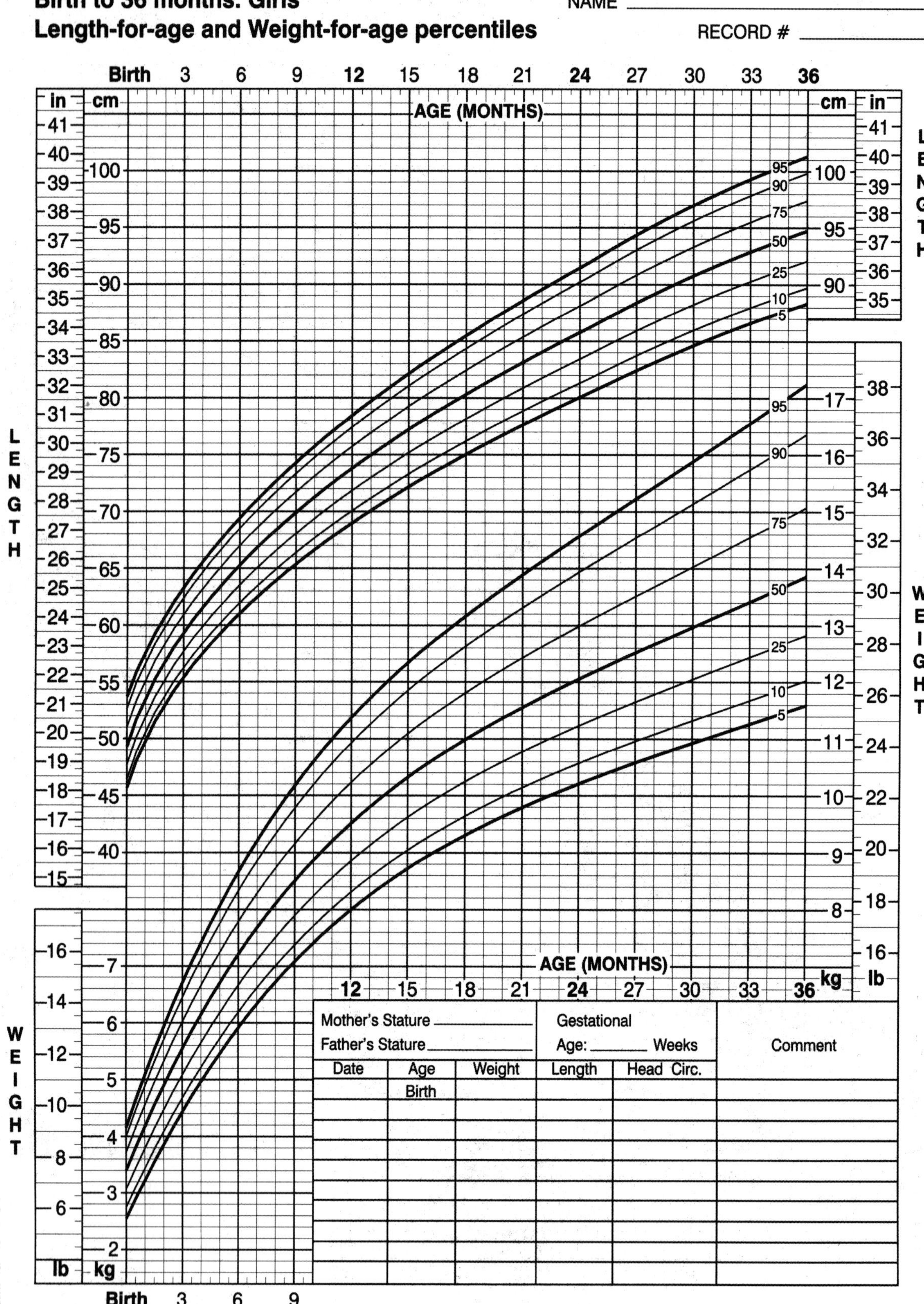

C

FIGURE 22.1. (*continued*) C: Height percentiles in girls from birth to 36 months.

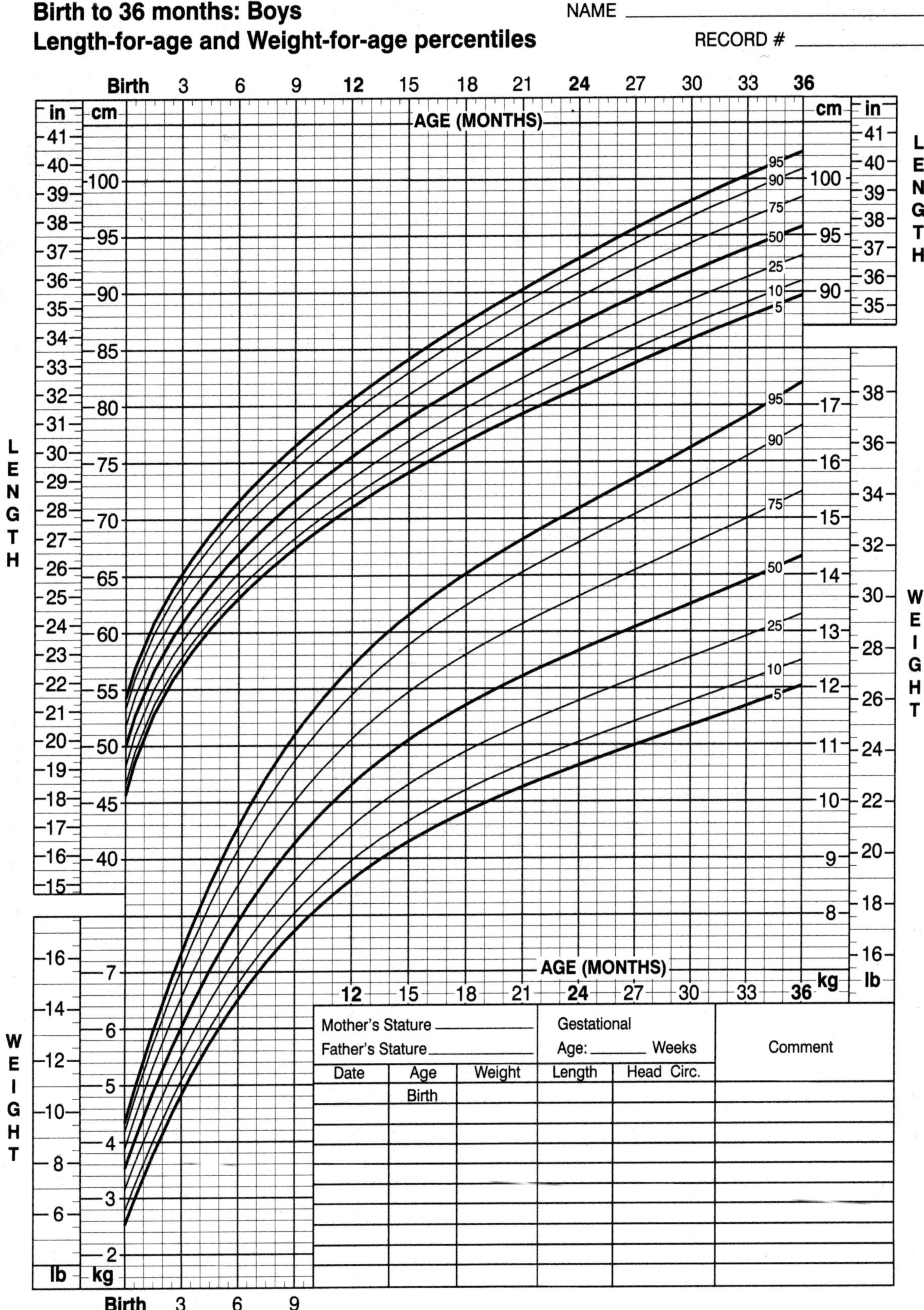

D

FIGURE 22.1. *(continued)* **D:** Height percentiles in boys from birth to 36 months. BMI, body mass index. (From Centers for Disease Control and Prevention Web site. Available at: http://www.cdc.gov. Accessed April 2003, with permission.)

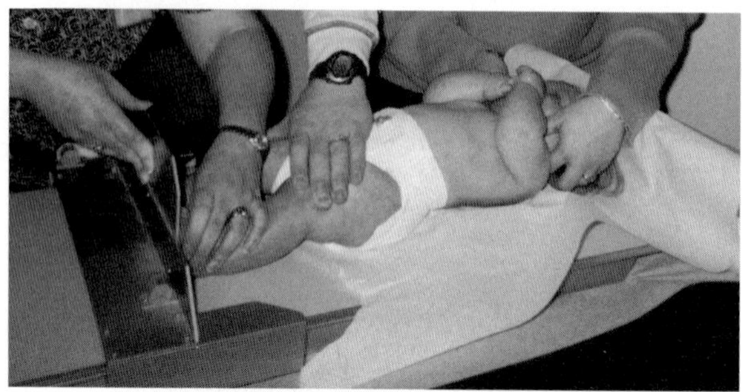

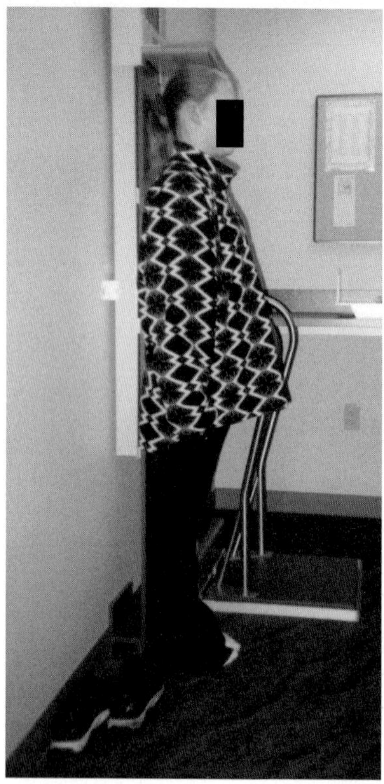

FIGURE 22.2. Proper positioning of an infant **(A)** and child **(B)** for accurate measurement.

Growth Velocity

Growth velocity is an extremely useful tool for assessing health and for determining the effectiveness of various therapies. The accuracy and interpretation of growth velocity calculations depend on the accuracy of the underlying measurement and on the choice of an appropriate interval for a velocity calculation. Growth velocity varies throughout the year in healthy children; thus, the most accurate calculation of growth rate is that done with measurements that are exactly a year apart. Sometimes practical considerations, such as availability of measurements and the need to make therapeutic decisions in a timely manner, preclude using measurements over a complete year. Because multiplying the time over which two measurements were taken by the appropriate factor to calculate an annual growth rate necessarily multiplies any measurement inaccuracy, extreme caution should be used in interpretation of growth rates calculated over less than a 6-month period. It is crucial when plotting growth velocities on charts to draw bars around the midpoint of the growth velocity as plotted to indicate the time over which the velocity was calculated. It is also important, especially when assessing therapies, to choose time intervals for growth velocity calculation that represent significant events. For example, the expectation and interpretation for a growth velocity in the first year of growth hormone (GH) treatment is different from the expectation for the second year of treatment and so forth. Intervals of treatment should not be mingled with intervals without treatment in calculation of growth velocities.

Growth velocity data that correspond to the height standards shown in Figure 22.1 are not available. Thus, standards for growth velocity that were derived from longitudinal data should be used (Fig. 22.3).

Interpretation of growth velocities differs from interpretation of absolute height. Because a growth velocity of around the fiftieth percentile is required to maintain an absolute height around the fiftieth percentile, a growth velocity that is consistently at the tenth percentile over years cannot be considered normal. That differs significantly from an absolute height that could be considered quite normal if it remained at the tenth percentile over years. A child who has a growth velocity at the tenth (or even twenty-fifth percentile) over many years will gradually fall lower on the percentiles for absolute height.

Sitting Height

Measurement of sitting height can be helpful when there is reason to suspect that the patient has a condition or disease that differentially affects either the spine or the long bones. Examples might be hypophosphatemic rickets or a patient with scoliosis or those who have had irradiation of the spine or spina bifida. Sitting height is best measured with a device specifically constructed for this purpose consisting of a box of appropriate width for comfortable sitting of a precise height. The patient can then sit on the box and position the upper body and head as for a standing measurement. The height of the box is subtracted from the stadiometer measurement. Standards for sitting height are provided in Figure 22.4. In circumstances in which it is informative to separately assess growth of the spine and long bones, height and sitting height can be measured. The difference between the two can be used to assess growth of long bones in conjunction with measurement of arm span.

Other Measurements of Linear Growth

To assess very small changes in growth over short periods of time, very precise methods have been devised for measurement of the lower leg. This technique is referred to as *knemometry.* Although the precision of the technique is very

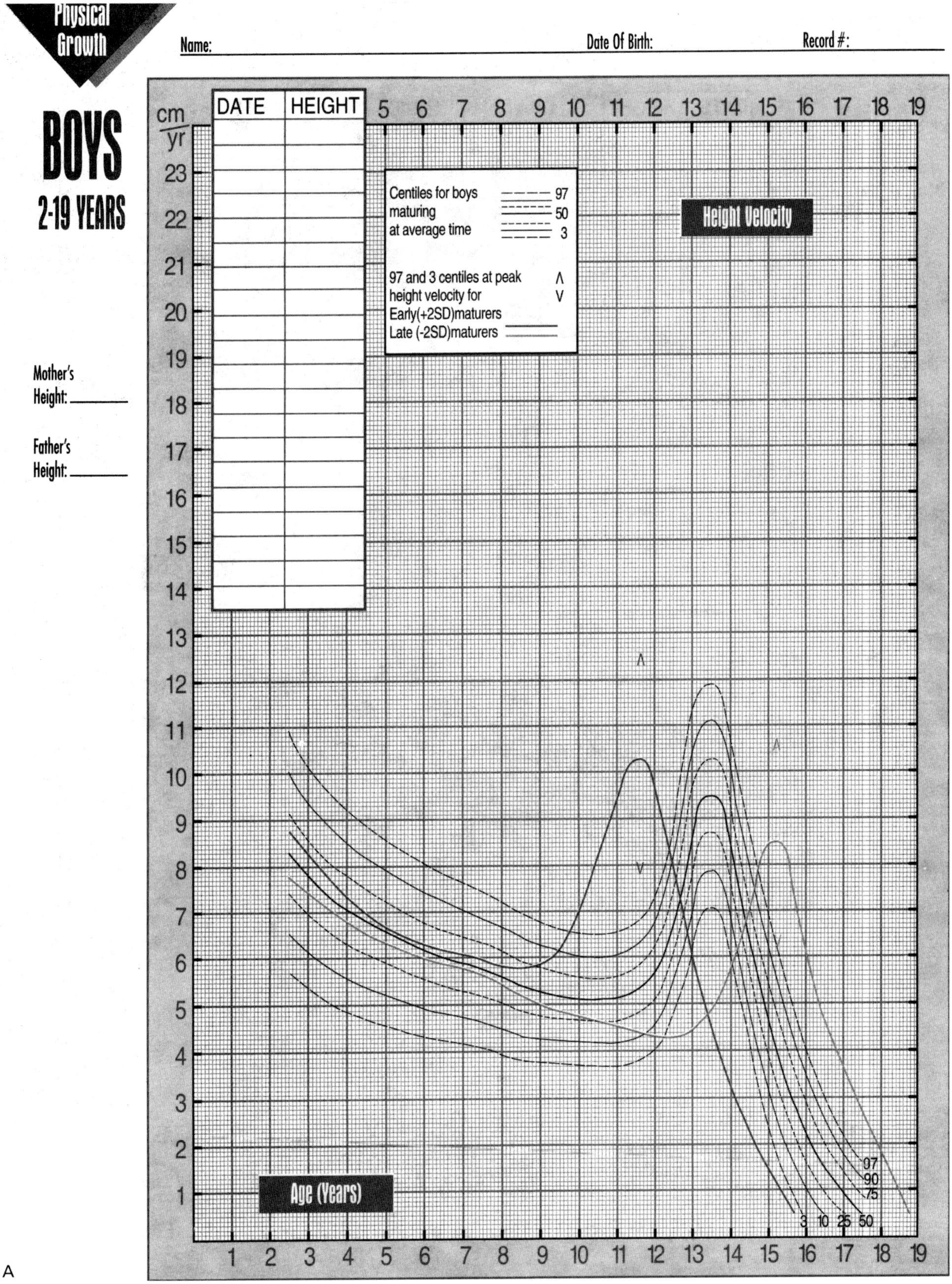

Physical Growth

BOYS

2-19 YEARS

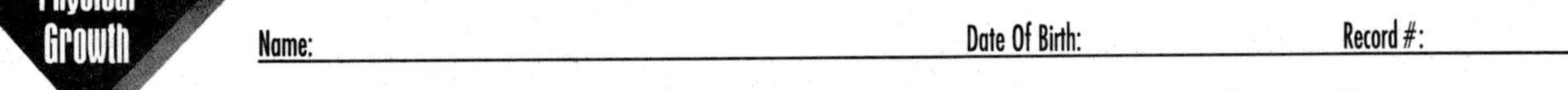

Mother's Height: ______

Father's Height: ______

DATE	HEIGHT

Height Velocity

cm/yr

23
22
21
20
19
18
17
16
15
14
13
12
11
10
9
8
7
6
5
4
3
2
1

5 6 7 8 9 10 11 12 13 14 15 16 17 18 19

Centiles for boys maturing at average time — 97, 50, 3

97 and 3 centiles at peak height velocity for Early(+2SD)maturers Λ, Late (-2SD)maturers V

97
90
75

3 10 25 50

Age (Years)

1 2 3 4 5 6 7 8 9 10 11 12 13 14 15 16 17 18 19

A

FIGURE 22.3. **A:** Height velocity in boys 2 to 19 years of age. (*continued*)

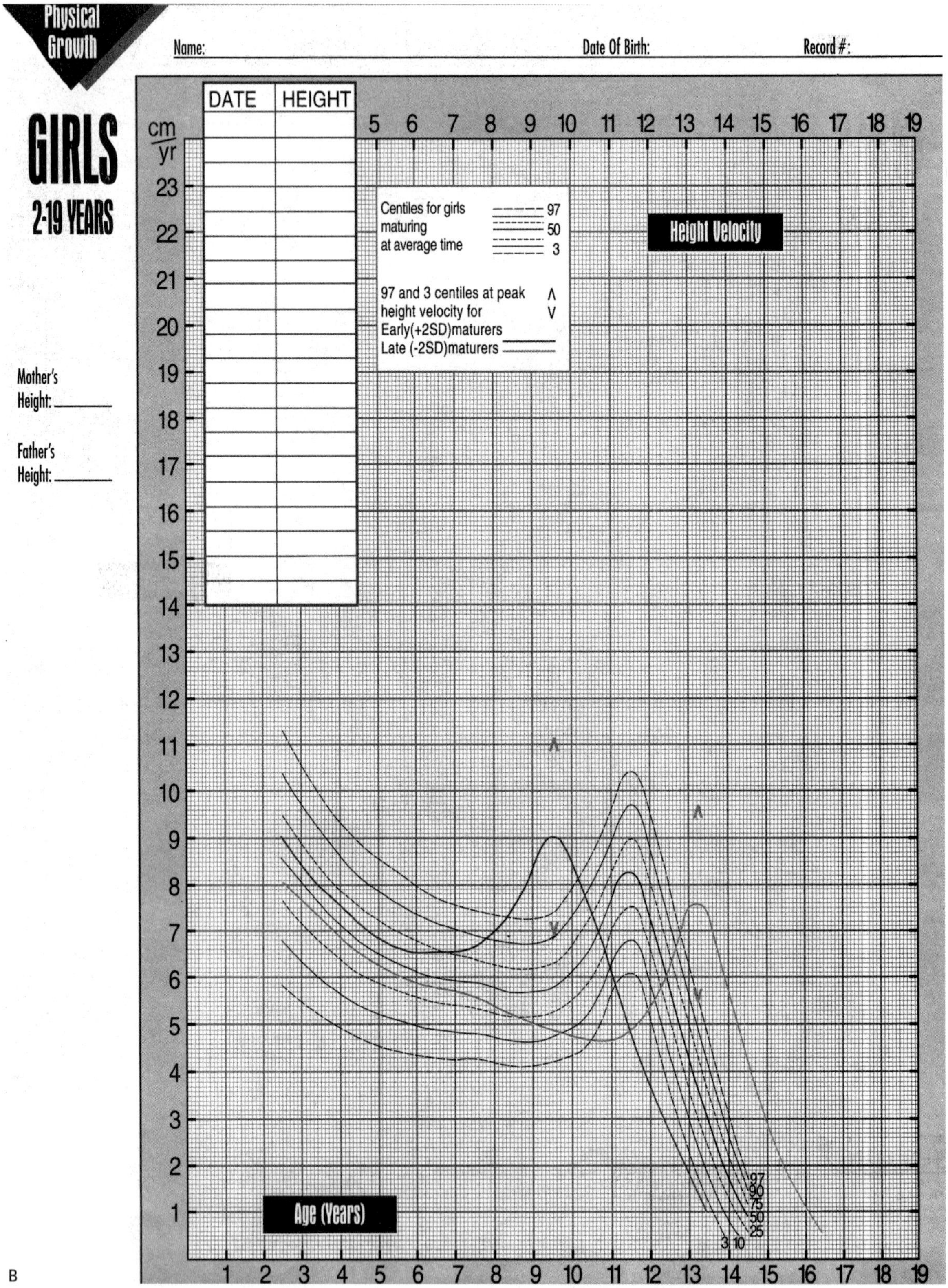

Physical Growth

Name: Date Of Birth: Record #:

GIRLS
2-19 YEARS

Mother's Height: ______

Father's Height: ______

DATE	HEIGHT

Height Velocity

Centiles for girls maturing at average time — 97, 50, 3

97 and 3 centiles at peak height velocity for Early(+2SD)maturers ∧ ∨
Late (-2SD)maturers

cm/yr

Age (Years)

B

FIGURE 22.3. (*continued*) **B:** Height velocity in girls 2 to 19 years of age. [From Tanner JM, Davies PS. Clinical longitudinal standards for height and height velocity for North American children. *J Pediatric* 1985;107(3):317–329, with permission.]

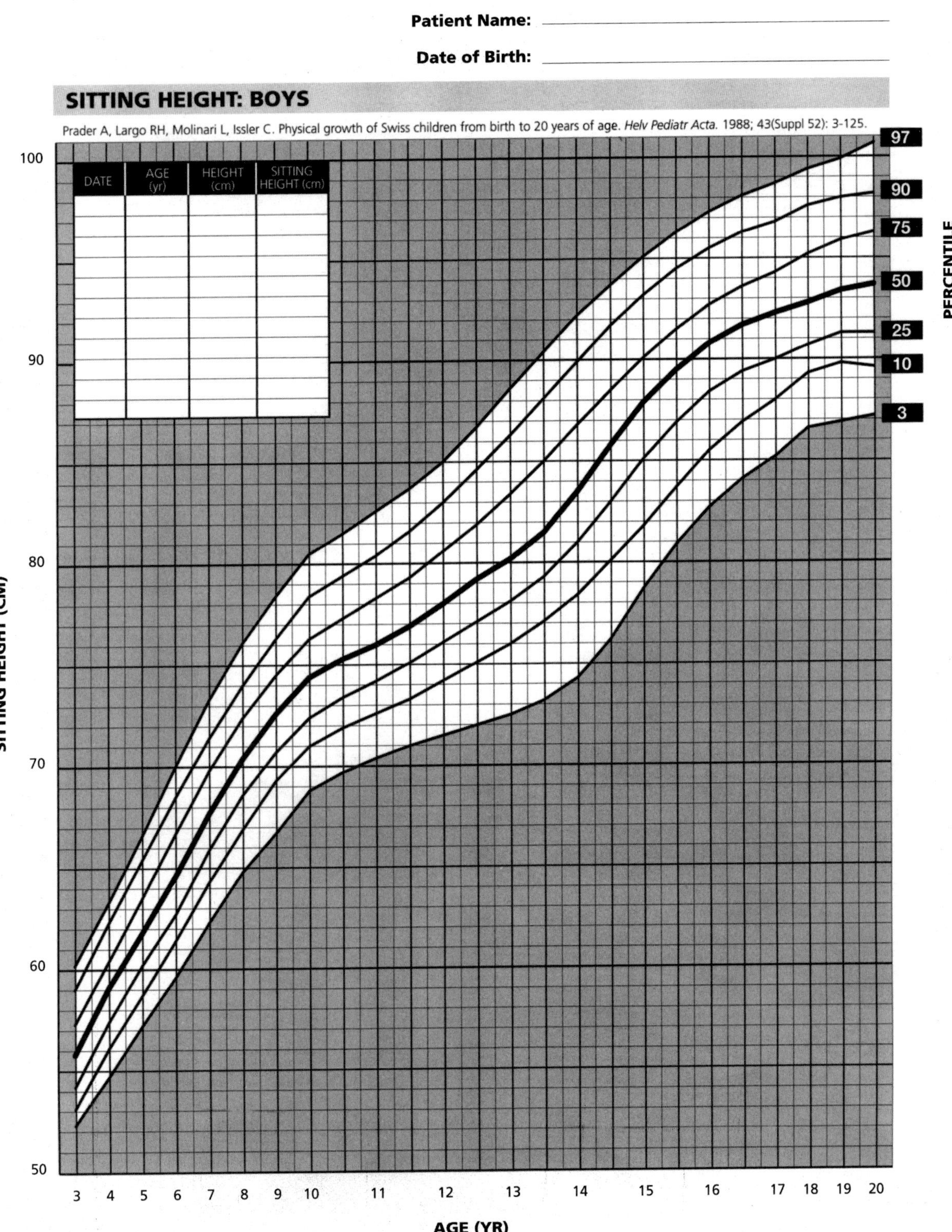

FIGURE 22.4. A: Standards for sitting height for boys. (*continued*)

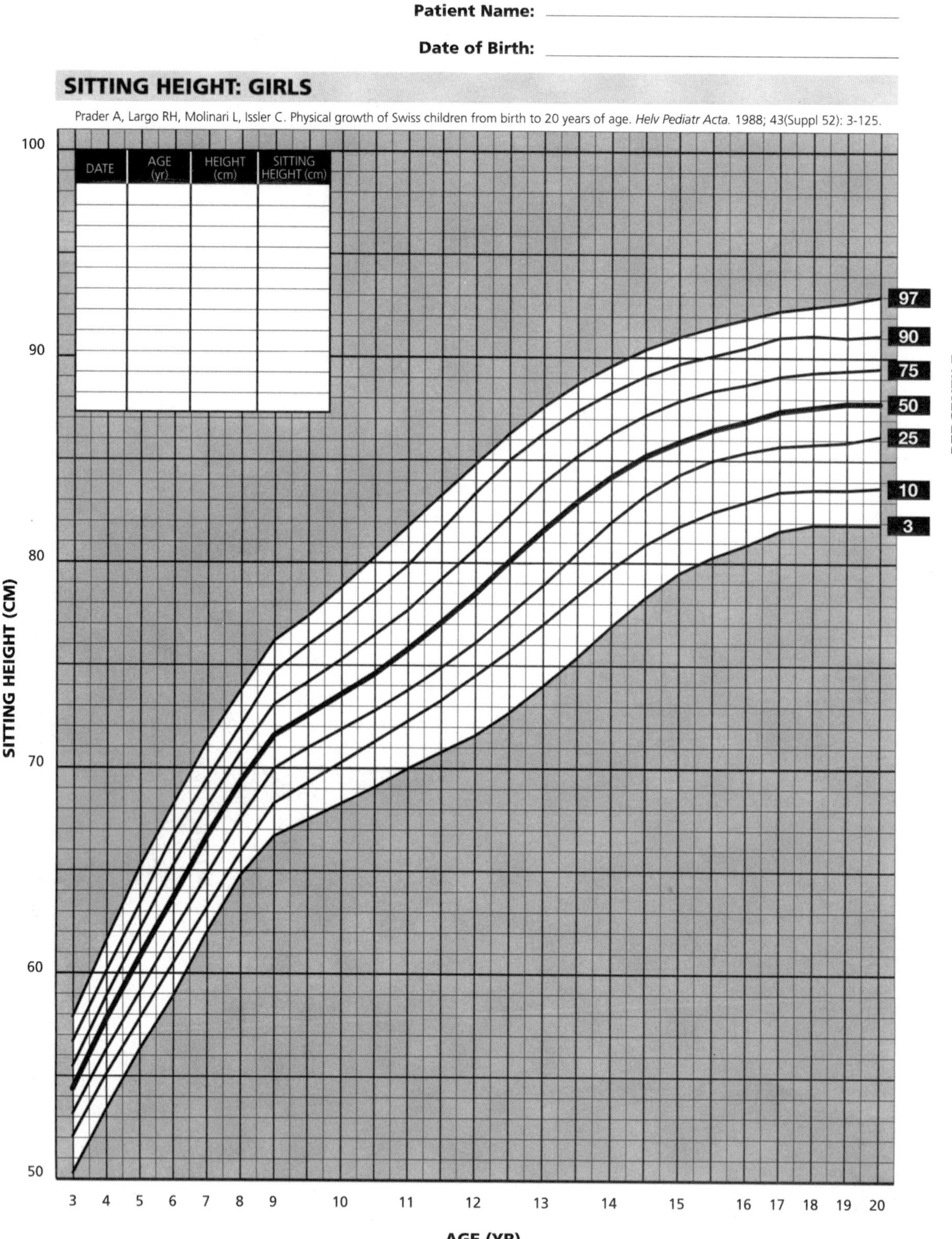

B

FIGURE 22.4. (*continued*) **B:** Standards for sitting height for girls. [From Prader A, Largo RH, Molinari L, et al. Physical growth of Swiss children from birth to 30 years of age. *Helv Pediatr Acta* 1988;43(Suppl 52):3–125, with permission.]

high, and significant advance in growth can be detected over time periods as brief as a single day, in practice, this technique is not widely applied in clinical settings and is mainly reserved for research use (1–3).

Head Circumference

Occipitofrontal circumference is an important measurement in young children up to about 3 years while brain size is increasing. Occipitofrontal circumference is affected by nutritional conditions and chronic illness only in extreme situations and generally does not give much insight into either the presence or progression of renal disease. As occipitofrontal circumference reflects brain growth, which is generally independent of somatic growth, it is an independent marker of whether an insult or multisystem disease that may have caused renal disease has also affected central nervous system development.

Body Mass Index

Weight is commonly measured, and the measurement is usually quite precise if care is taken to weigh the patient in a standard and minimum amount of clothing, such as a light hospital gown (or diaper for a young infant). Weight can be plotted for age and compared to height. Generally, it is thought to be optimum if the weight and height percentiles are the same. This is not the case for most patients, so an alternative measure of the weight to height relationship is needed to determine whether a patient is at risk from either too much or too little body mass (weight). BMI is calculated as weight in kg/height in m^2. Children who have a BMI higher than the seventy-fifth percentile or lower than the fifth percentile have increased health risks, which will be additive to any underlying renal disease (4–6). Thus, calculating BMI and either plotting or determining BMI SDS is another valuable health indicator. Standards for BMI percentiles are provided in Figure 22.5.

BMI is generally perceived to be a proxy for body composition, but there is significant variation in the weight of bone and muscle among individuals, making the correlation between BMI and other determinations such as fat mass are not precise. If techniques such as isotope dilution or quantitative dual-energy x-ray absorptiometry are not practical, a good approximation of fat mass can be determined by bioelectrical impedance. If it is important to document whether changes in weight are due to fat or fat-free mass, bioelectrical impedance can be quite helpful. It is important to use regression equations derived specifically for children, however, rather than relying on the immediate output of commercial machinery.

Bone Age

Physiologic maturity of the skeleton can be estimated by assessing specific radiologic findings that progress in an orderly fashion in specific bones. In clinical practice, the atlas by Greulich and Pyle is almost universally used (7). This method displays a series of standards for boys and girls at various ages. An accompanying text describes the changes in specific bones because the last standard is provided. The *bone age* is reported as the standard that looks most like the radiograph of the patient. To use this information appropriately, it is important to recognize that the standards were derived approximately 50 years ago and may not entirely reflect current secular trends. There are often gaps of an entire year between standards, making it difficult to assess less dramatic changes in bone maturation. Finally, this system does not take into account that not every bone in every patient matures at the same pace as the radiographic standards. It is quite common to find a significant discrepancy among the maturity of the bones of the hand and wrist.

A more precise and useful method for bone age assessment requires 20 bones to be scored into one of (usually) eight categories of maturity and a score given for each of the categories (8). The numerical sum of the scores for each of the 20 bones is translated to a bone age. This method has the first advantage of a validated weighting system to account for the fact that some bones are more reliable predictors of maturity than others. A second advantage is the ability to assess the bone age as an almost continuous variable of 0.1-year increments. Using this system, it is possible to detect more subtle changes in maturation. When applied by very experienced interpreters, these two methods give quite comparable results. In situations of discordant clinical and radiologic findings, it is sometimes advantageous to use both methods. The 20-bone method can be much more time consuming, however, and is unlikely to be commonly used by radiologists.

The issue of what a bone age means is both intuitively obvious, yet potentially open to misinterpretation. On the one hand, a delay in bone age can imply that the individual in question has more potential for growth than would be assumed by plotting a height measurement alone. On the other hand, the tendency of films to be interpreted as either *normal* or *abnormal* based on whether they fall within two SDs of a mean reading can cause unwarranted consternation. It is perhaps more helpful to think of a bone age as a descriptor of maturation that cannot be abnormal in and of itself. A bone age is only one clue contributing to a decision about whether a growth pattern is indicative or a consequence of an underlying abnormality or treatment.

Pubertal Stages

Just as accurate assessment of height and growth velocity informs assessment of health, accurate staging of the pubertal process and monitoring of the progression of pubertal development can be a good indicator of general health and adequacy of treatment for underlying renal disease. Figure 22.6 describes the pubertal staging method of Tanner that is the accepted method to quantify pubertal development. It should be noted that pubertal stage is not described in one number,

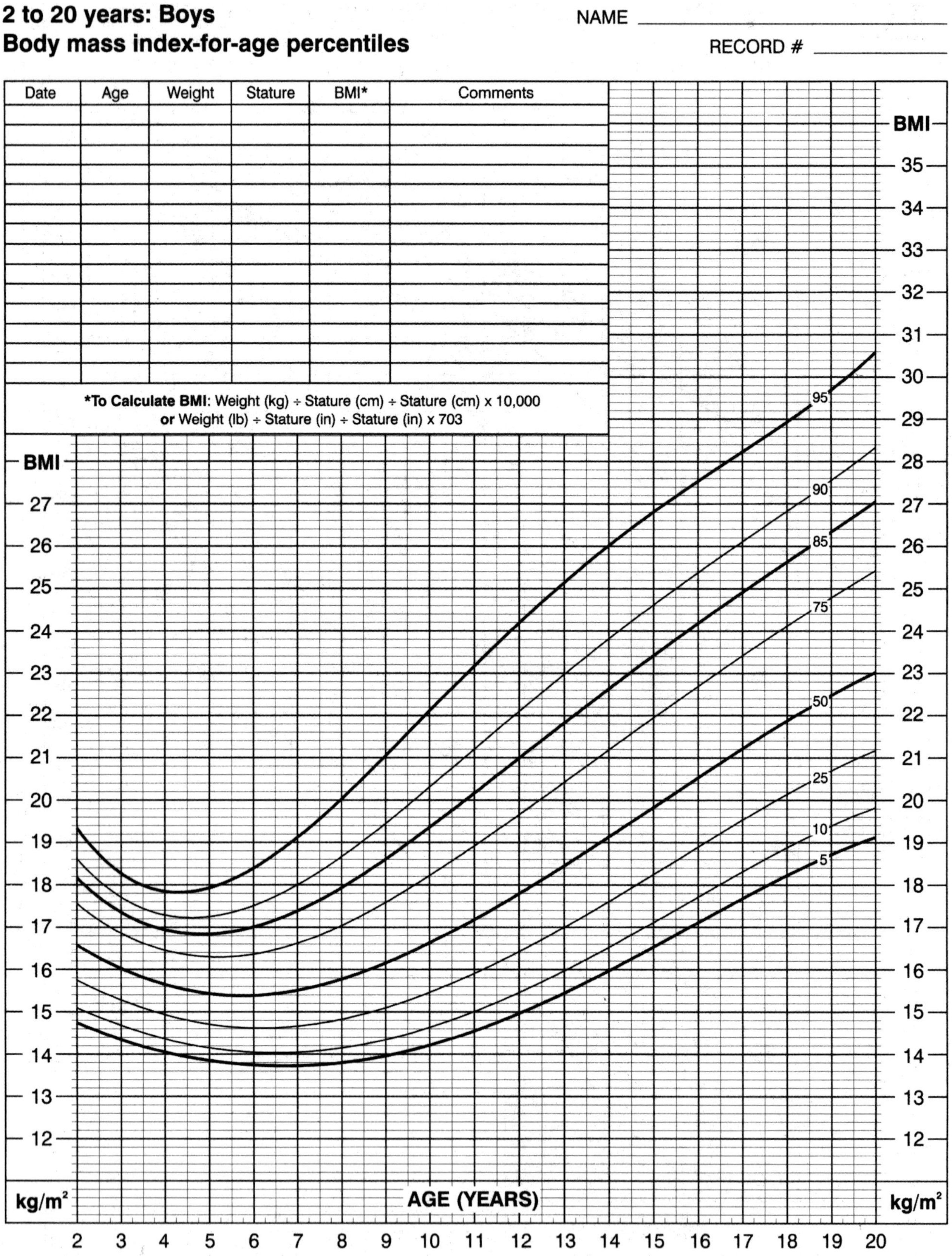

2 to 20 years: Boys
Body mass index-for-age percentiles

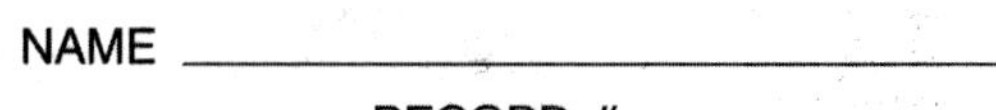

Date	Age	Weight	Stature	BMI*	Comments

***To Calculate BMI:** Weight (kg) ÷ Stature (cm) ÷ Stature (cm) x 10,000
or Weight (lb) ÷ Stature (in) ÷ Stature (in) x 703

BMI

35 34 33 32 31 30 29 28 27 26 25 24 23 22 21 20 19 18 17 16 15 14 13 12

95 90 85 75 50 25 10 5

kg/m² AGE (YEARS) kg/m²

A 2 3 4 5 6 7 8 9 10 11 12 13 14 15 16 17 18 19 20

FIGURE 22.5. A: Standards for body mass index (BMI) percentiles for boys. *(continued)*

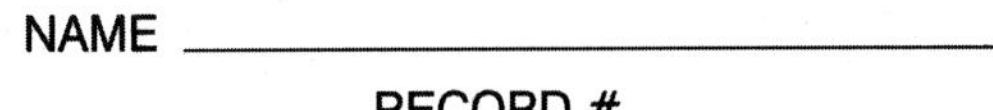

2 to 20 years: Girls
Body mass index-for-age percentiles

NAME ______________________

RECORD # ____________

Date	Age	Weight	Stature	BMI*	Comments

***To Calculate BMI**: Weight (kg) ÷ Stature (cm) ÷ Stature (cm) x 10,000
or Weight (lb) ÷ Stature (in) ÷ Stature (in) x 703

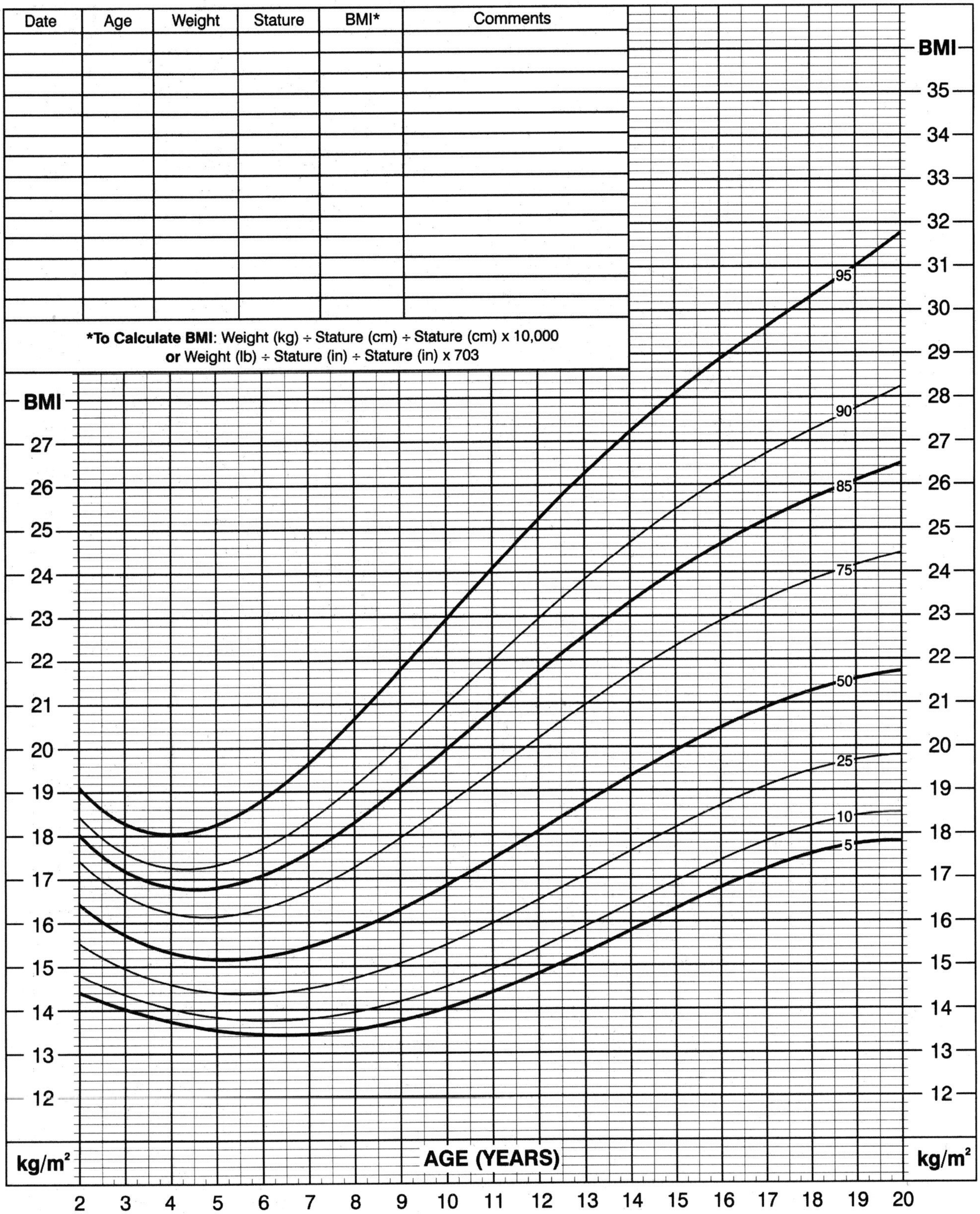

B

FIGURE 22.5. (*continued*) **B:** Standards for body mass index (BMI) percentiles for girls. (From Centers for Disease Control and Prevention Web site. Available at: http://www.cdc.gov. Accessed April 2003, with permission.)

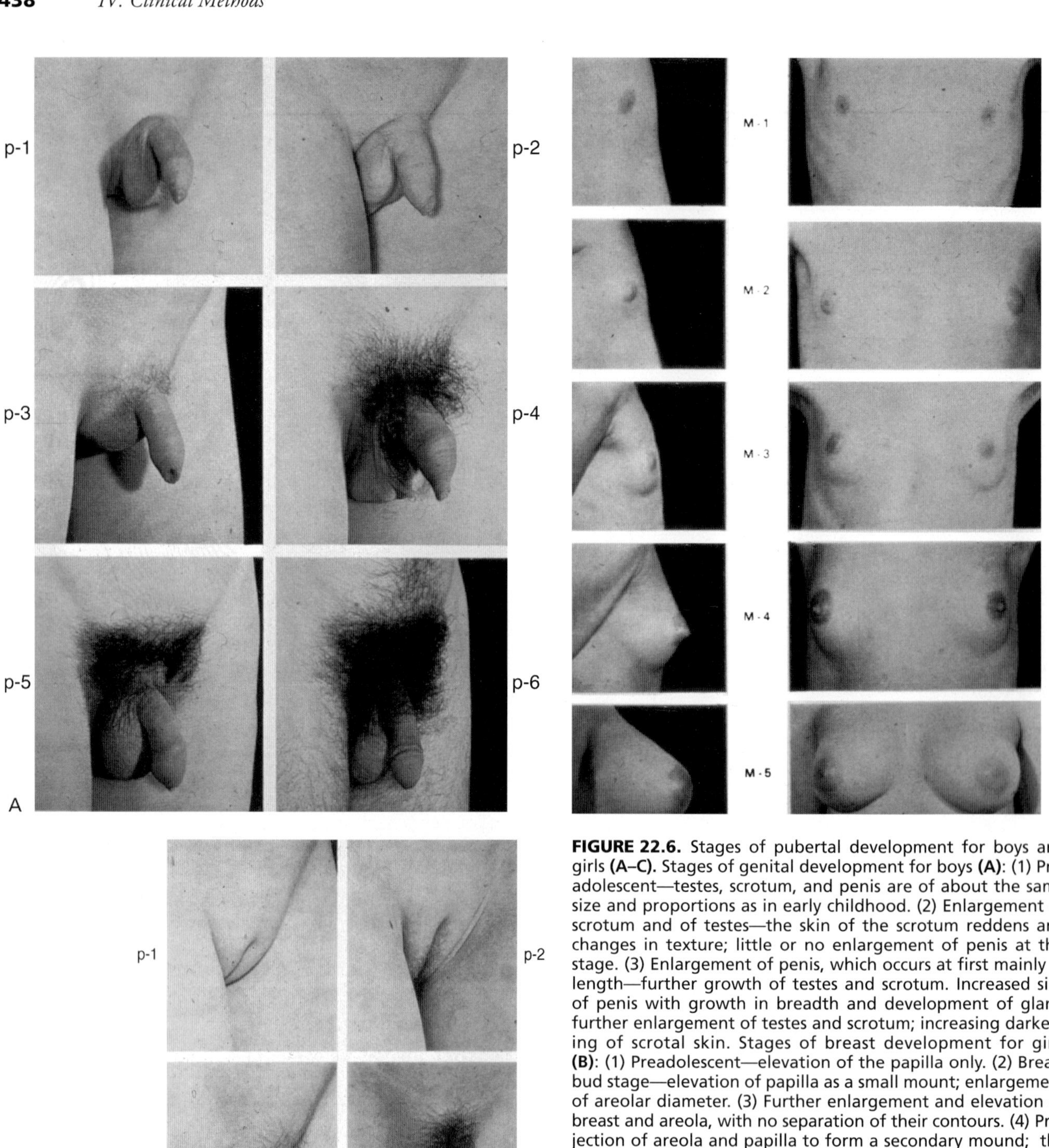

FIGURE 22.6. Stages of pubertal development for boys and girls **(A–C).** Stages of genital development for boys **(A)**: (1) Preadolescent—testes, scrotum, and penis are of about the same size and proportions as in early childhood. (2) Enlargement of scrotum and of testes—the skin of the scrotum reddens and changes in texture; little or no enlargement of penis at this stage. (3) Enlargement of penis, which occurs at first mainly in length—further growth of testes and scrotum. Increased size of penis with growth in breadth and development of glans; further enlargement of testes and scrotum; increasing darkening of scrotal skin. Stages of breast development for girls **(B)**: (1) Preadolescent—elevation of the papilla only. (2) Breast bud stage—elevation of papilla as a small mount; enlargement of areolar diameter. (3) Further enlargement and elevation of breast and areola, with no separation of their contours. (4) Projection of areola and papilla to form a secondary mound; the development of the areolar mound does not occur in all girls; in one-fourth it is absent and in a further one-fourth relatively slight. (5) Mature stage—projection of papilla only, caused by recession of the areola to the general contour of the breast. Stages of pubic hair development for boys and girls **(A,C):** (1) Preadolescent—the vellus over the pubes is not developed further than over the abdominal wall. (2) Sparse growth of long, slightly pigmented downy hair, or only slightly curled, appearing chiefly at the penis or along the labia. (3) Considerably darker, coarser, and more curled; the hair spreads sparsely over the junction of the pubes. (4) Hair now resembles adult in type but the area covered is still considerably smaller than in the adult; no spread to the medial surface of the thighs. (5) Adult in quantity and type with distribution of the horizontal (classically feminine) pattern; spread to the medial surface of thighs but not up linea alba or elsewhere above the base of the inverse triangle. (From Tanner J. *Growth at adolescence*. Oxford: Blackwell, 1962, with permission.)

but, rather, a separate stage should be given for pubic hair development and breast or genital development. In some situations, these numbers are discordant. It is particularly important to accurately assess testicular size by comparison to a standard orchidometer with a gradation of sizes from 1 to 25 mL. This volume should be recorded in addition to the pubic hair stage and the genital stage. A description of pubertal stage should be part of every physical examination.

NORMAL GROWTH—PHASES AND DRIVERS OF GROWTH

The first phase of growth is intrauterine growth. Although prenatal growth can be influenced by factors such as chromosomal constitution and fetal hormone production, the single most significant contributor to adequate fetal growth seems to be adequate nutrition. Adequate nutrition, in turn, depends on adequate maternal nutrition and adequate delivery of nutrients through a competent placenta. If either of these aspects of nutrition fails, intrauterine growth retardation or restriction (IUGR) results. Approximately 85% of children with intrauterine growth retardation or restriction exhibit catchup growth in the preschool years and ultimately achieve normal adult stature. The observation that approximately 15% of intrauterine growth retardation or restriction babies do not catch up has lead to the hypothesis of intrauterine growth programming. This hypothesis and the mechanisms that might be responsible for it are under active investigation (9).

The second phase of growth is the rapid growth in both length and weight that occurs during the first 2 years or so after birth. Through mechanisms that are poorly understood and may be related to nutritional programming of growth, this infantile growth also seems to be driven to a significant extent by intrauterine nutrition. During this phase of growth, a healthy baby would be expected to grow approximately 25 cm/year. During the later part of this growth phase, most commonly between approximately 9 and 24 months, many children who were well nourished *in utero* but whose genetics suggest they are likely to be shorter children cross percentiles in a downward fashion to bring their length more in line with genetic expectations. This is a normal growth adjustment in this phase and does not necessarily indicate an abnormality of growth.

There have been a number of studies associating growth during this phase with plasma growth factors, such as insulin-like growth factor (IGF)-1, IGF-2, IGF-binding protein (IGFBP) 3, and IGFBP1 (10–12). It is not clear, however, that these associations reflect a causative influence of the growth factors or a common driver of both growth and the growth factors, such as nutrition or programming of the growth factors by either nutrition or other unknown factors.

The third phase of growth lasts from approximately 2 years until the time of the pubertal growth spurt. During this phase, growth is driven by genetics with the permissive input of the child's own normal endocrine system. The growth velocity curves demonstrate well that growth velocity is constantly declining during this phase. Growth velocity for any given child is not always in a consistent percentile. In fact, a healthy child with a growth velocity with a negative SDS (i.e., below the mean) in 1 year is statistically most likely to have a growth velocity with a positive SDS (i.e., above the mean) in a subsequent year. Thus, in addition to the usefulness of calculating growth velocities over a full year, additional conclusions about the normality or abnormality of a growth pattern can require reliable data over several years.

The fourth phase of growth is the pubertal growth spurt. The time of onset of the pubertal growth spurt varies between genders but also among individuals of the same gender. Growth velocity increases dramatically and more in girls than in boys before declining as pubertal development is complete. Because the timing of the onset of puberty is variable, it is appropriate to take pubertal stage into consideration when assessing growth rate. If puberty has not begun, growth velocity will continue to decline until pubertal onset. Thus, growth velocity can be quite low in a child who has delayed onset of puberty at an age when most of his or her peers are having a pubertal growth spurt. This "dip before the spurt" phenomenon can be differentiated from a significant abnormality of growth by assessing pubertal stage and possibly bone age (see later).

After several years of exposure to sex steroids, the epiphyses of the long bones fuse, and linear growth is no longer possible. This effect on bones is believed to be mediated by estrogen in both boys and girls (13). It is this maturational effect that is responsible for the decline in growth velocity after the peak of the pubertal growth spurt and for the ultimate cessation in growth. Thus, individuals who have significant delay of their bone maturity (bone age) also have residual growth potential. If the delay in bone maturity is due to either the effect of serious illness or due to treatment with glucocorticoids or other medication, the growth potential inherent in a delayed bone age is not always completely achieved (14).

DETERMINATION OF GENETIC TARGET RANGE AND CORRECTION OF GROWTH EXPECTATIONS FOR PARENTAL HEIGHTS

In the third or childhood phase of growth, height is significantly impacted by genetics. Any assessment of absolute height must take into account the target height range, which is best estimated statistically by parental heights. To plot a genetic target range, the height of the same sex parent should be plotted on the right edge of the growth chart. The height of the opposite sex parent should be plotted either by transferring the percentile on the appropriate sex chart to the child's chart (i.e., plotting a twenty-fifth percentile mother at the twenty-fifth percentile on a boy's

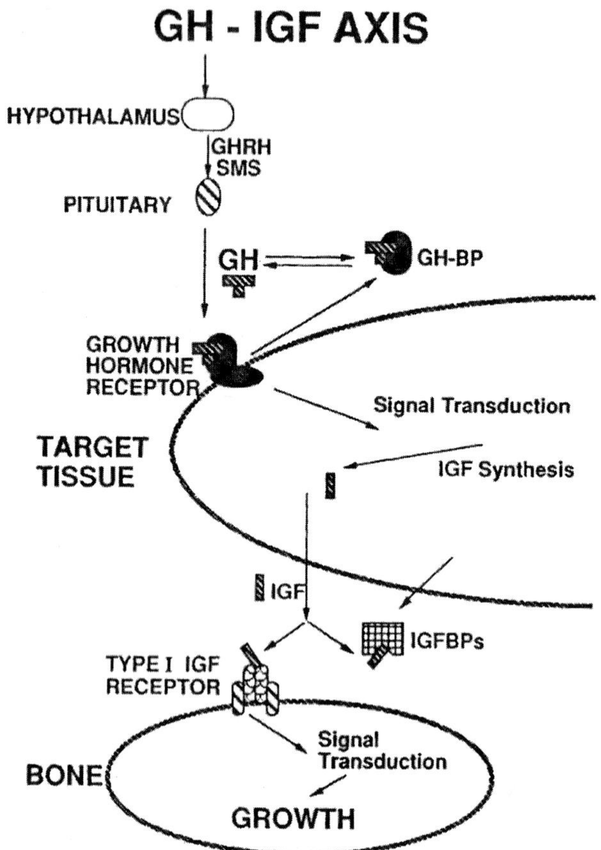

FIGURE 22.7. Normal physiology of the somatotropic axis. GHRH, growth hormone-releasing hormone; IGFBP, insulin-like growth factor-binding protein; SMS, somatostatin. (From Rosenfeld R, Rosembloom A, Guevara-Aguirre J. *Endocrine Reviews* 1995;15:369–390, with permission.)

chart) or by adding 13 cm to the mother's height and plotting it on a boy's chart or subtracting 13 cm from a father's height and plotting it on a girl's chart. Next, the midpoint of these two parental heights should be calculated and plotted. A range of 10 cm above and below this midpoint will include the fifth to ninety-fifth percentiles of the target range for that set of parents.

Further use can be made of these data to calculate a Z score adjusted for parental height. For example, if a child has a height Z score of –2 and the midpoint of the genetic target range has a Z score of –1.5, the child has a Z score of –0.5 when adjusted for genetic target range.

PHYSIOLOGY OF GROWTH HORMONE SECRETION

Although a comprehensive discussion of the physiology and pathophysiology of GH secretion is beyond the scope of this text, it is useful to bear in mind current understanding of the regulatory mechanisms of the somatotropic axis when assessing the growth of children with renal dysfunction.

A diagram of the functioning of the somatotropic axis is shown in Figure 22.7 (15). Multiple inputs from a variety of neurotransmitters and neuropeptides influence the hypothalamic output of GH releasing hormone, which stimulates, and somatostatin, which inhibits GH release from the pituitary. A newly described hormone, ghrelin, appears to be an additional stimulant to pituitary release of GH, but its role in physiologic regulation of growth is not yet clear (16).

GH combines with a specific GH receptor to initiate a signal transduction cascade in multiple tissues that leads to synthesis of IGF-1. IGF-1 in turn interacts with multiple IGFBPs and the type 1 IGF receptor to affect multiple other signal transduction cascades that ultimately lead to tissue growth and other metabolic effects of IGF-1. Thus, it is possible for perturbations in this axis at any point to cause an abnormality of growth. Increasing understanding of the complex interrelationship of nutrition and the somatotropic axis makes a clear distinction between primary nutritional abnormalities and primary abnormalities of the somatotropic axis very difficult. A recent review of the regulation and abnormalities of the somatotropic axis outlines the many subtleties of the interpretation of hormone levels in the context of nutritional perturbation (17).

GROWTH IN CHRONIC RENAL INSUFFICIENCY

Growth failure has long been recognized in children with chronic renal failure (18). Recent advances in dialysis and transplantation offer the potential for the child with end-stage renal disease to live well into adulthood. This magnifies the problem of growth failure, as they are unlikely to reach normal adult stature, leading to the need for investigation of the etiology of growth delay and development of strategies to overcome short stature in children with decreased renal function. The need for adequate, sustained growth is the single most important element that sets children apart from adults with chronic renal failure.

Most children with renal insufficiency exhibit profound growth retardation. The classic depiction of a typical growth pattern in a child with renal failure is shown in Figure 22.8 (19). Infants demonstrate severe statural height failure, whereas older children parallel the growth curve of the normal child but remain below it, and the adolescent again falls away from the curves demonstrating an attenuated pubertal growth spurt (19,20). The Growth Failure in Children with Renal Diseases Study looked at children with renal failure from 23 centers, grouped by degree of insufficiency and age (Table 22.1). Children with more severe renal failure and those with congenital disease and early onset of renal failure tended to have more growth delay (21).

In a study of children requiring dialysis (22), Fine found severe height delay with 70% of children below the age of 5 years more than 2 SD below the mean for age (Fig. 22.9). The effect of long-term dialysis on the growth of children with chronic renal failure was studied by Kleinknecht et al. in

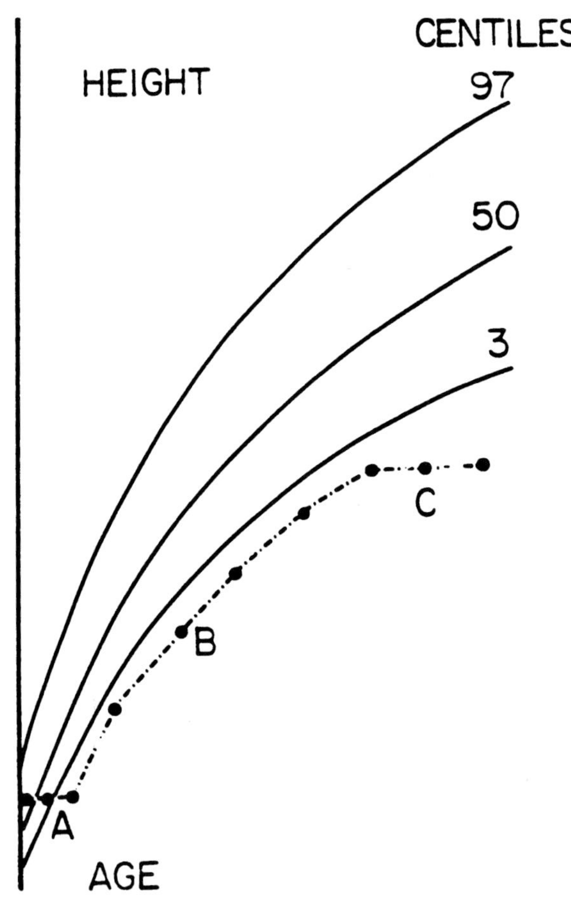

FIGURE 22.8. Schematic representation of growth in children with renal insufficiency. A represents the first 2 years of life. B represents 2 years of age until onset of puberty. C represents the pubertal period. (From Betts P, Magrath G. Growth pattern and dietary intake of children with chronic renal insufficiency. *BMJ* 1974;2:189–193, with permission.)

the 1970s (23). Seventy-six children were followed for 12 to 111 months (mean 30 months) on their individualized dialysis regimens (23). In the 50 prepubertal children there was a mean height loss of 0.38 SD/year. The mean height gain during puberty in 11 pubertal children was only 2 cm/year in girls and 2.7 cm/year in boys, although some subjects exhibited a prolonged growth period (up to age 21 years in one child). A more recent study by van Diemen-Steenvoorde and Donckerwolcke of 35 prepubertal children receiving hemodialysis for more than 1 year (mean, 2.5 years) revealed a loss of 0.31 SD/year (24). The pubertal growth spurt was 3.2 cm/year for boys and 2.1 cm/year for girls at this center. The multicenter report from the European Dialysis and Transplant Association in 1978 of prepubertal children followed for more than 4 years on hemodialysis cited a loss of 0.43 SD/year in height (25). More recent data from the North American Pediatric Renal Transplant Cooperative Study (26), a registry of children with renal failure in North America, continues to demonstrate a loss of 0.32 height SDS over a 2-year period in children receiving dialysis (27).

TABLE 22.1. GROWTH FAILURE IN CHILDREN WITH CHRONIC RENAL FAILURE

Category	No. of patients	Height SD score
Age (yr)		
1–3	31	−1.4
4–6	23	−1.0
7–10	28	−0.7
Disease		
Acquired	23	−0.9
Congenital	59	−1.1
Renal failure[a]		
Mild	34	−0.9
Moderate	29	−1.2
Severe	12	−1.1

[a]Mild, creatinine clearance 50–75 mL/min/1.73 m²; moderate, creatinine clearance 30–49 mL/min/1.73 m²; severe, creatinine clearance <30 mL/min/1.73 m².
Adapted from Abitbol C, Warady B, Massie M, et al. Linear growth and anthropometric and nutritional measurements in children with mild to moderate renal insufficiency: a report of the growth failure in children with renal diseases study. *J Pediatr* 1990;116:S46–S62.

Several studies indicate that children on chronic ambulatory peritoneal dialysis grow better than those receiving chronic hemodialysis or transplantation (28–34). However, these studies show little, if any, statistical significance of the data and are not controlled for age, underlying disease, nutritional intake, and other factors affecting health and growth. Often, the hemodialysis data are derived from historical controls. This can be misleading, as studies have shown general improvement in SD scores on hemodialysis when comparing successive time periods (35). Some of the children had experienced failure of peritoneal dialysis before the institution of hemodialysis, further confounding the analyses. Even under optimal conditions, children on peritoneal dialysis still do not exhibit catchup growth, with several studies showing more than one-half of the children continue to lose growth percentiles while on dialysis (30,36–38).

Transplantation remains the ultimate goal for the pediatric end-stage renal disease patient. Recent data from the North American Pediatric Renal Transplant Cooperative Study show a mean standardized height of −2.16 SDS in nearly 400 transplant recipients (26). Younger children tend to be more severely growth retarded, reflecting the impact of chronic renal failure during the early growth spurt. After transplantation, children younger than 5 years demonstrate some catchup growth, but children older than 6 years have no acceleration of growth rate and may even continue to lose ground, becoming more growth retarded (26,34,39). Thus, it is clear that growth failure cannot be corrected by transplantation and must be addressed earlier in the course of renal failure.

Final adult height is greatly affected by the growth failure seen with chronic renal failure in children. The European Dialysis and Transplant Association found in 1981 (40) that the mean height of adults who had suffered from

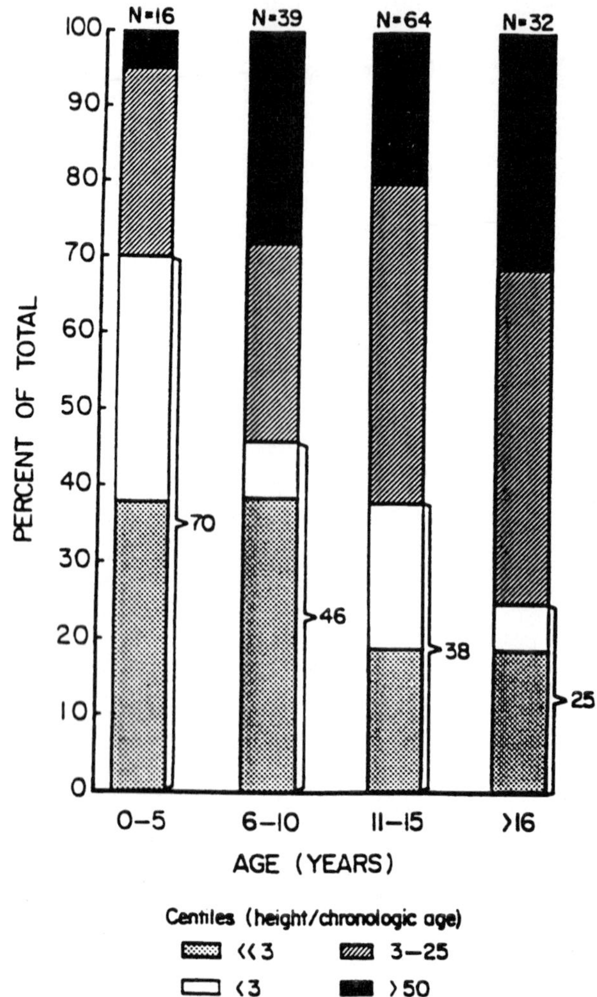

FIGURE 22.9. Relationship between degree of growth retardation and age at onset of renal insufficiency. (From Fine R. Growth in children with renal insufficiency. In: Nissenson AR, Gentile DE, eds. *Clinical dialysis*, 2nd ed. Norwalk, CN: Appleton & Lange, 1990:667–675, with permission.)

chronic renal failure during childhood was 3 SD below the mean (–3.0 SDS). In 1985, the European Dialysis and Transplant Association (35) further reported 62% of men and 41% of women who had renal replacement therapy before the age of 15 had final adult heights below the normal range. This confirms the expectation that children with renal failure at an early age never demonstrate catchup growth and thus reach adulthood significantly height compromised.

ETIOLOGY OF GROWTH DELAY IN CHRONIC RENAL FAILURE

Many factors, listed in Table 22.2, are thought to contribute to the growth failure associated with chronic renal insufficiency, but the mechanisms responsible for their effects are

TABLE 22.2. FACTORS CONTRIBUTING TO GROWTH FAILURE IN CHILDREN WITH RENAL INSUFFICIENCY

Age at onset of primary renal disease
Etiology of primary renal disease
Degree of renal impairment
Inadequate caloric and protein intake
Renal osteodystrophy
Metabolic acidosis
Tubular defects
  Polyuria
  Salt wasting
  Potassium depletion
  Other losses (calcium, phosphorous, etc.)
Corticosteroid administration
Anemia
Infection
Psychosocial factors
Uremic inhibitors of growth hormones and related proteins

Adapted from Stewart C, Fine R. Growth in children with renal insufficiency. *Semin Dial* 1993;6:37–45; Rigden S, Rees L, Chantler C. Growth and endocrine function in children with chronic renal failure. *Acta Paediatr Scand* 1990;370:S20–S27; and French C, Genel M. Pathophysiology of growth failure in chronic renal insufficiency. *Kidney Int* 1984;30:S59–S64.

poorly understood (41–43). As noted in Figure 22.9, children with onset of renal failure earlier in life have more severe growth impairment than those diagnosed later. Figure 22.10 depicts the severe growth failure of a group of children with obstructive uropathy, which is usually congenital, thus exerting an influence on growth from birth (22).

A correlation between degree of renal failure and growth dysfunction has been reported, although this correlation has not been demonstrated in all studies (21,35,42,44). Poor nutritional intake can certainly influence growth in any setting, and chronic renal failure is no exception (45). Some authors report improvement in height SD scores with nutritional intervention (42,46–48).

Renal osteodystrophy, intercurrent infections, metabolic acidosis, and tubular defects have been correlated to poor growth, and specific therapy for these defects can be growth enhancing (21,44,45,49). Corticosteroids are well known to inhibit statural growth, but are not usually required therapeutically once dialysis is initiated (50). Although chronic anemia was long thought to be a contributing factor to growth failure, early reports of correction of anemia with recombinant erythropoietin have been disappointing regarding improvement in nutrition or growth (51–54). Psychosocial factors have also been shown to affect the growth of children with impaired renal function (35).

EFFECTS OF UREMIA ON GROWTH HORMONE/INSULIN-LIKE GROWTH FACTOR AXIS

It was thought that abnormalities of GH and IGF-1 played no role in the pathogenesis of growth failure in renal insuf-

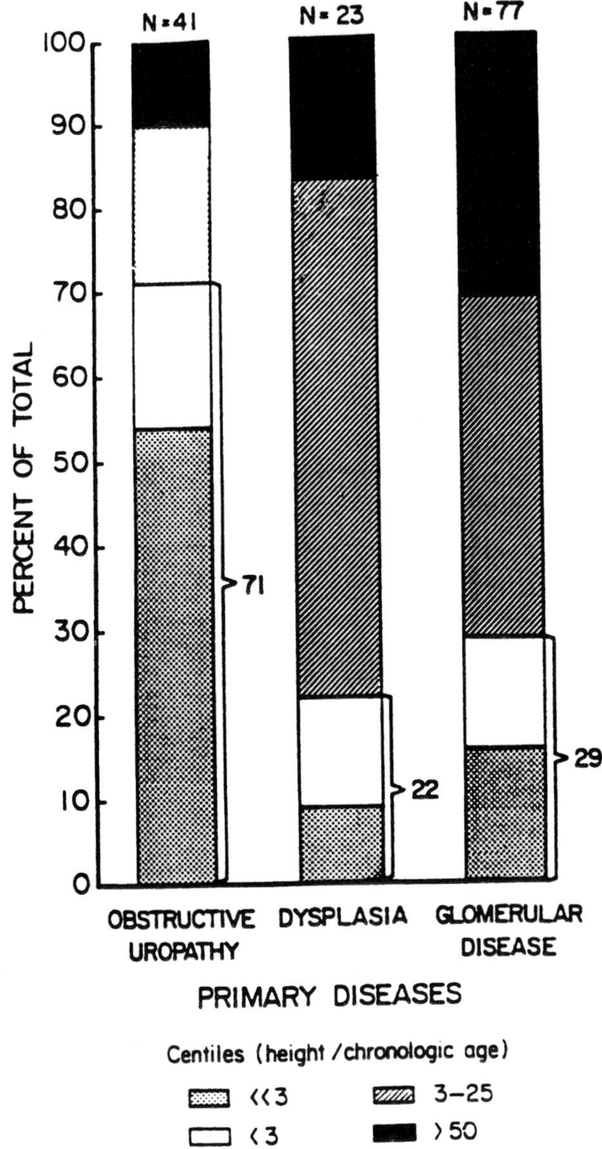

FIGURE 22.10. Relationship between degree of growth retardation and primary renal disease. (From Fine R. Growth in children with renal insufficiency. In: Nissenson AR, Gentile DE, eds. *Clinical dialysis*, 2nd ed. Norwalk, CN: Appleton & Lange, 1990:667–675, with permission.)

ficiency. However, recent studies have begun to elucidate perturbations of the GH axis in chronic renal failure, which brings this aspect of growth failure into focus and lays the groundwork for therapeutic interventions (55–64).

GH functions by stimulating production and release of IGF-1 as well as by more direct effects on target tissues (64,65). Early reports indicated reduced (66) or high (62) IGF-1 levels in uremia when measured by radioimmunoassay. Bioassays have also found reduced activity of IGF in uremia, with some investigators finding a slight rise in activity after a dialytic session and others demonstrating higher levels with transplantation, raising the possibility of uremic inhibitors (66–68). More recent reports, using improved extraction techniques, indicate that IGF-1 activity is near normal in uremia (64,69–71).

Current research is focusing on the physiology and pathophysiology of GH-binding proteins and IGFBPs in normal and abnormal growth (71–77). Uremic children have been shown to have a low serum level of GH-binding protein (75). This may play some role in end-organ effect. At least six IGFBPs have been identified and characterized (55,78). IGFBP1, IGFBP3, and IGFBP4 have been shown to be elevated in uremic children and the excess binding protein, especially IGFBP3, acts as an IGF-1 inhibitor (55,72,73,76,79).

TREATMENT OF THE GROWTH FAILURE OF CHRONIC RENAL INSUFFICIENCY

The alterations in GH-binding proteins and IGFBPs in chronic renal failure provide a rationale for the use of recombinant human growth hormone (rhGH) to treat the growth failure in prepubertal uremic children. Theoretically, excess ligand might be expected to overcome any inhibitory effect of increased binding. Landmark studies by Mehls and colleagues demonstrated a stimulatory effect of growth hormone on chondrocytes and longitudinal growth in uremic rats (80–82). Several other investigators confirmed the growth-enhancing effects of GH in this animal model (83–86). These studies also provided reassurance regarding stability of renal function and serum lipids (83,84,86), although concern has been raised regarding a trend toward reduced survival and glomerular hypertrophy with glomerulosclerosis in treated animals (83).

The favorable results of the use of rhGH in the rat model led to subsequent trials in uremic children. In 1988, Lippe et al. reported a twofold increase in height velocity in five growth-retarded, uremic children given rhGH (87). This center has since reported growth data from nine patients followed for up to 36 months on GH therapy (88–90). SD scores in these nine patients improved from mean −3.18 to −2.50 at 12 months, whereas the four subjects treated for 36 months improved from −2.78 to −1.29. The individual growth chart of a typical subject is shown in Figure 22.11. Bone age did not advance disproportionately to chronologic age in these patients. There were no significant changes in serum chemistries, calculated creatinine clearances, thyroid function tests, or glucose tolerance. IGF-1 levels increased in all patients (90).

These encouraging preliminary results have been supported by Tönshoff and the German Study Group who have now studied 61 uremic children (20 predialysis, 24 dialysis, 17 transplanted) receiving daily subcutaneous rhGH for 1 to 2 years (91,92). The 17 prepubertal, predialysis subjects improved from a pretreatment median SDS of −3.0 to −2.0 after 1 year of therapy. This study reports a

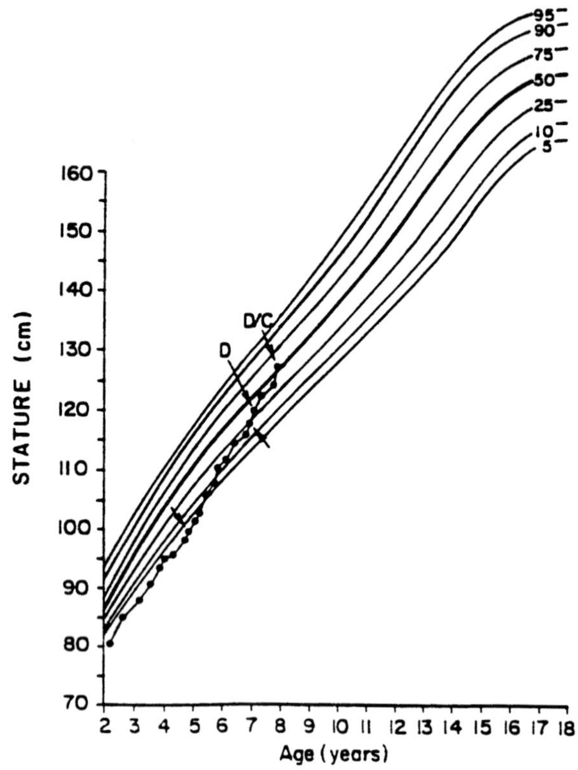

FIGURE 22.11. Growth of individual patient before and during treatment with recombinant human growth hormone (rhGH). ↓, rhGH thrice weekly; ↑, rhGH daily; D, dialysis initiated; D/C, rhGH discontinued. [From Fine R, Pyke-Grimm K, Nelson P, et al. Recombinant human growth hormone treatment of children with chronic renal failure: long-term (1- to 3-year) outcome. *Pediatr Nephrol* 1991;5:477–481, with permission.]

significant improvement in height in all patient groups with no untoward effects, except an elevation in insulin levels. This has been found to be a transient abnormality in the longer-term study (90). Mehls et al. also found an increase in IGF-1 after treatment, with no further rise in IGFBP3 concentration (55). Johansson et al. and Van Es and the European Study Group have followed 94 prepubertal children (41 predialysis and 53 transplanted) for up to 2 years of rhGH therapy (93,94). In children treated for 2 years, height SDS was improved from –2.8 to –1.8 in predialysis patients. No significant side effects were reported.

Multiple other reports have confirmed the effect of rhGH in overcoming the short stature associated with uremia in the pediatric population (95–101), including two reports of improved height in children with nephropathic cystinosis (100,101). Encouraging data exist about improvement in height SDS and head circumference in infants treated with GH. The role of the GH/IGF-1 axis in this age group still requires more clarification, especially whether treatment could relate to improved neurodevelopment (98,99). Although more difficult to assess, pubertal uremic children are also believed to respond favorably to GH treatment (92–95,97,102,103).

Concerns regarding potential long-term side effects have not been borne out by experimental data. Fine and colleague's randomized, placebo-controlled study should provide excellent data on both long-term effectiveness and adverse effects (99). Specific concerns raised regarding avascular necrosis of the femoral head, progression of renal failure, and lipid and insulin abnormalities have not been borne out in subsequent investigations (104–109).

Reports of the use of rhGH in growth-retarded children with renal allografts are encouraging with some improvement in height SDS despite the concomitant use of corticosteroids to suppress allograft rejection (92–95,110–114). However, concerns about a deleterious effect on the allograft demand caution in this patient population (115,116). Further randomized, controlled studies are necessary to determine the safety of treatment in this setting. Until then, the best approach appears to be normalization of height using growth hormone before transplantation, as final adult height is best predicted by height achieved before transplantation (39,117).

Many of the above studies included patients receiving dialysis. Fine et al. reported five children undergoing chronic cycling peritoneal dialysis who received rhGH (118). Only three showed improvement in height SDS, but length of treatment was less than 1 year in the other two. Tönshoff et al. found improvement in the height velocity SDS in eight children undergoing dialysis treated with rhGH (1 hemodialysis, 7 peritoneal dialysis), but the change was not as marked as in a single predialysis patient (91). This trend continued in the larger German study, with improvement in SDS from –3.2 to –2.7 in ten dialysis patients treated for 1 year (96). However, in Hokken-Koelega and colleagues' placebo-controlled, double-blind, crossover trial there was no difference found in the response of dialysis patients compared to conservatively managed predialysis patients, with mean increases in height velocity of 2.9 cm/6 months versus 3.0, respectively (96). An encouraging report by Tom et al. demonstrates some catchup growth in children on maintenance hemodialysis with increased intensity of hemodialysis and closely monitored nutritional intake, raising the possibility of overcoming the poor growth response in the dialysis population (119).

Significant controversy exists regarding the safety and efficacy of rhGH after transplantation. Thus, it remains to be seen whether any height deficit remaining after successful transplantation will be amenable to rhGH therapy.

Children treated with GH may have their growth limited by fusion of the epiphyses as a result of normal pubertal development. Because of some evidence that delaying puberty in children with GH deficiency can increase height prognosis (17), such therapy might be considered for children undergoing GH treatment for chronic renal insufficiency. The benefit to be derived from such treatment in patients with chronic renal insufficiency has yet to be documented.

There are early indications that therapy with GH can have a positive effect on ultimate adult height. Recently, the German

Study Group for Growth Hormone Treatment in Chronic Renal Failure demonstrated that mean final adult height for children with chronic renal failure treated with growth hormone was 1.6 SD below normal, a marked improvement over historical controls who were untreated (120).

CONCLUSION

The growth retardation of children with chronic renal failure is a major problem for the pediatric nephrologist. With the current success of dialysis and transplantation in minimizing the mortality of early-stage renal disease, these children should live well into adulthood. Allowing them to appreciate their full adult height potential is a realistic goal. The use of rhGH to enhance growth during the early years of renal insufficiency and during dialysis has been shown to be effective. Further long-term studies are needed to determine whether growth will continue and genetic potential for ultimate adult height will be attained. Potential long-term side effects also need to be continually monitored in a rigorous fashion. Concern still exists regarding growth and the use of rhGH after transplantation to maximize growth. Thus, preventing growth retardation and recovering lost growth during early renal insufficiency and the dialytic period may be the best way to maximize adult height in this population.

REFERENCES

1. Valk I, Langhout Chabloz A, Smals A, et al. Accurate measurement of the lower leg length and the ulnar leg length and its application in short term growth measurements. *Growth* 1983;47:53–66.
2. Wales J, Milner R. Knemometry in assessment of linear growth. *Arch Dis Child* 1987;62:166–171.
3. Dean H, Schentag C, Winter J, et al. Predictive value of short-term growth using knemometry in a large population of healthy children. *Acta Paediatr Scand* 1990;79:57–63.
4. Must A, Jacques P, Dallal G, et al. Long-term morbidity and mortality of overweight adolescents. *N Engl J Med* 1992; 327:1350–1355.
5. Javier Nieto F, Moyses S, Comstock G. Childhood weight and growth rate as predictors of adult mortality. *Am J Epidemiol* 1992;136:201–213.
6. Wong C, Gipson D, Gillen D, et al. Anthropometric measures and risk of death in children with end-stage renal disease. *Am J Kidney Dis* 2000;36:811–819.
7. Greulich W, Pyle S. *Radiographic atlas of skeletal development of the hand and wrist.* Stanford, CA: Stanford University Press, 1959.
8. Tanner J, Whitehouse R, Cameron N, et al. *Assessment of skeletal maturity and prediction of adult height (TW2 method)*, 2nd ed. London: London, Academic Press, 1983.
9. Phillips D. Endocrine programming and fetal origins of adult disease. *Trend Endocrinol Metab* 2002;13:363–408.
10. Fall C, Pandit A, Law, et al. Size at birth and plasma insulin line growth factor-1 concentrations. *Arch Dis Child* 1995; 73:287–293.
11. Ong K, Kratsch J, Kiess W, et al. Size at birth and cord blood levels of insulin, insulin-like growth factor I (IGF-I), IGF-II, IGF-Binding Protein-1 (IGFBP-1), IGFBP-3 and the soluble IGF-II/mannose-6-phosphate receptor in term human infants. *J Clin Endocrinol Metab* 2000;85:4266–4269.
12. Ong K, Kratzsch J, Kiess W, et al. Circulating IGF-I levels in childhood are related to both current body composition and early postnatal growth rate. *J Clin Endocrinol Metab* 2002;87:1041–1044.
13. Smith E, Boyd J, Frank G, et al. Estrogen resistance caused by a mutation in the estrogen receptor gene in a man. *N Engl J Med* 1994;331:1056–1061.
14. Ackland F, Preece M. Catch-up growth. *Pediatrician* 1987;14:226–233.
15. Rosenfeld R, Rosembloom A, Guevara-Aguirre J. Growth hormone (GH) insensitivity due to primary GH receptor deficiency. *Endocrine Reviews* 1995;15:369–390.
16. Muller A, Lamberts S, Janssen J, et al. Ghrelin drives GH secretion during fasting in man. *Eur J Endocrinol* 2002; 146:203–207.
17. Rosenfeld R, Cohem P. Disorders of growth hormone/insulin-like growth factor secretion and action. In: Sperling MA, ed. *Pediatric endocrinology*, 2nd ed. Philadelphia: Saunders, 2002:211–288.
18. Stickler G. Growth failure in renal disease. *Pediatr Clin North Am* 1976;23:885–894.
19. Betts P, Magrath G. Growth pattern and dietary intake of children with chronic renal insufficiency. *BMJ* 1974;2:189–193.
20. Schaefer F, Wingen A, Hennicke M, et al. Growth charts for prepubertal children with chronic renal failure due to congenital renal disorder. *Pediatr Nephrol* 1996;10:288–293.
21. Abitbol C, Warady B, Massie M, et al. Linear growth and anthropometric and nutritional measurements in children with mild to moderate renal insufficiency: a report of the growth failure in children with renal diseases study. *J Pediatr* 1990;116:S46–S62.
22. Fine R. Growth in children with renal insufficiency. In: Nissenson AR, Gentile DE, eds. *Clinical dialysis*, 2nd ed. Norwalk, CN: Appleton & Lange, 1990:667–675.
23. Kleinknecht C, Broyer M, Gagnadoux M-F, et al. Growth in children treated with long-term dialysis. In: Hamburger J, Crosnier J, Grünfeld JP, eds. *Advances in nephrology*. Chicago: Year Book Medical Publishers, 1980:133–163.
24. Van Diemen-Steenvoorde R, Donckerwolcke RA. Growth and sexual maturation in pediatric patients treated by dialysis and following kidney transplantation. *Acta Paediatr Scand* 1988;343:S109–S117.
25. Donckerwolcke R, Chantler C, Brunner F, et al. Combined report on regular dialysis and transplantation of children in Europe 1977. *Proc Eur Dialysis Transpl Assoc* 1978;15:77–114.
26. Avner E, Chavers B, Sullivan E, et al. Renal transplantation and chronic dialysis in children and adolescents: the 1993 annual report of the North American Renal Transplant Cooperative Study. *Pediatr Nephrol* 1995;9:61–73.

27. Neu A, Ho M, McDonald R, et al. Chronic dialysis in children and adolescents. The 2001 NAPRTCS Annual Report. *Pediatr Nephrol* 2002;17:656–663.
28. Fennell R, Orak J, Hudson T, et al. Growth in children with various therapies for end stage renal disease. *Am J Dis Child* 1984;138:28–31.
29. Baum M, Powell D, Calvin S, et al. Continuous ambulatory peritoneal dialysis in children. Comparison with Hemodialysis. *N Engl J Med* 1982;307:1537–1542.
30. Stefanidis D, Hewitt I, Balfe J. Growth in children receiving continuous ambulatory peritoneal dialysis. *J Pediatr* 1983;102: 681–685.
31. Kaiser B, Stover J, Polinsky M, et al. The effect of different dialysis modalities on growth in children with chronic renal failure (abstract). *Kidney Int* 1986;29:233.
32. Potter D. Comparison of CAPD and hemodialysis in children. In: Fine RN, ed. *Chronic ambulatory peritoneal dialysis (CAPD) and chronic cycling peritoneal dialysis (CCPD) in children.* Boston: Nijhoff, 1987:297.
33. Gruskin A, Alexander S, Baluarte H, et al. Issues in pediatric dialysis. *Am J Kidney Dis* 1986;4:306–311.
34. Iitaka K, Hojo M, Moriya S, et al. Comparison of growth during continuous ambulatory peritoneal dialysis and renal transplantation using conventional immunosuppressive drugs in children. *Perit Dial Int* 1998;18:395–401.
35. Rizzoni G, Broyer M, Brunner F, et al. Combined report on regular dialysis and transplantation of children in Europe. *Proc Eur Dial Transplant* Assoc 1985;82:66–95.
36. Fine R, Salusky I. CAPD/CCPD in children: four years' experience. *Kidney Int* 1986;30:S7–S10.
37. Warady B, Kriley M, Lovell H, et al. Growth and development of infants with end-stage renal disease receiving long-term peritoneal dialysis. *J Pediatr* 1988;112:714–719.
38. Von Lilien T, Salusky I, Boechat I, et al. Five years experience with continuous ambulatory and continuous cycling peritoneal dialysis. *J Pediatr* 1987;111:513–518.
39. Fine R. Growth post renal-transplantation in children: lessons from the North American Pediatric Renal Transplant Cooperative Study (NAPRTCS). *Pediatr Tranplant* 1997;1: 85–89.
40. Chantler C, Broyer M, Donckerwolcke R, et al. Growth and rehabilitation of long-term survivors of treatment for end-stage renal failure in childhood. *Proc Eur Dial Transplant Assoc* 1981;18:329–342.
41. Stewart C, Fine R. Growth in children with renal insufficiency. *Semin Dial* 1993;6:37–45.
42. Rigden S, Rees L, Chantler C. Growth and endocrine function in children with chronic renal failure. *Acta Paediatr Scand* 1990;370:S20–S27.
43. French C, Genel M. Pathophysiology of growth failure in chronic renal insufficiency. *Kidney Int* 1984;30:S59–S64.
44. Ray P, Holliday M. Growth rate in infants with impaired renal function. *J Pediatr* 1988;113:594–600.
45. Claris-Appiani A, Bianchi M, Bini P, et al. Growth in young children with chronic renal failure. *Pediatr Nephrol* 1989; 3:301–304.
46. Wassner S, Abitbol C, Alexander S, et al. Nutritional requirements for infants with renal failure. *Am J Kidney Dis* 1986;4:300–305.
47. Parekh R, Flynn J, Smoyer W, et al. Improved growth in young children with severe chronic renal insufficiency who use specified nutritional therapy. *J Am Soc Nephrol* 2001; 12:2418–2426.
48. Letermann S, Shaw V, Trompeter RS. Long-term enteral nutrition in infants and young children with chronic renal failure. *Pediatr Nephrol* 1999;13:870–875.
49. Chantler C. Growth and metabolism in renal failure. *J R Coll of Physicians Lond* 1988;22:69–73.
50. Travis L, Chesney R, McEnery P, et al. Growth and glucocorticoids in children with kidney disease. *Kidney Int* 1978; 14:365–368.
51. Dabbagh S, Fleischmann L. The long-term follow-up of the efficacy of recombinant human erythropoietin (rhEPO) in children with chronic renal failure (CRF): a prospective study (abstract). *Pediatr Res* 1992;31:331A.
52. Warady B, Sabath R, Smith C, et al. Recombinant human erythropoietin therapy in pediatric patients receiving long-term peritoneal dialysis. *Pediatr Nephrol* 1991;5:718–723.
53. Watkins S, Hickman R, Avner E. Erythropoietin in pediatric renal patients—long-term follow-up (abstract). *Pediatric Res* 1991;29:354A.
54. Rees L, Rigden S, Chantler C. The influence of steroid therapy and recombinant human erythropoietin on the growth of children with renal disease. *Pediatr Nephrol* 1991;5:556–558.
55. Mehls O, Tonshoff B, Blum W, et al. Growth hormone and insulin-like growth factor I in chronic renal failure-pathophysiology and rationale for growth hormone treatment. *Acta Paediatr Scand* 1990;370:S28–S35.
56. Schaefer F, Schärer K, Mehls O. Pathogenic mechanisms of pubertal growth failure in chronic renal failure. *Acta Paediatr Scand* 1991;379:S3–S11.
57. Veldhuis J, Johnson M, Wilkowski M, et al. Neuroendocrine alterations in the somatotrophic axis in chronic renal failure. *Acta Paediatr Scand* 1991;379:S12–S23.
58. Cappa M, del Balzo P, Rizzoni G, et al. Somatostatinergic tone in children on chronic haemodialysis and after renal transplantation. *Pediatr Nephrol* 1991;5:548–551.
59. Garcia R, Andrade A, Perez J, et al. Altered growth hormone response after growth hormone releasing hormone administration in chronic renal failure. *J Endocrinol Invest* 1991;14:383–389.
60. Metzger D, Kerrigan J, Krieg RJ J, et al. Alterations in the neuroendocrine control of growth hormone secretion in the uremic rat. *Kidney Int* 1993;43:1042–1048.
61. Samaan N, Freeman R. Growth hormone levels in severe renal failure. *Metabolism* 1970;19:102–113.
62. Perrone L, Sinisi A, Criscuolo T, et al. Plasma and urinary growth hormone and insulin-like growth factor I in children with chronic renal insufficiency. *Child Nephol Urol* 1990;10: 72–75.
63. Schaefer F, Hamill G, Stanhope R, et al. Pulsatile growth hormone secretion in peripubertal patients with chronic renal failure. *J Pediatr* 1991;119:568–577.
64. Hokken-Koelega A, Hackeng W, Stijnen T, et al. Twenty-four-hour plasma growth hormone (GH) profiles, urinary GH excretion, and plasma insulin-like growth factor-I and - II levels in prepubertal children with chronic renal insufficiency and severe growth retardation. *J Clin Endocrinol Metab* 1990; 71:688–695.

65. Schoenle E, Zapf T, Foresch E. Insulin-like growth factor I stimulates growth in hypophysectomised rats. *Nature* 1982; 296:252–253.
66. Goldberg A, Trivedi B, Delmez J, et al. Uremia reduces serum insulin-like growth factor I, increases insulin-like growth factor II, and modifies their serum protein binding. *J Clin Endocrinol Metab* 1982;55:1040–1045.
67. Phillips L, Kopple J. Circulating somatomedin activity and sulphate levels in adults with normal and impaired kidney function. *Metabolism* 1981;30:1091–1095.
68. Kapila P, Jones J, Rees L. Effect of chronic renal failure and prednisolone on the growth hormone-insulin-like growth factor axis. *Pediatr Nephrol* 2001;16:1099–1104.
69. Powell D, Rosenfeld R, Sperry J, et al. Serum concentrations of insulin-like growth factor (IGF-I), IGF-II and unsaturated somatomedin carrier proteins in children with chronic renal failure. *Am J Kidney Dis* 1987;10:287–292.
70. Phillips L, Fusco A, Unterman T, et al. Somatomedin inhibitor in uremia. *J Clin Endocrinol Metab* 1984;59:764–772.
71. Hodson E, Brown A, Roy L, et al. Insulin-like growth factor-1, growth hormone-dependent insulin-like growth factor-binding protein and growth in children with chronic renal failure. *Pediatr Nephrol* 1992;6:433–438.
72. Blum W, Ranke M, Kietzmann K, et al. Growth hormone resistance and inhibition of somatomedin activity by excess of insulin-like growth factor binding protein in uraemia. *Pediatr Nephrol* 1991;5:539–544.
73. Lee P, Hintz R, Sperry J, et al. IGF binding proteins in growth-retarded children with chronic renal failure. *Pediatric Res* 1989;26:308–315.
74. Postel-Vinay M, Tar A, Crosnier H, et al. Plasma growth hormone-binding activity is low in uraemic children. *Pediatr Nephrol* 1991;5:545–547.
75. Maheshwari H, Rifkin I, Butler J, et al. Growth hormone binding protein in patients with renal failure. *Acta Endocrinol* 1992;127:485–488.
76. Powell D, Liu F, Baker B, et al. Characterization of insulin-like growth factor binding protein-3 in chronic renal failure serum. *Pediatric Res* 1993;33:136–143.
77. Tönshoff B, Schaefer F, Mehls O. Disturbance of growth hormone-insulin-like growth factor axis in uraemia. *Pediatr Nephrol* 1990;4:654–662.
78. Powell D. Effects of renal failure on the growth hormone-insulin-like growth factor axis. *J Pediatr* 1997;131:S13–S16.
79. Ulinski T, Mohan S, Kiepe D, et al. Serum insulin-like growth factor binding protein (IGFBP)-4 and IGFBP-5 in children with chronic renal failure: relationship to growth and glomerular filtration rate. The European Study Group for Nutritional Treatment of Chronic Renal Failure in Childhood. German Study Group for Growth Hormone Treatment in Chronic Renal Failure. *Pediatr Nephrol* 2000;14:589–597.
80. Kreusser W, Weinkauf R, Mehls O, et al. Effect of parathyroid hormone, calcitonin and growth hormone on cAMP content of growth cartilage in experimental uremia. *Eur J Clin Invest* 1982;12:337–343.
81. Mehls O, Ritz E. Skeletal growth in experimental uremia. *Kidney Int* 1983;24:S53–S62.
82. Mehls O, Ritz E, Hunziker E, et al. Improvement of growth and food utilization by human recombinant growth hormone in uremia. *Kidney Int* 1988;33:45–52.
83. Allen D, Fogo A, el-Hayek R, et al. Effects of prolonged growth hormone administration in rats with chronic renal insufficiency. *Pediatr Res* 1992;31:406–410.
84. Kawaguchi H, Komatsu Y, Hattori M, et al. Potential effects of recombinant human growth hormone (rhGH) on somatic growth in uremic rats. *Acta Paediatr Jpn* 1991;33:6–14.
85. Powell D, Rosenfeld R, Hintz R. Effects of growth hormone therapy and malnutrition on the growth of rats with renal failure. *Pediatr Nephrol* 1988;2:425–430.
86. Santos F, Chan J, Hanna J, et al. The effect of growth hormone on the growth failure of chronic renal failure. *Pediatr Nephrol* 1992;6:262–266.
87. Lippe B, Fine R, Koch V, et al. Accelerated growth following treatment of children with chronic renal failure with recombinant human growth hormone (Somatrem): a preliminary report. *Acta Paediatr Scand* 1988;343:S127–S131.
88. Koch V, Lippe B, Nelson P, et al. Accelerated growth after recombinant human growth hormone treatment of children with chronic renal failure. *J Pediatr* 1989;115:365–371.
89. Fine R. Recombinant human growth hormone treatment of children with chronic renal failure: update 1990. *Acta Paediatr Scand* 1990;370:S44–S51.
90. Fine R, Pyke-Grimm K, Nelson P, et al. Recombinant human growth hormone treatment of children with chronic renal failure: long-term (1- to 3-year) outcome. *Pediatr Nephrol* 1991;5:477–481.
91. Tönshoff B, Mehls O, Heinrich U, et al. Growth-stimulating effects of recombinant human growth hormone in children with end-stage renal disease. *J Pediatr* 1990;116:561–566.
92. Tönshoff B, Dietz M, Haffner D, et al. Effects of two years of growth hormone treatment in short children with renal disease. *Acta Paediatr Scand* 1991;379:S33–S34.
93. Johansson G, Sietnieks A, Janssens F, et al. Recombinant human growth hormone treatment in short children with chronic renal disease, before transplantation or with functioning renal transplants: An interim report on five European studies. *Acta Paediatr Scand* 1990;370:S36–S43.
94. Van Es A. Growth hormone treatment in short children with chronic renal failure and after renal transplantation: combined data from European clinical trials. *Acta Paediatr Scand* 1991;379:S42–S49.
95. Rees L, Rigden S, Ward G, et al. Treatment of short stature in renal disease with recombinant human growth hormone. *Arch Dis Child* 1990;65:856–880.
96. Hokken-Koelega A, Stijnen T, de Muinck Keizer-Schrama S, et al. Placebo-controlled, double-blind, cross-over trial of growth hormone treatment in prepubertal children with chronic renal failure. *Lancet* 1991;338:585–590.
97. Ortiz A, Placida Garron M, Rovira A, et al. Effect of recombinant human growth hormone in a postpediatric hemodialysis patient with delayed growth. *Am J Nephrol* 1992;12:471–473.
98. van Renen M, Hogg R, Sweeney A, et al. Accelerated growth in short children with chronic renal failure with both strict dietary therapy and recombinant growth hormone. *Pediatr Nephrol* 1992;6:451–458.
99. Fine R, Kohaut E, Frane J, et al. Multicenter randomized double blind placebo—controlled study of recombinant human growth hormone (rhGH) in children with chronic renal failure (CRF) (abstract). *Pediatr Res* 1993;33:355A.

100. Wilson D, Jelley D, Stratton R, et al. Nephropathic cystinosis: Improved linear growth after treatment with recombinant human growth hormone. *J Pediatr* 1989;115:758–761.
101. Andersson H, Markello T, Schneider J, et al. Effect of growth hormone treatment on serum creatinine concentration in patients with cystinosis and chronic renal disease. *J Pediatr* 1992;120:716–720.
102. Yadin O, Kamil E, Pyke-Grimm K, et al. Recombinant human growth hormone in pubertal patients with chronic renal disease. *Contrib Nephrol* 1992;100:139–154.
103. Hokken-Koelega A, de Jong R, Donckerwolcke R, et al. Use of recombinant human growth hormone (rhGH) in pubertal patients with CRI/dialysis/post-transplant: Dutch data. Dutch Study Group on Growth in Children with Chronic Renal Disease. *Br J Clin Prac* 1996;85:S5–S6.
104. Watkins S, Johanson A, Winters W, et al. Legg-Perthes in children with chronic renal failure during growth (abstract). *J Am Soc Nephrol* 1990;1:344.
105. Catterall A, Roberts G. Association of Perthes' Disease with congenital anomalies of genitourinary tract and inguinal region. *Lancet* 1971;1:996–997.
106. Mehls O, Ritz E, Oppermann H. Femoral head necrosis in uremic children without steroid treatment or transplantation. *J Pediatr* 1981;99:926–929.
107. Tönshoff B, Tönshoff C, Mehls O, et al. Growth hormone treatment in children with preterminal chronic renal failure: no adverse effect on glomerular filtration rate. *Eur J Pediatr* 1992;151:601–607.
108. Jedrzejowshi A, Panczyk-Tomaszewska M, Roszkowska-Blaim M, et al. Growth hormone therapy and lipid profile in children on chronic peritoneal dialysis. *Pediatr Nephrol* 2002;17:830–836.
109. Fine R, Kohaut E, Brown D, et al. Long-term treatment of growth retarded children with chronic renal insufficiency, with recombinant human growth hormone. *Kidney Int* 1996;49:781–785.
110. Bartosh S, Kaiser B, Rezvani I, et al. Effects of growth hormone administration in pediatric renal allograft recipients. *Pediatr Nephrol* 1992;6:68–73.
111. Fine R, Yadin O, Nelson P, et al. Recombinant human growth hormone treatment of children following renal transplantation. *Pediatr Nephrol* 1991;5:147–151.
112. Fine R, Yadin O, Moulten L, et al. Extended recombinant human growth hormone treatment after renal transplantation in children. *J Am Soc Nephrol* 1992;2:S274–S283.
113. Van Dop C, Donohoue P, Bock G, et al. Enhanced growth with growth hormone therapy after renal transplantation. *Pediatr Nephrol* 1989;3:468–469.
114. Van Dop C, Jabs K, Donohoue P, et al. Accelerated growth rates in children treated with growth hormone after renal transplantation. *J Pediatr* 1992;120:244–250.
115. Benfield M, Aail A, Waldo F, et al. The effect of rhGH in vitro on donor-specific hyporesponsiveness in pediatric transplantation. Pediatr Transplant 1997;1:90–97.
116. Benfield M, Kohaut E. Growth hormone is safe in children after renal transplantation. *J Pediatr* 1997;131:S28–S31.
117. Rodiguez-Soriano J, Vallo A, Quintela M, et al C. Predictors of final adult height after renal transplantation during childhood: a single-center study. *Nephron* 2000;86:266–273.
118. Fine R, Koch V, Boechat M, et al. Recombinant human growth hormone (rhGH) treatment of children undergoing peritoneal dialysis. *Perit Dial Int* 1990;10:209–214.
119. Tom A, McCauley L, Bell L, et al. Growth during maintenance hemodialysis: Impact of enhanced nutrition and clearance. *J Pediatr* 1999;134:464–471.
120. Haffner D, Schaefer F, Nissel R. Effect of growth hormone treatment on the adult height of children with chronic renal failure. *N Engl J Med* 2000;343:923–930.

23

DIAGNOSTIC IMAGING

FRED E. AVNI
MICHELLE HALL

Imaging the urinary tract (UT) plays a significant role in the work-up of many nephrouropathies (1,2). The numbers of techniques that are available to image the UT are numerous; each has its advantages and drawbacks. The work-up must be tailored to every patient taking into account the type of disease, clinical data, and questions to be answered. Hazards related to the use of a specific technique, such as radiation hazards, allergy, or postprocedural infection, should also be taken into account. Whatever technique is chosen, a decision tree must be applied in accordance with the ALARA principle (*as low as reasonably achievable*). This concept implies that imaging techniques have to be chosen to provide the most accurate diagnosis using the most adequate and safest technique in a specific indication. Whenever possible, a radiating technique should be replaced by a nonradiating one (3).

DIAGNOSTIC PROCEDURES

Ultrasound

Ultrasound (US) is the central imaging modality for assessing the UT in children. It is easy to perform. The examination is very accurate in assessing the presence of a kidney and the degree of dilatation. It should include evaluation of the bladder and ureters (not visible under normal conditions) (4,5). Kidney size should be compared to normograms; established according to age, weight, or height; and expressed in standard deviation (6). On US, the kidneys appear with a corticomedullary differentiation (CMD); the cortex is relatively echogenic and the medulla appears hypoechoic (Fig. 23.1). In the newborn, the cortex is hyperechoic compared to the liver; this is more pronounced in the premature newborn.

Pulsed Doppler analysis provides information about the venous and arterial vascularization of the kidneys. Spectral analysis demonstrates the degree of renal vascular impedance by means of the resistive index (RI) and blood velocity (Fig. 23.2). Color Doppler and Doppler energy allow the mapping of renal vascularization (5) (Fig. 23.3).

The bladder shape, wall, and content are evaluated as well. The wall thickness should be inferior to 3 mm. The volume can be evaluated using the following formula (7):

$$0.6 \times \text{bladder height} \times \text{width} \times \text{transverse diameter}$$

US can be used as an alternative method to detect vesicoureteric reflux (VUR) with sonicated contrast media (Fig. 23.4). There is a good correlation with classic voiding cystogram for demonstrating reflux (8).

Voiding Cystourethrogram

Voiding cystourethrogram (VCUG) remains the best imaging technique to detect VUR (Fig. 23.5). It also allows an evaluation of the urethra. It can be performed by catheterizing the bladder or through suprapubic puncture. The procedure should be explained in detail to the parents and to the patient. It should be performed in a strictly sterile manner. To minimize radiation, pulsed fluoroscopy may be used. Repeated filling of the bladder (cyclic VCUG) increases the rate of detection of VUR, especially in infants. VUR is graded according to the international reflux study group (grades I to V) (Fig. 23.5). Prophylactic antibiotherapy given 2 days before and 2 days after the examination is controversial, but the examination should be performed only when the urine has been tested sterile. Postprocedural infection occurs in 1 to 3% of patients, and hematuria may develop (9).

Intravenous Pyelography

The use of intravenous pyelography (IVP) has markedly decreased in recent years (Fig. 23.6A). The technique is progressively replaced by US, nuclear medicine, magnetic resonance (MR) imaging (Fig. 23.6B), and even computed tomography (CT). Known allergic disease and renal failure are the main contraindications (10).

Computed Tomography

CT has gained popularity since the development of helical CT that allows very rapid assessment of the UT. It provides exquisite cross-sectional anatomic and functional details. Two- and three-dimensional reconstruction helps to better visualize various anomalies. Yet, it is a radiating technique and it necessitates contrast injection. Still, the method is

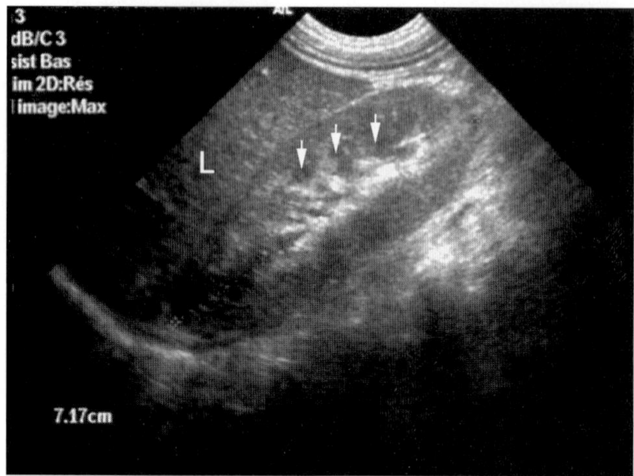

FIGURE 23.1. Normal ultrasound of the kidney in a child. Sagittal scan of the right kidney; the pyramids (*arrows*) are hypoechoic compared to the cortex. Cortical echogenicity is similar to that of the liver (L).

helpful in several conditions (tumors, urolithiasis, or abscess) (see below). Known allergic disease and renal failure are contraindications for contrast injection (11,12).

Magnetic Resonance Imaging

Thanks to the development of faster sequences, the use of MR imaging for the evaluation of the UT in children has rapidly extended. Structures are defined as appearing hyper- (white) or hyposignal (black). T2-weighted sequences (the so-called uro-MR sequences), allow the visualization of the collecting system. T1-weighted sequences provide more information on the renal parenchyma, especially after a gadolinium injection. The measurement of parenchymal enhancement provides information about the glomerular filtration (Fig. 23.6B).

MR imaging is progressively replacing IVP for the assessment of dilated UT, particularly for the evaluation of abnormal duplex systems or suspicion of ectopic extravesical ureteral insertion. Evaluation of tumoral extension or reflux nephropathy (RN) is another good indication. Another promising field is vascular investigation through MR angiography of the renal arteries, particularly in patients with hypertension (Fig. 23.7). The drawbacks of the method are its poor accessibility and the need for sedation in infants (13,14).

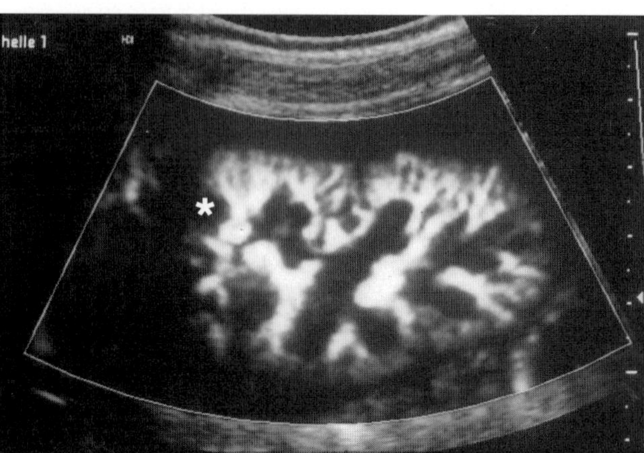

FIGURE 23.3. Power Doppler ultrasound of a normal kidney vascularization. Lack of vascularization of the upper pole is related to a rib artefact (*asterisk*).

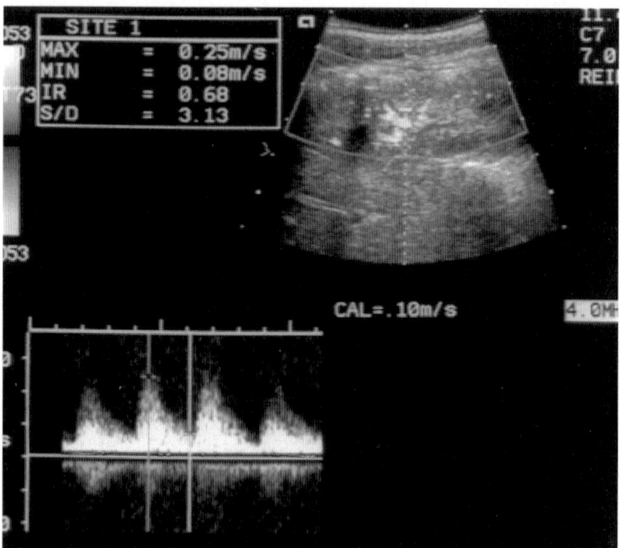

FIGURE 23.2. Duplex Doppler evaluation of normal renal vessels. Measurement of the resistive index (IR). The sample is measured at the level of the renal hilum. IR equals 0.68 (normal), maximum systolic velocity is 0.25 m/sec, and minimum diastolic velocity is 0.08 m/sec. CAL, calibration; S/D, systolic/diastolic.

Nuclear Medicine

Recent progress in nuclear medicine techniques includes production of new tracers, new applications of known tracers, development of various algorithms to determine renal function, and increased quality of instrumentation (15–18).

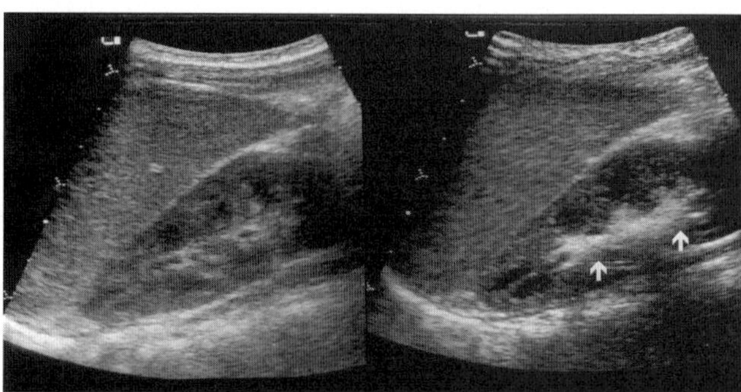

FIGURE 23.4. Sonographic voiding cystourethrogram. Sagittal scan of the right kidney before (*left*) and after (*right*) instillation of sonicated albumin. The contrast distends the renal pelvis (*arrows*) indicating vesicoureteric reflux. (Courtesy of K. Darge, M.D., Heidelberg, Germany.)

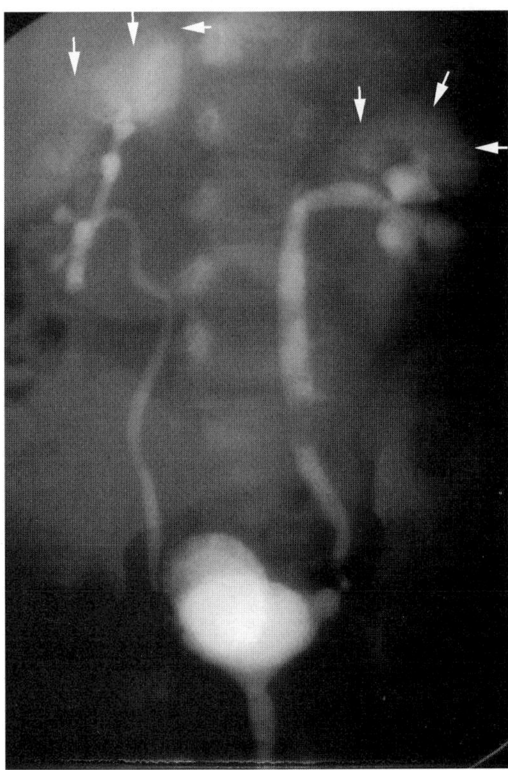

FIGURE 23.5. Radiologic voiding cystourethrogram. Bilateral vesicoureteric reflux [grade II (*right*) and grade III (*left*)] with intrarenal reflux enhancing the right upper and left upper parenchyma (*arrows*).

Renal Tracers

Chromium isotope–ethylenediaminetetraacetic acid, which is eliminated exclusively through glomerular filtration without tubular secretion or reabsorption, is a good tracer for the determination of glomerular filtration rate (GFR) using blood sampling.

Technetium 99m (^{99m}Tc)–diethylenetriamine pentaacetic acid is exclusively eliminated by glomerular filtration without tubular secretion or reabsorption. The energy of ^{99m}Tc–diethylenetriamine pentaacetic acid is adequate for gamma camera studies and allows studies of individual kidney renographic curves, relative and absolute GFR, determination of renal transit times, and furosemide-augmented tests.

Iodine 131– or iodine 123–hippurate is secreted mainly by the tubular cells and by the glomerular filtration (5 to 10%). Hippurate clearance is considered to reflect the renal plasma flow and is therefore called the *effective renal plasma flow*.

^{99m}Tc-mercaptotriglycylglycine (MAG-3) is eliminated almost completely by tubular secretion. The advantages of MAG-3 compared to ^{99m}Tc–diethylenetriamine pentaacetic acid are its higher extraction rate, higher signal to noise ratio, and better reproducibility for separate renal clearance measurements. ^{99m}Tc–MAG-3 offers the advantage of combining image with information about renal excretion (Fig. 23.7).

^{99m}Tc–dimercaptosuccinic acid (DMSA) is taken up by the proximal tubular cells and is only slightly excreted in the urine. DMSA provides interesting morphologic information in diseases affecting the renal cortex (Fig. 23.8).

By means of bladder instillation, ^{99m}Tc–pertechnetate anion can be used for direct cystography and detection of VUR (18).

Indications

Common indications are unilateral or bilateral hydronephrosis, UT infections with or without associated vesicoureteral reflux, small kidney, single kidney, urethral valves, pre- and postoperative follow-up, and follow-up of known VUR (15–21).

Study of Urinary Tract Obstruction (Standard and Diuretic Renography)

Two aspects of renal function are assessed: renal clearance and excretion of the tracer. Estimation of relative clearance (differential renal function) requires the measurement of GFR by injection of chromium isotope–ethylenediaminetetraacetic acid using a simple plasma sample technique. The most accurate method for evaluation of GFR is based on the plasma disappearance curve after a single bolus injection of a glomerular tracer.

The second parameter that may be obtained from a renographic curve is the evaluation of tracer molecule transport through the entire nephron, known as the *transit time*. A normal transit time (approximately 3 minutes) excludes renal obstruction. Abnormal transit time indicates urine stasis. It is not possible on the basis of a prolonged transit time to differentiate obstruction from simple dilatation of the collecting system.

The response to intravenous injection of furosemide provides additional information in cases of renal stasis. In cases of nonobstructive dilatation, the retained radioactivity in the UT is washed out rapidly by increased urine flow, whereas renal emptying is slow or nonexistent in the case of obstruction. However, the degree of washout depends on the degree of uptake of the tracer by the kidney. Poor response to furosemide may be observed in kidneys with impaired renal function in the absence of any obstruction (17).

Tubular tracers with a high extraction (e.g., iodine 123–hippurate, ^{99m}Tc–MAG-3, or ^{99m}Tc–ethylene dicysteine) are recommended. The response depends on the rate of tracer extraction. Postmicturition images should be acquired. During the first months of life, the response to furosemide is often equivocal despite the absence of obstruction because of the low extraction (low clearance values). In the presence of a full bladder, drainage from the kidney may be delayed even in the normal individual.

The interpretation of drainage in the presence of marked hydronephrosis is more difficult. Only good drainage is easily defined. The definitions of obstruction and risk factors of renal deterioration are still controversial.

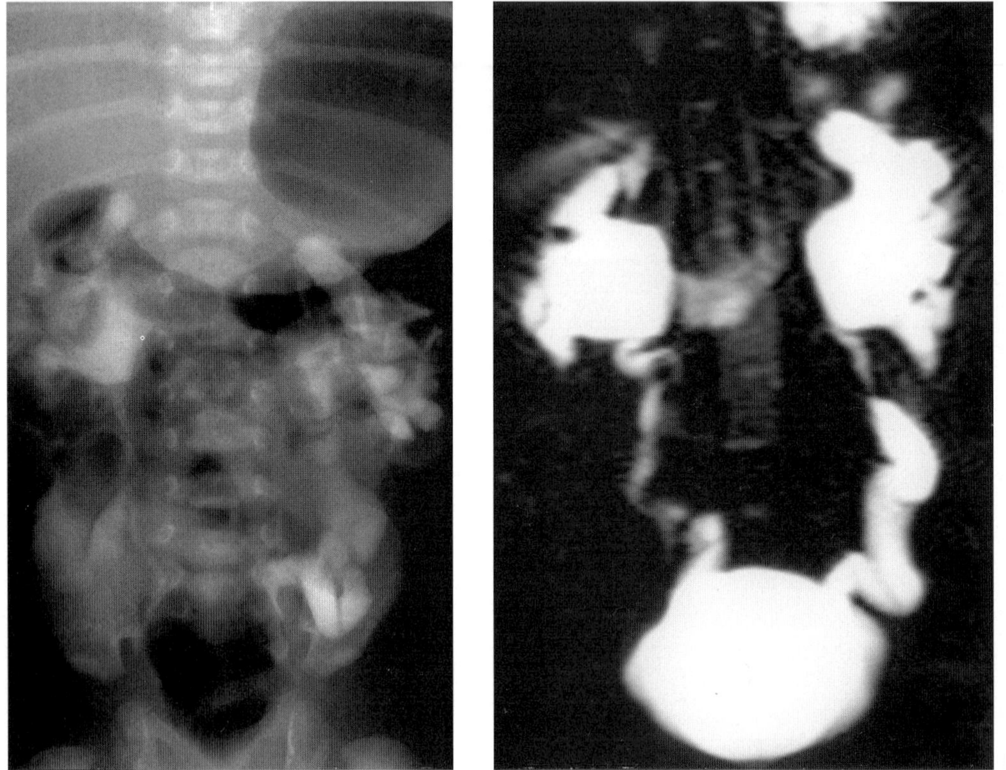

FIGURE 23.6. Bilateral urinary tract dilatation. **A:** Intravenous pyelography showing poor visualization of the right urinary tract. **B:** Magnetic resonance imaging showing uro–magnetic resonance sequence. There is good visualization of both ureters.

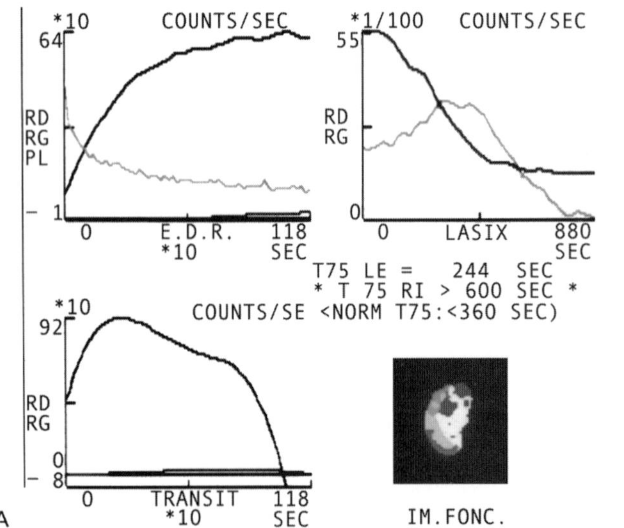

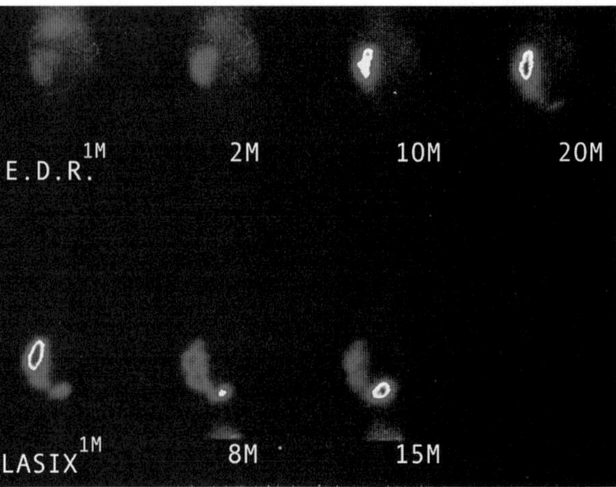

FIGURE 23.7. Mercaptotriglycine renogram in a 1-month-old boy with antenatal diagnosis of right hydronephrosis and left small cystic kidney. The renogram confirms a nonfunctioning left kidney and a ureterohydronephrosis with response to furosemide (megaureter on magnetic resonance). **A:** Curves corresponding to the function of the right kidney. **B:** Morphologic appearance of the dilated right urinary tract. (See Color Plate 23.7.)

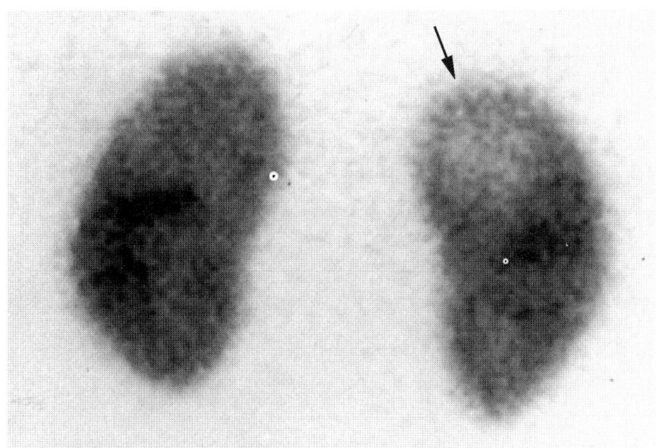

FIGURE 23.8. Technetium 99m–DMSA scan in a girl with acute pyelonephritis. There are defects in the upper pole of the right kidney (*arrow*).

Renal Morphology

^{99m}Tc-DMSA is the best agent for the demonstration of focal renal abnormalities because the tracer is retained mainly in the tubular cells. DMSA scintigraphy is the technique of choice for the detection of acute pyelonephritis (APN) and renal sequelae (Fig. 23.8). The DMSA technique is also indicated for the evaluation of small, ectopic, dysplastic, or infarct kidneys and for the confirmation of nonfunctional multicystic kidneys (19,21). Indirect cystogram is highly valuable for the follow-up of known VUR or in screening siblings (18).

IMAGING CONGENITAL URONEPHROPATHIES

Antenatal diagnosis has markedly modified the time of discovery of nephrouropathies. More and more cases are diagnosed *in utero* and evaluated at birth in asymptomatic patients. Obstetric US is able to diagnose accurately many uronephropathies. In some specific indications (maternal obesity, oligohydramnios, complex malformations), fetal MR imaging provides supplementary information (22,23).

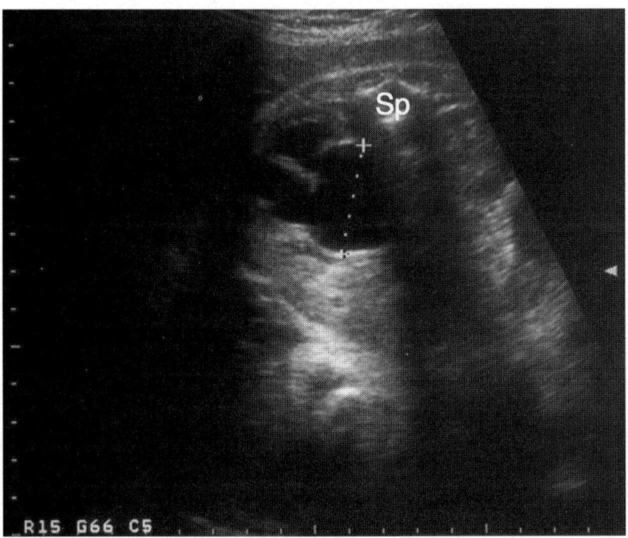

FIGURE 23.9. Ureteropyelic junction obstruction *in utero* (ultrasound). Transverse scan of the fetal abdomen at 34 weeks' gestation. Marked dilatation of the left renal pelvis and calyces (4 cm between crosses). Sp, fetal spine.

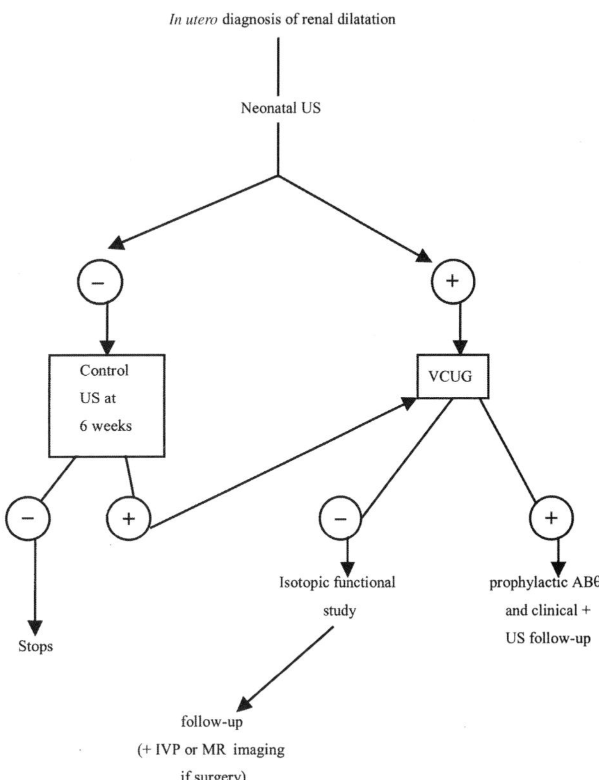

FIGURE 23.10. Neonatal work-up of *in utero* dilatation. +, normal US; –, abnormal US; AB, antibistherapy; IVP, intravenous pyelography; MR, magnetic resonance; US, ultrasound; VCUG, voiding cystourethrogram.

Neonatal Period

Because of the wider use of obstetric US, the evaluation of UT dilatation discovered *in utero* has been standardized (Figs. 23.9 and 23.10).

US is performed first—very rapidly if there is evidence of bilateral obstructive uropathy (i.e., pneumothorax, oligoanuria) or at the end of the first week in all other cases. If US examination is abnormal (Fig. 23.11 and Table 23.1), a VCUG is performed. If US is normal, a control examination is performed at 6 weeks. In the absence of VUR but with persisting dilatation, the degree of obstruction is evaluated with isotopes. Whenever surgery is elected, IVP or, rather, MR imaging should be performed to assess the morphology of the UT. When a conservative, nonsurgical approach is preferred, US allows the follow-up of the dilatation, which spontaneously resolves in many cases (22,24–26).

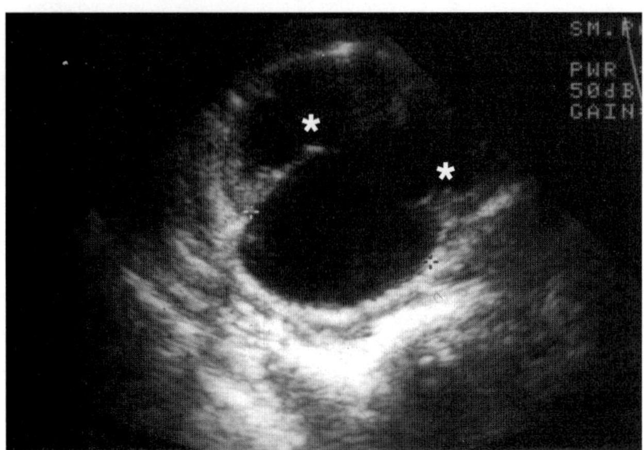

FIGURE 23.11. Ureteropyelic junction obstruction in a newborn (ultrasound). Marked dilatation—transverse scan 30 mm between crosses. The calyces (*asterisks*) are also dilated.

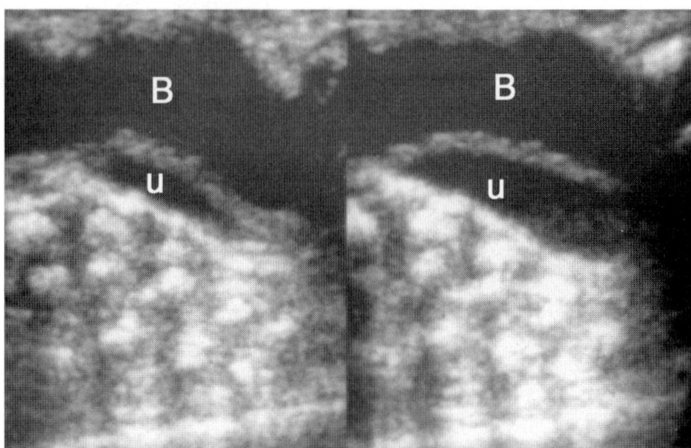

FIGURE 23.12. Dilated ureter (u) at ultrasound. Sagittal scans of the bladder (B). A dilated ureter is visible behind the bladder. Its caliber varies a few seconds apart, due to peristalsis.

Urinary Tract Dilatation

The role of imaging is to determine the level and degree of obstruction. Ureteropelvic junction (UPJ) obstruction is the main cause of UT dilatation *in utero* (Fig. 23.12) and at birth (Fig. 23.13). US shows a dilated renal pelvis above 7 mm (on a transverse scan of the kidney) (Figs. 23.12 and 23.13). Dilatations can be classified as mild (7 to 10 mm), moderate (10 to 15 mm), and marked (greater than 15 mm). Thinned, echogenic or cystic cortex suggests associated dysplasia. The degree of functional impairment is evaluated by isotopic studies. IVP or better MR imaging helps to demonstrate the degree of dilatation and the status of the remaining parenchyma (Fig. 23.14). On US, UPJ obstruction should be differentiated from multicystic dysplastic kidney (see later), ureterovesical junction obstruction, or dilating VUR.

A ureterovesical junction obstruction is characterized by the presence of a visible ureter (above 3 mm diameter). This dilatation is best evaluated behind a filled bladder (Fig. 23.12). The anomaly may be confirmed using MR imaging (Fig. 23.13).

The presence on US of a large bladder (above 6 cm height) suggests a bladder outlet obstruction. The main cause in boys is posterior urethral valves. The bladder is enlarged, its wall is thickened, and bilateral ureterohydronephrosis may be present already *in utero*. After birth, the anomaly is best demonstrated on the micturition phase of a VCUG (Fig. 23.14). Isotopes evaluate the degree of renal functional impairment. Other causes of bladder outlet obstruction include megalourethra, anterior valves, and urethral polyps, which are evaluated by a VCUG during the micturition phase (27,28).

Duplex kidneys are commonly found in newborns. On US, a band of parenchyma separates the two pelvic complexes. A nondilated duplex kidney should be considered as a normal variant. Complications may occur at the upper or lower poles and consist of obstruction or VUR. An extravesical ectopic insertion or ureterocele is classically found in rela-

TABLE 23.1. ULTRASOUND CRITERIA OF ABNORMAL URINARY TRACT POTENTIALLY ASSOCIATED WITH VESICOURETERIC REFLUX

Renal pelvis dilatation >7 mm
Ureteral dilatation >3 mm
Calyceal dilatation >2 mm
Pelvic wall thickening >1 mm
Dysplasia (small kidney, echogenic irregular cortex, cortical cysts)
Enlarged bladder >6 cm

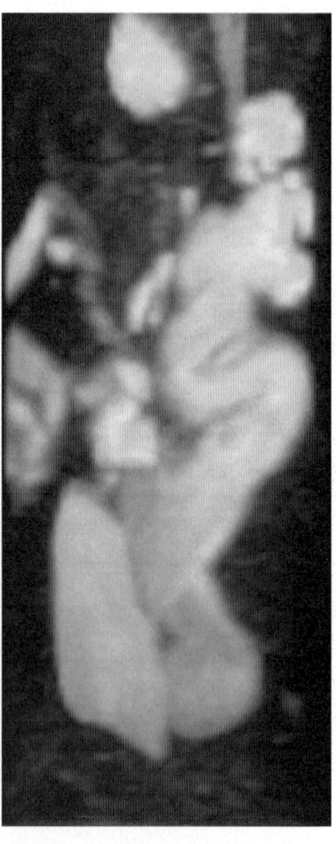

FIGURE 23.13. Magnetic resonance imaging of a left megaureter. Sagittal view. Uro–magnetic resonance sequence.

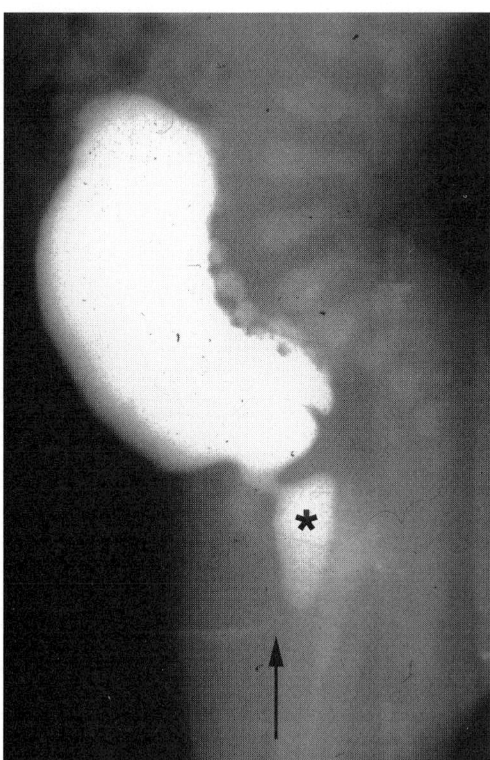

FIGURE. 23.14. Posterior urethral valves in a neonate—voiding cystourethrogram. Distended posterior urethra (*asterisk*) and narrow anterior urethra (*arrow*). Megabladder with diverticular wall.

tion to a dilated upper pole. The VCUG is performed after birth to visualize the ureterocele, which may prolapse within the urethra and induce bladder outlet obstruction. MR imaging has proved useful in the morphologic evaluation of complicated duplex systems (29,30) (Fig. 23.15).

In cases of nonsurgical management of urogenital uropathies, imaging allows a close follow-up. US confirms resolution of the dilatation and sufficient renal growth. Isotope techniques assess renal function.

Abnormal Kidney Number or Location

The role of imaging is either to confirm renal agenesis or to demonstrate an ectopic location. ^{99m}Tc-DMSA scanning is indicated when only one kidney has been identified. US can demonstrate pelvic ectopia. In the case of horseshoe kidney, a DMSA scan might better define the isthmus. In the case of cross ectopia and fusion, IVP or, rather, MR imaging is helpful to assess the exact anatomy and the potential complications (Fig. 23.16). US can find associated genital malformations in girls (31,32).

Kidney Dysplasia and Hypoplasia (Hypodysplasia)

US signs of hypodysplasia include small size, hyperechogenicity of the cortex, cysts within the parenchyma, and thinned parenchyma.

Cystic Renal Diseases

Cystic renal diseases discovered *in utero* or in the neonatal period encompass a large panel of diseases and US patterns (see the section Imaging of Renal Failure and Renal Graft).

Unilateral solitary cortical cyst is an uncommon finding. US follow-up is usually sufficient to exclude a cystic renal tumor.

In the case of unilateral multiple cysts, a multicystic dysplastic kidney is the most frequent finding (Fig. 23.17). In most cases, the US diagnosis is straightforward: a mass containing multiple cysts of varying size, without communication between them and without normal renal parenchyma. Contralateral anomalies are frequent, especially VUR. A ^{99m}Tc–MAG-3 diuretic renogram may assess the nonfunctioning multicystic dysplastic kidney and exclude an anomaly in the remaining functioning kidney. Involution may occur *in utero* or after birth (Fig. 23.17).

Bilateral cysts have to be separated between cases with medullary cysts and those with cortical cysts. In the case of medullary cysts, autosomal-recessive polycystic kidney disease is the first diagnosis to suspect. Affected kidneys are usually markedly enlarged (+2 to +4 standard deviation). The US pattern may be much more heterogeneous (Fig. 23.18A). Liver involvement is difficult to demonstrate in the neonatal period (33). Other causes of medullary cysts include many syndromes (e.g., Bardet Biedl syndrome).

The finding of bilateral cortical cysts is in favor of autosomal-dominant polycystic kidney disease (34). Yet, it is unusual to find significant cysts in the neonatal period (see below). Other causes of (large) neonatal bilateral renal cysts are tuberous sclerosis and von Hippel–Lindau disease.

Renal cystic disease is often detected *in utero* in fetuses with bilateral hyperechoic kidneys. Large (+4 standard deviation), poorly differentiated kidneys may correspond to autosomal recessive polycystic kidney disease (Fig. 23.18B) or autosomal dominant polycystic kidney disease. Hyperechoic kidneys with persisting CMD suggest autosomal dominant polycystic kidney disease and congenital nephrotic syndrome (35,36). US examination of the parents' and grandparents' kidneys may help with the diagnosis (37).

Congenital Nephrouropathies in Older Children

Some nephrouropathies are discovered later in childhood due to complications (infections, lithiasis, trauma, increasing obstruction) (see below). They are usually detected on US. CT, MR imaging, or VCUG is performed according to US findings and the complication. For instance, UPJ obstruction may be discovered after a trauma or lithiasis may develop in a previously unrecognized primary megaureter (38) (Fig. 23.19).

A dysplastic upper pole of a duplex system with an ectopic extravesical insertion may be discovered because of urinary

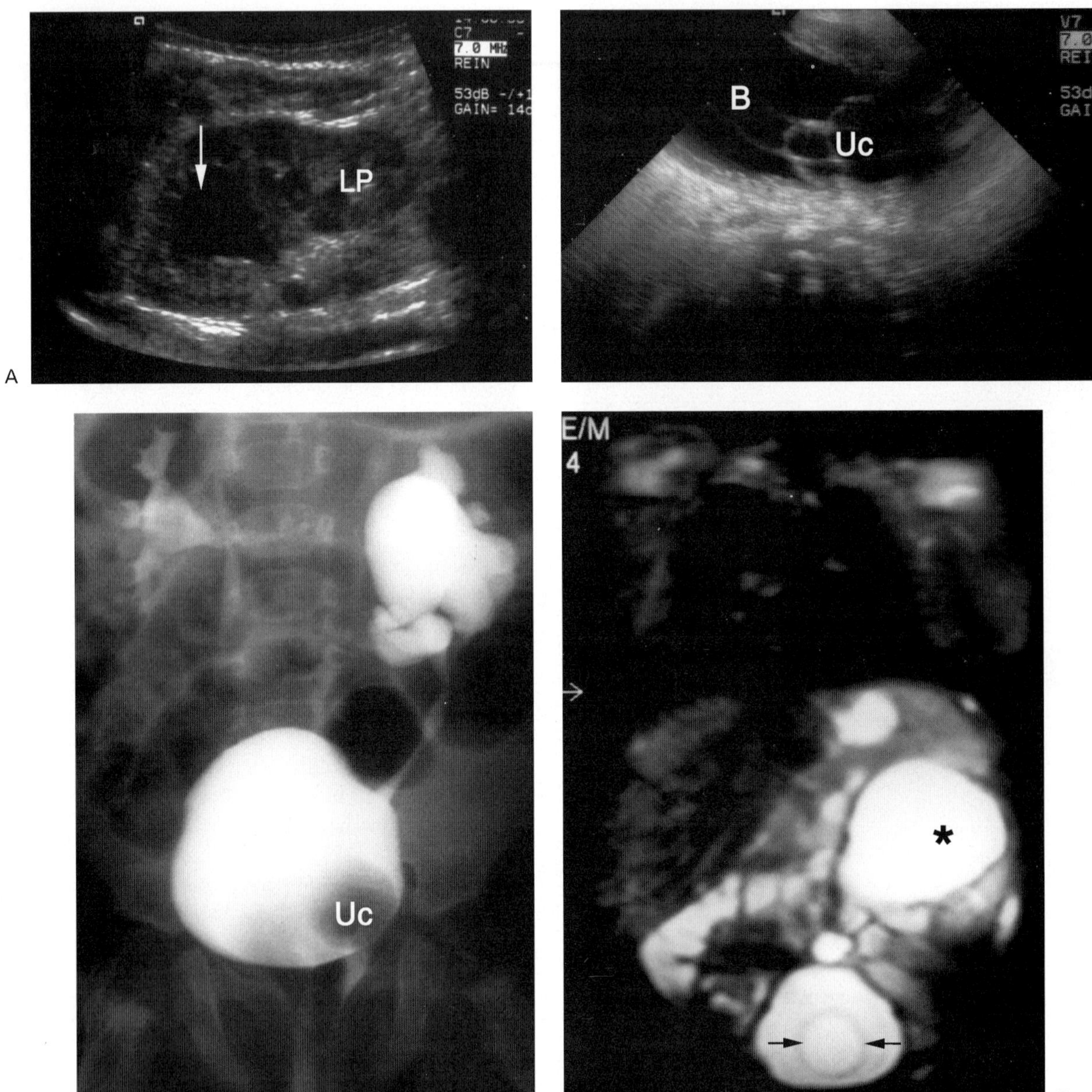

FIGURE 23.15. Complicated duplex kidney. **A:** Ultrasound of the left kidney. Sagittal scan showing significant dilatation of the upper pole (*arrow*). The lower pole (LP) is not dilated. **B:** Ultrasound of the bladder (B). A lobulated ureterocele (Uc) is visible within the bladder. **C:** Voiding cystourethrogram, showing intravesical Uc and vesicoureteric reflux into the left lower pole. Right grade II vesicoureteric reflux. **D:** Magnetic resonance imaging. Magnetic resonance urography sequence (coronal view). Dilated upper pole (*asterisk*) in relation to an intravesical ureterocele (*arrows*).

dribbling in a toilet-trained girl. The dysplastic upper pole may escape the US examination. An MR imaging examination (or a CT when MR imaging is not available), presently the most accurate technique for this indication (39) (Fig. 23.20), confirms the clinical suspicion.

INFECTIONS OF THE URINARY TRACT

The role of imaging in the case of UT infection is to determine whether there is an underlying favoring condition, whether the kidney is affected, and whether there is a VUR (Table 23.2). The US allows the detection of a congenital anomaly or a lithiasis. DMSA scintigraphy evaluates kidney involvement, and VCUG detects a VUR (40–42).

Acute Pyelonephritis

The main role of US is to detect a congenital anomaly. In addition, several features indicate acute renal infection: The main sign is an increased renal length or, more accurately, an

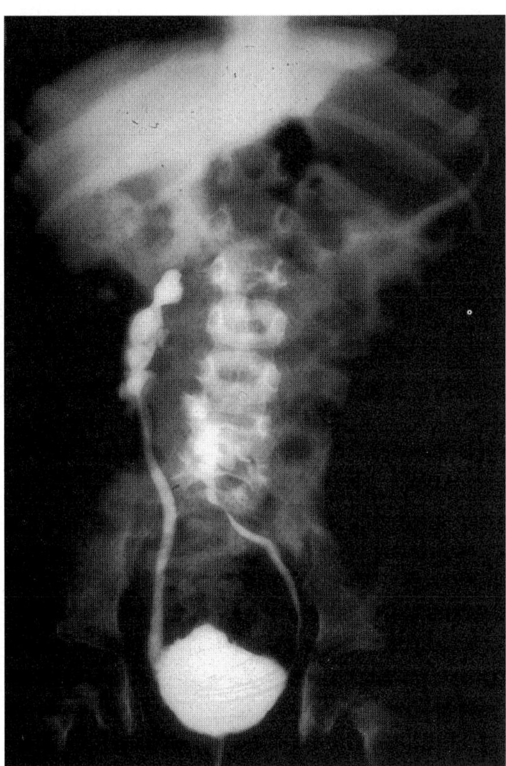

FIGURE 23.16. Intravenous pyelography of a right crossed fused ectopia of the left kidney.

increased renal volume (Fig. 23.21). Another sign is a thickening (above 1 mm) of the renal pelvis wall with a hyperechogenicity of the perihilar renal fat. These signs suggest pyelitis and ureteritis. The renal parenchyma may also show areas of increased or decreased echogenicity corresponding to an inflammatory edema and (hemorrhagic) necrosis. Such areas are typically undervascularized. This can be shown using color or power Doppler (Fig. 23.22). Echogenic urine with echogenic fluid level may correspond to pyonephrosis. It should be stressed that a normal US examination does not exclude APN (42,45–47).

Renal cortical lesions are detected by ^{99m}Tc-DMSA scintigraphy (Fig. 23.8). Decreased uptake is seen in areas of APN (47). The presence of a renal abnormality during the acute phase of infection seems to be the best predictor of renal sequelae. Conversely, the risk of developing scars is low when early scintigraphy is normal.

CT demonstrates very accurately renal involvement in cases of APN. It shows an increased renal volume and, after contrast enhancement, affected parenchymal areas. Yet, it is an irradiating technique, and it should not be used routinely (48) (see below). MR imaging has similar diagnostic performances to CT or DMSA scanning (Fig. 23.23).

A VCUG is performed to detect a VUR. Indirect cystography may be obtained by injecting contrast intravenously. It is also a valuable technique for detecting VUR under physiologic conditions without using a bladder catheterization. Children who are not toilet trained (younger than 3 years of age) may not be able to undergo this examination. The main indication is the follow-up of patients with known VUR.

Evolution of Acute Pyelonephritis

When treatment is adequate, the inflammatory infiltrates resolve progressively without sequelae; in such cases, the renal volume as measured on US returns to normal within 4 to 6

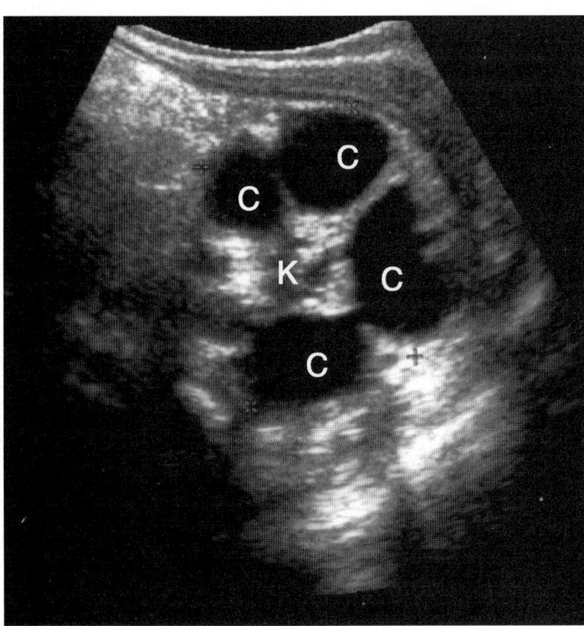

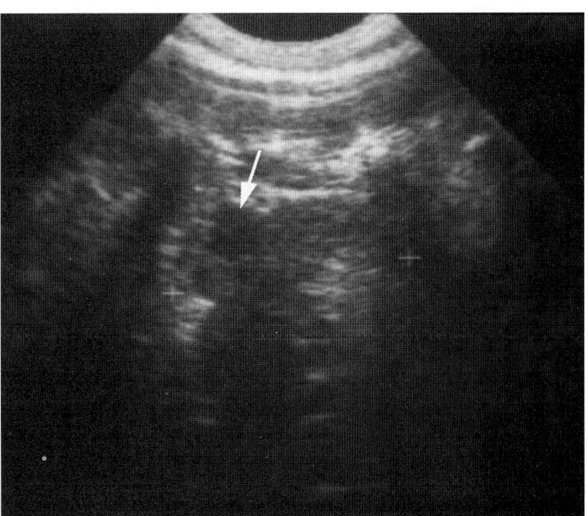

FIGURE 23.17. Involution of a multicystic dysplastic kidney (K). **A:** At birth; sagittal scan of the right kidney. Four cysts are visible (C). **B:** At 1 year of age, only one cyst has remained (*arrow*).

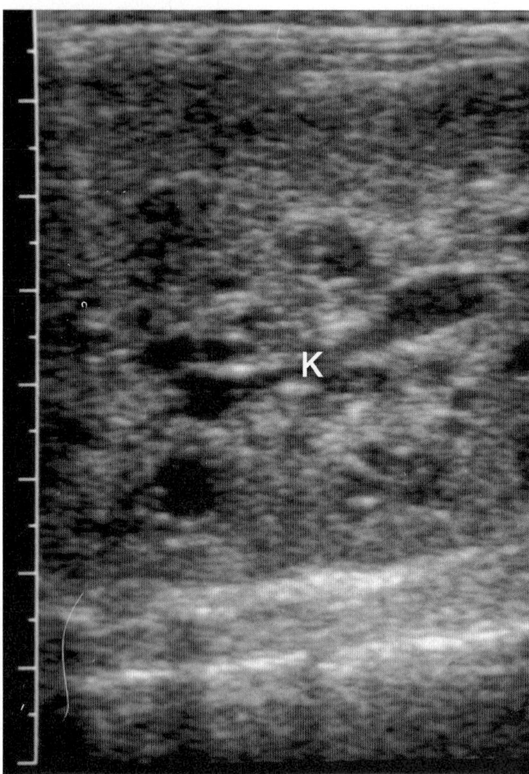

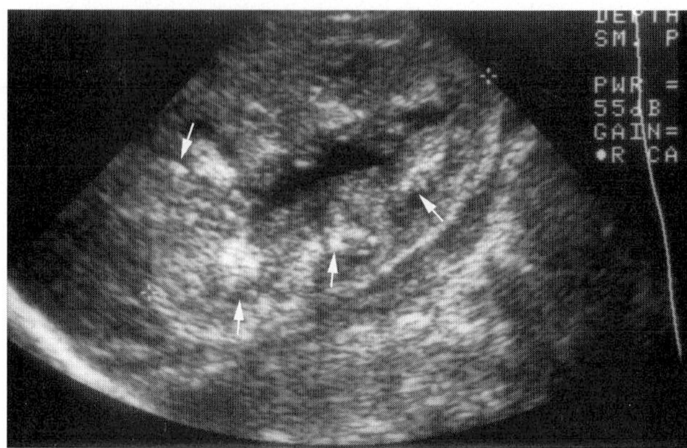

FIGURE 23.18. Neonatal autosomal-recessive polycystic kidney disease. Two different patterns at ultrasound. **A:** Sagittal scans of the left kidney (K) showing multiple medullary cysts. **B:** Left kidney in another patient. The pyramids appear hyperechoic (*arrows*).

weeks. This delay should be taken into account for planning follow-up examinations intended to assess renal growth (49).

In cases of late or inadequate treatment or resistance to antibiotherapy, the renal lesions may coalesce and form an abscess. US demonstrates the abscess as an inhomogeneous mass within the parenchyma; CT or MR imaging seems to be a better technique to demonstrate abscess formation, especially for bilateral lesions. These techniques better evaluate the extrarenal extension of the abscess than does US (46) (Fig. 23.21).

The rationale for early work-up and treatment of APN is to prevent recurrence and permanent lesions. Scintigraphy is performed at least 6 months to 1 year after the acute episode to detect renal scarring. Six months is the minimal time before one can consider a lesion as permanent (49,50) (Fig. 23.24A). US and IVP underestimate the number of scars. MR imaging is a promising technique for the evaluation of permanent renal damage and chronic renal scars (RN or chronic pyelonephritis) (Fig. 23.24B) (13,14).

Cystitis and Urethritis

The bladder is more commonly affected by infection than the kidneys; findings on US are not specific. The bladder wall may be thickened (above 3 mm), and urine may appear with echogenic debris. Of note, these findings may be present without infection (43,44). Urethritis is uncommon in children. On VCUG, during the micturition phase, the urethral lumen appears irregular.

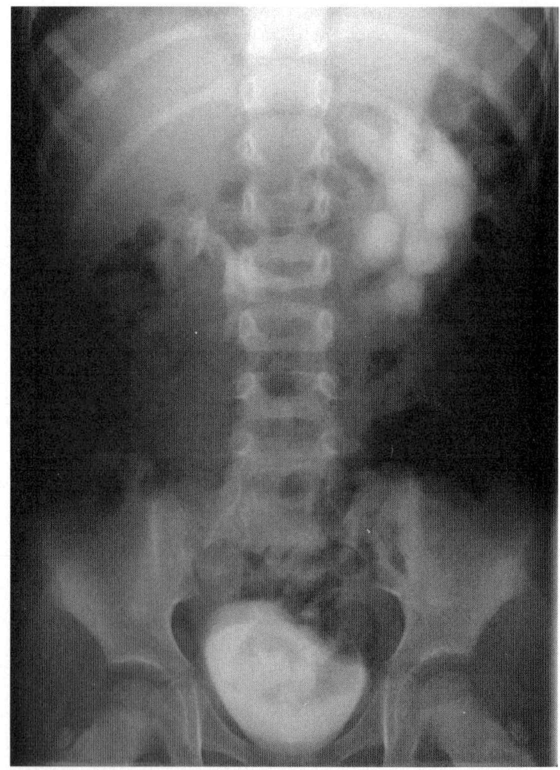

FIGURE 23.19. Horseshoe kidney with left ureteropyelic junction obstruction in a 9-year-old boy with acute left flank pain. Typical findings on an intravenous pyelography.

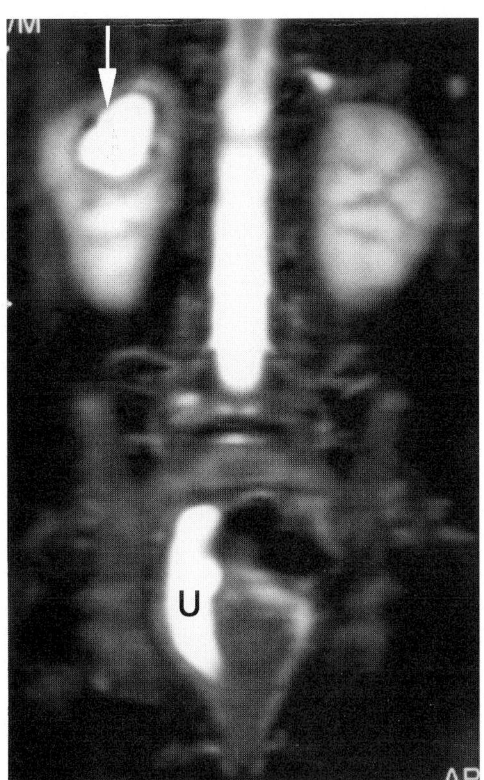

FIGURE 23.20. Four-year-old girl with urinary dribbling. Magnetic resonance imaging. Frontal view showing a right duplex kidney with dilated upper pole (*arrow*) associated with a dilated ectopic ureter (U).

Specific Organism Infections

Candidiasis

Candidiasis develops in immunocompromised patients, premature infants, and patients under chronic antibiotherapy. Candidiasis infection should be suspected on US case of: global renal hyperechogenicity, sludge distending the renal cavities, or the presence of fungus balls (echogenic masses partially filling the renal cavities) (51).

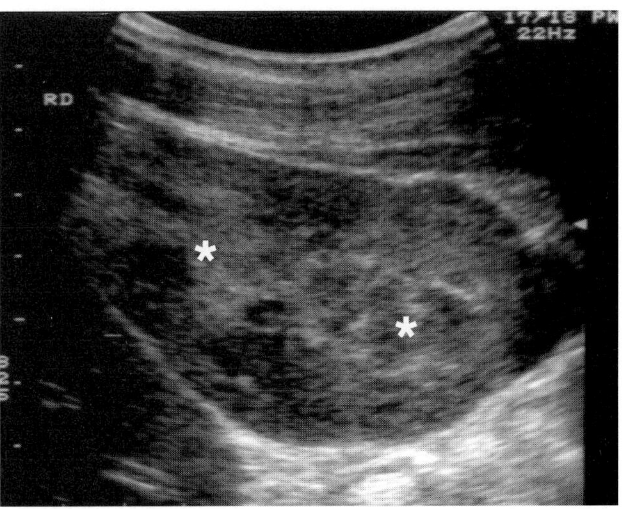

FIGURE 23.21. Acute right pyelonephritis. Sagittal scan of the right kidney that appears swollen, with patchy hyperechoic areas corresponding to inflammatory changes (*asterisks*).

Tuberculosis

The most typical features have been described on IVP: "drooping Lily" appearance of the pyelocalyceal system. In more advanced cases, the kidney is completely destroyed, small, and calcified (52).

VESICOURETERIC REFLUX

Primary VUR is a frequent cause of *in utero* dilatation of the UT (19). The most severe cases are detected in males. VUR may be associated with various congenital uropathies. Voiding dysfunction is another circumstance in which VUR is detected; in such cases, VUR is secondary to the bladder dysfunction. Although the relationship between UT infection and VUR is still debated, VUR is found in approximately 45% of cases with UT infection (53,54). Radiologic VCUG is the best method for the first assessment. VCUG confirms

TABLE 23.2 IMAGING IN URINARY TRACT INFECTION: RELATIVE CONTRIBUTION OF IMAGING EXAMINATIONS

Question	Ultrasound	Computed tomography	Magnetic resonance imaging	Intravenous pyelography	Voiding cystourethrogram	Dimercaptosuccinic acid
Underlying favoring condition?	++	++	++	+	0	0
Kidney affected?	+	+++	+++	+	0	+++
Vesicoureteric reflux?	0 but + with sonicated contrast	0	0	0	++	0
Scars	+	++	+++	+	0	+++

0, low; +, little; ++, moderate; +++, very contributive.

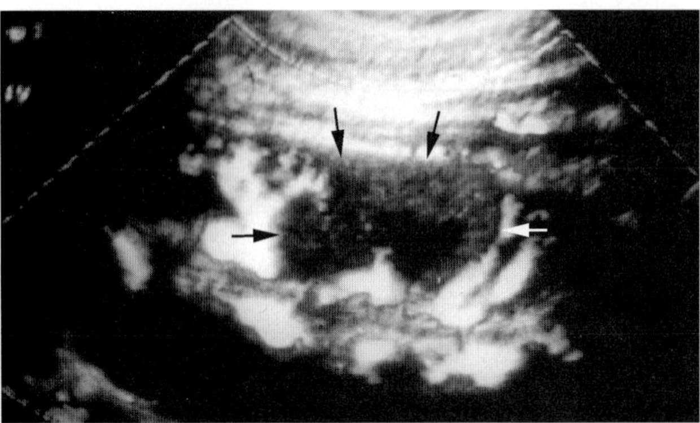

FIGURE 23.22. Acute pyelonephritis. Power Doppler ultrasound showing striking area of absent vascularization due to inflammatory involvement (*arrows*). (Courtesy of Dr. Dufour.) (See Color Plate 23.22.)

the VUR (including intrarenal VUR) and shows the morphology of the lower UT (including the urethra) (Fig. 23.5). It may also show bladder diverticula, reflux into ectopic ureters, or ureteroceles. Cyclic filling of the bladder has been shown to improve the rate of detection of VUR by 10 to 15%, especially in newborns. Tailored pulsed fluoroscopy and adapted filtration material (55) reduce radiation hazards. VUR is graded according to the international grading system. Higher grades of VUR are less likely to resolve spontaneously and are more often associated with dysplastic kidneys (56). Isotopic direct or indirect VCUG and cystosonography (using sonicated contrast media) are better suited for the follow-up of patients with known VUR or for screening siblings of patients with VUR (18,57,58). US is a poor predictor of a VUR. Yet, a completely detailed normal US examination of the UT is rarely associated with high-grade VUR (59). The parenchymal damage, the so-called RN, is best assessed by isotopes and MR imaging (Fig. 23.24B). It is present at birth in 20 to 30% of the cases (associated VUR and hypodysplasia), and acquired renal damage seems less frequent (60–62).

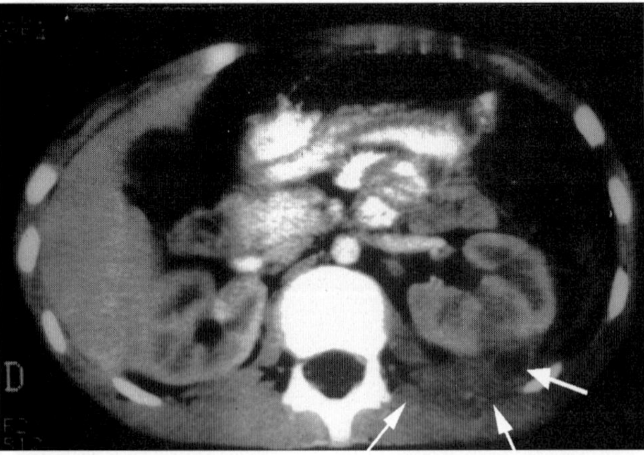

FIGURE 23.23. Acute pyelonephritis. Demonstration of a perirenal abscess on computed tomography (after contrast injection). A necrotic abscess has developed in the posterior surface of the left kidney and has extended into the posterior abdominal wall (*arrows*).

VOIDING DISORDERS

Voiding disorders are associated with a wide spectrum of anomalies. The role of imaging is to differentiate between organic and functional diseases.

Plain film of the abdomen evaluates constipation or associated vertebral malformations. US can exclude UT malformations and measure the bladder wall thickness and the vesical content pre- and postvoiding. VCUG is performed in the case of persisting symptoms. It detects a VUR and shows the bladder volume at maximum filling, the bladder contours, the type of micturition, and the appearance of the urethra. It may show a cause of obstruction in boys.

On VCUG, a transient opening of the bladder neck and opacification of the urethra up to the external sphincter, along with cessation of contrast material dripping, suggest an uninhibited detrusor contraction. A spinning-top urethra or a wide bladder neck anomaly suggests a bladder instability (63,64) (Fig. 23.25).

In the case of neurologic symptoms, MR imaging of the conus medullaris is helpful for the demonstration of a tethered, low-positioned cord; MR urography is efficient to demonstrate ectopic ureteral insertion associated with urinary dribbling (65).

A particular circumstance of voiding dysfunction is associated with neurogenic bladder. This anomaly is related, in most cases, to an open spina bifida. Typically, a neurogenic bladder has a pear-shape appearance, irregular diverticular margins, and a thickened wall (Fig. 23.26) (66).

IMAGING OF RENAL FAILURE AND RENAL GRAFT

In most patients with renal failure, US is important for diagnosis and follow-up. The contribution of US varies greatly from patient to patient. In some cases, US is insufficient and complementary examinations are necessary (e.g., obstructive tumoral infiltration of the ureters is evaluated with CT or MR imaging). All imaging findings must be analyzed according to the clinical findings and familial history.

Acute Renal Failure

Imaging is helpful in determining postrenal obstructive causes of acute renal failure; it is often informative for renal causes but seldom contributive for prerenal causes. The main US feature is an increased renal echogenicity (67). A completely normal US examination does not exclude renal lesions.

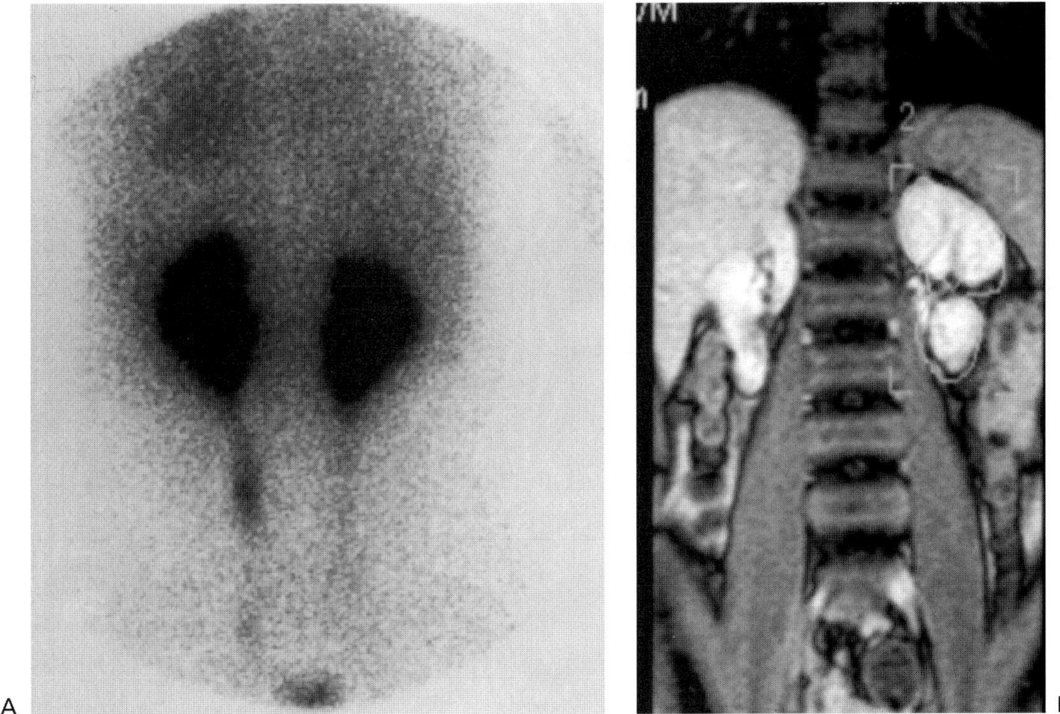

FIGURE 23.24. Pyelonephritic scars. **A:** Dimercaptosuccinic acid scan showing small, irregular kidneys. **B:** Magnetic resonance imaging showing bilateral small, irregular, scarred kidneys.

Hemolytic-Uremic Syndrome

During the acute phase, the renal cortex appears hyperechoic with increased CMD. During the oligoanuric phase, Doppler spectral analysis shows a high RI (approximately 1) (Fig. 23.27) that decreases with recovery. At a later phase, sequelae may appear as areas of medullar or cortical calcifications (related to necrosis), and global renal growth may be impaired (68). US examination helps to assess extrarenal lesions (digestive wall thickening, hemobilia). In

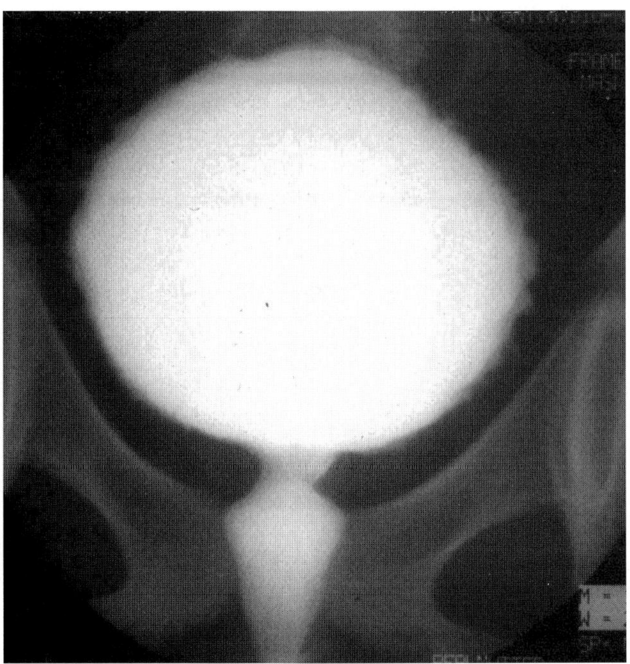

FIGURE 23.25. Spinning-top urethra on voiding cystourethrogram, typical for vesicourethral dyssynergia.

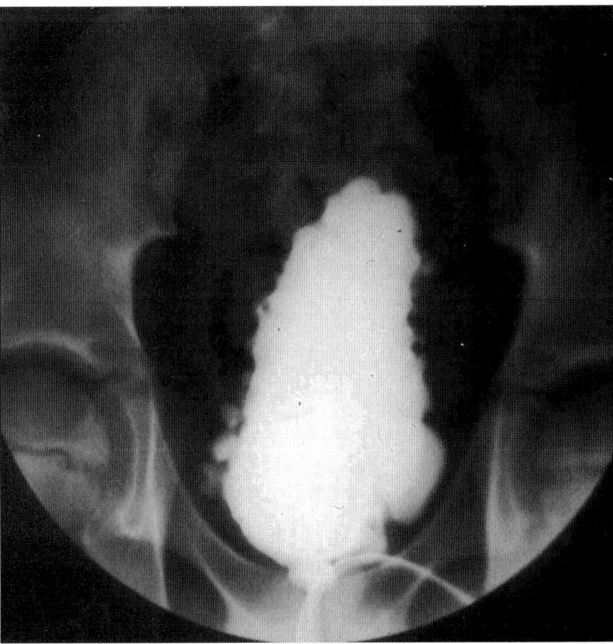

FIGURE 23.26. Neurogenic bladder on voiding cystourethrogram. Filling phase: trabeculated, diverticular bladder.

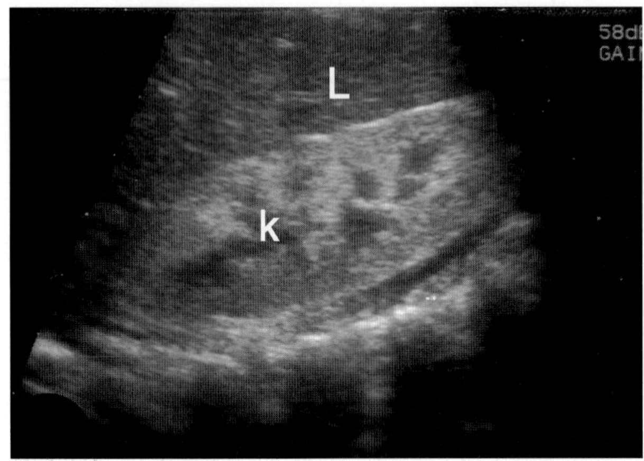

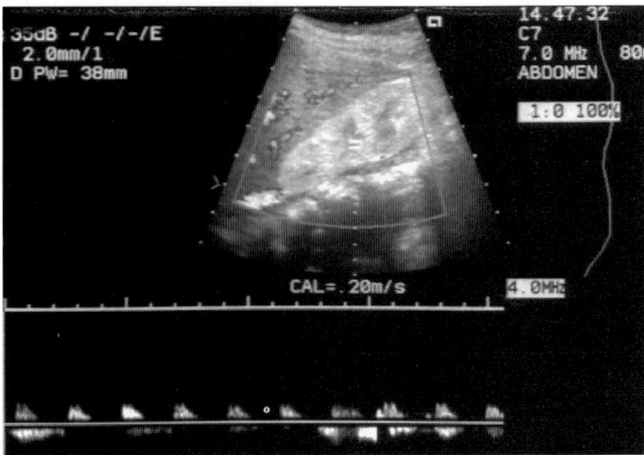

A B

FIGURE 23.27. Hemolysis (uremia syndrome), acute phase. **A:** Ultrasound of the right kidney (k). Striking hyperechogenicity of the cortex. **B:** Duplex Doppler ultrasound evaluation of the renal vessels. Resistive index equals 1; there is no diastolic flow. CAL, calibration; L, liver.

patients with neurologic symptoms, MR imaging of the brain may be necessary.

Medullar or Cortical Necrosis and Shock Kidneys

Medullar and cortical necrosis occur mainly in premature infants and are related to reduced arterial renal perfusion; during the acute phase, the renal cortex appears hyperechoic with persisting CMD, and spectral Doppler analysis demonstrates a high RI. In the case of medullar necrosis, calcifications may develop within the pyramids. In the case of severe cortical necrosis, the renal parenchyma shrinks, whereas in less severe cases, calcifications develop within the parenchyma. These conditions must be differentiated from the transient acute tubular blockade of a dehydrated neonate (Tamm-Horsfall proteinuria). The latter appears on US with hyperechoic pyramids, resolving within 2 to 3 days (69).

Renal Vein Thrombosis

Renal vein thrombosis most often occurs in the neonatal period and may develop *in utero*. At US, kidneys are enlarged and CMD is absent with hyperechoic streaks. Color Doppler may show the thrombus within the renal vein or the inferior vena cava (70).

Obstructive Uropathies

Several forms of obstructive uropathies may be associated with acute renal failure: the urethral prolapse of an ectopic ureterocele; congenital uropathy of a single kidney; and tumoral infiltration of the kidneys, ureters, or bladder neck. Bilateral urolithiases are all circumstances that may lead to acute renal failure.

Chronic Renal Failure

Chronic renal failure (CRF) interferes with statural and bone growth. Skeletal x-rays allow the evaluation of bone age. X-rays include (a) anteroposterior view of the hands and chest, including the claviculae, pelvis, long bones; and (b) dental view. Anomalies suggesting renal osteodystrophy include poor mineralization of the bones, osteolysis at the clavicular ends, phalangeal resorptions, and long bones with cortical thinning.

Renal Dysplasia and Hypoplasia

Renal dysplasia and hypoplasia may coexist, but dysplasia is only demonstrated on renal histology. At US, kidneys are small usually without CMD. Small cysts may be present within the parenchyma (71).

Cystic Renal Diseases

Among the diseases without genetic transmission, only bilateral obstructive uropathies may lead to CRF. In such conditions, on US, the kidneys are small, with a thin and hyperechoic cortex without CMD, and the renal cavities are dilated. Several cysts of varying sizes are visualized within the parenchyma.

Among the hereditary cystic diseases, some display characteristic patterns, and others are difficult to recognize (72). In autosomal recessive polycystic kidney disease, kidneys are enlarged, and the cystic lesions are mainly located in the medulla. The medulla may show macrocysts or may be hyperechoic due to multiple microcysts. With time, the cysts increase in size; some hyperechoic spots may appear and correlate with the development of CRF (Fig. 23.28). The periportal hepatic fibrosis may progress with periportal hyperechogenicity, and inhomogeneous liver echogenicity and signs of portal hypertension can be observed as well. In the case of autosomal dominant polycystic kidney disease, macrocysts are most often observed. In nephronophthisis, US changes are observed at approximately 10 to 12 years with the development of macrocysts (73). Peripheral cortical cysts

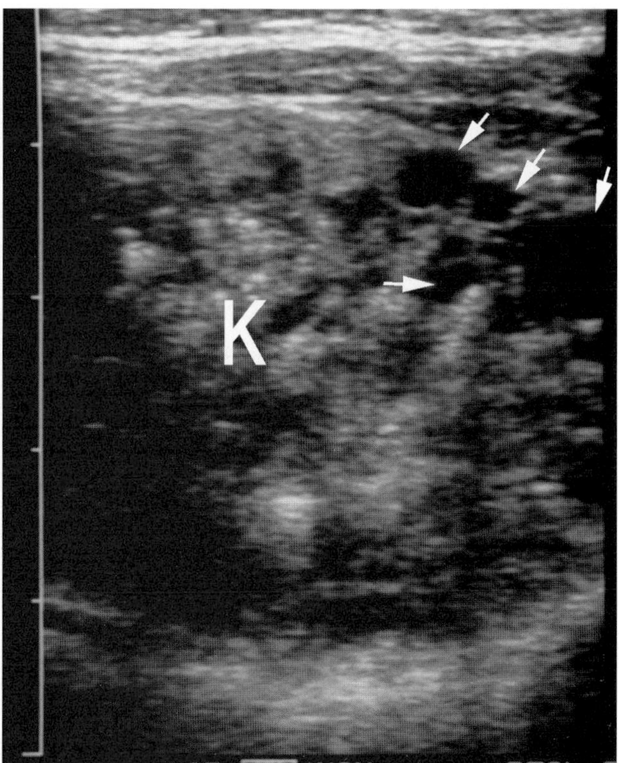

FIGURE 23.28. Autosomal-recessive polycystic kidney disease in a 10-year-old boy. The kidney (K) has a heterogeneous echogenicity. Some macrocysts have developed (*arrows*).

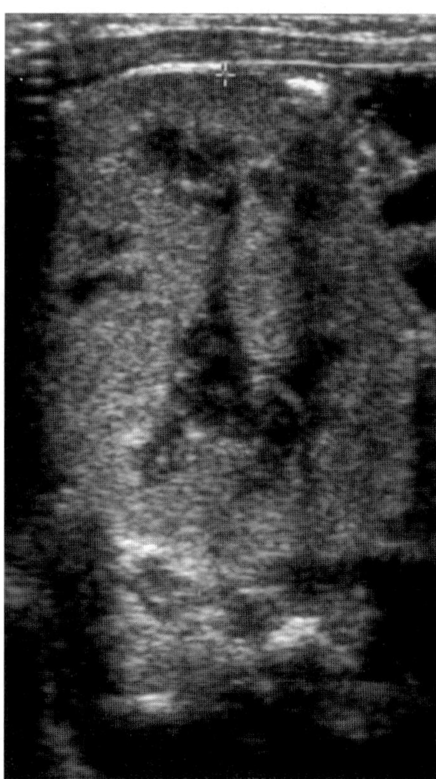

FIGURE 23.30. Congenital nephrotic syndrome of the Finnish type in a newborn with proteinuria. Enlarged kidney (6 cm between the *crosses*) with hyperechoic cortex and preserved corticomedullary differentiation.

can be found in glomerulocystic kidneys (Fig. 23.29). This entity can be isolated or part of syndromes (72). It is noteworthy that cysts may appear in patients on chronic dialysis.

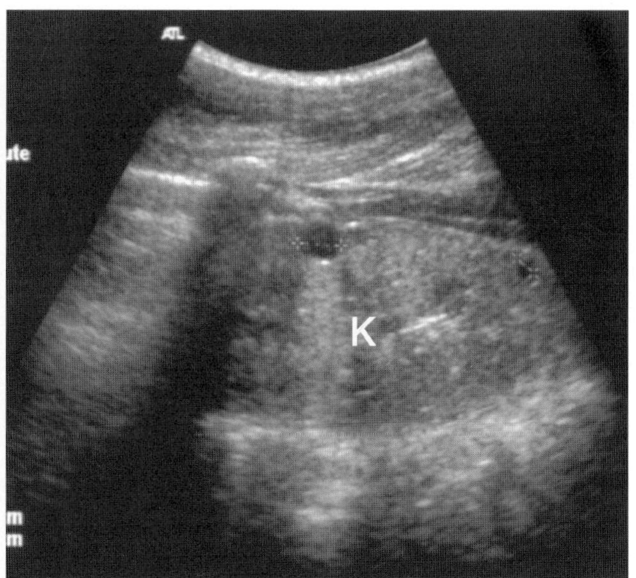

FIGURE 23.29. Glomerulocystic kidney. Sagittal scan of the left kidney (K). The parenchyma is hyperechoic without corticomedullary differentiation and with small peripheric cysts (between *crosses*).

Chronic Pyelonephritis or Reflux Nephropathy

The relationship between chronic pyelonephritis, RN, and CRF is controversial, as many parenchymal lesions may preexist already at birth. Whatever the cause of the lesions, the role of imaging is the detection of an underlying favoring condition. US may detect UT malformation, but the technique is less accurate for the demonstration of parenchymal lesions, which are best visualized on DMSA scans or MR imaging (74).

Congenital Nephrotic Syndromes

US shows enlarged kidneys with small hyperechoic pyramids in newborns with Finnish-type nephrotic syndrome. With time, the kidney size and echogenicity decrease and the pyramids disappear (Fig. 23.30). In patients with diffuse mesangial sclerosis, the US may show as diffusely heterogeneous with a patchy appearance. Other congenital nephrotic syndromes do not have typical US appearances (75).

Congenital Tubular Syndromes

Congenital tubular syndromes are numerous renal diseases that include primitive or secondary tubulopathies. Hypercalciuria is often present and is responsible for nephrocalcinosis that is detected by US (see below). US is also helpful in type I hyperoxaluria (see below) (76).

Renal Transplant

The renal transplant is easily evaluated by US. The kidney is very close to the abdominal surface; therefore, US is able to demonstrate its anatomy with good details. A CMD is always present. Examination includes an evaluation of the transplant volume (L × l × W × 0.52) and an analysis of the kidney echogenicity. Spectral analysis of the intrarenal vessels allows the evaluation of vascularization (77,78).

Complications may occur after surgery, during the first days, or later during follow-up. In the early posttransplant period, the role of imaging (mainly US) is to differentiate between postsurgical complications and early acute rejection (79).

Postsurgical Complications

US may demonstrate a fluid collection around the kidney. MR imaging is useful to differentiate a lymphocele, a hematoma, or a urinary leak. Doppler (duplex and color) is able to diagnose renal artery or vein thrombosis and, later, a renal artery stenosis (Fig. 23.31). Urologic complications may develop secondary to ureteral stenosis. An opacification may be necessary to show the exact site of obstruction (79).

Acute Rejection

In the case of acute rejection, the transplant volume is increased, echogenicity may become heterogeneous, and

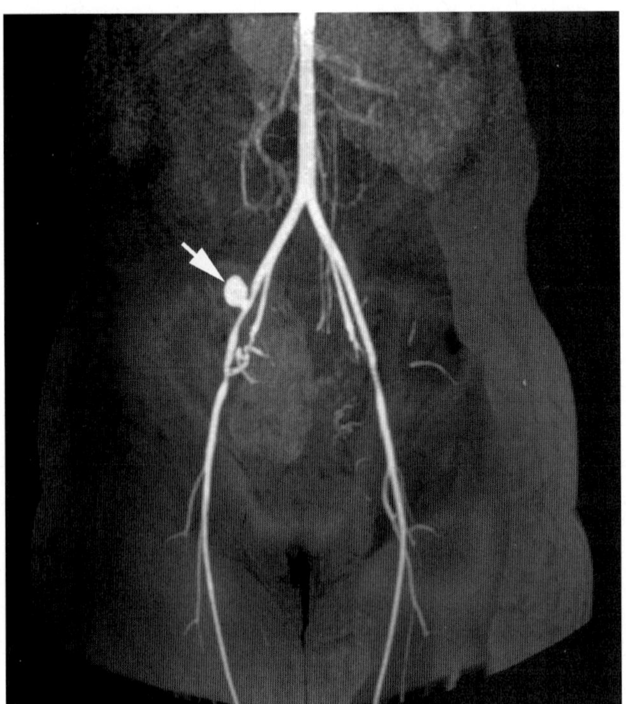

FIGURE 23.31. Aneurysm (*arrow*) on the vascular anastomotic site demonstrated by angio–magnetic resonance imaging.

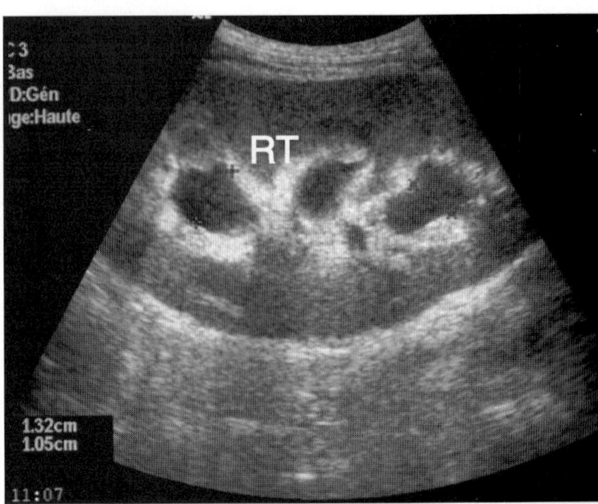

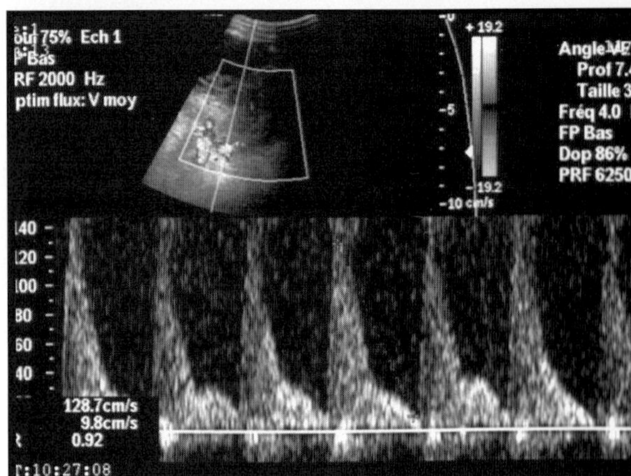

FIGURE 23.32. Acute rejection. **A:** Ultrasound. The renal transplant (RT) is swollen, the collecting system is distended, and there is perihilar hyperechogenicity. **B:** Doppler analysis. Increased vascular resistance (resistive index equals 0.85).

intrarenal RI may increase dramatically. In some cases, renal hilum becomes markedly hyperechoic, and the pelvic walls thicken (Fig. 23.32).

Other Complications

Other complications include infection and, rarely, calculi. Classical US signs usually accompany these complications. Lymphomas developing in immunocompromised patients may appear either as localized nodules or as an echogenic enlarged transplant.

UROLITHIASIS AND NEPHROCALCINOSIS

Urolithiasis

US is effective in detecting lithiasis, even tiny (2 to 3 mm), located in the kidney or the bladder. Urolithiasis determines, in most cases, a characteristic acoustic shadowing (Fig. 23.33). The role of imaging is to detect the lithiasis, to demonstrate a favoring underlying condition

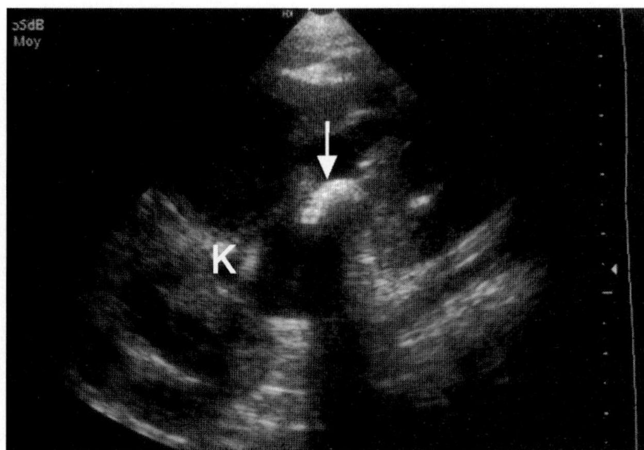

FIGURE 23.33. Urolithiasis—ultrasound. Sagittal scan of the left kidney (K). A lithiasis (*arrow*) is visible within the dilated collecting system.

(congenital malformation, nephrocalcinosis), and to follow the lithiasis under treatment. Plain film of the abdomen is helpful to demonstrate ureteral calcified stones that may be difficult to detect on US (80–82). In the case of renal colic, it might be useful to perform unenhanced CT with two- or three-dimensional reconstruction; this has been shown to be effective in demonstrating obstructive (multiple) ureteral stones (Fig. 23.34). Urethral stones may be more difficult to demonstrate; retrograde urethrography should be used to confirm the urethral stone. Whenever extracorporeal lithotripsy is applied, US and plain film of the abdomen can be used to follow the effects of treatment (83).

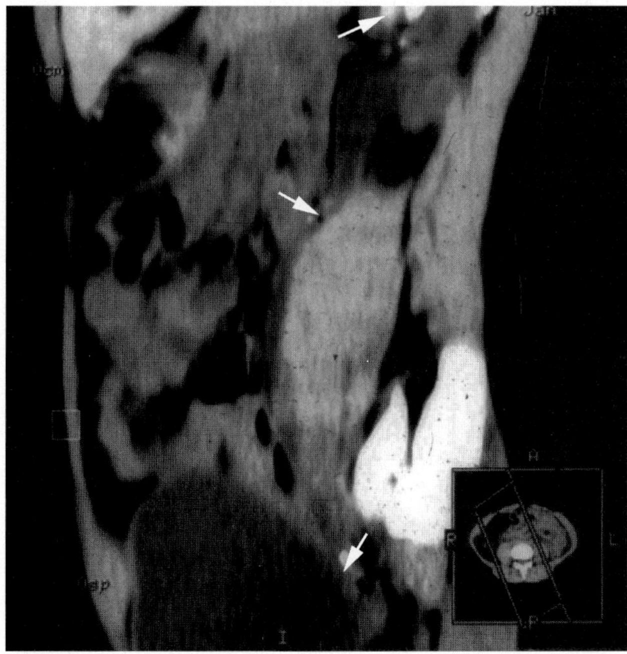

FIGURE 23.34. Urolithiasis—computed tomography: Reformatted two-dimensional images without contrast demonstrating multiple lithiasis (*arrows*) within the kidney and dilated ureter. The inset box indicates the scan plan.

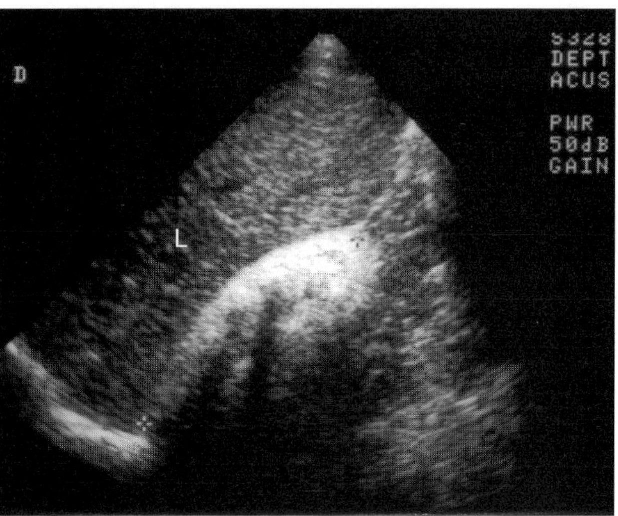

FIGURE 23.35. Cortical nephrocalcinosis. Highly echogenic kidney (between *crosses*) in a case of primary hyperoxaluria of type I. L, liver.

Nephrocalcinosis

Ultrasound Patterns

Nephrocalcinosis is suspected when hyperechogenic areas disturb the appearance of the kidney. Most cases of nephrocalcinosis are bilateral (84).

Cortical Nephrocalcinosis

Cortical nephrocalcinosis is rare in children. It can be extensive and determine acoustic shadowing behind the kidney as in neonatal hyperoxaluria of type I, or it can be more localized within areas of the parenchyma and correspond to sequelae of cortical necrosis or renal vein thrombosis (Fig. 23.35). In the case of vascular calcifications, the nephrocalcinosis can be unilateral.

Medullar Nephrocalcinosis

On US, medullar nephrocalcinosis (MNC) can be graded into three stages: diffuse and homogeneous, diffuse and inhomogeneous, or limited to the tip of the pyramids (Fig. 23.36). Grading helps to evaluate the effect of treatment in specific diseases. US is the best way to detect medullary nephrocalcinosis. Medullar hyperechogenicity is not always due to nephrocalcinosis. The differential diagnosis must, therefore, include the US features as well as clinical, biochemical, and genetic data (85,86).

Imaging Features of Specific Diseases

MNC is present and may be associated with urolithiasis and medullary cysts in patients with distal tubular acidosis (87). The severe neonatal form of primary hyperoxaluria

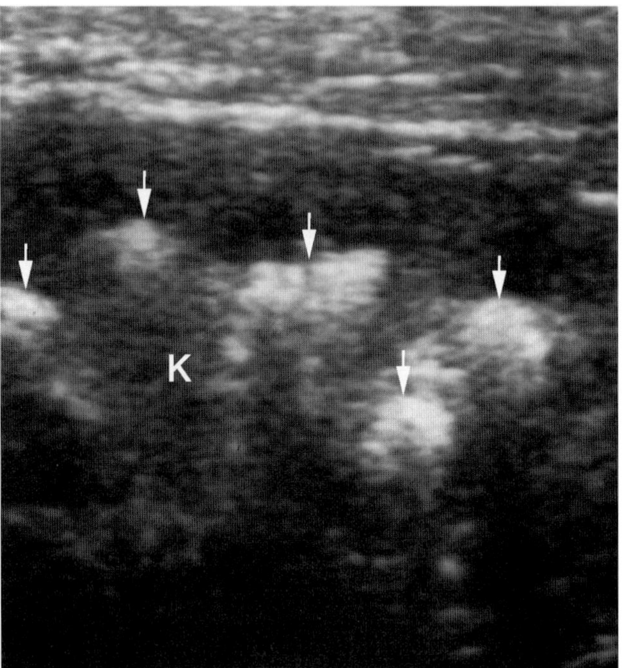

FIGURE 23.36. Medullary nephrocalcinosis. Sagittal scan of the kidney (K). Diffuse medullar, hyperechogenicity (*arrows*).

type I is associated with a cortical nephrocalcinosis that induces a markedly increased cortical echogenicity determining an acoustic shadowing. In later childhood, MNC is observed. Urolithiasis and renal colic are common complications demonstrated by US (88). Renal calcifications and skeletal lesions may be impressive (Fig. 23.37). The relationship between furosemide and MNC is unclear. The MNC is inhomogeneous and persists for a long period of time (89).

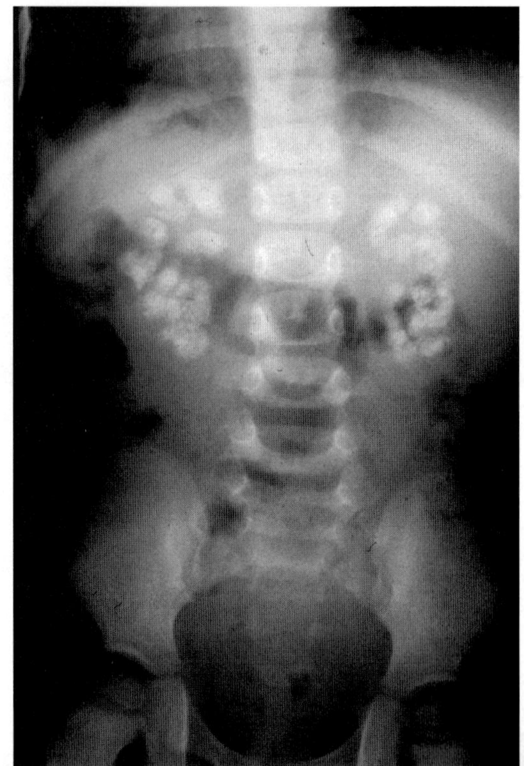

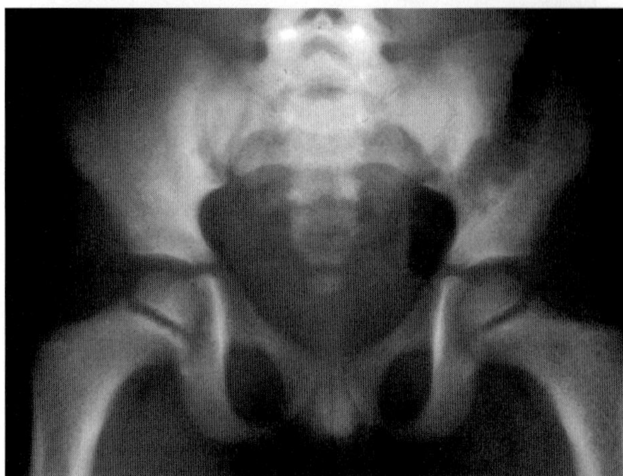

FIGURE 23.37. Primary hyperoxaluria of type I. **A:** Plain film of the abdomen. Impressive bilateral renal calcifications. **B:** Pelvic girdle. Densification and coarse trabeculation of the bones due to renal osteodystrophy.

TRAUMA TO THE URINARY TRACT

Kidney Trauma

Imaging, especially US and CT, has greatly modified the management of abdominal trauma in children. It allows more conservative, nonsurgical attitudes (90–92). US shows major renal damage and fluid collections (Fig. 23.38A). Color and duplex Doppler allows the evaluation of the vessels. Yet, the method has several limitations; because intestinal air may limit renal visibility, a normal US does not exclude parenchymal damage. Therefore, CT may be more suited for the first evaluation of children with suspected renal damage (Fig. 23.38B). CT is performed after contrast injection to demonstrate urinary leakage. CT angiography two-dimensional reconstruction allows an accurate evaluation of the renal vessels. A control examination may be useful if clinical evolution is unsatisfactory, suggesting persistent bleeding. Angiography must be limited to cases for which therapeutic intervention is likely.

Lower Urinary Tract

Bladder laceration is associated with bony pelvis fractures. Such laceration of the bladder should be suspected on US when large amounts of fluid are visualized in the cul-de-sac. VCUG can be performed if necessary to visualize the leakage site. The same mechanism explains the lesions to the urethra. Demonstration of the lesion may be difficult,

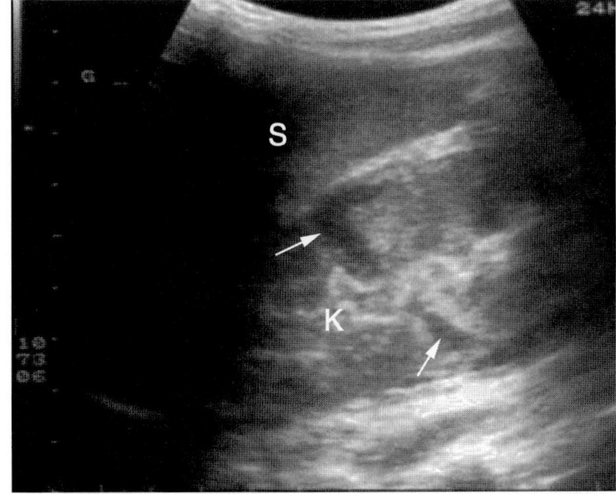

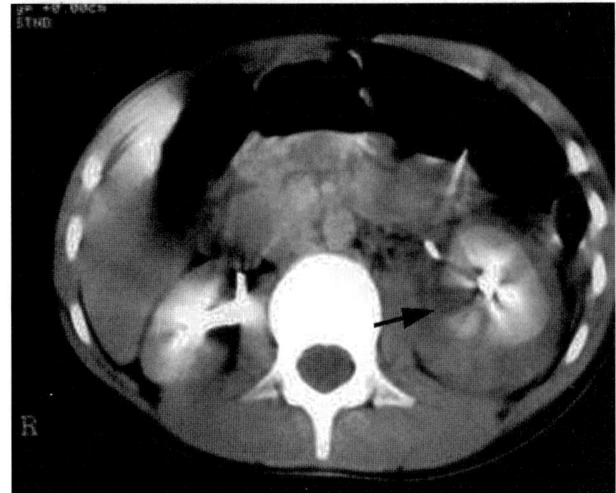

FIGURE 23.38. Left renal trauma. **A:** Ultrasound. Sagittal scan of the kidney (K). A renal fracture is visible (*arrows*). **B:** Computed tomography after contrast enhancement. Left perirenal hematic collection. The renal fracture is also visible (*arrow*). S, spleen.

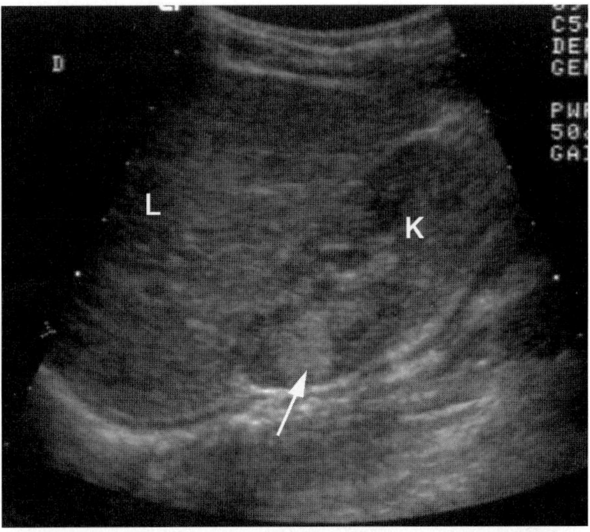

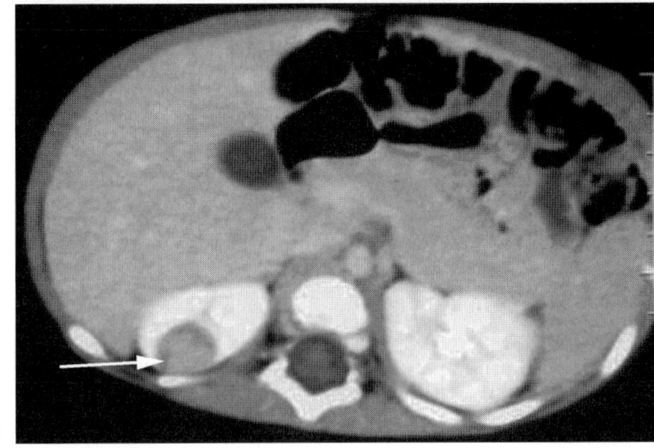

FIGURE 23.39. Renal tumors: small right Wilms' tumor in a case of hemihypertrophy. **A:** Ultrasound of echogenic area (*arrow*) in the upper pole of the right kidney (K). **B:** Computed tomography after contrast enhancement. The mass is less dense than the rest of the kidney (*arrow*) L, liver.

and a retrograde urethrogram should be performed very cautiously (93).

RENAL AND URINARY TRACT TUMORS

Role of Imaging

Imaging allows the detection and localization of the tumor, the analysis of its content and appearance, and the evaluation of the extent. Evaluation must be performed in conjunction with clinical and biologic data. It also has to fit into therapeutic protocols.

US easily localizes small tumors (Fig. 23.39). Large tumors are more difficult to delineate (Fig. 23.40). The technique easily differentiates cystic from solid-type tumors. CT and MR imaging are better suited for the evaluation of large tumors. Both are able to assess the tumor's relationship with the retroperitoneal vessels (Figs. 23.39 and 23.40). CT is performed without and with contrast enhancement. CT without contrast demonstrates the presence of calcifications within the tumor. Contrast enhancement is aimed to define the limits between normal parenchyma and tumor. Urographic-type images can be obtained at the end of the examination to visualize the ureters. During the same examination, an evaluation of the lungs can be obtained to exclude metastasis. A disadvantage of the technique is the irradiation hazards that can be associated. MR imaging may provide the same information as CT about the tumor without using x-rays (94–96).

Imaging of Specific Renal Tumors

Wilms' Tumor or Nephroblastoma

At diagnosis, the tumor is large but well demarcated from the normal parenchyma. On US, the tumor is echogenic

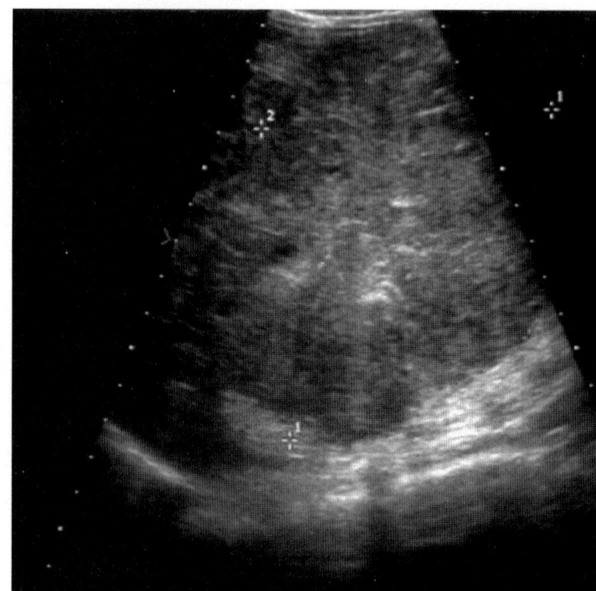

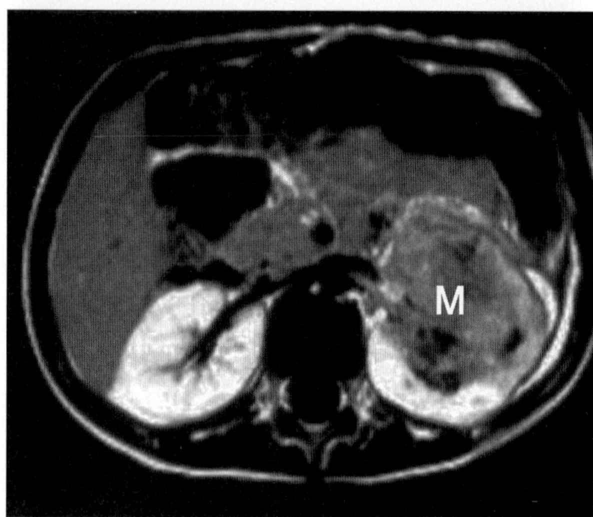

FIGURE 23.40. Renal tumors: large Wilms' tumor. **A:** Ultrasound. The tumor (between *crosses*) is difficult to delineate. **B:** Magnetic resonance imaging transverse scan after gadolinium. The mass (M) is better delineated.

with a solid content (Figs. 23.39 and 23.40). Areas of necrosis or hemorrhage are visible within the mass, especially after chemotherapy. Adenopathies can be seen next to the mass; extrarenal metastatic extent can be seen within the vena cava. The contralateral kidney should be checked for bilateral tumors. On CT or MR imaging, the tumor is more clearly delineated than with US, and bilateral tumors are easier to demonstrate (Figs. 23.39 and 23.40). The tumor appears heterogeneous due to areas of necrosis, but the solid content is enhanced after contrast injection. The tumor rarely contains calcifications or fat. It may appear partially or completely cystic.

The main differential diagnosis is neuroblastoma, Wilms' tumor tends to displace the abdominal vessels,

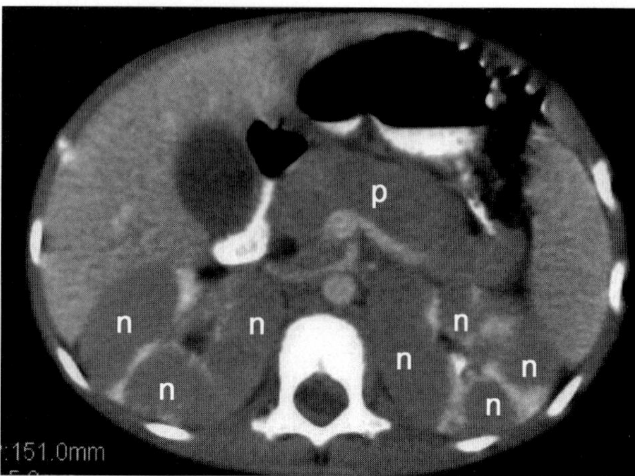

FIGURE 23.41. Renal lymphoma. Computed tomography with contrast. There is a bilateral nodular (n) involvement of both kidneys. The pancreas (p) was also affected.

whereas neuroblastoma tends to encase them; calcifications are more frequent in neuroblastoma.

Nephroblastomatosis

There is a loss of CMD on US in the diffuse form. On CT or MR imaging, the kidneys are large and there is a rim of thick cortical parenchyma that does not enhance after contrast injection. In the focal nodular form, one or more nodules are present; they do not enhance after contrast injection. They are more homogeneous than Wilms' tumor (97,98).

Lymphoma

Renal involvement occurs mainly in Burkitt's lymphoma and is usually bilateral. Other sites are often affected (e.g., ovaries, testicles). On US, lymphomatous nodules are hypoechoic compared to normal parenchyma; they enhance poorly on CT after contrast injection (99) (Fig. 23.41).

Other Malignant Tumors

Other malignant tumors are rare in children; their diagnosis is usually performed at histology rather than on imaging. Their rate of metastasis, particularly to the skeleton, is higher (100).

Screening Patients at Risk

As several syndromes (Denys-Drash, Beckwith-Wiedemann, Perlman, aniridia) are associated with a higher risk of Wilms' tumor, patients affected should be screened regularly by US (101) (Fig. 23.40).

Benign Renal Tumors

Mesoblastic nephroma is the most common tumor in the newborn and fetus. On imaging, the mass is well defined

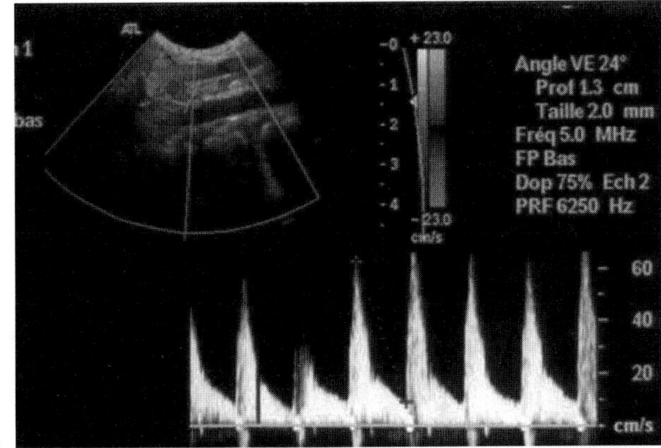

A

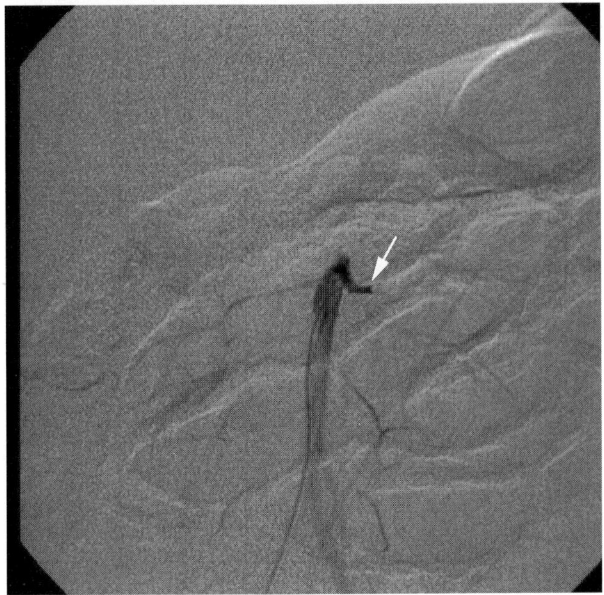

B

FIGURE 23.42. Hypertension in an 18-month-old boy with severe left renal artery stenosis. **A:** Doppler ultrasound. Increased resistive index and increased velocity at the ostium of the left renal artery. **B:** Angiography. Complete occlusion of the left renal artery (*arrow*). (Courtesy of F. Brunelle, M.D.)

from the normal parenchyma and is generally of solid type (102). Multilocular cystic nephroma appears as a cystic, septated mass on imaging; it cannot be differentiated from cystic nephroblastoma (103). Angiomyolipoma in children is invariably associated with tuberous sclerosis. The lesions are small and diffuse in early childhood, with a high fatty content; they are larger and fewer in adolescents and appear heterogeneous on US or CT (104).

Bladder Tumors

US is the easiest imaging method for the demonstration of a bladder tumor. Yet the method is unable to differentiate malignant from benign or inflammatory pseudotumors unless the tumor has extended beyond the bladder wall and metastases are present. CT and MR imaging are performed to evaluate the spreading of a malignant tumor (105–107).

RENOVASCULAR HYPERTENSION

Imaging may show scars, diffuse nephropathy, or diffuse sequelae of a vascular disease. Doppler US may show signs of renal artery stenosis (i.e., increased blood velocity at the renal artery ostium). A normal US examination does not exclude an anomaly. MR angiography has great potential for demonstrating renal vessel anomalies; the method is not yet standardized, and its accuracy has to be confirmed. ^{99m}Tc–MAG-3 or -DMSA before and after captopril stimulation can be a sensitive screening method for renovascular disease.

As fibromuscular hyperplasia and osteal stenosis are the most common causes of hypertension in children, arteriography remains the method of choice whenever the renal vascular origin of hypertension is highly probable. When a stenosis is present, an angioplasty can be performed immediately (108–110) (Fig. 23.42).

In a case of pheochromocytoma, metaiodobenzylguanidine scan, CT, or MR imaging should be performed to localize and delineate the mass.

INTERVENTIONAL IMAGING AND POSTOPERATIVE STUDIES

Interventional Imaging

Nephrostomy (Fig. 23.43) is the main interventional procedure in children. Pyonephrosis in a dilated collecting system is an indication (111).

Specific Postoperative Findings

US is the main imaging technique for the follow-up of surgical procedures (112). Isotopic evaluation allows detection of progression renal impairment.

Ureteropelvic Junction Obstruction

Nephrostomy of a very dilated congenital UPJ obstruction allows assessment of kidney function and helps the physician decide whether pyeloplasty or nephrectomy should be performed. Dilatation of the pelvicalyceal system may increase slightly after surgery due to edema; it decreases slowly thereafter within 6 to 8 weeks. Isotopic evaluation 6 months after surgery enables assessment of the evolution of renal function (113,114).

Ureterovesical Junction Obstruction

Leakage due to necrosis can occur at the site of the vesical reimplantation, and a hematoma or a urinoma may develop. The resolution of the ureteral dilatation can be monitored on US. At the level of the bladder, a characteristic posterior wall thickening can be observed at the level of the reimplantation (112,115).

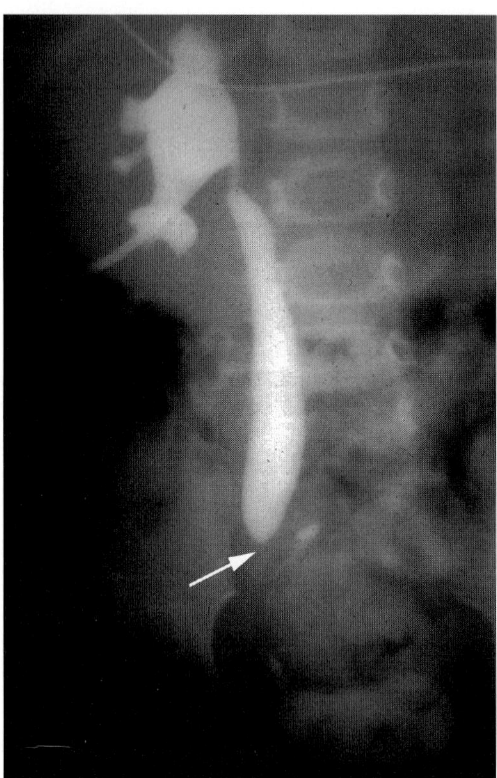

FIGURE 23.43. Right nephrostomy and opacification of the urinary tract in a case of ureteral stenosis (*arrow*).

Vesicoureteric Reflux

In cases of ureteral reimplantation, a thickening of the posterior bladder wall can be observed. Whenever the subureteric injection of Teflon (STING procedure) or other material is chosen, a small hyperechoic mass with acoustic shadowing can be seen at the level of the ureterovesical junction (Fig. 23.44). Transitory UT dilatation can also be observed. A control VCUG is useful 6 months after surgery to confirm the disappearance of the VUR (112,116).

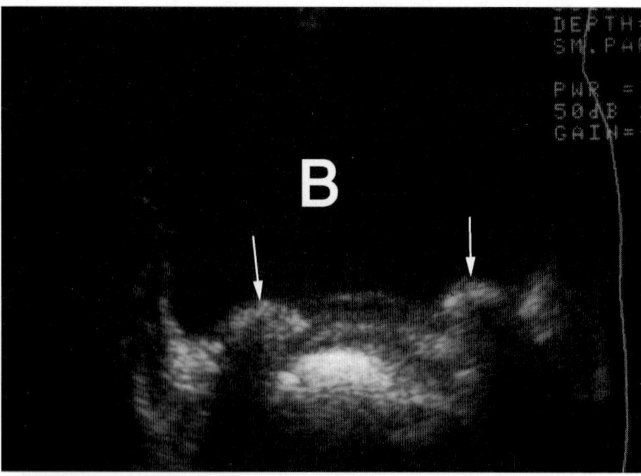

FIGURE 23.44. Bilateral Teflon injection. Transverse scan of the bladder (B). Teflon appears hyperechoic (*arrows*).

Duplex Collecting System

Unroofing of ectopic intravesical ureteroceles during endoscopy has been advocated to relieve obstruction and to allow functional improvement of the affected upper pole. The ureterocele collapses and appears as an intravesical pseudomass. The dilatation resolves and can be monitored by US. Secondary VUR may develop (112,117).

REFERENCES

1. Fotter R, ed. *Pediatric uroradiology*. Heidelberg, Germany: Springer-Verlag, 2001.
2. Fernback SK. Pediatric uroradiology—1997. *World J Urol* 1998;16:46–51.
3. Slovis TL. The ALARA concept in pediatric CT: myth or reality? *Radiology* 2002;222:5–6.
4. Yamazaki Y, Yagoritoma H. US characteristics of the urinary tract in healthy neonates. *J Urol* 2001;166:1054–1057.
5. Siegel M. The urinary tract. In: Siegel M, ed. *Pediatric sonography*, 3rd ed. New York: Lippincott–Raven Publishers 2001:385–392.
6. Zerin JM, Blane CE. US measurement of renal length in children: a reappraisal. *Pediatr Radiol* 1994;24:101–106.
7. Hiraoka M, Tsukahara H, Tsuchida S, et al. US evaluation of bladder volume in children. *Pediatr Nephrol* 1993;7:533–535.
8. Darge K, Troeger J, Duetting T, et al. Reflux in young patients. *Radiology* 1999;210:201–207.
9. Fernbach SK. Pediatric VCUG: a pictorial guide. *Radiographics* 2000;20:155–168.
10. Lebowitz RL. Excretory urography in children. *AJR Am J Roentgenol* 1994;163:990.
11. Siegel MJ. The kidney. In: Siegel MJ, ed. *Pediatric body CT*, 2nd ed. Philadelphia: Lippincott Williams & Wilkins, 1999:226–252.
12. Scheck RJ, Coppenrath EM, Kellner MW, et al. Radiation dose and image quality in spiral CT. *Br J Radiol* 1998;71:734–744.
13. Rodeigne LV, Spiekman D, Heifkens RJ, Shortliffe LD. MR imaging for the evaluation of hydronephrosis, reflux and renal scarring in children. *J Urol* 2001;166:1023–1027.
14. Avni FE, Balli MA, Regnault M, et al. MR urography in children. *Eur J Radiol* 2002;43:154–166.
15. Kraus SJ. Genitourinary imaging in children. *Ped Clin North Am* 2001;48:1381–1424.
16. Piepsz A, Colarinha P, Gordon I, et al. Guidelines for glomerular filtration rate determination in children. *Eur J Nucl Med* 2001;28:31–36.
17. Gordon I, Colarinha P, Piepz A, et al. Guidelines for standard and diuretic renography in children. *Eur J Nucl Med* 2001;28:BP21–BP30.
18. Gordon I. Guidelines for indirect radionuclide cystography. *Eur J Nucl Med* 2001;28:BP15–BP17.
19. De Bruyn R, Gordon I. Postnatal investigation of fetal renal disease. *Prenat Diagn* 2001;21:984–991.
20. Piepsz A. Cortical scintigraphy and urinary tract infection in children. *Nephrol Dial Transpl* 2002;17:560–562.
21. Piepsz A, Baufox MD, Gordon I, et al. Consensus on renal

cortical scintigraphy in children with urinary tract infection. *Semin Nucl Med* 1999;29:160–174.

22. Avni FE, Garel L, Hall M, et al. Perinatal approach to anomalies of the urinary tract. In: Avni FE, ed. *Perinatal imaging: from ultrasound to MR imaging.* Heidelberg, Germany: Springer-Verlag, 2002.
23. Poutama J, Vaminen R, Partamen K, Kirkainen P. Diagnosing fetal urinary tract anomalies: benefits of MRI compared to US. *Acta Obstet Gynecol Scand* 2000;79:65–71.
24. Ismaïli K, Avni FE, Hall M. Results of systematic VCUG in infants with antenatally diagnosed renal pelvis dilatation. *J Pediatr* 2002;9:726–733.
25. Maizels M, Reisman ME, Flom LS, et al. Grading nephroureteral dilatation detected in the first year of life. *J Urol* 1992;148:609–614.
26. Peters CA. Urinary tract obstruction in children. *J Urol* 1995;154:1874–1884.
27. Dinneen MD, Dhillon DK, Ward HC, et al. Antenatal diagnosis of PUV. *J Urol* 1993;72:364–369.
28. Dacher JN. Abnormalities of the lower urinary tract and urachus. In: Fotter R, ed. *Pediatric uroradiology.* Heidelberg, Germany: Springer-Verlag 2001:91–101.
29. Fernbach SK, Fenistein KA, Spencer K, et al. Ureteral duplications and its complications. *RadioGraphics* 1997;17:109–127.
30. Avni FE, Nicaise N, Hall M, et al. The role of MR imaging for the assessment of complicated duplex kidneys in children. *Pediatr Radiol* 2001;31:215–223.
31. Mandell J, Palhiel HJ, Peters CA, et al. Prenatal findings associated with a unilateral nonfunctioning or absent kidney. *J Urol* 1994;152:176–178.
32. Atiyeh B, Husman D, Baunn M. Contralateral renal abnormalities in patients with renal agenesis and noncystic renal dysplasia. *Pediatrics* 1993;91:812–815.
33. Zerres K, Mücher G, Becker J, et al. Prenatal diagnosis of ARPKD. *Am J Med Genet* 1998;76:137–144.
34. Fick GM, Duley IT, Johusin JD, et al. The spectrum of ADPKD in children. *J Am Soc Nephrol* 1994;4:1654–1660.
35. Carr MC, Benaceraf Br, Estroff JA, Mandell J. Prenatally diagnosed hyperechoic kidneys: postnatal outcome. *J Urol* 1995;53:442–444.
36. Savage M, Jaaskilaaien J, Koskimis O. Diagnostic US changes in the kidneys of 20 infants with congenital nephrotic syndrome. *Eur Radiol* 1995;5:49–54.
37. Avni EF, Guissard G, Hall M, et al. Hereditary polycystic kidney diseases in children. *Pediatr Radiol* 2002;32:169–174.
38. Avni EF, Hall M, Collier F, Schulman CC. Anomalies of the renal pelvis and ureter. In: Fotter R, ed. *Uroradiology in children.* Heidelberg, Germany: Springer-Verlag 2001:61–90.
39. Avni EF, Matos C, Rypens F, Schulman CC. Ectopic vaginal insertion of an upper pole ureter. *J Urol* 1997;158:1931–1932.
40. Pennington DJ, Zerin MJ. Imaging of the UTI. *Pediatr Ann* 1999;28:678–686.
41. Stark H. UTI in girls: the cost-effectiveness of currently recommended investigative routine. *Pediatr Nephrol* 1997;11: 174–177.
42. Mac Kenzie JR, Fonder K, Hollman AJ, et al. The value of US in the child with acute UTI. *Br J Urol* 1994;74:240–244.
43. Kaefer M, Barnewolt C, Retik AB, et al. The US diagnosis of intravesical obstruction. *J Urol* 1997;157:989–991.
44. Netto JMB, Perez LM, Kelly DR, et al. Pediatric inflammatory bladder tumors. *J Urol* 1999;162:1424–1429.
45. Dacher JN, Avni FE, Arnaud F, et al. Renal sinus hyperechogenicitiy in APN. *Pediatr Radiol* 1999;29:179–182.
46. Robben GF, Boesten M, Linmans J, et al. Significance of thickening of the wall of the collecting system. *Pediatr Radiol* 1999;29:736–740.
47. Hitzel A, Liard A, Vera P, et al. Color and power Doppler sonography versus DMSA scintigraphy in APN and in prediction of renal scarring. *J Nucl Med* 2002;43:27–32.
48. Dacher JN, Boillot B, Evni D, et al. Rationale use of CT in APN. *Pediatr Radiol* 1993;23:281–285.
49. Pickworth FE, Centin JB, Ditchfeld MR, et al. Sonographic measurement of renal enlargement in children with APN and time needed for resolution: implications for renal growth assessment. *AJR Am J Roentgenol* 1995;165:405–408.
50. Stokland E, Hellström M, Jacobsson B, et al. Renal damage one year after UTI: role of DMSA scanning. *J Pediatr* 1996;129:815–820.
51. Berman LH, Stringer DA, St Onge O, et al. An assessment of sonography in the diagnosis and management of neonatal renal candidiasis. *Clin Radiol* 1989;40:577–581.
52. Cremin BJ. Radiological imaging of urogenital tuberculosis in children with emphasis on ultrasound. *Pediatr Radiol* 1987;17:34–38.
53. Avni FE, Schulman CC. The origin of VUR in male newborns. *Br J Urol* 1996;78:454–459.
54. Zerin M, Ritchey M, Chang A. Incidental VUR in neonates with antenatally detected hydronephrosis and other renal abnormalities. *Radiology* 1993;187:157–160.
55. Hernandez RH, Goodsitt M. Reduction of radiation dose in pediatric patients using pulsed fluoroscopy. *AJR Am J Roentgenol* 1996;167:11247–1253.
56. Scott JES. Fetal VUR: a follow-up study. *Br J Urol* 1993;71:481–483.
57. Mentzel HJ, Vogt S, Patzer L, et al. Contrast enhanced sonography of VUR. *AJR Am J Roentgenol* 1999;173:737–740.
58. Chapman SJ, Chandler C, Haycock GB, et al. Radionuclide cystography in VUR. *Arch Dis Child* 1988;63:650–671.
59. Avni FE, Ayadi K, Rypens F, et al. Can careful US examination of the UT exclude VUR in the neonate? *Br J Radiol* 1997;70:977–982.
60. Chan Y, Chang K, Yeung C, et al. Potential utility of MRI in the evaluation of children at risk of renal scarring. *Pediatr Radiol* 1999;29:856–862.
61. Wemestrom M, Hanson S, Jodn U, et al. Primary and acquired renal scarring in boys and girls with UTI. *J Pediatr* 2000;136:30–34.
62. Marra G, Barbieri G, Dell'Agnda CA, et al. Congenital renal damage associated with VUR detected prenatally in male infants. *J Pediatr* 1994;124:726–730.
63. Jarvelin MR, Huttunen MP, Seffaren J, et al. Screening of urinary tract anomalies among day and night wetting children. *Scand J Urol Nephrol* 1990;24:181–189.
64. Sillen U. Bladder dysfunction in children with VUR. *Acta Paediatr* 1999;431:S40–S47.
65. Pippisalle JL, Capolicchio G, Houle AM, et al. MRI in children with voiding dysfunction. *J Urol* 1998;160:1080–1083.

66. Fotter R. Neurogenic bladder in children—a new challenge for the radiologist. *Abdom Imaging* 1996;21:534–550.
67. Kraus RA, Gaisie G, Young LW. Increased renal parenchymal echogenicity, causes in children. *Radiographics* 1990;10: 1009–1018.
68. Patriquin HB, O'Regan S, Robitaille P, et al. Hemolytic-uremic syndrome: intrarenal arterial Doppler patterns as a useful guide to therapy. *Radiology* 1989;172:625–628.
69. Hewlett DG, Greenwood KL, Jacosz JM, et al. The incidence of transient medullary hyperechogenicity in neonatal US examination. *Br J Radiol* 1997;70:140–143.
70. Lalmand B, Avni EF, Nasr A, et al. Perinatal renal vein thrombosis. *J Ultrasound Med* 1990;9:437–440.
71. Hintchcliffe SA, Chan Y, Jones H, et al. Renal hypoplasia and postnatal acquired cortical loss. *Pediatr Nephrol* 1992;6: 439–444.
72. de Bruyn R, Gordon I. Imaging in cystic renal disease. *Arch Dis Child* 2000;83:401–407.
73. Chuang YF, Tsai TC. Sonographic findings in familial juvenile nephronophthisis-medullary cystic disease complex. *J Clin Ultrasound* 1998;26:203–206.
74. Olbring H, Hirche H. Koskimies O, et al. Renal growth in children with severe vesicoureteral reflux: 10-year prospective study of medical and surgical treatment: the International Reflux Study in Children (European branch). *Radiology* 2000;216:731–737.
75. Sonaga M, Jaaskelainen J, Koskimies O. Diagnostic US findings in the kidneys of 20 children with CNS of the Finnish type. *Eur Radiol* 1995;5:49–54.
76. Kraaytel P, Robben SGF, Wolf ED, et al. Primary hyperoxaluria type I: renal US before and after treatment. *Pediatr Nephrol* 1997;11:491–493.
77. Pozniak MA, Kely F, Dodd GD. Renal transplant ultrasound: imaging and Doppler. *Semin Ultrasound CT MR* 1991;12:319–334.
78. Herz DB, Mc Lorie GA, Hagez AT, et al. High resolution US characterization of early allograft hemodynamics in pediatric living related renal transplantation. *J Urol* 2001;166:1853–1858.
79. Suratt JT, Siegel MJ, Middleton WD. US of complications of pediatric renal allografts. *Radiographics* 1990;10:687–699.
80. Kraus SJ, Lebowitz RL, Royal SA. Renal calculi in children. *Pediatr Radiol* 1999;29:624–630.
81. Broderick NI. Plain radiograph and renal tract ultrasound in the management of children with renal tract calculi—a reply. *Clin Radiol* 2002;57:151.
82. Smergel E, Curenberg SB, Crisci KL, et al. CT urograms in pediatric patients with ureteral calculi: do adult criteria work? *Pediatr Radiol* 2001;31:720–723.
83. Rodrigues Netto N, Longo JA, Ikonomidi JA, et al. ESWL in children. *J Urol* 2002;167:2164–2165.
84. Alkhan O, Oznen MN, Costam M, et al. Systemic oxalosis. *Pediatr Radiol* 1995;25:15–16.
85. Schulz PK, Strife JL, Strife CF, et al. Hyperechoic renal medullary pyramids in children. *Radiology* 1994;181:163–167.
86. Nayr A, Kadiogly A, Sini A, et al. Causes of increased renal medullary hyperechogenicity in Turkish children. *Pediatr Nephrol* 1995;9:729–733.
87. Igarashi T, Shibuya K, Kamoshita S, et al. Renal cyst formation as a complication of primary renal tubular acidosis. *Nephron* 1991;99:75–79.
88. Kraayeveld P, Robben SG, Wolff ED, Meradji M. Primary hyperoxaluria type I: renal ultrasound before and after treatment. *Pediatr Nephrol* 1997;11:491–493.
89. Saarela T, Vaouralla A, Lamming P, et al. Incidence, US patterns and resolution of NC in low birthweight infants. *Acta Pediatr* 1999;88:655–660.
90. Morey AF, Bruce JF, Mc Annick JW. Efficacy of radiographic imaging in pediatric blunt renal trauma. *J Urol* 1996;156:2014–2018.
91. Stein JP, Kaji DM, Eastham J, et al. Blunt renal trauma in the pediatric population. Indications for radiographic evaluation. *Urology* 1994;44:406–410.
92. Pershad J, Cirhmore B. Serial bedside emergency US in a case of pediatric trauma. *Pediatr Emerg Care* 2000;16:375–376.
93. Dokuce AI, Ozdenir E, Ozturlc H, et al. Urogenital injuries in childhood. *Int Urol Nephrol* 2000;32:3–8.
94. Lowe LH, Isuani BH, Heller RM, et al. Pediatric renal masses: Wilms tumor and beyond. *Radiographics* 2000;20: 1585–1603.
95. Goske MJ, Mitchell C, Reslan WA. Imaging patients with Wilms' tumor. *Semin Urol Oncol* 1999;17:11–20.
96. Navy JF, Royal SA, Vaid YN, et al. Wilms' tumor: unusual manifestations. *Pediatr Radiol* 1995;25:576–586.
97. Rohrschneider WK, Weirich A, Rieden K, et al. US, CT and MR characteristics of nephroblastomatosis. *Pediatr Radiol* 1998;28:435–443.
98. Lonergan GJ, Martinez-Leon MI, Agrons GA, et al. Nephrogenic rests, nephroblastomatosis and associated lesions of the kidney. *Radiographics* 1998;18:947–968.
99. Ng YY, Healy JC, Vincent JM, et al. The radiology of non-Hodgkin lymphoma in childhood. *Clin Radiol* 1994;49: 594–600.
100. Glass RB, Davidson AJ, Feinbach SK. Clear cell sarcoma of the kidney: CT, US and pathologic correlation. *Radiology* 1991;180:715–717.
101. Choyke PL, Siegel MJ, Craft AW, et al. Screening for Wilms' tumor in children with Beckwith-Wiedeman syndrome. *Med Pediatr Oncol* 1999;32:196–200.
102. Irsutti M, Puget C, Bauwin C, et al. Mesoblastic nephroma: prenatal US and MRI features. *Pediatr Radiol* 2000;30:147–150.
103. Agrons GA, Wagner BJ, Davidson AJ, et al. Multilocular cystic renal tumor in children. *Radiographics* 1995;15:663–669.
104. Van Baal JG, Smits NJ, Keeman JN, et al. The evolution of renal angiomyolipomas in patients with tuberous sclerosis. *J Urol* 1994;152:35–38.
105. Dennery MP, Rushdem HG, Belman AB. US for the detection and follow-up of primary non sarcomata bladder tumors in children. *Urology* 2000;59:119–121.
106. Schneider G, Ahlhelm F, Altmeyer K, et al. Rare pseudotumors of the urinary bladder in children. *Eur Radiol* 2001;11:1024–1029.
107. Quillin SP, Mc Allister WH. Transitional cell of the bladder in children. *Urol Radiol* 1991;13:107–109.
108. Broekhuizen-de Gast HS, tiel-Van Burel MM, Van Beek MJ. Severe hypertension in children with renovascular disease. *Clin Nucl Med* 2001;26:606–609.

109. Fossali E, Signorini E, Indermite RC, et al. Renovascular disease and hypertension in children with neurofibromatosis. *Pediatr Nephrol* 2000;14:806–810.
110. Hofbeek M, Singer H, Rupperecht T, et al. Successful percutaneous transluminal angioplasty for treatment of renovascular hypertension in a 5-month-old child. *Eur J Pediatr* 1998;157:512–514.
111. Matsumoto AM, Deyter SW, Barth KH, et al. Percutaneous nephrostomy drainage in the management of neonatal anuria secondary to renal candidiasis. *J Pediatr Surg* 1990;25:1295–1297.
112. Rypens F, Avni EF, Bank WO, et al. The ureterovesical junction in children: sonographic findings after surgical or endoscopic treatment. *AJR Am J Roentgenol* 1992;158:837–842.
113. Kis E, Verebely T, Kovi R, et al. The role of US in the follow-up of postoperative changes after pyeloplasty. *Pediatr Radiol* 1998;28:247–249.
114. Doraiswamy DV. Ureteroplasty using balloon dilatation in children with UPJ obstruction. *J Pediatr Surg* 1994;29:937–940.
115. Mezzacappa PM, Price AA, Kassner EG, et al. Cohen ureteral reimplantation: US appearance. *Radiology* 1987;165:851–852.
116. Gore MD, Fembach SK, Donaldson JS, et al. Radiographic evaluation of subureteric Teflon to correct VUR. *AJR Am J Roentgenol* 1989;152:115–119.
117. Blyth B, Passerini Glazel G, Camuffo C, et al. Endoscopic incision of ureteroceles. *J Urol* 1993;149:556–560.

24

RENAL PATHOLOGY

AGNES B. FOGO

This chapter reviews the usual circumstances in which biopsies are obtained, methods of obtaining the biopsy material and analyzing the tissue, and the distinct characteristic morphologic findings in various diseases. Finally, current experimental techniques that may provide important pathogenic, prognostic, or diagnostic information are discussed.

RENAL BIOPSY INDICATIONS

The indications for renal biopsy vary according to the ethnic and age characteristics of the population studied and the geographic location because these factors influence the incidence of various renal diseases. The indications discussed below present the most common settings in children for which renal biopsy is undertaken.

Hematuria

Isolated hematuria (i.e., without proteinuria and with normal function of the kidney) may be due to hypercalciuria, familial, or urologic disease (1–3). Once these disorders are ruled out, a glomerular origin of persistent isolated hematuria should be considered. When present, red blood cell casts or dysmorphic red blood cells indicate glomerular origin of hematuria. Renal biopsy may define the underlying abnormality in these patients. The most common findings are mesangial proliferative disease or immunoglobulin (Ig) A nephropathy (Berger's disease). Less common disorders include hereditary nephritis (Alport's syndrome) and thin basement membrane lesion. The latter may be familial (benign familial hematuria) or sporadic. One-fourth to nearly one-half of the patients with isolated hematuria have normal biopsies (1–4). Renal biopsy may, therefore, define the pathology and provide assurance of a benign prognosis in some patients or diagnose a possible hereditary disease, which initiates screening of other family members. Finally, the information obviously is of importance in avoiding further repeated invasive evaluation in the patient.

Proteinuria

Isolated proteinuria may be postural or due to tubulointerstitial disease. These possibilities should be evaluated completely over time before renal biopsy is considered. Any glomerular disease may cause mild to moderate proteinuria as the only manifestation, and biopsy may yield the diagnosis even at an early stage.

Nephrotic Syndrome

Numerous children with nephrotic syndrome (NS) were studied when renal biopsy first became available. The biopsies showed so-called minimal change disease (MCD) in the vast majority of cases. The efficacy of corticosteroids in this setting has obviated the need for renal biopsies in most of these cases. Therefore, young children with NS typically undergo a therapeutic trial of corticosteroids without a biopsy. However, in infants with NS, in older children, or in those with evidence of nephritis (hypertension, hematuria, low C3, or decreased renal function) or who do not respond to corticosteroid therapy, renal biopsy is often performed. In these patients, a disease other than MCD [e.g., focal segmental glomerulosclerosis (FSGS), membranoproliferative glomerulonephritis (MPGN), IgA nephropathy, membranous glomerulonephritis, or, more rarely in infants, Finnish-type NS or diffuse mesangial sclerosis] is often present (4–9).

Acute Nephritis

The child with acute glomerulonephritis may need a biopsy when the course is not typical of acute poststreptococcal disease or if urinary abnormalities persist. Although the primary disease process may be evident in systemic conditions [e.g., Henoch-Schönlein purpura or systemic lupus erythematosus (SLE)], renal biopsy often is indicated to assess severity of injury and to guide therapy and prognosis. Differentiation of specific types of proliferative lesions (e.g., MPGN type I and dense deposit disease) is made by renal biopsy. This distinction has important implications for eventual treatment because the morphologic lesions of dense deposit disease invariably recur in transplants, although the clinical course is less severe than in the native kidney (10,11).

Acute Renal Failure

The cause of acute renal failure may be clinically obvious, or there may be multiple potential culprits. When prerenal and obstructive causes are not apparent, renal parenchymal disease should be considered. When acute renal failure is associated with nephritis, NS, or evidence of vasculitis or systemic diseases, biopsy is usually performed. Other common causes include acute tubular necrosis or injury, often caused by drug or ischemic injury, vascular disease, and interstitial nephritis. These conditions can often be diagnosed without renal biopsy. However, when the cause remains uncertain after complete evaluation, renal biopsy may be necessary for diagnosis (12).

Rapidly Progressive Glomerulonephritis

Renal biopsy may be considered an urgent procedure in the patient with rapidly progressive glomerulonephritis. Various systemic vasculitides that may be distinguished only by specific serologic studies (see below) or renal biopsy must be treated urgently to avoid severe chronic renal damage. Although anti–glomerular basement membrane (GBM) antibody or antineutrophil cytoplasmic antibody (ANCA) titers may provide useful information, the ANCA test in particular is not diagnostic of a specific condition; rather, it is a screening test for necrotizing vasculitides (13,14). ANCA positivity, whether in a perinuclear ANCA or cytoplasmic ANCA pattern, was present in approximately 60% of patients with immune-complex glomerulonephritis with crescents in a study of more than 200 renal biopsies (15). Furthermore, these specialized assays may have a longer turn-around time than the renal biopsy, from which preliminary information from immunofluorescence (IF) and light microscopy (LM) studies can be available within hours after biopsy.

Chronic Renal Insufficiency

Patients with renal insufficiency of uncertain etiology are candidates for renal biopsy. Although renal biopsy of the small, shrunken kidney is riskier because of the greater incidence of bleeding complications, the diagnosis of primary disease can be important. This information allows assessment of existing severity of morphologic lesions, determination of risk of recurrence in eventual renal transplant, and suitability of cadaveric versus living-related donor transplantation. If the disease has a familial basis or recurs frequently with resultant graft loss, cadaveric transplantation may be preferable to living-related donor transplant (11).

Systemic Diseases

The severity of renal involvement in systemic disease [e.g., hemolytic-uremic syndrome (HUS)], Henoch-Schönlein purpura, diabetes mellitus, or SLE may not be apparent without renal biopsy. The trend is now toward early biopsy in patients with diabetes and renal abnormalities. Severity of lesions and stage of chronicity and activity impart prognostic information and may affect therapeutic decisions (see below). The most extensively studied disease in this regard is SLE. Differentiation of specific lupus nephritis World Health Organization (WHO) class (see below) may be difficult without renal biopsy (16,17). Overall, evidence indicates that renal biopsy findings may be more sensitive than clinical assessment alone in evaluating the severity of renal involvement in SLE (18,19).

Follow-Up of Disease

With improved therapeutic modalities available for intervention in chronic progressive renal disease, sequential or follow-up biopsies become increasingly necessary to evaluate therapeutic efficacy. On the other hand, additional cytotoxic therapy with its side effects may be withheld if the biopsy shows end-stage histology. Intervention with, for example, low-protein diets, angiotensin-converting enzyme inhibitors, or angiotensin type 1 receptor blockers has been shown to alter the course of chronic progressive renal disease (20).

Transplantation

Renal transplant biopsies are useful in assessing episodes of clinically suspected rejection, investigating the cause of decreased renal function or urine output, and detecting the development of *de novo* or recurrent disease. Occasionally, infection may be diagnosed by renal biopsy. Drug toxicity may be diagnosed by morphologic findings. The absence of lesions in a patient with a rise in creatinine supports cyclosporine toxicity because this drug commonly causes a decline in the glomerular filtration rate by vasoconstriction and not overt structural lesions. The absence of findings of acute rejection in renal biopsy or by needle aspiration (see below) can assist in avoiding unnecessary immunosuppressive therapy with its potential for increased morbidity and mortality. Even a diagnosis of chronic rejection, which is not amenable to therapy, has important therapeutic implications for the patient.

Diseases that recur in the transplant with high frequency include IgA nephropathy, MPGN type I, dense deposit disease (also known as *MPGN type II*), FSGS, HUS, and membranous glomerulonephritis. The latter two can occur *de novo* in the transplant. Metabolic diseases (e.g., oxalosis and diabetic nephropathy) can also cause recurrent disease in the renal transplant if liver or pancreas transplantation does not cure the primary abnormality (11). Alport's syndrome is caused by mutation in one of the type IV collagen genes, resulting in abnormal GBM assembly and structure. Patients may develop anti-GBM antibody disease in the transplant because of antibodies against its normal type IV basement membrane collagen (21,22).

OBTAINING TISSUE

General Considerations

Percutaneous renal biopsy is the most common method for obtaining tissue for the kidney. In large series, major complications are rare. The technique, first done in 1951 by Iverson and Brun, allows tissue yield in 93 to 95% of biopsies, with more than 87% of these being adequate (23–25). The biopsy

TABLE 24.1. DEFINITIONS OF COMMON MORPHOLOGIC TERMS

Term	Definition
Light microscopy	
Focal	Involving some glomeruli
Diffuse	Involving all glomeruli
Segmental	Involving part of glomerular tuft
Global	Involving total glomerular tuft
Lobular	Simplified, lobular appearance of capillary loop architecture (membranoproliferative glomerulonephritis)
Nodular	Acellular areas of mesangial matrix (diabetic nephropathy)
Sclerosis	Collapse and scarring of capillary loop
Crescent	Proliferation of parietal epithelial cells
Spikes	Projections of GBM intervening between subepithelial immune deposits (membranous glomerulonephritis)
Endocapillary proliferation	Increase in mesangial or endothelial cells
Hyaline	Descriptive of glassy, smooth-appearing material
Hyalinosis	Hyaline appearing insudation of plasma proteins (focal segmental glomerulosclerosis)
Mesangium	Stalk region of capillary loop with mesangial cells surrounded by matrix
Subepithelial	Between visceral epithelial cell and GBM
Subendothelial	Between endothelial cell and GBM
Tram-track	Double contour of GBM due to deposits or CMIP (see below)
Wire loop	Thick, rigid appearance of capillary loop due to subendothelial deposits
Activity	Score of possible treatment-sensitive lesions (e.g., based on extent of crescents, cellular infiltrate, necrosis, proliferation)
Chronicity	Score of probable irreversible lesions (e.g., based on extent of tubular atrophy, interstitial fibrosis, fibrous crescents, sclerosis)
Immunofluorescence	
Granular	Discontinuous flecks of staining along capillary loop producing granular pattern
Linear	Smooth continuous staining along capillary loop
Electron microscopy	
Foot process effacement	Flattening of foot processes so that they cover the basement membrane
Microvillous transformation	Small extensions of visceral epithelial cells with villus-like appearance
CMIP	Extension of mesangial cell cytoplasm with interposition between endothelial cell cytoplasm and basement membrane and underlying new basement membrane formation
Reticular aggregates	Organized arrays of membrane particles within endothelial cells
Immunotactoid GP	Large, organized microtubular deposits, >30 nm in diameter
Fibrillary GP	Fibrils 14–20 nm in diameter without organization

CMIP, circumferential mesangial interposition; GBM, glomerular basement membrane; GP, glomerulopathy.

findings altered diagnoses in half of the cases in one series, indicating different therapeutic approaches in approximately one-third of those cases (26). Although some renal diseases show diagnostic features by LM (Table 24.1), special studies add to the sensitivity of the study. For the renal biopsy to be most useful, it must be evaluated appropriately by an experienced renal pathologist. Biopsies must be examined by special LM, IF microscopy, and electron microscopy (EM) for the most accurate diagnosis (27). If the nephrologist's hospital does not provide these services, arrangements must be made to send tissue in appropriate fixatives (see below) to a reference laboratory with these capabilities. If such services cannot be provided, it is doubtful whether the institution should be undertaking renal biopsies.

Contraindications

Contraindications to percutaneous biopsy are solitary, ectopic, or horseshoe kidney; bleeding diathesis; abnormal renal vascular supply; and uncontrolled hypertension (23–25,28). Relative contraindications include obesity; uncooperative patients; hydronephrosis; ascites; and small, shrunken kidneys—all are associated with greater risk for complications. Open biopsy is preferable if the biopsy information is crucial in these conditions. Percutaneous biopsy is contraindicated if the kidney has tumors, large cysts, abscesses, or pyelonephritis because the needle track may facilitate spread of malignant cells or infection. Open biopsy allows selection of specific areas for biopsy in these situations.

Biopsy Technique

The patient may be admitted on the day of the biopsy. Before biopsy is done, ultrasound examination must confirm that there are two kidneys in normal position. Laboratory evaluation must include a complete blood cell count with normal platelet count, partial thromboplastin and prothrombin times, fibrinogen level, and bleeding time. The blood bank should type and hold one unit of blood. The biopsy optimally is timed so that an experienced technician or pathologist can attend to ensure prompt processing of the biopsy tissue.

Food and drink should be withheld for at least 6 hours before biopsy, and the child should be lightly sedated but still able to cooperate during the biopsy. The child lies in the prone position with a sandbag or rolled sheet under the abdomen, and the skin of the flank is prepped and draped in sterile fashion. Although the left kidney is usually preferred, either side can be chosen for biopsy. The lower pole of the kidney is marked on the skin with a pen after localization by any of several imaging techniques (e.g., fluoroscopy, radionuclide scanning, intravenous urography, computed tomography, or ultrasound—the last being the most commonly used method). Local anesthetic is infiltrated first in the skin and then in deeper tissues, taking care not to enter the kidney. A small incision is made through the skin and a spinal needle stylet inserted into the depth of the kidney while the patient holds his or her breath in midinspiration. When the kidney capsule is punctured, a loss of resistance can be felt. The needle moves with inspiration when the child is asked to breathe, confirming that it is within the renal parenchyma. Arterial pulsations can also be seen when the needle is within the kidney. The exact depth of the kidney and position of the needle are noted by ultrasound and marked on the stylet at the point where these respiratory movements are no longer transmitted to the stylet as it is slowly removed. Conventional or spring-loaded needles are used for renal biopsies. Most now use the spring-loaded, so-called biopsy gun. For conventional needles, the biopsy needle is inserted to the desired position as the patient again holds his or her breath, advancing the cannula over the obturator once the needle is in correct position. The entire needle with the core of tissue is then removed.

An automatic spring-loaded biopsy system has been used widely in the last several years because of the simplicity and ease of the technique (29,30). The kidney is localized with ultrasound guidance, and the depth of the kidney as judged by ultrasound and the spinal needle is used to place the biopsy needle to reach the kidney capsule. The patient holds his or her breath for only a few seconds while the spring-loaded needle is activated, causing the obturator to automatically advance into the kidney, and the entire needle is then removed with the tissue core. It is important to note that the caliber of the needle used with any of these techniques directly impacts the adequacy of the specimen (31). When 18-gauge needles are used with this method, the resulting cores are very small and there is artifact along the edges. The use of a 16-gauge needle, thus, is more likely to provide an adequate tissue sample without distortion and with fewer passes necessary to obtain adequate tissue.

Usually, two cores of tissue are necessary for optimum evaluation, or three cores if 18-gauge needles are used. If tissue cannot be obtained after several passes, the biopsy should be attempted on another day. After biopsy, a firm dressing is applied, and the child is kept supine in bed for 24 hours and monitored with frequent checks of vital signs and urine for hematuria. The hematocrit should be rechecked at 4 and 24 hours after the biopsy. The child may be discharged the next day if no complications arise (28). An evaluation of the impact of earlier discharge showed that observation for 8 hours or less after renal biopsy missed more than 20% of complications (32).

Open biopsy can be performed under local or general anesthesia. The kidney can be directly visualized even through a small incision. Although a larger sample may be obtained with a wedge biopsy, it is preferable to also perform a needle biopsy to sample deeper cortex and medulla for assessment of diseases that preferentially involve juxtamedullary glomeruli (see below).

Aspiration Biopsy

Fine-needle aspiration (FNA) biopsy technique is used most often in the transplant setting for analysis of immunologically activated cells. FNA is especially useful in evaluating acute rejection (33). FNA can also obtain material for culture. A modified FNA technique has been described for collection of glomeruli from either native or transplant kidneys to analyze glomerular lesions. This technique has limitations in sample size and is obviously not suitable for study of vascular, tubular, or interstitial processes. The less invasive nature of the procedure makes it amenable to serial monitoring of diffuse glomerular lesions in native or transplanted kidneys (34).

Complications

Important complications occur in 5 to 10% of patients (23,35–43). Major complications, usually bleeding, leading to nephrectomy occurred in five patients in a review of 8081 biopsies (41) and one patient in a series of 5120 biopsies. In a series totaling 1820 biopsies in children, one nephrectomy resulted (35–40). Transient microscopic hematuria is universal after biopsy, although macroscopic hematuria is seen in only 5.0% and requires transfusion in up to 2.3% of patients. Perirenal hematoma is most often asymptomatic and can be seen by computed tomography in up to 85% of biopsies. Symptomatic hematoma is rare, occurring in less than 2%. Arteriovenous fistulae are symptomatic with hematuria, hypertension, or cardiac failure in only 0.5% of biopsies, although bruits may be detected in as many as 75% of patients. Most fistulae heal within a few months. Other complications have been reported, including inadvertent puncture of other viscera or major renal vessels, sepsis, renal infection, and seeding of cancer. Death is rare, occurring in less than 0.1% in reviews of large series. Complication rates appear to be slightly higher in less developed countries (35,37). Complications for the spring-loaded needle biopsy system appear to be similar to conventional needles if the same gauge is used (44). Complications relate in part to the number of passes made to obtain tissue. Therefore, the lower rate of complication with an 18-gauge, spring-loaded needle in some studies is offset largely by the need for more passes for adequate samples and the distortion of tissue and edge artifact with use of an 18-gauge needle (see above).

ASSESSMENT OF THE RENAL BIOPSY

Adequacy of Sample

Cores of fat and connective tissue float when placed in saline, but a core of renal parenchyma sinks. The biopsy sample should also be visually inspected with a dissecting microscope or hand lens. Glomeruli are visualized as small red dots in the biopsy core. Scarred glomeruli may be difficult to identify because they are not perfused. In a diffuse disease, such as membranous glomerulonephritis, one glomerulus may be adequate for diagnosis. However, in other conditions (e.g., crescentic glomerulonephritis, FSGS, or lupus WHO class III glomerulonephritis), the lesions may be focal. The greater the number of glomeruli sampled, the lower the probability of missing a focally distributed lesion (45). If only 10% of glomeruli in the kidney are involved by the focal process, a biopsy sample of only ten glomeruli has a 35% probability of missing the lesion, decreasing to 12% if the biopsy contains 20 glomeruli. When one-fourth of glomeruli are involved in the kidney, there is only a 5% chance of missing the abnormal glomeruli in a biopsy of ten glomeruli. A biopsy of 20 to 25 glomeruli is sufficient to distinguish between mild disease (less than 20% of glomeruli involved), moderate disease (20 to 50% of glomeruli involved), or severe disease (more than 50% of glomeruli involved). However, the widespread use of small-gauge, spring-loaded biopsy needles often results in smaller samples, which make the above assessments of severity and extent of lesions difficult or impossible. The sample site must also be considered in evaluating the adequacy of tissue. Even a large biopsy consisting only of superficial glomeruli cannot exclude the presence of early FSGS in which the initial involvement is in the juxtamedullary glomeruli. Likewise, although nephronophthisis is most often diagnosed clinically, a juxtamedullary biopsy would be necessary for morphologic diagnosis.

Allotment of Tissue

Renal tissue should be studied by LM techniques with special stains [hematoxylin and eosin, modified silver stain (periodic acid and methenamine or Jones' stain), periodic acid-Schiff (PAS), IF, and EM] (26,27,46). The tissue is divided so that glomeruli are present in each portion of the sample. Optimally, the pathologist or an experienced histotechnologist attends the biopsy and inspects and allots tissue for each study. If this is impossible, tissue may be placed in saline and brought directly to the laboratory for prompt processing. It is important to handle the tissue gently so that artifacts do not occur. The fresh tissue must not be picked up with forceps because this crushes and distorts the morphology. The core can be handled carefully with a wooden stick or pipette. The core should not be placed on a sponge or gauze pad because this may cause a divot-like artifact as the unfixed tissue molds to the holes of the underlying surface. The biopsy specimen is therefore placed on a clean smooth surface, such as a wax board, for cutting.

It may be difficult to identify the cortical end of the specimen even after inspection with a hand lens or dissecting microscope when scarring or severe injury is present. Therefore, we recommend cutting two 1-mm pieces with a sharp blade from each end of the core for EM studies. The remaining core is then divided into specimens for IF and LM. Of note, use of an 18-gauge needle yields tissue cores that are too thin to divide lengthwise, leading to a greater chance of problems in allocation of tissue for each method of study. This tissue should be cut across into two pieces for IF and LM. When two cores are obtained, we prefer to duplicate this process, rather than allocating one complete core to one study to maximize chances of adequacy of tissue for each study. When the tissue sample obtained is very small, the nephrologist and the pathologist should consider the differential diagnosis and allocate tissue accordingly. For example, in a case of suspected IgA nephropathy, tissue for IF is most important. Although EM studies can be done on other portions of tissue (as long as mercury-based fixatives have not been used), IF studies cannot be done reliably on fixed tissue. When tissue for EM is inadequate, portions of the paraffin-embedded tissue left after LM examination may be cut out from the block and processed for EM. Although the quality is not optimal, diagnostic findings can still be discerned. In special circumstances, when no tissue remains in the paraffin block and a focal lesion in one section must be studied, one may attempt to process the tissue section from a glass slide for EM.

Light Microscopy

Numerous fixatives are used for LM examination, and they vary from institute to institute. Satisfactory results may be obtained with Zenker's, Bouin's, formalin, Carnoy's, or paraformaldehyde. Material for IF studies may be snap frozen immediately at 20°C in solutions of isopentane, dry ice, acetone, or freon and embedded in Tissue-tech, OCT, or other compounds for frozen sections. If tissue cannot immediately be snap frozen, it may be placed in Michel's tissue media, where it may be stored for up to 1 week before freezing. This allows tissue to be sent to reference laboratories for appropriate processing. Tissue for EM may be fixed in glutaraldehyde, formaldehyde, or other appropriate fixatives. Tissue placed in glutaraldehyde should be promptly processed or, if stored for future possible processing, should be transferred to an appropriate buffer solution within 1 week to avoid artifacts. Tissue for LM is routinely processed, embedded in paraffin, and cut into 2- to 3-μ thick sections and stained. Serial sections with multiple levels are then prepared for examination.

If water-soluble compounds are expected (e.g., as urate or uric acid), the tissue should be fixed in ethanol. Lipids are best detected in frozen sections because they are extracted during xylene processing for paraffin sections. Hematoxylin and eosin stains are most useful for overall assessment of the interstitium, allowing particularly good visualization of infiltrating cells, especially eosinophils. In addition, fibrin may be easily visualized by this stain. PAS stain accentuates basement membranes and matrix material and allows definition of the brush border of proximal tubular cells. Areas of hyalinosis and protein precipitation, including cryoglobulin, are also accentuated with PAS stain. The basement membrane and areas of deposits are best visualized by silver stain, usually the Jones' stain. Masson's trichrome stain may be used to accentuate areas of fibrosis and stains areas of collagen deposition bluish. Other special stains may be indicated. These include Congo red stain for amyloidosis and special stains for bacterial or fungal organisms and acid-fast bacilli. Special techniques may also be used on the LM material. These include polarization to detect crystals or foreign bodies and morphometry to assess glomerular size (see below) and severity of interstitial fibrosis quantitatively.

Immunofluorescence

IF studies are most commonly done by direct IF on frozen tissue sections, with application of fluorescein-conjugated antibodies directed against IgG, IgA, IgM, and complement component C3. Additional antisera may be used as clinically indicated. These include antisera to κ or λ light chain, antisera to hepatitis B antigen, thyroglobulin, fibrinogen, C1q, antisera to type IV collagen chains, and C4d. Some of these antigens are recognized by antisera even after fixation and can be detected by immunohistochemical techniques (e.g., immunoperoxidase) on the formalin-fixed tissue sections and then studied with a light microscope. This technique requires enzyme pretreatment of tissue, which must be tailored exactly depending on length and type of fixation, section thickness, and antigen one wishes to study. Direct observation of the digestion process, stopping when all plasma is removed from capillary loops, has been used to achieve reliable results (47). These challenges have prevented widespread use of this technique.

Frozen tissue sections stained by the commonly used method of fluorescein-conjugated antibodies are viewed by IF microscopy, evaluating staining in glomeruli, vessels, tubules, and interstitium. The pattern of glomerular staining is assessed to define granular or linear capillary basement staining or mesangial deposits. Arteriolar staining, especially with C3 in patients with hematuria, may be of diagnostic significance. Tubules may show deposits in lupus nephritis or light chain deposition disease. Nuclear staining can be seen in lupus or lupus-like diseases as a tissue manifestation of the patient's positive antinuclear antibodies. IF is more sensitive than EM in identifying immune deposits; however, EM provides more detailed information on the exact localization of those deposits (27,46). Lesions of interest should be photographed because fluorescence fades on storage and with light exposure.

Electron Microscopy

Tissue for EM is processed with postfixation in 1% osmium tetroxide, which enhances contrast of the tissue, and then dehydrated and embedded. With new, more rapidly polymerizing embedding media (e.g., Spurr), tissue may be ready for examination within 1 day. EM study was found to add information in 6 to 11% of renal biopsies in a study from 1983 (24). A more recent study showed that EM was needed to make a diagnosis in 21% of cases and provided important confirmatory data in approximately 20% of cases (27). EM showed diagnostic pathologic abnormalities in 18% of patients with normal LM findings. Larger, so-called thick sections (1 μ) are stained with toluidine blue to select smaller areas for thin sectioning for the electron microscope. Usually, the glomerulus containing the most representative lesion is chosen. If there are irregular or focal lesions, several glomeruli may be sampled. The 60- to 90-Å thin sections are stained with uranyl acetate and lead citrate before viewing to enhance contrast.

The characteristic immune deposits are denser than basement membrane or matrix materials. In specific diseases, such as cryoglobulinemia, amyloid, immunotactoid or fibrillary glomerulopathies, or lupus nephritis, specific substructure of deposits may be seen. Specific localization of immune complexes is done by EM examination, indicating whether deposits are subendothelial, subepithelial, mesangial, or in all of the above compartments. In some diseases, such as light chain deposition disease or lupus nephritis, deposition may also be seen in vessels and tubules. So-called fingerprint deposits, with substructures reminiscent of fingerprinting, are present in some cases of lupus nephritis. Reticular aggregates (or so-called tubular arrays) of membrane material in endothelial cell cytoplasm throughout the body are characteristically seen in large numbers in patients with SLE or human immunodeficiency virus (HIV) infection and are believed to reflect a response to high levels of interferon (46,48).

EM also delineates specific basement membrane abnormalities. For instance, small subepithelial deposits without surrounding new basement membrane material do not result in spikes and, therefore, cannot be visualized by Jones' stain on LM but can still be detected directly by EM. The lamina densa of the GBM is markedly thickened in diabetic nephropathy. Circumferential mesangial interposition is defined by extension of monocytes and mesangial cell cytoplasm into the subendothelial space, with newly formed basement membrane interpositioning between the advancing mesangial cells and the endothelium, thus providing the classic double contours with silver stain seen by LM in MPGN. Increased lucent material is present in the lamina rara interna in transplant glomerulopathy, HUS, toxemia, and other diseases presumed to involve coagulopathy. In these conditions, deposition of fibrin, fibrinogen, and their degradation products may also occur. Fibrin is recognizable by its dense, coarse, sheaf-like structure, with periodicity observed in favorable sections. Morphometry of the GBM from EM prints is used to diagnose thin basement membranes in hereditary nephritides. EM also allows structural assessment of changes of specific cells (see below). Diagnostic inclusions are seen in various storage or metabolic diseases (e.g., Fabry's disease).

BASIC RENAL LESIONS

Normal

The normal glomerulus consists of a complex branching network of capillaries originating at the afferent arteriole and draining into the efferent arteriole. The glomerulus contains three resident cell types: mesangial, endothelial, and epithelial cells (Fig. 24.1). The epithelial cells cover the urinary surface of the GBM with pseudopod-like extensions called *foot processes* with intervening filtration slits. Endothelial cells are opposed to the inner surface of the GBM and are fenestrated. At the stalk of the capillary, the endothelial cell is separated from the mesangial cells by intervening mesangial matrix. Because the endothelial cell nucleus most often lies in this stalk region, it may be difficult to distinguish from the mesangial cell nucleus by LM. The term *endocapillary* is used to describe proliferation filling up the capillary lumen, contributed to by proliferation of mesangial, endothelial, and infiltrating inflammatory cells. In contrast, *extracapillary proliferation* refers to proliferation of the parietal epithelial cells that line Bowman's capsule.

The mesangial cell is a contractile cell that also has phagocytic properties. It lies embedded in the mesangial matrix in the stalk region of the capillary loops, attached to anchor sites at the ends of the loop by thin extensions of its cytoplasm. Normally, up to three mesangial cell nuclei per lobule are present. The basement membrane consists of three layers distinct by EM, the central broadest lamina densa, and the less electron-dense zones of lamina rara externa and interna. Thickening occurs with maturational growth. Most investigators have found thicker basement membranes in boys, with normal range from 220 to 260

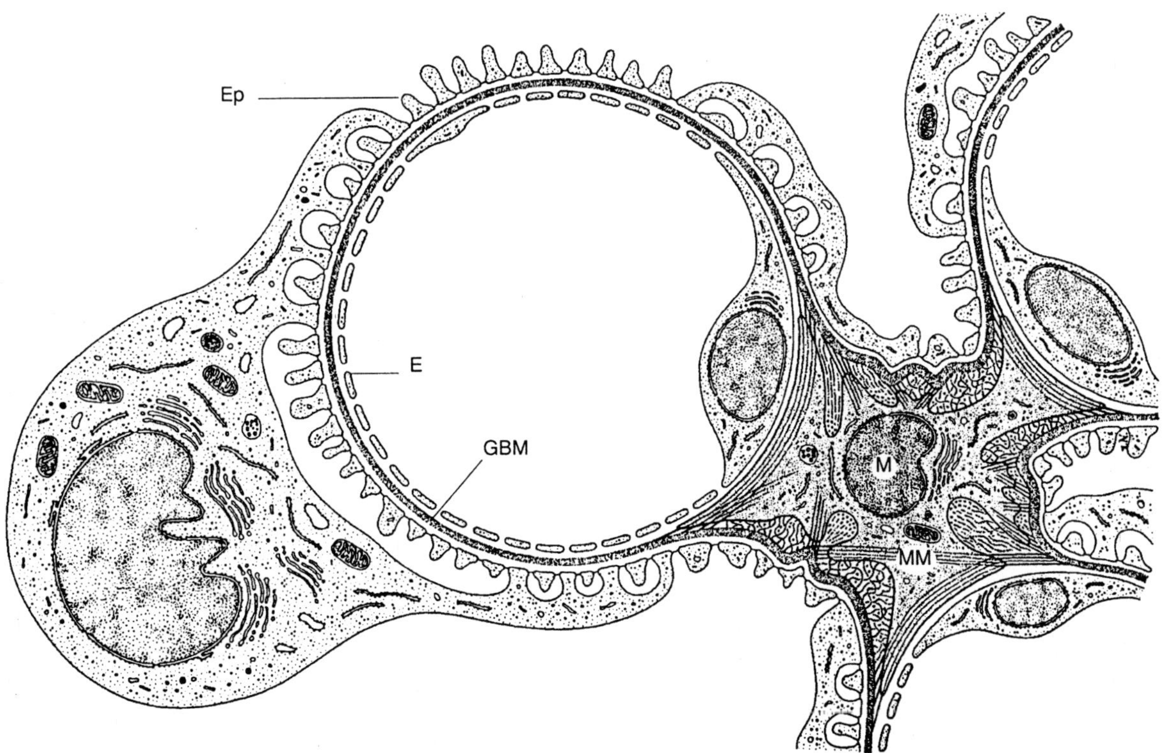

FIGURE 24.1. Schematic illustration of glomerulus with glomerular capillary attached to a mesangial stalk area. The glomerular endothelium (E) is fenestrated and lines the glomerular basement membrane (GBM), which covers the mesangium. The outside of the GBM is covered by the epithelial cell and its foot processes (Ep). The mesangial cell (M) is embedded within the mesangial matrix (MM), with processes connecting to the GBM. (Courtesy of Professor Wilhelm Kriz. From Venkatachalam MA, Kriz W. Anatomy of the kidney. In: Heptinstall RH, ed. *Pathology of the kidney*, 4th ed. Boston: Little, Brown and Company, 1992:1:35, with permission.)

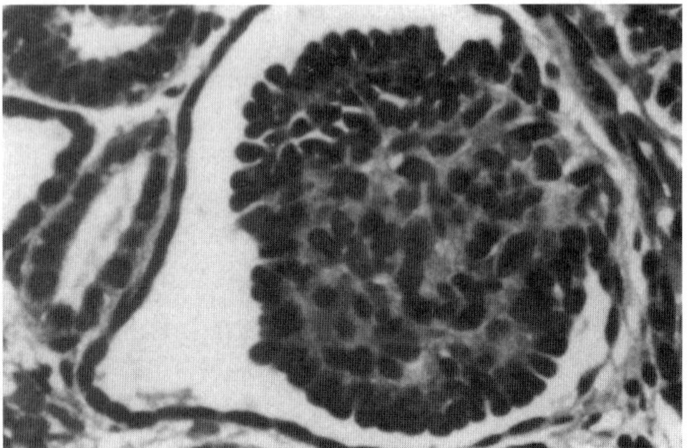

FIGURE 24.2. Immature glomerulus with plump, dark epithelial cells from biopsy of a baby at 29 weeks' gestation (periodic acid-Schiff stain, ×670).

nm at 1 year of age, 280 to 327 nm at 5 years of age, 329 to 370 nm at 10 years of age, and 358 to 399 nm at 15 years of age (49,50). In our laboratory, we found a range of GBM thickness in children with normal kidneys from approximately 110 nm at 1 year of age to 222 ± 14 nm at 7 years of age.

The glomerulus is surrounded by Bowman's capsule, which is lined by parietal epithelial cells. These are continuous with the proximal tubule, identifiable by its PAS-positive brush border. The efferent and afferent arterioles can be distinguished morphologically in favorably oriented sections or by tracing their origins on serial sections. Segmental, interlobular, and arcuate arteries may also be present in the renal biopsy specimen. The cortical biopsy also allows assessment of the tubulointerstitium. Proximal tubules are readily identified by their PAS-positive brush border lacking in the distal tubules. Collecting ducts show cuboidal, cobblestone-like epithelium. The medulla may also be included in the biopsy.

During fetal maturation, the glomerular capillary tufts are initially covered by large, cuboidal, darkly staining epithelial cells with only small lumina visible (Fig. 24.2). The cells lining Bowman's space undergo a similar change from initial tall columnar to cuboidal to flattened epithelial cells, except for those located at the opening of the proximal tubule, where cells remain taller. Immature nephrons may occasionally be seen in the superficial cortex of children up to 1 year of age. Glomerular growth continues until adulthood, with average normal glomerular diameter approximately 95 μ in a group of patients younger than 5 years of age (average age, 2.2 years) and 140 to 160 μ in adulthood (51,52).

Overall Pattern

Assessment of the biopsy specimen must include inspection of all sections from different levels because additional glomeruli may be sampled on deeper cuts of the biopsy core and many diseases are characterized by focal lesions. Assessment of severity and patterns of lesions is made, and normal and affected glomeruli are counted. Lesions are classified as focal if only some glomeruli are involved, diffuse if all glomeruli are involved, segmental if only portions of glomeruli are involved, and global if entire glomerular tufts are involved. Characteristic glomerular disease patterns include lobular proliferation in MPGN, nodular proliferation of mesangial matrix material with paucicellular areas in characteristic Kimmelstiel-Wilson lesions, focal and segmental sclerosis, and crescent formation (Table 24.1). The *crescent*, or proliferation of parietal epithelial cells, owes its name to its shape in well-established lesions. Fibrin and thrombosis are best assessed by Jones' stain.

Glomeruli are assessed for alterations in size (see below). It is important to compare with a normal control for a given age group because glomerular maturational growth is rapid in children. Glomerular hypertrophy may be an important predictor of increased risk of FSGS in children with apparent MCD (see below). Maturational pattern of glomeruli (see above) should be noted.

Glomeruli are assessed for glomerulosclerosis (i.e., the presence of segmental obliteration and scarring of glomerular capillary tufts). Sclerosis may be in a segmental or global pattern (Table 24.2). Previous studies suggested that up to 10% of glomeruli are normally globally sclerosed in people younger than 40 years of age (53). More recent work suggests that this number may be even smaller in children, with less than 1 to 3% global sclerosis expected normally up to age 40 or 56 years, respectively (54,55). These occasional globally sclerotic glomeruli are believed to represent errors of nephrogenesis. The incidence of global sclerosis increases with aging, up to half the patient's age minus 10 (55). Globally sclerosed glomeruli in a greater percentage indicate the possibility of renal disease (focal global sclerosis) (56).

The pattern of tubulointerstitial fibrosis, whether proportional to glomerular sclerosis, whether diffuse or present in a striped pattern after the medullary rays or in broad patchy zones, has diagnostic significance (see below).

Specific Glomerular Cells

Podocytes

The podocytes (glomerular visceral epithelial cells) may show vacuolization in various diseases with severe proteinuria. Although more extensive vacuolization of podocytes has been seen in FSGS compared with patients with MCD (57), these changes are seen only after established sclerotic lesions are identifiable by LM and do not permit distinction of these two disease processes in the early phase in which segmental sclerosis may be undetected. Hypertrophy of podocytes is prominent in MCD and FSGS. Effacement of the foot processes of the podocytes by EM is common to any disease with marked proteinuria, and the podocyte may also show microvillous transformation with long, attenuated pseudo-

TABLE 24.2. CHARACTERISTIC ABNORMALITIES OF GLOMERULAR DISEASES

Disease and typical clinical presentation	Light microscopy pattern	Immunofluorescence staining			EM, other findings
		Mesangial	Subepithelial	Subendothelial	
Hematuria/nephritis					
Alport's syndrome	Early: normal Late: sclerosis	–	–	–	Thin, split GBM
Lupus WHO class II (mesangial)	Normal or mesangial proliferation	+ All Igs, C3, C1q	–	–	Immune deposits by EM, reticular aggregates in endothelial cells
Lupus WHO class III (focal proliferative)	Proliferative, <50% of glomeruli	+	+ (few) All Igs, C3, C1q	+ (scattered)	Immune deposits by EM, reticular aggregates in endothelial cells
Lupus WHO IV (diffuse proliferative)	Proliferative, >50% of glomeruli	+	+ All Igs, C3, C1q	+ (wire loop)	Immune deposits by EM, reticular aggregates in endothelial cells
IgA nephropathy	Mesangial proliferation	+ Predominantly IgA	–	–	Immune deposits by EM
Henoch-Schönlein purpura	Mesangial proliferation, crescents	+	+/– Predominantly IgA	+/–	Immune deposits by EM
Postinfectious GN	Hypercellular, PMNs, endocapillary proliferation	+/–	+ Coarsely granular IgG, C3	–	Irregular, hump-like deposits on top of GBM by EM
Hemolytic-uremic syndrome	Arteriolar/glomerular thrombosis	–	–	–	Increased lucency and thickness of lamina rara interna by EM, swollen endothelial cells, no deposits by EM
MPGN I	Hypercellular, lobular double contour GBM	+	–	+ IgG, C3	Subendothelial, intramembranous immune deposits by EM, circumferential mesangial interposition
MPGN II (dense deposit disease)	Hypercellular, +/– lobular, ribbon-like capillary wall	± C3	Ribbon-like, discontinuous C3		Intramembranous nonimmune dense deposits by EM
Nephrotic syndrome					
Minimal change disease	Normal	–	–	–	Effacement of epithelial cell foot processes, no deposits by EM
Focal segmental glomerulosclerosis	Segmental glomerulosclerosis, glomerular hypertrophy	+/– IgM, C3	–	–	Effacement of epithelial cell foot processes, no deposits by EM
Diabetic nephropathy	Increased mesangial matrix, +/– nodular, thick GBM, hyalinized arterioles	–	–	–	Thick GBM without deposits
Lupus WHO class V (membranous)	Spikes on Jones' stain	Few	+ All Igs, C3, C4	–	Immune deposits by EM, reticular aggregates in endothelial cells
Idiopathic membranous GN	Spikes on Jones' stain	–	+ IgG, C3	–	Immune deposits by EM
Rapidly progressive glomerulonephritis					
Anti-GBM disease	Focal segmental necrosis of glomeruli, crescents	–	Linear IgG		No deposits by EM
Wegener's granulomatosis	Focal segmental necrosis of glomeruli, crescents	–	–	–	No deposits by EM
Microscopic polyangiitis	Focal segmental necrosis of glomeruli, crescents	–	–	–	No deposits by EM

+, present; –, absent; +/–, variably present; EM, electron microscopy; Ig, immunoglobulin; GBM, glomerular basement membrane; GN, glomerulonephritis; MPGN, membranoproliferative glomerulonephritis; PMNs, polymorphonuclear neutrophils; WHO, World Health Organization.

pods. Podocytes are limited in their ability to proliferate. However, the early sclerotic lesion of FSGS is characterized by prominence and apparent increase of the overlying podocytes often associated with endocapillary foam cells. The collapsing variant of FSGS or HIV-associated nephropathy both show prominent hyperplasia and protein droplets of the podocytes overlying segmental collapse of the glomerular capillary tuft. In the situation of recurrent FSGS in the renal transplant, NS and foot process effacement may be seen within weeks after biopsy, with sclerosis becoming apparent at a later date (58). In Fabry's disease, there is accumulation of glycosphingolipid because of deficiency of α-galactosidase. Podocytes show marked vacuolization by LM with characteristic whorled, laminated, electron-dense myelin bodies by EM. In Fabry's disease, these inclusions may also be present in endothelial cells, tubular epithelial cells, and some interstitial cells (24,46).

Mesangial Cells

Hyperplasia of mesangial cells is recognized by LM when more than three mesangial cell nuclei are present per mesangial region. Increased mesangial prominence may be due to increased cellularity, increased matrix, deposits, or a combination. Large mesangial deposits appear on Jones' stain as pinkish areas surrounded by the light silver-staining areas of mesangial matrix. So-called mesangial interposition results when the monocyte or mesangial cell cytoplasm extends outward between basement membrane and endothelial cells and new matrix accumulates between the mesangial and endothelial cell bodies.

Endothelial Cells

Extreme proliferation and swelling of endothelial cells can obliterate capillary lumina in conditions characterized by abnormalities of coagulation. Endothelial cells usually contain characteristic reticular aggregates in lupus nephritis and HIV-associated nephropathy (46,48). Endocapillary cell proliferation is characteristic of, for example, diffuse proliferative lupus nephritis and MPGN type I.

Crescents

Crescents consist primarily of proliferating parietal epithelial cells with some infiltrating macrophages and are a manifestation of severe glomerular injury. The name reflects the often crescent-shaped sheet of cells filling up part or nearly all of Bowman's space. Crescents result from injuries that break the GBM, leading to exudation of plasma protein and formation of fibrin within Bowman's space, which then induces proliferation of the parietal epithelial cells and infiltration of macrophages. When crescents are a prominent histologic feature, the patient most often presents clinically with a rapidly progressive glomerulonephritis.

Crescents may occur in a variety of diseases. Diseases with crescents as a primary manifestation include antibody-mediated injury (anti-GBM antibody disease), immune-complex diseases (e.g., lupus nephritis), and nonimmune diseases. The latter are often, but not invariably, associated with positive ANCA tests and may be associated with systemic disease or be renally limited. The perinuclear ANCA pattern is most often associated with microscopic polyangiitis, whereas the cytoplasmic ANCA pattern is typical in Wegener's granulomatosis. Of note, positive ANCA tests are not sensitive in distinguishing these categories (13–15). Renal biopsy is, therefore, critical for accurate diagnosis. Diagnosis and appropriate treatment must occur rapidly in this clinical situation to optimize chances of recovery of renal function. The early lesion of cellular crescents is responsive to cytotoxic therapy. Biopsy indications of irreversible renal damage include breaks of Bowman's capsule and fibrous transformation of the cellular crescents, periglomerular fibrosis, and scarred glomeruli and tubulointerstitium.

Glomerular Basement Membrane

GBM abnormalities are best evaluated by EM. The basement membrane is abnormally thick in diabetic nephropathy (46). Diffuse, abnormally thin GBMs, less than 250 nm in adults, are seen in familial hematuria (49–50). In children, the diagnosis of thin basement membranes is more difficult than in adults because GBM increases in thickness with normal maturation. GBM thickness should be compared with normal for age and sex (see above) (49,59,60). In Alport's syndrome, the basement membrane is characterized by irregular thickness, either very thin or very thick, with splitting and splintering of the basement membrane (22,61). The GBM in nail-patella syndrome is irregular, thickened, and split, with electron-lucent areas containing banded collagen type I fibers (46).

Immune deposits may localize on either side of the GBM. Subepithelial immune deposits are characteristically seen in membranous glomerulonephritis. Subendothelial immune deposits are seen, for example, in lupus proliferative nephritis or MPGN type I.

The basement membrane may appear split by LM in diseases other than MPGN type I or dense deposit disease. In transplant glomerulopathy, the split appearance results from varying degrees of mesangial interposition and widening with increased lucent material in the lamina rara interna. This is also a characteristic finding in preeclampsia, transplant glomerulopathy, and chronic HUS (46).

Tubules

Morphologically evident tubular necrosis correlates poorly with the clinical extent of acute tubular necrosis. The changes vary from nondiagnostic vacuolization to frank necrosis with sloughing of tubular epithelial cells and flattened epithelium characteristic of regeneration (24). In cortical necrosis, zones of cortex, including glomerular structures, are necrotic. Tubules are atrophied with dilation and flattened epithelium in chronic renal disease, presumably secondary to lesions affecting the glomerulus, although inherent interstitial factors may also be involved in these changes. Tubular atrophy is also present in primary tubulointerstitial diseases. Tubulointerstitial fibrosis is an important manifestation of cyclosporine toxicity. The fibrosis occurs along the medullary rays, resulting in a striped, rather than diffuse, pattern of fibrosis, with intervening preserved tubules.

Nonspecific casts of Tamm-Horsfall protein are seen in chronic renal disease. Other casts may have a diagnostic appearance, such as the giant cells surrounding tubular casts in light chain cast nephropathy (so-called myeloma kidney). Casts of myoglobin with characteristic reddish-brown appearance are seen in rhabdomyolysis, often with associated acute tubular necrosis. Crystals (e.g., oxalate) may be identified by examination under polarized light. Tubules contain characteristic inclusions in Fabry's disease.

Polymorphonuclear neutrophils within collecting ducts and proximal tubules are diagnostic of acute pyelonephritis. In chronic pyelonephritis, there is tubular atrophy and interstitial fibrosis, characteristically in a patchy, regional distribution. The combination of segmental glomerular sclerosis with ischemic changes of corrugation and thickening of the GBM and periglomerular fibrosis and patchy, regional interstitial fibrosis and tubular atrophy is characteristic of reflux nephropathy (62).

Cysts may be demonstrated by biopsy, although the diagnosis of specific cystic diseases is usually made by combination of clinical and ultrasound findings. The segment of the nephron giving rise to the cysts can be identified by histochemical stains (63). Areas of low cuboidal epithelial-lined structures surrounded by a cuff of immature mesenchyme are present in the dysplastic kidney, often with cartilage, fat, or abnormal blood vessels in the interstitium. The deep medullary cystic dilation characteristic of nephronophthisis can be identified with a deep biopsy. Dilation of proximal tubules with microcyst formation in conjunction with sclerosis is characteristic of congenital NS of Finnish type. FSGS in a collapsing pattern with podocyte hyperplasia, numerous reticular aggregates by EM, and tubular cystic dilation and interstitial fibrosis out of proportion to the severity of glomerular lesions is highly suggestive of HIV-associated nephropathy (48).

Interstitium

Interstitial edema is a nonspecific change present, for example, in early acute transplant rejection, renal vein thrombosis, or inflammatory processes. Identification of eosinophils in an infiltrate is suggestive of drug-induced interstitial nephritis, although eosinophils are also present in some cases of idiopathic interstitial nephritis (64). Eosinophils can also be part of acute cellular rejection in the transplant. Nonnecrotizing granulomas, with or without eosinophils, most often reflect drug-induced hypersensitivity reaction. Fibrosis results in increased spacing of tubules because of the accumulation of PAS-positive collagenous material. The connective tissue also stains specifically blue with Masson's trichrome stain. Fibrosis in a striped pattern suggests chronic cyclosporine toxicity (65,66). Occasionally, the interstitium is infiltrated by malignancy. Hematopoietic neoplasms are especially prone to involve the kidney.

Vessels

Arterioles and larger segmental and interlobular arteries are evaluated for changes in the intima and media; the presence of deposits, fibrin, hyalin, amyloid, or other material; or the presence of vasculitis. Larger vessels typically are not sampled by a biopsy, and diseases that affect these large vessels (e.g., classic polyarteritis nodosa) are, therefore, best evaluated by other methods (e.g., arteriography). Intimal fibrosis and medial thickening with hyperplasia and hypertrophy of media are characteristic of hypertensive injury. Specific eccentric patterns of medial necrosis with nodular protein deposition suggest acute cyclosporine nephrotoxicity (66). Fibrin thrombi, when present in glomeruli or arterioles, are the essential lesions of the thrombotic microangiopathies (e.g., HUS) (46). Fibrin localizes predominantly within glomerular lumina in disseminated intravascular coagulation and hyperacute rejection.

CLINICAL PATHOLOGIC CORRELATIONS

After evaluation of the structural changes of the renal biopsy in conjunction with the clinical history, a diagnosis may be obvious. In some cases, the biopsy specimen may show overlap features, or there may be elements that do not correlate clearly with the clinical setting. Close collaboration by nephrologists and pathologists is essential in arriving at the diagnosis. The pathologist must be familiar with clinical manifestations of renal disease, and the nephrologist should be familiar with the terminology used by the pathologist to describe the biopsy findings (Table 24.2).

When lesions are evaluated, the balance of all elements must be considered. When a typical disease pattern is not present, one must consider whether more than one process is taking place. For instance, drug-induced interstitial nephritis may be superimposed on other glomerular disease. This is especially true in the transplant setting in which multiple disease processes may occur at one time. In some instances, the biopsy findings do not correlate with the patient's renal function. When such apparent discrepancies are found, one possibility is that the biopsy specimen is not representative of all the nephrons of the kidney. The number of glomeruli necessary to estimate the severity of diseases that show focal distribution has been discussed above. However, the extent of glomerulosclerosis may in and of itself not correlate with renal function. Tubulointerstitial atrophy and fibrosis may be more closely correlated with extent of renal damage and renal function (67–69). One must also consider the elements other than structure that influence the patient's renal function (i.e., blood pressure, filtration properties of the GBM, and the glomerular filtering surface area). Patients with enlarged glomeruli, either caused by compensatory hypertrophy or by a primary pathologic process, may show less deterioration of renal function than expected based on the extent of glomerular scarring. Similarly, treatment of the patient with antihypertensive agents that affect glomerular filtration rate (e.g., angiotensin-converting enzyme inhibitors, which preferentially dilate efferent arterioles) may actually increase serum creatinine levels in the short term. Compensation by remaining nephrons may mask ongoing severe disease processes such that creatinine levels may remain near normal until late in the course of disease when therapy is less likely to have an impact on chronic progressive injury.

Diagnostic Findings in Selected Renal Diseases

Minimal Change Disease and Focal Segmental Glomerulosclerosis

MCD is diagnosed only after the exclusion of abnormal findings at the LM level, with diffuse foot process effacement as the only abnormality by EM. The disease is characteristically sensitive to glucocorticoid therapy. However, repeated renal biopsies in patients with apparent MCD initially have shown progression to FSGS, which has a high incidence of progression to end-stage renal disease (70,71). As discussed above, a small sample may not include the segmentally sclerotic glomerulus diagnostic of FSGS. In FSGS, there is often also hyalinosis, an insudation of plasma proteins and lipids with a glassy, smooth (hyaline) appearance on LM. There are no immune deposits, and foot process effacement is present in all glomeruli by EM (Fig. 24.3). Mesangial expansion in the native kidney biopsy may be associated with increased risk for recurrence in the transplant (72).

The presence of IgM in a biopsy that otherwise appears to be MCD (so-called IgM nephropathy) does not have prognostic value (73). Some variants of FSGS may have prognostic value (74). A recently proposed working classification of FSGS aims to examine whether morphologic patterns of FSGS have prognostic implications (Table 24.3) (75). The usual type is diagnosed when no special features are present. The collapsing type of FSGS—characterized by collapse of the glomerular tuft, either segmental or global with associated podocyte hypertrophy and/or hyperplasia—shows a rapid progression to end-stage disease (76). The cellular lesion, with endocapillary proliferation with frequent foam cells and often with podocyte hyperplasia, may represent an early stage of FSGS (77). The tip lesion (i.e., sclerosis localized to the proximal tubular pole) may have a better prognosis (78). The perihilar variant, with sclerosis and hyalinosis localized to the vascular pole, likely more often represents a secondary sclerosing process.

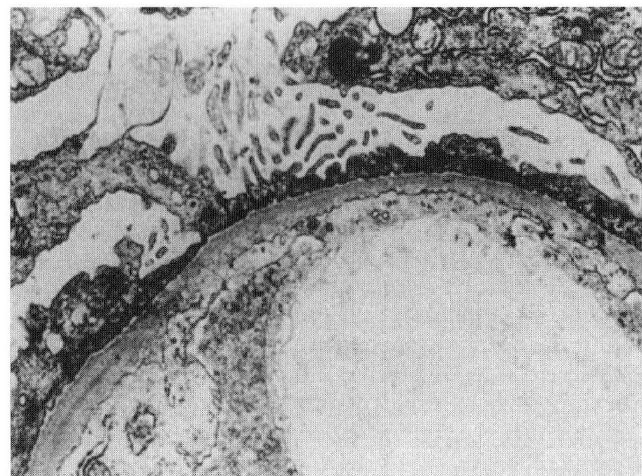

FIGURE 24.3. Minimal change disease. The foot processes are flattened and appear fused (×11,000).

C1q nephropathy is characterized by either no sclerosis or segmental glomerulosclerosis by LM, with mesangial C1q deposits and lesser Ig components without dominant or codominant IgA (79). EM shows mesangial and paramesangial dense deposits but a lack of reticular aggregates. Patients typically are adolescents, have steroid-resistant NS, and do not have clinical evidence of SLE. Although these

TABLE 24.3. WORKING CLASSIFICATION OF FOCAL SEGMENTAL GLOMERULOSCLEROSIS (FSGS)

Type	Key histologic feature	Possible prognostic implication
FSGS, not otherwise specified	Segmental sclerosis	Typical course
Collapsing FSGS	Collapse of tuft, GVEC hyperplasia	Poor prognosis
Cellular FSGS	Endocapillary proliferation, often GVEC hyperplasia	?Early stage lesion
Tip lesion	Sclerosis of tuft at proximal tubule pole	?Better prognosis
Perihilar variant	Sclerosis and hyalinosis at vascular pole	?May reflect a secondary type of FSGS

GVEC, glomerular visceral epithelial cell.

findings suggest a distinct clinicopathologic entity, the prognostic significance of these lesions has not yet been established. Progression to end-stage renal disease has occurred in some patients with sclerosis at biopsy, but long-term outcome of those without sclerosis at presentation has not yet been established.

Because therapy and prognosis are different for MCD versus FSGS, early distinction of these two entities is of primary interest. We studied pediatric patients with steroid-resistant NS and MCD on renal biopsies and compared them to patients with apparent MCD on biopsy who subsequently progressed to overt FSGS (51). Morphometric analysis of initial biopsies showed that glomerular size at the onset of disease, before sclerosis was apparent, was remarkably larger in patients who subsequently progressed to FSGS (Fig. 24.4) (80,81). There was a higher risk for development of FSGS in patients younger than 5 years of age with glomerular area greater than 1.5 times that of normal age-matched controls. On the other hand, glomerular size equal to or less than normal controls in this group of patients indicated a good prognosis. Calculated glomerular diameter for increased risk of FSGS in these patients younger than 5 years of age was more than 118 μ versus 95 μ glomerular diameter in age-matched controls. Depending on processing and fixation, these values may vary (our values are based on paraffin-embedded tissue fixation in formalin or Zenker's fixative). Normal ranges should be established in each laboratory assessing glomerular size.

From these studies, abnormal glomerular enlargement suggests a high probability of development of FSGS in pediatric patients with apparent MCD. Causes of abnormal glomerular enlargement other than idiopathic FSGS (e.g., diabetes mellitus, cyanotic cardiovascular disease, and massive obesity) must be excluded before such inferences can be made. It is interesting to note that the incidence of FSGS may be increased in these diseases. The association of abnormal glomerular growth with development of glomerulosclerosis may reflect a pathogenic linkage in that processes leading to excess matrix and sclerosis may be manifested as glomerular growth. This view is supported by the coexistence of these two processes in many other diseases, including sickle cell diseases, HIV infection, and reflux nephropathy (82).

Recently, specific gene mutations of podocyte-specific genes have been identified in some forms of familial FSGS. A gene for autosomal dominant FSGS has now been localized to ACTN-4 at chromosome 19q13. ACTN-4 encodes alpha-actinin-4, and a gain-of-function mutation with possible altered actin cytoskeleton interactions has been proposed (83). The prognosis of this form of familial FSGS has been poor, with progression to renal disease in 50% of patients by age 30 years. Recurrence in the transplant has been very rare in autosomal dominant forms of FSGS. Autosomal recessive FSGS with early onset and rapid progression to end stage is caused by mutations in NPHS2, which encodes podocin (84). Podocin is expressed only in podocytes and is an integral stomatin protein family member. Its function is not determined. Mutations in NPHS2 have been described in sporadic steroid-resistant FSGS. In both autosomal dominant and autosomal recessive forms of FSGS, there is genetic heterogeneity. These familial forms do not have specific morphologic features of the segmental sclerosis.

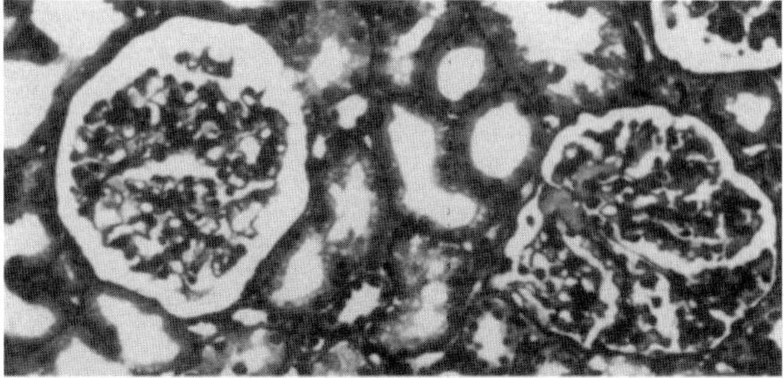

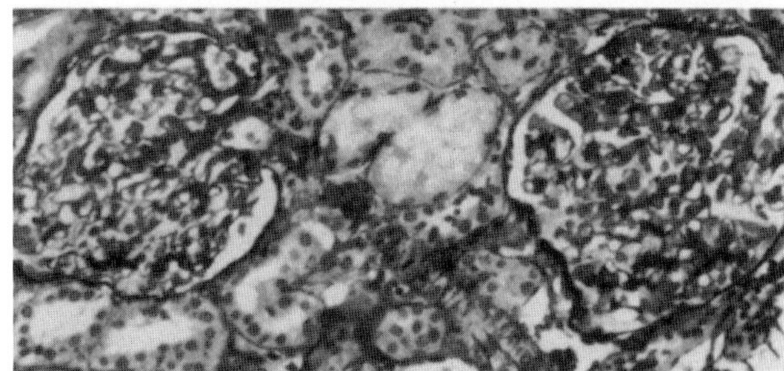

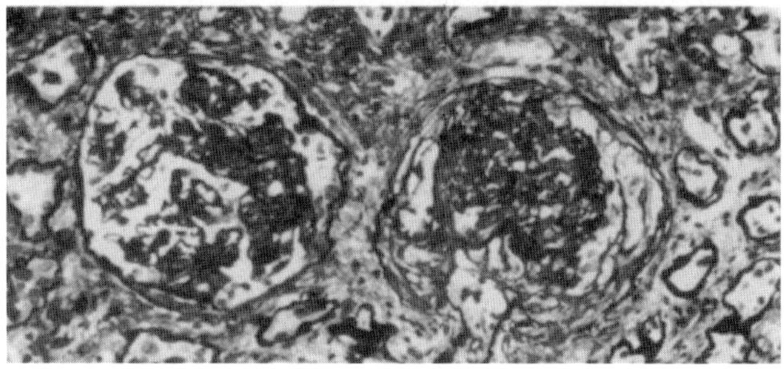

FIGURE 24.4. Apparent minimal change disease (MCD) with subsequent progression to focal segmental glomerulosclerosis (FSGS). The first biopsy from this 5-year-old girl **(middle)** was indistinguishable from MCD, except for marked glomerular hypertrophy versus age-matched typical MCD with subsequent benign clinical course **(top)**. The patient's later biopsy **(bottom)**, 50 months later, showed segmental sclerosis, diagnostic of FSGS (Jones' stain, ×160).

In contrast, congenital NS of Finnish type shows mesangial hypercellularity or no glomerular lesion, along with dilated proximal tubules by LM. The gene, NPHS1, also located in the 19q13 region, codes for nephrin and is mutated in this disease (85). Nephrin localizes to the slit diaphragm of the podocyte and is tightly associated with CD2-associated protein. Nephrin is believed to function as a zona occludens–type junction protein. CD2-associated protein plays a crucial role in receptor patterning and cytoskeletal polarity, and its absence resulted in sclerosis and foot process effacement in mice, supporting a role for CD2-associated protein in the function of the slit diaphragm. The slit diaphragms are crucial for regula-

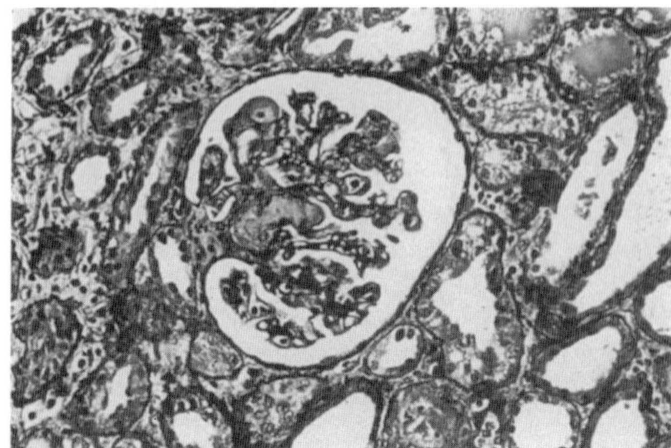

FIGURE 24.5. Arteriolar fibrin thrombi with minor areas of thrombi in capillary loops in hemolytic uremic syndrome (Jones' stain, ×270).

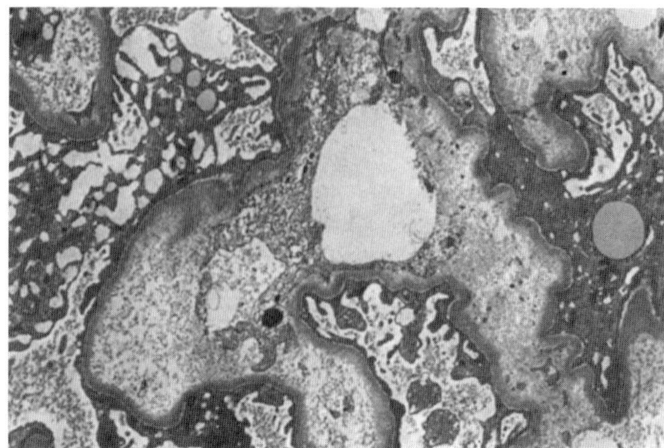

FIGURE 24.6. Hemolytic uremic syndrome. The lamina rara interna (endothelial side of the glomerular basement membrane) is widened with increased lucent material. No immune deposits are present (×3300).

tion of permselectivity and are decreased in density in proteinuric conditions.

FSGS associated with mitochondrial cytopathy, due to a mutation of mitochondrial DNA in tRNAleu(UUR), may show multinucleated podocytes and have abnormal mitochondria by EM examination. Patients also have unusual hyaline lesions in the arterioles. Some patients with FSGS without full-blown features of mitochondrial cytopathy (e.g., myopathy, stroke, encephalopathy, occasionally diabetes mellitus, hearing problems, and cardiomyopathy) have also been reported to have this mitochondrial mutation (86).

Hemolytic-Uremic Syndrome

HUS is the most common disease in children that is manifested by injury to the microvasculature. In adults, thrombotic thrombocytopenic purpura and postpartum renal failure may produce similar morphologic changes. By LM, thrombi in glomeruli and arterioles are present (Fig. 24.5). The renal biopsy findings, rather than clinical parameters, have recently been found to best predict long-term prognosis (87). Patients with cortical necrosis have a particularly ominous prognosis. The extent of glomerular versus arteriolar involvement is also of prognostic significance. Generally, both the long-term prognosis and the clinical presentation are more severe if larger vessels are involved. Arterial involvement was not seen in biopsies performed during the first 2 weeks of hospitalization (88). The glomerular endothelium is markedly swollen, nearly occluding capillary lumina. Fibrin thrombi are visualized easily. With chronicity, these areas may progress to segmental collapse with sclerosis, especially when arterioles are involved. The arterioles can become completely occluded by thrombi, with necrosis of vessel walls. IF shows occasional nonspecific entrapment of C3 and IgM in collapsed areas with fibrin and fibrinogen. EM shows extreme swelling of the glomerular endothelium with increased lucent material in the lamina rara interna of the basement membrane with entrapped platelets, fibrin, and red cell fragments without immune deposits (Fig. 24.6). *De novo* thrombotic microangiopathy in the renal transplant is indistinguishable morphologically from HUS in the native kidney. Cyclosporine and FK506 have both been implicated in its pathogenesis (89,90). For further discussion of HUS, see Chapter 47.

Henoch-Schönlein Purpura and Immunoglobulin A Nephropathy

Henoch-Schönlein purpura is often viewed as the systemic variant of IgA nephropathy (Berger's disease) (4,91). The glomerular manifestations are similar, with mild to moderate mesangial proliferation with predominance or codominance of mesangial IgA by IF studies. IgG, IgM, and C3 deposits may also be detected. The Ig deposits are present diffusely, even in glomeruli that appear normal by LM.

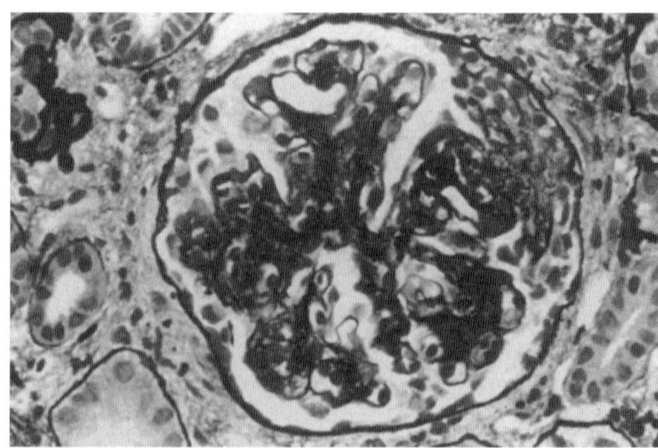

FIGURE 24.7. Mesangial prominence, segmental sclerosis, and small organizing crescent with adhesion in Henoch-Schönlein purpura. Immunofluorescence demonstrated immunoglobulin A mesangial deposits (Jones' stain, ×430).

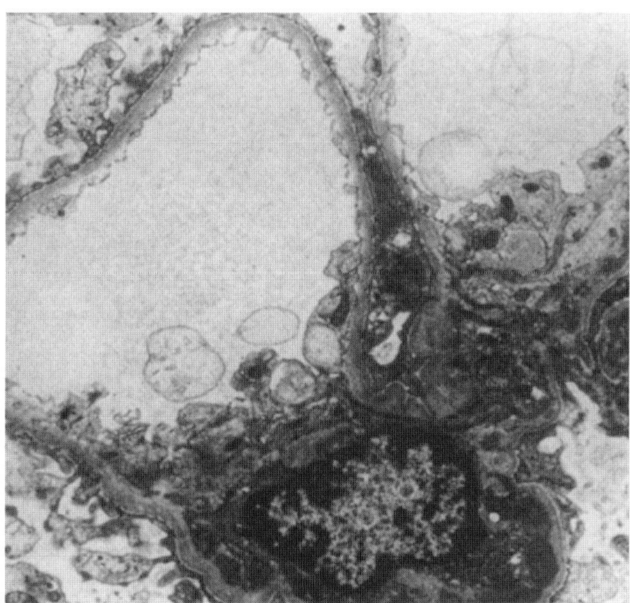

FIGURE 24.8. Dense deposits surrounding mesangial cell in Henoch-Schönlein purpura (×3400).

Early lesions show predominantly mesangial hypercellularity, with more prominence of matrix and even segmental sclerosis with progressive disease (92) (Fig. 24.7). In severe cases, there may be necrosis of glomerular tufts with crescents in Bowman's space. By EM, electron-dense mesangial deposits are present, with occasional spillover of deposits to subendothelial regions in the regions adjacent to the mesangium (Fig. 24.8). Deposits are decreased when clinical remission occurs (93). In Henoch-Schönlein purpura, deposits are often present in subepithelial areas as well as associated with more severe glomerular lesions, including crescents, and worse outcome (92). Classification schemas analogous to those for lupus nephritis have been proposed (94,95). For further discussion of Henoch-Schönlein purpura and IgA nephropathy, see Chapters 31 and 45.

Membranoproliferative Glomerulonephritis Type I

Type I MPGN is characterized by the tram-track appearance of the GBM on silver stain because of duplication around intramembranous and subendothelial deposits and interposition of mesangial cells and macrophages (Fig. 24.9). The glomeruli are enlarged and hypercellular with a lobular appearance by LM (Fig. 24.10). There is marked mesangial hypercellularity and occasional polymorphonuclear neutrophils, and mononuclear cells may be present. By IF, C3 predominates in a coarse granular pattern along basement membranes with moderate amounts of IgG and IgM. Subendothelial and occasional mesangial immune deposits are seen by EM (4,46). MPGN may be idiopathic or secondary to any of numerous chronic infections. Hepatitis C positivity, often with associated cryoglobulins, was present in approximately one-fourth of adult cases of MPGN type I in adults in Japan and the United States (96,97). This association has not been demonstrated in a study of children with apparent idiopathic MPGN (98). MPGN type I recurs in 20 to 30% of grafts and may lead to graft loss (11). Secondary MPGN more often demonstrates a focal segmental pattern of proliferation, contrasting the more diffuse involvement seen in idiopathic MPGN.

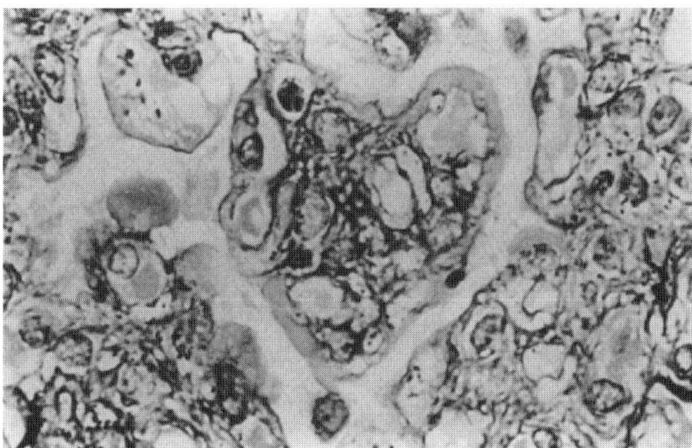

FIGURE 24.9. Split basement membrane (tram-tracking) in membranoproliferative glomerulonephritis type I caused by subendothelial/intramembranous deposits and mesangial interposition (Jones' stain, ×1125).

Dense Deposit Disease

In dense deposit disease (also called *type II MPGN*), the glomeruli may appear similar by LM to those of type I MPGN. However, the pathogenesis is entirely different. These patients show circulating IgG autoantibodies, also known as *C3 nephritic factor* (10,99,100). The basement membranes are deeply eosinophilic, often with a ribbon garland or sausage-shaped contour. By IF, smooth linear deposits of C3 are found, typically without Ig staining. The disease is named *dense deposit disease* because of the characteristic appearance by EM with strongly electron-dense deposits underlying the basement membrane. Studies of the dense deposits indicate that these are

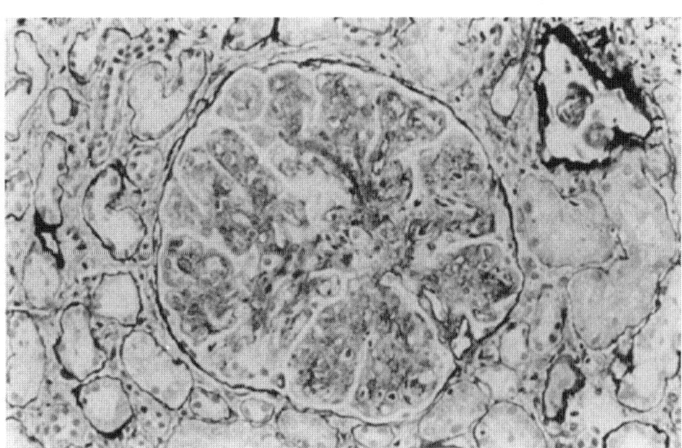

FIGURE 24.10. Lobular appearance of glomeruli in membranoproliferative glomerulonephritis type I (×430).

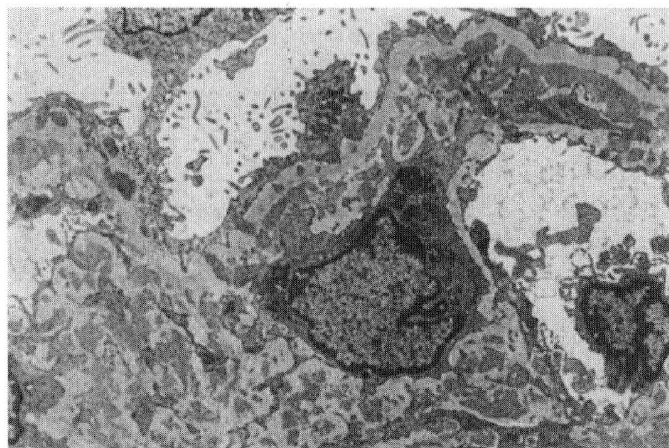

FIGURE 24.11. Lupus nephritis, diffuse proliferative with massive dense mesangial and subendothelial deposits and fewer deposits in subepithelial areas (×5600).

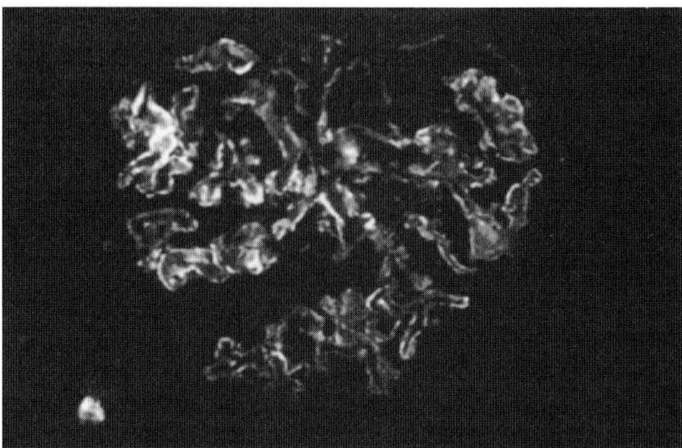

FIGURE 24.13. Immunofluorescence of granular capillary and small mesangial immunoglobulin G deposits in diffuse proliferative lupus nephritis. The larger segments of capillary loop staining correspond to subendothelial deposits, with a smooth outer edge where deposits are molded underneath the glomerular basement membrane (×250).

likely an alteration of basement membrane material and not deposition of circulating immune complexes. Although less specific than EM diagnosis, deposits can also be identified by their staining with the fluorescent dye thioflavin T in cases in which EM examination cannot be performed (100). Renal survival may be worse than in type I MPGN (median survival, 8.7 vs. 15.3 years) (101). The distinction between these two diseases is also important because dense deposit disease invariably recurs in renal transplantation, although loss of graft is not always the outcome (10).

Lupus Nephritis

Lupus nephritis is not a single disease but rather a spectrum of severity of involvement of the kidney by the immune complexes characteristic of SLE. Most patients with SLE have morphologic manifestation of renal immune deposition. However, patients who undergo renal biopsy most often have clinical renal manifestations and have more pronounced changes. Lupus nephritis is characterized by deposits in all anatomic compartments of the glomerulus (i.e., mesangial, subepithelial, and subendothelial regions) (17,18) (Figs. 24.11 and 24.12). All Ig classes, C3, and smaller amounts of C4 are usually found in lupus nephritis deposits (Fig. 24.13), and dense immune-complex deposits are seen by EM. Reticular aggregates (see above) are typically seen in endothelial cells in any class of lupus nephritis (4,46) (Fig. 24.14).

The WHO classifications, either the original or modified, are most commonly used (16,17). A recent meeting sponsored by the International Society of Nephrology and the Renal Pathology Society has put forth a revised lupus nephritis classification to clarify some areas of difficulty in the previous versions. In this new classification, class I has minimal mesangial deposits with normal LM. Class II is characterized by mesangial expansion and deposits with only scattered peripheral loop deposits. In class III, focal proliferative lupus nephritis, deposits are present in mesangial areas, focal endocapillary proliferation, and subendothelial deposits, with or without scattered subepi-

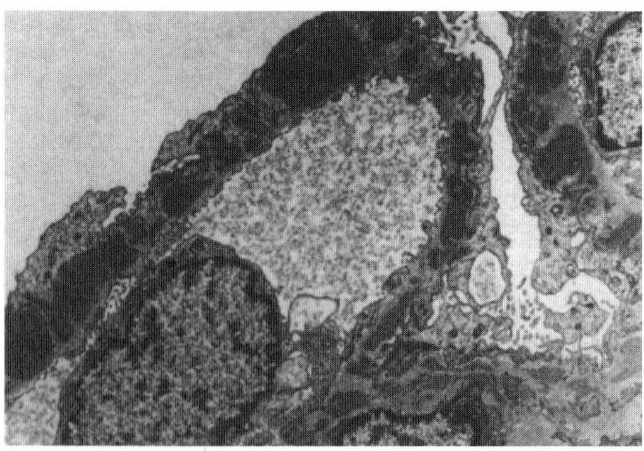

FIGURE 24.12. Membranous glomerulonephritis with subepithelial deposits and intervening lamina densa (seen as spikes by silver stain on light microscopy) (×15,580).

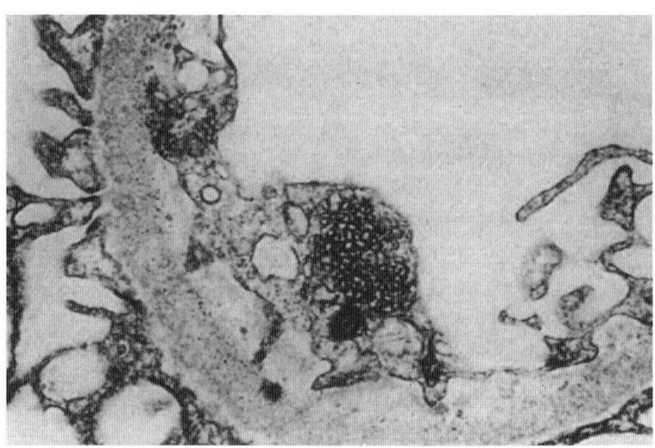

FIGURE 24.14. Endothelial cell containing tubular-shaped reticular aggregates in lupus nephritis (×20,000).

thelial deposits. The process, by definition, involves less than 50% of glomeruli. There is wide heterogeneity in the severity and activity of lesions, with varying amounts of proliferation. Foci of necrosis, cellular crescents (indices of activity), and cellular adhesions may be present, which over time may evolve to sclerosis and fibrous crescents (indicators of chronicity). The subendothelial deposits result in thick, rigid-appearing capillary basement membrane by LM, the so-called wire-loop lesions.

When lesions affect more than 50% of glomeruli, lupus nephritis is characterized as class IV diffuse proliferative glomerulonephritis. Findings are similar to those in class III but with more endocapillary proliferation and other active lesions. Hyaline thrombi (aggregates of immune complexes) may fill capillary lumina. IF demonstrates widespread distribution of immune complexes. EM confirms the massive and extensive immune complex deposition (Fig. 24.11). For classes III and IV, the extent of active versus chronic lesions is specified. Evidence indicates a particularly poor prognosis of segmental necrotizing lesions in class IV lupus nephritis; thus, the presence of these lesions versus global endocapillary proliferation is noted (102).

Class V membranous lupus nephritis is characterized by predominance of subepithelial deposits in a pattern similar to that of idiopathic membranous glomerulonephritis with added mesangial deposits (Fig. 24.12). Subendothelial deposits are minor components in class V. When there are superimposed focal or diffuse proliferative lesions in addition to membranous changes, both processes are diagnosed (e.g., combined diffuse proliferative and membranous lupus nephritis, WHO classes IV and V). Widespread chronic sclerosing lesions in a nonspecific pattern in a case of lupus nephritis are defined as *class VI.* Tubular basement membrane deposits can occur in any class of lupus nephritis and may account in part for the tubulointerstitial injury. Vascular lesions include immune deposits or thrombotic microangiopathy, often related to antiphospholipid antibodies. For further discussion of lupus nephritis, see Chapter 46.

Anti–Glomerular Basement Membrane Antibody Disease

LM examination shows crescentic glomerulonephritis with focal necrotizing lesions. Patients may not always show detectable serum levels of anti-GBM antibodies, especially after the acute phase of illness. Serology is positive in 95% of patients in the first 6 months after onset. However, in all patients, even those with negative serology, linear IgG staining by IF of capillary basement membrane is present (Fig. 24.15). EM shows no immune deposits. Patients with more than 50% crescents have a worse prognosis (103). For further discussion of anti-GBM antibody disease, see Chapter 34.

Wegener's Granulomatosis

By LM, the appearance of Wegener's granulomatosis is the same as for other crescentic necrotizing glomerulonephritides (e.g., microscopic polyangiitis or anti-GBM antibody disease) (Fig. 24.16). The lesions are focal and segmental. Granulomas are rare in the kidney, and arteritis is rarely found in the small sample inherent to the renal needle biopsy. IF studies allow differentiation of the lesion from anti-GBM antibody disease. It shows fibrin and fibrinogen in areas of necrosis and nonspecific trapping of Ig, especially IgM. By EM, immune deposits are not identified. Distinction from microscopic polyangiitis cannot usually be made by renal biopsy findings. Clinical manifestations must be used to distinguish between these two disorders. For further discussion of Wegner's granulomatosis, see Chapter 34.

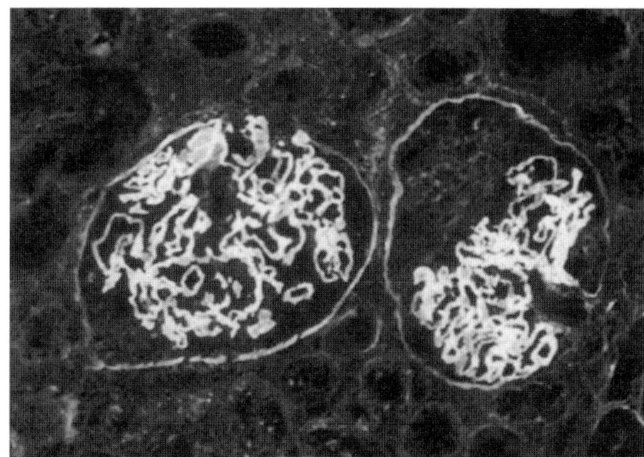

FIGURE 24.15. Antiglomerular basement membrane antibody disease with linear staining by immunofluorescence for immunoglobulin G. A crescent is present in the glomerulus on the right (×125).

Postinfectious Glomerulonephritis

Patients with typical poststreptococcal glomerulonephritis do not usually undergo renal biopsy. When the diagnosis remains in question, when abnormalities persist, or when the initial dis-

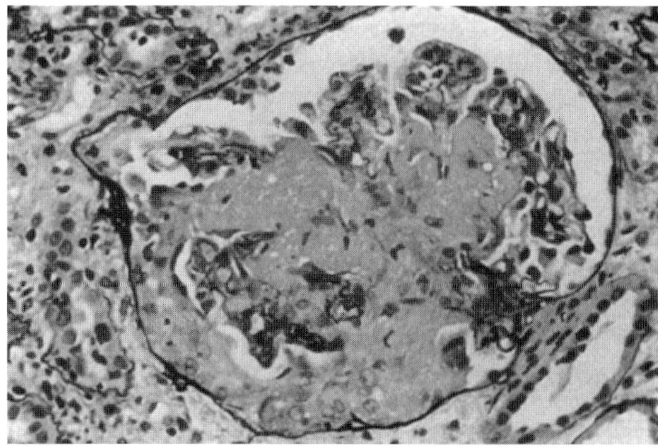

FIGURE 24.16. Segmental necrosis and crescent in Wegener's granulomatosis. Immunofluorescence was negative (Jones' stain, ×430).

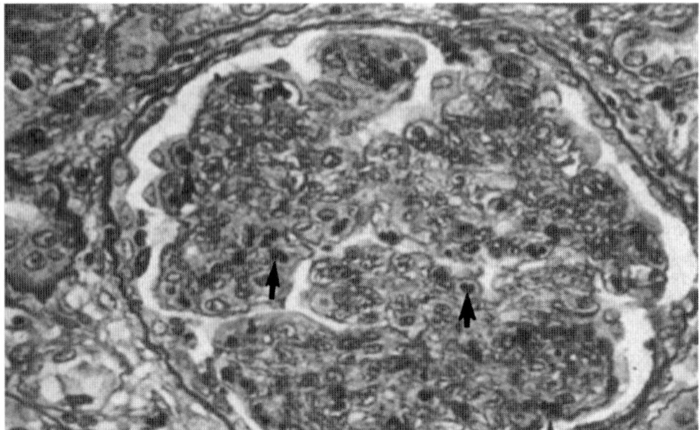

FIGURE 24.17. Postinfectious glomerulonephritis with endocapillary proliferation and polymorphonuclear neutrophil infiltration (*arrows*) (periodic acid-Schiff stain, ×430).

ease is severe, renal biopsy may be done. Glomeruli are enlarged and hypercellular with prominent endocapillary proliferation and infiltration by neutrophils and mononuclear cells (Fig. 24.17). In severe disease, crescents are present. Occasionally, large subepithelial deposits can be visualized by LM. These differ from those typical of membranous glomerulonephritis in being more unevenly distributed along the capillary basement membrane and larger in size. The deposits lie on top of the basement membrane, rather than being embedded within it (as in membranous glomerulonephritis); therefore, spikes are not usually present. By IF, there are coarsely granular, discontinuous areas of IgG and C3 along the capillary basement membrane. The capillary lumina can be obliterated by infiltrating mononuclear cells, swollen endothelial cells, and polymorphonuclear leukocytes. Electron-dense subepithelial deposits are large, variegated, dome-shaped or haystack-shaped, and irregularly spaced (Fig. 24.18). Occasional mesangial deposits are present in many biopsies. For further discussion of postinfectious glomerulonephritis, see Chapter 30.

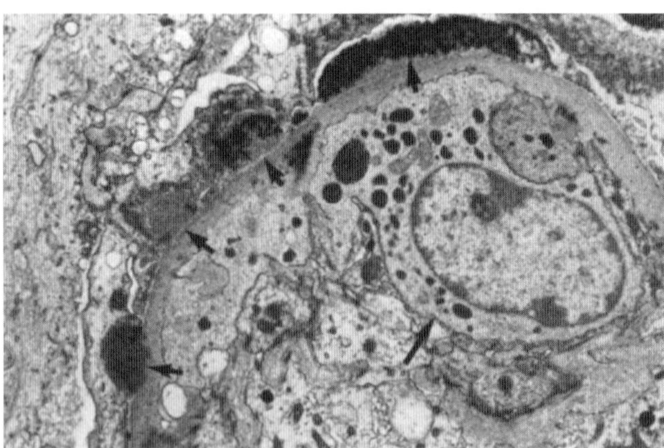

FIGURE 24.18. Electron micrograph of subepithelial large, irregularly spaced, dome-shaped subepithelial deposits in postinfectious glomerulonephritis. The deposits are variegated and lie on top of the glomerular basement membrane (*short arrows*). There is endocapillary proliferation with polymorphonuclear neutrophil (*long arrow*) infiltration (×7000).

Diabetic Nephropathy

Diabetic nephropathy affects 30 to 40% of patients with diabetes mellitus, either type 1 or type 2, with overt clinical nephropathy manifest 15 to 20 years after onset of diabetes. Therefore, diabetic nephropathy has been considered a disease of adults. However, recent studies in adolescents demonstrate that diabetic lesions may be present even after short duration of disease (104). In addition, obesity and type 2 diabetes mellitus are increasing in children. These structural changes included GBM thickening and mesangial expansion and were associated with proteinuria, hypertension, and decline in glomerular filtration rate. Overt diabetic nephropathy with nodular glomerulosclerosis and afferent and efferent arteriolar hyalinization was present in several of these patients. For further discussion of diabetic nephropathy, see Chapter 49.

Alport's Syndrome and Thin Basement Membrane Lesion

Early in life, in boys with Alport's syndrome and in female carriers, the renal biopsy may show no significant LM abnormalities. At later stages, glomerulosclerosis, interstitial fibrosis, and prominent foam cells are typical. These foam cells are not specific for this disease and are found in numerous proteinuric states. Glomeruli show varying stages of matrix expansion and sclerosis. IF may show nonspecific trapping of IgM. By EM, the diagnostic lesion consists of irregular thinned and thickened areas of the GBMs with splitting and irregular multilaminated appearance of the lamina densa, so-called basket weaving. In between these lamina, granular, mottled material is present. At early stages of disease (i.e., in children or women), the basement membrane may show only thinning. Some male patients with classic Alport's syndrome only have basement membrane thinning even at advanced clinical stages (22,105).

Immunostaining for type IV collagen chains can aid in the interpretation of thin basement membranes (105). Heterotrimers of α_3, α_4, and α_5 type IV collagen are normally present in the GBM. Mutation of α_5 type IV collagen in X-linked Alport's syndrome prevents incorporation of the other chains into the heterotrimer. In kidney biopsies, approximately 70 to 80% of male patients with X-linked Alport's syndrome lack staining of GBM; distal tubular basement membrane; and Bowman's capsule for α_3, α_4, and α_5 (type IV) chains. In autosomal recessive Alport's syndrome, due to mutations of either α_3 or α_4, the GBMs usually show no expression of α_3, α_4, or α_5 type IV collagen; however, in contrast to X-linked cases, there is strong expression of α_5 and α_6 type IV collagen in Bowman's capsule, distal tubular basement membrane, and skin. Female patients who are heterozygous for X-linked Alport's syndrome frequently show mosaic staining of GBM and distal tubular basement membrane for α_3, α_4, and α_5 type IV collagen chains and skin mosaic staining for α_5 type IV collagen. Patients with autosomal dominant Alport's syndrome have not been studied immunohistochemically. Of note, occasional cases with Alport's syndrome clinically and by renal biopsy showed apparent normal α_5 type IV pattern of skin IF staining, and approximately 20% of male X-linked Alport's syndrome patients and affected homozygous autosomal recessive Alport's syndrome patients show faint or even normal staining of the GBM for α_3 and α_5, likely because the antigenic site recognized by the antibody has not been altered by the mutation.

Thinning of the GBM is the characteristic finding in benign familial hematuria (59,60). The diagnosis of thin basement membranes is based on morphometric measurements from EM prints, revealing marked thinning of the lamina densa of the GBM. LM and standard IF are normal. The GBM thickness normally increases with age. Normal thickness in adults in one series was 373 ± 42 nm in men versus 326 ± 45 nm in women. GBM thickness less than 250 nm has been used as a cutoff in many series (106). In children, the diagnosis of thin basement membranes must be made with caution, establishing normal age-matched controls within each laboratory. In our laboratory, we found a range of GBM thickness in normal children, from approximately 110 nm in 1-year-olds to 222 ± 14 nm in 7-year-olds. As mentioned above, thin GBM (without lamellation) may also be an early or only manifestation in some kindreds with Alport's syndrome. Thus, the presence of thin GBM cannot per se be taken to categorically indicate a benign prognosis. Some patients with benign familial hematuria clinically have mutations of α4 type IV collagen, suggesting a continuum of autosomal recessive Alport's syndrome with benign familial hematuria (107). The immunostaining patterns in such benign familial hematuria patients have not been established.

PROGNOSTIC IMPLICATIONS OF BIOPSY FINDINGS

When the biopsy sample is adequate, extensive, severe, and irreversible lesions signify a dismal prognosis for the patient. Globally sclerotic glomeruli are not amenable to treatment, although evidence from human diabetic nephropathy and animal studies indicates that the earlier stages of sclerosis may be affected by some therapeutic interventions and may even be reversible (108–110). Similarly, active lesions with ongoing cellular crescents, necrosis, and inflammatory infiltrate are potentially dramatically modulated by therapy, allowing subsequent healing. There may be minimal irreversible damage to glomerular structures when intervention occurs early.

Although the renal biopsy may yield a diagnosis, there is less information of prognostic indicators in diseases that have a variable course. Extensive analysis aimed at determining histologic features associated with poor prognosis has been done in some diseases discussed below.

Classification schemes, especially for lupus nephritis and membranous glomerulonephritis, imply progression from one stage of disease to the next. Although sequential biopsies have illustrated progression from focal to diffuse proliferative glomerulonephritis in lupus nephritis, there is no clear-cut evidence that progression occurs among all WHO classes (16–18). In lupus nephritis, patients with less severe proliferative disease, especially segmental necrotizing lesions, appear to have better prognoses.

Although the presence of cellular crescents is associated with activity of disease clinically, the renal biopsy offers additional prognostic information beyond that gleaned from the clinical presentation (111). Focal and diffuse proliferative lesions (WHO classes III and IV) may present very similarly clinically, but only the latter appears to require intense, long-term immunosuppression. Lesions of activity in lupus nephritis include endocapillary proliferation, necrosis, cellular crescents, interstitial inflammatory cells, and acute tubular necrosis. Lesions that indicate chronicity include tubular atrophy, interstitial fibrosis, glomerular sclerosis, and fibrous crescents.

Although assessment of activity and chronicity indices is useful for population groups, these appear to have less absolute information to guide assessment in individual patients. Nonetheless, in large series, assessment of indices of activity and severity in patients with lupus nephritis or other diseases has shown some correlation with prognosis and response to therapy. Diffuse proliferative lesions, extensive crescents, segmental necrosis, and tubulointerstitial fibrosis are associated with progression to end-stage renal disease (111,112). The best prognostic indicator in a recent study was the proportion remaining of intact glomeruli (113).

IgA nephropathy was previously believed to have a benign prognosis. In a large series of adult patients with IgA nephropathy, poor prognosis was indicated by segmental glomerulosclerosis, adhesions or crescents, and tubulointerstitial fibrosis (114). Progression occurs in 11 to 15% of pediatric patients (4,92,115). Scoring of activity and chronicity of lesions has been correlated with clinical course. Activity is assessed by degrees of crescent formation, mesangial proliferation, and interstitial infiltrate. Chronicity is scored by degrees of fibrous crescents, segmental and global sclerosis, tubular atrophy, and interstitial fibrosis (116). High indices of chronic injury and focal segmental glomerular changes were associated with a worse prognosis (117,118). Histologic features that predicted progression in a recent multicenter study in children were crescents, tubulointerstitial fibrosis, and glomerulosclerosis in 20% or more of glomeruli (115). Predominance of matrix expansion appears to be a later stage of injury associated with a higher percentage of sclerosis and persistent proteinuria (93). Extension of deposits to glomerular basement areas has also been reported as a poor prognostic indicator (116).

Focal glomerulosclerosis superimposed on membranous glomerulonephritis has been associated with more severe tubulointerstitial nephritis and a worse outcome. This lesion was present in 20% of children with hepatitis B–associated membranous glomerulonephritis (119).

Renal Transplant Biopsy

The primary use of biopsy in the renal transplantation is to uncover the reason for altered renal function. Causes of renal dysfunction in the transplant can be broadly divided

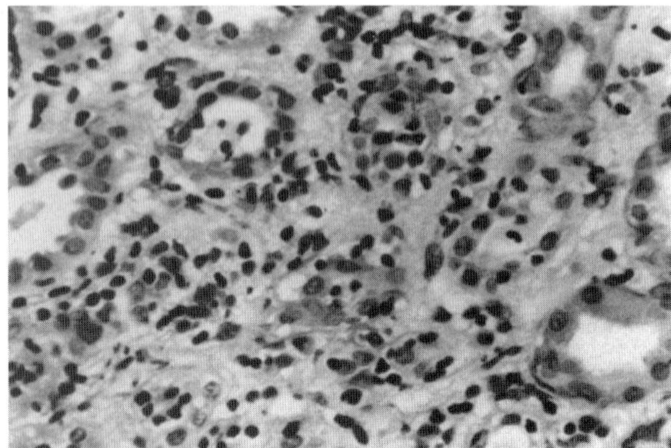

FIGURE 24.19. Acute rejection, classified as type I by Cooperative Clinical Trials in Transplantation criteria. There is interstitial lymphocytic infiltrate with tubulitis, activated lymphocytes, tubular cell injury, and interstitial edema (Jones' stain, ×220).

into (a) those related to rejection, drug toxicity, recurrent or *de novo* disease; and (b) those related to the procedure itself (e.g., acute tubular necrosis).

Rejection

Acute rejection is diagnosed by the presence of either interstitial inflammation with lymphocytes and plasma cells infiltrating tubules (tubulitis, the hallmark of acute interstitial type rejection) (Fig. 24.19) or, when more severe, by extension of this process to vessels, with subendothelial arterial or arteriolar infiltration by lymphocytes (endothelialitis, the hallmark of acute vascular rejection) (Fig. 24.20). The interstitial changes of acute rejection are not pathognomonic. In contrast, the finding of endothelialitis is highly specific for acute vascular rejection. Appropriate stains (e.g., PAS) must be used to allow visualization of the tubular basement membrane and identification of tubulitis. An adequate specimen for evaluation of possible rejection should contain at least two cores with at least seven glomeruli and two arteries (120).

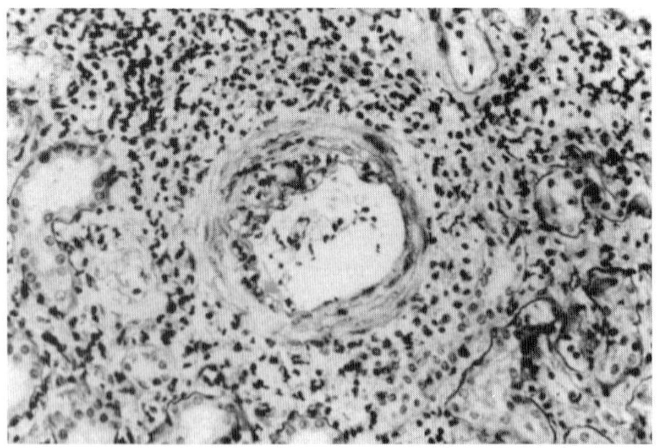

FIGURE 24.20. Acute vascular rejection, classified as type II by Cooperative Clinical Trials in Transplantation criteria. There is subendothelial infiltration by lymphocytes in this artery, so-called endothelialitis (Jones' stain, ×220).

Several schemes have been used to diagnose and classify rejection: the Banff scoring system, based on detailed scoring of various components of injury; and the Cooperative Clinical Trials in Transplantation criteria (120,121). In both classification schemes, acute rejection is based on the presence of tubulitis or endothelialitis (i.e., lymphocytes in the tubule under the tubular basement membrane or underneath the endothelium of arteries). Other inflammatory cells (e.g., eosinophils, neutrophils, and plasma cells), although much fewer in number than T lymphocytes, may also contribute to the infiltrate in acute rejection. Type I rejection in both schemas is diagnosed when interstitial lymphocytic infiltrate and tubulitis are present (greater than 25% of parenchyma infiltrated in Banff; greater than 5% in Cooperative Clinical Trials in Transplantation criteria) (Fig. 24.20). Infiltrate and tubulitis less than specified for type I is called borderline by Banff criteria (126). Acute vascular rejection is classified in the same manner in both schemas. Type II acute vacular rejection is diagnosed when there is mild or moderate endothelialitis (arteritis), and severe acute vascular rejection (type III) is diagnosed when there is transmural vascular inflammation or fibrinoid necrosis. These types are differentiated not only based on histologic pattern, but also on differences in underlying mechanisms and response to therapies; types I and II are T-cell dependent processes and are separated based on the likely greater severity of any rejection with endothelialitis, whereas antibody-mediated mechanisms contribute to type III changes.

Identification of acute rejection at earlier stages and, thus, initiation of treatment at milder levels of injury appear to be clinically important. Thus, mild tubulitis that is borderline by Banff criteria, even in normally functioning grafts, was found to be predictive of higher serum creatinine at follow-up. In contrast, treatment of such subclinical rejection in the early time period after transplantation resulted in better preserved renal function at 24 months (122).

There are no specific IF or EM immune complexes associated with acute rejection. The recent surge of exciting molecular studies indicates the possibility of earlier, more sensitive, and specific diagnosis of acute rejection using these techniques (see below) (123). In particular, the presence in peritubular capillaries of C4d, a complement breakdown product that binds covalently to tissue, is highly associated with antidonor antibodies (humoral rejection) (124). Diagnosis of humoral antibody-mediated rejection has important therapeutic and prognostic implications. C4d staining can be done on frozen tissue and, most recently, also on fixed paraffin-processed tissue (125).

The changes of chronic rejection include intimal fibrosis of arteries, interstitial fibrosis, and transplant glomerulopathy (121,126). A previous or baseline biopsy is necessary to prove that intimal fibrosis is *de novo* and potentially represents chronic rejection rather than a preexisting, nonspecific change in the graft. Interstitial fibrosis is also a nonspecific finding and may result from various injuries.

Transplant glomerulopathy is a more specific lesion indicative of chronic rejection. By LM, the glomeruli show basement membrane splitting, corrugation, and even segmental sclerosis with hyalinosis. The latter lesion likely resulted in erroneous reports of *de novo* idiopathic FSGS in the transplant. However, in transplant glomerulopathy, there is widening of the lamina rara interna of the GBM with mesangial cell interposition and new basement membrane formation by EM. Reduplication of basal lamina of peritubular capillaries is suggested to be more specific of transplant glomerulopathy but may also occur in some other glomerular diseases and HUS (127).

Cyclosporine and FK506 Toxicity

Cyclosporine toxicity may manifest in various ways. Tacrolimus (FK506) has much the same spectrum of toxicity as cyclosporine (126,128). The most common morphologic lesion in patients with a clinical diagnosis of cyclosporine toxicity, as verified by clinical follow-up, is that of a normal kidney biopsy morphologically. In these patients, renal dysfunction is due to reversible, cyclosporine-induced vasoconstriction and hypofiltration. Morphologic changes of cyclosporine toxicity include arteriolopathy with injury to the endothelium and vascular smooth muscle cells. In its classic form, this injury results in nodular IgM IF positivity along the apical side of the arteriole, with necrosis and smooth muscle cell injury demonstrated by EM (126,128). By LM, concentric hyalinosis is present, whereas typically eccentric, more segmental hyalinosis is associated with hypertension. Isometric tubular vacuolization in a patchy distribution, although not specific, is also indicative of cyclosporine toxicity. Chronic cyclosporine toxicity results in a striped distribution of interstitial fibrosis caused by injury along the medullary rays (126). This pattern often cannot be gleaned by small needle biopsies. FSGS with ischemic, corrugated GBMs in remaining glomeruli may also result from cyclosporine toxicity and can be associated with significant proteinuria (128).

Cyclosporine has also been associated with thrombotic microangiopathy lesions (see above) (126,128). Of note, thrombotic microangiopathy can occur in patients who are recipients of transplants of kidneys or other organs and after radiation, with or without cyclosporine treatment. In some patients, collapsing-type glomerulosclerosis may be associated with cyclosporine toxicity, likely representing a response to severe vascular injury and ischemia (129).

Recurrent and De Novo *Disease*

Recurrent and *de novo* diseases are important causes of renal allograft injury, affecting approximately 10% of renal allografts (126). Of all graft loss, 2 to 4% is due to recurrence of disease. IF microscopy should be performed in all transplant biopsies to rule out this possibility. When IF or LM findings in conjunction with the clinical setting indicate an undetermined lesion, EM study should also be performed.

In children, the most common recurrent diseases include, notably, IgA nephropathy, Henoch-Schönlein purpura, MPGN, dense deposit disease, and FSGS (130). Although SLE has been reported to recur only rarely, our experience indicates a recurrence rate of approximately 30% (131). However, morphologic recurrence of disease does not necessarily lead to graft loss (126,130). Dense deposit disease recurs morphologically in nearly all patients but with only 10 to 20% resultant graft loss. Although classic diarrhea-associated HUS recurs only very rarely, atypical HUS (which includes familial forms) has a recurrence rate of 15 to 25%, with 40 to 50% graft loss. Although IgA nephropathy recurs in approximately 50% of patients, only 10% of grafts with recurrent disease are lost. MPGN type I recurs in 20 to 30%, with 10 to 40% graft loss. FSGS recurs in 20 to 30% of cases, resulting in graft loss in 30 to 50% of these. Of note, in recurrent FSGS, the only morphologic change found in the first weeks after recurrence of proteinuria is foot process effacement, with early segmental sclerosis detectable at 6 to 8 weeks.

De novo disease may also affect the transplant. Membranous glomerulonephritis is the most common *de novo* glomerulonephritis in the transplant. The etiology remains unknown (126). Glomerulonephritis related to infections (e.g., hepatitis C–related MPGN) also can occur in the transplant. Early changes of diabetic nephropathy develop much more rapidly in the transplant than in the native kidney and may occur within a few years, whether diabetes preexisted or is corticosteroid induced. Thrombotic microangiopathy may be related to drug toxicity (see above) or be idiopathic in the transplant.

Posttransplant lymphoproliferative disease (PTLD) is due to the unrestrained proliferation of B lymphocytes, most often because of transformation by Epstein-Barr virus, and is an aggressive process, which if untreated, disseminates and may cause death (132). PTLD may respond to decreased immunosuppression. An expansile lymphoid infiltrate with atypical, transformed lymphocytes and serpiginous necrosis are features suggestive of PTLD (132).

Immunohistochemical studies can be used to detect Epstein-Barr virus to further support this diagnosis. Typing studies of the lymphocytic infiltrate are not often helpful because most PTLD is polytypic, rather than clonal. Of note, acute rejection and PTLD may be present concurrently.

Polyoma (BK) virus nephropathy has increased in the last years in the transplant and is perhaps related to increased immunosuppression (133). The biopsy shows a pleomorphic infiltrate with lymphocytes, plasma cells, and polymorphonuclear neutrophils and eosinophils, with enlarged tubular cells with smudgy nuclei. BK infection is confirmed by immunostaining. The prognosis is poor, although there may be some response to decreased immunosuppression and antiviral therapy.

NEW METHODS FOR THE FUTURE

With the recent surge of application of molecular biology techniques to the study of renal disease, candidate factors involved in pathogenesis and progression of disease are being studied in animal models. Studies in human beings have also commenced. With further development of such studies, we may identify specific abnormal processes and, thus, target therapy more specifically. Research techniques that have been advantageously applied to elucidate pathogenesis of disease include immunostaining; identifying specific antigen in deposits of membranous glomerulonephritis in some patients (thyroglobulin with Hashimoto's disease; hepatitis B, C antigen); identifying light chains or paraproteins in plasma cell dyscrasia–associated diseases; identifying specific type IV collagen abnormalities in Alport's syndrome and C4d as a marker of humoral rejection; and elucidating the pathogenesis of specific *Escherichia coli*–associated toxins in some forms of HUS.

Current studies are aimed at understanding disease etiologies and mechanisms at a molecular level and studying renal biopsies by laser capture microdissection, with real time or standard reverse transcription polymerase chain reaction (RT-PCR), and *in situ* hybridization techniques (134–136). Recent efforts have expanded use of these techniques to study mechanisms of injury and progression. Competitive RT-PCR has been used successfully on even single, isolated glomeruli from human biopsies (134). Modulation of growth factors, collagens, cytokines, chemokines, and their receptors have been investigated molecularly in renal biopsies. Cytokines and chemokines and their receptors were upregulated in diseases with macrophage influx and mesangial cell proliferation, supporting an important role in initiating and perpetuating injury. Such approaches can offer exciting new mechanistic insights into renal diseases.

In parallel, genetic studies are targeted at identifying patients at risk for progression in diseases with a variable course, such as diabetes and IgA nephropathy. Polymorphisms of the renin-angiotensin system genes have been implicated as risk factors for progression and also as indices for response to therapies that target this system (137,138).

Diagnostic use of RT-PCR and *in situ* hybridization has focused on detection of viruses, including hepatitis B and C, cytomegalovirus, polyoma virus, and Epstein-Barr virus. Increased expression of various immune-activated genes (e.g., perforin, granzyme, and fas ligand) quantified by competitive RT-PCR showed initial high predictive value for acute rejection, but subsequent studies have not been as clear cut (123).

Together, these approaches promise to map risks and mechanisms of disease initiation and progression and point to targets to achieve resolution of injury. Sequential biopsies with evaluation of changes in structure and patterns of abnormal factors and modulation by therapy may be necessary to fully understand pathogenesis. Instead of diagnoses of morphologic patterns recognized by current techniques in the renal biopsy specimen, molecular techniques may allow more precise diagnosis of the specific diseases and identification of injury mechanisms.

ACKNOWLEDGMENTS

The author wishes to thank Drs. Tina Kon and Aida Yared, for their suggestions, and the late Dr. Alan Glick, for his advice and photographic assistance.

REFERENCES

1. Hisano S, Kwano M, Hatae K, et al. Asymptomatic isolated microhaematuria: natural history of 136 children. *Pediatr Nephrol* 1991;5:578–581.
2. Turi S, Visy M, Vissy A, et al. Long-term follow-up of patients with persistent/recurrent, isolated haematuria: a Hungarian multicentre study. *Pediatr Nephrol* 1989;3:235–239.
3. Trachtman H, Weiss RA, Bennett B, et al. Isolated hematuria in children: indications for a renal biopsy. *Kidney Int* 1984;25:94–99.
4. Silva FG. Overview of pediatric nephropathology. *Kidney Int* 1988;33:1016–1032.
5. Sibley RK, Mahan J, Mauer SM, et al. A clinicopathologic study of forty-eight infants with nephrotic syndrome. *Kidney Int* 1985;27:544–552.
6. Habib R, Kleinknecht C. The primary nephrotic syndrome of childhood. Classification and clinicopathologic study of 406 cases. In: Sommers SC, ed. *Pathology annual.* New York: Appleton-Century-Crofts, 1971:417–474.
7. Cameron JS. Histology, protein clearances, and response to treatment in the nephrotic syndrome. *BMJ* 1968;4:352–356.
8. White RHR, Glasgow EF, Mills RJ. Clinicopathological study of nephrotic syndrome in childhood. *Lancet* 1970;1:1353–1359.
9. Rapola J. Congenital nephrotic syndrome. *Pediatr Nephrol* 1987;1:441–446.
10. Habib R, Gubler M-C, Loirat C, et al. Dense deposit disease: a variant of membranoproliferative glomerulonephritis. *Kidney Int* 1975;7:204–215.
11. Cameron JS. Recurrent primary disease and de novo nephritis following renal transplantation. *Pediatr Nephrol* 1991;5:412–421.
12. Mustonen J, Pasternack A, Helin H, et al. Renal biopsy in acute renal failure. *Am J Nephrol* 1984;4:27–31.
13. Jennette JC, Wilkman AS, Tuttle RH, et al. Frequency and pathologic significance of anti-proteinase 3 and anti-myeloperoxidase antineutrophil cytoplasmic autoantibodies (ANCA) in immune complex glomerulonephritis. *Lab Invest* 1996;74:167A(abst).
14. Rao JK, Weinberger M, Oddone EZ, et al. The role of antineutrophil cytoplasmic antibody (c-ANCA) testing in the diagnosis of Wegener granulomatosis. A literature

review and meta-analysis. *Ann Intern Med* 1995;123:925–932.

15. Jennette JC. Antineutrophil cytoplasmic autoantibody-associated disease: a pathologist's perspective. *Am J Kidney Dis* 1991;18:164–170.
16. McCluskey RT. Lupus nephritis. In: Sommers SC, ed. *Kidney pathology decennial 1966–1975.* East Norwalk, CT: Appleton-Century-Crofts, 1975:435.
17. Churg J, Sobin LH. *World Health Organization (WHO) Monograph: renal disease. Classification and atlas of glomerular diseases.* New York: Igaku-Shoin Medical Publishers, 1982.
18. Rush PJ, Baumal R, Shore A, et al. Correlation of renal histology with outcome in children with lupus nephritis. *Kidney Int* 1986;29:1066–1071.
19. Schwartz MM, Bernstein J, Hill GS, et al., and the Lupus Nephritis Collaborative Study Group. Predictive value of renal pathology in diffuse proliferative lupus glomerulonephritis. *Kidney Int* 1989;36:891–896.
20. Remuzzi G, Ruggenenti P, Perico N. Chronic renal diseases: renoprotective benefits of renin-angiotensin system inhibition. *Ann Intern Med* 2002;136:604–615.
21. van de Heuvel LPWJ, Schröder CH, Savage COS, et al. The development of anti-glomerular basement membrane nephritis in two children with Alport's syndrome after renal transplantation: characterization of the antibody target. *Pediatr Nephrol* 1989;3:406–413.
22. Kashtan CE, Michael AF. Alport syndrome. *Kidney Int* 1996;50:1445–1463.
23. Kark RM. Renal biopsy. *JAMA* 1968;205:220–226.
24. Gault MH, Muehrcke RC. Renal biopsy: current views and controversies. *Nephron* 1983;34:1–34.
25. Madaio MP. Renal biopsy. *Kidney Int* 1990;38:529–543.
26. Cohen AH, Nast CC, Adler SG, et al. Clinical utility of kidney biopsies in the diagnosis and management of renal disease. *Am J Nephrol* 1989;9:309–315.
27. Haas M. A reevaluation of routine electron microscopy in the examination of native renal biopsies. *J Am Soc Nephrol* 1997;8:70–76.
28. de Chadar Jvian JP, Kaplan BS. The kidney biopsy. In: Barakat AY, ed. *Renal disease in children. Clinical evaluation and diagnosis.* New York: Springer-Verlag, 1990:117–132.
29. Wiseman DA, Hawkins R, Numerow LM, et al. Percutaneous renal biopsy utilizing real time, ultrasonic guidance and a semiautomated biopsy device. *Kidney Int* 1990;38:347–349.
30. Donovan KL, Thomas DM, Wheeler DC, et al. Experience with a new method for percutaneous renal biopsy. *Nephrol Dialysis Transplant* 1991;6:731–733.
31. Oberholzer M, Trohorst E, Perret E, et al. Minimum sample size of kidney biopsies for semiquantitative and quantitative evaluation. *Nephron* 1983;34:192–195.
32. Marwah DS, Korbet SM. Timing of complications in percutaneous renal biopsy: what is the optimal period of observation? *Am J Kidney Dis* 1996;28:47–52.
33. Häyry P, von Willebrand E. Fine needle aspiration in transplantation pathology. In: Sale GE, ed. *The pathology of organ transplantation.* Boston: Butterworth, 1990:285–301.
34. Yussim A, Shapira Z, Shmueli D, et al. Use of modified fine needle aspiration for study of glomerular pathology in human kidneys. *Kidney Int* 1990;37:812–817.
35. Al Rasheed SA, Al Mugeiren MM, Abdurrahman MB, et al. The outcome of percutaneous renal biopsy in children: an analysis of 120 consecutive cases. *Pediatr Nephrol* 1990;4:600–603.
36. Edelmann CM Jr, Greifer I. A modified technique for percutaneous needle biopsy of the kidney. *J Pediatr* 1967;70:81–86.
37. Abdurraman MB. Percutaneous renal biopsy in a developing country: experience with 300 cases. *Ann Trop Paediatr* 1984;4:25–30.
38. Karafin L, Kendall AR, Fleisher DS. Urologic complications in percutaneous renal biopsy in children. *J Urol* 1970;103:332–335.
39. Carvajal HF, Travis LB, Srivastava RN, et al. Percutaneous renal biopsy in children: an analysis of complications in 890 consecutive biopsies. *Tex Rep Biol Med* 1971;29:253–264.
40. Colodny AH, Reckler JM. A safe, simple and reliable method for percutaneous (closed) renal biopsies in children: results in 100 consecutive patients. *J Urol* 1975;113:222–224.
41. Welt L. Questionnaire on renal biopsies. *JAMA* 1968;205:226.
42. McVicar M, Nicastri AD, Gauthier B. Improved renal biopsy technique in children. *N Y State J Med* 1974;74:830–831.
43. White RHR. Observations on percutaneous renal biopsy in children. *Arch Dis Child* 1963;38:260–266.
44. Burstein DM, Korbet SM, Schwartz MM. The use of the automatic core biopsy system in percutaneous renal biopsies: a comparative study. *Am J Kidney Dis* 1993;22:545–552.
45. Corwin HL, Schwartz MM, Lewis EJ. The importance of sample size in the interpretation of the renal biopsy. *Am J Nephrol* 1988;8:85–89.
46. Silva FG, Pirani CL. Electron microscopic study of medical diseases of the kidney. *Mod Pathol* 1988;1:292–315.
47. Furness PN, Boyd S. Electron microscopy and immunocytochemistry in the assessment of renal biopsy specimens: actual and optimal practice. *J Clin Pathol* 1996;49:233–237.
48. D'Agati V, Suh J-I, Carbone L, et al. Pathology of HIV-associated nephropathy: a detailed morphologic and comparative study. *Kidney Int* 1989;35:1358–1370.
49. Shindo S, Yoshimoto M, Kuriya N, et al. Glomerular basement membrane thickness in recurrent and persistent hematuria and nephrotic syndrome: correlation with sex and age. *Pediatr Nephrol* 1988;2:196–199.
50. Morita M, White RHR, Raafat F, et al. Glomerular basement membrane thickness in children. A morphometric study. *Pediatr Nephrol* 1988;2:190–195.
51. Fogo A, Hawkins EP, Berry PL, et al. Glomerular hypertrophy in minimal change disease predicts subsequent progression to focal glomerular sclerosis. *Kidney Int* 1990;38:115–123.
52. Hurley RM, Drummond KN. Glomerular enlargement in primary renal disease. A quantitative study. *Arch Pathol* 1974;97:389–391.
53. Kaplan C, Pasternack B, Shah H, et al. Age-related incidence of sclerotic glomeruli in human kidneys. *Am J Pathol* 1975;80:227–234.
54. Kappel B, Olsen S. Cortical interstitial tissue and sclerosed glomeruli in the normal human kidney, related to age and sex. A quantitative study. *Virchows Arch* 1980;387:271–277.
55. Smith SM, Hoy WE, Cobb L. Low incidence of glomerulosclerosis in normal kidneys. *Arch Pathol Lab Med* 1989;113:1253–1256.

56. Nash MA, Greifer I, Olbing H, et al. The significance of focal sclerotic lesions in glomeruli in children. *J Pediatr* 1976;88:806–813.
57. Chiang ML, Hawkins EP, Berry PL, et al. Diagnostic and prognostic significance of glomerular epithelial cell vacuolization and podocyte effacement in children with minimal lesion nephrotic syndrome and focal segmental glomerulosclerosis: an ultrastructural study. *Clin Nephrol* 1988;30:8–14.
58. Verani RR, Hawkins EP. Recurrent focal segmental glomerulosclerosis. *Am J Nephrol* 1986;6:263–270.
59. Yoshikawa N, Matsuyama S, Iijima K, et al. Benign familial hematuria. *Arch Pathol Lab Med* 1988;112:794–797.
60. Steffes MW, Barbosa J, Basgen JM, et al. Quantitative glomerular morphology of the normal human kidney. *Lab Invest* 1983;49:82–86.
61. Yoshioka K, Hino S, Takemura T, et al. Type IV collagen α5 chain: normal distribution and abnormalities in X-linked Alport syndrome revealed by monoclonal antibody. *Am J Pathol* 1994;144:986–996.
62. Heptinstall RH. Pyelonephritis: pathologic features. In: Heptinstall RH, ed. *Pathology of the kidney*, 4th ed. Boston: Little, Brown and Company, 1992:1489–1561.
63. Verani R, Walker P, Silva FG. Renal cystic disease of infancy: results of histochemical studies. A report of the Southwest Pediatric Nephrology Study Group. *Pediatr Nephrol* 1989;3:37–42.
64. Hawkins EP, Berry PL, Silva FG. Acute tubulointerstitial nephritis in children: clinical, morphologic, and lectin studies. A report of the Southwest Pediatric Nephrology Study Group. *Am J Kidney Dis* 1989;14:466–471.
65. Myers BD, Ross J, Newton L, et al. Cyclosporine-associated chronic nephropathy. *N Engl J Med* 1984;311:699–705.
66. Mihatsch MJ, Thiel G, Basler V, et al. Morphological patterns in cyclosporine-treated renal transplant recipients. *Transplant Proc* 1985;17(Suppl 1):101–116.
67. Böhle A, Mackensen-Haen S, Gise H. Significance of tubulointerstitial changes in the renal cortex for the excretory function and concentration ability of the kidney: a morphometric contribution. *Am J Nephrol* 1987;7:421–433.
68. Striker GE, Shainuck LI, Cutler RE, et al. Structural-functional correlations in renal disease. I. A method for assaying and classifying histopathologic changes in renal disease. *Hum Pathol* 1970;1:615–630.
69. Schainuck LI, Striker GE, Cutler RE, et al. Structural-functional correlations in renal disease. II. The correlations. *Hum Pathol* 1970;1:631–641.
70. Trainin EB, Gomez-Leon G. Development of renal insufficiency after long-standing steroid-responsive nephrotic syndrome. *Int J Pediatr Nephrol* 1982;3:55–58.
71. Southwest Pediatric Nephrology Study Group. Focal segmental glomerulosclerosis in children with idiopathic nephrotic syndrome. A report of the Southwest Pediatric Nephrology Study Group. *Kidney Int* 1985;27:442–449.
72. Senggutuvan P, Cameron JS, Hartley RB, et al. Recurrence of focal segmental glomerulosclerosis in transplanted kidneys: analysis of incidence and risk factors in 59 allografts. *Pediatr Nephrol* 1990;4:21–28.
73. Al-Eisa A, Carter JE, Lirenmann DS, et al. Childhood IgM nephropathy: comparison with minimal change disease. *Nephron* 1996;72:37–43.
74. Fogo A, Ichikawa I. Focal segmental glomerulosclerosis. *Pediatr Nephrol* 1996;10:374–391.
75. Devarajan P, Spitzer A. Towards a biological characterization of focal segmental glomerulosclerosis. *Am J Kidney Dis* 2002;39:625–636.
76. Detwiler RK, Falk RF, Hogan SL, et al. Collapsing glomerulopathy: a clinically and pathologically distinct variant of focal segmental glomerulosclerosis. *Kidney Int* 1994;45:1416–1424.
77. Schwartz MM, Evans J, Bain R, Korbet SM. Focal segmental glomerulosclerosis: prognostic implications of the cellular lesion. *J Am Soc Nephrol* 1999;10:1900–1907.
78. Howie AJ, Brewer DB. Further studies on the glomerular tip lesion: early and late stages and life table analysis. *J Pathol* 1985;147:245–255.
79. Iskandar SS, Browning MC, Lorentz WB. C1q nephropathy: a pediatric clinicopathologic study. *Am J Kidney Dis* 1991;18:459–465.
80. Suzuki J, Yoshikawa N, Nakamura H. A quantitative analysis of the glomeruli in focal segmental glomerulosclerosis. *Pediatr Nephrol* 1994;8:416–419.
81. Nyberg E, Bohman SO, Berg U. Glomerular volume and renal function in children with different types of the nephrotic syndrome. *Pediatr Nephrol* 1994;8:285–289.
82. Fogo AB. Glomerular hypertension, abnormal glomerular growth and progression of renal diseases. *Kidney Int* 2000;57(Suppl 75):S15–S21.
83. Kaplan JM, Kim SH, North KN, et al. Mutations in ACTN4, encoding alpha-actinin-4, cause familial focal segmental glomerulosclerosis. *Nat Genet* 2000;24:251–256.
84. Boute N, Gribouval O, Roselli S, et al. NPHS2, encoding the glomerular protein podocin, is mutated in autosomal recessive steroid-resistant nephrotic syndrome. *Nat Genet* 2000;24:349–354.
85. Khoshnoodi J, Tryggvason K. Congenital nephrotic syndromes. *Curr Opin Genet Dev* 2001;11:322–327.
86. Doleris LM, Hill GS, Chedin P, et al. Focal segmental glomerulosclerosis associated with mitochondrial cytopathy. *Kidney Int* 2000;58:1851–1858.
87. Gagnadoux MF, Habib R, Gubler MC, et al. Long-term (15–25 years) outcome of childhood hemolytic-uremic syndrome. *Clin Nephrol* 1996;46:39–41.
88. Argyle JC, Hogg RJ, Pysher TJ, et al. A clinicopathological study of 24 children with hemolytic uremic syndrome. *Pediatr Nephrol* 1990;4:52–58.
89. Van Buren D, Van Buren CT, Flechner SM, et al. De novo hemolytic uremic syndrome in renal transplant recipients immunosuppressed with cyclosporine. *Surgery* 1985;98:54–62.
90. Schwarz A, Krause P-H, Offerman G, et al. Recurrent and de novo renal disease after kidney transplantation with or without cyclosporine A. *Am J Kidney Dis* 1991;17:524–531.
91. Lévy M, Gonzalez-Burchard G, Broyer M, et al. Berger's disease in children: natural history and outcome. *Medicine* 1985;64:157–180.
92. Yoshikawa N, Ito H, Nakamura H. IgA nephropathy in children from Japan. *Child Nephrol Urol* 1989;9:191–199.
93. Yoshikawa N, Iijima K, Matsuyama S, et al. Repeat renal biopsy in children with IgA nephropathy. *Clin Nephrol* 1990;33:160–167.
94. Lee SM, Rao VM, Franklin WA, et al. IgA nephropathy:

morphologic predictors of progressive renal disease. *Hum Pathol* 1982;13:314–322.
95. Haas M. Histologic subclassification of IgA nephropathy: a clinicopathologic study of 244 cases. *Am J Kidney Dis* 1997;29:829–842.
96. Yamabe H, Johnson RJ, Gretch DR, et al. Hepatitis C virus infection and membranoproliferative glomerulonephritis in Japan. *J Am Soc Nephrol* 1995;6:220–223.
97. Johnson RJ, Gretch DR, Yamabe H, et al. Membranoproliferative glomerulonephritis associated with hepatitis C virus infection. *N Engl J Med* 1993;328:465–470.
98. Nowicki MJ, Welch TR, Ahmad N, et al. Absence of hepatitis B and C viruses in pediatric idiopathic membranoproliferative glomerulonephritis. *Pediatr Nephrol* 1995;9:16–18.
99. Galle P, Mahieu P. Electron dense alteration of kidney basement membranes. A renal lesion specific of a systemic disease. *Am J Med* 1975;58:749–764.
100. Churg J, Duffy JL, Bernstein J. Identification of dense deposit disease: a report for the international study of kidney diseases in children. *Arch Pathol Lab Med* 1979;103:67–72.
101. Schwertz R, de Jong R, Gretz N, et al., and Arbeitsgemeinschaft Padiatrische Nephrologie. Outcome of idiopathic membranoproliferative glomerulonephritis in children. *Acta Paediatr* 1996;85:308–312.
102. Najafi CC, Korbet SM, Lewis EJ, et al. Significance of histologic patterns of glomerular injury upon long-term prognosis in severe lupus glomerulonephritis. *Kidney Int* 2001;59:2156–2163.
103. Merkel F, Pullig O, Marx M, et al. Course and prognosis of anti-basement membrane antibody (anti-BM-Ab)-mediated disease: report of 35 cases. *Nephrol Dial Transplant* 1994;9:372–376.
104. Ellis EN, Pysher TJ. Renal disease in adolescents with type I diabetes mellitus: a report of the Southwest Pediatric Nephrology Study Group. *Am J Kidney Dis* 1993;22:783–790.
105. Pirson Y. Making the diagnosis of Alport's syndrome. *Kidney Int* 1999;56:760–775.
106. Gauthier B, Trachtman H, Frank R, et al. Familial thin basement membrane nephropathy in children with asymptomatic microhematuria. *Nephron* 1989;51:502–508.
107. Buzza M, Wang YY, Dagher H, et al. COL4A4 mutation in thin basement membrane disease previously described in Alport syndrome. *Kidney Int* 2001;60:480–483.
108. Fioretto P, Steffes MW, Sutherland DE, et al. Reversal of lesions of diabetic nephropathy after pancreas transplantation. *N Engl J Med* 1998;339:69–75.
109. Ikoma M, Kawamura T, Fogo A, et al. Cause of variable therapeutic efficiency of angiotensin converting enzyme inhibitor on the glomerular mesangial lesions. *Kidney Int* 1991;40:291–301.
110. Fogo A. Progression and potential regression of glomerulosclerosis. *Kidney Int* 2001;59:804–819.
111. Austin HA III, Boumpas DT, Vaughan EM, et al. High-risk features of lupus nephritis: importance of race and clinical and histological factors in 166 patients. *Nephrol Dial Transplant* 1995;10:1620–1628.
112. Baqi N, Moazami S, Singh A, et al. Lupus nephritis in children: a longitudinal study of prognostic factors and therapy. *J Am Soc Nephrol* 1996;7:924–929.
113. Hill GS, Delahousse M, Nochy D, et al. A new morphologic index for the evaluation of renal biopsies in lupus nephritis. *Kidney Int* 2000;58:1160–1173.
114. Katafuchi R, Oh Y, Hori K, et al. An important role of glomerular segmental lesions on progression of IgA nephropathy: a multivariate analysis. *Clin Nephrol* 1994;41:191–198.
115. Hogg RJ, Silva FG, Wyatt RJ, et al. Prognostic indicators in children with IgA nephropathy: report of the Southwest Pediatric Nephrology Study Group. *Pediatr Nephrol* 1994;8:15–20.
116. Andreoli SP, Yum MN, Bergstein JM. IgA nephropathy in children: significance of glomerular basement membrane deposition of IgA. *Am J Nephrol* 1986;6:28–33.
117. Andreoli SP, Bergstein JM. Treatment of severe IgA nephropathy in children. *Pediatr Nephrol* 1989;3:248–253.
118. Linn JT, Berg U, Bohman S-O, et al. Course and long-term outcome of idiopathic IgA nephropathy in children. *Pediatr Nephrol* 1991;5:383–386.
119. Hsu H-C, Wu C-Y, Lin C-Y, et al. Membranous nephropathy in 52 hepatitis B surface antigen (HBsAg) carrier children in Taiwan. *Kidney Int* 1989;36:1103–1107.
120. Colvin RB, Cohen AH, Saiontz C, et al. Evaluation of pathologic criteria for acute renal allograft rejection: reproducibility, sensitivity, and clinical correlation. *J Am Soc Nephrol* 1997;8:1930–1941.
121. Racusen LC, Solez K, Colvin RB, et al. The Banff 97 working classification of renal allograft pathology. *Kidney Int* 1999;55:713–723.
122. Rush D, Jeffery J, Trpkov K, et al. Effect of subclinical rejection on renal allograft histology and function at 6 months. *Transplant Proc* 1996;28:494–495.
123. Strehlau J, Pavlakis M, Lipman M, et al. Quantitative detection of immune activation transcripts as a diagnostic tool in kidney transplantation. *Proc Natl Acad Sci U S A* 1997;94:695–700.
124. Mauiyyedi S, Crespo M, Collins AB, et al. Acute humoral rejection in kidney transplantation: II. morphology, immunopathology, and pathologic classification. *J Am Soc Nephrol* 2002;13:779–787.
125. Bohmig GA, Exner M, Habicht A, et al. Capillary C4d deposition in kidney allografts: a specific marker of alloantibody-dependent graft injury. *J Am Soc Nephrol* 2002;13:1091–1099.
126. Colvin RB. The renal allograft biopsy. *Kidney Int* 1996;50:1069–1082.
127. Drachenberg CB, Steinberger E, Hoehn-Saric E, et al. Specificity of intertubular capillary changes: comparative ultrastructural studies in renal allografts and native kidneys. *Ultrastruct Pathol* 1997;21:227–233.
128. Mihatsch MJ, Ryffel B, Gudat F. The differential diagnosis between rejection and cyclosporine toxicity. *Kidney Int* 1995;(Suppl 52):S63–S69.
129. Meehan SM, Pascual M, Williams WW, et al. De novo collapsing glomerulopathy in renal allografts. *Transplantation* 1998;65:1192–1197.
130. Habib R, Gagnadoux M-F, Broyer M. Recurrent glomerulonephritis in transplanted children. *Contrib Nephrol* 1987;55:123–135.
131. Goral S, Ynares C, Shappell SB, et al. Recurrent lupus nephritis in renal transplant recipients revisited: it is not rare. *Transplantation* 2003;75:651–656.

132. Randhawa PS, Magnone M, Jordan M, et al. Renal allograft involvement by Epstein-Barr virus associated with post-transplant lymphoproliferative disease. *Am J Surg Pathol* 1996;20:563–571.
133. Randhawa PS, Finkelstein S, Scantlebury V, et al. Human polyoma virus-associated interstitial nephritis in the allograft kidney. *Transplantation* 1999;67:103–109.
134. Esposito C, Phillips CL, Liu ZH, et al. Molecular analysis of human glomerular disease. *Kidney Int* 1996;53(Suppl):S21–S25.
135. Barnes JL, Milani S. In situ hybridization in the study of the kidney and renal disease. *Semin Nephrol* 1995;15:9–28.
136. Kretzler M, Cohen CD, Doran P, et al. Repuncturing the renal biopsy: strategies for molecular diagnosis in nephrology. *J Am Soc Nephrol* 2002;13:1961–1972.
137. Hunley TE, Julian BA, Phillips JA, et al. Angiotensin converting enzyme gene polymorphism: potential silencer motif and impact on progression in IgA nephropathy. *Kidney Int* 1996;49:571–577.
138. Yoshida H, Mitarai T, Kawamura T, et al. Role of the deletion polymorphism of the angiotensin converting enzyme gene in the progression and therapeutic responsiveness of IgA nephropathy. *J Clin Invest* 1995;96:2162–2169.

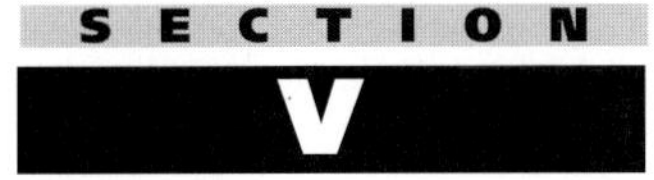

GLOMERULAR DISEASE

25

CONGENITAL NEPHROTIC SYNDROME

CHRISTER HOLMBERG
KARL TRYGGVASON
MARJO K. KESTILÄ
HANNU J. JALANKO

Renal diseases associated with nephrotic syndrome (NS) in the first year of life are uncommon and make up a heterogeneous group of disorders with different proposed causes, courses, and prognoses. *Congenital NS* (CNS) is defined as proteinuria leading to clinical symptoms soon after birth. An arbitrary age limit of 3 months has been proposed to separate CNS from "infantile" NS, which becomes manifest later during the first year of life (1). Although this age limit is useful for statistical purposes, it is not sufficient for the classification of early-onset NS (Fig. 25.1). The most common type of CNS is CNS of the Finnish type (CNF), with a clinical onset before the age of 1 month. The other early-onset NSs have a more widespread age of onset, from the first days of life to several months of age. The diagnosis of a patient with early manifestations of NS must be based on several criteria, including clinical presentation, family history, laboratory findings, and renal histology. In the coming years, the classification will be modified by the use of molecular genetics.

CNS and early-onset NS can be classified into primary and secondary or acquired forms (Table 25.1). CNF is considered the prototype of CNS, and in recent years progress has been made in the knowledge of the genetics, pathophysiology, and clinical aspects of CNF (2–4). In this chapter, management of CNF is presented more thoroughly.

PRIMARY NEPHROTIC SYNDROME

Congenital Nephrotic Syndrome of the Finnish Type

CNF originally referred to a severe form of CNS typically seen in Finnish newborns (5,6). After the gene (named *NPHS1*) responsible for this disorder was isolated in 1998, it became clear that not all cases of "typical" CNF are caused by mutations in *NPHS1* and, on the other hand, mutations in *NPHS1* may sometimes cause atypical (mild) forms of NS. This has led to some confusion in the nomenclature; both CNF and NPHS1 are used as abbreviations for the same disorder. In this text, CNF is used to denote the clinical entity. The term *NPHS1* can be used to refer to cases known to be caused by *NPHS1* mutations.

Epidemiology

CNF is an autosomal recessive disease first described by Hallman et al. (5). The disease is more frequent in Finland, the incidence being 1 in 8200 live births (7). However, patients with CNF have been reported all over the world among various ethnic groups (8–12). A high incidence of NPHS1 has been reported among the Old Order Mennonites in Lancaster County, Pennsylvania (9). In a subgroup of "Groffdale Conference" Mennonites, the incidence is 1 in 500, which is almost 20 times greater than that observed in Finland.

Clinical Features

The basic problem in CNF is severe loss of protein, beginning during the fetal period (7). The signs and symptoms are believed to be secondary to this protein deficiency (7,13,14). In a recent survey, more than 80% of the children were found to be born prematurely (before the thirty-eighth week), with a mean birth weight of 2600 g (1500 to 3500 g). However, only 2 of the 46 newborns were small for gestational age (14). Amniotic fluid is often meconium stained, but most neonates do not have major pulmonary problems. The placenta is larger than normal and almost invariably weighs more than 25% of the baby's birth weight. The mean ratio of placental to infant weight is 0.38 in babies with CNF, compared with 0.18 in normal babies. The reason for this is not known.

In typical CNF, edema and abdominal distention become evident soon after birth. NS was diagnosed within the first week in 82% of the Finnish patients and within 2 months in the remaining cases (14). In contrast to most

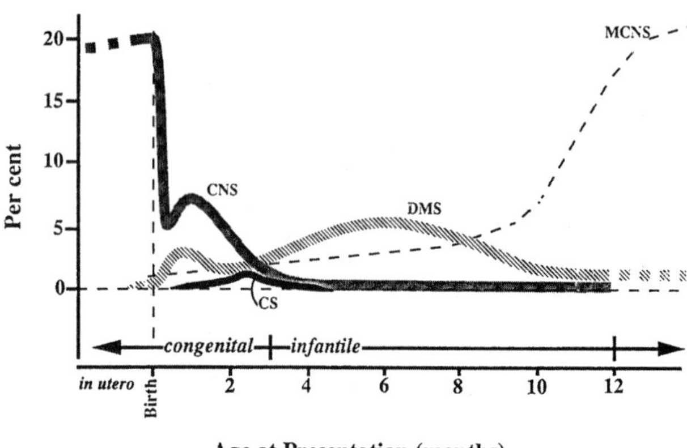

FIGURE 25.1. Schematic presentation of the age at presentation for 178 children with nephrotic syndrome detected in the first year of life. CNS, congenital nephrotic syndrome; DMS, diffuse mesangial sclerosis; MCNS, minimal-change nephrotic syndrome. (From Mauch TJ, Vernier RL, Burke BA, et al. Nephrotic syndrome in the first year of life. In: Holliday MA, Barratt TM, Avner ED, eds. *Pediatric nephrology*, 2nd ed. Baltimore: Williams & Wilkins, 1994:788–802, with permission.)

other CNS, the protein loss in CNF leads to severe hypoalbuminemia, and the serum albumin concentration is typically less than 10 g/L before protein substitution (15). Without albumin substitution and nutritional support, the classic picture of CNF develops: generalized edema, abdominal distention, ascites, umbilical hernias, and widened cranial sutures and fontanelles (5).

Infants with CNF do not have extrarenal malformations. Minor functional disorders in the central nervous system and heart, however, are quite common during the course of the disease. Most children have muscular hypotonia, and computed tomography or magnetic resonance imaging showed mild atrophic changes in the brain in a third of the Finnish patients (14). Dystonic cerebral palsy has been diagnosed in 8% of the Finnish patients; the etiology of this manifestation is not known. Minor cardiac findings, such as hypertrophy and mild functional pulmonary stenosis, have been reported in one-fourth of the Finnish patients (14). In a recent report form Malta, pulmonary valve stenosis was found in three cases and a subaortic stenosis in one patient (16).

TABLE 25.1. CLASSIFICATION OF CONGENITAL AND EARLY-ONSET NEPHROTIC SYNDROME (NS)

- Primary NS
  - Congenital nephrosis of the Finnish type
  - Isolated diffuse mesangial sclerosis
  - Denys-Drash syndrome
  - Congenital NS with brain and other malformations
  - Minimal-change NS
  - Focal segmental glomerulosclerosis
  - Membranous glomerulopathy
  - Unclassified
- Secondary NS
  - Infections
    - Congenital syphilis
    - Toxoplasmosis, rubella, cytomegalovirus
    - Hepatitis, human immunodeficiency virus
    - Malaria
  - Systemic lupus erythematosus

Laboratory Findings

In CNF, the first urine analysis already shows proteinuria, microscopic hematuria, and, often, some leukocyturia. The magnitude of proteinuria depends on the serum albumin concentration. The urinary protein concentration exceeds 20 g/L when the serum albumin concentration is above 15 g/L (15) and no medication reducing filtration pressure has been given. This is in contrast to CNS associated with diffuse mesangial sclerosis (DMS), in which patients usually have less severe proteinuria (Table 25.2). In addition to albumin, many other proteins are lost in the urine: immunoglobulin G (IgG), transferrin, apoproteins, lipoprotein lipase, antithrombin III (ATIII), ceruloplasmin, vitamin D–binding protein, and thyroid-binding globulin (17). The serum levels of these proteins and their ligands (e.g., thyroxin) are low, leading to secondary metabolic disturbances. The low thyroxine concentration leads to an increase in thyroid-stimulating hormone (TSH) (18). Low serum albumin and postheparin plasma lipoprotein lipase activities and high free fatty acid concentrations lead to hypertriglyceridemia. Total and low-density lipoprotein cholesterol levels are high, but high-density lipoprotein levels are low, and the low-density lipoprotein and high-density lipoprotein particles are enriched with triglycerides (17). These lipid abnormalities and arteriolar changes are seen already during the first year of life and may lead to an increased risk of arteriosclerosis (19). The characteristics of CNF are given in Table 25.2. Today, the diagnosis can be confirmed by the analysis of the *NPHS1* gene.

Radiologic Findings

Saraga et al. reported ultrasonographic measurements in 20 children with CNF (20). Kidney size was normal in most patients during the first 2 months. The renal cortex was hyperechogenic, and the medullary pyramids were echolucent in two-thirds of cases. Corticomedullary differentiation was preserved. The central echo was merged with the surrounding cortical echoes in most kidneys, and the pelvic areas were normal.

Between 2 and 12 months, the size of the kidneys was above two standard deviations in all children, but with a normal outline. The renal cortex was hyperechogenic, corticomedullary differentiation had mostly disappeared, and the medullary pyramids were still echolucent. After 12 months, there was a decrease in kidney size, and the parenchyma was hyperechogenic, with loss of corticomedullary differentia-

TABLE 25.2. TYPICAL FEATURES OF CONGENITAL NEPHROSIS OF THE FINNISH TYPE (CNF) AND DIFFUSE MESANGIAL SCLEROSIS (DMS)

Features	CNF	DMS
Proteinuria, onset	Starts intrauterinely	Can start at birth, but mostly during first year of life
Amniotic fluid alpha-feto-protein	Always increased	Usually normal
Placenta	>25% of birth weight	Usually normal
Proteinuria, magnitude	Severe (>20 g/L with a serum albumin >15 g/L)	Usually less severe
Glomerular filtration rate	Normal during the first 6–12 mo	End-stage renal disease within months after presentation
Histology	Radial dilation of proximal tubules after 3 mo	Mesangial sclerosis contracting the glomerular tuft; tubular atrophy; interstitial fibrosis
DNA analysis	Mutations in the *NPHS1* gene	Mutations of the *WT1* gene in Denys-Drash syndrome and some cases of isolated DMS

tion. These findings correlate with the histologic changes showing increased dilation of proximal tubules at first and interstitial fibrosis and glomerular sclerosis later on.

Pathology

CNF kidneys are smooth surfaced, and the renal cortex is somewhat thicker than normal. In an autopsy series, the mean kidney weight was almost twice that of age-matched control children (21). Older patients had smaller, "normal-sized" kidneys, probably because of atrophy and scarring of the renal parenchyma. Pathologic findings are confined to the renal cortex without medullary lesions. The changes are progressive with age, from occasional dilated tubules in the fetal kidneys to severe tubulointerstitial and glomerular abnormalities at the age of 1 to 2 years (21,22).

In the fetal period, the CNF kidneys develop quite normally. At 16 to 22 gestational weeks, the glomeruli show few changes by light microscopy, but occasional dilated tubules are seen in most cases (23,24). The dilations contain bright, eosinophilic, colloid material, and the epithelium is low and cuboidal. By electron microscopy, the mature glomeruli show effacement of podocyte foot processes and irregular foot processes. The slit pores between the foot processes are of various sizes, and the filamentous image of the slit diaphragm is completely missing in cases with severe *NPHS1* mutations (25). It is remarkable that also carriers of *NPHS1* mutations can have these "proteinuric" changes, making the pathologic diagnosis difficult (26).

The pathologic changes are subtle by light microscopy during the first month. The glomeruli show a slight to moderate mesangial cell proliferation. Irregular microcystic dilatations of proximal tubules are inconstantly found on renal biopsy specimens (Figs. 25.2 and 25.3). Thick-walled small arteries and fetal glomeruli are present, but they are also seen in normal kidneys of this age group. Electron microscopy shows effacement of foot processes (Fig. 25.4) and a thin glomerular basement membrane (GBM), which is already evident in the fetal kidneys (27).

Biopsies taken 3 to 8 months after birth usually show the most characteristic changes of CNF. Numerous radial dilations of the tubules are the most obvious feature (Fig. 25.2B). The glomeruli show moderate mesangial hypercellularity, but some degenerative changes, such as shrinking of the glomerular tuft, fibrotic thickening of the Bowman's capsule, and glomerular sclerosis, become evident (Fig. 25.3A). Interstitial fibrosis and scattered lymphocyte infiltrates begin to develop (14). The proportion of sclerotic and ischemic glomeruli increases. Some tubular dilatations increase in size, and their epithelium becomes atrophic. Interstitial fibrosis and inflammation increase.

Genetics

NPHS1 and Nephrin

CNF is inherited as an autosomal recessive trait (6). The gene responsible for most CNF cases has been localized to chromosome 19q13.1 (28) and named *NPHS1* (2). It has a size of 26 kb and contains 29 exons. *NPHS1* codes for nephrin, which is a 1241-residue, cell adhesion protein of the Ig family (Fig. 25.5). The extracellular part of nephrin contains eight Ig-like modules and one fibronectin type III domain. The intracellular domain has no significant homology with other known proteins but it has nine tyrosine residues, some of which may become phosphorylated during ligand binding. The expression of nephrin was first reported to be restricted to glomerular podocytes (2). Recent studies on the *NPHS1* promoter have confirmed this localization (29,30). The data obtained from mice, however, suggest that nephrin is also expressed in some areas of the central nervous system (e.g., cerebellum and spinal cord) and in pancreatic beta cells (31). The tissue expression of nephrin in humans is not clear. Pancreatic expression of nephrin has been reported (32), but our

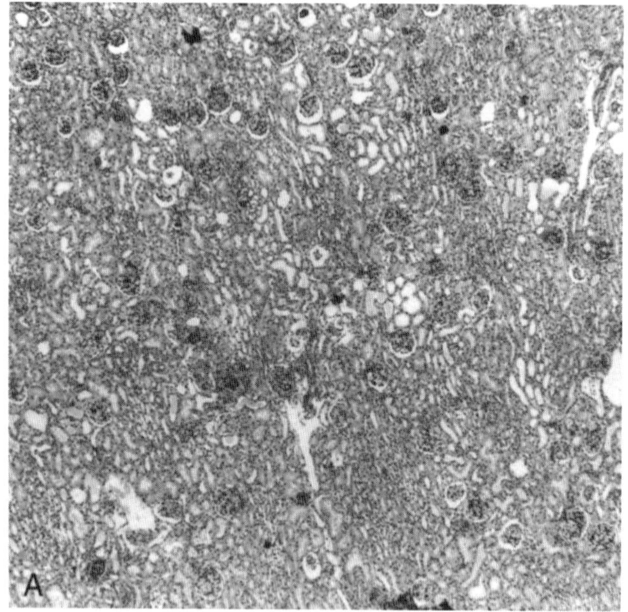

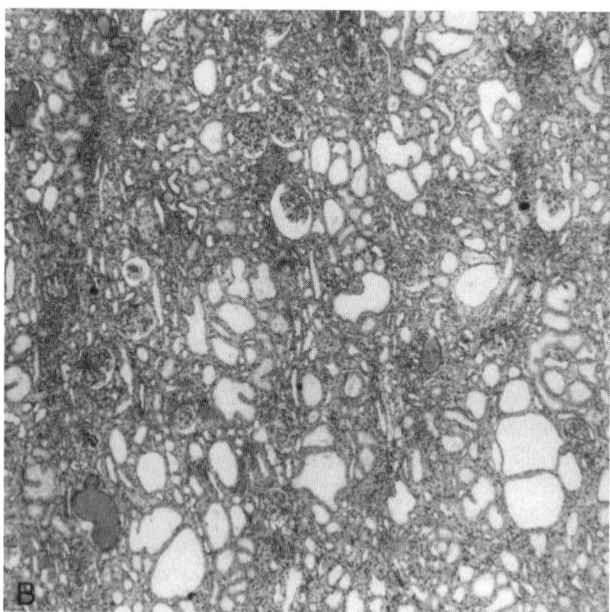

FIGURE 25.2. **A:** Histologic picture of the congenital nephrotic syndrome of the Finnish-type kidney at 4 weeks of age. **B:** Histologic picture of the congenital nephrotic syndrome of the Finnish-type kidney at 6 months of age. Note the increase of the dilated tubules (magnification, ×60).

results suggest that nephrin expression in humans is restricted to the glomerulus (33).

NPHS1 Mutations

Sequencing the *NPHS1* coding region has revealed two important mutations in more than 90% of the Finnish CNF patients (2). The first mutation, a 2–base pair deletion in exon 2, causes a frame shift resulting in a stop codon within the same exon (Fin-major mutation). The second is a nonsense mutation in exon 26 (Fin-minor). Fin-major leads

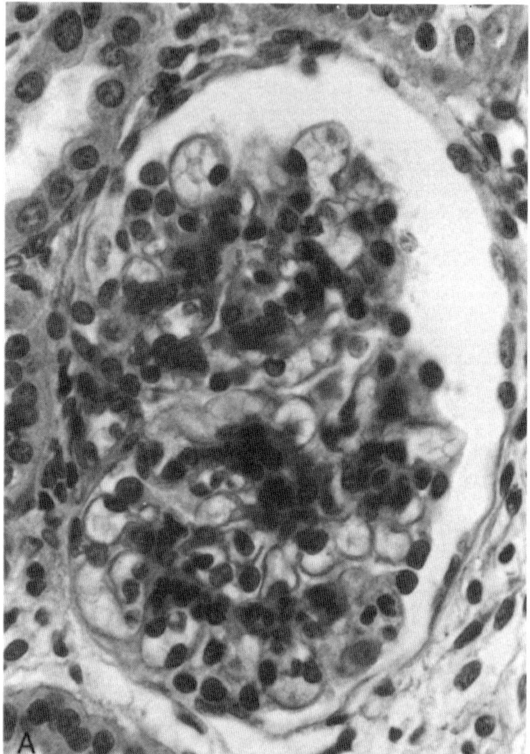

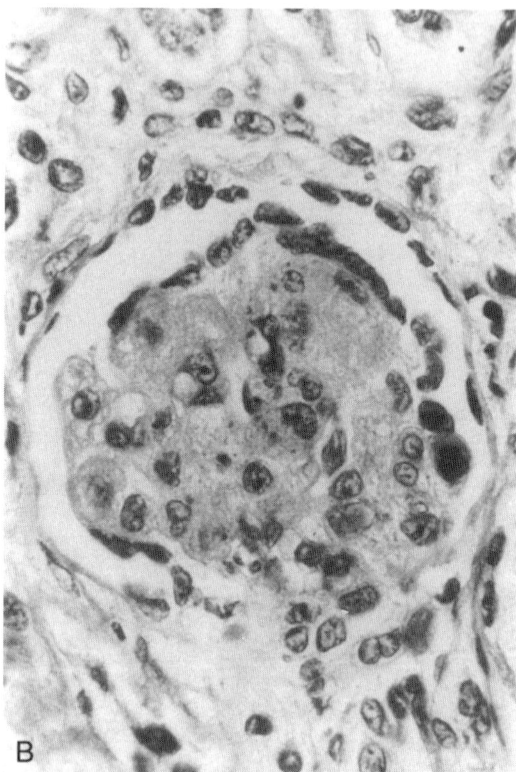

FIGURE 25.3. **A:** Congenital nephrotic syndrome of the Finnish type. Histologic picture of a glomerulus showing mesangial hypercellularity (×240). **B:** Diffuse mesangial sclerosis. Histologic picture of a contracted glomerulus. Note the ribbon of podocytes covering the glomerular tuft (×240).

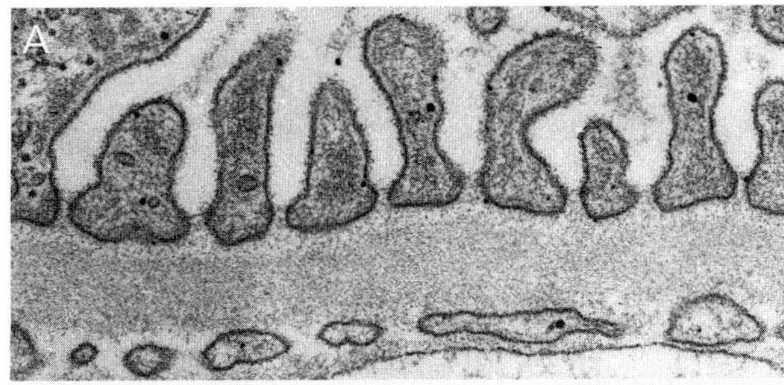

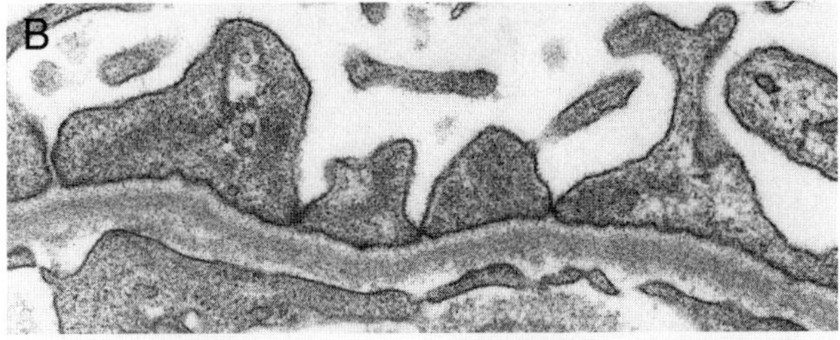

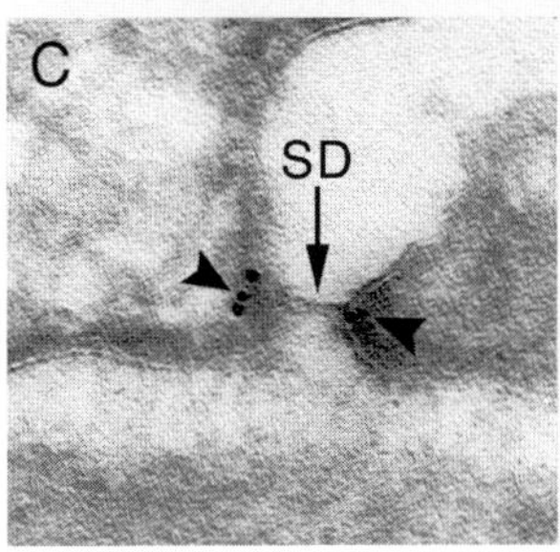

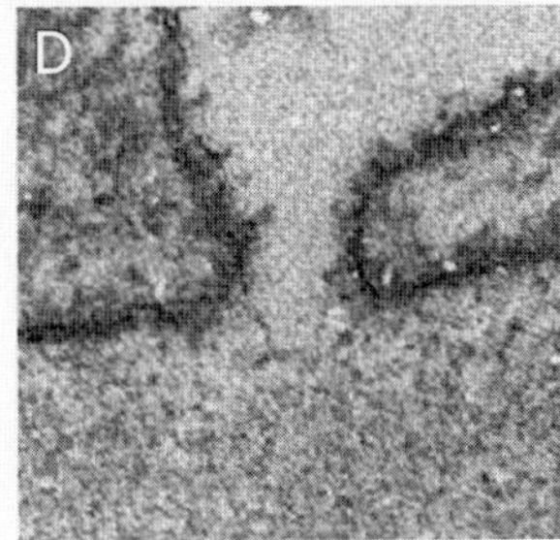

FIGURE 25.4. Electron microscopy of the glomerular capillary wall. **A:** Normal kidney showing the podocyte foot processes, the glomerular basement membrane, and the endothelium. **B:** Congenital nephrotic syndrome of the Finnish-type (CNF) kidney (Fin-major/Fin-major genotype) shows irregular podocyte foot processes. **C:** Immunoelectron microscopy of a podocyte pore in normal kidney. The filamentous image of the slit diaphragm (SD) is seen (*arrow*). Antibodies against the intracellular part of the nephrin show the localization of nephrin in the SD (gold particles, *arrowheads*). **D:** Immunoelectron microscopy of the podocyte slit pore in CNF kidney. No SD or nephrin is seen.

to a truncated 90-residue protein, and Fin-minor leads to a truncated 1109-residue protein. In addition to Fin-major and Fin-minor, a few missense mutations in the Finnish patients have been found (8). The uniform mutation pattern seen in the Finnish population can be explained by the founder effect.

Several reports on *NPHS1* mutations in non-Finnish patients have been published (8–12). The patients come from Europe, North America, North Africa, the Middle East, and Asia. In contrast to the Finnish patients, most non-Finns have "individual mutations." These include deletions, insertions, nonsense, missense, and splicing mutations spanning over the whole gene. For the moment, more than 60 mutations in *NPHS1* have been identified (Fig. 25.6). Missense mutations are all located within the extracellular part and cluster to exons coding for the Ig-like motifs two, four, and seven (8,11,12). The Fin-major and

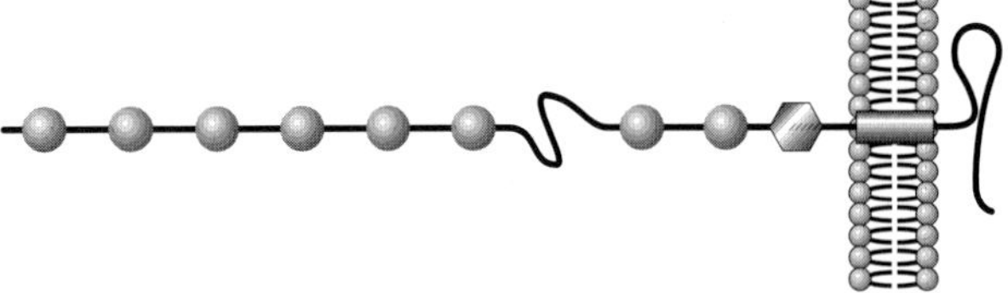

FIGURE 25.5. The structure of nephrin. The protein is a transmembrane cell adhesion receptor with small intracellular and a larger extracellular domain. The extracellular domain contains eight immunoglobulin-like modules (*circles*) and one fibronectin type III–like domain (*hexagon*) adjacent to the transmembrane domain. Nephrin is a major component on the podocyte slit diaphragm.

Fin-minor mutations are rare outside Finland. Enrichment of other mutations has been reported also in non-Finns. In Mennonites, the 1481delC mutation is common and leads to a truncated protein of 547 residues (9). On the other hand, a homozygous nonsense mutation R1160X in exon 27 has been found in all Maltese cases (12). Importantly, 6 of the 16 cases with this mutation had an atypically mild disease. The same mutation has been reported in six French CNF patients, and two of them had mild disease (34).

Congenital Nephrotic Syndrome of the Finnish Type Not Caused by *NPHS1* Mutations

In the report of Lenkkeri et al. (8), no mutations in *NPHS1* were found in 7 out of the 35 patients (20%) with classical CNF. Mutations may lie on important regulatory elements, which are not known yet, but it seems that *NPHS1* mutations are not the only cause of CNF. Koziell et al. (12) found no *NPHS1* mutations in 8 of 37 CNF cases. In two of these eight patients, mutations were found in the *NPHS2* gene, coding for another podocyte protein, podocin. Mutations in *NPHS2* normally lead to a recessive form of focal segmental glomerulosclerosis (FSGS) appearing later in life (35). Koziell et al. also reported three cases of CNS patients who had mutations both in *NPHS1* and *NPHS2*, indicating a functional interrelationship between the two genes (12). These patients showed FSGS on renal biopsy.

Pathogenesis

Normal Glomerular Filter

Sieving of the plasma occurs in kidney glomeruli through the capillary wall (glomerular filtration barrier). This barrier is composed of three layers: a fenestrated endothelium, the GBM, and visceral epithelial cells (podocytes) (3,36). The podocytes enclose the capillaries in a comb-like fashion, where the adjacent "spikes" (foot processes) form an interrupted sheet around the capillaries. The foot processes are connected just above the GBM by an extracellular structure, the slit diaphragm (Fig. 25.7). This structure bridges the filtration pores between the adjacent podocyte foot processes, and, by electron microscopy, it is seen as a

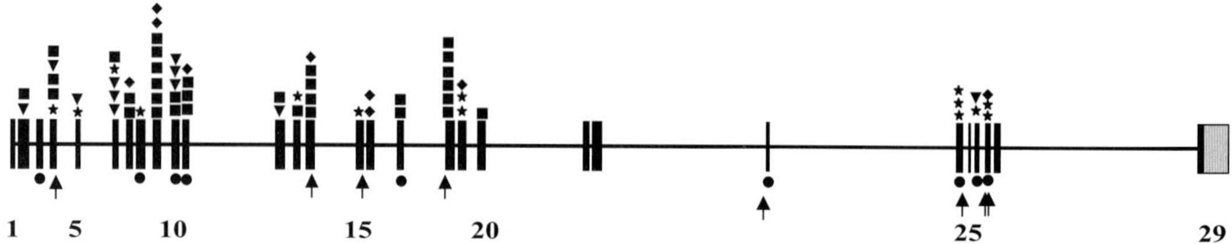

FIGURE 25.6. The *NPHS1* gene contains 29 exons (bars) at a size of 26 kb. For the moment, 65 different mutations have been reported in congenital nephrotic syndrome of the Finnish-type patients. These include 32 missense mutations, 11 deletions or insertions, 14 nonsense mutations, and eight splice-site mutations. In addition, nine amino acid changes without known phenotype effect and nine polymorphic changes have been detected. See text for references. [■], missense; [▼], deletion/insertion; [●], polymorphism; [↑], splice site; [★], nonsense; [♦], amino acid change without known phenotype effect.

thin line connecting the cell membranes. The filter serves both as a size-selective and a charge-selective sieve. It is believed that the GBM restricts the passage of macromolecules especially according to the charge, whereas the slit diaphragm forms a size-selective filter (36,37).

Immunoelectron microscopy revealed that nephrin was localized at the slit diaphragm area of human kidney glomerulus (38). Later, this localization was confirmed in mouse and rat (39–41). A hypothetical model was presented in which nephrin molecules from adjacent foot processes show a head-to-head assembly through homophilic interactions and form a backbone of the slit diaphragm (3,38). Recently, this model has been modified with other molecules such as NEPH1 and FAT interacting with nephrin in the slit diaphragm (42–44).

Slit Diaphragm in Congenital Nephrotic Syndrome of the Finnish Type

The Fin-major and Fin-minor mutations of the *NPHS1* gene lead to a complete absence of nephrin in the CNF kidney glomerulus (14). These kidneys also totally lack the filamentous image of podocyte slit diaphragms as studied by electron microscopy (Fig. 25.4). Similarly, nephrin knock-out mice, dying of severe proteinuria soon after birth, lack the slit diaphragm filaments by electron microscopy (31). These findings indicate that the absence of nephrin leads to distortion of the slit diaphragm and the leakage of plasma proteins into urine through the "empty" podocyte pores. Liu et al. (45) have shown that many missense *NPHS1* mutations seen in non-Finnish CNF patients lead to misfolding of the nephrin molecule and a defective intracellular nephrin transport in the podocyte. This most probably explains why even "mild" (missense) mutations cause heavy proteinuria and a typical clinical disease (12).

Role of Podocytes

It has become evident that podocytes play a crucial role in glomerular filtration (37,46,47), and mutations in genes coding for the other podocyte proteins probably lead to disorders resembling CNF (Fig. 25.7). Mutations in the gene coding for alpha-actinin-4 cause NS in humans (48), and lack of CD2-associated protein causes NS in neonatal mice (49,50). Nephrin, podocin, NEPH1, and CD2-associated protein are known to interact with each other and the actin cytoskeleton of the podocyte foot process, and defects in this interplay may cause proteinuria (37,43,51,52). Under-

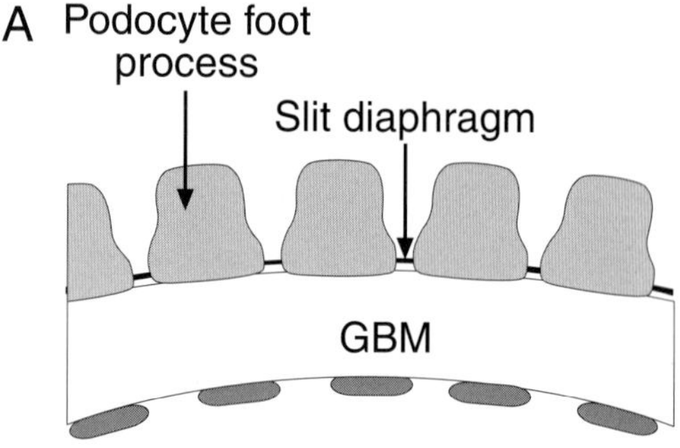

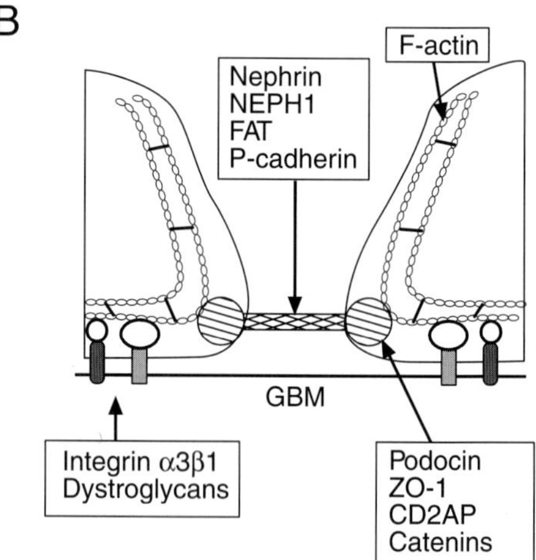

FIGURE 25.7. A: The structure of the glomerular capillary wall. The podocyte foot processes are connected by slit diaphragms. **B:** A model of the podocyte foot processes showing some of the known components of the slit diaphragm and the intracellular attachment proteins. The interplay between the different components is important in restricting the passage of plasma proteins into urine. GBM, glomerular basement membrane.

standing of the glomerular filtration barrier and its components is increasing rapidly, and it is to be expected that new "NS genes" will be identified in the near future.

Prenatal Diagnosis

Proteinuria in CNF starts *in utero*, and the measurement of alpha-fetoprotein (AFP) in the amniotic fluid and maternal serum has successfully been used for prenatal screening for CNF and in families with a previous CNF diagnosis (53,54). Fetal serum contains high levels of AFP, and leakage of fetal plasma proteins into amniotic fluid and further to maternal serum occurs in CNF as well as in neural tube defects. Elevated AFP levels and normal ultrasonographic findings of the fetus are considered diagnostic for CNF.

Amniotic fluid AFP levels exceeding five multiples of the normal median have traditionally been regarded as pathologic. The problem, however, is that heterozygous fetus carriers of *NPHS1* mutations may have elevated values (up to 50 multiples of the normal median) and a false-positive result in the AFP test (26,55). This may lead to termination of pregnancy on false grounds. The temporary proteinuria in carrier fetuses is also associated with tubular microcysts and podocyte foot process effacement (26). Thus, the differentiation of affected and carrier fetuses is quite difficult. In affected cases, the amniotic fluid AFP levels stay highly elevated, and repeated measurements of AFP levels during the second trimester are strongly recommended before making the diagnosis.

Analysis of *NPHS1* from placental biopsies or amniotic fluid cells is the method of choice for a precise diagnosis of CNF (2). In the Finnish population, analysis of the two major mutations is feasible. This is the case also when the disease-causing mutations are known in a family and can be specifically searched. If a fetus (without a family history of CNF) is suspected to have CNF based on elevated AFP values, sequencing of *NPHS1* is also possible, but due to the large size of the gene (29 exons) the analysis of the whole gene is time consuming and may not be done fast enough. *NPHS1* is mutation-rich and in almost all families, individual mutations have been found. In a case of missense mutation, a large number of control samples must be analyzed to find out if the amino acid substitution is a polymorphic change or a disease-causing mutation.

Management of Congenital Nephrotic Syndrome

The therapeutic decisions should usually aim at renal transplantation, which today is the only "curative" therapy in most cases (56). Immunosuppressive therapy with steroids or cyclophosphamide is not effective (1,57). The goals are to provide good nutrition, control edema, and prevent thrombosis and infections, allowing the child to reach a weight and body size allowing a successful kidney transplantation (58–60). With optimal therapy, growth and development are satisfactory, and after the first months patients can spend the daytime at home and receive their nightly albumin infusions in the hospital.

Antiproteinuric Medication

A clear reduction of protein excretion with captopril and indomethacin in CNF patients has been reported (61–63). On the other hand, Birnbacher et al. found that captopril had no effect on protein excretion in their patients (64). In our experience, patients with the Fin-major and Fin-minor mutations do not respond to captopril or indomethacin. Both of these mutations, as well as many of the missense mutations, lead to a situation in which no nephrin is expressed on the podocyte surface (14,45). In such cases, this therapy is probably not effective. On the other hand, if an *NPHS1* mutation leads to a single amino acid change and quite normal nephrin expression, a reduction in the protein excretion may be observed (14). Thus, treatment with angiotensin-converting enzyme inhibitor and indomethacin is worth trying in cases in which the *NPHS1* mutations or their biologic effect are not known. A kidney biopsy with immunohistochemistry of nephrin and electron microscopic evaluation of the podocyte slit diaphragm may help in making the decision of the treatment strategy.

Albumin Substitution

Proteinuria without substitution leads to protein malnutrition, reduced growth, and secondary symptoms of hypoproteinemia (15). Mahan et al. (56) first reported good results in CNS with a high-energy (120 kcal/kg/day), high-protein (3 to 4 g/kg/day), and low-sodium diet. Diuretics were given daily and intravenous albumin occasionally. Although this treatment substantially improved outcome, developmental delay and neurologic abnormalities were observed in 93% of the children, and all exhibited growth retardation. Broyer et al. (65) demonstrated substantial catch up growth with aggressive tube feeding in CNS, but their patients never reached the fourth percentile in growth.

Since the mid-1980s, we have adopted a more aggressive approach (15,17). Parenteral albumin infusions, 3 to 4 g albumin/kg/day, are started at birth. Indwelling deep-vein catheters are used from the age of 3 weeks. Albumin is given as a 20% solution together with intravenous furosemide (0.5 mg/kg). It is first divided into three or four 2-hour infusions, and after 1 month of age given as one infusion (over 6 to 8 hours) during the night. With this substitution, patients do not have substantial edema (15,17).

Nutrition

Patients with CNF should receive enterally 130 kcal/kg of energy and 4 g/kg of protein per day (in addition to parenteral albumin). Calorie intake is composed of 10 to 14% protein, 40 to 50% fat, and 40 to 50% carbohydrate. Rapeseed oil (10 to 15 mL) and fish oil (2 mL) are added to increase the ratio of monounsaturated and polyunsaturated fatty acids and the polyunsaturated to saturated ratio of the diet. The excess protein is given as a casein-based protein product and additional energy as glucose polymers. The daily water intake is 100 to 130 mL/kg (15). Many patients need a nasogastric tube to guarantee their energy intake. The children should also receive vitamin D_2 (2000 IU/day), vitamin E from the rapeseed oil (2.5 to 3.0 mg/day), and water-soluble vitamins, according to the recommended dietary allowances for healthy children of the same age. Supplementary magnesium (40 to 60 mg/day) and calcium (500 mg/day for patients younger than 6 months, 750 mg/day for patients 6 to 12 months, and 1000 mg/day for patients older than 12 months) are also given.

Additional Medication

Patients with CNF often have low levels of serum thyroid-binding globulin and thyroxine (66,67). McLean et al. (18) reported an increase in TSH in four of five patients with CNS and a positive response to thyroxine substitution. We have had a similar experience. Although serum thyroxine concentration is always low, TSH may be normal in the beginning but increases in most patients during the first months. Thus, we have adopted a policy of routinely giving thyroxine from birth, adjusting the dosage according to TSH.

Urinary excretion of plasminogen and ATIII is accompanied by increased levels of macroglobulin, fibrinogen, thromboplastin, and factors II, V, VII, X, and XII, contributing to hypercoagulopathy (68). Thromboses and severe coagulation problems have been reported in children with CNS (15,56,69), and the use of low-dose aspirin and dipyridamole therapy has been recommended (56). Our CNF patients are treated with sodium warfarin from 4 weeks of age, and no severe thrombotic complications have occurred since this therapy was commenced. Before surgical or vascular procedures, warfarin is stopped, and ATIII (50 IU/kg) is given to temporarily correct the ATIII deficiency.

Bacterial infections are a major complication in infants with CNF (7,56). Because of urinary losses of gamma globulin and complement factors B and D (70,71), nephrotic children are especially prone to infections caused by capsular bacteria, such as pneumococci, and prophylactic use of penicillin has been recommended (56). Ljungberg et al. retrospectively analyzed the incidence and type of infection in 21 infants with CNF during the first year of life (72). The infants had 63 verified and 62 suspected episodes of sepsis. The use of central venous lines had no effect on the incidence, and the prophylactic use of antibiotics or immunoglobulins did not reduce the incidence. Thus, we do not recommend prophylactic medication, but a high degree of suspicion of septic infections is warranted. The symptoms are often vague and masked by signs of focal infections occurring at the same time. Antibiotic therapy should be started promptly on suspicion and should cover the major hospital strains of bacteria. Response to treatment is usually excellent. Because of the urinary loss of IgG, no vaccinations are given.

Unilateral Nephrectomy

Some centers have adopted a routine of performing unilateral nephrectomy to reduce protein losses (73,74). This decreases the need and frequency of the albumin infusions and may help in the everyday management. We propose bilateral nephrectomy and peritoneal dialysis at an early age to avoid the many problems encountered during the nephrotic stage. Prolonged NS is also accompanied by lipid abnormalities, which leads to vascular changes already during infancy (19).

Dialysis and Transplantation

Although normal growth can be achieved with optimal therapy during the nephrotic stage, the patients are still malnourished and hypoproteinemic (15,17). To optimize treatment, we perform bilateral nephrectomy and commence continuous cyclical peritoneal dialysis when the weight reaches 7 kg. The aim is to improve the child's nutritional state before kidney transplantation (56,75). While receiving continuous cyclical peritoneal dialysis, the patient's general condition improves, muscle mass increases, and catch up growth can be documented (75–77). Transplantation can be performed also preemptively, and the results are satisfactory (78,79).

The first report of successful kidney transplantation in CNF dates back to 1973 (80), and in 1984 Mahan et al. reported excellent results with kidney transplantation in 17 children with CNS (56). Two-year patient and graft survival was 82 and 71%, respectively. Twelve of 15 surviving children had normal school and social performances, although two attended special education classes. Since 1987, 56 CNF patients have received a transplant kidney in Finland. Patient survival at 5 years is more than 90%, and graft survival is approximately 80%, with a mean glomerular filtration rate of 67 mL/min/1.73 m^2. Mean height standard deviation score was –1.4 at transplantation and improved to –0.9 after 5 years. Less than 20% of the patients are receiving growth hormone therapy. A great majority (72%) of those who have reached school age attend a normal class. The early patients who experienced thrombotic complications have neurologic handicaps (81–84).

Recurrence of Proteinuria

In CNF patients, a special risk after kidney transplantation is the recurrence of NS, which may lead to graft loss

(85–89). Recent findings indicate that at least half of the patients with recurrence have circulating antinephrin antibodies, which most probably react against the glomerular filter and induce protein leakage (89). Recurrence of NS has occurred in 13 Finnish patients, and all of them have a severe Fin-major/Fin-major genotype. These infants produce antibodies against the "novel antigen" in the graft. Treatment of recurrence with steroids, cyclophosphamide, and plasmapheresis often leads to remission (85,86,89).

Isolated Diffuse Mesangial Sclerosis

The term *diffuse mesangial sclerosis* denotes NS associated with the histologic change of DMS of the renal glomeruli (90,91). DMS can be isolated (IDMS) or associated with additional anomalies, especially Denys-Drash syndrome (DDS). In Habib's material, 26 patients with DMS were isolated, and 14 were associated with DDS (91). IDMS often occurs in females, but male patients have also been described (92,93). An autosomal recessive inheritance has been suggested in some cases (91,94,95). Mutations in the Wilms' tumor gene (*WT1*) have been described in children with IDMS (92,96). Recently, Yang et al. (97) described decreased podocyte expression of WT1 and strong expression of PAX2 in most IDMS patients, suggesting that one of the genes implicated in the cascade of *WT1* regulation (e.g., *PAX2*) could be involved in IDMS.

Pathology

The pathologic changes of DMS are characteristic (98). In the early phase, the glomeruli show increase of the mesangial matrix and podocyte hypertrophy. Then, the GBM becomes thickened, and the expanded mesangium shows a delicate PAS-positive mesh with embedded mesangial cells. The mesangial expansion and sclerosis causes obliteration of the capillary lumens and, finally, the contraction of the glomerular tufts. There is no cellular proliferation during the progression of IDMS, but a single layer of large podocytes often covers the sclerotic tufts (Fig. 25.3). A corticomedullary gradient of affected glomeruli is often present, the deepest glomeruli being the least affected. Tubulointerstitial lesions include atrophic tubules and interstitial fibrosis. Dilated tubules are also seen, but this feature is not as pronounced as in CNF.

By electron microscopy, the abundant mesangial matrix often contains filaments and collagenlike fibrils, and the GBM is thickened (98,99). Immunohistochemical analysis of DMS glomeruli shows deposits of disorganized collagen components and heparan sulfate proteoglycan, and absence of laminin and collagen IV in the hyalinized glomerular segments (100). There are no significant immune deposits, although some studies have shown variable amounts of IgM, C1q, and C3 in the mesangium or in the periphery of the glomeruli (91,94).

Clinical Features and Management

The pregnancy and delivery are usually normal, and the size of the placenta, when recorded, has been normal with rare exceptions (101). Proteinuria can manifest in the first 3 months of life, but it is more often detected later in infancy (96,101). Proteinuria is often moderate, and in contrast to CNF, the patients develop progressive renal insufficiency and end-stage renal disease (ESRD) within a few months or years (Table 25.2). A large proportion of patients develop hypertension.

Steroids and other immunosuppressive drugs are ineffective in IDMS. Early treatment is similar to that which has been outlined for CNF, but with less aggressive protein substitution. Renal transplantation is the only curative treatment of this disease.

Denys-Drash Syndrome

The triad of Wilms' tumor, male pseudohermaphroditism (XY), and progressive glomerulopathy is known as *DDS* (102,103). It often presents as congenital or early-onset NS, but the onset may range from the newborn period to childhood (91,104,105). The characteristic glomerular lesion is DMS.

Genetics

DDS is caused by mutations in the *WT1* gene, which is located at chromosome 11p13 and encodes a transcription factor of the zinc-finger family (106,107). Alternative splicing produces four transcripts of WT1. WT1 expression is important for normal fetal differentiation of the kidney and urinary organs (108,109). Heterozygous, *de novo* germline mutations in *WT1* are observed in nearly all patients with DDS. More than 60 mutations have been reported. Most are missense mutations in exons 8 and 9, encoding zinc-fingers 2 and 3 (110,111). The most prevalent is R394W located at zinc-finger 3. Also, deletions, insertions, and nonsense mutations that lead to a truncated protein have been described in DDS patients (93,111). Frasier syndrome, which is characterized by focal glomerular sclerosis, delayed kidney failure, and male pseudohermaphroditism with complete gonadal dysgenesis, is caused by point mutations in the donor splice site in intron 9, resulting in the loss of the +KTS isoform (112).

Clinical Features and Management

DDS can be divided into three clinical categories: (a) genotypic males with all three abnormalities, (b) genotypic males with nephropathy and ambiguous external and/or internal genitalia only, and (c) genotypic females with nephropathy and Wilms' tumor only (111,113). Male pseudohermaphroditism characterized by ambiguous genitalia or female phenotype with dysgenetic testes or streak gonads is observed in all 46,XY patients. By contrast, all 46,XX children reported had a normal female phenotype with normal ovaries when the information was available. The nephropathy may precede the tumor (104,113,114).

The nephropathy begins with proteinuria and NS. In contrast to CNF, renal failure is often observed at presentation (111). Progression to ESRD before the age of 4 years is the rule. No correlation between the genotype and the severity of renal disease has been observed (115). Kidney transplantation remains the only therapeutic alternative, and favorable results without recurrence of DMS have been reported (97). Because of the risk of developing Wilms' tumor, prophylactic nephrectomy at the time of ESRD or transplantation is usually performed (113).

Other Primary Nephrotic Syndromes

In 1968, Galloway and Mowat (116) described two siblings showing congenital microcephaly, NS, and hiatus hernia. Several subsequent reports showing various brain malformations and congenital or early-onset NS have been called *Galloway-Mowat syndrome* (117). The classic Galloway-Mowat syndrome is an autosomal recessive disorder, but the disease-causing gene has not been isolated (118). In patients with CNS and brain malformation, the histologic finding may be DMS (119). In several reports, the renal histology is not fully described, but pathologic changes other than DMS have been reported (119–121). A wide variety of additional anomalies have also been reported in patients with CNS and brain malformation, including dysmorphic facial features (122–124). Other defects include ocular, limb, cardiac, and diaphragmatic anomalies (121,125). Ocular abnormalities have also been described in siblings with DMS (93,101). Oculocerebrorenal (Lowe) syndrome (126) and the nail-patella syndrome (osteo-onychodysplasia) (127) have been shown to be associated in rare cases with CNS.

Idiopathic NS in the newborn is rare but becomes more common during the first year of life. Minimal changes or FSGS are more common (58,59,90,128) than diffuse mesangial hypercellularity or membranous glomerulonephritis (90,129). Diagnosis of minimal-change nephrotic syndrome (MCNS) in the very young infant may be difficult but is important because immunosuppressive treatment may be effective (130). MCNS in very young infants often carries a worse prognosis and shows more familial cases than MCNS in the older age groups (131). In some reports (132), clinicopathologic classification of congenital or infantile nephrosis has been difficult.

SECONDARY NEPHROTIC SYNDROMES

NS has been described secondary to some congenital and infantile disorders. Syphilis, toxoplasmosis, some viral infections, and the infantile form of systemic lupus erythematosus (SLE) are the most important secondary causes of congenital and infantile NS.

Infections

Congenital syphilis has long been known to cause CNS. It may cause a nephritic or nephrotic syndrome in the newborn (57). Proteinuria is common, but full-blown NS is less common. Hematuria is often present (133). NS may manifest in the newborn but is more often seen between 1 and 4 months of age (57,134). Syphilis causes a combination of glomerulonephritis and interstitial nephritis. Membranous glomerulonephritis appears to be common (135) and is a rare example of an immune complex–mediated glomerulonephritis in the newborn. Interstitial lymphocyte and plasma cell infiltration usually accompanies the glomerulonephritis. Antimicrobial therapy, usually penicillin, is curative, provided that irreversible renal lesions have not developed (136).

Toxoplasmosis has been associated with CNS in a few cases (137,138). Congenital rubella has been reported to cause CNS with membranous glomerulonephritis (139). An association of neonatal cytomegalovirus infection and CNS has also been reported (140,141). In these infections, manifestations other than NS lead to the correct diagnosis. Acquired immunodeficiency syndrome caused by the human immunodeficiency virus is associated with nephropathy, including NS (142). This disease usually affects children older than 1 year, but infants with nephropathy have been reported (143). Hepatitis B virus may cause membranous glomerulonephritis, and infants with NS associated with hepatitis B infection have been described (144).

Infantile Systemic Lupus Erythematosus

Although SLE is rarely diagnosed before 5 years of age, an infantile form of SLE has been reported (145–148). NS was the major clinical finding in five infants aged 6 weeks to 6 months with SLE. These patients had elevated antinuclear antibody titers, hypocomplementemia, and diffuse proliferative glomerulonephritis. Response to the immunosuppressive therapy was poor in many cases.

CONCLUSION

Congenital and early-onset NS forms a group of severe diseases, which so far have been mainly classified according to histology. The isolation of the *WT1*, *NPHS1*, *NPHS2*, and other podocyte genes will most probably lead to a new

CNS classification in the near future. If a child has proteinuria from birth and no signs of renal failure or extra renal malformations, the diagnosis of CNF is likely and can be confirmed by the analysis of *NPHS1*. If mutations in *NPHS1* are not found, sequencing of *NPHS2* may be indicated. On the other hand, analysis of *WT1* and *NPHS2* are indicated in infants with proteinuria and renal failure, especially if renal histology shows DMS or FSGS. Newborns and small infants with heavy proteinuria should have nutritional support and albumin substitution to guarantee normal growth and development. Antiproteinuric therapy with an angiotensin-converting enzyme inhibitor and indomethacin can be tried, especially in cases with CNF-type disease. In most CNS patients, renal transplantation is the only curative treatment, and patient and graft survival, as well as the quality of life of these patients, have greatly improved.

REFERENCES

1. Mauch TJ, Vernier RL, Burke BA, et al. Nephrotic syndrome in the first year of life. In: Holliday MA, Barratt TM, Avner ED, eds. *Pediatric nephrology*, 2nd ed. Baltimore: Williams & Wilkins, 1994:788–802.
2. Kestilä M, Lenkkeri U, Lamerdin J, et al. Positionally cloned gene for a novel glomerular protein—nephrin—is mutated in congenital nephrotic syndrome. *Mol Cell* 1998;1:575–582.
3. Tryggvason K. Unraveling the mechanism of glomerular ultrafiltration: nephrin, a key component of the slit diaphragm. *J Am Soc Nephrol* 1999;10: 2440–2445.
4. Jalanko H, Patrakka J, Tryggvason K, Holmberg C. Genetic kidney diseases disclose the pathogenesis of proteinuria. *Ann Med* 2001;33:526–533.
5. Hallman N, Hjelt L, Ahvenainen EK. Nephrotic syndrome in newborn and young infants. *Ann Pediatr Fenn* 1956;2:227–241.
6. Norio R. Heredity in congenital nephrotic syndrome. *Ann Pediatr Fenn* 1966;12[Suppl 27]:1–94.
7. Huttunen N-P. Congenital nephrotic syndrome of Finnish type. Study of 75 cases. *Arch Dis Child* 1976;51:344–348.
8. Lenkkeri U, Männikkö M, McCready P, et al. Structure of the gene for congenital nephrotic syndrome of the Finnish type (NPHS1) and characterization of mutations. *Am J Hum Genet* 1999;64:51–61.
9. Bolk S, Puffenberger EG, Hudson J, et al. Elevated frequency and allelic heterogeneity of congenital nephrotic syndrome, Finnish type, in the old order Mennonites. *Am J Hum Genet* 1999; 65:1785 1790.
10. Aya K, Tanaka H, Seino Y. Novel mutation in the nephrin gene of a Japanese patient with congenital nephrotic syndrome of the Finnish type. *Kidney Int* 2000;57:401–404.
11. Beltcheva O, Martin P, Lenkkeri U, Tryggvason K. Mutation spectrum in the nephrin gene (NPHS1) in congenital nephrotic syndrome. *Hum Mutat* 2001;17:368–373.
12. Koziell A, Grech V, Hussain S, et al. Genotype/phenotype correlations of NPHS1 and NPHS2 mutations in nephrotic syndrome advocate a functional inter-relationship in glomerular filtration. *Hum Mol Genet* 2002;11:379–388.
13. Hallman N, Norio R, Rapola J. Congenital nephrotic syndrome. *Nephron* 1973;11:101–110.
14. Patrakka J, Kestila M, Wartiovaara J, et al. Congenital nephrotic syndrome (NPHS1): features resulting from different mutations in Finnish patients. *Kidney Int* 2000;58:972–980.
15. Holmberg C, Antikainen M, Rönnholm K, et al. Management of congenital nephrotic syndrome of the Finnish type (Review). *Pediatr Nephrol* 1995;9:87–93.
16. Grech V, Chan M, Vella C, et al. Cardiac manifestations associated with the congenital nephrotic syndrome. *Pediatr Nephrol* 2000;14:1115–1117.
17. Antikainen M, Holmberg C, Taskinen MR. Growth, serum lipoproteins and apoproteins in infants with congenital nephrosis. *Clin Nephrol* 1992;38:254–263.
18. McLean RH, Kennedy TL, Rosoulpour M, et al. Hypothyroidism in the congenital nephrotic syndrome. *J Pediatr* 1982;101:72–75.
19. Antikainen M, Holmberg C, Taskinen MR. Short-term effects of renal transplantation on plasma lipids and lipoprotein lipase in children with congenital nephrosis. *Clin Nephrol* 1994;41:284–289.
20. Saraga M, Jääskeläinen J, Koskimies O. Diagnostic sonographic changes in the kidneys of 20 infants with congenital nephrotic syndrome of the Finnish type. *Eur Radiol* 1995;5:49–54.
21. Huttunen N-P, Rapola J, Vilska J, et al. Renal pathology in congenital nephrotic syndrome of Finnish type: a quantitative light microscopic study of 50 patients. *Int J Pediatr Nephrol* 1980;1:10–16.
22. Rapola J, Sariola H, Ekblom P. Pathology of fetal congenital nephrosis: immunohistochemical and ultrastructural studies. *Kidney Int* 1984;25:701–707.
23. Autio-Harmainen H, Rapola J. Renal pathology of fetuses with congenital nephrotic syndrome of the Finnish type. A qualitative and quantitative light microscopic study. *Nephron* 1981;29:158–163.
24. Rapola J. Renal pathology of fetal congenital nephrosis. *Acta Pathol Microbiol Immunol Scand* 1981;89:63–64.
25. Ruotsalainen V, Patrakka J, Tissari P, et al. Role of nephrin in cell junction formation in human nephrogenesis. *Am J Pathol* 2000;157:1905–1916.
26. Patrakka J, Martin P, Salonen R, et al. Proteinuria and prenatal diagnosis of congenital nephrosis in fetal carriers of nephrin gene mutations. *Lancet* 2002;359:1575–1577.
27. Autio-Harmainen H, Rapola J. The thickness of the glomerular basement membrane in congenital nephrotic syndrome of the Finnish type. *Nephron* 1983;34:48–50.
28. Kestilä M, Mannikkö M, Holmberg C, et al. Congenital nephrotic syndrome of the Finnish type maps to the long arm of chromosome 19. *Am J Hum Genet* 1994;54:757–764.
29. Moeller MJ, Kovari IA, Holzman LB. Evaluation of a new tool for exploring podocyte biology: mouse Nphs1 5' flanking region drives LacZ expression in podocytes. *J Am Soc Nephrol* 2000;11:2306–2314.
30. Wong MA, Cui S, Quaggin SE. Identification and characterization of a glomerular-specific promoter from the

human nephrin gene. *Am J Physiol Renal Physiol* 2000;279:F1027–1032.

31. Putaala H, Soininen R, Kilpeläinen P, et al. The murine nephrin gene is specifically expressed in kidney, brain and pancreas: inactivation of the gene leads to massive proteinuria and neonatal death. *Hum Mol Genet* 2001;10:1–8.
32. Palmén T, Ahola H, Palgi J, et al. Nephrin is expressed in the pancreatic beta cells. *Diabetologia* 2001;44:1274–1280.
33. Kuusniemi A-M, Kestila M, Lahdenkari A-T, et al. Tissue expression of nephrin in man and pig (*submitted*).
34. Antignac C. Inherited forms of steroid-resistant nephrotic syndrome. In: Clinical Nephrology Conferences Syllabus. 2002; ASN Philadelphia.
35. Boute N, Gribouval O, Roselli S, et al. NPHS2, encoding the glomerular protein podocin, is mutated in autosomal recessive steroid-resistant nephrotic syndrome. *Nat Genet* 2002;24:349–354.
36. Somlo S, Mundel P. Getting a foothold in nephrotic syndrome. *Nat Genet* 2000;24:333–335.
37. Mundel P, Shankland S. Podocyte biology and response to injury. *J Am Soc Nephrol* 2002;13:3005–3015.
38. Ruotsalainen V, Ljungberg P, Wartiovaara J, et al. Nephrin is located in the slit diaphragm of glomerular podocytes. *Proc Natl Acad Sci U S A* 1999;96:7962–7967.
39. Ahola H, Wang S, Luimula P, et al. Cloning and expression of the rat nephrin homolog. *Am J Pathol* 1999;155:907–913.
40. Holzman LB, St. John PL, Kovari IA, et al. Nephrin localizes to the slit pore of the glomerular epithelial cell. *Kidney Int* 1999; 56:1481–1491.
41. Putaala H, Sainio K, Sariola H, Tryggvason K. Primary structure of mouse and rat nephrin cDNA and structure and expression of the mouse gene. *J Am Soc Nephrol* 2000;11:991–1001.
42. Donoviel D, Freed D, Vogel H, et al. Proteinuria and perinatal lethality in mice lacking NEPH1, a novel protein with homology to nephrin. *Mol Cell Biol* 2001;21:4829–4836.
43. Sellin L, Huber TB, Gerke P, et al. NEPH1 defines a novel family of podocin-interacting proteins. *FASEB J* 2003;17:115–117.
44. Inoue T, Yaoita E, Kurihara H, et al. FAT is a component of glomerular slit diaphragms. *Kidney Int* 2001;59:1003–1012.
45. Liu L, Done S, Khoshnoodi J, et al. Defective nephrin trafficking by missense mutations in the NPHS1 gene: insight into the mechanisms of congenital nephrotic syndrome. *Hum Mol Genet* 2001;10:2637–2644.
46. Wickelgren I. First components found for key kidney filter. *Science* 1999;286:225–226.
47. Kerjaschki D. Caught flat-footed: podocyte damage and the molecular bases of focal glomerulosclerosis. *J Clin Invest* 2001;108:1583–1587.
48. Kaplan J, Kim S, Norrth K, et al. Mutations in ACTN4, encoding alpha-actinin-4, cause familial focal segmental glomerulosclerosis. *Nat Genet* 2000;24:251–256.
49. Shih NY, Karpitskii V, Nguyen A, et al. Congenital nephrotic syndrome in mice lacking CD2-associated protein. *Science* 1999;286:312–315.
50. Shih N-Y, Li J, Cotran R, et al. CD2AP localizes to the slit diaphragm and binds to nephrin via a novel C-terminal domain. *Am J Pathol* 2001;159:2303–2308.
51. Schwarz K, Simons M, Reiser J, et al. Podocin, a raft-associated component of the glomerular slit diaphragm, interacts with CD2AP and nephrin. *J Clin Invest* 2001;108:1621–1629.
52. Huber TB, Kottgen M, Schilling B, et al. Interaction with podocin facilitates nephrin signaling. *J Biol Chem* 2001; 276:41543–41546.
53. Seppälä M, Aula P, Rapola J, et al. Congenital nephrotic syndrome: prenatal diagnosis and genetic counselling by estimation of amniotic-fluid and maternal serum alphafetoprotein. *Lancet* 1976;2:123–124.
54. Ryynänen M, Seppälä M, Kuusela P, et al. Antenatal screening for congenital nephrosis in Finland by maternal serum alpha-fetoprotein. *Br J Obstet Gynaecol* 1983;90:437–442.
55. Männikkö M, Kestilä M, Lenkkeri U, et al. Improved prenatal diagnosis of the congenital nephrotic syndrome of the Finnish type based on DNA analysis. *Kidney Int* 1997;51:868–872.
56. Mahan J, Mauer S, Sibley R, et al. Congenital nephrotic syndrome: evolution of medical management and results of renal transplantation. *J Pediatr* 1984;105:549–557.
57. McDonald R, Wiggelinkhuitzen J, Kaschula OC. The nephrotic syndrome in very young infants. *Am J Dis Child* 1971;122:507–512.
58. Hamed R, Shomaf M. Congenital nephrotic syndrome: a clinico-pathologic study of thirty children. *J Nephrol* 2001;14:104–109
59. Licht C, Eifinger F, Gharib M, et al. A stepwise approach to the treatment of early onset nephrotic syndrome. *Pediatr Nephrol* 2000;14:1077–1082.
60. Savage JM, Jefferson JA, Maxwell AP, et al. Improved prognosis for congenital nephrotic syndrome of the Finnish type in Irish families. *Arch Dis Child* 1999;80:466–469.
61. Pomeranz A, Wolach B, Bernheim J, Korzets Z. Successful treatment of Finnish congenital nephrotic syndrome with captopril and indomethacin. *J Pediatr* 1995;126:140–142.
62. Guez S, Giani M, Melzi M, et al. Adequate clinical control of congenital nephrotic syndrome by enalapril. *Pediatr Nephrol* 1998;12:130–132.
63. Heaton PA, Smales O, Wong W. Congenital nephrotic syndrome responsive to captopril and indomethacin. *Arch Dis Child* 1999;81:174–175.
64. Birnbacher R, Furster E, Aufricht C. Angiotensin converting enzyme inhibitor does not reduce proteinuria in an infant with congenital nephrotic syndrome of the Finnish type. *Pediatr Nephrol* 1995;9:400–403.
65. Broyer M, Narcy P, Rault G, et al. Nutritional therapy in nephrotic children. *Contrib Infus Ther Clin Nutr* 1988;19:61–75.
66. Gavin LA, McMahon FA, Castle IN, et al. Alterations in serum thyroid hormones and thyroxin-binding globulin in patients with nephrosis. *J Clin Endocrinol Metab* 1978;46:125–130.
67. Chadha V, Alon U. Bilateral nephrectomy reverses hypothyroidism in congenital nephrotic syndrome. *Pediatr Nephrol* 1999;13:209–211.
68. Panicucci F, Sagripanti A, Vispi M, et al. Comprehensive study of haemostasis in nephrotic syndrome. *Nephron* 1983;33:9–13.
69. Llach F, Papper S, Massry SG. The clinical spectrum of renal vein thrombosis. *Am J Med* 1980;69:819–827.

70. Harris H, Umetsu D, Geha R, et al. Altered immunoglobulin status in congenital nephrotic syndrome. *Clin Nephrol* 1986;25:308–313.
71. Mathias R, Stecklein H, Guay-Woodford L, et al. Gamma globulin deficiency in newborns with congenital nephrotic syndrome. *N Engl J Med* 1989;320:398–399.
72. Ljungberg P, Holmberg C, Jalanko H. Infections in infants with congenital nephrosis of the Finnish type. *Pediatr Nephrol* 1997;11:148–152.
73. Mattoo TK, al-Sowailem AM, al-Harbi MS, et al. Nephrotic syndrome in 1st year of life and the role of unilateral nephrectomy. *Pediatr Nephrol* 1992;6:16–18.
74. Coulthard MG. Management of Finnish congenital nephrotic syndrome by unilateral nephrectomy. *Pediatr Nephrol* 1989;3:451–453.
75. Antikainen M. Protein and lipid metabolism in nephrotic infants on peritoneal dialysis after nephrectomy. *Pediatr Nephrol* 1993;7:428–433.
76. Hölttä TM, Rönnholm KA, Jalanko H, et al. Peritoneal dialysis in children under 5 years of age. *Perit Dial Int* 1997;17:573–580.
77. Hölttä T, Rönnholm K, Jalanko H, Holmberg C. Clinical outcome of pediatric patients on peritoneal dialysis under adequacy control. *Pediatr Nephrol* 2000;14:889–897.
78. Englund M, Berg U, Bohlin A-B, et al. Ten years' experience of renal transplantation in children in the cyclosporin era. *Transplantation* 1993;56:1124–1130.
79. Kim M, Stablein D, Harmon W. Renal transplantation in children with congenital nephrotic syndrome: a Report of the North American Pediatric Renal Transplant Cooperative Study (NAPRTCS). *Pediatr Transplant* 1998;2:305–308.
80. Hoyer JR, Kjellstrand CM, Simmons RL, et al. Successful renal transplantation in three children with congenital nephrotic syndrome. *Lancet* 1973;1:1410–1412.
81. Qvist E, Laine J, Rönnholm K, et al. Graft function 5–7 years after renal transplantation in early childhood. *Transplantation* 1999;67:1043–1049.
82. Qvist E, Krogerus L, Rönnholm K, et al. Course of renal allograft histopathology after transplantation in early childhood. *Transplantation* 2000;70:480–487.
83. Qvist E, Marttinen E, Rönnholm K, et al. Growth after renal transplantation in infancy or early childhood. *Pediatr Nephrol* 2002;17:438–443.
84. Qvist E, Pihko H, Fagerudd P, et al. Neurodevelopmental outcome in high-risk patients after renal transplantation in early childhood. *Pediatr Transplant* 2002;6:53–62.
85. Sigström L, Hansson S, Jodal U. Long-term survival of a girl with congenital nephrotic syndrome and recurrence of proteinuria after renal transplantation. *Pediatr Nephrol* 1989;3:C169.
86. Flynn JT, Schulman SL, deChadaverian J-P, et al. Treatment of steroid-resistant post-transplant nephrotic syndrome with cyclophosphamide in a child with congenital nephrotic syndrome. *Pediatr Nephrol* 1992;6:553–555.
87. Laine J, Jalanko H, Holthöfer H, et al. Post-transplantation nephrosis in congenital nephrotic syndrome of the Finnish type. *Kidney Int* 1993;44:867–874.
88. Barayan S, Al-Akash S, Malekzadeh M, et al. Immediate post-transplant nephrosis in a patient with congenital nephrotic syndrome. *Pediatr Nephrol* 2001;16:547–549.
89. Patrakka J, Ruotsalainen V, Qvist E, et al. Recurrence of nephrotic syndrome in patients with congenital nephrosis (NPHS1): role of nephrin. *Transplantation* 2002;73:394–403.
90. Habib R, Bois E. Heterogeneite des syndromes nephrotiques a debut precoce du nourrison (syndrome nephrotique "infantile"). *Helv Pediatr Acta* 1973;28:91–107.
91. Habib R. Nephrotic syndrome in the 1st year of life. *Pediatr Nephrol* 1993;7:347–353.
92. Jeanpierre C, Denamur E, Henry I, et al. Identification of constitutional WT1 mutations in patients with isolated diffuse mesangial sclerosis, and analysis of genotype/phenotype correlations by use of computerized mutation database. *Am J Hum Genet* 1998;62:824–833.
93. Salomon R, Gubler M, Niaudet P. Genetics of the nephrotic syndrome. *Curr Opin Pediatr* 2000;12:129–134.
94. Barakat A, Khoury L, Allam C, et al. Diffuse mesangial sclerosis and ocular abnormalities in two siblings. *Int J Pediatr Nephrol* 1982;3:33–35.
95. Ozen S, Tinaztepe K. Diffuse mesangial sclerosis: a unique type of congenital and infantile nephrotic syndrome. *Nephron* 1996;72:288–291.
96. Ito S, Takata A, Hataya H, Ikeda M, et al. Isolated diffuse mesangial sclerosis and Wilms tumor suppressor gene. *J Pediatr* 2001;138:425–427.
97. Yang Y, Jeanpierre C, Dressler G, et al. *WT1* and *PAX-2* podocyte expression in Denys-Drash syndrome and isolated diffuse mesangial sclerosis. *Am J Pathol* 1999;154:181–192.
98. Habib R, Gubler MC, Antignac C, et al. Diffuse mesangial sclerosis: a congenital glomerulopathy with nephrotic syndrome. *Adv Nephrol Necker Hosp* 1993;22:43–57.
99. Rumpelt H, Bachmann H. Infantile nephrotic syndrome with diffuse mesangial sclerosis: a disturbance of glomerular basement membrane development? *Clin Nephrol* 1980;13:146–150.
100. Nerlich AG, Wiest I, Schleicher ED. Localization of extracellular matrix components in congenital nephrotic syndromes. *Pediatr Nephrol* 1995;9:145–153.
101. Lennert T, Hörtling A, Mildenberger E, et al. Augenveränderungen be diffuser mesangialer Sklerose (DMS). *Monatschr Kinderheilk* 1997;145:209.
102. Denys P, Malvaux P, Van den Berghe H, et al. Association d'un syndrome anatomopathologique de pseudohermaphrodisme masculin, d'une tumeur de Wilms, d'une nephropathie parenchymateuse et d'un mosaicisme XX/XY. *Arch Fr Pediatr* 1967;24:729–739.
103. Drash A, Sherman F, Hartmann W, et al. A syndrome of pseudohermaphroditism, Wilms' tumor, hypertension and degenerative renal disease. *J Pediatr* 1970;76:585–593.
104. Eddy A, Mauer S. Pseudohermaphroditism, glomerulopathy and Wilms' tumor (Drash syndrome) frequency in end-stage renal failure. *J Pediatr* 1985;106:584–587.
105. Jadresic L, Leake J, Gordon I, et al. Clinicopathologic review of twelve children with nephropathy, Wilms tumor, and genital abnormalities. *J Pediatr* 1990;117:717–725.
106. Pelletier J, Bruening W, Kashtan CE, et al. Germline mutations in the Wilms' tumor suppressor gene are associated with abnormal urogenital development in Denys-Drash syndrome. *Cell* 1991;67:437–447.
107. Huff V. Genotype/phenotype correlations in Wilms' tumor. *Med Pediatr Oncol* 1996;27:408–414.

108. Pritchard-Jones K, Fleming S, Davidson D, et al. The candidate Wilms' tumour gene is involved in genitourinary development. *Nature* 1990;346:194–197.
109. Pitchard-Jones K. The Wilms tumor gene, WT1, in normal and abnormal nephrogenesis. *Pediatr Nephrol* 1999;13:620–625.
110. Coppes MJ, Campbell CE, Williams B. The role of WT1 in Wilms tumorigenesis. *FASEB J* 1993;7:886–895.
111. Schumacher V, Scharer K, Wuhl E, et al. Spectrum of early onset nephrotic syndrome associated with WT1 missense mutations. *Kidney Int* 1998; 53:1594–1600.
112. Barbaux S, Niaudet P, Gubler MC, et al. Donor splice site mutations in the *WT1* gene are responsible for Frasier syndrome. *Nat Genet* 1997;17:467–469.
113. Melocoton TL, Salusky IB, Hall TR, et al. A case report of Drash syndrome in a 46,XX female. *Am J Kidney Dis* 1991;18:503–508.
114. Barakat A, Papadopoulo Z, Chanda R, et al. Pseudohermaphroditism, nephron disorder and Wilms tumor: a unifying concept. *Pediatrics* 1974;54:366–369.
115. Denamur E, Andre J-L, Niaudet P, et al. Absence of correlation between genotype and the severity of diffuse mesangial sclerosis in Denys-Drash syndrome. *Pediatr Nephrol* 2000;14:439–440.
116. Galloway W, Mowat A. Congenital microcephaly with hiatus hernia and nephrotic syndrome in two sibs. *J Med Genet* 1968;5:319–321.
117. Cohen AH, Turner MC. Kidney in Galloway-Mowat syndrome: clinical spectrum with description of pathology. *Kidney Int* 1994;45:1407–1415.
118. Srivastava T, Whiting J, Carola R, et al. Podocyte proteins in Galloway-Mowat syndrome. *Pediatr Nephrol* 2001;16: 1022–1029.
119. Garty BZ, Eisenstein B, Sandbank J, et al. Microcephaly and congenital nephrotic syndrome owing to diffuse mesangial sclerosis: an autosomal recessive syndrome. *J Med Genet* 1994;31:121–125.
120. Palm L, Högerstrand I, Kristoffersson U, et al. Nephrosis and disturbances of neuronal migration in male siblings: a new hereditary disorder? *Arch Dis Child* 1986;61:545–548.
121. Cooperstone BG, Friedman A, Kaplan BS. Galloway-Mowat syndrome of abnormal gyral patterns and glomerulopathy. *Am J Med Genet* 1993;47:250–254.
122. Yalcinkaya F, Tumer N, Ekim M, et al. Congenital microcephaly and infantile nephrotic syndrome: a case report. *Pediatr Nephrol* 1994;8:72–73.
123. Sano H, Miyanoshita A, Watanabe N, et al. Microcephaly and early-onset nephrotic syndrome: confusion in Galloway-Mowat syndrome. *Pediatr Nephrol* 1995;9:711–714.
124. Meyers KVC, Kaplan P, Kaplan BS. Nephrotic syndrome, microcephaly, and developmental delay: three separate syndromes. *Am J Med Genet* 1999;82:257–260.
125. Mildenberger E, Lennert T, Kunze J, et al. Diffuse mesangial sclerosis: associated with unreported congenital anomalies and placental enlargement. *Acta Paediatr* 1998;87:1301–1305.
126. Nielsen KF, Steffensen GK. Congenital nephrotic syndrome associated with Lowe's syndrome. *Child Nephrol Urol* 1990;10:92–95.
127. Similä S, Vesa L, Wasz-Höckert O. Hereditary onycho-osteodysplasia (the Nail-Patella Syndrome) with nephrosis-like renal disease in a newborn boy. *Pediatrics* 1970;46:61.
128. Bensman A, Vasmant D, Mougenot B, et al. Syndrome nephrotique infantile cortico-sensible. *Arch Fr Pediatr* 1982;39:391–395.
129. Bachmann H, Rumpelt H, Thoenes W. Klinische and pathologisch-anatomische Befunde bei verschiedenen Formen des angeborenen nephrotischen Syndroms. *Monatschr Kinderheilk* 1980;128:465–471.
130. Larbre F, Guibaud P, Freycon M-T, et al. Evolution prolongue d'un syndrome nephrotique congenital lesions glomurulaires minimes. *Pediatrie* 1978;33:287–294.
131. Gonzales G, Kleinknecht C, Gubler M, et al. Syndromes nephrotiques familiaux. *Rev Pediatr* 1977;12:427–433.
132. Kleinknecht C, Lenoir G, Broyer M, et al. Coexistence of antenatal, infantile, and juvenile nephrotic syndrome in a single family. *J Pediatr* 1981;98:938–940.
133. Sanchez-Bayle M, Ecija J, Estepa R. Incidence of glomerulonephritis in congenital syphilis. *Clin Nephrol* 1983;20:27–35.
134. Niemsiri S. Congenital syphilitic nephrosis. *Southeast Asian J Trop Med Public Health* 1993;24:595–600.
135. Losito A, Buciarelli E, Massi-Benedetti F. Membranous glomerulonephritis in congenital syphilis. *Clin Nephrol* 1979;12:32–38.
136. Wiggelinkhuizen J, Kaschula R, Uys C, et al. Congenital syphilis and glomerulonephritis with evidence for immunopathogenesis. *Arch Dis Child* 1973;48:375–381.
137. Shahin B, Papadopoulou Z, Jenis E. Congenital nephrotic syndrome associated with congenital toxoplasmosis. *J Pediatr* 1974;85:366–342.
138. Beale M, Strayer D, Kissane J. Congenital glomerulosclerosis and nephrotic syndrome in two infants. Speculations and pathogenesis. *Am J Dis Child* 1979;133:842–847.
139. Esterly JR, Oppenheimer EH. Pathological lesions due to congenital rubella. *Arch Pathol* 1969;87:380–388.
140. Batisky DL, Roy SD, Gaber LW. Congenital nephrosis and neonatal cytomegalovirus infection: a clinical association. *Pediatr Nephrol* 1993;7:741–743.
141. Dandge VP, Dharnidharka VR, Dalwai W, et al. Congenital mesangioproliferative nephrotic syndrome associated with cytomegalovirus infection. *Indian Pediatr* 1993;30:665–667.
142. Ross M, Klotman P. Recent progress in HIV-associated nephropathy. *J Am Soc Nephrol* 2002;13:2997–3004.
143. Strauss J, Abitbol C, Zilleruelo G, et al. Renal disease in children with the acquired immunodeficiency syndrome. *N Engl J Med* 1989;321:625–630.
144. Gilbert R, Wiggelinkhuizen J. The clinical course of hepatitis B virus–associated nephropathy. *Pediatr Nephrol* 1994;8:11–14.
145. Sandborg C. Childhood systemic lupus erythematosus and neonatal lupus syndrome. *Curr Opin Rheumatol* 1998;10: 481–487.
146. Lam C, Imundo L, Hirsch D, et al. Glomerulonephritis in a neonate with atypical congenital lupus and toxoplasmosis. *Pediatr Nephrol* 1999;13:850–853.
147. Massengill S, Richard G, Donelly W. Infantile systemic lupus erythematosus with onset simulating congenital nephrotic syndrome. *J Pediatr* 1994;124:27–31.
148. Dudley J, Fenton T, Unsworth J, et al. Systemic lupus erythematosus presenting as congenital nephrotic syndrome. *Pediatr Nephrol* 1996;10:752–755.

26

INHERITED GLOMERULAR DISEASES

MARIE CLAIRE GUBLER
LAURENCE HEIDET
CORINNE ANTIGNAC

Inherited glomerular disease encompasses a large number of various unrelated disorders. A tentative classification may be suggested, taking into account clinical, morphologic, pathogenetic, and genetic features (Table 26.1), but it is of limited value because of our incomplete knowledge of basic defects and pathogenesis of conditions. Glomerular involvement may appear as the primary defect, either isolated, as in the congenital nephrotic syndrome of the Finnish type, or as part of a genetically determined syndrome, as in Alport's syndrome. Glomerular lesions may develop secondarily as a consequence of inherited metabolic diseases such as diabetes mellitus or familial amyloidosis.

The incidence of hereditary glomerulopathies is probably under evaluated because of diagnostic difficulties. In fact, the differences in the observed incidence of hereditary nephropathies between groups probably depend on the extent of family investigations. In the pediatric series of Necker-Enfants Malades Hospital, inherited glomerulopathies are responsible for approximatively 6.5% of end-stage renal failure (ESRF) occurring before the age of 16 years (1). According to the European Dialysis Transplantation Association registry, 15% of ESRF are due to hereditary glomerulopathies. Familial occurrence of glomerulopathies was observed by Waldherr in 7 to 8% of patients with biopsy-proven glomerulonephritis (2).

Since 1990, dramatic advances in molecular biology technology have led to an explosive growth in our knowledge of inherited disorders. New DNA-based diagnostic tests are possible when the disease genes have been localized or cloned. Recognition of the genetic nature of a given disease and its precise identification have become essential in offering patients and families the possibilities of accurate genetic counseling, presymptomatic testing, and prenatal diagnosis. However, in nephrology, and especially in pediatric nephrology, the gene defects responsible for several inherited conditions remain to be identified. The goal is now to precisely define the orphan syndromes on clinical, morphologic, and genetic criteria, this delineation being the first and obligatory step for further molecular genetic investigations and continuing progress.

STRUCTURE OF THE GLOMERULAR BASEMENT MEMBRANE

The glomerular filtration barrier consists of three layers: the fenestrated vascular endothelium, the glomerular basement membrane (GBM), and the podocyte slit diaphragm. The GBM is a highly specialized type of basement membrane (BM) (or basal lamina), between 310 and 380 nm in thickness in the mature human kidney, with a trilamellar structure composed of a thick lamina densa between two thin lamina rara. It plays an important role as a selective size and charge filtration barrier for macromolecules during the formation of primary urine.

As in every BM in the body, the major components of the GBM are type IV collagen, laminin, nidogen, and proteoglycans (3). Type IV collagen provides the structural framework and is responsible for the mechanical resistance of the BM and attachment of other glycoproteins. Laminin is involved in cell attachment, cell growth, and differentiation. Nidogen, which is always associated in equimolar proportion with laminin, seems to act as a connecting protein between laminin and type IV collagen. Heparan sulfate proteoglycans, the major proteoglycans present in the GBM, are characterized by strongly anionic heparan sulfate chains and are implicated in the charge-controlled macromolecular filtration through the GBM. Minor constituents found in the BM are osteonectin (BM-40, secreted protein, acidic and rich in cystein), fibronectin, and amyloid P. In the mesangial matrix, the major BM components are associated with type VI collagen, chondroitin sulfate proteoglycan, fibronectin, and tenascin.

The structure of type IV collagen, the scaffold of the GBM, is interesting because of its implication in acquired and hereditary glomerular diseases. Type IV collagen belongs to the large collagen family, comprising 21 different types of molecules encoded by at least 32 genes. Each collagen molecule is formed of three α-chains folded together to form a triple helix. Specific features of type IV collagen are its length, 400 nm, and the persistence at its C-

TABLE 26.1. CLASSIFICATION OF INHERITED GLOMERULOPATHIES

1. Hereditary disorders of the glomerular basement membrane
   - Alport's syndrome and variants
   - Familial benign hematuria
   - Collagen type III glomerulopathy
2. Hereditary disorders of the podocyte
   - Finnish-type nephrotic syndrome
   - Familial steroid resistant idiopathic nephrotic syndrome
   - Familial focal and segmental glomerulosclerosis
   - Diffuse mesangial sclerosis
   - Hereditary onychoosteodysplasia: the nail-patella syndrome
   - Epstein/Fechtner syndromes
3. Hereditary metabolic disorders with primary glomerular involvement
   - Adolescent-type cystinosis
   - Fabry disease
   - Other lysosomal diseases with glomerular involvement
4. Hereditary metabolic disorders with secondary glomerular involvement
   - Diabetes mellitus
   - Sickle-cell disease
   - Familial amyloidosis
   - Alpha-1 antitrypsin deficiency
   - Various hereditary complement defects/factor H deficiency
   - Alagille syndrome
   - Lecithin cholesterol acyltransferase deficiency
   - Lipoprotein glomerulopathy
   - Type III hyperlipoproteinemia
   - Familial juvenile megaloblastic anemia
5. Other hereditary diseases associated with glomerular involvement
   - Charcot-Marie-Tooth disease
   - Cockayne syndrome
   - Hereditary acroosteolysis
   - Bardet-Biedl syndrome
   - Alström syndrome
   - Familial dysautonomia
6. Hereditary glomerulopathies without extrarenal symptoms
   - Familial lobular glomerulopathy/familial glomerulopathy with giant fibrillar deposits; "fibronectin glomerulopathy"
   - Other familial glomerulopathies
7. Mitochondrial cytopathies with glomerular involvement
8. Rare and "bizarre" syndromes
   - Hirooka disease
   - Galloway syndrome
   - Hunter disease
   - Barakat disease
   - Edwards disease
   - Mattoo disease, etc.

terminal end of a noncollagenous (NC) 26- to 28-kDa globular domain, called NC (or NC1), which is a binding site between two type IV molecules. The other terminal domain, 7S, at the N terminus is the aggregation site for four molecules. In addition, frequent short interruptions in the repeated collagen-specific Gly-X-Y sequence are present in the type IV collagen chains and are responsible for the flexibility of the molecule. These features are the structural basis for the specific network organization of type IV collagen (3).

Six type IV collagen subunit components, the chains α_1–α_6(IV), have been identified, and their primary structure has been determined in human and for most of them in mouse (4,5). *COL4A1* and *COL4A2* genes coding for α_1(IV) and α_2(IV) have been cloned and mapped to the long arm of chromosome 13 as a contiguous group (6). They are the most abundant, have a ubiquitous distribution, and form heterotrimers consisting of two α_1(IV) chains and one α_2(IV) chain. Subsequently, two other chains, α_3(IV) and α_4(IV), have been identified, and their genes, *COL4A3* and *COL4A4*, have been located to chromosome 2 (7). Their complete sequence has been determined (8,9). The antigenic determinants responsible for autoimmunization in the Goodpasture syndrome have been localized to the 28-kDa NC domain of α_3(IV) (10,11). The *COL4A5* gene was mapped to the Xq22 region, the locus previously assigned to the X-linked Alport's syndrome, making it a good candidate gene for Alport's syndrome (12–14). Subsequently, the gene *COL4A6* was assigned to the same region and shown to be located head-to-head to *COL4A5* (Fig 26.1) (15,16).

Immunohistochemical studies have shown that the α_1 and α_2(IV) chains are present in nearly all BM. By contrast, the α_3 to α_6(IV) chains have a selective distribution within specialized BM of the kidney, eye, inner ear, choroid plexus, and lung (17). Within the kidney, mesangial areas, Bowman's capsules, and extraglomerular BM are strongly stained with antibodies to the α_1 and α_2(IV) chains, whereas restricted labeling of the GBM and of the distal tubular BM is obtained with anti-α_3, -α_4 and -α_5(IV) antibodies (18,19). The α_6(IV) chain is absent in the GBM but is co-distributed with the α_5(IV) chain in distal tubule and collecting duct BM and in Bowman's capsules (20,21). The

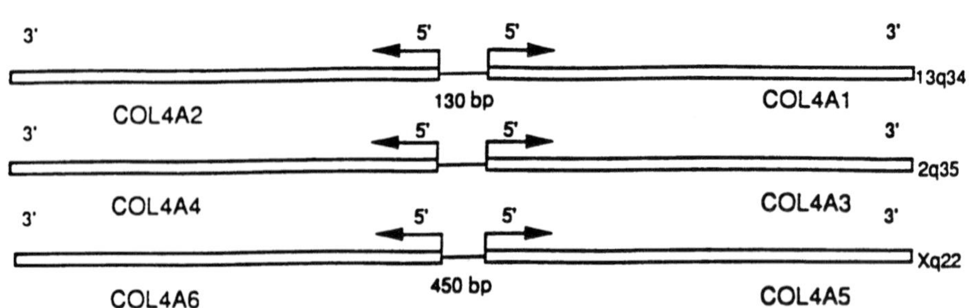

FIGURE 26.1. Schematic representation of the distribution of type IV collagen gene on chromosomes 13, 2, and X. bp, base pair.

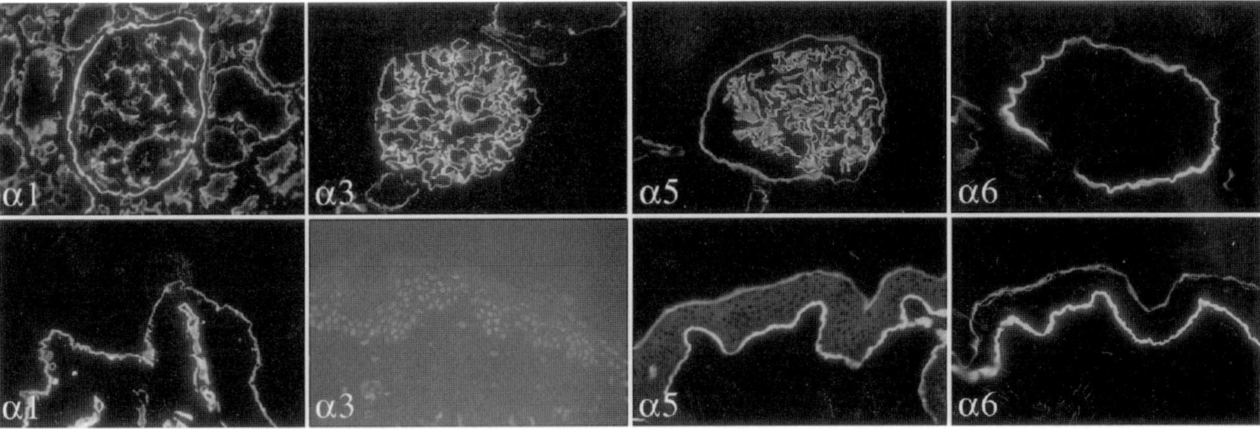

FIGURE 26.2. Immunofluorescence microscopy. Normal distribution of the α(IV) chains in renal and epidermal basement membranes. (See Color Plate 26.2.)

α_5 and α_6(IV) chains are co-distributed with the α_1 and α_2(IV) chains in epidermal BM (Fig. 26.2). In the GBM, the α(IV) chains are organized into two separate networks, one containing α_1(IV), and α_2(IV) is restricted to the subendothelial side of the GBM, and the other, the major one, consisting of α_3, α_4, and α_5(IV) chains, is distributed throughout the thickness of the GBM (17,18,22).

HEREDITARY DISORDERS OF THE GLOMERULAR BASEMENT MEMBRANE

Alport's Syndrome: A Hereditary Disorder of Basement Membrane Collagen

Classic Alport's syndrome (23) is an inherited renal disorder characterized by familial occurrence in successive generations of progressive hematuric nephritis, with ultrastructural changes of the GBM and sensorineural hearing loss. Ocular defects are commonly associated. Usually male patients have severe renal disease leading to ESRF before the fourth decade, whereas most female patients have a normal life span. Alport's syndrome has been reported in kindreds of all ethnic and geographic origins. Alport's syndrome is considered the cause of approximatively 0.6 to 2.3% of ESRF in Europe and the United States (24–26). This proportion is probably underestimated because of diagnostic difficulties. The Alport's syndrome gene frequency is estimated to be 1 per 5000 to 1 per 10,000 (24).

Over the last 20 years, successive observations and findings have led to better comprehension of the renal and extrarenal manifestations of Alport's syndrome and to the identification of the new collagen IV genes, mutations of which are responsible for the disease. Questions raised by the phenotypic heterogeneity of the syndrome are partly explained by the genetic and molecular heterogeneity of the condition.

The mode of transmission of Alport's syndrome has long been debated, as shown by the many hypotheses proposed to explain the transmission of the disease in the large Mormon family initially reported by Perkoff. The difficulty was essentially related to the insufficiency of the criteria accepted to identify affected subjects in the families. This problem has in large part been resolved because hematuria is considered an indispensable diagnostic criterion. With this condition, it has become clear that the disease was transmitted as an X-linked dominant trait in the "P" family (27).

Further family analyses have demonstrated the genetic heterogeneity of Alport's syndrome (24,28,29), with a particularly high frequency of dominant X-linked transmission (24). Autosomal dominant transmission confirmed by father-to-son transmission has been reported in some families with classic Alport's syndrome (28–30) or with progressive hematuric nephritis without deafness (31,32). Autosomal recessive transmission has been observed, especially in families with parental consanguinity and in which several siblings are affected and, regardless of gender, present severe Alport's syndrome, whereas parents are clinically unaffected (29). Last, in families having juvenile Alport's syndrome, the frequent absence of descendants from affected males makes it impossible to specify the exact mode of inheritance. Linkage studies using polymorphic markers situated on chromosome X have confirmed the frequency of X-linked dominant transmission and have allowed localization of the gene of the Alport's syndrome at Xq22 (33,34). Finally, identification of mutations in the *COL4A3* and *COL4A4* confirmed the genetic heterogeneity of the disease (see later).

X-Linked Alport's Syndrome

Clinical Presentation

First symptoms usually occur early in life, especially in males (35–38). In a group of 58 patients observed in a pediatric department, symptoms were detected before the age of 1 year in 14% of the children and before the age of 6 years in 72% (38). In childhood, macroscopic or microscopic hematuria is the major presenting symptom (35–40) and may be observed at birth (38). However, the disease may be first discovered in adulthood in patients presenting with proteinuria-microscopic hematuria, with or without hypertension or renal failure. Alport's syndrome may be revealed by routine urinalysis or by family screening in mildly affected female patients.

Clinical and Laboratory Findings

Renal Disease

Microscopic hematuria is present in all patients and is usually persistent. It may be intermittent in some girls and in younger boys (38). Single or recurrent episodes of macroscopic hematuria are observed in approximately one-half of the patients, often within the 2 days after an upper respiratory tract infection. In our experience, these episodes are common during the first years of life and disappear after the age of 10 to 15 years. The duration of macroscopic hematuria usually varies from 1 to 10 days but in some instances may persist for months. Proteinuria is a common finding in males (36,38,41) but is not necessarily present in younger patients. It increases progressively with age, often exceeding 1 g/24 hours after 10 to 15 years, with development of nephrotic syndrome in approximately 40% of cases. Proteinuria is often absent, mild, or intermittent in affected females. Leukocyturia and pyuria are incidental findings.

Long-term follow-up varies according to the gender of affected patients and to genetic factors. Male patients progress to terminal renal failure. They follow a similar pattern of evolution: mild and intermittent proteinuria during childhood, then persistent and increasing proteinuria with possible development of nephrotic syndrome, hypertension, and renal failure. Depending on the rate of progression to ESRF, two types of the syndrome have been distinguished: (a) a progressive or "juvenile" type in which ESRF occurs around the age of 20 years, always before 31 years according to Atkin et al. (24), and the course is highly stereotyped within a given family (24,38); and (b) a "nonprogressive" (42) or "adult" type (24) in which age at ESRF is around 40 years, and the course is much more diverse, making individual prognosis impossible. By contrast, most female carriers have mild disease. Some of them progress to ESRF but usually at a slower rate than males (26,28).

Hearing Defects

Sensorineural hearing loss is bilateral. It is never congenital. In our experience, the initial hearing defect, at 2000, 4000, or 8000 Hz, is recognized by audiometry before the age of 15 years in 85% of boys and in 18% of girls (38). Serial audiologic studies of young males often demonstrate progression of hearing loss and extension to other frequencies. Involvement of the conversational zones leads to hearing difficulties necessitating hearing aids. In female patients, but also in some of the males affected with the "adult" type Alport's syndrome, stable and mild hearing defect is detected only by audiometry. The progression of hearing loss roughly parallels that of renal impairment (42). Partial hearing improvement reported after transplantation might be due to the suppression of the superimposed consequences of uremia on hearing.

Ocular Defects

Various types of ocular defects involving the lens, retina, and cornea have been described (44–48). The anterior lenticonus is a regular, conical protrusion on the anterior aspect of the lens. This lesion is not detected at birth and develops progressively over the years, almost exclusively in male subjects (38,46). With the exception of traumatic lenticonus, it is specific to Alport's syndrome. It has been observed in 25% of patients examined in a pediatric series (38) and in 33% of cases in an adult series (46). Lenticonus can be complicated by subcapsular cataract, without diagnostic significance, but possibly leading to loss of visual acuity. The microspherophakia reported by Sohar was in fact anterior lenticonus, as revealed by histologic examination of the lens (49).

Retinal changes are asymptomatic but more frequent, observed in 37% of patients (46). They are always present when there is anterior lenticonus. They consist of bilateral, densely packed whitish-yellow granulations surrounding the foveal area. They are superficially located in the retina. The fovea itself, whose reflection is suppressed, is dark red. These lesions are also specific. In the child, they can be difficult to identify because changes in pigmentation of the macula and disappearance of the foveola reflex precede the appearance of perimacular granulations (38). The anterior lenticonus and macular lesions, although inconstant, are reliable diagnostic criteria for Alport's syndrome. They are observed in juvenile forms of Alport's syndrome and seem to portend poor prognosis (46).

Nonspecific corneal lesions have been recently described in Alport's syndrome patients. They consist in posterior polymorphic dystrophy (47) and in recurrent corneal ulceration (48).

Clinical Variants of X-Linked Alport's Syndrome

Associated changes, including platelet abnormalities, esophageal leiomyomatosis, cerebral dysfunction, polyneuropathy, hyperprolinuria, ichthyosis, and thyroid and parathyroid involvement, have been reported. They affect only a minority of kindreds. Except for two X-linked contiguous gene deletion syndromes, one resulting in esophageal leiomyomatosis, the other in the AMME (*A*lport syndrome, *m*ental retardation, *m*idface hypoplasia, and *e*lliptocytosis) syndrome (50), most of these anomalies seem to be coincidental associations or complications of renal failure. On the other hand, the syndromes characterized by the association of platelet disorder and nephritis are not caused by type IV collagen deficiency.

Diffuse Esophageal Leiomyomatosis and Alport's Syndrome

The association of esophageal, tracheobronchial, and genital leiomyomatosis (with vulvar and clitoral enlargement), first described by Garcia-Torrès et al. (51), has now been reported in more than 30 families (52–54). These patients have typical X-linked Alport's syndrome, often of juvenile type, in which a notable factor is the frequent association of bilateral congenital cataract of particular severity and type. Esophageal involvement is responsible for dysphagia and may be recognized by radiologic investigations. Accidental deaths caused by tracheobronchic lesions occurring during surgical operations have been reported. Interestingly, diffuse leiomyomatosis is fully penetrant and completely expressed in females (52). Approximately 20% of children with esophageal leiomyomatosis should be affected with Alport's syndrome.

Hereditary Nephritis without Deafness

In some families, hematuric nephritis resembling adult-type Alport's syndrome progresses to ESRF without sensorineural hearing loss (even at the audiometric level) or any other extrarenal symptom (24,55). Whether these observations constitute a different entity or a variant of Alport's syndrome has been debated. Genetic studies have provided new criteria for classifying these syndromes.

Pathology

By *light microscopy*, renal findings are not specific. In young children, renal biopsy specimens show no abnormalities, although an increased number of immature glomeruli have been reported (35). With increasing age, the mesangium shows a mild and irregular excess in matrix with areas of segmental proliferation, and the capillary walls may appear thickened and irregular. Advancing glomerular disease is characterized by increasing mesangial enlargement and occurrence of segmental sclerosis and hyalinosis. Tubulointerstitial changes appear early. The presence of interstitial foam cells has often been considered as suggestive of Alport's syndrome, but these cells are seen in most types of chronic glomerulonephritis.

Conventional *immunofluorescent studies* of renal tissue are usually negative. However, granular deposits of C3 or traces of immunoglobulin M (IgM) may be observed in the glomeruli of some patients (38). In advanced cases, deposits of immunoglobulins along some GBM segments and deposits of IgM and C3 within segmental glomerular lesions are present.

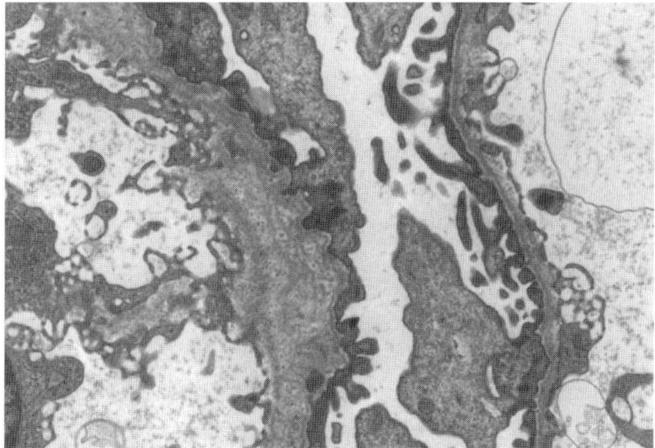

FIGURE 26.3. Electron micrograph. Lead citrate and uranyl acetate stain (×11,250). Alport's syndrome. Thickened glomerular basement membrane showing splitting of the lamina densa and presence of granulations.

The characteristic lesions of the GBM were demonstrated by *ultrastructural studies* (41,56,57). These lesions associate irregular thickening of the GBM with splitting and splintering of the lamina densa, thus delimiting clear zones containing microgranulations (Fig. 26.3). The external aspect of the GBM is irregularly festooned and bordered by hypertrophied podocytes. GBM thickening is usually diffuse in the adult, whereas in the child it is segmental and a second anomaly—thinning of the GBM with occasional ruptures—is associated and may be predominant (Fig. 26.4) (37,38,58,59). Segmental thickening occurs early as it has been observed in renal biopsy specimens from children 1 to 5 years old (31,37,38,40,57). Semiquantitative studies have shown that the percentage of thick segments is higher in boys than in girls, and in boys it progressively increases with age and level of proteinuria (60). Thick and split GBM has been observed in patients with classical Alport's syndrome and with Alport's syn-

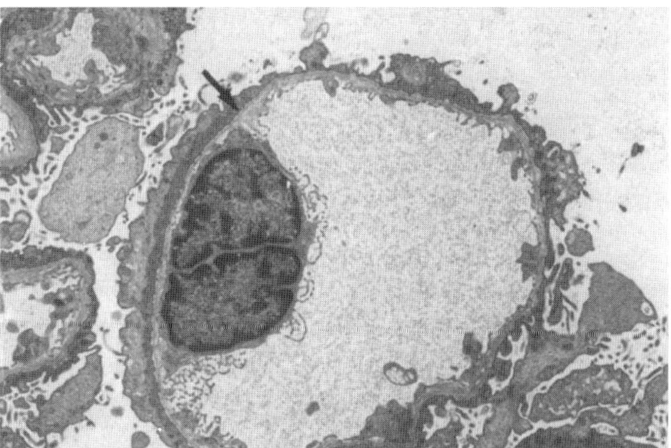

FIGURE 26.4. Electron micrograph. Lead citrate and uranyl acetate stain (×4800). Alport's syndrome. Thin and regular glomerular basement membrane (*arrow*) with attenuated lamina densa. Epithelial foot processes are extensively fused.

drome associated with leiomyomatosis (50,51). They have also been found in a few patients having progressive hereditary nephritis without deafness (31,40,56,60). In a family of Samoyed dogs, an animal model of Alport's syndrome, the GBM is normal at birth; thickening of the GBM and splitting of the lamina densa appear in the first weeks of life in the males, encompassing the whole GBM around the age of 3 months, whereas in the females the lesions remain segmental (61). Similar GBM changes were found in another canine family of Alport's syndrome (62).

The thick and split GBM lesion is specific (63). Its finding in children who have sporadic hematuria helps identify Alport's syndrome. However, this lesion can be absent, with the GBM appearing normal or presenting only nonspecific lesions (42,56,60,64) or uniformly thin (39,58,59,64,65). The GBM lesion can also appear late as reported in a family with progressive hematuric nephritis without deafness, in which lesions were observed in two brothers aged 19 and 21 years, 8 years after an initial renal biopsy that had shown normal GBM (32). Last, excessive thickening of the lamina rara interna without any change in the structure of the lamina densa has been reported in one of the families first described by Perkoff (66).

Concordance of ultrastructural lesions within families is usual. The lesion-associating thickening of the GBM and fragmentation of the lamina densa is both a marker in certain families and an index of severity (42,59). A few discordances have been reported. In a study of 100 patients—88 children and 12 adults belonging to 85 families with progressive hematuric nephritis with or without deafness—we found ultrastructural alterations of the GBM in all of them. The GBM was thickened and split in most of the patients having classic Alport's syndrome and thin in 10 of 14 patients having progressive hematuric nephritis without deafness. In 18 patients with classic Alport's syndrome, the GBM was uniformly thin (Fig. 26.3). In three of them, renal biopsy of another member of the family disclosed a thick and split GBM. On the contrary, in a large family in which seven affected members, aged 10 to 47 years, had been biopsied, the only GBM lesion observed was thinning. Thus, the existence of uniformly thin GBM in both the child and the adult is not always synonymous with benign familial hematuria and should be considered as a possible morphologic variant of Alport's syndrome (65).

In addition to GBM changes, focal thickening of Bowman's capsules and tubular BMs are observed. They are characterized by a marked bulging and splitting of the BMs delineating clear areas containing osmiophilic granules, lipid droplets, or vesicular formations. They are usually associated with the more severe GBM changes.

BM of retina and cochlea have not been studied by electron microscopy. Streeten et al. (67) demonstrated thinning and many dehiscences of the anterior lens capsule of patients with lenticonus. Epidermal BM was found to be multilamellated in one family, but this anomaly has not been confirmed by other investigators.

Immunohistochemical and Immunochemical Anomalies

In 1976, McCoy described the lack of fixation of an anti-GBM alloantibody developed in a transplanted Alport's syndrome patient on the GBM of Alport's syndrome patients (68). This observation was confirmed by other investigators using the same type of serum or serum from Goodpasture patients. The anomaly suggested the absence or the modification of GBM structural antigen(s). This hypothesis was confirmed by biochemical and immunochemical studies of GBM prepared from Alport's syndrome end-stage kidneys showing the absence of NC peptides that were targets for anti-GBM antibodies (69–70). The Goodpasture epitopes were subsequently localized to the 28-kDa NC domain of the α_3 chain of type IV collagen (10,11).

Parallel to the studies on the α_3(IV) chain, the Minneapolis group showed that the serum of one of their transplanted Alport's patients who had developed anti-GBM antibodies recognized a 26-kDa NC peptide different from the 28-kDa Goodpasture antigen and from the NC domain of the α(IV) collagen chains so far identified. This antigen had the same renal distribution as the α_3 and α_4(IV) chains but was also present in the epidermal BM (EBM) of normal subjects (71). They suggested that this antigen would correspond to the NC domain of a fifth type IV collagen chain, α_5(IV), and that anomaly in this chain would be the biochemical substrate of the Alport's syndrome (72), a hypothesis further confirmed by the identification of the *COL4A5* gene (12–14).

The distribution of α_1–α_6 chains of type IV collagen in X-linked Alport's syndrome has been studied by several groups (19,20,43,73–77). In most, but not all male patients, no expression of α_3(IV), α_4(IV), α_5(IV), and α_6(IV) is detected in renal BMs, whereas the distribution of the chains is discontinuous in female patients, a finding consistent with the random inactivation of one X in each female cell. In contrast, α_1(IV), α_2(IV), and collagen type VI are overexpressed in the GBM (78). Both α_5(IV) and α_6(IV) are also absent from the EBM in males and have a segmental distribution in females (Fig. 26.5) (19,71,73, 76,78) providing a simple approach for the diagnosis of X-linked Alport's syndrome. In a series of 78 patients—mostly children—with Alport's syndrome, the distribution of the α_3–α_5(IV) chains was abnormal in two-thirds of the patients with classic Alport's syndrome. On the contrary, in one-third of them and in eight patients who had hereditary nephritis without deafness, the distribution of the chains was normal in the GBM and/or the EBM. Two patients were studied in each of eight families, and the immunohistochemical results were concordant (43). Abnormal distribution of the α_3, α_4, and α_5(IV) chains has been observed

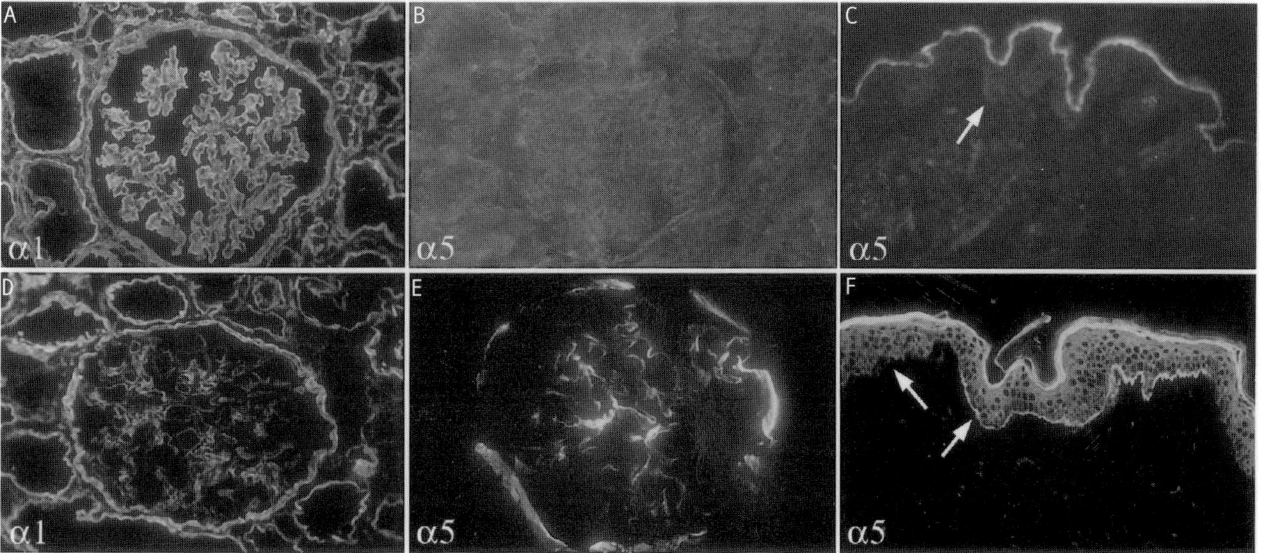

FIGURE 26.5. Immunofluorescent microscopy. Distribution of the α(IV) chains in renal and epidermal basement membranes of male **(A–C)** and female **(D–F)** patients affected with X-linked Alport's syndrome. **C:** Absence of epidermal basement membrane labeling (*arrow*). **F:** Discontinuous epidermal basement membrane labeling (*arrows*). (See Color Plate 26.5.)

in anterior lens capsules of one of the two patients with Alport's syndrome and anterior lenticonus who underwent capsulectomy for cataract extraction (79). The group of patients with abnormal distribution of the α_3–α_5(IV) chains is of particular interest. This anomaly appears to be a marker of severe juvenile forms of Alport's syndrome because: (a) the thickened and split GBM indicating poor prognosis was observed in 36 of the 37 α_3–α_5(IV)–negative patients studied, and (b) all males belonging to α_3–α_5(IV)–negative families progressed to ESRF before the age of 30 years (43).

Affected animals in both models of canine X-linked Alport's syndrome display the same immunohistologic anomalies as in humans (61,62). In addition, in dogs without any clinical evidence of extrarenal involvement, antigens were absent from the specialized membranes of the eye and internal ear.

Mutations in the COL4A5 *Gene: Molecular Heterogeneity of X-Linked Alport's Syndrome*

As soon as it was identified, the *COL4A5* gene, localized at Xq22, became the candidate gene for the Alport's syndrome and, a few months later, the description of the first mutations confirmed this hypothesis (80). Thus far, more than 300 different mutations have been identified by different groups, corresponding to a detection rate of 40 to 80% according to the screening method.

Deletions or other major rearrangements (duplication, insertion/deletion, inversion) of *COL4A5* have been detected by Southern blot analysis in 5 to 15% of cases (81–83). Deletions vary in size and location, ranging from the absence of a few exons to the complete absence of the gene, and involve various parts of the gene. They can result in total loss of expression of the gene, in a shortened α5(IV) chain, or in an aberrant gene product, within all cases a major effect on the organization of the collagen IV molecule and thus on the GBM structure.

All types of small mutations, distributed throughout the *COL4A5* gene, have been observed (80,84–94). Various consequences at the protein level may be expected from resulting changes in amino acid residues. The most common mutation found is glycine substitution by bulkier amino acid in the collagenous domain. It creates an interruption in the repeated collagen-specific gly-X-Y sequence and affects the formation of the triple helix. Removal of highly conserved cysteine in the NC domain could affect the correct conformation of the NC1 domain and influence the formation of the triple helix and of the intermolecular crosslinks (84). Nonsense mutations and small deletions or insertions resulting in a frame shift at the RNA level and in a premature stop codon lead to the synthesis of a putative truncated α5(IV) chain often lacking the NC domain. Splice site mutations are expected to alter the conformation of the protein or result in premature termination of the translation.

As indicated earlier, heterogeneity in the X-linked Alport's syndrome male phenotype has been documented widely. They are partly explained by the molecular heterogeneity of the disease. As shown in a European collaborative study, large deletions, nonsense mutations, or small mutations changing the reading frame confer to affected males a 90% probability of developing ESRF and hearing loss before 30 years of age, whereas the same risk is approx-

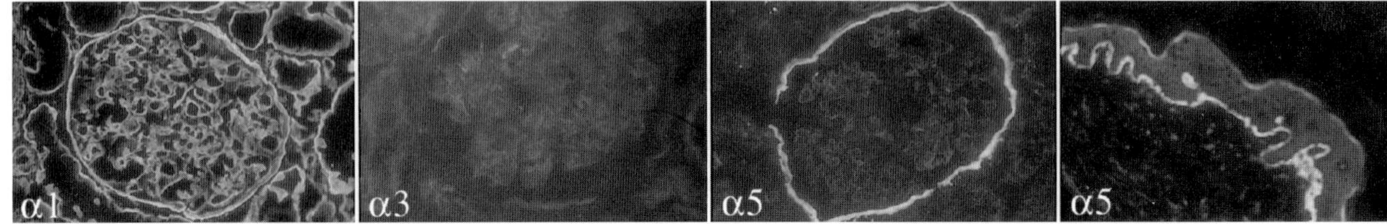

FIGURE 26.6. Immunofluorescent microscopy. Distribution of the α(IV) chains in renal and epidermal basement membranes of patients affected with autosomal recessive Alport's syndrome. (See Color Plate 26.6.)

imatively 50% for ESRF and 60% for hearing loss in patients with missense mutations (91).

At the protein level in most patients with a *COL4A5* mutation, there is a loss of the α_5(IV) chains in BMs. A striking feature is the co-absence of the α_3 and α_4 chains of type IV collagen. The mechanisms resulting in such a configuration are controversial. It is now established that α_3(IV) and α_4(IV) mRNA are expressed in male patients affected with X-linked Alport's syndrome, and thus *COL4A5* mutations probably result in defective molecular assembly and subsequent proteolysis of the chains (95,96).

Deletions of COL4A5 *and* COL4A6 *Genes in Alport's Syndrome Associated with Diffuse Esophageal Leiomyomatosis*

No isolated *COL4A6* mutation has been found in Alport's syndrome patients. But deletions removing the 5' end of both *COL4A5* and *COL4A6* genes are observed in all patients with Alport's syndrome associated with diffuse esophageal leiomyomatosis (51–54). Interestingly, in all cases, the deletion involves only the first two exons of *COL4A6*, whereas its extent in *COL4A5* is variable. In contrast, patients with *COL4A5* deletions associated with a larger deletion in *COL4A6* are affected with Alport's syndrome without diffuse esophageal leiomyomatosis (53,54). Dramatic changes in the composition of myocyte extracellular matrix was observed in the tumoral tissue. They include the co-absence of the α5 and α6(IV) chains contrasting with the high level of *COL4A6* transcripts, raising the question of a potential role for this RNA in the tumoral process (97).

Autosomal Recessive Alport's Syndrome

It is now recognized that 10 to 20% of Alport's syndrome patients are affected with the autosomal recessive form of the disease (29). Most features of the disease are identical to those observed in X-linked families. The nephritis usually progresses to early-onset ESRF, sensorineural hearing loss is often present, and ocular lesions, identical to those in X-linked families, may or may not be associated. Ultrastructural changes of the GBM in homozygotes are not distinguishable from those seen in classic Alport's syndrome. By contrast, some features suggest autosomal recessive inheritance—consanguinity, severe disease in affected females, and mild or no symptoms in the parents. As in X-linked Alport's syndrome, the GBM antigenicity is normal in a minority of patients and abnormal in most of them (98). A peculiar pattern of α_3–α_5(IV) distribution has been identified: It is characterized by the co-absence of the 3 chains in the GBM and the presence of the α_5(IV) chain in collecting ducts and EBM at places where the α_5(IV) chain is not associated with the α_3(IV) and α_4(IV) chains (Fig 26.6) (98). Mutations of the *COL4A3* or *COL4A4* genes have been identified in autosomal recessive Alport's syndrome (8,9,88,99–102). The status of heterozygote carriers is highly variable. Most of them are asymptomatic or have isolated microscopic hematuria with thin GBM, which are typical features of familial benign hematuria (8,9). In rare cases, heterozygotes have a slowly progressive nephritis. Murine models of autosomal recessive Alport's syndrome have been developed by knock-out of the *COL4A3* gene (103,104).

Autosomal Dominant Alport's Syndrome

A few cases of autosomal dominant Alport's syndrome with or without deafness have been reported (28–32). The renal prognosis in male patients is significantly better than in X-linked Alport's syndrome (28). In 2000, a *COL4A3* splice site mutation was identified in a large Irish family with autosomal dominant inheritance. This finding completes the spectrum of type IV collagen mutations in all genetic forms of Alport's syndrome (105). An autosomal dominant nephropathy with GBM changes similar to those occurring in Alport's syndrome has been described in bull terrier dogs (106).

Kidney Transplantation in Alport's Syndrome Patients and Anti-Glomerular Basement Membrane Nephritis

Favorable long-term results have been observed in most Alport's syndrome patients who have undergone kidney transplantation (107–109). However, approximately 3% of transplanted males affected with Alport's syndrome develop anti-GBM glomerulonephritis (88,91,110). This complication occurs within the first year after transplantation and leads to severe crescentic glomerulonephritis and subsequent graft loss. Patients are usually male and are affected with early-onset Alport's syndrome and deafness, progressing to ESRF before or around the age of 20 years. A few female patients, all affected with recessive Alport's syndrome, also developed anti-GBM nephritis (68,88,99, 101,102), but this complication has not been reported in females with X-linked disease. Recurrence of anti-GBM nephritis on a second transplant is common (111–113).

Nearly all patients who developed anti-GBM nephritis carry large deletions of the *COL43* or *COL4A5* genes or premature stop codon predicted to result in absent or truncated proteins without the NC domain of the molecule (88,91,99,101,102,114,115). The risk for these patients of developing anti-GBM nephritis reaches 15% (91).

The production of anti-GBM antibodies after kidney transplantation is induced by the exposure of GBM antigens for which the patient has not established immune tolerance. These antibodies recognize the NC domain of type IV collagen chains (72,116). Several types of specificities have been observed. Most patients with the *COL4A5* mutation develop antibodies against the 26-kDa NC domain of α_5(IV) (118), but antibodies against the α_3(IV)NC domain have also been observed (116,117,120). The serum of patients with the *COL4A3* mutation recognizes the NC domain of the α_3(IV) chain (102,118). In addition, transient linear IgG fixation along the GBM has been observed in approximatively 15% of transplanted patients in the absence of crescentic glomerulonephritis (119). More recently, this abnormal fixation has been shown to be associated with the presence of circulating anti-GBM antibodies with a wide spectrum of reactivity to the α_3, α_4, and α_5(IV) chains (120).

Factors other than the genetic defect are probably implicated in the occurrence of immunization, as suggested by the absence of anti-GBM posttransplant glomerulonephritis in most patients with major *COL4A5* mutations (43,88,91) and the intrafamilial discordance, with regard to the occurrence of GBM alloimmunization, observed in one family with a *COL4A5* deletion (82,113).

Diagnosis and Genetic Counseling

Diagnosis of Alport's syndrome is based on the finding of hematuria with or without proteinuria, hypertension, and renal failure in association with the following features: (a) familial hematuria, (b) sensorineural hearing loss present either in the proband or in one of the affected relatives, and (c) progression to renal failure occurring in at least one affected subject. Flinter et al. require one additional criterion—ocular changes or ultrastructural lesions of the GBM—for the diagnosis of Alport's syndrome (121). Diffuse esophageal leiomyomatosis and abnormal expression of the α_3, α_4, and α_5(IV) chains are other criteria (91). All hematuric patients fulfilling four criteria are actually affected with Alport's syndrome, but, from a practical point of view, diagnosis of Alport's syndrome is not always that easy. It has to be considered in every child who has persistent hematuria of glomerular origin, even in the absence of proven familial disease. The investigations to be performed are Addis counts in parents and siblings, regular audiograms, and ocular examinations seeking incipient anomalies (extrarenal symptoms are absent in very young children). Before performing renal biopsy, skin biopsy showing the absence or focal distribution of the α_5(IV) chain in the EBM can be used for rapid identification of X-linked Alport's syndrome (78). Renal biopsy with immunohistochemical and ultrastructural studies of the renal specimen allows one to exclude glomerulonephritis and especially IgA nephropathy, another frequent cause of microscopic and macroscopic hematuria, in children. Thick and split GBM, and abnormal GBM distribution of type IV collagen chains, are specific markers of the disease. However, normal immunohistochemistry of the GBM and/or the finding of thin BMs do not eliminate the diagnosis of Alport's syndrome. We never observed normal GBM ultrastructure in children affected with Alport's syndrome. Transmission of the disease by asymptomatic female carriers in X-linked Alport's syndrome or autosomal recessive transmission may explain the absence of evident family history. Another possibility is the occurrence of a neo-mutation, which accounts for up to 18% of patients with the syndrome.

Correct identification of the mode of inheritance is necessary for genetic counseling. Affected and unaffected subjects should be identified, making it crucial to detect asymptomatic carriers. In X-linked dominant Alport's syndrome, affected fathers will transmit the disease to all their daughters and to none of their sons. Half of the children—of either sex—of affected mothers will be affected. In autosomal dominant Alport's syndrome, affected parents transmit the disease to 50% of their offspring; father-to-son transmission is characteristic for this mode of inheritance.

Presymptomatic and prenatal diagnosis by linkage analysis or by direct *COL4A5* study are now possible in previously tested and informative families. In these families, DNA testing may allow the precise identification of asymptomatic female carriers, which is important in view of possible kidney donation and for genetic counseling.

Prognosis and Treatment

The prognosis of Alport's syndrome nephropathy is poor: All males progress to ESRF. Hearing impairment, ocular changes, and family history of juvenile-type Alport's syndrome have an ominous significance. In an individual male or female patient, regular increase in proteinuria is the most accurate clinical symptom indicating a poor prognosis. The presence of glomerular, tubular, and interstitial changes by light microscopy; the degree of GBM thickening and splitting; and the defect in GBM antigenicity are also indicative of severe disease. Severe *COL4A5* rearrangements are associated with juvenile-type nephritis.

The renal disease is progressive. However, recently, it has been shown that cyclosporin A could delay progression of ESRF (122). Angiotensin-converting enzyme inhibition decreases proteinuria and could also slow the rate of progression (123,124). Prospective controlled trials based on the precise clinical and genetic definition of the disease should be undertaken among larger series of patients to allow definitive conclusions. Also, therapeutic trials on animal models are now possible. Regular dialysis does not raise specific problems in Alport's syndrome patients. Most results indicate that posttransplant survival and renal function are as good as, or better than, in other groups of patients. The question of the selection of heterozygotes—asymptomatic or having isolated hematuria—as possible kidney donors is strongly debated (110). The development of anti-GBM glomerulonephritis in the transplanted kidney remains a rare possibility, but anti-GBM antibodies have to be sought in cases of rapid deterioration of kidney function.

Hearing loss has to be detected early and treated by hearing aid for a better comfort of the child and for preventing further degradation of the auditory center.

Familial Benign Essential Hematuria

Familial benign essential hematuria (FBEH) is defined by familial occurrence of persistent hematuria without proteinuria and without progression to renal failure or hearing defect. Diffuse attenuation of the GBM is usually considered the hallmark of the condition. However, thin GBM is not pathognomonic for familial benign hematuria. The incidence of this hematuric disorder has not been clearly evaluated. Recent data have shown that, at least in some families, type IV collagen is involved in the pathogenesis of the disorder (8,9,125).

Clinical and Laboratory Findings

Hematuria is often detected in childhood by routine urinalysis (58,59,126–128), but it may also be discovered in adults (129–131). It is usually microscopic and persistent. Episodes of gross hematuria have been reported, but we have never observed them in our series of patients. Clinical and laboratory investigations fail to disclose any other symptom: proteinuria is absent, there is no progression to renal failure, and no extrarenal manifestation.

Pathology

Few renal biopsies have been performed in this benign disease. By *light microscopy*, the renal tissue appears normal, except for the occasional presence of red blood cells within tubular lumens. No specific deposits are detected by *immunofluorescence*; small granular C3 deposits may be seen on the flocculus or the arteriolar wall. Diffuse and extreme attenuation of the GBM was first described by Rogers et al. in a well-documented family; it was the only lesion detected at the *ultrastructural level* in the five biopsied patients aged from 19 to 51 years (132). This finding has been confirmed by further observations (2,58,65,126–128,130,131), but, in some patients belonging to families affected with FBEH, the GBM has been found normal (2,128). Thinning of the GBM is usually regular and diffuse, but focal attenuation, involving at least 50% of capillary walls, may be observed. The structure and contours of the GBM are normal.

There is a wide discrepancy among investigators concerning the mode of identification of "thin" GBM. It may be based on subjective evaluation of GBM thickness followed by measurements of representative GBM segments or on systematic, numerous, random GBM measurements leading to the establishment of average values. The definition of thin GBM also varies among groups. In the first study by Rogers et al., the average thickness of the GBM was 150 nm (132). GBM thickness was between 100 and 200 nm in most pediatric series (65,127,128). In adult series, the mean GBM thickness values leading to the diagnosis of thin GBM varied from 206 to 319 nm. Overlaps between "abnormal" values and normal values measured in controls are observed in some series. Immunohistochemical studies of the GBM gave normal results in all patients tested (46,65,130,134).

Genetic Transmission

FBEH is usually considered to be transmitted as an autosomal dominant trait. In the family extensively studied by Rogers et al., in which eight members with persistent hematuria have been identified in four generations, the disease is clearly inherited as a dominant trait, but the autosomal dominant inheritance proposed by the authors is not demonstrated in the absence of father-to-son transmission (132). Male-to-male transmission was observed in two out of ten families in our series and in some kindreds in the series recently reported (130,135). Recent data have demonstrated that some patients with "familial benign hematuria" have *COL4A3* or *COL4A4* mutations and consequently are heterozygotes for autosomal recessive Alport's syndrome (8,9,136,137). However, genetic linkage to these genes has been excluded in some kindreds (138,139).

Sporadic cases of benign hematuria with thin GBM have been reported by different groups. Further analyses are still necessary to elucidate their relationship to FBEH.

Diagnosis and Prognosis

FBEH, when diagnosed in hematuric children, implicates a favorable short-term and long-term prognosis. Diagnosis is based on a series of negative symptoms (absence of proteinuria and of extrarenal involvement), on the results of family investigations demonstrating the absence of progression of the disease in adult males, and if necessary, on renal biopsy findings showing thin GBM with normal antigenicity. However, the distinction between FBEH and Alport's syndrome may be difficult, especially in young children. In both conditions, hematuria may be the only symptom. Thinning of the GBM is often prominent in children affected with Alport's syndrome and may constitute the only lesion, even in adulthood. Normal antigenicity of the GBM is observed in approximately 30% of Alport's syndrome patients. It is impossible to determine whether the course of the disease will be progressive or not when only adult females are affected in a kindred. In the absence of a pathognomonic marker, diagnosis of FBEH should be made with caution and reconsidered if proteinuria or extrarenal symptoms are detected in the proband or in family members during the follow-up.

Thin Basement Membrane Nephropathy

Thin GBM is frequently found in patients with FBEH, but the lesion that seems to represent approximately 11% of nontransplant renal biopsies in some groups (130) is not specific and is not the guarantee of benign disease. However, in recent years, various terms based on the ultrastructural finding of thin GBM have been used to describe, mostly in adults, the heterogeneous conditions characterized by hematuria and attenuation of the GBM (130,131,133) sometimes associated with proteinuria and progression to renal failure. The terms *thin glomerular basement membrane disease, thin basement membrane nephropathy, thin membrane nephropathy,* and *familial thin basement membrane nephropathy* are ambiguous because they suggest that the finding of thin GBM is a marker for a specific and common disorder with a uniformly good prognosis. In our opinion, thin GBM has to be viewed as a lesion and not a clinicopathologic entity. In children with this lesion, the diagnosis of Alport's syndrome has to be considered before any other possibility. The same ultrastructural lesion found in late adulthood in association with isolated microscopic hematuria probably has an overall favorable prognostic significance. However, substantial proteinuria and progression to ESRF have been reported in adult patients with thin GBM (131).

Hereditary Osteo-Onychodysplasia (Nail-Patella Syndrome)

Hereditary osteo-onychodysplasia (HOOD), or *nail-patella syndrome* (NPS), is a rare autosomal dominant disorder defined by the association of nail dysplasia, bone abnormalities, and renal involvement. Since the first description of the disease (140), more than 500 cases have been reported in kindreds from all geographic origins. This curious association and the presence of fibrillar collagen within the GBM have suggested that HOOD could be an inherited connective tissue disorder. However, recently, *LMX1B,* a transcription factor involved in limb and renal development has been shown to be the NPS protein.

Dysmorphic Syndrome

The dysmorphic features were first described in 1897 by Little, who reported on a family of 18 members in whom nails and patellae were absent (140). Several reports followed, and the typical, bilateral, and symmetric involvement of the nails, knees, elbows, and pelvis were put forth by Mino et al. (141).

Nail involvement is almost constant: It has been found absent in only 6 of 147 patients, despite the presence of other elements of the tetrad (142). It predominates on the hands, where the thumb and the index finger are more severely affected. Lesions range from hemidysplasia to total nail aplasia. Common features are longitudinal pterygium and absence or triangular appearance of the lunulae. Nail dysplasia is usually visible from birth.

The *knees* are abnormal in 95% of cases. The patellas are hypoplastic or even absent. They have a tendency to dislocate laterally, producing difficulties in learning to walk in children and in climbing stairs in adults (143). In fact, the functional disability is usually limited, and the most frequent complications are knee pains, recurring patella dislocations, and early onset of arthrosis. The dysplasia may also involve other structures of the knee.

Elbow dysplasia was mentioned in 94% of cases. The radial head may be small and dislocated in a posterolateral position. Associated anomalies include deformities of the distal humeral extremity, hypoplasia of the olecranon, and elongation of the radial neck. These anomalies may lead to mild to severe limitation of extension, pronation, and supination of the forearm, especially in cases of webbing of the skin at the anterior aspect of the elbow joint.

The presence of *iliac horns,* usually discovered on plain film or intravenous pyelogram, was reported in 70.7% of cases. They are asymptomatic, bilateral, triangular, and symmetric formations arising from the posterior aspect of the ilium (143). In some cases, they may be detected by palpation through the buttock muscles.

Various other bone abnormalities have been described but are not contributive to diagnosis. According to the severity of the dysmorphic syndrome, HOOD may be discovered at various ages, but the notion of family history strongly contributes to its early recognition. Some severely affected neonates with clubbed feet are misdiagnosed as arthrogryposis. Mild forms of the disease may remain undetected over decades.

Abnormal pigmentation of the inner margin of the iris is seen in approximately 50% of patients, and recently open-angle glaucoma has been recognized as an additional feature of the disorder (144).

Renal Involvement

Renal involvement was first reported in 1950 (145,146). Curiously enough, renal symptoms are not found in all patients or in all families. They seem to develop in approximately 30 to 40% of cases (142,147), but this evaluation is perhaps overestimated. Both genders are equally affected. The most common presenting feature is proteinuria with occasional nephrotic syndrome sometimes associated with microscopic hematuria.

Progression to ESRF occurs in approximatively 30% of patients with renal symptoms. Cases of rapid evolution to renal failure have been observed in the pediatric population. In fact, we lack precise knowledge of the long-term renal outcome in HOOD. A surprising evolution has been observed in a neonate with typical deformities belonging to a severely affected family: Nephrotic syndrome was present at birth, but proteinuria disappeared within 2 weeks and was still absent 8 months later (147). A striking feature of the disease is the total unpredictability of renal prognosis, even within a given family. It is illustrated by a personal observation in which a child developed ESRF at 15 years of age, whereas his monozygote twin had only intermittent proteinuria at 27 years. This suggests that superimposed factors, which remain to be identified, may be implicated in the rapid progression of the glomerulopathy in some patients. Goodpasture syndrome, membranous nephropathy, necrotizing angiitis, and IgA nephropathy have been observed in HOOD patients (142).

Pathology

Light microscopy is poorly contributive. The lesions of focal-segmental sclerosis, when present, are nonspecific and correlate with the severity of renal insufficiency. *Immunofluorescence* may show focal deposits of IgM and C3.

The specific glomerular lesion has been identified by *electron microscopy* (148). It is characterized by the presence of clusters of fibrillar collagen irregularly distributed within thick GBM segments and within the mesangial matrix. With standard staining techniques, the GBM and the mesangial matrix often have a "moth-eaten" appearance (149). Staining with phosphotungstic acid often is necessary to disclose the collagen bundles (Fig. 26.7). They have a fibrillar structure with a major periodicity of 40 to 60 nm, but, in some instances, no periodicity can be detected. The width of individual fibrils varies considerably. These lesions have been found within the GBM in all patients studied, mostly within the lamina densa (148,150–154). However, we could not detect any GBM collagen fiber in the first biopsy specimen from a child affected with HOOD and presenting with infantile nephrotic syndrome. The lesions were evident on the second renal specimen obtained 3 years later. By contrast, in the 2-year-old child reported by Browning et al. (154), diffuse thickening of the GBM was associated with focal subendothelial accumulation of fibrillar collagen. No tubular BM involvement has been described.

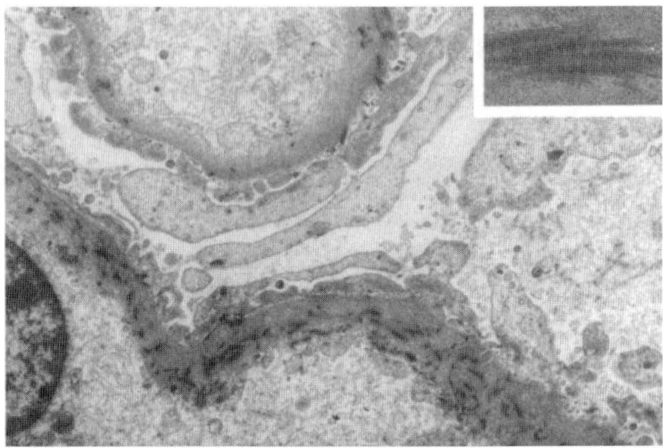

FIGURE 26.7. Electron microscopy. Phosphotungstic acid stain (×10,500). Nail patella syndrome. Irregular distribution of fibrillar collagen within the glomerular basement membrane. Inset shows the typical periodicity of interstitial collagen (×48,000).

There is a curious lack of correlation between the severity and the extension of ultrastructural GBM lesions on one hand, and the patient's age, the severity of proteinuria, or even the degree of renal failure on the other. Typical lesions have been found in patients who were not proteinuric (162,164).

Immunohistochemical studies of the GBM using antibodies against the NC domain of α_3(IV) gave conflicting results—normal labeling in three patients and no GBM labeling in two others (119). We detected type III collagen with an irregular mesangiocapillary localization and observed abnormal distribution of type VI collagen in glomeruli from several patients confirming the abnormal biochemical composition of the glomerular extracellular matrix.

Genetic Transmission: Mutations in the Gene LMX1B

HOOD is transmitted as an autosomal dominant trait. The gene located at 9q34 is closely linked to those coding for ABO blood groups and for adenylate kinase (155,156). Taking into account the absence of nephropathy in some kindreds, Lommen et al. suggested that there are two allelic mutations of the HOOD locus, one causing HOOD without nephropathy and one associated with the possible occurrence of nephropathy (157). The risks for affected parents of having a child with nephropathy, eventually leading to ESRF, should be different in these two types of families.

In 1998, *LMX1B* was shown to be the NPS gene by two groups using two different approaches. Positional cloning, candidate gene approach, and identification of mutations were used by the first group (158). For the second group, the resemblance between the phenotypes in mice inactivated for the *Lmx1b* gene and in NPS patients suggested that *LMX1B* might be the NPS gene (159). Further studies confirmed this finding, and more than 100 *LMX1B* mutations have now been reported in NPS patients (160–164). LMX1B is a transcription factor belonging to the LIM homeodomain protein family playing an important role during development. It establishes dorsoventral patterning of the limb in which it is expressed in a temporally and spatially restricted manner (165). Mice with a homozygous deletion of the gene exhibit nail and skeletal defects similar to those observed in patients and GBM abnormalities and die within 24 hours after birth (165). The previously known function of LMX1B provides a satisfactory explanation for the occurrence of nail and skeletal anomalies in NPS patients (159). On the other hand, the recent demonstration of the early and persistent expression of *lmx1b* in the podocyte, and the role of the protein in the regulation of the expression of type IV collagen α4 chain and other podocyte proteins opened new avenues for the understanding of the NPS nephropathy (166–168). The expression of the α3 and α4 chains of type IV collagen is strongly reduced in the GBM of $Lmx1b^{-/-}$ mice (166,168). Similarly, decreased expression of CD2AP and podocin—two markers of podocyte differentiation, responsible when mutated of proteinuria and nephrotic syndrome—was observed in *Lmx1b* null mice (167). Moreover, binding sites for Lmx1b were identified in both podocin and Cd2ap promoters and in an enhancer sequence in *COL4A4* intron 1 (166–168). These findings strongly suggest that defects in GBM type IV collagen and changes in podocyte phenotype contribute to glomerular disease in NPS. However, no renal symptom and no defects in the expression of these proteins were found in heterozygous mice.

Diagnosis and Treatment

As seen earlier, clinical diagnosis of nail-patella syndrome is easy and based on identification of the elements of the classic tetrad. At the ultrastructural level, the finding of collagen fibers within the GBM of nonsclerotic glomeruli is quite specific for the condition. One exception is the detection of similar lesions in a few patients without extrarenal anomalies of the HOOD series (see Collagen Type III Glomerulopathy).

Evolution of renal symptoms is unpredictable. No specific treatment is available. No recurrence of GBM lesions and no anti-GBM glomerulonephritis have so far been reported after kidney transplantation.

Collagen Type III Glomerulopathy

Massive accumulation of collagen fibers within the glomerular tuft has been reported in 22 patients with proteinuria unassociated with extrarenal symptoms (169–177). The glomerulopathy has been termed *primary glomerular fibrosis* (172), *collagenofibrotic glomerulonephropathy* (174,177), or *collagen type III glomerulopathy* (173,175,176). The glomerular involvement was initially considered as being an incomplete, purely renal form of HOOD (169). However, analysis of morphologic, clinical, and genetic data strongly suggests that they represent a new type (or new types) of glomerulopathy.

Pathology

By *light microscopy*, glomerular lesions are peculiar, contrary to the lesions observed in most patients affected with HOOD. The glomerular tuft is significantly enlarged because of both expansion of the mesangial matrix and thickening of the capillary walls owing to accumulation of poorly stained subendothelial material. There is no significant increase in the number of mesangial cells. Conventional *immunohistologic studies* are negative or show segmental and focal deposits of various immunoglobulins and complement factors. Expansion of the mesangial matrix and of the subendothelial aspect of the GBM by a heterogeneous electron-lucent material is confirmed by *electron microscopic studies*. The most characteristic finding is the detection (after selective stainings) of bundles of collagen fibers accumulated within the expanded mesangium and the subendothelial space of the GBM. The lamina densa is usually normal. Thus, changes in the glomerular structure and distribution of the collagen fibers are different from those observed in HOOD. Antibodies to type III collagen are strongly positive on the glomerular tuft.

Clinical Data

The disease has been described in both genders and in patients aged from 1 to 70 years. Persistent proteinuria with or without nephrotic syndrome is observed in all cases and is often the presenting symptom. Microscopic hematuria and hypertension are inconstant. Anemia has been noted in several patients (174–177).

Concerning the progression of the disease, a striking difference appears between adult and pediatric series. Stable renal function or slow progression to renal failure is observed in most adult patients (174,175), whereas a protracted course to ESRF is frequently described in children (171,179).

Genetic Data

Family investigations were negative in most patients reported to date. In two adult patients (170,171), the family history of renal disease is consistent with dominant transmission of the condition (170). By contrast, autosomal recessive transmission of the disease was suggested in the pediatric series on the finding of parental consanguinity, involvement of several siblings of both genders, and absence of renal and extrarenal symptoms in parents (171,175).

Further studies are necessary to clarify the actual incidence, the long-term evolution, and the basic mechanisms responsible for the massive overproduction of type III collagen. Of interest, in one young boy, collagen type III glomerulopathy was associated with autosomal recessive factor H (FH) deficiency (176), an inherited disorder possibly associated with the occurrence of glomerular lesions (see Factor H Deficiency). From a practical point of view, the typical ultrastructural and immunohistochemical anomalies have to be sought in proteinuric patients with atypical glomerular lesions that could mimic thrombotic microangiopathy of the glomerular type. Evaluation of C3 and factor-serum levels has to be systematically performed.

Hereditary Nephritis with Thrombopenia and Giant Platelets: Epstein/Fechtner Syndromes

The association of hereditary nephritis with macrothrombocytopenia (MTCP), first reported by Epstein et al. (178), has long been regarded as an Alport's syndrome variant. These authors studied two families with MTCP, deafness, and nephritis, a syndrome that appeared to be autosomal dominant. In Fechtner syndrome, patients are affected with nephritis and MTCP as well. However, they also display cataracts and small, pale blue cytoplasmic inclusions within the neutrophils and eosinophils that were not described in Epstein families (179). Leukocyte inclusions are also observed in two other autosomal dominant MTCPs without renal, ocular, or hearing defects: Sebastian syndrome and May-Hegglin anomaly.

The Epstein and Fechtner syndromes appear heterogeneous because of the variable severity of hematologic, renal, and auditory symptoms. Thrombopenia may be asymptomatic or responsible for hemorrhagic complications. Progression to ESRF is variable and does not generally occur before the fourth or fifth decade of life. It is absent in some families. On the contrary, rapid progression to ESRF during childhood has been reported (180). Early occurrence of deafness, particularly in females, is commonly observed. In addition, dissociation between the renal disease and the thrombopenia has been reported. Some males, both thrombopenic and deaf, who are obligatory transmitters of Alport's syndrome have no renal impairment (181), which is never observed in classic Alport's syndrome

Renal histology shows variable and nonspecific abnormalities, including variable degrees of mesangial cell proliferation and mesangial matrix expansion and some tubular atrophy. Electron microscopy shows mesangial alterations, focal or diffuse effacement of podocyte foot processes, and alterations of the GBM. GBM lesions reminiscent of ultrastructural GBM lesions observed in Alport's syndrome have been reported. However, GBM alteration in Fechtner and Epstein syndrome have mostly a focal distribution and, except from rare cases (180), are not specific of Alport's syndrome.

In 1999, the May-Hegglin anomaly, the Sebastian syndrome, and the Fechtner syndrome were shown to be genetically linked to chromosome 22q (182,183) suggesting that these three dominant MTCPs were allelic. Indeed, mutations in the *MYH9* gene, encoding the nonmuscle myosin heavy chain IIA, were subsequently identified in patients affected with one of these three diseases as well as in Epstein syndrome (184–186). This gene is expressed in the kidney from the early stages of nephrogenesis to adulthood, mainly in the podocytes and peritubular capillaries (186).

HEREDITARY METABOLIC DISORDERS WITH PRIMARY GLOMERULAR INVOLVEMENT

Fabry Disease

Anderson-Fabry disease is a rare X-linked recessive disorder of glycosphingolipid metabolism resulting from deficiency of the lysosomal hydrolase, α-galactosidase A (187). Clinical aspects of this disease are discussed in Chapter 50.

Characteristic glycolipid accumulation within every glomerular, vascular, and interstitial cell and within distal tubular cells has been observed in renal tissue from all hemizygous patients irrespective of their age at renal biopsy. In heterozygous females, a peculiar feature is the presence of two intermingled cell populations, one normal and one massively involved by the storage disease. Degenerative renal changes develop with age. They first affect vessels and are characterized by the presence of round fibrinoid deposits resulting from necrosis of smooth muscle cells. They are secondarily associated with nonspecific vascular, glomerular, and tubulointerstitial lesions (188). Of interest, the reported beneficial effect of enzyme replacement therapy seems to be linked to decrease glycolipid accumulation in the vascular endothelium (189).

Other Glomerular Lipidoses

Nephrosialidosis is a rare and severe form of oligosaccharidosis, or glucoproteinosis (previously classified as mucolipidosis type I). The condition is inherited as an autosomal recessive trait and is caused by neuraminidase deficiency. The clinical and radiologic features of the disease include dysmorphic facies, visceral storage disease, severe mental retardation, skeletal abnormalities, foam cells in the marrow, and cherry red spot on funduscopy. A specific feature is the early occurrence of progressive glomerular symptoms leading to ESRF in the first years of life (190). Podocytes and proximal tubular cells show severe vacuolization. At the electron microscopic level, membrane-bound vacuoles look empty because of the loss of the stored material during fixation.

Glomerular symptoms are rare in other lipidoses (191). They usually are mild or absent in patients affected with *Gaucher disease*, an autosomal recessive condition in which the accumulation of glucosylceramide within monocytes-macrophages results from deficient activity of the lysosomal enzyme glycosylceramidase. Severe symptoms, proteinuria, and progressive renal failure have been described in only a few adult patients, most often after splenectomy. Large "Gaucher" cells with abundant, pale, faintly fibrillar cytoplasm have been observed in endothelial and mesangial position within glomeruli and also in the interstitium.

In *Niemann-Pick disease, I-cell disease*, and *GM1 gangliosidosis*, silent accumulation of glycolipids or mucopolysaccharides within glomerular cells has been detected by examination of autopsy material (191).

HEREDITARY METABOLIC DISORDERS WITH SECONDARY GLOMERULAR INVOLVEMENT

Familial Amyloidosis

Hereditary amyloidosis encompasses a group of autosomal dominant disorders characterized by the extracellular accumulation of protein fibrils having β-pleated sheet conformation. They are now classified according to the type of protein composing amyloid fibrils and for some of them according to the type of mutation detected in the corresponding gene. Transthyretin variants have been found in most affected families, but systemic hereditary amyloidosis may be associated with variants of cystatin C, gelsolin, apolipoprotein A1, fibrinogen, or lysozyme (192). In hereditary amyloidosis, symptoms, usually of the neurologic series, develop during adulthood. Except for a few families with apolipoprotein A1, fibrinogen, or lysozyme variant, renal symptoms are not a prominent and early feature, but severe renal involvement may be observed in all types of familial amyloidoses and has an ominous significance.

Familial Mediterranean fever, an autosomal recessive disorder common in Mediterranean and Middle Eastern populations, especially in Sephardic Jews and Armenians, is characterized by recurrent episodes of fever, abdominal pain, joint pain, and less frequently, pleuritis or pericarditis. The prognosis of the disease depends on the development of amyloidosis of the AA type with prominent renal involvement. The gene involved in familial Mediterranean fever, designated *MEFV*, has been identified by positional cloning (193,194). Colchicine administration has been shown to reduce the number of attacks and to prevent amyloidosis (195).

Development of amyloid of the AA type occurs in other types of inflammatory disorders also characterized by recurrent attacks of fever with visceral, synovial, muscular, or cutaneous inflammation—the *Muckle-Well syndrome* and the *TRAPS syndrome* both transmitted on the autosomal dominant mode (196).

Alpha-1 Antitrypsin Deficiency

Alpha-1 antitrypsin (α1AT) is a major serine protease inhibitor synthesized by the liver. The gene responsible for α1AT deficiency has been localized on chromosome 14. α1AT deficiency, phenotype ZZ, may result in emphysema in adults (review in 197). Renal complications are rare in these patients. Conversely, approximately 25 cases of glomerulonephritis have been described in α1AT-deficient children with severe chronic liver disease (198–200), another possible and early complication of this autosomal dominant biochemical defect. Diffuse or focal segmental type I membranoproliferative glomerulonephritis was present in most cases, but diffuse endocapillary glomerulonephritis has also been observed. Immunofluorescence revealed the presence of immunoglobulins, often including IgA and complement components. The co-localization of PiZ protein with immunoproteins has been observed (200,201), but is not a constant finding (199). Expression of glomerular involvement varies from no disease to proteinuria, hypertension, and renal failure. Its severity roughly parallels that of renal lesions. A direct pathogenic link with α1AT deficiency has been suggested based on the presence of granular α1AT or PiZ subendothelial deposits and on the increased incidence of glomerular lesions in α1AT-deficient patients compared with a controlled cirrhotic population (200). Regression of nephrotic syndrome and glomerular lesions has been observed after liver transplantation (201). In adults, association of α1AT deficiency and systemic vasculitis, especially Wegener syndrome, has been described, suggesting involvement of the gene in the pathogenesis of these diseases (202).

Factor H Deficiency

Homozygous deficit in FH, a 150-kDa glycoprotein controlling the alternative pathway of complement activation, is usually responsible for increased susceptibility to infections. In several families, renal involvement consisting of atypical dense deposit disease, hemolytic uremic syndrome, or collagen type III glomerulopathy has been reported (203).

Dense deposit disease, observed in two brothers, was characterized by the early onset of glomerular symptoms, with recurrent macroscopic hematuria and the abundance of mesangial and parietal granular C3 deposits (204). FH deficiency has been shown in piglets with autosomal recessive dense deposit disease. The disease develops early after birth and progresses rapidly to ESRF. Transfusion of normal porcine plasma or injection of FH into affected pigs increases survival, demonstrating the role of FH deficiency and alternative complement activation in the pathogenesis of the disease (205).

Low C3 level has been described in several atypical, recurrent, and/or familial cases of *hemolytic uremic syndrome* and, recently, the role of FH deficiency and the identification of mutations of the FH gene have been reported by several groups (206–213). It appears now that FH deficiency is one major cause of familial hemolytic uremic syndrome associated with a high risk of recurrence in renal allografts. Within families, a striking feature is the absence of correlation between the degree of FH deficiency and the presence and severity of renal disease.

Extensive deposition of *type III collagen* has been identified in a young patient with progressive glomerulopathy and FH deficiency; the relationship between the two abnormalities is still unclear (181).

Alagille Syndrome

Alagille syndrome, or *syndromic paucity of interlobular ducts*, is an autosomal dominant disorder with variable penetrance, recognized as a common cause of severe cholestase is in children. Liver abnormalities are associated with a peculiar facial appearance, cardiovascular malformations, butterfly-like vertebral arch defect, embryotoxon, hypogonadism, growth retardation, and high-pitched voice. The disease is caused by mutations in *Jagged1*, which encodes a ligand for the Notch1 receptor, implicated in cell differentiation (214,215). Glomerular lesions of variable severity have been observed in some patients (216). They are characterized by the presence of clear vacuoles containing osmiophilic material within the mesangial matrix and sometimes within the GBM. Mesangial foam cells may be associated (Fig. 26.8). The extent of mesangio-lipidosis is related to the degree of cholestasis and is probably a consequence of the resulting abnormal lipid metabolism. A striking feature is the early occurrence of these lesions during the first years of life in some patients contrasting with the paucity of renal symptoms. Progression to renal failure in adulthood may be a major complication for patients with this syndrome.

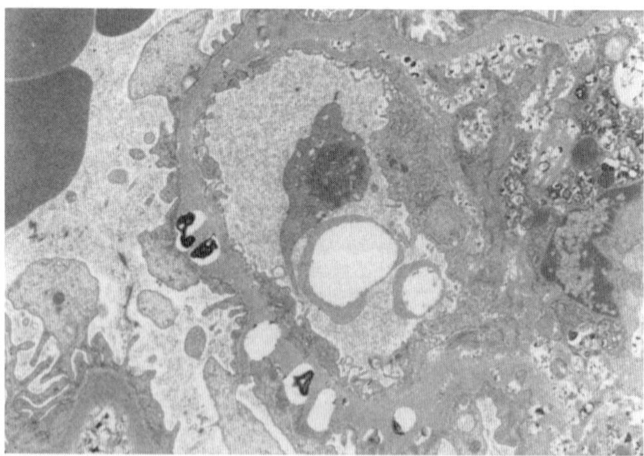

FIGURE 26.8. Electron microscopy. Lead citrate and uranyl acetate stain (×8600). Alagille syndrome. Massive accumulation of lipid vacuoles within mesangial cells and matrix. Irregular distribution of lipid vacuoles within the glomerular basement membrane.

Hereditary Lecithin-Cholesterol Acyltransferase Deficiency

Hereditary lecithin-cholesterol acyltransferase (L-CAT) deficiency, first described in Norway, is a rare autosomal recessive disorder characterized by an inability to esterify plasma cholesterol and by abnormal deposition of unesterified cholesterol in tissues, including the kidney (217,218). Progression to ESRF usually occurs in the fourth or fifth decade. Glomerular lesions resemble those seen in Alagille syndrome. They include accumulation of foam cells of endothelial and mesangial origin and massive deposition of lipids within the mesangial matrix and along the subendothelial aspect of the GBM (217). The *L-CAT* gene has been localized on chromosome 16, and different point mutations spread in all exons of the gene have been described in families of various geographic origins (218).

Lipoprotein Glomerulopathy

Lipoprotein glomerulopathy is a new type of renal disease characterized by intraglomerular lipoprotein thrombosis and high plasma concentration of apolipoprotein E. Since the first publication by Saito et al. in 1989 (219), numerous cases have been observed mostly, but not exclusively, in Japan (220–224). The disease, observed in both genders, usually is detected in adulthood; however, in some cases, first symptoms occurred in childhood (224). All patients have persistent proteinuria resulting in nephrotic syndrome in most of them. Some have mild to moderate proteinuria for a long period, whereas progression to ESRF has been observed. Transplantation has been followed by the recurrence of glomerular lesions (221,223). Curiously, systemic manifestations of lipidosis are consistently absent. The familial occurrence observed in some kindreds suggested a genetic basis for the disease, involving perhaps the isoform E_2 of apolipoprotein E. Actually, a variant of apolipoprotein E, apolipoprotein E Sendai, characterized by a missense mutation resulting in arginine-145 to proline substitution appears to be the most frequent mutation in the patients (222), but other mutations have been described (223).

Glomerular lipidosis has also been observed in patients with *familial hypercholesterolemia* resulting from defect in the receptor for low-density lipoproteins, in *type III hyperlipoproteinemia*, and in the rare cases of *cholesterolic polycoria*. In these diseases, clinical symptoms usually develop in adulthood.

Familial Juvenile Megaloblastic Anemia

Familial juvenile megaloblastic anemia, or *Imerslund-Gräsbeck syndrome*, is a rare autosomal recessive disorder caused by primary and selective vitamin B_{12} malabsorption. Anemia appearing in infancy or early childhood is nearly always associated with mild and nonprogressive proteinuria, usually considered of glomerular origin. Minor and nonspecific glomerular changes have been described by electron microscopy (225).

OTHER HEREDITARY DISEASES WITH GLOMERULAR INVOLVEMENT

Charcot-Marie-Tooth Disease

Charcot-Marie-Tooth (CMT) disease is a familial peripheral neuropathy resulting in progressive symmetric atrophy and weakness of distal muscles and sensory loss. Various clinical forms of the disease have been described according to nerve morphology and nerve conduction velocity, age at onset of symptoms, and presence or absence of associated symptoms. This clinical heterogeneity is explained by the genetic heterogeneity of the condition: Autosomal dominant, X-linked dominant, and X-linked recessive modes of inheritance have been described (226,227). In 1993, mutations in the myelin protein zero gene on chromosome 1, peripheral myelin protein 22 gene on chromosome 17 and connexin 32 on chromosome X were identified (228–230). Renal symptoms with focal glomerular sclerosis have been reported in a few patients and seem to segregate with the neuropathy in some families (231). They consist of long-standing proteinuria occurring in childhood or in adolescence, followed by rapid progression to ESRF. Because some of these patients are also deaf, CMT disease with renal involvement could have been considered a variant of Alport's syndrome. Deafness is a possible manifestation of peripheral involvement in CMT disease, and, except in one family with co-segregation of AS and CMT disease (232), no specific ultrastructural changes of the GBM have been observed in patients with CMT disease.

Cockayne Syndrome

Cockayne syndrome is an unusual autosomal recessive disorder. Characteristic symptoms are poor growth, neurologic abnormalities, premature aging, senile face, sensorineural hearing loss, cataracts, pigmentary retinopathy, sun sensitivity, and dental caries, as reported in a comprehensive review of 140 patients by Nance and Berry (233). Death occurs in most cases during the first or second decade. Increased cell sensitivity to the killing effect of ultraviolet radiation has been observed, caused by a specific defect in the DNA repair system. Renal symptoms consisting of hypertension, mild proteinuria, or renal insufficiency develop in approximately 10% of patients. The basic lesion seems to be diffuse and homogeneous thickening of the GBM (234,235). The syndrome is clinically and genetically heterogeneous (236).

Hereditary Acro-Osteolysis with Nephropathy

Hereditary acro-osteolysis is a rare disorder characterized by arthritis-like episodes and progressive resorption of carpal and tarsal bones. Inherited, dominant or recessive, and sporadic cases have been reported. Hypertension, proteinuria, and progressive renal failure may occur in some patients (237). Arteriolar thickening and sclerosis and focal glomerulosclerosis are the usual histopathologic findings.

Other Syndromes with Renal Involvement

Renal involvement is nearly constant in *Biedl-Bardet syndrome* (BBS), an autosomal recessive disorder, the cardinal features of which are obesity, polydactylia, mental retardation, retinal dystrophy, and hypogonadism (238). The disease is genetically heterogenous. Six genes have been localized, and the first one has been identified (239). BBS is responsible for severe renal disease in 15 to 55% of patients, according to different series. Glomerular symptoms, such as proteinuria, as well as questionable glomerular changes, have been described in only a few patients. Actually, tubular dysfunction and abnormal kidney structure detected by urography are the main renal symptoms in BBS. Cystic kidney dysplasia and/or tubulointerstitial lesions seem to be the most consistent lesions in this disease (240,241).

Alström syndrome is a rare autosomal recessive disorder, the gene of which has been recently identified. It is characterized by the association of profound childhood blindness, nerve deafness, obesity, and diabetes mellitus and differs from BBS by the absence of mental retardation and polydactyly. It is considered a classic cause of proteinuria. However, primary glomerular involvement has not been demonstrated, and tubular dysfunction and tubulointerstitial lesions have been observed in the few patients studied (242).

In *familial dysautonomia*, an autosomal recessive neuropathy that occurs in the Ashkenazi Jewish population, renal involvement seems to be primarily vascular with secondary development of glomerulosclerosis (243).

HEREDITARY GLOMERULOPATHIES WITHOUT EXTRARENAL SYMPTOMS

Familial Lobular Glomerulonephritis/ Fibronectin Glomerulopathy: A Heterogeneous Entity?

Several familial cases of atypical lobular glomerulopathies have been reported (244–247). They were characterized by extensive subendothelial and mesangial deposits in which immunoglobulins and complement components were inconstant or lacking. Patients had persistent proteinuria, hematuria, and hypertension. Slow progression to ESRF or severe cerebral vascular complications (in one family) occurred around the third decade of life. The disease is transmitted as an autosomal dominant trait. Recently, strong reactivity of deposits to fibronectin derived from the plasma was shown in patients previously reported and in additional families (248–252). The names "fibronectin glomerulopathy" or "familial glomerulonephritis with fibronectin deposits" were suggested for this glomerulopathy (220). However, the pathogenic significance of fibronectin deposition remains to be confirmed. It has been suggested that genetically altered fibronectin is trapped within the glomerular tuft, but fibronectin was excluded as a causative gene by linkage analysis in a large family (250). Linkage analysis of a large pedigree led to the localization of a gene at 1q32 (253).

The homogeneity of this new entity is not demonstrated. Clinical evolution varies between families with regard to the occurrence of cerebral vascular complications, progression to ESRF, evolution after transplantation, and ultrastructural appearance of deposits. One child developed nephrotic syndrome at 3 years of age (252). In some kindreds, deposits are homogeneous and granular with a restricted subendothelial and mesangial distribution (245, 248), whereas in others they are fibrillar (246,247,249) and also observed in subepithelial location (246). Of four patients from different families who were reported to have undergone kidney transplants, the disease recurred in one only (248,250).

Other Familial Glomerulopathies

A curious form of hereditary nephropathy has been described by Grottum et al. in 11 members of a large family (254). Persistent moderate proteinuria was abruptly followed by rapidly progressive renal failure, malignant hypertension, and microangiopathic anemia and thrombocytopenia occurring at the ages of 24 to 31 years (254). Diffuse vascular damages and ischemic glomeruli with IgM and C3 deposits were observed in all cases. A glomerular disease with a similar clinical course has been observed in another family. The presence of diffuse round mesangial deposits of C3 was the characteristic feature in this family (255). In both families, the disease appears to be autosomal dominant.

MITOCHONDRIAL CYTOPATHIES

Mitochondrial cytopathies are a heterogeneous group of diseases. They are due to genetic defects of one or several mitochondrial enzyme complexes that play a major role in oxidative phosphorylation and energy production. They have long been regarded as neuromuscular diseases only, but any organs dependent on mitochondrial energy supply may be affected by these disorders (256). For a long time, renal involvement was regarded as being rare, the most frequent manifestation, usually seen in children, being proximal tubulopathy manifested by a de Toni Debré Fanconi syndrome (257). More recently, several cases of glomerulopathy have been reported (257–273), and this expression is probably more frequent than initially thought.

Glomerular involvement has been initially described in three children who developed nephrotic syndrome with focal segmental glomerulosclerosis before the age of 5 years (258,259). These patients had mitochondrial cytopathies manifested by the association of myopathy, ophthalmoplegia, and deafness or pigmentary retinitis and hypoparathyroidism.

Since 1994, approximately 40 cases of glomerulopathies, initially isolated or associated with extrarenal symptoms, have been reported. The clinical presentation of the renal disease is nonspecific: occurrence of proteinuria at various ages between 1.6 and 35.0 years, progressive increase with age with eventual development of nephrotic syndrome, and variable rate of progression to ESRF. An important feature is the usual absence of hematuria. Steroid therapy is ineffective. Proteinuria was the revealing symptom of the disease in 12 patients aged 10 to 32 years who secondarily developed extrarenal symptoms. Proteinuria/nephrotic syndrome was also found in patients aged 17 to 34 years who have maternally inherited diabetes and/or deafness or, less frequently, complete or incomplete MELAS (*m*itochondrial *e*ncephalomyopathy with *l*actic *a*cidosis and *s*troke-like episodes) syndrome. This observation led to the identification of the mitochondrial DNA MELAS mutation in most patients with mitochondrial glomerulopathy.

Focal and segmental glomerulosclerosis was observed in nearly all renal biopsies. An increased number of abnormal mitochondria of various shapes and sizes was found in podocytes by Hotta et al. (271), but in most cases, no mitochondrial lesion was seen. Mitochondrial abnormalities appear to be more frequent and prominent in proximal tubular cells despite the absence of tubular symptoms. Arteriolar deposits have been described in the five biopsies examined by Doleris et al. (269). They could result from individual myocyte necrosis and participate in the progression of glomerular lesions.

RARE AND "BIZARRE" SYNDROMES

Several curious syndromes with a glomerular component have been described in single or few families (274–280). Their basic defect and final classification have not been determined. According to recent data on mitochondrial cytopathies, some of these disorders could be caused by mitochondrial defects.

ACKNOWLEDGMENTS

A. Beziau, Y. Deris, L. Guicharnaud, M. Lacoste, M. Sich, technical assistance. D. Bronner, B. Coupé, secretarial support. Institut National de la Santé et de la Recherche Scientifique (INSERM), Assistance Publique des Hôpitaux de Paris.

REFERENCES

1. Broyer M. Fréquence et causes de l'insuffisance rénale chez l'enfant. In: Royer P, Habib R, Mathieu H, Broyer M, ed. *Néphrologie Pédiatrique*. Paris: Flammarion Médecine-Sciences,1983:425–430.
2. Waldherr R. Familial glomerular disease. *Contrib Nephrol* 1982;33:104–121.
3. Timpl R. Structure and biological activity of basement membrane proteins. *Eur J Biochem* 1989;180:487–502.
4. Zhou J, Reeders ST. The α chains of type IV collagen. In: Tryggvason K, ed. *Molecular pathology and genetics of Alport syndrome*. Basel; New York: Karger, 1996:80–104.
5. Heikkilä P, Soininen R. The type IV collagen gene family. In: Tryggvason K, ed. *Molecular pathology and genetics of Alport syndrome*. Basel; New York: Karger, 1996:105–129.
6. Soininen R, Huotari M, Hostikka SL, et al. The structural genes for alpha1 and alpha2 chains of human type IV collagen are divergently encoded on opposite DNA strands and have an overlapping promoter region. *J Biol Chem* 1988;263:17217–17220.
7. Mariyama M, Zheng KG, Yang FT, Reeders ST. Colocalization of the genes for the alpha3(IV) and alpha4(IV) chains of type-IV collagen to chromosome 2 bands 2-q35-q37. *Genomics* 1992;13:809–813.
8. Boye E, Mollet G, Forestier L, et al. Determination of the genomic structure of the COL4A4 gene and of novel mutations causing autosomal recessive Alport syndrome. *Am J Hum Genet* 1998;63:1329–1340.
9. Heidet L, Arrondel C, Cohen-Solal L, et al. Structure of the human type IV collagen gene COL4A3 and mutations in autosomal Alport syndrome. *J Am Soc Nephrol* 2001;12:97–106
10. Hudson BG, Wieslander J, Wisdom BJ, Noëlken ME. Biology of disease. Goodpasture syndrome: molecular architecture and function of basement membrane antigen. *Lab Invest* 1989;61:256–269.
11. Turner N, Mason PJ, Brown R, et al. Molecular cloning of the human Goodpasture antigen demonstrates it to be the α3 chain of type IV collagen. *J Clin Invest* 1992;89:592–601.
12. Hostikka SL, Eddy RL, Byers MG, et al. Identification of a distinct type IV collagen α chain with restricted kidney distribution and assignment of its gene to the locus of X-linked Alport syndrome. *Proc Natl Acad Sci U S A* 1990;87:1606–1610.
13. Myers JC, Jones TA, Pohjolainen ER, et al. Molecular cloning of alpha5(IV) collagen and assignment of the gene to the region of the X chromosome containing the Alport syndrome locus. *Am J Hum Genet* 1990;46:1024–1033.
14. Pihlajaniemi T, Pohjolainen ER, Myers JC. Complete primary structure of the triple-helical region and the carboxy-terminal domain of a new type IV collagen chain, α5(IV). *J Biol Chem* 1990;265:13758–13766.
15. Sugimoto M, Oohashi T, Ninomiya Y. The genes COL4A5 and COL4A6, coding for basement membrane collagen chains α5(IV) and α6(IV), are located head-to-head in close proximity on human chromosome Xq22 and COL4A6 is transcribed from two alternative promoters. *Proc Natl Acad Sci U S A* 1994; 91:11679–11683.
16. Zhou J, Ding M, Zhao Z, Reeders ST. Complete primary structure of the sixth chain of human basement membrane collagen α(IV). Isolation of the cDNAs for α6(IV) and comparison with five other type IV collagen chains. *J Biol Chem* 1994;269:13193–13199.
17. Kleppel MM, Santi PA, Cameron JD, et al. Human tissue distribution of novel basement membrane collagen. *Am J Pathol* 1989;134:813–825.
18. Butkowski RJ, Wieslander J, Kleppel M, et al. Basement membrane in the kidney: regional localization of novel chains related to collagen IV. *Kidney Int* 1989;35:1195–1202.
19. Yoshioka K, Hino S, Takemura T, et al. Type IV collagen α5 chain. Normal distribution and abnormalities in X-linked Alport syndrome revealed by monoclonal antibodies. *Am J Pathol* 1994;144:986–996.
20. Peissel B, Geng L, Kalluri R, et al. Comparative distribution of the α1(IV), α5(IV) and α6(IV) collagen chains in normal human adult and fetal tissues and in kidneys from X-linked Alport syndrome patients. *J Clin Invest* 1995;96:1948–1957.
21. Ninomiya Y, Kagawa M, Iyama K, at al. Differential expression of two basement membrane collagen genes, COL4A6 and COL4A5, demonstrated by immunofluorescence staining using peptide-specific monoclonal antibodies. *J Cell Biol* 1994;130:1219–1229.
22. Gunwar S, Ballester F, Noelken ME, et al. Glomerular basement membrane. Identification of a novel disulfide-cross-linked network of alpha3, alpha4, and alpha5 chains of type IV collagen and its implication for the pathogenesis of Alport syndrome. *J Biol Chem* 1998;273:8767–8775.
23. Alport AC. Hereditary familial congenital haemorrhagic nephritis. *BMJ* 1927;1:504–506.
24. Atkin CL, Gregory MC, Border WA. Alport syndrome. In: Schrier RW, Gottschalk CW, eds. *Diseases of the kidney*, 4th ed. Boston: Little, Brown and Company 1988:617–641.
25. Milliner DS, Pierides AM, Holley KE. Renal transplantation in Alport's syndrome. Anti-glomerular basement membranes glomerulonephritis in the allograft. *Mayo Clin Proc* 1982;57:35–43.
26. Gretz N, Broyer M, Brunner FP, et al. Alport's syndrome as a cause of renal failure in Europe. *Pediatr Nephrol* 1987;1:411–415.
27. O'Neill W, Atkin CL, Bloomer HA. Hereditary nephritis: a re-examination of its clinical and genetic features. *Ann Intern Med* 1978;88:176–182.
28. Pochet JM, Bobrie G, Landais P, et al. Renal prognosis in Alport's and related syndromes: influence of the mode of inheritance. *Nephrol Dial Transplant* 1988;4:1016–1021.
29. Feingold J, Bois E, Chompret A, et al. Genetic heterogeneity of Alport syndrome. *Kidney Int* 1985;27:672–677.
30. Evans SH, Erickson RP, Kelsch R, Peirce JC. Apparently changing pattern of inheritance in Alport's hereditary nephritis: genetic heterogeneity versus altered diagnostic criteria. *Clin Genet* 1980;17:285–292.
31. Gaboardi F, Edefonti A, Imbasciati E, et al. Alport's syndrome (Progressive hereditary nephritis). *Clin Nephrol* 1974;2:143–156.
32. Beathard GA, Granholm NA. Development of the characteristic ultrastructural lesion of hereditary nephritis during the course of the disease. *Am J Med* 1977;62:751–756.

33. Atkin CL, Hasstedt SJ, Menlove L, et al. Mapping of Alport syndrome to the long arm of the X chromosome. *Am J Hum Genet* 1988;42:249–255.
34. Brunner H, Schröder C, Van Bennekom C, et al. Localization of the gene for X-linked Alport's syndrome. *Kidney Int* 1988;34:507–510.
35. Antonovych TT, Deasy PF, Tina LU, et al. Hereditary nephritis: early clinical functional and morphological studies. *Pediatr Res* 1969;3:545–556.
36. Kaufman DB, McIntosh RM, Smith FG, et al. Diffuse familial nephropathy: a clinico-pathological study. *J Pediatr* 1970;77:37–47.
37. Rumpelt HJ, Langer KH, Schärer K, et al. Split and extremely thin glomerular basement membranes in hereditary nephropathy (Alport's syndrome). *Virchows Arch A Pathol Anat Histol* 1974;364:225–233.
38. Gubler MC, Levy M, Broyer M, et al. Alport's syndrome: a report of 58 cases and a review of the literature. *Am J Med* 1981;70:493–505.
39. Farboody GH, Valenzuela R, McCormack LJ, et al. Chronic hereditary nephritis. A clinicopathologic study of 23 new kindreds and review of the literature. *Hum Pathol* 1979;10:655–668.
40. Yoshikawa N, White RHR, Cameron AH. Familial hematuria: clinicopathological correlations. *Clin Nephrol* 1982;17:172–182.
41. Hinglais N, Grünfeld JP, Bois E. Characteristic ultrastructural lesion of the glomerular lesion of the glomerular basement membrane in progressive hereditary nephritis (Alport's syndrome). *Lab Invest* 1972;27:473–487.
42. Grünfeld JP, Bois EP, Hinglais N. Progressive and non progressive hereditary chronic nephritis. *Kidney Int* 1973;4: 216–228.
43. Gubler MC, Antignac C, Deschênes G, et al. Genetic, clinical and morphologic heterogeneity in Alport's syndrome. *Adv Nephrol Necker Hosp* 1992;22:14–35.
44. Polack BCP, Hogewind BL. Macular lesions in Alport's disease. *Am J Ophthalmol* 1977;84:533–535.
45. Nielsen CE. Lenticonus anterior and Alport's syndrome. *Acta Ophthalmol* 1977;56:518–530.
46. Perrin D, Junger P, Grünfeld JP, et al. Perimacular changes in Alport's syndrome. *Clin Nephrol* 1980;13:163–167.
47. Teekhasaenee C, Nimmanit S, Wutthiphan S, et al. Posterior polymorphous dystrophy and Alport syndrome. *Ophthalmology* 1991;98:1207–1215.
48. Rhys C, Snyers B, Pirson Y. Recurrent corneal erosion associated with Alport's syndrome. *Kidney Int* 1997;52:208–211.
49. Arenberg JK, Dodson VN, Falls HF, et al. Alport's syndrome: reevaluation of the associated ocular abnormalities and report of a family study. *J Pediatr Ophtalmol* 1967;4:21–32.
50. Jonso JJ, Renieri A, Gallagher PG, et al. Alport syndrome, mental retardation, midface hypoplasia, and elliptocytosis: a new X linked contiguous gene deletion syndrome. *J Med Genet* 1998;35:273–278.
51. Garcia Torres R, Guarner V. Leiomiomatosis del esophago, traqueo bronquial y genital asociada con nefropatia hereditaria tipo Alport: un nuevo sindrome. *Rev Gastroenterol Mex* 1983;48:163–170.
52. Antignac C, Zhou J, Sanak M, et al. Alport syndrome and diffuse leiomyomatosis: deletions in the 5' end of the CO4A5 collagen gene. *Kidney Int* 1992;42:1178–1183.
53. Heidet L, Dahan K, Zhou J, et al. Deletions of both α5(IV) and α6(IV) collagen genes in Alport syndrome and in smooth muscle cell proliferation associated with Alport syndrome. *Hum Mol Genet* 1995;4:99–108.
54. Antignac C, Heidet L. Mutations in Alport syndrome associated with diffuse esophageal leiomyomatosis. In: Tryggvason K, ed. *Molecular pathology and genetics of Alport syndrome*. Basel; New York: Karger, 1996:172–182.
55. Grünfeld JP, Grateau G, Noël LH, et al. Variants of Alport's syndrome. *Pediatr Nephrol* 1987;1:419–421.
56. Churg J, Sherman RL. Pathologic characteristics of hereditary nephritis. *Arch Pathol* 1973;95:374–379.
57. Spear GS, Slusser RJ. Alport's syndrome: emphasizing electron microscopic studies of the glomerulus. *Am J Pathol* 1972;69:213–224.
58. Piel CF, Blava CG, Goodman JR. Glomerular basement membrane attentuations in familial nephritis and "benign" hematuria. *J Pediatr* 1982;101:358–365.
59. Yoshikawa N, Ito H, Matsuyama S, et al. Hereditary nephritis in children with and without characteristic glomerular basement membrane alterations. *Clin Nephrol* 1988;30: 122–127.
60. Rumpelt HJ. Hereditary nephropathy (Alport syndrome): correlations of clinical data with glomerular basement membrane alterations. *Clin Nephrol* 1980;13:203–207.
61. Baumal R, Thorner P, Valli VEO, et al. Renal disease in carriers female dogs with X-linked hereditary nephritis. *Am J Pathol* 1991;139:751–764.
62. Lee GE, Helman RG, Kashtan CE, et al. New form of X-linked dominant hereditary nephritis in dogs. *Am J Vet Res* 1999;60:373–383.
63. Kohaut EC, Singer DB, Nevels BK, Hill LL. The specificity of split renal membranes in hereditary nephritis. *Arch Pathol Lab Med* 1976;100:475–479.
64. Habib R, Gubler MC, Hinglais N, et al. Alport's syndrome: experience at Hospital Necker. *Kidney Int* 1982;21:S20–S28.
65. Gubler MC, Beaufils H, Noël LH, Habib R. Significance of thin glomerular basement membranes in hematuric children. *Contrib Nephrol* 1990;80:141–156.
66. O'Neill WM, Mennemeyer RP, Bloomer HA, Atkin CL. Early pathologic features of hereditary nephritis: a clinicopathologic correlation. *Path Res Pract* 1980;168:146–162.
67. Streeten BW, Robinson MR, Wallace R, Jones DB. Lens capsule abnormalities in Alport's syndrome. *Arch Ophtalmol* 1987;105:1693–1697.
68. McCoy RC, Johnson KH, Stone WJ, Wilson CB. Absence of nephritogenic GBM antigen(s) in some patients with hereditary nephritis. *Kidney Int* 1982;21:642–652.
69. Kleppel M, Kashtan CE, Butkowski RJ, et al. Alport familial nephritis. Absence of 28 kilodalton non-collagenous monomers of type IV collagen in glomerular basement membrane. *J Clin Invest* 1987;80:263–266.
70. Savage COS, Noël LH, Cashman S, et al. Hereditary nephritis: immunoblotting studies of the glomerular basement membrane. *Lab Invest* 1989;60:613–618.
71. Kashtan C, Fish AJ, Kleppel M, et al. Nephritogenic antigen determinants in epidermal and renal basement mem-

branes of kindreds with Alport-type familial nephritis. *J Clin Invest* 1986;78:1035–1044.
72. Kashtan CE, Michael AF. Alport syndrome. *Kidney Int* 1996;50:1445–1463.
73. Kashtan CE, Kleppel MM, Gubler MC. Immunohistochemical findings in Alport syndrome. In: Tryggvason K, ed. *Molecular pathology and genetics of Alport syndrome.* Basel; New York: Karger, 1996:142–153.
74. Kashtan CE, Kim Y. Distribution of the α1 and α2 chain of collagen IV and of collagens V and VI in Alport syndrome. *Kidney Int* 1992;42:115–126.
75. Naito I, Kawai S, Nomura S, et al, and the Japanese Alport Network. Relationship between COL4A5 gene mutation and distribution of type IV collagen in male X-linked Alport syndrome. *Kidney Int* 1996;50:304–311.
76. Nakanishi K, Yoshikawa N, Iijima K, et al. Immunohistochemical study of α1-5 chains of type IV collagen in hereditary nephritis. *Kidney Int* 1994;46:1413–1421.
77. Mazzucco G, Barsotti P, Muda AO, et al. Ultrastructural and immunohistochemical findings in Alport's syndrome: a study of 108 patients from 97 Italian families with particular emphasis on COL4A5 mutating correlations. *J Am Soc Nephrol* 1998;9:1023–1031.
78. van der Loop FT, Monnens LA, Schroder CH, et al. Identification of COL4A5 defects in Alport syndrome by immunohistochemistry of skin. *Kidney Int* 1999;55:1217–1224.
79. Cheong HI, Kashtan CE, Kim Y, et al. Immunohistologic studies of type IV collagen in anterior lens capsules of patients with Alport syndrome. *Lab Invest* 1994;70:553–557.
80. Barker DF, Hostikka SL, Zhou J, et al. Identification of mutations in the COL4A5 collagen gene in Alport syndrome. *Science* 1990;247:1224–1227.
81. Boye E, Vetrie D, Flinter F, et al. Major rearrangements in the alpha5(IV)collagen gene in three patients with Alport syndrome. *Genomics* 1991;11:1125–1132.
82. Ding J, Zhou J, Tryggvason K, Kashtan CE. COL4A5 deletions in three patients with Alport syndrome and posttransplant antiglomerular basement membrane nephritis. *J Am Soc Nephrol* 1994;5:161–168.
83. Antignac C, Knebelmann B, Drouot L, et al. Deletions in the COL4A5 collagen gene in X-linked Alport syndrome: characterization of the pathological transcripts in non renal cells and correlation with disease expression. *J Clin Invest* 1994;93:1195–1207.
84. Tryggvason K. Mutations in type IV collagen genes and Alport phenotypes. In: Tryggvason K, ed. *Molecular pathology and genetics of Alport syndrome.* Basel; New York: Karger, 1996:154–171.
85. Renieri A, Bruttini M, Galli L, et al. X-linked Alport syndrome: an SSCP-based mutation survey over all 51 exons of the COL4A5 gene. *Am J Hum Genet* 1996;58:1192–1204.
86. Knebelmann B, Breillat C, Forestier L, et al. Spectrum of mutations in the COL4A5 gene in X-linked Alport syndrome *Am J Hum Genet* 1996;59:1221–1232.
87. Kawai S, Nomura S, Harano T, et al. The COL4A5 gene in Japanese Alport syndrome patients: spectrum of mutations of all exons. *Kidney Int* 1996;49:814–822.
88. Lemmink HH, Schröder CH, Monnens LAH, Smeets HJM. The clinical spectrum of type IV collagen mutations. *Hum Mutat* 1997;9:477–499
89. Plant KE, Green PM, Vetrie D, Flinter FA. Detection of mutations in COL4A5 in patients with Alport syndrome. *Hum Mutat* 1999;13:124–132.
90. Inoue Y, Nishio H, Shirakawa T, et al. Detection of mutations in the COL4A5 gene in over 90% of male patients with X-linked Alport's syndrome by RT-PCR and direct sequencing. *Am J Kidney Dis* 1999;34:854–862.
91. Jais JP, Knebelmann B, Giatras I, et al. X-linked Alport syndrome. Natural history in 195 families and genotype-phenotype correlations in males. *J Am Soc Nephrol* 2000;11:649–657.
92. Martin P, Heiskari N, Pajari H, et al. Spectrum of COL4A5 mutations in Finnish Alport syndrome patients. *Hum Mutat* 2000;15:579.
93. Barker DF, Denison JC, Atkin CL, Gregory MC. Efficient detection of Alport syndrome COL4A5 mutations with multiplex genomic PCR-SSCP. *Am J Med Genet* 2001;98:148–160.
94. Hertz JM, Juncker I, Persson U, et al. Detection of mutations in the COL4A5 gene by SSCP in X-linked Alport syndrome. *Hum Mutat* 2001;18:141–148.
95. Nakanishi K, Yoshikawa N, Iijima K, Nakamura H. Expression of type IV collagen α3 and α4 chain mRNA in X-linked Alport syndrome. *J Am Soc Nephrol* 1996;7:938–945.
96. Heidet L, Cai Y, Guicharnaud L, et al. Glomerular expression of type IV collagen chains in normal and X-linked Alport syndrome kidneys. *Am J Pathol* 2000;156:1901–1910.
97. Heidet L, Cai Y, Sado Y, et al. Diffuse leiomyomatosis associated with X-linked Alport syndrome: extracellular matrix study using immunohistochemistry and in situ hybridization. *Lab Invest* 1997;76:233–243.
98. Gubler MC, Knebelmann B, Beziau A, et al. Autosomal recessive Alport syndrome. Immunohistochemical study of type IV collagen chain distribution. *Kidney Int* 1995;47:1142–1147.
99. Mochizuki T, Lemmink HH, Mariyama M, et al. Identification of mutations in the α3(IV) and α4(IV) collagen genes in autosomal recessive Alport syndrome. *Nat Genet* 1994;8:77–82.
100. Knebelman B, Forestier L, Drouot L, et al. Splice-mediated insertion of an Alu sequence in the COL4A3 mRNA causing autosomal recessive Alport syndrome. *Hum Mol Genet* 1994;4:675–679.
101. Ding J, Stitzel J, Berry P, et al. Autosomal recessive Alport syndrome: mutation in the COL4A3 gene in a woman with Alport syndrome and posttransplant antiglomerular basement membrane nephritis. *J Am Soc Nephrol* 1995;5:1714–1717.
102. Kalluri R, Van den Heuvel LP, Smeets HJM, et al. A COL4A3 gene mutation and posttransplant anti-α3(IV) collagen alloantibodies in Alport syndrome. *Kidney Int* 1995;47:1199–1204.
103. Miner JH, Sanes JR. Molecular and functional defects in kidneys of mice lacking collagen α3(IV): implications for Alport syndrome. *J Cell Biol* 1996;135:1403–1413.
104. Cosgrove D, Meehan DT, Grunkemeyer JA, et al. Collagen COL4A3 knockout: a mouse model for autosomal Alport syndrome. *Genes Dev* 1996;10:2981–2992.
105. van der Loop, Heidet L, Timmer ED, et al. Autosomal dominant Alport syndrome caused by a COL4A3 splice site mutation. *Kidney Int* 2000;58:1870–1875.

106. Hood JC, Savige J, Hendtlass A, et al. Bull terrier hereditary nephritis: a model for autosomal dominant Alport syndrome. *Kidney Int* 1995;47:758–765.
107. Göbel J, Olbricht CJ, Offner G, et al. Kidney transplantation in Alport's syndrome: long-term outcome and allograft anti-GBM nephritis. *Clin Nephrol* 1992;38:299–304.
108. Peten E, Pirson Y, Cosyns JP, et al. Outcome of thirty patients with Alport's syndrome after renal transplantation. *Transplantation* 1991;52:823–826.
109. Byrne MC, Budisavljecic MN, Fan Z, et al. Renal transplant in patients with Alport syndrome. *Am J Kidney Dis* 2002;39:769–775.
110. Kashtan CE. Alport syndrome: renal transplantation and donor selection. *Ren Fail* 2000;22:765–768.
111. Rassoul Z, Al-khader AA, Al-Sulaiman M, et al. Recurrent allograft antiglomerular basement membrane glomerulonephritis in a patient with Alport's syndrome. *Am J Nephrol* 1990;10:73–76.
112. Goldman M, Depierreux M, De Pauw L, et al. Failure of two subsequent renal grafts by anti-GBM glomerulonephritis in Alport's syndrome: case report and review of the literature. *Transpl Int* 1990;3:82–85.
113. Kashtan CE, Butkowski R, Kleppel MM, et al. Posttransplant antiglomerular basement membrane nephritis in related males with Alport syndrome. *J Lab Clin Med* 1990;116:508–515
114. Smeets HJM, Melenhorst JJ, Lemmink HH, et al. Different mutations in the COL4A5 gene in two patients with different features of Alport syndrome. *Kidney Int* 1992;42:83–88.
115. Netzer KO, Renders L, Zhou J, et al. Deletions of the COL4A5 gene in patients with Alport syndrome. *Kidney Int* 1992;42:1336–1344.
116. Hudson BG, Kalluri R, Gunwar S, et al. The pathogenesis of Alport syndrome involves type IV collagen molecules containing the α3(IV) chain: evidence from anti-GBM nephritis after transplantation. *Kidney Int* 1992;42:179–187.
117. Kalluri R, Weber M, Netzer KO, et al. COL4A5 deletion and production of posttransplant anti-α3(IV) collagen antibodies in Alport syndrome. *Kidney Int* 1994;45:721–726.
118. Brainwood D, Kashtan CE, Gubler MC, Turner AN. Targets of alloantibodies in Alport anti-glomerular basement membrane disease after renal transplantation. *Kidney Int* 1998;53:762–766.
119. Noël LH, Gubler MC, Bobrie G, et al. Inherited defects of renal basement membranes. *Adv Nephrol* 1989;18:77–94.
120. Kalluri R, Torre A, Shield CF III, et al. Identification of alpha3, alpha4, and alpha5 chains of type IV collagen as alloantigens for Alport posttransplant and anti-glomerular basement membrane antibodies. *Transplantation* 2000;69:679–683.
121. Flinter FA, Cameron JS, Chantler C, et al. Genetic of classic Alport's syndrome. *Lancet* 1988;2:1005–1007.
122. Callis L, Vila A, Carrera M, Nieto J. Long-term effect of cyclosporine A in Alport's syndrome. *Kidney Int* 1999;55:1051–1056.
123. Cohen EP, Leman J. In hereditary nephritis angiotensin converting enzyme inhibition decreases proteinuria and may slow the rate of progression. *Am J Kidney Dis* 1996;27:199–203.
124. Proesmans W, Knockaert H, Trouet D. Enalapril in pediatric patients with Alport syndrome: 2 years' experience. *Eur J Pediatr* 2000;159:430–433.
125. Lemmink HH, Nillesen WN, Mochizuki T, et al. Benign familial hematuria due to mutation of the type IV collagen α4 chain. *J Clin Invest* 1996;98:1114–1118.
126. Kobayashi O, Wada H, Okawa K, Maeda H. Renal H: renal glomerular changes of non familial and familial benign hematuria. *Int J Pediatr Nephrol* 1980;1:86–92.
127. Tina L, Jenis E, Jose P, et al. The glomerular basement membrane in benign familial hematuria. *Clin Nephrol* 1982;17:1–4.
128. Yoshikawa N, Hashimoto H, Katayama Y, et al. The thin glomerular basement membrane in children with hematuria. *J Pathol* 1984;142:253–257.
129. Abe S, Amagasaki Y, Konishi K, et al. Thin basement membrane syndrome in adults. *J Clin Pathol* 1987;40:318–322.
130. Aarons I, Smith PS, Davies RA, et al. Thin membrane nephropathy: a clinicopathological study, *Clin Nephrol* 1989;32:151–158.
131. Tiebosch ATMG, Frederik PM, van Breda Vriesman PJC, et al. Thin-basement-membrane nephropathy in adults with persistent hematuria. *N Engl J Med* 1989;320:14–18.
132. Rogers PW, Kurtzman NA, Bunn SM, White MG. Familial benign essential hematuria. *Arch Intern Med* 1973;131:257–262.
133. Perry GJ, George CRP, Field MJ, et al. Thin-membrane nephropathy, a common cause of glomerular hematuria. *Med J Aust* 1989;151:63642.
134. Petterson E, Törnroth T, Wieslander J. Abnormally thin glomerular basement membrane and the Goodpasture epitope. *Clin Nephrol* 1990;33:105–109.
135. Schröder CH, Bontemps CM, Assmann KJM, et al. Renal biopsy and family studies in 65 children with isolated hematuria. *Acta Paediatr Scand* 1990;79:630–636.
136. Buzza M, Wang YY, Dagher H, Babon JJ, et al. COL4A4 mutation in thin basement membrane disease previously described in Alport syndrome. *Kidney Int* 2001;60:480–483.
137. Badenas C, Praga M, Tazon B, et al. Mutations in the COL4A4 and COL4A3 genes cause familial benign hematuria. *J Am Soc Nephrol* 2002;13:1248–1254.
138. Yamazaki H, Nakagawa Y, Saito A, et al. No linkage to the COL4A3 locus in Japanese thin basement membrane disease families. *Nephrol* 1995;1:315–321
139. Buzza M, Wilson D, Savige J. Segregation of hematuria in thin basement membrane disease with haplotypes at the loci for Alport syndrome. *Kidney Int* 2001;59:1670–1676.
140. Little EM. Congenital absence or delayed development of the patella. *Lancet* 1897;2:781–784.
141. Mino RA, Mino VH, Livingstone RG. Osseous dysplasia and dystrophy of the nails review of literature and report of a case. *AJR Am J Roentgenol* 1948;60:633–641.
142. Meyrier A, Rizzo R, Gubler MC. The nail-patella syndrome. A review. *J Nephrol* 1990;2:133–140.
143. Lucas GL, Opitz JM. The nail-patella syndrome. Clinical and genetic aspects of 5 kindreds with 38 affected family members. *J Pediatr* 1966;68:273–288.
144. Lichter PR, Richards JE, Downs CA, et al. Cosegregation of open-angle glaucoma and the nail-patella syndrome. *Am J Ophthalmol* 1997;124:506–515.
145. Brixey AM, Burke RM. Arthro-onychodysplasia. *Am J Med* 1950;8:738–744.

146. Hawkins CF, Smith OE. Renal dysplasia in family with multiple hereditary abnormalities including iliac horns. *Lancet* 1950;1:803–811.
147. Simila S, Vesa L, Wasz-Hockert O. Hereditary onycho-osteodysplasia (the nail-patella syndrome) with nephrosis-like renal disease in a newborn boy. *Pediatrics* 1970;46:61–65.
148. Ben Bassat M, Cohen L, Rosenfield J. The glomerular basement membrane in the nail-patella syndrome. *Arch Pathol* 1971;92:350–355.
149. Del Pozo E, Lapp H. Ultrastructure of the kidney in the nephropathy of the nail-patella syndrome. *Am J Clin Pathol* 1970;54:845–851.
150. Hoyer JR, Michael AF, Vernier RL. Renal disease in nail-patella syndrome: clinical and morphologic studies. *Kidney Int* 1972;2:231–238.
151. Morita T, Laughlin LO, Kawano K, et al. Nail-patella syndrome. Light and electron microscopic studies of the kidney. *Arch Intern Med* 1973;131:271–277.
152. Bennet WM, Musgrave JE, Campbell RA, et al. The nephropathy of the nail-patella syndrome. Clinicopathologic analysis of 11 kindreds. *Am J Med* 1973;54:304–319.
153. Taguchi T, Takebayashi S, Nishimura M, Tsuru N. Nephropathy of nail-patella syndrome. *Ultrastruct Pathol* 1988;12:175–183.
154. Browning MC, Weidner N, Lorentz WB, Jr. Renal histopathology of the nail-patella syndrome in a two-year-old boy. *Clin Nephrol* 1988;29:210–213.
155. Renwick JH, Lawler SD. Genetical linkage between the ABO and nail patella loci. *Ann Hum Genet Lond* 1955;19:312–331.
156. McIntosh L, Clough MV, Schaffer AA, et al. Fine mapping of the nail-patella syndrome locus at 9q34. *Am J Hum Genet* 1997;60:133–142.
157. Lommen EJP, Hamel BCJ, te Slaa RL. Nephropathy in hereditary osteo-onychodysplasia (HOOD): variable expression or genetic heterogeneity? In: *Genetics of kidney disorders*. Alan R Liss, 1989:157–160.
158. Dreyer SD, Zhou G, Baldini A, et al. Mutations in LMX1B cause abnormal skeletal patterning and renal dysplasia in nail patella syndrome. *Nat Genet* 1998;19:47–50.
159. Vollrath D, Jaramillo-Babb VL, Clough MV, et al. Loss-of-function mutations in the LIM-homeodomain gene, LMX1B, in nail patella syndrome. *Hum Mol Genet* 1998; 7:1091–1098.
160. Clough MV, Hamlington JD, McIntosh I. Restricted distribution of loss-of-function mutations within the LMX1B genes of nail-patella syndrome patients. *Hum Mutat* 1999;14:459–465.
161. Seri M, Melchionda S, Dreyer S, et al. Identification of LMX1B gene point mutation in Italian patients affected with nail-patella syndrome. *Int J Mol Med* 1999;4:285–290.
162. Knoers NV, Bongers EM, van Beersum SE, et al. The nail-patella syndrome: identification of mutations in the LMX1B gene in Dutch families. *J Am Soc Nephrol* 2000;11:1762–1766
163. McIntosh I, Dreyer SD, Clough MV, et al. Mutation analysis of LMX1B gene in nail-patella syndrome patients. *Am J Hum Genet* 1998;63:1651–1658.
164. Hamlington JD, Jones C, McIntosh I. Twenty-two novel LMX1B mutations identified in nail patella syndrome (NPS) patients. *Hum Mutat* 2001;18:458.
165. Chen H, Lun Y, Ovchinnokov D, et al. Limb and kidney defects in Lmx1b mutant mice suggest an involvement of LMX1B in human nail patella syndrome. *Nat Genet* 1998;19:51–55.
166. Morello R, Zhou G, Dreyer SD, et al. Regulation of glomerular basement membrane collagen expression by LMX1B contributes to renal disease in nail patella syndrome. *Nat Genet* 2001;27:205–208.
167. Miner JH, Morello R, Andrews KL, et al. Transcriptional induction of slit diaphragm genes by Lmx1b is required in podocyte differentiation. *J Clin Invest* 2002;109:1065–1072.
168. Rohr C, Prestel J, Heidet L, et al. The LIM-homeodomain transcription factor Lmx1b plays a crucial role in podocytes *J Clin Invest* 2002;109:1073–1082
169. Sabnis SG, Antonovych TT, Argy WP, et al. Nail-patella syndrome. *Clin Nephrol* 1980;14:148–153.
170. Dombros N, Katz A. Nail patella like lesions in the absence of skeletal abnormalities. *Am J Kidney Dis* 1982;1:237–240.
171. Salcedo JR. An autosomal recessive disorder with glomerular basement membrane abnormalities similar to those seen in the nail-patella syndrome. Report of a kindred. *Am J Med Genet* 1984;19:579–584.
172. Ikeda K, Yokoyama H, Tomosugi N, et al. Primary glomerular fibrosis: a new nephropathy caused by diffuse intraglomerular increase in atypical type III collagen fibers. *Clin Nephrol* 1990;33:155–159.
173. Imbasciati E, Gherardi G, Morozumi K, et al. Collagen type III glomerulopathy: A new idiopathic glomerular disease. *Am J Nephrol* 1991;11:422–429.
174. Arakawa M, Yamanaka N, eds. *Collagenofibrinotic glomerulonephropathy*. Nigata: Nishimura; London: Smith-Gordon, 1991.
175. Gubler MC, Dommergues JP, Foulard M, et al. Collagen type III glomerulopathy: a new type of hereditary nephropathy. *Pediatr Nephrol* 1993;7:354–360
176. Vogt BE, Wyatt RJ, Burke BA, et al. Inherited factor H deficiency and collagen type III glomerulopathy. *Pediatr Nephrol* 1995;9:11–15.
177. Tamura H, Matsuda A, Kidoguchi N, et al. A family with two sisters with collagenofibrotic glomerulopathy. *Am J Kidney Dis* 1996;27:588–595.
178. Epstein CJ, Sahud MA, Piel CF, et al. Hereditary macrothrombocytopathia, nephritis and deafness. *Am J Med* 1972;52:299–310.
179. Peterson LC, Venkateswara Rao K, Crosson JT, White JG. Fechtner syndrome—a variant of Alport's syndrome with leucocyte inclusions and macrothrombocytopenia. *Blood* 1985;65:397–406.
180. Moxey-Mims MM, Young G, Silverman A, et al. End stage renal disease in two pediatric patients with Fechtner syndrome. *Pediatr Nephrol* 1999;13:782–789.
181. Eckstein JD, Filip DJ, Watts JC. Hereditary thrombocytopenia, deafness and renal disease. *Ann Intern Med* 1975;82:639–645
182. Kunishima S, Kojima T, Tanaka T, et al. Mapping of a gene for May-Hegglin anomaly to chromosome 22q. *Hum Genet* 1999;105:379–383.
183. Toren A, Amariglio N, Rozenfeld-Granot G, et al. Genetic linkage of autosomal dominant Alport syndrome with leu-

cocyte inclusions and macrothrombocytopenia (Fechtner syndrome) to chromosome 22q11–13. *Am J Hum Genet* 1999;65:1711–1717.
184. The May-Hegglin/Fechtner Syndrome Consortium. Mutations in MYH9 result in the May-Hegglin anomaly, and Fechtner and Sebastian syndromes. *Nat Genet* 2000;26: 103–105.
185. Kelly MJ, Jawien W, Ortel TL, Korczak JF. Mutation of the MYH9 gene, encoding non-muscle myosin heavy chain A, in May-Hegglin anomaly. *Nat Genet* 2000;26:106–108.
186. Arrondel C, Vodovar N, Knebelmann B, et al. Expression of the non-muscle myosin heavy chain IIA in the human kidney and screening for MYH9 mutations in Epstein and Fechtner syndromes. *J Am Soc Nephrol* 2002;13:65–74
187. Desnick RJ, Ioannou YA, Eng CM. α-Galactosidase A deficiency: Fabry disease. In: Scriver CR, Beaudet AL, Sly WS, Valle D, eds. *The metabolic and molecular bases of inherited disease,* 7th ed. New York: McGraw-Hill, 1995:2741–2774.
188. Gubler MC, Lenoir G, Grünfeld JP, et al. Early renal changes in hemizygous and heterozygous patients with Fabry's disease. *Kidney Int* 1978;13:223–235
189. Desnick RJ, Banikazemi M, Wasserstein M. Enzyme replacement therapy for Fabry disease, an inherited nephropathy. *Clin Nephrol* 2002;57:1–8.
190. Maroteaux P, Humbel R, Strecker G, et al. Un nouveau type de sialidose avec atteinte rénale: la néphrosialidose. *Arch Franç Pediat* 1978;35:819–829.
191. Faraggiana J, Churg J. Renal lipidoses: a review. *Hum Pathol* 1987;7:661–679.
192. Benson MD. Amyloïdosis. In: Scriver CR, Beaudet AL, Sly WS, Valle D, eds. *The metabolic bases of inherited disease,* 7th ed. New York: McGraw-Hill, 1995:4157–4194.
193. International FMF consortium. Ancient missense mutations in a new member of the RoRet gene family are likely to cause familial Mediterranean fever. *Cell* 1997;90:797–807.
194. French FMF consortium. A candidate gene for familial Mediterranean fever. *Nat Genet* 1997;17:25–31.
195. Zemer D, Pras M, Sohar E, et al. Colchicine in the prevention and treatment of the amyloidosis of familial Mediterranean fever. *N Engl J Med* 1986;314:1001–1005.
196. Dodé C, Hazenberg BPC, Pêcheux C, et al. Mutational spectrum in the *MEFV* and *TNFRSF1A* genes in patients suffering from AA amyloidosis and recurrent inflammatory attacks. *Nephrol Dial Transplant* 2002;17:1212–1217.
197. Cox DW. α1-antitrypsine deficiency. In: Scriver CR, Beaudet AL, Sly WS, Valle D, eds. *The metabolic bases of inherited disease,* 7th ed. New York: McGraw-Hill, 1995:4125–4158.
198. Morz SP, Cutz E, Balfe JW, et al. Membranoproliferative glomerulonephritis in childhood cirrhoses with alpha1-antitrypsin deficiency. *Pediatrics* 1976;57:232–238.
199. Lévy M, Gubler MC, Hadchouel M, et al. Déficit en alpha–1-antitrypsine et atteinte rénale. *Néphrologie* 1985;6:65–70.
200. Davis ID, Burke B Freese D, et al. The pathologic spectrum of the nephropathy associated with α1AT-antitrypsin deficiency. *Hum Pathol* 1992;23:57–62.
201. Elzouki AN, Lingren S, Nilsson S, et al. Severe alpha1-antitrypsin deficiency (PiZ homozygosity) with membranoproliferative glomerulonephritis and nephrotic syndrome, reversible after orthoptic liver transplantation. *J Hepatol* 1997;26:1403–1407.
202. Elzouki AN, Segelmark M, Wieslander J, et al. Strong link between the alpha 1-antitrypsin PiZ allele and Wegener's granulomatosis. *J Intern Med* 1994;236:543–548.
203. Ault BH. Factor H and the pathogenesis of renal diseases. *Pediatr Nephrol* 2000;14:1045–1053.
204. Levy M, Halbwachs-Mecarelli L Gubler MC, et al. H deficiency in two brothers with atypical dense intramembranous deposit disease. *Kidney Int* 1986;30:949–956.
205. Hogasen K, Jansen JH, Molines TE, et al. Hereditary porcine membranoproliferative glomerulonephritis type II is caused by factor H deficiency. *J Clin Invest* 1995;95:1054–1061.
206. Thompson R, Winterborn M. Hypocomplementemia due to a genetic deficiency of β1H globulin. *Clin Exp Immunol* 1981;46:110–119.
207. Pichette V, Quérin S, Schürch W, et al. Familial hemolytic uremic syndrome and homozygous factor H deficiency. *Am J Kidney Dis* 1994;24:936–941.
208. Warwicker P, Goodship THJ, Donne RL, et al. Genetic studies into inherited and sporadic hemolytic uremic syndrome. *Kidney Int* 1998;53:836–844.
209. Rougier N, Kazatchine MD, Roudier JP, et al. Human complement factor U deficiency associated with hemolytic uremic syndrome. *J Am Soc Nephrol* 1998;9:2318–2326.
210. Noris M, Ruggenenti P, Perna A, et al. Hypocomplementemia discloses genetic predisposition to hemolytic uremic syndrome and thrombotic thrombocytopenic purpura: role of factor H abnormalities. *J Am Soc Nephrol* 1999;10:281–293.
211. Richards A, Buddles MR, Donne RL, et al. Factor H mutations in hemolytic uremic syndrome cluster in exons 18–20, a domain important for host cell recognition. *Am J Hum Genet* 2001;68:485–490.
212. Caprioli J, Bettinaglio P, Zipfel PF, et al. The molecular basis of familial hemolytic uremic syndrome: mutation analysis of factor H reveals a hot spot in short consensus repeat 20. *J Am Soc Nephrol* 2001;12:297–307.
213. Pérez-Caballero D, Gonzalès-Rubio C, Gallardo ME, et al. Clustering of missense mutations in the C-terminal region of factor H in atypical hemolytic uremic syndrome. *Am J Hum Genet* 2001;68:478–484.
214. Li L, Krantz ID, Deng Y, et al. Alagille syndrome is caused by mutations in human *Jagged1*, which encodes a ligand for Notch1. *Nat Genet* 1997;16:243–251.
215. Oda T, Elkahloun AG, Pike BL, et al. Mutations in the human *Jagged1* gene are responsible for Alagille syndrome. *Nat Genet* 1997;16:235–242.
216. Habib R, Dommergues JP, Gubler MC, et al. Glomerular mesangio-lipidosis in Alagille syndrome (arteriohepatic dysplasia). *Pediatr Nephrol* 1987;1:455–464.
217. Gjone E. Familial lecithin: cholesterol acyltransferase deficiency. A new metabolic disease with renal involvement. *Adv Nephrol* 1981;10:167–186.
218. Glomset JA, Assmann G, Gjone E, et al. Lecithin: cholesterol acyltransferase deficiency and fish eye disease. In: Scriver CR, Beaudet AL, Sly WS, Valle D, eds. *The metabolic bases of inherited disease,* 7th ed. New York: McGraw-Hill, 1995:1933–1951.
219. Saito T, Sato H, Kudo K, et al. Lipoprotein glomerulopathy: Glomerular lipoprotein thrombi in a patient with hyperlipoproteinemia. *Am J Kidney Dis* 1989;13:148–153.

220. Abt AB, Cohen AH. Newer glomerular diseases. *Semin Nephrol* 1996;16:501–510.
221. Saito T, Sato H, Oikawa S. Lipoprotein glomerulopathy: a new aspect of lipid induced glomerular injury. *Nephrology* 1995;1:17–24.
222. Oikawa S, Matsunaga A, Saito T, et al. Apolipoprotein E Sendai (arginine145 proline): a new variant associated with lipoprotein glomerulopathy. *J Am Soc Nephrol* 1997;8:820–823.
223. Miyata T, Sugiyama S, Nangaku M, et al. Apolipoprotein E2/E5 variants in lipoprotein glomerulopathy recurred in transplanted kidney. *J Am Soc Nephrol* 1999;10:1590–1595.
224. Maruyama K, Arai H, Ogawa T, et al. Lipoprotein glomerulopathy: a pediatric report. *Pediatr Nephrol* 1997;11:213–214.
225. Rumpelt HJ, Michl W. Selective vitamin B12 malabsorption with proteinuria (Imerslund-Najman-Gräsbeck-syndrome): ultrastructural examinations on renal glomeruli. *Clin Nephrol* 1979;11:213–217.
226. Hentati A, Lamy C, Melki J, et al. Clinical and genetic heterogeneity of Charcot-Marie-Tooth Disease. *Genomics* 1992;12:155–157.
227. Murakami T, Garcia CA, Reiter LT, Lupski JR. Charcot-Marie-Tooth disease and related inherited neuropathies. *Medicine* 1996;75:233–250.
228. Su Y, Brooks DG, Li L, et al. Myelin protein zero gene mutated in Charcot-Marie-Tooth type 1B disease. *Genetics* 1993;90:10856–10860.
229. Roa BB, Garcia CA, Suter U, et al. Charcot-Marie-Tooth disease type 1A. Association with a spontaneous point mutation in the PMP22 gene. *N Engl J Med* 1993;329:96–101.
230. Bergoffen J, Scherer SS, Wang S, et al. Connexin mutations in X-linked Charcot-Marie-Tooth disease. *Science* 1993; 262:2039–2042.
231. Gherardi R, Belghiti-Deprez D, Hirbec G, et al. Focal glomerulosclerosis associated with Charcot-Marie-Tooth disease. *Nephron* 1985;40:357–361.
232. Gregory MC, Terreros D, Kashtan CE, et al. Ultrastructural and immunologic evidence of Alport syndrome in a kindred with Charcot-Marie-Tooth disease. *J Am Soc Nephrol* 1991;2:254.
233. Nance MA, Berry SA. Cockayne syndrome: review of 140 cases. *Am J Med Genet* 1992;42:68–84.
234. Hirooka M, Hirota M, Kamada M. Renal lesions in Cockayne syndrome. *Pediatr Nephrol* 1988;2:239–243.
235. Sato H, Saito T, Kurosawa K, et al. Renal lesions in Cockayne's syndrome. *Clin Nephrol* 1988;29:206–209.
236. Mahmoud AA, Youssef GM, Al-Hifzi I, Diamandis EP. Cockayne syndrome in three sisters with varying clinical presentation. *Am J Med Genet* 2002;111:81–85.
237. Shinohara O, Kubota C, Kimura M Nishimura G, Takahashi S. Essential osteolysis associated with nephropathy, corneal opacity, and pulmonary stenosis. *Am J Med Genet* 1991;41:482–486.
238. Harnett JD, Green JS, Cramer BC, et al. The spectrum of renal disease in Laurence-Moon-Bield syndrome. *N Engl J Med* 1988;319:615–618.
239. Mykytyn K, Nishimura GY, Searby CC, et al. Identification of the gene (BBS1) most commonly involved in Bardet-Biedl syndrome, a complex human obesity syndrome. *Nat Genet* 2002;31:435–438.
240. Gershoni-Baruch R, Nachlieli T, Leibo R, et al. Cystic kidney dysplasia and polydactyly in 3 sibs with Bardet-Biedl syndrome. *Am J Med Genet* 1992;44:269–273.
241. Tieder M, Levy M, Gubler MC, et al. Renal abnormalities in Bardet-Biedl syndrome. *Int J Pediatr Nephrol* 1982;3: 188–203.
242. Goldstein JL, Fialkow PJ. The Alström syndrome. Report of three cases with further delineation of the clinical, pathophysiological, and genetic aspects of the disorder. *Medicine* 1973;52:53–71.
243. Pearson J, Gallo G, Gluck M, et al. Renal disease in familial dysautonomia. *Kidney Int* 1980;17:102–112.
244. Tuttle SE, Sharma HM, Bay W, et al. A unique familial lobular glomerulopathy. *Arch Pathol Lab Med* 1987;11:726–731.
245. Abt AB, Wassner SJ, Moran JJ. Familial lobular glomerulopathy. *Hum Pathol* 1991;22:825–829.
246. Bürgin M, Hofmann E, Reutter FW, et al. Familial glomerulopathy with giant fibrillar deposits. *Virchows Arch A Pathol Anat Histol* 1980;388:313–326.
247. Mazzucco G, Maran E, Rollino C, et al. Glomerulonephritis with organized deposits: a mesangiopathic, not immune complex-mediated disease? A pathologic study of two cases in the same family. *Hum Pathol* 1992;23:63–68.
248. Strom EH, Banfi G, Krapf R, et al. Glomerulopathy associated with predominant fibronectin deposits: a newly recognized hereditary disease. *Kidney Int* 1995;48:163–170.
249. Assmann KJM, Koene RAP, Wetzels JFM. Familial glomerulonephritis characterized by massive deposits of fibronectin. *Am J Kidney Dis* 1995;25:781–791.
250. Gemperle O, Neuweiler J, Reutter FW, et al. Familial glomerulopathy with giant fibrillar (fibronectin-positive) deposits: 15 year follow-up in a large kindred. *Am J Kidney Dis* 1996;28:668–675.
251. Sato H, Matsubara M, Marumo J, et al. Familial lobular glomerulopathy: first case report in Asia. *Am J Kidney Dis* 1998;31:1–5.
252. Niimi K, Tsuru N, Uesugi N, et al. Fibronectin glomerulopathy with nephrotic syndrome in a 3-year-old male. *Pediatr Nephrol* 2002;17:363–366
253. Volmer M, Jung M, Ruschendorf F, et al. The gene for human fibronectin glomerulopathy maps to 1q32, in the region of the regulation of complement activation gene cluster. *Am J Med Genet* 1998;63:1724–1731.
254. Grottum KA, Flatmark A, Myhre E, et al. Immunological hereditary nephropathy. *Acta Med Scand* 1974;[Suppl] 571:1–28.
255. Kourilsky O, Gubler MC, Morel-Maroger L, et al. A new form of familial glomerulonephritis. *Nephron* 1982;30:97–105.
256. Munnich A, Rustin P. Clinical spectrum and diagnosis of mitochondrial disorders. *Am J Med Genet* 2001;106:4–17.
257. Niaudet P, Rötig A. The kidney in mitochondrial cytopathies. *Kidney Int* 1997;51:1000–1007
258. Brun P, Ogier H, Romero N, et al. Syndrome néphrotique avec hyalinose segmentaire et focale au cours d'une cytopathie mitochondriale. *Pédiatrie* 1992;47:231.
259. Feigenbaum A, Bergeron C, Richardson R, et al. Premature atherosclerosis with photomyoclonic epilepsy, deafness, dia-

betes mellitus, nephropathy and neurodegenerative disorder in two brothers: a new syndrome? *Am J Med Genet* 1994;49: 118–124.

260. Manouvrier S, Rotig A, Hannebique G, et al. Point mutation of the mitochondrial tRNA(Leu) gene (A3243G) in maternally inherited hypertrophic cardiomyopathy, diabetes mellitus, renal failure, and sensorineural deafness. *J Med Genet* 1995;32:654–656.
261. Mochizuki H, Joh K, Kawame H, et al. Mitochondrial encephalomyopathy preceded by de Toni-Debré-Fanconi syndrome or focal segmental glomerulosclerosis. *Clin Nephrol* 1996;46:347–352.
262. Yorifuji T, Kawai M, Momoi T, et al. Nephropathy and growth hormone deficiency in a patient with mitochondrial tRNA(leu(UUR)) mutation. *J Med Genet* 1996;33:621–622.
263. Jansen JJ, Maassen JA, van der Woude FJ, et al. Mutation in mitochondrial tRNA [Leu (UUR)] gene associated with progressive kidney disease. *J Am Soc Nephrol* 1997;8:1118–1124.
264. Shigemoto M, Yoshimasa Y, Yamamoto Y, et al. Clinical manifestations due to point mutation of the mitochondrial tRNAleu(UUR) gene in five families with diabetes mellitus. *Intern Med* 1998;37:265–272.
265. Kurogouchi F, Oguchi T, Mawatari E, et al. A case of mitochondrial cytopathy with a typical point mutation for MELAS, presenting with severe focal-segmental glomerulosclerosis as main clinical manifestation. *Am J Nephrol* 1998;18:551–556.
266. Damian MS, Hertel A, Seibel P, et al. Follow-up in carriers of the "MELAS" mutation without strokes. *Eur Neurol* 1998;39:9–15.
267. Cheong HI, Chae JH, Kim JS, et al. Hereditary glomerulopathy associated with a mitochondrial tRNA (Leu) gene mutation. *Pediatr Nephrol* 1999;13:477–480.
268. Nakamura S, Yoshinari M, Doi Y, et al. Renal complications in patients with diabetes mellitus associated with an A to G mutation of mitochondrial DNA at the 3243 position of leucine tRNA. *Diabetes Res Pract* 1999;44:183–189.
269. Doleris L, Hill GS, Chedin P, et al., Focal segmental glomerulosclerosis associated with mitochondrial cytopathy. *Kidney Int* 2000;58:1851–1858.
270. Yamagata K, Tomida C, Umeyama K, et al. Prevalence of Japanese dialysis patients with an A-to-G mutation at nucleotide 3243 of the mitochondrial $tRNA^{Leu\ (UUR)}$ gene. *Nephrol Dial Transpl* 2000;15:365–368.
271. Hotta O, Inoue CN, Miyabayashi S, et al. Clinical and pathologic features of focal segmental glomerulosclerosis with mitochondrial $tRNA^{Leu(UUR)}$ gene mutation. *Kidney Int* 2001;59:1236–1243.
272. Hameed R, Raafat F, Ramani P, et al. Mitochondrial cytopathy presenting with focal segmental glomerulosclerosis, hypoparathyroidism, sensorineural deafness, and progressive neurological disease. *Postgrad Med J* 2001;77:523–526.
273. van den Ouweland JMW, Lemkes HHPJ, Ruitenbeek W, et al. Mutation in mitochondrial $tRNA^{Leu(UUR)}$ gene in a large pedigree with maternally transmitted type II diabetes mellitus and deafness. *Nat Genet* 1992;1:11–15.
274. Hirooka M, Ohno T, Kubota N, et al. Hereditary hematuria associated with mental retardation, convulsions, abnormal EEG and ocular abnormalities. *Tohoku J Exp Med* 1969;98:199–211.
275. Galloway WH, Movat AP. Congenital microcephaly with hiatus hernia and nephrotic syndrome in two sibs. *J Med Genet* 1968;5:319–321.
276. Hunter AGW, Jurenka S, Thompson D, Evans JA. Absence of the cerebellar granular layer, mental retardation, tapetoretinal degeneration and progressive glomerulopathy: an autosomal recessive oculo-renal-cerebellar syndrome. *Am J Med Genet* 1982;11:383–395.
277. Barakat AY, D'Albora JB, Martin MM, Jose PA. Familial nephrosis, nerve deafness, and hypoparathyroidism. *J Pediatr* 1977;91:61–64.
278. Yasui M, Narahara K, Kobayashi M, et al. New familial nephropathy involving glomerular and tubular basement membranes. *Pediatr Nephrol* 1994;8:584–586.
279. Edwards BD, Patton MA, Dilly SA, Eastwood JB. A new syndrome of autosomal recessive nephropathy, deafness, and hyperparathyroidism. *J Med Genet* 1989;26:289–293.
280. Mattoo TK, Akhtar M. Familial glomerulopathy with proximal tubular dysfunction: a new syndrome? *Pediatr Nephrol* 1990;4:223–227.

27

STEROID-SENSITIVE IDIOPATHIC NEPHROTIC SYNDROME IN CHILDREN

PATRICK NIAUDET

In children, the most common cause of nephrotic syndrome is idiopathic nephrotic syndrome, also called *nephrosis*. Idiopathic nephrotic syndrome is defined by the association of a nephrotic syndrome and minimal changes on renal biopsy by light microscopy with foot process fusion of epithelial cells on electron microscopy. No immunoglobulin (Ig) or complement fraction deposit is seen on immunofluorescence examination. Patients with minimal change disease most often respond to corticosteroids. As renal biopsy is not usually performed when the patient responds to corticosteroids, the term *minimal change disease* has become synonymous with steroid-sensitive nephrotic syndrome.

However, in some patients who respond to corticosteroids, histologic examination shows diffuse mesangial proliferation or focal and segmental glomerular sclerosis (FSGS). In addition, IgM deposits may be found. Several authors believe that minimal change disease is a distinct disease and that diffuse mesangial proliferation, FSGS, and IgM nephropathy are also distinct entities. There is no doubt that patients with diffuse mesangial proliferation or FSGS are more frequently resistant to corticosteroids and have a significant propensity for progression to renal failure. Conversely, patients with minimal change disease rarely progress to end-stage renal failure. However, there is an overlap between these histologic variants, and a significant proportion of patients with FSGS responds to corticosteroids, whereas some patients with minimal change disease are resistant to corticosteroids. Moreover, in the early stages, FSGS and minimal change disease are indistinguishable (1).

Experience has shown that response to steroid therapy carries a greater prognostic weight than the histologic features seen on the initial renal biopsy. Therefore, two types of idiopathic nephrotic syndrome can be described according to the response to corticosteroids: steroid-responsive idiopathic nephrotic syndrome, in which proteinuria rapidly resolves, and steroid-resistant idiopathic nephrotic syndrome (see Chapter 29), in which the nephrotic syndrome persists despite the treatment. This distinction is also more helpful for the clinician, as the therapeutic options are more dependent on the initial response to corticosteroids than on the results of renal biopsy.

EPIDEMIOLOGY

The incidence of idiopathic nephrotic syndrome varies with age, race, and geography. The annual incidence in children in the United States has been estimated to be 2.0 to 2.7 per 100,000 (2), with a cumulative prevalence of 16 per 100,000. Geographic or ethnic differences are well known. In the United Kingdom, for example, the incidence of idiopathic nephrotic syndrome is sixfold greater in Asian than in European children (3); this is also true for Indians (4), Japanese, and Southwest Asians. Idiopathic nephrotic syndrome is rare in Africa, where most cases of nephrotic syndrome seem to be related to structural glomerular lesions unresponsive to steroids (5). Such differences underline the role of genetic as well as environmental factors in the pathogenesis of this disease.

Although idiopathic nephrotic syndrome accounts for only 25% of adult cases (6), it is by far the most common cause of nephrotic syndrome in children. Almost all nephrotic children between 1 and 6 years of age in Western countries have idiopathic nephrotic syndrome. The International Study of Kidney Disease in Children (ISKDC) found minimal change disease in 76.6% of children with primary nephrotic syndrome (7).

There is male preponderance in children, with a male to female ratio of 2:1 (7,8), but both sexes are similarly affected in adolescents. The familial occurrence of idiopathic nephrotic syndrome is well known. In a European survey, White found that 3.3% of 1877 patients with idiopathic nephrotic syndrome (excluding congenital nephrotic syndrome) had affected family members, mainly siblings (9). Nineteen of the 63 children had minimal change disease, and 18 of them had affected siblings, whereas the remaining child's father was affected with the disease. This incidence was greater than among the general population. Idiopathic nephrotic syndrome was also reported in identical twins (10). In one series of familial cases (11), the disease tended to develop in siblings at the same age, with the same renal histology and the same outcome. Another study reported 34 patients in 15 families; the response to corticosteroids was identical within members of individual families (12). The age and sex distribution, the relapsing course, and the absence of renal failure in 15 steroid-responsive familial cases were comparable to the sporadic cases.

ASSOCIATED DISORDERS

Idiopathic nephrotic syndrome is, by definition, a primary disease. Nevertheless, in a number of cases, an upper respiratory tract infection, an allergic reaction, or another factor may immediately precede the development or relapse of the disease.

Many agents or conditions have been reported to be associated with idiopathic nephrotic syndrome (e.g., infectious diseases, drugs, allergy, vaccinations, and malignancies) (Table 27.1). The question remains whether these factors are real causes, a simple coincidence, or precipitating agents.

Allergy is associated with up to 30% of cases (13,14). Among a list of anecdotal cases, the allergens reported include fungi, poison ivy, ragweed pollen, house dust, jellyfish stings, bee stings, and cat fur. A food allergen (i.e., cow's milk or egg) may be responsible for relapses of steroid-sensitive nephrotic syndrome. Laurent et al. evaluated the effect of an oligo-antigenic diet given for 10 to 15 days to 13 patients. This diet coincided with improvement of proteinuria in nine, including complete remission in five (15).

The association between minimal change disease and malignancies mainly concerns lymphomatous disorders: Hodgkin's disease and non-Hodgkin's lymphomas (16). The nephrotic syndrome may be the presenting feature of the disease. It usually disappears after successful treatment of the malignancy. Other types of neoplasias that have been associated with idiopathic nephrotic syndrome include colon carcinoma, bronchogenic neoplasia, and small cell carcinoma (17).

Eosinophilic lymphoid granuloma in Asians (Kimura's disease) has also been reported in association with steroid-responsive idiopathic nephrotic syndrome. Several cases of minimal change disease have been reported in association with the onset of insulin-dependent diabetes mellitus. The disease is usually responsive to corticosteroids and follows a relapsing course.

TABLE 27.1. CONDITIONS ASSOCIATED WITH IDIOPATHIC NEPHROTIC SYNDROME

Allergy
Pollen
Fungi
Cow's milk
House dust
Bee stings
Cat fur
Poison ivy
Drugs
Nonsteroidal antiinflammatory drugs
Ampicillin
Gold
Lithium
Mercury
Trimethadione
Malignancies
Hodgkin's disease
Non-Hodgkin's lymphoma
Colon carcinoma
Bronchogenic carcinoma
Others
Viral infection
Kimura's disease
Diabetes mellitus
Myasthenia gravis
Immunization

HISTOCOMPATIBILITY ANTIGENS AND IDIOPATHIC NEPHROTIC SYNDROME

A three- to fourfold increased incidence of HLA-DR7 in children with idiopathic nephrotic syndrome has been reported (18,19). Clark et al. found a strong association between HLA-DR7 and the *DQB1* gene of *HLA-DQW2* and steroid-sensitive nephrosis and suggested that the β-chains of DR7 and DQW2 contribute to disease susceptibility (20).

An association with HLA-B8 was reported in Europe. Children with atopy and HLA-B12 have a 13-fold increased risk of developing idiopathic nephrotic syndrome.

CLINICAL FEATURES

The disease is characterized by a sudden onset, with edema being the most frequent presenting symptom. Edema increases gradually and becomes clinically detectable when fluid retention exceeds 3 to 5% of body weight. It is often initially apparent around the eyes and misdiagnosed as an allergy. Edema is gravity dependent. During the day, periorbital edema decreases while it localizes to the lower extremities. In the reclining position, it localizes to the back. It is white, soft, and pitting. Edema of the scrotum and penis, or labia, may also be observed. Anasarca may develop. Blood pressure is usually normal but sometimes elevated. The abdomen may bulge with umbilical or inguinal hernias. When ascites build up rapidly, the child complains of abdominal pain and malaise. Abdominal pain may also result from severe hypovolemia, peritonitis, pancreatitis, thrombosis, or steroid-induced gastritis. Shock is not unusual after a sudden fall of plasma albumin, with abdominal pain and peripheral circulatory failure. Emergency treatment is needed.

The nephrotic syndrome is occasionally discovered during routine urine analysis. The disease may also be revealed by a complication. Peritonitis due to *Streptococcus pneumoniae* is a classical mode of onset. Deep vein or arterial thromboses and pulmonary embolism may also occur during the first attack or during a relapse.

LABORATORY FINDINGS

Urine Analysis

Nephrotic range proteinuria is defined as urinary protein excretion greater than 50 mg/kg/day or 40 mg/m^2/hr. It is higher at onset and decreases as plasma albumin concentration falls. In young children, it may be difficult to obtain a 24-hour urine collection, and urinary protein to creatinine ratio or albumin to creatinine ratio in untimed urine specimens is useful. For these two indices, the nephrotic range is 200 to 400 mg/mmol. In most cases, proteinuria is highly selective, consisting of albumin and lower-molecular-weight proteins. The selectivity of proteinuria may be appreciated by polyacrylamide gel electrophoresis or by the evaluation of the Cameron index that is the ratio of IgG to transferrin clearances. A favorable index would be below 0.05 to 0.10; a poor index is above 0.15 or 0.20. A poor Cameron index is often associated with FSGS. However, there is a considerable overlap in results, and the test has limited value. Microscopic hematuria is present in 20% of cases and has no influence on the response to steroid therapy. Conversely, macroscopic hematuria is exceptional and, in the context of idiopathic nephrotic syndrome, may be related to renal vein thrombosis. The urine sediment often contains fat bodies. Hyaline casts are also usually found in patients with massive proteinuria, but granular casts are not present unless there is associated acute renal failure and acute tubular necrosis. Urinary sodium is low, 1 to 2 mmol/day, resulting in sodium retention and edema.

Blood

Plasma protein levels are markedly reduced, less than 50 g/L, due to hypoalbuminemia. Plasma albumin level is usually lower than 25 g/L and may be less than 10 g/L. Electrophoresis shows a typical pattern with low albumin, increased α_2-globulins, and, to a lesser extent, β-globulins, whereas γ-globulins are decreased. IgG is considerably decreased, IgA slightly decreased, and IgM is increased. Lipid abnormalities include high levels of cholesterol, triglyceride, and lipoproteins. Total cholesterol and low-density lipoprotein cholesterol are elevated, whereas high-density lipoprotein cholesterol remains unchanged or low, particularly high-density lipoprotein 2, leading to an increased low-density lipoprotein to high-density lipoprotein cholesterol ratio. Patients with severe hypoalbuminemia have increased triglycerides and very-low-density lipoprotein. Apoproteins and apolipoproteins B, CII, and CIII are also elevated. The levels of lipoprotein(a) are elevated in nephrotic patients.

Serum sodium is often reduced due in part to hyperlipemia and in part to the dilution from renal retention of water due to hypovolemia and inappropriate antidiuretic hormone secretion. Hyperkalemia may be observed in cases of renal insufficiency. Hypocalcemia is related to hypoalbuminemia, and the level of ionized calcium is usually normal. Plasma creatinine is elevated in one-third of cases and returns to normal when remission occurs.

Hemoglobin levels and hematocrit are increased in patients with plasma volume contraction. Thrombocytosis is common and may reach 5×10^8/L or 10^9/L. Fibrinogen and factors V, VII, VIII, and X are increased, whereas antithrombin III, the heparin cofactor, and factors XI and XII are decreased. These abnormalities contribute to a hypercoagulable state.

COMPLICATIONS

Acute Renal Failure

Some patients have a reduction of the glomerular filtration rate (GFR) attributed to hypovolemia, with complete return to normal after remission. A reduced GFR may be found despite normal effective plasma flow (21,22). Bohman et al. showed a close relationship between the degree of foot-process effacement and both the GFR and the filtration fraction, suggesting that foot-process effacement leads to a reduction of the glomerular filtering area or of permeability to water and small solutes (23). This reduction is transitory, with a rapid return to normal after remission.

Marked oliguria may occur in children (24). Oliguric renal failure may be the presenting symptom. Renal failure may be secondary to bilateral renal vein thrombosis that can be diagnosed by sonography. Acute renal failure has also been reported with interstitial nephritis. Skin rash and eosinophilia are suggestive of this diagnosis, which is often associated with furosemide or other medication.

Acute renal failure is usually reversible, often with intravenous albumin and high-dose furosemide-induced diuresis (25). In some cases in which glomerular structure is normal on initial histology, renal failure may persist for as long as 1 year (21) and rarely be irreversible (26).

Infections

Bacterial infections are frequent in nephrotic children (Table 27.2). Sepsis may occur at the onset of the disease. The most common infection is peritonitis, often with *S. pneumoniae*. Other organisms may be responsible: *Escherichia coli*, *Streptococcus bovis*, *Haemophilus influenzae*, and other gram-negative

TABLE 27.2. INFECTIONS IN NEPHROTIC SYNDROME

Clinical syndrome	Risk factors
Pneumococcal peritonitis	Low immunoglobulin G
Haemophilus infection	Low factor B
Gram-negative sepsis	Edematous tissue
Staphylococcus cellulitis	Impaired lymphocyte function
	Corticosteroids
	Immunosuppressive drugs

organisms. Apart from peritonitis, children may develop meningitis, pneumonitis, or cellulitis. Several factors may explain the propensity of nephrotic children to develop bacterial infections: low IgG levels due to an impaired synthesis, urinary loss of factor B, and impaired T-lymphocyte function. Factor B is a cofactor of C3b in the alternative pathway of complement, which has an important role in opsonization of bacteria such as *S. pneumoniae.*

Viral infections may be observed in patients receiving corticosteroids or immunosuppressive agents. Varicella is often observed in these young children and may be life-threatening if acyclovir therapy is not promptly initiated. Of interest, measles infection may induce long-lasting remissions.

Thrombosis

Nephrotic patients are at risk of developing thromboembolic complications (Table 27.3). Several factors contribute to this increased risk of thrombosis: a hypercoagulable state, hypovolemia, immobilization, and infection. A number of hemostatic abnormalities have been described in nephrotic patients: an increase in platelet aggregability; an increase in fibrinogen and factors V, VII, VIII, X, and XIII, whereas the levels of antithrombin III (heparin cofactor), proteins C and S, and factors XI and XII are decreased; and an increase in fibrinolytic system components (e.g., tissue plasminogen activator and plasminogen activator inhibitor-1) (27). The incidence of thromboembolic complications in nephrotic children is reported to be approximately 3%. However, this percentage may underestimate the true incidence. In one series, systematic evaluation by ventilation-perfusion scans showed defects consistent with pulmonary embolism in 28% of all patients with steroid-dependent minimal change disease (28). Pulmonary embolism should be suspected in cases with pulmonary or cardiovascular symptoms and may be confirmed by angiography or angioscintigraphy. Renal vein thrombosis should be suspected in patients with nephrotic syndrome who develop sudden macroscopic hematuria or acute renal failure. In such cases, Doppler ultrasonography shows an increase in kidney size and the absence of blood flow in the renal vein. Thrombosis may also affect the arteries (e.g., pulmonary arteries or other deep veins).

TABLE 27.3. THROMBOSIS IN NEPHROTIC SYNDROME

Clinical syndrome	Risk factors
Pulmonary emboli	Hypovolemia
Pulmonary artery thrombosis	Hyperviscosity
Cerebral venous thrombosis	Low antithrombin III
Renal vein thrombosis	High fibrinogen
Peripheral venous and artery thrombosis	Platelet hyperaggregability
	Hyperlipemia

TABLE 27.4. NEPHROTIC HYPOVOLEMIA

Clinical features	Precipitating factors
Abdominal pain	Severe relapse
Hypotension	Infection
Sluggish circulation	Diuretics
Relative polycythemia	Paracentesis
Acute tubular necrosis	Diarrhea
Thrombosis	

Hypovolemia

Hypovolemia is common and typically observed early during a relapse (Table 27.4). Sepsis, diarrhea, or diuretics may precipitate hypovolemia. Hypovolemic children often have abdominal pain, low blood pressure, and cold extremities. Hemoconcentration with a raised hematocrit accompanies hypovolemia.

RENAL BIOPSY

Indications

Renal biopsy is not indicated at onset in a child 1 to 8 years of age with typical symptoms of idiopathic nephrotic syndrome. Complete remission induced by corticosteroid therapy strongly supports the diagnosis. A renal biopsy is indicated at disease onset in clinical settings suggesting another type of glomerular disease. These include moderate nephrotic syndrome, a long previous course of mild proteinuria, macroscopic hematuria, marked hypertension, and persistent renal insufficiency. A decreased plasma C3 fraction is also an indication for renal biopsy. Age younger than 12 months and older than 11 years is another indication, even in patients with a typical clinical picture.

In steroid-dependent patients, the therapeutic approach is not influenced by histology. Therefore, a renal biopsy is not necessary before initiating a course of alkylating agents but is recommended before starting cyclosporine treatment to allow assessment of nephrotoxicity on a later biopsy.

Pathology

Light microscopy shows minimal changes in the majority of children with steroid-responsive nephrotic syndrome. FSGS occurs in only 5 to 10% of such patients (Fig. 27.1) (29). Mesangial proliferation is present in a small number of

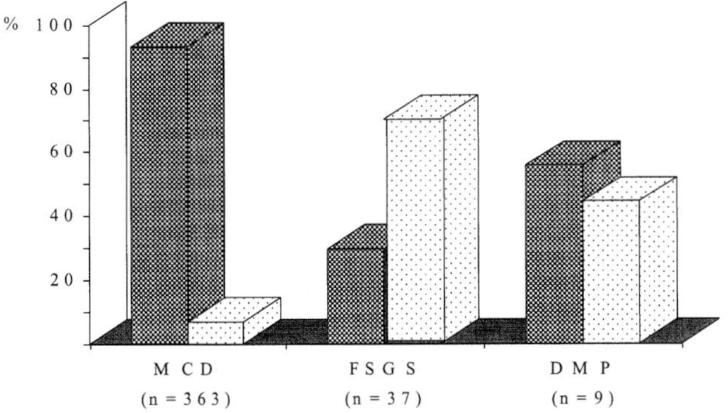

FIGURE 27.1. Responses to steroids in children with idiopathic nephrotic syndrome according to histology/responders (*checkered bars*) and nonresponders (*dotted bars*). DMP, diffuse mesangial proliferation; FSGS, focal and segmental glomerular sclerosis; MCD, minimal change disease.

patients. Immunofluorescence generally reveals no immune staining, but mesangial deposits of IgM and, more rarely, IgA, IgG, and C3 may be observed.

A complete description of the histopathology of minimal change disease, diffuse mesangial proliferation, focal and global sclerosis, FSGS, and IgM-associated nephropathy is presented in Chapter 29.

PATHOPHYSIOLOGY: MECHANISMS OF PROTEINURIA

In normal individuals, the clearance of albumin is approximately 1% of that of neutral proteins with similar molecular weight (e.g., polyvinylpyrrolidone or dextran). Similarly, the clearance of neutral dextran is higher than that of anionic sulfate dextran with similar molecular weight. These data indicate that the permeability of the glomerular basement membrane (GBM) is determined not only by the size but also by the charge of the protein. It is believed that the anionic charge of the GBM is responsible for the charge selectivity of filtration. The anionic (negative) charges of the GBM repulse negatively charged albumin molecules, which have an isoelectric point of 4.6.

The mechanism of proteinuria in the absence of histologic alterations on light microscopy has suggested an electrochemical disorder of the GBM. Indeed, it was shown that the glomerular K_f is diminished despite increased permeability to serum albumin. Using polyvinylpyrrolidone (30) or dextrans (31) with Einstein-Stokes radii between 2.0 and 4.8 nm as test macromolecules, the pore size of the GBM was shown to be reduced contrasting with massive albuminuria. This suggested a loss of glomerular negative charges. Kitano et al., using polyethylamine as a cationic probe, reported a decrease in the anionic charges of the GBM in minimal change disease (32). Carrie et al. studied renal biopsy sections stained by colloidal iron and showed that its glomerular uptake was markedly reduced (33). They postulated a reduced sialic acid content in the GBM, as sialic acid residues are responsible for glomerular negative charges (34).

Van den Born et al. produced a mouse monoclonal antibody to partially purified heparan sulfate proteoglycan isolated from rat glomeruli (35). By indirect immunofluorescence, the monoclonal antibody bound to the GBM on rat kidney sections. By electron microscopy, a diffuse staining of the GBM was observed. After intravenous injection, the monoclonal antibody was localized along the GBM with a granular staining and 1 day later in the mesangium with a concomitant decrease in staining along the GBM. By electron microscopy, 1 hour after injection, the antibody was bound mainly to the inner side of the GBM. Intravenous injection of this antibody in rats resulted in selective proteinuria. This model shows that neutralization of heparan sulfate anionic charges may contribute to albuminuria.

Levin et al. and Boulton-Jones et al. presented data indicating that loss of negative charges was not restricted to the glomeruli in patients with idiopathic nephrotic syndrome but was also found on erythrocyte and platelet membranes, as shown by reduced binding of Alcian blue, a cationic dye (36,37). A cationic protein is found in the plasma and the urine of patients in relapse.

IMMUNE SYSTEM IN STEROID-RESPONSIVE IDIOPATHIC NEPHROTIC SYNDROME

Cellular Immunity

In 1974, Shalhoub postulated that idiopathic nephrotic syndrome might be secondary to a disorder of T-lymphocyte function (38). He hypothesized that clonal expansion of a T-lymphocyte subpopulation might result in the production of lymphokines, which increased the permeability of the glomerular filtration barrier to proteins. Data supporting this hypothesis were the response of the disease to corticosteroids and alkylating agents; the remission occurring in association with measles, which depresses cell-mediated immunity; the susceptibility of patients to pneumococcal infections; and the occurrence of minimal change nephrotic syndrome in patients with Hodgkin's disease.

Peripheral blood T-lymphocyte subpopulations have been shown to be altered in children during a relapse, with an increase in memory T-cell subsets ($CD45RO^+CD4^+$ T cells and $CD45RO^+CD8^+$ T cells) (39). Increased expression of the interleukin (IL)-2 receptor on the T-lymphocyte surface is found in patients with minimal change disease during relapse but not during remission (40).

Cell-mediated immunity is depressed in patients with idiopathic nephrotic syndrome and returns to normal with remission. Their lymphocytes have an impaired response to mitogens (41,42). This decreased response is partly reversible when normal human serum is added to the culture medium instead of autologous serum, suggesting both intrinsic defects of the cells and the presence of inhibitory factors in the serum (43). Macrophages may be responsible for the impaired response of mononuclear cells to mitogens. The proliferative response of these cells returns to normal during remission. Therefore, a soluble factor may inhibit the proliferative response of T lymphocytes. Other abnormalities of cell-mediated immunity have been described in minimal change nephrotic syndrome. Skin reactivity to common antigens and recall response to common antigens are decreased during relapses and return to normal during remission (44).

Sahali et al. used a subtracted complementary DNA library screening to identify genes that might be differentially expressed in patients in relapse compared to those in remission (45). They found several upregulated genes, some of which are closely involved in T-cell activation. Relapsing patients display persistently high levels of nuclear factor-κB DNA-binding activity and downregulation of IκBα messenger (mRNA), which may account for increased production of several cytokines. In contrast, nuclear factor-κB binding activity returns to normal during remission with concomitant upregulation of IκBα and downregulation of most of the cytokines. An upregulation of c-maf expression and a downregulation of IL-12 recepter during relapse may suggest that T-cell activation in patients with minimal change disease evolves toward a T-helper-2 phenotype (46).

Humoral Immunity

Patients with minimal change disease have depressed serum IgG levels. This is more pronounced during relapses but persists during remission (47). Conversely, serum IgM is elevated. Altered serum levels of IgG and IgM may be secondary to abnormal T-cell regulation of Ig synthesis (48). Factors B and D are decreased during relapses but return to normal during remission. Specific antibodies to pneumococcal or streptococcal antigens are reduced in these patients up to 20 years after remission. This suggests that patients with minimal change nephrotic syndrome have a defect of the immune response that is not directly related to the nephrotic state. However, it does not imply that it is pathogenic.

Circulating Factors

Increased production of several lymphokines by activated T lymphocytes may alter glomerular permeability to albumin. Lagrue et al. described a vascular permeability factor, a lymphokine found in the supernatant of concanavalin A–activated lymphocytes from patients with minimal change disease that enhances vascular permeability when injected in guinea pigs (49,50). The vascular permeability factor is produced by T lymphocytes and is distinct from IL-2. Cyclosporine suppresses *in vitro* vascular permeability factor production. (51). Tanaka et al. found that supernatants of peripheral mononuclear cells stimulated with concanavalin injected in the renal artery of rats induced proteinuria along with reduction of the GBM anionic charges (52).

Koyama et al. found a glomerular permeability factor in the supernatant of a T-cell hybridoma derived from peripheral T lymphocytes from a patient with minimal change disease (53). The supernatant induced proteinuria when injected in the rat. Histology showed partial fusion of glomerular epithelial cell foot processes without immune deposits.

Several studies have shown increased *in vitro* production of IL-2, IL-4, and interferon-γ by lymphocytes and high plasma and urine concentrations of the soluble IL-2 receptor in patients during a relapse. The soluble IL-2 receptor suppresses lymphocyte proliferation. Patients in relapse have increased $CD4^+$ and $CD8^+$ IL-13 mRNA expression as compared to patients in remission or controls (54). The IL-13 and IL-4 cytokines are produced by stimulated Th2 lymphocytes. Activation of Th2 lymphocytes is known to play a key role in atopy. Glomerular epithelial cells express IL-4 and IL-13 receptors, and both cytokines increase transcellular ion transport in cultured cells as well as basolateral secretion of lysosomal proteinases (55,56). Such effects of IL-4 and IL-13 may explain an alteration of glomerular permeability.

Increased IL-2 concentrations have been found in supernatants of lymphocyte cultures from patients with idiopathic nephrotic syndrome, and IL-2 can induce proteinuria and a reduction of anionic sites of the GBM when injected into the rat kidney. Nephrotic syndrome has been observed in patients treated with recombinant IL-2 and interferon-α (57,58). Garin et al. reported an increased serum concentration of IL-8 and the presence of its mRNA in mononuclear cells from patients with minimal change disease during relapses (59). They also found that IL-8 may affect the metabolism of the GBM and postulated that it might alter glomerular permeability. Serum concentrations of tumor necrosis factor-α and its mRNA in peripheral mononuclear cells from patients with idiopathic nephrotic syndrome are increased in comparison with controls or patients in remission (60).

Schnaper and Aune (61–63) reported the presence of a lymphokine, the soluble immune response suppressor, in the urine and serum from patients with steroid-responsive nephrotic syndrome, including minimal change nephrotic syndrome and other histopathologic forms of nephrotic syndrome. The soluble immune response suppressor is produced by regulatory T lymphocytes and inhibits both delayed hypersensitivity reactions and antibody responses. The soluble immune response suppressor may contribute to the decreased immune responsiveness of patients with minimal change disease.

TREATMENT

Symptomatic Treatment

Diet

Diet includes a protein intake of 130 to 140% of the normal daily allowance according to statural age. Salt restriction is necessary for the prevention and treatment of edema. A very low salt diet is necessary in the case of edema. Fluid restriction is recommended for moderate to severe hyponatremia (plasma sodium concentration less than 125 mmol/L). A reduction of saturated fat is advisable. Carbohydrates are given preferentially as starch or dextrin-maltose, avoiding sucrose, which increases lipid disturbances.

Hypovolemia

Hypovolemia, a consequence of rapid loss of serum albumin, may be aggravated by diuretics. When symptomatic, this complication requires emergency treatment by rapid infusion of plasma (20 mL/kg) or albumin 20% (1 g/kg) administered with monitoring of heart rate, respiratory rate, and blood pressure.

Diuretics

Diuretics should only be used in cases of severe edema, after hypovolemia has been corrected. Patients with anasarca may be treated with furosemide (1 to 2 mg/kg) or, if necessary, furosemide and salt-poor albumin (1 g/kg infused over 4 hours) (25). This approach is effective immediately, but it is not long-lasting. Moreover, respiratory distress with congestive heart failure has been observed in some patients (64). Spironolactone (5 to 10 mg/kg) may be effective to minimize hypokalemia in patients with normal renal function. Diuretics must be used with caution. They may induce intravascular volume depletion with a risk of thromboemboli and acute renal failure as well as severe electrolyte imbalance. Refractory edema with serous effusions may require drainage of ascites or pleural effusions. Head-out immersion has been reported to be helpful in some cases (65).

Thromboemboli

Patients with severe hypoalbuminemia are at risk for thromboembolic complications. Prevention includes mobilization, avoiding hemoconcentration, and treating early sepsis or volume depletion. Prophylactic warfarin may be given to patients with a plasma albumin concentration below 20 g/L, a fibrinogen level greater than 6 g/L, or an antithrombin III level less than 70% of normal. Patients at risk may alternatively be treated with low-dose aspirin and dipyridamole, although no controlled trials have been performed to demonstrate their efficacy in preventing thrombosis (66). Heparin is given initially if thrombosis occurs alone or with thrombolytic agents. The heparin dose necessary to obtain a therapeutic effect is often greater than normal due to decreased antithrombin III levels.

Antihypertensive Drugs

Hypertension is treated using beta-blockers or calcium-channel blockers during acute episodes. In cases of persistent hypertension, an angiotensin-converting enzyme inhibitor or an inhibitor of angiotensin receptor 2 is preferred.

Infections and Immunizations

Prophylaxis of *S. pneumoniae* with oral penicillin is often prescribed to children during initial corticosteroid treatment. Although antibody response to pneumococcal vaccine is blunted in children with steroid-responsive nephrotic syndrome, vaccination with the conjugated pneumococcal vaccine (7vPCV) is recommended (67). In cases of peritonitis, antibiotics against both *S. pneumoniae* and gram-negative organisms are started after peritoneal fluid sampling. Varicella is a serious disease in patients receiving immunosuppressive treatment or daily corticosteroids. Varicella immunity status should therefore be assessed. In the case of exposure of an at-risk patient, acyclovir therapy should be initiated. Immunization with live virus vaccines is contraindicated in immunosuppressed patients.

Specific Treatment

Corticosteroid treatment should be initiated in all cases of idiopathic nephrotic syndrome regardless of histopathology. The majority of patients is steroid responsive: 89% of children studied by White et al. (68) and 98% of the patients with minimal changes on histology. Steroid responders may relapse, but the majority still responds to steroids throughout the subsequent course. Only 1 to 3% of patients initially steroid sensitive subsequently become steroid resistant and are defined as *late nonresponders* (69).

Initial Treatment

Steroids should not be started immediately, as spontaneous remission occurs in 5% of cases within the first 8 to 15 days. Some of these early spontaneous remissions are definitive. Infection must be treated before starting steroids, not only to prevent the risk of overwhelming sepsis during treatment, but also because occult infection may be responsible for steroid resistance (3). Patients should have a tuberculin test (i.e., purified protein derivative) before initiation of immunosuppressive therapy.

Glucocorticoid therapy is started when the diagnosis of idiopathic nephrotic syndrome is most likely in a child or after renal biopsy has been performed. Prednisone remains the cornerstone of therapy. Prednisolone has the advantage of being soluble in water, making treatment easier in young children, but it may fail to induce remission in some patients who respond quickly to the same dosage of prednisone. The differences in intestinal absorption and drug interactions (e.g., with aluminium gels) may explain decreased efficacy in some children.

The ISKDC regimen consists of prednisone, 60 mg/m^2/day, with a maximum of 80 mg/day in divided doses for 4 weeks, followed by 40 mg/m^2/day with a maximum of 60 mg/day in divided doses on 3 consecutive days per week for 4 weeks (70). The Arbeitsgemeinschaft für Pädiatrische Nephrologie showed that an alternate-day regimen (40 mg/m^2 every other day for 4 weeks) after initial daily therapy resulted in a significantly lower number of patients with relapses and fewer relapses per patient (71). It also showed that on alternate days, prednisone could be given in a single dose rather than in divided doses.

A response occurs in most cases within 10 to 15 days (median, 11 days). According to the ISKDC data, approximately 90% of responders enter remission within 4 weeks after starting glucocorticoids, whereas less than 10% go into remission after 2 to 4 more weeks of daily medication (70). A small number of patients go into remission after 8 to 12 weeks of daily steroids (6,72), but prolongation of daily steroid treatment beyond 4 or 5 weeks increases the risk of side effects. An alternative for patients who are not in remission after 4 weeks is to administer three to four pulses of methylprednisolone (1 g/1.73 m^2). This additional regimen seems to be associated with fewer side effects than prolongation of daily high-dose steroids and probably produces remission more rapidly in the few patients who would have entered the second month of daily therapy (73).

The duration of initial steroid therapy influences the risk of relapse. The Arbeitsgemeinschaft für Pädiatrische Nephrologie compared a standard regimen of 4-week daily prednisone and 4 weeks of alternate-day prednisone with a shorter course comprising prednisone given at a dose of 60 mg/m^2/day until the urine was protein free, followed by alternate-day prednisone until serum albumin returned to normal (74). Treatment lasted approximately 1 month in children receiving the short course. However, these children had twice the relapse rate so that, at the end of the trial, they had received an amount of prednisone significantly greater than had the standard treatment group.

After an 8-week steroid regimen, 50 to 70% of children experienced relapses. Several controlled studies have compared the 8-week regimen with longer duration of steroid regimen (3 to 7 months), including 4 to 8 weeks of daily prednisone followed by alternate-day prednisone (75–79). With a follow-up of 2 years, a significant reduction of 25 to 30% in the relapse rate was observed with a prednisone regimen of 3 months or more.

The number of children with frequent relapses is also decreased with a longer initial course of prednisone. Longer duration is more important than the cumulative dose of prednisone in reducing the risk of relapse. This relative risk decreases by 0.133 (13%) for every additional month of treatment up to 7 months (80). There are no data showing that treating for more than 7 months is beneficial. However, an alternate-day regimen over 1 year did not reduce the rate of relapse compared to a 5-month alternate-day regimen (81). Although the studies were not designed to analyze the side effects of glucocorticoids, the authors did not report increased toxicity with longer duration of treatment.

Treatment of Relapses

Approximately 30% of children experience only one attack and are definitively cured after a single course of steroids. Persistent remission for 18 to 24 months after stopping treatment is likely to reflect definitive cure, and the risk of later relapses is low. Ten percent to 20% of patients relapse several months after stopping treatment and are most often cured after three or four episodes, which respond to a standard course of corticosteroids. The remaining 50 to 60% experience relapses as soon as steroid therapy is stopped or when dosage is decreased. In some cases, exacerbation of proteinuria is only transient, and spontaneous remissions are observed (82). The risk of relapse is greater in children aged younger than 5 years at onset and in male patients. These steroid-dependent patients often raise difficult therapeutic problems.

Steroid-dependent patients may be treated with repeated courses of prednisone, 60 mg/m^2/day, continued 3 days after the urine has become protein free, followed by alternate-day prednisone, 40 mg/m^2, for 4 weeks as proposed by the ISKDC (70). Another option consists of treating relapses with daily prednisone, 40 to 60 mg/m^2, until proteinuria has disappeared for 4 to 5 days. Thereafter, prednisone is switched to alternate days, and the dosage is tapered to 15 to 20 mg/m^2 every other day, according to the steroid threshold (i.e., the dosage at which the relapse has occurred). Treatment is then continued for 12 to 18 months. The first approach allows better definition in terms of number of relapses but is associated with more relapses. The latter regimen is associated with fewer steroid side effects as the cumulative dosage is lower. Prolonged courses of alternate-day steroid therapy are often well tolerated by young children, and growth velocity is not affected. However, prednisone dosage must be as low as possible to minimize side effects. In adolescents, steroid therapy is often accompanied by decreased growth velocity.

A controlled trial has shown that deflazacort reduces the risk of relapse in comparison with equivalent doses of prednisone without additional side effects (83). However, deflazacort is not available in all countries.

The role of upper respiratory tract infections in exacerbating nephrotic syndrome has been highlighted in all series: 71% of relapses were preceded by such an event in a prospective study, although only 45% of respiratory infections were followed by an exacerbation of proteinuria (84). Mattoo et al. found that the risk of relapse was decreased during upper respiratory tract infections when prednisone was given daily for 5 days rather than on alternate days (85).

Leisti et al. suggested a role for postcorticosteroid adrenal suppression in triggering relapses (86), and some clinicians have suggested possible prevention by low-dose maintenance hydrocortisone (87,88) (Fig. 27.2).

Alternative Treatments

Alternative treatment is required in children who relapse on alternate-day prednisone therapy and experience severe glucocorticoid side effects (e.g., growth retardation, behavior

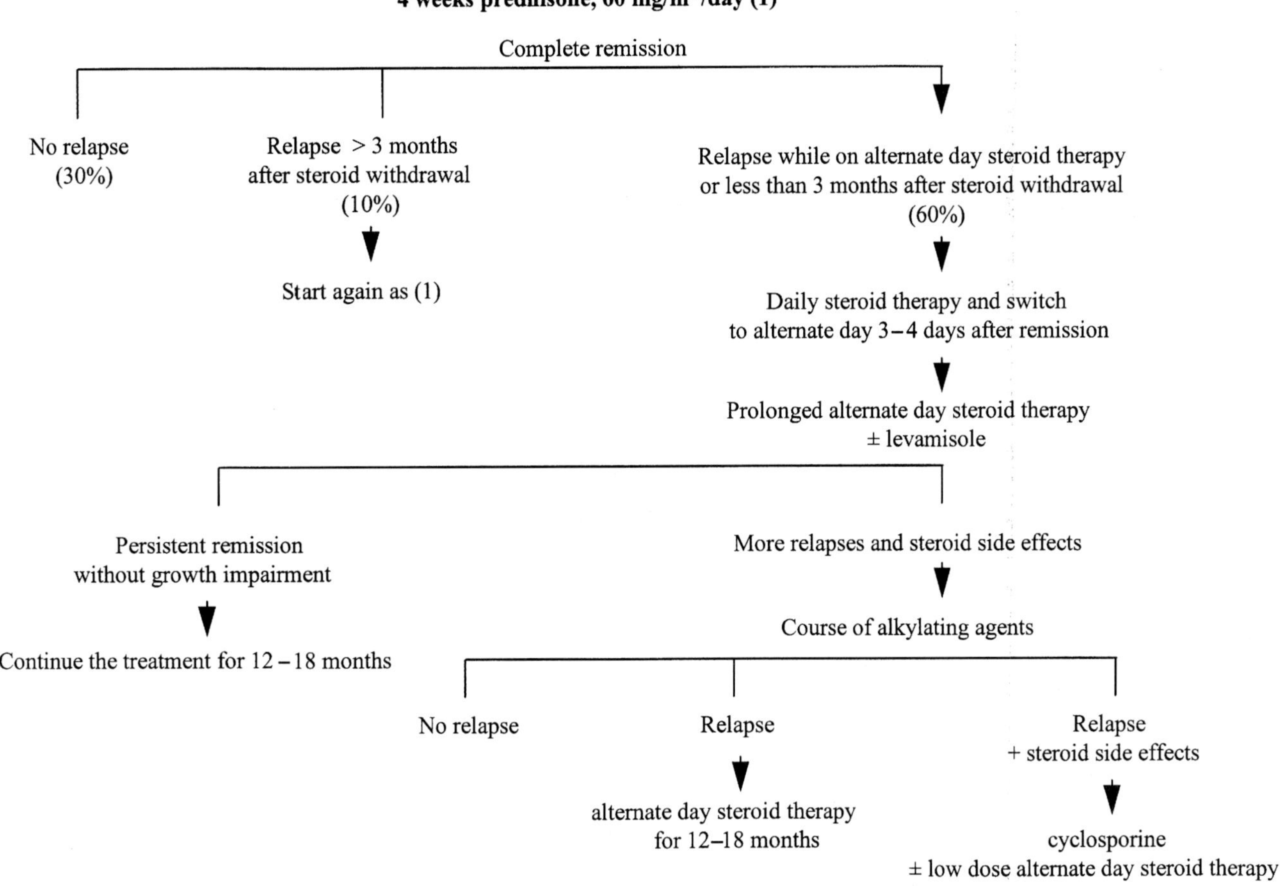

FIGURE 27.2. Treatment of idiopathic nephrotic syndrome regardless of histopathology.

disturbances, cushingoid features, hypertension, cataracts, or osteopenia). Alternative treatment is also indicated in children at risk of toxicity (e.g., diabetes or during puberty), in children with severe relapses accompanied by thrombotic complications, or severe hypovolemia and in those with poor compliance. Alternative treatments include levamisole, which has a weak steroid sparing effect, and alkylating agents (e.g., cyclophosphamide, chlorambucil, or cyclosporine).

Levamisole

The beneficial effect of levamisole was first described by Tanphaichitr et al. (89). Levamisole was subsequently reported to reduce the risk of relapse in steroid-dependent patients (90–93). A significant steroid-sparing effect at a dose of 2.5 mg/kg every other day was demonstrated in a prospective controlled trial of the British Association for Paediatric Nephrology (94). Another controlled study confirmed the efficacy of levamisole for preventing relapses (95). However, the beneficial effect of levamisole is not sustained after stopping treatment.

Levamisole given for 6 months was compared with cyclophosphamide given for 8 to 12 weeks in a retrospective study involving 51 children with steroid-dependent nephrotic syndrome (96). The relapse rate and the cumulative dose of prednisone were reduced to the same extent with both drugs.

Side effects include neutropenia, agranulocytosis, vomiting, cutaneous rash, and neurologic symptoms, including insomnia, hyperactivity, and seizures. However, levamisole is well tolerated in most children.

Alkylating Agents

Alkylating agents have been used for more than 40 years to achieve long-lasting remission in patients with idiopathic nephrotic syndrome.

Cyclophosphamide

The efficacy of cyclophosphamide for preventing relapses of idiopathic nephrotic syndrome was reported more than 20 years ago (97) and confirmed in a prospective study by Barratt and Soothill, who compared an 8-week course of cyclophosphamide to prednisone alone (98). An ISKDC trial found a 48% relapse rate after a mean follow-up of 22 months in children treated with a combination of cyclophosphamide and prednisone compared to a 88% relapse rate in patients on prednisone alone (99).

Several studies have addressed the relationship between dose, duration of treatment, and therapeutic efficacy. Treatment for 12 weeks at a daily dose of 2 mg/kg was found to be more effective than an 8-week course, with 67% as compared to 22% remaining in remission after 2 years (100). However, a randomized trial showed that prolonging the course of cyclophosphamide from 8 to 12 weeks did not further reduce the proportion of children experiencing relapses (101).

Cyclophosphamide is less effective in patients with steroid dependency compared to patients with frequent relapses (102). The incidence of relapse after cyclophosphamide is significantly higher in patients with FSGS (73%) or mesangial proliferation compared to 22% in children with minimal change disease (103).

Cyclophosphamide toxicity includes bone marrow depression, hemorrhagic cystitis, gastrointestinal disturbances, alopecia, and infection. Leukopenia is frequently observed, but weekly hematologic monitoring may limit its severity, and concomitant steroids help blunt marrow depression. Hemorrhagic cystitis rarely occurs. Alopecia, which is variably pronounced, remits a few weeks after stopping treatment. Viral infections can be overwhelming if cyclophosphamide is not stopped in due time.

Long-term toxicity includes malignancy, pulmonary fibrosis, ovarian fibrosis, and sterility. The risk of sterility is greater in boys than in girls. The cumulative threshold dose above which the risk of oligo- or azoospermia increases is between 150 and 250 mg/kg (104–106). Azoospermia is reversible in some patients (107). In girls, the cumulative dose associated with sterility is greater but not well defined. Pregnancies have been reported after treatment courses of longer than 18 months (108).

Chlorambucil

Beneficial results have also been achieved with chlorambucil in steroid-responsive idiopathic nephrotic syndrome. In 1973, Grupe demonstrated the efficacy of chlorambucil given for 2.5 to 12.0 weeks, with a relapse rate of only 13% (109). A controlled trial of chlorambucil for 6 to 12 weeks showed prolonged remissions of 1 to 3 years (110). Baluarte et al. obtained similar results in relapsing steroid-responsive nephrosis (111). Williams et al. showed that low daily doses are preferable: 91% of patients on a dose of 0.3 mg/kg and 80% of those on 3 mg/kg were still in remission 4 years later (112).

Acute toxic effects are less frequent with chlorambucil than with cyclophosphamide. Leukopenia and thrombocytopenia may occur and are reversible within 1 to 3 weeks. Severe microbial and viral infections have been reported, including malignant hepatitis and measles encephalitis.

Long-term toxic effects include the risk of developing malignancy, which has been reported in patients with prolonged therapeutic courses. Gonadal toxicity, as with cyclophosphamide, is more common in male patients. Azoospermia is total and probably irreversible at cumulative doses above 10 to 20 mg/kg. No case of azoospermia was reported in patients given less than 8 mg/kg.

Cyclosporine

In a number of uncontrolled studies, cyclosporine has been shown to reduce the incidence of relapses in 75 to 90% of patients with steroid-dependent idiopathic nephrotic syndrome (113). However, most patients experience relapses when the dosage is tapered or when cyclosporine is withdrawn. Relapse rate usually returns to the pretreatment rate. Hulton et al. found that patients in whom cyclosporine had been discontinued and later restarted had more relapses, requiring steroids in addition to cyclosporine to maintain remission (114).

The effects of cyclosporine have been evaluated in two comparative trials in steroid-sensitive patients. Cyclosporine at a dosage of 6 mg/kg/day for 3 months then tapered over 3 months was compared with chlorambucil given for 2 months. At 12 months, 30% of patients who had received chlorambucil and only 5% of those who received cyclosporine were still in remission (115). A multicenter randomized controlled trial compared cyclosporine for 9 months and then tapered over 3 months with oral cyclophosphamide for 2 months (116). After 2 years, 25% of the patients (50% of adults and 20% of children) who had received cyclosporine had not relapsed, whereas 63% of those treated with cyclophosphamide (40% of adults and 68% of children) were still in remission. During the year after treatment, the relapse rate (1.8 vs. 0.7) and the steroid dosage required (109 vs. 23 mg/kg/yr) were significantly higher in children who had received cyclosporine.

Tejani et al. performed a randomized controlled trial comparing low-dose prednisone and cyclosporine versus high-dose prednisone for 8 weeks as initial treatment in 28 children (117). Thirteen of the 14 children receiving the combined treatment went into remission compared to only 8 of the 14 receiving prednisone alone ($p < .05$). The duration of remission after ending treatment was comparable in both groups. Ingulli and Tejani reported that severe hypercholesterolemia may inhibit cyclosporine efficacy and that patients with severe hyperlipidemia require higher doses for maximal effectiveness (118).

Considering the high rate of cyclosporine dependency as well as its nephrotoxicity, steroid-dependent patients should first be treated with alkylating agents before resorting to cyclosporine (113,119). In patients being treated with cyclosporine, it is often difficult to determine if any observed changes in renal function are transient or due to the nephrotoxic effect of the drug. In these cases, it is advisable to reduce dosage or even stop cyclosporine treatment. Lesions of chronic cyclosporine-induced nephrotoxicity can develop without any appreciable decline of the GFR (120,121). As it is often necessary to use long therapeutic courses of cyclosporine, repeat renal biopsies are advised to detect lesions. They most often consist of tubulointerstitial injury, characterized by stripes of interstitial fibrosis containing clusters of atrophic tubules, as well as vascular lesions.

Other side effects of cyclosporine are of less concern: Hypertension, hyperkalemia, hypertrichosis, gum hypertrophy, and hypomagnesemia are common but easily manageable with standard therapies.

Azathioprine and Mycophenolate Mofetil

Abramowicz et al. (122) performed a controlled, multicenter trial in children with steroid-sensitive nephrotic syndrome that demonstrated that azathioprine had no effect in preventing relapses. Preliminary data suggest that mycophenolate mofetil treatment may have a beneficial effect in inducing and maintaining remission (123) in such patients. Such data must be confirmed in prospective clinical trials.

LONG-TERM OUTCOME

Steroid-dependent patients may have a prolonged course. However, if the patient continues to respond to steroids, the risk of progression to chronic renal failure is minimal.

Schärer and Minges found that 22% of patients had only one attack and 35% of the relapsing patients continued to relapse after 10 years (124). Trompeter et al. reported the late outcome of 152 children with steroid-responsive nephrotic syndrome after a follow-up of 14 to 19 years: 127 (83%) were in remission, 4 had hypertension, 10 were still relapsing, and 11 had died (125). The duration of the disease was longer in children who had their initial episode before the age of 6 years. Wynn et al. found that 15% of 132 patients had a persistent relapsing course with a mean follow-up of 27.5 years (126). Lewis et al. reviewed 26 patients older than age 20 years, five of whom were still relapsing during adulthood (127).

Koskimies et al. reported on the follow-up of children with idiopathic nephrotic syndrome in Finland from 1967 to 1976: 94 of 114 cases had responded to corticosteroids. Twenty-four percent of steroid responders had no relapse, 22% had infrequent relapses, and 54% had frequent relapses. More than two-thirds were in remission at time of report (128). None of these patients developed renal insufficiency, and none died from the disease.

Overall, this favorable long-term prognosis has also been observed in patients with steroid-responsive FSGS: 19 children reported by Arbus et al. remained responders, and none had renal insufficiency after a mean follow-up of 10 years (74).

Fakhouri et al. recently reported on the outcome in adulthood of 102 patients born between 1970 and 1975 (129). Forty-two percent presented at least one relapse in adulthood. A young age at onset and a high number of relapses during childhood were associated with a risk of relapse in adulthood.

REFERENCES

1. Kashgarian M, Hayslett JP, Seigel NJ. Lipoid nephrosis and focal sclerosis: distinct entities or spectrum of disease. *Nephron* 1974;13:105–108.
2. McEnery PT, Strife CF. Nephrotic syndrome in childhood. Management and treatment in patients with minimal change disease, mesangial proliferation, or focal glomerulosclerosis. *Pediatr Clin North Am* 1982;29:875–894.
3. Sharples PM, Poulton J, White RHR. Steroid responsive nephrotic syndrome is more common in Asians. *Arch Dis Child* 1985;60:1014–1017.
4. Srivastava RN, Mayekar G, Anand R, et al. Nephrotic syndrome in Indian children. *Arch Dis Child* 1975;50:626–680.
5. Coovadia HM, Adhikari M, Morel-Maroger L. Clinicopathological features of the nephrotic syndrome in South African children. *QJM* 1979;48:77–91.
6. Cameron JS, Turner DR, Ogg CS, et al. The nephrotic syndrome in adults with minimal change glomerular lesions. *Q JM* 1974;43:461–488.
7. International Study of Kidney Disease in Children. Nephrotic syndrome: prediction of histopathology from clinical and laboratory characteristics at time of diagnosis. *Kidney Int* 1978;13:159–165.
8. Hayslett JP, Kashgarian M, Bensch KG, et al. Clinicopathological correlation in the nephrotic syndrome due to primary renal disease. *Medicine* 1973;52:93–120.
9. White RHR. The familial nephrotic syndrome. A European survey. *Clin Nephrol* 1973;1:215–219.
10. Roy S, Pitcock JA. Idiopathic nephrosis in identical twins. *Am J Dis Child* 1971;121:428–439.
11. Moncrieff MW, White RHR, Glasgow EF, et al. The familial nephrotic syndrome II. A clinicopathological study. *Clin Nephrol* 1973;1:220–229.
12. Gonzalez G, Kleinknecht C, Gubler MC, Lenoir G. Nephrose familiale. *Rev Pédiatr* 1977;13:427–433.
13. Thomson PD, Barratt TM, Stokes CR, et al. HLA antigens and atopic features in steroid responsive nephrotic syndrome of childhood. *Lancet* 1976;2:765–768.
14. Meadow SR, Sarsfield JK. Steroid responsive nephrotic syndrome and allergy: clinical studies. *Arch Dis Child* 1981;56:5 09-516.
15. Laurent J, Rostoker G, Robeva R, et al. Is adult idiopathic nephrotic syndrome food allergy? *Nephron* 1987;47:7–11.
16. Eagen JW, Lewis EJ. Glomerulopathies of neoplasia. *Kidney Int* 1977;11:297–303.
17. Lee JC, Yamauchi H, Hopper J. The association of cancer and the nephrotic syndrome. *Ann Intern Med* 1966;64:41–51.
18. de Mouzon-Cambon A, Bouissou F, Dutau G, et al. HLA-DR7 in children with idiopathic nephrotic syndrome. Correlation with atopy. *Tissue Antigens* 1981;17:518–524.

19. Alfiler CA, Roy LP, Doran T, et al. HLA-DRW7 and steroid responsive nephrotic syndrome of childhood. *Clin Nephrol* 1980;14:71–74.
20. Clark AG, Vaughan RW, Stephens HA, et al. Genes encoding the beta-chains of HLA-DR7 and HLA-DQW2 define major susceptibility determinants for idiopathic nephrotic syndrome. *Clin Sci (Lond)* 1990;78:391–397.
21. Dorhout EJ, Roos JC, Boer P, et al. Observations on edema formation in the nephrotic syndrome in adults with minimal lesions. *Am J Med* 1979;67:378–384.
22. Bohlin AB. Clinical course and renal function in minimal change nephrotic syndrome. *Acta Paediatr Scand* 1984;73: 631–636.
23. Bohman SO, Jaremko G, Bohlin AB, Berg U. Foot process fusion and glomerular filtration rate in minimal change nephrotic syndrome. *Kidney Int* 1994;25:696–700.
24. Sakarlan A, Timmons C, Seikaly M. Reversible idiopathic acute renal failure in children with primary nephrotic syndrome. *J Pediatr* 1994;125:723–727.
25. Fliser D, Zurbruggen I, Mutschler E, et al. Coadministration of albumin and furosemide in patients with the nephrotic syndrome. *Kidney Int* 1999;55:629–634.
26. Raij L, Keane WF, Leonard A, Shapiro FL. Irreversible acute renal failure in idiopathic nephrotic syndrome. *Am J Med* 1976;61:207–214.
27. Andrew M, Brooker LA. Hemostatic complications in renal disorders of the young. *Pediatr Nephrol* 1996;10:88–99.
28. Hoyer PF, Gonda S, Barthels M, et al. Thromboembolic complications in children with nephrotic syndrome. *Acta Paediatr Scand* 1986;75:804–810.
29. Southwest Pediatric Nephrology Study Group. Focal segmental glomerulosclerosis in children with idiopathic nephrotic syndrome. *Kidney Int* 1985;27:442–449.
30. Robson AM, Giangiacomo J, Kienstra RA, et al. Normal glomerular permeability and its modification by minimal change nephrotic syndrome. *J Clin Invest* 1974;54:1190–1199.
31. Southwest Pediatric Nephrology Study Group. Association of IgA nephropathy with steroid-responsive nephrotic syndrome. *Am J Kidney Dis* 1985;5:157–164.
32. Kitano Y, Yoshikawa N, Nakamura H. Glomerular anionic sites in minimal change nephrotic syndrome and focal segmental glomerulosclerosis. *Clin Nephrol* 1993;40:199–204.
33. Carrie BJ, Salyer WR, Myers BD. Minimal change nephropathy: an electrochemical disorder of the glomerular membrane. *Am J Med* 1981;70:262–268.
34. Blau EB, Haaz JE. Glomerular sialic acid and proteinuria in human renal disease. *Lab Invest* 1973;28:477–481.
35. Van den Born J, Van den Heuvel LP, Bakker MA, et al. A monoclonal antibody against GBM heparan sulfate induces an acute selective proteinuria in rats. *Kidney Int* 1992;41:115–123.
36. Levin M, Walters MD, Smith C, et al. Steroid-responsive nephrotic syndrome: a generalized disorder of membrane negative charge. *Lancet* 1985;ii:239–242.
37. Boulton-Jones JM, McWilliams G, Chandrachud L. Variation in charge on red cells of patients with different glomerulopathies. *Lancet* 1986;ii:186–189.
38. Shalhoub RJ. Pathogenesis of lipoid nephrosis: a disorder of T cell function. *Lancet* 1974;ii:556–559.
39. Yan K, Nakahara K, Awa S, et al. The increase of memory T cell subsets in children with idiopathic nephrotic syndrome. *Nephron* 1998;79:274–278.
40. Topaloglu R, Saatci U, Arikan M, et al. T-cell subsets, interleukin-2 receptor expression and production of interleukin-2 in minimal change nephrotic syndrome. *Pediatr Nephrol* 1994;8:649-652.
41. Sasdelli M, Cagnoli L, Candi P, et al. Cell mediated immunity in idiopathic glomerulonephritis. *Clin Exp Immunol* 1981;46:27–34.
42. Taube D, Brown Z, Williams DG. Impaired lymphocyte and suppressor cell function in minimal change nephropathy membranous nephropathy and focal glomerulosclerosis. *Clin Nephrol* 1984;22:176–182.
43. Al-Azzawi YHM, Altawil NG, Alshamaa IA. Lymphocyte transformation test in adult patients with minimal change nephrotic syndrome. *Scand J Immunol* 1994;40:277–280.
44. Fodor P, Saitua MT, Rodriguez E, et al. T-cell dysfunction in minimal-change nephrotic syndrome of childhood. *Am J Dis Child* 1982;136:713–717.
45. Sahali D, Pawlak A, Le Gouvello S, et al. Transcriptional and post-transcriptional alterations of IkappaBalpha in active minimal-change nephrotic syndrome. *J Am Soc Nephrol* 2001;12:1648–1658.
46. Sahali D, Pawlak A, Valanciute A, et al. A novel approach to investigation of the pathogenesis of active minimal-change nephrotic syndrome using subtracted cDNA library screening. *J Am Soc Nephrol* 2002;13:1238–1247.
47. Giangiacomo J, Cleary TG, Cole BR, et al. Serum immunoglobulins in the nephrotic syndrome. A possible cause of minimal change nephrotic syndrome. *N Engl J Med* 1975;293:8–12.
48. Yokoyama H, Kida H, Abe T, et al. Impaired immunoglobulin G production in minimal change nephrotic syndrome in adults. *Clin Exp Immunol* 1987;70:110–115.
49. Lagrue G, Branellec A, Blanc C, et al. A vascular permeability factor in lymphocyte culture supernatants from patients with nephrotic syndrome. II. Pharmacological and physicochemical properties. *Biomedicine* 1975;23(2):73–75.
50. Sobel AT, Branellec AL, Blanc CJ, Lagrue GA. Physiochemical characterization of a vascular permeability factor, produced by Con A stimulated human lymphocytes. *J Immunol* 1977;119:1230–1234.
51. Heslan JM, Branellec AI, Pilatte Y, et al. Differentiation between vascular permeability factor and IL-2 in lymphocyte supernatants from patients with minimal-change nephrotic syndrome. *Clin Exp Immunol* 1991;86:157–162.
52. Tanaka R, Yoshikawa N, Nakamura H, Ito H. Infusion of peripheral blood mononuclear cell products from nephrotic children increases albuminuria in rats. *Nephron* 1992;60:35–41.
53. Koyama A, Fujisaki M, Kobayashi M, et al. A glomerular permeability factor produced by human T cell hybridoma. *Kidney Int* 1991;40:453–460.
54. Yap HK, Cheung W, Murugasu B, et al. Th1 and Th2 cytokine mRNA profiles in childhood nephrotic syndrome: evidence for increased IL-13 mRNA expression in relapse. *J Am Soc Nephrol* 1999;10:529–537.
55. Van Den Berg JG, Aten J, Chand MA, et al. Interleukin-4 and interleukin-13 act on glomerular visceral epithelial cells. *J Am Soc Nephrol* 2000;11:413–422.

56. Van Den Berg JG, Aten J, Annink C, et al. Interleukin-4 and -13 promote basolateral secretion of H+ and cathepsin L by glomerular epithelial cells. *Am J Physiol Renal Physiol* 2002;282:F26–F33.
57. Hisanaga S, Kawagoe H, Yamamoto Y, et al. Nephrotic syndrome associated with recombinant interleukin-2. *Nephron* 1990;54:277–278.
58. Traynor A, Kuzel T, Samuelson E, Kanwar Y. Minimal change glomerulopathy and glomerular visceral epithelial hyperplasia associated with alpha-interferon therapy for cutaneous T-cell lymphoma. *Nephron* 1994;67:94–100.
59. Garin EH, Blanchard DK, Matsushima K, Djeu JY. IL-8 production by peripheral blood mononuclear cells in nephrotic patients. *Kidney Int* 1994;45:1311–1317.
60. Bustos C, Gonzalez E. Muley R, et al. Increase of tumour necrosis factor alpha synthesis and gene expression in peripheral blood mononuclear cells of children with idiopathic nephrotic syndrome. *Eur J Clin Invest* 1994;24:799–805.
61. Schnaper HW, Aune TM. Identification of the lymphokine soluble immune response suppressor in urine of nephrotic children. *J Clin Invest* 1985;76:341–349.
62. Schnaper HW, Aune TM. Steroid-sensitive mechanism of soluble immune response suppressor production in steroid-responsive nephrotic syndrome. *J Clin Invest* 1987;79:257–264.
63. Schnaper HW. A regulatory system for soluble immune response suppressor production in steroid-responsive nephrotic syndrome. *Kidney Int* 1990;38:151–159.
64. Haws R, Baum M. Efficacy of albumin and diuretic therapy in children with nephrotic syndrome. *Pediatrics* 1993;91:1142–1146.
65. Rascher W, Tulassay T, Seyberth HW, et al. Diuretic and hormonal responses to head out water immersion in nephrotic syndrome. *J Pediatr* 1986;109:609–614.
66. McBryde KD, Kershaw DB, Smoyer WE. Pediatric steroid-resistant nephrotic syndrome. *Curr Probl Pediatr Adolesc Health Care* 2001;31:280–307.
67. Overturf GD. American Academy of Pediatrics. Committee on Infectious Diseases. Technical report: prevention of pneumococcal infections, including the use of pneumococcal conjugate and polysaccharide vaccines and antibiotic prophylaxis. *Pediatrics* 2000;106:367–376.
68. White RHR, Glasgow EF, Mills RJ. Clinicopathological studies of nephrotic syndrome in childhood. *Lancet* 1970;i:1353–1359.
69. Trainin EB, Boichis H, Spitzer A, et al. Late non responsiveness to steroids in children with the nephrotic syndrome. *J Pediatr* 1975;87:519–523.
70. International Study of Kidney Disease in Children. The primary nephrotic syndrome in children. Identification of patients with minimal change nephrotic syndrome from initial response to prednisone. *J Pediatr* 1981;98:561–564.
71. Arbeitsgemeinschaft für Pädiatrische Nephrologie. Alternate-day vs. intermittent prednisone in frequently relapsing nephrotic syndrome. *Lancet* 1979;i:401–403.
72. Schlesinger ER, Sultz HA, Mosher WE, Feldman JG. The nephrotic syndrome. Its incidence and implications for the community. *Am J Dis Child* 1968;116:623–632.
73. Murnaghan WM, Vasmant D, Bensman A. Pulse methylprednisolone therapy in severe idiopathic childhood nephrotic syndrome. *Acta Paediatr Scand* 1984;73:733–739.
74. Arbus GS, Poucell S, Bacheyie GS, Baumal R. Focal segmental glomerulosclerosis with idiopathic nephrotic syndrome: three types of clinical response. *J Pediatr* 1982;101:40–45.
75. Bagga A, Hari P, Srivastava RN. Prolonged versus standard prednisolone therapy for initial episode of nephrotic syndrome. *Pediatr Nephrol* 1999;13:824–827.
76. Ehrich JH, Brodehl J. Long versus standard prednisone therapy for initial treatment of idiopathic nephrotic syndrome in children. Arbeitsgemeinschaft fur pädiatrische Nephrologie. *Eur J Pediatr* 1993;152:357–361.
77. Ksiazek J, Wyszynska T. Short versus long initial prednisone treatment in steroid-sensitive nephrotic syndrome in children. *Acta Paediatr* 1995;84:889–893.
78. Norero C, Delucchi A, Lagos E, Rosati P. Initial therapy of primary nephrotic syndrome in children: evaluation in a period of 18 months of two prednisone treatment schedules. Chilean Co-operative Group of Study of Nephrotic Syndrome in Children. *Rev Med Chil* 1996;124:567–572.
79. Ueda N, Chihara M, Kawaguchi S, et al. Intermittent versus long-term tapering prednisolone for initial therapy in children with idiopathic nephrotic syndrome. *J Pediatr* 1988;112:122–126.
80. Hodson EM, Knight JF, Willis NS, Craig JC. Corticosteroid therapy in nephrotic syndrome: a meta-analysis of randomized controlled trials. *Arch Dis Child* 2000;83:45–51.
81. Kleinknecht C, Broyer M, Loirat C, et al. Comparison of short and long term treatment at onset of steroid sensitive nephrosis. Preliminary results of a multicentric controlled trial from the French Society of Pediatric Nephrology. *Int J Pediatr Nephrol* 1982;3:45.
82. Wingen AM, Muller-Wiefel DE, Scharer K. Spontaneous remissions in frequently relapsing and steroid dependent idiopathic nephrotic syndrome. *Clin Nephrol* 1985;23:35–40.
83. Broyer M, Terzi F, Lehnert A, et al. A controlled study of deflazacort in the treatment of idiopathic nephrotic syndrome. *Pediatr Nephrol* 1997;11:418–422.
84. McDonald NE, Wolfish N, McLaine P, et al. Role of respiratory viruses in exacerbation of primary nephrotic syndrome. *J Pediatr* 1986;108:378–382.
85. Mattoo TK, Mahmoud MA. Increased maintenance corticosteroids during upper respiratory infection decrease the risk of relapse in nephrotic syndrome. *Nephron* 2000;85:343–345.
86. Leisti S, Koskimies O, Rapola J, et al. Association of postmedication hypocortisolism with early first relapse of idiopathic nephrotic syndrome. *Lancet* 1977;ii:795–796.
87. Leisti S, Koskimies O, Perheentupa J, et al. Idiopathic nephrotic syndrome: prevention of early relapse. *BMJ* 1978;1:892.
88. Schoeneman MJ. Minimal change nephrotic syndrome: treatment with low doses of hydrocortisone. *J Pediatr* 1983;102:791–793.
89. Tanphaichitr P, Tanphaichitr D, Sureetanan J, Chatasigh S. Treatment of nephrotic syndrome with levamisole. *J Pediatr* 1980;96:490–493.
90. Niaudet P, Drachman R, Gagnadoux MF, Broyer M. Treatment of idiopathic nephrotic syndrome with levamisole. *Acta Paediatr Scand* 1984;73:637–641.
91. Mehta KP, Ali U, Kutty M, Kolhatkar U. Immunoregulatory treatment for minimal change nephrotic syndrome. *Arch Dis Child* 1986;61:153–158.
92. Drachman R, Schlesinger M, Alon U, et al. Immunoregula-

tion with levamisole in children with frequently relapsing steroid responsive nephrotic syndrome. *Acta Paediatr Scand* 1988;77:721–726.
93. Mongeau JG, Robitaille PO, Roy F. Clinical efficacy of levamisole in the treatment of primary nephrosis in children. *Pediatr Nephrol* 1988;2:398–401.
94. British Association for Pediatric Nephrology. Levamisole for corticosteroid dependent nephrotic syndrome in childhood. *Lancet* 1991;337:1555–1557.
95. Dayal U, Dayal AK, Shastry JC, Raghupathy P. Use of levamisole in maintaining remission in steroid-sensitive nephrotic syndrome in children. *Nephron* 1994;66:408–412.
96. Alsaran K, Grisaru S, Stephens D, Arbus G. Levamisole vs. cyclophosphamide for frequently-relapsing steroid-dependent nephrotic syndrome. *Clin Nephrol* 2001;56:289–294.
97. Coldbeck JH. Experience with alkylating agents in the treatment of children with the nephrotic syndrome. *Med J Aust* 1963;2:987–989.
98. Barratt TM, Soothill JF. Controlled trial of cyclophosphamide in steroid sensitive relapsing nephrotic syndrome of childhood. *Lancet* 1970;ii:479–482.
99. International Study of Kidney Disease in Children. Prospective controlled trial of cyclophosphamide therapy in children with the nephrotic syndrome. *Lancet* 1974;ii:423–427.
100. Arbeitsgemeinschaft für Pädiatrische Nephrologie. Cyclophosphamide treatment of steroid dependent nephrotic syndrome: comparison of eight week with 12 week course. *Arch Dis Child* 1987;62:1102–1106.
101. Ueda N, Kuno K, Ito S. Eight and 12 week courses of cyclophosphamide in nephrotic syndrome. *Arch Dis Child* 1990;65: 1147–1150.
102. Arbeitsgemeinschaft für Pädiatrische Nephrologie. Effect of cytotoxic drugs in frequently relapsing nephrotic syndrome with or without steroid dependence *N Engl J Med* 1982;306: 451–454.
103. Siegel N J, Gaudio KM, Krassner LS, et al. Steroid dependent nephrotic syndrome in children: histopathology and relapses after cyclophosphamide treatment. *Kidney Int* 1981;19:454–459.
104. Penso J, Lippe B, Ehrlich R, Smith FC. Testicular function in prepubertal and pubertal male patients treated with cyclophosphamide for nephrotic syndrome. *J Pediatr* 1994;84: 831–836.
105. Hsu AC, Folami AO, Bain J, Rance CP. Gonadal functions in males treated with cyclophosphamide for nephrotic syndrome. *Fert Steril* 1979;31:173–177.
106. Trompeter RS, Evans PR, Barratt TM. Gonadal function in boys with steroid responsive nephrotic syndrome treated with cyclophosphamide for short periods. *Lancet* 1981;i:1177–1180.
107. Buchanan JD, Fairley KF, Barris JU. Return of spermatogenesis after stopping cyclophosphamide therapy. *Lancet* 1975;ii:156–157.
108. Watson AR, Taylor J, Rance CP, Bain J. Gonadal function in women treated with cyclophosphamide for childhood nephrotic syndrome: a long term follow-up study. *Fert Steril* 1986;46:331–333.
109. Grupe WE. Chlorambucil in steroid dependent nephrotic syndrome. *J Pediatr* 1973;82:598–604.
110. Grupe WE, Makker SP, Ingelfinger JR. Chlorambucil treatment of frequently relapsing nephrotic syndrome. *N Engl J Med* 1976;295:746–749.
111. Baluarte HJ, Hiner L, Gruskin AB. Chlorambucil dosage in frequently relapsing nephrotic syndrome: a controlled clinical trial. *J Pediatr* 1978;92:295–298.
112. Williams SA, Makker SP, Ingelfinger JR, Grupe WE. Long term evaluation of chlorambucil plus prednisone in idiopathic nephrotic syndrome of childhood. *N Engl J Med* 1980;302:929–933.
113. Niaudet P, Habib R. Cyclosporine in the treatment of idiopathic nephrosis. *J Am Soc Nephrol* 1994;5:1049–1056.
114. Hulton SA, Neuhaus TJ, Dillon MJ, Barratt TM. Long-term cyclosporine A treatment of minimal-change nephrotic syndrome of childhood. *Pediatr Nephrol* 1994;8:401–403.
115. Niaudet P. Comparison of cyclosporin and chlorambucil in the treatment of steroid-dependent idiopathic nephrotic syndrome: a multicentre randomized controlled trial. The French Society of Paediatric Nephrology. *Pediatr Nephrol* 1992;6(1):1–3.
116. Ponticelli C, Edefonti A, Ghio L, et al. Cyclosporin versus cyclophosphamide for patients with steroid-dependent and frequently relapsing idiopathic nephrotic syndrome: a multicentre randomized controlled trial. *Nephrol Dial Transplant* 1993;8:1326–1332.
117. Tejani A, Suthanthiran M, Pomrantz A. A randomized controlled trial of low-dose prednisone and ciclosporin versus high-dose prednisone in nephrotic syndrome of children. *Nephron* 1991;59:96–99.
118. Ingulli E, Tejani A. Severe hypercholesterolemia inhibits cyclosporin A efficacy in a dose-dependent manner in children with nephrotic syndrome. *J Am Soc Nephrol* 1992;3:254-259.
119. British Association for Paediatric Nephrology. Consensus statement on management and audit potential for steroid responsive nephrotic syndrome. *Arch Dis Child* 1994;70:151–157.
120. Meyrier A, Noel LH, Auriche P, Callard P. Long-term renal tolerance of cyclosporine A treatment in adult idiopathic nephrotic syndrome. *Kidney Int* 1994;45:1446–1456.
121. Habib R, Niaudet P. Comparison between pre- and post-treatment renal biopsies in children receiving cyclosporine for idiopathic nephrosis. *Clin Nephrol* 1994;42:141–146.
122. Abramowicz M, Barnett HL, Edelmann CM Jr, et al. Controlled trial of azathioprine in children with nephrotic syndrome. A report for the international study of kidney disease in children. *Lancet* 1970;1(7654):959–961.
123. Choi MJ, Eustace JA, Gimenez LF, et al. Mycophenolate mofetil treatment for primary glomerular diseases. *Kidney Int* 2002;61:1098–1114.
124. Schärer K, Minges U. Long term prognosis of the nephrotic syndrome in childhood. *Clin Nephrol* 1973;1:182–187.
125. Trompeter RS, Hicks J, Lloyd BW, et al. Long term outcome for children with minimal change nephrotic syndrome. *Lancet* 1985;i:368–370.
126. Wynn SR, Stickler GB, Burke EC. Long term prognosis for children with nephrotic syndrome. *Clin Pediatr* 1988;27:63–68.
127. Lewis MA, Davis N, Baildom E, et al. Nephrotic syndrome from toddlers to twenties. *Lancet* 1989;i:255–259.
128. Koskimies O, Vilska J, Rapola J, Hallman N. Long-term outcome of primary nephrotic syndrome. *Arch Dis Child* 1982;57:544–548.
129. Fakhouri F, Bocquet N, Taupin P, et al. Steroid sensitive nephrotic syndrome: from childhood to adulthood. *Am J Kidney Dis* 2003;41:550–557.

28

STEROID-RESISTANT IDIOPATHIC NEPHROTIC SYNDROME IN CHILDREN

PATRICK NIAUDET

Idiopathic nephrotic syndrome is defined by the combination of nephrotic syndrome (proteinuria, hypoalbuminemia, hyperlipidemia, and edema) with nonspecific histologic abnormalities of the kidney, including minimal changes, focal segmental glomerulosclerosis (FSGS), and diffuse mesangial proliferation. Glomeruli show a fusion of epithelial cell foot processes on electron microscopy and no significant deposits of immunoglobulins (Igs) or complement on immunofluorescence.

Many authors consider minimal change disease (MCD), diffuse mesangial proliferation, and FSGS as separate diseases because of differences in response to corticosteroids and subsequent clinical course (1). Indeed, these various pathologic features carry prognostic significance. Patients with FSGS and those with diffuse mesangial proliferation more frequently have hematuria, are often resistant to corticosteroid treatment, progress more often to renal failure, and may have a recurrence of the nephrotic syndrome soon after transplantation. Recent data demonstrate differences between the basic pathophysiology of FSGS and MCD. FSGS appears to be a podocyte disease (2). The notion of podocyte dysregulation (3–5), the different expression of cyclin-dependent kinase inhibitors in MCD and in FSGS, the role of these cell cycle disturbances leading to podocyte proliferation and maturation (6), and the identification of parvovirus B19 in glomeruli of patients with FSGS (7,8) support the separation of minimal change nephrotic syndrome and FSGS as distinct entities. Moreover, Streulau et al. found transforming growth factor β1 (TGF-β1) gene expression in 18 of 20 patients with steroid-resistant FSGS and in only 3 of 14 steroid-sensitive patients (9). These data support a sequence of specific immunologically mediated events that contribute to progressive renal damage in children with FSGS.

In the early stages, FSGS and minimal change nephropathy are indistinguishable (10). A significant number of patients with FSGS respond favorably to glucocorticoid therapy (11), whereas some steroid-resistant patients have no sclerotic changes on systematic histopathologic evaluation (11,12). Therefore, some authors believe that, although histologic variants of the idiopathic nephrotic syndrome carry prognostic significance, they cannot at present be considered as separate entities (13).

The term *MCD* has become synonymous with steroid-sensitive idiopathic nephrotic syndrome, although renal biopsy is usually not performed in patients who respond to steroid therapy. Indeed, in many centers, renal biopsy is recommended only for those patients who do not respond to steroids. Consequently, renal biopsy findings in recent published series are not representative of the true incidence of various histopathologic categories seen in idiopathic nephrotic syndrome. It is, therefore, more appropriate to classify the patients according to their response to steroid therapy. Response to glucocorticoid therapy has greater prognostic value than the histologic features seen on initial renal biopsy. Thus, two types of nephrosis can be defined: *steroid-responsive* (see Chapter 27) and *steroid-resistant nephrotic syndrome* (SRNS).

In this chapter, we focus on the 10% of children with idiopathic nephrotic syndrome who do not respond to corticosteroids and are at risk for extrarenal complications of nephrosis as well as the development of end-stage renal disease (ESRD). Steroid-resistant idiopathic nephrotic syndrome accounts for more than 10% of children who progress to ESRD.

SRNS is a heterogeneous entity. In some patients, particularly those who experience a recurrence after renal transplantation, the disease is probably immunologically mediated by a cytokine that increases the permeability of the glomerular basement membrane (GBM) to proteins. In other cases (e.g., familial cases), the disease is related to a primary defect of the filtration barrier. Recent studies have highlighted the roles of newly identified podocyte proteins and demonstrated that mutations of corresponding genes may be responsible for SRNS (14).

CLINICAL AND BIOLOGIC FEATURES

SRNS may occur during the first year of life, but it usually starts between 2 and 7 years of age, with a male to female ratio of 2:1 (15). The disease is characterized by sudden onset, with edema being the major presenting symptom. Edema becomes clinically detectable when fluid retention exceeds 3 to 5% of body weight. Edema is gravity dependent and localized to the lower extremities in the upright position and to the dorsal part of the body in the reclining position. Edema is white, soft, and pitting, retaining the marks of clothes or finger pressure. Anasarca may develop with ascites and pleural and pericardial effusions. Although there may also be abdominal distention, dyspnea is rare. Periorbital edema may limit eye opening, and edema of the scrotum and penis or labia may be seen. Blood pressure is usually normal but is sometimes elevated. Rapid formation of ascites is often associated with abdominal pain and malaise, but these symptoms may also be related to concomitant hypovolemia. Abdominal pain is occasionally due to a complication such as peritonitis, thrombosis, or, rarely, pancreatitis. Cardiovascular shock is not unusual, secondary to the sudden fall of plasma albumin, with abdominal pain and symptoms of peripheral circulatory failure with cold extremities and hypotension.

The nephrotic syndrome is occasionally discovered during a routine urine analysis. Macroscopic hematuria is observed in a few cases. SRNS may present with an infectious or thrombotic complication.

Proteinuria during the Urinalysis

Nephrotic range proteinuria is defined as urinary protein excretion greater than 50 mg/kg/day or 40 mg/m^2/hr mean value. Proteinuria during the first days may be higher, as the urinary concentration of proteins also depends on the plasma albumin concentration. In young children, it may be difficult to perform accurate 24-hour urine collections, and urinary protein to creatinine ratio or urine albumin to urine creatinine ratio in untimed urine specimens is useful. For these two indices, the nephrotic range is 200 to 400 mg/mmol (16).

The amount of protein excreted in the urine does not reflect the quantity of protein crossing the GBM because a significant amount is reabsorbed in the proximal tubule. Typically, in severe nephrotic syndrome with glomerular lesions and resistance to steroid treatment, the urine contains not only albumin but also higher-molecular-weight proteins. This can be seen on polyacrylamide gel electrophoresis and can also be quantified by means of the selectivity index. The selectivity index is the ratio of IgG (molecular weight, 150 kDa) to albumin (70 kDa) or transferrin (80 kDa) clearances. A selectivity index above 0.15 or 0.20 is frequently observed in SRNS. However, the test is of limited clinical value because of its poor specificity. Some children with SRNS and tubulointerstitial lesions have both glomerular and tubular proteinuria with an increased excretion of β_2-microglobulin, retinol-binding protein, and lysozyme due to impaired protein reabsorption in the proximal tubule.

The urine sediment of patients with idiopathic nephrotic syndrome often contains fat bodies. Hyaline casts are also usually found in patients with massive proteinuria, but granular casts are not present unless there is associated acute renal failure and acute tubular necrosis. Macroscopic hematuria is rare, occurring in 3% of patients. Microscopic hematuria is far more common and may be observed in up to two-thirds of patients, particularly those with FSGS.

Urinary sodium excretion is low (less than 5 mmol per 24 hours), associated with sodium retention and edema. Kaliuresis is usually higher than natriuresis but may be reduced in oliguric patients.

Blood Chemistry

Serum proteins are markedly reduced, and serum lipid usually increased. Plasma protein levels are below 50 g/L in 80% of patients and below 40 g/L in 40% (17). Albumin concentration usually falls below 20 g/L and may be less than 10 g/L. Electrophoresis shows not only low albumin levels but also increased α_2-globulins and, to a lesser extent, β-globulins, whereas γ-globulins are decreased. IgG is markedly decreased, IgA is slightly reduced, IgM is increased, while IgE is normal or increased. Among other proteins, fibrinogen and β-lipoproteins are increased and antithrombin III is decreased.

Hyperlipidemia is a consequence of (a) an increased hepatic synthesis of cholesterol, triglycerides, and lipoproteins; (b) a decreased catabolism of lipoproteins due to a decreased activity of lipoprotein lipase that normally transforms very-low-density lipoprotein to low-density lipoprotein (LDL) via intermediate-density lipoprotein; and (c) decreased LDL receptor activity and an increased urinary loss of high-density lipoprotein (HDL) (18). Total cholesterol and LDL cholesterol are elevated, whereas HDL cholesterol remains unchanged or low, particularly HDL2, leading to an increased LDL to HDL cholesterol ratio. Patients with severe hypoalbuminemia have increased triglycerides and very-low-density lipoprotein. Apoproteins and apolipoproteins B, CII, and CIII are also elevated. The levels of lipoprotein(a) are elevated in nephrotic patients, which further contributes to an increased risk of cardiovascular and thrombotic complications.

Serum electrolytes are usually within the normal range. A low sodium level may be related to dilution from inappropriate renal retention of water due to hypovolemia and inappropriate antidiuretic hormone secretion. A mild reduction of plasma sodium concentration may be an artifact related to hyperlipidemia depending on reference laboratory methodology. Serum potassium may be high in oliguric patients. Serum calcium is consistently low as a result of hypoproteinemia. Ionized calcium is usually normal but may be decreased due to urinary loss of 25-hydroxyvitamin D3 (19) and normal but inappropriate levels of calcitriol (20). Blood urea nitrogen and creatinine concentrations are usually within the normal range or slightly increased, reflecting a modest reduction in glomerular filtration rate (GFR).

A few patients with FSGS and a poor subsequent outcome present with a Fanconi syndrome: glycosuria, aminoaciduria, urinary bicarbonate loss, and hypokalemia (21). A defect in urinary acidification has also been reported (22).

Hematology

Hemoglobin levels and hematocrit are increased in patients with plasma volume contraction. Anemia with microcytosis may be observed and is probably related to urinary loss of siderophilin. Thrombocytosis is common and may reach 5×10^8 or 10^9/L.

COMPLICATIONS

Acute Renal Failure

Renal function is usually within normal limits at presentation. A reduction of the GFR, secondary to hypovolemia, is frequent (23). A reduced GFR may be found in patients with normal effective plasma flow (24,25). Bohman et al. showed a close relationship between the degree of foot-process fusion and both GFR and filtration fraction, suggesting that fusion of foot processes could lead to a reduction of glomerular filtering area or of permeability to water and small solutes (26).

Acute renal failure may be secondary to bilateral renal vein thrombosis. Interstitial nephritis is another possible cause of acute renal failure, especially in association with furosemide administration.

Chronic Renal Failure

Patients with SRNS are at major risk of developing end-stage renal failure (ESRF), which is seen in less than 3% of patients with idiopathic nephritic syndrome who respond to glucocorticoid therapy. ESRD develops in at least 50% of patients with SRNS. As patients develop ESRD, all features of their nephritic syndrome may improve because a decrease in urinary protein excretion parallels their decreased GFR.

We have retrospectively analyzed in the Enfants Malades series the outcome of 181 children with SRNS who have been followed for at least 5 years. Eighty-five percent were primary nonresponders, 15% were late nonresponders, and 13% had a sibling affected by the same disease. Initial renal biopsy had shown MCD in 62 cases and FSGS in 119 cases. Renal survival rates were 65% at 5 years, 50% at 10 years, and 34% at 15 years. It is interesting to note that the rate of progression to ESRF was similar in patients with minimal changes or FSGS on initial biopsy.

Data reported in other series are difficult to compare, as most of them deal with patients with FSGS. The Southwest Pediatric Nephrology Study Group (27) reported 75 children with FSGS followed for periods of 7 to 217 months. Twenty-one percent had progressed to ESRF, 23% had decreased GFR, 37% had a persistent nephrotic syndrome, and 11% were in remission.

Progression to ESRF has been reported to be more rapid in patients of African or Hispanic descent when compared with whites. Ingulli and Tejani found that among 57 black and Mexican American children, 50% of them reached ESRF in 3 years, and 95% reached this stage after 6 years (28). In addition, among the children with idiopathic nephrotic syndrome, the proportion of those with steroid-resistant FSGS was increased in black and Mexican American children.

Growth

Growth may be severely affected in children with persistent nephrotic syndrome. Hypothyroidism related to urinary loss of iodinated proteins has been observed and may be treated. Low plasma IgF1 and IgF2 levels associated with urinary loss of carrier proteins have also been reported (29). The response of such patients to growth hormone therapy has not been studied.

Infections

Bacterial infections are frequent in nephrotic children. Sepsis may occur at the onset of the disease. The most common infection is peritonitis, often with *Streptococcus pneumoniae* (30). Other organisms may be responsible: *Escherichia coli*, *Streptococcus bovis*, *Haemophilus influenzae*, and other gram-negative organisms. Apart from peritonitis, children may develop meningitis, pneumonitis, and cellulitis. Several factors may explain the propensity of nephrotic children to develop bacterial infections: low IgG levels due to an impaired synthesis, urinary loss of factor B, and impaired T-lymphocyte function. Factor B is a cofactor of C3b of the alternative pathway of a complement that has an important role in opsonization of bacteria, such as *S. pneumoniae*.

Thrombosis

Nephrotic patients are at risk of developing thromboembolic complications. Several factors contribute to the increased risk of thrombosis: hypercoagulability state, hypovolemia, immobilization, and infection. A number of hemostatic abnormalities have been described in nephrotic patients: (a) increased platelet aggregability; fibrinogen; and factors V, VII, VIII, X, and XIII; and (b) decreased levels of antithrombin III, heparin cofactor, proteins C and S, and factors XI and XII. Furthermore, fibrinolytic system components (e.g., tissue plasminogen activator, plasminogen activator inhibitor-1) are increased (31). The incidence of thromboembolic complications in nephrotic children is close to 3%. However, this percentage may be underestimated as shown by systematic ventilation-perfusion scans, which have demonstrated defects consistent with pulmonary embolism in 28% of patients with steroid-dependent idiopathic nephrotic syndrome (32). Pulmonary embolism should be suspected in patients with SRNS who present with acute pulmonary or cardiovascular symptoms. The diagnosis may be confirmed by angiography or angioscintigraphy. Renal vein thrombosis should be suspected in cases with sudden macroscopic hematuria or acute renal failure. Doppler ultrasonography shows an increase in kidney size and the absence of blood flow in the renal vein. Thrombosis may affect the arteries (e.g., pulmonary arteries) or other deep veins.

RENAL BIOPSY

Light microscopic analysis of kidneys from patients with SRNS demonstrates three major morphologic patterns: minimal changes, diffuse mesangial proliferation, and FSGS.

Minimal Change Nephropathy

On light microscopy, glomeruli may be normal with normal capillary walls and normal cellularity. Swelling and vacuolation of epithelial cells and a slight increase in mesangial matrix are often observed. Mild mesangial hypercellularity may be noted (17,33,34) as well as scattered foci of tubular lesions and interstitial fibrosis.

Ultrastructural changes are always present, involving podocytes and mesangial stalks. Podocyte foot-process fusion is generalized and constant; its extent is closely related to the degree of proteinuria (35). Other epithelial changes consist of microvillus formation and the presence of numerous protein reabsorption droplets. The GBMs are normal, with no parietal deposits. The endothelial cells are often swollen (36). Mesangial alterations include mesangial cell hyperactivity, increased mesangial matrix, and occasionally finely granular, osmiophilic deposits located along the internal side of the basement membrane. These ultrastructural alterations are nonspecific and are probably related to massive proteinuria.

Diffuse Mesangial Proliferation

Some patients with steroid-resistant idiopathic nephrotic syndrome show a marked increase in mesangial matrix associated with hypercellularity (Fig. 28.1) (17,23,34, 37). However, peripheral capillary walls are normal, and immunofluorescence microscopy is negative. Electron microscopy shows foot-process fusion similar to the changes observed in MCD. The presence of mesangial hypercellularity has been reported to have prognostic significance with a higher rate of progression to renal failure (37), but these findings have not been confirmed by other authors (27,38).

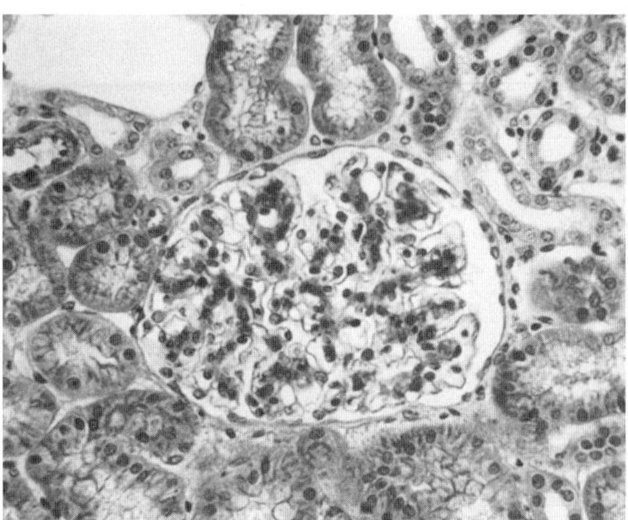

FIGURE 28.1. Diffuse mesangial proliferation without sclerosis. Light microscopy with trichrome light green (×400).

Focal and Segmental Glomerular Sclerosis

The glomerular lesions affect a variable proportion of glomeruli (11,17,34). The focal changes are limited to a part of the tuft, with the other capillary loops showing no modification. The lesions always predominate at the corticomedullary junction (39). The segmental lesion affects a few capillary loops that stick together either at the hilum or at the periphery of the tuft (Fig. 28.2) (40,41). The clinical course has been found to be more benign when the location of these sclerotic lesions is peripheral (the tip lesion), although such findings have not been confirmed by other authors (42,43). Hyaline material is often present within the sclerotic lesions. A clear halo zone is observed at the periphery of the sclerotic segments. The segmental lesion has a different aspect depending on whether it affects a group of capillary loops free in Bowman's space or is adherent to Bowman's cap-

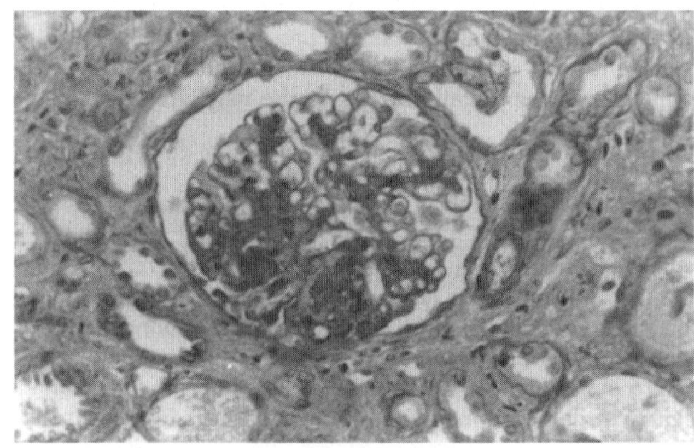

FIGURE 28.2. Focal and segmental glomerular sclerosis. Obliteration of capillary lumens by a combination of sclerosis and hyalinosis. Light microscopy with trichrome light green (×280).

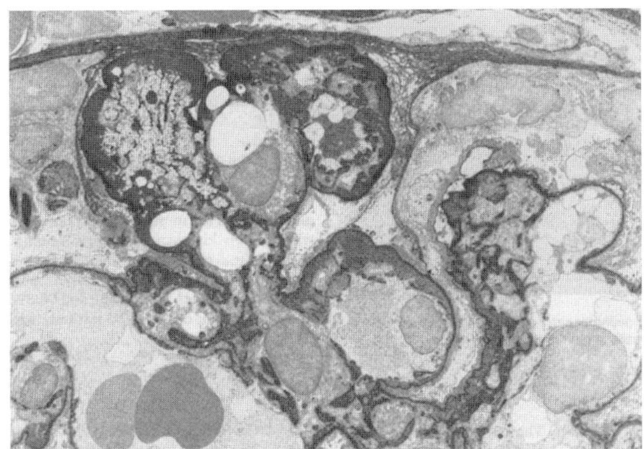

FIGURE 28.3. Focal and segmental glomerulosclerosis. Segmental lesion of the tuft is characterized by the obliteration of capillary lumens by granular and lipid deposits. Multilayered basement membrane material is seen around the lesion. Note the presence of focal detachment of podocytes along the adjacent capillary lumens. Electron microscopy with silver impregnation (×3900).

sule. The free sclerotic segments are always surrounded by a crown of flat or hypertrophied podocytes. The podocytes form a continuous layer overlying the damaged areas of the tuft and in close apposition to the clear halo. When the sclerotic lesion is adherent to Bowman's capsule, there is a direct synechia between the collapsed capillary loops and Bowman's basement membrane. The rest of the tuft and the nonsclerotic glomeruli show either minimal changes or diffuse mesangial proliferation, both with foot-process fusion. Glomerular hypertrophy is common in FSGS; when such hypertrophy is found in MCD, it is somewhat predictive of further development to FSGS (44,45).

Tubular atrophy and interstitial fibrosis are often present and apparently proportional to the glomerular damage (11,46). Focal glomerular lesions should therefore be suspected when focal tubular and interstitial changes are found associated with minimal glomerular changes. On immunofluorescence, the segmental lesions show strong staining with anti-IgM and anti-C3 antisera.

By electron microscopy, the lesion is characterized by the presence of paramesangial and subendothelial, finely granular, osmiophilic deposits (46–48), with either disappearance or swelling of endothelial cells, and an increase in mesangial matrix material (Fig. 28.3). Fatty vacuoles may be seen in the middle of the abnormal deposit or in the cytoplasm of endothelial and mesangial cells. The peripheral synechia, located between podocytes and basement membrane, is formed by the apposition of acellular material in which thin and irregular layers of newly formed basement membranes are visible. Modifications of the podocytes consist of focal cytoplasmic degeneration, breakdown of cell membranes, and detachment of epithelial cells from basement membranes, with filling of the resulting space by cell debris and new membranes (49).

A subgroup of patients has collapsing focal segmental glomerular sclerosis characterized by a global collapse of the glomerular capillaries with marked hypertrophy of epithelial cells (Fig. 28.4) (50). These patients rapidly progress to renal failure. Such features closely resemble those observed in human immunodeficiency virus–associated nephropathy (51). Many authors consider collapsing glomerulopathy to be a distinct form of FSGS that may be idiopathic, observed in renal transplants of patients with recurrent nephrotic syndrome, or associated with human immunodeficiency virus or parvovirus infection (52,53). Idiopathic collapsing glomerulopathy predominates in blacks and has a poor prognosis (54).

Recent studies on collapsing glomerulopathy and on patients with recurrence of nephrotic syndrome after renal transplantation have shown important changes in the podocytes with major cell cycle derangement (4,5). The normal, mature podocyte does not divide and does not express proliferative markers (e.g., proliferating cell nuclear antigen and Ki-67). The podocyte expresses several cell-surface proteins (e.g., WT-1, C3b receptor, glomerular epithelial protein-1, podocalyxin, synaptopodin, and vimentin). The first stages of FSGS are characterized by the loss of cell surface proteins and the expression of macrophage markers and cytokeratin. Proliferation markers (proliferating cell nuclear antigen and Ki-67) are expressed. This "podocyte dysregulation" is accompanied by podocyte detachment from the GBM.

FSGS is an irreversible scarring process in the glomeruli, as shown by the analysis of repeat biopsies (47,48,55). Studies in experimental animals (56) as well as in nephrotic patients have shown that proteinuria precedes the development of focal sclerotic lesions. The same sequence was reported in patients with recurrence of the disease

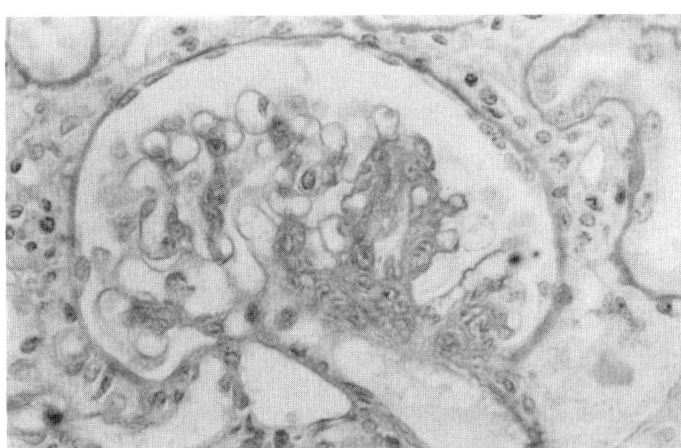

FIGURE 28.4. Collapsing glomerulopathy. Early glomerular lesion characterized by the irregular collapse of capillary loops. Light microscopy with periodic acid-Schiff (×320).

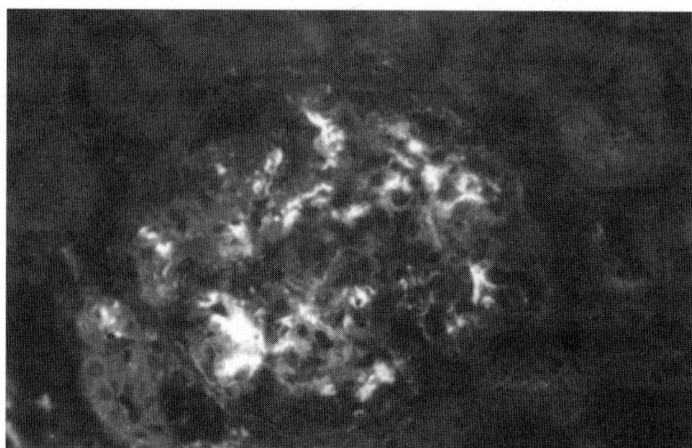

FIGURE 28.5. Idiopathic nephrotic syndrome with minimal changes. Diffuse mesangial deposits of immunoglobulin M. Immunofluorescence (×300).

after transplantation. Within weeks after recurrence of proteinuria, podocytes appear swollen and vacuolated by electron microscopy. The podocytes exhibit strong mitotic activity, with multinucleation and expression of the proliferating cell nuclear antigen and Ki-67 proliferation markers.

FSGS is not a specific histopathologic lesion: Similar alterations may be seen in persistent idiopathic proteinuria; heroin-associated nephropathy; and, independently, in association with acquired immunodeficiency syndrome, Alport's syndrome, hypertension, pyelonephritis, and obesity. FSGS has also been reported in renal hypoplasia with oligomeganephronia, after partial nephrectomy, and in other conditions associated with a reduction in nephron number, including reflux nephropathy and obstructive uropathy.

Immunoglobulin M–Associated Nephropathy

Immunofluorescence microscopy is usually negative (57,58). However, mesangial deposits of IgM, IgG, C3, and, more rarely, IgA have been reported (Fig. 28.5). Cohen et al. found that patients with IgM deposits in the mesangium had a poor response to corticosteroids (59). Other studies have not confirmed these findings. Habib et al. reported on immunofluorescence studies in a series of 222 children with idiopathic nephrotic syndrome (60). Although IgM was the Ig most frequently present in the glomeruli (54 of 222), there was no correlation between IgM deposits, the initial response to steroid therapy, or the final outcome. IgM deposits have also been described in association with diffuse mesangial proliferation and with FSGS.

Relationship between the Different Histologic Patterns

Repeat renal biopsies in patients with idiopathic nephrotic syndrome have shown morphologic transition between the three main histologic patterns. Some patients with clear evidence of minimal changes on initial biopsy have FSGS on a second biopsy. A high proportion of these patients are steroid resistant. Tejani found that FSGS lesions had developed in 60% of 48 patients with steroid-resistant MCD, in association with aggravation of symptoms (61). The progression to sclerosis may occur from minimal change or from mesangial proliferation (37,62). Conversely, some patients who show diffuse mesangial proliferation, regardless of whether it is associated with focal sclerosis on initial biopsy, may demonstrate minimal change or FSGS on repeat biopsy (27).

In conclusion, it may be considered that, at least in children, MCD, FSGS, and diffuse mesangial proliferation represent histologic variations of idiopathic nephrotic syndrome that may be found alone or in any combination on sequential biopsies in the same patient.

CLINICOPATHOLOGIC CORRELATIONS

The relative frequencies of the three histologic patterns differ in steroid-sensitive and steroid-resistant patients. A report of the International Study of Kidney Disease in Children showed that among 354 patients with idiopathic nephrotic syndrome who had an initial response to prednisone, 95.5% had MCD, 3.0% had FSGS, and 1.5% had diffuse mesangial proliferation. Conversely, among 55 patients who did not respond to prednisone, 45.5% had MCD, 47.5% had FSGS, and 7.0% had diffuse mesangial proliferation (63). This study also analyzed the numbers of responders and nonresponders within each histologic category. Among the 363 patients with minimal change, 193.1% were responders and 6.9% nonresponders, whereas among the 37 patients with FSGS, 29.7% responded to prednisone and 70.3% did not. Waldherr et al. found that only 2 out of 36 patients with diffuse mesangial proliferation responded to corticosteroids (37).

PATHOPHYSIOLOGY

In 1974, Shalhoub postulated that lymphokines may be responsible for the increased permeability of the GBM (64). Lagrue et al. first described the vascular permeability factor (VPF), a lymphokine found in the supernatant of concanavalin A–activated lymphocytes from patients with MCD that enhances vascular permeability when injected intradermally into the guinea pigs (65,66). Heslan et al. showed that VPF was produced by T lymphocytes and was distinct from interleukin (IL)-2 (67,68). Maruyama et al. showed that cyclosporine at concentrations ranging from 100 to 250 ng/mL was able to suppress the *in vitro* production of VPF by mononuclear cells from patients with MCD (69). VPF was also found in other diseases, such as IgA nephropathy. Tanaka et al. found that the supernatants of concanavalin A–activated lymphocytes from patients with MCD or FSGS induced a marked proteinuria when injected in the renal artery of rats together with a reduction of the anionic charges of the GBM (70). Boulton-Jones et al. infused lymphocyte culture supernatants into the renal artery of rats and found reduced colloidal iron staining in the kidneys, suggesting a loss of negative charges of the GBM (71). Similarly, Wilkinson et al. showed that the infusion of plasma from nephrotic patients to rabbits induced proteinuria and a reduction in the number of anionic sites on the GBM (72).

Koyama et al. described a glomerular permeability factor in the supernatant of T-cell hybridoma derived from the fusion between peripheral T lymphocytes of a patient with MCD and a T-cell line, CCRF-HSB2 (73). The glomerular permeability factor was identified by the ability of the supernatant to induce a proteinuria when injected intravenously (IV) in the rat. In addition, rats injected with the supernatants show a partial fusion of foot processes of glomerular epithelial cells and no immune deposits. Glomerular permeability factor is different from the other known lymphokines. Its molecular weight is between 60,000 and 160,000.

Other lymphokines may play a pathogenic role in SRNS (74). Increased IL-2 levels have been found in lymphocyte culture supernatants from patients with idiopathic nephrosis, and IL-2 can induce proteinuria and a reduction of the anionic sites of the GBM when injected into the rat kidney (68,75). A nephrotic syndrome has been described in several patients treated with recombinant IL-2 and interferon-α.

The rapid recurrence of proteinuria after renal transplantation in 30% of patients with SRNS is a strong argument for the presence of a circulating factor that increases the permeability of the GBM. Savin et al. identified a serum factor in some patients with FSGS that increases the albumin permeability of isolated rat glomeruli. The presence of the factor was strongly predictive of the recurrence of proteinuria after renal transplantation (76). A VPF, which induces proteinuria when injected into the renal artery of rats, was found in the serum from a transplanted patient who had recurrence of the nephrotic syndrome (77). However, subsequent attempts to isolate such a factor have failed. Dantal et al. treated patients who had recurrent nephrotic syndrome with plasma protein A adsorption (78). The administration to rats of material eluted from the protein A columns increased urinary albumin excretion. The active fraction had a molecular weight below 100,000. The factor or factors that may be responsible for recurrent nephrotic syndrome after transplantation appear to be bound to an Ig (79).

The Buffalo/Mna strain of rats spontaneously develops proteinuria with FSGS at 2 months of age. Le Berre et al. found that the nephrotic syndrome recurs when Buffalo/Mna rats receive a kidney from a healthy LEW.1W rat (80). Conversely, proteinuria and renal lesions regress when kidneys from a Buffalo/Mna rat are transplanted into normal LEW.1W rats. Although recurrence of proteinuria is not immediate after transplantation, this model may provide new insights into the pathogenesis of FSGS and the mechanisms of recurrence after transplantation in humans.

Two additional observations indicate that circulating factors, rather than innate kidney defects, render the GBM more permeable to proteins: Lagrue et al. reported the case of a woman with steroid-resistant FSGS who gave birth on two occasions to children who were proteinuric and hypoalbuminemic at birth. In both cases, proteinuria and nephrotic syndrome disappeared within 2 and 3 weeks, respectively (81). The second observation concerns the report of a 20-year-old man with MCD who died of cerebral hemorrhage and whose kidneys were transplanted into two recipients whose primary renal disease was not idiopathic nephrotic syndrome. In both cases, proteinuria and all features of MCD disappeared within 6 weeks of transplantation (82).

The pathogenesis of glomerulosclerosis is still unknown (83). Several factors, including hemodynamic factors, cytokines and growth factors, hyperlipidemia, and platelet activation, lead to an increase of mesangial matrix production by resident cells. Patients with lesions of FSGS have a significant glomerular hypertrophy. Experimental and clinical data demonstrate that abnormal glomerular growth is associated with glomerular sclerosis. Growth factors involved in the process include platelet-derived growth factor, TFG-β, angiotensin II, thromboxane A_2, macromolecule deposition, coagulation factors, and lipids (84–86). It is interesting to note that angiotensin regulates the expression of platelet-derived growth factor and TFG-β. This may explain the fact that angiotensin-converting enzyme inhibitors may prevent the decline of renal function in nephrotic patients.

Genetic Factors

In recent years, there have been several reports on the molecular basis of familial cases of idiopathic nephrotic syndrome with FSGS. Moreover, the discovery of molecular defects leading to FSGS has provided important insight in the critical role of newly identified podocyte proteins in the glomerular filtration barrier to proteins.

Mathis et al. performed linkage analysis in a large family in which FSGS followed an autosomal dominant mode of inheritance (87). Some patients developed severe proteinuria and ESRD by the fourth decade, whereas others had only mild proteinuria. The responsible gene, located on chromosome 19q13, encodes α-

actinin-4, an actin-filament cross-linking protein (88). Mutations in this gene were detected in affected patients (88). In vitro, mutant α-actinin-4 binds filamentous actin more strongly than does wild-type α-actinin-4. Regulation of the actin cytoskeleton of glomerular podocytes may be altered in this subpopulation of FSGS patients.

Another family with autosomal dominant FSGS was studied by linkage analysis (89,90). The disease was diagnosed during the third decade of life, with high-grade proteinuria progressing to ESRD in a relatively high percentage of cases. The authors detected a linkage to chromosome 11q21-q22 with a maximum lod score of 9.89. Winn et al. described another large family with autosomal dominant FSGS but no linkage to chromosome 11q21 or 19q13 (90).

Fuchshuber et al. mapped a locus to chromosome 1q25-q31 for autosomal recessive SRNS characterized by an early-onset steroid resistance, a rapid progression to renal failure, and the absence of recurrence after transplantation (91). Using a positional cloning approach, Boute et al. identified the causative gene, NPHS2, which is expressed only on podocytes and encodes an integral membrane protein, podocin (92). By immunoelectron microscopy, podocin is located at the foot processes, opposite the slit diaphragm (93). This 42-kDa protein is structurally related to human stomatin, an adapter protein that links mechanosensitive channels to the cytoskeleton on the cell surface. Podocin may link membrane proteins (e.g., nephrin) to the cytoskeleton. Ten different NPHS2 mutations comprising nonsense, frameshift, and missense mutations were found to segregate with the disease. Podocin mutations have also been identified in 15 to 30% of patients with sporadic SRNS (94,95).

CD2-associated protein (CD2AP), which anchors CD2 receptors of T lymphocytes to the cytoskeleton, is also expressed in the podocyte. Shih et al. observed that mutant mice lacking CD2AP develop proteinuria and renal failure (96). They showed that CD2AP and nephrin interact directly, suggesting an important role of this protein in the anchoring of nephrin to the slit diaphragm or into the signaling pathways (97). No mutations in the CD2AP gene associated with SRNS have been reported to date.

The Wilms' tumor suppressor gene, WT-1, encodes a transcription factor presumed to regulate the expression of numerous target genes through DNA binding. It plays a key role in renal and gonadal maturation. Mutations in WT-1 have been associated with nephroblastoma or glomerular diseases (Denys-Drash syndrome and Frasier syndrome). The WT-1 gene contains ten exons covering approximately 50 kb of genomic DNA. Exons 1 to 6 encode a proline/glutamine-rich transcriptional regulatory region, whereas exons 7 to 10 encode the four zinc-fingers of the DNA-binding domain. Two alternative splicing regions—one corresponding to the 17 amino acids encoded by exon 5 and the other to three amino acids [lysine-threonine-serine (KTS)] encoded by the 3' end of exon 9—lead to the synthesis of four isoforms with definite and stable proportions and different functions. The target genes potentially regulated, most often negatively, by WT-1 include genes coding for transcription factors (e.g., PAX2, PAX8, NovH, and WT-1) and for growth factors or their receptors (insulin-like growth factor-2, insulin-like growth factor-R, platelet-derived growth factor-A, TGF-β, and EGFR) (98). WT-1 is strongly expressed during embryofetal life (99). In the mature kidney, WT-1 expression persists only in podocytes and epithelial cells of Bowman's capsule. WT-1 gene disruption in mice results in the absence of kidneys and gonads, suggesting a key role of WT-1 in the maturation of the genitourinary tract.

Frasier syndrome is characterized by male pseudohermaphroditism and progressive glomerulopathy (100). Proteinuria is discovered during childhood, usually between 2 and 6 years of age or later. It increases progressively with time and does not respond to corticosteroids or to immunosuppressive agents. The disease runs a slow, progressive course to ESRD. Renal biopsy shows FSGS. No recurrence is observed after transplantation. Patients have female external genitalia, and it is often the evaluation of primary amenorrhea in nephrotic females that leads to the diagnosis of 46,XY gonadal dysgenesis, which is frequently complicated by gonadoblastoma.

Barbaux et al. detected point mutations in the donor splice site in intron 9 of the WT-1 gene (101). These mutations were heterozygous, and appeared *de novo* in the two patients whose parents were studied. The mutations result in loss of the +KTS isoform. Similar intronic mutations have been described by other authors (102,103). This indicates that donor splice-site mutations in WT-1 intron 9 are constant in Frasier syndrome. The former definition of Frasier syndrome included only 46,XY patients with a female phenotype. However, Frasier syndrome mutations may be responsible for isolated persistent glomerulopathy with focal sclerosis in genetically female patients and in patients with Denys-Drash syndrome (104,105).

Nephrotic syndrome with FSGS has been reported in patients with mitochondrial cytopathies (106–108). An A to G transition at position 3243 in mitochondrial DNA was reported in some of these patients who presented with isolated nephrotic syndrome or with nephrotic syndrome in association with mitochondrial myopathy, encephalopathy, lactic acidosis, stroke-like episodes, or progressive external ophthalmoplegia. Other patients develop diabetes mellitus or hearing loss.

Some familial cases of minimal change nephrotic syndrome are associated with other abnormalities (e.g., microcephaly and hiatus hernia), as in the Galloway-Mowat syndrome (109). Spondyloepiphyseal dysplasia was found in association with FSGS (110). Other syndromes, including microcephaly or disturbances of neuronal migration, have also been reported in association with early-onset nephrotic syndrome (111).

TREATMENT

Symptomatic Treatment

Symptomatic treatment—including dietary recommendations; use of diuretics; prevention and therapy of infectious and thromboembolic complications; and treatment of hypovolemia, hypertension, and hyperlipidemia—is identical to that recommended for the glucocorticoid-responsive patient with idiopathic nephrotic syndrome (see Chapter 27).

Immunosuppressive Therapy

By definition, patients with SRNS have not responded to standard glucocorticoid regimens (see Chapter 27).

Pulse Methylprednisolone

Methylprednisolone pulse therapy has been advocated for patients with SRNS. The protocol proposed by Mendoza et al. consists of methylprednisolone (30 mg/kg IV) administered every other day for 2 weeks; weekly for 8 weeks; every other week for 8 weeks; monthly for 9 months; and then every other month for 6 months in association with oral prednisone and, if necessary, cyclophosphamide or chlorambucil (112). At an average of over 6 years of follow-up, 21 of 32 children were in complete remission, and the 5-year incidence of ESRD was approximately 5% versus 40% in historic controls (113). Side effects included nausea during the infusion of pulse methylprednisolone in almost all, slowed growth in four patients, small cataracts that did not interfere with vision in five patients, and infections in two patients. There were no cases of abdominal striae, diabetes mellitus, or aseptic necrosis of bone.

Initial enthusiasm for usage of pulse methylprednisolone in patients with SRNS has been decreased by subsequent studies that have failed to produce similar results. A preliminary multicenter report of 15 children with FSGS was unable to confirm the efficacy of pulse corticosteroids (114). A mean of 15 pulses were given, and eight patients also received an alkylating agent. At the end of the study, only four patients maintained a complete remission, whereas five patients had a poor outcome with progression to ESRD or death. Waldo et al. did not observe complete remission in ten children who were treated with this protocol (115), whereas Hari et al. reported a 65% response rate (116).

Alkylating Agents

Although alkylating agents have little therapeutic effect in patients with SRNS, they are still widely used either alone or in combination with corticosteroids. Cyclophosphamide has been more often used than chlorambucil. The rate of full or partial remission is higher in patients with partial steroid resistance, those with late steroid resistance, or those in whom initial renal biopsy has shown MCD, by comparison with those showing initial resistance to corticosteroids or FSGS. The International Study of Kidney Disease in Children recently reported on 60 children with steroid-resistant FSGS who were randomly allocated to receive (a) prednisone, 40 mg/m^2 on alternate days for 12 months (control group) or (b) cyclophosphamide, 2.5 mg/kg body weight for 3 months plus prednisone, 40 mg/m^2, on alternate days for 12 months (117). Complete remissions were observed in 28% of children in the control group and in 25% of children who received cyclophosphamide. The authors concluded that there was no beneficial effect of cyclophosphamide in these patients. Geary et al. reported full or partial response to cyclophosphamide in 12 of 29 steroid-resistant patients with FSGS (118). Renal failure developed less frequently in partial responders (one of nine) than in those who did not respond at all (seven of eight). Siegel et al. observed complete remissions in six steroid-resistant patients with MCD, three of whom relapsed but became steroid responsive (119). Similarly, Bergstrand et al. reported that some patients with steroid-resistant nephrosis treated with cyclophosphamide had become steroid responsive (120). Conversely, White and Glasgow observed no improvement after cyclophosphamide treatment in 15 steroid-resistant children with focal sclerosis (121). Cameron et al. reported only 1 responder out of 13 children with steroid-resistant nephrosis and FSGS who received cyclophosphamide (122). Similarly, Tejani et al. reported no remission with cyclophosphamide in ten steroid-resistant children (123). In a controlled trial involving 13 children with steroid-resistant minimal change nephrotic syndrome, IV pulse cyclophosphamide was shown to be beneficial when compared to oral cyclophosphamide (124). Rennert et al. treated ten children with steroid-resistant FSGS with IV cyclophosphamide. Only two of the five patients who were initial nonresponders went into remission, whereas all five late nonresponders achieved complete reemission (125).

The side effects of cyclophosphamide include bone marrow depression, hemorrhagic cystitis, gastrointestinal tract symptoms, alopecia, and infection. Hemorrhagic cystitis occurs infrequently at the doses used in these patients.

Long-term toxic effects include the risk of cancer, pulmonary fibrosis, ovarian fibrosis, and sterility. Gonadal toxicity is well established, and the risk of sterility is greater in boys than in girls. The cumulative threshold dose above which oligo- or azoospermia may occur is above 250 mg/kg (126,127). Azoospermia is reversible in some patients (128). The risk of cancer is difficult to define with the short courses used to treat idiopathic nephrotic syndrome.

Chlorambucil has been used in a few studies. Baluarte et al. described remissions in 10 of 17 cases (129). Williams et al. treated six children who all went into remission with a follow-up of 1.3 to 9.4 years (130). We treated 74 steroid-resistant children with chlorambucil, 0.2 mg/kg, for 2 to 6 months, and only 14 (19%) achieved complete or partial remission.

Acute toxic effects are less frequent with chlorambucil than with cyclophosphamide. Leukopenia and thrombocytopenia may occur and are reversible within 1 to 3 weeks. Severe viral infections have been reported. Long-term toxic effects include an increased risk of malignancy (131). Gonadal toxicity, which predominantly affects male patients, is probably irreversible (azoospermia) at cumulative doses above 10 mg/kg.

Combined Immunosuppression

Trompeter proposed aggressive immunosuppression for a subgroup of patients with FSGS, refractory nephrotic syndrome, or rapid progression to renal failure (132). The regimen included vincristine, 1.5 mg/m²/wk in eight weekly IV doses; cyclophosphamide, 3 mg/kg/day for 8 weeks; and prednisolone, 2 mg/kg/day initially, with progressive tapering after 2 weeks. Lasting remissions were observed in 7 of 21 children, starting 6 months to 3 years from the onset of therapy. Almeida et al. observed a complete and stable remission in only two of the seven children who received this regimen (133).

Azathioprine

Azathioprine was considered to be ineffective in steroid-resistant patients after the report of Abramowicz et al., who found no difference between a 3-month course of azathioprine and placebo (134). However, Cade et al. reported complete remission in 13 adult patients with steroid-resistant idiopathic nephrotic syndrome (135).

Cyclosporine

Cyclosporine has been used to treat patients with SRNS. Initial reports showed that only 20% of 60 steroid-resistant children achieved complete remission (136–142). A partial response was observed in 13% of cases, but it was usually transient (143).

The Collaborative Study of Sandimmune in Nephrotic Syndrome analyzed the data from different clinical studies, including 226 steroid-resistant patients, adults, and children (144). The analysis demonstrated that the rate of complete remission was significantly higher when cyclosporine was given in combination with steroids: 24% compared to 14%.

The French Society of Pediatric Nephrology reported the results of a prospective trial, including 65 children treated with cyclosporine, 150 to 200 mg/m², and prednisone, 30 mg/m²/day for 1 month and on alternate days for 5 months thereafter (145). Twenty-seven patients (42%) went into complete remission and four (6%) partial remission, whereas 34 (52%) did not respond to the combined treatment. Complete remission occurred in more than one-half of the patients within the first 2 months of this treatment, which makes it likely that the treatment was responsible for the remission, although spontaneous remission cannot be excluded. It is interesting to note that eight patients who relapsed after cyclosporine treatment subsequently responded to steroids and experienced a steroid-dependent course. Progression to renal failure was observed only in patients who had not responded (12 patients) or had only a partial response (1 patient) to the combined treatment.

Ingulli et al. reported that prolonged cyclosporine treatment in children with steroid-resistant FSGS reduced proteinuria and slowed progression to ESRF (146). The dose of cyclosporine (4 to 20 mg/kg/day) was titrated to the serum cholesterol level to achieve a remission. In this study, only 5 of the 21 treated patients (24%) progressed to ESRF compared to 42 of 54 patients from a historical control group who had not received this treatment.

Ponticelli et al. compared cyclosporine to supportive therapy in a randomized trial (147). Seven of the 22 treated patients went into complete remission, six experienced partial remission, and nine did not respond. Only 38% of the patients who responded had sustained remissions. In the control group, only 3 of the 19 patients achieved partial remission. Tejani and Liberman compared cyclosporine and placebo in 25 children with steroid-resistant FSGS (148). All 12 patients who were treated demonstrated a decrease in proteinuria compared to two in placebo-treated patients.

Gregory et al. treated 15 children with SRNS cyclosporine combined with prednisone. They observed a remission in 13 children after a mean duration of treatment of 2 months (149).

Singh et al. recently reported the effect of cyclosporine in 42 children with steroid-resistant FSGS (150). The mean proteinuria decreased from 7.1 to 1.8 g/day, whereas the serum albumin increased from 2.1 to 3.5 g/dL. The mean serum creatinine increased from 0.85 to 1.26 mg/dL. Twenty-five patients responded with a complete remission.

Patients who respond to cyclosporine often relapse when the dose is tapered or discontinued (151). Many reports indicate that the prolonged use of cyclosporine is associated with chronic nephrotoxicity. The most prominent histologic feature of chronic cyclosporine nephrotoxicity is the presence of tubulointerstitial lesions, characterized by stripes of interstitial fibrosis containing groups of atrophic tubules. Cyclosporine-associated arteriolopathy is rarely observed. Classen et al. did not find significant changes on the renal biopsies of five patients treated for a mean period of 10 months (152). Habib and Niaudet performed repeat renal biopsies in 42 patients (153). There were no significant changes in 18 patients, several foci of atrophic tubules with thickened basement membranes within stripes of interstitial fibrosis in 15 patients, and extensive lesions of interstitial fibrosis with atrophic tubules in nine patients. In this study, 9 of the 15 patients with several foci of atrophic tubules and all nine patients with severe interstitial fibrosis had MCD on pre- and posttherapy biopsies without FSGS, suggesting that the lesions were secondary to cyclosporine and not to the natural course of the disease. At the time of most recent biopsy, all children, including the nine patients with the most severe tubulointerstitial lesions, had normal renal function. Thus, morphology is a more sensitive indicator of chronic cyclosporine nephrotoxicity than GFR.

Other side effects give less cause for concern and respond to standard therapy: elevation of blood pressure, hyperkalemia, hypertrichosis, gum hypertrophy, and hypomagnesemia.

FK506

A few patients have been treated with the immunophilin modulator FK506 with poor results (154).

Nonsteroidal Antiinflammatory Drugs

Nonsteroidal antiinflammatory drugs may decrease proteinuria. Several authors have used indomethacin in the treatment of idiopathic nephrotic syndrome with variable results. Donker et al. found a reduction of proteinuria in patients with focal sclerosis associated with a simultaneous reduction of GFR (155). Velosa et al. also reported a significant reduction in proteinuria in patients treated with meclofenamate (156).

The detrimental effect of nonsteroidal antiinflammatory drugs on renal function is well established, and patients with renal disease seem more vulnerable (157,158). Positive sodium balance, increased edema, and risk of arterial hypertension are recognized complications. The decreased GFR observed with nonsteroidal antiinflammatory drugs is usually reversible and marked only in salt-sodium–depleted patients. However, irreversible renal failure was reported with a high incidence in a prospective study in children with nonresponsive nephrotic syndrome and focal sclerosis (159).

Angiotensin-Converting Enzyme Inhibitors

The angiotensin-converting enzyme inhibitor captopril was reported to dramatically decrease nephrotic range proteinuria secondary to renovascular hypertension and secondary FSGS (160). A decrease in proteinuria and even complete remission have also been observed in patients with chronic glomerulopathies with or without hypertension (161). Reduction of proteinuria by 50% without a concomitant decrease in GFR was reported in children with SRNS (162). Further studies are needed to confirm these observations.

Lipid-Lowering Agents

Hyperlipidemia has been shown to accelerate the progression of glomerular sclerosis in experimental animals. Controlled trials in adult patients have shown that lipid-lowering agents can prevent the decline of renal function in a variety of chronic nephropathics. No such studies have been performed in children.

RECURRENCE OF IDIOPATHIC NEPHROTIC SYNDROME IN TRANSPLANTED KIDNEYS

A major problem in patients with idiopathic nephrotic syndrome who progress to ESRF and subsequently undergo renal transplantation is the risk of recurrent disease in the graft. The overall risk of recurrence is estimated at 25%. The risk appears to be different in children and adults. Senggutuvan et al. reported recurrence in 8 of 16 children compared to 3 of 27 adults (163). In children, recurrence is more frequent when the disease is diagnosed after 6 years of age (164,165). Similarly, a rapid progression of the disease to ESRF was a major factor associated with recurrence: In most series, when the duration of disease has been shorter than 3 years, the nephrotic syndrome recurs in one-half of the patients (166,167). The histopathologic pattern observed on the first biopsy during the course of the disease is also an important predictive factor (163,165,166,168,169). Recurrence occurs in 50 to 80% of patients in whom initial biopsy showed diffuse mesangial proliferation but in only 25% of patients with MCD on initial biopsy. Most patients who experience a recurrence in a first graft show recurrence in a second graft (170–173). Conversely, when a first graft has been lost due to rejection without recurrence, a second graft can be performed safely, as no recurrence has been described in this setting.

In children, recurrence of proteinuria occurs in most cases within the first hours or days after transplantation. A high proportion of patients with immediate recurrence show delayed graft function (164,170,174). In some patients, proteinuria recurs several months later. Proteinuria is most often associated with a nephrotic syndrome. Transplant biopsy, when performed early, usually shows minimal glomerular changes with foot-process fusion (175–177). Lesions of FSGS appear after several days or weeks (176).

Graft failure occurs in approximately 60% of patients with recurrence versus 23% of those without recurrence (163,164,170,178). Some patients may maintain adequate renal function for several years despite persistent nephrotic syndrome (164,167).

The role of cyclosporine in recurrent SRNS remains unclear. There is no evidence that cyclosporine can prevent the recurrence of nephrotic syndrome after transplantation (179–184). After the introduction of cyclosporine, the incidence of recurrence did not change, but graft survival improved (164,179,180,183). In patients who have recurrent disease, high doses of cyclosporine may be effective. Mowry et al. reported on 11 children who received 12 renal transplants and who had been treated with high-dose cyclosporine, plasma exchanges, or a combination of both (185). Remission was observed in 10 of the 12 recipients. Ingulli and Tejani reported two children with recurrent nephrotic syndrome who both achieved remission when cyclosporine dosage was gradually increased from 15 mg/kg/day to 27 and 35 mg/kg/day (186). A similar experience was reported by Srivastava et al. (187). In our group, 17 children with recurrence were treated with IV cyclosporine at an initial dose of 3 mg/kg/day, which was then adjusted to maintain whole blood levels between 250 and 350 ng/mL. In 14 of the 17 cases (82%), proteinuria completely disappeared after 20.8 ± 8.4 days (range, 12 to 40 days). The treatment was ineffective in the remaining three patients. Plasma exchanges were performed in four patients during the first 2 months, and proteinuria regressed in three cases and persisted in one. Persistent remission was observed in 11 patients with a follow-up of 3.7 ± 3.0 years. Actuarial graft survival was 92% and 70% at 1 and 5 years (188). We advocate the early use of IV cyclosporine as a first-line treatment in recurrent idiopathic nephrotic syndrome after renal transplantation. There is limited experience with the use of tacrolimus (FK506) in recurrent nephrotic syndrome after transplantation (189).

Plasma exchange has been performed in a number of patients and, in some cases, combined with increased immunosuppression (190–196) and associated with partial or transient remissions. Improved results were observed when the treatment was started early. Dantal et al. treated eight kidney transplant recipients with recurrent nephrotic syndrome with plasma protein adsorption (78). The treatment consistently decreased urinary protein excretion by an average of 82% at the end of a cycle. The effect of adsorption was short-lived, and protein excretion returned to pretreatment levels within a maximum of 2 months.

CONCLUSION

There is evidence to suggest that MCD and FSGS represent a spectrum of diseases (197). Indeed, it is likely that several disease entities are included in the term *steroid-resistant idiopathic nephrotic syndrome*. In many patients, circulating agents produced by immune cells increase GBM permeability to proteins. In these patients, cyclosporine may be effective. Recurrence posttransplantation is another feature of such patients. In other patients, the disease is genetically transmitted and is resistant to all treatments. Defects in podocyte proteins have been identified in some of these familial cases.

REFERENCES

1. Habib R, Churg J. Minimal change disease, mesangial proliferative glomerulonephritis and focal sclerosis: individual entities or a spectrum of disease. In: Robinson RR, ed. *Nephrology: proceedings of the IXth International Congress of Nephrology*, Los Angeles: Springer-Verlag, 1984:634–644.
2. Kriz W, Elger M, Nagata M, et al. The role of podocytes in the development of glomerular sclerosis. *Kidney Int Suppl* 1994;45:S64–S72.
3. Bariety J, Nochy D, Jacquot C, et al. Diversity and unity of focal and segmental glomerular sclerosis. *Adv Nephrol Necker Hosp* 1998;28:1–42.
4. Bariety J, Bruneval P, Hill G, et al. Posttransplantation relapse of FSGS is characterized by glomerular epithelial cell transdifferentiation. *J Am Soc Nephrol* 2001;12:261–274.
5. Barisoni L, Mokrzycki M, Sablay L, et al. Podocyte cell cycle regulation and proliferation in collapsing glomerulopathies. *Kidney Int* 2000;58:137–143.
6. Shankland SJ, Eitner F, Hudkins KL, et al. Differential expression of cyclin-dependent kinase inhibitors in human glomerular disease: role in podocyte proliferation and maturation. *Kidney Int* 2000;58:674–683.
7. Tanawattanacharoen S, Falk RJ, Jennette JC, Kopp JB. Parvovirus B19 DNA in kidney tissue of patients with focal segmental glomerulosclerosis. *Am J Kidney Dis* 2000;35:1166–1174.
8. Moudgil A, Nast CC, Bagga A, et al. Association of parvovirus B19 infection with idiopathic collapsing glomerulopathy. *Kidney Int* 2001;59:2126–2133.
9. Strehlau J, Schachter AD, Pavlakis M, et al. Activated intrarenal transcription of CTL-effectors and TGF-beta1 in children with focal segmental glomerulosclerosis. *Kidney Int* 2002;61:90–95.
10. Kashgarian M, Hayslett JP, Seigel NJ. Lipoid nephrosis and focal sclerosis: distinct entities or spectrum of disease. *Nephron* 1974;13:105–108.
11. Habib R. Focal glomerular sclerosis. *Kidney Int* 1973;4:355–361.
12. Siegel NJ, Gur A, Krassner LS. Minimal lesion nephrotic syndrome with early resistance to steroid therapy. *J Pediatr* 1975;377–380.
13. McAdams AJ, Valentini RP, Welch TR. The nonspecificity of focal segmental glomerulosclerosis. The defining characteristics of primary focal glomerulosclerosis, mesangial proliferation, and minimal change. *Medicine* 1997;76:42–52.
14. Antignac C. Genetic models: clues for understanding the pathogenesis of idiopathic nephrotic syndrome. *J Clin Invest* 2002;109:447–449.
15. International Study of Kidney Disease in Children. Nephrotic syndrome in children: prediction of histopathology from clinical and laboratory characteristics at time of diagnosis. *Kidney Int* 1978;13:159–165.
16. Elises JS, Griffiths PD, Hocking MD, et al. Simplified quantitation of urinary protein excretion in children. *Clin Nephrol* 1988;30:225–229.
17. Habib R, Kleinknecht C. The primary nephrotic syndrome of childhood. Classification and clinicopathologic study of 406 cases. *Pathol Annu* 1971;6:417–474.
18. Thabet MAE, Salcedo JR, Chan JCM. Hyperlipidemia in childhood nephrotic syndrome. *Pediatr Nephrol* 1993;7:559–566.
19. Sato KA, Gray RW, Lemann J. Urinary excretion of 25-hydroxy-vitamin D in health and the nephrotic syndrome. *J Lab Clin Med* 1982;99:325–330.

20. Freundlich M, Bourgoignie JJ, Zilleruelo G, et al. Calcium and vitamin D metabolism in children with nephrotic syndrome. *J Pediatr* 1986;108:383–387.
21. McVicar M, Exeni R, Susin M. Nephrotic syndrome and multiple tubular defects in children: an early sign of focal segmental glomerulosclerosis. *J Pediatr* 1980;97:918–922.
22. Rodriguez-Soriano J, Vallo A, Castillo G. Defect in urinary acidification in nephrotic syndrome and its correction by furosemide. *Nephron* 1982;32:308–313.
23. White R HR, Glasgow EF, Mills RJ. Clinicopathological studies of nephrotic syndrome in childhood. *Lancet* 1970;i:1353–1359.
24. Berg U, Bohlin AB. Renal hemodynamics in minimal change nephrotic syndrome in childhood. *Int J Pediatr Nephrol* 1982; 3:187–192.
25. Bohlin AB. Clinical course and renal function in minimal change nephrotic syndrome. *Acta Paediatr Scand* 1984;73: 631–636.
26. Bohman SO, Jaremko G, Bohlin AB, Berg U. Foot process fusion and glomerular filtration rate in minimal change nephrotic syndrome. *Kidney Int* 1984;25:696–700.
27. Southwest Pediatric Nephrology Study Group. Focal segmental glomerulosclerosis in children with idiopathic nephrotic syndrome. *Kidney Int* 1985;27:442–449.
28. Ingulli E, Tejani A. Racial differences in the incidence and outcome of idiopathic focal and segmental glomerulosclerosis in children. *Pediatr Nephrol* 1991;5:393–397.
29. Garin EH, Grant MB, Silverstein JH. Insulin-like growth factors in patients with active nephrotic syndrome. *Am J Dis Child* 1989;43:865–867.
30. Krensky A, Ingelfinger JR, Grupe WE. Peritonitis in childhood nephrotic syndrome 1970–1980. *Am J Dis Child* 1982;136: 732–736.
31. Andrew M, Brooker LA. Hemostatic complications in renal disorders of the young. *Pediatr Nephrol* 1996;10:88–99.
32. Hoyer PF, Gonda S, Barthels M, et al. Thromboembolic complications in children with nephrotic syndrome. *Acta Paediatr Scand* 1986;75:804–810.
33. Cameron JS, Turner DR, Ogg CS, et al. The nephrotic syndrome in adults with minimal change glomerular lesions. *Q JM* 1974;43:461–488.
34. Churg J, Habib R, White RHR. Pathology of the nephrotic syndrome in children. *Lancet* 1970;i:1299–1302.
35. Powell HR. Relationship between proteinuria and epithelial cell changes in minimal lesion glomerulopathy. *Nephron* 1976;16:310–317.
36. Kawano K, Wenzl J, McCoy J, et al. Lipoid nephrosis. A multifold blind study including quantitation. *Lab Invest* 1971;24:499–503.
37. Waldherr R, Gubler M, Levy M, et al. The significance of pure mesangial proliferation in idiopathic nephrotic syndrome. *Clin Nephrol* 1978;10:171–179.
38. Yoshikawa N, Itto H, Akamatsu R, et al. Focal segmental glomerulosclerosis with and without nephrotic syndrome in children. *J Pediatr* 1986;109:65–70.
39. Rich AR. A hitherto undescribed vulnerability of the juxtamedullary glomeruli in the lipoid nephrosis. *Bull John Hopkins Hosp* 1957;100:173–179.
40. Howie AJ, Brewer DB. The glomerular tip lesion: a previously undescribed type of segmental glomerular abnormality. *J Pathol* 1984;142:205–220.
41. Ito H, Yoshikawa N, Aozai F, et al. Twenty seven children with focal segmental glomerulosclerosis: correlation between the segmental location of the glomerular lesions and prognosis. *Clin Nephrol* 1984;22:9–14.
42. Huppes W, Hene RJ, Kooiker CJ. The glomerular location of segmental lesions in focal segmental glomerulonephrosclerosis. *Clin Nephrol* 1988;33:211–219.
43. Morita M, White RHR, Coad NAG, Faafat F. The clinical significance of the glomerular location of segmental lesions in focal segmental glomerulonephrosclerosis. *Clin Nephrol* 1990;33:211–219.
44. Fogo A, Hawkins EP, Berry PL, et al. Glomerular hypertrophy in minimal change disease predicts subsequent progression to focal glomerular sclerosis. *Kidney Int* 1990;38:115–123.
45. Muda AO, Feriozzi S, Cinotti G, Faraggiana T. Glomerular hypertrophy and chronic renal failure in focal segmental glomerulosclerosis. *Am J Kidney Dis* 1994;23:237–241.
46. Jenis EH, Teichman S, Briggs WA, et al. Focal segmental glomerulosclerosis. *Am J Med* 1974;57:695–705.
47. Nagi AH, Alexander F, Lanigan R. Light and electron microscopical studies of focal glomerular sclerosis. *J Clin Pathol* 1971;24:846–850.
48. Hyman LR, Burkholder PM. Focal sclerosing glomerulonephropathy with segmental hyalinosis. A clinicopathologic analysis. *Lab Invest* 1973;28:533–544.
49. Grishman E, Churg J. Focal glomerular sclerosis in nephrotic patients: an electron microscopy study of glomerular podocytes. *Kidney Int* 1975;7:111–122.
50. Weiss MA, Daquioag E, Margolin G, Pollack VE. Nephrotic syndrome, progressive irreversible renal failure and glomerular "collapse." A new clinicopathologic entity? *Am J Kidney Dis* 1986;7:20–28.
51. Detwiler RK, Falk RJ, Hogan SL, Jennette JC. Collapsing glomerulopathy: a clinically and pathologically distinct variant of focal segmental glomerulosclerosis. *Kidney Int* 1994;45:1416–1424.
52. Nagata M, Hattori M, Hamano Y, et al. Origin and phenotypic features of hyperplastic epithelial cells in collapsing glomerulopathy. *Am J Kidney Dis* 1998;32:962–969.
53. Toth CM, Pascual M, Williams WW Jr, et al. Recurrent collapsing glomerulopathy. *Transplantation* 1998;65:1009–1010.
54. Valeri A, Barisoni L, Appel GB, et al. Idiopathic collapsing focal segmental glomerulosclerosis: a clinicopathologic study. *Kidney Int* 1996;50:1734–1746.
55. Nash MA, Greifer I, Olbing H, et al. The significance of focal sclerotic lesions of glomeruli in children. *J Pediatr* 1976;88:806–813.
56. Couser WG, Stilmant MM. Mesangial lesion and focal glomerular sclerosis in the aging rat. *Lab Invest* 1975;33:491–501.
57. Michael AF, McLean RH, Roy LP, et al. Immunologic aspects of the nephrotic syndrome. *Kidney Int* 1973;3:105–115.
58. Jao W, Pollak VE, Norris SH, et al. Lipoid nephrosis. *Medicine* 1973;52:445–468.
59. Cohen AH, Border WA, Glassock RJ. Nephrotic syndrome with glomerular mesangial IgM deposits. *Lab Invest* 1978; 38:610–619.

60. Habib R, Girardin E, Gagnadoux MF, et al. Immunopathological findings in idiopathic nephrosis: clinical significance of glomerular "immune deposits." *Pediatr Nephrol* 1988;2: 402–408.
61. Tejani A. Morphological transitions in minimal change nephrotic syndrome. *Nephron* 1985;39:157–159.
62. Hirszel P, Yamase HT, Carney WR, et al. Mesangial proliferative glomerulonephritis with IgM deposits. Clinicopathologic analysis and evidence for morphologic transitions. *Nephron* 1984;38:100–108.
63. International Study of Kidney Disease in Children. The primary nephrotic syndrome in children. Identification of patients with minimal change nephrotic syndrome from initial response to prednisone. *J Pediatr* 1981;98:561–564.
64. Shalhoub RJ. Pathogenesis of lipoid nephrosis: a disorder of T cell function. *Lancet* 1974;ii:556–559.
65. Lagrue G, Branellec A, Blanc C, et al. A vascular permeability factor in lymphocyte culture supernatants from patients with nephrotic syndrome. II. Pharmacological and physicochemical properties. *Biomedicine* 1975;23:73–75.
66. Sobel AT, Branellec AL, Blanc CJ, Lagrue G. Physiochemical characterization of a vascular permeability factor, produced by Con A stimulated human lymphocytes. *J Immunol* 1977;119:1230–1234.
67. Heslan JM, Branellec AI, Laurent J, Lagrue G. The vascular permeability factor is a T lymphocyte product. *Nephron* 1986;42:187–188.
68. Heslan JMJ, Branellec AI, Pilatte Y, et al. Differentiation between vascular permeability factor and IL-2 in lymphocyte supernatants from patients with minimal-change nephrotic syndrome. *Clin Exp Immunol* 1991;86:157–162.
69. Maruyama K, Tomizawa S, Shimabukoro N, et al. Effect of supernatants derived from T lymphocyte culture in minimal change nephrotic syndrome on rat kidney capillaries. *Nephron* 1989;51:73–76.
70. Tanaka R, Yoshikawa N, Nakamura H, Ito H. Infusion of peripheral blood mononuclear cell products from nephrotic children increases albuminuria in rats. *Nephron* 1992;60:35–41.
71. Boulton-Jones JM, Tulloch I, Dore B, McLay A. Changes in the glomerular capillary wall induced by lymphocyte products and serum of nephrotic patients. *Clin Nephrol* 1983;20:72–77.
72. Wilkinson AH, Gillespie C, Hartley B, Williams DG. Increase in proteinuria and reduction in number of anionic sites on the glomerular basement membrane in rabbits by infusion of human nephrotic plasma in vivo. *Clin Sci* 1989;77:43–48.
73. Koyama A, Fujisaki M, Kobayashi M, et al. A glomerular permeability factor produced by human T cell hybridoma. *Kidney Int* 1991;40:453–460.
74. Bakker WW, Van Luijk WHJ. Do circulating factors play a role in the pathogenesis of minimal change nephrotic syndrome? *Pediatr Nephrol* 1989;3:341–349.
75. Kawaguchi H, Yamaguchi Y, Nagata M, Itoh K. The effects of human recombinant interleukin-2 on the permeability of glomerular basement membranes in rats. *Jap J Nephrol* 1987; 29:1–11.
76. Savin VJ, Sharma R, Sharma M, et al. Circulating factor associated with increased glomerular permeability to albumin in recurrent focal segmental glomerulosclerosis. *BMJ* 1996;334:878–883.
77. Zimmerman SW. Increased urinary protein excretion in the rat produced by serum from patient with recurrent focal glomerular sclerosis after renal transplantation. *Clin Nephrol* 1984;22:32–38.
78. Dantal J, Bigot E, Bogers W, et al. Effect of plasma protein adsorption on protein excretion in kidney-transplant recipients with recurrent nephrotic syndrome. *BMJ* 1994;330:7–14.
79. Dantal J, Godfrin Y, Koll R, et al. Antihuman immunoglobulin affinity immunoadsorption strongly decreases proteinuria in patients with relapsing nephrotic syndrome. *J Amer Soc Nephrol* 1998;9:1709–1715.
80. Le Berre L, Godfrin Y, Gunther E, et al. Extrarenal effects on the pathogenesis and relapse of idiopathic nephrotic syndrome in Buffalo/Mna rats. *J Clin Invest* 2002;109:491–498.
81. Lagrue G, Branellec A, Niaudet P, et al. Transmission d'un syndrome néphrotique à deux nouveau-nés. Régression spontanée. *La Presse Médicale* 1991;20:255–257.
82. Ali AA, Wilson E, Moorhead JF, et al. Minimal-change glomerular nephritis—normal kidneys in an abnormal environment? *Transplantation* 1994;58:849–852.
83. Ichikawa I, Fogo A. Focal segmental glomerulosclerosis. *Pediatr Nephrol* 1996;10:374–391.
84. Border WA, Noble NA, Ketteler M. TGF-β: a cytokine mediator of glomerulosclerosis and a target for therapeutic intervention. *Kidney Int* 1995;47:S59–S61.
85. Ichikawa I, Ikoma M, Fogo A. Glomerular growth promoters, the common key mediator for progressive glomerular sclerosis in chronic renal diseases. *Adv Nephrol* 1991;20:127–148.
86. Tanaka R, Sugihare K, Tatematsu A, Fogo A. Internephron heterogeneity of growth factors and sclerosis—Modulation of platelet-derived growth factor by angiotensin II. *Kidney Int* 1995;47:131–139.
87. Mathis BJ, Kim SH, Calabrese K, et al. A locus for inherited focal segmental glomerulosclerosis maps to chromosome 19q13. *Kidney Int* 1998;53:282–286.
88. Kaplan JM, Kim SH, North KN, et al. Mutations in ACTN4, encoding alpha-actinin-4, cause familial focal segmental glomerulosclerosis. *Nat Genet* 2000;24:251–256.
89. Winn MP. Not all in the family: mutations of podocin in sporadic steroid-resistant nephrotic syndrome. *J Am Soc Nephrol* 2002;13:577–579.
90. Winn MP, Conlon PJ, Lynn KL, et al. Clinical and genetic heterogeneity in familial focal segmental glomerulosclerosis. International Collaborative Group for the Study of Familial Focal Segmental Glomerulosclerosis. *Kidney Int* 1999;55:1241–1246.
91. Fuchshuber A, Jean G, Gribouval O, et al. Mapping a gene (SRN1) to chromosome 1q25-q31 in idiopathic nephrotic syndrome confirms a distinct entity of autosomal recessive nephrosis. *Hum Mol Genet* 1995;4:2155–2158.
92. Boute N, Gribouval O, Roselli S, et al. NPHS2, encoding the glomerular protein podocin, is mutated in autosomal recessive steroid-resistant nephrotic syndrome. *Nat Genet* 2000;24:349–354.
93. Roselli S, Gribouval O, Boute N, et al. Podocin localizes in the kidney to the slit diaphragm area. *Am J Pathol* 2002;160:131–139.
94. Fuchshuber A, Gribouval O, Ronner V, et al. Clinical and genetic evaluation of familial steroid-responsive nephrotic syndrome in childhood. *J Am Soc Nephrol* 2001;12:374–378.

95. Frishberg Y, Rinat C, Megged O, et al. Mutations in NPHS2 encoding podocin are a prevalent cause of steroid-resistant nephrotic syndrome among Israeli-Arab children. *J Am Soc Nephrol* 2002;13:400–405.
96. Shih NY, Li J, Karpitskii V, et al. Congenital nephrotic syndrome in mice lacking CD2-associated protein. *Science* 1999;286:312–315.
97. Shih NY, Li J, Cotran R, et al. CD2AP localizes to the slit diaphragm and binds to nephrin via a novel C-terminal domain. *Am J Pathol* 2001;159:2303–2308.
98. Reddy JC, Licht JD. The WT1 Wilms' tumor suppressor gene: How much do we really know? *Biochim Biophys Acta* 1996;1287:1–28.
99. Pritchard-Jones K, Fleming S, Davidson D, et al. The candidate Wilms' tumour gene is involved in genitourinary development. *Nature* 1990;346:194–197.
100. Frasier S, Bashore RA, Mosier HD. Gonadoblastoma associated with pure gonadal dysgenesis in monozygotic twins. *J Pediatr* 1964;64:740–745.
101. Barbaux S, Niaudet P, Gubler MC, et al. Donor splice-site mutations in WT1 are responsible for Frasier syndrome. *Nat Genet* 1997;17:467–470.
102. Kikuchi H, Takata A, Akasaka Y, et al. Do intronic mutations affecting splicing of WT1 exon 9 cause Frasier syndrome? *J Med Genet* 1998;35:45–48.
103. Klamt B, Koziell A, Poulat F, et al. Frasier syndrome is caused by defective alternative splicing of WT1 leading to an altered ratio of WT1 +/–KTS splice isoforms. *Hum Mol Genet* 1998;7:709–714.
104. Demmer L, Primack W, Loik V, et al. Frasier syndrome: a cause of focal segmental glomerulosclerosis in a 46,XX female. *J Amer Soc Nephrol* 1999;10:2215–2218.
105. Denamur E, Bocquet N, Mougenot B, et al. Mother-to-child transmitted WT1 splice-site mutation is responsible for distinct glomerular diseases. *J Am Soc Nephrol* 1999;10:2219–2223.
106. Doleris LM, Hill GS, Chedin P, et al. Focal segmental glomerulosclerosis associated with mitochondrial cytopathy. *Kidney Int* 2000;58:1851–1858.
107. Hotta O, Inoue CN, Miyabayashi S, et al. Clinical and pathologic features of focal segmental glomerulosclerosis with mitochondrial tRNALeu(UUR) gene mutation. *Kidney Int* 2001;59:1236–1243.
108. Kurogouchi F, Oguchi T, Mawatari E, et al. A case of mitochondrial cytopathy with a typical point mutation for MELAS, presenting with severe focal-segmental glomerulosclerosis as main clinical manifestation. *Am J Nephrol* 1998;18:551–556.
109. Galloway WH, Mowat AP. Congenital microcephaly and nephrotic syndrome in two sibs. *J Med Genet* 1968;5:319–321.
110. Ehrich JHH, Offner G, Shirg E, et al. Association of spondylo-epiphyseal dysplasia with nephrotic syndrome. *Pediatr Nephrol* 1990;4:117–212.
111. Bogdanovic R, Kuzmanovic M, Markovic-Lipkovski J, et al. Glomerular involvement in myelodysplastic syndromes. *Pediatr Nephrol* 2001;16:1053–1057.
112. Mendoza SA, Reznik VM, Griswold W, et al. Treatment of steroid resistant focal segmental glomerulosclerosis with pulse methyl prednisolone and alkylating agents. *Pediatr Nephrol* 1990;4:303–307.
113. Tune BM, Kirpekar RK, Reznik VM, et al. Intravenous methylprednisolone and oral alkylating agent therapy of prednisone-resistant pediatric focal segmental glomerulosclerosis: a long-term follow-up. *Clin Nephrol* 1995;43:84–88.
114. Guillot AP, Kim MS. Pulse steroid therapy does not alter the course of focal segmental glomerulosclerosis. *J Am Soc Nephrol* 1993;4:276.
115. Waldo FB, Benfield MR, Kohaut EC. Methylprednisolone treatment of patients with steroid-resistant nephrotic syndrome. *Pediatr Nephrol* 1992;6:503–505
116. Hari P, Bagga A, Jindal N, Srivastava RN. Treatment of focal glomerulosclerosis with pulse steroids and oral cyclophosphamide. *Pediatr Nephrol* 201;16:901–905.
117. Tarshish P, Tobin JN, Bernstein J, Edelman CM. Cyclophosphamide does not benefit patients with focal segmental glomerulosclerosis. A report of the International Study of Kidney Disease in Children. *Pediatr Nephrol* 1996;10:590–593.
118. Geary DF, Farine M, Thorner P, Baumal R. Response to cyclophosphamide in steroid resistant focal segmental glomerulosclerosis. *Clin Nephrol* 1984;22:109–113.
119. Siegel NJ, Gur A, Krassner LS. Minimal lesion nephrotic syndrome with early resistance to steroid therapy. *J Pediatr* 1975;87:377–380.
120. Bergstrand A, Bollgren I, Samuelson A. Idiopathic nephrotic syndrome of childhood. Cyclophosphamide induced conversion from steroid refractory to highly steroid sensitive disease. *Clin Nephrol* 1973;1:302–306.
121. White RHR, Glasgow EF. Focal glomerulosclerosis. A progressive lesion associated with steroid resistant nephrotic syndrome. *Arch Dis Child* 1971;46:877–886.
122. Cameron JS, Chantler C, Ogg CS, White RHR. A long term stability of remission in nephrotic syndrome after treatment with cyclophosphamide. *BMJ* 1974;4:7–11.
123. Tejani A, Nicastri AD, Sen D, et al. Long-term evaluation of children with nephrotic syndrome and focal segmental glomerular sclerosis. *Nephron* 1983;35:225–231.
124. Elhence R, Gulati S, Kher V, et al. Intravenous pulse cyclophosphamide—a new regime for steroid-resistant minimal change nephrotic syndrome. *Pediatr Nephrol* 1994;8:1–3
125. Rennert WP, Kala UK, Jacobs D, et al. Pulse cyclophosphamide for steroid-resistant focal segmental glomerulosclerosis. *Pediatr Nephrol* 1999;13:113–116.
126. Hsu AC, Folami AO, Bain J, Rance CP. Gonadal functions in males treated with cyclophosphamide for nephrotic syndrome. *Fertil Steril* 1979;31:173–177.
127. Trompeter RS, Evans PR, Barratt TM. Gonadal function in boys with steroid responsive nephrotic syndrome treated with cyclophosphamide for short periods. *Lancet* 1981;1:1177–1179.
128. Buchanan JD, Fairley KF, Barris JU. Return of spermatogenesis after stopping cyclophosphamide therapy. *Lancet* 1975;ii:156–157.
129. Baluarte HJ, Gruskin AB, Polinski MS, et al. Chlorambucil therapy in the nephrotic syndrome. In: Gruskin AB, Norman ME. *Pediatric nephrology: proceedings of the Fifth International Pediatric Nephrology Symposium.* Boston: Martinus Nijhoff, 1980:423–429.
130. Williams SA, Makker SP, Ingelfinger JR, Grupe WE. Long-term evaluation of chlorambucil plus prednisone in the nephrotic syndrome of childhood. *BMJ* 1980;302: 929–933.
131. Müller W, Brandis M. Acute leukemia after cytotoxic treat-

ment for non malignant disease in childhood. *Eur J Pediatr* 1981;136:105–108.

132. Trompeter RS. Steroid resistant nephrotic syndrome: a review of the treatment of focal segmental glomerulosclerosis in children. In: Murakami K, Kitagawa T, Yabuta K, Sakai T, eds. *Recent advances in pediatric nephrology*. Amsterdam: Excerpta Medica, 1987:363–371.
133. Almeida MP, Almeida HA, Rosa FC. Vincristine in steroid resistant nephrotic syndrome. *Pediatr Nephrol* 1994;8:79–80.
134. Abramowicz M, Barnett HL, Edelmann CM Jr, et al. Controlled trial of azathioprine in children with nephrotic syndrome. A report for the international study of kidney disease in children. *Lancet* 1970;I:959–961.
135. Cade R, Mars D, Privette M, et al. Effect of long-term azathioprine administration in adults with minimal change glomerulonephritis and nephrotic syndrome resistant to corticosteroids. *Arch Intern Med* 1986;146:737–741.
136. Capodicasa G, de Santo NG, Nuzzi F, Giordano C. Cyclosporine A in nephrotic syndrome of childhood: a 14 month experience. *Int J Pediatr Nephrol* 1986;7:69–72.
137. Brandis M, Burghard R, Leititis J, et al. Cyclosporine A for treatment of nephrotic syndromes. *Transplant Proc* 1988;20: S275–S279.
138. Brodehl J, Hoyer PF, Oemar BS, et al. Cyclosporine treatment of nephrotic syndrome in childhood. *Transplant Proc* 1988;22:S269–S274.
139. Garin EH, Orak JK, Hiott KL, Sutherland SE. Cyclosporin therapy for steroid resistant nephrotic syndrome. A controlled study. *Am J Dis Child* 1988;142:985–988.
140. Niaudet P, Habib R, Tête MJ, et al. Cyclosporin in the treatment of idiopathic nephrotic syndrome in children. *Pediatr Nephrol* 1987;1:566–573.
141. Tejani A, Butt K, Trachtman H, et al. Cyclosporine induced remission of relapsing nephrotic syndrome in children. *J Pediatr* 1987;111:1056–1062.
142. Waldo FB, Kohaut EC. Therapy of focal segmental glomerulosclerosis with cyclosporine A. *Pediatr Nephrol* 1987;1:180–182.
143. Niaudet P, Habib R. Cyclosporine in the treatment of idiopathic nephrosis. *J Am Soc Nephrol* 1994;5:1049–1056.
144. Collaborative Study Group of Sandimmun in Nephrotic Syndrome. Safety and tolerability of cyclosporine A (Sandimmun) in idiopathic nephrotic syndrome. *Clin Nephrol* 1991;35:S48–S60.
145. Niaudet P and The French Society of Pediatric Nephrology. Treatment of childhood steroid resistant idiopathic nephrosis with a combination of cyclosporine and prednisone. *J Pediatr* 1994;125:981–985.
146. Ingulli E, Singh A, Baqi N, et al. Aggressive, long-term cyclosporine therapy for steroid-resistant focal segmental glomerulosclerosis. *J Am Soc Nephrol* 1995;5:1820–1825.
147. Ponticelli C, Rizzoni G, Edefonti A, et al. A randomized trial of cyclosporine in steroid-resistant idiopathic nephrotic syndrome. *Kidney Int* 1993;43:1377–1384.
148. Lieberman K, Tejani A for the New York-New Jersey Pediatric Nephrology Collaborative Study Group. A randomized double blind placebo-controlled trial of cyclosporine in steroid resistant idiopathic focal segmental glomerulosclerosis in children. *J Am Soc Nephrol* 1996;7:56–63.
149. Gregory MJ, Smoyer WE, Sedman A, et al. TE Long-term cyclosporine therapy for pediatric nephrotic syndrome: a clinical and histologic analysis. *J Am Soc Nephrol* 1996;7:543–549.
150. Singh A, Tejani C, Tejani A. One-center experience with cyclosporine in refractory nephrotic syndrome in children. *Pediatr Nephrol* 1999;13:26–32.
151. Niaudet P, Broyer M. Cyclosporin in the therapy of idiopathic nephrotic syndrome in children. In: Andreucci VE, ed. *International yearbook of nephrology*. Boston: Kluwer Academic Publishers, 1989:155–168.
152. Clasen W, Kindler J, Mihatsch MJ, Sieberth HG. Long-term treatment of minimal change nephrotic syndrome with cyclosporin: a control biopsy study. *Nephrol Dial Transplant* 1988;3:733–737.
153. Habib R, Niaudet P. Comparison between pre- and post-treatment renal biopsies in children receiving ciclosporine for idiopathic nephrosis. *Clin Nephrol* 1994;42:141–146.
154. Mc Cauley J, Shapiro R, Ellis D, et al. Pilot trial of FK 506 in the management of steroid resistant nephrotic syndrome. *Nephrol Dial Transplant* 1993;8:1286–1290.
155. Donker AJM, Brentjens JRH, Van der Hem GK. Treatment of the nephrotic syndrome with indomethacin. *Nephron* 1978;22:374–381.
156. Velosa JA, Torres VE. Benefits and risks of nonsteroidal antiinflammatory drugs in steroid resistant nephrotic syndrome. *Am J Kidney Dis* 1986;8:345–350.
157. Bennett WM. The adverse renal effects of nonsteroidal anti-inflammatory drugs: increasing problems or overrated risk. *Am J Kidney Dis* 1983;2:477.
158. Clive DM, Stoff JS. Renal syndrome associated with nonsteroidal antiinflammatory drugs. *BMJ* 1984;310:563–572.
159. Kleinknecht C, Broyer M, Gubler MC. Irreversible renal failure after indomethacin in steroid-resistant nephrosis. *BMJ* 1980;302:691.
160. Martinez-Vea A, Garciaruiz C, Carrera M, et al. Effect of captopril in nephrotic range proteinuria due to renovascular hypertension. *Nephron* 1987;45:162–163.
161. Ferder LF, Inserra F, Daccordi H, Smith RD. Enalapril improved renal function and proteinuria in chronic glomerulonephritis. *Nephron* 1990;55:S90–S95.
162. Milliner D, Morgenstern BZ. Angiotensin converting enzyme inhibitor for reduction of proteinuria in children with steroid resistant nephrotic syndrome. *Pediatr Nephrol* 1991;5:587–590.
163. Senggutuvan P, Cameron JS, Hartley RB. Recurrence of focal segmental glomerulosclerosis in transplanted kidneys: analysis of incidence and risk factors in 59 allografts. *Pediatr Nephrol* 1990;4:21–28.
164. Gagnadoux MF, Broyer M, Habib R. Transplantation in children with idiopathic nephrosis. In: Murakami K, Kitagawa T, Yabuta K, Sakai T, eds. *Recent advances in pediatric nephrology*. New York: Excerpta Medica, 1987;351–356.
165. Rizzoni G, Ehrich JHH, Bunner FP, et al. Combined report on regular dialysis and transplantation of children in Europe, 1990. *Nephrol Dial Transplant* 1991;6:31–42.
166. Habib R, Hebert D, Gagnadoux MF, Broyer M. Transplantation in idiopathic nephrosis. *Transpl Proc* 1982;14:489–495.
167. Leumann EP, Briner J, Donckerwolcke RA, et al. Recurrence of focal segmental glomerulosclerosis in the transplant kidney. *Nephron* 1980;25:65–71.

168. Pinto J, Lacerda G, Cameron JS, et al. Recurrence of focal segmental glomerulosclerosis in renal allografts. *Transplantation* 1981;32:83–89.
169. Maizel SE, Sibley RK, Horstman JP, et al. Incidence and significance of recurrent focal segmental glomerulosclerosis in renal allograft recipients. *Transplantation* 1981;32:512–516.
170. Striegel JE, Sibley RK, Fryd DS, Mauer SM. Recurrence of focal segmental sclerosis in children following renal transplantation. *Kidney Int* 1986;30:S44–S50.
171. Cameron JS. Recurrent primary disease and de novo nephritis following renal transplantation. *Pediatr Nephrol* 1991;5:412–421.
172. Ramos EL, Tisher CC. Recurrent diseases in the kidney transplant. *Am J Kidney Dis* 1994;24:142–154.
173. Stephanian E, Matas AJ, Mauer SM, et al. Recurrence of disease in patients retransplanted for focal segmental glomerulosclerosis. *Transplantation* 1992;53:755–757.
174. Kim EM, Striegel J, Kim Y, et al. Recurrence of steroid-resistant nephrotic syndrome in kidney transplants is associated with increased acute renal failure and acute rejection. *Kidney Int* 1994;45:1440–1445.
175. Korbet SM, Schwartz MM, Edmund JL. Recurrent nephrotic syndrome in renal allograft. *Am J Kidney Dis* 1988;11:270–276.
176. Morales JM, Andres A, Prieto C, et al. Clinical and histological sequence of recurrent focal and segmental glomerulosclerosis. *Nephron* 1988;48:241–242.
177. Verani RR, Hawkins EP. Recurrent focal segmental glomerulosclerosis: a pathologic study of the early lesion. *Am J Nephrol* 1986;6:263–270.
178. Dantal J, Baatard R, Hourmant M, et al. Recurrent nephrotic syndrome following renal transplantation in patients with focal glomerulosclerosis: a one-center study of plasma exchange effects. *Transplantation* 1991;52;827–831.
179. Artero M, Biava C, Amend W, et al. Recurrent focal glomerulosclerosis: natural history and response to therapy. *Am J Med* 1992;92:375–383.
180. Banfi M, Colturi C, Montagnino G, Ponticelli C. The recurrence of focal segmental glomerulosclerosis in kidney transplant patients treated with cyclosporine. *Transplantation* 1990;50:594–596.
181. Pirson Y, Squifflet JP, Marbaix E, et al. Recurrence of focal glomerulosclerosis despite cyclosporin treatment after renal transplantation. *BMJ* 1986;292:1336.
182. Schwarz A, Krause PH, Offermann G, Keller F. Recurrent and de novo renal disease after renal transplantation with or without cyclosporine. *Am J Kidney Dis* 1991;17:524–531.
183. Vincenti F, Biava C, Tomalanovitch S, et al. Inability of cyclosporine to completely prevent the recurrence of focal glomerulosclerosis after kidney transplantation. *Transplantation* 1989;47:595–598.
184. Voets AJ, Hoitsma AJ, Koene RAP. Recurrence of nephrotic syndrome during cyclosporin treatment after renal transplantation. *Lancet* 1986;i:266–267.
185. Mowry J, Marik J, Cohen A, et al. Treatment of recurrent focal segmental glomerulosclerosis with high dose cyclosporine and plasmapheresis. *Transplant Proc* 1993;25:1345–1346.
186. Ingulli E, Tejani A, Butt KM, et al. High-dose cyclosporine therapy in recurrent nephrotic syndrome following renal transplantation. *Transplantation* 1990;49:219–221.
187. Srivastava RN, Kalia A, Travis LB, et al. Prompt remission of post-renal transplant nephrotic syndrome with high-dose cyclosporine. *Pediatr Nephrol* 1994;8:94–95.
188. Salomon R, Gagnadoux MF, Niaudet P. Intravenous cyclosporine therapy in recurrent nephrotic syndrome following renal transplantation in children. *Transplantation* 2003;75:810–814.
189. MacCauley J, Shapiro R, Jordan M, et al. FK506 in the management of nephrotic syndrome after renal transplantation. *Transplant Proc* 1993;25:1351–1354.
190. Artero ML, Sharma R, Savin VJ, Vincenti F. Plasmapheresis reduces proteinuria and serum capacity to injure glomeruli in patients with recurrent focal glomerulosclerosis. *Am J Kidney Dis* 1994;23:574–581.
191. Cochat P, Kassir A, Colon S, et al. Recurrent nephrotic syndrome after transplantation: early treatment with plasmaphaeresis and cyclophosphamide. *Pediatr Nephrol* 1993;7:50–54.
192. Dantal J, Baatard R, Hourmant M, et al. Recurrent nephrotic syndrome following renal transplantation in patients with focal glomerulosclerosis. A one-center study of plasma exchange effects. *Transplantation* 1991;52:827–831.
193. Li PKT, MacMoune LF, Leung CB, et al. Plasma exchange in the treatment of early recurrent focal glomerulosclerosis after renal transplantation. Report and review. *Am J Nephrol* 1993;13:289–292.
194. Munoz J, Sanchez M, Perez-Garcia R, et al. Recurrent focal glomerulosclerosis in renal transplants proteinuria relapsing following plasma exchange. *Clin Nephrol* 1985;24:213–214.
195. Solomon LR, Cairns SA, Lawler W, et al. Reduction of post-transplant proteinuria due to recurrent mesangial proliferative (IgM) glomerulonephritis following plasma exchange. *Clin Nephrol* 1981;16:44–50.
196. Zimmerman SW. Plasmapheresis and dipyridamole for recurrent focal glomerular sclerosis. *Nephron* 1985;40:241–245.
197. Cameron JS. The enigma of focal segmental glomerulosclerosis. *Kidney Int* 1996;50:S119–S131.

29

IMMUNE MECHANISMS OF GLOMERULAR INJURY

ALLISON A. EDDY

OVERVIEW

Immunologic pathways initiate and propagate glomerular injury. Over the past decade, major advances in cellular, molecular, genetic, and immunologic sciences have provided significant new insights into the pathogenesis of glomerulonephritis. For the purpose of review, the immunopathogenic mechanisms can be divided into two basic phases. Primary mechanisms of glomerulonephritis focus on those events that initiate glomerular injury. These initial events alone rarely produce significant and sustained damage. The role of the humoral immune system, dependent on B lymphocyte activation and antibody production, has been recognized for nearly a century (Fig. 29.1). Although two distinct antibody-mediated pathways have been proposed, current evidence suggests that antibody interaction with antigens *in situ* within the glomerulus (which may or may not lead to the formation of immune complexes) predominates, whereas glomerular trapping of immune complexes preformed within the circulation occurs rarely, if ever. The cellular immune system, dependent on T-lymphocyte activation, occasionally triggers glomerular injury. However, for many glomerular diseases, separation of B-cell and T-cell pathways is rather artificial as the cellular and humoral effector limbs of the immune system often collaborate.

The secondary immune mechanisms of glomerular injury implicate cascades of inflammatory mediators that are recruited to propagate renal damage after the primary glomerular attack. Some of these mediators play essential roles; others may modify disease severity, but their participation is not essential. The secondary mediators are variable depending on the nature of the primary injury, but they often include lymphohemopoietic cells [polymorphonuclear leukocytes (PMNs), monocytes, and platelets] and activated components of the complement cascade. Resident glomerular endothelial cells, mesangial cells, and epithelial cells may be activated and further contribute to the inflammatory response. Most of the secondary mediators that have been identified are products of lymphohemopoietic cells or resident glomerular cells and include cytokines and growth factors, reactive oxygen metabolites, bioactive lipids [platelet-activating factor (PAF) and eicosanoids], proteases, and vasoactive substances [endothelin (ET) and nitric oxide (NO)]. It is hoped that by understanding the immunopathogenesis of glomerulonephritis, new therapeutic strategies will emerge. Furthermore, future genetic studies may find that genotype-dependent expression and/or activity levels of certain key mediators predict risk and severity of glomerulonephritis.

STRUCTURE OF THE GLOMERULAR CAPILLARY WALL AND MESANGIUM

A basic understanding of the architecture of the glomerulus is necessary to appreciate the basis of the dynamic interactions between intrinsic components of the glomerular capillary wall and mesangium and the blood-borne mediators of glomerular injury. The *glomerular basement membrane* (GBM) is a specialized extracellular matrix lined by the endothelial and visceral epithelial cells. It acts as a filtration barrier with selective permeability, allowing passage of small plasma molecules but almost completely restricting filtration of molecules larger than albumin. It also plays a more dynamic role regulating the adhesion and behavior of adherent cells. Chemical analyses have shown the GBM to be 80% collagenous proteins, primarily collagen IV (α_3, α_4, and α_5 chains). A number of the other components have been identified such as laminin-11 and entactin/nidogen (1). The GBM also contains proteoglycans, the most abundant of which is agrin. Although constituting only 1% of the dry weight of the GBM, these anionic components contribute significantly to the charge-selective properties of the ultrafiltration unit. The onset of proteinuria is usually characterized by a loss of charge as well as size selectivity. At least four theories have been proposed to explain the alterations in the GBM charge: masking by immune complexes, depolymerization by oxygen radicals, alterations in proteoglycan synthesis, and proteolytic diges-

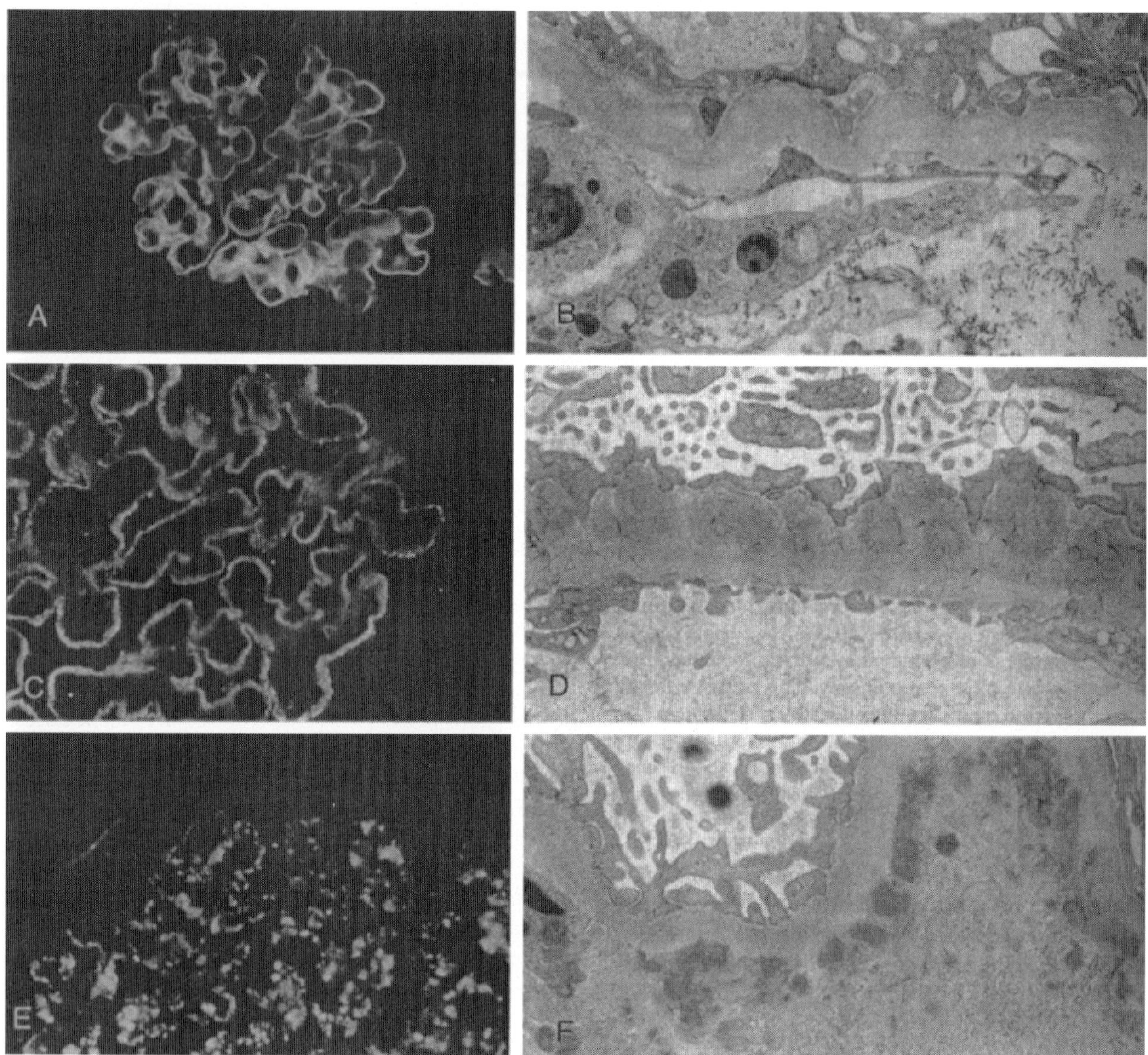

FIGURE 29.1. Immunofluorescence and electron microscopic features of three distinct patterns of immune-mediated glomerular injury. In anti–glomerular basement membrane (GBM) nephritis, immunoglobulin G (IgG) is deposited in a linear pattern along the GBM **(A)**. Although dense immune deposits are not detected by electron microscopy, there may be expanded lucent subendothelial areas **(B)**. Membranous nephropathy is characterized by granular deposits of IgG and C3 **(C)** along the epithelial aspect of the glomerular capillary wall, which correspond to the subepithelial deposits present on electron microscopy **(D)**. Immune complex–induced glomerulonephritis, illustrated by the renal biopsy of a patient with lupus nephritis, is characterized by the deposition of immunoglobulins and complement **(E)** along the glomerular capillary wall and within the mesangium. Electron microscopy reveals electron-dense deposits in similar locations **(F)**.

tion (2). On the other hand, exactly how erythrocytes traverse the GBM remains enigmatic. A recent ultrastructural study suggests that they may traverse through gaps in the GBM (3).

The *mesangium*, the region occupying the centrolobular position between the mesangial cells and the perimesangial basement membrane, is similar in composition but not identical to the peripheral GBM. It consists of a dense network of microfibrils; fibronectin appears to be the most abundant component. During the filtration process, some plasma enters the mesangial zone, gaining access through the mesangial "waist" or "angle," bypassing the GBM. Circulating immune complexes commonly become lodged in this area.

The intrinsic glomerular cells—specialized epithelial cells (podocytes), mesangial cells, and endothelial cells—play an active role in the regulation of both normal physiologic processes and pathologic states. *Mesangial cells* have

TABLE 29.1. GLOMERULAR MATRIX ADHESION MOLECULES

	Matrix ligand	Glomerular expression		
		Mesangial	Epithelial	Endothelial
β_1 integrins (VLA family of lymphocytes antigens)				
α_1	Laminin, collagens I and IV	+	–	+
α_2	Laminin, collagens I and IV	+	+	+
α_3	Fibronectin, laminin, collagen, entactin	+	+	+
α_5	Fibronectin, RGD peptide	+	–	+
α_8	Fibronectin, vitronectin, tenascin	+	–	–
β_3 integrins				
α_v	Vitronectin, fibronectin, fibrinogen	+	–	+
β_5 integrins				
α_v	Vitronectin, fibronectin	+	+	–

+, present; –, absent; RGD, arginine, glycine, aspartate, amino acid sequence; VLA, very late antigen.

smooth muscle cell–like characteristics and attach to the GBM at several sites. Consequently, mesangial cell contraction modifies glomerular filtration. In response to injury, these cells may change phenotypically, and presumably functionally, by expression of additional smooth muscle cell proteins such as α smooth muscle actin, desmin, and calponin and matrix-binding integrin receptors (Table 29.1) (4,5). Mesangial cells express receptors that may actively engage in antibody-mediated glomerular injury: receptors for the Fc fragment of immunoglobulin G (IgG) (FcγRIII or CD16) and IgA.

Mesangial cell proliferation, a common feature of glomerulonephritis, may replenish cells depleted by mesangiolysis, but proliferation may also have pathologic consequences by enhancing the production of proinflammatory and profibrotic substances. Most proliferating mesangial cells are resident glomerular cells, but precursor cells may also migrate in from the extraglomerular mesangium within the juxtaglomerular apparatus and from the bone marrow (6–8). Given the close association between mesangial hypercellularity and glomerular injury, understanding the mechanisms that regulate their number is important. Proliferation is controlled at multiple levels: mitogens and their receptors, intracellular signaling pathways, and intranuclear events. Many proteins are mesangial cell mitogens including platelet-derived growth factor (PDGF)-B and -C, insulin-like growth factor-1, epidermal growth factor (EGF), transforming growth factor α (TGFα), low-dose TGFβ, basic fibroblast growth factor (FGF), chemokines, insulin, interleukin-1 (IL-1), tumor necrosis factor (TNF), ET, serotonin, bradykinin, vasopressin, thrombin, fibronectin, and prostaglandin (PG)$F_2\alpha$.

Recent studies have identified several nuclear proteins that tightly regulate the mesangial cell cycle at multiple levels (Fig. 29.2). Their actions ultimately determine whether the retinoblastoma protein, a negative cell-cycle regulator, will be inactivated by phosphorylation. With retinoblastoma protein inactivation, transcription factors of the E2F family are released to promote transcription of several cell-cycle proteins that promote mitosis (9). Cell-cycle inhibitory agents such as E2F decoy oligonucleotides and cyclin-dependent kinase inhibitors have been used experimentally to prevent mesangial cell proliferation after immunologic injury, with beneficial outcomes (10,11).

Mesangial cells may produce several products that may contribute to acute and chronic glomerular damage such as vasoactive hormones (renin, angiotensin II, vasopressin, ET), bioactive lipids (PGs, leukotrienes, PAF), peptide growth factors and cytokines (PDGF, IL-1α, IL-1β, insulin-like growth factor-1, IL-8), matrix proteins (mainly collagen I but also types III, IV, and V; laminin; and fibronectin), glycosaminoglycans, thrombospondin, procoagulants, fibrinolytic factors (plasminogen activators), proteinases, and reactive oxygen species (ROS). Megsin is a recently identified serine protease inhibitor that is produced primarily by mesangial

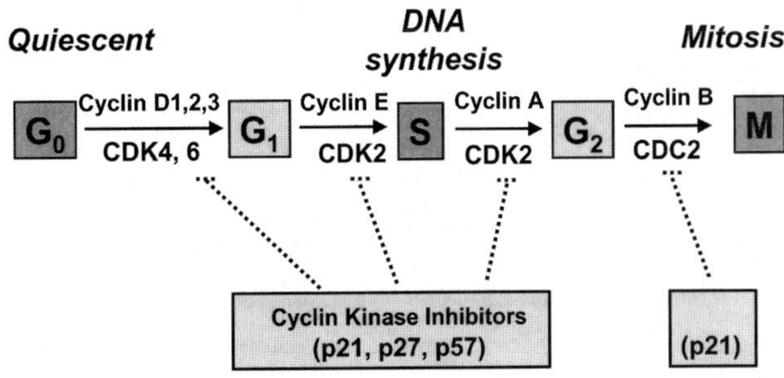

FIGURE 29.2. Cell-cycle regulatory proteins in glomerular cell proliferation. Cellular proliferation is characterized by the orderly progression of cells through sequential phases from the quiescence (G_0), resting (G_1), DNA synthesis (S), resting (G_2), and mitosis (M). Each step is regulated by cell-cycle proteins (cyclins) that bind and activate cyclin-dependent kinases (CDK). Each step may be blocked by negative cell-cycle proteins, CDK inhibitors. Recent studies indicate that the several CDK inhibitors are expressed in normal glomeruli and play a major role in the regulation of the glomerular cell proliferative responses to mitogens produced during injury. CDK inhibition has been shown to decrease mesangial cell proliferation, decrease matrix expansion, and improve renal function in rats with Thy 1 nephritis (11). (Courtesy of Dr. Stuart Shankland, University of Washington).

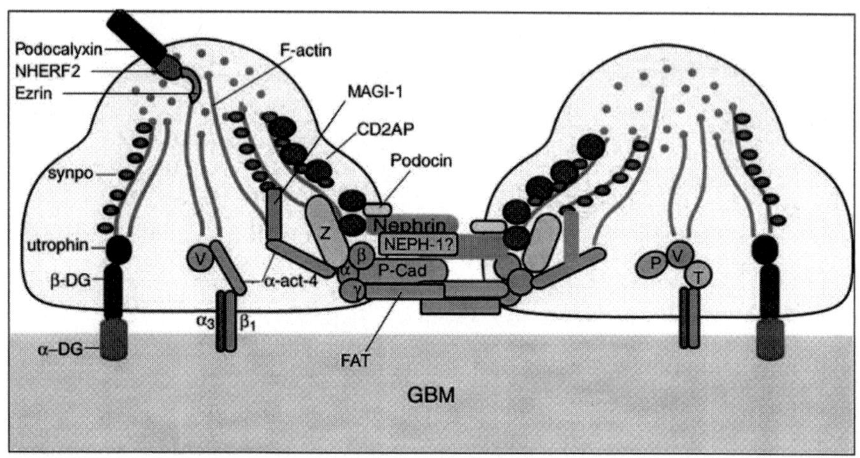

FIGURE 29.3. Molecular anatomy of the glomerular podocyte. The basal sole plate of the podocyte approximates the glomerular basement membrane (GBM) and is directly attached to it in areas of focal contact via $\alpha_3\beta_1$ integrin receptors and the α,β dystroglycan (α-, β-DG) complex. Adjacent podocytes are joined laterally by a modified adherens junction of "slit diaphragms." Genetic mutations in several slit diaphragm–associated proteins cause inherited nephrotic syndrome, including nephrin, CD2AP, podocin, and the nephrin homologue neph-1. The apical membrane extending from the slit diaphragm into Bowman's space is covered with an anionic glycoprotein coat made predominantly of podocalyxin. Each of these domains is connected to the intracellular actin cytoskeleton that functions to maintain podocyte structural integrity. The complexity of the contractile apparatus has become appreciated with the identification of several key subcomponents that interact with actin, including myosin II, α-actinin-4 (α-act-4), talin (T), vinculin (V), and synaptopodin (synpo). MAGI-1, membrane-associated guanylate kinase inverted-1; NHERF2, NA^+/H^+ exchanger regulatory factor 2; P, paxillin; P-Cad, P-cadherin. (From Mundel M, Shankland SL. Podocyte biology and response to injury. *J Am Soc Nephrol* 2002;13:3005–3015, with permission.)

cells and is associated with mesangial proliferation and matrix expansion when overproduced (12).

Glomerular *podocytes* serve several functions such as pinocytosis of proteins that have leaked through the GBM, synthesis of GBM matrix proteins, and restriction of passage of proteins at the level of the slit diaphragm. Epithelial cells synthesize many biologically active products, including extracellular matrix proteins [type IV collagen, heparan sulfate proteoglycan (HSPG), fibronectin], cyclooxygenase (COX), and lipoxygenase products; urokinase-type plasminogen activator and plasminogen activator inhibitor-1; and antioxidant enzymes, IL-1, and angiopoietin-1. Podocytes express C3b/C4b and Fc receptors that may interact directly with immune complexes. The outer podocyte cell membrane is differentiated into three structurally and functionally distinct regions that are illustrated in Figure 29.3 (13).

The functional hallmark of glomerular injury is proteinuria. The filtration barrier of the glomerular capillary wall is regulated at the level of the GBM and the slit diaphragm. Perturbations of podocyte slit diaphragm function underlie most if not all types of glomerulonephritis and are often associated with significant structural changes as well, namely, foot-process retraction or effacement. The cellular processes that cause foot-process effacement remain to be elucidated, but they may recapitulate embryonic development in reverse and an uncoupling of the actin cytoskeleton from membrane functional domains (13,14). Proteinuria can be rapidly induced in animals by injection of antibodies to slit diaphragm proteins such as nephrin (15). A parallel process has been observed in some congenital nephrotic syndrome patients who develop nephrotic syndrome after renal transplantation in association with antinephrin antibody production. In many glomerular diseases, podocytes completely detach from the GBM and are shed into the urinary space (16). Unlike mesangial cells, glomerular podocytes are terminally differentiated cells that, with a few exceptions, fail to proliferate in response to injury. The reasons for this are not yet entirely clear. Highly differentiated podocytes express high levels of cyclin-dependent kinase inhibitors, p21, p27, and p57 (Fig. 29.2). A proliferative phenotype can be restored by genetic deficiency of p21 or p27 (17,18). However, the complete answer to this question is likely to be more complex with evidence that injured podocytes can enter the cell cycle but arrest at the G2/M phase. This failure to proliferate and self-replenish is problematic, as podocyte loss is now recognized as a harbinger of progressive glomerular sclerosis (19).

Glomerular *endothelial cells* line the capillary wall. These cells assume a flattened profile and are densely perforated by transendothelial pores or fenestrae, water channels that may permit direct size-dependent access of blood-borne factors to the basement membrane (20). Endothelial cells can proliferate (21). Their integrity after renal injury is partially maintained by vascular endothelial growth factor (VEGF) and angiopoi-

TABLE 29.2. ENDOTHELIAL LEUKOCYTE ADHESION MOLECULES IN EXPERIMENTAL GLOMERULONEPHRITIS

Family	Member	Primary cellular distribution	Ligand
Selectins	L-selectin (leukocyte)	PMN, Mϕ, lymphocytes	Mucins (e.g., addressin, CD34, Gly-CAM)
	P-selectin (platelet)	Platelets, activated endothelium	Mucins (e.g., sLe^x)
	E-selectin (endothelial)	Activated endothelium	Mucins (e.g., sLe^x)
β_1 integrins (VLA proteins)	$\alpha_4\beta_1$ (VLA-4)	Mϕ, lymphocytes, eosinophils ± PMN	VCAM-1, fibronectin
β_2 (leukocyte) integrins	CD11a/CD18 (LFA-1)	All leukocytes	ICAM-1, 2, 3
	CD11b/CD18 (Mac-1)	PMN, Mϕ	ICAM-1, C3bi, fibrinogen, factor X
	CD11c/CD18 (p150, 95)	PMN, Mϕ	ICAM-1
	CD11d/CD18	Mϕ subset	?
IgG-like	ICAM-1 (CD54)	Endothelium, some leukocytes, mesangial cells	β_2 integrins
	ICAM-2	Endothelium, some leukocytes	CD11a/CD18
	ICAM-3 (CD50)	All leukocytes	?
	VCAM-1	Activated endothelium, glomerular parietal epithelium, ± mesangial cells	$\alpha_4\beta_1$ (VLA-4)

Gly-CAM, glycosylation-dependent cell adhesion mococule-1; ICAM, intercellular adhesion molecule; LFA, lymphocyte function-associated antigen; Mϕ, monocytes/macrophages; PMN, polymorphonuclear leukocytes; sLe, sialyl Lewis; VCAM, vascular cell adhesion molecule; VLA, very late antigen.

etin-1 that bind to their endothelial receptors, Flk-1 and Tie-2, respectively (22). Angiopoietin-2 also binds to the Tie-2 receptor, but it antagonizes and destabilizes capillary integrity (23). Glomerular endothelial cells appear unique in many respects compared to endothelial cells of other origin. Although less extensively studied than other glomerular cells, they also undergo specific alterations in structure, function, and metabolism during glomerular injury, making them active participants in injurious and reparative processes. Endothelial cells synthesize several coagulation proteins, growth factors, and cytokines; extracellular matrix proteins; and vasoactive molecules. The surface of endothelial cells expresses angiotensin-converting enzyme (ACE) and ET-converting enzymes that catalyze the formation of the vasoconstrictors angiotensin II and mature ET, respectively. They may express several different adhesion molecules that promote interactions with blood-borne leukocytes, platelets, and the third component of complement (Table 29.2). Other functions include synthesis of reactive oxygen metabolites and the potential to serve as antigen-presenting cells.

Cellular interactions with the GBM and extracellular matrix play an essential role in maintaining glomerular integrity and function. Among the numerous cell-matrix adhesion molecules, those of the β_1 integrin family of membrane glycoproteins (also known as *very late antigens*) have been most extensively studied in the glomerulus (Table 29.1). The β_1 chain associates with one of 12 different α chains, the most abundant glomerular isoform being $\alpha_3\beta_1$. In addition to maintaining glomerular capillary wall integrity, integrins can function as classical signal-transducing receptors to initiate a variety of cellular responses that may play a role in the glomerular response to injury: mitogenesis and synthesis of matrix proteins, reactive oxygen metabolites, and arachidonic acid (AA) metabolites. The identification of anti–β_1 integrin antibodies in polyclonal antisera against the tubular brush-border fraction Fx1A and GBM, which induce proteinuria in experimental animals, suggests that integrins play an important role in maintaining the permselectivity of the glomerular capillary wall. Recent studies suggest the $\alpha_1\beta_1$ may also play an important role in extracellular matrix remodeling during progressive glomerulosclerosis (24,25).

HUMORAL IMMUNE MECHANISMS OF INDUCTION OF GLOMERULAR INJURY

Antibody-mediated glomerular injury is the result of a B-lymphocyte–driven immune response. B-lymphocyte activation requires T-lymphocyte participation. The fact that helper T lymphocytes recognize antigen in the context of major histocompatibility complex (MHC) class II antigens (HLA DR in humans) has led to speculation that the risk of developing immune-mediated glomerulonephritis may be linked to the inheritance of certain MHC class II genes. Although beyond the scope of this review, several studies have suggested an association between various DR antigens and the risk of developing anti-GBM nephritis, IgA nephropathy, membranous nephropathy, and lupus nephritis (26–28).

Interaction of Antibodies with Intrinsic Matrix Components of the Glomerular Extracellular Matrix

Normal structural components of the GBM may be the target of an autoantibody attack leading to the development of anti-GBM nephritis, which in humans may occur with

(Goodpasture syndrome) or without pulmonary involvement. Experimentally, anti-GBM nephritis is induced by passive administration of heterologous antibodies (nephrotoxic serum nephritis) or by active immunization with heterologous GBM in an immunologic adjuvant (experimental autoimmune glomerulonephritis).

Glomerular Basement Membrane

The GBM target antigen(s) in the classic experimental model of nephrotoxic serum (or Masugi) nephritis has not been completely elucidated and is likely multiple. In contrast, the dominant human Goodpasture antigen is known to be part of the collagen IV molecule, and it has been further localized to a conformation-dependent epitope residing within the amino-terminal noncollagenous NC-1 globular domain of α3(IV) collagen (29,30). The gene encoding α3(IV) collagen is located in the q35-37 region of chromosome 2. Immunization with antibodies to α3(IV) collagen or dimers of α3(IV) induces mild nephritis in animals. Less common, other components of the GBM may also serve as antibody targets. In general, immunization with collagen IV, laminin, fibronectin, and HSPG or administration of their specific antisera alone produces minor morphologic changes without proteinuria, although more severe disease has occasionally been reported.

Anti-GBM antibodies may play a role in other forms of glomerulonephritis. For example, patients with poststreptococcal glomerulonephritis may develop circulating antibodies to type IV collagen, laminin, entactin/nidogen, and HSPG. Anti-DNA antibodies isolated from the sera of patients with systemic lupus erythematosus (SLE) cross-react with HSPG and type IV collagen, probably via antibody-bound DNA-histone complexes. Humans with X-linked dominant hereditary nephritis lack the α_5 chain of collagen IV, a gene that is encoded in the Xq region of the X chromosome. This genetic defect results in a secondary failure of α_3 and α_4 collagen IV chains to be integrated into the GBM. Primary mutations in the genes that encode the α_3 and α_4 chains of collagen IV are responsible for autosomal recessive hereditary nephritis. After renal transplantation, approximately 2 to 4% of the Alport syndrome recipients develop anti-GBM disease in the normal renal allograft due to the formation of anti-α_3, -α_4, and/or -α_5 collagen IV antibodies (31).

Mesangial Matrix

The antigenic composition of the mesangial matrix is similar to that of the GBM, yet it appears to be largely protected from immune attack in anti-GBM nephritis, presumably because the nephrotoxic antibodies bind avidly to the GBM before they gain access to the mesangium. It is possible that unique mesangial matrix antigens exist and are the target of immune attack. Injection of a monoclonal antibody to a rat mesangial matrix component (81 kDa) induces mesangial electron-dense deposit formation, although histologic changes and proteinuria do not develop. A glycoprotein [matrix metalloproteinase (MMP)-50/100] has been identified that is unique to rat glomerular mesangium, the expression of which is increased in several models of nephritis. A similar unique human mesangial antigen has been identified (32).

Antibody Interaction

After injection of heterologous anti-GBM antiserum (or nephrotoxic antiserum), the antibody binds to the GBM within minutes, gaining free access through the open glomerular endothelial fenestrae. By immunofluorescence microscopy, the antibody is observed in a linear pattern corresponding to the distribution of the GBM. Formation of electron-dense deposits along the glomerular capillary wall does not ensue (Fig. 29.1). Alterations in glomerular structure and function occur as a direct consequence of antibody binding to the GBM, leading to proteinuria and a decline in glomerular filtration rate (GFR). Ultrastructural changes include a rearrangement of GBM laminin, foot-process fusion, loss of GBM anionic–binding sites, and evidence of cellular injury. Some of these changes may be induced by the interaction of the antiserum with glomerular epithelial cell antigens such as the β_1 integrins and aminopeptidase A (33).

Secondary Mediators

Although antibody binding alone causes some alterations in glomerular structure and function, additional mediators are needed for the full expression of the injury, otherwise the initial damage subsides after 24 hours. This subsequent period of glomerular inflammation is associated with the infiltration of PMNs, chemoattracted by complement proteins C5a and C3b generated by interactions with the anti-GBM antibody. Depletion of PMNs or complement prevents proteinuria. There is some evidence that the membrane attack complex (MAC) of complement also plays a role in mediating cellular damage. In experimental models of anti-GBM nephritis induced by heterologous antiserum, a second phase of glomerular inflammation develops 5 to 7 days later as a result of the production of antibodies by the immunized animal (autologous antibodies) to the heterologous antibody, which is now acting as a foreign antigen planted along the GBM. In addition to antibody complement–induced damage, other mechanisms of injury are now recognized. T cells sensitized to GBM antigens play an important role and may even cause severe glomerulonephritis in the absence of nephritogenic antibodies (34). The complement-binding domain of IgG (as opposed to the antigen-binding domain) may also interact directly with mesangial cells, podocytes, and inflammatory cells through interactions with Fc receptors. Studies in mice demonstrated that deficiency of the γ chain (shared by Fc receptors

I, II, and III) was associated with significantly milder anti-GBM nephritis (35).

Interaction of Antibodies with Glomerular Cell–Surface Antigens

Experimental models involving the binding of antibodies to cell-surface antigens have now been described for the three cell types intrinsic to the glomerulus. Antibody attack is directed to the epithelial cells in Heymann nephritis and in glomerular diseases associated with the anti–slit diaphragm antibodies, to mesangial cells in anti–Thy 1 disease, and to endothelial cells when animals are injected with antibodies to ACE and possibly with antineutrophil cytoplasmic antibodies (ANCA). These interactions may produce glomerular injury associated with the formation of immune complexes (*in situ*) or associated with perturbations in normal cellular function but without the formation of immune complexes. Knowledge gained from investigation of these experimental models has revolutionized thinking about the immunopathogenesis of glomerular injury. *In situ* mechanisms now appear to play the dominant role in most forms of human glomerulonephritis.

Podocytes

The model of Heymann nephritis has been extensively studied because it resembles human membranous nephropathy (Fig. 29.1). Heymann nephritis can be induced in susceptible strains of rats by active immunization with the antigen. Proteinuria develops by 8 to 10 weeks in 30 to 80% of the immunized animals. A similar lesion can also be induced passively by injection of the appropriate antibody, producing proteinuria within 5 days.

Nephritogenic Antigen

Extensive work by several investigators has determined that the primary target antigen is a large 517-kDa glycoprotein named *megalin* (previously called *glycoprotein gp330* and *gp600*) (36). Megalin, a member of the low-density lipoprotein receptor gene family, is an endocytosis receptor for multiple ligands such as plasminogen, plasminogen activator complexes, apolipoprotein E–enriched β very-low-density lipoprotein, lipoprotein lipase, clusterin/apolipoprotein J, retinol-binding protein, insulin, β_2 microglobulin, thyroglobulin, and certain polybasic drugs, to name a few. Megalin is also present on other epithelial cells, including the brush border of proximal tubules where it serves an important role in albumin reabsorption, pneumocytes, and ependymal cells in the brain. Mice that lack megalin develop abnormalities in the kidneys, lungs, and central nervous system, and most die of respiratory failure shortly after birth. A second antigen is involved, a 44-kDa protein known as *RAP* (receptor-associated protein). This protein is homologous to human low-density lipoprotein receptor–related protein/α_2-macroglobulin receptor. RAP associates with megalin and may function in a regulatory role to control megalin-ligand interactions. Purified antibodies to either megalin or RAP induce subepithelial immune complex formation, but neither antibody alone produces the full renal disease spectrum that was first observed by Edgington and colleagues when they injected polyclonal anti-Fx1A antiserum into rats (36a). This has led to the notion that other antigen-antibody interactions may also be involved. Candidates include antibodies to dipeptidyl peptidase IV, β_1 integrin, laminin, and antibodies to complement regulatory proteins, Crry and CD59. The nephritogenic antigen(s) in idiopathic human membranous nephropathy is still unknown; megalin is not expressed by human podocytes. There is still speculation that circulating immune complexes involving exogenous antigens may also play a role in human membranous nephropathy (37).

Antibody Interaction

The primary interaction that initiates the formation of subepithelial immune deposits in passive Heymann nephritis is the binding *in situ* of antibodies to megalin on the foot processes of glomerular podocytes. *In vitro* studies suggest that cross linking of the antibodies redistributes the antigens into progressively larger aggregates that are subsequently shed into the subepithelial space. These complexes may then be modified by the addition of further megalin and/or RAP molecules (36).

Secondary Mediators

Induction of renal injury and proteinuria depends on the activation of complement, but inflammatory cells are not required. Immunofluorescence studies reveal early and prominent participation of the complement cascade (C3 and neoantigens of the MAC of complement) in the subepithelial deposits. Rats depleted of complement fail to develop proteinuria despite antibody deposition, although perturbations in glomerular flow can be detected by micropuncture studies. Neutralization of Crry and CD59, complement regulatory proteins expressed on the surface of podocytes (by antibodies naturally present in anti-Fx1A antiserum), promotes proteinuria (38). Sublethal podocyte attack by C5b-9 has several consequences, including the production of eicosanoids and ROS and disruption of focal adhesions that link the actin cytoskeleton to extracellular matrix (39,40). Disruption of slit diaphragms and reduction of the glomerular heparan sulfate agrin are other structural consequences associated with the development of proteinuria (41). Once glomerular damage is established, ongoing complement activation appears to be unnecessary because complement depletion at this time does not abolish proteinuria. After transplantation of a kidney with active Heymann nephritis into a normal syngenic rat, complement deposits begin to disappear within 2 to 4 weeks, but proteinuria persists much longer. These studies suggest that structural alterations to the glomerular filter are long-standing once damaged by the antibody complement-dependent pathway.

Mesangial Cells

The rat Thy 1 model of glomerulonephritis has proven to be an important investigative model as so many glomerular diseases are characterized by mesangial cell proliferation. Thy 1 is an 18-kDa membrane glycoprotein most notably expressed in the thymus and brain. It is also expressed on the surface of normal rat mesangial cells; circulating rat lymphocytes are negative. Mesangial cell injury is induced by the injection of heterologous antithymocyte serum or anti–Thy 1.1 monoclonal antibody. Anti–Thy 1 nephritis is a biphasic model of glomerular disease, the first phase characterized by mesangiolysis (1 hour to 2 days) and the second phase by mesangial cell proliferation and glomerular microaneurysm formation (4 to 14 days). Despite histologic and glomerular micropuncture evidence of significant glomerular injury, proteinuria is often mild. Mesangiolysis is the consequence of antibody-directed, complement-mediated injury to mesangial cells and can be abrogated by complement depletion but not by the elimination of leukocytes. Deposition of components of the terminal complement cascade within the mesangium suggests that cell lysis is mediated by the MAC of complement. The hypercellular phase is mainly due to the proliferation of the smooth muscle–type mesangial cells. It does not occur if the mesangiolytic phase is prevented by complement depletion. Lymphohemopoietic cells—PMNs, monocytes, and platelets—also invade the glomerulus during the initial phase of mesangial injury. Several mesangial cell mitogens have been identified, and their effects on mesangial cell cycle regulatory proteins are becoming clarified and offer the possibility of future therapeutic targeting (Fig. 29.2). Integrin-dependent interactions between mesangial cells and their matrix also modulate their proliferative response (25). Platelets and PDGF-B appear to play an important pro-mitotic role in the Thy 1 model. Although antimesangial cell antibodies appear to be uncommon in humans, they have been identified in a few patients with IgA nephropathy and lupus nephritis (42,43). Nonetheless, mesangial cells respond to and elicit a large variety of pathophysiologic events, whether initiated by an antibody or another form of injury.

Endothelial Cells

The ability of antiendothelial antibodies to cause glomerular damage is best exemplified by renal allograft rejection. Several antigen families may be targeted, especially MHC class I and II antigens. Antiendothelial antibodies have also been demonstrated in patients with SLE, systemic vasculitis, and thrombotic microangiopathy, although the relationship of these antibodies to the pathophysiology of the disease remains unclear. An animal model of antibody-induced renal thrombotic microangiopathy has recently been developed and some of the mediators of injury identified, but the target antigen(s) have yet to be determined (44).

There is increasing evidence that ANCA associated with pauciimmune necrotizing glomerulonephritis are pathogenic, although the specifics of the connection between the antibodies to the granulocyte proteins (proteinase 3 and myeloperoxidase) and endothelial injury are still unraveling. Classical "immune complexes" are not formed, but recent data support a direct link between antibody-mediated activation of neutrophils and monocytes and glomerular endothelial injury (45). Endothelial cells may also express and/or internalize proteinase 3 and become directly involved in the pathogenetic process—both ANCA-dependent and -independent (46,47). Recent studies in animal models provide convincing evidence that antimyeloperoxidase antibodies cause glomerular damage (48).

ACE present on endothelial cells has been used as an experimental target for antibody attack to induce epimembranous nephropathy in rabbits, but whether there is a human counterpart to this model is unknown. The anti-ACE antibody binds to and redistributes endothelial cell-surface ACE, followed by shedding of antigen-antibody complexes from the cell membrane in a sequence of events reminiscent of that proposed for Heymann nephritis. The reason that these complexes move from a subendothelial (days 1 to 2) to a subepithelial position (days 3 to 24) concentrated at filtration slits is not entirely clear, but it may be related to hydrodynamic factors as the plasma filtrate crosses the GBM. The glomerular lesion is characterized histologically by complement deposition and the presence of PMNs, but their respective roles in the pathogenesis of the glomerular disease remain to be defined.

Interaction of Antibodies with Exogenous Antigens Trapped or Planted within the Glomerulus

Exogenous macromolecules trapped or planted within the glomerulus may become antigenic targets for antibodies, resulting in the *in situ* formation of immune complexes. Although still unproven, this pathway may account for some forms of immune complex nephritis occurring in humans after exposure to certain drugs, toxins, or microorganisms or in association with malignancy. Endogenous antigens originating at extrarenal sites may also induce renal injury by a similar mechanism.

Antigen Candidates

Several experimental manipulations have been used to trap antigens in the glomerulus with glomerular injury ensuing as circulating antibodies bind *in situ* to the planted antigen. Several factors might promote antigen entrapment. Low (subnephritic) concentrations of antiglomerular antibodies may initially bind and serve as a magnet for further antibody recruitment (e.g., antiidiotypic antibodies, antirheumatoid factor antibodies or antiheterologous antibodies as occurs in animals injected with nephrotoxic serum produced in another animal). Other possibilities include electrostatic interactions (cationic antigens binding to GBM anionic sites such as streptococcal proteinase) (49), glomerular carbohydrate interactions with lectins (e.g., lectin-like domains on microbial pathogens), glomerular matrix interactions (e.g., DNA-histone complexes binding glomerular heparan sulfate and fibronectin), or mesangial entrapment of a molecule of colloidal size as they percolate through normal mesangial channels.

Glomerular Deposition of Circulating Immune Complexes

Since the recognition of the *in situ* mechanism of glomerular immune complex formation, the concept of the entrapment of immune complexes preformed in the circulation has been increasingly challenged. It is now believed that most immune complexes form *in situ* even in such classical diseases as lupus nephritis. Nonetheless, the "circulating immune complex" pathway likely contributes to some extent in the pathogenesis of human glomerulonephritis, and nearly 75 years of work using animal models of immune-complex glomerulonephritis have taught us a great deal about the immunopathogenesis of glomerular injury. With rare exception, the nature of the nephritogenic antigens in human glomerulonephritis are unknown. Putative antigens include foreign serum proteins, drugs, food antigens, infectious organisms (bacteria, parasites, viruses, fungi, and mycoplasma), and certain endogenous antigens (nucleic acids, thyroid antigens, tumor antigens, nuclear non-DNA antigens, erythrocyte antigens, and renal tubular antigens).

Animal Models of Immune Complex Glomerulonephritis

The classic model of immune complex–induced tissue injury is acute serum sickness, induced in rabbits by injecting heterologous plasma proteins such as albumin or ovalbumin. The clinicopathologic features resemble those of acute poststreptococcal glomerulonephritis. Glomerular injury begins abruptly during the phase of antibody-dependent immune elimination of the antigen coincident with the appearance of circulating immune complexes. Injury resolves again in 2 to 3 weeks. The most striking and extensively studied spontaneous models of immune complex occur in certain strains of mice and resemble lupus nephritis (NZB X NZW)F1, BXSB, and MRL/*lpr*/*lpr* mice.

Glomerular Immune Complex Deposition and Injury

Multiple factors influence the capacity of a circulating immune complex to remain soluble, lodge within, and initiate glomeruli injury. First, the antigen must be immunogenic and persist in the circulation long enough to allow antibody generation and binding. The size of the immune complex that is formed, determined primarily by the antigen-to-antibody ratio, has a major influence on its rate of clearance from the circulation (faster rates being associated with a lower risk of nephritis) and on the pattern of deposition within glomeruli. Large-latticed complexes formed near antigen:antibody equivalence are efficiently eliminated by the mononuclear phagocyte system and are minimally entrapped by glomeruli, mainly in the mesangium. The smallest immune complexes pass freely through the glomerulus without being trapped. It is the intermediate-size immune complexes (e.g., Ag2:Ab2) that are retained within glomeruli. In primates, soluble-circulating immune complexes are eliminated via a complement-dependent "erythrocyte shuttle" within the mononuclear phagocyte system. Within minutes of formation, circulating immune complexes bind complement and attach to the erythrocyte complement receptor 1 (CR1). This interaction protects peripheral organs such as the kidney from immune-complex deposition and injury. Erythrocytes bearing immune complexes circulate to the liver, where the complexes are transferred to Kupffer cell Fc receptors and catabolized.

Physicochemical properties such as net charge are important. Given the net negative charge of the glomerular capillary wall, cationic antigens are more nephrotoxic than neutral or anionic ones. Both size and charge also influence the location of trapping. Small highly cationic complexes (isoelectric point, 9.5 to 11.5) deposit along the glomerular capillary wall, whereas large cationic complexes tend to lodge in the mesangium. The high renal blood flow rates and transcapillary hydraulic pressure gradients are thought to explain why the kidney is particularly vulnerable to immune complex–mediated tissue injury. Alterations in glomerular hemodynamics may affect the severity of injury. For example, serum sickness is worse in hypertensive rabbits, a reduction in GFR decreases immune-complex deposition, and renal artery stenosis protects the kidney from immune-complex disease.

In Situ *Modification and Damage*

Trapped glomerular immune complexes are free to escape unless a series of events occur *in situ* to stabilize them. Intraglomerular immune complexes enlarge over time, the morphologic counterpart of the *in situ* interactions that rearrange, enlarge, and stabilize the lattice structure. In fact, the immune complex is in a state of dynamic equilibrium with its component parts in the circulation. The immune response typically involves polyclonal B-cell activation, involving a heterogeneous group of antibodies. The addition of antibodies of increasing affinity may provide further stability to the complex. The entire immune complex may act as a planted antigen, recruiting additional antibody systems such as rheumatoid factors (antibodies reactive with the Fc and occasionally Fab fragment of IgG), antiidiotypic antibodies binding to unique epitopes of the Fab antibody fragment, and immunoconglutinins, which are IgM antibodies that react with sites on activated fragments of C3 and C4. At other times, subsequent events dissolve the complexes. The addition of nonprecipitating antibodies, excess antigen, and/or complement proteins may decrease and ultimately dissolve glomerular immune deposits. Proteolytic enzymes may also accelerate complex removal.

Once nephritogenic immune complexes stabilize within the glomerulus, they trigger a sequence of events that induce glomerular inflammation and proteinuria. Marrow-derived monocytes are the key mediators of proteinuria in experimental models of acute serum sickness.

Unique Features of Immunoglobulin A Nephropathy

New insights into the pathogenesis of experimental IgA nephropathy have been made in recent years and are further discussed in Chapter 31. Only a few unique factors will be mentioned here. It appears that many antigens may be involved, although this remains speculation. One recent study identified *Haemophilus parainfluenzae* antigens in the mesangium of 31% with IgA nephropathy and 4% with other renal diseases, illustrating one example of a possible link between microbial pathogens in this disease (50). The IgA molecule is unique in that 10 to 20% circulates in a polymeric form, with monomers linked by J chain. Humans produce two isotypes—IgA1 and IgA2—but it appears that most of the glomerular deposits are monomeric IgA1. Despite a strong clinical correlation between acute mucosal infections (respiratory and gastrointestinal), and perhaps abnormal mucosal immunity, and nephritis exacerbations, most of the data point to the bone marrow and not the mucosal immune system as the origin of the glomerular IgA1 deposits. Bone marrow transplantation data, both human anecdotes and studies in the spontaneous ddY mouse model, suggest that IgA nephropathy is a primary stem cell disorder (51).

Several recent studies have focused on the biochemical structure of the IgA molecule and have consistently reported differences in the carbohydrate structure between patients and controls (52,53). The number of O-linked galactose sugars in the hinge region of IgA1 is significantly reduced in the patients. Although the metabolic basis of this galactose deficiency is not yet known, it is thought to be of primary pathogenetic significance. Relevant observations include its delayed rate of clearance from the circulation, increased binding to mesangial cells, and recognition as an antigenic determinant by naturally occurring IgA1 and IgG antibodies.

The ability of IgA to bind to fibronectin and certain lectins may facilitate glomerular uptake. After the observation that mice lacking uteroglobin, an antiinflammatory protein with high affinity for fibronectin, spontaneously develop IgA nephropathy, additional studies have yet to confirm its role in human IgA nephropathy (54). Mesangial deposition of IgA alone is insufficient to cause glomerular injury. IgA may also bind to mesangial cells and trigger subsequent effects, although the specific receptor involved remains to be identified—it appears to be distinct from the known receptors IgA FcαR1 (CD89), asialoglycoprotein receptor, and the polymeric Ig receptor (55).

Whereas C3 is almost always present in association with IgA immune deposits, IgA is an inefficient activator of the alternative pathway. The recent recognition that IgA can activate complement by the third or mannan-binding lectin pathway may be relevant to IgA glomerular injury (56). Alternatively it may be the co-deposited IgG or IgM molecules that activate complement and mediate renal injury. In most experimental IgA models, hematuria is C3 dependent, but the terminal components C5b-9 are not required.

CELLULAR IMMUNE MECHANISMS OF INDUCTION OF GLOMERULAR INJURY

T lymphocytes play an intricate role in the immune responses that cause glomerulonephritis, usually culminating in the generation of nephritogenic antibodies. Considerably less common, it has long been suspected that T cells may occasionally cause glomerular injury by recruiting monocytes in the absence of antibodies. Evidence that T cells alone, working in the absence of antibodies, can induce glomerular injury, has been convincingly demonstrated in animal models of autoimmune glomerulonephritis. Transfer of GBM-sensitized $CD4^+$ T cells to normal animals can induce glomerulonephritis (34,57). In a related model based on the injection of subnephritic doses of anti-GBM antibodies (that serves as the "planted" antigen for subsequent immunologic attack by the host immune system), crescentic glomerulonephritis develops even in antibody-deficient mice, whereas disease is attenuated in T-cell–depleted animals (58).

An alternative T-cell–dependent antibody-independent mechanism that may cause glomerular dysfunction involves T-cell activation and release of a "lymphokine" that alters the glomerular permselectivity barrier, causing proteinuria in the absence of glomerular inflammation (59). Such a mechanism, first proposed Shalhoub in 1974 (59a), is still the favored immunopathogenetic paradigm for idiopathic minimal change nephrotic syndrome and focal segmental glomerulosclerosis (FSGS) despite the lack of definitive evidence. The nature of the putative lymphocyte-derived glomerular permeability factor remains elusive despite several proposed candidates [reviewed in (60)]. Savin et al. identified a factor in the plasma of FSGS patients that exerts permeability changes in a rat glomerular bioassay and predicts the risk of allograft-recurrent FSGS in some patients (60a). The factor itself has not been isolated. Immunoabsorption to protein A suggests that it may circulate in association with IgG. Similar permeability activity has also been identified in the plasma of patients with

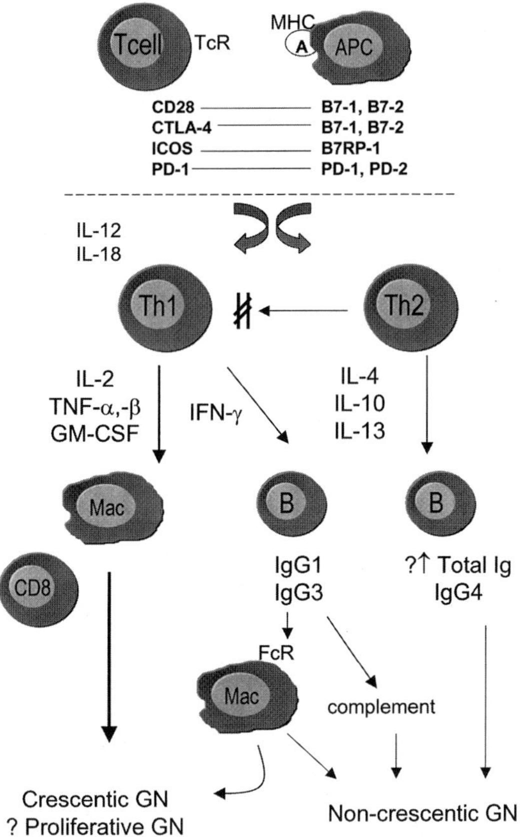

FIGURE 29.4. Antigen-dependent T-cell activation and functional polarization. When T cells encounter antigen-presenting cells (APC), at least two signals must be transmitted before an immune response is initiated. The first signal is emitted by ligation of the T-cell receptor with antigenic peptides bound to major histocompatibility complex (MHC) molecules on the APC. T-helper cells (CD4+) interact with MHC class II, and T-cytotoxic cells (CD8+) interact with MHC class I molecules. A second signal is required for full activation. It may be provided by CD28 that activates T cells after binding to its ligand, B7-1 or B7-2, on APCs. Once activated, T cells begin to express a CD28 homologue (CTLA-4) that binds B7-1 and B7-2 with higher affinity and inhibits T-cell activation. Therapeutic administration of CTLA-4 can decrease the severity of autoimmune nephritis. Two new members of the CD28 superfamily are ICOS (inducible costimulator) and PD-1 (programmed death-1) that interact with their respective APC ligands, B7RP-1, and PD-L1 or PD-L2. The second major costimulatory family is the tumor necrosis factor (TNF)–TNF-R family, which includes CD154 expressed by activated T cells and CD40 expressed by APCs, including B cells. The CD154-CD40 system appears to be particularly important in antibody-mediated diseases such as lupus nephritis. Several new TNF-TNF-R superfamily members have been identified and await investigation in glomerulonephritis (GN): 4-IBB/4-IBBL, CD134/CD134L, and CD27/CD70. Resident glomerular mesangial and epithelial cells may function as nonprofessional APCs to activate T cells, but it is unlikely that they can initiate a primary immune response. T-helper (Th) cells activated by antigen can be divided into two distinct subsets based on the cytokines they produce. Th1 cells synthesize interleukin-2 (IL-2), interferon-gamma (IFNγ), TNF, and granulocyte-macrophage colony stimulating factor (GM-CSF) and mediate delayed-type hypersensitivity reactions with monocyte and cytotoxic T-cell activation and immunoglobulin class switching to favor the production of complement-fixing immunoglobulin G (IgG) isotypes. The Th1 pathway predominates in hypercellular/proliferative forms of glomerulonephritis. In contrast, Th2 cells are characterized by the production of IL-4, -5, -10, and -13 and mediation of allergic, immediate-type hypersensitivity reactions associated with mast cells and production of IgE and the weaker complement-fixing IgG1. The Th2 cytokine profile is commonly associated with nonproliferative glomerular diseases such as minimal change nephrotic syndrome and membranous nephropathy. Cytokine therapy has been used experimentally to attenuate Th1-dependent proliferative diseases: either administration of Th2 cytokines or inhibition of Th1 cytokines/receptors. (Modified from Kitching AR. Cytokines, T cells and proliferative glomerulonephritis. *Nephrology* 2002;7:244–249.)

podocin mutations, indicating that this "factor" is not unique to idiopathic FSGS (61). Alternatively, it has been suggested that proteinuria may be the consequence of the loss of an inhibitory substance, perhaps a lipoprotein, which serves in normal individuals to block the permeability factor (62,63). Two fundamental aspects of T-lymphocyte biology have been extensively investigated in the past decade, yielding insights that bear relevance to the basic immunology and possible therapeutics of glomerulonephritis. The first is the identification of pairs of costimulatory molecules involved with MHC molecules in antigen recognition, and the second is the identification of functionally distinct subsets of T cells (64–66). These functions are reviewed in Figure 29.4.

SECONDARY MEDIATORS OF GLOMERULAR INJURY

After the primary immunopathogenic event that initiates glomerular injury, a series of secondary mediators are recruited and activated to execute the inflammatory response. Definitive proof that these pathways are involved in renal damage is usually based on the results of selective inhibition or depletion of the effector system under investigation and by studies in knock-out mice.

Polymorphonuclear Leukocytes

PMNs are present in several human and experimental glomerulonephritides in which they contribute to inflammation-associated injury. Depletion of PMNs during the heterologous phase of anti-GBM nephritis and in the Con A-anti–Con A model of immune-complex nephritis prevents proteinuria. In PMN-dependent lesions, the cells appear abruptly, and several factors may play a role in their recruitment, including chemoattraction to C3a, C5a, or alpha (C-X-C) chemokines; immune adherence to CR1 or CR3; and Fc receptor–dependent binding to antibodies. Among numerous toxic PMN secretory products, ROS and proteolytic enzymes (e.g., GBM-degrading serine proteases, neutral proteinases such as elastase and cathepsin G and matrix-degrading metalloproteinases) have been most frequently implicated in glomerular damage. Other PMN activities that may contribute include proteolytic activation of plasma protein cascades, such as the coagulation pathway; release of cationic proteins that may bind and neutralize GBM anionic charge sites; and the synthesis of phospholipid metabolites [PGs, thromboxanes (Tx), leukotrienes, and PAF], hydrogen peroxide, and vasoactive substances (histamines). Products derived from PMN granules that are targeted by ANCA have been implicated in the genesis of endothelial cell damage and focal necrotizing glomerulonephritis.

Monocytes and Macrophages

Monocytes and macrophages (Mϕ) are present in many glomerular diseases, particularly in crescentic and postinfectious glomerulonephritis. Although most of these cells migrate into glomeruli from the circulation, they may also proliferate *in situ* (67). Beginning with landmark studies in the late 1970s, the pivotal role played by Mϕ in the genesis of primary glomerulonephritis has clearly been established by numerous studies. Mϕ may also be recruited during a secondary wave of glomerular injury, associated with disease progression, as demonstrated in the remnant kidney model and in lipid-induced glomerular disease. Although unraveling the effector pathways of monocyte-dependent glomerular damage is challenging owing to their multifunctionality, several activities appear to be involved: (a) phagocytosis, which may eliminate immune reactants but may also activate pathways that promote damage; (b) antigen presentation to T cells after induction of MHC class II surface molecules; and (c) biosynthesis of numerous proinflammatory products: cytokines, procoagulant and fibrinolytic proteases and proteins, matrix-degrading enzymes, ROS, vasoactive substances, and cationic proteins. Although Mϕ express CRs (CR1 and CR3) and are chemoattracted to C5a *in vitro*, glomerular Mϕ recruitment is usually complement-independent in experimental models. Mϕ also express receptors for antibody Fc fragments that may participate in their recruitment and activation (68). It is also quite clear that activated Mϕ and PMN represent a highly heterogeneous population of cells, and even in glomerulonephritis some of these cells are programmed to be antiinflammatory and to terminate ongoing injury.

Glomerular Leukocyte Recruitment Mechanisms

To reach a site of inflammation, leukocytes must first adhere to and subsequently emigrate through retracted endothelial junctions and the basement membrane out into the surrounding tissue [reviewed in (69)]. This is accomplished by a multistep process involving a series of leukocyte surface adhesion molecules that bind to cognate receptors on the endothelium (Fig. 29.5; Table 29.2). Leukocyte migration to sites of inflammation is directionally regulated by chemoattractant molecules, especially chemokines (chemotactic cytokines). These small proteins (8 to 10 kDa) are subdivided into four major families (already more than 50 ligands and 17 different receptors identified) based on the position of the first two cysteine residues (Table 29.3) (70). Only two of the families have been extensively investigated. The α-chemokines share a common CXC structure (X denotes any intervening amino acid), and many are involved in the recruitment of PMN. They bind to G-protein–coupled CXC receptors and activate intracellular phosphatases. Each receptor typically binds more than one chemokine making for great pleiotropy and redundancy in the system. PMN are known to express CXCR1 and CXCR2. It has recently been reported that glomerular podocytes also express CXCR1, -3, -4, and -5, although their role here has yet to be determined (71). IL-8 (that binds to CXCR1 and 2) has been implicated

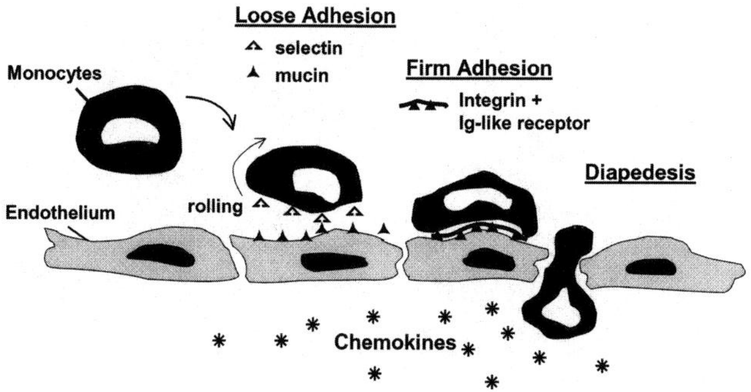

FIGURE 29.5. Mechanisms of glomerular leukocyte recruitment. The earliest and relatively transient adhesions, which cause leukocytes to "roll" along the endothelium, are mediated by surface receptors with lectin-like domains (selectins) that bind to specific glycoprotein ligands (mucins). Not expressed by normal glomeruli, P- and E-selectins have been detected in some diseased human glomeruli. Their only ligand in normal glomeruli is CD34. Selectin blocking and neutralization studies have not been shown to prevent leukocyte recruitment or proteinuria. In fact, in a study of P-selectin–deficient mice, anti–glomerular basement membrane (GBM) nephritis was more severe compared to wild-type mice (149). Once activated, leukocytes soon become firmly attached to the endothelium by engaging leukocyte integrins ($\alpha_1\beta_1$ and β_2) with their endothelial ligands, which are members of the immunoglobulin (Ig) gene superfamily: intercellular adhesion molecules (ICAM) and vascular cell adhesion molecules (VCAM) (reviewed in Table 29.2). Low-level glomerular ICAM-1 and ICAM-2 expression has been observed in some studies, whereas VCAM-1 appears limited to parietal epithelial cells of Bowman's capsule. Thus far, interventions designed to prevent leukocyte recruitment in acute glomerular disease by selectively blocking a single leukocyte integrin ligand have generally been ineffective. Whether this is due to overlapping functions of other receptors or whether other reactions promote leukocyte adherence to the glomerular endothelium remains to be determined. Galectins, osteopontin, and CD44 may be involved, for example. In addition to recruitment, leukocyte integrin-ligand interactions may activate several intracellular signaling pathways and alter leukocyte functions. These effects may partially explain why mice with genetic ICAM-1 deficiency and nephrotoxic serum nephritis develop milder chronic renal damage (150). Directed by chemokines, leukocytes ultimately migrate between endothelial cells to the site of injury.

in PMN recruitment in some inflammatory glomerular diseases. Additional CXC chemokines are chemoattractants for other cells but not PMN. These include interferon gamma (IFN-γ)–inducible protein of 10 kDa (IP-10) and monokine induced by IFN-γ (Mig); both have been detected in inflamed glomeruli (72).

The role of the second chemokine family in glomerulonephritis, the CC or β chemokines, has been more extensively investigated. In general, the CC chemokines recruit monocytes and other mononuclear cell lineages but not PMN. At least 10 CC receptors are known; monocytes express CCR1, -2, and -5. Monocyte chemoattractant protein-1 (MCP-1) has been most extensively investigated; MCP-2, -3, -4, and -5 also exist. MCP-1 binds to CCR2 and its expression is often detected in proliferative and crescentic glomerulonephritis. MCP-1 deficiency or neutralization usually decreases glomerular monocyte numbers and disease severity. RANTES (*r*egulated upon *a*ctivation, *n*ormal *T* cell *e*xpressed and *s*ecreted) binds to monocyte CCR1 and CCR5, and its inhibition has also been protective in experimental proliferative nephritis. However, neither MCP-1 nor RANTES blockade achieves sustained reversal of monocyte infiltration and proteinuria in any model. It has become evident that several of the chemokines have other effects, including cellular activation and generation of Th1 or Th2 responses. For example, inhibition of macrophage inflammatory proteins (MIP)-1α and -1β (CC chemokines) decreased proteinuria without affecting monocyte numbers. Rather surprising, despite the beneficial effect reported in experimental nephritis with either antireceptor antibody therapy or inhibition of MCP-1, genetic deletion of CCR1 and CCR2 has not been protective in the same disease model (73–76). In fact, both knock-out mice develop worse anti-GBM nephritis, perhaps due to a greater Th1 polarity and more aggressive crescent formation.

Fractalkine is the only known membrane-bound chemokine. It belongs to a third chemokine class, CXXXC, and binds to its own unique receptor (CX3CR1) that is expressed on natural killer cells, T cells, and mesangial cells (77,78). Chemokine expression is primarily induced by proinflammatory cytokines such as IL-1 and TNF-α. The transcription factor NF-κB is frequently involved, and NF-κB inhibition may be an effective strategy to reduce glomerular inflammation (79). In addition to lymphohematopoietic cells, mesangial cells may be an important source of chemokines in glomerulonephritis. Resident glomerular cells may also respond to chemokines via specific receptors. Mesangial cells express CCR1 and CX3CR and proliferate in response to IL-10 via an unknown receptor.

Platelets and Platelet-Activating Factors

Intraglomerular platelets or their degradation products are commonly observed in diseases such as membranoproliferative glomerulonephritis and lupus nephritis. Evaluation of circulating platelets isolated from such patients often shows evidence that they have been activated *in vivo*. Although antiplatelet therapy has been advocated in the diseases discussed earlier, its efficacy has not been clearly established. The role of platelets as inflammatory mediators in experimental glomerulonephritis has been investigated for several decades now, but results have been inconsistent because of the difficulties inherent in platelet depletion and nonspecific drug inhibition studies.

Mechanisms of glomerular platelet recruitment to the kidney are poorly characterized. Complement activation is critical in a model of *in situ* immune-complex nephritis (Con A-anti–Con A) and in anti–Thy 1 nephritis, but whether this is a result of immune adherence to CR1 or of chemoattraction to C5a is unknown. Platelets may adhere to and become activated by the GBM in a reaction reminiscent of the *in vitro* effects of collagen. Other factors that have been implicated in intraglomerular adherence or activation of platelets include immune adherence to Fc recep-

TABLE 29.3. CHEMOKINES IN GLOMERULAR DISEASE

Family	Members	Abbreviation		Receptors	Primary target cells
CXC (alpha)	Growth-related oncogene alpha	GRO-α	CXCL1	CXCR2	PMN
	Platelet factor 4	PF4	CXCL4	?	PMN, eosinophils
	Interleukin-8	IL-8	CXCL8	CXCR1, CXCR2	PMN
	Monokine induced by interferon gamma	Mig	CXCL9	CXCR3	T cells
	Interferon gamma–induced protein	IP-10	CXCL10	CXCR3	Th1 cells, NK cells
CC *(beta)*	Monocyte chemoattractant protein-1	MCP-1	CCL2	CCR2	Mϕ, dendritic cells, T cells, NK cells
	Macrophage inflammatory protein-1α	MIP-1α	CCL3	CCR1, CCR5	Mϕ, dendritic cells, Th1 cells, NK cells
	Macrophage inflammatory protein-1β	MIP-1β	CCL4	CCR5	Mϕ, dendritic cells, Th1 cells, NK cells
	Regulated on activation, normal T cell expressed and secreted	RANTES	CCL5	CCR1, CCR3, CCR5	Mϕ, dendritic cells, Th1 cells, NK cells
	Eotaxin		CL11	CCR3	Eosinophils, basophils, Th2 cells, dendritic cells
CX_3C	Fractalkine	FKN	CX3CL1	CX_3CR1	T cells, NK cells
C	Lymphotactin	LTN	XCL1	XCR1	T cells

Mϕ, monocytes/macrophages; NK, natural killer; PMN, polymorphonuclear leukocyte; Th, T helper.
Note: This is a partial listing, highlighting chemokines most frequently investigated in glomerular disease. CXCR4 is also a T-cell coreceptor for human immunodeficiency virus (HIV)-1; CCR5 is a coreceptor for HIV-1 strains that infect macrophages and activated T cells.

tors, activation of the coagulation cascade, TxA_2, and PAF. The role of platelet adhesion molecules, including P-selectin, glycoprotein Ib, platelet-endothelial cell adhesion molecule (PECAM-1), and β_3 integrins (e.g., glycoprotein IIb-IIIa) in glomerular disease has not yet been determined.

Several platelet products may be injurious to glomeruli such as bioactive lipids (PAF and TxA_2), platelet factor 4 (a cationic protein that participates in the coagulation cascade and is a CXC chemokine for leukocytes), and growth factors (PDGF, TGF-β1). PAF has a multitude of biologic effects that may be mediated by the phospholipid itself (leukocyte chemoattraction, altered vascular permeability) or indirectly by stimulating release of substances such as Tx, PGs, leukotrienes, lysosomal enzymes, superoxide, IL-1, MCP-1, and TNF. PAF is not only produced by platelets but also in turn triggers platelet aggregation, activation, and degranulation. Antagonists to PAF or its receptor have decreased disease severity in several experimental glomerulonephritis models. Platelets may further modulate glomerular injury by activating C3 and C5 of the complement cascade, activating the intrinsic coagulation cascade, or by synthesis of β-thromboglobulin (inhibits endothelial release of prostaglandin I_2) or vasoactive amines such as histamine and serotonin.

Soluble Secreted Peptides

Growth factors and cytokines are small polypeptide messengers (most approximately 6 to 30 kDa) that bind to target cells by specific surface receptors to initiate a variety of cellular responses (Table 29.4). Most of these factors can be produced by native glomerular cells as well as inflammatory cells.

Epidermal Growth Factor Family

One of the first circulating growth factors to be recognized, EGF was originally isolated from mouse submandibular glands and human urine. Most studies have failed to identify immunoreactive EGF in diseased glomeruli. *In vitro*, EGF stimulates mesangial cell contraction and PG synthesis; intrarenal EGF infusion decreases GFR and renal blood flow. TGFα shares 30% sequence homology with EGF and exerts its biologic action by binding to the EGF receptor. A newer family member, heparin-binding EGF-like growth factor, a mesangial cell mitogen, is expressed in disease models associated with mesangial cell proliferation (80). Heparin-binding EGF also has direct glomerular hemodynamic effects (81).

Fibroblast Growth Factor

FGF-2 or basic FGF (bFGF) is a potent angiogenic factor that also regulates matrix synthesis and is a mitogen for all intrinsic glomerular cells. FGF-2 has affinity for heparin and HSPG and may bind to basement membranes/extracellular matrix *in vivo*. In the Thy 1 nephritis model, production of bFGF increases during the phase of mesangial cell proliferation. Disease severity is enhanced by exogenous FGF and

TABLE 29.4. SOLUBLE SECRETED PEPTIDES IN ACUTE GLOMERULAR INJURY

Promotes injury	Prevents injury	Either (model-dependent)
Fibroblast growth factor-2	Interleukin-4	Granulocyte-colony stimulating factor
Granulocyte-macrophage colony stimulating factor	Interleukin-11	Interleukin-6
Heparin-binding epidermal growth factor–like growth factor	Interleukin-13	Interleukin-10
Interferon-gamma	Vascular endothelial growth factor	Interleukin-12
Interleukin-1		Transforming growth factor β
Interleukin-8		
Interleukin-18		
Macrophage colony stimulating factor		
Macrophage migration inhibition factor		
Platelet-derived growth factor		
Tumor necrosis factor-α		

attenuated by FGF-2 neutralization/antagonism (82). FGF may also contribute to the genesis of glomerulosclerosis as chronic administration causes podocyte damage in rats, and it enhances cytokine-induced endothelial cell apoptosis (83).

Colony-Stimulating Factors

Colony-stimulating factors (CSF) are a family of glycoproteins that not only regulate the development of hematopoietic progenitor cells but also promote the inflammatory response of mature cells such as macrophages. Increased CSF expression has been reported in several proliferative glomerular diseases. Mice deficient in granulocyte-macrophage (GM)–CSF develop less inflammation (PMN and Mϕ) after injection of nephrotoxic antiserum and membranoproliferative glomerulonephritis has been reported in a patient exposed to chronic GM-CSF treatment (84,85). The effects of G-CSF may be dose-dependent based on the observation that low-dose G-CSF promotes a Th2 response and worse nephritis in MRL-*lpr/lpr* mice, whereas high-dose therapy downregulated expression of the Fcγ receptor III and attenuated nephritis (86). Increased M-CSF has also been observed in proliferative nephritis. Macrophage migration inhibitory factor is another proinflammatory protein shown to be upregulated in glomerular diseases associated with a leukocyte infiltrate. Anti–migration inhibitory factor antibodies partially reverse glomerular injury induced with anti-GBM antiserum (87).

Interleukins

ILs are a large family of cytokines (at least 25) that play a central role in inflammatory and immunologic responses. The expression and function of several members have been examined in glomerulonephritis. In addition to the role played by ILs in the polarization and function of Th1/Th2 cells, several ILs are produced by and/or regulate the behavior of resident glomerular cells. IL-1, IL-8, and IL-18 have proinflammatory roles in most glomerular diseases. IL-1 induces mesangial cell proliferation and promotes synthesis of a variety of substances: eicosanoids, oxygen radicals, collagenase, cytokines, chemokines, and adhesion molecules. It also enhances collagen synthesis by glomerular epithelial cells. Renal IL-1 mRNA levels are increased in several glomerular diseases, and neutralization studies with a soluble IL-1 receptor antagonist diminish inflammation and proliferation in rats with anti–Thy 1 or nephrotoxic serum nephritis (88). IL-8 is an important mediator of granulocyte chemoattraction and activation. Mesangial cells produce IL-8 when stimulated with cytokines such as IL-1 and TNF-α. IL-8 neutralization prevents neutrophil infiltration in a model of immune complex glomerulonephritis. In humans, urinary IL-8 levels are higher in patients with glomerulonephritis associated with leukocyte infiltration. IL-18 treatment has been reported to exacerbate SLE nephritis and cell-mediated crescentic nephritis (89,90).

ILs with antiinflammatory effects that have been shown to attenuate glomerulonephritis include IL-4, IL-10, and IL-11. Promotion of a Th2 response and inhibition the proinflammatory effects of macrophages are effects of IL-4. Both mesangial cells and podocytes can produce IL-4. The protective role of IL-4 has been documented in the anti-GBM nephritis model, both by studies in IL-4–deficient mice that develop worse disease and by IL-4 therapy that attenuates disease (91–93). In this model, IL-11 therapy has also been protective (94). IL-10 suppresses the nephritogenic Th1 immune responses; IL-10–/– mice develop worse nephrotoxic serum nephritis than IL-10+/+ mice (95). In the Thy 1 nephritis and anti-GBM nephritis model, IL-10 therapy is protective (95,96).

Some ILs may have either pro- or antiinflammatory effects depending on the type of disease evaluated. For example, IL-6 is a cytokine produced by several blood-borne cells as well as glomerular endothelial and mesangial cells. IL-6 may be detectable in glomeruli and the urine in several proliferative glomerular diseases in animals and humans. Neutralizing anti–IL-6 antibodies and IL-6 receptor blockade decreased the severity of lupus nephritis, whereas IL-6 transgenic mice spontaneously develop glomerulonephritis (97). Yet, IL-6 recombinant protein therapy reduced disease severity in rats with anti-GBM nephritis (98). Anti-GBM nephritis is less severe in IL-12–deficient mice, whereas IL-12 DNA plasmid therapy reduces the severity of immune complex nephritis associated with graft-versus-host disease (99,100).

Interferon Gamma

IFN-γ is a member of a family of glycoproteins (α, β, and γ) with immunomodulatory, antiviral, and antineoplastic activity. IFN-γ has been shown to play a key role in several autoimmune diseases including lupus nephritis. Deletion of IFN-γ or its receptor or treatment with a neutralizing antibody or IFN-γR-Fc chimeric protein reduces renal disease in several SLE mouse models (101,102). Macrophages have been identified as an important source of IFN-γ, and IFN-γ expression regulates glomerular monocyte migration (103).

Platelet-Derived Growth Factor

PDGF is a dimeric glycoprotein of four known isoforms—PDGF-A, -B, -C, and -D. It has diverse biologic activities, including chemoattraction and activation of inflammatory cells, mitogenesis, and promotion of tissue repair. It also has vasoconstrictor properties. The mitogenic effect of PDGF on mesangial cells is especially remarkable, but it may also trigger a chemotactic and contractile response. Mesangial cells may also produce PDGF. During the mesangial proliferative phase of Thy 1 nephritis, PDGF neutralization by antibody, aptamers, PDGF receptor-IgG, or a PDGF receptor tyrosine kinase selective inhibitor is effective in blocking proliferation (104). Enhanced expression of PDGF and the PDGF-B receptor has been observed on human glomerulonephritis. The role of the more recently discovered PDGF-C and PDGF-D remains to be determined, although it has already been shown that PDGF-C can be made by podocytes and induce mesangial cell proliferation (105,106).

Transforming Growth Factor

TGFβ is a family of polypeptide growth factors with at least three distinct mammalian isoforms. TGFβ has diverse biologic actions that are relevant to glomerular disease, including its ability to modulate (sometimes in a dose-dependent manner) inflammatory and immunologic responses, cellular proliferation, apoptosis and differentiation, angiogenesis, and extracellular matrix metabolism. TGFβ appears to be the primary mediator of glomerulosclerosis. TGFβ production by resident and/or inflammatory cells may occur early in the course of glomerular injury, but its pathogenetic role in the acute phase of glomerulonephritis is still not clear. It is most commonly reported to have antiproliferative and proapoptotic effects. TGFβ also has striking immunosuppressive effects that may prove to be relevant to initiation of immune-mediated glomerular injury. Although TGFβ therapy has been reported to attenuate experimental autoimmune diseases such as arthritis and encephalitis, mice overexpressing Smad7, an inhibitor of TGFβ signaling, were found to have less severe anti-GBM nephritis (107).

Tumor Necrosis Factor

TNF-α is a proinflammatory cytokine primarily produced by monocytes and macrophages, although mesangial cells can also synthesize TNF-α. It is particularly important in the genesis of septic shock and the associated renal endothelial damage. TNF-α is also thought to play a role in proliferative glomerular diseases including anti-GBM nephritis, murine lupus nephritis, and serum sickness. Anti-GBM nephritis is less severe in TNF-α knock-out mice (108). TNF-α can induce mesangial cell contraction and synthesis of a variety of products such as IL-1, IL-8, GM-CSF, MCP-1, PGs, procoagulant, NO, and ROS.

Vascular Endothelial Growth Factor

VEGF, also known as vascular permeability factor, promotes capillary repair and angiogenesis through endothelial cell mitogenesis. Four isoforms have been identified: $VEGF_{121}$ and $VEGF_{165}$ (the most abundant) are soluble secreted forms, whereas the 189 and 206 isoforms are usually cell-bound. Within glomeruli, podocytes and activated mesangial cells produce VEGF, whereas its receptors, flt-1 and flk-1, are expressed on endothelial cells. Inhibition of VEGF exacerbates Thy 1 nephritis and results in the development of microaneurysms, whereas treatment with $VEGF_{165}$ promotes recovery from thrombotic microangiopathy (22,44,109).

Coagulation Cascade

The normal glomerulus is remarkably protected from the formation of thrombi, but fibrin deposition is frequently observed as a feature of three pathologic states: thrombotic microangiopathy, proliferative and necrotizing glomerulonephritis, and crescent formation. Earlier studies using anticoagulation with warfarin, heparin, or hirudin (a thrombin antagonist) yielded conflicting data on the potential for this intervention to diminish the severity of crescentic glomerulonephritis. Studies with fibrinolytic agents (ancrod, streptokinase or tissue plasminogen activator) have generally been more convincing with attenuated disease reported in models of anti-GBM nephritis, serum sickness, and lupus nephritis. The most compelling data that fibrin plays a significant role are based on a study of anti-GBM nephritis in fibrinogen-deficient mice (110). The number of intraglomerular monocytes, crescent formation, and serum creatinine levels were significantly reduced in the fibrinogen–/– mice. In proliferative glomerular diseases, fibrin's primary role may be monocyte recruitment to the glomerular tuft and to Bowman's space to the site of crescent formation. The pathways that regulate glomerular fibrin deposition and removal are reviewed in Figure 29.6.

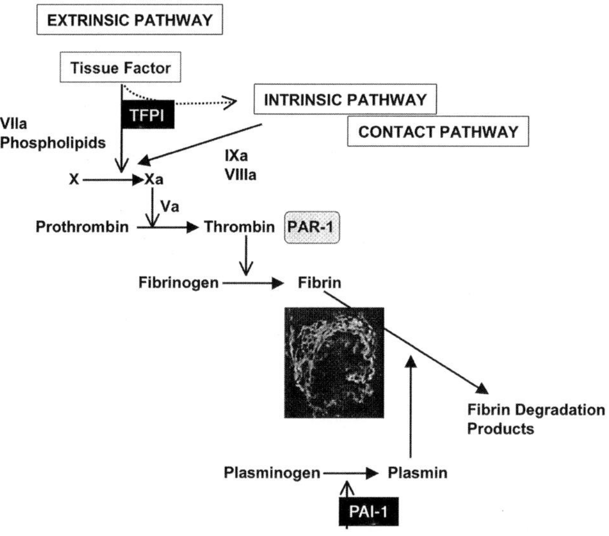

FIGURE 29.6. Regulation of glomerular fibrin deposition and removal. Fibrin deposition may be the consequence of intraglomerular activation of prothrombotic cascades and/or decreased endogenous fibrinolytic activity, primarily intraglomerular tissue plasminogen activator (tPA). Most of the fibrin associated with immunologic glomerular diseases is generated by activation of the extrinsic coagulation pathway that begins with the activation of factor VII by the tissue factor (TF) procoagulant to generate VIIa. TF can be produced by resident glomerular cells or monocytes/macrophages in response to several inflammatory stimuli. In addition, normal renal vessels constitutively express a TF inhibitor, tissue factor pathway inhibitor (TFPI), which is downregulated in many crescentic glomerular diseases. The importance of the TF pathway has been confirmed in experiments showing worse disease with TFPI neutralization and milder disease with recombinant TFPI therapy or TF inhibition (151). Several other factors contribute to the antithrombotic environment within normal glomerular such as PGI_2, nitric oxide, antithrombin III, and thrombomodulin (152,153). It is becoming apparent that certain coagulation proteins may themselves have proinflammatory effects that may contribute to glomerular injury. For example, mesangial cells express and can be activated by a thrombin receptor, protease-activated receptor-1 (PAR-1). The receptor is activated by the protease TRAP. Mice genetically PAR-1–deficient develop less severe anti-GBM nephritis, whereas PAR-1 activation by recombinant TRAP therapy causes worse disease but only in PAR-1–expressing mice (154). Mesangial cells proliferate after exposure to factor Xa, a VIIa cofactor for thrombin generation (155). Fibrin itself may also bind to cell surfaces through several potential mechanisms, especially by binding to $\alpha_v\beta_3$ integrin (156). Glomeruli produce plasminogen activators, mainly tPA, which normally protect the kidney from the damaging effects of fibrin accumulation. Mice with a genetic deficiency of tPA or plasminogen develop worse anti-GBM nephritis (157). Production of PA inhibitors, especially plasminogen activator inhibitor-1 (PAI-1) and perhaps protease nexin-1, may depress endogenous plasmin activity and promote glomerular fibrin deposition. In addition to its role in acute glomerular injury, it is now evident that the glomerular tPA/PAI-1 balance is involved in the chronic phase of injury and glomerulosclerosis through activities that regulate accumulation of not only fibrin but also extracellular matrix proteins [reviewed in (158)]. uPA, urokinase-type plasminogen activator.

Complement Cascade

Since the first description of complement proteins in diseased human glomeruli in 1956, the role of complement has been extensively investigated in experimental glomerular disease models. It is now evident that the complement cascade is multifunctional, somewhat paradoxically functioning systemically to prevent the formation and deposition of immune complexes but at a local level contributing to the inflammatory response through its intraglomerular effects. Most of the soluble complement components are made in the liver, but glomeruli may contribute to local production, especially during inflammation (111). The three pathways of complement activation are reviewed in Figure 29.7.

Complement-mediated glomerular injury may be a consequence of leukocyte recruitment, or complement itself may directly attack target cells. Complement activation generates the small chemoattractant peptides C3a and C5a that are especially effective in recruiting and activating PMN expressing C3a and C5a receptors. The latter fragment is unique for its chemotactic activity, which leads to the recruitment and activation of PMNs. Observations during the heterologous phase of anti-GBM nephritis provide the most compelling evidence for the complement PMN–dependent mechanism of glomerular injury. The MAC of complement may also activate the transcription factor NF-κB leading to further inflammation due to IL-8 and MCP-1 production (112). The importance of this pathway is illustrated by studies in complement-depleted or -neutralized animals that are protected from the early injury induced by anti-GBM antibodies. Despite the presence of C3a and C5a receptors on several other cells, including monocytes, the glomerular recruitment of monocytes is usually complement independent. Mesangial cells also express the C5a receptor that may lead to direct cellular activation in the absence of PMN (113).

Based on important observations in the models of passive Heymann nephritis and anti–Thy 1 nephritis, it was recognized that the terminal complement components C5b-C9 that form the MAC can directly induce glomerular injury without inflammatory cells. Many subsequent studies using different strategies to inhibit or deplete complement or experiments in rodents with genetic complement deficiencies have clearly established the requirement for C5b-9 formation within glomeruli as the key event that initiates glomerular cell damage. The nature of this injury is still an area of active investigation, but several possibilities have been recognized. Multiple C9 molecules of the MAC polymerize to form ring-like structures that insert into the lipid bilayer of cell membranes, forming channels. Insertion into erythrocyte cell membranes leads to hemolysis, but nucleated cells are more resilient. C5b-9 can induce cell death by apoptosis, and such a mechanism may explain the early phase of complement-dependent mesangiolysis in rats with Thy 1 nephritis and glomerular endothelial cell loss in antibody complement–dependent thrombotic microangiopathy (114). "Sublytic" levels of C5b-9 have been shown to significantly modify the

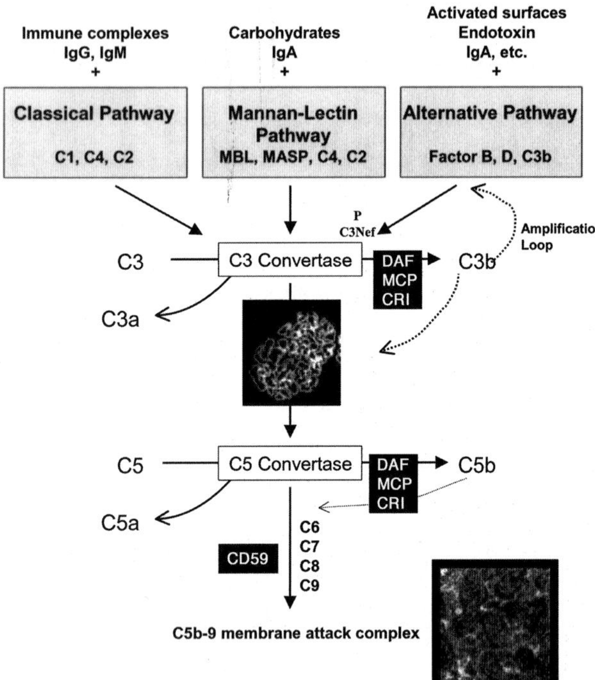

FIGURE 29.7. The complement cascade. The complement cascade is composed of at least 35 plasma proteins and several cell membrane receptors. The cascade is divided into three activation pathways: the classical, alternative, and mannan-lectin recognition pathways, which activate different early components, and a common terminal unit leading to the formation of C5b-9 and the membrane attack complex (MAC) of multiple C9 molecules. In humans, the classical pathway is activated by the binding of Clq to the Fc region of immunoglobulin G1 (IgG1), IgG2, IgG3, or IgM. The alternative pathway is usually triggered by immunoglobulin-independent interactions with substances such as damaged tissues, polysaccharides, or microorganisms. IgA may activate the alternative pathway, but it does not capture C3 molecules efficiently. GBM can also activate the alternative pathway. The recently identified lectin complement pathway leads to complement activation when the plasma protein mannan-binding lectin (MBL), which has a structure similar to C1q, binds to specific carbohydrate structures. MBL normally circulates as a complex with a family of serine protease (MBL-associated serine proteases-1, -2, -3) that becomes activated as a consequence of MBL-carbohydrate interactions. These proteases subsequently cleave C3 and C4. C3 nephritic factor (C3NeF) is an IgG autoantibody that reacts with the alternative pathway C3 convertase (C3bBb), an interaction that enhances enzyme activity leading to C3 consumption. The membrane attack complex of polymerized C9 molecules forms ring-like structures that may insert into cellular and basement membranes to cause dysfunction (illustrated within renal basement membrane in the lower-right immunoelectron photomicrograph). At least four cell surface proteins, highlighted in black boxes at their sites of action, inhibit complement activation and protect glomerular cells from complement-mediated damage: decay accelerating factor (DAF), membrane cofactor protein (MCP), complement receptor 1 (CR1), and CD59. (The MAC photomicrograph is from Falk et al. Ultrastructural localization of the membrane attack complex of complement in human renal tissues. *Am J Kidney Dis* 1987;9:121–128, with permission.)

behavior of the targeted cell. For example, several intracellular signaling pathways are activated in glomerular epithelial cells, leading to increased synthesis of eicosanoids and matrix protein; mesangial cells respond by increased synthesis of IL-1, ROS, and PG; and endothelial cells produce MCP-1 and IL-8 (112,115). At least some of these products are coupled to alterations in the glomerular capillary permselectivity barrier that lead to proteinuria. What remains perplexing is the mechanism by which MAC causes glomerular injury and proteinuria in immunologic diseases associated with noncellular antigens. Although the GBM lacks a lipid bilayer, C5b-9 does bind to it. In factor H–deficient Yorkshire piglets that spontaneously develop membranoproliferative glomerulonephritis type II (dense intramembranous deposit disease in the absence of immune complex deposition) and factor H knock-out mice with MPGN, deposits of C5b-9 can be seen along the GBM early in the course of the disease (116).

Glomerular cells are normally protected from complement-mediated injury due to a cell-surface defense mechanism that inhibits complement activation and/or function (117). In human glomeruli, three such molecules have been well characterized, but additional molecules exist. Decay accelerating factor (DAF or CD55) and membrane cofactor protein (MCP or CD46) regulate C3 and C5 activation. CD59 inhibits at the level of C8 activation, preventing MAC formation (Fig. 29.7). In glomeruli, MCP and CD59 are expressed by all three types of intrinsic cells, whereas DAF expression is minimal, sometimes found on podocytes. Studies based on human biopsies show that MCP and CD59 expression is increased, and DAF is expressed *de novo* in the mesangium in various forms of glomerulonephritis. Crry is the rodent homolog with activities similar to DAF and MCP. Not only does blockade of complement regulatory proteins such as DC59 or Crry exacerbate complement-dependent glomerulonephritis, but also soluble Crry and CD59 can effectively inhibit complement and attenuate renal injury (118,119).

Two additional complement regulatory proteins are of interest for their potential to attenuate glomerular injury. CR1 (CD35) preferentially binds to C3b and C4b and is expressed on glomerular podocytes. CR1 also functions as a regulatory molecule to protect cells from injury, and treatment with soluble CR1 has been shown to attenuate glomerular injury. Clusterin is a plasma protein that is frequently found within glomerular immune deposits in association with vitronectin and soluble C5b-9. Clusterin depletion enhances immune complex glomerulonephritis in mice (120).

Systemically, the primary function of the complement is one of defense and protection against infectious and autoimmune disease. This role is powerfully illustrated by the observation that individuals with genetic complement deficiencies have an increased incidence of infectious diseases and SLE that is often associated with glomerulonephritis. The risk is greatest with deficiencies of the early components of the classical pathway.

The complement cascade plays a role in the normal processing and elimination of immune complexes before they can deposit in tissues such as glomeruli. *In vitro* studies have shown that components of the classical pathway help to maintain circulating immune complexes soluble by interfering with their aggregation so that they can be eliminated by the mononuclear phagocytic system. In primates, the opsonization of immune complexes by complement facilitates hepatic elimination by the "erythrocyte shuttle." In the lupus-prone mouse, deficiency of C3, C4, and factor B causes worse renal disease (121–123). The alternative complement pathway is able to dissolve antigen-antibody complexes by intercalating C3 molecules into their lattice structure. This activity may help to clear immune complex deposits from glomeruli. Recent observations in C1q-deficient mice, which like deficient humans develop a lupus-like syndrome, suggest that complement plays an important role in the clearance of apoptotic cells (a potential source of nuclear autoantigens) (124).

Reactive Oxygen Species

ROS are partially reduced oxygen molecules containing an unpaired electron that are generated during oxygen metabolism and are capable of an independent existence. Oxygen normally accepts four electrons to be converted directly into water. Acceptance of one electron generates superoxide anion (O_2^-), two electrons produce hydrogen peroxide (H_2O_2), and three electrons generate the hydroxyl radical (OH·). Although H_2O_2 itself is not an oxygen radical, it is an important precursor. ROS may be generated by intrinsic glomerular cells (endothelial, mesangial, epithelial) or infiltrating leukocytes by a variety of stimuli, and they can cause glomerular damage. In experimental models of glomerular disease, alterations in glomerular permselectivity and proteinuria have been linked to ROS generation. Other effects relevant to the glomerulus include the ability of ROS to influence the susceptibility of the GBM to degradation directly or indirectly via the activation of latent proteases (collagenase, gelatinase) or by inactivation of collagenolytic enzyme inhibitors (α_1-protease inhibitor), halogenation and damage to glomerular structures via interactions with hypohalous acid derivatives (derived from PMN), mediation of cellular toxicity, vasodilation of the microcirculation, and altered metabolic activity of intrinsic glomerular cells. ROS may also be involved in the initiation phase of glomerular damage, for example, by altering the hexameric structure of collagen IV to expose the normally "hidden" Goodpasture antigen (125).

Several different ROS may cause glomerular injury. Superoxide anions are the most abundant species produced by the respiratory burst of PMNs, but they are poorly reactive in aqueous solution and are unlikely to mediate tissue injury. It is more likely that the toxic glomerular effects of O_2^- relate to its conversion to hydroxyl radicals via the Haber-Weiss reaction. Hydrogen peroxide appears to be an important mediator of PMN-dependent models of glomerular diseases. Infusion of H_2O_2 directly into the renal artery of rats causes dose-dependent proteinuria, and depletion of H_2O_2 with catalase therapy reduces PMN-dependent proteinuria. In addition to its potential role as an antigenic target in ANCA-associated vasculitis, myeloperoxidase catalyzes the formation of another toxic product by reaction of H_2O_2 with a halide, usually to produce hypochlorous acid. The role of highly toxic hydroxyl radicals in glomerular injury is less clearly defined. Both H_2O_2 and O_2^- may be converted to OH· via the Haber-Weiss reaction, and OH· scavenger therapy has been beneficial in several experimental models, but in general the agents used may have additional effects unrelated to OH· depletion. Analogous to atherosclerosis, lipid peroxidation products may also deposit in glomeruli with proinflammatory effects. Glomeruli are normally equipped with effective antioxidant defenses—catalase, superoxidase dismutase, and glutathione peroxidase. The response of these endogenous systems has not been extensively investigated in glomerulonephritis, but a recent study reported a decline in glomerular antioxidant activity during the phase of ROS generation in rats with Thy 1 nephritis (126).

Eicosanoids

Eicosanoids (*eicos* is the Greek word for 20 indicating their number of carbon atoms) are a family of biologically important autocoids derived from AA that are released from plasma membranes by cytosolic phospholipases (rate-limiting step). Two major pathways generate oxidized AA products of interest in glomerular disease: the COX and lipoxygenases (Fig. 29.8). Each pathway has its own receptors; some are expressed on glomerular cells. Whereas both resident glomerular cells and inflammatory cells are active in AA oxidation, most often resident cells produce COX

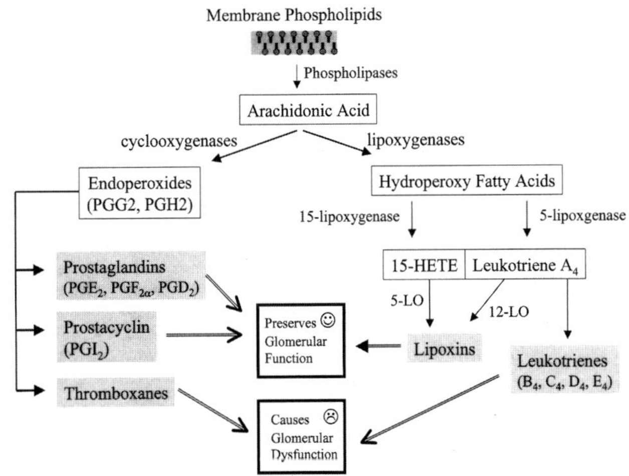

FIGURE 29.8. Glomerular effects of eicosanoids. Arachidonic acid released from plasma membranes by phospholipases is metabolized by cyclooxygenase and lipoxygenase enzymes to yield eicosanoids that can regulate glomerular hemodynamics and/or the intensity of inflammation. Some eicosanoids preserve renal blood flow and dampen inflammation, whereas others compromise glomerular blood flow and enhance inflammation. HETE, hydroxyeicosatetraenoic acid.

products, and leukocytes produce lipoxygenase products, with some overlap. Eicosanoids have profound effects on renal blood flow and leukocyte recruitment/activation that may either preserve renal blood flow and prevent inflammation (PGs and lipoxins) or decrease GFR and promote inflammation (Tx and leukotrienes).

Two COX genes have been identified that encode constitutive COX-1 (and the recently identified COX-3 splice variant) and the inducible COX-2, respectively (127). Neither isoform is easily detected in normal glomeruli, but several inflammatory stimuli induce COX-2 expression during glomerulonephritis. Mesangial cells are the most important intrinsic glomerular source of prostaglandin E_2; epithelial and endothelial cells produce some. Prostaglandin E_2 is often synthesized in response to acute glomerular injury in which it serves to preserve renal blood flow by vasodilation and mesangial cell relaxation. It may also have an antiinflammatory role, suppressing lymphocyte function and macrophage recruitment, preserving vascular permeability, and downregulating the synthesis of MCP-1, NO, and collagen (128,129). Prostaglandin I_2 or prostacyclin may also dampen the severity of acute glomerular injury through hemodynamic and antiinflammatory effects and by its ability to inhibit platelet activation.

Usually Tx are the most abundant eicosanoids produced by nephritic glomeruli. Elevated glomerular and/or urinary TxB_2 (the stable TxA_2 hydration product) levels have been reported in virtually every experimental model of glomerulonephritis examined, and inhibition therapy has been beneficial, especially in lupus nephritis. A relationship between TxB_2 and proteinuria has been proposed, but conflicting reports exist. A recent study reported that glomerular albumin permeability could be increased *in vitro* by incubation with TxA_2 (130). In addition to its ability to contract mesangial cells and to constrict blood vessels, TxA_2 also induces platelet aggregation, mediates the glomerular effects of PAF, and may stimulate matrix protein synthesis. TxA_2 may be synthesized by inflammatory cells (PMN, Mϕ, and platelets) as well as intrinsic glomerular cells.

Lipoxygenase products may also be produced during acute glomerulonephritis (Fig. 29.8). The 5-lipoxygenase products (5-HETE, LTB_4, and leukotrienes C_4, D_4, E_4) appear to originate from infiltrating leukocytes, whereas 12-lipoxygenase predominates in platelets. Elevated levels of LTB_4 have been reported in several experimental models and associated with worse glomerular damage due to both hemodynamic effects (vasoconstriction) and enhancement of leukocyte recruitment and activation. Although the functional significance of all of the products of AA lipoxygenation has not yet been determined, studies using LTB_4, LTC_4, and LTD_4 receptor antagonists have reduced glomerular disease severity (131).

Lipoxins are a family of more recently described eicosanoids that undergo dual lipoxygenation by either 5- and 15- or 5- and 12-lipoxygenases (132). They have significant antiinflammatory effects, particularly because of their ability to block leukotriene-mediated PMN chemotaxis and β_2 integrin–dependent adhesion. Within inflamed glomeruli, interaction between PMNs (a source of 5-lipoxygenase) and platelets (a source of 12-lipoxygenase) results in the generation of lipoxins. Mϕ are a rich source of 15-lipoxygenase. The antiinflammatory effects of 15-lipoxygenase were nicely demonstrated in an anti-GBM nephritis model by gene transfection (133).

Two dietary manipulations that induce changes in eicosanoid metabolism have been shown to attenuate glomerulonephritis severity. First, dietary supplementation with fish oil that contains omega-3 fatty acids (especially eicosapentaenoic acids and docosahexaenoic acid) modifies both COX and lipoxygenase metabolites. Second, dietary depletion of essential fatty acids impairs renal production of a specific lipid-derived Mϕ chemoattractant and eicosanoids such as LTB_4. In addition to alterations in eicosanoid biosynthesis, both fish oil supplementation and essential fatty acid deficiency have been shown to reduce macrophage production of TNF-α, ROS, and NO. Fish oil decreases mesangial cell proliferation in response to mitogens such as PDGF that have been implicated in the pathogenesis of mesangioproliferative glomerular disorders (134).

Endothelin and Nitric Oxide

ETs are a family of peptides first isolated in 1988. Three mammalian isoforms are known: ET-1, -2, and -3. ET, predominantly ET-1, is produced constitutively by intrinsic glomerular cells, most notably by endothelial cells. Several mediators of glomerular inflammation are reported to stimulate the production of ET-1 by mesangial cells *in vitro*, TGFβ, IL-1, TNF-α, PDGF, thrombin, and Tx, for example. Synthesis of ET-1 by mesangial cells and macrophages has also been documented *in vivo* in several human and animal models of glomerulonephritis. Evidence of a direct role for ET-1 in glomerular damage is based on the ability of ET-receptor blockade to attenuate experimental glomerulonephritis and the presence of glomerulosclerosis in ET-1 overexpressing mice. ET may function as a mesangial cell mitogen and a mediator of inflammation by upregulating adhesion molecules and by enhancing monocyte chemoattraction and activation. ET-1 may also stimulate matrix protein production.

Several endothelium-derived factors can mediate vascular relaxation, but the term *endothelium-derived relaxing factor* has become synonymous with NO. NO is a gaseous free radical that is liberated from the enzymatic conversion of L-arginine to citrulline by NO synthase. NO is an unstable molecule with a half-life of a few seconds; its stable oxidation products, nitrites and nitrates, or its secondary mediator, cyclic guanosine monophosphate, are used to estimate rates of NO generation. Three NO synthase isoforms have been identified: two constitutive, calcium-dependent enzymes originally described in the brain (nNOS) and endothelium (eNOS), respectively, and an inducible, calcium-independent enzyme first described in macrophages (iNOS). In normal glomeruli low levels of eNOS and sometimes iNOS may be present, but generally these enzymes are quiescent unless stimulated. The acute phase of glomerular disease is usually characterized by increased NO production, and several inflammatory stimuli have been shown to stimulate production, endotoxin, TNF-α, IL-1, cyclic adenosine monophosphate, and IFN, for example.

Despite great interest in the biologic role of NO, it remains unclear whether its enhanced expression during glomerulonephritis serves a primary beneficial or detrimental role because it elicits multiple effects. An emerging theme suggests that the origin of NO—both cellular source and generating enzyme isoform—may determine its fate and function. Enhanced eNOS activity has many protective outcomes, including vasodilation to preserve renal plasma flow, inhibition of platelet aggregation and thrombosis, and decreased leukocyte recruitment (135). In eNOS–/– mice, anti-GBM antibodies induce severe glomerular damage with worse inflammation and fibrosis than is observed in wild-type mice (136). Experimental thrombotic microangiopathy is also worsened by inhibition of endogenous eNOS (137).

In other models of glomerular injury, NO is produced by iNOS activity of inflammatory leukocytes and, less often, of mesangial cells and is often associated with glomerular damage. NO can be oxidized to peroxynitrite, a toxic ROS (138). NO may also bind directly to iron or thiol groups on proteins and modify their function. Heme oxygenase has been recognized as an important defense against oxidative injury, and one of its activities is to downregulate iNOS expression (139). NO has been ascribed other functions that may be relevant to glomerular injury but these still need further *in vivo* investigation—mitogenesis, apoptosis, vascular permeability changes, immune response modulation, and matrix synthesis (140). Pharmacologic blockade of iNOS using the inhibitor L-NIL has been beneficial in some but not all tested models, but genetic deficiency of iNOS does not alter the severity of anti-GBM nephritis (141,142).

RESOLUTION OR PROGRESSION OF GLOMERULAR INJURY

The immunologic events initiating glomerular injury are often self-limited. Yet, the outcome is extremely variable, ranging from the regeneration of an entirely normal glomerulus to global glomerulosclerosis. It is becoming evident that many genetic factors influence the glomerular response to injury (143). It is also clear that the events occurring simultaneously in the tubulointerstitium play a critical role in determining the long-term outcome in patients with primary glomerulonephritis. Although a discussion of issues relevant to the resolution of glomerular injury is beyond the scope of this chapter, a few recent observations merit presentation.

The difference between recovery and progression may be determined by the duration or intensity of the initial insult. This can be shown experimentally using nephritogenic antibodies in which the injection of a single dose induces injury followed by full recovery, whereas multiple injections may cause progressive fibrosis. Glomerular sclerosis is characterized by the progressive accumulation of extracellular matrix proteins. As damaged glomeruli repair themselves, matrix protein synthesis may be transiently increased, but in the absence of ongoing injury, this phase of mesangial matrix expansion often does not progress to the destructive phase of glomerulosclerosis. Matrix-degrading enzymes are produced by glomeruli. They include serine proteases (plasminogen activators, elastase) and the MMPs (interstitial collagenase, gelatinases, stromelysin, and membrane-type MMP). Each of these enzymes has a naturally occurring inhibitor(s). An increase in proteolytic enzyme secretion or a decrease in inhibitor activity could degrade early glomerular matrix protein deposits. It is increasingly recognized that many of these proteases/inhibitors are multifunctional proteins. For example, MMP-2 is a gelatinase that also activates mesangial cells, whereas the tissue inhibitor of metalloproteinase-1 inhibits mesangial cell apoptosis (144,145).

Mesangial cell proliferation is a feature of many acute glomerular diseases that progress to chronic disease, but it is not clear that mesangial hypercellularity per se predicts progression. More important is the phenotypic transformation of mesangial cells into smooth muscle–like cells (expressing alpha smooth muscle actin, non–smooth muscle myosin, and the intermediate filament, desmin). These cells are the primary source of the sclerosing matrix proteins. Innate genetic programs within mesangial precursor cells may determine their phenotypic and functional fate (8). The contribution of podocytes to the expanding pool of matrix proteins is unclear, although *in vitro* these cells synthesize several matrix proteins. During glomerular repair, novel interstitial matrix proteins may be synthesized that further modulate the function of glomerular cells through integrin-dependent signaling mechanisms (Table 29.1).

Apoptotic programs play a critical role (146). During the recovery phase, apoptosis has been shown to be important in the reversal of mesangial cell hypercellularity and perhaps in the elimination of inflammatory cells. Programmed cell death may further deplete all lines of intrinsic glomerular cell as glomeruli succumb to destruction by sclerosis. An important area of investigation is the study of the molecular pathways that program glomerular cell death and whether different mechanisms are involved in the beneficial effects of apoptosis that terminate inflammation compared to those that lead to acellular sclerotic glomeruli.

During the evolution of glomerular injury, several soluble factors may be produced that help dampen or even terminate disease progression. These may be products of intrinsic glomerular cells, inflammatory leukocytes, or T cells polarized to a Th2 phenotype. Examples include Th2 cytokines (Fig. 29.4), matrix-degrading proteases, fibrinolytic activity (Fig. 29.6), complement regulatory proteins (Fig. 29.7), antiinflammatory eicosanoids (Fig. 29.8) protective growth factors (Table 29.4), and NO. Some glycoproteins synthesized during the inflammatory phase may sequester and inhibit fibrosis-promoting cytokines. For example, SPARC (*s*ecreted *p*rotein *a*cidic and *r*ich in *c*ysteine) binds PDGF, HSPG binds bFGF, and small proteoglycans, including decorin and biglycan, block the actions of TGF-β1.

On the other hand, other products of glomerular inflammation have fibrogenic potential. The central role of TGFβ is undisputed based on data from many studies (147). Many other factors contribute, some working via TGFβ interactions and other independently such as angiotensin II and ET-1 [reviewed in (148)]. Numerous physical features associated with glomerular injury have been implicated in the genesis of glomerulosclerosis, but how they function at a molecular level is not fully understood. These include intraglomerular hypertension (which may cause glomerular mechanical stretch-induced TGF-β1 synthesis), mesangial overload, the glomerular hypertrophic response, podocyte protein overload, podocytopenia, hyperlipidemia, and secondary cellular immune responses to cryptic glomerular antigens exposed during injury.

ACKNOWLEDGMENTS

Grants supporting the author's research and academic efforts are greatly appreciated and acknowledged, from the National Institutes of Health (DK54500 and DK44757) and the Juvenile Diabetes Foundation. Most of the references cited have been published since the writing of this chapter for the 4th edition of *Pediatric Nephrology*. Readers are referred to Chapter 40 in the fourth edition and Chapter 32 in the third edition for a partial listing of earlier published work that is relevant to the immunopathogenesis of glomerular injury.

REFERENCES

1. Miner JH. Renal basement membrane components. *Kidney Int* 1999;56:2016–2024.
2. Raats CJ, Van Den Born J, Berden JH. Glomerular heparan sulfate alterations: mechanisms and relevance for proteinuria. *Kidney Int* 2000;57:385–400.
3. Collar JE, Ladva S, Cairns TD, et al. Red cell traverse through thin glomerular basement membranes. *Kidney Int* 2001;59:2069–2072.
4. Kuhara T, Kagami S, Kuroda Y. Expression of beta 1-integrins on activated mesangial cells in human glomerulonephritis. *J Am Soc Nephrol* 1997;8:1679–1687.
5. Sugenoya Y, Yoshimura A, Yamamura H, et al. Smooth-muscle calponin in mesangial cells: regulation of expression and a role in suppressing glomerulonephritis. *J Am Soc Nephrol* 2002;13:322–331.
6. Hugo C, Shankland SJ, Bowen-Pope DF, et al. Extraglomerular origin of the mesangial cell after injury. A new role of the juxtaglomerular apparatus. *J Clin Invest* 1997;100:786–794.
7. Imasawa T, Utsunomiya Y, Kawamura T, et al. The potential of bone marrow-derived cells to differentiate to glomerular mesangial cells. *J Am Soc Nephrol* 2001;12:1401–1409.
8. Cornacchia F, Fornoni A, Plati AR, et al. Glomerulosclerosis is transmitted by bone marrow-derived mesangial cell progenitors. *J Clin Invest* 2001;108:1649–1656.
9. Shankland SJ. Cell cycle regulatory proteins in glomerular disease. *Kidney Int* 1999;56:1208–1215.
10. Maeshima Y, Kashihara N, Yasuda T, et al. Inhibition of mesangial cell proliferation by E2F decoy oligodeoxynucleotide in vitro and in vivo. *J Clin Invest* 1998;101:2589–2597.
11. Pippin JW, Qu Q, Meijer L, et al. Direct in vivo inhibition of the nuclear cell cycle cascade in experimental mesangial proliferative glomerulonephritis with Roscovitine, a novel cyclin-dependent kinase antagonist. *J Clin Invest* 1997;100:2512–2520.
12. Miyata T, Inagi R, Nangaku M, et al. Overexpression of the serpin megsin induces progressive mesangial cell proliferation and expansion. *J Clin Invest* 2002;109:585–593.
13. Kerjaschki D. Caught flat-footed: podocyte damage and the molecular bases of focal glomerulosclerosis. *J Clin Invest* 2001;108:1583–1587.
14. Takeda T, McQuistan T, Orlando RA, et al. Loss of glomerular foot processes is associated with uncoupling of podocalyxin from the actin cytoskeleton. *J Clin Invest* 2001;108:289–301.
15. Topham PS, Kawachi H, Haydar SA, et al. Nephritogenic mAb 5-1-6 is directed at the extracellular domain of rat nephrin. *J Clin Invest* 1999;104:1559–1566.
16. Mundel P, Shankland SJ. Podocyte biology and response to injury. *J Am Soc Nephrol* 2002;13:3005–3015.
17. Ophascharoensuk V, Fero ML, Hughes J, et al. The cyclin-dependent kinase inhibitor p27Kip1 safeguards against inflammatory injury. *Nat Med* 1998;4:575–580.
18. Bariety J, Nochy D, Mandet C, et al. Podocytes undergo phenotypic changes and express macrophagic-associated markers in idiopathic collapsing glomerulopathy. *Kidney Int* 1998;53:918–925.
19. Kriz W. Podocyte is the major culprit accounting for the progression of chronic renal disease. *Microsc Res Tech* 2002;57:189–195.
20. Sorensson J, Fierlbeck W, Heider T, et al. Glomerular endothelial fenestrae in vivo are not formed from caveolae. *J Am Soc Nephrol* 2002;13:2639–2647.
21. Oda T, Yoshizawa N, Takeuchi A, et al. Glomerular proliferating cell kinetics in acute post-streptococcal glomerulonephritis (APSGN). *J Pathol* 1997;183:359–368.
22. Masuda Y, Shimizu A, Mori T, et al. Vascular endothelial growth factor enhances glomerular capillary repair and accelerates resolution of experimentally induced glomerulonephritis. *Am J Pathol* 2001;159:599–608.
23. Yuan HT, Tipping PG, Li XZ, et al. Angiopoietin correlates with glomerular capillary loss in anti-glomerular basement membrane glomerulonephritis. *Kidney Int* 2002;61:2078–2089.

24. Cook HT, Khan SB, Allen A, et al. Treatment with an antibody to VLA-1 integrin reduces glomerular and tubulointerstitial scarring in a rat model of crescentic glomerulonephritis. *Am J Pathol* 2002;161:1265–1272.
25. Kagami S, Urushihara M, Kondo S, et al. Effects of anti-alpha1 integrin subunit antibody on anti-Thy-1 glomerulonephritis. *Lab Invest* 2002;82:1219–1227.
26. Phelps RG, Rees AJ. The HLA complex in Goodpasture's disease: a model for analyzing susceptibility to autoimmunity. *Kidney Int* 1999;56:1638–1653.
27. Bhimma R, Hammond MG, Coovadia HM, et al. HLA class I and II in black children with hepatitis B virus-associated membranous nephropathy. *Kidney Int* 2002;61:1510–1515.
28. Akiyama F, Tanaka T, Yamada R, et al. Single-nucleotide polymorphisms in the class II region of the major histocompatibility complex in Japanese patients with immunoglobulin A nephropathy. *J Hum Genet* 2002;47:532–538.
29. Hellmark T, Burkhardt H, Wieslander J. Goodpasture disease. Characterization of a single conformational epitope as the target of pathogenic autoantibodies. *J Biol Chem* 1999;274: 25862–25868.
30. Borza DB, Netzer KO, Leinonen A, et al. The Goodpasture autoantigen. Identification of multiple cryptic epitopes on the NC1 domain of the alpha3(IV) collagen chain. *J Biol Chem* 2000;275:6030–6037.
31. Kalluri R, Torre A, Shield CF 3rd, et al. Identification of alpha3, alpha4, and alpha5 chains of type IV collagen as alloantigens for Alport posttransplant anti-glomerular basement membrane antibodies. *Transplantation* 2000;69:679–683.
32. Kagami S, Okada K, Funai M, et al. A monoclonal antibody (1G10) recognizes a novel human mesangial antigen. *Kidney Int* 1992;42:700–709.
33. Chugh S, Yuan H, Topham PS, et al. Aminopeptidase A: a nephritogenic target antigen of nephrotoxic serum. *Kidney Int* 2001;59:601–613.
34. Wu J, Hicks J, Borillo J, et al. CD4(+) T cells specific to a glomerular basement membrane antigen mediate glomerulonephritis. *J Clin Invest* 2002;109:517–524.
35. Park SY, Ueda S, Ohno H, et al. Resistance of Fc receptor-deficient mice to fatal glomerulonephritis. *J Clin Invest* 1998;102:1229–1238.
36. Farquhar MG, Saito A, Kerjaschki D, et al. The Heymann nephritis antigenic complex: megalin (gp330) and RAP. *J Am Soc Nephrol* 1995;6:35–47.
36a. Edgington TS, Glassock RJ, Watson JI, et al. Characterization and isolation of specific renal tubular epithelial antigens. *J Immunol* 1967;99:1199–1210.
37. Oliveira DB. Membranous nephropathy: an IgG4-mediated disease. *Lancet* 1998;351:670–671.
38. Cunningham PN, Hack BK, Ren G, et al. Glomerular complement regulation is overwhelmed in passive Heymann nephritis. *Kidney Int* 2001;60:900–909.
39. Peng H, Takano T, Papillon J, et al. Complement activates the c-Jun N-terminal kinase/stress-activated protein kinase in glomerular epithelial cells. *J Immunol* 2002;169:2594–2601.
40. Takano T, Cybulsky AV. Complement C5b-9-mediated arachidonic acid metabolism in glomerular epithelial cells: role of cyclooxygenase-1 and -2. *Am J Pathol* 2000;156:2091–2101.
41. Raats CJ, Luca ME, Bakker MA, et al. Reduction in glomerular heparan sulfate correlates with complement deposition and albuminuria in active Heymann nephritis. *J Am Soc Nephrol* 1999;10:1689–1699.
42. O'Donoghue DJ, Darvill A, Ballardie FW. Mesangial cell autoantigens in immunoglobulin A nephropathy and Henoch-Schönlein purpura. *J Clin Invest* 1991;88:1522–1530.
43. Chan TM, Leung JK, Ho SK, et al. Mesangial cell-binding anti-DNA antibodies in patients with systemic lupus erythematosus. *J Am Soc Nephrol* 2002;13:1219–1229.
44. Suga S, Kim YG, Joly A, et al. Vascular endothelial growth factor (VEGF121) protects rats from renal infarction in thrombotic microangiopathy. *Kidney Int* 2001;60:1297–1308.
45. Falk RJ, Jennette JC. ANCA are pathogenic—oh yes they are! *J Am Soc Nephrol* 2002;13:1977–1979.
46. Sibelius U, Hattar K, Schenkel A, et al. Wegener's granulomatosis: anti-proteinase 3 antibodies are potent inductors of human endothelial cell signaling and leakage response. *J Exp Med* 1998;187:497–503.
47. Yang JJ, Preston GA, Pendergraft WF, et al. Internalization of proteinase 3 is concomitant with endothelial cell apoptosis and internalization of myeloperoxidase with generation of intracellular oxidants. *Am J Pathol* 2001;158:581–592.
48. Xiao H, Heeringa P, Hu P, et al. Antineutrophil cytoplasmic autoantibodies specific for myeloperoxidase cause glomerulonephritis and vasculitis in mice. *J Clin Invest* 2002;110:955–963.
49. Parra G, Rodriguez-Iturbe B, Batsford S, et al. Antibody to streptococcal zymogen in the serum of patients with acute glomerulonephritis: a multicentric study. *Kidney Int* 1998;54: 509–517.
50. Ogura Y, Suzuki S, Shirakawa T, et al. *Haemophilus parainfluenzae* antigen and antibody in children with IgA nephropathy and Henoch-Schönlein nephritis. *Am J Kidney Dis* 2000;36:47–52.
51. Imasawa T, Nagasawa R, Utsunomiya Y, et al. Bone marrow transplantation attenuates murine IgA nephropathy: role of a stem cell disorder. *Kidney Int* 1999;56:1809–1817.
52. Tomana M, Novak J, Julian BA, et al. Circulating immune complexes in IgA nephropathy consist of IgA1 with galactose-deficient hinge region and antiglycan antibodies. *J Clin Invest* 1999;104:73–81.
53. Donadio JV, Grande JP. IgA nephropathy. *N Engl J Med* 2002;347:738–748.
54. Zheng F, Kundu GC, Zhang Z, et al. Uteroglobin is essential in preventing immunoglobulin A nephropathy in mice. *Nat Med* 1999;5:1018–1025.
55. Leung JC, Tsang AW, Chan DT, et al. Absence of CD89, polymeric immunoglobulin receptor, and asialoglycoprotein receptor on human mesangial cells. *J Am Soc Nephrol* 2000;11:241–249.
56. Roos A, Bouwman LH, van Gijlswijk-Janssen DJ, et al. Human IgA activates the complement system via the mannan-binding lectin pathway. *J Immunol* 2001;167:2861–2868.
57. Kalluri R, Danoff TM, Okada H, et al. Susceptibility to anti-glomerular basement membrane disease and Goodpasture syndrome is linked to MHC class II genes and the emergence of T cell-mediated immunity in mice. *J Clin Invest* 1997;100:2263–2275.
58. Rosenkranz AR, Knight S, Sethi S, et al. Regulatory interactions of alphabeta and gammadelta T cells in glomerulonephritis. *Kidney Int* 2000;58:1055–1066.

59. Sahali D, Pawlak A, Valanciute A, et al. A novel approach to investigation of the pathogenesis of active minimal-change nephrotic syndrome using subtracted cDNA library screening. *J Am Soc Nephrol* 2002;13:1238–1247.
59a. Shalhoub RJ. Pathogenesis of lipoid nephrosis: a disorder of T-cell function. *Lancet* 1974;2:556–560.
60. Glassock R. Circulating permeability factors in the nephrotic syndrome—a fresh look at an old problem. *J Am Soc Nephrol* 2003;14:541–543.
60a. Savin VJ, Sharma R, Sharma M, et al. Circulating factor associated with increased glomerular permeability to albumin in recurrent focal segmental glomerulosclerosis. *N Engl J Med* 1996;334:878–883.
61. Carraro M, Caridi G, Bruschi M, et al. Serum glomerular permeability activity in patients with podocin mutations (NPHS2) and steroid-resistant nephrotic syndrome. *J Am Soc Nephrol* 2002;13:1946–1952.
62. Candiano G, Musante L, Carraro M, et al. Apolipoproteins prevent glomerular albumin permeability induced in vitro by serum from patients with focal segmental glomerulosclerosis. *J Am Soc Nephrol* 2001;12:143–150.
63. Sharma R, Sharma M, McCarthy ET, et al. Components of normal serum block the focal segmental glomerulosclerosis factor activity in vitro. *Kidney Int* 2000;58:1973–1979.
64. Yamada A, Salama AD, Sayegh MH. The role of novel T cell costimulatory pathways in autoimmunity and transplantation. *J Am Soc Nephrol* 2002;13:559–575.
65. Holdsworth SR, Kitching AR, Tipping PG. Th1 and Th2 T helper cell subsets affect patterns of injury and outcomes in glomerulonephritis. *Kidney Int* 1999;55:1198–1216.
66. Mathieson PW. Cytokine polymorphisms and nephrotic syndrome. *Clin Sci (Lond)* 2002;102:513–514.
67. Yang N, Isbel NM, Nikolic-Paterson DJ, et al. Local macrophage proliferation in human glomerulonephritis. *Kidney Int* 1998;54:143–151.
68. Gomez-Guerrero C, Duque N, Casado MT, et al. Administration of IgG Fc fragments prevents glomerular injury in experimental immune complex nephritis. *J Immunol* 2000;164: 2092–2101.
69. Adler S, Brady HR. Cell adhesion molecules and the glomerulopathies. *Am J Med* 1999;107:371–386.
70. Luster AD. Chemokines—chemotactic cytokines that mediate inflammation. *N Engl J Med* 1998;338:436–445.
71. Huber TB, Reinhardt HC, Exner M, et al. Expression of functional CCR and CXCR chemokine receptors in podocytes. *J Immunol* 2002;168:6244–6252.
72. Romagnani P, Lazzeri E, Lasagni L, et al. IP-10 and Mig production by glomerular cells in human proliferative glomerulonephritis and regulation by nitric oxide. *J Am Soc Nephrol* 2002;13:53–64.
73. Topham PS, Csizmadia V, Soler D, et al. Lack of chemokine receptor CCR1 enhances Th1 responses and glomerular injury during nephrotoxic nephritis. *J Clin Invest* 1999;104:1549–1557.
74. Bird JE, Giancarli MR, Kurihara T, et al. Increased severity of glomerulonephritis in C-C chemokine receptor 2 knockout mice. *Kidney Int* 2000;57:129–136.
75. Mack M, Cihak J, Simonis C, et al. Expression and characterization of the chemokine receptors CCR2 and CCR5 in mice. *J Immunol* 2001;166:4697–4704.
76. Zernecke A, Weber KS, Erwig LP, et al. Combinatorial model of chemokine involvement in glomerular monocyte recruitment: role of CXC chemokine receptor 2 in infiltration during nephrotoxic nephritis. *J Immunol* 2001;166:5755–5762.
77. Ito Y, Kawachi H, Morioka Y, et al. Fractalkine expression and the recruitment of CX3CR1+ cells in the prolonged mesangial proliferative glomerulonephritis. *Kidney Int* 2002; 61:2044–2057.
78. Luo Y, Lloyd C, Gutierrez-Ramos JC, et al. Chemokine amplification in mesangial cells. *J Immunol* 1999;163:3985–3992.
79. Lopez-Franco O, Suzuki Y, Sanjuan G, et al. Nuclear factor-kappa B inhibitors as potential novel anti-inflammatory agents for the treatment of immune glomerulonephritis. *Am J Pathol* 2002;161:1497–1505.
80. Mishra R, Leahy P, Simonson MS. Gene expression profiling reveals role for EGF-family ligands in mesangial cell proliferation. *Am J Physiol Renal Physiol* 2002;283:F1151–1159.
81. Feng L, Garcia GE, Yang Y, et al. Heparin-binding EGF-like growth factor contributes to reduced glomerular filtration rate during glomerulonephritis in rats. *J Clin Invest* 2000;105:341–350.
82. Floege J, Burg M, Hugo C, et al. Endogenous fibroblast growth factor-2 mediates cytotoxicity in experimental mesangioproliferative glomerulonephritis. *J Am Soc Nephrol* 1998;9:792–801.
83. Messmer UK, Briner VA, Pfeilschifter J. Basic fibroblast growth factor selectively enhances TNF-alpha-induced apoptotic cell death in glomerular endothelial cells: effects on apoptotic signaling pathways. *J Am Soc Nephrol* 2000;11:2199–2211.
84. Kitching AR, Ru Huang X, Turner AL, et al. The requirement for granulocyte-macrophage colony-stimulating factor and granulocyte colony-stimulating factor in leukocyte-mediated immune glomerular injury. *J Am Soc Nephrol* 2002;13:350–358.
85. Magen D, Mandel H, Berant M, et al. MPGN type I induced by granulocyte colony stimulating factor. *Pediatr Nephrol* 2002;17:370–372.
86. Zavala F, Masson A, Hadaya K, et al. Granulocyte-colony stimulating factor treatment of lupus autoimmune disease in MRL-lpr/lpr mice. *J Immunol* 1999;163:5125–5132.
87. Yang N, Nikolic-Paterson DJ, Ng YY, et al. Reversal of established rat crescentic glomerulonephritis by blockade of macrophage migration inhibitory factor (MIF): potential role of MIF in regulating glucocorticoid production. *Mol Med* 1998;4:413–424.
88. Tesch GH, Lan HY, Atkins RC, et al. Role of interleukin-1 in mesangial cell proliferation and matrix deposition in experimental mesangioproliferative nephritis. *Am J Pathol* 1997;151:141–150.
89. Kitching AR, Tipping PG, Kurimoto M, et al. IL-18 has IL-12-independent effects in delayed-type hypersensitivity: studies in cell-mediated crescentic glomerulonephritis. *J Immunol* 2000;165:4649–4657.
90. Esfandiari E, McInnes IB, Lindop G, et al. A proinflammatory role of IL-18 in the development of spontaneous autoimmune disease. *J Immunol* 2001;167:5338–5347.
91. Tam FW, Smith J, Karkar AM, et al. Interleukin-4 ameliorates experimental glomerulonephritis and up-regulates glo-

merular gene expression of IL-1 decoy receptor. *Kidney Int* 1997;52:1224–1231.
92. Cook HT, Singh SJ, Wembridge DE, et al. Interleukin-4 ameliorates crescentic glomerulonephritis in Wistar Kyoto rats. *Kidney Int* 1999;55:1319–1326.
93. Kluth DC, Ainslie CV, Pearce WP, et al. Macrophages transfected with adenovirus to express IL-4 reduce inflammation in experimental glomerulonephritis. *J Immunol* 2001;166: 4728–4736.
94. Lai PC, Cook HT, Smith J, et al. Interleukin-11 attenuates nephrotoxic nephritis in Wistar Kyoto rats. *J Am Soc Nephrol* 2001;12:2310–2320.
95. Huang XR, Kitching AR, Tipping PG, et al. Interleukin-10 inhibits macrophage-induced glomerular injury. *J Am Soc Nephrol* 2000;11:262–269.
96. Chadban SJ, Tesch GH, Lan HY, et al. Effect of interleukin-10 treatment on crescentic glomerulonephritis in rats. *Kidney Int* 1997;51:1809–1817.
97. Suematsu S, Matsuda T, Aozasa K, et al. IgG1 plasmacytosis in interleukin 6 transgenic mice. *Proc Natl Acad Sci U S A* 1989;86:7547–7551.
98. Karkar AM, Smith J, Tam FW, et al. Abrogation of glomerular injury in nephrotoxic nephritis by continuous infusion of interleukin-6. *Kidney Int* 1997;52:1313–1320.
99. Timoshanko JR, Kitching AR, Holdsworth SR, et al. Interleukin-12 from intrinsic cells is an effector of renal injury in crescentic glomerulonephritis. *J Am Soc Nephrol* 2001;12:464–471.
100. Okubo T, Hagiwara E, Ohno S, et al. Administration of an IL-12-encoding DNA plasmid prevents the development of chronic graft-versus-host disease (GVHD). *J Immunol* 1999; 162:4013–4017.
101. Lawson BR, Prud'homme GJ, Chang Y, et al. Treatment of murine lupus with cDNA encoding IFN-gammaR/Fc. *J Clin Invest* 2000;106:207–215.
102. Haas C, Ryffel B, Le Hir M. IFN-gamma is essential for the development of autoimmune glomerulonephritis in MRL/Ipr mice. *J Immunol* 1997;158:5484–5491.
103. Carvalho-Pinto CE, Garcia MI, Mellado M, et al. Autocrine production of IFN-gamma by macrophages controls their recruitment to kidney and the development of glomerulonephritis in MRL/lpr mice. *J Immunol* 2002;169:1058–1067.
104. Gilbert RE, Kelly DJ, McKay T, et al. PDGF signal transduction inhibition ameliorates experimental mesangial proliferative glomerulonephritis. *Kidney Int* 2001;59:1324–1332.
105. Eitner F, Ostendorf T, Van Roeyen C, et al. Expression of a novel PDGF isoform, PDGF-C, in normal and diseased rat kidney. *J Am Soc Nephrol* 2002;13:910–917.
106. Changsirikulchai S, Hudkins KL, Goodpaster TA, et al. Platelet-derived growth factor-D expression in developing and mature human kidneys. *Kidney Int* 2002;62:2043–2054.
107. Kanamaru Y, Nakao A, Mamura M, et al. Blockade of TGF-beta signaling in T cells prevents the development of experimental glomerulonephritis. *J Immunol* 2001;166:2818–2823.
108. Le Hir M, Haas C, Marino M, et al. Prevention of crescentic glomerulonephritis induced by anti-glomerular membrane antibody in tumor necrosis factor-deficient mice. *Lab Invest* 1998;78:1625–1631.
109. Ostendorf T, Kunter U, Eitner F, et al. VEGF(165) mediates glomerular endothelial repair. *J Clin Invest* 1999;104:913–923.
110. Drew AF, Tucker HL, Liu H, et al. Crescentic glomerulonephritis is diminished in fibrinogen-deficient mice. *Am J Physiol Renal Physiol* 2001;281:F1157–F1163.
111. Zhou W, Marsh JE, Sacks SH. Intrarenal synthesis of complement. *Kidney Int* 2001;59:1227–1235.
112. Kilgore KS, Schmid E, Shanley TP, et al. Sublytic concentrations of the membrane attack complex of complement induce endothelial interleukin-8 and monocyte chemoattractant protein-1 through nuclear factor-kappa B activation. *Am J Pathol* 1997;150:2019–2031.
113. Wilmer WA, Kaumaya PT, Ember JA, et al. Receptors for the anaphylatoxin C5a (CD88) on human mesangial cells. *J Immunol* 1998;160:5646–5652.
114. Hughes J, Nangaku M, Alpers CE, et al. C5b-9 membrane attack complex mediates endothelial cell apoptosis in experimental glomerulonephritis. *Am J Physiol Renal Physiol* 2000; 278:F747–F757.
115. Takano T, Cybulsky AV, Yang X, et al. Complement C5b-9 induces cyclooxygenase-2 gene transcription in glomerular epithelial cells. *Am J Physiol Renal Physiol* 2001;281:F841–F850.
116. Pickering MC, Cook HT, Warren J, et al. Uncontrolled C3 activation causes membranoproliferative glomerulonephritis in mice deficient in complement factor H. *Nat Genet* 2002;31: 424–428.
117. Nangaku M. Complement regulatory proteins in glomerular diseases. *Kidney Int* 1998;54:1419–1428.
118. Quigg RJ, He C, Lim A, et al. Transgenic mice overexpressing the complement inhibitor crry as a soluble protein are protected from antibody-induced glomerular injury. *J Exp Med* 1998;188:1321–1331.
119. Bao L, Haas M, Boackle SA, et al. Transgenic expression of a soluble complement inhibitor protects against renal disease and promotes survival in MRL/lpr mice. *J Immunol* 2002;168:3601–3607.
120. Rosenberg ME, Girton R, Finkel D, et al. Apolipoprotein J/clusterin prevents a progressive glomerulopathy of aging. *Mol Cell Biol* 2002;22:1893–1902.
121. Sekine H, Reilly CM, Molano ID, et al. Complement component C3 is not required for full expression of immune complex glomerulonephritis in MRL/lpr mice. *J Immunol* 2001;166:6444–6451.
122. Watanabe H, Garnier G, Circolo A, et al. Modulation of renal disease in MRL/lpr mice genetically deficient in the alternative complement pathway factor B. *J Immunol* 2000; 164:786–794.
123. Einav S, Pozdnyakova OO, Ma M, et al. Complement C4 is protective for lupus disease independent of C3. *J Immunol* 2002;168:1036–1041.
124. Botto M, Dell'Agnola C, Bygrave AE, et al. Homozygous C1q deficiency causes glomerulonephritis associated with multiple apoptotic bodies. *Nat Genet* 1998;19:56–59.
125. Kalluri R, Cantley LG, Kerjaschki D, et al. Reactive oxygen species expose cryptic epitopes associated with autoimmune Goodpasture syndrome. *J Biol Chem* 2000;275:20027–20032.

126. Gaertner SA, Janssen U, Ostendorf T, et al. Glomerular oxidative and antioxidative systems in experimental mesangioproliferative glomerulonephritis. *J Am Soc Nephrol* 2002;13:2930–2937.
127. Chandrasekharan NV, Dai H, Roos KL, et al. COX-3, a cyclooxygenase-1 variant inhibited by acetaminophen and other analgesic/antipyretic drugs: cloning, structure, and expression. *Proc Natl Acad Sci U S A* 2002;99:13926–13931.
128. Lianos EA. Activation and potential interactions between the arachidonic acid and L-arginine:nitric oxide pathways in glomerulonephritis. *Kidney Int* 1998;53:540–547.
129. Schneider A, Harendza S, Zahner G, et al. Cyclooxygenase metabolites mediate glomerular monocyte chemoattractant protein-1 formation and monocyte recruitment in experimental glomerulonephritis. *Kidney Int* 1999;55:430–441.
130. McCarthy ET, Sharma M. Indomethacin protects permeability barrier from focal segmental glomerulosclerosis serum. *Kidney Int* 2002;61:534–541.
131. Suzuki S, Kuroda T, Kazama JI, et al. The leukotriene B4 receptor antagonist ONO-4057 inhibits nephrotoxic serum nephritis in WKY rats. *J Am Soc Nephrol* 1999;10:264–270.
132. Baud L, Fouqueray B, Bellocq A. Switching off renal inflammation by anti-inflammatory mediators: the facts, the promise and the hope. *Kidney Int* 1998;53:1118–1126.
133. Munger KA, Montero A, Fukunaga M, et al. Transfection of rat kidney with human 15-lipoxygenase suppresses inflammation and preserves function in experimental glomerulonephritis. *Proc Natl Acad Sci U S A* 1999;96:13375–13380.
134. Schmitz PG, Zhang K, Dalal R. Eicosapentaenoic acid suppresses PDGF-induced DNA synthesis in rat mesangial cells: involvement of thromboxane A2. *Kidney Int* 2000;57:1041–1051.
135. Heeringa P, Steenbergen E, van Goor H. A protective role for endothelial nitric oxide synthase in glomerulonephritis. *Kidney Int* 2002;61:822–825.
136. Heeringa P, van Goor H, Itoh-Lindstrom Y, et al. Lack of endothelial nitric oxide synthase aggravates murine accelerated anti-glomerular basement membrane glomerulonephritis. *Am J Pathol* 2000;156:879–888.
137. Shao J, Miyata T, Yamada K, et al. Protective role of nitric oxide in a model of thrombotic microangiopathy in rats. *J Am Soc Nephrol* 2001;12:2088–2097.
138. Heeringa P, van Goor H, Moshage H, et al. Expression of iNOS, eNOS, and peroxynitrite-modified proteins in experimental anti-myeloperoxidase associated crescentic glomerulonephritis. *Kidney Int* 1998;53:382–393.
139. Datta PK, Koukouritaki SB, Hopp KA, et al. Heme oxygenase-1 induction attenuates inducible nitric oxide synthase expression and proteinuria in glomerulonephritis. *J Am Soc Nephrol* 1999;10:2540–2550.
140. Cattell V. Nitric oxide and glomerulonephritis. *Kidney Int* 2002;61:816–821.
141. Cattell V, Cook HT, Ebrahim H, et al. Anti-GBM glomerulonephritis in mice lacking nitric oxide synthase type 2. *Kidney Int* 1998;53:932–936.
142. Reilly CM, Farrelly LW, Viti D, et al. Modulation of renal disease in MRL/lpr mice by pharmacologic inhibition of inducible nitric oxide synthase. *Kidney Int* 2002;61:839–846.
143. Fornoni A, Wang Y, Lenz O, et al. Association of a decreased number of d(CA) repeats in the matrix metalloproteinase-9 promoter with glomerulosclerosis susceptibility in mice. *J Am Soc Nephrol* 2002;13:2068–2076.
144. Turck J, Pollock AS, Lee LK, et al. Matrix metalloproteinase 2 (gelatinase A) regulates glomerular mesangial cell proliferation and differentiation. *J Biol Chem* 1996;271:15074–15083.
145. Lin H, Chen X, Wang J, et al. Inhibition of apoptosis in rat mesangial cells by tissue inhibitor of metalloproteinase-1. *Kidney Int* 2002;62:60–69.
146. Savill J. Regulation of glomerular cell number by apoptosis. *Kidney Int* 1999;56:1216–1222.
147. Bottinger EP, Bitzer M. TGF-beta signaling in renal disease. *J Am Soc Nephrol* 2002;13:2600–2610.
148. Eddy AA. Molecular basis of renal fibrosis. *Pediatr Nephrol* 2000;15:290–301.
149. Rosenkranz AR, Mendrick DL, Cotran RS, et al. P-selectin deficiency exacerbates experimental glomerulonephritis: a protective role for endothelial P-selectin in inflammation. *J Clin Invest* 1999;103:649–659.
150. Janssen U, Ostendorf T, Gaertner S, et al. Improved survival and amelioration of nephrotoxic nephritis in intercellular adhesion molecule-1 knockout mice. *J Am Soc Nephrol* 1998;9:1805–1814.
151. Cunningham MA, Ono T, Hewitson TD, et al. Tissue factor pathway inhibitor expression in human crescentic glomerulonephritis. *Kidney Int* 1999;55:1311–1318.
152. Westenfeld R, Gawlik A, de Heer E, et al. Selective inhibition of inducible nitric oxide synthase enhances intraglomerular coagulation in chronic anti-Thy 1 nephritis. *Kidney Int* 2002;61:834–838.
153. Ikeguchi H, Maruyama S, Morita Y, et al. Effects of human soluble thrombomodulin on experimental glomerulonephritis. *Kidney Int* 2002;61:490–501.
154. Cunningham MA, Rondeau E, Chen X, et al. Protease-activated receptor 1 mediates thrombin-dependent, cell-mediated renal inflammation in crescentic glomerulonephritis. *J Exp Med* 2000;191:455–462.
155. Monno R, Grandaliano G, Faccio R, et al. Activated coagulation factor X: a novel mitogenic stimulus for human mesangial cells. *J Am Soc Nephrol* 2001;12:891–899.
156. Xu Q, Chen X, Fu B, et al. Integrin alphavbeta3-RGDS interaction mediates fibrin-induced morphological changes of glomerular endothelial cells. *Kidney Int* 1999;56:1413–1422.
157. Kitching AR, Holdsworth SR, Ploplis VA, et al. Plasminogen and plasminogen activators protect against renal injury in crescentic glomerulonephritis. *J Exp Med* 1997;185:963–968.
158. Eddy AA. Plasminogen activator inhibitor-1 and the kidney. *Am J Physiol Renal Physiol* 2002;283:F209–220.

30

ACUTE PROLIFERATIVE GLOMERULONEPHRITIS

ENDRE SULYOK

Acute proliferative glomerulonephritis (GN) includes a variety of diseases with diverse etiologies and variable morphologic appearances clinically presenting with a nephritic syndrome. These include abrupt onset, gross or microscopic hematuria, proteinuria varying from minimal to nephrotic range, casts on urinalysis, fluid overload with hypertension, and variable degree of renal insufficiency with oliguria or anuria. The term *proliferative* implies glomerular hypercellularity, whatever the origin of cells. They may invade the glomeruli from the circulation or may originate from glomerular mesangial, endothelial, or epithelial cells. Glomerular involvement may be focal or diffuse, segmental or global, according to the number of glomeruli and extent of glomerular injury.

The underlying mechanism of acute proliferative GN is immune-mediated inflammation as evidenced by glomerular deposits containing immune complexes and complement components in most cases. In pauci-immune crescentic GN, the pathogenetic role of immune mechanisms is indicated by the high rate of positivity for antineutrophil cytoplasmic antibodies.

It is important to emphasize that the morphologic patterns are not specific of a distinct clinical entity, and a specific disease may have different histologic appearances (Table 30.1). GN may be primary or secondary to a systemic process, such as vasculitis (1). As the etiology, history, clinical manifestations, laboratory findings, morphologic patterns, and clinical course may be extremely variable, an evaluation is needed for an appropriate diagnosis and adequate therapeutic interventions.

In this chapter, the acute poststreptococcal GN (APSGN) is presented in detail because it serves as a prototype of postinfectious proliferative GN. It is the most commonly encountered and the best understood form of proliferative GN. The terms *diffuse intracapillary GN, diffuse endocapillary GN,* and *acute postinfection GN* are also used in the text as synonyms.

ACUTE POSTSTREPTOCOCCAL GLOMERULONEPHRITIS

Epidemiology

The major aspects of the epidemiology of APSGN have been summarized in comprehensive reviews by several authors (2–4). Sporadic cases have been reported to occur in clusters, but endemic and epidemic outbreaks have also been recognized. Most often, APSGN follows upper respiratory tract infections in temperate climates or skin infections in tropic and subtropic areas caused by group A streptococci or, occasionally, groups C and G streptococci. Only certain streptococcal strains are capable of causing GN; these are called *nephritogenic streptococci.* Nephritogenic strains have the cell wall M-protein serotypes 1, 2, 3, 4, 12, 18, 25, 49, 55, 57, and 60. Postpharyngitis GN is usually associated with M types 1, 3, 4, 12, 18, 25, and 49, whereas postpyoderma GN is related to specific M types 2, 49, 55, 57, and 60. The incidence of GN after infection with nephritogenic streptococci is variable and depends on the M serotype and the site of infection. It has been reported to range from 1 to 33% of the patients, with the overall risk of approximately 15%. Clinically apparent GN occurs in less than 2% of children infected with various streptococcal strains. Seasonal variation is characteristic for APSGN in the temperate climate because streptococcal throat infections are more common in winter and early spring, whereas streptococcal pyoderma mostly occurs in late summer and early fall.

The occurrence of APSGN is influenced by certain host factors, such as age, sex, socioeconomic background, and genetic predisposition. The disease is more frequent among children between the ages of 2 and 12 years, although 5% of the patients are younger than 2 years of age. Boys are more often affected with clinically overt GN than girls, with the ratio of 2:1.

Epidemic outbreaks tend to occur in closed communities and in densely populated areas where poor hygiene, malnutrition, anemia, and intestinal parasites are common. Since the 60s of the last century, marked steady declines have been noted in the prevalence of APSGN, although cyclic recurrences have been observed in certain communities. The reason for the apparent decline in the prevalence of the disease is not clear and may be attributed to the widespread use of antibiotics, improved hygienic conditions, changes in nephritogenic potential of streptococcus strains, or altered susceptibility of the host (5). After recovery from APSGN, protective immunity is acquired against

TABLE 30.1. HISTOLOGIC CATEGORIES OF ACUTE PROLIFERATIVE (HYPERCELLULAR) GLOMERULONEPHRITIS (GN)

Histologic pattern	Causes
Diffuse intracapillary proliferative (exudative) GN (with neutrophils)	Usually postinfectious Occasionally related to SLE or vasculitis
Diffuse proliferative GN (without neutrophils)	Postinfectious GN SLE

Mesangial proliferative GN	Primary forms of GN
	  Resolving postinfectious GN
	  IgA nephropathy
	  IgM nephritis
	Accompanying systemic disease
	  SLE
	  Infective endocarditis
	  Henoch-Schönlein purpura
	  Mixed connective tissue disease

Membranoproliferative (mesangiocapillary) GN	Idiopathic
	Systemic immune complex diseases
	  Mixed cryoglobulinemia
	  SLE
	  Sjögren's syndrome
	  Hereditary deficiencies of complement components
	Infectious diseases
	  Bacterial
	    Infected ventriculoatrial shunts
	    Endocarditis
	  Viral
	    Hepatitis B and C
	    Human immunodeficiency virus
	  Protozoal: malaria, schistosomiasis
	  Other: mycoplasma, mycobacteria
	Neoplasms
	Chronic liver diseases
	Miscellaneous

Diffuse extracapillary proliferative (crescentic) GN	

Diseases with crescent in majority of cases	Anti–glomerular basement membrane antibody diseases
	  With pulmonary hemorrhage (Goodpasture's syndrome)
	  Without pulmonary hemorrhage
	Antineutrophil cytoplasmic antibody–associated GN
	  Wegener's granulomatosis
	  Polyarteritis nodosa
	Hypersensitivity vasculitis
	Idiopathic crescentic GN

Diseases with crescent in minority of cases	Postinfectious GN SLE IgA nephropathy Henoch-Schönlein purpura Essential mixed cryoglobulinemia Membranoproliferative GN

Ig, immunoglobulin; SLE, systemic lupus erythematosus.
Adapted from Kern WF, Laszik ZG, Nadasdy T, et al. The true (hypercellular or "proliferative") glomerulonephritis. Diseases associated with the nephritic syndrome. In: Kern WF, Laszik ZG, Nadasdy T, et al., eds. *Atlas of renal pathology*. Philadelphia: WB Saunders, 1999:669–689.

the nephritogenic strains. This protective immunity is more likely related to the specificities and neutralizing capacity of antibodies rather than to the antibody titer itself (6).

Family studies have suggested genetic predisposition for APSGN by demonstrating its higher incidence in siblings of index cases with sporadic disease (38%) than the expected attack rate of children at risk in epidemics (4.5 to 28.0%) (7). The genetic aspects of APSGN are further supported by the reports of common association of the disease with HLA-DR1 and -DRw4, whereas patients with HLA-

DRw48 and -DRw8 appear to be less susceptible to development of primary GN (8,9).

Pathogenesis

APSGN is an immune-mediated disease associated with throat or skin infections with certain nephritogenic strains of group A streptococci. Streptococcal constituents or products that may trigger pathologic processes have not been fully defined. Furthermore, the exact mechanism of renal injury remains controversial, although several theories have been proposed: (a) trapping of circulating immune complexes in the glomeruli (10,11); (b) molecular mimicry between streptococcal and renal antigens (i.e., normal glomerular tissue acting as autoantigen reacts with circulating antibody formed against streptococcal antigens) (12–14); (c) *in situ* immune complex formation between antistreptococcal antibodies and glomerular planted antigens (15,16); and (d) direct complement activation by streptococcal antigens deposited in the glomeruli (17).

Streptococcal Factors Implicated in the Pathogenesis of Acute Poststreptococcal Glomerulonephritis

The group A streptococci are covered with an outer hyaluronic acid capsule required for resistance to phagocytosis and bacterial adherence to epithelial cells. Extracellular surface molecules further consist of a group A carbohydrate polymer, a mucopeptide, and an M protein. The M protein extends from the cell surface as an alpha-helical coiled-coil dimer, which appears as hair-like projections on the surface of streptococci (18).

M Protein and M-Like Proteins

Groups A and C and human isolates of group G streptococci possess M proteins, and more than 80 serotypes have already been identified. M proteins have the variable N-terminal region projected outward and the highly conserved C-terminal part anchored in the cell membrane. The genes encoding several types of M proteins, called *emm genes*, have been cloned, and their nucleotide sequences have been established. M proteins have a common structure: the heptad-repeating amino acid sequence motifs within each region of the molecule. M proteins have been divided into two classes based on their reactivity with antibodies against the C repeat region. Class I M proteins contain a surface-exposed epitope that reacts with these antibodies and are opacity-factor negative, whereas class II M-protein serotypes do not contain the class I epitope, do not react with anti–C repeat region antibodies, and are opacity-factor positive (19).

The nephrogenicity of group A streptococci appears to be related to specific M-protein serotypes, but not all strains of the same M-protein serotype are nephritogenic. There is an apparent difference in streptococcal strains leading to APSGN through pharyngeal or skin infection. The predominant M-protein serotypes associated with pyoderma and APSGN are M proteins 2, 42, 49, 56, 57, 60, whereas M proteins 1, 4, 12, and 25 are associated with throat infection and APSGN. In general, the pyoderma or skin strains belong to the class II M-protein serotypes with the capacity to produce opacity factor but having no reaction with antibodies against C repeat region (20).

The potential role of M proteins in inducing APSGN has been extensively studied. Markedly elevated immunoglobulin (Ig) G titers against the C-terminal region but not the N-terminal region of the M12 protein were found in patients with APSGN as compared to patients with pharyngitis or chronic GN or healthy individuals. Binding of IgG to bacteria is assumed to be of importance for the development of APSGN. Binding of IgG and IgA aggregates is frequently detected among nephritogenic streptococci. Fc regions of IgG and IgA may bind to the surface of certain group A streptococcus strains through M proteins or M-like proteins. Fc receptor–positive group A streptococci isolates elicit anti-IgG response and promote deposition of IgG and C3 in the rabbit kidney immunized with group A streptococcus. These findings suggest that Fc receptors of nephritogenic streptococci may induce anti-IgG molecules and, consequently, may contribute to the pathogenesis of APSGN by enhancing renal deposition of immune complexes (21,22).

The role of M proteins in inducing renal injury is further supported by the well-established cross-reactivity of M proteins with glomerular basement membrane (GBM) antigens. Antiglomerular antibodies have been shown to react with streptococcal M12 protein. A number of surface proteins from nephritogenic streptococci have been reported to bind constituents of GBM (e.g., heparan sulfate, laminin, and collagen IV). The streptococcal host factor-binding proteins share structural homologies with classical M proteins and are designated as *M-like proteins* (23).

Endostreptosin

Endostreptosin is a 40- to 50-kDa protein derived from the streptococcal cell cytoplasm. It was found to absorb antiglomerular antibodies from the sera of patients after APSGN. Endostreptosin has been detected in the glomeruli in the early phase of APSGN. In the late stages of the disease, it is not detectable, but increased serum antistreptosin titers are diagnostic of APSGN. Endostreptosin deposited in the GBM is considered to be an *in situ* activator of the alternative pathway of the complement system and immunologically distinct from other streptococcal enzymes or cell wall components (24,25).

Cationic Antigens

Cationic proteins of group A streptococci are known to have affinity for the polyanionic GBM. Antibodies raised against cationic proteins from nephritogenic group A streptococcus isolates were shown to bind to renal biopsy samples from patients with APSGN, and antibodies to these cationic antigens were detected in APSGN patients. Cationic antigens generate *in situ* immune complexes and initiate glomerular inflammation. As C3 deposition precedes that of IgG in APSGN, the cationic protein–related mechanisms are likely to be involved in the later phase of the disease (26).

Streptococcal Pyrogenic Exotoxin B

Streptococci isolated from patients with nephritis produce a 46-kDa extracellular protein not found in strains from patients without acute GN. This nephritis strain–associated protein was found to be a plasmin-binding protein and was later identified as *streptococcal pyrogenic exotoxin B* (SpeB) precursor, also known as the *streptococcal proteinase zymogen.* It is believed that the protease or superantigenic properties of this exotoxin/protease/plasmin binding may cause an activation of the immune system by cleaving several host factors that favor the release of active inflammatory mediators, vascular permeability factors, and biologically active fragments from the streptococcal wall (27). Antibody titers to SpeB are markedly elevated in APSGN as opposed to patients with acute rheumatic fever, scarlet fever, or healthy subjects. SpeB is detected in the glomeruli of 67% APSGN biopsy specimens as compared with only 16% of non-APSGN cases (28).

Streptokinase

Streptokinase, a 46-kDa, 414–amino acid, extracellular protein is considered to be involved in the pathogenesis of APSGN. Nine different genotypes of streptokinase have been identified, and ska-1, -2, -6, and -9 have been found to be associated with APSGN. The streptokinase genes are highly conserved, and a greater than 90% homology in the amino acid sequence is observed in nephritogenic strains as compared with less than 60% homology for nonnephritogenic strains (29). Streptokinase was found to be tightly bound to the glomeruli, and glomerular deposits of streptokinase could be detected with a highly sensitive staining technique. Streptokinase is known to form complexes with plasminogen and plasmin, and these complexes have the capacity to convert plasminogen to plasmin. Plasmin then activates the local complement cascade, causes degradation of extracellular matrix proteins, and induces the release of vasoactive bradykinin. In an experimental model, the deletion of the streptokinase gene was shown to eliminate the nephritogenic properties of the strain (30).

Neuraminidase

It has also been suggested that in APSGN, the autologous IgG becomes autoimmunogenic after being desialized by streptococcal neuraminidase. The modified antigenic IgG stimulates the anti-IgG rheumatoid factor response, which may lead to the formation of cryoglobulins. The pathogenic role of neuraminidase is further supported by the demonstration of free sialic acid and neuraminidase activity in the serum of APSGN patients and by experimental evidence that intravenous (IV) neuraminidase administration promotes renal infiltration of leukocytes and that neuraminidase-treated leukocytes preferentially accumulate in the kidney (31,32). However, neuraminidase is also produced by non-nephritogenic streptococcus strains. It has been proposed that the formation of autoantibody to IgG could be due to its incorporation into a streptococcal antigen-antibody complex rather than to its modification by neuraminidase.

Nephritis-Associated Plasmin Receptor

A 43-kDa protein designated as *nephritis-associated plasmin receptor* (NAPlr) has been isolated from nephritogenic streptococci. This antigen is present in glomeruli in the early stage of APSGN, and antibodies to NAPlr are detected in the serum of 92% of patients within 3 months of the onset of the disease. Soluble NAPlr could bind to the glomeruli and attack activated plasmin, which has a central role in the process of local inflammation. In addition, NAPlr directly contributes to alternative complement activation (33).

Complement Cascade

Humoral immunity initiated by nephritogenic streptococcal antigens is assumed to be mediated by *in situ* formation of antigen-antibody complexes and by glomerular deposition of circulating immune complexes. These processes lead to the activation of the classical and the alternative complement pathways as evidenced by the depressed serum levels and the glomerular localization of the components of complement cascade.

The classical pathway is primarily involved in the early stage of disease and is likely activated by immune complexes when IgG has become deposited. Several observations suggest that the alternative pathway is operating as well. These include (a) the glomerular presence of properdin; (b) C3 deposition precedes that of IgG, or even C3 may be present in the glomeruli without IgG; and (c) in the acute stage of APSGN serum levels of C3 and C5 are low, whereas the levels of early components of the classical activation pathway (e.g., C1q, C2, or C4) are normal or only slightly depressed (34–36). Other studies have revealed an activation of the terminal complement pathway and the generation of the terminal $C5_b$-C9 complex, also designated as *membrane attack complex*, by showing its elevated plasma level and colocalization with C3 deposits in glomerular capillaries and mesangium in patients with APSGN. The potential importance of this terminal complement complex implies its capacity to stimulate the production of vasoactive substances, proteolytic enzymes, and reactive oxygen radicals—all known to damage the integrity of glomerular capillary membrane. $C3_a$ and $C5_a$ also appear to be involved in tissue damage, as they function as chemotactic factors for infiltrating cells and cause histamine release and increased permeability (4). The early phase of APSGN may be associated with C3 nephritic factor and decreased plasma levels of C3. C3 nephritic factor is an autoantibody against the C3 convertase that stabilizes this inherently labile enzyme and induces a continuous activation of alternative pathways with subsequent C3 depletion (37).

During the course of GN, protective mechanisms have been identified against complement-mediated injury of glomerular cells. Surface-bound proteins expressed on glomerular cells are assumed to prevent complement activation, and soluble complement receptors and those on the glomerular visceral epithelial cells appear to attenuate glomerular injury (38).

Coagulation System

Intraglomerular deposition of fibrin or fibrinogen-related antigen is a constant finding in APSGN. The activation of the coagulation system is further indicated by the increased levels of plasma high-molecular-weight fibrinogen complexes, the development of hypo- or hyperfibrinogenemia, the depression of factor XIII, α_2-macroglobulin, and the activation of factor XII. Fibrinolysis is increased as shown by the elevation of serum and urinary fibrinogen or fibrin degradation products. Urinary excretion of these products is believed to reflect the degradation of glomerular fibrin deposits and the beginning of the recovery phase of the disease. It is interesting to note that there is no relationship between serum levels of C3 and fibrin degradation products. The possible involvement of platelet activation has also been proposed because of the diminished platelet survival time and the presence of platelet-activating factor and platelet-derived growth factor in APSGN (39).

Cellular Infiltration and Cytokine Production

APSGN is characterized by diffuse glomerular hypercellularity, primarily as a result of accumulation of polymorphonuclear leukocytes and monocytes, an increase in intrinsic glomerular cells, and a transient pathologic expansion of mesangial matrix. Resident endothelial and mesangial cells proliferate, and macrophages are believed to induce this proliferation. Glomerular macrophage infiltration appears to be mediated by complement-induced chemotaxis and by antigen-specific T-cell activation. Streptococcal superantigens cause a selective increase in T-cell receptor β and massive T-cell activation with the release of T-cell–derived lymphokines [e.g., interleukin (IL)-1 and IL-6] (40).

Hisano et al. found more infiltrating macrophages and the four macrophage subclasses—early-, acute-, chronic-stage inflammatory, and chronic-stage mature macrophages—in the glomeruli of patients with APSGN compared to patients with IgA nephropathy (41). The proportion of intraglomerular proliferating macrophages decreases with time during the course of the disease in APSGN, whereas it remains constant in IgA nephropathy. Infiltrating cells undergo apoptosis, which is a prerequisite for the elimination of these cells and the resolution of renal injury. Decreased apoptosis has been found to be associated with a progressive clinical course (42). In addition to macrophages, neutrophils and T lymphocytes are present in the glomeruli but not B lymphocytes (43). Recently, proinflammatory monocytes or macrophages expressing CD16 antigen have been demonstrated in the glomeruli and the urine of patients with active proliferative GN, and the number of these cells appears to correlate with the severity of acute glomerular inflammation (44). $CD16^+$ macrophages produce high levels of proinflammatory cytokines [e.g., tumor necrosis factor (TNF)], whereas antiinflammatory cytokines (e.g., IL-10) are absent or produced at a low level (45). Increased local production of proinflammatory cytokines may induce the expression of adhesion molecules (intercellular adhesion molecule-1) and lymphocyte function–associated molecule-1 on endothelial cells, and these molecules may facilitate the adhesion of circulating cells to the renal endothelium and their subsequent invasion into the parenchyma (46). In response to nephritogenic glomerular antigen, two subsets of fully differentiated T helper cells are activated. T helper-1 cells produce IL-2 and interferon-gamma, activate macrophages, and induce expression of MHC antigen, whereas T helper-2 cells secrete IL-4, -5, and -6, cofactors for B-cell proliferation, and stimulants for Ig production (47). IL-1 has the potential to increase glomerular inflammation, whereas antiinflammatory cytokines (e.g., IL-4, -6, -10, -13, and transforming growth factor β) reduce IL-1 synthesis by macrophages and suppress the generation of oxygen radicals and nitrogenous intermediates, the secretion of proteolytic enzymes, and the expression of Fc receptors (48). It is of note that IL-4 ameliorates experimental GN also by upregulating the glomerular gene expression of IL-1 decoy receptor (49). IL-8 is a selective activator and chemoattractant of polymorphonuclear leukocytes secreted by monocytes and intrinsic glomerular mesangial, endothelial, and epithelial cells. Glomerular immunoreactivity for IL-8 correlates with neutrophil infiltration and clinical activity in patients with APSGN. Transforming growth factors β1, β2, and β3, originating from infiltrating monocytes or macrophages or from mesangial cells, are also abundant in biopsy specimens of APSGN and appear to be responsible for the accumulation of mesangial matrix components, including collagens, proteoglycans, and fibronectin (50).

It has recently been shown that selective podocyte injury exacerbates mesangial cell proliferation and mesangial matrix expansion, which consequently contributes to the progression of experimental proliferative GN. Podocyte dysfunction is an important factor in the development of irreversible mesangial alterations. Basic fibroblast growth factor is also released by the podocytes, and it may further amplify podocyte damage and mesangial alterations (51).

Mesangial injury or activation may also be controlled by serine protease inhibitors. Megsin, a novel member of the superfamily of serine protease inhibitors, is predominantly expressed in mesangial cells, and its expression is upregulated at the peak of hypercellularity and matrix accumulation during various glomerular diseases. Imbalance between proteinases and their inhibitors may participate in the expansion of mesangial extracellular matrix by modulating the turnover of glomerular mesangial matrix compounds (52,53).

It is generally accepted that proinflammatory cytokines and chemokines originating from infiltrating cells or from resident glomerular cells are more expressed in proliferative GN. Their expression is differentially regulated by the presence of immune complexes, and there is a relationship between cytokine gene expression and clinical manifestations (54). In patients with APSGN, plasma levels of IL-6 have been shown to parallel the clinical course, whereas TNF-α is elevated in the acute phase and variable thereafter. Levels of platelet-derived growth factor always remain normal (55).

Free Oxygen Radicals

Recent studies have revealed some major features of oxygen stress and antioxidant defense mechanisms in children with APSGN. Lipid peroxidation is enhanced, as demonstrated by increased red blood cell osmotic fragility, elevated levels of malonyl dialdehyde, oxidized glutathione, and hemoglobin. Furthermore, the activities of major antioxidant enzymes including superoxide dismutase, catalase, glutation peroxidase, and glutation-*S*-transferase are markedly depressed in children with APSGN as compared with healthy control children. As a result, the levels of reduced glutathione are significantly lower and the reduced glutathione–oxidized glutathione redox system is depleted. APSGN children, therefore, have diminished antioxidant defense capacity and may suffer from prolonged oxidative stress with increased susceptibility to lipid peroxidation and osmotic lysis of red blood cells (56,57). There is evidence for a redox-sensitive regulation of transcription factors and gene expression of prooxidant and antioxidant mediators. The genetic shifting of superoxide to nitric oxide–dominated chemistry during the course of GN may alter the self-limited inflammatory responses of glomerular mesangial and endothelial cells to tissue injury (58).

Pathologic Changes

Microscopic Findings

Microscopic findings correspond to the infiltration with professional immune cells, activation, and proliferation of resident glomerular cells and matrix expansion.

Capillary tufts are enlarged and exhibit marked lobularity and hypercellularity with global and relatively uniform involvement of all glomeruli (Fig. 30.1). During the course of the disease, distinct patterns of cellular reaction can be recognized.

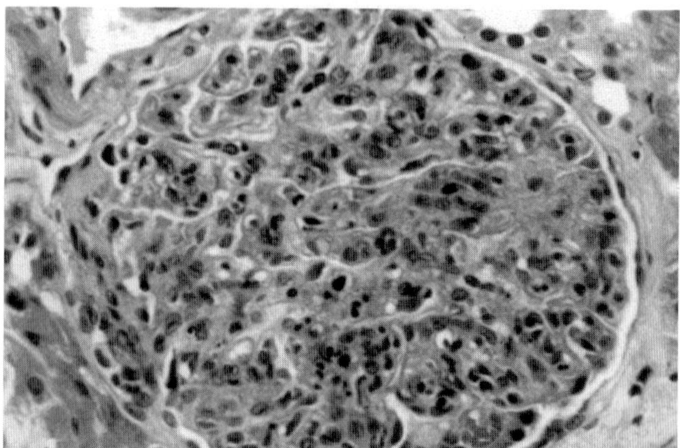

FIGURE 30.1. Acute postinfectious glomerulonephritis. The glomeruli show global intracapillary hypercellularity with large numbers of polymorphonuclear leukocytes in the glomerular capillary lumina (hematoxylin and eosin stain, ×400). (Courtesy of Peter Degrell, University of Pécs Faculty of Medicine, Nephrological Center, Pécs, Hungary.) (See Color Plate 30.1.)

At the early stage of the disease, glomerular hypercellularity is due to an influx of blood-borne polymorphonuclear leukocytes and monocytes, whereas in later stages, it is mainly caused by proliferation of intrinsic endothelial and mesangial cells. T-helper and T-suppressor lymphocytes also participate at the onset of APSGN. In addition to mesangial proliferation, mesangial matrix accumulation, growing mesangial fibers, mesangiolysis, and expression of molecules mediating the cross-communication between resident and invading cells, have been noted. Mesangial hypercellularity may persist long after apparent resolution of the disease. Extracapillary proliferation (i.e., crescents) may also be present in a minority of cases. Capillary walls are not thickened, but the lumens are frequently occluded. The GBMs may be irregular due to the characteristic humps observed on electron microscopy. Renal tubules are usually not involved, although protein resorption droplets have been noted in the proximal tubular cells and erythrocytes, sometimes mixed with eosinophilic cast-like material, and neutrophils may be present in the tubular lumen. Tubular vacuolation, dilatation, or atrophy is rarely observed.

Renal arteries and arterioles are generally spared or show minimal changes. There have been occasional reports of fibrinoid necrosis and necrotizing vasculitis that are usually associated with hypertension (3). The involvement of interstitium is not remarkable; interstitial edema and scattered inflammatory cells may be present.

Immunofluorescence Microscopy

Early in the clinical course, coarse granular staining for IgG and C3 can be detected in the glomerular capillary walls; IgM is found less frequently, and IgA and early complement

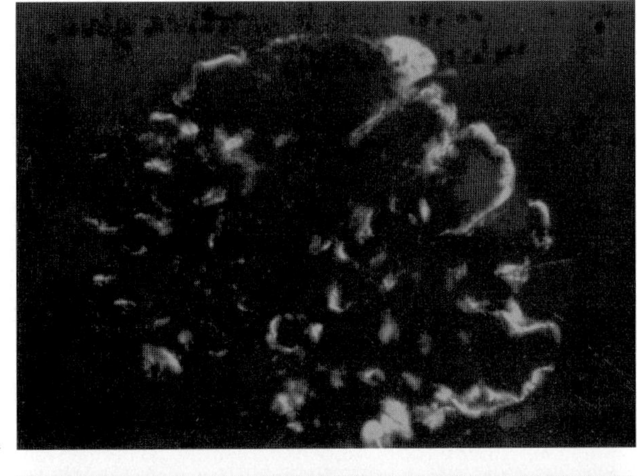
A

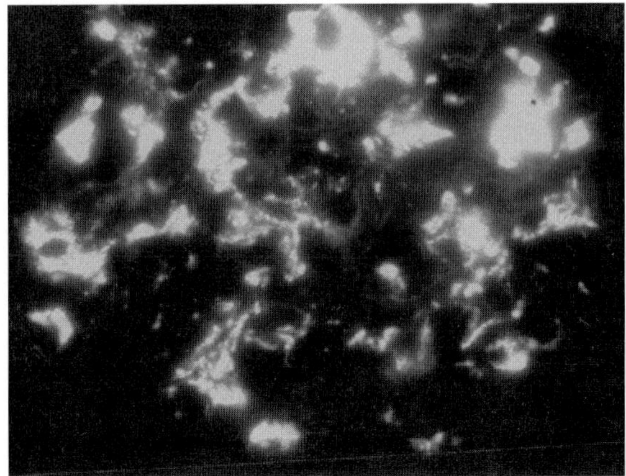
B

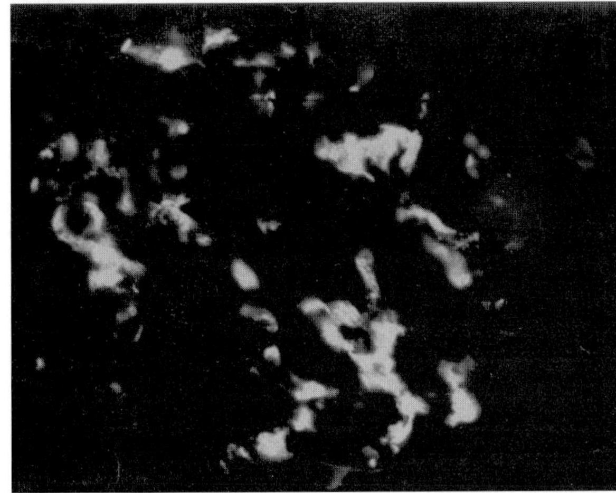
C

FIGURE 30.2. Acute postinfectious glomerulonephritis by immunofluorescence. **A:** Garland pattern. Large, subepithelial deposits of immunoglobulin G on the outer side of the glomerular basement membrane (×400). **B:** Starry sky pattern. There are fine and coarse granular deposits of immunoglobulin G in the glomerular capillary walls and in the mesangium (×400). **C:** Mesangial pattern. Predominantly mesangial, coarse granular deposits of C3 (×400). (Courtesy of Peter Degrell, University of Pécs Faculty of Medicine, Nephrological Center, Pécs, Hungary.) (See Color Plate 30.2.)

components (i.e., C1 and C4) are usually absent. As the disease evolves, staining for C3 predominates, whereas IgG staining becomes less apparent. Three distinct immunofluorescence patterns have been described and are designated as *garland*, *starry sky*, and *mesangial* patterns (Fig. 30.2). Garland pattern consists of discrete, densely packed, sometimes confluent capillary wall deposits often seen in patients with extracapillary proliferation and heavy proteinuria with worse prognosis. Starry sky pattern displays fine, granular IgG and C3 deposits in the capillary walls and mesangium and occurs mainly at the acute stage of the disease. The mesangial pattern is characterized by granular deposition of C3 and IgG predominantly in the mesangium, with the capillary walls being relatively spared. C3 deposits prevail over IgG, and this pattern appears to be closely related to the resolution of the disease. It is of note that although the distinct patterns of immunofluorescence staining and their clinical correlates are well established, combinations of these patterns and transitional forms are often observed (59,60).

Electron Microscopy

Ultrastructural examination shows a swelling of glomerular endothelial and mesangial cells with closure of the capillary lumen. The most consistent finding is the presence of large, electron-dense, immune-type deposits on the subepithelial surface of the GBM, classically referred to as *humps* (Fig. 30.3). These are most abundant during the first few weeks of APSGN and tend to disappear 6 weeks after the clinical onset of disease. The electron density of the deposits is variable and diminishes with time, and the appearance of electron-lucent regions in the deposit is regarded as a sign of morphologic resolution (61,62). Subendothelial, mesangial, and membranous deposits may also be present, but they are less consistent and smaller in size. GBMs are generally normal in contour and thickness, although patchy thickening and focal disruption may occasionally be identified. The glomerular capillary endothelium may also be partially disrupted, with neutrophils directly adjacent to the denuded GBM.

It has been suggested that several morphologic alterations—including glomerular hypercellularity, crescent formation, the degree of interstitial volume, the number of glomerular humps, and the intensity of immunofluorescent staining for IgG and C3—may influence the initial presentation, clinical course, and long-term outcome of APSGN. The combination of these morphologic features is likely to have greater prognostic value than any single finding alone (3).

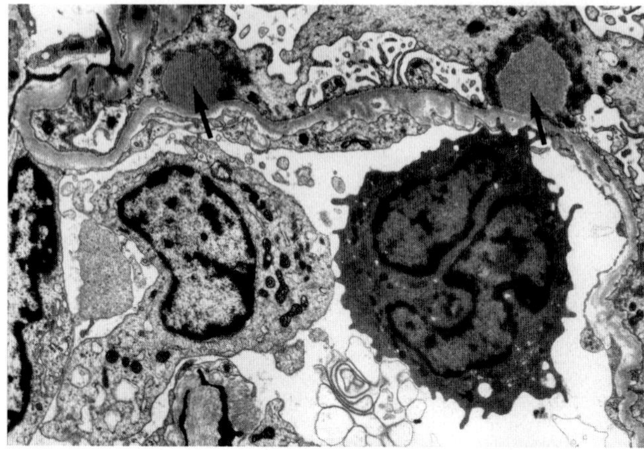

FIGURE 30.3. Acute postinfectious glomerulonephritis on electron micrograph. Hump-like, electron-dense subepithelial deposits (*arrows*) are seen in the glomerular capillary wall, with polymorphonuclear leukocytes in the capillary lumina (×6000). (Courtesy of Peter Degrell, University of Pécs Faculty of Medicine, Nephrological Center, Pécs, Hungary.)

TABLE 30.2. CLINICAL MANIFESTATIONS OF ACUTE POSTSTREPTOCOCCAL GLOMERULONEPHRITIS IN CHILDREN AND ELDERLY ADULTS

Symptom	Children (%)	Elderly patients (%)
Hematuria	100	100
Proteinuria	80	92
Edema	90	75
Hypertension	60–80	83
Oliguria	10–50	58
Dyspnea, heart failure	<5	43
Nephrotic proteinuria	4	20
Azotemia	25–40	83
Early mortality	<1	25

From Rodriguez-Iturbe B. Acute endocapillary glomerulonephritis. In: Davison AM, Cameron JS, Grunfeld J-P, et al. *Oxford textbook of clinical nephrology*. Oxford, UK: Oxford University Press, 1998:613–623, with permission.

Clinical Presentation

Typical APSGN is characterized by the abrupt onset of hematuria and proteinuria often in association with edema, hypertension, and mild to moderate renal functional impairment. The disease is usually preceded by group A β-hemolytic streptococcus infection of the throat or skin. The long-term prognosis is generally favorable, but some patients may have life-threatening acute complications or may slowly progress to renal failure.

Acute nephritic syndrome follows throat or skin infection after a latent period of 1 to 2 weeks or 3 to 6 weeks, respectively. During the latent period, microscopic hematuria may be detected. Some patients remain asymptomatic, and the ratio of subclinical to clinically overt disease is estimated to be 4 to 5:1 (7,63,64).

The most common presenting symptoms are hematuria, edema, proteinuria, and hypertension. Gross hematuria is present in 24 to 40% of children with APSGN. The urine is smoky or coke-colored, and the patients may have dysuria, frequency, and abdominal discomfort. Macroscopic hematuria may be present for up to 2 weeks, and microscopic hematuria may remain evident for months after illness resolution. Glomerular hematuria is characterized by dysmorphic red blood cells and red blood cell casts best seen in freshly prepared urine by phase-contrast microscopy. Mild to moderate proteinuria is common in APSGN, whereas proteinuria of nephrotic range is rare in children.

Transient oliguria occurs in approximately 50% of children with APSGN, but anuria is rare. Decreased urine output is the result of markedly decreased filtration fraction and glomerular filtration rate (GFR), diminished distal delivery of the filtrate, and maintained or even enhanced sodium and fluid reabsorption in the distal nephron.

Edema and vascular congestion results from salt and water retention. Edema may be mild and confined to the periorbital area or severe with pleural effusion, ascites, and hypertension. Periorbital edema may be apparent in the morning, but as the day progresses, edema localizes in the abdomen or lower extremities. In younger children, edema is usually generalized, whereas in adolescents and adults, it is limited to the face and legs. Congestive heart failure may complicate the clinical course of the acute nephritic syndrome presenting with orthopnea, dyspnea, cough, pulmonary crackles, and gallop rhythm.

Hypertension is observed in more than 80% patients. It is volume dependent in addition to the increased peripheral vascular resistance; plasma volume and cardiac output are invariably elevated. Hypertension can be associated with headaches, somnolence, changes in mental status, anorexia, nausea, and convulsion. Some patients present with *hypertensive emergency*, which is defined as blood pressure greater than 30% of normal for age and sex or any elevation with evidence of encephalopathy, heart failure, or pulmonary edema. Central nervous system involvement during the course of APSGN may be secondary to hypertensive encephalopathy, but it can also be attributed to cerebral vasculitis. In normotensive children presenting with severe neurologic symptoms, magnetic resonance imaging may show multiple bilateral supratentorial lesions in the white and gray matter—a finding consistent with vasculitic infarct (64–66).

Other nonspecific symptoms include nausea, vomiting, malaise, anorexia, weakness, lumbar pain, and abdominal discomfort. Clinical manifestations of APSGN in children are summarized and compared to those seen in adults in Table 30.2 (4).

Diagnostic Evaluation

Diagnostic work-up includes identification of nephritic syndrome, antecedent streptococcal infection, serologic markers of immune-mediated inflammation, and, when needed, renal histology.

Urine analysis reveals distorted, also termed *dysmorphic* or *crenated*, red blood cells and red blood cell casts indicative of glomerular hematuria (67,68). Proteinuria, usually moderate, reaches the nephrotic range in 5 to 10% of patients with APSGN. It lasts for approximately 6 months (69,70). Leukocyte, hyaline, and granular casts are also frequently seen (7). There is a transient elevation of blood urea nitrogen and serum creatinine due to a decreased GFR with normal or low renal plasma flow and markedly depressed filtration fraction. Tubular function is usually preserved or mildly reduced (3).

Recent streptococcal infection is confirmed by the demonstration of increased titers of antibodies against antigens of cell wall and extracellular products of group A streptococci. In clinical practice, repeated measurements of antistreptolysin, anti–deoxyribonuclease B, antihyaluronidase, antistreptokinase, and anti–nicotinamide adenine dinucleotidase are used to demonstrate streptococcal infection. The antistreptolysin and anti–nicotinamide adenine dinucleotidase titers are elevated in 80% of patients with postpharyngitis nephritis, whereas antihyaluronidase and anti–deoxyribonuclease B titers are elevated in 80 to 90% of patients after skin infections. Antibody titers are elevated 1 to 5 weeks after infections and return to their initial levels after several months (72). Antibiotic treatment may attenuate antibody response (73,74). IgG antibodies against the C region of streptococcal M protein have been claimed to be a more reliable diagnostic marker for APSGN because they remain significantly elevated long after the other streptococcal antibodies have normalized (21).

In patients with APSGN, the complement system is activated as assessed by measurement of the total hemolytic complement (CH 50), C3, and C4. More than 90% of APSGN patients have low levels of C3 and CH 50 and normal or mildly depressed C4 levels, indicating a preferential activation of the alternative pathways (4,71,75). In most cases, C3 returns to normal within 8 weeks, although a prolonged decrease of C3 has been reported (76).

Serum levels of IgG and IgM are elevated in 90% of patients (3). Circulating immune complexes can be detected in 58% of cases as compared to 4% in normal individuals (10), and 66% of patients have cryoglobulins (77). Serum IgG levels and glomerular IgG deposits are not directly correlated. A group of APSGN patients with elevated serum IgG was identified as being unable to form glomerular IgG deposits; in these cases, the severity of disease appeared to be independent of serum IgG levels (78). Increased circulating levels and urinary excretion of some cytokines during the acute phase of APSGN are found to be correlated with the clinical course (54,55). Of interest, antineutrophil cytoplasmatic autoantibodies were detected in 9% of APSGN patients, and their presence was significantly associated with a more severe glomerular disease as assessed by serum creatinine and crescent formation (79).

Because APSGN has a self-limited course with a good prognosis, renal biopsy is rarely indicated. It should be considered, however, for patients with atypical history or presentation, including nephrotic-range proteinuria in the acute stage, normal serum complement, progressively increasing serum creatinine, prolonged hypocomplementemia for more than 3 months, ongoing macroscopic hematuria, or long-lasting proteinuria (73).

Considering differential diagnosis, Figure 30.4 gives a simplified diagnostic work-up. Determination of serum complement levels has a critical role in the initial evaluation of acute nephritic syndrome and may discriminate between diseases with low or normal complement levels (80).

Treatment

The acute nephritic syndrome is treated with restricted salt and fluid intake. When significant edema or hypertension is present, furosemide or other loop diuretics should be given to initiate prompt diuresis and to correct fluid overload, volume-dependent hypertension, and cardiovascular congestion. In some patients, hypertensive emergencies may occur and antihypertensive agents are needed. Initial management of severe hypertension includes calcium-channel blockers (e.g., IV nicardipine), IV labetalol or dihydralazine followed by maintenance antihypertensive therapy with loop diuretics, and calcium-channel blockers (e.g., nifedipine). Administration of angiotensin-converting enzyme inhibitors is not recommended because they can cause hyperkalemia.

Occasionally, pulmonary edema may develop, which needs aggressive diuretic treatment, oxygen, and morphine administration. Hyperkalemia can be controlled by restriction of potassium intake, administration of potassium-binding resin, and, in more severe cases, IV salbutamol. Dialysis is indicated in cases of persistent electrolyte abnormalities, fluid overload, or severe azotemia.

Streptococcal infection has usually resolved before presentation, but patients with positive throat or skin cultures or clinical evidence of streptococcal pharyngitis should receive antibiotic therapy (e.g., penicillin or erythromycin). Preventive antimicrobial treatment is also indicated for the immediate family members and for those individuals who are in close contact with the affected persons. The spread of infection can also be limited if personal hygiene measures are taken (2,4,81).

In a subset of patients with progressive clinical course or with histologic evidence of extensive crescent formation, aggressive treatment with pulse methylprednisolone, with or without cytotoxic drugs, should be considered (82,83). The beneficial effect of this therapeutic intervention has been suggested by case reports.

Prognosis and Clinical Outcome

APSGN in children is a benign disease with an early mortality rate of less than 1%. Most children undergo complete

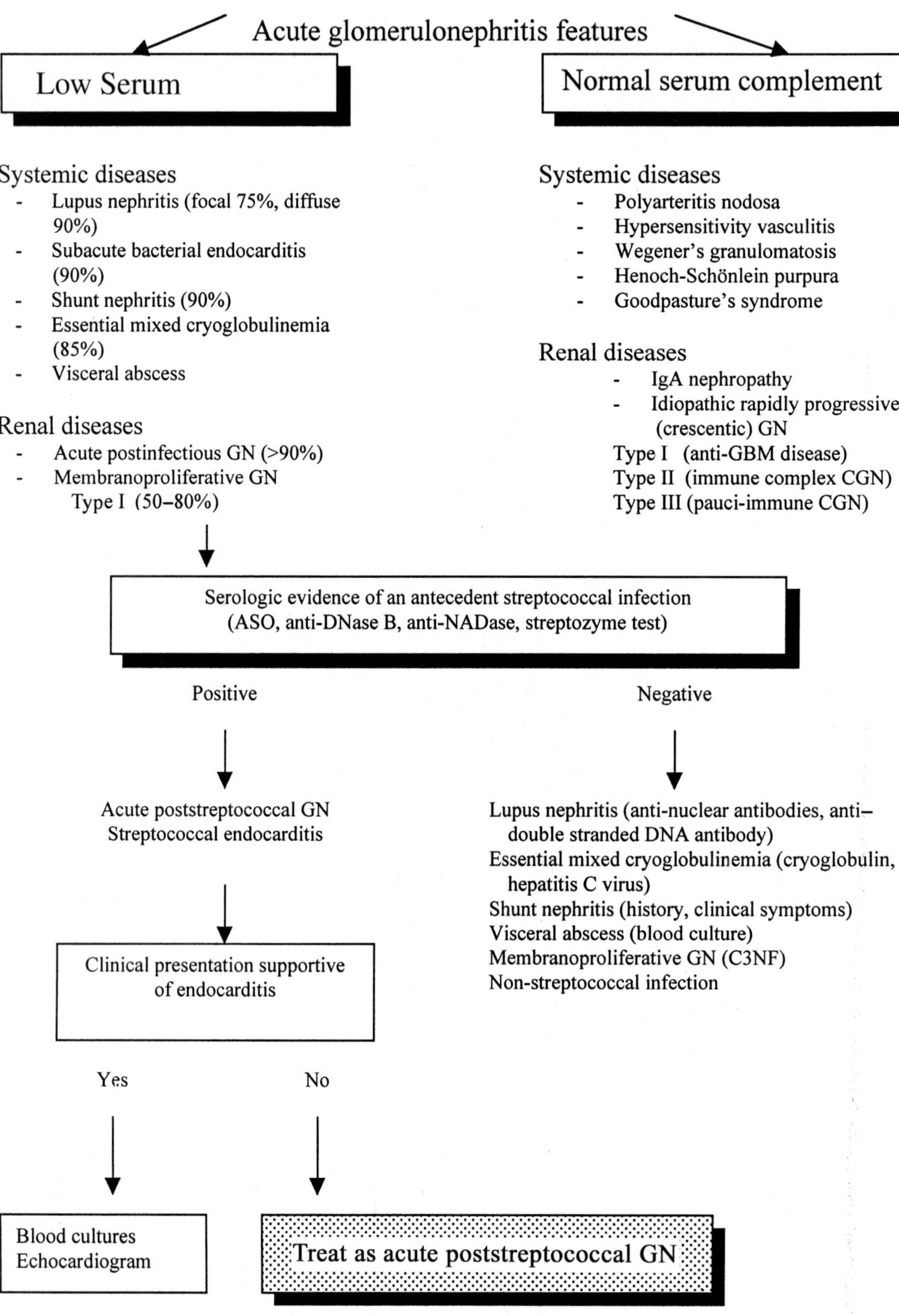

FIGURE 30.4. Diagnostic work-up and etiologic classification of acute glomerulonephritis. Number in parentheses indicates the frequency of low complement levels. CGN, crescent-forming glomerulonephritis; C3NF, C3 nephritis factor; GBM, glomerular basement membrane; GN, glomerulonephritis. (Adapted from Yoshizawa N. Acute glomerulonephritis. *Intern Med* 2000;39:687–694; and Lang MM, Fowers C. Identifying poststreptococcal glomerulonephritis. *Nurse Pract* 2001;34:37–47.)

remission; hypertension and gross hematuria usually resolve over several weeks, proteinuria may last for several months, and microscopic hematuria may persist for years. Less than 2% of the patients have been reported to progress to end-stage renal failure.

Attempts have been made to identify clinical features and morphologic markers that may serve as prognostic indicators. Nephrotic range proteinuria, persistent oliguria, and impaired renal function may have an adverse effect on clinical outcome. Similarly, morphologic changes (e.g., extensive crescent formation, atypical humps on electron microscopy, garland pattern on immunofluorescence or glomerular necroses, adhesions, thromboses, and sclerosis) have been found to be more often associated with poor prognosis (2,3). Follow-up studies have been undertaken to assess the long-term consequences of APSGN. The rate of morphologic healing increases steadily with the time elapsed from the clinical presentation of APSGN to the renal biopsy: 20% at 2 years after the onset of the disease, to 94% at 10 years after onset, and to 97% at 12 years after onset (84). There is a clear dissociation between histologic healing and clinical resolution. Despite the very low rate of histologic abnormalities, approximately 20% of the patients have persistent urine abnormalities or reduced GFR, and 8 to 13% have proteinuria and hypertension (4).

Healing, usually defined as the absence of persistent inflammation, does not exclude the fact that the reduced number of intact nephrons undergo hemodynamic changes over time, and the resulting hyperfiltration may cause further renal damage with urine abnormalities or hypertension. In fact, simultaneous measurements of GFR and effective renal plasma flow at the acute stage of the disease and at follow-up 2 to 12 years later revealed relative hyperperfusion of the kidney; the hypothesis has been put forward that in the remaining intact nephrons, significant damage may develop insidiously many years after apparent resolution of APSGN (85). This hypothesis appears to be supported by the observations that renal functional reserve, as assessed by acute protein loading test, is markedly reduced in patients who have recovered from APSGN (77,86).

APSGN is still considered a benign disease in children, with the vast majority of patients recovering without apparent long-term sequelae (87). It remains to be established whether the more severe clinical presentation and progression is related to older age or whether it may be attributed to specific *Streptococcus* strains.

Patients who have experienced APSGN have life-long protection against recurrence of the disease because of the intense immune response to nephritogenic streptococci (3). However, recurrent APSGN has been reported with an incidence of 0.7 to 7.0%. Occasional recurrence was attributed to the suppression of immune reaction due to early antibiotic therapy, although other mechanisms may also be implicated (88). NAPlr protein, a recently identified pathogenetic antigen in APSGN, is always detected in the glomerular mesangium and GBM in the early stage of the disease. Anti-NAPIr antibodies have been shown to be protective against a second attack of APSGN in most patients. When the disease recurred, antibodies against NAPlr were not present in the sera, indicating that failure to induce this specific immune response may contribute to recurrence of APSGN (89).

ACKNOWLEDGMENT

This work was supported by the Hungarian National Research Foundation, grant number OTKA T 030673.

REFERENCES

1. Kern WF, Laszik ZG, Nadasdy T, et al. The true (hypercellular or "proliferative") glomerulonephritis. Diseases associated with the nephritic syndrome. In: Kern WF, Laszik ZG, Nadasdy T, et al., eds. *Atlas of renal pathology*. Philadelphia: WB Saunders, 1999:14–37.
2. Cole BR, Salinas-Madrigal L. Acute proliferative glomerulonephritis and crescentic glomerulonephritis. In: Barratt TM, Avner ED, Harmon WE, eds. *Pediatric nephrology*. Baltimore: Lippincott Williams & Wilkins, 1999:669–689.
3. Silva FG. Acute postinfectious glomerulonephritis and glomerulonephritis complicating persistent bacterial infection. In: Jennette JC, Olson JL, Schwarz MM, Silva FG, eds. *Heptinstall's pathology of the kidney*. Philadelphia: Lippincott–Raven Publishers, 1998:389–453.
4. Rodriguez-Iturbe B. Acute endocapillary glomerulonephritis. In: Davison AM, Cameron JS, Grunfeld J-P, et al., eds. *Oxford textbook of clinical nephrology*. Oxford, UK: Oxford University Press, 1998:613–623.
5. Schwartz B, Facklam RR, Breiman RF. Changing epidemiology of group A streptococcal infection in the USA. *Lancet* 1990;336:1167–1171.
6. Norstrand A, Norgren M, Holm SE. Pathogenetic mechanism of acute post-streptococcal glomerulonephritis. *Scand J Infect Dis* 1999;31:523–537.
7. Rodriguez-Iturbe B, Rubio L, Garcia R. Attack rate of post-streptococcal glomerulonephritis in families. A prospective study. *Lancet* 1981;1(8217):401–403.
8. Layrisse Z, Rodriguez-Iturbe B, Garcia R, et al. Family studies of the HLA system in acute poststreptococcal glomerulonephritis. *Human Immunol* 1983;7:177–185.
9. Naito S, Hohara M, Arakawa K. Association of class II antigens of HLA with primary glomerulopathies. *Nephron* 1987;45:111–114.
10. Border WA. Immune complex detection in glomerular diseases. *Nephron* 1979;24:105–113.
11. Friedman J, van de Rijn I, Ohkuni H, et al. Immunological studies of post-streptococcal sequelae: evidence for presence of streptococcal antigens in circulating immune complexes. *J Clin Invest* 1984;74:1027–1034.
12. Lindberg LH, Vosti KL. Elution of glomerular bound antibodies in experimental streptococcal glomerulonephritis. *Science* 1969;166:1032–1033.
13. Goroncy-Bermes P, Dale JB, Beachey EH, et al. Monoclonal antibody to human renal glomeruli cross-reacts with streptococcal M protein. *Infect Immun* 1987;55:2416–2419.

14. Kraus W, Beachey EH. Renal autoimmune epitope of group A streptococci specified by M protein tetrapeptide: Ile-Arg-Leu-Arg. *Proc Natl Acad Sci U S A* 1988;85:4516–4520.
15. Treser G, Semar M, McVicar M, et al. Antigenic streptococcal components in acute glomerulonephritis. *Science* 1969;163: 676–677.
16. Lange K, Seligson G, Cronin W. Evidence for the in situ origin of streptococcal GN: glomerular localization of endostreptosin and the clinical significance of the subsequent antibody response. *Clin Nephrol* 1983;19:3–10.
17. Brady HR, Brenner BM. Pathogenetic mechanisms of glomerular injury. In: Fauci AS, ed. *Harrison's principles of internal medicine.* New York: McGraw-Hill, 1998:1529–1536.
18. Phillips GNP, Flicker PF, Cohen C, et al. Streptococcal M protein:α-helical coiled-coil structure and arrangements on the cell surface. *Proc Natl Acad Sci U S A* 1981;78:4689–4693.
19. Bessen DE, Fischetti VA. Differentiation between two biologically distinct classes of group A streptococci by limited substitutions of amino acids within the shared region of M protein-like molecules. *J Exp Med* 1990;172:1757–1764.
20. Cunningham MW. Pathogenesis of group A streptococcal infections. *Clin Microbiol Rev* 2000;13:470–511.
21. Mori K, Ito Y, Kamikawaji N, et al. Elevated titer against the C region of streptococcal M protein and its immunodeterminants in patients with poststreptococcal acute glomerulonephritis. *J Pediatr* 1997;131:293–299.
22. Heath DG, Cleary PP. Fc receptor and M-protein genes of group A streptococci are products of gene duplication. *Proc Natl Acad Sci U S A* 1989;86:4741–4745.
23. Glurich I, Winters B, Albini B, et al. Identification of *Streptococcus pyogenes* proteins that bind to rabbit kidney in vitro and in vivo. *Microb Pathog* 1991;10:209–220.
24. Lange K, Seligson G, Cronin W. Evidence for the in situ origin of poststreptococcal glomerulonephritis: glomerular localization of endostreptosin and the clinical significance of the subsequent antibody response. *Clin Nephrol* 1983;19:3–10.
25. Yoshizawa N, Oshima S, Sagel I, et al. Role of a streptococcal antigen in the pathogenesis of acute poststreptococcal glomerulonephritis. Characterization of the antigen and a proposed mechanism for the disease. *J Immunol* 1992;148:3110–3116.
26. Vogt A, Batsford S, Rodriguez-Iturbe B, et al. Cationic antigens in poststreptococcal glomerulonephritis. *Clin Nephrol* 1983;20:271–279.
27. Kotb M. Bacterial pyrogenic exotoxins as superantigens. *Clin Microbiol Rev* 1995;8:411–426.
28. Cu GA, Mezzano S, Bannan JD, et al. Immunohistochemical and serological evidence for the role of streptococcal proteinase in acute post-streptococcal glomerulonephritis. *Kidney Int* 1998;54:819–826.
29. Johnston KH, Chaiban JE, Wheeler RC. Analysis of the variable domain of the streptokinase gene from streptococci associated with poststreptococcal glomerulonephritis. In: Orefici G, ed. *New perspectives on streptococci and streptococcal infections.* Stuttgart, Germany: Gustav Fischer Verlag, 1992:339–341.
30. Nordstrand A, Norgren M, Ferretti JJ, et al. Streptokinase as a mediator of acute post-streptococcal glomerulonephritis in an experimental mouse model. *Infect Immun* 1998;66:315–321.
31. Mosquera JA, Rodriguez-Iturbe B. Extracellular neuraminidase production of streptococci with acute nephritis. *Clin Nephrol* 1984;21:21–28.
32. Marin C, Mosquera JA, Rodriguez-Iturbe B. Neuraminidase promotes neutrophil, lymphocyte and macrophage infiltration in the normal kidney. *Kidney Int* 1995;47:88–95.
33. Yoshizawa N. Acute glomerulonephritis. *Intern Med* 2000; 39:687–694.
34. Sorger K. Pathomorphological findings. In: Sorger K, ed. *Postinfectious glomerulonephritis. Subtypes, clinico-pathological correlations, and follow-up studies.* Stuttgart, Germany: Gustav Fisher Verlag, 1986:15–19.
35. Endre YH, Pussell BA, Charlesworth JA, et al. C3 metabolism in acute glomerulonephritis: implications for sites of complement activation. *Kidney Int* 1984;25:937–941.
36. Brentjens JR, Milgrom ML, Andrews GA. Classification and immunopathologic features of human nephritis. In: Wilson CB, Brenner BM, Stein JH, eds. *Contemporary issues in nephrology.* New York: Churchill Livingstone, 1979;3:214–254.
37. Williams DG. C3 nephritic factor and mesangiocapillary glomerulonephritis. *Pediatr Nephrol* 1997;11:96–98.
38. Couser WG, Johnson RJ, Young BA, et al. The effects of soluble recombinant complement receptor 1 on complement mediated experimental glomerulonephritis. *J Am Soc Nephrol* 1995;5:1888–1894.
39. Eddy AA. Immune mechanisms of glomerular injury. In: Barratt TM, Avner ED, Harmon WE, eds. *Pediatric nephrology.* Baltimore: Lippincott Williams & Wilkins, 1999:641–668.
40. Herman A, Kappler JW, Marrack P, et al. Superantigens: mechanisms of T-cell stimulation and role in immune responses. *Annu Rev Immunol* 1991;9:745–772.
41. Hisano S, Sasatomi Y, Kiyoshi Y, et al. Macrophage subclasses and proliferation in childhood IgA glomerulonephritis. *Am J Kidney Dis* 2001;37:712–719.
42. Soto H, Mosquera J, Rodriguez-Iturbe B, et al. Apoptosis in proliferative glomerulonephritis: decreased apoptosis expression in lupus nephritis. *Nephrol Dial Transplant* 1997;12:273–280.
43. Parra G, Platt JL, Falk RJ, et al. Cell population and membrane attack complex in glomeruli of patients with post-streptococcal glomerulonephritis: identification using monoclonal antibodies by indirect immunofluorescence. *Clin Immunol Immunopathol* 1984;33:324–332.
44. Hotta O, Ysua N, Ooyama M, et al. Detection of urinary macrophages expressing the CD16 (FcγRIII) molecule: a novel marker of acute inflammatory glomerular injury. *Kidney Int* 1999;55:1927–1934.
45. Frankenberger M, Sternsdorf T, Pechumer H, et al. Differential cytokine expression in human blood monocyte subpopulation: a polymerase chain reaction analysis. *Blood* 1996;87:373–377.
46. Parra G, Romero M, Henriquez-La Roche C, et al. Expression of adhesion molecules in poststreptococcal glomerulonephritis. *Nephrol Dial Transplant* 1994;9:1412–1417.
47. Stevens TL, Bossie A, Sanders VM, et al. Regulation of antibody secretion by subsets of antigen-specific helper T cells. *Nature* 1988;334:255–258.
48. Dinarello CA. Interleukin-1. In: Thomson AV, ed. *The cytokine handbook.* San Diego: Academic Press, 1994:186.
49. Tam FWK, Smith J, Karkar AM, et al. Interleukin-4 ameliorates experimental glomerulonephritis and up-regulates

glomerular gene expression of IL-1 decoy receptor. *Kidney Int* 1997;52:1224–1231.
50. Mezzano S, Burgos ME, Olavvaria F, et al. Immunohistochemical localization of IL-8 and TGF-β in streptococcal glomerulonephritis. *J Am Soc Nephrol* 1997;8:234–241.
51. Morioka Y, Koike H, Ikezumi Y, et al. Podocyte injuries exacerbate mesangial proliferative glomerulonephritis. *Kidney Int* 2001;60:2192–2204.
52. Nangaku M, Miyata T, Suzuki D, et al. Cloning of rodent megsin revealed its up-regulation in mesangioproliferative nephritis. *Kidney Int* 2001;60:641–652.
53. Miyata T, Inagi R, Nangaku M, et al. Overexpression of the serpin megsin induces progressive mesangial cell proliferation and expansion. *J Clin Invest* 2002;109:585–593.
54. Kim YS, Zheng S, Yang SH, et al. Differential expression of various cytokine and chemokine genes between proliferative and non-proliferative glomerulonephritides. *Clin Nephrol* 2001;56:199–206.
55. Soto HM, Parra G, Rodriguez-Iturbe B. Circulating levels of cytokines in poststreptococcal glomerulonephritis. *Clin Nephrol* 1997;47:6–12.
56. Devasena T, Lalitha S, Padma K. Lipid peroxidation, osmotic fragility and antioxidant status in children with acute post-streptococcal glomerulonephritis. *Clin Chim Acta* 2001;308:155–161.
57. Túri S, Németh I, Torkos A, et al. Oxidative stress and antioxidant defense mechanisms in glomerular diseases. *Free Radic Biol Med* 1997;22:161–168.
58. Pfeilschifter J, Beck K-F, Eberhardt W, et al. Changing gears in the course of glomerulonephritis by shifting superoxide to nitric oxide-dominated chemistry. *Kidney Int* 2002;61:809–815.
59. Sorger K, Gessler U, Hübner FK, et al. Subtypes of acute postinfectious glomerulonephritis: synopsis of clinical and pathological features. *Clin Nephrol* 1982;17:114–128.
60. Sorger K, Balun J, Hübner FK, et al. The garland type of acute postinfectious glomerulonephritis: morphological characteristics and follow-up studies. *Clin Nephrol* 1983;20:17–26.
61. Churg J, Grishman E. Ultrastructure of immune deposits in renal glomeruli. *Ann Intern Med* 1972;76:479–486.
62. Tornroth T. The fate of subepithelial deposits in acute poststreptococcal glomerulonephritis. *Lab Invest* 1976;35:461–474.
63. Dodge WF, Spargo BF, Travis LB. Occurrence of acute glomerulonephritis in siblings contacts of children with sporadic acute glomerulonephritis. *Pediatrics* 1967;40:1028–1030.
64. Glassock RJ, Adler SG, Ward HJ, Cohen AH. Primary glomerular diseases. In: Brenner BM, Rector FC, eds. *The kidney*. Philadelphia: WB Saunders, 1986:929–1013.
65. Rovang RD, Zawada ET, Santella RN, et al. Cerebral vasculitis associated with acute post-streptococcal glomerulonephritis. *Am J Nephrol* 1997;17:89–97.
66. Soylu A, Kavukcu S, Turkmen M, et al. Posterior leukoencephalopathy syndrome in poststreptococcal acute glomerulonephritis. *Pediatr Nephrol* 2001;16:601–603.
67. Birch DF, Fairley KF, Whitworth JA, et al. Urinary erythrocyte morphology in the diagnosis of glomerular hematuria. *Clin Nephrol* 1983;20:78–84.
68. Van Iseghem P, Hauglustaine D, Bollens W, et al. Urinary erythrocyte morphology in acute glomerulonephritis. *BMJ* 1983;287:1183.
69. Freedman P, Meister HP, Co BS, et al. Subclinical renal response to streptococcal infection. *N Engl J Med* 1966;275: 795–802.
70. Reinstein CR. Epidemic nephritis at Red Lake, Minnesota. *J Pediatr* 1955;47:25–34.
71. Berry PL, Brewer ED. Glomerulonephritis and nephrotic syndrome. In: Oski FA, ed. *Principles and practice of pediatrics*. Philadelphia: JB Lippincott Co, 1994:1785–1788.
72. Foster MH. Serologic evaluation of the renal patient. In: Jacobson HR, Striker GR, Klahr S, eds. *The principles and practice of nephrology*. New York: Mosby, 1995:71–84.
73. Pan CG. Glomerulonephritis in childhood. *Curr Opin Pediatr* 1997;9:154–159.
74. Madaio MP. Postinfectious glomerulonephritis. In: Jacobson HR, Striker GR, Klahr S, eds. *The principles and practice of nephrology*. New York: Mosby, 1995:122–125.
75. Levy M, Sich M, Pirotzky E, et al. Complement activation in acute glomerulonephritis in children. *Int J Pediatr Nephrol* 1985;6:17–24.
76. Dedeoglu IO, Springate JE, Waz WR, et al. Prolonged hypocomplementemia in poststreptococcal acute glomerulonephritis. *Clin Nephrol* 1996;46:302–305.
77. Rodriguez-Iturbe B. Epidemic post-streptococcal glomerulonephritis. *Kidney Int* 1984;25:129–136.
78. West CD, McAdams AJ. Serum and glomerular IgG in poststreptococcal glomerulonephritis are correlated. *Pediatr Nephrol* 1998;12:392–396.
79. Ardiles LG, Valderrama G, Moya P, et al. Incidence and studies on antigenic specificities of antineutrophil-cytoplasmic autoantibodies (ANCA) in poststreptococcal glomerulonephritis. *Clin Nephrol* 1997;47:1–5.
80. Lang MM, Fowers C. Identifying poststreptococcal glomerulonephritis. *Nurse Pract* 2001;8:34,37–42,44–47.
81. Johnson F, Carapetis J, Patel MS, et al. Evaluating the use of penicillin to control outbreaks of acute poststreptococcal glomerulonephritis. *Pediatr Infect Dis* J 1999;18:327–332.
82. Robson AM, Cole BR, Kienstra RA, et al. Severe glomerulonephritis complicated by coagulopathy. Treatment with anticoagulant and immunosuppressive drugs. *J Pediatr* 1997;90:881–892.
83. Roy S, Murphy WM, Arant BS. Poststreptococcal crescentic glomerulonephritis in children: comparison of quintuple therapy versus supportive care. *J Pediatr* 1981;98:403–410.
84. Roy S, Pitcock JA, Ettledorf JN. Prognosis of acute poststreptococcal glomerulonephritis in childhood: prospective study and review of the literature. *Adv Pediatr* 1976;23:35–69.
85. Herthelius M, Berg U. Renal function during and after childhood acute poststreptococcal glomerulonephritis. *Pediatr Nephrol* 1999;13:907–911.
86. Cleper J, Davidovitz M, Halevi R, et al. Renal functional reserve after acute poststreptococcal glomerulonephritis. *Pediatr Nephrol* 1997;11:473–476.
87. Pinto SWL, Sesso R, Vasconcelos E, et al. Follow-up of patients with epidemic poststreptococcal glomerulonephritis. *Am J Kidney Dis* 2001;38:249–255.
88. Roy S, Wall HP, Etteldorf JN. Second attacks of acute glomerulonephritis. *J Pediatr* 1969;75:758–767.
89. Watanabe T, Yoshizawa N. Recurrence of acute poststreptococcal glomerulonephritis. *Pediatr Nephrol* 2001;16:598–600.

31

IMMUNOGLOBULIN A NEPHROPATHY

NORISHIGE YOSHIKAWA

Immunoglobulin (Ig) A nephropathy was first described in 1968 by Berger and Hinglais (1) and is now recognized as a distinct clinicopathologic entity with a higher frequency worldwide than any other primary glomerulopathy (2). It was initially considered a benign condition, but extended follow-up of patients indicates that 20 to 50% of adults ultimately progress to end-stage renal failure (2,3). Likewise, the favorable prognosis initially attributed to children with IgA nephropathy must be questioned in the light of more recent studies (4–8).

EPIDEMIOLOGY

IgA nephropathy has been diagnosed all over the world, but its prevalence varies widely from one country to another. In the Pacific Rim (e.g., Japan, Singapore, Australia, and New Zealand), IgA nephropathy accounts for as many as one-half of cases of primary glomerulonephritis. In Europe, it accounts for between 20 and 30% of all primary glomerulonephritis, whereas in North America, it is responsible for only 2 to 10%. The explanation for this apparent variability in incidence is uncertain, but it may be due to a racial difference in the incidence of IgA nephropathy or to differences in biopsy selection practices (9).

Genetic factors and environmental influences could contribute to geographic differences in prevalence. A lower prevalence among blacks than whites has been reported in the United States. However, in American children, similar incidences of IgA nephropathy in white and black children from Shelby County, Tennessee, have been reported (10). In Australia (11), where the population is heterogeneous and includes many immigrants from Third World countries, all racial groups seem to be affected equally.

The high incidence of IgA nephropathy in certain countries may reflect the practice of routine urinalysis. In Japan, all children between the ages of 6 and 18 years are screened annually, and those found to have urinary abnormalities are referred for further investigation. Thus, IgA nephropathy is the most common primary glomerulopathy in children seen in Kobe University and Wakayama Medical University Hospitals, detected in approximately 30% of biopsy specimens obtained.

ETIOLOGY

Because of the frequent association between upper respiratory tract or gastrointestinal infection and the onset of macroscopic hematuria, it has been suggested that certain viral or bacterial infections may lead to IgA nephropathy. Considerable effort has been directed toward the search for antigens and for the antibody specificity of the mesangial IgA, but it has met with limited success. Many antigens, including herpes simplex virus, cytomegalovirus, Epstein-Barr virus nuclear antigen, adenovirus, and milk antigen, have been identified. The observation of numerous antigenic substances in the glomeruli indicates that the antigenic materials in IgA nephropathy may be heterogeneous. The presence of *Haemophilus parainfluenzae* antigens in a diffuse and global distribution in the glomerular mesangium and the presence of IgA antibody against *H. parainfluenzae* in sera of Japanese patients with IgA nephropathy have been demonstrated (12,13).

Predisposing Genetic Factors

Predisposing genetic factors have been suggested as important in the development of IgA nephropathy (14). Moreover, it has been suggested that genetic factors may not only determine susceptibility to glomerulonephritis but also influence the pathologic severity and natural course of IgA nephropathy (15,16).

Evidence for genetic factors being important in IgA nephropathy is provided by family studies (15–19). Rambausek et al. reported that 9.6% of patients with mesangial IgA nephropathy in Germany had one or more siblings with glomerulonephritis (15). Julian et al. described kindred from eastern Kentucky in which six patients with IgA nephropathy descended from one ancestor and eight other patients belonged to potentially related pedigrees (17). Moreover, they indicated that at least 48 (60%) of 80 IgA nephropathy patients who were born in same region were related to at least one other patient (18). Scolarim et al. reported that 26 (14%) of 185 patients with IgA nephropathy investigated in Italy were related to at least one other patient with the disease (19). These family studies suggest that familial predisposition is a very common finding and genetic factors are influenced in the pathogenesis of IgA nephropathy. Recently, Gharavi et al. (20) demonstrated linkage of IgA nephropathy to 6q22-23 under a dominant model of transmission with incomplete penetrance.

Genetic factors are implicated in both disease susceptibility and disease progression (21). Polymorphisms of Ig heavy-chain switch region gene (22), Iα1 germ-line transcript regulatory region gene (23), genes of the renin angiotensin system (24,25), and platelet activating factor acetylhydrolase gene (26) have been reported. Although some associations have emerged, they have been inconsistent (27). Some of the discrepancies may be caused by different sample sizes and different geographic regions of the patients included in the studies.

PATHOGENESIS

Although the pathogenesis of IgA nephropathy remains uncertain, there is substantial evidence that it is an immune complex disease (2,28). Granular electron-dense deposits are observed in the glomerular mesangial areas by electron microscopy and confirmed as containing IgA and C3 by immunofluorescence microscopy. Circulating IgA immune complexes have been detected by several different assays often associated with IgG immune complex. Many immunologic abnormalities that may lead to the formation of IgA immune complex have been reported in patients with IgA nephropathy. Recurrence of IgA nephropathy frequently occurs in allografts (29), and a rapid disappearance of glomerular IgA deposits is observed when kidneys with mesangial IgA deposits are transplanted to patients without IgA nephropathy. Although much of this work was performed in adults, there is no evidence to suggest that the findings cannot be extrapolated to children. Moreover, glomerular IgA deposits associated with histologic lesions similar to those of human IgA nephropathy can be induced in laboratory animals by passive administration of preformed IgA immune complex or by active immunization (30–34).

Nature of Mesangial Immunoglobulin A Deposits

IgA contributes to immunity at the level of the external secretory system. IgA exists in monomeric and polymeric forms. Monomeric IgA represents approximately 90% of the serum IgA and is produced mainly by the circulating lymphocytes and plasma cells in the spleen and bone marrow. Polymeric IgA is produced mostly by lymphocytes and plasma cells in the gastrointestinal and respiratory tracts, where it is synthesized as monomers and then secreted as dimers linked by the J-chain, which is also produced within the plasma cells. During the passage of dimeric IgA molecules through the mucosal epithelium toward the external lumen, the secretory component is attached through specific noncovalent interactions; this component appears to protect the dimeric IgA from the proteolytic enzymes present in the external secretions. IgA has two subclasses, IgA1 and IgA2. Approximately 90% of serum IgA is composed of IgA1 mostly produced in the bone marrow, whereas IgA2 is mostly derived from the local mucosa of the gastrointestinal and respiratory tracts. Both IgA1 and IgA2 are produced in the mucosa.

The most prominent finding in the glomeruli of renal biopsy specimens from patients with IgA nephropathy is mesangial IgA deposition. The majority of investigators has indicated that IgA1 is the predominant subclass present in the glomeruli (35). The J-chain has also been identified in the mesangium in patients with IgA nephropathy (36). Secretory component is not present in the mesangial deposits, but immunofluorescence studies of renal biopsy sections from patients with IgA nephropathy have indicated that it binds to the mesangial areas *in vitro* (37). These observations suggest that the mesangial IgA deposits are polymeric, a hypothesis further supported by the immunochemical characterization of IgA eluted from renal biopsy sections (38). Assessment of polymeric IgA1 production by *in situ* hybridization for J-chain messenger RNA in IgA plasma cells shows downregulation in the mucosa (39) and upregulation in the bone marrow (40). Impaired mucosal IgA responses allowing enhanced antigen challenge to the marrow shown by de Fijter et al. (41) could be the primary abnormality in IgA nephropathy, although this remains unproven (42).

A number of studies have suggested that the alternative complement pathway has a pathogenetic role in IgA nephropathy. This hypothesis is consistent with the typical immunohistologic demonstration of C3 and properdin in a pattern and distribution similar to that of IgA in the glomeruli, in the absence of C1q and C4. The detection of the membrane attack complex of complement further supports the pathogenetic role of complement activation in this disease (43). Certain types of IgA aggregates or IgA from patients with myeloma have been shown to activate complement *in vitro* (44). IgA has been reported to activate the complement system via the mannan-binding lectin pathway (45). However, there is no direct evidence that complement activation is mediated by IgA deposition in the glomeruli. Activation of C3 is observed in the majority of adult and pediatric patients with IgA nephropathy, but the mediator as well as the pathophysiologic significance of this complement activation remains to be determined. C3 is deposited in the kidney but is also produced by mesangial cells in IgA nephropathy (46).

With regard to antibody specificity, IgA eluted from cryostat sections of IgA nephropathy biopsies has been reported to react with mesangial areas of its own and other IgA nephropathy patients' biopsies, but not with normal kidney (47). Such eluates have also been shown to contain antibodies that react with tonsillar cells and cultured fibroblasts obtained from patients with IgA nephropathy (48).

In summary, the immunochemical nature of the mesangial deposits in IgA nephropathy is consistent with antigen-polymeric IgA complexes predominantly of A1 subclass and, perhaps, multispecific for ubiquitous mucosally derived antigens.

Immunoglobulin A Glycosylation

IgA glycosylation has received recent attention as a putative nonimmune feature of IgA, which may explain its abnormal behavior and glomerular deposition in IgA nephropathy (49). IgA1 subclass is prominent in IgA nephropathy. IgA1 is unique among all Igs in its possession of a hinge region rich in proline, serine, and threonine and characterized by five O-glycosylation sites (Fig. 31.1). These O-glycosylation sites consist of N-acetylgalactosamine O-linked to the serine residues of hinge region. Abnormal galactosylated IgA1 increases affinity for glomerular fibronectin, laminin, and collagen IV (50) and may lead to accumulation of IgA in the mesangium (51). Preliminary data indicate that deficient galactosylation of hinge-region glycans may be detected even in family members of patients with IgA nephropathy (52). Altered amino-acid sequence of the IgA1 hinge region is a possible mechanism to consider for abnormal galactosylation of IgA1. However, the hinge region is a highly conserved region of the IgA1 molecule. There is no evidence for any nucleotide sequence alteration or transcriptional abnormality of the hinge region in IgA nephropathy (53). It has also been postulated that altered galactosylated IgA1 in IgA nephropathy may be due to a deficiency or structural modification of β1,3-galactosyltransferase, the enzyme responsible for the terminal galactosylation of GalNAc on O-linked glycans (54). This structural or functional deficiency may be genetically determined. The recent sequence of β1,3-galactosyltransferase may help us to understand the genetic basis of these abnormalities (55,56). Circulating IgA1 has reduced terminal galactose on O-linked hinge-region sugars in IgA nephropathy (57), apparently because of a B-cell defect in β1,3-galactosyltransferase, the enzyme responsible for placing terminal galactose on O-linked sugars (58). The IgA1 O-glycan chains are truncated in IgA nephropathy (59). Circulating immune complexes in IgA nephropathy consist of IgA1 with a galactose-deficient hinge region, and the deficiency of galactose may result in the generation of antigenic determinants that are recognized by naturally occurring IgG and IgA1 antibodies (60). Sano et al. demonstrated that enzymatically deglycosylated human IgA1 molecules accumulate and induce inflammatory cell reaction (61); Amore et al. showed that glycosylation of circulating IgA modulates mesangial proliferation in IgA nephropathy (62).

Immunoglobulin A Immune System

There is a general agreement that serum levels of IgA are increased in 50 to 70% of patients with IgA nephropathy, with elevations in both monomeric and polymeric IgA. There is an increase in polymeric IgA1-producing plasma cells in the bone marrow (63) and in the tonsils (64) of patients with IgA nephropathy. The proportion of IgA-λ in serum IgA is also increased. Serum IgA is more anionic, owing to the increased anionicity of λ- compared with κ-light chain (65). The binding of IgA to mesangial cells is charge dependent, and anionic charge may play an important role in IgA1 deposition in the mesangium (66). In

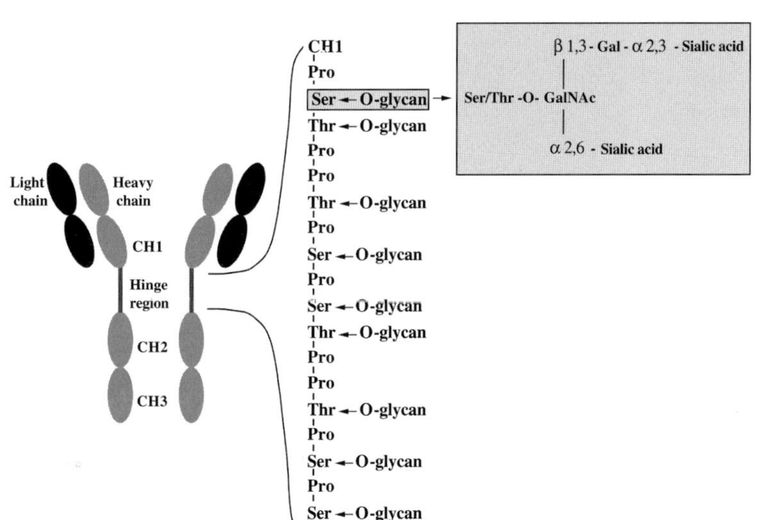

FIGURE 31.1. Immunoglobulin A1 (IgA1) molecule with hinge region O-glycosylation sites. IgA1 molecule with two heavy chains, each having three constant region domains, CH1 to CH3, and a hinge region between CH1 and CH2. Each serine (Ser) and threonine (Thr) residue is a potential site for O-glycan side chain. O-glycosylation sites consist of N-acetylgalactosamine (GalNAc) O-linked to the Ser or Thr residues of hinge region. Pro, proline.

addition to the increased levels of serum IgA, various types of autoantibodies of the IgA class have been recognized. These IgA autoantibodies include rheumatoid factor (67), antinuclear antibodies (68), and anticollagen antibodies (69). However, the IgA may be polyspecific, indicating a polyclonal increase rather than true antigen-specific autoantibodies (70). IgA immune complexes are frequently detected (71). Cultured peripheral blood lymphocytes from patients with the disease produce more IgA than do those of normal individuals, either spontaneously or after polyclonal stimulation *in vitro*. We also demonstrated an increased spontaneous and pokeweed mitogen-stimulated IgA production by peripheral blood lymphocytes in children with IgA nephropathy (72). This increased IgA production remained stable during the follow-up period in patients with persistent urinary abnormalities but decreased toward normal in patients with clinical remission.

IgA production is T-cell dependent, and the increased production in IgA nephropathy may indicate altered T-cell function. An increased circulating OKT4 to OKT8 cell ratio, due to increased OKT4 helper T lymphocytes and decreased OKT8 cytotoxic-suppressor T lymphocytes, has been reported in patients (73). Increased IgA-specific helper T-cell activity and decreased IgA-specific suppressor T-cell activity have also been reported (74,75).

Defective clearance of immune complexes from the circulation may also be important (76), but this seems more likely to be a consequence rather than the cause of the increased immune complex load.

Mechanism of Progression

IgA alone appears to be sufficient to provoke injury in susceptible individuals (77), and deposition of polymeric IgA, but not of monomeric IgA, can initiate glomerulonephritis (78). There is little to suggest that the mechanisms of mesangial proliferative glomerulonephritis, progression, and scarring are distinct in IgA nephropathy compared with other types of chronic glomerulonephritis. Studies *in vitro* and in animal models of mesangial proliferative glomerulonephritis have shown the key role of cytokines and growth factors, particularly platelet-derived growth factor and transforming growth factor β, in the induction and progression of mesangial injury, and there is evidence that these are also involved in IgA nephropathy (79–81). Studies in children with IgA nephropathy suggest that mesangial proliferation may in part be the result of local production of cytokines, interleukin-1, interleukin-6, tumor necrosis factor, platelet-derived growth factor, transforming growth factor β, vascular permeability factor, and endothelial growth factor (82–85). Although much has been learned about the basic abnormalities of IgA in IgA nephropathy, therapeutic interventions that may prevent glomerular IgA deposition or the subsequent inflammation and injury have to be found.

PATHOLOGY

Immunohistologic Findings

The diagnostic immunopathologic pattern of IgA nephropathy is the presence of IgA in the glomerular mesangium as the sole or predominant Ig. IgA deposits often extend just beyond the mesangiocapillary junctions into the adjacent capillary walls (Fig. 31.2). There are also deposits of IgG or IgM with the same staining pattern as IgA but with lesser intensity and frequency. In our series, mesangial IgA deposits were associated with IgG in 32% of patients, IgM in 8%, and both IgG and IgM in 11% (86). C3 deposits were observed in a similar distribution pattern in 64% of cases. The early components of the classical complement pathway, C4 or C1q, are absent. Fibrin- or fibrinogen-related antigens are found in a diffuse mesangial distribution in 25 to 70% of patients and are believed to be one of the injurious agents in the glomeruli (87). Although, in most patients, IgA is present only in the mesangial regions, in approximately 10% of patients it is also observed in the peripheral capillary walls. Such peripheral capillary wall deposits, whether documented by immunofluorescence or electron microscopy, have been associated with more severe clinical manifestations and a poor renal outcome (88–91).

Light Microscopic Findings

Various glomerular changes are observed. The most characteristic abnormality is mesangial enlargement, caused by various combinations of hypercellularity and increase in matrix (Fig. 31.3). Occasionally, small eosinophilic and PAS-positive fibrinoid mesangial deposits are also seen.

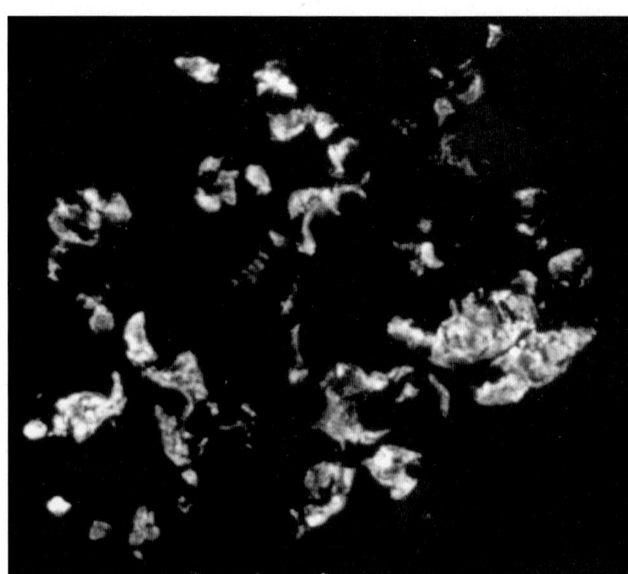

FIGURE 31.2. Immunofluorescence micrograph showing mesangial immunoglobulin A deposits in a patients with immunoglobulin A nephropathy.

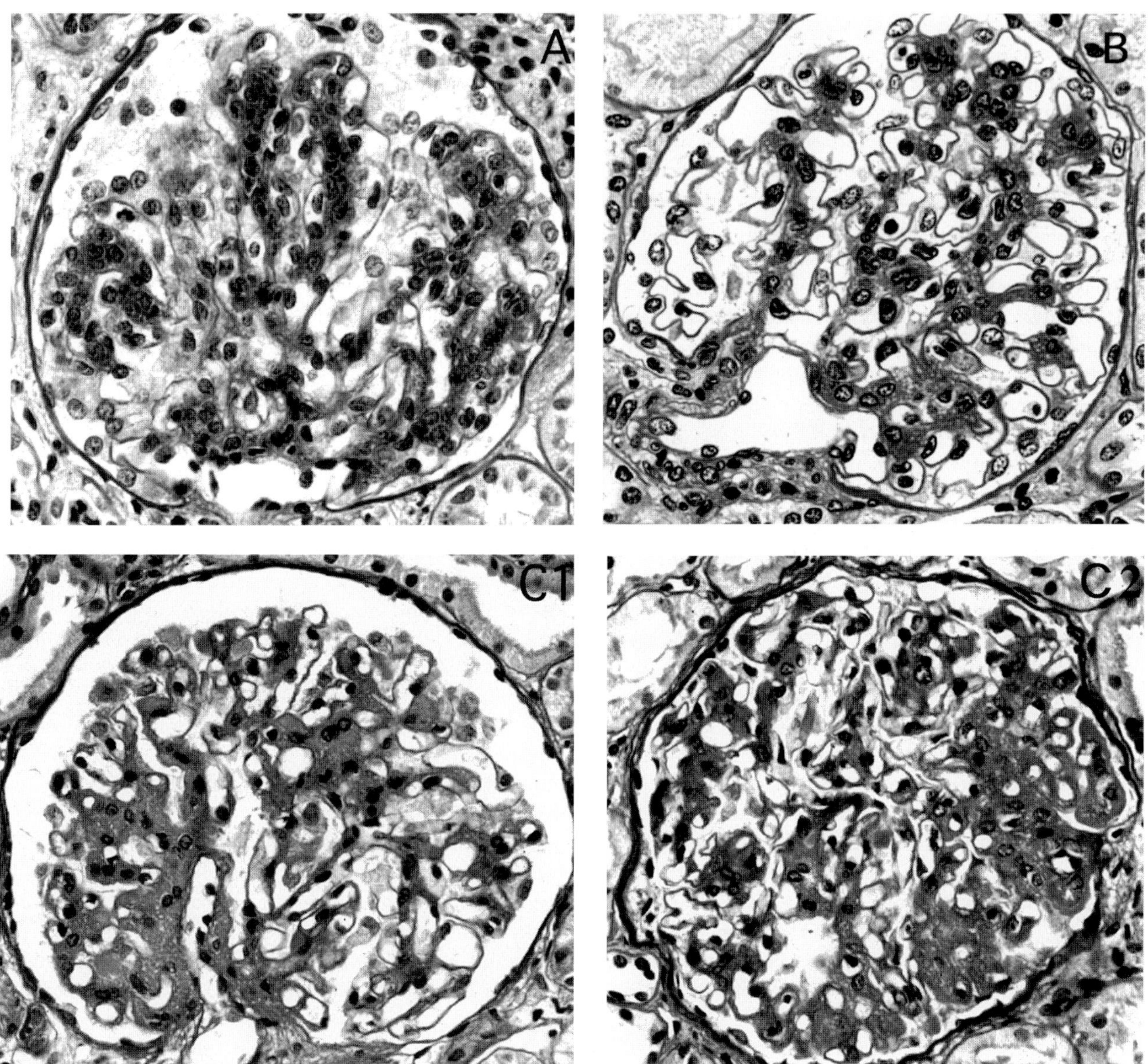

FIGURE 31.3. Light micrograph showing mesangial proliferation in patients with immunoglobulin A nephropathy. Three types of mesangial changes are identified: **A:** Mesangial hypercellularity is more prominent than the increase in matrix. **B:** The degrees of mesangial hypercellularity and matrix increase are similar. **C1,C2:** The increase in matrix is more prominent than the mesangial cellularity.

Biopsies can be graded according to the amount of mesangial cell proliferation on the basis of the World Health Organization criteria (92).

1. Minimal glomerular lesions. The majority of glomeruli appears optically normal, although a few may show a slight increase of mesangial matrix, with or without accompanying hypercellularity. The number of mesangial cells per peripheral mesangial area does not exceed three. There are also small foci of tubular atrophy and interstitial lymphocyte infiltration in some patients.
2. Focal mesangial proliferation. Up to 80% of glomeruli show moderate or severe mesangial cell proliferation (i.e., more than three cells per peripheral mesangial area). The degree of mesangial cell proliferation varies considerably among glomeruli as well as segmentally within individual glomeruli. The proliferation is usually associated with increased matrix. Small cellular or fibrocellular crescents are frequently found but rarely affect more than 20% of the glomeruli. Capsular adhesions are frequently seen overlying lobules showing mesangial proliferation. Segmental capillary collapse is often observed in association with crescents. A small number of glomeruli showing global sclerosis is often present. Tubular atrophy, interstitial fibrosis, and interstitial lymphocyte infiltration are frequently present but are not extensive.
3. Diffuse mesangial proliferation. More than 80% of glomeruli show moderate or severe mesangial cell prolifera-

tion, which varies in intensity in different regions of the mesangium in a given glomerulus as well as from one glomerulus to another. Mesangial cell proliferation is always accompanied by increased mesangial matrix. Cellular and fibrocellular crescents are often found, usually affecting less than 50% of the glomeruli, although in approximately 10% of patients, more than 50% are involved. Capsular adhesions are frequently seen in the absence of crescents. A small number of globally sclerosed glomeruli are often present. Tubular atrophy, interstitial fibrosis, and interstitial lymphocyte infiltration are frequently present and are extensive in 10% of patients.

Three types of mesangial changes are identified in children with IgA nephropathy (5) (Fig. 31.3): (a) Mesangial hypercellularity is more prominent than the increase in matrix, (b) the degrees of mesangial hypercellularity and matrix increase are similar, and (c) the increase in matrix is more prominent than the mesangial cellularity.

The first type of lesion is seen in biopsies in which the interval between onset of disease and biopsy is short. Serial pathologic observations reveal that prominent mesangial hypercellularity is almost exclusively seen in initial biopsies and disappears in follow-up biopsies. These observations suggest that predominant mesangial hypercellularity is characteristic of the early lesion of childhood IgA nephropathy and may disappear within a matter of months. An increase in mesangial cells, although sometimes present, is seldom striking in adult patients (93). In contrast, biopsies with a predominant matrix increase show a long interval between onset of disease and biopsy and a high percentage of glomerular sclerosis. Serial pathologic observations reveal that this type of change is usually seen in follow-up biopsies. An increase in the amount of mesangial matrix with duration of the disease has also been noted in adult patients (94). These findings suggest that progression of IgA nephropathy leads to gradual resolution of mesangial hypercellularity and an increase of matrix associated with the development of sclerosis (95).

The severity of tubulointerstitial changes usually reflects the severity of glomerular damage. Vascular lesions, such as arterial or arteriolar sclerosis, are reported to be common in adults (96) but are very unusual in children with IgA nephropathy (97). This difference may be related to the age at biopsy and the duration of disease before biopsy.

Electron Microscopy

Electron microscopic abnormalities are mainly observed in the mesangium, which is variably enlarged by a combination of increased cytoplasm and matrix. Electron-dense deposits in the mesangium are the most constant and prominent feature and are seen in almost all patients (Fig. 31.4). They are granular masses situated immediately beneath the lamina densa in the perimesangial region and expanded mesangium. The size and extent of mesangial deposits varies from patient to patient; in some patients, they are large and produce localized protrusions. Peripheral glomerular capillary wall deposits are also found in the subendothelial and subepithelial regions. Subendothelial deposits occur most frequently in the capillary wall adjacent to the mesangium, although they are also observed in the peripheral part of the loop. Subepithelial deposits are reported to be unusual in adult patients but are frequently found in children with IgA nephropathy. They are generally small and flat and localized to a few capillary loops; the humps typical of acute poststreptococcal glomerulonephritis are never observed. Lysis of the glomerular basement membrane is also seen quite frequently in children (98). In affected areas of the glomerular capillary walls, the lamina densa is thin and irregular, and the epithelial aspect of the glomerular basement membrane shows irregular segments of low electron density with an expanded, washed-out appearance. The epithelial foot processes are generally well preserved, but diffuse foot process effacement may be seen in patients with the nephrotic syndrome.

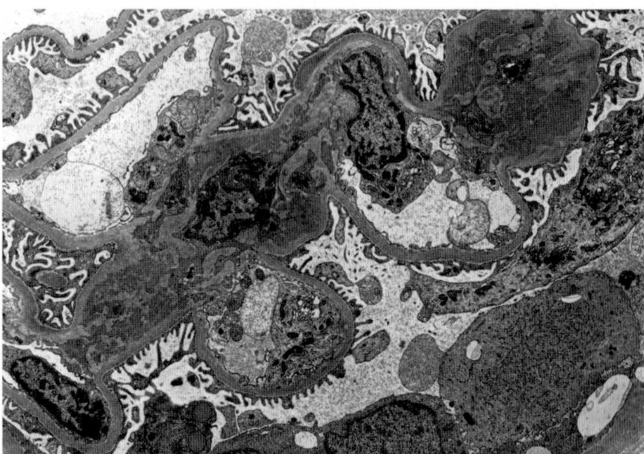

FIGURE 31.4. Electron micrograph showing numerous electron-dense deposits in the mesangium in a patient with immunoglobulin A nephropathy.

Repeat Renal Biopsy Findings

There have been only a few reports on the results of repeat renal biopsies (99,100). We previously reported our results in children with IgA nephropathy (6). At the time of the second biopsy, 23 patients had shown *clinical remission*, defined as complete disappearance of proteinuria and hematuria with normal renal function, whereas 38 had persistent urinary abnormalities with normal renal function. There were no differences between the two groups with regard to the initial clinical findings and the pathologic findings in the initial biopsy. The second biopsy in patients who were in clinical remission showed improvement of the glomerular lesions on light microscopy, a disappearance of or a decrease in mesangial IgA deposits, and a decreased amount of electron-dense deposits. Conversely, light microscopy showed a progression of histologic lesions and the persistence of both mesangial IgA deposits and electron-dense deposits in patients with persistent urinary abnormalities. Clinical remission and histologic regression have been reported in adults with IgA nephropathy (101).

CLINICAL FEATURES

IgA nephropathy occurs at all ages but is most common during the second and third decades of life; it affects boys more often than girls, with the reported male to female ratio varying from less than 2:1 to 6:1 (2). In a study of Japanese children (86), the mean age at presentation was 9.3 years in boys and 10.3 years in girls, and the male to female ratio was 3:2. The clinical presentation of IgA nephropathy varies. Some patients have asymptomatic microscopic hematuria with or without proteinuria. Other patients have recurrent episodes of macroscopic hematuria. Some patients present with acute nephritic syndrome and, more rarely, with acute renal failure.

Sixty-two percent of our 258 Japanese children were found to have microscopic hematuria or asymptomatic proteinuria (86). Twenty-six percent presented with macroscopic hematuria and 12% with an acute nephritic syndrome or nephrotic syndrome. Several studies from Europe and the United States reported that more than 80% of the patients have episodes of macroscopic hematuria, and recurrent macroscopic hematuria is traditionally regarded as the hallmark of childhood IgA nephropathy (102–105). However, it was the initial feature in only 26% of our series, presumably because of the school screening program that detected a high prevalence of asymptomatic urinary abnormalities rather than regional variation in the expression of IgA nephropathy. During the observation period, 60% of our patients had one or more episodes of macroscopic hematuria, whereas the other 40% remained asymptomatic.

Macroscopic hematuria often occurs in association with upper respiratory tract infections; less frequently, it occurs in association with other infections involving the mucosal system (e.g., diarrhea and sinusitis). Episodes of macroscopic hematuria are sometimes associated with loin pain. The interval between the precipitating infection and the appearance of hematuria ranges from 1 to 2 days compared with 1 or 2 weeks in acute postinfectious glomerulonephritis. Many patients have recurrent episodes of macroscopic hematuria—each often associated with the same type of infection. The number of recurrences and the intervals between different episodes are variable. The incidence of macroscopic hematuria is lower in adults (105,106).

Patients with a nephritic or nephrotic onset have the most severe glomerular damage. The most common presenting symptom is macroscopic hematuria. Hypertension is infrequent and usually mild to moderate. Nephrotic edema is reported in approximately 10% of patients. Acute renal failure is occasionally associated with episodes of macroscopic hematuria and is usually reversible. However, a number of investigators have documented a subset of patients with IgA nephropathy that is characterized by extensive crescents and a rapidly progressive course (107–109).

LABORATORY INVESTIGATIONS

Serum IgA levels are increased in 30 to 50% of adult patients but in only 8 to 16% in children with IgA nephropathy (86). For this reason, it is seldom of diagnostic significance. Serum complement component concentrations are usually normal, but the C3 level should be measured routinely if the patient has been referred for investigation after the first attack of hematuria to eliminate a diagnosis of postinfectious glomerulonephritis or membranoproliferative glomerulonephritis. Likewise, the antistreptococcal antibody titers should be determined after initial hematuria. The serum creatinine should be measured routinely to estimate renal function; if necessary, the glomerular filtration rate should be determined. If present, proteinuria should be quantified, as proteinuria is associated with histologic lesions and a risk of progression. The plasma proteins should be measured routinely in the presence of heavy proteinuria.

DIFFERENTIAL DIAGNOSIS

The diagnosis of IgA nephropathy is based on the presence of IgA as the sole or predominant Ig in the glomerular mesangium. Because diffuse mesangial IgA deposits are observed in a variety of other disorders (Table 31.1), the diagnosis of IgA nephropathy can be made only by exclusion.

Relationship between Immunoglobulin A Nephropathy and Henoch-Schönlein Purpura

There is a close relationship between IgA nephropathy and Henoch-Schönlein purpura (110). The morphologic and immunopathologic features are similar in the two conditions (110,111), which are characterized by various degrees of focal or diffuse mesangial proliferation, the diffuse deposition of IgA in the mesangium, and electron-dense deposits in the mesangium. Elevated serum IgA levels are found in both IgA nephropathy and Henoch-Schönlein purpura nephritis, and IgA-containing circulating immune complexes have been demonstrated in both conditions. Infective episodes precede Henoch-Schönlein purpura nephritis in 30 to 50% of patients, and the presence of *H. parainfluenzae* antigens in a diffuse and global distribution in the glomerular mesangium and the presence of IgA antibody against *H. parainfluenzae* in sera of Japanese children with Henoch-Schönlein purpura nephritis have also been demonstrated (13). The two disorders have been reported to coexist in different members of

TABLE 31.1. DISEASES ASSOCIATED WITH DIFFUSE MESANGIAL IMMUNOGLOBULIN A (IgA) DEPOSITS

IgA nephropathy (Berger's disease)
Multisystem disease
- Henoch-Schönlein purpura
- Systemic lupus erythematosus
- Cystic fibrosis
- Celiac disease
- Crohn's disease
- Dermatitis herpetiformis
- Ankylosing spondylitis

Neoplasms
- Carcinomas of the lung and colon
- Monoclonal IgA gammopathy
- Mucosis fungoides
- Non-Hodgkin's lymphoma

Infectious diseases
- Mycoplasma infections
- Leprosy
- Toxoplasmosis

Others
- Chronic liver disease
- Thrombocytopenia
- Pulmonary hemosiderosis
- Mixed cryoglobulinemia
- Polycythemia
- Scleritis

the same family, including a pair of monozygotic twins who developed the disorders simultaneously after a well-documented adenovirus infection (112–115). Moreover, the evolution of IgA nephropathy into Henoch-Schönlein purpura nephritis in the same patient is described in both adults and children (116–118). It has been suggested that the two conditions are variants of the same process and that IgA nephropathy is Henoch-Schönlein purpura nephritis without the rash. Although there are similarities in their pathologic and immunologic features, the two conditions are clinically different, and the pathogenesis is not clear. Our study suggests that Henoch-Schönlein purpura nephritis is an acute disease, with glomerular lesions nonprogressive after the onset (119). Therefore, in most patients, the prognosis is associated with the severity of glomerular change at the onset. In contrast, IgA nephropathy is a chronic, slowly progressive glomerular lesion, which may eventually lead to chronic renal failure, whatever the presentation. A few patients with Henoch-Schönlein purpura nephritis have recurrent episodes of macroscopic hematuria and a progressive renal disease on repeat renal biopsies. Finally, Henoch-Schönlein purpura nephritis occurs mostly in young children and is rare in adulthood, whereas IgA nephropathy affects mainly older children and younger adults.

Chronic Liver Disease

Glomerular IgA deposits may be observed in patients with various types of chronic liver diseases (120–122). Mesangial proliferation and IgA deposits are the most common findings. Most patients with chronic liver disease have clinically asymptomatic renal disease. The pathogenetic mechanisms that contribute to mesangial IgA deposition in chronic liver diseases remain unknown. Significant elevations of the serum monomeric and polymeric IgA levels have been reported. Impaired hepatic clearance and increased synthesis of polymeric IgA, abnormalities of IgA metabolism, and portosystemic shunting of antigens and immune complexes have been suggested as possible causes of mesangial IgA deposition (123).

Idiopathic Nephrotic Syndrome

A few patients with steroid-sensitive nephrotic syndrome show mesangial deposits of IgA on renal biopsy. They are classified by some as IgA nephropathy, whereas others consider that mesangial IgA in patients with minimal changes (i.e., without cellular proliferation) is coincidental. This probably applies to idiopathic nephrotic syndrome associated with mesangial IgA deposits occurring in Asians and explains a favorable response to steroids, which is not the case in true IgA nephropathy (124).

NATURAL HISTORY AND PROGNOSIS

In adult series, the incidence of renal insufficiency varies from less than 10% to as high as 45% in patients followed for more than 1 year. In long-term follow-up of adult patients, 30 to 35% have been found to develop progressive renal insufficiency 20 years after the initial discovery of disease (2,125–127). It can be estimated that 1 to 2% of adult patients will enter end-stage renal failure each year from time of diagnosis (128). The long-term prognosis of the 169 Japanese children with IgA nephropathy who were followed for more than 10 years indicates that 9% of the patients had developed chronic renal failure by 15 years (Fig. 31.5).

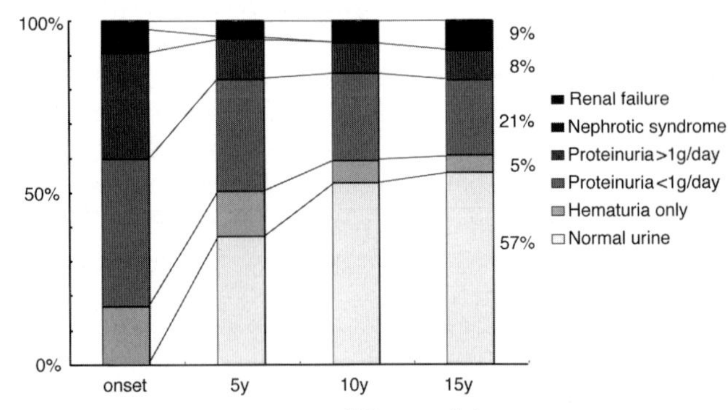

FIGURE 31.5. Long-term prognosis of the 169 Japanese children with immunoglobulin A nephropathy who were followed for more than 10 years.

Because of the variable rate of progression to chronic renal failure, there have been attempts to identify features present at the time of diagnosis that would predict the ultimate outcome. The following clinical findings are regarded as poor prognostic indicators in adult patients (2): persistent hypertension, persistent heavy proteinuria, and reduced glomerular filtration rate at presentation (125–127,129–134). In children, several studies have shown that the degree of proteinuria correlates with the severity of morphologic glomerular lesion (104,135–137) and heavy proteinuria at the time of biopsy predicts a poor outcome (91,138). In contrast, slight proteinuria or its absence at the time of biopsy predicts a favorable outcome. There is general agreement that hypertension and low glomerular filtration rate at presentation are significant factors in determining the outcome of adult patients with IgA nephropathy. In children, acute renal failure at onset is usually transient and associated with macroscopic hematuria and reversible tubular lesions. Male gender has also been considered an unfavorable prognostic feature by some investigators (126), but we (91) and others (89) could not confirm it in a large cohort of adult and pediatric patients. Schena et al. reported an increased risk of end-stage renal disease in familial IgA nephropathy (139).

Several pathologic features are associated with a poor outcome: diffuse mesangial proliferation; a high proportion of glomeruli showing sclerosis, crescents, or capsular adhesions; the presence of moderate or severe tubulointerstitial changes; the presence of subepithelial electron-dense deposits; and lysis of the glomerular basement membrane by electron microscopy (91). Patients with diffuse mesangial proliferation have been reported to have a significantly worse prognosis than those with focal proliferation or minimal lesions by light microscopy in adults (125,130,140). In many adult studies (89,125,133,141), glomerular sclerosis and crescents have also been associated with poor renal outcome. Levy and associates found that mesangial proliferative glomerulonephritis with crescents was associated with poor prognosis in children (135). Because the severity of the tubulointerstitial changes usually corresponds with the severity of the glomerular changes, tubulointerstitial changes in IgA nephropathy are believed to be secondary to the glomerular injury. Vascular lesions, such as arterial or arteriolar sclerosis, have been reported to play an important role in the progression of IgA nephropathy in adults. However, vascular changes are very unusual in children (5,105,108). This difference may be related to the age at biopsy and the duration of disease before biopsy.

TREATMENT

IgA nephropathy is a leading cause of chronic renal disease and end-stage renal disease in adult patients, and recent long-term studies assessing the prognosis in children have challenged earlier views that the condition represents a benign disorder. Thus, IgA nephropathy presents a therapeutic challenge in both adults and children. Because of the variable rate of progression to renal failure, and because of the probable multifactorial pathogenesis of the disease, the effectiveness of any treatment can only be properly evaluated by means of a randomized controlled trial (142). When considering treatment protocols, an issue of great importance is the selection of appropriate patients in whom the treatment is to be evaluated. Patients with heavy proteinuria at biopsy and the most severe glomerular lesions on renal biopsy appear to be at greatest risk of progressive renal deterioration and, therefore, the most appropriate candidates for specific therapeutic interventions. Patients with long-standing disease and extensive, irreversible glomerular damage are unsuitable for such treatments.

Controlled double-blind trials in adult patients with IgA nephropathy (143–145) showed that treatment with fish oil for 2 years retarded the rate at which renal function was lost, but a meta-analysis showed that there was only a 75% probability that fish oil was beneficial (146). Recent studies have indicated that angiotensin-converting enzyme inhibitors reduce urinary protein excretion and preserve renal function in adult patients with IgA nephropathy (147,148), but there is no randomized controlled study demonstrating that angiotensin-converting enzyme inhibitors preserve renal function in IgA nephropathy. High-dose intravenous methylprednisolone was shown to delay development of renal failure in a randomized controlled trial in adult patients (149). However, no convincing evidence has been published to date to support the use of fish oil, angiotensin-converting enzyme inhibitors, or high-dose intravenous methylprednisolone for the treatment of children with IgA nephropathy; at present, there is no curative therapy for IgA nephropathy (150).

Our recent controlled trial by the Japanese Pediatric IgA Nephropathy Treatment Study Group demonstrated that treatment of children with severe IgA nephropathy with prednisolone, azathioprine, heparin-warfarin, and dipyridamole for 2 years early in the course of disease prevents immunologic renal injury and progression of the disease (151). Seventy-eight children with newly diagnosed IgA nephropathy showing diffuse mesangial proliferation were randomly assigned to receive either the combined therapy of prednisolone, azathioprine, heparin-warfarin, and dipyridamole for 2 years (group 1) or the combination of heparin-warfarin and dipyridamole for 2 years (group 2). Urinary protein excretion was significantly reduced in group 1 patients but remained unchanged in group 2 patients. Serum IgA concentration was also significantly reduced in group 1 patients but was unchanged in group 2 patients. Blood pressure and creatinine clearance were normal at the end of the trial in all but one group 2 patient who developed chronic renal insufficiency. The percentage of glomeruli showing sclerosis was unchanged in group 1 patients but significantly increased in group 2 patients. The intensity of mesangial IgA deposits significantly decreased in group 1 patients but remained unchanged in group 2 patients. The beneficial effects of prednisolone, azathioprine, heparin-warfarin, and dipyridamole treatment were accompanied by relatively few serious side effects specifically attributable to the drugs.

Progression of IgA nephropathy leads to gradual resolution of mesangial hypercellularity and an increase of matrix and is associated with the development of sclerosis (5). The majority of patients with IgA nephropathy in our series are diagnosed early in the course of the disease, and the asymptomatic period before the discovery of urinary abnormalities is short. Patients with long-standing disease and extensive glomerulosclerosis are unsuitable for treatment. In our controlled trial, the average interval between onset and discovery of disease and start of treatment was 11 months, and no patient showed predominant matrix increase or extensive glomerulosclerosis. Early diagnosis and early treatment are very important in IgA nephropathy.

Recurrence of mesangial IgA deposits is often observed in transplant recipients whose original disease was IgA nephropathy (29,152). Clinically, such recurrences are mild or even asymptomatic; despite this risk of recurrent glomerulonephritis, graft survival in patients with IgA nephropathy is considered good (29).

REFERENCES

1. Berger J, Hinglais N. [Intercapillary deposits of IgA-IgG]. *J Urol Nephrol (Paris)* 1968;74:694–695.
2. D'Amico G. The commonest glomerulonephritis in the world: IgA nephropathy. *QJM* 1987;64:709–727.
3. Emancipator SN, Gallo GR, Lamm ME. IgA nephropathy: perspective on pathogenesis and classification. *Clin Nephrol* 1985;24:161–179.
4. Yoshikawa N, Ito H, Yoshiara S, et al. Clinical course of IgA nephropathy in children. *J Pediatr* 1987;110:555–560.
5. Yoshikawa N, Iijima K, Maehara K, et al. Mesangial changes in IgA nephropathy in children. *Kidney Int* 1987;32:585–589.
6. Yoshikawa N, Iijima K, Matsuyama S, et al. Repeat renal biopsy in children with IgA nephropathy. *Clinical Nephrol* 1990;33:160–167.
7. Wyatt RJ, Kritchevsky SB, Woodford SY, et al. IgA nephropathy: long-term prognosis for pediatric patients. *J Pediatr* 1995;127:913–919.
8. Hogg RJ, Silva FG, Wyatt RJ, et al. Prognostic indicators in children with IgA nephropathy-report of the Southwest Pediatric Nephrology Study Group. *Pediatr Nephrol* 1994;8:15–20.
9. Rodicio JL. Idiopathic IgA nephropathy. *Kidney Int* 1984:25: 717–729.
10. Sehic AM, Gaber LW, Roy S 3rd, et al. Increased recognition of IgA nephropathy in African-American children. *Pediatr Nephrol* 1997;11:435–437.
11. Clarkson AR, Woodroffe AJ, Aarons I. IgA nephropathy and Henoch-Schönlein purpura. In: Schrier RW, Gottschalk CW, eds. *Diseases of the kidney*. Boston: Little, Brown and Company, 1996:1645–1670.
12. Suzuki S, Nakatomi Y, Sato H, et al. *Haemophilus parainfluenzae* antigen and antibody in renal biopsy samples and serum of patients with IgA nephropathy. *Lancet* 1994;343:12–16.
13. Ogura Y, Suzuki S, Shirakawa T, et al. *Haemophilus parainfluenzae* antigen and antibody in children with IgA nephropathy and Henoch-Schönlein nephritis. *Am J Kidney Dis* 2000;36:47–52.
14. Hsu SI, Ramirez SB, Winn MP, et al. Evidence for genetic factors in the development and progression of IgA nephropathy. *Kidney Int* 2000;57:1818–1835.
15. Rambausek MH, Waldherr R, Ritz E. Immunogenetic findings in glomerulonephritis. *Kidney Int* 1993;43:S3–S8.
16. Schmidt S, Ritz E. Genetic factors in IgA nephropathy. *Ann Med Interne (Paris)* 1999;150:86–90.
17. Julian BA, Quiggins PA, Thompson JS, et al. Familial IgA nephropathy. Evidence for an inherited mechanism of disease. *N Engl J Med* 1985;312:202–208.
18. Wyatt RJ, Rivas ML, Julian BA, et al. Regionalization in hereditary IgA nephropathy. *Am J Hum Genet* 1987;41:36–50.
19. Scolari F, Amoroso A, Savoldi S, et al. Familial clustering of IgA nephropathy: further evidence in an Italian population. *Am J Kidney Dis* 1999;33:857–865.
20. Gharavi AG, Yan Y, Scolari F, et al. IgA nephropathy, the most common cause of glomerulonephritis, is linked to 6q22-23. *Nat Genet* 2000;26:354–357.
21. Hsu SI, Ramirez SB, Winn MP, et al. Evidence for genetic factors in the development and progression of IgA nephropathy. *Kidney Int* 2000;57:1818–1835.
22. Shimomura M, Yoshikawa N, Iijima K, et al. Polymorphism of immunoglobulin heavy chain switch region gene in children with severe IgA nephropathy. *Clin Nephrol* 1995;43:211–215.
23. Yano N, Asakura K, Endoh M, et al. Polymorphism in the $I\alpha_1$ germ-line transcript regulatory region and IgA productivity in patients with IgA nephropathy. *J Immunol* 1998;160:4936–4942.
24. Tanaka R, Iijima K, Murakami R, et al. ACE gene polymorphism in childhood IgA nephropathy: association with clinicopathological findings. *Am J Kidney Dis* 1998;31:774–779.
25. Maruyama K, Yoshida M, Shirakawa T, et al. Polymorphisms of renin-angiotensin system genes and proteinuria in children with IgA nephropathy. *Pediatr Nephrol* 2001;16:350–355.
26. Tanaka R, Xu H, Iijima K, et al. Role of platelet-activating factor acetylhydrolase gene mutation in Japanese childhood immunoglobulin A nephropathy. *Am J Kidney Dis* 1999;34: 289–295.
27. Schena FP, D'Altri C, Cerullo G, et al. ACE gene polymorphism and IgA nephropathy: an ethnically homogeneous study and a meta-analysis. *Kidney Int* 2001;60:732–740.
28. Sakai H. Current views on pathogenesis and treatment. In: Andreucci VE, ed. *International year book of nephrology*. Boston: Kluwer Academic Publisher, 1989:23–46.
29. Andresdottir MB, Hoitsma AJ, Assmann KJ, et al. Favorable outcome of renal transplantation in patients with IgA nephropathy. *Clin Nephrol* 2001;56:279–288.
30. Yoshikawa N, Iijima K, Ito H. IgA nephropathy in children. *Nephron* 1999;83:1–12.

31. Yoshikawa N, Iijima K, Ito H. Pathophysiology and treatment of childhood IgA nephropathy. *Pediatr Nephrol* 2001;16:446–457.
32. Rifai A, Small P, Ayoub EM. Experimental IgA nephropathy. Factors governing the persistence of IgA-antigen complexes in the circulation of mice. *Contrib Nephrol* 1984;40:37–44.
33. Isaacs K, Miller F. Dextran-induced IgA nephropathy. *Contrib Nephrol* 1984;40:45–50.
34. Emancipator S, Gallo G, Lamm M. Experimental IgA nephropathy induced by oral immunization. *J Exp Med* 1983;157: 572–582.
35. Conley ME, Cooper MD, Michael AF. Selective deposition of IgA1 in IgA nephropathy, anaphylactoid purpura nephritis, and systemic lupus erythematosus. *J Clin Invest* 1980;66:1432–1436.
36. Komatsu N, Nagaura H, Watanabe K, et al. Mesangial deposition of J chain-linked polymeric IgA in IgA nephropathy. *Nephron* 1983;33:61–64.
37. Valentijin RM, Radl J, Haayman JJ, et al. Macromolecular IgA in the circulation and mesangial deposits in patients with primary IgA nephropathy. *Contrib Nephrol* 1984;40:87–92.
38. Monteiro RC, Habwachs-Mecarelli L, Berger J, et al. Characterization of eluted IgA in primary IgA nephropathy. *Contrib Nephrol* 1984;40:107–111.
39. Harper SJ, Pringle JH, Wicks AC, et al. Expression of J chain mRNA in duodenal IgA plasma cells in IgA nephropathy. *Kidney Int* 1994;45:836–844.
40. Harper SJ, Allen AC, et al. Increased dimeric IgA producing B cells in the bone marrow in IgA nephropathy determined by in situ hybridisation for J chain mRNA. *J Clin Pathol* 1996;49:38–42.
41. de Fijter JW, Eijgenraam JW, Braam CA, et al. Deficient IgA1 immune response to nasal cholera toxin B in primary IgA nephropathy. *Kidney Int* 1996;50:952–961.
42. White RHR, Yoshikawa N, Feehally J. IgA nephropathy and Henoch-Schönlein nephritis. In: Barratt TM, Avner ED, Harmon WE, eds. *Pediatric nephrology*, 4th ed. Baltimore: Lippincott Williams & Wilkins, 1999:691–706.
43. Rauterberg EW, Lieberknecht HM, Wingen AM, et al. Complement membrane attack (MAC) in idiopathic IgA-glomerulonephritis. *Kidney Int* 1987;31:820–829.
44. Julian BA, Wyatt RJ, McMorrow RG, et al. Serum complement proteins in IgA nephropathy. *Clin Nephrol* 1983;20:251–258.
45. Roos A, Bouwman LH, van Gijlswijk-Janssen DJ, et al. Human IgA activates the complement system via the mannan-binding lectin pathway. *J Immunol* 2001;167:2861–2868.
46. Abe K, Miyazaki M, Koji T, et al. Expression of decay accelerating factor mRNA and complement C3 mRNA in human diseased kidney. *Kidney Int* 1998;54:120–130.
47. Tomino Y, Endoh M, Nomoto Y, et al. Specificity of eluted antibody from renal tissue of patients with IgA nephropathy. *Am J Kid Dis* 1982;1:276–280.
48. Tomino Y, Sakai H, Endoh M, et al. Cross-reactivity of IgA antibodies between renal mesangial areas and nuclei of tonsillar cell in patients with IgA nephropathy. *Clin Exp Immunol* 1983;51:605–610.
49. Allen AC, Feehally J. IgA1 glycosylation and the pathogenesis of IgA nephropathy. *Am J Kidney Dis* 2000;35:551–556.
50. Kokubo T, Hiki Y, Iwase H, et al. Protective role of IgA1 glycans against IgA1 self-aggregation and adhesion to extracellular matrix proteins. *J Am Soc Nephrol* 1998;9:2048–2054.
51. Allen AC, Bailey EM, Brenchley PE, et al. Mesangial IgA1 in IgA nephropathy exhibits aberrant O-glycosylation: observations in three patients. *Kidney Int* 2001;60:969–973.
52. Tomana M, Matousovic K, Julian BA, et al. Galactose-deficient IgA1 in sera of IgA nephropathy patients is present in complexes with IgG. *Kidney Int* 1997;52:509–516.
53. Greer MR, Barratt J, Harper SJ, et al. The nucleotide sequence of the IgA1 hinge region in IgA nephropathy. *Nephrol Dial Transplant* 1998;13:1980–1983.
54. Allen AC, Topham PS, Harper SJ, et al. Leucocyte. β1,3 galactosyltransferase activity in IgA nephropathy. *Nephrol Dial Transplant* 1994;12:701–706.
55. Amado M, Almeida R, Carneiro F, et al. A family of human beta3-galactosyltransferases. Characterization of four members of a UDP-galactose:beta-N-acetyl-glucosamine/betanacetyl-galactosamine beta-1,3-galactosyltransferase family. *J Biol Chem* 1998;273:12770–12778.
56. Zhou D, Berger EG, Hennet T. Molecular cloning of a human UDP-galactose: G1cNAcbete 1, 3 GalNAc betal, 3 galactosyltransferase gene encoding an O-linked core-elongation enzyme. *Eur J Biochem* 1999;263:571–576.
57. Allen AC, Harper SJ, Feehally J. Galactosylation of N- and O-linked carbohydrate moieties of IgA1 and IgG in IgA nephropathy. *Clin Exp Immunol* 1995;100:470–474.
58. Allen AC, Topham PS, Harper SJ, et al. Leucocyte beta 1,3 galactosyltransferase activity in IgA nephropathy. *Nephrol Dial Transplant* 1997;12:701–706.
59. Allen AC, Bailey EM, Barratt J, et al. Analysis of IgA1 O-glycans in IgA nephropathy by fluorophore-assisted carbohydrate electrophoresis. *J Am Soc Nephrol* 1999;10:1763–1771.
60. Tomana M, Novak J, Julian BA, et al. Circulating immune complexes in IgA nephropathy consist of IgA1 with galactose-deficient hinge region and antiglycan antibodies. *J Clin Invest* 1999;104:73–81.
61. Sano T, Hiki Y, Kokubo T, et al. Enzymatically deglycosylated human IgA1 molecules accumulate and induce inflammatory cell reaction in rat glomeruli. *Nephrol Dial Transplant* 2002;17:50–56.
62. Amore A, Cirina P, Conti G, et al. Glycosylation of circulating IgA in patients with IgA nephropathy modulates proliferation and apoptosis of mesangial cells. *J Am Soc Nephrol* 2001;12:1862–1871.
63. Harper SJ, Allen AC, Pringle JH, et al. Increased dimeric lgA producing B cells in the bone marrow in lgA nephropathy determined by in situ hybridization for J chain mRNA. *J Clin Pathol* 1996;49:38–42.
64. Harper SJ, Allen AC, Bene MC, et al. Increased dimeric lgA-producing B cells in tonsils in IgA nephropathy determined by in situ hybridization for J chain mRNA. *Clin Exp Immunol* 1995;101:442–448.
65. Harper SJ, Allen AC, Bene MC, et al. Increased dimeric IgA-producing B cells in tonsils in IgA nephropathy determined by in situ hybridization for J chain mRNA. *Clin Exp Immunol* 1995;101:442–448.
66. Leung JC, Tang SC, Lam MF, et al. Charge-dependent binding of polymeric IgA1 to human mesangial cells in IgA nephropathy. *Kidney Int* 2001;59:277–285.

67. Sinico RA, Fornasieri A, Oreni N, et al. Polymeric IgA rheumatoid factor in idiopathic IgA mesangial nephropathy (Berger's disease). *J Immunol* 1986;137:536–541.
68. Nomoto Y, Suga T, Miura M, et al. Characterization of an acidic nuclear protein recognized by autoantibodies in sera from patients with IgA nephropathy. *Clin Exp Immunol* 1986;65:513–519.
69. Cederholm B, Wieslander J, Bygren P, et al. Patients with IgA nephropathy have circulating anti-basement membrane antibodies reacting with structures common to collagen I, II, and IV. *Proc Natl Acad Sci U S A* 1986;83:6151–6155.
70. O'Donoghue DJ, Feehally J. Autoantibodies in IgA nephropathy. *Contrib Nephrol* 1995;111:93–103.
71. Hall RP, Stachura I, Cason J, et al. IgA-containing circulating immune complexes in patients with IgA nephropathy. *Am J Med* 1983;74:56–63.
72. Iijima K, Yoshikawa N, Shiozawa S, et al. Immune abnormalities and clinical course in childhood IgA nephropathy. *Nephron* 1990;56:255–260.
73. Kameda A, Yoshikawa N, Shiozawa S, et al. Lymphocyte subpopulations and function in childhood IgA nephropathy. *Nephron* 1991;59:546–551.
74. Sakai H, Nomoto Y, Arimori S. Decrease of IgA-specific suppressor T cell activity in patients with IgA nephropathy. *Clin Exp Immunol* 1979;38:243–248.
75. Sakai H, Endoh M, Tomino Y, et al. Increase of IgA specific helper T cells in patients with IgA nephropathy. *Clin Exp Immunol* 1982;50:77–82.
76. Roccatello D, Picciotto G, Torchio M, et al. Removal systems of immunoglobulin A and immunoglobulin A containing complexes in IgA nephropathy and cirrhosis patients. The role of asialoglycoprotein receptors. *Lab Invest* 1993;69:714–723.
77. Allen AC, Barratt J, Feehally J. Immunoglobulin A nephropathy. In: Neilson EG, Couser WG, eds. *Immunologic renal diseases,* 2nd ed. Philadelphia: Lippincott Williams & Wilkins, 2001:931–947.
78. Stad RK, Bruijn JA, van Gijlswijk-Janssen DJ, et al. An acute model for lgA-mediated glomerular inflammation in rats induced by monoclonal polymeric rat lgA antibodies. *Clin Exp Immunol* 1993;92:514–521.
79. Niemir ZI, Stein H, Noronha IL, et al. PDGF and TGF-beta contribute to the natural course of human IgA glomerulonephritis. *Kidney Int* 1995;48:1530–1541.
80. Stein-Oakley AN, Maguire JA, Dowling J, et al. Altered expression of fibrogenic growth factors in IgA nephropathy and focal and segmental glomerulosclerosis. *Kidney Int* 1997;51:195–204.
81. Taniguchi Y, Yorioka N, Masaki T, et al. Localization of transforming growth factors beta1 and beta2 and epidermal growth factor in IgA nephropathy. *Scand J Urol Nephrol* 1999;33:243–247.
82. Yoshioka K, Takemura T, Murakami K, et al. Transforming growth factor-beta protein and mRNA in glomeruli in normal and diseased human kidneys. *Lab Invest* 1993;68:154–163.
83. Yoshioka K, Takemura T, Murakami K, et al. In situ expression of cytokines in IgA nephritis. *Kidney Int* 1993;44:825–833.
84. Iijima K, Yoshikawa N, Connolly DT, et al. Human mesangial cells and peripheral blood mononuclear cells produce vascular permeability factor. *Kidney Int* 1993;44:959–966.
85. Noguchi K, Yoshikawa N, Kariya-Ito S, et al. Activated mesangial cells produce vascular permeability factor in early-stage mesangial proliferative glomerulonephritis. *J Am Soc Nephrol* 1998;9:1815–1825.
86. Yoshikawa N, Ito H, Nakamura H. IgA nephropathy in children from Japan. *Child Nephrol Urol* 1989;9:191–199.
87. Miura M, Tomino Y, Yagame M, et al. Immunofluorescent studies on alpha-2 plasmin inhibitor in glomeruli from patients with IgA nephropathy. *Clin Exp Immunol* 1985;62:380–386.
88. Yoshikawa N, Ito H, Nakahara C, et al. Glomerular electron-dense deposits in childhood IgA nephropathy. *Virchows Arch* 1985;406:33–43.
89. D'Amico G, Minetti L, Ponticelli C, et al. Prognostic indicators in idiopathic IgA mesangial nephropathy. *QJM* 1986;59: 363–378.
90. Andreoli SP, Yum MN, Bergstein JM. IgA nephropathy in children: significance of glomerular basement membrane deposition of IgA. *Am J Nephrol* 1986;6:28–33.
91. Yoshikawa N, Ito H, Nakamura H. Prognostic factors in childhood IgA nephropathy. *Nephron* 1992;60:60–67.
92. Churg J, Bernstein J, Glassock RJ. In: *Renal disease: classification and atlas of glomerular diseases,* 2nd ed. Tokyo: Igaku-Shoin Medical Publishers, 1995:86–88.
93. Zimmerman SW, Burkholder PM. Immunoglobulin A nephropathy. *Arch Intern Med* 1975;135:1217–1223.
94. Hara M, Endo Y, Nihei H, et al. IgA nephropathy with subepithelial deposits. *Virchows Arch* 1980;386:249–263.
95. Suzuki J, Yoshikawa N, Nakamura H. A quantitative analysis of the mesangium in children with IgA nephropathy: sequential study. *J Pathol* 1990;161:57–64.
96. Nicholls KM, Fairley KF, Dowling JP, et al. The clinical course of mesangial IgA-associated nephropathy in adults. *QJM* 1984;210:227–250.
97. Andreoli SP, Yum MN, Bergstein JM. IgA nephropathy in children: significance of glomerular basement membrane deposition of IgA. *Am J Nephrol* 1986;6:28–33.
98. Yoshikawa N, Yoshiara S, Yoshiya K, et al. Lysis of the glomerular basement membrane in children with IgA nephropathy and Henoch-Schönlein nephritis. *J Pathol* 1986;142:253–257.
99. Droz D. Natural history of primary glomerulonephritis with mesangial deposits of IgA. *Contrib Nephrol* 1976;2:150–156.
100. Ibels LS, Gyory AZ. IgA nephropathy: analysis of the natural history, important factors in the progression of renal disease, and a review of the literature. *Medicine (Baltimore)* 1994;73: 79–102.
101. Hotta O, Furuta T, Chiba S, et al. Regression of IgA nephropathy: a repeat biopsy study. *Am J Kidney Dis* 2002;39:493–502.
102. Michalk D, Waldherr R, Seelig HP, et al. Idiopathic mesangial IgA-glomerulonephritis in childhood. *Eur J Pediatr* 1980;134:13–22.
103. Linné T, Aperia A, Broberger O, et al. Course of renal function in IgA glomerulonephritis in children and adolescents. *Acta Paediatr Scand* 1982;71:735–743.
104. Lévy M, Gonzalez-Buschard G, Broyer M, et al. Berger's disease in children. *Medicine* 1985;64:157–180.
105. Southwest Pediatric Nephrology Study Group. A multicenter study of IgA nephropathy in children: report of the Southwest Pediatric Nephrology Study Group. *Kidney Int* 1982;22:643–652.
106. Ueda Y, Sakai O, Yamagata M, et al. IgA glomerulonephritis in Japan. *Contrib Nephrol* 1977;4:36–47.

107. Nakamoto Y, Asano Y, Dohi K, et al. Primary IgA glomerulonephritis and Schönlein-Henoch purpura nephritis: clinicopathological and immunohistological characteristics. *QJM* 1978;47:495–516.
108. Silva FG, Hogg RJ. IgA nephropathy. In: Tisher CC, Brenner BM, eds. *Renal pathology: with clinical and functional correlations*. Philadelphia: Lippincott, 1989:434–493.
109. Abuelo JG, Esparza AR, Matarese RA, et al. Crescentic IgA nephropathy. *Medicine (Baltimore)* 1984;63:396–406.
110. Davin JC, Ten Berge IJ, Weening JJ. What is the difference between IgA nephropathy and Henoch-Schönlein purpura nephritis? *Kidney Int* 2001;59:823–834.
111. Habib R, Niaudet P, Levy M. Schönlein-Henoch purpura nephritis and IgA nephropathy. In: Tisher C, Brenner B, eds. *Renal pathology: with clinical and functional correlations*, 2nd ed. Philadelphia: JB Lippincott Co, 1994:472–523.
112. Yoshikawa N, Nakanishi K, Iijima K. Henoch-Schönlein purpura. In: Neilson Eg, Couser WG, eds. *Immunologic renal diseases*, 2nd ed. Philadelphia: Lippincott Williams & Wilkins, 2001:1127–1140.
113. Levy M. Do genetic factors play a role in Berger's disease? *Pediatr Nephrol* 1987;1:447–454.
114. Montoliu J, Lens XM, Torras A, et al. Henoch-Schönlein purpura and IgA nephropathy in father and son. *Nephron* 1990;54:77–79.
115. Meadow SR, Scott DG. Berger disease: Henoch-Schönlein syndrome without the rash. *J Pediatr* 1985;106:27–32.
116. Araque A, Sanchez R, Alamo C, et al. Evolution of immunoglobulin A nephropathy into Henoch-Schönlein purpura. *Am J Kidney Dis* 1995;25:340–342.
117. Silverstein DM, Greifer I, Folkert V, et al. Sequential occurrence of IgA nephropathy and Henoch-Schönlein purpura: support for common pathogenesis. *Pediatr Nephrol* 1994;8: 752–752.
118. Weiss JH, Bhathena DB, Curtis JJ, et al. A possible relationship between Henoch-Schönlein syndrome and IgA nephropathy (Berger's disease): an illustrative case. *Nephron* 1978;22:582–591.
119. Yoshikawa N, Ito H, Yoshiya K, et al. Henoch-Schönlein nephritis and IgA nephropathy: a comparison of clinical course. *Clin Nephrol* 1987;27:233–237.
120. Manigand G, Morel-Maroger L, Simon J, et al. Lésions rénales glomérulaires et cirrhose du foie: note préliminaire sur les lésions histologiques de rein au cours des cirrhoses hépatiques, d'apres 20 prélevements biopsiques. *Rev Eur Etud Clin Biol* 1970;15:989–996.
121. Pouria S, Feehally J. Glomerular IgA deposition in liver disease. *Nephrol Dial Transplant* 1999;14:2279–2282.
122. Kalsi J, Delacroix DL, Hodgson HJF. IgA in alcoholic cirrhosis. *Clin Exp Immunol* 1983;52:499–504.
123. Sancho J, Egido J, Sanchez-Crespo M, et al. Detection of monomeric and polymeric IgA containing immune complexes in serum and kidney from patients with alcoholic liver disease. *Clin Exp Immunol* 1981;47:327–335.
124. Habib R, Girardin E, Gagnadoux MF, et al. Immunopathological findings in idiopathic nephrosis: clinical significance of glomerular "immune deposits." *Pediatr Nephrol* 1988;2:402–408.
125. D'Amico G, Imbasciati E, Barbiano di Belgioioso G, et al. Idiopathic IgA mesangial nephropathy: clinical and histological study of 374 patients. *Medicine* 1985;64:49–60.
126. Droz D, Kramar A, Nawar T, et al. Primary IgA nephropathy: prognostic factors. *Contrib Nephrol* 1984;40:202–207.
127. D'Amico G. Natural history of idiopathic IgA nephropathy: role of clinical and histological prognostic factors. *Am J Kidney Dis* 2000;36:227–237.
128. Glassock RJ, Adler SG, Ward HJ, et al. Primary glomerular diseases. In: Brenner BM, Rector FC Jr, eds. *The kidney*. Philadelphia: Saunders, 1991:1182–1279.
129. Hood SA, Velosa JA, Holley KE, et al. IgA-IgG nephropathy: predictive indices of progressive disease. *Clin Nephrol* 1981;16:55–62.
130. Kobayashi Y, Tateno S, Hiki Y, et al. IgA nephropathy: prognostic significance of proteinuria and histologic alterations. *Nephron* 1983;34:146–153.
131. Katz A, Walker JK, Landy PJ. IgA nephritis with nephrotic range proteinuria. *Clin Nephrol* 1983;20:67–71.
132. Chida Y, Tomura S, Takeuchi J. Renal survival rate of IgA nephropathy. *Nephron* 1985;40:189–194.
133. Neelakantappa K, Gallo GR, Baldwin DS. Proteinuria in IgA nephropathy. *Kidney Int* 1988;33:716–721.
134. Bartosik LP, Lajoie G, Sugar L, et al. Predicting progression in IgA nephropathy. *Am J Kidney Dis* 2001;38:728–735.
135. Levy M, Gonzalez-Buschard G, Broyer M, et al. Berger's disease in children. *Medicine* 1985;64:157–180.
136. Hattori S, Karashima S, Furuse A, et al. Clinicopathological correlation of IgA nephropathy in children. *Am J Nephrol* 1985;5:182–189.
137. Andreoli SP, Yum MN, Bergstein JM. IgA nephropathy in children: significance of glomerular basement membrane deposition of IgA. *Am J Nephrol* 1986;6:28–33.
138. Hogg RJ. Prognostic indicators and treatment of childhood IgA nephropathy. *Contrib Nephrol* 1995;111:194–200.
139. Schena FP, Cerullo G, Rossini M, et al. Increased risk of end-stage renal disease in familial IgA nephropathy. *J Am Soc Nephrol* 2002;13:453–460.
140. Haas M. Histologic subclassification of IgA nephropathy: a clinicopathologic study of 244 cases. *Am J Kidney Dis* 1997;29: 829–842.
141. Nicholls KM, Fairley KF, Dowling JP, et al. The clinical course of mesangial IgA-associated nephropathy in adults. *QJM* 1984;210:227–250.
142. Wyatt RJ, Hogg RJ. Evidence-based assessment of treatment options for children with IgA nephropathies. *Pediatr Nephrol* 2001;16:156–167.
143. Donadio JJ, Bergstralh EJ, Offord KP, et al. A controlled trial of fish oil in IgA nephropathy. Mayo Nephrology Collaborative Group. *N Engl J Med* 1994;331:1194–1199.
144. Donadio JV Jr, Grande JP, Bergstralh EJ, et al. The long-term outcome of patients with IgA nephropathy treated with fish oil in a controlled trial. Mayo Nephrology Collaborative Group. *J Am Soc Nephrol* 1999;10:1772–1777.
145. Donadio JV Jr, Larson TS, Bergstralh EJ, et al. A randomized trial of high-dose compared with low-dose omega-3 fatty acids in severe IgA nephropathy. *J Am Soc Nephrol* 2001;12:846–847.
146. Dillon JJ. Fish oil therapy for IgA nephropathy: efficacy and interstudy variability. *J Am Soc Nephrol* 1997;8:1739–1744.
147. Yoshida H, Mitarai T, Kawamura T, et al. Role of the deletion polymorphism of the angiotensin converting enzyme

gene in the progression and therapeutic responsiveness of IgA nephropathy. *J Clin Invest* 1995;96:2162–2169.
148. Perico N, Remmuzzi A, Sangalli F, et al. The antiproteinuric effect of angiotensin antagonism in human IgA nephropathy is potentiated by indomethacin. *J Am Soc Nephrol* 1998;9:2308–2317.
149. Pozzi C, Bolasco PG, Foggazzi GB, et al. Corticosteroids in IgA nephropathy: a randomised controlled trial. *Lancet* 1999;353:883–887.
150. Schlöndorff D, Dendorfer U, Brumberger V, et al. Limitations of therapeutic approaches to glomerular diseases. *Kidney Int* 1995;48(Suppl):19–25.
151. Yoshikawa N, Ito H, Sakai T, et al. A controlled trial of combined therapy for newly diagnosed severe childhood IgA nephropathy. *J Am Soc Nephrol* 1999;10:101–109.
152. Odum J, Peh CA, Clarkson AR, et al. Recurrent mesangial IgA nephritis following renal transplantation. *Nephrol Dial Transplant* 1994;9:309–312.

32

MEMBRANOPROLIFERATIVE GLOMERULONEPHRITIS

C. FREDERIC STRIFE
MICHAEL C. BRAUN
CLARK D. WEST

Membranoproliferative glomerulonephritis (MPGN) is characterized on histology by glomerular hypercellularity, increased mesangial matrix, thickening of the peripheral capillary walls, and a splitting of the glomerular basement membranes (GBMs) due to mesangial interposition in the capillary walls. The term *MPGN* was originally used by Habib et al. (1) in 1961 to describe the glomeruli in a group of patients with chronic nephritis. In 1965, this appearance was associated with hypocomplementemia (2). In 1973, a second chronic nephritis, originally called *dense deposit disease* by Berger and Galle (3), was classified as a variant of MPGN (4) and later designated *MPGN type II.* The more common type, in which subendothelial deposits predominate, was designated *type I.* The term *mesangiocapillary glomerulonephritis* has been used interchangeably with *membranoproliferative glomerulonephritis.* A nephritis morphologically similar to type I found in patients with chronic antigenemia or malignancies makes necessary the additional classification of secondary as opposed to idiopathic MPGN (Table 32.1). In the 1970s, several observers using silver-impregnated electron micrographs described a third type of MPGN with ultrastructural features distinct from MPGN types I or II (5–7). In MPGN type III, complex alterations of the GBM are revealed by the silver stain, together with deposits that are subendothelial and subepithelial as well as within the GBM. Although certain aspects of MPGN types I and III are similar, the clinical and morphologic differences between the two make their separation feasible. Because this distinction is not universally accepted, this chapter considers MPGN types I and III together, whereas type II is discussed separately.

MEMBRANOPROLIFERATIVE GLOMERULONEPHRITIS TYPES I AND III

Epidemiology and Genetics

The incidence of MPGN is difficult to ascertain; however, it is roughly estimated that there are one to two cases per 10^6 pediatric patients (8). In most series, MPGN type I has been found to be the most common form (Table 32.2). In those studies that distinguished MPGN type I and type III, the relative frequency of type III ranges from 14 to 37% (9–12) (Table 32.2). In our experience, type III is at least as common as type I (11). MPGN types I and III usually present in older children or adolescents. Occasionally, they have been observed in patients older than 30 years or younger than 5 years. The prevalence of MPGN type I has decreased in most series from 15 to 20% of primary glomerulonephritides in the 1970s to less than 5%.

Support for a genetic susceptibility for both MPGN types I and III was provided by the observation that an extended haplotype, B8,DR3,SC01,GLO2 is significantly more frequent in patients with these two types than in the general white population (13). Also, patients with MPGN types I and III have a similarly high frequency of inherited complement deficiencies (14). Finally, there are a number of reports of familial clustering of MPGN type I (15–19). Reports of familial type III are rare (20). Recently, however, an Irish family with eight affected members in four generations was reported. Significant evidence for linkage was observed on chromosome 1q31-32 (21).

Presentation and Clinical Manifestations

The presentation of MPGN generally falls into three categories: nephrotic syndrome, acute nephritic syndrome, or asymptomatic hematuria and proteinuria discovered by chance (Table 32.3). The specific MPGN type cannot be distinguished by the presenting clinical features because of extensive overlap (22).

Nephrotic Syndrome

Edema as the presenting symptom is present in approximately one-third of patients with either MPGN type I or

TABLE 32.1. CLASSIFICATION OF MEMBRANO–PROLIFERATIVE GLOMERULONEPHRITIS (MPGN)

MPGN type I
- Primary or idiopathic
- Secondary/chronic infections
  - Bacterial: endocarditis, visceral abscesses, infected ventricular shunts, osteomyelitis
  - Viral: hepatitis B and C, human immunodeficiency virus
  - Protozoal: malaria, schistosomiasis
  - Other: mycoplasma, fungal
- Immunologic (autoimmune) diseases
  - Systemic lupus erythematosus glomerulonephritis
  - Chronic active hepatitis
- Paraprotein deposition diseases
  - Cryoglobulinemia
  - Light chain disease
- Neoplastic
  - Leukemia or lymphoma
  - Neuroblastoma

MPGN type II
- Idiopathic
- Associated with partial lipodystrophy

MPGN type III
- Idiopathic

III (Table 32.3). These patients have significant proteinuria and usually microscopic hematuria with red cell and granular casts. Serum concentrations of albumin and immunoglobulin (Ig) G are typically low, and approximately 70 to 80% have a low serum C3 level. In the absence of effective treatment, a nephrotic syndrome is strongly associated with a poor prognosis.

Acute Nephritic Syndrome

Gross hematuria with an acute nephritic syndrome is the presenting feature in approximately 25% of patients with MPGN. Mild hypoalbuminemia is common. Although renal function is usually normal, a rare patient may have a rapidly progressive course. Such patients usually have a low serum level of C3, making distinction from acute poststreptococcal glomerulonephritis difficult. A biopsy is often not performed until it is apparent that the return of C3 concentration to a normal level is not occurring, as is typical for resolving acute poststreptococcal glomerulonephritis.

TABLE 32.2. RELATIVE FREQUENCY OF MEMBRANOPROLIFERATIVE GLOMERULONEPHRITIS BY TYPE

Series	Type I (%)	Type II (%)	Type III (%)	No. of patients
Iitaka (9)	78	5	17	41
ISKDC (10)	58	19	23	73
Braun (11)	36	23	41	78
Schwertz (12)	52	34	14	50
Totals	53	21	26	242

ISKDC, International Study of Kidney Disease in Children.

TABLE 32.3. CLINICAL PRESENTATION OF MEMBRANOPROLIFERATIVE GLOMERULONEPHRITIS TYPES I AND III

	Type I (%)	Type III (%)
Clinical presentation[a]		
Edema	19	32
Gross hematuria	28	24
Asymptomatic microhematuria or proteinuria	22	65
Additional common features at presentation		
Symptoms of systemic disease	26	0
Hypertension	60	21
Low serum C3	68	86
Acute infection before presentation	33	26

[a]Patients may present with more than one clinical feature.

Asymptomatic Microhematuria and Proteinuria

The diagnosis of MPGN is made in approximately 50% of patients because of the chance discovery of hematuria and proteinuria in the otherwise healthy child. This presentation is most common in MPGN type III patients (22). Renal function and serum albumin levels are usually normal.

Associated Clinical Features

Braun et al. (11) observed that glomerular filtration rate estimated from serum creatinine is lower at presentation in patients with MPGN type I when compared to those with MPGN type III. They speculated that the relatively greater glomerular proliferation in MPGN type I is likely related to the lower glomerular filtration rate. The higher frequency of hypertension at presentation in patients with MPGN type I may also relate to the greater degree of glomerular proliferation. Encephalopathy due to hypertension is rare at presentation but has been reported during follow-up in both treated and untreated patients (10). Antecedent constitutional complaints, including fatigue, lassitude, and weight loss, characterize the onset in approximately 25% of patients with MPGN type I but are not observed in those with MPGN type III (22). Table 32.3 lists these clinical features.

Laboratory Abnormalities

An occasional patient, especially with MPGN type I, has a normochromic, normocytic anemia out of proportion to the degree of renal insufficiency. However, the distinctive feature of the three MPGN types is hypocomplementemia (Fig. 32.1), caused in many by the presence of autoantibodies, called *nephritic factors* (NFs), directed at epitopes on comple-

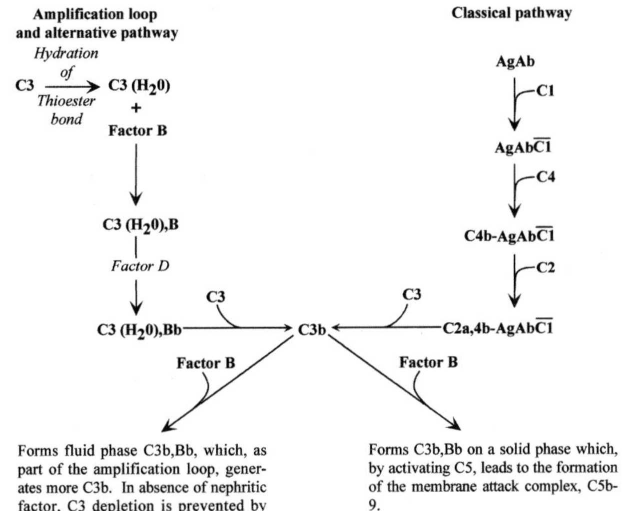

FIGURE 32.1. Activation of either the classical or alternative complement pathways produces activated C3, C3b, which can form fluid-phase or solid-phase C3b,Bb (convertase). Normally, both fluid-phase and solid-phase C3b,Bb are rapidly inactivated by complement control proteins. Both can be stabilized by the nephritic factor (see Fig. 32.2). C3b,Bb stabilized on a solid phase can activate C5 and form the membrane attack complex, C5-9. (Courtesy of John Bissler, M.D.)

ment proteins (Fig. 32.2). The serum C3 concentration is low in nearly 80% at their initial evaluation. In all, three mechanisms are believed to be responsible for the hypocomplementemia: circulating immune complexes activating the classical complement pathway, NFs that interfere with the normal control of the complement cascade, and inhibition of C3 synthesis mediated by circulating C3 breakdown products. A rare patient with hypocomplementemia as a result of a defect in the regulatory proteins of the complement system has an MPGN-like glomerulonephritis (23).

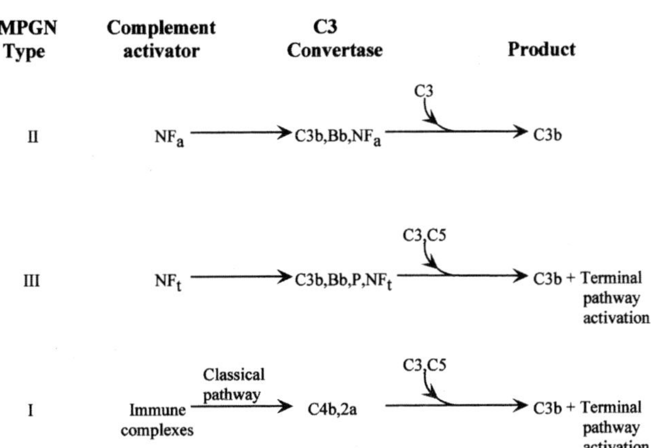

FIGURE 32.2. Fluid-phase activation of C3 in membranoproliferative glomerulonephritis (MPGN). In MPGN type II, the convertase stabilized by nephritic factor-a (NF_a) activates only C3. The convertase produced in type I by immune complexes and the nephritic factor complex produced in type III can form a C3,C5 convertase that activates both C3 and terminal components. This results in low C3 levels in type II, low C3 and C5 levels in type I, and low C3,C5, and terminal component levels in type III. On a solid phase such as the renal glomerulus, it is possible that in type I, a C3,C5 convertase is deposited and nephritogenesis is the result. Solid-phase events that are nephritogenic in types II and III are not clear. NF_t, nephritic factor of the terminal pathway; P, properdin. (Courtesy of John Bissler, M.D.)

Of patients with MPGN type I, approximately 40% of those with a low serum C3 level have in addition a low serum level of C4, suggesting classical complement pathway activation (Fig. 32.2) (22). A few also have low serum levels of C1q and C2, but these complement components may be low as a result of heavy proteinuria (24).

The complement perturbation in MPGN type III is distinct from that in both types I and II; C4 levels are typically normal, and severely hypocomplementemic patients (C3 less than or equal to 30 mg/dL) commonly have depressed levels of C5 and properdin and of one or more of the other terminal components, C6, C7, and C9 (25–27). Depression of the latter components is seen in only 10% of those with type I and is not seen in type II. The NF in MPGN type III is presumably responsible for the low levels of terminal components (Fig. 32.2). Known as the *NF of the terminal pathway* (NF_t), it differs from that found in type II in that *in vitro* it converts C3 slowly with maximum conversion in 4 hours rather than 30 minutes. The conversion is properdin dependent and activates terminal components (28). It is believed to stabilize a convertase with the composition $(C3b,Bb)_n$,P,NF_t. It is composed of properdin (P) and several convertase (C3b,Bb) complexes, which serve to activate C5.

Pathology

Glomeruli in MPGN type I by light microscopy (Fig. 32.3) usually have a uniform increase in cellularity due to an influx of leukocytes and mesangial proliferation. The mesangial proliferation causes glomerular enlargement and marked reduction in the number of open capillary lumens. With silver stain, capillary walls may show a double contour called *tram-tracking*. This is the result of new basement membrane formation at the site of mesangial interposition. With progression, the mesangial proliferation may become replaced by centrolobular hyalinization, giving the glomeruli a progressively more lobular appearance. In MPGN type III, the degree of mesangial proliferation is typically less in comparison to type I and often focal in distribution (Fig. 32.3). Glomerular size is usually normal. Double contoured capillary walls are rare, due to less mesangial interposition. These differences, however, cannot reliably distinguish MPGN type I from type III by light microscopy.

Immunofluorescent microscopy (29) usually can distinguish type I from types II or III (Table 32.4) in that C4 is usually present in type I; C3, C4, and IgG colocalize on the periphery of the glomerular lobules, the so-called fringe pattern (Fig. 32.4). In MPGN type III, C3 deposition is typically in a mesangial and capillary loop pattern, C4 is

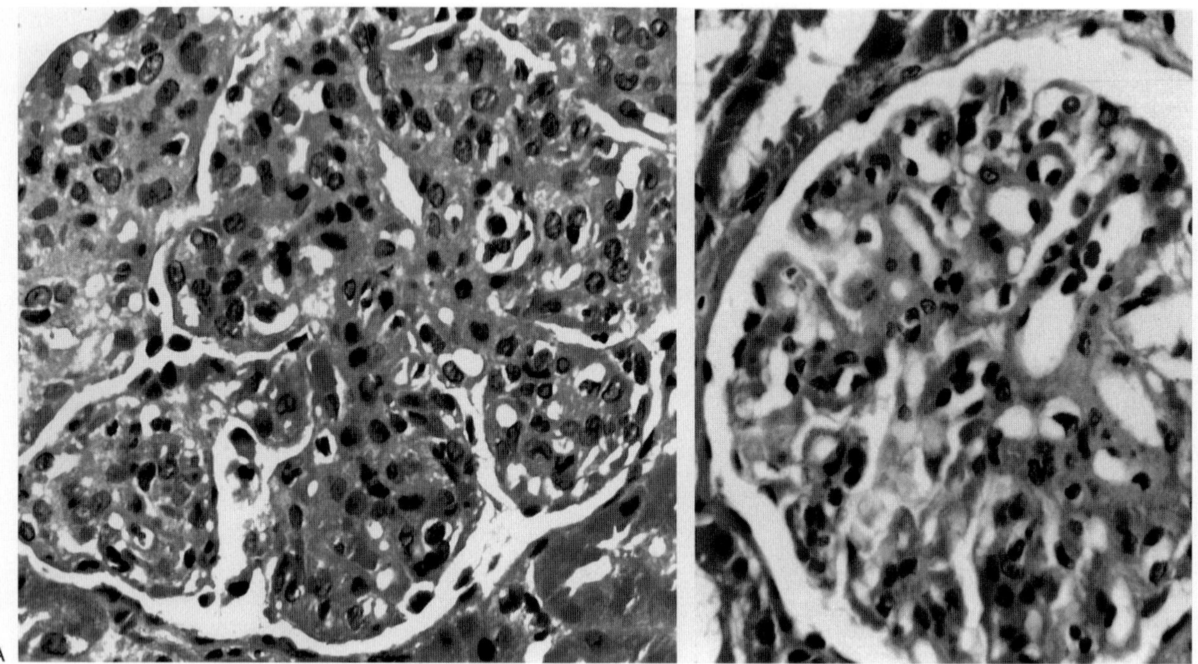

FIGURE 32.3. Light microscopic appearance of membranoproliferative glomerulonephritis (MPGN) types I and II. **A:** The glomerulus is enlarged, very cellular, and has a lobulated appearance. The mesangium is markedly expanded. The capillary walls are thickened in appearance, and, frequently, the capillary lumens are obscured by the mesangial expansion. In addition to the increase in mesangial cells, scattered neutrophils are also identified in many of the segments. **B:** The type III glomerulus is less cellular in appearance, and there is less expansion of the mesangium. Most of the capillary loops are patent; however, thickened capillary walls are evident. (Courtesy of Dr. David Witte.) (See Color Plate 32.3.)

rarely present, and IgG is present in small amounts in approximately 50% of cases (22).

Ultrastructural studies are essential to distinguish MPGN type I from type III (Table 32.5). In MPGN type I, uranyl-lead–stained micrographs typically demonstrate a completely intact GBM without breaks or laminations (Fig. 32.5). There is prominent mesangial proliferation with extension of the mesangium at least partially around the glomerular capillaries (interposition), which, with the subendothelial deposits, causes narrowing of the capillary lumen.

In MPGN type III, uranyl-lead stains typically demonstrate a complex thickening and irregularity of the GBM. However, the type III lesion—characterized by a discontinuous fragmented, laminated appearance of the GBM (Table 32.5)—is best seen with methenamine silver stains (Fig. 32.5). The distribution of deposits in this lesion has been shown to vary according to the C3 level at the time of the biopsy (Table 32.5).

Pathogenesis

Idiopathic MPGN type I is presumed to be secondary to circulating immune complexes composed of IgG (antibody)–unknown antigen–C3, which deposit in the subendothelial glomerular space, giving rise to a response that includes marked mesangial proliferation. Evidence for this hypothesis is based on the observation that indistinguishable renal pathology is present in glomerulonephritis secondary to identified infectious, oncogenic, and other antigens (Table 32.1). In addition, the pattern of complement activation is via the classical complement pathway in at least 40% of patients, favoring the presence of circulating immune complexes.

Little is known regarding the pathogenesis of MPGN type III. Normal serum C4 levels and the absence C4 in glomeruli suggest that immune complex formation does not play a major pathogenic role. West and associates have

TABLE 32.4. COMPARISON OF IMMUNOFLUORESCENT MICROSCOPY IN MEMBRANOPROLIFERATIVE GLOMERULONEPHRITIS TYPES I AND III

	C4 (%)	C3 (%)	C5 (%)	Immunoglobulin G (%)
Type I	75	100	100	100
Type III	0	100	100	50

Adapted from Wyatt RJ, McAdams AJ, Forristal J, et al. Glomerular deposition of complement-control proteins in acute and chronic glomerulonephritis. *Kidney Int* 1979;16:505–512.

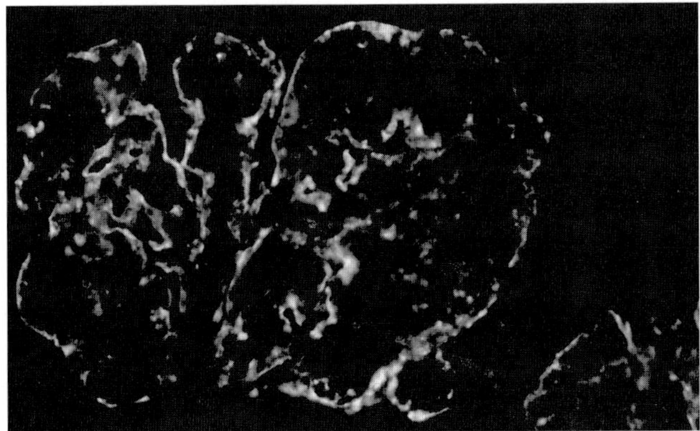

FIGURE 32.4. Immunofluorescence appearance of membranoproliferative glomerulonephritis type I. The prominent peripheral distribution of immunoglobulin G deposits in the capillary walls results in a fringe pattern. (Courtesy of Dr. David Witte.) (See Color Plate 32.4.)

reported a strong association between hypocomplementemia and the presence of paramesangial and subendothelial deposits (30,31). Subendothelial deposits, in particular, were never found in patients normocomplementemic at biopsy (Table 32.5). They suggest that NF_t may play a significant role in the development and perpetuation of the ultrastructural changes that define MPGN type III. Although this is a provocative and intriguing hypothesis, these findings must clearly be reconciled with other reports that have failed to demonstrate any relationship between the presence of NF, the duration or severity of hypocomplementemia, and either renal survival or disease progression in MPGN type III (11,32).

Natural History

The natural history of MPGN was described in detail by Cameron et al. (33) in a report comparing the long-term outcome of 69 children and adults with MPGN type I (type III, presumably, was included in this group) to 35 with type II (Fig. 32.6). The outcome was poor irrespective of type, with 50% losing renal function by 10 years and 90% by 20 years. Similar results have been observed by Habib et al. (4). Cameron et al. (33) noted that MPGN type I progressed more slowly in children than in adults during the first 10 years of follow-up. There are no reports that compare the courses of MPGN types I and III in the absence of effective treatment. Outcome has been shown to be adversely affected by the presence of nephrotic syndrome or renal insufficiency at onset and by the presence of crescents in the initial biopsy.

Treatment

The effectiveness of treatment regimens for MPGN has to be judged by the outcome of usually uncontrolled, retrospective observations on small numbers of patients. In several series, the basic regimen has been supplemented in some patients by other treatment modalities. Despite these shortcomings, some consensus has emerged.

Steroids

The treatment regimens that appear to improve outcome in patients with MPGN types I and III have used steroids. The Cincinnati group (11,34–36) has used high-dose (2 mg/kg to a maximum of 80 mg) alternate-day prednisone

TABLE 32.5. DIFFERENCES IN GLOMERULAR ULTRASTRUCTURE IN TYPE I AND TYPE III MEMBRANOPROLIFERATIVE GLOMERULONEPHRITIS AS VIEWED IN URANYL-LEAD– AND METHENAMINE-SILVER–STAINED PREPARATIONS

	Type I	Type III
Uranyl-lead staining		
Basement membrane	*Intact*	Thickened areas with patchy dense deposits
Methenamine-silver staining		
Basement membrane	*Intact*	*Type III lesion*[a] present with both ↓ [C3] and nl [C3]
Uranyl-lead and methenamine-silver staining		
Subendothelial deposits	*Always present with ↓ [C3]* *Present in 50% with nl [C3]*	*Present in 50% with ↓ [C3]* *Never present with nl [C3]*
Subepithelial paramesangial deposits	*Very rare; never with nl [C3]; in ~12% with ↓ [C3]*	*Present with ↓ [C3] and in those with nl [C3] if level has been low in past year*
Subepithelial loop deposits	Frequent, accompany subendothelial deposits	May be present; not clearly related to [C3]

↓ [C3], serum C3 level low at time of biopsy; nl [C3], serum C3 level normal at the time of biopsy.
Note: Correlations of deposits with serum C3 levels are taken from references (3) and (31). Italics indicate key features differentiating types I and III.
[a]Type III lesion is a complex lesion of the GBM that appears to originate from several generations of subepithelial and subendothelial deposits forming in conjunction with multiple interruptions of the lamina densa such that the deposits are partially confluent. Lesions develop a complex laminated appearance because each generation of deposit is covered by new lamina densa–like material.
From Braun MC, West CD, Strife CF. Differences between membranoproliferative glomerulonephritis types I and III in long-term response to an alternate-day prednisone regimen. *Am J Kidney Dis* 1999;34:1022–1032, with permission.

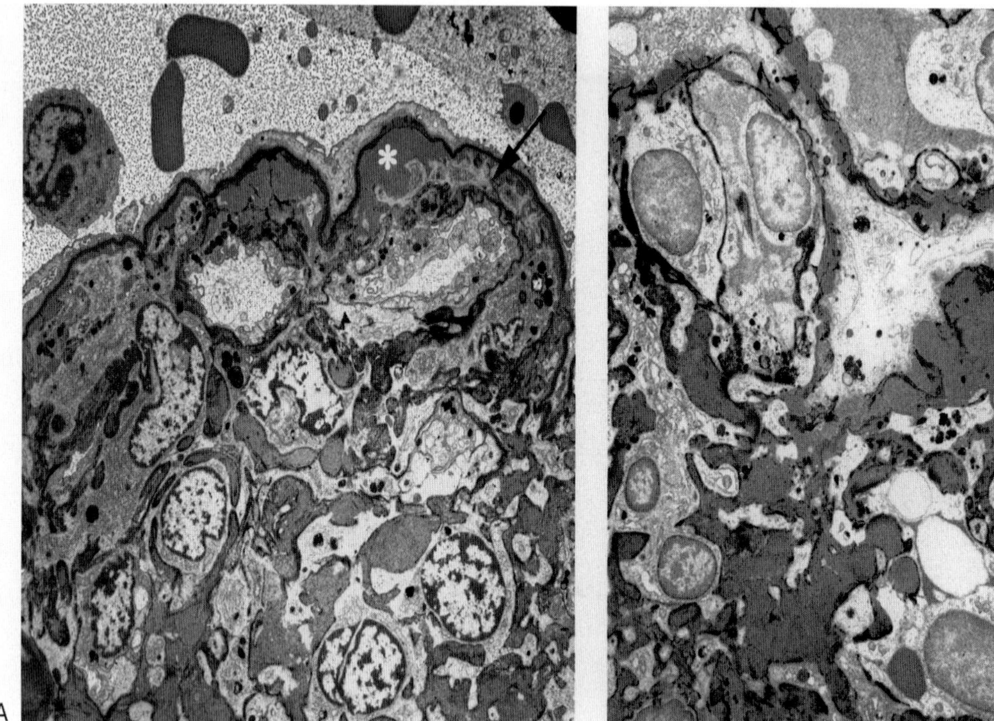

FIGURE 32.5. Ultrastructural features of membranoproliferative glomerulonephritis types I and II. **A:** An electron photomicrograph of a glomerulus with membranoproliferative glomerulonephritis type I. Note the prominent mesangial proliferation and deposits in the mesangium. The capillary walls are thickened due to extensive interposition (*arrow*) in addition to prominent subendothelial deposits (*asterisk*). In this silver-stained preparation, the lamina densa can be clearly identified and is generally intact. **B:** The glomerulus with the type III lesion also shows by silver stain extensive mesangial proliferation and deposits. The capillary walls show extensive disruptions of the lamina densa, with deposits that are subepithelial and subendothelial and, at times, completely obscure the lamina densa. (Courtesy of Dr. David Witte.)

for a minimum of 2 years. Dose reduction thereafter is based on improvement of clinical parameters (e.g., urinalysis, serum albumin, serum C3 level) and glomerular morphology (e.g., degree of mesangial proliferation, number of open capillary lumens). In the long term, prednisone dose is slowly reduced if there is no evidence of disease reactivation (e.g., increase in proteinuria or hematuria or decrease in serum C3 level). Because many, if not most, patients continue with at least some degree of proteinuria as a result of chronic glomerular damage, loss of microhematuria appears to be the best clinical indicator of disease remission (35). Most patients have continued on alternate-day steroids for at least 5 years and many for much longer periods.

Reports of outcome with this regimen have been encouraging but continue to be difficult to interpret because of small patient numbers, retrospective analysis of data, lack of a control group, and use in some patients of adjunctive therapies. Kidney survival at 10 years was 84% and, at 20 years, was 54%. In the most recent report (11) using the same alternate-day prednisone regimen, renal survival was 80% at 10 years in those with type I and 70% in those with type III. In addition to a lower renal survival, those with type III had, at 10 years, a significantly greater frequency of proteinuria and hematuria and a lower glomerular filtration rate.

Based on early reports of improved outcome with alternate-day prednisone, the International Study of Kidney Disease in Children sponsored a randomized, double-blind, placebo-controlled 5-year trial of alternate-day prednisone, 40 mg/m^2 versus placebo in 80 children with MPGN and heavy proteinuria (10). The study included 42 patients with MPGN type I and 17 with type III. Treatment failure was defined as an increase in serum creatinine of either greater than or equal to 30% over baseline or greater than 0.4 mg/dL. Outcome analysis evaluating patients with MPGN types I and III as a group showed that at last follow-up (mean 5.25 years), 33% of patients treated with prednisone and 58% in the placebo group were treatment failures (p = .07). The results favored treatment with prednisone.

Similar results were obtained by Mota-Hernandez et al. (37), who treated eight MPGN type I patients with alternate-day prednisone and ten with placebo. After an average follow-up of 6 years, treated patients had stable or improved renal function, whereas four of ten placebo-treated patients had progressed to end-stage renal disease.

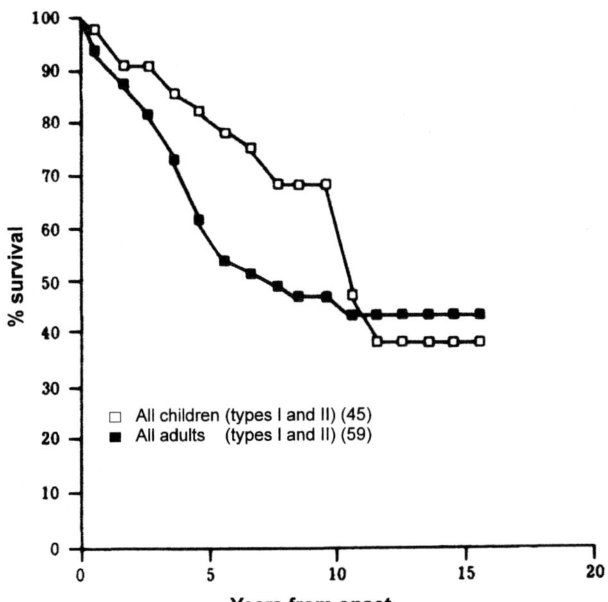

FIGURE 32.6. Comparison of renal survival between adults and children. (From Cameron JS, Turner DR, Heaton J, et al. Idiopathic mesangiocapillary glomerulonephritis. Comparison of types I and II in children and adults and long-term prognosis. *Am J Med* 1983;74:175–192, with permission.)

Additional uncontrolled reports have favored the use of alternate-day prednisone (9,38–40). The observation that, in the absence of treatment, the disease in patients not nephrotic at presentation progresses more slowly (4,33) has led to the recommendation that steroids be withheld in these patients (41) or used in a low dose (39,40). However, others have shown significantly better outcomes in patients treated with prednisone early in the course of the disease regardless of severity (9,35).

Long-term follow-up data on patients with MPGN type III have recently been published by a number of centers (11,12,42). The data should be viewed with caution, as less than 50% of the patients initially studied were available for long-term follow-up, and the numbers of patients studied were small. The report by Iitaka et al. (42) is by far the most promising, with 100% renal survival after 16 years of follow-up. However, it is uncertain if the universally good outcome was due to early identification and aggressive therapy or to an unknown factor that moderates the course of the disease in the Japanese population. Finally, the outcome reported by Braun et al. (11) and by Schwertz et al. (12) is less encouraging, with 70% renal survival at 10 years and 50% renal survival at 15 years, respectively.

Other Therapies

Other controlled prospective therapy trials have shown no long-term benefits with the antiplatelet agent dipyridamole (43) or with cyclophosphamide, warfarin, and dipyridamole (44). Uncontrolled reports have suggested no or limited benefit from treatment with other cytotoxic agents, antimalarials, or anticoagulants.

Disease Recurrence in Renal Transplant Recipients

The rate of recurrence in type I MPGN ranges between 20 and 30% (48). Patients with recurrence may remain asymptomatic or develop proteinuria or hematuria. Hypocomplementemia is inconstant. According to Briganti et al., the incidence of graft loss at 10 years due to recurrence is 15% (49). No therapy has been proven to be effective. The role of cyclosporine is uncertain, as some authors have found that the rate of recurrence had decreased from 30 to 10% after the introduction of cyclosporine, whereas other authors did not find any changes. Case reports have suggested that graft survival may be improved by the addition of cyclophosphamide to immunosuppressive drugs (45,50). There are two case reports of recurrent MPGN type III in adult cadaveric renal transplant patients (46,47).

MPGN TYPE II (DENSE DEPOSIT DISEASE)

Epidemiology and Genetics

MPGN type II is the least frequent of the three types (Table 32.2). It constitutes 19 to 34% of the cases in whites and 5% in Japanese. There is no evidence for a genetic basis for the disease. We have two families in which one of a pair of identical twins has the disease, and a similar family has been reported (51). Onset is most often in childhood.

Presentation and Clinical Manifestations

Symptoms and signs at presentation can include hematuria, proteinuria, hypertension, and edema. Hematuria is always present; in those with gross hematuria, the onset is that of an acute nephritic syndrome. Presentation with a nephrotic syndrome is common and has been associated with a poor prognosis (52,53). Even before onset of renal failure, hypertension can develop, but hypertensive encephalopathy is rarely a presenting event.

The clinical course is characterized by a nephrotic syndrome that persists or develops and increasingly severe hypertension (52,54,55). Occasionally, patients present with renal failure and have a rapidly progressive course (54,56). Conversely, a few may have periods after onset when their nephritis is silent (54); their urinary abnormalities completely disappear and only hypocomplementemia remains. Signs of nephritis may return, often associated with intercurrent infection, and persist.

There is increasing evidence that MPGN type II is a systemic disease. First, partial lipodystrophy and hypocomplementemia may be present for a considerable period before signs of glomerulonephritis appear (57). Second, renal transplants in almost every case quickly develop dense deposits in the GBM, often in the absence of manifestations of glomerulonephritis (58). Third, dense deposits similar to those in the GBM develop in the basement membranes of the sinusoids of the spleen (59) and in Bruch's membrane in the choriocapillaris of the eye (60). The eye lesion is associated with drusen, which resemble those seen in adults with macular degeneration. It is of interest that these spleen and eye membranes, like the GBM, are unique in that they are bathed in plasma.

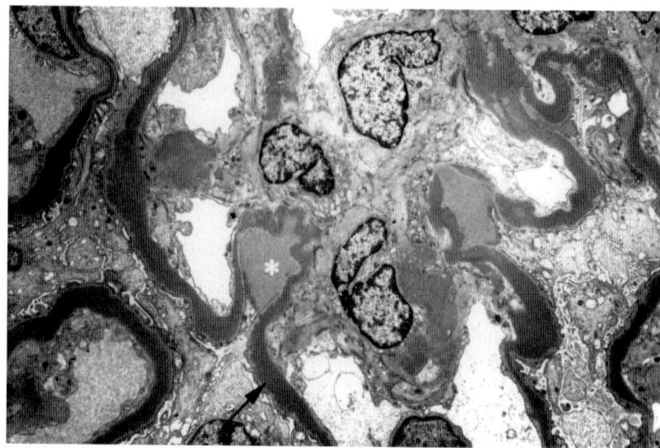

FIGURE 32.7. Ultrastructural features of membranoproliferative glomerulonephritis type II. In this electron photomicrograph of a uranyl-lead acetate–stained preparation, the lamina densa can be seen to be expanded by accumulation of electron-dense material (*arrow*), which has a fusiforme configuration. In addition to the dense deposit material, there are also large, discrete subepithelial deposits (*asterisk*) located in the paramesangial region. (Courtesy of Dr. David Witte.)

Laboratory Abnormalities

Distinctive features of the disease are the complement profile and the frequent presence of NF (Fig. 32.2). The profile is characterized by levels of C3, which may be markedly depressed with normal or near normal levels of other components (25). Thus, the depressed properdin and C5 levels seen in the other types of MPGN, in acute glomerulonephritis, and in the nephritis of systemic lupus are not present. The depressed C3 is produced by activation of native C3 by the alternative pathway convertase, C3b,Bb, which has been stabilized by the NF of the amplification loop, NF_a (Fig. 32.2). The stabilized convertase, C3b,Bb, NF_a, has a half-life more than 15 times that of the native convertase (61). The inactivated C3 it forms is quickly inactivated by factors H and I and is subsequently degraded to the ultimate C3 breakdown products, C3c and C3dg. All three of these derivatives may be found in the circulation (62–64). Contributing heavily to the hypocomplementemia is an inhibition of C3 synthesis attributed to a negative feedback produced by the circulating C3 breakdown products (65,66).

Pathology

In most cases, by light microscopy, the glomeruli are uniformly hypercellular with increased mesangial matrix, and the number of open capillary lumens is commensurately reduced. In contrast to MPGN type I, the proliferation is rarely great enough to increase glomerular size. The diagnosis of type II can occasionally be made by light microscopy of silver-stained preparations; the basement membrane is thickened, and at sites of the intramembranous deposits, argyrophilia is lost. The dense deposits may also be visualized by light microscopy by their ability to stain with thioflavin T (67). Deposits are located along the GBM, the Bowman's capsule, and the tubular basement membrane. By immunofluorescence, IgG, IgA, IgM, and C4 are rarely found in glomerular deposits, indicating that the classical pathway of complement is not activated.

C3 deposits are abundant. Kim et al. (68) found C3 to be present along the margin but not within the central portion of the dense deposits in the GBM, giving a double linear appearance (railroad tracks). They also observed C3 deposits within the mesangium outlining circular structures that represent shed fragments of the basement membrane (mesangial rings). The railroad tracks are visualized with labeled anti-C3c and -C3d, indicating that they are composed of C3b, iC3b, and C3dg, whereas the paramesangial deposits stain only with anti-C3c, indicating that they are formed from C3c deposited from the circulation (69).

The diagnostic intramembranous deposits are best seen by electron microscopy of uranyl-lead–stained specimens (Fig. 32.7). They usually occupy only the lamina densa but occasionally may be present only in the lamina interna (70). The deposits may be discontinuous. Similar deposits may also be found in Bowman's capsule and in the basement membranes of isolated groups of tubules. If searched for, subepithelial deposits can be found on the parts of the basement membrane that overlay the mesangium (paramesangial) if the patient was biopsied when hypocomplementemic (71). Occasionally, hump-like subepithelial deposits are present on the capillary loops.

Pathogenesis

The pathogenesis of the disease is not known. Many investigators find that the actual measurement of NF or of its surrogate, hypocomplementemia, does not show a straightforward correlation with activity of the disease. A few, however, have found a correlation between absence of hypocomplementemia or of NF and a benign course (72,73). Evidence that NF is more than an epiphenomenon is the observation that patients with several uncommon conditions—one of which is homozygous deficiency of factor H—are like those with MPGN type II in that they have convertase circulating in abnormally high concentration and have an unusual frequency of glomerulonephritis. How circulating convertase produces the nephritis is not clear (74).

It has been proposed that in consonance with the frequent association of deficiency of complement components with nephritis, the deficiency of C3 produced by NF is per se in some way nephritogenic. Another proposal is that it is an immune complex disease with the complexes generated by a subclinical infection, which in turn is a consequence of the hypocomplementemia. The absence of signs of classical pathway activation makes this concept unlikely.

Support for a role of complement in the pathogenesis of MPGN is provided by the observation that not only humans homozygous for deficiency in factor H can develop nephritis (23), but also that this deficiency in pigs (75) and mice (76) produces a lethal nephritis resembling MPGN type II. In mice, deposition of C3 and C9 antedating the deposition of IgG indicated that immune complexes do not initiate the glomerular injury. The disease was shown to be complement dependent in that glomerular damage can be prevented by the back-crossing of factor H–deficient mice with mice deficient in factor B, thus preventing convertase formation.

A possible link between NF and partial lipodystrophy is based on the fact that adipocytes are the only source of factor D, the enzyme that activates the convertase precursor, C3b,B, to form the alternative pathway convertase, C3b,Bb. NF has been shown to lyse adipocytes *in vitro*, and it is postulated that in certain individuals, the combination of NF and factor D in high concentrations fosters adipocyte destruction leading to partial lipodystrophy (77). This explanation requires that generation of NF antedate the onset of lipodystrophy.

Natural Course

In the absence of effective treatment, 50% renal survival after diagnosis is, in most series, 9 years. Survival is definitely shortened in patients presenting with a nephrotic syndrome. In one series, 10% of the patients went into remission.

Treatment

Because of the infrequency of the disease, a large experience with a single therapy has not been reported. Antiplatelet, anticoagulant, and immunosuppressive drugs have been used usually in combination with corticosteroids, but there is no evidence that such regimens are effective. Although not used in a clinical trial or in a large series, high-dose alternate-day prednisone is currently the most widely used treatment. We find that this regimen is not consistently effective and its effectiveness unpredictable. Of 14 patients who have received this regimen in this clinic, the disease in 5 is in remission. Serial renal biopsies have shown improvement in these patients to the extent that the dense deposit in the GBM is partially or completely lost (78).

Disease Recurrence in Renal Transplant Recipients

The rate of recurrence of dense deposits after renal transplantation is high, ranging from 50 to 100% in various series (83). Only a fraction of patients with recurrence develop proteinuria and, sometimes, nephrotic syndrome. A number of investigators have correlated disease recurrence with persistent or recurrent hypocomplementemia (58,80,84), whereas others could find no correlation with either low C3 levels or the presence of NF (81,85). The North American Pediatric Renal Transplant Cooperative Study group analyzed the 2-year kidney transplant survival and found an increased rate of graft loss for patients with MPGN type II; 45% were lost to disease recurrence. In published reports, graft loss due to recurrent MPGN type II varies widely from 0 to 100% (52,79,80–82).

REFERENCES

1. Habib R, Michielsen P, de Montera H, et al. Clinical, microscopic and electron microscopic data in the nephrotic syndrome of unknown origin. In: Wolstenholme GEW, Cameron CM, eds. *Renal biopsy*, vol. 1. London: Churchill, 1961:70.
2. West CD, McAdams AJ, McConville JM, et al. Hypocomplementemic and normocomplementemic persistent (chronic) glomerulonephritis; clinical and pathological characteristics. *J Pediatr* 1965;67:1089–1112.
3. Berger J, Galle P. Depots denses au sein des basales du rein. *Presse Med* 1963;71:2351–2354.
4. Habib R, Kleinknecht C, Gubler MC, et al. Idiopathic membranoproliferative glomerulonephritis in children. Report of 105 cases. *Clin Nephrol* 1973;1:194–214.
5. Strife CF, McEnery PT, McAdams AJ, et al. Membranoproliferative glomerulonephritis with disruption of the glomerular basement membrane. *Clin Nephrol* 1977;7:65–72.
6. Anders D, Thoenes W. Basement membrane-changes in membranoproliferative glomerulonephritis: a light and electron microscopic study. *Virchows Arch A Pathol Anat Histol* 1975;369:87–109.
7. Anders D, Agricola B, Sippel M, et al. Basement membrane changes in membranoproliferative glomerulonephritis. II. Characterization of a third type by silver impregnation of ultra thin sections. *Virchows Arch A Pathol Anat Histol* 1977; 376:1–19.
8. Coppo R, Gianoglio B, Porcellini MG, Maringhini S. Frequency of renal diseases and clinical indications for renal biopsy in children (report of the Italian National Registry of Renal Biopsies in Children). Group of Renal Immunopathology of the Italian Society of Pediatric Nephrology and Group of Renal Immunopathology of the Italian Society of Nephrology. *Nephrol Dial Transplant* 1998;13:293–297.
9. Iitaka K, Ishidate T, Hojo M, et al. Idiopathic membranoproliferative glomerulonephritis in Japanese children. *Pediatr Nephrol* 1995;9:272–277.
10. Tarshish P, Bernstein J, Tobin JN, et al. Treatment of mesangiocapillary glomerulonephritis with alternate-day pred-

nisolone: a report of the International Study of Kidney Disease in Children. *Pediatr Nephrol* 1992;6:123–130.
11. Braun MC, West CD, Strife CF. Differences between membranoproliferative glomerulonephritis types I and III in long-term response to an alternate-day prednisone regimen. *Am J Kidney Dis* 1999;34:1022–1032.
12. Schwertz R, de Jong R, Gretz N, et al. Outcome of idiopathic membranoproliferative glomerulonephritis in children. Arbeitsgemeinschaft Padiatrische Nephrologie. *Acta Paediatr* 1996;85:308–312.
13. Welch TR, Beischel L, Balakrishnan K, et al. Major-histocompatibility-complex extended haplotypes in membranoproliferative glomerulonephritis. *N Engl J Med* 1986;314:1476–1481.
14. Coleman TH, Forristal J, Kosaka T, et al. Inherited complement component deficiencies in membranoproliferative glomerulonephritis. *Kidney Int* 1983;24:181–190.
15. Berry PL, McEnery PT, McAdams AJ, et al. Membranoproliferative glomerulonephritis in two sibships. *Clin Nephrol* 1981;16:101–106.
16. Bakkaloglu A, Soylemezoglu O, Tinaztepe K, et al. Familial membranoproliferative glomerulonephritis. *Nephrol Dial Transplant* 1995;10:21–24.
17. Stutchfield PR, White RH, Cameron AH, et al. X-linked mesangiocapillary glomerulonephritis. *Clin Nephrol* 1986;26:150–156.
18. Sherwood MC, Pincott JR, Goodwin FJ, et al. Dominantly inherited glomerulonephritis and an unusual skin disease. *Arch Dis Child* 1987;62:1278–1280.
19. Power DA, Ng YC, Simpson JG. Familial incidence of C3 nephritic factor, partial lipodystrophy and membranoproliferative glomerulonephritis. *QJM* 1990;75:387–398.
20. Bogdanovic RM, Dimitrijevic JZ, Nikolic VN, et al. Membranoproliferative glomerulonephritis in two siblings: report and literature review. *Pediatr Nephrol* 2000;14:400–405.
21. Neary JJ, Colon PJ, Croke D, et al. Linkage of a gene causing familial membranoproliferative glomerulonephritis type III on chromosome 1. *J Am Soc Nephrol* 2002;13:2052–2057.
22. Jackson EC, McAdams AJ, Strife CF, et al. Differences between membranoproliferative glomerulonephritis types I and III in clinical presentation, glomerular morphology, and complement perturbation. *Am J Kidney Dis* 1987;9:115–120.
23. West CD. Nephritic factors predispose to chronic glomerulonephritis. *Am J Kidney Dis* 1994;24:956–963.
24. Strife CF, Jackson EC, Forristal J, et al. Effect of the nephrotic syndrome on the concentration of serum complement components. *Am J Kidney Dis* 1986;8:37–42.
25. Verade WS, Forristal J, West CD. Patterns of complement activation in idiopathic membranoproliferative glomerulonephritis, types I, II, and III. *Am J Kidney Dis* 1990;16:196–206.
26. Mollnes TE, Ng YC, Peters DK, et al. Effect of nephritic factor on C3 and on the terminal pathway of complement in vivo and in vitro. *Clin Exp Immunol* 1986;65:73–79.
27. Clardy CW, Forristal J, Strife CF, et al. Serum terminal complement component levels in hypocomplementemic glomerulonephritides. *Clin Immunol Immunopathol* 1989;50:307–320.
28. Clardy CW, Forristal J, Strife CF, et al. A properdin dependent nephritic factor slowly activating C3, C5, and C9 in membranoproliferative glomerulonephritis, types I and III. *Clin Immunol Immunopathol* 1989;50:333–347.
29. Wyatt RJ, McAdams AJ, Forristal J, et al. Glomerular deposition of complement-control proteins in acute and chronic glomerulonephritis. *Kidney Int* 1979;16:505–512.
30. West CD, McAdams AJ. Membranoproliferative glomerulonephritis type III: association of glomerular deposits with circulating nephritic factor-stabilized convertase. *Am J Kidney Dis* 1998;32:56–63.
31. West CD, McAdams AJ. Glomerular paramesangial deposits: association with hypocomplementemia in membranoproliferative glomerulonephritis types I and III. *Am J Kidney Dis* 1998;31:427–434.
32. Schwertz R, Rother U, Anders D, et al. Complement analysis in children with idiopathic membranoproliferative glomerulonephritis: a long-term follow-up. *Pediatr Allergy Immunol* 2001;12:166–172.
33. Cameron J, Turner D, Heaton J, et al. Idiopathic mesangiocapillary glomerulonephritis. Comparison of types I and II in children and adults and long-term prognosis. *Am J Med* 1983;74:175–192.
34. McEnery PT, McAdams AJ, West CD. Membranoproliferative glomerulonephritis: improved survival with alternate day prednisone therapy. *Clin Nephrol* 1980;13:117–124.
35. McEnery PT, McAdams AJ, West CD. The effect of prednisone in a high-dose, alternate-day regimen on the natural history of idiopathic membranoproliferative glomerulonephritis. *Medicine (Baltimore)* 1985;64:401–424.
36. McEnery PT. Membranoproliferative glomerulonephritis: the Cincinnati experience—cumulative renal survival from 1957 to 1989. *J Pediatr* 1990;116:S109–S114.
37. Mota-Hernandez F, Gordillo-Paniagua G, Munoz-Arizpe R, et al. Prednisone versus placebo in membranoproliferative glomerulonephritis: long-term clinicopathological correlations. *Int J Pediatr Nephrol* 1985;6:25–28.
38. Bergstein J, Andreoli S. Response of type I membranoproliferative glomerulonephritis to pulse methylprednisolone and alternate-day prednisone therapy. *Pediatr Nephrol* 1995;9:268–271.
39. Warady B, Guggenheim S, Sedman A, et al. Prednisone therapy of membranoproliferative glomerulonephritis in children. *J Pediatr* 1985;107:702–707.
40. Ford D, Briscoe D, Shanley P, et al. Childhood membranoproliferative glomerulonephritis type I: limited steroid therapy. *Kidney Int* 1992;41:1606–1612.
41. Somers M, Kertesz S, Rosen S, et al. Non-nephrotic children with membranoproliferative glomerulonephritis: are steroids indicated? *Pediatr Nephrol* 1995;9:140–144.
42. Iitaka K, Moriya S, Nakamura S, et al. Long-term follow-up of type III membranoproliferative glomerulonephritis in children. *Pediatr Nephrol* 2002;17:373–378.
43. Donadio JJ, Offord K. Reassessment of treatment results in membranoproliferative glomerulonephritis, with emphasis on life-table analysis. *Am J Kidney Dis* 1989;6:445–451.
44. Cattran DC, Cardella CJ, Roscoe JM, et al. Results of a controlled drug trial in membranoproliferative glomerulonephritis. *Kidney Int* 1985;27:436–441.
45. Lien Y-HH, Scott K. Long-term cyclophosphamide treatment for recurrent type I membranoproliferative glomerulonephritis after transplantation. *Am J Kidney Dis* 2000;35:539–543.
46. Morales JM, Martinez MA, Munoz de Bustillo E, et al. Recurrent type III membranoproliferative glomerulonephri-

tis after kidney transplantation. *Transplantation* 1997;63: 1186–1188.

47. Meyers KE, Finn L, Kaplan BS. Membranoproliferative glomerulonephritis type III. *Pediatr Nephrol* 1998;12:512–522.
48. Andresdottir MB, Assmann KJ, Hoitsma AJ, et al. Recurrence of type I membranoproliferative glomerulonephritis after renal transplantation: analysis of the incidence, risk factors, and impact on graft survival. *Transplantation* 1997;63:1628–1633.
49. Briganti EM, Russ GR, McNeil JJ, et al. Risk of renal allograft loss from recurrent glomerulonephritis *N Engl J Med* 2002;347:103–109.
50. Cahen R, Trolliet P, Dijoud F, et al. Severe recurrence of type I membranoproliferative glomerulonephritis after transplantation: remission on steroids and cyclophosphamide. *Transplant Proc* 1995;27:1746–1747.
51. Reichel W, Kobberling J, Fischbach H, et al. Membranoproliferative glomerulonephritis with partial lipodystrophy: discordant occurrence in identical twins. *Klin Wochenschr* 1976;54:75–81.
52. Lamb V, Tisher CC, McCoy RC, et al. Membranoproliferative glomerulonephritis with dense intramembranous alterations. A clinical pathologic study. *Lab Invest* 1977;36:607–617.
53. Bennett WM, Fassett RG, Walker RG, et al. Mesangiocapillary glomerulonephritis type II (dense-deposit disease): clinical features of progressive disease. *Am J Kidney Dis* 1989; 13:469–476.
54. Habib R, Gubler M-C, Loirat C, et al. Dense deposit disease: a variant of membranoproliferative glomerulonephritis. *Kidney Int* 1975;7:204–215.
55. Kashtan CE, Burke B, Burch G, et al. Dense intramembranous deposit disease: a clinical comparison of histological subtypes. *Clin Nephrol* 1990;33:1–6.
56. Rose GM, Cole BR, Robson AM. The treatment of severe glomerulopathies in children using high dose intravenous methylprednisolone pulses. *Am J Kidney Dis* 1981;1:148–156.
57. Sissons JGP, West RJ, Fallows J, et al. The complement abnormalities of lipodystrophy. *N Engl J Med* 1976;294:461–465.
58. Turner DR, Cameron JS, Bewick M, et al. Transplantation in mesangiocapillary glomerulonephritis with intramembranous dense "deposits": recurrence of disease. *Kidney Int* 1976;9: 439–448.
59. Thorner P, Baumal R. Extraglomerular dense deposits in dense deposit disease. *Arch Pathol Lab Med* 1982;106:628–631.
60. Duvall-Young J, MacDonald MK, McKechnie NM. Fundus changes in (type II) mesangiocapillary glomerulonephritis simulating drusen: a histopathological report. *Br J Ophthalmol* 1989;73:297–302.
61. Daha MR, Van Es LA. Further evidence for the antibody nature of C3 nephritic factor (C3 NeF). *J Immunol* 1979; 123:755–758.
62. West CD, Winter S, Forristal J, et al. Evidence for in vivo breakdown of beta1C-globulin in hypocomplementemic glomerulonephritis. *J Clin Invest* 1967;26:539–548.
63. Perrin LH, Lambert TH, Miescher PA. Complement breakdown products in plasma from patients with systemic lupus erythematosus and patients with membranoproliferative or other glomerulonephritides. *J Clin Invest* 1975;56:165–176.
64. Davis AE 3rd, Harrison RA, Lachmann PJ. Physiologic inactivation of fluid phase C3b: isolation and structural analysis of C3c, C3d,g (alpha 2D), and C3g. *J Immunol* 1984;132:1960–1966.
65. Alper CA, Rosen FS. Studies of the in vivo behavior of human C3 in normal subjects and patients. *J Clin Invest* 1967;46:2021–2034.
66. Charlesworth JA, Williams DG, Sherington E, et al. Metabolic studies of the third component of complement and the glycine-rich beta glycoprotein in patients with hypocomplementemia. *J Clin Invest* 1974;53:1578–1587.
67. Churg J, Duffy JL, Bernstein J. Identification of dense deposit disease: a report for the International Study of Kidney Diseases in Children. *Arch Pathol Lab Med* 1979;103:67–72.
68. Kim Y, Vernier RL, Fish AJ, et al. Immunofluorescence studies of dense deposit disease. The presence of railroad tracks and mesangial rings. *Lab Invest* 1979;40:474–480.
69. West CD, Witte DP, McAdams AJ. Composition of nephritic factor-generated glomerular deposits in membranoproliferative glomerulonephritis type 2. *Am J Kidney Dis* 2001;37:1120–1130.
70. Swainson CP, Robson JS, Thomson D, et al. Mesangiocapillary glomerulonephritis: a long-term study of 40 cases. *J Pathol* 1983;141:449–468.
71. West CD, McAdams AJ. Paramesangial glomerular deposits in membranoproliferative glomerulonephritis type II correlate with hypocomplementemia. *Am J Kidney Dis* 1995;25:853–861.
72. Schena FP, Pertosa G, Stanziale P, et al. Biological significance of the C3 nephritic factor in membranoproliferative glomerulonephritis. *Clin Nephrol* 1982;18:240–246.
73. Klein M, Poucell S, Arbus GS, et al. Characteristics of a benign subtype of dense deposit disease: comparison with the progressive form of this disease. *Clin Nephrol* 1983;20:163–171.
74. West CD, McAdams AJ. The alternative pathway C3 convertase and glomerular deposits. *Pediatr Nephrol* 1999;13:448–453.
75. Hogasen K, Jansen JH, Mollnes TE, et al. Hereditary porcine membranoproliferative glomerulonephritis type II is caused by factor H deficiency. *J Clin Invest* 1995;95:1054–1061.
76. Pickering MC, Cook HT, Warren J, et al. Uncontrolled C3 activation causes membranoproliferative glomerulonephritis in mice deficient in complement factor H. *Nat Genet* 2002; 31:424-428.
77. Mathieson PW, Wurzner R, Oliveria DB, et al. Complement-mediated adipocyte lysis by nephritic factor sera. *J Exp Med* 1993;177:1827–1831.
78. McEnery PT, McAdams AJ. Regression of membranoproliferative glomerulonephritis type II (dense deposit disease): observations in six children. *Am J Kidney Dis* 1988;12:138–146.
79. Galle P, Hinglais N, Crosnier J. Recurrence of an original glomerular lesion in three renal allografts. *Transplant Proc* 1971;3:368–370.

80. Eddy A, Sibley R, Mauer SM, et al. Renal allograft failure due to recurrent dense intramembranous deposit disease. *Clin Nephrol* 1984; 21:305–313.
81. Droz D, Nabarra B, Noel L, et al. Recurrence of dense deposits in transplanted kidneys: I. Sequential survey of the lesions. *Kidney Int* 1979;15:386–395.
82. Briner J. Glomerular lesions in renal allografts. *Ergeb Inn Med Kinderheilkd* 1982;49:1–76.
83. Aneresdottir M, Assman K, Hoitsma A, et al. Renal transplantation with dense deposit disease: morphological characteristics of recurrent disease and clinical outcome. *Nephrol Dial Transplant* 1999;14:1723–1731.
84. Berthoux F, Ducret F, Colon S, et al. Renal transplantation in mesangioproliferative glomerulonephritis (MPGN): relationship between the high frequency of recurrent glomerulonephritis and hypocomplementemia. *Kidney Int* 1975;7: S323–S327.
85. Habib R, Antignac C, Hinglais N, et al. Glomerular lesions in the transplanted kidney in children. *Am J Kidney Dis* 1987;10:198–207.

33

MEMBRANOUS NEPHROPATHY

SUDESH PAUL MAKKER

Membranous nephropathy (MN) is a chronic glomerular disease with distinct histopathologic features. The term *membranous glomerulitis* was first used by Bell in 1938, reporting a light microscopy study of autopsied kidneys from patients with nephrotic syndrome (NS) (1). In a subgroup whose glomeruli had no proliferation, he noted that some had essentially normal glomeruli, whereas others had diffuse thickening of the glomerular basement membrane (GBM). The latter cases were termed *membranous glomerulitis*. It is interesting to note that two of them were children. Later, Bell noted that the GBM had a vacuolated appearance (2).

In 1957, Jones introduced the periodic acid–silver methenamine stain to study kidney tissue of patients with NS and observed that the GBM in membranous glomerulitis had a peculiar appearance, with the thickened GBM resolving into a thinner membrane from which protruded many silver-positive projections (3). Between the projections, a silver-negative hyaline material was present in the form of droplets. Jones' description is now widely accepted as the pathognomic feature of MN, and his stain is routinely used in the processing of renal biopsy specimens. At approximately the same time, Movat and McGregor first used electron microscopy, and Mellors et al. used immunofluorescence microscopy in the study of this disease and further elucidated the ultrastructural and immunohistologic features of MN (4,5).

The characteristic histopathologic features of MN are (a) lack of proliferation in the glomerulus and a diffusely thickened glomerular capillary wall exhibiting silver-positive projections, or so-called spikes, with silver methenamine stain under light microscopy; (b) fine granular staining for immunoglobulin (Ig) G and complement along the periphery of the glomerular capillary wall on immunofluorescence microscopy; and (c) electron-dense deposits located exclusively in the subepithelial position along the GBM on electron microscopy.

Although the term *membranous glomerulitis* was used commonly in earlier medical literature, *membranaus nephropathy* is now the preferred term. *MN* is a histopathologic term used to describe a unique glomerular lesion and is not itself a clinical entity.

PATHOLOGY

Light Microscopy

Under light microscopy, the glomeruli are normal in size or slightly enlarged. Their cellularity appears normal, and there is no infiltration with inflammatory cells or proliferation of mesangial or endothelial cells. The epithelial cells may be normal or enlarged and prominent (Fig. 33.1). In most patients, no epithelial cell crescents are present, but occasionally such crescents are seen in association with a clinical picture of rapidly progressive glomerulonephritis. The mesangial matrix is not increased, and the glomerular tufts do not show excessive lobulation. The capillary loops are usually patent but may be occluded in advanced cases. The predominant change in MN is in the glomerular capillary walls, which show varying grades of diffuse thickening involving all capillary loops and all glomeruli. The thickened capillary wall is best visualized in the periodic acid–methenamine silver stained sections in which the GBM itself is stained black, and the subepithelial deposits in the GBM are not stained. Because of their location in the subepithelial space, these unstained deposits are surrounded by black-staining newly synthesized GBM that appears as small black spikes projecting from the GBM toward the urinary space (Fig. 33.2). In tangentially cut sections, it may give a vacuolated appearance. In the advanced stages, the subepithelial deposits are incorporated into the GBM, giving it a chain-like appearance. As the lesion progresses, the capillary walls increase in thickness, their lumen is occluded, and eventually the glomeruli become sclerosed.

In the early stages, the tubules, vessels, and interstitium are normal. As the disease advances, there is progressive tubular atrophy, accumulation of mononuclear cell infiltrate, and increasing interstitial fibrosis, and the kidney eventually develops the appearance of end-stage kidney disease (6,7).

Immunofluorescence Microscopy

With immunofluorescence microscopy, all cases of MN show bright, fine to coarse granular staining for IgG along the glomerular capillary wall (Fig. 33.3). Using monoclonal

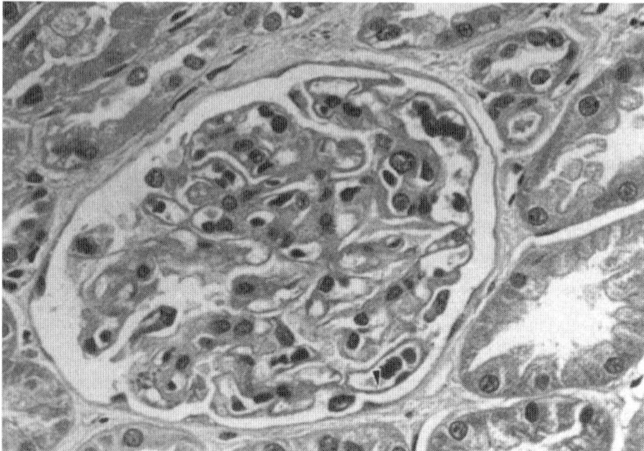

FIGURE 33.1. Early membranous nephropathy with mild diffuse thickening of capillary loop membranes (*arrowhead*) (hematoxylin and eosin stain, ×100). (Courtesy of Dr. John A. Wolfe, Sutter Hospitals, Sacramento, CA.)

antibodies against human IgG subclasses, it appears that the predominant IgG staining in the granules is for IgG4 (13). No staining for IgG is seen in the mesangium in idiopathic MN; if present, it should arouse the suspicion of systemic lupus erythematosus (SLE) as the underlying cause. The staining for IgA and IgM is variable and not intense and is in the same location as IgG. Staining for complement C3 is similar in character and distribution to that for IgG and is usually, but not always, of similar intensity. Staining for C1q and C4 is seen, but the intensity is much less than that for C3, and intense staining for C1q should arouse suspicion of SLE. Recently, staining for membrane attack component of complement C5b-9 has been noted in a similar location to that of IgG (14,15). Staining for fibrin is also commonly present.

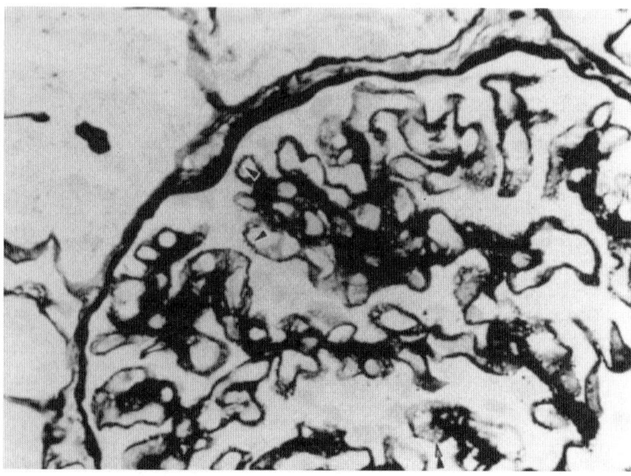

FIGURE 33.2. Membranous nephropathy, silver stain showing formation of spikes (*single arrowheads*) and a moth-eaten appearance with multiple small holes in the basement membranes when cut *en face* (*double arrowhead*) (Jones silver stain, approximately ×160). (Courtesy of Dr. John A. Wolfe, Sutter Hospitals, Sacramento, CA.)

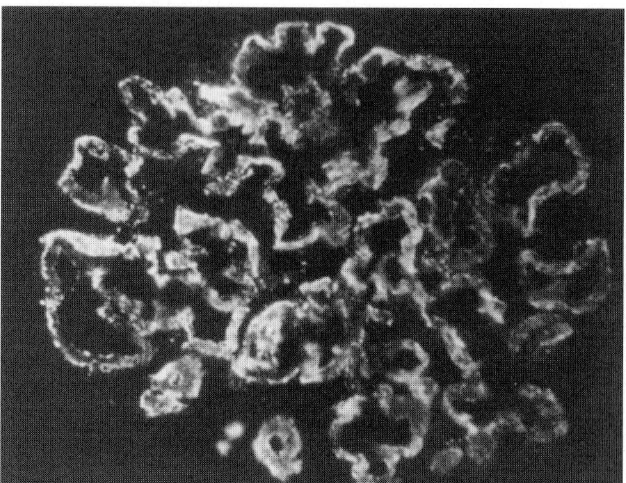

FIGURE 33.3. Membranous nephropathy, immunofluorescent study showing the typical brightly stained granular immune-complex deposits along the entire glomerular basement membrane (anti–immunoglobulin G, approximately ×100). (Courtesy of Dr. John A. Wolfe, Sutter Hospitals, Sacramento, CA.)

Electron Microscopy

The electron microscopy findings in MN are characteristic. The hallmark is the presence of electron-dense deposits, located exclusively in the subepithelial space along the capillary wall and corresponding to the granular IgG deposits seen on immunofluorescence microscopy (Fig. 33.4). No electron-dense deposits are seen in the subendothelial space or in the mesangium, and the mesangial cellularity is normal. An occasional mesangial deposit should arouse suspicion of MN associated with SLE. Four morphologic stages of MN are recognized:

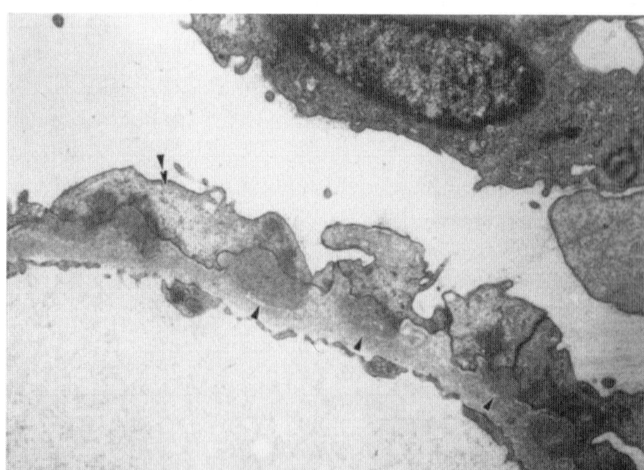

FIGURE 33.4. Electron micrograph showing the portion of glomerular peripheral capillary membrane with multiple, fairly evenly spaced, electron-dense immune-complex deposits located on the subepithelial side of the basement membrane (*arrowheads*). There is very early deposition of basement membrane between these deposits. Notice the loss of normal epithelial cell foot process architecture (*double arrowheads*) (×9700). (Courtesy of Dr. Richard R. Wilber, and Dr. John A. Wolfe, Sutter Hospitals, Sacramento, CA.)

1. In stage I, the GBM is normal in thickness and appearance. The electron-dense deposits are small to moderate in size but discrete. The smaller deposits are generally located at the site of the slit diaphragm. Moderate-size deposits cover a greater area of the subepithelial space, adjacent to where the foot processes of the visceral glomerular epithelial cells are usually fused.
2. In stage II, the deposits are numerous, larger, and confluent. Projections of GBM, corresponding to the spikes seen on light microscopy staining black with silver stains, are seen between the deposits. The GBM itself is generally not thickened.
3. In stage III, the deposits are larger and surrounded by the projections of GBM. The density of the deposits is decreased, and the GBM appears irregularly thickened.
4. In stage IV, the deposits have been incorporated into GBM and have become electron lucent and, thus, are sometimes difficult to differentiate from the surrounding GBM. The GBM is now severely altered and irregularly thickened.

Stage II is the most common type of lesion (10,11,16,17), whereas stages III and IV are considered as showing resolution. Because MN is a chronic disease, probably involving continuous or multiple generations of deposit formation, different stages of the lesion in a patient may be seen at any given time, as reported by Habib et al. in the largest series of children with MN (10). There is insufficient information in children to determine the correlation between the different histologic stages and the clinical manifestation or course of the disease (9,12,16).

CLASSIFICATION

MN in children may be divided into two categories based on cause: (a) idiopathic or primary; and (b) secondary, in which MN develops in association with another condition, such as SLE, or the patient has been exposed to certain infectious agents or drugs (Table 33.1) (8,18–39).

Compared with adults, a greater percentage of cases of MN in children are secondary (19). In the largest series, 43% had an associated condition (8,19). In several parts of the world—particularly Southeast Asia (20,21), Japan (40), Africa (41–43), and certain parts of Europe (44–46)—hepatitis B is a significant factor in the etiology of MN. Other infections, such as congenital syphilis (22,23), malaria (24), and filariasis (25), are also of etiologic significance in those areas where they are prevalent. Whether certain host factors predispose people to the development of MN in such infected children is unclear. Medications and neoplasms are rare causes of MN in children compared with adults (8,19).

The cause of the idiopathic type of MN is unknown, but several observations suggest immune dysregulation:

TABLE 33.1. CLASSIFICATION OF MEMBRANOUS GLOMERULONEPHROPATHY IN CHILDREN

Idiopathic or primary
Associated with other conditions—secondary
Infections
Hepatitis B (8,18–21)[a]
Congenital syphilis (22,23)[a]
Malaria? (24)
Filariasis (25)
Immunologic or autoimmune diseases
Systemic lupus erythematosus (8,12,18,19)[a]
Enteropathy (27)
Crohn's disease (28, 29)
Pemphigus (30)
Drugs
D-Penicillamine (8,17)[a]
Neoplastic
Ovarian tumor (33)
Neuroblastoma (34)
Gonadoblastoma (35)
Wilms' tumor? (36)
Miscellaneous
De novo occurrence in renal transplant (37)[a]
Fanconi's syndrome (8,26)
Sickle cell disease (8)
Diabetes mellitus? (38)
Associated with antitubular basement membrane (8,26) and antialveolar basement membrane antibodies (38)
Thrombocytopenia (8) and microangiopathic anemia (39)
Juvenile cirrhosis or alpha-1 antitrypsin deficiency (40)

[a]Accounts for majority of the cases.

1. The development of MN in certain patients (both children and adults) with SLE.
2. The development of MN in other autoimmune disorders [e.g., insulin-dependent diabetes mellitus in children (38) (S. P. Makker, *unpublished observation*, 1980) and adults (47), children with autoimmune enteropathy (27), Crohn's disease (28,29), multiple sclerosis (31) or pemphigus (29), adults with Graves' disease (6,48), primary biliary cirrhosis (6,49), Sjögren's syndrome (6), rheumatoid arthritis (6), Hashimoto's thyroiditis (6), dermatitis herpetiformis (6), and ankylosing spondylitis (6)].
3. MN can occur in association with the development of autoantibodies to other renal antigens [i.e., tubular basement membrane in children (26) and GBM in adults (50)].
4. An autoimmune MN indistinguishable from idiopathic MN in humans can be produced in rats by immunization with rat tubular antigens (Heymann nephritis).
5. Mercury is known to produce immune dysregulation and autoimmunity including MN in certain strains of rats (51), and mercury exposure in adult patients can also produce MN (6).

Genetic factors are also important in idiopathic MN. Strong associations of HLA-DR3 (52,53) and DQA1 allele

(54) have been reported with idiopathic MN in adults. MN has been reported in two HLA identical brothers (both children) (55) and, in another instance, in a father and son with HLA-DR3 (56). Based on the aforementioned observations, it may be hypothesized that idiopathic MN in humans is an autoimmune disease occurring in certain genetically predisposed individuals and precipitated by unknown exogenous or endogenous events.

IDIOPATHIC MEMBRANOUS NEPHROPATHY

Prevalence

Idiopathic MN may be discovered during evaluation of asymptomatic proteinuria or NS (8,19,57). Because all children with asymptomatic proteinuria do not come to the attention of physicians, and because renal biopsies are not performed on all patients with asymptomatic proteinuria or even those with NS, the exact prevalence of MN in children is unknown. In the International Study of Kidney Disease in Children, idiopathic MN was found in only 4 of 400 children with NS (58). The rarity of idiopathic MN as a cause of NS in children is supported by our experience and by others who have found that only 2 to 6% of those children with NS who are studied by renal biopsy have idiopathic MN (8,10,16,17,59). In contrast, idiopathic MN is a common glomerular disease in adults; it is responsible for 25 to 40% of cases of idiopathic NS (60,61).

Pathogenesis

The pathogenesis of idiopathic MN is unknown. Based on immunofluorescence and ultrastructural findings, it is clearly an immunologically mediated disease. The granular deposits containing IgG, which correspond to the subepithelial ultrastructural electron-dense deposits, are believed to represent antigen-antibody complexes. The antigen(s) in the deposits and the process by which they form, enlarge, and partially resolve are not known. Whether the antigen is exogenous or endogenous, renal or nonrenal, or the same or different in various cases of MN is also unclear. Based on studies of Heymann nephritis in the rat, both the active (62) and passive (63,64) types, it is possible that the deposits in idiopathic human MN, like the deposits of Heymann nephritis, are formed *in situ* after binding of an autoantibody to a glomerular antigen; a large (600-kDa) glycoprotein variously named as gp600/gp330/megalin (65,66) presents on the surface of the glomerular epithelial cell (67) (see Chapter 39). Recently, the pathogenic region on gp600/gp330/megalin has been localized to a small area in the N-terminal of this protein (68). Two case reports, one in a child (69) and another in an adult (70), and recent data (71,72) in a small number of patients support this concept of pathogenesis. An interesting case supporting the concept that MN can develop in a human by the binding of antibodies against at least one expressed podocyte protein, neutral endopeptidase, was reported recently (73). In this case, antibodies against neutral endopeptidase produced by a mother who herself had a deficiency of this protein were transferred to her fetus, producing a MN in the newborn. The mother apparently had been immunized against this protein during an earlier pregnancy.

Also, based on the studies in Heymann nephritis, it appears that (a) the subepithelial immune deposits come to lie in this unique position after capping and shedding of the antigen-antibody complexes formed *in situ* on the surface of the glomerular epithelial cell (74); and (b) after immune-deposit formation complement activation ensues, resulting in the generation of the terminal membrane attack component (C5b-9), which may be an important mediator of the resulting proteinuria (75,76). A critical threshold of the amount of the antigen-antibody complexes and the ensuing complement activation is required for the development of proteinuria (77). The generated C5b-9 is inserted into the cell membrane of the glomerular epithelial cell and then endocytosed, transported intracellularly, and finally excreted into the urinary space and urine (78). How the activation of complement and the formation of C5b-9 produce proteinuria in Heymann nephritis is not established, but reactive oxygen species (79), metalloproteinases (80), phospholipases, and protein kinases (81) appear to play a role. Whether a similar mechanism operates in human MN is unclear. However, C5b-9 can be demonstrated in the human idiopathic MN lesion (14,15) and is also excreted in the urine (82). *In situ* subepithelial antigen-antibody deposits in experimental animals can also result from the binding of antibodies to nonglomerular, cationic, exogenous antigens implanted experimentally in the lamina rara externa of the GBM (83).

Circulating immune complexes of appropriate size and charge, made *in vitro* by artificially covalently linking an exogenous antigen and antibody followed by intravenous infusion into an experimental animal, also localize in the subepithelial region (84) and produce the subepithelial deposits of MN. Whether such a mechanism operates in humans is unknown, but it appears to be unlikely.

In summary, human MN is an antibody-mediated disease of uncertain and imprecise pathogenesis. However, the hypotheses that it is an autoimmune disease of the kidney and that the subepithelial immune deposits are formed *in situ* with an endogenous glomerular antigen are attractive.

Clinical and Laboratory Findings

Clinical features of idiopathic MN at onset are summarized in Table 33.2. MN can occur at any age, including infancy. Habib et al. (10) reported two patients of 8 and 10 months of age, and the author has seen two infants present at 5 and 11 months. Sixty percent of the children are male; 40% are female (Table 33.2). The children may have overt features of

TABLE 33.2. CLINICAL FEATURES OF MEMBRANOUS GLOMERULONEPHRITIS

Clinical features	Habib et al. (10)	Southwest Pediatric Nephrology Study Group (12)	Latham et al. (11)	Ramirez et al. (16)	Trainin et al. (59)	Makker	Total number	Percent
No. of cases	50	54	14	22	14	9	163	
Boys	38	28	9	11	6	7	99	60
Girls	12	26	5	11	8	2	64	40
Onset								
Age (yr)	0.7–15.0	6.0–15.0	3.5–6.0	0.9–20.0	2.0–15.0	0.4–15.0	—	—
Asymptomatic proteinuria	26	8	3	5	3	0	45/162	28
Nephrotic syndrome	24	45	11	17	11	9	117/162	72
Hypertension	3	16	7	8	2	1	37/163	22
Macroscopic hematuria	3	0	0	0	0	0	3/163	2
Microscopic hematuria	30/46	30	8	14	14	9	111/159	70
Renal failure	0	—	—	1	1	1	2/73	3
Normal C3	11/11	—	—	14	14	9	45/47	98
Course								
Follow-up (yr)	1.0–10.0	0.2–14.0	1.0–16.0	1.0–11.0	0.8–7.0	1.0–14.0	—	—
No treatment	5	20	1	11	3	2	42	26
Treatment								
Prednisone	+	+	+	+	+	+	—	—
Cytotoxic drugs	+	+	+	+	–	+	—	—
Outcome								
Remission	26	13/50	4	7	6	6	62/159	39
Active disease	19	?	7	9	4	2	41/109	38
Chronic renal failure	5	10/44?	3	6	4	1	29/153	19

+, present; –, not present.

NS (e.g., anasarca) or asymptomatic proteinuria (57); presentation with NS is more common (69%). Although presentation with macroscopic hematuria is rare, it has been reported (10); however, microscopic hematuria at presentation is common (69%). Presentation with isolated microscopic hematuria without proteinuria or NS is extremely rare (16). Hypertension at onset is uncommon (21%). Renal failure at onset is rare (2.3%), but the author has seen a child present with rapidly progressive acute renal failure, whose glomerular histology showed MN with glomerular crescents. In patients with edema, laboratory findings of NS (i.e., hypoproteinemia, low serum albumin concentration, hyperlipidemia, and heavy proteinuria) are present. Serum complement levels CH50, C3, and C4 are normal in most patients (Table 33.2).

Diagnosis

No specific clinical finding or simple, routinely performed laboratory test is diagnostic for MN. The condition should be suspected when (a) features of a chronic glomerulonephropathy (i.e., proteinuria, hematuria, abnormal urine sediment, with or without hypertension, or renal failure) are present; and (b) the laboratory tests for more common glomerulonephritides are negative [i.e., normal serum complement, negative serology for syphilis, negative serologic test for hepatitis B surface antigen (HB_sAg), a negative antinuclear antibody test, and negative tests for poststreptococcal infection]. Lack of prompt response to corticosteroids in a nephrotic patient may also suggest MN. However, a definitive diagnosis can only be made by a histologic diagnosis on a renal biopsy specimen.

Treatment

Treatment consists of immunosuppressive drugs and renoprotective agents (e.g., angiotensin-converting enzyme inhibitors or angiotensin II receptor antagonists) and lipid-lowering drugs [e.g., hydroxymethylglutaryl coenzyme A reductase inhibitors (statins)]. Although there have been no reported studies employing renoprotective agents in children with MN, there are sufficient data in adults with MN (85) and other proteinuric renal diseases that it seems reasonable to use angiotensin-converting enzyme inhibitors or angiotensin II receptor antagonists in all patients with MN, except those with renal failure (86). Lipid-lowering drugs may be used in nephrotic patients (87).

There are no controlled clinical trials in children of treatment with corticosteroids or other immunosuppressive drugs. Therefore, no definitive approach to therapy is available at this time. However, based on uncontrolled studies (8,12,16,17,19,59,88), the following approach appears rational: Children with asymptomatic proteinuria and without hypertension, renal failure, or NS should be given angiotensin-converting enzyme inhibitors or angiotensin II receptor antagonists and not treated with corticosteroids or other immunosuppressive therapy because most are likely to go into remission and do well.

How to treat all other children with idiopathic MN remains a difficult decision at present. It is unlikely that sufficient numbers can be collected to conduct a prospective, randomized, double-blind controlled study because of the low prevalence of the disease in children. In the absence of such information, decisions have to be based on information available from controlled studies using immunosuppressive drugs performed in adults with idiopathic MN (Table 33.3).

Alternate-day corticosteroids alone have been used in three controlled trials (89–91). Two trials compared a 100- to 150-mg alternate-day dose of prednisone for 8 weeks with placebo. In the study from the United States (89), the treatment was associated with more complete and partial remissions of the NS. However, the follow-up period was short, and the rate of deterioration of renal function was unexpectedly high in the control group. The other study, from the United Kingdom (90), found no significant difference (p <.05) between the untreated and treated groups in plasma creatinine concentration, creatinine clearance, or 24-hour protein excretion. The third study, from Canada (91), using 45 mg/m^2 prednisone for 6 months, concluded that the therapy was of no benefit (p <.2).

In trials with corticosteroids and other immunosuppressive agents, a controlled study from Italy (92) used a 6-month course of daily corticosteroids alternating with chlorambucil (0.2 mg/kg/day) as follows: Methylprednisolone was first given intravenously, 1 g/day for 3 days, followed by daily oral prednisone, 0.4 mg/kg for 27 days. Prednisone was then discontinued and chlorambucil given at a dosage of 0.2 mg/kg/day for 1 month. These alternating courses of prednisone and chlorambucil were continued for 6 months. At 5 years of follow-up, there were significantly more remissions in treated than in untreated patients (p = .026). There was significant deterioration of renal function in the untreated group (p = .0002) but not in the treated group (p value was not significant). At 10 years of follow-up, these benefits were maintained (93). The same group from Italy performed another controlled trial comparing the same regimen of chlorambucil with steroids or with steroids alone (94). The authors found that the addition of chlorambucil was associated with more remissions of the NS and preservation of renal function. In another controlled trial of selected patients with progressive MN, cyclosporine (3.5 mg/kg/day for 12 months) was found to be beneficial (95). Significant reductions of proteinuria (p <.02) and a slower rate of decline of renal function (p <.02) were observed during therapy (95). Recently, in a controlled trial of adult steroid-resistant nephrotic patients treated for 26 weeks with prednisone (0.15 mg/kg/day) plus cyclosporine (3.5 mg/kg/day) or prednisone alone, 75% of the former and 22% of the latter groups achieved partial or complete remission of proteinuria (96).

The most promising results in the aforementioned studies were obtained in the Italian study using alternating courses of daily prednisone and chlorambucil. This treatment, or treatment with cyclosporine (95,96), may be tried in children who have persistent NS with or without other features of severe disease (i.e., renal failure or hypertension). Children generally tolerate corticosteroids well and are unlikely to develop severe side effects on dosages used in the Italian protocol, but there is a possibility of gonadal toxicity and oncogenic potential with chlorambucil and renal toxicity with cyclosporine. Newer therapies are emerging. In a preliminary

TABLE 33.3. RESULTS OF CONTROLLED TRIALS OF TREATMENT OF IDIOPATHIC MEMBRANOUS GLOMERULONEPHRITIS IN ADULTS

Study (reference)	No. of patients	Follow-up (mo)	Treatment	Conclusion
Collaborative Study Group (USA) (89)	Untreated—38 Treated—34	26–52	Prednisone, 125 mg (100–150 mg) every other d × 8 wk	"Less deterioration of renal function in treated patients."
Cattran et al. (Canada) (90)	Untreated—77 Treated—81	48 ± 3	Prednisone, 45 mg/m^2 every other d × 6 mo	"No benefit."
Cameron et al. (UK) (91)	Untreated—51 Treated—52	52 ± 6	Prednisone, 125–150 mg every other d × 8 wk	"No significant difference between treated and untreated groups in plasma creatinine, creatinine clearance or 24-h proteinuria."
Pontelli et al. (Italy) (92)	Untreated—39 Treated—42	60 median	Methylprednisolone, 1 mg IV × 3 d Prednisone, 0.4 mg/kg × 27 d Chlorambucil, 0.2 mg/kg × 30 d Three cycles; total: 6 mo	"Produces sustained remission of nephrotic syndrome and helps preserve renal function."

study, pentoxifylline (1200 mg/day for 6 months), which suppresses the tumor necrosis factor-α cytokine, reduced proteinuria in ten adult patients from 4.6 to 27.0 g/day to 0.0 to 10.9 g/day without causing side effects (97).

Patients with NS may develop deep vein thrombosis, particularly renal vein thrombosis. Whether prophylactic anticoagulants should be used in these patients remains unsettled.

Clinical Course

The clinical course of idiopathic MN is variable. Some patients (particularly those with asymptomatic proteinuria) achieve spontaneous remission, others continue with NS, and some develop end-stage renal failure. A review of the literature (10,12,16,59,88) (Table 33.2) shows that after a variable follow-up ranging from 1.0 to 15.8 years, irrespective of treatment, 18% of the children develop chronic renal failure, 41% achieve remission, and 37% continue to have active disease but without renal failure. These results, however, need to be interpreted in light of the uncontrolled and retrospective nature of the studies and the variable follow-up time, ranging from 2.0 months to 15.8 years. It is important to note that all 29 patients who went to chronic renal failure had NS at onset or subsequently during the course. Hypertension at onset is associated with a less favorable outcome (Makker SP, *unpublished observation*, 2003) (10,12,16,46,59,88). There is insufficient information to determine the frequency of spontaneous remission in a child presenting with NS who is not treated or to determine the relationship between sex, age at onset, and renal failure at onset and the final outcome.

Resolution

Idiopathic MN is a chronic disease and, therefore, most likely involves continuous or multiple generations of deposits. Do children achieving complete remission (normal urine) stop forming new deposits, completely resolve their previous deposits, and normalize their GBMs? If these changes do occur, how long does it take? It is difficult to answer these questions because sequential renal biopsies after complete remissions are not often performed. We have studied the problem in active Heymann nephritis of the rat (98). Proteinuric MN kidneys were transplanted into normal, unilaterally nephrectomized syngeneic Lewis rats to follow the course of the resolution of established MN in a normal host, thus preventing any new generation of deposits. Sequential renal biopsies were performed over time (Fig. 33.5). We found that the resolution of the process was very slow. At 38 weeks, the deposits were still positively stained for rat IgG by immunofluorescence, and electron microscopy showed thickened lamina densa, irregular subepithelial contour, and lucent deposits in the lamina densa of GBM. This suggests that if a comparable pace of resolution occurs in humans, complete resolution in children will take several years, even after the cessation of new deposits.

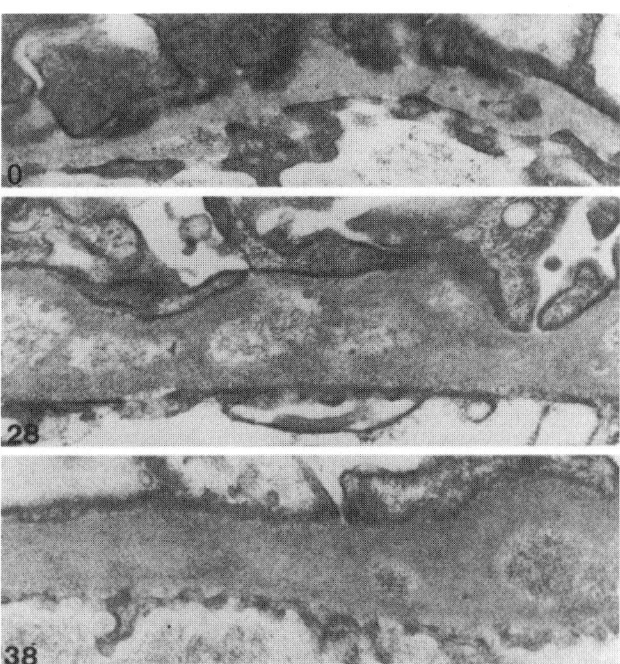

FIGURE 33.5. Ultrastructural findings in the transplanted Heymann nephritis rat kidney at weeks 0, 28, and 38 transplanted into a normal syngeneic Lewis rat. At 0 time, the subepithelial deposits are evident. After 28 weeks, the glomerular basement membrane is thickened, the subepithelial deposits have become lucent, and the subepithelial contour is irregular. At 38 weeks, the latter changes persist (×43,000). (Electron microscopy performed by Seymour Rosen, M.D., Harvard Medical School, Boston.)

MEMBRANOUS GLOMERULONEPHROPATHY ASSOCIATED WITH HEPATITIS B

Epidemiology

Many cases of MN associated with hepatitis B in children have been reported from several parts of the world, including the United States (99), Europe (8,44,46), Africa (41,43), and the Orient (20,21,39,100). The largest series of patients have come from Southeast Asia (20,21), consistent with the higher prevalence of HB$_s$Ag-carrier state. The prevalence of HB$_s$Ag carriers is approximately 0.3 to 1.0% in North America, 1.0% in western Europe, 7.0% in Africa, and 10.0% in Southeast Asia, where it is endemic (101). For instance, in Taiwan, 95% of all MN, excluding SLE, is due to hepatitis B (21). In these areas, vertical transmission from infected mothers to their children and horizontal transmission between siblings is likely because 33 to 36% of siblings of patients show a positive blood test for HB$_s$Ag (21). Transmission in adolescents through drug abuse or sex is also possible (102).

Clinical Features

Children with MN associated with hepatitis B, like the children with idiopathic MN, usually have NS or are detected during evaluation of persistent proteinuria (8,20,21,40–46,99,100).

Microscopic hematuria is common, and even macroscopic hematuria has occasionally been reported. Rarely, a patient may have only microscopic hematuria without proteinuria (20). In almost all large series, boys predominate overwhelmingly (75 to 80%) (8,20,21), as opposed to idiopathic MN, in which boys and girls are affected in approximately equal numbers (Table 33.2). Age at onset in large series has varied from 2 to 16 years. Retrospective analysis of symptomatology at onset reveals that patients start with flu-like illness consisting of low-grade fever, poor appetite, nausea, vomiting, and malaise, but usually no jaundice. After these symptoms subside, hematuria and proteinuria are noted (20). However, most come to attention because of the onset of edema as the result of MN, and evidence for hepatitis is discovered only during evaluation. The liver may be enlarged in some patients at onset.

Laboratory tests on serum for a profile of hepatitis B antigen and antibodies show a positive result for HB_sAg in all patients, usually a negative result for hepatitis B antibody, and a positive result for hepatitis B early antigen (HB_eAg) in more than 90% of patients (20,21). Serum levels of complement components C3 and C4 are usually low (21) at onset, but they may return to normal at some time during the course of the disease. Serum levels of liver transaminase enzymes may be elevated on presentation and, in some cases, persist chronically (8,20,40,44). Liver biopsies usually show chronic hepatitis (8,20). However, the long-term course of the liver disease remains to be studied. Hepatitis B–associated MN is suspected in a child with features of a glomerular disease (i.e., proteinuria, hematuria, or NS), who during laboratory evaluation is found to have a positive test result for HB_sAg in serum, and the diagnosis is established by renal biopsy. If serum complement C3 levels are low, it is an additional piece of evidence in favor of hepatitis B–associated MN versus idiopathic MN. On the basis of clinical manifestations alone at the time of presentation, the two conditions may be difficult to differentiate, and a high index of suspicion is necessary.

Pathology

The pathology of MN associated with hepatitis B is similar to that of idiopathic MN and is indistinguishable in most cases. The two conditions may be differentiated on the basis of demonstration of HB_eAg in the glomerular immune deposits by immunofluorescence microscopy. When Fab_2 portions of monoclonal antibodies to HB_sAg, hepatitis B core antigen (HB_cAg), and HB_eAg are used for detection, HB_eAg is present in most (90% or greater) patients with hepatitis-associated MN, but it is not seen in idiopathic MN (20,21,103). HB_sAg and HB_cAg were not detected in hepatitis-associated MN in these studies.

Pathogenesis

The exact pathogenesis of hepatitis B–associated MN is unknown, but a high frequency of HLA allele DQB1*0603 noted in South African children suggests a role for genetic factors (104). The presence of IgG in the subepithelial deposits shows that these deposits contain immune complexes. How the deposits are formed is unclear. Two hypotheses have been considered. According to the first, circulating immune complexes consisting of antigen(s) of hepatitis virus and their corresponding antibodies (elicited as the result of chronic infection) are trapped in the glomerulus and come to lie in the subepithelial space during the formation of glomerular ultrafiltrate. According to the second hypothesis, certain freely circulating hepatitis B virus antigens pass through the GBM during the process of ultrafiltration and are implanted in the subepithelial space. Theoretically, cationic antigens are more likely to pass through the GBM than anionic ones because of the anionic nature of the GBM. Once implanted, the deposits form by the binding of antibodies crossing the GBM from the circulation.

To prove either hypothesis, hepatitis antigen(s) must be demonstrated in the glomerular immune deposits. Indeed, hepatitis B antigens have been demonstrated in these deposits by immunofluorescence microscopy. Since the first study by Combes et al. (105), HB_sAg, HB_eAg, and HB_cAg have been detected by many investigators, but the findings have been inconsistent (41). Part of the explanation for the inconsistent results is the questionable specificity of the older reagents used in the earlier studies. Recent studies, as alluded to earlier, have used Fab_2 portions of the highly specific monoclonal antibodies (20,21,103) and have found that only HB_eAg (and not the other antigens) is present in the glomerular immune deposits, suggesting the importance of HB_eAg in pathogenesis. The molecular weight of free HB_eAg in circulation is approximately 100,000 daltons, and its isoelectric point is 4.8 (anionic). These physicochemical characteristics of HB_eAg probably do not favor the *in situ* hypothesis.

To substantiate the hypothetical circulating immune complex, complexes of the same antigen antibody specificity as those detected in the glomerular immune deposits and of a size and charge that would localize in subepithelial space must be demonstrated in circulation. The available information in this regard is limited and discordant (45). Takekoshi et al. (106) have demonstrated circulating immune complexes of HB_eAg and antibody of an approximate size greater than IgG in the serum of two children they studied. However, the problem is complicated by the fact that circulating immune complexes of hepatitis B antigens and antibody are present in patients with chronic hepatitis B infection without MN.

Treatment and Course

The course of hepatitis B–associated MN is variable, ranging from spontaneous recovery in some (106) to end-stage renal failure in others (42,107). Retrospective analysis of six studies (20,21,42,107–109) comprising a total of 82 children, most of whom had been treated with corticosteroids, showed that within 12 months after diagnosis, nearly 60% were in remission. The remainder had persistent disease, with 7.3% having chronic renal failure and 2.4% end-stage renal failure (103). In one large study of 52 patients from Taiwan (20), 38 of whom were treated with corticosteroids, 64% of the children were in remission at 1 year and 92% at 7 years after follow-up, and only one patient was in renal failure. Four children who received no treatment were in remission at 2 years. In another series of 70 patients from South Africa (110), 60 of whom were untreated, it was reported that the cumulative probability of remission was 64% at 4 years and 84% at 10 years; after 90 months of follow-up, three patients were still nephrotic, and two had developed end-stage renal failure. The average duration of proteinuria in these patients was 30 months, with remission of proteinuria usually occurring 6 months after clearance of HB_eAg from the serum. Overall, these two studies suggest that although there can be a prolonged period of morbidity, the eventual outcome in most of the children is favorable. On the other hand, in another study from Taiwan (20) of 32 patients treated with corticosteroids, 70.6% had persistent disease and 12.3% progressive disease after 2 years of follow-up, and HB_sAg in serum remained positive in most cases throughout the course of the disease, even among some who were in clinical remission (20,21). However, children whose serum became negative for HB_sAg were more likely to have remission than those whose serum remained positive for HB_sAg (20). The treatment for hepatitis-associated MN is evolving, but at present, there is no optimal and accepted treatment for hepatitis-associated MN in children. Corticosteroids do not appear to be beneficial and probably should not be used because they may enhance viral replication in mononuclear cells (111). Recently, recombinant human interferon-α (subcutaneous injections three times a week) has been reported to be beneficial (112). In this study, two groups of 20 patients each with persistent proteinuria and NS who had previously not shown a response to corticosteroids were either treated with recombinant human interferon-α for 1 year or given only supportive treatment. At the end of the study, all (20 of 20) treated patients were free of proteinuria; however, in the untreated patients, two were also free of proteinuria, 12 had mild proteinuria, and only six had persistent heavy proteinuria. Thus, without treatment, 70% of the patients showed improvement in proteinuria. All treated patients had flu-like symptoms in the first 2 weeks of therapy; later, 30% of the patients developed psychiatric problems. Longer follow-up of treated and untreated patients is needed to draw conclusions regarding the recommendation of this therapy.

MEMBRANOUS NEPHROPATHY ASSOCIATED WITH SYSTEMIC LUPUS ERYTHEMATOSUS

The histopathology of the renal lesion in some patients with SLE can have an appearance that is indistinguishable from the histology observed in idiopathic MN. In a large series of children from the United States who had renal involvement secondary to SLE, MN was present in nearly 10% (113). In another study from the United States, 10 of 64 patients evaluated for MN had SLE as the underlying cause (12). However, in a study from France (18), only 2 of 65 children with MN had SLE.

Children with MN associated with SLE commonly have features of a glomerular disease associated with other extrarenal manifestations of SLE. These usually include hematuria and proteinuria, with or without NS and with or without hypertension or renal failure. However, patients may have only a glomerular disease and no other manifestations of SLE. Laboratory tests on serum for SLE are usually positive (i.e., antinuclear antibodies, anti–double-stranded DNA antibodies, and low serum complement C3 and C4). However, occasionally all clinical manifestations may be absent, and the laboratory tests for SLE may be negative at presentation and become positive only later; in some cases, this may be years. Patients with inherited deficiency of the second component of complement are prone to develop SLE, and these patients may present initially with MN and later develop SLE. Renal biopsy findings of SLE-associated MN and idiopathic MN may be identical. However, presence of mesangial deposits and strong positive staining of the deposits for C1q and C4, as strong as the staining for C3, are suspicious of SLE. The treatment of MN associated with SLE is similar to the treatment of other SLE patients with renal involvement, including the use of corticosteroids and cytotoxic drugs.

MEMBRANOUS NEPHROPATHY IN RENAL ALLOGRAFTS

MN in a renal allograft may develop *de novo* or as a result of the recurrence of the original idiopathic MN. The recurrence rate in adults has been reported to vary from 26.3 (114) to 50.0% (115). Because of the paucity of cases, the recurrence rate in children is unknown. Several cases of *de novo* MN in the transplanted kidney have been reported (37). In children, the incidence of *de novo* occurrence of MN in transplanted kidneys is estimated to be approximately 1 to 2% (36,116), but in one large series from France, 9.3% of the renal transplants in children developed *de novo* MN (36). Part of the reason for the higher incidence in this report may be the greater frequency of routine renal transplant biopsies. MN was discovered in nine patients by the latter approach, with none of them having proteinuria, suggesting that the actual incidence of the condition is higher. In other patients, it is discovered during evaluation of proteinuria, NS, or a suspected rejection. The pathogenesis of *de novo* MN is not understood. However, there is a high rate of recurrence of the *de novo* MN in the second allograft, suggesting that host factors play a role

(36). No correlation between the development of *de novo* MN and age or sex of the patient, the original disease producing end-stage renal failure, and the time between the transplant and the onset of MN has been observed. However, ureteral obstruction (116,117) and a good histocompatibility match (118,119) could be possible predisposing factors. The course of *de novo* MN is variable. Some patients never even develop proteinuria, whereas others develop NS; in some, it may contribute to the deterioration of renal function in association with chronic rejection. In general, the demise of the graft is more often caused by the rejection process than the *de novo* MN.

MEMBRANOUS NEPHROPATHY ASSOCIATED WITH OTHER INFECTIONS

MN may be associated with a number of other infections (Table 33.1). Congenital syphilis should be considered in the differential diagnosis in any infant presenting with NS. Infants with congenital syphilis also often have other clinical features of congenital syphilis, and most have microscopic hematuria. The diagnosis can be confirmed by a positive serologic test result for syphilis. Complement levels of CH50, C3, and C4 are low at onset and return to normal after treatment with penicillin (21). Renal biopsy findings are similar to those of idiopathic MN, except that staining to C1q is commonly present (22). Treponema antigen has been demonstrated in the glomerular immune deposits (120). Early treatment with penicillin leads to complete recovery. This emphasizes that the physician needs to be aware that (a) a potentially curable condition can be the cause of NS in infants, and (b) once the offending agent has been eradicated, MN can resolve.

Other parasitic infections, such as malaria, filaria, and hydatid disease, can produce MN and should be considered in the differential diagnosis when exposure to these parasites is suspected. Leprosy and schistosomiasis have been associated with MN in adults (6).

MEMBRANOUS NEPHROPATHY ASSOCIATED WITH DRUGS AND TOXINS

MN has been reported in association with a number of drugs and toxins in adults, including gold, mercury, captopril, fenoprofen, penicillamine (6,18), and, more recently, mercaptopropionylglycine (121). A few cases in children associated with penicillamine used to treat cystinuria, Wilson's disease, and rheumatoid arthritis have also been reported (8,17). Generally, there is no relationship to the dose or duration of treatment, and proteinuria disappears once the drugs are withdrawn. Recently, in two children, MN was reported to be associated with exposure to formaldehyde (32).

MEMBRANOUS NEPHROPATHY ASSOCIATED WITH TUMORS

MN has been associated with a number of malignancies in adults (6,122)—the most common being bronchogenic carcinoma, gastric carcinoma, and adenocarcinoma of the colon. A few cases have also been reported in children (Table 33.1). In two cases reported in children (33,34), resolution of MN was observed after excision of the tumor.

MEMBRANOUS NEPHROPATHY ASSOCIATED WITH OTHER DISORDERS

In addition to SLE, MN has been reported with a number of other autoimmune and immunologic diseases. Cases in children have been reported with enteropathy (27), Crohn's disease (28,29), pemphigus (30), multiple sclerosis (31), immune thrombocytopenic purpura (123), and sarcoidosis (124). In a recent report of MN associated with enteropathy (27), autoantibodies to a 55-kDa epithelial cell protein common to intestine and kidney were detected in the serum of the child and were temporally related to the development of enteropathy and MN.

A distinct entity consisting of antitubular basement membrane–associated tubulointerstitial nephritis, Fanconi's syndrome, and MN has been recognized (26). All of the reported children except for one with this disease have been boys. The tubular autoantigen is a 58-kDa protein that is located in the basement membrane of the proximal tubule (125). The glomerular autoantigen is a 600-kDa protein (gp600/gp330/megalin/LRP II) (26). Isolated cases of MN are associated with a number of other conditions in children (Table 33.1).

REFERENCES

1. Bell ET. A clinical and pathological study of subacute and chronic glomerulonephritis, including lipoid nephrosis. *Am J Pathol* 1938;14:691–736.
2. Bell ET. *Renal diseases*, 2nd ed. Philadelphia: Lea & Febiger, 1950.
3. Jones DB. Nephrotic glomerulonephritis. *Am J Pathol* 1957; 33:313–329.
4. Movat HZ, McGregor DD. The fine structure of the glomerulus in membranous glomerulonephritis (lipoid nephrosis) in adults. *Am J Clin Pathol* 1959;32:109–127.
5. Mellors RC, Ortega LG, Holman HR. Role of gamma globulins in pathogenesis of renal lesions in systemic lupus erythematosus and chronic membranous glomerulonephritis, with an observation on the lupus erythematosus cell reaction. *J Exp Med* 1957;106:191–202.
6. Rosen S, Tornroth T, Bernard DB. Membranous glomerulonephritis. In: Tisher CC, Brenner BM, eds. *Renal pathology with clinical and functional correlations.* Philadelphia: JB Lippincott Co, 1989:196–227.

7. Heptinstall RH. Membranous glomerulonephritis. In: Heptinstall RH, ed. *Pathology of the kidney*. Boston: Little, Brown and Company, 1983:519–555.
8. Kleinknecht C, Habib R. Membranous glomerulonephritis. In: Holliday MA, Barratt TM, Vernier RL, eds. *Pediatric nephrology*. Baltimore: Williams & Wilkins, 1987:462–470.
9. Olbing H, Greifer I, Bennet BP, et al. Idiopathic membranous nephropathy in children. *Kidney Int* 1973;3:381–390.
10. Habib R, Kleinknecht C, Gubler MC. Extramembranous glomerulonephritis in children: report of 50 cases. *J Pediatr* 1973;82:754–766.
11. Latham P, Poucell S, Koresaar A, et al. Idiopathic membranous glomerulopathy in Canadian children: a clinicopathologic study. *J Pediatr* 1982;101:682–685.
12. Southwest Pediatric Nephrology Study Group. Comparison of idiopathic and systemic lupus erythematosus associated membranous glomerulonephritis in children. *Am J Kidney Dis* 1986;7:115–124.
13. Doi T, Mayumi M, Kanatsu K, et al. Distribution of IgG subclasses in membranous nephropathy. *Clin Exp Immunol* 1984;58:57–62.
14. Hinglais N, Kazatchkine MD, Bhakdi S, et al. Immunohistochemical study of the C5b-9 complex of complement in human kidneys. *Kidney Int* 1986;30:399–410.
15. Lai KN, Lo ST, Lai FM. Immunohistochemical study of the membrane attack complex of complement and S-protein in idiopathic and secondary membranous nephropathy. *Am J Pathol* 1989;135:469–476.
16. Ramirez F, Brouhard BH, Travis LB, et al. Idiopathic membranous nephropathy in children. *J Pediatr* 1982;101:677–681.
17. Locard-Bisot S, Cochat P, Gilly J, et al. Membranous glomerulonephritis in children: 20 cases. *Pediatrics* 1990;45:527–532.
18. Kleinknecht C, Levy M, Gagnadoux MF, et al. Membranous glomerulonephritis with extra-renal disorders in children. *Medicine* 1979;58:219–228.
19. Cameron JS. Membranous nephropathy in childhood and its treatment. *Pediatr Nephrol* 1990;4:193–198.
20. Hsu HC, Wu CY, Lin CY, et al. Membranous nephropathy in 52 hepatitis B surface antigen (HBsAg) carrier children in Taiwan. *Kidney Int* 1989;36:1103–1107.
21. Lin CY. Hepatitis B virus-associated membraneous nephropathy: clinical features, immunological profiles and outcome. *Nephron* 1990;55:37–44.
22. Sanchez-Bayle M, Ecija JL, Estepa R, et al. Incidence of glomerulonephritis in congenital syphilis. *Clin Nephrol* 1983;20:27–31.
23. Schillinger F, Montagnac R, Goclowski C, et al. Glomerulonephrite extra-membraneuse de la syphilis acquise chez un malade recemment par le virus de l'hepatite B. Mise en evidence au niveau du rein de l'antigene treponemique par immunofluorescence indirecte. *Presse Med* 1983;12:153–156.
24. Hendrickise RG, Adeniyi A. Quartan malarial nephrotic syndrome in children. *Kidney Int* 1979;16:67–74.
25. Ngu JL, Chatelanat F, Leke R, et al. Nephropathy in Cameroon: evidence for filarial derived immune-complex pathogenesis in some cases. *Clin Nephrol* 1985;24:128–134.
26. Makker S, Widstrom R, Huang J. Membranous nephropathy, interstitial nephritis, and Fanconi syndrome—glomerular antigen. *Pediatr Nephrol* 1996;10:7–13.
27. Colletti RB, Guillot AP, Rosen S, et al. Autoimmune enteropathy and nephropathy with circulating anti-epithelial cell antibodies. *J Pediatr* 1991;118:858–864.
28. O'Loughlin EV, Robson L, Scott B, et al. Membranous glomerulonephritis in a patient with Crohn's disease of the small bowel. *J Pediatr Gastroenterol Nutr* 1985;4:135–139.
29. Glasman M, Kaplan M, Spivak W. Immune-complex glomerulonephritis in Crohn's disease. *J Pediatr Gastroenterol Nutr* 1986;5:966–999.
30. Esterley NB, Gotoff SP, Lolekha S, et al. Bullous pemphigoid and membranous glomerulonephropathy in a child. *J Pediatr* 1973;83:466–470.
31. Campos A, Gieron M, Gunasakeran S, et al. Membranous nephropathy associated with multiple sclerosis. *Pediatr Nephrol* 1993;9:64–66.
32. Breysse P, Couser W, Alpers C, et al. Membranous nephropathy and formaldehyde exposure. *Ann Intern Med* 1994;120: 396–397.
33. Beauvais P, Vaudour G, Boccon Gibod L, et al. Membranous nephropathy associated with ovarian tumour in a young girl: recovery after removal. *Eur J Pediatr* 1989;148:624–625.
34. Zheng HL, Maruyama T, Matsuda S, et al. Neuroblastoma presenting with the nephrotic syndrome. *J Pediatr Surg* 1979; 14:414–419.
35. Lopez JA, Lario Munoz A, Rosa Arias J, et al. Wilms' tumor associated with membranous glomerulonephritis. *Arch Esp Urol* 1989;42:163–165.
36. Heidet L, Gagnadoux M, Beziau A, et al. Recurrence of de novo membranous glomerulonephritis in renal grafts. *Clin Nephrol* 1994;41:314–318.
37. Gallego N, Olivares F, Mampaso F, et al. Membranous nephropathy, antitubular basement membrane antibodies and alveolar hemorrhage in a diabetic child. *Child Nephrol Urol* 1990;10:154–157.
38. McDonald DT, Roy LP. Micro-angiopathic haemolysis, thrombocytopenia and nephrotic syndrome associated with membranous nephropathy in a Vietnamese boy. *Aust Paediatr J* 1988;24:311–313.
39. Rodriguez-Soriano J, Fidalgo I, Camarero C, et al. Juvenile cirrhosis and membranous glomerulonephritis in a child with alpha-1-antitrypsin deficiency PiSZ. *Acta Paediatr Scand* 1978; 67:793–796.
40. Takekoshi Y, Tanaka M, Shida N, et al. Strong association between membranous nephropathy and hepatitis B surface antigenaemia in Japanese children. *Lancet* 1978;2:1065–1068.
41. Levy J, Kleinknecht C. Membranous glomerulonephritis and hepatitis B infection. *Nephron* 1980;26:259–265.
42. Seggie J, Nathoo K, Davies PG. Association of hepatitis B (HBs) antigenaemia and membranous glomerulonephritis in Zimbabwean children. *Nephron* 1984;38:115–119.
43. Wiggelinkhuizen J, Sinclair Smith C, Stannard LM, et al. Hepatitis B virus associated membranous glomerulonephritis. *Arch Dis Child* 1983;58:488–496.
44. Brzosko WJ, Krawczynski K, Nazarewica T, et al. Glomerulonephritis associated with hepatitis B surface antigen immune complexes in children. *Lancet* 1974;2:478–482.
45. Navarro M, Meseguer CG, Larrausi M. Hepatitis B antigenemia and nephropathy in children. *Int J Pediatr Nephrol* 1982;3:136–139.

46. del Vecchio-Blanco C, Polito C, del Vaporaso Gado R, et al. Membranous glomerulopathy and hepatitis B virus (HBV) infection in children. *Int J Pediatr Nephrol* 1983; 4:235–238.
47. Yoshikawa Y, Truong LD, Mattioli CA, et al. Membranous glomerulonephritis in diabetic patients: a study of 15 cases and review of the literature. *Mod Pathol* 1990;3:36–42.
48. Sato Y, Sasaki M, Kan R, et al. Thyroid antigen-mediated glomerulonephritis in Graves' disease. *Clin Nephrol* 1989;31: 49–52.
49. Carella G, Marra L, Bevilacqua E. A case of membranous glomerulonephritis in the course of primary biliary cirrhosis. *Am J Gastroenterol* 1989;84:579–580.
50. Pettersson E, Tornroth T, Miettinen A. Simultaneous anti-glomerular basement membrane and membranous glomerulonephritis: case report and literature review. *Clin Immunol Immunopathol* 1984;31:171–180.
51. Druet P. Contribution of immunological reactions to nephrotoxicity. *Toxicol Lett* 1989;46:55–64.
52. Klouda PT, Acheson EJ, Goldby FS, et al. Strong association between idiopathic membranous nephropathy and HLA-DRw3. *Lancet* 1979;2:770–771.
53. Sachs S, Warner C, Campbell D, et al. Molecular mapping of HLA class II region in HLA-DR3 associated idiopathic membranous nephropathy. *Kidney Int* 1993;43(Suppl 39): 14–19.
54. Vaughan RW, Demaine AG, Welsh KI. A DQA1 allele is strongly associated with idiopathic membranous nephropathy. *Tissue Antigens* 1989;34:261–269.
55. Elshihabi I, Kaye C, Brzowski A. Membranous nephropathy in two human leukocyte antigen-identical brothers. *J Pediatr* 1993;123:940–942.
56. Mezzano S, Rojas G, Ardiles L, et al. Idiopathic membranous nephropathy, associated with HLA-DRw3 and not related to monocyte-phagocyte system Fc receptor dysfunction, in father and son. *Nephron* 1991;58:320–324.
57. Yoshikawa N, Kitagawa K, Ohta K, et al. Asymptomatic constant isolated proteinuria in children. *J Pediatr* 1991;119: 375–379.
58. Barnett H. The natural and treatment history of glomerular diseases in children—what can we learn from cooperative studies? Proceedings of the VIth Congress of the ISN 1976: 470–485.
59. Trainin EB, Boichis H, Spitzer A, et al. Idiopathic membranous nephropathy. Clinical course in children. *N Y State J Med* 1976;76:357–360.
60. Glasrock RJ, Adler SG, Ward HJ, et al. Primary glomerular diseases. In: Brenner BM, Rector FC Jr, eds. *The kidney.* Philadelphia: WB Saunders, 1991:1238–1244.
61. Coggins CH. Membranous nephropathy. In: Schrier RW, Gottschalk CW, eds. *Strauss and Welt's diseases of the kidney.* Boston: Little, Brown and Company 1988:2005–2033.
62. Makker SP, Moorthy B. In situ immune complex formation in isolated perfused kidney using homologous antibody. *Lab Invest* 1981;42:1–5.
63. Van Damme BJ, Fleuren GJ, Bakker WW, et al. Experimental glomerulonephritis in the rat induced by antibodies directed against tubular antigen. V. Fixed glomerular antigens in the pathogenesis of heterologous immune complex glomerulonephritis. *Lab Invest* 1978;38:502–510.
64. Couser WG, Steinmuller DR, Stillmant MM, et al. Experimental glomerulonephritis in the isolated perfused rat kidney. *J Clin Invest* 1978;62:1275–1287.
65. Makker SP, Singh AK. Characterization of the antigen (gp600) of Heymann nephritis. *Lab Invest* 1984;50:287–293.
66. Kerjaschki D, Farquhar MG. The pathogenic antigen of Heymann nephritis is a glycoprotein of the renal proximal tubule brush border. *Proc Natl Acad Sci U S A* 1982;79: 5557–5561.
67. Kerjaschki D, Farquhar MG. Immunocytochemical localization of the Heymann nephritis antigen (gp330) in glomerular epithelial cells of normal Lewis rats. *J Exp Med* 1983;157:667–686.
68. Olenikov AV, Brady F , Makker SP. A small N-terminal 60k-D fragment of gp600 (megalin), the major autoantigen of active Heymann nephritis can induce a full-blown disease. *J Am Soc Nephrol* 2000;11:57–64
69. Makker SP, Kirson I. Immune complex induced nephrotic syndrome (NS) with circulating brush border antibody (BBab) to human Fx1A in an infant immunopathologically similar to Heymann nephritis (HN) of rats. *Kidney Int* 1979; 16:912.
70. Douglas MFS, Rabideau DP, Schwartz MM, et al. Evidence on autologous immune complex nephritis. *N Engl J Med* 1981;305:1326–1329.
71. Niles J, Collins B, Baird L, et al. Antibodies reactive with a renal glycoprotein and with deposits in membranous nephritis. *Kidney Int* 1987;31:338.
72. Makker SP, Kanalas JJ. Autoantibodies to human gp330 in sera of patients with idiopathic membranous glomerulonephropathy. *Kidney Int* 1989;35:211.
73. Debiec H, Guigonis V, Mougenot B, et al. Antenatal membranous glomerulonephritis due to anti-neutral endopeptidase antibodies. *N Engl J Med* 2002;346:2053–2060.
74. Camussi G, Brentjens JR, Noble B, et al. Antibody-induced redistribution of Heymann antigen on the surface of cultured glomerular visceral epithelial cells: possible role in the pathogenesis of Heymann glomerulonephritis. *J Immunol* 1985;135:2409–2416.
75. Couser WG, Baker PJ, Adler S. Complement and the direct mediation of glomerular injury: a new perspective. *Kidney Int* 1985;28:879–891.
76. De Heer E, Daha MR, Bhakdi S, et al. Possible involvement of terminal complement complex in active Heymann nephritis. *Kidney Int* 1985;27:388–393.
77. Makker S. Analysis of glomeruli-eluted gp330 autoantibodies and of gp330 antigen of Heymann nephritis. *J Immunol* 1993;151:6500–6508.
78. Kerjaschki D, Matthias S, Binder S, et al. Transcellular transport and membrane insertion of the C5b-9 membrane attack complex of complement by glomerular epithelial cells on experimental membranous nephropathy. *J Immunol* 1989; 143:546–552.
79. Shah S. Evidence suggesting a role for hydroxyl radical in passive Heymann nephritis. *Am J Physiol* 1988;245:F337–F344.
80. McMillan J, Riordan J, Couser W, et al. Characterization of a glomerular epithelial cell metalloproteinase as matrix metalloproteinase-9 with enhanced expression in a model of

membranous nephropathy. *J Clin Invest* 1996;97;1094–1101.

81. Cybulsky AV, Papillon J, McTavish AJ. Complement activates phospholipases and protein kinases in glomerular epithelial cells. *Kidney Int* 1998;54:360–372.
82. Kon S, Coupes B, Short C, et al. Urinary C5b-9 excretion and clinical course in idiopathic membranous nephropathy. *Kidney Int* 1995;48:1953–1958.
83. Border WA, Ward JH, Kamil ES, et al. Induction of membranous nephropathy in rabbits by administration of an exogenous cationic antigen. Demonstration of a pathogenic role for electrical charge. *J Clin Invest* 1982;69:451–461.
84. Caulin-Glasser T, Gallo GR, Lamm ME. Nondissociating cationic immune complexes can deposit in glomerular basement membrane. *J Exp Med* 1983;158:1561–1572.
85. Gansevoort RT, Heeg JE, Vriesendorp R, et al. Antiproteinuric drugs in patients with idiopathic membranous glomerulopathy. *Nephrol Dial Transplant* 1992;7(Suppl 1):91–96.
86. Jafar TH, Schmid CH, Landa M, et al. Angiotensin-converting enzyme inhibitors and progression of nondiabetic renal diseases: a meta-analysis of patient-level data. *Ann Intern Med* 2001;135:73–87.
87. Fried LF, Orchard TJ, Kasiske BL. Effect of lipid reduction on the progression of renal disease: a meta-analysis. *Kidney Int* 2001;59:260–269.
88. Tsukahara H, Takahashi Y, Yoshimoto M, et al. Clinical course and outcome of idiopathic membranous nephropathy in Japanese children. *Pediatr Nephrol* 1993;7:387–391.
89. Collaborative study of the adult idiopathic nephrotic syndrome. A controlled study of short term prednisone treatment in adults with membranous nephropathy. *N Engl J Med* 1979;301:1301–1306.
90. Cattran DC, Delmore T, Roscoe J, et al. A randomized controlled trial of prednisone in patients with idiopathic membranous nephropathy. *N Engl J Med* 1989;320:210–215.
91. Cameron JS, Healy MJR, Adu D. The Medical Research Council trial of short term high dose alternate day prednisolone in idiopathic membranous nephropathy with a nephrotic syndrome in adults. *QJM* 1990;74:133–156.
92. Ponticelli C, Zucchelli P, Passerini P, et al. A randomized trial of methylprednisolone and chlorambucil in idiopathic membranous nephropathy. *N Engl J Med* 1989;320:8–13.
93. Ponticelli C, Zucchelli P, Passerini P, et al. A 10-year follow-up of a randomized study with methylprednisolone and chlorambucil in membranous nephropathy. *Kidney Int* 1995;48:1600–1604.
94. Ponticelli C, Zucchelli P, Passerin IP, et al. Methylprednisolone and chlorambucil as compared to methylprednisolone alone for the treatment of idiopathic membranous nephropathy. *N Engl J Med* 1992;327:599–603.
95. Cattran D, Greenwood C, Ritchie S, et al. A controlled trial of cyclosporine in patients with progressive membranous nephropathy. *Kidney Int* 1995;47:1130–1135.
96. Cattran DC, Appel GB, Hebert LA, etal. Cyclosporine in patients with steroid-resistant membranous nephropathy: a randomised trial. *Kidney Int* 2001;59:1484–1490.
97. Ducloux D, Bresson-Vautrin C, Chalopin JM. Use of pentoxifylline in membranous nephropathy. *Lancet* 2001;357:1672–1673.
98. Makker SP, Kanalas JJ. Course of transplanted Heymann nephritis kidney in normal host: implications for mechanism of proteinuria in membranous glomerulonephropathy. *J Immunol* 1989;142:3406–3410.
99. Southwest Pediatric Nephrology Study Group. Hepatitis B surface antigenemia in North American children with membranous glomerulonephropathy. *J Pediatr* 1985;106:571–578.
100. Yoshikawa N, Ito H, Yamada Y, et al. Membranous glomerulonephritis associated with hepatitis B antigen in children: a comparison with idiopathic membranous glomerulonephritis. *Clin Nephrol* 1985;23:28–34.
101. Szmuness W, Harley EJ, Ikram H, et al. Sociodemographic aspects of the epidemiology of hepatitis B. In: Vyas GN, Cohen SN, Schmid R, eds. *Viral hepatitis*. Philadelphia: Franklin Institute, 1978:297–320.
102. McCollum RW, Zuckerman AJ. Viral hepatitis: report on WHO informal consultation. *J Med Virol* 1981;8:1–29.
103. Lai KN, Li PKT, Lui SF, et al. Membranous nephropathy related to hepatitis B virus in adults. *N Engl J Med* 1991; 324:1457–1463.
104. Bhimma R, Hammond MG, Coovadia HM, et al. HLA class I and II in black children with hepatitis B virus-associated membranous nephropathy. *Kidney Int* 2002;61:1510-1515.
105. Combes B, Stastny P, Shorey J, et al. Glomerulonephritis with deposition of Australia antigen-antibody complexes in glomerular basement membrane. *Lancet* 1971;2:234–237.
106. Takekoshi Y, Tanaka M, Miyakawa Y, et al. Free "small" and IgG-associated "large" hepatitis B e antigen in the serum and glomerular capillary walls of two patients with membranous glomerulonephritis. *N Engl J Med* 1979;300:814–819.
107. Kleinknecht C, Levy M, Peix A, et al. Membranous glomerulonephritis and hepatitis B surface antigen in children. *J Pediatr* 1979;95:946–952.
108. Furuse A, Hattori S, Terashima T, et al. Circulating immune complex in glomerulonephropathy associated with hepatitis B virus infection. *Nephron* 1982;31:212–218.
109. Ito H, Hattori S, Matusda I, et al. Hepatitis B e antigen-mediated membranous glomerulonephritis. *Lab Invest* 1981; 44:214–220.
110. Gilbert R, Wiggenlinkuizen J. The clinical course of hepatitis B virus-associated nephropathy. *Pediatr Nephrol* 1994;8: 11–14.
111. Lin CY, Lo S. Treatment of hepatitis B virus-associated membranous nephropathy with adenine arabinoside and thymic extract. *Kidney Int* 1991;39:301–306.
112. Lin CY. Treatment of hepatitis B virus-associated membranous nephropathy with recombinant alfa-interferon. *Kidney Int* 1995;47:225–230.
113. Platt JL, Burke BA, Fish AJ, et al. Systemic lupus erythematosus in the first two decades of life. *Am J Kidney Dis* 1982; 2:212–222.
114 Couchoud C, Pouteil-Noble C, Colon S, et al. Recurrence of membranous nephropathy after renal transplantation. *Transplantation* 1995;59:1275–1279.
115. Marcen R, Mampaso F, Teruel J, et al. Membranous nephropathy occurrence after kidney transplantation. *Nephrol Dial Transplant* 1996;6:1129–1133.

116. Gomez-Campdera FJ, Niembro E. "De novo" membranous glomerulonephritis in renal allografts in children. *Clin Nephrol* 1989;31:279.
117. Hoitsma AJ, Kroon AA, Wetzels JF, et al. Association between ureteral obstruction and de novo membranous nephropathy in renal allografts. *Transplant Proc* 1990;22:1388–1389.
118. Cosyns JP, Pirson Y, Squifflet JP, et al. De novo membranous nephropathy in human renal allografts: report of 9 patients. *Kidney Int* 1982;22:177–183.
119. Bansal UK, Koseny GA, Fresco R, et al. De novo membranous nephropathy following renal transplantation between conjoint twins. *Transplantation* 1986;41:404–406.
120. O'Regan S, Fong JSC, de Chadarevian JP, et al. Treponemal antigens in congenital and acquired syphilitic nephritis. *Ann Intern Med* 1976;85:325–327.
121. Lindell A, Denneberg T, Enestrom S, et al. Membranous glomerulonephritis induced by 2-mercaptopropionylglycine (2-MPG). *Clin Nephrol* 1990;34:108–115.
122. Brueggemeyer CD, Ramirez G. Membranous nephropathy: a concern for malignancy. *Am J Kidney Dis* 1987;9:23–26.
123. Lande MB, Thomas GA, Houghton DC. Membranous nephropathy associated with chronic immune thrombocytopenic purpura in childhood. *Am J Kidney Dis* 2001;37:E40.
124. Dimitriades C, Shetty AK, Vehaskari M, et al. Membranous nephropathy associated with childhood sarcoidosis. *Pediatr Nephrol* 1999;13:444–447.
125. Katz A, Fish A, Santamaria P, et al. Role of tubulointerstitial nephritis antigen I human antitubular basement membrane nephritis associated with membranous nephropathy. *Am J Med* 1992;93:691–698.

34

CRESCENTIC GLOMERULONEPHRITIS

MICHAEL J. DILLON

Crescentic glomerulonephritis is the histopathologic correlate of the clinically defined condition of rapidly progressive glomerulonephritis (RPGN) (1). It is relatively rare in childhood (2–9) and is characterized by the presence of extensive crescents demonstrable on renal biopsy and by sudden and progressive decline in renal function. It can accompany most forms of primary glomerulonephritis in childhood and can be associated with various systemic disorders [e.g., systemic lupus erythematosus (SLE)] and several forms of systemic vasculitis (2,3,7,8). The severity of the condition, the multiple etiologies, and the well-recognized poor prognosis have resulted in the use of multiple treatment regimens, the efficacy of which have been difficult to assess (10), and there has been a lack of clarity in identifying variables with therapeutic and prognostic implications.

DEFINITION

There are a number of definitions of *crescentic glomerulonephritis*, and this varied nomenclature has created problems in data interpretation and comparing outcomes of treated patients. There is general agreement that crescentic glomerulonephritis is defined by the presence of large epithelial crescents within Bowman's space, but the appearance of the crescents and the number required for the diagnosis are arguable. In childhood, more than 75% (3), 50% or more (2,7), and occasionally as few as 20% of glomeruli affected have been considered to represent crescentic glomerulonephritis (5). In a series described by Neild et al. (11) of 39 patients with RPGN and extensive crescent formation, ten patients younger than 14 years of age had greater than 60% of glomeruli affected. However, in another series of 13 children with RPGN, Cunningham et al. (4) reported the number of glomeruli affected as varying from 10 to 100%. In other series with undoubtedly crescentic glomerulonephritis, the clinical factors have been emphasized irrespective of the number of crescents (12).

Jardim et al. (7) considered that crescentic glomerulonephritis was present when large epithelial crescents, filling Bowman's space, occurred in 50% or more of glomeruli present in a renal biopsy specimen, irrespective of any changes in the underlying glomerular tuft. In addition, crescents were divided into *cellular*, *fibrocellular*, or *fibrous* categories according to their histopathologic appearances and were further subcategorized according to other criteria, including changes in the glomerular tuft, immunochemical staining, and clinicopathologic correlations.

INCIDENCE

The real incidence of crescentic glomerulonephritis in children is unknown. It comprises 2 to 5% of all cases of glomerulonephritis in adults (13); Andrassy et al. (14) calculated the annual incidence in Germany to be 0.7 per 100,000 adults. Miller et al. (15) reported crescentic lesions in 56 of 372 children with glomerular pathology on renal biopsy; in 26, there was a clinical course compatible with RPGN. These data are not dissimilar to those quoted for adults, emphasizing the relative rarity of the condition in children.

CAUSES

There are a number of ways of considering the causes of crescentic glomerulonephritis. There are classifications that consider the immunofluorescence staining patterns on renal biopsy and subdivide disorders according to the appearances into (a) anti–glomerular basement membrane (GBM) antibody disease; (b) no staining or pauci-immune disease; and (c) immune complex disease (13,16). Using these criteria, the most frequently observed pattern in childhood (in contrast to adults) is immune complex disease, constituting 80% of cases, with pauci-immune and anti-GBM disease making up the remainder in a ratio of 2:1 (2,7,13).

Other classifications consider RPGN or crescentic glomerulonephritis under headings of disease category (e.g., anti-GBM disease), primary systemic vasculitis, other disorders (e.g., SLE), primary glomerulonephritis, infection-associated glomerulonephritis, and miscellaneous causes (Table 34.1).

In four large series of childhood patients with crescentic glomerulonephritis reported from the United States, France,

TABLE 34.1. CAUSES OF CRESCENTIC GLOMERULONEPHRITIS IN CHILDHOOD

Anti-GBM antibody disease
- Anti-GBM nephritis, Goodpasture's syndrome, with perinuclear antineutrophil cytoplasmic antibody–associated microscopic polyangiopathy, posttransplantation in Alport's syndrome

Primary systemic vasculitis
- Henoch-Schönlein purpura, microscopic polyarteritis or polyangiopathy, idiopathic crescentic nephritis, Wegener's granulomatosis, Churg-Strauss syndrome

Systemic disorders
- SLE, Behçet's syndrome, Weber-Christian disease, relapsing polychondritis, essential mixed cryoglobulinemia, mixed connective tissue disease, dermatomyositis, juvenile rheumatoid arthritis, Sjögren's syndrome, sarcoidosis

Primary glomerulonephritis
- Mesangiocapillary glomerulonephritis, IgA nephropathy, membranous nephropathy

Infection-related glomerulonephritis
- Poststreptococcal glomerulonephritis, legionella, mycoplasma, syphilis, hepatitis B and C, tuberculosis, human immunodeficiency virus, bacterial endocarditis, shunt nephritis, leprosy, visceral abscess

After medication
- Penicillamine, rifampicin and hydralazine, enalapril, interleukin-2, interferon-α, phenylbutazone, propylthiouracil, isoniazid

Miscellaneous causes
- Malignant tumors, leukemia and lymphomas, silicosis, alpha-1-antitrypsin deficiency, hyper-IgD syndrome

After transplantation
- Anti-GBM disease in Alport's syndrome (mentioned above), recurrence of IgA nephropathy and mesangiocapillary glomerulonephritis, anti-GBM, Henoch-Schönlein purpura, SLE

GBM, glomerular basement membrane; Ig, immunoglobulin; SLE, systemic lupus erythematosus.

the United Kingdom, and India, the pattern of disease was similar but there was variation, as might be expected, between centers (2,3,7,8).

The Southwest Pediatric Nephrology Study Group (2) reported on 50 children with histologically 50% or more glomeruli affected by crescents. Thirteen had nonspecified immune complex disease, nine had SLE, seven had idiopathic (nonimmune complex) crescentic glomerulonephritis, six had poststreptococcal glomerulonephritis, four had immunoglobulin (Ig) A nephropathy, three had Henoch-Schönlein purpura, three had vasculitis, three had possible anti-GBM disease, and two had dense deposit disease (Table 34.2).

Niaudet and Levy (3) reported the findings in 41 children with more than 75% crescents on biopsy. Eleven had Henoch-Schönlein purpura, nine had membranoproliferative glomerulonephritis, five had acute glomerulonephritis, three had anti-GBM disease, three had IgA nephropathy, three had polyarteritis, three had glomerulonephritis without evidence of deposits, two had immune complex glomerulonephritis, one had SLE, and one had shunt nephritis (Table 34.2).

Jardim et al. (7) described 30 children with 50% or more crescents on biopsy. Of these, nine had Henoch-Schönlein purpura, seven had mesangiocapillary glomerulonephritis (type I in six and type III in one), five had vasculitis (three had microscopic polyarteritis, one had polyarteritis nodosa, and one had Wegener's granulomatosis), four had idiopathic crescentic nephritis, two had poststreptococcal glomerulonephritis, two had anti-GBM disease, and one had SLE (Table 34.2).

Srivastava et al. (8) reported 43 children with crescents in more than 50% of glomeruli. Of these, 11 had poststreptococcal glomerulonephritis; six had an underlying

TABLE 34.2. CAUSES OF CRESCENTIC GLOMERULONEPHRITIS IN CHILDREN (PERCENTAGE)

	SPNSG[a] (N = 50)	Niaudet and Levy[b] (N = 41)	Jardim et al.[c] (N = 30)	Srivastava et al.[d] (N = 43)
Nonspecified immune complex disease	26	4.8	—	—
Systemic lupus erythematosus	18	2.4	3.3	2.3
Idiopathic crescentic glomerulonephritis	14	7.3	13.3	60.4
Poststreptococcal glomerulonephritis	12	12.1	6.6	25.5
Immunoglobulin A nephropathy	8	7.3	—	—
Henoch-Schönlein purpura	6	26.8	30.0	6.9
Vasculitis	6	7.3	16.6	—
Anti–glomerular basement membrane disease	6	7.3	6.6	2.3
Mesangiocapillary glomerulonephritis	4	21.9	23.3	—
Shunt nephritis	—	2.4	—	—
Juvenile chronic arthritis	—	—	—	2.3

N, number of patients.
[a]Data from SPNSG (Southwest Pediatric Nephrology Study Group). A clinico-pathological study of crescentic glomerulonephritis in 50 children. *Kidney Int* 1985;27:450–458.
[b]Data from Niaudet P, Levy M. Glomerulonéphritis à croissants diffus. In: Royer P, Habib R, Mathieu H, Broyer M, eds. *Néphrologie pédiatrique*, 3rd ed. Paris: Flammarion, 1983:381–394.
[c]Data from Jardim HMPF, Leake J, Risdon RA, et al. Crescentic glomerulonephritis in children. *Pediatr Nephrol* 1992;6:231–235.
[d]Data from Srivastava RN, Moudgil A, Bagga A, et al. Crescentic glomerulonephritis in children: a review of 43 cases. *Am J Nephrol* 1992;12: 155–161.

TABLE 34.3. CLINICAL FEATURES OF CRESCENTIC GLOMERULONEPHRITIS IN CHILDREN

Symptom	Incidence (%)
Hematuria (macroscopic)	50–90
Proteinuria	72–100
Oliguria	4–100
Edema	13–90
Anemia	~70
Hypertension	17–85
Renal impairment	100

Data from references 2–4, 7, and 8.

systemic disorder consisting of Henoch-Schönlein purpura in three, SLE in one, anti-GBM disease in one, and chronic rheumatoid arthritis in one; and in 26, the condition was classified as idiopathic (Table 34.2).

CLINICAL PRESENTATION

Most children with crescentic glomerulonephritis have an acute nephritis presentation with proteinuria, hematuria, volume overload, hypertension, and renal impairment. This may evolve quickly and initially give the impression of a postinfectious glomerulonephritis but can be associated with a more protracted clinical course that can be deceptive and may be the cause of a delay in diagnosis and introduction of appropriate treatment. In patients in whom the crescentic glomerulonephritis is secondary to or associated with a systemic disorder (e.g., lupus or vasculitis), clinical features of this may be present and helpful diagnostically. Pulmonary hemorrhage might suggest anti-GBM disease or vasculitis. However, in childhood, anti-GBM glomerulonephritis often occurs without lung involvement, and pulmonary hemorrhage is the exception rather than the rule.

In the series of 30 patients reviewed by Jardim et al. (7), all had hematuria (macroscopic in 15); all had proteinuria (nephrotic syndrome in 14); edema was present at the onset in 24; hypertension was present in 9; oliguria requiring dialysis for fluid control occurred in 15; and the glomerular filtration rate (GFR) was less than 30 mL/min/1.73 m^2 at presentation in 22 patients and between 30 and 60 mL/min per 1.73 m^2 in the remaining 8. These data are very similar to those recorded in other reports in the literature (2–4). However, it is important to emphasize that there is a fairly wide spectrum of presenting clinical features (Table 34.3).

LABORATORY FINDINGS

Laboratory investigations substantiate the clinical impression of renal impairment as well as confirming the presence of hematuria and proteinuria. The degree of renal failure can be deceptive with GFR findings, often substantially more impaired than might have been deduced from random plasma creatinine values. Anemia, which is frequently present, is more marked than anticipated (13) and is usually normochromic and normocytic.

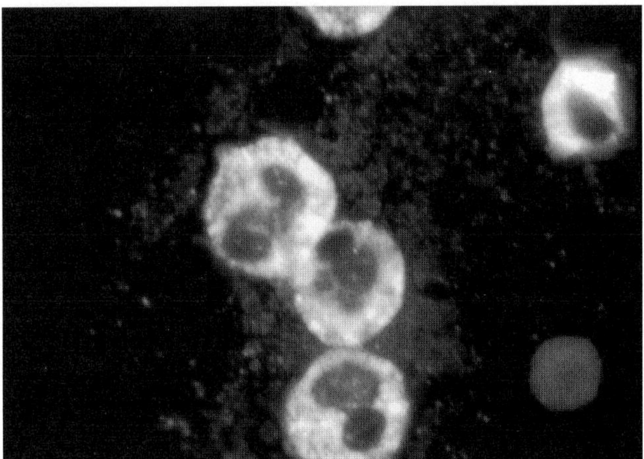

FIGURE 34.1. Cytoplasmic staining antineutrophil cytoplasmic antibody pattern in a standard indirect immunofluorescence assay.

Serologic abnormalities vary according to the underlying disease state. Hypocomplementemia is not uncommon in immune complex disease and SLE. Circulating anti-GBM antibodies would be expected in anti-GBM disease (17); if this condition is suspected, it is essential to have a rapid result from the laboratory, as initiation of early treatment is critically important. Circulating anti-GBM IgG antibodies can be demonstrated by indirect immunofluorescence or enzyme immunoassay. Enzyme immunoassay is more sensitive and specific as compared to indirect immunofluorescence.

Raised anti–streptolysin O levels with or without raised anti–deoxyribonuclease B are features of poststreptococcal glomerulonephritis, but they can be increased coincidentally in other forms of crescentic glomerulonephritis and may, therefore, not be diagnostically helpful. Antinuclear

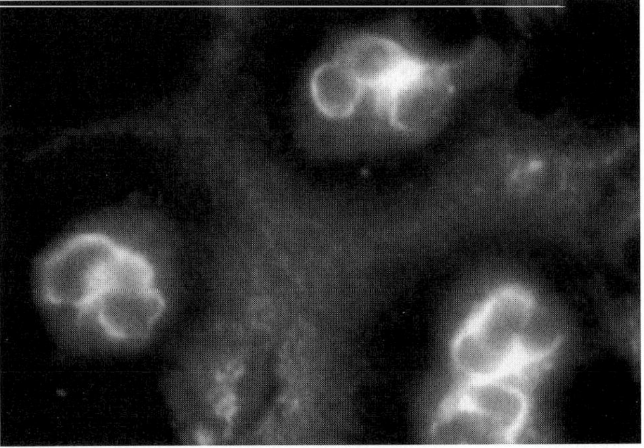

FIGURE 34.2. Perinuclear staining antineutrophil cytoplasmic antibody pattern in a standard indirect immunofluorescence assay.

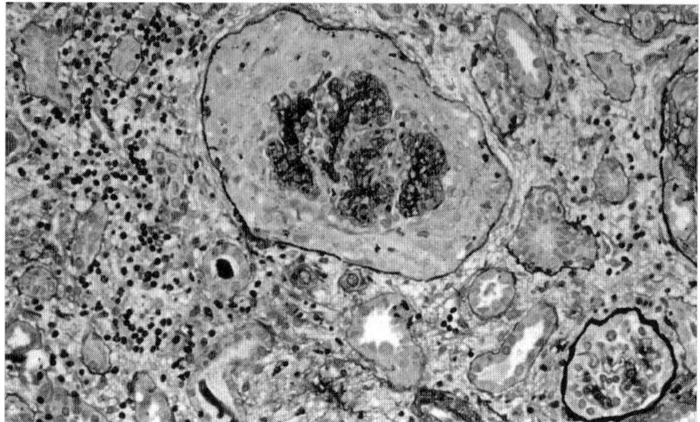

FIGURE 34.3. Cellular crescent.

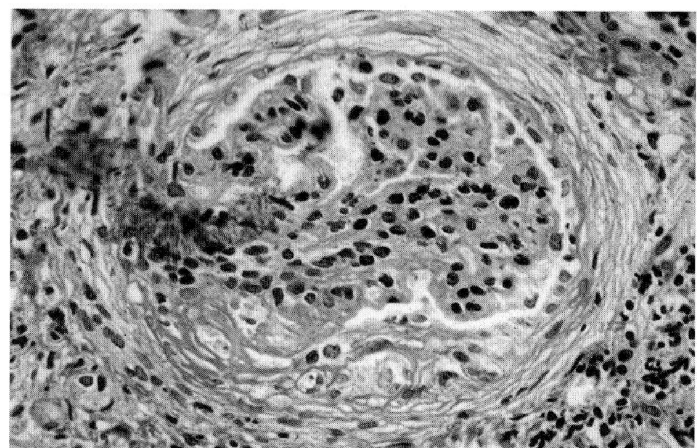

FIGURE 34.5. Fibrous crescent.

and anti–double-stranded DNA antibodies point to a diagnosis of SLE nephritis.

Elevated levels of antineutrophil cytoplasmic antibodies (ANCAs) may reflect an underlying vasculitic cause, such as Wegener's granulomatosis or microscopic polyarteritis (or polyangiopathy) (18,19). Two neutrophil primary-granule enzymes are the targets of the majority of ANCAs in systemic vasculitis. ANCAs directed against proteinase-3 are strongly associated with Wegener's granulomatosis and produce a cytoplasmic staining pattern in a standard indirect immunofluorescence assay (19,20) (Fig. 34.1). ANCA directed against myeloperoxidase, producing a perinuclear staining pattern, is often seen in microscopic polyangiopathy, but perinuclear ANCA may also be directed against other epitopes and is seen in other nonvasculitic conditions (19,21) (Fig. 34.2). The presence of circulating ANCA in a child with crescentic glomerulonephritis might be helpful diagnostically with a cytoplasmic pattern suggestive of Wegener's granulomatosis and a perinuclear pattern suggestive of microscopic polyangiopathy (22). In children with idiopathic disease, which is considered probably to be a form of microscopic polyarteritis, such a positive finding can be helpful, but negative results do not exclude Wegener's granulomatosis, nor do they exclude microscopic polyangiitis. ANCA-positive crescentic glomerulonephritis is also associated with propyl thiouracil treatment in children (23).

HISTOPATHOLOGY

Controversy exists as to how many glomeruli have to be associated with crescents to designate the disease as *crescentic glomerulonephritis.* As mentioned previously, authors vary in their views, and more than 75% (3), 50% or more (2,7,8), and occasionally even 20% of glomeruli affected have been considered to represent crescentic glomerulonephritis (5). There is, in addition, a need to characterize the nature of the crescents, and three categories are recognized. *Cellular crescents* are those in which there is prominent proliferation of epithelial cells, with some admixture of macrophages and occasionally neutrophils filling the urinary space and compressing the tuft (Fig. 34.3). *Fibrocellular crescents* are those in which strands of membrane-like material and collagen fibers are present among the cells forming the crescent (Fig. 34.4). *Fibrous crescents* are those in which the cells of the crescent have virtually all disappeared to be replaced by collagen (7) (Fig. 34.5).

The nature of the underlying disease causing the crescentic glomerulonephritis is based on various criteria: (a) the

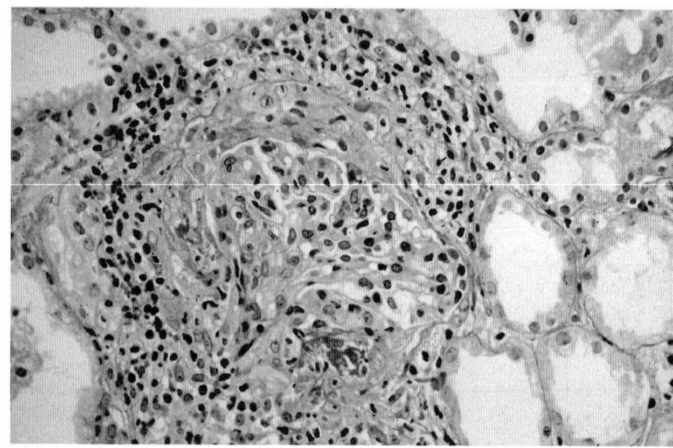

FIGURE 34.4. Fibrocellular crescent.

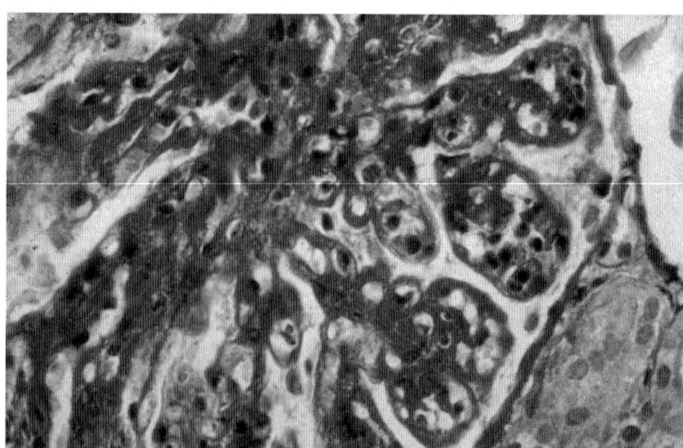

FIGURE 34.6. Mesangiocapillary glomerulonephritis.

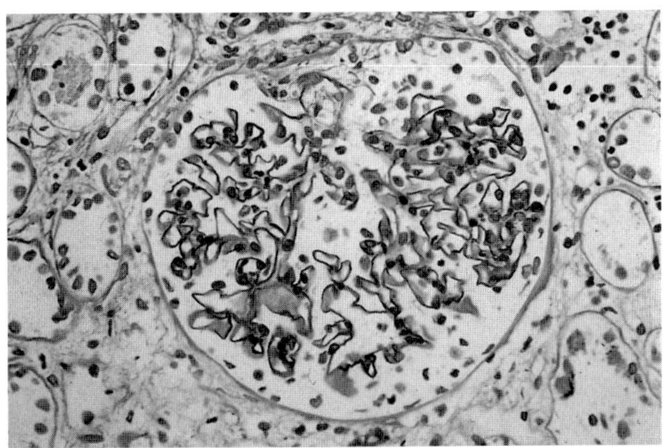

FIGURE 34.7. Anti–glomerular basement membrane glomerulonephritis with linear immunoglobulin G demonstrable by immunochemical staining.

associated changes in the glomerular tuft, such as those of mesangiocapillary glomerulonephritis (Fig. 34.6); (b) the immunochemical staining, such as the presence of linear IgG staining along the glomerular capillary walls in anti-GBM glomerulonephritis (Fig. 34.7); and (c) clinicopathologic factors, such as in polyarteritis nodosa, Wegener's granulomatosis, and microscopic polyarteritis (7). However, the identification of the underlying glomerulonephritis is often difficult, but immunofluorescence studies can prove helpful in, for example, mesangiocapillary glomerulonephritis, anti-GBM disease, IgA nephropathy, and Henoch-Schönlein purpura (Fig. 34.8).

It is clear that the number of crescents is not necessarily the most important factor in terms of subsequent outcome. This is much more closely related to the nature of the crescents, with fibrous crescents having a worse prognosis than cellular or fibrocellular crescents (7). It is also clear that the histopathologic appearances of the crescents can change quite rapidly from cellular to fibrous, especially if therapeutic intervention is delayed. The implication from this evolution is that the underlying glomeruli became seriously compromised with progression to glomerulosclerosis and irrecoverable renal impairment. This process leading to glomerulosclerosis is similar in most causes of crescentic glomerulonephritis, and at a late stage, it is usually not possible to distinguish the etiology from histopathologic examination.

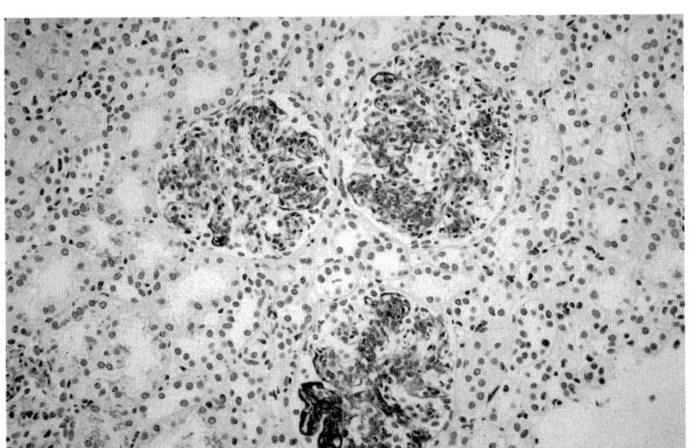

FIGURE 34.8. Henoch-Schönlein purpura mesangial deposition of immunoglobulin A demonstrable by immunochemical staining.

IMMUNOPATHOGENETIC MECHANISMS

In severe inflammatory glomerular injury, whatever the initial insult or injury, crescent formation may be the final pathway. A crescent is a proliferation of extracapillary cells within Bowman's space. There is evidence that crescent formation is initiated by cytokine-driven proliferation of the parietal glomerular epithelial cells (24–26). Associated with this, localized breaks in the GBM of Bowman's capsule (27–29), mediated by activated leukocytes, are followed by macrophage infiltration into Bowman's space with local fibrin formation (30). Current evidence suggests that crescent formation is a feature of cell-mediated rather than humoral immune mechanisms (31).

TREATMENT AND OUTCOME

The heterogeneity and poor outcome of childhood crescentic glomerulonephritis has led to multiple treatment regimens. Steroids (oral or high-dose intravenous), cytotoxic agents, anticoagulants, antiplatelet agents, and plasma exchange, alone or in different combinations, have all been described (2,3,7,8,10,11,32) (Table 34.4).

High-dose intravenous methylprednisolone, often recommended in adults (33), has been used in children with crescentic glomerulonephritis by Ferraris et al. (32), coupled with cyclophosphamide, with long-term renal recovery in five children after a mean follow-up of 35 months. Methylprednisolone has also been used alone in 29 children with severe proliferative glomerulonephritis (12), with a favorable outcome (GFR greater than 80 mL/min/1.73 m^2) observed in 18 (62%) after a mean follow-up of 35 months.

Combined immunosuppressive and anticoagulant therapy as reported by the Southwest Pediatric Nephrology Study Group (2) resulted in 24 of 47 (52%) patients recovering renal function. The importance of anticoagulants in this regimen has been emphasized by Cunningham et al. (4) who reported recovery of renal function in 7 of 13 (54%) patients with crescentic glomerulonephritis. A similar regime used by Niaudet and Levy (3) was associated with renal recovery of varying degree in 19 of 41 (46.3%) patients (Table 34.5).

Treatment regimens used in the study of Jardim et al. (7) included corticosteroids, cyclophosphamide, azathioprine, anticoagulant and antiplatelet agents, and plasma exchange in varying combinations. Despite these intensive therapeutic approaches, approximately 50% of patients eventually pro-

TABLE 34.4. TREATMENT OPTIONS FOR CRESCENTIC GLOMERULONEPHRITIS IN CHILDHOOD

Induction
- Prednisolone 2 mg/kg/d PO
- If fulminant disease, methyl prednisolone, 600 mg/m^2/d × 3 IV, followed by PO prednisolone in above dose
- Cyclophosphamide, 2 mg/kg/d PO (for 2–3 mos), or pulsed cyclophosphamide, 500–750 mg/m^2/dose IV every 3–4 wks × 6
- If fulminant or unresponsive disease or if anti-GBM disease, plasma exchange, two volume exchanges daily × 5–10 d
- Antiplatelet therapy ± anticoagulation
- Treatment for underlying disease (often covered by above) with antimicrobial therapy, removal of offending drugs, and treatment of malignant disease

Maintenance
- Alternate-day low-dose prednisolone (tapering from high induction dose)
- Azathioprine, 2 mg/kg/d, at least until remission maintained for >1 yr and in practice for approximately 18 mo
- Cyclosporin, methotrexate, and mycophenolate mofetil as alternative maintenance drugs if azathioprine incapable of controlling the disease

Refractory disease
- Humanized monoclonal antibodies [e.g., anti-CD4 and anti-CD52 or anti–tumor necrosis factor agents (e.g., infliximab)]

Supportive therapy
- Dialysis, diuretics, antihypertensives, and so forth

gressed to end-stage renal failure. Four children on long-term follow-up had GFRs greater than 80 mL/min per 1.73 m^2, six had GFRs of 30 to 80 mL/min per 1.73 m^2, and three had GFRs of less than 30 mL/min per 1.73 m^2. Patients with fibrous crescents did less well, and there was evidence to support the view that the longer the interval between disease onset and commencement of treatment, the worse the prognosis. All patients whose treatment was delayed to beyond 3 months after disease onset went into end-stage renal failure; those treated 1 to 3 months after onset had variable results (two out of five patients recovered renal function); and the 12 patients treated in the first month after onset responded well (7) (Table 34.5).

The benefits of plasma exchange in anti-GBM nephritis have been demonstrated in adult patients (34) and have led to its use in other disorders (e.g., immune complex–mediated RPGN) (34). The literature remains confusing in terms of the benefits of plasma exchange in RPGN from other causes, with some showing benefit (35) and others no effect (36). Pusey et al. (37) demonstrated that dialysis-dependent patients were more likely to recover renal function if treated with plasma exchange. Jardim et al. (7) treated 24 children by plasma exchange; although statistically there was no significant difference between patients who were and who were not exchanged, nine of the ten patients with a GFR of greater than 30 mL/min per 1.73 m^2 at latest follow-up received this treatment. However, the majority of the patients who progressed to renal failure despite plasma exchange had fibrous crescents on presentation. In the Niaudet and Levy report (3), plasma exchange was used in seven of 41 patients, and only the two patients not requiring dialysis on presentation recovered renal function. This emphasizes that the need for dialysis at onset is a predictor of worse outcome as has been shown in several series (3,7,11). Gianviti et al. (38) also showed that the addition of plasma exchange to other intensive therapy in patients with RPGN had beneficial effects.

Evidence-based data on treatment are very limited and unavailable in children. However, for adults, an analysis of evidence-based recommendations was published by Jindal in 1999 (39). In this report, early aggressive therapy was recommended despite weak supporting evidence because of the high risk of end-stage renal disease. Treatment for anti-GBM antibody-induced crescentic glomerulonephritis should be initiated early and should include pulsed methylprednisolone, a 2-week course of plasmapheresis, and 2 months' treatment with corticosteroids and cyclophosphamide. Treatment for pauci-immune crescentic glomerulonephritis should be pulsed methylprednisolone, followed by oral corticosteroids and cyclophosphamide for 6 to 12 months. Recurrences can be managed similarly along with appropriate supportive therapy.

In terms of prognosis, it is accepted that poststreptococcal crescentic glomerulonephritis has a better prognosis, with spontaneous improvement after supportive management (3,40). Roy et al. (41) found no advantage from immuno-

TABLE 34.5. OUTCOME IN CHILDREN WITH CRESCENTIC GLOMERULONEPHRITIS

	SPNSG[a] (N = 50)	Niaudet and Levy[b] (N = 41)	Jardim et al.[c] (N = 30)	Srivastava et al.[d] (N = 43)
Normal renal function	13 of 47 (27.6%)	13 (31.7%)	4 (13.3%)	6 (13.9%)
Chronic renal impairment	11 of 47 (23.4%)	6 (14.6%)	10 (33.3%)	14 (32.5%)
End-stage renal failure	23 of 47 (48.9%)	22 (53.6%)	16 (53.3%)	23 (53.4%)

N, number of patients.
[a]Data from SPNSG (Southwest Pediatric Nephrology Study Group). A clinico-pathological study of crescentic glomerulonephritis in 50 children. *Kidney Int* 1985;27:450–458.
[b]Data from Niaudet P, Levy M. Glomerulonéphritis à croissants diffus. In: Royer P, Habib R, Mathieu H, Broyer M, eds. *Néphrologie pédiatrique*, 3rd ed. Paris: Flammarion, 1983;381–394.
[c]Data from Jardim HMPF, Leake J, Risdon RA, et al. Crescentic glomerulonephritis in children. *Pediatr Nephrol* 1992;6:231–235.
[d]Data from Srivastava RN, Moudgil A, Bagga A, et al. Crescentic glomerulonephritis in children: a review of 43 cases. *Am J Nephrol* 1992;12:155–161.

suppression and anticoagulants over conservative management in children with poststreptococcal disease. However, progression to renal failure has been reported in children (3–5,7,8); hence, the outlook is not uniformly good.

Of other causes of crescentic glomerulonephritis, mesangiocapillary glomerulonephritis, microscopic polyangiitis, anti-GBM disease, and the idiopathic form seem to have a worse prognosis than, for example, Henoch-Schönlein purpura or SLE, which are among the more common causes of the condition (3,7). However, the outlook for any patient is very dependent on the need for dialysis at onset and the presence of fibrous crescents on biopsy (3,7,11).

In conclusion, it is clear that crescentic glomerulonephritis in childhood, as in adult practice, is caused by many different conditions with diverse pathogenetic mechanisms. These determine the natural history and the most appropriate treatment. Precise rapid diagnostic categorization and aggressive appropriate therapy are, in the majority of cases, indicated in light of the well-recognized poor prognosis in a substantial proportion of those affected.

REFERENCES

1. Heptinstall RH. Crescentic glomerulonephritis. In: Heptinstall RH, ed. *Pathology of the kidney*, 3rd ed. Boston: Little, Brown and Company, 1983:443–447.
2. SPNSG (Southwest Pediatric Nephrology Study Group). A clinico-pathological study of crescentic glomerulonephritis in 50 children. *Kidney Int* 1985;27:450–458.
3. Niaudet P, Levy M. Glomerulonéphritis à croissants diffus. In: Royer P, Habib R, Mathieu H, Broyer M, eds. *Néphrologie pédiatrique*, 3rd ed. Paris: Flammarion, 1983:381–394.
4. Cunningham RJ, Gilfoil M, Cavallo T, et al. Rapidly progressive glomerulonephritis in children: a report of thirteen cases and a review of the literature. *Pediatr Res* 1980;14:128–132.
5. Anand SK, Trygstad CW, Sharma HM, et al. Extracapillary proliferative glomerulonephritis in children. *Pediatrics* 1975; 56:434–442.
6. Dilma MG, Adhikari M, Coovadin HM. Rapidly progressive glomerulonephritis in black children: a report of 4 cases. *S Africa Med J* 1981;60:829–832.
7. Jardim HMPF, Leake J, Risdon RA, et al. Crescentic glomerulonephritis in children. *Pediatr Nephrol* 1992;6:231–235.
8. Srivastava RN, Moudgil A, Bagga A, et al. Crescentic glomerulonephritis in children: a review of 43 cases. *Am J Nephrol* 1992;12:155–161.
9. Tapaneya-Olarn W, Tapeneya-Olarn C, Boonpucknavig V, et al. Rapidly progressive glomerulonephritis in Thai children. *J Med Ass Thailand* 1992;75[Suppl 1]:32–37.
10. Haycock GB. The treatment of glomerulonephritis in children. *Pediatr Nephrol* 1988;2:247–255.
11. Neild GH, Cameron JS, Ogg CS, et al. Rapidly progressive glomerulonephritis with extensive glomerular crescent formation. *QJM* 1983;52:395–416.
12. Robson AM, Rose GM, Cole BR, et al. The treatment of severe glomerulopathies in children with methyl prednisolone pulses. Proceedings of 8th International Congress of Nephrology, Athens. Basel: Karger, 1981:305–311.
13. Rees AJ, Cameron JS. Crescentic glomerulonephritis. In: Davison AM, Cameron JS, Grünfeld J-P, et al., eds. *Oxford textbook of clinical nephrology*, 2nd ed. Oxford, UK: Oxford University Press, 1998:625–646.
14. Andrassy K, Kuster S, Waldherr R, et al. Rapidly progressive glomerulonephritis: analysis of prevalence and clinical course. *Nephron* 1991;59:206–212.
15. Miller MN, Baumal R, Poucell S, et al. Incidence and prognostic importance of glomerular crescents in renal disease of childhood. *Am J Nephrol* 1984;4:244–247.
16. Bidani AK, Lewis EJ. Idiopathic rapidly progressive glomerulonephritis and Goodpasture's syndrome. In: Edelmann CM, ed. *Pediatric kidney disease*, 2nd ed. Boston: Little, Brown and Company, 1992:1223–1245.
17. Levin M, Rigden SPA, Pincott JR, et al. Goodpasture's syndrome: treatment with plasmapheresis, immunosuppression and anticoagulation. *Arch Dis Child* 1983;58:697–702.
18. Walters MD, Savage COS, Dillon MJ, et al. Antineutrophil cytoplasm antibody in crescentic glomerulonephritis. *Arch Dis Child* 1988;63:814–817.
19. Dillon MJ, Tizard EJ. Antineutrophil cytoplasmic antibodies and antiendothelial cell antibodies. *Pediatr Nephrol* 1991;5:256–259.
20. Kallenberg CG, Brouwer E, Weening JJ, et al. Anti-neutrophil cytoplasmic antibodies: current diagnostic and pathophysiological potential. *Kidney Int* 1994;46:1–15.
21. Falk RJ, Jennette JC. Anti-neutrophil cytoplasmic autoantibodies with specificity for myeloperoxidase in patients with systemic vasculitis and idiopathic necrotizing and crescentic glomerulonephritis. *N Engl J Med* 1988;318:1651–1657.
22. Hattori M, Kurayama H, Koitabashi Y. Antineutrophil cytoplasmic autoantibody-associated glomerulonephritis in children. *J Am Soc Nephrol* 2001;12:1493–500.
23. Fujieda M, Hattori M, Kurayama H, et al. Clinical features and outcomes in children with anti-neutrophil cytoplasmic autoantibody-positive glomerulonephritis associated with propyl thiouracil treatment. *J Am Soc Nephrol* 2002;13:437–445.
24. Jeannette JC, Hipp CG. The epithelial cell antigen phenotype of glomerular crescent cells. *Am J Clin Pathol* 1985; 86:274–280.
25. Boucher A, Droz D, Adafer E, et al. Relationship between the integrity of Bowman's capsule and the composition of cellular crescents in human crescentic glomerulonephritis. *Lab Invest* 1987;5:526–533.
26. Muller GA, Muller CA, Markovic-Lipkovski J, et al. Renal major histocompatibility complex antigens and cellular components in rapidly progressive glomerulonephritis identified by monoclonal antibodies. *Nephron* 1988;49:132–139.
27. Burkholder PM. Ultra structure demonstration of injury and perforation of the glomerular basement membrane in acute proliferative glomerulonephritis. *Am J Pathol* 1969;56:251–265.
28. Bonsib SM. Glomerular basement membrane discontinuities: scanning election microscopic study of acellular glomeruli. *Am J Pathol* 1985;119:357–360.
29. Bonsib SM. Glomerular basement membrane necrosis and crescent organization. *Kidney Int* 1988;33:966–974.

30. Atkins RC, Holdsworth SR, Glasgow EF, et al. The macrophage in human rapidly progressive glomerulonephritis. *Lancet* 1976;i:830–832.
31. Bolton WK, Innes DJ, Sturgill BC, et al. T-cells and macrophages in rapidly progressive glomerulonephritis: clinicopathologic correlations. *Kidney Int* 1987;32:869–896.
32. Ferraris JR, Gallo GE, Ramires J, et al. "Pulse" methyl prednisolone therapy in the treatment of acute crescentic glomerulonephritis. *Nephron* 1983;34:207–208.
33. Bolton WK, Sturgill BC. Methyl prednisolone therapy for acute crescentic rapidly progressive glomerulonephritis. *Am J Nephrol* 1989;9:368–375.
34. Lockwood CM, Pinching AJ, Sweny P, et al. Plasma exchange and immunosuppression in the treatment of fulminating immune complex mediated crescentic nephritis. *Lancet* 1977;i:63–67.
35. Thysell H, Bygren P, Bengstsson U, et al. Immunosuppression and the additive effect of plasma exchange in treatment of rapidly progressive glomerulonephritis. *Acta Med Scand* 1982;212:107–114.
36. Glockner WH, Sieberth HG, Wichmann HE, et al. Plasma exchange and immunosuppression in rapidly progressive glomerulonephritis: a controlled, multi-centre study. *Clin Nephrol* 1988;29:1–8.
37. Pusey CD, Rees AJ, Evans DJ, et al. Plasma exchange in focal necrotizing glomerulonephritis without anti-GBM antibodies. *Kidney Int* 1991;40:757–763.
38. Gianviti A, Trompeter RS, Barratt TM, et al. Retrospective study of plasma exchange in patients with idiopathic rapidly progressive glomerulonephritis and vasculitis. *Arch Dis Child* 1996;75:186–190.
39. Jindal KK. Management of idiopathic crescentic and diffuse proliferative glomerulonephritis: evidence-based recommendations. *Kidney Int* 1999;(Suppl)70:S33–S40.
40. Whitworth JA, Morel-Maroger L, Mignon F, et al. The significance of extracapillary proliferation: clinico-pathological review of 60 patients. *Nephron* 1976;16:1–19.
41. Roy S, Murphy, WM, Arant BS. Poststreptococcal crescentic glomerulonephritis in children: comparison of quintuple therapy versus supportive care. *J Pediatr* 1981;98:403–410.

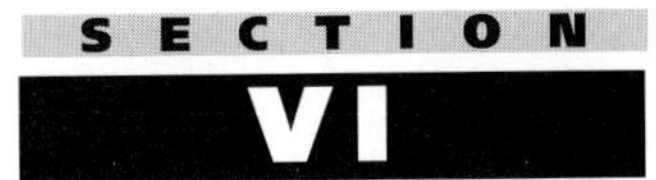

SECTION VI

TUBULAR DISEASE

35

NEPHRONOPHTHISIS-MEDULLARY CYSTIC KIDNEY DISEASE

FRIEDHELM HILDEBRANDT

DEFINITION OF THE NEPHRONOPHTHISIS-MEDULLARY CYSTIC DISEASE COMPLEX

The nephronophthisis-medullary cystic disease (NPH-MCKD) complex describes a distinct clinicopathologic entity of inherited diseases that lead to chronic renal failure on the pathologic basis of a chronic sclerosing tubulointerstitial nephropathy (1). Whereas NPH is an autosomal recessive disease with onset of end-stage renal disease in adolescence, the term *medullary cystic kidney disease* is used for autosomal dominant variants with onset in adulthood. NPH represents the most frequent genetic cause of chronic renal failure in the first two decades of life (6–8). Diseases of the NPH-MCKD complex are characterized clinically by a defect in urinary concentrating capacity, anemia, and progression into terminal renal failure in adolescence or young adulthood (2,3). On renal histology, NPH-MCKD exhibits a characteristic triad of disruption of renal tubular basement membranes (TBMs) with tubular cell atrophy, tubulo-interstitial fibrosis, and cyst formation (4,55). Extrarenal manifestations have been described in association with recessive NPH, but are absent from MCKD. After the first descriptions of NPH by Smith and Graham (2) and Fanconi et al. (3), more than 300 cases have been reported (4,5), and the disease complex has been extensively reviewed (1,6–8). The term *nephronophthisis* is used for the recessively inherited variants of the complex, and the term *medullary cystic kidney disease* denotes the autosomal dominant variants.

ETIOLOGY AND MOLECULAR GENETICS

To date, no aberrations of chromosome number have been reported in any disease of the NPH-MCKD complex, with the single exception of a partial monosomy of chromosome 3 described by Sarles et al. (9). Because little insight had been available into the pathogenesis of NPH-MCKD, a positional cloning approach was used toward the identification of genes for the complex. After chromosomal localization and gene identification by positional cloning, different disease variants can be distinguished on the basis of distinct gene loci (Table 35.1).

In juvenile NPH (NPH1), a gene locus has been mapped to chromosome 2q12.3 (10). This locus was further refined (11–16), and the gene (*NPHP1*) responsible for NPH1 was identified by positional cloning (17,18). Approximately 85% of patients with NPH1 carry large homozygous deletions of the *NPHP1* gene (19,20). Spontaneously occurring deletions of the *NPHP1* locus (20) as well as specific loss-of-function point mutations of *NPHP1* have been characterized (18,21,22). In a subset of patients with large deletions in *NPHP1*, there is an association with oculomotor apraxia type Cogan (23). Another subset shows an association with retinitis pigmentosa (22). No specific molecular characteristics have been detected that clearly identify the subgroup of NPH1 patients with extrarenal associations. The protein encoded by *NPHP1,* "nephrocystin," contains an *src*-homology 3 (SH3) domain with high sequence similarity to the *c-crk* proto-oncogene. This suggests that nephrocystin may play a role as a docking protein in cell-cell or cell-matrix signaling processes, or both. Nephrocystin is highly conserved in evolution, including the nematode *Caenorhabditis elegans*.

Infantile NPH (NPH2) is a distinct disease entity, in which end-stage renal failure occurs within the first 3 years of life (24,25). NPH2 differs from other forms of NPH by the presence of enlarged kidneys and cortical microcysts and the absence of medullary cysts. Histologically, there is no disruption of TBMs. A gene locus (*NPHP2*) for NPH2 was localized to 9q22-q31 in one Bedouin kindred (26). Morphologically, the disease phenotype encompasses features of both NPH and autosomal recessive polycystic kidney disease (ARPKD). Recently, recessive mutations in the *inversin* gene have been identified as the cause of *NPHP2* (26a).

In NPH type 3 (NPH3), a third NPH gene locus (*NPHP3)* for "adolescent NPH" has been localized to chromosome 3q21-q22 (27), and several candidate genes

TABLE 35.1. DISEASE VARIANTS, GENE LOCI, AND EXTRARENAL MANIFESTATIONS OF THE NEPHRONOPHTHISIS-MEDULLARY CYSTIC KIDNEY DISEASE (NPH-MCKD) COMPLEX

Disease	Inheritance	ESRD (median in yr)	Chromosome	Gene (product)	Extrarenal association
NPH					
NPHP1 (juvenile)	AR	13	2q12.3	*NPHP1* (nephrocystin)	SLS, OMA
NPHP2 (infantile)	AR	1–3	9q22-q31	*INV* (inversin)	*Situs inversus*, SLS
NPHP3 (adolescent)	AR	19	3q22	?	SLS
NPHP4	AR	20	1p36	*NPHP4* (nephroretinin)	SLS, OMA
MCKD					
MCKD1	AD	62	1q21	?	Hyperuricemia
MCKD2	AD	32	16p12	*UMOD* (Thamm-Horsfall protein)	Hyperuricemia

AR, autosomal recessive; AD, autosomal dominant; ESRD, end-stage renal disease; OMA, oculomotor apraxia type Cogan; SLS, Senior-Loken syndrome.

have been excluded (28,29). In addition, linkage to *NPHP3* was identified in families with Senior-Loken syndrome (SLS) (30).

The disease gene for NPH type 4 (NPH4) has been identified on chromosome 1p36 (31–33). The gene and its gene product nephroretinin are novel and highly conserved in evolution. Subsets of patients with mutations in the *NPHP4* gene exhibited SLS as well as Cogan syndrome (31,32).

The locus for MCKD type 1 (MCKD1) has been mapped to 1q21 (34–36). Microscopic and macroscopic pathology of dominant MCKD is indistinguishable from recessive NPH. The *MCKD1* locus has been refined to 4 centi-Morgan (cM) (37), and the gene (*NPR1*) for natriuretic peptide receptor-1 has been excluded as a candidate gene (38).

A second locus, MCKD type 2 (MCKD2), has been mapped to chromosome 16q12 (39–44). The *MCKD2* locus was refined to a 1.3-megabase (Mb) interval, demonstrating that it co-localizes with the locus for familial juvenile hyperuricemic nephropathy (45). The *UMOD* gene has very recently been identified as causative for MCKD2. There is evidence for existence of a third MCKD locus (46,47).

HISTOPATHOLOGY

Renal histopathology is similar in all variants of the NPH-MCKD complex, and has been described in 27 patients with NPH by Waldherr et al. (4). Kidney size is normal or moderately reduced. There is always bilateral renal involvement. Macroscopically, the kidney surface has a finely granular appearance, most likely due to the protrusion of dilated cortical collecting ducts. There are between 5 and approximately 50 cysts of 1 to 15 mm in diameter located preferentially at the corticomedullary border. The cysts arise primarily from the distal convoluted and medullary collecting tubules, as shown by microdissection (48), but may also appear in the papilla. Cysts are observed only in approximately 70% of autopsy cases and seem to arise late in the course of the disease (49). Therefore, the presence of cysts is not a prerequisite for diagnosis. No cysts are present in organs other than the kidney.

The histologic changes of NPH are characteristic but not specific for the disease and develop postnatally. Typically, there is pronounced thickening and multilayering of the TBM, which represents the most characteristic histologic feature of the NPH-MCKD complex (Fig. 35.1). By light microscopy, there appears to be a sequence of events. TBM disruption is followed by lymphocytic and histocytic peritubular infiltration. Subsequently, atrophic or dilated and tortuous tubules develop predominantly at the corticomedullary junction. In advanced stages, the picture

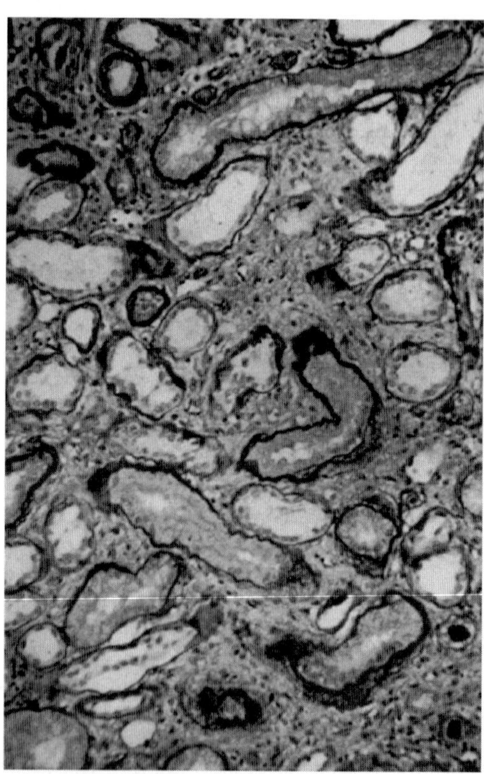

FIGURE 35.1. Renal histology of nephronophthisis-medullary cystic kidney disease. Note the characteristic triad of tubular basement membrane disruption, tubular cell atrophy with cysts, and interstitial infiltration and fibrosis. Hematoxylin-eosin stain. (Courtesy of Prof. R. Waldherr, Heidelberg, Germany.)

merges into a diffuse, sclerosing, tubulo-interstitial nephropathy. TBM changes and cyst formation are most prominent in distal tubules, where cysts are lined with a single layer of cuboidal or flattened epithelium (50–53). Glomeruli demonstrate periglomerular fibrosis with splitting and thickening of Bowman's capsule. Glomerular obsolescence is only present in nephrons that have been destroyed by tubular alterations. Leakage of Tamm-Horsfall protein from damaged collecting tubules into the interstitium has been demonstrated (54). On transmission electron microscopy, there is thickening, splitting, attenuation, and granular disintegration of the TBM without clear stages of transition (55). A marked increase of microfilaments is seen at the base of the tubular epithelial cells.

PATHOGENESIS

Changes in tubular function characterize NPH-MCKD and include decreased urinary concentration ability and aminoaciduria. Proteinuria is a rare finding. Histologic changes (see Histopathology) also emphasize the central role of altered tubular structure in the pathogenesis. Cysts do not seem to be important for disease progression (56). Cohen and Hoyer (57) have hypothesized that NPH results from a primary defect of TBM matrix components. Such abnormalities lead to reduced mechanical compliance of the distal tubule with consecutive cyst development. In SLS, both renal and retinal changes are thought to be degenerative rather than dysplastic (58).

Recent data suggest that NPH results from a primary defect in tubular cell-cell contacts (adherens junctions) or tubular cell-matrix interactions, or both (59). The *NPHP1* gene product, nephrocystin, is a docking protein that binds through multiple domains of protein-protein interaction to proteins of cell-cell signaling and cell-matrix signaling at adherens junctions and focal adhesions, respectively. The src-homology-3 domain of nephrocystin binds to proline-rich peptides on the protein p130cas (c-crk–associated substrate), which is known to be a major mediator of adherens junction and focal adhesion signaling (60–62). Nephrocystin, in MDCK cells, co-localizes to adherens junctions with p130Cas and with the integral adherens junction protein E-cadherin (61). Expression of an exogenous nephrocystin construct with a defective SH3 domain in MDCK cells decreased electrical resistance (63). In addition, it has been shown that targeting of nephrocystin to adherens junctions of MDCK cells was dependent on the nephrocystin homology domain (NHD). The NHD represents the C-terminal half of nephrocystin, which by secondary structure prediction is featureless and exhibits no homology with any known proteins. Binding of nephrocystin to the actin-organizing proteins filamin A and B occurs via the NHD domain (63).

Nephrocystin binds to the signaling proteins p130Cas (64), focal adhesion kinase 2 (Fak2, *alias* Pyk2), and tensin, which are integral components of focal adhesion signaling (62). Nephrocystin expression leads to phosphorylation of Pyk2 on tyrosine residue 402, which in turn activates the transcription factors ERK1 and ERK2 (extracellular signal–related kinases 1 and 2). Thus, nephrocystin helps recruit Pyk2 to cell-matrix adhesions, thereby initiating Pyk2-dependent signaling (62). Nephroretinin, the product of the *NPHP4* gene mutations that cause NPH4 and SLS type 4 (32), has been shown by co-immunoprecipitation to interact with nephrocystin (33). In patients with NPH, abnormal expression of the α_5 integrin fibronectin receptor has been demonstrated in renal TBMs (65). This leads to the hypothesis that renal tubular cells in NPH express α_5 integrin fibronectin receptor within focal adhesions as a compensatory mechanism for defective function of the α_6 integrin molecule. This, in turn, would lead to destruction of the TBM, which is a typical histologic finding early in the course of NPH. In addition, alterations in hepatocyte growth factor (66) and Pax2 (67) have been described in NPH.

ANIMAL MODELS

Further support for the hypothesis that a defect in tubular cell-cell or cell-matrix interaction is an important pathogenetic mechanism in NPH comes from the finding that targeted disruption of the mouse tensin gene leads to a renal phenotype closely resembling human NPH (68). Because tensin is a major component of focal adhesions, defects in these matricellular contact points might play a central role in the pathogenesis of NPH. Additional mouse models with features of NPH include kd/kd mice (69,70), angiotensin-converting enzyme knock-out mice (71), and Bcl-2 knock-out mice (72). Recently, strong synteny of the human *NPHP3* locus has been demonstrated to the locus pcy mouse whose renal histopathology closely resembles human NPH (73). Also, the RhoGDI-α-"knock-out"-mouse model exhibits a renal cystic phenotype, which shares certain histologic features with human NPH (74).

Recently, nephrocystin was shown to interact with inversin, the gene product defective in NPH2, and both nephrocystin and inversin have been demonstrated to co-localize to single cilia on MDKC cells (26a). This expression pattern provides a possible link between the pathogenesis of NPH and the pathogenesis of polycystic kidney disease because polycystin-1 and polycystin-2 have been shown to be expressed in cilia of renal epithelial cells, where they might exert a function as a mechanosensory renal tubular flow sensor (75).

CLINICAL PRESENTATION

Nephronophthisis

Diseases of the NPH-MCKD complex are characterized by the insidious onset of renal failure. In recessive NPH, the

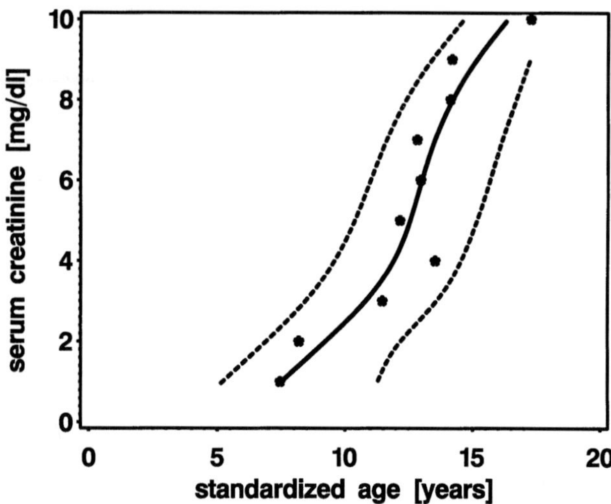

FIGURE 35.2. Progression chart representing the average course of deterioration of renal function in 19 patients of eight families with juvenile nephronophthisis as proven by deletion detection. Median (*solid line*) and quartile (*dashed lines*) curves were calculated from 308 serial serum creatinine values. (From Hildebrandt F, Strahm B, Nothwang HG, et al. Molecular genetic identification of families with juvenile nephronophthisis type 1: rate of progression to renal failure. *Kidney Int* 1997;51:261–269, with permission.)

symptoms of polyuria, polydipsia, decreased urinary concentrating ability, and secondary enuresis are the earliest presenting symptoms in more than 80% of cases (5) and occur at 4 to 6 years of age. The symptom of starting to regularly drink at night, once children are 6 to 10 years old, is rather characteristic of NPH. Pallor, weakness, and generalized pruritus are also common. Anemia and growth retardation occur later and are usually pronounced. All affected individuals progress to end-stage renal disease and therefore require renal replacement therapy. In a study conducted in 19 patients of eight families with deletion-positive NPH1, a serum creatinine of 5.5 mg/dL was reached at an average age of 13.1 years of age (range, 7 to 25 years) (76). From this study, charts for prediction of progression toward renal failure were derived (Fig. 35.2). A difference in age of progression to renal failure was shown between patients with deletion-positive NPH1 and patients from a Venezuelan kindred of adolescent NPH (NPH3), in which median age of onset of end-stage renal disease was 19 years (27). If renal failure has not developed by the age of 25 years, the diagnosis of recessive NPH should be questioned. A high concordance rate (77) of the development of renal failure has been noted in monozygotic twins (78). A characteristic early finding in NPH is the decreased ability to concentrate the urine above 800 mOsm/kg of water after an 8-hour water deprivation test or vasopressin administration (1). Published reports do not adequately answer the question of whether renal sodium loss is a typical finding in the disease complex. Typically, edema, hematuria, and urinary tract infections are absent in NPH. Hypertension is rare, particularly given the degree of chronic renal insufficiency. Due to the lack of specificity of the initial symptoms with absence of edema and hypertension, most children have already developed chronic renal failure when they first come to clinical attention. This presents a small but definite risk of sudden death from fluid and electrolyte imbalance. Disease recurrence has never been reported after renal transplantation for NPH (79,80).

Extrarenal manifestations occur only in recessive NPH, but are absent from MCKD. The most frequent extrarenal association is retinitis pigmentosa seen in SLS (81,82). SLS occurs in approximately 12% of all patients with the NPH-MCKD complex (83), which would be equivalent to 18% of all autosomal recessive cases. An early-onset and a late-onset type of SLS have been described. Intrafamilial dissociation of renal and eye involvement has never been demonstrated convincingly in any published pedigree. In the early-onset type, children present with coarse nystagmus and/or blindness at birth or within the first 2 years of life. Funduscopic alterations are present in all SLS patients by the age of 10 years. The late-onset form is characterized by development of blindness during school age after a variable period of night blindness. Other eye symptoms besides tapeto-retinal degeneration comprise nystagmus, myopia, coloboma of the chorioidea, strabismus, hyperopia, optical nerve atrophy, and amblyopia (5). Age of onset, symptoms, and histology of renal disease is identical to what is known from NPH patients without ocular involvement. In patients with recessive mutations in the *NPHP1* gene, no molecular difference in defects of the *NPHP1* gene have been identified that would distinguish patients with the purely renal form of NPH from patients with the association of NPH and retinitis pigmentosa. As in SLS, no specific molecular differences of the *NPHP1* gene distinguish patients with the purely renal form of NPH from patients with the association of NPH and Cogan syndrome (23). With ocular motor apraxia, infants with Cogan syndrome cannot move their eyes sideways, which leads to a pattern of compensatory head thrusts. This symptom resolves within the first few years of life. Additional forms of extrarenal involvement are congenital hepatic fibrosis (84,85) and developmental defects of bone, predominantly in the form of cone-shaped epiphyses (type 28 and 28A) (86). These can also occur in combination with retinal degeneration and cerebellar ataxia (87,88). In Joubert syndrome type B, a developmental disorder with multiple organ involvement, NPH occurs in association with coloboma of the eye or retinal degeneration; aplasia of the cerebellar vermis with ataxia; and the facultative symptoms of psychomotor retardation, polydactyly, and neonatal tachypnea/dyspnea (89,90). An NPH-like phenotype has also been observed in Sensenbrenner syndrome (91).

Medullary Cystic Kidney Disease

Goldman and associates were the first to report a large kindred with autosomal dominant, adult-onset MCKD (92).

This was followed by the publication of two large pedigrees from the United States by Gardner and Burke et al. (93,94). The dominant form of the disease complex differs from the recessive forms in that the onset of end-stage renal disease is in the third decade of life or even later (95), with an average at age 28.5 years (96). In MCKD, penetrance appears to be very high by the age of 45 years. The second feature distinguishing MCKD from NPH is the lack of extrarenal involvement in dominant disease, with the exception of hyperuricemia and gout. For MCKD1, an association of the renal symptoms with hyperuricemia and gout has been described (34,39), and MCKD2 has been found to localize to the same chromosomal region as familial juvenile hyperuricemic nephropathy (45).

EPIDEMIOLOGY

NPH and dominant MCKD seem to be distributed evenly among males and females. NPH has been reported from virtually all regions of the world (5). The incidence of the disease has been estimated to be 9 per 8.3 million patients in the United States (97) or 1 in 50,000 live births in Canada (98). The condition constitutes the most frequent genetic cause for end-stage renal disease in the first two decades of life and is a major cause of end-stage renal disease in children, accounting for 10 to 25% of these patients (5,99,100). In the North American pediatric end-stage renal disease population, pooled data indicate a prevalence of less than 5% (101,102). MCKD appears to be somewhat less infrequent.

DIAGNOSIS AND DIFFERENTIAL DIAGNOSIS

Laboratory Studies

Patients with NPH are usually diagnosed when an increased serum creatinine value is detected during evaluation for nonspecific complaints. History generally reveals prolonged nocturia since school age. Specific gravity of a morning urine specimen will be low. Renal ultrasound will then corroborate the diagnosis (see Imaging) (Fig. 35.3), which can be subsequently confirmed by molecular genetic diagnostics if NPH1, NPH2, or NPH4 is present (http://www.renalgenes.org). A diagnostic algorithm for NPH has been suggested (76). Hematuria, proteinuria, and bacteriuria are uncommon in NPH. In rare cases when proteinuria is present, it is usually mild and of the tubular type. Laboratory studies are needed to assess the severity of renal failure and generally demonstrate elevated serum creatinine, blood urea nitrogen, phosphorus, metabolic acidosis, hypocalcemia, and anemia. In SLS, retinitis pigmentosa is diagnosed by its specific findings on ophthalmoscopy, including increased pigment, attenuation of retinal vessels, and pallor of the optic disk. If retinitis pigmentosa is present, electroretinography and electro-oculography can be used to evaluate severity. Retinal degeneration is characterized by a constant and complete extinction of the electroretinogram, preceding the development of visual and funduscopic signs of retinitis pigmentosa (103). Ophthalmoscopy should be performed in any patient to evaluate for signs of SLS, as it may occur in patients with NPH1, NPH2, or NPH3. Liver function tests and hepatic ultrasonography are important to facilitate detection of patients with hepatic fibrosis.

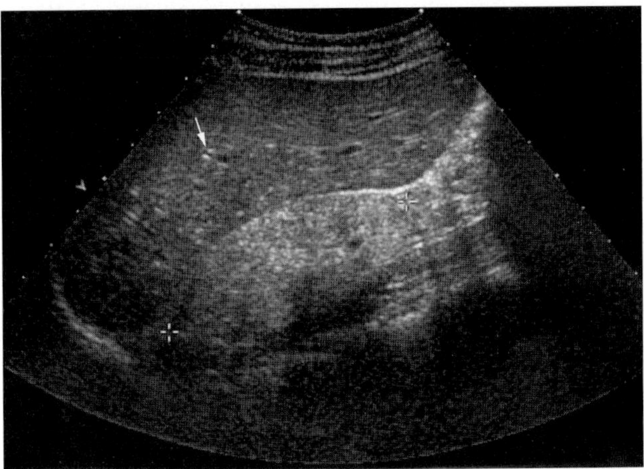

FIGURE 35.3. Renal ultrasound in nephronophthisis. Note loss of cortico-medullary differentiation, cysts at the cortico-medullary border of the kidney, and increased echogenicity, which renders the ultrasound pattern similar to the pattern of liver (*arrow*). In nephronophthisis, kidneys are typically normal in size. (Courtesy of Dr. U. Vester, Essen, Germany.)

Imaging

The most useful imaging technique in the NPH-MCKD complex is ultrasonography. Kidneys are of normal or moderately reduced size and show increased echogenicity (which renders the renal echo texture more echogenic than that of the liver), loss of cortico-medullary differentiation, and, in later stages, cyst formation at the cortico-medullary border of the kidneys (104) (Fig. 35.3). Garel et al. have seen medullary cysts in 13 of 15 children studied at the time of renal failure (mean age, 9.7 years) (105). Roentgenography contributes little to the diagnosis of the disease. Medullary cysts can sometimes also be demonstrated on magnetic resonance imaging or computed tomography (106,107). Histology is characteristic but not pathognomonic in NPH-MCKD because cysts may be absent, and tubulointerstitial disease can be relatively unspecific. Renal biopsy can be circumvented as an initial procedure due to the availability of molecular genetic diagnostics in NPH1, NPH2, and NPH4. If molecular genetic diagnostics do not detect a molecular defect, the diagnosis can be based on the combined results of typical history, with polyuria, polydipsia, and anemia; the classical appearance of the kidney on ultrasound; and renal histology. A thorough pedigree analysis should be documented for each of three successive generations to rule out autosomal dominant MCKD.

Molecular Genetic Diagnosis

Recently, molecular genetic diagnosis has become available for NPH1, NPH2, and NPH4 through identification of the respective genes (see Laboratory Studies) (http://www.renalgenes.org). A diagnostic algorithm should be followed to avoid unnecessary renal biopsy (76). Molecular genetic analysis is the only diagnostic procedure by which the diagnosis of NPH1, NPH2, and NPH3 can be made with certainty. However, due to the presence of additional loci for NPH, the lack of detection of mutations in the *NPHP1* gene does not exclude the diagnosis of NPH. If renal disease with features of the NPH-MCKD complex occurs in a person older than 25 years, its presence should be thoroughly sought in preceding generations. This may frequently result in detection of a pattern of autosomal dominant inheritance. In MCKD1, only indirect molecular genetic diagnosis by haplotype analysis is possible so far, as the respective genes have not yet been identified. For this purpose, a pedigree and blood samples from at least seven affected members and their first-degree relative will have to be obtained. In MCKD2, mutational analysis of the *UMOD* gene can be performed.

Molecular genetic testing should be performed only after consent within the guidelines of the National and International Societies for Human Genetics. Before genetic counseling, a thorough pedigree analysis to distinguish recessive (early-onset) from dominant (late-onset) disease is mandatory, and extrarenal organ involvement should be sought. Because nonsymptomatic potential carriers of recessive defects should not be examined by molecular genetic diagnostics, unaffected siblings younger than 13 years of age should be re-evaluated yearly for maximal urinary concentrating ability and renal ultrasound. If symptoms evolve and serum creatinine changes, molecular genetic diagnostics after informed consent is warranted to allow early prevention of complications from electrolyte disturbances, dehydration, anemia, and growth retardation. If a transplant recipient's renal histology suggests NPH and a living related donor is considered, molecular genetic diagnostics may help to exclude or detect renal disease within the family. Because there is genetic locus heterogeneity in diseases of the NPH-MCKD complex, prenatal diagnosis can only be performed by direct genetic testing. This requires a setting in which a specific mutation or deletion of the *NPHP1* gene has already been characterized in an affected sibling.

Differential Diagnosis

On histopathology, the NPH-MCKD complex has to be differentiated from other forms of interstitial nephropathies such as chronic pyelonephritis or drug injury. In oligomeganephronic dysplasia, kidney size is reduced, and histology is distinct from NPH. The paucity of urinary abnormalities, the frequent lack of hypertension, normal kidney size, and the localization of renal cysts (if present) readily differentiate variants of the NPH-MCKD complex from recessive or dominant polycystic kidney disease. Finally, medullary sponge kidney (108) can easily be distinguished from the complex, as it does not usually lead to chronic renal failure and shows calcifications and calculi on renal ultrasound.

PROGNOSIS AND THERAPY

There is no specific therapy for NPH or MCKD. Therapy is symptomatic and is directed toward the treatment of hypertension, if present, as well as the correction of disturbances of electrolyte, acid-base, and water balance. Hypokalemia may contribute to polyuria, and oral potassium supplementation may alleviate this symptom. Metabolic acidosis should be corrected and osteodystrophy and secondary hyperparathyroidism treated with adequate calcium supplementation, phosphorus restriction, non-magnesium–containing phosphate binders, and vitamin D therapy. Anemia should be treated with iron supplementation and erythropoietin, and growth retardation may require administration of growth hormone if the diagnosis is made early enough for an intervention. Adequate nutrition should be maintained with the help of a dietitian. Psychological counseling of the patients is an integral part of therapy because of the poor self-image associated with growth retardation and to alleviate pressures resulting from the need to comply with complicated medications and dietary prescriptions. All patients require renal replacement therapy by dialysis and renal transplantation during childhood, adolescence, or, in dominant disease, in early adult life.

REFERENCES

1. Gardner KD Jr. Juvenile nephronophthisis and renal medullary cystic disease. In: Gardner KD Jr, ed. *Cystic diseases of the kidney*. New York: Wiley, 1976.
2. Smith CH, Graham JB. Congenital medullary cysts of the kidneys with severe refractory anemia. *Am J Dis Child* 1945;69:369–377.
3. Fanconi G, Hanhart E, Albertini A, et al. Die familiäre juvenile Nephronophthise. *Hel Pediatr Acta* 1951;6:1–49.
4. Waldherr R, Lennert T, Weber HP, et al. The nephronophthisis complex: a clinicopathologic study in children. *Virchows Arch* 1982;394:235–254.
5. Kleinknecht C. The inheritance of nephronophthisis. In: Spitzer A, Avner ED, eds. *Inheritance of kidney and urinary tract diseases*. Boston: Kluwer Academic Publishers, 1989.
6. Hildebrandt F, Waldherr R, Kutt R, Brandis M. The nephronophthisis complex: clinical and genetic aspects. *Clin Investig* 1992;70:802–808.

7. Kleinknecht C, Habib R. Nephronophthisis. In: Cameron S, Davison AM, Grünfeld JP, et al., eds. *Oxford textbook of clinical nephrology*. Oxford: Oxford Press, 1992:2188–2197.
8. Hildebrandt F, Jungers P, Grünfeld J-P. Medullary cystic and medullary sponge renal disorders. In: Schreier WB, Gottschalk C, eds. *Diseases of the kidney*. Boston: Little, Brown and Co., 1996:499–519.
9. Sarles HE, Rodin AE, Poduska PR, et al. Hereditary nephritis, retinitis pigmentosa and chromosomal abnormalities. *Am J Med* 1968;45:312–321.
10. Antignac C, Arduy C, Beckmann JS, et al. A gene for familial juvenile nephronophthisis maps to chromosome 2p. *Nat Genet* 1993;3:342–345.
11. Hildebrandt F, Singh-Sawhney I, Schnieders B, et al. Mapping of a gene for familial juvenile nephronophthisis: refining the map and definition of flanking markers on chromosome 2. *Am J Hum Genet* 1993;53:1256–1261.
12. Spurr NK, Barton H, Bashir R, et al. Report of the third international workshop on human chromosome 2 mapping 1994. *Cytogenet Cell Genet* 1994;67:215–244.
13. Hildebrandt F, Cybulla M, Strahm B, et al. Physical mapping of the gene for juvenile nephronophthisis (NPH1) by construction of a complete YAC contig of 6.5 Mb on chromosome 2q13. *Cytogenet Cell Genet* 1996;73:235–239.
14. Spurr NK, Bashir R, Bushby K, et al. Report of the fourth International Workshop on Human Chromosome 2 Mapping. *Cytogenet Cell Genet* 1996;73:255–273.
15. Nothwang HG, Strahm B, Denich D, et al. Molecular cloning of the interleukin-1 gene cluster: construction of an integrated YAC, PAC and partial transcriptional map in the region of chromosome 2q13. *Genomics* 1997;41:370–378.
16. Nothwang HG, Stubanus M, Adolphs J, et al. Construction of a gene map of the nephronophthisis type 1 (NPH1) region on human chromosome 2q12. *Genomics* 1998;47:276–285.
17. Hildebrandt F, Otto E, Rensing C, et al. A novel gene encoding an SH3 domain protein is mutated in nephronophthisis type 1. *Nat Genet* 1997;17:149–153.
18. Saunier S, Calado J, Heilig R, et al. A novel gene that encodes a protein with a putative src homology 3 domain is a candidate gene for familial juvenile nephronophthisis. *Hum Mol Genet* 1997;6:2317–2323.
19. Saunier S, Calado J, Benessy F, et al. Characterization of the *NPHP1* locus: mutational mechanism involved in deletions in familial juvenile nephronophthisis. *Am J Hum Genet* 2000; 66:778–789.
20. Otto E, Betz R, Rensing C, et al. A deletion distinct from the classical homologous recombination of juvenile nephronophthisis type 1 (NPH1) allows exact molecular definition of deletion breakpoints. *Hum Mutat* 2000;16:211–223.
21. Hildebrandt F, Strahm B, Nothwang HG, et al. Molecular genetic identification of families with juvenile nephronophthisis type 1: rate of progression to renal failure. *Kidney Int* 1997;51:261–269.
22. Caridi G, Murer L, Bellantuono R, et al. Renal-retinal syndromes: association of retinal anomalies and recessive nephronophthisis in patients with homozygous deletion of the NPH1 locus. *Am J Kidney Dis* 1998;32:1059–1062.
23. Betz R, Rensing C, Otto E, et al. Children with ocular motor apraxia type Cogan carry deletions in the gene (*NPHP1*) for juvenile nephronophthisis. *J Pediatr* 2000;136:828–831.
24. Bodaghi E, Honarmand MT, Ahmadi M. Infantile nephronophthisis. *Int J Pediatr Nephrol* 1987;8:207–210.
25. Gagnadoux MF, Bacri JL, Broyer M, et al. Infantile chronic tubulo-interstitial nephritis with cortical microcysts: variant of nephronophthisis or new disease entity? *Pediatr Nephrol* 1989;3:50–55.
26. Haider NB, Carmi R, Shalev H, et al. A Bedouin kindred with infantile nephronophthisis demonstrates linkage to chromosome 9 by homozygosity mapping. *Am J Hum Genet* 1998;63:1404–1410.
26a. Otto E, Schermer B, O'Toole J, et al. Inversion mutations cause nephronophthisis type 2, linking renal cystic disease to the function of primary cilia and left-right axis determination. *Nat Genet* 2003;(*in press*).
27. Omran H, Fernandez C, Jung M, et al. Identification of a new gene locus for adolescent nephronophthisis, on chromosome 3q22 in a large Venezuelan pedigree. *Am J Hum Genet* 2000;66:118–127.
28. Omran H, Haffner K, Vollmer M, et al. Exclusion of the candidate genes ACE and Bcl-2 for six families with nephronophthisis not linked to the NPH1 locus. *Nephrol Dial Transplant* 1999;14:2328–2331.
29. Volz A, Melkaoui R, Hildebrandt F, et al. Candidate gene analysis of KIAA0678 encoding a DNA J-like protein for adolescent nephronophthisis and Senior-Loken syndrome type 3. *Cytogenet Genome Res* 2002;97:163–166.
30. Omran H, Sasmaz G, Haffner K, et al. Identification of a gene locus for Senior-Loken syndrome in the region of the nephronophthisis type 3 gene. *J Am Soc Nephrol* 2002;13:75–79.
31. Schuermann MJ, Otto E, Becker A, et al. Mapping of gene loci for nephronophthisis type 4 and Senior-Loken syndrome, to chromosome 1p36. *Am J Hum Genet* 2002;70:1240–1246.
32. Otto E, Hoefele J, Ruf R, et al. A gene mutated in nephronophthisis and retinitis pigmentosa encodes a novel protein, nephroretinin, conserved in evolution. *Am J Hum Genet* 2002; 71:1161–1167.
33. Mollet G, Salomon R, Gribouval O, et al. The gene mutated in juvenile nephronophthisis type 4 encodes a novel protein that interacts with nephrocystin. *Nat Genet* 2002;32:300–305.
34. Christodoulou K, Tsingis M, Stavrou C, et al. Chromosome 1 localization of a gene for autosomal dominant medullary cystic kidney disease. *Hum Mol Genet* 1998;7:905–911.
35. Stavrou C, Pierides A, Zouvani I, et al. Medullary cystic kidney disease with hyperuricemia and gout in a large Cypriot family: no allelism with nephronophthisis type 1. *Am J Med Genet* 1998;77:149–154.
36. Neumann HP, Zauner I, Strahm B, et al. Late occurrence of cysts in autosomal dominant medullary cystic kidney disease. *Nephrol Dial Transplant* 1997;12:1242–1246.
37. Fuchshuber A, Kroiss S, Karle S, et al. Refinement of the gene locus for autosomal dominant medullary cystic kidney disease type 1 (MCKD1) and construction of a physical and partial transcriptional map of the region. *Genomics* 2001;72:278–284.
38. Koptides M, Mean R, Stavrou C, et al. Novel NPR1 polymorphic variants and its exclusion as a candidate gene for medullary cystic kidney disease (ADMCKD) type 1. *Mol Cell Probes* 2001;15:357–361.

39. Scolari F, Ghiggeri GM, Amoroso A, et al. Genetic heterogeneity for autosomal dominant medullary cystic kidney disease (ADMCKD). *J Am Soc Nephrol* 1998;9:393A.
40. Scolari F, Ghiggeri GM, Casari G, et al. Autosomal dominant medullary cystic disease: a disorder with variable clinical pictures and exclusion of linkage with the NPH1 locus. *Nephrol Dial Transplant* 1998;13:2536–2546.
41. Scolari F, Puzzer D, Amoroso A, et al. Identification of a new locus for medullary cystic disease, on chromosome 16p12. *Am J Hum Genet* 1999;64:1655–1660.
42. Kamatani N, Moritani M, Yamanaka H, et al. Localization of a gene for familial juvenile hyperuricemic nephropathy causing underexcretion-type gout to 16p12 by genome-wide linkage analysis of a large family. *Arthritis Rheum* 2000;43:925–929.
43. Stiburkova B, Majewski J, Sebesta I, et al. Familial juvenile hyperuricemic nephropathy: localization of the gene on chromosome 16p11.2-and evidence for genetic heterogeneity. *Am J Hum Genet* 2000;66:1989–1994.
44. Hateboer N, Gumbs C, Teare MD, et al. Confirmation of a gene locus for medullary cystic kidney disease (MCKD2) on chromosome 16p12. *Kidney Int* 2001;60:1233–1239.
45. Dahan K, Fuchshuber A, Adamis S, et al. Familial juvenile hyperuricemic nephropathy and autosomal dominant medullary cystic kidney disease type 2: two facets of the same disease? *J Am Soc Nephrol* 2001;12:2348–2357.
46. Kroiss S, Huck K, Berthold S, et al. Evidence of further genetic heterogeneity in autosomal dominant medullary cystic kidney disease. *Nephrol Dial Transplant* 2000;15:818–821.
47. Fuchshuber A, Kroiss S, Karle S, et al. Refinement of the gene locus for autosomal dominant medullary cystic kidney disease type 1 (MCKD1) and construction of a physical and partial transcriptional map of the region. *Genomics* 2001;72:278–284.
48. Sherman FE, Studnicki FM, Fetterman GH. Renal lesions of familial juvenile nephronophthisis examined by microdissection. *Am J Clin Pathol* 1971;55:391.
49. Sworn MJ, Eisinger AJ. Medullary cystic disease and juvenile nephronophthisis in separate members of the same family. *Arch Dis Child* 1972;47:278.
50. Giselson N, Heinegard D, Holuster G, et al. Renal medullary cystic disease or familial juvenile nephronophthisis: a renal tubular disease. Biochemical findings in two siblings. *Am J Med* 1970;48:174–184.
51. Chamberlin BC, Hagge WW, Stickler GB. Juvenile nephronophthisis and medullary cystic disease. *Mayo Clin Proc* 1977;52:485–491.
52. Van Collenburg JJM, Thompson HW, Huber J. Clinical, pathological and genetic aspects of a form of cystic disease of the renal medulla: familial juvenile nephronophthisis (FNPH). *Clin Nephrol* 1978;9:55–62.
53. Ivemark BI, Ljungqvist A, Barry A. Juvenile nephronophthisis. Part II. A histologic and microangiographic study. *Acta Paediat (Uppsala)* 1960;49:480–487.
54. Resnick J, Sisson S, Vernier RL. Tamm-Horsfall protein. Abnormal localization in renal disease. *Lab Invest* 1978;38:550.
55. Zollinger HU, Mihatsch MJ, Edefonti A, et al. Nephronophthisis (medullary cystic disease of the kidney): a study using electron microscopy, immunofluorescence, and a review of the morphological findings. *Helv Paediatr Acta* 1980;35:509–530.
56. Bernstein J, Gardner KD. Hereditary tubulo interstitial nephritis. In: Cotran RS, Brenner BM, Stein JH, eds. *Oxford textbook of clinical nephrology*. Oxford: Oxford Press, 1992:2188–2197.
57. Cohen AH, Hoyer JR. Nephronophthisis. A primary tubular basement membrane defect. *Lab Invest* 1986;55:564–572.
58. Saraux H, Dhermy P, Fontaine J-C, et al. La dégéneréscence rétino-tubulaire de Senior et Löken. *Arch Ophthalmol* 1970;30:683–696.
59. Hildebrandt F. Identification of a gene for nephronophthisis. *Nephrol Dial Transplant* 1998;13:1334–1336.
60. Hildebrandt F, Otto E. Molecular genetics of nephronophthisis and medullary cystic kidney disease. *J Am Soc Nephrol* 2000;11:1753–1761.
61. Donaldson JC, Dempsey PJ, Reddy S, et al. Crk-associated substrate p130(Cas) interacts with nephrocystin and both proteins localize to cell-cell contacts of polarized epithelial cells. *Exp Cell Res* 2000;256:168–178.
62. Benzing T, Gerke P, Hopker K, et al. Nephrocystin interacts with Pyk2, p130(Cas), and tensin and triggers phosphorylation of Pyk2. *Proc Natl Acad Sci U S A* 2001;98:9784–9789.
63. Donaldson JC, Dise RS, Ritchie MD, et al. Nephrocystin-conserved domains involved in targeting to epithelial cell-cell junctions, interaction with filamins, and establishing cell polarity. *J Biol Chem* 2002;277:29028–29035.
64. Hildebrandt F, Otto E. Molecular genetics of nephronophthisis and medullary cystic kidney disease. *J Am Soc Nephrol* 2000;11:1753–1761.
65. Rahilly MA, Fleming S. Abnormal integrin receptor expression in two cases of familial nephronophthisis. *Histopathology* 1995;26:345–349.
66. Yorioka N, Taniguchi Y, Yamashita K, et al. Hepatocyte growth factor in nephronophthisis-medullary cystic disease complex. *Pediatr Nephrol* 1996;10:515–516.
67. Murer L, Caridi G, Della Vella M, et al. Expression of nuclear transcription factor PAX2 in renal biopsies of juvenile nephronophthisis. *Nephron* 2000;91:588–593.
68. Lo SH, Yu QC, Degenstein L, Chen LB, Fuchs E. Progressive kidney degeneration in mice lacking tensin. *J Cell Biol* 1997;136:1349–1361.
69. Lyon MF, Hulse EV. An inherited kidney disease of mice resembling human nephronophthisis. *J Med Genet* 1971;8:41–48.
70. Sibalic V, Sun L, Sibalic A, et al. Characteristic matrix and tubular basement membrane abnormalities in the CBA/Ca-kdkd mouse model of hereditary tubulointerstitial disease. *Nephron* 1998;80:305–313.
71. Esther CR, Howard TE, Marino EM, et al. Mice lacking angiotensin-converting enzyme have low blood pressure, renal pathology, and reduced male fertility. *Lab Invest* 1996;74:953–965.
72. Veis DJ, Sorenson CM, Shutter JR, Kersmeyer SJ. Bcl-2-deficient mice demonstrate fulminant lymphoid apoptosis, polycystic kidneys, and hypopigmented hair. *Cell* 1993;75:229–240.
73. Omran H, Haffner K, Burth S, et al. Human adolescent nephronophthisis: gene locus synteny with polycystic kid-

ney disease in pcy mice. *J Am Soc Nephrol* 2001;12:107–113.

74. Togawa A, Miyoshi J, Ishizaki H, et al. Progressive impairment of kidneys and reproductive organs in mice lacking Rho GDIalpha. *Oncogene* 1999;18:5373–5380.
75. Igarashi P, Somlo S. Genetics and pathogenesis of polycystic kidney disease. *J Am Soc Nephrol* 2002;13:2384–2398.
76. Hildebrandt F, Strahm B, Nothwang HG, et al. Molecular genetic identification of families with juvenile nephronophthisis type 1: rate of progression to renal failure. *Kidney Int* 1997;51:261–269.
77. Mongeau JG, Worthen HG. Nephronophthisis and medullary cystic disease. *Am J Med* 1967;43:345–355.
78. Makker SP, Grupe WE, Perrin E, et al. Identical progression of juvenile hereditary nephronophthisis in monozygotic twins. *J Pediatr* 1973;82:773–779.
79. Steele BT, Lirenman DS, Battie CW. Nephronophthisis. *Am J Med* 1980;68:531–538.
80. ASC/NIH Renal Transplantation Registry, 1975.
81. Senior B, Friedmann AI, Braudo JL. Juvenile familial nephropathy with tapetoretinal degeneration: a new oculorenal dystrophy. *Am J Ophthalmol* 1961;52:625–633.
82. Løken AC, Hanssen O, Halvorsen S et al. Hereditary renal dysplasia and blindness. *Acta Paediatr* 1961;50:177–184.
83. Gardner KD, Evan AP. The nephronophthisis-cystic renal medullary complex. In: Hamburger J, Crosnier J, Grünfeld J-P, eds. *Nephrology*. New York: Wiley, 1979:893–907.
84. Boichis H, Passwell J, David R, et al. Congenital hepatic fibrosis and nephronophthisis. A family study. *QJM* 1973; 42:221–233.
85. Delaney V, Mullaney J, Bourke E. Juvenile nephronophthisis, congenital hepatic fibrosis and retinal hypoplasia in twins. *QJM* 1978;New Series XLVII:281.
86. Mainzer F, Saldino RM, Ozonoff MB, et al. Familial nephropathy associated with retinitis pigmentosa, cerebellar ataxia and skeletal abnormalities. *Am J Med* 1970;49:556–562.
87. Fontaine JL, Boulestreix J, Saraux H, et al. Nephropathie tubulo-interstitielle de l'entfant avec degenerescence tapetoretinienne. *Arch Franc Pediatr* 1970;27:459–470.
88. Donaldson MDC, Warner AA, Trompeter RS, et al. Familial juvenile nephronophthisis, Jeune's syndrome and associated disorders. *Arch Dis Child* 1985;60:426–434.
89. Saraiva JM, Baraitser M. Joubert syndrome: a review. *Am J Med Genet* 1992;43:726–731.
90. Hildebrandt F, Nothwang HG, Vossmerbaumer U, et al. Lack of large, homozygous deletions of the nephronophthisis 1 region in Joubert syndrome type B. APN Study Group. Arbeitsgemeinschaft fur Padiatrische Nephrologie. *Pediatr Nephrol* 1998;12:16–19.
91. Costet C, Betis F, Berard E, et al. Pigmentosum retinitis and tubulo-interstitial nephronophthisis in Sensenbrenner syndrome: a case report. *J Fr Ophtalmol* 2000:23:158–160.
92. Goldman SH, Walker SR, Merigan TC, et al. Hereditary occurrence of cystic disease of the renal medulla. *N Engl J Med* 1966;274:984–992.
93. Gardner GD. Evolution of clinical signs in adult-onset disease of the renal medulla. *Ann Intern Med* 1971;74:47–54.
94. Burke JR, Inglis JA, Craswell KR, et al. Juvenile nephronophthisis and medullary cystic disease—the same disease (report of a large family with medullary cystic disease associated with gout and epilepsy). *Clin Nephrol* 1982;18:1–8.
95. Swenson RS, Kempson RL, Friedland GW. Cystic disease of the renal medulla in the elderly. *JAMA* 1972;228:1401.
96. Gardner KD. Evolution of clinical signs in adult-onset disease of the renal medulla. *Ann Intern Med* 1971;74:47–54.
97. Potter DE, Holliday MA, Piel CF, et al. Treatment of end-stage renal disease in children: a 15-year experience. *Kidney Int* 1980;18:103–109.
98. Waldherr R, Schärer K, Weber HP, Gretz N. Der Nephronophthise-Komplex. *Nieren- und Hochdruckkrankheiten* 1983;12:397–406.
99. Cantani A, Bamonte G, Ceccoli D et al. Familial juvenile nephronophthisis. *Clin Pediatr* 1986;25:90–95.
100. Betts PR, Forest-Hay I. Juvenile nephronophthisis. *Lancet* 1973;2:475–478.
101. Watkins SL, Avner ED. Renal dysplasia and cystic disease. In: Holliday MA, Barrat TM, Avner ED, eds. *Pediatric nephrology*. Baltimore: Williams and Wilkins, 1993.
102. Avner ED. Medullary cystic disease and medullary sponge kidney. In: Greenberg A, ed. *Primer on kidney diseases*. Boston: Academic Press, 1994.
103. Bernstein J. Hepatic involvement in hereditary renal syndromes. Genetic aspects of developmental pathology. *Birth Defects* 1987;23:115–130.
104. Blowey DL, Querfeld U, Geary D, et al. Ultrasound findings in juvenile nephronophthisis. *Pediatr Nephrol* 1996;10:22–24.
105. Garel LA, Habib, R, Pariente D, et al. Juvenile nephronophthisis: sonographic appearance in children with severe uremia. *Radiology* 1984;151:93.
106. McGregor AR, Bailey RR. Nephronophthisis-cystic renal medulla complex: diagnosis by computerized tomography. *Nephron* 1989;53:70.
107. Fyhrquiest FY, Klockars M, Gordin A, et al. Hyperreninemia, lysozymuria, and erythrocytosis in Fanconi syndrome with medullary cystic kidney. *Acta Med Scand* 1980;207:359.
108. Cacchi R, Ricci V. Sopra una rara e forse ancora non descritta effezione cistica della piramidi renali ("rene a spugna"). *Atti Soc Ital Urol* 1948;5:59.

36

POLYCYSTIC KIDNEY DISEASE

KATHERINE MacRAE DELL
RUTH A. McDONALD
SANDRA L. WATKINS
ELLIS D. AVNER

Polycystic kidney disease (PKD) is a heritable disorder with diffuse cystic involvement of both kidneys without dysplasia (1). All forms of PKD can have clinical manifestations in infants and children. The major clinical entities of autosomal recessive PKD (ARPKD) and autosomal dominant PKD (ADPKD) have considerable overlap in clinical presentation and radiographic features. Glomerulocystic kidney disease (GCKD) can be a feature of several inherited, sporadic, and syndromal conditions, as well as an expression of ADPKD.

PATHOPHYSIOLOGY OF CYST FORMATION IN POLYCYSTIC KIDNEY DISEASE

In the 1990s, major advances were made in understanding the molecular genetics of PKD. Through a combination of positional cloning, direct sequencing, and use of the rapidly expanding genome databases, the major causative genes for both ADPKD (*PKD1* and *PKD2*) as well as ARPKD (*PKHD1*) have been identified (2–5) (Table 36.1). Details specific to the molecular genetics of ARPKD and ADPKD are addressed in the respective sections that follow. Despite the advances in the identification of the PKD genes and proteins, the precise mechanisms by which these gene defects result in cyst formation have not yet been fully elucidated. Considerable insights into the understanding of cyst formation pathogenesis have been provided by many studies of the cellular pathophysiology of PKD. These studies complement the advances made in the genetics of the diseases and may form the basis for future therapeutic interventions.

On the basis of extensive *in vivo* and *in vitro* studies using human tissue and animal models of PKD, at least three basic processes are operative in renal cyst formation and progressive enlargement: (a) tubular cell hyperplasia; (b) tubular fluid secretion; and (c) abnormalities in tubular extracellular matrix (ECM), structure, and/or function (6–12) (Fig. 36.1). Delineating the extent to which these factors, singly or in combination, contribute to cyst development and enlargement in ADPKD and ARPKD remains an area of active investigation.

TUBULAR HYPERPLASIA

Tubular hyperplasia is a central morphologic feature of all described human renal cystic diseases (7,10). On the basis of mathematic modeling of cyst growth, it has been shown that tubular cell hyperplasia, with expansion of tubular wall segments to accommodate an increased cellular mass, is an essential factor in cyst formation and enlargement (12). Furthermore, cyst-derived epithelial cells from ADPKD and ARPKD demonstrate increased cell growth potential compared with controls (9,13). Unlike normal renal epithelia, ADPKD cystic epithelia respond to increased intracellular cyclic adenosine monophosphate (cAMP) with proliferation (14,15). Recent data demonstrate differences in cAMP-dependent protein kinase and proliferation in normal and polycystic kidney epithelia in a murine model of ARPKD (16). Additional *in vivo* data demonstrate increased renal tubular epithelial cell proliferation in both cystic and noncystic tubular epithelium from ADPKD and ARPKD kidneys (17).

A growing body of evidence implicates the epidermal growth factor receptor (EGFR) and its respective ligands, including epidermal growth factor (EGF) and transforming growth factor-α (TGFα), in proliferation of cystic epithelium. In both human ADPKD and ARPKD and in several murine models of PKD, cystic kidneys display characteristic alterations in EGFR expression. Quantitative abnormalities, including increased messenger RNA (mRNA) and protein, and qualitative differences, in particular, the appearance of "mislocalized" EGFR expressed on the apical surface of tubular epithelium, are seen (18–20). Apical EGFR is functional and capable of transmitting mitogenic signals *in vitro* (21).

TABLE 36.1. HUMAN POLYCYSTIC KIDNEY DISEASE GENES AND PROTEINS

Disease	Gene	Mode of inheritance	Chromosome location	Protein	Function/role
ADPKD	*PKD1*	AD	16p13.3–p13.12	Polycystin 1	?Receptor
ADPKD	*PKD2*	AD	4q21–q23	Polycystin 2	Cation channel
ARPKD	*PKHD1*	AR	6p21	Fibrocystin (polyductin)	?Receptor
GCKD (hypoplastic variant)	*HNF-1β*	AD	17cen–q21.3	Hepatocyte nuclear factor-1β	Transcription factor

ADPKD, autosomal dominant polycystic kidney disease; ARPKD, autosomal recessive polycystic kidney disease; GCKD, glomerulocystic kidney disease.

Inhibition of EGFR function *in vitro* by treatment with either an inhibitor of tyrosine kinase function or a blocking antibody inhibits formation of proximal tubule cysts and significantly decreases explant growth and distal nephron differentiation (22,23). Additional support for a central role for EGFR in the pathogenesis of cyst formation is provided by *in vivo* data. Inhibition or reduction of EGFR function, either by treatment with a novel tyrosine kinase inhibitor (24) or genetic manipulation (25), leads to a marked reduction in cyst formation and enlargement in animal models. Of note, EGFR is part of a larger family of receptors (the c-ErbB/HER receptors), and there are limited data on the expression and function of these related receptors in PKD. C-ErbB2 (HER2) overexpression is seen in some cysts of ADPKD kidneys but not in late-stage ARPKD kidneys (26). However, late-gestation/early postnatal human ARPKD samples showed increased ErbB-2 expression compared with normal human fetal and postnatal kidneys (27). The functional significance of altered ErbB2 expression in PKD remains to be determined. Studies in a murine models of ARPKD demonstrate that ErbB4 expression increases with progressive cystic disease, whereas a decrease is seen in normal (noncystic) age-matched controls (28).

Abnormalities in EGFR ligand expression have also been reported in both ARPKD and ADPKD. Renal cyst fluid contains EGF or EGF-like peptides in mitogenic concentrations, despite apparent reductions in EGF tissue expression (9,29–31). Treatment with EGF transiently improves renal function in murine models (32) but has no effect on histopathologic abnormalities, and continued EGF treatment worsens disease and shortens survival (33). TGFα and EGF are cystogenic in both murine embryonic organ cultures (34) and normal human kidney cells grown in a unique collagen gel system *in vitro* (35). ADPKD kidneys and cells derived from ADPKD have increased mRNA or protein levels of TGFα (18,36). Transgenic mice that overexpress TGFα develop cystic kidneys (37). Additional data suggest that inhibiting EGFR ligand function may also partially ameliorate disease. Treatment with an inhibitor of TGFα processing decreases cystic kidney disease in a murine model, although less effectively than EGFR inhibition. (38). Recent data demonstrate that combining inhibition of EGFR ligand function with EGFR inhibition may maximize therapeutic effectiveness while minimizing toxicity (39). Additional EGFR ligands, including amphiregulin and heparin-binding EGF, are abnormally expressed in PKD and may prove to also have a role in proliferation of cystic epithelium (40).

Epithelial cell hyperplasia may be mediated not only by factors that control cell proliferation (such as activation of the EGFR/EGFR ligand axis) but also by alterations of

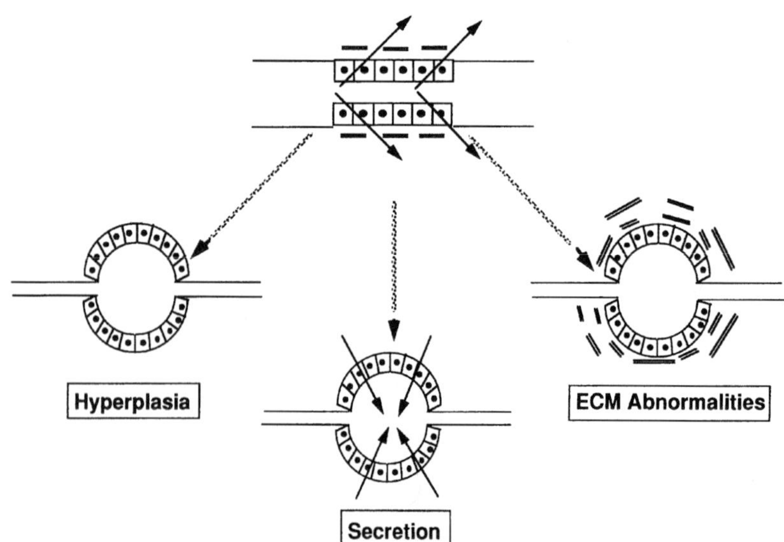

FIGURE 36.1. Pathophysiology of renal cyst formation. Studies in a variety of experimental models and human diseases implicate three major factors in renal cyst formation and progressive enlargement. Normal renal tubular absorptive epithelium can become cystic if (a) hyperplasia, localized to a distinct nephron segment, requires accommodation of an increased cell mass; (b) secretion, as opposed to absorption, leads to the net accumulation of intratubular fluid with low (or no) afferent tubular flow or efferent tubular obstruction; or (c) extracellular matrix (ECM) abnormalities alter the epithelial microenvironment such that abnormal cell-matrix interactions result in abnormal epithelial hyperplastic and secretory activity. These processes are not mutually exclusive, may reflect some characteristics of undifferentiated epithelium, and probably operate in concert during renal tubular cyst formation and progressive enlargement.

normal apoptotic mechanisms. Emerging evidence suggests that dysregulation of apoptosis, or the balance between apoptosis and proliferation, may contribute to the progression of ARPKD and ADPKD (41–43). Evidence in support of a role for apoptosis in the pathogenesis of PKD is provided by studies of various components of the apoptosis pathway, including several caspases and the bcl-2/bax family of proteins. Ali et al. (44) demonstrated a six- to sevenfold increase in caspase 3 and 4 activity in kidneys of *cpk* mice, a murine model of ARPKD. Unlike previous studies in which increased apoptosis was found in renal tubules, this study localized apoptosis primarily to the interstitium with little evidence of cell death in either cystic or noncystic tubules. Increased rates of apoptosis in a murine model of ARPKD were demonstrated in the interstitial cells surrounding cystic collecting tubules (CT) when compared to interstitial cells surrounding normal CT (45). Ecder et al. (46) have reported upregulation of caspase 3 in the Han/SPRD rat, a model of ADPKD.

Data regarding the antiapoptotic molecule, bcl-2, and its related proteins are somewhat conflicting. Mice deficient in bcl-2 develop severe multicystic hypoplasia characterized by proximal and distal tubular cysts and hyperproliferation of epithelium and interstitium (47). In contrast, increased bcl-2 expression has been demonstrated in animal models of both ARPKD and ADPKD (42,44,46). Of note, in one study, decreased expression of another antiapoptotic molecule, Bcl-X(L), suggests that the balance (rather than the absolute expression levels) of different components of the pro- and antiapoptotic pathways may be the critical factor in the development of cystic kidney disease (46). Abnormalities in the apoptotic pathway may also directly or indirectly impact on the normal cell-cell interactions (48–51). Alterations in apoptosis may also be mediated, in part, by abnormal expression of proto-oncogenes, in particular, c-myc. In both murine ARPKD and human ADPKD kidneys, c-myc is overexpressed in cystic tissue (42,52–54) and associated with a marked increase in both tubular cellular proliferation and apoptosis (55–57). Other genes, such as *pax2*, may also have a role in apoptosis in PKD (58).

FLUID SECRETION

In addition to epithelial hyperplasia, some data demonstrate a significant role for tubular fluid secretion in cyst formation and progressive enlargement (7,9,10). On a theoretical basis, tubular fluid secretion, in addition to hyperplasia, fulfills the requirements for cyst growth predicted by mathematic modeling (12). Cellular proliferation without tubular secretion would produce solid tumor nests of tubular cells rather than cysts. In ADPKD, more than 70% of cysts have no afferent or efferent tubular connections, and thus must fill by transepithelial secretion of solute and fluid (59,60).

Studies in a variety of model systems have evaluated possible mechanisms involved in PKD tubular fluid secretion. Work to date has identified a major role for cAMP-mediated chloride secretion during *in vitro* cyst formation (14,61–63). A putative lipid "secretagogue" isolated from cyst fluid of human ADPKD kidneys was found to stimulate intracellular cAMP and stimulate fluid secretion (64).

Additional *in vivo* and *in vitro* studies demonstrate a potential role for quantitative and qualitative alterations in Na^+-K^+-adenosine triphosphatase (ATPase) activity in mediating tubular fluid secretion in cystogenesis (65–70). In proximal tubules, it has been postulated that increases in Na^+-K^+-ATPase activity modulate tubular secretion and cyst formation through activation of a secondary active transport process (e.g., tubular organic anion secretion), which osmotically obligates intratubular fluid accumulation and cystogenesis (65–67). In collecting tubules, apical, as opposed to normal, basolateral cell surface Na^+-K^+-ATPase expression may mediate basal to apical vectorial sodium transport and thus directly drive fluid secretion in affected nephron segments in ADPKD and ARPKD (68–70). Apical Na^+-K^+-ATPase expression in murine ARPKD may reflect an exaggeration of the normal developmental profile of collecting tubule sodium pump expression (70). This, in association with the relatively undifferentiated ultrastructural and genetic profile of cystic tubular epithelium (11), suggests that abnormalities in the differentiation program of cystic tubular cells may be basic to the process of cystogenesis. Of note, however, apical Na^+-K^+-ATPase expression has not been a consistent finding in all PKD models (71).

It has been hypothesized that cAMP-stimulated chloride and fluid secretion occurs through activity of the cystic fibrosis transmembrane receptor (CFTR), the chloride channel mutated in cystic fibrosis (72). CFTR Cl^- channels exist in apical membranes of ADPKD and are major mediators of forskolin-stimulated chloride and fluid secretion by epithelial cells of human polycystic kidneys *in vitro* (72,73). CFTR is required for cAMP-dependent *in vitro* renal cyst formation (74). *In vivo* support for a role of CFTR in the pathogenesis of PKD was provided in a report of an ADPKD kindred in which cystic fibrosis was also present. Patients with ADPKD and CF (which results in a loss of functioning CFTR) were found to have less severe disease than those with ADPKD who did not have CF (75). However, a subsequent report failed to demonstrate such a protective effect (76). Because of the phenotypic variation within ADPKD families, it was difficult to determine if CFTR was, in fact, functioning as a significant modifying disease gene, or if the phenotypic differences were due to other modifying factors. This question was recently directly addressed in a murine model of ARPKD. Mice homozygous for the CFTR mutation (CFTR "knock-out" mice) were bred with the *bpk* mouse, a murine model of ARPKD. No improvement in cystic disease in resultant double mutants was found (77). These data suggest that CFTR activity does not play a central role in the pathogenesis of ARPKD, and that it is not necessary for cyst growth or enlargement. Chloride channels (other than CFTR) or abnormalities in amiloride-sensitive sodium transport may have roles in fluid secretion in cystic ARPKD epithelium (77). The role of CFTR in ADPKD remains to be determined.

EXTRACELLULAR MATRIX

The third major mediator of tubular cyst formation and progressive enlargement is abnormalities involving the ECM (7,9–11,68). Diffuse ultrastructural and biochemical abnormalities of tubular basement membranes have been demonstrated in human and animal models of PKD. Specific defects in the biosynthesis and transport of sulfated proteoglycans have also been identified (9,11,78–80). Renal tubular cells from patients with ADPKD grown *in vitro* produce increased amounts of ECM when compared with normal tubular epithelia (81).

It does not appear that matrix abnormalities mediate simple changes in the compliance or viscoelastic properties of tubular basement membranes, leading to distention under normal intratubular pressures (82). Rather, it would appear that altered matrix composition modulates cyst formation through altered tubular epithelial cell matrix interactions. These interactions regulate various aspects of cell growth, cell surface protein expression, cytodifferentiation, and gene expression (8,11). Conceivably, altered epithelial cell matrix interaction could modulate or amplify the processes of hyperplasia and fluid secretion discussed above.

Experimental evidence suggests that matrix metalloproteinases (MMPs) and tissue inhibitors of metalloproteinases may play a role in progression of disease in PKD (83–85). Elevated serum levels of MMPs, including MMP-1, tissue inhibitor of metalloproteinase-1, and MMP-9, have been demonstrated in a cohort of ADPKD patients when compared to normal controls (86). Although it is difficult to determine whether abnormal MMP expression is a reflection of a primary abnormality or a secondary effect, recent data suggest that inhibition of MMPs may have an impact on the severity of disease in animal models of ADPKD and ARPKD (38,87). Overexpression of other basement membrane, ECM, and cell adhesion components have also been demonstrated in PKD. Tenacin, an ECM glycoprotein, is abnormally expressed in human ARPKD and ADPKD fetal kidneys and in a murine model of ARPKD (88,89). Irregular expression of α-integrin subunits has also been demonstrated in fetal PKD kidneys (90).

Abnormal processes within the interstitium leading to interstitial inflammation and fibrosis contribute to progression in all cystic kidney diseases. For instance, monocyte chemoattractant protein-1, a chemoattractant and mediator of interstitial inflammation, is upregulated in ADPKD rats (91). In addition, oxidant stress is increased and protective effects of antioxidants decreased in the kidneys of animal models of both ARPKD and ADPKD models (92). Abnormalities in steroid and lipid metabolism have also been demonstrated in murine ARPKD (93–95). Angiogenesis may have a role in the pathogenesis of cyst expansion in ADPKD as well. When cysts enlarge, their nutrient requirements may outstrip their blood supply in a manner analogous to tumor progression in cancer. Recent studies demonstrate increased vascularity around cysts and evidence of ongoing angiogenesis (96). Whether angiogenesis has a role in cyst expansion in ARPKD remains to be determined.

Theories of renal cyst formation generated in experimental models are not mutually exclusive and are largely complementary. A mutant gene or environmental factors can directly lead to alterations in tubular epithelial metabolism. Some environmental factors can modulate the expression of a mutant gene or directly lead to tubular cell death. An induced alteration of tubular cell metabolism may subsequently lead directly to the abnormal sorting of transport proteins, growth factor receptors, or cell adhesion molecules, with resultant abnormal ECM production or production of growth factors mediating tubular hyperplasia. Induced changes in transtubular transport energetics may lead to hyperplasia secondary to increased transmembrane sodium flux, whereas programmed cell death may lead to further hyperplasia secondary to tubular regeneration. Alterations in sodium- or chloride-mediated transtubular transport could lead to net intratubular fluid accumulation. Subsequent increases in tubular wall tension may further increase stimulation of epithelial proliferation, leading to tubular hyperplasia. The presence of a particular pattern of tubular hyperplasia, along with necrotic debris from cell death, may lead to partial tubular obstruction and further increases in tubular wall tension. Finally, abnormal ECM production could alter the epithelial microenvironment, further increasing hyperplasia and transtubular transport, thereby contributing to cyst formation and progressive cyst enlargement. Such an overall hypothetical schema of renal cyst formation appropriately focuses future investigations on the molecular mechanisms by which tubular epithelial hyperplasia is controlled and tubular metabolism is altered in both experimental and human cystic diseases.

AUTOSOMAL RECESSIVE POLYCYSTIC KIDNEY DISEASE

ARPKD is an inherited disorder characterized by cystic dilations of renal collecting ducts and varying degrees of hepatic abnormalities consisting of biliary dysgenesis and periportal fibrosis (97). ARPKD has alternatively been referred to as *infantile PKD*. This term, however, is generally no longer used because of recognition that the disease can present any time from the prenatal period through adolescence. Furthermore, other forms of PKD, including ADPKD, can present in the neonatal period (98).

Epidemiology, Genetics, and Prenatal Diagnosis

Based on published reports, ARPKD occurs at an incidence of 1 in 10,000 to 1 in 40,000 pregnancies (99,100). The frequency of the gene in the population is estimated to be approximately 1 in 70 (101). However, the exact incidence is unknown, because published reports vary in the populations studied (e.g., autopsied patients vs. survivors), and affected children may die in the perinatal period without a definitive diagnosis. With improvements in neonatal management leading to improved survival rates, as well as formal reporting mechanisms (such as a newly developed ARPKD registry), more accurate incidence rates may become established. Consistent with autosomal recessive disease, heterozygotes (carriers) are unaffected. The recurrence risk for subsequent pregnancies is 25%, and unaffected siblings have a 66% risk of being a carrier for ARPKD (97). Males and females are affected equally, and ARPKD affects all racial and ethnic groups.

In 1994, Zerres et al. (102) localized *PKHD1* to a region on chromosome 6p21. To date, all kindreds with features typical of ARPKD have demonstrated linkage to the 6p21 locus (101). Thus, there is no evidence for genetic heterogeneity in patients with the typical features of ARPKD. However, a kindred with features of ARPKD as well as additional extrarenal abnormalities, including skeletal and facial anomalies, has recently been described, and linkage to the 6q21 locus excluded (103).

In 2002, the gene for ARPKD was cloned by two independent research groups (4,5). *PKHD1* spans a region of more than 400 kilobases (kb) of genomic DNA and contains at least 66 and possibly over 86 exons. The mRNA for the gene is produced as multiple alternative transcripts. The primary transcript of approximately 14 to 16 kb in length encodes a novel protein termed *fibrocystin* (alternatively named *polyductin*). Fibrocystin is a large protein with a predicted molecular weight of 447 kDa, similar in size to polycystin 1. The precise function of fibrocystin is unknown at present. However, protein modeling suggests that it is a membrane-bound protein with immunoglobulin-like properties, including the presence of several TIG/IPT domains (immunoglobulin-like folds shared by plexins and transcription factors). These motifs suggest that fibrocystin may function as a receptor. Several alternative transcripts described lack the transmembrane domain, suggesting that (if translated) they may result in production of secreted forms of fibrocystin as well (5). Northern analyses and reverse transcriptase-polymerase chain reaction demonstrate that *PKHD1* is expressed in both fetal and adult kidney, and to a much lesser extent in liver, pancreas, and lung. Expression in other organs was not seen (4,5).

Prenatal diagnosis may be made in a family with at least one known affected child through the technique of linkage analysis (see Chapter 18). Linkage analysis uses analysis of polymorphic markers that flank the location of a known disease gene to "track" the disease. This technique can also be used to identify whether the unaffected sibling is a carrier of the disease. In informative families, the accuracy of prenatal diagnosis using linkage analysis was greater than 95% (104). An accurate genetic diagnosis, however, is critically dependent on confirming the diagnosis of ARPKD in the affected sibling (104). Diagnostic criteria as modified from Dell and Avner and Zerres et al. (97,105) include

1. Ultrasonographic features typical of ARPKD, including enlarged, echogenic kidneys with poor corticomedullary differentiation
2. One or more of the following:
   a. Absence of renal cysts in both parents when ages older than 30 years
   b. Clinical, laboratory, or radiographic evidence of hepatic fibrosis
   c. Hepatic pathology demonstrating characteristic ductal plate abnormality
   d. Previous affected sibling with pathologically confirmed disease
   e. Parental consanguinity suggestive of autosomal recessive inheritance

Although *PKHD1* has been cloned and identified, direct mutation analysis is currently not available for clinical purposes due to its large size and the presence of multiple exons.

Pathogenesis

Despite recent advances in the understanding of the molecular genetics of ARPKD, the pathogenesis remains undefined. Analysis of *PKHD1* mutations in 14 probands demonstrated six truncating and 12 missense mutations throughout the gene (4). Eight affected patients were actually compound heterozygotes. However, because the actual function of fibrocystin has not been determined, the mechanism by which abnormalities in this protein produce renal cysts and hepatic fibrosis is unknown. It is anticipated that with greater understanding of the function of fibrocystin, genotype-phenotype studies in the future may be informative.

Insights provided by several murine models of ARPKD (Table 36.2), especially those for which the causative gene has been identified, may shed light on the pathogenesis of this disease.

The *pck* rat developed spontaneously in a colony of Sprague-Dawley rats and was initially reported to be a model of ADPKD in 2001 (106). Affected animals develop progressive cystic enlargement of the kidneys after the first week of life. Renal cysts develop from several nephron segments, including loop of Henle, distal tubules, and collecting ducts. Liver cysts are evident at birth. In addition, *pck* rats develop a liver lesion consistent with Caroli's disease (congenital hepatic fibrosis) (107). Segmental and saccular dilatation of the intrahepatic bile ducts is first seen *in utero* and progresses with age. A ductal plate abnormality with overgrowth of portal connective tissue is seen. Proliferative activity of biliary epithelium is increased compared to controls. Rates of apoptosis in biliary epithelium are lower than controls in the first week of life, then increase to greater than controls after 3 weeks (107). The severity of the kidney disease was found to be greater in males,

TABLE 36.2. MURINE MODELS OF POLYCYSTIC KIDNEY DISEASE (PKD)[a]

Species	Gene/mutant	Mode of inheritance	Chromosome location	Protein product	Function/role/comments
Mouse					
	Bpk	AR	10	Bicaudal	RNA-binding protein
	Cpk	AR	12	Cystin	Cilia-associated protein
	Inv	AR	4	Inversin	Role in left-right axis development
	Jck	AR	11	Nek8	Function unknown
	Kat	AR	8	Nek1	Function unknown
	Jcpk	AR	10	?	Allelic with *bpk*
	orpk (TgN737)	AR	14	Polaris	Role in left-right axis development; cilia-associated protein
	Pcy	AR	9	?	Phenotype consistent with ADPKD
Rat					
	Han-SPRD(*Cy*)	AD	5	?	Function unknown
	Pck	AR	9	Fibrocystin (polyductin)	Some clinical features of ADPKD
	Wpk	AR	5	?	Function unknown

AD, autosomal dominant; AR, autosomal recessive.
[a]Knock-out models for PKD are not included in this listing.

although the liver disease did not show a similar pattern. Although phenotypically similar to both ADPKD and ARPKD, the *pck* trait, which is inherited in an autosomal recessive fashion, was found to map to an area syntenic with the region for human ARPKD. Subsequent genetic studies led to the cloning of human *PKHD1* (see Epidemiology, Genetics, and Prenatal Diagnosis) and confirmed that the mutation in *pck* mice lies within the region of *PKDH1*, and, thus, *pck* is a genetic model for human ARPKD (4). The question of why this model displays features of both ARPKD and ADPKD remains unanswered at this time.

Recent studies of two murine ARPKD models, *cpk* and *orpk,* suggest that ARPKD may result, in part, from disruptions in some function or functions of cilia present on the apical surface of the renal tubule cells. The *cpk* (congenital PKD) mouse model arose from a spontaneous mutation in C57BL/6J mice (108) and is the most well-studied ARPKD murine model. *Cpk* mice appear normal at birth, but starting at postnatal day 5, progressive proximal tubule and collecting duct cystic enlargement occurs with prominent tubular cell hyperplasia (109,110). Animals die in renal failure at 3 to 4 weeks of age with massively enlarged kidneys (109,111,112). Although the renal abnormalities are consistently present on a number of genetic backgrounds, the liver phenotype and other extrarenal manifestations are highly influenced by genetic background effects (95,112,113).

By positional cloning, the *cpk* gene was localized to mouse chromosome 12, and the gene was recently cloned and identified (114). The *cpk* gene has five exons spanning approximately 14.4 kb of genomic DNA. The complementary DNA is 1,856 base pairs (bp) in length, and at least two splice variants are recognized. The mutation in *cpk/cpk* mice is a 12-bp and 19-bp deletion, resulting in a frame shift. The gene encodes a novel protein, cystin. Expression analysis demonstrates that cystin is a novel cilia-associated protein that localizes to the apical cilia of renal tubule epithelia (114). However, the mechanism by which the mutation results in polycystic kidneys remains unknown.

The *orpk* model (Oak Ridge PKD) arose as the result of large-scale mutagenesis project (6). The mutated gene, Tg737, has been localized to chromosome 13 (115). Mice homozygous for the *orpk* mutation develop polycystic kidneys and hepatic fibrosis. Functional correction ("rescue") of the renal but not the liver disease was accomplished by expression of cloned wild-type Tg737 in affected *orpk* animals (116,117). The Tg737 protein product, polaris, appears to have a key role in development, in particular left/right axis determination (118). Of note, however, polaris has also been found to localize to the cilia of Madin-Darby canine kidney cells, and cells derived from collecting tubules of *orpk* mice demonstrate abnormal cilia development (119). Whether the emerging "cilia hypothesis" of PKD pathogenesis will have relevance to human ARPKD (or to ADPKD) remains to be determined.

The pathogenesis of congenital hepatic fibrosis in ARPKD remains obscure. Increased expression of both the profibrotic molecules TGFβ and thrombospondin-1 have been demonstrated in human ARPKD livers (120). The study of the hepatic abnormality in the *pck* rat (discussed above) or the *bpk* mouse model of ARPKD may provide additional insights. The latter arose from a spontaneous mutation in an inbred colony of Balb/c mice and results, apparently, from a mutation in a gene encoding the mRNA and targeting protein, bicaudal C (121,122). These animals develop massively enlarged kidneys and die of renal failure in the first month of postnatal life. In addition to cystic kidneys, *bpk* animals develop hepatic abnormalities consisting of proliferative intrahepatic biliary tract ectasia and nonobstructive dilation of the common bile duct (121). Biliary epithelial hyperplasia, like renal tubule hyperplasia in this model, appears to be mediated by a mitogenic cycle driven by the TGFα/EGF/EGFR axis (123). In addition, both the renal and hepatic diseases of these mice are ameliorated by treatment with EGFR tyrosine kinase inhibitor (24).

Pathology

In the infant and young child, the kidneys are reniform but grossly enlarged. Pinpoint opalescent dots are visible on the capsular surface and correspond to cystic cortical collecting ducts (124). Microscopically (Fig. 36.2A), the cysts are usually smaller than 2 mm in size ("microcysts") and have been shown by microdissection (125), histochemical, and immunologic studies (126–128) to be dilated collecting ducts lined by low columnar or cuboidal epithelium. The glomeruli and other tubular structures appear to be decreased in number because of marked collecting duct ectasia and interstitial edema. In fetal kidneys, proximal tubular cystic lesions have also been identified (129), but are largely absent by birth. The pelvicaliceal system and renal vessels appear normal. Unlike ADPKD, in which the cysts become discontinuous with the tubule, the cystic tubules in ARPKD are fusiform in shape and remain in contact with the urinary stream. Microdissection studies and scanning electron microscopy demonstrate that obstruction of urinary flow is not a component of ARPKD (124,125). With increased patient survival, the development of larger renal cysts, interstitial fibrosis, and hyperplasia produces a pattern more like ADPKD (see later) (130). Gang and Herrin (131) described increasing fibrosis and inflammation in later specimens from patients who had typical collecting duct microcysts during infancy. It is unclear whether the fibrotic change is part of natural course of disease or caused by environmental factors such as toxins, hypertension, end-stage renal failure, or hemodialysis.

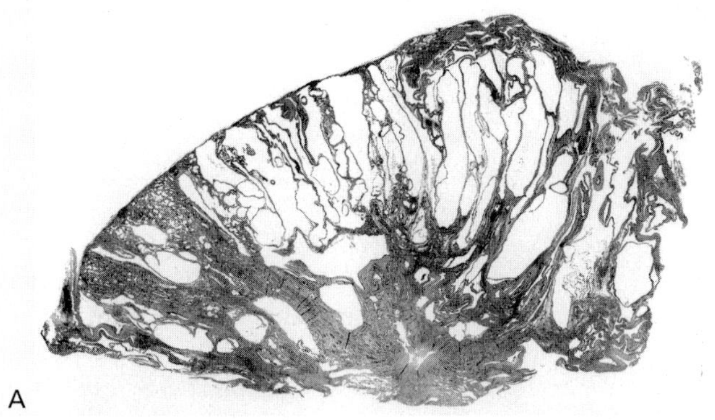

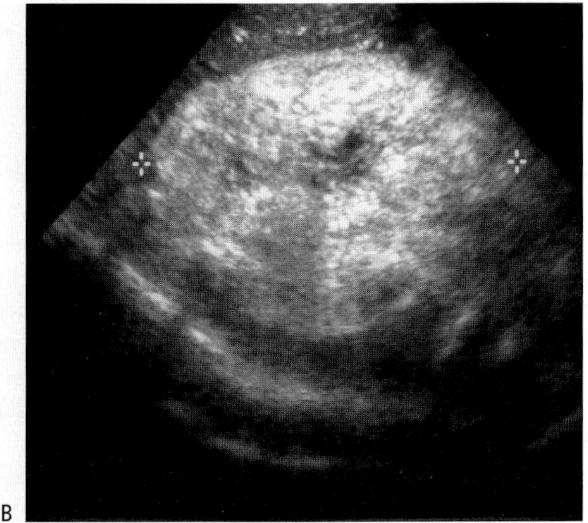

FIGURE 36.2. Kidney histology and ultrasonography of autosomal recessive polycystic kidney disease (ARPKD). **A:** Microscopic appearance of a kidney biopsy from a 7-month-old with ARPKD demonstrating multiple radially oriented collecting tubule cysts extending from the medulla to the peripheral cortex. A small amount of residual parenchyma contains glomeruli and noncystic tubules situated between the cysts. No glomerular cysts or signs of renal dysplasia are present. (Hematoxylin and eosin stain; original magnification ×1.) (Specimen kindly provided by Dr. Steven Emancipator, Case Western Reserve University.) **B:** Renal ultrasound (right kidney) of a newborn with ARPKD demonstrates the typical appearance of echogenic, enlarged kidneys (length = 6.5 cm; normal for age = 4.48 ± 0.62 cm) with poor corticomedullary differentiation.

Some degree of biliary dysgenesis and hepatic fibrosis is always present in ARPKD. Even in the newborn, the liver demonstrates microscopic abnormalities. The classic liver lesion shows a typical ductal plate abnormality consisting of portal fibrosis surrounding increased numbers of hyperplastic, ectatic biliary ducts with normal hepatocellular histology (130,132). With time, hepatomegaly and portal hypertension become evident in many patients. Intrahepatic biliary ectasia may result in macrocysts and dilation of extrahepatic bile ducts sometimes resulting in an enlarged gallbladder (133) or choledochal cysts (134). Although the combination of collecting tubule and biliary ectasia with periportal fibrosis is unique to ARPKD, portal fibrosis and bile duct proliferation may be associated with other types of renal diseases, including ADPKD (135,136) and cystic dysplasia.

Clinical and Radiographic Features

Historically, ARPKD was originally separated into four distinct clinical entities based on age at presentation and relative degrees of renal and hepatic involvement (137). Although such distinctions present a useful clinicopathologic classification, there is often much overlap between the degrees of renal and hepatic involvement present. ARPKD and congenital hepatic fibrosis with renal tubular ectasia are likely different phenotypic manifestations of the same genetic abnormality (138). In contrast to ADPKD (see later), intrafamilial variability in ARPKD disease phenotype is reportedly small (139).

The majority of patients with ARPKD present in infancy (105,140). In a series of 33 patients with ARPKD who survived the neonatal period, 11 were diagnosed in the first days of life, 18 between 1 and 18 months, and four between 6 and 11 years of age (141). Rare presentations late in adolescence and even into adulthood have been described (142). With the widespread use of prenatal ultrasound, many patients with ARPKD are detected *in utero*. Prenatal ultrasound may demonstrate the findings of oligohydramnios, large renal masses, or absence of fetal bladder filling (143).

At birth, patients usually present with large, palpable flank masses that may be large enough to complicate delivery. Urine output is usually normal; however, oliguric acute renal failure may occur (99). In that subset of patients, increased urine output and a corresponding improvement in renal function may be seen after improvement in respiratory status (144). Most patients (70 to 80%), even without overt renal failure, have evidence of impaired renal function in the newborn period (105,145). However, death from renal insufficiency is uncommon in that age group (137). Hyponatremia related to a urine dilution defect is often present, but usually resolves over time (105,140). Metabolic acidosis has also been reported (140,145). As might be predicted from a pathologic process that affects the collecting tubule, most patients have a urinary concentrating defect and symptoms of polyuria and polydipsia (130,140,141,145).

Hypertension, which may be severe, is common in both infants and children and can be a presenting feature (99,130). It can be present in patients with normal renal function and eventually affects almost all children with the disease (145). Although the pathophysiology of hypertension in ARPKD is not clearly understood, peripheral vein renin levels are not usually elevated (140,141). If not aggressively managed, hypertension can result in cardiac hypertrophy and congestive heart failure (CHF), which may be a factor in progression of underlying renal insufficiency.

Pulmonary insufficiency, as manifest by respiratory distress, is a major cause of morbidity and mortality in neonates with ARPKD. Pulmonary hypoplasia, resulting from oligohydramnios, may be complicated by respiratory embarrassment due to massively enlarged kidneys. Additional causes of respiratory distress in these patients include pneumothorax and atelectasis, or a variety of common neonatal pulmonary disorders such as surfactant deficiency, bacterial pneumonia, meconium aspiration, or persistent fetal circulation. Severely affected infants may demonstrate the full components of the oligohydramnios sequence, including pulmonary hypoplasia, abnormal extremities, and characteristic Potter's facies (146). Infants with true pulmonary hypoplasia often die soon after birth secondary to pulmonary insufficiency.

A subset of patients with ARPKD may present as older infants with abdominal enlargement secondary to enlarged kidneys or hepatosplenomegaly without the full spectrum of clinical symptoms outlined above. Although hepatic involvement is invariably present microscopically, it may be clinically absent in at least 50 to 60% of neonates (105). In contrast, the small percentage of patients who are diagnosed with ARPKD as older children often present primarily with signs and symptoms of hepatic fibrosis and portal hypertension, including hepatosplenomegaly (101,147). In fact, cystic renal disease in these patients may be detected as an incidental finding during abdominal imaging. Liver synthetic function is usually intact.

By ultrasonography, infants have characteristic large echogenic kidneys with poor corticomedullary differentiation (Fig. 36.2B). Macrocysts are usually not present, although they may be seen with worsening disease. Renal macrocysts smaller than 2 cm and increased medullary echogenicity have been reported in older children (130). In a study of sonographic features of adult patients with ARPKD, Nicolau et al. (148) noted the presence of multiple small cysts in a normal-sized kidney, increased cortical echogenicity, and loss of corticomedullary differentiation as common features.

Ultrasonographic findings in the liver include hepatomegaly, increased echogenicity, and poor visualization of the peripheral portal veins. Reversal of normal venous flow by Doppler study, suggestive of portal hypertension, may be seen. Macroscopic liver cysts are uncommon (149), although choledochal cysts have been reported (134). A smaller percentage of patients have overt evidence of biliary duct dilatation (Caroli's disease).

Diagnosis

Prenatal diagnosis may be suggested by antenatal ultrasound findings of enlarged kidneys, oligohydramnios, and absence of urine in the bladder (150). Sonographic features of ARPKD may present in the second trimester but usually are not apparent until after 30 weeks' gestation (151). Both false-positive and false-negative results have been reported (152). However, with newer high-resolution obstetric ultrasonography, it is probable that diagnostic sensitivity and detection rates will improve. Wisser et al. (153) reported a case of a fetus with pathologically confirmed ARPKD who demonstrated echogenic, normal-sized kidneys at 15 ± 4 weeks' gestation. Although less common, ADPKD in infants may have an antenatal sonographic appearance that is difficult to distinguish from ARPKD (98). Increased maternal alpha fetoprotein and amniotic fluid trehalase activity have been identified as potential markers for ARPKD, but neither has been confirmed as specific or sensitive for disease detection *in utero* (154,155).

Although specific clinical diagnostic criteria for ARPKD have not been established, the clinical constellation of bilateral palpable flank masses, respiratory distress, and history of oligohydramnios and hypertension in an infant is suggestive of ARPKD. Diagnostic criteria modified from Zerres et al. (105) are outlined in Epidemiology, Genetics, and Prenatal Diagnosis. For the minority of children who present later in childhood, renal ultrasonographic features may be less reliable. Kidneys are echogenic and large, but massive enlargement is generally not seen. The echogenicity of the kidneys in older children may be similar to that of ADPKD, and macrocysts more typical of ADPKD may be present (156). As noted, in the subset of patients who present as older children and adolescents, hepatic abnormalities are often the prominent presenting feature.

Magnetic resonance imaging (MRI) shows enlarged kidneys with hyperintense T2-weighted signals. A characteristic hyperintense, linear radial pattern in the cortex and medulla representing microcystic dilatation has been described on RARE-MR urography (17). Radionuclide studies, such as renal technetium-99m DMSA and liver HIDA imaging, may also aid in establishing the diagnosis of ARPKD (158). As noted previously, genetic testing is available at present only for families that already have an affected child. With the recent cloning and ongoing characterization of *PKHD1*, however, it is possible that direct mutation analysis may become available in the future.

Treatment and Complications

Survival of neonates with ARPKD has improved in concert with overall advances in neonatal artificial ventilation and intensive care. It is currently impossible to predict which neonates with ARPKD requiring immediate artificial ventilation have critical degrees of pulmonary hypoplasia incompatible with survival (1,145). In some instances, severe pulmonary distress may be secondary to potentially reversible fluid overload, neonatal lung disease, or restricted diaphragmatic motion secondary to massively enlarged kidneys. In selected cases, some authors have advocated continuous venovenous hemofiltration, unilateral nephrectomy, or bilateral nephrectomy coupled with peritoneal dialysis to allow optimal ventilation and thereby assess the long-term pulmonary prognosis of the patient (159–161).

Infants and young children without significant renal insufficiency must be followed closely. Because most children with ARPKD have a concentrating defect, significant dehydration is a particular risk during intercurrent illnesses that may increase insensible water loss (e.g., through fever), limit free water intake (e.g., through nausea), or increase extrarenal water loss (e.g., through vomiting or diarrhea). In patients with severe polyuria, thiazide diuretics may be of benefit to decrease distal nephron solute and water delivery. Supplemental bicarbonate therapy is required for those with metabolic acidosis.

Hypertension can be difficult to manage and may require multiple medications (99). Despite the fact that peripheral vein renin values are not usually elevated in hypertensive ARPKD patients, most patients respond well to angiotensin-converting enzyme (ACE) inhibitors, which are the treatment of choice. If additional medications are required, calcium channel blockers, β-blockers (in those without chronic lung disease or signs of CHF), and diuretics are appropriate choices.

Urinary abnormalities may be present or develop over the course of disease. Pyuria is a relatively common finding and can be seen in the absence of demonstrable bacteriuria or documented infection (130). Urinary tract infection (UTI) has been reported as a common complication in at least one uncontrolled series (145), but it is unclear whether children with ARPKD truly have an increased incidence of upper or lower UTIs when compared with appropriately age-matched controls. Thus, as in any child with an abnormal urinalysis, clinical features and appropriately obtained urine cultures must guide antibiotic therapy. If a UTI is documented, a voiding cystourethrogram and renal ultrasound should be performed to determine the possible presence of vesicoureteral reflux and rule out obstruction or superimposed upper tract structural abnormalities (131). Microscopic or gross hematuria and proteinuria may also be seen on occasion (99,145). In infants and children who develop renal insufficiency, the consequences of chronic renal failure (e.g., growth failure, anemia, and osteodystrophy) become apparent as renal function decreases.

Difficulties in feeding, even in patients without renal insufficiency, are often noted. This is presumably due to the presence of enlarged kidneys or liver, or both, interfering with normal gastrointestinal function. Supplemental feeding via nasogastric or gastrostomy tubes may be required to optimize weight gain and growth.

Dialysis or transplantation, or both, are indicated when children with ARPKD reach end-stage renal failure. Peritoneal dialysis in ARPKD is often successful even in the face of large kidneys and hepatosplenomegaly. Kidney transplantation offers definitive renal replacement therapy in children with ARPKD. Successful kidney transplantation prolongs survival and often accelerates growth and development in young uremic children. Nephrectomies may be indicated before, or at the time of, transplantation to control hypertension and/or to permit room for transplant placement in patients with massively enlarged kidneys.

With improved patient survival and advances in renal replacement therapy, hepatic complications progressively dominate the clinical picture of many patients with ARPKD (105,147,162). The older child may have complications of hepatic fibrosis and portal hypertension (130,137). These include hepatosplenomegaly, bleeding esophageal varices, portal thrombosis, and hypersplenism causing thrombocytopenia, anemia, and leukopenia.

A serious and potentially lethal complication in ARPKD patients with significant hepatic involvement is bacterial cholangitis, which has been reported as early as a few weeks of age (145). Fever or elevation of liver function tests at any time should lead to the suspicion of cholangitis and result in complete evaluation and appropriate antimicrobial therapy. However, patients may not present with the classic clinical findings of cholangitis, and the diagnosis should be strongly considered in ARPKD patients with unexplained recurrent sepsis with gram-negative organisms (163).

In infants and children with hepatic involvement, close monitoring for complications of portal hypertension is mandated, particularly as typical liver function tests (e.g., serum albumin and transaminases) are normal. Yearly ultrasonography to determine changes in liver or spleen size or identify portal hypertension by reversal of venous flow is noninvasive and may be of value. Endoscopy is necessary to evaluate suspected esophageal varices that can be treated by sclerotherapy or banding before life-threatening hemorrhage. Periodic monitoring should reveal the hematologic profile of hypersplenism. Sudden worsening of anemia should raise the possibility of occult gastrointestinal blood loss secondary to splenic sequestration or variceal bleeding. Portosystemic shunting may be indicated in some cases (140,164). However, Tsimaratos et al. (165) recently reported recurrent hepatic encephalopathy leading to death in two children with portocaval shunts who progressed to ESRD. It has been hypothesized that loss of kidney function results in impaired clearance of toxins that are shunted from the liver. This finding has raised concerns about whether liver transplantation should be considered as an alternative therapy for ARPKD patients with portal hypertension being evaluated for possible shunts. With the increased use and successful outcome of living-related partial liver transplants, this option may be more viable than previously considered. In fact, sequential liver and kidney living-related transplants have recently been reported (166).

In addition to the significant medical problems noted, the psychosocial stresses of ARPKD on the patient and family can be overwhelming. Social support measures and periods of respite care are often necessary. A team approach using the skills of pediatric nephrologists in concert with other pediatric medical subspecialists, specialized nurses, dietitians, social workers, psychiatrists, and other support staff is required to provide optimal comprehensive care for children with ARPKD.

Prognosis

Prognosis is difficult to assess, although it is now clear that survival of all but the most severely affected neonates who demonstrate pulmonary hypoplasia is possible (1,130). Published reports vary with respect to neonatal survival rates, but suggest that approximately 70% of patients survive the newborn period with aggressive neonatal intensive care (140,145,147). Actuarial survival rates calculated from birth for 55 patients with ARPKD referred to a pediatric tertiary care center revealed that 86% were alive at 3 months, 79% at 1 year, 51% at 10 years, and 46% at 15 years (140). Calculations based on patients who survived to 1 year of age showed that 82% were alive at 10 years and 79% at 15 years (140). Patients who survive the neonatal period usually have a decreased glomerular filtration rate (GFR), but studies have demonstrated subsequent improvement in renal function consistent with some degree of continued renal maturation (99). Indeed, GFR may be normal by 12 months of age, and those patients with neonatal presentations who survive past 1 month of age generally do not develop renal insufficiency until late childhood or early adolescence. Life-table analysis of a cohort of patients surviving the first month of life revealed a renal survival of 86% at 1 year and 67% at 15 years (147).

As noted, with the success of renal transplantation and improved survival of patients with ARPKD, morbidity and mortality of complications related to congenital hepatic fibrosis are more common and clinically relevant. Khan et al. recently reported the outcome of 14 patients with ARPKD after renal transplantation (167). With a mean follow-up of 14 years, the study showed 1-and 5-year patient survival rates of 93% and 86%, respectively. Overall, 36% of patients died, and in four of five of those patients, death was directly related to complications of hepatic disease. In those who survived, 63% had portal hypertension. Thus, complications of CHF developed in almost 80% of patients after renal transplantation for ARPKD.

AUTOSOMAL DOMINANT POLYCYSTIC KIDNEY DISEASE

ADPKD is a systemic inherited disease characterized by progressive cystic enlargement of the kidneys coupled with variable extrarenal manifestations involving the gastrointestinal tract, cardiovascular system, reproductive organs, and the brain (168). ADPKD has alternatively been called *adult PKD*. However, this term is a misnomer because ADPKD has been diagnosed in the fetus, newborn, and older child and adolescent (99,141,169,170).

Epidemiology, Genetics, and Prenatal Diagnosis

ADPKD is the most common inherited human kidney disease and occurs at an incidence of approximately 1 in 1000. It affects all races, and males and females are both affected; however, the phenotype may be more severe in males (171). ADPKD is a rare cause of ESRD in the pediatric population, but accounts for approximately 5 to 10% of ESRD in adults. The two major disease-causing genes are *PKD1* and *PKD2*. In the general population, *PKD1* accounts for approximately 85% of ADPKD, with *PKD2* accounting for the remaining 15%. A third ADPKD locus (*PKD3*, or non-PKD1 or PKD2) has been suggested by a few case reports (172–174). Mutations in *PKD1* and *PKD2* produce similar phenotypes; however, the age of onset of cystic disease, hypertension, and renal insufficiency is delayed in the latter (175–177).

PKD1 has been mapped to chromosome 16p13.3 (178). Its exact location was pinpointed because it was bisected by a chromosome translocation; members with the balanced exchange had PKD (2). Like *PKHD1*, *PKD1* is a very large gene, spanning 53 kb of genomic DNA, with 46 exons encoding a 14.5-kb transcript (179). A portion of the gene is duplicated in the proximal portion of chromosome 16.

The gene encodes a large 4304–amino acid protein product, polycystin-1, a novel 460-kDa protein that is predicted to be involved in cell-cell or cell-matrix interactions (180).

PKD2 has been linked to chromosome 4q13-q23 and was cloned and identified in 1996 (3,181). The *PKD2* gene expresses a 5.4-kb mRNA, which encodes a 968–amino acid polypeptide, polycystin-2 (3). Polycystin-2 has been recently shown to be a nonselective voltage-gated ion channel (182).

Prenatal genetic diagnosis is available for "informative" families with suitable pedigree structures using the technique of linkage analysis (141). In addition, techniques for accurate mutation screening by DHPLC for both PKD1 and 2 are currently being refined, but the mutation detection rate has not been fully determined (168,183). As with any prenatal genetic testing, the question arises as to whether termination of an affected pregnancy is an acceptable option for couples, especially given the wide clinical spectrum and the treatable nature of the disease (i.e., treatment of chronic renal failure and dialysis or transplantation) (184). In the majority of kindreds, fetuses harboring an ADPKD mutation will not show any obvious renal or other abnormalities, and patients may be asymptomatic for two to three decades. Potential benefits of prenatal diagnosis, either by genetic testing or ultrasonography, include early genetic counseling, careful preparation for management of an affected fetus at and after delivery (in the case of a fetus with clinical evidence of disease), and close follow-up of an affected child. However, diagnosing ADPKD years before the onset of symptoms has potential major adverse outcomes that must be considered, including psychological stress on the child and family and potential discrimination in employment, financial, and insurance matters (185,186). Surveys of ADPKD families indicate that only 4% would consider pregnancy termination if the fetus were affected (187). Genetic linkage analysis for *PKD1* or *PKD2* is not routinely performed for prenatal diagnosis in the United States or Europe (188).

Pathogenesis

Despite the extraordinary advances in the 1990s in defining the genetics of ADPKD, the precise mechanisms by which mutations in the *PKD1* and *PKD2* genes result in the formation of renal and extrarenal cysts is unknown (189).

PKD1

Polycystin-1 possesses a large extracellular domain, transmembrane spanning regions, and an intracellular carboxy-terminus (190,191). The extracellular domain is dominated by the presence of 16 copies of an 80–amino acid immunoglobulin-like repeat, the PKD domain. Although the function of this domain is unknown, PKD domains in several other proteins are located on their extracellular surface and are highly glycosylated. The amino-terminal domain of polycystin 1 also contains a leucine-rich repeat, an LDL-A domain, an REJ domain, and a calcium-dependent lectin domain. The presence of the REJ domain is particularly intriguing because it may be a potential regulatory site for the molecule (192). These structural components, taken as a whole, suggest that the extracellular portion of polycystin-1 may be capable of binding an as yet undefined ligand (191). Polycystin-1 is anchored to the cell membrane by 7 to 11 putative transmembrane domains. The carboxy-terminus (intracellular portion) of polycystin 1 contains several phosphorylation sites and a putative coiled-coil domain, which has been demonstrated to interact *in vitro* with the carboxy-terminus of the protein product of the *PKD2* gene (193,194). These numerous features suggest that polycystin-1 is a large, multifunctional molecule that is involved in carbohydrate motif recognition, ligand binding, and Ca^{2+} regulation. It may engage in cell-cell and/or cell-matrix interactions, which regulate signal transduction pathways mediated by cell-surface protein-protein interactions.

Defining the expression pattern of polycystin-1 has been hampered, in part, by discrepancies in the reported tissue and cellular localization of the protein. This is likely due to issues related to antibody specificities (191). However, it appears that polycystin-1 is expressed in multiple tissues, including kidney, liver, pancreas, intestine, and cerebral blood vessels (all sites of cystic changes in ADPKD), as well as in the lung, testis, and other tissues (195–198). The protein is overexpressed in the cystic epithelium of ADPKD kidneys (195), and these cells remain phenotypically immature. Immunohistochemistry studies located the protein in renal tubular epithelial cells of human fetuses, diminishing in abundance with age but with persistent expression into adulthood (195,199), suggesting a role in renal development. Further evidence of the importance of polycystin-1 in development was provided by knock-out mouse models in which a variety of mutations have been introduced that result in the loss of functional polycystin. Animals lacking polycystin-1 die *in utero* or soon after birth and demonstrate abnormalities in multiple organs, including the heart, blood vessels, kidneys, and pancreas (200–202). The subcellular localization of polycystin-1 in renal tubular epithelium appears to shift during development from a predominantly basal staining in fetuses to apical/lateral staining in adult kidneys (203).

Although the precise function of polycystin-1 is unknown, emerging data regarding its binding partners may shed light on its role in normal and cystic kidney epithelium. As noted, polycystin-1 has recently been shown to bind polycystin-2 at the coiled-coil domain. Polycystin-2 is a cation channel, and it has been suggested that polycystin-1 plays a role in regulation of that channel. Results of immunohistochemistry and functional studies suggest that polycystin co-localizes with and forms large complexes with a wide variety of proteins, including those involved with cell-matrix interactions (such as $\alpha_2\beta_1$ integrins and focal adhesion complexes) as well as cell-cell interactions (including E-cadherin-β-catenin complexes) (191,203,204). Additional data demonstrate that polycystin-1 induces resistance to apoptosis and spontaneous tubulogenesis in Madin-Darby canine kidney cells (205). Nickel et al. (206) reported that the C terminal of polycystin-1 triggers branching morphogenesis and migration of inner medullary collecting duct cells and supports *in vitro* tubule formation. These studies suggest a potential connection between altered polycystin-1 function and cystogenesis (204).

ADPKD is characterized by considerable intrafamilial phenotypic variation. By analyzing two closely linked polymorphic markers within the *PKD1* gene, Qian et al. revealed that the renal epithelia from single cysts are monoclonal, containing only the mutant haplotype (207). A subsequent study by Brasier et al. (208) confirmed these findings. These two studies suggest that patients harboring a germline mutation in the one allele of a PKD gene undergo a somatic "second hit," which results in the loss of the remaining normal allele and genetic homozygosity in the affected cell or cells. These studies provide a possible molecular explanation for both the focal nature of cysts (only 1 to 2% of tubules may be cystic in ADPKD) as well as the phenotypic variability within families harboring the same germline mutation.

To date, multiple different mutations throughout the *PKD1* gene have been identified in patients with ADPKD, with no particular "hot spots" for mutations identified (209). The majority of mutations are predicted to result in truncation of the polycystin-1 protein. Of note, several kindreds were identified that had tuberous sclerosis coexistent with severe childhood-onset ADPKD. These kindreds were subsequently found to have large deletions in an area containing both *PKD1* and adjacent tuberous sclerosis 2 (*TSC2*) genes, resulting in a contiguous gene syndrome (210). Another kindred has been identified exhibiting cosegregation of an overlapping connective tissue disorder and ADPKD 1 (211). Although consistent genotype/phenotype correlations have not been demonstrated to date, Rosetti et al. (212) recently found that even in light of significant inter- and intrafamilial phenotypic heterogeneity, patients with mutations in the 5' region of *PKD1* had significantly more severe disease than those with mutations in the 3' portion of the gene. The location, rather than the type of mutation, was found to be the factor that correlated with the onset of ESRD.

PKD2

Polycystin-2 contains six transmembrane regions and has intracellular domains at both its amino- and carboxy-termini. The transmembrane regions share significant homology with voltage-activated Ca^{2+}/Na^{+} channels, which suggests that polycystin-2 could be a channel protein. The carboxy-terminus contains an EF-hand domain that binds Ca^{2+}. The carboxy-terminus also contains several potential phosphorylation sites. By immunostaining of human and murine renal tissues, polycystin-2 was found to be widely expressed and was present in the kidney. The highest levels of expression within the kidney were the thick ascending loop of Henle and the distal convoluted tubule, where it localized to the basolateral plasma membrane of kidney tubular epithelium (213). Polycystin-2, like polycystin-1, is expressed in the vasculature, including porcine aorta and normal human elastic and intracranial arteries (214).

Recently, Koulen et al. (182) confirmed by single channel studies that polycystin-2 (a member of a subfamily of the transient receptor potential channel superfamily) functions as a calcium-activated intracellular ion release channel *in vivo* and hypothesized that PKD results from the loss of regulation of an intracellular calcium release signaling pathway.

Multiple mutations in *PKD2* have been identified in affected families, and as with *PKD1*, most families have unique mutations (215). These mutations truncate polycystin-2 and appear to be loss-of-function mutations. Similar to *PKD1*, mice homozygous for targeted mutations in *PKD2* die *in utero* or soon after birth and demonstrate cardiac defects in septum formation as well as kidney and pancreatic cysts (216). Although there is significant genetic and phenotypic variability in patients with PKD2 mutations, it has recently been suggested that certain clusters or groups of mutations may be associated with more severe clinical disease (217).

Pathology

In ADPKD (Fig. 36.3A), kidney cysts form in glomeruli and all tubular segments, although the proximal tubule is a common site of involvement. Glomerular cysts may be seen as a component of ADPKD or as a separate disease entity. Unlike ARPKD, in which the cystic dilatations are fusiform in nature and remain in connection with the tubular lumen, in ADPKD the enlarging cysts eventually "pinch off" and become disconnected from the tubular lumen and urinary space.

Clinical and Radiographic Features

Patients with ADPKD are usually diagnosed and become symptomatic in adulthood. However, children affected with ADPKD may become symptomatic or be diagnosed as an incidental finding. The clinical spectrum of pediatric ADPKD ranges from severe neonatal manifestations indistinguishable from ARPKD to renal cysts noted on ultrasound in asymptomatic children (1,98,99,141,169). The diagnosis of ADPKD has been made *in utero* by ultrasound, and affected newborns can present with Potter's phenotype and die from pulmonary hypoplasia. Affected infants can be born with large hyperechoic kidneys with or without macrocysts and variable degrees of renal insufficiency. As with ARPKD, hypertension can present during the newborn or infant periods and is common even in pediatric patients with normal renal function (141,169,218). Hypertension appears to be mediated by reduced renal blood flow, activation of the renin-angiotensin system, and increased sodium retention (219,220).

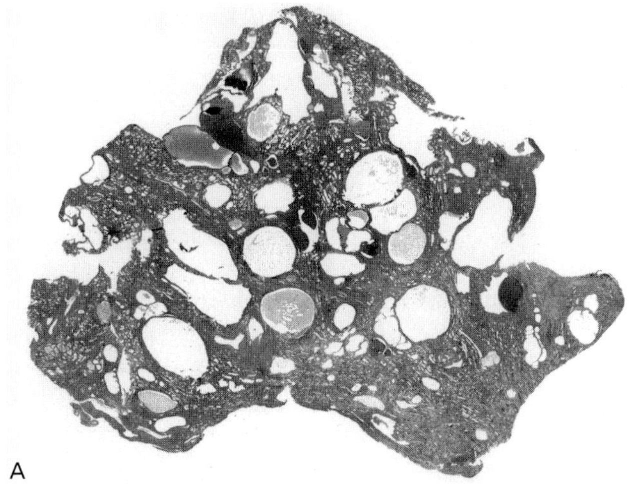

A

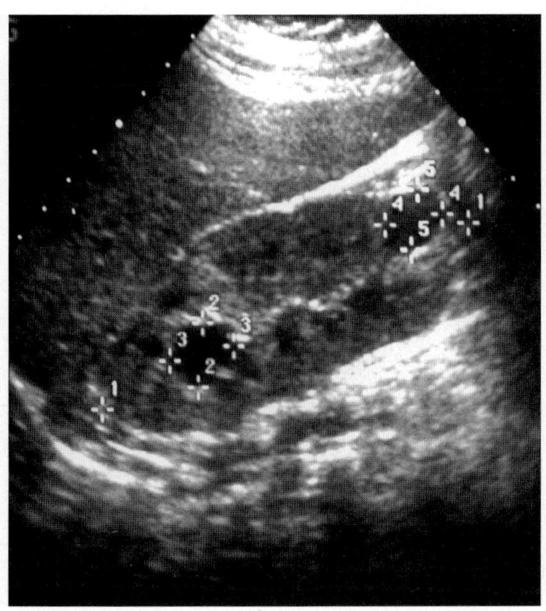

B

FIGURE 36.3. Kidney histology and ultrasonography of autosomal dominant polycystic kidney disease (ADPKD). **A:** Microscopic appearance of a kidney biopsy from an adult with ADPKD demonstrating multiple thin-walled cysts of varying sizes involving different nephron segments. Focal hemorrhage is noted within some cysts. (Hematoxylin and eosin stain; original magnification ×1.) (Specimen kindly provided by Dr. Steven Emancipator, Case Western Reserve University.) **B:** Renal ultrasound (right kidney) of a 13-year-old with ADPKD demonstrates several cysts (the largest measuring 1.5 cm × 1.6 cm). The left kidney also had several cysts not present on an ultrasound 2 years before this study. Kidneys are 11.4 cm (*right*) and 11.7 cm (*left*) (normal for age = 9.79 cm ± 1.5 cm).

In older children, presenting symptoms include abdominal pain, palpable abdominal masses, gross or microscopic hematuria, UTIs, abdominal or inguinal hernias, and hypertension. The occurrence of gross hematuria after seemingly minor trauma to the flank region should raise the possibility of ADPKD (or obstructive uropathy). Renal insufficiency is rare but can occur in childhood (169,221). A concentrating defect may be present, leading to polyuria and polydipsia, but this is more consistently a clinical feature of ARPKD than ADPKD (145,222). Renal infections are common in adult patients with ADPKD and can be a presenting feature in the affected infant and child (141). Potential complications of pediatric renal infection include pain, perinephric abscess, hemorrhage, chronic pyelonephritis, sepsis, and death. It has been reported that the risk of pyuria and bacteriuria in ADPKD increases progressively from 2% in the second decade to 32% in the seventh decade.

In families with known ADPKD, asymptomatic children may be identified by ultrasonographic examination (Fig. 36.3B) (169). In children at risk, the presence of even single cysts in normal-sized kidneys is highly predictive of future development of symptomatic ADPKD (169). In children with ADPKD, renal involvement is commonly asymmetric (including asymmetric kidney enlargement) and is unilateral in a small minority (223). The extrarenal features of ADPKD seen commonly in adults (224,225) are only rarely seen in pediatric patients. When present, they can sometimes help to clinically differentiate ADPKD from ARPKD. Although hepatic, pancreatic, or ovarian cysts are rarely detected before puberty, they have been reported in affected children in the first year of life (226,227). Liver cysts in children are not generally associated with pain, infection, and hepatomegaly as noted in adult patients. Congenital hepatic fibrosis with severe portal hypertension in children and adults with ADPKD has been reported (135,136). The presence of pancreatic cysts has been found exclusively in *PKD1* patients, and they do not appear to contribute to morbidity or mortality (228). Similarly, although rarely detected before the age of 20 years, there are reports of clinically significant cerebral vessel aneurysms in pediatric ADPKD patients (229). The increased incidence of cardiac valvular abnormalities, such as mitral valve prolapse, commonly seen in the adult ADPKD population (224,230), has also been reported in children with ADPKD (231). There have also been several reports of endocardial fibroelastosis in children with ADPKD (232,233). Increased left ventricular mass and Doppler abnormalities consistent with early diastolic dysfunction has been reported to occur in normotensive children and young adults with ADPKD (234). An increased risk of coronary aneurysms has been reported in adults, but no pediatric cases have been reported to date (235).

Diagnosis

There are no specific clinical diagnostic criteria for children with suspected ADPKD. Prenatal diagnosis is suggested by antenatal ultrasound findings of enlarged kidneys with or without cysts and absent urine in the bladder. However, these findings may not be evident until the third trimester. (236,237). In families not known to have ADPKD, diagnosis of ADPKD in the fetus or young child can lead to the diagnosis of ADPKD in asymptomatic adults after parental radiographic studies. Because simple cysts are extremely rare in childhood (238), the finding of even one renal cyst should alert the clinician to the possibility of ADPKD. In pediatric patients with a 50% risk of ADPKD, the finding of one cyst is considered diagnostic. Ultrasonographic screening of asymptomatic pediatric patients at risk is an issue of some debate. Because cysts may not be evident until adulthood, the finding of a negative ultrasound may be falsely reassuring (239). Conversely, there may be significant psychosocial and financial implications of a diagnosis of ADPKD in an asymptomatic patient who may not develop clinical signs of disease for several decades. If ADPKD is clinically suspected, family members (including the grandparents if the parents are younger than 30 years) should be considered for radiographic evaluation (240). As noted previously, genetic testing in the form of linkage analysis is available. Direct mutation screening is available, but accuracy has not been fully determined, particularly for *PKD1* mutations. An up-to-date listing of laboratories currently performing genetic testing for PKD for clinical or research purposes is available at www.geneclinics.org.

Treatment and Complications

At present, there are no disease-specific therapies for ADPKD. However, a number of interventions have been shown to slow progression of disease in animal models, including dietary flaxseed, soy protein or protein restriction, sodium citrate, caffeine restriction, and EGFR tyrosine kinase inhibition (241–247). To date, none has proven to significantly alter the clinical course of disease in humans (248).

Asymptomatic children at risk for ADPKD should be followed annually for the development of hematuria, hypertension, or palpable abdominal masses. Any of these findings is an indication for ultrasound examination and close clinical follow-up. Renal insufficiency and ESRD in the child with ADPKD is treated with standard medical management of chronic renal failure and renal replacement therapy as indicated (see Chapters 70 through 74). As with other forms of chronic kidney disease, hypertension management is essential in slowing progression to ESRD in PKD. It has been suggested that ACE inhibitors, angiotensin II receptor antagonists, and chymase inhibitors may offer benefits in addition to antihypertensive effects (249–251); however, this has not been confirmed. A longitudinal study of children with ADPKD treated with ACE inhibitors is currently under way, and a larger scale, multicenter National Institutes of Health trial is being planned to address the question in adults. Of note, reversible acute renal failure may be precipitated by ACE inhibitors in ADPKD patients with diminished kidney function and massive cystic involvement (252).

A number of renal and extrarenal complications may occur in patients with ADPKD. In pediatric patients, gross hematuria and UTI, in particular, cyst infection, are the more common. Flank pain may also be seen. Renal calculi, a common finding in adult patients with ADPKD (253), are rare in childhood. Although no data are available regarding specific features of UTIs or renal cyst infections in pediatric ADPKD patients, it is reasonable to assume that their clinical course is similar to that described for adult ADPKD patients (254). Sterile pyuria is common, and appropriate cultures are needed to determine whether an infection is present. Most renal infections are caused by gram-negative enteric organisms and can be complicated by cyst infection. Eradication of cyst infections is often difficult, despite *in vitro* sensitivity of responsible organisms; thus, the use of antibiotics that penetrate cyst walls is mandated (255). Antibiotics that generally penetrate cyst walls include ciprofloxacin (256) and sulfonamides. Penicillins and aminoglycosides (standard treatments for UTI) are generally ineffective in treating cyst infection (255,257). Aggressive antibiotic treatment is critical because recurrent or ineffectively treated UTIs appear to be a definite risk factor in progression of renal disease (258). Occasionally, cyst drainage may be required to control infection, and MRI may be a useful modality for identifying which cyst is infected (259). In extreme cases, nephrectomy may be indicated (255). Prophylactic antibiotics should be considered before the introduction of any urinary tract instrumentation in children with ADPKD.

Episodes of flank pain are unusual in pediatric patients with few cysts. With progressive disease, however, particularly in certain adolescents, flank pain may become a more prominent feature. In the majority of instances, the painful episodes resolve within a few days. Pain relief is accomplished with acetaminophen or brief courses of oral narcotics. Nonsteroidal antiinflammatory agents should be avoided. Long-term narcotic use is discouraged due to abuse potential. Nonpharmacologic interventions and referral to a chronic pain management center should be considered (260). In cases of severe pain, laparoscopic cyst decortications may be performed (261).

As noted, hepatic cysts are rare in the pediatric population. Patients with hepatic cysts may develop cyst infections. Typically, these infections present as right upper quadrant pain, fever, leukocytosis, and a rise in liver enzymes (262). Antibiotics alone may be ineffective, and the addition of surgical drainage is generally recommended (263). Intestinal diverticular disease (224) has not been reported in pediatric ADPKD patients.

Routine cerebral arteriography is not recommended for screening of possible intracranial aneurysms in pediatric ADPKD patients. The optimal age for screening and the natural history of aneurysm development are unknown in pediatric patients. Although aneurysms are found in patients with negative family histories, intrafamilial clustering of aneurysms has been reported in ADPKD populations (264,265). Thus, it may be reasonable to consider investigation of children with positive family histories of cerebral aneurysms or those with symptoms such as headache. Use of magnetic resonance angiography may permit effective, noninvasive detection of significant aneurysms (266). Even in adults, however, routine screening by magnetic resonance angiography is generally reserved for those patients with symptoms or a positive family history.

Prognosis

The prognosis of ADPKD presenting in the fetus or neonate is uncertain, given the small number of cases and short follow-up periods reported. Although neonatal ADPKD was once thought to have an ominous prognosis, small series suggest that it may be compatible with favorable long-term patient and renal survival (141,145,169,236). Prognosis in the older child generally better. Progression to ESRD in childhood is rare in this latter group, and the majority maintain normal renal function through adolescence (267). However, progression of disease does occur during childhood, especially in children with evidence of severe renal enlargement at a young age (267). Proteinuria has been identified as a potential early marker of severe cystic disease in children (268). Approximately 50% of adult patients with ADPKD progress to ESRD. On average, patients with PKD1 typically progress at an earlier age, with a mean age at ESRD of 53.0 years, whereas those with PKD2 progress to ESRD at a mean age of 69.1 years (176). In light of the significant inter- and intrafamilial phenotypic heterogeneity, it is difficult to predict at what age a given patient with ADPKD will develop renal failure.

Once renal insufficiency occurs, GFR typically decreases at a rate of approximately 2 to 3 mL/min/1.73 m^2 per year, with GFR declining at a faster rate in men than women (171). Decline in GFR correlates with an increase in renal cyst volume and a decrease in parenchymal volume as determined by CT (269,270). Moreover, increased renal volume growth rate positively correlates with decline in renal function in patients with early disease and preserved GFR (171). Thus, renal volumes and rate of renal growth may be markers for disease progression in ADPKD.

GLOMERULOCYSTIC KIDNEY DISEASE

The term *glomerulocystic kidney disease* (GCKD), coined by Taxy and Filmer in 1976, is used to describe the morphologic appearance of glomerular cysts, which occur in a variety of conditions (271). GCKD was first described clinically by Ross in 1941 (272). GCKD can be categorized into three major groups: (a) nonsyndromal heritable and sporadic forms of GCKD, (b) GCKD as the major component of heritable malformation syndromes, and (c) glomerular cysts as a minor component of abnormal or dysplastic kidney disease, some of which are syndromal.

Epidemiology, Genetics, and Prenatal Diagnosis

Primary GCKD with isolated renal involvement can be an autosomal dominant disease, a familial hypoplastic disease, or a sporadic occurrence. Reports exist of infants with GCKD who have family members affected with ADPKD, which raises the question of whether these two entities are different expressions of the same genetic defect. Sporadic GCKD and GCKD occurring in the context of familial ADPKD are clinically, sonographically, and histopathologically indistinguishable. The sporadic cases are conceivably new mutations of the same disease.

Reports of kindreds with GCKD suggest autosomal dominant inheritance in some cases (273). Carson et al. described a family of 18 first-degree relatives with six affected individuals (274). Their review of the literature for reported cases revealed several other such families, although sporadic cases constitute the bulk of patients with this diagnosis. An apparently distinct entity is hypoplastic GCKD, a dominantly inherited disease reported in only a few families (275,276). These kidneys, apart from being glomerulocystic, are small, and imaging studies show abnormal pyelocaliceal anatomy. Recently, mutations in the hepatocyte nuclear factor-1β gene were identified in four kindreds with this hypoplastic GCKD variant (277).

GCKD can be associated with such syndromes as orofaciodigital syndrome type I (278), brachymesomelia-renal syndrome (279), trisomy 13 (280), Majewski-type short rib polydactyly syndrome (280), and Jeune syndrome (281) and can be seen as a component of the renal abnormalities in nephronophthisis (282). Although tubular sclerosis generally includes tubular cysts, glomerular cysts can be present (282). Glomerular cysts also occur as a minor component in several other syndromes, including Zellweger cerebrohepatorenal syndrome (280,281) in which the cysts are typically present but rarely serious enough to affect renal function.

Other syndromes that may be associated with glomerular cysts as a component of renal dysplasia include Meckel syndrome, glutaric aciduria type II, and renal-hepatic-pancreatic dysplasia (282). The glomerular cysts are minor in comparison with the dysplastic components of the renal disease, although they may be present in sufficient numbers to create confusion with other glomerulocystic conditions.

Pathogenesis and Pathology

The pathogenesis of GCKD remains unknown. Clinically, GCKD can be difficult to distinguish from other cystic kidney diseases. The diagnosis can only be established by histologic examination of renal tissue. Sporadic GCKD in young infants is histopathologically indistinguishable from ADPKD-related GCKD. The kidneys in both the familial and sporadic forms are variably enlarged, with the degree of renal enlargement related to the degree of cyst formation (282). The cysts in both groups may be diffuse but can also be clustered, which may be responsible for asymmetric and asynchronous clinical presentations. Diffuse involvement is associated with interstitial edema, whereas patchy involvement is associated with better preservation of overall renal structure and function.

Characteristically, the cysts are dilated Bowman's spaces, comprising a sphere lined with cuboidal or columnar cells and containing abortive or primitive-appearing glomeruli (271), which occur as small scattered cysts separated by normal parenchyma. The cysts are located in the cortex, with preservation of the medulla. This lack of tubular involvement differentiates GCKD from other cystic diseases in which cysts generally arise from tubular dilation. In rare cases, they are more diffuse, surrounded by atrophic and fibrotic parenchyma. They may be found in association with tubular cysts and dysplasia (282).

The kidneys in sporadic GCKD and the GCKD form of ADPKD often contain abnormally differentiated pyramids, a type of medullary dysplasia. Both forms of GCKD are associated with biliary dysgenesis in approximately 10% of cases (282).

Clinical and Radiographic Features

Most GCKD patients described in the literature have some degree of renal failure, and many have hypertension at presentation. The typical presentation is that of an infant with abdominal masses, renal insufficiency, and enlarged cystic kidneys on sonography. GCKD may manifest in adulthood with hypertension, flank pain, and hematuria. Variable degrees of renal dysfunction are seen. Later detection may be consistent with a milder course (169,274). Clinically, hepatic cysts have also been described (282).

Patients with the familial hypoplastic GCKD variant have small kidneys with abnormal collecting systems and abnormal or absent papillae (275,276). Family studies show a pattern compatible with autosomal dominant inheritance. Most patients appear to have chronic renal failure early in life but subsequently have stable courses without progression to ESRD.

Several reports of GCKD describe patients with no clear familial or syndromic association (280,283,284). Histologically and clinically, these patients resemble familial cases with large, hyperechoic kidneys. It remains unclear whether these sporadic cases are a distinct entity or are associated with unrecognized syndromal or familial cases. Reports on an infant with GCKD and multiple cardiac rhabdomyomas and an infant with severe GCKD who later developed skin findings consistent with tuberous sclerosis strongly suggest an association of GCKD with tuberous sclerosis (285,286). This, together with the new information regarding the molecular basis of ADPKD and tuberous sclerosis and the reported familial association of GCKD and ADPKD, raises the possibility that autosomal dominant GCKD, ADPKD, and tuberous sclerosis are genetically linked in some kindreds. Single case studies have also reported GCKD in association with Henoch-Schönlein purpura (287), hepatoblastoma (288), and as a sequela of hemolytic-uremic syndrome (289,290).

Ultrasonography demonstrates bilateral renal enlargement without distortion of the renal contour, increased echogenicity of the cortex and medulla, loss of corticomedullary junction differentiation, and small cortical cysts (283,291). Radiographically, a feature that can help distinguish GCKD from ARPKD is abnormal medullary pyramids in the latter. In the future, CT and nuclear MRI may be of some value in differentiating between these two diseases (292). Reduced intensity of cortex on T1-weighted images and abnormalities of corticomedullary differentiation may help confirm the diagnosis.

In summary, GCKD represents a heterogeneous collection of heritable and nonheritable clinical entities. The clinical course and prognosis are quite variable and often dependent on the presence of associated disorders.

POLYCYSTIC KIDNEY DISEASE ASSOCIATED WITH CONGENITAL SYNDROMES

Many diseases can present with enlarged kidneys or cysts in the infant and young child and can initially be confused with PKD (Table 36.3). Abdominal ultrasound examination and nuclear isotope scanning help rule out multicystic renal dysplasia and obstructive uropathy. Multicystic dysplastic kidney is generally unilateral with macrocysts of varying sizes, differ-

TABLE 36.3. DIFFERENTIAL DIAGNOSIS OF POLYCYSTIC KIDNEY DISEASE IN THE PEDIATRIC PATIENT

Cystic diseases
Autosomal recessive polycystic kidney disease
Autosomal dominant polycystic kidney disease
Glomerulocystic kidney disease
Congenital and hereditary diseases
Tuberous sclerosis
Multicystic dysplastic kidney
Nephronophthisis complex
Glycogen storage disease
Congenital nephrosis
Syndromes
Meckel-Gruber syndrome
Jeune syndrome and other chondrodysplasia syndromes
Ivemark syndrome
Bardet-Biedl syndrome
Zellweger cerebrohepatorenal syndrome
Beckwith-Wiedemann syndrome
Trisomy 9 and 13
Neoplasia
Nephroblastomatosis
Bilateral Wilms' tumor
Leukemia or lymphoma
Miscellaneous
Pyelonephritis
Glomerulonephritis
Radiocontrast nephropathy
Bilateral renal vein thrombosis
Transient nephromegaly

Adapted from McDonald RA, Avner ED. Inherited polycystic kidney disease in children. *Semin Nephrol* 1991;11:632–642.

entiating it from ARPKD (see Chapter 5). On radionuclide scanning, it demonstrates no function, permitting differentiation from ADPKD. Most syndromic and other inherited disorders can usually be differentiated from ARPKD and ADPKD by associated clinical features, with the exception of GCKD, occasionally tuberous sclerosis, and von Hippel-Lindau disease (1,97,293). GCKD can be a feature of several inherited, sporadic, or syndromic conditions as discussed above. In addition, GCKD may be an early histopathologic expression of the ADPKD gene in young patients. Tuberous sclerosis is an autosomal dominant neurocutaneous disorder, in which hyperplastic cystic lesions may affect any portion of the nephron (285). Genetic linkage of the chromosome 16 loci for tuberous sclerosis and ADPKD1 has been demonstrated (294). The *TSC2* gene has been identified and encodes a novel protein, tuberin. Uncommonly, patients show polycystic renal involvement without clinical neurocutaneous involvement or positive family history. Several kindreds have been identified with tuberous sclerosis and severe childhood-onset ADPKD; they have large deletions in the area containing *PKD1* and adjacent *TSC2* gene (210). Analysis of the deletions indicates that they inactivate *PKD1*, in contrast to mutations reported in ADPKD patients in which abnormal transcripts have been detected. von Hippel-Lindau disease is a dominantly inherited cancer syndrome characterized by renal cell carcinoma, pheochromocytoma, and hemangioblastomas of the eye, spine, and cerebellum. Cystic kidneys and pancreas may be seen and, rarely, patients may present with "typical" features of ADPKD (295). To differentiate GCKD, tuberous sclerosis, and von Hippel-Lindau from ARPKD and ADPKD, detailed family history, physical examination, and close clinical follow-up are necessary.

DIFFERENTIAL DIAGNOSIS OF POLYCYSTIC KIDNEYS IN CHILDHOOD

In most clinical settings, the major problem in differential diagnosis of PKD in the pediatric patient is clearly delineating ARPKD from ADPKD. In fact, ADPKD presenting in the neonatal period may be indistinguishable clinically from ARPKD (98,145). In such instances, a staged evaluation, including careful history, physical examination, imaging, and histologic examination, is recommended. As noted in Table 36.4, certain clinical features can help differentiate between ARPKD and ADPKD, although no single finding is diagnostic. A complete family history is often the most important element in difficult cases. Parents should have renal and liver ultrasonography. If the parents of a child with undiagnosed PKD are younger than 30 years, the grandparents should also be evaluated because 4 to 5% of patients with ADPKD may not have visible renal cysts before age 30. Absence of any cystic disease in family members makes the diagnosis of ARPKD more likely because less than 5 to 8% of all ADPKD cases appear to result from new gene mutations (168). Radiographic studies may clearly distinguish ARPKD and ADPKD in some cases (Table 36.4). However, in clinical practice, 20 to 30% of all cases show certain features of both diseases on radiographic studies, making definitive diagnosis difficult if not impossible. If the constellation of physical and radiologic findings is equivocal, a tissue diagnosis may be required (Figs. 36.2 and 36.3). Renal biopsies, particularly when stained with segment-specific lectins (127,296), clearly differentiate the isolated fusiform cortical collecting tubular cysts of ARPKD (Fig. 36.2) from the heterogeneous cystic nephron involvement of ADPKD (Fig. 36.3). In certain instances, liver biopsy may provide additional information and reveal the characteristic biliary dysgenesis of ARPKD. However, hepatic portal fibrosis and bile duct ectasia have been associated with other types of renal cystic diseases, including ADPKD. In the future, further molecular analysis of ARPKD and ADPKD mutations will permit definitive genetic diagnosis and guide genetic counseling in childhood PKD.

TABLE 36.4. DIFFERENTIAL CLINICAL FEATURES OF CHILDHOOD POLYCYSTIC KIDNEY DISEASE

Major clinical features of both ARPKD and ADPKD
Enlarged kidneys
Hypertension
Concentrating defect
Sterile pyuria
Clinical features suggesting ARPKD rather than ADPKD
Neonatal presentation
Progression to end-stage renal disease as a child
Hepatosplenomegaly
Portal hypertension and esophageal varices
Bacterial cholangitis
Negative family history
Clinical features suggesting ADPKD rather than ARPKD
Positive family history
Extrarenal cysts
Cerebral aneurysms
Asymptomatic presentation
Unilateral renal presentation
Hematuria
Urinary tract infection

Adapted from Avner ED. Polycystic kidney disease. In: Drukker A, Grushkin A, eds. *Pediatric nephrology.* In: Branski D, series ed. Pediatric and adolescent medicine. Basel: AG Karger, 1993.

ACKNOWLEDGMENTS

Dr. Avner is the director and Dr. Dell a member of the National Institutes of Health–supported Rainbow Center for Childhood PKD (#P50-DK27306), Rainbow Babies and Children's Hospital, and Case Western Reserve University. Dr. Dell is supported by a Mentored Clinical Scientist Award (#K08 DK-59488). Dr. Avner is also supported in part by grants from the Polycystic Kidney Research Foundation and Wyeth-Ayerst Research.

REFERENCES

1. McDonald RA, Avner ED. Inherited polycystic kidney disease in children. *Semin Nephrol* 1991;11:632–642.
2. The European Polycystic Kidney Disease Consortium. The polycystic kidney disease 1 gene encodes a 14 kb transcript and lies within a duplicated region on chromosome 16. *Cell* 1994;77:881–894.
3. Mochizuki T, Wu G, Hayashi T, et al. PKD2, a gene for polycystic kidney disease that encodes an integral membrane protein. *Science* 1996;272:1339–1342.
4. Ward CJ, Hogan MC, Rossetti S, et al. The gene mutated in autosomal recessive polycystic kidney disease encodes a large, receptor-like protein. *Nat Genet* 2002;30:259–269.
5. Onuchic LF, Furu L, Nagasawa Y, et al. PKHD1, the polycystic kidney and hepatic disease 1 gene, encodes a novel large protein containing multiple immunoglobulin-like plexin-transcription-factor domains and parallel beta-helix 1 repeats. *Am J Hum Genet* 2002;70:1305–1317.
6. Murcia NS, Sweeney WE Jr, Avner ED. New insights into the molecular pathophysiology of polycystic kidney disease. *Kidney Int* 1999;55:1187–1197.
7. Avner ED, McAteer KA, Evan AP. Models of cysts and cystic kidneys. In: Gardner KD, ed. *The cystic kidney.* Dordrecht: Kluwer, 1990:55–98.
8. Orellana SA, Avner ED. Cystic maldevelopment in the kidney. *Semin Nephrol* 1995;15:341–352.
9. Wilson PD, Sherwood AC. Tubulocystic epithelium. *Kidney Int* 1991;39:450–463.
10. Grantham JJ. The etiology, pathogenesis, and treatment of autosomal dominant polycystic kidney disease: recent advances. *Am J Kidney Dis* 1996;28:788–803.
11. Calvet JP. Polycystic kidney disease: primary extracellular matrix abnormality or defective cellular differentiation. *Kidney Int* 1993;43:101–108.
12. Welling LW. Pathogenesis of cysts and cystic kidneys. In: Gardner KD, ed. *The cystic kidney.* Dordrecht: Kluwer, 1990:99–116.
13. Hjelle JT, Waters DC, Golinska BT, et al. Autosomal recessive polycystic kidney disease: characterization of human peritoneal and cystic kidney cells in vitro. *Am J Kidney Dis* 1990;15:123–136.
14. Hanaoka K, Guggino WB. cAMP regulates cell proliferation and cyst formation in autosomal polycystic kidney disease cells. *J Am Soc Nephrol* 2000;11:1179–1187.
15. Yamaguchi T, Pelling JC, Ramaswamy NT, et al. cAMP stimulates the in vitro proliferation of renal cyst epithelial cells by activating the extracellular signal-regulated kinase pathway. *Kidney Int* 2000;57:1460–1471.
16. Marfella-Scivittaro C, Quinones A, Orellana SA. cAMP-dependent protein kinase and proliferation differ in normal and polycystic kidney epithelia. *Am J Physiol Cell Physiol* 2002;282:C693–707.
17. Nadasdy T, Laszik Z, Lajoie G, et al. Proliferative activity of cyst epithelium in human renal cystic diseases. *J Am Soc Nephrol* 1995;5:1462–1468.
18. Klingel R, Dippold W, Storkel S, et al. Expression of differentiation antigens and growth-related genes in normal kidney, autosomal dominant polycystic kidney disease, and renal cell carcinoma. *Am J Kidney Dis* 1992;19:22–30.
19. Du J, Wilson PD. Abnormal polarization of EGF receptors and autocrine stimulation of cyst epithelial growth in human ADPKD. *Am J Physiol* 1995;269:C487–495.
20. Orellana SA, Sweeney WE, Neff CD, et al. Epidermal growth factor receptor expression is abnormal in murine polycystic kidney. *Kidney Int* 1995;47:490–499.
21. Sweeney WE, Avner ED. Functional activity of epidermal growth factor receptors in autosomal recessive polycystic kidney disease. *Am J Physiol* 1998;275:F387–394.
22. Sweeney WE, Futey L, Frost P, et al. In vitro modulation of cyst formation by a novel tyrosine kinase inhibitor. *Kidney Int* 1999;56:406–413.
23. Pugh JL, Sweeney WE Jr, Avner ED. Tyrosine kinase activity of the EGF receptor in murine metanephric organ culture. *Kidney Int* 1995;47:774–781.
24. Sweeney WE, Chen Y, Nakanishi K, et al. Treatment of polycystic kidney disease with a novel tyrosine kinase inhibitor. *Kidney Int* 2000;57:33–40.
25. Richards WG, Sweeney WE, Yoder BK, et al. Epidermal growth factor receptor activity mediates renal cyst formation in polycystic kidney disease. *J Clin Invest* 1998;101: 935–939.
26. Herrera GA. C-erb B-2 amplification in cystic renal disease. *Kidney Int* 1991;40:509–513.
27. Nakanishi K, Sweeney W Jr, Avner ED. Segment-specific c-ErbB2 expression in human autosomal recessive polycystic kidney disease. *J Am Soc Nephrol* 2001;12:379–384.
28. Dell KM, Nemo R, Sweeney W Jr, et al. Abnormalities in the heparin-binding EGF/ErbB4/EGFR axis in murine ARPKD (Abstract). *J Am Soc Nephrol* 2002;13:107A.
29. Wilson PD, Du J, Norman JT. Autocrine, endocrine and paracrine regulation of growth abnormalities in autosomal dominant polycystic kidney disease. *Eur J Cell Biol* 1993;61:131–138.
30. Horikoshi S, Kubota S, Martin GR, et al. Epidermal growth factor expression in the congenital polycystic mouse. *Kidney Int* 1992;39:57–62.
31. Gattone VH II, Calvet JP. Murine infantile polycystic kidney disease: a role for reduced renal epidermal growth factor. *Am J Kidney Dis* 1991;17:606–607.
32. Gattone VH II, Lowden DA, Cowley BD Jr. Epidermal growth factor ameliorates autosomal recessive polycystic kidney disease in mice. *Dev Biol* 1995;169:504–510.
33. Nakanishi K, Gattone VH II, Sweeney WE, et al. Renal dysfunction but not cystic change is ameliorated by neonatal epidermal growth factor in bpk mice. *Pediatr Nephrol* 2001;16:45–50.
34. Avner ED, Sweeney WE Jr. Polypeptide growth factors in metanephric growth and segmental nephron differentiation. *Pediatr Nephrol* 1990;4:372–377.
35. Neufield TK, Douglass D, Grant M, et al. In vitro formation and expansion of cysts derived from human renal cortex epithelial cells. *Kidney Int* 1992;41:1222–1236.
36. Lee DC, Chan KW, Chan SY. Expression of transforming growth factor alpha and epidermal growth factor receptor in adult polycystic kidney disease. *J Urol* 1998;159:291–296.
37. Lowden DA, Lindemann GW, Merlino G, et al. Renal cysts in transgenic mice expressing transforming growth factor-alpha. *J Lab Clin Med* 1994;124:386–394.

38. Dell KM, Nemo R, Sweeney WE Jr, et al. A novel inhibitor of tumor necrosis factor-alpha converting enzyme ameliorates polycystic kidney disease. *Kidney Int* 2001;60:1240–1248.
39. Hamahira K, Sweeney WE, Gatrell-Garcia M, et al. Tyrosine kinase inhibitor (EKB) alone or in combination with an inhibitor of TGF-a secretion ameliorates cyst progression in murine ARPKD (Abstract). *Pediatr Res* 2002;51:422A.
40. Dell KM, Nemo R, Sweeney WE Jr, et al. Evidence for a role of multiple epidermal growth factor receptor (EGFR) ligands in the pathogenesis of ARPKD (Abstract). *Pediatr Res* 2002;51:421A.
41. Woo DD, Miao SY, Pelayo JC, et al. Taxol inhibits progression of congenital polycystic kidney disease. *Nature* 1994;368:750–753.
42. Lanoix J, D'Agati V, Szabolcs M, et al. Dysregulation of cellular proliferation and apoptosis mediates human autosomal dominant polycystic kidney disease (ADPKD). *Oncogene* 1996;13:1153–1160.
43. Winyard PJ, Nauta J, Lirenman DS, et al. Deregulation of cell survival in cystic and dysplastic renal development. *Kidney Int* 1996;49:135–146.
44. Ali SM, Wong VY, Kikly K, et al. Apoptosis in polycystic kidney disease: involvement of caspases. *Am J Physiol Regul Integr Comp Physiol* 2000;278:R763–R769.
45. Hamahira K, Sweeney W, Avner ED. Role of apoptosis and proliferation in cyst formation in the bpk model of ARPKD (Abstract). *J Am Soc Nephrol* 2002;13:112A.
46. Ecder T, Melnikov VY, Stanley M, et al. Caspases, Bcl-2 proteins and apoptosis in autosomal-dominant polycystic kidney disease. *Kidney Int* 2002;61:1220–1230.
47. Veis DJ, Sorenson CM, Shutter JR, et al. Bcl-2–deficient mice demonstrate fulminant lymphoid apoptosis, polycystic kidneys and hypopigmented hair. *Cell* 1993;75:229–240.
48. Sorenson CM. Nuclear localization of beta-catenin and loss of apical brush border actin in cystic tubules of bcl-2 –/– mice. *Am J Physiol* 1999;276:F210–217.
49. Saadi-Kheddouci S, Berrebi D, Romagnolo B, et al. Early development of polycystic kidney disease in transgenic mice expressing an activated mutant of the beta-catenin gene. *Oncogene* 2001;20:5972–5981.
50. Moser M, Pscherer A, Roth C, et al. Enhanced apoptotic cell death of renal epithelial cells in mice lacking transcription factor AP-2beta. *Genes Dev* 1997;11:1938–1948.
51. Trudel M, Lanoix J, Barisoni L, et al. C-myc-induced apoptosis in polycystic kidney disease is Bcl-2 and p53 independent. *J Exp Med* 1997;186:1873–1884.
52. Cowley BD Jr, Smardo FL Jr, Grantham JJ, et al. Elevated c-myc protooncogene expression in autosomal recessive polycystic kidney disease. *Proc Natl Acad Sci U S A* 1987;84:8394–8398.
53. Cowley BD Jr, Chadwick LJ, Grantham JJ, et al. Elevated proto-oncogene expression in polycystic kidneys of the C57BL/6J (cpk) mouse. *J Am Soc Nephrol* 1991;1:1048–1053.
54. Harding MA, Gattone VH II, Grantham JJ, et al. Localization of overexpressed c-myc mRNA in polycystic kidneys of the cpk mouse. *Kidney Int* 1992;41:317–325.
55. Trudel M, Barisoni L, Lanoix J, et al. Polycystic kidney disease in SBM transgenic mice: role of c-myc in disease induction and progression. *Am J Pathol* 1998;152:219–229.
56. Trudel M, D'Agati V, Costantini F. C-myc as an inducer of polycystic kidney disease in transgenic mice. *Kidney Int* 1991;39:665–671.
57. Ricker JL, Mata JE, Iversen PL, et al. C-myc antisense oligonucleotide treatment ameliorates murine ARPKD. *Kidney Int* 2002;61:125–131.
58. Ostrom L, Tang MJ, Gruss P, et al. Reduced Pax2 gene dosage increases apoptosis and slows the progression of renal cystic disease. *Dev Biol* 2000;219:250–258.
59. Grantham JJ, Geiser JL, Evan AP. Cyst formation and growth in autosomal dominant polycystic kidney disease. *Kidney Int* 1987;31:1145–1152.
60. Ye M, Grantham JJ. The secretion of fluid by renal cysts from patients with autosomal dominant polycystic kidney disease. *N Engl J Med* 1993;329:310–313.
61. Mangoo-Karim R, Uchic M, Lechene C. Renal epithelial cyst formation and enlargement in vitro: dependence on cAMP. *Proc Natl Acad Sci U S A* 1989;86:6007–6011.
62. Macias WL, McAteer JA, Tanner GA, et al. NaCl transport by Madin Darby kidney cyst epithelial cells. *Kidney Int* 1992;42:308–319.
63. Grantham JJ, Ye M, Gattone VH II, et al. In vitro fluid secretion by epithelium from polycystic kidneys. *J Clin Invest* 1995;95:195–202.
64. Grantham JJ, Ye M, Davidow C, et al. Evidence for a potent lipid secretagogue in the cyst fluids of patients with autosomal dominant polycystic kidney disease. *J Am Soc Nephrol* 1995;6:1242–1249.
65. Avner ED, Sweeney WE Jr, Finegold DN, et al. Sodium-potassium ATPase activity mediates cyst formation in metanephric organ culture. *Kidney Int* 1985;28:447–455.
66. Avner ED, Sweeney WE Jr, Young MC, et al. Congenital murine polycystic kidney disease. II. Pathogenesis of tubular cyst formation. *Pediatr Nephrol* 1988;2:210–218.
67. Avner ED, Sweeney WE Jr, Ellis D. In vitro modulation of tubular cyst regression in murine polycystic kidney disease. *Kidney Int* 1989;36:960–968.
68. Wilson PD, Burrow CR. Autosomal dominant polycystic kidney disease: cellular and molecular mechanisms of cyst formation. *Adv Nephrol* 1992;21:125–142.
69. Wilson PD, Sherwood AC, Palla K, et al. Reversed polarity of Na(+)-K(+)-ATPase: mislocation to apical plasma membranes in polycystic kidney disease epithelia. *Am J Physiol* 1991;260:F420–F430.
70. Avner ED, Sweeney WE Jr, Nelson WJ. Abnormal sodium pump distribution during renal tubulogenesis in congenital murine polycystic kidney disease. *Proc Natl Acad Sci U S A* 1992;89:7447–7451.
71. Kawa G, Nagao S, Yamamoto A, et al. Sodium pump distribution is not reversed in the DBA/2FG-pcy, polycystic kidney disease model mouse. *J Am Soc Nephrol* 1994;4:2040–2049.
72. Hanaoka K, Devuyst O, Schwiebert EM, et al. A role for CFTR in human autosomal dominant polycystic kidney disease. *Am J Physiol* 1996;270:C389–C399.
73. Davidow CJ, Maser RL, Rome LA, et al. The cystic fibrosis transmembrane conductance regulator mediates transepithelial fluid secretion by human autosomal dominant polycystic kidney disease epithelium in vitro. *Kidney Int* 1996;50:208–218.

74. Sweeney WE, Avner ED, Elmer HL, et al. CFTR is required for cAMP-dependant in vitro renal cyst formation. *J Am Soc Nephrol* 1998;9:1954.
75. O'Sullivan DA, Torres VE, Gabow PA, et al. Cystic fibrosis and the phenotypic expression of autosomal dominant polycystic kidney disease. *Am J Kidney Dis* 1998;32:976–983.
76. Persu A, Devuyst O, Lannoy N, et al. CF gene and cystic fibrosis transmembrane conductance regulator expression in autosomal dominant polycystic kidney disease. *J Am Soc Nephrol* 2000;11:2285–2296.
77. Nakanishi K, Sweeney WE Jr, Macrae Dell K, et al. Role of CFTR in autosomal recessive polycystic kidney disease. *J Am Soc Nephrol* 2001;12:719–725.
78. Jin H, Carone FA, Nakamura S, et al. Altered synthesis and intracellular transport of proteoglycans by cyst-derived cells from human polycystic kidneys. *J Am Soc Nephrol* 1992; 2:1726–1733.
79. Liu ZZ, Carone FA, Nakumara S, et al. Altered synthesis of proteoglycans by cyst-derived cells from autosomal-dominant polycystic kidneys. *Am J Physiol* 1992;263:F697–F704.
80. Kovacs J, Carone FA, Liu ZZ, et al. Differential growth factor-induced modulation of proteoglycans synthesized by normal human renal versus cyst-derived cells. *J Am Soc Nephrol* 1994;5:47–54.
81. Candiano G, Gusmano R, Altieri P, et al. Extracellular matrix formation by epithelial cells from human polycystic kidney cysts in culture. *Virchows Arch B Cell Pathol Incl Mol Pathol* 1992;63:1–9.
82. Grantham JJ, Donoso VS, Evan AP, et al. Viscoelastic properties of tubule basement membranes in experimental renal cystic disease. *Kidney Int* 1987;32:187–197.
83. Rankin CA, Suzuki K, Itoh Y, et al. Matrix metalloproteinases and TIMPS in cultured C57BL/6J-cpk kidney tubules. *Kidney Int* 1996;50:835–844.
84. Rankin CA, Itoh Y, Tian C, et al. Matrix metalloproteinase-2 in a murine model of infantile-type polycystic kidney disease. *J Am Soc Nephrol* 1999;10:210–217.
85. Schaefer L, Han X, Gretz N, et al. Tubular gelatinase A (MMP-2) and its tissue inhibitors in polycystic kidney disease in the Han:SPRD rat. *Kidney Int* 1996;49:75–81.
86. Nakamura T, Ushiyama C, Suzuki S, et al. Elevation of serum levels of metalloproteinase-1, tissue inhibitor of metalloproteinase-1 and type IV collagen, and plasma levels of metalloproteinase-9 in polycystic kidney disease. *Am J Nephrol* 2000;20:32–36.
87. Obermuller N, Morente N, Kranzlin B, et al. A possible role for metalloproteinases in renal cyst development. *Am J Physiol Renal Physiol* 2001;280:F540–550.
88. Daikha-Dahmane F, Dommergues M, Narcy F, et al. Distribution and ontogenesis of tenascin in normal and cystic human fetal kidneys. *Lab Invest* 1995;73:547–557.
89. Ojeda JL. Abnormal tenascin expression in murine autosomal recessive polycystic kidneys. *Nephron* 1999;82:261–269.
90. Daikha-Dahmane F, Narcy F, Dommergues M, et al. Distribution of alpha-integrin subunits in fetal polycystic kidney diseases. *Pediatr Nephrol* 1997;11:267–273.
91. Cowley BD Jr, Ricardo SD, Nagao S, et al. Increased renal expression of monocyte chemoattractant protein-1 and osteopontin in ADPKD in rats. *Kidney Int* 2001;60:2087–2096.
92. Maser RL, Vassmer D, Magenheimer BS, et al. Oxidant stress and reduced antioxidant enzyme protection in polycystic kidney disease. *J Am Soc Nephrol* 2002;13:991–999.
93. Ogborn MR, Crocker JF, McCarthy SC. RU38486 prolongs survival in murine congenital polycystic kidney disease. *J Steroid Biochem* 1987;28:783–784.
94. Deshmukh GD, Radin NS, Gattone VH II, et al. Abnormalities of glycosphingolipid, sulfatide, and ceramide in the polycystic (cpk/cpk) mouse. *J Lipid Res* 1994;35:1611–1618.
95. Crocker JF, Blecher SR, Givner ML, et al. Polycystic kidney and liver disease and corticosterone changes in the cpk mouse. *Kidney Int* 1987;31:1088–1091.
96. Bello-Reuss E, Holubec K, Rajaraman S. Angiogenesis in autosomal-dominant polycystic kidney disease. *Kidney Int* 2001;60:37–45.
97. Dell KM, Avner ED. Autosomal recessive polycystic kidney disease. Edited by *GeneClinics: Clinical Genetic Information Resource* [database online]. Copyright, University of Washington, Seattle. Available at http://www.geneclinics.org. 2001.
98. Guay-Woodford LM, Galliani CA, Musulman-Mroczek E, et al. Diffuse renal cystic disease in children: morphologic and genetic correlations. *Pediatr Nephrol* 1998;12:173–182.
99. Cole BR, Conley SB, Stapleton FB. Polycystic kidney disease in the first year of life. *J Pediatr* 1987;111:693–699.
100. Kaariainen H. Polycystic kidney disease in children: a genetic and epidemiological study of 82 Finnish patients. *J Med Genet* 1987;24:474–481.
101. Zerres K, Rudnik-Schoneborn S, Steinkamm C, et al. Autosomal recessive polycystic kidney disease. *J Mol Med* 1998;76: 303–309.
102. Zerres K, Mucher G, Bachner L, et al. Mapping of the gene for autosomal recessive polycystic kidney disease (ARPKD) to chromosome 6p21–cen. *Nat Genet* 1994;7:429–432.
103. Hallermann C, Mucher G, Kohlschmidt N, et al. Syndrome of autosomal recessive polycystic kidneys with skeletal and facial anomalies is not linked to the ARPKD gene locus on chromosome 6p. *Am J Med Genet* 2000;90:115–119.
104. Zerres K, Mucher G, Becker J, et al. Prenatal diagnosis of autosomal recessive polycystic kidney disease (ARPKD): molecular genetics, clinical experience, and fetal morphology. *Am J Med Genet* 1998;76:137–144.
105. Zerres K, Rudnik-Schoneborn S, Deget F, et al. Autosomal recessive polycystic kidney disease in 115 children: clinical presentation, course and influence of gender. Arbeitsgemeinschaft fur Padiatrische, Nephrologie. *Acta Paediatr* 1996;85:437–445.
106. Lager DJ, Qian Q, Bengal RJ, et al. The pck rat: a new model that resembles human autosomal dominant polycystic kidney and liver disease. *Kidney Int* 2001;59:126–136.
107. Sanzen T, Harada K, Yasoshima M, et al. Polycystic kidney rat is a novel animal model of Caroli's disease associated with congenital hepatic fibrosis. *Am J Pathol* 2001;158:1605–1612.
108. Russell ES, McFarland EC. Cystic kidneys. *Mouse Newsletter* 1977;56:40–43.
109. Gattone VH II, Calvet JP, Cowley BD Jr, et al. Autosomal recessive polycystic kidney disease in a murine model. A gross and microscopic description. *Lab Invest* 1988;59:231–238.
110. Avner ED, Studnicki FE, Young MC, et al. Congenital murine polycystic kidney disease. I. The ontogeny of tubular cyst formation. *Pediatr Nephrol* 1987;1:587–596.

111. Mandell J, Koch WK, Nidess R, et al. Congenital polycystic kidney disease. *Am J Pathol* 1983;113:112–114.
112. Preminger GM, Koch WE, Fried FA, et al. Murine congenital polycystic kidney disease: a model for studying development of cystic disease. *J Urol* 1982;127:556–560.
113. Gattone VHI, MacNaughton KA, Kraybill AL. Murine autosomal recessive polycystic kidney disease with multiorgan involvement induced by the cpk gene. *Anat Rec* 1996;245: 488–499.
114. Hou X, Mrug M, Yoder BK, et al. Cystin, a novel cilia-associated protein, is disrupted in the cpk mouse model of polycystic kidney disease. *J Clin Invest* 2002;109:533–540.
115. Moyer JH, Lee-Tischler MJ, Kwon HY, et al. Candidate gene associated with a mutation causing recessive polycystic kidney disease in mice. *Science* 1994;264:1329–1333.
116. Yoder BK, Richards WG, Sommardahl C, et al. Differential rescue of the renal and hepatic disease in an autosomal recessive polycystic kidney disease mouse mutant. A new model to study the liver lesion. *Am J Pathol* 1997;150:2231–2241.
117. Yoder BK, Richards WG, Sommardahl C, et al. Functional correction of renal defects in a mouse model for ARPKD through expression of the cloned wild-type Tg737 cDNA. *Kidney Int* 1996;50:1240–1248.
118. Murcia NS, Richards WG, Yoder BK, et al. The Oak Ridge Polycystic Kidney (orpk) disease gene is required for left-right axis determination. *Development* 2000;127:2347–2355.
119. Yoder BK, Tousson A, Millican L, et al. Polaris, the protein disrupted in orpk mutant mice, is required for assembly of renal cilium. *Am J Physiol Renal Physiol* 2002;282:F541–F542.
120. El-Youssef M, Mu Y, Huang L, et al. Increased expression of transforming growth factor-beta1 and thrombospondin-1 in congenital hepatic fibrosis: possible role of the hepatic stellate cell. *J Pediatr Gastroenterol Nutr* 1999;28:386–392.
121. Nauta J, Ozawa Y, Sweeney WE Jr, et al. Renal and biliary abnormalities in a new murine model of autosomal recessive polycystic kidney disease. *Pediatr Nephrol* 1993;7:163–172.
122. Guay-Woodford LM. Mouse models of PKD: insights into disease pathogenesis. Edited by *NIH Strategic Planning Meeting for Polycystic Kidney Disease* Bethesda, MD, 2002
123. Nauta J, Sweeney WE, Rutledge JC, et al. Biliary epithelial cells from mice with congenital polycystic kidney disease are hyperresponsive to epidermal growth factor. *Pediatr Res* 1995;37:755–763.
124. Kissane JM. Renal cysts in pediatric patients. A classification and overview. *Pediatr Nephrol* 1990;4:69–77.
125. Osathanondh V, Potter EL. Pathogenesis of polycystic kidneys. Type I due to hyperplasia of interstitial portions of collecting tubules. *Arch Pathol* 1964;77:466–473.
126. Dalgaard OZ. Bilateral polycystic diseases of kidneys: a follow-up of two hundred and eighty-four patients and their families. *Acta Med Scand* 1957;328[Suppl]:1–255.
127. Faraggiana T, Bernstein J, Strauss L, et al. Use of lectins in the study of histogenesis of renal cysts. *Lab Invest* 1985;53:575–579.
128. Verani R, Walker P, Silva FG. Renal cystic disease of infancy: results of histochemical studies. A report of the Southwest Pediatric Nephrology Study Group. *Pediatr Nephrol* 1989;3:37–42.
129. Nakanishi K, Sweeney WE Jr, Zerres K, et al. Proximal tubular cysts in fetal human autosomal recessive polycystic kidney disease. *J Am Soc Nephrol* 2000;11:760–763.
130. Lieberman E, Salinas-Madrigal L, Gwinn JL, et al. Infantile polycystic disease of the kidneys and liver: clinical, pathological and radiological correlations and comparison with congenital hepatic fibrosis. *Medicine* 1971;50:277–318.
131. Gang DL, Herrin JT. Infantile polycystic disease of the liver and kidneys. *Clin Nephrol* 1986;25:28–36.
132. Bernstein J. Hepatic involvement in hereditary renal syndromes. *Birth Defects* 1987;23:115–130.
133. Alvarez F, Bernard O, Brunelle F, et al. Congenital hepatic fibrosis in children. *J Pediatr* 1981;99:370–375.
134. Kerr DN, Harrison CV, Sherlock S, et al. Congenital hepatic fibrosis. *QJM* 1961;30:91–117.
135. Lipschitz B, Berdon WE, Defelice AR, et al. Association of congenital hepatic fibrosis with autosomal dominant polycystic kidney disease. Report of a family with review of literature. *Pediatr Radiol* 1993;23:131–133.
136. Cobben JM, Breuning MH, Schoots C, et al. Congenital hepatic fibrosis in autosomal-dominant polycystic kidney disease. *Kidney Int* 1990;38:880–885.
137. Blyth H, Ockenden BG. Polycystic disease of the kidneys and liver presenting in childhood. *J Med Genet* 1971;8:257–284.
138. Kaplan BS, Kaplan P, de Chadarevian JP, et al. Variable expression of autosomal recessive polycystic kidney disease and congenital hepatic fibrosis within a family. *Am J Med Genet* 1988;29:639–647.
139. Deget F, Rudnik-Schoneborn S, Zerres K. Course of autosomal recessive polycystic kidney disease (ARPKD) in siblings: a clinical comparison of 20 sibships. *Clin Genet* 1995;47:248–253.
140. Kaplan BS, Fay J, Shah V, et al. Autosomal recessive polycystic kidney disease. *Pediatr Nephrol* 1989;3:43–49.
141. Gagnadoux MF, Habib R, Levy M, et al. Cystic renal diseases in children. *Adv Nephrol Necker Hosp* 1989;18:33–57.
142. Neumann HP, Zerres K, Fischer CL, et al. Late manifestation of autosomal-recessive polycystic kidney disease in two sisters. *Am J Nephrol* 1988;8:194–197.
143. Reuss A, Wladimiroff JW, Niermeyer MF. Sonographic, clinical and genetic aspects of prenatal diagnosis of cystic kidney disease. *Ultrasound Med Biol* 1991;17:687–694.
144. Kaplan BS, Kaplan P. Autosomal recessive polycystic kidney disease. In: Spitzer A, Avner ED, ed. *Inheritance of kidney and urinary tract diseases.* Dordrecht: Kluwer, 1990:265–276.
145. Kaarinnen H, Koskimies O, Norio R. Dominant and recessive polycystic kidney disease in children: evaluation of clinical features and laboratory data. *Pediatr Nephrol* 1988;2:296–302.
146. Potter EL. Facial characteristics of infants with bilateral renal agenesis. *Am J Obstet Gynecol* 1946;51:885–888.
147. Roy S, Dillon MJ, Trompeter RS, et al. Autosomal recessive polycystic kidney disease: long-term outcome of neonatal survivors. *Pediatr Nephrol* 1997;11:302–306.
148. Nicolau C, Torra R, Badenas C, et al. Sonographic pattern of recessive polycystic kidney disease in young adults. Differences from the dominant form. *Nephrol Dial Transplant* 2000;15:1373–1378.
149. Boal DK, Teele RL. Sonography of infantile polycystic kidney disease. *Am J Radiol* 1980;135:575–580.
150. Romero R, Cullen M, Jeanty P, et al. The diagnosis of congenital renal anomalies with ultrasound II. Infantile polycystic kidney disease. *Am J Obstet Gynecol* 1984;150:259–262.

151. Zerres K, Hansmann M, Mallmann R, et al. Autosomal recessive polycystic kidney disease. Problems of prenatal diagnosis. *Prenat Diagn* 1988;8:215–229.
152. Luthy DA, Hirsch JH. Infantile polycystic kidney disease: observations from attempts at prenatal diagnosis. *Am J Med Genet* 1985;20:505–517.
153. Wisser J, Hebisch G, Froster U, et al. Prenatal sonographic diagnosis of autosomal recessive polycystic kidney disease (ARPKD) during the early second trimester. *Prenat Diagn* 1995;15:868–871.
154. Morin PR, Potier M, Dallaire L, et al. Prenatal detection of autosomal recessive type of polycystic kidney disease by trehalase assay in amniotic fluid. *Prenat Diagn* 1981;1:75–79.
155. Townsend RR, Goldstein RB, Filly RA, et al. Sonographic identification of autosomal recessive polycystic kidney disease associated with increased maternal serum/amniotic fluid alpha-fetoprotein. *Obstet Gynecol* 1988;71:1008–1012.
156. Blickman JG, Bramson RT, Herrin JT. Autosomal recessive polycystic kidney disease: long-term sonographic findings in patients surviving the neonatal period. *AJR Am J Roentgenol* 1995;164:1247–1250.
157. Kern S, Zimmerhackl LB, Hildebrandt F, et al. Appearance of autosomal recessive polycystic kidney disease in magnetic resonance imaging and RARE-MR-urography. *Pediatr Radiol* 2000;30:156–160.
158. Zagar I, Anderson PJ, Gordon I. The value of radionuclide studies in children with autosomal recessive polycystic kidney disease. *Clin Nucl Med* 2002;27:339–344.
159. Bean SA, Bednarek FJ, Primack WA. Aggressive respiratory support and unilateral nephrectomy for infants with severe perinatal autosomal recessive polycystic kidney disease. *J Pediatr* 1995;127:311–313.
160. Munding M, Al-Uzri A, Gralneck D, et al. Prenatally diagnosed autosomal recessive polycystic kidney disease: initial postnatal management. *Urol* 1999;54:1097.
161. Spechtenhauser B, Hochleitner BW, Ellemunter H, et al. Bilateral nephrectomy, peritoneal dialysis and subsequent cadaveric renal transplantation for treatment of renal failure due to polycystic kidney disease requiring continuous ventilation. *Pediatr Transplant* 1999;3:246–248.
162. Fonck C, Chauveau D, Gagnadoux MF, et al. Autosomal recessive polycystic kidney disease in adulthood. *Nephrol Dial Transplant* 2001;16:1648–1652.
163. Kashtan CE, Primack WA, Kainer G, et al. Recurrent bacteremia with enteric pathogens in recessive polycystic kidney disease. *Pediatr Nephrol* 1999;13:678–682.
164. Benador N, Grimm P, Lavine J, et al. Transjugular intrahepatic portosystemic shunt prior to renal transplantation in a child with autosomal-recessive polycystic kidney disease and portal hypertension: a case report. *Pediatr Transplant* 2001; 5:210–214.
165. Tsimaratos M, Cloarec S, Roquelaure B, et al. Chronic renal failure and portal hypertension—is portosystemic shunt indicated? *Pediatr Nephrol* 2000;14:856–858.
166. Nakamura M, Fuchinoue S, Nakajima I, et al. Three cases of sequential liver-kidney transplantation from living-related donors. *Nephrol Dial Transplant* 2001;16:166–168.
167. Khan K, Schwarzenberg SJ, Sharp HL, et al. Morbidity from congenital hepatic fibrosis after renal transplantation for autosomal recessive polycystic kidney disease. *Am J Tranplant* 2002;2:360–365.
168. Harris PC, Torres VE. Autosomal dominant polycystic kidney disease. Edited by *GeneClinics: Clinical Genetic Information Resource* [database online]. Copyright, University of Washington, Seattle. Available at http://www.geneclinics.org. 2002.
169. Sedman A, Bell P, Manco-Johnson M, et al. Autosomal dominant polycystic kidney disease in childhood: a longitudinal study. *Kidney Int* 1987;31:1000–1005.
170. Milutinovic J, Rust PF, Fialkow PJ, et al. Intrafamilial phenotypic expression of autosomal dominant polycystic kidney disease. *Am J Kidney Dis* 1992;19:465–472.
171. Fick-Brosnahan GM, Belz MM, McFann KK, et al. Relationship between renal volume growth and renal function in autosomal dominant polycystic kidney disease: a longitudinal study. *Am J Kidney Dis* 2002;39:1127–1134.
172. Ariza M, Alvarez V, Marin R, et al. A family with a milder form of adult dominant polycystic kidney disease not linked to the PKD1 (16p) or PKD2 (4q) genes. *J Med Genet* 1997;34:587–589.
173. de Almeida S, de Almeida E, Peters D, et al. Autosomal dominant polycystic kidney disease: evidence for the existence of a third locus in a Portuguese family. *Hum Genet* 1995;96:83–88.
174. Daoust MC, Reynolds DM, Bichet DG, et al. Evidence for a third genetic locus for autosomal dominant polycystic kidney disease. *Genomics* 1995;25:733–736.
175. Ravine D, Walker RG, Gibson RN, et al. Phenotype and genotype heterogeneity in autosomal dominant polycystic kidney disease. *Lancet* 1992;340:1330–1333.
176. Hateboer N, v Dijk MA, Bogdanova N, et al. Comparison of phenotypes of polycystic kidney disease types 1 and 2. European PKD1–PKD2 Study Group. *Lancet* 1999;353:103–107.
177. Parfrey PS, Bear JC, Morgan J, et al. The diagnosis and prognosis of autosomal dominant polycystic kidney disease. *N Engl J Med* 1990;323:1085–1090.
178. Reeders ST, Breuning MH, Davies KE, et al. A highly polymorphic DNA marker linked to adult polycystic kidney disease on chromosome 16. *Nature* 1985;317:542–544.
179. The International Polycystic Kidney Disease Consortium. Polycystic kidney disease: the complete structure of the PKD1 gene and its protein. *Cell* 1995;81:289–298.
180. Harris PC. Autosomal dominant polycystic kidney disease: clues to pathogenesis. *Hum Mol Genet* 1999;8:1861–1866.
181. Peters DJ, Spruit L, Saris JJ, et al. Chromosome 4 localization of a second gene for autosomal dominant polycystic kidney disease. *Nat Genet* 1993;5:350–362.
182. Koulen P, Cai Y, Geng L, et al. Polycystin-2 is an intracellular calcium release channel. *Nat Cell Biol* 2002;4:191–197.
183. Rossetti S, Chauveau D, Walker D, et al. A complete mutation screen of the ADPKD genes by DHPLC. *Kidney Int* 2002;61:1588–1599.
184. Hodgkinson KA, Kerzin-Storrar L, Watters EA, et al. Adult polycystic kidney disease: knowledge, experience and attitudes to prenatal diagnosis. *J Med Genet* 1990;27:552–558.
185. Kielstein R, Sass H-M. Right not to know or duty to know? Prenatal screening for polycystic renal disease. *J Med Philos* 1992;17:395–405.
186. Frost N. Ethical implications of screening asymptomatic individuals. *FASEB J* 1992;6:2813–2817.

187. Sujansky E, Kreutzer SB, Johnson AM, et al. Attitudes of at-risk and affected individuals regarding presymptomatic testing for autosomal dominant polycystic kidney disease. *Am J Med Genet* 1990;35:510–515.
188. Zerres K, Rudnik-Schoneborn S, Deget F. Routine examination of children at risk for autosomal dominant polycystic kidney disease. *Lancet* 1992;339:1356–1357.
189. Wu G, Somlo S. Molecular genetics and mechanism of autosomal dominant polycystic kidney disease. *Mol Genet Metab* 2000;69:1–15.
190. Hughes J, Ward CJ, Peral B, et al. The polycystic kidney disease 1 (PKD1) gene encodes a novel protein with multiple cell recognition domains. *Nat Genet* 1995;10:151–160.
191. Wilson PD. Polycystin: new aspects of structure, function, and regulation. *J Am Soc Nephrol* 2001;12:834–845.
192. Moy GW, Mendoza LM, Schulz JR, et al. The sea urchin sperm receptor for egg jelly is a modular protein with extensive homology to the human polycystic kidney disease protein, PKD1. *J Cell Biol* 1996;133:809–817.
193. Qian F, Germino FJ, Cai Y, et al. PKD1 interacts with PKD2 through a probable coiled-coil domain. *Nat Genet* 1997;16:179–183.
194. Tsoikas L, Kim E, Arnould T, et al. Homo- and heterodimeric interactions between the gene products of PKD1 and PKD2. *Proc Natl Acad Sci U S A* 1997;94:6965–6970.
195. Ward CJ, Turley H, Ong AC, et al. Polycystin, the polycystic kidney disease 1 protein, is expressed by epithelial cells in fetal, adult, and polycystic kidney. *Proc Natl Acad Sci U S A* 1996;93:1524–1528.
196. Geng L, Segal Y, Peissel B, et al. Identification and localization of polycystin, the PKD1 gene product. *J Clin Invest* 1996;98:2674–2682.
197. Van Adelsberg JS, Frank D. The PKD1 gene produces a developmentally regulated protein in mesenchyme and vasculature. *Nat Med* 1995;1:359–364.
198. Ibraghimov-Beskrovnaya O, Dackowski WR, Foggensteiner L, et al. Polycystin: in vitro synthesis, in vivo tissue expression, and subcellular localization identifies a large membrane-associated protein. *Proc Natl Acad Sci U S A* 1997;94:6397–6402.
199. Geng L, Segal Y, Pavlova A, et al. Distribution and developmentally regulated expression of murine polycystin. *Am J Physiol* 1997;272:F451–F459.
200. Lu W, Peissel B, Babakhanlou H, et al. Perinatal lethality with kidney and pancreas defects in mice with a targeted Pkd1 mutation. *Nat Genet* 1997;17:179–181.
201. Boulter C, Mulroy S, Webb S, et al. Cardiovascular, skeletal, and renal defects in mice with a targeted disruption of the Pkd1 gene. *Proc Natl Acad Sci U S A* 2001;98:12174–12179.
202. Kim K, Drummond I, Ibraghimov-Beskrovnaya O, et al. Polycystin 1 is required for the structural integrity of blood vessels. *Proc Natl Acad Sci U S A* 2000;97:1731–1736.
203. Wilson PD, Geng L, Li X, et al. The PKD1 gene product, "polycystin-1," is a tyrosine-phosphorylated protein that colocalizes with alpha2beta1–integrin in focal clusters in adherent renal epithelia. *Lab Invest* 1999;79:1311–1323.
204. Huan Y, van Adelsberg J. Polycystin-1, the PKD1 gene product, is in a complex containing E-cadherin and the catenins. *J Clin Invest* 1999;104:1459–1468.
205. Boletta A, Qian F, Onuchic LF, et al. Polycystin-1, the gene product of PKD1, induces resistance to apoptosis and spontaneous tubulogenesis in MDCK cells. *Mol Cell* 2000;6:1267–1273.
206. Nickel C, Benzing T, Sellin L, et al. The polycystin-1 C-terminal fragment triggers branching morphogenesis and migration of tubular kidney epithelial cells. *J Clin Invest* 2002;109:481–489.
207. Qian F, Watnick TJ, Onuchic LF, et al. The molecular basis of focal cyst formation in human autosomal dominant polycystic kidney disease type I. *Cell* 1996;87:979–987.
208. Brasier JL, Henske EP. Loss of the polycystic kidney disease (PKD1) region of chromosome 16p13 in renal cyst cells supports a loss-of-function model for cyst pathogenesis. *J Clin Invest* 1997;99:194–199.
209. Rossetti S, Strmecki L, Gamble V, et al. Mutation analysis of the entire PKD1 gene: genetic and diagnostic implications. *Am J Hum Genet* 2001;68:46–63.
210. Brook-Carter PT, Peral B, Ward CJ, et al. Deletion of the TSC2 and PKD1 genes associated with severe infantile polycystic kidney disease—a contiguous gene syndrome. *Nat Genet* 1994;8:328–332.
211. Somlo S, Rutecki G, Giuffra LA, et al. A kindred exhibiting cosegregation of an overlap connective tissue disorder and the chromosome 16 linked form of autosomal dominant polycystic kidney disease. *J Am Soc Nephrol* 1993;4:1371–1378.
212. Rossetti S, Burton S, Strmecki L, et al. The Position of the Polycystic Kidney Disease 1 (PKD1) Gene mutation correlates with the severity of renal disease. *J Am Soc Nephrol* 2002;13:1230–1237.
213. Foggensteiner L, Bevan AP, Thomas R, et al. Cellular and subcellular distribution of polycystin-2, the protein product of the PKD2 gene. *J Am Soc Nephrol* 2000;11:814–827.
214. Torres VE, Cai Y, Chen X, et al. Vascular expression of polycystin-2. *J Am Soc Nephrol* 2001;12:1–9.
215. Veldhuisen B, Saris JJ, de Haij S, et al. A spectrum of mutations in the second gene for autosomal dominant polycystic kidney disease (PKD2). *Am J Human Genet* 1997;61:547–555.
216. Wu G, Markowitz GS, Li L, et al. Cardiac defects and renal failure in mice with targeted mutations in Pkd2. *Nat Genet* 2000;24:75–78.
217. Hateboer N, Veldhuisen B, Peters D, et al. Location of mutations within the PKD2 gene influences clinical outcome. *Kidney Int* 2000;57:1444–1451.
218. MacDermot KD, Saggar-Malik AK, Economides DL, et al. Prenatal diagnosis of autosomal dominant polycystic kidney disease (PKD1) presenting in utero and prognosis for very early onset disease. *J Med Genet* 1998;35:13–16.
219. Harrap SB, Davies DL, Macnicol AM, et al. Renal, cardiovascular and hormonal characteristics of young adults with autosomal dominant polycystic kidney disease. *Kidney Int* 1991;40:501–508.
220. Chapman AB, Schrier RW. Pathogenesis of hypertension in autosomal dominant polycystic kidney disease. *Semin Nephrol* 1991;11:653–660.
221. Fick GM, Duley IT, Johnson AM, et al. The spectrum of autosomal dominant polycystic kidney disease in children. *J Am Soc Nephrol* 1994;4:1654–1660.
222. Fick GM, Johnson AM, Strain JD, et al. Characteristics of very early onset autosomal dominant polycystic kidney disease. *J Am Soc Nephrol* 1993;3:1863–1870.

223. Fick-Brosnahan G, Johnson AM, Strain JD, et al. Renal asymmetry in children with autosomal dominant polycystic kidney disease. *Am J Kidney Dis* 1999;34:639–645.
224. Gabow P. Autosomal dominant polycystic kidney disease. *N Engl J Med* 1993;329:332–342.
225. Kaehny WD, Everson GT. Extrarenal manifestations of autosomal dominant polycystic kidney disease. *Semin Nephrol* 1991;11:661.
226. Everson GT. Hepatic cysts in autosomal dominant kidney disease. *Mayo Clin Proc* 1990;65:1020–1025.
227. Milutinovic J, Schabel SI, Ainsworth SK. Autosomal dominant polycystic kidney disease with liver and pancreatic involvement in early childhood. *Am J Kidney Dis* 1989;13:340–344.
228. Torra R, Nicolau C, Badenas C, et al. Ultrasonographic study of pancreatic cysts in autosomal dominant polycystic kidney disease. *Clin Nephrol* 1997;47:19–22.
229. Proesmans W, Van Damme B, Casaer P, et al. Autosomal dominant polycystic kidney disease in the neonatal period: association with cerebral arteriovenous malformation. *Pediatrics* 1982;70:971.
230. Lumiaho A, Ikaheimo R, Miettinen R, et al. Mitral valve prolapse and mitral regurgitation are common in patients with polycystic kidney disease type 1. *Am J Kidney Dis* 2001;38: 1208–1216.
231. Ivy DD, Shaffer EM, Johnson AM, et al. Cardiovascular abnormalities in children with autosomal dominant polycystic kidney disease. *J Am Soc Nephrol* 1995;5:2032–2036.
232. de Chadarevian JP, Kaplan BS. Endocardial fibroelastosis, myocardial scarring and polycystic kidneys. *Int J Pediatr Nephrol* 1981;2:273–275.
233. Mehrizi A, Rosenstine BH, Pusch A, et al. Myocardial infarction and endocardial fibroelastosis in children with polycystic kidneys. *Bull Johns Hopkins Hosp* 1964;115:95–98.
234. Bardaji A, Martinez Vea A, Gutierrez C, et al. Left ventricular mass and diastolic function in normotensive young adults with autosomal dominant polycystic kidney disease. *Am J Kidney Dis* 1998;32:970–975.
235. Hadimeri H, Lamm C, Nyberg G. Coronary aneurysms in patients with autosomal dominant polycystic kidney disease. *J Am Soc Nephrol* 1998;9:837–841.
236. Pretorius DH, Lee ME, Manco-Johnson ML, et al. Diagnosis of autosomal dominant polycystic kidney disease in utero and in the young infant. *J Ultrasound Med* 1987;6:249–255.
237. Main D, Mennuti MT, Cornfeld D, et al. Prenatal diagnosis of adult polycystic kidney disease. *Lancet* 1983;2:337–338.
238. McHugh K, Stringer DA, Hebert D, et al. Simple renal cysts in children: diagnosis and follow-up with US. *Radiology* 1991;178:383–385.
239. Gabow PA, Kimberling WJ, Strain JD, et al. Utility of ultrasonography in the diagnosis of autosomal dominant polycystic kidney disease in children. *J Am Soc Nephrol* 1997;8:105–110.
240. Bear JC, McManamon P, Morgan J, et al. Age at clinical onset and at ultrasonographic detection of adult polycystic kidney disease. *Am J Med Genet* 1984;18:45–53.
241. Ogborn MR, Nitschmann E, Weiler H, et al. Flaxseed ameliorates interstitial nephritis in rat polycystic kidney disease. *Kidney Int* 1999;55:417–423.
242. Ogborn MR, Bankovic-Calic N, Shoesmith C, et al. Soy protein modification of rat polycystic kidney disease. *Am J Physiol* 1998;274:F541–549.
243. Aukema HM, Housini I, Rawling JM. Dietary soy protein effects on inherited polycystic kidney disease are influenced by gender and protein level. *J Am Soc Nephrol* 1999;10:300–308.
244. Ogborn MR, Sareen S. Amelioration of polycystic kidney disease by modification of dietary protein intake in the rat. *J Am Soc Nephrol* 1995;6:1649–1654.
245. Tanner GA, Tanner JA. Citrate therapy for polycystic kidney disease in rats. *Kidney Int* 2000;58:1859–1869.
246. Tanner GA, Tanner JA. Chronic caffeine consumption exacerbates hypertension in rats with polycystic kidney disease. *Am J Kidney Dis* 2001;38:1089–1095.
247. Wang X, Sweeney W, Lager DJ, et al. The intraperitoneal administration of EKI-785 has opposing effects on the development of polycystic kidney disease in Han:SPRD and PCK rats (Abstract). *J Am Soc Nephrol* 2001;12:547A.
248. Davis ID, MacRae Dell K, Sweeney WE, et al. Can progression of autosomal dominant or autosomal recessive polycystic kidney disease be prevented? *Semin Nephrol* 2001;21:430–440.
249. Ecder T, Edelstein CL, Fick-Brosnahan GM, et al. Diuretics versus angiotensin-converting enzyme inhibitors in autosomal dominant polycystic kidney disease. *Am J Nephrol* 2001;21:98–103.
250. Watson ML, Macnicol AM, Allan PL, et al. Effects of angiotensin converting enzyme inhibition in adult polycystic kidney disease. *Kidney Int* 1992;41:206–210.
251. Weir MR, Dzau VJ. The renin-angiotensin-aldosterone system: a specific target for hypertension management. *Am J Hypertens* 1999;12:205S–213S.
252. Chapman AB, Gabow PA, Schrier RW. Reversible renal failure associated with angiotensin-converting enzyme inhibitors in polycystic kidney disease. *Ann Intern Med* 1991;115:769–773.
253. Gabow PA, Ikle DW, Holmes JH. Polycystic kidney disease: prospective analysis of non-azotemic patients and family members. *Ann Intern Med* 1984;101:238–247.
254. Gabow P. Autosomal dominant polycystic kidney disease. In: Gardner KD, ed. *The cystic kidney.* Dordrecht: Kluwer, 1990:295–326.
255. Schwab SJ, Bander SJ, Klahr S. Renal infection in autosomal dominant polycystic kidney disease. *Am J Med* 1987;82:714–718.
256. Rossi SJ, Healy DP, Savani DV, et al. High-dose ciprofloxacin in the treatment of a renal cyst infection. *Ann Pharmacother* 1993;27:38–39.
257. Gibson P, Watson ML. Cyst infection in polycystic kidney disease: a clinical challenge. *Nephrol Dial Transplant* 1998;13: 2455–2457.
258. Gabow PA, Johnson AM, Kaehny WD, et al. Factors affecting the progression of renal disease in autosomal-dominant polycystic kidney disease. *Kidney Int* 1992;41:1311–1319.
259. Chicoskie C, Chaoui A, Kuligowska E, et al. MRI isolation of infected renal cyst in autosomal dominant polycystic kidney disease. *Clin Imaging* 2001;25:114–117.
260. Bajwa ZH, Gupta S, Warfield CA, et al. Pain management in polycystic kidney disease. *Kidney Int* 2001;60:1631–1644.
261. Dunn MD, Portis AJ, Naughton C, et al. Laparoscopic cyst marsupialization in patients with autosomal dominant polycystic kidney disease. *J Urol* 2001;165:1888–1892.
262. Telenta A, Torres VE, Gross JB Jr, et al. Hepatic cyst infection in autosomal dominant polycystic kidney disease. *Mayo Clin Proc* 1990;65:933–942.

263. McDonald MI, Corey GR, Gallis HA, et al. Single and multiple pyogenic liver abscesses: natural history, diagnosis and treatment, with emphasis on percutaneous drainage. *Medicine* 1984;63:291–302.
264. Belz MM, Hughes RL, Kaehny WD, et al. Familial clustering of ruptured intracranial aneurysms in autosomal dominant polycystic kidney disease. *Am J Kidney Dis* 2001;38:770–776.
265. Chapman AB, Rubinstein D, Hughes R, et al. Intracranial aneurysms in autosomal dominant polycystic kidney disease. *N Engl J Med* 1992;327:916–920.
266. Huston J III, Torres VE, Sulivan PP, et al. Value of magnetic resonance angiography for the detection of intracranial aneurysms in autosomal dominant polycystic kidney disease. *J Am Soc Nephrol* 1993;3:1871–1877.
267. Fick-Brosnahan GM, Tran ZV, Johnson AM, et al. Progression of autosomal-dominant polycystic kidney disease in children. *Kidney Int* 2001;59:1654–1662.
268. Sharp C, Johnson A, Gabow P. Factors relating to urinary protein excretion in children with autosomal dominant polycystic kidney disease. *J Am Soc Nephrol* 1998;9:1908–1914.
269. King BF, Reed JE, Bergstralh EJ, et al. Quantification and longitudinal trends of kidney, renal cyst, and renal parenchyma volumes in autosomal dominant polycystic kidney disease. *J Am Soc Nephrol* 2000;11:1505–1511.
270. Sise C, Kusaka M, Wetzel LH, et al. Volumetric determination of progression in autosomal dominant polycystic kidney disease by computed tomography. *Kidney Int* 2000;58:2492–2501.
271. Taxy JB, Filmer RB. Glomerulocystic kidney. Report of a case. *Arch Pathol Lab Med* 1976;100:186–188.
272. Ross A. Polycystic kidney. Report of a case studied by reconstruction. *Am J Dis Child* 1941;61:116–127.
273. Sharp CK, Bergman SM, Stockwin JM, et al. Dominantly transmitted glomerulocystic kidney disease: a distinct genetic entity. *J Am Soc Nephrol* 1997;8:77–84.
274. Carson RW, Bedi D, Cavallo T, et al. Familial adult glomerulocystic kidney disease. *Am J Kidney Dis* 1987;9:154–165.
275. Rizzoni G, Loirat C, Levy M, et al. Familial hypoplastic glomerulocystic kidney. A new entity? *Clin Nephrol* 1982;18:263–268.
276. Kaplan BS, Gordon I, Pincott J, et al. Familial hypoplastic glomerulocystic kidney disease: a definite entity with dominant inheritance. *Am J Med Genet* 1989;34:569–573.
277. Bingham C, Bulman MP, Ellard S, et al. Mutations in the hepatocyte nuclear factor-1beta gene are associated with familial hypoplastic glomerulocystic kidney disease. *Am J Hum Genet* 2001;68:219–224.
278. Stapleton FB, Bernstein J, Koh G, et al. Cystic kidneys in a patient with oral-facial-digital syndrome type I. *Am J Kidney Dis* 1982;1:288–293.
279. Langer LO Jr, Nishino R, Yamaguchi A, et al. Brachymesomelia-renal syndrome. *Am J Med Genet* 1983;15:57–65.
280. Joshi VV, Kasznica J. Clinicopathologic spectrum of glomerulocystic kidneys: report of two cases and a brief review of literature. *Pediatr Pathol* 1984;2:171–186.
281. Bernstein J, Brough AJ, McAdams AJ. The renal lesion in syndromes of multiple congenital malformations: cerebrohepatorenal syndrome; Jeune asphyxiating thoracic dystrophy; tuberous sclerosis; Meckel syndrome. *Birth Defect* 1974;10:35–43.
282. Bernstein J. Glomerulocystic kidney disease—nosological considerations. *Pediatr Nephrol* 1993;7:464–470.
283. Fitch SJ, Stapleton FB. Ultrasonographic features of glomerulocystic disease in infancy: similarity to infantile polycystic kidney disease. *Pediatr Radiol* 1986;16:400–402.
284. Dosadeo S, Thompson AM, Abraham A. Glomerulocystic kidney disease. *Am J Clin Pathol* 1984;82:619–621.
285. Bernstein J, Robbins TO, Kissane JM. The renal lesions of tuberous sclerosis. *Semin Diagn Pathol* 1986;3:97–105.
286. Saguem MH, Laarif M, Remadi S, et al. Diffuse bilateral glomerulocystic disease of the kidneys and multiple cardiac rhabdomyomas in a newborn. Relationship with tuberous sclerosis and review of the literature. *Pathol Res Pract* 1992;188:367–373; discussion 373–364.
287. Miyazaki K, Miyazaki M, Yoshizuka N, et al. Glomerulocystic kidney disease (GCKD) associated with Henoch-Schönlein purpura: a case report and a review of adult cases of GCKD. *Clin Nephrol* 2002;57:386–391.
288. Greer ML, Danin J, Lamont AC. Glomerulocystic disease with hepatoblastoma in a neonate: a case report. *Pediatr Radiol* 1998;28:703–705.
289. Amir G, Rosenmann E, Drukker A. Acquired glomerulocystic kidney disease following haemolytic-uraemic syndrome. *Pediatr Nephrol* 1995;9:614–616.
290. Emma F, Muda AO, Rinaldi S, et al. Acquired glomerulocystic kidney disease following hemolytic uremic syndrome. *Pediatr Nephrol* 2001;16:557–560.
291. Cachero S, Montgomery P, Seidel FG, et al. Glomerulocystic kidney disease: case report. *Pediatr Radiol* 1990;20:491–493; discussion 494.
292. Egashira K, Nakata H, Hashimoto O, et al. MR imaging of adult glomerulocystic kidney disease. A case report. *Acta Radiol* 1991;32:251–253.
293. Chatha RK, Johnson AM, Rothberg PG, et al. Von Hippel-Lindau disease masquerading as autosomal dominant polycystic kidney disease. *Am J Kidney Dis* 2001;37:852–858.
294. Kandt RS, Haines JL, Smith M, et al. Linkage of an important gene locus for tuberous sclerosis to a chromosome 16 marker for polycystic kidney disease. *Nat Genet* 1992;2:37–41.
295. Browne G, Jefferson JA, Wright GD, et al. von Hippel-Lindau disease: an important differential diagnosis of polycystic kidney disease. *Nephrol Dial Transplant* 1997;12:1132–1136.
296. Holthofer H, Kumpulainer T, Rapola J. Polycystic disease of the kidney: evaluation and classification based on nephron segment and cell-type specific markers. *Lab Invest* 1990;62:363–369.

37

AMINOACIDURIA AND GLYCOSURIA

ISRAEL ZELIKOVIC

Only negligible amounts of amino acids and glucose are normally present in the final urine, reflecting very efficient reabsorption mechanisms for these organic solutes in the proximal tubule. Renal tubular transport defects or specific metabolic abnormalities result in excretion of significant quantities of amino acids or glucose in the urine. Although hereditary defects in renal tubular transport of most of these substances are uncommon, they are of major biologic importance. First, some of these membrane transport disorders [e.g., cystinuria, lysinuric protein intolerance (LPI), Hartnup disease] are associated with significant morbidity. Second, the study of these disorders has provided much insight into the physiology of renal tubular reclamation of amino acids and glucose and into the specific metabolic pathways that control their reabsorption and has been crucial in understanding the genetics of tubular transport systems.

This chapter summarizes the general characteristics of renal tubular transport of amino acids and glucose, reviews recent studies on the molecular biology of the transporters, describes the ontogeny of these transport processes, and discusses the specific hereditary membrane transport disorders that result in abnormal aminoaciduria and glycosuria. Special emphasis is given to classic cystinuria, including molecular genetic aspects of this disease. Not discussed in this chapter are overflow aminoaciduria and glucosuria, which occur when the filtered load of these solutes exceeds the transport capacity of the renal tubule. This tubular overload is characteristic of various inborn errors of amino acid metabolism and diabetes mellitus, which result in elevated plasma levels of amino acids and glucose, respectively. *Fanconi syndrome*, a proximal tubular disorder characterized by generalized aminoaciduria and urinary hyperexcretion of glucose, bicarbonate, phosphate, and other solutes, is discussed in Chapter 41.

AMINOACIDURIA

General Characteristics of Tubular Amino Acid Transport

Circulating free amino acids are derived from dietary protein that is hydrolyzed and absorbed in the intestine, from intracellular catabolism of peptides, and from *de novo* synthesis within cells. More than 99% of the load of free amino acid filtered by the kidneys of humans and other mammals is reabsorbed in the renal tubule and returned to plasma (1,2). Amino acid reabsorption occurs predominantly in the pars convoluta of the proximal tubule and, to a small extent, in the pars recta (1,2). Amino acids are reabsorbed primarily from tubular lumen by an active uphill transport across the luminal membrane (1). In studies using renal brush-border membrane vesicles (BBMV) from various animals to explore amino acid transport across this membrane, the rate of accumulation by vesicles and the magnitude of the overshoot, which indicates active concentrative transport, were greatly augmented by an external Na^+ gradient across the vesicle membrane (1). Hence, it is widely accepted that uptake of most amino acids at the brush-border surface occurs by Na^+-amino acid cotransport driven by the electrochemical Na^+ gradient from tubular lumen to cell (1,2) (Fig. 37.1). The energy maintaining the Na^+ gradient is established by the Na^+-K^+–adenosine triphosphatase (ATPase), which is located at the basolateral membrane and translocates Na^+ out and K^+ into the cell.

Active amino acid transport across the brush-border membrane is followed by efflux, mainly via carrier-mediated, Na^+-independent, facilitated diffusion or exchange from the cell into the peritubular space across the basolateral membrane (2–4) (Fig. 37.1). Thus, under normal conditions, net transepithelial movement of amino acids occurs from the tubular lumen to the peritubular space. However, net transepithelial flux of amino acids is composed of amino acid transport in both directions, namely lumen → interstitium and interstitium → lumen (3,4). Indeed, the basolateral membrane harbors active Na^+-dependent and Na^+-independent transport and exchange systems mediating amino acid uptake in the tubular cell (Fig. 37.1), and diffusional backflux of amino acids from cell into the tubular lumen is a well-documented phenomenon (3). Interstitium → lumen–oriented backflux through paracellular pathways also occurs. The sum of these vectorial fluxes determines the direction and the rate of transepithelial amino acid transport. This notion may be of major impor-

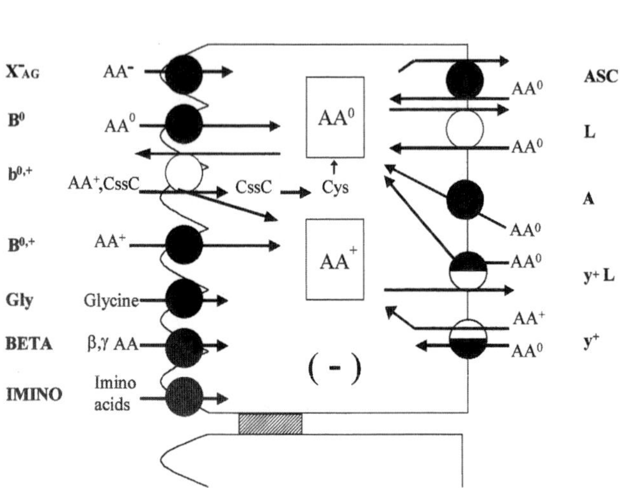

FIGURE 37.1. Summary of amino acid transport mechanisms in the proximal tubule. Filled circles indicate Na^+-dependent, active, carrier-mediated cotransport or antiport. Empty circles indicate Na^+-independent antiport or uniport (facilitated diffusion). Half-filled, half-empty circles indicate various combinations of the previously described circles. AA^0, neutral amino acids; AA^+, basic amino acids; AA^-, acidic amino acids; CssC, cystine; Cys, cysteine. See text for details.

tance in understanding renal tubular amino acid transport, particularly in disease states and during maturation (4,5).

Na^+-amino acid symport across the luminal membrane is a carrier-mediated saturable process obeying Michaelis-Menten kinetics (1,2). The effectiveness of the active reabsorption process for a specific amino acid depends on the ratio $V_{max}:K_m$ (1). A low V_{max} (decreased transport capacity) or a high K_m (diminished transporter-substrate affinity) for a given amino acid results in decreased reabsorption rate of this amino acid. Changes in efficiency or capacity of amino acid transport also play an important role in both neonatal aminoaciduria and hereditary aminoacidurias.

In analyzing the data obtained from microperfusion and micropuncture experiments and studies using BBMV for various amino acids (1), two or more Na^+-linked transport systems with different kinetic characteristics have been described. The demonstration of multiple transport systems for the same amino acid becomes meaningful if the reduced concentrations of filtered amino acid presented to the proximal straight tubule are considered. Thus, in the case of glycine, for example, two Na^+-dependent, active transport systems have been demonstrated along the luminal membrane of the isolated perfused proximal tubule (6): a low-affinity, high-capacity system in the convoluted segment and a high-affinity, low-capacity system in the straight segment. The latter system, which also operates in parallel to lower apical membrane backflux permeability in the proximal straight tubule (3), absorbs less glycine against a greater concentration gradient and probably permits the reduction of the luminal glycine concentration to lower levels than could be achieved in the proximal convoluted tubule (3,6). This axial heterogeneity of Na^+-linked amino acid uptake systems with respect to kinetic characteristics has been demonstrated for several amino acids (1) in BBMV derived from pars convoluta and pars recta of the proximal tubule. The recognition of several transport systems for the same amino acid as well as their axial heterogeneity is of major importance in understanding the pathophysiology of hereditary aminoaciduria.

One or more Na^+ ions are transported for each amino acid molecule translocated, and with most amino acids this process is electrogenic-positive favored by a negative cell interior (1,7). Na^+-amino acid stoichiometry determines the electrogenicity and efficiency of the transport system (3). Additional ions besides Na^+ are involved in the translocation of the amino acid carrier complex across the brush-border membrane (1). Taurine (8), glycine (9), and proline (10) transports, for example, operate by means of 2 or 3 Na^+:1 Cl^-:1 amino acid carrier complex.

Specificity of Transport

At least seven distinct group-specific Na^+-dependent transport systems exist in the tubular luminal membrane (1,2). Evidence for these systems is derived from a variety of microperfusion experiments and vesicle studies and, in humans, from the existence of inborn errors of renal tubular transport that can be explained only by defects in specific transport pathways (1,11). These include systems for dibasic amino acids, acidic amino acids, neutral α-amino acids, imino acids, glycine, β- and γ-amino acids, and cystine/cysteine.

There is good evidence to suggest that in addition to separate systems for L-cystine and the dibasic amino acids (L-lysine, L-arginine, and L-ornithine), these amino acids share a common transport pathway (12–14), as also suggested by the urinary hyperexcretion of all four amino acids in classic cystinuria (see Classic Cystinuria). Transport of L-cystine but not L-cysteine can also proceed via Na^+-dependent transport pathways for neutral amino acids (1,2). L-Cysteine is probably reabsorbed by an additional, separate, and specific transport system (2).

The broad-specificity transport pathway for neutral α-amino acids, which is a low-affinity, high-capacity system, is located in the proximal convoluted tubule (11). However, there are several alternative specific renal transport systems for neutral amino acids, including high-affinity systems located in the proximal straight tubule. The presence of such pathways is also suggested by the finding of isolated transport defects for neutral amino acids (see Neutral Aminoaciduria). The imino acids proline and hydroxyproline are reabsorbed by at least two systems, a low-affinity/high-capacity system in the proximal convoluted tubule shared with glycine and an imino acid–specific, high-affinity/low-capacity system in the proximal straight tubule (6,15). There also is a separate high-affinity/low-capacity system for glycine in the late proximal tubule (6).

TABLE 37.1. AMINO ACID TRANSPORT SYSTEMS OPERATING IN THE RENAL TUBULE

Amino acid transport system	Cloned cDNA	Amino acids transported	Mechanism of action	Localization
Neutral				
A	—	Short chain neutral	Na^+-AA cotransport	BLM
ASC	ASCT 1–2	Short chain neutral	Na^+-dependent AA antiport	BLM
B^0	ATB^0	Most neutral	Na^+-AA cotransport	BBM
Gly	GLYT 1–2	Glycine, sarcosine	2–3 Na^+/1Cl^-/1AA cotransport	BBM
IMINO	—	Proline, hydroxyproline	2–3 Na^+/1Cl^-/1AA cotransport	BBM
BETA	TAUT, GAT 1–3, BGT-1	Taurine, β-alanine, GABA, betaine	2–3 Na^+/1Cl^-/1AA cotransport	BBM
L	4F2hc/LAT-1, 4F2hc/LAT-2	Large, branched chain neutral	AA antiport	BLM
Cationic				
$B^{0,+}$	$ATB^{0,+}$ (?)	Cationic and neutral	Na^+/Cl^-/AA cotransport	BBM
$b^{0,+}$	rBAT/$b^{0,+}$AT	Cationic and neutral (including cystine)	AA antiport	BBM
y^+	CAT 1–4	Cationic and neutral (excluding cystine)	AA uniporter (facilitative transporter)	BLM
y^+L	4F2hc/y^+LAT-1 4F2hc/y^+LAT-2	Cationic and neutral (excluding cystine)	Na^+-dependent AA antiport	BLM
Anionic				
X^-_{AG}	EAAT 1-5	Anionic	3Na^+/AA cotransport, 1K^+-antiport	BBM

AA, amino acid; BBM, brush-border membrane; BLM, basolateral membrane; GABA, γ-aminobutyric acid.

The investigation of amino acid transport pathways in the plasma membrane of mammalian cells has delineated several transport systems (16–20) (Table 37.1; Fig. 37.1). Most of these transport systems also have been identified in the kidney (16,17,19,21). These systems include the Na^+-dependent concentrative A and ASC systems (for small neutral amino acids), B^0 (for most neutral amino acids), $B^{0,+}$ system (for dibasic and some neutral amino acids), X^-_{AG} system (for acidic amino acids), Gly system (for glycine and sarcosine), IMINO system (for proline and hydroxyproline), and β system (for taurine, β-alanine, and γ-aminobutyric acid), as well as the Na^+-independent nonconcentrative L system (for bulky neural, branched- chain amino acids and cysteine), y^+ system (for the dibasic amino acids lysine, arginine, and ornithine), y^+L system (for dibasic and neutral amino acids excluding cystine), and $b^{0,+}$ system (for dibasic and neutral amino acids including cystine). Systems A, ASC, L, y^+, and y^+L operate in the basolateral membrane (18,19,21) (Fig. 37.1). All these basolateral transporters (except for system A), as well as the luminal membrane-bound $b^{0,+}$ system, function as antiport (exchange) systems (19,20) (Fig. 37.1). Recent progress in molecular cloning of amino acid transporters has helped to characterize and define the nature and the role of most of these tubular amino acid transport mechanisms (see Molecular Structure of Amino Acid Transporters).

Adaptation and Regulation of Amino Acid Transport

Although the exact mechanisms regulating renal tubular amino acid reclamation have not been established, several factors are known to modulate transmembrane amino acid transport (1,22). These include ionic and voltage conditions (discussed earlier), as well as availability of amino acid substrate, osmotic changes, and protein phosphorylation.

Reabsorption of amino acids in the proximal tubule increases during periods of reduced amino acid intake and decreases with dietary excess (1). This renal adaptive response to diet is expressed at the tubular luminal membrane surface. It has been suggested (22,23) that both new synthesis of transporter protein and shuttling of preformed transporters are required for expression of the adaptive response. A recent expression study in *Xenopus* oocytes (24) has demonstrated that the rat renal taurine transporter is regulated by dietary taurine at the level of both messenger RNA (mRNA) accumulation and protein synthesis.

Amino acids are known to serve as regulatory osmolytes in mammalian cells, including kidney cells (25–27). The main amino acids involved in this function are taurine, proline, and glutamic acid (25,26,28). Studies using MDCK cells, a cell line of distal tubular origin, demonstrate changes in taurine transport in response to changes in osmolarity of the medium (29). It has been shown that osmotic regulation of taurine transport depends on changes in taurine transporter gene expression (30).

Serine/threonine protein kinases play a central role in signal transduction by phosphorylating and thereby activating effector proteins (31,32). Recent studies suggest that the three main groups of serine/threonine protein kinases, namely cyclic adenosine monophosphate–dependent protein kinase [protein kinase A (PKA)], Ca^{2+}- and phospholipid-dependent protein kinase [protein kinase C (PKC)], and multifunctional Ca^{2+}/calmodulin-dependent protein kinase II (CaMK II) alter amino acid transport across the tubular brush-border membrane (33–35). However, the exact role of protein kinase–induced phosphorylation in renal tubular amino acid transport remains to be established.

Molecular Structure of Amino Acid Transporters

Extensive efforts to isolate and identify the amino acid transport proteins in various tissues, including the kidney, have been largely unsuccessful. The isolation and molecular characterization of amino acid carrier proteins has been hindered by their very low abundance in the membrane, their poor stability *in vitro*, and the lack of specific tight-binding labels or inhibitors. Indirect approaches such as solubilization of proteins by organic solvents and incorporation into proteoliposomes, lectin-affinity chromatography, immunoprecipitation using monoclonal antibodies, and radiation inactivation analysis (36,37) have yielded little structural data. Since 1990, however, by using molecular biology techniques, much progress has been made in elucidating the molecular structure of various membrane-bound transport proteins, including amino acid transporters. This new area in the study of brush-border membrane transporters was pioneered by Hediger et al. (38), who cloned the small intestinal Na^+-glucose cotransporter using the powerful method of expression cloning in *Xenopus* oocytes. This strategy involves isolation of mRNA from the tissue of interest, microinjection into *Xenopus* oocytes, and analysis of expressed transport activity by measuring uptake of radiolabeled substrate. After size fractionation of mRNA, complementary (cDNA) synthesis, and DNA library screening by functional expression in oocytes, a single clone encoding the transporter activity is isolated. A similar approach has been used to clone, functionally express, and sequence various amino acid transporters.

The structural information and functional characteristics of amino acid transporters have led to their classification into four different gene families (19,20,39,40): Na^+- and Cl^--dependent transporters (the GAT family), the anionic/neutral amino acid transporters (the EAAT/ASCT family), cationic amino acid transporters (the CAT family), and cationic/neutral amino acid transporters [the rBAT/4F2 heavy chain (4F2hc) family]. Investigation of the primary structure of amino acid transporters has elucidated two main types of membrane proteins involved in amino acid transport (19): (a) members of the GAT, EAAT/ASCT, and CAT families, which present multiple transmembrane domains (Fig. 37.2) and are therefore considered putative carriers; and (b) members of the rBAT/4F2hc family, which do not fit this model (Figs. 37.3 and 37.4) and are known to function as components or subunits of heteromultimeric carriers.

GAT Family

The GAT family includes Na^+-Cl^-–γ-aminobutyric acid (GABA) (41), Na^+-Cl^--taurine (42), Na^+-Cl^--glycine (43), and Na^+-proline (44) cotransporters of the brain, which serve as neurotransmitters, as well as the Na^+-Cl^--taurine (45) cotransporter of the kidney. In addition to the taurine transporter of the kidney, Northern hybridization and polymerase chain reaction analysis have identified two GABA transporter isoforms, called *GAT 2* and *GAT 3* (46,47), as well as glycine transporter isoforms called *GLYT 1* and *GLYT 2* (48–50) in the kidney. The GAT family also includes the renal Na^+-Cl^--betaine transporter. All these transporters show high homology in sequence and structure, and most of them have an absolute requirement for Cl^-.

The proposed model of the GABA transporter (GAT 1) is shown in Figure 37.2. It is a 655-residue protein with a relative molecular mass of 73,925 d. The predicted secondary structure shows 12 hydrophobic, membrane-spanning domains with a large extracellular hydrophilic loop between spans 3 and 4. The molecular structure contains putative *N*-glycosylation and phosphorylation sites. The similarities between the family members may point toward domains important in Na^+, Cl^-, and substrate coupling (51). The Na^+-Cl^--betaine and Na^+-Cl^--taurine transporters are thought to play a major role in cell volume regulation in the renal medulla (26) (see Adaptation and Regulation of Amino Acid Transport).

EAAT/ASCT Family

The EAAT/ASCT family of transporters is made up of five Na^+- and K^+-dependent, Cl^--independent anionic amino acid transporters, and three neutral amino acid transporters (19,20). The anionic amino acid transporters include the GLAST (or EAAT1) (52), GLT (or EAAT2) (53), and EAAC1 (or EAAT3) (54), as well as EAAT4 (55) and EAAT5 (56), which serve as neurotransmitters and show marked similarity in sequence and structure. EAAC1, a neuronal and epithelial high-affinity glutamate transporter first cloned from rabbit small intestine (54), was also identified in the kidney by Northern hybridization analysis (54). *In situ* hybridization and immunofluorescence studies revealed that EAAC1 is expressed predominantly in the S2 and S3 segments of the proximal tubule (57).

The proposed model of EAAC1 (Fig. 37.2) shows a protein of 524 amino acids with a predicted molecular mass of 57,000 d and ten hydrophobic, membrane-spanning domains. The kinetics and specificity of this protein when expressed in *Xenopus* oocytes were similar to those of the X^-_{AG} transport system (see Specificity of Transport; Fig. 37.1). The gene for human EAAC1 (termed *SLC1A1*) has been localized to chromosome 9p24 (58). A defect in the EAAC1 gene is a likely cause of dicarboxylic aminoaciduria (see Dicarboxylic Aminoaciduria).

The neutral amino acid transports include the ASCT1 (or SATT) (59), ASCT2 (or AAAT) (60), and ATB^0 (61). ASCT1 and ASCT2, which were cloned from human brain (59) and mouse testis (60), respectively, have structural similarity to the anionic amino acid transporter gene family and appear to encode Na^+-dependent neutral amino acid trans-

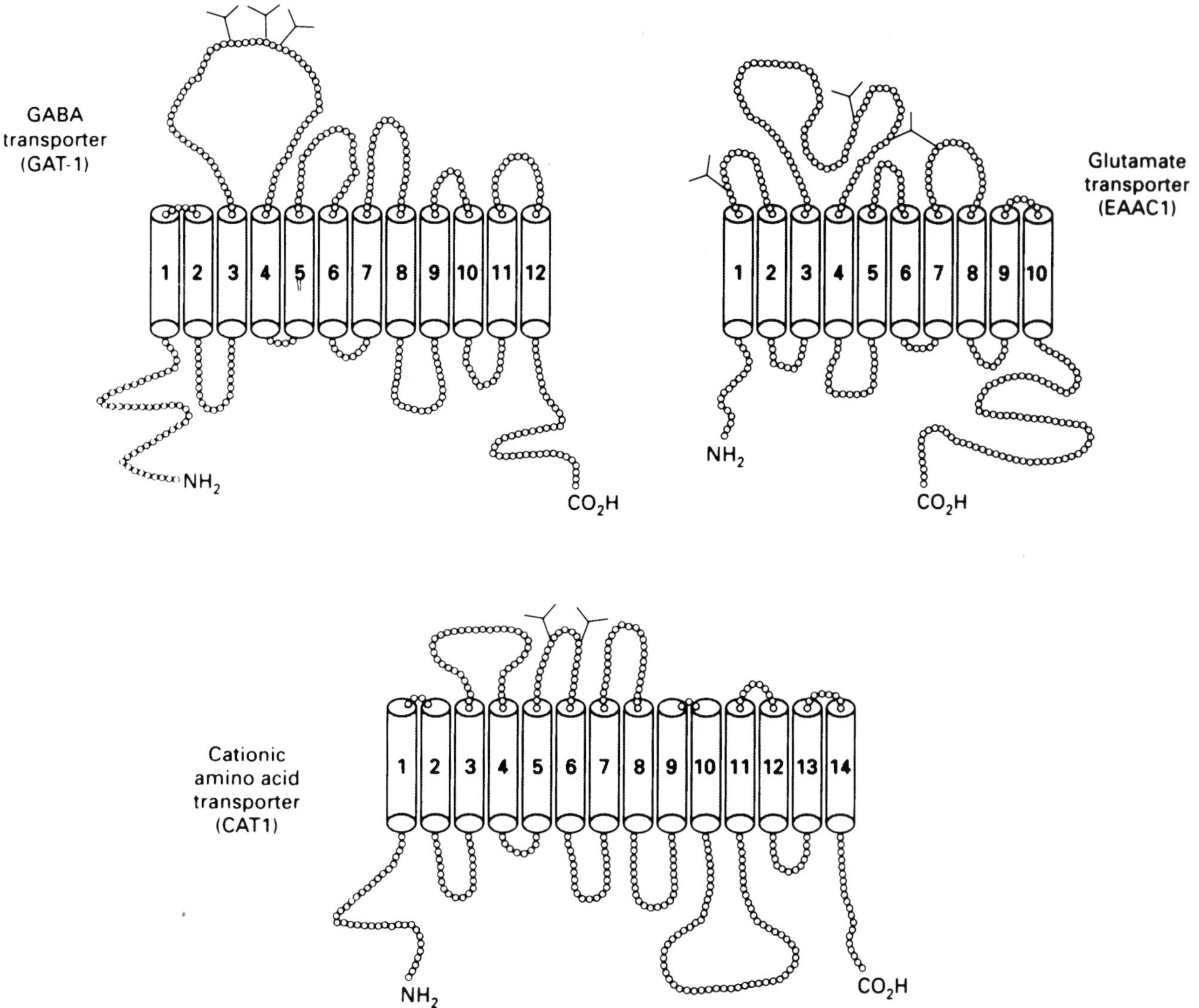

FIGURE 37.2. The putative transmembrane orientations of the γ-aminobutyric acid (GABA) transporter (GAT-1), the glutamate transporter (EAAC1), and the cationic amino acid transporter (CAT1) are shown as representative of three families of amino acid transporters. (Adapted from McGivan JD, Pastor-Anglada M. Regulatory and molecular aspects of mammalian amino acid transport. *Biochem J* 1994;299:321–334.)

porters with specificity characteristics of system ASC (see Specificity of Transport; Fig. 37.1). Northern blot analysis (59,60) revealed ubiquitous expression of these genes in several tissues, including expression in the kidney, consistent with the general metabolic role ascribed to system ASC. ATB^0 was cloned from human choriocarcinoma cells (61), and its transcripts were detected in the kidney among other tissues. Expression studies in the HeLa cells and oocytes showed an Na^+-dependent uptake of neutral amino acids with characteristics of the brush-border membrane system B^0 (see Specificity of Transport; Fig. 37.1). It is noteworthy that the transport systems EAAT1-5 (19,62), ASCT1 (63), and possibly ATB^0 (64) have a Cl^- channel mode of action in addition to their amino acid transport mode of activity.

CAT Family

The CAT genes were the first mammalian amino acid transporters cloned (40). Expression studies in *Xenopus* oocytes identified the ecotropic murine leukemia virus as the ubiquitous y^+ system (now called *CAT1*), an Na^+-independent transport system that accepts dibasic amino acids and excludes cystine (65,66). In addition, it catalyzes transport of neutral amino acids only in the presence of Na^+ (19) (Fig. 37.1). Northern hybridization analysis revealed the CAT1 gene in various mouse tissues, including the kidney (65). Since then, three other homologous murine cDNAs have been found to express a similar amino acid transport activity, CAT2, CAT3, and CAT4, all of which (except CAT3) are expressed in the kidney (19,67,68). The CAT

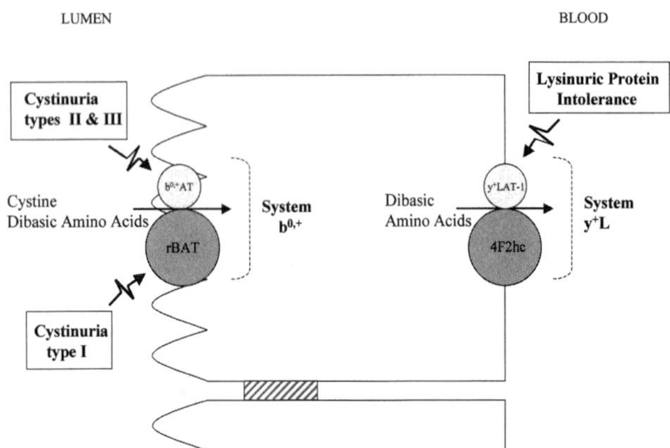

FIGURE 37.3. Transport pathways for cystine and dibasic amino acids at the luminal and basolateral membranes of a proximal tubular cell. Large circles represent the heavy subunits and small circles the light subunits of the heteromeric amino acid transporters $b^{0,+}$ and y^+L. Depicted are hereditary aminoacidurias caused by defects in these transporters. (Modified from Zelikovic I. Molecular pathophysiology of tubular transport disorders. *Pediatr Nephrol* 2001;16:919–935.)

transporters allow accumulation of cationic amino acids within the cell for general metabolic purposes. Also, it has been postulated that CAT-mediated arginine flux into cells could play a role in modulating nitric oxide synthesis in various cell types (67,69). This notion has been supported

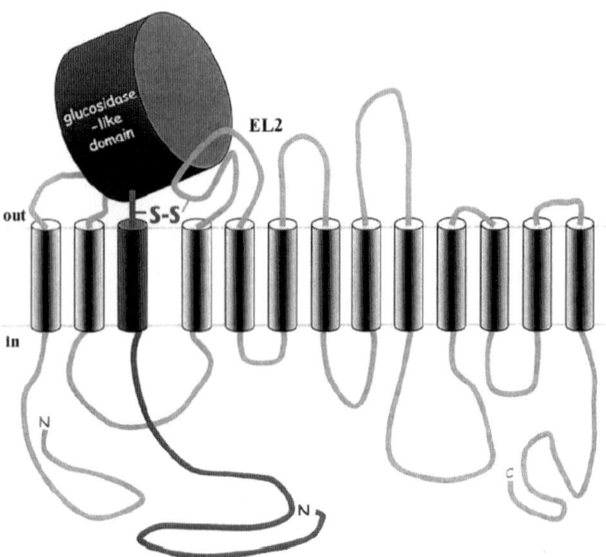

FIGURE 37.4. Schematic representation of the heteromeric amino acid transporters (HAT). The heavy subunit of HAT (HSHAT; *dark gray*) is linked by a disulfide bridge to the corresponding light subunit of HAT (LSHAT; *light gray*). The cysteine residues involved in this bond (S-S) are located extracellularly, just after the transmembrane (TM) domain of HSHAT and in the proposed extracellular loop 2 (EL2) of LSHAT. Loops and TM domains are not drawn to scale. See text for details. (Adapted from Chillaron J, Roca R, Valencia A, et al. Heteromeric amino acid transporters: biochemistry, genetics, and physiology. *Am J Physiol* 2001;281:F995–F1018.)

by studies demonstrating that CAT2 and nitric oxide synthase 2 transcripts are co-induced in concert with system y^+ activity (70). The CAT1 cDNA predicts a 629–amino acid protein with 14 membrane-spanning domains and a molecular mass of 68,000 d (Fig. 37.2).

rBAT/4F2 Heavy Chain Family

To gain insight into the transport defect in cystinuria, recent research has focused on the molecular structure of the family of carrier proteins responsible for transport of cystine and other dibasic amino acids. Several groups have demonstrated the expression of cystine (71) and dibasic and neutral amino acids (72–74) in *Xenopus* oocytes injected with mRNA of small intestine and kidney. In 1992 (75,76), kidney cortex cDNAs from rabbit and rat [named *rBAT* (75) and *D2* (76), respectively] have been cloned. On *in vitro* transcription to chromosomal RNA and injection into oocytes, they induce system $b^{0,+}$, the Na^+-independent transporter for neutral amino acids, dibasic amino acids, and cystine (see Specificity of Transport; Figs. 37.1 and 37.3). The predicted proteins for rBAT and D2 demonstrate significant homology with a family of the carbohydrate-metabolizing enzymes α-glucosidases. Similarly, chromosomal RNA from the human 4F2hc surface antigen, a glycoprotein highly regulated at the onset of cell proliferation, stimulated system y^+L amino acid transport (see Specificity of Transport; Figs. 37.1 and 37.3) in *Xenopus* oocytes (77).

The rBAT cDNA contains an open reading frame of 2049 nucleotides coding for a protein of 685 amino acids with a molecular mass of approximately 90,000 d (40). The predicted proteins for rBAT and D2, as well as the 4F2hc antigen (all of which show high structural similarity), were found to contain only one (19) or four (78) putative membrane-spanning domains, depending on different typologic models. This structure, which is atypical of the known membrane transport proteins, raised the possibility that these proteins function as activators of transport systems y^+L and $b^{0,+}$ or as regulatory subunits of these transporters. The functional promoter of the rat rBAT gene has been identified (79), and the gene for the human rBAT, named *D2H*, was localized to chromosome 2p21 (79,80). The human rBAT (D2H) gene has been called *SLC3A1* (see Classic Cystinuria).

In situ hybridization and immunolocalization studies have localized rBAT mRNA expression in the brush-border membrane of the proximal straight tubule (S3 segment) and the small intestinal mucosa (81,82). In contrast to rBAT, 4F2hc mRNA is almost ubiquitous with marked expression in kidney, where it localizes to the basolateral membrane of proximal tubular cells (19). Studies from several laboratories have demonstrated that both rBAT and 4F2hc are type II membrane glycoproteins, which constitute heavy subunits of heteromeric amino acid transporters (83–86). These studies showed that rBAT (90 kDa) and 4F2hc (85 kDa) associated by disulfide bridges with a light subunit (40 kDa) forming a heterodimeric complex of 125 kDa (85,86) (Fig. 37.4).

The light subunit of rBAT, termed *b^{0,+}AT*, and the light subunit of 4F2hc, termed *y^{+}LAT-1*, which were identified in 1998–1999 (87–89), are members of the family of light subunits of the heteromeric amino acid transporters (LSHAT) (85,86). As of 2000, seven members of the LSHAT family have been identified (85,86), to which the light subunits LAT-1 and LAT-2 that combine with 4F2hc to form the L system (see Specificity of Transport; Table 37.1; Fig. 37.1) also belong. Recent research on the characteristics of LSHATs (83,85) has revealed that they are unglycosylated proteins that contain 12 putative transmembrane domains (Fig. 37.4), they need coexpression with the corresponding heavy subunit to reach the plasma membrane, they confer the specific amino acid transport activity to the heteromeric complex, and, finally, all the amino acid transport activities associated with the LSHATs behave as amino acid exchangers (85,86). In the kidney, system $b^{0,+}$ (induced by rBAT and $b^{0,+}$AT; Figs. 37.1 and 37.3) acts as tertiary active exchange mechanism of tubular reabsorption of dibasic amino acids and cystine. This tertiary transport mechanism is linked to a high intracellular concentration of neutral amino acids (Fig. 37.1). System $b^{0,+}$-mediated efflux of neutral amino acids from renal epithelial cells is the driving force for cystine and cationic amino acid reabsorption from lumen to cell (84,90,91) (Fig. 37.1). Reabsorption of cystine and cationic amino acids is also favored by the intracellular-negative membrane potential and by the reduction of cystine to cysteine (Fig. 37.1) (84,91). System $y^{+}L$ (induced by 4F2hc and y^{+}LAT-1; Figs. 37.1 and 37.3) mediates an electroneutral exchange mechanism in which efflux of cationic amino acids (against the intracellular-negative voltage) is enhanced by the influx of neutral amino acids in the presence of Na^{+} (Fig. 37.1) (84,91). The tissue distribution of rBAT/$b^{0,+}$AT and 4F2hc/y^{+}LAT-1 and their role in renal uptake of cystine and dibasic amino acids have made them candidates for the defective genes in cystinuria and LPI, respectively (see Hereditary Aminoacidurias).

Future investigations into the molecular and biochemical characteristics of this expanding group of cloned amino acid transporters may yield important insight into the inherited human diseases that result from a defective transport of amino acids (see Hereditary Aminoacidurias).

Maturation of Tubular Amino Acid Transport

Urinary fractional excretion of almost all amino acids in humans (92) (Fig. 37.5) and animals (4) is higher in the newborn than later in life. A very high rate of urinary amino acid excretion is found in immature, very-low-birth-weight infants (93). Some amino acids, including glycine, alanine, proline, dibasic amino acids, and taurine (4,93), have been shown to contribute more to neonatal aminoaciduria than other amino acids. Theoretically, a structural, quantitative, or regulatory change in any one of the membrane-related events depicted in Figure 37.1 may underlie the diminished reabsorptive capacity of the renal tubule during early life (4,5).

As indicated earlier, proline and glycine reabsorption in the proximal tubule occurs predominantly by a shared low-affinity/high-capacity transport system in the proximal convoluted tubule as well as by two specific, high-affinity/low-capacity systems located in the proximal straight tubule—one for proline and one for glycine (1,6). Lasley and Scriver studied infants affected with familial renal iminoglycinuria to explore the ontogeny of proline and glycine reabsorption in the renal tubule (94). In iminoglycinuria, the shared transport system for proline and glycine is affected by mutation (see Iminoglycinuria). Using the occurrence of ontogeny and maturation together, Scriver's group provided evidence for the appearance of the two specific high-affinity transport systems in succession—the proline transporter by 3 months of age and the glycine transporter by 6 months of age (94). Similarly, earlier studies on glycine and proline transport in rat renal cortical slices (4) showed that the specific high-affinity transporters were not present at birth, yet appeared when

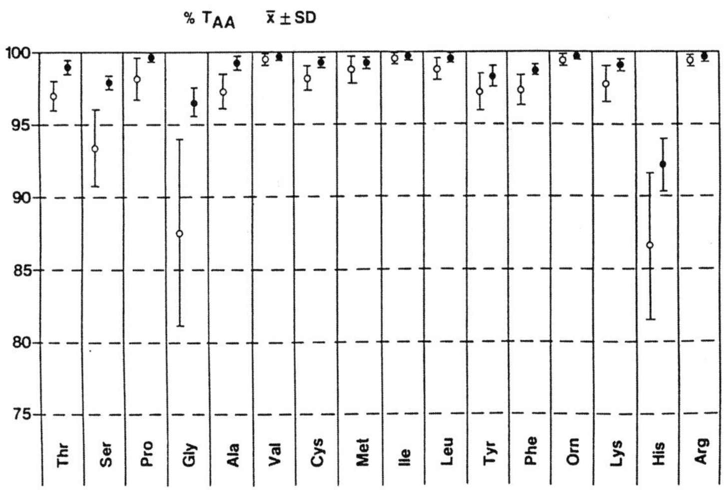

FIGURE 37.5. Tubular reabsorption of free amino acids (% T_{AA}) compared between infants (*open circles*) and children (*black dots*). Ala, alanine; Arg, arginine; Cys, cysteine; Gly, glycine; His, histidine; Ile, isoleucine; Leu, leucine; Lys, lysine; Met, methionine; Orn, ornithine; Phe, phenylalanine; Pro, proline; Ser, serine; Thr, threonine; Tyr, tyrosine; Val, valine. (Adapted from Brodehl J, Gellissen K. Endogenous renal transport of free amino acids in infancy and childhood. *Pediatrics* 1968;42:395–404.)

amino acid reabsorption reached adult levels. In contrast, subsequent animal studies demonstrated the existence of both low-affinity/high-capacity and high-affinity/low-capacity systems for several amino acids (4) in neonatal and adult kidneys; no new systems were acquired with maturation.

Studies using cortical slices and isolated tubules from several species have provided evidence for an impaired basolateral membrane exit step of amino acids from immature tubular cells (4). Decreased Na^+-dependent taurine transport has been demonstrated in basolateral membrane vesicles from hypertaurinuric mice (95). It remains to be established whether a similar alteration in basolateral membrane amino acid transport during early life contributes to neonatal hyperaminoaciduria.

Several studies explored the maturation of the first step of amino acid reabsorption, namely transport across the brush-border membrane. A gradual age-related increase in Na^+-coupled uptake of taurine (96) and proline (97) by rat renal BBMV and of cystine by isolated dog renal cortical tubules (98) has been demonstrated. Whereas the maturation of proline transport involved an increase in affinity (decrease in K_m) of transport (97), the maturation of cystine transport was associated with an increase in capacity (increased V_{max}) of transport (98).

Alterations in phospholipid composition have been documented during rat tubular brush-border membrane maturation (4), suggesting that changes in membrane fluidity may account for the observed maturational changes in Na^+-linked tubular amino acid transport. In addition, an increased permeability to Na^+ (97) and an enhanced amiloride-sensitive Na^+-H^+ exchange activity (99) have been demonstrated in neonatal rat renal BBMV. This alteration in ionic permeability and the increased luminal membrane Na^+-H^+ antiport [coupled with a diminished Na^+-K^+-ATPase activity known to exist in the basolateral membrane of the neonatal proximal tubular epithelium (100)] may result in a rapid dissipation of the electrochemical Na^+ gradient necessary for Na^+-amino acid cotransport, thereby contributing to the aminoaciduria of early life (97,99).

Protein kinases modulate renal tubular amino acid transport (see Adaptation and Regulation of Amino Acid Transport). Recent studies (32,101) demonstrate higher activity of PKC and CaMK II in the cytosol and the brush-border membrane derived from immature kidneys than in adult kidneys. Furthermore, the studies provide evidence for differential regulation of PKC (101) and CaMK II (32) isoenzymes during kidney development. Age-related changes in the activity and expression of protein kinases may underlie the developmental changes in tubular reclamation of amino acids and other solutes.

In summary, hyperaminoaciduria is a characteristic of the immature mammalian tubule. Although the mechanisms governing the developmental changes in tubular amino acid transport have not been fully established, evidence has accumulated that both luminal and antiluminal membrane-related events play a role in the maturation of amino acid transport. Most studies indicate that transport maturation does not represent the acquisition of new transport systems but rather a change in affinity or capacity of transporters. The role of protein kinase–induced phosphorylation in the maturation of renal tubular amino acid transport remains to be established. The exact cellular mechanisms and the biologic signals responsible for the observed developmental changes await future studies. Studies into the molecular structure of amino acid transporters will undoubtedly shed light on the mechanisms underlying the development of tubular amino acid reclamation.

Hereditary Aminoacidurias

Aminoacidurias are a group of disorders in which a single amino acid or a group of amino acids are excreted in excess amounts in the urine. The defective tubular reabsorption is assumed to result from a genetic defect in a specific transport system that directs the reabsorption of these amino acids under normal conditions. Some of these disorders also involve a similar transport abnormality in the intestine. As opposed to inborn errors of amino acid metabolism, in which plasma levels of amino acids are elevated, resulting in overflow aminoaciduria, plasma levels of amino acids in hereditary aminoacidurias are largely normal.

The aminoacidurias are generally categorized into five major groups according to the group-specific transport pathway presumed to be affected (Table 37.2). The groups are further subdivided into several disorders based on the profile of the affected amino acids within that group.

Cationic Aminoaciduria

Five distinct inborn errors of cationic amino acid transport have been identified: (a) classic cystinuria, (b) isolated cystinuria, (c) hyperdibasic aminoaciduria, (d) LPI, and (e) isolated lysinuria. These diseases differ in defined or putative transport systems affected, pathophysiology, organs involved, and clinical features. Classic cystinuria is the prototype for this group of hereditary aminoacidurias.

Classic Cystinuria

Cystinuria is a disorder of amino acid transport characterized by excessive urinary excretion of cystine and the dibasic amino acids lysine, arginine, and ornithine. The pathogenic mechanism of cystinuria is defective transepithelial transport of these amino acids in the proximal tubule and the small intestine (102). The very low solubility of cystine in the urine results in cystine stone formation in homozygous patients. Lysine, arginine, and ornithine do not form urinary stones. Urinary cystine calculi may produce considerable morbidity, including urinary obstruction, colic, infection, and in severe cases, loss of kidney function. Cystinuria accounts for 1 to 2% of all urolithiasis and 6 to 8% of urolithiasis in children

TABLE 37.2. HEREDITARY AMINOACIDURIAS

Disorder	Defective gene	Locus	Amino acid transport system defective	Individual amino acids affected	Localization of defect	Mode of inheritance	Prevalence	Clinical manifestations	Organs involved	OMIM no.[a]
Cationic aminoaciduria										
Classic cystinuria										
Type I	SLC3A1	2p16.3-21	rBAT (heavy subunit of $b^{0,+}$)	Cystine, lysine, arginine, ornithine	BBM	Autosomal recessive	1:7000–1:15,000	Urolithiasis	Kidney, intestine	220100
Type II and III	SLC7A9	19q13.1	$b^{0,+}$ AT (light subunit of $b^{0,+}$)	Cystine, lysine, arginine, ornithine	BBM	Incompletely autosomal recessive	1:7000–1:15,000	Urolithiasis	Kidney, intestine	600918
Isolated cystinuria	—	—	Cystine	Cystine	BBM	Autosomal recessive	Two siblings reported	Benign	Kidney	238200
Hyperdibasic aminoaciduria type I	—	—	Dibasic amino acids	Lysine, arginine, ornithine	BBM	Autosomal dominant	Two families reported	Mental retardation	Kidney, intestine	222690
Lysinuric protein intolerance (hyperdibasic aminoaciduria type II)	SLC7A7	14q11-13	y^{+}LAT-1 (light subunit of y^{+}L)	Lysine, arginine, ornithine	BLM	Autosomal recessive	1:60,000 (Finland)	Protein malnutrition, failure to thrive, hyperammonemia, seizures, coma	Kidney, intestine, liver	222700
Isolated lysinuria	—	—	Lysine (?)	Lysine	BBM (?)	Autosomal recessive	One patient reported	Failure to thrive, seizures, mental retardation	Kidney, intestine	—
Neutral aminoaciduria										
Hartnup disease	ATB^{0} (?)	19q13.3	B^{0} (neutral, monoamino monocarboxylic α-amino acids)	Alanine, serine, threonine, valine, leucine, isoleucine, phenylalanine, tyrosine, tryptophan, histidine, glutamine, asparagine	BBM	Autosomal recessive	1:20,000	Skin rash, cerebellar ataxia, psychiatric illnesses	Kidney, intestine	234500
Methioninuria	—	—	Methionine	Methionine	BBM	Autosomal recessive	Two cases reported	Edema, seizures, mental retardation	Kidney, intestine	250900
Histidinuria	—	—	Histidine	Histidine	BBM	Autosomal recessive	Four cases reported	Mental retardation	Kidney, intestine	235830
Imminoaciduria and glycinuria										
Imminoglycinuria	—	—	Immino acids and glycine	Proline, hydroxyproline, glycine	BBM	Autosomal recessive	1:15,000	Benign	Kidney, intestine	242600

(continued)

TABLE 37.2. *CONTINUED.*

Disorder	Defective gene	Locus	Amino acid transport system defective	Individual amino acids affected	Localization of defect	Mode of inheritance	Prevalence	Clinical manifestations	Organs involved	OMIM no.[a]
Isolated glycinuria	—	—	Glycine	Glycine	BBM	Autosomal recessive	Two families reported	Benign	Kidney	138500
Dicarboxylic aminoaciduria	EAAC1 (SLC1A1 ?)	9p24 (5p15 ?)	X^{-}_{AG} (acidic amino acids)	Glutamate, aspartate	BBM	Autosomal recessive	1:29,000 (French-Canadian)	Benign	Kidney, intestine	222730
β-amino aciduria (mouse)	—	—	β-amino acids	Taurine	BLM (?)	Autosomal recessive	—	Benign	Kidney	—

BBM, brush-border membrane; BLM, basolateral membrane.
[a]Online Mendelian Inheritance in Man (database at http://www.ncbi.nlm.nih.gov/omim).

(103,104). The defective gastrointestinal transport of cystine and dibasic amino acids in cystinuria does not result in intestinal disease.

The disease was first recognized in 1810 by Wollaston (105) and later by Berzelius (106), who called the stones "cystic oxide" and "cystine," respectively, assuming that the stones they analyzed originated in the bladder. In 1908, Garrod (107) postulated that cystinuria was an inborn error of cystine metabolism. In the 1950s, Dent and Rose (108) first recognized the true nature of the disease, suggesting that cystine and the dibasic amino acids lysine, arginine, and ornithine that have structural similarity (two amino groups separated by four to six chemical bonds) share a carrier protein in the brush-border membrane of the renal tubule and the small intestine. They postulated that this transport mechanism was defective in cystinuria.

Transport Defect. Normally, 1% of the filtered cystine and dibasic amino acids is excreted. In classic cystinuria, cystine clearance may be near or equal to the glomerular filtration rate (GFR), and in some patients even twice as high as the GFR, suggesting active cystine secretion (109). Lysine and ornithine clearance is 30 to 80% of the GFR, and arginine excretion is less abnormal.

Dent's postulate about a defective shared transport system for cystine and dibasic acids in cystinuria has been supported by the *in vivo* experiments of Kato (110) and Robson and Rose (111), demonstrating that in healthy subjects and cystinuric patients, increasing the filtered load of one of these amino acids decreased reabsorption of the others. However, this hypothesis was challenged by studies showing that cystine uptake was not impaired in kidney slices from cystinuric patients (112) and that cystine and dibasic amino acids did not share a common transport system in kidney slices of healthy and cystinuric patients (112). The reports of isolated cystinuria (113), isolated dibasic aminoaciduria (114), and isolated lysinuria (115) cast further doubts on Dent's hypothesis and suggested the existence of specific transport systems for these amino acids. Furthermore, the occurrence of several transport systems for cystine and dibasic amino acids was supported by the observations of Brodehl and Gellissen (92) and Scriver et al. (116) that tubular reabsorption capacity matures at different rates for different amino acids.

Subsequent studies using isolated cortical tubules and BBMV (12,13,117) have clarified the picture of tubular amino acid transport. These studies, coupled with the recognition that kidney slices preferentially expose the basolateral membrane, provided evidence for three brush-border membrane-bound and two basolateral membrane-bound carrier systems for cationic amino acids in the kidney. Transport at the brush-border membrane occurs by a system shared by cystine and the dibasic amino acids, a system specific for cystine, and a system specific for dibasic amino acids. It is the shared high-affinity, low-K_m system located in the S3 segment of the proximal tubule and identified as system $b^{0,+}$ (see Specificity of Transport; Figs. 37.1, and 37.3) that is defective in classic cystinuria. The low-affinity, high-K_m, unshared cystine system and the low-affinity, unshared dibasic amino acid system, both located in the S1-S2 segments of the proximal tubule, may be abnormal in isolated cystinuria and dibasic aminoaciduria, respectively. The antiluminal membrane harbors two specific systems, one for dibasic amino acids identified as *system* y^+L (see Specificity of Transport; Figs. 37.1 and 37.3) and one for cystine, but no shared system. These transport mechanisms mediate uptake and efflux of these amino acids across the basolateral membrane. The brush-border membrane of the intestinal cell has a single high-affinity, low-K_m, shared $b^{0,+}$ transport system for cystine and dibasic amino acids that is defective in classic cystinuria. Like kidney cells, intestinal cells have two basolateral membrane-bound, unshared specific transport systems; one (system y^+L) for dibasic amino acids; and one for cystine (5). The basolateral membrane-bound y^+L transporter for dibasic amino acids in the kidney and the intestine is defective in LPI (see Lysinuric Protein Intolerance). Amino acid transport in parenchymal cells and leukocytes from cystinuric patients is not impaired (5) because the defect is not expressed in the plasma membrane of these cells.

Genetics. Classic cystinuria is inherited in an autosomal recessive fashion. It is a common disorder with an overall prevalence of 1:7000 to 1:15,000 and estimated gene frequency of 0.01 (102). A very high prevalence, 1:2500, is observed in Israeli Jews of Libyan origin (118).

Although it is a recessive disease, phenotypic heterogeneity in homozygotes and heterozygotes is evident. The excretion patterns of cystine and dibasic amino acids in heterozygotes and analysis of amino acid transport in jejunal mucosa have delineated three cystinuric subtypes (119). In type I, the most common phenotype, heterozygotes have normal urinary amino acid excretion, and homozygotes have impaired intestinal transport of cystine and dibasic amino acids. In type II, heterozygotes have high excretion of cystine and dibasic amino acids, and homozygotes show impaired intestinal transport of dibasic amino acids but not of cystine. Type III heterozygotes have excretion rates intermediate between the other two, and homozygotes have normal intestinal transport of the four amino acids involved. The three subtypes were considered to be allelic, namely mild; moderate; and severe mutations at a single cystinuria gene locus (11). However, Goodyer et al. (120) provided evidence that type I and type III cystinuria mutations might involve two distinct genetic loci. This was demonstrated by the finding that type I/III compounds excreted less cystine than type I/I probands, although type III/N heterozygotes excrete higher levels of cystine than their type I/N counterparts. These findings could be explained by genetic complementation between nonallelic cystinuria genes. Subsequent genetic studies have supported this hypothesis (see Molecular Genetics). Whereas type I cystinuria is inherited as a fully recessive trait, type II and III (collectively termed *non-type I*) subtypes are inherited as incompletely recessive traits.

Renal ontogeny has important implications for genetic counseling in cystinuria. This was demonstrated by Scriver and colleagues' finding that heterozygous infants under 6 months of age who have immature tubular function can excrete cystine and dibasic amino acids at levels equivalent to those found in homozygous adults (116). Urinary excretion of these amino acids decreased steadily with age to reach the variant parental value in heterozygous infants but not in homozygotes. Hence, final classification of a cystinuric phenotype should not be done before the age of 6 months.

Molecular Genetics. The identification and characterization of the rBAT/D2H gene have led to the speculation that a defect in the human form of rBAT (SLC3A1) causes cystinuria. Pras et al. (121), using linkage analysis in 17 cystinuric families, demonstrated linkage between cystinuria and three genetic markers on chromosome 2p, providing strong evidence that SLC3A1 was indeed the gene causing the disease. Calonge et al. (122) identified six specific mutations in the SLC3A1 gene that segregated with a cystinuria phenotype, thereby establishing the rBAT gene as the cystinuria gene (Fig. 37.3). Subsequent studies have revealed additional mutations in SLC3A1 (123–125). As of 2000, more than 60 different rBAT mutations have been reported in patients with type I cystinuria (126). These mutations include nonsense, missense, splice site, frameshift mutations, and large deletions (102,126). Defective transport of cystine and dibasic amino acids has been demonstrated for many of these mutations when expressed in *Xenopus* oocytes (84). The most commonly occurring mutation is methionine 467 to threonine (M467T), which causes a defect in trafficking to the plasma membrane (127,128). This trafficking defect, which has also been demonstrated for other rBAT mutations (126,129), is consistent with the proposed role of rBAT as a "helper" of the corresponding light subunit in the heteromeric amino acid transporter. No SLC3A1 mutations have been found in type II or III patients (125,130).

In 1997, Wartenfeld et al. (131) and Bisceglia et al. (132) demonstrated that cystinuria type III (and possibly cystinuria type II) is linked to a locus on chromosome 19q13.1. In 1999, the International Cystinuria Consortium (133) identified the gene SLC7A9, which encodes the 487–amino acid protein $B^{0,+}$AT that belongs to the family of light subunits of amino acid transporters (see Molecular Structure of Amino Acid Transporters; Fig. 37.3). The gene localized to the non–type I cystinuria 19q locus. Cotransfection of $B^{0,+}$AT and rBAT in COS cells resulted in trafficking of rBAT to the plasma membrane and induced L-arginine uptake by cells. SLC7A9 mutations were found in Spanish, Italian, North American, and Libyan-Jewish cystinuria patients (133). The mutations in Jews of Libyan origin is valine 170 to methionine, which leads to complete loss of $B^{0,+}$AT amino acid

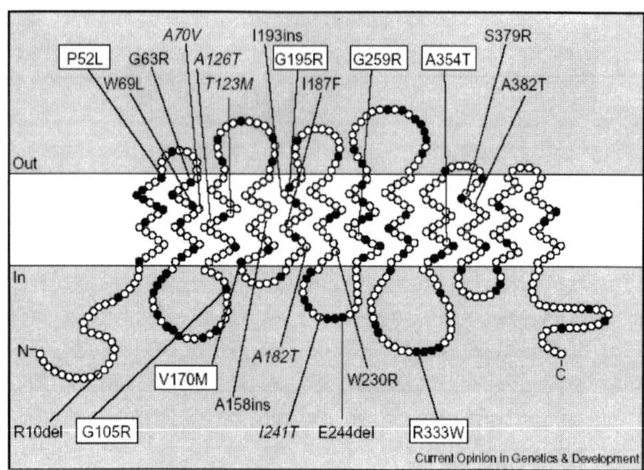

FIGURE 37.6. Representation of the cystinuria-specific missense or single amino acid point mutations identified in the $b^{0,+}$AT amino-acid transporter. Twenty-three missense or single amino acid point mutations in *SLC7A9* ($b^{0,+}$AT) are depicted. Amino acid residues conserved in all the human members of the light subunit of heteromeric amino acid transporter family are indicated in black. Mutations that are associated mainly with a severe urinary phenotype in heterozygotes (urine cystine levels similar to or below 200 µmol/g of creatinine and the sum of urine levels of cystine and the three dibasic amino acids similar to or below 1000 µmol/g of creatinine) are boxed. Mutations that are associated mainly with a mild urinary phenotype in heterozygotes (urinary levels of amino acids below the above indicated limits) are indicated in italics. The rest of mutations (with undefined or ambiguous phenotype) are indicated in smaller font. See text for details. (Adapted from Palacin M, Borsani G, Sebastio G. The molecular bases of cystinuria and lysinuric protein intolerance. *Curr Opin Gen Dev* 2001;11:328–335.)

uptake activity when cotransfected with rBAT in COS cells. As of 2000, more than 35 different $B^{0,+}$AT mutations have been identified in non–type I cystinuria patients (126,134) (Fig. 37.6). These mutations explain 79% of the alleles in 61 non–type I cystinuria patients included in the recent study by the International Cystinuria Consortium (134). The unexplained alleles might be due to mutations outside the open reading frame of the SLC3A1 gene, although mutations in other genes might cause non–type I cystinuria (85,126). One patient with I/III phenotype had a dual mutation in both SLC3A1 and SLC7A9, suggesting the existence of a digenic form of the disease (133).

Interestingly, although heterozygous for SLC7A9 mutation show type II or III trait, a minority have type I phenotype (84,135). These data have prompted the International Cystinuria Consortium to consider reclassification of cystinuria subtypes based on genotype rather than phenotype. This new classification includes the following:

Type A—due to two mutations on SLC3A1 on chromosome 2

Type B—due to two mutations on SLC7A9 on chromosome 19

Possible AB type—one mutation on each SLC3A1 and SLC7A9 (135)

Diagnosis and Clinical Features. The simplest diagnostic test is the microscopic examination of the urinary sediment of a freshly voided morning urine (102). The presence of typical flat hexagonal cystine crystals is diagnostic. Acidification of the urine precipitates cystine crystals and may improve the yield of the test. The best screening procedure is the cyanide-nitroprusside test (102). A positive reaction occurs with as little as 75 to 125 mg cystine per gram of creatinine, which is well below that of homozygotes, which excrete at least 250 mg/g creatinine. Some heterozygotes may also be detected by this procedure (105). The test is not specific and may detect acetone or homocystine as well. The definite test is a measurement of urine cystine and dibasic amino acid concentration by ion exchange chromatography. The upper limits of normal are 18, 130, 16, and 22 mg/g creatinine for cystine, lysine, arginine, and ornithine, respectively (104). In establishing the diagnosis of classic cystinuria, it is important to exclude other conditions associated with increased urinary cystine excretion, including isolated cystinuria, tubular immaturity in young infants, generalized aminoaciduria (Fanconi syndrome), and organic acidemias (102,104).

Cystine stones are radiopaque because of the density of the sulfur molecule, and on a roentgenogram, they appear smooth. Occasionally, they form staghorn calculi. Cystine also may act as a nidus for calcium oxalate so that mixed stones may be found (136). Factors contributing to mixed stone formation in cystinuria include alkalinization of urine and urinary tract infections.

The disease usually presents with renal colic. Occasionally, infection, hypertension, or renal failure may be the first manifestation (102). Cystinuria occurs with equal frequency in males and females, but males are more severely affected because of a greater likelihood of urethral obstruction in the male. Clinical manifestations usually occur in the second and third decades of life, with a 62% probability of stones by age 25 years (137). Most patients have recurrent stone formation. Cystinuric patients who receive a kidney transplant have normal urinary cystine and dibasic amino acid excretion after transplantation (138,139).

Treatment. Cystine crystalluria occurs when the cystine content of the urine exceeds 300 mg/L at pH 4.5 to 7.0. Cystine solubility increases sharply at a urine pH above 7 (104). The major therapeutic approaches to cystinuria are designed to increase the solubility of cystine, reduce excretion of cystine, and convert cystine to more soluble compounds (102). Therapies used in the management of cystinuria include the following:

- Increased oral fluid intake to increase urine volume and cystine solubility. Because cystinuric patients excrete 0.5 to 1.0 g cystine/day, intake of 3 to 4 L could be required to keep the urinary cystine concentration below 300 mg/L. Patients should develop a 24-hour schedule for drinking and voiding, with particular attention to nighttime hours, when urine may become supersaturated with cystine. Water should be taken at bedtime and whenever the patient awakens at night. Rigid adherence to fluid therapy is effective in approximately 70% of patients (102).
- Oral alkali in addition to high fluid intake to further increase cystine solubility in the urine (104). A urine pH of 7.5 to 8.0 can be maintained by the provision of 1 to 2 mEq/kg/day of bicarbonate or citrate in divided doses. Because high sodium intake increases cystine excretion (see Dietary Therapy), potassium citrate is preferred (104). Because urine alkalinization may result in formation of mixed calcium-containing stones, adherence to high fluid intake is crucial.
- Dietary therapy to reduce cystine production and excretion. Studies examining the effect of dietary restriction of methionine (a metabolic precursor to cystine) on urine cystine excretion have yielded variable results (104). Also, diets low in methionine are very difficult to follow and may be harmful to growing children. Therefore, dietary methionine restriction is not recommended (104). Urinary excretion of cystine and dibasic amino acids in cystinuric patients has been shown to correlate with urinary sodium excretion (140,141). Hence, dietary sodium restriction is recommended by some authors as a safe approach to the treatment of cystinuria (102). L-glutamine administered orally or intravenously in conjunction with low salt intake reduces cystine excretion (140,142), but this effect was not observed in patients receiving a normal salt diet (143). The mechanism of the anticystinuric effect of glutamine is unclear.
- Pharmacologic therapy to increase cystine solubility and decrease cystine excretion. The sulfhydryl-binding compound D-penicillamine (β-dimethylcysteine) leads to the formation of the mixed disulfide penicillamine-cysteine after a disulfide exchange reaction. This mixed disulfide is far more water-soluble than cystine. Hence, penicillamine acts by reducing cystine excretion as well as by permitting the excretion of a more soluble compound. Penicillamine, given at a dosage of 1 to 2 g/24 hours (30 mg/kg in children), is highly effective and reduces urinary cystine excretion to under 200 mg/g creatinine (144). Unfortunately, penicillamine produces serious side effects in 50% of patients (145). These reactions include rashes (including pemphigus), fever, arthralgia, nephrotoxicity (including nephrotic syndrome in up to 30% of patients and rapidly progressive glomerulonephritis), pancytopenia, and loss of taste. Penicillamine also increases copper and zinc excretion in the urine. The loss of taste may be reversed by copper administration (104). Pyridoxine metabolism may be impaired, and pyridoxine supplementation should be provided for patients receiving D-penicillamine. Most of these side effects revert to normal on discontinuation of the drug. Because of the serious side effects, D-penicillamine therapy should be reserved for patients unresponsive to conservative management, and

stepwise dosing is recommended (102). D-acetyl penicillamine, another anticystinuric sulfhydryl agent, has fewer side effects than D-penicillamine. Mercaptopropionyl glycine (MPG), another agent undergoing a disulfide exchange reaction, is as effective as D-penicillamine in the treatment of cystinuria (146). MPG has the same toxicity as D-penicillamine, but serious renal and hematologic reactions requiring cessation of therapy are much less common with MPG (146). Because of the lower incidence of side effects and because this compound can be used in patients who develop allergic reactions to D-penicillamine, MPG is the pharmacologic agent of choice in the therapy of cystinuria (146,147).

Several studies have examined the effect of captopril, an angiotensin-converting enzyme inhibitor, on urinary cystine excretion in cystinuric patients (148–150). This nontoxic sulfhydryl compound builds highly soluble captopril-cysteine disulfides. Although a reduction in cystine excretion has been demonstrated in some studies (148,149), others (150) have failed to show an effect. Further studies are needed to evaluate the efficacy of captopril therapy in cystinuria. It has been proposed that meso-1,3 dimercaptosuccinic acid (DMSA), an additional compound forming disulfide linkage with cysteine, might be a useful therapeutic agent in cystinuria (151). The efficacy of this agent in cystinuria remains to be established.

Ascorbic acid, which acts as a reducing agent to convert cystine to the more soluble cysteine, has been suggested as a therapeutic modality in patients with cystinuria (147). To date, the results of the use of this compound on a limited number of patients have been variable (104,147). Also, concerns have been raised that ascorbic acid therapy in cystinuria is potentially lithogenic because of the hyperoxaluric and hypocitraturic effect of this agent.

Several urologic procedures have been used to treat cystine stones:

- Chemolysis of stones by irrigation through a percutaneous nephrostomy. Successful dissolution of stones has been achieved using *N*-acetylcysteine, D-penicillamine, α-MPG, and a very alkaline agent, tromethamine (103,104).
- Extracorporal shock wave lithotripsy. This therapeutic modality has been only partially successful because of the organic nature and the uniform crystal structure of cystine stones (103,152). Percutaneous ultrasonic lithotripsy has been somewhat more effective (153).
- Lithotomy. Surgical removal of stones is necessary only in rare patients with obstructing or infected stones unresponsive to a more conservative approach.

In summary, the mainstays of therapy in cystinuria include hydration, alkalinization of the urine, and dietary sodium restriction. Full compliance with this regimen results in significantly reduced urinary cystine excretion and good long-term prognosis in most patients. Pharmacologic treatment with sulfhydryl agents should be reserved for patients in whom conservative therapy fails. Urologic intervention may be indicated in selected patients.

Isolated Cystinuria

Brodehl et al. (113) report two siblings who showed high urinary excretion rates of cystine but normal dibasic amino acid excretion. The children did not develop renal stones. This report, along with the detection of a similar abnormality in dogs (154), provides evidence of a separate cystine transporter not shared with dibasic amino acids in the tubular brush-border membrane, which appears to be defective in isolated cystinuria. The molecular nature of this proposed transporter is unknown.

Lysinuric Protein Intolerance (Hyperdibasic Aminoaciduria Type II)

LPI is a rare autosomal recessive disorder characterized by excessive urinary excretion of dibasic amino acids (especially lysine), normal cystine excretion, and poor intestinal absorption of dibasic amino acids (155–157). Plasma values of dibasic amino acids are subnormal. The disease is relatively common in Finland, where the prevalence of the disease is 1:60,000 (157). Approximately 100 patients, one-half of them Finns, have been described (157). Homozygous patients show massive dibasic aminoaciduria as well as hyperammonemia after a protein overload; heterozygotes have normal urinary amino acid excretion but impaired renal and intestinal transport of dibasic amino acids at increased loads. The clinical manifestations in homozygotes for LPI are those of protein malnutrition and postprandial hyperammonemia. They include failure to thrive, marked protein intolerance, anorexia, vomiting, diarrhea, hepatosplenomegaly, muscle hypotonia, interstitial lung disease, osteoporosis, seizures, and coma (157).

The pathogenic mechanism of LPI appears to be a defective transport of dibasic amino acids in the basolateral membrane of renal and intestinal epithelial cells, resulting in impaired efflux from cell to interstitium (158,159). This has been confirmed by a measurement of fluxes in jejunal biopsy specimens from LPI patients (158), as well as by the observation that infusion of citrulline to these patients results in massive argininuria and ornithinuria (159). Citrulline is reabsorbed from the tubular lumen by a neutral amino acid transport mechanism and is converted to arginine and ornithine in the renal cell. Impaired exit at the antiluminal membrane results in backflux of accumulated arginine and ornithine at the brush-border membrane surface. It is the high-affinity, specific dibasic amino acid transporter y^+L that is affected in this disease (84,128). Because basolateral membrane transporters of epithelial cells and plasma membrane transporters of parenchymal cells are homologous carriers, it is not surprising that hepatocytes (160), granulocytes (160), and cultured skin fibroblasts (161) from patients with LPI show impaired transport of dibasic amino acids. Erythrocytes from LPI patients, which do not have the y⁺L system, show normal cationic amino acid transport (162).

It is presumed that the defective hepatic transport of dibasic amino acids deprives hepatic cells of ornithine and arginine, which are necessary for urea production (157). This results in protein intolerance, hyperammonemia, and low urea formation. This notion is supported by the observation that L-citrulline supplements improve protein tolerance in LPI patients (159). This amino acid, a metabolic precursor of ornithine and arginine, is absorbed in the intestine, enters the hepatic cell via neutral amino acid transport mechanisms, is metabolized in the liver to ornithine and arginine, and restores the pathway for ammonia disposal (157).

In 1992, the rBAT homologous protein, the human cell surface glycoprotein 4F2hc (encoded by the gene CD98), was shown to induce y^+L cationic amino acid transport in *Xenopus* oocytes (77). Like rBAT, 4F2hc represents the heavy subunit of a disulfide-linked heteromeric amino acid transporter (163) (see Molecular Structure of Amino Acid Transporters; Figs. 37.3 and 37.4). Molecular analysis excluded CD98, which has been localized to chromosome 11, as a candidate gene for LPI (164). Linkage studies in Finnish and non-Finnish LPI families placed the gene of the disease to 14q11-13 (165,166).

In 1998, Torrents et al. (87) identified a human cDNA, SLC7A7, as encoding y^+LAT-1—a member of the family of light subunits that combine with 4F2hc to form heteromeric amino acid transporters (see Molecular Structure of Amino Acid Transporters; Fig. 37.3). The 4F2hc/y^+LAT-1 transporter has been shown to have the activity of amino acid transport system y^+L that is responsible for the efflux of basic amino acids at the basolateral plasma membrane of epithelial cells (128) (see Specificity of Transport; Figs. 37.1 and 37.3). The SLC7A7 gene localized to the LP1 locus (87). In 1999, the two groups (164,167) demonstrated that mutations in SLC7A7 cause LPI in Finnish, Italian, and Spanish patients. As of 2000, more than 25 SLC7A7 mutations, spread along the entire SLC7A7 gene, have been found in LPI patients from different ethnic groups (126). Expression studies in *Xenopus* oocytes showed that various LPI mutations result in proteins that fail to co-induce amino acid transport activity when expressed with 4F2hc (168). Two of the mutants reached the oocyte plasma membrane when coexpressed with 4F2hc, demonstrating that they are transport-inactivating mutations (168).

LPI is characterized by poor genotype/phenotype correlation. Even Finnish patients, who share the same founder mutation, show variation in thc clinical picture (168). Similarly, both interfamilial and intrafamilial phenotypic variability were observed in Italian LPI patient heterozygotes for the same mutation (169). This suggests that, in addition to SLC7A7 mutations, hitherto unknown factors play a role in the pathogenesis of LPI (126,128).

Therapy of LPI consists of protein restriction to prevent hyperammonemia, as well as oral supplements of arginine, ornithine, and, most important, citrulline (170). Administration of the latter amino acid, which corrects the hepatic deficiency in ornithine and arginine, results in clinical improvement and catch-up growth.

Hyperdibasic Aminoaciduria Type I

An autosomal dominant cationic aminoaciduria has been described in two families containing several heterozygotes and a single homozygote (114,171). This disease, called *hyperdibasic aminoaciduria type I*, is characterized by impaired renal reabsorption and intestinal absorption of the dibasic amino acids lysine, arginine, and ornithine but not of cystine. Plasma values of dibasic amino acids are normal, and there is no protein intolerance or hyperammonemia. The reported homozygous patient had mental retardation (171). Hyperdibasic aminoaciduria type I heterozygotes have modest cationic aminoaciduria, whereas LPI heterozygotes have no hyperaminoaciduria. It has been speculated that the brush-border membrane–bound, high-capacity transporter for dibasic amino acids, which excludes cystine, is defective in this disease. The molecular nature of this transporter is unknown.

Isolated Lysinuria

Omura et al. (115) reported a single child with increased urinary excretion of lysine; impaired intestinal absorption of this amino acid; low plasma lysine levels; and normal renal and intestinal transport of ornithine, arginine, and cystine. The patient did not have hyperammonemia but had failure to thrive and mental retardation, probably secondary to the deficiency of the essential amino acid, lysine. This case implies a defect in a selective transport system for lysine in the kidney and the intestine. Such a system has not been identified in physiologic or molecular studies.

Neutral Aminoaciduria

Three distinct disorders of neutral amino acid transport have been identified: Hartnup disorder, methioninuria, and histidinuria.

Hartnup Disease

Hartnup disease, which may have afflicted Julius Caesar and his family (172), was first recognized in two siblings in England in 1956 (173). This disease is characterized by intestinal malabsorption and massive aminoaciduria of the neutral monoamino monocarboxylic amino acids alanine, serine, threonine, valine, leucine, isoleucine, phenylalanine, tyrosine, tryptophan, histidine, glutamine, and asparagine (174). Most patients also have increased excretion of indolic compounds that originate in the gut from bacterial degradation of tryptophan (175). Transport of other neutral amino acids, including cystine, imino acids, glycine, and β-amino acids, is unaffected. The disease is inherited as an autosomal recessive trait and has an estimated incidence of 1:20,000 live births. Heterozygotes have normal urinary acid excretion under physiologic conditions. Clinical features in homozygotes may include photosensitive rash, cerebellar ataxia, and a variety of psychiatric manifestations, as in the features of pellagra (171). The pellagra-like manifestations are primarily caused by intestinal malabsorption and urinary loss of tryptophan, an amino acid that is required for niacin synthesis. The diagnosis should be suspected in any patient with pellagra who has no history of niacin or nicotinamide deficiency and should be made by chromatographic analysis of the urine (174).

A defect in the broad-specificity neutral α-amino acid transport mechanism in the renal and intestinal brush-border membrane is presumed to be the pathogenic mechanism underlying this disorder (11,176). Two lines of evidence support the hypothesis that the lesion is localized in the brush-border membrane (11). First, plasma amino acid response in patients with Hartnup disease was attenuated after oral feeding of free α-amino acids but not when appropriate dipeptides were given orally (177). The dipeptides are presumed to be reabsorbed by a dipeptide-specific brush-border membrane transporter and hydrolyzed in the enterocyte; the free amino acids exit the cell via a nondefective basolateral membrane-bound carrier. Second, tryptophan transport is normal in various parenchymal cells from patients with Hartnup disease, including leukocytes, placenta, and cultured skin fibroblasts (174,178). As indicated earlier, carriers in plasma membranes of parenchymal cells are homologous to basolateral membrane carriers in epithelial cells, which are supposed to be normal in Hartnup disease.

The transport characteristics and the epithelial distribution of the Na^+-dependent neutral amino acid transport B^o (see Specificity of Transport; Fig. 37.1), which is encoded by the recently identified ATB^o gene (61) (see Molecular Structure of Amino Acid Transporters), raise the possibility that this transporter is defective in Hartnup disorder. The role of this gene, which localizes to chromosome 19q13.3 (61), in the pathogenesis of Hartnup disorder has not been investigated.

The presence of alternative transport pathways for neutral amino acids in the renal tubule explains why the defect in the broad-specificity neutral amino acid transport in Hartnup disease results in only partial loss of some amino acids (e.g., phenylalanine) (11). These alternative systems, as well as the oligopeptide-preferring carriers in the kidney and intestine, are responsible for normal plasma amino acid values and lack of symptoms in most patients (179). As suggested by Scriver et al. (179), Hartnup disease is multifactorial in its pathogenesis, and only patients genetically predisposed to low plasma amino acid levels and impaired tryptophan metabolism develop symptoms.

Patients with Hartnup disease respond well to oral therapy with nicotinamide, 40 to 100 mg/day (180). More recently, oral administration of *tryptophan ethylester*, a lipid-soluble form of tryptophan, has been shown to increase serum tryptophan and reverse clinical symptoms in patients with Hartnup disease (181).

Methioninuria

There are two case reports of patients with isolated increased urinary excretion of methionine and its metabolic breakdown products (182,183). The patients had malodorous urine, edema, episodic hyperventilation, seizures, and mental retardation. The underlying defect appeared to be abnormal transport of methionine in the kidney and in the intestine. α-Hydroxybutyric acid, a bacterial degradation product of unabsorbed intestinal methionine, appeared in the urine of these patients. This organic acid may have been responsible for the neurologic manifestations in these patients. A low-methionine diet resulted in significant clinical improvement. These cases of isolated methioninuria, as well as the observation that methionine, which shares the broad-spectrum amino acid transport system with other neutral amino acids, are not hyperexcreted in Hartnup disease, provided evidence for the existence of a specific transport pathway for methionine in renal and intestinal epithelium.

Histidinuria

Two siblings (184) and two other patients (185,186) have been reported with isolated histidinuria. All showed significant mental retardation. Investigation revealed impaired transport of histidine in the kidney and intestine. Parents of the two affected siblings showed normal urinary histidine excretion under normal conditions but hyperhistidinuria after an oral histidine load. The mode of inheritance of this disease is uncertain, but autosomal recessive inheritance has been suggested (11). Although the broad-specificity transporter of neutral amino acids is the major carrier for histidine, as suggested by *in vitro* studies as well as by fractional excretion rates above 50% for this amino acid in Hartnup disease (11), the case reports of histidinuria suggest that an isolated histidine carrier is operating in the renal tubule and the intestine.

Iminoaciduria and Glycinuria

Two distinct disorders belong to this group of aminoacidurias: iminoglycinuria and isolated glycinuria.

Iminoglycinuria

Iminoglycinuria is an autosomal recessive membrane transport defect characterized by excretion of excessive amounts of proline, hydroxyproline, and glycine in the urine (187). Iminoglycinuria is a benign condition with an estimated incidence of 1:15,000 live births (187,188). It is the shared, brush-border membrane–bound, group-specific transport pathway for imino acids and glycine (see Specificity of Transport) that is defective in this condition (94,187). The selective glycine-specific and imino acid–specific transport systems are not affected. The activity of these selective transporters accounts for the normal plasma levels of glycine and imino acids observed in iminoglycinuria. As discussed earlier, the late maturation of these selective transporters in normal infants is responsible for neonatal physiologic iminoglycinuria (92,94). The absence of the selective transporters during early life also explains why infants with iminoglycinuria who lack the shared transporter have fractional excretion values for glycine and proline approaching 100%, which decline after the first months of life (11). Defective intestinal transport of proline has been found in some patients with iminoglycinuria (187). As expected, proline transport is not defective in leukocytes or skin fibroblasts because these cells do not possess carriers corresponding to a brush-border membrane carrier (11).

Iminoglycinuria is a genetically heterogenous condition with several mutant alleles (11,187). This view is supported by several observations. First, obligate heterozygotes may have hyperglycinuria (but not iminoaciduria) or may have normal urinary amino acid excretion (189). Second, some homozygous patients have an intestinal transport defect. Third, a variant exists with normal transport maximum (Tm) for proline and a defect affecting glycine transport more than proline transport, indicating a K_m defect (190).

The genetic defect responsible for iminoglycinuria is unknown. The transport characteristics of the amino acid transport system expected to be defective in this disorder fit those of the IMINO and/or the Na^+- and Cl^--dependent transporters of the GAT transporter family (see Specificity of Transport). The latter group includes GLYT1, GLYT2, and PROT, which transport glycine and/or proline. The GLYT transporters are expressed in the kidney and may be good candidates for the immunoglycinuria phenotype.

Differential diagnosis of iminoglycinuria includes neonatal iminoglycinuria; Fanconi syndrome, in which generalized aminoaciduria occurs; and hyperprolinemia, an inborn error of proline metabolism that exhibits overflow prolinuria as well as hydroxyprolinuria and glycinuria secondary to a proline-induced inhibition or hydroxyproline and glycine transport. This inhibition occurs at the shared luminal carrier for these amino acids.

Isolated Glycinuria

Isolated glycinuria without iminoaciduria has been reported in two families (190,191). It has been suggested that this condition is a manifestation of a mutation affecting the specific high-affinity carrier for glycine, the molecular identity of which remains to be established (11). It is possible, however, that hyperglycinuria represents a defect in the shared, imino acid-glycine transport system affecting affinity rather than capacity of the system (K_m variant). Because the condition appears to be inherited as an autosomal dominant trait, it also is possible that these cases represent hyperglycinuric heterozygotes for the iminoglycinuria allele. Glycinuria has also been reported in association with glycosuria, called *glycoglycinuria* (192). The defect underlying this autosomal dominant condition is unknown.

Dicarboxylic Aminoaciduria

Selective urinary hyperexcretion of the acidic amino acids glutamate and aspartate was first reported in two children (193,194). One of the children also had impaired intestinal absorption of these amino acids. The condition is inherited as an autosomal recessive trait and appears to be benign; screening in a French-Canadian population revealed a large number of healthy probands with hyperdicarboxylic aminoaciduria and an incidence of 1:29,000 live births (195).

The pathogenic mechanism appears to be a defect in the dicarboxylic amino acid transport system in the brush-border membrane. The excretion of dicarboxylic amino acids in homozygous patients may greatly exceed the GFR, suggesting tubular secretion or backflux of dicarboxylic amino acids from cell to lumen (11). Treatment with glutamate and aspartate corrected the hypoglycemia observed in one patient (193). This hypoglycemia probably resulted from the absence of these gluconeogenic amino acids.

The neuronal and peripheral anionic amino acid transporter EAAC1 (EAAT3) (see Molecular Structure of Amino Acid Transporters) is an obvious candidate for the transporters defective in dicarboxylic aminoaciduria. The transporter is highly expressed in the kidney and intestine (54). Peghini et al. (196) have shown that EAAC1-deficient mice develop dicarboxylic aminoaciduria, a finding that strongly suggests that the EAAC1 gene is a candidate gene for dicarboxylic aminoaciduria. In 2001, Nozaki et al. (197), by using homozygosity mapping, assigned the Hartnup disease locus to chromosome 5p15. Nevertheless, there are no functionally characterized genes mapped to this locus that seem to be obvious candidates for the Hartnup disorder.

An interesting feature of dicarboxylic aminoaciduria is the decreased uptake of anionic amino acids by cultured skin fibroblasts from patients with this condition (198). It has been shown that anionic amino acid–preferring carriers in epithelial brush-border and parenchymal cells have similar characteristics (11,198). As pointed out by Scriver and Tenenhouse (11), the apparent expression of the mutant gene in both the brush-border membrane of the epithelium and the plasma membrane of parenchymal cells is unique and contrary to the expected pattern of analogy between basolateral membrane-bound and plasma membrane-bound carriers (see Classic Cystinuria, Hartnup Disease, and Lysinuric Protein Intolerance). The possibility that the EAAC1 transporter, likely defective in dicarboxylic aminoaciduria, is expressed at both the luminal and basolateral membranes of the proximal tubule awaits future investigation.

β-Aminoaciduria

No inborn error of the β/γ-amino acid transport system that carries taurine, β-alanine, β-aminobutyric acid, and GABA has been reported in humans. An impaired taurine transport, however, has been found in an inbred mouse strain (C57BL/6J) (199). Studies using kidney slices (199) and isolated basolateral membrane vesicles (95) have localized the transport defect to the antiluminal membrane of the proximal tubular epithelium. In analogy with the defect in LPI, an impaired taurine exit across the basolateral membrane and backflux from cell to lumen may underlie the hypertaurinuria observed in the C57BL/6J mouse (95,199).

GLYCOSURIA

General Characteristics of Renal Glucose Transport

Under normal conditions, the reabsorption of filtered glucose by the renal tubule is almost complete. Less than 0.05% of the renal glucose load is excreted in the human urine (200); 90% of the filtered glucose is reabsorbed in the proximal convoluted tubule; and the rest is reclaimed in the proximal straight tubule, the loop of Henle, and, to some extent, the collecting duct (201).

Reabsorption of glucose across the proximal tubular brush-border membrane occurs by an active, carrier-mediated, concentrative, Na^+-dependent transport process (200,201). The Na^+ electrochemical gradient driving glucose transport across the brush-border membrane is maintained by the activity of the basolateral membrane-bound Na^+-K^+-ATPase that pumps Na^+ out and K^+ into the cell. Na^+-glucose cotransport across the luminal membrane is electrogenic positive and phlorizin inhibitable. Glucose exit from the cell occurs by an Na^+-independent–facilitated diffusion down the glucose concentration gradient (201). This diffusional exit of glucose is mediated by a carrier that is distinct from that found at the luminal membrane surface (see Facilitative Glucose Transporters).

The mammalian kidney is characterized by a limited capacity to reabsorb D-glucose (200). As plasma glucose concentration is progressively elevated, the amount of glucose reabsorbed increases linearly until a maximum value is reached (Fig. 37.7). Beyond this maximum rate of glucose reabsorption, further increases of filtered D-glucose are excreted in the urine. As shown in Figure 37.7, the glucose titration curve provides parameters of glucose transport such as minimum threshold (F_{min_G}), defined as the filtered glucose load at which 1 mg of glucose per minute appears in the urine, and the tubular maximum for glucose reabsorption (Tm_G). Reported Tm_G values for glucose in human adults and children have ranged between 260 and 350 mg/min/1.73 m^2 (202–204), with lower values in infants (204,205). When corrected for the GFR (Tm/GFR), Tm value for glucose in infants, children, and adults is approximately 2.5 mg/mL (204).

The glucose titration curve (Fig. 37.7) is characterized by a splay—a rounding of the curve during the transition from virtually complete reabsorption of filtered D-glucose to complete excretion of excess glucose load. This deviation from the theoretical curve is explained by the nephron functional heterogeneity (the gradual progression from the first to the last nephron to saturate), as well as by the variation in affinity for glucose or K_m values between carriers (the magnitude of the splay is inversely proportional to the affinity of the transporter for the D-glucose) (200).

Studies in isolated perfused tubules (206) and later experiments using isolated BBMV from pars convoluta (S1 and S2 segments) and pars recta (S3 segment) of the proximal tubule (207–209) demonstrate that the kinetic properties and stoichiometric relationships of D-glucose reabsorption change along the length of the nephron. These studies provide evidence for two Na^+-dependent transport mechanisms, a low-affinity/high-capacity cotransport system in the early proximal tubule and a high-affinity/low-capacity system in the late proximal tubule. The Na^+-glucose coupling ratio was found to be 1:1 in the convoluted proximal tubule and 2:1 in the straight proximal tubule (208,209).

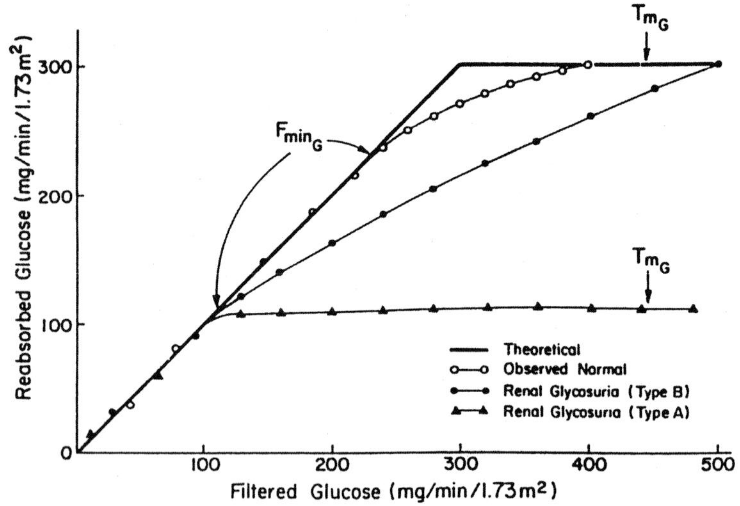

FIGURE 37.7. Renal glucose titration curves. Theoretical and observed normal curves are compared to abnormal curves observed in type A and type B renal glycosuria. Tm_G, maximum rate for glucose reabsorption; F_{min_G}, minimum threshold. (From Elsas LJ, Longo N. Glucose transporters. *Annu Rev Med* 1992;43:377–393, with permission.)

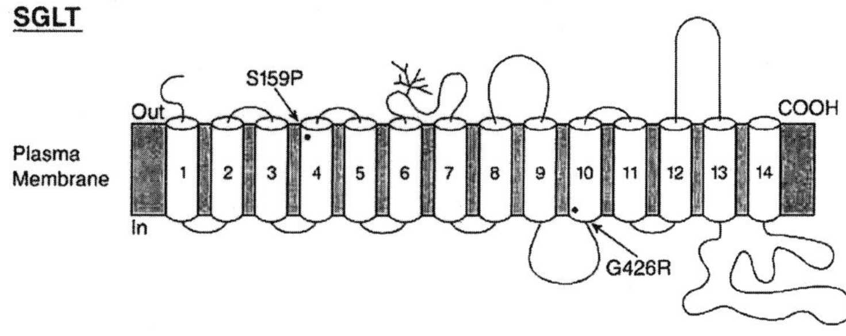

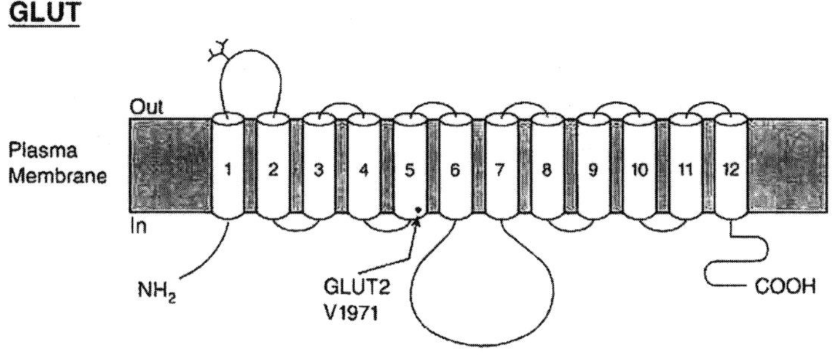

FIGURE 37.8. Schematic structure of the Na+/glucose cotransporter (SGLT) and the facilitative glucose transporter (GLUT). The two mutations shown in SGLT were identified in one of the original families with glucose-galactose malabsorption. (Adapted from Longo N. Human glucose transporters. *Adv Pediatr* 1998;45:293–313.)

The efficiency of a coupled carrier system increases as the power of the stoichiometry increases (201,209). Whereas the early proximal tubule glucose transporter is responsible for the reabsorption of the bulk of filtered D-glucose from the tubular lumen, the late proximal tubule glucose transporter is responsible for the removal of the last traces of glucose from the urine (209). The arrangement of transporters in series along the proximal tubule enables the kidney to reabsorb glucose from the urine in a more energy-efficient mechanism than can be achieved by either of the cotransporters acting alone.

Molecular Biology of Na$^+$-Glucose Cotransporters

Various approaches have been used to identify and isolate the Na$^+$-glucose cotransporters. Earlier methods, including solubilization and reconstitution techniques, semiselective and photoaffinity labeling, phlorizin affinity chromatography, radiation inactivation, and immunoaffinity absorption (201), have been inconclusive and yielded very limited biochemical data. However, considerable progress has been made in the past decade in elucidating the molecular structure of membrane proteins that catalyze sugar transport processes, including the Na$^+$-glucose cotransporter (51,210,211). Hediger et al., using expression cloning in *Xenopus* oocytes (see Molecular Structure of Amino Acid Transporters), cloned and sequenced the Na$^+$-dependent D-glucose transporter from rabbit (38) and human (212) intestine. Subsequently, molecular analysis revealed that rabbit intestinal and renal Na$^+$-glucose cotransporters are essentially identical (213). The Na$^+$-glucose cotransport proteins belong to the SGLT1 family of sodium cotransport proteins, which includes the renal Na$^+$-nucleoside, renal Na$^+$-myoinositol, and the *Escherichia coli* Na$^+$-proline cotransporters (51,211).

The SGLT1 transporter (Fig. 37.8) consists of 662 to 664 amino acids and has 14 membrane-spanning sequences that are presumed to be α-helical, with the NH_2 and COOH termini located on the cytoplasmic side of the membrane. A simple glycosylation site is found in the hydrophilic domain between transmembrane segments 5 and 6 (214). SGLT1 from rabbit (38), rat (216), pig (216), and human (212) show high homology in sequence and structure. The gene encoding the human intestinal SGLT1 has been recently localized to the q11.2lqter region of chromosome 22 (217). Recent studies using *Xenopus* oocytes (218) demonstrate that protein kinases (PKA and PKC) regulate SGLT1 activity by controlling the distribution of transporters between intracellular compartments and the plasma membrane and that this occurs by exocytosis and endocytosis.

Studies by Pajor et al. (219) and Lee et al. (215) using expression studies in *Xenopus* oocytes, Western and Northern analysis, and *in situ* hybridization and immunocytochemistry have provided evidence that the renal Na$^+$-glucose cotransporter SGLT1 is the high-affinity/low-capacity transporter found predominantly in the straight proximal tubule (S3 segment). Evaluation of the stoichiometry of SGLT1-mediated transport in *Xenopus* oocytes revealed an Na$^+$ to glucose coupling ratio of 2:1 (215).

A second low-affinity Na$^+$-glucose cotransporter named SGLT2 was isolated from rat (220) and human (221,222) kidney. The amino acid sequence of SGLT2 is 59% identical to that of SGLT1 (221). SGLT2 has an Na$^+$ glucose coupling ratio of 1:1, does not recognize galactose (which is a substrate for SGLT1), and is strongly expressed in proximal tubule S1 segments (222). Human SGLT2 gene was mapped to chromosome 16p11.2 close to the centromere (223).

A third Na^+-dependent glucose transporter, termed *SGLT3*, was isolated from an LLC-PK_1 pig renal cell line (224). It is a low-affinity, Na^+-glucose (not galactose) cotransporter (225). Human SGLT3 gene is located on chromosome 22 (211).

Facilitative Glucose Transporters

Glucose concentrated inside tubular epithelial cells flows to the interstitium down its concentration gradient through facilitative glucose transporters located in the basolateral membrane (200,226). The basolateral Na^+-independent and the luminal Na^+-dependent glucose transport systems also differ with respect to inhibition and specificity (201). The basolateral glucose transporter is inhibited by the mold metabolite cytochalasin-B but not by phlorizin. It also accepts D-glucose.

The basolateral membrane glucose transporters belong to a family of Na^+-independent facilitative glucose transporters, of which five different isoforms called *GLUT1*, *GLUT2*, *GLUT3*, *GLUT4*, and *GLUT5* have been identified (226–228). These subspecies have extensive structural homologies but differ in their tissue distribution, specific function, insulin sensitivity, sugar specificity, and kinetic characteristics. The human erythrocyte glucose transporter GLUT1 was the first glucose transporter to be cloned and sequenced (229). It is the most ubiquitously distributed of the transporter isoforms (227). Isoforms GLUT2 to GLUT5 have been cloned by screening cDNA libraries from various tissues and species with a GLUT1 DNA probe (226). The facilitative glucose transporters (Fig. 37.8) have 12 membrane-spanning domains, with both the NH_2 and the COOH termini of the protein facing the cytoplasm. A single glycosylation site is located between transmembrane domains 1 and 2.

GLUT2, a low-affinity transporter, is the predominant facilitative glucose transporter in hepatocytes and in the basolateral membrane of intestinal and renal tubular cells (230,231). In the kidney, GLUT2 is present only in the basolateral membrane of cells in the proximal convoluted tubule (S1 and S2 segments) (230,231). Studies using antipeptide antibodies specific for GLUT1 have detected this high-affinity transporter in the kidney (231,232). It was found in the basolateral membrane of cells forming the proximal straight tubule (S3 segment). GLUT5 has also been identified in the kidney (233).

Thus, it appears that transepithelial glucose transport in the proximal tubule occurs by two different pairs of apical Na^+-dependent and basolateral Na^+-independent glucose transporters (200,226) (Fig. 37.9). A luminal Na^+-dependent, low-affinity/high-capacity glucose transporter (designated SGLT2) and a basolateral Na^+-independent, low-affinity GLUT2 are responsible for the bulk of glucose reabsorption in the early part of the proximal tubule. A luminal Na^+-dependent, high-affinity/low-capacity SGLT1 coupled with the basolateral Na^+-independent, high-affinity GLUT1 reabsorb the remaining low concentration of glucose in the late part of the proximal tubule.

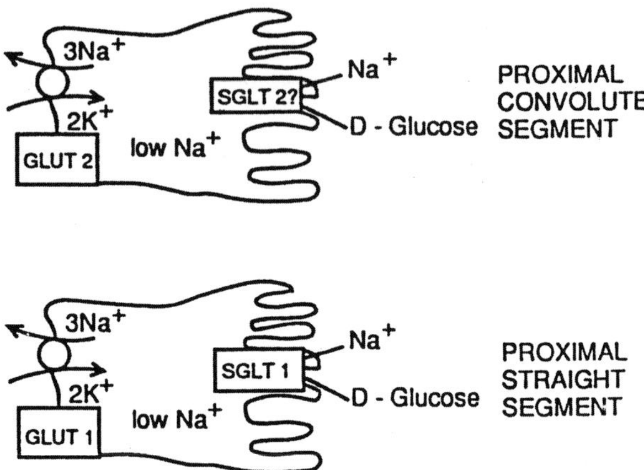

FIGURE 37.9. Schematic model for the distribution (luminal or basolateral) of cloned glucose transporters in renal tubular epithelium. Orientation permits net reabsorption from lumen to interstitium. (Adapted from Silverman M. Structure and function of hexose transporters. *Annu Rev Biochem* 1991;60:757–794.)

Maturation of Glucose Transport

The immature renal tubule in animals (234,235) and humans (204,236,237) is characterized by decreased ability to reabsorb glucose. Tubular reabsorption of glucose relates directly to postnatal age, and glycosuria occurs commonly in infants less than 30 weeks' gestational age (236–238). There are few data on the development of renal glucose transport mechanisms. The fetal kidneys of various animal species (234,239,240) have been shown to reabsorb glucose. In the fetal rat kidney (239), glucose reabsorption appeared to be Na^+ dependent and phlorizin inhibitable. A decreased initial rate uptake of α-methyl-D-glucoside was found in isolated renal tubules from neonatal rat (241) and dog (235). BBMV studies (242) demonstrated a concentrative, Na^+-dependent, electrogenic and phlorizin-sensitive glucose transport in the fetal rabbit kidney. The fetal glucose transport mechanism, however, had a significantly lower capacity than the adult glucose transport system. Recent experiments exploring the expression of SGLT1 and SGLT2 mRNAs in embryonic rat kidneys (220) revealed that the two Na^+-glucose cotransporters appeared early in gestation and that they were developmentally regulated. Recent evidence suggests that the increase in SGLT1 mRNA-accompanying cell differentiation in the pig kidney cell line LLC-PK_1 is regulated by PKA (243) and PKC (244).

Little is known about the maturation of the facilitative glucose transporters in the kidney. A study (245) examining the developmental pattern of these transporters in the rat kidney showed that renal GLUT1 and GLUT5 gene expression was unchanged throughout development, whereas

GLUT2 was most abundant before weaning. The latter finding may be related to the fact that the kidney alone seems to be responsible for gluconeogenesis before expression of gluconeogenic enzymes by the liver.

Further studies are needed to explore the activity, expression, and distribution of various glucose transporters during kidney development and to elucidate the molecular mechanisms underlying the maturation of renal tubular glucose transport.

Glycosuria

Hereditary renal glycosuria is an abnormality in which variable amounts of glucose are excreted in the urine at normal concentrations of blood glucose (246). The renal defect is specific for glucose, and there is no increase in the urinary excretion of other sugars. Renal glycosuria is a benign condition without symptoms or physical consequences except during pregnancy or prolonged starvation—when dehydration and ketosis may develop (246). The metabolism, storage, and use of carbohydrates as well as insulin secretion are normal. The condition exists from infancy throughout adult life, and diagnosis usually is done on routine urine analysis. The distinction between renal glycosuria and diabetes mellitus is made with a fasting blood glucose level and a glucose tolerance test. The genetic pattern in renal glycosuria is autosomal recessive, although glycosuria in some heterozygotes has led some investigators to postulate a dominant inheritance (246,247).

The underlying pathogenic mechanism appears to be an isolated, selective defect in proximal tubular glucose transport. Renal glycosuria is not associated with impaired D-glucose transport in the intestinal epithelium (248).

Renal glycosuria is a heterogeneous condition resulting from several mutations. Analysis of renal titration curves for glucose reabsorption reveals two types of renal glycosuria (246,249) (Fig. 37.7). In type A, or classic renal glycosuria, F_{minG} and Tm_G are reduced. In type B, F_{minG} is reduced, whereas Tm_G is normal but has an increased splay. It has been suggested that the type A mutation reflects reduction in the capacity of the glucose transport system, which might arise from a uniform defect in all nephrons, and type B reflects a decrease in the affinity of the transport system, which might also be a consequence of nephron heterogeneity (248,250). A third type of glycosuria, termed *type O*, was described by Oemar et al. (251). In this rare condition, tubular reabsorption of glucose is virtually absent, and all glucose filtered is excreted in the urine.

It is important to consider the relationships between renal glycosuria, a benign condition, and intestinal glucose-galactose malabsorption, a potentially lethal disease. Glucose-galactose malabsorption, an autosomal recessive disease, is characterized in homozygotes by a neonatal onset of severe watery diarrhea that results in death unless glucose and galactose are removed from the diet (246). Studies using jejunal biopsy specimens from affected patients have demonstrated a defect in intestinal Na^+-dependent glucose transport (252). In 1991, molecular genetic studies in two sisters afflicted with glucose-galactose malabsorption revealed a missense mutation that causes a change in residue 28 from aspartate to asparagine in the intestinal brush-border SGLT1 Na^+-glucose cotransporter (253). This made glucose-galactose malabsorption the first reported disease that is caused by a mutation in a membrane transport protein. As of 2000, more than 40 mutations have been identified in patients with glucose-galactose malabsorption (246). The mutant proteins, when expressed in *Xenopus* oocytes, cause a marked reduction in Na^+-glucose transport activity (246).

Patients with glucose-galactose malabsorption who have been studied show a mild defect in renal tubular reabsorption of glucose, with normal Tm for glucose but decreased minimal threshold (F_{minG}) (246,252). In contrast, patients with renal glycosuria show no defect in intestinal D-glucose absorption. This indicates that the SGLT1 Na^+-glucose cotransporter affected in glucose-galactose malabsorption is shared between the intestine and the kidney, as also suggested by the molecular studies of Pajor et al. (219) and Lee et al. (215) (see Molecular Biology of Na^+-Glucose Cotransporters). The glucose transporter impaired in glycosuria is not shared.

The accumulating clinical, physiologic, and molecular data on renal glucose transport have led to the following hypothesis of the pathogenesis of hereditary renal glycosuria (200,249). A defect in the low-affinity/high-capacity 1 Na^+:1 glucose cotransporter (SGLT2) of the early proximal tubule, which reabsorbs most renal tubular glucose, would produce type A classic renal glycosuria but has no effect on glucose absorption in the intestine. By contrast, SGLT1, the high-affinity/low-capacity 2 Na^+:1 glucose cotransporter of the late proximal tubule (which also carries galactose), mediates residual glucose reabsorption in the renal tubule, and when defective, as in glucose-galactose malabsorption, causes only mild type B renal glycosuria.

It is noteworthy that mutations in the gene for GLUT2, the facilitative glucose transporter, are also associated with glycosuria in the Fanconi-Bickel syndrome (254,255). This autosomal recessive disorder is characterized by hepatorenal glycogen accumulation, Fanconi syndrome, and impaired use of glucose and galactose. The renal loss of glucose is due to the transport defect for monosaccharides across the renal basolateral membrane. A recent study (256) has demonstrated that knock-out mice lacking the GLUT2 gene exhibit extreme glycosuria.

REFERENCES

1. Zelikovic I, Chesney RW. Sodium-coupled amino acid transport in renal tubule. *Kidney Int* 1989;36:351–359.
2. Silbernagl S, Gekle M. Amino acids and oligopeptides. In: Seldin DW, Giebisch G, eds. *The kidney: physiology and*

pathophysiology, 3rd ed. Philadelphia: Lippincott Williams & Wilkins, 2000:2179–2210.

3. Schafer JA, Barfuss DW. Membrane mechanisms for transepithelial amino acid absorption and secretion. *Am J Physiol* 1980;238:F335–F346.
4. Zelikovic I, Chesney RW. Development of renal amino acid transport systems. *Semin Nephrol* 1989;9:49–55.
5. Bergeron M, Goodyer PR, Gougoux A, et al. Pathophysiology of renal hyperaminoacidurias and glucosuria. In: Seldin DW, Giebisch G, eds. *The kidney: physiology and pathophysiology*, 3rd ed. Philadelphia: Lippincott Williams & Wilkins, 2000:2211–2233.
6. Barfuss DW, Schafer JA. Active amino acid absorption by proximal convoluted and proximal straight tubules. *Am J Physiol* 1979;236:F149–F162.
7. Zelikovic I, Budreau A. Cl^- and membrane potential dependence of amino acid transport across the rat renal brush border membrane. *Mol Genet Metab* 1999;67:236–247.
8. Zelikovic I, Stejskal-Lorenz E, Lohstroh P, et al. Anion dependence of taurine transport by rat renal brush border membrane vesicles. *Am J Physiol* 1989;256:F646–F655.
9. Scalera V, Corcellia A, Frassanito A, et al. Chloride dependence of the sodium-dependent glycine transport in pig kidney cortex brush-border membrane vesicles. *Biochim Biophys Acta* 1987;903:1–10.
10. Chesney RW, Zelikovic I, Budreau A, et al. Chloride and membrane potential dependence of sodium ion-proline symport. *J Am Soc Nephrol* 1991;2:885–893.
11. Scriver CR, Tenenhouse HS. Mendelian phenotypes as "probes" of renal transport systems for amino acids and phosphate. In: Windhager EE, ed. *Handbook of physiology: renal physiology*. New York: Oxford University Press, 1992:1977–2016.
12. McNamara PD, Pepe LM, Segal S. Cystine uptake by rat renal brush border vesicles. *Biochem J* 1981;194:443–449.
13. Segal S, McNamara PD, Pepe LM. Transport interaction of cystine and dibasic amino acid acids in renal brush border vesicles. *Science* 1977;197:169–171.
14. Völkl H, Silbernagl S. Reexamination of the interplay between dibasic amino acids and L-cystine/L-cysteine during tubular reabsorption. *Pflugers Arch* 1982;395:196–200.
15. Roigaard-Petersen H, Jacobsen C, Sheikh MI. Transport of L-proline by luminal membrane vesicles from pars recta of rabbit proximal tubule. *Am J Physiol* 1988;254:F628–F633.
16. Christensen HN. Role of amino acid transport and counter transport in nutrition and metabolism. *Physiol Rev* 1990;70:43–77.
17. Van Winkle LJ. Amino acid transport in developing animal oocytes and early conceptuses. *Biochim Biophys Acta* 1988;947:173–208.
18. Barker GA, Ellory JC. The identification of neutral amino acid transport systems. *Exp Physiol* 1990;75:3–26.
19. Palacin M, Estevez R, Bertran J, et al. Molecular biology of mammalian plasma membrane amino acid transporters. *Physiol Rev* 1998;78:969–1054.
20. Bröer S. Adaptation of plasma membrane amino acid transport mechanisms to physiological demands. *Pflügers Arch* 2002;444:457–466.
21. Rabito CA. Sodium cotransport processes in renal epithelial cell lines. *Miner Electrol Metab* 1986;12:32–41.
22. Chesney RW, Jones D, Zelikovic I. Renal amino acid transport: cellular and molecular events from clearance studies to frog eggs. *Pediatr Nephrol* 1993;7:574–584.
23. Chesney RW, Jolly K, Zelikovic I, et al. Increased Na^+-taurine symporter in rat renal brush border membranes: preformed or newly synthesized. *FASEB J* 1989;3:2081–2085.
24. Han X, Budreau AM, Chesney RW. Functional expression of rat renal cortex taurine transporter in *Xenopus laevis* oocytes: adaptive regulation by dietary manipulation. *Pediatr Res* 1997;41:624–631.
25. Chamberlin ME, Strange K. Anisosmotic cell volume regulation: a comparative view. *Am J Physiol* 1989;257:C159–C173.
26. Garcia-Perez A, Burg MB. Renal medullary organic osmolytes. *Physiol Rev* 1991;71:1081–1115.
27. Law RO. Amino acids as volume regulatory osmolytes in mammalian cells. *Comp Biochem Physiol* 1991;99A:263–277.
28. McGivan JD, Nicholson B. Regulation of high-affinity glutamate transport by amino acid deprivation and hyperosmotic stress. *Am J Physiol* 1999;277:F498–F500.
29. Uchida S, Nakanishi T, Moo Kwon H, et al. Taurine behaves as an osmolyte in Madin-Darby canine kidney cells. *J Clin Invest* 1991;88:656–662.
30. Uchida S, Kwon M, Preston A, et al. Expression of MDCK cell Na^+ and Cl^--dependent taurine transporter in *Xenopus laevis* oocytes. *J Biol Chem* 1991;266:9605–9609.
31. Nishizuka Y. The molecular heterogeneity of protein kinase C and its implication for cellular regulation. *Nature* 1988;334:661–665.
32. Zelikovic I, Przekwas J. The role of protein phosphorylation in renal amino acid transport. *Pediatr Nephrol* 1993;7:621–629.
33. Zelikovic I, Przekwas J. Ca^{++}-dependent protein kinases inhibit proline transport across the rat renal brush border membrane. *Am J Physiol* 1995;268:F155–F162.
34. Zelikovic I, Wager-Miller J. Regulation of proline transport in MDCK cells expressing a mutant regulatory subunit of cAMP-dependent protein kinase. *Mol Genet Metab* 2001;72:45;53.
35. Zelikovic I, Wager-Miller J. cAMP-dependent protein kinase inhibits proline transport across the rat renal tubular brush border membrane. *Biosci Rep* 2001;21:613–626.
36. Radian R, Bendahan A, Kanner BI. Purification and identification of the functional sodium- and chloride-coupled γ-aminobutyric acid transport glycoprotein from rat brain. *J Biol Chem* 1986;261:15437–15441.
37. Beliveau R, Demeule M, Jette M, et al. Molecular sizes of amino acid transporters in the luminal membrane from the kidney cortex, estimated by the radiation-inactivation method. *Biochem J* 1990;268:195–200.
38. Hediger MA, Coady MJ, Ikeda TS, et al. Expression cloning and cDNA sequencing of the Na^+/glucose cotransporter. *Nature* 1987;330:379–381.
39. McGivan JD, Pastor-Anglada M. Regulatory and molecular aspects of mammalian amino acid transport. *Biochem J* 1994;299:321–334.
40. Malandro MS, Kilberg MS. Molecular biology of mammalian amino acid transporters. *Annu Rev Biochem* 1996;65:305–336.
41. Guastella J, Nelson N, Nelson H, et al. Cloning and expression of a rat brain GABA transporter. *Science* 1990;249:1303–1306.
42. Liu QR, Lopez-Coprcuera B, Nelson H, et al. Cloning and expression of a cDNA encoding the transporter of taurine

and β-alanine in mouse brain. *Proc Natl Acad Sci U S A* 1992;89:12145–12149.
43. Guastella J, Brecha N, Weigmann C, et al. Cloning, expression, and localization of a rat brain high affinity glycine transporter. *Proc Natl Acad Sci U S A* 1992;89:7189–7193.
44. Fremeau RT, Caron MG, Blakely RD. Molecular cloning and expression of a high affinity L-proline transporter expressed in putative glutamatergic pathways of rat brain. *Neuron* 1992;8:915–926.
45. Uchida S, Kwon HM, Yamauchi A, et al. Molecular cloning of the cDNA for an MDCK cell Na^+- and Cl^--dependent taurine transporter that is regulated by hypertonicity. *Proc Natl Acad Sci U S A* 1992;89:8230–8234.
46. Liu QR, Lopez-Corcuera B, Mandiyan S, et al. Molecular characterization of four pharmacologically distinct γ-aminobutyric acid transporters in mouse brain. *J Biol Chem* 1993;268:2106–2112.
47. Plotkin M, Kojima R, Gullans SR. Colocalization of GABA transporter and receptor in rat kidney. *J Am Soc Nephrol* 1994; 5:318.
48. Liu QR, Lopez-Corcuera B, Mandiyan S, et al. Cloning and expression of a spinal cord-and brain-specific glycine transporter with novel structural features. *J Biol Chem* 1993; 268:22802–22808.
49. Kim KM, Kingsmore SF, Han H, et al. Cloning of the human glycine transporter type 1: molecular and pharmacological characterization of novel isoform variants and chromosomal localization of the gene in the human and mouse genomes. *Mol Pharmacol* 1994;45:608–617.
50. Plotkin M, Tang SS, Ingelfinger J, et al. GLYT2 glycine transporter expression and regulation in rat kidney and brain. *J Am Soc Nephrol* 1994;5:318.
51. Wright EM, Hager KM, Turk E. Sodium cotransport proteins. *Curr Opin Cell Biol* 1992;4:696–702.
52. Storck T, Schulte S, Hofmann K, et al. Structure, expression, and functional analysis of a Na^+-dependent glutamate/aspartate transporter from rat brain. *Proc Natl Acad Sci U S A* 1992;89:10955–10959.
53. Pines G, Danbolt NC, Bjoras M, et al. Cloning and expression of a rat brain L-glutamate transporter. *Nature* 1992;360:464–467.
54. Kanai Y, Hediger MA. Primary structure and functional characterization of a high affinity glutamate transporter. *Nature* 1992;360:467–471.
55. Fairman WA, Vandenberg RJ, Arriza JL, et al. An excitatory amino-acid transporter with properties of a ligand-gated chloride channel. *Nature* 1995;375:599–603.
56. Arriza JL, Eliasof S, Kavanaugh MP, et al. Excitatory amino acid transporter 5, a retinal glutamate transporter coupled to a chloride conductance. *Proc Natl Acad Sci U S A* 1997;94: 4155–4160.
57. Shayakul C, Kanai Y, Lee WS, et al. Localization of the high-affinity glutamate transporter EAAC1 in rat kidney. *Am J Physiol* 1997;273:F1023–F1029.
58. Smith CP, Weremowicz S, Kanai Y, et al. Assignment of the gene coding for the human high-affinity glutamate transporter EAAC1 to 9p24: potential role in dicarboxylic aminoaciduria and neurodegenerative disorders. *Genomics* 1994;20:335–336.
59. Arriza JL, Kavanaugh MP, Fairman WA, et al. Cloning and expression of a human neutral amino acid transporter with structural similarity to the glutamate transporter gene family. *J Biol Chem* 1993;268:15329–15332.
60. Utsunomiya-Tate N, Endou H, Kanai Y. Cloning and functional characterization of a system ASC-like Na^+-dependent neutral amino acid transporter. *J Biol Chem* 1996;271:14883–14890.
61. Kekuda R, Prasad PD, Fei YJ, et al. Cloning of the sodium-dependent, broad-scope, neutral amino acid transporter B^o from a human placental choriocarcinoma cell line. *J Biol Chem* 1996;271:18657–18661.
62. Fairman WA, Vandenberg RJ, Arriza JL, et al. An excitatory amino-acid transporter with properties of a ligand-gated chloride channel. *Nature* 1995;375:599–603.
63. Zerangue N, Kavanaugh MP. ASCT-1 is a neutral amino acid exchanger with chloride channel activity. *J Biol Chem* 1996;271:27991–27994.
64. Kekuda R, Torres-Zamorano V, Fei YJ, et al. Molecular and functional characterization of intestinal Na^+-dependent neutral amino acid transporter B^0. *Am J Physiol* 1997;272:G1463–G1472.
65. Kim JW, Closs EI, Albritton LM, et al. Transport of cationic amino acids by the mouse ecotropic retrovirus receptor. *Nature* 1991;352:725–728.
66. Wang H, Kavanaugh MP, North RA, et al. Cell-surface receptor for ecotropic murine retroviruses is a basic amino-acid transporter. *Nature* 1991;352:729–731.
67. Finley KD, Kakuda DK, Barrieux A, et al. A mammalian arginine/lysine transporter uses multiple promoters. *Proc Natl Acad Sci U S A* 1995;92:9378–9382.
68. Burger-Kentischer A, Muller E, Klein HG, et al. Cationic amino acid transporter mRNA expression in rat kidney and liver. *Kidney Int* 1998;67:S136–S138.
69. Kavanaugh MP. Voltage dependence of facilitated arginine flux mediated by the system y^+ basic amino acid transporter. *Biochemistry* 1993;32:5781–5785.
70. Stevens BR, Kakuda DK, Yu K, et al. Induced nitric oxide synthesis is dependent on induced alternatively spliced CAT-2 encoding L-arginine transport in brain astrocytes. *J Biol Chem* 1996;271:24017–24022.
71. McNamara PD, Rea CT, Segal S. Expression of rat jejunal cystine carrier in *Xenopus* oocytes. *J Biol Chem* 1991;266:986–989.
72. Coady MJ, Pajor AM, Toloza EM, et al. Expression of mammalian renal transporters in *Xenopus laevis* oocytes. *Arch Biochem Biophys* 1990;283:130–134.
73. Aoshima H, Tomita K, Sugio S. Expression of amino acid transport systems in *Xenopus* oocytes injected with mRNA of rat small intestine and kidney. *Arch Biochem Biophys* 1990;283:130–134.
74. Bertran J, Werner A, Stange G, et al. Expression of Na^+-independent amino acid transport in *Xenopus laevis* oocytes by injection of rabbit kidney cortex mRNA. *Biochem J* 1992;281:717–723.
75. Bertran J, Werner A, Moore ML, et al. Expression cloning of a cDNA from rabbit kidney cortex that induces a single transport system for cystine and dibasic and neutral amino acids. *Proc Natl Acad Sci U S A* 1992;89:5601–5605.
76. Wells RG, Hediger MA. Cloning of a rat kidney cDNA that stimulates dibasic and neutral amino acid transport and has sequence similarity to glucosidases. *Proc Natl Acad Sci U S A* 1992;89:5596–5600.

77. Bertran J, Magagnin S, Werner A, et al. Stimulation of system y^{+}-like amino acid transport by the heavy chain of human 4F2 surface antigen in *Xenopus laevis* oocytes. *Proc Natl Acad Sci U S A* 1992;89:5606–5610.
78. Mosckovitz R, Udenfriend S, Felix A, et al. Membrane topology of the rat kidney neutral and basic amino acid transporter. *FASEB J* 1994;8:1069–1074.
79. Yan N, Mosckovitz R, Gerber LD, et al. Characterization of the promoter region of the gene for the rat neutral and basic amino acid transporter and chromosomal localization of the human gene. *Proc Natl Acad Sci U S A* 1994;91:7548–7552.
80. Lee WS, Wells RG, Sabbag RV, et al. Cloning and chromosomal localization of a human kidney cDNA involved in cystine, dibasic, and neutral amino acid transport. *J Clin Invest* 1993;91:1959–1963.
81. Kanai Y, Stelzner MG, Lee WS, et al. Expression of mRNA (D2) encoding a protein involved in amino acid transport in S3 proximal tubule. *Am J Physiol* 1992;263:F1087–F1093.
82. Pickel VM, Nirenberg MJ, Chan J, et al. Ultrastructural localization of a neutral and basic amino acid transporter in rat kidney and intestine. *Proc Natl Acad Sci U S A* 1993;90:7779–7783.
83. Verrey F, Jack DL, Paulsen IT, et al. New glycoprotein-associated amino acid transporters. *J Membr Biol* 1999;172: 181–192.
84. Palacin M, Bertran J, Zorzano A. Heteromeric amino acid transporters explain inherited aminoacidurias. *Curr Opin Nephrol Hypertens* 2000;9:547–553.
85. Chillaron J, Roca R, Valencia A, et al. Heteromeric amino acid transporters: biochemistry, genetics, and physiology. *Am J Physiol* 2001;281:F995–F1018.
86. Wagner CA, Lang F, Bröer S. Function and structure of heterodimeric amino acid transporters. *Am J Physiol* 2001;281: C1077–C1093.
87. Torrents D, Estevez R, Pineda M, et al. Identification and characterization of a membrane protein (y^{+}L amino acid transporter-1) that associates with 4F2hc to encode the amino acid transport activity y^{+}L. A candidate gene for lysinuric protein intolerance. *J Biol Chem* 1998;273:32437–32445.
88. Feliubadalo L, Font M, Purroy J, et al. Non-type I cystinuria caused by mutations in SLC7A9, encoding a subunit ($b^{o,+}$AT) of rBAT. *Nat Genet* 1999;23:52–57.
89. Chairoungdua A, Segawa H, Kim JY, et al. Identification of an amino acid transporter associated with the cystinuria-related type II membrane glycoprotein. *J Biol Chem* 1999;274:28845–28848.
90. Busch AE, Herzer T, Waldegger S, et al. Opposite directed currents induced by the transport of dibasic and neutral amino acids in *Xenopus* oocytes expressing the protein rBAT. *J Biol Chem* 1994;269:25581–25586.
91. Chillaron J, Estevez R, Mora C, et al. Obligatory amino acid exchange via systems $b^{0,+}$-like and y^{+} L-like. A tertiary active transport mechanism for renal reabsorption of cystine and dibasic amino acids. *J Biol Chem* 1996;271:17761–17770.
92. Brodehl J, Gellissen K. Endogenous renal transport of free amino acids in infancy and childhood. *Pediatrics* 1968;42:395–404.
93. Zelikovic I, Chesney RW, Friedman AL, et al. Taurine depletion in very low birth weight infants receiving prolonged total parenteral nutrition: role of renal immaturity. *J Pediatr* 1990;116:301–306.
94. Lasley L, Scriver CR. Ontogeny of amino acid reabsorption in human kidney. Evidence for the homozygous infant with familial renal iminoglycinuria for multiple proline and glycine systems. *Pediatr Res* 1979;13:65–70.
95. Mandla S, Scriver CR, Tenenhouse HS. Decreased transport in renal basolateral membrane vesicles from hypertaurinuric mice. *Am J Physiol* 1988;255:F88–F95.
96. Chesney RW, Gusowski N, Zelikovic I, et al. Developmental aspects of renal β amino acid transport. V. Brush border membrane transport in nursing animals: effect of age and diet. *Pediatr Res* 1986;20:890–894.
97. Medow MS, Roth KS, Goldmann DR, et al. Developmental aspects of proline transport in rat renal brush border membranes. *Proc Natl Acad Sci U S A* 1986;7561–7564.
98. Foreman JW, Medow MS, Bovee KC, et al. Developmental aspects of cystine transport in the dog. *Pediatr Res* 1986;20:593–597.
99. Zelikovic I, Stejskal E, Lohstroh P, et al. Developmental maturation of Na^{+}-H^{+} exchange in rat renal tubular brush-border membrane. *Am J Physiol* 1991;261:F1017–F1025.
100. Schwartz GJ, Evan AP. Development of solute transport in rabbit proximal tubule. III. Na-K-ATPase activity. *Am J Physiol* 1984;246:F845–F852.
101. Mendez CF, Hansson A, Skoglund G, et al. Protein kinase C activity in rat renal proximal tubule cells. *Acta Physiol Scand* 1992;146:135–140.
102. Palacin M, Goodyer P, Nunes V, et al. Cystinuria. In: Scriver CR, Beaudet AL, Sly WS, et al., eds. *The metabolic and molecular bases of inherited disease.* New York: McGraw-Hill, 2001:4909–4932.
103. Singer A, Das S. Cystinuria: a review of the pathophysiology and management. *J Urol* 1989;142:669–673.
104. Milliner DS. Cystinuria. *Endocrinol Metab Clin North Am* 1990;19:889–907.
105. Wollaston WH. On cystic oxide. A new species of urinary calculus. *Trans R Soc Lond* 1810;100:223–230.
106. Berzelius D. Calculus urinaries. *Trait Chem* 1833;7:424.
107. Garrod AE. The Croonian lectures on inborn errors of metabolism. *Lancet* 1908;2:1, 73, 142, 214.
108. Dent CE, Rose GA. Amino acid metabolism in cystinuria. *QJM* 1951;20:205–218.
109. Frimpter GW, Horwith M, Furth E, et al. Inulin and endogenous amino acid renal clearances in cystinuria: evidence for tubular secretion. *J Clin Invest* 1962;41:281–288.
110. Kato T. Renal handling of dibasic amino acids and cystine in cystinuria. *Clin Sci Mol Med* 1977;53:9–15.
111. Robson EB, Rose GA. The effect of intravenous lysine on the renal clearances of cystine, arginine and ornithine in normal subjects, in patients with cystinuria and their relatives. *Clin Sci* 1957;16:75–91.
112. Fox M, Thier S, Rosenberg L, et al. Evidence against a single renal transport defect in cystinuria. *N Engl J Med* 1964; 270:556–561.
113. Brodehl J, Gellissen K, Kowalewski S. Isolierter Defekt der tubulren Cystinrckresorption in einer Familie mit idiopathischem Hypoparathroidismus. *Klin Wochenschr* 1967; 45:38–40.

114. Whelan DT, Scriver CR. Hyperdibasicaminoaciduria: an inherited disorder of amino acid transport. *Pediatr Res* 1968;2:525–534.
115. Omura K, Yamanaka N, Higami S, et al. Lysine malabsorption syndrome: a new type of transport defect. *Pediatrics* 1976;57:102–105.
116. Scriver CR, Clow L, Reade TM, et al. Ontogeny modifies manifestations of cystinuria genes: implications for counseling. *J Pediatr* 1985;106:411–416.
117. Foreman JW, Hwang SM, Segal L. Transport interactions of cystine and dibasic amino acids in isolated rat renal tubules. *Metabolism* 1980;29:53–61.
118. Weinberger A, Sperling O, Rabinovitz M, et al. High frequency of cystinuria among Jews of Libyan origin. *Hum Hered* 1974;24:568–572.
119. Rosenberg LE, Downing S, Durant JL, et al. Cystinuria: biochemical evidence of three genetically distinct diseases. *J Clin Invest* 1966;45:365–371.
120. Goodyer PR, Clow C, Reade T, et al. Prospective analysis and classification of patients with cystinuria identified in a newborn screening program. *J Pediatr* 1993;122:568–572.
121. Pras E, Arber N, Aksentijevich I, et al. Localization of a gene causing cystinuria to chromosome 2p. *Nat Genet* 1994;6:415–419.
122. Calonge MJ, Gasparini P, Chillaron J, et al. Cystinuria caused by mutations in rBAT, a gene involved in the transport of cystine. *Nat Genet* 1994;6:420–425.
123. Gasparini P, Calonge MJ, Bisceglia L, et al. Molecular genetics of cystinuria: identification of four new mutations and seven polymorphisms, and evidence for genetic heterogeneity. *Am J Hum Genet* 1995;57:781–788.
124. Pras E, Raben N, Golomb E, et al. Mutations in the SLC3A1 transporter gene in cystinuria. *Am J Hum Genet* 1995;56:1297–1303.
125. Horsford J, Saadi I, Raelson J, et al. Molecular genetics of cystinuria in French Canadians: identification of four novel mutations in type I patients. *Kidney Int* 1996;49:1401–1406.
126. Palacin M, Borsani G, Sebastio G. The molecular bases of cystinuria and lysinuric protein intolerance. *Curr Opin Genet Dev* 2001;11:328–335.
127. Chillaron J, Estevez R, Samarzija I, et al. An intracellular trafficking defect in type I cystinuria rBAT mutants M467T and M467K. *J Biol Chem* 1997;272:9543–9549.
128. Zelikovic I. Molecular pathophysiology of tubular transport disorders. *Pediatr Nephrol* 2001;16:919–935.
129. Saadi I, Chen XZ, Hediger M, et al. Molecular genetics of cystinuria: mutation analysis of SLC3A1 and evidence for another gene in type I (silent) phenotype. *Kidney Int* 1998;54:48–55.
130. Calonge MJ, Volpini V, Bisceglia L, et al. Genetic heterogeneity in cystinuria: the SLC3A1 gene is linked to type I but not to type III cystinuria. *Proc Natl Acad Sci U S A* 1995;92:9667–9671.
131. Wartenfeld R, Golomb E, Katz G, et al. Molecular analysis of cystinuria in Libyan Jews: exclusion of the SLC3A1 gene and mapping of a new locus on 19q. *Am J Hum Genet* 1997;60:617–624.
132. Bisceglia L, Calonge MJ, Totaro A, et al. Localization, by linkage analysis, of the cystinuria type III gene to chromosome 19q13.1. *Am J Hum Genet* 1997;60:611–616.
133. International Cystinuria Consortium. Non-type I cystinuria caused by mutations in SLC7A9, encoding a subunit ($b^{o,+}$AT) of rBAT. *Nat Genet* 1999;23:52–57.
134. International Cystinuria Consortium. Functional analysis of mutations in SLC7A9, and genotype-phenotype correlation in non-type I cystinuria. *Hum Mol Genet* 2001;10:305–316.
135. Dello Strologo L, Pras E, Pontesilli C, et al. Comparison between SLC3A1 and SLC7A9 cystinuria patients and carriers: a need for a new classification. *J Am Soc Nephrol* 2002;13:2547–2553.
136. Evans WP, Resnick MI, Boyce WH. Homozygous cystinuria: evaluation of 35 patients. *J Urol* 1982;127:707–709.
137. Smith A, Wilcken B. Homozygous cystinuria in New South Wales: a study of 110 individuals with cystinuria ascertained by methods other than neonatal screening. *Med J Aust* 1984;141:500–502.
138. Kelly S, Nolan EP. Postscript on excretion rates in posttransplant cystinuric patient. *JAMA* 1980;243:1897.
139. Krizek V, Erben J, Lazne M, et al. Disappearance of cystinuria after kidney transplantation. *Br J Urol* 1983;55:575.
140. Jaeger P, Portmann L, Saunders A, et al. Anticystinuric effects of glutamine and of dietary sodium restriction. *N Engl J Med* 1986;315:1120–1123.
141. Norman RW, Manetta WA. Dietary restriction of sodium as a means of reducing urinary cystine. *J Urol* 1990;1143:1193–1195.
142. Miyagi K, Nakada F, Ohshiro S. Effect of glutamine on cystine excretion in a patient with cystinuria. *N Engl J Med* 1979;301:196–198.
143. Skovby F, Rosenberg LE, Thier SO. No effect of L-glutamine on cystinuria. *N Engl J Med* 1980;302:236–237.
144. Halperin EC, Thier SO, Rosenberg LE. The use of D-penicillamine in cystinuria: efficacy and untoward reactions. *Yale J Biol Med* 1981;54:439–446.
145. Jaffe IA. Adverse effects profile of sulfhydryl compounds in man. *Am J Med* 1986;80:471–476.
146. Pak CYC, Fuller C, Sakhaee K, et al. Management of cystine nephrolithiasis with alpha-mercaptopropionylglycine. *J Urol* 1986;136:1003–1008.
147. Jaeger P. Cystinuria: pathophysiology and treatment. *Adv Nephrol* 1989;18:107–112.
148. Sloand JA, Izzo JL. Captopril reduces urinary cystine excretion in cystinuria. *Arch Intern Med* 1987;147:1409–1412.
149. Sandroni S, Stevens P, Barraza M, et al. Captopril therapy of recurrent nephrolithiasis in a child with cystinuria. *Child Nephrol Urol* 1988–89;9:347–348.
150. Coulthard M, Richardson J, Fleetwood A. Captopril is not clinically useful in reducing the cystine load in cystinuria or cystinosis. *Pediatr Nephrol* 1991;5:98.
151. Maiorino RM, Bruce DC, Aposhian HV. Determination and metabolism of dithiol chelating agents. VI. Isolation and identification of the mixed disulfides of meso-2,3-dimercaptosuccinic acid with L-cysteine in human urine. *Toxicol Appl Pharmacol* 1989;97:338–349.
152. Martin X, Salas M, Labeeuw M, et al. Cystine stones: the impact of new treatment. *Br J Urol* 1991;68:234–239.
153. Knoll LD, Segura JW, Patterson DE, et al. Long-term followup in patients with cystine urinary calculi treated by percutaneous ultrasonic lithotripsy. *J Urol* 1988;140:246–248.

154. Holtzapple PG, Bovee K, Rea CF, et al. Amino acid uptake by kidney and jejunal tissue from dogs with cystine stones. *Science* 1969;166:1525–1527.
155. Norio R, Perheentupa J, Kekomaki M, et al. Lysinuric protein intolerance, an autosomal recessive disease: a genetic study of 10 Finnish families. *Clin Genet* 1971;2:214–222.
156. Rajantie J, Simell O, Perheentupa J. Intestinal absorption in lysinuric protein intolerance: impaired for diamino acids, normal for citrulline. *Gut* 1980;21:519–524.
157. Simell O. Lysinuric protein intolerance and other cationic aminoacidurias. In: Scriver CR, Beaudet AL, Sly WS, et al., eds. *The metabolic and molecular bases of inherited disease.* New York: McGraw-Hill, 2001:4933–4956.
158. Desjeux JF, Rajantie J, Simell O, et al. Lysine fluxes across the jejunal epithelium in lysinuric protein intolerance. *J Clin Invest* 1980;65:1382–1387.
159. Rajantie J, Simell O, Perheentupa J. Lysinuric protein intolerance. Basolateral transport defect in renal tubuli. *J Clin Invest* 1981;67:1078–1082.
160. Simell O. Diamino acid transport into granulocytes and liver slices of patients with lysinuric protein intolerance. *Pediatr Res* 1975;9:504–508.
161. Smith DW, Scriver CR, Tenenhouse HS, et al. Lysinuric protein intolerance mutation is expressed in the plasma membrane of cultured skin fibroblasts. *Proc Natl Acad Sci U S A* 1987;84:7711–7715.
162. Smith DW, Scriver CR, Simell O. Lysinuric protein intolerance mutation is not expressed in the plasma membrane of erythrocytes. *Hum Genet* 1988;80:395–396.
163. Estevez R, Camps M, Rojas AM, et al. The amino acid transport system y+L/4F2hc is a heteromultimeric complex. *FASEB J* 1998;12:1319–1329.
164. Borsani G, Bassi MT, Sperandeo MP, et al. SLC7A7, encoding a putative permease-related protein, is mutated in patients with lysinuric protein intolerance. *Nat Genet* 1999;21:297–301.
165. Lauteala T, Sistonen P, Savontaus ML, et al. Lysinuric protein intolerance (LPI) gene maps to the long arm of chromosome 14. *Am J Hum Genet* 1997;60:1479–1486.
166. Lauteala T, Mykkanen J, Sperandeo MP, et al. Genetic homogeneity of lysinuric protein intolerance. *Eur J Hum Genet* 1998;6:612–615.
167. Torrents D, Mykkanen J, Pineda M, et al. Identification of SLC7A7, encoding $y^{+}LAT^{-1}$, as the lysinuric protein intolerance gene. *Nat Genet* 1999;21:293–296.
168. Mykkanen J, Torrents D, Pineda M, et al. Functional analysis of novel mutations in y^{+}LAT-1 amino acid transporter gene causing lysinuric protein intolerance (LPI). *Hum Mol Genet* 2000;9:431–438.
169. Sperandeo MP, Bassi MT, Riboni M, et al. Structure of the SLC7A7 gene and mutational analysis of patients affected by lysinuric protein intolerance. *Am J Hum Genet* 2000;66:92–99.
170. Rajantie J, Simell O, Rapola J, et al. Lysinuric protein intolerance: a two year trial of dietary supplementation therapy with citrulline and lysine. *J Pediatr* 1980;97:927–932.
171. Kihara H, Valente M, Porter MT, et al. Hyperdibasicaminoaciduria in a mentally retarded homozygote with a peculiar response to phenothiazines. *Pediatrics* 1978;51:223–229.
172. Dirckx JH. Julius Caesar and the Julian emperors: a family cluster with Hartnup disease? *Am J Dermatopathol* 1986;8:351–357.
173. Baron DN, Dent CE, Harris H, et al. Hereditary pellagra-like skin rash with temporary cerebellar ataxia, constant renal aminoaciduria and other bizarre biochemical features. *Lancet* 1956;1:421–428.
174. Levy HL. Hartnup disorder. In: Scriver CR, Beaudet AL, Sly WS, et al., eds. *The metabolic and molecular bases of inherited disease.* New York: McGraw-Hill, 2001:4957–4969.
175. Milne MD, Crawford MA, Girao CB, et al. The metabolic disorder in Hartnup disease. *QJM* 1960;29:407–421.
176. Shih VE, Bixby EM, Alpers DH, et al. Studies of intestinal transport defect in Hartnup disease. *Gastroenterology* 1971;61:445–453.
177. Asatoor AM, Cheng B, Edwards KDG, et al. Intestinal absorption of two dipeptides in Hartnup disease. *Gut* 1970;11:380–387.
178. Mahon BE, Levy HL. Maternal Hartnup disorder. *Am J Med Genet* 1986;24:513–518.
179. Scriver CR, Mahon B, Levy H, et al. The Hartnup phenotype: mendelian transport disorder, multifactorial disease. *Am J Hum Genet* 1987;40:401–412.
180. Halvorsen K, Halvorsen S. Hartnup disease. *Pediatrics* 1963;31:29–38.
181. Jonas AJ, Butler IJ. Circumvention of defective neutral amino acid transport in Hartnup disease using tryptophan ethyl ester. *J Clin Invest* 1989;84:200–204.
182. Smith AJ, Strang LB. An inborn error of metabolism with the urinary excretion of α-hydroxybutyric acid and phenylpyruvic acid. *Arch Dis Child* 1958;33:109–113.
183. Hooft C, Timmermans J, Snoeck J, et al. Methionine malabsorption syndrome. *Ann Pediatr* 1965;205:73–84.
184. Sabater J, Ferre C, Puliol M, et al. Histidinuria: a renal and intestinal histidine transport deficiency found in two mentally retarded children. *Clin Genet* 1976;9:117–124.
185. Holmgren G, Hambraeus L, De Chateau P. Histidinemia and "normohistidinemic histidinuria": report of three cases and the effect of different protein intakes on urinary excretion of histidine. *Acta Paediatr Scand* 1974;63:220–224.
186. Kamoun PP, Parvy P, Chathelineau L, et al. Renal histidinuria. *J Inherited Metab Dis* 1981;4:217–219.
187. Chesney RW. Iminoglycinuria. In: Scriver CR, Beaudet AL, Sly WS, et al., eds. *The metabolic and molecular bases of inherited disease.* New York: McGraw-Hill, 2001:4971–4981.
188. Turner B, Brown DA. Amino acid excretion in infancy and early childhood. A survey of 200,000 infants. *Med J Aust* 1972;1:62–65.
189. Scriver CR. Renal tubular transport of proline, hydroxyproline and glycine. III. Genetic basis for more than one mode of transport in human kidney. *J Clin Invest* 1968;47:823–835.
190. Greene ML, Lietman PS, Rosenberg LE, et al. Familial hyperglycinuria: new defect in renal tubular transport of glycine and imino acids. *Am J Med* 1973;54:265–271.
191. deVries A, Kochwa S, Lazebnik J, et al. Glycinuria, a hereditary disorder associated with nephrolithiasis. *Am J Med* 1957;23:408–415.
192. Kaser H, Cottier P, Antener I. Glucoglycinuria, a new familial syndrome. *J Pediatr* 1962;61:386–394.

193. Tiejema HL, Van Gelderen HH, Giesberts MAH, et al. Dicarboxylic aminoaciduria: an inborn error of glutamate and aspartate transport with metabolic implications in combination with hyperprolinemia. *Metabolism* 1974;23:115–123.
194. Melancon SB, Dallaire L, Lemieux B, et al. Dicarboxylic aminoaciduria: an inborn error of amino acid conservation. *J Pediatr* 1977;91:422–427.
195. Lemieux B, Aura-Blais C, Giguere R, et al. Newborn urine screening experience with over one million infants in the Quebec Network of Genetic Medicine. *J Inherited Metab Dis* 1988;11:45–55.
196. Peghini P, Janzen J, Stoffel W. Glutamate transporter EAAC-1–deficient mice develop dicarboxylic aminoaciduria and behavioral abnormalities but no neurodegeneration. *EMBO J* 1997;16:3822–3832.
197. Nozaki J, Dakeishi M, Ohura T, et al. Homozygosity mapping to chromosome 5p15 of a gene responsible for Hartnup disorder. *Biochem Biophys Res Commun* 2001;284:255–260.
198. Melancon SB, Grenier B, Dallaire L, et al. Dicarboxylic amino acid uptake in normal, Friedreich's ataxia, and dicarboxylic aminoaciduria fibroblasts. *J Can Sci Neurol* 1979;6:262–273.
199. Rozen R, Scriver CR, Mohyuddin F. Hypertaurinuria in the C57BL/6J mouse: altered transport at the renal basolateral membrane. *Am J Physiol* 1983;244:F150–F155.
200. Silverman M, Turner RJ. Glucose transport in the renal proximal tubule. In: Windhager EE, ed. *Handbook of physiology: renal physiology*. New York: Oxford University Press, 1992:2017–2038.
201. Sacktor B. Sodium-coupled hexose transport. *Kidney Int* 1989;36:342–350.
202. Smith HW, Goldring W, Chasis H, et al. The application of saturation methods to the study of glomerular and tubular functions in the human kidney. *J Mt Sinai Hosp* 1943;10:59–108.
203. Elsas LJ, Rosenberg LE. Familial renal glycosuria: a genetic reappraisal of hexose transport by kidney and intestine. *J Clin Invest* 1969;48:1845–1854.
204. Brodehl J, Franken A, Gellissen K. Maximal tubular reabsorption of glucose in infants and children. *Acta Paediatr Scand* 1972;61:413–420.
205. Tudvad F. Sugar reabsorption in prematures and full term babies. *Scand J Clin Lab Invest* 1949;1:281–283.
206. Barfuss DW, Schafer JA. Differences in active and passive glucose transport along the proximal nephron. *Am J Physiol* 1981;241:F322–F332.
207. Turner RJ, Moran A. Heterogeneity of sodium dependent D-glucose transport sites along the proximal tubule: evidence from vesicle studies. *Am J Physiol* 1982;242:F406–F414.
208. Turner RJ, Moran A. Stoichiometric studies of the renal cortical brush border membrane D-glucose transporter. *J Membr Biol* 1982;67:73–80.
209. Turner RJ, Moran A. Further studies of proximal tubular brush-border membrane. D-Glucose transport heterogeneity. *J Membr Biol* 1982;70:37–45.
210. Silverman M. Structure and function of hexose transporters. *Annu Rev Biochem* 1991;60:757–794.
211. Wright EM. Renal Na^+-glucose cotransporters. *Am J Physiol* 2001;280:F10–F18.
212. Hediger MA, Turk E, Wright EM. Homology of the human intestinal Na^+/glucose and *Escherichia coli* Na^+/proline cotransporters. *Proc Natl Acad Sci U S A* 1989;86:5748–5752.
213. Hirayama BA, Wong HC, Smith CD, et al. Intestinal and renal Na^+/glucose cotransporters share common structures. *Am J Physiol* 1991;261:C296–C304.
214. Hediger MA, Medlein J, Lee HS, et al. Biosynthesis of the cloned intestinal Na+/glucose cotransporter. *Biochim Biophys Acta* 1991;1064:360–364.
215. Lee WS, Kanai Y, Wells RG, et al. The high affinity Na^+/glucose cotransporter. Re-evaluation of function and distribution of expression. *J Biol Chem* 1994;269:12032–12039.
216. Ohta T, Isselbacher KJ, Rhoads DB. Regulation of glucose transporters and LLC-PK_1 cells: effects of D-glucose and monosaccharides. *Mol Cell Biol* 1990;10:6941–6499.
217. Hediger MA, Budard ML, Emanual BS, et al. Assignment of the human intestinal Na^+/glucose gene (SGLT 1) to the q11.2lqter regions of chromosome 22. *Genomics* 1989;4:297–300.
218. Hirsch JR, Loo DDF, Wright EM. Regulation of Na^+/glucose cotransporter expression by protein kinases in *Xenopus* laevis oocytes. *J Biol Chem* 1996;271:14740–14746.
219. Pajor AM, Hirayama BA, Wright EM. Molecular evidence for two renal Na^+/glucose cotransporters. *Biochim Biophys Acta* 1992;1106:216–220.
220. You G, Lee WS, Barros JG, et al. Molecular characteristics of Na^+-coupled glucose transporters in adult and embryonic rat kidney. *J Biol Chem* 1995;270:29365–29371.
221. Wells RG, Pajor AM, Kanai Y, et al. Cloning of a human kidney cDNA with similarity to the sodium-glucose cotransporter. *Am J Physiol* 1992;263:F459–F465.
222. Kanai Y, Lee WS, You G, et al. The human kidney low affinity Na^+/glucose cotransporter SGLT2, delineation of the major renal reabsorptive mechanism for D-glucose. *J Clin Invest* 1994;93:397–404.
223. Wells RG, Mohandas TK, Hediger MA. Localization of the Na^+/glucose cotransporter gene SGLT2 to human chromosome 16 close to the centromere. *Genomics* 1993;17:787–789.
224. Kong CT, Yet SF, Lever JE. Cloning and expression of a mammalian Na+/amino acid cotransporter with sequence similarity to Na+/glucose cotransporters. *J Biol Chem* 1993;268:1509–1512.
225. Mackenzie B, Panayotova-Heiermann M, Loo DD, et al. SAAT1 is a low affinity Na^+/glucose cotransporter and not an amino acid transporter. A reinterpretation. *J Biol Chem* 1994;269:22488–22491.
226. Thorens B. Facilitated glucose transporters in epithelial cells. *Annu Rev Physiol* 1993;55:591–608.
227. Mueckler M. Facilitative glucose transporters. *Eur J Biochem* 1994;219:713–725.
228. Longo N, Elsas LJ. Human glucose transporters. *Adv Pediatr* 1998;45:293–313.
229. Mueckler M, Caruso D, Baldwin SA, et al. Sequence and tissue distribution of a human glucose transporter. *Science* 1985;229:941–945.
230. Thorens B, Cheng ZQ, Brown D, et al. Liver glucose transporter: a basolateral protein in hepatocytes and intestine and kidney epithelial cells. *Am J Physiol* 1990;259:C279–C285.

231. Thorens B, Lodish HF, Brown D. Differential localization of two glucose transporter isoforms in kidney nephron. *Am J Physiol* 1990;259:C286–C295.
232. Takata K, Kasahara T, Kasahara M, et al. Localization of Na^+-dependent active type and erythrocyte/HepG2–type glucose transporters in rat kidney: immunofluorescence and immunogold study. *J Histochem Cytochem* 1991;39:287–298.
233. Kayano T, Burant CF, Fukumoto H, et al. Human facilitative transporters. *J Biol Chem* 1990;265:13276–13282.
234. Alexander DP, Nixon DA. Reabsorption of glucose, fructose and myoinositol by the foetal and post-natal sheep kidney. *J Physiol* 1963;167:480–486.
235. Foreman JW, Medow MS, Wald H, et al. Developmental aspects of sugar transport by isolated dog renal cortical tubules. *Pediatr Res* 1984;8:719–723.
236. Arant BS Jr. Developmental patterns of renal functional maturation compared in the human neonate. *J Pediatr* 1978;92:705–712.
237. Stonestreet BS, Rubin L, Pollak A, et al. Renal functions of low birth weight infants with hyperglycemia and glucosuria produced by glucose infusions. *Pediatrics* 1980;66:561–567.
238. Brodehl J, Oemar BS, Hoyer PF. Renal glucosuria. *Pediatr Nephrol* 1987;1:502–508.
239. Lelievre-Pegorier M, Geloso JP. Ontogeny of sugar transport in fetal rat kidney. *Biol Neonate* 1980;38:16–24.
240. Merlet-Benichou C, Pegorier M, Muffat-Joly M, et al. Functional and morphological patterns of renal maturation in the developing guinea pig. *Am J Physiol* 1981;241:F618–F624.
241. Roth KS, Hwang SM, Yudkoff M, et al. The ontogeny of sugar transport in kidney. *Pediatr Res* 1978;12:1127–1131.
242. Beck JC, Lipkowitz MS, Abramson RG. Characterization of the fetal glucose transporter in rabbit kidney. Comparison with the adult brush border electrogenic Na^+-glucose symporter. *J Clin Invest* 1988;82:379–387.
243. Peng H, Lever JE. Regulation of Na^+-coupled glucose transport in LLC-PK_1 cells. *J Biol Chem* 1995;270:23996–24003.
244. Shioda T, Ohta T, Isselbacher KJ, et al. Differentiation-dependent expression of the Na^+/glucose cotransporter (SGLT1) in LLC-PK_1 cells: role of protein kinase C activation and ongoing transcription. *Proc Natl Acad Sci U S A* 1994;91:11919–11923.
245. Chin E, Zhou J, Bondy C. Anatomical and developmental patterns of facilitative glucose transporter gene expression in the rat kidney. *J Clin Invest* 1993;91:1810–1815.
246. Wright E, Martin MG, Turk E,. Familial glucose-galactose malabsorption and hereditary glycosuria. In: Scriver CR, Beaudet AL, Sly WS, et al., eds. *The metabolic and molecular bases of inherited disease.* New York: McGraw-Hill, 2001: 4891–4908.
247. Elsas LJ, Busse D, Rosenberg LE. Autosomal recessive inheritance of renal glycosuria. *Metabolism* 1971;20:968–975.
248. Elsas LJ, Rosenberg LE. Familial renal glycosuria: a genetic reappraisal of hexose transport by kidney and intestine. *J Clin Invest* 1969;48:1845–1854.
249. Elsas LJ, Longo N. Glucose transporters. *Annu Rev Med* 1992;43:377–393.
250. Woolf LI, Goodwin BL, Phelps CE. Tm-limited renal tubular reabsorption and the genetics of renal glucosuria. *J Theor Biol* 1966;11:10–21.
251. Oemar BS, Byrd DJ, Brodehl J. Complete absence of tubular glucose reabsorption: a new type of renal glucosuria (type 0). *Clin Nephrol* 1987;27:156–160.
252. Elsas LJ, Hillman RE, Patterson JH, et al. Renal and intestinal hexose transport in familial glucose-galactose malabsorption. *J Clin Invest* 1970;49:576–585.
253. Turk E, Zabel B, Mundlos S, et al. Glucose/galactose malabsorption caused by a defect in the Na^+/glucose cotransporter. *Nature* 1991;350:354–356.
254. Manz F, Bickel H, Brodehl J, et al. Fanconi-Bickel syndrome. *Pediatr Nephrol* 1987;1:509–518.
255. Santer R, Schneppenheim R, Dombrowski A, et al. Mutations in GLUT2, the gene for the liver-type glucose transporter, in patients with Fanconi-Bickel syndrome. *Nat Genet* 1997;17:324–326.
256. Guillam MT, Hummler E, Schaerer E, et al. Early diabetes and abnormal postnatal pancreatic islet development in mice lacking Glut-2. *Nat Genet* 1997;17:327–330.

38

TUBULAR DISORDERS OF ELECTROLYTE REGULATION

JUAN RODRÍGUEZ-SORIANO

HYPOKALEMIC STATES

Hypokalemia may be due to a great number of causes, including inadequate dietary intake; increased losses by the gastrointestinal tract, skin, or kidney; and abnormal distribution of K in the body (see Chapter 8). In this section we discuss only the renal tubular disorders in which hypokalemia constitutes a prominent biochemical feature, as occurs in Bartter's and Gitelman's syndromes and in states of pseudohyperaldosteronism. For description of other hypokalemic tubulopathies, such as renal tubular acidosis or Fanconi's syndrome, the reader is referred to Chapters 39 and 42, respectively.

Bartter's-Like Syndromes

In 1962, Bartter and coworkers (1) reported two patients presenting with a new syndrome characterized by hypokalemia, metabolic alkalosis, hyperaldosteronism with normal blood pressure, decreased pressor responsiveness to infused angiotensin II, and hyperplasia of the juxtaglomerular complex. Since then, many reports, both in children and in adults, have appeared in the literature under the heading of Bartter's syndrome. It is now evident that this term encompasses a variety of inherited disorders of renal tubular transport that are characterized by a biochemical picture of hypokalemia, hypochloremia, metabolic alkalosis, hyperreninemia, normal blood pressure, and increased urinary excretion of Na, Cl, and K. Thus, the term *Bartter's-like syndromes* better defines this ensemble of closely related tubular disorders.

At the present time, patients with Bartter's-like syndromes can be divided into three different genetic and clinical entities (2–6): (a) neonatal Bartter's syndrome, (b) classic Bartter's syndrome, and (c) Gitelman's syndrome. Obviously, this classification may require modification in the future as new mutations are described and genotypic-phenotypic correlations are better known.

Neonatal Bartter's Syndrome

Genetics

The known appearance in the same sibship, with apparent normality of the parents and equal incidence in both sexes, points to an autosomal recessive inheritance. Recent findings have established the genetic heterogeneity of neonatal Bartter's syndrome (Table 38.1). In so-called type 1, frame shift, nonsense, and missense mutations in the gene locus SLC12A1 have been found (7–9). Probably these mutations are quite rare in the population because almost all patients studied to date are homozygous for an identical disease mutation in both chromosomes, as a consequence of parental consanguinity (7). The gene, located on 15q15-q21 and containing 26 exons, encodes the renal bumetanide-sensitive Na-K-2Cl cotransporter (also termed NKCC2) of the thick ascending limb of the loop of Henle.

Frame shift, nonsense, and missense mutations in the ROMK gene (locus symbol KCNJ1) have been demonstrated in patients affected with type 2 of the neonatal form (10–14). This gene, located on chromosome 11q24, encodes an adenosine triphosphate (ATP)-sensitive, inwardly rectifying K channel (ROMK) that recycles reabsorbed K back to the tubular lumen. There are 5 exons that are used in varying combinations to produce three isoforms of ROMK proteins that share a core of 372 amino acids encoded by exon 5. Most of the mutations causing neonatal Bartter's syndrome are located in this common exon 5 and disrupt an arginine-lysine-arginine triad necessary for the normal pH gating of the K_{ir} channels (15). However, there are reports showing that homozygous deletions removing exons 1 and 2 also result in neonatal Bartter's syndrome (13,16).

In some families, mutations in genes coding for NKCC2 or ROMK have not been found, reflecting further genetic heterogeneity. In fact, mutations in a third gene have been recently identified as a cause of a peculiar type of neonatal Bartter's syndrome that is associated with neurosensorial deafness and early chronic renal insufficiency (17). This gene, called BSND, is localized on 1p32.3 and is formed by

TABLE 38.1. GENETICS OF INHERITED DISORDERS OF ELECTROLYTE TRANSPORT

Inherited disorder	Type of inheritance	Gene localization	Gene symbol	Gene product
Neonatal Bartter's syndrome (type 1)	AR	15q15-21	SLC12A1	NKCC2
Neonatal Bartter's syndrome (type 2)	AR	11q24	KCNJ1	ROMK
Neonatal Bartter's syndrome with neurosensorial deafness (type 4)	AR	1p32.3	BSND	Barttin
Classic Bartter's syndrome (type 3)	AR	1p36	CLCNKB	ClC-Kb
Gitelman's syndrome	AR	16q13	SLC12A3	NCCT
Glucocorticoid-remediable aldosteronism	AD	8q22	CYP11B1/CYP11B2	11β-hydroxylase/aldo synthase
Liddle's syndrome	AD	16p12	SNCC1B, SCNN1G	β, γ ENaC
Apparent mineralocorticoid excess	AR	16q12	HSD11B2	11β-HSD2
Pseudohypoaldosteronism type 1				
AD renal form	AD	4q31.1	MLR	Mineralocorticoid receptor
AR multiple-organ form	AR	16p12	SNCC1B, SCNN1G	β, γ ENaC
	AR	12p13	SNCC1A	α ENaC
Pseudohypoaldosteronism type 2	AD	1q31-42, 12p13.3, 17p11-21	WKN1, WKN4	WNK1, WNK4 kinases
Hypomagnesemia with secondary hypocalcemia	AR	9q22	TRPM6	TRPM6
Isolated familial hypomagnesemia				
AD form	AD	11q23	FXYD2,	Na^+,K^+-adenosine triphosphatase γ subunit
AR form	AR	?	?	?
Familial hypomagnesemia and hypercalciuria	AR	3q	PCN1	Paracellin-1 (claudin-16)

AD, autosomal dominant; AR, autosomal recessive.

four exons and encodes a novel protein that has been termed *barttin* (18). This protein has two transmembrane α helices and is preferentially expressed in the ascending loop of Henle and inner ear. It acts as an essential β subunit for ClC-Ka and ClC-Kb chloride channels. It seems that heteromers formed by ClC-K channel and barttin are crucial for renal NaCl reabsorption and K recycling in the inner ear (19).

The correspondence between genotype and phenotype may not be as consistent as presented here, because there are patients with the hypercalciuric variant and abnormalities in the NKCC2 gene who have clinical onset beyond the neonatal period (9), and there are also occasional patients with classic Bartter's syndrome type 3, due to mutations or deletions in the CLCNKB gene, who may present with polyhydramnios and symptoms during the neonatal period (20).

Clinical and Biochemical Features

This subject has been reviewed by Proesmans (21). Clinical signs may be observed antenatally or immediately after birth and include marked polyhydramnios (appearing between 24 and 30 weeks' gestation and caused by intrauterine polyuria), premature delivery, massive polyuria, life-threatening episodes of dehydration, hypercalciuria, and early-onset nephrocalcinosis (Table 38.2). Urine output may be as great as 12 to 50 mL/kg/hr and continue to be greatly increased for at least 4 to 6 weeks after birth. Some patients have a distinctive appearance: they are thin, with small muscles and a triangular face characterized by prominent forehead, large eyes, protruding ears, and drooping mouth. Strabismus and sensorineural deafness have been reported (22,23). Failure to thrive and growth retardation are the rule, but appropriate therapy is followed by satisfactory growth (24). The presence of systemic manifestations such as osteopenia, fever, secretory diarrhea, convulsions, and increased susceptibility to infection has been noted (4).

Prenatal diagnosis can be made by the high Cl content of the amniotic fluid. Of interest, concentrations of amniotic fluid Na, K, Ca, and prostaglandin E_2 are normal (25). The biochemical examination of the mother's urine may also be useful for prenatal diagnosis because it may show very low concentrations of Na, Cl, and Ca (26). The definitive way to establish a prenatal diagnosis is through the mutational analysis of genomic DNA extracted from cultured amniocytes obtained by amniocentesis (27).

Patients with type 2 often present at birth with mild NaCl wasting and a biochemical picture that mimics primary pseudohypoaldosteronism type 1 (i.e., hyponatremia, hyperkalemia, and metabolic acidosis). Renal potassium wasting leading to hypokalemia and metabolic alkalosis may not be apparent until 3 to 6 weeks postnatally outside of the neonatal period, the biochemical features (hypokalemia, metabolic alkalosis, impaired concentrating ability, hyperreninism, and hyperaldosteronism) are identical to those later described with more detail in the section Classic Bartter's Syndrome.

Urinary Ca excretion always remains very elevated in spite of therapy. The presence of marked hypercalciuria and

TABLE 38.2. CLINICAL AND BIOCHEMICAL FEATURES OF BARTTER'S-LIKE SYNDROMES

Features	Neonatal Bartter's syndrome	Classic Bartter's syndrome	Gitelman's syndrome
Clinical onset	Neonatal	Infancy or childhood	Childhood or adulthood
Polyhydramnios/prematurity	Present	Often present	Absent
Polydipsia/polyuria	Present	Present	Absent
Salt craving	Present	Present	Absent
Growth retardation	Present	Present	Absent or occasional
Dehydration	Present	Often present	Absent
Muscle weakness/tetany	Absent	Occasionally present	Present
Nephrocalcinosis	Present	Absent	Absent
Sensorineural deafness	Occasionally present	Absent	Absent
Metabolic alkalosis	Present (it may be delayed)	Present	Present
Hypokalemia	Present (it may be delayed)	Present	Present
Hypomagnesemia	Absent or exceptional	Occasionally present?	Present
Urinary NaCl excretion	Very high	High	Normal or high
Urinary Ca excretion	Very high	Normal or high	Low
Urinary concentrating ability	Impaired	Impaired	Normal
Hyperrenin/hyperaldosteronism	Present	Present	Present
Hyperprostaglandinism	Present (it may be delayed)	Present	Absent
Hypertrophy of juxtaglomerular apparatus	Present	Present	Occasionally present

nephrocalcinosis in an infant or child with apparent Bartter's syndrome is consistent with the neonatal form beyond the neonatal period. Increased urinary excretion of prostaglandin E_2 has been considered a characteristic feature of neonatal Bartter's syndrome, but this is secondary to the basic defect of renal NaCl reabsorption and, therefore, may not be present in all patients, especially during the early neonatal period (28). Renal function is generally well preserved, but an occasional child may develop end-stage chronic renal disease.

Pathology

Placental pathology in two cases showed large placentas with extensive subtrophoblastic basal membrane mineralization (29). The cardinal renal biopsy finding is hyperplasia of the juxtaglomerular apparatus. Occasional absence of Tamm-Horsfall protein in the kidney probably represents a secondary phenomenon (30).

Pathophysiology

Seyberth et al. (4) suggested that the neonatal cases represented a different pathogenic entity, related to systemic overproduction of prostaglandins, so the term *hyperprostaglandin E_2 syndrome* was proposed. The increased renal and systemic prostaglandin E activity was indicated by symptoms such as fever, diarrhea, vomiting, osteopenia, and generalized convulsions, and by elevation of the urinary excretion of prostaglandin E-M metabolite (the major urinary metabolite of the E prostaglandins). However, molecular biology findings demonstrate abnormalities in the genes coding for either NKCC2 (genetic type 1) or ROMK (genetic type 2), and the prostaglandin abnormalities appear to be secondary phenomena.

The channels and transporters implied in NaCl reabsorption in the distal nephron are depicted in Figure 38.1. The absorptive Na-K-2Cl cotransporter or NKCC2 is a member of a family of four proteins also including secretory Na-K-2Cl, NaCl, and KCl cotransporters. All are structurally similar and are formed by 12 membrane-spanning helixes and long cytosolic amino- and carboxy-terminal segments (31). Structural abnormalities of this protein due to mutations of the encoding gene obviously lead to altered NaCl transport. The importance of NKCC2 in renal NaCl transport is underlined by findings in a knockout mouse model of Bartter's syndrome. These mice with an abated SLC12A1 gene manifest severe salt-wasting, which results in rapid neonatal death unless they are rescued by indomethacin treatment (32).

ROMK is a protein with two intramembranous domains containing the channel pore and two cytosolic amino- and carboxy-terminal segments. It is found along the distal nephron and is believed to be responsible for K secretion in the cortical collecting duct and K recycling in the thick ascending limb of the loop of Henle (33). Loss of ROMK function impairs the ability to recycle K from cells back into lumen, resulting in luminal K concentrations too low to permit continued Na-K-2Cl activity (34).

Normal function of the Na-K-2Cl cotransporter is responsible for the reabsorption of approximately 30% of filtered sodium. Therefore, it is not surprising that altered function of this cotransporter results in renal sodium wasting, volume contraction, hyperreninism, hyperaldosteronism, hyperkaluria, hypokalemia, metabolic alkalosis, and hyperprostaglandinism, thus closing the pathogenic circle (Fig. 38.2). As expected, patients with neonatal Bartter's syndrome exhibit a blunted natriuretic and hormonal response to furosemide when compared to controls (35). Elevated prostaglandin E_2 secretion aggravates the picture further by independent stimulation of the renin-aldosterone axis and inhibition of both ROMK channel activity and

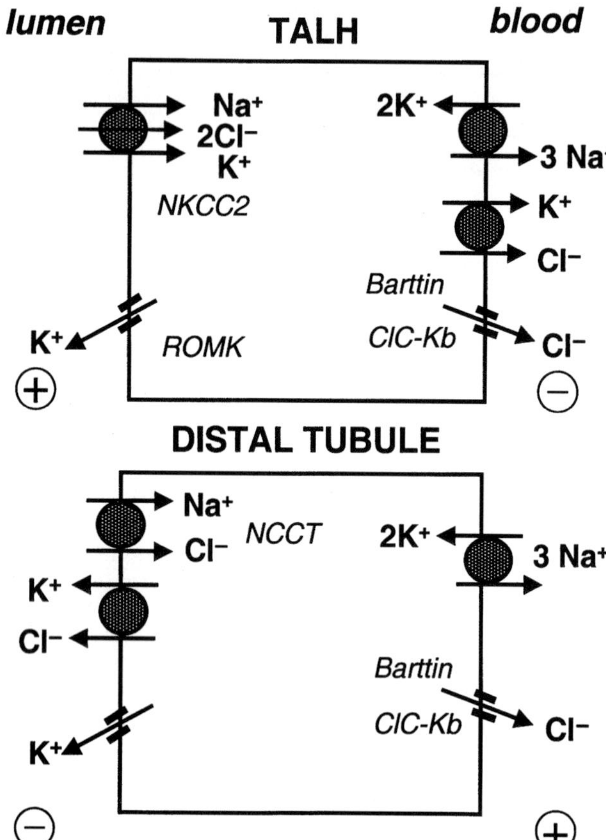

FIGURE 38.1. Schematic models of NaCl reabsorption in thick ascending limb of Henle (TALH) and convoluted distal tubule. In TALH, NaCl enters the cell from the lumen via an Na-2Cl-K cotransporter (NKCC2). K is recycled into the lumen via the K channel ROMK to permit the continuous functioning of this cotransporter. Cl leaves the cell across the basolateral membrane via a Cl channel (ClC-Kb) or in cotransport with K, while Na exits the cell through the Na,K-ATPase system. Barttin acts as an essential subunit of ClC-Kb. In the distal convoluted tubule, NaCl reabsorption in the luminal membrane is mediated by the NaCl cotransporter (NCCT) and leaves the cell through Cl channels and the Na,K-ATPase. A K-Cl cotransporter is also present at the luminal membrane.

NaCl transport in the thick ascending limb of Henle (36). However, although administration of prostaglandin synthetase inhibitors results in the impressive clinical and biochemical improvement, especially in type 2, it is not followed by complete correction of the tubular defect. Recent findings indicate that cyclooxygenase-2 is highly expressed in the macula densa of patients with salt-losing Bartter's syndrome and hyperreninemia (37) and that preferential inhibition of this enzyme by nimesulide in patients with neonatal Bartter's syndrome results in impressive improvement of hyperprostaglandinuria, secondary hyperaldosteronism, and hypercalciuria (38). These data would indicate that cyclooxygenase-2–derived prostaglandin E_2 is an important mediator for stimulation of the renin-angiotensin-aldosterone system in the kidney and that its preferential inhibition may offer a potential therapeutic benefit.

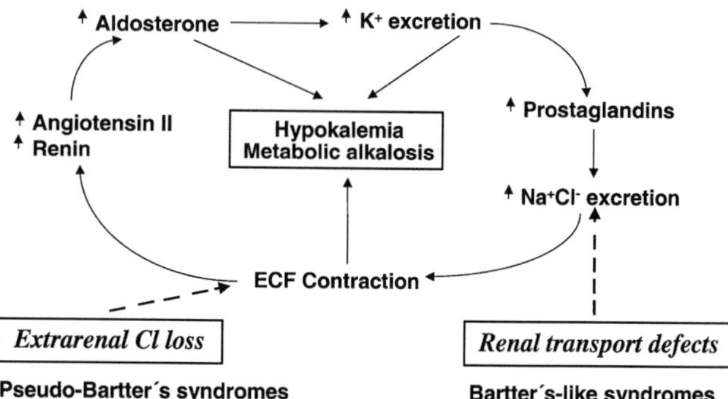

FIGURE 38.2. Schematic representation of pathophysiologic events leading to hypokalemia and metabolic alkalosis. Each of the biochemical and hormonal abnormalities observed in Bartter's syndrome could represent a proximate defect turning on the vicious circle. However, only extrarenal Cl loss (causing pseudo-Bartter's syndrome) and renal transport defects (causing Bartter's-like syndromes) appear as clinically relevant. ECF, extracellular fluid.

The presence of a primary NaCl transport defect in the loop of Henle was denied in the past by Seyberth et al. (4) on the basis that no abnormality in distal NaCl reabsorption could be demonstrated when children with this syndrome were studied beyond the neonatal period by oral hypotonic fluid administration. However, in our experience, when patients are studied after hypotonic saline infusion, a profound defect in distal NaCl reabsorption can be identified. The percent of distal NaCl reabsorption is dramatically low during infancy due to the increased distal NaCl delivery characteristic during this age.

The characteristic presence of hypercalciuria is not surprising because approximately 25% of filtered Ca is reabsorbed in the thick ascending limb of Henle coupled to Na-K-2Cl activity. Impaired electrogenic Cl transport impairs voltage-driven, paracellular Ca and Mg reabsorption. Hypercalciuria has also been related to an excessive synthesis of 1,25-dihydroxy-vitamin D (39) leading to augmented bone resorption and renal leak (40,41). Recent studies have shown that serum and urine of children with neonatal Bartter's syndrome contain excessive amounts of a heparin-like calciotropic factor closely related to basic fibroblastic growth factor, providing additional evidence that hypercalciuria is not solely due to an intrinsic renal leak (42,43).

Reabsorption of approximately 60% of filtered Mg also occurs in the loop of Henle and is dependent on the positive luminal voltage generated by the activity of the cotransporter. Absence of hypermagnesiuria in neonatal Bartter's syndrome may be explained by the compensatory Mg reabsorption taking place in distal convoluted tubules.

Differential Diagnosis

The clinical picture of neonatal Bartter's syndrome is so characteristic that diagnostic doubts rarely arise. A similar but apparently different syndrome has been described in a female infant, aged 5 weeks, who, in addition to the usual clinical features of neonatal Bartter's syndrome, had massive urinary excretion of prostaglandins E_2 and E-M metabolite, normal calcium metabolism, hyperphosphaturia, and severe hyperchloriduria and hyperkaluria with limited response to indomethacin. Molecular analysis determines if these findings really represent a new congenital renal tubular abnormality as proposed by the authors (44).

Type 2 neonatal Bartter's syndrome, due to mutations in the ROMK gene, may exhibit hyponatremia and hyperkalemia in the early neonatal period, thus mimicking the picture of primary pseudohypoaldosteronism type 1. The possible existence of prematurity, polyhydramnios, hypercalciuria, and nephrocalcinosis in the latter syndrome may contribute to the clinical confusion (45–48). The syndrome of familial hypomagnesemia-hypercalciuria with nephrocalcinosis may also be confused with neonatal Bartter's syndrome because hypercalciuria and nephrocalcinosis are already present, but significant hypomagnesemia may be absent in the early neonatal period.

Pseudo-neonatal Bartter's syndrome is rare, but biological abnormalities simulating Bartter's syndrome were observed in a preterm neonate with complex cyanotic heart disease, in whom the ductus arteriosus was maintained open by high doses of prostaglandin E_1 (49).

Treatment and Prognosis

In the immediate neonatal period, all therapeutic efforts should be directed to correct dehydration and electrolytic imbalance. Continuous saline infusion may be needed to attain this goal. Administration of indomethacin in the early postnatal period may not only be unnecessary but dangerous, given the risk of necrotizing enterocolitis. Prenatal treatment with indomethacin has been advocated when diagnosis is made prenatally (27). The apparent beneficial effects of indomethacin should be taken with extreme caution, however, and should be weighed against the potential therapeutic risks (50). Administering indomethacin to a mother whose fetus is known to have mutations characteristic of neonatal Bartter's syndrome may prevent progression of polyhydramnios, but may also be dangerous for the fetus.

At 4 to 6 weeks of life, patients greatly benefit from the administration of indomethacin and, eventually, of potassium chloride supplements. Although indomethacin has no direct effect on the inherited renal tubular abnormality, it is beneficial because it neutralizes the amplifying effect of prostaglandins on the features of Bartter's syndrome. In my experience, patients with the type 2 genetic defect are especially sensitive to indomethacin, and doses below 1 mg/kg/day may be sufficient to maintain plasma K levels within the normal range. In fact, a high dosage may lead to hyperkalemia, and K supplements may not be necessary with appropriate therapy.

In general, therapy permits clinical stabilization and catch-up growth. Bone age has been appropriate for chronological age, and pubertal and intellectual development have been normal. An occasional patient may even have a spontaneous resolution of all signs and symptoms at approximately 6 years of age (51). Although indomethacin may reduce the degree of hypercalciuria, renal calcium excretion remains greatly elevated, thus creating a real concern for the progression of the nephrocalcinosis. The use of preferential cyclooxygenase-2 inhibitors remains experimental. All coadjuvant therapies (e.g., amiloride, hydrochlorothiazide, potassium phosphate) have been ineffective, so one should expect a low decrease of glomerular filtration rate (GFR) over the years as a result of chronic tubulointerstitial nephropathy.

The neonatal form associated with neurosensorial deafness due to mutations in the BSND gene is resistant to therapy with indomethacin and always carries a bad long-term prognosis due to the progressive development of chronic renal insufficiency (52).

Classic Bartter's Syndrome

Genetics

The so-called classic form, or Bartter's syndrome type 3, is an autosomal recessive disease caused by large deletions or nonsense, missense, and splice mutations in a renal chloride channel gene (ClC-Kb) (20,53) (Table 38.1). In humans, there are two closely related voltage-gated chloride channels (ClC-Ka and ClC-Kb), proteins of 687 amino acids specifically expressed in mammalian kidney and encoded by two genes (locus symbols CLCNKA and CLCNKB), closely located on 1p36 where they are separated by only 11 kb (54). The fact that a certain number of patients with classic Bartter's syndrome do not demonstrate abnormalities in the CLCNKB gene indicates that other genes implicated in NaCl transport in the ascending loop of Henle may also be involved as a cause of this syndrome. A possible candidate gene could be the one encoding the synthesis of the basolateral KCl cotransporter.

Clinical Features

Frequently, there is a history of maternal hydramnios and premature delivery. Symptoms start during the first 2 years of life and include polyuria, polydipsia, vomiting, constipation, salt craving, tendency to dehydration, and failure to thrive (Table 38.2). Occasional cases may have a clinical onset during the neonatal period (20). Growth retardation occurs if early therapy is not instituted. However, normal adult height may be achieved with a delayed adolescent growth spurt. Associated growth hormone deficiency has been found in occasional patients (55). The clinical findings of fatigue, muscle weakness, cramps, and recurrent episodes of carpopedal spasm may be observed late in childhood but are more characteristically observed in Gitelman's syndrome. Some patients have a distinctive appearance: they are thin, with small muscles and a triangular face characterized by prominent forehead, large eyes, and drooping mouth. Other possible signs are developmental delay, minimal brain dysfunction with nonspecific electroencephalographic abnormalities, nephrocalcinosis, and polyuria-related ureterohydronephrosis. If hypokalemia is profound and prolonged, it may give rise to the formation of medullary cysts (56). Nephrocalcinosis is very rarely observed. Patients are always normotensive. On occasion, the diagnosis is suspected in an asymptomatic child because hypokalemia is found in a routine investigation.

Biochemical Features

The outstanding laboratory finding is hypokalemia, with K concentrations in blood ranging between 1.5 and 2.5 mEq/L. Hypokalemia is almost always accompanied by hypochloremia and metabolic alkalosis, although (exceptionally) the patient may present with metabolic acidosis (57). Hyperuricemia, induced by contraction of extracellular fluid volume, may be observed in approximately 50% of patients. Hypomagnesemia is rarely encountered, and its presence in a patient with features of Bartter's syndrome necessitates exclusion of the diagnosis of Gitelman's syndrome, in which hypomagnesemia is a cardinal finding. Other biochemical features rarely present are polycythemia, hypercalcemia, and hypophosphatemia.

The most characteristic urinary findings are the increased fractional excretion of K, Na, and Cl. The demonstration of a urinary Cl concentration above 10 mEq/L in a patient with hypochloremic metabolic alkalosis rules out extrarenal causes of Cl depletion (e.g., dietary deficiency, vomiting, cystic fibrosis) in which urinary Cl excretion is very low or even absent (58). Urinary Na wasting is also present, and it may be especially evident during dietary Na restriction. A very important urinary finding is the presence of normal or high urinary Ca excretion (59). Hypocalciuria is a characteristic finding of Gitelman's syndrome, but in exceptional cases it may also be observed in the follow-up of patients with classic Bartter's syndrome (60).

Defects in concentrating and diluting abilities are always present and are the result of both hypokalemia and impaired NaCl reabsorption in the ascending limb of the loop of Henle. The role played by prostaglandin oversecretion is probably secondary, because administration of prostaglandin synthetase inhibitors is not followed by complete correction of hyposthenuria. Another relevant finding is the inability to appropriately decrease urine pH during ammonium chloride loading. This is due to high rates of ammonium excretion, caused by both increased production and preferential diversion of ammonia into the urine. GFR is normal in early stages of the disease but may become impaired in untreated patients as a result of chronic hypokalemia. The sustained high levels of angiotensin II may theoretically cause progressive tubulointerstitial damage. However, if therapy is adequate, there is no long-term deterioration of renal function.

Hyperreninemia is constantly present and is accompanied, in most cases, by an elevated plasma concentration of aldosterone. In a few patients, however, aldosterone secretion is suppressed by K depletion. The renal K loss is not exclusively related to hyperaldosteronism, because it persists after renin suppression or adrenalectomy.

Paradoxically, blood pressure is normal despite increased blood levels of renin, angiotensin II, norepinephrine, and endothelin (61). In fact, stimulation of the renin-angiotensin-aldosterone axis might be necessary to maintain normotension, as administration of saralasin (a competitive inhibitor of angiotensin II) or captopril (a blocker of angiotensin-converting enzyme) induces a significant fall in blood pressure. The blunted increase in blood pressure after infusion of angiotensin II is not a constant diagnostic feature as initially reported by Bartter (1), because it improves after expansion of extracellular fluid volume or administration of prostaglandin synthetase inhibitors. The beneficial effect of indomethacin in this regard depends on its capacity not only to correct sodium depletion and thus suppress angiotensin production but also to normalize the pressor responsiveness to the latter hormone by inhibiting the secretion of prostaglandins. Indomethacin also corrects the hyperactivity of the adrenergic system, manifested by increased plasma levels of noradrenaline and vascular, but not metabolic, unresponsiveness to this hormone. Probably, the vascular hyporeactivity of Bartter's syndrome is a complex phenomenon dependent not only on vascular underfilling and increased prostaglandin synthesis but also on nitric oxide–mediated vasodilation. Increased urinary excretions of nitrites NO_2^- and NO_3^- and cyclic guanosine monophosphate all point to increased nitric oxide synthesis in vascular endothelial cells (62). Patients with Bartter's-like syndromes evidence a blunted Gq-mediated cell signaling that results in reduction in protein kinase C production and upregulation of the nitric oxide system (63).

A very important finding is the increased urinary excretion of prostaglandins, principally prostaglandin E_2 and 6-keto-prostaglandin F_{1a}, the main metabolite of prostaglandin I_2 or prostacyclin (64). Urinary excretion of prostaglandin F_{2a} is more variable. Urinary kallikrein excretion is also increased. Prostaglandin overproduction may cause defective platelet aggregation and inhibition of phytohemagglutinin-induced lymphocyte proliferation.

Pathology

The cardinal renal biopsy finding is hyperplasia of the juxtaglomerular apparatus, although it may be absent in occasional cases. Hyperplasia of interstitial renomedullary cells is observed more rarely. Glomerular hyalinization, apical vacuolization of proximal tubular cells, tubular atrophy, and interstitial fibrosis may be also observed as a long-term consequence of chronic K deficiency.

Pathophysiology

Different hypotheses (e.g., vascular resistance to angiotensin II, tubular defect in potassium secretion, primary hyperprostaglandinism, increased secretion of atrial natriuretic peptide) have been presented to explain the range of abnormalities seen in classic Bartter's syndrome, but it is now well established that most cases result from mutations in the renal Cl channel ClC-Kb or genetic defect type 3. Other patients who apparently have classic Bartter's syndrome may indeed have neonatal Bartter's syndrome with a delayed clinical onset, which may be caused by defects in NKCC2 or ROMK genes. The presence of nephrocalcinosis in the latter cases is an important clinical clue.

The ClC chloride channels are members of a single family originally defined by the voltage-gated Cl channel ClC-0, isolated from Torpedo electric organ and formed by at least nine different proteins (65). The members of this family, ClC-K1 and ClC-K2, were shown in the rat to be kidney-specific and expressed from the thin ascending limb of the loop of Henle onward (Fig. 38.1). The human homolog genes are called CLCNKA and CLCNKB. These genes encode the channels ClC-Ka and ClC-Kb, both formed of 687 amino acids and containing 12 transmembrane domains and cytosolic amino- and carboxy-terminal segments. Like other members of the family, these channels are gated by both voltage and chloride.

The Cl channel ClC-Kb is situated at the basolateral membrane of distal nephron segments and is mainly responsible for Cl exit from the cell into the bloodstream. It needs the β subunit barttin for functional expression. Therefore, it is not surprising that structural defects of the genes encoding both the channel itself and barttin are followed by defective NaCl reabsorption in the distal nephron. Alternative mechanisms of Cl transit across the basolateral membranes, such as a KCl cotransport, have also been proposed, so it must be assumed that overfunction of these other transporters cannot compensate completely for loss of function of the Cl channel. However, some compensation probably takes place because renal salt loss is not as massive as that observed in neonatal cases, and the phenotype of this genetic defect is quite variable.

The presence of a defective NaCl transport at the level of the ascending loop of Henle in classic Bartter's syndrome has long been suspected on the basis of the study of fractional clearances of Cl during hypotonic saline diuresis. The index of distal Cl reabsorption ($C_{H_2O} / C_{H_2O} + C_{Cl} \times 100$) is normally above 80% (66), whereas patients with this phenotype have values characteristically diminished, often below 60% (67). This defect is not observed in patients with hypokalemia of different etiologies (68). To reveal the tubular defect, the conditions of the study, especially NaCl intake, and route of administration must be rigorously standardized, and the diluting segment Cl reabsorption must be judged in relation to distal Cl delivery. In fact, distal Cl reabsorption is less affected or is even normal when renal clearance studies are performed after an oral water load instead of during hypotonic saline infusion (69,70).

It has long been postulated that the membrane ion transport defect was not limited to tubular cells but represented a generalized membrane transport defect, as intracellular Na concentration in erythrocytes or muscle cells was found to be consistently increased. The reasons proposed were either an increased Na permeability or a decreased passive Na efflux related to the low number of ouabain-sensitive Na-pumping sites (71). However, on the basis of recent data, it is more probable that these transport abnormalities are simple consequences of the hypokalemic state. The response to therapy has been variable; indomethacin corrects the intracellular action abnormalities but has little effect on the membrane transport defect, whereas complete correction of hypokalemia apparently normalizes all parameters (72).

Clinical Variants

Associated with Proximal Tubular Dysfunction. A few cases of Bartter's syndrome have been associated with signs of the Fanconi's syndrome (73–75). In a personal case and in the case reported by Fricker et al. (75), the renal biopsy showed hyperplasia of the juxtaglomerular apparatus but also marked interstitial fibrosis with hyalinized glomeruli and tubular atrophy. The interstitial fibrosis may not represent a differential finding and may only be the result of chronic hypokalemia (76). This entity should probably not be classified as a different syndrome, because in our case a homozygous missense mutation in the CLCNKB gene could be demonstrated. This clinical variant of Bartter's syndrome should be distinguished from the opposed situation (i.e., cases of primary Fanconi's syndrome) or cystinosis mimicking Bartter's syndrome due to the presence of hypokalemia and metabolic alkalosis (77–79). Patients with mitochondrial cytopathies often have signs of proximal tubular dysfunction but, exceptionally, a 10-year-old child with the Kearns-Sayre syndrome presented with signs of Bartter's syndrome (80).

Associated with Distal Tubular Defects Rather Than Loop of Henle Defects. Some adult patients reported as cases of Bartter's syndrome show a normal or near-normal capacity to form solute-free water after oral water loading and are therefore interpreted as having a distal tubular defect rather than a loop of Henle defect (81–84). Most of these patients exhibit hypocalciuria and should be considered to have Gitelman's syndrome and not a clinical variant of Bartter's syndrome (85).

Differential Diagnosis

Familial hypokalemic alkalosis with proximal tubulopathy (Güllner's syndrome) has been uniquely observed in three siblings of a sibship of four presenting with features very similar to Bartter's syndrome but with normal distal Cl reabsorption and characteristic focal histologic lesions consisting of dark staining of proximal tubular cells. Hypouricemia was the only biochemical abnormality that could be ascribed to impaired proximal tubular function (86,87).

Among the renal causes mimicking Bartter's syndrome, one should also consider the surreptitious use of loop diuretics such as furosemide (88,89). Although this situation is exceptional in children, the presence of diuretics in the urine may help to establish the diagnosis. There is a report of an 11-year-old boy presenting with a chronic salt-losing nephropathy manifested by volume depletion, hypodipsia, absence of salt appetite, normokalemic metabolic alkalosis, hyperreninemic hyperaldosteronism, hypertrophy of juxtaglomerular apparatus, highly conserved capacities to concentrate and dilute the urine, and paradoxically increased levels in plasma of atrial natriuretic peptide. Although this patient clinically resembles Bartter's syndrome, values of fractional NaCl reabsorption during hypotonic saline diuresis were normal, and no clinical amelioration was observed while on indomethacin therapy (90).

Bartter's syndrome should also be distinguished from states of Cl depletion from extrarenal causes: cyclical vomiting, laxative abuse, and cystic fibrosis. In these circumstances, the biochemical and histologic pictures may be identical to those present in Bartter's syndrome, but diagnosis is rapidly made if one measures urinary Cl excretion (58). States of mineralocorticoid excess should be easily excluded because all are associated with arterial hypertension.

Treatment and Prognosis

Treatment is designed primarily to correct the hypokalemia. Potassium supplementation in the form of KCl (1 to 3 mEq/kg/day or more) is always necessary. The amount needed changes according to the patient and must balance the amount of K lost by the kidney. However, in most cases, K supplementation alone is almost completely ineffective, as administered K is quickly lost into the urine. Addition of spironolactone (10 to 15 mg/kg/day) or triamterene (10 mg/kg/day) may be initially effective in the control of hypokalemia, but its effect is often transient. The administration of β-adrenergic inhibitors (e.g., propranolol) does not offer any additive advantage.

Therapy of Bartter's syndrome is today best accomplished by the use of prostaglandin synthetase inhibitors: indomethacin (2 to 5 mg/kg/day), acetylsalicylic acid (100 mg/kg/day), ibuprofen (30 mg/kg/day), or ketoprofen (20 mg/kg/day). Indomethacin is the drug most frequently used and is remarkably well tolerated. However, attention should be paid to signs of intolerance or toxicity (e.g., nausea, vomiting, abdominal pain, peptic ulcer, hematopoietic toxicity, or liver damage). The possibility of developing pseudotumor cerebri should also be considered, as it has been reported after both indomethacin and ketoprofen administration. The early effects of prostaglandin inhibition are spectacular, with improved well-being, strength and activity, diminution of polyuria and polydipsia, and reinstitution of normal, or even catchup, growth. There is an immediate increase in plasma K, which, however, rarely exceeds a concentration of 3.5 mEq/L. Plasma renin activity and aldosterone concentration decrease to normal, and the vascular response to angiotensin II or noradrenalin also normalizes. The distal tubular defect in Cl reabsorption remains unmodified. Addition of Mg salts should always be considered when hypomagnesemia is present because Mg deficiency may aggravate K wasting.

The efficacy of long-term use of prostaglandin synthetase inhibitors has been clearly established. When patients reach adulthood, clinical improvement is generally maintained, but there is some recurrence of hypokalemia and hyperreninemia, and there is a tendency to develop hypomagnesemia and hypocalciuria, thus mimicking the biochemical profile of Gitelman's syndrome (60). Tetanic episodes, which are always absent during childhood, may be observed in adults. Long-term prognosis remains guarded, however, and lack of rigorous therapeutic control may lead to slow progression to chronic renal failure (91). If the symptoms reappear, the dose of indomethacin should be readjusted, and a combined therapy with indomethacin and spironolactone should be initiated. In adults, the use of angiotensin-converting enzyme inhibitors (e.g., captopril, enalapril) has been tried with conflicting results (92,93). There are no data concerning their use in children with Bartter's syndrome, but one should be cautious given the risk of developing symptomatic hypotension.

Anesthetic procedures should be carefully managed in patients with Bartter's syndrome and special attention should be paid to maintain cardiovascular stability, control plasma K, and prevent renal damage (94). Maintenance of indomethacin therapy is mandatory when undergoing surgical procedures such as a percutaneous renal biopsy to avoid the risk of bleeding due to defective platelet aggregation.

Gitelman's Syndrome

The syndrome of familial hypokalemia-hypomagnesemia (Gitelman's syndrome) was first described by Gitelman, Graham, and Welt in 1966 (95). It is not as infrequent as reflected in the literature, because in the past it has been confused with Bartter's syndrome (96). Adult patients with Gitelman's syndrome are much more common than those with Bartter's syndrome. During childhood the incidence is probably similar (97).

Genetics

The equal incidence in both sexes and the lack of significant abnormalities in the parents suggest an autosomal recessive inheritance (Table 38.1). Molecular biology findings have established that almost all families studied have mutations in the gene locus SLC12A3 (98–102). This gene, located in 16q13 and containing 26 exons, encodes the renal thiazide-sensitive NaCl cotransporter (also variously abbreviated as TSC, NCC, NCCT, or ENCC1) that is mainly located in the distal convoluted tubule.

Clinical and Biochemical Features

Patients with Gitelman's syndrome are often asymptomatic, with the exception of transient episodes of weakness and tetany that are usually accompanied by abdominal pain, vomiting, and fever (Table 38.2). The disease-free intervals may be prolonged, and in many cases, diagnosis is only made during adult life. However, almost one-half of the patients complain of salt craving, musculoskeletal symptoms (e.g., cramps, muscle weakness, and aches), and constitutional symptoms (e.g., fatigue, dizziness, nocturia, and polydipsia) (103). In children, growth retardation is usually absent, but occasional cases may present evidence of associated growth hormone deficiency that improves with recombinant human growth hormone therapy (104,105). Chondrocalcinosis has been occasionally reported in adult patients and is due to deposition of calcium pyrophosphate dehydrate crystals (106,107). Ophthalmic examination may show choroidal calcifications (108).

The outstanding biochemical features are hypomagnesemia, hypokalemia, and moderate metabolic alkalosis. A modest elevation in uric acid may be present, although, on the whole, renal function is normal. The presence of hyperreninism and hyperaldosteronism may contribute to the confusion with classic Bartter's syndrome. However, a normal urinary excretion of prostaglandin E_2 has been reported (109). Generally, no abnormal findings are present at renal biopsy, although hypertrophy of juxtaglomerular apparatus may be occasionally observed.

The most characteristic finding in the urine, besides the presence of hypermagnesuria and hyperkaluria, is the striking diminution of urinary Ca excretion, which rarely exceeds 0.5 mg/kg/day. Plasma levels of parathyroid hormone and urinary excretion of cyclic adenosine monophosphate are normal. The study of distal tubular function reveals normal or only slightly impaired concentrating and acidifying mechanisms, but modestly reduced distal fractional Cl reabsorption during hypotonic saline diuresis. Values obtained are intermediary between normal values and values present in children with classic Bartter's syndrome (110). A striking finding is the increased natriuretic and kaliuretic response to the intravenous administration of furosemide and a blunted natriuretic response to hydrochlorothiazide (111). This suggests that the defect in NaCl reabsorption is in the distal tubule rather than in the ascending loop of Henle. The calciuric response to furosemide is blunted. This readily permits differentiation from patients with Bartter's syndrome, who exhibit an enhanced calciuric response to furosemide (112).

Pathophysiology

Gitelman's syndrome results from diminished NaCl transport in the distal convoluted tubule caused by defective function of the thiazide-sensitive NaCl cotransporter NCCT (Fig. 38.1). This was the first member of the Na-K-Cl cotransporter family to be identified and, as other members of this family, is formed by 12 membrane-spanning helixes and long cytosolic amino- and carboxy-terminal segments (31). Structural abnormalities of this transporter due to mutations of the encoding gene lead to defective processing with retention of the protein in the endoplasmic reticulum and lack of activity at the plasma membrane (113). As in Bartter's syndrome, the NaCl cotransporter defect directly leads to NaCl wasting, mild hypovolemia, metabolic alkalosis, and stimulation of the renin-angiotensin axis.

The exact mechanisms underlying hypocalciuria and hypomagnesemia are not yet fully elucidated, but both abnormalities may be direct consequences of the primary defect. In fact, they are also observed after administration of thiazide diuretics, which inhibit the distal luminal NaCl cotransporter. Hypocalciuria may result from increased tubular reabsorption of filtered Ca via a basolateral NaCa exchanger. No obvious abnormalities are found in plasma levels of parathyroid hormone or 1,25-dihydroxy vitamin D_3 levels (114,115). Hypermagnesuria also results from decreased tubular reabsorption of filtered Mg due to inhibition of an apical NaMg exchanger. Metabolic alkalosis may play an important role in the pathogenesis of hypermagnesuria by making the distal tubule cells resistant to Mg uptake (116). A study of renal tubular reabsorption of Mg, performed in three children with Gitelman's syndrome (96), revealed normal rates of Mg reabsorption when the amount filtered exceeded 1.2 mg/dL glomerular filtrate. However, in contrast to normal children, Mg excretion was also evident at levels of filtered Mg below 1.2 mg/dL GF, indicating a low renal Mg threshold. These data are compatible with the known fact that the bulk of filtered Mg is reabsorbed in the thick ascending loop of Henle and that the distal convoluted tubule only reabsorbs approximately 5% of filtered Mg (117).

Differential Diagnosis

Hypomagnesemia and hypocalciuria are universal in Gitelman's syndrome, thus allowing an easy differentiation from other hypokalemic syndromes (Table 38.2). Gitelman's syndrome should be differentiated from a rare entity described in an adult man who presented with a clinical syndrome of a probable proximal tubular origin, associating moderate glomerular impairment, hypokalemia, metabolic alkalosis, hypomagnesemia, glycosuria, hypocalciuria, and relative hypomagnesuria (118). Surreptitious diuretic ingestion may also mimic Gitelman's syndrome. Besides the urinary determination of diuretics, the molecular genetic diagnosis may also help to establish the correct diagnosis (119).

Treatment and Prognosis

Patients with Gitelman's syndrome are best treated with Mg salts alone, with no need, in most cases, to add either K salts or prostaglandin inhibitors. Many Mg salts have been used in the treatment of hypomagnesemic states (e.g., Mg oxide, Mg chloride, Mg pidolate, Mg lactate, Mg pyrrolidone carboxylate). In Gitelman's syndrome, we recommend the use of Mg chloride ($MgCl_2$) that also compensates for ongoing urinary Cl losses. Magnesium chloride has a high Mg content, is very soluble, and is not dependent on gastric acidity for absorption. Also, its administration is less often followed by diarrhea, although this complication may still develop with increasing dosage. We use a 5% solution that contains approximately 0.5 mEq (0.6 mg) Mg^{2+}/mL. The total dose should be individualized for each patient and given at 6- to 8-hour intervals. In our experience, regular administration of $MgCl_2$ not only partly corrects the hypomagnesemia and prevents the appearance of tetanic episodes, but also normalizes plasma K concentration, acid-base equilibrium, the renin-aldosterone axis, and urinary Ca excretion. However, there is some disagreement whether the K wasting may or may not be exclusively attributed to hypomagnesemia (120,121). In fact, occasional cases may require the additional administration of potassium salts or antialdosterone drugs (e.g., spironolactone or amiloride) to correct the hypokalemia (122). High-dosage indomethacin may be especially indicated in exceptional cases with growth retardation and bad tolerance to Mg supplementation (123).

The long-term prognosis of Gitelman's syndrome, in terms of preserving renal function and maintaining growth, appears to be excellent, but sustained lifelong Mg supplementation remains necessary to reduce the risk of tetanic episodes (124). There is a single report of an adult patient who developed end-stage renal disease (125).

Hyperaldosteronism

Although the common adult syndromes of primary hyperaldosteronism (e.g., renin-secreting tumor and Conn disease due to adrenal adenoma, carcinoma, or micronodular hyperplasia) (126) are outside the scope of this chapter, we will refer to one rare disorder, which may be observed during the pediatric age, the so-called glucocorticoid-remediable aldosteronism.

Glucocorticoid-Remediable Aldosteronism

Glucocorticoid-remediable aldosteronism, also called *familial hyperaldosteronism type 1*, represents a rare cause of low-renin hypertension in children and adults.

Genetics

Glucocorticoid-remediable aldosteronism, an autosomal dominant disease, arises due to a chimeric gene formed at meiosis after genetic recombination between two homologues, adjacent genes on chromosome 8q22, CYP11B1 and CYP11B2, encoding the enzymes 11β-hydroxylase and aldosterone synthase involved, respectively, in the final pathways of cortisol and aldosterone synthesis within the adrenal cortex (127) (Table 38.1). The final 11β-hydroxylation in the synthesis of cortisol in the zona fasciculata is regulated by 11β-hydroxylase, which depends on adrenocorticotropic hormone (ACTH) secretion. The final stages of aldosterone synthesis are catalyzed by the P-450 enzyme aldosterone synthase, whose expression is limited to the zona glomerulosa and is regulated by angiotensin II and K.

Clinical and Biochemical Features

Glucorticoid-remediable aldosteronism manifests clinically by the presence of familial low-renin hypertension. In affected family members, hypertension is already observed in those younger than 21 years of age and often during childhood (128). Hypertension is especially severe and may lead to cardiovascular complications (e.g., hemorrhagic stroke) in almost 20% of cases. Characteristic biochemical findings are metabolic alkalosis and very low plasma renin activity. Hypokalemia may be present but is not an obligatory finding.

Pathophysiology

Hypertension results from aldosterone excess, with aldosterone being under the control of ACTH rather than the normal secretagogue, angiotensin II. The chimeric gene possesses the 5' 11β-hydroxylase and the 3' aldosterone synthase sequences, and although it promotes the synthesis of aldosterone, it is under the regulatory control of ACTH and not of angiotensin II.

Diagnosis

The ratio between urinary concentrations of C-18 oxidation products (18-oxotetrahydrocortisol and 18-hydrocortisol) and tetrahydroaldosterone is characteristically increased, but given the technical difficulty of these analytical procedures, the diagnosis is generally established by the use of the dexamethasone suppression test, which is based on the decrease of aldosterone production after ACTH suppression. A value of plasma aldosterone below 4 ng/dL postdexamethasone correctly diagnoses glucocorticoid-remediable aldosteronism with high sensitivity and specificity (129). However, definitive diagnosis is established by the use of molecular biology techniques (130). There are a few patients who present with a positive dexamethasone suppression test without any evidence of abnormalities in CYP11B1 and CYP11B2 genes. The pathogenesis of these rare cases of glucocorticoid-remediable aldosteronism not linked to a chimeric CYP11B1/CYP11B2 gene remains unknown (131).

Therapy

Hypertension is refractory to therapy with the usual antihypertensive drugs but quickly resolves after administration of K-retaining diuretics such as spironolactone or amiloride. Occasionally, patients may require a combined therapy with nifedipine (132). Although administration of dexamethasone may also ameliorate the hypertension, its prolonged use is not recommended in childhood given its deleterious effect on growth.

Pseudohyperaldosteronism

Under the term *pseudohyperaldosteronism,* we include a few syndromes that present clinical and biochemical findings similar to those observed in primary hyperaldosteronism but without evidence of increased secretion of mineralocorticoids. In fact, plasma aldosterone levels are often undetectable.

Liddle's Syndrome

Liddle's syndrome is a very rare disorder of tubular transport, simulating primary hyperaldosteronism but with negligible aldosterone secretion. It was described in 1963 by Liddle, Bledsoe, and Coppage (133) in eight individuals of the same family.

Genetics

A pattern of autosomal dominant inheritance has been described, although some cases appear to be sporadic (134–136) (Fig. 38.1). Recent studies have demonstrated that this entity is caused by mutations of the genes encoding two of the three constitutive subunits of the amiloride-sensitive epithelial sodium channel (ENaC). Mutations of the genes encoding β subunit (βENaC) (137,138) and γ subunit (γENaC) (139) have been described. Both genes SNCC1B and SNCC1G are located on 16p12. No abnormalities have been noted in the gene SNCC1A, located at 12p13, or in encoding the α subunit (αENaC).

Clinical and Biochemical Features

Characteristic clinical and laboratory findings start in infancy and early childhood and include polyuria, polydipsia, failure to thrive, arterial hypertension, hypokalemic metabolic alkalosis, and almost absent renin and aldosterone secretion. Hypercalciuria, nephrocalcinosis, and renal medullary cysts have been noted in a few cases. Aldosterone secretion is not stimulated by salt restriction, and improvement is observed after administration of triamterene but not after administration of spironolactone.

Pathophysiology

Liddle's syndrome results from excessive renal tubular Na absorption through activation of the renal epithelial sodium channel. As mentioned above, this channel is formed by three subunit proteins (α, β, and γ) having short cytosolic termini, two transmembrane domains, and a large extracellular loop (140). The α subunit appears to be required for the assembly or function of the whole complex. The three ENaC subunits are homologous to each other and have approximately 35% amino acid identity. A possible membrane topology of the heterotetrameric complex is formed by two α subunits, one β subunit, and one γ subunit, because this complex maintains a high amiloride sensitivity and a very Na^+-selective pore (Fig. 38.3). The ENaC is not only present in the kidney but also in other organs (e.g., lung, colon, exocrine glands, skin and hair follicles). The C terminal of each ENaC subunit contains a xPPxY motif, which is necessary for interaction with the WW domains of the ubiquitin-protein ligase, Nedd4 (141). Nedd4 regulates ENaC function by controlling the number of channels at the cell surface. Liddle's mutations, leading to truncated C-terminus of the β or γ subunits,

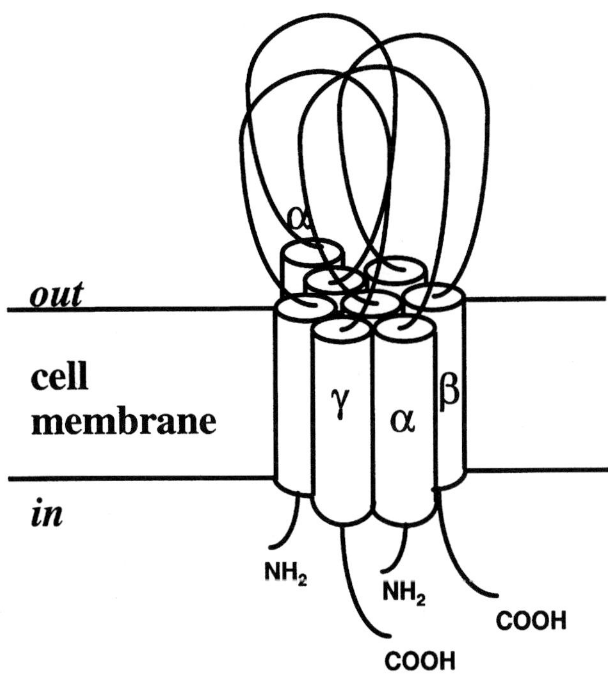

FIGURE 38.3. Membrane topology of the epithelial Na^+ channel. The proposed model is a heterotetrameric structure formed by two α subunits, one β subunit, and one γ subunit. Each subunit is formed by two membrane-spanning domains, a large extracellular loop, and cytoplasmic amino- and carboxytermini.

alter or delete the xPPxY motif, interrupt the interaction with Nedd4 protein, and lead to an increased number of Na channels in the apical membrane, increased Na reabsorption, expanded plasma volume with resulting hypertension, and inhibited renin-aldosterone axis with secondary potassium wasting (142–144). A transgenic mouse model for Liddle's syndrome reproduces, to a large extent, a human form of salt-sensitive hypertension (145). It is possible that polymorphisms of the β and γ subunits of the ENaC are related to variations of blood pressure in humans (146) and may contribute to the high incidence of salt-related hypertension in blacks (147).

Diagnosis

Diagnosis is mainly established with the syndrome of apparent mineralocorticoid excess. The presence of hypertensive individuals in successive generations is very suggestive of Liddle's syndrome. The lack of hypotensive effect of spironolactone or dexamethasone administration also suggests the diagnosis. Nowadays, genetic testing allows a sure and rapid diagnosis (148).

Therapy and Prognosis

Therapy consists of the combined administration of K supplementation (as KCl) and triamterene (10 mg/kg/day). Improvement is manifest by normalization of Na and K balances, resolution of hypertension, and reinstitution of normal growth. However, catch-up growth rarely occurs, and patients may remain significantly growth-retarded if the syndrome has been manifest early in infancy. If the diagnosis is not firmly established, a therapeutic trial with spironolactone or dexamethasone should also be considered given the clinical similarity with 11β-hydroxysteroid dehydrogenase (11β-HSD) deficiency.

Apparent Mineralocorticoid Excess

This entity, identified by Ulick and New (149), gives rise to a state of apparent mineralocorticoid excess (AME), which is clinically and biochemically very similar to Liddle's syndrome. Approximately 40 affected patients have been described worldwide (150).

Genetics

There are two isoenzymes of 11β-HSD: NADP(+)-dependent isoenzyme 1 (11β-HSD1), isolated from liver but widely expressed in many tissues; and NADP(+)-dependent isoenzyme 2 (11β-HSD2), highly expressed in kidney, placenta, and adrenal gland (151) (Table 38.1). The genes encoding both isoenzymes have been recently cloned. The gene HSD11B1, encoding 11β-HSD1 (liver isoenzyme), contains 6 exons and is located in chromosome 1, whereas the gene HSD11B2, encoding 11β-HSD2 (renal isoenzyme), contains 5 exons and is located in 16q12 (152,153).

AME is caused by autosomal recessive mutations in the HSD11B2 gene, which results in a deficiency of 11β-HSD2 (154–158). Most patients are homozygotes for one of the different mutations, and few compound heterozygotes have been identified.

Clinical and Biochemical Features

AME usually presents early in life and is characterized by polyuria, polydipsia, failure to thrive, hypertension, hypokalemic alkalosis, suppressed plasma renin activity, and absence of adrenal secretion of any known mineralocorticoid. Renal cysts, nephrocalcinosis, rickets, and hyperparathyroidism have been sporadically reported (159). Damage of many organs (e.g., kidneys, retina, heart, central nervous system) universally follows long-standing hypertension. Intrauterine growth retardation is a common finding and is probably secondary to placental 11β-HSD2 deficiency. The human placenta contains abundant 11β-HSD2, which has an important regulatory role of fetal growth (160).

A mild form of AME has been described in a 12.5-year-old girl presenting with mild hypertension and suppressed renin and aldosterone secretion but lacking hypokalemia and low birth weight. Despite these mild symptoms, it was proven that this girl was homozygous for a missense mutation in the HSD11B2 gene (150).

Pathophysiology

11b-HSD (EC 1.1.1.146) plays a critical role in determining the specificity of type I receptors. In the normal state, cortisol is converted by 11β-HSD to cortisone, thus allowing the preferential binding of aldosterone to type I receptors. In cases of 11β-HSD deficiency, there is a high intrarenal cortisol concentration that facilitates binding to the type I receptor, thus resulting in AME (161). Transgenic mice lacking 11β-HSD2 present all major features of human AME (162).

Diagnosis

Biochemical diagnosis can be made by measuring the ratio of cortisol to cortisone metabolites (tetrahydrocortisol plus allotetrahydrocortisol or tetrahydrocortisone). The optimal diagnostic test is to measure the generation of titrated water in plasma samples when 11-titrated cortisol is injected. Conversion of cortisol to cortisone is only 0 to 6% in AME patients, whereas the normal conversion is 90 to 95% (150).

Therapy

Therapy consists of the administration of the mineralocorticoid receptor blocker, spironolactone. After the administration of spironolactone, hypertension disappears, natriuresis ensues, and plasma renin activity becomes detectable. The daily dose of spironolactone ranges between 2 and 10 mg/kg. As hypercalciuria and nephrocalcinosis are consistent features of the disease, a thiazide diuretic may be added. Thiazide diuretics may not only contribute to improve hypercalciuria but also may aid to lower blood pressure and allow for the dose of spironolactone to be reduced (157). Renal transplantation, performed in exceptional cases, completely normalizes the clinical and biochemical picture (163).

Hypertension Secondary to Activated Mineralocorticoid Receptor

Geller et al. (164) have reported on a family whose propositus, a 15-year-old boy, had severe hypertension and suppressed plasma aldosterone levels. This patient and 11 of 21 at-risk relatives, all hypertensive, were heterozygous for a missense mutation substituting leucine for highly conserved serine at codon 810 of the mineralocorticoid receptor. This mutation resulted in a gain of function of the receptor and alteration of its specificity because it was also activated by progesterone. Carriers not only presented with severe early-onset hypertension but also, although normokalemic, tended to have lower plasma K values and manifested severe hypertension during episodes of pregnancy.

Secondary Pseudohyperaldosteronism

An acquired syndrome of pseudohyperaldosteronism, in all ways identical to 11β-HSD2 deficiency, has been observed after chronic ingestion of licorice (165). Natural licorice, an extract of *Glycyrrhiza glabra* root, contains glycyrrhizinic acid, which is a potent inhibitor of 11β-HSD2. This complication is exceptionally observed in children (166). Carbenoxolone, an antiulcer drug, also competitively inhibits 11β-HSD and causes sodium retention as a relevant side effect. The possibility that a syndrome of AME is secondary to creams or nasal sprays containing 9α-fluorinated corticoids should also be considered.

HYPERKALEMIC STATES

A situation of hyperkalemia may be caused by increased intake or endogenous liberation of K, decreased renal output, or abnormal distribution of K in the body (see Chapter 8). Most children with persistent hyperkalemia, in the absence of oversupplementation, demonstrate decreased renal excretion of K. In such cases, one must differentiate extrinsic causes, such as mineralocorticoid deficiency due to primary adrenal disorders, from intrinsic causes, such as renal failure or tubular renal disorders limiting K transport. The term *renal tubular hyperkalemia* has been proposed to describe a group of isolated renal tubular defects of K secretion in which hyperkalemia constitutes the outstanding biochemical feature (167).

To examine whether sustained hyperkalemia is due to a tubular defect of K secretion, it is necessary to challenge the mechanisms of tubular transport and to study the functioning of the renin-aldosterone system. Although sulfate infusion has been widely used to test the functioning of the cortical distal nephron, identical results can be obtained by acute intravenous administration of furosemide (1 mg/kg body weight). This diuretic blocks NaCl reabsorption in the ascending limb of the loop of Henle and thus increases the delivery of fluid and NaCl to the cortical collecting tubule. By enhancing Na reabsorption in excess of Cl reabsorption in this cortical segment, it creates a favorable electric gradient (lumen-negative) and facilitates the exit of K and H. Furosemide, by causing volume depletion, also enhances the secretion of renin and aldosterone. A summary of the results obtained by our group in a study of normal children is presented in Table 38.3 (167).

When assessing urinary K excretion, one must take into account that as GFR decreases, fractional K excretion increases exponentially. Because many patients with renal tubular hyper-

TABLE 38.3. RENAL RESPONSE OF CHILDREN (N = 20) TO ACUTE FUROSEMIDE ADMINISTRATION (MEAN ± STANDARD DEVIATION)

	UpH	$U_{TA}V$ (μEq/dL GF)	$U_{NH4}V$ (μEq/dL GF)	FE_{Na} (%)	FE_{Cl} (%)	FE_K (%)	PRA (ng/mL/h)	Paldo (ng/dL)
Basal values before furosemide	5.93 ±0.57	13.1 ±6.1	19.6 ±6.7	0.7 ±0.7	1.1 ±1.1	11.5 ±4.6	3.1 ±3.5	18.3 ±12.2
Peak values after furosemide[b]	4.96 ±0.32	22.7 ±10.7	30.9 ±8.0	8.4 ±3.5	12.6 ±4.9	35.4 ±8.9	8.6[a] ±5.9	32.5[a] ±18.6

FE_{Cl}, fractional excretions of chloride; FE_K, fractional excretions of potassium; FE_{Na}, fractional excretions of sodium; GF, glomerular filtrate; Paldo, plasma aldosterone concentration; PRA, plasma renin activity; $U_{NH4}V$, urinary excretions of ammonium; UpH, urine pH; $U_{TA}V$, urinary excretions of titratable acid.
[a]Values obtained 180 minutes after administration of furosemide.
[b]Mean of peak values obtained in each subject.
Adapted from Rodríguez-Soriano J, Vallo A. Renal tubular hyperkalaemia in childhood. *Pediatr Nephrol* 1988;2:498–509.

kalemia may exhibit some degree of renal insufficiency, it is necessary to relate values of fractional K excretion to the corresponding values for GFR. To study the action of aldosterone at the level of distal and collecting tubules, it is useful to calculate the so-called transtubular K concentration gradient (TTKG) by the formula proposed by West et al. (168):

$$\text{TTKG} = \frac{\text{K urine}/(\text{U/P})\text{ osmolality}}{\text{K blood}}$$

This index provides a ratio of the estimated concentration of K in the cortical collecting tubule (or urine K concentration adjusted for medullary water abstraction) to that of K in the peritubular fluid in the renal cortex. Values in normal children follow a nongaussian distribution, with a median of 6.0 and a range of 4.1 to 10.5. Transtubular K concentration gradient is significantly higher in infants, with a median value of 7.8 and a range of 4.9 to 15.5 (169). Any value below these limits should be interpreted as indicating mineralocorticoid deficiency or mineralocorticoid unresponsiveness.

MINERALOCORTICOID DEFICIENCY

Hyperreninemic Hypoaldosteronism

Several adrenal disorders are associated with a primary defect in aldosterone secretion that is accompanied by a secondary increase in plasma renin activity. This situation is almost always accompanied by salt-wasting and hyperkalemia, and, therefore, it should be distinguished from tubular resistance to aldosterone or pseudohypoaldosteronism. A detailed description of adrenal disorders is beyond the scope of this chapter.

Adrenal Insufficiency (Addison's Disease)

When adrenal insufficiency occurs in infancy, it is usually due to congenital adrenal hypoplasia, a condition that may be sporadic or inherited in an autosomal recessive or a sex-linked pattern. The X-linked adrenal hypoplasia is often associated with gonadotrophin deficiency, progressive hearing loss, glycerokinase deficiency, and muscular dystrophy. In older children and adults, other causes may be observed: autoimmune adrenalitis and, more rarely today, tuberculosis, amyloidosis, and acute adrenal hemorrhage or infarction. Adrenal leukodystrophy (Addison's-Schilder's disease) is a rare sex-linked inherited condition characterized by progressive neurologic damage associated with primary adrenal insufficiency.

Hereditary enzymatic defects may also cause mineralocorticoid deficiency. Salt-wasting is present in approximately two-thirds of patients with the classic form of congenital adrenal hyperplasia resulting from 21-hydroxylase deficiency (150,170). Salt-wasting occurs usually during the first weeks of life and results from inadequate synthesis of aldosterone. Patients become suddenly dehydrated, with signs of extracellular fluid volume depletion. Hyponatremia and hyperkalemia are present, and urinary NaCl excretion is inappropriately high. Urgent therapy is mandatory and includes NaCl supplementation and administration of hydrocortisone and 9α-fludrocortisone. Glucocorticoid and mineralocorticoid therapy should be maintained for life.

Isolated Defects of Aldosterone Biosynthesis

Aldosterone biosynthetic defects other than 21-hydroxylase deficiency can also cause salt-wasting and hyperkalemia (171). The conversion of 11-desoxycorticosterone to aldosterone requires the successive steps of 11 β-hydroxylation, 18-hydroxylation, and 18-oxidation, all catalyzed by a single enzyme, aldosterone synthase (P450c11AS) (172). There are two inborn errors caused by different mutations in the CYP11B2 gene encoding aldosterone synthase, the so-called corticosterone methyloxidase type I and type II defects (173). Infants with both defects, but especially with type I, present with failure to thrive, recurrent episodes of dehydration and salt-wasting, and hyperkalemia (174,175). Simultaneous serum determination of aldosterone and 18-hydroxycorticosterone levels permits differentiation between type I and type II defects (176). As in salt-wasting congenital adrenal hyperplasia, mineralocorticoid replacement therapy should be maintained for life.

Hyporeninemic Hypoaldosteronism

Hyporeninemic hypoaldosteronism is a syndrome characterized by inappropriately low aldosterone secretion without an associated impairment in the synthesis of cortisol but with low plasma renin activity. In fact, hypoaldosteronism apparently results from insufficient stimulation of the adrenal gland by the renin-angiotensin system. This condition was first reported by Hudson et al. (177), and since then, a great number of cases have been documented in the literature, particularly in adults with moderate chronic renal insufficiency due to diabetic nephropathy or chronic tubulointerstitial disorders. Hyperkalemia and metabolic acidosis constitute the cardinal biochemical features. Salt-wasting is not generally present. This syndrome has been rarely reported in children, but its frequency is probably higher than is usually recognized in patients with moderate chronic renal insufficiencies of various etiologies (178). This condition appears to be especially frequent in children with lupus nephritis or with chronic nephropathy secondary to methylmalonic acidemia.

The pathogenesis of hyporeninemic hypoaldosteronism in patients with chronic renal insufficiency is not yet elucidated. The hyperkalemia may be ascribed solely to hypoaldosteronism, but pharmacologic doses of mineralocorticoids are often needed to correct it. This indicates associated tubular resistance to aldosterone's action. Metabolic acidosis may

TABLE 38.4. CHARACTERISTICS OF TWO MAJOR FORMS OF PRIMARY TYPE I PSEUDOHYPOALDOSTERONISM

Characteristics	Renal	Multiple
Affected organs	Kidney	Kidney, sweat and salivary glands, colon
Mode of inheritance	Autosomal dominant	Autosomal recessive
Genetic defect	Mutations in the gene encoding the mineralocorticoid receptor	Mutations in the genes encoding the α, β, or γ subunits of epithelial Na channel
Salt-wasting	Variable	Severe
Catchup growth on NaCl supplements	Common	Rare
PRA and aldosterone concentration	Very high, PRA decreases with age	Very high
Sweat and salivary electrolytes	Normal	Very high
High-salt diet	1–3 yr	Lifelong?
Improvement with age	Common	Absent?

PRA, plasma renin activity.
Adapted from Hanukoglu A. Type I pseudohypoaldosteronism includes two clinically and genetically distinct entities with either renal or multiple target organ defects. *J Clin Endocrinol Metab* 1991;73:936–944.

result from selective aldosterone deficiency and from the direct inhibitory action of hyperkalemia on renal ammonia genesis and tubular transport of ammonia. Hypoaldosteronism appears to be the consequence of hyporeninemia, but the reason for this is unclear. Chronic extracellular fluid expansion, damage to the juxtaglomerular apparatus, reduced activity of the adrenergic system, impaired formation of active renin, or decreased synthesis of prostacyclin have all been advocated as possible causes (179).

Specific therapy is often not required if attention is paid to avoidance of renin-suppressing agents (i.e., beta-blockers, calcium channel blockers, and nonsteroidal antiinflammatory agents), or K-retaining drugs (i.e., amiloride, spironolactone, heparin, captopril, trimethoprim, tacrolimus, or cyclosporine) (180). However, when dangerous hyperkalemia or severe metabolic acidosis is present, therapeutic measures become necessary. Good results have been reported with the sustained administration of furosemide, either alone or combined with 9α-fludrocortisone.

The syndrome of hyporeninemic hypoaldosteronism may be occasionally observed as an isolated or familial entity, not necessarily in association with chronic renal insufficiency (181–183). An interesting feature of all these cases is the presence of salt-wasting, a condition rarely observed in cases of hyporeninemic hypoaldosteronism associated with chronic renal insufficiency.

Apparent Mineralocorticoid Unresponsiveness

The term *pseudohypoaldosteronism* has been coined to describe disorders of electrolyte homeostasis characterized by an apparent state of renal tubular unresponsiveness to the action of aldosterone and manifested by salt-wasting, hyperkalemia, and metabolic acidosis. Recent molecular biology studies have shown that these syndromes do not always result from target-organ unresponsiveness to mineralocorticoids but more often are caused by inherited abnormalities of renal Na transport.

Primary Type 1 Pseudohypoaldosteronism

Type 1 pseudohypoaldosteronism (PHA1) is a hereditary condition characterized by salt-wasting, hyperkalemia, and metabolic acidosis in the presence of markedly elevated plasma renin activity and aldosterone concentrations. Since its first description by Cheek and Perry in 1958 (184), many cases have been reported. In recent years, it has become clear that PHA1 is a heterogeneous syndrome that includes at least two clinically and genetically distinct entities with either *renal* or *multiple* target-organ defects (185) (Table 38.4). An exceptional case with apparent resistance to aldosterone limited to sweat and salivary glands without associated salt-wasting has also been reported (186).

Renal Type 1 Pseudohypoaldosteronism

Genetics

Renal PHA1 represents the most frequent form of PHA1 (Table 38.1). The mode of inheritance is autosomal dominant, with variable expression. Many cases appear as sporadic, but familial studies reveal high plasma levels of aldosterone in one of the apparently asymptomatic parents. The pathogenesis of renal PHA1 has been greatly clarified with the identification of heterozygous mutations in the mineralocorticoid receptor gene (187–189). The structure of the gene encoding the human mineralocorticoid receptor (MLR) has been elucidated. It is formed by 9 exons and is located at 4q31.1. Two different isoforms have been identified. Each isoform is expressed in approximately equivalent levels in kidney, colon, and sweat glands.

Clinical and Biochemical Features

Clinical features are extremely variable. In general, symptoms appear in early infancy with failure to thrive, weight loss, vomiting, and dehydration. Salt-wasting and polyuria may be already present in fetal life and manifested by maternal hydramnios. Occasional patients may present also with hypercalciuria and nephrocalcinosis. If therapy is delayed, patients may become severely undernourished. During the salt-wasting episodes, which may be triggered by intercurrent infections, patients appear shocked and comatose. A partial form with mild course of the disease and almost absent salt-wasting may be observed (190). Sweat and salivary electrolytes are characteristically normal. In exceptional cases, diagnosis can be made in asymptomatic newborn babies or even in cord blood on the basis of a positive family history.

The outstanding laboratory findings are hyponatremia and hyperkalemia. Metabolic acidosis may be also present. Hyponatremia may be masked by the hemoconcentration. Hyperkalemia varies from moderately to greatly increased values for plasma K concentration. Urinary Na excretion is inappropriately high, given the presence of hyponatremia. On the contrary, urinary K excretion is very low, with decreased values of fractional K excretion and transtubular K concentration gradient. GFR is normal after sodium depletion is corrected. Renal biopsy findings are usually negative, but in a few cases, hypertrophy of the juxtaglomerular apparatus has been reported. Although plasma electrolyte findings are very similar to those seen in defects of aldosterone biosynthesis, both plasma renin activity and aldosterone concentration are markedly elevated, urinary excretion of aldosterone and tetrahydroaldosterone are elevated, and a urinary pattern of aldosterone metabolites conforms to a normal pattern (i.e., a normal 18-hydroxy-tetrahydrocompound A to tetrahydroaldosterone ratio) (191). There is also a characteristic lack of improvement despite administration of large doses of mineralocorticoids.

The observation that many adult gene carriers have elevated aldosterone levels but no history of clinical disease raises the possibility that only a fraction of such carriers develop clinically evident disease (192). The reasons for the phenotype differences are unknown, but they may be related to intercurrent volume-depleting events or to dietary habits of salt ingestion. Also, the coexistence of polymorphisms or mutations in the gene encoding ENaC could play a potential contributory role. Polymorphisms and mutations that lead to either loss of function or gain of function of the epithelial Na^+ channel may aggravate or attenuate, respectively, the consequences of deficient mineralocorticoid receptor function.

Pathophysiology

The pathogenesis of renal pseudohypoaldosteronism type 1 is related to the loss of function of the mineralocorticoid receptor. The mineralocorticoid receptor is a protein of 984 amino acids belonging to the superfamily of steroid receptors. It contains an immunogenic domain, a zinc-finger DNA-binding domain, and a hormone-binding domain (193). At variance with glucocorticoid receptor that is almost ubiquitous, mineralocorticoid receptor expression is restricted to specific cells of kidney distal and collecting tubules, colonic epithelium, and sweat and salivary gland ducts. In all these epithelia, aldosterone stimulates Na reabsorption. Mineralocorticoid receptor–deficient mice have been generated by gene targeting technology. These knockout mice develop symptoms of pseudohypoaldosteronism soon after birth, which can be compensated by abundant NaCl administration. These NaCl-rescued mice display a strongly enhanced fractional renal excretion of Na, hyperkalemia, a persistently activated renin-angiotensin-aldosterone system, and very reduced ENaC activity in the kidney and colon (194).

Treatment and Prognosis

Renal PHA1 is treated with NaCl supplementation (3 to 6 g/day), which is followed by marked clinical and biochemical improvement. The expansion of extracellular fluid volume results in an increase of tubular flow and NaCl delivery to the distal nephron, thus creating a favorable gradient for K secretion despite the lack of mineralocorticoid action. The amount of NaCl required is deduced from the normalization of plasma K concentration and renin activity. Although the primary defect persists for life, improvement may occur beyond 1 or 2 years of age, due to maturation of proximal tubular transport, development of salt appetite, and improvement in the renal tubular response to mineralocorticoids (195). Older children with renal PHA1 are generally asymptomatic when eating a normal salt intake, but plasma aldosterone concentrations remain elevated. In contrast to aldosterone levels, plasma renin activity decreases into the normal range with advancing age. The discrepancy between renin and aldosterone secretion may be explained by the development of autonomous, tertiary hyperaldosteronism, as demonstrated by the increased excretion of 18-hydroxy-compound B (a characteristic marker of the functioning of the zona glomerulosa). Exceptionally, subtle symptoms leading to growth failure or even overt salt-wasting may persist to late childhood.

Multiple Type 1 Pseudohypoaldosteronism

Genetics

A few kindreds have been reported with multiple end-organ PHA1 since its original description (196,197) (Table 38.1). mineralocorticoid resistance is evident in kidney, lung, colon, and sweat and salivary glands. This variant is inherited as an autosomal recessive disorder, with uniform expression. The parents of affected children are asymptomatic and evidence normal plasma aldosterone levels. It has been demonstrated that this entity is caused by loss-of-function mutations of genes encoding one of the three constitutive subunits (i.e., α, β, and γ) of the ENaC (198–201). Critical hot spots for loss-of-function mutations seem to be the cysteine-reach domains in the large extracellular loop of the proteins (202).

Clinical and Biochemical Features

The multiple PHA1 presents with more severe salt-wasting and has a poorer outcome than the renal form. These patients manifest salt-wasting episodes early after birth, and death may ensue during the neonatal period. Sweat and salivary electrolytes are markedly elevated, and active Na transport in the rectal mucosa is impaired. Neither abnormality is corrected by the administration of exogenous mineralocorticoids. The high incidence of lower respiratory tract involvement may contribute to the confusion with cystic fibrosis (203,204). As in the renal form, hypercalciuria may be present.

Pathophysiology

Multiple target-organ PHA1 is due to defective Na transport in many organs containing the ENaC: kidney, lung, colon, and exocrine glands. Multiple PHA1 is allelic to Liddle's syndrome, but the mutations present result in loss of the channel activity with ensuing renal and rectal Na loss and increased sweat and saliva electrolyte values. The frequent lower respiratory involvement may be explained by the dysfunction of the ENaC of the respiratory epithelia (205). The impaired bacterial killing may be due to increased NaCl concentration in the airway surface fluid (206). The state of secondary hyperreninism and hyperaldosteronism is not caused by peripheral resistance to mineralocorticoids but derives from sustained extracellular fluid volume depletion.

Insights into pathogenesis have been facilitated by the development of transgenic mouse models in which expression of the α, β, or γ subunits of ENaC has been ablated. Of interest, only the αENaC-deficient mice present marked failure to clear the fetal lung fluid that leads to early neonatal death (207). If the mice are rescued from death by the engineered expression of the α subunit gene in the lung, they develop a full-blown picture of PHA, with salt-wasting and hyperkalemia (208). The βENaC- and γENaC-deficient mice do not die of neonatal respiratory failure but develop a very severe picture of neonatal salt-wasting and hyperkalemia from birth, similar to human PHA1 (209–211).

The neonatal lung findings present in αENaC-deficient mice are only exceptionally observed in humans (212), despite impressive truncations of the α subunit in some kindreds. However, some impairment in Na transport across airway epithelia may persist throughout life. In fact, pulmonary symptoms in patients with autosomal recessive PHA1 are not always related to infection and may be secondary (especially in young patients) to failure to absorb liquid from airway surfaces (213). The defect in Na transport can be demonstrated by measurement of transepithelial voltage across the nasal epithelium (214).

Treatment and Prognosis

There is a poor response to NaCl supplementation alone, and rectal administration of exchange resins and dietary manipulation reducing the intake of K are often necessary. Administration of indomethacin or hydrochlorothiazide or both may be useful in occasional patients (215). Improvement with age is less apparent, and therapy must be maintained throughout childhood and probably throughout life (216).

Early-Childhood Hyperkalemia

McSherry (217) described 13 infants and young children who presented with failure to thrive or growth retardation and frequent vomiting. The only biochemical abnormalities were hyperkalemia and metabolic acidosis. Clinical salt-wasting or hypertension was absent. Functional evaluation revealed a normal ability to acidify the urine, low NH_4 and K excretion, and a mild defect in HCO_3 reabsorption (i.e., functional markers of type 4 renal tubular acidosis). Plasma renin activity and aldosterone excretion were consistently normal or elevated. McSherry speculated that this entity could be due to a primary or idiopathic unresponsiveness of the distal nephron to aldosterone that manifested itself by defects in K and H excretion with integrity of Na reabsorption. However, Appiani et al. (218) reported five infants with similar clinical features who demonstrated a significantly increased fractional Na excretion. As in the cases communicated by McSherry, no clinical evidence of salt-wasting was observed.

Early-childhood hyperkalemia represents a variant of the renal form of PHA1. Therapy is generally required during the first years of life in the form of sodium bicarbonate alone or associated with caption-exchange resin. With treatment, growth accelerates and normal height is achieved within 6 months. The disorder appears to be transient, and at approximately 5 years of age, therapy is no longer needed.

Secondary Type 1 Pseudohypoaldosteronism

Secondary forms of PHA1 have been rarely reported. A partial tubular insensitivity to aldosterone may account for the hyperkalemia observed in some infants after unilateral renal vein thrombosis or for the salt-wasting and hyperkalemia that follow neonatal medullary necrosis. A syndrome of apparent renal tubular resistance to aldosterone was first documented in 1983 by Rodríguez-Soriano et al. in young infants with urinary tract infection and associated urinary tract malformations (219). Since then, 62 cases have been reported (220). After medical or surgical therapy, all abnormalities generally disappear, although, in cases of severe obstructive uropathy, renal sodium loss may become transiently more severe during the early obstructive period (221,222). The picture of hyponatremia or hyperkalemia may be also observed in infants and children with acute pyelonephritis, even in the absence of associated uropathy (223–225). All these observations indicate that renal ultrasonography and urine culture should be performed in any infant or child presenting with salt-wasting or hyperkalemia to exclude structural renal lesions or infection as the cause of the electrolyte disturbances.

Type 2 Pseudohypoaldosteronism (Gordon's Syndrome)

A familial syndrome (type 2 pseudohypoaldosteronism) of arterial hypertension, hyperkalemia, metabolic acidosis, suppressed plasma renin activity, and normal glomerular function was first described by Paver and Pauline in 1964 (226), although it was characterized as a new clinical entity by Gordon et al. in 1970 (227). Approximately 100 cases of so-called Gordon's syndrome have been reported in the literature (228). Hypertension represents a feature limited to adolescent or adult individuals. A similar condition has been reported in children with short stature, hyperkalemia, and metabolic acidosis but with normal blood pressure (Spitzer-Weinstein syndrome) (229–232). The finding in the same family of affected siblings with and without hypertension supports the conclusion that both syndromes are indeed the same genetic entity.

Genetics

Type 2 pseudohypoaldosteronism is inherited as an autosomal dominant entity. Linkage analysis has demonstrated genetic heterogeneity of the trait with involvement of at least three different loci in chromosomes 1q31-42, 12p13.3, and 17p11-q21 (233–235) (Table 38.1). Recently, mutations in two different genes belonging to the WNK family of serine-theonine kinases have been identified as a cause of type 2 pseudohypoaldosteronism (236). The WNK1 gene, formed by 28 exons and located in chromosome 12p, encodes the WNK1 kinase. Disease-causing mutations in WNK1 are large intronic deletions that increase WNK1 expression. WNK4 gene, formed by 19 exons and located in chromosome 17p, encodes the WNK4 kinase. The mutations in WNK4 are gain-of-function missense and cluster in a short, highly conserved segment of the encoded protein.

Clinical and Biochemical Features

Short stature and arterial hypertension are the cardinal signs in children and adults, respectively. Muscle weakness has also been reported. The relevant laboratory findings are hyperkalemia, hyperchloremic metabolic acidosis, hyporeninemic hypoaldosteronism, and normal GFR. Exceptionally, the metabolic manifestations may be already apparent in early infancy. Although not mentioned by most authors, hypercalciuria may be present and give rise to the formation of calcium oxalate stones.

Pathophysiology

Schambelan et al. (237) proposed the name of *chloride-shunt* syndrome (or type 2 pseudohypoaldosteronism), according to the hypothesis that the primary abnormality was a tubular hyperreabsorption of NaCl such that the mineralocorticoid-induced, charge-dependent K and H secretion would be attenuated by a voltage-shunting defect. Increased NaCl reabsorption would lead to expansion of plasma volume, suppressed secretion of renin and aldosterone, and eventual development of hypertension. In favor of this hypothesis was the complete reversal of the defect when distal NaCl delivery was increased by sodium sulfate or bicarbonate infusions or by the acute administration of furosemide.

Molecular biology studies have confirmed that increased distal tubular reabsorption of NaCl is the primary pathologic event in this syndrome. Both WNK1 and WNK4 kinases localize to the distal nephron segments known to play a key role in the homeostasis of Na reabsorption and H and K secretion. WNK1 is cytoplasmic, whereas WNK4 localizes to tight junctions. The gain-of-function mutations in these kinases may serve to increase transcellular or paracellular Cl conductance in the collecting duct, thereby increasing NaCl reabsorption and intravascular volume, while concomitantly dissipating the electrical gradient and diminishing H and K secretion (236).

Treatment and Prognosis

Diuretic therapy results in complete reversal of both clinical and biochemical abnormalities, with return of blood pressure to normal levels (when it is elevated), rise in plasma renin activity and aldosterone concentration, and correction of hyperkalemia and metabolic acidosis. Furosemide administration is very effective, but it aggravates the hypercalciuria and thus increases the risk of urolithiasis. In our opinion, the best treatment is the administration of hydrochlorothiazide (1.5 to 2.0 mg/kg/day) that is as effective as furosemide in the reversal of biochemical abnormalities and also corrects the hypercalciuria. Long-term prognosis remains uncertain because follow-up data are still limited.

HYPOMAGNESEMIC STATES

Chronic hypomagnesemia may be caused by inadequate dietary intake, defective gastrointestinal absorption, or increased urinary excretion and may be associated with hypocalcemia and hypokalemia. Mg depletion due to excessive urinary losses may occur as an acquired entity, in postobstructive diuresis; the diuretic phase of renal transplantation or acute tubular necrosis; states of hyperparathyroidism or hyperaldosteronism; or administration of diuretics (e.g., loop diuretics, thiazides), antiinfectious agents (e.g., aminoglycosides, capreomycin, amphotericin B, pentamidine), antineoplastic agents (e.g., cisplatinum), or immunosuppressive drugs (e.g., cyclosporine) (238). Cisplatinum may not only cause an acute renal Mg loss but also a chronic disorder that persists after withdrawal of the drug and may be associated with hypokalemia, metabolic alkalosis, and hypocalciuria (239,240).

Hypomagnesemia may also have a hereditary renal origin. This syndrome, known as *familial* or *congenital magnesium-losing kidney*, was first described by Freeman and Pearson in 1966 (241) and includes several different conditions, including familial hypokalemia or hypomagnesemia or Gitelman's syndrome, as discussed above (242,243). To differentiate between primary renal loss from intestinal loss of Mg, a 24-hour urinary Mg excretion or the fractional excretion of Mg in a random urine specimen should be obtained. Daily excretion of more than 30 mg of Mg per 1.73 m^2 or a fractional excretion of Mg above 2% in an individual with normal renal function points to renal Mg wasting (243).

Hypomagnesemia with Secondary Hypocalcemia

Hypomagnesemia with secondary hypocalcemia is an autosomal recessive disorder that manifests in the newborn period by very low plasma Mg and Ca concentrations (244). Patients usually present with restlessness, tremor, tetany, and overt seizures. In older children, clouded sensorium, disturbed speech, and choreoathetoid movements have been described. The hypocalcemia is secondary to parathyroid failure and peripheral parathyroid hormone resistance as a result of Mg deficiency. Hypokalemia is occasionally present and is corrected after normalization of plasma Mg. The disease appears to be fatal unless treated with very high oral intakes of Mg or, preferably, with continuous nocturnal nasogastric infusion of Mg (245).

Mg deficiency seems to depend on a double intestinal and renal transport defect (246). Genetic linkage to chromosome 9q22 was found in inbred Beduin families (247), and, recently, two groups of investigators have found independently that the disease is due to mutations in a new gene, TRPM6, belonging to the TRPM family (248,249) (Table 38.1). The TRPM6 gene, formed by 39 exons, encodes a protein with 2022 amino acids, which acts as a putative ion channel that is highly similar to the transient receptor potential channel family. These channels are characterized by six transmembrane domains, a conserved pore-forming region, and a Pro-Pro-Pro motif after the last transmembrane segment (250). TRPM6 is highly expressed in intestinal epithelia and kidney tubules and shows great similarity with TRPM7, a bifunctional protein that combines Ca and Mg-permeable action channel properties with protein kinase activity.

Isolated Familial Hypomagnesemia

Isolated hypomagnesemia, caused by congenital impairment of renal tubular Mg reabsorption, is a rare inherited disorder for which both autosomal dominant and autosomal recessive modes of inheritance have been described. Clinical features are variable, from asymptomatic cases to occurrence of carpopedal spasm or generalized convulsions. The nosologic classification of all these patients is difficult at present, but the absence of hypokalemia or nephrocalcinosis clearly separates them from the other entities discussed.

Autosomal Recessive Form

In the autosomal recessive form, the patients also have variable symptoms, but the urinary Ca excretion is normal (251,252). It probably represents a distinct disease because no linkage to any known previously reported loci has been found (243).

Autosomal Dominant Form

The autosomal dominant form is also associated with few symptoms other than chondrocalcinosis. Patients always have hypocalciuria and variable but usually mild hypomagnesemic symptoms (253,254). The disease locus, HOMG2, has been mapped to chromosome 11q23 in two Dutch families (255), but not in an American family (256), pointing out the existence of genetic heterogeneity. In the Dutch families, the disease was due to dominant-negative mutations in the gene FXYD2, encoding the Na^+,K^+-ATPase γ subunit (257) (Table 38.1). This mutation leads to a routing defect of the protein to the plasma membrane, thus decreasing the activity of Na^+,K^+-ATPase. Depolarization, reduced intracellular K, or increased intracellular Na could then determine a reduced Mg influx and secondary Mg wasting (257).

Familial Hypomagnesemia with Hypercalciuria and Nephrocalcinosis

The syndrome of familial hypomagnesemia with hypercalciuria and nephrocalcinosis should also be distinguished from other hereditary renal conditions leading to chronic hypomagnesemia. The first description was made by Michelis et al. in 1972 (258), but it was further characterized by Castrillo et al. in 1983 (259) (Michelis-Castrillo syndrome) and by Rodríguez-Soriano et al. in 1987 (96). Although only approximately 50 cases have been reported (260), the disease may be more common than usually appreciated.

Genetics

Hypomagnesemia with hypercalciuria and nephrocalcinosis behaves as an autosomal recessive disorder (Table 38.1). In favor of this type of inheritance is the fact that two sisters were transplanted with their parents' kidneys without reappearance of the disease (261). However, a study of 26 relatives belonging to four families is more suggestive of autosomal dominant inheritance with variable clinical expression in affected members (262). In the relatives, neither hypomagnesemia nor nephrocalcinosis or ocular abnormalities were present, but 11 of the 26 relatives (42%) exhibited isolated hypercalciuria. Praga et al. speculate that isolated hypercalciuria may represent a milder clinical expression of the disease, whereas the syndrome of hypomagnesemia with hypercalciuria and nephrocalcinosis could be the complete expression of this familial disorder.

Recent studies have demonstrated that this disease is caused by mutations in a novel gene, PCLN-1, located in chromosome 3q and encoding a novel renal tight junction protein involved in Mg and Ca transport, which was named *paracellin-1*, that belongs to the claudin family (claudin-16) (263–266).

Clinical and Biochemical Features

The cardinal clinical finding, besides episodic tetany or convulsions, is the development of nephrocalcinosis. This is constantly associated with polyuria and, more occasionally, with urinary tract infection or arterial hypertension. Nephrolithiasis has also been documented in several cases. Growth retardation is rarely present and, when observed, is more dependent on the nephrocalcinosis-related renal insufficiency than on the hypomagnesemia itself. An outstanding feature is the presence of ocular abnormalities such as myopia magna, horizontal nystagmus, chorioretinitis, and macular coloboma. Hearing impairment has also been occasionally reported. In some cases with profound hypomagnesemia, hypocalcemia, or a picture of vitamin D–resistant rickets may be observed, thus contributing to diagnostic confusion with distal renal tubular acidosis.

In contrast to Gitelman's syndrome, hypomagnesemia is not accompanied by hypokalemia, and there is a normal acid-base equilibrium or a tendency to metabolic acidosis instead of metabolic alkalosis. Hyperuricemia is manifest and may occasionally lead to gouty arthritis. The presence of variable degrees of renal insufficiency is related to the progression of the tubulointerstitial nephropathy induced by the nephrocalcinosis.

Hypermagnesuria occurs to a greater degree than with Gitelman's syndrome, despite a similar degree of hypomagnesemia. Documentation of marked hypercalciuria is the rule. Asymptomatic family members may exhibit isolated hypercalciuria, without hypomagnesemia. Defects in concentrating and acidifying mechanisms are probably secondary to nephrocalcinosis and contribute to the confusion with primary distal renal tubular acidosis (267). However, hypermagnesuria (but not hypomagnesemia) is only transiently observed in acidotic patients with distal renal tubular acidosis and rapidly corrects with alkali therapy. Thus, the association of hypomagnesemia and defective distal urinary acidification should strongly suggest the diagnosis of the syndrome of hypomagnesemia-hypercalciuria. Distal fractional Cl reabsorption, studied during hypotonic saline diuresis, is normal or very mildly impaired.

Pathophysiology

The primary defect is related to impaired tubular reabsorption of Ca and Mg in the thick ascending limb of Henle (Fig. 38.4). The study of tubular Mg reabsorption during continuous Mg sulfate infusion revealed a marked impairment of Mg reabsorption at all levels of filtered Mg, indicating that both renal threshold and renal tubular maximal reabsorption were decreased in this condition (96). These data strongly suggested the existence of a defect in Mg reabsorption at the level of the ascending limb of the loop of Henle, where most of filtered Mg is reabsorbed via the paracellular pathways and driven by the lumen-positive transepithelial electrical gradient (268). Recent molecular biology findings have shown that paracellin-1 plays a critical role in the control of Ca and Mg reabsorption in this nephron segment.

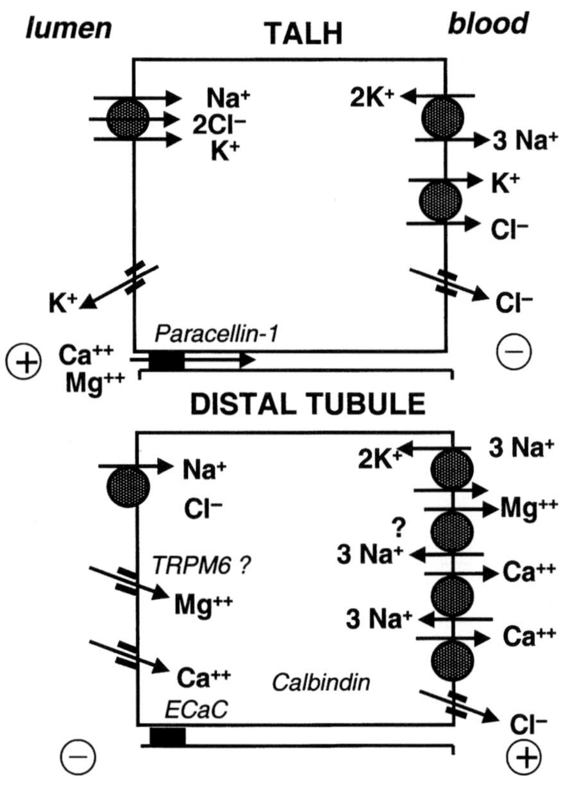

FIGURE 38.4. Schematic models of Ca and Mg reabsorption in thick ascending limb of Henle (TALH) and convoluted distal tubule. In TALH, Ca and Mg are exclusively reabsorbed via paracellular pathway through the action of paracellin-1 (claudin-16). In the distal convoluted tubule, Ca enters the cell from the lumen via an epithelial Ca channel (ECaC) and leaves the cell through a Ca ATPase and in exchange with Na. Mg absorption in the luminal membrane is mediated by an Mg channel (TRPM6?) and probably leaves the cell in exchange with Na. The functional integrity of Na^+,K^+-ATPase subunit appears to be essential for Mg reabsorption in the distal tubule.

Paracellin-1 belongs to the claudin family, and it has been renamed *claudin-16*. It shows sequence and structural similarity to other members of the claudin family. More than a dozen members of this family have been identified; all localize to tight junctions and appear to bridge the intercellular space by homo- or heterotypic interactions (269). Paracellin-1 is constituted by 305 amino acids with four transmembrane domains and intracellular N and C termini and is exclusively expressed in the kidney at the level of the thick ascending limb and distal tubule (263). Although almost 50% of Na reabsorption in the ascending loop of Henle also occurs via the paracellular pathways, it is likely that paracellin-1 only selectively mediates the barrier to divalent but not monovalent cations (270).

Treatment and Prognosis

The therapeutic results are poor. Combined therapy with Mg salts and hydrochlorothiazide permits some correction of the hypercalciuria, but the level of plasma Mg remains virtually the same. As the progression of the disease appears to be related to the worsening of the nephrocalcinosis, the administration of potassium citrate in the hope of arresting Ca deposition has been recommended (271,272).

Progressive renal impairment appears to be almost universal, and end-stage renal failure develops between 10 and 25 years of age. Treatment with Mg salts and thiazides for the majority of patients apparently failed to prevent the progression of the disease (264). At least 14 patients [five from our own series and nine from the literature (261,262)] have been successfully transplanted without recurrence of the disease, a fact strongly suggesting the existence of an intrinsic defect in Mg and Ca reabsorption of the native kidneys.

REFERENCES

1. Bartter FC, Pronove P, Gill JR, et al. Hyperplasia of juxtaglomerular complex with hyperaldosteronism and hypokalemic alkalosis. *Am J Med* 1962;33:811–828.
2. Rodríguez-Soriano J. Bartter's and related syndromes. The puzzle is almost solved. *Pediatr Nephrol* 1998;12:315–327.
3. Guay-Woodford LM. Bartter syndrome: unraveling the pathophysiologic enigma. *Am J Med* 1998;105:151–161.
4. Seyberth HW, Rascher W, Schweer W, et al. Congenital hypokalemia with hypercalciuria in preterm infants: a hyperprostaglandinuric tubular syndrome different from Bartter syndrome. *J Pediatr* 1985;107:694–701.
5. Clive DM. Bartter's syndrome: the unsolved puzzle. *Am J Kidney Dis* 1995;25:813–823.
6. McCredie DA. Variants of Bartter's syndrome. *Pediatr Nephrol* 1996;10:419–421.
7. Simon DB, Karet FE, Hamdan JM, et al. Bartter's syndrome, hypokalaemic alkalosis with hypercalciuria, is caused by mutations in the Na-K-2Cl cotransporter NKCC2. *Nat Genet* 1996;13:183–188.
8. Vargas-Poussou R, Feldmann D, Vollmer, et al. Novel molecular variants of the Na-K-2Cl cotransporter gene are responsible for antenatal Bartter syndrome. *Am J Hum Genet* 1998;62:1332–1340.
9. Bettinelli A, Ciarmatori S, Cesareo L, et al. Phenotypic variability in Bartter syndrome type I. *Pediatr Nephrol* 2000;14: 940–945.
10. Simon DB, Karet FE, Rodríguez-Soriano J, et al. Genetic heterogeneity of Bartter's syndrome revealed by mutations in the K^+ channel, ROMK. *Nat Genet* 1996;14:152–156.
11. International Collaborative Study Group for Bartter-like Syndromes. Mutations in the gene encoding the inwardly-rectifying renal potassium channel, ROMK, cause the antenatal variant of Bartter syndrome: evidence for genetic heterogeneity. *Hum Mol Genet* 1997;6:17–26.
12. Vollmer M, Koehrer M, Topaloglu R, et al. Two novel mutations in the gene for K_{ir} 1.1 *(ROMK)* in neonatal Bartter syndrome. *Pediatr Nephrol* 1997;12:69–71.
13. Jeck N, Derst C, Wischmeyer E, et al. Functional heterogeneity of ROMK mutations linked to hyperprostaglandin E syndrome. *Kidney Int* 2001;69:1803–1811.
14. Starremans PGJ, van der Kemp AW, Knoers NV, et al. Functional implications of mutations in the human renal outer medullary potassium channel (ROMK2) identified in Bartter syndrome. *Pflugers Arch* 2002;443:466–472.
15. Schulte U, Hahn H, Konrad M, et al. pH gating of ROMK (K_{ir} 1.1) channels: control by an arg-lys-arg triad disrupted in antenatal Bartter syndrome. *Proc Natl Acad Sci U S A* 1999;96:15298–15303.
16. Feldmann D, Alessandri JL, Deschênes G. Large deletion of the 5' end of the ROMK1 gene causes antenatal Bartter syndrome. *J Am Soc Nephrol* 1998;9:2357–2359.
17. Vollmer M, Jeck N, Lemmink HH, et al. Antenatal Bartter syndrome with sensorineural deafness: refinement of the locus on chromosome 1p31. *Nephrol Dial Transplant* 2000; 15:970–974.
18. Birkenhäger R, Otto E, Schürman M, et al. Mutation of BSND causes Bartter syndrome with sensorineural deafness and kidney failure. *Nat Genet* 2001;29:310–314.
19. Estevez R, Boettger T, Stein V, et al. Barttin is a Cl^- channel beta-subunit crucial for renal Cl^- reabsorption and inner ear K^+ secretion. *Nature* 2001;414:502–503.
20. Konrad M, Vollmer M, Lemmink HH, et al. Mutations in the chloride channel gene CLCNKB as a cause of classic Bartter syndrome. *J Am Soc Nephrol* 2000;11:1449–1459.
21. Proesmans W. Bartter syndrome ands its neonatal variant. *Eur J Pediatr* 1997;156:669–679.
22. Landau D, Shalev H, Ohaly M, Carmi R. Infantile variant of Bartter syndrome and sensorineural deafness: a new autosomal recessive disorder. *Am J Med Genet* 1995;59:454–459.
23. Madrigal G, Saborio P, Mora F, et al. Bartter syndrome in Costa Rica: a description of 20 cases. *Pediatr Nephrol* 1997;11:296–301.
24. Proesmans W, Massa G, Vanderschueren-Lodeweyckx M. Growth from birth to adulthood in a patient with the neonatal form of Bartter syndrome. *Pediatr Nephrol* 1988;2:205–209.
25. Proesmans W, Massa G, Vanderberghe K, et al. Prenatal diagnosis in Bartter syndrome. *Lancet* 1987;1:394.

26. Matsushita Y, Suzuki Y, Oya N, et al. Biochemical examination of the mother's urine is useful for prenatal diagnosis of Bartter syndrome. *Prenat Diagn* 1999;19:671–673.
27. Konrad M, Leonhardt A, Hensen P, et al. Prenatal and postnatal management of hyperprostaglandin E_2 syndrome after genetic diagnosis from amniocytes. *Pediatrics* 1999;103:678–683.
28. Moudgil A, Bagga A, Germain BM, et al. Neonatal Bartter's syndrome with hyperkalemia and normal urinary prostaglandin E_2. *Pediatr Nephrol* 1997;11:387–388.
29. Ernst LM, Parkash V. Placental pathology in fetal Bartter syndrome. *Pediatr Dev Pathol* 2002;5:76–79.
30. Schröter J, Timmermans G, Seyberth HW, et al. Marked reduction of Tamm-Horsfall protein synthesis in hyperprostaglandin E-syndrome. *Kidney Int* 1993;44:401–410.
31. Delpire E, Kaplan MR, Plotkin MD, et al. The Na-(K)-Cl cotransporter family in the mammalian kidney: molecular identification and function(s). *Nephrol Dial Transplant* 1996;11:1967–1973.
32. Takahashi N, Chernavvsky DR, Gómez RA, et al. Uncompensated polyuria in a mouse model of Bartter syndrome. *Proc Natl Acad Sci U S A* 2000;97:5434–5439.
33. Hebert SC. An ATP-regulated, inwardly rectifying potassium channel from rat kidney (ROMK). *Kidney Int* 1995;48:1010–1016.
34. Derst C, Konrad M, Köckerling L, et al. Mutations in the ROMK gene in antenatal Bartter syndrome are associated with impaired K^+ channel function. *Biochem Biophys Res Commun* 1997;230:641–645.
35. Köckerling A, Reinalter SC, Seyberth HW. Impaired response to furosemide in hyperprostaglandin E syndrome: evidence for a tubular defect in the loop of Henle. *J Pediatr* 1996;129:519–528.
36. Macica CM, Yang Y, Hebert SC, Wang WH. Arachidonic acid inhibits activity of cloned renal K+ channel, ROMK1. *Am J Physiol* 1996;271:F588–F594.
37. Komhoff M, Jeck ND, Seyberth HW, et al. Cyclooxygenase-2 expression is associated with the renal macula densa of patients with Bartter-like syndrome. *Kidney Int* 2000;58:2420–2424.
38. Nusing RM, Reinalter SC, Peterts M, et al. Pathogenetic role of cyclooxygenase-2 in hyperprostaglandin E syndrome/antenatal Bartter syndrome: therapeutic use of cyclooxygenase-2 inhibitor nimesulide. *Clin Pharmacol Ther* 2001;70:384–390.
39. Restrepo de Rovetto C, Welch TR, Hug G, et al. Hypercalciuria with Bartter's syndrome: evidence for an abnormality of vitamin D metabolism. *J Pediatr* 1989;115:397–404.
40. Leonhardt A, Timmermanns G, Roth B, et al. Calcium homeostasis and hypercalciuria in hyperprostaglandinism E syndrome. *J Pediatr* 1992;120:546–554.
41. Shoemaker LR, Welch TR, Bergstrom W, et al. Calcium kinetics in the hyperprostaglandin E_2 syndrome. *Pediatr Res* 1992;33:92–96.
42. Shoemaker LR, Bergstrom W, Ragosta K, et al. Humoral factor in children with neonatal Bartter syndrome reduces bone calcium uptake in vitro. *Pediatr Nephrol* 1998;12:371–376.
43. Williams WJ, Shoemaker LR, Schurman SJ, et al. Conjunctive effects of fibroblastic growth factor and glycosaminoglycan on bone metabolism in neonatal Bartter syndrome. *Pediatr Res* 1999;45:726–732.
44. Meyburg J, Mayatepek E, Hoffman GF, et al. Severe hyperchloriduria-hyperkaliuria: a new congenital renal tubular abnormality? *J Pediatr* 1996;128:376–378.
45. Abramson O, Zmora E, Mazor M, Shinwell ES. Pseudohypoaldosteronism in a preterm infant: intrauterine presentation as hydramnios. *J Pediatr* 1992;120:129–132.
46. Greenberg D, Abramson O, Phillip M. Fetal pseudohypoaldosteronism: another cause of hydramnios. *Acta Paediatr* 1992;84:582–584.
47. Shalev H, Ohali M, Abramson O, et al. Nephrocalcinosis in pseudohypoaldosteronism and the effect of indomethacin therapy. *J Pediatr* 1994;125:246–248.
48. Stone RC, Vale P, Rosa FC. Effect of hydrochlorothiazide in pseudohypoaldosteronism with hypercalciuria and severe hyperkalemia. *Pediatr Nephrol* 1994;10:501–503.
49. Langhendries JP, Thiry V, Bodart E, et al. Exogenous prostaglandin administration and pseudo-Bartter syndrome. *Eur J Pediatr* 1989;149:208–209.
50. Rodríguez-Soriano J. Bartter's syndrome comes of age. *Pediatrics* 1999;13:663–664.
51. Reinalter S, Declieger H, Proesmans W. Neonatal Bartter syndrome: spontaneous resolution of all signs and symptoms. *Pediatr Nephrol* 1998;12:186–188.
52. Jeck N, Reinalter BC, Henne T, et al. Hypokalemic salt-losing tubulopathy with chronic renal failure and sensorineural deafness. *Pediatrics* 2001;108:E5.
53. Simon DB, Bindra RS, Nelson-Williams C, et al. Mutations in the chloride channel *ClC-Kb* cause Barrett's syndrome type III. *Nat Genet* 1997;17:171–178.
54. Saito-Ohara F, Uchida S, Takeuchi Y, et al. Assignment of the genes encoding the human chloride channels, CLCNKA and CLCNKB, to 1p36 and of CLCN3 to 4q32-q33 by *in situ* hybridization. *Genomics* 1996;36:372–374.
55. Ruvalcaba RH, Martínez FE. Case report: familial growth hormone deficiency associated with Bartter's syndrome. *Am J Med Sci* 1992;303:411–414.
56. Torres VE, Young WF Jr, Offord KP, et al. Association of hypokalemia, aldosteronism and renal cysts. *N Engl J Med* 1990;322:345–351.
57. Rodríguez-Soriano J, Vallo A, Oliveros R. Bartter's syndrome presenting with features resembling renal tubular acidosis. Improvement of renal tubular defects by indomethacin. *Helv Paediatr Acta* 1978;33:141–151.
58. Mersin SS, Ramelli GP, Laux-End R, et al. Urinary chloride excretion distinguishes between renal and extrarenal metabolic alkalosis. *Eur J Pediatr* 1995;154:979–982.
59. Bettenelli A, Bianchetti MG, Girardin E, et al. Use of calcium excretion values to distinguish two forms of primary renal tubular hypokalemic alkalosis: Bartter and Gitelman syndromes. *J Pediatr* 1992;120:38–43.
60. Jeck N, Konrad M, Peters M, et al. Mutations in the chloride channel gene, CLCNKB, leading to a mixed Bartter-Gitelman phenotype. *Pediatr Res* 2000;48:754–758.
61. Caló L, Davis PA, Milani M, et al. Bartter's syndrome and Gitelman's syndrome: two entities sharing the same abnormality in vascular reactivity. *Clin Nephrol* 1998;50:65–67.
62. Caló L, Davis PA, Milani M, et al. Increased endothelial nitric oxide synthase mRNA level in Bartter's and Gitelman's syndrome. Relationship to vascular reactivity. *Clin Nephrol* 1999;51:12–17.

63. Caló L, Ceolotto G, Milani M, et al. Abnormalities of Gq-mediated cell signaling in Bartter and Gitelman syndromes. *Kidney Int* 2001;60:882–886.
64. Caló L, Cantaro S, Piccoli A, et al. Full pattern of urinary prostaglandins in Bartter's syndrome. *Nephron* 1990;56:451–452.
65. Jentsch TJ, Friedrich T, Schriever A, et al. The CLC chloride channel family. *Pflugers Arch* 1999;437:783–795.
66. Rodríguez-Soriano J, Vallo A, Castillo G, et al. Renal handling of water and sodium in infancy and childhood: a study using clearance methods during hypotonic saline diuresis. *Kidney Int* 1981;20:700–704.
67. Hené RJ, Koomans HA, Dorhout Mees EJ. Suppressed diluting segment reabsorption in Bartter's syndrome: studies in 1 patient and synthesis of literature. *Am J Nephrol* 1988;8:402–409.
68. Rodríguez Portales JA, Delea CS. Renal tubular reabsorption of chloride in Bartter's syndrome and other conditions with hypokalemia. *Clin Nephrol* 1986;6:269–272.
69. Ferreira SR, Kater CE. Comparative study of two tests of renal diluting ability in Bartter's syndrome. *Braz J Med Biol Res* 1994;27:1181–1191.
70. Garrick R, Ziyadeh FN, Jorkasky D, Goldfarb S. Bartter's syndrome: a unifying hypothesis. *Am J Nephrol* 1985;5:379–384.
71. Sechi LA, Melis A, Faedda R, et al. Heterogeneous derangement of cellular sodium metabolism in Bartter's syndrome. Description of two cases and review of the literature. *Panminerva Med* 1992;34:85–92.
72. Korff JM, Siebens AW, Gill JR. Correction of hypokalemia corrects the abnormalities in erythrocyte sodium transport in Bartter's syndrome. *J Clin Invest* 1984;74:1724–1729.
73. Dillon MJ, Shah V, Mitchell MD. Bartter's syndrome: 10 cases in childhood. Results of long-term indomethacin therapy. *QJM* 1979;48:429–446.
74. Sann L, Moreau P, Longin B, et al. Un syndrome de Bartter associant un hypercortisolisme, un diabète phosphoré et magnésien et une tubulopathie d'origine familiale. *Arch Fr Ped* 1975;32:349–366.
75. Fricker H, Frey K, Valloton MB, et al. Bartter-Syndrom und tubuläre Funktionsstörungen. *Helv Paediatr Acta* 1975;30:61–77.
76. Potter WZ, Trygstad CW, Helmer OM, et al. Familial hypokalemia associated with renal interstitial fibrosis. *Am J Med* 1974;57:971–977.
77. Houston IB, Boichis H, Edelmann CM Jr. Fanconi syndrome with renal sodium wasting and metabolic alkalosis. *Am J Med* 1968;44:638–646.
78. O'Regan S, Mongeau JG, Robitaille P. A patient with cystinosis presenting with the features of Bartter syndrome. *Acta Paediatr Belg* 1980;33:51–52.
79. Whyte P, Shaheb S, Schnaper H. Cystinosis with features suggesting Bartter's syndrome. *Clin Pediatr* 1985;24:447–451.
80. Goto Y, Itami N, Kajii N, et al. Renal tubular involvement mimicking Bartter syndrome in a patient with Kearns-Sayre syndrome. *J Pediatr* 1990;116:904–910.
81. Uribarri J, Alveranga D, Oh MS, et al. Bartter's syndrome due to a defect in salt reabsorption in the distal convoluted tubule. *Nephron* 1985;40:52–56.
82. Stein H. The pathogenic spectrum of Bartter's syndrome. *Kidney Int* 1985;28:85–93.
83. Puschett JB, Greenberg A, Mitro T, et al. Variant of Bartter's syndrome with distal tubular rather than loop of Henle defect. *Nephron* 1988;50:205–211.
84. Soupart A, Unger J, Debieve MF, et al. Bartter's syndrome with a salt reabsorption defect in the cortical part of Henle's loop. *Am J Nephrol* 1988;8:309–315.
85. Sutton RAL, Mavichak V, Halabe A, et al. Bartter's syndrome: evidence suggesting a distal tubular defect in a hypocalciuric variant of the syndrome. *Miner Electrolyte Metab* 1992;18:43–51.
86. Güllner MG, Gill JR, Bartter FC, et al. A familial disorder with hypokalemic alkalosis, hyperreninemia, aldosteronism, high urinary prostaglandins and normal blood pressure that is not "Bartter's syndrome." *Trans Assoc Am Physicians* 1979;92:175–188.
87. Güllner HG, Bartter FC, Gill JR, et al. A sibship with hypokalemic alkalosis and renal proximal tubulopathy. *Arch Intern Med* 1983;143:1534–1540.
88. Colussi G, Rambolá G, Airaghi C, et al. Pseudo-Bartter's syndrome from surreptitious diuretic intake: differential diagnosis with true Bartter's syndrome. *Nephrol Dial Transplant* 1992;7:896–901.
89. D'Avanzo M, Santinelli R, Tolone C, et al. Concealed administration of furosemide simulating Bartter's syndrome in a 4.5 year-old boy. *Pediatr Nephrol* 1995;9:749–750.
90. Rodríguez-Soriano J, Vallo A. Salt-losing nephropathy associated with inappropriate secretion of atrial natriuretic peptide—a new clinical syndrome. *Pediatr Nephrol* 1997;11:565–572.
91. Arant B, Brackett N, Young R, Still W. Case studies of siblings with juxtaglomerular hyperplasia and secondary hyperaldosteronism associated with severe azotemia and renal rickets-Bartter's syndrome or disease. *Pediatrics* 1970;46:344–361.
92. Hené RJ, Koomans HA, Dorhout Mees EJ, et al. Correction of hypokalemia in Bartter's syndrome by enalapril. *Am J Kidney Dis* 1987;9:200–205.
93. Scherling B, Verder H, Nielsen MD, et al. Captopril treatment in Bartter's syndrome. *Scand J Urol Nephrol* 1990;214:123–125.
94. Kannan S, Delph Y, Moseley HS. Anaesthetic management of a child with Bartter's syndrome. *Can J Anaesth* 1995;42:808–812.
95. Gitelman HJ, Graham JB, Welt LG. A new familial disorder characterized by hypokalemia and hypomagnesemia. *Trans Assoc Am Physicians* 1966;79:221–233.
96. Rodríguez-Soriano J, Vallo A, García-Fuentes M. Hypomagnesaemia of hereditary renal origin. *Pediatr Nephrol* 1987;1:465–472.
97. Gladziwa U, Schwarz R, Gitter AH, et al. Chronic hypokalaemia in adults: Gitelman's syndrome is frequent but classical Bartter's syndrome is rare. *Nephrol Dial Transplant* 1995;10:1607–1613.
98. Simon DB, Nelson-Williams C, Bia MJ, et al. Gitelman's variant of Bartter's syndrome, inherited hypokalaemic alkalosis, is caused by mutations in the thiazide-sensitive Na-Cl cotransporter. *Nat Genet* 1996;12:24–30.
99. Mastroianni N, Betinelli A, Bianchetti M, et al. Novel molecular variants of the Na-Cl cotransporter gene are

responsible for Gitelman syndrome. *Am J Hum Genet* 1996; 59:1019–1026.
100. Lemmink HH, Knoers N, Karolyi L, et al. Novel mutations in the thiazide-sensitive Na-Cl cotransporter gene in patients with Gitelman syndrome with predominant localization to the C-terminal domain. *Kidney Int* 1998;54:720–730.
101. Monkawa T, Kurihara I, Kobayashi JK, et al. Novel mutations in thiazide-sensitive Na-Cl cotransporter gene on patients with Gitelman syndrome. *J Am Soc Nephrol* 2000; 11:65–70.
102. Melander O, Ohro-Melander M, Bengtsson K, et al. Genetic variants of thiazide-sensitive NaCl cotransporter in Gitelman's syndrome and primary hypertension. *Hypertension* 2000;36:389–394.
103. Cruz DN, Shaer AJ, Bia MJ, et al. Gitelman's syndrome revisited: an evaluation of symptoms and health-related quality of life. *Kidney Int* 2001;59:710–717.
104. Bettinelli A, Rusconi R, Ciarmatori S, et al. Gitelman disease associated with growth hormone deficiency, disturbances in vasopressin secretion and empty sella: a new hereditary renal tubular-pituitary syndrome? *Pediatr Res* 1999;46:232–238.
105. Ko CW, Koo JK. Recombinant human growth hormone and Gitelman's syndrome. *Am J Kidney Dis* 1999;33:778–781.
106. Smilde TJ, Haverman JF, Schipper P, et al. Familial hypokalemia/hypomagnesemia and chondrocalcinosis. *J Rheumatol* 1994;21:1515–1519.
107. Calò L, Punzi L, Semplicini A. Hypomagnesemia and chondrocalcinosis in Bartter's and Gitelman's syndrome: review of the pathogenetic mechanisms. *Am J Nephrol* 2000;20: 347–350.
108. Vezzoli G, Soldati L, Jansen A, et al. Choroidal calcifications in patients with Gitelman's syndrome. *Am J Kidney Dis* 2000;36:855–858.
109. Lüthy C, Betinelli A, Iselin S, et al. Normal prostaglandinuria E_2 in Gitelman's syndrome, the hypocalciuric variant of Bartter's syndrome. *Am J Kidney Dis* 1995;25:824–828.
110. Zarraga Larrondo S, Vallo A, Gainza J, et al. Familial hypokalemia-hypomagnesemia or Gitelman's syndrome: a further case. *Nephron* 1992;62:340–344.
111. Colussi G, Romboli G, Brunati C, et al. Abnormal reabsorption of Na^+/Cl^- by the thiazide-inhibitable transporter of the distal convoluted tubule in Gitelman's syndrome. *Am J Nephrol* 1997;17:103–111.
112. Rodríguez-Soriano J, Vallo A. Familial hypokalemia-hypomagnesemia (Gitelman's syndrome). *Pediatr Nephrol* 1990; 4:C22.
113. Kunchaparty S, Palcso M, Berkman J, et al. Defective processing and expression of thiazide-sensitive Na-Cl cotransporter as a cause of Gitelman's syndrome. *Am J Physiol* 1999;277:F643–F649.
114. Colussi G, Macaluso M, Brunati C, et al. Calcium metabolism and calciotropic hormone levels in Gitelman's syndrome. *Miner Electrolyte Metab* 1994;20:294–301.
115. Bianchetti MG, Betinelli A, Casez JP, et al. Evidence for disturbed regulation of calciotropic hormone metabolism in Gitelman syndrome. *J Clin Endocrinol Metab* 1995;80:224–228.
116. Dai L-J, Friedman PA, Quamme GA. Acid-base changes alter Mg^{2+} uptake in mouse distal convoluted tubule cells. *Am J Physiol* 1997;272:F759–F766.
117. De Rouffignac C, Quamme G. Renal magnesium handling and its hormonal control. *Physiol Rev* 1994;74:305–322.
118. Mehrotra R, Nolph KD, Kathuria P, et al. Hypokalemic metabolic alkalosis with hypomagnesuric hypermagnesemia and severe hypocalciuria: a new syndrome? *Am J Kidney Dis* 1997;29:106–114.
119. Schepkens H, Hoeben H, Vanholder R, et al. Mimicry of surreptitious diuretic ingestion and the ability to make a genetic diagnosis. *Clin Nephrol* 2001;55:233–237.
120. Kamel S, Harvey E, Douek K, et al. Studies on the pathogenesis of hypokalemia in Gitelman's syndrome: role of bicarbonaturia and hypomagnesemia. *Am J Nephrol* 1998; 18:42–49.
121. Bettinelli A, Basilico E, Metta MG, et al. Magnesium supplementation in Gitelman syndrome. *Pediatr Nephrol* 1999;13:311–314.
122. Liaw LC, Banerjee K, Coiulthard MG. Dose related growth response to indomethacin in Gitelman syndrome. *Arch Dis Child* 1999;81:508–510.
123. Colussi G, Rombolà G, De Ferrari ME, et al. Correction of hypokalemia with antialdosterone therapy in Gitelman's syndrome. *Am J Nephrol* 1994;14:127–135.
124. Betinelli A, Metta MG, Perini A, et al. Long-term follow-up of a patient with Gitelman's syndrome. *Pediatr Nephrol* 1993;7:67–68.
125. Bonfante L, Davis PA, Spinello M, et al. Chronic renal failure, end-stage renal disease, and peritoneal dialysis in Gitelman's syndrome. *Am J Kidney Dis* 2001;38:165–168.
126. Ganguly A. Primary aldosteronism. *N Engl J Med* 1998; 339:1828–1834.
127. Lifton RP, Dluhy RG, Powers M, et al. A chimaeric 11-hydroxylase/aldosterone synthase gene causes glucocorticoid-remediable hyperaldosteronism and human hypertension. *Nature* 1992;355:262–265.
128. Dluhy RG, Anderson N, Harlin B, et al. Glucocorticoid-remediable aldosteronism is associated with severe hypertension in childhood. *J Pediatr* 2001;138:715–720.
129. Litchfield WR, New MI, Coolidge C, et al. Evaluation of dexamethasone suppression test for the diagnosis of glucocorticoid-remediable aldosteronism. *J Clin Endocrinol Metab* 1997;82:3570–3573.
130. MacConnachie AA, Kelly KF, McNamara A, et al. Rapid diagnosis and identification of cross-over sites in patients with glucocorticoid remediable aldosteronism. *J Clin Endocrinol Metab* 1998;83:4328–4331.
131. Fardella PE, Pinto M, Mosso L, et al. Genetic study of patients with dexamethasone suppressible aldosteronism without the chimeric CYP11B1/CYP11B2 gene. *J Clin Endocrinol Metab* 2001;86:4805–4807.
132. Dluhy RG, Lifton RP. Glucocorticoid remediable aldosteronism. *J Clin Endocrinol Metab* 1999;84:4341–4244.
133. Liddle GW, Bledsoe T, Coppage WS. A familial renal disorder simulating primary aldosteronism but with negligible aldosterone secretion. *Trans Assoc Am Physicians* 1963;76: 199–213.
134. Warnock DG. Liddle syndrome: an autosomal dominant form of human hypertension. *Kidney Int* 1998;53:18–24.

135. Palmer BF, Alpern RJ. Liddle's syndrome. *Am J Med* 1998; 104:301–309.
136. Yamashita Y, Koga M, Takeda Y, et al. Two sporadic cases of Liddle's syndrome caused by de novo ENaC mutations. *Am J Kidney Dis* 2001;37:499–504.
137. Shimkets RA, Warnock DG, Bositis CM, et al. Liddle's syndrome: heritable human hypertension caused by mutations in the beta subunit of the epithelial sodium channel. *Cell* 1994;79:407–414.
138. Tamura H, Schild L, Enomoto N, et al. Liddle's disease caused by a missense mutation of beta subunit of the epithelial sodium channel gene. *J Clin Invest* 1996;97:1780–1784.
139. Hansson JH, Nelson-Williams C, Suzuki H, et al. Hypertension caused by a truncated epithelial sodium channel gamma subunit: genetic heterogeneity of Liddle syndrome. *Nat Genet* 1995;11:76–82.
140. Benos DJ, Awayda MS, Ismailov II, et al. Structure and function of amiloride-sensitive Na^+ channels. *J Membr Biol* 1995;143:1–18.
141. Harvey KF, Dinudom A, Komwatana P, et al. All three WW domains of murine Nedd4 are involved in the regulation of epithelial sodium channels by intracellular Na^+. *J Biol Chem* 1999;274:12525–12530.
142. Abriel H, Loffing J, Rebhun JGF, et al. Defective regulation of the epithelial Na+ channel by Nedd4 in Liddle's syndrome. *J Clin Invest* 1999;103:667–673.
143. Snyder PM, Olson DR, McDonald FJ, et al. Multiple WW domains, but not the C2 domain, are required for inhibition of the epithelial Na+ channel by human Nedd4. *J Biol Chem* 2001;276:28321–28326.
144. Kamynina E, Debonneville C, Bens M, et al. A novel mouse Nedd4 protein suppresses the activity of the epithelial Na^+ channel. *FASEB J* 2001;15:204–214.
145. Pradervand S, Wang Q, Burnier M, et al. A mouse model for Liddle's syndrome. *J Am Soc Nephrol* 1999;10:2527–2533.
146. Wong ZY, Stebbing M, Ellis JA, et al. Genetic linkage of beta and gamma subunits of epithelial sodium channel to systolic blood pressure. *Lancet* 1999;353:1222–1225.
147. Su YR, Rutkowski MP, Klanke CA, et al. A novel variant of the beta-subunit of the amiloride-sensitive sodium channel in African Americans. *J Am Soc Nephrol* 1996;7:2543–2549.
148. Findling JW, Raff H, Hansson JH, et al. Liddle's syndrome: prospective genetic screening and suppressed aldosterone secretion in an extended kindred. *J Clin Endocrinol Metab* 1997;82:1071–1074.
149. New MI, Levine LS, Biglieri EG, et al. Evidence for an unidentified steroid in a child with apparent mineral corticoid hypertension. *J Clin Endocrinol Metabol* 1977;44:924–933.
150. New MI, Wilson RC. Steroid disorders in children: congenital adrenal hyperplasia and apparent mineralocorticoid excess. *Proc Natl Acad Sci U S A* 1999;96:12790–12797.
151. Albiston AL, Obeyesekere VR, Smith RE, et al. Cloning and tissue distribution of the human 11 beta-hydroxysteroid dehydrogenase type II enzyme. *Mol Cell Endocrinol* 1994;105:R11–R17.
152. Agarwal AK, Rogerson FM, Mune T, et al. Analysis of the human gene encoding the kidney isoenzyme of 11 beta-hydroxysteroid dehydrogenase. *J Steroid Biochem Mol Biol* 1995;55:473–479.
153. Agarwal AK, Rogerson FM, Mune T, et al. Gene structure and chromosomal localization of the human HSD11K gene encoding the kidney (type 2) isoenzyme of 11 beta-hydroxysteroid dehydrogenase. *Genomics* 1995;29:195–199.
154. Mune T, Rogerson FM, Nikkilä H, et al. Human hypertension caused by mutations in the kidney isoenzyme of 11 β-hydroxysteroid dehydrogenase. *Nat Genet* 1995;10:394–399.
155. Wilson RC, Harbison MD, Krozowski ZS, et al. Several homozygous mutations in the gene for 11 beta-hydroxysteroid dehydrogenase type 2 in patients with apparent mineral corticoid excess. *J Clin Endocrinol Metab* 1995;80: 3145–3150.
156. White PC, Mune T, Agarwal AK. 11 Beta-hydroxysteroid dehydrogenase and the syndrome of apparent mineral corticoid excess. *Endocr Rev* 1997;18:135–156.
157. Dave-Sharma AS, Wilson RC, Harbison MD, et al. Examination of genotype and phenotype relationships in 14 patients with apparent mineral corticoid excess. *J Clin Endocrinol Metab* 1998;83:2244–2254.
158. Odermatt A, Dick B, Arnold P, et al. A mutation in the cofactor-binding domain of 11 beta-hydroxysteroid dehydrogenase type 2 associated with mineral corticoid excess. *J Clin Endocrinol Metab* 2001;86:1247–1252.
159. Moudgil A, Rodich G, Jordan SC, et al. Nephrocalcinosis and renal cysts associated with apparent mineral corticoid excess. *Pediatr Nephrol* 2000;15:60–62.
160. McTernan CL, Draper N, Nicholson H, et al. Reduced placental 11beta-hydroxysteroid dehydrogenase type 2 mRNA levels in human pregnancies complicated by intrauterine growth restriction? An analysis of possible mechanisms. *J Clin Endocrinol Metab* 2001;86:4979–4983.
161. Benedicktsson R, Walker BR, Edwards CRW. Cellular selectivity of aldosterone action: role of 11 beta-hydroxysteroid dehydrogenase. *Curr Opin Nephrol Hypertens* 1995;4:41–46.
162. Holmes MC, Kotelevtsev Y, Mulling JJ, et al. Phenotypic analysis of mice bearing targeted deletions of 11beta-hydroxysteroid dehydrogenase 1 and 2 genes. *Mol Cell Endocrinol* 2001;171:15–20.
163. Palermo M, Delitala G, Sorba G, et al. Does kidney transplantation normalize cortisol metabolism in apparent mineral corticoid excess syndrome? *J Endocrinol Invest* 2000;23: 457–462.
164. Geller DS, Farhi A, Pinkerton N, et al. Activating mineral corticoid receptor mutation in hypertension exacerbated by pregnancy. *Science* 2000;289:119–123.
165. Walker BR, Edwards CR. Licorice-induced hypertension and syndromes of apparent mineral corticoid excess. *Endocrinol Metab Clin North Am* 1994;23:359–377.
166. Burgio E, Zammardi E, Vierucci A, et al. Un caso di pseudoiperaldosteronismo da ingestione di liquirizia. *Riv Ital Pediatr* 1980;6:391–392.
167. Rodríguez-Soriano J, Vallo A. Renal tubular hyperkalaemia in childhood. *Pediatr Nephrol* 1988;2:498–509.
168. West ML, Mardsen PA, Richardson RMA, et al. New clinical approach to evaluate disorders of potassium excretion. *Miner Electrolyte Metab* 1985;12:234–238.

169. Rodríguez-Soriano J, Ubetagoyena M, Vallo A. Transtubular potassium concentration gradient: a useful test to estimate renal aldosterone bio-activity in infants and children. *Pediatr Nephrol* 1990;4:105–110.
170. White PC, Speiser PW. Congenital adrenal hyperplasia due to 21-hydroxylase deficiency. *Endocr Rev* 2000;21:245–291.
171. Peter M, Fawaz L, Drop SLS, et al. Hereditary defect in biosynthesis of aldosterone: aldosterone synthase deficiency 1964–1997. *J Clin Endocrinol Metab* 1997;82:3525–3528.
172. Ulick S. Correction of the nomenclature and mechanism of the aldosterone biosynthetic defects. *J Clin Endocrinol Metab* 1996;81:1299–1300.
173. Ulick SA, Wang JZ, Morton LH. The biochemical phenotypes of two inborn errors in the biosynthesis of aldosterone. *J Clin Endocrinol Metab* 1992;72:1415–1420.
174. Geley S, Jöhrer K, Peter M, et al. Amino acid substitution R384P in aldosterone synthase causes corticosterone methyloxidase type I deficiency. *J Clin Endocrinol Metab* 1995; 80:424–429.
175. Picco P, Garibaldi L, Cotellessa M, et al. Corticosterone methyloxidase type II deficiency: a cause of failure to thrive and recurrent dehydration in early infancy. *Eur J Pediatr* 1992;151:170–173.
176. Peter M, Partsch C-J, Sippell WG. Multisteroid analysis in children with terminal aldosterone biosynthesis defects. *J Clin Endocrinol Metab* 1995;80:1622–1627.
177. Hudson JB, Chobanian AV, Relman AS. Hypoaldosteronism: a clinical study of a patient with an isolated adrenal mineral corticoid deficiency resulting in hyperkalemia and Stokes-Adams attacks. *N Engl J Med* 1957;257:529–536.
178. Rodríguez-Soriano J, Vallo A, Sanjurjo P, et al. Hyporeninemic hypoaldosteronism in children with chronic renal failure. *J Pediatr* 1986;109:476–482.
179. Williams GH. Hyporeninemic hypoaldosteronism. *N Engl J Med* 1986;314:1041–1042.
180. Clark BA, Brown RS. Potassium homeostasis and hyperkalemic syndromes. *Endocrinol Metab Clin North Am* 1995; 3:573–591.
181. Shuper A, Eisenstein B, Stark H, et al. Hyporeninemic hypoaldosteronism in a child with lactic acidosis, deafness, and mental retardation. *J Pediatr* 1982;100:769–772.
182. Monnens L, Fiselier T, Bos B, et al. Hyporeninemic hypoaldosteronism in infancy. *Nephron* 1983;35:140–142.
183. Landier F, Guyene TT, Boutignon H, et al. Hyporeninemic hypoaldosteronism in infancy: a familial disease. *J Clin Endocrinol Metab* 1984;58:143–148.
184. Cheek DB, Perry JA. A salt wasting syndrome in infancy. *Arch Dis Child* 1958;33:252–256.
185. Hanukoglu A. Type I pseudohypoaldosteronism includes two clinically and genetically distinct entities with either renal or multiple target organ defects. *J Clin Endocrinol Metab* 1991;73:936–944.
186. Anand SK, Froberg L, Northway JD, et al. Pseudohypoaldosteronism due to sweat gland dysfunction. *Pediatr Res* 1976;10:677–682.
187. Geller DS, Rodríguez-Soriano J, Vallo A, et al. Mutations in the mineral corticoid receptor gene cause autosomal dominant pseudohypoaldosteronism type I. *Nat Genet* 1998;19:279–281.
188. Tajima T, Kitagawa H, Yokoya S, et al. A novel missense mutation of mineral corticoid receptor gene in one Japanese family with a renal form of pseudohypoaldosteronism type 1. *J Clin Endocrinol Metab* 2000;85:4690–4694.
189. Vieman M, Peter M, López-Siguero JP, et al. Evidence for genetic heterogeneity of pseudohypoaldosteronism type 1: identification of a novel mutation in the human mineral corticoid receptor in one sporadic case and no mutations in two autosomal dominant kindreds. *J Clin Endocrinol Metab* 2001;86:2056–2059.
190. Ballauf A, Wendel U, Kupke I, et al. A partial form of pseudohypoaldosteronism type I without sodium wasting. *J Pediatr Endocrinol* 1994;7:57–60.
191. Wolthers BG, Kraan GP, van der Molen JC, et al. Urinary profile of a newborn suffering from pseudohypoaldosteronism. *Clin Chim Acta* 1995;236:33–43.
192. Vallo A, Geller DS, Rodríguez-Soriano J, et al. Phenotype-genotype correlations in two Spanish kindred with renal pseudohypoaldosteronism type 1. *Pediatr Nephrol* 1999;13:C28(abst).
193. Evans RM. The steroid and thyroid hormone receptor superfamily. *Science* 1988;240:889–895.
194. Berger S, Bleich M, Schmid W, et al. Mineralocorticoid receptor knock-out mice: lessons on Na+ metabolism. *Kidney Int* 2000;57:295–298.
195. Rossler A. The natural history of salt-wasting disorders of adrenal and renal origin. *J Clin Endocrinol Metab* 1984;59:689–700.
196. Oberfield SE, Levine LS, Carey RM, et al. Pseudohypoaldosteronism: multiple target organ unresponsiveness to mineral corticoid hormones. *J Clin Endocrinol Metab* 1979;48:228–234.
197. Savage MO, Jefferson IG, Dillon MJ, et al. Pseudohypoaldosteronism: severe salt wasting in infancy caused by generalized mineral corticoid unresponsiveness. *J Pediatr* 1982;101:239–242.
198. Chang SS, Grunder S, Hanukoglu A, et al. Mutations of the epithelial sodium channel cause salt wasting with hyperkalaemic acidosis, pseudohypoaldosteronism type 1. *Nat Genet* 1996;12:248–253.
199. Strautnieks SS, Thompson RJ, Gardiner RM, et al. A novel splice-site mutation in the γ subunit of the epithelial sodium channel gene in three pseudohypoaldosteronism type 1 families. *Nat Genet* 1996;3:248–250.
200. Bonny O, Chraibi A, Loffing J, et al. Functional expression of pseudohypoaldosteronism type I mutated epithelial Na^+ channel lacking the pore-forming region of its a subunit. *J Clin Invest* 1999;104:967–974.
201. Adachi M, Tachibana K, Asakura Y, et al. Compound heterozygous mutations in the gamma subunit gene of ENaC (1627delG and 1570-1G→A) in one sporadic Japanese patient with a systemic form of pseudohypoaldosteronism type 1. *J Clin Endocrinol Metab* 2001;86:9–12.
202. Firsov D, Robert-Nicoud M, Gruender S, et al. Mutational analysis of cysteine-rich domains of the epithelium sodium channel (ENaC). Identification of cysteines essential for channel expression at the cell surface. *J Biol Chem* 1999;274:2743–2749.
203. Hanukoglu A, Bistritzer T, Rakover Y, et al. Pseudohypoaldosteronism with increased saliva electrolyte values and frequent lower respiratory tract infections mimicking cystic fibrosis. *J Pediatr* 1994;125:752–755.
204. Marthinsen L, Kornfalt R, Aili M, et al. Recurrent *Pseudomonas* bronchopneumonia and other symptoms as in

cystic fibrosis in a child with type I pseudohypoaldosteronism. *Acta Paediatr* 1998;87:472–474.

205. Schaedel C, Marthinsen L, Kristofferson AC, et al. Lung symptoms in pseudohypoaldosteronism type I are associated with deficiency of the α subunit of the epithelial sodium channel. *J Pediatr* 1999;135:739–745.
206. Smith JJ, Travis SM, Greenberg EP, Welsh MJ. Cystic fibrosis airway epithelia fail to kill bacteria because of abnormal airway surface fluid. *Cell* 1996;85:229–236.
207. Hummler E, Barker P, Gatzy J, et al. Early death due to defective neonatal lung clearance in αENaC-deficient mice. *Nat Genet* 1996;12:325–328.
208. Hammler E, Barker P, Talbot C, et al. A mouse model for the renal salt-wasting syndrome pseudohypoaldosteronism. *Proc Natl Acad Sci U S A* 1997;94:11710–11715.
209. McDonald FJ, Yang B, Hrstka RF, et al. Disruption of the β subunit of the epithelial Na^+ channel in mice: hyperkalemia and neonatal death associated with a pseudohypoaldosteronism phenotype. *Proc Natl Acad Sci U S A* 1999;96:1727–1731.
210. Pradervand S, Barker PM, Wang Q, et al. Salt restriction induces pseudohypoaldosteronism type 1 in mice expressing low levels of the β-subunit of the amiloride-sensitive epithelial sodium channel. *Proc Natl Acad Sci U S A* 1999;96:1732–17371.
211. Barker PM, Nguyen MS, Gatzy JT, et al. Role of γENaC subunit in lung liquid clearance and electrolyte balance in newborn mice. Insights into perinatal adaptation and pseudohypoaldosteronism. *J Clin Invest* 1998;102:1634–1640.
212. Malagon-Rogers M. A patient with pseudohypoaldosteronism type 1 and respiratory distress syndrome. *Pediatr Nephrol* 1999;13:484–486.
213. Kerrem E, Bistritzer T, Hanukoglu A, et al. Pulmonary epithelial sodium-channel dysfunction and excess airway liquid in pseudohypoaldosteronism. *N Engl J Med* 1999;341:156–162.
214. Prince LS, Launspach JL, Geller DS, et al. Absence of amiloride-sensitive sodium absorption in the airway of an infant with pseudohypoaldosteronism. *J Pediatr* 1999;135:786–789.
215. Mathew PM, Manasra KB, Hamdan JA. Indomethacin and cation-exchange resin in the management of pseudohypoaldosteronism. *Clin Pediatr* 1993;32:58–60.
216. Hogg RJ, Marks JF, Marker D, et al. Long-term observations in a patient with pseudohypoaldosteronism. *Pediatr Nephrol* 1991;5:205–210.
217. McSherry E. Renal tubular acidosis in childhood. *Kidney Int* 1981;20:799–809.
218. Appiani AC, Marra G, Tirelli SA, et al. Early childhood hyperkalaemia: variety of pseudohypoaldosteronism. *Acta Paediatr Scand* 1986;75:970–974.
219. Rodríguez-Soriano J, Vallo A, Oliveros R, et al. Transient pseudo-hypoaldosteronism secondary to obstructive uropathy in infancy. *J Pediatr* 1983;103:375–380.
220. Bulchmann G, Schuster T, Heger A, et al. Transient pseudohypoaldosteronism secondary to posterior urethral valves. A case report and review of the literature. *Eur J Pediatr Surg* 2001;11:277–279.
221. Terzi F, Assael BM, Appiani AC, et al. Increased sodium requirement following early postnatal surgical correction of congenital uropathies in infants. *Pediatr Nephrol* 1990;4:581–584.
222. Tobias JD, Brock JD 3rd, Lynch A. Pseudohypoaldosteronism following operative correction of unilateral obstructive uropathy. *Clin Pediatr* 1995;34:327–330.
223. Rodríguez-Soriano J, Ubetagoyena M, Vallo A. Normokalaemic pseudohypoaldosteronism is present in children with acute pyelonephritis. *Acta Paediatr* 1992;81:402–406.
224. Gerigk M, Glanzmann R, Rascher W, et al. Hyponatremia and hyperkalaemia in acute pyelonephritis without urinary tract anomalies. *Eur J Pediatr* 1995;154:582–584.
225. Schoen EJ, Bhatia S, Ray GT, et al. Transient pseudohypoaldosteronism with hyponatremia-hyperkalemia in infant urinary tract infection. *J Urol* 2002;167:680–682.
226. Paver WKA, Pauline GJ. Hypertension and hyperpotassemia without renal disease in a young male. *Med J Aust* 1964;2:305–306.
227. Gordon RD, Geddes RA, Pawsey GK, et al. Hypertension and severe hyperkalaemia associated with suppression of renin and aldosterone and completely reversed by dietary sodium restriction. *Aust Ann Med* 1970;4:287–294.
228. Achard JM, Diese-Nicodème S, Fiquet-Kempf B, et al. Phenotypic and genetic heterogeneity of familial hyperkalemic hypertension (Gordon syndrome). *Clin Exp Pharmacol Physiol* 2001;28:1048–1052.
229. Spitzer A, Edelmann CM Jr, Goldberg L, et al. Short stature, hyperkalemia, and acidosis: a defect in renal transport of potassium. *Kidney Int* 1973;3:251–257.
230. Weinstein SF, Allan DME, Mendoza SA. Hyperkalemia, acidosis, and short stature associated with a defect in renal potassium excretion. *J Pediatr* 1974;85:355–358.
231. Farfel Z, Iaim A, Levi J, et al. Proximal renal tubular acidosis. Association with familial normoaldosteronemic hyperpotassemia and hypertension. *Arch Intern Med* 1978;138:1837–1840.
232. Rodríguez-Soriano J, Vallo A, Domínguez MJ. "Chloride-shunt" syndrome: an overlooked cause of renal hypercalciuria. *Pediatr Nephrol* 1989;3:113–121.
233. Mansfield TA, Simon DB, Farfel Z, et al. Multilocus linkage of familial hyperkalaemia and hypertension, pseudohypoaldosteronism type II, to chromosomes 1q31-42 and 17p11-q21. *Nat Genet* 1997;16:202–205.
234. Disse-Nicodème S, Achard J-M, Dessiter I, et al. A new locus on chromosome 12p13.3 for pseudohypoaldosteronism type II, an autosomal dominant form of hypertension. *Am J Hum Genet* 2000;67:302–310.
235. Disse-Nicodème S, Dessiter I, Fiquet-Kempf B, et al. Genetic heterogeneity of familial hyperkalaemic hypertension. *J Hypertens* 2001;19:1957–1964.
236. Wilson FH, Disse-Nicodème S, Choate KA, et al. Human hypertension caused by mutations in WNK kinases. *Science* 2001;293:1107–1112.
237. Schambelan M, Sebastian A, Rector FC Jr. Mineralocorticoid resistant renal hyperkalemia without salt wasting (type II pseudohypoaldosteronism): role of increased renal chloride reabsorption. *Kidney Int* 1981;19:716–727.
238. Al-Ghamdi SMG, Cameron EC, Sutton RAL. Magnesium deficiency: pathophysiological and clinical overview. *Am J Kidney Dis* 1994;24:737–752.

239. Bianchetti MG, Kanaka C, Ridolfi-Luthy A, et al. Chronic renal magnesium loss, hypocalciuria and mild hypokalaemic metabolic alkalosis after cisplatin. *Pediatr Nephrol* 1990;4: 219–222.
240. Ariceta G, Rodríguez-Soriano J, Vallo A, et al. Acute and chronic effects of cisplatin therapy on renal magnesium wasting. *Med Pediatr Oncol* 1997;28:35–40.
241. Freeman RM, Pearson E. Hypomagnesemia of unknown etiology. *Am J Med* 1966;41:645–656.
242. Meij IC, van den Heuvel LPWJ, Knoers NVAM. Inherited hypomagnesemia. *Adv Nephrol Necker Hosp* 2000;30:163–176.
243. Cole DEC, Quamme GA. Inherited disorders of renal magnesium handling. *J Am Soc Nephrol* 2000;11:1937–1947.
244. Shalkev H, Phillip M, Galil A, et al. Clinical presentation and outcome in primary familial hypomagnesemia. *Arch Dis Child* 1998;78:127–130.
245. Cole DEC, Kooh SW, Vieth R. Primary infantile hypomagnesemia: outcome after 21 years and treatment with continuous nocturnal nasogastric magnesium infusion. *Eur J Pediatr* 2000;159:38–43.
246. Matzkin H, Lotan D, Boichis H. Primary hypomagnesemia with a probable double magnesium transport defect. *Nephron* 1989;52:83–86.
247. Walder RY, Shalev H, Brennan TMH, et al. Familial hypomagnesemia maps to chromosome 9q, not to the X chromosome: genetic linkage mapping and analysis of a balanced translocation breakpoint. *Hum Mol Genet* 1997;6: 1491–1497.
248. Schlingmann KP, Weber S, Peters M, et al. Hypomagnesemia with secondary hypocalcemia is caused by mutations in TRPM6, a new member of the TRPM gene family. *Nat Genet* 2002;31:166–170.
249. Walder RY, Landau D, Meyer P, et al. Mutation in TRPM6 causes hypomagnesemia with secondary hypocalcemia. *Nat Genet* 2002;31:171–174.
250. Harteneck C, Plant TD, Schultz G. From worm to man: three subfamilies of TRP channels. *Trends Neurosci* 2000;23: 159–166.
251. Milazzo SC, Ahern MJ, Cleland LG, et al. Calcium pyrophosphate dehydrate deposition disease and familial hypomagnesemia. *J Rheumatol* 1981;8:767–771.
252. Geven WB, Monnens LM, Willems JL, et al. Isolated autosomal recessive renal magnesium loss in two sisters. *Clin Genet* 1987;32:398–402.
253. Geven W, Monnens L, Willems H, et al. Renal magnesium wasting in two families with autosomal dominant inheritance. *Kidney Int* 1987;31:1140–1144.
254. Meij IC, Illy KE, Monnens L. Severe hypomagnesemia in a neonate with isolated renal magnesium loss. *Nephron* 2000; 84:198.
255. Meij IC, Saar K, van den Heuvel LPWJ, et al. Hereditary isolated renal magnesium loss maps to chromosome 11q23. *Am J Hum Genet* 1999;64:180–188.
256. Kantorovich V, Adams JS, Gaines JE, et al. Genetic heterogeneity in familial renal magnesium wasting. *J Clin Endocrinol Metab* 2002;87:612–617.
257. Meij IC, Koenderink JB, van Bokhoven H, et al. Dominant isolated renal magnesium loss is caused by misrouting of the Na^+,K^+-ATPase gamma-subunit. *Nat Genet* 2000;26:265–266.
258. Michelis MF, Drash AL, Linarelli LG, et al. Decreased bicarbonate threshold and renal magnesium wasting in a sibship with distal renal tubular acidosis (evaluation of the pathophysiologic role of parathyroid hormone). *Metabolism* 1972;21:905–920.
259. Castrillo JM, Rapado A, Traba ML, et al. Nefrocalcinosis con hipomagnesemia. *Nefrología (Madrid)* 1983;3:159–165.
260. Benigno V, Canonica CS, Bettinelli A, et al. Hypomagnesemia-hypercalciuria-nephrocalcinosis: a report of nine cases and a review. *Nephrol Dial Transplant* 2000;15: 605–610.
261. Nicholson JC, Jones CL, Powell HR, et al. Familial hypomagnesemia-hypercalciuria leading to end-stage renal failure. *Pediatr Nephrol* 1995;9:74–76.
262. Praga M, Vara J, González-Parra E, et al. Familial hypomagnesemia with hypercalciuria and nephrocalcinosis. *Kidney Int* 1995;47:1419–1425.
263. Simon DB, Lu Y, Choate KA, et al. Paracellin-1, a renal tight junction protein required for paracellular Mg^{2+} resorption. *Science* 1999;285:103–106.
264. Weber S, Schneider L, Peters M, et al. Novel paracellin-1 mutations in 25 families with familial hypomagnesemia with hypercalciuria and nephrocalcinosis. *J Am Soc Nephrol* 2001;12:1872–1881.
265. Blanchard A, Jeunemaitre X, Coudol P, et al. Paracellin-1 is critical for magnesium and calcium reabsorption in the human ascending limb of Henle. *Kidney Int* 2001;59:2206–2215.
266. Kuwertz-Broking E, Frund S, Bulla M, et al. Familial hypomagnesemia-hypercalciuria in 2 siblings. *Clin Nephrol* 2001; 56:155–161.
267. Rodríguez-Soriano J, Vallo A. Pathophysiology of the renal acidification defect present in the syndrome of familial hypomagnesaemia-hypercalciuria. *Pediatr Nephrol* 1994;8:432–435.
268. Dai LJ, Ritchie G, Kerstan D, et al. Magnesium transport in the renal convoluted tubule. *Physiol Rev* 2001;81:51–84.
270. Tsukita S, Furuse M. Occludin and claudins in tight junctions strands: leading or supporting players? *Trends Cell Biol* 1999;9:268–273.
271. Leumann E, Hoppe B, Neuhaus T. Management of primary oxaluria: efficacy of oral citrate administration. *Pediatr Nephrol* 1993;7:207–210.
272. Pak CYC. Citrate and renal calculi: new insights and future directions. *Am J Kidney Dis* 1991;17:420–425.

39

RENAL TUBULAR ACIDOSIS

JOHN T. HERRIN

Renal tubular acidosis (RTA) is a clinical syndrome in which either an inherited or acquired renal tubular defect leads to failure to maintain a normal plasma bicarbonate concentration in the presence of a normal rate of acid production from the diet and metabolism. Systemic metabolic acidosis (MA) results from a decrease in net acid excretion (NAE) occurring as a defect in handling bicarbonate reabsorption or defect in hydrogen ion secretion.

RTA, clinically, is characterized by a normal anion gap, MA with hyperchloremia, bicarbonaturia, reduced urinary excretion of titratable acid (TA) and ammonia, and an elevated urinary pH. Disorders of bicarbonate reclamation by the proximal tubule are classified as *proximal* or *type 2 RTA*, whereas disorders resulting from a primary defect in distal tubular net proton secretion or from reduced buffer trapping in the tubular lumen (decreased generation of new bicarbonate for reabsorption) are called *distal* or *type 1 RTA*. Distal RTA (DRTA) results in low ammonium (NH_4^+) or in low TA excretion (1–8). Hyperkalemic RTA may occur as a result of aldosterone deficiency or tubular insensitivity to its effects (RTA type 4) (9–17). Low potassium excretion in the absence of aldosterone abnormalities may also lead to a hyperkalemic DRTA in obstructive uropathy and sickle cell anemia (18,19). In children with type 1 RTA, nonspecific symptoms occur early. If the acidosis is not corrected, electrolyte abnormalities, growth retardation, rickets, and nephrocalcinosis may follow. Growth retardation is a consistent feature of RTA in infants. Experimentally, MA in rats leads to inhibition of growth hormone secretion, decreased caloric intake, and decreased levels of hepatic insulin-like growth factor I expression (20,21). Similar abnormalities have been observed during systemic acidosis in childhood. Identification and correction of acidosis are important in preventing symptoms and guide approved genetic counseling and testing.

CLASSIFICATION AND TERMINOLOGY

The somewhat confusing nomenclature in RTA reflects the history of disease identification. Type 1, classic, or DRTA was the first recognized syndrome. Type 2, or proximal RTA (PRTA), was subsequently identified, then appreciated as the result of defective bicarbonate reabsorption. The hybrid nature of the infantile variant of DRTA, in which a distal tubular defect is coupled with an increased fractional excretion of bicarbonate, was initially believed to represent a distinct disease entity and was designated *type 3 RTA*. This term was subsequently applied to the mixed defects of proximal and distal tubular acidification, which result from a deficit in carbonic anhydrase (CA) 2 in osteopetrosis. The term *type 3 RTA* was later dropped from classification schemes, but only after aldosterone-dependent RTA type 4 was described. The present terminology in which type 1 = DRTA, type 2 = PRTA, and type 4 = aldosterone-dependent RTA is thus historically, rather than pathophysiologically, based (Table 39.1) (3,20,22).

Although DRTA is characterized by a low NH_4^+ excretion, some clinical syndromes with proximal tubular defects also demonstrate low NH_4^+ excretion. Bicarbonaturia most commonly results from proximal tubular loss but can also result from distal H^+ secretion. Because of such overlap syndromes, classification of RTA based on pathophysiology of the disorders is preferred (20,23,24).

The classification of RTA into primary defects in bicarbonate reabsorption, defects in net hydrogen ion excretion, or defects in aldosterone-sensitive acid secretion is shown in Table 39.1. Combined defects in proximal HCO_3^- reabsorption and H^+ ion secretion have been described and separate patients or families have variations of standard patterns; a subgroup of adolescents and adult patients with apparent DRTA can lower urinary pH in response to acidosis but cannot increase urinary partial pressure of carbon dioxide (PCO_2) in response to alkalinization of the urine by bicarbonate titration (25). Two patterns of combined or hybrid RTA have been described: (a) infants and young children with DRTA show high FE_{HCO_3} of 5 to 15% that clears with treatment and growth—bicarbonate loss is rare in older children but may occur with prolonged periods of untreated RTA with concurrent hyperparathyroidism (4,26); and (b) adult patients with Sjögren's syndrome and renal amyloidosis (2,27,28) show significant

TABLE 39.1. CLASSIFICATION AND NOMENCLATURE IN RENAL TUBULAR ACIDOSIS (RTA): CLINICAL AND PATHOPHYSIOLOGIC CRITERIA

Primary defect in bicarbonate reabsorption (proximal RTA, type 2)
- Mild to moderate metabolic acidosis or acid loading lowers the urine pH below 5.5. Low bicarbonate threshold FE_{HCO_3} above 10% by titration.

Primary defect in distal net H⁺ secretion
- Inability to lower urine pH below 5.5 if FE_{HCO_3} exceeds 5%; suspect an associated bicarbonate leak and test the ability to increase urinary Pco_2 during bicarbonate loading
  - Inability to maximally acidify urine (DRTA, type 1)
    - Diminished Na^+ to distal tubule; functional RTA (exchange defect)
    - Inability to secrete H^+ (secretory defect)
    - Increased back diffusion H^+ (gradient defect)
    - Abolition of the electrical gradient for H^+ ion secretion (short circuit or voltage defect) with concurrent impairment to K^+ secretion, furosemide decreases U_{pH} to normal
  - Hyperkalemic DRTA: hyperkalemia with U_{pH} above 5.5
  - Combined defects in proximal HCO_3 reabsorption and H^+ ion secretion (hybrid RTA type 1 = type 3, incomplete RTA) FE_{HCO_3} above 5%
  - RTA secondary to deficits in aldosterone activity or chloride reabsorption: type 4 RTA
  - Hyperkalemia, U_{pH} below 5.5, further differentiation by assessment volume status, renin-aldosterone
  - Subtypes
    - Aldosterone deficiency
      - High renin hypoaldosteronism = primary adrenal abnormality with normal renal function
      - Low renin hypoaldosteronism = primary renal disease with secondary mineralocorticoid deficit
    - Attenuated renal response to aldosterone with relative aldosterone deficiency
      - Chloride shunting (pseudohypoaldosteronism type 2); abnormal Na^+-K^+-$2Cl^-$ exchange
      - Deficient renin
    - Attenuated renal response: pseudohypoaldosteronism
      - Pseudohypoaldosteronism (infancy)
      - Primary transient early RTA4

DRTA, distal renal tubular acidosis; U_{pH}, urine PH.
Note: Incomplete DRTA syndrome: low NH^+_4, high U_{pH}, patient is not acidotic unless stressed.

reduction in tubular reabsorption of bicarbonate at normal plasma levels (i.e., a low threshold similar to type 2 RTA), combined with an inability to acidify maximally even with severe acidosis (25). A similar defect occurs in patients with Leigh's syndrome and osteopetrosis (29,30).

Incomplete RTA is a condition in which normal plasma bicarbonate is maintained despite decreased ability to acidify the urine (5). It is possible that a high rate of NH_4^+ excretion compensates for a decrease in TA excretion. Initially, the condition was described in patients with nephrocalcinosis or recurrent nephrolithiasis (5), or in families in which a propositus had complete RTA (31). It has been suggested that this latter condition represents a developmental stage of RTA (32).

RENAL CONTROL OF ACID-BASE BALANCE

The following brief review of the kidney's role in acid-base metabolism and renal acidification provides an outline to permit appropriate investigation, classification, and understanding of the pathophysiologic basis of symptomatology and treatment in RTA.

The activity of almost all body enzyme systems is dependent on hydrogen ion concentration; hence, the balance of hydrogen ion is tightly regulated. Normal body defenses against inappropriate changes in hydrogen ion concentration include (a) body buffering of generated or administered H^+, (b) respiratory excretion of volatile acid as carbon dioxide, and (c) renal reabsorption of filtered bicarbonate and generation of new bicarbonate by excretion of hydrogen ion from nonvolatile acid, produced as a result of protein metabolism. Excretion of protons provides for reabsorption of filtered bicarbonate and regeneration of bicarbonate when secreted hydrogen ion combines with a buffer other than bicarbonate (33).

Initial defense against change in pH occurs within seconds through the combination of H^+ with chemical buffers. These buffers do not remove the hydrogen ion from the body, but rather bind it until secondary excretion can occur as a result of respiration (within minutes) or renal excretion (within hours or days). Bicarbonate is the major extracellular fluid buffer, whereas phosphate acts as the major buffer in intracellular fluid and the urine, to increase H^+ excretion as TA.

In normal individuals, net acid production is balanced by NAE. In an average American diet (34,35), net endogenous noncarbonic acid production averages approximately 1 mEq/kg/day in adults and 1 to 3 mEq/kg/day (1 to 3 mEq per 100 calories) in healthy infants and children (36). Children generate as much as 2 to 3 mEq H^+/Kg, particularly during active growth, as a result of combination of OH^- and phosphate to form hydroxyapatite during bone formation. NAE results from excretion of ammonia and TA minus excreted bicarbonate ($NAE = U_{NH4}V + U_{TA}V$). $U_{NH4}V$ may be measured chemically or estimated clinically as U_{AG}, or urinary net charge. If U_{pH} is low (6.1 to 6.5), bicarbonate excretion may be omitted from calculations. $U_{TA}V$ is proportional to urinary phosphorus (31,33,37).

Each day, the kidney prevents loss of a large amount of filtered bicarbonate (i.e., 180 L/day × 25 mEq HCO_3^-/L = 4500 mEq/day in an adult). This is accomplished by secretion of H^+ into the tubular lumen by secondary active transport in tubular segments where filtered bicarbonate ions are reabsorbed by interaction with H^+ in the tubule to form H_2CO_3 in the presence of CA. Renal acid excretion is regulated by hormones that concurrently control sodium reabsorption and thus volume control (e.g., angiotensin II in the proximal tubule and aldosterone, antidiuretic hormone, and endothelin 1 in the distal tubule) (39). In addition, renal acid excretion is affected by factors that regulate bicarbonate reabsorption Pco_2 and by potassium balance, because hypokalemia increases H^+ distally by decreasing potassium exchange for NH_4^+ at the Na^+-K^+-$2Cl^-$ antiporter. K^+ and $NH4^+$ compete for a common site in the triporter of the thick ascending loop of Henle and for secretion in conjunction with basolateral Na^+ pumps (39,40).

Primary H^+ secretion occurs actively in the intercalated cells of the late distal tubule and collecting ducts, whereas excess H^+ combines in the tubule with phosphate and ammonia buffers (plus urate, creatinine, and citrate), generating new bicarbonate ions (37,38). In chronic acidosis, ammonia production and excretion increase (33,41–43). This pH balance is linked to sodium and water balance, with aldosterone stimulation of intercalated cells leading to excretion of hydrogen ion (44,45). Changes in plasma PCO_2 are linked to renal H^+ excretion, with increased PCO_2 leading to increased hydrogen ion secretion. Acid balance requires that dietary H^+ (which results from the metabolism of methionine, cysteine, and the chloride salts of lysine, arginine, and histidine) be removed by combination with bicarbonate to form an acid salt, water, and CO_2 (46). As CO_2 is exhaled (respiration), a deficit of bicarbonate is sustained. When reduced excretion of a metabolizable anion (e.g., ketones, hydroxy butyric acid) occurs in the presence of acid loading, there is an increased output of NH_4^+ with Cl^- (47,48). Retained anions are metabolized to neutral end products (48).

NAE results in the generation of new bicarbonate, which exits the cell by electroneutral chloride exchange. The bicarbonate generated is equal to that lost in buffering the endogenous load of noncarbonic (nonvolatile) acid generated from dietary intake and metabolism. If the diet is high in acid, increased acid excretion occurs, the urine is free of bicarbonate, and urinary pH approaches 4.5. In the presence of an alkaline load, the tubule rejects excess filtered bicarbonate, and urinary pH may approach 8 or 9. Phosphate buffer activity, and hence TA, is limited by dietary intake and reabsorption (22,38). Ammonium, on the other hand, is generated in the presence of acidosis. RTA is predominantly the result of either excess bicarbonate excretion or low NH_4^+ excretion (22).

RENAL ACIDIFICATION MECHANISM

The schema for normal acidification and sites of potential inherited or acquired defects are presented in Figure 39.1 and Table 39.2. Genetic control of H^+ excretion is mediated through control of the expression of membrane transporters in α-intercalated cells of the distal nephron, where luminal H^+ secretion occurs by an adenosine triphosphatase (ATPase)-dependent proton pump in the apical membrane that is linked to basolateral anion exchange (bicarbonate-chloride) AEI 3 (49). AEI mutations have been in DRTA (49,50). Enzyme defects in the CA2 system explain common pathophysiology of bone and ear in addition to both proximal and distal tubules in osteoporosis, as well as ear and kidney abnormalities in ATP6B1-β1 subunit mutations in DRTA with deafness (49,52). Mutations in the gene encoding NBC 1 (Na-HCO_3 transporter) lead to autosomal recessive PRTA (53).

TABLE 39.2. SUMMARY OF ACIDIFICATION MECHANISMS (39,40)

Glomerular filtration
- Delivery of bicarbonate and anions from food metabolism

Proximal tubule
- Apical H^+ secretion (leads to reabsorption bicarbonate)
  - H^+-ATPase
  - Coupled Na^+-H^+ exchange (NHE3 antiporter)
  - Back leakage from Cl^- (base exchange)
- Na^+ cotransporters (amino acid, glucose, phosphate, citrate)
  - Luminal CA4 enhances buffering and CO_2 reabsorption
  - Intracellular
  - Production of NH_3 and HCO_3 (from metabolism of glutamate and α ketoglutarate)
  - CA2 intracellular production H^+ and HCO_3^-
- Basolateral
  - Electrogenic Na^+-3 HCO_3^- cotransport (Na-HCO_3^--CO_3^-) NBC1
  - Na^+,K^+-ATPase (produce sodium gradient allowing Na^+ reabsorption)
  - Na^+-H^+ antiporter

Thick ascending loop of Henle
- Water reabsorption leads to bicarbonate reabsorption
- H^+ secretion (NHE3 activity)
- $NH4^+$ substitution for K^+ in the Na^+-K^+-$2Cl^-$ cotransporter

Distal nephron
- Apical
- H^+ secretion
  - H^+-ATPase intercalated cells (ATP6B1)
  - H^+,K^+-ATPase
- HCO_3^- secretion intercalated cells
- H^+ back leak (amphotericin B)
- Mineralocorticoids
- Stimulate H^+ secretion by the distal nephron in a sodium-dependent fashion
- Stimulate H^+ secretion in the cortical collecting duct and outer medullary collecting duct in a sodium-independent fashion
- Basolateral
  - Cl^--HCO_3^- (AE1)
  - CA luminal (buffering)
  - CA2 intracellular production H^+ and HCO_3^-

ATPase, adenosine triphosphatase; CA2, carbonic anhydrase 2.

Renal NH_4^+ Production and Transport

Ammonium is the source of H^+ for reabsorption of bicarbonate in the proximal tubule. Ammonia generation and excretion is the expected response to acidosis and the key to understanding RTA. At physiologic pH, NH_3, and NH_4^+ production from glutamine is regulated through glutaminase and phosphoenol-pyruvate carboxykinase with the production of α-ketoglutarate as a byproduct, which leads to the generation of two bicarbonate molecules (37,54,55).

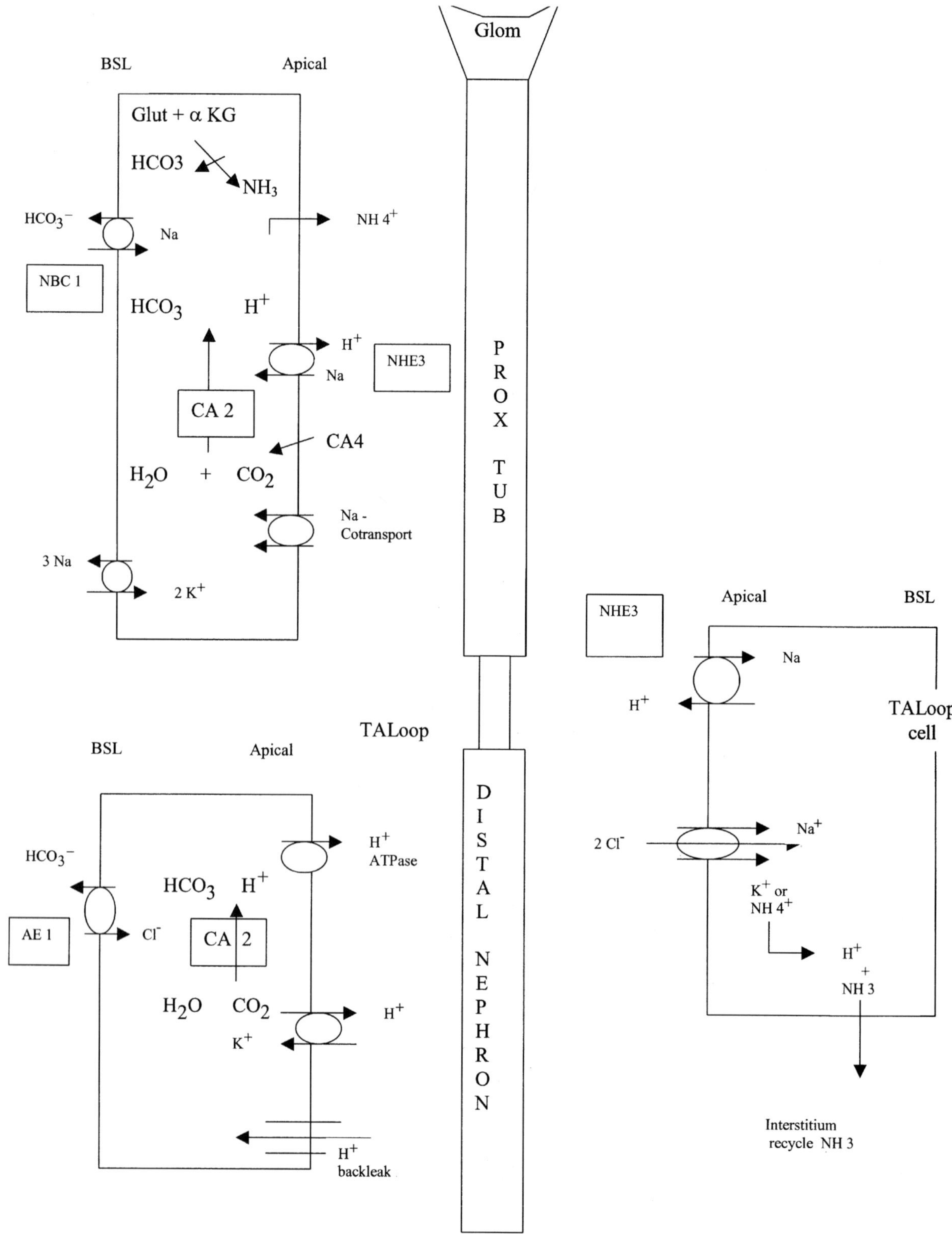

FIGURE 39.1. The schema outlines the major mechanism of acidification and the nephron site of activity for inherited and acquired defects in acidification. α KG, α-ketoglutarate; AE 1, anion exchanger Cl⁻ and HCO_3^-; Apical, apical surface (lumen) of cell; ATPase, adenosine triphosphatase; BSL, basolateral surface of the cell; CA 2, carbonic anhydrase 2; CA 4, carbonic anhydrase 4; Glom, glomerulus; Glut, glutamine; Na-Cotransport, Na cotransport at the apical surface of the cell with H^+ (includes Na⁻amino acid, Na⁻ phosphate, Na⁻ glucose, and Na⁻ citrate); NBC 1, Na, bicarbonate cotransporter; NHE 3, sodium hydrogen ion exchanger; PROX TUB, proximal tubule; TALoop, thick ascending loop of Henle.

In chronic MA, an increase in formation of ammonia from glutamine occurs with little change in phosphate excretion (phosphate released from bone is used in blood buffering during acidosis). NH_4^+ is secreted into the first portion of proximal tubule, substituting for H^+ in the Na^+-H^+-antiporter on the apical membrane (43,56,57). Increase in direct proximal convoluted tubule (PCT) ammonium secretion increases delivery distally. In the S3 segment of the proximal straight tubule, ammonium is increased by an acid disequilibrium pH. As fluid leaves the PCT to the loop of Henle, ammonium and ammonia efflux leads to an increased medullary gradient for ammonia. As fluid is removed from the thin loop, leading to alkalinization, efflux of ammonia can occur as a result of nonionic diffusion (58,59).

Direct ammonium transport across the medullary thick ascending limb apical membrane occurs by substitution of NH_4^+ for K^+ in the Na^+-K^+-$2Cl^-$ cotransporter (46). Countercurrent reentry of NH_4^+ in the proximal straight tubule thus correlates with flow. Ammonium is secreted from the interstitium into the medullary collecting ducts by a combination of diffusion of ammonia and H^+ secretion (active transport by H^+ ATPase and H^+,K^+-ATPase) (39,59,60).

Relationship of K^+ and NH_4^+

Hyperkalemia is a determinant of changes in acid-base balance by both direct and indirect effects on distal acidification. Serum potassium is a determinant of aldosterone secretion and thus of distal proton secretion (45). Chronic potassium deficiency increases NH_4^+ secretion, whereas hyperkalemia suppresses ammonium production (59). Hyperkalemia has no effect on ammonium transport in the PCT but impairs absorption from the thick ascending limb where NH_4^+ may substitute for K^+ in the Na^+-K^+-$2Cl^-$ exchanger (59,60).

Interactions of Sodium and Potassium Handling

Sodium and potassium handling are homeostatically regulated processes. Potassium secretion across the apical membrane of principal cells in the cortical collecting duct is tightly regulated (61). Quantitative potassium secretion depends on the apical membrane potassium conductance and the electrochemical driving force (EDF) across the apical membrane. Potassium conductance is the sum of the collective K channels in the apical membrane, so K secretion is regulated by urine flow and Na delivery and by factors that regulate EDF (e.g., K balance, transepithelial potential difference, pH and bicarbonate concentration of tubular fluid, systemic acid balance, and aldosterone) (61). The EDF for K^+ exchange is maintained by the basolateral Na^+,K^+-ATPase. The sodium pump generates a negative luminal potential and a high intracellular potassium concentration that augments potassium secretion. Na^+ absorption through the apical Na^+-selective channel (affected by aldosterone) maintains the negative potential difference in the tubular lumen. Aldosterone increases apical Na-selective channel activity, and with time, aldosterone can also increase the basolateral Na^+,K^+-ATP to produce changes, which parallel systemic K balance. Measurement of the transtubular K^+ gradient can thus be a clinical tool to assess K^+ excretion and direct therapy.

Factors Influencing Reabsorption of Bicarbonate

Nearly all of the bicarbonate filtered at the glomerulus is reabsorbed. Urinary excretion of acid results in generation of new bicarbonate equal in amount to that lost in buffering the endogenous load of noncarbonic acid generated from diet and metabolism.

In the proximal tubule, secretion of H^+ results in absorption of 80 to 90% of filtered bicarbonate, by combining with H^+ to form carbonic acid, which, in the presence of CA (isoenzyme 4 in the brush border), dissociates to form CO_2 and H_2O (62–64). Luminal CO_2 diffuses into the cells. In the presence of cytoplasmic CA (isoenzyme 2), hydroxylation occurs to form bicarbonate (63,64). Bicarbonate exits the basolateral membrane of the cell by a sodium-coupled mechanism (39). Hydrogen ion secretion in the proximal tubule is mediated by electroneutral Na^+ H^+ exchange at the luminal membrane. This exchange is driven by the lumen to cytoplasm sodium concentration gradient maintained by the basolateral Na^+,K^+-ATPase activity. In the presence of acetazolamide, carbonic acid (H_2CO_3) accumulates in the lumen, with an increase in H^+ concentration, leading to a decrease in H^+ secretion and bicarbonate reabsorption. Because factors that regulate sodium reabsorption alter bicarbonate reabsorption as a secondary effect, luminal bicarbonate concentration and pH, luminal flow rate, peritubular PCO_2, and angiotensin II are important determinants of bicarbonate reabsorption. H^+ secretion proximally varies inversely with peritubular bicarbonate, pH, and, to a lesser extent, potassium balance.

Factors Influencing Hydrogen Ion Secretion

In the distal nephron, H^+ secretion is responsible for reabsorption of the remaining 10 to 15% of filtered bicarbonate (not absorbed proximally), decreasing the pH to less than 6.1. As the luminal pH decreases further, secreted H^+ is titrated to the urinary buffers (phosphate and ammonium), completing a process initiated in the proximal tubule (33). In the adjacent cortical and medullary collecting tubules (MCTs), secretion of H^+ is mediated by a proton translocating ATPase (H^+ ATPase) located on the luminal surface of the α-intercalated cells (46). In the cortical collecting tubules (CCTs), principal cells mediate electrogenic transfer of sodium, thus creating a transepithelial electrical potential difference that is lumen negative and favors H^+ secretion. The principal cells are responsible for the secretion of potassium. Sodium transfer does not occur in the MCT. Secretion of H^+ by the distal tubule is influenced by aldosterone, sodium delivery, buffer delivery, changes in pH and PCO_2, luminal pH, and potassium (65–67). Aldosterone directly stimulates H^+ ATPase in the intercalated cells and sodium reabsorption by principal cells. The resulting luminal electronegativity further stimulates H^+ secretion. [Increased sodium delivery to the distal tubule when the avidity for sodium is high (e.g., volume depletion; administration of mineralocorticoid hormone) leads to sodium reabsorption, or when sodium is excreted with poorly absorbed anions such as sulfate, phosphate, ferrocyanide, or penicillin, an increased luminal negativity is generated.] If sodium is accompanied by chloride, the stimulus for H^+ secretion is lower because the chloride is passively reabsorbed by the paracellular pathway, dissipating the electrical gradient. An increase in distal delivery of buffer (e.g., phosphate loading or β-hydroxy butyrate during ketoacidosis) leads to stimulation of H^+ secretion and an increased formation of TA. H^+ secretion is stimulated by acidosis and inhibited by alkalosis. H^+ secretion is inhibited when the luminal pH reaches 4.5. Potassium depletion directly stimulates intercalated cells to secrete H^+ and stimulates ammonia production, distal delivery, and H^+ ion excretion.

CLINICAL SPECTRUM

Patients with RTA may have nonspecific symptoms such as anorexia, vomiting, constipation, polyuria, and polydipsia. Untreated children are characteristically growth retarded. Hyperchloremic MA (HCMA) with increased urinary pH, a lack of ammonia secretion ($+U_{AG}$), and even life-threatening acidosis, may occur in infants and young children. Nephrocalcinosis (68), renal calculi (69), and musculoskeletal complaints (myalgia, arthralgia) (70) are the most common presentations of adult type 1 RTA. Rickets may occur in type 1 (71) classic DRTA, although this is more commonly seen in association with PRTA resulting from Fanconi syndrome (72,73). A subgroup of children present with RTA in the course of adrenal insufficiency (aldosterone deficiency or tubular resistance) with signs of volume depletion. In adults, hyporeninemia and hypoaldosteronism more commonly occur in patients with decreased renal function in the presence of diabetes mellitus and interstitial disease (59).

Proximal Renal Tubular Acidosis Type 2

Symptoms

Characteristic symptoms include growth retardation, failure to thrive (FTT), and recurrent vomiting.

Epidemiology

PRTA occurs in a variety of conditions, most often associated with multiple tubular dysfunction (e.g., Fanconi syndrome) as part of cystinosis, galactosemia, tyrosinemia, Wilson's disease, Lowe's syndrome, and mitochondrial myopathies. Isolated transient or persistent proximal tubular defects in bicarbonate reabsorption have been described, predominantly in males (71,74).

Adult-onset persistent type 2 RTA and isolated PRTA defects have been associated with cyanotic congenital heart disease (75) and renal vascular accidents (76). A familial autosomal dominant form that presents in early childhood (74) and a congenital form associated with growth retardation, mental retardation, and ocular and dental abnormalities in two brothers has been described (77).

Genetics

Genetically transmitted forms include persistent PRTA (both autosomal dominant and autosomal recessive forms), an isolated familial transmitted PRTA (74), or as a PRTA syndrome in association with mental retardation and ocular and dental abnormalities (77). PRTA may also be associated with other genetically transmitted disorders (Table 39.3) such as osteopetrosis with CA2 deficiency (30), pyruvate carboxylase deficiency, familial forms associated with other hereditary dysfunction of proximal tubules (hereditary fructose intolerance) (2), mitochondrial myopathies, and glycogen storage disease.

Pathophysiology and Complications

Mechanisms suggested for the defective bicarbonate absorption include abnormality of the Na^+-H^+ exchanger, an impaired basolateral Na^+ HCO_3^- exchanger, decreased Na^+,K^+-ATPase activity attenuating the sodium gradient from lumen to cell, and inhibition of CA activity. Decrease in bicarbonate reabsorption in the proximal tubule results in increased delivery of bicarbonate to the distal tubule, overwhelming the distal tubular reabsorption capacity (normally approximately 15% of the filtered load) (26). Bicarbonate loss results in a decrease in NAE and secondary MA. As MA increases and plasma bicarbonate levels fall, the filtered load of bicarbonate falls below the distal tubular capacity and bicarbonate losses cease so that the urinary pH falls below 5.5 (2). Therefore, PRTA is characterized by MA, with a urinary pH above 5.5 under mild to moderate MA, and the ability to lower urinary pH below 5.5 under maximal stress.

In the isolated proximal lesion, other proximal tubular functions are intact (i.e., glycosuria, phosphaturia, and aminoaciduria, which characterize Fanconi syndrome, are absent); sodium bicarbonate losses stimulate aldosterone secretion, and loss of potassium by the principal cells in the CCT results in hypokalemia. Renin and aldosterone levels

TABLE 39.3. PRIMARY DEFECT IN BICARBONATE REABSORPTION [PROXIMAL RENAL TUBULAR ACIDOSIS (PRTA) TYPE 2]

Primary
- Sporadic
  - Transient childhood (71)
  - Persisting (adult onset) (73)
- Genetically determined
  - Primary PRTA (74)
  - Sporadic transient (71)
  - Genetic
    - Autosomal dominant
    - Autosomal recessive
  - Isolated PRTA with mental retardation and ocular and dental abnormalities (75)
  - Pyruvate carboxylase deficiency (118,119)
  - Mitochondrial myopathies (82,83)
  - Osteopetrosis (30,72,80)
- Carbonic anhydrase deficiency (120)
  - Sporadic
  - Genetic
  - Drug-induced (acetazolamide, sulfanilamide, mafenide acetate)

Secondary
- Hereditary multiple proximal tubular dysfunction, Fanconi syndrome
  - Cystinosis
  - Galactosemia
  - Glycogen storage disease type 1
  - Hereditary fructose intolerance (with fructose exposure)
  - Tyrosinemia
  - Wilson's disease
  - Heavy metals
  - Drugs and toxins
  - Carbonic anhydrase inhibitors
  - 6-Mercaptopurine
  - Streptozotocin
  - Ifosfamide
  - Outdated tetracycline
  - Sulfonamides
  - Mafenide acetate
  - Valproic acid
  - Heavy metals (Cd, Pb, Hg)
- Associated with other metabolic disorders
  - Primary or secondary hyperparathyroidism
  - Vitamin D deficiency and dependency
  - Leigh's syndrome (11,29,119)
  - Metachromatic leukodystrophy
  - Osteopetrosis (30,72)
  - Pyruvate carboxylase deficiency (118,119)
  - Lowe's syndrome (81)

Miscellaneous
- Amyloidosis (28)
- Cyanotic congenital heart disease
- Fallot tetralogy (75)
- Hereditary nephritis
- Hyperkalemia
- Multiple myeloma
- Nephrotic syndrome
- Renal cystic disease
- Renal transplant
- Renal vascular accident (76)
- Sjögren's syndrome (92,93)

Note: References are indicated in parentheses.

generally are elevated as a result of volume contraction (78). Hypokalemia, although common, is less prominent in isolated PRTA. Polyuria is common and appears early in the disorder with hypokalemia and solute diuresis (bicarbonate and sodium loss) (79). Acidosis leads to vomiting, lower caloric intake, and a decrease in growth rate that is reversed when acidosis is corrected (21). Bone age may be retarded.

Serum calcium, phosphorus, and vitamin D levels usually are normal despite persistent acidosis and rickets or osteomalacia (71,74). Abnormalities do not occur in primary isolated RTA unless vitamin D or calcium intake is marginal (73), but disturbances are common in secondary forms of RTA with multiple tubular defects (Fanconi syndrome) and in patients with osteopetrosis and a mixed RTA pattern (80). Nephrocalcinosis and nephrolithiasis are rare in PRTA as increased citrate excretion occurs together with increased calcium reabsorption in the distal tubule.

Treatment and Prognosis

Alkali supplement should be provided in amounts sufficient to offset the losses, which are variable and may be as high as 2 to 20 mmol/kg/day (59). Sodium restriction or hydrochlorothiazide, 1.5 to 2 mg/kg/day, may decrease alkali requirements by enhancing proximal reabsorption of sodium and bicarbonate.

Patients with Fanconi syndrome may require potassium, phosphate, and vitamin D supplementation in addition to specific therapy aimed at the underlying cause, such as cysteamine in cystinosis, chelating agents (i.e., penicillamine) in Wilson's disease, or dietary manipulation in galactosemia and tyrosinemia.

Prognosis in PRTA depends on the etiology. In transient DRTA, supplementation to preserve growth is all that is required. Adequate chronic alkali therapy protects against growth abnormalities in those with persistent lesions. Outcome in secondary lesions is determined by the underlying process and its response to treatment. Early treatment of galactosemia has an excellent prognosis, whereas patients with Lowe's syndrome (81) or mitochondrial myopathies (82,83) have less favorable outcomes.

Renal Tubular Acidosis Type 4

Symptoms

RTA type 4 is the most common nonazotemic form of RTA and may result from a number of disorders (Table 39.4). Patients usually present with hyperkalemia and mild MA. Ability to acidify the urine to a urinary pH below 5.5 is intact and signs of aldosterone deficiency or resistance may be present. Infants may have FTT, hyperkalemic MA with associated salt wasting (in aldosterone deficit), or resistance (pseudohypoaldosteronism) (13,16). In pseudohypoaldosteronism, renal sodium loss and potassium retention usually

TABLE 39.4. DISTAL RENAL TUBULAR ACIDOSIS (RTA): ALDOSTERONE-SENSITIVE TUBULAR DEFECTS (RTA 4)

- **Primary**
  - Early childhood transient (56)
- **Secondary**
  - Aldosterone deficiency
    - Aldosterone deficiency without intrinsic renal disease (primary adrenal insufficiency)
      - Addison's disease
      - Bilateral adrenalectomy
      - Congenital adrenal hyperplasia syndrome (21 hydroxylase deficiency) (11)
      - Isolated hypoaldosteronism (121–124)
      - Isolated hypoaldosteronism of critical illness?
      - Inherited corticosterone methyloxidase deficiency (123)
    - Hyporeninemia (hypoaldosteronism syndrome) (10,59,85)
      - Diabetes mellitus
      - Gout
      - Pyelonephritis
      - Interstitial nephritis
      - Nephrosclerosis (17)
  - Attenuated renal response to aldosterone
    - Pseudohypoaldosteronism
      - Pseudohypoaldosteronism (infancy) (13)
      - Chronic tubulointerstitial nephritis with salt wasting
      - Obstructive uropathy in infancy
    - Drugs
      - Spironolactone
      - Heparin
      - Amiloride
      - Prostaglandin inhibitors
      - Triamterene
      - Captopril
      - Cyclosporine
  - Attenuated renal response to aldosterone with relative aldosterone deficiency
    - Selective tubular dysfunction with hypertension and impaired renin
      - Synonyms (chloride shunt syndrome; pseudohypoaldosteronism type 2) (17)
    - With associated renin deficiency
      - Chronic tubulointerstitial nephritis with chronic renal insufficiency associated with deficient renin secretion
      - Obstructive uropathy
      - Renal transplant
      - Lupus erythematosus
      - Acute glomerulonephritis
      - Renal amyloidosis
  - Unclassified type 4
    - Distal tubular disease/interstitial disease
    - Renal amyloidosis
    - Lupus nephritis with antitubular basement membrane antibodies
    - Renal venous thrombosis
    - Drugs (methicillin)
  - Contributing or aggravating factors in RTA 4
    - KCl supplements
    - Heparin
    - Potassium-sparing diuretics
    - Prostaglandin inhibitors
    - Captopril
    - Cyclosporine

Note: References are indicated in parentheses.

remit by 4 or 5 years of age, although renin and aldosterone levels remain elevated. In adults, mild renal insufficiency and hyperkalemic acidosis out of proportion to the renal functional abnormalities is common (59). In the rare syndrome of chloride shunt-associated disorder (9,10,15,17), infants have FTT (16), whereas adolescents have hypertension and increased blood volume associated with hyporeninemia and lowered aldosterone levels (15,17).

In critically ill patients, a new syndrome of isolated hypoaldosteronism has been noted. This is believed to follow hypoxia, cytokine release, and atrial natriuretic peptide inhibition of aldosterone synthase. It is characterized by elevated adrenocorticotropic hormone and cortisol levels with decreased aldosterone and hyperkalemic MA, which is potentiated by K^+-sparing diuretics, K^+ load from parenteral nutrition, and heparin (54).

Genetics

Inherited defects resulting in type 4 RTA include absence of aldosterone and glucocorticoid hormones (e.g., congenital adrenal hypoplasia with salt wasting) (11) and isolated hypoaldosteronism (Table 39.4). Possible inheritance is suggested by familial cases of a form of early childhood hyperkalemic RTA (27).

Pathophysiology

RTA 4 results from deficiency of aldosterone or tubular unresponsiveness to its effects. Aldosterone stimulates H^+ secretion by intercalated cells and sodium absorption in the principal cells. This process increases luminal electronegativity, further enhancing sodium and potassium secretion. Increased potassium secretion by principal cells leads to enhanced ammonium production and distal delivery. In experimental aldosterone deficiency there is a decrease in NAE secondary to decreased ammonium formation; studies in human subjects after adrenalectomy confirm decreased ammonium secretion, which is corrected with mineralocorticoid supplementation (84). This suggests that renal acidification is under tonic stimulation by physiologic levels of mineralocorticoids (84).

As a result of aldosterone deficiency, hyperkalemia results from decreased potassium excretion (59,85). Bicarbonate excretion is reduced if plasma bicarbonate is returned to normal by supplementation. Reduced bicarbonate excretion allows a urinary pH of 5.5 to be attained under acidotic stimulation. Exclusion of other proximal tubular dysfunction is necessary to differentiate between PRTA and RTA 4. However, a decrease in urinary ammonium secretion leads to decreases in NAE and MA, with marked hyperkalemia after any increase in dietary potassium intake.

Citrate excretion usually is high in patients with RTA 4, and nephrocalcinosis and nephrolithiasis do not occur despite the acidosis. In patients with the early childhood form of RTA 4, calcium reabsorption is increased, further protecting against nephrocalcinosis (86).

Treatment of hyperkalemic RTA includes exclusion of excess dietary potassium intake or removal of potential offending drugs and correction of volume contraction. If restriction of dietary potassium intake does not produce correction, a trial of furosemide to ameliorate the acidosis and hyperkalemia should be undertaken (59,87). In an emergency, mineralocorticoid (fluorohydrocortisone) or sodium bicarbonate may be necessary to correct the acidosis, promote intracellular translocation of potassium, and increase potassium excretion. However, long-term use of sodium bicarbonate in mild renal insufficiency leads to volume overload and hypertension (6). In adrenal insufficiency, mineralocorticoid supplementation leads to correction of underlying pathophysiology. With pseudohypoaldosteronism, sodium chloride supplementation alone most often leads to correction; however, some patients additionally require sodium bicarbonate (86). In the small subgroup with a chloride shunt, possibly as a result of a defective Na^+-K^+-$2Cl^-$ transporter system, concurrent hypertension is present. Treatment includes salt restriction and thiazide or furosemide administration to correct both the hypertension and hyperkalemia by increasing sodium delivery to the distal tubule, resulting in increased H^+, K^+, and water excretion.

Prognosis

Prognosis depends on the underlying cause. Pseudohypoaldosteronism appears to result from a relative decrease in receptor number, leading to end-organ resistance that remits by 4 to 5 years of age (86). Primary adrenal lesions usually require permanent supplementation. Drug-induced changes may remit with removal of the drug and further avoidance of such agents. Hyporeninemic hypoaldosteronism from tubulointerstitial nephritis occurs in adult patients with diabetes or hyperuricemia and is likely to be associated with progressive renal insufficiency.

Distal Renal Tubular Acidosis Type 1, Classic Renal Tubular Acidosis

Symptoms

Symptoms differ in children and adults. Childhood presentation includes vomiting, FTT, and life-threatening acidosis. Nephrocalcinosis, renal calculi, or bone disease, including rickets or osteomalacia, are less common as presenting symptoms in younger children but are regularly present in older untreated patients (87). Adults have recurrent renal calculi and musculoskeletal complaints such as arthralgia, myalgia, and bone pain (70).

Genetics

A reduced rate of H^+ secretion may occur as a primary condition—DRTA inherited as either an autosomal dominant or autosomal recessive trait (26)—or secondary to nephrocalcinosis (88,89–91), autoimmune disease (84–86), or exposure to drugs such as amphotericin (91) (Table 39.5). The inherited forms may be present as an isolated defect (68) or associated with genetically transmitted systemic disease, such as CA2 deficiency (76,80), erythrocyte CA B deficiency, Ehlers-Danlos syndrome, hereditary elliptocytosis, hereditary fructose intolerance with nephrocalcinosis, Marfan's syndrome, sickle cell anemia, osteopetrosis (30), sensorineural deafness, carnitine palmitoyl transferase type 1 deficiency, and idiopathic hypercalciuria (89).

Pathophysiology

Disordered H^+ secretion in the CCT and MCT leads to decreased bicarbonate reabsorption in the distal tubule with consequent decrease in TA and ammonium secretion. The subsequent decrease in NAE leads to MA. Disordered H^+ secretion results in the inability to reduce urinary pH even with spontaneous or induced acidosis. Bicarbonate excretion in early childhood is greater than in adults, and FE_{HCO_3} may range from 5 to 15% (4,78). This large bicarbonate loss, in addition to the inability to secrete H^+, leads to potentially life-threatening acidosis and a much larger requirement for bicarbonate supplementation in the younger age group. Functional immaturity of the proximal tubule has been suggested as the cause for this increased bicarbonate loss (4,26). Further increases in bicarbonate requirements may occur during periods of subsequent growth when H^+ is produced during bone formation. At approximately 4 to 5 years of age, there is usually a decrease in bicarbonate supplementation to levels similar to those required for correction in adults. Bicarbonate excretion does not vary with filtered load over a wide range of plasma bicarbonate levels and results from the inability to reduce urinary pH below 7, even with severe acidosis. This phenomenon is consistent with impaired distal tubular bicarbonate reabsorption (26).

Most adults show a constant FE_{HCO_3} below 5% over a wide range of serum bicarbonate levels. However, some patients have been described with net base excretion resulting from FE_{HCO_3} exceeding TA + NH_4^+ (26).

Concurrent sodium and potassium wasting occur. Sodium wasting is a result of decreased reabsorption in both proximal and distal tubules with bicarbonate or other anions (94,95). Volume depletion stimulates renin-aldosterone secretion and leads to increased delivery of bicarbonate and poorly absorbed anions such as sulfate to the distal tubule. This promotes sodium and potassium wasting and consequent hypokalemia. Supplementation with alkali increases urinary pH and decreases the EDF for H^+ secretion, allowing correction of acidosis. Urinary sodium and potassium excretion subsequently fall, leading to improvement in electrolyte

TABLE 39.5. DISTAL RENAL TUBULAR ACIDOSIS (RTA)

Inability to secrete H^+ (secretory defect)
Primary distal RTA (persistent classic syndrome)
In infancy, associated HCO_3 wasting
In adolescence, secondary hyperparathyroidism
Nerve deafness develops in adolescence
Transient infantile form
Genetics (26,68,125)
Sporadic (8,26,27)
Endemic (8)
Secondary
Disorders of calcium metabolism with nephrocalcinosis or hypercalciuria
Primary hyperparathyroidism
Hyperthyroidism
Vitamin D intoxication
Genetics
Idiopathic hypercalciuria (89)
Hyperthyroidism (with nephrocalcinosis)
Medullary cystic disease—familial juvenile nephronophthisis
Hereditary fructose intolerance with fructose exposure
Associated with genetically transmitted disease
CA type 2 (30,80)
Erythrocyte CA B deficiency (126)
Ehlers-Danlos syndrome (127)
Hereditary elliptocytosis (128)
Marfan's syndrome (129)
Sickle cell anemia (130,131)
Osteopetrosis (30)
With associated deafness (125,132–136)
Carnitine palmitoyl transferase deficiency type 1 (137)
Autoimmune disorders
Hypergammaglobulinemia (91)
Sjögren's syndrome (92,93)
Chronic active hepatitis
Primary biliary cirrhosis
Thyroiditis
Fibrosing alveolitis
Systemic lupus erythematosus
Polyarteritis nodosa
Rheumatoid arthritis
Drug or toxin
Amphotericin B
Toluene
Analgesic abuse
Lithium
Cyclamate
Mercury
Associated with other renal disease
Obstructive uropathy
Pyelonephritis
Renal transplant rejection
Sickle cell disease
Leprosy
Associated with endocrine disease
Hypothyroidism
Salt-losing congenital adrenal hyperplasia
Functional RTA (exchange defect)
Marked volume depletion
Hyponatremic states (hepatic cirrhosis/nephrotic syndrome)
Sodium depletion
Increased back-diffusion H^+ (gradient defect)
Amphotericin B
Abolition of the electrical gradient for H^+ ion secretion
Short-circuit or voltage defect
Combined defects in proximal HCO_3 reabsorption and H^+ ion secretion
Infantile form type 1 RTA
Incomplete RTA

CA, carbonic anhydrase.

balance. Volume correction decreases aldosterone secretion and leads to retention of potassium and correction of the hypokalemia (51). A small group of patients have continued potassium wasting despite correction of the acidosis, a condition that may be associated with persisting hyperaldosteronism. MA is associated with an increased excretion of calcium and phosphorus (88) and a decrease in citrate excretion (5,31,96,97). In acidosis (spontaneous or induced by ammonium chloride), citrate enters the mitochondria through stimulation of a citrate carrier in the inner mitochondrial membrane (96,97). This leads to a decrease in cytosolic citrate and a gradient for reabsorption from lumen to cell. Medullary nephrocalcinosis and recurrent calcium phosphate or oxalate nephrolithiasis occur in the alkaline urine as a result of hypercalciuria and the reduced intraluminal citrate.

Nephrocalcinosis, which was, historically, a universal finding in patients with DRTA, has become rare with recognition and early institution of adequate alkali therapy. Persisting MA leads to buffering of hydrogen ion by bone (alkaline buffer salts) with development of metabolic bone disease (98). Correction of the acidosis leads to correction of bone disease, whereas nephrocalcinosis and nephrolithiasis tend to persist (69,99).

Some patients with DRTA appear to have impaired gastrointestinal absorption of calcium (100), as well as increased renal excretion of calcium, leading to hypocalcemia, hyperparathyroidism, hypophosphatemia, and rickets. This occurs in patients with untreated disease and is uncommon in patients receiving adequate alkali supplementation (68). MA itself may impair vitamin D metabolism and lead to intestinal malabsorption of calcium, with secondary bone disease with RTA. In acidotic children and adults with RTA and radiographic evidence of rickets (101,102), serum levels of 1,25-dihydroxyvitamin D (1,25-OH vitamin D) have been reported to be normal (101,102). However, in phosphorus-restricted healthy men, in whom basal levels of 1,25-OH vitamin D were increased twofold, a decrease occurred when acidosis was induced with ammonium chloride (103). The decrease was mediated by decreased production and increased clearance of 1,25-OH vitamin D (101). Thus, acidosis in humans can impair the renal production of 1,25-OH vitamin D.

Polyuria is always present in patients with DRTA and has been attributed to hypokalemia, nephrocalcinosis, solute excretion in untreated patients (e.g., hypercalciuria, phosphaturia, excess sodium, potassium, and bicarbonate excretion), or a primary tubular defect (79).

Treatment

Therapy is directed at correction of acidosis at a rate commensurate with risk of electrolyte and acid-base abnormality. Severe hypokalemia presents a risk to cardiac and respiratory muscle function (104) and should be at least partially corrected before correction of the acidosis (because the latter can aggravate the degree of hypokalemia) (3). Sodium and potassium supplementation may be supplied as citrate or bicarbonate, with one-third to one-half of the supplement provided as the potassium salt. Increased growth velocity is expected to follow appropriate therapy in 2 to 3 weeks in the infant, and increased bone formation is followed by an increase in acid production (68). Increased supplementation is required until stabilization occurs with normal growth rate (68). A longer period of therapy is required to restore growth in previously untreated older children. After age 4 to 5 years, there is reduced bicarbonate loss, and, therefore, lower dosages of alkali supplementation (1 to 2 mEq/kg/day or 2 to 4 mEq per 100 calories) maintain correction.

Prognosis

Growth rates can be restored and bone disease prevented by early and consistent therapy. Early treatment is also necessary to prevent nephrocalcinosis, which can lead to chronic interstitial nephritis with scarring and glomerulosclerosis (105).

DIAGNOSIS OF RTA

Diagnosis of RTA is based on clinical findings, assessment of plasma acid-base status, assessment of urine acidification (urinary pH), urinary ammonia or urine anion gap, and urine PCO_2. Tools for characterization are outlined in Table 39.6 and include acid loading (106), bicarbonate titration (107), urine to blood carbon dioxide tension during bicarbonate titration (18,108), neutral sodium phosphate infusion (101), and furosemide challenge (18,59,108). Urine-blood

TABLE 39.6. FEATURES OF RENAL TUBULAR ACIDOSIS (RTA)

	Proximal RTA	With bicarbonate wasting	Distal classic RTA	HyperK distal RTA	RTA 4 with GFR normal	Low GFR
Diagnostic testing	Bicarbonate Response		Acid load Bicarbonate response		Renin—Aldosterone	Renin—Aldosterone
S_{HCO_3} untreated	Usually 15–20 mmol/L		10–15 mmol/L	10–15 mmol/L	15–20 mmol/L	15–20 mmol/L
Features with metabolic acidosis						
SK^+	N/L	N/L	N/L	I	I	I
Min U_{pH}	<5.5	>5.5	>5.5	>5.5	<5.5	<5.5
Unstressed U_{pH}	>7.0	6.0–7.5	5.8–7.0	>5.5	<5.5	<5.5
Urine excretion						
NH_4	N	D	D	D	D	MD
K^+	N/I	I	I	D	D	D
Ca^{2+}	N	I	I	I	N	D
Citrate	N/I	D	D	?	N	N/D
$\%FE_{HCO_3}$ at normal S_{HCO_3}	>10–15%	>5–15%	<3–5%	<5%	>5–15%	<3–15%
U—B PCO_2 (alkaline urine)	N/I >20	L <15	L <15	L <15	N >20	L —
Nephrocalcinosis (renal stones)	–/+	++	++	+	–	–
Rickets	+	—	–/+	—	—	—
Bicarbonate to correct S_{pH} (mmol/kg/d)	4–10	10–15	1–2 adult 4–15 child	2–3	2–4	1–2
Response to bicarbonate (2 mEq/kg)	Refractory	Refractory	Good	Good	Variable	Good

+, often; ++, very common association; –, rare or absent; ?, unknown; D, decrease; GFR, glomerular filtration rate; I, increase; L, low; MD, marked decrease; N, normal; N/D, normal or decreased; N/I, normal or increased; S_{pH}, serum pH; U_{pH}, urine pH.

TABLE 39.7. PATHOPHYSIOLOGY OF DISTAL RENAL TUBULAR ACIDOSIS (RTA)

Physiologic disorder	Clinical condition	Plasma K^+	U–B PCO_2 with HCO_3 load	U–B PCO_2 with phosphate load	Na_2SO_4 loading U_{pH}	Furosemide K excretion
Secretory[a] defect	Classic RTA	N/L	L	L	>5.5	N/I
	Transplant rejection	—	—	—	—	—
Voltage-dependent defect[b]						
Severe distal Na transport defect	Obstructive uropathy	—	—	—	—	—
	Congenital adrenal hyperplasia	I	L	L	>5.5	D
Mild distal Na transport defect	Sickle hemoglobinopathy	I	L	N	<5.5	N
Impaired distal Na delivery	Hepatic cirrhosis	—	—	—	—	—
		N	?	?	<5.5	N/I
Gradient defect[c]	Nephrotic syndrome amphotericin B	N/L	N/L	?	D	N/I

?, unknown; D, decreased; I, increased; N, normal; N/I, normal or increased; N/L, normal or low; L, low; U_{pH}, urine pH.
[a]Failure to secrete H^+.
[b]Failure to generate luminal electronegativity, which occurs as a result of impaired distal Na transport or delivery.
[c]Increased back-diffusion of secreted H^+.

carbon dioxide tension may be used as a specialized laboratory test to define impaired H^+ secretion by the collecting tubule. Urine-blood PCO_2 is the most sensitive test for distal tubular H^+ excretion. Impaired excretion is associated with a urinary CO_2 tension (PCO_2) that does not increase to expected higher-than-plasma values after loading with sodium bicarbonate. Under normal circumstances, urinary pH and bicarbonate are increased by administration of sodium bicarbonate, and urinary PCO_2 rises to values considerably higher than those of blood (normally more than 20 mm above blood levels) (109,110). The difference in PCO_2 between urine and blood (U PCO_2 to B PCO_2 gradient) varies directly with the urine bicarbonate concentration. Increase in PCO_2 in alkaline urine reflects an increase in H^+ secretion in the collecting tubule, augmented by the high, intraluminal bicarbonate concentration (18). The secreted H^+ and luminal bicarbonate combine to form carbonic acid, which dissociates to carbon dioxide and water at an uncatalyzed rate (CA is not present in the lumen of the distal nephron). Because carbon dioxide generation occurs in the distal segments of the collecting duct, where medullary trapping of carbon dioxide can occur, and in the renal pelvis and bladder, where conditions are unfavorable for reabsorption of carbon dioxide into blood, carbon dioxide appears in increased amounts in the urine. Similar findings follow the administration of neutral sodium phosphate, which enhances the distal delivery of buffer. This stimulates H^+ secretion and increases the U PCO_2 to B PCO_2 gradient. This can also be used as a test of distal tubular H^+ secretion. Furosemide challenge (Table 39.7) may be used to assist in differentiation of site and mechanism of the defect in acidification (18). Delivery of sodium and reabsorption in the CCT is followed by an increase in luminal electronegativity. A similar increase in negativity can be produced by sodium sulfate infusion, which increases the sodium delivery; because the sulfate ion is impermeable, the gradient is maintained. In normal subjects with MA acid, urinary pH is further lowered by furosemide or sodium sulfate infusion and potassium excretion is increased.

Patients with diffuse impairment of H^+-ATPase from a decrease in glomerular filtration rate (GFR) or nephron number have a persistent alkaline urine with increased potassium excretion because principal cell function is usually intact (Table 39.7). Patients with a pump defect limited to the MCT have a normal increase in both H^+ and K^+ because cortical function is stimulated by intraluminal electronegativity. Patients with impairment in cortical sodium reabsorption (voltage defect) have baseline hyperkalemia and after challenge there is no increase in H^+ or K^+ because there is no increased intraluminal electronegative gradient.

Differential Diagnosis

1. Other causes of metabolic acidosis

(a) Gastrointestinal bicarbonate loss (e.g., diarrhea, fistula) or administration of drugs [e.g., $CaCl_2$, $MgSO_4$, cholestyramine (U Cl greater than Na + K)] (Fig. 39.2).

In chronic MA, ammonia generation from glutamine is stimulated with little change in phosphate excretion (phosphate released from bone is used in blood buffering during acidosis). Thus, it is helpful to focus on ammonia generation and excretion as the expected response in acidosis, and review of ammonia excretion is the key to understanding RTA. Urinary pH values taken alone may be misleading in chronic MA from gastrointestinal loss, particularly if hypokalemia is present. Here the increase in ammonia excretion buffers most of the secreted H^+, leading to a urinary pH of 5.5 to 6.0. Thus, if pH alone is considered

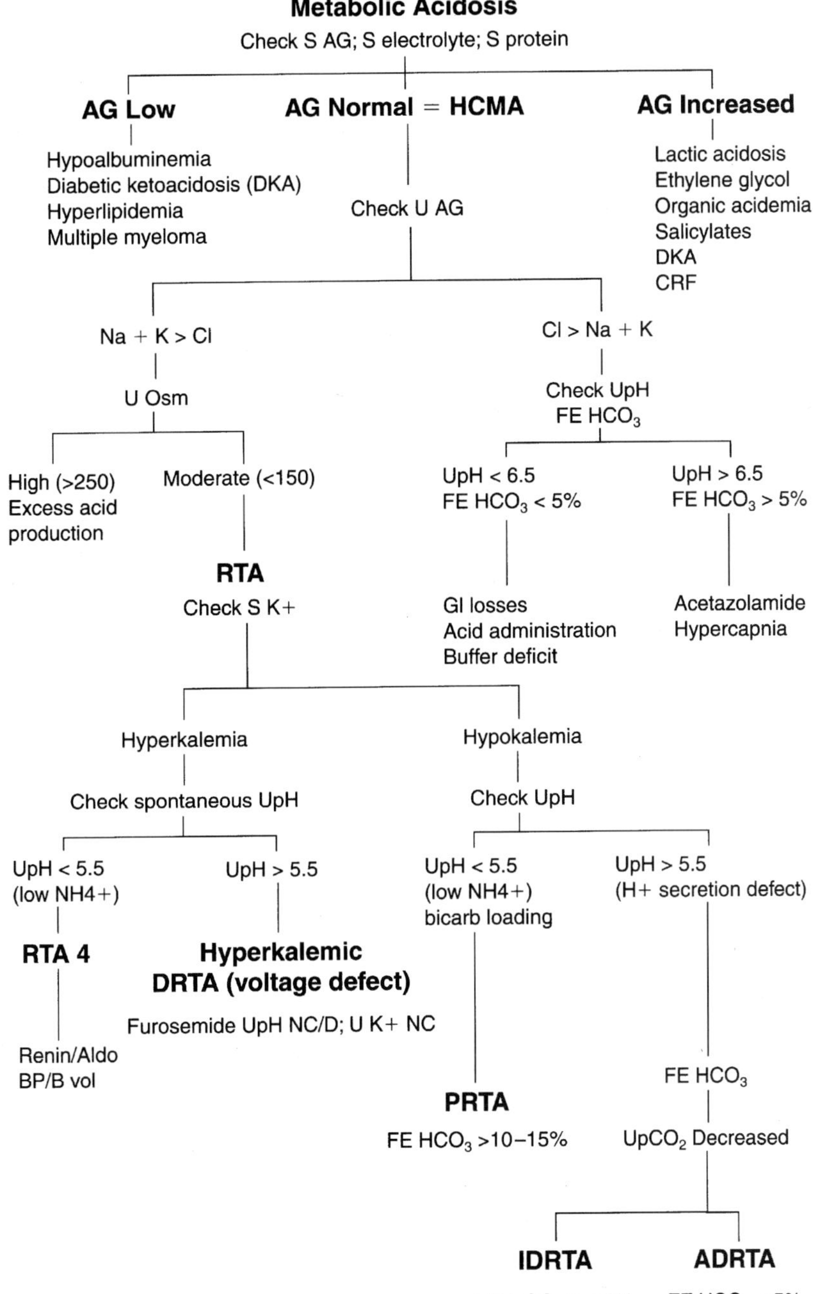

FIGURE 39.2. This algorithmic approach to the patient with metabolic acidosis illustrates the differential features leading to a diagnosis of renal tubular acidosis (RTA). Useful confirmatory tests and features of differing types of RTA are outlined at the steps in which they are used clinically. ADRTA, adult distal renal tubular acidosis; AG, anion gap; Aldo, aldosterone; BP, blood pressure; B Vol, blood volume; CRF, chronic renal failure; GI, gastrointestinal tract; HCMA, hyperchloremic metabolic acidosis; IDRTA, infantile distal renal tubular acidosis; PRTA, proximal renal tubular acidosis; S, serum; UpH, urine pH.

without consideration of urine AG, DRTA is suggested (24,111). In aldosterone deficiency, ammonia secretion is significantly impaired and H^+ secretion as ammonium is reduced. Here, incomplete buffering of secreted H^+ leads to low urinary pH even in patients with DRTA (112,113).

(b) Acid loading that may occur with NH_4Cl, acidic amino acids in parenteral nutrition, or ingestion of acid ingestion (e.g., HCl, NH_4Cl, lysine, arginine, sulfur, and phosphorus from food). HCMA is associated with a negative U_{AG}.

2. Anion gap acidosis (Fig. 39.2)

3. Pseudo-RTA: In malnourished patients, the catabolic state produces increased acid, ketones, a decrease in GFR, and a decrease in phosphate output. This limits both TA (decreased capacity to excrete H^+ with an acid urine), a decreased generation of ammonia from a glutamine deficit that further limits H^+ excretion, and increased ketone excretion (or potential loss of bicarbonate), thereby producing a pseudo-RTA syndrome.

4. Urinary diversion or augmentation of the bladder using segments of ileum or colon leads to hypokalemia with severe acidosis, particularly if there is poor drainage leading to prolonged mucosal contact with urine.

5. Uremic acidosis usually is associated with an increased anion gap (from phosphate and sulfate retention), whereas reduced nephron number is followed by severely decreased ammonium excretion and reduced bicarbonate reabsorption (associated with a relative solute diuresis in remaining nephrons) (114).

6. Urinary infection with urea-splitting organisms (e.g., *Proteus*), an alkaline urine, and, if there is parenchymal infection, MA. Urinalysis and culture are necessary to exclude such factitious RTA patterns, particularly in patients with obstructive uropathy.

7. Hyperkalemic DRTA is a condition in which low K^+ excretion is present together with a decreased ability to acidify the urinary pH to less than 5.5 during spontaneous or induced acidosis (18). Concurrent sodium wasting is common, so salt-losing congenital adrenal hyperplasia, pseudohypoaldosteronism, must be considered in the differential diagnosis. Furosemide or sodium sulfate testing demonstrates typical low potassium excretion.

8. Abnormal anions, certain drugs, or toxic substances may lead to decrease in value of U AG (e.g., ketonuria), and D lactic acidosis and toluene (glue sniffing) are associated with a (+) net charge, which may be misinterpreted. Formal measurement of NH_3 may be necessary to check anion gap if the history suggests these are potential causes. Glue sniffing leads to a high NH_3, U AG, and U osmolar gap (from conversion of toluene to hippurate). Check for D lactic acidosis if MA is associated with central nervous system confusion, particularly if there is history of bowel disease or resection. A trial of antibiotics to decrease production is then warranted.

9. Functional RTA secondary to marked decrease in sodium delivery (U_{Na} less than 10) limits distal H^+ excretion.

Other considerations in differential diagnosis include tubular dysfunction (which may occur as a result of extrinsic renal factors such as hyperkalemia, extracellular fluid expansion, and loss of potential bicarbonate during recovery from chronic hypocapnia), with volume expansion (dilutional) acidosis, or secondary hyperparathyroidism.

Practical Approach to Diagnosis

Symptoms often are nonspecific and a high index of suspicion is necessary. If HCMA with a normal anion gap is present, RTA should be suspected. Initial studies should include repeat blood gas, S_K, U_{AG}, urinary pH (by pH electrode measurement, not indicator strips, which are notoriously inaccurate), and urinalysis to identify proximal tubular dysfunction (e.g., proteinuria glycosuria, aminoaciduria) (Figs. 39.2 and 39.3).

Serum K^+ is helpful in classification because hypokalemia occurs in PRTA (type 2) and DRTA (type 1). Hyperkalemia suggests aldosterone deficit or resistance (type 4), voltage defect, or obstructive uropathy. Normal S K^+ occurs in RTA with renal insufficiency, uremia, and the McSherry syndrome (86).

If preliminary studies suggest HCMA with RTA, serum, and urine, chemistries should be evaluated with blood gases to rule out respiratory alkalosis and other potential causes of bicarbonate loss. Additional history should be obtained to check for potential HCl administration (e.g., parenteral nutrition, drug administration), renal or gastrointestinal losses of bicarbonate, or the presence of a bowel segment augmenting bladder capacity or used as a urinary diversion. Exclude concurrent or underlying renal disease with uremia or retention rather than tubular acidosis. In the patient with HCMA, urinary pH and urinary ammonia excretion should be evaluated by direct measurement or U_{AG} (calculate urinary net charge, U_{AG} + U_{Na} + U_K − U_{Cl} − UH_{CO3}) to evaluate the site of renal tubular lesion. A positive U_{AG} reflects low H^+ secretion and low ammonium excretion, whereas a negative U_{AG} reflects urinary bicarbonate loss.

Low NH_4^+ production (U_{AG} +) suggests DRTA, PRTA with low NH_4^+ production, D lactic acidosis, or failure to lower NH_4^+ in the lumen of the collecting duct because of excess distal delivery of HCO_3^- from the PCT (22).

High NH_4^+ production with acidosis makes it necessary to check for loss of metabolizable organic anions in the urine (these equal potential HCO_3^-). Here, the cause of acidosis is overproduction of organic acids, and the renal lesion does not cause the acidosis, which may be U_{AG}^+. Loss of metabolizable anion is suspected when there is an excessive rate of urinary excretion of organic anions shown by Na^+ + K^+ greater than Cl^- (22,48).

If there is a low NH_4^+ excretion, urinary pH should be evaluated. If the urinary pH is above 6.0, bicarbonate excretion should be evaluated by examining the urinary P_{CO_2} in alkaline urine to examine for distal lesions and fractional excretion of bicarbonate for proximal lesions. Evaluation for other features of Fanconi syndrome should be performed.

Low ammonium secretion is rare. It may occur with a urinary pH of 4 to 5 and a defect in NH_3 availability in the renal medullary interstitium with a decrease in buffering ability (22). This occurs with a low GFR (22), hyperkalemia (22), decreased levels of blood glutamine (e.g., decreased substrate for ammoniagenesis) (115), or high levels of fat-derived fuels (e.g., total parenteral nutrition)

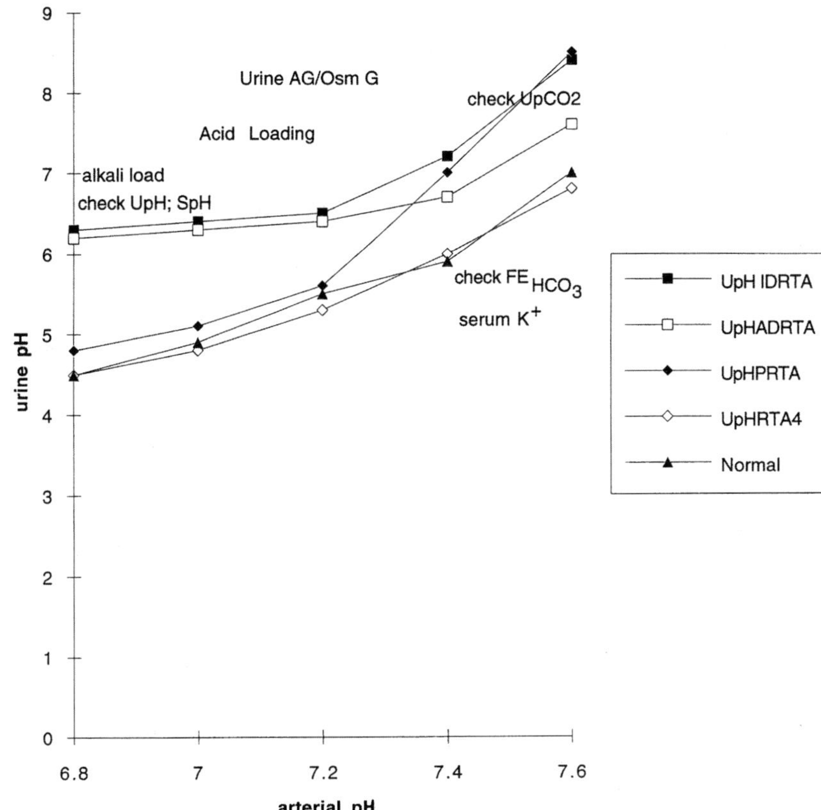

FIGURE 39.3. The figure shows the expected correlation between urine pH (UpH) and arterial pH. Captions highlight the most useful testing at different points in the spectrum. Alkali loading is most useful in the patient with marked acidosis; here comparison of the serum and urine pH allows differentiation between normals, proximal renal tubular acidosis (PRTA), and renal tubular acidosis (RTA) type 4. Acid loading is most useful in patients with normal serum pH (SpH) or mild acidosis. Estimations of net acid excretion from urine anion gap (Urine AG) are most helpful with urinary pH of approximately 6; urine osmolar gap (Osm G) or ammonium excretion measurement is most useful at serum pH below 7.4. Urinary Pco_2 measurement requires an alkaline urine. Fractional excretion of bicarbonate is helpful in differentiating between PRTA and the infantile form of distal RTA. Serum K^+ is helpful in differentiating RTA type 4 from other forms. ADRTA, adult distal renal tubular acidosis; IDRTA, infantile distal renal tubular acidosis.

competing with glutamine as a source for regeneration of ATP in the cells of the PCT with decrease in ammoniagenesis and in the hypothetical alkaline cell pH (22). The pH falls even with minimal H^+ transfer (22). A high urinary NH_4^+ or a negative net charge, negative U_{AG}, is consistent with normal distal acidification occurring in the older child (116).

Advantage should always be taken of any episode of spontaneous acidosis to screen for H^+ excretion. Standard treatment in RTA is base replacement; careful selection of testing during correction makes it possible to obtain information, which otherwise requires bicarbonate titration and correction of sodium deficit. This often allows characterization of RTA without the need for formal provocative testing. Formal testing, if subsequently required, should be delayed after correction of acidosis and a period of caloric adjustment to avoid the confounding effects of malnutrition, volume depletion, and other acid-base abnormalities.

The patient suspected of having RTA (Fig. 39.3) who is not overtly acidotic requires formal acid loading to induce an acidosis. A dose of 0.1 g/kg ammonium chloride (110 mEq/m^2) or 2.0 mEq/kg calcium chloride is administered orally or intravenously. Ammonia excretion and urinary pH are measured at 1, 2, and 8 hours. If secondary RTA from a metabolic disorder is possible, hyperammonemic syndromes must be excluded before administration of ammonium chloride to prevent life-threatening complications of hyperammonemia.

If the initial urinary pH is above 6.5 and serum bicarbonate is normal or only mildly depressed, evaluation for PRTA is necessary. Proximal tubular function should be evaluated because the defect (failure of bicarbonate reabsorption) in PRTA is, more commonly, part of a multiple defect syndrome (Fanconi syndrome) than an isolated defect.

If MA is present and the serum potassium is high (above 5 mEq/L) with a urinary pH below 5.5, one must consider RTA 4 (Table 39.8). Evaluation includes review of serum AG and U_{AG} (NAE), pH, assessment of volume and circulatory status (e.g., blood pressure, pulse, weight), and plasma renin and aldosterone measurement under stress (e.g., volume depletion or furosemide challenge). Persistently high urinary sodium loss suggests hypoaldosteronism or pseudohypoaldosteronism (117). Urine osmolality should be greater than isotonic and U_{Na} greater than 20 mmol/L for transtubular potassium gradient to be valid in assessing response to mineralocorticoid administration and furosemide challenge.

If U_{Na} is below 15 mmol/L, it is important to exclude an exchange defect because reduced H^+ may result from reduced sodium delivery. This is sometimes called *functional RTA* because of its transient nature and relationship to limited H^+ ion secretion by sodium delivery and poten-

TABLE 39.8. RENAL TUBULAR ACIDOSIS TYPE 4, HYPERKALEMIC ACIDURIA PHYSIOLOGIC SUBTYPING

Subtype	Plasma renin activity	Urine aldosterone/ serum aldosterone	Clinical blood pressure	Finding blood volume/plasma volume	Salt-wasting
Aldosterone deficiency ± renal disease					
Primary mineralocorticoid deficiency (Addison's congenital adrenal hyperplasia syndrome, isolated aldosterone deficiency)	S/E	L	L/N	L/N	E
Aldosterone deficit (hyporeninemia)					
Primary hyporenin-hypoaldosterone diabetes mellitus, gout, pyelonephritis, interstitial nephritis, nephrosclerosis	L	L	E/N	E/N	L
Adolescent hyperkalemia syndrome	L/N	L/N	E	E	L
Reduced tubular response					
Pseudohypoaldosteronism	M/E	M/E	L	L	E
Early childhood type 4	E	E	N	L/N	L

E, elevated; E/N, elevated or normal; L, low; L/N, low or normal; M/E, markedly elevated; N, normal; S/E, significantly elevated.

tial aldosterone effect rather than a true tubular defect. If this defect is suspected, the patient should be carefully assessed for dehydration, severe cardiac failure, and sodium chloride (deficit from vomiting, diuretic abuse, or overuse). If present, dehydration or sodium deficit should be corrected with appropriate hydration or salt supplementation before U_{pH} and U_{AG} are reassessed. If volume deficit is not apparent, a trial dose of furosemide or response to sodium sulfate infusion to increase sodium delivery to the distal tubule (with the consequent enhanced transepithelial voltage) should be administered. Expected response to furosemide administration in healthy subjects includes a decrease in urinary pH and increase in ammonia and U_K excretion. In patients with hyporeninemic hypoaldosteronism, urinary pH is decreased.

Therapy

In the patient with significant spontaneous acidosis, initial correction based on an exact diagnosis is not necessary, nor is it necessary to delay therapy until investigation is complete. Bicarbonate administration and titration are effective in correcting the acidosis with RTA regardless of type. However, in DRTA type 1 with hypokalemia, and likely hypocalcemia, partial correction of potassium and calcium should be carried out before total correction of serum bicarbonate to prevent muscle weakness, respiratory failure, arrhythmia, or painful tetany. Care should be taken to obtain appropriate diagnostic samples of blood and urine under spontaneous acidosis and during base supplementation to allow diagnosis without the need for formal acid loading or bicarbonate.

Acute Correction of Acidosis

First, serum potassium and calcium should be assessed and significant deficits should be partially replaced before correcting bicarbonate deficit. The bicarbonate deficit is replaced over 1 to 2 days depending on presenting symptoms. Initial correction to serum pH 7.25 to 7.30 is made using the Henderson equation ($H^+ = 24\ PCO_2/HCO_3$) to assess the desired bicarbonate supplementation. Remaining deficits should be calculated after equilibration with bicarbonate space of 0.6 body weight/kg (i.e., HCO_3 required = 0.6 – body weight/kg – [desired HCO_3 – measured HCO_3]), to which maintenance dosing is added. The adequacy of replacement is checked and the dosage of administered bicarbonate is titrated.

Maintenance Therapy

Once a deficit is corrected, it is necessary to provide sufficient base supplementation to balance nonvolatile acid production (DRTA) and to replace any continuing losses (PRTA). Base may be supplied as sodium bicarbonate (55 mEq/teaspoon), sodium citrate, or mixed sodium and potassium citrate depending on the presence or absence of continuing potassium losses. The aim is to maintain CO_2 greater than 20 to 22 mEq/L.

In DRTA, replacement covers the production of 2 to 4 mEq of acid/kg from the diet equivalent to 2 mEq per 100 kcal (Table 39.6). In young children, after treatment is commenced, an extra 2 to 3 mEq/kg acid may be generated from bone formation, as hydroxyl and phosphate groups are incorporated into hydroxyapatite. In PRTA, dosages as high as 4 to 15 mEq/kg/day are sometimes required to compensate for continuing losses secondary to the low tubular bicarbonate threshold.

Patients with RTA 4 require treatment for hyperkalemia (59). This may include correction of acidosis, sodium repletion, mineralocorticoid replacement, and, in some patients, glucocorticoid replacement (59,87). It is particularly important to review drug and dietary intake in patients with RTA type 4. Common contributing factors to hyperkalemia include low urine flow; decreased sodium delivery; rapid decline in GFR, particularly in acute or chronic renal failure; hyperglycemia or hyperosmolality; and unsuspected intake of potassium salt supplements or medications. Calculation of transtubular potassium gradient and response to furosemide and fluorohydrocortisone allow clinical correction of hyperkalemic syndromes while awaiting formal assessment of renin-aldosterone status. If there is a low transtubular potassium gradient (below 5) in a patient with hyperkalemia and no response to mineralocorticoid supplementation, a furosemide challenge and treatment with sodium or bicarbonate to increase excretion is appropriate.

REFERENCES

1. Simpson DP. Control of hydrogen ion homeostasis and renal acidosis. *Medicine* 1971;50:503–541.
2. Morris RC Jr. Renal tubular acidosis: mechanisms, classification and implications. *N Engl J Med* 1969;281:1405–1413.
3. Halperin M, Goldstein M, Haig A, et al. Studies on the pathogenesis of type 1 (distal) renal tubular acidosis as revealed by the urinary PCO_2 tensions. *J Clin Invest* 1974;53:669–677.
4. Rodriguez-Soriano J, Vallo A, et al. Distal renal tubular acidosis in infancy: a bicarbonate wasting state. *J Pediatr* 1975;86:524–532.
5. Wrong O, Davies HEF. The excretion of acid in renal diseases. *QJM* 1959;28:259–313.
6. Elkington JR, Huth EM, Webster GD Jr, et al. The renal excretion of hydrogen ion in renal tubular acidosis. *Am J Med* 1960;29:554–575.
7. Reynolds TB. Observations on the pathogenesis of renal tubular acidosis. *Am J Med* 1958;25:503–515.
8. Lightwood R, Payne WW, Black JA. Infantile renal acidosis. *Pediatrics* 1953;12:628–644.
9. Carroll HJ, Farber SJ. Hyperkalemia and hyperchloremic acidosis in chronic pyelonephritis. *Metabolism* 1964;13:808–817.
10. Sebastian A, McSherry E, Schambelan M, et al. Renal tubular acidosis in patients with hypoaldosteronism caused by renin deficiency. *Clin Res* 1973;21:706.
11. Oetliker OH, Zurbugg RP. Renal regulation of fluid, electrolyte and acid-base homeostasis in the salt losing syndrome of congenital adrenal hyperplasia (SL-CAH). ECF volume a compensating factor in aldosterone deficiency. *J Clin Endocrinol Metab* 1978;46:543–551.
12. David R, Golan S, Drucker W. Familial aldosterone deficiency: enzyme defect diagnosis, and clinical course. *Pediatrics* 1968;41:403–412.
13. Cheek DB, Perry JW. A salt wasting syndrome in infancy. *Arch Dis Child* 1958;33:252–256.
14. Dillon MJ, Leonard JV, Buckler JM, et al. Pseudo hypoaldosteronism. *Arch Dis Child* 1980;55:427–434.
15. Arnold JE, Healy JK. Hyperkalemia, hypertension and systemic acidosis without renal failure associated with a tubular defect in potassium excretion. *Am J Med* 1969;47:461–472.
16. Spitzer A, Edelmann CM, Goldberg LD, et al. Short stature, hyperkalemia and acidosis: a defect in renal transport of potassium. *Kidney Int* 1973;3:251–257.
17. Schambelan M, Sebastian A, Rector FC Jr. Mineralocorticoid-resistant renal hyperkalemia without salt wasting (type 2 pseudo-hypoaldosteronism). Role of increased renal chloride reabsorption. *Kidney Int* 1981;19:716–727.
18. Battle DC. Segmental characterization of defects in collecting tubule acidification. *Kidney Int* 1986;30:546–554.
19. Battle DC. Hyperkalemic hyperchloremic metabolic acidosis associated with selective aldosterone deficiency and distal renal tubular acidosis. *Semin Nephrol* 1981;1:260–274.
20. Krieg RJ Jr, Santos F, Chan JCM. Growth hormone, insulin-like growth factor and the kidney (Editorial review). *Kidney Int* 1995;48:321–336.
21. Challa A, Krieg RJ Jr, Thabet MA, et al. Metabolic acidosis inhibits growth hormone secretion in the rat. Mechanisms of growth retardation. *Am J Physiol* 1993;265:E547–E553.
22. Kamel KS, Briceno LF, Sanchez MD, et al. A new classification for renal defects in net acid excretion. *Am J Kidney Dis* 1997;29:136–146.
23. Vasuvattakul S, Nimmannit S, Shayakul C, et al. Should the urine PCO_2 or the rate of excretion of NH_4^+ be the gold standard to diagnose distal renal tubular acidosis? *Am J Kidney Dis* 1992;19:72–75.
24. Carlisle EJF, Donnelly SM, Halperin ML. Renal tubular acidosis (RTA): recognize the ammonium defect and pH or get the urine pH. *Pediatr Nephrol* 1991;5:242–246.
25. Battle D, Grupp M, Gaviria M, et al. Distal renal tubular acidosis with intact capacity to lower urinary pH. *Am J Med* 1982;72:751–758.
26. McSherry E, Sebastian A, Morris RC Jr. Renal tubular acidosis in infants: the several kinds, including bicarbonate wasting, classic renal tubular acidosis. *J Clin Invest* 1972;51:499–514.
27. Morris RC Jr, Sebastian A, McSherry E. Renal acidosis. *Kidney Int* 1972;1:322–340.
28. Sebastian A, McSherry E, Ueki I, et al. Renal amyloidosis, nephrotic syndrome, and impaired renal tubular reabsorption of bicarbonate. *Ann Intern Med* 1968;60:541–548.
29. Hirschman GH, Chan JCM. Complex acid-base disorders in subacute necrotizing encephalomyelopathy (Leigh's syndrome). *Pediatrics* 1978;61:278–281.
30. Sly WS, Hewett-Emmett D, Whyte MP, et al. Carbonic anhydrase 2 deficiency in 12 families with the autosomal recessive syndrome of osteopetrosis with renal tubular acidosis and cerebral calcification. *N Engl J Med* 1985;313:139–145.
31. Gyory AZ, Edwards KDG. Renal tubular acidosis. *Am J Med* 1968;45:43–62.
32. Elkington JR, Huth EJ, Webster GD, et al. The renal excretion of hydrogen ion in renal tubular acidosis. 1. Quantitative assessment of the response to ammonium chloride as an acid load. *Am J Med* 1960;29:554–573.
33. Pitts RF, Lotspeich WD, Scheiss WA, et al. The renal regulation of acid-base balance in man. 1. The nature of the mechanism for acidifying the urine. *J Clin Invest* 1947;26:48–56.
34. Lennon EJ, Lemann J Jr, Litzow JR. The effects of diet and stool composition on the net external balance of normal subjects. *J Clin Invest* 1996;45:1601–1607.

35. Kildeberg P. Disturbances of hydrogen ion balance occurring in premature infants. II. Late metabolic acidosis. *Acta Paediatr* 1964;53:517–526.
36. Chan JCM. Calcium and hydrogen ion metabolism in children with classic (type 1/distal) renal tubular acidosis. *Ann Nutr Metab* 1981;25:65–78.
37. Vallo A, Rodriguez-Soriano J. Oral phosphate loading test for assessment of distal renal tubular acidification in children. *Miner Electrolyte Metab* 1984;10:387–390.
38. Aruda JAL, Julka NK, Rubinstein H, et al. Distal acidification defect induced by phosphate deprivation. *Metabolism* 1980;29:826–836.
39. Hamm LL, Alpern RJ. Cellular mechanisms of renal tubular acidification. In: Seldin DW, Giebish G, eds. *The kidney: physiology and pathophysiology*, 3rd ed. Philadelphia: Lippincott, Williams & Wilkins, 2000:1935–1979.
40. Dubose TD, Alpern RJ. Renal tubular acidosis. In: Scriver CR, Beaudet AI, Sly WS, Valle D, eds. *Metabolic basis of inherited disease*, 8th ed. New York: McGraw-Hill, 2001:4983–5021.
41. Good DW, DuBose TD Jr. Ammonia transport by early and late proximal convoluted tubule of the rat. *J Clin Invest* 1987;79:689–691.
42. Pitts RF. Renal production and excretion of ammonia. *Am J Med* 1964;36:720–742.
43. Nagami GT, Sonu CM, Kurokawa K. Ammonia production by isolated mouse proximal tubule perfused in vitro. Effect of metabolic acidosis. *J Clin Invest* 1986;78:124–129.
44. Schwartz GJ, Al-Awqati Q. Carbon dioxide causes exocytosis of vesicles containing H^+ ion pumps in isolated perfused proximal and collecting tubules. *J Clin Invest* 1985;75:1638–1644.
45. Brown D, Hirsch S, Gluck S. Localization of a proton pumping ATPase in the rat kidney. *J Clin Invest* 1988;82:2114–2126.
46. Cogan MG, Quan AH. Renal acidification: integrated tubular responses. In: Winrager EE, ed. *Renal physiology*. New York: Oxford University Press, 1992:969–1016.
47. Edelmann C Jr, Soriano J, Boichis H, et al. Renal bicarbonate reabsorption and hydrogen ion excretion in normal infants. *J Clin Invest* 1967;46:1309–1317.
48. Kamel K, Ethier J, Stinebaugh B, et al. The removal of an inorganic acid load in subjects with ketoacidosis of chronic fasting: the role of the kidney. *Kidney Int* 1990;38:507–511.
49. Karet FE. Inherited renal tubular acidosis. In: Grünfeld J-P, Bach JF, Kreis H, eds. *Advances in nephrology*, vol 30. St Louis: Mosby, 1998:147–162.
50. Jarolim P, Shayakul C, Prabakaran D, et al. Autosomal dominant distal renal tubular acidosis is associated in three families with heterozygosity for R589H mutation in AE1 (band 3) Cl^- /$HCO3^-$ exchanger. *J Biol Chem* 1998;273:6380–6388.
51. Han JS, Kim GH, Kim J, et al. Secretory-defect distal renal tubular acidosis is associated with transporter defect in H(+)-ATPase and anion exchanger-1. *J Am Soc Nephrol* 2002;13: 1425–1432.
52. Bastani B, Gluck SL. New insights into the pathogenesis of distal renal tubular acidosis. *Miner Electrolyte Metab* 1996;22: 396–409.
53. Karet FE, Gainza FJ, Gyory AZ, et al. Mutations in the chloride-bicarbonate exchanger gene autosomal dominant but not autosomal recessive distal renal tubular acidosis. *Proc Natl Acad Sci U S A* 1998;95:6337–6342.
54. Hwang J-J, Curthoys NP. Effect of acute alterations in acid-base balance on rat phosphoenolpyruvate carboxykinase and glutaminase gene expression. *J Biol Chem* 1991;266:9392–9396.
55. Dubose TD Jr, Good DW, Hamm LL, et al. Ammonium transport in the kidney: new physiologic concepts and their implications. *J Am Soc Nephrol* 1991;1:1193–1203.
56. Kinsella JL, Aronson PS. Interaction of NH_4^+ and Li^+ with the renal microvillous membrane Na^+-H^+ exchanger. *Am J Physiol* 1981;241:C220–C226.
57. Kurtz I, Star R, Balaban RS, et al. Spontaneous luminal disequilibrium pH in S3 proximal tubules. Role of ammonia and bicarbonate transport. *J Clin Invest* 1986;78:989–996.
58. Dubose TD Jr, Good DW. Role of the thick ascending limb and inner collecting duct in the regulation of urinary acidification. *Semin Nephrol* 1991;11:120–128.
59. Dubose TD. Hyperkalemic hyperchloremic metabolic acidosis: pathophysiologic insights. *Kidney Int* 1997;51:591–602.
60. Watts BA, Good DW. Effects of ammonium on intracellular pH in rat medullary thick ascending limb: mechanism of apical membrane NH_4^+ transport. *J Gen Physiol* 1994;103:917–936.
61. Wright FS, Giebisch G. Regulation of potassium excretion. In: Seldin DW, Giebisch G, eds. *The kidney: physiology and pathophysiology*. New York: Raven Press, 1992:2209–2247.
62. Wistrand P, Knuttila KG. Renal membrane bound carbonic anhydrase. Purification and properties. *Kidney Int* 1989;35: 851–859.
63. Wistrand PJ. Human renal cytoplasmic carbonic anhydrase: tissue levels and kinetic properties under near physiological conditions. *Acta Physiol Scand* 1980;109:239–248.
64. Preisig PA, Toto RD, Alpern RJ. Carbonic anhydrase inhibitors. *Ren Physiol* 1987;10:136–159.
65. Gill JR Jr, Bell NH, Bartter FC. Impaired conservation of sodium and potassium in renal tubular acidosis and its correction by buffer anions. *Clin Sci* 1967;33:577–592.
66. Liu FY, Cogan MG. Angiotensin 2 stimulation of hydrogen ion secretion in the rat early proximal tubule. *J Clin Invest* 1987;80:272–275.
67. Liu FY, Cogan MG. Angiotensin 2 stimulates early proximal bicarbonate absorption in the rat by decreasing cyclic adenosine monophosphate. *J Clin Invest* 1989;84:83–91.
68. McSherry E, Morris RC Jr. Attainment and maintenance of normal stature with alkali therapy in infants and children with classic renal tubular acidosis. *J Clin Invest* 1978;61:509–527.
69. Coe FL, Parks JH. Stone disease in hereditary distal renal tubular acidosis. *Ann Intern Med* 1980;93:60–61.
70. Harrington TM, Bunch TW, Van den Berg CJ. Renal tubular acidosis: a new look at the treatment of musculoskeletal and renal disease. *Mayo Clinic Proc* 1983;58:354–360.
71. Nash MA, Torrado AD, Griefer I, et al. Renal tubular acidosis in infants and children. *J Pediatr* 1972;80:738–748.
72. Ohlsson A, Stark G, Sakati N. Marble brain disease: recessive osteopetrosis, renal tubular acidosis and cerebral calcification in three Saudi Arabian families. *Dev Med Child Neurol* 1980;22:72–96.
73. York SE, Yendt ER. Osteomalacia associated with renal bicarbonate loss. *Can Med Assoc J* 1966;94:1329–1342.
74. Brenes LG, Brenes JN, Hernandez MM. Familial proximal tubular acidosis. *Am J Med* 1977;63:244–252.

75. Rodríguez-Soriano J, Vallo A, Chouza M, et al. Proximal renal tubular acidosis in tetralogy of Fallot. *Acta Paediatr Scand* 1975;64:671–674.
76. Stark H, Geiger R. Renal tubular dysfunction following vascular accidents of the kidneys in the newborn period. *J Pediatr* 1973;83:933–940.
77. Wisnes A, Monn E, Stokke O, et al. Congenital, persistent proximal type renal tubular acidosis in two brothers. *Acta Paediatr Scand* 1979;68:861–868.
78. Rodríguez-Soriano J, Vallo A, Castillo G, et al. Natural history of primary distal renal tubular acidosis treated since infancy. *J Pediatr* 1982;101:669–676.
79. Rodríguez-Soriano J, Vallo A, Castillo G, et al. Pathophysiology of primary distal renal tubular acidosis. *Int J Pediatr Nephrol* 1985;6:71–78.
80. Bregman H, Brown J, Rogers A, et al. Osteopetrosis with combined proximal and distal renal tubular acidosis. *Am J Kidney Dis* 1982;2:357–362.
81. Oetliker O, Rossi E. The influence of ECF volume on the renal bicarbonate threshold: a study of two children with Lowe's syndrome. *Pediatr Res* 1969;3:140–148.
82. Egger J, Lake BD, Wilson J. Mitochondrial cytopathy. A multisystemic disease with ragged red fibres on muscle biopsy. *Arch Dis Child* 1981;56:741.
83. Sengers RCA, Stadhonders AM, Trijbels JMF. Mitochondrial myopathies. Clinical, morphological and biochemical aspects. *Eur J Pediatr* 1984;141:192–207.
84. Sebastian A, Sutton JM, Hutler HN, et al. Effect of mineralocorticoid replacement therapy on renal acid-base homeostasis in adrenalectomized patients. *Kidney Int* 1980;18:762–773.
85. Knochel JP. The syndrome of hyporeninemic hypoaldosteronism. *Annu Rev Med* 1979;30:145–153.
86. McSherry E. Current issues in hydrogen ion transport. In: Gruskin AB, Norman ME, eds. *Pediatric nephrology*. Hingham, MA: Martinus Nijhoff, 1981:403–415.
87. DuBose TD Jr, Cogan MG, Rector FC Jr. Acid-base disorders. In: Brenner BM, Rector FC, eds. *The kidney*, 5th ed. Philadelphia: WB Saunders, 1995:929–998.
88. Lemann J Jr, Litzow JR, Lennon EJ. Studies of the mechanism by which chronic acidosis augments urinary calcium excretion in man. *J Clin Invest* 1967;46:1318–1328.
89. Hamed JA, Czerwinski AW, Coates B, et al. Familial absorptive hypercalciuria and renal tubular acidosis. *Am J Med* 1979;67:385–391.
90. Parfitt AM, Higgins BA, Nassim JR, et al. Metabolic studies in patients with hypercalcemia. *Clin Sci* 1964;27:463–482.
91. Morris RC Jr, Fudenberg HH. Impaired renal acidification in patients with hypergammaglobulinemia. *Medicine* 1967;46:57–69.
92. Talal N. Sjögren's syndrome, lymphoproliferation and renal tubular acidosis. *Ann Intern Med* 1971;74:633–634.
93. Cohen EP, Bastani B, Cohen MR, et al. Absence of H^+-ATPase in cortical collecting tubules of a patient with Sjögren's syndrome and distal renal tubular acidosis. *J Am Soc Nephrol* 1992;3:264–271.
94. McCurdy DK, Frederic M, Elkington JR. Renal tubular acidosis due to amphotericin B. *N Engl J Med* 1968;278:124–131.
95. Reynolds TB. Observation on the pathogenesis of renal tubular acidosis. *Am J Med* 1958;25:503–515.
96. Norman ME, Feldman NI, Cohn RM, et al. Urinary citrate excretion in the diagnosis of distal renal tubular acidosis. *J Pediatr* 1978;92:394–400.
97. Simpson DP. Citrate excretion: a window on renal metabolism. *Am J Physiol* 1983;244:F223–F234.
98. Goodman AD, Lemann J Jr, Lennon EJ, et al. Production, excretion and net balance of fixed acid in patients with renal acidosis. *J Clin Invest* 1965;44:495–506.
99. Richards P, Chamberlain MJ, Wrong OM. Treatment of osteomalacia of renal tubular acidosis by sodium bicarbonate alone. *Lancet* 1972;2:994–997.
100. Greenberg AJ, McNamara H, McCrory WW. Metabolic balance studies in primary renal tubular acidosis: effects of acidosis on external calcium and phosphorus balances. *J Pediatr* 1966;69:610–618.
101. Chesney RW, Kaplan BS, Phelps M, et al. Renal tubular acidosis does not alter circulating values of calcitriol. *J Pediatr* 1984;104:51–55.
102. Cunningham J, Fraher LJ, Clemens TL, et al. Chronic acidosis with metabolic bone disease. *Am J Med* 1982;73:199–204.
103. Portale AA, Halloran BP, Harris ST, et al. Metabolic acidosis reverses the increase in serum $1,25(OH)_{2D}$ in phosphorus restricted men. *Am J Physiol* 1992;263:E1164–E1170.
104. Knochel JP. Neuromuscular manifestations of electrolyte disorders. *Am J Med* 1982;72:521–535.
105. Feest TG, Lockwood CM, Morley AR, et al. Renal histology and immunopathology in distal renal tubular acidosis. *Clin Nephrol* 1978;10:187–190.
106. Edelmann CM Jr, Boichis H, Rodriguez-Soriano J, et al. The renal response of children to acute ammonium chloride acidosis. *Pediatr Res* 1967;1:452–460.
107. Oster JR, Hotchkiss JL, Carbon M, et al. A short duration renal acidification test using calcium chloride. *Nephron* 1975;14:281–292.
108. Rodríguez-Soriano J, Vallo A, Castillo G, et al. Pathophysiology of primary distal renal tubular acidosis. *Int J Pediatr Nephrol* 1985;6:71–78.
109. Steinbaugh BJ, Schloeder FX, Tam SC, et al. Pathogenesis of distal renal tubular acidosis. *Kidney Int* 1981;19:1–7.
110. Battle D, Kurtzman NA. Distal renal tubular acidosis: pathogenesis and classification. *Am J Kidney Dis* 1982;1:328–344.
111. Halperin ML, Kamel K, Ethier J, et al. Biochemistry and physiology of ammonium excretion. In: Seldin D, Giebisch G, eds. *The kidney: physiology and pathophysiology*. New York: Raven Press, 1992:2645–2685.
112. Halperin ML, Margolis BL, Robinson LA, et al. The urine osmolal gap: a clue to estimate ammonium in "hybrid" types of metabolic acidosis. *Clin Invest Med* 1988;11:198–202.
113. Dyck R, Asthana S, Kalra J, et al. A modification of the urine osmolal gap: an improved method for estimating urine ammonium. *Am J Nephrol* 1990;10:359–362.
114. Pitts RF. Renal production and excretion of ammonia. *Am J Med* 1964;36:720–742.
115. Halperin ML, Chen CB. Plasma glutamine and renal ammoniagenesis in dogs with chronic metabolic acidosis. *Am J Physiol* 1987;252:F474–F479.
116. Kamel K, Ethier J, Richardson R, et al. Urine electrolytes and osmolality and how to use them. *Am J Nephrol* 1990;10:89–102.

117. West ML, Marsden PA, Richardson MA, et al. New clinical approach to evaluate disorders of potassium excretion. *Miner Electrolyte Metab* 1986;12:234–238.
118. Gruskin AB, Patel MS, Linshaw M, et al. Renal function studies and kidney pyruvate carboxylase in subacute necrotizing encephalomyelopathy (Leigh's syndrome). *Pediatr Res* 1973;7:832–841.
119. Atkin BM, Buist NRM, Utter MF, et al. Pyruvate carboxylase deficiency and lactic acidosis in a retarded child without Leigh's disease. *Pediatr Res* 1979;13:109–116.
120. Donckerwolke RA, Van Steckelenberg GJ, Tiddens HA. A case of bicarbonate-losing renal tubular acidosis with defective carboanhydrase activity. *Arch Dis Child* 1970;45:769–773.
121. David R, Golan S, Drucker W. Familial aldosterone deficiency: enzyme defect diagnosis, and clinical course. *Pediatrics* 1968;41:403–412.
122. Ulick S. Diagnosis and nomenclature of the disorders of the terminal potion of the aldosterone biosynthetic pathway. *J Clin Endocrinol Metab* 1976;44:279–291.
123. Veldhuis JD, Kulin HE, Santen RJ, et al. Inborn error in the terminal step of aldosterone biosynthesis: corticosterone methyl oxidase type 2 deficiency in a North American pedigree. *N Engl J Med* 1980;303:117–121.
124. Curtis JA, Monaghan HP, New MI, et al. Selective hypoaldosteronism in infancy. Report of a case. *Am J Dis Child* 1983;137:633–636.
125. Caldas A, Broyer M, Dechaux M, et al. Primary distal tubular acidosis in childhood: clinical study and long-term follow-up of 28 patients. *J Pediatr* 1992;121:233–241.
126. Shapira E, Ben-Yoseph Y, Eyal FG, et al. Enzymatically inactive red cell carbonic anhydrase B in a family with renal tubular acidosis. *J Clin Invest* 1978;53:59–63.
127. Levine AS, Michael AF Jr. Ehlers-Danlos syndrome with renal tubular acidosis and medullary sponge kidneys. *J Pediatr* 1967;71:107–113.
128. Baehner RI, Gilchrist GS, Anderson FJ. Hereditary elliptocytosis and primary renal tubular acidosis in a single family. *Am J Dis Child* 1968;115:414–419.
129. Takeda R, Morimoto S, Kuroda M, et al. Renal tubular acidosis, presenting as a syndrome resembling Bartter's syndrome, in a patient with arachnodactyly. *Acta Endocrinol* 1973;73:531–542.
130. Goosens JP, Van Eps LWS, Schouten H, et al. Incomplete renal tubular acidosis in sickle cell disease. *Clin Chim Acta* 1972;41:149–156.
131. Kong HH-P, Alleyne GAO. Defect in urinary acidification in adults with sickle cell anemia. *Lancet* 1968;2:954–955.
132. Cohen T, Brand-Auraban A, Karashi C, et al. Familial infantile renal tubular acidosis and congenital nerve deafness: an autosomal recessive syndrome. *Clin Genet* 1973;4:275–278.
133. Donckerwolcke RA, Van Biervliet JP, Koorevaar G, et al. The syndrome of renal tubular acidosis with nerve deafness. *Acta Pediatr Scand* 1976;65:100–104.
134. Simon H, Orive B, Zamora I, et al. The acidification defect in the syndrome of renal tubular acidosis with nerve deafness. *Acta Pediatr Scand* 1979;68:291–295.
135. Dungar DB, Brenton DP, Cain AR. Renal tubular acidosis and nerve deafness. *Arch Dis Child* 1980;55:221–225.
136. Cremers WRJ, Monnens LAH, Marres HMA. Renal tubular acidosis and sensorineural deafness. *Arch Otolaryngol* 1980;106:287–289.
137. Falik-Borenstein AC, Jordan SC, Saudubray JM, et al. Renal tubular acidosis in carnitine palmitoyltransferase type 1 deficiency. *N Engl J Med* 1992;327:24–27.

40

NEPHROGENIC DIABETES INSIPIDUS

NINE V. A. M. KNOERS
LEO A. H. MONNENS

HISTORY

The renal type of diabetes insipidus was appreciated as a separate entity more than 50 years ago, when it was described independently by two investigators: Forssman (1) in Sweden and Waring et al. (2) in the United States. Families with this type of defect, however, had been described previously (3) without clear differentiation of nephrogenic diabetes insipidus (NDI) from the central or neurohormonal form of the disorder. In 1947, Williams and Henry (4) noticed that injection of antidiuretic hormone (ADH) in doses sufficient to induce systemic side effects could not correct the renal concentrating defect in some patients. They coined the term *NDI.* Subsequent studies revealed active hormone in the serum and urine of affected persons and lent further support to the theory of renal unresponsiveness to vasopressin. NDI is synonymous with the terms *vasopressin-* or *ADH-resistant diabetes insipidus* and *diabetes insipidus renalis.*

DEFINITION AND CLINICAL MANIFESTATIONS

Congenital NDI is a rare inherited disorder, characterized by insensitivity of the distal nephron to the antidiuretic effects of the neurohypophyseal ADH, arginine vasopressin (AVP). As a consequence, the kidney loses its ability to concentrate urine, which may lead to severe dehydration and electrolyte imbalance (hypernatremia and hyperchloremia). The defect in NDI is present from birth, and manifestations of the disorder generally emerge within the first weeks of life. With breast milk feedings, infants usually thrive and do not develop signs of dehydration. This is because human milk has a low salt and protein content, and therefore a low renal osmolar load. With cows' milk formula feedings, the osmolar load to the kidney increases, resulting in an increased demand for free water. If cow's milk feedings are not supplemented by hypotonic fluids in infants with NDI, hypernatremic dehydration appears. Irritability, poor feeding, and poor weight gain are usually the initial symptoms (5). Patients are eager to suck but may vomit during or shortly after the feeding. Dehydration is evidenced by dryness of the skin, loss of normal skin turgor, recessed eyeballs, increased periorbital folding, depression of the anterior fontanelle, and a scaphoid abdomen. Intermittent high fever is a common complication of the dehydrated state, particularly in very young children. Body temperature can be normalized by rehydration. Seizures can occur but are rare and most often seen during therapy, particularly if rehydration proceeds too rapidly. Obstipation is a common symptom in children with NDI. Nocturia and enuresis are common complaints later in childhood.

Untreated, most patients fail to grow normally. In a retrospective study of 30 male NDI patients, most children grew below the 50th percentile, most of them having standard deviation (SD) scores lower than −1 and showing no clear catch up growth after the first year of life. Weight for height SD scores were initially low, followed by global normalization at school age (6). The exact reasons for the failure to thrive seen in NDI are unknown. Initial feeding problems and the ingestion of large amounts of low-caloric fluid resulting in a decreased appetite may play roles (7,8). Furthermore, it is possible that repeated episodes of dehydration have some as yet undetermined negative effects on growth.

Mental retardation has long been considered an important complication of untreated NDI and assumed to be a consequence of recurrent episodes of severe brain dehydration and cerebral edema caused by overzealous attempts at rehydration (9,10). Additional evidence underscoring the assumption that NDI has adverse effects on the cerebrum is provided by several reports describing intracranial calcifications in NDI patients (11,12). Such lesions are generally considered to be the result of hemorrhage or necrosis. Most of the reported patients with cerebral calcifications were mentally retarded.

Currently, mental retardation is considered to be rare due to earlier recognition and treatment of NDI. The frequency of mental retardation under modern treatment regimens is

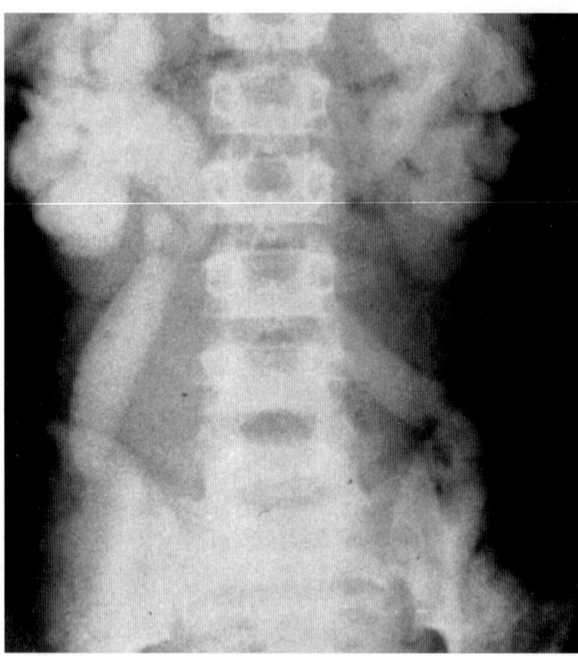

FIGURE 40.1. Intravenous pyelogram of a patient with congenital nephrogenic diabetes insipidus and severe hydronephrosis.

unknown, but in the largest psychometric study ever reported, only 2 of the 17 male NDI patients (aged 3 to 30 years) tested had a total intelligence quotient more than 2 SDs below the norm. Fourteen patients had an intelligence score within or above the normal range, and one patient had a general index score between –1 and –2 SD (13).

The psychological development of patients with NDI is influenced by a persistent desire for drinking and the need for frequent voiding, which compete with playing and learning. Therefore, many NDI patients are characterized by hyperactivity, distractibility, short attention span, and restlessness. In the psychometric study mentioned earlier, the criteria for attention deficit hyperactivity disorder were met in 8 of 17 tested NDI patients (13).

Persistent polyuria can result in the development of megacystis, hydroureter, and hydronephrosis (14) (Fig. 40.1). We have recently found that this complication is rare in patients with NDI. Dilation of the urinary tract occurred in only 2 of 30 patients studied (6).

DIAGNOSTIC PROCEDURES

The observation of polyuria in a dehydrated infant, together with the finding of a high serum sodium concentration, provides presumptive evidence of a renal concentrating defect. To confirm the concentrating defect and to distinguish the renal from the central form of diabetes insipidus, a vasopressin test is performed with 1-desamino-8-D-arginine vasopressin (DDAVP), a synthetic analogue of natural AVP that produces a high and prolonged antidiuretic effect. In the test, DDAVP (10 mg for infants, 20 mg for children) is administered intranasally. Urine is collected during the subsequent 5.5 hours. The first collected portion of the urine should be discarded. The maximal urine osmolality in any collected aliquot is chosen as a measure of the concentrating capacity (15). After DDAVP administration, NDI patients are unable to increase urinary osmolality, which remains below 200 mOsm/kg H_2O (normal greater than or equal to 807 mOsm/kg H_2O) and cannot reduce urine volume or free-water clearance.

Plasma vasopressin levels are normal or only slightly increased in affected children. Other laboratory findings have been described, which mainly result from chronic dehydration. Serum sodium concentration is generally elevated and may be as high as 170 mmol/L. There is also an increase in serum chloride concentration and retention of urea and creatinine. All values are normalized by adequate rehydration. In addition, reduced glomerular filtration rate and renal blood flow return to normal when a state of normal hydration has been achieved.

The primary congenital form of NDI must be differentiated from the secondary or acquired forms, which are much more common. In our experience, the urinary osmolality obtained after DDAVP administration in these disorders is always higher than in NDI. Several secondary causes, some of which are discussed later, are listed in Table 40.1.

TABLE 40.1. COMMON CAUSES OF ACQUIRED OR SECONDARY NEPHROGENIC DIABETES INSIPIDUS

Amyloidosis
Analgesic nephropathy
Chronic pyelonephritis
Chronic renal failure
Drug-induced
Lithium
Tetracyclines
Hypercalcemia/nephrocalcinosis
Hypokalemia
Juvenile nephronophthisis
Obstructive uropathy
Renal dysplasia
Sarcoidosis
Sickle cell anemia and trait

CELLULAR PHYSIOLOGY OF ARGININE VASOPRESSIN'S ANTIDIURETIC ACTION IN THE DISTAL NEPHRON

The physiologic action of vasopressin on the renal collecting duct has been one of the most intensively studied processes in the kidney. AVP (ADH) is synthesized on the ribosomes of the magnocellular neurons of the supraoptic and paraventricular nuclei of the hypothalamus as a large, biologically inactive bound form, and transported down the neuronal axons to the posterior pituitary where it is stored. After appropriate

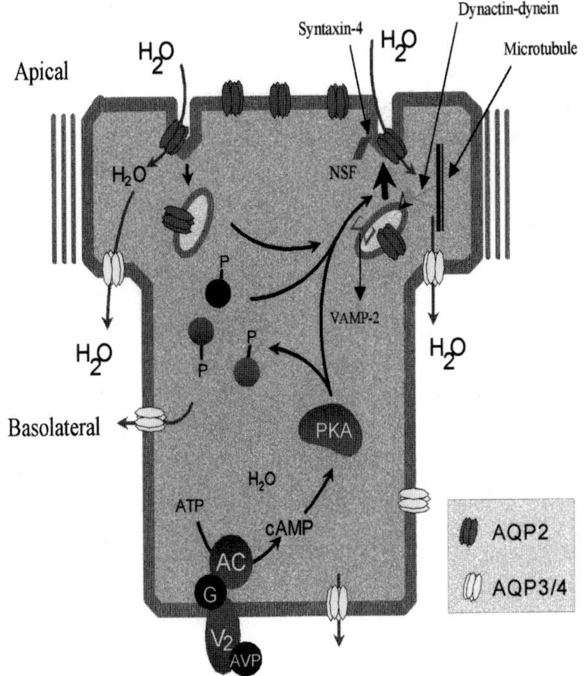

FIGURE 40.2. Schematic view of the antidiuretic arginine vasopressin (AVP) signaling pathway in collecting duct cells and the proteins (microtubule, dynactin-dynein) and vesicle targeting receptors (VAMP-2, syntaxin-4, NSF) that might participate in the specificity of aquaporin-2 (AQP2) water channel targeting to the luminal plasma membrane. AC, adenylate cyclase; AQP3, aquaporin-3 water channel; AQP4, aquaporin-4 water channel; G, stimulatory guanine nucleotide binding protein; NSF, *N*-ethylmaleimide–sensitive fusion protein; PKA, protein kinase A; V_2, vasopressin type-2 receptor. (See Color Plate 40.2.)

stimuli, AVP is secreted from the posterior pituitary into the circulation as biologically active hormone. AVP release is primarily regulated by changes in plasma osmolality (by more than 2%) but can also occur in response to nonosmotic stimuli. These nonosmotic stimuli are generally related to changes in either total blood volume or the distribution of extracellular fluid. In addition, physical pain, emotional stress, and certain drugs (e.g., nicotine) influence the release of AVP. In its effector organ, the kidney, AVP binds to vasopressin type-2 receptors (V_2Rs) on the basolateral membrane of the principal inner medullary collecting duct cells and of the arcade cells (Fig. 40.2). The arcades are long, highly branched renal tubule segments that connect distal convoluted tubules of several deep and midcortical nephrons to the origin of cortical collecting ducts. V_2R occupancy results, via the intermediacy of a stimulatory G protein (G_s), in activation of adenylate cyclase and an increase in intracellular cyclic adenosine monophosphate (cAMP) from adenosine triphosphate. The elevated cAMP levels stimulate protein kinase A (PKA), which in turn initiates a redistribution of aquaporin (AQP)-2 water channels from intracellular vesicles to the apical plasma membrane, rendering this membrane water permeable. Phosphorylation of a PKA consensus site in AQP2 (serine at position 256 in the cytoplasmic carboxy terminus) has been shown to be essential for AQP2 delivery to the apical membrane (16,17). In addition, it has been shown that anchoring of PKA to PKA-anchoring proteins, which ensures targeting of PKA to AQP2-bearing vesicles, is another prerequisite for AVP-mediated AQP2 translocation (18). The identity of the PKA-anchoring proteins involved has not yet been elucidated. The increase in apical membrane permeability allows water to flow from the tubule lumen, via AQP2 in the apical membrane and via AQP3 and AQP4, constitutive water channels in the basolateral membrane, to the hypertonic medullary interstitium. This then leads to the formation of concentrated urine. Withdrawal of vasopressin triggers the endocytosis of AQP2-containing vesicles and restores the water-impermeable state of the apical side of the cell.

The molecular machinery for the docking and fusion of AQP2-containing vesicles with the apical membrane is most likely similar to the process of synaptic vesicle fusion with the presynaptic membrane and involves vesicle (v) SNAREs (soluble NSF attachment protein receptors) and target membrane (t) SNAREs (Fig. 40.2). Thus, in subcellular fractions from rat kidney, enriched for AQP2-containing vesicles, the v-SNARE synaptobrevin (VAMP-2) was found, as well as the fusion-mediating protein SNAP23 (19–22). The potential t-SNARE syntaxin-4 was identified at the apical plasma membrane of rat kidney collecting duct principal cells (23). Rab3A, a member of the Rab family of guanosine triphosphatases, involved in exo- and endocytotic membrane trafficking, is also believed to play a role in AQP2 translocation to the apical membrane (21,24). In addition, it has been shown that both the microtubule-associated motor protein dynein and the associated dynactin-complex, which catalyze transport of vesicles along microtubules, are important in vasopressin-regulated trafficking of these vesicles (Fig. 40.2) (25). Recently, a critical role for calcium as an intracellular mediator of the vasopressin-induced trafficking of AQP2 has been established (26). The translocation of AQP2 from the intracellular vesicle to the plasma membrane can also be stimulated by cAMP-independent pathways. Thus, Bouley et al. have shown that nitric oxide and atrial natriuretic factor stimulate the insertion of AQP2 into renal epithelial cell membranes via a cyclic guanosine monophosphate–dependent pathway (27). The importance of this pathway is as yet unclear.

Long-term adaptation to circulating AVP levels, for instance, in a dehydrated state, is accomplished by increasing the expression of AQP2 messenger RNA (mRNA) and protein. A cAMP-responsive element in the AQP2 promotor has proven to be a key element in cAMP-dependent transcriptional regulation of this gene, and as such for the long-term regulation of water permeability (28).

GENETICS

Three different inheritance patterns of NDI have been recognized. In most cases (approximately 90%), NDI is transmitted as an X-linked recessive trait (MIM304800). In these families, female carriers who are clinically unaffected transmit the disease to sons, who display the complete clinical picture (1,4,29). In 1988, the major NDI locus was mapped to the distal region of the long arm of the X chromosome (Xq28) (30), and in 1992, mutations in the V_2R gene were shown to underlie X-linked NDI (31–33). In a minority of families (approximately 10%), the transmission and phenotypic characteristics of NDI are not compatible with an X-linked trait. In these families, females display the complete clinical picture of NDI and are clinically indistinguishable from affected male family members (34–36). In addition, linkage analysis in these families has excluded linkage between NDI and polymorphic DNA markers from the Xq28 region. Family pedigrees suggested the existence of both an autosomal recessive (MIM 222000) and an autosomal dominant form (MIM 125800) of NDI. In recent years, it has been demonstrated that both autosomal forms of NDI are caused by mutations in the AVP-sensitive AQP2 water channel (37,38). The prevalence of NDI is not exactly known, but the disease is assumed to be rare. Even in large pediatric and nephrology clinics, it is observed infrequently. In the Dutch population of approximately 15 million, 35 different families are known.

X-LINKED NEPHROGENIC DIABETES INSIPIDUS: MUTATIONS IN THE VASOPRESSIN TYPE-2 RECEPTOR GENE

The V_2R had long been considered a prime candidate for the defective step in the AVP-mediated response in X-linked NDI. The reason for this belief was the observation that in patients with X-linked NDI, not only the antidiuretic but also the vasodilatory coagulation and fibrinolytic responses to the V_2R-specific agonist DDAVP were lacking (39). This finding suggested a general V_2R defect in these patients. Independent support for the V_2R being involved in X-linked NDI was provided by the finding that a gene conferring V_2-like binding activity colocalized with the NDI locus in the subterminal region of the X chromosome long arm (Xq28) (40). Soon after the identification of the human V_2R gene and complementary DNA in 1992 (41), the role of the V_2R in the pathogenesis of NDI was finally proven by the demonstration of mutations in the encoding gene in affected individuals (31–33,42,43). The V_2R gene (AVPR2; Genbank association number L22206) is relatively small and consists of three exons separated by two short intervening sequences (introns). The mRNA has been found exclusively in the kidney, specifically in the cortical and medullary collecting ducts. The complementary DNA encodes a receptor protein of 371 amino acids, has a predicted molecular mass of approximately 41 kDa, and shares the general structure of a G protein–coupled receptor consisting of seven hydrophobic transmembrane helices, connected by extracellular and intracellular loops. The receptor contains one unique consensus sequence site for N-linked glycosylation in the extracellular amino-terminus (44) and phosphorylation sites for G protein–coupled receptor kinases represented by a serine cluster in the carboxy-terminus (45,46). The amino-terminal part of the protein including the first transmembrane domain and the positively charged first intracellular loop are important for proper insertion and orientation in the membrane (47). A conserved glutamate or dileucine motif in the intracellular carboxy terminal part of the receptor is essential for receptor transport from the endoplasmic reticulum (ER) to the Golgi apparatus (48). Two conserved adjacent cysteines in the C-terminus are palmitoylated, thereby anchoring the carboxy-tail to the plasma membrane and controlling the tertiary structure of this region of the receptor (49).

To date, more than 180 distinct putative disease-causing mutations in the V_2R gene have been detected in families with X-linked NDI (see http://www.medicine.mcgill.ca/nephros). Remarkably, the mutations are not clustered in one domain of the V_2R but are scattered throughout the protein, except for the part coding for the N- and C-terminal tails of the receptor. Approximately 50% of the mutations are missense mutations. Nucleotide deletions and insertions causing frame shifts (27%), nonsense mutations (12%), large deletions (5%), in-frame deletions or insertions (4%), and splice-site mutations (2%) account for the remainder of mutations (42). Several mutations are recurrent, as evidenced by the fact that these mutations were found on different haplotypes in ancestrally independent families. The most frequent of these recurrent mutations (D85N, V88M, R113W, R137H, S167L, R181C, and R202C) occur at potential mutational hotspots.

The impact of more than 80 mutations on the function of the V_2R has been studied in *in vitro* expression systems, such as COS-7 cells (monkey kidney cells), allowing further classification of the genotypes based on the cell-biologic outcome, similar to what has been done for other proteins (50–52). The first class of mutations (class I) yields defects in the synthesis of stable mRNA, which precludes the formation of sufficient amounts of protein. Mutations resulting in aberrant splicing, frame shifts, and premature termination of translation belong to this first category. Most of the truncated receptor proteins found in NDI patients result in a complete lack of receptors present on the cell surface and, consequently, preclude specific function of the receptor. The majority of mutations found in X-linked NDI belong to the second class (class II), in which the translation of the protein is completed, but the abnormal protein is misfolded or improperly assembled and trapped in the ER.

Subsequently, such mutant proteins are often targeted to proteosomes for degradation. Therefore, class II mutations also lead to severely reduced or absent receptor expression on the cell surface. Most missense mutations and in-frame deletions and some nonsense mutations in the V_2R fall in class II, and, except for some mutations in the extra- and intracellular loops (R104C, R113W, R143P, G201D, R337stop, E242stop), most of these mutations are located in transmembrane domains (L44P, I46K, L59P, L62P, L62-64del, L83P, L83Q, A84D, I130F, R137H, R143P, W164S, S167T, S167L, S167A, I209F, V287del, Y280C, L292P, A294P) (43,53–60). Recently, Morello et al. demonstrated a prolonged interaction time between the molecular chaperone calnexin and several class II V_2R mutant proteins and suggested that calnexin could play a role in the intracellular retention of misfolded V_2R proteins (61). This finding is consistent with the dual role proposed for calnexin. On the one hand, this chaperone is believed to assist folding of neosynthesized wild-type proteins, whereas on the other hand it targets the incompletely synthesized or misfolded proteins toward the degradation pathway (62).

A few of the missense and frame-shift mutations, however, have been shown not to significantly alter protein abundance at the cell surface, but either impair the coupling efficiency of the receptor to the stimulating G protein (class III mutations) or reduce AVP-binding affinity (class IV mutations). As yet, only a few mutations have been identified that belong to class III. These mutations are found in the lower half of the transmembrane regions (D85N, P322S/P) and within the second intracellular loop (R137H) (58,63). The study by Rosenthal et al. (63) demonstrating disturbed G protein activation of the *in vitro*–expressed R137H mutation, stresses the importance of the highly conserved DRY/H motif in the second intracellular loop for G protein activation, which is also known for other G protein–coupled receptors (64). In conflict with the study by Rosenthal, others have reported that the R137H mutant is almost completely retained in the cell interior (55).

Class IV mutations are mainly found in the first, second, sixth, and seventh transmembrane domains (L44F, A84D, V88M, Y128S, P286R, F287L, V277A, S315R) and in the first and second extracellular loops (W99R, R106C, F105V, R181C, G185C, ΔR202, R202C, T204N, Y205C, V206D, R113W) (43,53,56,59,61,65). It is well known that the conserved disulfide bridge between Cys112 in the first and Cys192 in the second extracellular loop ensures correct folding of these loops and, as a consequence, the establishment of the ligand-binding domain. It is assumed that the introduction of additional cysteine residues as a result of mutations found in NDI (R106C, R181C, G185C, R202C, Y205C) might impair receptor function by altering disulfide bonding of the conserved cysteine residues (58) or, more likely, by introducing an additional disulfide bond (66). Based on the finding of class IV mutations in transmembrane domains (I, II, VI), it can be concluded that several amino acids in these domains are involved in forming the conformation of the receptor for agonist binding.

Genotype-Phenotype Correlations in X-Linked Nephrogenic Diabetes Insipidus?

Almost all mutations in the V_2R gene result in a uniform clinical NDI phenotype with polyuric manifestations in the first weeks of life and poor growth. There are, however, a few exceptions to this rule. Three mutations (D85N, G201D, and P322S) are associated with a milder form of NDI, characterized by a later clinical presentation, around the age of 10, and without growth retardation. Functional studies of these mutations by *in vitro* expression systems have confirmed the partial phenotype of the NDI. P322S is the most remarkable of these three mutations, since another mutation substituting proline 322, namely P322H, is associated with a severe phenotype. By *in vitro* expression of both P322H and P322S in COS-7 cells, Ala et al. (58) have shown that the P322H mutant had totally lost the ability to stimulate the Gs/adenylate cyclase system, whereas the P322S mutant was able to stimulate adenylate-cyclase, albeit less than the wild-type receptor. Thus, the *in vitro* experiments closely correspond to the clinical phenotype. On the basis of three-dimensional modeling of the P322H and P322S mutant receptors, a plausible hypothesis to explain the molecular basis for the mild phenotype of the P322S has been proposed. Based on this modeling it is suggested that complete loss of function of the P322H receptor could be due, in part, to hydrogen bond formation between the His322 side chain and the carboxyl group of Asp85, which does not occur in the P322S receptor (58).

Recently, a family was reported in which the R137H mutation was associated with severe NDI in the proband but with very mild NDI in his affected brother (67). Genetic or environmental modifying factors are likely to account for this intrafamilial phenotype variability.

AUTOSOMAL RECESSIVE AND AUTOSOMAL DOMINANT FORMS OF NEPHROGENIC DIABETES INSIPIDUS: MUTATIONS IN THE AQUAPORIN-2 WATER CHANNEL

Both the autosomal recessive and the autosomal dominant types of NDI are caused by mutations in the AQP2 water channel gene (Genbank accession number z29491). The human AQP2 gene is a small gene consisting of 4 exons, comprising 5 kb genomic DNA. The 1.5-kb mRNA encodes a protein of 271 amino acids, which has a predicted molecular weight of 29 kDa (68). AQP2 belongs to a family of membrane integral proteins, AQPs, which function as selective water transporters throughout the plant and animal kingdom. In mammals, ten different AQPs have been identified to date, seven of which (AQPs 1 to 4 and 6 to 8) are highly expressed in the kidney. Like other AQPs, AQP2 is assembled in the membrane as a homotetramer in which each 29-kDa monomer, consisting of six membrane-spanning α-helical domains and intracellular

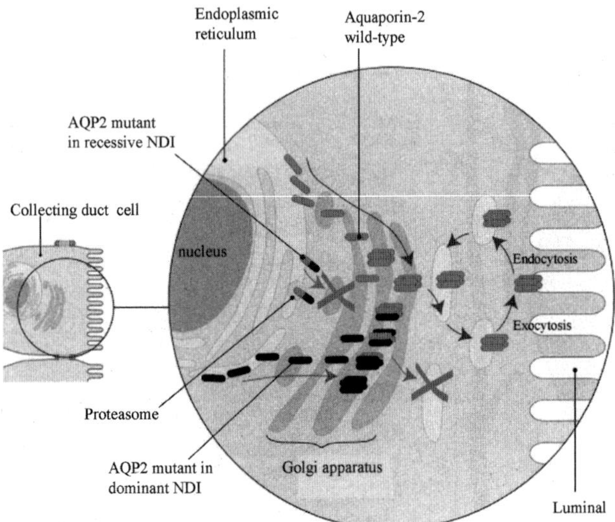

FIGURE 40.3. Schematic representation of the postulated mechanisms in a collecting duct cell to explain recessive and dominant forms of nephrogenic diabetes insipidus (NDI) caused by aquaporin-2 (AQP2) water channel mutations. Normal AQP2 proteins are transported from the endoplasmic reticulum via the Golgi apparatus to the luminal side of the cell. In case of a recessive NDI mutation, AQP2 is retained in the endoplasmic reticulum due to misfolding and is subsequently broken down by proteosomes. In case of a dominant NDI mutation, there is a change in the transport signal of the AQP2 protein and consequent misrouting to the Golgi network or late endosomes/lysosomes. (Adapted from Knoers NVAM, Deen PMT. Van Gen naar Ziekte; van vasopressine-V2-receptor en aquaporine-2 naar nefrogene diabetes insipidus. *Dutch J Med* 2000;144:2402–2404.) (See Color Plate 40.3.)

N- and C-termini, is a functional water channel. The six transmembrane domains are connected by five loops (A through E). In the hourglass hypothesis, loops B and E are assumed to fold back into the membrane and to interact via their highly conserved motifs asparagine-proline-alanine (NPA boxes) to form the water pore (69). Cryo-EM analysis of AQP1 crystals at atomic resolution revealed that this was indeed the case (70). AQP2 is exclusively localized in the apical membrane and a subapical compartment of collecting duct cells. It is upregulated by dehydration or AVP, indicating that it is the AVP-regulated water channel.

To date, 29 putative disease-causing mutations in AQP2 have been identified in families with autosomal recessive NDI (42,43,71,72). These include 23 missense mutations, two nonsense mutations, two small deletions, and two splice-site mutations. Approximately one-half of these mutations are found in the B and E loops of the protein, where it is likely that they will destroy the pore function of the protein. Expression studies in *Xenopus laevis* oocytes have revealed that all 23 AQP2 missense mutations that cause recessive NDI are class II mutations. Thus, these mutations lead to misfolding of the mutant protein and retention in the ER (71,73,74) (Fig. 40.3). At high expression levels in oocytes and Chinese hamster (CHO) cells, six of these AQP2 mutants (A147T, T126M, G64R, L22V, A47V, and T125M) confer water permeability (71,73,75,76). This indicates that at high expression levels, these AQP2 mutant proteins escape from the ER and are routed to the plasma membrane, where they are functional.

Several families have been described with autosomal dominant NDI, based on the transmission of the disease from father to son. In one of these families, a point mutation (G866A) in one allele of the AQP2 gene, resulting in the substitution of a lysine for a glutamic acid at position 258 (E258K) in the C-terminal tail of AQP2, was identified. Expression studies in *X. laevis* oocytes have shown that this E258K–AQP2 mutant is a properly folded functional water channel but is retained in the Golgi region (38) (Fig. 40.3). In coexpression studies with wild-type AQP2, a dominant-negative effect was observed, caused by impaired routing of wild-type AQP2 to the plasma membrane after hetero-oligomerization with the E258K mutant (77). Subsequently, a similar impairment of wild-type AQP2 in its routing to the plasma membrane of oocytes was reported for three other dominant AQP2 mutants (721delG, 763-772del, 812-818del) (78). Very recently, a novel AQP2 mutant (727delG) identified in a family with dominant NDI was shown to interfere with the routing of wild-type AQP2 to the apical membrane by its mistargeting to the late endosomes or lysosomes (79).

Remarkably, all mutations causing dominant NDI are located in the C-terminal tail of AQP2. The cell-biologic basis of dominant NDI, as revealed by *in vitro* expression of the mutations, underscores the importance of the C terminus of AQP2 in trafficking to the cell surface.

Kanno et al. (80) showed that AQP2 is detectable in the urine of normal individuals and, after treatment with DDAVP, in the urine of patients with central diabetes insipidus but not in that of patients with NDI. These initial findings, together with additional examinations of AQP2 excretion (81), raised the possibility of assessing AQP2 levels in the kidney by the measurement of urinary AQP2 levels. However, because the amount of AQP2 in the urine appears to be determined largely by trafficking of AQP2 to the apical membrane of collecting duct cells in response to vasopressin, rather than their content of AQP2 (82), AQP2 excretion in the urine must be interpreted with caution with respect to predicting AQP2 expression levels.

Differential Diagnosis between the X-Linked and the Autosomal Forms of Nephrogenic Diabetes Insipidus

Patients with X-linked NDI can be discriminated from patients with autosomal NDI on the basis of their extrarenal reaction to administration of the synthetic V_2-vasopressin analogue 1-DDAVP. Patients with autosomal NDI show normal increases in von Willebrand factor, factor VIII, and tissue-type plasminogen activator levels, whereas in patients with X-linked NDI, these extrarenal responses are absent as a result of an extrarenal mutant V_2R (83).

NEPHROGENIC DIABETES INSIPIDUS IN FEMALES

Several families have been described in which females show classic clinical and laboratory features of NDI. After the identification of AQP2 mutations as a cause for autosomal recessive NDI, and in some cases for autosomal dominant NDI, a satisfying explanation for the complete manifestation of the disease in some females had been found. However, several families have been reported in which symptomatic females do not have an AQP2 defect but are heterozygous for a V_2R defect (84–87). In some of these women, maximal urinary osmolality after DDAVP administration does not exceed 200 mOsmol/L. Of interest, in some of the reported families, asymptomatic female family members shared the same V_2R mutation with the manifesting females (84,88). The most likely explanation for the existence of different phenotypes in carriers of a V_2R mutation, varying from no symptoms to complete manifestation of the disorder, is skewed X-inactivation. This hypothesis was underlined by the study of Nomura et al., investigating the X-inactivation patterns of female carriers belonging to one family via the detection of a methylated trinucleotide repeat in the human androgen receptor gene (88). The V_2R mutation carriers in this family displayed different degrees of manifestation of NDI. One woman, who had no symptoms at all, showed random X-inactivation, whereas her grandmother with complete NDI showed extremely skewed methylation of one X chromosome. One should keep in mind that this skewed X-inactivation pattern in blood cells does not necessarily reflect the situation in renal collecting duct cells.

ACQUIRED NEPHROGENIC DIABETES INSIPIDUS

Although the hereditary forms of NDI are relatively rare, a wide range of pathologic conditions and drug treatments can lead to acquired NDI (Table 40.1). In a variety of these acquired forms of NDI, AQP2 expression is downregulated. For example, it has been shown that prolonged treatment of rats with therapeutic doses of lithium causes a 95% reduction in AQP2 expression in the inner medullary collecting duct principal cells, concomitant with the development of severe polyuria (89,90). Cessation of lithium infusion or DDAVP treatment for 1 week only partially reversed this downregulation, consistent with the clinical observation of slow recovery from induced NDI in patients treated with lithium. It is assumed that the inhibition of vasopressin-induced adenylate cyclase activity by lithium is the cause of the reduced expression of AQP2.

It has recently been demonstrated that there is also marked downregulation of AQP3, but not of AQP4, expression in kidneys of rats treated with lithium (90). It is assumed that reduced AQP3 expression also plays a crucial role in the development of lithium-induced polyuria. The mechanism of AQP3 downregulation remains to be elucidated.

Other polyuric states that have been associated with downregulation of *AQP2* expression in rat renal medulla include chronic hypokalemia, hypercalcemia, bilateral ureteral obstruction, low-protein diet, chronic renal failure, and puromycin aminonucleoside- or doxorubicin-induced nephrotic syndrome (91–95).

In some families with autosomal primary nocturnal enuresis, linkage analysis has revealed cosegregation of this disorder with polymorphic microsatellite markers from 12q, in the region where the AQP2 gene maps (96). Deen et al. sequenced the AQP2 coding region in affected primary nocturnal enuresis individuals from these dominant families but did not identify any significant mutations. Thus, the AQP2 gene could be excluded as a candidate for autosomal primary nocturnal enuresis. (97).

TREATMENT

The treatment of NDI has been challenging since the original description of the disorder. Replacement of urinary water losses by adequate supply of fluid is the most important component of therapy. However, most infants with NDI cannot drink the required amounts of fluid. One approach to reduce urine output is provision of a low-solute diet to reduce the renal osmolar load and decrease obligatory water excretion. Initially, a diet low in sodium (1 mmol/kg/day) as well as protein (2 g/kg/day) was recommended. However, severe limitations of dietary protein may introduce serious nutritional deficiencies. Therefore, it is preferable to prescribe dietary restriction of sodium only.

Diuretics, such as hydrochlorothiazide (2 to 4 mg/kg per 24 hours), were the first class of drugs shown to be effective in lowering the urine volume in NDI (98). When combined with a reduction of salt intake, hydrochlorothiazide reduces urine volume by 20 to 50% of baseline values. However, thiazide-induced hypokalemia may cause further impairment of urine-concentrating ability in patients with NDI. Another possible risk associated with hypokalemia is cardiac arrhythmia. Simultaneous administration of potassium salt is therefore advised in most cases.

There is ample evidence that the combined administration of hydrochlorothiazide with either a prostaglandin-synthesis inhibitor such as indomethacin (2 mg/kg/24 hr), or the potassium-sparing diuretic amiloride, is much more effective in reducing urine volume than the thiazide diuretic alone (99–103). Prolonged use of prostaglandin-synthesis inhibitors, however, is often complicated by gastrointestinal and hematopoietic side effects. Gastrointestinal complaints and complications include anorexia, nausea, vomiting, abdominal pain, ulceration, perforation, and hemorrhage. Hematopoietic reactions include neutropenia, thrombocytopenia, and, rarely, aplastic anemia. In addition, renal dysfunction has been described during indomethacin therapy, most often consisting of a slight reduction in glomerular filtration rate.

Amiloride counterbalances the potassium loss from prolonged use of thiazides and thus prevents hypokalemia. Because amiloride appears to have only minor long-term side effects, the combination of hydrochlorothiazide (2.0 to 4.0 mg/kg/24 hr) with amiloride (0.3 mg/kg/24 hr) is the treatment of choice for most patients. Our personal experience of more than 12 years with the amiloride-hydrochlorothiazide combination, however, indicates that amiloride is less well tolerated in young children below the age of 4 to 6 years because of persistent nausea. Therefore we recommend the use of the combination of indomethacin-hydrochlorothiazide in these young children.

For a long time, the following mechanism for the paradoxic effect of thiazides in NDI has been proposed; thiazides reduce sodium reabsorption in the distal tubule by inhibition of the NaCl cotransporter. This subsequently results in increased sodium excretion, extracellular volume contraction, decreased glomerular filtration rate, and increased proximal sodium and water reabsorption. Consequently, less water and sodium reach the collecting tubules, and less water is excreted (104,105). Recently, this long-standing hypothesis has been challenged by Magaldi, who reported new insights into the possible mechanism of thiazide action, based on microperfusion studies in rat inner medullary collecting duct (106,107). In these studies it was shown that in the absence of vasopressin, luminal hydrochlorothiazide increased osmotic and diffusional water permeabilities. Increased permeability facilitates water reabsorption in the collecting duct, and, thus, decreases water excretion. When prostaglandins were added, the effect of thiazides decreased. This finding may explain why indomethacin potentiates the effect of thiazides in NDI. The results of these microperfusion studies indicate that thiazides may act in nephron segments beyond the distal tubule. Because the effect of thiazides was only seen when they were applied to the luminal side of the inner medullary collecting duct, they do not apparently interact with the basolaterally located V_2R directly. Magaldi proposed that these drugs act at some point in the vasopressin cascade inside the cell, because an inhibitor of PKA blocked thiazide effects (107).

Because the majority of V_2R mutations found in X-linked NDI and all AQP2 mutations found in autosomal recessive NDI result in protein retention within the ER (class II mutations), a treatment aimed at restoring the plasma membrane routing of ER-retained, but otherwise functional, V_2R or AQP2 mutants becomes an interesting potential. Indeed, Morello et al. have recently shown *in vitro* that selective, nonpeptide cell-permeant V_2R antagonists increased cell-surface expression and rescued the function of V_2R mutants by promoting their maturation and targeting to the plasma membrane (108). Thus, these V_2R antagonists function as pharmacologic chaperones. The fact that eight distinct mutants could be rescued by the same treatment is promising, given the diversity of mutations identified in NDI.

Similarly, it has been shown that treatment of cells expressing ER-retarded AQP2 mutants with chemical chaperones, such as glycerol, facilitated the translocation of these mutants to the plasma membrane (76). The feasibility of treatment with pharmacologic and chemical chaperones awaits *in vivo* testing. It is important to appreciate that the exact ER-retention mechanisms of NDI causing V_2R and AQP2 mutants remain to be elucidated. *In vitro* studies have suggested that, in the future, gene therapy for NDI may become technically feasible (109). There are, however, questions as to whether gene therapy would be the treatment of choice for this disorder. Development of gene-transfer vectors and gene-delivery techniques as well as analysis of gene-therapy safety need to be pursued. Such studies determine the feasibility of gene therapy in renal diseases such as NDI. In this respect, recently developed transgenic mice carrying a functionally inactive V_2R receptor protein (110) and AQP2 knock-in mice (111) will be important reagents for preclinical testing.

REFERENCES

1. Forssman H. On hereditary diabetes insipidus with special regard to a sex-linked form. *Acta Med Scand* 1945;153:3–196.
2. Waring AJ, Kajdi L, Tappan V. A congenital defect of water metabolism. *Am J Dis Child* 1945;69:323–324.
3. McIlraith CH. Notes on some cases of diabetes insipidus with marked family and hereditary tendencies. *Lancet* 1892; ii:767–768.
4. Williams RH, Henry C. Nephrogenic diabetes insipidus: transmitted by females and appearing during infancy in males. *Ann Intern Med* 1947;27:84–95.
5 Kaplan SA. Nephrogenic diabetes insipidus. In: Holliday MA, Barratt TM, Vernier RL, eds. *Pediatric nephrology*. Baltimore: Williams & Wilkins, 1987:623–625.
6. van Lieburg AF, Knoers NVAM, Monnens LAH. Clinical presentation and follow-up of thirty patients with congenital nephrogenic diabetes insipidus. *J Am Soc Nephrol* 1999; 10:1958–1964.
7. Hillman DA, Neyzi O, Porter P, et al. Renal (vasopressin-resistant) diabetes insipidus: definition of the effects of homeostatic limitation in capacity to conserve water on the physical, intellectual, and emotional development of a child. *Pediatrics* 1958;21:430–435.
8. Vest M, Talbot NB, Crawford JD. Hypocaloric dwarfism and hydronephrosis in diabetes insipidus. *Am J Dis Child* 1963;105:175–181.
9. Forssman H. Is hereditary diabetes insipidus of nephrogenic type associated with mental deficiency? *Acta Psychol Neurol Scand* 1955;30:577–587.
10. Macaulay D, Watson M. Hypernatremia in infants as a cause of brain damage. *Arch Dis Child* 1967;42:485–491.
11. Kanzaki S, Omura T, Miyake M, et al. Intracranial calcification in nephrogenic diabetes insipidus. *JAMA* 1985;254:3349–3350.

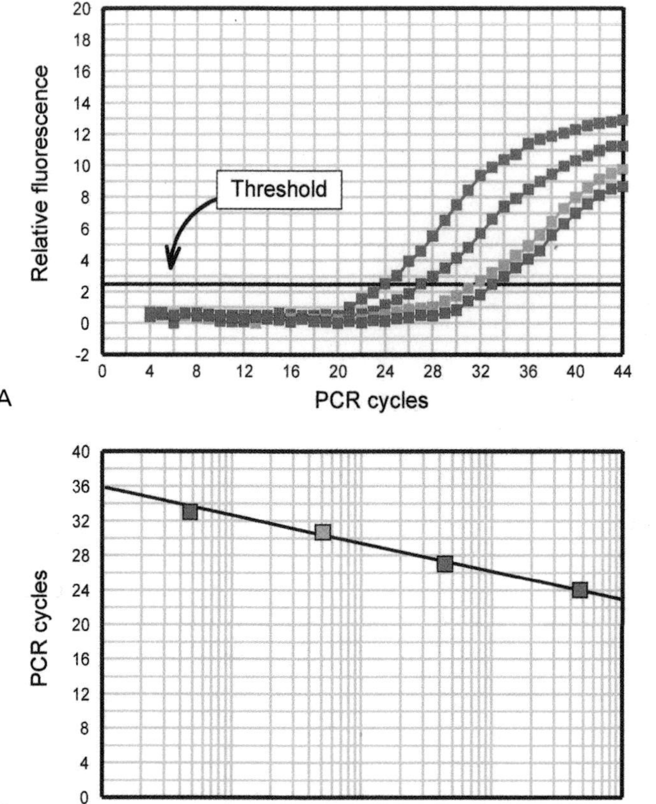

COLOR PLATE 14.4. Real-time reverse transcription polymerase chain reaction (PCR). The figure illustrates an actin calibration curve. Total RNA was extracted from HK2 cells and loaded in increasing concentrations in the sample reaction. Fluorescence was measured in real time as primers were incorporated in newly synthesized PCR fragments with an ABI Prism 7700. The number of cycles required to cross a given fluorescence threshold **(A)** is proportional to the initial amount of loaded messenger RNA **(B)**.

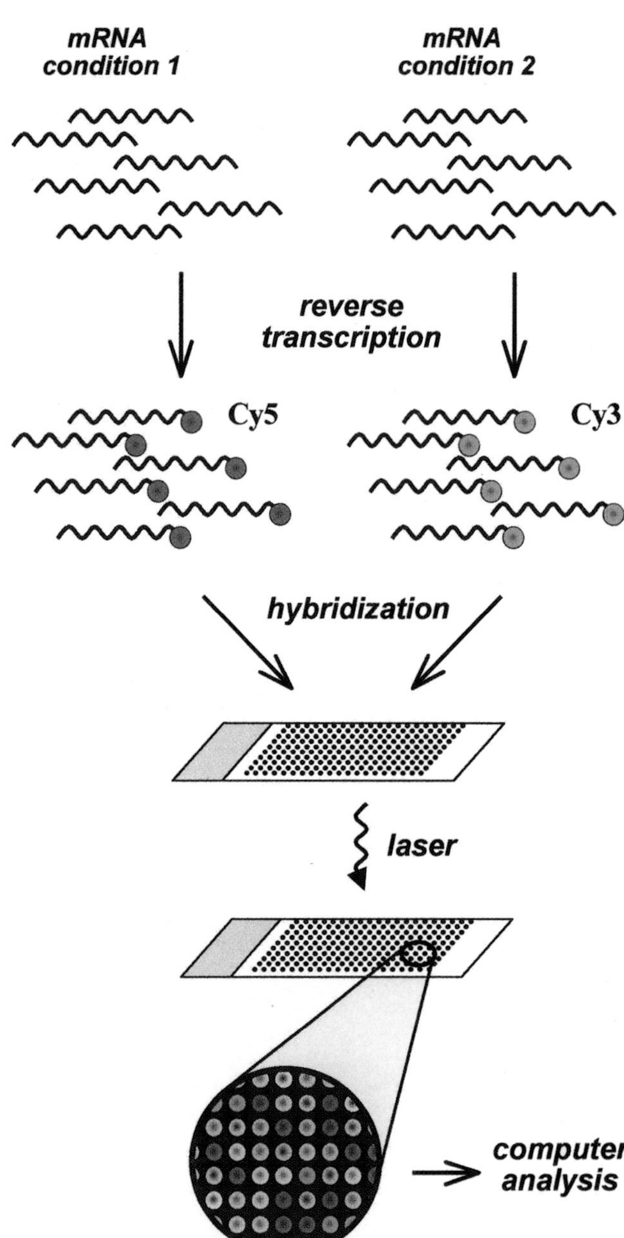

COLOR PLATE 14.5. Differential display on DNA microarrays. Messenger RNA (mRNA) obtained from two different samples are labeled with two fluorescent cyanine dyes with one round of reverse transcription. The fluorescent targets are then pooled and hybridized under stringent conditions to the clones on the microarray chip. The emission light is measured with a scanning confocal laser microscope at two different wavelengths that are specific for each dye. Monochrome images are then pseudo-colored, combined, and analyzed with suitable computer software.

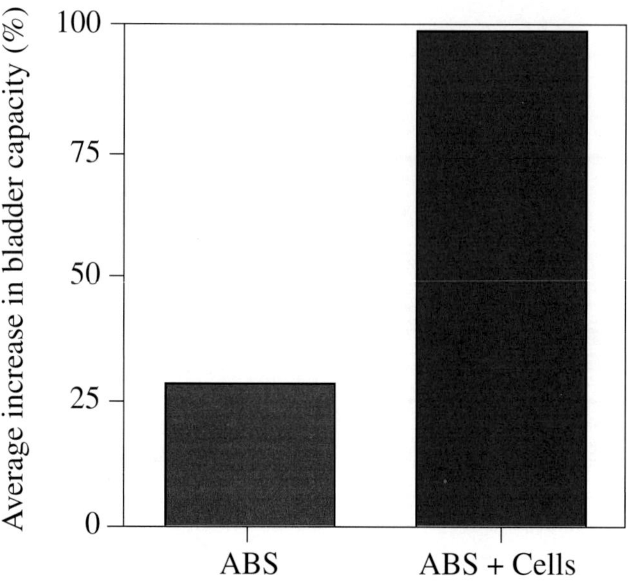

COLOR PLATE 19.2. Bladders augmented with a collagen matrix derived from bladder submucosa seeded with urothelial and smooth muscle cells [allogenic bladder submucosa (ABS) + cells] showed a 100% increase in capacity compared to bladders augmented with the cell-free ABS, which showed only a 30% increase in capacity within 3 months after implantation.

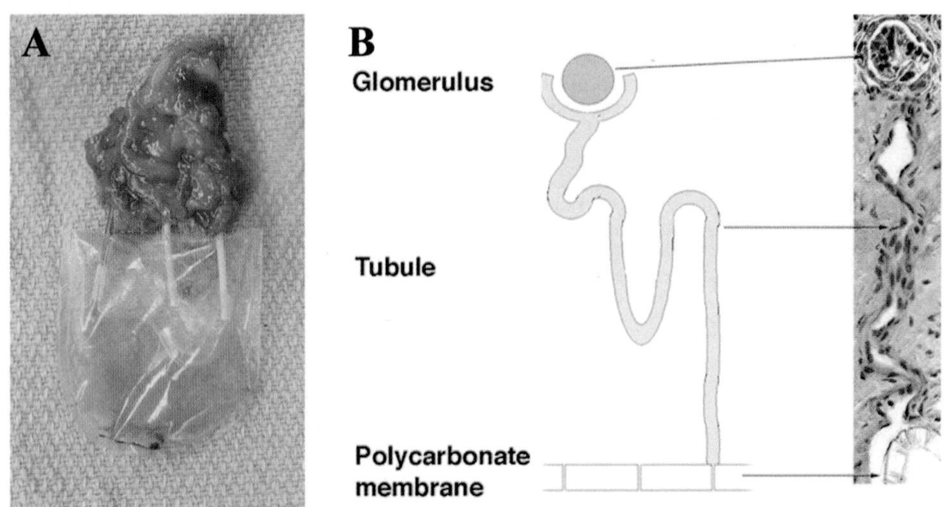

COLOR PLATE 19.4. Tissue-engineered renal units. **A:** Retrieved tissue-engineered renal unit shows the excretion of yellow fluid in the reservoir. **B:** The engineered tissue showed a clear unidirectional continuity between the mature glomeruli, their tubules, and the reservoir.

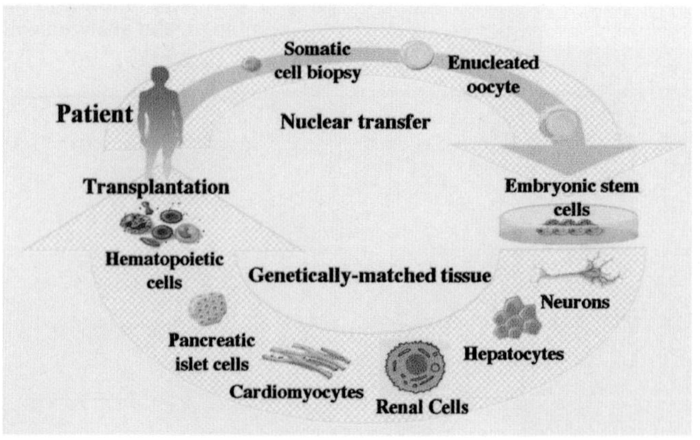

COLOR PLATE 19.6. Schematic diagram of therapeutic cloning approach for the isolation of genetically matched tissues.

A

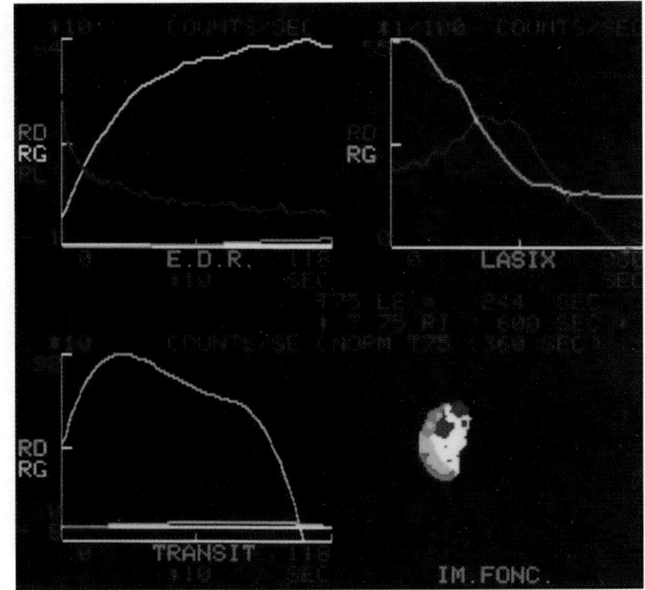

B

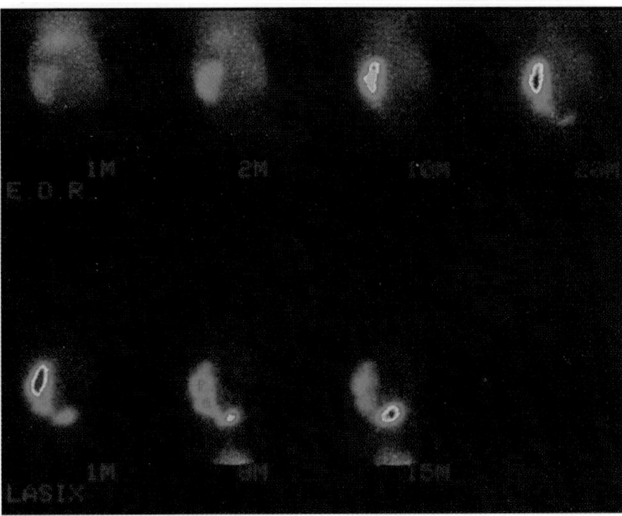

COLOR PLATE 23.7. Mercaptotriglycine renogram in a 1-month-old boy with antenatal diagnosis of right hydronephrosis and left small cystic kidney. The renogram confirms a nonfunctioning left kidney and a ureterohydronephrosis with response to furosemide (megaureter on magnetic resonance). **A:** Curves corresponding to the function of the right kidney. **B:** Morphologic appearance of the dilated right urinary tract.

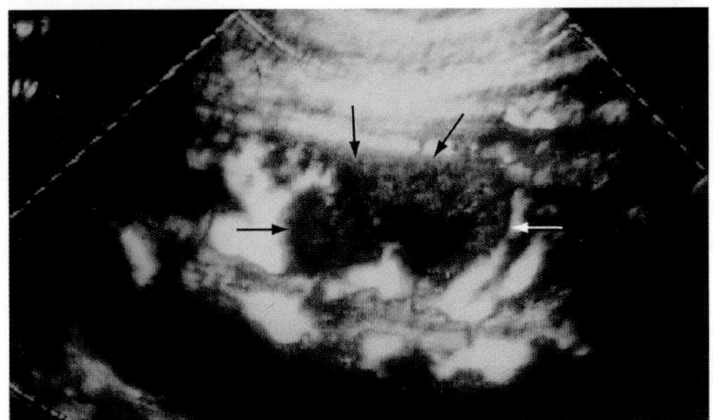

COLOR PLATE 23.22. Acute pyelonephritis. Power Doppler ultrasound showing striking area of absent vascularization due to inflammatory involvement (*arrows*). (Courtesy of Dr. Dufour.)

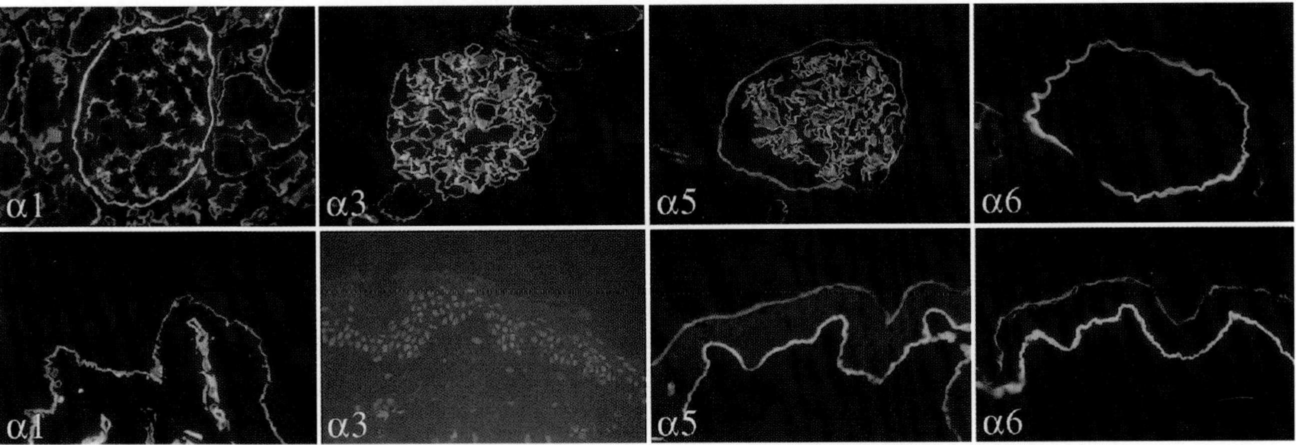

COLOR PLATE 26.2. Immunofluorescence microscopy. Normal distribution of the α(IV) chains in renal and epidermal basement membranes.

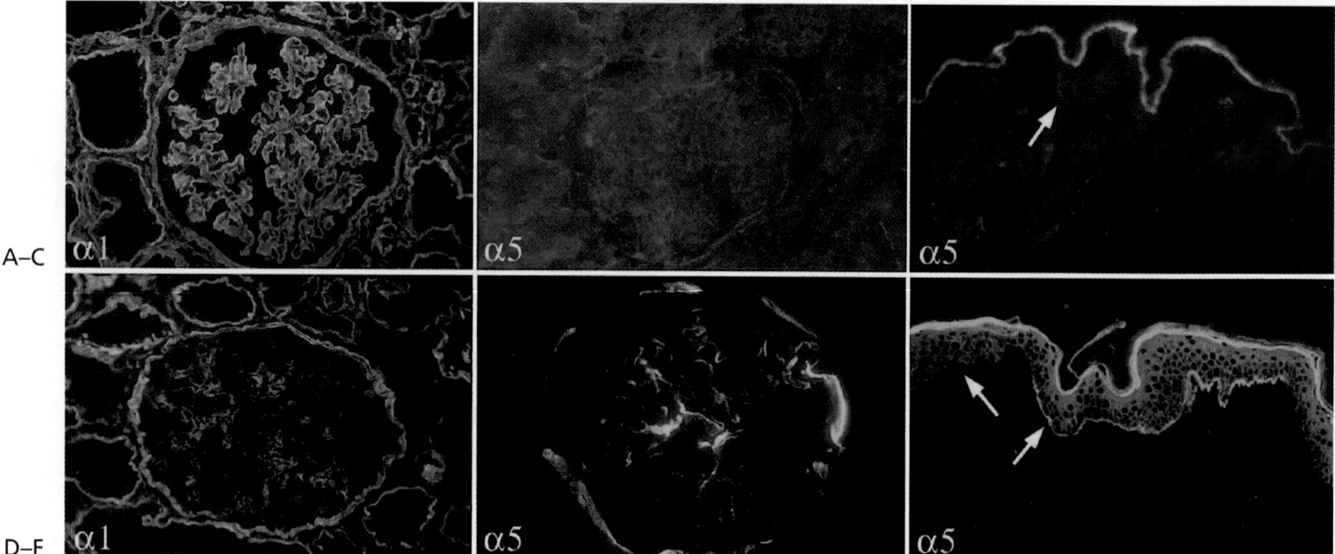

COLOR PLATE 26.5. Immunofluorescent microscopy. Distribution of the α(IV) chains in renal and epidermal basement membranes of male **(A–C)** and female **(D–F)** patients affected with X-linked Alport syndrome. **C:** Absence of epidermal basement membrane labelling (*arrow*). **F:** Discontinuous epidermal basement membrane labeling (*arrows*).

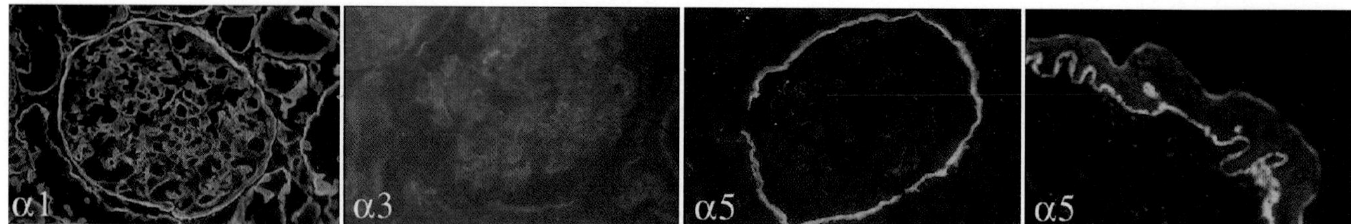

COLOR PLATE 26.6. Immunofluorescent microscopy. Distribution of the α(IV) chains in renal and epidermal basement membranes of patients affected with autosomal recessive Alport's syndrome.

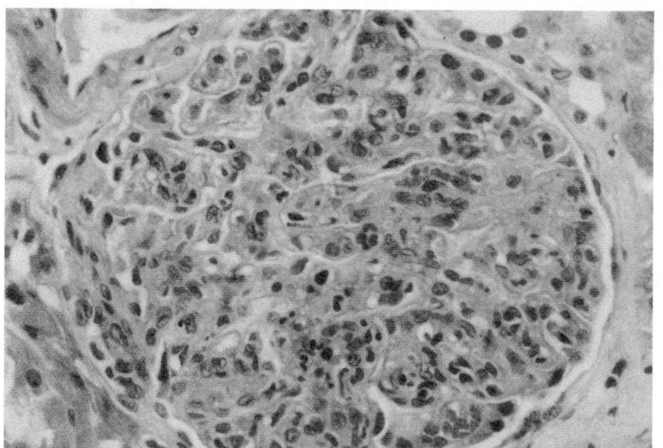

COLOR PLATE 30.1. Acute postinfectious glomerulonephritis. The glomeruli show global intracapillary hypercellularity with large numbers of polymorphonuclear leukocytes in the glomerular capillary lumina (hematoxylin and eosin stain, ×400). (Courtesy of Peter Degrell, University of Pécs Faculty of Medicine, Nephrological Center, Pécs, Hungary.)

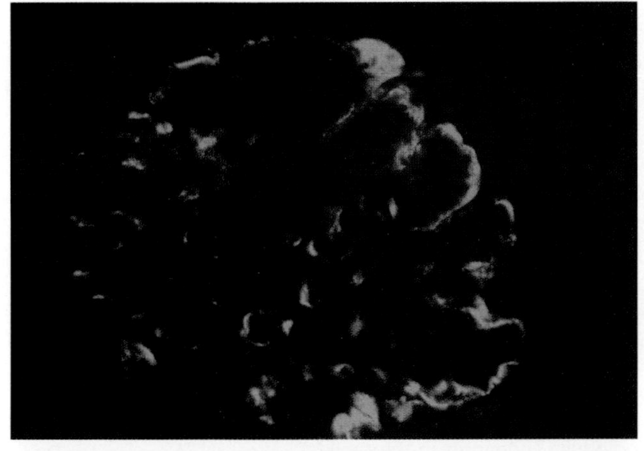

A

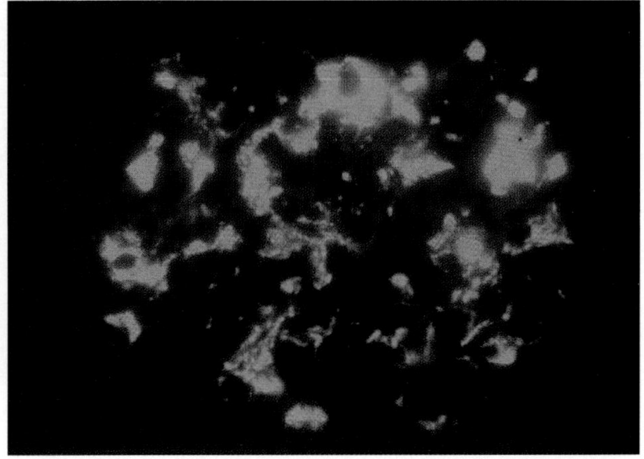

B

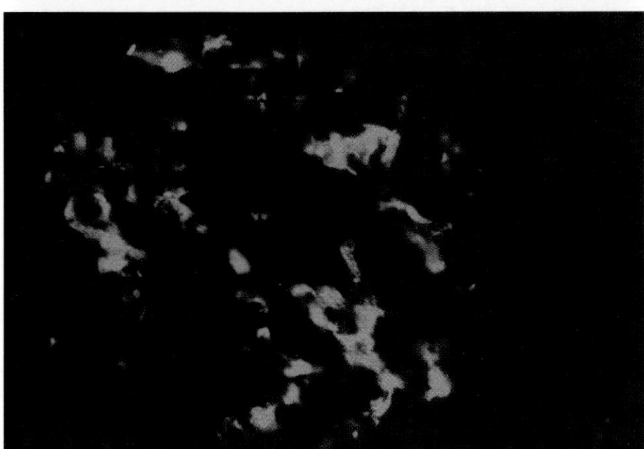

C

COLOR PLATE 30.2. Acute postinfectious glomerulonephritis by immunofluorescence. **A:** Garland pattern. Large, subepithelial deposits of immunoglobulin G on the outer side of the glomerular basement membrane (×400). **B:** Starry sky pattern. There are fine and coarse granular deposits of immunoglobulin G in the glomerular capillary walls and in the mesangium (×400). **C:** Mesangial pattern. Predominantly mesangial, coarse granular deposits of C3 (×400). (Courtesy of Peter Degrell, University of Pécs Faculty of Medicine, Nephrological Center, Pécs, Hungary.)

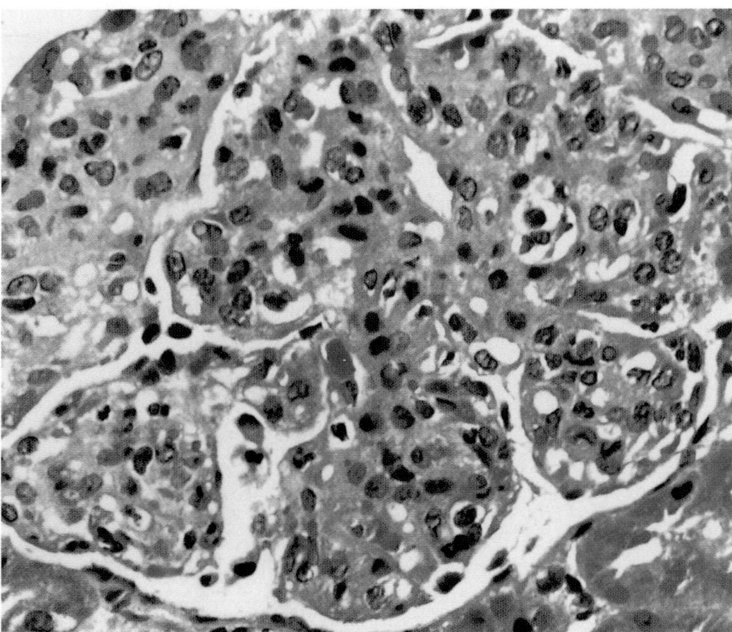

A

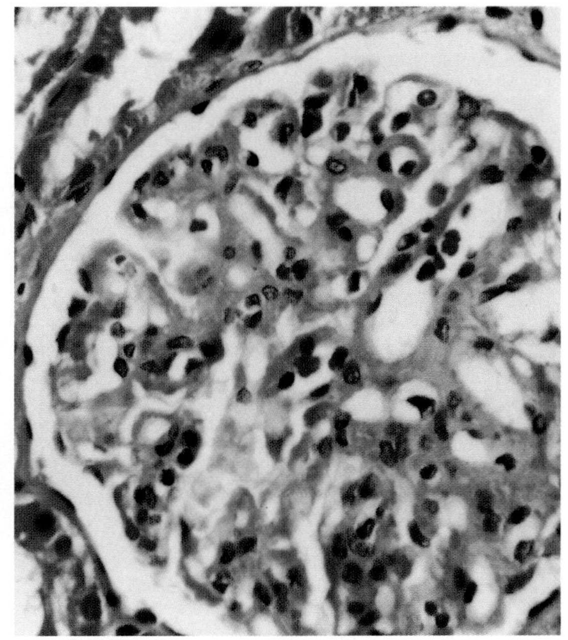

B

COLOR PLATE 32.3. Light microscopic appearance of membranoproliferative glomerulonephritis types I and III. **A:** The glomerulus is enlarged, very cellular, and has a lobulated appearance. The mesangium is markedly expanded. The capillary walls are thickened in appearance; frequently, the capillary lumens are obscured by the mesangial expansion. In addition to the increase in mesangial cells, scattered neutrophils are also identified in many of the segments. **B:** The type III glomerulus is less cellular in appearance, and there is less expansion of the mesangium. Most of the capillary loops are patent; however, thickened capillary walls are evident. (Courtesy of Dr. David Witte.)

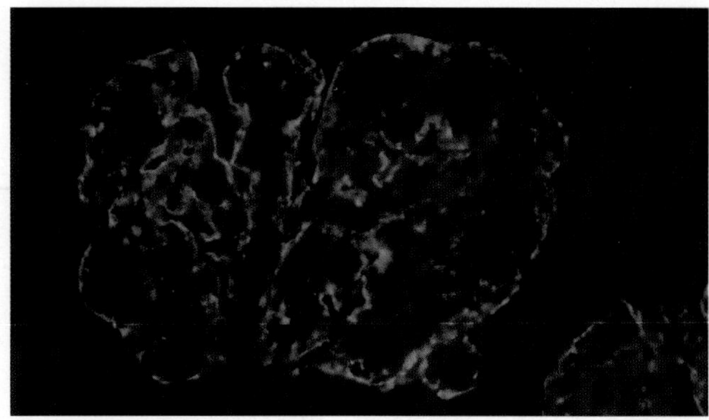

COLOR PLATE 32.4. Immunofluorescence appearance of membranoproliferative glomerulonephritis type I. The prominent peripheral distribution of immunoglobulin G deposits in the capillary walls results in a fringe pattern. (Courtesy of Dr. David Witte.)

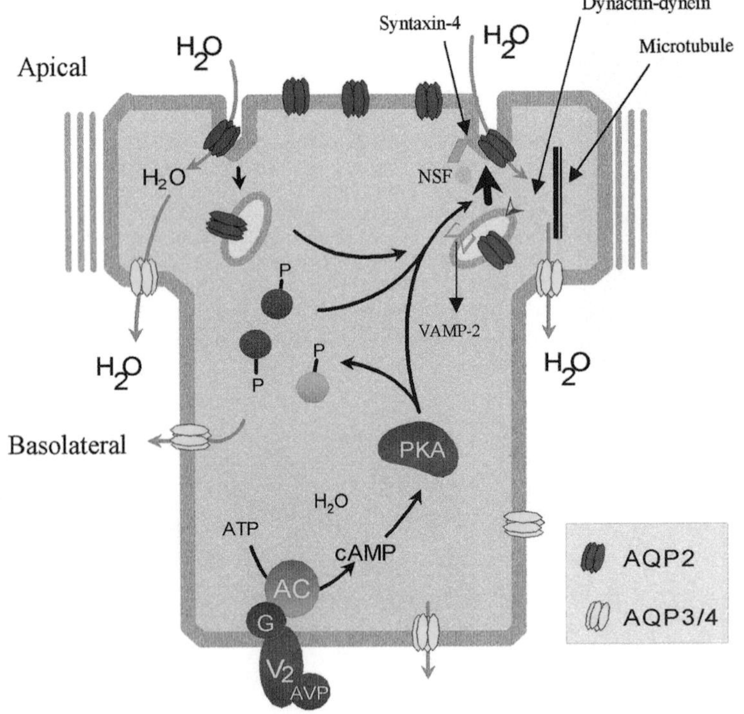

COLOR PLATE 40.2. Schematic view of the antidiuretic arginine vasopressin (AVP) signaling pathway in collecting duct cells and the proteins (microtubule, dynactin-dynein) and vesicle targeting receptors (VAMP-2, syntaxin-4, NSF) that might participate in the specificity of aquaporin-2 water channel (AQP2) targeting to the luminal plasma membrane. AC, adenylate cyclase; AQP3, aquaporin-3 water channel; AQP4, aquaporin-4 water channel; G, stimulatory guanine nucleotide binding protein; NSF, N-ethylmaleimide-sensitive fusion protein; PKA, protein kinase A; V_2, vasopressin type-2 receptor.

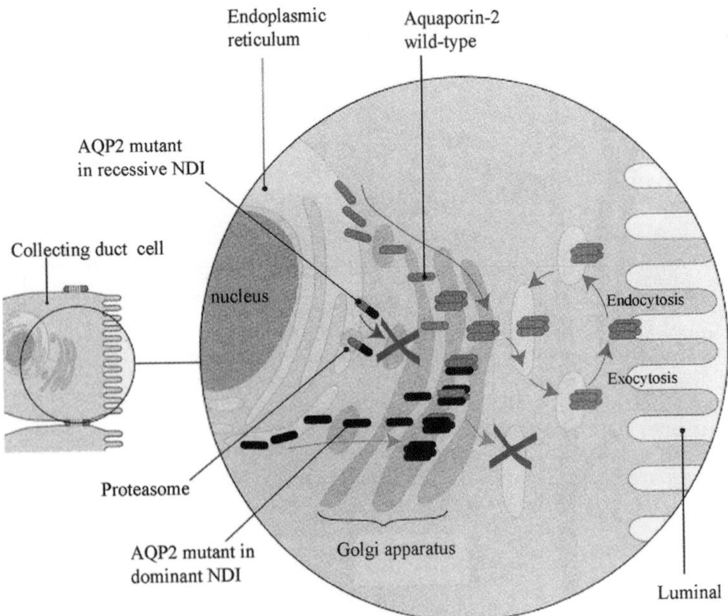

COLOR PLATE 40.3. Schematic representation of the postulated mechanisms in a collecting duct cell to explain recessive and dominant forms of nephrogenic diabetes insipidus (NDI) caused by aquaporin-2 (AQP2) water channel mutations. Normal AQP2 proteins are transported from the endoplasmic reticulum via the Golgi apparatus to the luminal side of the cell. In case of a recessive NDI mutation AQP2 is retained in the endoplasmic reticulum due to misfolding and subsequently broken down by proteosomes. In case of a dominant NDI mutation there is a change in the transport signal of the AQP2 protein and consequent misrouting to the Golgi network or late endosomes/lysosomes. (Adapted from Knoers NVAM, Deen PMT. Van Gen naar Ziekte; van vasopressine-V2-receptor en aquaporine-2 naar nefrogene diabetes insipidus. *Dutch J Med* 2000;144:2402–2404.)

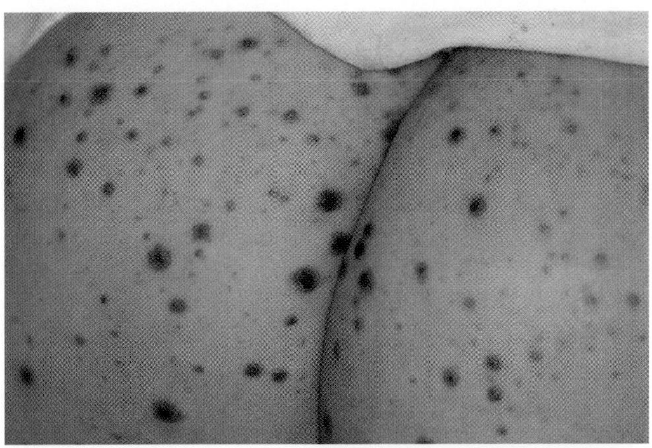

COLOR PLATE 45.2. Purpuric rash of Henoch-Schönlein purpura over the sides of the buttocks.

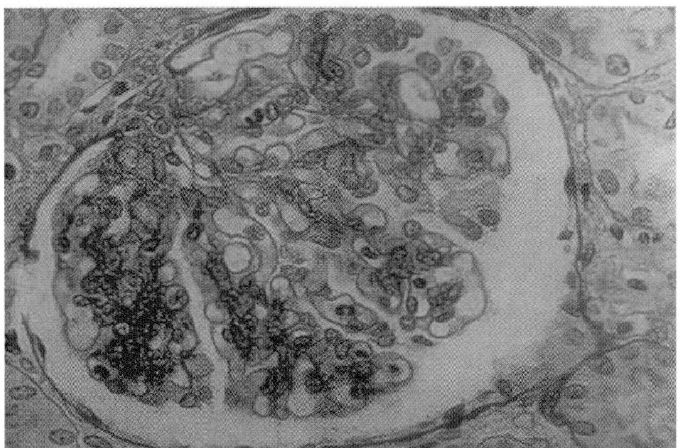

COLOR PLATE 45.5. Renal biopsy specimen from a patient with nephritis of Henoch-Schönlein purpura showing expansion of the mesangial matrix and increase in mesangial cellularity (periodic acid-Schiff ×250).

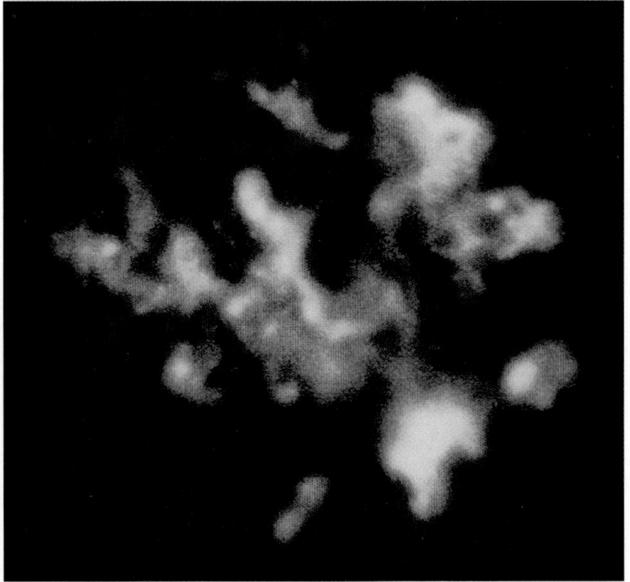

COLOR PLATE 45.7. Immunopathology of Henoch-Schönlein nephritis. Mesangial deposits of immunoglobulin A (antiimmunoglobulin A ×250).

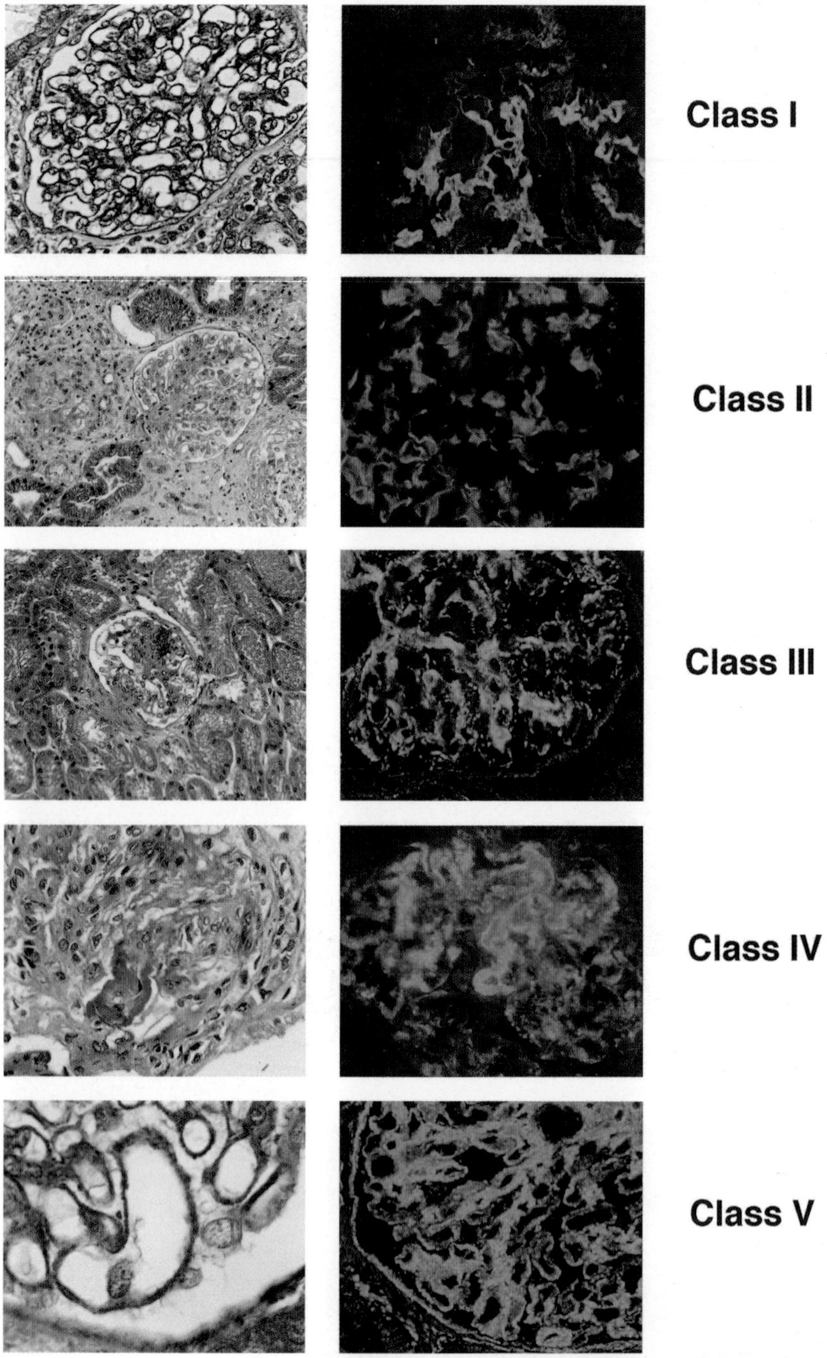

Class I

Class II

Class III

Class IV

Class V

COLOR PLATE 46.1. Class I: Normal glomerulus by light microscopy (*right-hand side*) but mesangial immune deposits by immunofluorescence (*left-hand side*) study. Class II: Purely mesangial hypercellularity and mesangial matrix expansion in glomerulus by light microscopy, with mesangial immune deposits by immunofluorescence study. Class III: Segmental endo- and extracapillary proliferation involving 50% of all glomeruli by light microscopy with mesangial and some subendothelial immune deposits by immunofluorescence study. Class IV: Global endo- and extracapillary proliferation and subendothelial deposits by light microscopy and numerous immune deposits by immunofluorescence study. Class V: Membranous glomerulonephritis, with subepithelial deposits by light microscopy, clearly defined by immunofluorescence study.

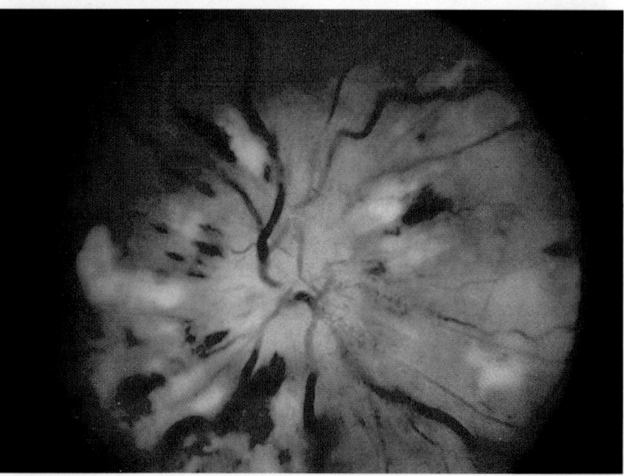

COLOR PLATE 61.2. Severe hypertensive retinopathy in a child with long-standing untreated hypertension showing arteriolar narrowing, hemorrhages and exudates, and papilledema.

12. Schofer O, Beetz R, Kruse et al. Nephrogenic diabetes insipidus and intracerebral calcification. *Arch Dis Child* 1990;65:885–887.
13. Hoekstra JA, van Lieburg AF, Monnens LAH, et al. Cognitive and psychosocial functioning of patients with nephrogenic diabetes insipidus. *Am J Med Genet* 1996;61:81–88.
14. Uribarri J, Kaskas M. Hereditary nephrogenic diabetes insipidus and bilateral nonobstructive hydronephrosis. *Nephron* 1993;65:346–349.
15. Monnens L, Smulders Y, van Lier H, et al. DDAVP test for assessment of renal concentrating capacity in infants and children. *Nephron* 1991;29:151–154.
16. Fushimi K, Sasaki S, Muramo F. Phosphorylation of serine 256 is required for cAMP-dependent regulatory exocytosis of the aquaporin-2 water channel. *J Biol Chem* 1997;272:14800–14804.
17. Katsura T, Gustafson CE, Ausiello DA. Protein kinase A phosphorylation is involved in regulated exocytosis of aquaporin-2 in transfected LCC-PK1 cells. *Am J Physiol* 1997;272:F816–F822.
18. Klussmann E, Maric K, Wiesner B, et al. Protein kinase A anchoring proteins are required for vasopressin-mediated translocation of aquaporin-2 into cell membranes of renal principal cells. *J Biol Chem* 1999;274:4934–4938.
19. Inoue T, Nielsen S, Mandon B, et al. SNAP-23 in rat kidney: co-localization with aquaporin-2 in collecting duct vesicles. *Am J Physiol* 1998;275:F752–F760.
20. Jo I, Harris HW, Amendt Raduege AM, et al. Rat kidney papilla contains abundant synaptobrevin protein that participates in the fusion of antidiuretic hormone-regulated water channel-containing endosomes in vitro. *Proc Natl Acad Sci U S A* 1995;92:1876–1880.
21. Liebenhoff U, Rosenthal W. Identification of Rab3-, Rab5a-, and synaptobrevin II-like proteins in a preparation of rat kidney vesicles containing the vasopressin-regulated water channel. *FEBS Lett* 1995;365:209–213.
22. Nielsen S, Marples D, Birn H, et al. Expression of VAMP2-like protein in kidney collecting duct intracellular vesicles. Colocalization with aquaporin-2 water channels. *J Clin Invest* 1995;96:1834–1844.
23. Mandon B, Chou C-L, Nielsen S, et al. Syntaxin-4 is localized to the apical plasma membrane of rat renal collecting duct cells: possible role in aquaporin-2 trafficking. *J Clin Invest* 1996;98:906–913.
24. Maric K, Oksche A, Rosethal W. Aquaporin-2 expression on primary cultured rat inner medullary collecting duct cells. *Am J Physiol* 1998;275:F796–F801.
25. Marples D, Schroer TA, Ahrens N, et al. Dynein and dynactin colocalize with aqp2 water channels in intracellular vesicles from kidney collecting duct. *Am J Physiol* 1998;43:F384–F394.
26. Chou C-L, Yip K-P, Michea L, et al. Regulation of aquaporin-2 trafficking by vasopressin in renal collecting duct: roles of ryanodine-sensitive Ca^{2+} stores and calmodulin. *J Biol Chem* 2000;275:36839–36846.
27. Bouley R, Breton S, Sun TX, et al. Nitric oxide and atrial natriuretic factor stimulate cGMP-dependent membrane insertion of aquaporin 2 in renal epithelial cells. *J Clin Invest* 2000;106:1115–1126.
28. Matsumura Y, Uchida S, Rai T, et al. Transcription regulation of aquaporin-2 water channel gene by cAMP. *J Am Soc Nephrol* 1997;8:861–867.
29. Carter C, Simpkiss M. The "carrier" state in nephrogenic diabetes insipidus. *Lancet* 1956;ii:1069–1073.
30. Knoers N, van der Heyden H, van Oost BA, et al. Nephrogenic diabetes insipidus: close linkage with markers from the distal long arm of the human X chromosome. *Hum Genet* 1988;80:31–38.
31. van den Ouweland AMW, Dreesen JCFM, Verdijk M, et al. Mutations in the vasopressin type-2 receptor gene associate with nephrogenic diabetes insipidus. *Nat Genet* 1992;2:99–102.
32. Pan Y, Metzenberg A, Das S, et al. Mutations of the V2 receptor are associated with X-linked nephrogenic diabetes insipidus. *Nat Genet* 1992;2:103–106.
33. Rosenthal W, Seibold A, Antamarian A, et al. Molecular identification of the gene responsible for congenital nephrogenic diabetes insipidus. *Nature* 1992;359:233–235.
34. Schreiner RL, Skafish PR, Anand SK, et al. Congenital nephrogenic diabetes insipidus in a baby girl. *Arch Dis Child* 1978;53:906–915.
35. Langley JM, Balfe JW, Selander T, et al. Autosomal recessive inheritance of vasopressin-resistant diabetes insipidus. *Am J Med Genet* 1991;38:90–94.
36. Brodehl J, Braun L. Familiarer nephrogener diabetes insipidus mit voller auspragung bei einer weiblichen saugling. *Klin Wochenschr* 1964;42:563.
37. Deen PMT, Verdijk MAJ, Knoers NVAM, et al. Requirement of human renal water channel aquaporin-2 for vasopressin-dependent concentration of urine. *Science* 1994;264:92–95.
38. Mulders SM, Bichet DG, Rijss JPL, et al. An aquaporin-2 water channel mutant which causes autosomal dominant nephrogenic diabetes insipidus is retained in the Golgi complex. *J Clin Invest* 1998;102:57–66.
39. Bichet DG, Razi M, Lonergan M, et al. Hemodynamic and coagulation responses to 1-desamino[8-D-arginine] vasopressin in patients with congenital nephrogenic diabetes insipidus. *N Engl J Med* 1988;318:881–887.
40. van den Ouweland AMW, Knoop MT, Knoers NVAM, et al. Colocalization of the gene for nephrogenic diabetes insipidus (DIR) and the vasopressin type-2 receptor (AVPR2) in the Xq28 region. *Genomics* 1992;13:1350–1353.
41. Birnbaumer M, Seibold A, Gilbert S, et al. Molecular cloning of the receptor for human antidiuretic hormone. *Nature* 1992;357:333–335.
42. Morello J-P, Bichet DG. Nephrogenic diabetes insipidus. *Annu Rev Physiol* 2001;63:607–630.
43. Knoers NVAM, Deen PMT. Molecular and cellular defects in nephrogenic diabetes insipidus. *Pediatr Nephrol* 2001;16:1146–1152.
44. Innamorati G, Sadeghi H, Birnbaumer M. A full active non-glycosylated V2 vasopressin receptor. *Mol Pharmacol* 1996;50:467–473.
45. Innamorati G, Sadeghi H, Eberle AN, et al. Phosphorylation of the V2 vasopressin receptor. *J Biol Chem* 1997;271:2486–2492.
46. Innamorati G, Sadeghi HM, Tran NT, et al. A serine cluster prevents recycling of the V2 vasopressin receptor protein. *Proc Natl Acad Sci U S A* 1998;95:2222–2226.
47. Schülein R, Rutz C, Rosenthal W. Membrane targeting and determination of transmembrane topology of the human vasopressin V2 receptor. *J Biol Chem* 1996;271:28844–28852.

48. Krause G, Hermosilla R, Oksche A, et al. Molecular and conformational features of a transport-relevant domain in the C-terminal tail of the vasopressin V2 receptor. *Mol Pharmacol* 2000;57:232–242.
49. Schülein R, Liebenhoff U, Muller H, et al. Properties of the human arginine vasopressin V2 receptor after site-directed mutagenesis of its putative palmitoylation site. *J Biol Chem* 1996;313:611–616.
50. Pind S, Riordan JR, Williams DB. Participation of the endoplasmic reticulum chaperone calnexin (p88, IP90) in the biogenesis of the cystic fibrosis transmembrane conductance regulator. *J Biol Chem* 1994;269:12784–12788.
51. Brooks DA. Protein processing: a role in the pathophysiology of genetic disease. *FEBS Lett* 1997;409:115–120.
52. Kuznetsor G, Nigam SK. Folding of secretory and membrane proteins. *N Engl J Med* 1998;339:688–695.
53. Albertazzi E, Zanchetta D, Barbier P, et al. Nephrogenic diabetes insipidus: functional analysis of new AVPR2 mutations identified in Italian families. *J Am Soc Nephrol* 2000;11:1033–1043.
54. Schöneberg T, Yun J, Wenkert D, et al. Functional rescue of mutant V2 vasopressin receptors causing nephrogenic diabetes insipidus by a coexpressed receptor polypeptide. *EMBO J* 1996;15:1283–1291.
55. Schöneberg T, Sculz A, Biebermann H, et al. V2 vasopressin receptor dysfunction in Nephrogenic diabetes insipidus caused by different molecular mechanisms. *Hum Mutat* 1998;12:196–205.
56. Pasel K, Schulz A, Timmermann K, et al. Functional characterization of the molecular defects causing nephrogenic diabetes insipidus in eight families. *J Endocrinol Metab* 2000;85:1703–1710.
57. Sadeghi HM, Innamorati G, Birnbaumer M. An X-linked NDI mutation reveals a requirement for cell surface V2R expression. *Mol Endocrinol* 1997;11:706–713.
58. Ala Y, Morin D, Sabatier N, et al. Functional studies of twelve mutant V2 vasopressin receptors related to nephrogenic diabetes insipidus: molecular basis of a mild phenotype. *J Am Soc Nephrol* 1998;9:1861–1872.
59. Postina R, Ufer E, Pfeiffer R, et al. Misfolded vasopressin V2 receptors caused by extracellular point mutations entail congenital nephrogenic diabetes insipidus. *Mol Cell Endocrinol* 2000;164:31–39.
60. Inaba S, Hatekeyama H, Taniguchi N, et al. The property of a novel V2 receptor mutant in a patient with nephrogenic diabetes insipidus. *J Clin Endocrinol Metabol* 2001;86:381–385.
61. Morello J-P, Salahpour A, Petäjä-Repo UE, et al. Association of calnexin with wild-type and mutant AVPR2 that cause nephrogenic diabetes insipidus. *Biochem* 2001;40:6766–6775.
62. Bross P, Corydon TJ, Andresen BS, et al. Protein misfolding and degradation in genetic diseases. *Hum Mutat* 1999;14:186–198.
63. Rosenthal W, Antamarian A, Gilbert S, et al. Nephrogenic diabetes insipidus. A V2 vasopressin receptor unable to stimulate adenylyl cyclase. *J Biol Chem* 1993;268:13030–13033.
64. Savarese TM, Fraser CM. In vitro mutagenesis and search for structure-function relationships among G-protein-coupled receptors. *Biochem J* 1992;283:1–19.
65. Chen C-H, Chen W-Y, Liu H-L, et al. Identification of mutations in the arginine vasopressin receptor 2 gene causing nephrogenic diabetes insipidus in Chinese patients. *J Hum Genet* 2002;47:66–73.
66. Schulein R, Zühlke K, Krause G, et al. Functional rescue of the nephrogenic diabetes insipidus-causing V2 receptor mutants G1185C and R202C by a second site receptor suppressor mutation. *J Biol Chem* 2001;276:8384–8392.
67. Kalenga K, Persu A, Goffin E, et al. Intrafamilial phenotype variability in nephrogenic diabetes insipidus. *Am J Kidney Dis* 2002;39:737–743.
68. Fushimi K, Uchida S, Harra Y, et al. Cloning and expression of apical membrane water channel of rat kidney collecting tubule. *Nature* 1993;361:549–552.
69. Jung JS, Preston GM, Smith BL, et al. Molecular structure of the water channel through aquaporin-CHIP. *J Biol Chem* 1994;269:14648–14654.
70. Murata K, Mitsuoka K, Hirai T, et al. Structural determinants of water permeation through aquaporin-1. *Nature* 2000;407:599–605.
71. Marr N, Bichet DG, Hoefs S, et al. Cell-biological and functional analysis of five new Aquaporin-2 missense mutations that cause recessive nephrogenic diabetes insipidus. *J Am Soc Nephrol* 2002;13:2267–2277.
72. Lin SH, Bichet DG, Sasaki S, et al. Two novel aquaporin-2 mutations responsible for congenital nephrogenic diabetes insipidus in chinese families. *J Clin Endocrinol Metab* 2002;87:2694–2700.
73. Mulders SM, Knoers NVAM, van Lieburg AF, et al. New mutations in the AQP2 gene in nephrogenic diabetes insipidus resulting in functional but misrouted water channels. *J Am Soc Nephrol* 1997;8:242–248.
74. Deen PMT, Croes H, van Aubel RAMH, et al. Water channels encoded by mutant aquaporin-2 genes in nephrogenic diabetes insipidus are impaired in their cellular routing. *J Clin Invest* 1995;95:2291–2296.
75. Marr N, Kamsteeg EJ, van Raak M, et al. Functionality of aquaporin-2 missense mutants in recessive nephrogenic diabetes insipidus. *Pflugers Arch* 2001;442:73–77.
76. Tamarappoo BK, Verkman AS. Defective aquaporin-2 trafficking in nephrogenic diabetes insipidus and correction by chemical chaperones. *J Clin Invest* 1998;101:2257–2267.
77. Kamsteeg E-J, Wormhoudt TAM, Rijss JPL, et al. An impaired routing of wild-type aquaporin-2 after tetramerization with an aquaporin-2 mutant explains dominant nephrogenic diabetes insipidus. *EMBO J* 1999;18:2394–2400.
78. Kuwahara M, Iwai K, Ooeda T, et al. Three families with autosomal dominant nephrogenic diabetes insipidus caused by aquaporin-2 mutations in the C-terminus. *Am J Hum Genet* 2001;69:738–748.
79. Marr N, Bichet DG, Lonergan M, et al. Heteroligomerization of an aquaporin-2 mutant with wild-type aquaporin-2 and their misrouting to late endosomes/lysosomes explains dominant nephrogenic diabetes insipidus. *Hum Mol Genet* 2002;11:779–789.
80. Kanno K, Sasaki S, Hirata Y, et al. Urinary excretion of aquaporin-2 in patients with diabetes insipidus. *N Engl J Med* 1995;332:1540–1545.
81. Deen PMT, van Aubel RAMH, van Lieburg AF, et al. Uri-

nary content of aquaporin-1 and 2 in nephrogenic diabetes insipidus. *J Am Soc Nephrol* 1996;7:1–7.

82. Wen H, Frokiaer J, Kwon TH, et al. Urinary excretion of aquaporin-2 in rat is mediated by a vasopressin-dependent apical pathway. *J Am Soc Nephrol* 1999;10:1416–1429.
83. van Lieburg AF, Knoers NVAM, Mallman R, et al. Normal fibrinolytic responses to 1-desamino-8-D-arginine vasopressin in patients with nephrogenic diabetes insipidus caused by mutations in the aquaporin-2 gene. *Nephron* 1996;72:544–546.
84. van Lieburg AF, Verdijk MAJ, Schoute F, et al. Clinical phenotype of nephrogenic diabetes insipidus in females heterozygous for a vasopressin type-2 receptor mutation. *Hum Genet* 1995;96:70–78.
85. Sato K, Fukuno H, Taniguchi T, et al. A novel mutation in the vasopressin V2 receptor gene in a woman with congenital nephrogenic diabetes insipidus. *Intern Med* 1999;38: 808–812.
86. Arthus M-F, Lonergan M, Crumley MJ, et al. Report of 33 novel AVPR2 mutations and analysis of 117 families with X-linked nephrogenic diabetes insipidus. *J Am Soc Nephrol* 2000;11:1044–1054.
87. Chan Seem CP, Dossetor JF, Penney MD. Nephrogenic diabetes insipidus due to a new mutation of the arginine vasopressin V2 receptor gene in a girl presenting with non-accidental injury. *Ann Clin Biochem* 1999;36:779–782.
88. Nomura Y, Onigata K, Nagashima T, et al. Detection of skewed X-inactivation on two female carriers of vasopressin type 2 receptor gene mutation. *J Clin Endocrinol Metab* 1997;82:3434–3437.
89. Marples D, Christensen S, Christensen EI, et al. Lithium-induced down-regulation of aquaporin-2 water channel expression in rat kidney medulla. *J Clin Invest* 1995;95: 1838–1845.
90. Kwon T-H, Laursen UH, Marples D, et al. Altered expression of renal AQPs and Na+ transporters in rats with lithium-induced NDI. *Am J Physiol* 2000;279:F552–F564.
91. Marples D, Dorup J, Knepper MA, et al. Hypokalemia-induced downregulation of aquaporin-2 water channel expression in rat kidney medulla and cortex. *J Am Soc Nephrol* 1996;97:1960–1968.
92. Frokiaer J, Marples D, Knepper M, et al. Bilateral ureteral obstruction downregulates expression of the vasopressin-sensitive aquaporin-2 water channel in rat kidney medulla. *J Am Soc Nephrol* 1995;6:1012.
93. Teitelbaum I, Strasheim A, McGuinness S. Decreased aquaporin-2 content in chronic renal failure. *J Am Soc Nephrol* 1996;7:1273.
94. Sands JM, Naruse M, Jacobs JD, et al. Changes in aquaporin-2 protein contribute to the urine concentrating defect in rats fed a low protein diet. *J Clin Invest* 1996;97:2807–2814.
95. Apostel E, Ecelbarger CA, Terris J, et al. Reduced renal medullary water channels expression in puromycin-aminonucleoside-induced nephrotic syndrome. *J Am Soc Nephrol* 1997;8:15–24.
96. Arnell H, Hjalmas K, Jagervall M, et al. The genetics of primary nocturnal enuresis: inheritance and suggestion of a second major gene on chromosome 12q. *J Med Genet* 1997;34:360–365.
97. Deen PM, Dahl N, Caplan MJ. The aquaporin-2 water channel in autosomal dominant primary nocturnal enuresis. *J Urol* 2002;167:1451–1452.
98. Crawford JD, Kennedy GC. Chlorothiazide in diabetes insipidus renalis. *Nature* 1959;193:891–892.
99. Monnens L, Jonkman A, Thomas C. Response to indomethacin and hydrochlorothiazide in nephrogenic diabetes insipidus. *Clin Sci* 1984;66:709–715.
100. Rasher W, Rosendahl W, Henricho IA, et al. Congenital nephrogenic diabetes insipidus: vasopressin and prostaglandins in response to treatment with hydrochlorothiazide and indomethacin. *Pediatr Nephrol* 1987;1:485–490.
101. Jakobsson B, Berg U. Effect of hydrochlorothiazide and indomethacin on renal function in nephrogenic diabetes insipidus. *Acta Paediatr* 1994;83:522–525.
102. Alon U, Chan JCM. Hydrochlorothiazide-amiloride in the treatment of congenital nephrogenic diabetes insipidus. *Am J Nephrol* 1985;5:9–13.
103. Knoers N, Monnens LAH. Amiloride-hydrochlorothiazide in the treatment of congenital nephrogenic diabetes insipidus. *J Pediatr* 1990;117:499–502.
104. Early LE, Orloff J. The mechanism of antidiuresis associated with the administration of hydrochlorothiazide to patients with vasopressin-resistant diabetes insipidus. *J Clin Invest* 1962;52:2418–2427.
105. Shirley DG, Walter SJ, Laycock JF. The antidiuretic effect of chronic hydrochlorothiazide treatment in rats with diabetes insipidus. *Clin Sci* 1982;63:533–538.
106. Cesar KR, Magaldi AJ. Thiazide induces water reabsorption in the inner medullary collecting duct of normal and Brattleboro rats. *Am J Physiol* 1999;277:F750–F756.
107. Magaldi AJ. New insights into the paradoxical effect of thiazides in diabetes insipidus therapy. *Nephrol Dial Transplant* 2000;15:1903–1905.
108. Morello J-P, Salahpour A, Laperriere A, et al. Pharmacological chaperones rescue cell-surface expression and function of misfolded V2 vasopressin receptor mutants. *J Clin Invest* 2000;105:887–895.
109. Schöneberg T, Sandig V, Wess J, et al. Reconstitution of mutant V2 vasopressin receptors by adenovirus-mediated gene transfer of a receptor fragment: molecular basis and clinical implication. *J Clin Invest* 1997;100:1547–1556.
110. Yun J, Schoneberg T, Liu J, et al. Generation and phenotype of mice harboring a nonsense mutation in the V2 vasopressin receptor gene. *J Clin Invest* 2000;106:1361–1371.
111. Yang B, Gillespie A, Carlson EJ, et al. Neonatal mortality in an aquaporin-2 knock-in model of recessive nephrogenic diabetes insipidus. *J Biol Chem* 2001;276:2775–2779.

41

CYSTINOSIS AND FANCONI SYNDROME

JOHN W. FOREMAN

In the 1930s, de Toni (1), Debré et al. (2), and Fanconi (3) independently described several children with the combination of renal rickets, glucosuria, and hypophosphatemia. The name of this clinical entity has been shortened to *Fanconi syndrome.* Fanconi syndrome is a dysfunction of the proximal tubule leading to excessive urinary excretion of amino acids, glucose, phosphate, bicarbonate, and other solutes handled by this nephron segment. These losses lead to the clinical problems observed in this syndrome (e.g., acidosis, dehydration, electrolyte imbalance, rickets, and growth failure). Numerous disorders, ranging from inborn errors of metabolism to exogenous toxins, are associated with Fanconi syndrome.

PATHOPHYSIOLOGY

Currently, the sequence of events underlying Fanconi syndrome is incompletely defined. A number of possible mechanisms exist that could lead to diminished net solute reabsorption in the proximal tubule (Fig. 41.1). At the membrane level, at least six possibilities exist:

1. An intrinsic defect in carrier function could be the cause. Because there are many different carriers, this is unlikely except for a defect in sodium binding common to most or all of the carriers.
2. There may be a generalized defect in the insertion or recycling of these carriers into the brush-border membrane or in a membrane lipid-protein carrier interaction necessary for their complete function.
3. Solute reabsorption may be normal, but the resorbed solute quickly leaks back into the lumen. This mechanism has been implicated in the experimental Fanconi syndrome induced by maleic acid (4).
4. There may be impairment in solute movement out of the cell at the basolateral membrane—this would lead to solute accumulation intracellularly, which would augment solute efflux across the luminal membrane, decreasing net transepithelial transport.
5. Dysfunction of the Na^+,K^+–adenosine triphosphatase (ATPase) pump would increase the intracellular Na concentration, diminishing the electrochemical gradient for Na influx at the luminal membrane and its coupling to other solute transport.
6. Finally, there could be a significant paracellular backflux of solute from increased permeability of the tight junctions between proximal tubule cells.

In addition to membrane defects, abnormalities in cellular organelle function could impair net solute reabsorption. Examples include the apical endosome in Dent's disease and the lysosome in cystinosis. Numerous filtered proteins are reabsorbed through binding to the endocytic receptors, megalin and cubilin (Fig. 41.2). The protein-receptor complex is then incorporated into an endosome. In the endosome, the ligand and the receptor are disassociated and the receptor is recycled back to the luminal membrane and the reabsorbed protein into lysosomes for further processing. This disassociation process is dependent on acidification of the endosome by an H^+-ATPase and the ClC-5 chloride channel. The importance of this pathway in Fanconi syndrome is underscored by the finding of low urinary levels of megalin in patients with Fanconi syndrome due to Dent's disease and Lowe syndrome but not all causes of Fanconi syndrome (5). An abnormal endocytic pathway may affect the recycling of transport proteins, other than megalin, back to the luminal membrane, leading to decreased solute reabsorption. Furthermore, disturbances in energy generation could impair net transepithelial transport. Energy is necessary for operation of the Na^+-K^+-ATPase pump and intracellular Na^+ regulation and may be involved with solute reabsorption in other undefined ways as well. A defect in energy generation has been raised as the underlying cause of Fanconi syndrome observed in a diverse group of disorders, including hereditary fructose intolerance (HFI), galactosemia, cytochrome-*c*-oxidase deficiency, and heavy metal poisoning. In experimental models of Fanconi syndrome (including those induced by maleic acid, succinylac-

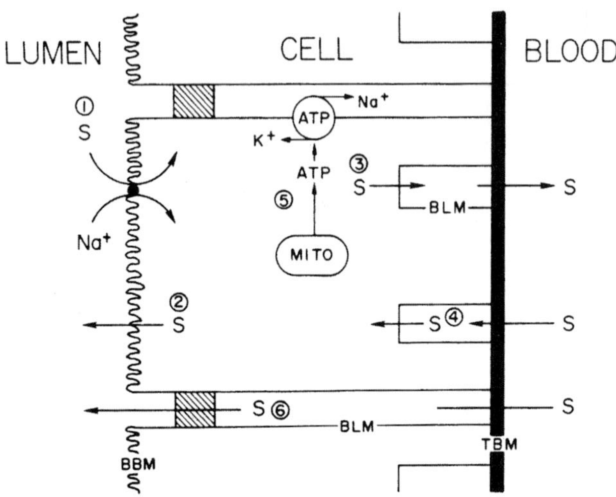

FIGURE 41.1. Model of solute (S) transport by the human renal proximal tubule cell. S uptake by the brush-border membrane (BBM) from the lumen is coupled to Na^+ influx. A favorable electrochemical driving force for luminal Na^+ is maintained by the Na^+-K^+–adenosine triphosphatase pump. Transported S is then either used by the cell or returned to the blood across the basolateral membrane (BLM). Fanconi syndrome could arise because of a defect of influx (1), leakage back into the lumen after influx (2), decreased flux out of the cell across the BLM (3), a defect in energy generation or transduction to the plasma membrane (4), an increase in backflux across the tight junctions between the cells (5), and, finally, defective transporter recycling (6). ATP, adenosine triphosphate; TBM, tubular basement membrane; MITO, mitochondrion.

etone, and cystine dimethylester), decreased adenosine triphosphate (ATP) production has been related to impaired solute reabsorption.

Experimental Models of Fanconi Syndrome

Maleic acid, the *cis* isomer of fumaric acid, has been used extensively to produce an experimental model of Fanconi syndrome (4,6–9). Injection of maleic acid in dogs and, especially, rats leads to a reversible Fanconi syndrome with aminoaciduria, glucosuria, phosphaturia, proteinuria, and bicarbonaturia. Maleic acid has been shown to inhibit Na^+-K^+-ATPase (6,7) and decrease cellular ATP levels (6–8). The low ATP levels were associated with low kidney tissue coenzyme A levels (8), leading to the speculation that maleic acid irreversibly bound to coenzyme A and impaired tricarboxylic acid cycle function. Maleic acid also has been shown to impair the incorporation of phosphate into the cell membrane (7). Maleic acid also disrupts the apical endocytic pathway of the renal tubule mediated by megalin, a receptor for a number of filtered proteins (9) (Fig. 41.2). Whether any or all of these effects underlies Fanconi syndrome induced by maleic acid is unclear.

Cadmium (10), lead (11,12), mercury (13), and uranium (14) have been used to induce experimental Fanconi syndrome. Animals given cadmium or lead have abnormal ATP levels and decreased Na^+-K^+-ATPase levels. Pathologically, experimental heavy metal toxicity is associated with significant abnormalities in renal tubule mitochondria. Outdated tetracycline, with the formation of anhydro-4-epitetracycline, causes reversible experimental Fanconi syndrome (15) associated with decreased mitochondrial respiration (16).

An experimental model of cystinosis and Fanconi syndrome has been created by injecting rats and incubating renal tubule cells with cystine dimethylester. Treated tubules had significantly increased cystine levels, decreased tubular transport, decreased metabolic fuel and O_2 consumption, decreased ATP levels, increased intracellular K^+ concentrations, and decreased mitochondrial respiration (17–19). ATP added to the incubation media partially restored the tubular transport function of the cystine-loaded cells, suggesting that cystine storage in cystinosis impairs mitochondrial function and ATP generation, leading to Fanconi syndrome. Succinylacetone has been proposed as the presumed toxin in tyrosinemia because of its structural similarity to maleic acid. Normal rats injected with this compound develop proteinuria, glucosuria, and aminoaciduria (20). Renal tubules incubated with succinylacetone have reduced amino acid, sugar, and phosphate transport; ATP levels; and O_2 consumption. Succinylacetone inhibits renal brush-border membrane transport and alters membrane fluidity (21). Thus, succinylacetone may be the cause of Fanconi syndrome in tyrosinemia.

Spontaneous Fanconi syndrome has been observed in several dog breeds, especially the Basenji (22,23). These dogs developed polyuria, polydipsia, glucosuria, aminoaciduria, and acidosis. The glomerular filtration rate (GFR) was normal in most of the dogs, although some went on to develop renal failure. Renal biopsies from affected dogs were normal except for large nuclei in a few tubular cells. Solute uptake by renal cortical slices from the affected dogs was also decreased. This model resembles the idiopathic human Fanconi syndrome.

SIGNS AND SYMPTOMS

Hyperaminoaciduria

Aminoaciduria is one of the major characteristics of Fanconi syndrome (Table 41.1). Virtually every amino acid is found in excess in the urine, giving rise to the designation of *generalized aminoaciduria.* Reabsorption rates vary for each amino acid, with some approaching the GFR. The easiest method for determining the renal handling of amino acids is to assess the percentage of tubular reabsorption (T_{aa}):

$$T_{aa} = 1 - \left[\frac{U_{aa} \times P_{aa}}{U_{cr}/P_{cr}}\right] \times (100\%)$$

where U_{aa} and P_{aa} are the urine and plasma amino acid concentrations and U_{cr} and P_{cr} are the urine and plasma creati-

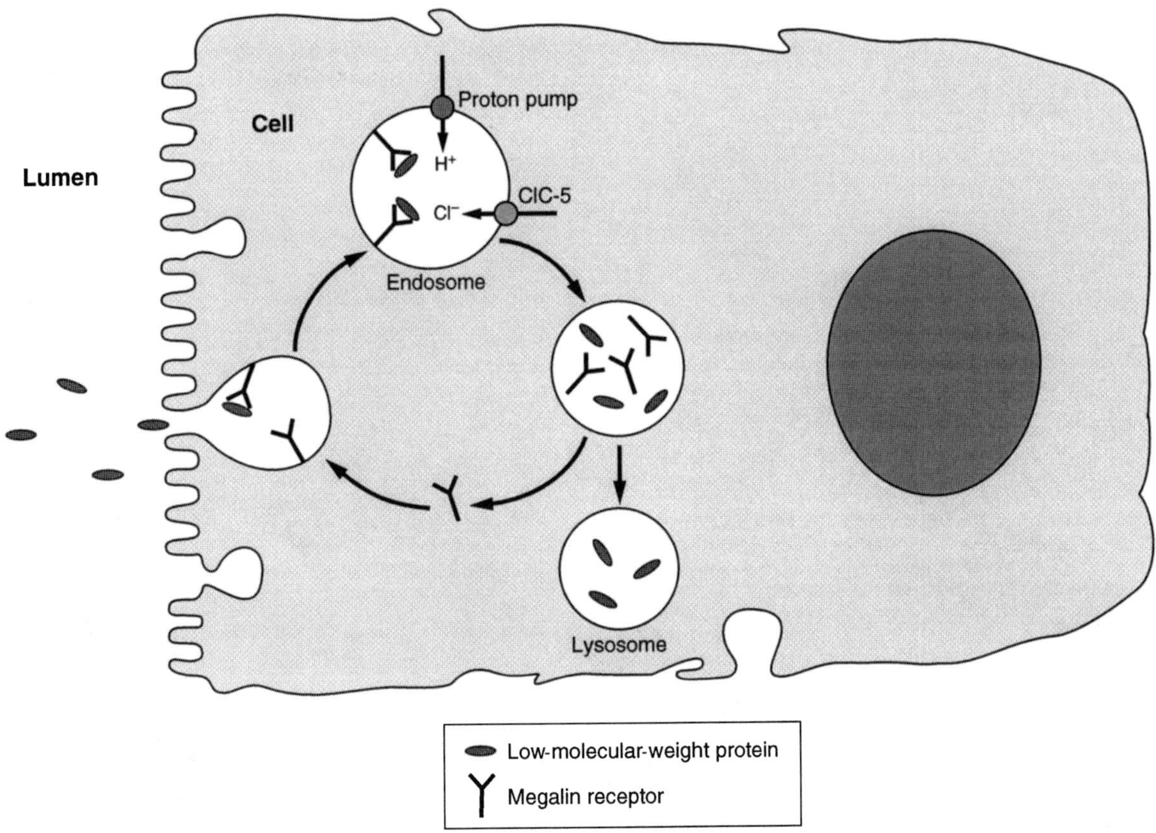

FIGURE 41.2. Megalin-endocytic pathway. Low-molecular-weight proteins in the luminal fluid bind to megalin and are endocytosed. The recycling of megalin and further catabolism of these proteins are dependent on acidification of the vesicle by a proton pump. The ClC-5 chloride channel provides an electrical shunt for efficient functioning of the proton pump. This endocytosis pathway may also play a role in membrane transporter recycling, and disruption of this pathway could interfere with absorption of other luminal solutes.

nine concentrations. Normally, T_{aa} for most amino acids is more than 98%, except for glycine (95%) and histidine (92%). The urinary amino acid losses in Fanconi syndrome do not cause any clinical consequences because the losses are trivial in relation to dietary intake. However, plasma amino acid levels tend to be lower than normal.

Glucosuria

Glucosuria is one of the originally recognized features of Fanconi syndrome. Glucosuria is the result of impaired tubular reabsorption of glucose and is present despite normal plasma glucose concentrations. It is often an early feature of Fanconi syndrome and indicates that the renal threshold (i.e., the plasma level of a solute when it first appears in the urine) is reduced.

Hypophosphatemia

Hypophosphatemia secondary to impairment in phosphate reabsorption is another important feature of Fanconi syndrome. Impaired phosphate reabsorption is usually not reflected by the excessive excretion of phosphate, except when Fanconi syndrome first develops. At a steady state, urinary phosphate excretion simply reflects dietary intake similar to that observed in X-linked hypophosphatemic rickets, vitamin D deficiency, and normals. Excessive phosphate excretion is observed only when plasma phosphate is above its steady-state level. Phosphate handling can be assessed by measuring the percentage of tubular reabsorption of phosphate, as described for amino acids. The tubular reabsorption of phosphate ranges from 80 to 95% in normal children (24), with much lower values in patients with Fanconi's syndrome. A preferred way of estimating the

TABLE 41.1. FEATURES OF FANCONI SYNDROME

Acidosis	Hypokalemia
Dehydration	Hypophosphatemia
Glucosuria	Hypouricemia
Growth retardation	Polyuria
Hyperaminoaciduria	Proteinuria
Hypocarnitinemia	Rickets

renal handling of phosphate is to derive the tubular maximal rate of phosphate reabsorption (Tm_p) related to GFR:

$$Tm_p/GFR = S_p - (U_p \times S_{cr}/U_{cr})$$

where S_p is serum phosphate, U_p is urine phosphate, S_{cr} is serum creatinine, and U_{cr} is urine creatinine, determined on simultaneous blood and urine specimens (25).

Phosphate handling by the kidney is affected by a number of factors, including parathyroid hormone (PTH) and vitamin D levels. PTH levels have been found to be both normal and elevated in patients with Fanconi syndrome (26,27). Low levels of 1,25-dihydroxy vitamin D have been found in some patients with Fanconi syndrome (28,29). Furthermore, patients with the Fanconi syndrome appear to have impaired conversion of 25 vitamin D to 1,25-dihydroxy vitamin D (30). Metabolic acidosis, another feature of Fanconi syndrome, also impairs the conversion of 25 vitamin D to 1,25-dihydroxy vitamin D. This may, in part, explain why alkali therapy may heal rickets in some patients with Fanconi syndrome. Bone disease is common in patients with long-standing untreated Fanconi syndrome (31).

Acidosis

Hyperchloremic acidosis, another feature of Fanconi syndrome, results from impaired bicarbonate reabsorption by the proximal tubule [proximal renal tubular acidosis (RTA)]. In Fanconi syndrome, more than 30% of the normal filtered bicarbonate load may be excreted when plasma levels are normal, leading to low plasma bicarbonate levels (usually between 12 and 18 mEq/L), and a reduction in extracellular fluid volume. Occasionally, there is an associated defect in distal acidification, usually in association with long-standing hypokalemia or nephrocalcinosis. Ammoniagenesis usually is normal or increased because of the hypokalemia and acidosis, unless there is associated impairment of GFR.

Sodium and Potassium Losses

Na^+ and K^+ losses may give rise to major clinical problems in patient's with Fanconi syndrome. Far less than the normal 60 to 80% of the filtered Na^+ load is reabsorbed in the proximal tubule in Fanconi syndrome. Part of this loss is related to impaired bicarbonate reabsorption, with the subsequent urinary excretion of $NaHCO_3$ and $KHCO_3$. In some cases, Na^+ and K^+ losses are so great that metabolic alkalosis and hyperaldosteronism result, simulating Bartter's syndrome despite the lowered bicarbonate threshold (32). The clearance of K^+ may be twice that of the GFR, and resultant hypokalemia has caused sudden death (33).

Dehydration

Polyuria, polydipsia, and frequent bouts of severe dehydration are common symptoms in patients with Fanconi syndrome. Despite dehydration, the urine is typically dilute. Recurrent febrile episodes, as a consequence of the dehydration, are often the first sign of Fanconi syndrome in infants with cystinosis. Polyuria is secondary to the osmotic diuresis from the excessive urinary solute losses. In some patients, there also appears to be an associated defect in renal concentrating ability, especially with prolonged hypokalemia.

Growth Retardation

Growth retardation is another common feature of Fanconi syndrome in children (34). The cause is multifactorial. Hypophosphatemia, disordered vitamin D metabolism, and acidosis can impair growth. Chronic hypokalemia and extracellular volume contraction may be additional factors, but glucosuria and aminoaciduria probably are not. However, even with correction of all of these metabolic abnormalities, most patients fail to grow, especially those with cystinosis.

Uricosuria

Impairment in renal handling of urate is often present in Fanconi syndrome, leading to hypouricemia, especially in adults. Urolithiasis from the uricosuria has rarely been reported (35). This is probably because the urine flow and pH are increased, inhibiting uric acid crystallization.

Proteinuria

Proteinuria, another feature of Fanconi syndrome, is usually minimal, except when the Fanconi syndrome develops in association with the nephrotic syndrome. The proteins lost in Fanconi syndrome (e.g., enzymes, immunoglobulin light chains, and hormones) are of low molecular weight (1900 to 30,000 d) (36).

ETIOLOGIES

Patients with Fanconi syndrome can be classified into two main categories: inherited and acquired (Table 41.2). In adults, the most common cause of a persistent Fanconi syndrome is an exogenous toxin, such as a heavy metal, whereas in children, the most common cause is an inborn error of metabolism, such as cystinosis.

Inherited Fanconi Syndrome

Cystinosis

Cystinosis, or cystine storage disease, is an enigmatic disorder characterized biochemically by excessive storage of cystine in the lysosomes of numerous organs, including the kidney (37). Three different types of cystinosis have been distinguished on the basis of the clinical course and the

TABLE 41.2. CAUSES OF FANCONI SYNDROME

Inherited	Acquired
Cystinosis	Amyloidosis
Galactosemia	Azathioprine
Glycogenosis	Chinese medicine
Hereditary fructose intolerance	Cisplatin
Idiopathic	Diachrome poisoning
Lowe syndrome	Gentamicin
Mitochondrial cytopathies	Glue sniffing
Tyrosinemia	Heavy metal poisoning
Wilson's disease	Ifosfamide
Dent's disease	Light-chain proteinuria
	Mesenchymal tumors
	Multiple myeloma
	Nephrotic syndrome
	Ranitidine
	Renal transplantation
	Sjögren's syndrome
	Streptozotocin
	Suramin

intracellular cystine content (38). Benign or ocular cystinosis is associated with cystine crystals only in the cornea and bone marrow and the smallest increase in intracellular cystine levels (39). There is no renal disease. Infantile or nephropathic cystinosis is most common and is associated with the highest intracellular levels of cystine (5 to 10 nmol/mg protein) in leukocytes or cultured fibroblasts. Autopsy kidney specimens contained 150 to 2000 nmol/mg protein of 0.5 cystine (40). Children with nephropathic cystinosis develop renal failure by late childhood. Patients with adolescent cystinosis tend to have intracellular cystine levels between those of the infantile and the ocular forms. Renal involvement occurs but does not appear until later and progresses more slowly (41).

Cystinosis arises from a defect in the egress of cystine from lysosomes (42). Heterozygotes for cystinosis have rates of lysosomal cystine egress that are one-half as fast as those from normal individuals, while homozygotes for nephropathic cystinosis have very low rates (42). This is due to a mutation in the CTNS gene, encoding the protein cystinosin, which is located on the short arm of chromosome 17 (43). Cystinosin is an integral lysosomal membrane protein composed of 367 amino acids with seven transmembrane domains and a C-terminal GYDQL sorting motif that directs it to the lysosomal membrane (43). It mediates the egress of cystine from the lysosome (44). Cystine transport is stimulated by an outwardly directed pH gradient (44). ATP also stimulates cystine egress through lysosomal acidification (45). The origin of lysosomal cystine in cystinosis is mainly from lysosomal protein degradation (46), but it is also from plasma cystine (47). There is no defect in cystine reduction or degradation in cystinosis (48).

Nephropathic cystinosis, with an estimated incidence of 1 in 200,000 births, is caused by a severe mutation on both chromosomes that leads to no functional protein (43). The most common mutation is a 57-kb deletion, but numerous other mutations have also been described. Ocular cystinosis is associated with one severe and one mild mutation leading to the production of some functional protein (49). Presumably there is enough lysosomal cystine transport to prevent the kidney and other organ dysfunction, but not enough to prevent corneal crystal formation. Patients with later onset or slower disease progression have been shown to have mutations that result in some functional protein, which results in less lysosomal cystine transport than occurs in ocular cystinosis (50).

The mechanism(s) by which increased intracellular cystine levels lead to renal injury and dysfunction remains unexplained in cystinosis. Lysosomal cystine concentration rises to levels sufficient to form crystals, which presumably cause cell injury and death. Foreman et al. (17) have shown that loading normal rat renal tubules with cystine impairs solute transport. Furthermore, cystine-loaded tubules have reduced metabolic fuel and O_2 consumption, ATP levels, and mitochondrial oxidation (18,19,51). These studies suggest that the intracellular storage of cystine may impair energy generation, which leads to defects in solute reabsorption.

In nephropathic cystinosis, high intracellular cystine concentrations can be found in virtually every cell and organ, including bone marrow, leukocytes, cornea, conjunctiva, retina, lymph nodes, liver, spleen, intestine, thyroid, muscle, and kidney. The brain was previously believed not to be affected in cystinosis, but a few patients surviving into their 20s have developed neurologic disorders in association with increased cystine levels in brain tissue (52,53). The definitive method of making the diagnosis of cystinosis is the demonstration of elevated intracellular levels of cystine, usually in polymorphonuclear leukocytes or fibroblasts. A prenatal diagnosis can be made by measuring the cystine content of amniotic cells (54). Finding needle-shaped, tinsel-like refractile opacities in the cornea by slit-lamp examination is also usually diagnostic (Fig. 41.3). Such ocular findings are invariably present after 2 years of age.

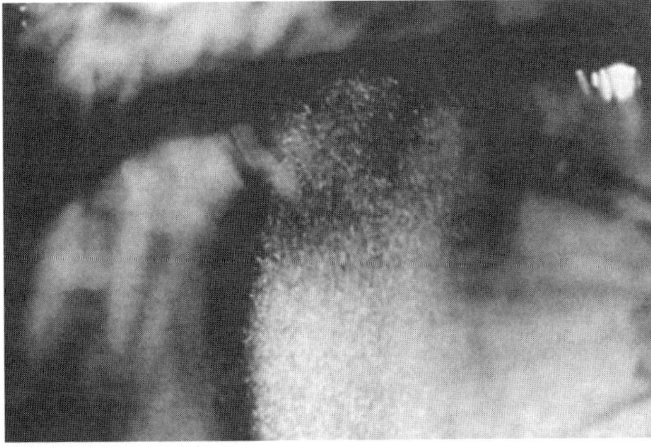

FIGURE 41.3. Tinsel-like refractile opacities in the cornea of a patient with cystinosis under slit lamp examination.

The first clinical signs and symptoms of cystinosis are polyuria, polydipsia, anorexia, failure to thrive, dehydration, and hyperchloremic metabolic acidosis, which usually appear in the latter half of the first year of life (55). Subtle abnormalities of tubular function can be demonstrated earlier in families with index cases, including glucosuria, generalized aminoaciduria, and mild proteinuria. Tubular reabsorption of phosphate is decreased with the development of hypophosphatemia and rickets. The renal threshold for bicarbonate is usually between 12 and 15 mEq/L. Hypokalemia and hypouricemia are common. Rarely, hyponatremia and metabolic alkalosis have been observed (32). Medullary calcinosis detected by renal ultrasound is relatively common (56), and a few patients have developed renal calculi (35). Children with cystinosis usually have fair complexion and blond hair, but this is not uniform. Cystinosis occurs in blacks but is less common than in whites.

Before the use of cysteamine, the GFR always declined in patients with nephropathic cystinosis, and end-stage renal disease developed between 7 and 10 years of age. Chronic dialysis and transplantation are well tolerated by children with cystinosis. Successful renal transplantation reverses the renal failure but does not improve the other symptoms of cystinosis (57). Cystine accumulates in the monocytes and interstitial cells of transplanted kidneys, but symptoms of proximal tubule dysfunction typical of cystinosis have not been noted. Photophobia is common and usually appears between 3 and 6 years of age. The severity of this symptom increases with age. In addition to corneal and conjunctival crystal deposits, a peripheral retinopathy can occur. The appearance of this is variable, with either hyperpigmented areas or the juxtaposition of hypopigmented and hyperpigmented areas in a salt-and-pepper pattern. Retinopathy affects the temporal more than the nasal side but occurs symmetrically in both eyes. Retinopathy tends to appear later in the course of the disease and to be progressive, although it has been observed in the first year of life. A few patients have developed visual impairment and blindness (55,57).

Growth failure is another major feature of cystinosis and, usually, is evident during the first year of life and before a significant decline in GFR. It occurs despite careful attention to electrolyte and mineral deficiencies. The appearance of renal failure and hypothyroidism further aggravates growth failure. Some patients have had improved growth after renal transplantation; however, the final height of patients with cystinosis is reduced. Recombinant growth hormone has improved linear growth (58), as has reducing intracellular cystine levels with cysteamine (59).

The morphologic features of the kidney in cystinosis vary with the stage of the disease (60). Early in the disease, cystine crystals are present in tubular epithelial cells, interstitial cells, and, rarely, glomerular epithelial cells. A swan-neck deformity or thinning of the first part of the proximal tubule can be observed, but this is not unique to cystinosis. Later in the course of the disease, pronounced tubular atrophy, interstitial fibrosis, and abundant crystal deposition occur. In the glomerulus, there is giant-cell formation of the visceral epithelium, segmental sclerosis, and eventual obsolescence. Hyperplasia and hypertrophy of the juxtaglomerular apparatus have been noted and probably are related to abnormalities of the renin-angiotensin system. Electron microscopy studies have demonstrated crystalline inclusions surrounded by a single limiting membrane, which electron diffraction has shown to be cystine. Peculiar dark cells, unique to the cystinotic kidney, have also been observed. These cells have a uniform darkening of their cytoplasm, probably reflecting a reaction between osmium tetroxide and cystine. These cells appear principally in the interstitium and visceral glomerular epithelium, but also in the loop of Henle, collecting duct, capillary endothelium, mesangium, and arteriolar smooth muscle layer.

Symptomatic treatment of nephropathic cystinosis involves early management of the tubulopathy and later management of renal failure. Acidosis and hypokalemia can be treated with potassium citrate. Rickets responds to vitamin D and phosphate supplementation. Low plasma and muscle carnitine levels have improved with prolonged supplementation (61). Careful attention to fluid and electrolyte replacement during gastroenteritis is particularly important.

The specific therapy for cystinosis is to lower tissue cystine levels. The best agent for this is cysteamine, which has been shown to lower intracellular cystine levels (Fig. 41.4) and to slow the decline in GFR, particularly in children with normal renal function treated before 2 years of age (59,62) (Fig. 41.5). Cysteamine therapy also improves linear growth (59,62) but does not improve the Fanconi syndrome. The most common problems associated with cysteamine are nausea, vomiting, and a foul odor and taste. These problems preclude its use in some patients. The best formulation is cysteamine bitartrate (Cystagon). Absorption of this formulation is equal to cysteamine

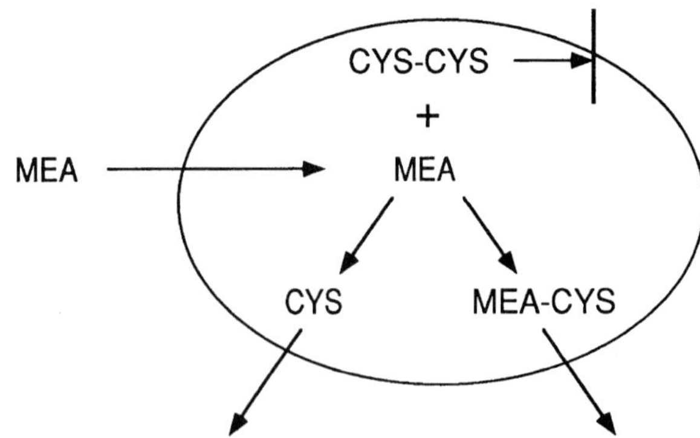

FIGURE 41.4. Effect of cysteamine (MEA) on lysosomal cystine (CYS-CYS). In cystinosis, the transporter for cystine egress from the lysosome is defective. Cysteamine can easily enter the lysosome and combine with cystine, forming cysteine (CYS) and the mixed disulfide cysteamine–cysteine (MEA-CYS). Both of these compounds can exit the lysosome via a transporter different from the cystine carrier.

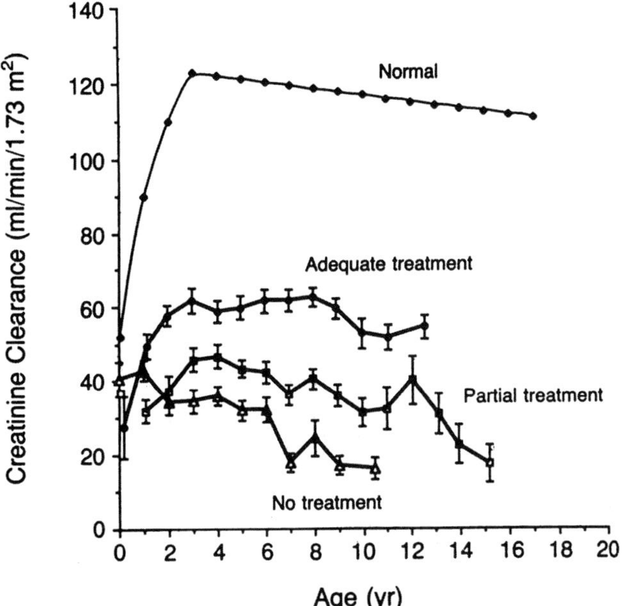

FIGURE 41.5. Mean creatinine clearance as a function of age in normal subjects, 17 patients with cystinosis who had received adequate therapy with cysteamine (started before 2 years of age and leukocyte cystine level less than or equal to 2 nmol of 0.5 cystine/mg protein), 32 who had received partial treatment, and 67 who had not received treatment. (From Markello TC, Bernardini IM, Gahl WA. Improved renal function in children with cystinosis treated with cysteamine. *N Engl J Med* 1993;328:1157–1162, with permission.)

HCl, and leukocyte cystine levels were lower after 3 weeks of therapy compared with cysteamine HCl, possibly reflecting better patient compliance with this formulation (63). The current recommendation for treatment of cystinosis is to initiate cysteamine soon after the diagnosis is made and to increase dosage over 4 to 6 weeks to 1.3 g/m^2/day in four divided doses. Slowly increasing the dosage minimizes the risk of a serum sickness–like reaction. Leukocyte cystine levels should be checked every 3 to 4 months to monitor effectiveness and compliance. The goal of therapy is to maintain cystine levels below 1.0 nmol 0.5 cystine/mg protein (63).

With the use of dialysis and renal transplantation to improve survival, a number of new complications of cystinosis have been recognized (57). Common problems include hypothyroidism, splenomegaly, hepatomegaly, decreased visual acuity, and corneal ulcerations. A few patients have developed insulin-dependent diabetes mellitus after renal transplantation in association with cystine crystal deposition in the pancreas (64). Of greater concern, several patients have developed progressive neurologic disorders (52,53). Cortical atrophy has also been noted (65). A generalized myopathy and swallowing difficulties attributed to muscular dysfunction have been observed in most patients older than 20 years (66). Patients also have a restrictive ventilatory defect attributable to this myopathy (67). Hypogonadism is common in adult male patients with cystinosis (68). These late-onset complications highlight the need to continue cysteamine therapy throughout life.

Galactosemia

Galactosemia is an autosomal recessive inherited disorder of galactose metabolism. The most common type is the result of deficient activity of the enzyme galactose-1-phosphate uridyl-transferase, known as *transferase deficiency galactosemia*, with an incidence of 1 in 62,000 live births. The gene for galactose-1-phosphate uridyl-transferase is found on the short arm of chromosome 9 (69). This enzyme catalyzes the reaction of galactose-1-phosphate (Gal-1-PO_4) plus uridine diphosphate glucose to uridine diphosphate galactose plus glucose-1-phosphate. Uridine diphosphate galactose can then be further metabolized to either glucose or CO_2 and H_2O via glycolysis. Deficiency of this enzyme leads to the intracellular accumulation of galactose-1-phosphate with damage to the liver, proximal renal tubule, ovary, brain, and lens. A less common cause of galactosemia is a deficiency of galactose kinase, which forms galactose-1-phosphate from galactose. Cataracts are the only manifestation of this form of galactosemia.

Affected infants ingesting milk containing lactose, the most common source of galactose in the diet, rapidly develop vomiting, diarrhea, and failure to thrive. Most also manifest jaundice and unconjugated hyperbilirubinemia and may have severe hemolysis. Continued intake of galactose leads to hepatomegaly and cirrhosis. Cataracts appear within days after birth, although they often are detectable only by a slit-lamp examination. Mental retardation may develop within a few months. Fulminant *Escherichia coli* sepsis has been described in a number of infants (70); it may be a result of inhibition of leukocyte bactericidal activity.

In addition to these clinical findings, galactose intake in patients with galactosemia leads, within days, to hyperaminoaciduria and albuminuria. Melituria, which is a cardinal feature of Fanconi syndrome, is principally a result of galactosuria and not glucosuria. There seems to be little or no impairment in glucose handling by the renal tubule. Galactosemia should be suspected when there is a urinary reducing substance that does not react in a glucose oxidase test. However, finding galactose in the urine does not establish the diagnosis because it can be seen in severe liver disease, in the first week of life in normal newborns (71) and even for longer periods in premature infants (72), and in some children with a high consumption of milk (73). Galactosuria disappears in affected infants after the withdrawal of galactose, which can obscure the diagnosis. Confirmation of a suspected diagnosis should be made by demonstrating deficient transferase activity in red blood cells, fibroblasts, leukocytes, or hepatocytes.

The relationship of biochemical abnormalities to specific symptoms of galactosemia is not clear. Accumulation of Gal-1-PO_4 with the ingestion of galactose can inhibit a number of pathways for carbohydrate metabolism and correlates with some clinical symptoms. Defective galactosylation of proteins has also been postulated. Formation of galactitol from galactose by aldose reductase has been proposed as a pathogenetic mechanism and is at least responsible for cataract formation. As to the renal tubular abnormalities, aminoaciduria has been induced in normal rats fed a high-galactose diet (74) and in normal human subjects given galactose intravenously (75). Experimentally, galactose inhibits amino acid uptake by slices of kidney cortex (76).

Galactosemia is treated by eliminating galactose from the diet. Acute symptoms and signs resolve within a few days. Cataracts also regress to some extent. However, even with early elimination of galactose, developmental delay, speech impairment, ovarian dysfunction, and growth retardation are common outcomes in galactosemia. Profound intellectual deficits are rare even in suboptimally treated infants (77).

Hereditary Fructose Intolerance

HFI is another disorder of carbohydrate metabolism associated with Fanconi syndrome (78,79). Patients with HFI experience nausea, vomiting, and symptoms of hypoglycemia shortly after ingesting fructose, sucrose, or sorbitol. These symptoms may progress to convulsions, coma, and even death, depending on the amount consumed. Concomitant serum biochemical findings include decreases in serum in glucose, phosphate, and bicarbonate and increases in serum uric acid and lactic acid after fructose ingestion. Chronic exposure to fructose leads to failure to thrive, hepatomegaly, jaundice, hepatic cirrhosis, and nephrocalcinosis.

HFI is inherited as an autosomal recessive trait with an incidence estimated to be 1 in 20,000. It is caused by a deficiency of the enzyme fructose-1-phosphate aldolase B, which cleaves fructose-1-phosphate into D-glyceraldehyde and dihydroxyacetone phosphate for further conversion into glucose or CO_2 and H_2O. The gene for aldolase B is found on the long arm of chromosome 9 (79). Aldolase B is present in liver, small intestine, and proximal renal tubule cells. Symptoms of HFI appear at weaning when fruit, vegetables, and sweetened cereals that contain fructose or sucrose are introduced. Symptoms appear in the newborn period if the infant is fed a formula containing sucrose. Young infants with this disorder may have a catastrophic illness, with severe dehydration, shock, acute liver impairment, bleeding, or acute renal failure, with exposure to fructose. The diagnosis should be suspected when characteristic symptoms develop after the ingestion of fructose. Confirmation can be made either by performing a fructose tolerance test or by assaying the activity of fructose-1-phosphate aldolase in a liver biopsy specimen.

Abnormalities associated with Fanconi syndrome appear rapidly after the ingestion of fructose (80,81). Proximal bicarbonate reabsorption falls by 20 to 30%, leading to RTA. The development of lactic acidosis adds significantly to the metabolic acidosis (82). Chronic fructose ingestion may lead to nephrocalcinosis, impairing distal tubular function as well. Although the onset of proximal tubule dysfunction is rapid after fructose loading, resolution of these symptoms may take days or weeks (83).

Acute fructose loading in the rat has been used as a model for HFI (84–86). Fructose loading leads to depletion of intracellular phosphate as fructose-1-phosphate accumulates and adenine deaminase is activated. Adenine deaminase converts adenosine monophosphate to inosinic monophosphate and ultimately to uric acid. A fall in adenosine monophosphate causes a drop in adenosine diphosphate and ATP, because these levels are maintained at or near equilibrium by adenylate kinase. Therefore, a drop in intracellular phosphate can cause a depletion of ATP. Furthermore, phosphate depletion impairs ATP regeneration by mitochondria. Fructose infusion induces a fall in tissue ATP in normal humans as well (87), and to an even greater extent in patients with HFI. This fall in ATP may be the cause of Fanconi syndrome because, experimentally, ATP depletion impairs substrate reabsorption in the proximal tubule.

Treatment of this disorder is strict avoidance of foods containing fructose and sucrose. Most patients develop a strong aversion to such foods, making this interdiction easy. The greatest risk occurs during infancy.

Glycogenesis

A number of patients have been described with Fanconi syndrome and glycogen storage in the liver and kidney (88–91). The syndrome is inherited as an autosomal recessive trait and is characterized by heavy glucosuria along with other features of Fanconi syndrome. This has led to the name *renal glucose losing syndrome* or *Fanconi-Bickel syndrome* because the glucose losses can be massive. Fanconi syndrome may appear in the first few months of life and precede the development of hepatomegaly from glycogen storage. The degree of renal tubular dysfunction is often severe, and rickets, osteoporosis, and growth retardation are common. Glucose tolerance tests are diabetic in pattern, but glucagon stimulation leads only to a slight increase in blood sugar. Galactose metabolism also is impaired, but the activities of the enzymes associated with galactose metabolism are normal. Ketonemia, ketonuria, elevations in plasma lactate and pyruvate, and hyperlipidemia are also observed as in type I glycogen storage disease. A few patients with type I glycogen storage disease have been described with mild Fanconi syndrome (92).

Fanconi-Bickel syndrome is caused by a deficiency of the transporter, GLUT2, that facilitates the exit of glucose and other hexoses from the basolateral side of the proximal tubule and intestinal cell and the entry and exit of these sugars from the hepatocyte and pancreatic β-cell (93). The therapy of this disorder is directed at the renal solute losses;

treatment of rickets, which can be severe; and frequent feeding to prevent ketosis. Uncooked cornstarch has been shown to lessen hypoglycemia and improve growth (94).

Tyrosinemia

Hereditary tyrosinemia type I, also known as *hepatorenal tyrosinemia*, is an autosomally inherited defect of tyrosine metabolism affecting the liver, kidneys, and peripheral nerves (95). The liver is the major organ affected in tyrosinemia, and liver dysfunction may be evident in the first month of life. Clotting abnormalities can be the initial sign of liver disease, with little elevation in transaminases. Infants may also have obvious and severe signs of liver disease, and those presenting at younger than 2 months of age have a high likelihood of dying during the first year of life. Some children are not diagnosed until after infancy; they have more indolent liver disease but are at risk for acute exacerbations of liver dysfunction. All children eventually develop macronodular cirrhosis, and many develop hepatocellular carcinoma. Acute, painful peripheral neuropathy may appear and can lead to transient paralysis. Autonomic dysfunction with hypertension and tachycardia can be associated with this acute neuropathy. Some renal tubular dysfunction is evident in all patients with tyrosinemia, especially those presenting after infancy. Rickets, secondary to the renal phosphate loss, can be severe. Generalized aminoaciduria, renal tubular acidosis, and mild proteinuria are also often seen, whereas glucosuria is less common because plasma glucose levels are usually low. Nephromegaly is common, and nephrocalcinosis may be seen. Glomerulosclerosis and impaired GFR may be seen with time. Plasma tyrosine and methionine levels usually are elevated in untreated patients. The hypermethioninemia imparts a cabbage-like odor to affected patients. In association with these amino acid abnormalities, *p*-hydroxyphenolic compounds, as a result of *p*-hydroxyphenyl pyruvate dioxygenase inhibition, are elevated in the urine. The presence of succinylacetone in blood or urine is diagnostic of hereditary tyrosinemia type I.

A deficiency of fumarylacetoacetate hydrolase activity is the cause of hereditary tyrosinemia type I (96). The gene coding for this enzyme resides on the long arm of chromosome 15 (97,98). Patients with early onset of severe symptoms tend to have no immunologically detectable fumarylacetoacetate hydrolase peptide, whereas patients with a more chronic course usually have detectable peptide. Decreased or absent activity of fumarylacetoacetate hydrolase leads to accumulation of maleylacetoacetate and fumarylacetoacetate in affected tissues. These compounds can react with free sulfhydryl groups and reduce intracellular levels of glutathione. They also may be capable of acting as alkylating agents. Maleylacetoacetate and fumarylacetoacetate are not detectable in plasma or urine but are converted to succinylacetoacetate. Succinylacetone, a metabolite of succinylacetoacetate, is structurally similar to maleic acid, which is known to induce Fanconi syndrome and may be the cause of the tubular dysfunction of tyrosinemia. Experimentally, succinylacetone administration to rats leads to Fanconi syndrome (20,21). Succinylacetone is also a potent inhibitor of D-aminolevulinic acid dehydratase, leading to the accumulation of D-aminolevulinic acid. This compound is neurotoxic and probably causes the acute porphyria-like symptoms of tyrosinemia.

Treatment with a low-phenylalanine and low-tyrosine diet dramatically improves the renal tubule dysfunction (99). In chronic cases, this diet leads to a rise in plasma phosphate, healing of rickets, a decrease in aminoaciduria, and the disappearance of glucosuria and proteinuria. However, its efficacy in halting the liver disease is uncertain. There is a risk of inducing deficiencies of phenylalanine or tyrosine. There is evidence for hepatic involvement prenatally, before any elevations of tyrosine or methionine are evident, and this raises doubt that elevated levels of these amino acids are the cause of liver injury (100). Liver transplantation has been successfully used to treat patients with severe liver failure and to prevent the development of hepatoma. Liver transplantation leads to rapid correction of Fanconi syndrome (101). Nitrotrifluorobenzoylcyclohexadione, which blocks *p*-hydroxyphenyl pyruvate dioxygenase and the formation of maleylacetoacetate and fumarylacetoacetate, dramatically improves the renal and hepatic dysfunction (95).

Wilson's Disease

Wilson's disease is a disorder of copper metabolism that affects numerous organ systems. Approximately 40% of patients present with liver disease, 40% with extrapyramidal symptoms, and 20% with psychiatric or behavioral abnormalities (102). Although symptoms rarely occur before 6 years of age, the most common presentation in children is with chronic active hepatitis or cirrhosis with little or no neurologic findings except those ascribable to hepatic failure. Greenish-brown rings at the limbus of the cornea, independently described by Kayser (103) and Fleischer (104), are usually present and are pathognomonic of Wilson's disease.

The underlying problem in Wilson's disease is a defect in a P-type copper transporting ATPase in the liver. This leads to a severe impairment in biliary copper excretion, the major excretory route for copper, and in the incorporation of copper into ceruloplasmin (105). These abnormalities cause excessive intracellular accumulation of copper in the liver, with subsequent overflow into other tissues such as brain, cornea, and renal proximal tubule. The gene for this enzyme has been localized to chromosome 13q14.3, and multiple mutations have been described in patients with Wilson's disease (105).

Excessive storage of copper in the kidney leads to renal tubular dysfunction in most patients and a full-blown Fanconi syndrome in some (106). Hematuria also has been noted. Renal plasma flow and GFR decrease as the disease progresses, but death from extrarenal causes occurs before the onset of renal failure. Tubular dysfunction overshadows the glomerular disease. Fanconi syndrome usually appears before the onset of hepatic failure and is characterized by intermittent glucosuria; aminoaciduria; decreased phosphate reabsorption leading to hypophosphatemia, osteomalacia, and rickets; and mild proteinuria. Hypouricemia secondary to a significant uricosuria is common and is a clue to the diagnosis (107,108). Hypercalciuria (109), with the development of renal stones and nephrocalcinosis (110), also has been reported. Besides proximal tubular dysfunction, abnormalities in distal tubular function, decreased concentrating ability, and distal RTA have also been observed.

Histologically, the kidney in untreated Wilson's disease shows either no alterations on light microscopy or only flattened proximal tubule cells without recognizable brush borders (107). Electron microscopy shows loss of the brush border, disruption of the apical tubular network, electron-dense bodies (probably representing metalloproteins) in the subapical region of tubule cell cytoplasm, and cavitation of the mitochondria with disruption of the normal cristae pattern. Rubeanic acid staining shows intracytoplasmic copper granules. The copper content of kidney tissue is significantly elevated.

The diagnosis of Wilson's disease should be suspected in children and young adults with unexplained neurologic disease, chronic active hepatitis, acute hemolytic crisis, behavioral or psychiatric disturbances, or the appearance of Fanconi syndrome. In such patients, the presence of Kayser-Fleischer rings is an important clue in making the diagnosis, but slit lamp examination may be necessary. Serum ceruloplasmin levels are decreased in 96% of patients with Wilson's disease, making this a useful screening test. However, normal values may be seen in young children with severe liver disease. A significantly increased urinary copper level is also useful in making the diagnosis, especially if it increases significantly with D-penicillamine. Liver copper levels are increased in untreated patients; however, in advanced cirrhosis this may not be the case.

Treatment with D-penicillamine reverses the renal dysfunction and may reverse the hepatic and neurologic disease, depending on the degree of damage before the onset of therapy (111). Recovery, however, is slow. Trientine can also chelate copper and is indicated in patients who cannot tolerate penicillamine. Tetrathiomolybdate is a potent agent in removing copper from the body and may be the drug of choice for patients with neurologic disease to prevent the immediate worsening of symptoms that can occur with penicillamine. Zinc salts, which induce intestinal metallothionein and blockade of intestinal absorption of copper, are useful in maintenance therapy. Liver transplantation has been successful in some patients but should be reserved for those with liver failure (112).

Lowe Syndrome

Lowe syndrome (oculocerebrorenal syndrome) is characterized by congenital cataracts and glaucoma, severe mental retardation, hypotonia with diminished to absent reflexes, and renal abnormalities (113,114). Initially, the renal abnormalities are those of Fanconi syndrome but, later, GFR is impaired. The disorder is transmitted as an X-linked recessive trait mapped to Xp24-p26 (115). This gene codes for a phosphatidylinositol bisphosphate phosphatase (116) localized in the Golgi complex (117). A few females have been reported (118,119). This may be explicable by the Lyon hypothesis, or there are several modes of inheritance. Cataracts and punctuate lens opacities have been noted in mothers of affected males, and these findings have been proposed as a method of carrier detection (120). Generalized aminoaciduria with relative sparing of the branched-chain amino acids is a constant feature of Lowe syndrome after the first several months of life. Proteinuria is present from infancy and often exceeds 1 g/m^2 body surface area per day. Glucosuria is minimal and only intermittently present. Phosphate reabsorption is variably impaired, but this impairment appears to worsen with age. Potassium reabsorption is also impaired and some patients require supplementation. Proximal RTA, polyuria, and impaired concentrating ability are common. The GFR usually only slowly declines with the appearance of end-stage renal failure in the fourth decade of life.

The histology of the kidney by light microscopy is normal early in the disorder (121,122). Swelling of endothelial cells with thickening and splitting of the glomerular basement membrane and fusion of the epithelial foot processes were observed by electron microscopy. In the proximal tubule cells, there was shortening of the brush border and enlargement of the mitochondria, with distortion and loss of the cristae. With progression of the disease, there was further thickening of the basement membrane, increased cellularity of the glomeruli, glomerular fibrosis, tubular atrophy, dilation, and interstitial fibrosis.

Treatment of Lowe syndrome is only symptomatic. The eye abnormalities usually require therapy early in infancy. Electrolyte and vitamin D supplements are needed by many patients for treatment of Fanconi syndrome. Renal insufficiency usually develops in adulthood.

Dent's Disease

Dent's disease is an X-linked recessive disorder characterized by low-molecular-weight proteinuria, hypercalciuria, nephrolithiasis, nephrocalcinosis, and, in some cases, rickets (123). Affected males also have aminoaciduria, phosphaturia, and glucosuria. They also excrete β_2-microglobulin in amounts that are 100-fold greater than normal. Another characteristic of affected males is severe hypercalciuria that leads to recurrent stone formation. These stones are usually made up of calcium phosphate or a mixture of calcium phosphate and oxalate. In addition, most affected males and some females have medullary nephrocalcinosis. Rickets is a frequent problem in children and osteomalacia in adults. Hypokalemia is also common. Renal failure is common and may occur by late childhood. The renal pathology is not pathognomonic and mainly shows interstitial nephritis with scattered calcium deposits. Hemizygous females usually only have low-molecular-weight proteinuria and mild hypercalciuria.

X-linked recessive hypophosphatemic rickets, X-linked recessive nephrolithiasis, and Japanese idiopathic low-molecular-weight proteinuria have similar features, and all are part of the clinical spectrum of an absent or inactive renal ClC-5 chloride channel from a mutation in the CLCN-5 gene located at Xp11.22 (124). A number of mutations have been described, and the same mutation may result in a different phenotype in different patients, indicating that there are other genetic or environmental modifiers. The ClC-5 chloride channel resides in the membrane of endocytic vesicles just below the luminal membrane of the proximal tubule. Entry of Cl^- via this channel is necessary for acidification of the vesicle by the H^+-ATPase pump. Inactivation of this channel interferes with protein reabsorption and cell surface receptor recycling, which may explain the hypercalciuria, phosphaturia, glucosuria, and aminoaciduria. Targeted disruption of the ClC-5 channel in a mouse led to a phenotype that was quite similar to that of patients with Dent's disease (125).

Treatment of Dent's disease is largely supportive. High fluid intake is helpful for the stone disease. Calcium restriction reduces calcium excretion but probably adds to the bone disease. A pharmacologic dose of vitamin D heals the rickets but may worsen the hypercalciuria. Thiazide diuretics reduce the hypercalciuria, but these patients are quite sensitive to them and may develop dehydration and hypotension.

Mitochondrial Cytopathies

In 1977, Biervliet et al. (126) described a family in which three infants died from a mitochondrial myopathy in association with lactic acidemia and Fanconi syndrome. Subsequent to this report, two more infants with similar clinical presentations were reported (127,128). The infants were noted to have weak cries and a poor suck, with generalized hypotonia in the neonatal period. The hypotonia and weakness progressed in all affected infants, leading to respiratory failure and death. Examination of muscle cells from these babies showed lipid-filled vacuoles in type I fibers and swollen mitochondria with abnormal cristae. Cytochrome-*c*-oxidase activity, an important enzyme in the electron-transport chain, was very low in both muscle and kidney. This deficiency, with its consequent impairment of oxidative phosphorylation, appeared to underlie the myopathy and renal tubulopathy.

After these reports, it has been recognized that there is a diverse group of diseases related to dysfunction of mitochondria in various tissues, termed *mitochondrial cytopathies* (129,130). Most are caused by abnormalities in mitochondrial DNA that lead to impaired oxidative phosphorylation.

TABLE 41.3. MITOCHONDRIAL CYTOPATHIES

MERRF	Myoclonic epilepsy with ragged red fibers
NARP	Neuropathy, ataxia, and retinitis pigmentosa
MELAS	Mitochondrial encephalopathy, lactic acidosis, and stroke-like episodes
LHON	Leber hereditary optic neuropathy
Leigh syndrome	Maternally inherited Leigh syndrome (somnolence, blindness, deafness, peripheral neuropathy, degeneration of brainstem)
Pearson syndrome	Pancytopenia, exocrine pancreatic deficiency, hepatic dysfunction
Kearns Sayre syndrome	Ophthalmoplegia, pigmentary retinopathy, heart block, ataxia
Alpers syndrome	Intractable epilepsy, liver disease, neuronal degeneration

The mitochondrion has its own DNA, which encodes for 13 protein subunits of 4 biochemical complexes; 2 ribosomal RNAs; 22 transfer RNAs; and machinery for DNA replication, transcription, and translation. Mitochondrial DNA mutates ten times more often than nuclear DNA; has no introns, so mutations are more likely to affect DNA coding sequences; lacks protective histones; and has an ineffective repair system. Mitochondria with their DNA are inherited maternally and multiple mitochondria are present in each egg. Therefore, normal and mutant mitochondria can coexist within a cell, a condition termed *heteroplasmy*, and this proportion can vary from cell to cell and tissue to tissue. This allows otherwise lethal mutations to exist and gives rise to the variation in the phenotype of a particular mutation. Some mitochondrial DNA mutations, mainly missense mutations, can be homoplasmic (i.e., affecting every mitochondrion).

Mitochondrial cytopathies most often present with neurologic disorders such as myopathy, myoclonus, ataxia, seizures, external ophthalmoplegia, stroke-like episodes, and optic neuropathy. Other manifestations include pigmentary retinitis, diabetes mellitus, exocrine pancreatic insufficiency, siderocrestic anemia, sensorineural hearing loss, pseudoobstruction of the colon, hepatic disease, cardiac conduction disorders, and cardiomyopathy. These various manifestations tend to group together in specific syndromes and reflect specific mutations in mitochondrial DNA (Table 41.3).

The most common renal manifestation associated with mitochondrial cytopathies is Fanconi syndrome, although a few patients have had focal segmental glomerulosclerosis with nephrotic syndrome. All of the patients with renal abnormalities have had extrarenal disorders, mainly neurologic diseases. Most patients presented in the first months of life and died soon after.

A clue to these disorders is an elevated serum or cerebrospinal fluid lactate level, especially if associated with an altered lactate to pyruvate ratio, suggesting a defect in mitochondrial respiration. The presence of ragged red fibers, a manifestation of abnormal mitochondria, in a muscle biopsy is another clue, especially with large abnormal mitochondria on electron microscopy of muscle tissue. Specific abnormalities of respiratory chain enzyme activity are best made by spectrographic analysis of isolated mitochondria, tissue homogenates, circulating lymphocytes, or cultured fibroblasts. Analysis of the mitochondrial DNA for deletions, duplications, or point mutations adds further insight into the nature of the abnormality.

There is little to offer these patients in terms of definitive therapy (131). Low electron transport chain complex III activity can be treated with menadione or ubidecarenone. Deficient complex I activity may be treated with riboflavin and ubidecarenone. Ascorbic acid has been used to minimize oxygen free-radical injury. A high-lipid, low-carbohydrate diet has been tried in cytochrome-*c*-oxidase deficiency.

Idiopathic Fanconi Syndrome

A number of patients develop complete Fanconi syndrome in the absence of any known cause. These cases have been called *idiopathic* or *primary Fanconi syndrome* (26–28,34,132–139). Originally, only adults were believed to be affected; hence, it was called *adult Fanconi syndrome*. However, it is now clear that idiopathic Fanconi syndrome occurs in children as well. All of the features of Fanconi syndrome may not be present when the patients are first studied. Idiopathic Fanconi syndrome can be inherited in an autosomal dominant (27,132), autosomal recessive (29), and even an X-linked pattern (134). However, most cases occur sporadically, without any evidence of genetic transmission. The possibility of an underlying enzymatic or other abnormality that has not yet been described as causing Fanconi syndrome should be kept in mind, especially in those in whom the syndrome is inherited. A number of patients, in whom the known causes of Fanconi syndrome have been excluded, still appear to have an underlying metabolic abnormality (136,137). Deal et al. (138) described six infants from consanguineous marriages with idiopathic Fanconi syndrome, ichthyosis, dysmorphism, jaundice, and diarrhea who failed to thrive and died in infancy.

Children with idiopathic Fanconi syndrome usually exhibit growth failure, recurrent dehydration, and rickets, despite an adequate intake of vitamin D. They often have the other features of Fanconi syndrome, including polyuria, polydipsia, hypokalemia, hypophosphatemia, RTA, aminoaciduria, glucosuria, and proteinuria. The GFR, usually, is normal in childhood. The prognosis is variable. These patients require careful management to prevent death from dehydration and electrolyte imbalance. However, some develop chronic renal failure 10 to 30 years after the onset of symptoms (26,132,135,139).

Renal morphologic descriptions of such cases are scanty. In some reports, no abnormalities were found, and others reported tubular atrophy with interstitial fibrosis interspersed with areas of tubular dilation. Significantly dilated proximal tubules with swollen epithelium and grossly enlarged mitochondria with displaced cristae have also been noted.

Therapy for idiopathic Fanconi syndrome remains symptomatic. Careful follow-up of these patients is necessary to prevent serious dehydration and electrolyte imbalance as well as severe bone disease. Renal transplantation has been done in a few patients who have reached end-stage renal disease (140). Fanconi syndrome has recurred in the allograft without evidence of rejection, suggesting that in some cases, there is an extrarenal cause of idiopathic Fanconi syndrome.

Acquired Causes

Exogenous Intoxications

Numerous substances can injure the proximal renal tubule, and this injury can range from an incomplete Fanconi syndrome to acute tubular necrosis and renal failure. The extent of the tubular damage is variable and depends on the type of toxin, the amount, and the host. A detailed history, therefore, is important in patients with tubular dysfunction to discover whether a toxin is the cause.

A major cause of proximal tubular dysfunction is heavy metal intoxication. Lead poisoning induces Fanconi syndrome, principally in children (141,142). However, the tubular dysfunction usually is overshadowed by the involvement of other organs, especially the central nervous system. Generalized aminoaciduria is regularly present in children with moderate lead poisoning. Glycosuria and hypophosphatemia with impaired phosphate reabsorption can also occur, but not as often. There is a rough correlation between the severity of the intoxication and the completeness of Fanconi syndrome. In acute lead poisoning, the alterations in renal histology are mainly in the proximal tubule and include eosinophilic intranuclear inclusions with mitochondrial swelling (143).

Cadmium intoxication also leads to Fanconi syndrome (142,144), usually after a long exposure to the toxin. This poisoning was dramatized by a large number of cases appearing in the Jintsu River Basin in Japan after World War II. It was characterized by severe bone pain, which gave rise to the name *Itai-Itai* (*ouch-ouch*) disease. Aminoaciduria, glucosuria, hypophosphatemia with impaired phosphate reabsorption, hyposthenuria, and RTA were also observed. The cause was traced to industrial contamination of the soil and water with cadmium.

Certain organic compounds cause Fanconi syndrome in humans. Outdated tetracycline causes a reversible Fanconi syndrome even in therapeutic doses (15,145,146). Affected patients experience dizziness, muscular weakness, acidosis, and, occasionally, neurologic symptoms. They have a generalized aminoaciduria, renal glucosuria, hypophosphatemia,

RTA, hypokalemia, proteinuria, and hypouricemia. The GFR is moderately reduced in some. Recovery is rapid when the degraded drug is stopped. The compound responsible for the tubular dysfunction is anhydro-4-tetracycline formed from tetracycline by heat, moisture, and a low pH.

A number of other compounds also may give rise to Fanconi syndrome, often in association with a reduced GFR, but the renal injury usually is reversible. For example, a few patients ingesting methyl-3-chromone (diachrome) (147), 6-mercaptopurine (148), toluene (glue sniffing) (149), Chinese medicine (150), valproate (151), suramin (152), and Lysol (153) have developed Fanconi syndrome. Gentamicin (154), streptozotocin (155), and ranitidine (156) have caused Fanconi syndrome and renal failure. Tubular dysfunction during recovery from acute renal failure from any cause can occur, diminishing the significance of some toxins as inducers of Fanconi syndrome.

A number of cancer chemotherapy agents have been associated with Fanconi syndrome and renal tubule dysfunction, especially cisplatin and ifosfamide. The nephrotoxicity of cisplatin is dose dependent and often irreversible (157). Renal cisplatin toxicity is manifested by tubular proteinuria, aminoaciduria, hypercalciuria, hyperphosphaturia, and, especially, hypermagnesuria. The hypermagnesuria can be severe, persistent, and difficult to treat. Reductions in GFR are common with prolonged use of cisplatin. Cisplatin principally affects the tubule, especially the proximal and distal tubules at the corticomedullary junction. Strict attention to hydration and avoidance of other nephrotoxins are helpful in preventing cisplatin nephrotoxicity.

Ifosfamide is another useful chemotherapeutic agent against solid tumors. However, nephrotoxicity is a well-documented side effect of this drug (158–162). Fanconi syndrome may appear at any time but seems more likely to appear after doses greater than 60 g/m^2 body surface area in children under 2 years of age, in those with reduced renal mass, and in those treated previously with cisplatin. Hypophosphatemic rickets as a consequence of Fanconi syndrome has occurred in a number of these children long after cessation of the drug, as has a reduced GFR. Experimentally, the perfusion of isolated rat kidneys with chloroacetaldehyde, a metabolite of ifosfamide, caused Fanconi syndrome, although this was not observed with ifosfamide or acrolein, another metabolite of ifosfamide (163).

Other Acquired Disorders

Dysproteinemia associated with a number of diseases is a cause of Fanconi syndrome. This cause is mainly observed in adults because the diseases are rare in children. Dysproteinemia and Fanconi syndrome are associated with multiple myeloma (164), light-chain proteinuria (165), Sjögren's syndrome (166), and amyloidosis (167). The appearance of tubular dysfunction is correlated with specific light chains or light-chain fragments (Bence Jones proteins) that crystallize within the tubule cells (164,168).

Hypophosphatemia has been well described in patients with benign and malignant mesenchymal tumors of bone. A single patient was also reported who had Fanconi syndrome, as well as hypophosphatemia, in association with a nonossifying fibroma of bone (169). Removal of the tumor led to resolution of the tubular dysfunction, indicating a humoral substance that impaired tubular transport.

The nephrotic syndrome has rarely been associated with Fanconi syndrome (170). The renal pathology in most cases is focal segmental glomerulosclerosis, and Fanconi syndrome heralds a poor prognosis. These patients have hypokalemia, RTA, rickets, and growth retardation. Hypocalcemia and tetany can be significant problems in these children.

Fanconi syndrome has appeared rarely after renal transplantation (171). The pathogenesis probably is multifactorial (e.g., sequels of acute tubular necrosis, rejection, nephrotoxic drugs, ischemia from renal artery stenosis, and residual hyperparathyroidism) (172).

THERAPY

Therapy, when possible, should be directed at the underlying cause, such as avoidance of the offending nutrient in galactosemia, HFI, and tyrosinemia. Wilson's disease can be treated with penicillamine and other copper chelators. Heavy metal intoxication can be treated with chelation therapy. In these cases, resolution of Fanconi syndrome usually is complete.

In other instances, therapy is directed at the biochemical abnormalities secondary to the renal solute losses and the bone disease often present in these patients. Proximal RTA usually requires high dosages of alkali (2 to 10 mEq/kg/day given in divided doses throughout the day) for correction. Some patients require even higher dosages that may lead to volume expansion and further bicarbonate wasting. In this situation, 1 to 3 mg/kg/day of hydrochlorothiazide to prevent volume expansion may lessen the dose of alkali needed. Hydrochlorothiazide aggravates the potassium losses, however. Potassium supplementation is also commonly needed, especially if there is significant RTA. The use of potassium citrate, lactate, or acetate corrects hypokalemia as well as acidosis. A few patients require sodium supplementation, as well as potassium. Again, the use of a metabolizable anion aids in the correction of the acidosis. Rare patients require NaCl supplementation. Usually these patients manifest alkalosis when untreated because of large urinary NaCl losses leading to volume contraction, which overrides the RTA. Magnesium supplementation is required in those patients who manifest hypomagnesemia. Ensuring adequate fluid intake is essential, especially during gastrointestinal diseases. This is of greater importance in the infant who does not have free access to fluid. Correction of hypokalemia and its effect on the concentrating ability of the distal tubule may decrease polyuria.

Bone disease is another important aspect of managing patients with Fanconi syndrome. Often, complaints referable to this problem (e.g., pain, fractures, rickets, or growth failure) are the presenting feature. Factors implicated in bone disease include hypophosphatemia, decreased synthesis of calcitriol, hypercalciuria, and chronic acidosis. Both low and normal plasma levels of calcitriol have been found in patients with Fanconi syndrome. Moreover, healing of rickets has occurred in patients receiving supplemental vitamin D without phosphate and in some receiving phosphate without supplemental vitamin D. In the presence of hypophosphatemia, oral phosphate should be started with the goal of normalizing serum phosphate levels. This often requires 1 to 3 g/day of supplemental phosphate. This is best given in divided doses, and the dosage should be slowly increased over several weeks to reduce the gastrointestinal intolerance. With regard to vitamin D supplementation, it is unclear whether standard vitamin D (i.e., ergocalciferol) or a vitamin D metabolite is better. Currently, most clinicians would use a vitamin D metabolite, such as calcitriol or dihydrotachysterol. This obviates concern of inadequate hydroxylation by proximal tubule mitochondria and reduces the risk of prolonged hypercalcemia because of the shorter half-life of these metabolites. Vitamin D therapy improves the hypophosphatemia and lessens the risk of hyperparathyroidism. Supplemental calcium is indicated in those with hypocalcemia after supplemental vitamin D has been started.

Hyperaminoaciduria, glucosuria, proteinuria, and hyperuricosuria usually do not lead to clinical symptoms and do not require specific treatment. Carnitine supplementation has been utilized in patients with Fanconi syndrome to improve muscle function and lipid profiles (61). Urinary carnitine is incompletely reabsorbed in patients with Fanconi syndrome, leading to both low plasma and muscle levels of carnitine (173).

Despite correction of all of these metabolic factors, some patients continue to grow poorly, especially those with cystinosis. Supplemental growth hormone has been used successfully in a few such patients. Although there is concern that growth hormone therapy may hasten renal failure, growth hormone therapy in children with renal failure from a variety of causes does not appear to worsen their renal function (174).

REFERENCES

1. de Toni G. Remarks on the relations between renal rickets (renal dwarfism) and renal diabetes. *Acta Paediatr* 1933;16:479–484.
2. Debré R, Marie J, Cléret F, et al. Rachitisme tardif coexistánt avec une nephrite chronique et une glycosurie. *Arch Med Enf* 1934;37:597–606.
3. Fanconi G. Die nicht diabetischen glykosurien und hyperglykamien des alterm kindes. *Jahrb Kinderheikld* 193;133:257–300.
4. Rosenberg LE, Segal S. Maleic acid-induced inhibition of amino acid transport in rat kidney. *Biochem J* 1964;92:345–352.
5. Norden AGW, Lapsley M, Igarashi T, et al. Urinary megalin deficiency implicates abnormal tubular endocytic function in Fanconi syndrome. *J Am Soc Nephrol* 2002;13:125–133.
6. Kramer HJ, Gonick HC. Experimental Fanconi syndrome. I. Effect of maleic acid on renal cortical Na-K-ATPase activity and ATP levels. *J Lab Clin Med* 1970;76:799–808.
7. Eiam-Ong S, Spohn M, Kurtzman NA, Sabatini S. Insight into the biochemical mechanism of maleic acid-induced Fanconi syndrome. *Kidney Int* 1995;48:1542–1548.
8. Szczepanska M, Angielski S. Prevention of maleate-induced tubular dysfunction by acetoacetate. *Am J Physiol* 1980;239:F50–F56.
9. Bergeron M, Mayers P, Brown D. Specific effect of maleate on an apical membrane glycoprotein (gp330) in the proximal tubule of the rat. *Am J Physiol* 1996;271:F908–F916.
10. Gonick HC, Indraprasit S, Rosen VJ, et al. Experimental Fanconi syndrome: III. Effect of cadmium on renal tubular function, the ATP-Na-K-ATPase transport system and renal tubular ultrastructure. *Min Electro Metab* 1980;3:21–35.
11. van Studnitz W, Haeger-Aronsen B. Urinary excretion of amino acids in lead poisoned rabbits. *Acta Pharmacol Toxicol* 1962;19:35–42.
12. Goyer RA. The renal tubule in lead poisoning: I. Mitochondrial swelling and aminoaciduria. *Lab Invest* 1968;19:712–777.
13. Gyrd-Hansen N, Helleberg A. Methoxyethyl mercury toxicity in pigs: kidney functions and mercury distribution. *Acta Pharmacol Toxicol* 1976;38:229–240.
14. Nomiyama K, Foulkes EC. Some effects of uranyl acetate on proximal tubular functions in rabbit kidney. *Toxicol Appl Pharmacol* 1968;13:89–98.
15. Lindquist RR, Fellers FX. Degraded tetracycline nephropathy: functions, morphologic and histochemical observations. *Lab Invest* 1966;15:864–876.
16. DuBuy HG, Showacre JL. Selective localization of tetracycline in mitochondria of living cells. *Science* 1961;133:196–197.
17. Foreman JW, Bowring MA, Lee J, et al. Effect of cystine dimethylester on renal solute handling and isolated renal tubule transport in the rat: a new model of the Fanconi syndrome. *Metabolism* 1987;36:1185–1191.
18. Coor C, Salmon R, Quigly R, et al. Role of adenosine triphosphate (ATP) and Na, K ATPase in the inhibition of proximal tubule transport with intracellular cystine loading. *J Clin Invest* 1991;87:955–961.
19. Foreman JW, Benson L. Effect of cystine loading on substrate oxidation by rat renal tubules. *Pediatr Nephrol* 1990;4:236–239.
20. Roth KS, Carter BE, Higgins ES. Succinylacetone effects on renal tubular phosphate metabolism: A new model for experimental Fanconi syndrome. *Proc Soc Exp Biol Med* 1991;196:428–431.
21. Spencer PD, Medow MS, Moses LC, et al. Effects of succinylacetone on the uptake of sugars and amino acids by brush border vesicles. *Kidney Int* 1988;34:671–677.

22. Bovee KC, Segal S. Canine models of human renal transport disorders. In: Hommes FA, ed. *Models for the study the inborn errors of metabolism.* Amsterdam: Elsevier, 1979.
23. Bovee KC, Joyce T, Reynolds R, et al. The Fanconi syndrome in Basenji dogs: a new model for renal transport defects. *Science* 1978;201:1129–1131.
24. Kruse K, Kracht U, Gopfert G. Renal threshold phosphate concentration. *Arch Dis Child* 1982;57:217–233.
25. Brodehl J, Kruse A, Hoyer PF. Assessment of maximal tubular phosphate reabsorption: comparison of direct measurement with the nomogram of Bijvoet. *Pediatr Nephrol* 1988;2:183–189.
26. Clarke BL, Wynne AG, Wilson DM, et al. Osteomalacia associated with adult Fanconi's syndrome: clinical and diagnostic features. *Clin Endocrinol* 1995;43:479–490.
27. Tolaymat A, Sakarcan A, Neiberger R. Idiopathic Fanconi syndrome in a family. Part I. Clinical aspects. *J Am Soc Nephrol* 1992;2:1310–1317.
28. Chesney RW, Rosen JF, Hamstra AJ, et al. Serum 1,25-dihydroxyvitamin D levels in normal children and in vitamin D disorders. *Am J Dis Child* 1980;134:135–139.
29. Tieder M, Arie R, Modai D, et al. Elevated serum 1,25-dihydroxyvitamin D concentrations in siblings with primary Fanconi's syndrome. *N Engl J Med* 1988;319:845–849.
30. Brewer ED, Tsai HC, Morris RC. Evidence for impairment of metabolism of 25-hydroxyvitamin D_3 in children with Fanconi syndrome. *Clin Res* 1976;24:154A.
31. Brodehl J. Tubular Fanconi syndrome with bone involvement. In: Bickel H, Stern J, eds. *Inborn errors of calcium and bone metabolism.* Lancaster, United Kingdom: MTP Press, 1976;191–213.
32. O'Regan S, Mongeau J-G, Robitaille PO. A patient with cystinosis presenting with features of Bartter's syndrome. *Acta Paediatr Belg* 1980;33:51–52.
33. Brodehl J, Hagge W, Gellissen K. die Veränderungen der nierenfunktion bei der cystinose. Teil 1: Die Inulin-, PAH-, und elektrolyt-clearance in verschiedenen stadien der erkrankung. *Ann Paediatr (Basel)* 1965;205:131–154.
34. Haffner D, Weinfurth A, Seidel C, et al. Body growth in primary de Toni-Debre-Fanconi syndrome. *Pediatr Nephrol* 1997;11:40–45.
35. Black J, Stapleton FB, Roy S, et al. Varied types of urinary calculi in a patient with cystinosis without renal tubular acidosis. *Pediatrics* 1986;78:295–297.
36. Waldmann TA, Strober W, Mogielnicki RP. The renal handling of low molecular weight proteins. II. Disorders of serum proteins. Catabolism in patients with tubular proteinuria, the nephrotic syndrome of uremia. *J Clin Invest* 1972;51:2162–2174.
37. Schneider JA, Katz B, Melles RB. Update on nephropathic cystinosis. *Pediatr Nephrol* 1990;4:645–653.
38. Schneider JA, Wong V, Bradley KH, et al. Biochemical comparisons of the adult and childhood forms of cystinosis. *N Engl J Med* 1968;279:1253–1257.
39. Brubaker RF, Wong VG, Schulman JD, et al. Benign cystinosis: the clinical, biochemical, and morphological findings in a family with two affected siblings. *Am J Med* 1970;49: 546–550.
40. Schulman JD. Cystine storage disease: investigations at the cellular and subcellular levels. In: Carson NAJ, Raine DN, eds. *Inherited disorders of sulphur metabolism.* Edinburgh: Churchill Livingstone, 1971:123–140.
41. Goldman H, Scriver CR, Aaron K, et al. Adolescent cystinosis: comparisons with infantile and adult forms. *Pediatrics* 1971;47:979–988.
42. Gahl WA, Tietz F, Bashan N, et al. Defective cystine exodus from isolated lysosome rich fractions of cystinotic leukocytes. *J Biol Chem* 1982;257:9570–9575.
43. Town M, Jean G, Cherqui S, et al. A novel gene encoding an integral membrane protein is mutated in nephropathic cystinosis. *Nat Genet* 1998;18:319–324.
44. Kalatzis V, Cherqui S, Antignac C, Gasnier B. Cystinosin, the protein defective in cystinosis, is a H^+-driven lysosomal cystine transporter. *EMBO J* 2001;20:5940–5949.
45. Greene AA, Clark KF, Smith ML, Schneider JA. Cystine exodus from normal leukocytes is stimulated by MgATP. *Biochem J* 1987;246:547–549.
46. Thoene JG, Oshima RG, Ritchie DG, et al. Cystinotic fibroblasts accumulate cystine from intracellular protein degradation. *Proc Natl Acad Sci U S A* 1977;74:4505–4507.
47. Scarlett L, Lloyd JB. Mechanism of cystine reaccumulation by cystinotic fibroblasts in vitro. *Biosci Rep* 1990;10:225–229.
48. Tietz F, Bradley KH, Schulman JD. Enzymatic reduction of cystine by subcellular fractions of cultured and peripheral leukocytes from normal and cystinotic individuals. *Pediatr Res* 1972;6:649–658.
49. Anikster Y, Lucero C, Guo J, et al. Ocular nonnephropathic cystinosis: clinical, biochemical, and molecular correlations. *Pediatr Res* 2000;47:17–23.
50. Attard M, Jean G, Forestier, L et al. Severity of phenotype in cystinosis varies with mutations in the CTNS gene: predicted effect on the model of cystinosin. *Human Molec Genet* 1999;8:2507–2514.
51. Foreman JW, Benson LL, Wellons M, et al. Metabolic studies of rat renal tubule cells loaded with cystine: the dimethylester model of cystinosis. *J Am Soc Nephrol* 1995;6:269–272.
52. Jonas AJ, Conley SB, Marshall R, et al. Nephropathic cystinosis with central nervous system involvement. *Am J Med* 1987;83:966–970.
53. Vogel DG, Malezadeh MH, Cornford ME, et al. Central nervous system involvement in nephropathic cystinosis. *J Neuropathol Exp Neurol* 1990;49:591–599.
54. Schneider JA, Verroust FM, Kroll WA, et al. Prenatal diagnosis of cystinosis. *N Engl J Med* 1974;290:878–882.
55. Broyer M, Guillot M, Gubler MC, et al. Infantile cystinosis: a re-appraisal of early and late symptoms. *Adv Nephrol* 1981;11:137–166.
56. Theodoropoulos DS, Shawker TH, Heinreichs C, Gahl WA. Medullary nephrocalcinosis in nephropathic cystinosis. *Pediatr Nephrol* 1995;9:412–418.
57. Gahl WA, Schneider JA, Thoene JG, et al. Course of nephropathic cystinosis after 10 years. *J Pediatr* 1986;109:605–608.
58. Wilson DP, Jelley D, Stratton R, et al. Nephropathic cystinosis: improved linear growth after treatment with recombinant growth hormone. *J Pediatr* 1989;115:758–761.
59. Gahl WA, Reed GF, Thoene JG, et al. Cysteamine therapy for children with nephropathic cystinosis. *N Engl J Med* 1987;316:971–977.

60. Spear GS. The pathology of the kidney. In: Schulman JD, ed. *Cystinosis*. Washington, DC: US Government Printing Office, 1973:37–53.
61. Gahl WA, Bernardini IM, Dlakas MC, et al. Muscle carnitine repletion by long-term carnitine supplementation in nephropathic cystinosis. *Pediatr Res* 1993;34:115–119.
62. Markello TC, Bernardini IM, Gahl WA. Improved renal function in children with cystinosis treated with cysteamine. *N Engl J Med* 1993;328:1157–1162.
63. Schneider JA, Clark KF, Greene AA, et al. Recent advances in the treatment of cystinosis. *J Inherit Metab Dis* 1995;18:387–397.
64. Fivush B, Green OC, Porter CC, et al. Pancreatic endocrine insufficiency in post-transplant cystinosis. *Am J Dis Child* 1987;141:1087–1089.
65. Nichols SL, Press GA, Schneider JA, et al. Cortical atrophy and cognitive performance in infantile nephropathic cystinosis. *Pediatr Neurol* 1990;6:379–381.
66. Sonies BC, Ekman EF, Andersson HC, et al. Swallowing dysfunction in nephropathic cystinosis. *N Engl J Med* 1990;323:565–570.
67. Anikster Y, Lacbawan F, Brantly M, et al. Pulmonary dysfunction in adults with nephropathic cystinosis. *Chest* 1995;119:394–401.
68. Boyer M, Tete MJ. Delayed complications of cystinosis: a review of 33 patients older than 18 years. *Anal Pediatric* 1995;42:635.
69. Tyfield L, Reichardt J, Fridovich-Keil J, et al. Classical galactosemia and mutations at the galactose-1-uridyl transferase (GALT) gene. *Hum Mutat* 1999;13:417–430.
70. Levy HL, Sepe SJ, Shih VE, et al. Sepsis due to *Escherichia coli* in neonates with galactosemia. *N Engl J Med* 1977;297:828–825.
71. Dahlquist A, Svenningsen NW. Galactose in the urine of newborn infants. *J Pediatr* 1969;75:454–462.
72. Haworth JC, MacDonald MS. Reducing sugars in urine and blood of premature babies. *Arch Dis Child* 1957;32:417–421.
73. Hall WK, Cravey CE, Chen PT, et al. An evaluation of galactosuria. *J Pediatr* 1970;77:625–630.
74. Rosenberg L, Weinberg A, Segal S. The effect of high galactose diets on urinary excretion of amino acids in the rat. *Biochim Biophys Acta* 1961;48:500–505.
75. Fox M, Thier S, Rosenberg L, et al. Impaired renal tubular function induced by sugar infusion in man. *J Clin Endocrinol Metab* 1964;24:1318–1327.
76. Thier S, Fox M, Rosenberg L, et al. Hexose inhibition of amino acid uptake in the rat-kidney-cortex slice. *Biochim Biophysics Acta* 1964;93:106–115.
77. Waggoner DD, Buist NRM, Donnel GN. Long term prognosis in galactosemia: results in a survey of 350 cases. *J Inherit Metab Dis* 1990;13:802–818.
78. Odievre M, Gentil C, Gautier M, et al. Hereditary fructose intolerance in childhood. *Am J Dis Child* 1978;132:605–608.
79. Ali M, Rellos P, Cox T. Hereditary fructose intolerance. *J Med Genet* 1998;35:353–365.
80. Morris RC Jr. An experimental renal acidification defect in patients with hereditary fructose intolerance: I. Its resemblance to renal tubular acidosis. *J Clin Invest* 1967;47:1389–1398.
81. Morris RC Jr. An experimental renal acidification defect in patients with hereditary fructose intolerance. II. Its distinction from classic renal tubular acidosis and its resemblance to the renal acidification defect associated with the Fanconi syndrome of children with cystinosis. *J Clin Invest* 1968;47:1648–1663.
82. Richardson RMA, Little JA, Pattern RL, et al. Pathogenesis of acidosis in hereditary fructose intolerance. *Metabolism* 1979;28:1133–1138.
83. Levin B, Snodgrass GJAI, Oberholzer VG, et al. Fructosemia. Observations in seven cases. *Am J Med* 1968;45:826–838.
84. Burch HB, Lowry OH, Meinhardt L, et al. Effect of fructose, dihydroxyacetone, glycerol and glucose on metabolites and related compounds in the liver and kidney. *J Biol Chem* 1970;245:2092–2102.
85. Morris RC Jr, Nigon K, Reed EB. Evidence that depletion of inorganic phosphate determines the severity of the disturbance of adenine nucleotide metabolism in the liver and renal cortex of the cortex of the fructose-loaded rat. *J Clin Invest* 1978;61:209–220.
86. Bade JC, Zelder O, Rumpelt HF, et al. Depletion of liver adenine phosphates and metabolic effects of intravenous infusion of fructose or sorbitol in man and in the rat. *Eur J Clin Invest* 1973;3:436–441.
87. Hultman E, Nilsson LH, Sahlin K. Adenine nucleotide content of human liver. Normal values and fructose induced depletion. *Scand J Clin Lab Invest* 1975;35:245–251.
88. Fanconi G, Bickel H. Die chronische Aminoacidurie (Aminosaurediabetes oder nephrotisch-glukosurischer Zwergwuchs) bei de Glykogenose und der Cystinkrankheit. *Helv Paediatr Acta* 1949;4:359–366.
89. Brodehl J, Gelissen K, Hagge W. The Fanconi syndrome in hepato-renal glycogen storage disease. In: Peters G, Roch-Ramel F, eds. *Progress in nephrology*. Berlin: Springer Verlag, 1969;241–243.
90. Hurvitz H, Elpeleg ON, Barash V, et al. Glycogen storage disease, Fanconi nephropathy, abnormal galactose metabolism and mitochondrial myopathy. *Eur J Pediatr* 1989;149:48–51.
91. Sanjad SA, Kaddoura RE, Nazer HM, et al. Fanconi's syndrome with hepatorenal glycogenosis associated with phosphorylase b kinase deficiency. *Am J Dis Child* 1993;147:957–959.
92. Chen Y-T, Scheinman JI, Park HK, et al. Amelioration of proximal renal tubular dysfunction in type I glycogen storage disease with dietary therapy. *N Engl J Med* 1990;323:590–593.
93. Santer R, Schneppenheim R, Dombrowski A, et al. Mutations in GLUT2, the gene for the liver-type glucose transporter, in patients with Fanconi-Bickel syndrome. *Nat Genet* 1997;17:324–326.
94. Lee PJ, van't Hoff WG, Leonard JV. Catch-up growth in Fanconi-Bickel syndrome with uncooked cornstarch. *J Inherit Metab Dis* 1995;18:153–156.
95. Holme E, Lindstedt S. Diagnosis and management of tyrosinemia type I. *Curr Opin Pediatr* 1995;6:726–732.
96. Kvittingen EA, Halvorsen S, Jellum E. Deficient fumarylacetoacetate funarylhydrolase activity in lymphocytes and fibroblasts from patient with hereditary tyrosinemia. *Pediatr Res* 1983;14:541–544.
97. Phaneuf D, Labelle Y, Berube D, et al. Cloning and expression of the cDNA encoding human fumarylacetoacetate

hydrolase, the enzyme deficient in hereditary tyrosinemia: assignment of the gene to chromosome 15. *Am J Hum Genet* 1991;48:525–535.
98. Rootwelt H, Berger R, Gray G, et al. Novel splice, missense, and nonsense mutations in the fumarylacetoacetase gene causing tyrosinemia type I. *Am J Hum Genet* 1994;55:653–658.
99. Fairney A, Francis D, Ersser RS, et al. Diagnosis and treatment of tyrosinosis. *Arch Dis Child* 1968;43:540–547.
100. Hosteter MK, Levy HL, Winter HS, et al. Evidence for liver disease preceding amino acid abnormalities in hereditary tyrosinemia. *N Engl J Med* 1983;308:1265–1267.
101. Shoemaker LR, Strife CF, Balistreri WF, et al. Rapid improvement of the renal tubular dysfunction associated with tyrosinemia after hepatic replacement. *Pediatrics* 1992;89:251–255.
102. Scheinberg IH, Sternlieb I. *Wilson's disease*. Philadelphia: WB Saunders, 1984.
103. Kayser B. Ueber einen fall von angeborener grünlieber verfärbung der cornea. *Klin Monatsbl Augenheilkd* 1902;40:22–25.
104. Fleischer B. Die periphere braun-grünliche hornhautverfärbung der cornea. allgemeinerkrankung. *Münch Med Wochenschr* 1909;56:1120–1123.
105. Bull PC, Thomas GR, Rommens JM, et al. The Wilson's gene. *Nat Genet* 1993;5:327–337.
106. Reynolds ES, Tannen RL, Tyler HR. The renal lesion in Wilson's disease. *Am J Med* 1966;40:518–537.
107. Leu ML, Strickland GT, Gutman RA. The renal lesion on Wilson's disease: response to penicillamine therapy. *Am J Med Sci* 1970;260:381–398.
108. Mahoney JP, Sandberg AA, Gabler CJ, et al. Uric acid metabolism in hepatolenticular degeneration. *Proc Soc Exp Biol Med* 1955;88:427–430.
109. Litin RB, Randall RV, Goldstein NP, et al. Hypercalciuria in hepatolenticular degeneration (Wilson's disease). *Am J Med Sci* 1959;238:614–620.
110. Fulop M, Sternlieb I, Scheinberg IM. Defective urinary acidification in Wilson's disease. *Ann Intern Med* 1968;68:770–777.
111. Brewer GJ. Practical recommendations and new therapies for Wilson's disease. *Drugs* 1995;50:240–249.
112. Ede RJ, Nazer H, Mowat AP, et al. Wilson's disease: clinical presentation and use of prognostic index. *Gut* 1986;27:1377–1381.
113. Charnas LR, Bernardini I, Rader D, et al. Clinical and laboratory findings in the oculocerebrorenal syndrome of Lowe, with special reference to growth and renal function. *N Engl J Med* 1991;324:1318–1325.
114. Lowe CU, Terrey M, MacLachlan EA. Organic-aciduria, decreased renal ammonia production, hydrophthalmos and mental retardation: a clinical entity. *Am J Dis Child* 1952;83:164–184.
115. Silver DN, Lewis RA, Nussbaum RL. Mapping the Lowe oculocerebrorenal syndrome to Xq24-q26 by use of restriction fragment length polymorphisms. *J Clin Invest* 1987;79:282–285.
116. Zhang W, Jefferson AM, Auethavekiat V, et al. The protein deficient in Lowe's syndrome is a phosphatidylinositol-4,5-bisphosphate 5-phosphatase. *Proc Natl Acad Sci U S A* 1995;92:4853–4856.
117. Olivos-Glander IM, Janne PA, Nussbaum RL. The oculocerebrorenal syndrome gene product is a 105-kD protein localized to the Golgi complex. *Am J Hum Genet* 1995;57:817–823.
118. Svorc I, Masopust I, Komarkowa A, et al. Oculo-cerebro-renal syndrome in a female child. *Am J Dis Child* 1967;114:186–190.
119. Sagel I, Ores RO, Yuceoglu AM. Renal function and morphology in a girl with oculo-cerebro-renal syndrome. *J Pediatr* 1970;77:124–127.
120. Brown N, Gardner RJM. Lowe syndrome: identification of the carrier state. *Birth Defects Orig Artic Ser* 1976;12:579–591.
121. Witzleben CL, Schoen EJ, Tu WE, et al. Progressive morphologic renal changes in the oculo-cerebro-renal syndrome of Lowe. *Am J Med* 1968;44:319–324.
122. Ores RP. Renal changes in oculo-cerebro-renal syndrome of Lowe. *Arch Pathol* 1970;89:221–225.
123. Thakker RV. Pathogenesis of Dent's disease and related syndromes of X-linked nephrolithiasis. *Kidney Int* 2000;57:787–793.
124. Scheinman SJ. X-linked hypercalciuric nephrolithiasis: clinical syndromes and chloride channel mutations. *Kidney Int* 1998;53:3–17.
125. Wang SS, Devuyst O, Courtoy PJ, et al. Mice lacking renal chloride channel, ClC-5, are a model for Dent's disease, a nephrolithiasis disorder associated with defective receptor-mediated endocytosis. *Hum Mol Genet* 2000;9:2937–2945.
126. Biervliet JPAM, Bruinvis L, Ketting D, et al. Hereditary mitochondrial myopathy with lactic acidemia, a de Toni-Fanconi-Debre syndrome, and a defective respiratory chain in voluntary striated muscle. *Pediatr Res* 1977;11:1088–1093.
127. DiMauro S, Mendell JR, Sahenk Z, et al. Fatal infantile mitochondrial myopathy and renal dysfunctions due to cytochrome-c-oxidase deficiency. *Neurology* 1980;30:795–803.
128. Heiman-Patterson TD, Bonilla E, DiMauro S, et al. Cytochrome-c-oxidase deficiency in a floppy infant. *Neurology* 1982;32:898–900.
129. Johns DR. Mitochondrial DNA and disease. *N Engl J Med* 1995;333:638–644.
130. Niaudet P, Rotig A. Renal involvement in mitochondrial cytopathies. *Pediatr Nephrol* 1996;10:368–373.
131. Hammans SR, Morgan-Hughes AJ. Mitochondrial myopathies: clinical features, investigation, treatment, and genetic counseling. In: Schapire AVH, DiMauro S, eds. *Mitochondrial disorders in neurology*. Oxford, United Kingdom: Butterworth Heinemann, 1996;49–74.
132. Friedman AL, Trygstad CW, Chesney RW. Autosomal dominant Fanconi syndrome with early renal failure. *Am J Clin Genet* 1978;2:225–232.
133. Christiaens L, Biserte G, Farriaux J, et al. La forme idiopathique du syndrome de Toni-Debre-Fanconi. *Semin Hop Paris Ann Pediatr* 1965;41:49–62.
134. Neimann N, Pierson M, Marchal C, et al. Nephropathie familiale glomerulotubulaire avec syndrome de Toni-Fanconi. *Arch Fr Pediatr* 1968;25:43–69.
135. Hunt DD, Stearns G, McKinley JB, et al. Long-term study of a family with the Fanconi syndrome without cystinosis (de Toni-Debre-Fanconi syndrome). *Am J Med* 1966;40:492–510.

136. Chesney RW, Kaplan BS, Teitel D, et al. Metabolic abnormalities in the idiopathic Fanconi syndrome: studies of carbohydrate metabolism in two patients. *Pediatrics* 1981;67:113–118.
137. Aperia A, Bergqvist G, Linne T, et al. Familial Fanconi syndrome with malabsorption and galactose intolerance, normal kinase and transferase activity. *Acta Paediatr Scand* 1981;70:527–533.
138. Deal JE, Barratt TM, Dillon MJ. Fanconi syndrome, ichthyosis, dysmorphism, jaundice and diarrhea: a new syndrome. *Pediatr Nephrol* 1990;4:308–313.
139. Patrick A, Cameron JS, Ogg CS. A family with a dominant form of idiopathic Fanconi syndrome leading to renal failure in adult life. *Clin Nephrol* 1981;16:289–292.
140. Briggs WA, Kominami N, Wilson RE, et al. Kidney transplantation in Fanconi syndrome. *N Engl J Med* 1972;286:25.
141. Chisolm JJ, Harrison HC, Eberlein WE, et al. Aminoaciduria, hypophosphatemia and rickets in lead poisoning. *Am J Dis Child* 1955;89:159–168.
142. Goyer RA, Tsuchuja K, Leonard DL, et al. Aminoaciduria in Japanese workers in the lead and cadmium industries. *Am J Clin Pathol* 1972;57:635–642.
143. Galle P, Morel-Maroger L. Les lesions renales du saturnisme humain et experimental. *Nephron* 1965;2:273–286.
144. Kazantzis G, Glynn FV, Spowage JS, et al. Renal tubular malfunction and pulmonary emphysema in cadmium pigment workers. *QJM* 1963;32:165–192.
145. Cleveland WW, Adams WC, Mann JB, et al. Acquired Fanconi syndrome following degraded tetracycline. *J Pediatr* 1965;66:333–342.
146. Brodehl J, Gellisson K, Hagge W, et al. Reversibles renales Fanconi-Syndrome durch toxisches abbauprodukt des tetrazyklins. *Helv Paediatr Acta* 1968;23:373–383.
147. Otten J, Vis HL. Acute reversible renal tubular dysfunction following intoxication with methyl-3-chromone. *J Pediatr* 1968;73:422–425.
148. Butler HE, Morgan JM, Smythe CM. Mercaptopurine and acquired tubular dysfunction in adult nephrosis. *Arch Intern Med* 1965;116:853–856.
149. Moss AH, Gabow PA, Kaehny WD, et al. Fanconi syndrome and distal renal tubular acidosis after glue sniffing. *Ann Intern Med* 1980;92:69–70.
150. Izumotani T, Ishimura E, Tsumura K, et al. An adult case of Fanconi syndrome due to a mixture of Chinese crude drugs. *Nephron* 1993;65:137–140.
151. Lande MB, Kim MS, Bartlett C, et al. Reversible Fanconi syndrome associated with valproate therapy. *J Pediatr* 1993;123:320–322.
152. Rago RP, Miles JM, Sufit RL, et al. Suramin-induced weakness from hypophosphatemia and mitochondrial myopathy. *Cancer* 1994;73:1954–1959.
153. Spencer AG, Granglen GT. Gross aminoaciduria following a Lysol burn. *Lancet* 1952;1:190–192.
154. Russo JC, Adelman RD. Gentamicin-induced Fanconi syndrome. *J Pediatr* 1980;96:151–153.
155. Schein P, Hahn R, Gordon P, et al. Streptozotocin for malignant insulinomas and carcinoid tumors. *Arch Intern Med* 1973;132:555–561.
156. Neelakantappa K, Gallo G, Lowenstein J. Ranitidine-associated interstitial nephritis and Fanconi syndrome. *Am J Kidney Dis* 1993;22:333–336.
157. Madias NE, Harrington JT. Platinum nephrotoxicity. *Am J Med* 1978;65:307–314.
158. Skinner R, Pearson ADJ, Price L, et al. Nephrotoxicity after ifosfamide. *Arch Dis Child* 1990;65:732–738.
159. Burk CD, Restaino I, Kaplan BS, et al. Ifosfamide-induced renal tubular dysfunction and rickets in children with Wilms tumor. *J Pediatr* 1990;117:331–335.
160. Goren M, Wright RK, Pratt CB, et al. Potentiation of ifosfamide neurotoxicity, hematoxicity, and tubular nephrotoxicity from prior cis-diamminedichloroplatinum (11) therapy. *Cancer Res* 1987;47:1457–1460.
161. Suarrez A, McDowell H, Niaudet P, et al. Long-term follow-up of ifosfamide renal toxicity in children treated for malignant mesenchymal tumors: an International Society of Pediatric Oncology report. *J Clin Oncol* 1991;9:2177–2182.
162. Raney B, Ensign LG, Foreman J, et al. Renal toxicity of ifosfamide in pilot regimens of the intergroup rhabdomyosarcoma study for patients with gross residual tumor. *Am J Pediatr Hematol Oncol* 1994;16:286–295.
163. Zamlauski-Tucker MJ, Morris ME, Springate JE. Ifosfamide metabolite chloroacetaldehyde causes Fanconi syndrome in the perfused rat kidney. *Toxicol Appl Pharmacol* 1994;129:170–175.
164. Solomon A, Weiss DT, Kattine AA. Nephrotoxic potential of Bence Jones proteins. *N Engl J Med* 1991;324:1845–1857.
165. Smithline N, Kassirer JP, Cohen JJ. Light-chain nephropathy: renal tubular dysfunction associated with light-chain proteinuria. *N Engl J Med* 1976;294:71–74.
166. Shearn MA, Tu WH. Nephrogenic diabetes insipidus and other defects in renal tubular function in Sjögren syndrome. *Am J Med* 1965;39:312–318.
167. Finkel PN, Kronenberg K, Pesce AJ, et al. Adult Fanconi syndrome, amyloidosis and marked light chain proteinuria. *Nephron* 1973;10:124.
168. Aucouturier P, Bauwens M, Khamlichi AA, et al. Monoclonal lg L chain V domain fragment crystallization in myeloma-associated Fanconi's syndrome. *J Immunol* 1993;150:3561–3568.
169. Leehey DJ, Ing T, Daugirdas JT. Fanconi syndrome associated with a non-ossifying fibroma of bone. *Am J Med* 1985;78:708–710.
170. McVicar M, Exeni R, Susin M. Nephrotic syndrome and multiple tubular defects in children: an early sign of focal segmental glomerulosclerosis. *J Pediatr* 1980;97:918–922.
171. Friedman AL, Chesney R. Fanconi's syndrome in renal transplantation. *Am J Nephrol* 1981;1:145–147.
172. Better OS. Tubular dysfunction following kidney transplantation. *Nephron* 1980;25:209–213.
173. Bernardini I, Rizzo WB, Dalaks M, et al. Plasma and muscle free carnitine deficiency due to renal Fanconi syndrome. *J Clin Invest* 1985;75:1124–1130.
174. Tonshoff B, Tonshoff C, Mehls O, et al. Growth hormone treatment in children with preterminal chronic renal failure: no adverse effect on glomerular filtration rate. *Eur J Pediatr* 1992;151:601–607.

42

PRIMARY HYPEROXALURIA

PIERRE COCHAT
LAURE B. D. E. COLLARD

First report on oxalosis by Lepoutre, reprinted from *Journal d'Urologie Médicale et Chirurgicale* 1927;20:424, with permission.

> *Calculs multiples chez un enfant; infiltration du parenchyme rénal par des dépôts cristallins.* — Chez un enfant de quatre ans et demi, opéré ou soigné pour calculs multiples de l'urètre, de l'uretère et des deux reins, une biopsie fait découvrir un parenchyme rénal bourré de concrétions cristallines d'oxalate de chaux. Ce cas réalise en clinique l'expérience d'Ebstein et Nicolaier, qui, faisant ingérer de l'oxamide à des chiens, voyaient de développer des calculs urinaires et de multiples formations cristallines dans le parenchyme rénal.

Primary hyperoxaluria (PH) results from endogenous overproduction of oxalic acid, as opposed to secondary hyperoxaluria, which is attributable to increased intestinal absorption or excessive intake of oxalate. Such derangement leads to accumulation of oxalate within the body. The main target organ is the kidney because oxalate cannot be metabolized and is excreted in the urine, leading to nephrocalcinosis, recurrent urolithiasis, and subsequent renal impairment. Hyperoxaluria, the hallmark of any kind of PH, is associated with increased urinary excretion of either glycolate in PH type 1 (PH1) or L-glycerate in PH type 2 (PH2).

OXALATE METABOLISM

Oxalate is a poorly soluble end-product of the metabolism of a number of amino acids, particularly glycine, and of other compounds such as sugars and ascorbic acid (Fig. 42.1). The immediate precursors of oxalate are glyoxylate and glycolate. The main site of synthesis of glyoxylate and oxalate is the liver peroxisome, which can also detoxify glyoxylate by reconversion into glycine, catalyzed by alanine:glyoxylate aminotransferase (AGT). In the cytosol, glyoxylate can be converted into oxalate by lactic acid dehydrogenase. It can also be converted into glycolate by glyoxylate reductase (GR) and into glycine by glutamate:glyoxylate aminotransferase. Glycolate can also be formed from hydroxypyruvate, a catabolite of glucose and fructose. Hydroxypyruvate can be converted into L-glycerate by lactic acid dehydrogenase, and into D-glycerate by hydroxypyruvate reductase (HPR), which also has a GR activity.

PRIMARY HYPEROXALURIA TYPE 1

PH1, the most common form of PH, is an autosomal recessive disorder caused by the functional defect of the hepatic, peroxisomal, pyridoxal phosphate–dependent enzyme AGT, the protein product of a gene that has been identified on chromosome 2q37.3. The disease occurs because AGT activity is undetectable or because AGT is mistargeted to mitochondria, which may explain clinical and enzymatic heterogeneity.

Metabolic Derangement

PH1 is due to a deficiency of the liver-specific pyridoxal phosphate–dependent enzyme AGT (EC 2.6.1.44, 392 amino acids, 43 kDa) (Fig. 42.1) (1). The resulting decreased transamination of glyoxylate into glycine leads to subsequent increase in its oxidation to oxalate, a poorly soluble end-product. In patients with a presumptive diagnosis of PH, 10 to 30% are identified as non-PH1 because AGT enzymatic activity and immunoreactivity are normal (2). Among PH1 patients, 75% have undetectable enzyme activity (*enz–*) and the majority of these also have no immunoreactive protein (cross-reacting material, *crm–*). In the rare *enz–/crm+* PH1 patients, a catalytically inactive but immunoreactive AGT is found within the peroxisomes. The remaining PH1 patients have AGT activity in the range of 5 to 50% of the mean normal activity (*enz+*), and the level of immunoreactive protein parallels the level of enzyme activity (*crm+*) (2). In *enz+/crm+* patients, the disease is caused by a mistargeting of AGT: approximately 90% of the immunoreactive AGT is localized in the mitochondria instead of in the peroxisomes, where only 10% of the activity is found; almost all patients who are pyridoxine-responsive are in this group (3,4). Of interest, human hepatocyte AGT, which is

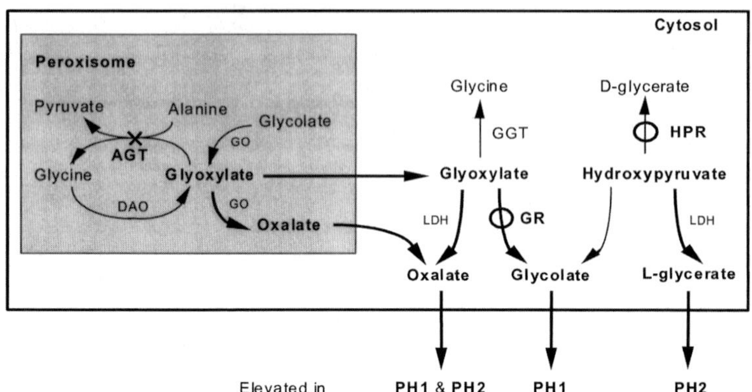

FIGURE 42.1. Human hepatocyte. Major reactions involved in oxalate, glyoxylate, and glycolate metabolism in the human hepatocyte. AGT, alanine:glyoxylate aminotransferase; DAO, D-amino oxidase; GGT, glutamate: glyoxylate aminotransferase; GO, glycolate oxidase; GR, glyoxylate reductase; HPR, hydroxypyruvate reductase; LDH, lactate dehydrogenase; PH1, primary hyperoxaluria type 1; PH2, primary hyperoxaluria type 2; X, metabolic block in PH1; O, metabolic block in PH2.

normally exclusively localized within the peroxisomes, is unable to function when diverted to the mitochondria, its normal localization in several other species (e.g., cat, dog, frog) (3). In addition, patients with a primary peroxisomal disorder (e.g., Zellweger syndrome) do not exhibit hyperoxaluria (5).

Different AGT crystal forms have been recently obtained for some polymorphic variants [AGT, AGT (P11L), AGT (P11L, I340M)] (6).

Genetics

PH1 is the most common form of PH (1:60,000 to 1:120,000 live births) (7,8). Due to autosomal recessive inheritance, it is much more frequent when parental consanguinity is present (9–11). Indeed, it is responsible for less than 0.5% of pediatric end-stage renal failure (ESRF) in Europe versus 13% in Tunisia (7).

Human liver AGT complementary DNA and genomic DNA have been cloned and sequenced; the normal AGT gene (*AGXT*) is a single copy gene, which maps to chromosome 2q37.3 (11 exons spanning approximately 10 kb) (2). Polymorphic variations have been identified in *AGXT* (2); the two best-studied polymorphic variants are those encoded by the major *AGXT* allele (80% frequency in the European and North American populations) and the minor *AGXT* allele, which has a frequency of 20%.

More than 40 mutations in the *AGXT* gene have been identified to date. However, some of them are more frequent and may play a role either in enzyme trafficking or in expression of a specific clinical or biochemical phenotype (12–16). The G630A mutation leading to a G170R substitution is found in one-third of European and North American patients and appears to act together with the P11L polymorphism leading to peroxisome-to-mitochondrion AGT mistargeting. Double heterozygous patients seem to present at a younger age and demonstrate a more aggressive disease. The T444C mutation is more frequent in the severe forms; the G630A mutation is more frequent in less severe cases (17). In addition, G630A mutation homozygotes have higher AGT residual activity (17). In any condition, the P11L polymorphism, which has a high allelic frequency (approximately 20%) plays an important role in determining the phenotypic manifestations of specific mutations (15).

DNA analysis among different ethnic groups has revealed the presence of specific mutations, founder effects, and phenotype-genotype correlations among North African, Japanese, Turkish, and Pakistani populations (2,18,19).

Prenatal diagnosis using a combination of linked polymorphism and detection of the two most common mutations has an accuracy of more than 99% and can be performed from chorionic villi or amniocytes according to gestational age (20).

Clinical Presentation

PH1 has four general clinical presentations: (a) a rare infantile form with early nephrocalcinosis and rapid kidney failure, (b) a rare late-onset form with occasional stone passage in late adulthood, (c) the most common form with recurrent urolithiasis and progressive renal failure leading to a diagnosis of PH1 in childhood or adolescence, and (d) a rare condition where PH1 is diagnosed after the prompt recurrence of the disease after kidney transplantation (7,21,22). In addition, some patients are asymptomatic, and PH1 may be discovered by family history.

Renal Involvement

PH1 presents with symptoms referable to the urinary tract in more than 90% of cases [e.g., loin pain, hematuria, urinary tract infection, passage of stones, evidence of nephrocalcinosis (Fig. 42.2), uremia, metabolic acidosis, growth delay, anemia]. Calculi—multiple, bilateral, and radiopaque—are composed of calcium oxalate. Nephrocalcinosis, best demonstrated by ultrasound, is evident on plain abdomen x-ray at an advanced stage. The median age at presentation is 5 years, ranging from birth to the sixth decade; ESRF is reached by the age of 25 years in one-half of patients (23). The infantile form of PH1 often presents as a life-threatening condition because of rapid progression to ESRF due to both early oxalate load and immature glomerular filtration rate (GFR); one-half of the patients experience ESRF at the time of diagnosis, and 80% develop ESRF by the age of 3 years (9).

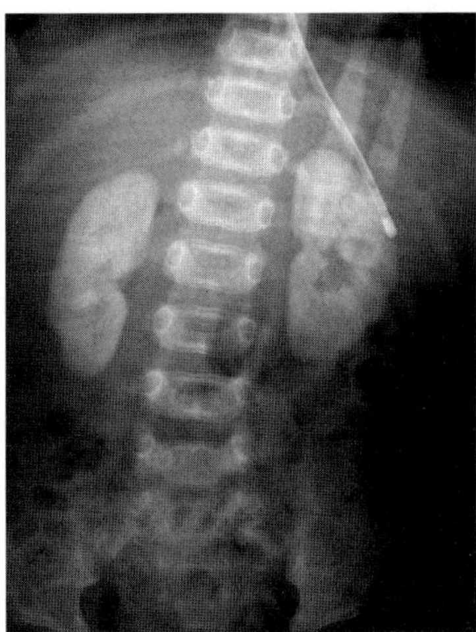

FIGURE 42.2. Plain abdomen x-ray in a 20-month-old primary hyperoxaluria type 1 boy: bilateral nephrocalcinosis, 13 months after starting hemodialysis (5 × 3/wk).

Extrarenal Involvement

When GFR falls to below 40 to 50 mL/min per 1.73 m^2, continued overproduction of oxalate by the liver along with reduced oxalate excretion by the kidneys leads to a critical saturation point for plasma oxalate (plasma oxalate concentration greater than 30 to 50 μmol/L) so that oxalate deposition occurs in many organs (24,25). Bone is the major compartment of the insoluble oxalate pool (Fig. 42.3), and bone oxalate content is higher (15 to 910 μmol oxalate per gram bony tissue) than that observed in ESRF patients without PH1 (2 to 9 μmol/g) (26). Calcium oxalate crystals accumulate first in the metaphyseal area and form characteristic, dense suprametaphyseal bands on x-ray (27). Later on, oxalate osteopathy leads to pain, erythropoietin-resistant anemia, and spontaneous fractures, sometimes in infancy (Fig. 42.4). Along with the skeleton, systemic involvement includes many organs because of progressive vascular lesions—heart (e.g., cardiomyopathy, arrhythmias, heart block), nerves (e.g., polyradiculoneuropathy, mononeuritis multiplex), joints (e.g., synovitis, chondrocalcinosis), skin (e.g., ulcerating calcium oxalate nodules, calcinosis cutis, livedo reticularis), soft tissues (e.g., peripheral gangrene), retina (e.g., flecked retinopathy, choroidal neovascularization), and other visceral lesions (e.g., intestinal infarction, hypothyroidism) (7,28–33).

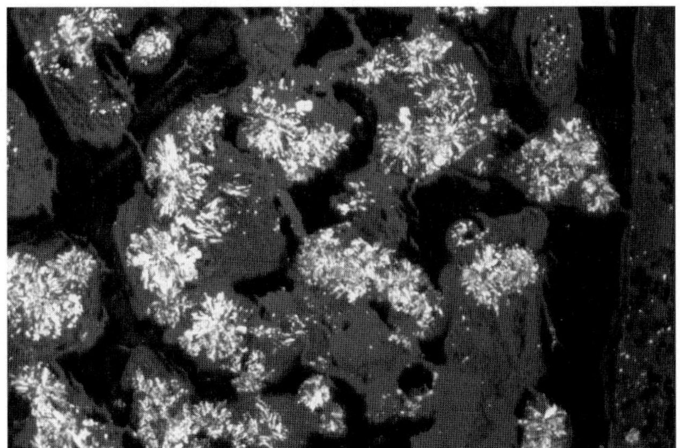

FIGURE 42.3. Bone histology from a 13-year-old girl with primary hyperoxaluria type 1 on hemodialysis for 2 years: oxalate crystals on polarized light microscopy.

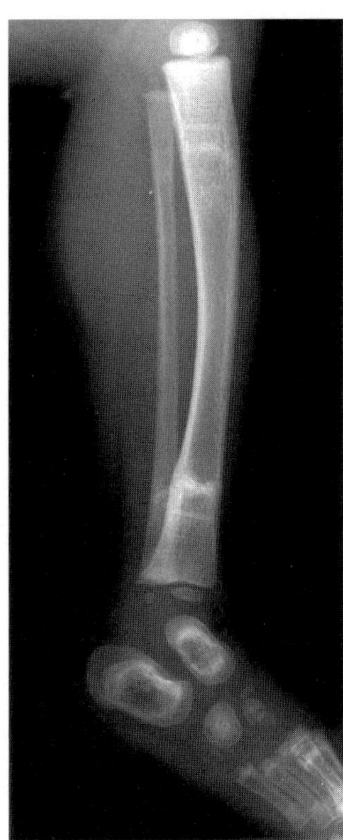

FIGURE 42.4. Spontaneous fracture of the left tibia in a 25-month-old boy on hemodialysis.

Systemic involvement, named *oxalosis*, is responsible for poor quality of life leading to both disability and severe complications. Indeed, PH1 is one of the most life-threatening hereditary renal diseases, mainly in developing countries where the mortality rate approaches 100% in the absence of adequate treatment (34).

Diagnosis

The combination of both clinical and radiologic presentation is a strong argument for PH1 in a large number of patients. In addition, family history may bring additional information (e.g., other affected siblings, parental consanguinity, and unexplained death in siblings) (34). Physicochemical investigation is of major interest in diagnosis, and infrared spectroscopy is helpful for the identification and the quantitative analysis of stones, showing calcium oxalate monohydrate crystals (type Ic whewellite, $CaC_2O_4.H_2O$) (35). Such crystals can also be identified in urine or biopsy

TABLE 42.1. PLASMA AND URINE CONCENTRATIONS OF OXALATE, GLYCOLATE, AND L-GLYCERATE: NORMAL VALUES

Urine	Oxalate per day	Child	<0.46 mmol/1.73 m^2
		Adult	<0.40 mmol/1.73 m^2
	Oxalate: creatinine	<1 yr	<0.15 mmol/mmol
		1–4 yr	<0.13 mmol/mmol
		5–12 yr	<0.07 mmol/mmol
		Adult	<0.08 mmol/mmol
	Glycolate per day	Child	<0.55 mmol/1.73 m^2
		Adult	<0.26 mmol/1.73 m^2
	Glycolate: creatinine	<1 yr	<0.07 mmol/mmol
		1–4 yr	<0.09 mmol/mmol
		5–12 yr	<0.05 mmol/mmol
		Adult	<0.04 mmol/mmol
	L-glycerate: creatinine	Child	<0.03 mmol/mmol
Plasma	Oxalate	Child	<7.40 μmol/L
		Adult	<5.40 μmol/L
	Oxalate: creatinine	Child	<0.19 μmol/μmol
		Adult	<0.06 μmol/μmol

Note: Oxalate (COOH-COOH): 1 mmol = 90 mg; glycolate (COOH-CH_2OH): 1 mmol = 76 mg.
From Barratt TM, Danpure CJ. Hyperoxaluria. In: Barratt TM, Avner ED, Harmon WE, eds. *Pediatric nephrology*, 4th ed. Baltimore: Williams & Wilkins, 1999:609–619; Leumann E, Hoppe B. The primary hyperoxalurias. *J Am Soc Nephrol* 2001;12:1986–1993; and Gaulier JM, Cochat P, Lardet G, et al. Serum oxalate microassay using chemiluminescence detection. *Kidney Int* 1997;52:1700–1703, with permission.

tissues (e.g., kidney, bone, marrow) by polarized light microscopy or infrared spectroscopy (36). Funduscopy may also show flecked retina as early as infancy. In patients with normal or significant residual renal function, concomitant hyperoxaluria and hyperglycoluria are indicative of PH1 (Table 42.1), but 20 to 30% of PH1 patients do not present with hyperglycoluria (37). In dialysis patients, the biochemical assessment may include plasma oxalate or glycolate to creatinine ratio, and oxalate or glycolate measurement in dialysate (34,35,22).

A definitive diagnosis requires assessments of AGT activity and immunoreactivity in hepatic tissue (from a freshly frozen liver biopsy specimen, minimum of 4 mg). Nevertheless, there is controversial information about the relationship between AGT activity and the severity of the disease (17). Liver biopsy is mandatory if liver transplantation is being considered (see below). In selected populations, a direct molecular diagnosis can be performed, such as the search for the I244T mutation in patients from Maghreb (Basmaison, *submitted*). However, in most clinical settings, the search for frequent mutations (G630A, T853C, G170R) cannot currently replace enzymology in the diagnosis of PH1 (34,38). Prenatal diagnosis can be performed from DNA obtained from chorionic villi (10 to 12 weeks' gestation) or amniocytes (13 to 17 weeks' gestation). It is based on either mutational analysis using polymerase chain reaction amplification, or linkage analysis using the various intragenic and extragenic polymorphisms; the latter is more generally applicable, provided DNA from the index case and parents is available (20). Such a procedure identifies normal, affected, and carrier fetuses. In the absence of identified mutations in an index case, the two most common mutations (G170R and I144T) can be checked (2). The detection of *AGXT* mutations using simplified reliable technology can be proposed to identify healthy carriers among family members, and sometimes for screening of polymorphisms in patients with nephrolithiasis (16).

Treatment and Prognosis

Supportive Treatment

Conservative measures should be started as soon as the diagnosis of PH1 has been made or even suspected. The aims are to decrease oxalate production and to increase the urinary solubility of calcium oxalate. The risk of stone formation is increased when urine oxalate exceeds 0.4 to 0.6 mmol/L, especially if urine calcium exceeds 4 mmol/L. Therefore, therapy should keep the concentrations of oxalate and calcium below these limits (39). This should be accomplished by maintaining a high fluid intake (greater than 2 L/m^2/day), sometimes requiring a nasogastric tube or gastrostomy in infants, complemented by administration of calcium-oxalate crystallization inhibitors. Citrate (potassium or sodium), 100 to 150 mg/kg/day in three to four divided doses (8,40,41), has been shown to be effective in PH1 patients. When it is not available, crystallization inhibition may be accomplished by sodium bicarbonate (aiming at keeping pH greater than or equal to 7), magnesium or orthophosphate (20 to 60 mg/kg body weight per day) administration (40). Diuretics require careful management: furosemide maintains a high urine output but increases the risk of calciuria, whereas the diuretic effect of hydrochlorothiazide is less marked but is associated with an appreciable decrease of calcium excretion. The combination of both loop agents and thiazides is recommended in most instances.

Restriction of dietary oxalate intake (e.g., beet roots, strawberries, rhubarb, spinach, coffee, tea, nuts) has very limited influence on the disease because dietary oxalate contributes very little to hyperoxaluria in PH (40). Calcium restriction is not recommended, because dietary calcium is required to bind oxalate and form insoluble calcium oxalate complexes in the gut. Vitamin C supplementation is not recommended because ascorbic acid is a precursor of oxalate. The effects of conservative measures can be assessed by serial determinations of crystalluria score and calcium oxalate supersaturation software (41,42).

Pyridoxine (cofactor of AGT, see Fig. 42.1) sensitivity is found in 10 to 40% of patients, so that it must be tested early at a daily dose of 2 to 5 mg/kg with stepwise increase up to 10 to 20 mg/kg (8). Response to pyridoxine may delay the progression to ESRF. Pyridoxine sensitivity can be detected by monitoring of both oxalate and glycolate and can be tested at any stage of the disease (2,3,41). However, one should keep in mind that large doses of pyridoxine might induce sensory neuropathy. Patients most likely to respond are those with residual AGT activity (43), but pyridoxine responsiveness is still poorly understood at the molecular level. An attempt to inhibit hepatic synthesis of oxalate by using (L)-2-oxothiazolidine-4-carboxylate has been reported without clinically significant changes in urinary oxalate excretion (44).

The treatment of stones should avoid open and percutaneous surgery because further renal parenchymal damage alters the GFR (45). The use of extracorporeal shock wave lithotripsy may be an available option in selected patients, but the presence of nephrocalcinosis may be responsible for parenchymal damage. Bilateral nephrectomy is recommended in most patients on renal replacement therapy to limit the risk of infection, obstruction, and passage of stones.

Renal Replacement Therapy

Dialysis

Conventional dialysis is unsuitable for PH1 patients who have reached ESRF because it cannot clear sufficient amounts of oxalate (3). In such patients, plasma oxalate levels range between 80 and 160 μmol/L (normal is less than 7 μmol/L) (Table 42.1). Therefore, daily hemodialysis (6 to 8 hours per session) using high-flux membranes would be required. Such a strategy cannot be routinely used (46). A reasonable therapeutic goal is to keep predialysis plasma oxalate concentration below 50 μmol/L to limit the progression of systemic oxalosis. Daily hemodialysis in infants raises major technical and developmental problems and its association with nighttime peritoneal dialysis may be sometimes proposed. Conventional long-term hemodialysis is generally regarded as contraindicated because it prolongs a deteriorating quality of life because of unabated progression of extrarenal oxalate deposition.

The benefit of pre- and posttransplantation hemodialysis is still debated and should be limited to patients with either oliguria or severe systemic oxalate loads.

Kidney Transplantation

Successful kidney transplantation allows significant removal of soluble oxalate. However, because the biochemical defect is in the liver, overproduction of oxalate and subsequent deposition in tissues continues unabated. High urinary oxalate excretion originates from both ongoing oxalate production from the native liver and oxalate deposits in tissues. Due to oxalate accumulation in the transplanted kidney, overall graft survival is limited. Therefore, isolated kidney transplantation is no longer recommended in most pyridoxine-unresponsive patients (see later). The long-term outcome of PH1 after renal transplantation remains uncertain, with a 5- to 10-year patient survival rate ranging from 10 to 50% (47). In addition, renal transplantation does not prevent the progression of skeletal and vascular complications. Outcome of renal transplantation is unrelated to residual AGT activity (48), but graft survival is improved if transplantation is performed when there is substantial renal function (i.e., a GFR ranging from 20 to 30 mL/min/1.73 m^2), and in the absence of major extrarenal involvement. In selected patients, good results have been reported after early renal transplantation and vigorous perioperative dialysis (49,50). However, at this point in time, living-related donors should be avoided because the overall results are poor (47). Isolated kidney transplantation may be a temporary solution for PH in developing countries before managing the patient in a specialized center for further (combined) liver, if required, kidney transplantation. Even with previous pyridoxine resistance, it is recommended to retest vitamin B_6 responsiveness after isolated renal transplantation (49).

Enzyme Replacement Therapy

Ideally, any kind of transplantation should precede accumulation of large systemic oxalate loads. Assessment of the oxalate burden therefore needs to be regularly monitored by measurement of serial GFR, plasma oxalate (Table 42.1), calcium oxalate saturation, and systemic involvement (assessment of bone mineral density by quantitative measures, such as bone histology and computed tomography) (34,51–54).

Rationale for Liver Transplantation

Because the liver is the only organ responsible for glyoxylate detoxification by AGT, the excessive production of oxalate continues as long as the native metabolically defective liver is left in place. Therefore, any form of enzyme replacement succeeds only when the deficient host liver is concomitantly removed (55). Successful liver transplantation can supply the missing enzyme in the correct organ (e.g., liver), cell (e.g., hepatocyte), and intracellular compartment (e.g., peroxisome) (2,55). The ultimate goal of organ replacement is to reduce endogenous oxalate synthesis and provide good oxalate clearance via either the native or the transplanted kidney.

Of interest, the removed native liver from a PH1 patient has been used for domino transplantation in a high-risk 69-year-old marginal recipient with initially a favorable postoperative clinical outcome but evolution toward progressive renal insufficiency due to hyperoxaluria (56).

Combined Liver-Kidney Transplantation

In Europe, eight to ten combined liver-kidney transplantations per year have been reported in the PH1 Transplant Registry Report (47). The results are encouraging. Patient survival approximates 80% at 5 years and 65 to 70% at 10 years. In addition, despite the potential risks for the grafted kidney due to oxalate release from body stores, kidney survival is approximately 95% at 3 years posttransplantation, and the GFR ranges between 40 and 60 mL/min/1.73 m^2 after 5 to 10 years (47,54,55).

Isolated Liver Transplantation

Isolated liver transplantation might be the considered initial therapy in selected patients before advanced chronic renal failure has occurred (i.e., at a GFR between 60 and 40 mL/min/1.73 m^2) (18,58). Such a strategy has a strong rationale but raises ethical controversies. Approximately 20 patients have received an isolated liver transplant to date. Overall outcome is difficult to evaluate because the course of the disease is unpredictable and a sustained improvement can follow a phase of rapid decrease in GFR (57–59).

Posttransplantation Reversal of Renal and Extrarenal Involvement

Deposits of calcium oxalate in tissues can be remobilized according to the accessibility of oxalate burden to the blood stream (55). After combined liver-kidney transplantation, plasma oxalate returns to normal before urine oxalate does, and oxaluria can remain for several months posttransplantation (3,47,49). Therefore, there is still a risk of recurrent nephrocalcinosis or renal calculi that might jeopardize renal graft function. Glycolate, which is more soluble than oxalate and does not accumulate, is excreted in normal amounts immediately after liver transplantation. Thus, independent of the transplantation strategy, the kidney must be protected from damage induced by the systemic oxalate load suddenly released from tissues. Forced fluid intake (3 to 5 L/1.73 m^2/day) supported by diuretics and the use of crystallization inhibitors is the most important strategy. Plasma oxalate concentration, crystalluria, and calcium oxalate saturation are helpful tools in renal graft management after combined liver-kidney transplantation (42,53,60). The benefit of daily high-efficiency pre- and posttransplant hemodialysis or filtration is still debated; it provides a rapid drop in plasma oxalate but also an increased risk of urinary calcium-oxalate supersaturation and therefore should be limited to patients with anuria or with evidence of significant systemic oxalate involvement (34,52,60).

Combined transplantation should be planned when the GFR ranges between 20 and 40 mL/min/1.73 m^2 because, at this level, oxalate retention increases rapidly (22,59). In patients with ESRF, vigorous hemodialysis should be started and urgent liver-kidney transplantation should be performed. Even at these late stages, damaged organs other than the kidney, such as the skeleton or the heart, do benefit from enzyme replacement from the donor liver (57,60,61), which results in an appreciable improvement in quality of life.

Donors for Combined Liver-Kidney Transplantation

The type of donor (i.e., cadaver or living related) depends mainly on the physician and the country where the patient is treated (34,62,63) (Table 42.2). A living related donor must be considered because of the restricted number of potential biorgan donors. A living related donor can be proposed in a preemptive procedure using either isolated liver or synchronous liver-kidney transplantation. In patients with end-stage renal disease and systemic involvement, a metachronous transplantation procedure might be an option because a first-step liver transplantation will then allow oxalate clearance by vigorous hemodialysis before considering further kidney transplantation from the same (living related) donor.

Fate of Primary Hyperoxaluria Type 1 in Infants

PH1 in early childhood raises specific problems due to (a) the severity of the disease in infants (approximately 50% death rate), (b) the access to available diagnostic procedures in this age group, and (c) the adequacy of management, which directly reflects local economic particulars. Infantile PH1 presents two different issues worldwide. It is

TABLE 42.2. SUGGESTIONS FOR TRANSPLANTATION STRATEGIES IN PRIMARY HYPEROXALURIA TYPE 1 PATIENTS ACCORDING TO RESIDUAL GLOMERULAR FILTRATION RATE (GFR), SYSTEMIC INVOLVEMENT, AND LOCAL FACILITIES[a]

GFR (mL/min/1.73 m^2)	Estimated oxalate burden	Proposed transplantation strategy	Comments
60–40	±	Preemptive CAD liver Tx?	Hazardous, limited experience Raises ethical problems Do not reject LRD (in case of further kidney Tx)
30–10	++	Preemptive synchronous CAD liver-kidney Tx	No advantage with LRD HD only if post-Tx acute tubular necrosis/delayed graft function
End-stage renal disease	+++	Metachronous LRD Tx procedure: 1. Liver Tx 2. Aggressive HD to clear oxalate 3. Ox store assessment 4. Kidney Tx using the same donor	Avoid synchronous CAD Tx: Renal risk ++ Pre- and post-Tx HD required? Avoid metachronous CAD Tx: Needs two different donors See synchronous

±, mild; ++, moderate; +++, important; CAD, cadaver; HD, hemodialysis; LRD, living related donor; Tx, transplantation.
[a]Authors' personal opinion.

a very rare disease in developed countries where combined liver-kidney transplantation is available in children older than 6 months of age (or 5 to 6 kg body weight). Yet, it is a frequent cause of early end-stage renal disease in developing countries, often due to consanguinity, where therapeutic withdrawal is widely applied (9,58). Management of PH1 is, therefore, a major example of ethical, epidemiologic, technical, and financial dilemmas, which may be raised by recessive, inherited diseases with early life-threatening onset presenting in different socioeconomic contexts.

Future Trends

Although gene therapy has been advocated, many years of research will be required before its potential may be actualized (3). Amino acid changes found in AGT may affect its stability (6). A better understanding of such changes will facilitate design pharmacologic agents that stabilize AGT, leading to appropriate targeting of functional proteins in the potential of PH1 without the need for organ transplantation (Danpure, *personal communication*, 1999).

NON–TYPE 1 PRIMARY HYPEROXALURIA

In patients with overt hyperoxaluria, the pattern of urinary metabolites is indicative but not diagnostic of PH. In patients with a clinical picture of PH1, 10 to 30% have normal AGT activity that may lead to a diagnosis of PH2 or of another disorder causing hyperoxaluria. Enzyme activity measurement in a single-needle liver biopsy can confirm or exclude PH1 and PH2.

Primary Hyperoxaluria Type 2

PH2 is another rare inherited defect of oxalate metabolism causing raised urine oxalate and L-glycerate (Fig. 42.1).

Metabolic Derangement

PH2 is characterized by the absence of an enzyme with GR, HPR, and D-glycerate dehydrogenase activities (Fig. 42.1) (64–66). Analysis of liver and lymphocyte samples from patients with PH2 showed that GR activity was either very low or undetectable, whereas D-glycerate dehydrogenase activity was reduced in liver but within the normal range in lymphocytes (67).

Genetics

There is evidence for autosomal recessive transmission, and the gene encoding the enzyme GR or HPR (*GRHPR*) has been located on chromosome 9q11 (68). Several missense, nonsense, and deletion mutations have been identified (66).

Clinical Presentation

PH2 has been documented in less than 40 published patients (65,69). Median age at onset of first symptoms is 1 to 2 years, and the classical presentation is urolithiasis, including hematuria and obstruction. However, stone-forming activity is lower than in PH1 so that nephrocalcinosis and urinary tract infection are less frequent (41). Glomerular filtration rate is usually maintained during childhood, and systemic involvement is therefore exceptional (69).

Diagnosis

In the presence of hyperoxaluria without hyperglycoluria, a diagnosis of PH2 should be considered, especially when AGT activity is normal. However, hyperoxaluria in PH2 tends to be less pronounced than in PH1. The biochemical hallmark is the increased urinary excretion of L-glycerate (Table 42.1) (70), but the definitive diagnosis requires measurement of GR activity in a liver biopsy (71) as some PH2 patients have normal L-glycericaciduria (72).

Treatment and Prognosis

The overall long-term prognosis in PH2 is better than for PH1. ESRF occurs in 12% of patients between 23 and 50 years of age (69). As in PH1, supportive treatment includes high fluid intake, crystallization inhibitors, and prevention of complications; there is no rationale to use pyridoxine. Kidney transplantation has been performed in some end-stage renal disease patients, often leading to recurrence (nephrocalcinosis), including hyperoxaluria and L-glycerate excretion (69,73,74). The concept of liver transplantation has therefore been suggested, but more data are needed concerning the tissue distribution of the deficient enzyme and the biochemical impact of hepatic GR/HPR deficiency before such a strategy can be recommended.

Non–Type 1 Non–Type 2 Primary Hyperoxaluria

Few reports have shown a possible association of PH (a) without AGT or GR/HPR deficiency, and (b) with hyperglycoluria in the absence of AGT deficiency (75–77). It is therefore likely that there is at least another form of PH yet to be identified; hepatic glycolate oxidase is a candidate enzyme for a third form of inherited hyperoxaluria.

CONCLUSION

Children with nephrocalcinosis or urolithiasis should be screened for hyperoxaluria. Those patients with hyperoxaluria or recurrent calcium oxalate urolithiasis should be referred for diagnosis and management to specialized clinical centers with interest and experience in the conditions and access to the appropriate biochemical and molecular biologic facilities. Major advances in biochemistry, enzymology, genetics, and management of PH have been achieved during recent years. Further steps will assess genotype-phenotype relationships and underlying metabolic defects of atypical PH. The ongoing analysis of data from multicenter databases will improve transplantation/enzyme replacement strategies and subsequent patient survival and quality of life.

Foundations dealing with hyperoxaluria include http://www.ohf.org and http://www.airg-france.org.

REFERENCES

1. Danpure CJ, Jennings PR. Peroxisomal alanine:glyoxylate aminotransferase deficiency in primary hyperoxaluria type 1. *FEBS Lett* 1986;201:20–24.
2. Danpure CJ, Rumsby G. Enzymological and molecular genetics of primary hyperoxaluria type 1. Consequences for clinical management. In: Khan SR, ed. *Calcium oxalate in biological systems.* Boca Raton, FL: CRC Press, 1995:189–205.
3. Barratt TM, Danpure CJ. Hyperoxaluria. In: Barratt TM, Avner ED, Harmon WE, eds. *Pediatric nephrology*, 4th ed. Baltimore: Williams & Wilkins, 1999:609–619.
4. Danpure CJ, Cooper PJ, Wise PJ, et al. An enzyme trafficking defect in two patients with primary hyperoxaluria type 1: peroxisomal alanine: glyoxylate aminotransferase rerouted to mitochondria. *J Cell Biol* 1989;108:1345–1352.
5. Danpure CJ. Primary hyperoxaluria. In: Scriver CR, Beaudet AL, Sly WS, et al., eds. *The metabolic and molecular bases of inherited disease.* New York: McGraw-Hill, 2001:3323–3367.
6. Zhang X, Roe SM, Pearl LH, et al. Crystallization and preliminary crystallographic analysis of human alanine:glyoxylate aminotransferase and its polymorphic variants. *Acta Crystallogr D Biol Crystallogr* 2001;57:1936–1937.
7. Cochat P, Rolland MO. Primary hyperoxaluria. In: Fernandes J, Saudubray JM, van den Berghe G, eds. *Inborn metabolic diseases and treatment*, 3rd ed. Heidelberg, Germany: Springer Verlag, 2000:441–446.
8. Leumann E, Hoppe B. The primary hyperoxalurias. *J Am Soc Nephrol* 2001;12:1986–1993.
9. Cochat P, Koch Nogueira PC, Mahmoud AM, et al. Primary hyperoxaluria in infants: medical, ethical and economic issues. *J Pediatr* 1999;135:746–750.
10. Madani K, Otoukesh H, Rastegar A, et al. Chronic renal failure in Iranian children. *Pediatr Nephrol* 2001;16:140–144.
11. Rinat C, Wanders RJA, Drukker A, et al. Primary hyperoxaluria type 1: a model for multiple mutations in a monogenic disease within a distinct ethnic group. *J Am Soc Nephrol* 1999;10:2352–2358.
12. Basmaison O, Rolland MO, Cochat P, et al. Identification of 5 novel mutations in the AGXT gene. *Hum Mutat* 2000;15:577.
13. Danpure CJ, Purdue PE, Fryer P, et al. Enzymological and mutational analysis of a complex primary hyperoxaluria type 1 phenotype involving alanine:glyoxylate aminotransferase peroxisome-to-mitochondrion mistargeting and intraperoxisomal aggregation. *Am J Hum Genet* 1993;53:432–438.
14. Nogueira PK, Vuong TS, Bouton O, et al. Partial deletion of the AGXT gene (EX1_EX7del): a new genotype in hyperoxaluria type 1. *Hum Mutat* 2000;15:384–385.
15. Lumb MJ, Danpure CJ. Functional synergism between the most common polymorphism in human alanine:glyoxylate aminotransferase and four of the most common disease-causing mutations. *J Biol Chem* 2000;275:36415–36422.
16. Pirulli D, Giordano M, Lessi M, et al. Detection of AGXT gene mutations by denaturing high-performance liquid chromatography for diagnosis of hyperoxaluria type 1. *Clin Exp Med* 2001;1:99–104.
17. Amoroso A, Pirulli D, Florian F, et al. AGXT gene mutations and their influence on clinical heterogeneity of type 1 primary hyperoxaluria. *J Am Soc Nephrol* 2001;12:2072–2079.
18. Latta A, Müller-Wiefel DE, Sturm E, et al. Transplantation procedures in primary hyperoxaluria type 1. *Clin Nephrol* 1996;46:21–23.
19. von Schnakenburg C, Hulton SA, Milford DV, et al. Variable presentation of primary hyperoxaluria type 1 in 2 patients homozygous for a novel combined deletion and insertion mutation in exon 8 of the *AGXT* gene. *Nephron* 1998;78:485–488.
20. Rumsby G. Experience in prenatal diagnosis of primary hyperoxaluria type 1. *J Nephrol* 1998;11(Suppl 1):13–14.
21. Blaschke S, Grupp C, Haase J, et al. A case of late-onset primary hyperoxaluria type 1. *Am J Kidney Dis* 2002;39:E11.
22. Wong PN, Tong GM, Lo KY, et al. Primary hyperoxaluria: a rare but important cause of nephrolithiasis. *Hong Kong Med J* 2002;8:202–206.
23. Cochat P, Deloraine A, Rotily M, et al. Epidemiology of primary hyperoxaluria type 1. *Nephrol Dial Transplant* 1995;10 (Suppl 8):3–7.
24. Toussaint C, De Pauw L, Vienne A, et al. Radiological and histological improvement of oxalate osteopathy after combined liver-kidney transplantation in primary hyperoxaluria type 1. *Am J Kidney Dis* 1993;2:54–63.
25. Morgan SH, Purkiss P, Watts RWE, et al. Oxalate dynamics in chronic renal failure. Comparison with normal subjects and patients with primary hyperoxaluria. *Nephron* 1987;46:253–257.
26. Marangella M, Vitale C, Petrarulo M, et al. Bony content of oxalate in patients with primary hyperoxaluria or oxalosis-unrelated renal failure. *Kidney Int* 1995;48:182–187.
27. Schnitzler C, Kok JA, Jacobs DWC, et al. Skeletal manifestations of primary oxalosis. *Pediatr Nephrol* 1991;5:193–199.
28. Frishberg Y, Feinstein S, Rinat C, Drukker A. Hypothyroidism in primary hyperoxaluria type 1. *J Pediatr* 2000;136:255–257.
29. Furby A, Mourtada R, Charasse C, et al. [Polyradiculoneuropathy in an adult with primary hyperoxaluria] in French. *Rev Neurol (Paris)* 2000;156:62–64.
30. Maldonado I, Prasad V, Reginato AJ. Oxalate crystal deposition disease. *Curr Rheumatol Rep* 2002;4:257–264.
31. Marconi V, Mofid MZ, McCall C, et al. Primary hyperoxaluria: report of a patient with livedo reticularis and digital infarcts. *J Am Acad Dermatol* 2002;46:S16–S18.
32. Theodossiadis PG, Friberg TR, Panagiotidis DN, et al. Choroidal neovascularization in primary hyperoxaluria. *Am J Ophtalmol* 2002;134:134–137.

33. Yoshioka J, Park YD, Tanaka Y, et al. Echocardiographic features in a patient with primary hyperoxaluria. *Echocardiography* 2001;18:599–602.
34. Cochat P, Basmaison O. Current approaches to the management of primary hyperoxaluria. *Arch Dis Child* 2000;82:470–473.
35. Quy Dao N, Daudon M. *Infrared and Raman spectra of calculi*. Paris: Elsevier, 1997.
36. Daudon M, Estepa L, Lacour B, et al. Unusual morphology of calcium oxalate calculi in primary hyperoxaluria. *J Nephrol* 1998;11(Suppl 1):51–55.
37. Latta K, Brodehl J. Primary hyperoxaluria type 1. *Eur J Pediatr* 1991;149:518–522.
38. Rumsby G. Biochemical and genetic diagnosis of the primary hyperoxalurias: a review. *Mol Urol* 2000;4:349–354.
39. Hallson PC. Oxalate crystalluria. In: Rose GA, ed. *Oxalate metabolism in relation to urinary stone*. London: Springer Verlag, 1988:131–166.
40. Leumann E, Hoppe B, Neuhaus T. Management of primary hyperoxaluria: efficacy of oral citrate administration. *Pediatr Nephrol* 1993;7:207–211.
41. Milliner DS, Wilson DM, Smith LH. Phenotypic expression of primary hyperoxaluria: comparative features of types I and II. *Kidney Int* 2001;59:31–36.
42. Jouvet P, Priquelier L, Gagnadoux MF, et al. Crystalluria: a clinically useful investigation in children with primary hyperoxaluria post-transplantation. *Kidney Int* 1998;53:1412–1416.
43. Marangella M. Transplantation strategies in type 1 primary hyperoxaluria: the issue of pyridoxine responsiveness. *Nephrol Dial Transplant* 1999;14:301–303.
44. Holmes RP, Assimos DG, Wilson DM, et al. (L)-2-oxothiazolidine-4-carboxylate in the treatment of primary hyperoxaluria type 1. *BJU Int* 2001;88:858–862.
45. Gambaro G, Favaro S, D'Angelo A. Risk for renal failure in nephrolithiasis. *Am J Kidney Dis* 2001;37:233–243.
46. Yamauchi T, Quillard M, Takahashi S, et al. Oxalate removal by daily dialysis in a patient with primary hyperoxaluria type 1. *Nephrol Dial Transplant* 2001;16:2407–2411.
47. Jamieson NV. The results of combined liver/kidney transplantation for primary hyperoxaluria (PH1) 1984–1997. The European PH1 transplant registry report. European PH1 Transplantation Study Group. *J Nephrol* 1998;11(Suppl 1):36–41.
48. Katz A, Freese D, Danpure CJ, et al. Success of kidney transplantation in oxalosis is unrelated to residual hepatic enzyme activity. *Kidney Int* 1992;42:1408–1411.
49. Monico CG, Milliner DS. Combined liver-kidney and kidney-alone transplantation in primary hyperoxaluria. *Liver Transpl* 2001;11:954–963.
50. Scheinman JI, Najarian JS, Mauer SM. Successful strategies for renal transplantation in primary oxalosis. *Kidney Int* 1984;25:804–811.
51. Behnke B, Kemper MJ, Kruse HP, et al. Bone mineral density in children with primary hyperoxaluria type 1. *Nephrol Dial Transplant* 2001;16:2236–2239.
52. Hoppe B, Kemper MJ, Bokenkamp A, et al. Plasma calcium oxalate supersaturation in children with primary hyperoxaluria and end-stage renal failure. *Kidney Int* 1998;56:268–274.
53. Kuo LW, Horton K, Fishman EK. CT evaluation of multisystem involvement by oxalosis. *AJR Am J Roentgenol* 2001;177:661–663.
54. Watts RWE, Morgan SH, Danpure CJ, et al. Combined hepatic and renal transplantation in primary hyperoxaluria type I: clinical report of 9 cases. *Am J Med* 1991;90:179–188.
55. Danpure CJ. Scientific rationale for hepato-renal transplantation in primary hyperoxaluria type 1. In: Touraine JL, et al., eds. *Transplantation and clinical immunology XXII*. Amsterdam, The Netherlands: Elsevier, 1991:91–95.
56. Donckier V, El Nakadi I, Closset J, et al. Domino hepatic transplantation using the liver from a patient with primary hyperoxaluria. *Transplantation* 2001;71:1346–1348.
57. Cochat P, Shärer K. Should liver transplantation be performed before advanced renal insufficiency in primary hyperoxaluria type 1? *Pediatr Nephrol* 1993;7:212–218.
58. Ellis SR, Hulton SA, McKiernan PJ, et al. Combined liver-kidney transplantation for primary hyperoxaluria in young children. *Nephrol Dial Transplant* 2001;16:348–354.
59. Shapiro R, Weismann I, Mandel H, et al. Primary hyperoxaluria type 1: improved outcome with timely liver transplantation: a single center report of 36 children. *Transplantation* 2001;72:428–432.
60. Gagnadoux MF, Lacaille F, Niaudet P, et al. Long term results of liver-kidney transplantation in children with primary hyperoxaluria. *Pediatr Nephrol* 2001;16:946–950.
61. Detry O, Honoré P, DeRoover A, et al. Reversal of oxalosis cardiomyopathy after combined liver and kidney transplantation. *Transpl Int* 2002;15:50–52.
62. Nakamura M, Fuchinoue S, Nakajima I, et al. Three cases of sequential liver-kidney transplantation from living related donors. *Nephrol Dial Transplant* 2001;16:166–168.
63. Nolkemper D, Kemper MJ, Burdelski M, et al. Long-term results of pre-emptive liver transplantation in primary hyperoxaluria type 1. *Pediatr Transplant* 2000;4:177–181.
64. Giafi CF, Rumsby G. Primary hyperoxaluria type 2: enzymology. *J Nephrol* 1998;11(Suppl 1):29–31.
65. Mistry J, Danpure CJ, Chalmers RA. Hepatic D-glycerate dehydrogenase and glyoxylate reductase deficiency in primary hyperoxaluria type 2. *Biochem Soc Trans* 1988;16:626–627.
66. Webster KE, Ferree PM, Holmes RP, et al. Identification of missense, nonsense, and deletion mutations in the GRHPR gene in patients with primary hyperoxaluria type 2. *Hum Genet* 2000;107:176–185.
67. Giafi CF, Rumsby G. Kinetic analysis and tissue distribution of human D-glycerate dehydrogenase/glyoxylate reductase and its relevance to the diagnosis of primary hyperoxaluria type 2. *Ann Clin Biochem* 1998;35:104–109.
68. Cramer SD, Ferree PM, Lin K, et al. The gene encoding hydroxypyruvate reductase (GRHPR) is mutated in patients with primary hyperoxaluria type II. *Hum Mol Genet* 1999;8:2063–2069.
69. Kemper MJ, Conrad S, Müller-Wiefel DE. Primary hyperoxaluria type 2. *Eur J Pediatr* 1997;156:509–512.
70. Rashed MS, Aboul-Enein HY, Al Amoudi M, et al. Chiral liquid chromatography tandem mass spectrometry in the determination of configuration of glyceric acid in urine of

patients with D-glyceric and L-glyceric acidurias. *Biomed Chromatogr* 2002;16:191–198.
71. Marangella M, Petrarulo M, Cossedu D, et al. Detection of primary hyperoxaluria type 2 (L-glyceric aciduria) in patients with end-stage renal failure. *Nephrol Dial Transplant* 1995;10:1381–1385.
72. Rumsby G, Sharma A, Cregeen DP, et al. Primary hyperoxaluria type 2 without L-glyceraciduria: is the disease under-estimated? *Nephrol Dial Transplant* 2001;16:1697–1699.
73. Law CW, Yuen YP, Lai CK, et al. Novel mutation in the GRHPR gene in a Chinese patient with primary hyperoxaluria type 2 requiring renal transplantation from a living related donor. *Am J Kidney Dis* 2001;38:1307–1310.
74. Johnson SA, Rumsby G, Cregeen D, et al. Primary hyperoxaluria type 2 in children. *Pediatr Nephrol* 2002;17:597–601.
75. Monico CG, Persson M, Ford GC, et al. Potential mechanisms of marked hyperoxaluria not due to primary hyperoxaluria I or II. *Kidney Int* 2002;62:392–400.
76. van Acker KJ, Eyskens FJ, Espeel MF, et al. Hyperoxaluria with hyperglycoluria not due to alanine: glyoxylate aminotransferase defect: a novel type of primary hyperoxaluria. *Kidney Int* 1996;50:1747–1752.
77. Kist-van Holthe JE, Onkenhout W, van der Heijden AJ. Pyridoxine-responsive nephrocalcinosis and glycolic aciduria in two siblings without hyperoxaluria and with normal alanine:glyoxylate aminotransferase activity. *J Inherit Metab Dis* 2000;23:91–92.

43

TUBULOINTERSTITIAL NEPHRITIS

URI S. ALON

Involvement of the tubulointerstitial compartment in renal diseases can be either primary or even more commonly secondary to glomerular, vascular, or structural disease (Table 43.1). However, even in the latter disorders the magnitude of involvement and damage to the tubulointerstitium can have a significant effect on the outcome of the primary disease (1,2). This chapter addresses primary tubulointerstitial nephritis (TIN), which is a syndrome in which there is a spectrum ranging from acute to chronic diseases. TIN is characterized histologically by inflammation and damage of tubulointerstitial structures, with relative sparing of glomerular and vascular elements (3,4). Acute TIN is typically associated with marked tubulointerstitial inflammation, varying degrees of edema and tubular epithelial cell damage, and mononuclear cell infiltration (5). In contrast, chronic lesions generally are characterized by evidence of tubular epithelial cell damage and atrophy, with tubulointerstitial fibrosis (5). Although there are important clinical and pathophysiologic distinctions between acute and chronic TIN, they are best viewed as a continuum of manifestations of renal injury (6,7). Acute TIN is often reversible; however, progression to chronic renal disease can occur (8,9).

STRUCTURE AND FUNCTION OF THE TUBULOINTERSTITIAL COMPARTMENT

The tubulointerstitial compartment comprises approximately 80% of the renal parenchyma with the majority of its volume contributed by the tubules (10). The interstitium is made of matrix and cells. Two main types of cells are recognized:

1. Type I interstitial cells are fibroblast-like cells that are able to produce and degrade extracellular matrix, with a subgroup residing in the inner medulla producing prostaglandins.
2. Type II interstitial cells include dendritic antigen-presenting cells located mainly in the cortex.

In addition, a few monocyte-derived macrophages capable of phagocytosis are found in all renal zones (11,12). The matrix is composed of a fibrillar net of basement membrane and interstitial collagens, glycoproteins, and proteoglycans, as well as interstitial fluid (12). The interstitium provides structural support for the nephrons and capillaries and plays an important role in the transport of solutes. It is also the site of production of cytokines and hormones such as prostaglandins and erythropoietin. The roles of the tubules in maintaining homeostasis of fluid, electrolytes, minerals, and acid-base balance are described in previous chapters. Damage to different segments of the tubules result in metabolic abnormalities related to the affected segments.

PATHOPHYSIOLOGY

The similarity of tubulointerstitial lesions in all forms of TIN, which is characterized by predominantly T-cell lymphocytic infiltrates, suggests immune-mediated mechanisms of renal injury (6,13). Such mechanisms are likely important in either initiating tubular injury or amplifying damage induced by both immune and nonimmune causes. Studies from experimental models of tubulointerstitial disease indicate that both cell-mediated and humoral immune mechanisms are relevant pathways that induce renal injury (14,15).

CELL-MEDIATED IMMUNITY

Historically, abnormalities in cell-mediated immune response have been implicated as central to the pathophysiology of TIN. Analysis of infiltrating mononuclear cells in human TIN of various etiologies demonstrated the majority of them to be T lymphocytes (16–18). The T-cell lymphocytic ($CD4^+$ and $CD8^+$) interstitial infiltrates generally occur in the absence of antibody deposition (5). Immunohistochemical studies conducted on biopsies obtained in drug-induced TIN also indicate the importance of cell-cell interactions in intrarenal inflammation because there is a significant increase in interstitial expression of cellular adhesion molecules. In human forms of acute TIN, increased expression of lymphocyte function–associated antigen-1 and very late antigen-4 cell-surface receptors, as well

TABLE 43.1. CLASSIFICATION OF TUBULOINTERSTITIAL NEPHRITIS (TIN)

Primary TIN
Infection (bacterial pyelonephritis, hantavirus, leptospirosis)
Immune-mediated (antitubular basement membrane disease)
Drug-induced (antimicrobials, analgesics, lithium, cyclosporine, Chinese herbs)
Toxins (lead)
Hereditary (cystinosis, hyperoxaluria, Wilson disease)
Metabolic disorders (hypercalcemia, hyperkalemia, hyperuricosuria)
Hematologic disorders (sickle cell disease)
Miscellaneous (Balkan nephropathy)
Secondary TIN
Glomerular disease
Vascular disease
Structural disease
Cystic diseases
Obstructive disease
Reflux

Modified from Rastegar A, Kashgarian M. The clinical spectrum of tubulointerstitial nephritis. *Kidney Int* 1998;54:313–327.

as their respective ligands intercellular adhesion module-1 and vascular cell adhesion molecule-1, is seen in areas of mononuclear cell infiltration (19). Further support of cell-mediated events in human disease is derived from the observation of *in vivo* and *in vitro* activation of lymphocytes isolated from affected patients after repeat exposure to specific inciting agents of TIN (20,21). In view of these observations, the role of cell-mediated events in TIN has been extensively studied in murine models of anti-TBM disease and spontaneous TIN (15,22,23). In both of these models, the effector T-cell (T_e) lymphocytes that differentiate in diseased animals are $CD8^+$ renal tubular antigen–specific T cells. Nephritogenic $CD8^+$ T_e cells induce renal injury in genetically susceptible animals and adoptively transfer renal disease to naïve hosts (14,15,22,23).

Cell-mediated responses are initiated by T-cell recognition of relevant antigen presented in the context of appropriate major histocompatibility complex (MHC) molecules. Class I MHC molecules primarily direct $CD8^+$ T cell responses, and class II MHC determinants direct $CD4^+$ T cell responses (24). *In vitro* studies show that resident renal cells, such as renal tubular epithelial cells, glomerular epithelial cells, and mesangial cells, have the potential to present a variety of antigens (25,26). Correlation of *in vitro* antigen-presenting activity to disease activity *in vivo*, however, has not been established (27). It is noteworthy that renal tubular epithelial cells express class II MHC determinants in inflammatory renal disease and in culture when stimulated by proinflammatory cytokines such as interferon-gamma and tumor necrosis factor-α (28,29). Moreover, class II MHC expression on renal tubular epithelial cells induces *in vitro* proliferation of antigen-specific T-cell clones and hybridomas and promotes autoimmune renal disease *in vivo*. These findings suggest that induced class II MHC expression on renal tubular epithelial cells promotes autoimmune injury by facilitating presentation of a self (tubular)-antigen by nonlymphoid cells (27). The cause for antigen expression by the tubular cells is unknown. Tubular epithelial cells normally do not express costimulatory molecules such as CD80 and CD86, which likely limits their ability to present antigen under physiologic conditions (30). Genetic susceptibility may play a factor in antigen expression and consequent immune response (15). Other mechanisms, such as drugs or infectious agents, may serve as inciting antigens of cell-mediated responses targeting the kidney (31,32). In addition, degenerate recognition of peptide antigens by autoreactive T cells in autoimmune disease has been reported (31,33). The potential relevance of such molecular mimicry in autoimmune T-cell activation to renal immune responses, however, awaits further investigation. There is a large body of research focused on analysis of the interaction between effector and suppressor T cells in the inflammatory process in the renal interstitium. However, their definitive role in the pathogenesis of TIN is still unclear (9,10).

ANTIBODY-MEDIATED IMMUNITY

Antibody-mediated TIN is occasionally seen. When antibodies are present on immunofluorescence investigation they are usually associated with the tubulointerstitial cells, along the basement membrane or as immune complexes. Anti-TBM staining often occurs as part of anti-GBM disease but at times it appears to be a primary phenomenon resembling experimental anti-TBM disease. Anti-TBM antibodies can be seen at times in association with drug-induced TIN and more commonly in the setting of renal transplantation due to the presence of foreign antigens in the transplanted kidney (34,35).

Primary immune deposit–mediated TIN is rare. It seems that in such instances the complexes are formed *in situ*, as circulating complexes would have been entrapped in the glomeruli. Indeed, in cases in which immune complexes are detected in the interstitium, they are also observed in the glomeruli as in systemic lupus erythematosus (SLE), immunoglobulin A (IgA) nephropathy, and membranous nephropathy. It is believed that in these disorders immune reactants are delivered to the interstitium through the process of glomerular proteinuria. The presence of interstitial immune complexes might still require cellular immune response genes for the development for complete inflammatory reaction. Most studied experimentally is anti-TBM disease. Other animal models for experimental antibody- and immune complex–mediated TIN include the Heymann nephritis antigen complex in the brush-border disorder (36) and reaction to Tamm-Horsfall protein (37).

LOCAL AND EXTRARENAL ANTIGENS

Antigens presented to the immune system may be derived from resident cells or arrive at the tubulointerstitial compartment from an extrarenal origin. As mentioned previously, resident cells of the tubulointerstitial component and, in particular, tubular epithelial cells have the potential to present antigens. In addition, local antigens may be related to Tamm-Horsfall protein or uromodulin, which is a glycoprotein secreted by the cells of the ascending loop of Henle. The glycoprotein can cause immune deposits at the base of the tubular cell and the lymphatic drainage of the ascending limb and result in binding of neutrophils to the cell-surface anchored glycoprotein (38,39). In Heymann nephritis, antibodies reacting to the tubular brush border have been detected, at times associated with interstitial infiltration (40,41). Most extensively studied is the antigen in antitubular basement membrane (anti-TBM) disease, named *3M-1* (42,43). It was detected both in humans and rodents, showing extensive polymorphic expression (44,45).

Extrarenal antigens may present to the interstitium as isolated antigens or as part of an immune complex. Antigens arriving at the tissue like those originally derived from drugs such as penicillin, cephalosporin, and phenytoin, combine with antibodies and inflammatory cells that initiate the interstitial disease. Another mechanism by which outside antigens initiate an immune response is by mimicking of epitopes. For instance, some antibodies to *Escherichia coli* cross-react with Tamm-Horsfall protein (46). It is also possible that a similar mechanism operates in TIN that follows certain viral illnesses (47,48). It has also been hypothesized that noninfectious, shared epitopes may instigate the immune process, as might be the case in anti-DNA antibodies (49,50).

Circulating immune deposits that settle in the interstitium can cause TIN. This might be the case in SLE, IgA nephropathy, and possibly some cases of chronic idiopathic human tubulointerstitial nephritis (51,52). Experimentally, a model of chronic serum sickness disease in the rabbit results in immune deposits in the interstitium (53).

CYTOKINES AND AMPLIFICATION OF INJURY

Events resulting from infiltration of T cells, deposition of specific antibodies, or immune complexes that augment inflammation and injury are part of the *amplification process*. These processes include the release of cytokines and proteases from T cells; the attraction and activation of nonspecific immune effector cells, including eosinophils and macrophages (18), which release various effector products; and the activation of the complement cascade. Interestingly, the presence of complement in TIN is inconsistent and when present is usually associated with deposition of IgG and immune complexes (53–55) or IgE and eosinophils (53,55,56). Even more important seems to be the activation of the alternative passway by ammonia in the absence of antibodies (57). This process may be instrumental in the process of progressive local injury in nonimmune-mediated TIN. It may also indicate the importance of correction of metabolic acidosis in the prevention of progressive damage to the kidneys by diminishing ammonia production. It is possible that both resident epithelial cells and infiltrating cells further amplify the damage by expressing chemokines. This subclass of structurally related cytokines selectively promotes the chemotaxis, adhesion, and activation of leukocytes (58). After obstruction in the mouse, the most potent recruiter of macrophages is monocyte chemoattractant peptide-1, which is expressed in tubular epithelium (59). The chemokines induce their effect by binding to specific cell-surface receptors on target cells. The various types of leukocytes are activated by different chemokines binding to different receptors. The pharmacologic blockage of chemokines and their receptors may have a potential in controlling the inflammatory response (60). In humans with ureteropelvic junction obstruction, urinary monocyte chemoattractant peptide-1 is increased and decreases after surgical alleviation of the obstruction (61).

FIBROGENESIS AND ATROPHY

Interstitial fibrosis is the final common pathway for a variety of glomerular and tubular disorders, particularly when associated with massive glomerular proteinuria or the presence of inflammatory cells in the tubulointerstitial component (62,63). It seems that both processes induce local cytokines that transform and activate several types of resident cells in the tubulointerstitial compartment to produce new or modified extracellular matrix (64). Some of the activated cells probably change phenotype (65–67). It is unclear why what is usually a self-limited wound repair process continues unabated. It is possible that homeostatic regulatory mechanisms fail to stop or reverse fibrosis during the continuous inflammatory process of chronic TIN.

Tubulointerstitial scars are primarily composed of collagen types I and III, fibronectin, and tenascin (68,69). Other glycoproteins may participate as well. Early in the development of a scar, the fibrotic tissue may contain monocytes, tubular cells, and fibroblasts (63). It seems that the local monocytes release cytokines affecting the activity of their neighboring fibroblasts. The phenotypic expression of the fibroblast and hence the renal glycoprotein synthesized by it may be related to the type of cytokine stimulating the cell (70). Among the strongest morphogenic cytokines driving TIN fibrosis is angiotensin II (71).

The source of the fibroblasts in the tubulointerstitium is yet unknown. There are several lines of evidence that suggest they may arise from transformation of resident cells like the tubular epithelium. This mechanism is called *epithelial-mesenchymal transformation* (72–74). The transformation is probably activated by immune-mediated mechanisms and various cytokines that result in changes in the basement membrane of the tubular epithelial cell. Once transformed to a mesenchymal cell, it acquires motility and becomes responsive to growth factor stimuli (75). Several local chemoattractants stimulate the migration of the newly formed fibroblasts. These chemoattractants are released by macrophages or the fibroblasts themselves (76,77). Fibroblasts secrete transforming growth factor β (TGFβ), which amplifies the process (78). Once fibroblasts migrate to their new location, they begin to deposit fibronectin matrix, which serves as a skeleton for the deposition of other glycoproteins. Concomitantly with the transformation process, the effect of cytokines on tubular cells can result in their atrophy by disturbing their basement membrane synthesis. Additional damage to the tubular cell can be caused by T-cell clones, with cytotoxic activity resulting in tubular cell destruction and atrophy. Thus, tubular atrophy and interstitial fibrosis coexist.

ACUTE TUBULOINTERSTITIAL NEPHRITIS

Epidemiology

Acute TIN accounts for 10 to 25% of reported cases of acute renal failure (ARF) in adults (3) and up to 7% of children with ARF (79). However, in both children and adults, acute TIN may be underreported because many patients with ARF recover spontaneously after removal of the suspected offending agent, and definitive diagnosis based on a renal biopsy is not routinely established (7). Lower reported incidences of acute TIN in children than in adults may reflect more common use of nephrotoxic pharmacologic agents and greater prevalence of preexisting renal abnormalities in older patients.

Clinical, Laboratory, and Radiologic Features

The clinical manifestations of TIN are variable, and many of them are seen in both acute and chronic TIN (Table 43.2). The severity of renal impairment ranges from mild azotemia and asymptomatic urinary abnormalities to oliguric ARF (80). The nonspecific nature of the clinical findings in TIN emphasizes the need for a renal biopsy to make a definitive diagnosis in questionable cases (4,81). In one series of 13 children with biopsy-proven acute TIN, only 6 were suspected of having the diagnosis before the procedure (82). However, in a child suspected to have acute TIN, if improvement in kidney function is noticed after withholding the suspected offending agents and starting treatment, there is no need for a biopsy.

Systemic manifestations of a hypersensitivity reaction, such as fever, rash, and arthralgias, are variable findings. Although these symptoms are more likely to occur in drug-induced acute TIN (79,83), in a series of nine adults with acute TIN caused by medications, components of this classic triad were presenting symptoms in only approximately one-half of the patients (84). The rash may be maculopapular, morbilliform, or urticarial, and it often is fleeting (84–87). Arthralgias are seldom a prominent feature (84). Acute TIN associated with infection may present with extrarenal manifestations of disease, such as fever and sore throat (82). Nonspecific constitutional symptoms of fatigue, anorexia, weight loss, nausea and vomiting, and flank pain with macroscopic hematuria may occur (85,87). Oliguria can occur, but 30 to 40% of patients with acute TIN have nonoliguric ARF (3). Hypertension and edema are seldom noted,

TABLE 43.2. CLINICAL PRESENTATION OF TUBULOINTERSTITIAL NEPHRITIS

History
Exposure to toxic substances
Family history of tubulointerstitial nephritis
Nephrotoxic drug use
Past or family history of vesicoureteral reflux
Recurrent urinary tract infections
Uveitis
Symptoms
Abdominal pain
Anorexia[a]
Arthralgias
Diarrhea
Dysuria
Edema
Emesis[a]
Eye tenderness (seen in TINU syndrome)
Fatigue[a]
Fever[a]
Flank or loin pain
Headache
Lymphadenopathy
Malaise
Myalgia
Nocturia
Polydipsia
Polyuria
Rash
Sore throat[a]
Weight loss[a]
Signs
Abdominal pain
Arthritis
Costovertebral tenderness
Edema
Evidence for left ventricular hypertrophy
Fever[a]
Hypertension
Hypertensive retinopathy
Lacrimation (seen in TINU syndrome)
Lethargy
Pallor[a]
Pharyngitis
Poor growth[a]
Rachitic changes[a]
Rash (may be maculopapular, morbilliform, or urticarial)
Volume depletion

TINU, tubulointerstitial nephritis with uveitis.
[a]Common finding in children.

TABLE 43.3. PATTERNS OF RENAL TUBULAR DYSFUNCTION IN TUBULOINTERSTITIAL NEPHRITIS

Nephron site	Functional defect	Clinical manifestation
Proximal tubule	Decreased HCO_3, PO_4, amino acid, uric acid, and glucose reabsorption	Fanconi syndrome, hyperchloremic metabolic acidosis
Loop of Henle	Defective NaCl reabsorption, decreased magnesium reabsorption	Polyuria (polydipsia), salt wasting, magnesium losses
Distal tubule	Defective NaCl reabsorption and potassium and hydrogen ion secretion	Hyperkalemia, hyperchloremic metabolic acidosis, salt wasting
Collecting tubule	Defective water reabsorption	Nephrogenic diabetes insipidus

Modified from Toto RD. Review: acute tubulointerstitial nephritis. *Am J Med Sci* 1990;299:392–410.

except in specific drug-induced lesions, such as the nephrotic syndrome associated with nonsteroidal antiinflammatory drugs (NSAIDs) (88) or in TIN secondary to glomerular disease (8,80).

Acute and chronic TIN have quite similar laboratory findings (7). Renal tubular epithelial cell damage is the predominant finding in all forms of TIN, and biochemical abnormalities observed in patients with TIN may reflect injury to specific nephron segments involved in the inflammatory process (Table 43.3) (89). In general, cortical damage may affect mainly the proximal and distal tubules, whereas medullary lesions may affect mainly the loop of Henle and the collecting duct. Proximal tubule injury results in Fanconi syndrome with impaired urinary reabsorption of glucose, bicarbonate, phosphorus, amino acids, and uric acid (90). Damage to the loop of Henle may result in magnesium and sodium losses. Distal tubular lesions result in renal tubular acidosis, impaired potassium excretion, and sodium wasting (91). Biochemical abnormalities in TIN include an elevated serum creatinine concentration with hyperchloremic metabolic acidosis (3,82). If proximal tubular involvement is prominent, serum phosphorus, bicarbonate, uric acid, and potassium concentrations may be decreased. Many patients have nonoliguric renal failure, a urine concentrating defect, and relatively bland changes on urine microscopic examination.

Relevant serologic studies in the investigation of TIN are listed in Table 43.4. Normochromic, normocytic anemia is often associated with TIN (79,89). Hemolytic anemia has also been reported in acute TIN induced by allopurinol, penicillins, and rifampin (4,89). Leukocytosis may occur, and some but not all patients with drug-induced TIN have a peripheral eosinophilia (83,84,87). Drug-induced liver damage is reflected in elevated hepatic enzymes (92,93). Elevated serum IgE titers have been reported in up to 50% of biopsy-proven cases and is suggestive but not diagnostic of drug-induced TIN (80,84). Anti-DNA antibodies, antinuclear antibodies, and complement levels are normal in most forms of TIN, unless associated with a systemic autoimmune disorder (3,85). Circulating anti-TBM antibodies are detected on rare occasions (86).

TABLE 43.4. SERUM AND URINE ABNORMALITIES OFTEN FOUND WITH TUBULOINTERSTITIAL NEPHRITIS (TIN)

Serum abnormalities
Anemia
  Hemolytic
  Nonhemolytic[a]
Circulating immune complexes (may be seen in immune-mediated TIN)
Elevated hepatic enzymes (in patients with associated drug-induced liver damage)
Eosinophilia[a]
Hyperchloremic metabolic acidosis (normal anion gap)[a]
Hypernatremia
Hypokalemia
Hypoaldosteronism
Hypophosphatemia
Hyporeninemia
Hypouricemia
Increased erythrocyte sedimentation rate[a]
Increased immunoglobulin E level
Increased immunoglobulin G level
Increased blood urea nitrogen[a]
Increased creatinine[a]
Leukocytosis (with or without eosinophilia)
Urine abnormalities
Aminoaciduria
Bacteriuria
Bicarbonaturia
Eosinophiluria (seen usually in drug-induced TIN)
Glucosuria (in absence of hyperglycemia)
Hematuria (usually microscopic)[a]
Hyposthenuria
Leukocyturia
Magnesium wasting
Phosphaturia
Proteinuria (usually mild to moderate)[a,b]
Casts
  Granular
  Hyaline
  Red blood cells (seen occasionally in drug-induced TIN)
  White blood cells (seen in infection-mediated acute or chronic TIN)
Salt-wasting

[a]Common finding in children.
[b]Can be massive with nonsteroidal antiinflammatory drugs and less commonly with other drugs.

Urinary abnormalities vary considerably (Table 43.4). Microscopic hematuria is commonly detected, and macroscopic hematuria and sterile pyuria also occur (79,87). Mild to moderate proteinuria (less than 1 g/day) is detected in most patients with TIN (82). Nephrotic range proteinuria is not characteristic of TIN but has been associated with acute TIN induced by certain medications, including NSAIDs, lithium, ampicillin, and rifampin (5,94). Urinary sediment analysis shows granular, hyaline, and white blood cell casts (5). Red blood cell casts are rarely seen in acute TIN (82). *Eosinophiluria*, defined as greater than 1% of urinary leukocytes stained positively with Hansel's or Wright's stain, is suggestive of acute TIN and has been reported in 50 to 90% of patients with drug-induced acute TIN (84,95). However, eosinophiluria can be seen in many inflammatory renal diseases (96). In a study of 51 patients, eosinophiluria had a sensitivity of 40% and specificity of 72%, with a positive predictive value for TIN of only 38% (96).

Renal ultrasound examination usually demonstrates normal or enlarged kidneys, depending on the extent of tubulointerstitial inflammation and edema (3,79). Gallium citrate scanning may be useful in distinguishing acute TIN from other common causes of ARF (84). However, increased uptake on gallium scan is a relatively nonspecific finding and may be seen in cases of allograft rejection, acute pyelonephritis, and severe minimal change nephrotic syndrome (3). A definitive diagnosis of TIN can be made only by renal biopsy (3,4).

Pathology

Typical light microscopy findings in acute TIN consist of tubulointerstitial mononuclear cell infiltration and edema, with varying abnormalities in renal tubular epithelial cells (Fig. 43.1) (80,81). In general, vessels and glomerular structures are unaffected (80,84). Mild mesangial hypercellularity or periglomerular inflammation and fibrosis occasionally are seen (82). Cellular infiltrates, primarily of lymphocytes, often are patchy and are variably distributed throughout the kidney (5,84). Monocytes, macrophages, and plasma cells are also commonly noted in affected areas (82,85). Eosinophils are most commonly seen with drug-induced acute TIN and can comprise up to 10% of the infiltrate (86). Interstitial granulomas occasionally are seen, particularly in drug-induced or infection-related acute TIN (97). Complement and immunoglobulin deposition is not characteristic of acute TIN (5,98,99) but has been noted in children with acute TIN because of SLE, syphilis, hepatitis B, shunt nephritis, and some drug-induced lesions (100).

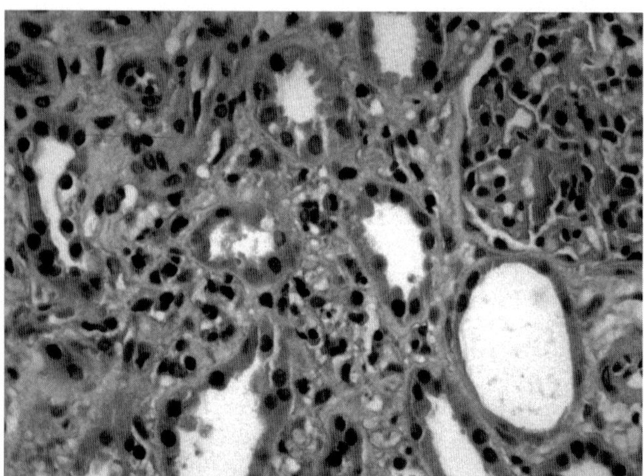

FIGURE 43.1. Acute tubulointerstitial nephritis (TIN). Light microscopy of idiopathic TIN in a 14-year-old girl. Cortical renal parenchyma showing a normal glomerulus, extensive interstitial edema, infiltration by lymphocytes and eosinophils, and cellular epithelial tubular degenerative changes.

Tubular epithelial cell damage varies from minimal histologic changes to frank necrosis (83,98). Most often there is flattening of renal tubular cells with atrophy, degeneration, and loss of the brush border in proximal convoluted tubules (5,8). Renal tubules are commonly dilated, with splitting or fracturing of the basolateral membrane. The tubule lumens may contain desquamated cells or blood (8,82). In some instances, infiltrating lymphocytes are observed between tubular epithelial cells (84). Electron microscopy typically reveals striking renal tubular epithelial cell mitochondrial damage, cytoplasmic vacuoles, and significantly dilated rough endoplasmic reticulum (81,82,84).

Etiology

The causes of acute TIN can be grouped into four broad categories: medications, infections, immunologic diseases, or idiopathic processes (Table 43.5). As described in the Pathology section of this chapter, all forms of acute TIN have similar pathologic features. Unique features of distinct forms of acute TIN are described in more detail.

Medications

Medications, rather than infection, are now the leading cause of acute TIN in children (8). An ever-increasing list of medications is implicated as causing acute TIN (Table 43.6). Establishing a clear link between a medication and acute TIN may be difficult, however, because many case reports of drug-induced acute TIN are in patients who have received several medications simultaneously. Nevertheless, a few categories of drugs are consistently associated with acute TIN in both children and adults: antibiotics, NSAIDs, anticonvulsants, and diuretics (83,84,87). Although symptoms of acute TIN caused by a specific drug can occur within hours or months after starting a medication, they are usually seen 2 to 3 weeks after starting therapy (4). Antimicrobials and NSAIDs are the most common drugs causing acute TIN in children (83,87). The incidence of acute TIN caused by methicillin, which is no longer used, was 16% (87). The incidence of acute TIN with currently available

TABLE 43.5. ETIOLOGIC CLASSIFICATION OF ACUTE TUBULOINTERSTITIAL NEPHRITIS

Immune-mediated[a]
Drug hypersensitivity (see Table 43.6)
β-Lactam antibiotics[a]
Other antibiotics
Diuretics
Nonsteroidal antiinflammatory drugs
Other drugs
Immunologic diseases
Usually associated with glomerulonephritis
Immunoglobulin A nephropathy
Membranous glomerulonephritis
Syphilis
Systemic lupus erythematosus[a]
Usually *not* associated with glomerulonephritis
Allograft rejection
Tubulointerstitial nephritis with uveitis syndrome
Infection-mediated[a] **(see Table 43.7)**
Direct infection of renal parenchyma (infectious agents identified in the interstitium)
Reactive (sterile) interstitial nephritis (infectious agents *not* identified in the interstitium)
Idiopathic

[a]Common cause in children.

penicillins is significantly less than that previously observed with methicillin. Systemic manifestations of hypersensitivity with fever, rash, and eosinophilia in the setting of ARF can occur in up to 30% of patients with penicillin-induced acute TIN (4). By contrast, these hypersensitivity manifestations are not typically associated with NSAID-induced acute TIN (88). NSAID-induced TIN may be associated with minimal change nephrotic syndrome (94). Although NSAID-induced acute TIN in children occurs less often than in adults, the increasing availability of over-the-counter NSAID preparations for children may result in an increase in cases in that age group.

Drug-induced acute TIN is an idiosyncratic reaction, and, as such, it is difficult to predict which patients will be affected. No specific risk factors have been consistently identified. Acute TIN has been reported with various routes of administration, including oral, intravenous, intramuscular, and rectal (83,87,98,101). Duration and the dosage of therapy also do not correlate well with the development of disease, although several reports suggest that acute TIN is more common with high-dose therapy (7,87).

The association of drug-induced acute TIN with fever, rash, and eosinophilia suggests an underlying allergic reaction to administered drugs. Reports of accelerated, recurrent TIN on drug rechallenge also implicate drug hypersensitivity (101,102). Administration of structurally similar medications may induce cross-reactivity as evidenced by recurrent acute TIN after cephalosporin administration in individuals with previous penicillin-induced TIN (87).

Drug-induced acute interstitial nephritis was found to be a cause for graft dysfunction in kidney transplant recipients. Early diagnosis and treatment prevented permanent damage (103).

Infections

In the preantibiotic era, infection, especially streptococcal, was the predominant cause of acute TIN in children. Councilman's initial postmortem findings of TIN involved 42 children who succumbed to scarlet fever (104). With the development of effective antimicrobial therapy, the incidence of *Streptococcus*-associated acute TIN has decreased. Other infectious organisms have become important causes of acute TIN. These include unusual bacteria such as *Rickettsia* species, *Yersinia*, and mycoplasma. Viruses, such as adenovirus and human immunodeficiency virus, and parasites are also causes of acute TIN (Table 43.7) (5,105–107). Infections may induce acute TIN by two distinct processes. Organisms may directly invade the renal parenchyma, producing local renal infection and inflammation. This form of acute TIN may respond to treatment of the underlying infection. Alternatively, organisms may induce "reactive" intrarenal inflammation without evidence of renal infection. The latter mechanism is implicated by the observation that group A streptococcal infections can cause acute TIN in children, even with appropriate antibiotic therapy (82). Mechanisms for the renal inflammatory reaction in the absence of renal infection are not clearly elucidated but are presumed to be immunologically mediated (82).

Immunologic Diseases

Immunologic diseases elicit acute TIN in two distinct settings (Table 43.5). TIN occurs with either a primary glomerular lesion or, less commonly, as an isolated primary TIN. SLE is the most important cause of acute TIN seen in association with glomerulonephritis in children. Tubulointerstitial immune deposits may be present in up to 60% of SLE patients who are biopsied and correlate with both severity of interstitial inflammation and degree of functional renal impairment (108,109). As is the case with other glomerular diseases, severe tubulointerstitial involvement with fibrosis is a poor prognostic indicator for renal function (100). Acute TIN occasionally is seen in children with membranous nephropathy, postinfectious glomerulonephritis, and shunt nephritis (100). IgA nephropathy was associated with significant TIN in 37% of 51 patients (110). At follow-up, patients with renal tubular deposits had significantly worse renal function than those with isolated glomerular findings (110). Immunologic diseases that present with isolated tubulointerstitial involvement are tubulointerstitial nephritis with uveitis (TINU) syndrome, allograft rejection, and rarely SLE (111,112). Allograft rejection is discussed in detail in Chapter 75.

TINU syndrome was first described in 1975 in a report of two adolescent girls who developed ARF with eosino-

TABLE 43.6. DRUGS ASSOCIATED WITH ACUTE TUBULOINTERSTITIAL NEPHRITIS

Anticonvulsants
Carbamazepine[a]
Lamotrigine
Phenobarbital[a]
Phenytoin[a]
Sodium valproate[a]
Antiinflammatory drugs and analgesics
Benoxaprofen
Diclofenac
Diflunisal
Fenoprofen
Floctafenine
Ibuprofen
Indomethacin
Ketoprofen
Mefenamic acid
Naproxen[a]
Niflumic acid[a]
Phenazone
Phenylbutazone
Piroxicam
Rofecoxib
Sulfasalazine
Sulfinpyrazone
Sulindac
Suprofen
Tolmetin[a]
Zomepirac
β-Lactam antibiotics
Cephalosporins
  Cefaclor
  Cefotaxime
Cefoxitin
Cephalexin
Cephaloridine
Cephalothin
Cephradine
Penicillins and derivatives
  Amoxicillin
  Ampicillin[a]
  Carbenicillin
  Cloxacillin[a]
  Flucloxacillin
  Methicillin[a]
  Mezlocillin
  Nafcillin[a]
  Oxacillin
  Penicillin G[a]
Other antibiotics
  p-Acyclovir
  Azithromycin
  Aztreonam
  Chloramphenicol
  Ciprofloxacin
  Clarithromycin
  Clotrimazole
  Erythromycin[a]
  Gentamicin
  Indinavir
  Isoniazid
  Lincomycin
  Loracarbef[a]
  Nitrofurantoin
  Norfloxacin
  p-Aminosalicylic acid
  Piromidic acid
  Polymyxin sulfate
  Rifampin
  Spiramycin
  Sulfonamides[a]
  Sulfadiazine
  Trimethoprim-sulfamethoxazole[a]
  Tetracyclines
  Minocycline[a]
  Vancomycin
Diuretics
Chlorthalidone
Ethacrynic acid
Furosemide
Thiazides
Ticrynafen
Tienilic acid
Triamterene
Other drugs
Aldomet
Allopurinol
Amlodipine
Amphetamine
Anti-CD4 antibodies
Aspirin
Azathioprine
Captopril
Chlorprothixene
Cimetidine
Clofibrate
Clozapine
Coumadin
Crack cocaine
Creatine
Cyclosporin[a]
Cytosine-Arabinoside
Diazepam
Doxepin
Ethambutol
Haloperidol
Heroin
Herbal medicines
Imipramine
Interleukin-2
Mesalamine[a]
Omeprazole
Phenazone
Phenindione[a]
Phenylpropanolamine[a]
Propranolol
Propylthiouracil
Quinine
Radiographic contrast agents
Ranitidine
Recombinant interferon-alpha
Streptokinase

[a]Cases reported in children.

philic TIN associated with anterior uveitis and bone marrow granulomas (113). Subsequent reports have highlighted the significant adolescent female predominance (111). The pathogenesis of this syndrome remains unclear, and preliminary evidence suggests roles for both humoral- and cell-mediated immune mechanisms. Circulating or deposited immune complexes were detected in up to 60% of patients (114,115). A significant number of patients, however, have no evidence of tubulointerstitial immune deposits on renal biopsy. Analysis of the lymphocytic infiltrates on biopsies of patients with TINU demonstrated a predominance of activated memory T-helper cells, thus providing further evidence for cell-mediated events (111). A genetic predisposition is suggested by the occurrence of TINU in identical twins within the same year (116). Patients usually have anorexia, fever, weight loss, abdominal pain, and polyuria. Eye tenderness may not be evident at presentation, as uveitis could occur at any time with respect to the onset of renal disease (117). Laboratory abnormalities include an elevated erythrocyte sedimentation rate, increased serum IgG levels, azotemia, and nonhemolytic anemia. Urinary abnormalities include proteinuria, glucosuria, and sterile pyuria. The interstitial nephritis resolves completely, either spontaneously or after steroid therapy in most cases. In a study of 21 children with acute TIN, TINU patients required a longer period of time for the renal function to recover in comparison with other etiologies (118). The uveitis often requires multiple steroid courses and other immunosuppressives, like methotrexate, azathioprine, and cyclosporin A, and may relapse (100,119).

TABLE 43.7. CLASSIFICATION OF TUBULOINTERSTITIAL NEPHRITIS ASSOCIATED WITH INFECTION

Direct infection of renal parenchyma (infectious agents identified in the interstitium)
Bacteria
Leptospira spp.[a]
Mycobacteria
Various species commonly associated with pyelonephritis[a]
Viruses
Adenovirus[a]
Cytomegalovirus[a]
Hantaviruses[a]
Polyoma virus (BK type)
Fungi
Histoplasma
Various species commonly associated with pyelonephritis
Rickettsia
Rickettsia diaporica (Q fever)
Rickettsia rickettsii
Reactive (sterile) interstitial nephritis (infectious agents not identified in the interstitium)
Bacteria
Brucella spp.
Corynebacterium diphtheriae
Francisella tularensis[b]
Group A-hemolytic streptococcus[a]
Legionella pneumophila
Mycoplasma hominis
Salmonella typhi
Streptococcus pneumoniae[a]
Treponema pallidum[b]
Yersinia pseudotuberculosis[a]
Viruses
Epstein-Barr virus[a]
Hepatitis B virus[b]
Human immunodeficiency virus (HIV)
Mumps[a]
Rubella virus[b] (togavirus)
Rubeola virus (paramyxovirus)
Parasites
Ascaris[b]
Leishmania donovani
Toxoplasma gondii[a]
Other
Kawasaki disease

[a]Cases reported in children.
[b]Incompletely documented or isolated cases.
Modified from Colvin RB, Fang LST. Interstitial nephritis. In: Tischer CC, Brenner BM, eds. *Renal pathology*. Philadelphia: JB Lippincott, 1994:723–768.

Recent case reports described the association of TINU with granulomatous hepatitis (120), hyperthyroidism (121), and Epstein-Barr virus infection (122).

Idiopathic

Idiopathic cases of acute TIN are uncommon in childhood. In a series of 12 children with biopsy-proven acute TIN, only 1 had idiopathic disease (8). These cases are diagnosed by exclusion of the previously described entities and usually are not associated with hypersensitivity symptoms of fever, rash, or eosinophilia (3).

Treatment and Prognosis

The initial treatment of acute TIN is primarily supportive, with dialysis therapy as indicated (3,4). It is important to immediately discontinue all possible offending medications, which in many patients might be multiple. When replacing the suspected medications, it is important to select medications that are not potentially cross-reactive (e.g., a cephalosporin to replace a β-lactam penicillin) or other potentially nephrotoxic agents (87). In infection-related acute TIN, specific treatment of the underlying infection is indicated (82).

The use of corticosteroid therapy for acute TIN remains controversial (7). Anecdotal case reports and uncontrolled trials with small numbers of patients suggest a therapeutic benefit (9,79,82). However, prospective controlled studies of corticosteroids or other cytotoxic agents in acute TIN are lacking, and it is possible that many reported patients would have recovered merely from the withdrawal of the inciting agent. Various steroid treatment regimens for acute TIN have been reported, primarily in the adult literature (84,123). Some children have been treated with daily prednisone at a dosage of 2 mg/kg/day, which is tapered rapidly over 2 to 4 weeks (82). Pulse methylprednisolone followed by high-dose daily or alternate-day prednisone has also been used in adults (123). In idiopathic cases and in those in whom removal of the offending agent do not result in improvement, we use a similar protocol of pulse methylprednisolone followed by daily oral prednisone of 2 mg/kg (maximum dose, 80 mg) for 4 weeks, then change to alternate day treatment and taper over a period of several months depending on the response.

Prognosis for recovery of renal function in children with acute TIN is excellent (8,79,82,87). Most affected patients recover renal function completely within weeks to months of onset of ARF. The mean renal recovery time of 13 children with acute TIN from various causes was 69.5 ± 34.7 days (82). All patients had normal serum creatinine and urinalysis at follow-up examination 1.5 to 10.0 years after presentation. Of note, the clinical or histologic severity of disease at presentation did not correlate with rate of recovery of renal function. Another study of seven children with acute TIN, 42% of who required dialysis, reported a renal recovery rate of 86% (79). In two studies of adults with acute TIN, poor prognostic factors included the severity of the interstitial inflammation on renal biopsy and the duration of ARF (124,125).

CHRONIC INTERSTITIAL NEPHRITIS

Epidemiology

Chronic TIN in children occurs primarily in the setting of obstructive uropathy, vesicoureteral reflux, and inherited conditions (3,9). Obstructive uropathy accounts for almost 20% of all children who develop end-stage renal disease (126). Primary chronic TIN from other causes accounts for only 2 to 4% of children with chronic renal failure (126). In a few families, chronic TIN has been described in association with cholestatic liver disease (92,93) and in others with mitochondrial abnormalities (127,128).

Clinical, Laboratory, and Radiologic Features

Chronic TIN tends to progress more slowly than other forms of chronic renal diseases, and therefore, affected individuals often have no clinical evidence of disease until late in the course of renal insufficiency (3). Many patients have nonspecific constitutional symptoms characteristic of chronic renal failure, with weight loss, growth retardation, fatigue, anorexia, vomiting, and occasionally polyuria and polydipsia (129). Hypertension may also occur (130). Patients with the syndrome of chronic TIN associated with cholestatic liver disease may also have symptoms of hepatic dysfunction, such as pruritus and scleral icterus (131). Naturally, in children with chronic TIN, a major manifestation may include growth failure.

The clinical, laboratory, and radiologic findings in chronic TIN are in essence similar to those observed in acute TIN. However, as in other cases of chronic kidney failure, the deterioration in kidney function is insidious, and the medical history might extend back to a longer period. In contrast to some patients with acute TIN, patients with chronic TIN do not have oliguria; on the contrary, some may be polyuric. In advanced cases, renal ultrasonography shows small and hyperechogenic kidneys. Skeletal radiographs may show renal osteodystrophy and in the case of Fanconi syndrome rickets and osteomalacia.

Pathology

Histologic findings in chronic TIN are characterized by tubulointerstitial fibrosis with a lymphocytic infiltrate, as well as tubular atrophy and thickening of the TBM (3,132). When renal damage is associated with high intratubular pressure, as occurs with vesicoureteral reflux and urinary tract obstruction, dilated renal tubules are particularly evident (81). In primary chronic TIN, glomeruli are often normal until late in the course of disease, when periglomerular fibrosis and global sclerosis are seen (Fig. 43.2) (131,132).

Etiology

The causes of chronic TIN are summarized in Table 43.8. Of note, acute TIN from any cause can progress to chronic TIN if the disease process is not abated by removal of the inciting agent or steroid therapy. Secondary chronic TIN associated with primary glomerular or vascular disorders, especially focal segmental glomerulosclerosis and hemolytic uremic syndrome, is a common histologic finding in patients with progressive renal disease (133).

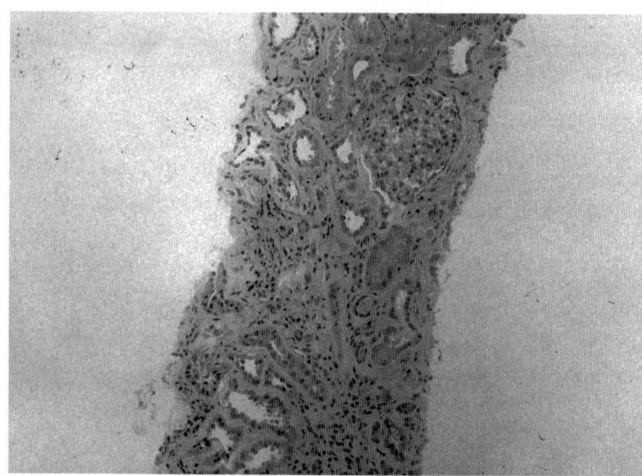

FIGURE 43.2. Chronic tubulointerstitial nephritis (TIN). Light microscopy of idiopathic chronic TIN in a 12-year-old boy. Renal cortex showing moderate interstitial fibrosis, tubular atrophy, and tortuosity. The interstitium is infiltrated by scattered mononuclear cells. A preserved glomerulus with periglomerular fibrosis is seen.

Chronic TIN in children most commonly is due to obstructive uropathy or high-grade vesicoureteral reflux, especially when associated with urinary tract infections (126). Urinary tract obstruction of only a few weeks' duration may result in irreversible renal damage (7). Isolated vesicoureteral reflux without obstruction might also be associated with chronic TIN in children. Interstitial damage and progressive fibrosis in these disorders may result from renal immune responses that amplify tubulointerstitial injury initially induced by high urinary tract pressures in the setting of infection. Persistent and progressive renal inflammation and damage can occur, however, despite relief of the obstruction or surgical correction of the vesicoureteral reflux (127,134,135).

Treatment and Prognosis

There is currently no known effective therapy for chronic TIN. Naturally, when an offending agent is detected, it should be removed. However, even in such cases the damage may be irreversible and its progression self-perpetuating. Some experimental data indicate the potential for pharmacotherapy in stopping or slowing the inflammatory, apoptotic, and fibrotic mechanisms by blocking their stimulating signals and activity. For instance, in the mouse model of unilateral obstruction, injury to the kidneys starts with increased angiotensin II production, which activates TGFβ in a cascade, leading to tubulointerstitial inflammation and fibrosis (59). The use of angiotensin-converting enzyme (ACE) inhibitors in this model dimin-

TABLE 43.8. ETIOLOGIC CLASSIFICATION OF CHRONIC INTERSTITIAL NEPHRITIS

Drug-related
- Acetaminophen
- Aspirin
- *cis*-Platinum
- Cyclosporine[a]
- Lithium
- L-Lysine
- Methoxyflurane
- Nitrosoureas (streptozotocin, CCNU, BCNU)
- Phenacetin
- Phenylbutazone
- Propylthiouracil

Heavy metal–related
- Arsenic
- Bismuth
- Cadmium
- Copper
- Gold
- Iron
- Lead
- Mercury
- Uranium

Hereditary
- Acute intermittent porphyria
- Alport syndrome
- Cystinosis
- Lesch-Nyhan syndrome
- Medullary cystic disease–Juvenile nephronophthisis complex
- Medullary sponge kidney
- Oxalosis
- Methylmalonic acidemia
- Fabry disease
- Polycystic kidney disease
- Sickle cell disease
- Wilson disease

Idiopathic

Infection-mediated (see Table 43.7)
- Direct infection of renal parenchyma (chronic or recurrent acute pyelonephritis)
- Reactive (sterile) interstitial nephritis

Immune-mediated
- Diseases usually associated with glomerulonephritis
  - Systemic lupus erythematosus[a]
  - Antiglomerular basement membrane disease
  - Mixed cryoglobulinemia
  - Polyarteritis nodosa
  - Wegener granulomatosis
- Diseases *not* usually associated with glomerulonephritis
  - Allograft rejection
  - Chronic active hepatitis
  - Familial immune complex interstitial nephritis
  - Sjögren syndrome
  - Tubulointerstitial nephritis and uveitis syndrome

Radiation-induced (induces cytotoxic reactive oxygen molecules)

Metabolic
- Hypercalcemia
- Hypercalciuria
- Hyperphosphatemia
- Hyperuricemia
- Hyperoxaluria
- Hyperparathyroidism
- Hypokalemia (potassium-losing nephropathy)

Miscellaneous
- Anorexia nervosa
- Balkan nephropathy
- Hemorrhagic fever
- Syndrome of tubulointerstitial nephritis and chronic cholestatic liver disease
- Hypoxic disorders
- Sarcoidosis

Neoplastic
- Leukemia
- Lymphoma
- Multiple myeloma

Urologic[a]
- Urinary tract obstruction
  - Calculi
  - Congenital
  - Posterior urethral valves[a]
  - Prune belly syndrome[a]
  - Ureteropelvic junction obstruction[a]
  - Surgery
  - Tumor
- Vesicoureteral reflux[a]

[a]Common cause in children.

ished transformation of renal cells to interstitial myofibroblasts and decreased migration of inflammatory cells into the interstitium. However, ACE inhibitors do not affect tubular atrophy (59).

In a recent study in the mouse model of unilateral ureteral obstruction, injection of exogenous hepatocyte growth factor blocked myofibroblast activation and dramatically prevented interstitial fibrosis (136). The study suggested that blockage of the transition of tubular epithelial cells to myofibroblasts may provide a novel therapeutic approach in halting fibrosis. In another study on the same animal model, administration of bone morphometric protein-7 prevented tubulointerstitial fibrosis and inhibited tubular atrophy by prevention of apoptosis. The exact mechanism of action by which bone morphometric protein-7 provides a renoprotective effect is yet unknown (59). Several studies have demonstrated the potential of 3-hydroxy-3-methylglutaryl CoA reductase inhibitors, like simvastatin and fluvastatin, in ameliorating interstitial fibrosis in animal models (137,138). Other studies examined the effect of blocking TGFβ and its mediators, like connective tissue growth factor in tissue fibrosis (139). A different direction of investigation is focused on the potential protective effect of nitric oxide in chronic TIN (61,140,141).

At the moment, patients with chronic TIN are treated with supportive therapy. Whether the use of angiotensin-converting enzyme inhibitors or 3-hydroxy-3-methylglutaryl CoA reductase inhibitors in human chronic TIN is effective as it is in some glomerular diseases associated with proteinuria has yet to be proven.

The prognosis for normalization of renal function in chronic TIN is less favorable than in acute disease. In specific forms of chronic TIN, such as juvenile nephronophthisis, progression to end-stage renal disease is almost inevitable (129,130). By contrast, patients with chronic TIN in the setting of obstructive uropathy have a more variable clinical course (127,134).

ACKNOWLEDGMENT

Supported by the Sam and Helen Kaplan Research Fund in Pediatric Nephrology.

REFERENCES

1. Eknoyan G, McDonald MA, Appel D, et al. Chronic tubulo-interstitial nephritis: correlation between structural and functional findings. *Kidney Int* 1990;38:736–743.
2. Nath KA. Tubulointerstitial changes as a major determinant in the progression of renal damage. *Am J Kidney Dis* 1992;20:1–17.
3. Eknoyan G. Tubulointerstitial nephropathies. In: Massry SG, Glassock RJ, eds. *Textbook of nephrology*, 3rd ed. Baltimore: Williams & Wilkins, 1995:1036–1046.
4. Appel GB. Acute interstitial nephritis. In: Neilson EG, Couser WG, eds. *Immunologic renal diseases*. Philadelphia: Lippincott–Raven, 1997:1221–1234.
5. Colvin RB, Fang LST. Interstitial nephritis. In: Tischer CC, Brenner BM, eds. *Renal pathology*. Philadelphia: JB Lippincott, 1994:723–768.
6. Neilson EG. Pathogenesis and therapy of interstitial nephritis. *Kidney Int* 1989;35:1257–1270.
7. Jones CL, Eddy AA. Tubulointerstitial nephritis. *Pediatr Nephrol* 1992;6:572–586.
8. Hawkins EP, Berry PL, Silva FG. Acute tubulointerstitial nephritis in children: clinical, morphologic, and lectin studies. A report of the Southwest Pediatric Nephrology Study Group. *Am J Kidney Dis* 1989;14:466–471.
9. Dell KM, Kaplan BS, Meyers CM. Tubulointerstitial nephritis. In: Barrat TM, Avner ED, Harmon WE, eds. *Pediatric nephrology*, 4th ed. Baltimore: Lippincott Williams & Wilkins, 1999:823–834.
10. Rastegar A, Kashgarian M. The clinical spectrum of tubulo-interstitial nephritis. *Kidney Int* 1998;54:313–327.
11. Wolgast MA, Larson M, Nygren K. Functional characteristics of renal interstitium. *Am J Physiol* 1981;241:F105–F111.
12. Lemley KV, Kriz W. Anatomy of the renal interstitium. *Kidney Int* 1991;39:370–381.
13. Meyers CM, Neilson EG. Immunopathogenesis of tubulo-interstitial disease. In: Massry S, Glassock R, eds. *Textbook of nephrology*, 3rd ed. Baltimore: Williams & Wilkins, 1995:671–677.
14. Meyers CM, Kelly CJ. Effector mechanisms in organ-specific autoimmunity I. Characterization of a CD8+ T cell line that mediates murine interstitial nephritis. *J Clin Invest* 1991;88:408–416.
15. Neilson EG, Phillips SM. Murine interstitial nephritis I. Analysis of disease susceptibility and its relationship to pleomorphic gene products defining both immune response genes and a restrictive requirement for cytotoxic T cells at H-2K. *J Exp Med* 1982;125:1075–1085.
16. Bender WL, Whelton A, Beschorner WE, et al. Interstitial nephritis, proteinuria, and renal failure caused by nonsteroidal anti-inflammatory drugs: immunologic characterization of the inflammatory infiltrate. *Am J Med* 1984;76:1006–1012.
17. Boucher A, Droz D, Adafer E, et al. Characterization of mononuclear cell subsets in renal cellular interstitial infiltrates. *Kidney Int* 1986;29:1043–1049.
18. Rosenberg ME, Schendel PB, McCurdy FA, et al. Characterization of immune cells in kidneys from patients with Sjögren's syndrome. *Am J Kidney Dis* 1988;11:20–22.
19. Mampaso F, Sanchez-Madrid F, Molina A, et al. Expression of adhesion receptor and counterreceptors from the leukocyte-endothelial adhesion pathways LFA-1/ICAM-1 and VLA-4/VCAM-1 on drug-induced tubulointerstitial nephritis. *Am J Nephrol* 1992;12:391–392.
20. Appel GB, Kunis CL. Acute tubulointerstitial nephritis. *Contemp Issues Nephrol* 1983;10:151–185.
21. McLeish KR, Senitzer D, Gohara AF. Acute interstitial nephritis in a patient with aspirin hypersensitivity. *Clin Immunol Immunopathol* 1979;14:64–69.
22. Neilson EG, McCafferty E, Mann R, et al. Murine interstitial nephritis III. The selection of phenotypic (Lyt and L3T4) and idiotypic (RE-Id) T cell preferences by genes in Igh-1 and H-2K characterize the cell-mediated potential for disease expression: susceptible mice provide a unique effector T cell repertoire in response to tubular antigen. *J Immunol* 1985;134:2375–2382.
23. Kelly CJ, Korngold R, Mann R, et al. Spontaneous nephritis in kdkd mice. II. Characterization of a tubular antigen-specific, H-2K restricted Lyt-2+ effector T cell that mediates destructive tubulointerstitial injury. *J Immunol* 1986;136:526–531.
24. Swain SI. T cell subsets and the recognition of MHC class. *Immunol Rev* 1983;74:129–142.
25. Hagerty DT, Allen PM. Processing and presentation of self and foreign antigens by the renal proximal tubule. *J Immunol* 1992;148:2324–2330.
26. Radeke HH, Emmendorffer A, Uciechowski P, et al. Activation of autoreactive T-lymphocytes by cultured syngeneic glomerular mesangial cells. *Kidney Int* 1993;45:763–774.
27. Meyers CM. T-cell regulation of renal immune responses. *Curr Opin Nephrol Hypertens* 1995;4:270–276.
28. Halloran PF, Jephthat-Ochola J, Urmson J, et al. Systemic immunologic stimuli increase class I and II antigen expression in mouse kidney. *J Immunol* 1985;135:1053–1060.
29. Wuthrich RP, Glimcher LH, Yui MA, et al. MHC class II, antigen presentation, and tumor necrosis factor in renal tubular epithelial cells. *Kidney Int* 1990;37:783–792.
30. Hagerty DT, Evavold BD, Allen PM. Regulation of the costimulator B7, not class II major histocompatibility complex, restricts the ability of murine kidney tubule cells to stimulate CD4+ T cells. *J Clin Invest* 1994;93:1208–1215.
31. Kelly CJ, Roth DA, Meyers CM. Immune recognition and response to the renal interstitium. *Kidney Int* 1991;31:518–530.

32. Mori S, Nose M, Miyazawa M, et al. Interstitial nephritis in Aleutian mink disease. Possible role of cell-mediated immunity against virus-infected tubular epithelial cells. *Am J Pathol* 1994;144:1326–1333.
33. Bhardwaj V, Kumar V, Geysen HM, et al. Degenerate recognition of a dissimilar antigenic peptide by myelin basic protein-reactive T cells. Implications for thymic education and autoimmunity. *J Immunol* 1993;151:5000–5010.
34. Border WA, Lehman DH, Egan JD, et al. Antitubular basement membrane antibodies in methicillin-associated interstitial nephritis. *N Engl J Med* 1974;291:381–384.
35. Wilson CB, Lehman DH, McCoy RC, et al. Antitubular basement membrane antibodies after renal transplantation. *Transplantation* 1974;18:447–452.
36. Salant DJ, Quigg RJ, Cybulsky AV. Heymann nephritis: mechanisms of renal injury. *Kidney Int* 1989;35:976–984.
37. Hoyer JR. Tubulointerstitial immune complex nephritis in rats immunized with Tamm-Horsfall protein. *Kidney Int* 1980;17:284–292.
38. Thomas DBL, Davies M, Williams JD. Tamm-Horsfall protein. An aetiological agent in tubulointerstitial disease? *Exp Nephrol* 1993;1:281–284.
39. Cavallone D, Malagolini N, Serafini-Cessi F. Binding of human neutrophils to cell-surface anchored Tamm-Horsfall glycoprotein in tubulointerstitial nephritis. *Kidney Int* 1999; 55:1787–1799.
40. Noble B, Mendrick DL, Brentjens JR, et al. Antibody-mediated injury to proximal tubules in the rat kidney induced by passive transfer of homologous anti-brush border serum. *Clin Immunol Immunopathol* 1981;19:289–301.
41. Gronhagen-Riska C, von-Willebrand E, Honkanen E, et al. Interstitial cellular infiltration detected by fine-needle aspiration biopsy in nephritis. *Clin Nephrol* 1990;34:189–196.
42. Clayman MD, Martinez-Hernandez A, Michaud L, et al. Isolation and characterization of the nephritogenic antigen producing antitubular basement membrane disease. *J Exp Med* 1985;161:290–305.
43. Clayman MD, Michaud L, Brentjens J, et al. Isolation of the target antigen of human anti-tubular basement membrane antibody-associated interstitial nephritis. *J Clin Invest* 1986;77:1143–1147.
44. Wilson CB. Individual and strain differences in renal basement membrane antigens. *Transplant Proc* 1980;12(suppl 1):69–73.
45. Lehman DH, Lee S, Wilson CB, Dixon FJ. Induction of antitubular basement membrane antibodies in rats renal by transplantation. *Transplantation* 1974;17:429–431.
46. Fasth A, Ahlstedt S, Hanson LA, et al. Cross-reactions between the Tamm-Horsfall glycoprotein and *Escherichia coli*. *Int Arch Allergy Appl Immunol* 1980;63:303–311.
47. Platt JL, Sibley RK, Michael AF. Interstitial nephritis associated with cytomegalovirus infection. *Kidney Int* 1985;28: 550–552.
48. van-Ypersele-de-Strihou C, Mery JP. Hantavirus-related acute interstitial nephritis in western Europe: Expansion of a world-wide zoonosis. *Q J Med* 1989;73:941–950.
49. Madaio MP, Carlson J, Cataldo J, et al. Murine monoclonal anti-DNA antibodies bind directly to glomerular antigens and form immune deposits. *J Immunol* 1987;138:2883–2889.
50. Faaber P, Rijke TPM, Van de Putte LBA, et al. Cross-reactivity of human and murine anti-DNA antibodies with heparan sulfate. *J Clin Invest* 1986;77:1824–1830.
51. Wilson CB. Nephritogenic tubulointerstitial antigens. *Kidney Int* 1991;39:501–517.
52. Makker SP. Tubular basement membrane antibody-induced interstitial nephritis in systemic lupus erythematosus. *Am J Med* 1980;69:949–952.
53. Brentjens JR, O'Connell DW, Pawlowski IB, et al. Extra glomerular lesions associated with deposition of circulating antigen-antibody complexes in kidneys of rabbits with chronic serum sickness. *Clin Immunol Immunopathol* 1974; 3:112–126.
54. Lehman DH, Wilson CB, Dixon FJ. Extraglomerular immunoglobulin deposits in human nephritis. *Am J Med* 1975;58:765–796.
55. Couser WG. Mechanisms of glomerular injury: an overview. *Semin Nephrol* 1991;11:254–258.
56. Hyun J, Galen MA. Acute interstitial nephritis: a case characterized by increase in serum IgG, IgM, and IgE concentrations: Eosinophilia, and IgE deposition in renal tubules. *Arch Intern Med* 1981;141:679–681.
57. Nath KA, Hostetter MK, Hostetter TH. Pathophysiology of chronic tubulo-interstitial disease in rats. Interactions of dietary acid load, ammonia, and complement C3. *J Clin Invest* 1985:76;667–675.
58. Segerer S, Nelson PJ, Schlondorff D. Chemokines, chemokine receptors, and renal disease: from basic science to pathophysiologic and therapeutic studies. *J Am Soc Nephrol* 2000;11:152–176.
59. Hruska K. Treatment of chronic tubulointerstitial disease: a new concept. *Kidney Int* 2002;61:1911–1922.
60. Luster AD. Chemokines—chemotactic cytokines that mediate inflammation. *N Engl J Med* 1998;338:436–445.
61. Harris DC. Tubulointerstitial renal disease. *Curr Opin Neph Hyperten* 2000;10:303–313.
62. Remuzzi G, Bertani T. Mechanisms of disease: pathophysiology progressive nephropathies. *N Engl J Med* 1998;339: 1448–1456.
63. Strutz F, Neilson EG. The role of lymphocytes in the progression of interstitial disease. *Kidney Int* 1994;45(suppl 45):S106–S110.
64. Kuncio GS, Neilson EG, Haverty TP. Mechanisms of tubulointerstitial fibrosis. *Kidney Int* 1992;39:550–556.
65. Muller GA, Rodemann HP. Characterization of human renal fibroblasts in health and disease: I. Immunophenotyping of cultured tubular epithelial cells and fibroblasts derived from kidneys with histologically proven interstitial fibrosis. *Am J Kidney Dis* 1991;17:680–683.
66. Rodemann HP, Muller GA. Characterization of human renal fibroblasts in health and disease: II. In vitro growth, differentiation, and collagen synthesis of fibroblasts from kidneys with interstitial fibrosis. *Am J Kidney Dis* 1991;17: R684–R686.
67. Tang WW, Ulich TR, Lacey DL, et al. Platelet-derived growth factor-BB induces renal tubulointerstitial myofibroblast formation and tubulointerstitial fibrosis. *Am J Pathol* 1996;148:1169–1180.
68. Rulz-Ortega M, Gomez-Garre D, Alcazar R, et al. Involvement of angiotensin II and endothelin in matrix protein

production and renal sclerosis. *J Hypertens* 1994;12(suppl 4):S51–S58.

69. Tang WW, Van GY, Qi M. Myofibroblasts and alpha 1 (III) collagen expression in experimental tubulointerstitial nephritis. *Kidney Int* 1997;51:926–931.
70. Freundlich B, Bomalaski JS, Neilson EG, Jimenez SA: Immune regulation of fibroblast proliferation and collagen synthesis by soluble factors from mononuclear cells. *Immunol Today* 1986;7:303–307.
71. Ishidoya S, Morrissey J, McCracken R, et al. Angiotensin II receptor antagonists ameliorates renal tubulointerstitial fibrosis caused by unilateral ureteral obstruction. *Kidney Int* 1995;47:1285–1294.
72. Strutz F, Okada H, Lo CW, et al. Identification and characterization of a fibroblast marker: FSP1. *J Cell Biol* 1995;130:393–405.
73. Okada H, Danoff TM, Kalluri R, et al. An early role to FSP1 in epithelial-mesenchymal transformation. *Am J Physiol* 1997;273:563–574.
74. Ng Y-Y, Huang T-P, Yang W-C, et al. Tubular epithelial-myofibroblast transdifferentiation in progressive tubulointerstitial fibrosis in 5/6 nephrectomized rats. *Kidney Int* 1998;54:864–877.
75. Alvarez RJ, Haverty TP, Watanabe M, et al. Biosynthetic and proliferative heterogeneity of anatomically distinct fibroblasts probed with paracrine cytokines. *Kidney Int* 1992;41:14–23.
76. Wahl LM, Winter CC. Regulation of guinea pig macrophage collagenase production by dexamethasone and colchicine. *Arch Biochem Biophys* 1984;230:661–667.
77. Wahl S, Hunt D, Wakefield L, et al. Transforming growth factor beta (TGF-β) induces monocyte chemotaxis and growth factor production. *Proc Natl Acad Sci U S A* 1987;84:5788–5792.
78. Heeger P, Neilson EG. Treatment of interstitial nephritis. In: Glassock R, ed. *Current therapy in nephrology and hypertension*, vol. 3. Philadelphia: Dekker, 1992:108–113.
79. Greising J, Trachtman H, Gauthier B, et al. Acute interstitial nephritis in adolescents and young adults. *Child Nephrol Urol* 1990;10:189–195.
80. Ooi BS, Jao W, First MR, et al. Acute interstitial nephritis: a clinical and pathologic study based on renal biopsies. *Am J Med* 1975;59:614–629.
81. Zollinger HU, Mihatsch MJ. Renal pathology in biopsy. Berlin: Springer-Verlag, 1978:118–146, 407–410.
82. Ellis D, Fried WA, Yunis EJ, et al. Acute interstitial nephritis in children: a report of 13 cases and review of the literature. *Pediatrics* 1981;67:862–870.
83. Lantz B, Cochat P, Bouchet JL, et al. Short-term niflumic-acid-induced acute renal failure in children. *Nephrol Dial Transplant* 1994;9:1234–1239.
84. Linton AL, Clark WF, Driedger AA, et al. Acute interstitial nephritis due to drugs. *Ann Intern Med* 1980;93:735–741.
85. Ruley EJ, Lisi LM. Interstitial nephritis and renal failure due to ampicillin. *J Pediatr* 1974;6:878–881.
86. Hyman LR, Ballow M, Knieser MR. Diphenylhydantoin interstitial nephritis. Roles of cellular and humoral immunologic injury. *J Pediatr* 1978;92:915–920.
87. Sanjad SA, Haddad GG, Nassar VH. Nephropathy, an underestimated complication of methicillin therapy. *J Pediatr* 1974;84:873–877.
88. Kleinknecht D. Interstitial nephritis, the nephrotic syndrome, and chronic renal failure secondary to nonsteroidal anti-inflammatory drugs. *Semin Nephrol* 1995;15:228–235.
89. Toto RD. Review: acute tubulointerstitial nephritis. *Am J Med Sci* 1990;299:392–410.
90. Cogan MG. Tubulointerstitial nephropathies: a pathophysiologic approach. *West J Med* 1980;132:134–142.
91. Cogan MC, Arieff AI. Sodium wasting, acidosis, and hyperkalemia induced by methicillin interstitial nephritis. *Am J Med* 1978;65:500–507.
92. Neuhaus TJ, Stallmach T, Leumann E, et al. Familial progressive tubulo-interstitial nephropathy and cholestatic liver disease—a newly recognized entity? *Eur J Pediatr* 1997;156: 723–726.
93. Montini G, Carasi C, Zancan L, et al. Chronic cholestatic liver disease with associated tubulointerstitial nephropathy in early childhood. *Pediatrics* 1997;100:e10.
94. Brezin JH, Katz SM, Schartz AB, et al. Reversible renal failure and nephrotic syndrome associated with nonsteroidal anti-inflammatory drugs. *N Engl J Med* 1979;301:1271–1273.
95. Nolan CRF, Anger MS, Kelleher SP. Eosinophiluria—a new method of detection and definition of the clinical spectrum. *N Engl J Med* 1986;315:1516–1520.
96. Ruffing KA, Hoppes P, Blend A, et al. Eosinophils in the urine revisited. *Clin Nephrol* 1994;41:163–166.
97. Korzets Z, Elis A, Bernheim J, et al. Acute granulomatous interstitial nephritis due to nitrofurantoin. *Nephrol Dial Transplant* 1994;9:713–715.
98. Thieme RE, Caldwell SA, Lum GM. Acute interstitial nephritis associated with loracarbef therapy. *J Pediatr* 1995; 127:997–1000.
99. Okada K, Okamoto Y, Kagami S, et al. Acute interstitial nephritis and uveitis with bone marrow granulomas and anti-neutrophil cytoplasmic antibodies. *Am J Nephrol* 1995; 15:337–342.
100. Levy M, Guesry P, Loirat C, et al. Immunologically mediated tubulointerstitial nephritis in children. *Contrib Nephrol* 1979;16:132–140.
101. Saltissi D, Pusey CD, Rainford DJ. Recurrent acute renal failure due to antibiotic-induced interstitial nephritis. *BMJ* 1979;1:1182–1183.
102. Assouad M, Vicks SL, Pokroy MV, et al. Recurrent acute interstitial nephritis on rechallenge with omeprazole. *Lancet* 1994;344:549.
103. Josephson MA, Chiu MY, Woodle ES, et al. Drug-induced acute interstitial nephritis in renal allografts: Histopathologic features and clinical course in six patients. *Am J Kid Dis* 1999;34:540–548.
104. Councilman WT. Acute interstitial nephritis. *J Exp Med* 1898;3:393–420.
105. Ito M, Hirabayashi N, Uno Y, et al. Necrotizing tubulointerstitial nephritis associated with adenovirus infection. *Hum Pathol* 1991;22:1225–1231.
106. Nochy D, Glotz D, Dosquest P, et al. Renal disease associated with HIV infection: a multicentric study of 60 patients from Paris hospitals. *Nephrol Dial Transplant* 1993;8:11–19.
107. Koo JW, Park SN, Choi SM, et al. Acute renal failure associated with *Yersinia pseudotuberculosis* infection. *Pediatr Nephrol* 1996;10:582–586.

108. Magil AB, Tyler M. Tubulointerstitial disease in lupus nephritis. *Histopathology* 1984;8:81–87.
109. Park MH, D'Agati V, Appel GB, et al. Tubulointerstitial disease in lupus nephritis: relationship to immune deposits, interstitial inflammation, glomerular changes, renal function, and prognosis. *Nephron* 1986;44:309–319.
110. Frasca GM, Vangelista A, Biagini G, et al. Immunological tubulointerstitial deposits in IgA nephropathy. *Kidney Int* 1982;22:184–191.
111. Rodriguez-Perez JC, Cruz-Alamo V, Perez-Aciego P, et al. Clinical and immune aspects of idiopathic acute tubulointerstitial nephritis and uveitis syndrome. *Am J Nephrol* 1995; 15:386–391.
112. Singh AK, Ucci A, Madias NE. Predominant tubulointerstitial lupus nephritis. *Am J Kidney Dis* 1996;27:273–278.
113. Dobrin RS, Vernier RL, Fish AL. Acute eosinophilic interstitial nephritis and renal failure with bone marrow lymph node granulomas and anterior uveitis, a new syndrome. *Am J Med* 1975;59:325–333.
114. Vanhaesebrouck P, Carton D, De Bel C, et al. Acute tubulo-interstitial nephritis and uveitis syndrome (TINU syndrome). *Nephron* 1985;40:418–422.
115. Iida H, Terada Y, Nishino A, et al. Acute tubulointerstitial nephritis with bone marrow granulomas and uveitis. *Nephron* 1985;40:108–110.
116. Gianviti A, Greco M, Barsotti P, et al. Acute tubulointerstitial nephritis occurring with 1-year lapse in identical twins. *Pediatr Nephrol* 1994;8:427–430.
117. Vohra S, Eddy A, Levin AV, et al. Tubulointerstitial nephritis and uveitis in children and adolescents. *Pediatr Nephrol* 1999;13:426–432.
118. Kobayashi Y, Honda M, Yoshikawa N, Ito H. Acute tubulo-interstitial nephritis in 21 Japanese children. *Clin Nephrol* 2000;54:191–197.
119. Gion N, Stavrou P, Foster CS. Immunomodulatory therapy for chronic tubulointerstitial nephritis-associated uveitis. *Am J Ophthal* 2000;129:764–768.
120. Segev A, Ben-Chitrit S, Orion Y, et al. Acute eosinophilic interstitial nephritis and uveitis (TINU syndrome) associated with granulomatous hepatitis. *Clin Nephrol* 1999;51: 310–313.
121. Paul E, Why SV, Carpenter TO. Hyperthyroidism: a novel feature of the tubulointerstitial nephritis and uveitis syndrome. *Pediatrics* 1999;104:314–317.
122. Grefer J, Santer R, Ankermann T, et al. Tubulointerstitial nephritis and uveitis in association with Epstein-Barr virus infection. *Pediatr Nephrol* 1999;13:336–339.
123. Pusey CD, Saltissi D, Bloodworth L, et al. Drug-associated acute interstitial nephritis: clinical and pathological features and the response to high-dose steroid therapy. *Q JM* 1983; 52:194–211.
124. Kida H, Abe T, Tomosugi N, et al. Prediction of the long-term outcome in acute interstitial nephritis. *Clin Nephrol* 1984;22:55–60.
125. Laberke HG, Bohle A. Acute interstitial nephritis: correlations between clinical and morphological findings. *Clin Nephrol* 1980;14:263–273.
126. Kohaut EC, Tejani A. The 1994 annual report of the North American Pediatric Renal Transplant Cooperative Study. *Pediatr Nephrol* 1996;10:422–434.
127. Ormos J, Zsurka G, Turi S, et al. Familial mitochondrial tubulointerstitial nephropathy. *Nephrol Dial Transplant* 1999; 14:785–786.
128. Tzen, CY, Tsai JD, Wu TY, et al. Tubulointerstitial nephritis associated with a novel mitochondrial point mutation. *Kidney Int* 2001;59:846–854.
129. Hildebrandt F, Waldess R, Kutt R, et al. The nephronophthisis complex: clinical and genetic aspects. *Clin Invest* 1992;70:802-808.
130. Gagnadoux MF, Bacri JL, Broyer M, et al. Infantile chronic tubulo-interstitial nephritis with cortical microcysts: variant of nephronophthisis or new disease entity? *Pediatr Nephrol* 1989;3:50–55.
131. Popovic-Rolovic M, Kostic M, Sindjic M, et al. Progressive tubulointerstitial nephritis and chronic cholestatic liver disease. *Pediatr Nephrol* 1993;7:396–400.
132. Helczynski L, Landing BH. Tubulointerstitial renal diseases of children: pathologic features and pathogenetic mechanisms in Fanconi's familial nephronophthisis, antitubular basement membrane antibody disease, and medullary cyst disease. *Pediatr Pathol* 1984;2:1–24.
133. D'Amico G, Ferrario F, Rastaldi MP. Tubulointerstitial damage in glomerular disease: its role in the progression of renal damage. *Am J Kidney Dis* 1995;26:124–132.
134. Tejani A, Butt K, Glassberg K, et al. Predictors of eventual end-stage renal disease in children with posterior urethral valves. *J Urol* 1986;136:857–860.
135. Hodson J, Maling JMJ, McManamon PJ, et al. Reflux nephropathy. *Kidney Int* 1975;8:S50–S58.
136. Yang J, Liu Y. Blockage of tubular epithelial to myofibroblast transition by hepatocyte growth factor prevents renal interstitial fibrosis. *J Am Soc Nephrol* 2002;13:96–107.
137. Johnson DW, Saunders HJ, Field MJ, Pollock CA. In vitro effects of simvastatin on tubulointerstitial cells in a human model of cyclosporin nephrotoxicity. *Am J Physiol* 1999; 276:F467–F475.
138. Mroiyama T, Kawada N, Nagatoya K, et al. Fluvastatin suppresses oxidative stress and fibrosis in the interstitium of mouse kidneys with unilateral ureteral obstruction. *Kidney Int* 2001;59:2095–2103.
139. Gupta S, Clarkson MR, Duggan J, et al. Connective tissue growth factor: Potential role in glomerulosclerosis and tubulointerstitial fibrosis. *Kidney Int* 2000;58:1389–1399.
140. Kelly CJ, Gold DP. Nitric oxide in interstitial nephritis and other autoimmune diseases. *Semin Nephrol* 1999;19:288–295.
141. Gabbai FB, Hammond TC, Thomson SC, et al. Effect of acute iNOS inhibition on glomerular function in tubulointerstitial nephritis. *Kidney Int* 2002;61:851–854.

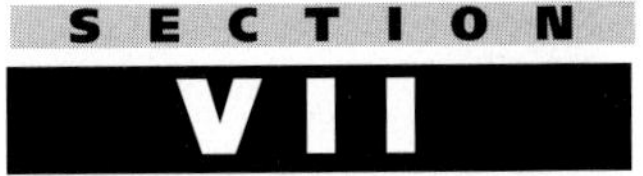

SYSTEMIC DISEASE

44

RENAL VASCULITIS

RUDOLPH P. VALENTINI
WILLIAM E. SMOYER

Renal vasculitis, or inflammation of the blood vessels involving the kidney, is a process mediated by neutrophilic infiltration of vessel walls resulting in fibrinoid necrosis. Its consequences include compromise of the vascular lumen and tissue ischemia. *Renal vascular involvement* is defined as a process affecting the blood supply to the kidney and its vessels within. Therefore, this consists of vessels of various sizes such as the aorta, renal artery, renal arterioles, or glomerular capillaries. Typically, renal manifestations of vasculitis include hypertension and glomerulonephritis.

Pediatric diseases associated with renal vasculitis may be renal-limited, but are more commonly systemic. Those with systemic manifestations may involve other large, medium, and small vessels outside of the renovascular system, such as the subclavian arteries, coronary arteries, alveolar capillaries, and postcapillary venules of the dermis. Depending on the organ systems involved, sinopulmonary, dermatologic, gastrointestinal (GI), and/or musculoskeletal symptoms may develop. In an effort to afford clinicians an easier way to differentiate the various forms of systemic vasculitis, a few classification schemes have been developed. Because no one classification scheme is complete, a combination of various schemata is typically needed.

A clinical classification scheme based on the organs involved can be used to develop a differential diagnosis. For example, a child presenting with glomerulonephritis and pulmonary hemorrhage is considered to have a pulmonary renal syndrome. The differential diagnosis for this clinical entity includes Wegener granulomatosis (WG), microscopic polyangiitis (MPA), anti–glomerular basement membrane (anti-GBM) disease, systemic lupus erythematosus (SLE), and Henoch-Schönlein purpura (HSP) (Table 44.1). This differential diagnosis can be further narrowed after considering further clinical and laboratory data.

Another vasculitis classification scheme relates to the caliber of the vessel(s) involved. The differential diagnosis can be separated into diseases involving small, medium, or large vessels. The small vessel vasculitides with renal involvement (e.g., HSP, SLE, WG, MPA, Churg-Strauss disease, and anti-GBM disease) typically affect the glomerular capillaries and manifest clinically as glomerulonephritis. The vasculitides involving larger vessels such as classic polyarteritis nodosa (cPAN) (medium vessels) or Takayasu's arteritis (TA) (large vessels) are more apt to result in renal ischemia and hypertension.

Further characterization of a child with a small vessel vasculitis manifesting as a pulmonary renal syndrome requires laboratory testing and in many instances a tissue biopsy. Serologic testing includes C3 and C4, antinuclear antibodies (ANAs), anti–double-stranded DNA antibodies, anti-GBM antibodies, antineutrophil cytoplasmic autoantibodies (ANCAs), anti-proteinase 3 (PR3) antibodies, and anti-myeloperoxidase (MPO) antibodies.

A histologic classification scheme uses features of the renal biopsy to differentiate disease states. Light microscopy can point out the presence of a necrotizing glomerulonephritis as can be seen in the small vessel vasculitides. In addition, the presence of granulomas would point further toward WG or Churg-Strauss disease (1). Unfortunately, granulomas, when present, are less likely to be seen on a renal biopsy when compared to a lung biopsy (2,3).

Immunofluorescence is the most useful part of the renal biopsy when classifying forms of renal vasculitis. Immune complex diseases such as HSP and lupus have characteristic glomerular staining patterns. Linear immunoglobulin G staining along the GBM is characteristic of anti-GBM disease. Minimal or absent immunofluorescence staining is seen in the pauciimmune glomerulonephritides, such as WG, MPA, Churg-Strauss disease, and ANCA (+) pauci-immune crescentic glomerulonephritis. A summary of the above classification systems can be seen in Table 44.2.

This background is used as a foundation on which to develop a more detailed comparison of these various forms of renal vasculitis. The reader should note that anti-GBM antibody disease (Goodpasture disease) is not always classified with vasculitis, although it is an immune-mediated process resulting in a focal necrotizing and crescentic glomerulonephritis and pulmonary hemorrhage. For further discussion of anti-GBM antibody disease, see Chapter 34. The forms of vasculitis are discussed by the size of the vessel involved beginning with the small vessel vasculitides.

TABLE 44.1. PULMONARY RENAL SYNDROMES IN CHILDREN

Antineutrophil cytoplasmic autoantibody–associated diseases
Wegener granulomatosis
Microscopic polyangiitis
Churg-Strauss syndrome
Immune complex diseases
Systemic lupus erythematosus
Henoch-Schönlein purpura
Anti–glomerular basement membrane disease (Goodpasture disease)
Other
Legionella infection
Renal vein thrombosis with pulmonary embolus

SMALL VESSEL VASCULITIS

By definition, the *small vessel vasculitides* are diseases with a predilection for involvement of small arteries, arterioles, capillaries, and postcapillary venules. The differential diagnosis for this disease category is quite extensive. As mentioned earlier, the types of small vessel vasculitis can be further classified using immunopathology. When glomerulonephritis is present, the immunofluorescence component of the renal biopsy reveals the presence or absence of significant immunostaining and results in classification as immune complex–mediated disease, anti-GBM disease, or pauciimmune disease.

Immune Complex–Mediated Disease

The two most common systemic forms of immune complex–mediated small vessel vasculitis with renal involvement in pediatrics are HSP and SLE. These two topics are dealt with in Chapters 45 and 46.

TABLE 44.2. RENAL VASCULITIS IN CHILDREN

Systemic diseases with renal involvement
Large vessel vasculitis
Takayasu's arteritis
Medium vessel vasculitis
Polyarteritis nodosum
Kawasaki disease
Small vessel vasculitis
Immune complex diseases
Systemic lupus erythematosus
Henoch-Schönlein purpura
Pauciimmune diseases
Granulomatous
Wegener granulomatosis
Churg-Strauss Disease
Non-granulomatous
Microscopic polyangiitis
Anti–glomerular basement membrane disease
Renal-limited disease
Antineutrophil cytoplasmic autoantibodies (+) pauciimmune crescentic glomerulonephritis

Pauciimmune-Mediated Disease

By definition, pauciimmune vasculitis is a small vessel vasculitis that features minimal or no immune deposits on immunofluorescence on a renal biopsy. Most varieties are ANCA associated, but a small number are ANCA negative (4,5). Based on the Chapel Hill Consensus Conference, ANCA-associated vasculitis is comprised of three systemic diseases and one renal limited disease (1). MPA is an ANCA-associated systemic vasculitis that often involves the skin, lungs, and kidneys. It is characterized by a positive ANCA test [perinuclear ANCA (pANCA) or cytoplasmic ANCA (cANCA)], absence of airway symptoms, and absence of granulomas on biopsy. WG is a systemic vasculitis with multiorgan involvement, including the respiratory tract; is usually cANCA positive; and is characterized by the presence of granulomas on biopsy. Churg-Strauss disease is the third ANCA-associated systemic vasculitis and is characterized by the presence of granulomas on biopsy and clinical asthma and eosinophilia. The renal limited ANCA (+) vasculitis is known as *pauciimmune crescentic glomerulonephritis*. These four entities are described in greater detail later beginning with the granulomatous ANCA (+) systemic vasculitides.

Wegener Granulomatosis

WG is a clinicopathologic entity that is uncommon in children. The triad of generalized WG consists of necrotizing granulomatous lesions of the upper or lower respiratory tract, generalized necrotizing vasculitis involving both small- and medium-sized vessels, and focal necrotizing glomerulonephritis (6,7). Regional WG is distinguished from generalized WG by the absence of renal disease. While the largest case series have been reported in adults, scattered reports of WG exist in the pediatric literature (8–10). Since the advent of ANCA testing, the definitions of WG have been revised. This has enabled clinicians to better distinguish it from MPA, a disease with which it shares much in common.

The definition of WG, as determined by the Chapel Hill Consensus Conference on the Nomenclature of Systemic Vasculitis, requires evidence of granulomatous inflammation (1). This "new" definition is contrasted from that previously used by the National Institute of Health (NIH) studies of WG patients. At the NIH, patients were required to have a clinical history compatible with WG and histologic evidence of either a vasculitis or granulomatous inflammation in a typical organ system (10). The absence of an absolute need for evidence of granulomatous inflammation in the NIH studies suggests that their WG patient population also included patients who are today classified as MPA. This distinction makes comparison of older studies to more modern ones difficult.

This section focuses on renal manifestations of WG and their treatment. The extrarenal symptoms are discussed

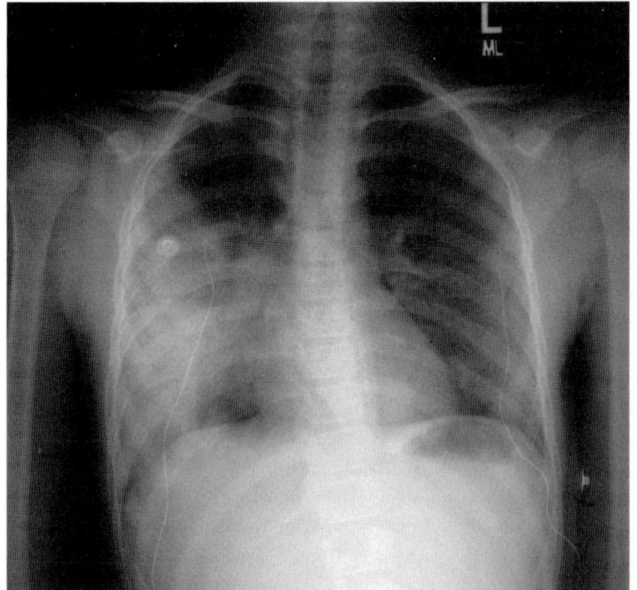

A

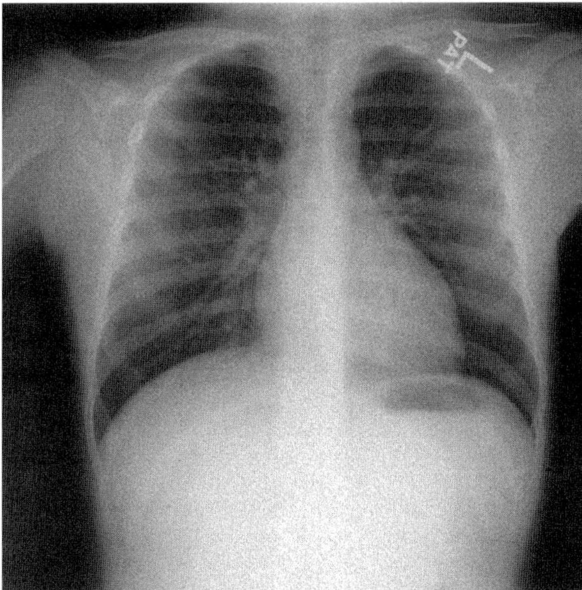

B

FIGURE 44.1. **A:** A 10-year-old boy with a history of fever, rash, and arthritis presented with hemoptysis accompanied by hematuria and proteinuria. His c-antineutrophil cytoplasmic autoantibody was positive at 1:512. Chest x-ray revealed opacification of the middle and lower lung fields on the right side. **B:** Ten weeks later, a follow-up chest x-ray showed complete resolution of the pulmonary infiltrates.

only briefly, as more comprehensive reports exist in the otolaryngology and ophthalmology literature (12,13).

From the outset of its initial descriptions in the literature, the prognosis of patients afflicted with WG was grim. Untreated adults with WG survived an average of only 5 months, with 82% succumbing to the disease within the first year and 90% by the second year (14). Corticosteroid treatment only increased the mean survival time to 12.5 months. The advent of cytotoxic therapy for WG, however, resulted in markedly improved patient survival. At a mean follow-up of 51 months, Fauci et al. reported a patient survival rate of 88% in 85 patients with WG (2).

The most comprehensive report on children with WG was published from the NIH (8). This study did not include any data on ANCA testing but described the clinical presentation, clinical course, and morbidity of children classified as having WG. Affected children were predominantly adolescent (mean age of onset, 15.4 years) and female (16 of 23 patients). There was a median of 8 months from onset of symptoms until a definitive diagnosis was secured. Clinical features at presentation were largely sinopulmonary, followed later by renal symptoms.

Children with WG usually sought medical attention for symptoms related to the upper and lower respiratory tract. Ear, nose, and throat pathology was present in 87% of patients, with sinusitis occurring most commonly (61%) (8). Large numbers of children developed large airway disease early on and subglottic stenosis later in their courses. The 48% of pediatric patients with subglottic stenosis far exceeded the 10% occurrence reported in adults (11). Pulmonary involvement in WG can range from asymptomatic to severe and fulminant. Pulmonary infiltrates (61%), pulmonary nodules (43%), and hemoptysis (26%) were the most common lung abnormalities. Radiographic abnormalities may occur in the absence of symptoms. In its most severe form, WG may present as life-threatening diffuse alveolar hemorrhage, which is often accompanied by progressive glomerulonephritis (Fig. 44.1).

Constitutional symptoms at disease onset included fever and weight loss. Other systemic symptoms at presentation included arthalgia/arthritis in approximately one-third of patients and rash in 9%. Eye disease was common and included dacrocystitis, proptosis, eye pain, and episcleritis.

The neurologic and cardiovascular systems can be involved as well. The adult literature states that 4% of patients with WG present with nervous system involvement, but it eventually develops in 10 to 34% (15). A peripheral neuropathy such as mononeuritis multiplex has been the most frequent neurologic manifestation described in adults with WG. Cardiac involvement is rarely detected antemortem but includes pericarditis and coronary arteritis in 10 to 20% of cases. Necrotizing vasculitis of the coronary vessels can result in a myocardial infarction or sudden death (15).

In this same large pediatric WG series, glomerulonephritis was present in only 9% of children at disease presentation, although it ultimately developed in 61% during the course of their disease (8). Hematuria, proteinuria, and renal insufficiency were common, whereas hypertension and gross hematuria were unusual. Fifty-seven percent of children with renal involvement developed chronic renal insufficiency, and 14% required dialysis.

The incidence of WG in children is difficult to determine, but it is known to occur much less frequently than in adults. According to the 1999 United States Renal Data Systems Annual Data Report, WG was the underlying cause of end-stage renal disease (ESRD) in 40 pediatric patients (age younger than 20) over 5 years (1993 to 1997). The median age of these patients was 16 years. Forty-eight percent were male and 82% were white (16).

Pathogenesis

Necrotizing vasculitis of small arteries and veins together with granuloma formation are the hallmark lesions of WG. Granulomatous necrotizing lesions are most commonly found in the respiratory tract. Lung involvement may include bilateral nodular cavitary infiltrates (15). The renal biopsy lesion is that of a pauciimmune-necrotizing and crescentic glomerulonephritis.

The pathogenesis of WG is still unknown. The role of ANCAs has not yet been determined. An autoimmune mechanism seems likely, but direct evidence does not yet exist *in vivo*. It is known that *in vitro* neutrophils from patients with active WG express PR3 on their surface, thus increasing their accessibility to circulating PR3 antibodies. Furthermore, "primed" neutrophils from patients with WG have increased basal superoxide anion production, which enhances their inflammatory potential (17). In addition, *in vitro* tests have shown that neutrophils activated by ANCA are retained within the vessel longer owing to increased endothelial adhesion and reduced transendothelial migration, thereby increasing their ability to induce endothelial injury (18). Finally, ANCA induces endothelial injury *in vitro* through the activation of neutrophils that release reactive oxygen radicals and inflammatory cytokines and proteases (reviewed in 18). Respiratory infections may be part of the inciting event for both the initial onset of disease, as well as for relapses. There is also an increased association of WG and the HLA-B8 and HLA-DR2 gene loci (19,20).

Laboratory Features

General

Nonspecific laboratory abnormalities in WG include anemia, thrombocytosis, and leukocytosis in 30 to 60% of adults. Marked eosinophilia is rare. Rheumatoid factor is positive in a low titer in two-thirds of patients, whereas ANA is present in 10 to 20% of patients. Serum complement levels are normal or increased. Westergren erythrocyte sedimentation rate and C-reactive protein are elevated in 90% of patients with active and generalized disease (15).

Antineutrophil Cytoplasmic Autoantibodies

The most specific serologic test for WG is autoantibodies directed against cytoplasmic constituents of neutrophils and monocytes. A cytoplasmic staining pattern on indirect immunofluorescence (cANCA) is characteristic of WG. More specific antibody assays, such as enzyme-linked immunosorbent assay (ELISA), have determined that PR3 is the antigen to which the cANCA in WG is most often directed. Although the cANCA test in WG is not specific for PR3, in patients with vasculitis approximately 90% of cytoplasmic ANCA are PR3-ANCA (4). It should be noted that neither cANCA nor anti-PR3 antibodies are specific for WG, as they are found in other forms of vasculitis, including MPA. Therefore, it is generally recommended that both indirect immunofluorescence ANCA testing and more specific ANCA testing be done in the clinical setting of vasculitis.

The likelihood of obtaining a positive ANCA test in patients with WG varies depending on severity and activity of disease. Circulating cANCA are detected in 90% of patients with active, generalized (sinopulmonary and renal) WG and also in 40 to 70% of those with active, regional (sinopulmonary) disease. In contrast, approximately 30 to 40% of patients in remission still have a positive cANCA (15). This emphasizes the need to treat patients based on their clinical findings rather than just the ANCA test.

Differential Diagnosis

The differential diagnosis for regional WG includes acute infectious processes that lead to sinopulmonary symptoms alone. The differential diagnosis for patients with glomerulonephritis and pulmonary hemorrhage (pulmonary-renal syndrome) includes anti-GBM disease, SLE, HSP, and the other ANCA-associated diseases such as MPA and Churg-Strauss disease. Other rarer causes are listed in Table 44.1. Those with skin involvement, abdominal pain, arthralgias, and glomerulonephritis could have HSP, SLE, or an ANCA-associated disease.

Workup

A routine evaluation should start with a complete blood count, electrolytes, blood urea nitrogen, creatinine, albumin, urinalysis, Westergren sedimentation rate, and chest radiograph. Depending on the clinical indication, indirect immunofluorescence ANCA and ELISA ANCA testing for anti-PR3 and anti-MPO antibodies, ANA, C3, C4, and anti-GBM antibody, should be performed. Consideration should also be given to obtaining computed tomography of the sinuses and orbits.

A renal biopsy is essential for proper diagnosis if hematuria, proteinuria, or azotemia is present. It allows the clinician to classify the glomerulonephritis as immune complex mediated, anti-GBM disease, or pauciimmune. In many centers, the biopsy results return more rapidly than immunologic serologies, thereby allowing a more prompt diagnosis. Moreover, approximately 10% of patients with WG are ANCA negative, so serologic testing cannot be relied on exclusively (4). It

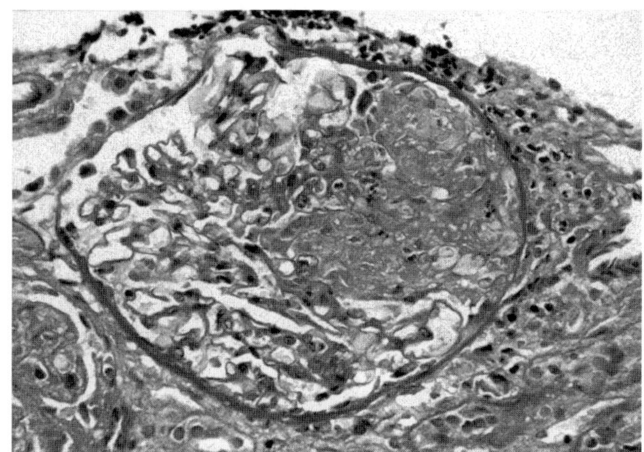

FIGURE 44.2. Segmental necrotizing and crescentic glomerulonephritis. (Periodic acid-Schiff stain ×125.)

should be noted that, unlike a biopsy of the lungs or sinuses, a renal biopsy in a patient with WG rarely shows the presence of granulomas (2,15). A kidney biopsy typically shows a pauciimmune-necrotizing and crescentic glomerulonephritis. Immunofluorescence shows scant immunostaining and few, if any, electron-dense deposits on electron microscopy (21). A renal biopsy documenting the focal, necrotizing, and crescentic glomerulonephritis of WG is shown in Figure 44.2.

In a patient with minimal renal disease, another tissue biopsy site may be needed. In the presence of nodules or infiltrates on chest radiograph or computed tomography, lung biopsy is often diagnostic, with patchy necrosis, granulomatous inflammation, and vasculitis seen. In the setting of pulmonary hemorrhage, surgical lung biopsy is much riskier. Fiberoptic bronchoscopy with bronchoalveolar lavage can confirm the presence of blood and/or hemosiderin-laden macrophages. Stains and cultures can be obtained to rule out infection (15,22).

Churg-Strauss Syndrome

Churg-Strauss syndrome (CSS) is a systemic necrotizing vasculitis with hypereosinophilia and extravascular granulomas that occurs almost exclusively in patients with asthma (23). It is also characterized as a pauciimmune small vessel vasculitis, being distinguished from MPA and WG by the presence of granulomatous inflammation and asthma, respectively (24). It is a systemic vasculitis that affects the lungs, skin, peripheral nerves, GI tract, heart, and kidneys (25). Unlike WG, CSS is extremely uncommon in children, with only an occasional case report in the literature and no pediatric case series. As a result, most information presented is adult data used in an effort to prepare pediatricians to recognize the rare patient with this disorder.

It has been postulated that CSS occurs in three clinical phases: a prodromal, allergic phase (asthma and/or allergic rhinitis); an eosinophilic phase (tissue and peripheral eosinophilia); and a vasculitic phase (with multiorgan involvement) (26). Six criteria were developed by the American College of Rheumatology in an effort to standardize the diagnosis of CSS for study purposes. The criteria included asthma, eosinophilia (greater than 10% or absolute eosinophil count greater than 1500), mononeuropathy or polyneuropathy, histologic evidence of a vasculitis, paranasal sinusitis, and nonfixed pulmonary infiltrates on chest x-ray.

Two adult studies have helped characterize this disorder (3,25). Asthma was present at the time of presentation in nearly all cases. Mononeuritis multiplex was present in 44 to 77%; constitutional symptoms (weight loss, fever, and myalgias), sinusitis, and allergic rhinitis all occurred in approximately 60% of cases. Skin involvement occurred in 50 to 70% of cases, with palpable purpura being the most common manifestation. Cardiac involvement occurred at presentation in 12.5 to 28.1%, and existed as pericardial effusion, pericarditis, myocarditis, ischemic cardiomyopathy, and conduction abnormalities. The GI tract was involved in 31 to 38% of patients. Abdominal pain was the most common symptom; more severe involvement included intestinal perforation, GI bleeding, and pancreatitis.

Renal involvement (proteinuria, glomerulonephritis, hypertension, renal insufficiency, and renal infarct) was evident in 26% of cases of CSS in one study. A second study reported that 12.5% of CSS patients had renal involvement that included glomerulonephritis, renal insufficiency, and hematuria. Hypertension was present in 16% of patients (3,25).

Laboratory findings consisted of leukocytosis with eosinophilia, and elevated erythrocyte sedimentation rate was present in 80 to 100% of cases, ANA greater than 1:160 was present in 11 to 15%, rheumatoid factor in 24% of patients, and less than 1% had a positive anti–double-stranded DNA with clinical manifestations of lupus (3,25). ANCA testing was positive in 48% of sera from CSS patients using indirect immunofluorescence and was pANCA in the majority of cases (3). ELISA revealed ANCA specificity toward MPO in 10 of 11 cases (3). In another study, IIF ANCA were negative in eight patients with CSS who were in remission and in 78% who were positive during the acute phase of illness (25). It was also noted that only 50% of patients had a positive ANCA in association with a clinical relapse. Chest x-rays revealed patchy infiltrates in 38 to 75% (3,25).

Histologic findings included necrotizing vasculitis (64%), vascular and perivascular eosinophil infiltrates (55%), and extravascular granulomas (15%) in one study (25). Because extravascular granulomas are only infrequently seen on biopsy specimens, it is recommended that this feature of the disease not be required to make the diagnosis. Renal biopsy specimens have shown segmental proliferative glomerulonephritis in some and necrotizing vasculitis with crescents in others; immunofluorescence has been negative (3,25,27).

Treatment consisted of prednisone alone or usually in accompaniment with cyclophosphamide (CYP). CYP treatment lasted 1.0 to 1.5 years and was most often given orally. Plasma exchange has been studied and does not appear to have additional benefit to that of corticosteroids and CYP (28).

Clinical outcome in adults was favorable. In one study of 32 patients, the patient survival was 94% at 1 year and 90% at 5 years. Four deaths occurred—three directly related to vasculitis (intestinal perforation in two patients and severe cardiac, GI, and renal involvement) and one related to a nosocomial infection. Remissions occurred in all patients, and relapses occurred in 28% of patients; approximately one-half of these relapses occurring in the first year of therapy (25). Long-term prognosis in another study correlated with myocardial involvement, proteinuria greater than 1 g/24 hr, and severe GI tract involvement including GI hemorrhage, intestinal perforation, pancreatitis, or laparotomy (3).

Microscopic Polyangiitis

The distinction between MPA and the other ANCA-associated diseases has been discussed. In brief, it is a nongranulomatous, multisystem, pauciimmune, small vessel vasculitis without upper airway involvement. There is significant overlap with WG in terms of organ system involvement. It is associated with ANCA in more than 80% of patients. pANCA on indirect immunofluorescence is most common and more specifically on MPO. Owing to the small number of ANCA-associated diseases reported in pediatrics, most specifics are derived from adult studies. As previously mentioned, because the Chapel Hill Conference has set stricter diagnostic criteria, future pediatric studies are likely to attempt to more carefully distinguish the various ANCA-associated small vessel vasculitides.

MPA can often mimic cPAN histologically, as both diseases are capable of producing a necrotizing arteritis. The key distinction is in the size of the vessels involved. Because MPA is a small vessel vasculitis, it is capable of affecting arterioles, capillaries, and postcapillary venules. This clinically results in alveolar capillaritis (pulmonary hemorrhage), glomerular capillary inflammation (glomerulonephritis), and inflammation of the dermal postcapillary venules (leukocytoclastic angiitis resulting in purpura). By definition, MPA can affect medium vessels, but cPAN is restricted from affecting vessels smaller than this size (1, reviewed in 4).

A study from Chapel Hill of 107 patients with necrotizing glomerulonephritis who met criteria for MPA was followed prospectively for an average of 2.5 years. Indirect immunofluorescence revealed that 65% were pANCA (+) and 35% cANCA (+) are ANCA positive. Twelve disease-related deaths occurred, and 46 patients reached ESRD. The patients had pulmonary involvement in 36% of cases and cutaneous involvement in 12%. Mortality risk factors were analyzed and revealed that those patients presenting with pulmonary hemorrhage had a relative risk (RR) of death of 8.6. Other risk factors of statistical significance included increased mortality when cANCA pattern was present (as compared to pANCA; RR, 3.8). A protective effect of CYP treatment was seen when compared to corticosteroids alone (RR, 0.18; $p = .012$). Predictors of need for renal replacement therapy were statistically associated with serum creatinine at the time of study entry and African American race (29). This study thus clearly highlighted the potential morbidity and mortality of this disease.

In another adult study using Chapel Hill criteria, patients with WG (N = 56) were compared to those with MPA (N = 67). ANCA testing on patients with WG revealed 87% were PR3 (+), 11% MPO (+), and 2% ANCA negative. Those with MPA showed that 39% were PR3 (+), 56% MPO (+), and 5% ANCA negative. Patients with WG were more likely to have upper respiratory and pulmonary disease. Relapses and renal outcomes were similar in both groups (30).

Finally, the French Vasculitis Study Group conducted a recent retrospective study of 85 adults meeting Chapel Hill criteria for MPA. ANCA testing was positive in 75%; 65% were pANCA (+) and 10% were cANCA (+). Constitutional symptoms were prevalent with fever in 55% and anorexia or weight loss in 73% of patients. Renal disease was present in 79%, skin involvement in 62% (purpura in 41%), and mononeuritis multiplex in 58%. Deaths occurred in nearly one-third of patients followed 70 months, most owing to vasculitis or infection (31).

In another study looking at causes of pulmonary renal syndromes in adult patients, serologic testing found that 48 of 88 patients were ANCA positive (PR3—19 patients; MPO—29 patients), 6 patients had exclusively anti-GBM disease, 7 others had both ANCA and anti-GBM antibodies, and 27 patients had neither antibody. The authors noted that only eight of these patients had clinical or histologic evidence to support a diagnosis of WG (32). By Chapel Hill criteria, then, MPA was the most common identifiable cause of pulmonary renal syndrome in adults.

Pediatric reports of this entity are rare. Similar to adults, pediatric patients can present with life-threatening pulmonary hemorrhage as part of the pulmonary renal syndrome. In addition to these organ systems, a recent case report was published of an adolescent female with a pANCA (+) pauciimmune crescentic glomerulonephritis who presented in renal failure with cerebral vasculitis (seizures with multifocal ischemic defects on magnetic resonance imaging). The CNS manifestations of this patient's disease responded to CYP and plasma exchange (33).

In summary, the prognosis of MPA appears similar to WG. Although granulomatous inflammation does not occur, it is often the sinopulmonary symptoms of WG that result in patients seeking medical attention. The relative reduction of these symptoms means patients with MPA may be more apt to present with advanced disease. Because patients with advanced disease tend to have a poor outcome, a high index of suspicion for MPA (ANCA disease) is needed to minimize long-term morbidity.

Treatment of Antineutrophil Cytoplasmic Autoantibody–Associated Glomerulonephritis and Vasculitis—Wegener Granulomatosis, Microscopic Polyangiitis, and Churg Strauss Disease

The mainstay of treatment for ANCA-associated diseases includes a combination of corticosteroids and cytotoxic agents. Because the dosages and the manner of administration can vary according to the stage of treatment, the treatment section is separated into three parts: acute supportive treatment, induction therapy, and maintenance therapy.

Acute Supportive Treatment

From an immunosuppressive standpoint, most centers treat adults and children with ANCA diseases with either oral prednisone or intravenous (IV) methylprednisolone. Pulse methylprednisolone at a dose of 7 to 15 mg/kg/dose is often given in three successive daily doses followed by daily prednisone at 1 to 2 mg/kg/day (4,28,34–38). CYP is given in one of two ways. Many centers prefer oral CYP to induce a remission and optimally reduce the incidence of relapses (30,39). Others prefer IV CYP, which is as efficacious at inducing a remission as the oral preparation (4,28,34). IV CYP can be given safely with aggressive hydration along with sodium 2-mercaptoethane sulfonate (MESNA) to minimize the risk of hemorrhagic cystitis. In addition, the cumulative dose tends to be much lower with the IV preparation, which should theoretically result in a reduction in dose-related, long-term malignancy risks. In our pediatric cohort of ANCA (+) glomerulonephritis and vasculitis, those children with a history of pulmonary hemorrhage (defined as life-threatening disease) were treated with oral CYP for fear of the consequences of a catastrophic relapse. All others were treated with IV CYP, except for one child who was changed from IV to oral due to lack of response to IV (38).

Other empiric treatments that have been tried but have not been well studied include plasma exchange and IV immunoglobulin (IVIG) (28,36,40). The former treatment has the theoretical advantage of removing a circulating agent that may be causative, whereas the latter may be immunomodulating (41). Additional supportive treatments such as oxygen, assisted ventilation, transfusion, extracorporeal membrane oxygenation, and dialysis have been used as life-saving measures.

Induction Immunosuppressive Therapy

This phase of treatment has been arbitrarily defined as that occurring between 2 weeks and 6 months after diagnosis (38). Prednisone is given typically as 1 to 2 mg/kg/day initially divided b.i.d., which is continued for 1 to 3 months before being tapered. Some centers taper to alternate day prednisone at a dose of 1 to 2 mg/kg/q.o.d. after 2 months of treatment, while others slowly reduce the dose of steroids, which are continued on a daily basis. With regard to the CYP dose, those centers giving monthly IV CYP give an initial dose of 500 to 600 mg/m^2/dose with a nadir white blood cell count 10 to 14 days later being used to determine the next dose. Dose increases in increments of 250 mg/m^2/dose are then used up to a maximum dose of 1000 mg/m^2/dose. Oral CYP is given at a starting dose of 2 mg/kg/day (maximum dose of 150 mg). Dosage reductions are made based on the presence of leukopenia/neutropenia on complete blood cell counts, monitored weekly.

Maintenance Immunosuppressive Therapy

This period has been arbitrarily defined as the period that follows the first 6 months of treatment. The optimal duration of treatment remains debatable. Many adult centers are now stopping corticosteroids 3 to 4 months into therapy and discontinuing all treatment as early as 6 months (42). Other centers use the 6-month cutoff as a time to transition patients to a less toxic regimen and substitute azathioprine (AZA) for CYP at this point. Rottem et al. chose to treat children with oral CYP for 1 year after a remission was achieved before reducing the dosage by 25 mg every 2 months as tolerated (8). Their median treatment time with oral CYP was 28 months. In our cohort of children with ANCA-associated vasculitis and glomerulonephritis, we chose to transition patients to AZA after an approximate 6-month treatment period with IV CYP. A select group of patients who had either a poor response to IV CYP or life-threatening disease at presentation were treated instead with oral CYP, which was continued for 1 year. Those treated with oral CYP were changed at 1 year to either AZA or methotrexate (MTX) in an effort to provide sufficient immunosuppressive therapy while avoiding long-term use of CYP (38).

Newer Therapeutic Regimens

MTX has been used as a substitute for CYP during the induction stage of WG treatment of children and adults (9,43). This agent appears to be reasonably effective (71% remission rate) if selectively used in patients with non–life-threatening forms of WG and when used in conjunction with corticosteroids. MTX dosages in WG range from 0.15 to 0.30 mg/kg/wk in adults, to as high as 0.6 mg/kg/wk in children (9,11). Although AZA has been proven to be inferior to CYP during the induction phase of treatment, it may have its greatest role in "maintaining" a remission state, as has been discussed (2,38). Its main advantage is that it is far less toxic than CYP and is usually well tolerated.

Mycophenolate mofetil (MMF) is a newer antiproliferative immunosuppressive medication that possesses a relatively favorable toxicity profile and a lymphocyte selective mode of action, through inhibition of IMPDH (*i*nosine *m*ono*p*hosphate *deh*ydrogenase). In a study of 11 adults with ANCA-associated systemic vasculitis (WG = 9, MPA = 2), MMF was substituted for CYP during the maintenance phase of treatment and used with corticosteroids to maintain a remission in 10 of 11 patients followed for 15 months (44). No pediatric reports of MMF usage in WG exist at this time. Certainly, larger studies are needed during the maintenance phase to determine whether MMF will prove efficacious.

Treatment Summary

At the present time, our typical approach to a patient with ANCA (+) vasculitis and glomerulonephritis is to treat with prednisone (1 to 2 mg/kg/day; maximum, 80 mg) for 1 to 2 months before tapering to alternate day dosing schedule. In addition, CYP is given for 6 to 12 months before changing over to AZA. The decision on the duration of CYP is related to the severity of disease at presentation, with patients with non–life-threatening disease typically receiving monthly IV CYP for 6 months in conjunction with corticosteroids. If in remission, the patient is then transitioned to AZA at 2 mg/kg/day while steroids continue to be tapered slowly. Those patients with pulmonary hemorrhage (life-threatening disease) are treated with oral CYP for 1 year in conjunction with corticosteroids. At that point, AZA is again substituted for CYP if the patient is in remission. *Remission* is defined as lack of symptoms, stable renal function, benign urinalysis (except for some proteinuria), and a stable erythrocyte sedimentation rate. A repeat renal biopsy looking for histologic confirmation of inactive disease is usually performed before transitioning a patient off of CYP.

Trimethoprim/sulfamethoxazole has become a mainstay of WG treatment, as it can be used as prophylaxis for *Pneumocystis carinii* pneumonia, which occurred in approximately 4% of adult WG patients from the NIH (11). An additional advantage is its efficacy in reducing respiratory relapses in adults with WG, a fact that may be secondary to treatment of nasal carriage of *Staphylococcus aureus*, which was associated with serious sinopulmonary infections in the early NIH studies (2,45).

Outcome of Antineutrophil Cytoplasmic Autoantibody-Associated Vasculitis and Glomerulonephritis

Despite high remission rates in childhood WG (87%), relapses were frequent (53%) (7). In addition, morbidity from either the disease or its treatment was extremely high (87%). Nasal deformity was common (48%), as was subglottic stenosis (35%), which necessitated subglottic dilatation in two patients and tracheostomy in six others. Renal insufficiency was present in approximately one-third of patients. Treatment-induced morbidity included cystitis (50%) and infertility (28%). Steroid side effects included cataracts and aseptic necrosis. Infections requiring hospitalization and IV antibiotics occurred in 43% of patients. The frequency of infections correlated with the degree of immunosuppression. The lowest rate occurred while off immunosuppression and increased twofold with steroids alone and increased twelvefold during combined steroid and CYP therapy (8). Although no malignancies were reported, longer-term follow-up is clearly needed. Two pediatric deaths were reported (8.7%), occurring 2.2 and 15 years after disease onset. Adult studies have reported a marked increase in bladder carcinomas (11- to 33-fold increased risk) after successful treatment of WG with CYP for at least 1 year (11,30,46). The risk of bladder carcinoma is higher in patients having had hemorrhagic cystitis, again making a case for the use of IV CYP in whom this complication can be largely eliminated by using IV hydration and MESNA.

Outcomes from other more recent studies have been slightly better, but patient selection criteria and treatment protocols have been modified. Of those pediatric cases with ANCA-associated vasculitis and glomerulonephritis, a cumulative incidence of ESRD of 30% has occurred in 20 patients from six clinical reports (9,35,38,47–49). Because these reports are of children with coexisting glomerulonephritis, all patients had renal disease at presentation. Those developing ESRD typically presented with very advanced disease. Seven of these patients were reported from a single center, and a lower incidence of ESRD (14%) was found. Of the remaining 13 patients, the incidence of ESRD was 38%.

Until recently, children with ANCA (+) glomerulonephritis were believed to have an ESRD risk of 30%. This figure was corroborated by a large recent retrospective series of 31 pediatric patients with ANCA (+) glomerulonephritis conducted by members of the Japanese Society for Pediatric Nephrology. All patients were ANCA (+) and had renal biopsy–proven pauciimmune necrotizing and crescentic glomerulonephritis. Ten had renal-limited, necrotizing crescentic glomerulonephritis, and 21 (68%) were classified as MPA. Twenty-six patients (84%) received treatment with corticosteroids and CYP, and five patients with corticosteroids alone; 84% of patients achieved remission, and 39% of responders relapsed in a median of 24 months. Nine of 31 patients (29%) progressed to ESRD; an additional 6 (19.4%) had reduced renal function, whereas nearly one-half (48.4%) had normal renal function at a median follow-up of 42 months. Life-table analysis showed 75% renal survival at 39 months. Patients who subsequently developed ESRD (N = 9) had significantly higher average peak serum creatinine levels and more chronic pathologic lesions at diagnosis compared with patients with favorable renal outcome (N = 15) (50).

With regard to renal transplantation, disease recurrence has occurred and is estimated to be approximately 17%, with the time to relapse at an average of 31 months (51). Disease recurrence has been successfully treated with CYP (52). The presence of a positive ANCA test, however, is not a contraindication to transplantation, which has occurred as early as 6 months after the development of ESRD (53).

Conclusions

WG and other forms of ANCA-associated small vessel vasculitis continue to be diagnosed in the pediatric population. The renal prognosis is difficult to estimate when comparing patients with WG who have mild if any renal disease at presentation versus those who present to pediatric nephrology units with advanced renal failure. The largest report of children with WG, in which only 9% presented with renal disease, estimated that 14% went on to ESRD (8). This is contrasted to published reports of children presenting with renal disease to a pediatric nephrology center, where the incidence of ESRD ranges from 14 to 60%, with the largest series reporting 29%. The speed with which the children are diagnosed and treated is likely to affect both the short- and long-term outcomes. The long-term outcome can be further improved by finding less toxic treatment regimens capable of achieving disease remission with fewer side effects. Long-term follow-up of these patients is necessary, for even those in sustained remission have the potential to relapse.

POLYARTERITIS NODOSA

cPAN is a necrotizing vasculitis of medium-sized vessels without involvement of arterioles, capillaries, and venules. These medium-sized vessels are defined as main visceral arteries, such as the coronary, hepatic, mesenteric, and renal arteries. Focal-necrotizing injury to the vessel wall leads to aneurysm formation. The clinical features are tissue infarction, hemorrhage, and organ dysfunction (54). It is important that cPAN be distinguished from MPA, a disease with which it is often confused. The confusion dates back to the early descriptions of polyarteritis nodosa when it was believed to occur as two types: polyarteritis with extraglomerular vasculitis (cPAN) and that with glomerulonephritis, which they named *microscopic polyarteritis* (55). These two types of PAN were redefined by the Chapel Hill Consensus Conference. In short, cPAN is a medium vessel vasculitis, which is limited to medium vessels. This distinguishes cPAN from patients with MPA whose necrotizing vasculitis is usually limited to small vessels but can overlap into the medium vessels (1). This means a patient presenting with a systemic vasculitis whose renal involvement is manifested as glomerulonephritis cannot be classified as cPAN.

Unlike patients with MPA, cPAN is typically ANCA negative (56). It has been associated with hepatitis B infection in adults and children (57–59). Classic PAN is a multisystem disease that can lead to GI, nervous system, musculoskeletal system, cutaneous, and renal involvement. Cutaneous features include livedo reticularis or inflammatory nodules, with or without gangrene. Musculoskeletal symptoms consist of severe myalgias and/or arthritis/arthralgias. Nervous system involvement includes both peripheral neuropathy (mononeuritis multiplex) and encephalopathy. GI symptoms include abdominal pain and blood in the stool. Renovascular hypertension occurs in approximately one-third of adults; renal involvement is usually flank pain and hematuria and, more rarely, retroperitoneal hemorrhage from aneurysmal rupture (54,60,61). Hypertension and renal involvement were present in 65% of patients in one pediatric study, but this study predated Chapel Hill criteria and ANCA testing and almost certainly included a mixture of pediatric patients now classified as having cPAN and MPA (57).

Renal involvement in cPAN, as defined by Chapel Hill criteria, was analyzed in an adult patient cohort from Kuwait. Chronic renal failure with (38%) or without proteinuria (31%) was frequently seen. Less frequently seen were nephrotic syndrome (6%) and rapidly progressive renal failure (6%) (62). A recent pediatric case report of severe renal impairment in a child with cPAN demonstrated the need to use histology to discern necrotizing glomerulonephritis versus necrotizing arteritis of the renal vascular bed (56). Either form of vasculitis is capable of inducing renal failure; the latter form, although less common, occurs through renal ischemia.

The diagnosis of cPAN is often made with the aid of a kidney biopsy, in which a necrotizing vasculitis without a crescentic or necrotizing glomerulonephritis is seen. Angiography of vessels involving the kidney or intestinal vessels often shows aneurysms. The high-resolution technique of selective renal angiography is often required to detect very small peripheral aneurysms (63). The interlobar and arcuate arteries are most commonly involved, with the main renal artery occurring on rare occasions (54). Although aneurysms in the medium-sized renal arteries are seen in cPAN, they are not specific for this entity as they can be seen in TA, Kawasaki disease (KD), WG, MPA, and Churg-Strauss disease (54). Aneurysms of the renal vessels can be seen on an arteriogram done in a child presenting with hypertension who was diagnosed with cPAN (Fig. 44.3).

Treatment consists of corticosteroids and usually an alkylating agent such as CYP or AZA (54,56,59). Plasma exchange has not proven beneficial in this disease (64). The prognosis of this disease has been examined in adults, and it was found that patients with more than 1 g of protein excretion in 24 hours, renal insufficiency, cardiomyopathy, CNS involvement, or severe GI involvement had a worse prognosis (65). Prognosis in children appears to be improving with more aggressive immunosuppressive treatment. A recent series of 11 children from Saudi Arabia reported 100% survival. All of these patients were treated with steroids, and nine children also received cytotoxic agents (66).

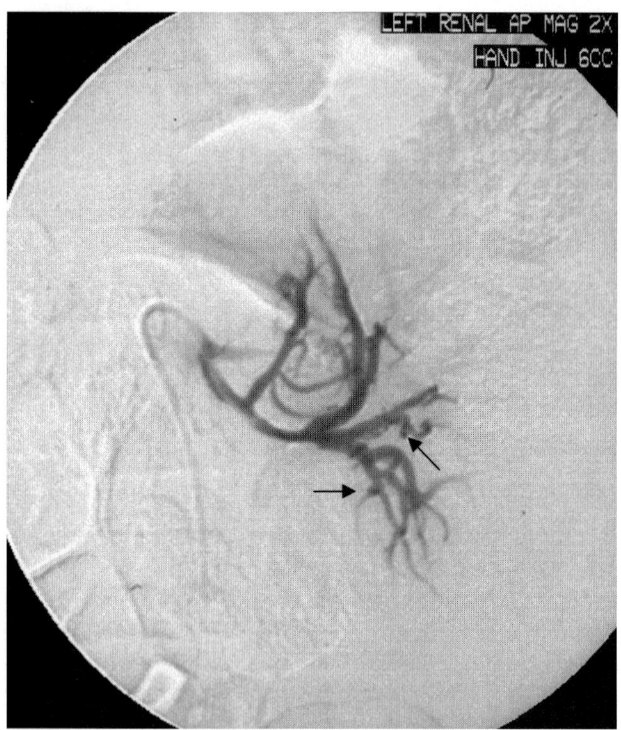

FIGURE 44.3. Renal arteriogram of a 5-year-old child presenting with hypertension. Selective injection of left renal artery showed small aneurysms arising from the interlobar and interlobular arteries (*arrows*). This study aided in the diagnosis of classic polyarteritis nodosa in this child.

This is contrasted to earlier reports in which cytotoxic immunosuppressive treatment was used more sparingly and mortality was as high as 16% (57,67).

KAWASAKI DISEASE

Tomisaku Kawasaki's initial report in English of 50 Japanese children with an illness characterized by fever, rash, conjunctival injection, swelling of the hands and feet, and cervical lymphadenopathy appeared in 1974 (68). This illness would later become known as *Kawasaki disease* or *mucocutaneous lymph node syndrome*. Coronary artery vasculitis is the most important feature of this disease. KD is the second most common form of vasculitis in childhood, behind HSP (69). This disease occurs worldwide but is much more common in Japan where the finest epidemiologic studies exist. This disease is 1.3 times more common in males than females (70). In Japan, KD incidence rates peak at 3 to 5 months of age in females, with two peaks occurring in males—at 3 to 5 months and a second peak at 9 to 11 months of age. This recent survey also revealed that 82% of cases occurred in children younger than 4 years of age (70). It is also the most common cause of acquired heart disease in children in the United States, the United Kingdom, and Japan (69,71). An infectious etiology is suspected but is as yet unproven.

The diagnostic criteria for KD includes six signs and symptoms: fever of 5 days or more; bilateral nonpurulent, conjunctival injection; mucous membrane changes of the upper respiratory tract (injected pharynx, injected, fissured lips, and strawberry tongue); peripheral extremity changes (peripheral edema and erythema, and periungual desquamation); polymorphous rash; and cervical lymphadenopathy (at least one node more than 1.5 cm in diameter) (72). Typical cases have fever of 5 days or more and four of the five criteria without any other known disease process. Atypical cases are characterized by coronary aneurysms and at least four other criteria (73).

KD is a systemic medium vessel vasculitis, and its primary morbidity involves the coronary arteries, in which coronary artery aneurysms have been reported to occur in 20 to 25% of untreated children (74). Renovascular involvement also occurs, albeit less commonly, and typically involves the interlobar arteries of the kidney (75). Recently, a previously normotensive child was reported to develop renovascular hypertension 6 months after an episode of KD. Arteriography revealed unilateral ostial stenosis of the main renal artery (76).

Renal parenchymal involvement has also been noted in KD. Veiga et al. reported a child with acute renal failure associated with biopsy-proven acute interstitial nephritis during the acute phase of illness (77). Nardi et al. performed ultrasonography in 7 children with KD. They found a correlation between enlarged, echogenic kidneys with increased corticomedullary differentiation in affected children and abnormal renal function, hematuria, proteinuria, and pyuria (78). Lande et al. reported a patient with KD who presented with acute renal failure requiring 1 week of hemodialysis before renal function normalized (79).

Laboratory findings in KD include leukocytosis, thrombocytosis, sterile pyuria, and pleocytosis of the cerebrospinal fluid. ANCAs and antiendothelial cell antibodies have been reported to be present in KD (80,81). Two subsequent studies using control patients with nonspecific febrile illnesses revealed that neither ANCA nor antiendothelial cell antibodies were of diagnostic value when attempting to distinguish early KD from other childhood illnesses and, therefore, were unlikely to be involved in the pathogenesis of KD (82,83). Because of the high incidence of coronary aneurysms in KD, echocardiography and ECG are recommended for all patients at the time of diagnosis (69).

After diagnosis of KD is made, the standard of care is IVIG and high-dose aspirin, which have been shown to reduce the risk of coronary aneurysms to less than 5% (84,85). A single dose of 2 g/kg of IVIG is superior to lower doses (400 mg/kg/dose) given on 4 consecutive days (85). IVIG treatment is ideally administered within the first 10 days of illness (85,86). It should be noted that IVIG can be given beyond this 10-day window, and failure to respond to single-dose IVIG may necessitate administration of a second dose later if the patient remains symptomatic (87). Aspirin dosing is recommended at 30 to 50 mg/kg/day in four divided doses until fever resolves, then 2 to 5 mg/kg/day for a minimum of 6 weeks (69). The role of corticosteroids in KD is controversial but, in general, their use is discouraged.

Long-term outcome of KD largely depends on the presence of coronary artery aneurysms. Follow-up echocardiography is recommended at 10 to 14 days and again in 6 to 8 weeks in an effort to closely monitor for the development of aneurysms or follow up the status of previously diagnosed aneurysms. It is recommended to discontinue aspirin in those without aneurysms 6 weeks into the illness. Most mild coronary artery aneurysms (3 to 4 mm) regress within 2 years, but those who have giant aneurysms (greater than 8 mm) are unlikely to resolve. Persistent aneurysms are prone to stenosis, which can lead to thrombosis, myocardial infarction, or death (69). Indeed, KD is the most common cause of myocardial infarction in childhood (54).

The overall prognosis for KD, however, is quite good. Those with giant aneurysms require the closest follow-up, but it is recommended that all children with KD receive lifelong follow-up (69).

TAKAYASU'S ARTERITIS

TA is the most common large vessel vasculitis in the pediatric age group. It is a granulomatous inflammatory condition that usually begins in the subclavian vessels and progressively involves the carotids, aorta, and possibly the renal arteries. It is known as the *pulseless disease*, owing to its involvement with the aortic arch and subclavian vessels resulting in arterial narrowing and decreased brachial pulses (54,88). Six diagnostic criteria have been established and include age of onset of 40 years or less, claudication of an extremity, decreased brachial pulse, greater than 10 mm Hg difference in systolic blood pressure between arms, bruit over the subclavian artery, and narrowing or occlusion of the aorta, its primary branches or major arteries of the extremities not caused by atherosclerosis, fibromuscular dysplasia, or other causes (89). The diagnosis is most likely when three of these six criteria are met.

Hypertension is the most common renal manifestation and can be attributed to coarctation of the aorta and, less often, renal artery stenosis (90,91). Another renal manifestation is ischemic kidney disease (92). TA occurs predominantly in females. The female to male ratio is 9:1, with most cases being diagnosed between 10 and 20 years of age (54). It is more frequently seen in the Japanese population but does occur worldwide. The pathogenesis of this disorder is poorly understood.

Clinical features are divided into a prepulseless phase and a pulseless phase. Constitutional symptoms (fever, malaise, headache, myalgias, arthralgias, and weight loss) occur during the prepulseless phase. As arterial involvement advances, end-organ–ischemic symptoms occur (93). Adult patients present with symptoms of claudication, abdominal pain, and/or ischemic changes to the hands. Pediatric patients more often present with symptoms attributed to hypertension and its complications, namely hypertensive encephalopathy and congestive heart failure (93). Other features of TA include dermatologic manifestations (erythema nodosum and pyoderma gangrenosum of the lower extremities in some cases) and symptoms attributable to compromised cerebral blood flow (dizziness, headaches, syncope, and stroke). Hemoptysis, shortness of breath, and pulmonary hypertension can occur due to pulmonary arterial involvement, and angina can occur due to compromised coronary blood flow attributable to either aortic or coronary arteritis. Signs of disease at presentation include hypertension in approximately 50% of cases, asymmetrical pulses, and bruits over the subclavian, brachial, and abdominal vessels (94,95).

Laboratory findings include anemia, elevated erythrocyte sedimentation rate, and elevated C-reactive protein (93,95). Serologic markers, including ANA and ANCA, are typically negative. Arteriography often shows involvement of the aortic arch, its branches, and/or the distal aorta and its branches (95) (Fig. 44.4).

Treatment of TA has consisted of corticosteroids initially in most settings. Steroid-resistant cases have been treated with CYP (96). More recently, MTX has been used in conjunction with corticosteroids and resulted in a higher remission rate and lower maintenance steroid dosage compared to historical con-

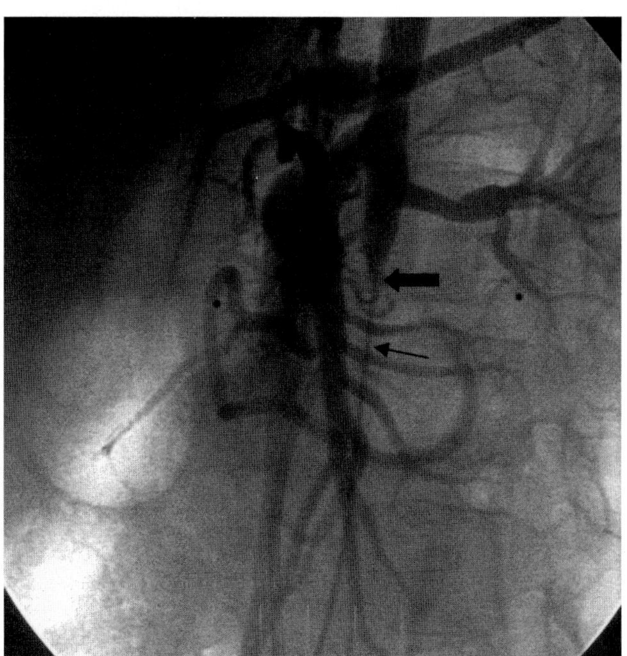

FIGURE 44.4. Aortogram obtained at cardiac catheterization in a child with Takayasu's arteritis. The small arrow indicates the catheter within the descending aorta. The large arrow indicates an abrupt tapering of the descending aorta with extensive collateral vessels. (Courtesy of Dr. Thomas J. Forbes, Pediatric Cardiology, Children's Hospital of Michigan, Detroit, Michigan.)

trols (97). Strategies to manage severe hypertension in childhood TA have included the use of vasodilators, beta blockers, and diuretics. Angiotensin-converting enzyme inhibitors have been used but must be used with great caution in those with renovascular involvement due to the risk of precipitating acute renal failure (90). Percutaneous transluminal angioplasty for treatment of stenosis of the descending thoracic and/or abdominal aorta has been used with moderate success (98). The long-term prognosis of TA is generally quite good, with 5-year survival rates of approximately 95% (95,97).

DRUG-ASSOCIATED VASCULITIS

Several drugs have been associated with ANCA positive vasculitis, with hydralazine and propylthiouracil (PTU) being the two most commonly reported (99). In one study, the authors analyzed the 30 patients with the highest titers of anti-MPO antibodies from a pool of 250 patients with ANCA-positive vasculitis and anti-MPO antibodies. Of these 30 patients, 10 patients (33%) were exposed to hydralazine and 3 patients (10%) to PTU. An additional 17% were exposed to other agents such as penicillamine, allopurinol, or sulfasalazine (99).

Patients in the hydralazine group had multisystem disease with renal, sinopulmonary, and dermatologic manifestations. Nine of ten patients had glomerulonephritis, and all five biopsied patients had pauciimmune necrotizing and crescentic glomerulonephritis. Pulmonary abnormalities included pulmonary infiltrates (five patients), hemoptysis (four patients), and alveolar hemorrhage with granulomatous changes in one patient with hemoptysis. Dermatologic manifestations were noted in three patients, with leukocytoclastic vasculitis in two; ear, nose, and throat findings occurred in two patients as well (99). In all ten patients, hydralazine was discontinued and corticosteroids were administered. CYP was also added to the treatment regimen in eight of these patients. Although two patients died, the remainder did well.

PTU exposure was noted in three patients, with only one developing renal involvement—a pauciimmune necrotizing glomerulonephritis. Dermatologic involvement included leukocytoclastic vasculitis in two patients. Treatment consisted of withdrawal of PTU and a combination of topical and systemic corticosteroids, with CYP usage in one patient. The authors concluded that a causal link between exposure to hydralazine or PTU and the development of an ANCA-positive vasculitis was likely.

Another study of childhood-onset Graves disease found that 16 of 25 patients (64%) treated with PTU had a positive ANCA when compared to 6% of untreated patients and none of ten patients treated with methimazole (100). These authors concluded that PTU induces MPO antibody production but speculated that other factors such as patient race and severity of Graves disease may be important cofactors as well. They suggested that methimazole should be considered as first-line therapy for Graves disease.

There is one report of two children on PTU who subsequently developed pauciimmune-necrotizing and crescentic glomerulonephritis associated with ANCA (+) serology. Both patients had hyperthyroidism and were exposed to PTU for 34 months and 1 month, respectively. Indirect immunofluorescence demonstrated pANCA, and ELISA demonstrated antibodies to MPO (101). Both patients were treated with corticosteroids and CYP, with one patient improving and the other developing ESRD.

A recent report of seven children from Japan described an additional cohort of children with PTU-associated ANCA (+) glomerulonephritis. All patients were positive for MPO-ANCA, and had biopsy-proven pauciimmune-necrotizing and crescentic glomerulonephritis. They were a mean age of 14 years and were exposed to PTU for a mean of 37 months (102). Treatment consisted of corticosteroids in all patients, with CYP added in two. Only one of seven patients presented with rapidly progressive glomerulonephritis. Nearly 5-year mean follow-up showed that renal function was normal in all patients; as such, the authors concluded that PTU-associated ANCA (+) glomerulonephritis has a better prognosis than nondrug-induced ANCA (+) glomerulonephritis, such as WG and MPA.

In light of the previously mentioned reports, it behooves the caregiver to take a detailed medication exposure history in all patients with vasculitis. Although hydralazine and PTU are the most commonly associated agents, isolated reports of a number of other medications associated with vasculitis currently exist (penicillamine, allopurinol, and minocycline), and additional medications are likely to be added to this list in the future (103–105).

CONCLUSION

Renal vasculitis should be considered in all patients presenting with glomerulonephritis, especially in those with other systemic symptoms. Those patients with renal-limited disease may be more difficult to diagnose. Serologic tests and renal biopsy optimize the clinician's chances at achieving an early diagnosis. Early diagnosis and aggressive treatment afford the patient with the best chance at a favorable outcome. Continued research into the pathogenesis of these disorders and the development of more specific therapies should lead to better long-term results in this challenging patient population.

REFERENCES

1. Jennette JC, Falk RJ, Andrassy K, et al. Nomenclature of systemic vasculitides: proposal of an international consensus conference. *Arthritis Rheum* 1994;37:187–192.
2. Fauci AS, Haynes BF, Katz P, et al. Wegener's granulomatosis: prospective clinical and therapeutic experience with 85 patients for 21 years. *Ann Intern Med* 1983;98:76–85.

3. Guillevin L, Cohen P, Gayraud M, et al. Churg-Strauss syndrome. Clinical study and long-term follow-up of 96 patients. *Medicine* 1999;78:26–37.
4. Jennette JC, Falk RJ. Small-vessel vasculitis. *N Engl J Med* 1997;337:1512–1523.
5. Cohen BA, Clark WF. Pauci-immune renal vasculitis: natural history, prognostic factors, and impact of therapy. *Am J Kidney Dis* 2000;36:914–924.
6. Wegener F. Über eine eigenartige rhinogene Granulomatose mit besonderer Beiteligung des Arteriensystems und der Nieren. Beitrage zur Pathologischen Anatomie und zur Allgemeinen Pathologie 1939;102:36–38.
7. Godman GC, Churg J. Wegener's Granulomatosis: pathology and review of the literature. *Arch Pathol* 1954;58:533–553.
8. Rottem M, Fauci AS, Hallahan MS, et al. Wegener granulomatosis in children and adolescents: clinical presentation and outcome. *J Pediatr* 1993;122:26–31.
9. Gottlieb BS, Miller LC, Ilowite NT. Methotrexate treatment of Wegener granulomatosis in children. *J Pediatr* 1996;129:604–607.
10. Stegmayr BG, Gothefors L, Malmer B, et al. Wegener granulomatosis in children and young adults. A case study of ten patients. *Pediatr Nephrol* 2000;14:208–213.
11. Hoffman GS, Kerr GS, Leavitt RY, et al. Wegener granulomatosis: an analysis of 158 patients. *Ann Intern Med* 1992; 116:488–498.
12. Haynes BF, Fishman ML, Fauci AS, et al. The ocular manifestations of Wegener's granulomatosis. Fifteen years experience and review of the literature. *Am J Med* 1977;63:131–141.
13. Lawson VG, Reid AJ, Cardella CJ, et al. Wegener's granulomatosis and the respiratory system. *J Otolaryngol* 1982;11: 60–64.
14. Walton EW. Giant-cell granuloma of the respiratory tract (Wegener's granulomatosis). *BMJ* 1958;2:265–270.
15. Lynch JP and Hoffman GS. Wegener's granulomatosis: controversies and current concepts. *Comp Ther* 1998;24:421–440.
16. Pediatric End-Stage Renal Disease. United States Renal Data Services 1999 Annual Data Report. 1999:113–130.
17. Harper L, Cockwell P, Adu D, et al. Neutrophil priming and apoptosis in anti-neutrophil cytoplasmic autoantibody-associated vasculitis. *Kidney Int* 2001;59:1729–1738.
18. Savage COS. ANCA-associated renal vasculitis. *Kidney Int* 2001;60:1614–1627.
19. Katz P, Alling DW, Haynes BF, et al. Association of Wegener's granulomatosis with HLA-B8. *Clin Immunol Immunopathol* 1979;14:268–270.
20. Elkon KB, Sutherland DC, Rees AJ, et al. HLA antigen frequencies in systemic vasculitis: increase in HLA-DR2 in Wegener's granulomatosis. *Arthritis Rheum* 1983;26:102–105.
21. Jennette JC. Crescentic glomerulonephritis. In: Jennette JC, Olson JL, Schwartz MM, et al., eds. *Heptinstall's pathology of the kidney*, 5th ed. Philadelphia: Lippincott–Raven, 1998:625–656.
22. Valentini RP, Toder DS. Wegener Granulomatosis. In: Neish SR, ed. *Emedicine—pediatrics*. Emedicine, Inc. 2002:(*in press*).
23. Churg J, Strauss L. Allergic granulomatosis, allergic angiitis and periarteritis nodosa. *Am J Pathol* 1951;27:277–301.
24. Jennette JC, Falk RJ. Antineutrophil cytoplasmic autoantibodies and associated diseases: a review. *Am J Kidney Dis* 1990;6:517–529.
25. Solans R, Bosch JA, Perez-Bocanegra C, et al. Churg-Strauss syndrome: outcome and long-term follow-up of 32 patients. *Rheumatology* 2001;40:763–771.
26. Lanham JG, Elkon KB, Pusey CD, et al. Systemic vasculitis with asthma and eosinophilia: a clinical approach to the Churg-Strauss syndrome. *Medicine* 1984;63:65–81.
27. Minami J, Ishibashi-Ueda H, Okano Y, et al. Crescentic glomerulonephritis and elevated antimyeloperoxidase antibody in a patient with Churg-Strauss syndrome. *Nephron* 1997;77:105–108.
28. Guillevin L, Lhote F, Cohen P, et al. Corticosteroids plus pulse cyclophosphamide and plasma exchanges versus corticosteroids plus pulse cyclophosphamide alone in the treatment of polyarteritis nodosa and Churg-Strauss syndrome patients with factors predicting poor prognosis. A prospective, randomized trial in sixty-two patients. *Arthritis Rheum* 1995;38:1638–1645.
29. Hogan SL, Nachman PH, Wilkman AS, et al. Prognostic markers in patients with antineutrophil cytoplasmic autoantibody-associated microscopic polyangiitis and glomerulonephritis. *J Am Soc Nephrol* 1996; 7:23-32.
30. Westman KW, Bygren PG, Olsson H, et al. Relapse rate, renal survival, and cancer morbidity in patients with Wegener's granulomatosis or microscopic polyangiitis with renal involvement. *J Am Soc Nephrol* 1998;9:842–852.
31. Guillevin L, Durand-Gasselin B, Cevallos R, et al. Microscopic polyangiitis: clinical and laboratory findings in eighty-five patients. *Arthritis Rheum* 1999;42:421–430.
32. Niles JL, Böttinger EP, Saurina GR, et al. The syndrome of lung hemorrhage and nephritis is usually an ANCA associated condition. *Arch Intern Med* 1996;156:440–445.
33. Deshpande PV, Gilbert R, Alton H, et al. Microscopic polyarteritis with renal and cerebral involvement. *Pediatr Nephrol* 2000;15:134–135.
34. Falk RJ, Hogan S, Carey TS, et al. Clinical course of antineutrophil cytoplasmic autoantibody-associated glomerulonephritis and systemic vasculitis. *Ann Intern Med* 1990;113:656–663.
35. Nash MC, Jones CL, Walker RG, et al. Anti-neutrophil cytoplasmic antibody-associated glomerulonephritis in children. *Pediatr Nephrol* 1993;7:11–14.
36. Nachman PH, Hogan SL, Jennette JC, et al. Treatment response and relapse in antineutrophil cytoplasmic autoantibody-associated microscopic polyangiitis and glomerulonephritis. *J Am Soc Nephrol* 1996;7:33–39.
37. Jayne DRW, Rasmussen N. Treatment of antineutrophil cytoplasm autoantibody-associated systemic vasculitis: initiatives of the European Community Systemic Vasculitis Clinical Trials Study Group. *Mayo Clin Proc* 1997;72:737–747.
38. Valentini RP, Smoyer WE, Sedman AB, et al. Outcome of antineutrophil cytoplasmic autoantibodies-positive glomerulonephritis and vasculitis in children: a single center experience. *J Pediatr* 1998;132:325–328.
39. Hoffman GS, Leavitt RY, Fleisher TA, et al. Treatment of Wegener's granulomatosis with intermittent high-dose intravenous cyclophosphamide. *Am J Med* 1990;89:403–410.
40. Jayne DRW, Esnault VLM, Lockwood CM. ANCA anti-idiotype antibodies and the treatment of systemic vasculitis

with intravenous immunoglobulin. *J Autoimmun* 1993;6: 207–219.
41. Kazatchkine MD and Kaveri SV. Immunomodulation of autoimmune and inflammatory diseases with intravenous immune globulin. *N Engl J Med* 2001;345:747–755.
42. Falk RJ and Jennette JC. ANCA small-vessel vasculitis. *J Am Soc Nephrol* 1997; 8:314–322.
43. Hoffman GS, Leavitt RY, Kerr GS, et al. The treatment of Wegener's granulomatosis with glucocorticoids and methotrexate. *Arthritis Rheum* 1992;35:1322–1329.
44. Nowack R, Gobel U, Klooker P, et al. Mycophenolate mofetil for maintenance therapy of Wegener's granulomatosis and microscopic polyangiitis: a pilot study in 11 patients with renal involvement. *J Am Soc Nephrol* 1999;10:1965–1971.
45. Stegeman CA, Cohen Tervaert JW, de Jong PE, et al. Trimethoprim-sulfamethoxazole (co-trimoxazole) for the prevention of relapses of Wegener's granulomatosis. *N Engl J Med* 1996;335:16–20.
46. Talar-Williams C, Hijazi YM, Walther MC, et al. Cyclophosphamide-induced cystitis and bladder cancer in patients with Wegener granulomatosis. *Ann Intern Med* 1996;124:477–484.
47. Baldree LA, Gaber LW, McKay CP. Anti-neutrophil cytoplasmic autoantibodies in a child with pauci-immune necrotizing and crescentic glomerulonephritis. *Pediatr Nephrol* 1991;5: 296–299.
48. Walters MDS, Savage COS, Dillon MJ, et al. Antineutrophil cytoplasm antibody in crescentic glomerulonephritis. *Arch Dis Childhood* 1988;63:814–817.
49. Ellis EN, Wood EG, Berry P. Spectrum of disease associated with anti-neutrophil cytoplasmic autoantibodies in pediatric patients. *J Pediatr* 1995;126:40–43.
50. Hattori M, Kurayama H, Koitabashi Y. Antineutrophil cytoplasmic autoantibody-associated glomerulonephritis in children. *J Am Soc Nephrol* 2001;12:1493–1500.
51. Nachman PH, Segelmark M, Westman K, et al. Recurrent ANCA-associated small vessel vasculitis after transplantation: a pooled analysis. *Kidney Int* 1999;56:1544–1550.
52. Grotz W, Wanner C, Rother E, et al. Clinical course of patients with antineutrophil cytoplasm antibody positive vasculitis after kidney transplantation. *Nephron* 1995;69:234–236.
53. Frasca GM, Neri L, Martello M, et al. Renal transplantation in patients with microscopic polyarteritis and antimyeloperoxidase antibodies: report of three cases. *Nephron* 1996;72:82–85.
54. Jennette JC and Falk RJ. Renal involvement in systemic vasculitis. In: Greenberg A, Cheung AK, Coffmann TM, et al., eds. *Primer on kidney diseases*, 2nd ed. San Diego, Academic Press, 1998:200–207.
55. Davson J, Ball J, and Platt R. The kidney in periarteritis nodosa. *QJM* 1948;17:175–202.
56. Bakkaloglu SA, Ekim M, Tumer N, et al. Severe renal impairment in the case of classic polyarteritis nodosa. *Pediatr Nephrol* 2001;16:148–150.
57. Ozen S, Besbas N, Saatci U, et al. Diagnostic criteria for polyarteritis nodosa in childhood. *J Pediatr* 1992;120:206–209.
58. Guillevin L, Lhote F, Cohen P, et al. Polyarteritis nodosa related to hepatitis B virus. A prospective study with long-term observation of 41 patients. *Medicine* 1995;74:238–253.
59. Duzova A, Bakkaloglu A, Yuce A, et al. Successful treatment of polyarteritis nodosa with interferon alpha in a nine-month old girl. *Eur J Pediatr* 2001;160:519–520.
60. Smith DL, Wernick R. Spontaneous rupture of a renal artery aneurysm in polyarteritis nodosa: critical review of the literature and report of a case. *Am J Med* 1989;87:464–467.
61. Lhote F, Guillevin L. Polyarteritis nodosa, microscopic polyangiitis, and Churg-Strauss syndrome. Clinical aspects and treatment. *Rheum Dis Clin North Am* 1995;21:911–947.
62. El-Reshaid K, Kapoor M, El-Reshaid W, et al. The spectrum of renal disease associated with microscopic polyangiitis and classic polyarteritis nodosa in Kuwait. *Nephrol Dial Transplant* 1997;12:1874–1882.
63. Mindell HJ, Fairbank J. Renal imaging techniques. In: Greenberg A, Cheung AK, Coffmann TM, et al., eds. *Primer on kidney diseases*, 2nd ed. San Diego: Academic Press, 1998:47–53.
64. Guillevin L, Fain O, Lhote F, et al. Lack of superiority of steroids plus plasma exchange to steroids alone in the treatment of polyarteritis nodosa and Churg-Strauss syndrome. A prospective, randomized trial in 78 patients. *Arthritis Rheum* 1992;35:208–215.
65. Guillevin L, Lhote F, Gayraud M, et al. Prognostic factors in polyarteritis nodosa and Churg-Strauss syndrome. A prospective study in 342 patients. *Medicine* 1996;75:17–28.
66. Al Mazyad AS. Polyarteritis nodosa in Arab children in Saudi Arabia. *Clin Rheumatol* 1999;18:196–200.
67. Blau EB, Morris RF, Yunis EJ. Polyarteritis nodosa in older children. *Pediatrics* 1977;60:227–234.
68. Kawasaki T, Kosaki F, Okawa S, et al. A new infantile acute febrile mucocutaneous lymph node syndrome (MLNS) prevailing in Japan. *Pediatrics* 1974;54:271–276.
69. Brogan PA, Bose A, Burgner D, et al. Kawasaki disease: an evidence based approach to diagnosis, treatment, and proposals for future research. *Arch Dis Childhood* 2002;86:286–290.
70. Yanagawa H, Nakamura Y, Yashiro M, et al. Incidence survey of Kawasaki disease in 1997 and 1998 in Japan. *Pediatrics* 2001;107(3). Available at: http://www.pediatrics.org/cgi/content/full/107/3/e33. Accessed June 2003.
71. Burns JC, Kushner HI, Bastian JF, et al. Kawasaki disease: a brief history. *Pediatrics* 2000;106(2). Available at: http://www.pediatrics.org/cgi/content/full/106/2/e27. Accessed June 2003.
72. Dajani AS, Taubert KA, Takahashi M, et al. Diagnosis and treatment of Kawasaki disease in children. *Circulation* 1993; 87:1760–1780.
73. Yanagawa H, Nakamura Y, Yashiro M, et al. Results of the nationwide epidemiologic survey of Kawasaki disease in 1995 and 1996 in Japan. *Pediatrics* 1998;102(6). Available at: http://www.pediatrics.org/cgi/content/full/102/6/e65. Accessed June 2003.
74. Kato H, Koike S, Yamamoto M, et al. Coronary aneurysms in infants and young children with acute febrile MCLNS. *J Pediatr* 1975;86:892–898.
75. Naoe S, Takahashi K, Masuda H, et al. Kawasaki disease: with particular emphasis on arterial lesions. *Acta Pathologica Japonica* 1991;41:785–797.

76. Foster BJ, Bernard C, Drummond KN. Kawasaki disease complicated by renal artery stenosis. *Arch Dis Childhood* 2000;83:253–255.
77. Veiga PA, Pieroni D, Baier W, et al. Association of Kawasaki disease and interstitial nephritis. *Pediatr Nephrol* 1992;6:421–423.
78. Nardi PM, Haller JO, Friedman AP, et al. Renal manifestations of Kawasaki's disease. *Pediatr Radiol* 1985;15:116–118.
79. Lande MB, Gleeson JG, Sundel RP. Kawasaki disease and acute renal failure. *Pediatr Nephrol* 1993;7:593.
80. Savage CO, Tizard J, Jayne D, et al. Antineutrophil cytoplasm antibodies in Kawasaki disease. *Arch Dis Childhood* 1989;64:360–363.
81. Tizard EJ, Baguley E, Hughes GR, et al. Antiendothelial cell antibodies detected by a cellular based ELISA in Kawasaki disease. *Arch Dis Childhood* 1991;66:189–192.
82. Guzman J, Fung M, Petty RE. Diagnostic value of antineutrophil cytoplasmic and anti-endothelial cell antibodies in early Kawasaki disease. *J Pediatr* 1994;124:917–920.
83. Nash MC, Shah V, Reader JA, et al. Anti-neutrophil cytoplasmic antibodies and anti-endothelial cell antibodies are not increased in Kawasaki disease. *Br J Rheumatol* 1995;34: 882–887.
84. Newburger JW, Tekahashi M, Burns JC, et al. The treatment of Kawasaki syndrome with intravenous γ globulin. *N Engl J Med* 1986;315:341–347.
85. Durongpisitkul K, Gururaj VJ, Park JM, et al. The prevention of coronary artery aneurysm in Kawasaki disease: a meta-analysis on the efficacy of aspirin and immunoglobulin treatment. *Pediatrics* 1995;96:1057–1061.
86. Terai M, Shulman ST. Prevalence of coronary artery abnormalities in Kawasaki disease is highly dependent on gamma globulin dose but independent of salicylate dose. *J Pediatr* 1997;131:888–893.
87. Han RK, Silverman ED, Newman A, et al. Management and outcome of persistent or recurrent fever after initial intravenous gamma globulin therapy in acute Kawasaki disease. *Arch Pediatr Adolesc Med* 2000;154:694–699.
88. Fauci A. The vasculitis syndromes. In: Wilson JD, Braunwald E, Isselbacher KJ, et al., eds. *Harrison's principles of internal medicine*, 12th ed. New York: McGraw-Hill, 1991: 1456–1463.
89. Arend WP, Michel BA, Block DA, et al. The American College of Rheumatology 1990 criteria for the classification of Takayasu arteritis. *Arthritis Rheum* 1990;33:1129–1134.
90. Milner LS, Jacobs DW, Thomson PD, et al. Management of severe hypertension in childhood Takayasu's arteritis. *Pediatr Nephrol* 1991;5:38–41.
91. Munir I, Uflacker R, Milutinovic J. Takayasu's arteritis associated with intrarenal vessel involvement. *Am J Kidney Dis* 2000;35:950–953.
92. Chugh KS, Sakhuja V. Takayasu's arteritis as a cause of renovascular hypertension in Asian countries. *Am J Nephrol* 1992;12:1–8.
93. Muranjan MN, Bavdekar SB, More V, et al. Study of Takayasu's arteritis in children: clinical profile and management. *J Postgrad Med* 2000;46:3–8.
94. Lupi-Herrera E, Sanchez-Torres G, Marcushamer J, et al. Takayasu's arteritis. Clinical study of 107 cases. *Am Heart J* 1977;93:94–103.
95. Hall S, Barr W, Lie JT, et al. Takayasu arteritis. A study of 32 North American patients. *Medicine* 1985;64:89–99.
96. Shelhamer JH, Volkman DJ, Parillo JE, et al. Takayasu's arteritis and its therapy. *Ann Intern Med* 1985;103:121–126.
97. Hoffman GS, Leavitt RY, Kerr GS, et al. Treatment of glucocorticoid-resistant or relapsing Takayasu arteritis with methotrexate. *Arthritis Rheum* 1994;37:578–582.
98. Rao SA, Mandalam KR, Rao VR, et al. Takayasu arteritis: initial and long-term follow-up in 16 patients after percutaneous transluminal angioplasty of the descending thoracic and abdominal aorta. *Radiology* 1993;189:173–179.
99. Choi HK, Merkel PA, Walker AM, et al. Drug-associated antineutrophil cytoplasmic antibody-positive vasculitis: prevalence among patients with high titers of antimyeloperoxidase antibodies. *Arthritis Rheum* 2000;43:405–413.
100. Sato H, Hattori M, Fujieda M, et al. High prevalence of antineutrophil cytoplasmic antibody positivity in childhood onset Graves' disease treated with propylthiouracil. *J Clin Endocrinol Metabol* 2000;85:4270–4273.
101. Vogt BA, Kim Y, Jennette JC, et al. Antineutrophil cytoplasmic autoantibody-positive crescentic glomerulonephritis as a complication of treatment with propylthiouracil in children. *J Pediatr* 1994;124:986–988.
102. Fujieda M, Hattori M, Kurayama H, et al. Clinical features and outcomes in children with antineutrophil cytoplasmic autoantibody-positive glomerulonephritis associated with propylthiouracil treatment. *J Am Soc Nephrol* 2002;13:437–445.
103. Gaskin G, Thompson EM, Pusey CD. Goodpasture-like syndrome associated with anti-myeloperoxidase antibodies following penicillamine treatment. *Nephrol Dial Transplant* 1995;10:1925–1928.
104. Choi HK, Merkel PA, Niles JL. ANCA-positive vasculitis associated with allopurinol therapy. *Clin Exp Rheumatol* 1998;16:743–744.
105. Elkayam O, Yaron M, Caspi D. Minocycline-induced autoimmune syndromes: an overview. *Semin Arthritis Rheum* 1999;28:392–397.

45

HENOCH-SCHÖNLEIN PURPURA

ROSANNA COPPO
ALESSANDRO AMORE

HISTORY AND DIAGNOSTIC CRITERIA

At the beginning of the nineteenth century, Heberden reported the observation of a child presenting with petechial hemorrhages on the lower limbs, joint and abdominal pain, bloody stools, and gross hematuria (1). The syndrome was named after the description by Schönlein of the clinical entity characterized by purpura and joint pain (2) and by Henoch of the frequent association of gastrointestinal symptoms and renal involvement (3). Henoch-Schönlein purpura (HSP) is a small vessel vasculitis with multiorgan involvement including skin, gastrointestinal tract, joints, and kidneys with variable clinical expression (4,5). The syndrome frequently begins after an infectious episode. The past ambiguous definitions of hypersensitivity angiitis, anaphylactoid purpura, or streptococcal rheumatic peliosis indicate the frequent relationship between HSP and either allergy or infections.

The differential diagnosis is sometimes difficult in adults because HSP overlaps other forms of systemic vasculitides, which are more common in adult age. Conversely, in subjects younger than 20 years, palpable purpura and bowel angina are most often due to HSP (5). Skin biopsy may be helpful, as it shows granulocytes in the small arteriole or venule walls (leukocytoclastic vasculitis) and immunoglobulin (Ig) A vascular deposits. The 1994 Consensus Conference on Nomenclature of Systemic Vasculitides defined HSP as a *small vessel vasculitis* (involving capillaries, arterioles, and venules) with IgA-dominant immune deposits, typically involving skin, gut, and glomeruli and associated with arthralgias or arthritis (6).

PATHOGENESIS

The finding of IgA deposits in the vessel wall as well as in the glomerular mesangial area allows a clear-cut distinction between HSP and other systemic vasculitides or collagen diseases with similar multiorgan involvement.

IgA is found in serum and mostly in external secretions. It plays a major role in mucosal immunity. There are two distinct subclasses of IgA—IgA1 and IgA2—differing with the insertion of 19 amino acids, present in IgA1 and absent in IgA2 subclass (7). Either subclass is synthesized by plasma cells as a 155-kDa protein consisting of two α heavy chains and two κ or λ light chains, or as dimers or polymers of the basic 4-chain Ig structure, with molecular weights multiple of 155 kDa. Dimers are joined by a J chain and can be transported from the basolateral to the luminal surface of secretory epithelia via a specialized glycoprotein receptor, the secretory component. In human serum, IgA is predominantly monomeric, of the IgA1 subclass, and is derived from plasmocytes within the bone marrow and the spleen. Mucosal-derived plasmocytes produce predominantly dimeric IgA containing J chain (8). Glomerular deposits in HSP as well as in primary IgA nephropathy (IgAN) are made of polymeric IgA1, leaving open the possibility of either bone-marrow or mucosal origin, by a somehow disturbed synthetic pathway (9).

HSP and IgAN can be triggered by mucosal infections. Because IgA is the prominent Ig in mucosal secretions acting as a defense against viral and bacterial agents, several authors have tried to identify the eliciting antigen(s). HSP could be secondary to an immune response because eluted mesangial IgA cross-react with the mesangial area of other biopsy samples from different HSP patients (10). The concept of HSP as an antigen-dependent process was further emphasized by the experimental observation that most closely reproduces HSP: a systemic vasculitis with nephritis can be induced by injecting animals with a complement-activating carbohydrate antigen (11,12). Food antigens or infectious organisms have been suspected (13–15), but the possibility of a single eliciting antigen remains unproven (16,17).

The accumulation of IgA immune complexes (ICs) within glomeruli has been considered the major pathogenic mechanism for HSP nephritis as for idiopathic IgAN. High levels of IgA-ICs have been detected during clinically active phases of purpuric rashes or HSP nephritis (18–21). However, IgA-ICs are not detected in all patients with renal involvement, which means that other pathogenic mechanisms may be involved.

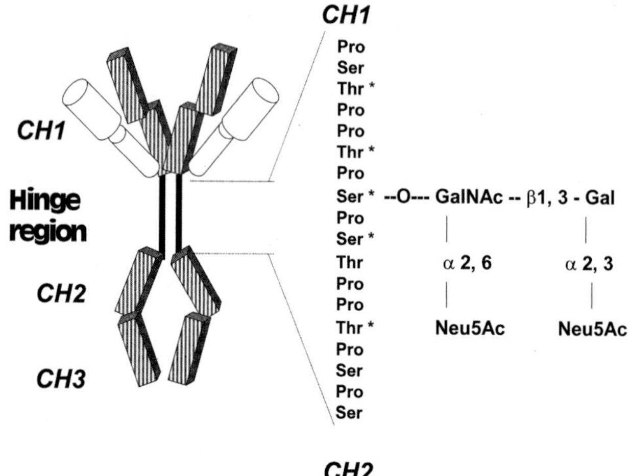

FIGURE 45.1. Human immunoglobulin A1 is highly glycosylated, as it contains five short O-linked oligosaccharide chains composed of *N*-acetylgalactosamine acid (GalNAc), galactose (Gal), and neuraminic acid (Neu5Ac). These oligosaccharides are coupled to serine (Ser) or threonine (Thr) residues in the hinge region, connecting the CH1 and CH2 domains.

In HSP patients, and particularly in those with nephritis, circulating IgA molecules react with α-galactosyl residues (21), fibronectin (22) or gluten-derived molecules (17) or mesangial matrix glycoproteins (23), and endothelial cells (24). Hence, it was postulated that these effects were not due to true antigen-antibody reactions but to some kind of affinity of circulating IgA to various molecules, mostly glycoproteins.

Attention has been focused on the carbohydrate moieties of IgA molecules. Human IgA1, the predominant subclass deposited in both HSP nephritis and primary IgAN, is highly glycosylated (7) (Fig. 45.1). In addition to the N-linked oligosaccharides typically present in the carboxyl terminal portion of all classes of Ig heavy chain, IgA1 contains five short O-linked oligosaccharide chains composed of *N*-acetylgalactosamine, galactose, and sialic acid. These oligosaccharides are coupled to serine or threonine residues, which lie in the hinge region connecting the CH1 and CH2 domains, at the junction between the Fab and the Fc portions of the IgA molecule (7).

Several data support an aberrant IgA1 glycosylation, not only in patients with primary IgAN but also in patients with HSP (25–27). A genetic defect leading to an inadequate activity of β1-3 galactosyltransferase in B cells has been postulated as for primary IgAN (28). An imbalance in lymphocyte function, with a prevalence of T-helper 2 over T-helper 1 T-cell subsets, can lead to altered IgA glycosylation in mice (29). *In vitro* desialylated or degalactosylated IgA show a high tendency for self-aggregation resulting in the formation of macromolecules with a molecular weight similar to IgA-ICs (30). Hence, aberrantly glycosylated IgA can circulate in monomeric form or participate in the formation of self-aggregates or true ICs.

Whether present in ICs or in self-aggregates, such aberrantly glycosylated IgA likely escape clearance by hepatic receptors for asialoglycoproteins (31) because of the lack of galactose and possibly because of the size of the aggregates, which excludes them from the space of Disse. Abnormally glycosylated IgA1 may deposit in glomeruli more readily than normal IgA1 by virtue of enhanced lectin-like reactivity with the fibronectin, laminin, and collagen within the mesangial matrix (23). Finally, mesangial catabolism of aberrantly glycosylated IgA may be diminished. In combination, these factors can lead to the accumulation or a prolonged persistence of IgA deposits in the mesangium.

An enhanced interaction of IgA with Fcα receptors on mesangial cells results in cellular activation and phlogistic mediator synthesis. We demonstrated an increased expression of integrin adhesion molecules (32) and of the inducible form of nitric oxide synthase in mesangial cells (33) after incubation with aggregates of desialylated or degalactosylated IgA. The resultant increase in the production of intraglomerular nitric oxide may lead to peroxidative damage, apoptosis, and sclerosis. The effect can be further enhanced by the concomitant depressed expression of vascular endothelial growth factor induced by aberrantly glycosylated IgA on mesangial cells, leading to an impaired repair process (34). Aggregates of IgA also stimulate the synthesis of a variety of cytokines (e.g., interleukin-6, platelet-derived growth factor, interleukin-1, tumor necrosis factor-α, transforming growth factor-β), vasoactive factors (e.g., prostaglandins, thromboxane, leukotrienes, endothelin, platelet-aggregating factor, nitric oxide), or chemokines (monocyte chemotactic protein-1; interleukin-8; macrophage inflammatory protein-1; HRANTES) by mesangial cells (35,36).

Complement activation may have a role in the pathogenesis of HSP nephritis. It is of interest that aberrantly glycosylated IgA can activate complement more efficiently than normal IgA (37).

Antineutrophil cytoplasmic antibodies of the IgA isotype [IgA-antineutrophil cytoplasmic antibodies (ANCA)] have been found in adults with HSP, but other reports failed to confirm these findings (38,39). We demonstrated that IgA molecules from children and adults with HSP nephritis show an increased binding to sonicated neutrophil extracts and to purified myeloperoxidase but not to serine protease 3 (26). Of interest, this reactivity was never observed in sera from patients with primary IgAN, even though they have aberrantly glycosylated IgA. This binding is affected by electrical charge and carbohydrate interactions. Both fibronectin and the lectin jacalin, which can bind IgA and the carbohydrate moieties of other glycoproteins, enhance the binding of IgA to myeloperoxidase. These data are consistent with a lectin-like binding of IgA to neutrophil cytoplasmic antigens. We speculate that the aberrant glycosylation of IgA1 in HSP patients explains several abnormal reactivities and a high affinity for ANCA antigens. These antigens may be released in excess during phlogistic processes, leading to circulating IgA1-ANCA complexes, which, in the presence of increased levels of eosinophilic cationic proteins (40) as well as other phlogistic mediators (41,42), may favor vascular deposition of IgA1. The vascular affinity for circulating IgA-containing immune material leads to purpura and systemic vasculitis.

B cells synthesizing IgA are increased during acute phases of the disease, and abnormalities of T-suppressor activity have been observed during the acute phase (43). Transforming growth factor-β–secreting T cells have been detected in circulation during the phases of clinical activity of HSP, but they resolve during recovery (44). In patients with HSP nephritis, a reduction in Fcγ, C3b, and fibronectin receptor function of mononuclear phagocytes has been reported (45). These abnormalities were transient, probably secondary to saturation of receptors more than a primary event.

Plasma IgE levels are increased in HSP and are significantly higher than in IgAN (46). This increase could be consequent to a prevalence of T-helper 2 lymphocytes. Serum eosinophil cationic proteins are elevated in HSP (40), again suggesting an activation of the IgE-system allergy. Serum C3 and C4 values are within the normal ranges, even though CH50 and properdin levels are often reduced. These data, together with the frequent increase in C3d (19,42) in young patients with active HSP nephritis, suggest C3 activation, possibly via the alternative pathway, balanced by enhanced factor synthesis, thus masking the complement consumption.

Several reports indicate that some HLA class II gene polymorphisms can be a risk factor for HSP. A positive association with DRB1*01 and DRB1*11 (64 vs. 48% in the controls) as well as a negative association with HLA-DRB1*07 was first reported by our group in an Italian cohort (47,70) and confirmed in another study (48). An increase of DQA1*0301 was found in Japanese children (49). An increased frequency of homozygous C4A or C4B null phenotype was observed in whites (50) and in Japanese patients (49). No association of angiotensin-converting enzyme genes, polymorphism and manifestations, or progression of HSP nephritis was found (51). The risk of developing severe gastrointestinal complications is negatively associated with polymorphism of the intracellular adhesion molecule 1, and it has been suggested that it might also reduce the risk of renal involvement (52).

CLINICAL DATA

Epidemiology

HSP is the most frequent vasculitis in childhood. Its annual incidence is approximately 14 cases of 100,000 children (53). HSP is frequent in the first decade of life; however, it rarely affects children younger than 2 years of age. The median age at onset is 4 to 5 years (54). The sex ratio shows a male preponderance (male to female ratio, 1.4–1.7:1) (55). Renal involvement is more frequent between 6 and 10 years of age (56–58). The geographic distribution of HSP is similar to that of primary IgAN. HSP is common in Europe [particularly in France, Italy, Spain, UK (4), and Finland] and Asia (e.g., Japan, Singapore, and China) (59), whereas it is less common in North America and Africa. The disease may be favored by racial factors, as HSP rarely affects blacks and Indians (60).

Factors Triggering Henoch-Schönlein Purpura

The disease may be triggered by a peculiar event, most often an infectious disease, in approximately two-third of patients (56). *Streptococcus* β, *Yersinia, Mycoplasma, Toxoplasma,* varicella, measles, rubella, adenovirus, HIV, and several other agents have been recorded among the triggering factors but without direct evidence of causality (44). There is a peak incidence of HSP in winter in North Europe and in June in Italy (58). Some epidemic clusters and familial cases of HSP have been reported (61).

The role of allergic reactions has been questioned, as well as the role of vaccinations (e.g., against smallpox or influenza), drugs (e.g., including ciprofloxacin, vancomycin, minocycline, carbamazepine), or other allergens (44).

Systemic Manifestations

HSP syndrome is characterized by a multiorgan involvement (56,58,62).

Skin

The characteristic skin lesions consist of slightly raised, palpable, purpuric macules that do not disappear on pressure with normal platelet count. They mostly begin with erythematous macules, some of which evolve into slightly raised urticarial papules, which soon become purpuric and eventually take a fawn color as they fade. Individual petechiae often become confluent in large patches. The purpuric rash often has a symmetric distribution over the extensor surfaces of the lower limbs and forearms and the buttock sides (Fig. 45.2). The purpura is present in the ankle area and in the milder cases it can be present only there. It also affects pressure areas (e.g., belt and pants) and occasionally affects earlobes, nose, and genitalia. Sometimes the rash is accompanied by fever and general malaise, with a clinical picture of infectious purpura or allergic reaction. At microscopic examination of skin biopsy, leukocytoclastic vasculitis of dermal vessels is observed with IgA deposits in the vascular wall.

Purpura is concomitant with renal involvement in two-thirds of the cases (58). In 25% of children, purpura pre-

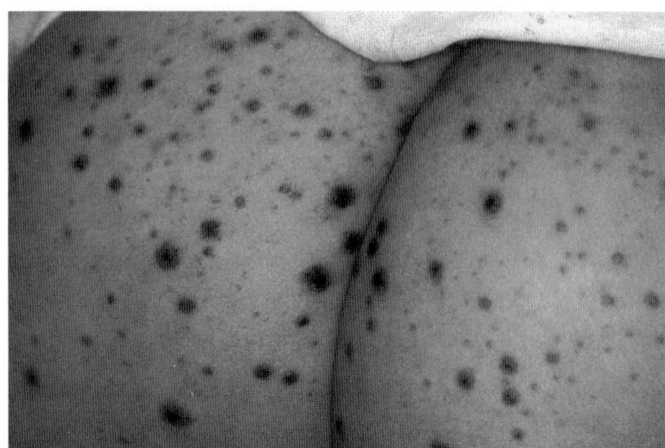

FIGURE 45.2. Purpuric rash of Henoch-Schönlein purpura over the sides of the buttocks. (See Color Plate 45.2.)

cedes and in 8% follows the urinary abnormalities by 3 to 12 months.

The purpura lasts for a few days but often relapses. Subsequent flare-up of purpura occur in 26% of children with severe renal disease (62). Relapses of purpura may be accompanied by macroscopic hematuria and a transient increase in proteinuria, although the extent and duration of purpuric rash are not correlated with the severity of the renal lesions.

Gastrointestinal Tract

Gastrointestinal symptoms are reported in 50 to 70% of patients (4), more frequently in children than in adults (58). The most typical manifestation is diffuse abdominal pain, increasing after meals, referred to as *bowel angina*. Vomiting, hematemesis, and hematochezia or melena is frequent (5). Major abdominal complications, like intussusception, intestinal infarction, and bowel perforation are rare events. The pain is often severe and mimics an acute surgical emergency. Steroid therapy may be useful in relieving bowel-wall edema and pain.

Joints

Transient arthralgia is reported in 50 to 70% of cases (4). They mostly involve lower limb articulations, ankles, and knees, with a picture of oligoarticular synovitis. A periarticular edema may be present. The articular involvement does not lead to joint erosions, deformities, or functional limitations.

Kidney

The selection of HSP patients strongly affects the data concerning the prevalence of renal involvement (4,53,55,59,63). Variations in the prevalence of renal involvement among different series may also depend on the methods of detection of

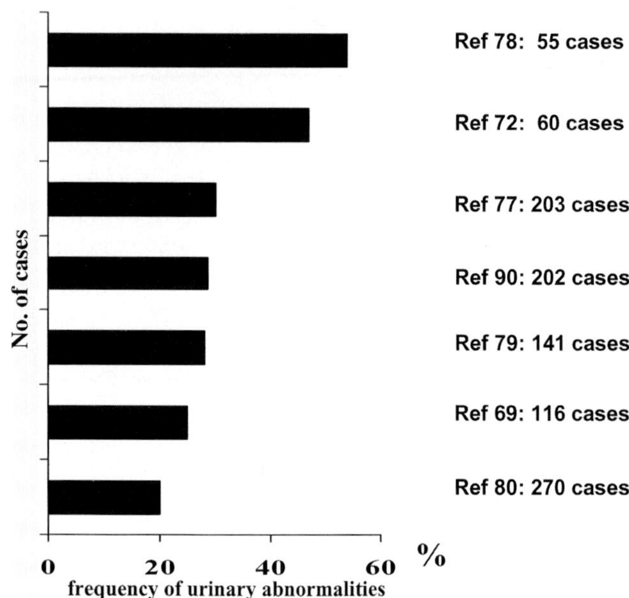

FIGURE 45.3. Renal involvement detected by urinalysis in unselected cohorts of children with Henoch-Schönlein purpura.

nephritis. The prevalence may increase if serial urinalyses are performed. The percentage of renal involvement among children with HSP increases progressively to 35% at 1 year (64). In unselected cohorts of children, the prevalence of the renal involvement during the course of HSP is approximately 33%, ranging from 20 to 55% (57) (Fig. 45.3).

In cohorts of children with severe renal disease, as in the cohort of the Italian register of renal biopsies in children (65), the prevalence of glomerulonephritis related to HSP is 11.6% of all renal diseases.

The preselection of children investigated also affects the clinical picture. General pediatricians often report a systemic disease with modest and transient urinary abnormalities (66), whereas in pediatric nephrology departments the renal disease is more severe (56,67,68).

The manifestations of glomerulonephritis secondary to HSP include isolated microscopic or macroscopic hematuria, mild or heavy proteinuria with or without nephrotic syndrome, renal failure, and hypertension (57). The most frequent clinical presentation of HSP nephritis in nonselected pediatric series is an isolated microscopic hematuria (66,69). In 80% of cases, it is detected within 4 weeks after the onset of the disease. It is often transient, detectable only by routine urinalysis during the acute phase, followed by a complete recovery. In some patients, proteinuria of variable amount is present (Fig. 45.4). A nephrotic syndrome is more common in referral centers but is rare in unselected series. Renal function is normal in most children but may be impaired in children with nephrotic syndrome. It is most often a moderate renal failure, which rarely requires dialysis. Hypertension is rare at onset of the disease and has been reported in children with minimal urinary abnormalities.

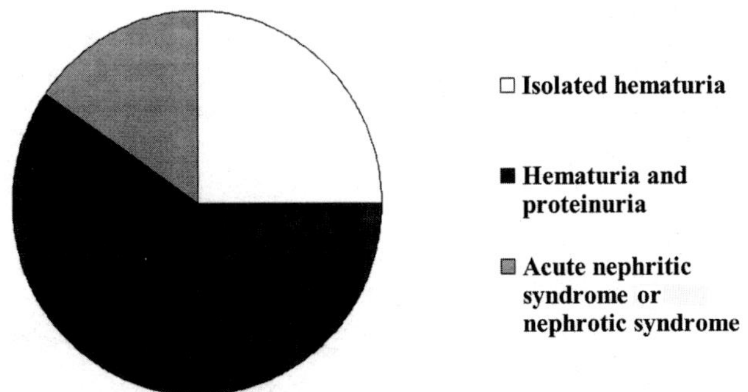

FIGURE 45.4. Clinical presentation of children with nephritis of Henoch-Schönlein purpura. Cumulative data from 666 children (63,69,72,78–80,90).

Other Nonrenal Manifestations

HSP can be complicated by a cerebral vasculitic process resulting in convulsions, encephalopathy, chorea, or blindness (63).

Other rare manifestations include hemorrhage in the calf or subcutaneously, pulmonary-renal syndrome, pancreatitis, adrenal bleeding, or testicular involvement, mimicking torsion (44).

The vasculitic process can affect the ureter (70). In these cases, it is generally associated with loin pain. The ureteral lesions of necrotizing vasculitis may evolve into sclerotic lesions and progress to stenosis, requiring correction (71,72).

LABORATORY DATA

In HSP, as in idiopathic IgAN, serum IgA levels are increased in up to 50 to 70% of patients, but the increase is often limited to the acute initial phase, and when the disease heals, serum IgA returns within normal values, confirming a pivotal role of IgA abnormalities in pathogenesis of HSP. The subclass mostly increased is polymeric IgA1 (44).

IgA-ICs and IgA-fibronectin aggregates have been detected mostly during the acute phase or during clinical relapses (19–22). IgA antibodies to endogenous or exogenous antigens have been reported, including IgA rheumatoid factor (73). High levels of IgA reacting with sonicated neutrophil extracts (IgA-ANCA) and with purified cytoplasmatic antigens (myeloperoxidase) have also been detected in children with HSP nephritis (38,26).

Platelet count is in the normal range, and the activity of the clotting factors is normal. Conversely, abnormalities in fibrin-stabilizing factor (factor XIII) have been reported as well as increased von Willebrand factor plasma levels (74), indicating an endothelial damage that favors fibrin deposition and crescent formation.

PATHOLOGY

Light Microscopy Features

HSP nephritis is characterized by mesangial damage with different degrees of hypercellularity (Fig. 45.5), ranging from isolated mesangial proliferation to focal and segmental proliferation and severe crescentic glomerulonephritis.

Light microscopic examination shows a wide range in terms of the type and severity of glomerular involvement from one patient to another and also within the same biopsy, from glomerulus to glomerulus (56). Classifications of HSP nephritis are mostly based on the severity of the proliferative lesions (4,60). Six histologic classes are distinguished according to the presence or absence and the extension of extracapillary proliferation, with subclasses defining the degree of the endocapillary proliferation (Table 45.1). The distribution of histologic grades in an analysis of 270 children showed 50% in class III, with almost even representation of the other classes, but class VI, pseudomembranoproliferative lesions, is far less common (Fig. 45.6).

Adhesions of the tuft to Bowman's capsule can be found in coincidence with segmental proliferative lesions, often with splitting and duplication of glomerular basement membranes. In rare cases, there is a severe mesangial proliferation associated with mesangial interposition in which cells and matrix migrate into the capillary walls, between the basement membrane and endothelial cytoplasm, mimicking a membranoproliferative glomerulonephritis. Polymorphonuclear cells may infiltrate the glomerular tufts, sometimes as severely as in acute poststreptococcal glomerulonephritis. Segmental necrosis of the glomerular tuft is often present at onset. It is not rare to detect intracapillary glomerular thrombi.

It is common to find crescent formation varying in size from a limited segment to circumferential crescents. At onset, crescents are cellular, then evolve into fibrous cres-

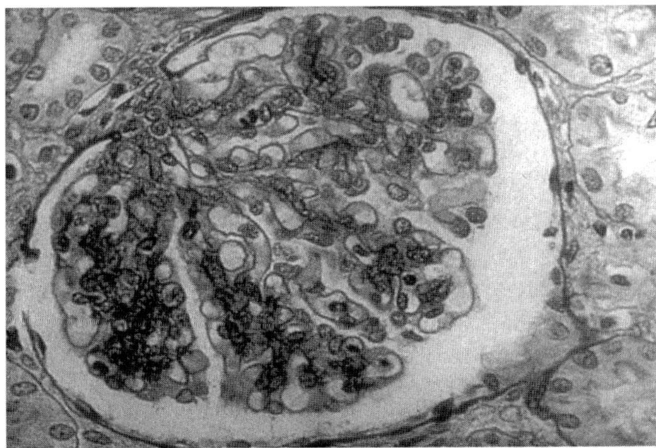

FIGURE 45.5. Renal biopsy specimen from a patient with nephritis of Henoch-Schönlein purpura showing expansion of the mesangial matrix and increase in mesangial cellularity (periodic acid-Schiff ×250). (See Color Plate 45.5.)

TABLE 45.1. CLASSIFICATION OF HENOCH-SCHÖNLEIN NEPHRITIS LESIONS ACCORDING TO EMANCIPATOR

Class I: minimal glomerular lesions and absence of crescents
Class II: no crescents
IIa: pure mesangial proliferation
IIb: focal-segmental endocapillary proliferation
IIc: diffuse endocapillary proliferation
Class III: presence of extracapillary cellular proliferation in less than 50% of glomeruli
IIIa: in association with focal and segmental endocapillary proliferation
IIIb: with diffuse endocapillary proliferation
Class IV: florid extracapillary proliferation in 50–75% of glomeruli
IVa: in association with focal and segmental endocapillary proliferation
IVb: with diffuse endocapillary proliferation
Class V: extracapillary proliferation in more than 75% of glomeruli
Va: in association with focal and segmental endocapillary proliferation
Vb: with diffuse endocapillary proliferation
Class VI: pseudomembranoproliferative glomerulonephritis

Adapted from Emancipator SN. IgA nephropathy and Henoch-Schönlein purpura. In: Jennette JC, Olson JL, Schwartz MM, et al., eds. *Heptinstall's pathology of the kidney.* Philadelphia: Lippincott–Raven publishers, 1998.

cents, generating segmental scars or global sclerosis. The most common histologic feature is a predominance of small crescents. In children with severe renal symptoms, extracapillary proliferation is detected in more than one-half of the cases (59,62). In these cases, crescents often involve less than 50% of glomeruli (class III). Some biopsies show periglomerular inflammatory infiltrates, mostly associated with crescents (15% of the children) (62).

Hyalin change or accumulation of fibrinoid material or necrosis with inflammatory infiltration and clear findings of vasculitis are present in approximately 10% of children. Blood vessels may show medial hypertrophy and intimal fibroelastosis. Necrosis of the capillary tuft has been reported in 8% of children, coincident with extracapillary proliferation.

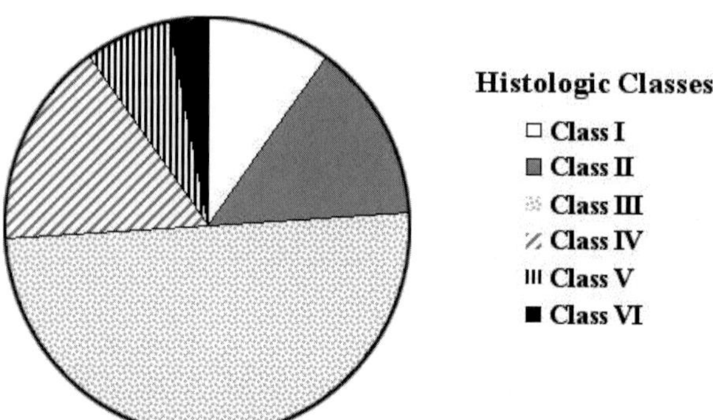

FIGURE 45.6. Distribution of histologic grades in Henoch-Schönlein purpura nephritis. Cumulative data from 270 renal biopsies (59,81,106).

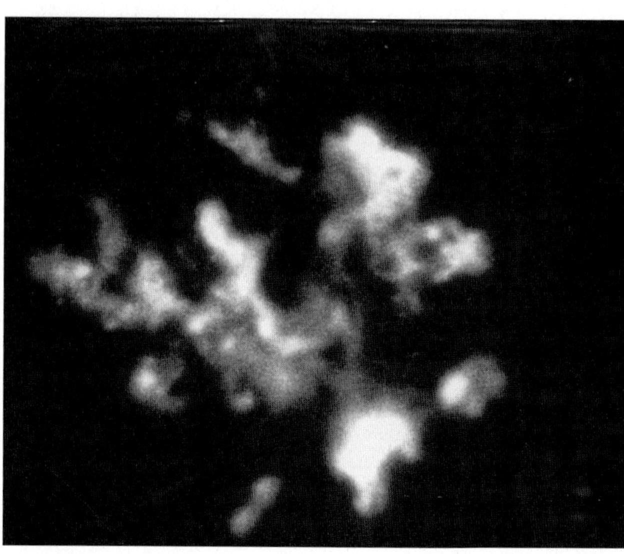

FIGURE 45.7. Immunopathology of Henoch-Schönlein nephritis. Mesangial deposits of IgA (antiimmunoglobulin A ×250). (See Color Plate 45.7.)

The renal biopsies from children with HSP nephritis show degenerative tubular alterations with flattening, vacuolization, desquamation, and focal loss of the brush-border microvilli in the cortex (60). Tubular cylinders and blood casts are detected in 30% of patients.

Immunohistochemistry

Mesangial IgA granular deposits are the hallmark of the disease, which, in contrast with the frequent focal and segmental proliferative changes, is always diffuse as in primary IgAN (Fig. 45.7). IgA1 is the dominant subclass with equal distribution of light chains. The J chain is detectable, indicating that IgA in deposits is dimeric, but it is not identical to secretory IgA because the secretory component is absent. Extensive subendothelial deposits are associated with the most severe histologic forms with endocapillary proliferation or crescents.

C3 is codeposited in 75 to 85% of the cases similarly to idiopathic IgAN. The membrane attack complex C5-C9 and the alternative complement pathway components are always detected. Early classical pathway complement components C1q and C4 are present only rarely and stain with low intensity (60). IgG and IgM codeposits are present in 40% of the cases. Fibrin or fibrinogen deposits are found in 60 to 70% of patients, both in mesangial and in parietal areas, often coincident with mesangial proliferation, suggesting a role of the clotting cascade activation. Glomerular fibrin-related deposits are much more frequently present in HSP nephritis than in IgAN (55) and are often related to active phases with extracapillary proliferation. Deposits of IgA and C3 can be found in arterioles or cortical peritubular capillaries in children with severe glomerular changes.

Electron Microscopy

Electron-dense deposits are detectable in a setting of mesangial matrix expansion and variable degree of cellular hyperplasia (60). The deposits, initially paramesangial and small, become larger and of nonuniform density, in strict connection with the mesangial matrix. Most deposits have a mesangial localization with parietal extensions (in 60% of the cases) and are purely mesangial in 30% of cases. The parietal, paramesangial electron-dense material is generally subendothelial, more rarely subepithelial. Sometimes, electron-dense deposits, hump-like with garland shape or fluffy aspects, are detectable. In other cases, deposits show with a woolly aspect in the external rara lamina, placed in the periphery of the capillary loops and delimited by a thick layer of new basement membrane. As a possible consequence of the membrane reactivity to immune deposits, the presence of parietal deposits modifies the capillary basal membrane profile because of the widening of the rara internal and external lamina, with neoformed layers.

Follow-Up Renal Biopsies

Studies of serial biopsies in children with HSP showed a good correlation between the histologic changes, clinical data, and outcome (75). When patients undergo clinical resolution, mesangial proliferation disappears and crescents regress, while others evolve into segmental synechiae. IgA deposits substantially decrease and sometimes completely disappear. Conversely, when repeat biopsies are performed in patients with persistently active or progressing nephritis, the proliferation continues to be severe, and evolution into fibrotic lesions is detected. The importance of careful clinical monitoring during the follow-up of children with HSP nephritis must be stressed also on the basis of the good correlation between clinical and histologic data reported by this study.

Nonrenal Lesions

The typical lesion of HSP, either in skin, gut, or in kidney vessels, is leukocytoclastic vasculitis with fragmentation of leukocyte nuclei in and around arterioles, capillaries, and venules, surrounded by infiltrating neutrophils and monocyte cells in the presence of nuclear residues (nuclear dust) in the wall of arterioles. Fibrin deposits and arteriolar and venular necrosis can be found. Deposits of IgA and C3 are present in the dermal capillaries in purpuric lesions and uninvolved skin and are considered a valid diagnostic criterion, with 100% specificity in combination with leukocytoclastic vasculitis. IgG and IgM can be codeposited in approximately 20% of the cases, whereas C1q and C4 are absent. Similar deposits have been reported in superficial derma capillaries of IgAN patients. In dermatitis herpetiformis, IgA deposits are found as well, but they are located on the top of the derma papilla. In systemic lupus erythematosus, the dermal-epidermal junction is mostly positive for IgG, C1q, and C4.

The diagnosis may be difficult in the rare cases in which skin eruption entirely consists of urticaria lesions without purpura. Hypersensitivity vasculitis is sometimes overlapping, but the dermal IgA vascular deposits are specific for HSP lesions.

Correlations between Clinical and Pathologic Data

In the Italian HSP series of 74 children (58,62), patients with minimal proteinuria had a higher prevalence of class I and II lesions (92%), without crescents. In cases with significant proteinuria, more severe renal lesions were frequently found. Extracapillary proliferation was also often found in children with nonnephrotic proteinuria (33% of class III and IV). Gross hematuria at presentation was associated with crescent formations in the 22% of the children. The clinical feature mostly predictive for severe histologic lesions is the onset with renal function impairment, as 62% of children with severe acute nephritic syndrome and severe kidney function impairment had crescents, and other authors reported similar findings (76).

CLINICAL COURSE AND PROGNOSIS

HSP nephritis accounts for 5% of children with end-stage renal failure in Europe (4,56). The clinical course and long-term outcome vary according to the cohorts examined, particularly when unselected cohorts are compared with children followed by pediatric nephrology units. In unselected series, HSP is a mild disease, with renal involvement in a minority of cases, mostly presenting with isolated hematuria or minimal proteinuria and with long-term sequelae concerning no more than 1% of patients (80). Reports of series of children admitted into general pediatric hospitals indicate a prevalence of urinary sediment abnormalities of 20 to 28%, generally lasting for more than 1 month (73,77–80). With a follow-up of more than 10 years, a progression to end-stage renal failure is observed in approximately 2 to 3% of the children with initial signs of renal involvement (81).

The remission rates reported by tertiary reference centers are below 50%, with poor outcome in 10 to 25% of children (56,68). In cohorts of children with a severe disease, long-term prognosis is poorer, as 15 to 30% of them progress to renal failure with wide variability depending on the duration of follow-up (57). In a long-term follow-up study, a late progression was observed after 25 years in 25% of children, not only in cases with persistently active renal disease but also in others having experienced clinical improvement after the acute phase (68). These authors reported persistent urinary

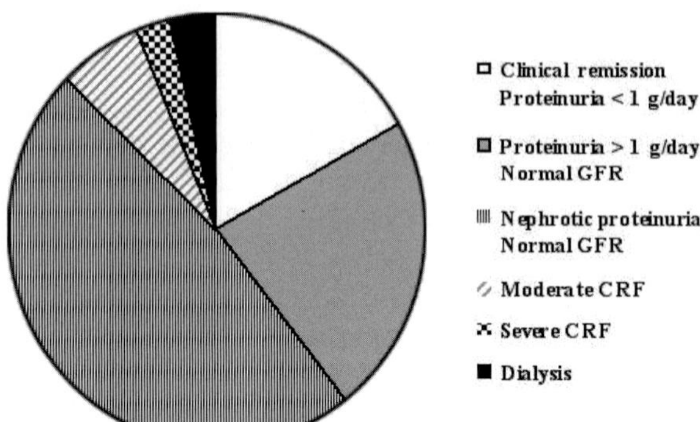

FIGURE 45.8. Long-term renal outcome of patients with Henoch-Schönlein nephritis. Mean 5-year follow-up of 57 children with severe Henoch-Schönlein nephritis, warranting renal biopsy. CFR chronic renal failure; GFR, glomerular filtration rate. (Adapted from Coppo R, Mazzucco G, Cagnoli L, for the Italian Group of Renal Immunopathology. Long-term prognosis of Henoch-Schönlein nephritis in adults and in children. *Nephrol Dial Transplant* 1997;12:2277–2283.)

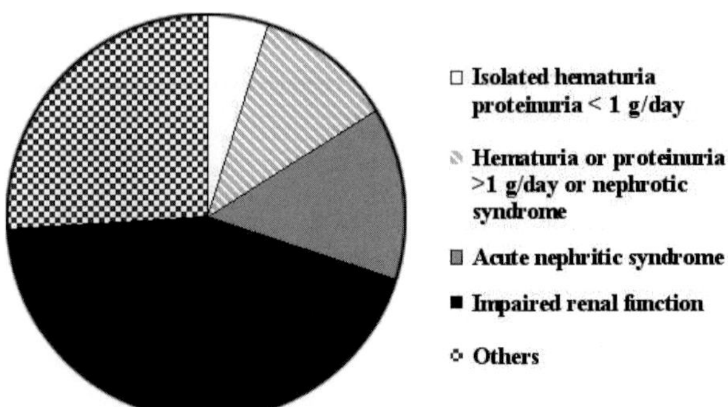

FIGURE 45.9. Risk factors for progression of renal disease in Henoch-Schönlein purpura nephritis. Cumulative data of 77 children (63,69,72,78,79,90).

abnormalities in 15% of children with a nephritic onset or persistent heavy proteinuria, 40% of those with a nephritic presentation and 50% of those with mixed nephritic-nephrotic syndrome at onset. Some of these patients ended in chronic renal failure. It is clear that renal function may deteriorate during the follow-up even in patients who apparently completely recovered 2 years after onset (68), perhaps due to sequences of glomerular hypertension.

The presence and extent of extracapillary proliferation is certainly important to identify children with potentially progressive renal disease. There is a close relationship between the extent of crescents and long-term sequela in patients with class IV and V, with extensive glomerular involvement by crescents in more than 50% and more than 75% of glomeruli, respectively. In a Japanese series, 33% of class IV and 83% of class V ended with chronic renal failure (59). In the Italian multicenter study (62), after 1 to 20 (mean, 5) years, one-third of the children who had had a renal biopsy were in remission (Fig. 45.8). In 40% of the cases, only minimal or moderate proteinuria was left. Chronic renal failure or end-stage renal disease occurred in 12% of children. The delay between onset and end-stage renal failure varied from a few days to 20 years, with an average of 10 years. When comparing children and adults with a HSP nephritis, the outcomes were substantially similar, with loss of renal function in 26% of adults and in 27% of children after 10 years (62).

Children at Risk for Progression

It is of paramount importance to identify children with potentially progressive renal disease. As reported above, the clinical presentation is, in general terms, indicative of the long-term outcome (69). In some reports, nephrotic syndrome or renal insufficiency at onset were risk factors (44%) for renal failure after two decades of follow-up (68) (Fig. 45.9).

Conversely, in the Italian cohort (62), no significant prognostic factor was found, including renal function impairment at presentation or hypertension. Mild proteinuria or, at the opposite, nephrotic-range levels, were associated with high frequency of remission or functional deterioration. However, children with mild proteinuria also frequently displayed severe histologic lesions with extracapillary proliferation, and nephrotic and nonnephrotic children had similar outcomes.

The percentage of glomeruli involved by extracapillary proliferation, the extent of Bowman's space occupied by individual crescents, the fresh or fibrous crescent ratio and are important risk factors (67). The predictive value of mild extracapillary proliferation was low when crescents involved less than 50% of glomeruli (class III) (renal failure in 18% of children with crescents on renal biopsy), also because some cases without crescents experienced an unfavorable outcome (23% of cases).

Renal Transplantation in Children with Henoch-Schönlein Purpura Nephritis

Recurrence of IgA mesangial deposits may occur after renal transplantation, even though the recurrence of clinical symptoms of HSP is rare. The actuarial risk for histologic or immunofluorescent recurrence is 35% at 5 years, with graft loss in 11% (82,83). In most patients, no clinical manifestations or minimal hematuria accompany histologic recurrence in grafted kidneys (84). Recurrence is not prevented by triple therapy, including cyclosporine, and is more frequent in rapidly progressive cases. Delaying transplantation of 1 year after the last systemic signs was not effective in decreasing the rate of recurrence (82). The recurrence rate appears to be increased in recipients of living-related grafts, suggesting a role for genetic factors. This is controversial, however, and the issue of using living donors for renal transplantation in HSP is still debated (85,86).

THERAPY

Mild cases do not require treatment, provided urine monitoring is ensured to detect anomalies mostly during the first 2 to 3 months after onset of the purpuric rash.

The abdominal pain is generally controlled by small doses of steroids, which favor a rapid resolution. Patients with recurrent necrotizing purpura or severe abdominal pain have been successfully treated by intravenous Ig infusions (87).

Because in most cases the purpuric rash precedes by days or weeks the detection of urinary abnormalities, attempts have been made to prevent the development of the nephropathy by giving prednisone (1 to 2.5 mg/kg/day for 1 to 3 weeks). A beneficial effect was not observed in retrospective studies, which compared treated versus untreated patients. However, the treatment was often reserved to the more active cases, thus introducing a selection bias, which may have influenced the outcome (88,89). Conversely, a prospective trial (albeit not strictly randomized) suggested a protective effect of a 2-week course of prednisone (90). The prevention consisted in avoiding the appearance of microscopic hematuria, which is not associated with a high risk for progression to renal failure.

Once the nephritis has developed, it is possible either to treat or to wait for a spontaneous remission. Based on observations dating decades ago, oral corticosteroids were believed to be ineffective for treating HSP nephritis. Indeed, retrospective analyses failed to demonstrate any benefit of prednisone in children with HSP nephritis (91). However, again a selection bias favoring treatment of more severe cases was likely, because the severity of the disease was a major determinant in the decision to treat. More recently, a 1-year treatment with oral prednisone and azathioprine in patients with moderately severe renal involvement gave positive results in comparison with historical, untreated cases (92,56). However, as the historical group included particularly severe cases, no recommendation for treatment of moderately severe HSP nephritis is presently possible (93).

Tonsillectomy has been proposed for HSP nephritis, as for primary IgAN, with the aim of limiting the mucosal immune response. The overall analysis does not support the recommendation for this intervention in HSP nephritis (94).

There is a need for an efficient treatment for children with severe endocapillary and extracapillary proliferation and clinical presentation of nephrotic or nephritic syndrome with impaired renal function. An aggressive therapeutic regimen resulted in a favorable clinical outcome in 11 of 12 children with 60 to 90% glomeruli with crescent formation. This regimen consisted in a triple therapy of three methylprednisolone pulses followed by a 6-month course of prednisone, dipyridamole, and cyclophosphamide for 3 months (95). More than 60% of these patients experienced a complete remission. Similar positive results have been reported using high-dose steroids in association with oral cyclophosphamide (96).

A larger French series confirmed that methylprednisolone pulses followed by a 3-month course of oral prednisone and, in some patients, with a 2-month course of oral cyclophosphamide, resulted in clinical recovery in 71% of children with nephritic syndrome or crescentic involvement in greater than 50% of the glomeruli, versus 40% in a historical group of untreated children (97). Similarly, in children with greater than 50% glomeruli involved with crescents, good results were reported with oral prednisone for 4 months in association with a 2-month course of cyclophosphamide and heparin or warfarin for 4 months (98). A combination of prednisone, azathioprine, or cyclophosphamide also gave positive results (99).

Our group (100), and more recently others (101), successfully treated children with rapidly progressive HSP nephritis with plasma exchanges, corticosteroids, and cytotoxic drugs. In our series, even though some cases experienced a complete remission, most had subsequent relapses and, despite a new cycle of plasma exchanges, renal function did not improve, and patients progressed to end-stage renal failure. The progression was delayed by 1 to 4 years. In the Japanese series, 60% of the treated patients had a complete remission of renal disease after 10 years. A German series showed that aggressive treatment including PE may delay the rate of progression in the majority of patients with severe crescentic HSP nephritis, but the treatment was unable to definitely prevent the progression to end-stage renal failure (102).

The analysis of uncontrolled studies with a combination of corticosteroids (e.g., either intravenous pulses or oral), immunosuppressive drugs (e.g., cyclophosphamide or azathioprine) sometimes in association with anticoagulation (e.g., warfarin or dipyridamole) in children with nephrotic range proteinuria, or major extracapillary proliferation on biopsy allows us to conclude that aggressive therapeutic regimens are effective in decreasing the rapidity of progression to chronic renal failure. However, these treatments should be started early during the course of the disease before the crescents become fibrotic. At this late stage, the treatments are ineffective.

In patients with heavy proteinuria, favorable results with decrease in proteinuria and improvement of histologic index of renal activity have been reported using intravenous Ig infusions (103,104). However, a rebound was noticed shortly after the therapeutic cycles, which somehow banished the positive results obtained (103). On the contrary, Ig infusion may be useful in cases with severe recurrent purpuric rash and mild urinary symptoms.

RELATIONSHIP BETWEEN HENOCH-SCHÖNLEIN PURPURA AND PRIMARY IMMUNOGLOBULIN A NEPHROPATHY

The main reason for which a relationship between HSP and IgA nephropathy has been suggested is that these two conditions are indistinguishable by renal histopathology. Furthermore, other features are in favor of an unifying concept. Occasional patients with IgA nephropathy have extrarenal symptoms. A few patients may present with IgA nephropathy and develop a purpuric rash months or years later. In the following years, some patients with HSP may develop episodes of macroscopic hematuria suggestive of IgA nephropathy, in the following years. The occurrence of both diseases in the same family is not uncommon. In a French national survey on 40 families with two or more members affected by primary IgAN, five had members presenting with complete HSP syndrome, confirming a possible genetic link between the two diseases (105). Most patients with HSP nephritis who undergo renal transplantation have a recurrence of IgA deposits in the graft in the absence of extrarenal symptoms, as do patients with IgA nephropathy. Last, a male preponderance is seen in both diseases, and the high prevalence of both conditions is observed in the same geographic areas (e.g., Europe, Asia).

HSP and primary IgAN share similar disturbances in the IgA system. Both diseases present with high levels of serum IgA, as well as high levels of circulating IgA-ICs, IgA1-IC, and IgA-fibronectin aggregates, as discussed above, even though the levels in acute phases of HSP are generally higher than in primary IgAN (20,22). Both diseases have aberrantly glycosylated IgA in circulation.

REFERENCES

1. Heberden W. *Commentaria di morboriana: historia and curatione.* London: Payne, 1801.
2. Schönlein JL. *Allgemeine und specielle pathologie und therapie.* Wurtzberg, Germany: Etlinger, 1832.
3. Henoch, EH. Verhandlungen arztlicher gesellschaffen. *Berliner Klin Wochenschr* 1868;5:517–530.
4. Meadow SR, Glasgow EF, White RHR. Schoenlein-Henoch nephritis. *QJM* 1972;41:241–258.
5. Mills JA, Michel BA, Bloch DA, et al. The American College of Rheumatology 1990 criteria for the classification of Henoch-Schoenlein purpura. *Arthritis Rheum* 1990;33:1114–1121.
6. Jennette JC, Falk RJ, Andrassy K, et al. Nomenclature of systemic vasculitides. Proposal of an International Consensus Conference. *Arthritis Rheum* 1994;2:187–192.
7. Kerr MA. The structure and function of human IgA. *Biochem J* 1990;271:285–296.
8. Mestecky J, McGhee JR. Immunoglobulin A (IgA): molecular and cellular interactions involved in IgA biosynthesis and immune response. *Adv Immunol* 1987;40:153–168.
9. Emancipator SN. Immunoregulatory factors in the pathogenesis of IgA nephropathy. *Kidney Int* 1990;38:1216–1229.
10. Tomino Y, Sakai H, Endoh M, et al. Cross-reactivity of eluted antibodies from renal tissues of patients with Henoch-Schoenlein nephritis and IgA nephropathy. *Am J Nephrol* 1983;3:218–223.
11. Rifai A, Chen A, Imai H. Complement activation in experimental IgA nephropathy: an antigen-mediated process. *Kidney Int* 1987;32:838–844.
12. Montinaro V, Esparga AR, Cavallo T, et al. Antigen as mediator of glomerular injury in experimental IgA nephropathy. *Lab Invest* 1991;64:508–519.
13. Ackroyd JF. Allergic purpura, including purpura due to food, drugs and infections. *Am J Med* 1953;14:605–614.
14. Miescher PA, Reymond A, Ritter O. Le rôle de l'allergie bactérienne dans la pathogénèse de certaines vasculites. *Schweiw Med Wochensch* 1956;86:799–808.
15. Coppo R. The pathogenetical potential of environmental antigens in IgA nephropathy. *Am J Kidney Dis* 1988;5:420–424.
16. Coppo R, Amore A, Roccatello D. Dietary antigens and primary immunoglobulin A nephropathy. *J Am Soc Nephrol* 1992;2:S173–S180.
17. Coppo R, Amore A, Roccatello D, et al. IgA antibodies to dietary antigens and lectin-binding IgA in sera from Italian, Australian and Japanese IgA nephropathy patients. *Am J Kidney Dis* 1991;17:468–487.
18. Kauffmann RH, Herrmann WA, Meyer CD, et al. Circulating immune complexes in Henoch-Schoenlein purpura. A longitudinal study of their relationship to disease activity and vascular deposition of IgA. *Am J Med* 1980;69:859–866.
19. Coppo R, Basolo B, Martina G, et al. Circulating immune complexes containing IgA, IgG and IgM in patients with primary IgA nephropathy and with Henoch-Schoenlein nephritis. Correlation with clinical and histologic signs of activity. *Clin Nephrol* 1982;18:230–239.
20. Coppo R, Basolo B, Piccoli G, et al. IgA1 and IgA2 immune complexes in primary IgA nephropathy and Henoch-Schoenlein nephritis. *Clin Exp Immunol* 1984;57:583–590.
21. Davin JC, Malaise M, Foidart J, et al. Anti-alpha-galactosyl antibodies and immune complexes in children with Henoch-Schönlein purpura or IgA nephropathy. *Kidney Int* 1987;31:1132–1139.
22. Jennette JC, Wieslander J, Tuttle R, et al. Serum IgA-fibronectin aggregates in patients with IgA nephropathy and Henoch-Schoenlein purpura: diagnostic value and pathogenic implications. The Glomerular Disease Collaborative Network. *Am J Kidney Dis* 1991;18:466–471.
23. Coppo R, Amore A, Gianoglio B, et al. Serum IgA and macromolecular IgA reacting with mesangial matrix components. *Contr Nephrol* 1993;104:162–171.
24. Fornasieri A, Pinerolo C, Bernasconi P, et al. Anti-mesangial and anti-endothelial cell antibodies in IgA mesangial nephropathy. *Clin Nephrol* 1995;44:71–79.
25. Saulsbury FT. Alteration in the O-linked glycosylation of IgA1 in children with Henoch-Schönlein purpura. *J Rheumatol* 1997;24:2246–2249.
26. Coppo R, Cirina P, Amore A, et al. Properties of circulating IgA molecules in Henoch-Schoenlein purpura nephritis with focus on neutrophil cytoplasmic antigen IgA binding (IgA-ANCA): new insight into a debated issue. *Nephrol Dial Transplant* 1997;12:2269–2276.
27. Allen AC, Willis FR, Beattie TJ, et al. Abnormal IgA glycosylation in Henoch-Schönlein purpura restricted to patients with clinical nephritis. *Nephrol Dial Transplant* 1998;13:930–934.
28. Allen AC, Topham PS, Harper SJ, et al. Leucocyte beta 1,3 galactosyltransferase activity in IgA nephropathy. *Nephrol Dial Transplant* 1997;12:701–706.

29. Chintalacharuvu SR, Emancipator SN. The glycosylation of IgA produced by murine B cells is altered by Th2 cytokines. *J Immunol* 1997;159:2327–2333.
30. Kokubo T, Hiki Y, Iwase H, et al. Protective role of IgA1 glycans against IgA1 self aggregation and adhesion to extracellular matrix proteins. *J Am Soc Nephrol* 1998;9:2048–2054.
31. Roccatello D, Picciotto G, Torchio M, et al. Removal systems of immunoglobulin A and immunoglobulin A containing complexes in IgA nephropathy and cirrhosis patients. The role of asialoglycoprotein receptors. *Lab Invest* 1993;69:714–723.
32. Peruzzi L, Amore A, Cirina P, et al. Integrin expression and IgA nephropathy: in vitro modulation by IgA with altered glycosylation and macromolecular IgA. *Kidney Int* 2000;58:2331–2340.
33. Amore A, Cirina P, Conti G, et al. Glycosylation of circulating IgA in patients with IgA nephropathy modulates proliferation and apoptosis of mesangial cells. *J Am Soc Nephrol* 2001;12:1862–1871.
34. Amore A, Conti G, Cirina P, et al. Aberrantly glycosylated IgA molecules downregulate the synthesis and secretion of vascular endothelial growth factor in human mesangial cells. *Am J Kidney Dis* 2000;36:1242–1252.
35. Gesualdo L, Di Paolo S, Milani S, et al. Expression of platelet-derived growth factor receptors in normal and diseased human kidneys. An immunochemistry and in situ hybridization study. *J Clin Invest* 1994;94:50–58.
36. Grandaliano G, Gesualdo L, Ranieri E, et al. Monocyte chemoattractant peptide-1 expression in acute and chronic human nephritides: a pathogenetical role in interstitial monocyte recruitment. *J Am Soc Nephrol* 1996;7:906–913.
37. Nikolova EB, Tomana M, Russell MW. The role of the carbohydrate chains in complement (C3) fixation by solid-phase-bound human IgA. *Immunol* 1994;82:321–327.
38. Ronda N, Esnault VL, Layward L, et al. Antineutrophil cytoplasm antibodies (ANCA) of IgA isotype in adult Henoch-Schönlein purpura. *Clin Exp Immunol* 1994;95:49–55.
39. Sinico RA, Tadros M, Radice A, et al. Lack of IgA antineutrophil cytoplasmic antibodies in Henoch-Schönlein purpura and IgA nephropathy. *Clin Immunol Immunopathol* 1994;73:19–26.
40. Namgoong MK, Lim B, Kim JS. Eosinophil cationic protein in Henoch-Schönlein purpura and in IgA nephropathy. *Pediatr Nephrol* 1997;11:703–706.
41. Ranieri E, Gesualdo L, Petrarulo F, et al. Urinary IL6/EGF ratio: a useful prognostic marker for the progression of renal damage in IgA nephropathy. *Kidney Int* 1996;50:1990–2001.
42. Smith GC, Davidson JF, Hughes DA, et al. Complement activation in Henoch-Schoenlein purpura. *Pediatr Nephrol* 1997;11:477–480.
43. Casanueva B, Rodriguez-Valverde V, Farinas MC, et al. Autologous mixed lymphocyte reaction and T-cell suppressor activity in patients with Henoch-Schönlein purpura and IgA nephritis. *Nephron* 1990;54:224–228.
44. Davin JC, Berge IJ, Weening JJ. What is the difference between IgA nephropathy and Henoch-Schönlein purpura nephritis? *Kidney Int* 2001;59:823–834.
45. Davin JC, Vandenbroeck MC, Foidart JB, et al. Sequential measurements of the reticulo-endothelial system function in Henoch-Schoenlein disease in childhood. Correlation with various immunological parameters. *Acta Pediatr Scand* 1985;74:201–206.
46. Davin JC, Pierard G, Dechenne C, et al. Possible pathogenetic role of IgE in Henoch-Schoenlein purpura. *Pediatr Nephrol* 1994;8:169–171.
47. Amoroso A, Berrino M, Canale L, et al. Immunogenetics of Henoch-Schoenlein disease. *Eur J Immunogenetics* 1997;2:323–333.
48. Amoli MM, Thomson W, Hajeer AH, et al. HLA-DRB1*01 association with Henoch-Schönlein purpura in patients from Northwest Spain. *J Rheumatol* 2001;28:1266–1270.
49. Jin DK, Kohsaka T, Koo JW, et al. Complement 4 locus II gene deletion and DQA1*0301 gene: genetic risk factors for IgA nephropathy and Henoch-Schoenlein nephritis. *Nephron* 1996;73:390–395.
50. Mc Lean RH, Wyatt RJ, Julian BA. Complement phenotypes in glomerulonephritides: increased frequency of homozygous null C4 phenotypes in IgA nephropathy and Henoch-Schoenlein purpura. *Kidney Int* 1984;26:855–860.
51. Amoroso A, Danek G, Vatta S, et al. Polymorphism in angiotensin-converting enzyme gene and severity of renal disease in Henoch-Schoenlein patients. *Nephrol Dial Transplant* 1998;13:3184–3188.
52. Amoli MM, Mattey DL, Calvino MC, et al. Polymorphism at codon 469 of the intercellular adhesion molecule-1 locus is associated with protection against severe gastrointestinal complications in Henoch-Schönlein purpura. *J Rheumatol* 2001;28:1014–1018.
53. Nielsen HE. Epidemiology of Schoenlein-Henoch purpura. *Acta Paediatr Scand* 1988;77:125–131.
54. Cameron J. Henoch-Schoenlein purpura: clinical presentation. *Contr Nephrol* 1984;40:246–256.
55. Habib R, Cameron JS. Schoenlein-Henoch purpura. In: Bacon PA, Hadler MN, eds. *The kidney: rheumatic disease.* London, Butterworth Scientific, 1982.
56. Lévy, Broyer M, Arsan A. Anaphylactoid purpura nephritis in childhood natural history and immunopathology. In: Hamburger J, Crosnier J, Maxwell MH, eds. *Advances in nephrology from the Necker Hospital.* Chicago: Year Book, 1976:183–228.
57. Rieu P, Noel LH. Henoch-Schoenlein nephritis in children and adults. *Ann Med Int* 1999;150:151–158.
58. Coppo R, Amore A, Gianoglio B. Clinical features of Henoch-Schoenlein purpura. *Ann Med Int* 1999;150:143–150.
59. Habib R, Levy M. Les néphropathies du purpura rhumatoide chez l'enfant. Etude clinique et anatomique de 60 observations. *Arch Fr Ped* 1972;29:305–324.
60. Emancipator SN. IgA nephropathy and Henoch-Schönlein purpura. In: Jennette JC, Olson JL, Schwartz MM, et al., eds. *Heptinstall's pathology of the kidney.* Philadelphia: Lippincott–Raven, 1998.
61. Farley TA, Gillespies S, Rasoulpour M, et al. Epidemiology of a cluster of Henoch-Schoenlein purpura. *Am J Dis Child* 1989;143:798–803.
62. Coppo R, Mazzucco G, Cagnoli L, for the Italian Group of Renal Immunopathology. Long-term prognosis of Henoch-Schoenlein nephritis in adults and in children. *Nephrol Dial Transplant* 1997;12:2277–2283.

63. Yoshikawa N. Henoch-Schoenlein purpura. In: Neilson EG, Couser WG. *Immunologic renal diseases.* Philadelphia: Lippincott–Raven, 1997:1119–1131.
64. Kaku Y, Nohara K, Honda S. Renal involvement in Henoch-Schoenlein purpura: a multivariate analysis of prognostic factors. *Kidney Int* 1998;53:1755–1759.
65. Coppo R, Gianoglio B, Porcellini MG, et al. Frequency of renal diseases and clinical indications for renal biopsy in children (report of the Italian National Registry of Renal Biopsies in Children). *Nephrol Dial Transplant* 1998;13: 293–297.
66. Farine M, Poucell S, Geary DL, et al. Prognostic significance of urinary findings and renal biopsies in children with Henoch-Schoenlein nephritis. *Clin Paediatrics* 1986;25:257–259.
67. Yoshikawa N, White RH, Cameron AH. Prognostic significance of the glomerular changes in Henoch-Schönlein nephritis. *Clin Nephrol* 1981;5:223–229.
68. Goldstein AR, White RH, Akuse R, et al. Long-term follow-up of childhood Henoch-Schönlein nephritis. *Lancet* 1992;339:280–282.
69. Blanco R, Martinez-Taboada VM, Rodriguez-Valverde V, et al. Henoch-Schoenlein purpura in adulthood and childhood: two different expressions of the same syndrome. *Arthritis Rheum* 1997;40:859–864.
70. Kher KK, Sheth KJ, Makker SP. Stenosing ureteritis in Henoch-Schoenlein purpura. *J Urol* 1983;129:1040–1041.
71. Bruce RG, Bishof NA, Jackson EC, et al. Bilateral ureteral obstruction associated with Henoch-Schoenlein purpura. *Pediatr Nephrol* 1997;11:347–349.
72. Michel BA, Hunder GG, Bloch DA, et al. Hypersensitivity vasculitis and Henoch-Schoenlein purpura: a comparison between the two disorders. *J Rheumatol* 1992;19:721–728.
73. Saulsbury FT. IgA rheumatoid factor in Henoch-Schoenlein purpura. *J Pediatrics* 1986;108:71–76.
74. De Mattia D, Penza R, Giordano P, et al. Von Willebrand factor XIII in children with Henoch-Schoenlein purpura. *Pediatr Nephrol* 1995;9:603–605.
75. Niaudet P, Levy M, Broyer M, et al. Clinicopathologic correlations in severe forms of Henoch-Schoenlein purpura nephritis based on repeat biopsies. *Contr Nephrol* 1984;40:250–254.
76. Droz D. La biopsie rénale dans les glomérulopathies à dépots mésangiaux d'IgA. In: Droz D, Lantz B, eds. *Maladie de Berger et purpura rhumatoide. Biopsie rénale.* Paris: INSERM, 1955:151–166.
77. Haar J, Thomsen K, Spaarrevohn S. Renal involvement in Henoch-Schoenlein purpura. *BMJ* 1974;2:405–406.
78. Niaudet P, Lenoir GD, Habib R. *La néphropathie du purpura rhumatoide chez l'enfant: journee Parisienne de pediatrie.* Paris: Flammarion Médecine-Sciences, 1986:145–150.
79. Koskimies O, Rapola J, Savilahti E, et al. Renal involvement in Schoenlein-Henoch purpura. *Acta Pediatr Scand* 1974;63: 357–363.
80. Stewart M, Savage JM, McCord D. Long term renal prognosis of Henoch-Schönlein purpura in an unselected childhood population. *Eur J Paediatr* 1988;147:113–115.
81. Hotta O, Taguma Y, Yoshizawa N, et al. Long-term effects of intensive therapy combined with tonsillectomy in patients with IgA nephropathy. *Acta Otolaryngol Suppl* 1996;523:165–168.
82. Meulders Q, Pirson Y, Cosyns JP, et al. Course of Henoch-Schoenlein nephritis after renal transplantation: report on ten patients and review of the literature. *Transplantation* 1994;58:1179–1186.
83. Kessler M, Hiesse C, Hestin D, et al. Recurrence of immunoglobulin A nephropathy after renal transplantation in the cyclosporine era. *Am J Kid Dis* 1996;28:99–104.
84. Cameron JS. Recurrent diseases in renal allografts. *Kidney Int Suppl* 1993;43:S91–S94.
85. Ramos EL. Recurrent diseases in the renal allograft. *J Am Soc Nephrol* 1991;2:109–121.
86. Muller T, Sikora P, Offner G, et al. Recurrence of renal disease after kidney transplantation in children: 24 years of experience in a single center. *Clin Nephrol* 1998;49:272–274.
87. Heldrich FJ, Minkin S, Gatdula CL. Intravenous immunoglobulin in Henoch-Schoenlein purpura: a case study. *Medical J* 1993;42:577–579.
88. Buchanec J, Galanda V, Belakova S, et al. Incidence of renal complications in Schoenlein-Henoch purpura syndrome in dependence on an early administration of steroids. *Int J Urol Nephrol* 1988;20:409–412.
89. Saulsbury FT. Corticosteroid therapy does not prevent nephritis in Henoch-Schoenlein purpura. *Pediatr Nephrol* 1993;7:69–71.
90. Mollica F, Li Volti S, Garozzo R, et al. Effectiveness of early prednisone treatment in preventing the development of nephropathy in anaphylactoid purpura. *Eur J Paediatr* 1992;151:140–144.
91. Counahan R, Winterborn MH, White RH, et al. Prognosis of Henoch-Schoenlein purpura nephritis in children *BMJ* 1977;2:11–14.
92. Foster BJ, Bernard C, Drummond KN, et al. Effective therapy for Henoch-Schoenlein purpura nephritis with prednisone and azathioprine: a clinical and histopathologic study. *J Paediatrics* 2000;36:370–375.
93. Wyatt RJ, Hogg RJ. Evidence-based assessment of treatment options for children with IgA nephropathies. *Pediatr Nephrol* 2001;16:156–167.
94. Sanai A, Kudoh F. Effects of tonsillectomy in children with IgA nephropathy, purpura nephritis, or other chronic glomerulonephritides. *Acta Otolaryngol Suppl* 1996;523:172–174.
95. Oner A, Tinaztepe K, Erdogan O. The effect of triple therapy on rapidly progressive type of Henoch-Schoenlein purpura nephritis. *Pediatr Nephrol* 1955;9:6–10.
96. Flynn JT, Smoyer WE, Bunchman TE, et al. Treatment of Henoch-Schoenlein purpura glomerulonephritis in children with high-dose corticosteroids plus oral cyclophosphamide. *Am J Nephrol* 2001;21:128–133.
97. Niaudet P, Habib R. Methylprednisone pulse therapy in the treatment of severe forms of Schoenlein-Henoch purpura nephritis. *Pediatr Nephrol* 1998;12:238–243.
98. Iijima K, Ito-Kariya S, Nakamura H, et al. Multiple combined therapy for severe Henoch-Schoenlein nephritis in children. *Pediatr Nephrol* 1998;12:244–248.
99. Bergstein J, Leiser J, Andreoli SP. Response of crescentic Henoch-Schoenlein purpura nephritis to corticosteroid and azathioprine therapy. *Clin Nephrol* 1998;49:9–14.
100. Coppo R, Basolo B, Amore A, et al. Plasma exchange in primary IgA nephropathy and Henoch-Schoenlein syndrome nephritis. *Plasma Ther Trans Tech* 1985;6:705–723.

101. Hattori M, Ito K, Konomoto T, et al. Plasmapheresis as the sole therapy for rapidly progressive Henoch-Schoenlein purpura nephritis in children. *Am J Kidney Dis* 1999;33:427–433.
102. Scharer K, Krmar R, Querfeld U, et al. Clinical outcome of Schoenlein-Henoch purpura nephritis in children. *Pediatr Nephrol* 1999;13:816–823.
103. Rostoker G, Desvaux-Belghiti D, Pilatte Y, et al. High dose immunoglobulin therapy for severe IgA nephropathy and Henoch-Schoenlein purpura. *Ann Intern Med* 1994;120 476–484.
104. Kasuda A, Migita K, Tsuboi M, et al. Successful treatment of adult-onset Henoch-Schoenlein purpura nephritis with high-dose immunoglobulins. *Intern Med* 1999;38:376–379.
105. Lévy M. Familial cases of Berger's disease and anaphylactoid purpura. *Kidney Int* 2001;60:1611–1612.
106. Yoshikawa N, Ito H, Yoshiya K, et al. Henoch-Schoenlein nephritis and IgA nephropathy in children: a comparison of clinical course. *Clin Nephrol* 1987;27:233–237.

46

SYSTEMIC LUPUS ERYTHEMATOSUS

PATRICK NIAUDET
RÉMI SALOMON

Systemic lupus erythematosus (SLE) is a chronic inflammatory disease characterized by highly diverse clinical manifestations and the presence in the serum of antibodies reacting with different cell nuclei components. The skin, joints, lungs, heart, kidneys, nervous system, and other organs are involved. The role of autoantibodies in the pathogenesis of the disease is subject to debate. Certain autoantibodies, such as those reacting with cell surface determinants or circulating proteins, are directly responsible for specific clinical manifestations of the disease. The clinical course of the disease is characterized by flares, periods of chronic disease, and periods of remissions.

The American Association of Rheumatology developed diagnostic criteria of SLE (1,2) to establish with certainty the diagnosis of SLE and to distinguish it from other rheumatic diseases (Table 46.1). When four of these criteria are present, the sensitivity of the diagnosis of SLE is 95% and the specificity is 96%. Some patients with the disease may not satisfy the criteria initially but may develop other manifestations later and then develop the full criteria for the diagnosis of SLE. For example, some patients may have isolated nephritis, such as membranous nephropathy, without serologic evidence of SLE at first.

The prevalence of SLE is approximately 40 per 100,000 in Europe and North America (3). SLE is three times more frequent in blacks than in whites but is exceptional in blacks from Africa (4,5). In a recent survey of pediatric lupus in the United Kingdom, the relative risk was 6.7 in Asian populations and 6.1 in black populations compared with the white population (6). The frequency of the principal risk factors for SLE does not differ in blacks compared to whites (7). In more than 80% of cases, SLE affects females after puberty. The female to male ratio increases from 2:1 in prepubertal children to 4.5:1.0 in adolescents and 8:1 in adults (8). In children, most cases of lupus occur after age 5, with a peak incidence in late childhood and adolescence (9). Twenty percent of SLE cases begin in childhood.

The presentation of the disease in children varies both in terms of the gravity of symptoms and the diversity of clinical manifestations. However, the disease is often more acute and severe, affecting multiple organs in children compared to adults (10–13). In addition to the organ damage, SLE has a major detrimental impact on growth and psychological development. It is important to promote a multidisciplinary approach to SLE to assure better individual treatment of patients.

PATHOGENESIS

The etiology of the SLE remains unknown, despite the progress that has been made during the recent years in understanding the pathogenic mechanisms of the disease. SLE is characterized by the development of autoantibodies directed against a variety of self-components, and, contrary to other autoimmune diseases, there are no stigma of organ-specific autoimmunity.

Genetic Factors

The evidence for a genetic susceptibility to SLE in humans is based on familial aggregation. The prevalence of SLE is estimated to be 2.6 to 3.5% in first-degree relatives of SLE probands compared with 0.3 to 0.4% in relatives of matched controls. Moreover, an increase in concordance rate is observed in monozygotic twins (24 to 56%) compared to dizygotic twins (2 to 5%). The risk of developing the disease in siblings of SLE patients is 10 to 40 times higher than that in the general population. A French analysis of 125 families that included at least two individuals with SLE demonstrated a nonmendelian inheritance, suggesting a complex multifactorial inheritance pattern with several genes interacting together in a single individual (14). Population-based studies have shown associations of SLE with numerous polymorphic alleles of several major histocompatibility complex class II genes and of various complement components (C1q, C2, C4). Further association with Fcγ on chromosome 1q23, mannose binding ligand, interleukin-6 and -10, and tumor necrosis factor has been demonstrated. Genetic linkage studies have identified 60 susceptibility loci with varying degrees

TABLE 46.1. THE 1982 REVISED AMERICAN ASSOCIATION OF RHEUMATOLOGY CRITERIA FOR CLASSIFICATION OF SYSTEMIC LUPUS ERYTHEMATOSUS

Malar rash
Discoid rash
Photosensitivity
Oral ulcers
Arthritis
Serositis (pleuritis or pericarditis)
Proteinuria >0.5 g/d or red blood cell casts
Psychosis or seizures
Hemolytic anemia or leukopenia (<4000/mm^3) or lymphopenia (<1500/mm^3) or thrombopenia (<100,000/mm^3)
Antinuclear antibodies
Anti–double-stranded DNA antibodies or anti-Sm antibodies or false-positive TPI/VDRL or positive lupus erythematosus cell test

TPI, *Treponema pallidum* immobilization.

of evidence for linkage in humans. Seven of these met or exceeded the threshold for significant linkage at 1q22-23, 1q41, 2q37, 4p16, 6p21-11, 16q13, and 17p13. An interaction between 16q12 and 1q23 loci has been demonstrated in a cohort of 115 multiethnic families. This interaction is more pronounced in nonwhites (15). Recently, a polymorphism in a gene encoding an immunoreceptor named *programmed cell death 1* (PD-1) has been associated with development of lupus in Europeans and Mexicans (16). Because lupus is a multifactorial disease with multigenic inheritance, it is highly likely that many more polymorphisms with subtle functional impact will be described. Studies in various mouse models suggest that lupus may be mediated by a multitude of genetic abnormalities that impact on specific checkpoints, starting with a loss of immunologic tolerance to nuclear antigens and progressing to a pathogenic autoimmunity and to organ targeting. Several studies suggest that increased liberation or disturbed clearance of nuclear DNA-protein complexes after cell death may initiate the disease. DNAse1-deficient mice, generated by gene targeting, exhibit a phenotype very similar to classic human SLE (17). Moreover, mutations responsible for a loss of function of this enzyme have been found in patients with SLE (18). Table 46.2 shows several gene variants that have been associated with SLE in humans and in mice (16–27).

Environmental and Infectious Factors

Based on twin concordance studies, the induction of SLE requires more than genetic factors. Environmental, hormonal, toxic, and infectious factors have been proposed. The high degree of homology between a small peptide sequence of the Epstein-Barr virus (EBV) nuclear antigen-2 and the SmD1 ribonucleoprotein, a target of autoantibodies in SLE patients, suggests that antibodies elicited by the viral antigen may cross-react with SmD1. EBV-specific immune responses may play a role in the production of SmD1 autoantibodies in SLE patients (28). Seroconversion against EBV was observed in 99% of children with SLE as compared to only 70% of their controls. Thus, EBV may be a causative factor in SLE (29). Photosensitivity is a common feature of SLE, and the disease is aggravated by sun exposure in 40 to 70% of patients. Ultraviolet light induces apoptosis of keratinocytes, which may, in turn, develop

TABLE 46.2. MOUSE AND HUMAN GENES THAT CAUSE LUPUS

Categories	Mouse with null mutation	Patients with systemic lupus erythematosus (SLE)	References
Regulatory machinery			
Activation threshold of lymphocytes			
PD-1	Autoimmune cardiomyopathy	A polymorphism in intron 1 is more frequent in patients than in control (12 vs. 5%)	16,19
Lyn	Autoreactive antibodies and severe glomerulonephritis	Lyn is significantly decreased in B cells at the messenger RNA and protein levels	20,21
Deletion of autoreactive T cells			
P21	Anti–double-stranded DNA, glomerulonephritis	Reduced expression of p21 in lymphocytes	22,23
Scavenger machinery			
C1q	High autoantibody titers, 25% had glomerulonephritis with great numbers of glomerular apoptotic bodies	C1q deficiency is strongly associated with SLE	24,25
DNAse1	Antinuclear autoimmunity and glomerulonephritis	Heterozygous nonsense mutation and decreased DNAse1 activity in serum of patients	17,18
Serum amyloid P (SAP)	Antinuclear autoimmunity and severe glomerulonephritis	Low levels of SAP-DNA complexes in serum of patients	26,27

small surface blebs containing lupus autoantigens such as the Ro particle (30). Similarly, drugs (e.g., chlorpromazine) (31) and environmental toxins (e.g., silica dust) are capable of inducing apoptosis.

Hormonal Factors

The female predominance in SLE is particularly strong during childbearing ages, suggesting that hormonal differences may contribute to the increased risk of the disease (32,33). Reduced androgen levels and increased estradiol and prolactin levels have been reported in SLE patients. Moreover, whereas administration of androgens leads to improvement, estrogen and prolactin exacerbate disease severity. On the other hand, a population-based study of 240 female SLE patients found little evidence that estrogen- or prolactin-related exposures were associated with an increased risk of lupus (34).

Role of T and B Lymphocytes

In SLE, autoantibodies, immune complexes, and autoreactive T cells may cause tissue damage. The loss of self-tolerance in the periphery appears to be critical in the pathogenesis of SLE (35). Self-antigen can trigger autoimmunity by several ways. The level of autoantigens may be increased by an impaired clearance of immune complexes or of apoptotic cells. Defects in the complement system or lymphocyte Fc receptor alterations may enhance the level of available autoantigen (36–38). Perturbations of the cytokine network could activate antigen-presenting cells and thereby reduce the signaling threshold to a given concentration of autoantigen in self-reactive peripheral T or B cells (39). Alterations in these different regulatory pathways have been described in lupus-prone natural and knockout mouse models (Table 46.2). Moreover, polymorphisms or mutations of several genes implicated in these processes have been reported in lupus patients.

The production of autoantibodies against components of the cell nucleus is a hallmark of SLE. The most prominent of these autoantibodies is directed against double-stranded (ds) DNA and histones. There is growing evidence that the nucleosome, the fundamental unit of chromatin, composed of histones and dsDNA, is a major autoantigen that drives a T-cell–dependent autoimmune response. The implication of the nucleosome in the pathogenesis of SLE seems to be related closely to an abnormal regulation of apoptosis and an impaired clearance of apoptotic products. High levels of these products and particularly of nucleosomes themselves have been observed in lupus patients in comparison to controls (40).

Dendritic cells are key regulators of the immune system. These professional antigen-presenting cells induce the activation of naïve T cells and stimulate growth and proliferation of B cells. The serum of patients induces monocytes to differentiate into dendritic cells able to capture dying allogeneic cells and present their antigens to autologous $CD4^+$ T cells leading to proliferation. Furthermore, this capacity to induce dendritic cell differentiation is correlated with disease activity (41), and the capacity is abolished by blocking interferon-gamma, suggesting that this cytokine is the major mediator of monocyte to dendritic cell differentiation. One scenario proposes that dendritic cells might capture apoptotic cells and nucleosomes present in the blood of SLE patients. Subsequent presentation of autoantigens by these dendritic cells to $CD4^+$ T cells could initiate the expansion of autoreactive T cells, followed by differentiation of autoantibody-producing B cells.

Complement Deficiency

Activation of the complement system is implicated in the defense against microbes and in the adaptive immune response and inflammation. The complement system plays a paradoxic role in the development and expression of SLE. While the activation of complement is involved in tissue damage, inherited deficiencies of components of the classic pathway are strongly associated with the development of SLE. Lupus develops in many patients with complete deficiencies in C1q (90%) and C4 (75%), suggesting that these molecules have a protective role against the development of the disease (42). The protective role of C1q has been confirmed by the observation of severe lupus nephritis in C1q-deficient mice.

CLINICAL MANIFESTATIONS

Lupus is often acute in onset and includes general symptoms of fever and fatigue associated with cutaneous and articular symptoms (11,43). SLE may also begin with an isolated symptom such as a hemolytic anemia, a nephritic syndrome with hematuria, chorea, or pericarditis. The performance of systematic serologic tests permits the linkage of these manifestations to SLE (44).

General symptoms, particularly weight loss, anorexia, and asthenia, are virtually constant in SLE. Episodic fever is frequent during acute phase of the disease or during infection. Pulmonary or urinary tract infections are frequent during the course of SLE. Opportunistic infections may be life threatening. A number of factors may favor a relapse of the disease, including exposure to ultraviolet light (45), infection (46), stress (47), surgery, or pregnancy.

Joints and Muscles

Arthralgia is the most common manifestation of SLE, observed in 80% of cases during the evolution of the disease (48). Both large and small articulations, especially of the hands, are affected, causing moderate pain and articular swelling. The damage of periarticular tissues is often more pronounced than synovial damage, especially in the form of tendinitis. Arthritis is very rarely deforming, and synovial fluid contains relatively few cells. Myalgia is less frequent. Avascular osteonecrosis, which often affects femoral heads, may occur in the absence of treatment with corticosteroids.

Skin

The most classic skin lesion of SLE is the butterfly rash over the cheeks and nose, which is present in one-third of cases. The rash often appears after sun exposure. Maculopapular eruptions on the upper portion of the trunk as well as any areas exposed to light are the most common. Papular lesions and squamous lesions on the trunk, face, and palms of the hands can be observed in the less severe cutaneous forms of the disease, often linked to the presence of anti-Ro antibodies. Raynaud's phenomena of the extremities causes painful white marble-like lesions, leg ulcers, and periungual or finger-pad erythema. Urticarial eruptions and pigmentation anomalies are sometimes observed. Cutaneous photosensitivity is noted, especially in white patients. Mucosal lesions, particularly in the form of oral ulcerations, are common. Alopecia is observed in some children, especially those with active forms of the disease.

Lungs

Pulmonary involvement occurs in more than 75% of children. Pleuritis, observed in 40% of children, is often asymptomatic or may be present as thoracic pain. The pleural fluid is an exudate, containing a large number of neutrophils and lymphocytes. The levels of C3 and C4 in the fluid are diminished, and the level of antinuclear antibodies (ANA) is elevated. Anomalies in diaphragmatic function have been reported and can be responsible for dyspnea. Pulmonary damage may be manifested as an acute pneumonitis with thoracic pain, dyspnea, and fever. Poorly defined opacities can be observed on x-ray. Histologically, these lesions consist of infiltrates of lymphocytes and plasma cells. Chronic fibrosing alveolitis has been described. Pulmonary arterial hypertension is a rare but a severe problem that may be secondary to repeated pulmonary embolism (49). Acute pulmonary hemorrhage during the acute phase of the disease or during infections may be life threatening.

Heart

Pericarditis is frequent in SLE and is often diagnosed on echocardiography. Myocarditis with congestive heart failure is rare. Endocarditis of Liebman-Sachs, which often affects the mitral valve and is associated with antiphospholipid (APL) antibodies, is rare (50).

Nervous System

Neuropsychiatric symptoms are present in 30 to 45% of children with SLE. (51,52). These symptoms can either be a direct result of SLE or secondary to arterial hypertension, renal insufficiency, infectious complication, hemostasis abnormalities, or various treatments, particularly corticosteroids (53). Mood disorders or behavior disturbances are often difficult to interpret in this chronic disease. Headache is the most frequent neurologic manifestation of SLE and is often accompanied by localized or generalized seizures. Symptoms suggestive of a cerebral tumor have been described. Chorea is frequent in children, sometimes in association with APL antibodies. Cranial nerve palsies have been described, particularly ptoses and hemiparesis. Psychiatric symptoms consist of difficulties with attention or memory, disorientation, behavioral problems, depression, or psychotic states with hallucinations and delirium (54,55). These symptoms can occur in an acute, transitory manner, during a flare of the disease, or may be more prolonged. They are often linked to ischemic cerebral vascular lesions that can be visualized by magnetic resonance imaging. Damage to the large arteries is rare. The role of antineuronal antibodies that are found in up to one-half of patients in the pathophysiology of these lesions is uncertain. Thrombotic phenomena secondary to the antiphospholipid antibodies may also play a role in the pathogenesis of neurologic manifestations (56). Behavioral problems and a decrease in academic achievement are often noted in children with SLE. These problems could be linked to the disease itself, to treatment with corticosteroids, or to the psychological response to a serious chronic illness. If these problems are secondary to SLE, the symptoms can respond favorably to an increase in corticosteroid doses.

Eye

Both the retina and the cornea can be affected by SLE. Keratoconjunctivitis sicca is the most common ocular manifestation. The retinal lesions consist of white, cotton-like exudative lesions of the optic nerve, papillary edema, or thrombosis of the central retinal artery.

Hematopoietic System

Hematologic manifestations are common in SLE. Inflammatory cervical or diffuse adenopathies occur in children with SLE. Anemia, observed in more than one-half of cases, is usually normochromic and normocytic, and its degree reflects the activity of the disease. Hemolytic anemia is present, and is often, in less than 10% of cases, accompanied by reticulocytosis, a positive Coombs' test, an increase in free bilirubin levels, and a decrease in haptoglobin levels. Aplastic anemia has been reported and responds to treatment with corticosteroids. Leukopenia, noted in more than 50% of cases, is partially responsible for an increased sensitivity to infections. Neutropenia may be linked to medullary suppression, hypersplenism, or antineutrophil antibodies. Lymphopenia affects both T and B lymphocytes. Thrombopenia, noted in 10 to 25% of cases, is accompanied by an increase in megakaryocytes in the marrow, indicating peripheral destruction of platelets. The acute, severe forms of thrombocytopenia are often observed during an acute phase of the disease and are responsive to treatment with corticosteroids, while more chronic forms are less symptomatic and less responsive.

Antiphospholipid Antibodies

APL antibodies may be directed against epitopes on oxidized phospholipids complexed with a glycoprotein, beta 2-glycoprotein I, or against the glycoprotein itself. The principal APL antibodies include anticardiolipin antibodies, beta 2-glycoprotein I antibodies, and the lupus anticoagulant. These APL antibodies are responsible for thrombosis *in vivo*. Conversely, they prolong phospholipid-dependent coagulation tests *in vitro* (57). Patients with SLE have a high incidence of APL antibodies with a consequent high risk of thrombosis.

A patient with the APL syndrome must meet at least one of the two clinical criteria (e.g., vascular thrombosis or complications of pregnancy) and at least one of two laboratory criteria (e.g., anticardiolipin antibodies or lupus anticoagulant antibodies). Patients with APL antibodies develop arterial or venous thromboses, thrombocytopenia, and the experience of repeated abortions. Primary APL syndrome occurs in patients without clinical evidence of another autoimmune disease, whereas secondary APL occurs in association with autoimmune or other diseases. The prevalence of APL antibodies is 1 to 5% among apparently healthy subjects in the young and increases with age. Among patients with SLE, the prevalence of APL is much higher, ranging from 12 to 30% for anticardiolipin antibodies and 15 to 34% for lupus anticoagulant antibodies (58). The APL syndrome develops in 50 to 70% of patients with SLE and APL antibodies within 20 years of the initial diagnosis.

Patients with primary and secondary APL syndrome have similar consequences of APL antibodies. The clinical hallmark of the APL syndrome is the presence of vascular thrombosis. Venous thromboses are more frequent than arterial thrombosis. Involvement of the small vessels, particularly in the kidneys, can mimic the hemolytic-uremic syndrome or thrombotic thrombocytopenic purpura. APL syndrome may also occur as a more chronic process, resulting in progressive loss of organ function (59).

In a cross-sectional cohort study in 59 consecutive SLE patients, 13 thrombotic events occurred in 10 of the 59 patients (17%). There was a direct relationship between the presence of a lupus anticoagulant and a thrombotic event (60). Similar findings were reported in a retrospective study in 36 children with lupus nephritis. No difference in the incidence of APL positivity was detected between the eight children who experienced thrombotic complications and the others (61).

Altered fibrinolysis, secondary to an increase of the inhibitor of the plasminogen activator and a decrease of protein S, has also been described in patients with SLE. Other more rare circulating anticoagulants have been observed. They are true *in vivo* anticoagulants, including antifactor VIII, antifactor XI, and antifactor XII.

Endocrine Manifestation

An autoimmune thyroiditis, including antithyroid and antimicrosome antibodies, may be responsible for symptoms of hypothyroidism and, less often, hyperthyroidism. A recent study found a high frequency of antithyroid antibodies in children with SLE, but most often without clinical manifestations. Diabetes mellitus is often secondary to high doses of corticosteroids, but it may be secondary to SLE with the presence of antiinsulin receptor antibodies. Hormonal contraception may promote lupus activity and thromboses, particularly in patients with APL antibodies. Therefore, it is important that appropriate contraception is adapted when necessary, and patients must be informed of the risks of future pregnancy, which would need specialized monitoring (62).

Gastrointestinal Manifestations

Gastrointestinal manifestations are often secondary to the side effects of treatments. Gastritis and peptic ulcers may be secondary to the use of nonsteroidal antiinflammatory agents or corticosteroids. Oral ulcers are frequent during the course of SLE, and patients may complain of dysphagia. Esophageal reflux or ulceration may occur. Abdominal pain is a frequent complaint in patients with SLE, and it may be related to serositis, peritonitis, intestinal vasculitis, intraabdominal thrombosis, small intestinal bacterial overgrowth, or pancreatitis (63). Vascular lesions can cause intestinal ischemia or perforations. Clinical manifestations linked to these gastrointestinal lesions can be masked by corticosteroids. Pancreatitis may be directly related to SLE or secondary to corticosteroid therapy.

Hepatomegaly is frequent but rarely accompanied by significant liver dysfunction. The presence of liver abnormalities with ANA is more likely to be due to chronic active hepatitis, also called *lupoid hepatitis*, than to SLE.

RENAL DISEASE IN SYSTEMIC LUPUS ERYTHEMATOSUS

Pathogenesis of Lupus Nephritis

Genetic or acquired susceptibility factors are probably associated with the onset of renal disease. Numerous mouse models have improved our understanding of the pathogenesis of lupus nephritis.

Nucleosome plays a central role in the pathogenesis of SLE. There is increasing evidence that increased apoptosis and impaired clearance of apoptotic cells facilitate the emergence of anti-DNA antibodies and immune complexes. Nucleosomes are also important for triggering tissue lesions, including glomerular lesions. There are at least two mechanisms that explain how autoantibodies mediate tissue damage: (a) deposition of preformed immune complexes in the kidney or *in situ* formation of these complexes via the interaction between nucleosome already deposited in the glomerulus and anti-dsDNA or (b) cross-reactivity of antibodies with glomerular basement membrane components. α-Actinin has recently been identified as a cross-reactive target bound by nephritogenic anti-dsDNA in a lupus mouse model (64). α-Actinin is an actin-bundling protein expressed in podocytes, monocytes, capillaries, and larger vessels. Mutations of the gene encoding the isoform α-actinin-4 have been identified in familial focal and segmental glomerulosclerosis. α-Actinin may also be a target for anti-dsDNA in humans. Other cell-surface and matrix receptors on various cell types, including mesangial cells, fibroblasts, and monocytes, could bind nucleosomes in the kidney.

Inherited deficiencies of the early components of the complement classic pathway are the strongest susceptibility genes for the development of SLE in humans. C1q-deficient mice have been generated by homologous recombination (24). The presence of multiple apoptotic bodies in the altered glomeruli suggests a critical role for C1q in the clearance of apoptotic cells. This finding is consistent with the report that C1q binds to apoptotic keratinocyte (65). Apoptotic cells are believed to be a major source of the autoantigens of the SLE, and impairment of their removal by complement may explain the link between hereditary complement deficiency and the development of SLE.

Another study on the lupus-prone New Zealand black and New Zealand white mouse has shown that the γ chain of the T-lymphocyte receptor is mandatory for the initiation of the inflammatory cascade in the kidney. Indeed, when the New Zealand black and New Zealand white mice were backcrossed with FcγR-deficient mice, glomeruli were not affected despite the deposition of immune complexes and C3 (66). In humans, decreased binding affinity of the FcγRIIIA-158F allele may result in ineffective clearance of antigen-antibody complexes, resulting in an increased susceptibility to immune-complex–mediated nephritis (67). Of interest, another polymorphism in the gene coding for the FcγRIIIA receptor represents a significant risk factor for SLE but has no clear effect on susceptibility for lupus nephritis (68).

Clinical Findings

Clinical symptoms of renal involvement are noted in 40 to 80% of patients, appearing most often during the first years (8). Renal involvement is variable, with some patients showing minimal urinary anomalies and others having nephritic syndrome with rapidly progressive renal failure. Proteinuria is the most frequent symptom. Proteinuria is frequently abundant, accompanied by a nephrotic syndrome. Microscopic hematuria is frequently associated with proteinuria and is rarely seen in isolation. The urinary sediment contains granular and red blood cell casts. Patients with severe nephritis are often hypertensive and have reduced renal function. Up to 50% of children with lupus nephritis have a decreased glomerular filtration rate (GFR). Signs of renal tubular dysfunction may be observed and are related to immune deposits along the tubular basement membranes and to interstitial cellular infiltrates. Increased excretion of β_2-microglobulin is frequently found. Renal tubular acidosis with hyperkalemia has been reported.

Histologic Classification

Most nephrologists believe that the presence of urinary abnormalities or impairment of renal function is an indication for renal biopsy, especially to guide the initial treatment (69). There is no correlation between symptoms and the class of glomerular lesions (focal or diffuse proliferative glomerulonephritis with varying degrees of severity or membranous glomerulonephritis). The type of histologic lesion is most important in deciding the best therapy and in determining prognosis. A renal biopsy may be indicated in a patient with glomerular disease in which there are no extrarenal manifestations of SLE. It is more difficult to decide whether to perform a renal biopsy in patients with no clinical evidence of renal disease. Indeed, glomerular lesions may be found in this setting, most often with mesangial deposits and mild mesangial proliferation. Although the clinical evidence of renal involvement is present in only 40 to 75% of SLE patients, renal biopsy studies show nearly universal histologic changes. The majority of clinically asymptomatic patients will show moderate histologic damage, but some may have more severe histologic lesions, such as focal and segmental glomerulonephritis, or, very rarely, diffuse proliferative glomerulonephritis.

Histologic anomalies are present in virtually all SLE patients, and immune deposits are almost always found on immunofluorescence examination or by electron microscopy. There is a wide diversity of glomerular damage in SLE. Moreover, tubulointerstitial and vascular lesions can be observed in addition to glomerular lesions. Numerous classifications have been proposed based primarily on the histologic damage observed by light microscopy. One such system was developed by the International Study of Kidney Disease in Children. The classification of the World Health Organization is now widely accepted (Table 46.3) (70,71). An adequate renal specimen, containing at least ten glomeruli, must be obtained for light microscopy analysis. Immunofluorescence examination is also mandatory. Electron microscopy may aid the classification but is not necessary for diagnosing

TABLE 46.3. WORLD HEALTH ORGANIZATION CLASSIFICATION OF LUPUS NEPHRITIS

I. Normal glomeruli
  A. No deposit
  B. Normal by light microscopy but deposits by immunofluorescence or electron microscopy
II. Mesangiopathic glomerulonephritis
  A. Mesangial widening and/or mild hypercellularity
  B. Moderate hypercellularity
III. Focal and segmental glomerulonephritis (with mesangial alterations)
  A. With active necrotizing lesions
  B. With active and sclerosing lesions
  C. With sclerosing lesions
IV. Diffuse proliferative glomerulonephritis (with severe mesangial and endocapillary proliferation and subendothelial deposits)
  A. Without segmental lesions
  B. With active necrotizing lesions
  C. With active and sclerosing lesions
  D. With sclerosing lesions
V. Membranous glomerulonephritis
  A. Pure membranous glomerulonephritis
  B. Associated with class II lesions (A or B)
  C. Associated with class III lesions (A, B, or C)
  D. Associated with class IV lesions (A B, C, or D)
VI. Advanced sclerosing glomerulonephritis

lupus nephritis. The study of renal biopsies has allowed for the definition of several histopathologic aspects of lupus nephritis (Fig. 46.1). Furthermore, biopsies have permitted clinicopathologic correlations with the natural outcome of the disease. Of importance, the histologic categories of the biopsies guide therapeutic decisions (72,73).

The World Health Organization classification of lupus nephritis includes six classes:

In class I, the glomeruli appear normal on light microscopy. Immunofluorescence and electron microscopic examinations are negative or show slight mesangial deposits. In these cases, patients generally show no clinical or biologic signs of renal damage. Class I is rarely observed on biopsy specimens of SLE patients and is present only in patients without clinical manifestation of renal disease.

In class II, there is a hypertrophy of the mesangial matrix, with a proliferation of mesangial cells. This is called a *mesangial proliferative lupus glomerulonephritis* and is observed in 20% of patients. Immunofluorescence and electron microscopy examination show mesangial deposits, whereas the glomerular walls are normal. Urine examination can be normal or may reveal a microscopic hematuria and moderate proteinuria. The prognosis is excellent except in cases of transformation to a more severe form (74).

Class III is observed in 10 to 20% of patients. These lesions appear as focal lupus glomerulonephritis in which the proportion of glomeruli presenting focal lesions is less than 50%. Class III can range from focal proliferative and necrotic lesions affecting a limited proportion of glomeruli to more diffuse lesions affecting a higher proportion of glomeruli. In the latter cases, tubulointerstitial lesions are often present in addition to glomerular lesions. Immunofluorescence and electron microscopy examination reveal diffuse mesangial deposits and focal deposits along the glomerular capillary walls.

When less than 20% of glomeruli are affected by small segmental lesions, patients usually have mild renal symptoms with low-grade proteinuria without nephrotic syndrome and normal GFR. The long-term prognosis is favorable, with probably less than 5% risk of progression to end-stage renal failure after 5 years (75). Conversely, when cellular proliferation, necrosis, and large subendothelial deposits involve more than 40% of the glomeruli, the clinical symptoms are more severe with active urine sediment, nephrotic syndrome, hypertension, and moderate renal insufficiency in some patients. The prognosis is the same as for diffuse proliferative glomerulonephritis (72,75).

Class IV corresponds to diffuse proliferative lupus glomerulonephritis, the most common and severe form of lupus nephritis, in which more than 50% of glomeruli present a marked hypercellularity. Hypercellularity may affect a segment of the glomerulus or may be global, involving more than one-half of the glomerular tuft. In addition, active lesions are often seen including necrotic lesions, karyorrhexis, hematoxylic bodies, leukocytic infiltrates, wire loops, and hyaline thrombi. The proportion of glomeruli with epithelial crescents is an important factor in determining the prognosis of this type of glomerulonephritis. Tubulointerstitial lesions with mononuclear cell infiltrates are common. Immunofluorescence and electron microscopy examination show diffuse mesangial and extensive subendothelial immune deposits. Deposits are also found frequently along the tubular basement membranes and the capillary walls. The clinical symptoms are often severe: hematuria with casts, nephrotic syndrome, hypertension, and moderate or severe renal insufficiency. Patients with class IV glomerulonephritis are at high risk of progression to end-stage renal disease if adequate therapy is not undertaken.

Class V corresponds to membranous lupus glomerulonephritis, characterized by a thickening of the glomeruli capillary walls and the presence of global or segmental continuous subepithelial immune deposits separated by "spikes." There is little or no cellular proliferation, and mesangial deposits are almost constant in SLE. In some patients, the membranous lesions are associated with lesions of class II, III, or IV. The latter category resembles clinically diffuse proliferative glomerulonephritis. Membranous glomerulonephritis may precede other manifestations of lupus. Moderate proteinuria is accompanied by hematuria in 50% of patients. Nephrotic syndrome often develops. Moderate renal failure and hypertension are observed in 25% of patients.

Class VI corresponds to an advanced stage of lupus nephritis where most glomeruli are sclerotic but without evidence of active glomerular lesions.

By immunofluorescence, the composition of deposits is remarkable no matter where they are located. In these

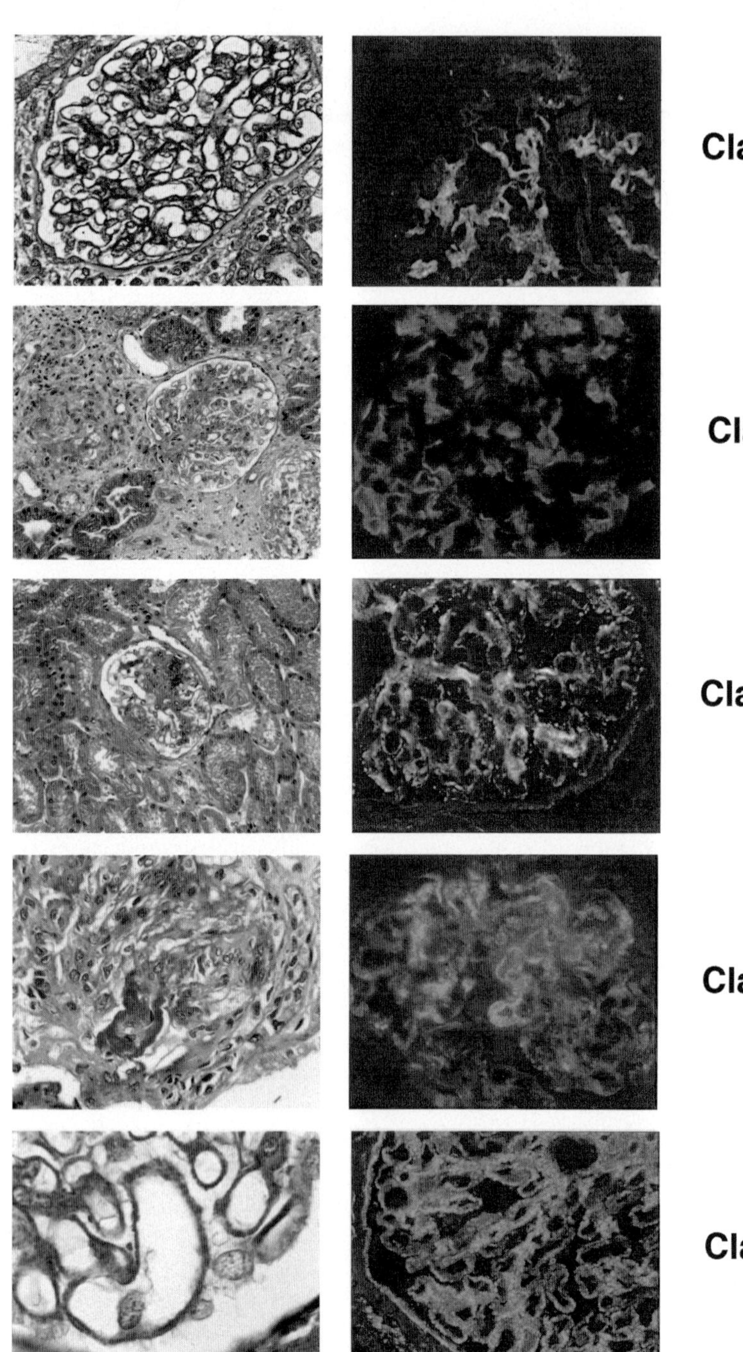

FIGURE 46.1. Class I: Normal glomerulus by light microscopy (*right-hand side*) but mesangial immune deposits by immunofluorescence (*left-hand side*) study. Class II: Purely mesangial hypercellularity and mesangial matrix expansion in glomerulus by light microscopy, with mesangial immune deposits by immunofluorescence study. Class III: Segmental endo- and extracapillary proliferation involving 50% of all glomeruli by light microscopy with mesangial and some subendothelial immune deposits by immunofluorescence study. Class IV: Global endo- and extracapillary proliferation and subendothelial deposits by light microscopy and numerous immune deposits by immunofluorescence study. Class V: Membranous glomerulonephritis, with subepithelial deposits by light microscopy, clearly defined by immunofluorescence study. (See Color Plate 46.1.)

deposits, IgG is dominant, mostly IgG1 and IgG3. IgA and IgM are also present, as well as early complement components, C4 and C1q, along with C3. Such positivity for all three Ig classes and C3, C4, and C1q is called *full house* and is found only in lupus nephritis. Fibrin deposits are also found, particularly in class IV biopsies.

Activity and Chronicity Indexes

Pirani et al. and Morel-Maroger et al. introduced the concept of histologic signs of activity and chronicity (76,77). Later, Austin et al. introduced the activity and the chronicity indices, which may help to define the prognosis (78). Active histologic lesions include cellular crescents, endocapillary proliferation, fibrinoid necrosis, karyorrhexis, thrombi, wire loops with subendothelial immune deposits, glomerular leucocyte infiltration, and interstitial mononuclear cell infiltration (Table 46.4). These active lesions are each graded 0 to 3 (with both necrosis and cellular crescents graded 0 to 6) to give an activity index graded 0 to 24. Active lesions are potentially reversible with the treatment. Recent studies have shown that glomerular capillary

TABLE 46.4. ACTIVE AND CHRONIC HISTOLOGIC RENAL LESIONS

Active lesions
- Glomerular
  - Endocapillary hypercellularity
  - Fibrinoid necrosis
  - Karyorrhexis
  - Hyaline thrombi
  - Wire loops (subendothelial deposits)
  - Hematoxylic bodies
  - Cellular crescents
  - Leukocyte infiltrates
- Tubulointerstitial
  - Mononuclear cell infiltrates
  - Tubular necrosis

Chronic lesions
- Glomerular
  - Glomerular sclerosis (segmental or global)
  - Fibrous crescents
  - Fibrous adhesions
  - Extramembranous deposits
- Tubulointerstitial
  - Interstitial fibrosis
  - Tubular atrophy

wall necrosis is associated with poor outcome, especially when these lesions affect a high percentage of glomeruli (79). Extramembranous deposits are not considered as active lesions. Conversely, irreversible lesions, including glomerular sclerosis, fibrous crescents, tubular fibrosis, and interstitial fibrosis, permit the definition of chronicity index. These lesions do not respond to treatment. If the activity and the chronicity indices are important to decide the best therapy for individual patients, their prognostic significance is still debated. The National Institutes of Health group found that an activity index greater than 12 of 24 or an elevated chronicity index were indicative of a poor renal prognosis (78). A chronicity index less than 2 was associated with a 10-year renal survival rate of 100%, whereas a chronicity index between 2 and 4 was associated with a 10-year renal survival rate of only 70%. The renal survival rate at 10 years was only 35% in patients with a chronicity index greater than 4. However, a more recent study including unselected patients with lupus nephritis found that activity and chronicity indices were not well correlated with renal outcome (80).

Repeat Renal Biopsies

Repeat biopsies have shown that transformations from one class to another are possible, either via aggravation or amelioration of the histologic lesions. A mesangiopathic glomerulonephritis can transform into focal and segmental glomerulonephritis or diffuse proliferative glomerulonephritis. These, in turn, are susceptible to improvement under treatment. In contrast, transformation is rare in cases of membranous glomerulonephritis. Repeat renal biopsies allow for the evaluation of the efficiency of treatment and are useful in considering therapeutic changes, particularly in cases of worsening clinical symptoms (e.g., proteinuria, renal insufficiency). In some cases, clinical aggravation may be secondary to sclerotic lesions, for which treatment is ineffective. Sclerotic lesions are especially seen in patients who have had insufficient treatment for an active nephropathy. In other cases, clinical deterioration may be related to active histologic lesions, which require a more aggressive treatment. Also, deterioration of renal function may be related to nephrotoxic treatments, such as nonsteroidal antiinflammatory drugs, cyclosporine, or antibiotics, rather than to SLE itself. Hill et al. recently reported that a repeat renal biopsy at 6 months after a change of treatment carries great prognostic significance (81).

Prognostic Factors in Patients with Severe Lupus Nephritis

Some patients with diffuse proliferative glomerulonephritis are at higher risk of progression, particularly those with extensive crescent formation and necrotizing glomerular lesions (82–87). In addition to these histologic signs of severity, other factors may be of prognostic significance, including age, gender, race, hypertension, initial serum creatinine concentration, the delay between onset of renal disease and treatment, the occurrence of exacerbations of the nephropathy, and the response to therapy after the first year (78,84,88–92). Thus, despite numerous controlled and uncontrolled therapeutic studies, there is still no general agreement on the best course of therapy in these patients.

An analysis of these prognostic factors is important in proposing the most effective and safest therapy for individual patients. Several studies have shown that lupus nephritis has a worse prognosis in men compared to women. Renal survival in black Americans with diffuse proliferative glomerulonephritis is poorer compared to white patients (93). Renal survival rate in black patients was 58% at 5 years, compared to 95% in white patients who retained renal function after pulse cyclophosphamide therapy. Several possible reasons for the significance of race in the poorer prognosis in lupus nephritis have been proposed and include socioeconomic effects, different HLA phenotypes, and inherited susceptibility for progression to renal failure.

Levey et al. identified several risk factors for progression to renal failure in 86 patients with severe class III or class IV lupus glomerulonephritis who were treated with prednisone and oral cyclophosphamide (94). An elevation of serum creatinine was the only initial feature predictive of progression to renal failure. Of interest, the same authors found that the subsequent clinical course in response to therapy supplemented prognosis based on initial serum creatinine. The risk of progression to renal failure was higher in those patients who did not show resolution of renal abnormalities within 48 weeks of follow-up. Patients with normal initial serum creatinine and patients with resolution of initial serum creatinine elevations to normal had a similar and much lower risk of progression to renal failure. Other authors have also reported the poor prognostic significance of elevated serum creatinine at presentation (78,84,89,95,96). However, these findings were not confirmed in several studies with longer periods of follow-up (72,83,92,97).

Esdaile et al. studied the impact of the delay between the onset of renal disease, the renal biopsy, and initiation of therapy (98). They found that the duration of renal disease before renal biopsy was a statistically significant predictor for renal failure or death due to renal disease. The most likely explanation for these findings is that early treatment of renal disease is associated with better outcome. There was a significant increase in serum creatinine, in urinary protein excretion, and in activity and chronicity indexes on renal biopsy in those patients in whom the treatment was delayed. Lim et al. found that chronicity index, male gender, and initial renal insufficiency were prognostic factors for diffuse proliferative lupus nephritis (99). Similarly, Conlon et al. analyzed, retrospectively, a cohort of 43 patients, one-half of which progressed to end-stage renal disease and were treated with IV cyclophosphamide. Elevated serum creatinine and a high degree of interstitial fibrosis on renal biopsy before treatment were associated with a worse renal prognosis (100).

Moroni et al. studied the prognostic significance of renal flares, defined as a rapid increase of serum creatinine or proteinuria, in a retrospective study of 70 patients with lupus nephritis (92). Patients with renal flares had a higher probability of having a persistent doubling of serum creatinine compared to those who had no renal flares. The relative risk of having a persistent doubling of serum creatinine was 27 times higher in patients with rapid increases in serum creatinine. This outcome was more frequent in patients who did not respond rapidly to therapy. These data support the need for aggressive treatment of lupus nephritis exacerbations.

Several reports have claimed a poorer prognosis of lupus nephritis in children as compared to adults. However, Cameron et al. reported a renal survival rate of 85% at 5 years and 82% at 10 years in a series of 80 patients with onset of disease under the age of 20 years (101). Platt et al. found 5- and 10-year survival rates of 85 and 81%, respectively, in a series of 70 patients (9). A few reports in recent years have identified the risk factors for renal failure in children with lupus nephritis. Yang et al. retrospectively evaluated the clinical course, histopathology, and prognosis of 167 children (102). Patients with persistent hypertension, anemia, increased serum creatinine concentration at the time of biopsy, and low titer of CH50 were more prone to develop renal failure. The overall renal and patient 5-year survival rates were 87.7% and 91.1%, respectively. McCurdy et al. reported on a group of 71 children, of whom 22% progressed to end-stage renal failure (96). They also found that persistent hypertension, anemia, abnormalities of the urinalysis, and elevated serum creatinine levels were associated with progression to renal failure. Emre et al. found that the prognosis of lupus nephritis in children is primarily dependent on the histopathologic lesions. Moreover, the severity of the clinical renal disease at admission and the presence of persistent hypertension were the main poor prognostic factors (103). Baqi et al. analyzed the risk factors for renal failure in 56 children with lupus nephritis (104). Univariate analysis revealed that an elevated serum creatinine level, a decreased C3 complement level, hypertension, and class IV lupus nephritis were associated with the rate of progression to renal failure. Multivariate analysis showed that progression to renal failure was independently associated with class IV lupus nephritis, hypertension at presentation, and low C3 complement level in association with elevated serum creatinine levels. These three reports, as well as other studies in adults, found that hypertension was virtually always a significant risk factor for renal failure. Therefore, children with hypertension should be treated appropriately with antihypertensive drugs, as control of blood pressure may be as important as antiinflammatory treatment.

Prognostic Factors in Patients with Membranous Lupus Nephritis

Patients with pure membranous nephropathy without mesangial hypercellularity have a good prognosis with a 5-year renal survival close to 85% (105,106). Conversely, Sloan et al. found that when membranous nephropathy was associated with segmental endocapillary proliferation or necrosis in less than 50% of glomeruli, the 5-year renal survival was 72% and only 49% when more than 50% of glomeruli were affected (106). Therefore, associated glomerular inflammation and necrosis are important prognostic factors in membranous lupus nephritis. Elevation of initial serum creatinine or worsening renal function and severe nephrotic syndrome are also risk factors for poor renal outcome.

LABORATORY INVESTIGATIONS

SLE is characterized by a large variety of autoantibodies, of which some, such as anti-DNA antibodies, are found almost exclusively in patients suffering from this disease (107). Such autoantibodies associate with the corresponding antigen and form immune complexes, which activate the classic complement pathway. These immune complexes can be detected in the circulation or are deposited in different tissues where they are detectable by immunofluorescence techniques.

The detection of ANA by indirect immunofluorescence is a simple and sensitive test in which the serum is incubated with a tissue section. ANA are present in significant titer in 95% of patients with SLE, and the diagnosis is unlikely in their absence (108). The pattern of fluorescence gives an indication of the specificity of the antibodies. A homogenous or diffuse aspect of fluorescence is related to the presence of antidesoxyribonucleoprotein antibodies and is strongly associated with SLE. The same antibodies are responsible for the formation of Hargraves cells (lupus erythematosus cells). After the reaction of the antibodies with the nucleus of leukocytes, the chromatin pattern is altered, and the DNA forms a large mass with the antibodies and complement that is then ingested by a phagocyte. A peripheral aspect of the fluorescence points to the presence of antinative DNA antibodies, characteristic of active SLE. A speckled aspect of the fluorescence is related to the presence of antibodies reacting with various nuclear antigens, such as anti-Sm or antiribonucleoprotein antibodies. Such a pattern of fluorescence may be observed in SLE or mixed connective tissue disease but is more frequently associated with scleroderma. The nucleolar pattern is observed in only 25% of patients with SLE.

The presence of ANA is not unique to SLE because they can be detected in other rheumatologic disorders such as chronic juvenile arthritis, scleroderma or mixed connective tissue disease, autoimmune hepatitis, thyroiditis, or after taking certain medications. ANA titers should be determined, as low levels can be found in up to 2% of the general population. High levels of ANA are highly suggestive of SLE. A small number of patients with SLE do not have ANA, but more than one-half of these do have anti-SSA antibodies. Anti-SSA antibodies cannot be detected by indirect immunofluorescence tests. Clinically, patients with anti-SSA antibodies generally have photosensitivity, arthralgia, and serous effusions.

Antinative dsDNA antibodies are more specific to SLE (109–111). They can be detected in the serum by measuring their capacity to bind radiolabeled native DNA (Farr test) or by an immunoenzymatic technique. Anti-DNA antibodies can also be detected by indirect immunofluorescence on the microorganism *Crithidia luciliae*, which have a kinetoplast in their cytoplasm containing native DNA. The Farr assay detects high-avidity antibodies, whereas the immunoenzymatic technique also detects low-avidity antibodies. The enzyme-linked immunosorbent assay is of interest for screening diagnosis. The Farr assay is better correlated to the presence and the severity of the nephritis. Moreover, the Farr assay gives estimation on the level of antibodies, which is used to monitor disease activity. Normal or stable levels are positively correlated to a stability of the disease, whereas an increase often precedes the reappearance or aggravation of clinical manifestations of the disease.

Anti-Sm antibodies are specific to SLE but are only found in 30% of patients and are often associated with a less severe form of the disease (112). Antiribonucleoprotein antibodies, present in 35% of SLE cases, are not specific for SLE. Antierythrocyte antibodies, detected by the Coombs' test, can be responsible for severe hemolytic anemia. Antiplatelet antibodies are often present, sometimes causing thrombocytopenia. Antilymphocyte antibodies, directed against T lymphocytes, may play a role in the pathogenesis of the disease. Siegert et al. found a correlation between the levels of anti-C1q antibodies and the occurrence of nephritis, the titers of anti-DNA antibodies, and hypocomplementemia (113). The increase of anti-C1q titers was correlated with the development of proliferative glomerulonephritis. Thus, the serial measurements of these antibodies may be useful to predict relapses of nephritis. Because C1q is found in glomerular immune deposits, C1q may act as a planted antigen for anti-C1q antibodies, thus increasing the inflammatory reaction (114).

APL antibodies, including anticardiolipin and the lupus anticoagulant, may be found in SLE and are responsible for an increased risk of thrombotic complications.

Many of these autoantibodies can be responsible for the formation of immune complexes, either in the serum or localized in tissues. Circulating immune complexes can be detected by several tests, but these tests are not useful in the diagnosis or the monitoring of SLE, as many other conditions can be accompanied by circulating immune complexes. Immune complexes deposited in tissues are detected by direct immunofluorescence techniques. Deposits are frequently found in the kidneys. Skin biopsy may show immunoglobulin, principally IgG, and complement fraction deposits at the dermoepidermic junction. This is the lupus band test that is highly suggestive of SLE (115).

Hypocomplementemia is observed in 75% of cases at presentation, particularly in patients with nephritis. Decreased levels of CH50, C1q, and C4 are related to the activation of the classic pathway of the complement system. A permanently low C4 level may also be secondary to null C4 alleles. A deficiency of other complement factors may also be observed. Levels of C4, C1q, and C3 are used to monitor disease activity in conjunction with anti-DNA antibodies. In most patients with nephritis, flares are preceded by a decrease of these complement components. Concentrations of properdin and factor B are also depressed due to the activation of the alternative pathway.

Regular testing of biologic parameters (blood cell count, erythrocyte sedimentation rate, serum albumin, proteinuria, urinary sediment, GFR, anti-DNA antibodies, CH50, C4, and C3) every 3 to 6 months is important during the evolution of the disease. This testing allows for the detection of hematologic or renal involvement as well as a serologic evidence of disease activity before the appearance of clinical manifestations (116).

DRUG-INDUCED LUPUS

Several drugs, particularly those that are metabolized by acetylation in the liver, such as procainamide or hydralazine, can induce a lupus-like syndrome (117,118). The syndrome is more likely to develop in slow acetylators, which have a genetically determined deficit in hepatic *N*-acetyltransferase (119).

One characteristic of drug-induced lupus is the presence of antihistone antibodies that are found in 95% of such patients. Other autoantibodies, such as anti-DNA antibodies, are rarely found in those with drug-induced lupus. These autoantibodies are formed against a complex between DNA and a histone dimer of H2A and H2B. Of interest, although the drugs responsible for drug-induced lupus are quite heterogeneous, all of these antibodies are directed against the same epitope (120). With hydralazine, the complex is composed of H1 and H3-H4 and DNA.

Procainamide, hydralazine, penicillamine, isoniazid, interferon-alpha, methyldopa, chlorpromazine, and diltiazem are all likely causes of lupus. Anticonvulsants (e.g., phenytoin, mephenytoin, trimethadione, ethosuximide), quinidine, antithyroid drugs, and antimicrobial agents (e.g., sulfonamides, rifampin) may possibly induce lupus. Clinical manifestations associated with drug-induced lupus include fever, cutaneous rash, arthralgia, and serositis, whereas renal, hematologic, or neurologic symptoms are rare. Anti-DNA antibodies are often absent, and the levels of complement fractions are normal.

The differentiation between SLE and lupus syndrome secondary to a medication is not always clear. The principal criterion is the spontaneous recovery from the syndrome within 6 months after withdrawal of the suspected medication.

NEONATAL LUPUS

Neonatal lupus occurs in 1 to 2% of children born to mothers with lupus and is due to passively transferred autoantibodies. The main complication of neonatal lupus is a total and irreversible atrioventricular block secondary to anti-SSA (Ro) and anti-SSB antibodies, which interfere with the development of the conduction system (121). Some infants require insertion of a pacemaker. The incidence of congenital heart block in children from mothers with anti-SSA (Ro) antibodies ranges from 0.2 to 7.5% (122).

Other newborns, particularly girls, may present with erythematous rash that often develops after exposure to ultraviolet light. The rash regresses totally after 6 months. Other manifestations may include anemia, moderate leukopenia and thrombocytopenia, or hepatomegalia with cytolysis (123).

TREATMENT OF LUPUS NEPHRITIS

Therapeutic options for patients with lupus nephritis vary depending on the histologic lesions observed on renal biopsy.

Therapy of Patients with Mild Renal Lesions

Patients with class II mesangial proliferative lupus glomerulonephritis do not need specific therapy, as there is little probability of progression (74). Nevertheless, careful follow-up of the patient is necessary, as transformation to a more severe renal disease is possible.

Therapy of Patients with Focal and Segmental Glomerulonephritis

Patients with focal and segmental glomerulonephritis who have less than 20% of the glomeruli affected by small segmental lesions have a favorable long-term outcome. These patients may require treatment for extrarenal lesions, but they do not need specific therapy for these renal lesions. Conversely, when cellular proliferation and necrosis involve more than 40% of the glomeruli, the course of the disease is similar to that of diffuse proliferative glomerulonephritis, and the same aggressive therapy is needed (72,75).

Therapy of Patients with Diffuse Proliferative Glomerulonephritis

Patients with active and extensive focal proliferative glomerulonephritis and those with diffuse proliferative glomerulonephritis are at high risk of progression to end-stage renal disease if adequate therapy is not undertaken (124). The therapeutic regimen for class IV lupus nephritis has changed over the years (125). Although there are a large number of reports on this topic, there are only a few randomized studies. Most of these studies do not indicate the long-term outcome after 10 years of follow-up. Pollak et al. showed that high doses of corticosteroids could improve the course of diffuse proliferative glomerulonephritis, whereas low doses were ineffective (126). Most nephrologists treat these patients with prednisone, 1 to 2 mg/kg/day for several months, followed by a slow dose reduction when the disease is controlled. However, high doses of oral prednisone alone may give poor long-term results and are often associated with serious side effects. Many authors have proposed initial therapy with IV methylprednisolone pulses that have potent and rapid antiinflammatory and immunosuppressive effects (127–131). After methylprednisolone pulses, extrarenal symptoms disappear rapidly, and serum creatinine rapidly returns to normal. Furthermore, these pulses frequently permit initiation of oral prednisone at a lower dose, thus reducing the complications of long-term treatment.

Some patients with diffuse proliferative glomerulonephritis are well controlled with corticosteroids alone. However, several studies have shown that renal survival is significantly better when cyclophosphamide or azathioprine is added to corticosteroids (132–136). A metaanalysis of eight trials published between 1971 and 1983 compared the outcome of 113 patients treated by corticosteroids alone with the outcome of 137 other patients who received cyclophosphamide or azathioprine in addition to corticosteroids with a follow-up of 2 to 82 months (137). The addition of cyclophosphamide or azathioprine lowered the incidence of progression to renal failure by 40% compared to a treatment with corticosteroids alone. There was no difference in terms of mortality between both groups. The metaanalysis could not determine whether cyclophosphamide or azathioprine was superior.

In studies performed at the National Institutes of Health, 111 patients with lupus nephritis were randomized in five groups and received either high-dose prednisone alone or moderate doses of prednisone in association with azathioprine, oral cyclophosphamide, oral cyclophosphamide and azathioprine, or cyclophosphamide given as IV boluses (138). There was no difference in outcome during the first 5 years, but after 5 years, the incidence of renal failure was significantly higher in the group receiving prednisone alone compared to patients given IV cyclophosphamide. There was a trend to a better outcome in patients who received IV cyclophosphamide compared to those given oral cyclophosphamide alone or in combination with azathioprine, although the differences were not statistically significant. Patients receiving azathioprine did better during the first decade than those treated with prednisone alone, but the incidence of renal failure was not statistically different after 10 years in these two groups. The results of these studies have greatly influenced nephrologists in their therapeutic decisions. Many of them use IV cyclophosphamide for the treatment of diffuse proliferative glomerulonephritis (139,140). However, the interpretation of the results of the National Institutes of Health trials should take into account several points. First, among the 111 patients enrolled in the studies, 6 had no renal biopsy, 7 had a mesangiopathic glomerulonephritis, and 16 had pure membranous glomerulonephritis. Second, some of the patients included in the prednisone group were from a historical group. Third, the number of at-risk patients after 10 years was only 8 to 12 in each group. Aggressive therapy, including cytotoxic agents, is indicated in those patients at high risk for progression to renal failure, including an elevated serum creatinine level at the time of renal biopsy, a severe nephrotic syndrome, hematocrit below 25%, crescent formation, severe tubulointerstitial disease, and vascular changes (86).

Cyclophosphamide given as monthly boluses at a starting dose of 750 mg/m^2 may be less toxic than given orally every day at a dose of 2 mg/kg body weight. The dose of cyclophosphamide given as boluses is increased to 1000 mg/m^2 if the white blood cell count remains above 3000/mm^3 (141). The optimal duration of cyclophosphamide pulse therapy has not been determined. Another National Institutes of Health trial was performed in 65 patients with severe lupus nephritis defined by an impairment of renal function or a high-activity index on renal biopsy (135). Three regimens were compared. The first regimen consisted of 6 monthly pulses of cyclophosphamide, the second of the same regimen followed cyclophosphamide pulses every 3 months for an 2 additional years, and the third of 6 monthly pulses of methylprednisolone without cyclophosphamide. Oral prednisone was given to all patients at a starting dose of 0.5 mg/kg/day and then tapered. The probability of doubling serum creatinine after 5 years of follow-up was higher in patients treated with methylprednisolone pulses compared to those receiving cyclophosphamide (48 vs. 25%). The probability of relapse of lupus nephritis was significantly higher in patients receiving cyclophosphamide pulses for 6 months compared to those receiving the long-course cyclophosphamide regimen (55 vs. 10% after 5 years of observation). The conclusions were that cyclophosphamide pulses are more effective than methylprednisolone pulses in preserving renal function and that maintenance cyclophosphamide pulses reduce the risk of relapse. Recent studies have shown that a combination of methylprednisolone pulses and cyclophosphamide pulses are more effective in the long-term follow-up and no more toxic than either therapy alone (131,142).

The data on the efficacy of cyclophosphamide pulses remain scant in children with active lupus nephritis (143). Lehman et al. treated 16 children with cyclophosphamide monthly for 6 months and then every 3 months (144). They reported significant improvement at 1 year in urine protein excretion, hemoglobin levels, C3 and C4, and creatinine clearance despite a significant reduction in prednisone dosage. Baqi et al. compared the results of two treatment modalities in children with class II and class IV lupus nephritis: high-dose pulse methylprednisolone for 10 days, followed by oral prednisone (20 patients) or IV cyclophosphamide given monthly for 6 months and then every 3 months for a period of 3 years with oral prednisone (30 patients) (104). The authors did not find any difference in outcome for the two treatment modalities.

Other authors have reported on the potential to control the disease with shorter courses of therapy. The Euro-Lupus Nephritis Trial performed a randomized trial in 90 adult patients with diffuse proliferative lupus nephritis to compare the efficacy and the toxicity of a high-dose IV cyclophosphamide regimen (6 monthly pulses and 2 quarterly pulses) and a low-dose IV cyclophosphamide regimen (6 fortnightly pulses at a fixed dose of 500 mg) (145). The regimen of low-dose cyclophosphamide followed by azathioprine achieved similar clinical results compared to the high-dose cyclophosphamide regimen. Levey et al. reported the results of the Lupus Nephritis Collaborative Study, in which patients with severe lupus nephritis were treated with oral prednisone at a starting dose of 60 to 80 mg/day and oral cyclophosphamide for 8 weeks (94). Exacerbations were treated using increased doses of corticosteroids. Only 16% of the 31 patients who had normal serum creatinine concentration at the start of the treatment had a rise of serum creatinine at latest follow-up. Only two of them (6.5%) progressed to renal failure. Conversely, 16 of the 55 patients (29%) with elevated initial serum creatinine levels progressed to renal failure during the follow-up period. Patients with severe lupus nephritis and normal initial serum creatinine may thus achieve excellent outcome without cyclophosphamide pulses, although the duration of follow-up in this study was rather short. Lim et al. suggested that treatment with oral corticosteroid could induce remission in patients who have mild histologic and clinical features and recommended an evaluation of the prognostic factors before the selection of treatment modality (146).

After the observations of the improvement of nephritis in murine lupus with the use of mycophenolate mofetil (MMF) (147–149), several uncontrolled studies in adults and in children confirmed the potential benefits of this drug in lupus nephritis (150–154). A controlled trial involving 42 patients with diffuse proliferative lupus nephritis compared the efficacy and side effects of a regimen of prednisolone and MMF given for 12 months with those of a regimen of prednisolone and cyclophosphamide given for 6 months, followed by prednisolone and azathioprine for 6 months. At 1 year, both groups showed similar rates of complete or partial remissions, relapses, and treatment discontinuations (155). Adverse effects of treatment were more frequent in the group of patients receiving cyclophosphamide. Two other controlled trials comparing MMF and IV cyclophosphamide found no significant differences with a follow-up of 1 to 2 years (156,157). Ongoing trials are being performed in the United States, and long-term follow-up of these patients is important to confirm whether MMF is as efficient as IV cyclophosphamide.

An effective treatment should be associated with control of the extrarenal manifestations of SLE, a normalization of complement levels and anti-DNA antibody titers, as well as a decrease in the activity of the urine sediment, a decrease of proteinuria, and a decrease or stabilization of plasma creatinine. Our current protocol for patients with severe lupus nephritis is to start with 3 methylprednisolone pulses followed by oral prednisone 1.5 mg/kg/day and 6 monthly pulses of cyclophosphamide. In children with milder disease, we may begin the treatment with IV methylprednisolone pulses followed by oral prednisone at moderate doses, 1.0 to 1.5 mg/kg body weight per day before deciding to add cytotoxic agents. A second renal biopsy is performed, and when the disease is controlled, the patient may be maintained on azathioprine or mycophenolate while the prednisone dosage is slowly tapered. This regimen may have a lower risk of neoplasia and gonadal toxicity than prolonged cyclophosphamide therapy (158). There is a risk of flare of SLE if the immunosuppressive treatment is stopped before 2 years or in case of significant proteinuria (159). Therefore, corticosteroids and immunosuppressive drugs should only be stopped after 3 years if the patient shows normal GFR, proteinuria less than 1 g/day, and inactive urine sediment.

Treatment of Relapses

Relapse of the disease may be defined by a worsening of renal symptoms. Some patients may present with an increase in serum creatinine associated with active urinary sediment and often increased proteinuria (160). The presence of red-cell or white-cell casts is predictive of a renal relapse. In other patients, increase in proteinuria is the only renal symptom. In such cases, serologic abnormalities are important. An elevation in the titer of anti-DNA antibodies and a decrease in the complement levels (C4 and C3) are most often associated with renal flares. These serologic parameters should be checked regularly, as their changes often precede clinical relapse (161,162). In cases with worsening of renal symptoms, repeat renal biopsy may also be of help before deciding a change in the therapy. Patients who show active lesions on repeat renal biopsy may need aggressive treatment. Other patients with increased serum creatinine may have extensive tubulointerstitial lesions with mild glomerular lesions, which do not respond to therapy. Other patients treated initially for diffuse proliferative glomerulonephritis and who responded well to therapy may have an increased proteinuria several months later. A repeat renal biopsy is useful in this situation, as it may show active lesions or pure membranous nephropathy, which require different therapeutic decisions. We believe that a repeat renal biopsy is often needed in patients with renal relapses to decide the best therapy and to avoid unnecessary aggressive treatments. Some authors treat renal exacerbations with methylprednisolone pulses followed by oral prednisone with tapering doses (163).

Treatment of Patients with Membranous Nephropathy

Patients with pure membranous nephropathy, mild proteinuria, and normal renal function have a good prognosis, and there is general agreement that no specific treatment is needed (105,106). The treatment of patients with nephrotic syndrome is controversial. These patients are at risk of thrombotic complications. Moroni et al. performed a trial in which patients were randomly assigned to receive either a 6-month regimen consisting of corticosteroids (3 methylprednisolone pulses followed by oral prednisone 0.5 mg/kg/day during months 1, 3, and 5) and chlorambucil (0.2 mg/kg/day during months 2, 4, and 6) or treatment based on symptoms (164). The probability of surviving without developing renal failure at 10 years was 92% in the treated group versus 60% in the control group. Complete or partial remissions were significantly more frequent in the treated group. Radhakrishnan et al. treated 10 nephrotic patients with cyclosporine for periods up to 43 months (165). Proteinuria decreased to less than 1 g/day in six patients and between 1 and 2 g/day in two patients. Repeat renal biopsies in five patients showed a decrease in the histologic activity index but a rise in the chronicity index. Serum creatinine levels were not significantly increased at the end of the study.

Patients with a worsening of renal function should have a repeat renal biopsy, as patients with membranous nephropathy may develop proliferative glomerulonephritis. In this setting, aggressive treatment must be undertaken rapidly.

Other Therapeutic Approaches

Plasma exchange has been proposed with the goal of removing immune complexes that may be involved in the pathogenesis of lupus nephritis. A randomized controlled trial of 86 patients with severe lupus nephritis compared a standard therapy with prednisone and oral cyclophosphamide to the same treatment with plasma exchanges, three times a week for 4 weeks (166). The mean follow-up was 136 weeks. There were no differences between both groups in terms of patient survival, renal survival, clinical activity of the disease, and complications. However, plasma exchange may not be of help in individual patients (167,168). A multicenter trial of the effects of synchronized plasma exchanges and cyclophosphamide pulses in patients with very severe lupus is currently in progress.

Intravenous immunoglobulins have been reported to be effective in individual patients, including patients with proliferative lupus nephritis (169–171). Cyclosporine has been given to patients who were not well controlled by standard therapy. The treatment was followed by a decrease of proteinuria and an improvement of renal function, and the dose of prednisone could be tapered (172). These results suggest that cyclosporine may be used as a steroid-sparing agent in some patients. Several biologic agents have recently been studied in SLE. LJP-394, which consists of four linked oligonucleotides, has been shown to decrease anti-DNA titers (173). Anti-CD40 ligand monoclonal antibodies improve renal disease in murine lupus (174). However, studies in humans were abandoned because of thrombotic complications (175).

PROGNOSIS AND COMPLICATIONS

Until 30 years ago, the prognosis of patients with lupus nephritis was very poor. Better management of lupus has improved the prognosis with a 10-year survival rate exceeding 80% (176). The disease is often marked by flares and periods of remission. The prognosis of SLE must also take into consideration iatrogenic complications, because they are often linked with flares of the disease, particularly infections, vascular complications, osteonecrosis, or thrombosis.

Infectious complications are a significant cause of death during the course of SLE (177). These are favored by leukopenia and the reduction of the phagocytic functions, functional asplenia, hypocomplementemia, and, more important, by treatment with corticosteroids and immunosuppressive agents (178–180). Some authors have recommended systematic preventive antibiotherapy and antipneumococcal vaccination. Sepsis may be difficult to distinguish from a relapse of lupus. Herpes zoster is very common among the viral complications (9,181). Early treatment with acyclovir avoids dissemination.

Accelerated atherosclerosis is now recognized as a frequent cause of morbidity and mortality in young adults with lupus, and the process may start during childhood (181–186). Myocardial infarction has been reported in very young patients (187). The pathogenesis is probably multifactorial and includes inflammatory vascular disease, APL antibodies, hypertension, lipid abnormalities associated with the nephrotic syndrome or renal insufficiency, and corticosteroids (188–193). The risk of coronary disease is multiplied nine times during the course of SLE and increases with age and the duration of the disease.

Thrombosis is another common complication of SLE (194). The risk factors include APL antibodies, decreased levels of plasminogen activator, decreased levels of protein S, and in some patients, the additional risks related to the nephrotic syndrome (195–200). Arterial thromboses are observed in lupus patients with APL antibodies and often involve cerebral arteries (201). Venous thromboses are more common (202). Pulmonary embolism is frequent and may be complicated by pulmonary hypertension.

End-stage renal failure occurs in 10 to 20% of patients with severe renal disease after a mean period of 5 years (203,204). While lupus nephritis progresses to renal insufficiency, the activity of SLE often diminishes in terms of other clinical manifestations and biologic symptoms (205). Dialysis can be started and these patients do as well as non-lupus patients with end-stage renal disease. Some patients, however, have a rapid course to renal failure, maintaining clinical and serologic signs of activity. Therapeutic decisions are difficult as aggressive treatments may allow a recovery of renal function and discontinuation of dialysis. On the other hand, these patients are at higher risk of iatrogenic complications, particularly infection, which may be life-threatening (206,207). Clinical and biologic symptoms of the disease most often improve in patients on chronic dialysis, thus allowing stopping of corticosteroids and immunosuppressive therapy. However, clinical manifestations can persist or even appear at this stage.

Renal transplantation is the treatment of choice for those who progress to renal failure. The outcome after renal transplantation in these patients is similar to that of patients with other diseases in adults (208–211) and children (212). However, it is advisable to wait before proposing transplantation until the clinical and serologic activity of lupus has decreased for a few months. Moreover, a period without corticosteroids and immunosuppressive agents may be beneficial to the child. After renal transplantation, the activity of the disease declines, and recurrence in the graft is unusual. The very low rate of recurrence of the disease after transplantation is a strong argument against a direct role of circulating immune complexes in the pathogenesis of the nephropathy.

Ischemic thrombosis of the bone is a rare complication of lupus in children. Several factors may be involved, including the presence of APL antibodies and corticosteroid therapy. It may affect any bone, but the femoral head and the femoral condyle are more commonly involved (213). Bone mineral density measurements may show osteoporosis, and a recent study found an inverse correlation between bone mineral density and the cumulative dosage of corticosteroid but no significant correlation between bone mineral density and duration or activity of the disease (214).

Growth retardation is a major concern in children treated for several years with corticosteroids, particularly those who need to maintain on daily steroid therapy. Other complications of corticosteroids include cataracts, gastrointestinal hemorrhage, and diabetes mellitus. A cushingoid aspect is frequent and often badly tolerated by adolescent girls. It may explain poor compliance leading to severe relapses.

Side effects of cytotoxic drugs are common. The incidence of hemorrhagic cystitis after IV cyclophosphamide is very low, provided adequate hydration using the IV route is given (141). To minimize the risk of hemorrhagic cystitis, mesna, which binds to cyclophosphamide metabolites in the urine, may be helpful. Nausea and vomiting may be in part prevented by the concomitant use of antiemetic agents such as ondansetron (Zofran). Cyclophosphamide pulses often result in neutropenia with a serious risk of infection, which may be life-threatening (180). Children and their families should be aware of the risk of transient alopecia. Ovarian toxicity is another serious complication (215,216). The risk of amenorrhea depends on the age of the patient at the start of treatment and the total number of pulses (217). When treatment is given for 6 months, the risk of amenorrhea is very low if the patient is younger than 25 years, whereas 25% of patients older than 30 years will develop this complication. When the total number of pulses exceeds 15, the probability of developing amenorrhea is 17% for patients younger than 25 years and nearly 100% for those older than 30 years. Gonadotropin-releasing hormone antagonist may preserve ovarian function (218). There are no published data on long-term gonadal toxicity of cyclophosphamide pulses given to prepubertal girls. The gonadal toxicity of pulse cyclophosphamide in men has not been studied. However, studies in children with idiopathic nephrotic syndrome suggest that this toxicity may occur if the cumulative dosage is higher than 200 mg/kg. Severe infections have been reported in children with lupus nephritis after IV cyclophosphamide (219). It should be noted that no disseminated malignancies have been reported in patients treated with cyclophosphamide pulses, although longer follow-up periods are needed before any definite conclusions may be drawn.

REFERENCES

1. Tan EM, Cohen AS, Fries JF, et al. The 1982 revised criteria for the classification of systemic lupus erythematosus. *Arthritis Rheum* 1982;25:1271–1277.
2. Hochberg MC. Updating the American College of Rheumatology Revised criteria for the classification of systemic lupus erythematosus. *Arthritis Rheum* 1997;40:1725.
3. Hochberg MC. Systemic lupus erythematosus. *Rheum Dis Clin North Am* 1990;16:617–639.
4. Citera G, Wilson WA. Ethnic and geographic perspectives in SLE. *Lupus* 1993;2:351–353.
5. Symmons DP. Frequency of lupus in people of African origin. *Lupus* 1995;4:176–178.
6. Gardner-Medwin JM, Dolezalova P, Cummins C, et al. Incidence of Henoch-Schönlein purpura, Kawasaki disease, and rare vasculitides in children of different ethnic origins. *Lancet* 2002;360:1197–1202.
7. Parks C, Cooper G. Explaining racial disparity in systemic lupus erythematosus. Environmental and genetic risk factors in the Carolina lupus study. *Ann Epidemiol* 2002;12:62.
8. Cameron JS. Lupus nephritis. *J Am Soc Nephrol* 1999;10:413–424.
9. Platt JL, Burke BA, Fish AJ, et al. Systemic lupus erythematosus in the first two decades of life. *Am J Kidney Dis* 1982;11:S212–S222.
10. Tucker LB, Menon S, Schaller JG, et al. Adult- and childhood-onset systemic lupus erythematosus: a comparison of onset, clinical features, and outcome. *Br J Rheumatol* 1995;34:866–872.
11. Hood MJ, tenCate R, van Suijlekom Smit LWA, et al. Childhood-onset systemic lupus erythematosus—clinical presentation and prognosis in 31 patients. *Scand J Rheumatol* 1999;28:222–226.
12. Carreno L, Lopes-Longo FJ, Montaegudo I, et al. Immunological and clinical differences between juvenile and adult onset systemic lupus erythematosus. *Lupus* 1999;8:287–292.
13. Font J, Cervera R, Espinosa G, et al. Systemic lupus erythematosus (SLE) in childhood: analysis of clinical and immunological findings in 34 patients and comparison with SLE characteristics in adults. *Ann Rheum Dis* 1998;57:456–459.
14. Michel M, Johanet C, Meyer O, et al. Familial lupus erythematosus. Clinical and immunologic features of 125 multiplex families. *Medicine (Baltimore)* 2001;80:153–158.
15. Tsao BP. An update on genetic studies of systemic lupus erythematosus. *Curr Rheumatol Rep* 2002;4:359–367.
16. Prokunina L, Castillejo-Lopez C, Oberg F, et al. A regulatory polymorphism in PDCD1 is associated with susceptibility to systemic lupus erythematosus in humans. *Nat Genet* 2002;32:666–669.
17. Napirei M, Karsunky H, Zevnik B, et al. Features of systemic lupus erythematosus in Dnase1-deficient mice. *Nat Genet* 2000;25:177–181.
18. Yasutomo K, Horiuchi T, Kagami S, et al. Mutation of DNASE1 in people with systemic lupus erythematosus. *Nat Genet* 2001;28:313–314.
19. Nishimura H, Okazaki T, Tanaka Y, et al. Autoimmune dilated cardiomyopathy in PD-1 receptor-deficient mice. *Science* 2001;291:319–322.
20. Hibbs ML, Tarlinton DM, Armes J, et al. Multiple defects in the immune system of Lyn-deficient mice, culminating in autoimmune disease. *Cell* 1995;83:301–311.
21. Liossis SN, Solomou EE, Dimopoulos MA, et al. B-cell kinase lyn deficiency in patients with systemic lupus erythematosus. *J Investig Med* 2001;49:157–165.

22. Balomenos D, Martin-Caballero J, Garcia MI, et al. The cell cycle inhibitor p21 controls T-cell proliferation and sex-linked lupus development. *Nat Med* 2000;6:171–176.
23. Ho CY, Wong CK, Li EK, et al. Expression of cyclin B1 and cyclin dependent kinase inhibitor p21 in lymphocytes in patients with systemic lupus erythematosus. *J Rheumatol* 2002;29:2537–2544.
24. Botto M, Dell'Agnola C, Bygrave AE, et al. Homozygous C1q deficiency causes glomerulonephritis associated with multiple apoptotic bodies. *Nat Genet* 1998;19:56–59.
25. Walport MJ, Davies KA, Botto M. C1q and systemic lupus erythematosus. *Immunobiology* 1998;199:265–285.
26. Bickerstaff MC, Botto M, Hutchinson WL, et al. Serum amyloid P component controls chromatin degradation and prevents antinuclear autoimmunity. *Nat Med* 1999;5:694–697.
27. Sorensen IJ, Holm Nielsen E, Schroder L, et al. Complexes of serum amyloid P component and DNA in serum from healthy individuals and systemic lupus erythematosus patients. *J Clin Immunol* 2000;20:408–415.
28. Incaprera M, Rindi L, Bazzichi A, et al. Potential role of the Epstein-Barr virus in systemic lupus erythematosus autoimmunity. *Clin Exp Rheumatol* 1998;16:289–294.
29. James JA, Neas BR, Moser KL, et al. Systemic lupus erythematosus in adults is associated with previous Epstein-Barr virus exposure. *Arthritis Rheum* 2001;44:1122–1126.
30. Casciola-Rosen LA, Anhalt G, Rosen A. Autoantigens targeted in systemic lupus erythematosus are clustered in two populations of surface structures on apoptotic keratinocytes. *J Exp Med* 1994;179:1317–1330.
31. Hieronymus T, Grotsch P, Blank N, et al. Chlorpromazine induces apoptosis in activated human lymphoblasts: a mechanism supporting the induction of drug-induced lupus erythematosus? *Arthritis Rheum* 2000;43:1994–2004.
32. Lahita RG. Sex hormones and systemic lupus erythematosus. *Rheum Dis Clin North Am* 2000;26:951–968.
33. McMurray RW. Sex hormones in the pathogenesis of systemic lupus erythematosus. *Front Biosci* 2001;6:E193–E206.
34. Cooper GS, Dooley MA, Treadwell EL, et al. Hormonal and reproductive risk factors for development of systemic lupus erythematosus: results of a population-based, case-control study. *Arthritis Rheum* 2002;46:1830–1839.
35. Shlomchik MJ, Craft JE, Mamula MJ. From T to B and back again: positive feedback in systemic autoimmune disease. *Nat Rev Immunol* 2001;1:147–153.
36. Prodeus AP, Goerg S, Shen LM, et al. A critical role for complement in maintenance of self-tolerance. *Immunity* 1998;9:721–731.
37. Nash JT, Taylor PR, Botto M, et al. Immune complex processing in C1q-deficient mice. *Clin Exp Immunol* 2001;123:196–202.
38. Scott RS, McMahon EJ, Pop SM, et al. Phagocytosis and clearance of apoptotic cells is mediated by MER. *Nature* 2001;411:207–211.
39. Janeway CA Jr, Bottomly K. Signals and signs for lymphocyte responses. *Cell* 1994;76:275–285.
40. Amoura Z, Koutouzov S, Piette JC. The role of nucleosomes in lupus. *Curr Opin Rheumatol* 2000;12:369–373.
41. Blanco P, Palucka AK, Gill M, et al. Induction of dendritic cell differentiation by IFN-alpha in systemic lupus erythematosus. *Science* 2001;294:1540–1543.
42. Pickering MC, Botto M, Taylor PR, et al. Systemic lupus erythematosus, complement deficiency, and apoptosis. *Adv Immunol* 2000;76:227–324.
43. Rosenberg AM. Systemic lupus erythematosus in children. *Springer Semin Immunopathol* 1994;16:261–279.
44. Cervera R, Khamashta MA, Font J, et al. Systemic lupus erythematosus: clinical and immunologic patterns of disease expression in a cohort of 1,000 patients. The European Working Party on Systemic Lupus Erythematosus. *Medicine* 1993;72:113–124.
45. Nived O, Johansen PB, Sturfelt G. Standardized ultraviolet-A exposure provokes skin reaction in SLE. *Lupus* 1993;2:247–250.
46. Duffy KN, Duffy CM, Gladman DD. Infection and disease activity in SLE: a review of hospitalized patients. *J Rheumatol* 1991;18:1180–1184.
47. Adams SG Jr, Dammers PM, Saia TL, et al. Stress, depression, and anxiety predict average symptom severity and daily symptom fluctuation in SLE. *J Behav Med* 1994;17:459–477.
48. Pistiner M, Wallace DJ, Nessim S, et al. Lupus erythematosus in the 1980s: a survey of 570 patients. *Semin Arthritis Rheum* 1991;21:55–64.
49. Pan TL, Thumboo J, Boey ML. Primary and secondary pulmonary hypertension in systemic lupus erythematosus. *Lupus* 2000;9:338–342.
50. Leung WH, Wing KL, Lau CP, et al. Association between antiphospholipid antibodies and cardiac abnormalities in patients with systemic lupus erythematosus. *Am J Med* 1990;89:411–419.
51. Quintero-Del-Rio AI, Van M. Neurologic symptoms in children with systemic lupus erythematosus. *J Child Neurol* 2000;15:803–807.
52. Steinlin MI, Blaser SI, Gilday DL, et al. Neurologic manifestations of childhood lupus erythematosus. *Pediatr Neurol* 1995;13:191–197.
53. Denburg SD, Carbotte RM, Denburg JA. Corticosteroids and neuropsychological functioning in patients with systemic lupus erythematosus. *Arthritis Rheum* 1994;37:1311–1320.
54. Iverson GL, Anderson KW. The etiology of psychiatric symptoms in patients with systemic lupus erythematosus. *Scand J Rheumatol* 1994;23:277–282.
55. Miguel EC, Pereira RM, Pereira CA, et al. Psychiatric manifestations of systemic lupus erythematosus: clinical features, symptoms, and signs of central nervous system activity in 43 patients. *Medicine* 1994;73:224–232.
56. Karassa FB, Ioannidis JP, Touloumi G, et al. Risk factors for central nervous system involvement in systemic lupus erythematosus. *QJM* 2000;93:169–174.
57. Levine JS, Branch W, Rauch J. The antiphospholipid syndrome. *N Engl J Med* 2002;346:752–763.
58. Lee T, von Scheven E, Sandborg C. Systemic lupus erythematosus and antiphospholipid syndrome in children and adolescents. *Curr Opin Rheumatol* 2001;13:415–421.
59. Daugas E, Nochy D, Huong du LT, et al. Antiphospholipid syndrome nephropathy in systemic lupus erythematosus. *J Am Soc Nephrol* 2002;13:42–52.
60. Berube C, Mitchell L, Silverman E, et al. The relationship of antiphospholipid antibodies to thromboembolic events

in pediatric patients with systemic lupus erythematosus: a cross-sectional study. *Pediatr Res* 1998;44:351–356.
61. Massengill SF, Hedrick C, Ayoub EM, et al. Antiphospholipid antibodies in pediatric lupus nephritis. *Am J Kidney Dis* 1997;29:355–361.
62. Mok CC, Wong RW. Pregnancy in systemic lupus erythematosus. *Postgrad Med J* 2001;77:157–165.
63. Hallegua DS, Wallace DJ. Gastrointestinal manifestations of systemic lupus erythematosus. *Curr Opin Rheumatol* 2000; 12:379–385.
64. Deocharan B, Qing X, Lichauco J, et al. Alpha-actinin is a cross-reactive renal target for pathogenic anti-DNA antibodies. *J Immunol* 2002;168:3072–3078.
65. Korb LC, Ahearn JM. C1q binds directly and specifically to surface blebs of apoptotic human keratinocytes: complement deficiency and systemic lupus erythematosus revisited. *J Immunol* 1997;158:4525–4528.
66. Clynes R, Dumitru C, Ravetch JV. Uncoupling of immune complex formation and kidney damage in autoimmune glomerulonephritis. *Science* 1998;279:1052–1054.
67. Seligman VA, Suarez C, Lum R, et al. The Fcgamma receptor IIIA-158F allele is a major risk factor for the development of lupus nephritis among Caucasians but not non-Caucasians. *Arthritis Rheum* 2001;44:618–625.
68. Karassa FB, Trikalinos TA, Ioannidis JP. Role of the Fcgamma receptor IIa polymorphism in susceptibility to systemic lupus erythematosus and lupus nephritis: a meta-analysis. *Arthritis Rheum* 2002;46:1563–1571.
69. Ponticelli C, Moroni G. Renal biopsy in lupus nephritis—what for, when and how often? *Nephrol Dial Transplant* 1998;13:2452–2454.
70. McCluskey RT. Lupus nephritis. In: Summers SC, ed. *Kidney pathology: Decennial.* New York: Appleton & Lange, 1975:456–459.
71. Churg J, Berstein J, Glassock RJ. Lupus nephritis. In: Churg J, Berstein J, Glassock RJ, eds. *Renal diseases. Classification and atlas of glomerular diseases.* New York: Igaku-Shoin, 1995:151.
72. Appel GB, Cohen DJ, Pirani CL, et al. Long-term follow-up of lupus nephritis: a study based on the WHO classification. *Am J Med* 1987;83:877–885.
73. Balwin. Clinical usefulness of the morphological classification of lupus nephritis. *Am J Kidney Dis* 1982;2:142–149.
74. Lee HS, Mujais SK, Kasinath BS, et al. Course of renal pathology in patients with systemic lupus erythematosus. *Am J Med* 1984;77:612–620.
75. Schwartz MM, Kawala KS, Corwin H, et al. The prognosis of segmental glomerulonephritis in systemic lupus erythematosus. *Kidney Int* 1987;32:274–279.
76. Pirani CL, Salinas-Madrigal L. Evaluation of percutaneous renal biopsy. In: Sommers SC, ed. *Pathology annual,* Vol 3. New York: Appleton Century Crofts, 1968:249–254.
77. Morel-Maroger L, Mery JP, Droz D, et al. The course of lupus nephritis: contribution of serial renal biopsies. *Adv Nephrol* 1976;6:79–86.
78. Austin HA, Munez LR, Joyce KM, et al. Prognostic factors in lupus nephritis. Contribution of renal histological data. *Am J Med* 1983;75:382–391.
79. Najafi CC, Korbet SM, Lewis EJ, et al. Significance of histologic patterns of glomerular injury upon long-term prognosis in severe lupus glomerulonephritis. *Kidney Int* 2001; 59:2156–2163.
80. Schwartz MM, Lan SP, Bernstein J, et al. The role of pathology indices in the management of severe lupus glomerulonephritis. *Kidney Int* 1992;42:743–748.
81. Hill GS, Delahousse M, Nochy D, et al. Predictive power of the second renal biopsy in lupus nephritis: significance of macrophages. *Kidney Int* 2001;59:304–316.
82. Austin HA, Munez LR, Joyce KM. Diffuse proliferative lupus nephritis: identification of specific pathologic features affecting renal outcome. *Kidney Int* 1984;25:689–695.
83. Esdaile JM, Levinton C, Federgreen W, et al. The clinical and renal biopsy predictors of long-term outcome in lupus nephritis: a study of 87 patients and review of the literature. *QJM* 1989;72:779–833.
84. Gruppo Italiano Per Lo Studio Della Nefrite Lupica (GISNEL). Lupus nephritis: prognostic factors and probability of maintaining life-supporting renal function 10 years after the diagnosis. *Am J Kidney Dis* 1992;19:473–479.
85. Donadio JV, Hart GM, Bergtal H, et al. Prognostic determinants in lupus nephritis: a long-term clinicopathologic study. *Lupus* 1995;4:109–115.
86. Austin HA, Boumpas DT, Vaughan EM, et al. Predicting renal outcomes in severe lupus nephritis: contributions of clinical and histologic data. *Kidney Int* 1994;45:544–550.
87. Appel GB, Valeri A. The course and treatment of lupus nephritis. *Ann Rev Med* 1994;45:525–537.
88. Iseki K, Miyasato F, Oura T, et al. An epidemiologic analysis of end-stage lupus nephritis. *Am J Kidney Dis* 1994;23:547–554.
89. Austin HA, Boumpas DT, Vaughan EM, et al. High-risk features of lupus nephritis: importance of race and clinical and histological factors in 166 patients. *Nephrol Dial Transplant* 1995;10:1620–1628.
90. Baqi N, Moazami S, Singh A, et al. Lupus nephritis in children—a longitudinal study of prognostic factors and therapy. *J Am Soc Nephrol* 1996;7:924–929.
91. Colon PJ, Fischer CA, Levesque MC, et al. Clinical, biochemical and pathological predictors of poor response to intravenous cyclophosphamide in patients with proliferative lupus nephritis. *Clin Nephrol* 1996;46:170–175.
92. Moroni G, Quaglini S, Maccario M, et al. "Nephritic flares" are predictors of bad long-term outcome in lupus nephritis. *Kidney Int* 1996;50:2047–2053.
93. Dooley MA, Hogan S, Jennette C, et al., for the Glomerular Disease Collaborative Network. Cyclophosphamide therapy for lupus nephritis: poor renal survival in black Americans. *Kidney Int* 1997;51:1188–1195.
94. Levey AS, Lan SP, Corwin HL, et al. Progression and remission of renal disease in the Lupus Nephritis Collaborative Study. Results of treatment with prednisone and short-term oral cyclophosphamide. *Ann Intern Med* 1992;116:114–123.
95. Magil AB, Puterman ML, Ballon HS, et al. Prognostic factors in diffuse proliferative lupus glomerulonephritis. *Kidney Int* 1998;34:511–517.
96. McCurdy DK, Lehman TJA, Berstein B, et al. Lupus nephritis: prognostic factors in children. *Pediatrics* 1992;89:240–246.
97. Ginzler EM, Diamond HS, Weiner M, et al. A multicenter study on outcome in systemic lupus erythematosus. I. Entry

variables as predictors of prognosis. *Arthritis Rheum* 1982; 25:601–611.
98. Esdaile JM, Joseph L, MacKenzie T, et al. The benefit of early treatment with immunosuppressive agents in lupus nephritis. *J Rheumatol* 1994;21:2046–2051.
99. Lim CS, Chin HJ, Jung YC, et al. Prognostic factors of diffuse proliferative lupus nephritis. *Clin Nephrol* 1999;52:139–147.
100. Conlon PJ, Fischer CA, Levesque MC, et al. Clinical, biochemical and pathological predictors of poor response to intravenous cyclophosphamide in patients with proliferative lupus nephritis. *Clin Nephrol* 1996;46:170–175.
101. Cameron JS. Lupus nephritis in childhood and adolescence. *Pediatr Nephrol* 1994;8:230–249.
102. Yang LY, Chen WP, Lin CY. Lupus nephritis in children—a review of 167 patients. *Pediatrics* 1994;94:335–340.
103. Emre S, Bilge I, Sirin A, et al. Lupus nephritis in children: prognostic significance of clinicopathological findings. *Nephron* 2001;87:118–126.
104. Baqi N, Moazami S, Singh A, et al. Lupus nephritis in children: a longitudinal study of prognostic factors and therapy. *J Am Soc Nephrol* 1996;7:924–929.
105. Pasquali S, Banfi G, Zucchelli A, et al. Lupus membranous nephropathy: long-term outcome. *Clin Nephrol* 1993;39: 175–182.
106. Sloan RP, Schwartz MM, Korbet SM, et al. Long-term outcome in systemic lupus erythematosus membranous glomerulonephritis. *J Am Soc Nephrol* 1996;7:299–305.
107. Pisetsky DS. Anti-DNA and autoantibodies. *Curr Opin Rheumatol* 2000;12:364–368.
108. von Muhlen CA, Tan EM. Autoantibodies in the diagnosis of systemic rheumatic diseases. *Semin Arthritis Rheum* 1995; 24:323–358.
109. Hahn BH. Antibodies to DNA. *N Engl J Med* 1998;338: 1359–1368.
110. Smeenk R, Brinkman K, van den Brink H, et al. Antibodies to DNA in patients with SLE. Their role in the diagnosis, the follow-up and the pathogenesis of the disease. *Clin Rheumatol* 1990;9:S100–S110.
111. Eaton RB, Schneider G, Schur PH. Enzyme immunoassay for antibodies to nDNA. Specificity and quality of antibodies. *Arthritis Rheum* 1983;26:52–62.
112. Munves EF, Schur PH. Antibodies to Sm and RNP: prognosticators of disease involvement. *Arthritis Rheum* 1983; 26:848–853.
113. Siegert CEH, Daha MR, Tseng C, et al. Predictive value of IgG autoantibodies against C1q for nephritis in systemic lupus erythematosus. *Ann Rheum Dis* 1993;52:851–856.
114. Siegert CE, Kazatchkine MD, Sjoholm A, et al. Autoantibodies against C1q: view on clinical relevance and pathogenic role. *Clin Exp Immunol* 1999;116:4–8.
115. Cardinali C, Caroni M, Fabbri P. The utility of the lupus band test on sun-protected non-lesional skin for the diagnosis of systemic lupus erythematosus. *Clin Exp Rheumatol* 1999;17:427–432.
116. Spronk PE, Limburg PC, Kallenberg CG. Serological markers of disease activity in systemic lupus erythematosus. *Lupus* 1995;4:86–94.
117. Hess E. Drug-induced lupus. *N Engl J Med* 1988;318: 1460–1462.
118. Fritzler MJ. Drugs recently associated with lupus syndromes. *Lupus* 1994;3:455–459.
119. Grant DM, Morike K, Eichelbaum M, et al. Acetylation pharmacokinetics. The slow acetylator phenotype is caused by decreased or absent arylamine *N*-acetyltransferase in human liver. *J Clin Invest* 1990;85:968–872.
120. Rubin RL, Bell SA, Burlingame RW. Autoantibodies associated with lupus induced by diverse drugs target a similar epitope in the (H2A-H2B)-DNA complex. *J Clin Invest* 1992;90:165–173.
121. Julkunen H, Kurki P, Kaaja R, et al. Isolated congenital heart block. Long-term outcome of mothers and characterization of the immune response to SS-A/Ro and to SS-B/La. *Arthritis Rheum* 1993;36:1588–1598.
122. Buyon JP, Kim MY, Copel JA, et al. Anti-Ro/SSA antibodies and congenital heart block: necessary but not sufficient. *Arthritis Rheum* 2001;44:1723–1727.
123. Lee LA. Neonatal lupus: clinical features, therapy, and pathogenesis. *Curr Rheumatol Rep* 2001;3:391–395.
124. Austin HA, Balow JE. Natural history and treatment of lupus nephritis. *Semin Nephrol* 1999;19:2–11.
125. Zimmerman R, Radhakrishnan J, Valeri A, et al. Advances in the treatment of lupus nephritis. *Annu Rev Med* 2001;52: 63–78.
126. Pollak VE, Pirani CL, Kark RM. Effects of large doses of prednisone on the renal lesions and life span of patients with lupus glomerulonephritis. *J Lab Clin Med* 1961;57:495–511.
127. Cathcart ES, Idelson BA, Scheinberg MA, et al. Beneficial effects of methylprednisolone "pulse" therapy in diffuse proliferative lupus nephritis. *Lancet* 1976;1:63–66.
128. Kimberly RP, Lockshin MD, Sherman RL, et al. High-dose intravenous methylprednisolone pulse therapy in systemic lupus erythematosus. *Am J Med* 1981;70:817–824.
129. Barron KS, Person DA, Brewer EJ, et al. Pulse methylprednisolone therapy in diffuse proliferative lupus nephritis. *J Pediatr* 1982;101:137–141.
130. Ponticelli C, Zucchelli P, Moroni G, et al. Long-term prognosis of diffuse lupus nephritis. *Clin Nephrol* 1987;28:263–271.
131. Gourley MF, Austin HA, Scott D, et al. Methylprednisolone and cyclophosphamide, alone or in combination, in patients with lupus nephritis. A randomized, controlled trial. *Ann Intern Med* 1996;125:549–557.
132. Donadio JV, Holley KE, Ferguson RH, et al. Treatment of diffuse proliferative lupus nephritis with prednisone and combined prednisone and cyclophosphamide. *N Engl J Med* 1978;299:1151–1155.
133. Steinberg AD. The treatment of lupus nephritis. *Kidney Int* 1986;30:769–787.
134. Austin HA, Klippel JH, Balow JE, et al. Therapy of lupus nephritis. *N Engl J Med* 1986;314:614–619.
135. Boumpas DT, Austin HA, Vaughn EM, et al. Controlled-trial of pulse methylprednisolone versus two regimen of pulse cyclophosphamide in severe lupus nephritis. *Lancet* 1992;340:741–745.
136. Appel GB. Cyclophosphamide therapy of severe lupus nephritis (Journal club). *Am J Kidney Dis* 1997;30:872–878.
137. Felson DT, Anderson J. Evidence for the superiority of immunosuppressive drugs and prednisone over prednisone

alone in lupus nephritis. Results of a pooled analysis. *N Engl J Med* 1984;311:1528–1533.
138. Steinberg AD, Steinberg SC. Long-term preservation of renal function in patients with lupus nephritis receiving treatment that includes cyclophosphamide versus those treated with prednisone only. *Arthritis Rheum* 1991;34:945–950.
139. McCune WJ, Golbus J, Zeldes W, et al. Clinical and immunologic effects of monthly administration of intravenous cyclophosphamide in severe systemic lupus erythematosus. *N Engl J Med* 1988;318:1423–1431.
140. Valeri A, Radhakrishnan J, Estes D, et al. Intravenous pulse cyclophosphamide treatment of severe lupus nephritis: a prospective five-year study. *Clin Nephrol* 1994;42:71–78.
141. Balow JE, Boumpas DT, Fessler BJ, et al. Management of lupus nephritis. *Kidney Int* 1996;49:S88–S92.
142. Illei GG, Austin HA, Crane M, et al. Combination therapy with pulse cyclophosphamide plus pulse methylprednisolone improves long-term renal outcome without adding toxicity in patients with lupus nephritis. *Ann Intern Med* 2001;135:248–257.
143. Niaudet P. Treatment of lupus nephritis in children. *Pediatr Nephrol* 2000;14:158–166.
144. Lehman TJA, Sherry DD, Wagner-Weiner L. Intermittent intravenous cyclophosphamide therapy in lupus nephritis. *J Pediatr* 1989;114:1055–1060.
145. Houssiau FA, Vasconcelos C, D'Cruz D, et al. Immunosuppressive therapy in lupus nephritis: the Euro-Lupus Nephritis Trial, a randomized trial of low-dose versus high-dose intravenous cyclophosphamide. *Arthritis Rheum* 2002;46:2121–2131.
146. Lim CS, Chin HJ, Jung YC, et al. Prognostic factors of diffuse proliferative lupus nephritis. *Clin Nephrol* 1999;52:139–147.
147. Van Bruggen MC, Walgreen B, Rijke TP, et al. Attenuation of murine lupus nephritis by mycophenolate mofetil. *J Am Soc Nephrol* 1998;9:1407–1415.
148. Zoja C, Benigni A, Noris M, et al. Mycophenolate mofetil combined with a cyclooxygenase-2 inhibitor ameliorates murine lupus nephritis. *Kidney Int* 2001;60:653–663.
149. Jonsson CA, Svensson L, Carlsten H. Beneficial effect of the inosine monophosphate dehydrogenase inhibitor mycophenolate mofetil on survival and severity of glomerulonephritis in systemic lupus erythematosus (SLE)-prone MRLlpr/lpr mice. *Clin Exp Immunol* 1999;116:534–541.
150. Dooley MA, Cosio FG, Nachman PH, et al. Mycophenolate mofetil therapy in lupus nephritis: clinical observations. *J Am Soc Nephrol* 1999;10:833–839.
151. Glicklich D, Acharya A. Mycophenolate mofetil therapy for lupus nephritis refractory to intravenous cyclophosphamide. *Am J Kidney Dis* 1998;32:318–322.
152. Kingdon EJ, McLean AG, Psimenou E, et al. The safety and efficacy of MMF in lupus nephritis: a pilot study. *Lupus* 2001;10:606–611.
153. Buratti S, Szer IS, Spencer CH, et al. Mycophenolate mofetil treatment of severe renal disease in pediatric onset systemic lupus erythematosus. *J Rheumatol* 2001;28:2103–2108.
154. Gaubitz M, Schorat A, Schotte H, et al. Mycophenolate mofetil for the treatment of systemic lupus erythematosus: an open pilot trial. *Lupus* 1999;8:731–736.
155. Chan TM, Li FK, Tang CS, et al. Efficacy of mycophenolate mofetil in patients with diffuse proliferative lupus nephritis. Hong Kong-Guangzhou Nephrology Study Group. *N Engl J Med* 2000;343:1156–1162.
156. Li LS, Hu WX, Chen HP, et al. Mycophenolate mofetil vs cytoxan pulse for induction of DPLN (Abstract). *J Am Soc Nephrol* 2000;11:A486.
157. Ye ZZ, Tan YH, Hong XP. Mycophenolate mofetil versus cyclophosphamide in the treatment of severe SLE patients. *Lupus* 2001;10(Suppl 1):S99.
158. Mok CC, Ho CT, Chan KW, et al. Outcome and prognostic indicators of diffuse proliferative lupus glomerulonephritis treated with sequential oral cyclophosphamide and azathioprine. *Arthritis Rheum* 2002;46:1003–1013.
159. Ponticelli C, Moroni G, Banfi G. Discontinuation of therapy in diffuse proliferative lupus nephritis. *Am J Med* 1988;85:275.
160. Hebert LA, Dillon JJ, Middendorf DF, et al. Relationship between appearance of urinary red blood cell/white blood cell casts and onset of renal relapse in systemic lupus erythematosus. *Am J Kidney Dis* 1995;26:432–438.
161. ter Borg EJ, Horst G, Hummel EJ, et al. Measurement of increases in anti-double-stranded DNA antibody levels as a predictor of disease exacerbation in systemic lupus erythematosus. A long-term, prospective study. *Arthritis Rheum* 1990;33:634–643.
162. Leblanc BA, Gladman DD, Urowitz MB. Serologically active, clinically quiescent systemic lupus erythematosus—long-term followup. *J Rheumatol* 1994;21:174–175.
163. Ponticelli C. Treatment of lupus nephritis—the advantages of a flexible approach. *Nephrol Dial Transplant* 1997;12:2057–2059.
164. Moroni G, Maccario M, Banfi G, et al. Treatment of membranous lupus nephritis. *Am J Kidney Dis* 1998;31:681–686.
165. Radhakrishnan J, Kunis CL, Dagati V, et al. Cyclosporine treatment of lupus membranous nephropathy. *Clin Nephrol* 1994;42:147–154.
166. Lewis EJ, Hunsicker LG, Lan SP, et al. A controlled trial of plasmapheresis therapy during severe lupus nephritis. *N Engl J Med* 1992;326:1373–1379.
167. Jordan SC, Ho W, Ettenger R, et al. Plasma exchange improves glomerulonephritis of systemic lupus erythematosus in selected pediatric patients. *Pediatr Nephrol* 1987;1:276–280.
168. Dau PC, Callaghan J, Parker R, et al. Immunologic effects of plasmapheresis synchronized with pulse cyclophosphamide in systemic lupus erythematosus. *J Rheumatol* 1991;18:227–276.
169. Lin CY, Hsu HC, Chiang H. Improvement of histological and immunological change in steroid and immunosuppressive drug-resistant lupus nephritis by high-dose intravenous gamma globulin. *Nephron* 1989;53:303–310.
170. Oliet A, Hernandez E, Gallar P, et al. High-dose intravenous gamma-globulin in systemic lupus erythematosus. *Nephron* 1992;62:465.
171. Boletis JN, Ioannidis JP, Boki KA, et al. Intravenous immunoglobulin compared with cyclophosphamide for proliferative lupus nephritis. *Lancet* 1999;354:569–570.
172. Favre H, Miescher PA, Huang YP, et al. Cyclosporin in the treatment of lupus nephritis. *Am J Nephrol* 1989;9:S57–S60.

173. Tumlin J. Lupus nephritis: novel immunosuppressive modalities and future directions. *Semin Nephrol* 1999;19:67–76.
174. Kalled SL, Cutler AH, Datta SK, et al. Anti-CD40 ligand antibody treatment of SNF1 mice with established nephritis: preservation of kidney function. *J Immunol* 1998;160:2158–2165.
175. Kawai T, Andrews D, Colvin RB, et al. Thromboembolic complications after treatment with monoclonal antibodies against CD40 ligand. *Nat Med* 2000;6:114–115.
176. Trager J, Ward MM. Mortality and causes of death in systemic lupus erythematosus. *Curr Opin Rheumatol* 2001;13:345–351.
177. Petri M. Infection in systemic lupus erythematosus. *Rheum Dis Clin North Am* 1998;24:423–456.
178. Ginsler E, Sharon E, Diamond H, et al. Computer analysis of factors influencing frequency of infection in systemic lupus erythematosus. *Arthritis Rheum* 1978;21:37–44.
179. Paton NI, Cheong IK, Kong NC, et al. Risk factors for infection in Malaysian patients with systemic lupus erythematosus. *QJM* 1996;89:531–538.
180. Pryor BD, Bologna SG, Kahl LE. Risk factors for serious infection during treatment with cyclophosphamide and high-dose corticosteroids for systemic lupus erythematosus. *Arthritis Rheum* 1996;39:1475–1482.
181. Bono L, Cameron JS, Hicks JA. The very long-term prognosis and complications of lupus nephritis and its treatment. *QJM* 1999;92:211–218.
182. Farhey Y, Hess EV. Accelerated atherosclerosis and coronary disease in SLE. *Lupus* 1997;6:572–577.
183. Urowitz M, Gladman D, Bruce I. Atherosclerosis and systemic lupus erythematosus. *Curr Rheumatol Rep* 2000;2:19–23.
184. Ilowite NT. Premature atherosclerosis in systemic lupus erythematosus. *J Rheumatol* 2000;27(Suppl)58:15–19.
185. Karrar A, Sequeira W, Block JA. Coronary artery disease in systemic lupus erythematosus: a review of the literature. *Semin Arthritis Rheum* 2001;30:436–443.
186. Salmon JE, Roman MJ. Accelerated atherosclerosis in systemic lupus erythematosus: implications for patient management. *Curr Opin Rheumatol* 2001;13:341–344.
187. Ishikawa S, Segar WE, Gilbert EF, et al. Myocardial infarct in a child with lupus erythematosus. *Am J Dis Child* 1978; 132:696–699.
188. Aranow C, Ginzler EM. Epidemiology of cardiovascular disease in systemic lupus erythematosus. *Lupus* 2000;9:166–169.
189. Svenungsson E, Jensen-Urstad K, Heimburger M, et al. Risk factors for cardiovascular disease in systemic lupus erythematosus. *Circulation* 2001;104:1887–1893.
190. Koike T. Antiphospholipid antibodies in arterial thrombosis. *Ann Med* 2000;32(Suppl)1:27–31.
191. Ostrov BE, Min W, Eichenfield AH, et al. Hypertension in children with systemic lupus erythematosus. *Semin Arthritis Rheum* 1989;19:90–98.
192. Ilowite NT, Samual P, Ginzler E, et al. Dyslipoproteinemia in pediatric systemic lupus erythematosus. *Arthritis Rheum* 1998;31:859–863.
193. Bulkley HB, Roberts WC. The heart in systemic lupus erythematosus and the changes induced in it by corticosteroid therapy. *Am J Med* 1975;58:243–264.
194. Montes de Oca MA, Babron MC, Blétry O, et al. Thrombosis in systemic lupus erythematosus: a French collaborative study. *Arch Dis Child* 1991;66:713–717.
195. Qushmaq K, Esdaile J, Devine DV. Thrombosis in systemic lupus erythematosus: the role of antiphospholipid antibody. *Arthritis Care Res* 1999;12:212–219.
196. Esmon NL, Smirnov MD, Safa O, et al. Lupus anticoagulants, thrombosis and the protein C system. *Haematologica* 1999;84:446–451.
197. Galli M, Finazzi G, Norbis F, et al. The risk of thrombosis in patients with lupus anticoagulants is predicted by their specific coagulation profile. *Thromb Haemost* 1999;81:695–700.
198. Male C, Lechner K, Eichinger S, et al. Clinical significance of lupus anticoagulants in children. *J Pediatr* 1999;134:199–205.
199. Angles-Cano E, Sultan Y, Clavel J. predisposing factors to thrombosis in systemic lupus erythematosus: possible relation to endothelial cell damage. *J Lab Clin Med* 1979;94:312–323.
200. Haselaar P, Derksen RHWM, Blokzijl L, et al. Risk factors for thrombosis in lupus patients. *Ann Rheum Dis* 1989;48:933–940.
201. Asherson RA, Khamashra MA, Gil A, et al. Cerebrovascular disease and antiphospholipid antibodies in systemic lupus erythematosus, lupus-like disorders and the primary antiphospholipid syndrome. *Am J Med* 1991;86:391–399.
202. Appel G, Williams GS, Melzer JI, et al. Renal vein thrombosis, nephrotic syndrome and systemic lupus erythematosus. *Ann Intern Med* 1976;85:310–317.
203. Cheigh JS, Stenzl KH. End-stage renal disease in systemic lupus erythematosus. *Am J Kidney Dis* 1993;21:2–8.
204. Berden JHM. Lupus nephritis. *Kidney Int* 1997;52:538–558.
205. Bruce IN, Hallett DC, Gladman DD, et al. Extrarenal disease activity in systemic lupus erythematosus is not suppressed by chronic renal insufficiency or renal replacement therapy. *J Rheumatol* 1999;26:1490–1494.
206. Leaker B, Fairley KF, Dowling J, et al. Lupus nephritis: clinical and pathological correlation. *QJM* 1987;238:163–179.
207. Nossent JC, Swaak AJG, Berden JHM. Systemic lupus erythematosus: analysis of disease activity in 55 patients with end stage renal failure with hemodialysis or continuous ambulatory peritoneal dialysis. *Am J Med* 1990;89:169–174.
208. Nossent JC, Swaak AJG, Berden JHM. Systemic lupus erythematosus after renal transplantation: patient and graft survival and disease activity. *Ann Intern Med* 1991;114:183–188.
209. Goss JA, Cole BR, Jendrisak MD, et al. Renal transplantation for systemic lupus erythematosus and recurrent lupus nephritis. A single center experience and review of the literature. *Transplantation* 1991;52:805–810.
210. Mojcik CF, Klippel JH. End-stage renal disease and systemic lupus erythematosus. *Am J Med* 1996;101:100–107.
211. Ward MM. Outcomes of renal transplantation among patients with end-stage renal disease caused by lupus nephritis. *Kidney Int* 2000;57:2136–2143.
212. Bartosh SM, Fine RN, Kenneth Sullivan E. Outcome after transplantation of young patients with systemic lupus erythematosus: a report of the north American pediatric renal transplant cooperative study. *Transplantation* 2001;72:973–978.
213. Bergstein JM, Wiens C, Fish AJ. Avascular necrosis of bone in systemic lupus erythematosus. *J Pediatr* 1974;85:31–35.

214. Trapani S, Civinini R, Ermini M, et al. Osteoporosis in juvenile systemic lupus erythematosus: a longitudinal study on the effect of steroids on bone mineral density. *Rheumatol Int* 1998;18:45–49.
215. Mcdermott EM, Powell RJ. Incidence of ovarian failure in systemic lupus erythematosus after treatment with pulse cyclophosphamide. *Ann Rheum Dis* 1996;55:224–229.
216. Mok CC, Lau CS, Wong RW. Risk factors for ovarian failure in patients with systemic lupus erythematosus receiving cyclophosphamide therapy. *Arthritis Rheum* 1998;41:831–837.
217. Boumpas DT, Austin HA, Vaughan EM, et al. Risk of sustained amenorrhea in patients with systemic lupus erythematosus treated with intermittent pulse cyclophosphamide therapy. *Ann Intern Med* 1993;119:366–369.
218. Blumenfeld Z, Shapiro D, Shteinberg M, et al. Preservation of fertility and ovarian function and minimizing gonadotoxicity in young women with systemic lupus erythematosus treated by chemotherapy. *Lupus* 2000;9:401–405.
219. Tangnararatchakit K, Tapaneya-Olarn C, Tapaneya-Olarn W. The efficacy of intravenous pulse cyclophosphamide in the treatment of severe lupus nephritis in children. *J Med Assoc Thai* 1999;82(Suppl)1:S104–S110.

47

HEMOLYTIC UREMIC SYNDROMES

CHANTAL LOIRAT
C. MARK TAYLOR

DEFINITIONS OF HEMOLYTIC UREMIC SYNDROME AND THROMBOTIC THROMBOCYTOPENIC PURPURA

The syndromes known as *hemolytic uremic syndrome* (HUS) and *thrombotic thrombocytopenic purpura* (TTP) share similar clinical features and pathology. Both are defined by hemolytic anemia with fragmented red cells and thrombocytopenia, an association commonly referred to as *microangiopathic hemolytic anemia* (MAHA). The underlying pathology is thrombotic microangiopathy (TMA), a microvascular occlusive disorder of capillaries, arterioles, and, less frequently, arteries. In TTP, microvascular aggregation of platelets causes ischemic lesions mainly in the brain, less frequently in the kidney and other organs. By contrast, in HUS, platelet-fibrin thrombi mostly affect the kidney. TTP was initially described by Moschcowitz in 1925 (1) and HUS by Gasser et al. in 1955 (2). TTP, which occurs most often in adults, is characterized by the clinical pentad of fever, MAHA, thrombocytopenia, neurologic abnormalities, and variable renal dysfunction. HUS is characterized by the triad of MAHA, thrombocytopenia, and acute renal failure, although brain involvement may complicate the disease. Clearly, the clinical description of both syndromes overlaps. In general, nephrologists call the syndrome they see HUS, whereas hematologists call it TTP.

Both disorders remained mysterious until the 1980s. In 1982, Moake et al. (3) reported that unusually large multimers of von Willebrand factor (VWF) released from endothelial cells were present in the plasma of patients with chronic relapsing TTP and proposed that a failure to process these multimers explained the disorder. In 1985, Karmali et al. (4) demonstrated that HUS in children was associated with enteric infection by *Escherichia coli* that produce verocytotoxin (VT) (Shiga-like toxin). Subsequent investigations clarified the mechanisms of both disorders (5).

VARIOUS TYPES OF HEMOLYTIC UREMIC SYNDROMES IN CHILDREN

Twenty years ago it was recognized that childhood HUS could be divided into two main groups according to the clinical presentation and outcome. The importance of a prodrome of diarrhea associated with HUS (D+ HUS) was recognized as a distinguishing feature of the main group (6). Its infectious origin was confirmed a few years later (7). D+ HUS represents approximately 90% of cases in children, usually younger than 3 years of age, and is an acquired disease related to the endothelial toxicity of infectious agents, mainly VT-producing *Escherichia coli* (VTEC).

In contrast, HUS not associated with a prodrome of diarrhea (D– HUS) can occur at any age, including the newborn. D– HUS may be familial, with autosomal dominant or, more frequently in children, autosomal recessive transmission. A similar distinction between acquired and intrinsic forms applies in adults (8). In children, various pathogenic mechanisms, corresponding to distinct subgroups of D– HUS, are described (9). A neonatal form is associated with methylmalonic acidemia due to intracellular vitamin B_{12} deficiency. Some D– HUS cases are associated with abnormalities of the complement regulator factor H (fH) or its gene. Another subgroup of children with HUS, often of neonatal onset and running a recurrent TTP-like course, has been shown to have constitutional deficiency of the VWF-cleaving protease (VWF-cp). In spite of these advances, the pathogenesis in many cases of D– HUS remains unknown.

SOME PROBLEMS OF TERMINOLOGY

The D+ HUS/D– HUS terminology is simple and clinically useful, but it can mislead. Occasionally, some patients with VTEC infection do not have diarrhea (10,11). On the other hand, a diarrheal disease may trigger HUS in a patient with a constitutional predisposition to HUS. Thus, classifying patients only according to the presence or absence of diarrhea can lead to erroneous management.

D+ HUS is commonly referred to as *typical*, and D– HUS as *atypical*. This terminology, although criticized, remains useful for the rough classification of patients.

TABLE 47.1. A CLASSIFICATION OF HEMOLYTIC UREMIC SYNDROME (HUS) IN CHILDREN

Infection-induced HUS
- Enterohemorrhagic *Escherichia coli* producing verocytotoxin
- Shigella dysenteriae type 1 producing Shiga toxin
- *Streptococcus pneumoniae* producing neuraminidase
- Human immunodeficiency virus

Genetic HUS
- Complement abnormalities: factor H deficiency, factor H-gene mutations
- von Willebrand factor–cleaving protease constitutional deficiency
- Defects of vitamin B_{12} intracellular metabolism

Drug-induced HUS
- Calcineurin inhibitors
- Mitomycin C, cytotoxic drugs, gemcitabine
- Ticlopidine, clopidogrel
- Quinine

HUS superimposed to other pathologies
- *De novo* posttransplantation HUS
- After bone marrow transplantation
- Systemic lupus erythematosus and antiphospholipid syndrome
- Collagen type III glomerulopathy

HUS of unknown etiology
- Autosomal recessive HUS of unknown mechanism
- Autosomal dominant HUS of unknown mechanism
- HUS of unknown mechanism without a prodrome of diarrhea

However, the terms *epidemic* and *sporadic*, implying D+ HUS and D– HUS, are irrelevant. D+ HUS may occur in an outbreak of VTEC infection, but most cases occur in isolation. Ideally, the classification of the various forms of HUS should rely on etiology and pathogenesis, rather than on overlapping clinical criteria.

In all cases, a thorough inquiry of recent and past history of the patient and the family members is indicated. Unexplained anemia or thrombocytopenia at birth or later, bleeding or thrombotic events, complications of pregnancy, hematuria or proteinuria, and renal disease or unexplained death in family members, particularly in infancy, are important pointers to underlying mechanisms.

In this chapter, we have used an etiologic classification whenever there is good evidence for it. Table 47.1 is an attempt to classify pediatric HUS, to guide the clinician towards a diagnosis. Table 47.2 summarizes the currently recommended investigations.

DIAGNOSIS OF HEMOLYTIC UREMIC SYNDROME

Microangiopathic Hemolytic Anemia

MAHA, a consistent feature of HUS, is a Coombs' test–negative hemolytic anemia in which red cells become fragmented (schizocytes). The hemolysis is intravascular and plasma lactate dehydrogenase is elevated, whereas haptoglobin is very low in the acute phase and during relapse. Haptoglobin is often the last abnormality to normalize in remission, and persistently low haptoglobin

TABLE 47.2. DIAGNOSTIC APPROACH OF THE VARIOUS SUBGROUPS OF HEMOLYTIC UREMIC SYNDROME

Subgroup	Clinical features	Investigations
VT-producing *Escherichia coli*–induced hemolytic uremic syndrome	Age <3, but not neonatal Prodromic diarrhea Sudden onset	Stool culture on MacConkey's sorbitol medium; serotyping of colonies; VT detection in stools by polymerase chain reaction Detection of immunoglobulin M antibodies in the serum (O157 and other selected serotypes)
Streptococcus pneumoniae infection	Concomitant infection by *S. pneumoniae*	Erythrocytes polyagglutination detected during attempted blood group determination (false-positive Coombs' test) Confirm by peanut lectin *Arachis hypogea* test
Complement anomalies	Any age, including neonates Relapsing course Familial, several years apart (siblings or parents)	Factor H deficiency, factor H gene mutations Complement C3 may be low due to alternative pathway activation
VWF-cp deficiency	Severe neonatal hemolytic anemia and thrombocytopenia treated by exchange transfusions Later onset also observed Thrombotic thrombocytopenic purpura–like relapsing course Familial (siblings)	Total VWF-cp deficiency, without anti–VWF-cp antibodies
Inborn errors of vitamin B_{12} metabolism	Generally neonatal onset with failure to thrive and neurologic deterioration Also observed in older children without neurologic symptoms	Increased serum and urine methylmalonic acid, low serum homocysteine, high urine homocysteine
Antiphospholipid syndrome	Malignant antiphospholipid syndrome	Measure antiphospholipid and anticardiolipin antibodies and lupus anticoagulant

VWF, von Willebrand factor; VWF-cp, von Willebrand factor–cleaving protease; VT, verocytotoxin.

levels may indicate ongoing chronic hemolysis in some cases. There is no correlation between the severity of anemia and the renal impairment. Often, the reverse is seen, in that children with prolonged anuria exhibit only mild hemolysis. The correction of MAHA by nephrectomy in chronic D– HUS cases suggests that red cell fragmentation occurs in the renal microcirculation, an idea supported 40 years ago by Brain et al. (12).

Thrombocytopenia

Thrombocytopenia associated with MAHA is another common feature of all types of HUS. It is variable in severity. Petechia and surgical bleeding rarely occur unless the platelet count is below 20×10^9/L. Thrombocytopenia is due to consumption. Plasma fibrinogen and factor V levels are normal, prothrombin and partial thromboplastin times are normal or shortened. Thrombin-antithrombin III complexes, prothrombin fragments, and D-dimers are increased, indicating localized thrombus formation and dissolution, although the overall fibrinolytic activity of plasma is reduced (13,14).

Acute Renal Failure

Sudden anuria is observed in approximately 50% of children with D+ HUS (11,15). Most other children with D+ HUS have oliguria. Rarely, high urine output renal failure occurs. Microscopic hematuria is usual in the acute phase. Urine may be red either because of hematuria or because of hemoglobinuria in severe hemolysis. Proteinuria is also common at the acute phase. By contrast, renal involvement in D– HUS often has an insidious onset with proteinuria, hematuria, and a progressive increase of serum creatinine over a few days or weeks.

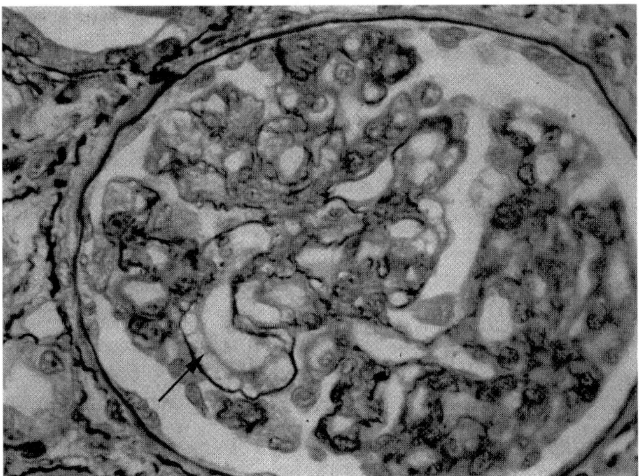

FIGURE 47.1. Glomerular thrombotic microangiopathy with double contour appearance of glomerular capillary wall and widening of the subendothelial space (*arrow*).

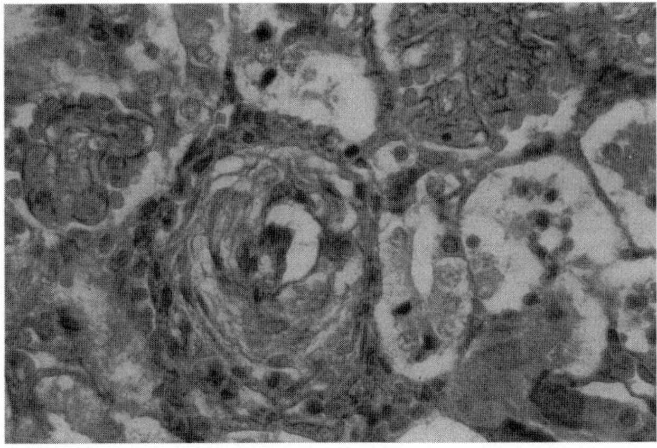

FIGURE 47.2. Preglomerular arteriole in glomerular thrombotic microangiopathy, showing the widening and swelling of the endothelial and subendothelial layers, with narrowing of the arteriolar lumen.

Hypertension may be observed transiently in the acute phase of D+ HUS. This may relate to volume overload. Renin-mediated hypertension may also occur in the severe forms of D+ HUS, either early or months or years after the acute phase. In D– HUS, severe renin-dependent

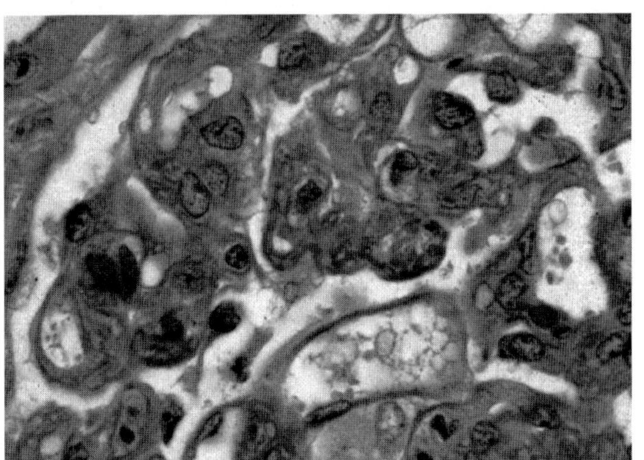

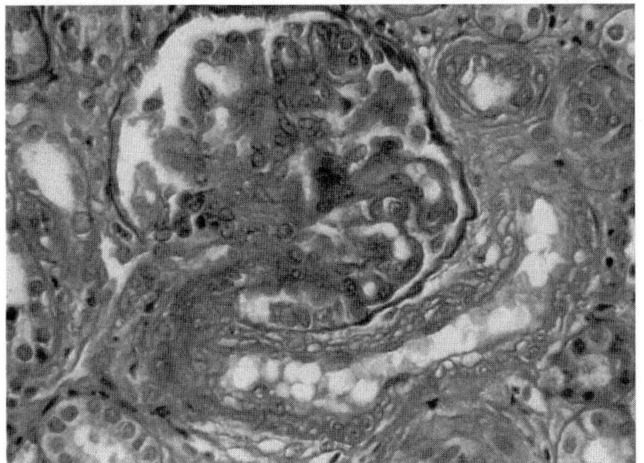

FIGURE 47.3. Glomerular thrombotic microangiopathy. **A:** Fibrin thrombi in glomerular capillaries. **B:** Obliteration of the preglomerular arteriole by fibrin thrombus.

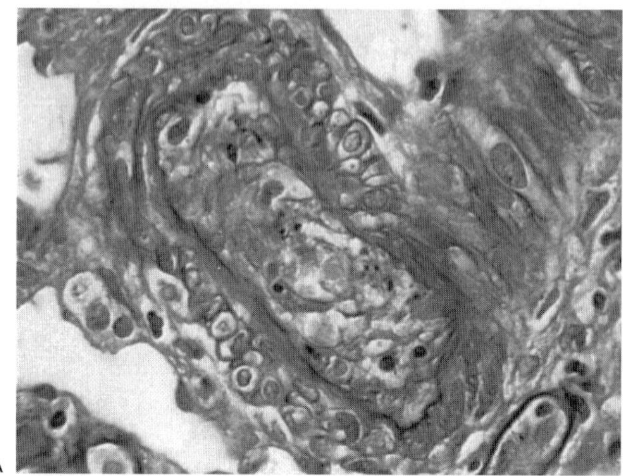

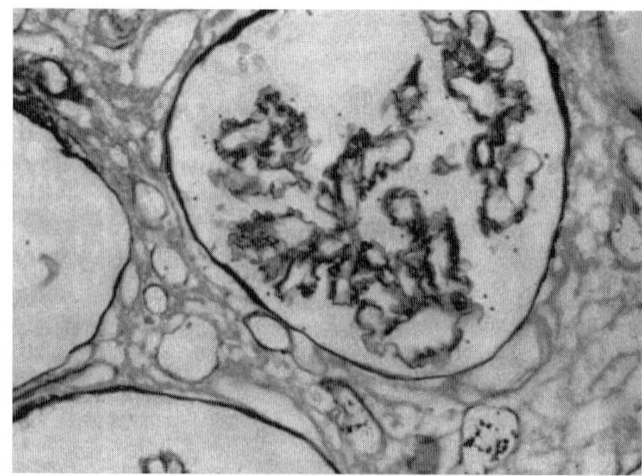

FIGURE 47.4. Arterial thrombotic microangiopathy. A: Arteriolar obliteration by a fibrin thrombus. B: Shrinkage of the tuft and wrinkling of the basement membranes.

hypertension is frequent, both at onset and in relapse, and generally persists.

PATHOLOGY

Renal biopsies, undertaken more commonly 20 years ago than today, demonstrate three main types of lesions as identified by Habib et al. (16,17).

Glomerular Thrombotic Microangiopathy

Glomerular TMA is characterized by the thickening of glomerular capillary walls, with widening of the subendothelial space, and frequent double contour appearance (Fig. 47.1). Endothelial cells may appear swollen, obstructing the capillary, or detached from the basement membrane. These lesions are observed mainly in glomerular capillaries and preglomerular arterioles (Fig. 47.2), whereas larger arteries are only rarely involved. The mesangial matrix often has a fibrillar appearance. The glomeruli may be enlarged, with capillaries distended by red cells and platelet-fibrin thrombi (Fig. 47.3A) that may also be observed in the afferent arterioles (Fig. 47.3B). Immunofluorescence microscopy shows fibrin deposits in the subendothelial spaces and in capillary and arteriole thrombi. This pattern is typical of D+ HUS (15–19).

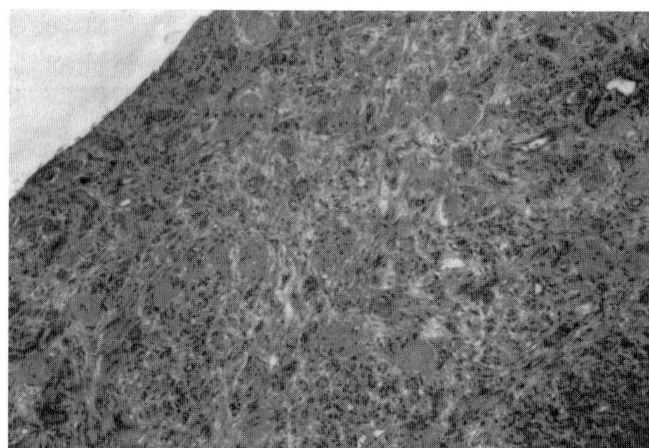

FIGURE 47.5. Cortical necrosis with diffuse glomerular and tubulointerstitial fibrosis.

Arterial Thrombotic Microangiopathy

Arterial TMA involves arterioles and interlobular arteries. Intimal edema and proliferation, necrosis of the arterial wall, luminal narrowing, and thrombosis are observed (Fig. 47.4A). Glomeruli appear ischemic and shrunken, with wrinkling of the basement membranes of the collapsed capillaries (Fig. 47.4B). Arterial TMA is typical of D– HUS and is generally associated with severe hypertension and poor renal prognosis (17,20).

Cortical Necrosis

Cortical necrosis (Fig. 47.5), patchy or rarely diffuse to the whole superficial cortex, is due to acute cortical ischemia after obstruction of the local microcirculation. It is mainly observed in the most severe forms of D+ HUS and is generally associated with prolonged anuria at the acute phase, with a high risk of chronic renal failure.

INFECTION-INDUCED HEMOLYTIC UREMIC SYNDROME

Verocytotoxin-Producing *Escherichia coli* Infection and Hemolytic Uremic Syndrome

HUS is the most severe manifestation of VTEC infection in humans. At least 80% of childhood HUS in developed countries is attributable to this zoonosis, and from the early

1980s, HUS has become a leading cause of pediatric acute renal failure in developed countries.

Verocytotoxin-Producing Escherichia coli

Most strains of *E. coli* pose no risk to human health and reside as commensal organisms in the colon. However, in 1977, it was recognized that certain *E. coli* produced a potent exotoxin that caused lysis of vero cells, a primate kidney cell line with epithelial characteristics (21). The toxin, VT-1, was subsequently shown to be homologous to Shiga toxin produced by *Shigella dysenteriae* type 1 (22) and a member of a family of toxins with similar structure. The toxins produced by *E. coli* are referred to by two interchangeable terms, VT or Shiga-like toxin.

VTEC infection was associated with hemorrhagic colitis in 1982 (23) and with childhood HUS 1 year later (4,24). There followed a number of epidemiologic reports that confirmed VTEC as a cause of human disease (5,25–27), and with this came the recognition that other members of the Shiga toxin family, VT-2 and VT-2c, were involved (see later).

In outbreaks of human VTEC infection, the causative strains have frequently been traced to animal sources, predominantly cattle (28,29). Contaminants include meat and bovine products, fruit, vegetables, and surface water. VTEC can survive for long periods in soil and water. However, bacteriologic surveillance of apparently healthy humans, for example, those working in the meat industry, has shown that VTEC excretion is not uncommon, and the strains identified differ from those associated with disease (30). Likewise, the strains of VTEC that colonize animals usually have different properties from those affecting humans, even though they produce the same toxins (31). This suggests that, although the toxin or certain variants of it are necessary for inducing human disease, they are not sufficient by themselves. Other bacterial cofactors are usually needed.

The most important virulence cofactor found in human pathogenic VTEC is the ability to form an attaching and effacing lesion on enterocytes. This is a characteristic of enteropathogenic *E. coli* (EPEC) (32). The genes responsible for this reside in the locus for enterocyte effacement, a 35.6-kB pathogenicity island in the bacterial chromosome that includes the genes for intimin and the translocated intimin receptor, *eaeA* and *tir*, respectively. EPEC inject their own bacterial receptor, the translocated intimin receptor, into the host enterocyte by a type 3 secretion system as outlined in Figure 47.6. This becomes incorporated into the apical membrane of the colonocyte. The *E. coli* can then bind to the host cell via surface expression of the adhesion protein intimin. In so doing, the translocated intimin receptor causes signaling events in the host cell, leading to cytoskeletal changes such as loss of the normal villous structure and a condensation of actin to form a nest-like pedicle beneath the adherent bacterium (33).

Enterohemorrhagic *E. coli* (EHEC) can be considered as those that combine both VT production and the adhesion properties of EPEC. Unlike *S. dysenteriae* type 1, neither EPEC nor EHEC invade the intestinal mucosa. However, EHEC deliver exotoxin in the immediate vicinity of the enterocyte. Not all VTEC are EHEC. In an extensive review of the bacterial properties of VTEC isolated from humans, the strains that induced hemorrhagic colitis and HUS were more likely to produce VT-2 or VT-2c and to express intimin and hemolysin than organisms from asymptomatic individuals (34).

VTEC O157:H7/H– is the predominant cause of HUS in the Americas and western Europe (*O* refers to the lipopolysaccharide serotype of *E. coli*, and *H* to the flagella type). VTEC O157 more often bears VT-2 than VT-1—occasionally both—and consistently contains the locus for enterocyte effacement. Many other serotypes of VTEC also exhibit adhesion and are pathogenic. Each may have its own geographic distribution. O111 is more prevalent in southern Europe and Australia. O118 was recently reported in Germany with two patterns emerging (35). In the first, the organism produced VT-1, bore the genes for intimin and hemolysin, and was associated with colitis and HUS. This strain was traced back to cattle on two farms. The second was the identification of a similar O-serotype that produced VT-2d but neither intimin nor hemolysis. This was found in patients with minor or no symptoms.

Organisms hitherto naïve for VT can acquire the plasmid for VT production by lysogenic phage transfer. If this occurs in a strain with existing covirulence factors, such as enterocyte attachment, humans may be at risk. However, phage transfer is not restricted to *E. coli*. One outbreak of HUS was traced to infection by a VT-2–producing *Citrobacter freundii* (36).

Shiga Toxin Family

All members of the Shiga toxin family have varying degrees of sequence homology and a common structure of an A subunit linked to a pentamer of B subunits. Whereas Shiga toxin is encoded in the chromosome of *S. dysenteriae* type 1, VT is encoded in plasmids. Shiga toxin and VT-1 are identical except for one amino acid in the A subunit, and there is approximately 55% homology between VT-1 and VT-2. VT-1, VT-2, and VT-2c are associated with human disease, VT-2 being the most important. Other VT-2 variants have been recovered from asymptomatic humans, mammals, and birds.

VT needs to be internalized to cause direct cellular toxicity (Fig. 47.6). The B subunit is responsible for cell recognition and uptake by binding the terminal carbohydrate moiety, galactose α1-4β galactose of globotriaosylceramide (Gb3) (CD77) expressed on the cell surface (37). Whether a species is susceptible to the toxin, and to some extent the pattern of disease, is determined by the distribution of VT receptors. Gb3 is strongly expressed in primates, mostly on

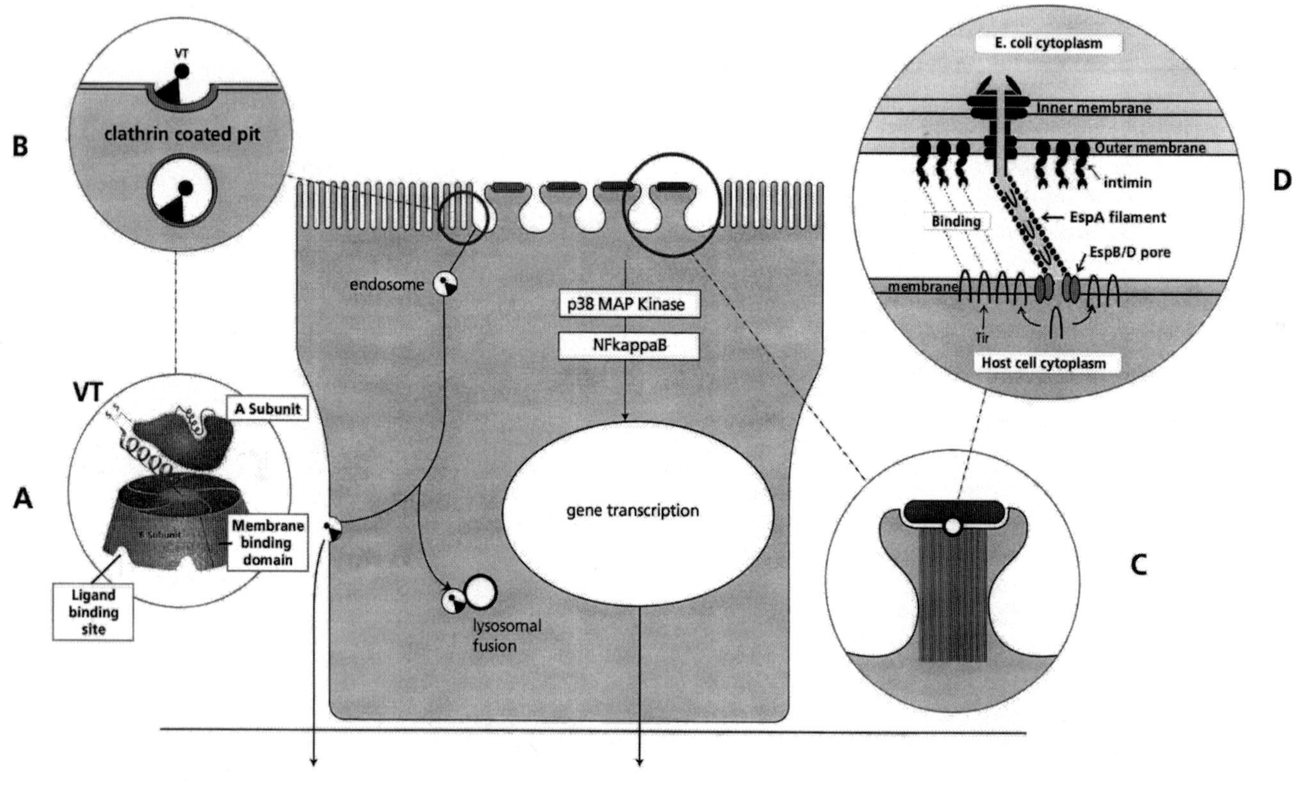

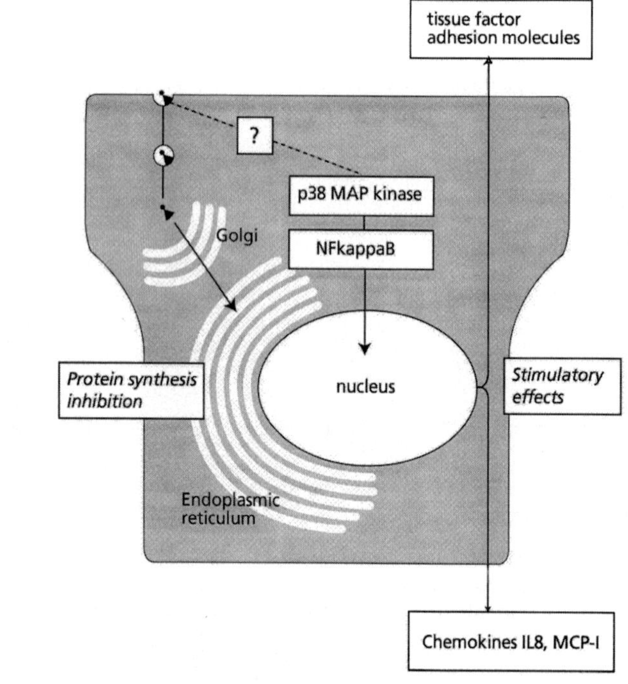

FIGURE 47.6. **A:** Effect of verocytotoxin (VT) on colonic epithelial cells. Main cartoon shows the attachment of VT-producing *Escherichia coli* to the colonocyte. Locally released VT is taken up into endosomes and either digested by lysosomes, transported across the epithelial monolayer, or released into the cytoplasm. *A*: The A-5B structure of VT. (Inset *A* from Donnelly JJ, Rappuoli R. Blocking bacterial enterotoxins. *Nat Med* 2000;6:257–258, with permission.) *B*: Endocytosis within a clathrin-coated pit after binding of B subunit to Gb3 ligand. *C:* Attaching and effacing lesion showing *Escherichia coli* bound to a pedestal-like structure with reorganization of the underlying cytoskeleton. *D:* Type 3 secretion by which the intimin receptor is injected into the host cell membrane to permit firm attachment. (Courtesy of Dr. S. Knutton.) **B:** Effect of VT on endothelial cells. High levels of toxin exposure induce protein synthesis inhibition, the toxin being transported in a retrograde fashion from the Golgi apparatus to the endoplasmic reticulum and cleaving ribosomal RNA. Low exposure to VT causes cell signaling as shown in the outline. The proximal signaling pathways are unknown. IL, interleukin; MCP, monocyte chemoattractant protein.

renal tubular epithelial cells and gut. Many species, such as domestic cattle, have little expression of Gb3 and are consequently unaffected by the toxin.

After binding to the receptor within a clathrin-coated pit, the intact toxin is endocytosed. From here it may be reexported or fused with a lysosome for degrading. However, some is routed to various intracellular destinations, including the nucleus and the cytosol (38,39). During this, the toxin is cleaved by either furin or calpain to release the A subunit into the cytosol. The A subunit contains an enzyme that depurinates a specific adenine residue near the 3' end of the 28S ribosomal RNA at a point where aminoacyl transfer RNA is assembled within the 60S ribosome (40). The rate of ribosomal depurination exceeds the ability for repair so that only a very small amount of free A subunit is needed to prevent peptide assembly and arrest protein synthesis.

Effect of Verocytotoxin on Cells

Verotoxins appear to have two different actions on cells, cytotoxicity and stimulatory effects. Experimentally, cytotoxicity requires a higher dosage of toxin or longer exposure than the stimulatory effects.

Cytotoxicity

Cell killing is generally held to be the consequence of protein synthesis inhibition. To some extent, cytotoxicity depends on the stage of the cell cycle (41). VT causes apoptosis in vero cells (42) and cultured foreskin microvascular endothelial cells (43), both of which bear the Gb3 receptor. Primary cultures of human renal epithelial cells are exquisitely sensitive to VT-1 (44) but die through necrosis (45). Both human umbilical and glomerular endothelial cells are comparatively resistant to VT, but pretreatment with the inflammatory cytokines tumor necrosis factor (TNF)-α, interleukin (IL)-1β, or bacterial lipopolysaccharide makes them sensitive through the upregulation of Gb3 (46,47). Human mesangial cells are resistant to the cytocidal effects of VT (48). *In vitro*, VT-1 kills cells at a lower concentration than VT-2, although in animal models VT-2 often appears to be more injurious.

Stimulatory Effects

VT induces the release of proinflammatory cytokines and chemokines from various cells at low concentrations that cause neither cell death nor decreased protein synthesis. In human enterocytes, VT induces the production of IL-8 and other members of the C-X-C chemokine family (49,50). VT-2 at sublethal dosage on human endothelial cells upregulates messenger RNA for IL-8 and monocyte chemoattractive protein-1, causing a marked increase in leukocyte adhesion and migration into the endothelial monolayer (51). Moreover, sublethal doses of VT-1 induce the production of tissue factor messenger RNA and the total procoagulant activity of human endothelial cells (52). Given that tissue factor is the primary regulator of coagulation and that coagulation precedes the onset of acute renal failure in HUS, this may be a very important observation. Monocytes have also been shown to produce TNF-α and other cytokines in response to VT (53).

In all these studies, the cell-signaling pathways appear to be similar. They involve the p38/mitogen-activated protein kinase pathway, the primary response gene *c-jun* and the transcription factor NFκB. How VT initiates the signaling process remains unknown (Fig. 47.6).

Ribotoxin administration to animal models confirms the early and massive release of proinflammatory cytokines and chemokines, an effect that is augmented if there is an independent stimulus such as bacterial lipopolysaccharide (54–56). The site of production of cytokines has not been fully investigated, but in some experiments there is evidence that TNF-α is produced in the kidney itself (54,57,58).

Pathogenesis of Verocytotoxin-Induced Hemolytic Uremic Syndrome

VT is released by adherent VTEC on the apical surface of the colonic epithelium and is delivered to the submucosa by transcytosis. Here it is responsible, either in part or in whole, for causing the microvascular lesion of the colon. There are edema, hemorrhage, thrombosis, and neutrophil infiltration affecting all layers of the bowel wall, and the overlying mucosa is shed.

In the glomerulus, it is widely assumed that direct endothelial cell injury by VT is an initiating event. Early animal studies of VT intoxication showed that sites of endothelial damage, albeit not renal, correlate with receptor expression in the target tissue (59). Human kidneys strongly express Gb3, but on tubular cells rather than vascular. Glomeruli have weak expression, except perhaps in young children (60). This detracts from the idea that toxin is preferentially taken up by glomerular endothelium to cause cell death. However, endothelial Gb3 expression is promoted by TNF-α and IL-1β, and there is evidence that TNF-α is increased early in human HUS (61), offering some support to the hypothesis.

A previous problem with the hypothesis was that VT could not be identified freely in plasma, raising questions about its systemic distribution. The finding that VT binds to the surface of neutrophils via a receptor with a lower affinity than Gb3 and that it is not internalized raises the possibility that neutrophils might transport VT to target sites outside the colon (62).

Neutrophils may have other important roles in the disease. Neutrophil traffic in the colonic mucosa appears to increase the transport of toxin across the epithelial border (63). Neutrophilia occurs very early in VTEC infection, and higher peripheral blood neutrophil counts predict both the progression to HUS (64) and its severity (65). HUS plasma contains high concentrations of elastase, which suggests that neutrophils are activated within the circulation (66), and there is an excess of neutrophils in the glomeruli of patients coming to postmortem examination in the early phase of the disease (19). This is in keeping with Zoja's observation that very low dosage of VT-2 induces leukocyte adhesion on vascular endothelium (51).

It is now clear that procoagulant events precede the onset of renal impairment, making it almost certain that renal impairment is the consequence of intraglomerular thrombosis, microvascular obstruction, and nephron ischemia (67).

This is in keeping with the *in vitro* findings that VT can induce procoagulant changes in human endothelium (68) and upregulate tissue factor expression (52). It may also be relevant that VT-1 has been shown to exert a proaggregatory effect on platelets (69).

Histopathology

The typical histologic features of VTEC infection are of glomerular TMA, with glomerular capillary thrombosis causing distension of the capillary loops with or without extension into the afferent arteriole (18,19). The distension suggests that thrombosis starts in the glomerular capillaries themselves or at their junction with the efferent arteriole. Cortical necrosis, when present, is patchy, but may be extensive. There is no doubt that glomerular TMA is a destructive process leading to nephron loss. In a follow-up study by Habib (16), the proportion of glomeruli showing fibrosis at 1 year correlated with the proportion of glomeruli with TMA lesions in the acute phase of the illness. In keeping with this, Moghal et al. found marked compensatory glomerular hypertrophy in HUS survivors with ongoing proteinuria 5 years after onset, which fits with the hypothesis of adaptation to a reduced number of functioning nephrons (70).

Epidemiology

Less than 10% of individuals with VTEC-induced diarrhea develop HUS (71,72). The reason for the low risk of disease after exposure is not known. It seems unlikely to be simply a dose effect, as even a small inoculum can induce illness. It was previously assumed that humans did not produce anti-VT antibodies after infection. With more accurate assays, this has been shown to be incorrect and it has been shown that approximately one-half of healthy adults have immunoglobulin (Ig) G antibodies to VT2 (73). Although it is as yet unclear whether VT-2 antibodies are protective, the observation accords with the epidemiology. The lowest prevalence of antibody is seen in early childhood, the period of greatest incidence of HUS. Waning antibody titers in the elderly may explain the greater severity of disease in this age group. The peak age of onset of HUS is 1 to 2 years. In North America and western Europe, it is rare before 9 months, but in some communities, Argentina, for example, a younger onset is seen, probably reflecting different feeding practices.

The annual incidence of VT-induced HUS in children younger than 5 years is as high as 3.4 per 100,000 children in Scotland and approximately four times this in Argentina. However, in western Europe and in Australia and North America, the figure is on the order of 1 to 2. The incidence for children younger than 15 years of age is approximately one-half that of those younger than 5 years of age (7,11,74–76).

Most cases of infection are sporadic, making it difficult to locate the environmental source. Outbreaks provide the opportunity to trace the contaminant. Secondary person-to-person spread is well recognized, and early sanitary advice is needed to prevent it.

Laboratory Investigation for Verocytotoxin-Producing Escherichia coli

The most important VTEC serotype in the Americas and much of Europe is O157 with or without the flagella-type H7. However, a wide range of serotypes are reported in central Europe and Australia. These are usually O-serotypes already known to be EPEC (e.g., O26, O55, O111). Geography, therefore, has implications for the investigative strategy. Where O157 is the prevalent VTEC serotype, selective culture of stool samples on sorbitol MacConkey's agar is used. O157, characteristically, does not induce sorbitol fermentation. Colonies can then be identified serologically. Although practical, this is not the most sensitive approach. VTEC excretion is transient, usually a few days. In many cases, both the diarrhea and the excretion of VTEC have resolved by the time the diagnosis of HUS is made. Culture enrichment techniques for O157 and serologic tests for O157 lipopolysaccharide antibodies will not detect other strains. A rising antibody titer to a relevant VTEC O-serotype can be diagnostic in patients whose stools no longer contain the pathogen.

A more assured technique for identifying VTEC in stool samples, although laborious, is to use polymerase chain reaction for the relevant VT genes. With this technique, one can identify strains that have more than one VT plasmid. Probe-positive colonies are then cultured, and their O-serotypes can be determined.

In epidemics, it is important to confirm the link between the human cases and the source of infection, for example, in food or cattle. This is achieved by further characterizing the VTEC strains, either by relatively simple lytic bacteriophage typing or by using more sophisticated techniques such as pulse field gel electrophoresis (77). One has to recognize that, at present, negative results are obtained even in carefully investigated outbreaks of D+ HUS.

Clinical Features

Diarrhea and vomiting are typical of VTEC-induced HUS although, rarely, a patient with evidence of infection will develop HUS without intestinal symptoms. It is therefore important that investigation for VTEC is conducted in all cases of HUS, regardless of whether they present with diarrhea. The majority of patients experiences abdominal cramps and diarrhea, which is bloody in more than 70% of cases. Rectal prolapse, intussusception, toxic dilatation of colon, and perforation can occur. Early surgical referral is needed so that if laparotomy proves necessary, the timing is carefully adjudicated.

Hydration at the time of the diagnosis of HUS is variable between cases. Fifty percent appear normally hydrated, but

25% have clinical evidence of vascular volume overload, and the remainder have various degrees of dehydration. Hypovolemic shock occurs in approximately 2% of children. Low plasma sodium concentrations are common at diagnosis and tend to be lower in those with clinical hypovolemia. Low plasma albumin concentrations are common, particularly in hypovolemic and shocked patients, indicating a capillary leak.

The onset of oligoanuria appears between 1 and 14 days after the onset of diarrhea, typically between days 4 and 7, and is preceded by thrombocytopenia and anemia. Anemia is usually maximal approximately 1 day after the onset of oliguria, with 90% of cases being anemic and 95% thrombocytopenic at presentation. Jaundice occurs in 35%. A mild, transient increase in the plasma concentration of liver enzymes occurs in 40%. Approximately one-half of children are anuric at that stage, and up to 75% need dialysis soon after admission (11,15). Hypertension occurs in one-third of patients, usually as a transient feature at approximately the time of the resolution of the oliguric phase.

The most common extrarenal manifestation is central nervous system (CNS) disturbance affecting up to 20% of cases. This usually consists of seizures, typically occurring within the first 48 hours of diagnosis, accompanied by hyponatremia but rarely arterial hypertension. Devastating cerebral edema and encephalopathy can occur suddenly. Children may appear agitated, confused, drowsy, or express hallucinations. This is followed by seizures, coma, cranial nerve palsy, decerebrate posturing, and hindbrain herniation causing respiratory arrest. The speed of progression can be rapid so that a child with early signs of a confusional state should be transferred to an intensive care setting for close monitoring. Rarely, patients will have focal CNS signs and stroke-like events implying large arterial occlusions. Fluctuating neurologic signs are also described in TTP and are not typical of VTEC-induced HUS. CNS imaging is useful in distinguishing microvascular damage and cerebral edema from intracranial hemorrhage. Magnetic resonance imaging (MRI) is more sensitive than tomodensitometry to detect early structural lesions. When these are limited or absent, recovery without sequelae is very likely. Extensive necrotic lesions (Fig. 47.7) are predictive of fatal outcome or of severe neurologic deficit.

Cardiomyopathy and diabetes mellitus due to necrotizing pancreatitis affect less than 5% of patients (78–81).

Treatment

VTEC are sensitive to a wide range of antibiotics, and it has been tempting to consider antibiotic treatment. However, retrospective reviews suggest that antibiotics are associated with an increased risk of HUS (64,82,83). The rationale for this is that certain antibiotics cause increased toxin release from VTEC *in vitro* (84). However, in a Japanese report, the use of an oral form of fosfomycin appeared protective (85). Although the recent metaanalysis of the literature by

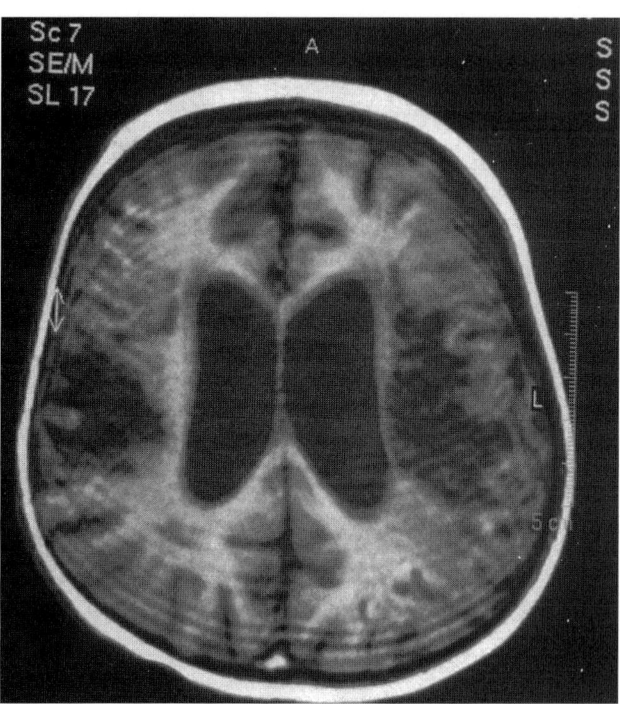

FIGURE 47.7. Extensive cerebral necrotic lesions demonstrated by magnetic resonance imaging.

Safdar et al. (86) indicates no definite answer to the question of whether antibiotics do or do not increase the risk of HUS in patients with O157 *E. coli* infection, as a general rule, they should not be given. Antidiarrheal agents may also be harmful and should be avoided (87).

Binding free toxin in the intestine to prevent its absorption is an attractive idea that has not, so far, proved clinically successful. For example, Synsorb, a resin with a moderately high affinity for VT, has not yet been clinically proven. Newer, soluble agents with more increased toxin binding characteristics, such as "starfish," have yet to be tested. Experimentally, passive immunization with anti-VT antibody can ameliorate disease models and may in the future become a human therapy.

Clinical management is supportive, and patients need close monitoring. Vascular volume, electrolyte disturbance (hyponatremia, hyperkalemia, and acidosis), hypertension, and anemia require correction. Blood transfusion may be required to keep the hemoglobin above 8 g/dL. In undertaking blood transfusion, there must be control of vascular volume and any resulting hyperkalemia. In a few oliguric patients, a high dose of furosemide will induce a diuresis, allowing dialysis to be avoided. Platelet infusions should only be given if there is bleeding not controllable by simple local measures.

There is no evidence that early dialysis improves outcome. If a surgical complication of the colitis is suspected, peritoneal dialysis is contraindicated, and vascular access should be secured for hemodialysis. Anticoagulation and thrombolytic therapy with streptokinase or urokinase are ineffective. Plasma therapy is unproven, although some use plasma exchange (PE) in cases with encephalopathy.

Confusional states, drowsiness, irritability, hallucination, and seizure are ominous signs and may be the first indication of raised intracranial pressure or an evolving neurologic catastrophe. Management at this point should involve neurologists or intensivists. Seizures require immediate treatment with anticonvulsants, and electroencephalogram monitoring is a helpful guide to therapy.

Outcome

Using D+ HUS as a surrogate for VTEC, the early mortality in children is less than 3% with the exception of epidemics, in which it is sometimes higher. In recent surveys in the United Kingdom (manuscript in preparation) and France (11), in which 80% and 86% of D+ HUS was attributable to VTEC O157 infection, an acute mortality of 1.5% was recorded. Death was due to CNS involvement. Less than 5% of patients do not regain independent renal function.

In the first decade after D+ HUS, up to 30% of survivors experienced adverse renal outcome consisting of proteinuria, hypertension, or renal impairment, including end-stage renal failure in 5 to 10% (15,75,88–90). This percentage may increase up to 60% during the second and third decade after D+ HUS (91–94). These sequelae are more likely if the patient is anuric more than 1 week or requires more than 14 days of dialysis during the acute stage. However, the penalty of reduced nephron mass and increased single nephron filtration in the lifetime of the patient is difficult to predict. Occasionally, individuals who were shown to have normal plasma creatinine protein excretion and blood pressure 5 or more years after onset start to develop albuminuria. Later, some of these patients have evidence of declining renal function (95). It is therefore advisable to follow up patients, especially if there was prolonged anuria at the acute phase, for signs of incipient nephropathy by checking for albuminuria and hypertension. Such changes occur well in advance of any rise of plasma creatinine. Although not formally tested, there is a general view that patients with proteinuria are likely to benefit from angiotensin-converting enzyme inhibitors or receptor antagonists.

Posttransplant Course

The evolution after renal transplantation is known from the literature in 132 children who received 154 kidney transplants after D+ HUS. In most series, no recurrence of HUS was observed (75,96–99). Three patients reported by Eijjenraam et al. had possible recurrence of HUS, although the authors considered the diagnosis between HUS recurrence and rejection as uncertain (100). Finally, only one patient reported by Miller et al. with D+ HUS at 1 year of age had definite recurrence 7 days after transplantation and at 12 years of age, with hemolysis, thrombocytopenia, TMA on graft biopsy, and graft loss due to recurrence (101). Thus, the incidence of definite HUS recurrence after transplantation in children with D+ HUS appears to be less than 1%. Cyclosporine was used in more than one-half of these transplants. Moreover, renal transplantation in children with D+ HUS was not associated with an increased risk of graft failure compared to non-HUS patients (75,97,99,100).

Shigella Dysenteriae Type 1 Dysentery-Associated Hemolytic Uremic Syndrome

S. dysenteriae type 1 dysentery-associated HUS is frequent in endemic areas such as India, Bangladesh, and southern Africa. It may also be encountered in industrialized countries in children returning from these areas. The pathogenesis is similar to that of VTEC-induced HUS. However, *S. dysenteriae* is enteroinvasive, and the overall severity of the disease is greater than that of VTEC-induced HUS. Severe dysentery, high fever, and massive leukocytosis (greater than 30,000 to 40,000/mm^3) are common (102–105). In their series of 81 cases from 1994 to 1996 in Kwazulu-Natal, South Africa, Bhimma et al. (105) observed that 18.5% of patients had positive blood culture and 21.0% had disseminated intravascular coagulation. Ninety percent of patients had acute oliguric renal failure. Complications included encephalopathy in 35% of patients, seizures in 15%, and hemiplegia in 2%. Protein-losing enteropathy was observed in 32% of patients, gastrointestinal perforation in 10%, rectal prolapse in 6%, and toxic megacolon in 5%. Myocarditis occurred in 6% of patients, congestive cardiac failure in 4%, and cardiomyopathy in 4%. Mortality was 17%. Only 39% of patients had no sequelae, whereas 42% had chronic renal failure and 1% had end-stage renal failure. The high incidence of cortical necrosis in postdysenteric HUS has been formerly noted (104,106,107).

These patients need urgent appropriate antibiotic therapy, which has been shown to reduce the incidence of HUS (103), and life-support measures.

Streptococcus pneumoniae–Associated Hemolytic Uremic Syndrome

Pneumococcus, *Neuraminidase, and Red Cell Polyagglutination*

A rare but distinctive form of HUS occurs as a complication of pneumococcal infection. With hindsight, it seems very likely that one of Gasser's original cases had this form of the syndrome (2). Typically, it is accompanied by red cell polyagglutination, the laboratory finding that a patient's red cells are agglutinated *in vitro* by blood group ABO-compatible serum. It is sometimes during an attempt to crossmatch blood for a patient with HUS or pneumococcal infection that this comes to light.

Pathogenesis

On healthy human cells, the membrane-associated Thomsen-Friedenreich (T) antigen is masked by sialic acid of the cell glycocalyx and therefore not exposed. The T epitope bears the motif galactose-β-1-3-galactose-*N*-acetylglucosamine that is recognized by an IgM antibody normally present in plasma. T is also recognized by the peanut lectin *Arachis hypogea*, which is the basis of a useful laboratory test when investigating polyagglutination.

Neuraminidase is produced by various pathogens including *S. pneumoniae*, *Clostridia* species, and influenza viruses. Neuraminidase, released during infection, cleaves *N*-acetylneuraminic (sialic) acid from the cell glycocalyx to reveal the T-cryptantigen. There is good evidence of T-antigen exposure on red cells, platelets, and endothelium in this form of HUS (108). It was originally believed that the T-antigen antibody reaction might explain the pathogenesis. However, the naturally occurring anti-T is a cold antibody and unlikely to cause agglutination *in vivo* (109). The true pathogenesis is unknown. It is of interest that neuraminidase has been shown to remove the complement inhibitory effect of complement factor (fH) on human red cells, making them vulnerable to complement-induced lysis (110).

Clinical Features

Patients are usually infants and preschool-aged children; however, adult cases have been described. More than 50 cases have appeared in the literature; the largest two series only describe 11 and 12 cases, respectively (111,112). To this can be added eight cases from a national survey of childhood HUS in the United Kingdom conducted through the years 1997 to 2001 (C. M. Taylor, *personal communication*).

The diagnosis should be suspected in any child with an MAHA associated with sepsis but normal coagulation. Typically, there is an underlying pneumococcal infection, usually pneumonia and empyema, less often meningitis or septicemia. Pneumococcal infection usually precedes the onset of HUS by not more than a few days. Anemia, thrombocytopenia, and oliguric renal failure occur abruptly with a profound deterioration in the child's clinical condition. HUS can be distinguished from disseminated, consumptive, intravascular coagulation, which can also complicate pneumococcal sepsis, in that the prothrombin and partial thromboplastin times are not prolonged, and plasma fibrinogen concentrations are normal. T antigen exposure on red cells is confirmed by testing with the peanut lectin *A. hypogea*. The histology in this form of HUS shows glomerular thrombosis with or without patchy cortical necrosis.

The microangiopathic process is more severe and more prolonged than in D+ HUS. For example, the average duration of thrombocytopenia is 11.6 days as against the usual 7.0 in D+ HUS (112). Extrarenal manifestations include pancreatitis, elevated plasma concentrations of liver enzymes, cerebrovascular disease, and cardiac dysfunction. It is important to eradicate the underlying infection promptly. Management is otherwise supportive. It is traditional advice to avoid the administration of plasma products that contain the naturally occurring IgM. For example, if transfusions are required, red cells or platelets are washed to remove plasma. There is no evidence of benefit from this approach, which is now questioned.

The acute mortality remains high. Combining the review in the contemporary report of Brandt et al. (112) and the experience of the recent United Kingdom survey in which two of the eight children died, the acute mortality for cases reported since 1990 is in the order of 20%. Survivors often regain renal function, although there are a number of cases that progress to chronic renal failure. Because the disease is an acquired single episode, relapse does not occur, and one can expect that transplantation would not be complicated by disease recurrence (113).

Human Immunodeficiency Virus 1–Associated Hemolytic Uremic Syndrome

TMA has been reported in several hundred human immunodeficiency virus cases worldwide (114). These patients, some of them children (115,116), often present with HUS or TTP (manifest as acute or rapidly progressing renal failure), MAHA, thrombocytopenia, and, frequently, neurologic symptoms. Most patients progress to end-stage renal failure. In a multicenter autopsy study, 7% of 214 patients whose death was attributable to acquired immunodeficiency syndrome had evidence of TMA (117). In a study from France (118), 32 of 92 human immunodeficiency virus–infected patients with acute or rapidly progressing renal failure had HUS, TMA being confirmed histologically in most cases. The pathogenesis of TMA involves endothelial damage with local activation of coagulation (114), and a role for antiphospholipid autoantibodies has been postulated. Complete deficiency of VWF-cp due to the presence of an IgG1 inhibitor has also been observed in an acquired immunodeficiency syndrome patient (119).

The incidence of human immunodeficiency virus–associated TMA appears to have decreased since the introduction of antiviral therapy.

GENETIC FORMS OF HEMOLYTIC UREMIC SYNDROME

Hemolytic Uremic Syndrome Associated with Complement Factor H Deficiency

Complement abnormalities have been reported in cases of HUS for more than 25 years. Broadly, two patterns have emerged. The first is a transient reduction of plasma C3 with activation of the alternative pathway. This is quite often seen in the acute presentation of infection-related forms of HUS, including that induced by *S. dysenteriae* and D+ HUS

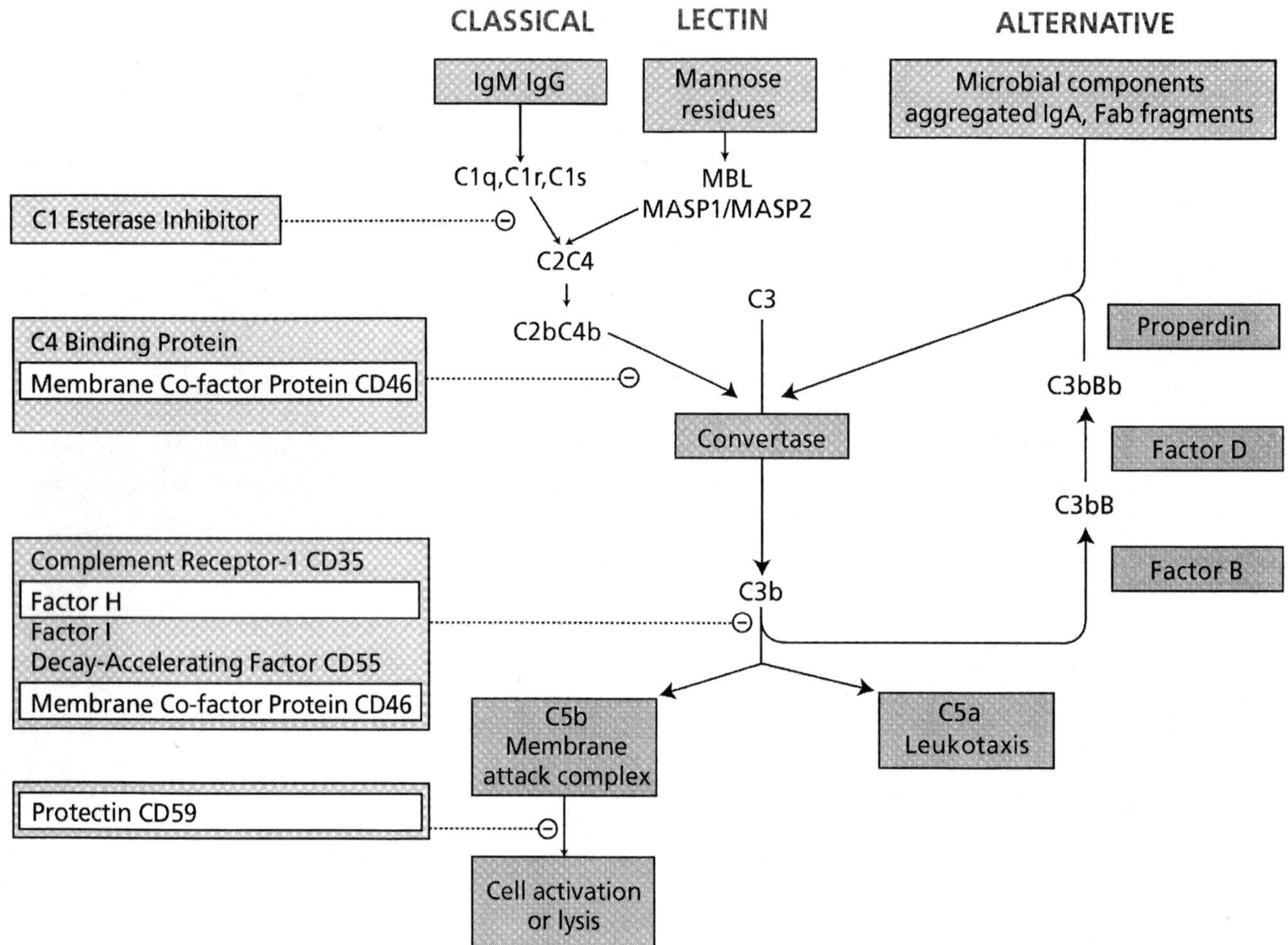

FIGURE 47.8. Regulation of the complement pathways. Regulators known to be located in human renal vasculature are shown in a clear surround. Fab, fragment antigen binding; Ig, immunoglobulin; MBL, Mannose binding lectin.

(102,120). On recovery from the acute episode, the complement profile returns to normal. It is not clear to what extent complement participates in the pathogenesis of infection-related forms of HUS.

The second pattern is one of persistent hypocomplementemia. This points to an innate defect in complement regulation and a rare and distinctive HUS subgroup with deficiency of the complement regulator fH. Furthermore, genetic studies in patients with HUS have found various mutations in the fH gene that extend this phenotype. In this extension, many cases of HUS with fH mutations have normal concentrations of plasma C3. The plasma concentration of fH may be normal or reduced, but the mutations predict loss of fH function.

Pathogenesis

Complement is an integral part of the innate immune system. The alternative and lectin pathways activate immediately on contact with invading organisms, thus recognizing them as "foreign." Host cells are defended against the indiscriminate activity of complement by a number of downregulators, both soluble and mounted on the cell surface (Fig. 47.8). Different cells and organs have their own specific distribution of complement regulators.

fH plays a central role in the regulation of complement, both in the fluid phase and on the surface of cells. It is a glycoprotein with a molecular weight of 155 kDa produced mainly in the liver. It circulates in plasma and binds to polyanionic sites on vascular endothelium and red cells. The molecule is a single peptide and consists of 20-fold globular domains known as *short consensus repeat* (SCR). There are three binding regions for C3b, each being specific for a different part of the molecule. These appear in SCRs 1 to 4, the site also responsible for factor I cofactor activity, SCRs 6 to 10, and the terminal SCRs 16 to 20 (121,122). fH competes with factor B for freshly generated C3b and acts as a cofactor for factor I in C3b degradation. This arrests both the amplification step of C3 convertase and the generation of downstream products, leukotactic C5a, and the membrane attack complex C5b–C9.

There are also three binding sites for heparin and other polyanions by which fH becomes attached to cell surfaces. The tertiary structure of the molecule leaves the C-terminal SCR 20 exposed. This suggested an important function for this site, particularly when combined with the observation that this part of the molecule is a hot spot for mutations in HUS (123–125). Confirmation came from functional *in vitro* studies of mutated fH (126) and by mapping of known mutations to models of the fH molecule (127). Moreover, certain C-terminal mutants show impaired binding to both heparin and the C3d component of C3b (128). In summary, the C-terminal mutations of fH implicated in HUS create a molecule that may bind C3b in the fluid phase but cannot attach to anionic sites on cell surfaces to protect them.

How fH deficiency causes HUS is not clear. The fact that some fH-deficient patients do not present until middle age or have long remissions suggests that fH deficiency predisposes patients to HUS but is an insufficient cause by itself. A second hit is needed. As with other forms of HUS, interest has focused on vascular endothelial injury. Any retraction or detachment of endothelial cells reveals sites in the subendothelial space that activate complement (129). Perhaps endothelial injuries that in normal circumstances would resolve lead to complement activation that propagates in the absence of cell-associated fH.

Complement is an essential component of certain models of glomerular TMA that in some respects resemble HUS. One example is the generalized Shwartzman reaction in rabbits in which the injection of bacterial lipopolysaccharide caused glomerular thrombosis. Another is a rat model of immune glomerular injury accelerated by lipopolysaccharide in which the roles of the membrane attack complex C5–9 and the complement regulator CD59 are strongly implicated (44,130). fH deficiency in other species has not, so far, been linked to HUS, but there is an association with mesangiocapillary glomerulonephritis type II in pigs (131), and perhaps humans (132).

Genetics

The first report linking fH deficiency to HUS was of a child with relapsing HUS and low C3. He was found to have homozygous fH deficiency and plasma fH less than 10% of normal, whereas his consanguineous parents had approximately one-half the normal concentrations. A sibling of the index case who did not have signs of disease also had very low concentrations, indicating a homozygous state (133).

Since then, there have been several reports of patients with very low fH concentrations, implying homozygous inheritance (134–137), although some may be compound heterozygotes as has been later shown in the case described by Warwicker et al. (138) (T. H. J. Goodship, *personal communication*). In these, complement C3 is usually depressed in the range of 0.2 to 0.5 g/dL. HUS is mostly reported in infancy or early childhood, but sometimes there are adult family members with similar fH depletion who have not disclosed disease.

In 1998, Warwicker et al. showed linkage between chromosome 1q32, the site of a gene cluster of complement regulators that includes fH, and HUS in three well-described families (139). Subsequently, mutation analysis confirmed defects in a number of cases of both familial and sporadic, childhood and adult (138,140,141). These include frame shifts introducing stop codons that truncate the fH protein, mutations that appear to affect the tertiary form of the molecule and its export from the endoplasmic reticulum, and a "hot spot" for mutations in the C-terminal, predicted to impair the ability of fH to bind polyanions and C3b.

Many of these patients are heterozygous and have moderate or normal levels of fH and normal levels of C3 and factor B. Although hypocomplementemia and a low fH point to this disease mechanism, normal fH and C3 do not exclude it. It is therefore advisable to carry out genetic investigations in all cases of HUS apart from those with evidence of VTEC infection. It seems very likely that some cases of HUS hitherto associated with pregnancy or use of the contraceptive pill may be related to fH deficiency, reinforcing the need for appropriate molecular investigation. In patients with familial or relapsing HUS, a genetic diagnosis is mandatory.

Clinical Features

These patients present either sporadically or sometimes with a family history (132,142,143). When inquiring after the health of family members, one needs to be suspicious of histories of unexplained anemia or infant deaths, as these may represent undiagnosed cases. The age of onset ranges from the neonatal period to adulthood. There is often a precipitating event, such as an infective illness, often an upper respiratory tract infection. The MAHA is marked in the early stages and in relapse but tends to resolve once anuric end-stage renal failure is reached. However, the plasma haptoglobin often remains suppressed, suggesting ongoing low levels of hemolysis. The clinical course is complicated by persistent severe hypertension, with the attendant problems of end-organ damage, particularly hypertensive encephalopathy. Although individual episodes may resolve, relapse is common, and with each attack, recovery is less certain. Historically, the majority of patients progressed to end-stage renal failure or died, but survival rate for contemporary cases is probably more favorable.

Renal histology typically shows mesangial proliferation with increased matrix giving the glomeruli a solid, lobulated appearance. Mesangial cell interposition leads to the reduplication of the basement membrane and double contours to the capillary walls on silver staining. There may be arterial as well as arteriolar changes. Immunohistochemistry reveals complement deposition in the capillary walls but it is not usually extensive.

Treatment

Treatment of HUS with fresh frozen plasma (FFP) or PE was undertaken empirically long before the role of fH deficiency was proposed. There is now at least some logic behind its use for this subgroup, although experience is fragmentary. Normal plasma contains fH at a concentration of 0.5 g/L. The dose required to regulate complement is not known. Landau et al. (144) showed benefit from biweekly infusions of plasma at a dose of up to 20 mL/kg/day, similar to Nathanson's experience (145). In the case previously reported by Warwicker (138), a PE using 100 mL/kg body weight of FFP was needed to improve the concentration of C3 and normalize factor B, an effect that lasted for approximately 5 days (J. Cansick, *personal communication*). However, fluid phase activity in plasma may not be in itself protective, as fH needs to be bound to cell surfaces to operate.

Posttransplant Course

The outcome of transplantation in patients with this form of HUS is not well documented, but approximately one-third experience recurrence. Of 11 patients in whom the transplant course was documented (124,138–140,144, 146; three cases in Hôpital des Enfants Malades, P. Niaudet, and one in Hôpital Robert Debré, C. Loirat, *unpublished*), 5 lost their graft due to recurrence [sporadic case in (139), patient F34 and F39; and sporadic case in (124), previously published in (140); familial case in (144)].

Seven patients with normal C3 and fH concentrations, but with mutations in the fH gene, have been transplanted (139). Two of them from one family have had HUS recurrence leading to graft loss [family 1 in (139)]. No recurrence was seen in the other five [family 2b and family 3, previously published in (147)] (139).

At present it is not clear why certain individuals relapse, whereas others do not. Most clinicians are wary of using drugs that are associated with HUS, such as cyclosporine and tacrolimus. When considering live donation by a family member, one needs to ensure that the donor does not have undisclosed fH mutations. Liver (148) or combined liver and kidney transplantation (149) have been undertaken in two cases, with encouraging results.

Hemolytic Uremic Syndrome and Thrombotic Thrombocytopenic Purpura Associated with von Willebrand Factor–Cleaving Protease (ADAMTS 13) Deficiency

von Willebrand Factor and von Willebrand Factor–Cleaving Protease

VWF is a multimeric glycoprotein with two hemostatic functions (150–152). It acts as a carrier protein for blood-clotting factor VIII in the circulation and is required for both platelet adhesion to sites of vascular damage and platelet aggregation at high shear rates of blood flow present in the microcirculation. VWF is synthesized by vascular endothelial cells and megakaryocytes as a precursor subunit of 275 kDa. Tail-to-tail dimers of VWF precursor subunits are formed by disulfide bonding near the C-terminals. Additional head-to-head disulfide bonds between the N-termini of the dimers creates multimers with up to 40 dimeric subunits and a molecular mass in excess of 20,000 kDa (Fig. 47.9). The multimers are stored in the endothelial Weibel-Palade bodies and the alpha granules of platelets. The larger the VWF multimers, the more effective they are in acting as a bridge between platelets and forming platelet aggregates. However, VWF does not normally circulate in these very large multimeric forms. A specific plasma protease, VWF-cp, physiologically cleaves the largest multimers of VWF released from endothelial cells and platelets (151,154). It does so at a specific site between Tyr 842 and Met 843 to form the smaller multimers normally found in plasma (155) (Fig. 47.9).

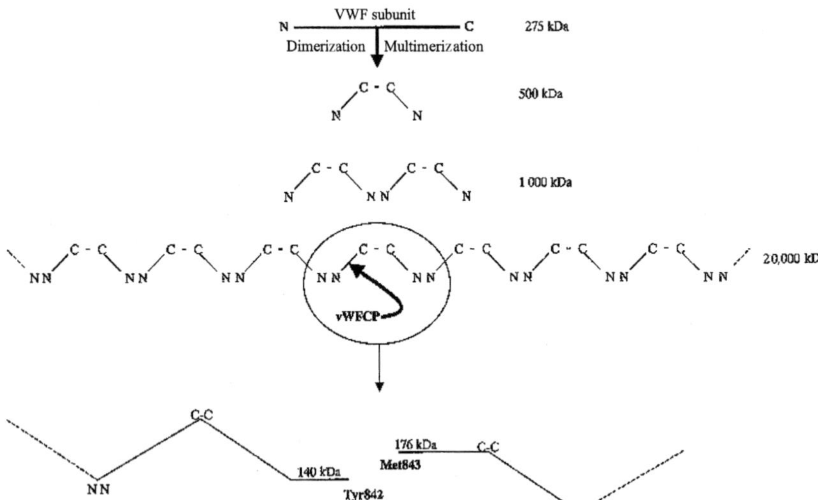

FIGURE 47.9. Multimeric structure of von Willebrand factor (VWF) and physiologic proteolysis of multimers by VWF-cleaving protease (VWFCP). (Modified from Girma J, Veyradier A, Meyer D. ADAMTS 13, la protéase spécifique du facteur von Willebrand. *Med Sci* 2002;18:15–17.)

VWF-cp is a metalloprotease synthesized in the liver that has been identified as the thirteenth member of the ADAMTS (*a* *d*esintegrin-like *a*nd *m*etalloprotease with *t*hrombo*s*pondin type 1 motif) family (156–159). The gene for VWF-cp has been identified on chromosome 9 and the amino acid sequence determined (158). Plaimauer et al. (160) recently demonstrated the functional activity of ADAMTS 13 gene product (i.e., recombinant VWF-cp), opening the way to the production of a recombinant protein.

von Willebrand Factor–Cleaving Protease in Adults with Thrombotic Thrombocytopenic Purpura and Hemolytic Uremic Syndrome

Most studies of VWF-cp have been performed in adults with TTP. They demonstrated that many cases are linked to a profoundly deficient activity of VWF-cp, typically less than 5% of normal. VWF-cp deficiency is occasionally constitutional and probably inherited by autosomal recessive transmission. Much more commonly, it is induced by an acquired inhibitory autoantibody (160–164). By allowing the persistence of unusually large multimers of VWF in plasma, severe VWF-cp deficiency promotes the formation of platelet thrombi in the microcirculation and is responsible for the microangiopathic disease and its ischemic manifestations. Adults with HUS, unlike TTP, were generally found not to be associated with a VWF-cp defect (161–163). The exception being a case of D+ HUS in a woman with a transient total deficiency of VWF-cp in the acute phase and no anti–VWF-cp antibodies (165). In a recent study from the Italian Registry of Recurrent and Familial HUS/TTP, Remuzzi et al. confirmed that most TTP adult patients have VWF-cp deficiency due to the presence of an inhibitor, whereas some have a constitutional and familial deficiency (166). However, these authors also observed that among 28 adult patients with recurrent or familial HUS (with onset in childhood in 16), 5 had VWF-cp constitutional deficiency. None of these had VWF-cp inhibitor.

von Willebrand Factor–Cleaving Protease in Pediatric Hemolytic Uremic Syndrome Associated with a Prodrome of Diarrhea

Hunt et al., Tsaï et al., and Schneppenheim et al. studied VWF-cp activity in a total of 62 D+ HUS children (167–169). Only one child had a total VWF-cp deficiency (167). Of interest, this patient had clinical features of TTP requiring plasma therapy, and his VWF-cp deficiency was related to an inhibitor. Veyradier et al. (170) studied 41 children with D+ HUS and found an undetectable VWF-cp in the acute phase in only 1 child who had a VTEC-induced HUS and a clinical presentation and outcome similar to the other patients. In this case, VWF-cp deficiency was not due to an inhibitor and completely recovered after the acute phase of HUS. This is similar to the adult patient with D+ HUS mentioned above (165). The mechanism of these transient VWF-cp deficiencies in D+ HUS remains unclear, as they had none of the other recognized explanations (171).

von Willebrand Factor–Cleaving Protease in Pediatric Thrombotic Thrombocytopenic Purpura and Hemolytic Uremic Syndrome without a Prodrome of Diarrhea

Antibody-induced VWF-cp deficiency has been reported in a few cases of childhood TTP. In addition to the child with D+ HUS, a TTP-like course and anti–VWF-cp autoantibody mentioned above (167), Robson and Tsaï (172) reported an 8-year-old boy with severe VWF-cp deficiency linked to an inhibitor. Among nine children with TTP studied by Schneppenheim et al. (169), all with VWF-cp below 5% of normal, four had antibodies against VWF-cp. These children, aged between 11 months and 11 years, had mild symptoms of TTP. In the remaining five, VWF-cp deficiency was due to mutation in ADAMTS 13 gene.

Constitutional deficiency in VWF-cp due to mutations in the ADAMTS 13 gene accounts for a subgroup of patients with so-called atypical D– HUS. Out of 23 children with D– HUS, Veyradier et al. (170) observed undetectable VWF-cp activity in six, both acutely and in remission, and in the absence of inhibitors. The clinical presentation of these patients appears similar to that of the original patients described in 1960 by Schulman et al. (173) and in 1978 by Upshaw (174), now revisited as congenital TTP due to hereditary VWF-cp deficiency (175). In 20 of 29 reported cases, the disease started at birth with jaundice, severe hemolytic anemia, and thrombocytopenia, needing treatment by exchange blood transfusions (169,170,174,176–183). Nine children with later onset had their first hemolytic crisis between 6 and 56 months of age (169,174,176–178,180,182). All cases relapsed, often after intercurrent infection. The frequency of relapses is unpredictable, with a disease-free interval varying from 1 month to several years. Nevertheless, in some patients, relapses become increasingly frequent, finally occurring every 3 to 4 weeks (170). Some patients have persistent hemolysis and thrombocytopenia.

In the first years of life, the disease is limited to hematologic symptoms, although transient increases of serum creatinine may be seen during hemolytic crises. Later, progressive renal involvement may appear. Proteinuria was observed at 23 months and 3 years of age in two children, respectively (179,183), with chronic renal failure at 4 years of age in one (183). Another patient developed renal failure during a relapse at 16 years of age (181). The six patients reported by Veyradier et al. (170) also had mild proteinuria when they were 2 to 8 years old. Hypertension developed in two of them at 7 and 9 years of age, with progressive renal insufficiency at 10 years of age in one, who reached end-stage renal disease at 14 years of age. Renal histology showed severe glomerular and arteriolar TMA lesions (170,184). In addition, five patients have been reported with CNS involvement (170,176,181) with episodes of coma, seizures, hemiparesis, and ischemic lesions on cerebral MRI angiography or tomodensitometry, one of them with severe intellectual sequelae (176). Two children also had retinal ischemia, and one had myocardial ischemia (170).

The phenotype of constitutional VWF-cp deficiency can be so variable that 2 of 50 patients classified as idiopathic thrombocytopenic purpura and one classified as Evans syndrome had complete VWF-cp deficiency (169), and a 16-year-old girl who never had TMA but did have neonatal hemolysis/thrombocytopenia had only mild fluctuating thrombocytopenia (60 to 80 × 10^9/L) (170). This variability is in agreement with the results of Furlan's group, which described an age-dependent clustering of congenital TTP (185). Indeed, one-half of all subjects became symptomatic in childhood, whereas the other one-half had their first bout of TTP as adults, mostly between 30 and 40 years. On the other hand, neonatal death from massive hemolysis or death during childhood with multivisceral TMA can also be observed (169,170). The association in one family (170) of a stillborn child and of a propositus with lobster-claw deformity of the hand, an anatomic detail also described in the case-report of Upshaw in 1978 (174), may indicate an ischemic process *in utero*.

The ADAMTS 13 gene has been studied in three series of VWF-cp deficient patients, with a total of 16 patients and 12 pedigrees so far (169,180,186). Twenty-three different mutations have been described, which were missense, nonsense, or truncating mutations. The mutation sites were located throughout the molecule. Most of the patients were compound heterozygotes for two different mutations, and only a few were homozygotes. Of interest, Kokame et al. showed that some mutations abrogated activity of the enzyme, whereas others retained low but significant activity (186). As yet, a correlation between phenotype and genotype cannot be established, but this may change with a larger number of subjects.

Treatment of von Willebrand Factor–Cleaving Protease Deficiency

Patients with the hereditary form can be treated by FFP infusions to replace active VWF-cp. Virus-inactivated plasma contains the same amount of VWF-cp as untreated plasma (165,181). FFP effectively reverses hemolytic crises, prevents relapse when given prophylactically, and limits the progression of organ damage (170,184,187,188). VWF-cp has a half-life of 2 to 3 days (187) and is effective at low concentrations. Plasma infusions (10 mL/kg body weight) every 2 to 4 weeks seem sufficient to maintain remission, whereas increasing the interval beyond 4 weeks risks relapse (170,182). The ideal interval between infusions (i.e., from 2 to 4 weeks) may be established for an individual patient by monitoring the platelet count after plasma therapy. Plasma infusions are best used preventively as rescue plasma infusions, even given early in a relapse, may not prevent CNS involvement (170).

Plasma treatment, started long before the association with VWF-cp deficiency was known, has maintained its clinical effectiveness in some cases for more than 20 years (170,174,179). These patients have developed neither resistance to plasma therapy nor, as far as is known, anti–VWF-cp antibodies.

The administration of 1-desamino-8-D-arginine vasopressin is contraindicated in patients with VWF-cp deficiency as symptomatic relapse of TTP has been reported within 1 hour of 1-desamino-8-D-arginine vasopressin infusion (189). In 10 healthy volunteers and 3 patients with type 1 von Willebrand disease, Reiter et al. (190) recently demonstrated a decrease of VWF-cp activity to approximately one-half the initial value and the appearance of large VWF multimers 60 minutes after the administration of desmopressin, suggesting a consumption of VWF-cp after desmopressin induced release of larger VWF multimers. Thus, even nasal or oral 1-desamino-8-D-arginine vasopressin to our opinion is contraindicated in VWF-cp–deficient enuretic patients. The question of which prophylaxis to avoid triggering factors of TMA is raised when an asymptomatic sibling is diagnosed in a family and in patients with bouts of TTP. In women, VWF-cp deficiency probably has to be considered as a contraindication to estroprogestatives.

Patients with acquired VWF-cp inhibitors may need more aggressive therapy, including PE, and, in some cases, immunosuppressive treatment, vincristine, or splenectomy (187). Low inhibitor titers can be overcome by the VWF-cp of FFP, and this may explain why plasma therapy or PE (between 1.0 and 2.5 times the plasma volume) is effective in most cases of TTP. Patients with high inhibitor titers are less likely to respond to PE by the end of 9 days (191). Nevertheless, in many cases, VWF-cp activity eventually returns to normal (162). This suggests that in these patients, the inhibitors represent a temporarily deranged immune response to VWF-cp. In some patients, the immune reaction persists, leading to a chronic or refractory disease. These cases may benefit from measures that suppress or block the inhibitor.

Posttransplant Course in Hemolytic Uremic Syndrome and Thrombotic Thrombocytopenic Purpura Associated with Constitutional von Willebrand Factor–Cleaving Protease Deficiency

Only one patient with constitutional VWF-cp deficiency has had renal transplantation (170,184). MAHA, thrombocytopenia, and renal failure recurred 5 days after transplantation, with arterial TMA lesions in the graft. The child also had transient amaurosis related to retinal ischemia and seizures and coma 35 days after transplantation, with ischemic lesions on cerebral tomodensitometry. PE with FFP was started empirically on day 7 posttransplantation, which corrected hemolysis and thrombocytopenia and stabilized graft function. Twice-monthly PE was continued during the 9 subsequent years without recurrence. After VWF-cp deficiency was identified in this patient, a second renal transplantation was performed at 24 years of age, under FFP cover. No recurrence has occurred during the year of follow-up after grafting, and the patient is well with twice-monthly FFP infusions (H. Nivet, *personal communication*).

Hemolytic Uremic Syndrome Associated with Congenital Intracellular Defects of Vitamin B_{12} Metabolism

HUS may occur in children with inherited abnormalities of the intracellular metabolism of vitamin B_{12} [cobalamin (Cbl)] (192–194). Considering the generally poor prognosis of these diseases and the possibility of prenatal diagnosis, detection is crucial.

Metabolism of Cobalamin

Cbl in the diet binds to intrinsic factor produced by gastric cells. Absorption is effected by binding of the intrinsic factor–Cbl complex to ileal receptors, followed by endocytosis and lysosomal digestion of the complex, releasing Cbl, which attaches to transcobalamin II. The complex Cbl-transcobalamin II is released from the cells into the portal blood stream and is captured by specific receptors of the Cbl-transcobalamin II complex at the surface of a number of cells. Within cells, Cbl follows two different metabolic pathways (Figs. 47.10 and 47.11). In the first one, cytosolic, Cbl is transformed to methylCbl (CH3-Cbl), the coenzyme of methionine synthase, which catalyzes the methylation of homocysteine to methionine. The second pathway occurs within mitochondria and consists of the adenylation of Cbl to form adenyl-Cbl (Ado-Cbl). Ado-Cbl is the coenzyme of methylmalonyl-CoA mutase that catalyzes the transformation of methylmalonyl-CoA to succinyl-CoA. So far, seven genetic defects have been demonstrated, which disturb the intracellular metabolism of Cbl (193). Defects in the early steps of these pathways, CblC, CblD, and CblF, result in deficient activity of both coenzymes, Ado-Cbl and CH3-Cbl, inducing deficient activity of both Cbl-requiring enzymes, methylmalonyl-CoA mutase and methionine synthase. These patients have homocystinuria, hyperhomocysteinemia, hypomethioninemia combined with methylmalonic aciduria, and hypermethylmalonic acidemia. CblE and CblG, due to defective CH3-Cbl synthesis, induce a functional deficiency of methionine synthase. These patients have homocystinuria without methylmalonic aciduria. CblA and CblB defects both impair the synthesis of Ado-Cbl, leading to a deficient activity of methylmalonic-CoA mutase. These patients have methylmalonic aciduria without homocystinuria. All these diseases have an autosomal recessive transmission.

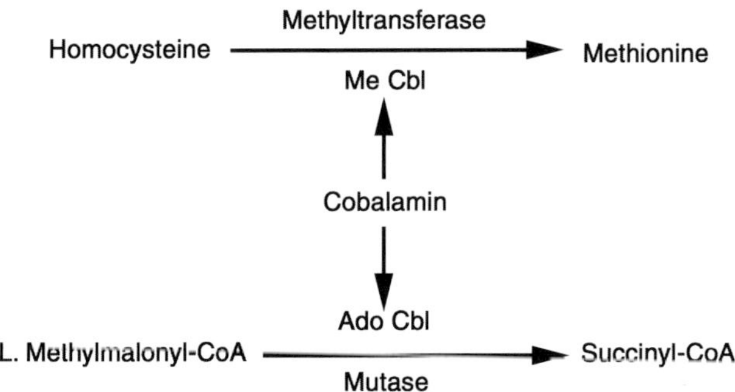

FIGURE 47.10. The two major chemical reactions catalyzed by cobalamin: the conversion of homocysteine to methionine and of methylmalonyl-CoA to succinyl-CoA. (From Russo P, Doyon J, Sonsino E, et al. Inborn errors of cobalamin metabolism and the hemolytic uremic syndrome. In: Kaplan B, Trompeter S, Moake J, ed. *The hemolytic uremic syndrome and thrombotic thrombocytopenic purpura*. New York: Marcel Dekker, 1992:255–270, with permission.)

Hemolytic Uremic Syndrome in Cobalamin C Defect

HUS has been reported mainly in CblC defect. Among a total of 44 CblC patients from the literature and from their personal experience, Ogier de Baulny et al. in 1998 reported the occurrence of HUS in 17 (194), mainly in the neonatal form of the disease. Out of 32 CblC patients who had clinical symptoms in the neonatal period or early infancy (younger than 3 months), 12 developed full-blown HUS before 3 months of age, and 4 additional patients from the literature had renal signs compatible with HUS before 3 months of age (194). Another CblC patient with HUS at 28 days of age has recently been reported (196). These children display feeding difficulties with anorexia, poor sucking, vomiting, weight loss associated with hypotonia, and lethargy early after birth. Megaloblastic anemia is frequent. Quite often, the diagnosis remains uncertain until the occurrence of HUS. At this stage, MAHA is severe and recurrent, with schizocytosis and thrombocytopenia. Renal involvement consists of hematuria, proteinuria, renal failure of variable severity, and hypertension. HUS is most often associated with multisystem deterioration, including cardiac failure due to cardiomyopathy, respiratory failure due to interstitial lung disease, hepatocellular failure, diarrhea, and gastrointestinal bleeding and further neurologic deterioration with seizures and coma. Tomodensitometry shows nonspecific cortical and subcortical atrophy; MRI shows periventricular demyelinization. Retinopathy with visual impairment is frequent. Treatment with hydroxycobalamin (greater than or equal to 1 mg/day initially), oral betaine, and folic acid normalize the metabolic anomalies within a few days, but mortality is extremely high. Among the 16 CblC cases with HUS reviewed by Ogier de Baulny et al. (194), only 2 were alive at 10 years of age (H. Ogier

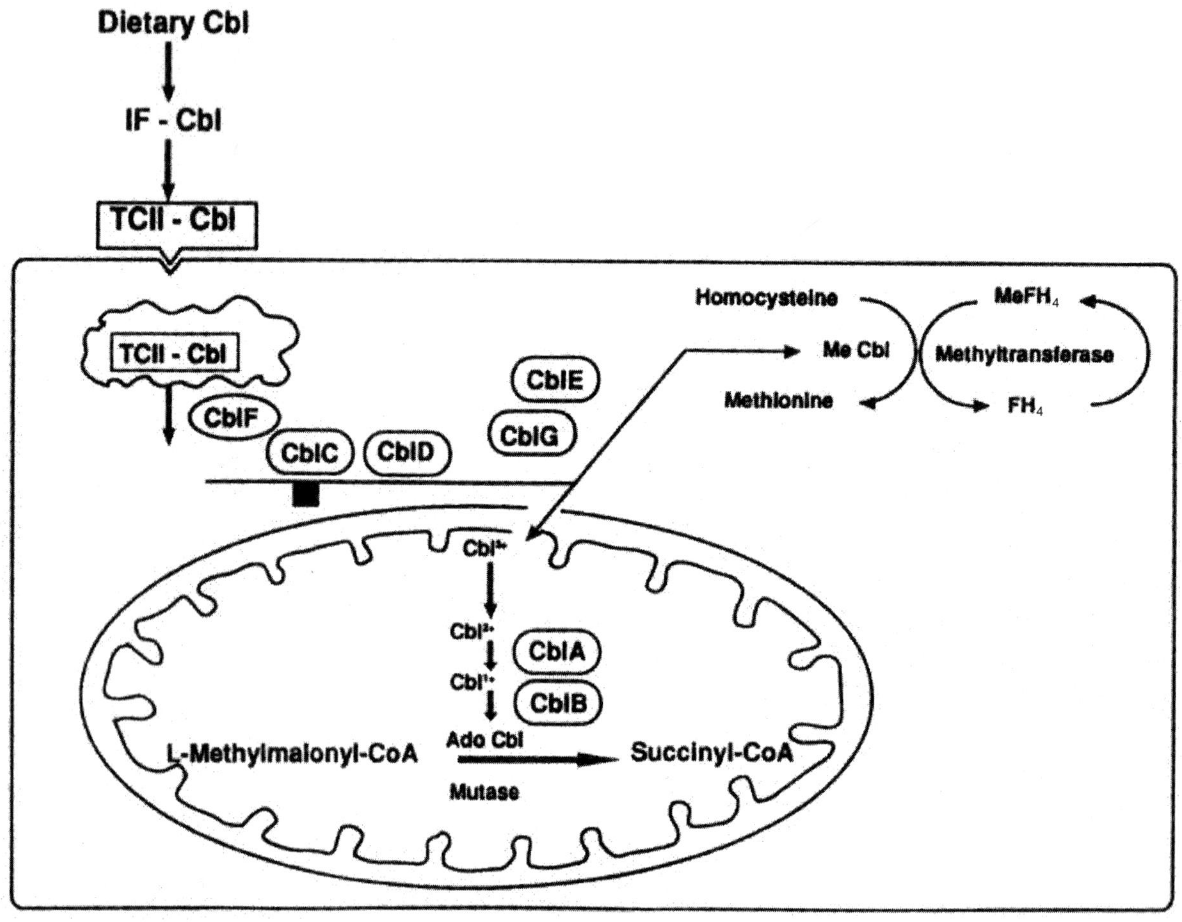

FIGURE 47.11. The intracellular conversion of cobalamin to either methylcobalamin or adenosylcobalamin. (From Russo P, Doyon J, Sonsino E, et al. Inborn errors of cobalamin metabolism and the hemolytic uremic syndrome. In: Kaplan B, Trompeter S, Moake J, ed. *The hemolytic uremic syndrome and thrombotic thrombocytopenic purpura*. New York: Marcel Dekker, 1992:255–270, with permission.)

de Baulny, *personal communication*) and 7 months of age (197), with severe visual and neurologic impairment. The patient reported by Kind et al. also was alive at 6 months of age, with visual and neurologic sequels (196).

Thus, the diagnosis of CblC defect must be considered whenever HUS occurs in an infant with feeding difficulties and neurologic impairment preceding the HUS and atypical features like megaloblastosis and leukoneutropenia with hypersegmentation of neutrophils.

At autopsy, widespread TMA with glomerular and arteriolar thrombosis is observed in the kidneys, and possibly in the brain, heart, lungs, and liver. Total atrophy of the gastric mucosa with extensive cystic changes is also characteristic.

Occurrence of HUS in CblC patients with symptoms in late infancy and early childhood is quite exceptional. One child with HUS at 9 months of age has been reported (194). Von Hove et al. (198) reported 2 siblings, a 12 year-old boy and his 4-year-old sister, who presented with proteinuria and hematuria, hypertension, and chronic hemolytic anemia. The boy developed an episode of severe hypertensive encephalopathy and transient renal failure. Neither child had neurologic symptoms, only minimal pigmentary retinal abnormalities were seen. Renal biopsy showed chronic TMA lesions. Both patients had hyperhomocysteinemia and mild methylmalonic aciduria. Fibroblasts showed decreased Cbl uptake and reduced methyl and adenosyl Cbl formation compatible with the Cbl group, but milder than that found in cells of most patients. After treatment with high doses of hydroxycobalamin (5 mg/day) and betaine, homocysteine levels normalized, hemolysis and hematuria disappeared, proteinuria almost normalized, and creatinine clearance has been stable after 1 year of follow-up.

Hemolytic Uremic Syndrome in Methionine Synthase (Cobalamin G) Defect

One CblG patient with HUS has been reported (199). This 18-month-old girl born from consanguineous parents had macrocytic megaloblastic anemia followed by HUS with schistocytosis, renal failure, and hypertension. Renal biopsy showed glomerular and arteriolar TMA. Methioninemia and the activity of methionine synthase were decreased, indicating that the patient had CblG defect. Treatment with hydroxycobalamin and folic acid corrected the anemia, but the child progressed to end-stage renal failure at 13 years of age and had pulmonary hypertension at 6 years of age. Most likely, the pulmonary hypertension was due to vascular lesions similar to those observed in the kidney and in some neonatal forms of CblC with pulmonary involvement.

Mechanisms of Hemolytic Uremic Syndrome in Remethylation Defects

The mechanism of HUS in inborn errors of Cbl metabolism is uncertain. TMA is probably secondary to vascular endothelial damage caused by the high homocysteine concentrations. Hyperhomocysteinemia induces endothelium lesions in rats (200) and pulmonary thrombi in mice (201). Hyperhomocysteinemia is a well-established risk of vascular disease in humans (202,203). However, homocysteine alone cannot be the only risk factor, because HUS has not been described in patients with cystathionine synthase, whose plasma homocysteine concentrations are higher than those encountered in Cbl-mutant patients.

DRUG-INDUCED HEMOLYTIC UREMIC SYNDROME

Calcineurin Inhibitors (Cyclosporine, Tacrolimus)

HUS associated with cyclosporine A (CsA) therapy was first reported after bone marrow transplantation. Subsequently, it was reported after liver, kidney, or heart transplantation (204). The syndrome generally occurs during the first few weeks of transplantation and is associated with high blood concentrations of CsA. Most often, there is no full-blown HUS, but TMA lesions at renal pathology, with or without deterioration of renal function (205). Tacrolimus-induced posttransplant HUS cases have also been recognized (206), with a reported incidence of approximately 1% in recipients of renal transplants (207).

Chemotherapy

Several cytotoxic drugs can induce HUS, probably due to toxicity to endothelial cells, mainly mitomycin C, given alone or in association with 5-fluorouracil and doxorubicin (208), bleomycin, epirubicin, cisplatin, and, more recently, the antimetabolite gemcitabine (209).

Ticlopidine, Clopidogrel

HUS/TTP was first reported in patients receiving ticlopidine for 2 to 12 weeks, with an estimated incidence of 1 case in 1600 to 5000 patients (210). Clopidogrel has largely replaced ticlopidine in clinical practice because it has a more favorable safety profile. Nevertheless, TTP has also developed in some patients receiving clopidogrel (approximately 10 to 15 cases per 3 million people treated). TTP occurred within 2 weeks after initiation of treatment. Antibodies against VWF-cp, inducing a severe VWF-cp deficiency, have been demonstrated in most cases of ticlopidine-induced TTP and PE are efficient both clinically and on the activity of VWF-cp (210,211). This antibody-mediated mechanism was also found in some patients with clopidogrel-induced TTP, but not all (212). Although almost all patients with ticlopidine-associated TTP had a response to PE within seven or fewer sessions and have had no relapses, some patients with clopidogrel-associated TTP require up to 30 PE, and some of them may have relapses up to 7 months after the discontinuation of clopidogrel (210).

Quinine

Patients presensitized to quinine may develop TTP/HUS, sometimes triggered by a single tablet taken many months after a previous exposure. They present with chills, fever, MAHA, thrombocytopenia, and possibly neurologic abnormalities. Renal involvement may be mild or asymptomatic, but acute renal failure is also possible. Out of 17 patients reported by Kojouri et al. (213), four died and seven had chronic renal failure. These patients with quinine-induced TTP/HUS have been shown to have developed quinine-dependent antibodies to erythrocytes, granulocytes, and the glycoprotein Ib/IX and IIb/IIIa expressed on the platelet surface (214).

HEMOLYTIC UREMIC SYNDROME SUPERIMPOSED TO OTHER PATHOLOGIES

De Novo Posttransplantation Hemolytic Uremic Syndrome

De novo posttransplant HUS occurring in renal or nonrenal transplant recipients is usually triggered by calcineurin inhibitors (207), or in exceptional cases, by OKT3 (215) or viral infections, especially cytomegalovirus (216). Influenza A virus (217) and parvovirus B19 (218) have also been reported as triggering a few cases of HUS after renal transplantation. Renal TMA associated with anticardiolipin antibodies has been reported in hepatitis C–positive renal transplant recipients (219). Last, undetectable VWF-cp activity secondary to the presence of inhibitors has been reported in a patient with HUS and TMA after renal transplantation. Discontinuation of CsA and PE increased the VWF-cp activity, which was followed by resolution of MAHA and improvement of graft function. Thus, the role of calcineurin inhibitors in the formation of autoantibodies to VWF-cp remains to be explored (220).

Hemolytic Uremic Syndrome after Bone Marrow Transplantation

A clinical picture resembling HUS may develop after bone marrow transplantation (BMT) (204,221–224). MAHA, thrombocytopenia, renal failure, frequently severe hypertension, and possibly seizures occur several months (e.g., at least 3 months, mean 8 months) after BMT. Pretransplant total body irradiation probably plays a role through its toxicity toward endothelial cells. However, HUS has been described in patients exposed to cytotoxic chemotherapy without renal irradiation (225). Some patients with post-BMT/HUS have also received high doses of CsA. However, in rats, CsA does not appear to exacerbate radiation nephropathy (226), and HUS is well documented in BMT recipients who have never received CsA (227, 228). Besides radiotherapy, the presence of graft versus host disease appears as another risk factor (229).

Renal histology in post-BMT/HUS shows striking glomerular mesangiolysis and diffuse endothelial cells damage with subendothelial expansion and capillary loop occlusion (224,225,230).

In adult patients, the cumulative risk of BMT-induced HUS/TTP is approximately 25%, mainly observed in the first 12 months after BMT (231). Subclinical renal dysfunction is even more frequent (232).

An increase of the plasma levels of IL-8, thrombomodulin, and plasminogen activator inhibitor has been demonstrated in patients with HUS or TTP after BMT, with a close relationship between improvement in symptoms and a decrease of IL-8 levels, suggesting a role of this cytokine (233). VWF-cp levels were normal in six patients with BMT-associated TMA (234). The very low turnover of endothelial cells, with cell death delayed until the cell divides, may explain why radiation HUS/TTP is a late phenomenon, occurring months after the exposure (224).

Hemolytic Uremic Syndrome Associated with Systemic Lupus Erythematosus or Antiphospholipid Syndrome

The coexistence of systemic lupus erythematosus (SLE) and HUS/TTP is rare in adults and has only been reported in approximately 20 children (235–237). Serum haptoglobin concentration must be measured whenever a child with SLE shows thrombocytopenia, Coombs'-negative anemia, and schizocytes. Correct diagnosis is important, as treatment with plasmapheresis and FFP is necessary to control the disease.

HUS/TTP has also been described in the context of catastrophic antiphospholipid syndrome (238), in association with lupus anticoagulant or anticardiolipin or anti-B2 glycoprotein I antibodies. An acquired deficiency of VWF-cp due to an inhibitor has been reported both in SLE patients with (239) or without (240) antiphospholipid antibodies.

Hemolytic Uremic Syndrome Superimposed to Collagen Type III Glomerulopathy

The occurrence of HUS has been reported in children with a hereditary (autosomal recessive) glomerulopathy called *collagen type III glomerulopathy* or *complex basalopathy* (241). This glomerulopathy is characterized by an increase of mesangial matrix, thickening of capillary walls, and double contour appearance of glomerular basement membranes, due to the accumulation of collagen type III. The association with fH deficiency reported in one child (134) raises the question of the role of fH deficiency in the pathogenesis of the glomerular anomalies.

HEMOLYTIC UREMIC SYNDROME OF UNKNOWN MECHANISM

Even when fully investigated, no etiologic diagnosis is found in a high proportion of children with D– HUS. This includes cases with clear indication that there must be an inherited cause.

Autosomal Recessive Hemolytic Uremic Syndrome Not Associated with Prodrome of Diarrhea of Unknown Mechanism

D– HUS with presumed autosomal recessive inheritance is mainly observed in children (242), although the age of onset ranges from neonates (243) to adults (244,245). Age at onset of HUS tends to be similar in siblings. A recurrent course is common. Many patients die, especially those with early onset. Progression to end-stage renal disease is almost constant. The course after renal transplantation is not documented in those with childhood onset. Eleven patients in four families reported by Kaplan et al. (246) had HUS at 17 to 36 years of age and received 14 renal transplants. Recurrence occurred in 9 out of the 14 grafts. The use of CsA or the type of donor had no role in the risk of recurrence. In one family, one patient had HUS posttransplant recurrence, but not his sibling (246). Most probably, the risk of recurrence in children with autosomal recessive HUS is as high as in adults.

Autosomal Dominant Hemolytic Uremic Syndrome Not Associated with Prodrome of Diarrhea of Unknown Mechanism

Autosomal dominant HUS generally starts during adulthood (242,247). Among the 68 patients from 16 families reviewed by Kaplan and Leonard, 18 were children in whom HUS started between 5 months and 17 years of age (247). A recurrent course of HUS has been reported in only 3 cases out of 62. Twenty-eight patients (45%) died, 6 were alive and well (19%) without renal failure, and 28 (45%)

had end-stage renal failure. Twenty patients received 32 kidney grafts. Recurrence occurred in 17 (65%). The nephrectomy of native kidney did not appear to influence the outcome.

Hemolytic Uremic Syndrome of Unknown Mechanism without a Prodrome of Diarrhea

Clinical Course

The clinical pattern of these patients can be gleaned from the main pediatric reviews. A total of approximately 100 cases can be analyzed (15,242,248–251). Age at onset varied from 3 days to 14 years, with several patients developing HUS as neonates. The onset of renal involvement is often insidious. Between 13 (250) and 54% (249) of patients have oligoanuria at onset, but at least one-half have a nonoliguric progressive increase of serum creatinine with proteinuria and hematuria. Thus, the interval between the onset of renal symptoms and the need for dialysis may vary from a few days to several months with three-fourths of patients finally requiring dialysis (15,248,250). Severe hypertension is associated in one-half to 75% of patients. Relapses with exacerbation of MAHA have been reported in 18% of patients of Siegler's series (249), 32 to 55% in 3 other series (15,248,250). The incidence of CNS involvement is highly variable, from 0% (251) to 8 to 13% (15,249), up to 30 to 48% (248) and 48% (250). This, and the variability of the overall severity of the disease, most probably reflects the heterogeneity of patients regrouped under the eponym of unexplained D– atypical HUS. Thus, in the group of patients reported by Siegler et al. (249), mortality rate was 0%, evolution to end-stage renal disease was observed in only 12% of patients (mainly in those with relapses), and recovery without renal sequels in 47%. Other series had mortality rates varying from 13% (251) to 20 to 26% (15,248,250), and end-stage renal disease rates from 21 to 27% (15,248) to 42 to 56% (250,251). Thus, full renal recovery was observed in only 7 to 26% of patients in these series (15,248,250,251).

Treatment

Some rare cases of D– HUS of unknown mechanism have a positive response to FFP infusion or PE (252,253), justifying this empirical approach. The recommended amount of FFP infused is 10 mL/kg over 6 to 7 consecutive days, which cannot be done without PE if the child is anuric. During PE sessions, one or two plasma volumes (40 to 80 mL/kg) are exchanged daily or on alternate days over 1 week. Efficacy is judged on the platelet count, the correction of MAHA, the normalization of haptoglobin, and, eventually, neurologic improvement. Renal function may take several weeks to show an improvement.

Posttransplant Course

The incidence of HUS recurrence can be analyzed from the literature in 59 children with atypical D– HUS of unknown mechanism who received 73 kidney transplants (75,97,98,101,248,250). Thirteen of the 59 children (22%) had recurrence of HUS on one or several grafts, with a total of 18 recurrences on 73 grafts (25%). In addition, there are 7 individual case reports with 11 grafts and 9 recurrences (254–260). Therefore, a total of 27 grafts with HUS recurrence can be analyzed. The time between initial HUS and renal transplantation does not appear to affect the risk of recurrence. In most cases, HUS recurred during the first month after transplantation, but late occurrence several years after transplantation has also been observed. The role of calcineurin inhibitors is unclear. The type of donor, cadaveric or living related, does not appear to have a role in the risk of recurrence. The outcome after HUS recurrence is poor, with graft loss within a few days or weeks in most cases. Those with recurrence in a first graft usually experience recurrence in subsequent grafts. However, there are exceptions to this, and a few who show no recurrence on a first graft will do so on subsequent grafts.

CONCLUSION

Despite its rarity, great progress has been made in understanding the mechanisms of HUS in recent years. However, the high proportion of D– HUS for which no etiology can be found suggests that there may be diagnostic categories still to be discovered. Collaboration between many clinical centers and laboratories will be needed to keep up this momentum.

REFERENCES

1. Moschcowitz E. An acute febrile pleiochromic anemia with hyalin thrombosis of the terminal arterioles and capillaries. An undescribed disease. *Arch Intern Med* 1925;36:89–93.
2. Gasser C, Gautier E, Steck A, et al. Hämolytisch-urämische syndrome: bilaterale nierenrinden nekrosen bei akuten erworbenen hämolytischen anämien. *Schweitz Med Wochenschr* 1955;85:905–909.
3. Moake J, Rudy C, Troll J, et al. Unusually large plasma factor VIII: von Willebrand factor multimers in chronic relapsing thrombotic thrombocytopenic purpura. *N Engl J Med* 1982;307:1432–1435.
4. Karmali MA, Petric M, Lim C, et al. The association between idiopathic hemolytic uremic syndrome and infection by verotoxin-producing *Escherichia coli. J Infect Dis* 1985;151:775–782.
5. Moake J. Thrombotic microangiopathies. *N Engl J Med* 2002;347:589–600.
6. Levin M, Barratt JM. Haemolytic uraemic syndrome. *Arch Dis Child* 1984;59:397–400.

7. Milford D, Taylor C, Guttridge B, et al. Haemolytic uraemic syndromes in the British Isles 1985–1988: association with verocytotoxin producing *Escherichia coli*. Part 1: clinical and epidemiological aspects. *Arch Dis Child* 1990; 65:716–721.
8. Melnyk AM, Solez K, Kjellstrand CM. Adult hemolytic-uremic syndrome. A review of 37 cases. *Arch Intern Med* 1995;155:2077–2084.
9. Ruggenenti P, Noris M, Remuzzi G. Thrombotic microangiopathy, hemolytic uremic syndrome, and thrombotic thrombocytopenic purpura. *Kidney Int* 2001;60:831–846.
10. Milford D, Taylor C. New insights into the haemolytic uraemic syndromes. *Arch Dis Child* 1990;65:713–715.
11. Decludt B, Bouvet P, Mariani-Kurkdjian P, et al. Haemolytic uraemic syndrome and Shiga toxin-producing Escherichia coli infection in children in France. The Societe de Nephrologie Pediatrique. *Epidemiol Infect* 2000;124:215–220.
12. Brain M, Dacie J, Hourihane D. Microangiopathic haemolytic anaemia: possible role of vascular lesions in pathogenesis. *Br J Haematol* 1962;8:358–374.
13. Nevard C, Jurd K, Lane D, et al. Activation of coagulation and fibrinolysis in childhood diarrhoea-associated haemolytic uraemic syndrome. *Thromb Haemost* 1997;78:1450–1455.
14. Chandler W, Jelacic S, Boster D, et al. Prothrombotic coagulation abnormalities preceding the hemolytic-uremic syndrome. *N Engl J Med* 2002;346:23–32.
15. Loirat C, Baudouin V, Sonsino E, et al. Hemolytic-uremic syndrome in the child. *Adv Nephrol Necker Hosp* 1993;22:141–168.
16. Habib R, Levy M, Gagnadoux M, et al. Prognosis of the hemolytic uremic syndrome in children. *Adv Nephrol Necker Hosp* 1982;11:99–128.
17. Habib R. Pathology of the hemolytic uremic syndrome. In: Kaplan B, Trompeter R, Moake J, eds. *Hemolytic uremic syndrome and thrombotic thrombocytopenic purpura.* New York: Marcel Dekker, 1992:315–353.
18. Richardson S, Karmali M, Becker L, et al. The histopathology of the hemolytic uremic syndrome associated with verocytotoxin-producing *Escherichia coli* infections. *Hum Pathol* 1988; 19:1102–1108.
19. Inward CD, Howie AJ, Fitzpatrick MM, et al. Renal histopathology in fatal cases of diarrhoea-associated haemolytic uraemic syndrome. British Association for Paediatric Nephrology. *Pediatr Nephrol* 1997;11:556–559.
20. Thoenes W, John H. Endotheliotropic (hemolytic) nephroangiopathy and its various manifestation forms (thrombotic microangiopathy, primary malignant nephrosclerosis, hemolytic-uremic syndrome). *Klin Wochenschr* 1980;58: 173–184.
21. Konowalchuk J, Speirs J, Stavric S. Vero response to a cytotoxin of *Escherichia coli. Infect Immun* 1977;18:775–779.
22. O'Brien A, La Veck G. Purification and characterization of a *Shigella dysenteriae* 1-like toxin produced by *Escherichia coli. Infect Immun* 1983;40:675–683.
23. Riley LW, Remis RS, Helgerson SD, et al. Hemorrhagic colitis associated with a rare *Escherichia coli* serotype. *N Engl J Med* 1983;308:682–685.
24. Karmali MA, Petric M, Lim C, et al. *Escherichia coli* cytotoxin, haemolytic-uraemic syndrome, and haemorrhagic colitis. *Lancet* 1983;2:1299–1300.
25. Crump J, Sulka A, Langer A, et al. An outbreak of *Escherichia coli* O157:H7 infections among visitors to a dairy farm. *N Engl J Med* 2002;347:555–560.
26. O'Brien S, Adak G. *Escherichia coli* O157:H7—piecing together the jigsaw puzzle. *N Engl J Med* 2002;347:555–560.
27. Andreoli S, Trachtman H, Acheson D, et al. Hemolytic uremic syndrome: epidemiology, pathophysiology, and therapy. *Pediatr Nephrol* 2002;17:293–298.
28. Kobayashi H, Shimada J, Nakazawa M, et al. Prevalence and characteristics of shiga toxin-producing *Escherichia coli* from healthy cattle in Japan. *Appl Environ Microbiol* 2001;67:484–489.
29. Meyer-Broseta S, Bastian SN, Arne PD, et al. Review of epidemiological surveys on the prevalence of contamination of health cattle with *Escherichia coli* serogroup O157:H7. *Int J Hyg Environ Health* 2001;203:347–361.
30. Stephan R, Ragettli S, Untermann F. Prevalence and characteristics of verotoxin-producing *Escherichia coli* (VTEC) in stool samples from asymptomatic human carriers working in the meat processing industry in Switzerland. *J Appl Microbiol* 2000;88:335–341.
31. Morabito S, Dell'Omo G, Agrimi U, et al. Detection and characterization of Shiga toxin-producing *Escherichia coli* in feral pigeons. *Vet Microbiol* 2001;82:275–283.
32. Kaper JB. Enterohemorrhagic *Escherichia coli. Curr Opin Microbiol* 1998;1:103–108.
33. Frankel G, Phillips A, Rosenshine I, et al. Enteropathogenic and enterohaemorrhagic *Escherichia coli*: more subversive elements. *Mol Microbiol* 1998;30:911–921.
34. Friedrich AW, Bielaszewska M, Zhang WL, et al. *Escherichia coli* harboring Shiga toxin 2 gene variants: frequency and association with clinical symptoms. *J Infect Dis* 2002;185:74–84.
35. Beutin L, Bulte M, Weber A, et al. Investigation of human infections with verocytotoxin-producing strains of *Escherichia coli* (VTEC) belonging to serogroup O118 with evidence for zoonotic transmission. *Epidemiol Infect* 2000;125: 47–54.
36. Schmidt H, Montag M, Bockemuhl J, et al. Shiga-like toxin II-related cytotoxins in *Citrobacter freundii* strains from humans and beef samples. *Infect Immun* 1993;61:534–543.
37. Stein P, Boodhoo A, Tyrrell G, et al. Crystal structure of the cell-binding B oligomer of verotoxin-1 from *E. coli. Nature* 1992;355:748–750.
38. Sandvig K, Van Deurs B. Endocytosis, intracellular transport, and cytotoxic action of Shiga toxin and ricin. *Physiol Rev* 1996;76:949–966.
39. Arab S, Murakami M, Dirks P, et al. Verotoxins inhibit the growth of and induce apoptosis in human astrocytoma cells. *J Neurooncol* 1998;40:137–150.
40. Furutani M, Kashiwagi K, Ito K, et al. Comparison of the modes of action of a Vero toxin (a Shiga-like toxin) from *Escherichia coli*, of ricin, and of alpha-sarcin. *Arch Biochem Biophys* 1992;293:140–146.
41. Pudymaitis A, Lingwood C. Susceptibility to verotoxin as a function of the cell cycle. *J Cell Physiol* 1992;150:632–639.
42. Inward CD, Williams J, Chant I, et al. Verocytotoxin-1 induces apoptosis in vero cells. *J Infect* 1995;30:213–218.
43. Pijpers A, van Setten P, van den Heuvel L, et al. Verocytotoxin-induced apoptosis of human microvascular endothelial cells. *J Am Soc Nephrol* 2001;12:767–778.

44. Hughes AK, Stricklett PK, Schmid D, et al. Cytotoxic effect of Shiga toxin-1 on human glomerular epithelial cells. *Kidney Int* 2000;57:2350–2359.
45. Williams J, Boyd B, Nutikka A, et al. A comparison of the effects of verocytotoxin-1 on primary human renal cell cultures. *Toxicol Lett* 1999;105:47–57.
46. van de Kar N, Monnens L, Karmali M, et al. Tumor necrosis factor and interleukin-1 induce expression of the verocytotoxin receptor globotriaosylceramide on human endothelial cells: implications for the pathogenesis of the hemolytic uremic syndrome. *Blood* 1992;80:2755–2764.
47. van Setten P, van Hinsbergh V, van der Velden T, et al. Effects of TNF alpha on verocytotoxin cytotoxicity in purified human glomerular microvascular endothelial cells. *Kidney Int* 1997;51:1245–1256.
48. van Setten PA, van Hinsberg VW, van den Heuvel LP, et al. Verocytotoxin inhibits mitogenesis and protein synthesis in purified human glomerular mesangial cells without affecting cell viability: evidence for two distinct mechanisms. *J Am Soc Nephrol* 1997;8:1877–1888.
49. Thorpe C, Hurley B, Lincicome L, et al. Shiga toxins stimulate secretion of interleukin-8 from intestinal epithelial cells. *Infect Immun* 1999;67:5985–5993.
50. Thorpe C, Smith W, Hurley B, et al. Shiga toxins induce, superinduce, and stabilize a variety of C-X-C chemokine mRNAs in intestinal epithelial cells, resulting in increased chemokine expression. *Infect Immun* 2001;69:6140–6147.
51. Zoja C, Angioletti S, Donadelli R, et al. Shiga toxin-2 triggers endothelial leukocyte adhesion and transmigration via NF-kappaB dependent up-regulation of IL-8 and MCP-1. *Kidney Int* 2002;62:846–856.
52. Ishii H, Takada K, Higuchi T, et al. Verotoxin-1 induces tissue factor expression in human umbilical vein endothelial cells through activation of NF-kappaB/Rel and AP-1. *Thromb Haemost* 2000;84:712–721.
53. van Setten P, Monnens L, Verstraten R, et al. Effects of verocytotoxin-1 on nonadherent human monocytes: binding characteristics, protein synthesis, and induction of cytokine release. *Blood* 1996;88:174–183.
54. Taylor CM, Williams JM, Lote CJ, et al. A laboratory model of toxin-induced hemolytic uremic syndrome. *Kidney Int* 1999;55:1367–1374.
55. Siegler RL, Pysher TJ, Lou R, et al. Response to Shiga-toxin-1, with and without lipopolysaccharide, in a primate model of hemolytic uremic syndrome. *Am J Nephrol* 2001; 21:420–425.
56. Palermo M, Alves-Rosa F, Rubel C, et al. Pretreatment of mice with lipopolysaccharide (LPS) or IL-1beta exerts dose-dependent opposite effects on Shiga toxin-2 lethality. *Clin Exp Immunol* 2000;119:77–83.
57. Harel Y, Silva M, Giroir B, et al. A reporter transgene indicates renal-specific induction of tumor necrosis factor (TNF) by shiga-like toxin. Possible involvement of TNF in hemolytic uremic syndrome. *J Clin Invest* 1993;92:2110–2116.
58. Hughes AK, Stricklett PK, Kohan DE. Shiga toxin-1 regulation of cytokine production by human glomerular epithelial cells. *Nephron* 2001;88:14–23.
59. Richardson S, Rotman T, Jay V, et al. Experimental verocytotoxemia in rabbits. *Infect Immun* 1992;60:4154–4167.
60. Lingwood CA. Verotoxin-binding in human renal sections. *Nephron* 1994;66:21–28.
61. Lopez EL, Contrini MM, Devoto S, et al. Tumor necrosis factor concentrations in hemolytic uremic syndrome patients and children with bloody diarrhea in Argentina. *Pediatr Infect Dis J* 1995;14:594–598.
62. te Loo D, Monnens L, van Der Velden T, et al. Binding and transfer of verocytotoxin by polymorphonuclear leukocytes in hemolytic uremic syndrome. *Blood* 2000;95:3396–3402.
63. Hurley BP, Thorpe CM, Acheson DW. Shiga toxin translocation across intestinal epithelial cells is enhanced by neutrophil transmigration. *Infect Immun* 2001;69:6148–6155.
64. Pavia AT, Nichols CR, Green DP, et al. Hemolytic-uremic syndrome during an outbreak of *Escherichia coli* O157:H7 infections in institutions for mentally retarded persons: clinical and epidemiologic observations. *J Pediatr* 1990;116:544–551.
65. Walters M, Matthei I, Kay R, et al. The polymorphonuclear leucocyte count in childhood haemolytic uraemic syndrome. *Pediatr Nephrol* 1989;3:130–134.
66. Fitzpatrick MM, Shah V, Filler G, et al. Neutrophil activation in the haemolytic uraemic syndrome: free and complexed elastase in plasma. *Pediatr Nephrol* 1992;6:50–53.
67. Chandler WL, Jelacic S, Boster DR, et al. Prothrombotic coagulation abnormalities preceding the hemolytic-uremic syndrome. *N Engl J Med* 2002;346:23–32.
68. Morigi M, Galbusera M, Binda E, et al. Verotoxin-1-induced up-regulation of adhesive molecules renders microvascular endothelial cells thrombogenic at high shear stress. *Blood* 2001;98:1828–1835.
69. Karpman D, Papadopoulou D, Nilsson K, et al. Platelet activation by Shiga toxin and circulatory factors as a pathogenetic mechanism in the hemolytic uremic syndrome. *Blood* 2001;97:3100–3108.
70. Moghal N, Ferreira M, Howie A, et al. The late histologic findings in diarrhea-associated hemolytic uremic syndrome. *J Pediatr* 1998;133:220–223.
71. Griffin P, Tauxe R. The epidemiology of infections caused by *Escherichia coli* O157:H7, other enterohemorrhagic *E. coli*, and the associated hemolytic uremic syndrome. *Epidemiol Rev* 1991;13:60–98.
72. Rowe P, Orrbine E, Lior H, et al. Risk of hemolytic uremic syndrome after sporadic *Escherichia coli* O157:H7 infection: results of a Canadian collaborative study. Investigators of the Canadian Pediatric Kidney Disease Research Center. *J Pediatr* 1998;132:777–782.
73. Ludwig K, Karmali MA, Sarkim V, et al. Antibody response to Shiga toxins Stx2 and Stx1 in children with enteropathic hemolytic-uremic syndrome. *J Clin Microbiol* 2001;39: 2272–2279.
74. Rowe PC, Orrbine E, Wells GA, et al. Epidemiology of hemolytic-uremic syndrome in Canadian children from 1986 to 1988. The Canadian Pediatric Kidney Disease Reference Centre. *J Pediatr* 1991;119:218–224.
75. Repetto HA. Epidemic hemolytic-uremic syndrome in children. *Kidney Int* 1997;52:1708–1719.
76. Elliot EJ, Robins-Browne RM, O'Loughlin EV, et al. Nationwide study of haemolytic uraemic syndrome: clinical, microbiological, and epidemiological features. *Arch Dis Child* 2001;85:125–131.

77. Bender JB, Hedberg CW, Besser JM, et al. Surveillance by molecular subtype for *Escherichia coli* O157:H7 infections in Minnesota by molecular subtyping. *N Engl J Med* 1997;337: 388–394.
78. Siegler R. Spectrum of extrarenal involvement in postdiarrheal hemolytic-uremic syndrome. *J Pediatr* 1994;125:511–518.
79. Gallo E, Gianantonio C. Extrarenal involvement in diarrhoea-associated haemolytic-uraemic syndrome. *Pediatr Nephrol* 1995;9:117–119.
80. Robitaille P, Gonthier M, Grignon A, et al. Pancreatic injury in the hemolytic-uremic syndrome. *Pediatr Nephrol* 1997;11:631–632.
81. Walker A, Benson L, Wilson G, et al. Cardiomyopathy: a late complication of hemolytic uremic syndrome. *Pediatr Nephrol* 1997;11:221–222.
82. Proulx F, Turgeon J, Delage G, et al. Randomized, controlled trial of antibiotic therapy for *Escherichia coli* O157:H7 enteritis. *J Pediatr* 1992;121:299–303.
83. Wong C, Jelacic S, Habeeb R, et al. The risk of the hemolytic-uremic syndrome after antibiotic treatment of *Escherichia coli* O157:H7 infections. *N Engl J Med* 2000;342:1930–1936.
84. Molbak K, Mead PS, Griffin PM. Antimicrobial therapy in patients with *Escherichia coli* O157:H7 infection. *JAMA* 2002;288:1014–1016.
85. Ikeda K, Ida O, Kimoto K, et al. Effect of early fosfomycin treatment on prevention of hemolytic uremic syndrome accompanying *Escherichia coli* O157:H7 infection. *Clin Nephrol* 1999;52:357–362.
86. Safdar N, Said A, Gangnon RE, et al. Risk of hemolytic uremic syndrome after antibiotic treatment of *Escherichia coli* O157:H7 enteritis: a meta-analysis. *JAMA* 2002;288:996–1001.
87. Cimolai N, Basalyga S, Mah DG, et al. A continuing assessment of risk factors for the development of *Escherichia coli* O157:H7-associated hemolytic uremic syndrome. *Clin Nephrol* 1994;42:85–89.
88. Fitzpatrick MM. Long-term outcome of the hemolytic uremic syndrome in children. In: Kaplan B, Trompeter R, Moake J, (eds). *Hemolytic uremic syndrome and thrombotic thrombocytopenic purpura.* New York: Marcel Dekker, 1992:441–451.
89. Kelles A, Van Dyck M, Proesmans W. Childhood haemolytic uraemic syndrome: long-term outcome and prognostic features. *Eur J Pediatr* 1994;153(1):38–42.
90. Huseman D, Gellermann J, Vollmer I, et al. Long-term prognosis of hemolytic uremic syndrome and effective renal plasma flow. *Pediatr Nephrol* 1999;13(8):672–677.
91. Fitzpatrick M, Shah V, Trompeter R, et al. Long term renal outcome of childhood haemolytic uraemic syndrome. *BMJ* 1991;303:489–492.
92. Gagnadoux MF, Habib R, Gubler MC, et al. Long-term (15–25 years) outcome of childhood hemolytic-uremic syndrome. *Clin Nephrol* 1996;46:39–41.
93. Spizzirri F, Rahman R, Bibiloni N, et al. Childhood hemolytic uremic syndrome in Argentina: long-term follow-up and prognostic features. *Pediatr Nephrol* 1997;11:156–160.
94. Blahova K, Janda J, Kreisinger J, et al. Long-term follow-up of Czech children with D+ hemolytic-uremic syndrome. *Pediatr Nephrol* 2002;17:400–403.
95. Milford D, White R, Taylor C. Prognostic significance of proteinuria one year after onset of diarrhea-associated hemolytic-uremic syndrome. *J Pediatr* 1991;118:191–194.
96. Pirson Y, Leclercq B, Squifflet J, et al. Good prognosis of the hemolytic uremic syndrome after renal transplantation. *Nephrol Dial Transplant* 1986;1:134.
97. Gagnadoux MF, Habib R, Niaudet P, et al. Results of renal transplantation in childhood hemolytic-uremic syndrome. *J Am Soc Nephrol* 1996;7:1908.
98. Müller N, Sikora P, Offner G, et al. Recurrence of renal disease after kidney transplantation in children: 24 years of experience in a single center. *Clin Nephrol* 1998;49:82–90.
99. Ferraris JR, Ramirez JA, Ruiz S, et al. Shiga toxin-associated hemolytic uremic syndrome: absence of recurrence after renal transplantation. *Pediatr Nephrol* 2002;17:809–814.
100. Eijgenraam FJ, Donckerwolcke RA, Monnens LA, et al. Renal transplantation in 20 children with hemolytic-uremic syndrome. *Clin Nephrol* 1990;33:87–93.
101. Miller R, Burke B, Schmidt W, et al. Recurrence of haemolytic-uraemic syndrome in renal transplants: a single-centre report. *Nephrol Dial Transplant* 1997;12:1425–1430.
102. Koster F, Levin J, Walker L, et al. Hemolytic-uremic syndrome after shigellosis. Relation to endotoxemia and circulating immune complexes. *N Engl J Med* 1978;298:927–933.
103. Butler T, Islam MR, Azad MA, et al. Risk factors for development of hemolytic uremic syndrome during shigellosis. *J Pediatr* 1987;110:894–897.
104. Srivastava R, Moudgil A, Bagga A, et al. Hemolytic uremic syndrome in children in northern India. *Pediatr Nephrol* 1991;5:284–288.
105. Bhimma R, Rollins NC, Coovadia HM, et al. Post-dysenteric hemolytic uremic syndrome in children during an epidemic of Shigella dysentery in Kwazulu/Natal. *Pediatr Nephrol* 1997;11:560–564.
106. Koster FT, Boonpucknavig V, Sujaho S, et al. Renal histopathology in the hemolytic-uremic syndrome following shigellosis. *Clin Nephrol* 1984;21:126–133.
107. Badami KG, Srivastava RN, Kumar R, et al. Disseminated intravascular coagulation in post-dysenteric haemolytic uraemic syndrome. *Acta Paediatr Scand* 1987;76:919–922.
108. Klein PJ, Bulla M, Newman RA, et al. Thomsen-Friedenreich antigen in haemolytic-uraemic syndrome. *Lancet* 1977;2: 1024–1025.
109. Eder A, Manno C. Does red-cell T activation matter? *Br J Haematol* 2001;114:25–30.
110. Fearon D. Regulation by membrane sialic acid of beta1H-dependent decay-dissociation of amplification C3 convertase of the alternative complement pathway. *Proc Natl Acad Sci U S A* 1978;75:1971–1975.
111. Nathanson S, Deschenes G. Prognosis of *Streptococcus pneumoniae*-induced hemolytic uremic syndrome. *Pediatr Nephrol* 2001;16:362–365.
112. Brandt J, Wong C, Mihm S, et al. Invasive pneumococcal disease and hemolytic uremic syndrome. *Pediatrics* 2002;110: 371–376.
113. Krysan DJ, Flynn JT. Renal transplantation after *Streptococcus pneumoniae*-associated hemolytic uremic syndrome. *Am J Kidney Dis* 2001;37:E15.
114. Alpers C. Light at the end of the TUNEL: HIV-associated thrombotic microangiopathy. *Kidney Int* 2003;63:385–396.

115. Jorda M, Rodriguez MM, Reik RA. Thrombotic thrombocytopenic purpura as the cause of death in an HIV-positive child. *Pediatr Pathol* 1994;14:919–925.
116. Turner M, Kher K, Rakusan T, et al. A typical hemolytic uremic syndrome in human immunodeficiency virus-1-infected children. *Pediatr Nephrol* 1997;11:161–163.
117. Gadallah MF, el-Shahawy MA, Campese VM, et al. Disparate prognosis of thrombotic microangiopathy in HIV-infected patients with and without AIDS. *Am J Nephrol* 1996;16:446–450.
118. Peraldi M, Maslo C, Akposso K, et al. Acute renal failure in the course of HIV infection: a single-institution retrospective study of ninety-two patients and sixty renal biopsies. *Nephrol Dial Transplant* 1999;14:1578–1585.
119. Sahud M, Claster S, Liu L, et al. von Willebrand factor-cleaving protease inhibitor in a patient with human immunodeficiency syndrome-associated thrombotic thrombocytopenic purpura. *Br J Haematol* 2002;116:909–911.
120. Monnens L, Hendrickx G, van Wieringen P, et al. Letter: Serum-complement levels in haemolytic-uraemic syndrome. *Lancet* 1974;2:294.
121. Zipfel P. Complement factor H: physiology and pathophysiology. *Semin Thromb Hemost* 2001;27:191–199.
122. Zipfel P. Hemolytic uremic syndrome: how do factor H mutants mediate endothelial damage? *Trends Immunol* 2001; 22:345–348.
123. Richards A, Buddles M, Donne R, et al. Factor H mutations in hemolytic uremic syndrome cluster in exons 18–20, a domain important for host cell recognition. *Am J Hum Genet* 2001;68:485–490.
124. Caprioli J, Bettinaglio P, Zipfel PF, et al. The molecular basis of familial hemolytic uremic syndrome: mutation analysis of factor H gene reveals a hot spot in short consensus repeat 20. *J Am Soc Nephrol* 2001;12:297–307.
125. Perez-Caballero D, Gonzalez-Rubio C, Gallardo M, et al. Clustering of missense mutations in the C-terminal region of factor H in atypical hemolytic uremic syndrome. *Am J Hum Genet* 2001;68:478–484.
126. Pangburn M. Cutting edge: localization of the host recognition functions of complement factor H at the carboxyl-terminal: implications for hemolytic uremic syndrome. *J Immunol* 2002;169:4702–4706.
127. Perkins S, Goodship T. Molecular modelling of the C-terminal domains of factor H of human complement: a correlation between haemolytic uraemic syndrome and a predicted heparin binding site. *J Mol Biol* 2002;316:217–224.
128. Hellwage J, Jokiranta TS, Friese MA, et al. Complement C3b/C3d and cell surface polyanions are recognized by overlapping binding sites on the most carboxyl-terminal domain of complement factor H. *J Immunol* 2002;169:6935–6944.
129. Hindmarsh E, Marks R. Complement activation occurs on subendothelial extracellular matrix in vitro and is initiated by retraction or removal of overlying endothelial cells. *J Immunol* 1998;160:6128–6136.
130. Nangaku M, Alpers C, Pippin J, et al. CD59 protects glomerular endothelial cells from immune-mediated thrombotic microangiopathy in rats. *J Am Soc Nephrol* 1998;9:590–597.
131. Hogasen K, Jansen J, Mollnes T, et al. Hereditary porcine membranoproliferative glomerulonephritis type II is caused by factor H deficiency. *J Clin Invest* 1995;95:1054–1061.
132. Ault BH. Factor H and the pathogenesis of renal diseases. *Pediatr Nephrol* 2000;14:1045–1053.
133. Thompson R, Winterborn M. Hypocomplementaemia due to a genetic deficiency of beta 1H globulin. *Clin Exp Immunol* 1981;46:110–119.
134. Vogt B, Wyatt R, Burke B, et al. Inherited factor H deficiency and collagen type III glomerulopathy. *Pediatr Nephrol* 1995;9:11–15.
135. Pichette V, Querin S, Schurch W, et al. Familial hemolytic-uremic syndrome and homozygous factor H deficiency. *Am J Kidney Dis* 1994;24:936–941.
136. Ohali M, Shalev H, Schlesinger M, et al. Hypocomplementemic autosomal recessive hemolytic uremic syndrome with decreased factor H. *Pediatr Nephrol* 1998;12:619–624.
137. Rougier N, Kazatchkine M, Rougier J, et al. Human complement factor H deficiency associated with hemolytic uremic syndrome. *J Am Soc Nephrol* 1998;9:2318–2326.
138. Warwicker P, Donne R, Goodship J, et al. Familial relapsing haemolytic uraemic syndrome and complement factor H deficiency. *Nephrol Dial Transplant* 1999;14:1229–1233.
139. Warwicker P, Goodship T, Donne R, et al. Genetic studies into inherited and sporadic hemolytic uremic syndrome. *Kidney Int* 1998;53:836–844.
140. Noris M, Ruggenenti P, Perna A, et al. Hypocomplementemia discloses genetic predisposition to hemolytic uremic syndrome and thrombotic thrombocytopenic purpura: role of factor H abnormalities. Italian Registry of Familial and Recurrent Hemolytic Uremic Syndrome/Thrombotic Thrombocytopenic Purpura. *J Am Soc Nephrol* 1999;10:281–293.
141. Buddles MR, Donne RL, Richards A, et al. Complement factor H gene mutation associated with autosomal recessive atypical hemolytic uremic syndrome. *Am J Hum Genet* 2000;66: 1721–1722.
142. Taylor C. Complement factor H and the haemolytic uraemic syndrome. *Lancet* 2001;358:1200–1202.
143. Taylor C. Hemolytic-uremic syndrome and complement factor H deficiency: clinical aspects. *Semin Thromb Hemost* 2001;27:185–190.
144. Landau D, Shalev H, Levy-Finer G, et al. Familial hemolytic uremic syndrome associated with complement factor H deficiency. *J Pediatr* 2001;138:412–417.
145. Nathanson S, Fremeaux-Bacchi V, Deschenes G. Successful plasma therapy in hemolytic uremic syndrome with factor H deficiency. *Pediatr Nephrol* 2001;16:554–556.
146. Roodhooft A, McLean R, Elst E, et al. Recurrent haemolytic uraemic syndrome and acquired hypomorphic variant of the third component of complement. *Pediatr Nephrol* 1990;4:597–599.
147. Pirson Y, Lefebvre C, Arnout C, et al. Hemolytic uremic syndrome in three adult siblings: a familial study and evolution. *Clin Nephrol* 1987;28:250–255.
148. Cheong HI, Lee BS, Kang HG, et al. Treatment of factor H deficiency-associated hemolytic uremic syndrome with liver transplantation. A case report [Abstract]. *J Am Soc Nephrol* 2001;12:550A.
149. Remuzzi G, Ruggenenti P, Codazzi D, et al. Combined kidney and liver transplantation for familial haemolytic uraemic syndrome. *Lancet* 2002;359:1671–1672.
150. Furlan M. Von Willebrand factor: molecular size and functional activity. *Ann Hematol* 1996;72:341–348.

151. Tsai H. Physiologic cleavage of von Willebrand factor by a plasma protease is dependent on its conformation and requires calcium ion. *Blood* 1996;87:4235–4244.
152. Ruggeri Z. Structure and function of von Willebrand factor. *Thromb Haemost* 1999;82:576–584.
153. Reference deleted.
154. Furlan M, Robles R, Lamie B. Partial purification and characterization of a protease from human plasma cleaving von Willebrand factor to fragments produced by in vivo proteolysis. *Blood* 1996;87:4223–4234.
155. Dent J, Berkowitz S, Ware J, et al. Identification of a cleavage site directing the immunochemical detection of molecular abnormalities in type IIA von Willebrand factor. *Proc Natl Acad Sci U S A* 1990;87:6306–6310.
156. Fujikawa K, Suzuki H, McMullen B, et al. Purification of human von Willebrand factor-cleaving protease and its identification as a new member of the metalloproteinase family. *Blood* 2001;98:1662–1666.
157. Gerritsen HE, Robles R, Lammle B, et al. Partial amino acid sequence of purified von Willebrand factor-cleaving protease. *Blood* 2001;98:1654–1661.
158. Zheng X, Chung D, Takayama T, et al. Structure of von Willebrand factor-cleaving protease (ADAMTS13), a metalloprotease involved in thrombotic thrombocytopenic purpura. *J Biol Chem* 2001;276:41059–41063.
159. Soejima K, Mimura N, Hirashima M, et al. A novel human metalloprotease synthesized in the liver and secreted into the blood: possibly, the von Willebrand factor-cleaving protease? *J Biochem* 2001;130:475–480.
160. Plaimauer B, Zimmermann K, Volkel D, et al. Cloning, expression, and functional characterization of the von Willebrand factor-cleaving protease (ADAMTS13). *Blood* 2002; 100:3626–3632.
161. Furlan M, Robles R, Galbusera M, et al. von Willebrand factor-cleaving protease in thrombotic thrombocytopenic purpura and the hemolytic-uremic syndrome. *N Engl J Med* 1998;339:1578–1584.
162. Tsai H, Lian E. Antibodies to von Willebrand factor-cleaving protease in acute thrombotic thrombocytopenic purpura. *N Engl J Med* 1998;339:1585–1594.
163. Veyradier A, Obert B, Houllier A, et al. Specific von Willebrand factor-cleaving protease in thrombotic microangiopathies: a study of 111 cases. *Blood* 2001;98:1765–1772.
164. Furlan M, Lammle B. Assays of von Willebrand factor-cleaving protease: a test for diagnosis of familial and acquired thrombotic thrombocytopenic purpura. *Semin Thromb Hemost* 2002; 28:167–172.
165. Veyradier A, Brivet F, Wolf M, et al. Total deficiency of specific von Willebrand factor-cleaving protease and recovery following plasma therapy in one patient with hemolytic-uremic syndrome. *Hematol J* 2001;2:352–354.
166. Remuzzi G, Galbusera M, Noris M, et al. von Willebrand factor cleaving protease (ADAMTS13) is deficient in recurrent and familial thrombotic thrombocytopenic purpura and hemolytic uremic syndrome. *Blood* 2002; 100:778–785.
167. Hunt BJ, Lammle B, Nevard CH, et al. von Willebrand factor-cleaving protease in childhood diarrhoea-associated haemolytic uraemic syndrome. *Thromb Haemost* 2001;85: 975–978.
168. Tsai H, Chandler W, Sarode R, et al. von Willebrand factor and von Willebrand factor-cleaving metalloprotease activity in *Escherichia coli* O157:H7-associated hemolytic uremic syndrome. *Pediatr Res* 2001;49:653–659.
169. Schneppenheim R, Budde U, Oyen F, et al. Von Willebrand factor cleaving protease and ADAMTS13 mutations in childhood TTP. *Blood* 2003;101:1845–1850.
170. Veyradier A, Obert B, Haddad E, et al. Severe deficiency of the specific von Willebrand factor-cleaving protease (ADAMTS 13) activity in a subgroup of children with atypical hemolytic uremic syndrome. *J Pediatr* 2003;142:310–317.
171. Mannucci PM, Canciani MT, Forza I, et al. Changes in health and disease of the metalloprotease that cleaves von Willebrand factor. *Blood* 2001;98:2730–2735.
172. Robson W, Tsai H. Thrombotic thrombocytopenic purpura attributable to von Willebrand factor-cleaving protease inhibitor in an 8-year-old boy. *Pediatrics* 2002;109:322–325.
173. Schulman I, Pierce M, Lukens A, et al. Studies on thrombopoietin I. A factor in normal human plasma required for platelet production: chronic thrombocytopenia due to its deficiency. *Blood* 1960;16:943–957.
174. Upshaw J. Congenital deficiency of a factor in normal plasma that reverses microangiopathic hemolysis and thrombocytopenia. *N Engl J Med* 1978;298:1350–1352.
175. Fujimura Y, Matsumoto M, Yagi H, et al. Von Willebrand factor-cleaving protease and Upshaw-Schulman syndrome. *Int J Hematol* 2002;75:25–34.
176. Haberle J, Kehrel B, Ritter J, et al. New strategies in diagnosis and treatment of thrombotic thrombocytopenic purpura: case report and review. *Eur J Pediatr* 1999;158:883–887.
177. te Loo D, Levtchenko E, Furlan M, et al. Autosomal recessive inheritance of von Willebrand factor-cleaving protease deficiency. *Pediatr Nephrol* 2000;14:762–765.
178. Allford SL, Harrison P, Lawrie AS, et al. Von Willebrand factor–cleaving protease activity in congenital thrombotic thrombocytopenic purpura. *Br J Haematol* 2000;111:1215–1222.
179. Barbot J, Costa E, Guerra M, et al. Ten years of prophylactic treatment with fresh-frozen plasma in a child with chronic relapsing thrombotic thrombocytopenic purpura as a result of a congenital deficiency of von Willebrand factor-cleaving protease. *Br J Haematol* 2001;113:649–651.
180. Levy GG, Nichols WC, Lian EC, et al. Mutations in a member of the ADAMTS gene family cause thrombotic thrombocytopenic purpura. *Nature* 2001;413:488–494.
181. Kentouche K, Budde U, Furlan M, et al. Remission of thrombotic thrombocytopenic purpura in a patient with compound heterozygous deficiency of von Willebrand factor-cleaving protease by infusion of solvent/detergent plasma. *Acta Paediatr* 2002;91:1056–1059.
182. Stark G, Wallis J, Allford S, et al. Chronic relapsing thrombotic thrombocytopenic purpura due to a deficiency of von Willebrand factor-cleaving protease activity. *Br J Haematol* 2002;117:251–252.
183. te Loo D, Levtchenko E, Furlan M, et al. Autosomal recessive inheritance of von Willebrand factor-cleaving protease deficiency. *Pediatr Nephrol* 2000;14:762–765.
184. Deschenes G, Veyradier A, Cloarec S, et al. Plasma therapy in von Willebrand factor protease deficiency. *Pediatr Nephrol* 2002;17:867–870.

185. Furlan M, Lammle B. Aetiology and pathogenesis of thrombotic thrombocytopenic purpura and haemolytic uraemic syndrome: the role of von Willebrand factor-cleaving protease. *Best Pract Res Clin Haematol* 2001;14:437–454.
186. Kokame K, Matsumoto M, Soejima K, et al. Mutations and common polymorphisms in ADAMTS13 gene responsible for von Willebrand factor-cleaving protease activity. *Proc Natl Acad Sci U S A* 2002;99:11902–11907.
187. Furlan M, Robles R, Morselli B, et al. Recovery and half-life of von Willebrand factor-cleaving protease after plasma therapy in patients with thrombotic thrombocytopenic purpura. *Thromb Haemost* 1999;81:8–13.
188. George JN. How I treat patients with thrombotic thrombocytopenic purpura-hemolytic uremic syndrome. *Blood* 2000;96:1223–1229.
189. Hara T, Kitano A, Kajiwara T, et al. Factor VIII concentrate-responsive thrombocytopenia, hemolytic anemia, and nephropathy. Evidence that factor VIII: von Willebrand factor is involved in its pathogenesis. *Am J Pediatr Hematol Oncol* 1986;8:324–328.
190. Reiter R, Knoebl P, Varadi K, et al. Changes in von Willebrand factor-cleaving protease (ADAMTS13) activity after infusion of desmopressin. *Blood* 2003;101:946–948.
191. Tsai HM, Li A, Rock G. Inhibitors of von Willebrand factor-cleaving protease in thrombotic thrombocytopenic purpura. *Clin Lab* 2001;47:387–392.
192. Rosenblatt D, Fenton W. Inherited disorders of folate and cobalamin transport and metabolism. In: Scriver CR, Beaudet AL, Sly NS, et al., eds. *The metabolic and molecular basis of inherited disease*, 8th ed. New York: McGraw-Hill, 2001:3897–3933.
193. Fowler B. Genetic defects of folate and cobalamin metabolism. *Eur J Pediatr* 1998;157(Suppl 2):S60–S66.
194. Ogier de Baulny H, Gerard M, Saudubray J, et al. Remethylation defects: guidelines for clinical diagnosis and treatment. *Eur J Pediatr* 1998;157(Suppl 2):S77–S83.
195. Reference deleted.
196. Kind T, Levy J, Lee M, et al. Cobalamin C disease presenting as hemolytic-uremic syndrome in the neonatal period. *J Pediatr Hematol Oncol* 2002;24:327–329.
197. Carmel R, Bedros A, Mace J, et al. Congenital methylmalonic aciduria—homocystinuria with megaloblastic anemia: observations on response to hydroxocobalamin and on the effect of homocysteine and methionine on the deoxyuridine suppression test. *Blood* 1980;55:570–579.
198. Van Hove J, Van Damme-Lombaerts R, Grunewald S, et al. Cobalamin disorder Cbl-C presenting with late-onset thrombotic micro-angiopathy. *Am J Med Genet* 2002;111:195–201.
199. Labrune P, Zittoun J, Duvaltier I, et al. Haemolytic uraemic syndrome and pulmonary hypertension in a patient with methionine synthase deficiency. *Eur J Pediatr* 1999;158:734–739.
200. Hladovec J. Experimental homocystinemia, endothelial lesions and thrombosis. *Blood Vessels* 1979;16:202–205.
201. McCully K, Vezeridis M. Histopathological effects of homocysteine thiolactone on epithelial and stromal tissues. *Exp Mol Pathol* 1989;51:159–170.
202. Macy P. Homocysteine: predictor of thrombotic disease. *Clin Lab Sci* 2001;14:272–275.
203. Stranger O, Weger M, Renner W, et al. Vascular dysfunction in hyperhomocyst(e)inemia. Implication for atherothrombotic disease. *Clin Chem Lab Med* 2001;39:725–733.
204. Ruggenenti P. Post-transplant hemolytic-uremic syndrome. *Kidney Int* 2002;62:1093–1104.
205. Zarifian A, Meleg-Smith S, O'Donovan R, et al. Cyclosporine-associated thrombotic microangiopathy in renal allografts. *Kidney Int* 1999;55:2457–2466.
206. Holman M, Gonwa T, Cooper B, et al. FK506-associated thrombotic thrombocytopenic purpura. *Transplantation* 1993;55:205–206.
207. Pham P, Peng A, Wilkinson A, et al. Cyclosporine and tacrolimus-associated thrombotic microangiopathy. *Am J Kidney Dis* 1999;36:556–560.
208. Giroux L, Bettez P. Mitomycin-C nephrotoxicity: a clinicopathologic study of 17 cases. *Am J Kidney Dis* 1985;6:28–39.
209. Walter R, Joerger M, Pestalozzi B. Gemcitabine-associated hemolytic-uremic syndrome. *Am J Kidney Dis* 2002;40:E16.
210. Bennett CL, Connors JM, Carwile JM, et al. Thrombotic thrombocytopenic purpura associated with clopidogrel. *N Engl J Med* 2000;342:1773–1777.
211. Sugio Y, Okamura T, Shimoda K, et al. Ticlopidine-associated thrombotic thrombocytopenic purpura with an IgG-type inhibitor to von Willebrand factor-cleaving protease activity. *Int J Hematol* 2001;74:347–351.
212. Evens AM, Kwaan HC, Kaufman DB, et al. TTP/HUS occurring in a simultaneous pancreas/kidney transplant recipient after clopidogrel treatment: evidence of a non-immunological etiology. *Transplantation* 2002;74:885–887.
213. Kojouri K, Vesely SK, George JN. Quinine-associated thrombotic thrombocytopenic purpura-hemolytic uremic syndrome: frequency, clinical features, and long-term outcomes. *Ann Intern Med* 2001;135:1047–1051.
214. Glynne P, Salama A, Chaudhry A, et al. Quinine-induced immune thrombocytopenic purpura followed by hemolytic uremic syndrome. *Am J Kidney Dis* 1999;33:133–137.
215. Abramowicz D, Pradier O, Marchant A, et al. Induction of thromboses within renal grafts by high-dose prophylactic OKT3. *Lancet* 1992;339:777–778.
216. Waiser J, Budde K, Rudolph B, et al. De novo hemolytic uremic syndrome postrenal transplant after cytomegalovirus infection. *Am J Kidney Dis* 1999;34:556–559.
217. Asaka M, Ishikawa I, Nakazawa T, et al. Hemolytic uremic syndrome associated with influenza A virus infection in an adult renal allograft recipient: case report and review of the literature. *Nephron* 2000;84:258–266.
218. Murer L, Zacchello G, Bianchi D, et al. Thrombotic microangiopathy associated with Parvovirus B 19 infection after renal transplantation. *J Am Soc Nephrol* 2000;11:1132–1137.
219. Baid S, Pascual M, Williams WW Jr, et al. Renal thrombotic microangiopathy associated with anticardiolipin antibodies in hepatitis C-positive renal allograft recipients. *J Am Soc Nephrol* 1999;10:146–153.
220. Pham P, Danovitch GM, Wilkinson A, et al. Inhibitors of ADAMTS13: a potential factor in the cause of thrombotic

microangiopathy in a renal allograft recipient. *Transplantation* 2002;74:1077–1080.
221. Cohen EP, Lawton CA, Moulder JE, et al. Clinical course of late-onset bone marrow transplant nephropathy. *Nephron* 1993;64(4):626–635.
222. Kondo M, Kojima S, Horibe K, et al. Hemolytic uremic syndrome after allogeneic or autologous hematopoietic stem cell transplantation for childhood malignancies. *Bone Marrow Transplant* 1998;21(3):281–286.
223. Rossi R, Kleta R, Ehrich J. Renal involvement in children with malignancies. *Pediatr Nephrol* 1999;13:153–162.
224. Cohen E. Radiation nephropathy after bone marrow transplantation. *Kidney Int* 2000;58:903–918.
225. Hebert M, Fish D, Madore F, et al. Mesangiolysis associated with bone marrow transplantation: new insights on possible etiogenic factors. *Am J Kidney Dis* 1994;23:882–883.
226. Lawton C, Fish B, Moulder J. Effect of nephrotoxic drugs on the development of radiation nephropathy after bone marrow transplantation. *Int J Radiat Oncol Biol Phys* 1994; 28:883–889.
227. Chappell M, Keeling D, Prentice H, et al. Haemolytic uraemic syndrome after bone marrow transplantation: an adverse effect of total body irradiation? *Bone Marrow Transplant* 1988;3:339–347.
228. Verburgh C, Vermeij C, Zijlmans J, et al. Haemolytic uraemic syndrome following bone marrow transplantation. Case report and review of the literature. *Nephrol Dial Transplant* 1996;11:1332–1337.
229. Miralbell R, Bieri S, Mermillod B, et al. Renal toxicity after allogeneic bone marrow transplantation: the combined effects of total-body irradiation and graft-versus-host disease. *J Clin Oncol* 1996;14:579–585.
230. Antignac C, Gubler MC, Leverger G, et al. Delayed renal failure with extensive mesangiolysis following bone marrow transplantation. *Kidney Int* 1989;35:1336–1344.
231. Leblond V, Sutton L, Jacquiaud C, et al. Evaluation of renal function in 60 long-term survivors of bone marrow transplantation. *J Am Soc Nephrol* 1995;6:1661–1665.
232. Patzer L, Hempel L, Ringelmann F, et al. Renal function after conditioning therapy for bone marrow transplantation in childhood. *Med Pediatr Oncol* 1997;28:274–283.
233. Takatsuka H, Wakae T, Mori A, et al. Thrombotic thrombocytopenic purpura and hemolytic uremic syndrome following allogeneic bone marrow transplantation. *Bone Marrow Transplant* 2002;29:907–911.
234. Arai S, Allan C, Streiff M, et al. Von Willebrand factor-cleaving protease activity and proteolysis of von Willebrand factor in bone marrow transplant-associated thrombotic microangiopathy. *Hematol J* 2001;2:292–299.
235. Caramaschi P, Riccetti M, Pasini A, et al. Reply to the letter: about systemic lupus erythematosus and thrombotic thrombocytopenic purpura. *Lupus* 1998;7:571.
236. Sakarcan A, Stallworth J. Systemic lupus erythematosus and thrombotic thrombocytopenic purpura: a case and review. *Pediatr Nephrol* 2001;16:672–674.
237. Tsao C, Hsueh S, Huang J. Initial presentation of hemolytic uremic syndrome in a boy with systemic lupus erythematosus. *Rheumatol Int* 2002;21:161–164.
238. Asherson R, Cervera R, Piette J, et al. Catastrophic antiphospholipid syndrome: clues to the pathogenesis from a series of 80 patients. *Medicine* 2001;80:355–377.
239. Matsuda J, Sanaka T, Gohchi K, et al. Occurrence of thrombotic thrombocytopenic purpura in a systemic lupus erythematosus patient with antiphospholipid antibodies in association with a decreased activity of von Willebrand factor-cleaving protease. *Lupus* 2002;11:463–464.
240. Gungor T, Furlan M, Lammle B, et al. Acquired deficiency of von Willebrand factor-cleaving protease in a patient suffering from acute systemic lupus erythematosus. *Rheumatology (Oxford)* 2001;40:940–942.
241. Gubler M, Dommergues J, Foulard M, et al. Collagen type III glomerulopathy: a new type of hereditary nephropathy. *Pediatr Nephrol* 1993;7:354–360.
242. Niaudet P, Gagnadoux M, Broyer M, et al. Hemolytic-uremic syndrome: hereditary forms and forms associated with hereditary diseases. *Adv Nephrol Necker Hosp* 2000;30: 261–280.
243. Wilson B, Flynn J. Familial, atypical hemolytic-uremic syndrome in a premature infant. *Pediatr Nephrol* 1998;12:782–784.
244. Hellman RM, Jackson DV, Buss DH. Thrombotic thrombocytopenic purpura and hemolytic-uremic syndrome in HLA-identical siblings. *Ann Intern Med* 1980;93:283–284.
245. Bergstein J, Michael A Jr, Kellstrand C, et al. Hemolytic-uremic syndrome in adult sisters. *Transplantation* 1974;17: 487–490.
246. Kaplan BS, Papadimitriou M, Brezin JH, et al. Renal transplantation in adults with autosomal recessive inheritance of hemolytic uremic syndrome. *Am J Kidney Dis* 1997;30: 760–765.
247. Kaplan B, Leonard M. Autosomal dominant hemolytic uremic syndrome: variable phenotypes and transplant results. *Pediatr Nephrol* 2000;14:464–468.
248. Fitzpatrick MM, Walters MD, Trompeter RS, et al. Atypical (non-diarrhea-associated) hemolytic-uremic syndrome in childhood. *J Pediatr* 1993;122:532–537.
249. Siegler R, Pavia A, Hansen F, et al. Atypical hemolytic-uremic syndrome: a comparison with postdiarrheal disease. *J Pediatr* 1996;128:505–511.
250. Neuhaus T, Calonder S, Leumann E. Heterogeneity of atypical haemolytic uraemic syndromes. *Arch Dis Child* 1997;76: 518–521.
251. Salomon R, Gagnadoux M, Niaudet P, et al. *Syndrome hémolytique et urémique atypique de l'enfant.* Paris: Flammarion, Médecine Sciences, Journées Parisiennes de Pédiatrie, 1998:9–18.
252. Gianviti A, Perna A, Caringella A, et al. Plasma exchange in children with hemolytic-uremic syndrome at risk of poor outcome. *Am J Kidney Dis* 1993;22:264–266.
253. Magen D, Oliven A, Shechter Y, et al. Plasmapheresis in a very young infant with atypical hemolytic uremic syndrome. *Pediatr Nephrol* 2001;16:87–90.
254. Folman R, Arbus GS, Churchill B, et al. Recurrence of the hemolytic uremic syndrome in a 3 1/2-year-old child, 4 months after second renal transplantation. *Clin Nephrol* 1978;10:121–127.
255. Strom T, McClusket R. Case records of the Massachussetts General Hospital. *N Engl J Med* 1986;314:1032–1040.

256. Springate J, Fildes R, Anthone S, et al. Recurrent hemolytic syndrome after renal transplantation. *Transplant Proc* 1988;20:559–561.
257. Goodman DJ, Walker RG, Birchall IE, et al. Recurrent haemolytic uraemic syndrome in a transplant recipient on orthoclone (OKT 3). *Pediatr Nephrol* 1991;5:240–241.
258. Mochon M, Kaiser B, deChadarevian J, et al. Cerebral infarct with recurrence of hemolytic-uremic syndrome in a child following renal transplantation. *Pediatr Nephrol* 1992;6:550–552.
259. Scantlebury V, Shapiro R, McCauley J, et al. Renal transplantation under cyclosporine and FK 506 for hemolytic uremic syndrome. *Transplant Proc* 1995;27:842–843.
260. Davin JC, Gruppen M, Bouts AH, et al. Relapse of atypical haemolytic uraemic syndrome after kidney transplantation: role of ATG and failure of mycophenolate mofetil as rescue therapy. *Nephrol Dial Transplant* 1999;14:984–987.

48

SICKLE CELL NEPHROPATHY

JON I. SCHEINMAN

The major clinical consequences of sickle cell disease (SCD) are vascular obstruction by sickled cells and anemia because of red blood cell (RBC) destruction. The sickling process may cause hematuria, renal papillary necrosis (RPN), and a urinary concentrating defect. There also is a chronic sickle cell glomerulopathy, which is less directly related to sickling, as well as unusual susceptibility to infections and to a recently reported specific form of malignancy.

Sickle hemoglobin (HbS) differs from normal hemoglobin (HbA) by the substitution of valine for glutamine in the 6 position of the β-globin chain (1). Under low oxygen tension in concentrated solution, HbS aggregates and forms intracellular fibers. These fibers prevent RBCs from deforming normally, so they do not pass easily through the microcirculation and thus cause occlusion. Repeated cycles make some cells irreversibly sickled, and even in well-oxygenated blood they cause abnormal viscosity. In addition, these abnormal cells are easily lysed, which causes anemia.

HEMATURIA AND RENAL PAPILLARY NECROSIS

Clinical Features

Gross hematuria may be the most dramatic clinical event in SCD (2). It is often painless and usually unilateral, more commonly on the left side (3), which is explained by increased venous pressure due to the greater length of the left renal vein. Hematuria can occur at any age. It is more often reported with sickle trait (HbAS), probably because of the higher genetic frequency of HbAS than of HbSS (4). RPN is usually discovered in patients with painless gross hematuria (5). Hematuria is not invariably present, however, and RPN can occur even in young children (3). When it was sought systematically, 40% of patients in one Nigerian series were found to have RPN (6). In another series, there was no difference in the incidence of RPN in symptomatic patients (65%) and in asymptomatic (62%) patients (7). The frequency of RPN on urography therefore suggests that the process develops subclinically without gross hematuria.

Pathogenesis

The pathology associated with isolated hematuria is rarely examined. In the past, kidneys removed from patients with uncontrolled bleeding in SCD showed relatively insignificant changes, primarily medullary congestion (4). The hematuria probably results from the sequence of renal medullary sickling, vascular obstruction, and RBC extravasation. This is precipitated by those factors present in the renal medulla that lead to sickling: The PaO_2 (35 to 40 mm Hg) is below the threshold (45 mm Hg) for sickling (8); the high osmolality of the medulla draws water from the RBC, which leaves the HbS concentrated, promoting the formation of hemoglobin polymers. The acidic environment of the renal medulla further increases the likelihood of sickling. This mechanism of microvascular occlusion explains many of the complications of SCD but is overly simplistic. The distortion of the cell is also partly explained by dehydration of the cell by enhanced KCl co-transport, induced by cell swelling and acidification (9). Furthermore, K^+ and water efflux are enhanced by transiently increased SS cell cytosolic Ca, induced by the membrane distortion.

Pathology

The pathology of RPN in SCD is a focal process, with some collecting ducts surviving within a diffuse area of fibrosis. Within the medullary fibrosis the vasa recta are destroyed, after initial dilation and engorgement (10). The dependence of the papilla on that circulation results from repeated small focal infarctions of the papilla (11). This differs from the RPN found in analgesia abuse, in which the vasa recta typically are spared, and most lesions occur in peritubular capillaries (11). These same factors are present in sickle trait, although with a smaller proportion of sickling cells. Because calyces are affected separately and sequentially in SCD, acute obstruction and renal failure are uncommon (7).

Diagnosis

Continued gross hematuria likely represents a form of renal "sickle crisis" in a patient with known HbSS or HbAS. Other

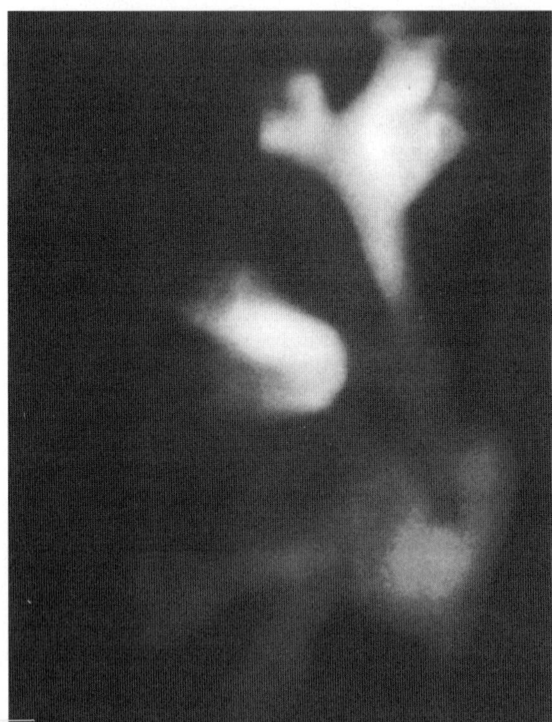

FIGURE 48.1. Tomographic pyelography of an 18-year-old patient with abdominal pain and hematuria. Papillary necrosis is evident from blunted medullary cavities, especially the upper pole. The bases of the calyces are preserved. The middle pole calyx has a possible sinus tract.

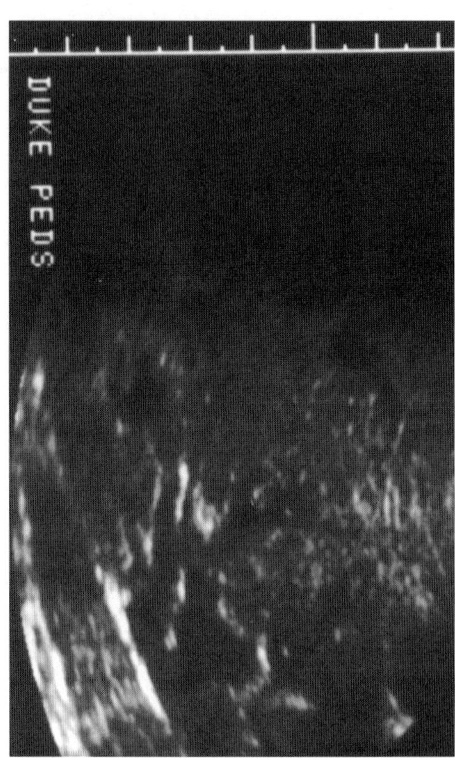

FIGURE 48.2. Ultrasonographic visualization of the same kidney as in Figure 48.1. The middle pole exhibits deep extensions into the papilla, likely sinus tracts, typical of the "papillary" form of renal papillary necrosis.

treatable causes of hematuria, including the distinctive renal medullary carcinoma in patients with sickle hemoglobin, must be excluded (12). Severe pain makes the diagnosis of renal sickle crisis less likely, whereas moderate discomfort often lateralizes the bleeding. Renal and bladder ultrasonography can rule out bleeding from a stone or tumor and diagnose RPN (see later). The increased echodensity of medullary pyramids on ultrasonography is typical of SCD, and in the absence of hypercalciuria, medullary echodensity in a patient with hematuria should suggest a sickle hemoglobinopathy (13). Walker (14) reviewed ultrasonographic reflectivity in young SCD patients (age 10 to 20 years) and found diffuse echogenicity in 9% and medullary echodensity in 3%. Surprisingly, these findings were greater in the milder genotypes, 37% in SC patients and 79% in Sβ^+ thalassemia patients. These findings are unexplained but are unlikely to represent RPN. The echodensity was found overall in 20% of patients with sickling processes and was interpreted to suggest subclinical nephrocalcinosis or iron deposition.

The diagnosis of RPN in SCD was traditionally made by urography. In the series of McCall et al., 39% of 189 patients had calyceal clubbing, including 23% with definite RPN (15). Cortical scarring as found in pyelonephritis does not accompany the calyceal clubbing of SCD (16). Other urographic findings of RPN in SCD are distinctive. A "medullary" form in which an irregular medullary cavity is present, often with sinus tracts, is common (7). The base of the calyx and its normal outline are preserved (16). Sonography can sometimes identify the early medullary form of papillary necrosis (17). A later finding is calcification of the medullary pyramids in a "garland" pattern surrounding the pelvis. This pattern of "shadowing" echodensity may be distinctive. The progression to the "papillary" form results in clubbing and caliectasis (Figs. 48.1 and 48.2). This is more common in analgesic nephropathy, in which an area of sequestration is often found, which results from infarction of a large area of the papilla (18). A prospective survey of symptomatic SCD patients (7) found that 11 of 18 SA patients had a form of RPN, but 8 of these 11 had evidence of infection. Nine of 11 symptomatic SS patients had RPN, of which 5 had evidence of infection. Asymptomatic patients included 16 of 22 SS patients with RPN, 1 of 3 SA patients, 3 of 4 SC patients, and 5 of 8 Sβ^+ patients. It is probably not necessary to perform contrast urography to visualize the renal architecture in SCD.

Treatment

In view of the benign pathology in SCD hematuria, conservative management is appropriate (4). Bed rest is often recommended to avoid dislodging hemostatic clots. It is advisable to maintain high rates of urine flow by both hypotonic fluid intake (4 L/1.73 m^2 surface area per day) and administration of diuretics (a thiazide or a loop diuretic such as furosemide), which should help clear clots from the bladder (3). In addition, a diuresis reduces medullary osmolarity and may therefore help alleviate sickling in the vasa recta. Some caution is necessary in the administration of sodium-containing fluids because of potential sodium retention (see later).

The combination of vasopressin and administration of hypotonic fluid to reduce plasma osmolality has been suggested. Hyponatremia induces water uptake by RBCs *in vitro*, thereby reducing the effective HbS concentration and making the cells less likely to sickle (4). This treatment is neither safe nor proven effective (4). Saline volume expansion would be especially ineffective and, coupled with hypertransfusion, would predispose to congestive heart failure. It would also be surprising if vasopressin were to increase the patient's urine concentration sufficiently to inhibit water diuresis (see later).

Because sickling is increased in an acid environment, alkalinization of the urine by 8 to 12 g $NaHCO_3$ (per 1.73 m^2) per day may reduce sickling in a urine environment, but this may not be relevant for medullary sickling (3). Alkalinizing the patient to increase the oxygen affinity of hemoglobin is theoretically valid but not of proven value in practice (4). Transfusions may be necessary for blood loss and could be helpful by increasing the proportion of normal HbAA cells and thus reducing sickling cells.

Epsilon aminocaproic acid (EACA) inhibits fibrinolysis, allowing clots to mediate hemostasis. The effective dosage in an adult is 8 g/day. In one series, 4 of 12 cases required EACA after failure of treatment with fluid administration and alkalinization (3). Unless other measures have failed, the risk of thrombosis should impose some caution in use of EACA. Lower dosages may be adequate to arrest hematuria, starting with 1 g (per 1.73 m^2) orally three times daily and increasing the dose until hemostasis occurs (4). Nephrectomy is rarely required for uncontrolled bleeding. Arteriographic localization and local embolization of the involved renal segment may avoid nephrectomy.

RPN can be prevented experimentally by either diabetes insipidus or water diuresis, which thereby eliminates the medullary concentration gradient (19). Thus the fluid administration prescribed for gross hematuria is also appropriate to prevent RPN. Angiotensin-converting enzyme (ACE) inhibition can experimentally induce a 50% increase in papillary blood flow (19). This may help prevent RPN, but it could aggravate hematuria acutely by increasing blood flow to a bleeding area.

TUBULAR DYSFUNCTION

The relevant medullary pathology in SCD is found in the region of the collecting ducts, the inner medulla, and the papilla. This results in dysfunction of the collecting duct and juxtamedullary nephrons (19). Sickling and vascular congestion of the medulla, seen in gross hematuria (4), are probably responsible for reversible concentrating defects. The basis of irreversible medullary dysfunction in RPN is likely the medullary fibrosis and destruction of vasa recta. Juxtamedullary nephrons and collecting ducts are destroyed, as is found in the model of RPN induced by bromoethylene-hydrobromide in rats (20).

Clinicopathologic Features

Urinary Concentration

The most common tubular abnormality in SCD is a urinary concentrating defect. Typically, HbSS patients achieve a urine concentration of 414 mOsm/kg after 8 to 10 hours of thirst, compared with 911 mOsm/kg in controls (21). Patients with sickle trait may have a diminished urinary concentrating capacity (22). This concentrating defect in children with SCD may result in enuresis (1) and an increased risk of dehydration during water deprivation.

The ability to concentrate urine depends on an intact collecting duct. The collecting ducts of juxtamedullary nephrons extend deepest into the medulla and are capable of generating the highest urine concentration. Poor sodium reabsorption in the collecting duct can result if the sluggish blood flow does not remove the reabsorbed sodium (19). The continued low-grade sickling and medullary congestion result in loss of the normal medullary concentration necessary for water reabsorption. This defective urine concentration can be transiently reversed by transfusion (23,24). The permanent destruction of collecting ducts by medullary fibrosis in humans with SCD (10) and in rats (20) results in an irreversible concentrating defect.

Vasopressin generation is normal in SCD, and the concentrating defect is not responsive to vasopressin. The concentrating defect is unique to sickling hemoglobinopathies, in that there is no concentrating defect in other anemias (25).

Diluting Capacity

Urinary dilution depends on the solute reabsorption in the ascending loop of Henle of cortical nephrons, which are not involved in SCD patients. They can usually dilute the urine normally (21,23).

Hydrogen Ion and Potassium Excretion

A proton gradient from tubular cell to lumen underlies acid excretion. Proton secretion is associated with the "intercalated" collecting duct cells, most prominent in the cortical segment of the collecting duct (19). Damage to the papillary segment is therefore unlikely to cause a severe acidification defect. However, juxtamedullary nephrons, which reabsorb HCO_3^-, are also severely involved in SCD. On this basis, some defect in acid excretion may occur (19).

An incomplete distal renal tubular acidosis (RTA) may complicate SCD, but it is usually not a clinical problem (23). The minimum urine pH achieved in response to NH_4Cl loading is not as low as in controls (5.8 vs. 5.1), but total NH_4 excretion is normal. Consequently, titratable acidity is reduced (26). Kurtzman has also described a "type IV RTA" in SCD, with a reduced ability to lower urine pH in response to Na_2SO_4 and inadequate K^+ secretion, especially in patients with decreased renal function (27). In one series, six of nine nephrotic SCD patients were reported to have type IV RTA (28).

Plasma renin and aldosterone levels may be increased in the face of medullary fibrosis (23). A protective mechanism likely exists: in the presence of inadequate K^+ secretion, a shift of K^+ to intracellular compartments probably occurs. Because this shift is under β_2 stimulation, beta-blockers or ACE inhibition may result in hyperkalemia (23). The electrolyte abnormalities resemble those in type IV RTA but actually result from an aldosterone-independent end-organ failure secondary to medullary fibrosis.

Proximal Tubular Reabsorption

An increased capacity for sodium reabsorption and a decreased sodium excretion with loop diuretics is seen in SCD (21,29). De Jong and Statius van Eps have proposed that the alterations in renal cortical function are adaptive, compensating for defects in medullary sodium and water conservation (10). The increased proximal sodium reabsorption results in decreased distal sodium delivery. Diuretic response is poor, because it depends on this more distal sodium delivery. Proximal tubular phosphate reabsorption, which usually parallels sodium reabsorption, is also increased. This may cause hyperphosphatemia, especially in the presence of an increased phosphate load generated by hemolysis (23).

Tubular Secretion

A significant disparity is found between creatinine clearance (CCr) and inulin clearance (CIn) in SCD. For example, in a small group of patients with SCD and an increased glomerular filtration rate (GFR) as measured by CIn (119 mL/min versus 97 mL/min for individuals without SCD), CCr was significantly higher than CIn in SCD patients (154 versus 119 mL/min) but not in those without SCD (114 vs. 97 mL/min) (21). This is an expression of increased tubular secretion of creatinine in SCD (23).

Uric acid secretion is similarly increased and is a functional adaptation to high uric acid generation (5). In patients with decreasing total GFR (and increasing GFR per nephron), fractional excretion of urate is further increased by decreased reabsorption (30).

Experimental Models of Tubular Dysfunction in Sickle Cell Disease

The rat model of RPN induced by bromoethylene-hydrobromide exemplifies distal tubule physiologic disturbances (20). As a baseline, these rats have a more dilute urine than controls. The juxtamedullary nephrons are nonfunctional. Sodium excretion changes little in response to hypervolemia. Although the measured atrial natriuretic peptide (ANP) level increases appropriately, an additional high-dose infusion of ANP can generate a normal response. The normal response to hypervolemia is likely mediated through inner medullary interstitial pressure, damaged in this model (and in SCD). In contrast, the response to salt loading generates a normal increased sodium excretion in experimental RPN, regulated by a more cortical mechanism (20).

Role of Prostaglandins in Tubular Dysfunction in Sickle Cell Disease

A series of studies begun by de Jong and Statius van Eps explored the effects of prostaglandin (PG) inhibition on renal function (10,31). The effect of PG inhibition on tubular function is especially revealing: there was a greater fall (42%) in the fractional excretion of Na in response to PG inhibition by indomethacin in SCD patients than in individuals without SCD (16%). This reflects a greater than normal effect of PGs on the delivery of sodium to the distal diluting segment. Although normal urinary dilution is not affected by PG inhibition, PG inhibition decreases urinary dilution in SCD (21).

PGs increase proximal sodium reabsorption. Under PG inhibition, more solute is delivered to and then reabsorbed by the thick ascending limb of the loop of Henle, which thereby increases interstitial hypertonicity. More free water is then absorbed in the relatively solute-impermeable descending limb, which results in a decreased response to water loading (21). Thus, although urinary diluting capacity is normal in SCD, it is being maintained only by PG and will be decreased by indomethacin (10). PG inhibition increases distal delivery, preventing the appropriate effect of vasopressin suppression during water diuresis in SCD (10). Increased proximal sodium reabsorption in SCD results in a decreased natriuretic response to loop diuretics (20), and PG inhibition restores that response.

Unlike in those without SCD, in SCD patients net acid excretion fails to increase in response to inhibition of PG synthesis by indomethacin (26) because of decreased NH_4^+ excretion. It is likely that NH_4^+ excretion is maintained at a maximum by endogenous PGs.

In summary, the tubular dysfunction of SCD manifests a defect in urine concentration, while dilution is maintained. Hydrogen ion and potassium secretion functions are only mildly affected, and proximal tubular mechanisms are exaggerated.

Treatment

Treatment of tubular disorders in SCD is usually unnecessary if renal function is normal. The risk of dehydration caused by decreased urinary concentrating ability requires earlier treatment of diarrhea or vomiting. There should be a cautious approach to volume expansion as treatment for sickle crises; administration of large volumes of standard sodium-containing fluids to significantly anemic patients with increased sodium reabsorption may result in congestive heart failure. Acidosis may require earlier treatment in the patient with SCD. Hyperuricemia, resulting from increased urate production, may be aggravated by diuretics (especially thiazides) that inhibit urate secretion. The edema accompanying severe anemia may be difficult to treat because the response to diuretics is diminished. Severe hemolysis may exceed the patient's ability to excrete potassium, especially if there is renal insufficiency. Beta-blockers or ACE inhibition can aggravate hyperkalemia (23), especially in the presence of some degree of renal impairment (27).

SICKLE CELL GLOMERULOPATHY

Clinical Features

The association of significant proteinuria with SCD has been recognized sporadically and usually described as a nephritic process. As early as 1959 (32), nephrotic syndrome was recognized in SCD. Proteinuria was identified in 17 of 54 patients (32). A population study found proteinuria in 20% of 284 patients at a single center, with a prevalence of 29% in adults but only 5% in children younger than 10 years of age (33). Bakir et al. recognized nephrotic syndrome in 12 of 240 adults with SCD, with proteinuria of 2 to 20 g/24 hr (28). In our series, 87 (26%) of 381 adult patients had significant proteinuria, with 12 in the nephrotic range (more than 2.5 g/24 hr) (34). In a more recent study of 34 adult patients with SCD, 7 had albuminuria with normal GFR and 17 had chronic renal failure, with glomerular injury and loss of ultrafiltration coefficient (35). In this series, GFR was related to hematocrit (36).

Lonsdorfer et al. (37) found that 40 to 45% of 31 SS patients aged 16 to 40 years had abnormal proteinuria, mostly selective (albumin). Twelve percent of the 17 patients who were younger than age 16 had abnormal proteinuria. Of 52 SA patients older than age 16, approximately 18% had abnormal proteinuria. Those with $S\beta^+$ were similar to SS patients, whereas those with SC disease fell between SS and SA patients.

The definition of sickle cell nephropathy that is most accepted is associated with nephrotic-range proteinuria. Although long-term studies have not been done, it appears to have a more rapid course than nephrotic syndrome due to other causes. In the experience of Bakir et al. (28), two-thirds of patients developed renal failure within 2 years. The onset of renal failure was heralded by increasingly inadequate erythropoiesis (38), and survival time after diagnosis was 4 years.

Pathology

The usual finding in sickle cell nephropathy is focal segmental glomerulosclerosis (FSGS), which is intimately associated with glomerular hypertrophy. Glomerular engorgement and hypertrophy were recognized as part of SCD by Berman and Tublin in 1960 (32). FSGS was reported in a 9-year-old nephrotic SCD patient in 1959 (32). Ten of our adult HbSS patients without significant renal impairment underwent renal biopsy because of proteinuria (34). Eight had FSGS involving a mean of 27% of glomeruli, and the other two had focal global sclerosis. There was focal tubulointerstitial fibrosis adjacent to sclerotic glomeruli. The nonsclerotic glomeruli were all enlarged, with diameters of 186 ± 14.5 μm versus 137.9 ± 19.3 μm in ten control biopsies. Immunofluorescence gave positive results only for immunoglobulin M, C3, and C1q irregularly in sclerotic segments. Electron microscopy confirmed the absence of immune complex–type dense deposits. There was focal electron-lucent expansion of the subendothelial zone in six specimens, with occasional mesangial cell interposition. No new mesangial matrix material was observed to suggest membranoproliferative glomerulonephritis (MPGN).

These findings agree with the description by Zamurovic and Churg (39). Glomerular hypertrophy was documented previously in adults with measured glomerular diameter (median, 257 μm; range, 220 to 316 μm) greater than in controls (median, 193 μm; range, 142 to 253 μm) (40). Bakir et al. described both the nonimmune MPGN-like lesion in nine patients, and FSGS (in 8% of glomeruli) or global sclerosis (in 14% of glomeruli) (28). In addition to FSGS, focal cortical infarcts have been described as a late finding in sickle cell nephropathy (8).

A report on the renal pathology in six HbSS patients with proteinuria described two patterns of FSGS: a "collapsing" and an "expansive" sclerosis (41). Glomeruli were significantly hypertrophied, with diameters of 233 ± 25.3 μm, compared with 158 ± 12.7 μm in subjects without SCD. Glomeruli were more hypertrophied in HbSS disease than in idiopathic FSGS (188.2 ± 17.9 μm). The glomeruli from HbSS patients without clinical evidence of renal disease (243.5 ± 12.5 μm) were the same size as in those with proteinuria.

Renal Function in Sickle Cell Glomerulopathy

Hyperfiltration

An increased GFR has been a recognized feature of SCD, especially in children, in studies dating from the 1950s (10). Renal plasma flow, as estimated by *p*-aminohippurate (PAH) clearance, is elevated in excess of GFR, which results in a lower than normal filtration fraction (12.9 vs. 17.5) (21). The extraction ratio of PAH (normally 90 to 95%) is also lower (24). The cause and mechanism of this physiologic alteration are unclear, although it is likely that increased cortical blood flow itself can cause decreased secretion by limiting diffusion from rapidly flowing plasma (24). A more recent analysis suggests a distinctive pattern of increased glomerular permeability (to dextrans) in SCD nephropathy, an increase in pore radius, which is not explained by purely hemodynamic changes. When chronic renal failure develops, the total number of membrane pores is reduced and a size-selectivity defect occurs.

Role of Prostaglandins in Glomerulopathy

The suggestion has been made that hyperfiltration and proximal tubular "hyperfunction" in SCD are a compensation for the distal tubular injury, mediated by the PG systems (10,20). In the studies by de Jong and Statius van Eps (see Tubular Dysfunction) (10), indomethacin decreased GFR and the estimated renal plasma flow (ERPF) in SCD patients but did not alter that of controls, which suggests that the PG system might be responsible for maintaining the GFR in SCD. Measured prostaglandin E_1 (PGE_1) excretion did not differ from that in controls, but prostaglandin F_2 (PGF_2) excretion was lower (42), which thus increased the ratio of the vasodilator PGE_1 to the vasoconstrictor PGF_2. Allon et al. (21) found that indomethacin decreased PGF_1 (prostacyclin, a vasodilator hormone) more in SCD patients (46%) than in control subjects (15%). GFR was decreased 16% by indomethacin in SCD but was unchanged in control subjects. The more dramatically increased ERPF and decreased filtration fraction of SCD were returned toward normal, and the net effect of PG inhibition was to reverse hyperfiltration.

Pathogenesis

Immunopathogenetic Mechanisms

In 1975, Strauss et al. (43) described an SCD membranoproliferative (MPGN) nephropathy in seven patients—four with nephrotic syndrome, and three of these under 15 years of age—with immunopathologic studies suggesting an immunocomplex disease. One proposed cause for the sickle cell nephropathy has been immunologic reaction to renal tubular epithelial cell complexes (10). Most now agree that evidence of immunocomplex deposition is usually lacking in SCD patients with heavy proteinuria.

Relationship to Other Glomerulopathies

The relationship of the pathologic findings of SCD to those of other nephropathies is unclear. Glomerular hypertrophy with FSGS is also found in the setting of reduced renal mass. Examples are reflux nephropathy, severe obesity (44), and rat models of renoprival glomerulosclerosis (45). In FSGS associated with idiopathic nephrotic syndrome, the glomeruli that develop sclerosis are hypertrophied (1). The nephropathy associated with type 1 glycogen-storage disease (GSD-1) includes both hyperfiltration and FSGS (46). The nephropathy associated with cyanotic congenital heart disease may arise from mechanisms similar to those operating in SCD: low oxygenation and increased blood viscosity from polycythemia (23,47).

Possible Mechanisms of Sickle Cell Disease Nephropathy

Hyperfiltration, in concert with direct endothelial damage by occlusion with sickled cells, might lead to endothelial hyperplasia and ultimately fibrosis (10,23). The iron deposited in tubular cells as hemosiderin has been suspected to have a role in the chronic nephropathy of SCD (8). The non–immune complex deposits found in SCD might derive from iron–protein complexes (8). Experimentally, saturated-iron complexes can induce a nephrotic syndrome in rabbits (24). Lande et al. found decreased renal cortical spin-echo signal by magnetic resonance imaging in SCD, which suggests an abnormal renal cortical iron metabolism (48). This does not occur in β-thalassemia, despite similar iron overload.

It is possible that FSGS is the consequence rather than the cause of interstitial fibrosis, which might obstruct the efferent glomerular capillaries, raising intraglomerular pressure and resulting in progressive (reactive) sclerosis (49). In SCD, in which medullary fibrosis is most prominent, the vasa recta supplying the juxtamedullary nephrons would be most affected by FSGS. Bhathena et al. (41) suggested that the "collapsing" pattern of FSGS, superimposed on already maximally hypertrophied glomeruli, might be a consequence of sickling and ischemic collapse, similar to the glomerular "microinfarcts" suggested by Chauhan et al. (8). The "expansive" form of FSGS is viewed as a mesangial cell reaction to capillary collapse.

Both the pathophysiologic and pathologic findings in sickle cell nephropathy resemble those in the rodent model of glomerular hypertension induced by renal mass reduction (50). Thus hyperfiltration, glomerular enlargement, and focal and segmental glomerulosclerosis could be a result of an increase in intraglomerular pressure as a consequence of efferent arteriolar vasoconstriction. In that model, and in others, the glomerular hypertension and the pathologic consequences are attenuated by angiotensin II–converting enzyme inhibition.

Any hypothesis should take into account the glomerular hypertrophy that is always present in SCD, probably related to the anemia itself. Proteinuria is not invariable in SCD and appears to be unrelated to the number and severity of SCD crises or the presence of hematuria, RPN, and so on. Therefore some other factors are likely to be operative in those at greatest risk of proteinuria and FSGS. Systemic hypertension is notably absent in these patients (34). The presence of hyperfiltration, glomerular hypertrophy, and FSGS does not imply that these findings are sequential or causative. A common stimulus may be operative, such as the growth-promoting hormones and cytokines (57), to which the glomerulus may be sensitive.

Diagnosis

Hyperfiltration

The upper limit of the normal range for GFR is not certain, even with CIn, the gold standard. The reliability of the clearance methods that can substitute for CIn have not been validated in the elevated range. In adult SCD subjects aged 40 to 75 years, CCr correlated well with the clearance of chromium-51 ethylenediaminetetra-acetic acid (^{51}Cr-EDTA) when clearance did not exceed 110 mL/min, although ^{51}Cr-EDTA exceeded CCr by almost 30% (23). In those without SCD, the urinary clearance of ^{51}Cr-EDTA is 85 to 95% that of CIn, whereas the clearances of technetium-99m diethylenetriamine penta-acetic acid and iodine 125 iothalamate are nearly identical to that of inulin (51). Because CCr usually exceeds CIn in healthy individuals, its validity in SCD is uncertain. The simplest estimation of GFR, by several formulas, uses plasma creatine (PCr) alone (52), but an additional problem in the use of these formulas is the greater overestimation of GFR by CCr in SCD patients than in those without SCD. The plasma clearance of ^{51}Cr-EDTA after bolus injection approximates CIn in healthy individuals (53) but at high clearances is far less accurate (54).

For most clinical purposes, an accurate measure of GFR is unnecessary. A decrease in GFR, particularly when accompanied by proteinuria, is ominous (55). However, the effects of treatment are difficult to assess in other than a clinical research environment, although simplified methods for nonisotopic iothalamate and PAH measurement are now available (56).

Proteinuria

Proteinuria detected by dipstick in a patient with SCD should be quantified and renal function assessed. Diseases other than sickle cell glomerulopathy should be considered. If hematuria is present, RBC casts may point to pathology other than sickle cell glomerulopathy. Hypertension, hypocomplementemia, and the presence of antinuclear antibodies also suggest other diagnoses. Judging from the relatively uniform findings in our series (34), few other additional studies are indicated.

Treatment

The course of the progression of FSGS to chronic renal insufficiency (CRI) in SCD remains difficult to assess, in part because of the difficulties in quantitation of renal function described earlier (56). Unless the cause is known, it is difficult to prescribe a treatment for the nephropathy of SCD. The patients with proteinuria in our series (34) were not those with the most frequent sickle crises or the severest anemia. Nevertheless, some factors in the sickle cell condition must predispose to the nephropathy. Therefore it is reasonable to attempt to minimize sickling and those factors known to promote FSGS in other primary diseases or in animal models, but whether hemodynamic alterations can change the progression of FSGS to CRI is controversial (57).

Protein Restriction

A high protein intake accelerates the development of FSGS in uninephrectomized rats without necessarily causing glomerular hyperperfusion (58). It is therefore attractive to consider protein restriction in the management of SCD nephropathy, as is being tried in several forms of renal disease. In children, restriction of protein intake may carry unreasonable risks (59). Delayed growth and development is already a particular risk in the SCD patient. Therefore, we advise only the avoidance of an unusually high protein intake (greater than the recommended dietary allowance).

Angiotensin-Converting Enzyme Inhibition

Glomerular hyperperfusion and proteinuria could be mediated through increased glomerular capillary pressure, reduction of which by ACE inhibition might protect the glomerulus from FSGS.

In a 2-week trial of enalapril treatment of 10 patients with mild SCD nephropathy, blood pressure, GFR (CIn), and ERPF (PAH clearance) did not change significantly, whereas proteinuria diminished by 57%, rebounding after treatment withdrawal (34). A more recent 6-month controlled trial of enalapril therapy in 22 SCD patients with microalbuminuria showed a significant decrease in the treatment group, whereas microalbuminuria increased in the control group (60). Whether long-term ACE inhibitor therapy has a salutary effect in preventing renal insufficiency is untested.

CHRONIC RENAL INSUFFICIENCY

Clinical Features

Renal failure is one of the major organ failures that occurs in SCD, almost certainly the consequence of the progression of FSGS. Of 22 patients with nephrotic syndrome, 68% developed CRI (28). Population studies of SCD have all shown a significant incidence of CRI. Of 368 patients in one sickle cell center, 4.6% had CRI (61) associated with proteinuria and increased age. In our series of 375 patients, 6.7% had CRI (34). In a series of 785 patients from California, 33 had CRI (4.2%) (62). Overall, 5 to 18% of SCD patients develop CRI (63).

The epidemiology of renal involvement in SCD may depend on other genetic characteristics that affect the levels of fetal hemoglobin (HbF), the tendency to sickle, and other factors. Powars et al. (64) initially reported the association of β-globin gene cluster haplotypes with renal involvement: the Central African Republics (CAR) haplotypes (Bantu, Cameroon) or Benin (intermediate involvement) versus non-CAR (Senegalese and Arab-Indian) phenotypes. Guasch et al. (65) found no association with these haplotypes, but instead an association with microdeletions in the α-globin gene. Microalbuminuria was found in 22 of 76 (29%) adult SCD patients but only 13% with the microdeletions, versus 40% without those microdeletions ($p < .01$). Those factors that affect the interactions of RBCs with endothelium may be equally important (see later).

Treatment

Specific treatment of the patient with SCD and renal failure has been poorly explored, and the problems of CRI are only magnified by SCD. Patients with renal failure, even if it is mild, sometimes have symptomatic anemia requiring transfusion. In some of these patients, treatment with erythropoietin can variably restore hemoglobin concentrations to higher levels (66). A few patients have been treated with hydroxyurea plus erythropoietin with apparent benefit (67).

Dialysis and Transplantation

The U.S. Renal Data System reported the causes of renal failure for 255,573 patients treated from 1989 through 1993 (54). Overall, 235 were SCD patients. This is far fewer than the 1% expected from the incidence of HbSS in the total population. It is possible that physicians do not offer treatment to many SCD patients who develop CRI, assuming that the other problems are insurmountable.

Ojo et al. (68) reviewed the transplant results in SCD and found 82 patients. There was no difference in the 1-year cadaveric graft survival [SCN, 78%; other causes of end-stage renal disease (ESRD), 77%], and the multivariable adjusted 1-year risk of graft loss indicated no significant effect of SCN [relative risk (RR) = 1.39, $p = .149$]. However, the 3-year cadaveric graft survival tended to be lower in the SCN group (48% vs. 60%, $p = .055$) and their adjusted 3-year risk of graft loss was significantly higher (RR = 1.60, $p = .003$). There was a trend toward higher survival in the SCN transplant recipients than in their dialysis-treated, wait-listed counterparts (RR = 0.14, $p = .056$). In comparison to the other-ESRD group (RR = 1.00), the adjusted mortality risk in the SCN group was higher both at 1 year (RR = 2.95, $p = .001$) and at 3 years (RR = 2.82, $p = .0001$) after renal transplantation. A trend was also found toward better patient survival with renal transplantation than with dialysis in end-stage sickle cell nephropathy.

In an analysis of the United Network of Organ Sharing registry from 1987 to 1996 (69), 54 patients were found with SCD and renal failure and for whom data were available on first renal transplant outcome. Patient survival for individuals with SCD was 90% at 1 year and (of 30 patients) 75% at 3 years. The proportional risk ratio (compared to those with immunoglobulin A nephropathy) was 7.8, the highest for any condition. First-graft survival for SCD patients was 82.5% at 3 years and 54% at 3 years. The proportional risk ratio for graft survival was 1.77, but after correction for deaths of patients with functioning grafts, was only 1.06 (barely an increased risk).

We have explored (J. I. Scheinman and R. Payne, *unpublished data*, 2002) the U.S. Renal Data System data files (2000) for evidence of the effect of SCD on the outcome of chronic renal failure. Although the diagnostic code for sickle cell nephropathy (assigned at the time of renal failure) yielded 904 patients, further exploration of patients discovered by hospitalization codes to have SS disease yielded a total of 1656 patients—237 undergoing transplantation and 1419 not undergoing transplantation. Even after other causes of renal failure (diabetes mellitus, etc.) were eliminated, SCD patients were compared to all other African American patients in life-table survival. Without transplantation, the groups differed significantly, with vastly different numbers, and projected 10-year survival was poor for both groups: 25% for African Americans and 15% for SCD patients.

Furthermore, the 36,264 African American patients undergoing transplantation had better survival rates than the 210 SCD patients, but the life-table projected survivals were still quite close, with approximately 50% survival at 15 years (Fig. 48.3). When an age-adjusted cohort of African American patients were used as controls, the difference

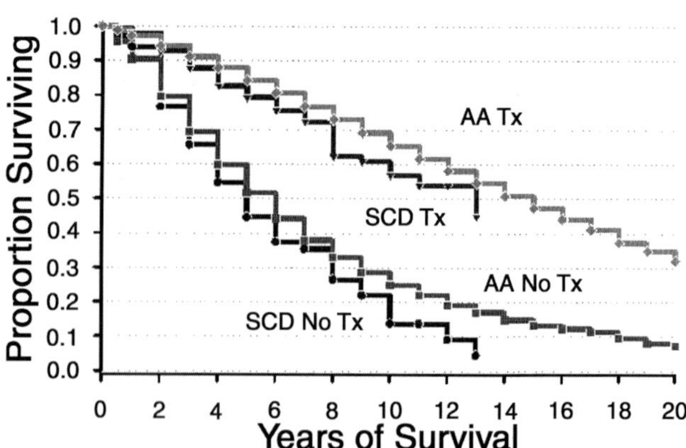

FIGURE 48.3. Life-table analysis of patient survival for end-stage renal failure patients with sickle cell disease (SCD) and age-matched African-American (AA) controls, treated with kidney transplantation or dialysis alone. All curves differ significantly due to the vastly greater numbers of AA patients (J. I. Scheinman and R. Payne, *unpublished data*, 2002). Tx, transplantation.

statistically disappeared (p <.19). Among those who did not undergo transplantation, comparison of the African American patients with the SCD patients yielded different findings, but projected survival rates for both groups were extremely poor: 25% for African American patients and 14% for SCD patients at 10 years.

A comparison of the 153 SCD patients undergoing transplantation with those who received no transplant showed a far better survival curve: 56% versus 14% at 10 years. Survival of SCD transplanted patients was also significantly better than the 133 nontransplanted patients who were on the waiting list. This was similar to the difference between all African American patients undergoing transplantation and nontransplanted African American patients assigned to the transplant waiting list. Of 957 patients listed since 1991, essentially the cyclosporin era, only 53 SCD patients received transplants whereas 898 did not undergo transplantation; survival of the patients receiving transplants is projected to be 67% at 7 years compared with 83% for the African American cohort.

These results continue to make the case that transplantation is a better option for the SCD patient with renal failure. Results may be less satisfactory than those for other African American patients, however, and grafts have been lost due to demonstrable massive sickling events.

The problems that have occurred in SCD patients after transplantation, especially the recurrent sickle crises, could have been aggravated by the increased blood viscosity associated with a rising hematocrit. These have been treated with frequent partial exchange transfusions (70). In one early series, seven of eight patients had frequent sickle crises after transplantation (71). Renal venous thrombosis and infarction have been reported (72). In one patient with HbAS, the transplanted kidney was unfortunately removed for an apparently irreversible acute rejection that was actually intrarenal sickling (71).

The management of renal transplantation in SCD patients should then focus on potential immediate problems. It is reasonable to warm the kidney with 37°C saline, to infuse dopamine at 4 μg/kg/min during and immediately after surgery, and to provide 40% oxygen and intravenous fluids to decrease viscosity. Partial exchange transfusion may be provided at 4-week intervals (71). It is possible that before an adequate erythropoietin response occurs from the transplanted kidney, recombinant erythropoietin should be given.

Sickle cell nephropathy has been reported to recur in as little as 3 years, although other factors contributed (73). Accelerated recurrence of native disease has been noted in the transplanted kidney in other diseases, notably diabetic nephropathy (74). It is possible that the use of hydroxyurea, in itself likely to interact with other immunosuppressants, can be used to prevent this. Bone marrow transplantation can cure SCD, and the possibility of coupling it with other transplantations will undoubtedly be explored. Caution will be needed, in view of the possible increase in infection with parvovirus (75), a common agent of aplastic crises that might be especially dangerous in the transplant patient.

OTHER PROBLEMS IN SICKLE CELL DISEASE RELATED TO NEPHROLOGY

Anemia

In the presence of continued hemolysis, the patient with SCD depends on continued erythropoiesis, which determines the level of anemia. Erythropoiesis can be measured by erythron transferrin uptake (76), independent of iron or transferrin saturation. A heme protein in the kidney senses a decreased level of oxygen delivery to the kidney and stimulates erythropoietin production (77). The SCD patient with renal failure loses this normal homeostatic mechanism and becomes far more anemic. Even in the presence of a competent bone marrow and erythropoietic stimulus, adequate iron is necessary. Patients with ulcers may subtly lose iron (8).

The hemoglobin level should probably be maintained at 50 to 60% of normal in patients with SCD, in view of the serious cardiac consequences of more severe anemia (78). Although an intrinsic cardiomyopathy has been suspected in SCD, a careful autopsy study of 52 patients with a mean age of 17 years concluded that anemia alone caused heart failure (78).

Sickle Crises—Clinical Features

Sickle cell crises (1) are painful episodes of vasoocclusion, often accompanied in the second or third day by fever without documented infection. Neither abnormal blood viscosity nor the number of sickle cells absolutely predicts the frequency of crises (2). The incidence of pain crises is 0.8/yr in SS disease and 1/yr in Sβ+ thalassemia (79). With greater degrees of anemia, there is less pain, probably because of diminished blood viscosity. With increasing HbF, there are proportionally fewer painful crises, which suggests a beneficial effect of even modest increases in HbF (79).

Crises may manifest in infants as the hand-foot syndrome because of poorly developed collateral circulation. The chest syndrome is accompanied by radiologic "white-out" and is life-threatening (80). The abdominal crisis is like a "surgical abdomen" but usually without rebound tenderness. In the presence of hematuria, the origin of the pain could be assumed to be the kidney. Neuromeningitis, multiinfarct dementia, or large-vessel occlusion (stroke) can occur (81), especially in infants and children (8). A sudden anemia may be caused by sequestration crises in the spleen in the first 2 years of life; thereafter, after development of splenic fibrosis, it occurs more often in the liver. Aplastic crises arise from vasoocclusion and hemolysis without compensatory erythropoiesis, often induced by a parvovirus-like agent.

Priapism

Priapism is a specialized vasoocclusion of the penis, which was found in as many as 42% of cases in one series (1). Painful, hot, tender erection, most often on waking, lasts up to 3 hours. This can be preceded by days or weeks of "stuttering." The engorgement is of the corpus cavernosa, usually not the spongiosum in children, with the glans flaccid (8). The pain is referred to the perineum and to the abdomen; analgesia, and often exchange transfusion, is necessary. Few patients require surgical drainage or placement of a shunt. Fibrosis may result, with consequent impotence (8).

Pathophysiology of Sickling

The clinical heterogeneity of SCD is further determined by recently described aggravators of sickling related to oxidative stress. Hemoglobin from RBCs of SCD patients has increased auto-oxidation and increased generation of superoxide and H_2O_2, OH^-, and lipid peroxidation products (82). In a transgenic model of SCD, increased oxidant stress extends renal sickling from a more limited area in the renal medulla to a more extensive distribution to the cortex (83). The aggravating factors of sickling are likely to include the agents of microvascular inflammation and constriction, and inhibitors of relaxation. Reactive species can divert vasoactive NO from mechanisms of vascular relaxation to agents of inflammation and constriction (82). Integrins ($\alpha_4\beta_1$) of the sickled RBC bind to both fibronectin (an acute-phase reactant) and vascular cell adhesion molecule-1 on endothelial cells, which is increased by inflammatory cytokines such as tumor necrosis factor-α.

Hemoxygenase-1 (HO-1) defends against and degrades heme, a lipophilic pro-oxidant, formed from the splitting of hemoglobin (83), studied in a transgenic sickle mouse. In the HO-1 "knock-out" model, administration of heme protein induces monocyte chemoattractive protein-1, mediated by nuclear factor-κB, and results in renal interstitial cell inflammation (84).

Thus increased induced oxidative stress from the sickling process precipitates acute vasoocclusive disease by mechanisms that affect the endothelium, and adhesion to it, as well as vasoconstriction.

The distorted sickle cell is partly explained by dehydration of the cell by enhanced KCl co-transport, induced by cell swelling and acidification (9). Furthermore, K^+ and water efflux are enhanced by transiently increased SS cell cytosolic Ca, induced by the membrane distortion.

Acute Renal Failure

A doubling or more of PCr was found in 12 of 116 patients with SCD admitted to the hospital. It was seen most often with infections and evidence of rhabdomyolysis, and in patients with lower hemoglobin levels (mean of 6.4 vs. 8.7 g/dL) (85). Volume depletion was the most common precipitating cause. In that study patient survival rate was an 83%, with recovery of function in all patients who survived, without progression to ESRD. It is likely that nonsteroidal antiinflammatory agents are partly responsible for some episodes of acute renal failure (86), in view of the likely maintenance of GFR by PG mechanisms in SCD.

Rhabdomyolysis with acute renal failure and disseminated intravascular coagulation has been seen (rarely) in patients with sickle trait after rigorous military training (87). Similarly, there is an apparently increased risk of sudden unexplained death in patients with sickle trait (88).

Hypertension

Hypertension is unusual in SCD (2 to 6%) compared to the published incidence of 28% for the African American population in the United States at all age ranges, as found by the Cooperative Study of Sickle Cell Disease (89).

In our series (34), hypertension was rare and was found only in one patient with nephrotic-range proteinuria without renal insufficiency. The one-third incidence of hypertension in Powars et al.'s patients with renal insufficiency is unexplained (38). Nevertheless, she found a positive association between blood pressure, stroke, and increased mortality in SCD patients (90).

Infections

Infections occur in HbSS disease as a result of vascular sequestration with tissue necrosis (e.g., osteomyelitis associated with avascular necrosis, or *Salmonella* infection with cholelithiasis) and the immune susceptibility of the splenectomized patient (1). The organisms most commonly found are *Diplococcus pneumoniae, Haemophilus influenzae, Mycoplasma,* and parvovirus (8). Prophylactic penicillin therapy is essential, as for any splenectomized patient. *H. influenza B* vaccination is also appropriate.

Urinary infections are uncommon in SCD, except perhaps in pregnancy. Technetium 99m diphosphonate scan shows an increased renal localization in HbSS. This apparently is not caused by infection but more likely by regional stasis or tubular ischemia, which leads to peritubular extravasation (91).

GENERAL TREATMENT STRATEGIES FOR SICKLE CELL DISEASE

Institution of frequent transfusion can reduce the risk of recurrence of cerebral vasculopathy (81) by decreasing the proportion of rheologically abnormal cells. Because of the risks, transfusion should be reserved for patients at greatest risk of sickling sequelae. Most recently, Doppler ultrasonography has helped identify cerebral vessels at risk of stroke (92).

Other hemoglobins modify the tendency of HbS RBCs to sickle. HbF inhibits sickling. The agent 5-azacitidine can increase HbF levels, probably by recruitment of HbF cells, but may be a carcinogen (93). The only agent able to significantly decrease sickling by myelosuppression of HbSS cells, thus increasing HbF, is hydroxyurea. Hydroxyurea is a cytotoxic agent that inhibits the growth of erythroid burst-forming units (94). In SCD, it is the SS cells that are suppressed, which allows an increase in HbF.

Charache et al. (95) achieved 8 to 18% HbF levels that were maintained over 2 years. It has been deduced that a 20% level of HbF is likely needed to produce a definitive clinical change with regard to either hemolysis or vasoocclusion (96). A trial involving 59 patients (97) suggested that a mean HbF level of 15% could be achieved. Trials of hydroxyurea therapy in adults and children (98) have shown that it provides a safe reduction in acute episodes and allows normal growth and development (99). In addition to its effect on RBC generation, hydroxyurea induces oxidative damage to SS cells that is greater than that to AA cells, even more than to HbF (100). Antioxidants such as α-tocopherol and ascorbate are protective *in vitro* and may enhance the safety of hydroxyurea.

Other mechanisms that can minimize the tendency to sickling and vasoocclusion have been investigated. Reversing the cellular dehydration in SCD has been explored by blocking cation-transport channels in erythrocyte membranes, which can shift cellular cation content and cell density toward normal. Clotrimazole, an antifungal drug, reduced cellular dehydration *in vitro* in transgenic mice with SCD and in patients with sickle cell anemia. Magnesium salts also interfere with cation transport and cause cell rehydration (101).

Whether the cellular changes induced by clotrimazole or magnesium salts are of clinical value is not known. Combinations of hydroxyurea plus clotrimazole and erythropoietin to prevent sickling have been studied in transgenic mice.

Bone marrow transplantation can cure SCD, and the possibility of combining it with other transplantations will doubtless be investigated. Less ablative conditioning for bone marrow transplantation is being explored (102). Because of the possible increase in infection with parvovirus (75), a common agent of aplastic crisis that might be especially dangerous in the transplant patient, caution is in order.

REFERENCES

1. Weatherall DF, Cleg SB, Higs DR, et al. The hemoglobinopathies. In: Scriver CR, Beaudet AL, Sly WS, et al., eds. *The metabolic basis of inherited disease*, 6th ed. New York: McGraw-Hill, 1992:2293–2335.
2. Oksenhendler E, Bourbigot B, Desbazeille F, et al. Recurrent hematuria in four white patients with sickle cell trait. *J Urol* 1984;132:1201–1203.
3. Osegbe DN. Haematuria and sickle cell disease. A report of 12 cases and review of the literature. *Trop Geograph Med* 1990;42:22–27.
4. Statius van Eps LAW, de Jong PE. Sickle cell disease. In: Scherer WR, Gottschalk KW, eds. *Diseases of the kidney*, 4th ed. Boston: Little, Brown, 1988:2561–2681.
5. Davies SC, Dewitt PE. Sickle cell disease. *Br J Hosp Med* 1984;31:440–444.
6. Audit JC, Ugbodaga CI, Okafor LA, et al. Urographic changes in homozygous sickle cell disease. *Diagn Imag* 1983;52:259–263.
7. Pandya KK, Koshy M, Brown N, et al. Renal papillary necrosis in sickle cell hemoglobinopathies. *J Urol* 1976;115: 497–501.
8. Chauhan PM, Kondlapoodi P, Natta CL. Pathology of sickle cell disorders. *Pathol Ann* 1983;18:253–276.
9. Bunn HF. Mechanisms of disease—pathogenesis and treatment of sickle cell disease. *N Engl J Med* 1997;337:762–769.
10. de Jong PE, Statius van Eps LW. Sickle cell nephropathy: new insights into its pathophysiology. *Kidney Int* 1985;27: 711–717.
11. Burry A, Cross R, Axelsen R. Analgesic nephropathy and the renal concentrating mechanism. *Pathol Ann* 1977;12:1–31.
12. Avery RA, Harris JE, Davis CJ, et al. Renal medullary carcinoma: clinical and therapeutic aspects of a newly described tumor. *Cancer* 1996;78:128–132.
13. Schultz PK, Strife JL, Strife CF, et al. Hyperechoic renal medullary pyramids in infants and children. *Radiology* 1991;181: 163–167.
14. Walker TM, Serjeant GR. Increased renal reflectivity in sickle cell disease: prevalence and characteristics. *Clin Radiol* 1995;50:566–569.
15. McCall IW, Moule N, Desai P, et al. Urographic findings in homozygous sickle cell disease. *Radiology* 1978;126:99–104.
16. Mapp E, Karasick S, Pollack H, et al. Uroradiological manifestations of S-hemoglobinopathy. *Semin Roentgenol* 1987; 22:186–194.
17. Braden GL, Kozinn DR, Hampf FE, et al. Ultrasound diagnosis of early renal papillary necrosis. *J Ultrasound Med* 1991;10:401–403.
18. Eknoyan G, Qunibi WY, Grissom RT, et al. Renal papillary necrosis: an update. *Medicine* 1982;61:55–73.
19. Sabatini S. Pathophysiologic mechanisms of abnormal collecting duct function. *Semin Nephrol* 1989;9:179–202.
20. Keeler R, Wilson N. Natriuretic response to hypervolemia is absent in rats with papillary necrosis. *Am J Physiol* 1989;257: R422–R426.
21. Allon M, Lawson L, Eckman JR, et al. Effects of nonsteroidal antiinflammatory drugs on renal function in sickle cell anemia. *Kidney Int* 1988;34:500–506.
22. Beutler E. Erythrocyte disorders: anemias related to abnormal globulin. In: Williams WJ, Beutler E, Erslev AJ, et al., eds. *Hematology*, 4th ed. New York: McGraw-Hill, 1992:613–626.
23. Allon M. Renal abnormalities in sickle cell disease. *Arch Intern Med* 1990;150:501–504.
24. Buckalew VM, Someren A. Renal manifestations of sickle cell disease. *Arch Intern Med* 1974;133:660–669.

25. Devereux S, Knowles SM. Rhabdomyolysis and acute renal failure in sickle cell anaemia. *BMJ* 1985;290:1707.
26. de Jong PE, de Jong-van den Berg LT, Schouten H, et al. The influence of indomethacin on renal acidification in normal subjects and in patients with sickle cell anemia. *Clin Nephrol* 1983;19:259–264.
27. Kurtzman NA. Acquired distal renal tubular acidosis. *Kidney Int* 1983;24:807–819.
28. Bakir AA, Hathiwala SC, Ainis H, et al. Prognosis of the nephrotic syndrome in sickle glomerulopathy. A retrospective study. *Am J Nephrol* 1987;7:110–115.
29. DeFronzo RA, Taufield PA, Black H, et al. Impaired renal tubular potassium secretion in sickle cell disease. *Ann Intern Med* 1979;90:310–316.
30. Morgan AG, de Ceulaer K, Serjeant GR. Glomerular function and hyperuricemia in sickle cell disease. *J Clin Pathol* 1984;37:1046–1049.
31. de Jong PE, de Jong-van den Berg LT, Donker AJ, et al. The role of prostaglandins and renin in sickle-cell nephropathy. A hypothesis. *Neth J Med* 1978;21:67–72.
32. Berman LB, Tublin I. The nephropathies of sickle-cell disease. *Arch Intern Med* 1959;103:602–606.
33. Sklar AH, Campbell H, Caruana RJ, et al. A population study of renal function in sickle cell anemia. *Int J Artif Organs* 1990;13:231–236.
34. Falk RJ, Scheinman JI, Phillips G, et al. Prevalence and pathologic features of sickle cell nephropathy and response to inhibition of angiotensin-converting enzyme. *N Engl J Med* 1992;326:910–915.
35. Guasch A, Cua M, Mitch WE. Early detection and the course of glomerular injury in patients with sickle cell anemia. *Kidney Int* 1996;49:786–791.
36. Guasch A, Cua M, You W, et al. Sickle cell anemia causes a distinct pattern of glomerular dysfunction. *Kidney Int* 1997;51: 826–833.
37. Lonsdorfer A, Comoe L, Yapo AE, et al. Proteinuria in sickle cell trait and disease: an electrophoretic. *Clin Chim Acta* 1989;181:239–248.
38. Powars DR, Elliott-Mills DD, Chan L, et al. Chronic renal failure in sickle cell disease: risk factors, clinical course, and mortality. *Ann Intern Med* 1991;115:614–620.
39. Zamurovic D, Churg J. Idiopathic and secondary mesangiocapillary glomerulonephritis. *Nephron* 1984;38:145–153.
40. Morgan AG, Shah DJ, Williams W. Renal pathology in adults over 40 with sickle-cell disease. *West Indian Med J* 1987;36:241–250.
41. Bhathena DB, Sondheimer JH. The glomerulopathy of homozygous sickle hemoglobin (SS) disease: morphology and pathogenesis. *J Am Soc Nephrol* 1991;1:1241–1252.
42. de Jong PE, Saleh AW, de Zeeuw D, et al. Urinary prostaglandins in sickle cell nephropathy: a defect in 9-ketoreductase activity? *Clin Nephrol* 1984;22:212–213.
43. Strauss J, Pardo V, Koss MN, et al. Nephropathy associated with sickle cell anemia: an autologous immune complex nephritis. I. Studies on nature of glomerular-bound antibody and antigen identification in a patient with sickle cell disease and immune deposit glomerulonephritis. *Am J Med* 1975;58:382–387.
44. Jennette JC, Charles L, Grubb W. Glomerulomegaly and focal segmental glomerulosclerosis associated with obesity and sleep-apnea syndrome. *Am J Kidney Dis* 1987;10:470–472.
45. Olson JL, Hostetter TH, Rennke HG, et al. Altered glomerular permselectivity and progressive sclerosis following extreme ablation of renal mass. *Kidney Int* 1982;22:112–126.
46. Chen YT, Coleman RA, Scheinman JI, et al. Renal disease in type I glycogen storage disease. *N Engl J Med* 1988;318:7–11.
47. Spear G. Glomerular alterations in cyanotic congenital heart disease. *Bull Johns Hopkins Hosp* 1960;106:347–367.
48. Lande IM, Glazer GM, Sarnaik S, et al. Sickle-cell nephropathy: MR imaging. *Radiology* 1986;158:379–383.
49. Yoshida Y, Fogo A, Ichikawa I. Glomerular hemodynamic changes vs. hypertrophy in experimental glomerular sclerosis. *Kidney Int* 1989;35:654–660.
50. Hostetter TH, Olson JL, Rennke HG, et al. Hyperfiltration in remnant nephrons: a potentially adverse response to renal ablation. *Nephron* 1981;241:F85-F93.
51. Haycock G. Creatinine, body size and renal function. *Pediatr Nephrol* 1989;3:22–24.
52. Schwartz GJ, Haycock GB, Edelmann CM, et al. A simple estimate of glomerular filtration rate in children derived from body length and plasma creatinine. *Pediatrics* 1976;58:259–263.
53. Mulhern JG, Perrone RD. Accurate measurement of glomerular filtration rate. *Int Yearb Nephrol* 1990;277–291.
54. Excerpts from the United States Renal Data System 1996 Annual Data Report. *Am J Kidney Dis* 1996;28:S1–165.
55. Walser M. Progression of chronic renal failure in man. *Kidney Int* 1990;37:1195–1210.
56. Coakley DF, Roland CL, Falk RJ, et al. Renal function assessment with HPLC analysis of iothalamate (IOTH) and para-aminohippurate (PAH) compared to inulin, PAH, and creatinine as measured by standard analytical methods. *Pharmacotherapy* 1991;11:265.
57. Woolf AS, Fine LG. Do glomerular hemodynamic adaptations influence the progression of human renal disease? *Pediatr Nephrol* 1991;5:88–93.
58. Morozumi K, Thiel G, Gudat F, et al. Studies on morphological outcome of cyclosporine-associated arteriolopathy after discontinuation of cyclosporine in patients with renal allografts. *Transplant Proc* 1993;25:537–539.
59. Raymond NG, Dwyer JT, Nevins P, et al. An approach to protein restriction in children with renal insufficiency. *Pediatr Nephrol* 1990;4:145–151.
60. Foucan L, Bourhis V, Bangou J, et al. A randomized trial of captopril for microalbuminuria in normotensive adults with sickle cell anemia. *Am J Med* 1998;104:339–342.
61. Heeg JE, de Jong PE, van der Hem GK, et al. Reduction of proteinuria by angiotensin converting enzyme inhibition. *Kidney Int* 1987;32:78–83.
62. Murthy VS, Haywood J. Survival analysis by sex, age, group and hemotype in sickle cell disease. *J Chronic Dis* 1981;34:3 13–319.
63. Thomas AN, Pattison C, Serjeant GR. Causes of death in sickle-cell disease in Jamaica. *BMJ* 1982;285:633–635.
64. Powars DR, Meiselman HJ, Fisher TC, et al. Beta-S gene cluster haplotypes modulate hematologic and hemorheologic expression in sickle cell anemia. Use in predicting clinical severity. *Am J Pediatr Hematol Oncol* 1994;16:55–61.
65. Guasch A, Zayas CF, Eckman JR, et al. Evidence that microdeletions in the alpha globin gene protect against the

development of sickle cell glomerulopathy in humans. *J Am Soc Nephrol* 1999;10:1014–1019.

66. Tomson CR, Edmunds ME, Chambers K, et al. Effect of recombinant human erythropoietin on erythropoiesis in homozygous sickle-cell anaemia and renal failure. *Nephrol Dial Transplant* 1992;7:817–821.
67. Rodgers GP, Dover GJ, Uyesaka N, et al. Augmentation by erythropoietin of the fetal-hemoglobin response to hydroxyurea in sickle cell disease [see comments]. *N Engl J Med* 1993;328:73–80.
68. Ojo AO, Govaerts TC, Schmouder RL, et al. Renal transplantation in end-stage sickle cell nephropathy. *Transplantation* 1999;67:291–295.
69. Bleyer AJ, Donaldson LA, McIntosh M, et al. Relationship between underlying renal disease and renal transplantation outcome. *Am J Kidney Dis* 2001;37:1152–1161.
70. Spector D, Zachary JB, Sterioff S, et al. Painful crises following renal transplantation in sickle cell anemia. *Am J Med* 1978;64:835–839.
71. Chatterjee SN, Lundberg GD, Berne TV. Sickle cell trait: possible contributory cause of renal allograft failure. *Urology* 1978;11:266–268.
72. Donnelly PK, Edmunds ME, O'Reilly K. Renal transplantation in sickle cell disease [Letter]. *Lancet* 1988;2:229.
73. Miner DJ, Jorkasky DK, Perloff LJ, et al. Recurrent sickle cell nephropathy in a transplanted kidney. *Am J Kidney Dis* 1987;10:306–313.
74. Mauer SM, Steffes MW, Connett J, et al. The development of lesions in the glomerular basement membrane and mesangium after transplantation of normal kidneys to diabetic patients. *Diabetes* 1983;32:948–952.
75. Khamashta MA, Williams FM, Hunt BJ. Anticoagulation for venous thromboembolism [Letter]. *N Engl J Med* 1999; 341:539–540.
76. Cazzola M, Pootrakul P, Huebers HA, et al. Erythroid marrow function in anemic patients. *Blood* 1987;69:296–301.
77. Goldberg JS, Dunning SP, Bunn HF. Regulation of the erythropoietin gene: evidence that the oxygen sensor is a heme protein. *Science* 1988;242:1412–1415.
78. Sztajzel J, Ruedin P, Stoermann C, et al. Effects of dialysate composition during hemodialysis on left ventricular function. *Kidney Int* 1993;41:S60–S66.
79. Platt OS, Thorington BD, Brambilla DJ, et al. Pain in sickle cell disease. Rates and risk factors. *N Engl J Med* 1991;325: 11–16.
80. Ponez M, Kane E, Gill FM. Acute chest syndrome in sickle cell disease: etiology and clinical correlates. *J Pediatr* 1985; 107:861–866.
81. Powars DR. Sickle cell anemia and major organ failure. *Hemoglobin* 1990;14:573–598.
82. Aslan M, Thornley-Brown D, Freeman BA. Reactive species in sickle cell disease. *Ann N Y Acad Sci* 2000;899:375–391.
83. Nath KA, Grande JP, Haggard JJ, et al. Oxidative stress and induction of heme oxygenase-1 in the kidney in sickle cell disease. *Am J Pathol* 2001;158:893–903.
84. Nath KA, Vercellotti GM, Grande JP, et al. Heme protein-induced chronic renal inflammation: suppressive effect of induced heme oxygenase-1. *Kidney Int* 2001;59:106–117.
85. Sklar AH, Perez JC, Harp RJ, et al. Acute renal failure in sickle cell anemia. *Int J Artif Organs* 1990;13:347–351.
86. Simckes AM, Chen SS, Osorio AV, et al. Ketorolac-induced irreversible renal failure in sickle cell disease: a case report. *Pediatr Nephrol* 1999;13:63–67.
87. Koppes GM, Daly JJ, Coltman CA, et al. Exertion-induced rhabdomyolysis with acute renal failure and disseminated intravascular coagulation in sickle cell trait. *Am J Med* 1977;63:313–317.
88. Kark JA, Posey DM, Schumacher HR, et al. Sickle-cell trait as a risk factor for sudden death in physical training. *N Engl J Med* 1987;317:781–787.
89. Johnson CS, Giorgio AJ. Arterial blood pressure in adults with sickle cell disease. *Arch Intern Med* 1981;141:891–893.
90. Pegelow CH, Colangelo L, Steinberg M, et al. Natural history of blood pressure in sickle cell disease: risks for stroke and death associated with relative hypertension in sickle cell anemia. *Am J Med* 1997;102:171–177.
91. Sty JR, Babbitt DP, Sheth K. Abnormal Tc-99m-methylene diphosphonate accumulation in the kidneys of children with sickle cell disease. *Clin Nucl Med* 1980;5:445–447.
92. Adams RA, McKie V, Nichols F, et al. The use of transcranial ultrasonography to predict stroke in sickle cell disease. *N Engl J Med* 1992;326:605–610.
93. Shannon KM. Recombinant erythropoietin in pediatrics: a clinical perspective. *Pediatr Ann* 1990;19:197–206.
94. Baliga BS, Pace BS, Chen HH, et al. Mechanism for fetal hemoglobin induction by hydroxyurea in sickle cell erythroid progenitors. *Am J Hematol* 2000;65:227–233.
95. Charache S, Dover GJ, Moyer MA, et al. Hydroxyurea-induced augmentation of fetal hemoglobin production in patients with sickle cell anemia. *Blood* 1987;69:109–116.
96. Noguchi CT, Rodgers GP, Serjeant G, et al. Current concepts: levels of fetal hemoglobin necessary for treatment of sickle cell disease. *N Engl J Med* 1988;318:96–99.
97. Charache S, Dover GJ, Moore RD, et al. Hydroxyurea: effects on hemoglobin F production in patients with sickle cell anemia. *Blood* 1992;79:2555–2565.
98. Ferster A, Tahriri P, Vermylen C, et al. Five years of experience with hydroxyurea in children and young adults with sickle cell disease. *Blood* 2001;97:3628–3632.
99. Wang WC, Helms RW, Lynn HS, et al. Effect of hydroxyurea on growth in children with sickle cell anemia: results of the HUG-KIDS Study. *J Pediatr* 2002;140:225–229.
100. Iyamu EW, Fasold H, Roa D, et al. Hydroxyurea-induced oxidative damage of normal and sickle cell hemoglobins in vitro: amelioration by radical scavengers. *J Clin Lab Anal* 2001;15:1–7.
101. Steinberg MH. Management of sickle cell disease. *N Engl J Med* 1999;340:1021–1030.
102. Schleuning M, Stoetzer O, Waterhouse C, et al. Hematopoietic stem cell transplantation after reduced-intensity conditioning as treatment of sickle cell disease. *Exp Hematol* 2002; 30:7–10.

49

DIABETIC NEPHROPATHY

LEONARD G. FELD

Insulin-dependent diabetes mellitus (IDDM) is an epidemic in our communities. The burden to diagnose and treat is growing as this group of patients continues to expand, and coincident with the disease is the profound morbidity and mortality. It is estimated that 30 to 50% of all patients with IDDM develop renal disease after 5 to 15 years of having the disorder (1). Diabetic nephropathy is characterized by progressive loss of renal function and systemic disturbances, including hypertension, proteinuria, and the numerous sequelae of chronic renal insufficiency. Renal involvement in IDDM typically follows a progressive course to end-stage renal disease (ESRD). IDDM is the most common cause of chronic renal failure requiring dialysis or transplantation in the United States (2). The prevalence of diabetes and chronic renal failure in the entire Medicare medical population is approximately 1.6% or 406,800 individuals (3). With an incidence rate of diabetic ESRD in pediatric patients (0 to 19 years of age) of 15.2 per 1 million population (4) and an incidence rate of diabetes mellitus in children 19 years of age or younger of 16.7 per 100,000 (4), it is essential to implement strategies such as strict control of blood glucose level and blood pressure and monitoring for microalbuminuria to decrease the risk of complications in the pediatric population and improve long-term survival (5). Not only does renal failure represent a significant health problem and affect the quality of life, the yearly costs of care for diabetic patients with renal failure are estimated to total over $6 billion.

PATHOGENESIS AND RISK FACTORS OF DIABETIC NEPHROPATHY

Despite the lack of a unifying hypothesis to explain the high incidence of renal disease in IDDM, a number of risk factors for the development of nephropathy have been identified. These include increased glomerular filtration rate (GFR) (glomerular hyperfiltration) (6–8), systemic and/or glomerular hypertension (9,10), vascular (endothelial) dysfunction (11–13), poor metabolic control (elevated levels of glycosylated hemoglobin), biochemical alterations in the glomerular basement membrane (GBM) resulting in increased vascular permeability and structural changes (14–16), genetic factors (predisposition to hypertension, familial clustering) (17,18), and dietary factors (high protein, sodium, and/or fat intake) (19–21).

Renal Hemodynamics

In some experimental animal models of diabetes, increased GFR associated with elevations in glomerular pressures has been implicated in the development and progression of kidney damage (10,22,23). Increased GFR, or glomerular hyperfiltration, is observed in 25 to 50% of patients in the early stages of IDDM. This glomerular hyperfunction may contribute to the initiation of diabetic nephropathy and may predict and/or contribute to its progression. Multiple mediators may initiate hyperfiltration. Although the precise mechanism is not understood, the diabetic milieu (hyperglycemia, insulinopenia, sorbitol accumulation) results in an increased GFR (24–26). The early hyperfiltration may be reversed with normalization of blood glucose concentrations. Whether glomerular hyperfiltration alone is a risk factor for overt nephropathy in humans remains controversial.

Hemodynamic studies have revealed that vasodilation of the resistance vessels in the kidney render glomerular capillaries vulnerable to pressure-related injury (22). Because the resistance in the preglomerular and postglomerular arterioles and systemic blood pressure determine glomerular capillary resistance, the combination of increased systemic blood pressure and the relative dilation (or decreased resistance) of afferent compared with efferent arterioles results in increased glomerular capillary pressure or glomerular hypertension. This abnormal regulation of intrarenal vascular resistance has been postulated to be an important factor in the glomerular injury in diabetes (19,22,27). Under normal circumstances, vascular tone is regulated through the production of potent vasoconstrictor substances (endothelin, angiotensin II, prostaglandin H_2, platelet-activating factor, platelet-derived growth factor) and vasodilatory mediators, namely endothelium-derived relaxing factor (or nitric oxide) and prostacyclin (28,29). In IDDM, vascular endothelial damage may shift the balance of vasoreactive factors toward vasoconstriction with a resultant increase in efferent (postglomerular) arteriolar resistance, increased glomerular capillary pressure (intrarenal hypertension), and progressive kidney dysfunction.

Metabolism

Glycemic Control

Many studies demonstrate the correlation between blood glucose (glycemic) control and the development of complications from diabetes mellitus (30–32). The Diabetes Control and Complications Trial (DCCT) conducted from 1983 to 1993 and the observational follow-up Epidemiology of Diabetes Interventions and Complications (EDIC) study of the DCCT cohort (30,32) have demonstrated the effect of intensive glycemic control on reducing the microvascular complications of IDDM. The DCCT involved 1441 patients with IDDM at 29 centers in the United States and Canada, and the EDIC study extended the follow-up of 1298 patients for an additional 7 years. The studies compared the effects of standard insulin therapy with intensive control (testing of blood glucose concentrations four or more times per day, four daily insulin injections, diet control, and exercise) on two cohorts. Cohort 1 (primary prevention trial) had no complications and a urinary albumin excretion rate of less than 28 μg/min. Cohort 2 (secondary intervention trial) had background retinopathy, a urinary albumin excretion rate higher than or equal to 28 μg/min or 40 mg/day (microalbuminuria), and normal GFR.

In the primary prevention trial of the DCCT, the intensive therapy group had a cumulative incidence of microalbuminuria of 16% after 9 years compared with 27% in the conventional treatment group. Overall, there was a 34% reduction in risk for the development of microalbuminuria in the intensive therapy group. In the EDIC, the prevalence of microalbuminuria in patients who did not have it at the end of the DCCT study remained significantly lower in the intensive treatment group than in the conventional therapy group (4.5 vs. 12.3%, $p < .001$). In the secondary prevention trial, the intensive therapy group had a cumulative incidence of microalbuminuria of 26% after 9 years compared with 42% in the conventional therapy arm. The reduction in risk for the development of microalbuminuria in the intensive therapy group was 43%. In the secondary intervention trial, the cumulative incidence of the development of clinical or overt nephropathy was more than two times higher in patients treated conventionally than in those receiving intensive treatment. This 56% reduction in absolute risk with intensive glycemic control at the end of the DCCT rose to 86% in the final years of the EDIC study.

The progression to chronic renal disease (serum creatinine level of greater than or equal to 2 mg/dL) or ESRD (dialysis and/or transplantation) was reached in 6 patients under intensive glycemic control compared to 17 individuals under conventional therapy. As discussed later, hypertension worsened in the conventional treatment group (33%) than in the intensive treatment patients (25%) by the end of the EDIC study. The DCCT and the EDIC follow-up study have provided compelling evidence that strict control of blood glucose concentration and near normalization of glycosylated hemoglobin levels reduce the risk of developing microalbuminuria, decrease the development of hypertension, and delay or prevent the progression to overt nephropathy/ESRD in IDDM.

Advanced Glycosylation End Products

An increasing body of information supports the role of advanced glycosylation end products (AGEs) as an important etiologic factor in diabetic nephropathy (33–35). As mentioned earlier, poor glycemic control is a prerequisite for diabetic nephropathy and is related to the accumulation of AGEs, the products of a glucose-protein interaction. A reversible or nonenzymatic glycation occurs as glucose and amino acids form a Schiff base. Over weeks to months, these products continue to be rearranged into irreversibly glycated AGEs. AGEs and their reaction with the receptors of AGE (RACE) in the blood vessels and within the kidney of patients with diabetes may cause renal damage by increasing the synthesis of basement membrane collagen and mesangial matrix, raising vascular permeability, and increasing growth factor secretion (36–38). This sequence of events leads to glomerular hypertrophy and eventual glomerulosclerosis. AGEs also may contribute to diabetic atherosclerosis through cellular activation and inflammation, cytokine and growth factor release, and increased vascular matrix and endothelial permeability. In addition, AGEs formed in the vascular matrix may limit vasodilation by interfering with the action of endothelium-derived relaxing factor (39). The decreased clearance of these products may contribute to ongoing diabetic tissue injury. In animal studies, the use of an inhibitor of AGEs, aminoguanidine or OPB 9195, can diminish overexpression of type IV collagen, laminin, vascular endothelial growth factor (VEGF), transforming growth factor β (TGF-β), and platelet-derived growth factor (27,40,41), which results in reduced glomerular proliferation and capillary permeability. The clinical implications of AGE inhibition or reduction are obvious, but additional studies are required.

Protein Kinase C

In the hyperglycemic state, enhanced synthesis of diacylglycerol (DAG) results from phosphatidylcholine by phospholipase D. DAG then activates protein kinase C (PKC) on its C1 regulatory domain (42). PKC activation influences expression of inducible nitric oxide within the mesangium, leading to glomerular vasodilation. In rats with streptozotocin-induced diabetes, activation of DAG kinase decreased

PKC activity, which led to restoration of renal hemodynamics. PKC activation may also lead to diabetes-induced renal structural and permeability changes. VEGF induces endothelial cell proliferation and vasopermeability in the microvasculature in diabetes. VEGF expression may be enhanced by hyperglycemia-induced PKC activation, and its proposed effect on glomerular permeability and albuminuria may be mitigated by PKC inhibition.

Activation of PKC stimulates transcription of TGF-β, which leads to mesangial expansion. In studies using a murine model of diabetes, PKC inhibition reduced TGF-β, which significantly reduced mesangial expansion and albuminuria (43).

In diabetes or chronic hyperglycemia, accumulation of DAG and activation of PKC have adverse effects on renal functional and structural changes.

Genetic Predisposition

Genetic approaches are being used to understand the susceptibility to or genesis of diabetic nephropathy. Anchored in the work of Pirart (43a), this research has found limited concordance between diabetic nephropathy and neuropathy or retinopathy. The probability of developing nephropathy is only approximately 25% in patients with neuropathy or retinopathy, whereas a patient with diabetic nephropathy has more than an 85% probability of developing neuropathy or retinopathy (44). Evidence suggests that selected individuals with diabetes mellitus have a genetic predisposition to developing nephropathy (18,45–47). Familial clustering studies of diabetic nephropathy show that, if a proband has nephropathy, the cumulative risk of nephropathy in siblings (72%) is almost 50% higher than in siblings (25%) of a proband without incipient or overt nephropathy (48).

The role of hypertension and the predisposition to diabetic nephropathy is supported by familial clustering, sodium-lithium countertransport activity, and hypertension and nephropathy susceptibility genes. Patients with hypertensive parents who also have hypertension themselves are at greater risk of nephropathy and have higher age-adjusted blood pressures in adolescence (49,50).

Modulations of the renin-angiotensin system (RAS) have been shown to influence the development and progression of changes in renal function and morphology in patients with diabetic kidney disease. This has led to the examination of genes controlling the components of the RAS as candidate genes for the association of hypertension and/or diabetic nephropathy. A relationship has been suggested between an insertion/deletion polymorphism of the angiotensin-converting enzyme (ACE) gene and diabetic nephropathy. Using a candidate gene approach, Doria et al. found a significant variation in the risk for developing diabetic nephropathy associated with the haplotypes at the ACE locus in IDDM patients with disease duration of 16 to 21 years (51). The variants of the ACE gene are in linkage disequilibrium with one or more ACE haplotypes and contribute to an increased susceptibility to nephropathy. A relationship between RAS gene polymorphism and increased urinary albumin excretion has also been observed in patients with noninsulin-dependent diabetes mellitus (type 2) (52). Deletion polymorphism in the ACE gene may reduce the long-term beneficial effect of ACE inhibition on retarding the progression of diabetic nephropathy (53).

Moczulski et al. performed a linkage study using pairs of siblings with IDDM discordant for diabetic nephropathy. Theoretical considerations supported by simulation studies indicated that discordant pairs, rather than concordant pairs, would be more effective in detecting a major susceptibility gene for diabetic nephropathy. These researchers found that in the regions containing ACE and angiotensinogen genes, loci were not linked with diabetic nephropathy, whereas the region containing the angiotensin II type 1 receptor locus showed linkage with diabetic nephropathy. This provides very strong evidence that a region (20-cM) around the angiotensin II type 1 receptor gene contains a major locus for susceptibility to diabetic nephropathy (54).

Polymorphisms in the endothelial nitric oxide synthase gene may be implicated in the development of nephropathy in patients with IDDM. Using the transmission disequilibrium test, a family-based design to test association and case-control studies, researchers found that DNA sequence differences in the endothelial nitric oxide synthase gene appear to influence the risk of advanced nephropathy in IDDM (55).

In 1999, the National Institute of Diabetes and Digestive and Kidney Diseases developed a consortium to identify genes or genomic regions that are associated with differential risks for the expression or progression of diabetic nephropathy. The consortium will combine multiple genetic strategies with complementary approaches using genetic material in an attempt to decipher the genes that contribute to the development of diabetic nephropathy (56).

NATURAL HISTORY OF NEPHROPATHY: FUNCTION AND STRUCTURE

The annual incidence of diabetic nephropathy reaches a peak after 15 years' duration of IDDM (57). Analysis of the cumulative incidence of persistent albuminuria in patients who have had diabetes for 25 years demonstrated a substantial reduction from 28% (1961 to 1965) to 5.8% (1971 to 1975). This change reflects improved glycemic control (58). In patients fated to develop diabetic nephropathy, the increasing duration of diabetes is associated with a progressive decline in glomerular filtration, increasing albuminuria followed by massive proteinuria, and eventual ESRD (Fig. 49.1) (59).

Renal involvement in patients with IDDM is classified into five stages according to the degree of changes in renal function and morphology. With the onset of diabetes, or

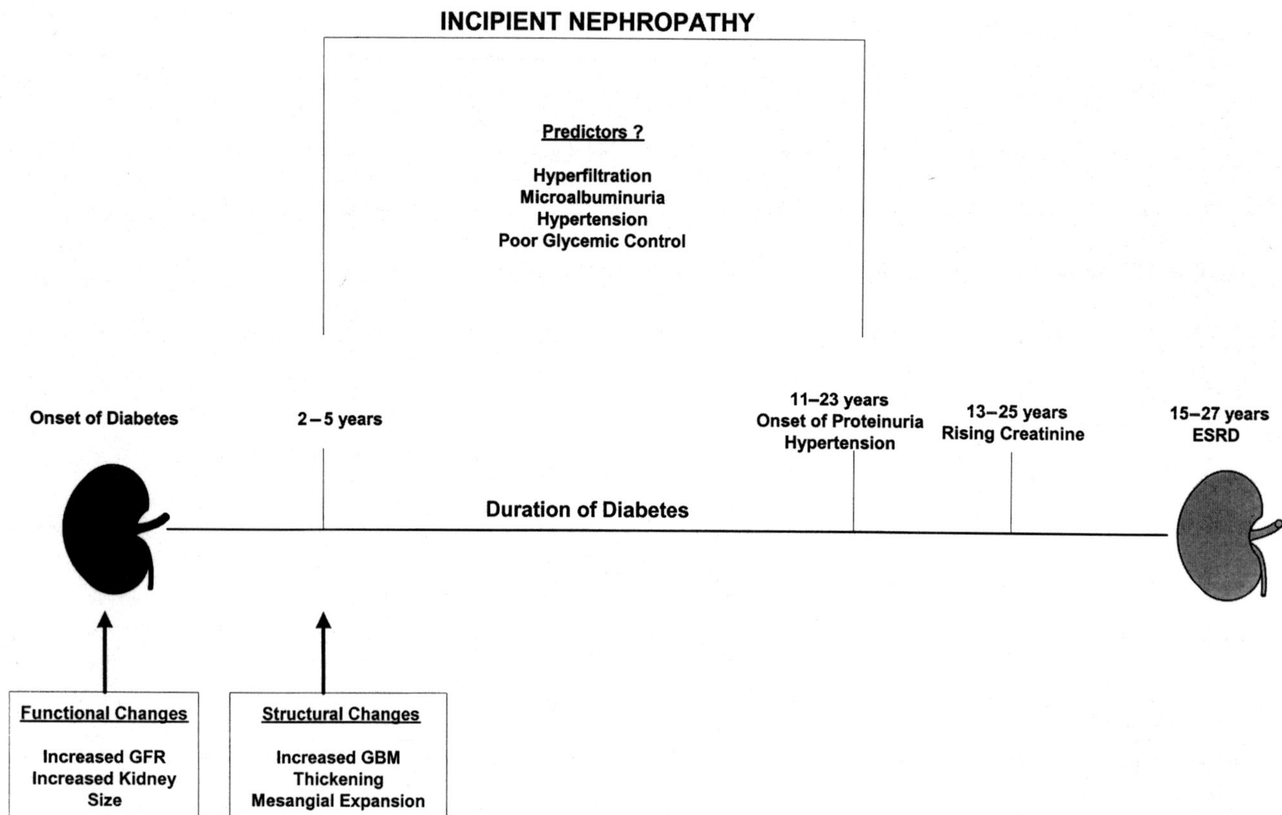

FIGURE 49.1. Natural history of diabetic nephropathy. ESRD, end-stage renal disease; GBM, glomerular basement membrane; GFR, glomerular filtration rate. (Modified from Breyer JA. Diabetic nephropathy in insulin-dependent diabetes. *Am J Kidney Dis* 1992;20:533–547.)

stage 1 nephropathy, the only findings are enlarged kidneys and glomerular hyperfiltration. There is no evidence of histologic lesions in glomeruli or vascular structures. In stage 2, the findings occur over 2 to 5 years and are similar to those in stage 1 except that histopathologic abnormalities can be found on renal biopsy (biopsy is not indicated for patients at this stage). On microscopic examination, basement membranes are thickened and mesangial areas show expansion.

Stage 3, or incipient diabetic nephropathy, is termed the *microalbuminuria phase.* It generally occurs during the second decade of diabetes. At this stage, renal function is normal and the routine dipstick test is negative for protein. Normal urinary albumin excretion is less than 20 μg/min (median, 2.3 to 6.4 μg/min) or less than 30 mg/day. Microalbuminuria is defined as more than 20 μg/min but less than 200 μg/min. In comparison, significant albuminuria or overt nephropathy (dipstick-positive proteinuria) is a value higher than 200 μg/min or 300 mg/day. Given the inherent difficulties of a 24-hour collection, microalbumin level can be indexed to the urinary creatinine concentration in an early morning specimen. The predictive value of the random urine sample albumin to creatinine index of 30 to 300 mg/g in predicting microalbuminuria has a sensitivity between 88 and 100% and a specificity between 81 and 100% (60). With the onset of microalbuminuria, the GFR begins to decrease, usually when the albumin excretion exceeds 70 μg/min. The decrease in the GFR is 3 to 4 mL/min/yr (61). With the onset of stage 3 nephropathy, systemic blood pressure increases and there is a progressive decline in the GFR. Anemia and disturbances in calcium-phosphorus homeostasis start to develop. In addition, patients with IDDM and microalbuminuria have a higher risk of extrarenal atherogenic abnormalities than individuals without microalbuminuria. The risk profile includes proliferative retinopathy; decreased left ventricular function; increased levels of total, very-low-density, and low-density lipoprotein cholesterol; and increased transcapillary escape of albumin.

The onset of stage 4 nephropathy is a harbinger of the need for renal replacement therapy by dialysis or transplantation within 10 years. This is the phase of dipstick-positive proteinuria, rapid decline in the GFR, significant to severe hypertension, and the other sequelae of moderate to severe renal insufficiency. As discussed later, strict glycemic control and effective control of blood pressure with ACE inhibition may slow the rate of decline in renal function. With the progression of renal failure, the stage of dialysis and transplantation (stage 5) is reached.

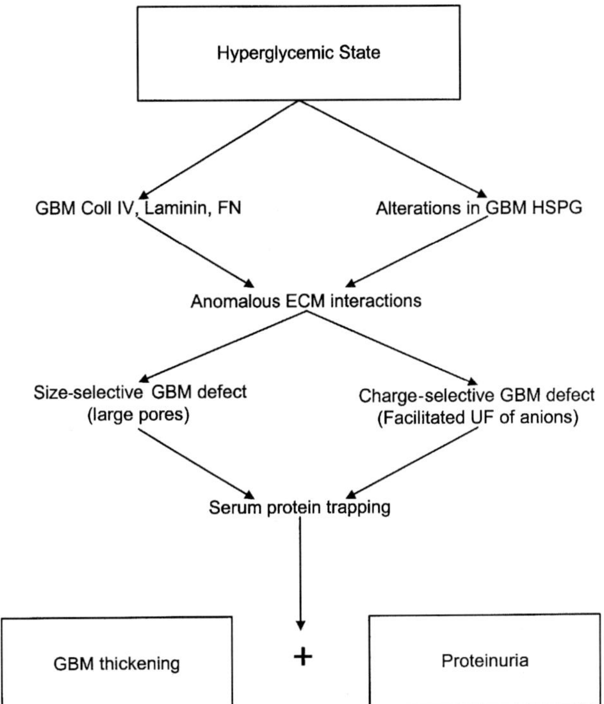

FIGURE 49.2. Hypothetical algorithm linking biochemical changes in the diabetic glomerular basement membrane (GBM) to the observed changes of GBM thickening and proteinuria. Coll, collagen; ECM, extracellular matrix; FN, fibronectin; HSPG, heparin sulfate proteoglycan; UF, ultrafiltration. (From Adler S. Structure-function relationships associated with extracellular matrix alterations in diabetic glomerulopathy. *J Am Soc Nephrol* 1994;5:1165–1172, with permission.)

With established diabetic nephropathy (microalbuminuria, decreased GFR), there is progression of histopathologic changes (renal extracellular basement membrane and mesangial expansion) within the kidney (62). Although Mauer et al. were unable to find a close relationship between duration of IDDM and GBM thickness or mesangial expansion, mesangial expansion (diffuse glomerulosclerosis) was inversely correlated to capillary filtering surface area (63). Based on studies showing an increased content of collagen types IV and V, serum proteins, and laminin in the thickened GBM (64) and alterations in the GBM content of heparan sulfate proteoglycan (HSPG), Alder hypothesized that these changes in the GBM may initiate a series of events leading to changes in the sieving properties of the GBM that result in proteinuria and loss of glomerular filtering surface area (65) (Fig. 49.2).

Although numerous studies exist of the functional, biochemical, and structural relationships in patients with diabetic nephropathy, additional studies are needed to answer the many remaining questions. What is the basis for the significant variability in the expression of diabetic nephropathy? Why does one group of patients with a duration of hyperglycemia of less than 20 years develop renal failure, whereas another group with a duration of 40 years of hyperglycemia never develops clinical nephropathy?

DETECTION AND MANAGEMENT OF DIABETIC NEPHROPATHY

The management of diabetes mellitus encompasses strict glycemic control, adherence to dietary guidelines established by the American Diabetes Association, lifestyle changes (no alcohol use or smoking), and an exercise program (66). As discussed earlier, the DCCT and other research confirms and extends the results of many other studies that intensive glycemic control reduces microalbuminuria and overt nephropathy. It is intuitive that normalizing the aberrant metabolic state will limit vascular injury in patients with diabetes. With the convenience of home glucose monitoring, office measurements of glycosylated hemoglobin, rapid-acting insulin, and insulin pumps, there are no valid reasons (on the part of patient or physician) that preclude consistent control of stable blood glucose concentrations.

Screening for Microalbuminuria

Measurement of urinary microalbumin excretion rate (UAER) by determination of a 24-hour or early morning albumin/creatinine index should be performed yearly for IDDM patients with disease duration of longer than 5 years. If the UAER value exceeds 20 μg/min (30 mg/day) or the albumin/creatinine index is higher than 30 μg/mg, a repeat test should be performed in 3 to 6 months to substantiate the diagnosis of microalbuminuria. If the results of the repeat test are below 20 μg/min, the patient returns to annual testing. If the value is increased, however, the initiation of ACE inhibitor therapy to delay progression of nephropathy is indicated (see later). Ketoacidosis, diuresis, acute illnesses, severe cardiac disease, urinary tract infections, menstrual bleeding, severe hypertension, poor glycemic control, vigorous exercise, and coincident nondiabetic renal disease influence the UAER. A diurnal variation in urinary albumin excretion is also seen in all stages of diabetic nephropathy. Postexercise albuminuria occurs in children with IDDM duration of longer than 5 years and normal preexercise UAER (67). Although dipsticks have been introduced to detect microalbuminuria, the radioimmunoassay test is still the most accurate method. In patients with persistent microalbuminuria and acceptable glycemic control or in patients with no reduction in microalbuminuria despite improved glycemic control, consideration should be given to the use of ACE inhibitors (see later) (68,69).

Numerous studies have demonstrated that the use of ACE inhibitors delays the progression of diabetic nephropathy. Animal studies initially demonstrated that ACE inhibitors could retard glomerular damage by normalizing glomerular capillary pressure independently of their antihypertensive effect. A large multicenter, randomized, prospective study of 409 patients who had IDDM of at least 7 years' duration, serum creatinine concentration of 2.5 mg/dL or lower, and urinary protein excretion higher than 500 mg/day has extended the known benefits of ACE inhibitors. The study found that treatment with an ACE inhibitor (captopril) reduced progression of diabetic nephropathy, improved the clinical outcome by reducing the number of patients requiring dialysis and/or transplantation, and provided renal protection independent of the antihypertensive effect (70). This study also found that 64% of the patients who died and 61% of the patients who required dialysis or transplantation were in the placebo group. Only 25 patients in the captopril group had a doubling of serum creatinine level compared with 43 in the placebo group. This was a 48% reduction in risk in the captopril group. The captopril group had a 50% risk reduction in the combined end points of death, dialysis, and transplantation. Last, significantly less proteinuria was seen in the captopril group than in the placebo-treated group. The study showed that the ACE inhibitor captopril significantly retarded the rate of loss of renal function in patients with stage 4 diabetic nephropathy.

In additional studies, the ACE inhibitor enalapril decreased UAER in IDDM patients with microalbuminuria at rest (incipient nephropathy, stage 3) and after exercise (71). Based on an extensive review of these and other studies, the Ad Hoc Committee of the Council on Diabetes Mellitus of the National Kidney Foundation published recommendations for the screening and management of microalbuminuria, or stage 3 nephropathy (72). Their conclusions and my recommendations follow (Tables 49.1 and 49.2).

It is appropriate to start at the lowest dosage and titrate the final dosage to blood pressure response. To increase compliance, the use of a long-acting ACE inhibitor may be considered. The recommended monitoring of ACE inhibitor therapy is to (a) measure the UAER every 6 months, and (b) monitor the serum creatinine and potassium concentrations 7 to 10 days after starting therapy and then every 3 months. If the microalbumin value is reduced by a lower-than-recommended dosage of an ACE inhibitor and blood pressure and creatinine level are stable, there is no reason to alter the dosage. However, if the microalbuminuria value is increasing, an upward dosage adjustment is appropriate.

TABLE 49.1. RECOMMENDATIONS FOR ANGIOTENSIN-CONVERTING ENZYME (ACE) INHIBITOR THERAPY[a] (THE FOLLOWING ARE SUGGESTED ADULT DOSAGES ONLY)

Incipient nephropathy
- Captopril: 12.5–25.0 mg twice daily (maximum, 50 mg twice daily)
- Enalapril: 5–20 mg daily (daily or divided twice daily)

Overt nephropathy
- Captopril: 25 mg three times daily
- Enalapril: 5–20 mg daily (daily or divided twice daily)

[a]Because the benefit of ACE Inhibitors is a class effect, other agents in this category may be considered.

TABLE 49.2. RECOMMENDATIONS FOR ANGIOTENSIN-CONVERTING ENZYME (ACE) INHIBITION AND ANTIHYPERTENSIVE THERAPY

Monitoring of ACE inhibitor therapy
- Obtain serum creatinine concentration at baseline and within 7–10 days after therapy is started, then at least every 3 months.
- If creatinine concentration increases by 0.5 mg/dL, refer to nephrologist.
- Obtain serum potassium concentration at baseline and within 7–10 days after therapy is started, then at least every 3 months.
- If potassium concentration ≥5 mEq/L, refer to nephrologist.
- Obtain complete blood count every 3 months.
- Check urinary albumin excretion rate every 6 months.

Therapy for hypertension
- Initial therapy
  - ACE inhibitor
- Second-line therapy
  - Low-dose diuretic (up to 25 mg)
  - α-Receptor blocker
  - Calcium channel blocker
- Problem drugs—use with caution or avoid
  - Beta-blockers
  - Potassium-sparing diuretics

Insufficient evidence exists to recommend the use of an ACE inhibitor in patients with normoalbuminuria and normotension.

In patients with non–insulin dependent diabetes mellitus (type 2), treatment with angiotensin II receptor antagonists has demonstrated renal protection independent of the blood pressure changes (73–75), whereas use of ACE inhibitors has not demonstrated a consistent beneficial effect. Although there are some data to support the use of angiotensin II receptor antagonists in patients with IDDM (76), their use should be reserved for patients unable to tolerate an ACE inhibitor due to the side effect of cough.

BLOOD PRESSURE CONTROL

Studies using ambulatory blood pressure monitoring in adolescents and young adults with normoalbuminuria and normal blood pressure suggest that an increase in nighttime systolic blood pressure may precede the development of microalbuminuria (77). If nocturnal elevations in blood pressure do identify a cohort of patients with IDDM and a predilection to microalbuminuria, then ACE inhibitor therapy may have value before the development of incipient nephropathy (78).

Effective control of blood pressure delays the progression of chronic renal disease. Numerous studies have demonstrated the efficacy of antihypertensive treatment in slowing the progression of diabetes-induced renal disease.

The approach to antihypertensive therapy for patients with diabetes is no different from that for nondiabetic subjects. Initial therapy should be an ACE inhibitor. The major risk is acute reduction in renal function or acceleration in deterioration of renal function in patients with bilateral renal artery stenosis. Hyperkalemia may occur secondary to renal insufficiency or hyporeninemic hypoaldosteronism (renal tubular acidosis type IV).

Second-line therapy includes calcium channel blocking (CCB) agents, α-receptor blockers, or a low-dose diuretic (hydrochlorothiazide, up to 25 mg/day). The major side effects of CCBs in patients with IDDM are orthostatic hypotension, constipation, edema, and headaches. Some studies report increased blood glucose concentrations with nifedipine secondary to lowering of insulin levels. The CCBs do not adversely effect lipid concentrations or renal function. To prevent electrolyte abnormalities and to limit adverse effects on carbohydrate metabolism, only low-dose diuretics should be prescribed. Diuretics are effective and may be synergistic with ACE inhibitor therapy.

Both potassium-sparing diuretics and beta-blocking agents should be used with caution in patients with IDDM. Beta-blocking agents, such as propranolol, may aggravate glycemic control, limit recognition of hypoglycemic episodes and delay recovery, adversely affect lipoprotein concentrations, and potentiate hyperkalemia after exercise.

SUMMARY

The goals of monitoring and therapy for children, adolescents, and adults with IDDM are to maintain good glycemic control, monitor UAERs after 5 years of diabetes, aggressively control blood pressure, use ACE inhibitors for persistent microalbuminuria, provide dietary and/or pharmacologic treatment of dyslipidemia, and maximize patient and family education regarding the complications of this chronic illness. Management of IDDM in children and adolescents requires the dedicated efforts of an interdisciplinary health care team, which includes the primary care practitioner, pediatric endocrinologist, pediatric nephrologist, dietitian, social worker, and ophthalmologist.

REFERENCES

1. Kussman MJ, Goldstein HH, Gleason RE. The clinical course of diabetic nephropathy. *JAMA* 1976;236:1861–1863.
2. U.S. Renal Data System, *USRDS 2001 annual data report: atlas of end-stage renal disease in the Unites States.* Bethesda, MD, National Institutes of Health, National Institute of Diabetes and Digestive and Kidney Diseases, 2001.
3. U.S. Renal Data System, *2001 ASN Symposium: The Epidemic of Diabetes Mellitus in the ESRD Population,* Bethesda, MD, National Institutes of Health, National Institute of Diabetes and Digestive and Kidney Diseases, 2001.
4. Libman IM, Laporte RE, Becker D, et al. Was there an epidemic of diabetes in nonwhite adolescents in Allegheny County, Pennsylvania *Diabetes Care* 1998;21:1278–1281.
5. Couper JJ, Clarke CF, Byrne GC, et al. Progression of borderline increases in albuminuria in adolescents with insulin-dependent diabetes mellitus. *Diabet Med* 1997;14:766–771.
6. Krolewski AS, Warram JH, Christlieb AR, et al. The changing natural history of nephropathy in type I diabetes. *Am J Med* 1985;78:785–794.
7. Mogensen CE. Early glomerular hyperfiltration in insulin-dependent diabetics and late nephropathy. *Scand J Clin Lab Invest* 1986;46:201–206.
8. Molitch ME, Steffes MW, Cleary PA, et al. Baseline analysis of renal function in the Diabetes Control and Complications Trial. *Kidney Int* 1993;43:668–674.
9. Christiansen CK, Mogensen CE. Effect of antihypertensive treatment on progression of incipient diabetic nephropathy. *Hypertension* 1985;7[Suppl II]:II-109–II-113.
10. Hostetter TH, Rennke HG, Brenner BM. The case for intrarenal hypertension in the initiation and progression of diabetic and other glomerulopathies. *Am J Med* 1982;72: 375–380.
11. Goligorsky MS, Chen J, Brodsky S. Endothelial cell function leading to diabetic nephropathy. Focus on nitric oxide. *Hypertension* 2001;37:744–748.
12. Meraji S, Jayakody L, Senaratne MPJ, et al. Endothelium-dependent relaxation in aorta of BB rat. *Diabetes* 1987;36: 978–981.
13. Gupta S, Sussman I, McArthur CS, et al. Endothelium-dependent inhibition of Na+–K+ ATPase activity in rabbit aorta by hyperglycemia: possible role of endothelium-derived nitric oxide. *J Clin Invest* 1992;90:727–732.
14. Brownlee M, Vlassara H, Cerami A. Nonenzymatic glycosylation and the pathogenesis of diabetic complications. *Ann Intern Med* 1984;101:527–537.
15. Makita Z, Radoff S, Rayfield EJ, et al. Advanced glycosylation end products in patients with diabetic nephropathy. *N Engl J Med* 1991;325:836–842.
16. Singh R, Barden A, Mori T et al. Advanced glycation end-product: a review. *Diabetologia* 2001;44:129–146.
17. Quinn M, Angelico MC, Cross A, et al. Concordance for kidney complications in siblings with IDDM. *Diabetes* 1992;41[Suppl 1]:121A(abst).
18. Seaquist ER, Goetz FC, Rich S, et al. Familial clustering of diabetic kidney disease: evidence for genetic susceptibility to diabetic nephropathy. *N Engl J Med* 1989;320:1161–1165.
19. Zatz R, Meyer TW, Rennke HG, et al. Predominance of hemodynamic rather than metabolic factors in the pathogenesis of diabetic nephropathy. *Proc Natl Acad Sci U S A* 1985; 82:5963– 5967.
20. Feldt-Rasmussen B, Mathiesen ER, Deckert T, et al. Central role for sodium in pathogenesis of blood pressure changes independent of angiotensin, aldosterone, and catecholamines in type I (insulin-dependent) diabetes mellitus. *Diabetologia* 1987;30:610–617.
21. Goldberg RB, Capuzzi D. Lipid disorders in type 1 and type 2 diabetes. *Clin Lab Med* 2001;21:147–172.

22. Hostetter TH, Troy JL, Brenner BM. Glomerular hemodynamics in experimental diabetes mellitus. *Kidney Int* 1981;19: 410–415.
23. Gartner K. Glomerular hyperfiltration during the onset of diabetes mellitus in two strains of diabetic mice. *Diabetologia* 1978;15:59–63.
24. Anderson S, Vora JP. Current concepts of renal hemodynamics in diabetes. *J Diabetes Complications* 1995;9:304–307.
25. Christiansen JS, Gammelgaard J, Orskov H, et al. Kidney functions and size in diabetics before and during insulin treatment. *Kidney Int* 1982;21:683–688.
26. Goldfarb S, Ziyadeh FNN, Kern EFO, et al. Effects of polyol-pathway inhibition and dietary myoinositol on glomerular hemodynamic function in experimental diabetes mellitus in rats. *Diabetes* 1991;40:465–471.
27. Zatz R, Dunn BR, Meyer TW, et al. Prevention of diabetic glomerulopathy by pharmacological amelioration of glomerular capillary hypertension. *J Clin Invest* 1986;77:1925–1930.
28. Luscher TF, Boulanger CM, Dohi Y, et al. Endothelium-derived contracting factors. *Hypertension* 1992;19:117–130.
29. Shepherd JT, Katusic ZS. Endothelium-derived vasoactive factors: I. Endothelium-dependent relaxation. *Hypertension* 1991;18[Suppl III]:III-76–III-85.
30. Diabetes Control and Complications Trial Research Group. The effect of intensive treatment of diabetes on the development and progression of long-term complications in insulin-dependent diabetes mellitus. *N Engl J Med* 1993;329: 977–986.
31. U.K. Prospective Diabetes Study Group. Intensive blood-glucose control with sulfonylureas or insulin compared with conventional treatment and risk of complications in patients with type 2 diabetes (UKPDS 33). *Lancet* 1998;352:837–853.
32. Writing Team for the Diabetes Control and Complications Trial/Epidemiology of Diabetes Interventions and Complications Research Group. Effect of intensive therapy on the microvascular complications of type 1 diabetes mellitus. *JAMA* 2002;287:2563–2569.
33. Vlassara H. Protein glycation in the kidney in diabetes and aging. *Kidney Int* 1996;49:1795–1804.
34. Brownlee M, Cerami A, Vlassara H. Advanced glycosylation end products in tissue and the biochemical basis of diabetic complications. *N Engl J Med* 1988;318:1315–1321.
35. Cohen MP, Ziyadeh FN. Role of amadori-modified nonenzymatically glycated serum proteins in the pathogenesis of diabetic nephropathy. *J Am Soc Nephrol* 1996;7:183–190.
36. Skolnik EY, Yang Z, Makita Z, et al. Human and rat mesangial cell receptors for glucose-modified proteins: potential role in kidney tissue remodeling and diabetic nephropathy. *J Exp Med* 1991;174:931–938.
37. Doi T, Vlassara H, Kirstein M, et al. Receptor-specific increase in extracellular matrix production in mouse mesangial cells by advanced glycosylation end products is mediated via platelet-derived growth factor. *Proc Natl Acad Sci U S A* 1992;89:2873–2877.
38. Bucala R, Vlassara H. Advanced glycosylation end products in diabetic renal and vascular disease. *Am J Kidney Dis* 1995; 26:875–888.
39. Bucala R, Tracey KJ, Cerami A. Advanced glycosylation products quench nitric oxide and mediate defective endothelium-dependent vasodilatation in experimental diabetes. *J Clin Invest* 1191;87:432–438.
40. Tuschida K, Makita Z, Yamagishi S, et al. Suppression of transforming growth factor beta and vascular endothelial growth factor in diabetic nephropathy in rats by a novel advanced glycation end-product inhibitor OPB-9195. *Diabetologia* 1999;42:577–588.
41. Sharma K, Ziyadeh FN. Hyperglycemia and diabetic kidney disease. The case for transforming growth factor beta as a key mediator. *Diabetes* 1995;44:1139–1146.
42. Ways DK, Sheetz MJ. The role of protein kinase C in the development of the complications of diabetes. *Vitam Horm* 2001;60:149–193.
43. Koya D, Jirousek MR, Lin Y-W, et al. Characterization of protein kinase beta-isoform activation on the gene expression of transforming growth factor β, extracellular matrix components and prostanoids in the glomeruli of diabetic rats. *J Clin Invest* 1997;100:115–126.
43a. Pirart J. Diabete et complications degeneratives. Presentation d'une etude prospective portant sur 4400 cas observes entre 1947 et 1973 (troisieme et derniere partie). *Diabete et Metabolisme* 1977;3:245–256.
44. Marre M. Genetics and the prediction of complications in type 1 diabetes. *Diabetes Care* 1999;22[Suppl 2]:B3–B58.
45. Krolewski AS, Warram JH, Christlieb AR, et al. The changing natural history of nephropathy in type I diabetes. *Am J Med* 1985;78:785–794.
46. Borch-Johnsen K, Norgaard K, Hommel E, et al. Is diabetic nephropathy an inherited complication? *Kidney Int* 1992;41: 719–722.
47. Viberti G. Why do we have to invoke genetic susceptibility for diabetic nephropathy? *Kidney Int* 1999;55:2526–2527.
48. Quinn M, Angelico MC, Warram JH, et al. Familial factors determine the development of diabetic nephropathy in patients with IDDM. *Diabetologia* 1996;39:940–945.
49. Barzilay J, Warram JH, Bak M, et al. Predisposition to hypertension: risk factor for nephropathy and hypertension in IDDM. *Kidney Int* 1992;41:723–730.
50. Roglic G, Colhoun HM, Stevens LK, et al. Parental history of hypertension and parental history of diabetes and microvascular complications in insulin-dependent diabetes mellitus: the EURODIAB IDDM Complications Study. *Diabet Med* 1998;15:418–427.
51. Doria A, Warram JH, Krolewski AS. Genetic predisposition to diabetic nephropathy. Evidence for a role of the angiotensin I converting enzyme gene. *Diabetes* 1994;43: 690–695.
52. Dudley CRK, Keavney B, Stratton IR, et al. Prospective diabetes study XV: relationship of renin-angiotensin system gene polymorphisms with microalbuminuria in NIDDM. *Kidney Int* 1995:48;1907–1911.
53. Parving H-H, Jacobsen P, Tarnow L, et al. Effect of deletion polymorphism of angiotensin converting enzyme gene on progression of diabetic nephropathy during inhibition of angiotensin converting enzyme: observational follow-up study. *BMJ* 1996;313:591–594.
54. Moczulski DK, Rogus JJ, Antonellis A, et al. Major susceptibility locus for nephropathy in type 1 diabetes chromo-

some 3q: results of novel discordant sib-pair analysis. *Diabetes* 1998;47:1164–1169.
55. Zanchi A, Moczulski DK, Hanna LS, et al. Risk of advanced diabetic nephropathy in type 1 is associated with endothelial nitric oxide synthase gene polymorphism. *Kidney Int* 2000;57:405–413.
56. Adler SG, Pahl M, Seldin MF. Deciphering diabetic nephropathy: progress using genetic strategies. *Curr Opin Nephrol Hypertens* 2000;9:99–106.
57. Dorman JS, Laporte RE, Kuller LH. The Pittsburgh Insulin dependent diabetes mellitus (IDDM) morbidity and mortality study. *Diabetes* 1984;33:271–276.
58. Bojestig M, Arnqvist HJ, Hermansson G, et al. Declining incidence of nephropathy in insulin-dependent diabetes mellitus. *N Engl J Med* 1994;330:15–18.
59. Mogensen CE, Christensen CK, Vittinghus E. The stages of diabetic renal disease with emphasis on the stage of incipient nephropathy. *Diabetes* 1983;32[Suppl 2]:64–78.
60. Marshall SM. Screening for microalbuminuria: which measurement *Diabet Med* 1991;8:706–711.
61. Feldt-Rasmussen B, Borch-Johnsen K, Deckert T, et al. Microalbuminuria: an important diagnostic tool. *J Diabetes Complications* 1994;8:137–145.
62. Mauer SM, Goetz FC, McHugh CE, et al. Long-term study of normal kidneys transplanted into patients with type 1 diabetes. *Diabetes* 1989;38:516–523.
63. Mauer SM, Steffes MW, Ellis EN, et al. Structural-functional relationships in diabetic nephropathy. *J Clin Invest* 1984;74:1143–1155.
64. Falk RJ, Scheinman JI, Mauer SM, et al. Polyantigenic expansion of basement membrane constituents in diabetic nephropathy. *Diabetes* 1983;32:4–9.
65. Alder S. Structure-function relationships associated with extracellular matrix alterations in diabetic glomerulopathy. *J Am Soc Nephrol* 1994;5:1165–1172.
66. Nutrition recommendations and principles for people with diabetes mellitus (position statement). *Diabetes Care* 1997;20 [Suppl 1]:106–108.
67. Kruger M, Gordjani N, Burghard R. Postexercise albuminuria in children with different duration of type-1 diabetes mellitus. *Pediatr Nephrol* 1996;10:594–597.
68. Travis LB. Prevention of renal disease in insulin-dependent diabetes mellitus: a responsibility for the pediatrician? *J Pediatr* 1991;117:273–274.
69. Casani A, Bangstad H-J, Chiarelli F. Detection and management of diabetic glomerulopathy in children and adolescents with insulin-dependent diabetes mellitus: need for improved knowledge and better care. *J Pediatr Endocrinol Metab* 2000;13:467–474.
70. Lewis EJ, Hunsicker LG, Bain RP, et al. The Collaborative Study Group: the effect of angiotensin-converting-enzyme inhibition on diabetic nephropathy. *N Engl J Med* 1993;329: 1456–1462.
71. Inserra F, Daccordi H, Ippolito JL, et al. Decrease of exercise-induced microalbuminuria in patients with type I diabetes by means of an angiotensin-converting enzyme inhibitor. *Am J Kidney Dis* 1996;27:26–33.
72. Bennett PH, Haffner S, Kasiske BL, et al. Screening and management of microalbuminuria in patients with diabetes mellitus. Recommendations to the Scientific Advisory Board of the National Kidney Foundation from an Ad Hoc Committee of the Council on Diabetes Mellitus of the National Kidney Foundation. *Am J Kidney Dis* 1995;25:107–112.
73. Lewis EJ, Hunsicker LG, Clarke WR, et al. Renoprotective effect of the angiotensin-receptor antagonist irbesartan in patients with nephropathy due to type 2 diabetes. *N Engl J Med* 2001;345:851–860.
74. Brenner BM, Cooper ME, deZeeum D, et al. Effects of losartan on renal and cardiovascular outcomes in patients with type 2 diabetes and nephropathy. *N Engl J Med* 2001; 345:861–869.
75. Parving H-H, Lehnert H, Brochner-Mortensen, et al. The effect of irbesartan on the development of diabetic nephropathy in patients with type 2 diabetes. *N Engl J Med* 2001;345: 870–878.
76. Andersen S, Tarnow L, Rossing P, et al. Renoprotective effects of angiotensin II receptor blockade in type 1 diabetic patients with diabetic nephropathy. *Kidney Int* 2000;57:601–606.
77. Lurbe E, Redon J, Kesani A, et al. Increase in nocturnal blood pressure and progression to microalbuminuria in type 1 diabetes. *N Engl J Med* 2002;347:797–805.
78. Ingelfinger JR. Ambulatory blood-pressure monitoring as a predictive tool. *N Engl J Med* 2002;347:778–779.

50

RENAL MANIFESTATIONS OF METABOLIC DISORDERS

WILLIAM G. van't HOFF

Although the majority of children with renal dysfunction have a structural, immunologic, or infective disorder, some have a metabolic defect arising from an abnormality in the biochemical pathways of cell metabolism. In many metabolic disorders, substrate accumulation or an enzyme deficiency can be documented in the kidney but without evidence of renal dysfunction (e.g., some of the lysosomal storage disorders). This review concentrates on those disorders in which there is a clear renal functional or structural abnormality. Several of these conditions are described in detail elsewhere in this book; this chapter highlights a number of other metabolic disorders and provides, in tabular form, the various metabolic causes of renal symptomatology (Tables 50.1 to 50.6). Many metabolic disorders can cause acute or chronic renal failure. It is rare for this to be the sole manifestation, however; therefore, these conditions are listed under the most important renal feature.

The proximal renal tubule has a very high-energy expenditure and is therefore sensitive to metabolic disorders that interfere with the generation of adenosine triphosphate (ATP). Mitochondrial dysfunction and reduced ATP levels are felt to be important in the pathogenesis of Fanconi syndrome, which is one of the most common renal manifestations of metabolic disease (Table 50.1); a fuller description is given in Chapter 41. Nephrocalcinosis and urolithiasis are also common manifestations of metabolic dysfunction, usually arising from defective reabsorption of a solute (e.g., cystine in cystinuria) or as a result of the urinary excretion of abnormally elevated plasma constituents (e.g., oxalate in hyperoxaluria). Renal glomerular involvement is less common but can occur as a result of abnormal deposition of storage material or a defect in the synthesis of the glomerular components (Table 50.4). As a result of improvements in the care of children with metabolic disorders, longer term manifestations are becoming more apparent. Cystinosis was once described as a renal disorder, and it was only as a result of renal transplantation that patients survived into adulthood and were then observed to develop extrarenal problems (1). In addition, in some disorders increased survival has led to the development of renal dysfunction [e.g., methylmalonic acidemia (MMA)]. Thus pediatric nephrologists need to remain vigilant to the possibility of a metabolic disorder, especially in children with extrarenal symptoms.

METHYLMALONIC ACIDEMIA

MMA is an autosomal recessive disorder of the metabolism of methylmalonyl coenzyme A (CoA) caused either by a defect of methylmalonyl CoA mutase or of the cofactor adenosyl cobalamin (2). Patients usually present in the neonatal period or early infancy with lethargy, vomiting, poor feeding, failure to thrive, and recurrent metabolic acidosis. Patients deficient in the cofactor respond favorably to cobalamin supplementation, but for those who have a partial or complete deficiency of the apoenzyme, the prognosis is poor with a mortality of approximately 50% within the first decade. In cobalamin-unresponsive patients, there is a significant incidence of neurologic and renal manifestations.

Renal Tubular and Glomerular Dysfunction

Children with MMA have evidence of renal tubular dysfunction, which becomes very profound during episodes of metabolic decompensation (usually triggered by intercurrent infection) with massive renal salt and bicarbonate losses. In a study of seven cobalamin-unresponsive patients, five had defects in urine concentration, two had impaired urine acidification, and several had hyporeninemic hypoaldosteronism (3). Chronic renal impairment has also been documented in cobalamin-unresponsive MMA patients. Walter et al. documented a low glomerular filtration rate (GFR) in 8 of 12 such children, 5 of whom had a GFR of less than 40 mL/min/1.73 m^2 (4). In a retrospective survey of patients with *all* forms of MMA, Baumgartner and Viar-

TABLE 50.1. FANCONI SYNDROME

Disorder	Main features	Renal features	References
Cystinosis	Poor growth; vomiting; rickets; often blond, fair hair; corneal cystine crystals; multisystem involvement	Fanconi syndrome, chronic renal failure, rarely urinary tract dilatation, calculi (urate/calcium oxalate)	See Chapter 41 (87)
Tyrosinemia type 1	Hepatomegaly, liver disease, rickets, neurologic crises	Fanconi syndrome, nephromegaly, nephrocalcinosis, calculi, chronic renal impairment	See Chapter 41 (88,89)
Mitochondrial disorders	Myopathy, poor growth, cardiomyopathy, liver dysfunction, neuropathy, retinopathy, ophthalmoplegia, endocrinopathy	Fanconi syndrome, Bartter's syndrome–like features, proteinuria, tubulointerstitial nephritis, cysts	See Chapter 41 (43–59)
Galactosemia	Vomiting, diarrhea, poor growth, jaundice, liver disease, hypotonia, cataracts	Fanconi syndrome	See Chapter 41
Dent's disease	Hypercalciuria, tubular proteinuria, X-linked	Fanconi syndrome, nephrocalcinosis/nephrolithiasis, chronic renal failure	90
Wilson's disease	Liver disease, neurologic symptoms, Kayser-Fleischer rings, cardiomyopathy	Fanconi syndrome, proteinuria, rarely acute renal failure, distal renal tubular acidosis, hypercalciuria, calculi	See Chapter 41 (91,92)
Glycogen-storage disease type 1	Hepatomegaly, hypoglycemia, seizures, poor growth, lactic acidosis	Fanconi syndrome, hypercalciuria, hyperfiltration, rarely distal tubular acidosis, renal calculi, proteinuria, focal segmental glomerulosclerosis, chronic renal impairment	See Chapter 41 (24–36)
Fanconi-Bickel syndrome	Hepatomegaly, rickets, poor growth, hypoglycemia	Fanconi syndrome, hyperfiltration, "diabetic-like" nephropathy	See Chapter 41 (37–41)
Oculocerebrorenal (Lowe) syndrome	Congenital cataracts, other ocular abnormalities, hypotonia, delayed development, X-linked transmission	Fanconi syndrome, chronic renal failure, nephrocalcinosis, rarely calculi	See Chapter 41
Fructosemia	Acute onset after fructose ingestion: poor feeding, vomiting, poor growth, hypoglycemia, liver failure	Fanconi syndrome, rarely acute renal failure	See Chapter 41 (93)

Note: See Chapter 41 for full description.

TABLE 50.2. OTHER TUBULAR DYSFUNCTION

Disorder	Main features	Renal features	References
Carbonic anhydrase II deficiency	Osteopetrosis, fractures, cerebral calcification, mental retardation, poor growth	Mixed type of renal tubular acidosis	94,95
Methylmalonic acidemia	Vomiting, acidosis, hypotonia, poor growth	Type IV renal tubular acidosis, tubulointerstitial changes, chronic renal failure	3
Pyruvate carboxylase deficiency (some forms)	Metabolic acidosis, neurologic symptoms, hepatomegaly	Tubular acidosis, renal impairment	96
Ehlers-Danlos syndrome	Skin fragility, joint hypermobility, visceral or vascular dilatation and rupture	Renal tubular acidosis, medullary sponge kidney, diverticula, hypoplasia	97,98
Carnitine palmitoyltransferase deficiency type I	Fasting or illness leading to encephalopathy, seizures, hepatomegaly	Renal tubular acidosis	99
Adenosine deaminase deficiency	Severe combined immunodeficiency	Transient renal tubular acidosis, proteinuria, mesangial sclerosis	100
Lysinuric protein intolerance	See Table 50.4	Renal tubular acidosis, aminoaciduria, glomerulonephritis, renal failure	101
Nephrogenic diabetes insipidus	Polyuria, polydipsia, hyposthenuria	Hydronephrosis, hydroureter, megacystis (in long term)	See Chapter 40
Kearns-Sayre syndrome	Ophthalmoplegia, retinal degeneration, heart block, ataxia, hyperparathyroidism	Bartter's-like syndrome, hypomagnesemia	49–51
Fabry disease	See text and Table 50.4	Hyposthenuria, renal tubular acidosis, proteinuria, chronic renal failure	75–77
Metachromatic leukodystrophy	Neurologic and intellectual regression, spasticity, incontinence	Renal tubular acidosis, mild aminoaciduria, mild renal impairment	102

TABLE 50.3. NEPHROCALCINOSIS AND UROLITHIASIS

Disorder	Main features	Other renal features	References
Cystinuria	Calculi	—	See Chapter 57
Primary hyperoxaluria	Calculi and nephrocalcinosis	Acute or chronic renal failure (presentation in infants)	See Chapter 42
Familial hyperuricemic nephropathy	Gout, chronic renal failure		66,68
Hypoxanthine-guanine phosphoribosyltransferase deficiency	Lesch-Nyhan syndrome (complete deficiency): developmental delay, choreoathetoid movements, self-mutilation Partial deficiency: gouty arthritis	Acute or chronic renal failure	66,68
Adenine phosphoribosyltransferase deficiency	Calculi (2,8-dihydroxyadenine)	Acute or chronic renal failure	68
Hereditary renal hypouricemia	Urolithiasis (urate/calcium oxalate), hyperuricemia, hypercalciuria	Uric acid nephropathy, acute renal failure	69–72,103
Blue diaper syndrome	Hypercalcemia, hypercalciuria, indicanuria → blue discoloration urine	Nephrocalcinosis	104
Xanthinuria	Calculi, myopathy, arthropathy	Acute or chronic renal failure	See Chapter 57
Hereditary orotic aciduria	Megaloblastic anemia, orotic acid crystalluria, hematuria, immunodeficiency	Crystalluria, obstructive uropathy	105–107
Glycogen-storage disease type 1	See Table 50.1	Tubular dysfunction, nephrocalcinosis, proteinuria, chronic renal impairment	29–30
Wilson's disease	See Table 50.1	Acute renal failure, tubular dysfunction	91
Congenital lactase deficiency	Watery diarrhea, poor weight gain	Nephrocalcinosis, hypercalciuria, hypercalcemia	108
Glucose-galactose malabsorption	Watery diarrhea	Calculi, nephrocalcinosis, hypercalcemia	109
Cystinosis	See Table 50.1	Rarely calculi	See Chapter 41 (87)
Dent's disease/X-linked nephrolithiasis	See Table 50.1	Nephrocalcinosis, aminoaciduria, Fanconi syndrome, chronic renal failure	90
Hypophosphatasia (infantile form)	Rickets, developmental delay, hypercalcemia, craniosynostosis	Hypercalciuria, nephrocalcinosis	110
Cystic fibrosis	Chronic lung disease, poor growth, pancreatic dysfunction	Microscopic nephrocalcinosis, calculi, proteinuria, rarely nephrotic syndrome (amyloidosis), chronic renal failure	111–114
Tyrosinemia type 1	See Table 50.1	Nephrocalcinosis, Fanconi syndrome, nephromegaly, chronic renal impairment	See Chapter 41 (88,89)
McCune-Albright syndrome	Fibrous bony dysplasia, café-au-lait pigmentation, precocious puberty	Nephrocalcinosis	115
Apparent mineralocorticoid syndrome	Hypertension, hypokalemia, alkalosis, reduced plasma renin	Nephrocalcinosis, medullary cysts	116

dot found that 20% of patients had a GFR of less than 60 mL/min/1.73 m^2 (5). This may be an underestimate of the incidence of renal impairment, because in some patients GFR had to be estimated from plasma creatinine concentrations. Long-term renal function in nine children with early-onset cobalamin-unresponsive MMA, in whom GFR was studied by a single-injection chromium ethylenediaminetetra-acetic acid slope-clearance method, is shown in Figure 50.1. With one exception, every GFR value is below the normal range and every child surviving to 12 years has a GFR of less than 40 mL/min/1.73 m^2 (6). The mainstay of treatment is a low-protein, high-calorie diet, and many such children have poor growth and reduced muscle bulk. Consequently, plasma creatinine concentrations do not accurately reflect glomerular function in MMA (4). Proteinuria and hematuria are absent and renal histopathology shows changes of tubulointerstitial nephritis (4,7,8). It is likely that the tubular dysfunction noted in MMA is related to hyporeninemic hypoaldosteronism observed in patients with tubulointerstitial nephritis and renal impairment (3).

The mechanism of nephrotoxicity in MMA is not yet known. Patients with MMA have hyperuricemia, which might lead to renal damage. Urate crystals have not been observed in renal biopsy material, however, and plasma urate is easily controlled in these patients with allopurinol (3). There is structural similarity between methylmalonate (which accumulates as a result of the enzyme deficiency) and maleic acid, used experimentally in animals to create a model of the renal Fanconi syndrome. However, the tubular manifestations of MMA do not correspond to generalized proximal tubular dysfunction. Accumulation of methylmalonate may interfere with mitochondrial function (2,9).

TABLE 50.4. PROTEINURIA AND GLOMERULONEPHRITIS

Disorder	Main features	Renal features	References
Fabry disease	See text; sensory changes in extremities, angiokeratoma, hyperhidrosis, corneal, lens opacities	Hyposthenuria, renal tubular acidosis, proteinuria, chronic renal failure	75–77
Imerslünd-Graesbeck syndrome	See text	Proteinuria, urinary tract abnormalities	20,21,23
Lecithin-cholesterol acyltransferase deficiency	See text	Proteinuria, hematuria, renal failure	83,84
Galactosialidosis (early infantile form)	Hydrops, edema, coarse facies, inguinal hernias, visceromegaly, spinal involvement, corneal and fundal abnormalities, cardiomyopathy, developmental delay, telangiectasias	Proteinuria, nephrotic syndrome	117–120
Glutamyl ribose-5-phosphate glycoproteinosis	Coarse facies, optic atrophy, muscle wasting, failure to thrive, seizures, neurologic deterioration	Proteinuria, chronic renal failure	121
Mucopolysaccharidosis type I (Hurler syndrome)	Coarse facies, corneal clouding, visceromegaly, dysostosis multiplex, developmental delay	Nephrotic syndrome, hypertension (due to aortic luminal narrowing)	122
Congenital disorder of glycosylation type I	See text and Table 50.5	Proteinuria (congenital nephrotic syndrome), microcysts	60–65
Infantile sialic acid storage disease	Hydrops, edema, dysmorphism, hepatosplenomegaly, hypotonia, poor growth	Proteinuria, nephrotic syndrome	123
Cystic fibrosis	See Table 50.3	Proteinuria, nephrotic syndrome (amyloidosis), microscopic nephrocalcinosis, calculi, chronic renal failure	111–114
Alpha-1 antitrypsin deficiency	Liver and lung disease	Hematuria, membranoproliferative glomerulonephritis (only seen with advanced liver disease), chronic renal failure	124,125
Lipoprotein glomerulopathy	Elevated apolipoprotein E	Nephrotic syndrome (resistant to treatment), hematuria, hypertension, renal failure, glomerular lipoprotein thrombi	126,127
Lysinuric protein intolerance	Vomiting, diarrhea after weaning, poor appetite and growth, hypotonia, visceromegaly, interstitial pneumonitis, encephalopathy	Proteinuria, hematuria, nephrotic syndrome, immune complex glomerulonephritis, tubulointerstitial nephritis, renal tubular acidosis, renal failure	101,128
Prolidase deficiency	Rash, dysmorphism, anemia, splenomegaly, recurrent infections	Systemic lupus erythematosus	129
Cobalamin C deficiency	See text	Hemolytic uremic syndrome, glomerulopathy	17–19
Mitochondrial disorders	See text and Table 50.1	Fanconi syndrome; rarely proteinuria, nephrotic syndrome, tubulointerstitial nephritis	43–59
Gaucher disease	Hepatosplenomegaly, hypersplenism	Proteinuria, hematuria, acute glomerulonephritis; calculi (*personal communication*)	130,131

Management of End-Stage Renal Failure in Methylmalonic Acidemia

A few reports exist of the management of end-stage renal failure (ESRF) in MMA patients. Plasma methylmalonate appears to rise in association with plasma creatinine, either due to reduced filtration or because it is nephrotoxic (10,11). Hemodialysis clearly reduces plasma methylmalonate levels and may improve metabolic and nutritional status (10). Because the deficient methylmalonyl CoA mutase is expressed in liver, a liver transplant should provide replacement enzyme. Several patients with MMA have now received liver transplants, either as an isolated organ in young children or in combination with a kidney transplant in older patients in chronic renal failure. The first patient who received a combined liver-kidney transplant (10) remains well with good renal and hepatic function 6 years after surgery (W. van't Hoff, *personal communication*). Other patients have died shortly after the procedure, however, and it is a worry that liver transplantation does not seem to protect the child from further neurologic toxicity (12,13). A 24-year-old patient demonstrated improved clinical and metabolic control after an isolated renal transplantation, although she developed diabetes mellitus and suffered marked cyclosporin toxicity (14). A similarly favorable outcome with an improvement in urine methylmalonate excretion has been demonstrated in a 17-year-old patient after renal

TABLE 50.5. METABOLIC CAUSES OF RENAL CYSTS

Disorder	Main features	Renal features	References
Zellweger syndrome	Facial dysmorphism, hypotonia, severe developmental delay, hepatomegaly	Microcysts and large cortical cysts	132
Alagille syndrome	Intrahepatic cholestasis, dysmorphism, posterior embryotoxon, butterfly vertebrae, hypogonadism, peripheral pulmonary stenosis	Cysts, multicystic dysplastic kidney, unilateral agenesis, hypoplasia, urinary concentration defect, calculi, glomerular mesangiolipidosis, renal failure	133,134
Carbohydrate-deficient glycoprotein syndrome type I	See text and Table 50.4	Cysts, proteinuria	60–65
Glutaric aciduria type II (neonatal onset)	Prematurity, hepatomegaly, dysmorphism, genitourinary abnormalities, hypotonia, odor, metabolic acidosis, hypoglycemia	Cystic change (microcysts/polycystic kidneys), nephromegaly, renal dysgenesis	135–138
Nephronophthisis	Can be associated abnormalities (Leber amaurosis, retinopathy, liver disease, neurologic and skeletal abnormalities)	Hyposthenuria, chronic renal failure	See Chapter 35
Smith-Lemli-Opitz syndrome	Facial dysmorphism; hypotonia; mental retardation; abnormalities of limbs, brain, genitalia; cholesterol biosynthesis defect	Cystic dysplasia, hypoplasia, agenesis, duplication, pelviureteric junction obstruction, vesicoureteral reflux	139,140
Cystinosis	See Table 50.1	Cysts are very rare	141
Pearson syndrome	Pancytopenia, pancreatic dysfunction, tubulopathy See text (Mitochondrial Disorders section)	Cortical cysts	57,58
Apparent mineralocorticoid syndrome	Hypertension, hypokalemia, alkalosis, reduced plasma renin	Nephrocalcinosis, medullary cysts	116

transplantation (15). In view of the late neurologic complications in those patients receiving liver transplants, the long-term prognosis for any patient with MMA receiving a transplant remains uncertain (16).

Cobalamin Defects

Early-onset hemolytic uremic syndrome has been reported in a number of patients with cobalamin C or G deficiency (17,18), in which defects are seen in the synthesis of adenosylcobalamin and methylcobalamin (cobalamin C defect) or of methionine synthase (cobalamin G defect). Patients with cobalamin C deficiency have defective function of the two enzymes dependent on these cofactors (methylmalonyl CoA mutase and N5-methyltetrahydrofolate:homocysteine methyltransferase). These children therefore have homocystinuria, hypomethioninemia, and cystathioninuria in addition to methylmalonic aciduria. Most present in

TABLE 50.6. OTHER MANIFESTATIONS

Disorder	Main features	Renal features	References
Menkes syndrome, Ehlers-Danlos syndrome type IX, occipital horn syndrome (OHS)	X-linked disorders Abnormal hair and facies, developmental delay and regression OHS patients have lax skin, herniae, no neurologic features	Bladder or ureteric diverticula	142,143
Homocystinuria	Ectopia lentis, skeletal abnormalities, neuropsychiatric symptoms, thromboembolism	Renal infarction, hypertension	144
Carnitine palmitoyltransferase deficiency type II	Neonatal-onset encephalopathy, hepatomegaly, cardiomyopathy	Renal dysgenesis	145
Glucose-6-phosphatase deficiency	Hemolytic anemia, jaundice	Acute renal failure	146
Porphyria (acute intermittent)	Recurrent abdominal pain, neurologic crises	Acute or chronic renal failure, urinary retention, acute hypertension	147,148
Exercise intolerance and myoglobinuria syndrome (various causes)	Myalgia, limb weakness, raised serum creatine phosphokinase	Recurrent myoglobinuria, acute renal failure	149,150

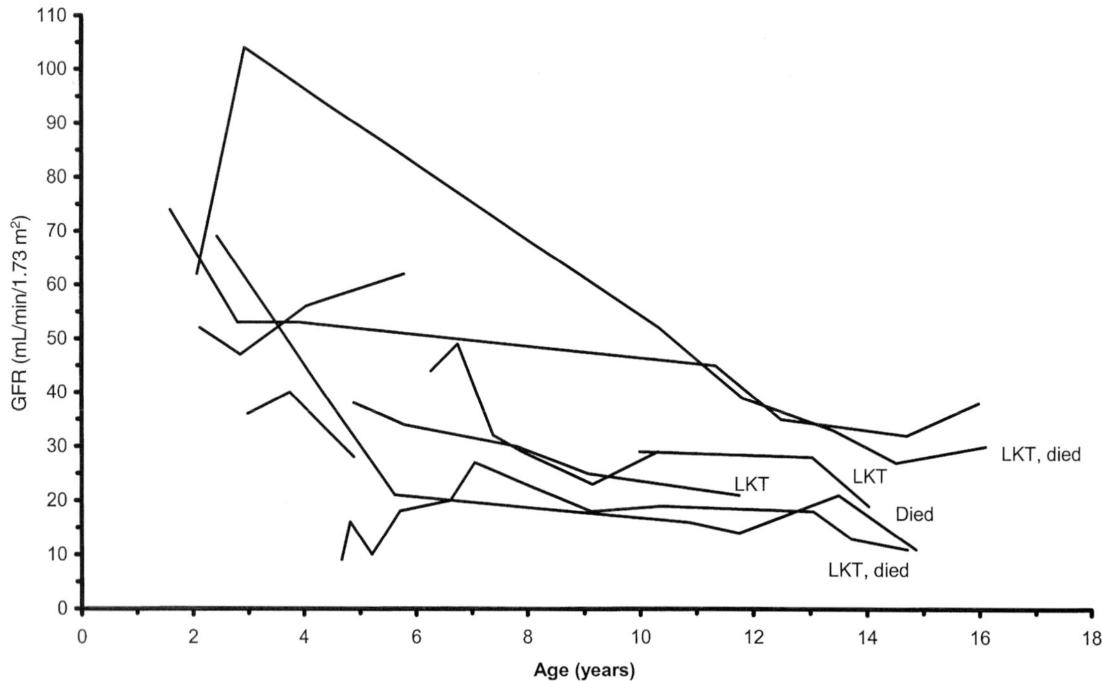

FIGURE 50.1. Glomerular filtration rate (GFR), determined by single-injection chromium ethylenediaminetetra-acetic acid slope-clearance method, in nine children with early-onset (cobalamin-unresponsive) methylmalonic acidemia. Four children underwent combined liver-kidney transplantation (LKT). Two of these and one other child have died. (From Van't Hoff W, McKiernan PJ, Surtees RA, et al. Liver transplantation for methylmalonic acidaemia. *Eur J Pediatr* 1999;158;S2:S70–S74, with permission.)

early infancy with poor feeding, failure to thrive, hypotonia, retinitis, respiratory distress, and cardiomyopathy. Investigation shows a megaloblastic anemia, pancytopenia, and liver dysfunction. Generally the prognosis has been poor. There have been rare case reports of older children with cobalamin C deficiency who developed hypertension, proteinuria, and chronic renal impairment, in association with focal segmental glomerulosclerosis or an unclassified glomerulopathy (18).

A number of patients with defective absorption of the cobalamin–intrinsic factor complex (Imerslünd-Grasbeck syndrome) have persistent proteinuria (20). The cobalamin–intrinsic factor complex binds to cubilin in the intestinal brush border. Cubilin is also expressed in the renal proximal tubule, where it interacts with megalin to form a tandem endocytic receptor complex (21). Cubilin is the major receptor for proximal tubular albumin reabsorption; thus, patients with Imerslünd-Grasbeck syndrome, in which the cubilin gene is defective, have albuminuria (22). Other manifestations include megaloblastic anemia and, biochemically, homocystinuria, homocystinemia, and methylmalonic aciduria (20). In addition to the metabolic abnormalities, two children with this disorder were reported as suffering from recurrent urinary tract infections secondary to neuropathic bladders (23).

GLYCOGEN-STORAGE DISEASES

Clinical Features

The glycogen-storage diseases (GSDs) are genetic disorders of the metabolism and regulation of glycogen. Two forms of GSD have significant renal manifestations: GSD type 1 (GSD-1) and the Fanconi-Bickel syndrome. GSD-1 is characterized by a deficiency of glucose-6-phosphatase in the liver, kidney, and intestine, which causes excessive glycogen storage, hepatomegaly, hypoglycemia, lactic acidosis, hyperuricemia, hyperlipidemia, and poor growth. Long-term complications include delayed puberty, hepatic adenomata, and renal disease. Chen and colleagues drew attention to the complication of ESRF in older GSD patients (24). In their review in 1988, 18 children under 10 years of age had normal renal function, whereas 14 of 20 patients aged 13 to 47 years had renal dysfunction (proteinuria, hypertension, or chronic renal failure). Subsequent investigators have demonstrated renal tubular and glomerular abnormalities. Ultrasonography demonstrates the renal enlargement secondary to glycogen deposition (25–28).

Renal Tubular Dysfunction

Proximal tubular dysfunction occurs as an early feature in GSD-1 but is generally subclinical, and a frank Fanconi syndrome is rare. Although tubular proteinuria (retinol-binding protein, β2M) and enzymuria (*N*-acetyl glucosaminidase) is significantly elevated in GSD-1 patients, plasma electrolytes are less disturbed (26,27). Distal tubular function is also perturbed with hypercalciuria and hypocitraturia, which predisposes GSD-1 patients to nephrolithiasis (29,30). A Gitelman-like syndrome of hypomagnesemia and hypocalciuria has also been described in a patient with GSD type 2 (31).

Glomerular Dysfunction

Patients with GSD-1 develop albuminuria and hyperfiltration (26,27,32). In a Dutch study, mean GFR and effective renal plasma flow were 188 and 927 mL/min/1.73 m^2, respectively (normal values for adult controls were 90 to 145 and 327 to 697 mL/min/1.73 m^2, respectively) in a group of 23 patients with GSD-1 aged 2 to 22 years (26). Persistent hyperfiltration leads to focal and global glomerulosclerosis and a decline in GFR (32,33). Other histologic abnormalities include glycogen deposition in proximal tubules, glomerular enlargement, and thickening and lamellation of GBM (34,35). Management of the metabolic abnormalities, which includes frequent feedings and the use of uncooked cornstarch, are the mainstays of treatment of GSD nephropathy. Antiproteinuric and lipid-lowering agents may have a role (36).

Fanconi-Bickel Syndrome

Fanconi-Bickel syndrome is a very rare autosomal recessive disorder of monosaccharide transport, manifesting in the first year of life with hepatomegaly (due to glycogen storage), hypoglycemia, and a severe generalized proximal tubulopathy leading to rickets. The Fanconi syndrome can be equal in magnitude to that in disorders such as cystinosis or tyrosinemia but is particularly characterized by heavy glycosuria and galactosuria (37–39). Treatment includes frequent feedings (and the use of uncooked cornstarch) together with management of the tubulopathy. The condition arises due to mutations in the GLUT2 facilitative glucose transporter, which is expressed in hepatocytes, pancreatic beta cells, and the basolateral membranes of intestinal and renal tubular epithelial cells (40). Decreased monosaccharide uptake by the liver explains the postprandial hyperglycemia and hypergalactosemia, which is exacerbated by inappropriately low insulin secretion due to abnormal glucose-sensing by pancreatic beta cells. The inability of the liver to transport glucose, together with heavy losses of glucose from the renal tubule, contributes to preprandial hypoglycemia (40). Renal glomerular hyperfiltration, microalbuminuria, and diffuse mesangial expansion have been reported in one child (41), and reduced GFR has been observed in some adults.

MITOCHONDRIAL DISORDERS

Description

Mitochondrial disorders are caused by defects in the respiratory chain enzymes that are located in this organelle. The respiratory chain is responsible for the process of oxidative phosphorylation in which electrons are transferred to oxygen, which generates a proton gradient. The flow of protons back through the mitochondrial membrane releases energy, which allows for the formation of ATP. The respiratory chain enzyme complexes are encoded partly by mitochondrial and partly by nuclear DNA. Mitochondrial DNA (mtDNA) differs from nuclear DNA: it is much smaller, has a unique genetic code, exists as a double-stranded loop, and is inherited exclusively from the mother. In contrast to nuclear DNA, mtDNA is randomly segregated during cell division. The proportion of mutant and wild-type mtDNA can therefore vary from tissue to tissue and can also change over time, which explains the enormous heterogeneity of mitochondrial disorders (42). The classification of mitochondrial disorders has been based on clinical, biochemical, and molecular phenotypes. The clinical features are extremely heterogeneous and often change with time, but virtually all patients have neurologic symptoms at some point. Frequent manifestations include myopathy, encephalopathy, seizures, developmental delay, ophthalmoplegia, retinal degeneration, cardiomyopathy, endocrinopathy, and liver disease.

Renal Manifestations

The most common renal manifestation is the Fanconi syndrome. It usually occurs in an infant with multisystem dysfunction, in which case the prognosis is poor (43,44). Generalized proximal tubular dysfunction has also been reported in children with other mitochondrial syndromes, including Kearns-Sayre, Pearson, and Leigh encephalopathy (43,45–49). In some children, hypomagnesemia and hypocalcemia are the predominant electrolyte abnormalities (48–50). Other tubular manifestations include a Bartter-like syndrome (51), renal tubular acidosis, and hypercalciuria (52,53). Renal glomerular involvement with proteinuria, focal segmental glomerulosclerosis, chronic tubulointerstitial nephritis, and chronic renal impairment are rarer associations of mitochondrial disorders (43,54–56). Renal cysts have been reported in both adults and children with mitochondrial disorders (57,58). In most children the renal lesion is part of multisystem dysfunction, but there are occasional reports of patients presenting with focal segmental glomerulosclerosis and later developing other manifestations of mitochondrial disease (54,59). A high index of suspicion is therefore required to diagnose a mitochondrial disorder. Unfortunately, measurement of the plasma lactate/pyruvate ratio, which is the first investigation of a child with mitochondrial dysfunction, may give a normal result in a patient with a renal tubulopathy due to loss of organic acids in the urine (43). In such a case, careful delineation of other system involvement, biopsy, and detailed biochemical and molecular studies may be required to confirm a defect in mitochondrial function.

CONGENITAL DISORDERS OF GLYCOSYLATION

The congenital disorders of glycosylation (CDGs) are a group of multisystem disorders in which there is defective glycosylation of glycoproteins (60). Several subtypes have been described, and the presentation is very heterogeneous, ranging from developmental delay in older children to a fatal multisystem disorder in infancy (60). In infancy, typical features of CDG type I include dysmorphism, hypotonia, failure to thrive, diarrhea, abnormal fat pads, inverted nipples, abnormal eye movements, hepatomegaly, and cardiomyopathy. Investigations often show hypothyroidism, olivopontocerebellar atrophy, and, diagnostically, abnormal isoelectric focusing of serum transferrin with an increase in asialo- and disialotransferrin and a decrease in tetra- and pentasialotransferrin.

The most common renal manifestation is the presence of microcysts, which produce a hyperechoic picture on ultrasonography (61,62). The cysts are located in the cortex and probably arise from the tubules (63). The kidneys may be enlarged, and single cysts have also been reported (62). Microcysts are not seen in all patients; even within a pair of affected siblings, only one had renal cysts (61). Proteinuria has been recorded in several cases and may contribute to the severe edema and ascites that these infants can develop (62). There have also been reports of nephrotic syndrome occurring within the first 2 months of life (63–65). One of these infants also developed renal failure, and at postmortem the kidneys showed features of diffuse mesangial sclerosis (64). Transferrin isoelectric focusing should be added to the list of investigations required to exclude a metabolic cause of nephrotic syndrome in infants [the test is not affected by the nephrotic state or by renal failure (64)].

DISORDERS OF PURINE METABOLISM AND TRANSPORT

Children who develop renal calculi, acute renal failure in the neonatal period, or crystal nephropathy require investigation of their purine metabolism. Purines are involved in the synthesis of nucleotides and coenzymes, in signal transduction (e.g., cyclic adenosine monophosphate), and in the generation of ATP. The metabolic end product, uric acid, and its immediate precursor (xanthine) are insoluble in urine, so that overproduction can predispose to the development of crystal formation. Urate is normally extensively reabsorbed in the proximal tubule. The process is age and sex dependent, with children reabsorbing less of the filtered urate and consequently having lower plasma urate concentrations (66). As GFR declines, the fractional excretion of urate increases (67).

Urolithiasis is the most common renal manifestation of a disorder of purine production (see Chapter 57). Children may or may not have typical features of calculi (pain, hematuria, infection). In some the diagnosis is made following family studies or during investigation of crystalluria. Anuric acute renal failure in an infant is a well-described presentation of purine overproduction, for example, adenine phosphoribosyltransferase (APRT) deficiency and hypoxanthine-guanine phosphoribosyl transferase (HGPRT) deficiency (68). In both APRT and HGPRT deficiencies, the urinary urate/creatinine ratio is normal. The plasma urate level is also normal in APRT deficiency but is grossly elevated in HGPRT deficiency (68). In these cases detailed investigation of purine metabolism is required. Both conditions are treated with a high fluid intake, restriction of dietary purines, and administration of allopurinol, which inhibits xanthine oxidase production.

Hyperuricemia with subsequent hyperuricosuria is also a feature of GSD-1. Calculi and renal failure can also occur as a result of disorders of urate transport in the renal tubule. Hyperuricosuria and hypouricemia can occur as a result of generalized proximal tubular dysfunction (e.g., Fanconi syndrome) but has also been described as an isolated transport defect associated with hypercalciuria, decreased bone density, and the development of calculi composed of a mixture of calcium oxalate and urate (69–72).

Familial juvenile hyperuricemic nephropathy is a disorder of unknown cause in which patients develop hyperuricemia, gout, and progressive renal failure (66,67). The onset is frequently in childhood or early adult life. Many families have been described with males and females equally affected and male-to-male transmission supporting the concept of an autosomal dominant pattern of inheritance (66). The disorder is characterized biochemically by hyperuricemia due to a reduced fractional excretion of urate. There is evidence that hyperuricemia predates renal impairment, and it is known that allopurinol reduces the progression of the nephropathy, which suggests that renal damage is related to hyperuricemia (73,74). The genetic defect of this disorder is under investigation, and it is thought likely to be due to an abnormality in urate transport.

FABRY DISEASE

Fabry disease is an X-linked disorder in which glycosphingolipids (predominantly globotriaosylceramide) accumulate in plasma and tissues as a result of a deficiency of α galactosidase A (75). Affected males usually present in late childhood with recurrent painful crises of the hands and feet, a characteristic skin rash (angiokeratoma corporis), and hypohidrosis. Slit-lamp examination reveals corneal and lenticular opacities.

Progressive glycosphingolipid deposition in the heart, blood vessels, and kidneys leads to the development of valvular and conduction abnormalities, angina, cerebrovascular disease, and progressive renal damage, usually in adult life. However, proteinuria, chronic renal failure, and even ESRF can occur by 15 years of age (76,77). The urine may show casts and desquamated cells containing lipid globules (78). Subsequently, polyuria and polydipsia indicate defective tubular function, and ESRF occurs typically around the fourth decade (76,77). Histologic examination of the kidney will demonstrate inclusions with a characteristic "onion skin" appearance in tubular epithelia, glomerular cells (especially podocytes), and endothelium (79). Glycosphingolipid deposits are seen in endothelial and epithelial cells of the glomeruli, in Bowman capsules, and in the distal tubules (79). The renal prognosis may bear some relationship to the level of detectable α galactosidase A activity. Onset of chronic renal failure was significantly later in those with more than 1% activity compared to those with undetectable activity (77). Studies indicate that approximately 1% of adult males with undiagnosed causes of ESRF have Fabry disease (80,81). Affected females (heterozygotes) generally have much milder manifestations, although, as a result of random X inactivation, these can be variable (76). There are some reports of proteinuria and hyposthenuria; renal failure has been described in a rare variant (75,76). Fabry patients with ESRF can be treated with dialysis and renal transplantation as for other causes of renal failure. Peritoneal dialysis may be preferable in view of the potential endothelial and cardiac complications of the disorder. There is some evidence of amelioration of the nonrenal manifestations after kidney transplantation. However, a more promising therapeutic approach is with recombinant α galactosidase A, which has been shown in a placebo-controlled double-blind study to reduce microvascular deposits of globotriaosylceramide in many organs, including the kidney (82).

LECITHIN-CHOLESTEROL ACYLTRANSFERASE DEFICIENCY

Lecithin-cholesterol acyltransferase (LCAT) is required for the esterification of cholesterol with unsaturated fatty acid derived from lecithin. Patients with LCAT deficiency accumulate unesterified cholesterol and phosphatidylcholine in plasma and tissues (83). Sequelae of tissue accumulation occur during childhood and include grayish corneal opacities, a hemolytic anemia, and proteinuria (sometimes in the nephrotic range) leading to progressive renal failure in adulthood (83–85). Tendon xanthomata and atherosclerosis have been described in a few cases. Biochemically, LCAT deficiency is characterized by a low total cholesterol concentration, variable triglyceride concentration, and abnormalities of lipoprotein structure and composition. The histology of the kidney shows mesangial hypercellularity and expansion with foam lipid deposits, holes and vacuolization in the glomerular basement membrane, arteriolar narrowing due to intimal thickening, and subendothelial lipid deposits (85). Creation of an LCAT "knock-out" mouse has provided further information on the pathogenesis of this disorder (86). Some of the null mice accumulated lipoprotein X and developed proteinuria secondary to glomerulosclerosis. Biochemically, although high-density lipoproteins were markedly reduced, aortic atheroma was attenuated in the "knock-out" mice, which suggests a role for other lipoproteins in generating atheroma.

REFERENCES

1. Theodoropoulos DS, Krasnewich D, Kaiser-Kupfer MI, et al. Classic nephropathic cystinosis as an adult disease. *JAMA* 1993;270:2200–2204.
2. Fenton WA, Gravel RA, Rosenblatt DS. Disorders of propionate and methylmalonate metabolism. In: Scriver CR, Beaudet AL, Sly WS, et al., eds. *The metabolic and molecular bases of inherited disease,* 8th ed. New York: McGraw-Hill, 2001:6257–6266.
3. D'Angio CT, Dillon MJ, Leonard JV. Renal tubular dysfunction in methylmalonic acidemia. *Eur J Pediatr* 1991;150:259–263.
4. Walter JH, Michalski A, Wilson WM, et al. Chronic renal failure in methylmalonic acidemia. *Eur J Pediatr* 1989;148:344–348.
5. Baumgartner ER, Viardot C. Long-term follow-up of 77 patients with isolated methylmalonic acidemia. *J Inherit Metab Dis* 1995;18:138–142.
6. Van't Hoff W, McKiernan PJ, Surtees RAH, et al. Liver transplantation in methylmalonic acidaemia. *Eur J Pediatr* 1999;158[S2]:S70–S74.
7. Rutledge SL, Geraghty M, Mroczet E, et al. Tubulointerstitial nephritis in methylmalonic acidemia. *Pediatr Nephrol* 1993;7:81–82.
8. Ohura T, Kikuchi M, Abukawa D, et al. Type 4 renal tubular acidosis (subtype 2) in a patient with methylmalonic acidaemia. *Eur J Pediatr* 1990;150:115–118.
9. Toyoshima S, Watanabe F, Saido H, et al. Methylmalonic acid inhibits respiration in rat liver mitochondria. *J Nutr* 1995;125:2846–2850.
10. Van't Hoff WG, Dixon M, Taylor J, et al. Combined liver-kidney transplantation in methylmalonic acidemia. *J Pediatr* 1998;132:1043–1044.
11. Rasmussen K, Vyberg B, Pedersen KO, et al. Methylmalonic acid in renal insufficiency: evidence of accumulation and implications for diagnosis of cobalamin deficiency [Letter]. *Clin Chem* 1990;36:1523–1524.
12. Chakrapani A, Sivakumar P, McKiernan PJ, et al. Metabolic stroke in methylmalonic acidemia five years after liver transplantation. *J Pediatr* 2002;140:261–263.

13. Nyhan WL, Gargus JJ, Boyle K, et al. Progressive neurologic disability in methylmalonic acidemia despite transplantation of the liver. *Eur J Pediatr* 2002;161:377–379.
14. Van Calcar SC, Harding CO, Lyne P, et al. Renal transplantation in a patient with methylmalonic acidaemia. *J Inherit Metab Dis* 1998;21:729–737.
15. Lubrano R, Scoppi P, Barsotti P, et al. Kidney transplantation in a girl with methylmalonic acidemia and end stage renal failure. *Pediatr Nephrol* 2001;16:848–851.
16. Leonard JV, Walter JH, McKiernan PJ. The management of organic acidaemias: the role of transplantation. *J Inherit Metab Dis* 2001;24:309–311.
17. Geraghty MT, Perlman EJ, Martin LS, et al. Cobalamin C defect associated with hemolytic-uremic syndrome. *J Pediatr* 1992;120:934–937.
18. Kind T, Levy J, Lee M, et al. Cobalamin C disease presenting as hemolytic-uremic syndrome in the neonatal period. *J Pediatr Hematol Oncol* 2002;24:327–329.
19. Brunelli SM, Meyers KEC, Guttenberg M, et al. Cobalamin C deficiency complicated by atypical glomerulopathy. *Pediatr Nephrol.* 2002;17:800–803.
20. Broch H, Imerslund O, Monn E, et al. Imerslünd-Grasbeck anemia: a long-term follow-up study. *Acta Paediatr Scand* 1984;73:248–253.
21. Verroust PJ, Birn H, Nielsen R, et al. The tandem endocytic receptors megalin and cubilin are important proteins in renal pathology. *Kidney Int* 2002;62:745–756.
22. Birn H, Fyfe JC, Jacobsen C, et al. Cubilin is an albumin binding protein important for renal tubular albumin reabsorption. *J Clin Invest* 2000;105;1353–1361.
23. Sandoval C, Bolten P, Franco I, et al. Recurrent urinary tract infections and genitourinary tract abnormalities in the Imerslünd-Grasbeck syndrome. *Pediatr Hematol Oncol* 2000;17: 331–334.
24. Chen YT, Coleman RA, Scheinman JI, et al. Renal disease in type I glycogen storage disease. *N Engl J Med* 1988;318:7–11.
25. Pozzato C, Botta A, Melgara C, et al. Sonographic findings in type I glycogen storage disease. *J Clin Ultrasound* 2001;29: 456–461.
26. Reitsma-Bierens WC, Smit GP, Troelstra JA. Renal function and kidney size in glycogen storage disease type I. *Pediatr Nephrol* 1992;6:236–238.
27. Lee PJ, Dalton RN, Shah V, et al. Glomerular and tubular function in glycogen storage disease. *Pediatr Nephrol* 1995; 9:705–710.
28. Wolfsdorf JI, Laffel LM, Crigler JF Jr. Metabolic control and renal dysfunction in type I glycogen storage disease. *J Inherit Metab Dis* 1997;20:559–568.
29. Weinstein DA, Somers MJ, Wolfsdorf JI. Decreased urinary citrate excretion in type 1a glycogen storage disease. *J Pediatr* 2001;138:378–382.
30. Restiano I, Kaplan BS, Stanley C, et al. Nephrolithiasis, hypocitraturia, and a distal renal tubular acidification defect in type I glycogen storage disease. *J Pediatr* 1993;122:392–396.
31. Oktenli C. Renal magnesium wasting, hypomagnesemic hypocalcemia, hypocalciuria and osteopenia in a patient with glycogenosis type II. *Am J Nephrol* 2000;20:412–417.
32. Chen YT, Coleman RA, Scheinman J, et al. Renal disease in type I glycogen storage disease. *N Engl J Med* 1988;318:7–11.
33. Baker L, Dahlem S, Goldfarb S, et al. Hyperfiltration and renal disease in glycogen storage disease, type I. *Kidney Int* 1989;35:1345–1350.
34. Verani R, Bernstein J. Renal glomerular and tubular abnormalities in glycogen storage disease type I. *Arch Pathol Lab Med* 1988;112:271–274.
35. Yokoyama K, Hayashi H, Hinoshita F, et al. Renal lesion of type Ia glycogen storage disease: the glomerular size and renal localization of apolipoprotein. *Nephron* 1995;70:348–352.
36. Pela I, Donati MA, Zammarchi E. Effect of ramipril in a patient with glycogen storage disease type I and nephrotic-range proteinuria. *J Inherit Metab Dis* 2001;24:681–682.
37. Manz F, Bickel H, Brodehl J, et al. Fanconi-Bickel syndrome. *Pediatr Nephrol* 1987;1:509–518.
38. Santer R, Schneppenheim R, Dombrowski A, et al. Mutations in GLUT2, the gene for the liver-type glucose transporter, in patients with Fanconi-Bickel syndrome. *Nat Genet* 1997;17:324–326.
39. Santer R, Schneppenheim R, Suter D, et al. Fanconi-Bickel syndrome—the original patient and his natural history, historical steps leading to the primary defect, and a review of the literature. *Eur J Pediatr* 1998;157:783–797.
40. Santer R, Steinmann B, Schaub J. Fanconi-Bickel syndrome—a congenital defect of facilitative glucose transport. *Curr Mol Med* 2002;2:213–227.
41. Berry GT, Baker L, Kaplan FS, et al. Diabetes-like renal glomerular disease in Fanconi-Bickel syndrome. *Pediatr Nephrol* 1995;9:287–291.
42. Shoffer JM. Oxidative phosphorylation diseases. In: Scriver CR, Beaudet AL, Sly WS, et al., eds. *The metabolic and molecular bases of inherited disease,* 8th ed. New York: McGraw-Hill, 2001:2367–2423.
43. Niaudet P, Rötig A. Renal involvement in mitochondrial cytopathies. *Pediatr Nephrol* 1996;10:368–373.
44. Morris AMM, Taylor RW, Birch-Machin MA, et al. Neonatal Fanconi syndrome due to a deficiency of complex III of the respiratory chain. *Pediatr Nephrol.* 1995;9:407–411.
45. Mori K, Narahara K, Nimomiya S, et al. Renal and skin involvement in a patient with Kearns-Sayre syndrome. *Am J Med Genet* 1991;38:583–587 .
46. Niaudet P, Heidet L, Munnich A, et al. Deletion of mitochondrial DNA in a case of de Toni-Debré-Fanconi syndrome and Pearson syndrome. *Pediatr Nephrol* 1994;8:164–168.
47. Ogier H, Lombes A, Scholte HR, et al. De Toni-Debré-Fanconi syndrome with Leigh syndrome revealing severe muscle cytochrome *c* oxidase deficiency. *J Pediatr* 1988;112:734–739.
48. Neiberger RE, George JC, Perkins LA, et al. Renal manifestations of congenital lactic acidosis. *Am J Kidney Dis* 2002; 39:2–23.
49. Katsanos KH, Elisaf M, Bairaktari E, et al. Severe hypomagnesemia and hypoparathyroidism in Kearns-Sayre syndrome. *Am J Nephrol* 2001;21:150–153.
50. Lee YS, Yap HK, Barshop BA, et al. Mitochondrial tubulopathy: the many faces of mitochondrial disorders. *Pediatr Nephrol* 2001;16:710–712.
51. Goto Y, Itami N, Kajii N, et al. Renal tubular involvement mimicking Bartter's syndrome in a child with Kearns-Sayre syndrome. *J Pediatr* 1990;116:904–910.

52. Pitkanen S, Feigenbaum A, Laframboise R, et al. NADH-coenzyme Q reductase (complex I) deficiency: heterogeneity in phenotype and biochemical findings. *J Inherit Metab Dis* 1996;19:675–686.
53. Egger J, Lake BD, Wilson J. Mitochondrial cytopathy. A multisystem disorder with ragged red fibres on muscle biopsy. *Arch Dis Child* 1981;56:741–752.
54. Doleris LM, Hill GS, Chedin P, et al. Focal segmental glomerulosclerosis associated with mitochondrial cytopathy. *Kidney Int* 2000;58:1851–1858.
55. Mochizuki H, Joh K, Kawame H, et al. Mitochondrial encephalomyopathies preceded by de Toni-Debré-Fanconi syndrome or focal segmental glomerulosclerosis. *Clin Nephrol* 1996;46:347–352.
56. Rotig A, Goutieres F, Niaudet P, et al. Deletion of mitochondrial DNA in a patient with chronic tubulo-interstitial nephritis. *J Pediatr* 1995;126:597–601.
57. Yamakawa T, Yoshida F, Kumagai T, et al. Glomerulocystic kidney associated with subacute necrotizing encephalomyelopathy. *Am J Kidney Dis* 2001;37:E14–E25.
58. Gurgey A, Ozalp I, Rotig A, et al. A case of Pearson syndrome associated with multiple renal cysts. *Pediatr Nephrol* 1996;10:637–638.
59. Hameed R, Raafat F, Ramani P, et al. Mitochondrial cytopathy presenting with focal segmental glomerulosclerosis, hypoparathyroidism, sensorineural deafness, and progressive neurological disease. *Postgrad Med J* 2001;77:523–526.
60. Jaeken J, Matthijs G, Carchon H, et al. Defects of *N*-glycan synthesis. In: Scriver CR, Beaudet AL, Sly WS, et al., eds. *The metabolic and molecular bases of inherited disease,* 8th ed. New York: McGraw-Hill, 2001:1601–1622.
61. Horslen SP, Clayton PT, Harding BN, et al. Olivopontocerebellar atrophy of neonatal onset and disialotransferrin developmental deficiency syndrome. *Arch Dis Child* 1991;66:1027–1032.
62. Strom EH, Stromme P, Westvik J, et al. Renal cysts in the carbohydrate-deficient glycoprotein syndrome. *Pediatr Nephrol* 1993;7:253–255.
63. Huthcesson ACJ, Gray RGF, Spencer DA, et al. Carbohydrate-deficient glycoprotein syndrome: multiple abnormalities and diagnostic delay. *Arch Dis Child* 1995;72:445–446.
64. Van der Knaap MS, Wevers RA, Monnens L, et al. Congenital nephrotic syndrome: a novel phenotype of type I carbohydrate-deficient glycoprotein syndrome. *J Inherit Metab Dis* 1996;19:787–791.
65. de Vries BB, van't Hoff WG, Surtees RA, et al. Diagnostic dilemmas in four infants with nephrotic syndrome, microcephaly and severe developmental delay. *Clin Dysmorphol* 2001;10:115–121.
66. Cameron JS, Moro F, Simmonds HA. Gout, uric acid and purine metabolism in paediatric nephrology. *Pediatr Nephrol* 1993:105–118.
67. Calabrese G, Simmonds HA, Cameron JS, et al. Precocious gout with reduced fractional urate clearance and normal purine enzymes. *Q J Med* 1990;75:441–450.
68. Simmonds HA, Cameron JS, Barratt TM, et al. Purine enzyme defects as a cause of acute renal failure in childhood. *Pediatr Nephrol* 1989;3:433–437.
69. Takeda E, Kuroda Y, Ito M, et al. Hereditary renal hypouricemia in children. *J Pediatr* 1985;107:71–74.
70. Greene ML, Marcus R, Aurbach GD, et al. Hypouricemia due to isolated renal tubular defect. *Am J Med* 1972;53:361–367.
71. Sperling O, Weinberger A, Oliver I, et al. Hypouricemia, hypercalciuria and decreased bone density: a hereditary syndrome. *Ann Intern Med* 1974;80:482–487.
72. Benjamin D, Sperling O, Weinberger A, et al. Familial hypouricemia due to isolated renal tubular defect. *Nephron* 1977;18:220–225.
73. Moro F, Ogg CS, Cameron JS, et al. Familial juvenile gouty nephropathy with renal urate hypoexcretion preceding renal disease. *Clin Nephrol* 1991;35:263–269.
74. Fairbanks LD, Cameron JS, Venkat-Raman, et al. Early treatment with allopurinol in familial hyperuricaemic nephropathy (FJHN) ameliorates the long-term progression of renal disease. *QJM* 2002;95:597–607.
75. Desnick RJ, Ioannou YA, Eng CM. α-Galactosidase A deficiency: Fabry disease. In: Scriver CR, Beaudet AL, Sly WS, et al., eds. *The metabolic and molecular bases of inherited disease,* 8th ed. New York: McGraw-Hill, 2001:3733–3774.
76. Grünfeld J-P, Lidove O, Joly D, et al. Renal disease in Fabry patients. *J Inherit Metab Dis* 2001;24[Suppl 2]:71–74.
77. Schiffman R. Natural history of Fabry disease in males: preliminary observations. *J Inherit Metab Dis* 2001;24[Suppl 2]:15–17.
78. Desnick RJ, Dawson G, Desnick SJ, et al. Diagnosis of glycosphingolipidoses by urinary sediment analysis. *N Engl J Med* 1971;284:739–744.
79. Sessa A, Meroni M, Battini G, et al. Renal pathological changes in Fabry disease. *J Inherit Metab Dis* 2001;24[Suppl 2]:66–70.
80. Desnick RJ. Fabry disease: unrecognised ESRD patients and effectiveness of enzyme replacement on renal pathology and function. *J Inherit Metab Dis* 2002;25[Supp 1]:P116,232–O(abst).
81. Thadhani R, Wolf M, West ML, et al. Patients with Fabry disease on dialysis in the United States. *Kidney Int* 2002;61:249–255.
82. Eng CM, Guffon N, Wilcox WR, et al. International Collaborative Fabry Disease Study Group. Safety and efficacy of recombinant human alpha-galactosidase A—replacement therapy in Fabry's disease. *N Engl J Med* 2001;345:9–16.
83. Glomset JA, Assmann G, Gjone E, et al. Lecithin:cholesterol acyltransferase deficiency and fish eye disease. In: Scriver CR, Beaudet AL, Sly WS, et al., eds. *The metabolic and molecular bases of inherited disease,* 8th ed. New York: McGraw-Hill, 2001:2817–2833.
84. Gjone E. Familial lecithin:cholesterol acyltransferase deficiency: a clinical survey. *Scand J Clin Lab Invest* 1974;33[Suppl 137]: 73–82.
85. Imbasciata E, Paties C, Scarpioni L, et al. Renal lesions in familial lecithin:cholesterol acyltransferase deficiency. Ultrastructural heterogeneity of glomerular changes. *Am J Nephrol* 1986;6:66–70.
86. Lambert G, Sakai N, Vaisman BL, et al. Analysis of glomerulosclerosis and atherosclerosis in lecithin cholesterol acyltransferase-deficient mice. *J Biol Chem* 2001;276:15090–15098.
87. Black J, Stapleton FB, Roy S III, et al. Varied types of urinary calculi in a patient with cystinosis without renal tubular acidosis. *Pediatrics* 1986;78:295–297.

88. Laine J, Salo MK, Krogerus L, et al. The nephropathy of type I tyrosinaemia after liver transplantation. *Pediatr Res* 1995;37:640–645.
89. Freese DK, Tuchman M, Schwarzenberg SJ, et al. Early liver transplantation is indicated for tyrosinaemia type I. *J Pediatr Gastoenterol Nutr* 1991;13:10–15.
90. Wrong OM, Norden AGW, Feest TG. Dent's disease: a familial proximal renal tubular syndrome with low molecular weight proteinuria, hypercalciuria, metabolic bone disease, progressive renal failure and a marked male preponderance. *QJM* 1994;87:473–493.
91. Wiebers DO, Wilson DM, McLeod RA, et al. Renal stones in Wilson's disease. *Am J Med* 1979;67:249–254.
92. Sozeri E, Feist D, Ruder H, et al. Proteinuria and other renal functions in Wilson's disease. *Pediatr Nephrol* 1997;11:307–311.
93. Odievre M, Gentil C, Gautier M, et al. Hereditary fructose intolerance in childhood. *Am J Dis Child* 1978;132:605–608.
94. Vainsel M, Fondu P, Cadranel S, et al. Osteopetrosis associated with proximal and distal tubular acidosis. *Acta Paediatr Scand* 1972;61:429–434.
95. Sly WS, Lang R, Avioli L, et al. Recessive osteopetrosis: new clinical phenotype. *Am J Hum Genet* 1972;24[Suppl]:34a (abst).
96. Atkin BM, Buist NRM, Utter M, et al. Pyruvate carboxylase deficiency and lactic acidosis in a retarded child without Leigh's disease. *Pediatr Res* 1979;13:109–116.
97. Levine AS, Michael AF. Ehlers-Danlos syndrome with renal tubular acidosis and medullary sponge kidneys. *J Pediatr* 1967;71:107–113.
98. Ghosh AK, O'Bryan T. Ehlers-Danlos syndrome and reflux nephropathy [Letter]. *Nephron* 1995;70:266.
99. Falik-Borenstein ZC, Jordan SC, Saudubray J-M, et al. Renal tubular acidosis in carnitine palmitoyltransferase type I deficiency. *N Engl J Med* 1992;327:24–27.
100. Ratech H, Greco MA, Gallo G, et al. Pathologic findings in adenosine deaminase-deficient severe combined immunodeficiency. *Am J Pathol* 1985;120:157–169.
101. DiRocco M, Garibotto G, Rossi GA, et al. Role of haematological, pulmonary and renal complications in the long-term prognosis of patients with lysinuric protein intolerance. *Eur J Pediatr* 1993;152:437–440.
102. Rodriguez-Soriano J, Rivera JM, Vallo A, et al. Proximal renal tubular acidosis in metachromatic leukodystrophy. *Helv Paediatr Acta* 1978;33:45–52.
103. Yeun JY, Hasbargen JA. Renal hypouricemia: prevention of exercise-induced acute renal failure and a review of the literature. *Am J Kidney Dis* 1995;25:937–946.
104. Drummond KN, Michael AF, Ulstrom RA, et al. The blue diaper syndrome: familial hypercalcemia with nephrocalcinosis and indicanuria. *Am J Med* 1964;37:928–948.
105. Huguley CM, Bain JA, Rivers SL, et al. Refractory megaloblastic anaemia associated with excretion of orotic acid. *Blood* 1959;14:615–634.
106. Girot R, Durandy A, Perignon J-L, et al. Hereditary orotic aciduria: a defect of pyrimidine metabolism with cellular immunodeficiency. *Birth Defect Orig Artic Ser* 1983;19:313–316.
107. Webster DR, Becroft DMO, Suttle DP. Hereditary orotic aciduria and other disorders of pyrimidine metabolism. In: Scriver CR, Beaudet AL, Sly WS, et al., eds. *The metabolic and molecular bases of inherited disease,* 8th ed. New York: McGraw-Hill, 2001.
108. Saarela T, Simila S, Koivisto M. Hypercalcaemia and nephrocalcinosis in patients with congenital lactase deficiency. *J Pediatr* 1995;127:920–923.
109. Abdullah AM, Abdullah MA, Abdurrahman MB, et al. Glucose-galactose malabsorption with renal stones in a Saudi child. *Ann Trop Paediatr* 1992;12:327–329.
110. Teree TM, Klein L. Hypophosphatasia: clinical and metabolic studies. *J Pediatr* 1968;72:41–50.
111. Melzi ML, Costantini D, Giani M, et al. Severe nephropathy in three adolescents with cystic fibrosis. *Arch Dis Child* 1991;66:1444–1447.
112. Katz SM, Krueger LJ, Falkner B. Microscopic nephrocalcinosis in cystic fibrosis. *N Engl J Med* 1988;319:263–266.
113. Allen JL. Progressive nephropathy in a patient with cystic fibrosis [Letter]. *N Engl J Med* 1986;315:764.
114. Matthews LA, Doershuk CF, Stern RC, et al. Urolithiasis and cystic fibrosis. *J Urol* 1996;155:1563–1564.
115. Kirk JM, Brain CE, Carson DJ, et al. Cushing's syndrome is caused by nodular hyperplasia in children with McCune-Albright syndrome. *J Paediatr* 1999;134;789–792.
116. Moudgil A, Rodich G, Jordan SC, et al. Nephrocalcinosis and renal cysts associated with apparent mineralocorticoid syndrome. *Pediatr Nephrol* 2000;15:60–62.
117. Gravel RA, Lowden JA, Callahan JW, et al. Infantile sialidosis: a phenocopy of type 1 GM1 gangliosidosis distinguished by genetic complementation and urinary oligosaccharides. *Am J Hum Genet* 1979;31:669–679.
118. Maroteaux P, Humbel R, Strecker G, et al. Un nouveau type de sialidose avec atteinte renal: la nephrosialidose, 1. Etude clinique, radiologique et nosologique. *Arch Fr Pediatr* 1978;35:819–829.
119. Aylsworth AS, Thomas GH, Hood JL, et al. A severe infantile sialidosis: clinical, biochemical and microscopic features. *J Pediatr* 1980;96:663–668.
120. Sewell AC, Pontz BF, Weitzel D, et al. Clinical heterogeneity in infantile galactosialidosis. *Eur J Pediatr* 1987;146:528–531.
121. Williams JC, Butler IJ, Rosenberg HS, et al. Progressive neurological deterioration and renal failure due to storage of glutamyl ribose-5-phosphate. *N Engl J Med* 1984;311:152–155.
122. Taylor J, Thorner P, Gerary DF, et al. Nephrotic syndrome and hypertension in two children with Hurler syndrome. *J Pediatr* 1986;108:726–729.
123. Sperl W, Gruber W, Quatacker J, et al. Nephrosis in two siblings with infantile sialic acid storage disease. *Eur J Pediatr* 1990;149:477–482.
124. Moroz SP, Cutz E, Balfe JW, et al. Membranoproliferative glomerulonephritis in childhood cirrhosis associated with $alpha_1$-antitrypsin deficiency. *Pediatrics* 1976;57:232–238.
125. Strife CF, Hug G, Chuck G, et al. Membranoproliferative glomerulonephritis and α_1-antitrypsin deficiency in children. *Pediatrics* 1983;71:88–92.
126. Koitabashi Y, Ikoma M, Miyahira T, et al. Long-term follow-up of a paediatric case of lipoprotein glomerulopathy. *Pediatr Nephrol* 1990;4:122–128.
127. Maruyama K, Arai H, Ogawa T, et al. Lipoprotein glomerulopathy: a pediatric case report. *Pediatr Nephrol* 1997;11:213–214.

128. Parsons H, Snyder F, Bowen T, et al. Immune complex disease consistent with systemic lupus erythematosus in a patient with lysinuric protein intolerance. *J Inherit Metab Dis* 1996;19:627–634.
129. Shrinath M, Walter JH, Haeney M, et al. Prolidase deficiency and systemic lupus erythematosus. *Arch Dis Child* 1997;76:441–444.
130. Brito T, Gomes dos Reis V, Penna DO, et al. Glomerular involvement in Gaucher's disease. A light, immunofluorescent, and ultrastructural study based on kidney biopsy specimens. *Arch Pathol* 1973;95:1–7.
131. Chander PN, Nurse HM, Pirani CL. Renal involvement in adult Gaucher's disease after splenectomy. *Arch Pathol Lab Med* 1979;103:440–445.
132. Wilson GN, Holmes RG, Custer J, et al. Zellweger syndrome: diagnostic assays, syndrome delineation, and potential therapy. *Am J Med Genet* 1986;24:69–82.
133. Martin SR, Garel L, Alvarez F. Alagille's syndrome associated with cystic renal disease. *Arch Dis Child* 1996;74:232–235.
134. Habib R, Dommergues JP, Gubler MC, et al. Glomerular mesangiolipidosis in Alagille syndrome (arteriohepatic dysplasia). *Pediatr Nephrol* 1987;1:455–464.
135. Sweetman L, Nyhan WL, Trauner DA, et al. Glutaric aciduria type II. *J Pediatr* 1980;96:1020–1026.
136. Lehnert W, Wendel U, Lindenmaier S, et al. Multiple acyl-CoA dehydrogenase deficiency (glutaric aciduria type II), congenital polycystic kidneys, and symmetric warty dysplasia of the cerebral cortex in two brothers. I. Clinical, metabolical, and biochemical findings. *Eur J Pediatr* 1982;139:56–59.
137. Bohm N, Uly J, Kiesling M, et al. Multiple acyl-CoA dehydrogenation deficiency (glutaric aciduria type II), congenital polycystic kidneys, and symmetric warty dysplasia of the cerebral cortex in two newborn brothers. II. Morphology and Pathogenesis. *Eur J Pediatr* 1982;139:60–65.
138. Mitchell G, Saudubray JM, Gubler MC, et al. Congenital anomalies in glutaric aciduria type 2 [Letter]. *J Pediatr* 1984;104:961.
139. Joseph JD, Uehling DT, Gilbert E, et al. Genitourinary abnormalities associated with Smith-Lemli-Opitz syndrome. *J Urol* 1987;137:719–721.
140. Cunniff C, Kratz LE, Moser A, et al. Clinical and biochemical spectrum of patients with RSH/Smith-Lemli-Opitz syndrome and abnormal cholesterol metabolism. *Am J Med Genet* 1997;68:263–269.
141. Strife CF, Strife JL, Wacksman J. Acquired structural genitourinary abnormalities contributing to deterioration of renal function in older patients with nephropathic cystinosis. *Pediatrics* 1991;88:1238–1241.
142. Byers PH, Siegel RC, Holbrook KA, et al. X-linked cutis laxa: defective cross-link formation in collagen due to decreased lysyl oxidase activity. *N Engl J Med* 1980;303:61–65.
143. Sartoris DJ, Luzzatti L, Weaver DD, et al. Type IX Ehlers-Danlos syndrome: a new variant with pathognomonic radiographic features. *Radiology* 1984;152:665–670.
144. Cusworth DC, Dent CE. Homocystinuria. *Br Med Bull* 1969;25:42–47.
145. Zinn AB, Zurcher VL, Kraus F, et al. Carnitine palmitoyltransferase B (CPT B) deficiency: a heritable cause of neonatal cardiomyopathy and dysgenesis of the kidney. *Pediatr Res* 1991;29:73A(abst).
146. Owusu SK, Addy J, Foli AK, et al. Acute reversible renal failure associated with glucose-6-phosphate dehydrogenase deficiency. *Lancet* 1972;1:1255–1257.
147. Whitelaw AGL. Acute intermittent porphyria, hypercholesterolaemia and renal impairment. *Arch Dis Child* 1974;49:406–447.
148. Yeung Laiwah AAC, Mactier R, McColl KEL, et al. Early-onset renal failure as a complication of acute intermittent porphyria. *QJM* 1983;52:92–98.
149. Tein I, Di Mauro S, De Vivo DC. Recurrent childhood myoglobinuria. *Adv Pediatr* 1990;37:77–117.
150. Kreuder J, Borkhardt A, Repp R, et al. Brief report: inherited metabolic myopathy and hemolysis due to a mutation in aldolase A. *N Engl J Med* 1996;334:1100–1104.

51

INFECTIOUS DISEASES AND THE KIDNEY

AMITAVA PAHARI
SAM WALTERS
MICHAEL LEVIN

The kidney is involved in a wide range of bacterial, viral, fungal, and parasitic diseases. In most systemic infections, renal involvement is a minor component of the illness, but in some, renal failure may be the presenting feature and the major problem in management. Although individual infectious processes may have a predilection to involve the renal vasculature, glomeruli, interstitium, or collecting systems, a purely anatomic approach to the classification of infectious diseases affecting the kidney is rarely helpful because most infections may involve several different aspects of renal function. In this chapter, a microbiologic classification of the organisms affecting the kidney is adopted. Although they are important causes of renal dysfunction in infectious diseases, urinary tract infections and hemolytic uremic syndrome (HUS) are not discussed in detail because they are considered separately in Chapters 53 and 47, respectively.

Elucidation of the cause of renal involvement in a child with evidence of infection must be based on a careful consideration of the geographic distribution of infectious diseases in different countries. A history of foreign travel; exposure to animals, insects, or unusual foods or drinks; outdoor activities such as swimming or hiking; and contact with infectious diseases must be sought in every case. The clinical examination should include a careful assessment of skin and mucous membranes and a search for insect bites, lymphadenopathy, and involvement of other organs. A close collaboration with a pediatric infectious disease specialist and hospital microbiologist will aid the diagnosis and management of the underlying infection.

A tantalizing clue to the pathogenesis of glomerular disease is the marked difference in the incidence of nephrosis and nephritis in developed and underdeveloped areas of the world. In several tropical countries, glomerulonephritis (GN) accounts for up to 4% of pediatric hospital admissions; the incidence in temperate climates is 10- to 100-fold less. This difference might be explained by a complex interaction of several different factors, including nutrition, racial and genetically determined differences in immune responses, and exposure to infectious diseases. A growing body of evidence, however, suggests that long-term exposure to infectious agents is a major factor in the increased prevalence of glomerular diseases in developing countries.

Renal involvement in infectious diseases may occur by a variety of mechanisms: direct microbial invasion of the renal tissues or collecting system may take place in conditions such as staphylococcal abscess of the kidney as a result of septicemic spread of the organism or as a consequence of ascending infection; damage to the kidney may be caused by the systemic release of endotoxin or other toxins and activation of the inflammatory cascade during septicemia or by a focus of infection distant from the kidney; ischemic damage may result from inadequate perfusion induced by septic shock; the kidney may be damaged by activation of the immunologic pathways or by immune complexes resulting from the infectious process. In many conditions, a combination of these mechanisms may be operative. In the assessment of renal complications occurring in infectious diseases, the possibility of drug-induced nephrotoxicity caused by antimicrobial therapy should always be considered. The nephrotoxic effects of antibiotics and other antimicrobial agents are not addressed in this chapter but are covered in Chapter 52.

BACTERIAL INFECTIONS

Bacterial infections associated with renal disease and the likely mechanisms causing renal dysfunction are shown in Table 51.1.

Systemic Sepsis and Septic Shock

Impaired renal function is a common occurrence in systemic sepsis (1). Depending on the severity of the infection and the organism responsible, the renal involvement may vary from insignificant proteinuria to acute renal failure requiring dialysis. The organisms causing acute renal failure as part of systemic sepsis vary with age and geographic location and also differ in normal and immunocompromised children. In the

TABLE 51.1. LIKELY MECHANISMS CAUSING RENAL DYSFUNCTION IN BACTERIAL INFECTIONS

Organism	Site/infection	Infection localized to kidney	Systemic infection; toxin/ inflammation	Ischemia/ hypoperfusion; vasomotor nephropathy	Distant infection; "immunologic/ delayed"	Others
Neisseria meningitidis	Septicemia		++	++		
	Chronic meningococcemia				+	
Staphylococcus aureus	Renal abscess	++				
	Distant abscess/endocarditis (see Table 51.2)				++	
	Sepsis		++	++		
	Toxic shock		++	++		
Staphylococcus epidermidis	Shunt infection (see Table 51.2)				++	
Group A *Streptococcus*	Sepsis		++	++		
	Toxic shock		++	++		
	APSGN				++	
Haemophilus influenzae (new biotype)	Brazilian purpuric fever		++	++		
Leptospira interrogans	Leptospirosis, Weil disease	++		++		
Streptococcus pneumoniae	Sepsis		++	++		
	Pneumonia					+ (HUS)
Escherichia coli and *Shigella*	Sepsis		++	++		
	Diarrhea			++		
	Colitis					++ (HUS)
Salmonella species	Sepsis		++?	++	+	
	Diarrhea			++		+ (HUS)
Vibrio species	Cholera			++		
Klebsiella	Sepsis		++	++		
Yersinia species	Enteritis				+	+ (HUS)
Campylobacter jejuni	Enteritis				+	
Mycobacteria tuberculi	Tuberculosis	+			+	
Treponema pallidum	Syphilis				+	
Mycoplasma pneumoniae	Pneumonia				+	+ (HUS)
Legionella	Pneumonia	+?				Rhabdomyolysis
Rickettsia rickettsii	Rocky Mountain spotted fever	+		+		
Coxiella burnetii	Q fever				+	

++, frequent complication of infection; +, uncommon but recognized complication; APSGN, acute poststreptococcal glomerulonephritis; HUS, hemolytic uremic syndrome.

neonatal period, group B streptococci, coliforms, *Staphylococcus aureus*, and *Listeria monocytogenes* are the organisms usually responsible. In older children, *Neisseria meningitidis*, *Streptococcus pneumoniae*, and *S. aureus* account for most of the infections. In people who are immunocompromised, a wide range of bacteria are seen, and, similarly, in tropical countries other pathogens, including *Haemophilus influenzae*, *Salmonella* species, and *Pseudomonas pseudomallei*, must be considered. Where *H. influenzae* type B vaccine has been introduced, however, the incidence of severe systemic infections due to this organism has shown a sharp fall.

Systemic sepsis usually presents with nonspecific features: fever, tachypnea, tachycardia, and evidence of skin and organ underperfusion. The pathophysiology of renal involvement in systemic sepsis is multifactorial (1,2). Hypovolemia with diminished renal perfusion is the earliest event and is a consequence of the increased vascular permeability and loss of plasma from the intravascular space. Hypovolemia commonly coexists with depressed myocardial function because of the myocardial depressant effects of endotoxin or other toxins. The renal vasoconstrictor response to diminished circulating volume and reduced cardiac output further reduces glomerular filtration, and oliguria is thus a consistent and early event in severe sepsis (1,3). The plasma kallikrein-kinin system is a potent vasodilator pathway, activated by endotoxin. Vasodilation of capillary beds leading to warm shock is common in adults with sepsis due to Gram-negative organisms but is less commonly seen in children, in whom intense vasoconstriction is the usual response to sepsis. If renal underperfusion and vasoconstriction are persistent and severe, the reversible prerenal failure is followed by established renal failure with the characteristic features of vasomotor nephropathy or acute tubular necrosis. Other mechanisms of renal damage in systemic sepsis include direct effects of endotoxin and other toxins on the kidney, and release of inflammatory mediators such as tumor necrosis factor (TNF) and other cytokines, arachidonic acid metabolites, and proteolytic enzymes (3). Nitric oxide (NO) is postulated to play a key role in the pathophysiology of renal failure in sepsis. Whether the renal effects of increased NO are beneficial or harmful remains unclear. Trials of selective NO synthetase inhibition did not offer any advantages over saline resuscitation (4). NO in endotoxemia is possibly beneficial because it maintains renal blood flow and glomerular filtration.

The renal findings early in septic shock are oliguria, with high urine/plasma urea and creatinine ratios, low urine sodium concentration, and a high urine/plasma osmolarity ratio. Once established, renal failure supervenes, and the urine is of poor quality with low urine/plasma urea and creatinine ratios, elevated urine sodium concentration, and low urine osmolarity. Proteinuria is usually present, and the urine sediment may contain red cells and small numbers of white cells (1).

Management of Acute Renal Failure in Systemic Sepsis

The management of acute renal failure in systemic sepsis depends on early diagnosis and administration of appropriate antibiotics to cover the expected pathogens. In addition, management is directed at improving renal perfusion and oxygenation. Volume replacement with crystalloid or colloid should be undertaken to optimize preload. Central venous pressure or pulmonary wedge pressure monitoring is essential to guide volume replacement in children in severe shocked (1,2). The use of low-dose (2 to 5 µg/kg/min) dopamine to reduce renal vasoconstriction together with administration of inotropic agents such as dobutamine or epinephrine to improve cardiac output may reverse prerenal failure. Early elective ventilation should be undertaken in patients with severe shock. If oliguria persists despite volume replacement and inotropic therapy, dialysis should be instituted early, because septic and catabolic patients may rapidly develop hyperkalemia and severe electrolyte imbalance.

In most children who develop acute renal failure as part of systemic sepsis or septic shock, the renal failure is of short duration, and recovery can be expected within a few days of achieving cardiovascular stability and eradication of the underlying infection. Occasionally, renal cortical necrosis or infarction of the kidney may result in prolonged or permanent loss of renal function.

Specific Infections Causing the Systemic Sepsis Syndrome

Meningococcus

N. meningitidis continues to be a major cause of systemic sepsis and meningitis in both developed and underdeveloped parts of the world (5). In developed countries, most cases are caused by group B strains, particularly after introduction of meningococcal C vaccination, whereas epidemics of *Meningococcus* groups A and C continue to occur in many underdeveloped regions of the world (5,6). Infants and young adults are most commonly affected, but cases in adolescents and young children are also common. There are two major presentations of meningococcal disease (5): Meningococcal meningitis presents with features indistinguishable from those of other forms of meningitis, including headaches, stiff neck, and photophobia. Lumbar puncture is required to identify the causative agent and distinguish this from other forms of meningitis. Despite the acute nature of the illness, the prognosis is good, and most patients with the purely meningitic form of the illness recover without sequelae.

Meningococcemia with purpuric rash and shock is the second and more devastating form of the illness. Affected patients present with nonspecific symptoms of fever, vomiting, abdominal pain, and muscle ache. The diagnosis is only obvious once the characteristic petechial or purpuric rash appears. Patients with a rapidly progressive purpuric rash, hypotension, and evidence of skin and organ underperfusion have a poor prognosis, with a mortality of 10 to 60%. Adverse prognostic features include hypotension, a low white cell count, absence of meningeal inflammation, thrombocytopenia, and disturbed coagulation indices (7).

Renal failure was seldom reported in early series of patients with meningococcemia, perhaps because most patients died rapidly of uncontrolled septic shock. With advances in intensive care, however, more children are surviving the initial period of profound hemodynamic derangement, and renal failure is more often seen as a major management problem. Approximately 10% of children with fulminant meningococcemia develop renal failure, which usually occurs 24 to 48 hours after the onset of illness (8).

The pathophysiology of meningococcal septicemia involves the activation of cytokines and inflammatory cells by endotoxin (5,6). Mortality is directly related to both the plasma endotoxin concentration and the intensity of the inflammatory response, as indicated by levels of TNFs and other inflammatory markers (9). Patients with meningococcemia have a profound capillary leak leading to severe hypovolemia. Loss of plasma proteins from the intravascular space is probably the major cause of shock (10). However, intense vasoconstriction further impairs tissue and organ perfusion, and vasculitis with intravascular thrombosis and consumption of platelets and coagulation factors is also present (5).

Oliguria is invariably present in children with meningococcemia during the initial phase of the disorder. This is prerenal in origin and may respond to volume replacement and inotropic support. If cardiac output cannot be improved and renal underperfusion persists, established renal failure supervenes. Occasionally, cortical necrosis or infarction of the kidneys occurs. Children with meningococcemia should be aggressively managed in a pediatric intensive care unit, with early administration of antibiotics (penicillin or a third-generation cephalosporin), volume replacement, hemodynamic monitoring, and the use of inotropic agents and vasodilators. If oliguria persists despite measures to improve cardiac output, elective ventilation and dialysis should be instituted early (5,6). Because activation of coagulation pathways occurs, severe acquired protein-C deficiency may result and is usually associated with substantial mortality (11). In survivors, end-organ failure including renal failure is not uncommon. Protein C is a natural anticoagulant which also has important antiinflammatory activity. Early replacement therapy with activated protein-C concentrate together with supportive treatment in meningococcemia may have an important role in reducing the complications, including the renal manifestations (12). Most patients who survive the initial 24 to 48 hours of the illness and regain hemodynamic stability will ultimately recover renal function.

The least common presentation of meningococcal sepsis is chronic meningococcemia. Patients with this form of the illness present insidiously with a vasculitic rash, arthritis, and evidence of multiorgan involvement. The features may overlap those of Henoch-Schönlein purpura or subacute bacterial endocarditis (SBE), and the diagnosis must be considered in patients presenting with fever, arthritis, and vasculitic rash, often accompanied by proteinuria or hematuria. Response to antibiotic treatment is good, but some patients may have persistent symptoms for many days resulting from an immune-complex vasculitis.

Staphylococcus aureus

Staphylococcal infections may affect the kidneys by direct focal invasion during staphylococcal septicemia, forming a renal abscess; by causing staphylococcal bacteremia; or by toxin-mediated mechanisms, as in the staphylococcal toxic shock syndrome.

Staphylococcal Abscess. Staphylococcal renal abscess presents with fever, loin pain and tenderness, and abnormal urine sediment, as do abscesses caused by other organisms (13). The illness often follows either septicemia or pyelonephritis. The diagnosis is usually considered only when a patient with clinical pyelonephritis shows an inadequate response to antibiotic treatment. The diagnosis is confirmed by ultrasonography or computed tomographic scan, which shows swelling of the kidney and intrarenal collections of fluid. Antibiotic therapy alone may result in cure, but if the patient remains unwell with evidence of persistent inflammation despite use of appropriate antibiotics, surgical intervention may be required. Percutaneous drainage under ultrasonographic or computed tomographic scan guidance is often effective and may avoid the need for a more direct surgical approach (13,14).

Staphylococcal Toxic Shock Syndrome. The staphylococcal toxic shock syndrome is a systemic illness characterized by fever, shock, erythematous rash, diarrhea, confusion, and renal failure. The disorder was first described by Todd et al. in 1978 in a series of seven children (15). During the 1980s, thousands of cases were reported in the United States, mostly cases in menstruating women associated with tampon use. Although most cases worldwide are seen in women and are associated with menstruation, children of both sexes and of all ages are affected (16).

The illness usually begins suddenly with high fever, diarrhea, and hypotension, together with a diffuse erythroderma (17). Mucous membrane involvement with hyperemia and ulceration of the lips and oral mucosa or vaginal mucosa, strawberry tongue, and conjunctival injection are usually seen. Desquamation of the rash occurs in the convalescent phase of the illness. Confusion is often present in the early stages of the illness and may progress to coma in severe cases. Multiple organ failure with evidence of impaired renal function, elevated levels of hepatic transaminases, thrombocytopenia, and disseminated intravascular coagulation (DIC) is often seen.

The diagnosis is made on the basis of the clinical features of fever, rash, hypotension, and subsequent desquamation along with deranged function of three or more of the following organ systems: gastrointestinal (GI), mucous membranes, renal, hepatic, hematologic, central nervous system, and muscle. Other disorders causing a similar picture, such as Rocky Mountain spotted fever, leptospirosis, measles, and streptococcal infection, must be excluded.

The staphylococcal toxic shock syndrome is now known to be due to infection or colonization with strains of *S. aureus* that produce one or more protein exotoxins (18). Most cases in adults are associated with toxic shock toxin I; in children, many of the isolates associated with the syndrome produce other enterotoxins (A to F). The staphylococcal enterotoxins appear to induce disease by acting as superantigens (19), which activate T cells bearing specific Vβ regions of the T-cell receptor; this causes proliferation and cytokine release (20). The systemic illness and toxicity are believed to result largely from an intense inflammatory response induced by the toxin. The site of toxin production is often a trivial focus of infection or simple colonization, and bacteremia is rarely observed.

Renal failure in toxic shock syndrome is usually caused by shock and renal hypoperfusion. In the early stages of the illness, oliguria and renal impairment are usually prerenal and respond to treatment of shock and measures to improve perfusion. In severe cases and in patients in whom treatment is delayed, acute renal failure develops as a consequence of prolonged renal underperfusion, and dialysis may be required. In addition to underperfusion, direct effects of the toxin or inflammatory mediators may also contribute to the renal damage. Recovery of renal function usually occurs, but in severe cases with cortical necrosis or intense renal vasculitis, prolonged dialysis may be required.

The management of staphylococcal toxic shock syndrome depends on early diagnosis and aggressive cardiovascular support with volume replacement, inotropic support, and, in severe cases, elective ventilation. If oliguria persists despite optimization of intravascular volume and administration of inotropic agents, dialysis should be commenced early (17).

Antistaphylococcal antibiotics should be started as soon as the diagnosis is suspected and the site of infection identified. Initial empiric antimicrobial therapy should include an antistaphylococcal antibiotic effective against β-lactamase–resistant organisms and a protein synthesis–inhibiting antibiotic such as clindamycin to stop further toxin production (21). If there is a focus of infection such as a vaginal tampon, surgical wound, or infected sinuses, the site should be drained early to prevent continued toxin release into the circulation. The intravenous administration of immune globulins may be considered when infection is refractory to several hours of aggressive therapy, an undrainable focus is present, or persistent oliguria with pulmonary edema occurs (21). With aggressive intensive care, most affected patients survive, and renal recovery is usual, even in patients who have had severe shock and multiorgan failure. Relapses and recurrences of staphylococcal toxic shock syndrome occur in a proportion of affected patients because immune responses to the toxin are ineffective in some individuals.

Streptococcus pyogenes

The group A streptococci (GAS) are a major worldwide cause of renal disease, usually as poststreptococcal nephritis. However, in addition to this postinfection immunologically mediated disorder, in recent years there have been increasing reports of GAS's causing acute renal failure as part of an invasive infection with many features of the staphylococcal toxic shock syndrome (22).

Acute Poststreptococcal Glomerulonephritis. Acute poststreptococcal GN (APSGN) is a delayed complication of pharyngeal infection or impetigo with certain nephritogenic strains of GAS. Different strains can be serotyped according to the antigenic properties of the M protein found in the outer portion of the bacterial wall. APSGN after pharyngeal infection is most commonly associated with serotype M12. In contrast, in APSGN after impetigo, serotype M49 is most commonly identified (23). On occasions, other serotypes and nontypeable strains have been described as causing GN.

The pathology and pathogenesis of the disorder is discussed in detail in Chapter 30. APSGN has a worldwide distribution. Epidemiologic differences are observed between pharyngitis-associated and impetigo-associated streptococcal infections. Pharyngitis-associated APSGN is most common during school age and has an unexplained male/female ratio of 2:1. It occurs more often in the cooler months, and familial occurrences are commonly described. The latent period is 1 to 2 weeks, in notable contrast to impetigo-associated cases, which have a latent period of 2 to 6 weeks. In many developing countries, children have chronic skin infections, and it may be difficult to establish the latent period with accuracy. Impetigo-associated cases are more common in the warmer months, sex distribution is equal, and children tend to be younger. Introduction of a nephritogenic strain into a family often results in the occurrence of several cases within that family, and in some cases, attack rates of up to 20% have been described (24). The incidence is linked to poor socioeconomic conditions.

Renal involvement in APSGN can be mild, and in many patients, the disease may not be manifested clinically. Studies of epidemics with nephritogenic strains of streptococci have shown that up to 50% of those infected had subclinical evidence of renal disease (24,25). In a typical case a sudden onset of facial or generalized edema occurs. Hypertension is usually modest but is severe in 5% of cases, and occasionally may lead to encephalopathy or left ventricular failure. The urine is smoky or tea colored in 30 to 50% of cases. Pallor, headache, backache, lethargy, malaise, anorexia, and weakness are all common nonspecific features.

The urine volume is decreased. Proteinuria is present (up to 100 mg/dL), and microscopy shows white cells, red cells, and granular and hyaline casts. Urea, electrolyte, and creatinine levels are normal in subclinical cases but show features of acute renal failure in severe cases. It may be possible to culture GAS from the skin or the throat in some patients. Other evidence of infection with a GAS can be obtained through the antistreptolysin-O titer (ASOT), which is increased in 60 to 80% of cases. Early antibiotic treatment can reduce the proportion of cases with elevated ASOT to 30%. Anti–deoxyribonuclease B and antihyaluronidase testing has been shown to be of more value than ASOT in confirming group A streptococcal infection in impetigo-associated cases. Measurement of anti–M protein antibodies is of more value for epidemiologic purposes than for the diagnosis of individual cases (25). Decreased C3 and total hemolytic complement levels are found in 90% of cases during the first 2 weeks of illness and return to normal after 4 to 6 weeks.

Penicillin should be given to eradicate the GAS organisms. Erythromycin, clindamycin, or a first-generation cephalosporin can be given to patients allergic to penicillin. Antibiotic treatment probably has no influence on the course of renal disease but will prevent the spread of a nephritogenic strain (26). Close contacts and family members who are culture-positive for GAS should also be given penicillin, although antibiotic treatment is not always effective in eliminating secondary cases. Recurrent episodes are rare, and immunity to the particular nephritogenic strain that caused the disease is probably lifelong. Antibiotic prophylaxis is therefore unnecessary.

Most studies suggest that the prognosis for children with APSGN is extremely good, with more than 90% making a complete recovery. However, 10% of cases may have a prolonged and more serious course with long-term chronic renal failure (27).

Other Streptococci. APSGN has also been described after outbreaks of group C *Streptococcus* infection (28). This has occurred after consumption of unpasteurized milk from cattle with mastitis. Patients developed pharyngitis followed by APSGN. Endostreptosin was found in the cytoplasm of these group C strains, and during the course of the illness, patients developed antiendostreptosin antibodies. This antigen has been postulated to be the nephritogenic component of GAS.

In addition, strains of group G streptococci have been implicated in occasional cases of APSGN (29). Isolates possessed the type M12 protein antigen identical to the nephritogenic type M12 antigen of some group A streptococcal strains.

Streptococcal Toxic Shock Syndrome and Invasive Group A Streptococcal Infection. Since 1988, there have been several reports of an illness with many similarities to the staphylococcal toxic shock syndrome, occurring in both children (30) and adults, associated with invasive group A streptococcal disease (26,31,32). Patients with this syndrome present acutely with high fever, erythematous rash, mucous membrane involvement, hypotension, and multiorgan failure. Unlike staphylococcal toxic shock syndrome, in which the focus of infection is usually trivial and bacteremia is seldom seen, the streptococcal toxic shock syndrome is usually associated with bacteremia or a serious focus of infection such as septic arthritis, myositis, or osteomyelitis (30,32). Laboratory findings of anemia, neutrophil leukocytosis, thrombocytopenia, and DIC are often present, together with impaired renal function, hepatic derangement, and acidosis. Acute renal failure requiring dialysis occurs in a significant proportion of cases.

The reason for the emergence of streptococcal toxic shock syndrome and the increasing numbers of cases with invasive disease caused by the GAS is unclear. Strains causing toxic shock syndrome and invasive disease appear to differ from common isolates of GAS in producing large amounts of pyrogenic toxins that may have superantigen-like activity. The pathophysiology of streptococcal toxic shock syndrome and that of the streptococcal toxins are similar in that both organisms produce superantigen toxins that induce release of cytokines and other inflammatory mediators.

Treatment of streptococcal toxic shock syndrome depends on the administration of appropriate antibiotics, aggressive circulatory support, and treatment of any multiorgan failure. Surgical intervention to drain the infective focus in muscle, bone, joint, or body cavities is often required. Recovery of renal function occurs in patients who respond to treatment of shock and the eradication of the infection.

Leptospira

Leptospirosis is an acute generalized infectious disease caused by spirochetes of the genus *Leptospira* (33). It is primarily a disease of wild and domestic animals, and humans are infected only occasionally through contact with animals. Most human cases occur in summer or autumn and are associated with exposure to leptospire-contaminated water or soil during recreational activities such as swimming or camping. In adolescents and adults, occupational exposure through farming or other contact with animals is the route of infection.

The spirochete penetrates intact mucous membranes or abraded skin and disseminates to all parts of the body, including the cerebrospinal fluid (CSF). Although leptospires do not contain classic endotoxins, the pathophysiology of the disorder has many similarities to that of endotoxemia. In severe cases, jaundice occurs because of hepatocellular dysfunction and cholestasis. Renal functional abnormalities may be profound and out of proportion to the histologic changes in the kidney (34). Renal involvement is predominantly a result of tubular damage, and spirochetes are commonly seen in the tubular lesions. The inflammatory changes in the kidney may result from either a direct toxic effect of the organism or immune-complex nephritis. However, hypovolemia, hypotension, and reduced cardiac output caused by myocarditis may contribute to the development of renal failure. In severe cases, a hemorrhagic disorder caused by widespread vasculitis and capillary injury also occurs (34,35).

The clinical manifestations of leptospirosis are variable. Of affected patients, 90% have the milder anicteric form of the disorder, and only 5 to 10% have severe leptospirosis with jaundice. The illness may follow a biphasic course. After an incubation period of 7 to 12 days, a nonspecific flu-like illness lasting 4 to 7 days occurs, associated with septicemic spread of the spirochete. The fever then subsides, only to recur for the second, "immune," phase of the illness. During this phase, the fever is low grade and there may be headache and delirium caused by meningeal involvement, as well as intense muscular aching. Nausea and vomiting are common. Examination usually reveals conjunctival suffusion, erythematous rash, lymphadenopathy, and meningism.

The severe form of the disease (Weil disease) presents with fever, impaired renal and hepatic function, hemorrhage, vascular collapse, and altered consciousness. In one series the most common organs involved were the liver (71%) and kidney (63%). Cardiovascular (31%), pulmonary (26%), neurologic (5%), and hematologic (21%) involvements were less common (36). Vasculitis, thrombocytopenia, and uremia are considered important factors in the pathogenesis of hemorrhagic disturbances and the main cause of death in severe leptospirosis (37). Urinalysis results are abnormal during the leptospiremic phase with proteinuria, hematuria, and casts. Uremia usually appears in the second week, and acute renal failure may develop once cardiovascular collapse and DIC are present (35).

The clinical features of leptospirosis overlap with those of several other acute infectious diseases, including Rocky Mountain spotted fever, toxic shock syndrome, and streptococcal sepsis. The diagnosis of leptospirosis should be considered in febrile patients with evidence of renal, hepatic, and mucous membrane changes and rash, particularly if a history of exposure to fresh water is found. Diagnosis can be confirmed by isolation of the spirochetes from blood or CSF in the first 10 days of the illness or from urine in the second week (35). The organism may be seen in biopsy specimens of the kidney or skin or in the CSF by dark-field microscopy or silver staining. Serologic tests to detect leptospirosis are now sensitive and considerably aid the diagnosis. Immunoglobulin M (IgM) antibody may be detected as early as 6 to 10 days into the illness, and antibody titers rise progressively over the next 2 to 4 weeks. Some patients remain seronegative, and negative serologic test results do not completely exclude the diagnosis. In one series levels of IgM and IgG anticardiolipin concentrations were significantly increased in leptospirosis patients with acute renal failure (37). Leptospirosis is treated with intravenous penicillin or other β-lactam antibiotics. The severity of leptospirosis is reduced by antibiotic treatment, even if started late in the course of the illness (38). Supportive treatment with volume replacement to correct hypovolemia, administration of inotropics, and correction of coagulopathy is essential in severe cases. Dialysis may be required in severe cases and may be needed for prolonged periods until recovery occurs.

Streptococcus pneumoniae

Infection with *S. pneumoniae* is one of the most common infections in humans and causes a wide spectrum of disease, including pneumonia, otitis media, sinusitis, septicemia, and meningitis. Despite the prevalence of the organism, significant renal involvement is relatively rare but is seen in two situations: Pneumococcal septicemia in asplenic individuals or in those with other immune deficiencies presents with fulminant septic shock in which renal failure may occur as part of a multisystem derangement. The mortality from pneumococcal sepsis in asplenic patients is high, even with early antibiotic treatment and intensive support.

The second nephrologic syndrome associated with *S. pneumoniae* is a rare form of HUS. In 1955, Gasser and colleagues described HUS as a clinical entity in children, and they included two infants with pneumonia among the five patients they described (39). HUS associated with *Pneumococcus* infection is induced by the enzyme neuraminidase released from *S. pneumoniae* (40,41). Thomsen-Friedenrich antigen (T antigen) is present on the surface of red blood cells, platelets, and glomerular capillary endothelia against which antibodies are present in normal serum. Neuraminidase causes desialation of red blood cells, and possibly other blood cells and endothelium, by the removal of terminal neuraminic acid, which leads to unmasking of the T antigen. The resultant widespread agglutination of blood cells causes intravascular obstruction, hemolysis, thrombocytopenia, and renal failure. Results of the direct Coombs test are frequently positive, either from bound anti-T IgM or from anti-T antibodies. The diagnosis of Thomsen-Friedenrich antibody–induced HUS should be suspected in patients with acute renal failure and hemolysis after an episode of pneumonia or bacteremia caused by *S. pneumoniae.*

Association with *S. pneumoniae* is defined by culture of pneumococci from a normally sterile site within a week before or after onset of signs of HUS. Clues to a pneumococcal cause, in addition to culture results, include severe clinical disease, especially pneumonia, empyema, pleural effusion, or meningitis; hemolytic anemia without a reticulocyte response; positive results on a direct Coombs test; and difficulties in ABO crossmatching or a positive minor crossmatch incompatibility (42). However, when renal disease is seen in the context of severe pneumococcal infection, it is important to maintain a broad diagnostic perspective, because the occurrence of acute tubular necrosis due to septic shock and DIC is well described (43,44).

Therapy for this syndrome should be with supportive treatment and antibiotics (usually penicillin); dialysis may be required if renal failure occurs. Because normal serum contains antibodies against the Thomsen-Friedenrich antigen, blood transfusion should be undertaken with washed red blood cells resuspended in albumin rather than plasma (40,41). Exchange transfusion and plasmapheresis have been used in some patients, with the rationale that these procedures may improve outcome by eliminating circulating neuraminidase (40,44,45). Intravenous IgG has been used in a patient and was shown to neutralize neuraminidase present in the patient's serum (46).

In comparison to patients with the more common diarrhea-associated HUS, *S. pneumoniae*–induced HUS patients have a more severe renal disease. They are more likely to require dialysis. Their long-term outcome may be affected by the severity of the invasive streptococcal disease itself, and a significant proportion of surviving patients (30 to 70%) develop end-stage renal failure (47,48).

Gastrointestinal Infections (*Escherichia coli, Salmonella, Campylobacter, Yersinia, Shigella, Vibrio cholerae*)

The diarrheal diseases caused by *Escherichia coli*, *Salmonella*, *Shigella*, *Campylobacter*, vibrios, and *Yersinia* remain important and common bacterial infections of humans. Although improvements in hygiene and living conditions have reduced the incidence of bacterial gastroenteritis in developed countries, these infections remain common in underdeveloped areas of the world, and outbreaks and epidemics continue to occur in both developed and underdeveloped countries. Renal involvement in the enteric infections may result from any of four possible mechanisms.

Severe Diarrhea and Dehydration

Regardless of the causative organism, diarrhea results in hypovolemia, abnormalities of plasma electrolyte composition, and renal underperfusion. If severe dehydration occurs and is persistent, oliguria from prerenal failure is followed by vasomotor nephropathy and established renal failure.

Systemic Sepsis and Endotoxemia

E. coli, *Shigella*, and *Salmonella* (particularly *Salmonella typhi*) may invade the bloodstream and induce septicemia or septic shock. Acute renal failure is commonly seen in infants with *E. coli* sepsis but is also reported with *Klebsiella*, *Salmonella*, and *Shigella* infections. Its pathophysiology and treatment were discussed previously.

Enteric Pathogen–Associated Nephritis

Enteric infections with *E. coli*, *Yersinia*, *Campylobacter*, and *Salmonella* have been associated with several different forms of GN, including membranoproliferative GN (MPGN), interstitial nephritis, diffuse proliferative GN, and IgA nephropathy (49–51).

In typhoid fever, GN ranging from mild asymptomatic proteinuria and hematuria to acute renal failure may occur (50,52–54). Renal biopsy findings show focal proliferation of mesangial cells, hypertrophy of endothelial cells, and congested capillary lumina. Immunofluorescent studies show IgM, IgG, and C3 deposition in the glomeruli, with *Salmonella* antigens detected within the granular deposits in the mesangial areas. In the IgA nephropathy after typhoid fever, *Salmonella* vi antigens have been demonstrated within the glomeruli.

Yersinia infection has been reported as a precipitant of GN in several studies (51,55). Transient proteinuria and hematuria are found in 24% of patients with acute *Yersinia* infection, and elevated creatinine levels in 10%. Renal biopsy reveals mild mesangial GN or IgA nephropathy. *Yersinia* antigens, immunoglobulin, and complement have been detected in the glomeruli. *Yersinia pseudotuberculosis* is well recognized as one of the causes of acute tubulointerstitial nephritis causing acute renal failure, especially in children; patients have histories of drinking untreated water in endemic areas (56–58). The illness begins with the sudden onset of high fever, skin rash, and GI symptoms. Later in the course, periungual desquamation develops, mimicking Kawasaki disease. Elevated erythrocyte sedimentation rate, C-reactive protein level, and thrombocytosis are noticeable, and mild degrees of proteinuria, glycosuria, and sterile pyuria are common. Acute renal failure, which typically develops 1 to 3 weeks after the onset of fever, follows a benign course with complete recovery. Renal biopsy mainly reveals findings of acute tubulointerstitial nephritis. Antibiotic therapy, although recommended, does not alter the clinical course, but reduces the fecal excretion of the organism (59,60).

Enteric Pathogen–Induced Hemolytic Uremic Syndrome

HUS is characterized by three distinct clinical signs: acute renal failure, thrombocytopenia, and microangiopathic hemolytic anemia. It was first described in 1955 and was associated with infection by Shiga toxin–producing *Shigella dysenteriae*. A major breakthrough in the search for the cause of HUS occurred in the 1980s when Karmali et al. reported that 11 of 15 children with diarrhea-associated HUS had evidence of infection with a strain of *E. coli* that produced a toxin active on vero cells (61). In diarrhea-associated HUS in the United States and most of Europe, *E. coli* O157:H7 is the most important of these strains. *E. coli* O157:H7 occurs naturally in the GI tract of cattle and other animals, and humans become infected through contaminated food products. Most outbreaks have been associated with consumption of undercooked meat, but unpasteurized milk and cider, drinking water, and poorly chlorinated water for recreational use have also been implicated as vehicles for bacterial spread. HUS is discussed in detail in Chapter 47.

Mycobacterium tuberculosis

The global epidemic of *Mycobacterium tuberculosis* is growing. Several factors have contributed to this increase, including the emergence of the human immunodeficiency virus (HIV) infection epidemic, large influxes of immigrants from countries in which tuberculosis (TB) is common, the emergence of multiple-drug–resistant *M. tuberculosis*, and breakdown of the health services for effective control of TB in various countries. It is generally estimated that, overall, one-third of the world's population is currently infected with the TB bacillus. There are more than 8 million cases of TB, which result in the death of approximately 2 million people each year. Furthermore, 5 to 10% of people who are infected with the TB bacillus develop TB disease or become infectious at some time during their lives (62,63). After respiratory illness in children, mycobacteria are widely distributed to many organs of the body during the lymphohematogenous phase of childhood TB (64). Tubercle bacilli can be recovered from the urine in many cases of miliary TB. Hematogenously spread tuberculomata develop in the glomeruli, which results in caseating, sloughing lesions that discharge bacilli into the tubules. In most cases, the renal lesions are asymptomatic and manifest as mycobacteria in the urine or as sterile pyuria.

Tuberculomata in the cortex may calcify and cavitate or may rupture into the pelvis, discharging infective organisms into the tubules, urethra, and bladder. Dysuria, loin pain, hematuria, and pyuria are the presenting features of this complication, but in many cases, the renal involvement is asymptomatic, even when radiologic and pathologic abnormalities are very extensive. Continuing tuberculous bacilluria may cause cystitis with urinary frequency and, in late cases, a contracted bladder (65). The intravenous urogram is abnormal in most cases. Early findings are pyelonephritis with calyceal blunting and calyceal-interstitial reflux. Later, papillary cavities may be seen, indicating papillary necrosis. Ureteric strictures, focal calcification, hydronephrosis, and cavitation may also be seen. Renal function is usually well preserved, and hypertension is uncommon. In some cases, either the infection itself or reactions to the chemotherapeutic agents may result in renal failure with evidence of an interstitial nephritis (65–67).

Classic symptomatic renal TB is a late and uncommon complication in children, rarely occurring less than 4 or 5 years after the primary infection, and therefore is most commonly diagnosed after adolescence (64,66). Adult studies have shown that 26 to 75% of renal TB coexists with active pulmonary TB and 6 to 10% of screened sputum-positive pulmonary TB patients have renal involvement.

The diagnosis is established by isolation of mycobacteria from the urine or by the presence of the characteristic clinical and radiographic features in a child with current or previous TB. Renal TB is treated with drug regimens similar to those used for other forms of TB, with isoniazid, rifampicin, and pyrazinamide administered initially for 2 months, and isoniazid and rifampicin then continued for a further 7 to 10 months. Late scarring and urinary obstruction may occur in cases with extensive renal involvement, and such patients should be followed by ultrasonography or intravenous urogram.

Mycobacteria, both *M. tuberculosis* and atypical mycobacteria, have also emerged as important causes of opportunistic infection in immunocompromised patients undergoing dialysis and in patients undergoing renal transplantation. The possibility of mycobacterial disease must be considered in patients with fever of unknown origin or unexplained disease in the lungs or other organs. Results of the Mantoux test are usually negative, and diagnosis depends on maintaining a high index of suspicion and isolating the organism from the infected site.

Treponema pallidum

Renal involvement has been well documented in both congenital and acquired syphilis, with an estimated occurrence of 0.3% in patients with secondary syphilis and up to 5% in those with congenital syphilis (68,69). The most common manifestation of renal disease in congenital syphilis is the nephrotic syndrome, with proteinuria, hypoalbuminemia, and edema. In some patients, hematuria, uremia, and hypertension may be seen. The renal disease is usually associated with other manifestations of congenital syphilis, including hepatosplenomegaly, rash, and mucous membrane findings.

Nephritis in congenital syphilis is usually associated with evidence of complement activation, with depressed levels of C1q, C4, C3, and C5. Histologic findings are a diffuse proliferative GN or a membranous nephropathy. The interstitium shows a cellular infiltrate of polymorphonuclear and mononuclear cells (70). Immunofluorescent microscopy reveals diffuse granular deposits of IgG and C3 along the glomerular basement membrane (GBM). Mesangial deposits may also contain IgM. On electron microscopy, scattered subepithelial electron-dense deposits are seen, with fusion of epithelial cell foot processes (70).

Good evidence exists that renal disease is due to an immunologically mediated reaction to treponemal antigens. Antibodies reactive against treponemal antigens can be eluted from the glomerular deposits, and treponemal antigens are present in the immune deposits. Treatment of both congenital and acquired syphilis with antibiotics results in rapid improvement in the renal manifestations (68,70).

Mycoplasma pneumoniae

Renal involvement is surprisingly rare in *Mycoplasma pneumoniae* infection considering the prevalence of this organism and its propensity to trigger immunologically mediated diseases such as erythema multiforme, arthritis, and hemolysis. Acute nephritis associated with *Mycoplasma* infection may occur 10 to 40 days after the respiratory tract infection (71,72). Renal histopathologic findings include type 1 MPGN, proliferative endocapillary GN, and minimal change disease (73). Antibiotic treatment of the infection does not appear to affect the renal disease, which is self-limited in most cases (71,72).

RICKETTSIAL DISEASES

The rickettsial diseases are caused by a family of microorganisms that have characteristics common to both bacteria and viruses and that cause acute febrile illnesses associated with widespread vasculitis. With the exception of Q fever, all are associated with erythematous rashes. There are four groups of rickettsial diseases:

1. The typhus group includes louse-borne and murine typhus, spread by lice and fleas, respectively.
2. The spotted fever group includes Rocky Mountain spotted fever, tick typhus, and rickettsial pox, which

are spread by ticks and mites, with rodents as the natural reservoir.
3. Scrub typhus is spread by mites.
4. Q fever is spread by inhalation of infected particles from infected animals.

Rickettsial diseases have a worldwide distribution and vary widely in severity, from self-limited infections to fulminant and often fatal illnesses (74). In view of the widespread vasculitis associated with these infections, subclinical renal involvement probably occurs in many of the rickettsial diseases. However, in Rocky Mountain spotted fever, tick typhus, and Q fever, the renal involvement may be an important component of the illness.

Rocky Mountain Spotted Fever

Rocky Mountain spotted fever is the most severe of the rickettsial diseases (75,76). The onset occurs 2 to 8 days after the bite of an infected tick. High fever develops initially, followed by the pathognomonic rash, which occurs between the second and sixth days of the illness. The rash initially consists of small erythematous macules, but later these become maculopapular and petechial, and in untreated patients, confluent hemorrhagic areas may be seen. The rash first appears at the periphery and spreads up the trunk. Involvement of the palms and soles is a characteristic feature (74).

Headache, restlessness, meningism, and confusion may occur together with other neurologic signs. Cardiac involvement with congestive heart failure and arrhythmia are common. Pulmonary involvement occurs in 10 to 40% of cases. Infection is associated with an initial leukopenia, followed by neutrophil leukocytosis. Thrombocytopenia occurs in most cases.

Histopathologically, the predominant lesions are in the vascular system (77). Rickettsiae multiply in the endothelial cells, which results in focal areas of endothelial cell proliferation, perivascular mononuclear cell infiltration, thrombosis, and leakage of red cells into the tissues. The renal lesions involve both blood vessels and interstitium, and acute tubular necrosis may occur. Acute GN with immune-complex deposition has been reported (78), but in most cases the pathology appears to be a direct consequence of the invading organism on the renal vasculature (76,79).

Renal dysfunction is an important complication of Rocky Mountain spotted fever. Elevation of urea and creatinine levels occurs in a significant proportion of cases, and acidosis is common. Prerenal renal failure caused by hypovolemia and impaired cardiac function may respond to volume replacement and inotropic support, but acute renal failure may subsequently occur, necessitating dialysis.

Rocky Mountain spotted fever is diagnosed by the characteristic clinical picture, the exclusion of disorders with similar manifestations (e.g., measles, meningococcal disease, and leptospirosis), and detection of specific antibodies in convalescence. Culture of *Rickettsia rickettsii*, immunofluorescent staining, and polymerase chain reaction (PCR) testing of blood and skin biopsy specimens are available only in reference laboratories. Antibiotics should be administered in suspected cases without awaiting confirmation of the diagnosis (79). Doxycycline is the drug of choice for children of any age. Chloramphenicol is also effective (80). Intensive support of shock and multiorgan failure may be required in severe cases, and peritoneal dialysis or hemodialysis may be required until renal function returns. Before the advent of specific therapy, mortality was 25%. Today the overall mortality in the United States is still 5 to 7%. Death predominantly occurs in cases in which the diagnosis is delayed.

Q Fever

Q fever is caused by *Coxiella burnetii* and has a worldwide distribution, with the animal reservoir being cattle, sheep, and goats. Human infection follows inhalation of infected particles from the environment. The clinical manifestations range from an acute self-limited febrile illness with atypical pneumonia to involvement of specific organs that causes endocarditis, hepatitis, osteomyelitis, and central nervous system disease (81).

Proliferative GN may be associated with either Q fever endocarditis or a chronic infection elsewhere in the body (82). Renal manifestations range from asymptomatic proteinuria and hematuria to acute renal failure, hypertension, and nephrotic syndrome. Renal histologic findings are those of a diffuse proliferative GN, focal segmental GN, or mesangial GN. Immunofluorescent studies reveal diffuse glomerular deposits of IgM in the mesangium, together with C3 and fibrin. *C. burnetii* antigen has not been identified within the renal lesions.

Treatment of the underlying infection may result in remission of the renal disease, but prolonged treatment may be required for endocarditis. Tetracycline has been used in conjunction with rifampicin, co-trimoxazole, or a fluoroquinolone.

Legionnaires' Disease

Since its recognition in 1976, Legionnaires' disease, caused by *Legionella pneumophila*, has emerged as an important cause of pneumonia. The disease most commonly affects the elderly but has been reported in both normal and immunocompromised children (83,84). Renal dysfunction occurs in a minority of patients (84). Patients who develop renal impairment present with oliguria and rising urea and creatinine levels. They are usually severely ill, with bilateral pulmonary infiltrates, fever, and leukocytosis. Shock may be present, and the renal impairment has been associated with acute rhabdomyolysis with high levels of creatine phosphokinase and myoglobinuria. Renal histologic examination usually shows a tubulointerstitial nephritis or acute tubular necrosis (84,85). The pathogenesis of the renal impairment is uncertain, but the organism has been detected within the kidney on electron microscopy and immunofluorescent studies, which suggests a direct toxic effect. Myoglobinuria and decreased perfusion may also be contributing factors, however. Mortality has been high in reported cases of Legionnaires' disease complicated by renal failure. Treatment is based on dialysis, intensive care, and antimicrobial therapy with erythromycin (84). Steroid therapy may be effective for tubulointerstitial nephritis (85).

INTRAVASCULAR AND FOCAL INFECTIONS

Nephritis has been reported in association with the presence of a wide range of microorganisms that cause chronic or persistent infection (Table 51.2) (49,86). It is likely that any infectious agent that releases foreign antigens into the circulation, including those of very low virulence, can cause renal injury either by deposition of foreign antigens in the kidney or by the formation of immune complexes in the circulation, which are then deposited within the kidney. Nephritis is most commonly seen in association with intravascular infections such as SBE or infected ventriculoatrial shunts, but it is also seen after focal extravascular infections; ear, nose, and throat infections; and abscesses.

TABLE 51.2. FOCAL INFECTIONS CAUSING GLOMERULONEPHRITIS

Site of infection	Organism
Infective endocarditis	Coagulase-negative staphylococci
	Staphylococcus aureus
	Pneumococci
	Viridans streptococci
	Enterococci
	Anaerobic streptococci
	Diphtheroids
	Haemophilus influenzae
	Coliforms
	Bacteroides
	Coxiella burnetii
	Legionella
	Candida albicans
Shunt infections	Coagulase-negative staphylococci
	S. aureus
	Diphtheroids
	Gram-negative bacilli
	Anaerobes
Focal abscess	*S. aureus*
	Gram-negative bacilli
Osteomyelitis	*S. aureus*/streptococci
Pyelonephritis	Coliforms
Pneumonia	*Streptococcus pneumoniae*
	Klebsiella
	S. aureus
	Mycoplasma
Otitis media	Pneumococcus/*S. aureus*
Gastrointestinal infection	*Yersinia, Campylobacter*
	Salmonella, Shigella

Bacterial Endocarditis

Renal involvement is one of the diagnostic features of bacterial endocarditis. Virtually all organisms that cause endocarditis also produce renal involvement (Table 51.2). Although endocarditis caused by bacteria is the most common and is readily diagnosed by blood culture (86), unusual but important causes of culture-negative endocarditis include Q fever (87) and *Legionella* infection (88). In the immunocompromised individual, opportunistic pathogens such as fungi and mycobacteria are important causes.

The usual renal manifestations of SBE are asymptomatic proteinuria, hematuria, and pyuria. Loin pain, hypertension, nephrotic syndrome, and renal failure may occur in more severe cases.

The renal lesions occurring in endocarditis are variable, and focal embolic and immune-complex–mediated features may coexist (86,89,90). Embolic foci may be evident as areas of infarction, intracapillary thrombosis, or hemorrhage. More commonly, there is a focal necrotizing or diffuse proliferative GN. Immunofluorescent studies show glomerular deposits of IgG, IgM, IgA, and C3 along the GBM and within the mesangium. Electron microscopy reveals typical electron-dense deposits along the GBM and within the mesangium (86,89,90).

Early reports suggested that the renal lesions were caused by microemboli from infected vegetations depositing in the kidney, a hypothesis supported by the occasional presence of bacteria within the renal lesions. Most subsequent evidence, however, indicates that immunologic mechanisms rather than emboli are involved in the pathogenesis in most cases: bacteria are rarely found within the kidney, and renal involvement occurs with lesions of the right side of the heart, which would not be likely to embolize to the kidney. Immune complexes containing bacterial antigens are present in the circulation, and both bacterial antigens and bacteria-specific antibodies can be demonstrated within the immune deposits in the kidney. Serum C3 level is usually low, and complement can be found within both the circulating and the deposited immune complexes. These features all support an immune-complex–mediated pathogenesis of the renal injury (86,89,90).

Treatment of the endocarditis with antibiotics usually results in resolution of the GN and is associated with the disappearance of immune complexes from the circulation and return of C3 levels to normal. The prognosis of the renal lesions in SBE generally depends on the response of the underlying endocarditis to antibiotics or, in cases of antibiotic failure, to surgical removal of the infective vegetations (91).

Shunt Nephritis

The well-documented association of GN with infected ventriculoatrial shunts is another example of an immune-complex nephritis similar to that seen in endocarditis (92). Coagulase-negative staphylococci are the causative organisms in 75% of cases. The clinical and pathologic findings are similar to those in SBE. Presenting features are proteinuria, hematuria, and pyuria, and they may progress to renal failure. Immune complexes containing the bacterial antigens and complement are present in the serum, and C3 is depressed. Histologic findings are those of a diffuse mesangiocapillary GN. Immunofluorescent microscopy demonstrates deposits of immunoglobulin and C3 along the GBM, and bacterial antigen can be demonstrated in the renal lesions (93).

The prognosis for the renal lesion is good if the infection is treated early. This usually involves removal of the infected shunt and administration of appropriate antibiotics (92,94). The possible progression to end-stage renal disease requires frequent nephrologic monitoring of patients with ventriculoatrial shunts (92). There are a few reports in the literature of a similar renal complication occurring in chronic infection of ventriculoperitoneal shunts.

Other Focal Infections

GN has been reported after chronic abscesses (49), osteomyelitis, otitis media, pneumonia, and other focal infections (Table 51.2). Acute renal failure has been the presenting feature of focal infections in various sites, including the lung, pleura, abdominal cavity, sinuses, and pelvis. Many different organisms have been responsible, including *S. aureus, Pseudomonas, E. coli,* and *Proteus* species. This is probably another example of immune-complex GN. C3 level is decreased in approximately one-third of reported cases, and immunofluorescent studies reveal diffuse granular deposits of C3 in the glomeruli of all reported instances, with a variable presence of immunoglobulin. The renal lesion is that of MPGN and crescentic nephritis. The renal outcome is reported to be good with successful early treatment of the underlying infection.

VIRAL INFECTIONS

The role of viral infections in the causation of renal disease has been less well defined than that of bacterial infections. Clearly defined associations of renal disease have been made with hepatitis B virus (HBV), hepatitis C virus (HCV), HIV, and hantaviruses, but the role of most other viruses in the pathogenesis of renal disease is not clearly defined. Most viruses causing systemic infection may trigger immunologically mediated renal injury. With increasing application of molecular techniques, it may be that a significant proportion of GNs currently considered to be idiopathic will ultimately be shown to be virus induced. In children with immunodeficiency states and those undergoing renal transplantation, viruses such as cytomegalovirus (CMV) and polyoma virus have been recognized to be associated with nephropathy.

Hepatitis B Virus

Since the discovery of hepatitis B surface antigen (HB_sAg) in 1964, hepatitis virus has been shown to infect more than 5% of the world's population and is a major cause of chronic hepatitis, cirrhosis, and hepatocellular carcinoma worldwide. Some 150 million to 200 million people have HB_sAg in the circulation. The infection is most common in Africa and the Orient, where it is acquired in childhood by vertical transmission from infected mothers or by horizontal transmission from other children or adults. In developed countries, transmission in adults occurs more often by blood product exposure, sexual contact, or intravenous drug use.

HBV is a complex DNA virus with an outer surface envelope (HB_sAg) and an inner nucleocapsid core containing the hepatitis B core antigen (HB_cAg), DNA polymerase, protein kinase activity, and viral DNA. Incomplete spherical and filamentous viral particles consisting solely of HB_sAg are the major viral products in the circulation and may be present in concentrations of up to 10^{14} particles per milliliter of serum. Hepatitis B e antigen (HB_eAg) can be released from HB_cAg by proteolytic treatment and may be found in the circulation either free or complexed to albumin or IgG antibodies. The presence of HB_eAg correlates with the presence of complete viral particles and the infectivity of the individual (95).

Infection with HBV may result in either a self-limited infectious hepatitis followed by clearance of the virus and complete recovery, or a chronic or persistent infection in which the immune response is ineffective in eliminating the virus. Chronic HBV infection with continued presence of viral antigens in the circulation caused by an ineffective host immune response provides the best-documented example of immunologically mediated renal injury caused by persistent infection (96).

Patterns of Hepatitis B Virus Immunologically Mediated Renal Disease

Serum Sickness

A serum sickness–like illness occurs in 10 to 25% of patients in the early prodromal phase of HBV hepatitis. Fever, maculopapular or urticarial rash, and transient arthralgias or arthritis are common. Occasionally, proteinuria, hematuria, or sterile pyuria are observed. The syndrome usually lasts 3 to 10 days and often resolves before the onset of jaundice (96,97). There have been no histologic studies of the renal changes during HBV serum sickness.

Hepatitis B Virus–Associated Polyarteritis Nodosa

Since 1970, numerous reports have linked HBV infection with polyarteritis nodosa (PAN). Most of these cases have been in adults, but the disorder has also been reported in children (98,99). HBV-associated PAN most commonly occurs after intravenous acquisition of the virus, often during intravenous drug usage. HBV PAN appears to be uncommon in Africa and the Orient, where infection is usually acquired in childhood.

HBV PAN presents weeks to months after a clinically mild hepatitis but may occasionally predate the hepatitis. After a serum sickness–like illness, frank vasculitis affecting virtually any organ appears. Abdominal pain, fever, mononeuritis multiplex, and pulmonary and renal involvement may occur. The renal involvement may appear as hypertension, hematuria, proteinuria, or renal failure (see Chapter 44). Laboratory investigations reveal a florid acute-phase response, leukocytosis, and anemia. Transaminase levels are usually elevated, and HB_sAg is present in the circulation. The pathology consists of focal inflammation of small and medium-sized arteries, with fibrinoid necrosis, leukocyte infiltration, and fibrin deposition. Renal pathology may be limited to the medium-sized arteries or may coexist with GN (96,100).

Circulating immune complexes containing HB_sAg and anti-HB_s antibodies are usually present in the circulation (96,100). C3, C4, and total hemolytic complement levels are depressed. HB_sAg, IgG, and IgM antibodies to HBV and C3 have been identified by immunofluorescence in the blood vessels (100). Although most evidence suggests that the pathogenesis involves an immune-complex–mediated vasculitis, autoantibody or cell-mediated vascular injury may coexist. If the condition is untreated, the mortality is high (98). Most studies suggest that steroids or immunosuppressants help to suppress the vasculitis but potentially predispose to chronic infection or progressive liver disease (96,98). Successful treatment of hepatitis B–associated PAN with lamivudine, a nucleoside analogue, either alone or in combination with interferon-alpha and conventional immunosuppressive therapy, have been reported (101–103).

Hepatitis B Virus–Associated Membranous Glomerulonephritis

HBV is now the major cause of membranous GN (MGN) in children worldwide. The proportion of patients with MGN caused by HBV is directly related to the incidence of HB_sAg in the population, with 80 to 100% of all cases of MGN in some African and Oriental countries being associated with HBV (96,104) (see Chapter 33).

HBV MGN usually presents in children aged 2 to 12. There is a striking male predominance; in the United States, 80% of patients are males (105). The virus is usually acquired by vertical transmission from infected mothers or horizontally from infected family members. Unlike adults with HBV MGN, children do not usually have a history of hepatitis or of active liver disease, but liver function test results are generally mildly abnormal. Liver biopsy specimens may show minimal abnormalities, chronic persistent hepatitis, or (occasionally) more severe changes (105).

The renal manifestations are usually of proteinuria, nephrotic syndrome, microscopic hematuria, or (rarely) macroscopic hematuria. Hypertension occurs in less than 25% of cases, and renal insufficiency is rare.

HB_sAg and HB_cAg are usually present in the circulation, and HB_e antigenemia is seen in a high proportion of cases. Occasionally, HB_sAg may be found in the glomeruli but is absent from the circulation. C3 and C4 levels are often low, and circulating immune complexes are found in most cases.

Immunohistologic study reveals deposits of IgG and C3 and (less commonly) IgM and IgA in subepithelial, subendothelial, or mesangial tissue. HBV particles may be seen on electron microscopy, and all the major hepatitis B antigens, including HB_sAg, HB_cAg, and HB_eAg, have been localized in the glomerular capillary wall on immunofluorescence.

Immunologic deposition of HBV and antibody in the glomerular capillary wall is clearly involved in the glomerular injury, but the underlying immunologic events are incompletely understood (96,106). Passive trapping of circulating immune complexes may be involved, but the circulating immune complexes containing HB_sAg are usually larger than would be expected to penetrate the basement membrane. HB_sAg and HB_cAg are anionic and are therefore unlikely to penetrate the glomerular capillary wall. In contrast, HB_eAg forms smaller complexes with anti-HB_e antibodies and may readily penetrate the GBM. This may explain the observation that HB_eAg in the circulation frequently correlates with the severity of the disease (96). An alternative mechanism for immune-mediated glomerular injury is the trapping of HBV antigens by antibody previously deposited in the kidney. Anti-HB_e antibodies are cationic and may readily localize in the glomerulus and subsequently bind circulating antigen and complement. The third possibility is that the depositions of HBV and antibodies are consequences of glomerular injury by cellular mechanisms or autoantibodies. Little evidence supports this view at present (96).

Other Hepatitis B Virus Glomerulonephritides

HBV infection has been associated with a variety of other forms of GN in both adults and children. In a recent series in children MPGN was found to be equal in incidence to MGN in the spectrum of HBV-associated GNs (107). Both MPGN and mesangial proliferative GN may be triggered by HBV. In several countries where HBV is common, the proportion of patients with these forms of nephritides who test positive for HBV greatly exceeds the incidence of positivity in the general population (106). As with MGN and HBV-associated PAN, circulating immune complexes and localization of HBV antigens in the glomeruli have been reported in both MPGN and mesangial proliferative GN, and it is likely that similar mechanisms are occurring (96,108). Several other forms of GN have been associated with HBV, including IgA nephropathy, focal glomerulosclerosis, crescentic nephritis, and systemic lupus erythematosus, but the evidence for these associations is less consistent than for the entities discussed earlier (108).

Treatment of Hepatitis B Virus Glomerulonephritis

HBV is normally cleared as a result of cell-mediated responses in which cytotoxic T cells and natural killer cells eliminate infected hepatocytes. It is not surprising, therefore, that the administration of steroids and immunosuppressive agents either may have no effect on HBV disease or may increase the risk of progressive disease (109). Children with HBV MGN have a good prognosis, and two-thirds undergo spontaneous remission within 3 years of diagnosis. Steroid therapy does not appear to provide any additional benefit (96,104,110). Antiviral therapy with interferon-alpha and lamivudine shows promise in facilitating clearance of HBV, and reports of elimination of the infection with antiviral therapy in both children and adults, together with improvement or resolution of the coexisting renal disease, are increasing (110–113).

Hepatitis C Virus

HCV is an enveloped, single-stranded RNA virus of approximately 9.4 kilobases in the Flaviviridae family. There are six major HCV genotypes. Hepatitis C is a common disease affecting approximately 400 million people worldwide. In the United States, 3.9 million persons are estimated to be anti-HCV positive, and 2.7 million may be chronically infected (114). An estimated 240,000 children in the United States have antibody to HCV and 68,000 to 100,000 are chronically infected (115). Children become infected through receipt of contaminated blood products or through vertical transmission. The risk of vertical transmission increases with higher maternal viremia and maternal co-infection with HIV.

Acute HCV infection is rarely recognized in children outside of special circumstances such as a known exposure from an HCV-infected mother or after blood transfusion. Most chronically infected children are asymptomatic and have normal or only mildly abnormal alanine aminotransferase levels. Although the natural history of HCV infection during childhood seems benign in the majority of instances, the infection can take an aggressive course in a proportion of children, leading to cirrhosis and end-stage liver disease during childhood. The factors responsible for this more aggressive course are unidentified (115). Even in adults, the natural history of HCV infection has a variable course, but a significant proportion of patients will develop some degree of liver dysfunction, and 20 to 30% will eventually have end-stage liver disease as a result of cirrhosis. The risk of hepatocellular carcinoma is significant for those who have established cirrhosis. Hepatitis C is currently the most common condition leading to liver transplantation in adults in the Western world.

GN has been described as an important complication of chronic infection with HCV in adults. The clinical presentation is usually of nephrotic syndrome or proteinuria, hypertension, or hematuria, with or without azotemia (116). MPGN, with or without cryoglobulinemia, and MGN are most commonly described. Isolated case reports of other, more unusual patterns of glomerular injury, including IgA nephropathy, focal segmental glomerulosclerosis, crescentic GN, fibrillary GN, and thrombotic microangiopathy, have also been associated with HCV infection (116,117). Glomerular deposition of hepatitis antigens and antibodies has been described and is believed to play a role in pathogenesis. Cryoglobulinemia is a common accompaniment of GN that is associated with the depression of serum complement levels (116). Renal failure may develop in 40 to 100% of patients who have MPGN (116,118). The presence of virus-like particles as well as viral RNA within the kidney sections of patients with HCV-associated glomerulopathies has been reported (119).

The diagnosis should be suspected if glomerular disease is associated with chronic hepatitis, particularly with the presence of cryoglobulins, but renal biopsy is necessary to establish a definitive diagnosis.

HCV infection is relatively common in children with end-stage renal disease and is an important cause of liver disease in this population. Acquisition of HCV infection continues to occur in dialysis patients because of nosocomial spread (120). Elevation of transaminase level is not a sensitive marker of infection in children and HCV enzyme-linked immunosorbent assay or PCR testing should be used to increase sensitivity (121). HCV-infected renal transplant recipients had higher mortality and hospitalization rates than other transplant recipients (122), and HCV infection has been reported to be associated with de novo immune-mediated GN, especially type 1 MPGN, in renal allografts, resulting in accelerated loss of graft function (123,124).

No large randomized, controlled trials of treatment of children with chronic hepatitis C have been performed. Small heterogeneous studies of interferon monotherapy have reported sustained virologic response rates of 35 to 40% (115). In adults, improvement of proteinuria and renal function often follows interferon-alpha treatment (116,118), but relapses are common after cessation of treatment. Combination of interferon with ribavirin in patients with chronic liver disease has been shown to increase the rate of sustained response in these patients (125). As yet, however, there are few data regarding the use of combination therapy with interferon and ribavirin in children. Moreover, interferon-alpha therapy is associated with acute or subacute renal failure in more than one-third of the patients with renal transplants (126).

Herpes Viruses

Cytomegalovirus

CMV is one of the eight human herpes viruses. Transmission of the virus requires exposure to infected body fluids such as breast milk, saliva, urine, or blood. Individuals initially infected with CMV may be asymptomatic or display nonspecific flu-like symptoms. After the initial infection CMV, like all herpes viruses, establishes latency for life but will be periodically excreted by an asymptomatic host. CMV replicates within renal cells, and on biopsy samples from immunocompromised hosts, viral inclusions can be visualized by light microscopy in cells of the convoluted tubules and collecting ducts (127). Glomerular cells and shed renal tubular cells may have characteristic inclusions, but clinically evident renal disease is rare and is seen virtually only in immunocompromised or congenitally infected children (127,128).

The clinical manifestations of CMV-induced renal disease in congenitally infected infants are variable and range from asymptomatic proteinuria to nephrotic syndrome and renal impairment. In congenital CMV infection, histologic changes of viral inclusions commonly occur in the tubules. In addition, proliferative GN has been reported, with evidence on electron microscopy of viral immune deposits in glomerular cells (128,129). In CMV-infected immunocompromised patients, immune-complex GN has been documented with mesangial deposits of IgG, IgA, C3, and CMV antigens within glomeruli. Eluted glomerular immunoglobulins have been shown to contain CMV antigens (130).

CMV is the most common viral infection after kidney transplantation. Experience with pediatric kidney transplant recipients suggests a 67% incidence of CMV infection (131). The direct and indirect effects of CMV infection result in significant morbidity and mortality among kidney transplant recipients. CMV-negative patients who receive a CMV-positive allograft are at risk for primary infection and graft dysfunction. Patients who are CMV seropositive at the time of transplantation are also at risk of reactivation and superinfection. Tubulointerstitial nephritis is a well-characterized pathologic feature of renal allograft CMV disease, which can be difficult to distinguish from injury caused by rejection. Histologic evidence of endothelial cell injury and mononuclear cell infiltration in the glomeruli has been reported (130). CMV glomerular vasculopathy in the absence of tubulointerstitial disease, causing renal allograft dysfunction, has also been reported (132). Beyond the acute allograft nephropathy associated with CMV viremia, CMV is known to cause chronic vascular injury. This may adversely affect the long-term outcome of the allograft and may be the explanation for the observed association with chronic allograft nephropathy (133).

Newer techniques for rapidly diagnosing CMV infection are becoming widely available and include shell vial culture, pp65 antigenemia assay, PCR, and the hybrid-capture RNA-DNA hybridization assay for qualitative detection of CMV PCR. Quantitative plasma PCR testing (PCR viral load) is increasingly used for diagnosis and monitoring of CMV viremia in renal transplant recipients.

Antiviral agents that have been shown to be effective against CMV include ganciclovir, valganciclovir, foscarnet, and cidofovir. Ganciclovir remains the drug of choice for treating established disease. Intravenous ganciclovir therapy is preferred in children because of the erratic absorption of oral ganciclovir. Major limitations of ganciclovir therapy are the induction of renal tubular dysfunction and bone marrow toxicity, principally neutropenia and thrombocytopenia. Dosage adjustments are necessary for recipients with renal dysfunction. Recent studies suggest that valganciclovir given orally is at least as good as ganciclovir in preventing CMV infection (134). Use of other antiviral agents such as foscarnet and cidofovir is limited because of nephrotoxicity and difficulty of administration. A number of reports have demonstrated the effectiveness of high-titer CMV immune globulin therapy in reducing severe CMV-associated disease when used in combination with ganciclovir (131,135).

Varicella-Zoster Virus

The association of varicella with nephritis has been known for more than 100 years since Henoch reported on four children with nephritis that occurred after the appearance of varicella vesicles. Varicella, however, is rarely associated with renal complications (136). In fatal cases with disseminated varicella and in the immunocompromised individual, renal involvement is more common. Cases in which varicella infection caused GN in renal transplant recipients have been reported (137). Histologic findings in fatal cases include congested hemorrhagic glomeruli, endothelial cell hyperplasia, and tubular necrosis. In mild and nonfatal cases and in nonimmunocompromised individuals, varicella is occasionally associated with a variety of renal manifestations, ranging from mild nephritis to nephrotic syndrome and acute renal failure (138). Histologic findings include endocapillary cell proliferation, epithelial and endothelial cell hyperplasia, and inflammatory cell infiltration (136). Rapidly progressive nephritis has also been reported. Immunohistochemical studies reveal glomerular deposition of IgG, IgM, IgA, and C3. On electron microscopy, granular electron-dense deposits have been found in the paramesangial region, and varicella antigens may be deposited in the glomeruli. The features suggest an immune-complex nephritis. Elevated circulating levels of IgG and IgA immune complexes and depressed C3 and C4 levels support this possibility (136).

Fulminant disseminated varicella and varicella in immunocompromised patients should be treated with intravenous acyclovir.

Epstein-Barr Virus

Renal involvement is common during acute infectious mononucleosis, usually manifesting as an abnormal urine sediment, with hematuria in up to 60% of cases. Hematuria, either microscopic or macroscopic, usually appears within the first week of the illness and lasts for a few weeks to a few months. Proteinuria is usually absent or low grade. More severe renal involvement with proteinuria, nephrotic syndrome, or acute nephritis with renal failure is much less common. Acute renal failure may be seen during the course of fulminant infectious mononucleosis with associated hepatic failure, thrombocytopenia, and encephalitis. It is usually caused by interstitial nephritis that is likely the result of immunopathologic injury precipitated by Epstein-Barr virus (EBV) infection. However, the identification of EBV DNA in the kidney raises the possibility that direct infection might play a role (139). The renal involvement must be distinguished from myoglobinuria caused by rhabdomyolysis, which may occur in infectious mononucleosis, and from bleeding into the renal tract as a result of thrombocytopenia.

Renal histologic findings in EBV nephritis are an interstitial nephritis with mononuclear cell infiltration and foci of tubular necrosis. Glomeruli may show varying degrees of mesangial proliferation. On immunohistochemical study, EBV antigens are seen in glomerular and tubular deposits. The prognosis for complete recovery of renal function is good. Treatment with corticosteroids may have a role in the management of EBV-induced acute renal failure and may shorten the duration of renal failure (140).

EBV-associated posttransplantation lymphoproliferative disease is a recognized complication in renal transplant recipients. Latent infection of EBV in renal proximal tubular epithelial cells has recently been described as causing idiopathic chronic tubulointerstitial nephritis (141).

Herpes Simplex Virus

The herpes simplex virus (HSV) causes persistent infection characterized by asymptomatic latent periods interspersed with acute relapses. As in other chronic and persistent infections, immunologically mediated disorders triggered by HSV are well recognized, and it is perhaps surprising that HSV has rarely been linked to nephritis. Acute nephritis and nephrotic syndrome have been associated with herpes simplex encephalitis. Renal histology shows focal segmental GN with mesangial and segmental deposits of IgM, C3, and HSV antigens. As with other herpes viruses, HSV has been suggested as a trigger for IgA nephritis, MPGN, and membranous nephropathy. Elevated levels of HSV antibodies have been reported in patients with a variety of forms of GN, but no conclusive evidence exists of an etiologic role for HSV (142).

Adenovirus, Enterovirus, and Influenza Virus

Adenovirus, enterovirus, and influenza virus are unrelated ubiquitous pathogens that infect large proportions of the population annually and yet are rarely associated with renal disease. The literature contains scattered reports of acute nephritis after infection with each of these viruses.

Adenovirus is a major cause of hemorrhagic cystitis and was implicated as the cause of hemorrhagic cystitis in 23 to 51% of children with this disorder (143). Boys are affected more often than girls, and hematuria persists for 3 to 5 days. Microscopic hematuria, dysuria, and frequency may occur for longer periods. Adenovirus types 11 and 21 are the usual strains isolated.

Influenza virus and enteroviruses, including echovirus and coxsackievirus, have been linked with acute nephritis and acute renal failure associated with rhabdomyolysis. In the newborn, enteroviruses cause fulminant disease with DIC, shock, and liver failure, and acute renal failure may occur.

Measles Virus

Renal involvement from measles virus is uncommon, although measles virus can be cultured from the kidney in fatal cases. An acute GN has been reported to follow measles with evidence of immune deposits containing measles virus antigen within the glomeruli. The nephritis is generally self-limiting (144).

Mumps Virus

Mild renal involvement is common during the acute phase of mumps infection. One-third of children with mumps have abnormal urinalysis results, with microscopic hematuria or proteinuria. Mumps virus may be isolated from urine during the first 5 days of the illness, at a time when urinalysis findings are abnormal. Plasma creatinine concentrations usually remain normal, despite the abnormal urine sediment, but more severe cases in adults have been associated with evidence of acute nephritis with impaired renal function. Renal biopsy specimens demonstrate an MPGN with deposition of IgA, IgM, C3, and mumps virus antigen in the glomeruli, which suggests an immune-complex–mediated process (145).

Human Immunodeficiency Virus

The World Health Organization estimated that there were 38.9 million adults and 3.2 million children living with HIV infection and acquired immunodeficiency syndrome (AIDS) in December 2002. Nearly 800,000 children were infected with HIV in 2002, mostly through their mothers before or during birth or through breast feeding (vertical transmission). A total of 610,000 children died of HIV/AIDS in 2002. Renal involvement in HIV infection was first described in 1984 in adults (146–148) and in children (149), and renal involvement occurs in 2 to 15% of HIV-infected children in the United States (150–152). Since the development of highly active antiretroviral therapy (HAART), however, the incidence of renal disease in HIV infection in both adults and children in industrialized countries has declined.

HIV-associated nephropathy (HIVAN) is characterized by both glomerular and tubular dysfunction, the pathogenesis of which is not entirely known. HIVAN is a clinicopathologic entity that includes proteinuria, azotemia, focal segmental glomerulosclerosis or mesangial hyperplasia, and tubulointerstitial disease (152). In adults in the United States, there is a markedly increased risk of nephropathy among African American persons with HIV infection. This appears to be true in children as well, but the data are sparse. The spectrum of HIVAN seems to be coincident with the degree of AIDS symptomatology. It is thought that HIVAN can present at any point in HIV infection, but most patients with HIVAN have CD4 counts of less than $200 \times 10^6/200$ cells/mL, which suggests that it may be primarily a manifestation of late-stage disease (153).

Although a spectrum of clinicopathologic entities including mesangial hyperplasia, focal segmental glomerulosclerosis, minimal change disease, and systemic lupus erythematosus nephritis has been described, the classic pathologic feature of HIVAN is the collapsing form of focal and segmental glomerulosclerosis (154). In the affected glomeruli, visceral epithelial cells are hypertrophied and hyperplastic, and contain large cytoplasmic vacuoles and numerous protein resorption droplets. There is microcystic distortion of tubule segments, which contributes to increasing kidney size. Podocyte hyperplasia can become so marked that it causes obliteration of much of the urinary space, forming "pseudocrescents" (155). Capillary walls are wrinkled and collapsed with obliteration of the capillary lumina. The interstitium is edematous with a variable degree of T-cell infiltration (156). The Bowman capsule can also be dilated and filled with a precipitate of plasma protein that represents the glomerular ultrafiltrate. One of the most distinctive features of HIVAN, however, is the presence of numerous tubuloreticular inclusions within the cytoplasm of glomerular and peritubular capillary endothelial cells (155).

Immunofluorescence testing is positive for IgM and C3 in capillary walls in a coarsely granular to amorphous pattern in a segmental distribution (154,156).

The presence of the HIV genome in glomerular and tubular epithelium has been demonstrated using complementary DNA probes and *in situ* hybridization. Proviral DNA has been detected by PCR in the glomeruli, tubules, and interstitium of microdissected kidneys from patients who had pathologic evidence of HIVAN, but it has also been detected in the kidneys of HIV-positive patients with other glomerulopathies (157). A combination of both proliferation and apoptosis of renal cells may cause the loss of nephron architecture. Apoptosis has been demonstrated in cells in the glomerulus, tubules, and interstitium of biopsy specimens from HIV-positive patients with focal segmental glomerulosclerosis. In addition, the role of various cytokines and growth factors, specifically transforming growth factor β (TGF-β), in the development of sclerosis has been studied (158,159).

Transgenic murine models provide some of the strongest evidence for a direct role of HIV-1 in the induction of HIVAN. These mice do not produce infectious virus but express the HIV envelope and regulatory genes at levels sufficient to re-create the HIVAN that is seen in humans (158). The kidneys of these transgenic mice have also been found to have elevated levels of TGF-β messenger RNA and protein (159). Additional factors such as genetic predisposition may explain the fact that African Americans have a greater likelihood of developing HIVAN than other racial groups.

HIV infection is also associated with other forms of renal disease. Glomerular syndromes other than HIVAN include MGN that resembles lupus nephritis and immune-complex GN, with IgA nephropathy and HCV-associated MPGN being the most common forms. There have also been several case reports of amyloid kidney (152,155,160). The kidneys may be affected by various other mechanisms. Opportunistic infections with organisms such as BK virus (BKV) that give rise to nephropathy and hemorrhagic cystitis have been reported in association with HIV infection (161). Systemic infections accompanied by hypotension can cause prerenal failure leading to acute tubular necrosis. Acute tubular necrosis has also been reported in HIV patients after the use of nephrotoxic drugs such as pentamidine, foscarnet, cidofovir, amphotericin B, and aminoglycosides. Intratubular obstruction with crystal precipitation can occur with the use of sulfonamides and intravenous acyclovir. Indinavir is well recognized to cause nephropathy and renal calculi (162). MPGN associated with mixed cryoglobulinemia and thrombotic microangiopathy/atypical HUS in association with HIV infections have been reported (163,164).

HIVAN can manifest as mild proteinuria, nephrotic syndrome, renal tubular acidosis, hematuria, and/or acute renal failure (149–152). Nephrotic syndrome and chronic renal insufficiency are late manifestations of HIVAN. Children with HIVAN are likely to develop transient electrolytic disorders, heavy proteinuria, and acute renal failure due to systemic infectious episodes or nephrotoxic drugs.

Early stages of HIVAN can be identified by the presence of proteinuria and "urine microcysts" along with renal sonograms showing enlarged echogenic kidneys. Urinary renal tubular epithelial cells are frequently grouped together to form these microcysts, which were found in the urine of children with HIVAN who had renal tubular injury (152). Advanced stages of HIVAN typically present with nephrotic syndrome with edema, heavy proteinuria, hypoalbuminemia, and few red or white blood cells in urinary sediments. Hypertension may be present, but usually blood pressure is within or below the normal range. HIVAN in adults follows a rapidly progressive course, with end-stage renal disease developing within 1 to 4 months, but in children this rapid progression does not necessarily occur. Definitive diagnosis of HIVAN should be based on biopsy results, and biopsy should be performed if significant proteinuria is present, because in approximately 50% of HIV-infected patients with azotemia and/or proteinuria (>1 g/24 hr) who undergo renal biopsy, the specimen will have histologic features consistent with other renal diseases (153).

When available, HAART should be given to children with symptomatic HIV disease. Specific treatment of HIVAN remains controversial. Several studies have looked at the role of HAART, angiotensin I–converting enzyme (ACE) inhibitors, steroids, and even cyclosporin with somewhat encouraging results. However, as yet no randomized case-controlled trials have been undertaken. Most of the studies have been small and retrospective, and many have included patients both with and without renal biopsy–proven HIVAN. Cyclosporin has been used to treat HIVAN in children with remission of nephrotic syndrome (150). Similar responses have been reported to treatment with corticosteroids in various studies (165–168). ACE inhibitors have been used with encouraging results (169).

The general regimen used to treat patients with HIV, including HAART, should be applied to children with HIVAN. The dosages of some medications must be adjusted to the patient's glomerular filtration. There are reports of spontaneous regression of HIVAN with supportive management and treatment with HAART, particularly with regimes containing protease inhibitors (170–173). It should be emphasized that the improvement reported with other modalities of treatment such as corticosteroids, cyclosporin, and ACE inhibitors always occurs when these agents are given in conjunction with antiretroviral therapy.

Several other therapeutic options have been suggested, aimed specifically at the presumed role of TGF-β in the pathogenesis of HIVAN. Treatment directed at its synthesis using gene therapy to block TGF-β gene expression is being explored. Therapy directed at decreasing the activity of TGF-β using anti–TGF-β antibodies or other inhibitory substances is also an area of investigation. In addition, blocking renal receptors for chemokines such as RANTES (*r*egulated upon *a*ctivation, *n*ormal *T* cell *e*xpressed and *s*ecreted), interleukin-8, and monocyte-chemoattractant protein-1 has been proposed as another possible treatment alternative (174).

Most reports of HIV-infected patients on hemodialysis have shown poor prognosis, with mean patient survival times ranging from 14 to 47 months. Mortality is therefore still close to 50% within the first year of dialysis. In general, improved survival is associated with younger age at initiation of hemodialysis and with higher CD4 counts. Access complications such as infection and thrombosis tend to occur at a higher rate in HIV-infected hemodialysis patients. Cross infection with HIV in dialysis patients is very rare. No patient-to-patient HIV transmission has yet been reported in a hemodialysis unit in the United States, although several such cases have occurred in South America (174,175).

Peritoneal dialysis is an alternative for HIV-infected patients. The incidence of peritonitis varies across studies, but some studies did report a higher incidence of *Pseudomonas* and fungal peritonitis in the HIV-positive population (174). Infections with unusual organisms such as *Pasteurella multocida*, *Trichosporon beigelii*, and *Mycobacterium avium-intracellulare* complex have also been reported. Several studies, however, have suggested that there is no significant difference between the HIV-infected and non–HIV-infected populations. Of note is that virus capable of replication *in vitro* has been recovered from the peritoneal dialysis effluent, and it can be recoverable for up to 7 days in dialysis bags at room temperature and for up to 48 hours in dry exchange tubing (174).

In general, long-term dialysis is thought to be preferable to renal transplantation, primarily because of the concern that the immunosuppressive therapy required after transplantation could promote progression of HIV/AIDS. The safety and efficacy of organ transplantation in the HAART era have not been described. A multicenter prospective study has been initiated to address these questions (176). However, a preliminary report presented at the Conference on Retroviruses and Opportunistic Infections in 2002 noted that the survival and graft function rates for HIV-infected transplantation recipients appeared to be good and that the rate of development of opportunistic infections is low in those with well-controlled HIV and relatively high CD4 counts (177).

Human Polyoma Virus

The human polyoma viruses (HPV) are members of the papovavirus family and have received increasing attention as pathogens in immunocompromised patients. They are nonenveloped viruses ranging in size from 45 to 55 nm, with a circular, double-stranded DNA genome that replicates in the host nucleus. The best-known species in this genus are the BKV, the JC virus (JCV), and the simian virus SV40. BKV was first isolated from the urine of a 39-year-old man who developed ureteral stenosis 4 months after renal transplantation (178). The name of the virus refers to the first patient's initials, which is also true of JCV. BKV establishes infection in the kidney and the urinary tract, and its activation causes a number of disorders, including nephropathy and hemorrhagic cystitis. BKV-associated nephropathy has become an increasingly recognized cause of renal dysfunction in renal transplantation patients (179–183). JCV establishes latency mainly in the kidney, and its reactivation can result in the development of progressive multifocal leukoencephalopathy. Recent studies have reported SV40 in the allografts of children who received renal transplants and in the urine, blood, and kidneys of adults with focal segmental glomerulosclerosis, which is a cause of end-stage renal disease and an indication for kidney transplantation (184).

BKV infection is endemic worldwide. Seroprevalence rates as high as 60 to 80% have been reported among adults in the United States and Europe. The peak incidence of primary infection (as measured by acquisition of antibody) occurs in children 2 to 5 years of age. BKV antibody may be detected in as many as 50% of children by 3 years of age, and in 60 to 100% of children by 9 or 10 years of age; antibodies wane thereafter. BKV infection may be particularly important in the pediatric transplantation population, in whom primary infection has a high probability of occurring while the children are immunosuppressed (185).

Primary infection with BKV in healthy children is rarely associated with clinical manifestations. Mild pyrexia, malaise, vomiting, respiratory illness, pericarditis, and transient hepatic dysfunction have been reported with primary infection. Investigators hypothesize that after an initial round of viral replication at the site of entry, viremia follows with dissemination of the virus to distant sites at which latent infection is established. The most frequently recognized secondary sites of latent infection are renal and uroepithelial cells. Secondary infection has been reported to cause tubulointerstitial nephritis and ureteral stenosis in renal transplantation patients. It may be that renal impairment in immunocompromised patients and in nonrenal solid organ transplant recipients is found to be frequently associated with BKV infection.

BK Virus Nephropathy in Patients Undergoing Renal Transplantation

The reported prevalence of BKV nephropathy in renal allografts is between 1 and 8% (179,180,183,186). Asymptomatic infection is characterized by viral shedding without any apparent clinical features. Viruria, resulting from either primary or secondary infection, can persist from several weeks to years. Tubulointerstitial nephritis associated with BKV in renal transplant recipients is accompanied by histopathologic changes, with or without functional impairment. "Infection" and "disease" must be differentiated carefully. BKV infection (either primary or reactivated) can progress to BKV disease, but will not always do so (185). Furthermore, not all cases of BKV disease lead to renal impairment. However, infection can progress to transplant dysfunction and graft loss, although the diagnosis may be complicated by the coexistence of active allograft rejection.

BKV nephritis is reported to have a bimodal distribution, with 50% of BKV-related interstitial nephritis cases occurring 4 to 8 weeks after transplantation and the remainder of patients developing disease months to years after transplantation (187). Allograft failure is due mainly to extensive viral replication in tubular epithelial cells leading to frank tubular necrosis (181). Although damage is potentially fully reversible early in the disease, persisting viral damage leads to irreversible interstitial fibrosis. Tubular atrophy and allograft loss has been observed in 45% of affected patients (181,188).

In most cases, BKV nephropathy in adult renal transplant recipients represents a secondary infection associated with rejection and its treatment. In children, however, primary BKV infection giving rise to allograft dysfunction may occur (185).

The definitive diagnosis of BKV nephropathy requires renal biopsy. Histopathologic features include severe tubular injury with cellular enlargement, marked nuclear atypia, epithelial necrosis, denudation of tubular basement membranes, focal intratubular neutrophilic infiltration, and mononuclear interstitial infiltration, with or without concurrent tubulitis. This constellation of histologic features, particularly severe tubulitis, is often misinterpreted as rejection, even by the experienced pathologist. The presence of well-demarcated basophilic or amphophilic intranuclear viral inclusions, primarily within the tubular and parietal epithelium of the Bowman capsule, can help distinguish BKV disease from rejection (180,181,183). Additional tests such as immunohistochemistry, PCR analysis, or electron microscopy of biopsied tissue aimed at the identification of BKV may be required.

A practical diagnostic approach for identifying BKV in renal transplant patients is summarized in Table 51.3.

Ureteral Stenosis in Renal Transplantation

BKV infection may cause ureteral obstruction due to ureteral ulceration and stenosis at the ureteric anastomosis. BKV-associated ureteral stenosis has been reported in 3% of renal transplant patients and usually occurs between 50 and 300 days after transplantation. Ulceration due to inflammation, proliferation of the transitional epithelial cells, and smooth muscle proliferation may lead to partial or total obstruction.

Hemorrhagic Cystitis in Bone Marrow Transplantation

BKV may be involved in acute, late-onset, long-duration hemorrhagic cystitis after bone marrow transplantation (189).

Treatment

Whether patients with asymptomatic viremia or viruria need specific therapeutic intervention is not certain. Review of the literature suggests that careful reduction of immune suppression, combined with active surveillance for rejection, will result in clinical improvement. Reduction in immunosuppression may precipitate episodes of acute cellular rejection, which need to be judiciously treated with corticosteroids. The outcome of BKV nephropathy is unpredictable, and stabilization of renal function may occur regardless of whether maintenance immunotherapy is altered or not (190).

Some reports favor the use of cidofovir. Cidofovir has important nephrotoxic side effects in the usual therapeutic dosage recommended for the treatment of CMV infection, and for BKV nephropathy a reduced dosage regime is generally used. The efficacy of cidofovir in reducing viremia

TABLE 51.3. DIAGNOSIS OF BK VIRUS (BKV) IN RENAL TRANSPLANT RECIPIENTS

Tests	Comments
Urine:	
Cytology: decoy cells BKV PCR	Presence of BKV by PCR or decoy cells in urine signifies BKV replication. Decoy cells are caused by infection of the urinary epithelial cells with HPV. The nuclei are enlarged and nuclear chromatin is completely homogenized by viral cytopathic effect. Positive PCR results for BKV viruria and presence of decoy cells have poor predictive value. Specificity is increased if >10 cells/ Cytospin along with presence of inflammatory cells.
Serum:	
Antibody assays BKV	Presence of antibody is usually indicative of previous infection; however, positive results for BKV DNA PCR on serum signifies BK viremia. BKV PCR testing of plasma has proven to be a sensitive (100%) and specific (88%) means to identify BKV–associated nephropathy in adults. Viral load has also been used to monitor infection and clearance. However, because primary infection occurs in childhood, it might not be applicable to the pediatric population.
Tissue:	
Histopathology Electron microscopy BKV PCR	The definitive diagnosis of BKV nephropathy requires renal biopsy. Histopathology might mimic rejection or drug toxicity. However, characteristic findings have been described. Electron microscopy and immune staining are helpful in confirming the diagnosis. PCR assays of viral load in tubular cells have been reported to be a sensitive marker for diagnosis and monitoring.

HPV, human polyoma virus; PCR, polymerase chain reaction.

has been demonstrated (191). However, spontaneous clearance of viral infection after reduction of immunosuppression (without cidofovir) has also been reported.

Viral Hemorrhagic Fever

Viral hemorrhagic fever involves at least 12 distinct RNA viruses that share the propensity to cause severe disease with prominent hemorrhagic manifestations (Table 51.4). The viral hemorrhagic fevers, widely distributed throughout both temperate and tropical regions of the world, are important causes of mortality and morbidity in many countries. Most viral hemorrhagic fevers are zoonoses (with the possible exception of dengue virus), in which the virus is endemic in animals and human infection is acquired through the bite of an insect vector. Aerosol and nosocomial transmissions from infected patients are important for Lassa, Junin, Machupo, and Congo-Crimean hemorrhagic fevers, and Marburg and Ebola viruses (192).

Viral hemorrhagic fevers have many clinical similarities but also important differences in their severity, major organs affected, prognosis, and response to treatment. In all viral hemorrhagic fevers, severe cases occur in only a minority of those affected; subclinical infection or nonspecific febrile illness occurs in the majority. Fever, myalgia, headache, conjunctival suffusion, and erythematous rash occur in all the viral hemorrhagic fevers (193). Hemorrhagic manifestations range from petechiae and bleeding from venipuncture sites to severe hemorrhage into the GI tract, kidney, and other organs. A capillary leak syndrome, with evidence of hemoconcentration, pulmonary edema, oliguria, and ultimately shock, occurs in the most severely affected patients (193). Renal involvement occurs in all the viral hemorrhagic fevers, proteinuria is common, and prerenal failure is seen in all severe cases complicated by shock. However, in Congo-Crimean hemorrhagic fever and hemorrhagic fever with renal syndrome (HFRS), an interstitial nephritis, which may be hemorrhagic, is characteristic, and renal impairment is a major component of the illness.

Dengue

Dengue is endemic and epidemic in tropical America, Africa, and Asia, where the mosquito vector *Aedes aegypti* is present (194). Classic dengue is a self-limited nonfatal disease; dengue hemorrhagic fever and dengue shock syndrome, which occur in a minority of patients, have a high mortality. After an incubation period of 5 to 8 days, the illness begins with fever, headache, arthralgia, weakness, vomiting, and hyperesthesia. In uncomplicated dengue the fever usually lasts 5 to 7 days. Shortly after onset a maculopapular rash appears, sparing the palms and the soles, and is occasionally followed by desquamation. Fever may reappear at the onset of the rash.

In dengue hemorrhagic fever and dengue shock syndrome, the typical febrile illness is complicated by hemorrhagic manifestations, ranging from a positive tourniquet test result or petechiae to purpura, epistaxis, and GI bleeding with thrombocytopenia and evidence of a consumptive coagulopathy. Increased capillary permeability is suggested by hemoconcentration, edema, and pleural effusions (194). In severe cases, hypotension and shock supervene, largely as a result of hypovolemia. Renal manifestations include oliguria, proteinuria, hematuria, and rising urea and creatinine. Acute renal failure occurs in patients with severe shock, primarily as a result of renal underperfusion. However, glomerular inflammatory changes may also occur. Children with dengue hemorrhagic fever show hypertrophy of endothelial and mesangial cells, mononuclear cell infiltrate, thinning of basement membranes, and deposition of IgG, IgM, and C3. Electron microscopy shows viral particles within glomerular mononuclear cells (195).

The diagnosis of dengue is made by isolation of the virus from blood or by serologic testing. There is no specific antivi-

TABLE 51.4. VIRAL HEMORRHAGIC FEVERS (HF)

Virus	Geographic distribution	Source of human infection	Incubation period (d)	Renal involvement	Renal pathology	Treatment
Dengue	Tropical Africa, South America, Asia	Mosquito	5–8	Rare, only in Dengue HF or shock	Vasomotor nephropathy, immune complex	Supportive
Yellow fever	Africa, South America	Mosquito	3–6	Common	Vasomotor nephropathy	Supportive
Congo-Crimean	Eastern Europe, Africa, Asia	Tick, nosocomial	2–7	In severe cases	Vasomotor nephropathy	Supportive ? Ribavirin
Hantaan viruses (Puumala, Seoul strains)	Europe, Asia, Africa, America	Rodents	4–42	HF and renal syndrome (Korean, Chinese, and Japanese epidemic HF, nephropathia epidemica)	Vasomotor nephropathy	Supportive
					Interstitial nephropathy	? Ribavirin
Rift Valley fever	Sub-Saharan Africa	Mosquito, contact with infected animals	3–7	Rare, only in fulminant cases	Vasomotor nephropathy	Supportive
Lassa fever	West Africa	Rodents, nosocomial	3–16	In cases with shock	Vasomotor nephropathy	Supportive and ribavirin
Junin, Argentine HF	Argentina	Rodents, nosocomial	5–19	In cases with shock	Vasomotor nephropathy	Supportive
Machupo, Bolivian HF	Bolivia	Rodents, nosocomial	5–19	In cases with shock	Vasomotor nephropathy	Supportive
Marburg	Africa	?, nosocomial	5–10	In cases with shock	Vasomotor nephropathy	Supportive
Ebola	Africa	?, nosocomial	5–10	In cases with shock	Vasomotor nephropathy	Supportive
Omsk	Eastern Europe	Tick	2–4	In cases with shock	Vasomotor nephropathy	Supportive
Kyasanur forest	India	Tick	3–8	In cases with shock	Vasomotor nephropathy	Supportive

ral treatment, and management of patients with dengue shock syndrome or dengue hemorrhagic fever depends on aggressive circulatory support and volume replacement with colloid and crystalloid. With correction of hypovolemia, renal impairment is usually reversible, but dialysis may be required in patients with established acute renal failure.

Yellow Fever

Yellow fever remains an important public health problem in Africa and South America. Renal manifestations are common and include albuminuria and oliguria. Over the next few days after first manifestation of infection, shock, delirium, coma, and renal failure develop, and death occurs 7 to 10 days after onset of symptoms. Laboratory findings include thrombocytopenia and evidence of hemoconcentration, rising urea and creatinine levels, hyponatremia, and deranged liver function test results. Pathologic findings include necrosis of liver lobules, cloudy swelling and fatty degeneration of the proximal renal tubules, and, often, petechiae in other organs. The oliguria appears to be prerenal and is due to hypovolemia; later, acute tubular necrosis supervenes. At present, there is no effective antiviral agent for yellow fever.

Congo-Crimean Hemorrhagic Fever

Congo-Crimean hemorrhagic fever, first recognized in the Soviet Union, is now an important human disease in Eastern Europe, Asia, and Africa (196). Severely affected patients become stuporous or comatose 5 to 7 days into the illness, with evidence of hepatic and renal failure and shock. Proteinuria and hematuria are often present. The disease is fatal in 15 to 50% of cases. The virus is sensitive to ribavirin, but there have been no clinical trials to confirm its efficacy.

Rift Valley Fever

Rift Valley fever is found in many areas of sub-Saharan Africa. In humans, most infections follow mosquito bites or animal exposure. The infection may present as an uncomplicated febrile illness, with muscle aches and headaches. In 10% of patients, encephalitis or retinal vasculitis occurs as a complication. In a small proportion of cases, a fulminant and often fatal hemorrhagic illness occurs with hematemesis, melena, epistaxis, and evidence of profound DIC. Severe hepatic derangement, renal failure, and encephalopathy are often present. Despite intensive care, mortality is high.

*Hemorrhagic Fever and Renal Syndrome (*Hantavirus*)*

The viruses causing HFRS all belong to the *Hantavirus* genus in the Bunyaviridae family. The hantaviruses are distributed worldwide and are maintained in nature through chronic infection of rodents and small mammals. Transmission to humans is by aerosolized infectious excreta. Human disease usually occurs in summer among rural populations with exposure to rodent-infested barns or grain stores. Urban transmission can occur, however. At least five hantaviruses are known to cause HFRS: Hantaan, Seoul, Puumala, Porogia, and Belgrade viruses (197). HFRS is endemic in a belt from Norway in the west through Sweden, Finland, the Soviet Union, China, and Korea to Japan in the east. The clinical severity of HFRS varies throughout this belt (198). Clinical entities include Korean hemorrhagic fever, nephropathia epidemica in Scandinavia, and epidemic hemorrhagic fever in Japan and China.

In general, HFRS due to Hantaan, Porogia, and Belgrade viruses is more severe and has higher mortality than that due to Puumala virus (nephropathia epidemica) or Seoul virus. Hantaan is predominant in the Far East, Porogia and Belgrade in the Balkans, and Puumala in Western Europe; Seoul has a worldwide distribution (197). The clinical features of the disease vary. The incubation period is 4 to 42 days. Although HFRS occurs with the same clinical picture in children as in adults, both incidence rates and antibody prevalence rates are very low in children under 10 years of age. Men of working age make up the bulk of clinical cases (198). Mild cases are indistinguishable from other febrile illnesses. In more severe cases, fever, headache, myalgia, abdominal pain, and dizziness are associated with the development of periorbital edema, proteinuria, and hematuria. There is often conjunctival injection, pharyngeal injection, petechiae, and epistaxis or GI bleeding. The most severely affected patients develop shock and renal failure. The disease usually passes through five phases: febrile, hypotensive, oliguric, diuretic, and convalescent. Laboratory findings include anemia, lymphocytosis, thrombocytopenia, prolonged prothrombin and bleeding times, and elevated levels of fibrin degradation products. Liver enzyme levels are elevated, and urea and creatinine levels are elevated during the oliguric phase. Proteinuria and hematuria are consistent findings.

The renal histopathologic findings are those of an interstitial nephritis with prominent hemorrhages in the renal medullary interstitium and renal cortex. Acute tubular necrosis may also be seen. Immunohistochemical analysis reveals deposition of IgG and C3, and the GBM, mesangial, and subendothelial deposits may be seen on electron microscopy (199).

Recovery from *Hantavirus*-associated disease is generally complete, although chronic renal insufficiency is a rare sequela of HFRS. In mildly affected patients, the disease is self-limiting and spontaneous recovery occurs. However, in severe cases, with shock, bleeding, and renal failure, dialysis and intensive circulatory support may be required (200). Mortality rates vary depending on the strain of virus; rates are 5 to 15% for hemorrhagic fever and renal syndrome in China and significantly lower for the milder Finnish form associated with the Puumala virus strain.

Ribavirin is active against Hantaan viruses *in vitro*, and clinical trials indicate that both mortality and morbidity can be reduced by treatment with this antiviral agent if it is administered early in the course of illness. Dosages of 33 mg/kg followed by 16 mg/kg every 6 hours for 4 days and then 8 mg/kg every 8 hours for 3 days have been used (201).

Lassa Fever

Lassa fever is a common infection in West Africa and usually manifests as a nonspecific febrile illness. In 10% of cases, a fulminant hemorrhagic disease occurs. In severe cases, proteinuria and hematuria are usually present, and renal failure may occur. Ribavirin is effective in decreasing mortality. As in other hemorrhagic fevers, intensive hemodynamic support and correction of the hemostatic derangements are important components of therapy (202).

Argentine and Bolivian Hemorrhagic Fevers

Junin and Machupo viruses, the agents of Argentine and Bolivian hemorrhagic fever, respectively, cause hemorrhagic fevers with prominent neurologic features and systemic and hemorrhagic features similar to those of Lassa fever. Oliguria, shock, and renal failure occur in the most severe cases.

Marburg Disease and Ebola Hemorrhagic Fever

Marburg and Ebola viruses have been associated with outbreaks of nosocomially transmitted hemorrhagic fever. Both viruses cause fulminant hemorrhagic fever. Onset is with high fever, headache, sore throat, myalgia, and profound prostration. An erythematous rash on the trunk is followed by hemorrhagic conjunctivitis, bleeding, impaired renal function, shock, and respiratory failure. The mortality rate is high. Renal histopathologic findings in fatal cases are of tubular necrosis, with fibrin deposition in the glomeruli. There is no specific treatment for these disorders.

PARASITIC INFECTIONS

Chronic exposure to infectious agents is a major factor in the increased prevalence of glomerular diseases in developing countries. Malaria is the best-documented parasitic infection associated with glomerular disease, but other parasitic infections including schistosomiasis, filariasis, leishmaniasis, and possibly helminth infections may also induce nephritis or nephrosis.

Malaria and Renal Disease

Malaria is estimated to cause up to 500 million clinical cases of illness and more than 1 million deaths each year (203). The association of quartan malaria and nephritis has been well known in both temperate and tropical zones since the end of the nineteenth century.

Epidemiologic studies provide the most conclusive evidence for a role of *Plasmodium malariae* in glomerular disease (204,205). Chronic renal disease was a major cause of morbidity and mortality in British Guiana in the 1920s. The frequent occurrence of *P. malariae* in the blood of these patients led to detailed epidemiologic studies that implicated malaria as a cause of the nephrosis. After the eradication of malaria from British Guiana, chronic renal disease ceased to be a major cause of death in that country (204).

The link between malaria and nephrotic syndrome was strengthened by studies in West Africa in the 1950s and 1960s that demonstrated a high prevalence of nephrotic syndrome in the Nigerian population (206). The pattern of nephrotic syndrome differed from that in temperate climates, with an older peak age, extremely poor prognosis, and unusual histologic features. The incidence of *P. malariae* parasitemia in patients with the nephrotic syndrome in Nigeria was vastly in excess of that occurring in the general population, whereas the incidence of *Plasmodium falciparum* parasitemia was similar to that in the general population. The age distribution of nephrotic syndrome also closely paralleled that of *P. malariae* infection (206). In some affected patients, circulating immune complexes and immunoglobulin, complement, and antigens were present in the glomeruli that were recognized by *P. malariae*–specific antisera.

Clinical and Histopathologic Features of Quartan Malaria Nephropathy

Most patients have poorly selective proteinuria and are unresponsive to treatment with steroids or immunosuppressive agents. The characteristic lesions of *P. malariae* nephropathy are capillary wall thickening and segmental glomerular sclerosis, which lead to progressive glomerular changes and secondary tubular atrophy (206). Cellular proliferation is conspicuously absent. Electron microscopy shows foot-process fusion, thickening of the basement membrane, and increase in subendothelial basement membrane–like material. Immunofluorescent studies show granular deposits of immunoglobulin, complement, and *P. malariae* antigen in approximately one-third of patients.

In addition to the histologic pattern, termed *quartan malaria nephropathy*, *P. malariae* infection is associated with a variety of other forms of histologic appearance, including proliferative GN and MGN (207).

Although quartan malaria nephropathy has been clearly linked to *P. malariae* infection in Nigeria, a number of studies from other regions in Africa have not revealed the typical histopathologic findings described in the Nigerian studies (208). Furthermore, quartan malaria nephropathy may be seen in children with no evidence of *P. malariae* infection or deposition of malaria antigens in the kidney. This, together with the fact that antimalarial treatment does not affect the progression of the disorder, raises the possibility that factors other than malaria might be involved in the initiation and perpetuation of the disorder. Although there is undoubtedly a strong association between *P. malariae* infection and nephrotic syndrome on epidemiologic grounds, the direct causal link is not proven. Most likely, a number of different infectious processes, including malaria, hepatitis B, schistosomiasis, and perhaps other parasitic infections that cause chronic or persistent infections and often occur concurrently in malaria areas, may all result in glomerular injury and a range of overlapping histopathologic features. The prognosis for the nephrotic syndrome in most African studies has been poor, regardless of whether the histologic findings were typical of quartan malaria nephropathy or whether *P. malariae* parasitemia was implicated. Treatment with steroids and azathioprine is generally ineffective, and a significant proportion of patients progress to renal failure.

Renal Disease Associated with Plasmodium falciparum *Infection*

P. falciparum appears to be much less likely to cause significant glomerular pathology. Epidemiologic studies have failed to show a clear association between *P. falciparum* parasitemia and the nephrotic syndrome. Whereas renal failure appears to be a common complication of severe malaria in adults, it seldom occurs in children.

Renal biopsy specimens from adult patients with acute *P. falciparum* infections who have proteinuria or hematuria show evidence of glomerular changes, including hypercellularity, thickening of basement membranes, and hyperplasia and hypertrophy of endothelial cells (209). Electron microscopy reveals electron-dense deposits in the subendothelial and paramesangial areas. Deposits of IgM, with or without IgG, are localized mainly in the mesangial areas. *P. falciparum* antigens can be demonstrated in the mesangial areas and along the capillary wall, which suggests an immune-complex GN. The changes, generally mild and transient, are probably unrelated to the acute renal failure that may complicate severe *P. falciparum* infection (209). Renal failure occurring in severe *P. falciparum* malaria is usually associated with acute intravascular hemolysis or heavy parasitic infection that leads to acute tubular necrosis. Heavily parasitized erythrocytes play a central role in the various pathologic factors (210). Although renal failure is usually associated with infection by *P. falciparum*, acute renal failure has been described with *Plasmodium vivax* infection and mixed infections (211).

Blackwater Fever

The term *blackwater fever* refers to the combination of severe hemolysis, hemoglobinuria, and renal failure. It was more common at the start of the twentieth century in nonimmune individuals receiving intermittent quinine therapy for *P. falciparum* malaria. Blackwater fever has become rare since 1950, when quinine was replaced by chloroquine. However, the disease reappeared in the 1990s, after the reuse of quinine because of the development of chloroquine-resistant organisms. Since then, several cases have been described after therapy with halofantrine and mefloquine, two new molecules similar to quinine (amino-alcohol family) (212). Renal failure generally occurred in the context of severe hemolytic anemia, hemoglobinuria, and jaundice. The pathophysiology of the disorder is unclear; however, it appears that a double sensitization of the red blood cells to the *P. falciparum* and to the amino-alcohols is necessary to provoke the hemolysis. Histopathologic findings include swelling and vacuolization of proximal tubules, necrosis and degeneration of more distal tubules, and hemoglobin deposition in the renal tubules. Recent studies indicates a better outcome with earlier initiation of intensive care and dialysis combined with necessary changes in antimalarial medications.

Schistosomiasis

Schistosomiasis affects 200 million people living in endemic areas of Asia, Africa, and South America (213). The infection is usually acquired in childhood, but repeated infections occur throughout life. *Schistosoma japonicum* is found only in the Orient, whereas *Schistosoma haematobium* occurs throughout Africa, the Middle East, and areas of southwest Asia. *Schistosoma mansoni* is widespread in Africa, South America, and southwest Asia.

Human infection begins when the cercarial forms invade through the skin, develop into *schistosomula*, and move to the lungs via the lymphatics or blood. They then migrate to the liver and mature in the intrahepatic portal venules. Sexual multiplication of adult worms takes place in the venules of the mesenteric venous system of the large intestine (*S. mansoni*) or in the venules of the urinary tract (*S. haematobium*). The females release large numbers of eggs, which may remain embedded in the tissues, embolize to the liver or lungs, or pass into the feces or urine.

Clinical manifestations may occur at any stage of the infection. Cercarial invasion may cause an intense itchy papular rash. Katayama fever is an acute serum sickness–like illness that occurs several weeks after infection, as eggs are being deposited in the tissues. Deposition of the eggs in tissues results in inflammation of the intestines, fibrosis of the liver, and portal hypertension. With *S. haematobium*, chronic inflammation and fibrosis of the ureters and bladder may lead to obstructive uropathy (214).

Renal manifestations of schistosomiasis occur most commonly in *S. mansoni* infection. Schistosomal nephropathy usually presents with symptoms including granulomatous inflammation in the ureters and bladder, but glomerular disease (probably on an immune-complex basis) may also occur. Renal disease usually occurs in older children or young adults with long-term infection, but serious disease may also occur in young children (214).

The early renal tract manifestations of schistosomiasis are suprapubic discomfort, frequency, dysuria, and terminal hematuria. In more severe cases, evidence of urinary obstruction appears. Poor urinary stream, straining on micturition, a feeling of incomplete bladder emptying, and a constant urge to urinate may be severely disabling symptoms. The fibrosis and inflammation of ureters, urethra, and bladder may be followed by calcification and may result in hydroureter, hydronephrosis, and bladder neck obstruction. Renal failure may ultimately develop, and there is a suspicion that carcinoma of the bladder may be linked to the chronic infective and inflammatory process. Secondary bacterial infection is common within the obstructed and inflamed urinary tract (213).

The hepatosplenic form of *S. mansoni* infection may be accompanied by a glomerulopathy in 12 to 15% of cases, manifested in the majority as nephrotic syndrome (215). Histopathologic findings include mesangioproliferative GN, focal segmental glomerulosclerosis, mesangiocapillary GN, MGN, and focal segmental hyalinosis (216). Immune complexes may be detected in the circulation of these patients, and glomerular granular deposition of IgM, C3, and schistosomal antigens are seen on immunofluorescence. Usually *Schistosoma*-specific nephropathy is a progressive disease and is not influenced by antiparasitic or immunosuppressive therapy (217), but isolated case reports of remission after treatment with praziquantel have been reported (218).

The diagnosis is confirmed by the detection of *Schistosoma* eggs in feces, urine, or biopsy specimens. Eggs are shed into the urine with a diurnal rhythm, and urine collected between 11 AM and 1 PM is the most useful. Urinary sediment obtained by centrifugation or filtration through a Nuclepore membrane should be examined.

In cases in which studies of urine and feces yield negative results in patients in whom the diagnosis is suspected, rectal biopsy specimens taken approximately 9 cm from the anus have a high diagnostic yield for both *S. mansoni* and *S. haematobium* infection. Biopsy of liver or bladder may be required to establish the diagnosis.

Antibodies indicating previous infection can be detected using enzyme-linked immunosorbent assay or radioimmunoassay. The tests are sensitive but lack specificity and may not differentiate between past exposure and current infection.

Praziquantel is the drug of choice for treatment of schistosomiasis. A single oral dose of 40 mg/kg is effective in *S.*

haematobium and *S. mansoni* infection and is usually well tolerated. The alternative drug for *S. mansoni* infection is oxamniquine. Complete remission of urinary symptoms may occur in renal disease of short duration, but in late disease with extensive fibrosis, scarring, and calcification, obstructive uropathy and renal failure may persist after the infection has been eradicated. There are reports of a drastic decrease in the number of severe hepatosplenic forms of *S. mansoni* infection after mass treatment of the population in endemic areas with oxamniquine. This also reduced schistosomal nephropathy (215).

Leishmaniasis

Visceral leishmaniasis is a chronic protozoon infection characterized by fever, hepatosplenomegaly, anemia, leukopenia, and hyperglobulinemia. Proteinuria and/or microscopic hematuria or pyuria have been reported in 50% of patients with visceral leishmaniasis (219). Acute renal failure in association with interstitial nephritis has also been reported (220). Renal histologic analysis in patients with visceral leishmaniasis reveals glomerular changes, with features of a mesangial proliferative GN or a focal proliferative GN, or a generalized interstitial nephritis with interstitial edema, mononuclear cell infiltration, and focal tubular degeneration. Immunofluorescence reveals deposition of IgG, IgM, and C3 within the glomeruli, as well as electron-dense deposits in the basement membrane and mesangium on electron microscopy (219). Circulating immune complexes together with immunoglobulin and complement deposition in the glomeruli suggests an immune-complex cause.

Renal disease in leishmaniasis is usually mild and may resolve after treatment of the infection. Renal dysfunction may be associated with treatment for visceral leishmaniasis with antimony compounds.

Filariasis

Proteinuria is more common in filarial hyperendemic regions of West Africa than in nonfilarial areas. Renal histologic analysis has shown a variety of different histopathologic appearances; the most common is diffuse mesangial proliferative GN with C3 deposition in the glomeruli (221). Renal biopsy specimens also demonstrate large numbers of eosinophils in the glomeruli, and microfilariae may be seen in the lumen of glomerular capillaries. Filarial antigens have been detected within immune deposits within the glomeruli.

Hydatid Disease

Echinococcus granulosus causes chronic cysts within a variety of organs. In addition, nephrotic syndrome in association with hydatid disease has been reported. Membranous nephropathy, minimal change lesions, and mesangiocapillary GN have been described in association with hydatid disease (222,223). Immunofluorescence reveals deposits of immunoglobulin, complement, and hydatid antigens within the glomeruli. Remission of nephrotic syndrome has been reported with treatment by antiparasitic agents such as albendazole (222,223).

Trypanosomiasis

Few reports have been published of renal disease occurring in patients with trypanosomiasis. The trypanosomal antigens can induce GN in a variety of experimental animals (224).

Toxoplasmosis

Nephrotic syndrome has occasionally been reported as a manifestation of congenital toxoplasmosis.

Dissemination of previously latent *Toxoplasma* infection in patients undergoing treatment with immunosuppressive drugs has been increasingly recognized in recent years. Reactivation of toxoplasmosis or progression of recently acquired primary infection should be considered in patients undergoing renal transplantation or immunotherapy for renal disease who develop unexplained inflammation of any organ.

FUNGAL INFECTIONS

Fungal infections of the kidneys and urinary tract occur most commonly as part of systemic fungal infections in patients with underlying immunodeficiency, as focal urinary tract infections in patients with obstructive lesions, or as a result of indwelling catheters. Although *Candida* infection is the most common fungal infection in both immunocompromised and nonimmunocompromised hosts, virtually all other fungal pathogens may invade the renal tract during severe immunocompromise.

Urinary infection with *Candida albicans* is most commonly a component of systemic candidiasis in patients who are severely immunocompromised. Systemic candidiasis is also seen in premature and term infants with perinatally acquired invasive candidiasis. Presentation is usually with systemic sepsis, fever or hypothermia, hepatosplenomegaly, erythematous rash, and thrombocytopenia. Systemic candidiasis may be seen on ophthalmologic investigation as microemboli in the retina. The first clue to the underlying diagnosis may be the presence of yeasts in the urine (225).

Candida involvement of the urinary tract may affect all structures including the glomeruli, tubules, collecting system, ureters, and bladder. Microabscesses may form within the renal parenchyma, and large balls of fungi may completely obstruct the urinary tract at any level. Acute renal failure caused by systemic candidiasis or obstruction of the renal tracts with fungal hyphae is a well-recognized complication of systemic candidal infection (225,226).

Indwelling catheters (which form a nidus for persistent infection) should be removed. Successful treatment of nonobstructing bilateral renal fungal balls by fluconazole either alone or in combination with liposomal amphotericin B has been reported (227,228). In the presence of obstruction, however, percutaneous nephrostomy to relieve the obstruction with antegrade amphotericin B irrigation, coupled with systemic antifungal therapy, is the mainstay of treatment (226). Amphotericin B is the most effective antifungal agent, but it is not excreted in the urine. Local irrigation via nephrostomy provides good results, however. For treatment of urinary tract candidiasis, it is usually combined with fluconazole or 5-flucytosine, both of which are excreted in high concentrations in the urine. Treatment is required for weeks to months to ensure complete elimination of the fungus, and the ultimate outcome is largely dependent on whether there is a permanent defect in immunity.

MISCELLANEOUS CONDITIONS

Hemorrhagic Shock and Encephalopathy

In 1983, Levin et al. first described hemorrhagic shock and encephalopathy, which appeared to be distinct from previously recognized pediatric disorders (229). Other cases have subsequently been reported from several centers in the United Kingdom, Europe, Israel, the United States, and Australia, and the syndrome is now recognized as a new and relatively common severe childhood disorder (230).

Hemorrhagic shock and encephalopathy usually affect infants in the first year of life, with a peak onset at 3 to 4 months of age. A prodromal illness with fever, irritability, diarrhea, or upper respiratory infection occurs 2 to 5 days before the onset in two-thirds of cases. Affected infants develop profound shock, coma, convulsions, bleeding and evidence of DIC, diarrhea, and oliguria. Laboratory findings include acidosis, falling hemoglobin and platelet levels, elevated urea and creatinine levels, and elevated levels of hepatic transaminases. Despite vigorous intensive care, the prognosis is poor, and most affected infants die or are left severely neurologically damaged (230,231). A small number of patients have been reported to survive without residual sequelae.

The renal impairment appears to be largely prerenal in origin, and when aggressive volume replacement and treatment of the shock results in improved renal perfusion, rapid improvement in renal function is usually observed. In patients with profound shock unresponsive to initial resuscitation, vasomotor nephropathy supervenes and dialysis may be required. Myoglobinuria in association with hemorrhagic shock and encephalopathy has been reported.

Kawasaki Disease

Following the description of the mucocutaneous lymph node syndrome by Kawasaki in 1968, Kawasaki disease has been recognized as a common and serious childhood illness with a worldwide distribution. Although the etiology remains unknown, epidemiologic features clearly suggest an infective cause. The disease occurs in epidemics, and wavelike spread has been demonstrated during outbreaks in Japan (see Chapter 44).

Amyloidosis

Deposition of amyloid within the kidney is an important complication of chronic and persistent infection. Amyloidosis is most common in patients with chronic osteomyelitis and chronic pulmonary infections such as bronchiectasis and is seen occasionally in those with persistent infections such as leprosy or malaria.

REFERENCES

1. Levin M. Shock. In: Black JA, ed. *Paediatric emergencies.* 2nd ed. London: Butterworth, 1987:87–116.
2. Parkin RM, Levin DL. Shock in the paediatric patient. *J Pediatr* 1982;101:163–169.
3. Cumming AD, Driedgen AA, McDonald JWD, et al. Vasoactive hormones in the renal response to systemic sepsis. *Am J Kidney Dis* 1988;11:23–32.
4. Cohen RI, Hassell AM, Marzouk K, et al. Renal effects of nitric oxide in endotoxemia. *Am J Respir Crit Care Med* 2001; 164:1890–1895.
5. Nadel S, Levin M, Habibi P. Treatment of meningococcal disease in childhood. In: Cartwright K, ed. *Meningococcal disease.* New York: John Wiley and Sons, 1995.
6. Heyderman R, Klein N, Levin M. Pathophysiology and management of meningococcal septicaemia. In: David T, ed. *Recent advances in paediatrics.* 11th ed. London: Churchill Livingstone, 1993:1–18.
7. Gedde-Dahl TW, Bjark P, Hoiby EA, et al. Severity of meningococcal disease: assessment by factors and scores and implications for patient management. *Rev Infect Dis* 1990; 12:973–991.
8. Case records of the Massachusetts General Hospital, case 4. *N Engl J Med* 1988;318:234–242.
9. Brandzaeg P, Kierulf P, Gaustad P, et al. Plasma endotoxin as a predictor of multiple organ failure and death in systemic meningococcal disease. *J Infect Dis* 1989;159:195–204.
10. Mercier JC, Beaufils F, Hartman JF, et al. Hemodynamic patterns of meningococcal shock in children. *Crit Care Med* 1988;16:27–33.
11. Faust SN, Levin M, Harrison OB, et al. Dysfunction of endothelial protein C activation in severe meningococcal sepsis. *N Engl J Med* 2001;345:408–416.
12. Smith OP, White B, Vaughan D, et al. Use of protein-C concentrate, heparin, and haemodiafiltration in meningococcus-induced purpura fulminans. *Lancet* 1997;350:1590–1593.
13. Wippermann CF, Schofer O, Beetz R, et al. Renal abscess in childhood: diagnostic and therapeutic progress. *Pediatr Infect Dis J* 1991;10:446–450.

14. Deyoe LA, Cronan JJ, Lambiase RE, et al. Percutaneous drainage of renal and perirenal abscesses: results in 30 patients. *Am J Roentgenol* 1990;155:81–83.
15. Todd J, Fishaut MI, Kapral F, et al. Toxic shock syndrome associated with phage group 1 staphylococci. *Lancet* 1978;ii:1116–1118.
16. Reingold AL, Shands KL, Dann BB, et al. Toxic shock syndrome not associated with menstruation: a review of 54 cases. *Lancet* 1982;i:1–4.
17. Buchdahl R, Levin M, Wilkins B, et al. Toxic shock syndrome. *Arch Dis Child* 1985;60:563–567.
18. Todd JK, Franco-Buff A, Lowellin DW, et al. Phenotypic distinctiveness of *Staphylococcus aureus* strains associated with toxic shock syndrome. *Infect Immun* 1984;45:339–344.
19. Marrack P, Kappler J. The staphylococcal enterotoxins and their relatives. *Science* 1990;248:705–711.
20. Fast DJ, Schlievert PM, Nelson RD. Toxic shock syndrome: associated staphylococcal and streptococcal pyrogenic toxins are potent inducers of tumour necrosis factor. *Infect Immun* 1989;57:291–294.
21. Toxic shock syndrome. In: Pickering LK, ed. *2000 Red Book: Report of the Committee on Infectious Diseases*. 25th ed. Elk Grove Village, IL: American Academy of Pediatrics, 2000:576–581.
22. Cone LA, Woodward DR, Schlievert PM, et al. Clinical and bacteriologic observations of a toxic shock–like syndrome due to *Streptococcus pyogenes*. *N Engl J Med* 1987;317:146–149.
23. Rodriguez-Iturbe B, Castillo L, Valbuena R. Acute post-streptococcal glomerulonephritis. A review of recent developments. *Paediatrician* 1979;8:307–324.
24. Dodge WF, Spargo BF, Travis LB. Occurrence of acute glomerulonephritis in sibling contacts of children with sporadic acute glomerulo-nephritis. *Pediatrics* 1967;40:1028–1030.
25. Lasch EE, Frankel V, Vardy PA. Epidemic glomerulonephritis in Israel. *J Infect Dis* 1971;124:141–147.
26. Weinstein L, LeFrock J. Does antimicrobial therapy of streptococcal pharyngitis or pyoderma alter the risk of glomerulonephritis? *J Infect Dis* 1971;124:229–231.
27. Popovic RM, Kostic M. Medium and long-term prognosis of patients with acute post-streptococcal glomerulonephritis. *Nephron* 1991;58:393–399.
28. Barnham M, Thornton T, Lange K. Nephritis caused by *Streptococcus zooepidemicus* (Lancefield group C). *Lancet* 1983;1:945–948.
29. Gnann JW, Gray BM, Griffin FM, et al. Acute glomerulonephritis following group G *Streptococcus* infection. *J Infect Dis* 1987;156:411–412.
30. Torres-Martinez C, Mehta D, Butt A, et al. *Streptococcus* associated toxic shock. *Arch Dis Child* 1992;67:126–130.
31. Stollerman GH. Changing group A *Streptococcus*: the reappearance of streptococcal "toxic shock." *Arch Intern Med* 1988; 148:1268–1270.
32. Stevens DL, Tanner MH, Winship J. Severe group A *Streptococcus* infections associated with a toxic shock-like syndrome and scarlet fever toxin A. *N Engl J Med* 1989;321:1–7.
33. Feigin RD, Anderson DC. Leptospirosis. In: Feigin RD, Cherry JD, eds. *Textbook of paediatric infectious diseases*. 4th ed. Philadelphia: WB Saunders, 1998:1529–1542.
34. Lai KN, Aarons I, Woodroffe AJ, et al. Renal lesions in leptospirosis. *Aust N Z J Med* 1982;12:276–279.
35. Kennedy ND, Pusey CD, Rainford DJ, et al. Leptospirosis and acute renal failure: clinical experiences and a review of the literature. *Postgrad Med J* 1979;55:176–179.
36. Clerke AM, Leuva AC, Joshi C, et al. Clinical profile of leptospirosis in South gujarat. *J Postgrad Med* 2002;48:117–118.
37. De Francesco Daher E, Oliveira Neto FH, Ramirez SM. Evaluation of hemostasis disorders and anticardiolipin antibody in patients with severe leptospirosis. *Rev Inst Med Trop Sao Paulo* 2002;44:85–90.
38. Watt G, Tuazon ML, Santiago E. Placebo controlled trial of intravenous penicillin for severe and late leptospirosis. *Lancet* 1988;1:433–435.
39. Gasser VC, Gautier E, Steck A, et al. Hämolytich-urämiche Syndrome: bilaterale Nierenrindennekrosen bei akuten erworbenen hämolytischen Anämien. *Schweiz Med Wochenschr* 1955;85:905.
40. Seger R, Joller P, Baerlocher K. Hemolytic-uremic syndrome associated with neuraminidase-producing micro-organism: treatment by exchange transfusion. *Helv Paediatr Acta* 1980; 35:359–367.
41. Moorthy B, Makker SP. Hemolytic uremic syndrome associated with pneumococcal sepsis. *J Pediatr* 1979;95:558–559.
42. Kaplan BS, Cleary TG, Obrig TG. Recent advances in understanding the pathogenesis of the hemolytic uremic syndromes. *Pediatr Nephrol* 1990;4:276–283.
43. Schenk EA, Panke TW, Cole HA. Glomerular and arteriolar thrombosis in pneumococcal septicemia. *Arch Pathol* 1970;89: 154–159.
44. Cabrera GR, Fortenberry JD, Warshaw BL, et al. Hemolytic uremic syndrome associated with invasive *Streptococcus pneumoniae* infection. *Pediatrics* 1998;101:699–703.
45. Seger R, Joller P, Baerlocher K, et al. Hemolytic-uremic syndrome associated with neuraminidase-producing microorganisms: treatment by exchange transfusion. *Helv Paediatr Acta* 1980;35:359–367.
46. Eber SW, Polster H, Quentin SH, et al. Hämolytisch-urämisches Syndrome bei pneumokok-ken-menigitis und -sepsis. Bedeutung der T-transformation. *Monatsschr Kinderheilkd* 1993;141:219–222.
47. Nathanson S, Deschenes G. Prognosis of *Streptococcus pneumoniae*-induced hemolytic uremic syndrome. *Pediatr Nephrol* 2001;16:362–365.
48. Brandt J, Wong C, Mihm S, et al. Invasive pneumococcal disease and hemolytic uremic syndrome. *Pediatrics* 2002;110: 371–376.
49. Beaufils M, Morel Maroger L, Sraer JD, et al. Acute renal failure of glomerular origin during visceral abscess. *N Engl J Med* 1976;295:185–189.
50. Sitprija V, Pipatanagul V, Boonpucknavig V, et al. Glomerulitis in typhoid fever. *Ann Intern Med* 1974;81:210–213.
51. Awunor-Renner C, Lawande RV. *Yersinia* and chronic glomerulopathy in the Savannah region of Nigeria. *BMJ* 1982;285:1464.
52. Buka I, Coovadia HM. Typhoid glomerulonephritis. *Arch Dis Child* 1980;55:305–307.
53. Dhawan A, Marwaha RK. Acute glomerulonephritis in multi-drug resistant *Salmonella typhi* infection. *Indian Pediatr* 1992;29:1039–1041.

54. Srivastava RN. Acute glomerulonephritis in *Salmonella typhi* infection. *Indian Pediatr* 1993;30:278–279.
55. Korpela M, Mustonen J, Pasternack A, et al. Urinary tract and renal findings in acute *Yersinia* infection. *Acta Med Scand* 1986;220:471–476.
56. Fukumoto Y, Hiraoka M, Takano T, et al. Acute tubulointerstitial nephritis in association with *Yersinia* pseudotuberculosis infection. *Pediatr Nephrol* 1995;9:78–80.
57. Koo JW, Park SN, Choi SM, et al. Acute renal failure associated with *Yersinia* pseudotuberculosis infection in children. *Pediatr Nephrol* 1996;10:582–586.
58. Cheong HI, Choi EH, Ha IS, et al. Acute renal failure associated with *Yersinia* pseudotuberculosis infection. *Nephron* 1995;70:319–323.
59. Sato K, Ouchi K, Komazawa M. Ampicillin vs. placebo for *Yersinia* pseudotuberculosis infection in children. *Pediatr Infect Dis J* 1988;7:686–689.
60. *Yersinia enterocolitica* and *Yersinia* pseudotuberculosis infections. In: Pickering LK, ed. *2000 Red Book: Report of the Committee on Infectious Diseases.* 25th ed. Elk Grove Village, IL: American Academy of Pediatrics, 2000:642–643.
61. Karmali MA, Petric M, Steele BT. Sporadic cases of haemolytic uraemic syndrome associated with faecal cytotoxin and cytotoxin producing *Escherichia coli* in stools. *Lancet* 1983;1:619–620.
62. World Health Organization, *Tuberculosis,* Fact Sheet No. 104. Revised. Geneva: World Health Organization, August 2002.
63. Dye C, Scheele S, Dolin P, et al, for the WHO Global Surveillance and Monitoring Project. Global burden of tuberculosis: estimated incidence, prevalence, and mortality by country. *JAMA* 1999;282:677–686.
64. Des Pres RM, Heim CR. *Mycobacterium tuberculosis.* In: Mandell GL, Douglas RG, Bennett JE, eds. *Principles and practice of infectious diseases.* 3rd ed. London: Churchill Livingstone, 1990:1877–1906.
65. Cos LR, Cockett AT. Genitourinary tuberculosis revisited. *Urology* 1982;20:111–117.
66. Ehrlich RM, Lattimen J. Urogenital tuberculosis in children. *J Urol* 1971;105:461–465.
67. Christensen WI. Genitourinary tuberculosis: review of 102 cases. *Medicine* 1974;53:377–390.
68. Kaplan BS, Wiglesworth FW, Marks MI. The glomerulopathy of congenital syphilis: an immune deposit disease. *J Pediatr* 1972;81:1154–1156.
69. Bhorades MS, Caray HB, Lee HJ. Nephropathy of secondary syphilis: a clinical and pathological spectrum. *JAMA* 1971;216:1159–1166.
70. Gamble CN, Reardan JB. Immunopathogenesis of syphilitic glomerulo-nephritis. *N Engl J Med* 1975;292:449–454.
71. Cochat P, Colon S, Bosshard S, et al. Membranoproliferative glomerulonephritis and *Mycoplasma pneumoniae* infection. *Arch Fr Pediatr* 1985;42:29–31.
72. Vitullo BB, O'Regan S, de Chadaneuian JP. *Mycoplasma pneumoniae* associated with acute glomerulonephritis. *Nephron* 1978;21:284–287.
73. Said MH, Layani MP, Colon S, et al. *Mycoplasma pneumoniae*–associated nephritis in children. *Pediatr Nephrol* 1999;13:39–44.
74. Edwards MS, Feigin RD. Rickettsial disease. In: Feigin RD, Cherry JD, eds. *Textbook of pediatric infectious diseases.* 4th ed. Philadelphia: WB Saunders, 1998:2239–2258.
75. Helmick CG, Bernard KW, Dangelo LJ. Rocky Mountain spotted fever: clinical, laboratory and epidemiological features in 262 cases. *J Infect Dis* 1984;150:480–486.
76. Walker DH, Mattern WD. Acute renal failure in Rocky Mountain spotted fever. *Arch Intern Med* 1979;139:443–448.
77. Bradford WD, Croker BP, Tisher CL. Kidney lesion in Rocky Mountain spotted fever. *Am J Pathol* 1979;97:381–392.
78. Quigg RJ, Gaines R, Wakely PE Jr, et al. Acute glomerulonephritis in a patient with Rocky Mountain spotted fever. *Am J Kidney Dis* 1991;17:339–342.
79. Dimmit SK, Millen DK. Rocky Mountain spotted fever. *Am J Clin Pathol* 1982;78:131–134.
80. Rocky Mountain spotted fever. In: Pickering LK, ed. *2000 Red Book: Report of the Committee on Infectious Diseases.* 25th ed. Elk Grove Village, IL: American Academy of Pediatrics, 2000:491–493.
81. Sawyer LA, Fishbein DB, McDade JE. Q fever: current concepts. *Rev Infect Dis* 1987;9:935–946.
82. Dathan JRE, Heyworth MF. Glomerulonephritis associated with *Coxiella burnetii* endocarditis. *BMJ* 1975;1:376.
83. Cutz E, Thonner PS, Raoc P. Disseminated *Legionella pneumophila* infection in an infant with severe combined immunodeficiency. *J Pediatr* 1982;100:760–762.
84. Shah A, Check F, Baskin S, et al. Legionnaire's disease and acute renal failure: case report and review. *Clin Infect Dis* 1992;14:204–207.
85. Nishitarumizu K, Tokuda Y, Uehara H, et al. Tubulointerstitial nephritis associated with Legionnaires' disease. *Intern Med* 2000;39(2):150–153.
86. Gutman RA, Striker GE, Gililand BC. The immune complex glomerulonephritis of bacterial endocarditis. *Medicine* 1972;51:1–5.
87. Perez-Fontan M, Huarte E, Tellez A, et al. Glomerular nephropathy associated with chronic Q fever. *Am J Kidney Dis* 1988;4:298–306.
88. Tompkins LS, Roessler BJ, Redd SC, et al. *Legionella* prosthetic-valve endocarditis. *N Engl J Med* 1988;318:530–535.
89. Neugarten N, Baldwin DS. Glomerulonephritis in bacterial endocarditis. *Am J Med* 1984;77:297–304.
90. Levy RL, Hong R. The immune nature of subacute bacterial endocarditis (SBE) nephritis. *Am J Med* 1973;54:645–652.
91. Baltimore RS. Infective endocarditis in children. *Pediatr Infect Dis J* 1992;11:903–907.
92. Haffner D, Schindera F, Aschoff A, et al. The clinical spectrum of shunt nephritis. *Nephrol Dial Transplant* 1997;12:1143–1148.
93. Dobrin RS, Day NK, Quie PG, et al. The role of complement, immunoglobulin and bacterial antigen in coagulase-negative staphylococcal shunt nephritis. *Am J Med* 1975;59:660–673.
94. Zunin C, Castellani A, Olivetti G, et al. Membranoproliferative glomerulonephritis associated with infected ventriculoatrial shunt: report of two cases recovered after removal of the shunt. *Pathologica* 1977;69:297–305.
95. Tiollais P, Pourcel C, Dejean A. The hepatitis B virus. *Nature* 1985;317:489–495.

96. Johnson RJ, Couser WG. Hepatitis B infection and renal disease: clinical, immunopathogenetic and therapeutic considerations. *Kidney Int* 1990;37:663–676.
97. Gocke DJ. Extrahepatic manifestations of viral hepatitis. *Am J Med Sci* 1975;270:49–52.
98. Sergent JS, Lockshin MD, Christian CL, et al. Vasculitis with hepatitis B antigenemia. Long term observation in nine patients. *Medicine* 1976;55:1–17.
99. Reznik VM, Mendoza SA, Self TW, et al. Hepatitis B-associated vasculitis in an infant. *J Pediatr* 1981;98:252–254.
100. Michalak T. Immune complexes of hepatitis B surface antigen in the pathogenesis of periarteritis nodosa. A study of seven necropsy cases. *Am J Pathol* 1978;90:619–632.
101. Avsar E, Savas B, Tozun N, et al. Successful treatment of polyarteritis nodosa related to hepatitis B virus with interferon alpha as first-line therapy. *J Hepatol* 1998;28:525–526.
102. Gupta S, Piraka C, Jaffe M. Lamivudine in the treatment of polyarteritis nodosa associated with acute hepatitis B. *N Engl J Med* 2001;344:1645–1646.
103. Erhardt A, Sagir A, Guillevin L, et al. Successful treatment of hepatitis B virus associated polyarteritis nodosa with a combination of prednisolone, alpha-interferon and lamivudine. *J Hepatol* 2000;33:677–683.
104. Wiggelinkhuizen J, Sinclair SC. Membranous glomerulonephropathy in childhood. *S Afr Med J* 1987;72:184–187.
105. Southwest Pediatric Nephrology Study Group. Hepatitis B surface antigenemia in North American children with membranous glomerulonephropathy. *J Pediatr* 1985;106:571–577.
106. Lai KN, Lai FM. The clinico-pathologic features of hepatitis B virus–associated glomerulonephritis. *QJM* 1987;63:323–333.
107. Ozdamar SO, Gucer S, Tinaztepe K. Hepatitis-B virus associated nephropathies: a clinicopathological study in 14 children. *Pediatr Nephrol* 2003;18:23–28.
108. Lai KN, Lai FM. Strong association between IgA nephropathy and hepatitis B surface antigenemia in endemic areas. *Clin Nephrol* 1988;29:229–234.
109. Thomas HC, Lever AML, Scully LJ, et al. Approaches to the treatment of hepatitis B virus and delta-related liver disease. *Semin Liver Dis* 1986;6:34–40.
110. Lisker MM, Webb D, Di-Bisceylie AM, et al. Glomerulonephritis caused by chronic hepatitis B virus infection: treatment with recombinant human alpha-interferon. *Ann Intern Med* 1989;111:479–483.
111. Dienstag JL, Schiff ER, Wright TL, et al. Lamivudine as initial treatment for chronic hepatitis B in the United States. *N Engl J Med* 1999;341:1256–1263.
112. Chung DR, Yang WS, Kim SB, et al. Treatment of hepatitis B virus associated glomerulonephritis with recombinant human alpha interferon. *Am J Nephrol* 1997;17:112–117.
113. Lin CY. Treatment of hepatitis B virus–associated membranous nephropathy with recombinant alpha-interferon. *Kidney Int* 1995;47:225–230.
114. Alter MJ, Kruszon-Moran D, Nainan OV, et al. The prevalence of hepatitis C virus infection in the United States, 1988 through 1994. *N Engl J Med* 1999;341:556–562.
115. Jonas MM. Children with hepatitis C. *Hepatology* 2002;36: S173–S178.
116. Stehman-Breen C, Willson R, Alpers CE, et al. Hepatitis C virus–associated glomerulonephritis. *Curr Opin Nephrol Hypertens* 1995;4:287–294.
117. Stehman-Breen C, Alpers CE, Fleet WP, et al. Focal segmental glomerular sclerosis among patients infected with hepatitis C virus. *Nephron* 1999;81:37–40.
118. Johnson RJ, Gretch DR, Couser WG, et al. Hepatitis C virus–associated glomerulonephritis. Effect of alpha-interferon therapy. *Kidney Int* 1994;46:1700–1704.
119. Sabry AA, Sobh MA, Irving WL, et al. A comprehensive study of the association between hepatitis C virus and glomerulopathy. *Nephrol Dial Transplant* 2002;17:239–245.
120. Fabrizi F, Poordad FF, Martin P. Hepatitis C infection and the patient with end-stage renal disease. *Hepatology* 2002;36:3–10.
121. Molle ZL, Baqi N, Gretch D, et al. Hepatitis C infection in children and adolescents with end-stage renal disease. *Pediatr Nephrol* 2002;17:444–449.
122. Batty DS Jr, Swanson SJ, Kirk AD, et al. Hepatitis C virus seropositivity at the time of renal transplantation in the United States: associated factors and patient survival. *Am J Transplant* 2001;1:179–184.
123. Roth D, Cirocco R, Zucker K, et al. De novo membranoproliferative glomerulonephritis in hepatitis C virus–infected renal allograft recipients. *Transplantation* 1995;59:1676–1682.
124. Cruzado JM, Carrera M, Torras J, et al. Hepatitis C virus infection and de novo glomerular lesions in renal allografts. *Am J Transplant* 2001;1:171–178.
125. Sabry AA, Sobh MA, Sheaashaa HA, et al. Effect of combination therapy (ribavirin and interferon) in HCV-related glomerulopathy. *Nephrol Dial Transplant* 2002;17:1924–1930.
126. Rostaing L, Modesto A, Baron E, et al. Acute renal failure in kidney transplant patients treated with interferon alpha 2b for chronic hepatitis C. *Nephron* 1996;74:512–516.
127. Myerson D, Hackman RC, Nelson JA, et al. Widespread presence of histologically occult cytomegalovirus. *Hum Pathol* 1984;15:430–439.
128. Beneck D, Greco MA, Feinder HD. Glomerulonephritis in congenital cytomegalic inclusion disease. *Hum Pathol* 1986;17: 1054–1059.
129. Stagno S, Volanakis JE, Reynolds DW, et al. Immune complexes in congenital and natal cytomegalovirus infection of man. *J Clin Invest* 1977;60:838–845.
130. Richardson WP, Colvin RB, Cheeseman SH, et al. Glomerulopathy associated with cytomegalovirus viremia in renal allografts. *N Engl J Med* 1981;305:57–63.
131. Breinig MK, Zitelli B, Starzl TE, et al. Epstein-Barr virus, cytomegalovirus and other viral infections in children after transplant. *J Infect Dis* 1999;156:273–279.
132. Onuigbo M, Haririan A, Ramos E, et al. Cytomegalovirus-induced glomerular vasculopathy in renal allografts: a report of two cases. *Am J Transplant* 2002;2:684–688.
133. Tong CY, Bakran A, Peiris JS, et al. The association of viral infection and chronic allograft nephropathy with graft dysfunction after renal transplantation. *Transplantation* 2002;74:576–578.
134. Pescovitz MD, Rabkin J, Merion RM, et al. Valganciclovir results in improved oral absorption of ganciclovir in liver transplant recipients. *Antimicrob Agents Chemother* 2000;44:2811–2815.
135. Fishman JA, Rubin RH. Infection in organ transplant recipients. *N Engl J Med* 1998;338:1741–1751.
136. Minkowitz S, Wenk R, Friedman E, et al. Acute glomerulone-

phritis associated with varicella infection. *Am J Med* 1968;44:489–492.
137. Os I, Strom EH, Stenehjem A, et al. Varicella infection in a renal transplant recipient associated with abdominal pain, hepatitis, and glomerulonephritis. *Scand J Urol Nephrol* 2001;35:330–333.
138. Lin CY, Hsu HC, Hung HY. Nephrotic syndrome associated with varicella infection. *Pediatrics* 1985;75:1127–1131.
139. Cataudella JA, Young ID, Iliescu EA. Epstein-Barr virus–associated acute interstitial nephritis: infection or immunologic phenomenon? *Nephron* 2002;92:437–439.
140. Verma N, Arunabh S, Brady TM, et al. Acute interstitial nephritis secondary to infectious mononucleosis. *Clin Nephrol* 2002;58:151–154.
141. Okada H, Ikeda N, Kobayashi T, et al. An atypical pattern of Epstein-Barr virus infection in a case with idiopathic tubulointerstitial nephritis. *Nephron* 2002;92:440–444.
142. Sinniah R, Khan TN, Dodd S. An in situ hybridization study of herpes simplex and Epstein Barr viruses in IgA nephropathy and non-immune glomerulonephritis. *Clin Nephrol* 1993;40:137–141.
143. Mufson MA, Belshe RB. A review of adenoviruses in the aetiology of haemorrhagic cystitis. *J Urol* 1976;115:191–194.
144. Lin CY, Hsu HC. Measles and acute glomerulonephritis. *Pediatrics* 1983;17:398–401.
145. Lin CY, Chen WP, Chiang H. Mumps associated with nephritis. *Child Nephrol Urol* 1990;10:68–71.
146. Rao TKS, Filippone EJ, Nicastri AD, et al. Associated focal and segmental glomerulosclerosis in the acquired immunodeficiency syndrome. *N Engl J Med* 1984;310:669–673.
147. Gardenswartz MH, Lerner CW, Seligson GR, et al. Renal disease in patients with AIDS: a clinicopathologic study. *Clin Nephrol* 1984;21:197–204.
148. Pardo V, Aldana M, Colton RM, et al. Glomerular lesions in the acquired immunodeficiency syndrome. *Ann Intern Med* 1984;101:429–434.
149. Strauss J, Montane B, Scott G, et al. Urinary and renal histological changes in children with the acquired immunodeficiency syndrome (AIDS). *Pediatr Res* 1984;18:371A.
150. Ingulli E, Tejani A, Fikrig S, et al. Nephrotic syndrome associated with acquired immunodeficiency syndrome in children. *J Pediatr* 1991;119:710–716.
151. Strauss J, Zilleruelo G, Abitbol C, et al. Human immunodeficiency virus nephropathy. *Pediatr Nephrol* 1993;7:220–225.
152. Ray PE, Rakusan T, Loechelt BJ, et al. Human immunodeficiency virus (HIV)–associated nephropathy in children from the Washington, D.C. area: 12 years' experience. *Semin Nephrol* 1998;18:396–405.
153. Winston JA, Klotman ME, Klotman PE. HIV-associated nephropathy is a late, not early, manifestation of HIV-1 infection. *Kidney Int* 1999;55:1036–1040.
154. Cohen AH. HIV-associated nephropathy: current concepts. *Nephrol Dial Transplant* 1998;13:540–542.
155. D'Agati V, Appel GB. Renal pathology of human immunodeficiency virus infection. *Semin Nephrol* 1998;18:406–421.
156. Cohen AH, Cohen GM. HIV-associated nephropathy. *Nephron* 1999;83:111–116.
157. Kajiyama W, Kopp JB, Marinos NJ, et al. Glomerulosclerosis and viral gene expression in HIV-transgenic mice: role of nef. *Kidney Int* 2000;58:1148–1159.
158. Schwartz EJ, Klotman PE. Pathogenesis of human immunodeficiency virus (HIV)–associated nephropathy. *Semin Nephrol* 1998;18:436–445.
159. Yamamoto T, Noble NA, Miller DE, et al. Increased levels of transforming growth factor-[beta] in HIV-associated nephropathy. *Kidney Int* 1999;55:579–592.
160. Dellow E, Unwin R, Miller R, et al. Protease inhibitor therapy for HIV infection: the effect on HIV-associated nephrotic syndrome. *Nephrol Dial Transplant* 1999;14:744–747.
161. Nebuloni M, Tosoni A, Boldorini R, et al. BK virus renal infection in a patient with the acquired immunodeficiency syndrome. *Arch Pathol Lab Med* 1999;123:807–811.
162. Kopp JB, Falloon J, Filie A, et al. Indinavir-associated interstitial nephritis and urothelial inflammation: clinical and cytologic findings. *Clin Infect Dis* 2002;34:1122–1128.
163. Dimitrakopoulos AN, Kordossis T, Hatzakis A, et al. Mixed cryoglobulinemia in HIV-1 infection: the role of HIV-1. *Ann Intern Med* 1999;130:226–230.
164. Turner ME, Kher K, Rakusan T, et al. A typical hemolytic uremic syndrome in human immunodeficiency virus-1–infected children. *Pediatr Nephrol* 1997;11:161–163.
165. Appel RG, Neill J. A steroid responsive nephrotic syndrome in a patient with human immunodeficiency virus infection. *Ann Intern Med* 1990;113:892–895.
166. Briggs WA, Tanawattanacharoen S, Choi MJ, et al. Clinicopathologic correlates of prednisone treatment of human immunodeficiency virus–associated nephropathy. *Am J Kidney Dis* 1996;28:618–621.
167. Eustace JA, Nuermberger E, Choi M, et al. Cohort study of the treatment of severe HIV-associated nephropathy with corticosteroids. *Kidney Int* 2000;58:1253–1260.
168. Smith MC, Austen JL, Carey JT, et al. Prednisone improves renal function and proteinuria in human immunodeficiency virus–associated nephropathy. *Am J Med* 1996;101:41–48.
169. Burns GC, Paul SK, Toth IR, et al. Effect of angiotensin-converting enzyme inhibition in HIV-associated nephropathy. *J Am Soc Nephrol* 1997;8:1140–1146.
170. Morales E, Martinez A, Sanchez-Ayuso J, et al. Spontaneous improvement of the renal function in a patient with HIV-associated focal glomerulosclerosis. *Am J Nephrol* 2002;22:369–371.
171. Wali RK, Drachenberg CI, Papadimitrou JC, et al. HIV-1–associated nephropathy and response to highly-active antiretroviral therapy. *Lancet* 1998;352:783–784.
172. Dellow E, Unwin R, Miller R, et al. Protease inhibitor therapy for HIV infection: the effect on HIV-associated nephrotic syndrome. *Nephrol Dial Transplant* 1999;14:744–747.
173. Ifudu O, Rao TK, Tan CC, et al. Zidovudine is beneficial in human immunodeficiency virus associated nephropathy. *Am J Nephrol* 1995;15:217–221.
174. Kimmel PL, Bosch JP, Vassalotti JA. Treatment of human immunodeficiency virus (HIV)–associated nephropathy. *Semin Nephrol* 1998;18:446–458.
175. Dave MB, Shabih K, Blum S. Maintenance hemodialysis in patients with HIV-associated nephropathy. *Clin Nephrol* 1998;50:367–374.
176. HIV+ Solid Organ Transplant Multi-Site Study. Clinical, immunologic and pharmacologic consequences of kidney transplantation in people with HIV infection. Available at: http://spitfire.emmes.com/study/hiv-k/. Accessed December 2002.

177. Roland M, Stock P, Carlson L, et al. Liver and kidney transplantation in HIV-infected patients: a preliminary multisite experience. Presented at: Ninth Conference on Retroviruses and Opportunistic Infections; February 24–28, 2002; Washington, DC. Session 86, Poster 655–M.
178. Gardner SD, Field AM, Coleman DV, et al. New human papovavirus (BK) isolated from urine after renal transplantation. *Lancet* 1971;1:1253–1257.
179. Binet I, Nickeleit V, Hirsch HH, et al. Polyomavirus disease under new immunosuppressive drugs: a cause of renal graft dysfunction and graft loss. *Transplantation* 1999;67:918–922.
180. Howell DN, Smith SR, Butterly DW, et al. Diagnosis and management of BK polyomavirus interstitial nephritis in renal transplant recipients. *Transplantation* 1999;68:1279–1288.
181. Nickeleit V, Hirsch HH, Binet IF, et al. Polyomavirus infection of renal allograft recipients: from latent infection to manifest disease. *J Am Soc Nephrol* 1999;10:1080–1089.
182. Nickeleit V, Klimkait T, Binet IF, et al. Testing for polyomavirus type BK DNA in plasma to identify renal-allograft recipients with viral nephropathy. *N Engl J Med* 2000;342:1309–1315.
183. Randhawa PS, Demetris AJ. Nephropathy due to polyomavirus type BK. *N Engl J Med* 2000;342:1361–1363.
184. Kwak EJ, Vilchez RA, Randhawa P, et al. Pathogenesis and management of polyomavirus infection in transplant recipients. *Clin Infect Dis* 2002;35:1081–1087.
185. Lin PL, Vats AN, Green M. BK virus infection in renal transplant recipients. *Pediatr Transplant* 2001:5:398–405.
186. Hirsch HH, Knowles W, Dickenmann M, et al. Prospective study of polyomavirus type BK replication and nephropathy in renal-transplant recipients. *N Engl J Med* 2002;347:488–496.
187. Arthur RR, Shah KV. Occurrence and significance of papovaviruses BK and JC in the urine. *Prog Med Virol* 1989:36:44–61.
188. Mathur VS, Olson JL, Darragh TM, et al. Polyoma-virus induced interstitial nephritis in two renal transplant recipients: case reports and review of the literature. *Am J Kidney Dis* 1997;29:754–758.
189. Apperley JF, Rice SJ, Bishop JA, et al. Late-onset hemorrhagic cystitis associated with urinary excretion of polyomaviruses after bone marrow transplantation. *Transplantation* 1987;43:108–112.
190. Ramos E, Drachenberg CB, Papadimitriou JC, et al. Clinical course of polyoma virus nephropathy in 67 renal transplant patients. *J Am Soc Nephrol* 2002;13:2145–2151.
191. Vats A, Randhawa PS, Shapiro R, et al. Quantitative viral load monitoring and cidofovir therapy for the management of BK virus associated nephropathy in children and adults. *Transplantation* 2003;75:105–112.
192. LeDuc JW. Epidemiology of haemorrhagic fever viruses. *Rev Infect Dis* 1989;11:5730–5735.
193. Cosgriff TM. Virus and hemostasis. *Rev Infect Dis* 1989;11: S677–S688.
194. Hayes EB, Gubler DJ. Dengue and dengue haemorrhagic fever. *Pediatr Infect Dis J* 1992;11:311–317.
195. Boonpucknavig V, Bhamarapravati N, Boonpucknavig S, et al. Glomerular changes in dengue haemorrhagic fever. *Arch Pathol Lab Med* 1976;100:206–212.
196. Swanepoel R, Shepherd AJ, Leman PA, et al. Epidemiology and clinical features of Crimean-Congo haemorrhagic fever in Southern Africa. *Am J Trop Med Hyg* 1987;36:130–142.
197. Hart CA, Bennett M. Hantavirus: an increasing problem? *Ann Trop Med Parasitol* 1994;88:347–358.
198. Niklasson BS. Haemorrhagic fever with renal syndrome, virological and epidemiological aspects. *Pediatr Nephrol* 1992;6: 201–204.
199. Grcevska L, Polenakovic M, Oncevski A, et al. Different pathohistological presentations of acute renal involvement in Hantaan virus infection: report of two cases. *Clin Nephrol* 1990;34:197–201.
200. Peco Antic A, Popovic Rolovic M, Gligic A, et al. Clinical characteristics of haemorrhagic fever with renal syndrome in children. *Pediatr Nephrol* 1992;6:335–338.
201. Huggins JW. Prospects for treatment of viral haemorrhagic fever with ribavirin, a broad spectrum antiviral drug. *Rev Infect Dis* 1989;11:S750–S761.
202. McCormick JB, King IJ, Webb PA, et al. Lassa fever: effective therapy with ribavirin. *N Engl J Med* 1986;314:20–26.
203. Greenwood B, Mutabingwa T. Malaria in 2002. *Nature* 2002;415:670–672.
204. Giglioli C. Malaria and renal disease with special reference to British Guiana. II. The effect of malaria eradication on the incidence of renal disease in British Guiana. *Ann Trop Med Hyg* 1962;56:225–241.
205. Marsh K, Greenwood BM. Immunopathology of malaria. *Clin Trop Med Commun Dis* 1986;1:91–125.
206. Hendrickse RG, Gilles HM. The nephrotic syndrome and other diseases in children in Western Nigeria. *East Afr Med J* 1963;40:186–201.
207. Abdurrahman MB, Aikhionbare HA, Babaoye FA, et al. Clinicopathological features of childhood nephrotic syndrome in northern Nigeria. *QJM* 1990;75:563–576.
208. Hendrickse RG, Adeniyi A, Edington GM, et al. Quartan malarial nephrotic syndrome. *Lancet* 1972;1:1143–1148.
209. Boonpucknavig V, Sitprua V. Renal disease in acute *Plasmodium falciparum* infection in man. *Kidney Int* 1979;16:44–52.
210. Eiam-Ong S. Current knowledge in falciparum malaria-induced acute renal failure. *J Med Assoc Thai* 2002;85:S16–S24.
211. Mehta KS, Halankar AR, Makwana PD, et al. Severe acute renal failure in malaria. *J Postgrad Med* 2001;47:24–26.
212. Van den Ende J, Coppens G, Verstraeten T, et al. Recurrence of blackwater fever: triggering of relapses by different antimalarials. *Trop Med Int Health* 1998;3:632–639.
213. Kline MW, Sullivan T. Schistosomiasis. In: Feign RD, Cherry JD, eds. *Textbook of paediatric infectious diseases.* 3rd ed. Philadelphia: WB Saunders, 1992:2112–2119.
214. Sobh MA, Moustafa FE, El-Housseini F, et al. Schistosomal specific nephropathy leading to end-stage renal failure. *Kidney Int* 1987;31:1006–1011.
215. Correia EI, Martinelli RP, Rocha H. Is glomerulopathy due to schistosomiasis mansoni disappearing? *Rev Soc Bras Med Trop* 1997;30:341–343.
216. Sobh MA, Moustafa FE, Sally SM, et al. Characterisation of kidney lesions in early schistosomal-specific nephropathy. *Nephrol Dial Transplant* 1988;3:392–398.
217. Martinelli R, Noblat AC, Brito E, et al. *Schistosoma mansoni*–induced mesangiocapillary glomerulonephritis: influence of therapy. *Kidney Int* 1989;35:1227–1233.
218. Turner I, Ibels LS, Alexander JH, et al. Minimal change glomerulonephritis associated with *Schistosoma haematobium*

infection—resolution with praziquantel treatment. *Aust N Z J Med* 1987;17:596–598.
219. Dutra M, Martinelli R, Marcelino de Carvalho E, et al. Renal involvement in visceral leishmaniasis. *Am J Kidney Dis* 1985;6:22–27.
220. Caravaca F, Munoz A, Pizarro JL, et al. Acute renal failure in visceral leishmaniasis. *Am J Nephrol* 1991;11:350–352.
221. Yap HK, Woo KT, Yeo PP, et al. The nephrotic syndrome associated with filariasis. *Ann Acad Med Singapore* 1982;11:60–63.
222. Gelman R, Brook G, Green J, et al. Minimal change glomerulonephritis associated with hydatid disease. *Clin Nephrol* 2000;53:152–155.
223. Covic A, Mititiuc I, Caruntu L, et al. Reversible nephrotic syndrome due to mesangiocapillary glomerulonephritis secondary to hepatic hydatid disease. *Nephrol Dial Transplant* 1996;11:2074–2076.
224. Costa RS, Monteiro RC, Lehuen A, et al. Immune complex–mediated glomerulopathy in experimental Chagas' disease. *Clin Immunol Immunopathol* 1991;58:102–114.
225. Eckstein CW, Kass EJ. Anuria in a newborn secondary to bilateral ureteropelvic fungus balls. *J Urol* 1982;127:109–112.
226. Bartone FF, Hurwitz RS, Rojas EL, et al. The role of percutaneous nephrostomy in the management of obstructing candidiasis of the urinary tract in infants. *J Urol* 1988;140: 338–341.
227. Stocker M, Caduff JH, Spalinger J, et al. Successful treatment of bilateral renal fungal balls with liposomal amphotericin B and fluconazole in an extremely low birth weight infant. *Eur J Pediatr* 2000;159:676–678.
228. Weintrub PS, Chapman A, Piecuch R. Renal fungus ball in a premature infant successfully treated with fluconazole. *Pediatr Infect Dis J* 1994;13:1152–1154.
229. Levin M, Kay JDS, Gould JG. Haemorrhagic shock and encephalopathy: a new syndrome with high mortality in young children. *Lancet* 1983;2:64–67.
230. Chesney PJ, Chesney RW. Haemorrhagic shock and encephalopathy: reflections about a new devastating disorder that affects normal children. *J Pediatr* 1989;114:254–256.
231. Levin M, Pincott JR, Hjelm M. Haemorrhagic shock and encephalopathy: clinical, pathologic, and biochemical features. *J Pediatr* 1989;114:194–203.

52

NEPHROTOXINS

RUSSELL W. CHESNEY
DEBORAH P. JONES

Because of its vital role as an excretory organ, the kidney is responsible for the elimination and metabolism of many foreign organic compounds, including pharmacologic agents. Ultimately these agents reach the urinary space for excretion via glomerular filtration or tubular secretion (Fig. 52.1). In some instances drugs must undergo transformation into metabolites, a reaction that may actually take place within tubular cells before secretion into the tubular lumen. Unfortunately, while performing its role as an excretory and metabolic organ, the kidney may undergo anatomic or functional changes as a result of drug-induced toxicity.

Factors that contribute to the distinct susceptibility of the kidney to injury include exposure to potentially harmful compounds, given the magnitude of blood flow through glomeruli and peritubular vessels; the large surface area available for uptake of potentially harmful compounds; the concentration of toxic species within the tubular lumen to promote accumulation of the toxin within the renal tubular cell; dependence of the renal tubular cell on a high metabolic rate to maintain function; and the distribution of unique transport systems that concentrate drugs or toxins within the tubular cell (1).

Certain nephrotoxins may preferentially damage specific nephron segments, depending on the area of maximal exposure, the location of specific uptake systems, and the nephronal location of specific intracellular sites that are susceptible to the toxin (1). The concentration of a drug within the renal tubular cell may be affected by the dissociation constant of the compound, its lipid solubility, tubular secretory or reabsorptive activity, water handling, competitive tubular transport mechanisms, urinary pH, and urinary flow rate. The concentration also may be affected by the distribution of enzymes that metabolize individual drugs and intracellular protective systems important in the maintenance of normal cell metabolism.

Potential mechanisms for drug-induced renal dysfunction include alterations in renal perfusion and glomerular filtration, tubular cell damage, and tubular obstruction (Fig. 52.2) (1). Toxic nephropathy, or drug-induced renal dysfunction, is primarily a disorder of the renal tubule; however, significant tubular damage eventually results in alterations in glomerular function as well. In addition, drugs or their metabolites may alter glomerular blood flow through vasoconstriction of the glomerular capillaries (1). This may be a primary event through actions on the endothelial cell or a secondary event via activation of tubuloglomerular feedback after tubular damage allows increased distal delivery of solute and fluid.

Drugs may undergo redox recycling, which results in oxidative stress within the cell and alters the normal antioxidant defense mechanisms. The elaboration of reactive oxygen species by the cytochrome P-450 system may enable reactive intermediates to initiate damage directly or to combine with glutathione (GSH) to deplete available GSH (2). GSH protects cells from oxidant stress as it participates in detoxification reactions during vital cell processes such as protein and nucleic acid synthesis. Depletion of cellular levels of GSH is a common pathway for nephrotoxic injury (2). Drugs or metabolites may either directly conjugate GSH or be metabolized to compounds that are reactive and may bind to GSH. Ultimately, reactive species promote injury, which interferes with normal cellular functions such as energy production, detoxification, transport, and macromolecular synthesis. Although they may come from widely different chemical classes and have different renal distributions, toxic compounds may ultimately affect renal integrity and function through inhibition of cellular energy production, disruption of membrane integrity, perturbation of vital cell functions such as protein or nucleic acid synthesis, or alteration in intracellular calcium homeostasis (Fig. 52.3).

This chapter focuses on the clinical characteristics, mechanisms of injury, if known, and potential methods to reduce or prevent drug-associated renal damage and dysfunction. The most common offending agents have been chosen; this discussion is not meant to be all inclusive.

NEPHROTOXICITY FROM ANTIBIOTICS

The concentration of antibiotics by renal tissue exposes them to a toxicity that other organs do not experience (3).

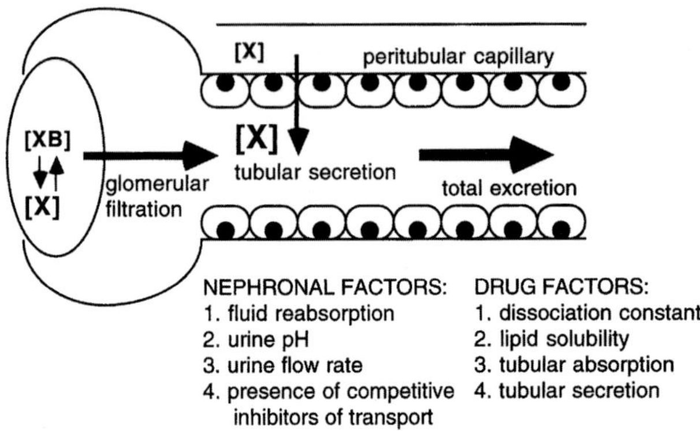

FIGURE 52.1. Renal drug elimination is a combination of glomerular filtration and tubular secretion. Many factors have an impact on renal cell accumulation and nephronal excretion.

Nephrotoxic clinical syndromes include acute tubular necrosis (ATN), acute interstitial nephritis (AIN), direct tubular effects on transport systems (electrolytes, protons leading to acidosis, concentration defects, or the full-blown Fanconi syndrome), and tubular obstruction from drug precipitation. Other mechanisms of antimicrobial toxicity include the induction of rhabdomyolysis or hemolytic anemia, which leads to release of cell products—myoglobin, phosphate, or hemoglobin. Macrolide antibiotics, which interfere with the metabolism of calcineurin inhibitors, may indirectly lead to renal damage (4).

Aminoglycosides

Aminoglycoside antibiotics are widely used antimicrobials that are particularly nephrotoxic (5). Although ATN is the most common mechanism of toxicity, a variety of tubular dysfunction states have been noted, including hypomagnesemia, hypocalcemia, hypokalemia, and full-blown Fanconi syndrome (3). Certain risk factors predispose to aminoglycoside toxicity: drug dosage, timing, and duration of administration; age group (especially neonates and geriatric populations); preexisting renal insufficiency, which may not be recognized by the caretaker; concomitant administration of other nephrotoxic agents, such as amphotericin B, certain cephalosporins, and cyclosporin; extracellular volume depletion; and potassium depletion. Other risk factors include use of a contrast medium, presence of shock or liver disease, and excessive use of diuretics (5).

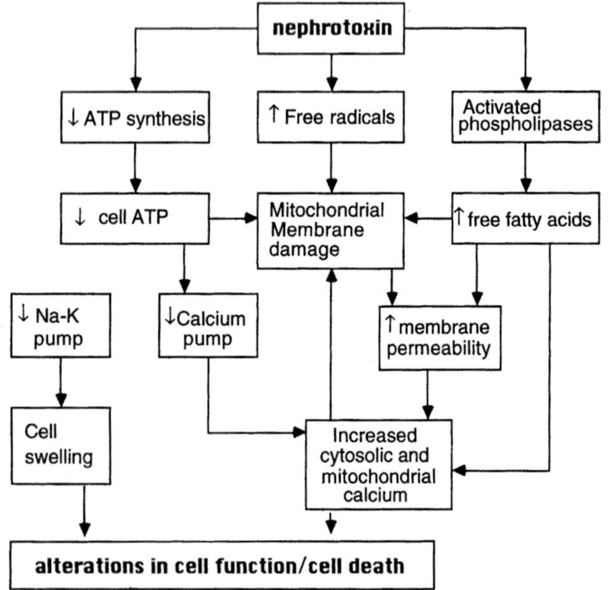

FIGURE 52.2. Biochemical pathways resulting in cell injury and dysfunction. ATP, adenosine triphosphate.

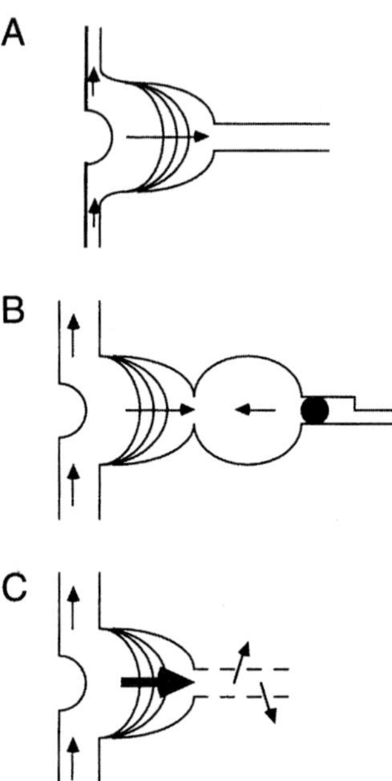

FIGURE 52.3. Mechanisms whereby drugs induce renal functional changes at the glomerulus and tubule. **A:** Vasoconstriction, which may be a primary or secondary event (drug examples are amphotericin B and cyclosporine). **B:** Tubular obstruction (drug examples are acyclovir and contrast media). **C:** Tubular cell injury and necrosis with backleak from loss of epithelial integrity (drug examples include aminoglycosides, amphotericin B, cisplatin, and ifosfamide).

Aminoglycosides are excreted primarily by glomerular filtration. Reabsorption by the proximal tubule cell occurs after charge interaction and binding of aminoglycosides, which are strongly cationic, with the brush-border membrane of the proximal tubule, followed by transport into the cell by pinocytosis into vesicles directed to lysosomes (6,7). Although less significant, reabsorption from the basolateral surface of the tubular cell may also contribute to total intracellular uptake (8). Accumulation of the drug within the lysosome results in phospholipid hydrolysis and the formation of electron-dense myeloid bodies, which are membranous structures found within lysosomes (5). Aminoglycosides appear to have a generalized effect on phospholipid membranes, which results in decreased surface charge and alterations in fluidity and permeability of tubular cell membranes (3,5).

Pathologic alterations have been reported after a single dose of aminoglycoside, but most animal models of aminoglycoside toxicity use multiple doses over several days to produce a model of toxic nephropathy. Once appreciable injury occurs, lysosomal membranes release sequestered aminoglycosides as well as lysosomal enzymes, which cause generalized cell injury and eventual necrosis (9,10).

The main pathologic finding in aminoglycoside nephrotoxicity is tubular cell necrosis, involving principally the most proximal segments of the nephron: the convoluted tubule and pars recta (S1 and S2) (1,11). The earliest pathologic finding is an increased number of lysosomes, followed by alterations in the brush-border architecture and mitochondrial swelling (12). This process may be focal or diffuse. Of interest, even during continued aminoglycoside administration, tubular cell regeneration can be evident. One component of the insensitivity of the regenerating tubule cell is the inhibition of aminoglycoside uptake across the apical membranes of S1 and S2 cells (13). Gentamicin also interferes with mitochondrial respiration by enhancing hydrogen peroxide generation, which includes iron mobilization from the mitochondria. Hydroxyradical scavengers and iron chelators are protective in the rat model of aminoglycoside toxicity (2).

Clinical features of aminoglycoside nephrotoxicity initially include subtle indications of tubular or glomerular dysfunction, and the nephrotoxicity occasionally progresses to oliguria and renal failure. The earliest clinically detectable abnormality is enzymuria, which results from loss of brush-border membrane segments bearing the enzymes (14). Tubular damage may rarely produce a Fanconi syndrome with proximal tubular wasting of glucose, phosphate, amino acids, and bicarbonate as well as numerous ions including magnesium (5,11). Urine volume initially may be increased with mild to moderate tubular toxicity because of a vasopressin-resistant concentrating defect. Renal dysfunction is most commonly detected after a rise in serum creatinine concentration or elevated aminoglycoside trough levels. Although it is rare, severe, sustained renal dysfunction has been described with peak serum creatinine levels at 3 to 10 days after cessation of aminoglycoside therapy and full recovery in weeks (15).

Glomerular filtration rate (GFR) may decrease after gentamicin administration in the absence of tubular necrosis from angiotensin II–mediated afferent arteriolar vasoconstriction. Prostaglandin synthetase inhibitors potentiate the vasoconstriction and hypofiltration, which provides indirect evidence of a palliative role of locally produced vasodilatory prostaglandins in this form of nephrotoxic injury (16). In addition to the microvascular and tubular changes, K_f (glomerular capillary ultrafiltration coefficient) is decreased because of a decrease in the number and density of glomerular capillary wall fenestrae (17,18).

The relative toxicity of the aminoglycosides, in order from most toxic to least, is neomycin, gentamicin, tobramycin, and amikacin (11). This order is dependent on the number of ionizable amino groups, which affects brush-border membrane binding: six for neomycin, five for gentamicin, four for amikacin and kanamycin, and three for streptomycin (19). Several factors may contribute to or predispose to aminoglycoside nephrotoxicity. Drug dosage and duration of therapy, particularly repeated and prolonged courses, determine the severity of the tubular toxicity. Concomitant administration of other nephrotoxic drugs, concomitant administration of cationic amino acids, volume depletion, potassium depletion, endotoxemia, hypokalemia, and hyperphosphatemia further potentiate renal injury (6,11,20). Nephrotoxicity may be attenuated by increased intake of dietary calcium, alkalinization of the urine, solute diuresis, and use of calcium-channel blockers or captopril (6).

Prevention of aminoglycoside toxicity involves the prudent use of aminoglycosides and alertness to iatrogenic potential. Careful dosing schedules reduce toxicity. The time of aminoglycoside administration also may affect toxicity. Both animal and human studies indicate that clearance is slower during periods of inactivity such as sleep (20). In addition, once-daily dosing has been adopted by some practitioners as a means of reducing toxicity without interfering with efficacy (21). Although not yet adopted by all pediatric centers, once-daily dosing proved to be effective, with higher peak levels and no difference in toxicity among a group of neonates (22). Animal studies also support this mode of therapy as a means of reducing the risk of nephrotoxicity while maintaining or even increasing bactericidal activity (23). It is prudent to avoid standard aminoglycoside dosages and administration intervals during periods of volume contraction or after vigorous diuresis. Blood levels of aminoglycosides should be monitored during administration with a target for the trough level of less than 2.0 μg/mL. Recognition of the interaction of certain drugs with each other allows anticipation of renal toxicity. For example, furosemide enhances renal aminoglycoside toxicity by leading to volume contraction. Cephalothin, not currently available in the United States, is the most potent interacting cephalosporin (3).

β-Lactam Antibiotics

The β-lactam antibiotics are related to the penicillins. Structurally, they are bicyclic compounds that acylate bacterial wall proteins and penetrate the bacterium to inactivate vital enzymes. Whereas most penicillin-like compounds are not nephrotoxic, certain cephalosporins and carbapenem compounds are associated with renal toxicity (24).

The β-lactams are extracted from renal venous blood by the organic acid transport system located on the basolateral surface of the tubular cell (organic anion transporter I, II, III). Intracellular accumulation results because of the limited ability of the proximal tubular cell to secrete the β-lactam at the luminal membrane into the luminal fluid (urine). Differences in organic acid transporter characteristics between basolateral and apical membranes result in marked accumulation with high intracellular levels, sometimes a thousand times higher than the levels found in plasma or other types of cells (24). Because of the very specific distribution of *p*-aminohippuric acid–sensitive organic acid transporters, renal injury in the form of tubular cell necrosis is limited to the proximal tubule (24). The initial event is thought to be lipid peroxidation with particular damage to the mitochondrial membrane, possibly through acylation of important membrane-associated transporters. Mitochondrial damage interferes with energy production, which leads to decreased levels of adenosine triphosphate and subsequent cell damage and death. Replacement of deficient cellular substrates can reverse toxicity (10). Damage secondary to β-lactams is related to decreased mitochondrial respiration and decreased succinate uptake by mitochondria within hours after drug administration (24).

The original compounds cephaloridine and cephaloglycin are no longer used; the new compound imipenem, which is a carbapenem, is nephrotoxic and is used only in combination with cilastin, an inhibitor of brush-border dehydropeptidase I. Cilastin inhibits the metabolism of imipenem to metabolites with structural similarity to cephaloridine (25). Meropenem, another agent in the carbapenem class, is not metabolized to an appreciable degree and therefore does not require co-administration with cilastin.

Clinical characteristics of β-lactam–associated nephrotoxicity include ATN with or without oliguria, which lasts days to weeks. Drug dosage should be adjusted according to the patient's renal function. Administration of organic anion transporter inhibitors (probenecid) may help to prevent injury. However, because these agents also impair tubular secretion, and thus drug elimination, blood levels of the β-lactam would be expected to be higher in the presence of organic anion inhibitors.

Renal toxicity from β-lactams can also result from hypersensitivity reactions. The molecular weights of all β-lactams are insufficient to be directly immunogenic. These antibiotics or their metabolites can bind to larger molecules, which then act as haptens. Although exposure to many penicillins and cephalosporins can result in AIN, AIN is most common with methicillin (26,27). This syndrome consists of fever, rash, oliguria, and, rarely, arthralgias. Laboratory findings are prominent in the urine with pyuria, eosinophiluria, and proteinuria with azotemia. The main therapy is discontinuation of the β-lactam, but glucocorticoids have been used and may enhance recovery (28).

Other Antibiotics

Because antibiotics are concentrated in tubules and urine, the opportunity for toxicity is great. *Sulfonamides* and their acetylated metabolites are poorly soluble in aqueous solutions and may lead to intrarenal obstruction. The use of sulfonamide mixtures, particularly the inclusion of *trimethoprim*, reduces this danger (3). Trimethoprim, which blocks bacterial and protozoal dihydrofolate reductases to inhibit tetrahydrofolic acid synthesis, has an amiloride-like influence on the distal tubule, which can result in hyperkalemia and metabolic acidosis (29,30).

Macrolide antibiotics, including *erythromycin, clarithromycin, azithromycin,* and *dirithromycin,* inhibit the cytochrome P-450 isoenzyme CYP 3A4, which interferes with the metabolism of cyclosporin or tacrolimus and results in indirect renal toxicity (31).

Although *vancomycin* was initially felt to be extremely nephrotoxic, this was likely the result of impurities when it was introduced in the 1950s, and its direct toxicity is difficult to demonstrate (3).

Tetracyclines have an interesting profile of nephrotoxicity. AIN along with nephrogenic diabetes insipidus has been described after use of demeclocycline. In cirrhotic patients, tetracyclines can potentiate acute renal failure. Use of outdated tetracyclines can lead to Fanconi syndrome. This latter result was due to a degradation product, anhydro-4-epitetracycline. Finally, syndromes of inappropriate secretion of antidiuretic hormone and phosphaturia have been described (3). Because of tooth staining, this class of agents is little used in children.

The polypeptide antibiotics polymyxin B, polymyxin E (*colostin*), and *bacitracin* are lipophilic agents that readily bind to plasma membranes. They have a mode of toxicity similar to that of aminoglycosides. This potential for nephrotoxicity has largely prevented their parenteral use. In the United States only topical preparations remain available (3).

ANTIFUNGAL AGENTS

Amphotericin B

Amphotericin B is an antifungal agent that exerts its effect by interaction with membrane sterols. This chemical interaction is the basis for its antifungal action as well as renal toxicity (11). Amphotericin B has two major pathophysiologic effects on the kidney: renal tubular cell injury, which is manifest as hypokalemia, hypomagnesemia, and acidosis; and decreased GFR secondary to afferent arteriolar vasoconstriction (5,32).

Unlike in most other drug-associated renal tubular toxicity, the primary tubular site of amphotericin B–induced injury is the distal tubule (11). The interaction of this drug with membrane cholesterol leads to the formation of aqueous pores, which greatly increase the permeability of the normally tight epithelium of the distal tubule; this results first in a backleak of H^+, Na^+, and Cl^-, and then to a vasopressin-resistant polyuria (11,33). Use of this agent will result in the formation of pores in all patients exposed. Increased permeability to Cl^- may stimulate increased tubuloglomerular feedback and reduce GFR, which ultimately results in renal ischemia and azotemia. In a canine model, amphotericin administration led to a decrease in urine flow and GFR within 1 hour, accompanied by increased renal vascular resistance as a result of afferent arteriolar constriction (34). Aminophylline blocks amphotericin B–induced vasoconstriction, which suggests a role for adenosine as a potential mediator (35). Verapamil also protects the kidney from vasoconstriction, which indicates that increased calcium in vascular smooth muscle may mediate the acute effects (36).

Amphotericin B nephrotoxicity may become clinically evident as a reduction in GFR, usually detected as an increase in plasma creatinine level or as distal tubular dysfunction with metabolic acidosis (secondary to the distal type of renal tubular acidification defect), salt wasting, polyuria, hypomagnesemia, or hypokalemia (6,11). Nephrotoxicity is predictable and usually reversible, although irreversible azotemia has been observed at large dosages. The severity of tubular toxicity and hypofiltration is proportional to the cumulative dose. In adults, a cumulative dose exceeding 5 g was associated with significant renal dysfunction, whereas patients who received less than a 600-mg cumulative dose rarely suffered renal toxicity (37). Newborn infants are equally susceptible to amphotericin nephrotoxicity (38). Concomitant use of diuretics, cyclosporine, or aminoglycoside antibiotics and abnormal pretreatment renal function increase the risk of amphotericin toxicity (11,37). This is especially true in the bone marrow transplant patient.

Sodium loading appears to have a beneficial effect on amphotericin B–induced nephrotoxicity by maintaining intravascular volume and reducing renal vasoconstriction (11,37). Mannitol has been shown to ameliorate nephrotoxicity in animal studies, but the benefit of this agent in humans has not been consistently demonstrated (39,40).

Lipid formulations of amphotericin B have been developed in an attempt to reduce renal toxicity and deliver more drug to treat serious fungal sepsis or resistant fungal disease. The aim of the lipid preparations of amphotericin B is to direct the drug to preferentially bind to fungal membranes rather than mammalian membranes. Several formulations of lipid-associated amphotericin B have been tested. Efficacy and toxicity vary depending on which lipid compounds are used. Neutropenic rabbits treated with Ambisome (5 mg/kg/day), which is a unilamellar vesicle formulation, did not exhibit the increased creatinine levels observed in animals given standard amphotericin B (41). Amphotericin B lipid complex was used in 228 immunocompromised patients with refractory mycoses or toxicity from standard amphotericin B. Renal toxicity was minimal. A prospective study comparing administration of regular amphotericin B with and without co-administration of lipid emulsion found that approximately two-thirds of those who received regular amphotericin B alone exhibited signs of renal toxicity, whereas minimal renal toxicity was seen in the group who received amphotericin B with lipid emulsion (42). In the setting of established renal insufficiency from administration of the standard amphotericin B formulation, renal function may not appreciably improve with use of liposomal or lipid-associated amphotericin B. Comparative clinical trials need to be performed to define the best preparation and dosage for various clinical situations.

Azoles

The azole antifungals consist of the imidazole ketoconazole and the two triazoles fluconazole and itraconazole (3). Each acts to inhibit ergosterol synthesis by blockade of the fungal cytochrome P-450 system.

These azoles are not directly toxic. Each—and ketoconazole, in particular—may lead to indirect nephrotoxicity in patients treated with calcineurin inhibitors by inhibiting CYP 3A4 metabolism of cyclosporin or tacrolimus (43).

Griseofulvin

Griseofulvin actually enhances cytochrome P-450 metabolism, so that it could theoretically increase calcineurin-inhibitor metabolism and lead to transplant rejection (3).

NONSTEROIDAL ANTIINFLAMMATORY DRUGS

Nonsteroidal antiinflammatory drugs (NSAIDs) inhibit cyclooxygenase and inhibit prostaglandin synthesis from arachidonic acid. The kidney synthesizes and metabolizes prostaglandins. Cortical prostaglandins modify regional blood flow, glomerular filtration, and renin release (44). Medullary prostaglandins regulate medullary blood flow, tubular response to arginine vasopressin, and sodium chloride reabsorption in the loop of Henle. Prostaglandin production can be stimulated by angiotensin II, arginine vasopressin, catecholamines, and renal sympathetic nerve stimulation. Stimulation of prostaglandin synthesis occurs by hormone-mediated activation of phospholipases, which release arachidonic acid from membrane-associated phospholipids (44).

Under normal conditions prostaglandins exert minimal effect on renal blood flow. Under conditions such as impaired GFR, alterations in renal hemodynamics, and sodium depletion, however, the compensatory release of vasodilatory prostaglandins I_2 and E_2 helps to maintain renal blood flow and GFR, and modifies the effect of local vasoconstrictive substances such as angiotensin II (44). Therefore, it is in the presence of such altered physiologic states that renal functional alterations associated with NSAIDs are likely to occur, because the normal compensatory mechanisms are blocked. NSAIDs potentiate prerenal ischemia, increasing sodium reabsorption by the proximal tubule and the ascending limb of the loop of Henle. NSAIDs also increase the sensitivity of the collecting tubule to vasopressin, which further adds to salt and water retention and may produce a hyporeninemic hypoaldosteronism through reduction of renin release (44).

Acute renal failure secondary to NSAIDs results from excessive vasoconstriction at the level of the afferent arteriole. An acute phenomenon often associated with oliguria, NSAID-induced acute renal failure usually is reversible. Risk factors include volume depletion from states such as dehydration, hemorrhage, congestive heart failure, hepatic failure with ascites, and hypoalbuminemia (44).

In addition to having physiologic actions that produce renal functional changes, NSAIDs also may produce a tubulointerstitial nephritis. Arising after 2 to 18 months of therapy, this syndrome is associated with an interstitial mononuclear cell infiltrate and occasionally epithelial cell podocyte fusion on electron microscopy (45). NSAIDs are also associated with polyuric acute renal failure with nephrotic syndrome. Renal functional recovery typically occurs when the agent is discontinued.

Long-term use of NSAIDs may cause papillary necrosis as well as chronic renal insufficiency through chronic ischemia (45). The risk of chronic renal disease (serum creatinine level above 1.5 mg/dL) in daily users of NSAIDs was 2.1% (34). Although most epidemiologic studies were performed in adults, children also are at risk for renal failure (46). Prenatal exposure may lead to renal failure–associated deaths after administration of 140 to 400 mg of indomethacin per day for anywhere between 2 and 11 weeks of therapy (47). Risk factors for renal functional changes are underlying volume depletion and renal disease (44). Acute administration of NSAIDs to patients with chronic renal insufficiency results in decreased renal plasma flow, decreased GFR, decreased fractional excretion of sodium, and decreased fractional free water clearance (48). Most healthy, normal subjects who take NSAIDs for a limited duration tolerate these agents without adverse events, but a subset of individuals appears to be at risk. Because ibuprofen is now commercially available for treatment of fever in children, the incidence of NSAID-related renal disease may increase. Febrile children often have reduced fluid intake in the face of increased insensible fluid losses with clinically mild but significant hypovolemia, which places them at risk for NSAID toxicity.

ANTIVIRAL AGENTS

Acyclovir and ganciclovir are active against herpes viruses and cytomegalovirus (CMV). Acyclovir is excreted primarily by the kidney. Anywhere from 30 to 90% of the drug is excreted unchanged in the urine in patients with normal glomerular filtration. Acyclovir is probably excreted by both glomerular filtration and tubular secretion (49). Pretreatment with probenecid decreases renal clearance of the drug by 32%, which supports a role for tubular secretion as a partial mechanism of excretion. The dosing interval must be adjusted in the setting of a decreased GFR (49).

Acyclovir administration is complicated by renal, hepatic, and neurologic dysfunction (49). Renal toxicity is associated with plasma concentrations of acyclovir exceeding 20 μg/mL. Renal levels of acyclovir can be 20 times the plasma levels. The solubility of acyclovir in water is 2.5 mg/mL, but solubility in urine is lower. Crystals form within the renal tubule (usually the collecting duct), which leads to intratubular obstruction followed by a rise in the serum creatinine concentration within 24 to 48 hours (50,51). Needle-shaped crystals may form in the urine even in those who do not have clinical evidence of renal dysfunction. In most cases, renal failure is not associated with oliguria and GFR returns to normal within 1 week. Urinary findings include hematuria, pyuria, proteinuria, and crystalluria. Histologically, ATN may be observed along with patchy interstitial infiltration (51).

Renal toxicity was noted in rats during preclinical toxicology studies. An obstructive nephropathy developed, with associated drug crystallization within the collecting ducts. The development of crystalluria was dosage related. Acyclovir administration to rats was accompanied by a reduction in GFR and significant increase in total renal vascular resistance without changes in urinary flow rate (52). Acute changes appeared to be secondary to increased arteriolar resistance, whereas chronic toxicity was associated with a decline in K_f in addition to vasoconstriction. Ganciclovir administration did not induce a decrease in GFR or change in renal vascular resistance in this rat model (52).

In a large series of patients who received acyclovir for serious infections, 58 of 354 adult patients experienced elevations of the serum creatinine level. In a separate study, 12% of children given acyclovir had elevated serum creatinine concentrations. Some of the elevations were transient, with improvement in the creatinine levels during continued administration of the drug. In most patients renal function returns to normal after discontinuation of the drug. Most importantly, one must adjust dosing intervals in the face of decreased GFR.

Risk factors for renal toxicity include high peak concentrations after rapid intravenous administration, dehydration (or conditions in which urine flow is diminished), and preexisting renal disease (53). Therefore, consideration of the individual's renal function, adequate hydration, and slow infusion rates (over a minimum of 1 hour) should lower the risk for renal toxicity.

Ganciclovir is excreted entirely by glomerular filtration, with 99% of the dose appearing in the urine (49). In addition, plasma clearance is highly correlated with creatinine clearance and is approximately twice that of creatinine clearance, which indicates significant elimination by proximal tubular secretion. Ganciclovir is seldom associated with renal insufficiency or damage except in the setting of impaired GFR and concomitant administration of nephrotoxic agents.

Foscarnet is an antiviral agent with promising results against herpes viruses. Foscarnet is a pyrophosphate analogue that interferes with viral replication by binding to a site on the herpes virus DNA polymerase or human immunodeficiency virus (HIV) reverse transcriptase (54,55). Foscarnet most commonly is used to treat CMV infection alone or in combination with ganciclovir, usually in the setting of CMV prophylaxis, CMV retinitis, or disease after bone-marrow transplantation or in immunodeficient states.

Foscarnet appears to be excreted primarily by glomerular filtration, with little contribution by tubular secretion (54). Foscarnet causes reversible decreases in GFR in 20 to 60% of patients. The incidence of acute renal failure is dependent on the definition used by the investigators (55). Two mechanisms for renal damage have been reported: tubular necrosis and crystallization within glomerular capillaries with crescentic glomerulonephritis. Hydration at the time of administration is thought to reduce the incidence of acute renal failure considerably.

Functional renal tubular effects of foscarnet include hypophosphatemia, hypokalemia, renal tubular acidosis, and vasopressin-resistant diabetes insipidus (56). Alterations in mineral metabolism associated with foscarnet therapy include hyperphosphatemia, hypocalcemia, and transient increases in parathyroid hormone level (57). Explanation of these alterations is difficult because animal studies demonstrated inhibition of proximal tubular reabsorption of phosphate and would have predicted hypophosphatemia. One group of investigators postulated that direct binding of foscarnet with ionized calcium is responsible for the acute hypocalcemia and that reducing the dosage may allow continued therapy.

In a series of bone marrow transplant recipients, increased creatinine levels occurred in 17 of 19 patients, with 4 requiring hemodialysis (58). Hypocalcemia was reported in 16, and hypophosphatemia in 17. When 26 courses of foscarnet were given to patients with HIV infection, two patients experienced a creatinine level higher than 3.0 mg/dL, six had hyperphosphatemia, three had hypophosphatemia, three had hypocalcemia, and two had hypokalemia (59). Acute renal failure associated with foscarnet also has been reported (60). Hydration with saline may reduce the risk of nephrotoxicity. An increase in the serum creatinine level (defined as more than 25% above baseline) occurred in 66% of nonhydrated adults but only 13% of hydrated adults. Even those with abnormal pretreatment GFR tolerated foscarnet therapy if the drug was given along with hydration (61). Protocols using a combination of foscarnet and ganciclovir at lower dosages have not been complicated with renal toxicity or electrolyte abnormalities (62).

Cidofovir is a nucleoside analogue of cytosine and an antiviral agent with activity against herpes viruses and potentially the BK virus (polyoma virus). The drug is filtered in its parent state without significant biotransformation. It causes increased creatinine concentration and proteinuria by direct proximal tubular toxicity characterized by proximal tubular necrosis. Although the precise mechanism of renal damage is not known, one theory proposed that cidofovir may interfere with synthesis or degradation of membrane phospholipids (63). Cidofovir (as well as adefovir) uses the basolateral organic anion transporter for tubular secretory elimination. Renal toxicity of cidofovir is dependent on its uptake into the proximal tubular cells via this organic acid exchanger (63).

Administration of saline and probenecid are thought to reduce renal toxicity. Renal damage is occasionally irreversible (64). In the days before the administration of protective treatment, acute renal insufficiency was reported in one-third of patients.

CYCLOSPORINE

Cyclosporine is a cyclic peptide extracted from the fungus *Tolypocladium inflatum.* Cyclosporine is an immunosuppressive agent used in posttransplantation combination therapy and treatment of nephrotic syndrome and several autoimmune diseases. It is highly lipophilic, which makes its administration problematic from the standpoint of formulation and absorption. A newer formulation known as Neoral has replaced the previous form Sandimmune in most centers. Cyclosporine is metabolized by the cytochrome P-450 system. Concomitant administration of compounds that stimulate the hepatic cytochrome P-450 system can result in increased plasma clearance, whereas those that inhibit cytochrome P-450 increase cyclosporine plasma levels and potentiate toxicity (65). Numerous drug interactions with cyclosporine have been reported and are listed in Table 52.1.

In addition, metabolism is age related, with younger children having faster metabolic clearance (66). Because infants and children have a more rapid clearance and larger volume of distribution than adults, children require larger dosages to achieve comparable blood concentrations.

TABLE 52.1. DRUGS THAT INTERACT WITH CYCLOSPORINE

Increase cyclosporine level	Decrease cyclosporine level	Increase toxicity
Azithromycin	Carbamazepine	Acyclovir
Cimetidine	Methylprednisolone	Aminoglycosides
Diltiazem	Nafcillin	Amphotericin B
Doxycycline	Phenobarbital	Ciprofloxacin
Erythromycin	Phenytoin	Clotrimazole
Ketoconazole	Rifampin	NSAIDs
Metoclopramide		Trimethoprim
Nicardipine		
Verapamil		

NSAIDs, nonsteroidal antiinflammatory drugs.

Cyclosporine-related renal toxicity may be detected in the form of a proximal tubulopathy with proteinuria, bicarbonate or electrolyte wasting, and enzymuria, or as glomerular dysfunction. Glomerular effects of cyclosporine result in a reduction of GFR and hypertension. Early functional changes include vasoconstriction of the afferent arteriole accompanied by an increase in serum creatinine level and blood pressure, and positive fluid balance. The toxicity appears to be dosage related. Intravenous administration and the rate of intravenous infusion also have an impact on renal toxicity (67).

Proximal tubule functional defects include impaired secretion of urea and uric acid; reduced fractional excretion of sodium, potassium, and phosphate; and reduced bicarbonate reabsorption with hyperchloremic metabolic acidosis. Acute nephrotoxicity is manifested by decreased urinary flow rate, usually in the setting of a cadaveric renal transplant or intravenous administration (68). Administration of other nephrotoxic agents, particularly amphotericin B, catecholamines, NSAIDs, and radiocontrast agents, may potentiate acute toxicity. Subacute injury, which is reversible, may be difficult to distinguish from renal transplant rejection, so that a renal biopsy is required.

Chronic nephrotoxicity, defined as a 20% or greater irreversible reduction in the GFR, is characterized by morphologic changes, including tubular atrophy, interstitial fibrosis, and vascular hyalinosis and sclerosis (69). Analysis of data from the North American Pediatric Renal Transplant Cooperative Study revealed that pediatric transplant recipients who were given higher cyclosporine dosages tended to have higher yet stable plasma creatinine levels 2 years after transplantation. Graft survival among children receiving higher cyclosporine dosages was better, however, which has led most transplant centers to tolerate a modest reduction in GFR to achieve better long-term graft survival. Most centers monitor whole blood trough levels to avoid overdosing and to ensure adequate immunosuppression. Since the introduction of Neoral, which was anticipated to reduce dosage requirements, reports of increased toxicity in the form of reduced graft function and hypertension indicate that targeting similar trough levels for Neoral as were targeted for Sandimmune results in greater total area under the curve, or greater cyclosporine exposure; this makes adjustment of the dosage independently of trough levels necessary in selected children (70).

Calcium-channel blockers such as diltiazem may prevent the renal vascular changes associated with cyclosporine (71). Although diltiazem interacts with the cytochrome P-450 system, which results in increased blood levels of the drug, it does appear to prevent delayed graft function in cadaveric transplants and to reduce the vasoconstrictive effects.

Endothelin may play a significant role in cyclosporine-associated vasoconstriction as a result of increased release and increased receptor density (71). Cyclosporine induces endothelin release from endothelial, mesangial, and renal tubular cells. Urinary excretion of endothelin is increased as well. In addition, endothelin receptors appear to be upregulated in a rat model of cyclosporine nephrotoxicity. Part of the protective effect of the calcium-channel blockers may be related to their attenuation of endothelin release. Endothelin receptor antagonists have also shown protective effects in cyclosporine-mediated toxicity.

RADIOCONTRAST AGENTS

Radiographic contrast agents are triiodinated benzoic acid derivatives, usually the sodium or methylglucamine salts of diatrizoate or iothalamate. Contrast agents are freely filtered at the glomerulus and are excreted primarily by the kidney. Some concentration of the drug may occur within the renal tubular cell, but most of a bolus of contrast material is excreted directly and rapidly into the urine (11).

The incidence of nephrotoxicity after administration of radiocontrast agents is difficult to assess accurately because of differences in the definition of contrast nephropathy and the populations included in the clinical studies. Studies of adults indicate that between 1 and 20% of the general population may be at risk for acute renal failure after radiocontrast administration, with a somewhat higher incidence among hospitalized or critically ill patients (72). Studies in children are lacking. Certainly, one might view contrast agents as potentially harmful, although not usually so unless other contributing factors are present. Risk factors include preexisting renal insufficiency, diabetes mellitus, multiple myeloma, dehydration, and hyperuricemia (72). Preexisting renal dysfunction is associated with a much greater risk of acute renal failure. Of patients who have renal insufficiency after radiocontrast administration, 50 to 75% had preexisting renal dysfunction, defined as a serum creatinine level of 2 to 3 mg/dL (11). These situations are less likely in children than in elderly adults.

Nephrotoxicity may be mild, with minimal clinical symptoms. Most cases are manifested as nonoliguric acute renal dysfunction, although renal injury may be more severe with typical oliguric renal failure. The peak rise in the serum creatinine level usually occurs 3 to 5 days after contrast administration, with return to baseline by 10 to 14 days. If nephrotoxicity is severe, pronounced oliguria may be evident within 24 hours of the injection (11). Pathologic changes are localized to the proximal tubular cell in the form of pronounced vacuolization, termed *osmotic nephrosis* (11). This form of acute tubular toxicity is characterized by a low fractional excretion of sodium.

Mechanisms responsible for the development of radiocontrast-induced renal dysfunction are not entirely understood. Several factors may interact to induce injury: tubular obstruction, direct tubular toxicity, and ischemia (72,73). Contrast agents induce the precipitation of intratubular proteins such as the myeloma proteins and urinary mucoproteins (Tamm-Horsfall protein), which potentially leads to tubular obstruction by casts (74). Although this theory often has been proposed as a mechanism for renal toxicity after contrast agent administration, studies have failed to support a significant role of cast formation and secondary tubular obstruction in the development of contrast nephropathy (75). Contrast agents are uricosuric and lead to urate crystal formation within renal tubular lumens, especially if urine flow or pH is reduced (76).

In support of a direct tubular toxicity, pathologic changes after radiocontrast administration include vacuolization of the proximal tubules, interstitial edema and inflammation, and tubular cell necrosis (72). Many studies demonstrate increased urinary excretion of enzymes and tubular proteins after administration of contrast agents. This is indicative of nonspecific renal tubular damage. Exposure of isolated proximal tubule segments to diatrizoate-containing contrast media resulted in cellular injury, and this effect was potentiated by hypoxia and addition of meglumine, a cationic compound often combined with diatrizoate (72). In addition, selected studies suggest altered renal tubular cell function secondary to the inhibition of tubular cell metabolism (11,77). Both organic acid transport and sodium transport are reduced in experimental forms of contrast nephropathy. A direct tubulotoxic effect was found when renal tubular cells in culture were incubated in various concentrations of contrast agent (77).

The renal hemodynamic response to intravenous radiocontrast administration is transient vasodilation (increased renal blood flow) followed by vasoconstriction and a decrease in the renal blood flow and GFR (72,78). The vasoconstriction occurs within minutes after injection of contrast agents and lasts for 10 to 20 minutes. This biphasic response in blood flow appears to be unique to the renal vasculature. The diminished filtration rate observed after administration of contrast agents cannot be mediated entirely by hypoperfusion because GFR remains decreased even after normalization of renal blood flow. Vasoconstriction is mediated by increased lipid peroxidation from the increased production and local release of oxygen free radicals and adenosine, a potent vasoconstrictor (72,78). If there is a role for the renin-angiotensin system, it has not been consistently demonstrated (72,73,78). Reduced renal production of prostacyclin is associated with contrast-induced injury (78). Additional vasoconstrictive forces may involve endothelin, because plasma and urinary levels of endothelin are increased after administration of high-osmolar contrast media. Recent studies demonstrate attenuation of contrast-induced vasoconstriction with administration of endothelin receptor antagonists (79). Contrast agents may induce structural and functional alterations in the erythrocyte, which results in hyperviscosity with sludging in small blood vessels and hypoxemia (80). This phenomenon could explain the preferential distribution of ischemia to the medulla.

Prevention of contrast nephropathy requires identification of potential risk factors. These include dehydration, NSAID use, diabetes, and conditions associated with decreased effective plasma volume, such as congestive heart failure, nephrosis, or cirrhosis, in which renal perfusion may already be compromised (72,73). Hydration has been said to be completely effective in prevention of injury. Administration of furosemide did not appear to offer protection. Mannitol administration was protective in nondiabetic patients but may have potentiated injury in diabetic patients (72). Likewise, dopamine afforded some renal protection in nondiabetic patients, yet offered no benefit in diabetic patients (72). Administration of agents that prevent the formation of oxygen free radicals attenuates the decline in GFR observed after the administration of radiocontrast in a canine model (72). Calcium-channel blockers also provide protection against this form of injury, which raises the possibility that increased intracellular calcium may mediate the hypofiltration (72).

The use of more expensive but less toxic nonionic contrast media has been proposed as a means to avoid the renal risk of standard contrast media, but there is insufficient evidence to justify their use in patients with normal renal function. These agents may prove beneficial to patients with impaired GFR (72).

IFOSFAMIDE

Ifosfamide is a cancer chemotherapeutic agent with impressive activity against a wide variety of solid tumors in children, including neuroblastoma, osteosarcoma, rhabdomyosarcoma, soft tissue sarcomas, testicular tumors, and Wilms' tumor (81). Ifosfamide is a structural isomer of cyclophosphamide. The tumoricidal action of these compounds is related to the alkylation and cross-linking of DNA to inhibit cell replication. Although both ifosfamide and cyclophosphamide are associated with hemorrhagic cystitis as well as myelosuppression, alopecia, and gastrointestinal symptoms, ifosfamide is associated with significant renal toxicity, which is not observed after administration of cyclophosphamide.

Ifosfamide may induce tubular wasting of glucose, amino acids, protein, and phosphate as well as decreased GFR (81,82). Although there is a great deal of interpatient variability in the pattern of ifosfamide-induced renal toxicity, in general ifosfamide toxicity is initially manifest as subclinical tubular damage with increased urinary excretion of brush-border enzymes from cell membrane loss, and a transient increase in urinary excretion of amino acids, phosphate, glucose, and protein. A progressive increase in renal tubular toxicity was observed in 11 patients after the initial three or four courses of ifosfamide treatment, with return to normal in between courses (82). Subsequent courses were characterized by failure to return to pretreatment levels between courses, with fixed tubular functional changes. In addition, glomerular damage and decreased GFR (presumably secondary to chronic tubular damage and fibrosis) were observed in five of seven patients at the end of therapy. Although less commonly observed, distal tubular dysfunction may occur after ifosfamide administration. Skinner reported a concentrating defect in 50% of the 12 patients in his series (81), and hypokalemia occurred in 4 patients reported by Husband et al. (83). In some patients a sign that ifosfamide has significantly affected renal function is a delay in the clearance of drugs such as methotrexate. In some patients tubulopathy becomes fixed, and in many of these, glomerular function also is affected. One should be reminded that, even in patients with obvious renal toxicity, the plasma creatinine level is often within normal limits because it is an insensitive marker of glomerular function in these patients. In general, patients do not manifest reductions in GFR in the absence of established tubular injury.

Not only are there acute effects of ifosfamide administration, but a subset of patients experience continued renal dysfunction, manifest as tubular wasting syndromes, or reduced GFR. The incidence of chronic renal failure secondary to ifosfamide therapy is reported to be 1 to 4% (82). Another late complication of ifosfamide administration is the occurrence of rickets caused by chronic hypophosphatemia (84–86). Of 12 children on whom Skinner reported, 8 had what was considered to be significant renal damage, 6 had reduced GFR, 4 had hypophosphatemia, 5 had glycosuria, 10 had generalized aminoaciduria, and 3 had radiographic evidence of rickets (87).

The incidence of ifosfamide-associated renal injury is highly variable, depending on the cumulative dosage, rapidity of administration, previous or concomitant administration of platinums or other nephrotoxic drugs or radiation, presence of a unilateral kidney, and age. Ifosfamide nephrotoxicity seems to be dose dependent and is more likely to occur in younger children or those who have undergone nephrectomy (81,84,88). Previous or sequential administration of other nephrotoxic agents increases the likelihood that renal toxicity will be observed with ifosfamide treatment. Most notably, patients who have previously been treated with cisplatin are at a greater risk for ifosfamide nephrotoxicity (88,89). Carboplatin administration also increases the risk of tubular toxicity after ifosfamide therapy (90). This phenomenon is interesting, because the major site of injury after the platinums is the late proximal and collecting duct, whereas that after ifosfamide appears to be the early proximal tubule.

The clinical pattern of renal injury is one of initially transient, reversible tubular wasting of glucose, potassium, bicarbonate, phosphate, and amino acids as well as low-molecular-weight proteins such as β_2-microglobulin. With early toxicity, tubular function tends to return nearly to baseline at the time of the next course. A few long-term follow-up studies have been published. These suggest that the renal defect in many of these children is chronic and may be progressive in nature. This is in contrast with results of long-term follow-up of cisplatin injury, in which GFR may improve over time although tubular defects may persist.

Numerous studies have looked at the incidence and pattern of renal injury associated with ifosfamide. Findings are highly variable, and partly this reflects the aggressiveness with which the studies of renal tubular and glomerular function were performed. If serum creatinine or creatinine clearance is used to assess the presence of decreased GFR, the incidence of glomerular dysfunction is underestimated, as evidenced by the study of Ashraf et al., who found that 7 of 20 patients had abnormal GFR values as assessed by chromium ethylenediaminetetra-acetic acid (Cr-EDTA) clearance, yet none of these had elevated plasma creatinine levels compared to age-related controls (91). In addition, nine children demonstrated increased fractional excretion of phosphate, six had decreased tubular threshold for phosphate, and only two had overt hypophosphatemia.

The activation of ifosfamide to its tumoricidal metabolites, 4-hydroxyifosfamide (4-OH-IF) and aldoifosfamide, occurs in the liver, with further metabolism to either isophosphoramide or carboxyifosfamide. The parent drug and its metabolites are excreted in the urine (92). When attempts are made to contrast the metabolites of cyclophosphamide and ifosfamide to incriminate the nephrotoxic species, ifosfamide metabolism is found to produce significantly greater quantities of chloracetaldehyde than cyclophosphamide. Because this compound has been noted to be toxic to cells and is found in high concentration in both the urine and plasma, it may play a role in the renal toxicity after ifosfamide therapy.

The mechanism of the renal tubular injury secondary to ifosfamide administration is unknown. Studies in which cultured proximal tubular cells are incubated in the parent drug or metabolites have been performed (93). The parent drug, ifosfamide, did not have an effect on amino acid or glucose transport, but the metabolite 4-OH-IF clearly inhibited transport of both substrates after 24 hours in 100 μmol/L. Another potentially active metabolite, chloracetaldehyde, stimulated uptake at low concentrations (<200 μmol/L) and shorter incubations but inhibited uptake at higher concentrations and longer exposure times. In low concentrations, 4-OH-IF stimulated phosphate transport, but transport was decreased at higher dosages (100 μmol/L). At even higher concentrations (300 to 400 μmol/L), Na^+-K^+–adenosine triphosphatase (Na^+-K^+-ATPase) activity was inhibited. Chloracetaldehyde (at concentrations greater than 175 μmol/L), reduced phosphate transport and the activity of the mitochondrial enzyme succinate cytochrome *c* oxidoreductase.

The bladder toxicity of the oxazaphosphorine compounds results primarily from the metabolite acrolein, although 4-OH-IF has also been implicated (81). Mesna, sodium-2 mercaptoethane sulfonate, has been used to reduce ifosfamide- and cyclophosphamide-related bladder toxicity without alteration of tumoricidal effects. Mesna binds to acrolein, chloracetaldehyde, and 4-OH-IF (94). Unfortunately, mesna does not seem to offer protection against tubular toxicity, although its failure to do so has been postulated to be related to the availability of mesna at the site of tubular injury (95). Mesna is oxidized to dimesna, which has no protective action. Dimesna can be converted back to mesna by renal tubular cells, but at the dosages currently used in clinical practice, free mesna levels may not be adequate or may be highly variable and thus inadequate for tubular protection.

PLATINUM COMPOUNDS

Cisplatin (*cis*-diaminedichloroplatinum II) is an inorganic platinum compound that may induce both acute and chronic renal toxicity with magnesium, sodium, and potassium wasting as well as decreased GFR (96). The drug contains a platinum atom surrounded by two chloride atoms and two ammonia molecules in the *cis* position. Carboplatin (*cis*-diamine-1,1-cyclobutane-dicarboxylate) platinum (II) has been introduced as a less nephrotoxic form of platinum, although it is now known that this compound also may cause renal injury. Cisplatin and carboplatin may undergo aquation with substitution of the chloride ions with hydroxyl groups, a reaction favored by low chloride concentrations such as are found in the cell, to form positively charged complexes that are likely to be the active form of the drug. Platinum compounds are excreted by the kidney via glomerular filtration. Platinum is concentrated in the renal cortex, with levels higher than in plasma, and appears to be accumulated via some transport process. Data suggest that elimination of the drug is delayed in the setting of a decreased GFR.

Proximal tubular cells are believed to accumulate platinum compounds by an energy-requiring mechanism or possibly by the organic base transport system (96). Differences in uptake of the platinum compounds might be related to stereospecificity or relative solubility and reactivity. Shortly after intravenous injection of cisplatin into rats, accumulation can be observed in the juxtamedullary region and outer stripe. This pattern is consistent with localization within the S3 portion of the proximal convoluted tubule, which is thought to be particularly susceptible to platinum. Acute changes in renal function occur after cisplatin administration, and these appear to be hemodynamically mediated, with reduced renal blood flow as well as tubular injury. Histologically, platinum-induced renal toxicity is characterized by tubular dilation, cytoplasmic vacuolization, nuclear pyknosis, and hydropic degeneration of cells in the corticomedullary region or S3 segment of the proximal tubule.

In a series of 22 children receiving cisplatin, 18 demonstrated GFR of less than 80 mL/min/1.73 m^2 as assessed by Cr-EDTA clearance (97). There was a mean decrease in GFR of 8% per course, but a great deal of individual variability was seen. In addition, the authors noted that neither plasma creatinine nor creatinine clearance was reliable in screening patients with significant reductions in GFR.

Long-term outcome for children who received cisplatin (median cumulative dose of 500 mg/min, range of 120 to 1860 mg/min) as part of their anticancer chemotherapy was studied by Brock et al. (98). Of 40 children available for study at the completion of therapy, 16 had a GFR above 80 mL/min/1.73 m^2, 13 had a GFR of 60 to 80 mL/min/1.73 m^2, and 11 had a GFR below 60 mL/min/1.73 m^2. Clearance measurements were repeated a mean of 2 years and 6 months from the end of therapy. A statistically significant improvement in GFR was found. Children with a GFR between 60 and 80 mL/min/1.73 m^2 at the end of treatment had a better chance of regaining a normal GFR; however, all of the 11 children with a GFR below 60 mL/min/1.73 m^2 improved, and 3 had normal GFR at last follow-up. Hypomagnesemia was found in 6 of 21 children at last follow-up.

The mechanism of platinum-related renal injury is being debated. It has been suggested that cisplatin is a direct tubular toxin and must be present in the tubular lumen at a minimum concentration of 1 mmol/L or 200 µg/mL (96). Several cellular perturbations have been identified in renal proximal tubular cells. These include inactivation of Na^+-K^+-ATPase, impaired mitochondrial function, altered gluconeogenesis, impaired substrate transport, lipid peroxidation, oxidation of sulfhydryl groups, and inhibition of nucleic acid and protein synthesis (99). The nephrotoxicity of cisplatin, transplatin, and carboplatin was examined in two continuous proximal tubular cell lines: primary cultures of rabbit cortical cells and OK cells (a continuous proximal tubular cell line). OK cells were spared from injury, probably because of decreased cellular uptake of the compounds. The rabbit proximal cells exhibited reduced viability at concentrations of cisplatin approximating 100 fmol/L, similar to peak levels in cancer patients. Toxicity was related to intracellular levels of platinum (99).

Isolated S3 segments of proximal tubules from rats given either transplatin or cisplatin were examined for alterations in oxygen consumption and respiration. No consistent abnormalities were detected, which makes mitochondria unlikely candidates for early nephrotoxicity (96). Other studies noted changes in mitochondrial function. Cisplatin also increased the oxidation of mitochondrial sulfhydryl groups, depleting GSH and leading to perturbations in mitochondrial calcium uptake and membrane potential (100). Antioxidants did not prevent the associated nephrotoxicity, which indicates that platinum probably exerts its effect by interacting directly with thiol groups rather than by inducing lipid peroxidation. Unfortunately, the concentrations of cisplatin used were considerably higher than would be expected from *in vivo* dosing. DNA synthesis was significantly inhibited by small concentrations of cisplatin, whereas greater concentrations of the other compounds were required. Cisplatin in the concentration range of 30 to 100 μmol/L induced a decrease in the activity of Na^+-K^+-ATPase as well as glucose uptake; the effect on glucose transport is probably secondary to a reduction in Na^+-K^+-ATPase activity because the sodium gradient would be decreased. Other experiments have shown that cisplatin may decrease glucose as well as phosphate transport. Similar findings were observed with carboplatin, but concentrations 20 times higher were necessary to induce the same alterations in cell functions (99).

Many favor inhibition of DNA synthesis as the primary biochemical effect. Cisplatin damages DNA by inducing interstrand and intrastrand cross-links and preventing normal replication. The amount of platinum cross-linkage correlates with toxicity as well as mutagenicity (96). Intrastrand cross-links are not found with transplatin, which is a much less toxic form of this class of agent.

Polyuria is a common finding after cisplatin administration and appears in two phases: urine osmolality falls over the first 24 to 48 hours after administration, and the second phase of increased urine volume and decreased osmolality occurs between 72 and 96 hours and is accompanied by decreased GFR as well (96). During the early phase, blood vasopressin levels are low and the kidney may concentrate urine in response to large doses of vasopressin. The latter phase of polyuria is thought to be secondary to the dilution of the medullary urea gradient, possibly related to abnormal urea recycling in the loop of Henle. In a model of chronic cisplatin nephrotoxicity, rats received three doses over 3 weeks. Polyuria, increased urinary sodium excretion, and decreased GFR along with decreased urinary cyclic adenosine monophosphate (cAMP) excretion were observed in the cisplatin-treated animals (101). Production of cAMP by inner medullary collecting duct cells was decreased after vasopressin stimulation in cisplatin-treated rats. Forskolin, a direct activator of adenyl cyclase, induced similar cAMP production in treated and control rats. In contrast, cAMP production after administration of sodium fluorescein, an agent that stimulates cAMP production via the guanine nucleotide regulatory protein, was significantly lower in cisplatin-treated animals than in controls. These results led the investigators to conclude that the polyuria associated with cisplatin is caused by an abnormality in signal transduction at the level of the G-protein component of the vasopressin receptor (101).

Hypomagnesemia is another common manifestation of cisplatin-induced renal toxicity and commonly persists long after therapy ceases (102). Rats receiving intraperitoneal cisplatin (2.5 mg/kg) for 3 weeks developed hypomagnesemia by the second week, which persisted to the eighth week after therapy (103). Urinary excretion of magnesium was inappropriately elevated. In addition, gut absorption of magnesium was decreased. Calcium and magnesium transport by the superficial proximal and distal tubules appeared to be unaffected when measured at 7 weeks, even though urinary excretion was elevated. Bone and muscle magnesium levels were significantly reduced at the end of the eighth week, which suggests depletion of mineral stores. Cisplatin increases distal tubular sodium conductance. Infusion of cisplatin into rat distal tubular segments caused an attenuation of the normally negative luminal charge generated by active sodium reabsorption in this segment (104). The effect of cisplatin on the luminal charge was reversed by addition of amiloride, a diuretic that blocks sodium channels. The authors conclude that cisplatin may interact with distal tubular Na^+ channels to increase potassium and magnesium excretion and that this is attenuated by co-administration of amiloride (104).

Therapeutic intervention to reduce renal toxicity associated with cisplatin has been aimed at reduced production and enhanced excretion of highly reactive metabolites (104,105). Infusion of mannitol and saline is the clinical intervention most commonly used to reduce cisplatin nephrotoxicity. In addition to providing optimal hydration before, during, and after administration, the co-administration of saline may reduce the spontaneous aquation reaction. In addition, these maneuvers may enhance excretion of the drug and minimize the period of contact between the renal tubule and toxin. The compound sodium thiosulfate reverses cisplatin-induced DNA cross-links and has been reported to reduce cisplatin injury in animals and humans (106,107). This compound is believed to protect the renal tubule through chelation of the drug and/or active metabolites. The concern that tumoricidal activity will be reduced has prevented widespread use of thiosulfates or other thiol compounds. Disulfiram, the disulfide dimer of diethyldithiocarbamate, differs from other chelating agents in that it offers protection when given after cisplatin, and it does not appear to alter chemotherapeutic efficacy (105,108). Despite some promising preliminary findings, co-administration of thiol compounds is not yet standard practice. One study used a novel method for reduction of cisplatin-induced renal toxicity in the rat. Administration of erythropoietin to rats after development of acute cisplatin-induced renal failure enhanced histologic and functional recovery primarily by improving tubular regeneration (109). The results observed with erythropoietin might potentially be applicable to other hemopoietic growth factors now commonly administered in coordination with cancer chemotherapeutic agents to speed bone marrow recovery. Human studies using growth factors in this setting are lacking.

Another potential method for minimizing renal toxicity is to avoid increasing the exposure to renal toxins by detecting reduced GFR early and by taking the GFR into account in dosing. Dosing of carboplatin based on the patient's GFR has been practiced by many centers and may potentially prevent toxicity by allowing dosage modifications in patients who have experienced otherwise undetectable reductions in GFR.

COMBINATION CHEMOTHERAPY

The combination of ifosfamide and cisplatin potentiates renal injury (110). One study compared glomerular function (unfortunately, creatinine clearance was used as the measure) and tubular function after either low-dose ifosfamide or a combination of ifosfamide and cisplatin and then high-dose cisplatin. Tubular functions such as amino acid excretion and albuminuria were comparable for the high-dose ifosfamide and combination groups, but phosphate wasting was more pronounced in the combination group (110). Despite delivering a much lower cumulative ifosfamide dose, combination therapy resulted in lower phosphate reabsorption in significantly more patients and a trend toward more frequent occurrence of tubular dysfunction. The aminoglycoside gentamicin did not appear to contribute significantly to observed renal toxicity. Of the 14 children with overt renal tubular wasting syndrome, eight had received combination therapy. Experience with combination therapy reveals that acute toxicity from ifosfamide is higher when carboplatin is administered within the same week than when a period of months elapses between these toxic therapies (90).

In conclusion, renal dysfunction as a result of drug administration may be manifest as a reduction of GFR or tubular dysfunction, most commonly of the proximal tubule. In most cases, this form of renal injury is reversible. Occasionally, there may be long-term renal dysfunction, as in the case of amphotericin B, cisplatin, and ifosfamide. The clinician must be aware of the potential for renal toxicity and must be prepared to make adjustments in the dosage or discontinue the offending agent. Anticipation of potential renal toxicity allows for maneuvers that may prevent renal damage and subsequent functional changes. Drug-induced renal dysfunction provides a model for acute renal failure and provides insight into renal injury in the general sense, which gives hope that in the future it will be possible to prevent injury or enhance recovery.

NATURAL NEPHROTOXINS

Marine animals, reptiles, and insects produce a number of biologic nephrotoxins (111) (Table 52.2).

Many of these toxins result in acute renal failure either directly or indirectly. The main indirect mechanism of nephrotoxicity is biologic-toxin–induced rhabdomyolysis (112). Although these natural nephrotoxins are uncommon causes of acute renal failure, they are of considerable interest.

Marine Animal Nephrotoxins

Fish poisons include at least three forms of biotoxins that result in ATN. First, there is an association between the ingestion of raw bile from the gall bladder of carp and acute renal failure. The belief that the raw bile of carp improves vision and rheumatism is found in Asia (113). Many of these Asian carp species have been introduced into the United States, and at least five species of carp have been implicated (114). All five carp species have ichthyogallotoxin in their bile, and this may represent the toxin. Alternatively, A C-27 bile alcohol, termed *cyprinol* and found in carp bile, is nephrotoxic in animals (111).

TABLE 52.2. COMMON BIOLOGIC NEPHROTOXINS PRODUCED BY ANIMALS AND PLANTS

Snake
Phospholipase A_2
Myotoxins
Procoagulant activating factors V and X
Spider
Sphingomyelinase D (*Loxosceles*)
Neurotoxins (*Latrodectus*)
Bee
Melittin
Phospholipase A_2
Mast cell degranulating protein
Wasp
Antigen 5
Mastoparans
Carp
Ichthyogallotoxin
Cyprinol

A second toxin as yet unidentified is responsible for Haff disease. Haff disease, characterized by acute rhabdomyolysis, can occur in humans and other animals that eat eels and burbot fish. Rhabdomyolysis can be found in subjects who ingest buffalo fish, a member of the carp family (115). These myotoxins or icthyosarcotoxins are unidentified.

A third agent is the palytoxin of the blue humphead parrotfish. Ingestion of this toxin can also result in cardiac muscle damage (116). Factors contributing to the pathogenesis of acute renal failure from rhabdomyolysis include the quality of myoglobin in nephrons, an acidic, highly concentrated urine, and delayed recognition of the disease.

Envenomation-Induced Acute Renal Failure

Snake Venoms

Four families of venomous snake are responsible for 40,000 deaths/yr, and 5 to 30% of subjects bitten by these snakes develop acute renal failure. Two families are responsible for most deaths and cases of renal failure: (a) the cobras, African mambas, and coral snakes, and (b) the vipers, adders, moccasins, and rattlesnakes (117). Approximately 90% of venoms are proteins that are proteolytic enzymes, phospholipases, and hyaluronidases. Other enzymes include ribonucleases, deoxyribonucleases, nucleotidases, and acidic and basic phosphatases. Procoagulants that activate the clotting cascade via factors V and X are also present. Myotoxins can also lead to rhabdomyolysis and myocardial damage, which reduce cardiac contractility, and pigment nephropathy.

Patients may show ATN, hypersensitivity reactions, extracapillary glomerulonephritis, AIN, and necrotizing arteritis of interlobular arteries on histologic studies (118,119). Laboratory investigations show evidence of intravascular hemolysis, disseminated intravascular coagulation, and azotemia (120). A number of snakebites lead mainly to rhabdomyolysis, including those of the king brown snake, sea snakes, diamondback rattler, canebrake rattler, and several vipers (112).

Spider Venoms

Two groups of spiders produce venom responsible for acute renal failure: the recluse spiders and the widow spiders (112). The mechanism of toxicity of the venom of the 56 recluse species is the presence of sphingomyelinase D, which leads to necrotic skin lesions, edema, erythema, chills, nausea, and myalgias (121). The main recluse spider in the United States is the brown recluse. These bites are generally more serious in young children.

The widow spiders excrete neurotoxins that produce cramping and muscle spasms. These toxins can lead to a neurogenic bladder with urinary obstruction. The venom of the black widow spider of the United States can also lead to rhabdomyolysis.

Bee and Wasp Venoms

Acute renal failure due to bee and wasp venoms requires massive numbers of stings, usually more than 100, which generally follows disturbance of a hive or nest (111). The toxins include melittin and other hemolysins, hyaluronidase, and others (Table 52.2). The toxins in wasps differ and consist of active amines, kinins, and antigen 5. The mechanisms of renal failure include hemolysis, rhabdomyolysis, direct toxic effects, and dehydration. The venom of the dark scorpion of the southwest United States may also cause rhabdomyolysis (112). Hypersensitivity reactions to bee and wasp venoms may also occur. The treatment of acute renal failure is symptomatic and dialysis may be required.

Chinese Herb Nephropathy

Chinese herb nephropathy, initially described in the early 1990s by Vanherweghem et al. in Belgium, is characterized by a tubulointerstitial disease (122). Proximal tubular dysfunction with a Fanconi syndrome or, more commonly, insidious chronic renal failure has been described (123). Aristolochic acids are the likely etiologic agent. Substitution of *Aristolochia fangchi* for *Stephania tetrandra*, herbs which differ in name in Chinese by only one character, is thought to have been the historical event leading to the increased incidence of this indolent renal disorder. These herbs were generally taken for the purpose of weight loss.

Aristolochic acids are naturally occurring compounds with carcinogenic and nephrotoxic effects. Although there is still debate as to whether they are solely responsible for all of the reported cases of Chinese herbal nephropathy (124), they have been shown to cause an interstitial nephropathy in the rabbit (125) but not the rat (126). Isolated case reports also describe proximal tubular dysfunction with hypokalemia, abnormal urinary excretion of low-molecular-weight proteins, and glycosuria as the presenting features in several adults (127–129).

Pathologic evidence of renal injury was demonstrated in the rabbit model. As with human pathologic changes, there was a distinct corticomedullary gradient of acellular interstitial fibrosis. Three patterns of injury were described: (a) restriction of fibrosis to the medullary ray (S3 segments), (b) extension to the outer cortical labyrinth (convoluted proximal tubules, S1 and S2 segments), and (c) extension to the inner cortical labyrinth and outer medulla (proximal tubules of deep nephrons) (125). The exact mechanism of aristolochic acid–induced injury is not known.

Renal function continues to deteriorate despite cessation of consumption of herbal remedies. Oral corticosteroid therapy may slow the progression of renal insufficiency. A group of 81 adults with Chinese herb nephropathy were subdivided according to pattern of renal failure (130). Thirty-nine demonstrated moderate renal failure with progression. Of these, 14 received oral prednisone initiated at 1 mg/kg for 1 month and then tapered to 0.15 mg/kg. The rate of increase in the serum creatinine level was less in the steroid-treated group.

Pediatric cases have not been reported.

ENVIRONMENTAL TOXINS

Organic Solvents: Ethylene Glycol, Diethylene Glycol, Propylene Glycol

Ethylene glycol is a major constituent of antifreeze and may be accidentally ingested because it has a sweet taste. It is metabolized initially by alcohol dehydrogenase to glycoaldehyde and eventually to oxalate. Intermediate metabolites include glycolic acid and glyoxylic acid, which contribute to the associated metabolic acidosis. A change in the ratio of the unreduced form of nicotinamide adenine dinucleotide to the reduced form favors the accumulation of lactic acid. Central nervous system symptoms and cardiovascular instability precede the onset of renal disease. Renal toxicity takes two forms: crystallization of oxalate within the renal tubules and direct tubular damage resulting in acute renal failure. Metabolic acidosis with elevated anion gap and altered mental status should prompt the consideration of this poisoning. Examination of the urine sediment early in the course may reveal either needle-shaped calcium oxalate monohydrate crystals or octahedral calcium oxalate dihydrate crystals. An elevated plasma osmolar gap may also be an indirect clue. Treatment is aimed at clearance of the toxic metabolites and may include hemodialysis in the case of renal failure or severe metabolic acidosis.

Diethylene glycol has been responsible for accidental poisoning associated with acute renal failure in the form of medication contamination. Recently, an outbreak of renal failure in Haiti resulted after two acetaminophen preparations were inadvertently contaminated with diethylene glycol during manufacture using contaminated glycerin. The mechanism of renal toxicity is thought to be proximal tubular damage and necrosis. Other organ systems, including the liver, pancreas, and brain, are often severely injured and contribute to the overall mortality of this accidental poisoning.

Propylene glycol (PG) may be responsible for ATN. The renal failure is usually the result of intravenous administration of medication solubilized in PG (131). Parenteral medications that contain PG include diazepam, digoxin, esmolol, hydralazine, nitroglycerin, pentobarbital, phenobarbital, phenytoin, and sulfamethoxazole/trimethoprim. Vitamin preparations may also contain PG. Clinical manifestations are similar to those of ethylene glycol toxicity, including metabolic acidosis with increased anion gap. A potential mechanism for toxicity has been postulated to be the inhibition of proximal tubular transport processes and membrane disruption (132).

Heavy Metals (Excluding Platinum)

Lead, mercury, gold, bismuth, and copper are uncommon but serious causes of nephrotoxicity. They have common mechanisms of renal tubular toxicity, and chronic exposure may lead to presentation with an acute syndrome or dysfunction. The primary site of injury is the proximal renal tubule, where heavy metals cause impaired mitochondrial function and secondary alterations in membrane integrity. Exposure to mercury and lead is generally accidental due to environmental contamination and is much less common now than several decades ago. The reader is referred to previously published comprehensive reviews of heavy metal renal toxicity (133,134).

REFERENCES

1. Weinberg JM. The cellular basis of nephrotoxicity. In: Schrier RW, Gottshalk CW, eds. *Diseases of the kidney.* 4th ed. Boston: Little, Brown, 1988:1137.
2. Ueda N, Walder PD, Shah SV. Oxidant stress in acute renal failure. In: Goligorsky MS, Stein JH, eds. *Contemporary issues in nephrology: acute renal failure.* New York: Churchill Livingstone, 1995;30:45–74.
3. Dillon JJ. Nephrotoxicity from antibacterial, antifungal, and antiviral drugs. In: Molitoris BA, Finn WF, eds. *Acute renal failure: a companion to Brenner and Rector's the kidney.* Philadelphia: WB Saunders, 2001:349–364.
4. Spicer ST, Liddle C, Chapman JR, et al. The mechanism of cyclosporine toxicity induced by clarithromycin. *Br J Clin Pharmacol* 1997;43:194–196.
5. Porter GA, Bennett WM. Nephrotoxic acute renal failure due to common drugs. *Am J Physiol* 1981;241:F1–F8.
6. Mendoza SA. Nephrotoxic drugs. *Pediatr Nephrol* 1988;2: 466–476.
7. Wedeen RP, Batuman V, Cheeks C, et al. Transport of gentamicin in rat proximal tubule. *Lab Invest* 1983;48:212–223.
8. Senekjian HO, Knight TF, Weinman EJ. Micropuncture study of the handling of gentamicin by the rat kidney. *Kidney Int* 1981;19:416–423.
9. Kaloyanides GJ. Drug-phospholipid interactions: role in aminoglycoside nephrotoxicity. *Ren Fail* 1992;14:351–357.
10. Tune BM, Reznik VM, Mendoza SA. Renal complications of drug therapy. In: Holliday MA, Barratt TM, Avner ED, eds. *Pediatric nephrology.* 3rd ed. Baltimore: Williams and Wilkins, 1994:1212–1226.
11. Coggins CH, Fang LS-T. Acute renal failure associated with antibiotics, anesthetic agents and radio-contrast agents. In: Brenner BM, Lazarus JM, eds. *Acute renal failure.* 2nd ed. New York: Churchill Livingstone, 1988:295.
12. DeBroe ME, Paulus GJ, Verpooten GA, et al. Early effects of gentamicin, tobramycin and amikacin on the human kidney. *Kidney Int* 1984;25:643–652.
13. Sundin DP, Meyer C, Dahl R, et al. Cellular mechanism of aminoglycoside tolerance in long-term gentamicin treatment. *Am J Physiol* 1997;272:C1309–C1318.
14. Beck PR, Thomson RB, Chaudhuri AK. Aminoglycoside antibiotics and renal function: changes in urinary gamma-glutamyltransferase excretion. *J Clin Pathol* 1977;30:432–437.
15. Cronin RE. Aminoglycoside nephrotoxicity: pathogenesis and prevention. *Clin Nephrol* 1979;11:251–256.
16. Higa EM, Schor N, Boim MA, et al. Role of the prostaglandin and kallikrein-kinin systems in aminoglycoside-induced acute renal failure. *Braz J Med Biol Res* 1985;18:355–365.
17. Humes HD. Aminoglycoside nephrotoxicity. *Kidney Int* 1988;33:900–911.
18. Baylis C, Rennke HR, Brenner BM. Mechanisms of the defect in glomerular ultrafiltration associated with gentamicin administration. *Kidney Int* 1977;12:344–353.
19. Williams PD, Bennett DM, Gleason CR, et al. Correlation between renal membrane binding and nephrotoxicity of aminoglycosides. *Antimicrob Agents Chemother* 1987;31:570–574.
20. Zager RA. Gentamicin nephrotoxicity in the setting of acute renal hypoperfusion. *Am J Physiol* 1988;254:F574–F581.
21. Hatala R, Dinh T, Cook DJ. Once-daily aminoglycoside dosing in immunocompetent adults: a meta-analysis. *Ann Intern Med* 1996;124:717–725.
22. Hayani KC, Hatzopoulos FK, Frank AL, et al. Pharmacokinetics of once-daily dosing of gentamicin in neonates. *J Pediatr* 1997;131:76–80.
23. Powell SH, Thompson WL, Luthe MA, et al. Once-daily vs. continuous aminoglycoside dosing: efficacy and toxicity in animal and clinical studies of gentamicin, netilmicin, and tobramycin. *J Infect Dis* 1983;147:918–932.
24. Tune BM. Nephrotoxicity of beta-lactam antibiotics: mechanisms and strategies for prevention. *Pediatr Nephrol* 1998;11: 768–772.
25. Balfour JA, Bryson HM, Brogden RN. Imipenem/cilastatin: an update of its antibacterial activity, pharmacokinetics and

therapeutic efficacy in the treatment of serious infections. *Drugs* 1996;51:99–136.
26. Al Shohaib S, Satti MS, Abunijem Z. Acute interstitial nephritis due to cefotaxime. *Nephron* 1996;73:725.
27. Shibasaki T, Ishimoto F, Sakai O, et al. Clinical characterization of drug-induced allergic nephritis. *Am J Nephrol* 1991;11:174–180.
28. Galpin JE, Shinaberger JH, Stanley TM, et al. Acute interstitial nephritis due to methicillin. *Am J Med* 1978;65:756–765.
29. Reiser IW, Chou S-Y, Brown MI, et al. Reversal of trimethoprim-induced antikaliuresis. *Kidney Int* 1996;50:2063–2069.
30. Porras MC, Lecumberri JN, Castrillon JL. Trimethoprim/sulfamethoxazole and metabolic acidosis in HIV-infected patients. *Ann Pharmacother* 1998;32:185–189.
31. Watkins VS, Polk RE, Stotka JL. Drug interactions of macrolides: emphasis on dirithromycin. *Ann Pharmacother* 1997;31:349–356.
32. Cheng JT, Witty RT, Robinson RR, et al. Amphotericin B nephrotoxicity: increased renal resistance and tubule permeability. *Kidney Int* 1982;22:626–633.
33. Andreoli TE. On the anatomy of amphotericin B-cholesterol pores in lipid bilayer membranes. *Kidney Int* 1973;4:337–345.
34. Butler WT, Hill GJ, Szwed CF, et al. Amphotericin B renal toxicity in the dog. *J Pharmacol Exp Ther* 1964;143:47–56.
35. Gerkens JF, Heidemann HT, Jackson EK, et al. Effect of aminophylline on amphotericin B nephrotoxicity in the dog. *J Pharmacol Exp Ther* 1983;224:609–613.
36. Tolins JP, Raij L. Adverse effect of amphotericin B administration on renal hemodynamics in the rat. Neurohumoral mechanisms and influence of calcium channel blockade. *J Pharmacol Exp Ther* 1988;245:594–599.
37. Fisher MA, Talbot GH, Maislin G, et al. Risk factors for amphotericin B–associated nephrotoxicity. *Am J Med* 1989; 87:547–552.
38. Baley JE, Kliegman RM, Fanaroff AA. Disseminated fungal infections in very low birth weight infants: clinical manifestations and epidemiology. *Pediatrics* 1984;73:144–152.
39. Bullock WE, Luke RG, Nuttall CE, et al. Can mannitol reduce amphotericin B nephrotoxicity? Double-blind study and description of a new vascular lesion in kidneys. *Antimicrob Agents Chemother* 1976;10:555–563.
40. Hellebusch AA, Salama F, Eadie E. The use of mannitol to reduce the nephrotoxicity of amphotericin B. *Surg Gynecol Obstet* 1972;134:241–243.
41. Sorkine P, Nagar H, Winbroum A, et al. Administration of amphotericin B in lipid emulsion decreases nephrotoxicity: results of a prospective, randomized, controlled study in critically ill patients. *Crit Care Med* 1996;24:1311–1315.
42. Walsh TJ, Gonzalez C, Lyman CA, et al. Invasive fungal infections in children. In: Aronoff SC, eds. *Advances in pediatric infectious diseases.* St. Louis: CV Mosby, 1996;11:240–246.
43. Canafax DM, Graves NM, Hilligoss DM, et al. Interaction between cyclosporine and fluconazole in renal allograft recipients. *Transplantation* 1991;51:1014–1018.
44. Bennett WM, Henrich WL, Stoff JS. The renal effects of nonsteroidal antiinflammatory drugs, summary and recommendations. *Am J Kidney Dis* 1996;28[Suppl 1]:S56–S62.
45. Seyberth HW, Leonhardt T, Tönshoff B, et al. Prostanoids in paediatric kidney diseases. *Pediatr Nephrol* 1991;5:639–649.
46. Primack WA, Rahman SM, Pullman J. Acute renal failure associated with amoxicillin and ibuprofen in an 11-year-old boy. *Pediatr Nephrol* 1997;11:125–126.
47. Blowey DL, Ben-David S, Koren G. Interactions of drugs with the developing kidney. *Pediatr Clin North Am* 1995;42:1415–1431.
48. Toto RD, Anderson SA, Brown-Cartwright D, et al. Effects of acute and chronic dosing of NSAIDs in patients with renal insufficiency. *Kidney Int* 1986;30:760–768.
49. Hammond PSG, Forland SC, Cutler RE. Antiviral agents in clinical nephrology. Part I: acyclovir, desciclovir, ganciclovir and vidarabine. *Dialysis Transplant* 1991;Feb:74–94.
50. Becker BN, Fall P, Hall C, et al. Rapidly progressive acute renal failure due to acyclovir: case report and review of the literature. *Am J Kidney Dis* 1993;22:611–615.
51. Sawyer MH, Webb DE, Balow JE, et al. Acyclovir-induced renal failure: clinical course and histology. *Am J Med* 1988;84: 1067–1071.
52. Dos Santos MDF, Dos Santos OFP, Boim MA, et al. Nephrotoxicity of acyclovir and ganciclovir in rats: evaluation of glomerular hemodynamics. *J Am Soc Nephrol* 1997;8:361–367.
53. Bianchetti MG, Rocult C, Oetliker OH. Acyclovir-induced renal failure: course and risk factors. *Pediatr Nephrol* 1991; 5:238–239.
54. Noormohamed FH, Youle MS, Higgs CJ, et al. Renal excretion and pharmacokinetics of foscarnet in HIV sero-positive patients: effects of probenecid pretreatment. *Br J Clin Pharmacol* 1997;43:112–115.
55. Maurice-Estepa L, Daudon M, Katlama C, et al. Identification of crystals in kidneys of AIDS patients treated with foscarnet. *Am J Kidney Dis* 1998;32:392–400.
56. Navarro JF, Quereda C, Quereda C, et al. Nephrogenic diabetes insipidus and renal tubular acidosis secondary to foscarnet therapy. *Am J Kidney Dis* 1996;27:431–434.
57. Jacobson MA, Gambertoglio JG, Aweeka FT, et al. Foscarnet-induced hypocalcemia and effects of foscarnet on calcium metabolism. *J Clin Endocrinol Metab* 1991;72:1130–1135.
58. Reusser P, Gambertoglio JG, Lilleby K, et al. Phase I-II trial of foscarnet for prevention of cytomegalovirus infection in autologous and allogeneic marrow transplant recipients. *J Infect Dis* 1992;66:473–479.
59. Safrin S, Assaykeen T, Follansbee S, et al. Foscarnet therapy for acyclovir-resistant mucocutaneous herpes simplex virus infection in 26 AIDS patients: preliminary data. *J Infect Dis* 1990;161:1078–1084.
60. Deray G, Martinez F, Katlama C, et al. Foscarnet nephrotoxicity: mechanisms, incidence and prevention. *Am J Nephrol* 1989;9:316–332.
61. Devay G, Katlama C, Dohin E. Prevention of foscarnet nephrotoxicity. *Ann Intern Med* 1996;113:332.
62. Aweeka FT, Gambertoglio JG, Kramer F, et al. Foscarnet and ganciclovir pharmacokinetics during concomitant or alternating maintenance therapy for AIDS-related cytomegalovirus retinitis. *Clin Pharmacol Ther* 1992;57:403–412.
63. Ho ES, Lin DC, Mendel DB, et al. Cytotoxicity of antiviral nucleotides adefovir and cidofovir is induced by the expres-

sion of human renal organic anion transporter. *J Am Soc Nephrol* 2000;11:383–393.
64. Lalezari JP, Stagg RJ, Kuppermann BD, et al. Intravenous cidofovir for peripheral cytomegalovirus retinitis in patients with AIDS. *Ann Intern Med* 1997;126:257–263.
65. Hoyer PF, Brodehl J, Ehrich JHH, et al. Practical aspects in the use of cyclosporin in paediatric nephrology. *Pediatr Nephrol* 1991;5:630–638.
66. Yee GC, Lennon TP, Gmur DJ, et al. Age dependent cyclosporine: pharmacokinetics in marrow transplant recipients. *Clin Pharmacol Ther* 1986;40:438–443.
67. Finn WF, McCormack AJ, Sullivan BA, et al. Influence of the rate of infusion on cyclosporin nephrotoxicity in the rat. *Ren Fail* 1989;11:3–15.
68. Bennett WM, Norman DJ. Action and toxicity of cyclosporine. *Annu Rev Med* 1986;37:215–224.
69. Myers BD, Ross J, Newton L, et al. Cyclosporine-associated chronic nephropathy. *N Engl J Med* 1984;311:699–705.
70. Kabasakul SC, Clarke M, Kane H, et al. Comparison of Neoral and Sandimmune cyclosporin A pharmacokinetic profiles in young renal transplant recipients. *Pediatr Nephrol* 1997;11:318–321.
71. Fassi A, Colombi F, Perico N, et al. Beneficial effects of calcium channel blockage on acute glomerular hemodynamic changes induced by cyclosporine. *Am J Kidney Dis* 1999;33:267–275.
72. Barrett BJ. Contrast nephrotoxicity. *J Am Soc Nephrol* 1994;5: 125–137.
73. Vari RC, Natarajan LA, Whitescarver SA, et al. Induction, prevention and mechanisms of contrast media-induced acute renal failure. *Kidney Int* 1988;33:699–707.
74. Dawnay AB, Thornley C, Nockler I, et al. Tamm-Horsfall glycoprotein excretion and aggregation during intravenous urography: relevance to acute renal failure. *Invest Radiol* 1985;20:53–57.
75. Bakris GL, Lass N, Gaber AO. Radiocontrast medium–induced declines in renal function: a role for oxygen free radicals. *Am J Physiol* 1990;258:F115–F120.
76. Postlethwaite AE, Kelley WN. Uricosuric effect of radiocontrast agents. A study in man of four commonly used preparations. *Ann Intern Med* 1971;74:845–852.
77. Humes HD, Hunt DA, White MD. Direct toxic effect of the radiocontrast agent diatrizoate on renal proximal tubule cells. *Am J Physiol* 1987;252:F246–F255.
78. Workman RJ, Shaff MI, Jackson RV. Relationship of renal hemodynamics and functional changes following intravascular contrast to the renin-angiotensin system and renal prostacyclin in the dog. *Invest Radiol* 1983;18:160–166.
79. Parnes E, Chou S-Y, Porush JG. Endothelial control of renal vascular response to radiocontrast dye. *J Am Soc Nephrol* 1992; 3:549(abst).
80. Schiantarelli P, Peroni F, Tirone P. Effects of iodinated contrast media on erythrocytes. I. Effects of canine erythrocytes on morphology. *Invest Radiol* 1973;8:199–204.
81. Skinner R, Sharkey IM, Pearson ADJ, et al. Ifosfamide, mesna and nephrotoxicity in children. *J Clin Oncol* 1993;11: 173–190.
82. Heney D, Wheeldon J, Rushworth P, et al. Progressive renal toxicity due to ifosfamide. *Arch Dis Child* 1991;66:966–970.
83. Husband DJ, Watkin SW. Fatal hypokalaemia associated with ifosfamide/mesna chemotherapy. *Lancet* 1988;1:1116.
84. Burk CD, Restaino I, Kaplan BS, et al. Ifosfamide-induced renal tubular dysfunction and rickets in children with Wilms' tumor. *J Pediatr* 1990;117:331–335.
85. Pratt CB, Meyer WB, Jenkins JJ, et al. Ifosfamide, Fanconi's syndrome and rickets. *J Clin Oncol* 1991;9:1495–1499.
86. Skinner R, Pearson ADJ, Price L, et al. Hypophosphatemic rickets after ifosfamide treatment in children. *BMJ* 1989; 298:1560–1561.
87. Skinner R, Pearson ADJ, Price L, et al. Nephrotoxicity of ifosfamide in children. *Lancet* 1989;2:159.
88. Rossi R, Godde A, Kleinebrand A, et al. Unilateral nephrectomy and cisplatin as risk factors of ifosfamide-induced nephrotoxicity: analysis of 120 patients. *J Clin Oncol* 1994;12: 159–165.
89. Goren MP, Wright RK, Pratt CP, et al. Potentiation of ifosfamide neurotoxicity, hematoxicity, and tubular nephrotoxicity by prior cis-diamide-dichloroplatinum(ii) therapy. *Cancer Res* 1987;47:1457–1460.
90. Marina NM, Poquette CA, Cain AM, et al. Comparative renal tubular toxicity of chemotherapy regimens including ifosfamide in patients with newly diagnosed sarcomas. *J Pediatr Hematol Oncol* 2000;22:112.
91. Ashraf MS, Brady J, Breatnach F, et al. Ifosfamide nephrotoxicity in paediatric cancer patients. *Eur J Pediatr* 1994;153:90–94.
92. Lewis LD, Fitzgerald DL, Mohan P, et al. The pharmacokinetics of ifosfamide given as short and long intravenous infusions in cancer patients. *Br J Clin Pharmacol* 1991;31:77–82.
93. Mohrmann M, Pauli A, Walkenhorst H, et al. Effect of ifosfamide metabolites on sodium-dependent phosphate transport in a model of proximal tubular cells (LLC-PK1) in culture. *Renal Physiol Biochem* 1993;16:285–298.
94. Hilgard P, Burkert H. Sodium 2-mercaptoethane sulfonate (mesna) and ifosfamide nephrotoxicity. *Eur J Cancer Clin Oncol* 1984;1:1353–1354.
95. Goren MP, Wright RK, Horowitz ME, et al. Ifosfamide induced subclinical tubular nephrotoxicity despite mesna. *Cancer Treat Rep* 1987;71:127–130.
96. Safirstein R, Winston J, Goldstein M, et al. Cisplatin nephrotoxicity. *Am J Kidney Dis* 1986;8:356–367.
97. Womer RB, Pritchard J, Barratt TM. Renal toxicity of cisplatin in children. *J Pediatr* 1985;106:659–663.
98. Brock PR, Koliouskas DE, Barratt TM, et al. Partial reversibility of cisplatin nephrotoxicity in children. *J Pediatr* 1991;118:531–534.
99. Courjault F, Leroy D, Coquery I, et al. Platinum complex–induced dysfunction of cultured renal proximal tubule cells: a comparative study of carboplatin, and transplatin with cisplatin. *Arch Toxicol* 1993;67:338–346.
100. Zhang JG, Lindup WE. Cisplatin nephrotoxicity: decreases in mitochondrial protein sulfhydryl concentration and calcium uptake by mitochondria from rat renal cortical slices. *Biochem Pharmacol* 1994;47:1127–1135.
101. Wong NLM, Walker VR, Wong EFC, et al. Mechanism of polyuria after cisplatin therapy. *Nephron* 1993;65:623–627.
102. Daugaard G, Abildgaard U, Holstein-Rathlou NH, et al. Renal tubular function in patients treated with high-dose cisplatin. *Clin Pharmacol Ther* 1988;44:164–172.
103. Mavichak V, Wong NLM, Quamme GA, et al. Studies on the pathogenesis of cisplatin-induced hypomagnesemia in rats. *Kidney Int* 1985;28:914–921.

104. Allen GG, Barratt LJ. Effect of cisplatin on the transepithelial potential difference of rat distal tubule. *Kidney Int* 1985;27: 842–847.
105. Walker EM, Gale GR. Methods of reduction of cisplatin nephrotoxicity. *Ann Clin Lab Sci* 1981;11:397–410.
106. Markman M, D'Acquisto R, Iannotti N. Phase I trial of high dose intravenous cisplatin with simultaneous intravenous sodium thiosulfate. *J Cancer Res Clin Oncol* 1991;117:151–155.
107. Wong NLM, Mavichak V, Magil AB. Sodium thiosulfate prevents cisplatin-induced hypomagnesemia. *Nephron* 1988;50: 308–314.
108. Erlanger H, Cutler RE. Cisplatin nephrotoxicity. *Dialysis Transplant* 1992;Sep:559–566.
109. Vaziri ND, Zhou XJ, Liao SY. Erythropoietin enhances recovery from cisplatin-induced acute renal failure. *Am J Physiol* 1994;266:F360–F366.
110. Rossi RM, Kist C, Wurster U, et al. Estimation of ifosfamide/cisplatinum-induced renal toxicity by urinary protein analysis. *Pediatr Nephrol* 1994;8:151–156.
111. Wang HY, Wang C, Cui T, et al. Biological nephrotoxins. In: Molitoris BA, Finn WF, eds. *Acute renal failure: a companion to Brenner and Rector's the kidney*. Philadelphia: WB Saunders, 2001:383–389.
112. Knochel JP. Nontraumatic rhabdomyolysis. In: Molitoris BA, Finn WF, eds. *Acute renal failure: a companion to Brenner and Rector's the kidney*. Philadelphia: WB Saunders, 2001:220–226.
113. Chen WY, Yen TS, Cheg JT, et al. Acute renal failure due to ingestion of raw bile of grass carp (*Ctenopharyngodon idellus*). *J Formos Med Assoc* 1976;75:149–157.
114. Centers for Disease Control and Prevention. Acute hepatitis and renal failure following ingestion of raw carp gallbladders—Maryland and Pennsylvania, 1991 and 1994. *JAMA* 1995;274:604.
115. Centers for Disease Control and Prevention. Haff disease associated with eating buffalo fish—United States 1997. *MMWR Morb Mortal Wkly Rep* 1998;47:1091–1093.
116. Okano H, Masuoka H, Kamei S, et al. Rhabdomyolysis and myocardial damage induced by palytoxin, a toxin of blue hump-head parrotfish. *Intern Med* 1998;37:330–333.
117. Warrell DA. Venomous bites and stings in the tropical world. *Med J Aust* 1993;159:773–779.
118. Soe S, Win MM, Htwe TT, et al. Renal histopathology following Russell's viper (*Vipera russellii*) bite. *Southeast Asian J Trop Med Public Health* 1993;24:193–197.
119. Sitprija V, Boonpucknavig V. Extracapillary proliferative glomerulonephritis in Russell's viper bite. *BMJ* 1980;2:1417.
120. Than-Than, Francis N, Tin-Nu-Swe, et al. Contribution of focal hemorrhage and microvascular fibrin deposition to fatal envenoming by Russell's viper (*Vipera russellii siamensis*) in Burma. *Acta Trop* 1989;46:23–28.
121. Futrell JM. Loxoscelism. *Am J Med Sci* 1992;304:261–267.
122. Vanherweghem JL, Depierreaux M, Tielemans C, et al. Rapidly progressive interstitial renal fibrosis in young women: association with slimming regimen including Chinese herbs. *Lancet* 1993;341:387–391.
123. Izumotani T, Ishimura E, Tsumura D, et al. An adult case of Fanconi syndrome due to a mixture of Chinese crude drugs. *Nephron* 1993;65:137–140.
124. Yang CS, Lin CH, Hsu HC. Rapidly progressive fibrosing interstitial nephritis associated with Chinese herbal drugs. *Am J Kidney Dis* 1994;35:313–318.
125. Cosyns JP, Dehouz JP, Guiot Y, et al. Chronic aristolochic acid toxicity in rabbits: a model for Chinese herbs nephropathy? *Kidney Int* 2001;59:2164–2173.
126. Cosyns JP, Goebbels RM, Liberton V, et al. Chinese herbs nephropathy–associated slimming regimen induces tumours in the forestomach but no interstitial nephropathy in rats. *Arch Toxicol* 1998;72:738–743.
127. Yang SS, Chu P, Lin YF, et al. Aristolochic acid–induced Fanconi's syndrome and nephropathy presenting as hypokalemic paralysis. *Am J Kidney Dis* 2002;39:E14.
128. Lee CT, Wu MS, Lu K, et al. Renal tubular acidosis, hypokalemic paralysis, rhabdomyolysis and acute renal failure—a rare presentation of Chinese herbal nephropathy. *Ren Fail* 1999;21:227.
129. Krumme B, Endmeir R, Vanhaelen M, et al. Reversible Fanconi syndrome after ingestion of a Chinese herbal "remedy" containing aristolochic acid. *Nephrol Dial Transplant* 2001;16: 400–402.
130. Vanherweghem JL, Abramowicz D, Tielemans C, et al. Effects of steroids on the progression of renal failure in chronic interstitial renal fibrosis: a pilot study in Chinese herbs nephropathy. *Am J Kidney Dis* 1996;27:209–215.
131. O'Brien KL, Selanikio JD, Hecdivert C, et al. Epidemic of pediatric deaths from acute renal failure caused by diethylene glycol poisoning. *JAMA* 1998;279:1175–1180.
132. Yorgin PD, Theodorou AA, Al-Uzri A, et al. Propylene glycol-induced proximal tubular cell injury. *Am J Kidney Dis* 1997;30:134–139.
133. Cafruny DJ, Feinfeld DA, Schwartz GJ, et al. Effects of drugs, toxins and heavy metals on the kidney. In: Edelmann CM Jr, ed. *Pediatric kidney disease.* 2nd ed. Boston: Little, Brown, 1992:1707–1726.
134. Bach PH. Acute renal failure associated with occupational and environmental settings. In: Molitoris BA, Finn WF, eds. *Acute renal failure: a companion to Brenner and Rector's the kidney*. Philadelphia: WB Saunders, 2001:414–424.

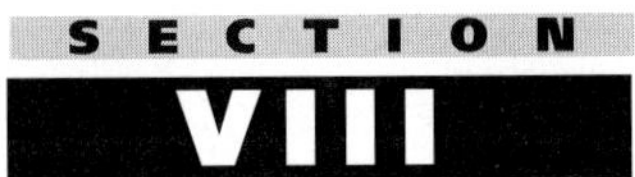

URINARY TRACT DISORDERS

53

URINARY TRACT INFECTION

SVERKER HANSSON
ULF JODAL

At the beginning of the twentieth century, the mortality rate of neonates and infants hospitalized because of acute pyelonephritis was approximately 20% (1–3). With the advent of antibiotics and modern aggressive diagnostic and therapeutic approaches, the mortality today is close to zero. However, long-time consequences of urinary tract infection (UTI) such as progressive renal deterioration to uremia, development of hypertension, and pregnancy complications remain. Most children with UTI have no such problems, so it is important to identify those at risk. Most of those at risk have anomalies within the urinary tract, such as obstruction or vesicoureteral reflux with dilatation of the upper tract. It is important to detect these anomalies early and to institute preventive measures promptly. The ideal goal is to diagnose the very first UTI, especially in infants, and to identify risk factors for subsequent complications. There is also great value in identifying children with a low risk of future problems so that the investigations and follow-up in these patients can be kept to a minimum, with a low frequency of invasive procedures.

Our knowledge of the natural history of UTI in childhood is still incomplete. Most children with UTI are treated at the primary care level, with each practitioner handling a limited number of children. It is, therefore, difficult to create the population-based registries necessary for large epidemiologic studies. Furthermore, the course of UTI often runs over several decades, and it is difficult to follow patients over such long periods. Finally, there is continuous change in management that influences and ideally improves the long-term prognosis but can make comparisons between different time periods difficult. An example is the switch from urography to dimercaptosuccinic acid (DMSA) scanning to study renal damage (4,5).

TERMINOLOGY

Urinary tract infection is the common term for the heterogeneous group of conditions in which there is growth of bacteria in the urinary tract.

Bacteriuria is presence of bacteria in bladder urine. Growth of 100,000 colony-forming units (CFU) in freshly voided urine is mostly used as the cutoff point between contamination and true bacteriuria. However, considerably higher levels occur because of contaminated urine, especially in small children. The optimal method for obtaining urine in small children is suprapubic aspiration. Any growth with this method signifies UTI.

Symptomatic UTI can be classified into *acute pyelonephritis* (with fever as the major symptom), which are infections involving the renal parenchyma, and *acute cystitis* (with acute voiding symptoms as the major feature), which are infections limited to the lower urinary tract. Such a classification is of practical importance, because renal infection carries a risk of renal scarring and requires more aggressive treatment, investigation, and follow-up than an infection restricted to the lower urinary tract. The 10 to 20% of the symptomatic infections that cannot be classified as either pyelonephritis or cystitis by history and simple laboratory investigations are called *unspecified UTIs.* For practical purposes, children with unspecified UTIs are best treated as having pyelonephritis.

Asymptomatic (or covert) bacteriuria (ABU) is the term used when bacteriuria is found in repeated samples from a child who does not report symptoms, usually at a health investigation or routine checkup.

There are major differences in sensitivity between the methods that can be used to identify renal parenchymal damage. It is, therefore, important to state the technique by which the investigation has been performed. *Pyelonephritic renal scarring* (often called *reflux nephropathy*) is focal or generalized damage of a kidney as seen on urography with reduction of the parenchyma, usually with related calyceal clubbing or blunting (6). This scarring is often associated with past or present vesicoureteral reflux, but renal damage can develop without demonstrable reflux. The more sensitive scintigraphic techniques, such as the DMSA scan, can visualize acute inflammation as well as permanent uptake defect. Acute inflammatory changes may be transient and disappear within 6 months of the acute infection.

The term *chronic pyelonephritis* has been used with varying meanings, which has led to a great deal of confusion; it should be used only in cases with typical histologic findings verified in biopsy specimens.

CLINICAL PRESENTATION

The symptoms of UTI depend not only on the intensity of the inflammatory reaction (host-parasite interaction) but also on the level of the infection and the age of the patient. High fever often is the only symptom of acute pyelonephritis. Children usually cannot report back or loin pain until they are 4 to 5 years old or even older, but renal tenderness can sometimes be found in small children who cooperate well at the physical examination.

Children with acute bacterial cystitis often have a temperature of around 38°C, but fever of 38.5°C or more should be taken as a sign of upper urinary tract involvement. Symptoms from the lower urinary tract such as pain at micturition and frequency are not often recognized before the age of 1.5 to 2.0 years and are frequently lacking in children with acute pyelonephritis. On the other hand, acute voiding problems are not synonymous with acute bacterial cystitis. Inspection of the genital area may reveal local inflammation such as vulvitis or balanitis.

In the newborn, the ability to prevent bacterial dissemination is poorly developed, and it is not unusual for children with malformations of the urinary tract to develop septicemia, sometimes in combination with meningitis. During the first month of life, the symptoms of infection may be nonspecific with low or no fever in about one-half of the cases. Thereafter, high fever is the most important symptom of acute pyelonephritis. In the newborn, a subnormal or only slightly elevated body temperature or symptoms such as apathy, anorexia, grayish color, and body tenderness can indicate a serious infection. UTI in infancy may also lead to failure to thrive.

EPIDEMIOLOGY

UTI is one of the most common bacterial diseases in children. Of 3556 7-year-old school entrants in Göteborg, Sweden, 7.8% of the girls and 1.6% of the boys had had symptomatic UTIs verified by urine culture (7). In one-half, the UTI had been associated with high fever, according to the original records from hospital or outpatient clinics, and, in most of these, a diagnosis of acute pyelonephritis was supported by laboratory tests.

The incidence of first-time UTI is highest during the first year of life. This is most marked for boys but also evident for girls. The numbers shown in Figure 53.1 represent approximately 90% of children with febrile UTI diagnosed in the population and approximately 50% of those with nonfebrile symptomatic UTI. Infections diagnosed during the first year of life are mostly acute pyelonephritis. A first-time UTI classified as acute cystitis occurs especially in girls 2 to 6 years of age.

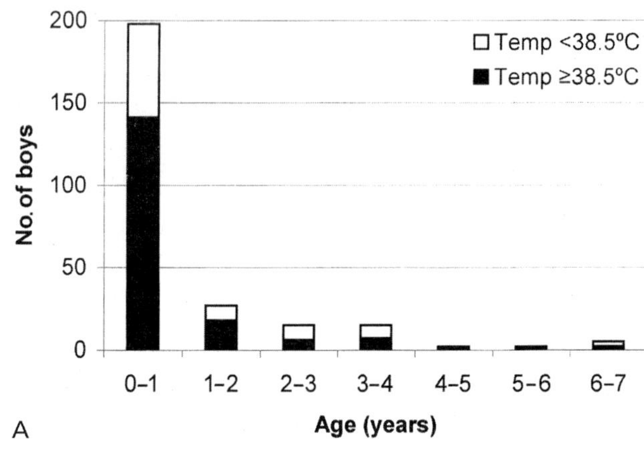

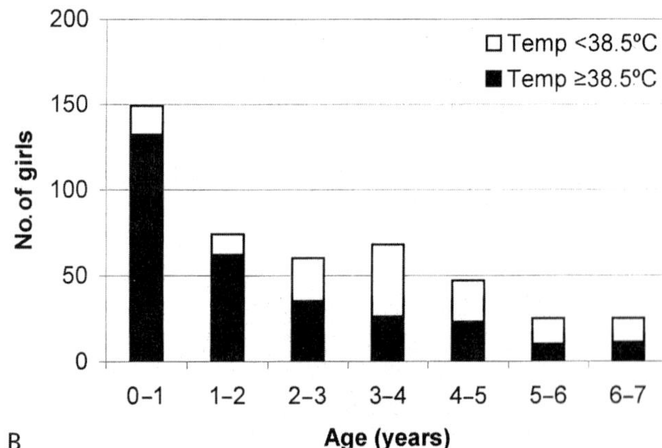

FIGURE 53.1. All children [264 boys **(A)** and 448 girls **(B)**] below 7 years of age with first-time symptomatic urinary tract infection identified at the Children's Hospital in Göteborg 1992–1995 according to age and temperature.

Figure 53.2 shows in more detail the difference between boys and girls during the first year of life. This material is taken from the Swedish UTI study in children carried out during the years 1993 to 1995 (8,9). There were many more boys than girls during the first months of life; after 6 months of age, girls became the majority. UTI without high fever occurred predominantly during the first few months of life. From this study, the minimal incidence of UTI during the first 2 years of life was estimated. The cumulative incidence was 2.5% in both boys and girls (9).

Identifying an epidemiologic pattern, such as that in the figures, requires that clinicians at the primary care level be highly aware of the high incidence of UTI in infants and small children. If these infections are undetected, many of the children will have UTI later and may already have permanent renal damage by that time. An example of a skewed epidemiologic pattern is given in a study from the Aber-

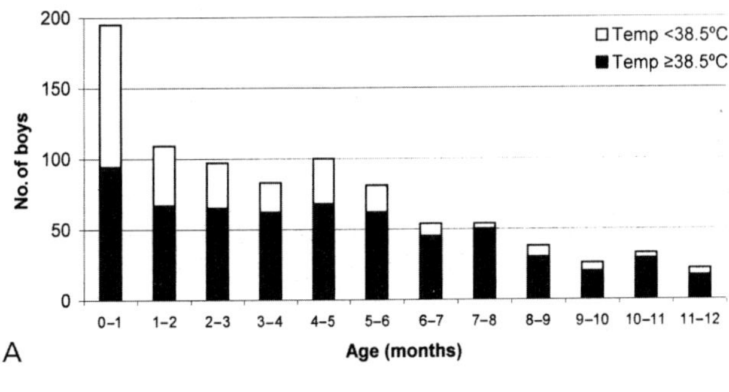

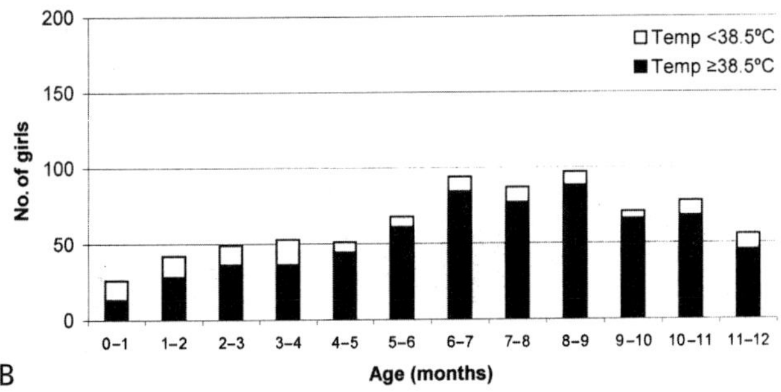

FIGURE 53.2. All children [892 boys **(A)** and 772 girls **(B)**] below 1 year of age with first-time symptomatic urinary tract infection (UTI) identified in the Swedish UTI study 1993–1995 according to age (months) and temperature.

deen area (10). Only 38 of 572 children (7%) referred for radiologic investigation during a 10-year period were under 2 years of age; comparative figures for Göteborg, with a similar child population of approximately 80,000, were 431 of 1177 (37%) (11).

In epidemiologic studies from the 1960s, 30% of girls with a first-time UTI were found to have a repeat infection within 1 year and 50% within 5 years; some had a long series of recurrences (12). However, these figures included symptomatic as well as asymptomatic recurrences, the latter having been detected by culturing of urine at frequent controls. Because it is now well known that ABU is principally an innocent condition (see later), urine cultures today are performed mainly in children with symptoms and not for screening purposes. The rate of new infections is also influenced by the use and duration of low-dose long-term antibacterial prophylaxis to prevent recurrences in high-risk patients. In our material, the overall recurrence rate in girls is approximately 15%. In boys, the recurrence rate is 15% during the first year of life; after 1 year of age, boys have few recurrences, and repeated infections are uncommon.

Obstructive malformations are found in 2% of girls and 10% of boys investigated because of UTI (12). In the previously mentioned Swedish UTI study in 1993 to 1995 there were 1953 children younger than 2 years with first-time UTI who were investigated by voiding cystourethrography. Vesicoureteral reflux was seen in 36% of the girls and 24% of boys; dilatation of the upper urinary tract was seen in one-half of them (8).

CAUSES AND PATHOGENESIS

The urinary tract normally is sterile, with the exception of the distal part of the urethra. Yet, UTI is one of the most common bacterial infections in children. Some individuals have a marked tendency to get repeated UTIs, and their defense against bacterial entry, persistence, and growth within the urinary tract is deficient.

Escherichia coli causes 80 to 90% of first-time UTIs in children; other commonly found bacteria are *Klebsiella, Proteus*, and *Staphylococcus saprophyticus*. *Proteus* species are found in approximately 30% of boys with uncomplicated cystitis, and *S. saprophyticus* is found in a similar proportion of adolescents of both sexes with acute UTI. However, patients with malformation or dysfunction of the urinary tract may become infected by other bacterial species that have low virulence for the urinary tract (e.g., enterococci, *Pseudomonas, Staphylococcus aureus* or *epidermidis, Haemophilus influenzae*, and group B streptococci) (12,13).

Bacteria causing recurrence in the first several months after antibiotic treatment frequently are resistant to the previously used drug. The reason for this is an antibiotic-induced change in the normal bowel flora and not persistence of resistant bacteria within the urinary tract (14). Bacteria that invade the urinary tract usually originate in the bowel. Boys also have a reservoir under the prepuce.

Periurethral Bacterial Flora

The periurethral area is colonized by both anaerobic and aerobic bacteria. These bacteria are part of the normal defense barrier against pathogenic microorganisms. A first step in the development of UTI is often a disturbance of the normal flora and colonization by Gram-negative strains, mostly *E. coli* (15). Such a change can be induced by antibiotic treatment. During the first years of life, however, the periurethral area mostly contains bacteria from the bowel, and enterobacteria and enterococci are indeed part of the normal periurethral flora of healthy children of this age (16). This colonization with such bacteria starts to decrease during the first year of life, and, after the age of 5 years, enterobacteria and enterococci are rarely present. In small girls, *E. coli* is the dominating Gram-negative periurethral species. In boys, *E. coli* dominates during the first 0.5 year of life; later, *Proteus* is as common. Because of this periurethral colonization in children aged 0 to 5 years, the bacterial prerequisites for ascending infections are often present. In older girls with high susceptibility to UTI, daily sampling has shown that periurethral colonization of Gram-negative bacteria precedes the development of bacteriuria (17).

Ascending Bacteria

The bacteria enter the urinary tract by ascending up the urethra. The importance of the ascending route is emphasized by the fact that the rate of UTI in infant boys circumcised at birth is only 10 to 30% of that in the noncircumcised (18,19).

The marked greater susceptibility of girls to UTI after the first 6 months of life can be explained by the difference in urethral length; the short female urethra provides an easy access to the bladder. Temporary ascent of bacteria to the bladder is probably not uncommon in the female; transient bacteriuria occurred in 5 of 23 healthy infant girls prospectively followed by weekly cultures for 10 weeks (Jodal et al., *unpublished data*, 1986). The reason why boys have a high frequency of UTI during the first 6 months of life is unclear.

Further ascent of bacteria from the bladder to the kidneys is facilitated through vesicoureteral reflux. Invasion of the upper urinary tract in children without demonstrable abnormalities may be explained by the capacity of some *E. coli* to adhere to uroepithelial cells (see later) (20).

Bacterial Properties

E. coli isolated from patients with different types of infections or from the fecal flora of healthy children express different virulence factors. These factors are lipopolysaccharides of certain serogroups (O antigens or endotoxin), capsular or K antigens, resistance to the bactericidal effect of serum, and adhesive capacity (21). The O-antigen is toxic and induces fever and inflammation, the K antigen enhances bacterial survival in tissues by conferring resistance to phagocytosis, resistance to killing by the bactericidal effect of serum improves bacterial survival in tissues, and adhesive capacity enhances bacterial persistence in the urinary tract.

The uropathogenic *E. coli* strains are a selected subset of the bacteria that colonize the bowel. They express a limited number of O:K:H surface antigen combinations as well as other virulence factors. These include adherence factors such as fimbriae and toxins. The bacteria causing acute pyelonephritis stimulate epithelial and other cells to produce cytokines and other proinflammatory factors (22). The systemic spread of cytokines such as interleukin-6 induces fever and activation of an acute phase response. The chemotactic cytokines such as interleukin-8 recruit polymorphonuclear granulocytes to the mucosal surface, and, in parallel, the bacteria are eliminated. A specific immune response to the infection follows later.

The severity of UTI correlates with the capacity of the infecting *E. coli* strain to adhere to epithelial cells. In 70% of girls with pyelonephritis, the *E. coli* isolated from urine have adhesins that specifically bind to receptors on the surface of epithelial cells in the urinary tract (23,24). Approximately 10% of healthy children have such *E. coli* in feces. Strains causing ABU rarely have binding ability. The factor that is most characteristic for the pyelonephritogenic *E. coli* clones is its adhesive capacity, which facilitates the bacterial invasion and which is especially important in individuals without anatomic or functional abnormalities (25). Bacterial adhesion triggers inflammation by activating the epithelial cells to which they attach (26). When this happens at the ureteral orifice, ureteritis is induced, leading to a functional disturbance with impaired flow of urine and increased chances for the bacteria to ascend further and cause renal infection (20,27).

The adherence of *E. coli* to epithelial cells is a specific process in which bacterial fimbriae bind to glycoconjugate receptors. Most pathogens express adhesins with several specificities, and most cells carry more than one potential receptor molecule. P-fimbriae recognize receptors that are antigens in the P blood group system and are associated with acute pyelonephritis. The receptor-specific part is located at the tip of the fimbrial rod. The binding depends on recognition of the Galα1-4Galβ-disaccharide, which is common to the globoseries of glycolipid receptors. Such receptors are expressed on epithelial cells in the colon and P-fimbriated *E. coli* were shown to become resident and to persist longer in the large intestine than other *E. coli* strains (28). It was also shown that of *E. coli* strains in the fecal flora, those carrying the genetic code for P-fimbriae (*pap*-positive) outcompeted other strains to cause UTI (29). Furthermore, adhesin-positive P-fimbriae stimulated cells to secrete significantly more interleukin-6 than adhesin-negative P-fimbriae (30).

Type 1 fimbriae bind to mannose-containing receptors, which are found on cells but also on secreted glycoproteins such as the Tamm-Horsfall protein and secretory immunoglobulin A (31). When these substances coat uroepithelial cells, they may provide receptor epitopes for bacterial surface colonization. When secreted, they may eliminate type 1 fimbriated *E. coli* strains and prevent colonization or infection. Type 1 fimbriae have been shown to increase the persistence of virulent *E. coli* in the kidneys and bladders of mice; the inflammatory response was increased compared to type 1 negative strains (32).

Tissue Properties

Uroepithelial cells from children with recurrent UTI have a higher receptivity for attaching bacteria than do cells from healthy controls (33,34). Several mechanisms have been proposed as explanations for this increased receptivity, all supported by some evidence, but relative importance and clinical relevance remain uncertain. The globoseries of glycolipids that are antigens in the P blood group system are present on cells all along the urinary tract. The structural prerequisites for fimbrial-receptor interactions are, therefore, present. The expression of these receptors on uroepithelial cells varies depending on P blood group, ABH blood group, and secretor state of the individual. Those who belong to the P blood group phenotype are unable to synthesize Galα1-4Galβ containing glycolipids; they lack functional receptors for P-fimbriated *E. coli*. However, the low frequency of P individuals in the population has precluded an evaluation of the relative morbidity in infections by P-fimbriated *E. coli* in individuals of the P compared to the P1 and P2 blood group phenotypes. P1 individuals were shown to have an 11 times increased risk of attracting recurrent episodes of acute pyelonephritis with P-fimbriated *E. coli* compared to P2 individuals (35). This risk was not related to a greater number of specific receptors in the children of the P1 compared to the P2 blood group; instead it was shown that P1 individuals had a greater tendency to carry P-fimbriated *E. coli* strains in the fecal flora (36). The mechanism of this increased carriage is not clear but a possibility is that P1 individuals express more or better receptors for P-fimbriated *E. coli* in the large intestine.

Host Resistance

Bladder Defense Mechanisms

Urine is an excellent medium for bacterial growth. Once bacteria reach the bladder, they multiply easily unless they are eliminated by defense mechanisms; however, the normal bladder is resistant to infection. This resistance is provided by at least two mechanisms: elimination of bacteria by bladder emptying and killing by epithelial cells (37).

Bacteria are washed out of the urinary bladder by repeated voiding. In animal experiments, more than 99.9% of inoculated bacteria were eliminated by voiding (38). Although most bacteria are cleared out by the emptying process, some remain in the film of urine lining the bladder epithelium. These organisms are eliminated by the antibacterial activity of the bladder wall. The nature of this activity is not known; however, it has been shown that a significant proportion of bacteria attaching to uroepithelial cells were killed within 15 minutes in normal children (39). Uroepithelial cells from girls with recurrent bacteriuria lacked this killing ability. The capacity of this local defense is limited, and it will have little effect if the volume of remaining urine is high.

Incomplete bladder emptying with residual urine means an ineffective hydrokinetic defense mechanism. In patients with vesicoureteral reflux and obstructive malformations, the disturbance of the urinary flow is evident. Most children with UTIs have no such abnormality demonstrable by the commonly used visualizing techniques. Instead, functional disturbance of the urinary bladder and residual urine are probably major factors in their recurring UTIs. In schoolgirls with ABU, approximately one-half had more than 5 mL of residual urine (40). Those with more than 5 mL residual urine had a recurrence rate of 75% within 1 year, compared with 17% in those with 0 to 5 mL. More than one-half of children with acute cystitis had residual urine at the time of the infection as well as 6 months later (41). This suggests that the inability to empty the bladder is a primary defect in these children and not a secondary one induced by the bacterial toxins.

Incomplete bladder emptying may be a factor in infants with a high frequency of UTIs. Most children younger than 2 years have around 5 mL of residual urine, a high proportion of their total bladder capacity of 20 to 100 mL (42). Bladder storing and emptying ability increased during the third year of life, when children normally start to achieve bladder control. The residual volume in schoolchildren usually is less than 5 mL (43).

Antiadherence Mechanisms

The susceptibility to infection with attaching bacteria can be modified by the secretion of antiadhesive receptor molecules or by individual differences in receptor expression.

Urine contains glycoproteins that interact with type 1 fimbriae. The Tamm-Horsfall glycoprotein and secretory immunoglobulin A express terminal mannose residues. Binding to these molecules hinders the attachment of type 1 fimbriated *E. coli* strains to the mucosal surface (44). However, antiadhesive Galα1-4Galβ–containing receptor analogs have not been described in human urine. It has been suggested that the special role of the globoseries of glycolipid receptors for the virulence of *E. coli* arises in part from the lack of secreted antiadhesive analogs in the urine (26).

Another possible mechanism to block the binding of bacteria to epithelial cells is specific antibodies against surface structures on bacteria. Acute pyelonephritis results in a specific immune response approximately 1 week after the first infection. However, the importance of the specific immunity in the defense against UTI is unclear, largely because of the considerable variability of antigenic expression on uropathogenic bacteria. Nevertheless, a vaccine against UTI is being developed. Preliminary results in monkeys suggest that a vaccine based on the FimH adhesin of *E. coli* type 1 pili may have use in preventing cystitis in humans (45).

Inflammation

Bacteria elicit an inflammatory response in the urinary tract. The magnitude and localization of this inflammatory response may explain many of the clinical features of UTI. Patients with acute pyelonephritis have inflammation of the kidneys combined with a generalized inflammatory response [fever, C-reactive protein (CRP), and leukocytes]. Patients with acute cystitis have an inflammatory reaction restricted to the lower urinary tract. Patients with ABU may show signs of local inflammation of the urinary tract (i.e., follicular cystitis seen at cystoscopy), but the magnitude of the reaction is not sufficient to make them symptomatic (46).

The binding of bacteria to uroepithelial cells is the first step in the cascade of events leading to inflammation that is important for both protection and damage of the urinary tract. Svanborg et al. have proposed that P fimbriae use the globoseries of glycosphingolipids as the primary receptors for adherence to epithelial cells and that they activate these cells by recruiting Toll-like receptor 4 as co-receptors for signal transduction (47). In experiments with mice they showed that Toll-like receptor 4–signaling deficiency disrupts the inflammatory response. The mice failed to develop symptoms and were unable to clear the infection, but no renal damage was seen. This carrier state resembled the situation in ABU patients. Further studies will show whether genetic variation in the receptor repertoire is of importance for development of symptomatic disease or asymptomatic carriage in humans.

The activation of uroepithelial cells by bacteria triggers the synthesis and secretion of inflammatory mediators and increases chemokine receptor expression by epithelial cells (48). A chemotactic gradient is created, and, in the response to the gradient, neutrophil cells leave the bloodstream, migrate through the tissues, and cross the epithelial barrier into the lumen of the urinary tract. These molecular and cellular interactions explain the emergence of leukocytes in urine—that is, pyuria (47). Interleukin-8 appears to be the main driving force for neutrophils to cross the human urinary tract epithelium, and the most important chemokine receptor seems to be CXCR1 (49). The blocking of this receptor in infected mice resulted in dysfunctional neutrophil migration with failure to cross the epithelium. The neutrophils accumulated under the epithelial barrier and abscesses were formed in the kidney parenchyma. The result was severe tissue damage with fibrosis and other signs of renal scarring (50,51). In control mice, neutrophils appeared in the kidneys within a few hours after infection and were seen crossing the epithelial barrier into the lumen. In the process, infection was cleared with no evidence of tissue damage. To test whether the CXCR1 genotype could be of relevance in human UTI, children with at least one episode of pyelonephritis were compared with age-matched controls with no history of UTI. The CXCR1 expression was lower in the patients than in the controls (51). These results suggest that children with UTI have a reduced neutrophil function caused by a low chemokine receptor expression. Further studies are required to define the importance of this deficiency.

PERMANENT RENAL DAMAGE

UTI is associated with permanent renal damage. The process of scarring after acute pyelonephritis is slow; it takes 1 to 2 years for a scar to develop fully as seen by urography (52). Children with unilateral damage, which accounts for approximately 85% of those with damage, have a compensatory hypertrophy of the other kidney, and the total glomerular filtration remains within the normal range. In children with bilateral damage, the glomerular filtration rate (GFR) often is decreased, and there is risk of progressive deterioration.

The frequency with which damage is found in children that have had febrile UTI depends on the sensitivity of the imaging technique used to reveal the damage, and also on the timing of the investigation. This variation can be illustrated by a study of 157 children (median age, 0.4 years; range, 5 days to 5.8 years) assessed at the time of their first symptomatic UTI and 1 year later by DMSA scintigraphy as well as urography (53). At the time of the UTI, 68 (43%) of the children had abnormal findings on scintigraphy and 10 (6%) on urography. One year later, the corresponding figures were 59 (38%) and 18 (11%). DMSA scintigraphy has a higher sensitivity to detect renal damage, but some of the early acute uptake defects seen with this test disappear. Urography, on the other hand, demonstrates additional cases with damage after 1 year as the scarring process progresses.

However, permanent damage (often described as reflux nephropathy although reflux is not a prerequisite for damage) may have developed *in utero* (congenital maldevelopment or renal dysplasia) or be acquired as a sequel of renal infection. When permanent renal damage is detected in older children and adults, it is usually not possible to distinguish between congenital and acquired damage, especially when there have been recurrent UTIs. Although this distinction may be difficult to determine, there are some important differences between the two conditions. Risdon demonstrated that among those with permanent renal damage detected in the early postnatal period, there was a close association with gross reflux, damaged kidneys tended to be small with smooth outlines rather than segmentally scarred, and the majority of the affected infants were boys (54,55). These results were corroborated in a study of an unselected group of 1221 children prospectively followed from their first symptomatic UTI. In this cohort, 74 children were ultimately found to have permanent renal damage by urography (renal scarring). There were significant differences between the 21 boys and 53 girls with damage (56). The median age at the first UTI was 0.3 years in the boys and 2.8 years in the girls. Damage was present already at the first urography in 18 of the 21 boys, and the damage was generalized in 15. Vesicoureteral reflux with dilatation was seen in 12 of the boys with damage on the first urography. Damage was seen on the first urography in 16 of the 53 girls and was generalized in 6. Reflux with dilatation was seen in only three of the girls with damage on the first urography. Thus, the damage was congenital in the majority of the boys, whereas it was acquired in most girls. Furthermore, the most important factor associated with development of renal scarring in the girls was the number of attacks of febrile UTI. There is also a gender difference, with a male predominance among infants with primary reflux detected after a prenatal diagnosis of hydronephrosis (57,58). Yeung et al., in children with antenatally diagnosed hydronephrosis, found that boys had dilated reflux and renal damage, whereas girls had mild reflux but normal kidneys (59).

LONG-TERM CONSEQUENCES

UTI cause significant morbidity and suffering for children, inconvenience and anxiety for families, and considerable consumption of medical resources. Although most children with UTIs have an excellent long-term prognosis, there is an important risk of serious complications in a small group, especially in those with hypoplastic or dysplastic congenital anomalies and dilated reflux. There may be impaired renal function, sometimes leading to chronic renal failure and even end-stage renal disease, hypertension, and complications of pregnancy.

Chronic Renal Failure

The more aggressive diagnostic and therapeutic approaches used in infancy and early childhood during the last decades seem to have decreased the risk of UTI leading to chronic renal failure. In a British report reflecting the management of the 1960s and 1970s, the major cause of end-stage renal failure was pyelonephritis with or without reflux accounting for 21% (60). In a French study covering the years 1975 to 1990, pyelonephritis with reflux was given as the etiology of 12% of children with chronic renal failure (61). For the period 1986 to 1995, only 1 of 102 children reaching end-stage renal disease in Kansas had a primary diagnosis of UTI with reflux (62). In Sweden, with a total population of 8.5 million, the situation is even better: Not a single child with chronic renal insufficiency, defined as GFR below 30 mL/min/1.73 m^2, because of UTI has been detected since 1986 (63).

Smellie et al. studied a group of 226 adults after a follow-up of 10 to 35 years (64). They were originally referred to a UTI clinic because of symptomatic UTI during childhood. Most of these had recurrent UTI and vesicoureteral reflux. Of the 226 patients, 85 had radiologic renal scarring by the age of 10 years, and no scars were detected later. Among the 72 adults with renal scarring that were reinvestigated at a mean age of 27 years, 18 (25%) had raised or borderline levels of plasma creatinine; three of them had reached end-stage renal disease.

In Göteborg, we recently performed a follow-up study 16 to 26 years after the first recognized UTI in childhood in 57 patients with renal scarring and 51 matched patients without scarring (65). They were a subgroup of an unselected cohort of 1221 cases with first-time UTI in the community during the years 1970 to 1979. The median GFR measured by chromium-51–edetic acid clearance was 99 mL/min/1.73 m^2 in both groups. There were eight subjects with GFR below 80 mL/min/1.73 m^2, and the lowest value was 69 mL/min/1.73 m^2. In patients with unilateral scarring, the total GFR remained unchanged over the years, whereas the individual GFR of the scarred kidneys declined significantly from 46 to 39 mL/min/1.73 m^2. In seven patients with bilateral scarring, GFR was significantly lower at follow-up than in those with unilateral scarring—84 and 101 mL/min/1.73 m^2, respectively. Thus, the renal function was well preserved, and the risk of renal impairment in these young adults was lower than previously described, most likely as a consequence of early detection and close supervision during childhood.

Hypertension

In Australian and British studies, development of hypertension has been shown in 10% of children and young adults with pyelonephritic renal scarring (reflux nephropathy) (66,67). The risk correlated to the extent of damage; 15 to 30% of children with bilateral scarring developed hypertension within 10 years (66). In a study 27 years after identification of nonobstructive focal renal scarring, 30 adults were reinvestigated; seven (23%) had hypertension >140/90 mm Hg (68). Smellie et al. in their long-term follow-up demonstrated hypertension in 14 (19%) of the 72 with radiologic renal scarring (64).

However, there is reason to believe that the frequency of hypertension in these studies is higher than we would find in unselected materials treated according to principles used during the last decades. In a population-based study from Göteborg, 54 women with renal scarring were followed continuously for a median of 23 years from the 1950s and 1960s; three (6%) developed hypertension (69). In the recent follow-up study from Göteborg described earlier (65), we also performed ambulatory 24-hour blood pressure monitoring 16 to 26 years after the first UTI in childhood (70). There was no difference between the two groups with and without renal scarring, not even when patients with more extensive or bilateral scarring were analyzed separately. These promising results indicate that at least in the perspective of 20 years from childhood, good care may be effective to minimize long-term risks.

Complications of Pregnancy

Women who had a tendency to recurrent UTIs as girls have an increased risk of new infections during pregnancy (71–73). Women with renal scarring have a significant rise of blood pressure during pregnancy. In women with severe reflux nephropathy, most pregnancies are complicated (74,75). Female patients with renal scarring should be followed carefully into adulthood and through the reproductive period.

DIAGNOSIS

The diagnostic procedure is based on urinalysis, with culture as the most important investigation. Urine in the normal bladder is sterile, but urine frequently becomes contaminated by bacteria during the passage from the bladder to the sampling container, especially in infants and small children. If this leads to a false diagnosis of UTI, the child is subjected to unnecessary treatment, investigations, and follow-up. On the other hand, failure to identify the child with UTI is associated with a risk of progressive renal damage. Therefore, the quality of the urine sample is crucial.

Methods of Urine Collection

The ideal sample of voided urine is a midstream specimen with a long bladder time, collected after uncovering the urethral orifice. A long interval between micturitions allows the bacteria to multiply and reach high counts, which decreases the overlap between samples representing contamination and true bacteriuria. The midstream technique means that the first urine containing most of the contaminating bacteria in the periurethral region is omitted. This method should always be used in children with adequate bladder control.

In infants and small children, urine is mostly obtained as a bag sample. The use of adhesive bags carries a high risk of contamination, however, and approximately 10% of such samples from healthy infants grow at least 50,000 CFU/mL (76). The skin should be dried thoroughly after cleaning the periurethral area, the child kept in an upright position to prevent having urine come in contact with the skin or entering the vagina, and the bag removed immediately after the child has voided. A single bag specimen should not be relied on for a diagnosis of UTI, even if there is pure growth of more than 100,000 CFU/mL urine; verification by a repeat sample is essential, preferably one obtained by suprapubic aspiration or catheterization.

Another technique to obtain urine for screening purposes is to use an absorbent pad placed inside the diaper (77). As soon as the child has voided, urine is recovered with the help of a syringe. The pad must be of the older fluffy type since it is not possible to extract urine from the modern gel-containing super-absorbing pads. The main advantage of the pad technique is that there are no skin reactions, which is a common problem with adhesive bags. The risk of getting a contaminated urine sample is as high with pads as with adhesive bags.

The best technique for obtaining an uncontaminated urine specimen is direct aspiration from the bladder by a suprapubic puncture. This is a simple procedure in infants, because the bladder is an intraabdominal organ during the first years of life. With the child in supine position, a thin needle attached to a syringe or a vacuum container is inserted vertically in the midline, 1 to 2 cm above the symphysis. Urine is usually obtained at a depth of 2 to 3 cm. The trick is to know when there is urine in the bladder. The chance is best when the diaper has been dry for at least 30 minutes, especially after the baby has been fed and the diuresis is high. The presence of bladder dullness by percussion over the suprapubic area or the demonstration of a bladder diameter of at least 30 mm by ultrasonography is associated with a high success rate (78,79).

Suprapubic aspiration causes no more pain to the child than any other needle puncture. Complications are rare; transient macroscopic hematuria occurs in approximately 2%, but microscopic hematuria is present in most suprapubic aspirations, making this technique unsuitable for evaluation of hematuria. Accidental penetration of the bowel does not lead to any problems beyond contamination of the sample. There are few problems of interpretation, however, because bowel aspiration results in growth of colonies of many different types, which is typical of contamination; more than 99% of children with true bacteriuria have growth of only one type of bacteria. Suprapubic aspiration is the preferred method to obtain urine for verification of UTI in small children. For patients older than 1 year, needle aspirations may be difficult for psychological reasons, although the anatomic prerequisites remain until the age of 4 or 5 years.

Catheterization of the bladder is another method of obtaining urine with minimal contamination. In many centers, this technique is rarely used, mainly because of the risk of introducing infection and of the negative psychological effects on children older than 1 year of age. Other centers use catheterization more commonly. We prefer catheterization if suprapubic aspiration has failed, especially if the child is severely ill and a reliable urine sample is needed before antibacterial treatment is started.

Culture of Urine

Urine should always be immediately refrigerated at 4°C until cultured to prevent growth of contaminating bacteria. It is essential that this temperature be maintained during transport.

Most bacteriologic laboratories use a calibrated loop containing approximately 0.002 mL of urine for routine culture. This means that growth of one colony of bacteria on the culture medium is equivalent to 500 CFU/mL. To obtain higher sensitivity, a larger volume of urine has to be cultured.

A dipslide culture has approximately the same sensitivity as the calibrated loop technique. With proper training, dipslides can be used and interpreted locally, provided that the staff uses them regularly to retain the skill of evaluating growth. It is possible to perform sensitivity testing on a dipslide, but it is usually better if the bacteriologic laboratory performs this analysis.

Two possible pitfalls with the dipslide should be mentioned. The most common problem is confluent growth of colonies of different types. This usually indicates contamination but may be caused by massive numbers of one bacterial strain combined with only a few contaminating bacteria. Such quantitative differentiation is hardly possible on the dipslide but is usually easy in a traditional culture. Instead of sending the positive dipslides to the laboratory for characterization of the bacteria, it is usually better to send the urine, provided that it has been kept overnight in the refrigerator and that it can remain cooled during the transportation. The other pitfall with the dipslide is that some bacteria that can cause UTI do not grow on cystine-lactose electrolyte-deficient or McConkey agar, which are most commonly used. Such bacteria are not common but should be considered in infants with sepsis, especially during the first months of life, and in those with recognized malformations of the urinary tract. Most of these bacteria are identified by a laboratory using blood agar or other rich culture media.

The interpretation of culture depends on the method of urine collection and on the clinical background. In urine obtained by suprapubic aspiration, any growth is considered significant. In catheter urine, the level of significance is mostly given as 1000 to 10,000 CFU/mL, but more precise reference values are lacking. Hoberman et al. have suggested a cutoff point of 50,000 CFU/mL (80). For voided specimens, the traditional cutoff level of 100,000 CFU/mL is roughly valid, but the probability of true bacteriuria in a single culture is not higher than 70 to 80%. However, in combination with acute localizing symptoms from the urinary tract such as marked dysuria and frequency together with pyuria, one urine sample with bacteriuria can be considered adequate for a diagnosis of UTI. A similar evaluation can be made in a child presenting with high fever and back pain together with pyuria. For all patients lacking symptoms specific for the urinary tract, a second urine specimen should be obtained before antibacterial treatment is started; when suprapubic aspiration is used, one urine sample is adequate. Another advantage with the latter technique is the absence of equivocal results. Low bacterial counts may occur; 20% of urine samples obtained with suprapubic aspiration had counts of 1000 to 50,000 CFU/mL (81). With such a finding, it is difficult to discriminate between true bacteriuria and contamination using any other sampling technique.

A diagnosis of ABU requires repeated samples over a period of several days in a child without fever or acute urinary symptoms within the preceding 2 weeks.

Other Urine Findings

Pyuria is measured most precisely by microscopy of unspun urine using a counting chamber; more than 10 leukocytes/μL in a boy and 50 in a girl is abnormal. A more crude but mostly adequate estimate of pyuria is obtained by analysis of urine sediment or by the use of test strips that react to granulocyte esterase activity in the urine.

Determination of pyuria is a helpful rapid investigation in a child suspected of having symptomatic UTI. Pyuria is present in 80 to 90% of episodes of symptomatic UTI; a urine sample without pyuria speaks against but does not exclude symptomatic UTI. However, the presence of leukocytes in the urine is not diagnostic of UTI. It may be found in febrile children with infections outside the urinary tract (82), in inflammatory diseases of other types in or near the urinary tract, and as a contamination from the vagina. Pyuria should be taken as an indication to obtain a urine sample of high quality for culture.

The *nitrite test* is based on the ability of most uropathogens to reduce nitrate to nitrite. The reduction is time dependent, and a positive test requires a long bladder time, often more than 4 hours, or significant residual urine. Therefore, the sensitivity of the nitrite test is low in infants and small children with frequent voiding. The sensitivity was only 11% with bacterial counts less than 100,000 CFU/mL in suprapubic aspirates in infants, whereas with higher counts the sensitivity was 44% (81). The predictive value of a positive test is more than 99% in girls and, thus, practically equivalent to bacteriuria. In small boys, the nitrite test is less reliable because nitrite-producing bacteria may accumulate under the prepuce and give a false-positive result. Another reason for a false-positive reaction is macroscopic hematuria, which can cause discoloration of the test strip. Furthermore, the test must be performed on a fresh urine sample or one that has been refrigerated immediately, because growing contaminating bacteria produce nitrite.

Hematuria is common in children with symptomatic UTI and is macroscopic in 20 to 25% of those with acute cystitis (83). However, determination of hematuria or albuminuria is of no value in establishing a diagnosis of UTI.

Site of Infection

A number of tests for defining the site of infection or level of UTI have been described. Some of these tests are complicated and require special facilities or skills; others are simple but may be nonspecific. Unfortunately, there is no universally accepted test that is applicable in everyday practice. One of the major obstacles to development of such a test is that there is no gold standard for establishing the true character of UTI. Localization of bacteria by ureteral catheterization (84) or bladder washout (85) has been used, but these tests are difficult in infants and small children. Pitfalls of diagnostic testing include intermittent discharge of bacteria from the kidney, resulting in false-negative results, and vesicoureteral reflux, which may lead to false-positive findings (86).

Another principle used to evaluate the site of infection is the measurement of host reactions to renal inflammation. An example of this principle is temporary tubular dysfunction leading to decreased renal concentrating capacity for several weeks after renal infection (87). Another is determination of antibodies to the infecting bacteria; this has a high predictive value for renal involvement, but the infecting bacteria must be available (88). Yet another is detection of antibody-coated bacteria in urine using fluorescein-labeled antiimmunoglobulin; this technique is unreliable in children, because there is a delay of several days before antibody is produced (89,90).

Renal imaging may reveal an inflammatory process in the kidney. Swelling of the kidney and dilatation of the collecting system may be seen on urography (91). General swelling can be seen on ultrasonography; this requires measurement and comparison with age-matched reference values for renal volume (92,93).

Another technique that shows an inflammatory process in the kidney is scintigraphy (e.g., technetium-99m DMSA scanning). Affected areas are seen as uptake defects. A metaanalysis of animal studies of acute pyelonephritis showed an overall sensitivity of 86% and a specificity of 91% (94). In clinical practice, a problem with the scintigraphic techniques is the difficulty of distinguishing between acute inflammatory changes and already established renal scars (95–97). Acute inflammatory changes may disappear shortly after start of treatment but may also persist for up to 4 to 5 months before they disappear; thus, timing of the investigation is important (98,99).

In primary care, a method for determining the site of infections should be rapid and inexpensive. White cell casts in urinary sediment are a classic finding indicating renal infection. However, these casts are easily overlooked if pyuria is massive, and they are easily dissolved, especially in alkaline urine. The sensitivity of this method, therefore, is low. Serum CRP level and sedimentation rate may be high in any inflammatory reaction with significant tissue involvement. Even though these methods lack specificity for kidney involvement, we find them to be of value in identifying those children with UTI who have marked host reactions (86). In acute cystitis, the infection is mostly superficial, involving only the bladder mucosa, and a generalized host reaction is not elicited. Another test that has recently attracted attention as a potential marker of bacterial disease is determination of procalcitonin in plasma. High concentrations were found to correlate with the severity of the acute renal lesions in children with pyelonephritis (100,101). Because these tests are all unspecific, they are usually of no help in patients with diseases in several organ systems.

In typical cases of acute pyelonephritis, there is little reason to perform tests for determining the site of infection in routine medical care. These patients should be treated immediately; most clinicians agree that diagnostic imaging and follow-up are indicated. Diagnostic tests designed to determine the site of infection are needed primarily in patients older than 1 to 2 years with no or equivocal signs of renal involvement to identify low-risk patients who can be excluded from investigations and further follow-up. These tests are also of value in children with suspected UTI who concurrently have symptoms and signs suggesting infections in other organs.

TREATMENT

Antibiotic Treatment

Children with symptomatic UTIs should be given antibiotics without delay but not until a urine sample of high quality has been acquired. The drug is chosen on the basis of the resistance pattern of uropathogens in the area as well as of recent antibacterial treatment received by the patient. With adequate treatment, the urine usually is sterile after 24 hours. Persisting growth indicates bacterial resistance or a severe abnormality of the urinary tract.

Oral medication is effective in most children with febrile UTI. Intravenous therapy may be needed, especially when vomiting prevents effective oral treatment or in infants with suspected septicemia. However, in this field, local traditions and beliefs guide the choice of treatment strategy; controlled studies are few indeed. The largest clinical trial using random allocation to different treatment modalities is by Hoberman et al. (102). A total of 306 children aged 1 to 24 months with fever and UTI were given either oral cefixime for 14 days or initial intravenous cefotaxime for 3 days followed by oral cefixime for 11 days. There was no difference between the groups regarding time to sterilization of the urine (24 hours in all children), time to defervescence, incidence of reinfection, and incidence and extent of permanent renal damage as evaluated by DMSA scintigraphy after 6 months. Two smaller studies of children with febrile UTI resulted in similar findings. In one, 3 and 7 days of intravenous temocillin were compared in both arms followed by oral amoxicillin with or without clavulanic acid until day 21 (103). In the other, one group of children was given a single intramuscular dose of ceftriaxone followed by 10 days of oral co-trimoxazole and the other 10 days of oral co-trimoxazole (104). Further studies addressing the efficacy of different routes of administration of the antibiotics are needed, but, so far, there is no evidence that parenteral is superior to oral treatment.

The most common drugs or groups of drugs for treating children with UTI are given in Table 53.1, which also includes the resistance pattern of bacteria isolated from children with UTI in 1992 to 1995 in Göteborg. There has been a marked

TABLE 53.1. ANTIBACTERIAL DRUGS IN CHILDHOOD URINARY TRACT INFECTION (UTI)

	Frequency of resistant bacteria in children with Primary UTI in Göteborg 1992–1995 (%)			
Drug	*Escherichia coli*	Non–*E. coli*	All	Serious adverse reactions
Ampicillin derivatives	27	61	31	—
Cephalosporins	1	29	4	—
Trimethoprim (with or without sulfonamide)	10	13	10	Bone marrow depression, mucocutaneous syndromes
Nitrofurantoin	1	61	7	Pulmonary
Ciprofloxacin	1	15	2	Cartilage (before puberty)
Aminoglucosides	1	1	1	Ototoxicity, renal toxicity

increase in resistance to ampicillin to approximately 30%, making this group of agents inappropriate as first choice; the combination with clavulanic acid may solve this problem. The resistance to the other drugs was 1 to 10%. However, there are considerable geographic variations in bacterial patterns and resistance properties (e.g., depending on local habits regarding prescription of antibacterial drugs). Rapid emergence of strains resistant to trimethoprim to a level of approximately 50% of urine isolates has been reported (105). Therefore, the choice of antibiotic must be based on knowledge of the local situation rather than on international reports.

Treatment of a child with an antibacterial drug for 10 days eradicates sensitive bacteria, irrespective of the localization of the UTI. In children with renal infections, the main objectives are to relieve symptoms and to prevent permanent renal damage. In children with infections limited to the lower urinary tract, the main objective is to relieve discomfort. Many patients with acute cystitis are free from symptoms after one or two doses of an antibiotic. Treatment for 5 days is adequate in children with cystitis (83).

Some have speculated that uptake defects on DMSA scintigraphy should lead to a more aggressive antibacterial treatment (106). There is no evidence to support this hypothesis. It is true that there is a correlation between extent of inflammation and uptake defect on scintigraphy. However, killing of the bacteria is usually a rapid process, and prolonged antibacterial treatment is not likely to influence the inflammatory process that can cause renal damage. Rather, we need the methodology to moderate inflammation to be able to decrease or prevent development of permanent renal damage. It is important to start antibacterial treatment without delay, because there is a correlation between duration of infection and extent of inflammation.

Antibacterial Prophylaxis

Low-dose, long-term prophylaxis has been traditionally used in patients at high risk for developing renal scarring, those with vesicoureteral reflux with dilatation of the upper urinary tract, and those who are prone to develop recurrent acute pyelonephritis. In these patients, prophylaxis sometimes is used for several years (107). It should be pointed out, however, that controlled studies comparing the long-term results of renal function in children given prophylaxis or immediate treatment at recurrences have not been performed. Probably, the most important measure in preventing deterioration of renal function is to inform the parents to seek medical advice early when the child gets fever and to have urine tested for bacteriuria. The efficacy of antibacterial treatment may be questioned. In the Swedish national UTI study, the recurrence rate in children with reflux grade IV to V was 45% in boys and 71% in girls (Esbjörner et al., *unpublished*, 2003).

Another indication for prophylaxis may be repeated attacks of cystitis. The frequency and severity of infections must be balanced against the difficulty of taking the drug regularly and the likelihood of adverse reactions. The duration of prophylaxis in this type of patient is mostly a subjective decision. However, the first measure should be to ensure regular bladder and bowel emptying.

TABLE 53.2. ANTIBIOTICS FOR LOW-DOSE PROPHYLAXIS AGAINST URINARY TRACT INFECTION

Antibiotic	Recommended dosage (mg/kg/24 h)	Resistant bacteria that may cause breakthrough infections	Rate of breakthrough infections/yr (%)
Nitrofurantoin	1	*Klebsiella*	26
Trimethoprim	0.5	*Staphylococcus epidermidis*	26
Trimethoprim-sulfonamide	0.5[a]	Enterobacteria	18
Cefadroxil	3–5	Enterococci	Unknown
Ciprofloxacin	1	Enterococci	Unknown

[a]Expressed as trimethoprim component.

Drugs that tend to select resistant bacteria in the bowel are not suitable for long-term prophylaxis. Antibiotics that have a minimal risk of selecting resistant strains and are effective in preventing recurrent UTI are given in Table 53.2. The drug is typically administered as a single bedtime dose. A high frequency of resistant uropathogens in an area makes a drug unsuitable for prophylaxis. The pharmacokinetic properties of the drugs are important. Antibiotics that are rapidly excreted (serum half-life of approximately 1 hour) have no antibacterial activity in urine after 8 to 12 hours; examples are nitrofurantoin and cefadroxil. However, one dose per day is effective, but failure to take the drug for 1 to 2 days increases the risk of reinfection. Examples of drugs with a longer excretion time are trimethoprim and ciprofloxacin, which usually give effective antibacterial activity in the urine for more than 24 hours.

Compliance is crucial to prophylaxis. The patient and family must be motivated and understand why it is important to take the drug every day, sometimes for several years. Repeated discussions on this subject are usually needed. Patient acceptance of the drug is necessary for successful prophylaxis; a medication that the child opposes has a low chance of being taken regularly. During prophylaxis, recurrences caused by bacteria sensitive to the drug usually indicate noncompliance; insufficient dosage is uncommon.

Breakthrough infections caused by resistant bacteria are seen with all drugs. The bacterial pattern varies, however, and the most commonly encountered bacteria are given in Table 53.2. These bacteria can cause pyelonephritis in the compromised host. In Göteborg, the rate of breakthrough infections with these drugs was 18 to 26% per treatment year. Double antimicrobial prophylaxis with nitrofurantoin and trimethoprim-sulfamethoxazole has been reported to be effective in girls with a high rate of breakthrough infections on a single-drug schedule (108).

RISK EVALUATION

It is essential that children with an increased risk of progressive renal deterioration be identified early; detection of malformations such as obstruction and renal hypoplasia and dysplasia is most important. Many of the children with these types of congenital problems have reduced renal function already from birth; superimposed UTIs may lead to further loss of function and chronic renal failure.

A number of risk factors are associated with permanent pyelonephritic renal damage (Table 53.3). Vesicoureteral reflux is detected by voiding cystourethrography; it is evaluated on a 5-grade scale (109). In studies using urography to detect renal scarring, the severity of reflux was related to the frequency of scarring of 444 children with first-time pyelonephritis (Table 53.4) (11). When the more sensitive DMSA technique was used for identification of permanent damage, more than one-half of the damaged kidneys were not related to reflux (53,110,111). These findings show that reflux is not a prerequisite for permanent renal damage. Still, reflux remains an important risk factor for renal damage; the extent of acute as well as permanent renal involvement has been reported to be higher in children with dilating reflux (24,53,111,112).

Malformations and reflux are diagnosed by imaging the urinary tract. The practical problems are deciding which patients should be investigated and timing the procedures. At first evaluation in the emergency room, it is often possible to identify the serious infections with a greater likelihood of underlying abnormalities that call for prompt investigation. The severely sick infant only a few months old and the child with sepsis are examples. The physical examination may reveal abnormalities that require rapid workup (e.g., hypertension, abdominal mass, or genital or lumbosacral midline anomalies). Similarly, laboratory findings such as hyponatremia, acidosis, or increased serum creatinine and bacteriologic findings such as uncommon bacteria or continued growth in urine obtained 24 hours after start of treatment indicate a more serious background.

Another factor that relates to the development of scarring is the time between the start of symptoms and the initiation of antibacterial treatment. This means that in suspected acute pyelonephritis there should be no unnecessary delay in starting treatment; antibiotics should be given as soon as adequate urine samples have been obtained, without awaiting report from the bacteriologic laboratory.

TABLE 53.3. RISK FACTORS ASSOCIATED WITH PERMANENT PYELONEPHRITIC RENAL DAMAGE

Obstruction
Reflux with dilatation
Age
Delay of treatment
Number of pyelonephritic attacks
Uncommon bacteria (non–*Escherichia coli*)

TABLE 53.4. RENAL SCARRING DETECTED BY UROGRAPHY DURING FOLLOW-UP IN 444 CHILDREN WITH FIRST URINARY TRACT INFECTION DIAGNOSED AS ACUTE PYELONEPHRITIS IN RELATION TO REFLUX STATUS

Reflux grade	Number of children	Number with renal scarring (%)
0	278	15 (5)
1	29	3 (10)
2	99	17 (17)
≥ 3	38	25 (66)

The severity of the permanent renal damage is associated with the number of pyelonephritic attacks (Table 53.5) (11,56,113). Therefore, early and prompt treatment of recurrences is essential. Prevention of new infections by antibacterial prophylaxis can be used in children with high risk of recurrences.

Low age has been related to an increased risk for renal scarring as detected by urography (114,115). Based on findings using DMSA scintigraphy for renal evaluation, the importance of low age for the development of damage has been challenged; the frequency of permanent damage was found to be higher in children older than 2 years (116). There may be several explanations for these divergent findings. Urography and scintigraphy have different sensitivity to detect permanent renal damage; the extent of the damage has to be taken into account and not just presence or absence of damage. In infants, especially in boys, the number of patients with prenatally acquired damage is higher, and there is often an association with gross reflux (54–56). The latter group was probably included in the older studies but may now be detected prenatally by ultrasound screening and thereby prevented from having the UTI needed for inclusion. A major problem is to ascertain that the patient materials are representative and not unintentionally selected; there is a definite risk that young children are referred for investigation more liberally and that there is a higher proportion of severely sick children in the older ones subjected to imaging procedures. Further studies are needed on this issue, but it is evident that pyelonephritic renal damage can develop also after the first

TABLE 53.5. RENAL SCARRING DETECTED BY UROGRAPHY DURING FOLLOW-UP IN 664 CHILDREN IN RELATION TO NUMBER OF PYELONEPHRITIC ATTACKS

Number of attacks	Number of children	Number with renal scarring (%)
0	141	7 (5)
1	366	32 (9)
2	98	15 (15)
3	38	12 (35)
≥ 4	24	14 (58)

year of life and that there is a considerable risk at least through the preschool years (111,113,117,118).

However, most children with UTI do not develop permanent renal damage. Children older than 2 years with single episodes of acute cystitis (i.e., with acute dysuria, without high fever, and with normal concentrating capacity) constitute a group with low risk of urinary tract anomalies in whom renal scarring is rare. In these cases, investigations may be omitted if there is no suspicion of UTI in the history and a high detection rate of pyelonephritis in infants in the community.

INVESTIGATIONS

The aim of the imaging investigations is early detection of patients at risk of progressive renal damage. Ultrasonography reveals dilatation of the upper urinary tract, severe loss of renal parenchyma, and major bladder anomaly. Urography shows obstructive malformation and established renal scarring; it also gives information about renal function and bladder status. Voiding cystourethrography can reveal vesicoureteral reflux and infravesical obstruction, especially posterior urethral valves in boys. Isotope cystography is useful for detection of reflux but cannot visualize the urethra. DMSA scintigraphy shows areas of acute inflammation as uptake defects in the early phase of renal infection; 6 months after an infection uptake, defects represent areas of permanent renal damage. DMSA scans also show the side-distribution of the renal function. Mercaptoacetyltriglycine (MAG3) renography visualizes the passage of the tracer through the urinary tract, gives a crude picture of the function of the kidneys that can be used to identify areas of major acute or permanent damage, and shows the side distribution of the renal function. After the initial study, the tracer substance can be followed during a micturition (indirect cystography).

Consideration of which techniques to use in routine care of patients should include the availability of the method and, perhaps most importantly, the experience and skill of the diagnostic department. Ultrasonography is the first investigation of choice because of its availability and noninvasiveness; severe abnormalities of the urinary tract are rapidly revealed. However, at the present level of technical development, an isolated ultrasonographic investigation is not sufficient to detect reflux or renal scarring.

For the choice of additional investigations and their timing, there are several possibilities. If DMSA scintigraphy is not available, voiding cystourethrography is recommended as most appropriate for risk evaluation (dilating reflux and urethral obstruction in boys), with a follow-up urography after 1 to 2 years. When DMSA scintigraphy is available, the identification of risk patients should be done with this technique. A normal scan means a low risk and no need for further investigations, provided there are no pyelonephritic recurrences (99,110,119).

There is also discussion of whether to investigate all children with UTI or use a selective approach (120,121). Our policy is to reserve imaging studies for all infants with UTI and to older children (older than 1 year) with acute pyelonephritis. The policy of not performing imaging studies in children older than 2 years with a clinical diagnosis of acute cystitis is based on our observation that radiologic abnormalities are rarely found in this group. Although this may be true in a community with a very high detection rate of UTIs in infants and small children, it must be emphasized again that children with previous undetected UTI and renal scarring may present later with afebrile symptomatic infections.

Another important aspect of UTI is an evaluation of the bladder and bowel functions. A detailed history of voiding and defecation habits often reveals abnormal patterns that warrant further investigation. A simple step is to register a flow curve and measure residual urine. Some children need a more complete urodynamic investigation.

MONITORING

A standardized protocol for treating children with UTIs has many advantages. Relevant diagnostic information is obtained, imaging and other investigations are carried out with less personal bias, and follow-up is easier when the patient and family understand the proposed schedule. Because there are differences in organizations, local facilities, and medical tradition, it is impossible to design a universally acceptable protocol. The one described here is a modification of the Göteborg model.

In the Emergency Room

Important points in the history are previous UTIs, recent episodes of high fever, and bladder- and bowel-emptying habits. It is essential to perform a full physical examination to exclude another focus of infection, lumbosacral or genital anomalies, abdominal mass (hydronephrosis or bladder distention), and hypertension. Urine is obtained, preferably by suprapubic aspiration or midstream technique, and is cultured and investigated for nitrite and pyuria. Serum is taken for analysis of CRP and creatinine. Further management depends on the diagnosis and the age of the child. All infants (younger than 1 year) with a UTI and older children with acute pyelonephritis are investigated with ultrasonography within a few days. In infants, we also perform a voiding cystourethrography and a DMSA scintigraphy. In older children, voiding cystourethrography is used selectively in those with dilatation at the ultrasound or in whom DMSA scintigraphy reveals renal damage.

Early Follow-Up

By early checkup, children with abnormal primary healing may be detected. Within 24 hours, the urine should be sterile; signs of inflammation persist longer. Fever and other symptoms should be normalized within 2 to 3 days and CRP below 20 mg/L after 4 to 5 days. The sedimentation rate may remain elevated for 2 to 3 weeks and the concentrating capacity decreased for some weeks to 2 to 3 months after start of treatment. After 4 to 5 days, children treated as outpatients are seen to ascertain that healing is uneventful.

Further Follow-Up

The schedule should be adapted to local traditions and resources. In our unit, there is only one checkup of children with an uneventful cystitis, but all other children are followed for at least 1 year after the UTI. At the visits, educational information is repeated, and the patient is encouraged to return whenever symptoms occur that can be related to UTI.

Repeat radiologic investigations or alternative procedures are primarily performed to detect development or progress of renal scarring. This routine is recommended after 1 to 2 years in patients considered to be at risk (Table 53.3).

Long-time follow-up of patients with renal scarring into adulthood is essential, with at least yearly blood pressure measurements. The patient is provided with immediate service at suspected recurrences and other complications.

ASYMPTOMATIC BACTERIURIA

The introduction of the quantitative culture during the 1950s resulted in a marked interest in silent urinary infections. These were believed to cause renal scarring, and many screening programs were started with the intention of early detection, treatment, and cure. The objective was prevention of both symptomatic UTI and damage to the kidneys. It was shown that pregnant women with untreated ABU had a considerable risk of developing acute pyelonephritis and that this risk could be avoided by detection and treatment of the bacteriuria.

During the 1960s, Kunin et al. conducted a long-term study of the epidemiology and natural history of UTI in schoolchildren in Virginia (122–124). They found significant bacteriuria in 1.2% of girls and 0.03% of boys. An annual incidence of 0.3% in girls was seen at repeated screening, and the accumulated risk for girls to acquire bacteriuria during school age was calculated as 5%. Vesicoureteral reflux was detected in 19%, and renal abnormalities with blunting of calyces were detected in 13% of these with UTI. All patients with bacteriuria were treated using short courses of antibacterial therapy for each episode of bacteriuria. Recurrences occurred in 80%, and pyelonephritis was seen in 10% of the cases, even when carefully followed and treated.

During the 1970s, prospective studies on ABU in schoolgirls were initiated using both treatment and nontreatment (125–129). Prevalence figures of 1.2 to 1.8% were found. The marked tendency to recurrence after treatment shown by Kunin et al. was confirmed. However, the main interest was in the practicality of nontreatment. In contrast to the situation in pregnant women, there was no evidence of a higher risk of acute pyelonephritis in untreated patients than in those who were treated. In addition, there was no impairment of renal growth or GFR in untreated patients (130–132). In girls with renal scarring, progression was seen equally among treated and untreated patients. Thus, no evidence suggested that ABU left untreated was detrimental to the kidneys or that antibacterial treatment had any beneficial effect.

Instead, studies during the 1980s indicate that treatment increases the risk of complications (131). Elimination of bacteria of low virulence in asymptomatic children resulted in recurrences in 80%; these recurrences were in the form of acute pyelonephritis in 15% of the children with normal kidneys and in 30% of those with renal scarring. In girls left untreated, the original strain usually remained in the urinary tract for many years without development of symptoms (133). An established bacterial strain in the urinary tract seems to prevent invasion by other bacteria, thus functioning as a biologic prophylaxis against colonization by potentially virulent bacteria.

Bacteriuria in Infancy

Mass screening for bacteriuria in infancy has been discussed as a means of preventing pyelonephritic renal scarring. Studies of bacteriuria in infancy pose problems of reaching a relevant population of adequate size and difficulties in obtaining uncontaminated urine samples. In an unselected group of 3581 newborn infants repeatedly screened for bacteriuria during the first year of life, ABU was confirmed by suprapubic aspiration in 36 (2.5%) of the boys and 14 (0.9%) of the girls (76). In the boys, bacteriuria was found almost exclusively during the first 6 months of life; in the girls, it was found throughout the first year. Two infants developed pyelonephritis within 2 weeks of the verification of bacteriuria, and the others remained free of symptoms. The bacteriuria cleared spontaneously within a few months in 36 of 45 untreated infants and in response to antibiotics given for infections in the respiratory tract in a further eight (134). Recurrences of bacteriuria were observed in 20% of the children, but only one had pyelonephritis (135).

Radiologic abnormalities were uncommon. Of the boys, three (9%) had vesicoureteral reflux, all without dilation, and none had renal anomalies. Of the girls, one had a scarred duplex kidney with reflux and another had moderate hydronephrosis. During a 6-year follow-up, no indications of renal damage were found; a repeat urography performed in 36 of the 50 children did not reveal development of renal scarring in any child (135). Mass screening for bacteriuria in infancy seems to result primarily in the detection of innocent bacteriuric episodes and is not recommended. Although screening for bacteriuria in healthy children has no place in any age group, it is important to perform urine cultures freely in symptomatic children, especially in infants with high fever or failure to thrive (136,137).

Symptoms in Schoolgirls with Asymptomatic Bacteriuria

Although the schoolgirls with ABU had not complained of symptoms that lead to medical consultation, most of them did give a history of symptoms such as urgency, urge incontinence, and difficult micturition when asked specific questions about voiding habits. This finding was emphasized by Savage et al. when they proposed the term *covert bacteriuria* as more appropriate than *asymptomatic bacteriuria* (138). Bladder dysfunction is common among girls with ABU (139). The pathogenesis is probably multifactorial, and it is difficult to know whether the bladder dysfunction is the cause of the bacteriuria or the bacteriuria is the cause of the abnormal bladder function. However, the symptoms do not seem to be temporally related to the acquisition of bacteriuria. Furthermore, there is no evidence that antibacterial treatment affects the lower urinary tract symptoms in these children. In a controlled study, Savage et al. found no improvement of enuresis, frequency, or urgency after antibacterial treatment (125). These patients probably have an underlying functional disturbance of the lower urinary tract and a secondary liability to urinary infections corresponding to the situation in children with neurogenic bladder disorders. This dysfunction may have been initiated by a previous symptomatic UTI or an inflammation of the genital area such as vulvitis. Painful voiding may have started a cycle of lower urinary tract dysfunction and recurrent UTIs. Bladder rehabilitation programs have been shown to be effective in children with dysfunctional voiding (140,141).

Relationship between Symptomatic and Asymptomatic Bacteriuria

Untreated symptomatic urinary infections may heal spontaneously or they may turn into ABU. How often this happens is not yet known. Recurrences after treated infections were asymptomatic in approximately one-third of the cases if the previous infection was symptomatic (12) but in two-thirds if it was asymptomatic (127). The explanation may be that the new bacteria are of low virulence or that the defense mechanisms of the child prevent the bacteria from attaching by blocking the binding sites (e.g., by antifimbriae antibodies induced by the previous infection).

Of greater practical interest perhaps is the frequency with which ABU develops into symptomatic infection. During follow-up of schoolgirls with untreated ABU, the risk of developing symptomatic pyelonephritis was found to be small. In most girls the same bacterial strain persisted within the urinary tract (133). In the few who developed them, acute symptoms were associated with a change from one bacterial strain to another with greater virulence. This change was often brought about by antibacterial treatment of upper respiratory infections, which eliminated the urinary bacteria (142). The urinary tract was thereby left open to new colonization, and development of symptoms depended on the properties of the bacteria that happened to invade.

In the Göteborg study of infants with screening bacteriuria, only 2 of 45 untreated infants developed acute pyelonephritis; the others remained symptom free (134). The study population contained another 20 (1.1%) girls and 22 (1.3%) boys with verified bacteriuria who were investigated because of symptoms. Of those with symptomatic bacteriuria diagnosed after 1 month of age, all had participated in the screening program with normal results before the diagnosis (76). These findings suggest that infants with primary asymptomatic and symptomatic bacteriuria make up two subpopulations with little overlap.

Treatment of Children with Asymptomatic Bacteriuria

There is no evidence that screening for bacteriuria in healthy children is of value in preventing renal disease, and general screening programs should be discontinued (143). Still, bacteriuria may be found accidentally or during follow-up after treatment of symptomatic UTI. Before a diagnosis of ABU is made in such cases, it is essential to confirm the bacteriuria in repeat urine samples and to ascertain that the child really is symptom free. Obtaining a detailed history is mandatory, including recent febrile episodes and failure to thrive. Specific questions about voiding and bowel habits are given in Table 53.6.

The physical examination includes the same points as in children with symptomatic UTI (e.g., abdominal palpation, inspection of the genitals and back for abnormalities, and blood pressure measurement).

Our general policy is to avoid the use of antibiotics in children with ABU, provided that there are no symptoms or signs indicating renal involvement (144). In children without such indications in the history or physical status, we use a normal CRP (below 20 mg/L) and a normal concentrating

TABLE 53.6. BLADDER AND BOWEL FUNCTION HISTORY

Voiding frequency
Urgency
Squatting or other holding maneuvers
Day wetting
Poor or fractionated stream
Prolonged voiding
Straining during voiding
Constipation, soiling

capacity for age as further support for a nontreatment policy. In every such child, we do an imaging procedure of the kidneys to rule out renal anomalies. The bladder function is studied by measuring residual urine by ultrasonography, and the flow pattern is visualized using a flow meter.

REFERENCES

1. Göppert-Kattowitz F. Über die eitrigen Erkrankungen der Harnwege im Kindesalter. *Ergebnisse der Inneren Medizin und Kinderheilkunde* 1908;2:30–73.
2. Thomson J, McDonald S. On acute pyelitis due to bacillus coli as it occurs in infancy with pathological reports on two fatal cases of pyelonephritis. *QJM* 1909–1910;3:251–268.
3. Jeffreys WM. Infection of the urinary tract in children by coliform organisms. *QJM* 1911;4:267–282.
4. Goldraich NP, Goldreich IH. Update on dimercaptosuccinic acid renal scanning in children with urinary tract infection. *Pediatr Nephrol* 1995;9:221–226.
5. Rushton HG. The evaluation of acute pyelonephritis and renal scarring with technetium 99m-dimercaptosuccinic acid renal scintigraphy: evolving concepts and future directions. *Pediatr Nephrol* 1997;11:108–120.
6. Hodson CJ, Wilson S. Natural history of chronic pyelonephritic scarring. *BMJ* 1965;II:191–194.
7. Hellström A, Hanson E, Hansson S, et al. Association between urinary symptoms at 7 years old and previous urinary tract infection. *Arch Dis Childhood* 1991;66:232–234.
8. Hansson S, Bollgren I, Esbjörner E, et al. Urinary tract infections in children below two years of age: a quality assurance project in Sweden. *Acta Paediatrica* 1999;88:270–274.
9. Jakobsson B, Esbjörner E, Hansson S. Minimum incidence and diagnostic rate of first urinary tract infection. *Pediatrics* 1999;104:222–226.
10. McKerrow W, Davidson-Lamb N, Jones PF. Urinary tract infection in children. *BMJ* 1984;289:299–303.
11. Jodal U. The natural history of bacteriuria in childhood. *Infect Dis Clin North Am* 1987;1:713–729.
12. Winberg J, Andersen HJ, Bergström T, et al. Epidemiology of symptomatic urinary tract infection in childhood. *Acta Paediatrica Scand* 1974;suppl 252:1–20.
13. Jodal U, Winberg J. Management of children with unobstructed urinary tract infection. *Pediatr Nephrol* 1987;1:647–656.
14. Bergström T, Lincoln K, Ørskov F, et al. Studies of urinary tract infections in infancy and childhood. VIII. Reinfection vs. relapse in recurrent urinary tract infections. Evaluation by means of identification of infecting organisms. *J Pediatr* 1967;71:13–20.
15. Stamey TA, Timothy M, Millar M, et al. Recurrent urinary infections in adult women. The role of introital enterobacteria. *Calif Med* 1971;115:1–19.
16. Bollgren I, Winberg J. The periurethral aerobic bacterial flora in healthy boys and girls. *Acta Paediatrica Scand* 1976;65:74–80.
17. Bollgren I, Winberg J. The periurethral aerobic flora in girls highly susceptible to urinary infections. *Acta Paediatrica Scand* 1976;65:81–87.
18. Wiswell TE, Roscelli JD. Corroborative evidence for the decreased incidence of urinary tract infections in circumcised male infants. *Pediatrics* 1986;78:96–99.
19. To T, Agha M, Dick PT, et al. Cohort study on circumcision of newborn boys and subsequent risk of urinary-tract infection. *Lancet* 1998;352:1813–1816.
20. Källenius G, Svensson SB, Hultberg H, et al. P-fimbriae of pyelonephritogenic *Escherichia coli:* significance for reflux and renal scarring—a hypothesis. *Infection* 1983;11:73–76.
21. Svanborg Edén C, de Man P, Jodal U, et al. Host parasite interaction in urinary tract infection. *Pediatr Nephrol* 1987;1:623–631.
22. Hedges S, Agace W, Svanborg C. Epithelial cytokine responses and mucosal cytokine networks. *Trends Microbiol* 1995;3:266–270.
23. Svanborg Edén C, Eriksson B, Hanson LÅ, et al. Adhesion to normal human uroepithelial cells of *Escherichia coli* from children with various forms of urinary tract infection. *J Pediatr* 1978;93:398–403.
24. Majd M, Rushton HG, Jantausch B, et al. Relationship among vesicoureteral reflux, P-fimbriated *Escherichia coli,* and acute pyelonephritis in children with febrile urinary tract infection. *J Pediatr* 1991;119:578–585.
25. Svanborg-Edén C, de Man P. Bacterial virulence in the urinary tract. *Infect Dis Clin North Am* 1987;1:731–750.
26. Svanborg C, Agace H, Hedges S, et al. Bacterial adherence and mucosal cytokine production. *Ann N Y Acad Sci* 1994;730:162–181.
27. Roberts JA, Suarez GM, Kaack B, et al. Experimental pyelonephritis in the monkey. VII. Ascending pyelonephritis in the absence of vesicoureteral reflux. *J Urol* 1985;133:1068–1075.
28. Wold A, Caugant D, Lidin-Janson G, et al. Resident colonic *Escherichia coli* strains frequently display uropathogenic characteristics *J Infect Dis* 1992;165:46–52.
29. Plos K, Carter T, Hull S, et al. Frequency and organisation of *pap* homolougus DNA in relation to clinical origin of uropathogenic *Escherichia coli. J Infect Dis* 1990;161:518–524.
30. Hedges S, Svensson M, Svanborg C. Interleukin-6 response of epithelial cell lined to bacterial stimulation *in vitro. Infect Immun* 1992;60:1295–1301.
31. Parkkinen J, Virkola R, Korhonen T. Identification of factors in human urine that inhibit the binding of *Escherichia coli* adhesins. *Infect Immun* 1988;56:2623–2629.
32. Connell A, Agace W, Klemm P, et al. Type 1 fimbrial adhesion enhances *Escherichia coli* virulence for the urinary tract. *Proc Natl Acad Sci U S A* 1996;93:9827–9832.
33. Källenius G, Winberg J. Bacterial adherence to periurethral epithelial cells in girls prone to urinary tract infection. *Lancet* 1978;2:540–542.
34. Svanborg-Edén C, Jodal U. Attachment of *Escherichia coli* to urinary sediment cells from urinary tract infection prone and healthy children. *Infect Immun* 1979;26:837–840.
35. Lomberg H, Hanson LÅ, Jacobsson B, et al. Correlation of P blood group phenotype, vesicoureteral reflux and bacterial attachment in patients with recurrent pyelonephritis. *N Engl J Med* 1983;308:1189–1192.
36. Plos K, Connell H, Jodal U, et al. Intestinal carriage of P fimbriated *Escherichia coli* and the susceptibility to urinary tract infection. *J Infect Dis* 1995;171:625–631.

37. Cox CE, Hinman F. Experiments with induced bacteriuria, vesical emptying and bacterial growth on the mechanisms of bladder defense to infection. *J Urol* 1961;86:739–748.
38. Norden CW, Green GH, Kass EH. Antibacterial mechanisms of the urinary bladder. *J Clin Invest* 1968;47:2689–2700.
39. Schulte-Wissermann H, Mannhardt W, Schwartz J, et al. Comparison of the antibacterial effect of uroepithelial cells from healthy donors and children with asymptomatic bacteriuria. *Eur J Pediatr* 1985;144:230–233.
40. Lindberg U, Bjure J, Haugstvedt S, et al. Asymptomatic bacteriuria in schoolgirls. III. Relation between residual urine volume and recurrence. *Acta Paediatrica Scand* 1975;64:437–440.
41. Lidefelt KJ, Erasmie U, Bollgren I. Residual urine in children with acute cystitis and in healthy children: assessment by sonography. *J Urol* 1989;141:916–917.
42. Jansson UB, Hanson M, Hanson E, et al. Voiding pattern in healthy children 0 to 3 years old: a longitudinal study. *J Urol* 2000;164:2050–2054.
43. Hjälmås K. Micturition in infants and children with normal lower urinary tract. *Scand J Urol Nephrol* 1976;suppl 37:1–106.
44. Wold A, Mestecky J, Tomana M, et al. Secretory immunoglobulin-A carries oligosaccharide receptors for *Escherichia coli* type 1 fimbrial lectin. *Infect Immun* 1990;58:3073–3077.
45. Langermann S, Möllby R, Burlein JE, et al. Vaccination with FimH adhesin protects cynomolgus monkeys from colonization and infection by uropathogenic *Escherichia coli*. *J Infect Dis* 2000;181:774–778.
46. Hansson S, Hanson E, Hjälmås K, et al. Follicular cystitis in girls with untreated asymptomatic or covert bacteriuria. *J Urol* 1990;143:330–332.
47. Svanborg C, Bergsten G, Fischer H, et al. The innate host response protects and damages the infected urinary tract. *Ann Med* 2001;33:563–570.
48. Godaly G, Proudfoot A, Offord R, et al. Role of epithelial interleukin-8 (IL-8) and neutrophil IL-8 receptor A in *Escherichia coli*-induced transuroepithelial neutrophil migration. *Infect Immun* 1997;65:3451–3456.
49. Godaly G, Hang L, Frendeus B, et al. Transepithelial neutrophil migration is CXCR1 dependent in vitro and is defective in IL-8 receptor knockout mice. *J Immunol* 2000; 165:5287–5294.
50. Hang L, Frendeus B, Godaly G, et al. Interleukin-8 receptor knockout mice have subepithelial neutrophil entrapment and renal scarring following acute pyelonephritis. *J Infect Dis* 2000;182:1738–1748.
51. Frendeus B, Godaly G, Hang L, et al. Interleukin-8 receptor deficiency confers susceptibility to acute experimental pyelonephritis and may have a human counterpart. *J Exp Med* 2000;192:881–890.
52. Filly R, Friedland GW, Govan DE, et al. Development and progression of clubbing and scarring in children with recurrent urinary tract infections. *Radiology* 1974;113:145–153.
53. Stokland E, Hellström M, Jacobsson B, et al. Evaluation of DMSA scintigraphy and urography in assessing both acute and permanent renal damage in children. *Acta Radiologica* 1998;39:447–452.
54. Risdon RA. The small scarred kidney of childhood. A congenital or an acquired lesion? *Pediatr Nephrol* 1987;1:632–637.
55. Risdon RA. The small scarred kidney in childhood. *Pediatr Nephrol* 1993;7:361–364.
56. Wennerström M, Hansson S, Jodal U, et al. Primary and acquired renal scarring in boys and girls with urinary tract infection. *J Pediatr* 2000;136:30–34.
57. Najmaldin A, Burge DM, Atwell JD. Reflux nephropathy secondary to intrauterine vesicoureteric reflux. *J Pediatr Surg* 1990;25:387–390.
58. Gordon AC, Thomas DFM, Arthur RJ, et al. Prenatally diagnosed reflux: a follow up study. *Br J Urol* 1990;65:407–412.
59. Yeung CK, Godley ML, Dhillon HK, et al. The characteristics of primary vesicoureteric reflux in male and female infants with pre-natal hydronephrosis. *Br J Urol* 1997;80:319–327.
60. Chantler C, Carter JE, Bewick M, et al. 10 years' experience with regular haemodialysis and renal transplantation. *Arch Dis Childhood* 1980;55:435–445.
61. Deleau J, Andre J-L, Briancon S, et al. Chronic renal failure in children: an epidemiological survey in Lorraine (France) 1975-1990. *Pediatr Nephrol* 1994;8:472–476.
62. Sreenarasimhaiah S, Hellerstein S. Urinary tract infections per se do not cause end-stage kidney disease. *Pediatr Nephrol* 1998;12:210–213.
63. Esbjörner E, Berg U, Hansson S. Epidemiology of chronic renal failure in children: a report from Sweden 1986–1994. *Pediatr Nephrol* 1997;11:438–442.
64. Smellie JM, Prescod NP, Shaw PJ, et al. Childhood reflux and urinary infection: a follow-up of 10-41 years in 226 adults. *Pediatr Nephrol* 1998;12:727–736.
65. Wennerström M, Hansson S, Jodal U, et al. Renal function 16-26 years after the first urinary tract infection in childhood. *Arch Pediatr Adolesc Med* 2000;154:339–345.
66. Heale WF. Hypertension and reflux nephropathy [Abstract]. *Aust Paediatr J* 1977;13:56.
67. Wallace DMA, Rothwell DL, Williams DI. The long-term follow-up of surgically treated vesicoureteric reflux. *Br J Urol* 1978;50:479–484.
68. Jacobson S, Eklöf O, Lins LE, et al. Long-term prognosis of post-infectious renal scarring in relation to radiological findings in childhood—a 27-year follow-up. *Pediatr Nephrol* 1992;6: 19–24.
69. Martinell J, Lidin-Janson G, Jagenburg R, et al. Girls prone to urinary infections followed into adulthood. Indices of renal disease. *Pediatr Nephrol* 1996;10:139–142.
70. Wennerström M, Hansson S, Hedner T, et al. Ambulatory blood pressure 16–26 years after the first urinary tract infection in childhood. *J Hypertens* 2000;18:485–491.
71. Sacks SH, Roberts R, Verrier-Jones K, et al. Effect of symptomless bacteriuria in childhood on subsequent pregnancy. *Lancet* 1987;2:991–994.
72. Martinell J, Jodal U, Lidin-Janson G. Pregnancies in women with and without renal scarring after urinary infections in childhood. *BMJ* 1990;300:840–844.
73. Mansfield JT, Snow BW, Cartwright PC, et al. Complications of pregnancy in women after childhood reimplantation for vesicoureteral reflux: an update with 25 years followup. *J Urol* 1995;154:787–790.

74. Kincaid-Smith P, Becker GJ. Reflux nephropathy in the adult. In: Hodson J, Kincaid-Smith P, eds. *Reflux nephropathy*. New York: Masson, 1979:21–28.
75. Jungers P, Houillier P, Chauveau D, et al. Pregnancy in women with reflux nephropathy. *Kidney Int* 1996;50:593–599.
76. Wettergren B, Jodal U, Jonasson G. Epidemiology of bacteriuria during the first year of life. *Acta Paediatrica Scand* 1985;74:925–933.
77. Liaw LCT, Nayar DM, Pedler SJ, et al. Home collection of urine for culture from infants by three methods: survey of parents' preferences and bacterial contamination rates. *BMJ* 2000;320:1312–1313.
78. Chu RWP, Wong YC, Luk SH, et al. Comparing suprapubic urine aspiration under real-time ultrasound guidance with conventional blind aspiration. *Acta Paediatrica* 2002;91:512–516.
79. Jodal U. Suprapubic aspiration of urine in the diagnosis of urinary tract infection in infants. *Acta Paediatrica* 2002;91:497–498.
80. Hoberman A, Wald ER, Reynolds EA, et al. Pyuria and bacteriuria in urine specimens obtained by catheter from young children with fever. *J Pediatr* 1994;124:513–519.
81. Hansson S, Brandström P, Jodal U, et al. Low bacterial counts in infants with urinary tract infection. *J Pediatr* 1998;132:180–182.
82. Turner GM, Coulthard MG. Fever can cause pyuria in children. *BMJ* 1995;311:924.
83. Abrahamsson K, Hansson S, Larsson P, et al. Antibiotic treatment for five days is effective in children with acute cystitis. *Acta Paediatrica* 2002;91:55–58.
84. Whitaker J, Hewstone AS. The bacteriologic differentiation between upper and lower urinary tract infection in children. *J Pediatr* 1969;74:364–369.
85. Fairley KF, Grounds AD, Carson NE, et al. Site of infection in acute urinary tract infection in general practice. *Lancet* 1971;2:615–618.
86. Jodal U, Lindberg U, Lincoln K. Level diagnosis of symptomatic urinary tract infections in childhood. *Acta Paediatrica Scand* 1975;64:201–208.
87. Winberg J. Renal function studies in infants and children with acute, nonobstructive urinary tract infections. *Acta Paediatrica Scand* 1959;48:577–589.
88. Jodal U. The immune response to urinary infections in childhood. I. Serological diagnosis of primary symptomatic infection in girls by indirect hemagglutination. *Acta Paediatrica Scand* 1975;64:96–104.
89. Hellerstein S, Kennedy E, Nussbaum L, Rice K. Localization of the site of urinary tract infections by means of antibody-coated bacteria in the urinary sediments. *J Pediatr* 1978;92:188–193.
90. Pylkkänen J. Antibody-coated bacteria in the urine of infants and children with their first two urinary tract infections. *Acta Paediatrica Scand* 1978;67:272–279.
91. Hellström M, Jodal U, Mårild S, et al. Ureteral dilatation in children with febrile urinary tract infection or bacteriuria. *Am J Radiol* 1987;148:483–486.
92. Dinkel E, Ertel M, Dittrich M, et al. Kidney size in childhood. Sonographical growth charts for kidney length and volume. *Pediatr Radiol* 1985;15:38–43.
93. Dinkel E, Orth S, Dittrich M, et al. Renal sonography in the differentiation of upper from lower urinary tract infection. *Am J Radiol* 1986;146:775–780.
94. Craig JC, Wheeler DM, Irwig L, et al. How accurate is dimercaptosuccinic acid scintigraphy for the diagnosis of acute pyelonephritis? A meta-analysis of experimental studies. *J Nuclear Med* 2000;41:986–993.
95. Goldraich NP, Ramos OL, Goldraich IH. Urography versus DMSA scan in children with vesicoureteric reflux. *Pediatr Nephrol* 1989;3:1–5.
96. Smellie JM. The DMSA scan and intravenous urography in the detection of renal scarring; editorial comment. *Pediatr Nephrol* 1989;3:6–8.
97. Goldraich NP, Goldraich IH. Update on dimercaptosuccinic acid renal scanning in children with urinary tract infection. *Pediatr Nephrol* 1995;9:221–226.
98. Stokland E, Hellström M, Jacobsson B, et al. Early 99mTc dimercaptosuccinic acid (DMSA) scintigraphy in symptomatic first-time urinary tract infection. *Acta Paediatrica* 1996;85: 430–436.
99. Jakobsson B, Svensson L. Transient pyelonephritic changes on ^{99m}technetium-dimercaptosuccinic acid scan for at least five months after infection. *Acta Paediatrica* 1997;86:803–807.
100. Benador N, Siegrist C-A, Gendrel D, et al. Procalcitonin is a marker of severity of renal lesions in pyelonephritis. *Pediatrics* 1998;102:1422–1425.
101. Smolkin V, Koren A, Raz R, et al. Procalcitonin as a marker of acute pyelonephritis in infants and children. *Pediatr Nephrol* 2002;17:409–412.
102. Hoberman A, Wald ER, Hickey RW, et al. Oral versus initial intravenous therapy for urinary tract infections in young febrile children. *Pediatrics* 1999;104:79–86.
103. Levtchenko E, Lahy C, Levy J, et al. Treatment of children with acute pyelonephritis: a prospective randomized study. *Pediatr Nephrol* 2001;16:878–884.
104. Baker PC, Nelson DS, Schunk JE. The addition of ceftriaxone to oral therapy does not improve outcome in febrile children with urinary tract infections. *Arch Pediatr Adolesc Med* 2001;155:135–139.
105. Madrigal G, Odio C, Mohs E, et al. Single dose antibiotic therapy is not as effective as conventional regimens for management of acute urinary tract infections in children. *Pediatr Infect Dis J* 1988;7:316–319.
106. Conway JJ, Cohn RA. Evolving role of nuclear medicine for the diagnosis and management of urinary tract infection. *J Pediatr* 1994;124:87–90.
107. Smellie JM, Grüneberg RN, Bantock HM, et al. Prophylactic co-trimoxazole and trimethoprim in the management of urinary tract infection in children. *Pediatr Nephrol* 1988;2:12–17.
108. Smith EM, Elder JS. Double antimicrobial prophylaxis in girls with breakthrough urinary tract infections. *Urology* 1994;43:708–712.
109. Report of the International Reflux Study Committee. Medical versus surgical treatment of primary vesicoureteral reflux: a prospective international reflux study in children. *J Urol* 1981;125:277–283.
110. Rosenberg AR, Rossleigh MA, Brydon MP, et al. Evaluation of acute urinary tract infection in children by dimercaptosuccinic acid scintigraphy: a prospective study. *J Urol* 1992; 148:1746–1749.
111. Jakobsson B, Berg U, Svensson L. Renal scarring after acute pyelonephritis. *Arch Dis Childhood* 1994;70:111–115.

112. Jakobsson B, Nolstedt L, Svensson L, et al. ^{99m}Tc-dimercaptosuccinic acid (DMSA) in the diagnosis of acute pyelonephritis in children: relation to clinical and radiological findings. *Pediatr Nephrol* 1992;6:328–334.
113. Martinell J, Hansson S, Claesson I, et al. Detection of urographic scars in girls with pyelonephritis followed for 13–38 years. *Pediatr Nephrol* 2000;14:1006–1010.
114. Pylkkänen J, Vilska J, Koskimies O. The value of level diagnosis of childhood urinary tract infection in predicting renal injury. *Acta Paediatrica Scand* 1981;70:879–883.
115. Berg UB, Johansson SB. Age as a determinant of renal functional damage in urinary tract infection. *Arch Dis Childhood* 1983;58:963–969.
116. Benador D, Benador N, Slosman D, et al. Are younger children at highest risk of renal sequelae after pyelonephritis? *Lancet* 1997;349:17–19.
117. Smellie JM, Ransley PG, Normand IC, et al. Development of new renal scars: a collaborative study. *BMJ* 1985;290:1957–1960.
118. Rushton HG, Majd M, Jantausch B, et al. Renal scarring following reflux and nonreflux pyelonephritis in children: evaluation with ^{99m}technetium-dimercaptosuccinic acid scintigraphy. *J Urol* 1992;147:1327–1332.
119. Ditchfield MR, de Campo JF, Cook DJ, et al. Vesicoureteral reflux: an accurate predictor of acute pyelonephritis in childhood urinary tract infection? *Radiology* 1994;190:413–415.
120. Welch TR, Forbes PA, Drummond KN, et al. Recurrent urinary tract infection in girls. Group with lower tract findings and a benign course. *Arch Dis Childhood* 1976;51:114–119.
121. Stark H. Urinary tract infections in girls: the cost-effectiveness of currently recommended investigative routines. *Pediatr Nephrol* 1997;11:174–177.
122. Kunin CM, Deutscher R, Paquin A. Urinary tract infection in school children: an epidemiologic, clinical and laboratory study. *Medicine* 1964;43:91–130.
123. Kunin CM. A ten-year study of bacteriuria in schoolgirls: final report of bacteriologic, urologic and epidemiologic findings. *J Infect Dis* 1970;122:382–393.
124. Gillenwater JY, Harrison RB, Kunin CM. Natural history of bacteriuria in schoolgirls. *N Engl J Med* 1979;301:396–399.
125. Savage DCL, Howie G, Adler K, Wilson MI. Controlled trial of therapy in covert bacteriuria in childhood. *Lancet* 1975;1:358–361.
126. McLachlan M, Meller S, Verrier-Jones E, et al. Urinary tract in schoolgirls with covert bacteriuria. *Arch Dis Childhood* 1975;50:253–258.
127. Lindberg U, Claesson I, Hanson LÅ, et al. Asymptomatic bacteriuria in schoolgirls. VIII. Clinical course during a 3-year follow-up. *J Pediatr* 1978;92:194–199.
128. Cardiff-Oxford Bacteriuria Study Group. Sequelae of covert bacteriuria in schoolgirls. *Lancet* 1978;1:889–893.
129. Newcastle Covert Bacteriuria Research Group. Covert bacteriuria in schoolgirls in Newcastle upon Tyne: a 5-year follow-up. *Arch Dis Childhood* 1981;56:585–592.
130. Verrier-Jones K, Asscher AW, Verrier-Jones ER, et al. Glomerular filtration rate in schoolgirls with covert bacteriuria. *BMJ* 1982;285:1307–1310.
131. Hansson S, Jodal U, Norén L, et al. Untreated bacteriuria in asymptomatic girls with renal scarring. *Pediatrics* 1989;84:964–968.
132. Aggarwal VK, Verrier Jones K, Asscher AW, et al. Covert bacteriuria: long term follow up. *Arch Dis Childhood* 1991;66:1284–1286.
133. Hansson S, Caugant D, Jodal U, et al. Untreated asymptomatic bacteriuria in girls. I–Stability of the urinary isolates. *BMJ* 1989;298:853–855.
134. Wettergren B, Jodal U. Spontaneous clearance of asymptomatic bacteriuria in infants. *Acta Paediatrica Scand* 1990;79:300–304.
135. Wettergren B, Hellström M, Stokland E, et al. Six year follow up of infants with bacteriuria on screening. *BMJ* 1990;301:845–848.
136. Roberts KB, Charney E, Sweren RJ, et al. Urinary tract infection in infants with unexplained fever: a collaborative study. *J Pediatr* 1983;103:864–867.
137. Hogg RJ. A search for the "elusive" urinary tract infection in febrile infants. *Pediatr Infect Dis J* 1987;6:233–234.
138. Savage DCL, Wilson MI, McHardy M, et al. Covert bacteriuria of childhood. A clinical and epidemiological study. *Arch Dis Childhood* 1973;48:8–20.
139. Hansson S, Hjälmås K, Jodal U, et al. Lower urinary tract dysfunction in girls with untreated asymptomatic or covert bacteriuria. *J Urol* 1990;143:333–335.
140. van Gool JD, Kuitjen RH, Donckerwolcke RA, et al. Bladder-sphincter dysfunction, urinary infection and vesicoureteral reflux with special reference to cognitive bladder training. *Contrib Nephrol* 1984;39:190–210.
141. Hellström A-L, Hjälmås K, Jodal U. Rehabilitation of the dysfunctional bladder in children: method and 3-year followup. *J Urol* 1987;138:847–849.
142. Hansson S, Jodal U, Lincoln K, et al. Untreated asymptomatic bacteriuria in girls: II—Effect of phenoxymethylpenicillin and erythromycin given for intercurrent infections. *BMJ* 1989;298:856–859.
143. Kemper KJ, Avner ED. The case against screening urinalyses for asymptomatic bacteriuria in children. *Am J Dis Child* 1992;146:343–346.
144. Linshaw M. Asymptomatic bacteriuria and vesicoureteral reflux in children. *Kidney Int* 1996;50:312–329.

54

VESICOURETERAL REFLUX AND SCARRING

H. GIL RUSHTON, JR.

Vesicoureteral reflux (VUR) is the backup of urine from the bladder into the ureters. Normally, a flap-valve mechanism at the ureterovesical junction prevents this reflux. Inadequate development of this flap is the underlying cause of reflux. The recognition of VUR and its significance has evolved only over the past 30 years. It is now evident that the anatomy of the ureterovesical junction is an inherited trait and that VUR is a familial phenomenon.

VUR is a risk factor for pyelonephritis. VUR alone does not cause renal damage, but intrarenal reflux (IRR) in combination with bacilluria permits invasion of the renal parenchyma by bacteria. Identifying children with VUR at an early age offers an opportunity to prevent episodes of acute pyelonephritis and the resultant renal scarring that leads to reflux nephropathy, hypertension, and renal insufficiency. Urinary tract infection (UTI) is the most common factor leading to recognition of VUR. Because it is usually the combination of UTI and reflux that leads to renal damage, it is important to perform cystography in children who develop UTI to identify those at risk.

CAUSES AND DEFINITIONS

Primary VUR is congenital and is not associated with any underlying neuromuscular or obstructive phenomenon. The antireflux mechanism is the result of a flap-valve mechanism (reviewed in reference 1). The submucosal portion of the ureter abuts bladder musculature and collapses during bladder emptying. Intravesical pressure plays a role in coapting the lumen during voiding. The orifice of a refluxing ureter tends to be located laterally and more cephalad in the bladder, resulting in shortening of the intravesical ureter (Fig. 54.1) (2). Efficiency of the antireflux mechanism correlates directly with the length of the submucosal ureter. This length may be genetically dictated. A number of specific uroepithelial genes and genetic polymorphisms have been causally related to primary VUR (3,4).

The grading of reflux was standardized when the International Reflux Study (IRS) was initiated (5). *Grade I* reflux fills the ureter only, whereas *grade II* fills the ureter and collecting system without dilation (Fig. 54.2). These are often called mild reflux. *Grade III* or *moderate reflux* causes mild blunting of the calyces with loss of the sharp delineation of the forniceal angles. *Grade IV* reflux has more than 50% of calyces blunted to the extent that the forniceal angles are no longer evident. *Grade V* reflux is defined by all calyces being blunted and papillary impressions lost. With each grade, ureteral dilation becomes more severe; in grades IV and V reflux, often called *severe* or *high-grade reflux*, the ureter is also tortuous.

Duplication of the collecting system plays a role in the incidence of VUR. The lower segment ureteral orifice of a duplicated system commonly is abnormally located; this increases the risk for VUR. Duplication also is an inherited trait (6). Although the incidence of reflux is greater and tends to be higher grade in patients with duplication, the prognosis, as with primary reflux, correlates well with orifice position and grade of reflux (7–9).

Secondary VUR is the consequence of pathologic bladder dynamics. Urethral obstruction, neuromuscular disease, or abnormal voiding patterns may be the underlying cause for VUR in those who might otherwise have no intrinsic ureterovesical abnormality. The classic obstructive state associated with reflux is a posterior urethral valve. VUR occurs in approximately one-half of boys with urethral obstruction secondary to a valve. However, approximately one-half of that reflux ultimately resolves with treatment of the obstruction.

In 1952, Hutch recognized the association of neuropathology with VUR (10). Abnormally high intravesical pressure may distort the ureterovesical junction, disrupting the normal antireflux mechanism. This may be associated with outpouching of bladder mucosa at the ureteral hiatus (paraureteral diverticulum). As is true in patients with a urethral valve, treatment of the neuropathic bladder also may result in resolution of reflux (11). Cohen et al. report that reflux resolved in 62% of 72 patients who were treated nonsurgically with clean intermittent catheterization and oxybutynin (Ditropan), when indicated, to reduce uninhibited bladder contractions (12). Similar results are reported by other groups (13–15).

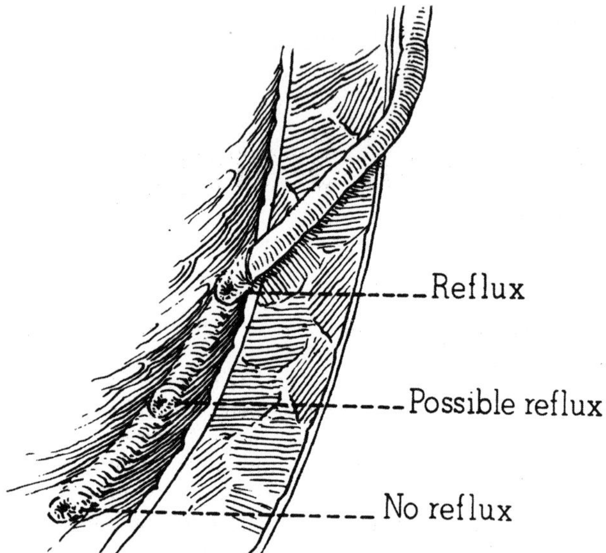

FIGURE 54.1. Normal and refluxing ureterovesical junctions. Refluxing ureterovesical junction has the same anatomic features as nonrefluxing orifice, except for inadequate length of intravesical submucosal ureter. Some orifices with borderline submucosal tunnels reflux intermittently. (From Glenn J, ed. *Urologic surgery*, 2nd ed. New York: Harper & Row, 1975, with permission.)

More recently, the relationship between dysfunctional voiding and VUR has been emphasized (16–18). Increased intravesical pressure from dyssynergic voiding (voluntary sphincter contraction instead of relaxation during detrusor contractions) can cause secondary reflux. Mayo and Burns report a significantly higher incidence of VUR (50%) in 30 children with dyssynergia (73% with UTI) compared with 24% of 97 wet children with bladder instability alone (45% with UTI) and only 8% of 64 children with normal urodynamic findings (31% with UTI) (19). However, as evidenced in this study, the relationship between reflux and voiding dysfunction is clouded because most studies of children with voiding dysfunction include a significant number of children with UTIs—a group known to have a high incidence of VUR (30 to 50%). Nevertheless, in a prospective study of 308 children with day and night wetting, reflux was detected in 23% of children with no history of UTI. In contrast, reflux was present in 34% of those with wetting and a history of UTI (20). Scholtmeijer et al. suggest that urodynamic evaluation be used to plan better treatment regimens for all children with reflux (21). That is probably impractical, because urodynamic studies in small children are difficult and often unreliable. Furthermore, most children with persistent underlying bladder instability after toilet training can be identified with a good voiding history, allowing one to be more selective with urodynamic evaluation. Once identified, instituting better voiding habits and reducing intravesical pressure with an anticholinergic may lead to resolution of reflux and reduction in UTIs (22,23).

The most severe form of dysfunctional voiding, the *Hinman syndrome* (24), often is associated with reflux. In this group, voluntary sphincter spasm is severe enough to produce a picture of true outlet obstruction. Enuresis, encopresis, incomplete bladder emptying, UTI, hydronephrosis, reflux, and renal failure sometimes result from this syndrome, which is thought to be emotionally induced. Failure to recognize dysfunctional voiding is one of the major causes of complications after ureteral reimplantation (25).

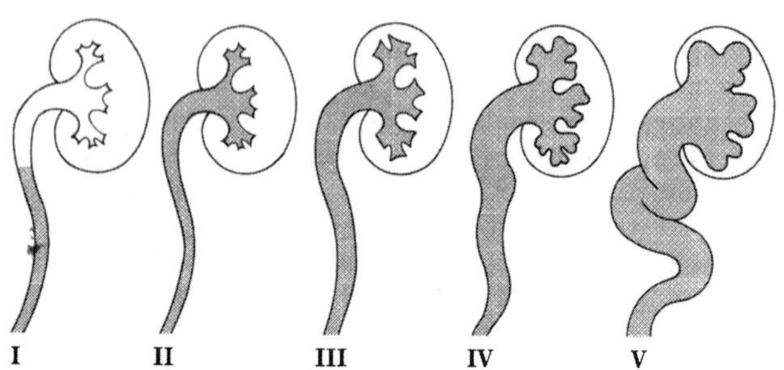

FIGURE 54.2. International classification of vesicoureteral reflux (VUR). Grade I: ureter only. Grade II: ureter, pelvis, calyces; no dilation, normal calyceal fornices. Grade III: mild or moderate dilation or tortuosity of the ureter, and mild or moderate dilation of the pelvis, but no or slight blunting of the fornices. Grade IV: moderate dilation or tortuosity of ureter and mild dilation of renal pelvis and calyces; complete obliteration of sharp angle of fornices but maintenance of papillary impressions in most calyces. Grade V: gross dilation and tortuosity of ureter; gross dilation of renal pelvis and calyces; papillary impressions are no longer visible in most calyces. (Modified from International Reflux Committee. Medical versus surgical treatment of primary vesicoureteral reflux. *Pediatrics* 1981;67:392.)

EPIDEMIOLOGY

The prevalence of VUR in healthy individuals is unknown. Ransley, in a compilation of several publications, reports reflux in 7 of 535 (1.3%) presumably healthy children (26). Because most patients evaluated have had UTI, most of the information about reflux has been gathered from that group. Reflux has been identified in 29 to 50% of children, mostly white girls, evaluated after UTI (27,28). In another study, only one-third as many African American as white girls with UTI had reflux (29). The incidence of UTI in African American girls also was reduced, resulting in a frequency of reflux in African American girls approximately one-tenth of that in whites.

As early as 1966, it was recognized that reflux associated with UTI was more common in younger children (30). In this review, reflux was present in 70% of children younger than 1 year, 25% of those younger than 4 years, 15% of those younger than 12 years, and 5% of adults. Despite this age-related incidence of VUR, Smellie et al. found no age-related difference between children with or without VUR who presented with UTI (31).

Stratification of the incidence of UTI by gender is difficult because the incidence of UTI (the presenting cause for evaluation) is so much greater in females than in males. Snodgrass found an equal incidence of reflux in males and females evaluated for dysfunctional voiding, approximately 12% in each (32). Scott found equal numbers of boys and girls with high-grade reflux (33). In the European branch of the IRS, females only slightly outnumbered males; in the U.S. branch, females outnumbered males by 10:1. The difference may be attributed to different circumcision practices in Europe and the United States and the higher incidence of UTI associated with the uncircumcised penis (34,35). In one retrospective review, only 14% of 545 patients with reflux were male (36); in another, 15% of 281 patients with reflux were male (37).

INHERITANCE AND SIBLING REFLUX

There has been increasing recognition of the familial occurrence of VUR. The mode of inheritance is poorly understood; it has been suggested that it is inherited in an autosomal-dominant manner, making it one of the most common inherited disorders (38). In several reviews, the relationship in siblings has been clearly identified. VUR has been identified consistently in 27 to 33% of siblings of index patients with VUR (39–41). The reflux in siblings was not associated with a history of UTI or with the severity of reflux, age, or incidence of renal scarring in the index case. An even higher incidence has been reported in children of parents who had reflux (42). Resolution of sibling VUR has been reported in up to 53% after a mean follow-up of 18.5 months (43). However, in one study, 27% of affected siblings were older than 10 years at the time of diagnosis (41). The inheritance of reflux is further supported by its significantly reduced incidence in African Americans.

DIAGNOSIS

VUR generally is detected during radiographic evaluation of children with UTI. Prompt evaluation of UTIs in children is predicated on the high prevalence of VUR in children with UTIs: Approximately one-third of white girls with UTI have reflux (27). Clinical features have proven unreliable in distinguishing children with UTI who have reflux from those who do not (31,44).

When should a child with UTI be evaluated radiographically? The signs and symptoms that typically accompany UTIs in infants and toddlers are not specific, making it difficult to determine whether an infection represents the first episode in those at greatest risk for renal damage (Table 54.1). Renal scarring may occur after a single episode of kidney infection (45–47). Up to 80% of all white girls and 60% of all African American girls experience reinfection within 18 months of their initial UTI (48,49). The incidence of renal scarring is higher in children with recurrent UTIs than in those with a single infection (31,50,51).

TABLE 54.1. PROMINENT SYMPTOMS IN NEONATAL NONOBSTRUCTIVE URINARY TRACT INFECTION

Symptom	Percentage
Weight loss[a]	76
Fever	49
Cyanosis or gray color	40
Distended abdomen	16
Central nervous system symptoms (purulent meningitis not included)	23
Generalized convulsions	7
Purulent meningitis	8
Jaundice (conjugated bilirubin increased)	7
Other	16

Note: N = 75, 0 to 30 days old.
[a]Registered for only 46 patients falling ill on days 0 to 10. Weight loss was not explained by vomiting, diarrhea, or refusal to eat.
Modified from Bergström T, Larson H, Lincoln K, et al: Studies of urinary tract infections in infancy and childhood. XII: Eighty consecutive patients with neonatal infection. *J Pediatr* 1972;80:858.

Taken together, all of the aforementioned factors warrant early evaluation of young children after their first documented UTI. Waiting until the child has two or more infections before proceeding with evaluation clearly increases the risk for permanent scarring. Most authorities agree that evaluation should be carried out after the first culture-documented UTI in children younger than 3 years; many suggest that this policy should be followed up to age 5 years. Any child with a febrile UTI and boys of any age should be evaluated (44). Because of the low incidence of VUR, evaluation of African American girls with UTIs might be reserved for infants and those with febrile UTIs or recurrences.

VUR is also detected when screening siblings for reflux and when infants who had hydronephrosis on prenatal ultrasonography are evaluated postnatally. In fact, recent studies suggest that VUR is one of the most common causes of prenatally detected hydronephrosis, occurring in up to one-third of patients evaluated postnatally (52–54). Patients with prenatal hydronephrosis should be evaluated with a cystogram even if the postnatal sonogram is negative, because as many as 25% of patients with grade III to V VUR have normal postnatal sonograms (55). VUR is also found more commonly in children with functional or structural anomalies such as neuropathic bladders, severe voiding dysfunction, prune-belly syndrome, multicystic kidneys, imperforate anus, unilateral renal agenesis, ureteropelvic junction obstruction, and other obstructive uropathies. Therefore, cystographic evaluation is recommended in the evaluation of patients with any of these findings.

Cystography

Both direct and indirect cystography techniques are used. Direct cystography involves filling the bladder by urethral

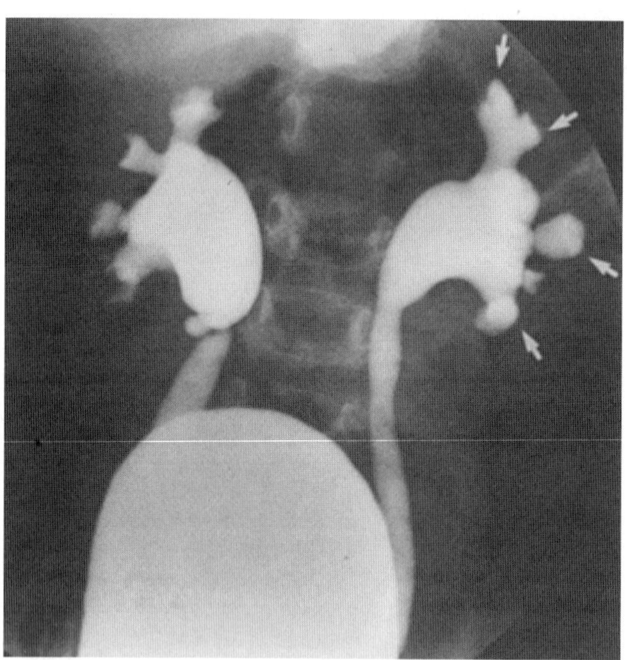

FIGURE 54.3. Contrast cystogram demonstrates bilateral vesicoureteral reflux, grade III (*right*) and grade IV (*left*). Ureteral and pelvic dilation are similar on both sides, but the sharp forniceal angles in the left kidney have been lost (*arrows*).

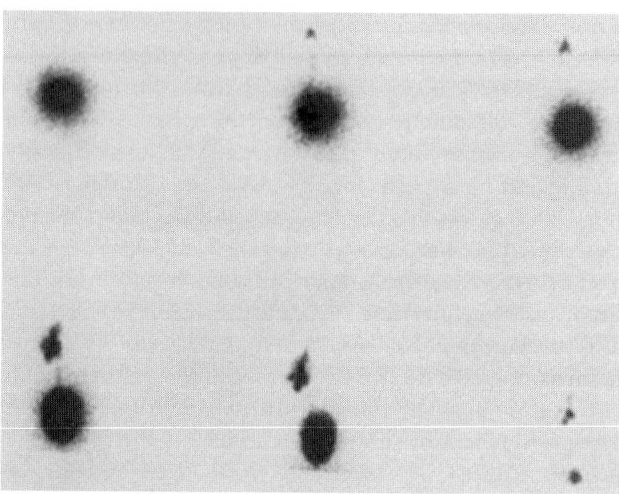

FIGURE 54.4. Sequential posterior images from a direct radionuclide cystogram demonstrate left vesicoureteral reflux during the filling, voiding, and postvoiding phases of the study. Reflux in the filling phases **(upper panel)** is mild but becomes moderate immediately before and during voiding **(lower panel)**.

catheterization or percutaneous suprapubic infusion. Both standard contrast medium and radiolabeled nuclides are satisfactory. In boys, contrast cystography is preferred because it allows the clinician to visualize the urethra and grade reflux (Fig. 54.3). It is also more reliable for detecting duplication, ureteral ectopia with or without ureteroceles, posterior urethral valves, bladder trabeculation, bladder diverticula, and foreign bodies. Many also prefer its use for the initial examination in girls because the grade of reflux can be determined. Several methods for grading are used (37); the IRS method is most widely accepted (Fig. 54.2) (5).

The reliability of contrast voiding cystography for demonstrating VUR is affected by a number of variables related to technique or patient. These include the size and type (straight vs. Foley) of catheter, rate of bladder filling, height of the column of contrast media, state of hydration, whether reflux is transient, and the volume, temperature, and concentration of the contrast medium (56). Jequier evaluated the reliability of contrast cystography for detection of VUR in children undergoing evaluation for first-time UTIs by using multiple fillings of the bladder (57). In patients with no reflux on the initial filling, VUR was demonstrated on repeat filling of the bladder in only 4%. Greater variation was observed in the grade of VUR detected when multiple fillings were used. A disadvantage of standard contrast cystography is the high gonadal radiation dosage it entails, particularly with multiple studies or fluoroscopic monitoring. The recent addition of digital fluoroscopy reduces gonadal radiation exposure (58). When a low-dose fluoroscopic system is combined with a computer-based video frame grabber, the ovarian radiation dosage compares favorably to radionuclide cystography (59,60).

Direct radionuclide cystography allows continuous monitoring for reflux throughout the study without additional radiation exposure. It is reported to be more sensitive than contrast cystography for the diagnosis of reflux (61,62). In a recent study, contrast cystography had a sensitivity of only 65% compared with radionuclide studies and did not detect any additional VUR not seen by nuclear cystography (63). Whereas precise grading of VUR is limited, it usually can be categorized as mild, moderate, or severe (Fig. 54.4). Although radionuclide cystography has been criticized for being unable to detect grade I VUR, a recent study found that direct radionuclide cystography demonstrated VUR to the renal pelvis in all 17 kidneys studied with grade I VUR on contrast cystography (64). The radiation dosage from radionuclide cystography is 50 to 200 times less than that with standard techniques using contrast cystography, making it ideal for the follow-up of children with VUR and for following results of antireflux surgery (65). It also helps confirm the absence of transient VUR when clinically suspected reflux has not been demonstrated by contrast voiding cystography (66). There is little justification for carrying out cystography with the child under anesthesia. The risk and cost of anesthesia cannot be justified, and the information derived from the static cystogram is vastly inferior to that obtained from the dynamic voiding study (67).

Indirect radionuclide cystography uses technetium-99m (^{99m}Tc)–diaminotetraethylpentacetic acid, which is excreted by glomerular filtration. Most of the radioisotope is in the bladder within 20 minutes. The presence of reflux can be assumed when radioisotope counts increase in the renal areas after voiding. Indirect cystography is less reliable for the detection of VUR than direct radionuclide cystography (68). Furthermore, significant patient cooperation in allowing adequate bladder filling and being able to void on command is required with indirect cystography (69). More recently, indirect radionuclide cystography using ^{99m}Tc-mercaptoacetyltriglycine (MAG-3) was reported to be unreliable for the detection of VUR, missing approximately two-thirds of reflux (70).

The interval between the UTI and lower tract evaluation has been controversial. A waiting period of 4 to 6 weeks after an acute infection has been suggested before the cystogram is obtained to avoid demonstrating transient, mild reflux secondary to inflammatory changes of the ureterovesical junction. However, reflux detected at the time of infection, which then immediately disappears after treatment, is rare (71). Furthermore, because the significance of VUR is greatest at the time of bacterial infection, demonstration of even transient reflux at that time may be meaningful. Of course, the urine should be sterile at the time of the study. One potential disadvantage of obtaining a cystogram early in the course of a febrile infection is that ureteral dilation resulting from the smooth-muscle paralyzing effects of *Escherichia coli* endotoxins may result in overestimation of the reflux grade (72–74). Nevertheless, waiting several weeks to obtain a cystogram is not required. Regardless of timing, antibiotic prophylaxis should be maintained in all patients until evaluation is completed (74).

Upper Tract Imaging

Recommendations for evaluation of the upper urinary tract in children with infection vary. The ideal study should be painless, safe, cost-effective, and associated with minimal or no radiation and yet be capable of detecting clinically significant structural malformations and renal scarring. Unfortunately, no such all-encompassing study exists. A tailored approach to the evaluation of children with UTI, beginning with a cystogram, is recommended (Fig. 54.5) (75–77). At the time of the cystogram, a renal ultrasound is obtained to exclude hydronephrosis or other major upper tract malformations. If both studies are normal, further imaging is usually not pursued. Certainly, cystoscopy is *not* indicated. However, if reflux is demonstrated, a renal cortical scan using ^{99m}Tc-DMSA (dimercaptosuccinic acid) is recommended to detect renal scarring. If renal scanning is unavailable, intravenous pyelography (IVP) is acceptable.

The unreliability of routine clinical and laboratory findings for confirming the diagnosis of pyelonephritis suggests the necessity for renal isotope scanning in some children with febrile UTIs (78,79). Both experimental studies in the pig and clinical studies have proven that cortical scintigraphy is highly reliable and useful for the detection of both acute and chronic inflammatory changes of pyelonephritis (79–81). DMSA scintigraphy should be the primary upper tract imaging modality in neonates and infants with febrile UTIs.

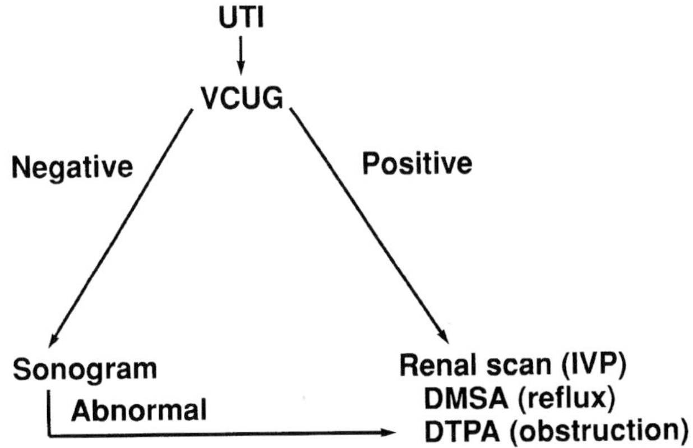

FIGURE 54.5. Algorithm for evaluation of children with urinary tract infection (UTI). DMSA, dimercaptosuccinic acid (renal scan); DTPA, diethylenetriamine–pentaacetic acid (renal scan); IVP, intravenous pyelogram; VCUG, voiding cystourethrogram. (From Rushton HG. Genitourinary infections: nonspecific infections. In: Kelalis PP, King LR, Belman AB, eds. *Clinical pediatric urology,* 3rd ed. Philadelphia: WB Saunders, 1992, with permission.)

Paradoxically, recent clinical studies reveal that most children (60 to 68%) with DMSA scan–documented acute pyelonephritis do not have VUR (78,79). Therefore, infants with febrile UTIs should be considered for evaluation by DMSA scintigraphy regardless of the presence or absence of VUR (78,79,82). Sonography is also indicated in the acutely ill child to exclude upper tract obstruction, particularly in those who do not respond to appropriate treatment.

PYELONEPHRITIS AND RENAL SCARRING

Renal scarring refers to the spectrum of radiographic abnormalities in the kidney, often called chronic atrophic pyelonephritis, which is associated with focal or diffuse areas of irreversible parenchymal damage. The term *chronic pyelonephritis* is actually a misnomer because renal scarring generally is not associated with indolent infection of the kidney. In 1973, Bailey recommended that the term *chronic atrophic pyelonephritis* be replaced by *reflux nephropathy* (83). The acceptance of this term underscores the consensus that VUR is the primary prerequisite for renal scarring in the absence of obstruction. The critical role that infection coupled with VUR plays in renal scarring was initially demonstrated in piglets with surgically induced VUR (84). Recent clinical studies report that renal scarring may also occur after pyelonephritis in the absence of demonstrable reflux (47,79,85). In one study, 62% of kidneys with new postpyelonephritic scarring were drained by nonrefluxing ureters (85). However, renal scarring was still significantly more common in kidneys with grade III or higher VUR than in kidneys with no or mild VUR. In other studies, VUR was present in only 20 to 50% of kidneys that developed new renal scarring after DMSA scan–documented acute pyelonephritis (79).

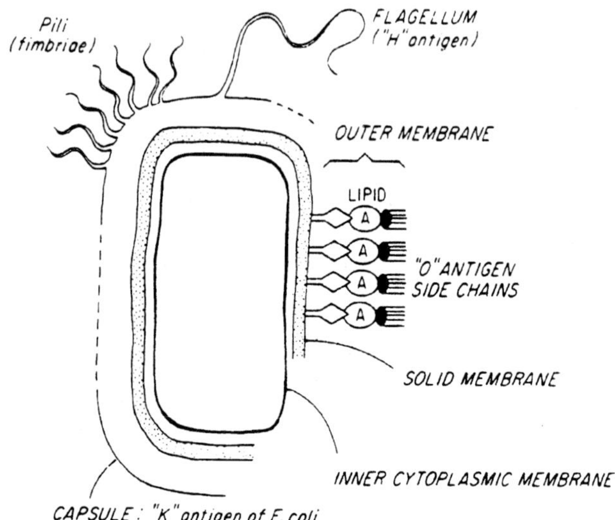

FIGURE 54.6. Schematic presentation of the antigenic structure of gram-negative enteric bacteria. (Modified from Young LS, Martin WJ, Meyer RD, et al. Gram-negative rod bacteremia: microbiologic, immunologic, and therapeutic considerations. *Ann Intern Med* 1977;86:456.)

These and other reports emphasize the role of bacterial virulence and host defense factors in acute pyelonephritis (86). The most prominent of these bacterial virulence factors is adherence of bacteria to specific urothelial receptors, mediated by the attachment of P-fimbriae located on the bacterial surface (Fig. 54.6) (87). Attachment to urothelial cells allows bacteria to ascend into the upper urinary tract, even in the absence of VUR. Supporting this conclusion, a disproportionately high percentage of P-fimbriated *E. coli* strains are isolated from patients with clinical acute pyelonephritis, compared with isolates from patients with cystitis or asymptomatic bacteriuria (Table 54.2) (88,89). *However, when present, VUR remains the most significant host risk factor for acute pyelonephritis and renal scarring.* When VUR is present, 80 to 90% of patients with febrile UTIs have abnormal DMSA renal scan findings (79). This is particularly true for kidneys with grade III to V VUR, which are at least twice as likely to have DMSA scan defects as are kidneys with no VUR or grade I or II VUR (90,91). When

TABLE 54.2. RELATIONSHIP OF P-FIMBRIATED *ESCHERICHIA COLI* AND TYPE OF URINARY TRACT INFECTION IN CHILDREN

Type	N[a]	% *E. coli* strains with P-fimbriae
Pyelonephritis	102	76–94
Cystitis	86	19–23
Asymptomatic bacteriuria	96	14–18
Fecal flora[b]	132	7–16

[a]Combined results from (88) and (89).
[b]Healthy controls.

VUR is present, attachment properties such as P-fimbriae are less important in causing acute pyelonephritis (92). Furthermore, the significance of P-fimbriae in the development of postpyelonephritic renal scarring has been questioned (93).

Diagnosis

Renal Scarring

In the past, renal scars have been detected primarily by IVP, which shows the affected area as focal thinning of the renal parenchyma with a corresponding calyceal deformity or clubbing. For reasons discussed later, renal scars are more often found in the upper and lower poles of the kidney. Scarring varies in severity. It can be limited to a single papilla in the pole of the kidney or it may be extensive, resulting in a small, shrunken, end-stage kidney with little or no function. For an IVP to detect renal scarring reliably, high-quality delineation of the renal outlines and calyceal systems is mandatory. This is difficult to achieve in young children (the group at greatest risk for renal scarring) with overlying bowel gas, stool, and poor renal concentrating ability and in children with bony abnormalities such as spina bifida (12). Tomography may increase the accuracy but also increases radiation exposure. Other limitations of IVP include the risk of contrast-induced reactions, fluid and electrolyte disturbances (particularly in infants), and an inability to detect acute pyelonephritis (94). Pyelographic evidence of renal scarring may not be evident for up to 2 years after the acute episode (95).

In many centers, ^{99m}Tc-DMSA renal scintigraphy has replaced IVP for the detection and assessment of renal scars. DMSA localizes in the proximal tubular cells; excretion is minimal. It is the preferred method for visualizing functioning renal parenchyma (96,97). DMSA can also provide quantitative assessment of differential renal function. Additional advantages over IVP include reduced gonadal radiation exposure and avoidance of contrast-induced reactions. Visualization is not hampered by overlying bowel gas, stool, or bony abnormalities or by renal position.

Renal scars detected by DMSA scintigraphy appear as focal or generalized areas of diminished uptake in the renal cortex. This may appear as thinning or flattening of the cortex in some kidneys; in others, renal scars appear as discrete wedge-shaped parenchymal defects (Fig. 54.7) (98). In more severe cases, generalized damage may be associated with multifocal or diffusely scarred kidneys and reduced differential renal function. A grading system for the severity of renal scarring as depicted by DMSA renal scans has been suggested (Table 54.3) (99).

DMSA scan is more sensitive than IVP for detecting renal scarring. Merrick et al. compared the findings in 79 children who had proven UTI and had been followed for 1 to 4 years (100). The sensitivity of IVP for the detection of renal scars was 80%, and specificity was 92%, whereas cortical scintigraphy had a sensitivity of 92% and specificity of 98%. Greater

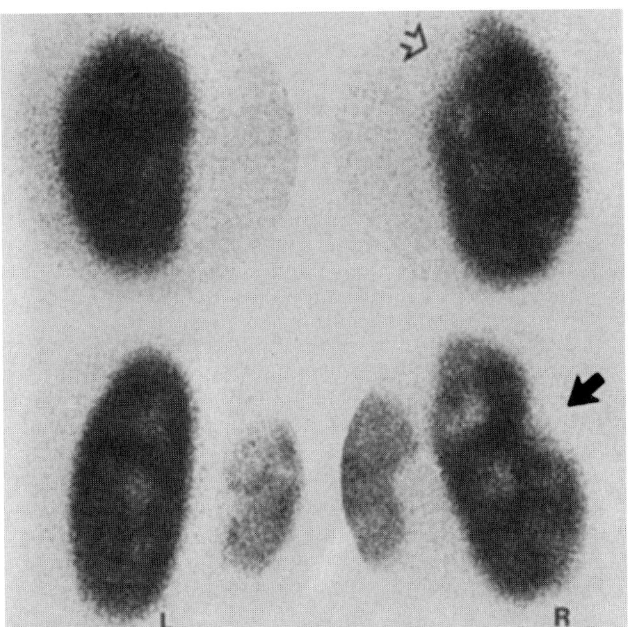

FIGURE 54.7. Posterior **(upper)** and posterior oblique **(lower)** views of a technetium-99m–dimercaptosuccinic acid renal scan in a 3.5-year-old girl with right grade III vesicoureteral reflux. Posterior view of right kidney reveals scarring in the upper pole evidenced by thinning of the cortex (*open arrow*). Posterior oblique view demonstrates a classic wedge-shaped scar in the midzone of the right kidney (*closed arrow*). Left kidney is normal.

sensitivity of the DMSA scan for the detection of renal scarring has been reported by others (99,101,102). When both IVP and DMSA scintigraphy demonstrate scars, an excellent correlation on a site-by-site basis has been reported (99–102). Nevertheless, some investigators citing examples in which each modality failed to detect renal scars demonstrated by the other suggest that both IVP and DMSA renal scintigraphy are necessary in the evaluation of renal scarring (103,104). That recommendation is not widely supported.

Pyelonephritis

Another major advantage of DMSA scintigraphy in the evaluation of children with reflux is its ability to detect acute pyelonephritic changes in the renal parenchyma (78–82). As opposed to the characteristic defects of renal scarring that are associated with loss or contraction of functioning cortex, the defects on DMSA scintigraphy caused by acute pyelonephritis are typically focal or diffuse areas of diminished uptake that are associated with preservation (or at times even bulging) of the renal cortical outline (78). Differentiating defects caused by acute pyelonephritis from those caused by renal scarring is difficult when acute pyelonephritis is superimposed over an area of cortical scarring. In 1995 and 1996, some authors advocated the application of single-photon emission computed tomography to DMSA scintigraphy, reporting greater sensitivity when compared to traditional planar imaging (105,106). However, in these clinical studies, histologic confirmation of acute pyelonephritis was not possible. In an experimental study in pigs with surgically induced VUR of infected urine, these two techniques were directly compared with histology (107). The sensitivity of single-photon emission computed tomography was higher than planar imaging (96 vs. 87%), but the specificity was lower (71 vs. 100%). Overall, agreement was 90% for both when compared with histology.

DMSA changes associated with acute pyelonephritis usually resolve after antibiotic treatment (Fig. 54.8) (79). Acute lesions may resolve as early as 2 weeks after treatment of acute pyelonephritis (108). However, they may persist for up to 4 months. Acute defects result in scarring in 36 to 52% of kidneys (Fig. 54.9) (47,79,85). The pathophysiologic mech-

TABLE 54.3. GRADING SYSTEM FOR RENAL SCARRING DETECTED BY DIMERCAPTOSUCCINIC ACID (DMSA) RENAL SCINTIGRAPHY

Type 1: No more than two scarred areas
Type 2: More than two scars with some areas of normal parenchyma between them
Type 3: Generalized damage to the whole kidney similar to obstructive nephropathy (i.e., contraction of the whole kidney without or with very few scars in the outline)
Type 4: End-stage "shrunken" (kidney with little or no uptake of DMSA; i.e., <10% of the overall function)

From Goldraich NP, Rames OL, Goldraich IH. Urography versus DMSA scan in children with vesicoureteral reflux. *Pediatr Nephrol* 1989;3:1.

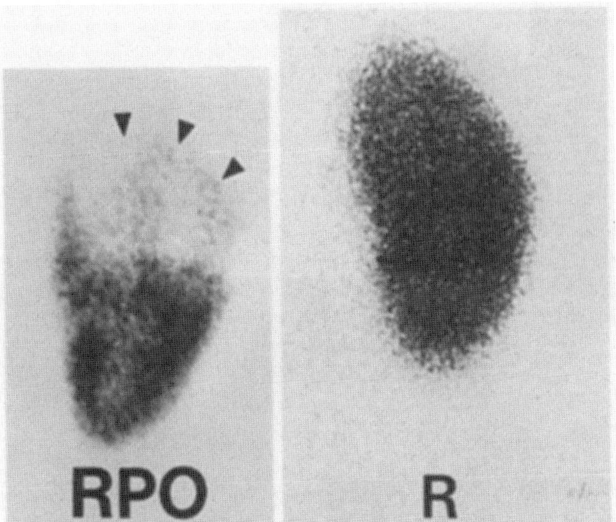

FIGURE 54.8. Technetium-99m–dimercaptosuccinic acid (DMSA) renal scan obtained during the evaluation of a 6-month-old uncircumcised boy with suspected acute pyelonephritis. Posterior oblique (RPO) image reveals severe acute inflammatory changes of the entire upper moiety of the right kidney. Follow-up DMSA renal scan 18 months later reveals complete resolution of inflammatory changes without residual scarring (posterior view). (From Rushton HG. Genitourinary infections: nonspecific infections. In: Kelalis PP, King LR, Belman AB, eds. *Clinical pediatric urology*, 3rd ed. Philadelphia: WB Saunders, 1992, with permission.)

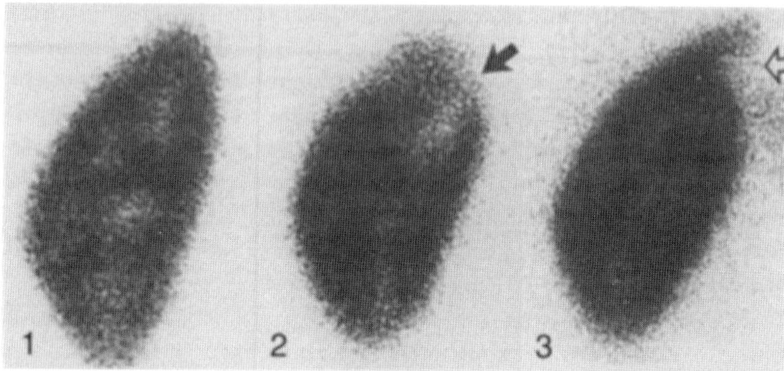

FIGURE 54.9. Serial technetium-99m–dimercaptosuccinic acid (DMSA) renal scans in a 3-year-old girl with previous febrile urinary tract infections associated with right vesicoureteral reflux and severe scarring of the right kidney. **1:** Previously normal left kidney. **2:** Acute pyelonephritis in the left upper pole (*closed arrow*) after successful right ureteral reimplantation. Repeat cystogram confirmed the *absence* of reflux on either side. **3:** Follow-up DMSA renal scan 15 months later shows progression to renal scarring (*open arrow*).

anisms that account for the DMSA changes caused by acute infection include changes in intrarenal blood flow and proximal tubular cell membrane transport function (109,110). Both of these result in diminished uptake.

Pathogenesis of Renal Scarring

Renal scarring is a term that applies to both congenital or embryologic and acquired or postnatal renal abnormalities (111). Most cases of scarring associated with reflux are detected during evaluation of children with UTI. However, recent reports of infants with prenatally detected hydronephrosis associated with reflux have confirmed cases of congenital renal functional abnormalities documented by DMSA scan even in the absence of known infection (112–115). There is also a high prevalence of renal functional abnormalities and scarring in children with reflux secondary to functional or anatomic bladder outlet obstruction. Lumping the renal sequelae from all of these pathophysiologic entities under the terms *renal scarring* or *reflux nephropathy* has hampered attempts at understanding the pathogenic mechanisms involved.

Renal pathology associated with reflux has been explained in several ways: an embryonic ectopic ureteral bud inducing abnormal renal development with subsequent dysplasia or a primary developmental arrest inducing dysplasia; renal damage resulting from sterile reflux and its water-hammer effects, perhaps mediated by an immunologic response; or IRR of infected urine into susceptible renal papilla, resulting in an inflammatory response and damage to the renal parenchyma.

Embryologic Dysplasia

Mackie and Stephens propose that renal dysplasia or hypoplasia is related to abnormal development of the embryonic ureteral bud (116). They propose that a ureteral bud that arises abnormally from the most caudal end of the wolffian duct is associated with an ectopic orifice located laterally on the trigone. As a consequence, a short or absent intramural tunnel results in a refluxing ureter. Meanwhile, the abnormally arising ureteral bud fails to penetrate the normal, central renal blastema, resulting in a hypoplastic or dysplastic kidney (Fig. 54.10). This theory, initially proposed to explain abnormalities in duplicated kidneys, was later extended to include single-system kidneys associated with reflux (117). Although this theory may explain renal pathology in selected cases of severe reflux or duplication anomalies with ectopic ureters, most kidneys associated with primary VUR do not exhibit histologic evidence of dysplasia (118).

Developmental theories may explain some of the functional abnormalities found in kidneys in which high-grade primary VUR was detected initially by the finding of hydronephrosis on prenatal sonography (112–115). Many of these infants with reflux detected by prenatal sonography were evaluated by renal scintigraphy before any known episodes of infection. Renal functional abnormalities in those kidneys suggest a congenital fetal nephropathy rather than an acquired abnormality. One study compared renal parenchymal damage demonstrated by DMSA renal scans in 17 infants with VUR detected after UTI, with 19 detected by prenatal sonography who were maintained on prophylaxis to prevent infection (119). A higher percentage of the chil-

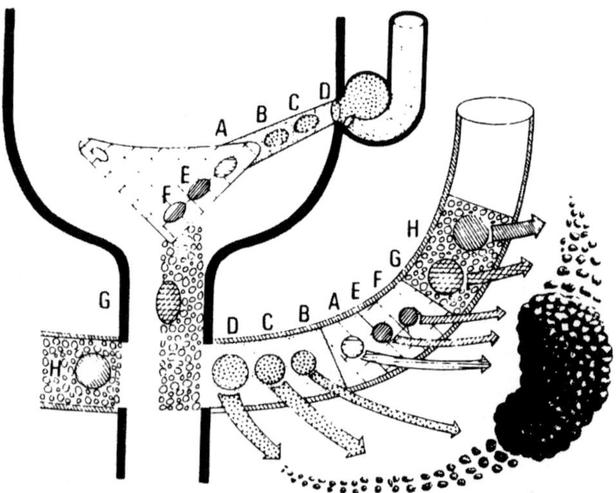

FIGURE 54.10. Relationship of ureteral bud positions on wolffian duct to nephrogenic blastema and orifice zones in bladder and urethra. (From Mackie GG, Stephens FD. Duplex kidneys: a correlation of renal dysplasia with position of the ureteral orifice. *J Urol* 1975;114:274, with permission.)

dren studied post-UTI had renal damage than did those who were detected prenatally and placed on prophylaxis before any UTI. Similarly, Crabbe et al. categorized typical patterns of DMSA abnormalities in a group of patients with prenatally uninfected primary VUR (15 children, 24 kidneys) compared with a group of patients with infected primary VUR (8 children, 15 kidneys) (115). In the uninfected group 4 of 24 kidneys (17%) were abnormal and these demonstrated global loss (i.e., small kidneys without focal scars). In contrast, 4 of 15 kidneys (27%) in the infected group were abnormal, and these all demonstrated evidence of focal renal scarring. A third group of patients with noninfected VUR associated with obstruction, including seven patients (nine kidneys) with posterior urethral valves and two with ureteropelvic junction obstruction, demonstrated total or near total loss of function in 9 of 11 kidneys (82%).

One must be cautious in extrapolating findings in these studies to the general population of children with reflux. Infants with reflux detected prenatally represent a select group of patients characterized by male predominance and a high incidence of severe reflux. Urodynamic evaluation has demonstrated hypercontractility with markedly elevated voiding pressures in most of these boys, which resolved within 1 to 2 years (120–122). Coincident with this, a higher than expected percentage of VUR resolved in this select group of patients. In contrast, children with reflux detected postnatally are predominantly female, and most have less severe reflux and a history of UTI. However, it is clear that not all reflux-associated renal abnormalities are acquired postnatally.

Sterile versus Infected Reflux

The theory that sterile reflux might produce renal scarring was proposed by Hodson et al., based on their experimental piglet model, in which reflux was produced by unroofing the intramural ureter (123). However, to potentiate reflux, obstruction of the bladder outlet was also created by placing a constricting ring around the urethra. Renal scarring was produced from reflux of sterile urine, with the most intense areas of scarring corresponding to areas shown by cystography to have IRR (pyelotubular backflow or urine from the renal pelvis into the collecting ducts). Previous clinical observations had also suggested a relationship between renal scarring and IRR in young children with moderate and severe VUR (124).

Evidence arguing against a role for sterile reflux in the pathogenesis of renal scarring comes from the studies of Ransley and Risdon, again using the multipapillary piglet model (84). As in Hodson and colleagues' model, VUR of urine was induced by unroofing the intramural ureter. However, bladder outlet obstruction was not created. In contrast to the findings of Hodson et al. (123), Ransley and Risdon did not find scarring in their animals with reflux of sterile urine. Instead, they found that when voiding pressure is normal, as in primary reflux, scarring occurred only when urinary infection was present in association with VUR and IRR.

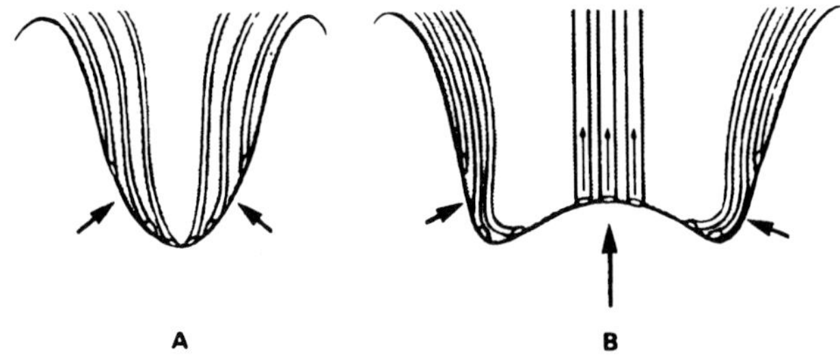

FIGURE 54.11. Papillary configuration in intrarenal reflux. **A:** Convex papilla (nonrefluxing papilla): crescentic or slit-like openings of collecting ducts opening obliquely onto the papilla. **B:** Concave or flat papilla (refluxing papilla): round collection ducts opening at right angles onto flat papilla. (From Ransley PG. Intrarenal reflux: anatomical, dynamic, and radiological studies. *Urol Res* 1977;5:61, with permission.)

IRR in the multipapillary kidneys of piglets occurs only in renal papillae that have specific morphologic features. With piglets, as with children, Ransley and Risdon discovered two basic types of renal papillae (Fig. 54.11) (125,126). Some are simple, conical structures with a convex calyceal surface onto which the papillary ducts open obliquely with slit-like orifices. These papillae do not allow IRR to occur. In contrast, papillae that fuse into larger papillae with flat or concave tips and have papillary ducts opening onto the calyx with gaping orifices do allow IRR to occur. These fused or compound papillae are most commonly found in the polar regions of the kidney, where scarring is noted most often. Postmortem studies performed on children dying from other causes revealed that approximately two-thirds of all human kidneys contain at least one potentially refluxing papilla (126). In one-fifth of all human kidneys, 30% of the papillae are potentially refluxing. Transformation of marginally competent nonrefluxing to incompetent refluxing papillae may result from reflux of infected urine or from scarring in adjacent papillae (80,84). This exposes a greater proportion of the kidney to IRR, increasing the risk for pyelonephritis and progressive renal scarring if UTI recurs. In contrast, kidneys that are populated entirely by nonrefluxing papillae may be protected from renal scarring, even if UTI and VUR are present.

In subsequent studies in pigs with varying degrees of bladder outlet obstruction, Ransley et al. demonstrated that renal scarring in the absence of infection could be produced only by *sustained* high intravesical pressure (127). These changes were associated with detrusor decompensation, defined by elevated resting pressures between voids and ineffective bladder emptying associated with large postvoid residuals. The clinical correlates to this type of sustained high-pressure reflux are few, primarily some boys with posterior urethral valves and some children with noncompliant neuropathic bladders and severe nonneuropathic voiding

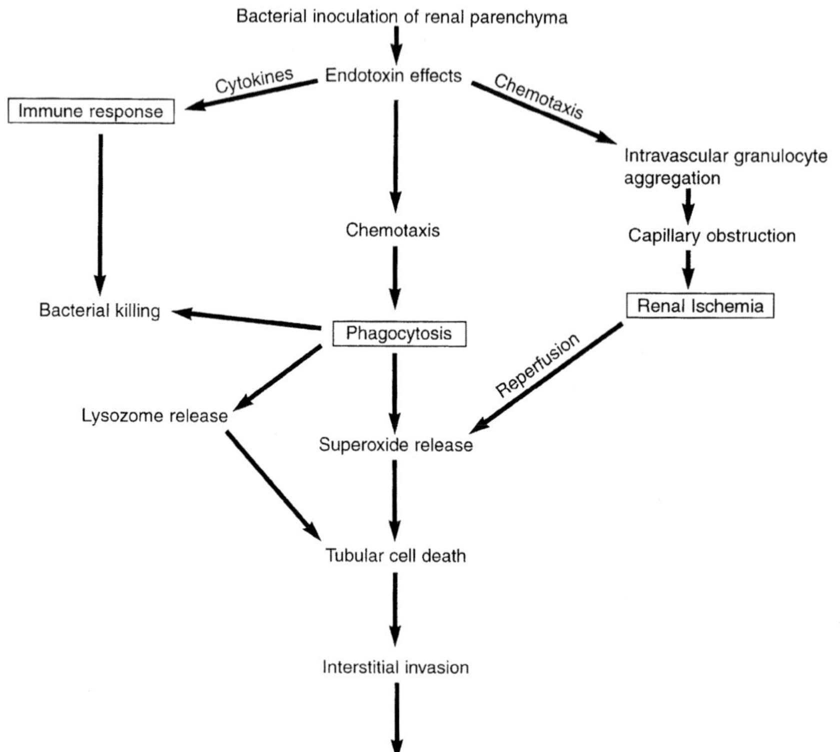

FIGURE 54.12. Hypothesis for the pathogenetic chain of events in acute pyelonephritis. [Modified from Roberts JA. Mechanisms of renal damage in chronic pyelonephritis (reflux nephropathy). *Curr Top Pathol* 1995;88:265–287.]

dyssynergia (Hinman's syndrome). In contrast, intermittent high voiding pressure in the absence of infection was not sufficient to produce scarring. Therefore, one can conclude that the water-hammer effect of VUR is not a contributor to renal damage in the absence of bladder outlet obstruction.

Role of Infection

Experimental studies by Roberts and others suggest that the acute inflammatory response that is responsible for the eradication of bacteria is also responsible for the early pyelonephritic damage to renal tissue and subsequent renal scarring (128). Using the primate model, Roberts developed a unified theory of the events that ultimately lead to renal scarring (Fig. 54.12). The initiating event is bacterial inoculation of the renal parenchyma, which elicits both immune and inflammatory responses. Whereas the immune response can be elicited by either live or heat-killed bacteria, the acute inflammatory response occurs only after inoculation with live bacteria (129). Because inoculation with heat-killed bacteria does not cause renal scarring, it appears that the acute inflammatory response is critical to the development of permanent renal damage.

The inflammatory response of pyelonephritis is triggered by complement activation from bacterial lipopolysaccharides (endotoxin). This leads to chemotactic migration of granulocytes to the site of infection. Experimentally, either complement depletion (induced by cobra venom) or granulocyte depletion (induced by nitrogen mustard) decreases the acute inflammatory response of pyelonephritis; this reduces renal tissue damage (130,131). Chemotaxis of granulocytes to the site of infection is followed by phagocytosis of bacteria, initiating the sequence of events that leads to renal injury. Granulocytes kill bacteria, releasing toxic enzymes (lysozymes) both within the granulocyte and into the lumen of renal tubules, which causes renal cell damage. The respiratory burst releasing superoxides occurs. This phenomenon, universal to acute inflammatory responses, generates oxygen radicals that are toxic not only to bacteria but also to the granulocytes and surrounding renal tubular cells (132). Tubular cell death releases the toxic inflammatory agents into the interstitium, causing further damage. Superoxides are also produced by cell reaction during reperfusion of ischemic tissue. Focal parenchymal ischemia, resulting from intravascular granulocyte aggregation and edema, occurs with bacterial infection of the renal parenchyma (90,133,134). In ischemic tissue, hypoxanthine is produced during anaerobic metabolism of adenosine monophosphate. During reperfusion, hypoxanthine in the presence of xanthine oxidase and oxygen yields superoxides and hydrogen peroxide (135). Treatment with allopurinol, an inhibitor of xanthine oxidase, protects against tissue damage from reperfusion injury and from that associated with bacteria in the renal parenchyma (136). It appears that the interstitial damage associated with the acute inflammatory response of pyelonephritis results from ischemia-related injury and from toxic enzymes. This leads to renal scarring.

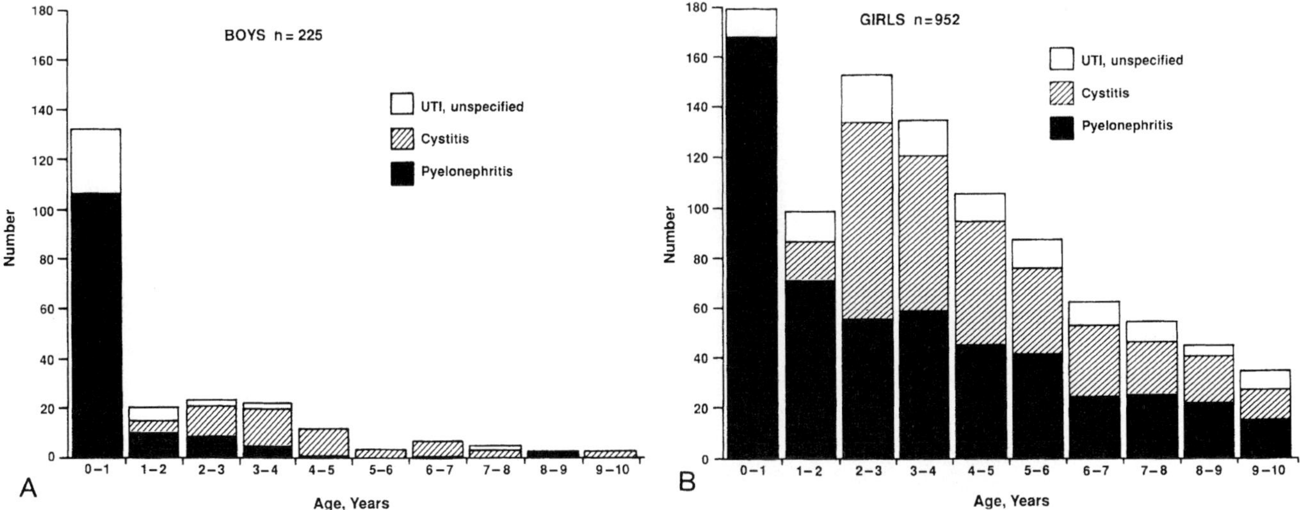

FIGURE 54.13. Children with first-time diagnosis of urinary tract infections (UTI) at the Children's Hospital in Göteborg, Sweden, from 1970 to 1979, according to age and clinical diagnosis. [From Jodal U. Host risk factors in pyelonephritis. In: Rushton HG, guest ed. Pyelonephritis: pathogenesis and management update. Ehrlich RM, ed. *Dialogues in pediatric urology*. Pearl River, NY: William J Miller, 1990;13(2):4–5, with permission.]

Clinical Studies

Most clinical knowledge about renal scarring comes from studies of patients with VUR. Clinical studies confirm the close association between UTI, VUR, and renal scarring (137–142). Older studies reported that 30 to 60% of children with VUR and a history of symptomatic UTIs have renal scarring at the time of their initial studies. More recent investigations suggest that the incidence of scarring may not be so high, perhaps reflecting the current trend toward earlier diagnosis and management (36). The onset of renal scarring is thought to occur early in life, usually before age 5 years and most often before 3 years of age (143,144). Although less common, new renal scarring may be acquired in older children (46).

The increased risk of renal scarring in infant kidneys is probably multifactorial. First, clinical pyelonephritis complicates UTIs much more commonly in infants (both boys and girls) younger than 1 year than in older children (Fig. 54.13) (51). In fact, approximately one-half of all febrile UTIs in childhood occur in infants 1 year old or younger (79). This may be in part the consequence of a higher incidence of IRR (145). Another contributing factor in infants is an incompletely developed immune system, which allows bacteria access to the urinary tract and reduces bactericidal activity. Finally, the diagnosis of UTIs is often delayed in infants, who typically have nonspecific signs and symptoms (143). All these factors increase the risk of damage and scarring.

New or progressive scarring is almost always associated with a prior UTI, most often clinical pyelonephritis (46,140–143,146). The correlation between the severity of VUR and renal scarring is well established (27,36,51,142,146–148) (Table 54.4). However, both new and preexisting renal scarring have been reported in some children who have had symptomatic urinary infection even without VUR (47,85,143, 150). A clear association between the number of pyelonephritic attacks and the incidence of renal scarring has been reported (Fig. 54.14) (46,145). Furthermore, both clinical and experimental studies have documented acute pyelonephritic damage, often associated with the presence of P-fimbriated *E. coli*, in the absence of demonstrable reflux (68,75,146). Renal scarring may be prevented or diminished in some instances by early antibiotic treatment of acute pyelonephritis (Fig. 54.8) (78,79,82,91,149). When reflux is present, new renal scarring is prevented by keeping the patient free of infection using low-dose antibiotic prophylaxis (36,148,151). This contrasts with the 10 to 20% incidence of new scarring and 62 to 66% incidence of progressive scarring reported in earlier studies in which recurrent UTIs in children were treated only with intermittent antibiotic therapy (140,152).

TABLE 54.4. RENAL SCARRING COMPARED WITH GRADE OF REFLUX

Grade of reflux	Percentage with scarring[a]
1	5
2	6
3	17
4	25
5	50

[a]Total number of kidneys evaluated, 804; total number of kidneys with scarring, 97 (12%).
Modified from Skoog SJ, Belman AB, Majd M. A nonsurgical approach to the management of primary vesicoureteral reflux. *J Urol* 1987;138:441.

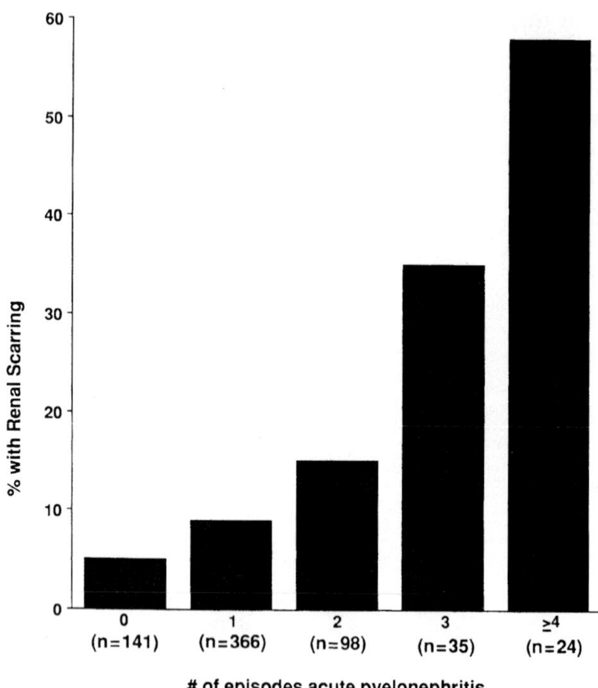

FIGURE 54.14. Relationship of renal scarring to number of episodes of acute pyelonephritis. (Modified from Jodal U. The natural history of bacteriuria in childhood. *Infect Dis Clin North Am* 1987;1:713.)

Martinell et al. prospectively studied 87 females with either renal scarring (45) or recurrent UTI (42) followed for a mean of 23 years after their first UTI in childhood (153). The attack rate (number of UTIs per patient per observation year) was highest in the first year of life (1.9), with a gradual decrease to the lowest rate (0.2) at age 11 to 15 years. Pyelonephritic episodes correlated with the presence of VUR, and renal scarring correlated with young age at the time of initial UTI, total number of pyelonephritic attacks, and the presence of reflux. Females with renal scarring continued to have a high number of pyelonephritic episodes after 10 years of age, implying that they should be followed closely into adulthood.

Additional clinical support for the role of infection in the development of acquired renal scarring is derived from prospective studies of children with acute pyelonephritis demonstrated by DMSA scintigraphy (47,85). Follow-up DMSA scans demonstrated new scarring in kidneys both with reflux and without reflux. All new scarring occurred at sites that exactly corresponded to areas of acute inflammation on the initial DMSA scans (Fig. 54.9). Areas of uninvolved parenchyma in pyelonephritic kidneys and contralateral normal kidneys remained normal on follow-up DMSA renal scans. It appears that once acute pyelonephritis had occurred, as demonstrated by DMSA scintigraphy at the time of infection, scarring is independent of reflux.

SEQUELAE OF RENAL SCARRING

Hypertension

Pyelonephritic scarring is the most common cause of unilateral renal parenchymal disease (nonvascular small kidneys) in patients and is a common cause of hypertension in children and young adults (154–157). The risk of hypertension in patients with renal scarring varies, based on length of follow-up and severity of scarring. In follow-up studies of children with renal scarring, approximately 6 to 13% of children with scarring develop hypertension (158–161). In some cases, it may be associated with progressive renal insufficiency (162). A recently reported long-term follow-up of an older cohort of 294 patients (mean age at presentation 17.3 years) with reflux nephropathy noted that the risk of hypertension increased with age and length of follow-up (163). Whereas 8.5% of these patients had hypertension at presentation, 38% were hypertensive at last follow-up (mean age, 34.2 years). Hypertension was significantly more common in those with severe bilateral parenchymal scarring. Similarly, in another series, 13% (11 of 83) of children with renal scarring were hypertensive at initial evaluation and another 17% (14 of 83) developed hypertension over the subsequent 4 to 20 years (164).

The development of hypertension associated with renal scarring is controversial. Some investigators report no evidence that the renin-angiotensin-aldosterone system (165,166) contributes; others report that it does (167–170). Although plasma renin activity levels are higher in patients with renal scarring than in controls, they are individually not predictive of the development of hypertension (160). Controversy also exists regarding the value of selective renal vein renin studies in hypertensive patients with scarred kidneys. In one study, segmental renal vein renin tests helped to localize sites of renin production (171). Others report that these tests are often falsely negative in hypertensive patients with unilateral nonvascular disease (154,164,172). In a prospective randomized study of the effect of nephrectomy on hypertension in patients with unilateral reflux nephropathy, nephrectomy was beneficial (173). Nephrectomy should be considered in young patients with hypertension associated with unilateral scarring when the contralateral kidney is normal and the involved kidney has less than 10 to 15% relative differential function (157,165). Despite these controversies, all would agree that the risk for hypertension in patients with reflux nephropathy is significant, and long-term follow-up is mandatory because hypertension may take 10 to 20 years to develop.

Renal Insufficiency

Reflux nephropathy also causes chronic renal insufficiency (174). It is reported in 5 to 10% of patients with end-stage renal disease (ESRD) presenting for dialysis or renal transplantation and in an even higher percentage of patients younger than 16 years (175–178). In one study, the incidence of renal insufficiency in 30 adults who were diagnosed with severe renal scarring as children was 10% (161). A more recent study of an older cohort of 294 patients (mean age at presentation, 17.2 years) with reflux nephropathy found that a 2% incidence of renal insufficiency [glomerular filtration rate (GFR) below 40 to 69 mL/min] at presentation had increased to 24% at last follow-up (mean age, 34.2 years). The more extensive the renal scarring, the higher the proportion with renal insufficiency (162). The current rate of patients presenting with ESRD associated with reflux nephropathy in Australia and New Zealand is 3.9 and 4.89 per million population each year, respectively (177).

The development of chronic renal insufficiency in children with reflux nephropathy is incompletely understood. Progression is almost always associated with proteinuria (179–181). In one review, ESRD developed in patients at a mean age of 21 years (175). Most patients who develop ESRD with reflux nephropathy have had hypertension at some time during their clinical course (176,180). The clinical course resulting in ESRD does not appear to be altered by either late surgical correction of VUR or control of UTI and hypertension (175,180,182). In one report, 4% (37 of 908) of children with reflux had reduced renal function, some of whom had secondary reflux associated with posterior urethral valves (183). GFR declined over a 5-year follow-up period in those with proteinuria and an initial creatinine clearance below 25 mL/min/m^2 (178). Chronic renal failure in women with reflux nephropathy may be exacerbated by pregnancy, particularly in those with hypertension and reduced GFR in the initial stage of pregnancy (184–186). In one study, 36% of women with moderate renal insufficiency developed hypertension, and 8% had accelerated deterioration of renal function during pregnancy (187).

Most patients (90 to 100%) with reflux nephropathy and ESRD have focal segmental glomerulosclerosis, almost always associated with proteinuria (179–181,187). A number of recent studies report elevated levels of a variety of protein markers in the urine of children with VUR and renal scarring, including β_2-microglobulin, retinol-binding protein, microalbumin, *N*-acetyl-β-D-glucosaminidase, and α_1-microglobulin (188–191). One such study that compared several of these protein markers reported that elevated urinary α_1-microglobulin was more predictive of abnormal renal function in children with reflux nephropathy, even before the appearance of significant proteinuria (188).

The pathogenesis of proteinuria and glomerulosclerosis in patients with reflux nephropathy and progressive renal insufficiency is controversial. At least four mechanisms have been proposed to explain these findings: immunologic injury, macromolecular trapping and mesangial dysfunction, vascular alterations and hypertension, and adaptive hemodynamic alterations that lead to glomerular hyperfiltration (192). The evidence at this time seems to favor the latter explanation, although the precise mechanism that leads to progressive glomerulosclerosis remains unknown (192–194). As of 1991, it was suggested that a common mechanism for hypertension and renal functional deterioration in patients with reflux nephropathy may be altered intrarenal or glomerular hemodynamics thought to be mediated, at least in part, by the intrarenal renin-angiotensin system (195). It was postulated that the selective use of angiotensin-converting enzyme inhibitors in these patients may not only control systemic blood pressure but also modify intrarenal hemodynamics to preserve renal function.

MANAGEMENT

Nonsurgical

It should have been obvious, with recognition that incidence of reflux diminished with increasing age, that reflux was a self-limiting process (30). An early series of patients followed nonsurgically was marred by the fact that these patients were not on continuous prophylaxis (152). Progression of scarring occurred in many of these patients and, in a commentary by one of the authors (152), was attributed to recurrent UTI. Subsequently, numerous reports showed the ability to prevent renal scarring by maintaining sterile urine (36,148,151). Smellie et al. found that renal growth was proportionate to somatic growth in 100 of 111 refluxing kidneys when infection was prevented (196). In the other 11, renal growth impairment was attributed to recurrent UTI. Sterile reflux was not thought to play a role in upper urinary tract scarring.

Large retrospective reviews confirm that moderate grades of reflux (I to III) resolve (36,148). In one study, 80% of reflux that resolved did so within 5 years of diagnosis (36). However, no data are available to predict the absolute resolution of reflux by grade. Smellie and Normand report resolution of reflux in 80% of renal units when reflux occurred into nondilated ureters (corresponding to grades I and II/V) (164). However, reflux resolved in only 40% of those with dilated systems (grades III to V). The report by the European Branch of the IRS found a significant difference in resolution between those with bilateral grades III and IV reflux and those with unilateral reflux of the same grades (34). Spontaneous resolution occurred in 60% of those with unilateral grade III reflux and 40% of those with grade IV. In those with bilateral grade III or IV reflux, spontaneous resolution occurred in only 10%. Whereas Skoog et al. found a significantly improved spontaneous resolution rate in children younger than 1 year ($p < .05$) (36), the European IRS branch found that to be true for boys but not for girls (34). In the American branch of the IRS, spontaneous resolution occurred within 5 years in only 25% of patients (35). Grade IV reflux accounted for 87% of the total group, influencing the low resolution rate.

Current management is predicated on the realizations that uninfected primary reflux does not initiate new renal damage and that most reflux will resolve. Therefore, children should be maintained on an antibiotic until evaluation is carried out. When VUR is identified, continuous prophylaxis using low-dose trimethoprim-sulfamethoxazole, nitrofurantoin, trimethoprim alone, or in the young infant, amoxicillin or cefaclor, once daily, generally prevents UTI (197). Nalidixic acid twice daily is also effective, but it is generally reserved for those who cannot tolerate or have had allergic reactions to the more commonly used medications. Using trimethoprim-sulfamethoxazole, only 1.5 breakthrough infections per 100 treatment months occurred in one study of 44 girls (198). Some children with breakthrough UTIs benefit from double antimicrobial prophylaxis using a combination of trimethoprim-sulfamethoxazole and nitrofurantoin (199).

As reported by both the European and American branches of the IRS, there was no difference in the incidence of UTIs in surgically and medically treated children (34,35). However, in those treated medically the infections were, by definition, breakthrough UTIs on prophylaxis, whereas most of those who had had surgical correction were no longer on prophylaxis. Furthermore, the incidence of clinically diagnosed pyelonephritis was three times higher in the nonsurgically treated group ($p < .01$) in the American branch (35).

Quarterly urine cultures are recommended as a routine, and urine culture at the time of any urinary symptoms or unexplained fever is mandatory. We recommend annual isotope cystograms and measurement of blood pressure, height, weight, and serum creatinine level. Our practice is to obtain an initial DMSA renal scan to detect preexistent scarring and determine baseline renal function, particularly in those with moderate or severe reflux and those with a history of a febrile UTI. DMSA scans are repeated after any breakthrough UTI and on the cessation of reflux. New scarring or loss of renal function can almost exclusively be attributed to breakthrough UTI (36,46,152).

Although retrospective reports suggest that renal growth as a consequence of surgical correction of reflux was more favorably affected than reflux treated nonsurgically (138,200), prospective studies suggest that there is no difference in renal growth or new renal scarring between medically and surgically treated groups and nonsurgically treated groups (201). Both the European and American branches of the IRS noted no difference in new renal scarring between medically and surgically treated patients (34,35). Younger patients were more likely to develop new scars, as were boys. Goldraich and Goldraich, using the more sensitive DMSA renal scan to evaluate kidneys, found new scars in only 7 of 202 children treated nonsurgically; all were associated with breakthrough UTI (202). Their study was confined to children who met their criteria for close follow-up. Measurement of renal mass by IVP, as reported by the European branch of the IRS, also demonstrated no difference between medically and surgically treated groups (203). Small kidneys with moderate and severe reflux (grades above II) grew poorly in both groups, whereas more normal sized kidneys grew normally.

Increased somatic growth has also been reported after surgical treatment of reflux (204,205), but it was also reported to be normal in girls treated with long-term prophylactic antibiotics for VUR (206). There is no evidence that growth is affected by sterile reflux. However, short stature associated with renal tubular acidosis has been reported in some patients with VUR and renal scarring (207,208).

Children with VUR who are dysfunctional voiders often become a difficult treatment group. For those who have this problem, gaining an understanding of coordinating voiding may be a complex task. Management must be tailored to the type of voiding abnormality (209). The mainstay of treatment of children with underlying bladder instability involves the long-term use of anticholinergics, primarily oxybutynin 2.5 to 5.0 mg two to three times a day. They can be helped by instituting a nonhurried, timed voiding schedule (five times daily). In contrast, many older girls with dysfunctional voiding and VUR are infrequent voiders (also called the *lazy bladder syndrome*). Treatment of these children is directed primarily toward the establishment of a regular or timed voiding schedule (every 2 to 3 hours). Multialarm wristwatches can be a useful and inexpensive reminder for school-aged children. These children also tend to be constipated. A high-fiber diet, including fiber supplements, as well as a daily toilet habit are part of the overall treatment program if voiding dysfunction is to be improved. Biofeedback therapy has also been used successfully in the management of cases of detrusor-sphincter dyssynergia (210).

Surgical

Probably no other topic in pediatric urology and nephrology has been so hotly debated as the surgical management of VUR. All would agree that antireflux surgery was performed too often during the 1960s and early 1970s. It is also clear that there are a number of highly successful surgical techniques for correcting VUR, each with its own advantages and disadvantages. Success rates exceeding 95% can be anticipated by those with experience performing the various procedures (35). However, the unanimity of opinion is lost when discussing the indications for and effects of surgical correction of reflux, in part because of the controversy about the goal of management in patients with reflux. Those whose ultimate goal of treatment is the cure of reflux commonly recommended surgery. Those whose primary goal is the prevention of pyelonephritis and new renal damage recommend surgery less commonly. Other alleged goals of successful surgery, including improved renal growth and function, improved statural growth, and prevention of scarring and UTI, have not been realized in prospective randomized studies comparing surgery with medical management (34,35,201). However, antireflux surgery does reduce pyelonephritic episodes (34,211). Today, most would agree that medical management is appropriate for patients with mild to moderate (grades I to III) VUR and reflux of any grade in the child younger than 1 year. The primary indications for surgery in this group of patients are uncontrolled breakthrough and symptomatic UTI. Some would restrict this indication to episodes of breakthrough acute pyelonephritis because persistent asymptomatic bacteriuria does not appear to be associated with progressive renal damage (212–214). Other reasons for surgical consideration include poor compliance with medical management or intolerance of medication, problems that are probably much more common than generally recognized (215).

Most also would agree that severe primary reflux (grade V) persisting beyond 1 or 2 years of age should be surgically corrected. These ureters are often associated with urinary stasis, creating an increased risk for upper tract infection. Preoperative evaluation includes differential renal function and drainage using renal scintigraphy. Small, poorly functioning kidneys (less than 10 to 15% total functional contribution) should be removed. Ureteral tailoring or tapering is often necessary when reimplanting ureters with grade V VUR. In experienced hands, success rates using these reconstructive techniques are 90 to 95% (216).

Greater controversy surrounds the optimal management of grade IV VUR. Medical management in these patients is as effective as surgery in the maintenance of renal function. However, the spontaneous resolution rate of grade IV is less than 40% after a follow-up of 5 years (34,35,217). Therefore, the decision for surgical intervention in these patients must be individualized, taking into account the need for continuous prophylaxis and repeated examinations. The age of the patient at presentation, patient compliance, the character of previous UTIs, and the presence or absence of renal scarring all play a role in the decision. Persistent grade IV reflux in children older than 3 years is unlikely to resolve; surgical management is probably the best treatment if it fails to improve after 2 years of medical management.

Another unanswered question remaining at this juncture centers around the ideal treatment of the child who approaches adolescence with continued mild to moderate reflux. Many urologists recommend surgical correction of VUR in any child with persistent reflux before puberty. The concern relates to the assumed increased risk of pyelonephritis in pregnancy with its affect on both mother and fetus. However, the patient who had UTI in childhood continues to be at risk for UTI in the future, regardless of whether reflux has resolved spontaneously, has been surgically corrected, or persists. During pregnancy, the prevalence for UTI in the general population is reported to range from 2 to 8%, compared with 37% in those with a history of childhood UTI (218,219). In one review, 41 women who had UTIs in childhood were followed up through 65 pregnancies (219). Nineteen had renal scarring, and 22 did not. They were compared with matched controls. The incidence of bacteriuria in pregnancy was higher in those with renal scarring (47%) than in those without scarring (27%) but both were significantly greater (less than .001 and less than .01, respectively) than in the controls without a history of UTI (2%). However, the incidence of pyelonephritis was higher in the group who had not had resolution of reflux at the time of their last follow-up (three of eight) than in those who had resolution of reflux (2 of 33, $p = .08$).

Treated UTI, including pyelonephritis, appears to have little negative effect on pregnancy or fetal outcome if renal function is normal (220–222). In the absence of preexisting bilateral renal scarring or impaired renal function, persistent VUR is not associated with increased fetal loss or maternal risk (223). However, there is an increased risk of preeclampsia and hypertension in those with preexisting renal scarring (218).

Correction of VUR does not guarantee prevention of problems in the future. Mansfield et al. reported on 104 women followed for an average of 25 years (224). Sixty-seven had surgical reimplantation of refluxing ureters, and 37 had persisting reflux at the time of last evaluation. Bacteriuria of pregnancy occurred in 40% of those with surgical correction and 15% of those whose reflux was not corrected. Eighteen percent of those surgically corrected had pyelonephritis of pregnancy, whereas only 1.5% with persisting reflux had pyelonephritis during pregnancy. These results should not be interpreted as a condemnation of surgery. Instead, these findings are probably a function of the patients who came to surgical correction as compared with those who did not. Those who underwent surgery were probably more susceptible to febrile infection, leading to more aggressive management during childhood.

Although many urologists recommend surgical correction of persisting VUR in the older child, some advocate stopping prophylaxis in the older child who has persistent mild or moderate VUR (225). Surgical correction is then reserved for those who might benefit from it, such as the girl who returns after cessation of prophylaxis with clinical evidence of pyelonephritis, ideally proven by renal cortical scan. Others would recommend this approach only in patients without significant renal scarring. Prospective study is needed to further validate this philosophy. Regardless, long-term follow-up and screening for bacteriuria during pregnancy should be emphasized for all girls with a history of recurrent UTIs.

Endoscopic Correction

Endoscopic correction of reflux is a new development that may be useful in some patients. Matouchek introduced this method, using Polytef paste injected under the ureteral orifice (226) (Fig. 54.15). O'Donnell and Puri subsequently popularized this technique, using 0.2 to 0.8 mL of Teflon paste injected subureterically at the ureterovesical junction (227). Results from a recent multicenter European survey involving 975 boys and 3191 girls report that 76% of refluxing ureters are cured with one injection, increasing to 85% after a second injection (228). Another 10.7% of refluxing ureters showed

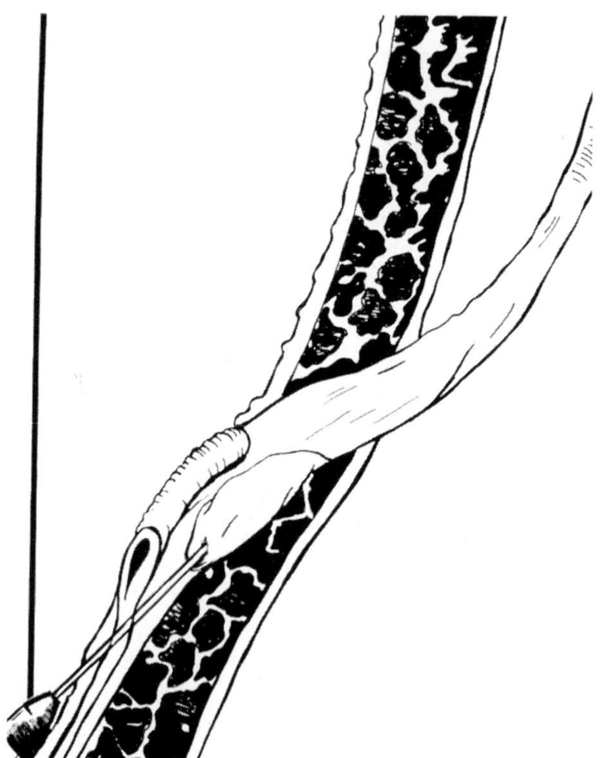

FIGURE 54.15. Endoscopic injection of Teflon paste beneath the intramural segment of ureter.

significant improvement. Ureteral obstruction was rare, occurring in only 0.32%. Lower success rates have been reported in cases of duplex systems, severe VUR, and neuropathic bladders (229–233). Long-term (2.0 to 5.5 years) follow-up has revealed recurrences in 12% of both low- and high-grade reflux (234). Concern about the long-term safety of injected Polytef in children has limited its acceptance by pediatric urologists in the United States and has resulted in increasing concern about its use in Europe. Animal studies have demonstrated that Polytef paste injected periurethrally for treatment of incontinence migrates to lymph nodes as well as lungs and brain, where it produces a foreign-body giant cell reaction with multinucleated giant cells (235). Similar migration has been reported in primates after subureteric injection. Large granulomatous reactions have been found at the injection sites (236). Isolated instances of distant (including pulmonary) migration and local giant cell response with granulomas at the injection site have also been reported (237–239). Concerns have been raised regarding risks in children who carry the Teflon implant for many decades. Longer-term clinical follow-up of children treated with Polytef paste will determine whether these concerns are warranted.

Although the actual long-term consequences of the migration and associated histologic changes are unknown, these safety concerns have stimulated a search for alternative substances. Several groups report results of endoscopic injection of glutaraldehyde cross-linked bovine dermal collagen in patients with VUR. Initial cessation of VUR has been reported in 63 to 75% after one injection (240,241). However, recurrence has been seen in up to 40% after 6 to 12 months (240,242). Results seem to be stable after 2 years of follow-up (243). Success rates were even lower in duplicated systems and ureters with high-grade reflux (240,243). However, minimal localized inflammatory reaction at the injection site without granuloma formation has been reported by these investigators (244). A variety of alternative substances are currently being investigated, including polyvinyl alcohol, silicone, autologous fat and cartilage, bioglass, dextranomer microspheres, and a self-detachable balloon system. A safe and effective substance for endoscopic correction of reflux is likely. At that time, the indications and pros and cons of medical, endoscopic, and surgical management of VUR will surely be the topic for renewed debate.

SUMMARY

Most laboratory and clinical evidence strongly supports the concepts that both VUR and urinary infection are underlying conditions in most cases of acquired renal scarring and that this damage is irreversible. It occurs primarily in regions of the kidney associated with IRR. The acute inflammatory response associated with renal parenchymal infection is the prerequisite for acquired renal scarring. VUR, when present, is the single most significant host risk factor for acute pyelonephritis and subsequent renal scarring. Renal scarring can be decreased or prevented by early treatment of initial episodes of acute pyelonephritis. Most kidneys with VUR are not scarred, despite a history of UTI. However, new scarring does occur in some patients after acute pyelonephritis, and it appears to be more likely in infants or children younger than 3 years. Therefore, it is often present at the time of initial investigation. Although scarring is more often associated with higher grades of reflux, it can occur with lower grades and in the absence of VUR after an episode of pyelonephritis. Kidneys with higher grades of VUR are at significantly greater risk for acute pyelonephritis than are kidneys with no or mild VUR.

Undoubtedly, some kidneys associated with high-grade VUR are congenitally abnormal (hypoplasia and dysplasia), which is easily confused radiographically with acquired postinfective renal scarring. Because most renal scarring is established at the time of initial investigation, it may be difficult to know whether preexistent scarring represents postinfective damage or developmental abnormalities. Finally, sterile primary VUR has not been shown to produce renal scarring, but sterile secondary VUR associated with obstruction and sustained high intravesical pressures may occasionally result in scarring. Clinical examples of this are uncommon but may include some boys with posterior urethral valves and some children with noncompliant bladders associated with neuropathic conditions (spina bifida, spinal cord injury) and severe voiding dyssynergia.

REFERENCES

1. Dillon MJ, Goonasekera CD. Reflux nephropathy. *J Am Soc Nephrol* 1998;9:2377–2383.
2. Mackie CG, Awang H, Stephens FD. The ureteric orifice: the embryologic key to radiologic status of the ureter. *J Pediatr Surg* 1975;10:473–481.
3. Hu P, Deng FM, Liang FX, et al. Ablation of uroplakin III gene results in small urothelial plaques, urothelial leakage, and vesicoureteral reflux. *J Cell Biol* 2000;151:961–971.
4. Ohtomo Y, Nagaoka R, Kaneko K, et al. Angiotensin converting enzyme gene polymorphism in primary vesicoureteral reflux. *Pediatr Nephrol* 2001;16:648–652.
5. International Reflux Study Committee. Medical versus surgical treatment of primary vesicoureteral reflux. *Pediatrics* 1981;67:392–400.
6. Babcock JR, Belman AB, Shkolnick A, et al. Familial ureteral duplication and ureterocele. *Urology* 1977;9:345.
7. Kaplan WE, Nasrallah P, King LR. Reflux in complete duplication in children. *J Urol* 1978;120:220.
8. Ben-Ami T, Gayer G, Hertz M, et al. The natural history of reflux in the lower pole of duplicated collecting systems: a controlled study. *Pediatr Radiol* 1989;19:308–310.
9. Peppas DS, Skoog SJ, Canning DA, et al. Nonsurgical management of primary vesicoureteral reflux in complete ureteral duplication: Is it justified? *J Urol* 1991;146:1594.
10. Hutch JA. Vesico-ureteral reflux in the paraplegic: cause and correction. *J Urol* 1952;68:457.
11. Kaplan WE. Firlit CF. Management of reflux in the myelodysplastic child. *J Urol* 1983;129:1195.
12. Cohen RA, Rushton HG, Belman AB, et al. Renal scarring and vesicoureteral reflux in children with myelodysplasia. *J Urol* 1990;144:541.
13. Kass EJ, Koff SA, Diokno AC. Fate of vesicoureteral reflux in children with neuropathic bladders managed by intermittent catheterization. *J Urol* 1981;125:63.
14. Agarwal SK, Khoury AE, Abramson RP, et al. Outcome analysis of vesicoureteral reflux in children with myelodysplasia. *J Urol* 1997;157:980–982.
15. Flood HD, Ritchey ML, Bloom DA, et al. Outcome of reflux in children with myelodysplasia managed by bladder pressure monitoring. *J Urol* 1994;152:1574–1577.
16. Seruca H. Vesicoureteral reflux and voiding dysfunction: a prospective study. *J Urol* 1989;142:494.
17. Greenfield SP, Wan J. The relationship between dysfunctional voiding and congenital vesicoureteral reflux. *Curr Opin Urol* 2000;10:607–610.
18. Koff SA. Relationship between dysfunctional voiding and reflux. *J Urol* 1992;148:1703–1705.
19. Mayo ME, Burns MW. Urodynamic studies in children who wet. *Br J Urol* 1990;65:641.
20. Williams MA, Noe HN, Smith RA. The importance of urinary tract infection in the evaluation of the incontinent child. *J Urol* 1994;151:188–190.
21. Scholtmeijer RJ, Griffiths DJ. The role of videourodynamic studies in diagnosis and treatment of vesicoureteral reflux. *J Pediatr Surg* 1990;25:669–671.
22. Homsy YC, Nsouli I, Hamburger B, et al. Effects of oxybutynin on vesicoureteral reflux in children. *J Urol* 1985;134:1168–1171.
23. Scholtmeijer RJ, Nijamn RJ. Vesicoureteric reflux and videourodynamic studies: results of a prospective study after three years of followup. *Urology* 1994;43:714–718.
24. Hinman F, Baumann FW. Vesical and ureteral damage from voiding dysfunction in boys without neurologic or obstructive disease. *J Urol* 1973;109:727.
25. Noe HN. The role of dysfunctional voiding in failure or complication of ureteral reimplantation for primary reflux. *J Urol* 1985;134:1172–1175.
26. Ransley PG. Vesicoureteric reflux. continuing surgical dilemma. *Urology* 1978;12:246–255.
27. Smellie JM, Edwards D, Hunter N, et al. Vesicoureteral reflux and renal scarring. *Kidney Int* 1975;8:S-65.
28. Levitt SB, Weiss RA. Vesicoureteral reflux: natural history, classification, and reflux nephropathy. In: Kelalis PP, King LR, Belman AB, eds. *Clinical pediatric urology*, 2nd ed. Philadelphia: WB Saunders, 1985:355–380.
29. Askari A, Belman AB. Vesicoureteral reflux in black girls. *J Urol* 1982;127:747.
30. Baker R, Maxfed W, Maglath J, et al. Relation of age, sex and infection to reflux: data indicating high spontaneous cure rate in pediatric patients. *J Urol* 1966;95:27.
31. Smellie JM, Normand ICS, Katz G. Children with urinary infection: a comparison of those with and those without vesicoureteral reflux. *Kidney Int* 1981;20:717.
32. Snodgrass W. Relationship of voiding dysfunction to urinary tract infection and vesicoureteral reflux in children. *Urology* 1991;38:341.
33. Scott JES. The management of ureteric reflux in children. *Br J Urol* 1977;49:109–118.
34. Tamminen-Mobius T, Brunier E, Ebel KD, et al. Cessation of vesicoureteral reflux for 5 years in infants and children allocated to medical treatment. The International Reflux Study in children; European branch. *J Urol* 1992;148(2):1662–1666.
35. Weiss R, Duckett J, Spitzer A. Results of randomized clinical trial of medical vs. surgical management of infants and children with grades III and IV primary vesicoureteral reflux (United States). *J Urol* 1992;148(2):1667–1673.
36. Skoog SJ, Belman AB, Majd M. A nonsurgical approach to the management of primary vesicoureteral reflux. *J Urol* 1987;138:941–946.
37. Dwoskin JY, Perlmutter AD. Vesicoureteral reflux in children: a computerized review. *J Urol* 1973;109:888.
38. Anonymous. Report of a meeting of physicians at the Hospital for Sick Children, Great Ormond Street, London. Vesicoureteric reflux: all in the genes? *Lancet* 1996;348:725–728.
39. Hollowell JG, Greenfield SP. Screening siblings for vesicoureteral reflux. *J Urol* 2002;168:2138–2141
40. Jerkins GR, Noe HN. Familial vesicoureteral reflux: a prospective study. *J Urol* 1982;128:774.
41. Wan J, Greenfield SP, Ng M, et al. Sibling reflux: a dual center retrospective study. *J Urol* 1996;156:677–679.
42. Noe HN, Wyatt RJ, Peeden JN Jr, et al. The transmission of vesicoureteral reflux from parent to child. *J Urol* 1992;148:1869.
43. Connolly LP, Treves ST, Zurakowski D, et al. Natural history of vesicoureteral reflux in siblings. *J Urol* 1996;156:1805–1807.
44. Hoberman A, Charron M, Hickey RW, et al. Imaging studies after a first febrile urinary tract infection in young children. *N Engl J Med* 2003;348:195–202.

45. Ransley PG, Risdon RA. Reflux nephropathy: effects of antimicrobial therapy on the evolution of the early pyelonephritic scar. *Kidney Int* 1981;20:733.
46. Smellie JM, Ransley PG, Normand ICS, et al. Development of new renal scars: a collaborative study. *BMJ* 1985;290:1957.
47. Rushton HG, Majd M, Jantausch B, et al. Renal scarring following reflux and nonreflux pyelonephritis: evaluation with 99m-technetium–dimercaptosuccinic acid scintigraphy. *J Urol* 1992;147:1327–1332.
48. Kunin CM. The natural history of recurrent bacteriuria in school girls. *N Engl J Med* 1970;282:1443.
49. Govan DE, Friedland GW, Fair WR, et al. Management of children with urinary tract infections. *Urology* 1975;6:273.
50. Winberg J, Bergstom T, Jacobsson B. Morbidity, age and sex distribution, recurrences and renal scarring in symptomatic urinary tract infection in childhood. *Kidney Int* 1975;8:S-101.
51. Jodal U. The natural history of bacteriuria in childhood. *Infect Dis Clin North Am* 1987;1:713.
52. Stocks A, Richards D, Frentzen B, et al. Correlation of prenatal renal pelvic anteroposterior diameter with outcome in infancy. *J Urol* 1996;155:1050–1052.
53. Adra AM, Mejides AA, Dennaoul MS, et al. Fetal pyelectasis: is it always "physiologic"? *Am J Obstet Gynecol* 1995;173:1263–1266.
54. Marra G, Barbieri G, Moiolo C, et al. Mild fetal hydronephrosis indicating vesicoureteric reflux. *Arch Dis Child Fetal Neonatal Ed* 1994;70:F147–F149.
55. Tibballs JM, De Bruyn R. Primary vesicoureteric reflux: how useful is postnatal ultrasound? *Arch Dis Child* 1996;75:444–447.
56. Friedland GW. The voiding cystogram: an unreliable study. In: Hodson J, Kincaid-Smith P, eds. *Reflux nephropathy*. New York: Masson, 1979:93–99.
57. Jequier S. Reliability of voiding cystourethrography to detect reflux. *AJR Am J Roentgenol* 1989;157:807.
58. Cleveland RH, Constantinou C, Blickman J, et al. Voiding cystourethrography in children: value of digital fluoroscopy in reducing radiation dose. *AJR Am J Roentgenol* 1991;158:137.
59. Kleinman PK, Diamond DA, Karellas A, et al. Tailored low-dose fluoroscopic voiding cystourethrography for the reevaluation of vesicoureteral reflux in girls. *AJR Am J Roentgenol* 1994;162:1151–1154.
60. Diamond DA, Kleinman PK, Spevak M, et al. The tailored low-dose fluoroscopic voiding cystogram for familial reflux screening. *J Urol* 1996;155:681–682.
61. Conway JJ, King LR, Belman AB. Detection of vesicoureteral reflux with radionuclide: a comparison study with roentgenographic cystography. *AJR Am J Roentgenol* 1972;115:720.
62. Nasrallah PF, Sreeramulu N, Crawford J. Clinical applications of nuclear cystography. *J Urol* 1982;128:550.
63. Jaya G, Bal CS, Padhy AK, et al. Radionuclide studies in the evaluation of urinary tract infections. *Indian Pediatr* 1996;33:635–640.
64. Saraga M, Stanicic A, Markovic V. The role of direct radionuclide cystography in evaluation of vesicoureteral reflux. *Scand J Urol Nephrol* 1996;30:367–371.
65. Willi UV, Treves ST. Radionuclide voiding cystography. In: Treves ST, ed. *Pediatric nuclear medicine*. New York: Springer-Verlag, 1985:105–120.
66. Kogan SS, Sigler L, Levitt SB, et al. Elusive vesicoureteral reflux in children with normal contrast cystograms. *J Urol* 1986;136:325.
67. Lebowitz RL. The detection of vesicoureteral reflux in the child. *Invest Radiol* 1986;21:519.
68. Majd M, Kass EJ, Belman AB. The accuracy of the indirect (intravenous) radionuclide cystogram in children. *J Nucl Med* 1983;24:23.
69. Conway JJ, Belman AB, Kind LR. Direct and indirect radionuclide cystography. *Semin Nucl Med* 1974;4:197.
70. De Sadeleer C, De Boe V, Keuppens F, et al. How good is technetium-99m mercaptoacetylglycine indirect cystography? *Eur J Nucl Med* 1994;21:223–227.
71. Gross GW, Lebowitz RK. Infection does not cause reflux. *AJR Am J Roentgenol* 1981;137:929.
72. Hellstrom M, Judal U, Marild S, et al. Ureteral dilatation in children with febrile urinary tract infection or bacteriuria. *AJR Am J Roentgenol* 1987;148:483.
73. Roberts JA. Experimental pyelonephritis in the monkey. III. Pathophysiology of ureteral malfunction induced by bacteria. *Invest Urol* 1975;13:117.
74. Lebowitz RL, Mandell J. Urinary tract infection in children: putting radiology in its place. *Radiology* 1987;165:1.
75. Ben Ami T, Rozin M, Hertz M. Imaging of children with urinary tract infection: a tailored approach. *Clin Radiol* 1989;40:64.
76. Blickman JG, Taylor GA, Lebowitz RL. Voiding cystography as the initial radiologic study in the child with urinary tract infection. *Radiology* 1985;156:659.
77. Belman AB. Urinary imaging in children. *Pediatr Infect Dis J* 1989;8:548.
78. Majd M, Rushton HG, Jantausch B, et al. Relationship among vesicoureteral reflux, P-fimbriated *Escherichia coli*, and acute pyelonephritis in children with febrile urinary tract infection. *J Pediatr* 1991;119:578.
79. Rushton HG. The evaluation of acute pyelonephritis and renal scarring with ^{99m}Tc-dimercaptosuccinic acid renal scintigraphy: evolving concepts and future directions. *Pediatr Nephrol* 1997;11:108–120.
80. Rushton HG, Majd M, Chandra R, et al. Evaluation of 99m-technetium-dimercapto-succinic acid renal scans in experimental acute pyelonephritis in piglets. *J Urol* 1988;140:1169.
81. Parkhouse HF, Godley ML, Cooper JM, et al. Renal imaging with ^{99m}Tc-labelled DMSA in the detection of acute pyelonephritis: an experimental study in the pig. *Nucl Med Commun* 1989;10:63.
82. Tappin DM, Murphy AV, Mocan MH, et al. A prospective study of children with first acute symptomatic *E. coli* urinary tract infection. *Acta Paediatr Scand* 1989;78:723.
83. Bailey RR. The relationship of vesicoureteric reflux to urinary tract infection in chronic pyelonephritis: reflux nephropathy. *Clin Nephrol* 1973;1:132.
84. Ransley PG, Risdon RA. Reflux and renal scarring. *Br J Radiol* 1978;51(Suppl 14):1.
85. Jakobsson B, Berg U, Svensson L. Renal scarring after acute pyelonephritis. *Arch Dis Child* 1994;70:111–115.
86. Kass EH, Svanborg-Eden C, eds. *Host-parasite interactions in urinary tract infections*. Proceedings of the Fourth International Symposium on Pyelonephritis. Chicago: University of Chicago Press, 1989.

87. Svanborg-Eden C, Hausson S, Jodal U, et al. Host-parasite interactions in the urinary tract. *J Infect Dis* 1988;157:421.
88. Kallenius G, Svennsson SB, Hultberg H, et al. Occurrence of P-fimbriated *Escherichia coli* in urinary tract infections. *Lancet* 1981;2:1369.
89. Vaisanen-Rhen V, Elo J, Vaisanen E, et al. P-fimbriated clones among uropathogenic *Escherichia coli* strains. *Infect Immun* 1984;43:149.
90. Majd M, Rushton HG. Renal cortical scintigraphy in the diagnosis of acute pyelonephritis. *Semin Nucl Med* 1992;22:98–111.
91. Jakobsson B, Soderlundh S, Berg U. Diagnostic significance of ^{99m}Tc-dimercaptosuccinic acid (DMSA) scintigraphy in urinary tract infection. *Arch Dis Child* 1992;67:1338–1342.
92. Lomberg H, Hellstrom M, Jodal U. Virulence associated traits in *Escherichia coli* causing first and recurrent episodes of urinary tract infection in children with or without reflux. *J Infect Dis* 1984;150:561.
93. Lomberg H, Hellstrom M, Jodal U, et al. Properties of *Escherichia coli* in patients with renal scarring. *J Infect Dis* 1989;159:579.
94. Silver TM, Kass EJ, Thornbury JR, et al. The radiological spectrum of acute pyelonephritis in adults and adolescents. *Radiology* 1976;118:65.
95. Filly RA, Friedland GW, Govan DE, et al. Development and progression of clubbing and scarring in children with recurrent urinary tract infections. *Radiology* 1974;113:145.
96. Moretti JH, Rapin JR, Le Poncin M, et al. Dimercaptosuccinic acid complexes: their structure, biological behavior and renal localization. In: Joekes AM, Constable AR, Brown NJG, et al., eds. *Radionuclides in nephrology*. London: Academic Press, 1982:25–31.
97. Bingham JB, Maisey MN. An evaluation of the use of ^{99m}Tc-dimercaptosuccinic acid (DMSA) as a static renal imaging agent. *Br J Radiol* 1978;51:599.
98. Rushton HG, Majd M. Dimercaptosuccinic acid renal scintigraphy for evaluation of pyelonephritis and scarring: review of experimental and clinical studies. *J Urol* 1992; 148:1726–1732.
99. Goldraich NP, Ramos OL, Goldraich IH. Urography vs. DMSA scan in children with vesicoureteric reflux. *Pediatr Nephrol* 1989;3:1.
100. Merrick MV, Uttley WS, Wild SR. The detection of pyelonephritic scarring in children by radioisotope imaging. *Br J Radiol* 1980;53:544.
101. Mansour M, Azmy AF, MacKenzie JR. Renal scarring secondary to vesicoureteral reflux. Critical assessment and grading. *Br J Urol* 1987;60:320.
102. Farnsworth JH, Rossleigh MA, Leighton DM, et al. Detection of reflux nephropathy in infants by 99m-technetium dimercaptosuccinic acid studies. *J Urol* 1991;145:542.
103. McLorie GA, Alibadi H, Churchill BM, et al. 99m-technetium-dimercapto-succinic acid renal scarring and excretory urography in diagnosis of renal scars in children. *J Urol* 1989;142:790.
104. Smellie JM, Prescod N, Shaw P, et al. Comparison of radiology and nuclear imaging in the assessment of patients with renal scarring. In: Kass EH, Svanborg-Eden C, eds. *Host-parasite interactions in urinary tract infections*. Chicago: University of Chicago Press, 1989:280–284.
105. Yen TC, Chen WP, Chang SL, et al. Technetium-^{99}m-DMSA renal SPECT in diagnosing and monitoring pediatric acute pyelonephritis. *J Nucl Med* 1996;37:1349–1353.
106. Itoh K, Yamashita T, Tsukamoto E, et al. Qualitative and quantitative evaluation of renal parenchymal damage by ^{99m}Tc-DMSA planar and SPECT scintigraphy. *Ann Nucl Med* 1995;9:23–28.
107. Majd M, Rushton HG, Chandra R, et al. ^{99m}Tc-DMSA renal cortical scintigraphy for the detection of experimental pyelonephritis in piglets: comparison of planar (pinhole) and SPECT imaging. *J Nucl Med* 1996;37:1731–1734.
108. Stokland E, Hellstrom M, Jacobsson B, et al. Early ^{99m}Tc dimercaptosuccinic acid (DMSA) scintigraphy in symptomatic first-time urinary tract infection. *Acta Paediatr* 1996;85:430–436.
109. DeLange MJ, Piers DA, Kosternik JGW, et al. Renal handling of technetium-99m DMSA: evidence for glomerular filtration and peritubular uptake. *J Nucl Med* 1989;30:1219–1223.
110. Goldraich NP, Alvarenga AR, Goldraich IH, et al. Renal accumulation of ^{99m}Tc-DMSA in the artificially perfused isolated rat kidney. *J Urol* 1985;134:1282.
111. Risdon RA. The small scarred kidney in childhood. *Pediatr Nephrol* 1993;7:361–364.
112. Anderson PAM, Rickwood AMK. Features of primary vesicoureteric reflux detected by prenatal sonography. *Br J Urol* 1991;67:267.
113. Gordon AC, Thomas DFM, Arthur RJ, et al. Prenatally diagnosed reflux: a follow-up study. *Br J Urol* 1990;65:407.
114. Najmaldin A, Burge DM, Atwell TD. Reflux nephropathy secondary to intrauterine vesicoureteric reflux. *J Pediatr Surg* 1990;25:387–390.
115. Crabbe DCG, Thomas DFM, Gordon AC, et al. Use of 99m-technetium-dimercaptosuccinic acid to study patterns of renal damage associated with prenatally detected vesicoureteral reflux. *J Urol* 1992;148:1229–1231.
116. Mackie GG, Stephens FD. Duplex kidneys: a correlation of renal dysplasia with position of the ureteral orifice. *J Urol* 1975;114:274.
117. Sommer JT, Stephens SD. Morphogenesis of nephropathy with partial ureteral obstruction and vesicoureteral reflux. *J Urol* 1981;125:67.
118. Ambrose SS, Parrott TS, Woodward JR, et al. Observations on the small kidney associated with vesicoureteral reflux. *J Urol* 1980;123:349.
119. Sheridan M, Jewkes F, Gaugh DCS. Reflux nephropathy in the first year of life: the role of infection. *Pediatr Surg Int* 1991;6:214.
120. Sillen U, Hjalmas K, Aili M, et al. Pronounced detrusor hypercontractility in infants with gross bilateral reflux. *J Urol* 1992;148:598–599.
121. Sillen U, Bachelard M, Hermanson G, et al. Gross bilateral reflux in infants: gradual decrease of initial detrusor hypercontractility. *J Urol* 1996;668–672.
122. Chandra M, Maddix H, McVicar M. Transient urodynamic dysfunction of infancy: relationship to urinary tract infections and vesicoureteral reflux. *J Urol* 1996;155:673–677.
123. Hodson CJ, Maling TM, McManmon TJ. The pathogenesis of reflux nephropathy (chronic atrophic pyelonephritis). *Br J Radiol* 1975;48(Suppl 13):1.

124. Rolleston TL, Maling TMJ, Hodson CJ. Intrarenal reflux and the scarred kidney. *Arch Dis Child* 1974;49:531.
125. Ransley PG, Risdon RA. Renal papillary morphology and intrarenal reflux in the young pig. *Urol Res* 1975;3:105.
126. Ransley PG, Risdon RA. Renal papillary morphology in infants and young children. *Urol Res* 1975;3:111.
127. Ransley PG, Risdon RA, Godley ML. High pressure sterile vesicoureteral reflux and renal scarring: an experimental study of the pig and mini-pig. *Contrib Nephrol* 1984;39:320.
128. Roberts JA. Mechanisms of renal damage in chronic pyelonephritis. *Curr Top Pathol* 1995;88:265–287.
129. Roberts JA, Dominique GJ, Martin LN, et al. Immunology of pyelonephritis in the primate model: live vs. heat-killed bacteria. *Kidney Int* 1981;19:297.
130. Roberts JA, Roth JK, Dominque G, et al. Immunology of pyelonephritis in the primate model. VI. Effect of complement depletion. *J Urol* 1983;129:193.
131. Shimamura T. Mechanisms of renal tissue destruction in an experimental acute pyelonephritis. *Exp Mol Pathol* 1981;34:34.
132. Roberts JA, Roth JK, Dominque G, et al. Immunology of pyelonephritis in the primate model. V. Effect of superoxide dismutase. *J Urol* 1982;128:1394.
133. Kaack MV, Dowling KJ, Patterson GM, et al. Immunology of pyelonephritis. VIII. *E. coli* causes granulocyte aggregation and renal ischemia. *J Urol* 1986;136:117.
134. Androulakakis PA, Ransley PG, Risdon RA, et al. Microvascular changes in the early stage of reflux pyelonephritis. An experimental study in the pig kidney. *Eur Urol* 1987;13: 219.
135. McCord JM. Oxygen-derived free radicals in postischemic tissue injury. *N Engl J Med* 1985;312:159.
136. Roberts JA, Kaack MB, Fussell EN. Immunology of pyelonephritis. VII. Effect of allopurinol. *J Urol* 1986;136:960.
137. Smellie JM, Normand ICS. Bacteriuria, reflux and renal scarring. *Arch Dis Child* 1975;50:581.
138. Scott JES, Stansfield JM. Ureteric reflux and kidney scarring in children. *Arch Dis Child* 1968;43:468.
139. Rolleston GL, Shannon FT, Utley WLF. Relationship with infantile vesicoureteric reflux to renal damage. *BMJ* 1970;1: 460.
140. Filly R, Friedland GW, Govan DE, et al. Development and progression of clubbing and scarring in children with recurrent urinary tract infections. *Radiology* 1974;113:145.
141. Huland H, Busch R. Pyelonephritis scarring in 213 patients with upper and lower tract infections: long-term follow-up. *J Urol* 1984;132:936.
142. Heale WF, Ferguson RS. Pathogenesis of renal scarring. In: Kass ED, Brumfitt W, eds. *Infections of the urinary tract: proceedings of the Third International Symposium on Pyelonephritis.* Chicago: University of Chicago Press, 1975;201–204.
143. Winberg J, Bollgren I, Kallenius G, et al. Clinical pyelonephritis and focal renal scarring: a selected review of pathogenesis, prevention and prognosis. *Pediatr Clin North Am* 1982;22:801.
144. Goldraich NP, Goldraich IH, Anselmi OE, et al. Reflux nephropathy: the clinical picture in South Brazilian children. *Contrib Nephrol* 1984;39:52.
145. Funston MR, Cremin BJ. Intrarenal reflux: papillary morphology and pressure relationships in children's necropsy kidneys. *Br J Radiol* 1978;51:665.
146. Shah KJ, Robins DG, White RHR. Renal scarring and vesicoureteric reflux. *Arch Dis Child* 1978;53:210.
147. Rolleston GL, Shannon FT, Utley WLF. Follow-up of vesicoureteric reflux in the newborn. *Kidney Int* 1975;8:S-59.
148. Bellinger MF, Duckett JW. Vesicoureteral reflux: a comparison of non-surgical and surgical management. *Contrib Nephrol* 1984;39:133.
149. Roberts JA, Suarez GM, Kaack B, et al. Experimental pyelonephritis in the monkey. VII. Ascending pyelonephritis in the absence of vesicoureteral reflux. *J Urol* 1985;133:1068.
150. Glauser MP, Lyons JM, Braude AI. Prevention of chronic experimental pyelonephritis by suppression of acute suppuration. *J Clin Invest* 1978;61:403.
151. Edwards D, Normand ICS, Prescod N, et al. Disappearance of vesicoureteric reflux during long-term antibiotic prophylaxis of urinary tract infection. *BMJ* 1977;2:285.
152. Lenaghan D, Whitaker JG, Jensen F, et al. The natural history of reflux and long-term effects of reflux on the kidney. *J Urol* 1976;115:728.
153. Martinell J, Claesson I, Lidin-Janson G, et al. Urinary infection, reflux and renal scarring in females continuously followed for 13–38 years. *Pediatr Nephrol* 1995;9:131–136.
154. Wanner C, Lusher T, Groth H, et al. Unilateral parenchymatous kidney disease and hypertension: results of nephrectomy and medical treatment. *Nephron* 1985;41:250–257.
155. Gill DG, Mendes da Costa B, Cameron JS, et al. Analysis of 100 children with severe and persistent hypertension. *Arch Dis Child* 1976;51:951.
156. Still JL, Cottom D. Severe hypertension in childhood. *Arch Dis Child* 1967;42:34–39.
157. Londe S. Cause of hypertension in the young. *Pediatr Clin North Am* 1978;25:55–65.
158. Wallace DMA, Rothwell DL, Williams DI. The long-term follow-up of surgically treated vesicoureteric reflux. *Br J Urol* 1978;50:479–484.
159. Heale WF. Hypertension and reflux nephropathy. *Aust Paediatr J* 1977;13:56–61.
160. Goonasekera CD, Shah V, Wade AM, et al. 15-year follow-up of renin and blood pressure in reflux nephropathy. *Lancet* 1996;347:640–643.
161. Martinell J, Lidin-Janson G, Jagenburg R, et al. Girls prone to urinary infections followed into adulthood. Indices of disease. *Pediatr Nephrol* 1996;10:139–142.
162. Jacobson SH, Eklof O, Eriksson CG, et al. Development of hypertension and uraemia after pyelonephritis in childhood: twenty-seven year follow-up. *BMJ* 1989;299:703.
163. Zhang Y, Bailey RR. A long-term follow-up of adults with reflux nephropathy. *N Z Med J* 1995;108:142–144.
164. Smellie JM, Normand ICS. Reflux nephropathy in childhood. In: Hodson J, Kincaid-Smith P, eds. *Reflux nephropathy.* New York: Masson, 1979:14–20.
165. Bailey RR, McRae CU, Maling TMJ, et al. Renal vein renin concentration in the hypertension of unilateral reflux nephropathy. *J Urol* 1978;120:21.
166. Bailey RR, Lynn KL, McRae CU. Unilateral reflux nephropathy and hypertension. *Contrib Nephrol* 1984;39:116.
167. Savage JM, Koh CT, Shah V, et al. Five year prospective study of plasma renin activity and blood pressure in patients with longstanding reflux nephropathy. *Arch Dis Child* 1987;62:678.

168. Jacobson SH, Kjellstrend CM, Lins LE. Role of hypervolaemia and renin in the blood pressure control of patients with pyelonephritic renal scarring. *Acta Med Scand* 1988; 224:47.
169. Holland NH, Kotchen T, Bhathena D. Hypertension in children with chronic pyelonephritis. *Kidney Int* 1975;8:S-243.
170. Luscher TF, Wanner C, Hauri D, et al. Curable renal parenchymatous hypertension: current diagnosis and management. *Cardiology* 1985;72(Suppl 1):33–45.
171. Dillon MJ, Smellie JM. Peripheral plasma renin activity, hypertension and renal scarring in children. *Contrib Nephrol* 1984;39:68.
172. Laberton RP, Noth RH, Glickman M. Frequent falsely negative renal vein renin test in unilateral renal parenchymal disease. *J Urol* 1981;125:477.
173. Bailey RR, Lynn KL, McRae CU, et al. Prospective randomised study of the effect of nephrectomy on blood pressure of patients with unilateral reflux nephropathy. In: Bailey RR, ed. *Second CJ Hodson Symposium on Reflux Nephropathy.* Christchurch, NZ: Design Printing Services, 1991: 37–40.
174. Arant BS Jr. Vesicoureteric reflux and renal injury. *Am J Kidney Dis* 1991;17:491.
175. Salvatierra O, Tanagho EA. Reflux as a cause of end stage kidney disease: report of 32 cases. *J Urol* 1977;117:441.
176. Bailey RR, Lynn KL, Buttimore AL, et al. End-stage reflux nephropathy. In: Bailey RR, ed. *Second CJ Hodson Symposium on Reflux Nephropathy.* Christchurch, NZ: Design Printing Services, 1991:49–52.
177. Disney APS. Reflux nephropathy in Australia and New Zealand: prevalence, incidence and management: 1975–1989. In: Bailey RR, ed. *Second CJ Hodson Symposium on Reflux Nephropathy.* Christchurch, NZ: Design Printing Services, 1991:53–56.
178. Bailey RR, Lynn KL, Robson RA. End-stage reflux nephropathy. *Ren Fail* 1994;16:27–35.
179. Zimmerman SW, Uehling DT, Burkholder PM. Vesicoureteral reflux nephropathy: evidence for immunologically mediated glomerular injury. *Urology* 1973;2:534–538.
180. Torres VE, Velosa JA, Holley KE, et al. Progression of vesicoureteral reflux nephropathy. *Ann Intern Med* 1980;92:776–784.
181. Bhathena DB, Weiss JH, Holland NH, et al. Focal and segmental glomerulosclerosis in reflux nephropathy (chronic pyelonephritis). *Am J Med* 1980;68:886.
182. Senekjian HO, Stinebaugh BJ, Mattioli CA, et al. Irreversible renal failure following vesicoureteral reflux. *JAMA* 1979;241:160.
183. Berger RE, Ansell JS, Shurtleff DB, et al. Vesicoureteral reflux in children with uremia: prognostic indicators for treatment and survival. *JAMA* 1981;246:56–59.
184. Weaver E, Craswell P. Pregnancy outcome in women with reflux nephropathy: a review of experience at the Royal Women's Hospital Brisbane, 1977–1986. *Aust N Z J Obstet Gynaecol* 1987;27:106.
185. Becker GJ, Ihle BU, Fairley KF, et al. Effect of pregnancy on moderate renal failure and reflux nephropathy. *BMJ* 1986; 292:796.
186. Kincaid-Smith P, Fairley KF. Renal disease in pregnancy. Three controversial issues: mesangial IgA nephropathy, focal glomerular sclerosis (focal and segmental hyalinosis and sclerosis), and reflux nephropathy. *Am J Kidney Dis* 1987;9:328.
187. Kincaid-Smith P. Glomerular lesions and atrophic pyelonephritis in reflux nephropathy. *Kidney Int* 1975;8:S-81.
188. Konda R, Sakal K, Ota S, et al. Followup study of renal function in children with reflux nephropathy after resolution of vesicoureteral reflux. *J Urol* 1997;157:975–979.
189. Assadi FK. Urinary β_2-microglobulin as a marker for vesicoureteral reflux. *Pediatr Nephrol* 1996;10:642–644.
190. Tomlinson PA, Smellie JM, Prescod N, et al. Differential excretion of urinary proteins in children with vesicoureteric reflux and reflux nephropathy. *Pediatr Nephrol* 1994;8:21–25.
191. Miyakita H, Puri P. Urinary levels of N-acetyl-β-D-glucosaminidase: a simple marker for predicting tubular damage in higher grades of vesicoureteric reflux. *Eur Urol* 1994;25:135–137.
192. Cotran RS. Glomerulosclerosis in reflux nephropathy. *Kidney Int* 1982;21:528–534.
193. Steinhardt GF. Reflux nephropathy. *J Urol* 1985;134:855.
194. Morita M, Yoshiara S, White RHR, et al. The glomerular changes in children with reflux nephropathy. *J Pathol* 1990; 162:245.
195. Arant BS. Inhibition of angiotensin converting enzyme (ACE) alters the clinical course of reflux nephropathy. Presented at the International Workshop on Reflux and Pyelonephritis. Tulane Regional Primate Research Center. Covington, LA Oct. 24–25, 1991.
196. Smellie JM, Edwards D, Normand ICS. Effect of vesicoureteral reflux on renal growth in children with urinary tract infection. *Arch Dis Child* 1981;56:593.
197. Greenfield SP, Management of vesicoureteral reflux in children. *Curr Urol Rep* 2001;2:113–121.
198. Hanson E, Hansson S, Jodal U. Trimethoprim-sulfadiazine prophylaxis in children with vesicoureteral reflux. *Scand J Infect Dis* 1989;21:201–204.
199. Smith EM, Elder JS. Double antimicrobial prophylaxis in girls with breakthrough urinary tract infections. *Urology* 1994;43:712–713.
200. Atwell JD, Vijay MR. Renal growth following reimplantation of the ureters for reflux. *Br J Urol* 1978;50:367.
201. Birmingham Reflux Study Group. Prospective trial of operative vs. nonoperative treatment of severe vesicoureteral reflux: five year observation. *BMJ* 1987;295:237–241.
202. Goldraich NP, Goldraich IH. Follow-up of conservatively treated children with high and low grade vesicoureteral reflux: prospective study. *J Urol* 1992;148(2):1683–1687.
203. Wikstad I, Claesson I, Olbing H, et al. Renal mass under medical vs surgical treatment in the European branch. Presented at the International Workshop on Reflux and Pyelonephritis, Covington, LA, Oct. 24–25, 1991.
204. Merrell RW, Mowad JJ. Increased physical growth after successful antireflux operation. *J Urol* 1979;122;523.
205. Sutton R, Atwell JD. Physical growth velocity during conservative treatment and following subsequent surgical treatment for primary vesicoureteric reflux. *Br J Urol* 1989;63:245.
206. Smellie JM, Priece MA, Patton AM. Normal somatic growth in children receiving low-dose prophylactic cotrimoxazole. *Eur J Pediatr* 1983;140:301.
207. Polito C, La Manna A, Capacchione A, et al. Height and weight in children with vesicoureteric reflux and renal scarring. *Pediatr Nephrol* 1996;10:564–567.

208. Guizar JM, Kornhauser C, Malacara JM, et al. Renal tubular acidosis in children with vesicoureteral reflux. *J Urol* 1996;156:193–195.
209. Rushton HG. Wetting and functional voiding disorders. *Urol Clin North Am* 1995;22:75–94.
210. Sugar EC, Firlit CF. Urodynamic feedback: a new therapeutic approach for childhood incontinence/infection (vesical voluntary sphincter dyssynergia). *J Urol* 1982;128:1253.
211. Elo J, Tallgren LG, Alfthan O, et al. Character of urinary tract infections and pyelonephritic renal scarring after antireflux surgery. *J Urol* 1983;129:343.
212. Aggarwal VK, Verrier-Jones K, Asscher AW, et al. Covert bacteriuria: long term follow-up. *Arch Dis Child* 1991;66:1284.
213. Hansson SA, Jodal U, Noren L, et al. Untreated bacteriuria in asymptomatic girls with renal scarring. *Pediatrics* 1989; 84:964.
214. Linshaw M. Asymptomatic bacteriuria and vesicoureteral reflux in children. *Kidney Int* 1996;50:312–329.
215. Wan J, Greenfield SP, Talley M, et al. An analysis of social and economic factors associated with followup of patients with vesicoureteral reflux. *J Urol* 1996;156:668–672.
216. Parrott TS, Woodard JR, Wolbert JJ. Ureteral tailoring: a comparison of wedge resection with infolding. *J Urol* 1990; 144:328.
217. McLorie GA, McKenna PH, Jumper BM, et al. High grade vesicoureteral reflux: analysis of observational therapy. *J Urol* 1990;144:537.
218. McGladdery SL, Aparicio S, Verrier-Jones K, et al. Outcome of pregnancy in an Oxford-Cardiff cohort of women with previous bacteriuria. *QJM* 1992;83(303):533–599.
219. Martinell J, Jodal U, Lidin-Janson G. Pregnancies in women with and without renal scarring after urinary infections in childhood. *BMJ* 1990;300(6728):840–844.
220. Romero R, Oyarzun E, Mazor M, et al. Meta-analysis of the relationship between asymptomatic bacteriuria and preterm delivery/low birth weight. *Obstet Gynecol* 1989;73:576–582.
221. Gilstrap LC, Leveno KJ, Cunningham FG, et al. Renal infection and pregnancy outcome. *Am J Obstet Gynecol* 1981; 141:709–716.
222. Fan YD, Pastorek JG, Miller JM Jr, et al. Acute pyelonephritis in pregnancy. *Am J Perinatol* 1987;4:324–326.
223. el-Khatib M, Packham DK, Becker GJ, et al. Pregnancy-related complications in women with reflux nephropathy. *Clin Nephrol* 1994;41:50–55.
224. Mansfield JT, Snow BW, Cartwright PC, et al. Complications of pregnancy in women after childhood reimplantation for vesicoureteral reflux: an update with 25 years of follow-up. *J Urol* 1995;154:787.
225. Belman AB. A perspective on vesicoureteral reflux. *Urol Clin North Am* 1995;22:139–150.
226. Matouchek E. Die behandlung des vesikorenalen reflukes durch transurethrale einspritzung von Teflonpaste. *Urologe* 1981;20:263.
227. O'Donnell B, Puri P. Endoscopic correction of primary vesicoureteric reflux. *Br J Urol* 1986;58:601.
228. Puri P, Ninan GK, Suranda R. Subureteric Teflon injection (STING). Results of a European survey. *Eur Urol* 1995; 27:71–75.
229. Dewan PA, O'Donnell B. Polytef paste injection of refluxing duplex ureters. *Eur Urol* 1991;19:35.
230. Merckx L, De Boe V, Braeckman J, et al. Endoscopic submucosal Teflon injection (STING): an alternative treatment of vesicoureteric reflux in children. *Eur J Pediatr Surg* 1995; 5:34–36.
231. Steinbrecher HA, Edwards B, Malone PS. The STING in the refluxing duplex system. *Br J Urol* 1995;76:165–168.
232. Puri P, Guiney EJ. Endoscopic correction of vesicoureteric reflux secondary to neuropathic bladder. *Br J Urol* 1986; 58:504.
233. Dewar PA, Guiney EJ. Endoscopic correction of vesicoureteric reflux in children with spina bifida. *Br J Urol* 1990;65:646.
234. Puri P. Endoscopic correction of primary vesicoureteric reflux by subureteric injection of polytetrafluoroethylene. *Lancet* 1990;335:1320.
235. Malizia AA Jr, Reiman HM, Myers RP, et al. Migration and granulomatous reaction after periurethral injection of Polytef (Teflon). *JAMA* 1984;251:3277.
236. Malizia AA, Rushton HG, Woodard JR, et al. Migration and granulomatous reaction after intravesical/subureteric injection of Polytef (Abstract 74). *J Urol* 1987;137(2):122A.
237. Mittleman RE, Marracini JV. Pulmonary Teflon granulomas following periurethral Teflon injection for urinary incontinence. *Arch Pathol Lab Med* 1983;107:611.
238. Claes H, Stroobants D, Van Meerbeck JV, et al. Pulmonary migration following periurethral polytetrafluoroethylene injection for urinary incontinence. *J Urol* 1989;142:821.
239. Brown S, Stewart RJ, O'Hara MD, et al. Histological changes following submucosal Teflon injection in the bladder. *J Pediatr Surg* 1991;26:546.
240. Leonard MP, Canning DA, Peters CA, et al. Endoscopic injection of glutaraldehyde cross-linked bovine dermal collagen for correction of vesicoureteral reflux. *J Urol* 1991; 145:115.
241. Frey P, Lutz, Jenny P, et al. Endoscopic subureteral collagen injection for the treatment of vesicoureteral reflux in infants and children. *J Urol* 1995;154:804–807.
242. Gordjani N, Frankenschmidt A, Zimmerhackl LB, et al. Subureteral collagen injection versus antireflux surgery in primary vesico-ureteral reflux grade III. *Eur J Pediatr* 1996; 155:491–494.
243. Reunanen M. Correction of vesicoureteral reflux in children by endoscopic collagen injection: a prospective study. *J Urol* 1995;154:2156–2158.
244. Leonard MP, Canning DA, Epstein JI, et al. Local tissue reaction to the subureteral injection of glutaraldehyde cross-linked bovine collagen in humans. *J Urol* 1990;143: 1209.

55

OBSTRUCTIVE UROPATHY

ROBERT L. CHEVALIER
JONATHAN A. ROTH

Urinary tract obstruction initiates a complex sequence of events resulting in impaired renal function (1). In early development, chronic urinary tract obstruction impairs renal growth and development. In view of its clinical importance, the pathophysiology of urinary tract obstruction has been studied intensively, leading to the development of numerous experimental models, including complete and partial ureteral obstruction, unilateral and bilateral obstruction, and acute and chronic obstruction. Most experiments have been performed in adult animals; therefore, comparisons with obstructive nephropathy in human infants and children must be made with caution. In this chapter, attention is focused on studies of the effects of urinary tract obstruction on the developing kidney and are compared to those in the adult. The functional effects of obstruction are directly dependent on the cellular responses, with the resultant effects on renal growth. The latter are of particular importance in the period of rapid somatic growth.

EFFECTS OF URINARY TRACT OBSTRUCTION ON RENAL GROWTH AND MATURATION

Unlike the human and guinea pig, in which nephrogenesis is completed before parturition, only 10% of nephrons are present in the rat at birth, with the remainder being formed by 14 days of age (2). Thus, the early postnatal period in the rat may be analogous to the midgestational period in the human. The rat, therefore, serves as a model for urinary tract obstruction during the critical period of rapid nephrogenesis.

A number of studies indicate that the developing kidney is uniquely susceptible to impaired growth from chronic ipsilateral unilateral ureteral obstruction (UUO). Complete UUO in the neonatal rat impairs the normal maturational increase in renal mass and DNA content of the ipsilateral kidney (Fig. 55.1A) (3). In the adult, in contrast, kidney DNA content is significantly increased by UUO (4). Chronic UUO in the neonatal rat results in prolonged renal expression of Wnt-4 and impairs the normal differentiation of mesenchyme to epithelium (5). Three weeks of partial UUO in the neonatal rat increases interstitial collagen deposition (primarily types I, III, and V), with an increase in type IV in the thickened and tortuous tubular basement membrane (6). The quantity of collagen deposited is directly correlated with the degree of pelvic distention (6).

Number of Nephrons

In both human studies and animal models, fetal and neonatal urinary tract obstruction is associated with a significant reduction in nephron number. Two days of UUO in the fetal rabbit reduces the number of nephrons by one-third, whereas UUO in the fetal sheep can decrease the number of nephrons by 50% (7–9). In the human fetus, urinary tract obstruction also reduces the number of nephrons (10). After partial UUO in neonatal pigs, the number of glomeruli is reduced by 28% (11). Either partial or complete UUO in the neonatal rat decreases the number of nephrons, with the magnitude of reduction being dependent on the duration of obstruction (12,13). Interestingly, UUO in the neonatal rat in the period immediately after the completion of nephrogenesis also significantly reduces the number of nephrons, most likely owing to massive cystic tubular dilatation that compresses neighboring nephrons (13). Severe tubular dilatation also contributes to nephron loss in human obstructive nephropathy (14).

Renal Vascular Development

Chronic UUO in the neonatal rat leads to a marked increase in renal renin expression and persistence of the fetal pattern of renin distribution (Figs. 55.1B and 55.2B) (3,15). It is now clear that renin expression by the renal microvasculature is a marker of vascular immaturity rather than of terminal differentiation (16). As described in Glomerular Development, relief of obstruction reduces the extent of renin distribution along afferent arterioles of the neonatal rat (17) and normalizes the renin content of the postobstructed kidney of the neonatal guinea pig (18).

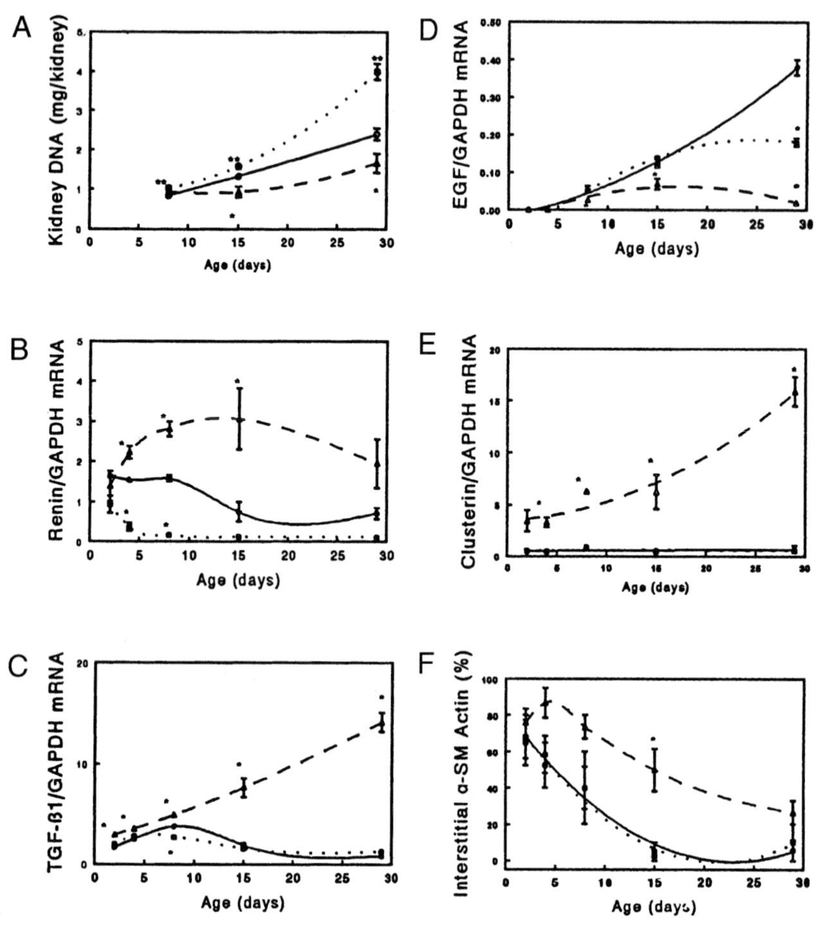

FIGURE 55.1. Effects of unilateral ureteral obstruction on the kidney of the neonatal rat: relation to postnatal age. **A:** Kidney DNA contents. **B:** Relative abundance of renal renin messenger RNA (mRNA). **C:** Relative abundance of renal transforming growth factor β1 (TGF-β1) mRNA. **D:** Relative abundance of renal prepro-epidermal growth factor (EGF) mRNA. **E:** Relative abundance of renal clusterin mRNA. **F:** Relative distribution of renal immunoreactive α-smooth muscle (α-SM) actin. Dashed line, kidney subjected to unilateral ureteral obstruction at birth; dotted line, intact opposite kidney; GAPDH, glyceraldehyde phosphate dehydrogenase; solid line, sham-operated rats. (From Chung KH, Chevalier RL. Arrested development of the neonatal kidney following chronic ureteral obstruction. *J Urol* 1996;155:1139–1144; and Chevalier RL. Growth factors and apoptosis in neonatal ureteral obstruction. *J Am Soc Nephrol* 1996;7:1098–1105, with permission.)

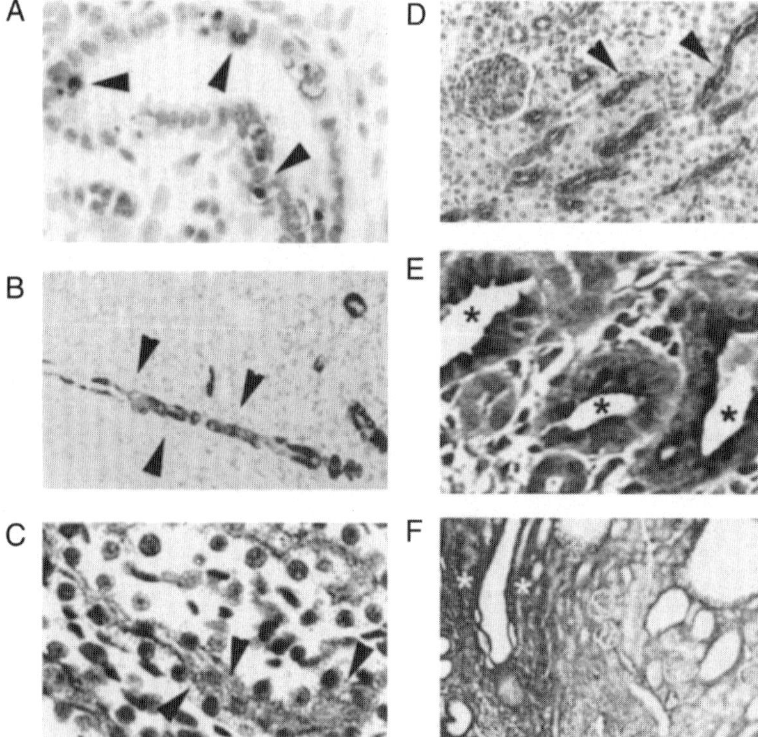

FIGURE 55.2. Effects of unilateral ureteral obstruction on the kidney of the neonatal rat. **A:** Apoptotic renal tubular epithelial cells (*arrowheads*) in 3-day-old rat kidney, subjected to ipsilateral ureteral obstruction since birth. **B:** Immunoreactive renin along the length of an interlobular renal artery (*arrowheads*). **C:** Immunoreactive transforming growth factor β1 (*arrowheads*) is increased in tubules of 14-day-old rat subjected to ipsilateral ureteral obstruction since birth. **D:** Immunoreactive epidermal growth factor (*arrowheads*) is decreased in tubules of 14-day-old rat subjected to ipsilateral ureteral obstruction since birth. **E:** Immunoreactive clusterin (*asterisks*) is increased in tubules of 14-day-old rat subjected to ipsilateral ureteral obstruction since birth. **F:** Immunoreactive α-smooth muscle actin (*asterisks*) is increased in the interstitium of 14-day-old rat subjected to ipsilateral ureteral obstruction since birth. (**A–D** From Chung KH, Chevalier RL. Arrested development of the neonatal kidney following chronic ureteral obstruction. *J Urol* 1996;155:1139–1144; Chevalier RL, Chung KH, Smith CD, et al. Renal apoptosis and clusterin following ureteral obstruction: the role of maturation. *J Urol* 1996;156:1474–1479; and Chevalier RL. Growth factors and apoptosis in neonatal ureteral obstruction. *J Am Soc Nephrol* 1996;7:1098–1105, with permission.)

Glomerular Development

After the induction of glomeruli, glomerular capillaries increase in number, associated with flattening of podocytes and increasing surface area for filtration (19). Chronic UUO in the neonatal rat either during nephrogenesis or during the subsequent maturational phase delays glomerular maturation (13,17)—a response that can be prevented by the administration of exogenous epidermal growth factor (EGF) (20).

Tubular Development

Tubular maturation can be measured by the progressive disappearance of markers normally expressed only in early development, such as Wnt-4 and clusterin (glycoproteins) (5,21) or KS (a kidney-specific gene with unknown function) (22). Chronic UUO in the neonatal rat leads to persistent tubular expression of clusterin (Figs. 55.1E and 55.2E), Wnt-4 (5), and KS (4,22). In addition, chronic UUO in the neonatal rat suppresses the normal maturational increase in tubular expression of EGF (Figs. 55.1D and 55.2D) (3), whereas administration of exogenous EGF reduces clusterin expression (23).

Renal Interstitial Development

The normal maturation of renal interstitial fibroblasts is reflected by the transformation of myofibroblasts to fibroblasts, such that fibroblasts lose their expression of vimentin and α-smooth muscle actin (24). Chronic UUO in the neonatal rat causes prolonged expression of α-smooth muscle actin by interstitial fibroblasts (Figs. 55.1F and 55.2F) (3), and dilated tubules from infants with severe congenital obstructive nephropathy are also surrounded by myofibroblasts (25).

Summary

The effects of chronic UUO on maturation of the developing kidney are shown in Figure 55.3. During normal renal development, nephrogenesis proceeds with increasing numbers of glomeruli and progressive glomerular maturation with proliferation of capillary loops. The maturing renal vasculature is characterized by the disappearance of renin from the length of the afferent arteriole, such that its localization is restricted to the juxtaglomerular region. Tubular maturation is reflected by the disappearance of vimentin and the increasing expression of EGF, whereas interstitial fibroblasts lose their expression of α-smooth muscle actin and vimentin. Chronic UUO causes a delayed or arrested maturation of the entire nephron.

ROLE OF APOPTOSIS

Urinary tract obstruction results in distal tubular epithelial cell apoptosis, characterized by condensed chromatin and cytoplasmic blebs (Fig. 55.2A) (26,27). UUO in the neonatal rat results in greater ipsilateral renal apoptosis compared to the adult (4). This may account at least in part for the fall in renal DNA content in the neonatal kidney (Fig. 55.1A) (4). Apoptosis has also been reported in renal tubules of fetuses and infants with obstructive nephropathy (28,29). Because renal tubular apoptosis leads to tubular atrophy (26), attention has focused on factors regulating apoptosis in the hydronephrotic kidney.

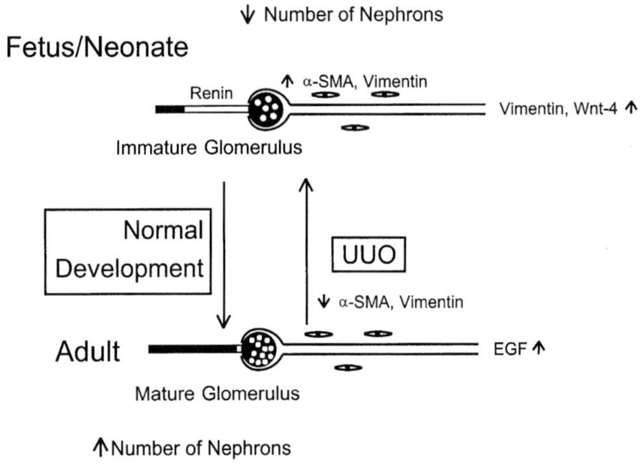

FIGURE 55.3. Effects of unilateral ureteral obstruction (UUO) on the developing kidney. The fetal/neonatal nephron is shown in the upper panel and the adult nephron in the lower panel. With normal maturation, the number of nephrons increases, and the glomeruli develop increased numbers of capillary loops. In addition, whereas renin extends along the afferent arteriole in the fetal kidney, renin is localized to the juxtaglomerular region of the mature kidney. During maturation, renal tubular vimentin and Wnt-4 expression disappears, and epidermal growth factor (EGF) expression increases. Whereas fetal interstitial fibroblasts express vimentin and α-smooth muscle actin (α-SMA), fibroblasts normally lose these markers with maturation. As a consequence of chronic UUO, the immature pattern of renal development persists. (Adapted from Chevalier RL. Molecular and cellular pathophysiology of obstructive nephropathy. *Pediatr Nephrol* 1999;13:612–619.)

Chronic UUO in the neonatal mouse results in necrosis of renal proximal tubular cells and apoptosis of distal tubular and collecting duct cells (30). Because proximal tubules undergo significant hypoxia after UUO, it is likely that necrosis of this tubular segment is consequent to decreased oxygen tension, as is the case after ischemic acute renal failure. Whereas the proximal tubule undergoes minimal dilatation after UUO, the collecting duct is significantly dilated (30). Moreover, tubular apoptosis is directly related to the magnitude of dilatation. Because apoptosis can be triggered by mechanical stretch of tubular cells and is proportional to the magnitude of axial strain, it is likely that the greater compliance of distal tubules contributes to the greater apoptosis of this tubular segment.

Growth Factors

Ureteral obstruction in the adult rat decreases the expression of ipsilateral renal prepro-EGF (31,32). Although EGF does not appear in the kidney until after birth (33), it

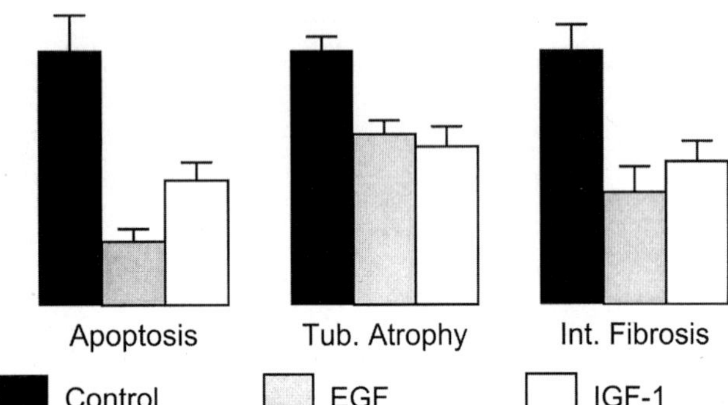

FIGURE 55.4. Relative renal tubular apoptosis, tubular (Tub.) atrophy, and interstitial (Int.) fibrosis in 1-week-old rats subjected to unilateral ureteral obstruction in the first 48 hours of life. The results have been normalized to control animals receiving vehicle injections (*black bars*). Experimental groups of rats received daily injections of epidermal growth factor (EGF, *gray bars*), or insulin-like growth factor-1 (IGF-1, *white bars*). For each parameter, experimental groups differ significantly from controls. (Data from Chevalier RL, Goyal S, Wolstenholme JT, et al. Obstructive nephropathy in the neonate is attenuated by epidermal growth factor. *Kidney Int* 1998;54:38–47; and Chevalier RL, Goyal S, Kim A, et al. Renal tubulointerstitial injury from ureteral obstruction in the neonatal rat is attenuated by IGF-1. *Kidney Int* 2000;57:882–890.)

is likely that activation of the EGF receptor plays a role in perinatal renal development (34). The normal developmental increase in renal EGF expression is prevented by ipsilateral UUO in the neonatal rat (Figs. 55.1D and 55.2D) (3). Administration of exogenous EGF to neonatal rats with UUO decreases tubular apoptosis in the obstructed kidney by 80% (Fig. 55.4) (23). In addition, EGF treatment reduces clusterin expression by renal tubular cells and significantly reduces tubular atrophy (23). Moreover, short-term administration of EGF markedly attenuates both tubular and interstitial renal injury 1 month after the release of UUO in the neonatal rat (35). Although the renal expression of insulin-like growth factor-1 (IGF-1) or its receptor is not altered by UUO in the neonatal rat, the administration of exogenous IGF-1, like EGF, significantly reduces renal tubular apoptosis, tubular atrophy, and interstitial fibrosis (36) (Fig. 55.4). Chronic UUO induces transient tubular expression of heparin-binding EGF, which can be induced in tubular cells subjected to stretch (37). Because heparin-binding EGF is also antiapoptotic, it is likely that expression of this growth factor serves to minimize apoptotic damage in the hydronephrotic kidney.

The mechanism whereby growth factors reduce apoptosis in the hydronephrotic kidney has been localized to the phosphorylation state of BAD, a pro-apoptotic molecule. When stretched, rat tubular cells undergo apoptosis, which can be reduced by 50% by treatment with either EGF or IGF-1 (38). Either UUO *in vivo* or cell stretch *in vitro* decreases tubular cell BAD phosphorylation, which is inhibited by the growth factors (38). As shown in Figure 55.5, when dephosphorylated, BAD dissociates from cytoplasmic chaperone proteins and complexes with BclX on

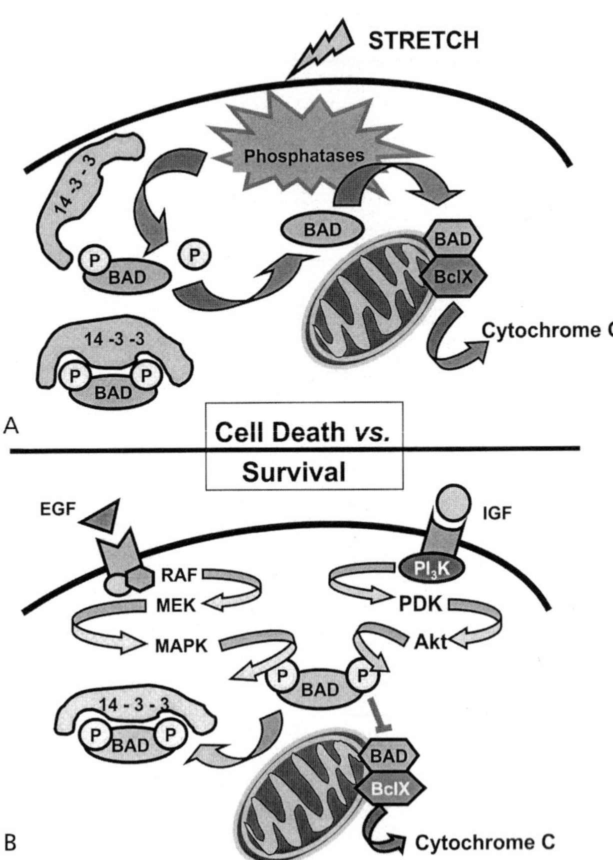

FIGURE 55.5. Shifting the balance between cell death and survival. **A:** Mechanical stretch injury induces activation of phosphatases, which dephosphorylate BAD, causing it to dissociate from chaperone proteins. Dephosphorylated BAD then forms a complex with BclX on the outer mitochondrial membrane, leading to release of cytochrome C into the cytoplasm, initiating apoptosis. **B:** The administration of growth factors [epidermal growth factor (EGF) or insulin-like growth factor-1 (IGF-1)], increases MAPK and Akt kinase activity to levels that compensate for the stretch-induced phosphatase action on BAD. As a result, BAD is phosphorylated and sequestered by the chaperone proteins to maintain cell survival. [From Kiley SC, Thornhill BA, Tang SS, et al. Growth factor-mediated phosphorylation of propapoptotic BAD reduces tubule cell death *in vitro* and *in vivo*. *Kidney Int* 2003;63(1):33–42, with permission.]

the mitochondrial membrane, resulting in the release of cytochrome C and the initiation of apoptosis. EGF and IGF-1 activate their respective kinases to maintain BAD phosphorylation and thereby increase cell survival.

Although transforming growth factor β1 (TGF-β1) is generally considered a fibrogenic cytokine (see Fibroblasts and Transforming Growth Factor-β), it also plays a significant role in promoting apoptosis in the hydronephrotic kidney (39). Stretching of tubular epithelial cells stimulates their expression of TGF-β1 and induces their apoptosis—a response that can be inhibited by antibody to TGF-β1 (40). The stretch-induced apoptotic response may, therefore, result at least in part from increased production of this pro-apoptotic cytokine. The action of TGF-β1 can be attenuated by an endogenous renal proteoglycan, decorin.

Mice lacking a functional decorin gene manifest increased tubular apoptosis and tubular atrophy after UUO (41).

Other Molecules Modulating Apoptosis

Chronic UUO induces the renal expression of a number of apoptosis-promoting molecules, including Fas, Fas ligand, tumor necrosis factor-R1, TRAIL, TRADD, RIP, caspases, FADD, and FAP (42,43). The rise and fall of expression of these molecules parallel changes in renal apoptosis in the hydronephrotic kidney. The presence of a nonfunctioning Fas receptor in C57B16/lpr mice reduces distal tubular apoptosis resulting from chronic UUO (44). Similarly, p53-deficient mice exhibit a significant reduction in apoptosis after UUO (45). These findings underscore the importance of apoptosis-regulatory molecules in the hydronephrotic kidney. Complete UUO in the fetal opossum kidney induces tubular apoptosis that is associated with an increase in Bax, a pro-apoptotic molecule, and a decrease in Bcl-2, an antiapoptotic molecule (46). In the neonatal rat subjected to UUO, renal tubular Bcl-2 expression is reduced in dilated apoptotic tubules but not in nondilated tubules (47). This is consistent with endogenous Bcl-2 normally inhibiting tubular apoptosis, which is dysregulated in the obstructed kidney.

While tubular cells themselves generate molecules regulating their own apoptosis, infiltrating cells can do so as well. Chronic UUO in mice deficient in selectin (an adhesion molecule) leads to reduced interstitial macrophage infiltration, along with decreased tubular apoptosis and tubular atrophy (48). The tubular cell apoptosis is due to soluble factors released by macrophages adjacent to the tubules in the hydronephrotic kidney.

In 1997, the sphingolipid ceramide was shown to induce apoptosis in the kidney (49). The very high prevalence of renal apoptosis in the developing rat is associated with similarly elevated levels of intrarenal ceramide, and both ceramide production and endogenous renal apoptosis decrease to adult levels during the first month of life (50). Prolonged UUO in the neonatal rat (but not the adult rat) increases endogenous renal ceramide and likely contributes to the prolonged renal apoptotic response of the neonatal obstructed kidney (51).

Summary

As shown in Figure 55.6, the regulation of tubular apoptosis in the hydronephrotic kidney is extremely complex and represents a balance between factors promoting apoptosis and countering survival factors. Stimuli for apoptosis include mechanical stretching of tubular cells, which results from the initial increase in hydrostatic pressure in a compliant tubular segment. Infiltrating macrophages contribute to apoptosis of tubular cells. Enhanced renal production of ceramide may also contribute to the increased susceptibility of the developing kidney to apoptosis. Apoptosis can be activated by TGF-β1, FAS, p53, or caspases. In contrast, growth factors such as EGF, IGF-1, hepatocyte growth factor, and heparin-bound EGF can inhibit apoptosis and tilt the balance in favor of survival. A better understanding of the renal cell biology of apoptosis should lead to improved means of preserving renal mass in patients with obstructive nephropathy.

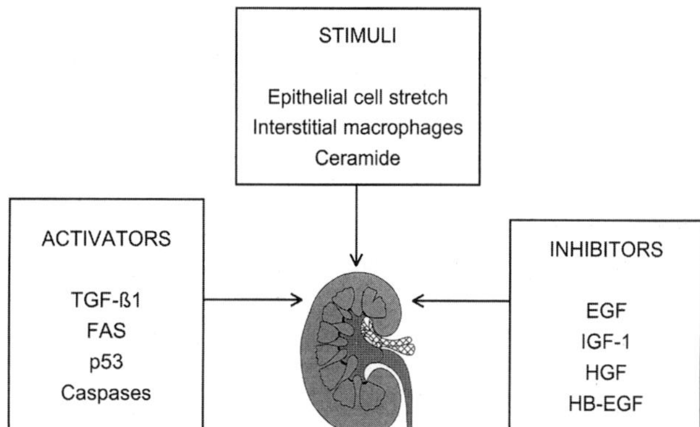

FIGURE 55.6. Regulation of apoptosis in the hydronephrotic kidney. Renal tubular cell apoptosis is enhanced by a variety of stimuli in the immature hydronephrotic kidney, including mechanical stretch of dilated tubular segments, release of pro-apoptotic molecules by infiltrating macrophages, and increased renal generation of ceramide. The ultimate fate of the cell is decided by the balance of signals mediating cell death [transforming growth factor β1 (TGF-β1), FAS, p53, caspases], and those acting as survival factors [epidermal growth factor (EGF), insulin-like growth factor-1 (IGF-1), hepatocyte growth factor (HGF), and heparin-bound epidermal growth factor (HB-EGF)].

INTERSTITIAL INFILTRATION AND FIBROSIS

After UUO in the adult rat, the renal interstitium of the ipsilateral kidney is infiltrated with leukocytes, beginning after 4 hours and becoming maximal at 24 hours (52). The cells produce a variety of vasoactive compounds, including prostaglandins, thromboxanes, and leukotrienes (53,54).

Macrophages

Although lymphocyte infiltration is not required for progressive tubular atrophy and interstitial fibrosis after UUO (55), macrophages appear to play a major role. Adhesion molecules, such as selectins, play a significant role in localizing macrophages to the renal interstitium in the developing kidney subjected to UUO (48). The macrophages, in turn, induce apoptosis of adjacent tubular epithelial cells (48). Infiltrating macrophages may produce tissue inhibitors of metalloproteinase, which in turn prevent degradation of extracellular matrix (56,57). After partial UUO in juvenile rats, renal expression of monocyte chemoattractant protein-1 is increased (58). Because urinary excretion follows renal expression of monocyte chemoattractant protein-1, and levels parallel the severity of obstruction, this molecule shows promise as a prognostic marker for infants and children with congenital hydronephrosis (59). Moreover, therapeutic inhibition of such chemokines may attenuate interstitial cellular influx and interstitial fibrosis in the hydronephrotic kidney (60,61). Whereas plasminogen activator inhibitor-1 contributes to interstitial fibrosis resulting from UUO (62,63), tissue inhibitor of metalloproteinase-1 does not (64).

Fibroblasts and Transforming Growth Factor-β

The source of interstitial fibroblasts appearing in the obstructed kidney is not clear at this time. Possibilities include proliferation of resident interstitial fibroblasts, pericytes, or transdifferentiation of renal tubular epithelial cells (65). Myofibroblast transformation, in which fibroblasts express α-smooth muscle actin, takes place in the interstitium of the obstructed kidney (66). Whereas α-smooth muscle actin normally disappears from the interstitium in the neonatal rat, this process is delayed by ipsilateral UUO (3). Myofibroblasts appear to be involved in extracellular matrix accumulation (67) and may play a role in the enhanced contractility of the renal cortex after UUO (68).

TGF-β1, a cytokine, stimulates extracellular matrix synthesis, inhibits its degradation, and induces the expression of α-smooth muscle actin in myofibroblasts (69,70). It is possible that expression of α-smooth muscle actin by fibroblasts is controlled by the increased generation of TGF-β1 in the obstructed kidney (66,67,71). TGF-β1 has been localized to renal tubular epithelial cells (72) and renal interstitial cells (73,74). Chronic UUO results in a significant increase in renal TGF-β1 expression (Figs. 55.1C and 55.2C) (3,32,72,73). TGF-β1 inhibits collagen degradation, and UUO results in a tenfold reduction in interstitial collagenolytic activity (75). Administration of a cyclooxygenase-2 inhibitor reduces TGF-β1 and interstitial fibrosis in the obstructed kidney (76). The role of TGF-β1 in mediating renal interstitial fibrosis after UUO has been elegantly demonstrated by the introduction of TGF-β1 antisense oligodeoxynucleotides into interstitial fibroblasts (77). Administration of exogenous hepatocyte growth factor to mice with UUO markedly reduces endogenous TGF-β1 expression, myofibroblast activation, and interstitial fibrosis in the hydronephrotic kidney (78,79). Although it appears likely that apoptosis of renal tubular epithelial cells contributes to the development of tubular atrophy, apoptosis may also be beneficial in countering fibrosis by clearing myofibroblasts from the interstitium (80,81). Although interstitial cells play a role in progressive interstitial fibrosis resulting from UUO, tubular cells also contribute to the fibrotic process. Administration of osteogenic protein-1 inhibits tubular apoptosis in rats with UUO, as well as inhibiting interstitial cellular infiltration (82).

Oxidative Stress

As a consequence of UUO, oxidative stress increases in the renal interstitium of the hydronephrotic kidney (83). Inhibition of oxidative stress reduces interstitial fibrosis resulting from UUO (84). After UUO, endogenous renal antioxidant enzyme activity is reduced (85). Whereas sodium depletion stimulates renal antioxidant enzyme production in the intact kidney, UUO inhibits this normal adaptive response (85). The impaired antioxidant production by the hydronephrotic kidney is a maladaptive response that presumably contributes to the progressive renal injury resulting from urinary tract obstruction.

RENIN-ANGIOTENSIN SYSTEM

Cellular and Molecular Role of Angiotensin in Hydronephrosis

The increased generation of a pressor material in the kidney with ipsilateral UUO has been known for more than 50 years. Beckwith reported that extracts of kidneys from rats with UUO induce hypertension when injected into normal animals (86). More recent detailed studies of the intrarenal renin-angiotensin system have been performed in rats subjected to complete UUO during the first 48 hours of life. In contrast to kidneys from sham-operated rats, in which 55% of juxtaglomerular apparatuses contain immunoreactive renin, the fraction is increased to approximately 75% of glomeruli in kidneys of 4-week-old rats with chronic ipsilateral UUO (15). Moreover, in contrast to the pattern of distribution in sham-operated rats, in which immunoreactive renin is localized to the juxtaglomerular apparatus, renin protein extends along the length of the afferent arteriole of 4-week-old rats with UUO (Fig. 55.2B) (15). This pattern is similar to that of the late gestational normal rat fetus (87). While renal renin content is increased in the kidney with ipsilateral UUO, it is suppressed in the intact opposite kidney (15). In contrast to the neonate, UUO in the adult rat does not result in redistribution of immunoreactive renin along the renal microvasculature.

Studies of renin secretion *in vivo* or in isolated perfused kidneys generally rely on measurements of plasma renin activity. The hemolytic plaque assay, however, permits direct measurement of hormone secretion by isolated cells (88). This technique has been used to determine whether renin secretion is increased by cortical cells from the rat kidney with ipsilateral UUO since birth. Rather than there being an increased amount of renin secretion per cell, the obstructed neonatal rat kidney demonstrates a recruitment of cortical cells secreting renin (89). It is likely that the enhanced secretion results from the increased transcription and storage of renin in the microvasculature of the immature kidney.

After acute UUO in the adult rat, renin expression is increased after only 1 hour (90). After 24 hours of UUO in the adult rat, blood vessels of the postobstructed kidney overexpress angiotensin-converting enzyme and angiotensinogen (91). In addition to increased renin production, these changes may contribute to increased intrarenal angiotensin II production after ipsilateral UUO. The adult rat responds differently to 4 weeks of UUO, because the distribution of renin messenger RNA and protein is not altered in the ipsilateral kidney (15,92). These studies reveal that the profound effects of UUO on the renin-angiotensin system of the immature kidney are markedly attenuated in the adult, presumably as a result of the developmental decrease in the activity of the renin-angiotensin system.

Additional studies in the neonatal rat with UUO have addressed the mechanism of activation of the renin-angiotensin system in both ipsilateral and intact opposite kidneys. Renal denervation ("chemical sympathectomy" produced by chronic administration of guanethidine) in developing rats with UUO prevents the expected increased proportion of juxtaglomerular apparatuses containing detectable immunostaining renin, as well as extension of renin along afferent arterioles (93). In addition, denervation also suppresses the increased renin gene expression of the immature kidney with ipsilateral UUO, indicating that renal nerves modulate renin gene expression (93). Although renal nerves do not mediate the vasoconstriction of the obstructed kidney, they modulate vascular tone of the intact opposite kidney (94). Renal nerves have also been shown to play a role in the enhanced renin gene expression normally observed at the time of birth in the fetal sheep (95). Chronic UUO in the guinea pig increases angiotensin-dependent vasoconstriction in the obstructed kidney independent of renal innervation (96). However, UUO decreases angiotensin-dependent vasoconstriction of the opposite kidney, an effect unmasked by sympathectomy (96).

Modulation of growth by ANG II depends on the type of receptor present on the cell (97). Whereas the angiotensin AT1 receptor appears to mediate many forms of renal vascular and tubular growth (98,99), activation of the AT2 receptor has been shown to inhibit cell growth (97,100) and even to induce apoptosis (101,102). AT1 receptors are present along the afferent and efferent arterioles, proximal tubules, and the luminal surface of the distal nephron (103). Although renal AT1 and AT2 receptors are downregulated after acute UUO in the neonatal rat, the AT1 receptor is upregulated after 28 days of UUO, at a time when intrarenal angiotensin II is increased (104). El-Dahr et al. have shown that renal angiotensinogen, angiotensin-converting enzyme, and ANG II are also increased in the obstructed kidney (105). It is possible that increased ANG II levels contribute to upregulation of AT1 receptor levels, as has been described in the proximal tubule (106). UUO in the neonatal rat reduces proliferation and stimulates apoptosis at least in part through the activation of AT2 receptors (107). In addition, ANG II stimulation of AT2 receptors promotes clusterin expression in the neonatal obstructed kidney (108).

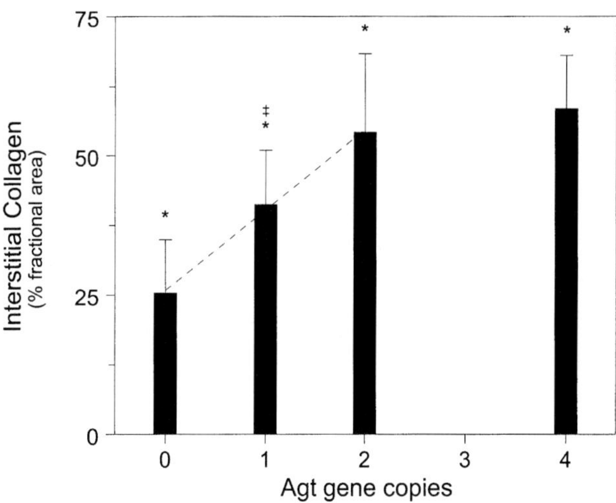

FIGURE 55.7. Renal interstitial collagen deposition in the hydronephrotic kidney is dependent on angiotensin II. Shown is the relative distribution of renal interstitial collagen in kidneys from neonatal mice with ipsilateral unilateral ureteral obstruction. There is a linear relationship between interstitial collagen deposition in the hydronephrotic kidney and the number of copies of functional angiotensinogen for 0 to 2 copies. There is no additive effect of additional copies of angiotensinogen (3 or 4 copies). Dashed line represents linear regression of individual data points. *, $p < .05$ vs. sham; ‡, $p < .05$ vs. other Agt genotypes. (From Fern RJ, Yesko CM, Thornhill BA, et al. Reduced angiotensinogen expression attenuates renal interstitial fibrosis in obstructive nephropathy in mice. *J Clin Invest* 1999;103:39–46, with permission.)

The quantitative contribution of angiotensin to interstitial fibrosis resulting from neonatal UUO has been demonstrated using mice having zero to four functional copies of the angiotensinogen gene (109). Renal interstitial collagen in neonatal mice with chronic UUO increases linearly with angiotensinogen expression, from a fractional area of 25% in zero-copy mice to 54% in two-copy mice (Fig. 55.7) (109). Thus, angiotensin regulates at least 50% of the renal interstitial fibrotic response in obstructive nephropathy. The remaining fibrotic response may be due in part to endogenous renal production of tumor necrosis factor-α (110), whose expression is greater in the neonatal kidney than the adult kidney after UUO (111).

Angiotensin-Induced Molecules

In addition to its direct actions as a growth factor, angiotensin also stimulates other growth-related compounds, including TGF-β1 (112), platelet-derived growth factor (113), osteopontin (114), adhesion molecules (115), and α-smooth muscle actin (113). These are associated with deposition of collagen, the development of interstitial fibrosis, and tubular atrophy and dilatation (113).

The increase in TGF-β1 in the obstructed adult kidney is regulated by ANG II (72,74,116,117), and inhibition of angiotensin AT1 receptors by losartan in neonatal rats with UUO reduces the expression of TGF-β1 in the obstructed kidney (118). In addition, ANG II has been shown to convert TGF-β1 to its active form (119). Thus, delayed treatment with enalapril reduces TGF-β1 expression and halts tubulointerstitial fibrosis in the obstructed kidney (117).

Whereas α-smooth muscle actin normally disappears from the interstitium in the neonatal rat, this process is delayed by ipsilateral UUO (3). Because ANG II exerts transcriptional regulation of the human α-smooth muscle actin gene (120), the persistent α-smooth muscle actin expressed by the interstitial vasculature of the neonatal obstructed kidney may be due to greater generation of tissue angiotensin resulting from recruitment of renin-secreting cells (89). It is also possible that expression of α-smooth muscle actin by fibroblasts is controlled by increased generation of TGF-β1 in the obstructed kidney (66,67,71).

Angiotensin and the Genesis of Obstructive Nephropathy

Although the AT2 receptor mediates apoptosis induced by ANG II, this receptor also appears to be important in limiting renal interstitial myofibroblast transformation in the hydronephrotic kidney (121). Moreover, there is evidence that by interfering with the apoptosis of undifferentiated mesenchymal cells, mutations in the AT2 receptor may underlie a variety of urinary tract malformations, including obstructive nephropathy (122). However, such mutations could not be confirmed in all populations (123).

In addition to the importance of ANG II in mediating the renal response to UUO, this peptide may also play a role in the development of the lower urinary tract. Mice lacking a functional AT1 receptor develop functional urinary tract obstruction similar to wild-type mice subjected to complete UUO (124). The renin-angiotensin system clearly plays a critical role in many of the processes involved in congenital obstructive nephropathy, and many of its protean effects remain to be elucidated.

RENAL FUNCTIONAL EFFECTS OF URETERAL OBSTRUCTION

Ureteral ligation initially causes increased ureteral pressure and a transient increase in renal blood flow (RBF), followed 12 to 24 hours later by decreased RBF (125,126). A decrease in glomerular filtration rate (GFR) follows the decline in RBF due to ipsilateral ureteral obstruction (127). Ureteral obstruction does not affect all nephrons equally: Deeper nephron function is lost at the expense of compensation by cortical nephrons (128). After the release of 18 hours of UUO in the weanling rat, however, superficial nephron GFR is reduced to a greater extent than that of juxtamedullary nephrons (129). After either UUO or bilateral ureteral obstruction (BUO), the number of filtering nephrons increases steadily during the first hours after relief of obstruction (130).

The chromium EDTA technique has been used to measure GFR in adult rats with complete UUO (131). GFR is reduced more severely than RBF, and, after relief of obstruction of 7 to 14 days, recovery of GFR diminishes with the duration of obstruction (131). Scanning electron microscopic examination of the rat kidney 24 hours after release of 2 weeks of UUO reveals ballooning of tubular epithelial cells, resulting in obliteration of the lumen despite relief of obstruction (132). After 2 weeks of recovery, the epithelial lining normalizes in some tubules but deteriorates further in others, indicating a marked heterogeneity in nephron injury (132). Tubular fluid flow is present in most nephrons 5 to 7 weeks after relief of 2 to 35 days of UUO and subsequent contralateral nephrectomy in the adult rat (133). However, the number of nephrons capable of recovery decreases with the duration of obstruction (133).

Hemodynamic Effects of Urinary Tract Obstruction

In all mammalian species studied to date, complete postnatal ipsilateral UUO results in significant renal vasoconstriction. Complete UUO in the neonatal rat reduces RBF by 77% (94). It is likely that at least some of the renal consequences of UUO are the result of ischemia secondary to afferent arteriolar vasoconstriction, which develops even after single nephron obstruction (134). However, there is no catchup growth of the ipsilateral kidney despite improved RBF after relief of partial UUO in the neonatal guinea pig (135). The dissociation of renal growth from renal vasoconstriction resulting from neonatal UUO suggests that hemodynamic factors alone cannot account for the impaired renal growth. Alterations in renal growth factors (discussed earlier) likely contribute to these effects.

Eicosanoids

The severity of reduced RBF resulting from ureteral obstruction has prompted a thorough investigation of potential mediators of renal vasoconstriction. Much attention is focused on eicosanoids as mediators of vascular tone, and the initial increase in RBF resulting from ipsilateral UUO is shown to be associated with increased renal production of vasodilator prostaglandins (136). The later increase in vasoconstriction, on the other hand, has been ascribed in the past to increased production of the vasoconstrictor prostanoid, thromboxane A2 (137–139). Glomeruli from rats with BUO produce increased amounts of prostaglandin E_2, 6-keto–prostaglandin F_{1a}, and TxB2, all of which can be suppressed by angiotensin-converting enzyme inhibition (140). This suggests that phospholipase A2 or cyclooxygenase is stimulated by enhanced angiotensin II formation by glomeruli from kidneys with BUO. In rats with congenital unilateral hydronephrosis, the reduction in single nephron GFR is due to a reduction in the ultrafiltration coefficient mediated by both angiotensin II and thromboxane A_2 (141). Urinary excretion of prostaglandin E_2 and thromboxane B_2 is increased in human neonates and infants with congenital obstructive uropathy (142). A balance between vasoconstrictors and vasodilators may play an important role in determining the vascular tone of kidneys with ureteral obstruction. Increased glomerular phospholipase A_2 and cyclooxygenase activity are reduced to normal when animals with BUO are treated with either angiotensin or thromboxane inhibitors (143).

There is an increased production of vasodilator prostanoids by glomeruli from the intact kidney (as well as the obstructed kidney) of rats with UUO (144). This increased prostaglandin synthesis could be suppressed by angiotensin-converting enzyme inhibition and restored by angiotensin II, suggesting that the prostaglandin production is angiotensin dependent (144). The reverse may also be the case: The increased renin release by glomeruli from kidneys with UUO can be abolished by prostaglandin inhibition (136).

Angiotensin

The role of the renin-angiotensin system in mediation of vasoconstriction resulting from ureteral obstruction is of particular interest in the maturing animal, because the activity of this system is markedly enhanced in early development. The involvement of the angiotensin in renal vasoconstriction is suggested by a doubling of the renin content of the obstructed kidney during partial UUO and its normalization after relief of obstruction (18). Chronic administration of enalapril (an angiotensin converting enzyme inhibitor) to neonatal guinea pigs with partial UUO prevents the decrease in RBF and glomerular contraction normally resulting from obstruction (145,146). This confirms the dependence of vasoconstriction on angiotensin. The effect of angiotensin can also be demonstrated during chronic obstruction of individual nephrons, in which angiotensin blockade by captopril or saralasin improves glomerular blood flow (147).

Although RBF does not return to normal after relief of 5 or 10 days of partial UUO in the neonatal guinea pig, enalapril has no additional salutary effect (18). Although enalapril has no effect on RBF of the intact kidney of neonatal guinea pigs with persistent contralateral UUO, after relief of obstruction, enalapril reduces renal vascular resistance of the intact kidney by 40% (18). Moreover, the vasoconstrictor response of the intact kidney to exogenous angiotensin II infusion is increased, suggesting an increased sensitivity of angiotensin II receptors in the intact kidney in response to relief of obstruction in the contralateral kidney. Thus, other factors are presumably responsible for the persistently depressed RBF of the postobstructed neonatal kidney. However, administration of captopril to rats during 1 to 3 weeks of UUO resulted in better preservation of kidney weight and GFR of the postobstructed kidney 3 months after relief of obstruction (148).

Atrial Natriuretic Peptide

Plasma concentration of atrial natriuretic peptide (ANP) is increased in adult rats with BUO, but not in those with UUO (149). ANP has been shown to act as a potent vasodilator in obstructed kidneys, and part of this effect is through stimulation of prostacyclin (150). These experiments suggest that the greater RBF of kidneys subjected to BUO compared to UUO may be due to higher circulating levels of ANP. Of particular interest is a report that infusion of ANP may have salutary effects on GFR of the kidney after relief of 24 hours of UUO (151). Saline loading has a similar beneficial effect, possibly through stimulation of secretion of endogenous ANP (151). Circulating ANP may also alter the vascular resistance of the obstructed kidney by inhibition of renin.

Arginine Vasopressin

Plasma levels of vasopressin are elevated in rats with 24 hours of BUO but not in those with UUO (152). The increase in vasopressin in rats with BUO is most likely due to hypernatremia and hyperosmolality. Treatment of animals with a specific antagonist of vasopressin V1 receptors increases GFR of the postobstructed kidney by 60%, and effective renal plasma flow more than doubles (152). These results suggest that vasopressin contributes to the vasoconstriction and renal functional impairment resulting from BUO.

Kininogen-Kinin System

Earlier studies of the adult rat after relief of 24 hours of UUO showed that administration of either carboxypeptidase B (which destroys kinins) or an inhibitor of kinin synthesis does not diminish the salutary effect of captopril on RBF of the postobstructed kidney (137). This suggests that angiotensin-converting enzyme inhibition does not act through potentiation of vasodilator kinins in this model. In fact, inhibition of kallikrein by aprotinin further decreases renal vasoconstriction after relief of 24 hours of UUO (153). This action appears to be due to stimulation of thromboxane and angiotensin by kinins in the postobstructed kidney (153). However, kallikrein messenger RNA and protein are significantly reduced by chronic ipsilateral UUO in the rat (154). The role of the kininogen-kinin system in ureteral obstruction therefore remains to be clarified.

Endothelial Factors

There has been much recent interest in the role of endothelial factors in the regulation of vascular tone. After unilateral release of BUO in adult rats, infusion of L-arginine, the substrate for nitric oxide synthase, increases effective renal plasma flow and GFR (155). Because nitric oxide is known to be an endothelium-derived relaxing factor (EDRF), it appears that in the setting of BUO EDRF activity is decreased. This contrasts with the UUO model, in which endogenous EDRF activity appears to be increased and is not limited by availability of substrate (156). Enhanced production of EDRF by the kidney with UUO reduces the renal vasoconstriction resulting from UUO (156,157). This may be due in part to inhibition of renin release by EDRF. Treatment of rats subjected to UUO with enalapril prevents many of the sequelae of obstruction in part by an increase in nitric oxide generation (158). Additional effects of UUO include an increase in glomerular soluble guanylyl cyclase activity (through angiotensin II stimulation) while blocking phosphodiesterase activity (159). By increasing the production of cyclic guanosine monophosphate, a vasodilator, these actions would serve to counter angiotensin-dependent vasoconstriction. Endogenous nitric oxide production also counters tubular apoptosis triggered by tubular stretch secondary to UUO (160) and attenuates interstitial fibrosis resulting from UUO (161).

Endothelial cells also produce endothelin—a potent vasoconstrictor. After relief of temporary UUO in the rat, abnormal responses of the postobstructed kidney to angiotensin II are mediated by endogenous endothelin (162).

Summary

Urinary tract obstruction induces marked changes in the activity of local vasoconstrictors and vasodilators, with a shift in the balance toward vasoconstriction. The role of angiotensin and eicosanoids appears to be clearly established, whereas that of other compounds, such as kinins and endothelial factors, remains to be elucidated. Interpretation of studies is made more difficult by the complex interactions among the vasoactive compounds, including stimulation of vasoconstrictors by vasodilators and vice-versa. In addition, the protean effects of many vasoactive compounds include the regulation of cell proliferation, apoptosis, and fibrogenesis, all of which are profoundly affected by urinary tract obstruction.

TUBULAR RESPONSES TO URINARY TRACT OBSTRUCTION

Postobstructive Diuresis

After the relief of BUO, natriuresis and diuresis are increased—a phenomenon described as *postobstructive diuresis*. Much of the effect is presumably due to an osmotic diuresis resulting from excretion of accumulated solutes. However, in addition to changes in tubular transport characteristics, altered circulating factors, such as increased circulating ANP and enhanced synthesis of prostaglandins, may play a role (149,163). In addition, altered sensitivity of the tubuloglomerular feedback mechanism also contributes to the diuresis (164). It is of interest that in addition to BUO, relief of UUO in neonates can be associated with postobstructive diuresis (165). This may be due to a relative glomerulotubular imbalance.

Sodium

Ureteral obstruction results in decreased reabsorption of sodium and water in juxtamedullary proximal tubules (129). After relief of obstruction, sodium reabsorption is decreased in the thick ascending limb of Henle, which contributes to a reduction in medullary tonicity. Sodium transport is reduced also in the medullary-collecting duct (166). It appears that the impaired sodium transport can be explained at least in part by alteration in the lipid environment of the basolateral membrane, leading to reduced Na-K-ATPase activity (167,168). Another factor implicated in postobstructive diuresis is a "functional denervation" of the kidney after relief of BUO (169). Acutely, postobstructive natriuresis may be beneficial in providing mobilization of extracellular fluid and reducing hypertension. However, prolonged salt wasting in some patients can lead to severe volume contraction and circulatory impairment. Chronic sodium depletion can also aggravate renal interstitial fibrosis resulting from UUO (85). Whereas sodium depletion normally stimulates endogenous renal antioxidant enzyme activity, UUO impairs this response, thereby contributing to the fibrogenic stimulus of renal oxidant injury that results from UUO (83,85). Because infants and children with severe obstructive uropathy frequently have significant salt wasting, adequate sodium supplementation may be beneficial in slowing progression of renal interstitial fibrosis.

Urinary Concentration

As indicated earlier, reduced removal of solute from the thick ascending limb of Henle leads to decreased solute content of the papillary interstitium and reduces the urinary concentrating capacity. A relative increase in blood flow to the papilla increases washout of solute, contributing further to loss of concentrating capacity. A third factor leading to impaired concentrating capacity is a reduced response of the cortical collecting duct to vasopressin. This occurs at a site distal to the generation of cyclic adenosine monophosphate (170). Frokiaer et al. have demonstrated that BUO and release of obstruction in the rat is associated with downregulation of the vasopressin-regulated water channel aquaporin (171,172). The maximal urinary concentration after administration of deamino-8-D-arginine vasopressin to young rabbits with UUO and contralateral nephrectomy is inversely proportional to the degree of hydronephrosis (173). This may be due at least in part to distortion of the medullary architecture: loops of Henle are splayed and tortuous 3 to 4 days after UUO in the rabbit (174). Temporary ureteral occlusion in the adult rat results in ischemic tubular necrosis in the inner and outer

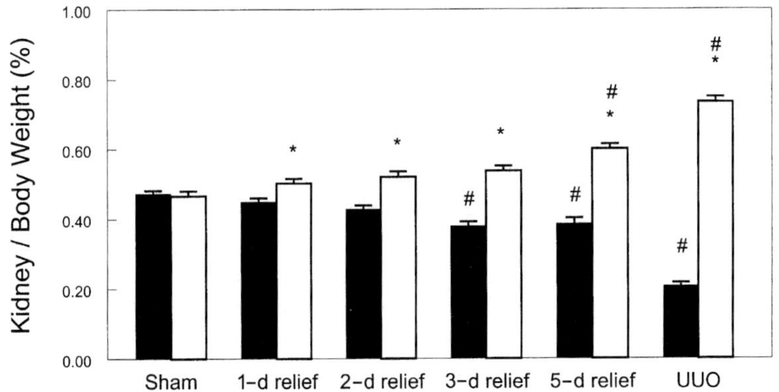

FIGURE 55.8. Kidney weight (factored for body weight) of obstructed (*black bars*) and contralateral (*white bars*) kidneys of neonatal rats 28 days after sham operation, after relief of 1 to 5 days' ureteral obstruction, or with persistent ureteral obstruction (UUO). There is a fine balance between the growth of the obstructed and opposite kidneys, such that combined renal mass remains constant. *, $p < .05$ vs. opposite kidney; #, $p < .05$ vs. sham. (From Chevalier RL, Thornhill BA, Wolstenholme JT, et al. Unilateral ureteral obstruction in early development alters renal growth: dependence on the duration of obstruction. *J Urol* 1999;161:309–313, with permission.)

medulla, which also presumably contributes to the concentrating defect (175). In addition, there is a disproportionate loss of juxtamedullary nephrons. The severity of the renal concentrating defect in children with obstructive nephropathy is highly variable but in some patients can approach that of nephrogenic diabetes insipidus, leading to episodes of hypernatremia in affected infants (176). Chronic polyuria secondary to obstructive nephropathy may accelerate renal injury: In weanling rats with partial UUO, chronic high urine flow rates induced by osmotic diuresis resulted in a significant decrease in GFR (177).

Potassium and Hydrogen Ion Handling

Obstructive nephropathy leads frequently to defective distal tubular potassium and hydrogen ion secretion (*type 4* renal tubular acidosis) (178,179). This can be due to impaired turnover of the sodium/potassium pump, diminished sensitivity of the distal tubule to aldosterone, or the loss of H+-ATPase in the apical surface of intercalated cells. Clinically, these changes lead to hyperkalemia and metabolic acidosis, even with unilateral obstruction, and may not resolve after surgical correction of obstruction (179–181).

Calcium and Phosphorus Handling

Experimental UUO results in reduced urinary calcium and phosphorus excretion due in part to a decreased renal response to parathyroid hormone. In patients with distal renal tubular acidosis due to obstructive nephropathy (*type 1*), urinary calcium excretion can be increased. Release of UUO in thyroparathyroidectomized dogs results in hypophosphaturia due to reduced filtered load of phosphate and increased tubular phosphate reabsorption (182).

RENAL COUNTERBALANCE

Although the UUO model represents an extreme case of asymmetrical kidney function, the severity of urinary tract obstruction in clinical practice is often unequally distributed between the two sides. Partial UUO in the immature guinea pig results in a compensatory increase in GFR of the intact opposite kidney; the younger the animal at the time of ureteral obstruction, the greater the response (183). The concept of "counterbalance" by the intact kidney in response to loss of function by the obstructed kidney was developed by Hinman in 1923 (184). The exaggerated adaptive response by the intact kidney of animals undergoing UUO in early development is also demonstrated by the remaining kidney after loss of renal mass in the neonate (185,186). The dynamic nature of the response is illustrated by the attenuation of compensatory hypertrophy of the intact kidney after relief of UUO in the guinea pig at 10 days of age (135). Temporary UUO in the neonatal rat inhibits growth of the obstructed kidney and accelerates growth of the opposite kidney in direct proportion to the duration of obstruction (Fig. 55.8) (187). This demonstrates clearly the very fine-tuning of the counterbalance mechanism in early development. Also demonstrating the plasticity of the counterbalance phenomenon is the maintenance of normal RBF and glomerular volume in kidneys of neonatal guinea pigs with ipsilateral UUO, if the contralateral kidney is removed at the time of birth (188).

EFFECTS OF URINARY TRACT OBSTRUCTION ON THE FETAL KIDNEY

Although the models described earlier have elucidated a number of mechanisms underlying the renal response to urinary tract obstruction, they do not address the intrauterine changes in the developing kidney with congenital obstruction. A question of primary clinical importance is the effect of relief of fetal urinary tract obstruction on functional development of the kidney. Moreover, in view of the association of pulmonary hypoplasia and oligohydramnios, the effect of severe urinary tract obstruction on development of the lung is of more immediate importance to the neonatal infant. Several laboratories have attempted to develop such models in the fetus or embryo (189). Ureteral obstruction in the chick embryo results in hydronephrosis but not in dysplastic changes, as are present in infants with severe degrees of obstruction (190). Ureteral ligation in the fetal rabbit results in a rapid decrease in the number of glomeruli, whereas relief of obstruction partially restores them (7,191). The opossum has also been studied because it is a marsupial, and most "fetal" development is completed in the maternal pouch rather than while attached to a placenta *in utero*. Obstruction in the fetal opossum results in tubular atrophy and interstitial fibrosis, with interstitial fibroblasts appearing similar to undifferentiated mesenchyme (192). In this model, relief of UUO does not affect weight or function of the ipsilateral kidney (193). In fact, relief of obstruction tends to decrease further the weight and function of the kidney, an effect that is ascribed to a renal inflammatory response (193). In addition, growth of the intact opposite kidney is also greater after relief of obstruction (193), results that are the reverse of those after relief of partial UUO in the postnatal guinea pig (135). As in the neonatal rat (36), the administration of IGF ameliorates the development of interstitial fibrosis in the fetal opossum subjected to complete UUO (194). This supports the role of growth factors in mediating or modulating the renal cellular response to UUO in the fetus as well as postnatally.

Because of their larger size and presumed greater similarity to the human fetus, a number of investigators have studied urinary tract obstruction in the fetal sheep. Initial studies in this species revealed that urethral obstruction before closure of the urachus results in a persistent umbilical fistula that prevents the development of hydronephrosis (195). Ureteral ligation performed during the first half of gestation results in dysplastic changes, whereas delay in obstruction until the last half of gestation results in preservation of renal architecture with little interstitial fibrosis or inflammation (196). It is likely that the dependence of the renal response to the timing of obstruction in the fetus relates to the changing rate of cellular proliferation, which is maximal near the midpoint of gestation (197). Partial bladder outlet obstruction in the fetal sheep increases renal renin expression and increases renal expression of the AT2 receptor (198). A greater abundance of the AT2 receptor is expected to enhance the apoptotic response to endogenous angiotensin.

Harrison and his colleagues have described an elegant model of bladder outlet obstruction in the fetal sheep, in which the urachus as well as the urethra are obstructed (199). Relief of obstruction at 112 to 124 days' gestation after 15 to 27 days' obstruction in the fetus lessens the degree of hydronephrosis and of pulmonary hypoplasia, resulting in a marked improvement in viability (199). Ureteral obstruction in the first trimester (43 to 45 days' gestation) or early midtrimester (58 to 66 days' gestation) results in marked interstitial fibrosis, primitive epithelial structures, and parenchymal disorganization typical of dysplasia (200,201). One animal developed a wrinkled, distended abdomen; deficient abdominal wall musculature; and undescended testes, comparable to the prune belly syndrome in humans. Recovery of renal function after relief of obstruction was found to be directly proportional to the duration of intrauterine decompression and inversely proportional to the duration of obstruction (202). As in the fetal rabbit model, relief of obstruction before the completion of nephrogenesis in the fetal sheep can lead to preservation of nephrons (203).

Chronic partial bladder obstruction in midtrimester in the sheep actually increases RBF and GFR, while renal architecture appears normal despite thinning of the cortex (204). These findings, which are the reverse of those described in postnatal animals, underscore the importance of the degree of obstruction in the determination of the renal response in the fetus. As with the results in the opossum described earlier, the response of the fetal kidney to obstruction *in utero* may differ significantly from the postnatal effects.

Complete UUO in the fetal sheep decreases RBF but not as severely as in adults (205). Peters et al. (9) report that UUO early in gestation results in compensatory growth of the opposite kidney in the fetal lamb. This finding illustrates the operation of counterbalance in the fetus, which indicates that compensatory renal growth is not dependent on functional demand.

Experimental ureteropelvic junction (UPJ) obstruction in the fetal monkey impairs growth of the kidney, which exhibits cystic dysplastic changes, interstitial expansion, and collecting duct apoptosis (206). A novel observation in this model is the prominent glomerular abnormality, with significant podocyte apoptosis (206). Although data are limited, congenital human obstructive nephropathy is also associated with glomerular changes (207).

CLINICAL IMPLICATIONS OF EXPERIMENTAL STUDIES OF URINARY TRACT OBSTRUCTION

The results of the fetal studies described earlier have important implications for the management of infants found to have severe obstructive nephropathy *in utero*: Prenatal intervention may allow preservation of renal mass before completion of nephrogenesis, as well as improved pulmonary development. The major problem is the lack of accurate prognostic criteria for identification of infants who would benefit from intervention. The primary limiting factor at present is the difficulty in visualizing the developing kidneys by ultrasonography before 18 weeks' gestation (208). In a report of a 10-year experience with prenatal intervention for hydronephrosis, successful vesicoamniotic shunt placement may aid pulmonary development, but does not prevent renal insufficiency (209). Significant technical advances are required to allow the development of a required anatomic definition, as well as the development of reliable functional parameters. Most needed, however, is a better understanding of the molecular and cellular mechanisms leading to the anomalies themselves. One promising approach is the study of a mouse strain with congenital progressive bilateral UPJ obstruction and hydronephrosis, a characteristic that is inherited as an autosomal recessive trait (210). Identification of the genetic basis for the abnormality may reveal some of the underlying developmental processes.

The lack of reliable markers of significant urinary tract obstruction is a critical issue. The numerous experimental studies showing renal activation of TGF-β1 in the hydronephrotic kidney may provide an index of obstruction: Urinary TGF-β is increased in children with severe urinary tract obstruction, and the correlation provides 90% sensitivity (211). Suppression of renal EGF is also a hallmark of experimental hydronephrosis, and urinary EGF concentration is markedly reduced in children with severe UPJ obstruction (59).

One of the primary concerns in the management of infants with obstructive nephropathy is the expected recoverability of renal mass and renal function after relief of the obstruction. Temporary UUO in the neonatal rat impairs renal growth proportional to the duration of obstruction before relief (Fig. 55.8) (187). Although relief of obstruction attenuates the renal cellular injury, alterations persist in the renal vasculature, tubules, and interstitium (17). Although relief of obstruction does not reverse a 40% reduction in the number of nephrons, the GFR of the postobstructed kidney is normal 1 month after relief (17). This suggests that remaining nephrons undergo hyperfiltration. One year after relief of obstruction, GFR is decreased by 80%, and proteinuria has developed (212). Importantly, glomerular sclerosis, tubular atrophy, macrophage infiltration, and interstitial fibrosis are increased not only in the postobstructed kidney but also in the opposite kidney (212). Fibrosis in the opposite kidney may be due in part to the increased renal expression of TGF-β receptors in both obstructed and opposite kidneys after UUO (213). These findings suggest that despite normal early postoperative GFR in infancy, children undergoing pyeloplasty for UPJ obstruction should be followed into adulthood. After relief of 5 days' UUO immediately after the completion of nephrogenesis, renal damage and loss of renal function are even more severe than those after relief of UUO during nephrogenesis (13). This suggests that if significant urinary tract obstruction is diagnosed in the prenatal or neonatal period, its relief should not be delayed.

Timing the relief of obstruction in the postnatal period is complicated by differences in available experimental models. As described earlier, severe partial UUO in the neonatal guinea pig leads to arrested growth of the ipsilateral kidney, which is not improved by relief of obstruction after 10 days (135). This suggests that any delay in relief of neonatal obstruction results in irreversible damage. In contrast, based on studies of the effects of partial UUO in the neonatal rat, Claesson and associates have concluded that early release of obstruction can prevent the reduction in ipsilateral kidney weight (214,215). However, the reduction in GFR in this model is only 10% when measured 9 to 12 weeks later (216), and the morphologic changes appear to stabilize after 3 weeks of UUO (217). Measurement of renal function by nuclear scintigraphy in rats studied up to 1 year after neonatal UUO reveals a 40% reduction in function and a similar reduction in kidney weight (218). If weanling rats are subjected to partial UUO, the morphologic effects are less severe than those resulting from UUO within the first 2 days of life (219). If partial UUO is delayed even longer (performed at 6 weeks of age), the impairment in GFR is minimal and does not progress over 15 weeks despite the presence of hydronephrosis (220). Thus, in the rat, as in the guinea pig, susceptibility of the kidney to injury from ipsilateral ureteral obstruction decreases with age. In the adult dog, complete recovery of renal function is possible after relief of UUO for 7 days (221). With 2 weeks of obstruction, there is 70% recovery 6 months after relief of obstruction (221). These experiments demonstrate the importance of the duration of obstruction in determining the capacity for recovery.

The dependence of recovery on the degree of obstruction has also been demonstrated in adult rats. Two to 6 weeks after the induction of partial UUO, there is a progressive decrease in the ratio of dry kidney weight to body weight, with the severity of loss of renal mass being proportional to the degree of obstruction (222). Six weeks after relief of obstruction of 8 weeks' duration, no enhancement of growth was observed (222). This indicates that the timing of relief of obstruction is critical, even in the adult.

Whereas all agree that the infant with bladder outlet obstruction should have prompt relief of obstruction, management of unilateral UPJ obstruction is not as clear. A major problem is the variability in the severity of obstruction in these patients and the difficulty in reliably assessing the degree of functional obstruction. Although a large proportion of infants with equivocal hydronephrosis identified prenatally appear to have normal renal functional development without intervention (223), others may demonstrate progressive impairment (224). Peters has, therefore, defined obstruction as "a condition of impaired urinary drainage, which, if uncorrected, will limit the ultimate functional potential of a developing kidney" (225).

The solution to this dilemma depends on improved methods for imaging the developing kidney, as well as more reliable means of monitoring renal function. In view of the exaggeration of renal "counterbalance" in early development, the greater adaptation of intact nephrons may mask the deterioration of obstructed ones, necessitating the accurate measurement of differential renal function. Such advances, along with improved understanding of the mechanisms underlying the renal response to urinary tract obstruction during maturation, should allow intervention before the development of irreversible changes in remaining nephrons.

Complete urinary tract obstruction has been clearly shown to cause renal deterioration. The natural history of partial urinary tract obstruction in humans is less well defined; however, basic science observations support early surgical intervention over a nonoperative approach when obstruction exists. Although a common radiologic technique such as ultrasonography accurately describes dilation of the upper urinary tract in both the pre- and postnatal settings, it cannot determine mechanical obstruction, which is a functional characteristic. The finding of hydronephrosis, then, can be a clinical challenge to the physician caring for infants and children. The purpose of early detection and accurate diagnosis of upper urinary tract obstruction is to determine which patient may benefit from surgical therapy or, in other words, to determine when dilation of the renal collecting system indicates the existence of worrisome pathology (a process of renal damage or deterioration). It is hoped that the loss of nephrons can be prevented or minimized.

CAUSES OF OBSTRUCTIVE UROPATHY: SPECIFIC CLINICAL DISEASES

Ureteropelvic Junction Obstruction

Classic *ureteropelvic junction obstruction* is defined as congenital hydronephrosis characterized by impaired urine flow from the renal pelvis into the proximal ureter. An intrinsic or extrinsic narrowing or blockage at the UPJ, this lesion causes progressive dilation of the renal pelvis and calyces and the potential for nephron loss. This is a common renal anomaly in children, with an incidence of 1 in 1500, and is the most common cause of hydronephrosis detected prenatally (226,227). It has been classified as extrinsic, intrinsic, or secondary. Historically, it was usual for children to present between 5 and 15 years of age with symptoms of infection, flank pain, abdominal mass, renal nephrolithiasis, or hematuria (Figs. 55.9 and 55.10). Because these children had abnormal imaging studies and were symptomatic, surgery was routinely performed. Today, hydronephrosis secondary to presumed UPJ obstruction is much more commonly detected during prenatal ultrasonography, as is discussed in

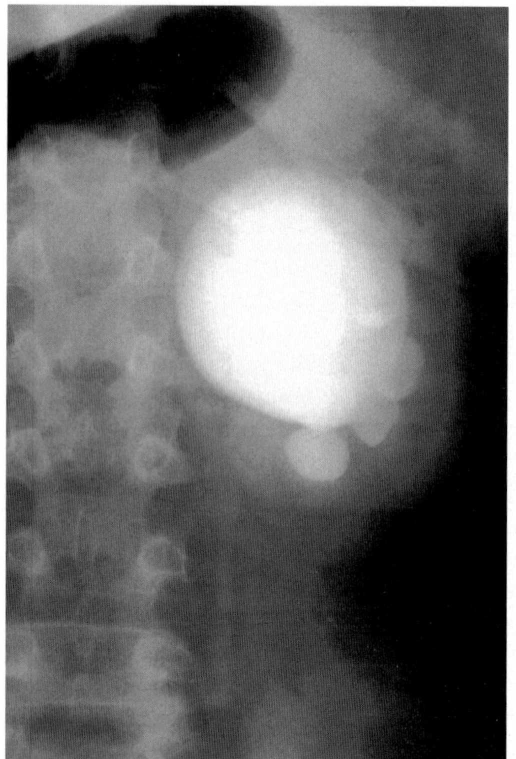

A

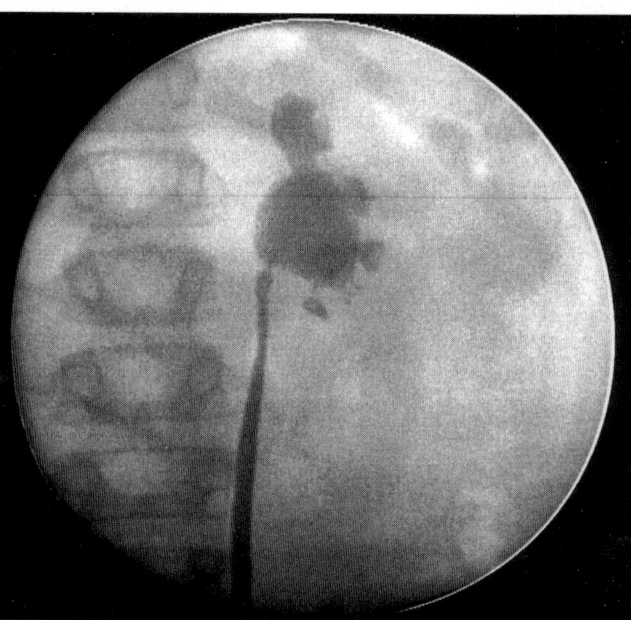

B

FIGURE 55.9. A: Seven-year-old girl with a 2-year history of intermittent left flank pain with nausea and vomiting. This intravenous urogram (here, 60 minutes postinjection of contrast) was performed while the patient was actively symptomatic and demonstrates a distended renal pelvis and calyces in comparison to the normal caliber ureter. The ureteropelvic junction (UPJ) is not well delineated. **B:** Left retrograde pyelogram performed several days later in the same patient at time when she was asymptomatic. Note the marked decrease in pelvicaliectasis (relative to the normal caliber ureter), as well as the concentric filling defect at the UPJ, highly suggestive of extrinsic compression. Open exploration with surgical repair later during the same procedure revealed extrinsic compression of the left UPJ due to a lower pole, crossing vessel. Dismembered pyeloplasty was performed.

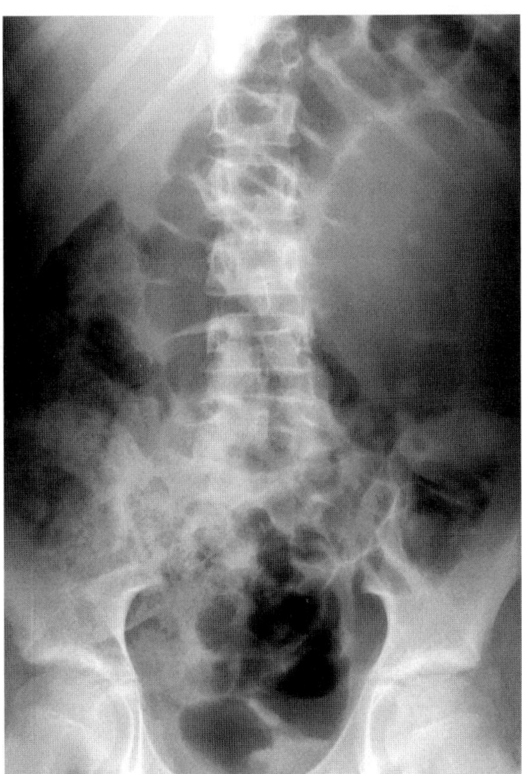

FIGURE 55.10. Twelve-year-old girl with a history of intermittent left flank pain and nausea. This plain film demonstrates a large, left abdominal opacity that pushes the colon medially. This markedly distended renal pelvis is palpable on physical examination.

Ultrasonography. UPJ obstruction is more commonly found on the left side, occurring in 60%; is more common in males than females (2:1); and occurs bilaterally in lesions in 10 to 40% of affected neonates in some reported series (228–230).

If the lumen of the ureter is narrow at the UPJ either in the presence or absence of ureteral kinking, then the obstruction is generally considered to be *intrinsic*. The ureteral wall is generally characterized by reduced amounts of smooth muscle with excess collagen deposition. Other findings with light microscopy include muscular disorientation, thickened adventitia, and inflammation, although it is not known which is causative of the other—the obstruction versus the histologic changes (231,232). It is also not known whether intrinsic UPJ obstruction is due to incomplete recanalization of the ureter, which begins at 42 days' gestation in the middle of the ureter and continues both distally and proximally, such that the very last parts of the ureter to recanalize are the ureterovesical junction (UVJ) and UPJ. Persistent muscular folds or kinks during recanalization have been described, as well as ureteral polyps and dysfunctional ureteropelvic muscular contractions (233–239).

The resistance to urine flow may cause a relatively constant partial obstruction or one that is intermittent (or flow-dependent). In other words, a particular flow rate may produce a configurational change at the UPJ that causes increased resistance (240).

If there is a dynamic character to flow across the UPJ, then obstruction may be episodic in nature due to intermittent kinking. This pattern is more commonly seen in older children or even adults, as opposed to classic neonatal UPJ obstruction. If an acute increase in urine output is not well compensated by the renal pelvis anatomically, then acute, transient flank pain with nausea may result. This has been called Dietl's crisis when bilateral (241,242).

Intermittent obstruction may also be caused by proximal ureteral compression by accessory or abnormal lower pole renal vasculature. These *extrinsic* lesions have been described as a compression of the proximal ureter between a crossing vessel and the fixed UPJ or a flattening of the ureter as it passes over a crossing vessel (233,243).

In high-grade vesicoureteral reflux (VUR), a very tortuous and dilated ureter may obstruct proximally, secondary to kinking—a phenomenon called *secondary UPJ obstruction*. VUR has been reported in 15% of children with UPJ obstruction; however, the percentage of those children in whom the upper tract obstruction is directly caused by the reflux is not clear (244–246).

Surgical repair of UPJ obstruction is an effective procedure with success rates of more than 90% and with low complication rates. Whereas some pediatric urologists approach the UPJ from the patient's flank, others approach more posteriorly via a dorsal lumbotomy incision. At the time of reconstruction, the diseased segment is excised (or transected and brought to the opposite side of the obstructing, crossing vessel), and the pelvis and spatulated ureter are reanastomosed. The redundant renal pelvis may also be trimmed, if necessary. To date, endoscopic (retrograde endopyelotomy) and percutaneous treatment of UPJ obstruction has been better established in adults than in children.

Ureterovesical Junction Obstruction

Ureterovesical junction obstruction is also an obstructive lesion of the ureter; however, it is characterized by pathology where the distal ureter meets the bladder. UVJ obstruction may be a primary process, or it may be a secondary process due to extrinsic compression of the ureter by a thickened bladder wall from other diseases, such as posterior urethral valves (PUVs) or neurogenic bladder dysfunction. UVJ obstruction has commonly been called an *obstructed megaureter*. Congenital megaureter is just that, a dilated ureter, and it accounts for approximately 20% of cases of hydronephrosis in the newborn. Its types include nonrefluxing-nonobstructed (idiopathic), refluxing-nonobstructed, nonrefluxing-obstructed, and refluxing-obstructed.

Obstructed megaureter is thought to be due to an abnormality in the distal ureteral muscle that causes an aperistaltic segment. UVJ obstruction may share a similar etiology with UPJ obstruction, and spontaneous improvement has been observed in both diseases, suggesting a maturational process in peristaltic function (247,248).

Ultrasonography may detect the presence of upper tract dilation in UVJ obstruction; however, additional studies are required to determine its etiology and importance, as outlined in Posterior Urethral Valves. If the UVJ obstruction is thought to be secondary to other diseases, such as PUV, VUR, or neurogenic bladder dysfunction, then treatment is directed toward the underlying cause. If obstruction is present, then surgical treatment is directed toward removing the aperistaltic lower ureteral segment, tapering the dilated distal ureter, and reimplanting the tailored ureter back into the bladder in an antirefluxing manner.

Posterior Urethral Valves

Posterior urethral valves are obstructing membranous folds within the lumen of the prostatic (posterior) urethra. They occur only in male infants and are the most common congenital cause of bladder outlet obstruction. PUV account for approximately 10% of cases of hydronephrosis in the newborn (249). The incidence of PUV has been estimated to be approximately 1 in 5000 to 8000. The pathophysiologic effects of lower urinary tract obstruction on the developing kidney are similar to those of upper tract obstruction; however, congenital bladder outlet obstruction can have immediate life-threatening consequences, as well as long-term, deleterious effects on both renal and bladder function.

There is no known genetic or familial predisposition toward the development of PUV, and their etiology has not been established. Some authors have theorized that the wolffian ducts in patients with PUVs have integrated abnormally into the prostatic urethra, which develops from the urogenital sinus by the eighth week of life (250).

PUVs typically appear as two thin leaflets running between the urethral floor and roof, causing a high-grade obstruction. Elevated pressures are transmitted to the kidneys as the developing bladder becomes thickened, trabeculated, and noncompliant as it carries out high-pressure work to empty. Normal bladder cycling does not occur, which may result in oligohydramnios prenatally. Elevated voiding pressures cause dilation of the posterior urethra and distortion of the bladder neck. The noncompliant bladder transmits elevated pressures to the renal parenchyma during filling and urine storage. Upper tract findings include pelvicaliectasis, ureterectasis, urinary stasis, parenchymal compression, and renal dysplasia. Bilateral hydroureteronephrosis may be present with or without high-grade VUR. Elevated upper tract pressure may cause urinary extravasation from a forniceal rupture resulting in a retroperitoneal urinoma or urinary ascites, if urine crosses the peritoneum. It is believed that pop-off mechanisms that relieve bladder pressure, such as VUR, may have a protective effect on renal function (251,252). It has been observed that contralateral renal function is preserved in patients with unilateral reflux into a nonfunctioning kidney, and this has been called the *VURD syndrome* (*v*alves, *u*nilateral reflux, *r*enal *d*ysplasia). Bladder diverticulae and renal urinary extravasation are less commonly occurring pop-off mechanisms than VUR.

The majority of patients with PUV are diagnosed prenatally, which permits treatment of the obstruction in the first few days of life; however, there is a wide clinical spectrum of progressive renal failure depending on the degree of *in utero* obstruction and bladder dysfunction. Some infants are diagnosed postnatally with conditions of respiratory distress (secondary to pulmonary hypoplasia from oligohydramnios), sepsis, azotemia, failure to thrive, or abdominal distention. The presence of a distended, palpable bladder may suggest PUV, as well as the failure to void in the first 24 hours of life or an abnormal urine stream. A good urine stream, however, does not rule out PUV. A tense abdomen may suggest the presence of urinary ascites or markedly hydronephrotic upper tracts. A voiding cystourethrogram (VCUG) is necessary to make the diagnosis of PUV before surgical intervention, with typical radiologic findings of a thick-walled, trabeculated bladder; an elongated, dilated posterior urethra; and an elevated bladder neck (Fig. 55.11).

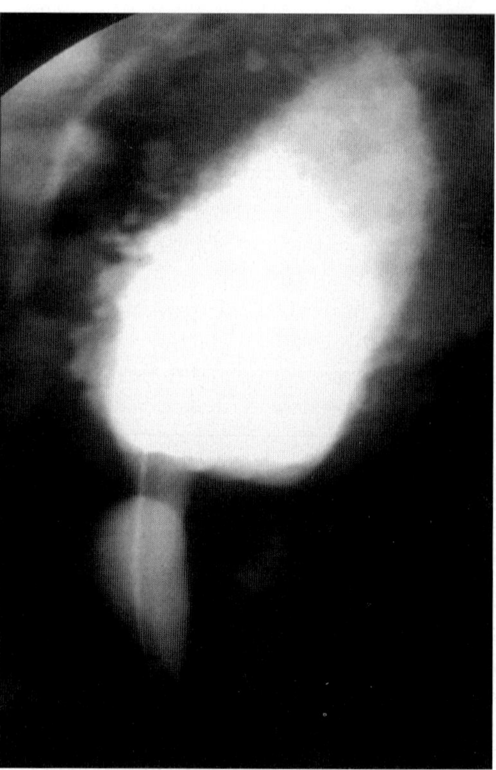

FIGURE 55.11. One-day-old boy with a history of bilateral hydroureteronephrosis and a thickened bladder wall detected prenatally. This voiding cystourethrogram demonstrates a markedly thickened and trabeculated bladder wall with dilation of the posterior urethra secondary to posterior urethral valves. A 5 French feeding tube was placed per urethra, and the boy was taken to the operating room before discharge for cystoscopy and transurethral resection of the valves.

Older boys have been diagnosed with PUV during a workup for urinary tract infections or symptoms such as frequency, daytime incontinence, and straining to void. These symptoms may be a result of bladder wall thickening, decreased detrusor compliance, or a renal concentrating defect with polydipsia and polyuria.

Once the diagnosis of PUV is suspected or made, initial management includes treatment of acute illness (respiratory distress, sepsis, dehydration, electrolyte abnormalities) and temporary drainage of the urinary tract with a small urethral catheter, such as a 5 French feeding tube. A Foley catheter is not recommended, as the balloon may fall back into the dilated posterior urethra, preventing the bladder from draining completely. Ultrasonography can confirm proper position of the urethral catheter in the bladder. Serial serum creatinine measurements over 7 to 10 days of total bladder decompression define the preoperative creatinine nadir before primary endoscopic ablation of the valves. Creatinine levels in the first few days of life reflect maternal levels. Secondary obstruction at the UVJ may coexist because of severe bladder thickening, and this may be reflected by persistent azotemia or sepsis despite adequate bladder decompression. Temporary supravesical urinary diversion (cutaneous ureterostomies) may then be required. A cutaneous vesicostomy may be required if the caliber of the urethra is too small for endoscopic ablation of the PUV.

Many patients with PUV have significant lower urinary tract dysfunction (incontinence) or worsening hydronephrosis despite successful primary valve ablation. Loss of bladder compliance, incontinence, and deterioration of renal function with poor renal concentrating ability are all part of a spectrum of the *valve bladder syndrome*. Long-term urodynamic follow-up as well as upper tract surveillance are required to ensure preservation of renal function, avoidance of infection, compliant low-pressure urine storage, and urinary continence. Whereas some authors have described a poor outcome (renal failure) with late presentation of PUV, others have demonstrated that a presentation before 1 year of age is a poor prognostic sign, as well as bilateral VUR at that time or incontinence after the age of 5 years (253–257).

DIAGNOSIS OF OBSTRUCTIVE UROPATHY

A diagnosis of obstructive uropathy is investigated further when hydronephrosis or hydroureteronephrosis is discovered on ultrasonography during either routine prenatal screening or during a clinical workup postnatally for the child with flank pain, hematuria, an abdominal mass, urinary tract infection, or incontinence. Hydronephrosis is the most common congenital condition that is detected by prenatal ultrasound and represents 50% of all abnormalities. Patients with imperforate anus, contralateral multicystic dysplastic kidney, congenital heart disease, VATER (*v*ertebral, *a*nus, *t*racheo*e*sophageal, *r*adial and renal) syndrome, or esophageal atresia should be screened with a renal ultrasound to rule out associated hydronephrosis.

Ultrasonography

Initial prenatal sonography is usually performed between 16 and 20 weeks of gestation. Approximately 20% of abnormalities evident *in utero* are not present after birth (258). When prenatal hydronephrosis is detected, the degree of dilation is calculated by measuring the anteroposterior diameter of the renal pelvis in the transverse plane of the kidney and is correlated with the current gestational age. Although there is no generally agreed-on definition of prenatal hydronephrosis, persistent postnatal renal abnormalities have been described when the anteroposterior diameter of the fetal renal pelvis measures greater than 6 mm at less than 20 weeks, greater than 8 mm at 20 to 30 weeks, and greater than 10 mm at more than 30 weeks of gestation (259). Prenatally or postnatally, the ultrasonographer should determine not only the degree of dilation but also whether it is unilateral or bilateral, if the ipsilateral ureter is dilated, and if the contralateral kidney is normal (parenchyma echotexture, presence of cystic disease). Prenatally, amniotic fluid volume is quantified carefully, because oligohydramnios can determine prognosis. Fetal urine comprises up to 90% of the amniotic fluid, and its contribution progressively increases from 16 to 20 weeks of gestation. The bladder of the fetus or child is imaged to assess its thickness, distention, and ability to empty. Lesions within the bladder, such as ureterocele, are assessed, as well as relevant lesions of other organ systems, such as spinal dysraphism. The gender of the fetus or child is also important to determine, because many congenital abnormalities causing hydronephrosis have a strong gender association, as most of the obstructive urologic malformations occur in males, with a male to female ratio of 3 to 4:1 (260). Duplication anomalies and ectopic ureterocele are more common in females.

Obstructive and nonobstructive processes can both cause dilation of the urinary tract. In the prenatal setting, obstructive etiologies include UPJ obstruction (44%), UVJ obstruction (21%), multicystic dysplastic kidney, ureterocele/ureteral ectopia, duplex kidney (12%), PUV (9%), urethral atresia, sacrococcygeal teratoma, and hydrometrocolpos. Nonobstructive etiologies include VUR (14%), physiologic dilation, prune belly syndrome, renal cystic disease, and megacalicosis (congenitally dilated calyces without pelviectasis and obstruction) (260).

On ultrasound, UPJ obstruction is characterized by pelvicaliectasis, no ipsilateral ureteral dilation, and normal bladder thickness and emptying. Measuring bladder thickness can differentiate potential PUV from megacystis or megaureter. The most important diagnosis to be made prenatally is PUV in the male fetus, because, as described earlier, surgical correction is needed in the early postnatal period (and in select cases may even be indicated prenatally). If the ipsilateral ureter is visualized (and therefore by definition is dilated) and pelvicaliectasis detected, then the following diagnoses are considered: VUR, PUV, megaureter, or ureterocele/ectopic ureter. Hydroureteronephrosis in the male with a thin-walled bladder and normal renal parenchyma is most likely not PUV but rather VUR.

Unilateral or bilateral hydroureteronephrosis with a trabeculated/thick-walled bladder and abnormal renal parenchyma (hyperechoic, cystic changes), with or without oligohydramnios (prenatal setting) in the male, is PUV until proven otherwise with a cystogram. If a ureterocele is visualized in the bladder and/or there is asymmetric upper pole caliectasis, then a duplication anomaly is suspected (261).

Renal duplex Doppler ultrasonography can be used to calculate the renal resistive index (RI). It is hypothesized that measuring changes in intra-RBF can distinguish between obstructive and nonobstructive hydronephrosis (262). The addition of furosemide to the Doppler protocol may help further discriminate between obstructive and nonobstructive hydronephrosis (263). An RI equal to or greater than 1.1 as well as an RI difference with furosemide diuresis of 70% or more are both Doppler sonographic variables that may correlate with obstruction (264). However, the use of the RI to determine obstruction is limited due to variability in technique, interpretation, and established normal variables of infants and children.

Ultrasonography, then, can correctly identify hydronephrosis, and specific findings of increased echogenicity, severe calyceal dilation, contralateral hypertrophy, or ipsilateral parenchymal loss can be worrisome for potential obstruction. However, physiologic assessment is not possible until functional studies are performed, typically with excretory urography or renography.

Excretory Urography

The intravenous urogram is an excellent study for evaluation of the older child with intermittent flank pain; however, it is most useful when performed while the child is symptomatic (Fig. 55.9A). Pelvicaliectasis with delayed excretion of contrast and poor visualization of the ipsilateral ureter are findings consistent with UPJ obstruction, especially when compared to a normal intravenous urogram or ultrasound performed when the child is asymptomatic. The finding of a delayed nephrogram may be consistent with obstruction; however, when excretion and antegrade flow are prolonged, then delayed imaging is necessary to visualize the ureter and its caliber to distinguish a UVJ lesion versus one at the UPJ. Obtaining postvoid views can help rule out bladder dysfunction as a contributing factor to the columnation of contrast, especially when a lesion at the UVJ is suspected. Urography can be a superior modality in preparation for surgery—when it is necessary to clarify complex anatomy—particularly in duplication anomalies.

Nuclear Renography

Nuclear medicine renal scans are more commonly used than urography as the method of choice to diagnose obstruction in the setting of hydronephrosis. Renography can quantitate individual and relative renal function, cortical transit time, and the antegrade drainage of the collecting systems before and after the administration of furosemide. Functional nuclear medicine studies are best performed after 1 month of age when renal concentrating ability has matured. The radiopharmaceuticals used include technetium-99m diethylenetriamine pentaacetic acid and mercaptoacetyltriglycerine (MAG-3), and a bladder catheter should be inserted for the test, especially if VUR is present.

Obstruction at the UPJ or UVJ is reflected by the half-time to washout of radioisotope-labeled urine and percentage of tracer retained within the renal pelvis or distal ureter beyond approximately 20 minutes (Fig. 55.12). In the hydronephrotic system, if the washout is quick after the furosemide is given, then the patient is said to have a dilated, nonobstructed system. Prolonged washout times in otherwise satisfactorily functioning kidneys may support the diagnosis of physiologically significant obstruction; however, no gold standard for obstruction exists. Some reports have described stable renal function despite impaired drainage on renography in some infants with hydronephrosis; however, this is not well established (265).

Upper Tract Urodynamics: Whitaker Test

Whereas imaging modalities such as ultrasonography and renography delineate the renal effects of impedance to urine flow, upper tract urodynamic studies demonstrate the pressure-flow characteristics of the upper urinary tract collecting system itself. The pressure changes described by antegrade perfusion pressure-flow studies (Whitaker test) are dependent on the compliance (the change in volume or flow over the change in pressure) and capacity of the renal pelvis, as well as the degree of outlet resistance. For this reason, upper tract urodynamic studies can be helpful in measuring the response of the renal pelvis to distention in equivocal cases of UPJ obstruction. Percutaneous access of the hydronephrotic renal collecting system is obtained, and perfusion of the kidney at a flow rate to mimic diuresis (10 mL/min) is performed. Pressures greater than 22 cm H_2O have been called obstructive, and those less than 15 cm H_2O have been described as nonobstructive, with a gray area in between (266–268). Because this flow rate may not be physiologic and because UPJ resistance changes as the pelvis distends, the traditional Whitaker test is somewhat limited. Great advances have been made to standardize urodynamics and to define obstruction in the hydronephrotic upper urinary tract; however, these studies are not able to predict future improvement or deterioration in function (269–272).

Cystography

Cystography is typically performed to rule out VUR and/or PUV. In the infant the study, it is usually accomplished through retrograde bladder filling via a 5 French feeding tube or similar Foley catheter. In general, a feeding tube is prefera-

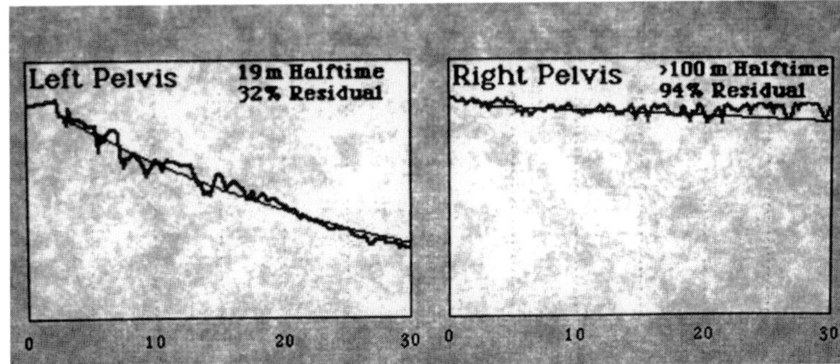

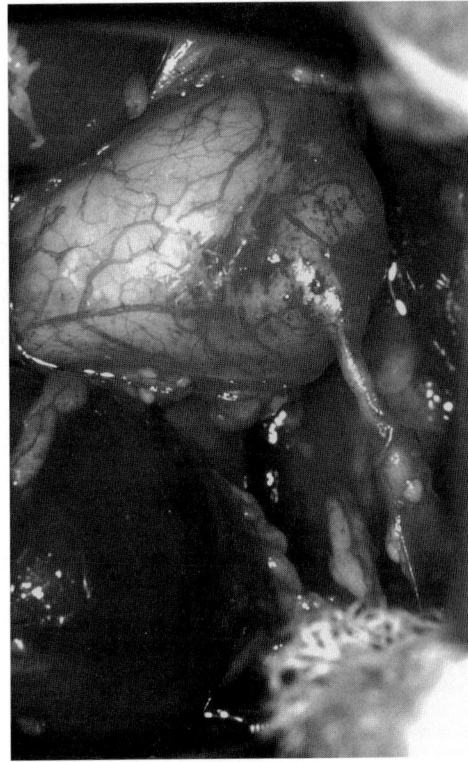

FIGURE 55.12. **A:** Diuretic renogram in a 3-month-old boy with a history of bilateral, prenatally detected hydronephrosis (right greater than left). Furosemide was injected at time 0. Whereas the right kidney demonstrates an obstructed pattern, the left side is indeterminate. **B:** Same patient during right flank exploration for high-grade ureteropelvic junction (UPJ) obstruction. Intraoperative findings demonstrate an intrinsic lesion at the UPJ.

ble, because it is less likely to obscure the diagnosis of a ureterocele. Cyclical filling and emptying of the bladder is necessary to distend the bladder and urethra (to rule out PUV) or to visualize VUR (when an ectopic ureter to the bladder neck or urethra refluxes only with cycles of voiding). If there is high-grade VUR, then the bladder may not fully distend until refluxed contrast drops back down. In this situation, obtaining delayed views may visualize antegrade flow across the UPJ and UVJ, which may help distinguish an obstructive component to the hydronephrosis.

Retrograde Pyelography

If the anatomy of the distal ureter has not been defined in the workup for UPJ obstruction, then cystoscopy with a retrograde pyelogram can be performed at the time of open surgical correction to determine the location and length of the obstruction (Fig. 55.9B). This helpful technique can exclude distal ureteral disease, but it should only be performed in conjunction with upper tract surgery for fear of introducing lower urinary tract bacteria into an obstructed or partially obstructed system.

MANAGEMENT OF OBSTRUCTIVE UROPATHY

Although hydronephrosis is not necessarily equivalent to obstruction (a process of potential renal deterioration), neither is it a normal finding (273). There is great interest, then, in the prognostic significance of findings associated with hydronephrosis. Various studies have proposed the factors that independently predict an adverse outcome. One report followed prospectively 148 children with a history of prenatal hydronephrosis for a mean of 39 months. Oligohydramnios, prematurity, and postnatal GFR lower than 20 mL/min were independent predictors of chronic renal failure by multivariate analysis (274). In a second multivariate study of prenatal hydronephrosis, oligohydramnios and megacystis (distended bladder) were highly predictive of fetal urethral obstruction on postnatal follow-up (275).

A pediatric urologist should evaluate and follow the infant with a history of prenatal hydronephrosis or the child with a history of flank pain, gross hematuria, nephrolithiasis, or febrile urinary tract infection. The physical examination is usually normal, and most of these children with unilateral hydronephrosis and a contralateral normal kidney appear entirely healthy.

Evaluation with VCUG, radionuclide imaging, and/or excretory urography further characterize the abnormality detected by ultrasound, as described earlier. Initial postnatal imaging includes ultrasonography in the first week of life to confirm the prenatal diagnosis if bilateral hydronephrosis was detected and at 3 to 4 weeks if unilateral hydronephrosis was noted prenatally. Follow-up prenatal ultrasonography is shown to give some false-negative results, thus supporting the need for postnatal scanning (276). Early postnatal dehydration and oliguria (first 24 to 48 hours of

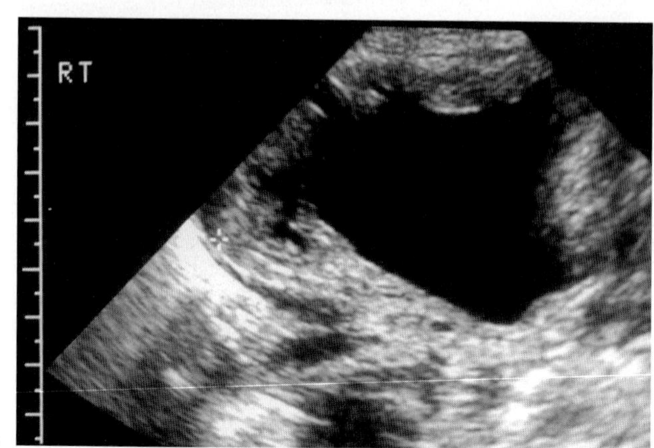

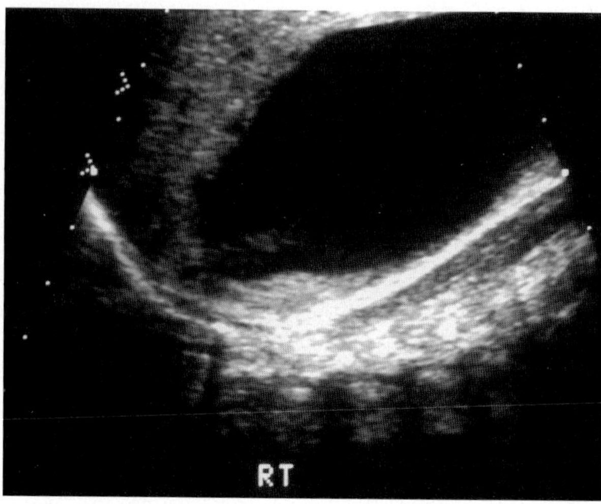

FIGURE 55.13. A: Renal ultrasound on day of life number 1 for this term boy with a history of prenatally detected, right hydronephrosis. Note the severe pelvicaliectasis. The ipsilateral ureter is not visualized and, therefore, by definition, not dilated. **B:** Same patient on day of life number 4 after a period of rehydration. Note the marked increase in dilation of the pelvis and blunting of the calyces, as well as thinning of the renal cortex.

life) may transiently mask the high-grade lesion in moderate to severe hydronephrosis (Fig. 55.13). Therefore, a normal or moderately abnormal ultrasound performed within the first 2 to 3 days of life for an infant with a history of higher-grade prenatal hydronephrosis may give a false sense of security and will need to be repeated after adequate rehydration. An immediate cystogram is performed in any infant with suspected bladder outlet obstruction before discharge from the hospital. In males, the most important early diagnosis to be made is PUV, because catheter drainage is necessary. In females, an obstructing ectopic ureterocele may need to be ruled out. Prenatal bladder outlet obstruction secondary to ureterocele requires early postnatal endoscopic decompression; however, the affected upper tract renal pole may not necessarily be salvaged (277).

All infants or children with hydronephrosis are placed on antibiotic prophylaxis pending the outcome of further evaluation. An infection in the setting of ureteral obstruction can cause significant morbidity in the uroseptic infant, and renal damage is a potential comorbidity. Oral amoxicillin (10 mg/kg/day) is the most commonly used prophylactic antibiotic. Trimethoprim-sulfamethoxazole, however, is not used in the early postnatal setting, because the neonate has only limited ability to metabolize the drug by acetylation in the liver.

When to obtain postnatal VCUG with a history of prenatal hydronephrosis is controversial, with some authors recommending VCUG in all infants and others only when there is bilateral hydronephrosis, ureteral dilation, or variable hydronephrosis (278–280). If VUR is noted, then antibiotic prophylaxis is started or continued with appropriate radiologic follow-up. Approximately 10 to 15% of prenatal cases of hydronephrosis result in the postnatal diagnosis of VUR. The majority of these infants are boys with bilateral, high-grade disease, and early circumcision has been hypothesized by some authors to decrease the incidence of breakthrough urinary tract infection in this subpopulation (278).

Because the natural history of prenatal hydronephrosis due to UPJ or UVJ obstruction remains to be well defined, it can be difficult to know whether to intervene surgically to potentially maximize renal function or to observe and allow for spontaneous resolution of hydronephrosis without risking normal renal growth and development. Some have argued that 85% of infants with prenatally detected hydronephrosis do not have a true obstruction (but rather a temporary physiologic impedance) and do not require surgery, as they will improve spontaneously (281,282). However, there are no prospective randomized studies comparing operative and nonoperative treatments of UPJ obstruction for comparable degrees of hydronephrosis. There are longitudinal follow-up studies on prenatal hydronephrosis that allow for crossover from observation to surgery when relative renal function is reduced by 10% or more or symptoms of UPJ obstruction occur. In one review of 321 patients with prenatal hydronephrosis, surgery did not significantly improve renal function in those with both UPJ obstruction and abnormal preoperative renal function (defined by decreased relative function on nuclear renography). However, in those patients with prenatal UPJ obstruction managed with observation alone, there was a small but significant risk of a modest loss of renal function as measured by MAG-3 (283). Overall, in series taking a nonoperative approach to patients with good initial relative renal function, a 25% crossover to surgery over long-term follow-up has been recognized.

It has been argued that renal function does not improve regardless of the initial level of relative renal function (284). A second study has concluded that poor renal function may not improve after obstruction is relieved (285).

Other authors, however, recommend early surgical treatment to prevent obstructive damage to the immature infant kidney, because better recovery of function may be possible when surgery is done in the first year of life (286,287). Furthermore, it has been shown in another series that only 18% of patients with obstructive parameters on nuclear renography resolved with conservative management (288). Concerns about conservative management are also raised in a review of 121 children in which renal function did improve in those undergoing early surgery but less so in those who were initially observed before surgery (289). Chertin et al. have described significant improvement in hydronephrosis and nuclear renography parameters in all 113 patients undergoing surgery for UPJ obstruction detected prenatally (290). These observations support early surgical intervention over a nonoperative approach for UPJ obstruction.

The long-term morbidity of mild hydronephrosis (pelviectasis without calyceal dilation) is low—rarely is surgery required. Moderate hydronephrosis (dilated pelvis and calyces without parenchymal thinning) may be associated with gradual improvement in severity of dilation and drainage parameters, without loss of relative renal function. It is severe hydronephrosis (pelvic dilation, calyceal blunting, and parenchymal thinning) that commonly requires surgical intervention for declining renal function, infection, or symptoms.

LONG-TERM FOLLOW-UP

The long-term prognosis for infants and children with congenital obstructive nephropathy is poorly defined. Unfortunately, many children undergoing pyeloplasty for UPJ obstruction and found to have a satisfactory immediate postoperative course are lost to follow-up after several years. In light of the experimental evidence, as well as the limited clinical data available, it is likely that some of these patients will eventually develop proteinuria, hypertension, or chronic renal insufficiency. The prognosis for children with PUV is more grim: A majority of patients diagnosed in fetal or neonatal life develop renal insufficiency by age 10 years (291,292). At a minimum, all children with obstructive nephropathy should have regular measurement of blood pressure, plasma creatinine, urinalysis, and periodic renal ultrasound. Every attempt must be made to maintain normotension and to minimize proteinuria. Nonsteroidal antiinflammatory drugs should be avoided. In the transition of care from pediatrician to internist, this follow-up should be maintained throughout adulthood.

ACKNOWLEDGMENTS

National Institutes of Health grants DK40558, DK44756, DK52612, and DK45179 supported original studies by Dr. Chevalier.

REFERENCES

1. Klahr S, Harris K, Purkerson ML. Effects of obstruction on renal functions. *Pediatr Nephrol* 1988;2:34–42.
2. Merlet-Benichou C, Gilbert T, Muffat-Joly M, et al. Intrauterine growth retardation leads to a permanent nephron deficit in the rat. *Pediatr Nephrol* 1994;8:175–180.
3. Chung KH, Chevalier RL. Arrested development of the neonatal kidney following chronic ureteral obstruction. *J Urol* 1996;155:1139–1144.
4. Chevalier RL, Chung KH, Smith CD, et al. Renal apoptosis and clusterin following ureteral obstruction: the role of maturation. *J Urol* 1996;156:1474–1479.
5. Nguyen HT, Thomson AA, Kogan BA, et al. Expression of the *Wnt* gene family during late nephrogenesis and complete ureteral obstruction. *Lab Invest* 1999;79:647–658.
6. Haralambous-Gasser A, Chan D, Walker RG, et al. Collagen studies in newborn rat kidneys with incomplete ureteric obstruction. *Kidney Int* 1993;44:593–605.
7. McVary KT, Maizels M. Urinary obstruction reduces glomerulogenesis in the developing kidney: a model in the rabbit. *J Urol* 1989;142:646–651.
8. Peters CA, Carr MC, Lais A, et al. The response of the fetal kidney to obstruction. *J Urol* 1992;148:503–509.
9. Peters CA, Gaertner RC, Carr MC, et al. Fetal compensatory renal growth due to unilateral ureteral obstruction. *J Urol* 1993;150(2 PT 2):597–600.
10. Gasser B, Mauss Y, Ghnassia JP, et al. A quantitative study of normal nephrogenesis in the human fetus: its implication in the natural history of kidney changes due to low obstructive uropathies. *Fetal Diagn Ther* 1993;8:371–384.
11. Eskild-Jensen A, Frokiaer J, Djurhuus JC, et al. Reduced number of glomeruli in kidneys with neonatally induced partial ureteropelvic obstruction in pigs. *J Urol* 2002;167:1435–1439.
12. Josephson S. Experimental obstructive hydronephrosis in newborn rats. III. Long-term effects on renal function. *J Urol* 1983;129:396–400.
13. Chevalier RL, Thornhill BA, Chang AY, et al. Recovery from release of ureteral obstruction in the rat: relationship to neprhogenesis. *Kidney Int* 2002;61:2033–2043.
14. Shibata S, Shigeta M, Shu Y, et al. Initial pathological events in renal dysplasia with urinary tract obstruction in utero. *Virchows Arch Int J Pathol* 2001;439:560–570.
15. El-Dahr SS, Gomez RA, Gray MS, et al. In situ localization of renin and its mRNA in neonatal ureteral obstruction. *Am J Physiol* 1990;258:F854–F862.
16. Lopez MLSS, Pentz ES, Robert B, et al. Embryonic origin and lineage of juxtaglomerular cells. *Am J Physiol Renal Physiol* 2001;281:F345–F356.
17. Chevalier RL, Kim A, Thornhill BA, et al. Recovery following relief of unilateral ureteral obstruction in the neonatal rat. *Kidney Int* 1999;55:793–807.
18. Chevalier RL, Gomez RA. Response of the renin-angiotensin system to relief of neonatal ureteral obstruction. *Am J Physiol* 1989;255:F1070–F1077.
19. Fogo A, Ichikawa I. Angiogenic action of angiotensin II is important for the glomerular growth of maturing kidneys. *Kidney Int* 1991;39:S37–S38.
20. Chevalier RL. Molecular and cellular pathophysiology of obstructive nephropathy. *Pediatr Nephrol* 1999;13:612–619.

21. French LE, Chonn A, Ducrest D, et al. Murine clusterin: molecular cloning and mRNA localization of a gene associated with epithelial differentiation processes during embryogenesis. *J Cell Biol* 1993;122:1119–1130.
22. Hilgers KF, Nagaraj SK, Karginova EA, et al. Molecular cloning of KS, a novel rat gene expressed exclusively in the kidney. *Kidney Int* 1998;54:1444–1454.
23. Chevalier RL, Goyal S, Wolstenholme JT, et al. Obstructive nephropathy in the neonate is attenuated by epidermal growth factor. *Kidney Int* 1998;54:38–47.
24. Marxer-Meier A, Hegyi I, Loffing J, et al. Postnatal maturation of renal cortical peritubular fibroblasts in the rat. *Anat Embryol (Berl)* 1998;197:143–153.
25. Daikha-Dahmane F, Dommergues M, Muller F, et al. Development of human fetal kidney in obstructive uropathy: correlations with ultrasonography and urine biochemistry. *Kidney Int* 1997;52:21–32.
26. Gobe GC, Axelsen RA. Genesis of renal tubular atrophy in experimental hydronephrosis in the rat. *Lab Invest* 1987;56: 273–281.
27. Kennedy WA II, Stenberg A, Lackgren G, et al. Renal tubular apoptosis after partial ureteral obstruction. *J Urol* 1994;152:658–664.
28. Poucell-Hatton S, Huang M, Bannykh S, et al. Fetal obstructive uropathy: patterns of renal pathology. *Pediatr Devel Pathol* 2000;3:223–231.
29. Winyard PJD, Nauta J, Lirenman DS, et al. Deregulation of cell survival in cystic and dysplastic renal development. *Kidney Int* 1996;49:135–146.
30. Cachat F, Lange-Sperandio B, Chang AY, et al. Ureteral obstruction in neonatal mice elicits segment-specific tubular cell responses leading to nephron loss. *Kidney Int* 2003;63:564–575.
31. Storch S, Saggi S, Megyesi J, et al. Ureteral obstruction decreases renal prepro-epidermal growth factor and Tamm-Horsfall expression. *Kidney Int* 1992;42:89–94.
32. Walton G, Buttyan R, Garcia-Montes E, et al. Renal growth factor expression during the early phase of experimental hydronephrosis. *J Urol* 1992;148:510–514.
33. Raaberg L, Nexo E, Mikkelsen JD, et al. Immunohistochemical localization and developmental aspects of epidermal growth factor in the rat. *Histochemistry* 1988;89:351–356.
34. Cybulsky AV, Goodyer PR, McTavish AJ. Epidermal growth factor receptor activation in developing rat kidney. *Am J Physiol* 1994;267:F428–F436.
35. Chevalier RL, Goyal S, Thornhill BA. EGF improves recovery following relief of unilateral ureteral obstruction in the neonatal rat. *J Urol* 1999;162:1532–1536.
36. Chevalier RL, Goyal S, Kim A, et al. Renal tubulointerstitial injury from ureteral obstruction in the neonatal rat is attenuated by IGF-1. *Kidney Int* 2000;57:882–890.
37. Nguyen HT, Bride SH, Badawy AB, et al. Heparin-binding EGF-like growth factor is up-regulated in the obstructed kidney in a cell- and region-specific manner and acts to inhibit apoptosis. *Am J Pathol* 2000;156:889–898.
38. Kiley SC, Thornhill BA, Tang SS, et al. Growth factor-mediated phosphorylation of propapoptotic BAD reduces tubule cell death *in vitro* and *in vivo. Kidney Int* 2003;63(1):33–42.
39. Miyajima A, Chen J, Lawrence C, et al. Antibody to transforming growth factor-β ameliorates tubular apoptosis in unilateral ureteral obstruction. *Kidney Int* 2000;58:2301–2313.
40. Ma LJ, Nakamura S, Whitsitt JS, et al. Regression of sclerosis in aging by an angiotensin inhibition-induced decrease in PAI-1. *Kidney Int* 2000;58:2425–2436.
41. Schaefer L, Macakova K, Raslik I, et al. Absence of decorin adversely influences tubulointerstitial fibrosis of the obstructed kidney by enhanced apoptosis and increased inflammatory reaction. *Am J Pathol* 2002;160:1181–1191.
42. Choi YJ, Baranowska-Daca E, Nguyen V, et al. Mechanism of chronic obstructive uropathy: increased expression of apoptosis-promoting molecules. *Kidney Int* 2000;58:1481–1491.
43. Truong LD, Choi YJ, Tsao CC, et al. Renal cell apoptosis in chronic obstructive uropathy: the roles of caspases. *Kidney Int* 2001;60:924–934.
44. Hughes J, Johnson RJ. Role of Fas (CD95) in tubulointerstitial disease induced by unilateral ureteric obstruction. *Am J Physiol* 1999;277:F26–F32.
45. Choi YJ, Mendoza L, Rha SJ, et al. Role of p53-dependent activation of caspases in chronic obstructive uropathy: evidence from p53 null mutant mice. *J Am Soc Nephrol* 2001;12:983–992.
46. Liapis H, Yu H, Steinhardt GF. Cell proliferation, apoptosis, Bcl-2 and Bax expression in obstructed opossum early metanephroi. *J Urol* 2000;164:511–517.
47. Chevalier RL, Smith CD, Wolstenholme JT, et al. Chronic ureteral obstruction in the rat suppresses renal tubular bcl-2 and stimulates apoptosis. *Exp Nephrol* 2000;8:115–122.
48. Lange-Sperandio B, Cachat F, Thornhill BA, et al. Selectins mediate macrophage infiltration in obstructive nephropathy in newborn mice. *Kidney Int* 2002;61:516–524.
49. Serlachius E, Svennilson J, Schalling M, et al. Protein kinase C in the developing kidney: isoform expression and effects of ceramide and PKC inhibitors. *Kidney Int* 1997;52:901–910.
50. Malik RK, Thornhill BA, Chang AY, et al. Apoptosis parallels ceramide content in the developing rat kidney. *Pediatr Nephrol* 2000;15:188–191.
51. Malik RK, Thornhill BA, Chang AY, et al. Renal apoptosis parallels ceramide content following chronic ureteral obstruction in the neonatal rat. *Am J Physiol* 2001;281:F86–F61.
52. Schreiner GF, Harris KPG, Purkerson ML, et al. Immunological aspects of acute ureteral obstruction: immune cell infiltrate in the kidney. *Kidney Int* 1991;34:487–493.
53. Okegawa T, Jonas PE, Deschryver K, et al. Metabolic and cellular alterations underlying the exaggerated renal prostaglandin and thromboxane synthesis in ureter obstruction in rabbits: inflammatory response involving fibroblasts and mononuclear cells. *J Clin Invest* 1983;71:81–89.
54. Reyes AA, Lefkowith J, Pippin J, et al. Role of the 5-lipooxygenase pathway in obstructive nephropathy. *Kidney Int* 1992;41:100–106.
55. Shappell SB, Gurpinar T, Lechago J, et al. Chronic obstructive uropathy in severe combined immunodeficient (SCID) mice: lymphocyte infiltration is not required for progressive tubulointerstitial injury. *J Am Soc Nephrol* 1998;9:1008–1017.
56. Engelmyer E, Van Goor H, Edwards DR, et al. Differential mRNA expression of renal cortical tissue inhibitor of metalloproteinase-1, -2, and -3 in experimental hydronephrosis. *J Am Soc Nephrol* 1995;5:1675–1683.
57. Diamond JR, Kees-Folts D, Ricardo SD, et al. Early and persistent up-regulated expression of renal cortical osteopontin in experimental hydronephrosis. *Am J Pathol* 1995;146:1455–1466.

58. Stephan M, Conrad S, Eggert T, et al. Urinary concentration and tissue messenger RNA expression of monocyte chemoattractant protein-1 as an indicator of the degree of hydronephrotic atrophy in partial ureteral obstruction. *J Urol* 2002;167:1497–1502.
59. Grandaliano G, Gesualdo L, Bartoli F, et al. MCP-1 and EGF renal expression and urine excretion in human congenital obstructive nephropathy. *Kidney Int* 2000;58:182–192.
60. Vielhauer V, Anders HJ, Mack M, et al. Obstructive nephropathy in the mouse: progressive fibrosis correlates with tubulointerstitial chemokine expression and accumulation of CC chemokine receptor 2-and 5-positive leukocytes. *J Am Soc Nephol* 2001;12:1173–1187.
61. Anders HJ, Vielhauer V, Frink M, et al. A chemokine receptor CCR-1 antagonist reduces renal fibrosis after unilateral ureter ligation. *J Clin Invest* 2002;109:251–259.
62. Oda T, Jung YO, Kim HS, et al. PAI-1 deficiency attenuates the fibrogenic response to ureteral obstruction. *Kidney Int* 2001;60:587–596.
63. Ishidoya S, Ogata Y, Fukuzaki A, et al. Plasminogen activator inhibitor-1 and tissue-type plasminogen activator are up-regulated during unilateral ureteral obstruction in adult rats. *J Urol* 2002;167:1503–1507.
64. Kim HS, Oda T, López-Guisa J, et al. TIMP-1 deficiency does not attenuate interstitial fibrosis in obstructive nephropathy. *J Am Soc Nephrol* 2001;12:736–748.
65. Okada H, Strutz F, Danoff TM, et al. Possible pathogenesis of renal fibrosis. *Kidney Int* 1996;49:S-37–S-38.
66. Diamond JR, Van Goor H, Ding G, et al. Myofibroblasts in experimental hydronephrosis. *Am J Pathol* 1995;146:121–129.
67. Schmitt-Graff A, Desmouliere A, Gabbiani G. Heterogeneity of myofibroblast phenotypic features: an example of fibroblastic cell plasticity. *Virchows Arch* 1994;425:3–24.
68. Nagle RB, Evans LW, Reynolds DG. Contractility of renal cortex following complete ureteral obstruction. *Proc Soc Exp Biol Med* 1975;148:611–614.
69. Roberts AB, McCune BK, Sporn MB. TGF-B: regulation of extracellular matrix. *Kidney Int* 1992;41:557–559.
70. Desmouliere A, Geinoz A, Gabbiani F, et al. Transforming growth factor-beta 1 induces alpha-smooth muscle actin expression in granulation tissue myofibroblasts and in quiescent and growing cultured fibroblasts. *J Cell Biol* 1993;122: 103–111.
71. Desmouliere A, Gabbiani G. Modulation of fibroblastic cytoskeletal features during pathological situations: the role of extracellular matrix and cytokines. *Cell Motil Cytoskel* 1994;29:195–203.
72. Kaneto H, Morrissey J, Klahr S. Increased expression of TGF-beta 1 mRNA in the obstructed kidney of rats with unilateral ureteral ligation. *Kidney Int* 1993;44:313 321.
73. Diamond JR, Kees-Folts D, Ding G, et al. Macrophages, monocyte chemoattractant peptide-1, and TGF-beta1 in experimental hydronephrosis. *Am J Physiol* 1994;266:F926–F933.
74. Pimentel JL Jr, Sundell CL, Wang SS, et al. Role of angiotensin II in the expression and regulation of transforming growth factor-Beta in obstructive nephropathy. *Kidney Int* 1995;48:1233–1246.
75. Gonzalez-Avila G, Vadillo-Ortega F, Perez-Tamayo R. Experimental diffuse interstitial renal fibrosis: a biochemical approach. *Lab Invest* 1988;59:245–252.
76. Miyajima A, Ito K, Asano T, et al. Does cyclooxygenase-2 inhibitor prevent renal tissue damage in unilateral ureteral obstruction? *J Urol* 2001;166:1124–1129.
77. Isaka Y, Tsujie M, Ando Y, et al. Transforming growth factor-β1 antisense oligodeoxynucleotides block interstitial fibrosis in unilateral ureteral obstruction. *Kidney Int* 2000;58:1885–1892.
78. Mizuno S, Matsumoto K, Nakamura T. Hepatocyte growth factor suppresses interstitial fibrosis in a mouse model of obstructive nephropathy. *Kidney Int* 2001;59:1304–1314.
79. Yang J, Liu Y. Blockage of tubular epithelial to myofibroblast transition by hepatocyte growth factor prevents renal interstitial fibrosis. *J Am Soc Nephrol* 2002;13:96–107.
80. Darby I, Skalli O, Gabbiani G. Alpha-smooth muscle actin is transiently expressed by myofibroblasts during experimental wound healing. *Lab Invest* 1990;63:21–29.
81. Tang WW, Ulich TR, Lacey DL, et al. Platelet-derived growth factor-BB induces renal tubulointerstitial myofibroblast formation and tubulointerstitial fibrosis. *Am J Pathol* 1996;148:1169–1180.
82. Hruska KA, Guo GJ, Wozniak M, et al. Osteogenic protein-1 prevents renal fibrogenesis associated with ureteral obstruction. *Am J Physiol Renal Physiol* 2000;279:F130–F143.
83. Kawada N, Moriyama T, Ando A, et al. Increased oxidative stress in mouse kidneys with unilateral ureteral obstruction. *Kidney Int* 1999;56:1004–1013.
84. Moriyama T, Kawada N, Nagatoya K, et al. Fluvastatin suppresses oxidative stress and fibrosis in the interstitium of mouse kidneys with unilateral ureteral obstruction. *Kidney Int* 2001;59:2095–2103.
85. Kinter M, Wolstenholme JT, Thornhill BA, et al. Unilateral ureteral obstruction impairs renal antioxidant enzyme activation during sodium depletion. *Kidney Int* 1999;55:1327–1334.
86. Beckwith JR. The effect of the time factor on the amount of pressor material present in kidney after unilateral ligation of renal pedicle and after unilateral ligation of ureter. *Am J Physiol* 1941;132:1–4.
87. Gomez RA, Lynch KR, Sturgill BC, et al. Distribution of renin mRNA and its protein in the developing kidney. *Am J Physiol* 1989;257:F850–F858.
88. Ice KS, Geary KM, Gomez RA, et al. Cell and molecular studies of renin secretion. *Clin Exp Hypertens* 1988;10:1169–1187.
89. Norwood VF, Carey RM, Geary KM, et al. Neonatal ureteral obstruction stimulates recruitment of renin-secreting renal cortical cells. *Kidney Int* 1994;45:1333–1339.
90. Pimentel JL Jr, Montero A, Wang SS, et al. Sequential changes in renal expression of renin-angiotensin system genes in acute unilateral ureteral obstruction. *Kidney Int* 1995;48:1247–1253.
91. Pimentel JL Jr, Martinez-Maldonado M, Wilcox JN, et al. Regulation of renin-angiotensin system in unilateral ureteral obstruction. *Kidney Int* 1993;44:390–400.
92. El Dahr S, Gomez RA, Khare G, et al. Expression of renin and its mRNA in the adult rat kidney with chronic ureteral obstruction. *Am J Kidney Dis* 1990;15:575–582.
93. Busse R, Mülsch A. Induction of nitric oxide synthase by cytokines in vascular smooth muscle cells. *FEBS Lett* 1990;275:87–90.
94. Chevalier RL, Thornhill BA. Ureteral obstruction in the neonatal rat: renal nerves modulate hemodynamic effects. *Pediatr Nephrol* 1995;9:447–450.

95. Robillard JE, Page WV, Smith FG, et al. Renal nerves increase renin gene expression and renin secretion at birth. *J Am Soc Nephrol* 1991;2:482.
96. Chevalier RL, Thornhill BA. Ureteral obstruction in the neonatal guinea pig: interaction of sympathetic nerves and angiotensin. *Pediatr Nephrol* 1995;9:441–446.
97. Stoll M, Steckelings UM, Paul M, et al. The angiotensin AT2-receptor mediates inhibition of cell proliferation in coronary endothelial cells. *J Clin Invest* 1995;95:651–657.
98. Tufro-McReddie A, Romano LM, Harris JM, et al. Angiotensin II regulates nephrogenesis and renal vascular development. *Am J Physiol* 1995;269:F110–F115.
99. Wolf G. Regulation of renal tubular cell growth: effects of angiotensin II. *Exp Nephrol* 1994;2:107–114.
100. Nakajima M, Hutchinson HG, Fujinaga M, et al. The angiotensin II type 2 (AT2) receptor antagonizes the growth effects of the AT1 receptor: gain-of-function study using gene transfer. *Proc Natl Acad Sci U S A* 1995;92:10663–10667.
101. Tanaka M, Ohnishi J, Ozawa Y, et al. Characterization of angiotensin II receptor type 2 during differentiation and apoptosis of rat ovarian cultured granulosa cells. *Biochem Biophys Res Commun* 1995;207:593–598.
102. Yamada T, Horiuchi M, Dzau VJ. Angiotensin II type 2 receptor mediates programmed cell death. *Proc Natl Acad Sci U S A* 1996;93:156–160.
103. Paxton WG, Runge M, Horaist C, et al. Immunohistochemical localization of rat angiotensin II AT1 receptor. *Am J Physiol* 1993;264:F989–F995.
104. Yoo KH, Norwood VF, El-Dahr SS, et al. Regulation of angiotensin II AT1 and AT2 receptors in neonatal ureteral obstruction. *Am J Physiol* 1997;273:R503–R509.
105. El-Dahr SS, Gee J, Dipp S, et al. Upregulation of renin-angiotensin system and downregulation of kallikrein in obstructive nephropathy. *Am J Physiol* 1993;264:F874–F881.
106. Cheng HF, Becker BN, Burns KD, et al. Angiotensin II upregulates type-1 angiotensin II receptors in renal proximal tubule. *J Clin Invest* 1995;95:2012–2019.
107. Chevalier RL, Thornhill BA, Wolstenholme JT. Renal cellular response to ureteral obstruction: role of maturation and angiotensin II. *Am J Physiol* 1999;277:F41–F47.
108. Yoo KH, Thornhill BA, Chevalier RL. Angiotensin stimulates TGF-beta 1 and clusterin in the hydronephrotic neonatal rat kidney. *Am J Physiol* 2000;278:R640–R645.
109. Fern RJ, Yesko CM, Thornhill BA, et al. Reduced angiotenisnogen expression attenuates renal interstitial fibrosis in obstructive nephropathy in mice. *J Clin Invest* 1999;103:39–46.
110. Guo G, Morrissey J, McCracken R, et al. Contributions of angiotensin II and tumor necrosis factor-alpha to the development of renal fibrosis. *Am J Physiol* 2001;280:F777–F785.
111. Nguyen HT, Thomson AA, Kogan BA, et al. Growth factor expression in the obstructed developing and mature rat kidney. *Lab Invest* 1999;79:171–184.
112. Kim S, Ohta K, Hamaguchi A, et al. Contribution of renal angiotensin II type I receptor to gene expressions in hypertension-induced renal injury. *Kidney Int* 1994;46:1346–1358.
113. Johnson RJ, Alpers CE, Yoshimura A, et al. Renal injury from angiotensin II-mediated hypertension. *Hypertension* 1992;19:464–474.
114. Diamond JR, Kreisberg R, Evans R, et al. Regulation of proximal tubular osteopontin in experimental hydronephrosis in the rat. *Kidney Int* 1998;54:1501–1509.
115. Ricardo SD, Levinson ME, DeJoseph MR, et al. Expression of adhesion molecules in rat renal cortex during experimental hydronephrosis. *Kidney Int* 1996;50:2002–2010.
116. Kaneto H, Morrissey J, McCracken R, et al. Enalapril reduces collagen type IV synthesis and expansion of the interstitium in the obstructed rat kidney. *Kidney Int* 1994;45:1637–1647.
117. Ishidoya S, Morrissey J, McCracken R, et al. Delayed treatment with enalapril halts tubulointerstitial fibrosis in rats with obstructive nephropathy. *Kidney Int* 1996;49:1110–1119.
118. Chung KH, Gomez RA, Chevalier RL. Regulation of renal growth factors and clusterin by angiotensin AT1 receptors during neonatal ureteral obstruction. *Am J Physiol* 1995;268:F1117–F1123.
119. Gibbons GH, Pratt RE, Dzau VJ. Vascular smooth muscle cell hypertrophy vs. hyperplasia. Autocrine transforming growth factor-Beta1 expression determines growth response to angiotensin II. *J Clin Invest* 1992;90:456–461.
120. Andrawis NS, Ruley EH, Abernethy DR. Angiotensin II regulates human vascular smooth muscle alpha-actin gene expression. *Biochem Biophys Res Commun* 1993;196:962–968.
121. Ma J, Nishimura H, Fogo A, et al. Accelerated fibrosis and collagen deposition develop in the renal interstitium of angiotensin type 2 receptor null mutant mice during ureteral obstruction. *Kidney Int* 1998;53:937–944.
122. Pope JC, Brock JW III, Adams MC, et al. Congenital anomalies of the kidney and urinary tract—role of the loss of function mutation in the pluripotent angiotensin type 2 receptor gene. *J Urol* 2001;165:196–202.
123. Hiraoka M, Taniguchi T, Nakai H, et al. No evidence for *AT2R* gene derangement in human urinary tract anomalies. *Kidney Int* 2001;59:1244–1249.
124. Miyazaki Y, Tsuchida S, Fogo A, et al. The renal lesions that develop in neonatal mice during angiotensin inhibition mimic obstructive nephropathy. *Kidney Int* 1999;55:1683–1695.
125. Moody TE, Vaughan ED, Jr., Gillenwater JY. Relationship between renal blood flow and ureteral pressure during 18 hours of total unilateral ureteral occlusion. *Invest Urol* 1975;13:246–251.
126. Felsen D, Loo MH, Vaughan ED Jr. Effect of ureteral obstruction on renal hemodynamics. *Semin Urol* 1991;5:160–166.
127. Harris RH, Gill JM. Changes in glomerular filtration rate during complete ureteral obstruction in rats. *Kidney Int* 1981;19:603–608.
128. Wilson DR. Micropuncture study of chronic obstructive nephropathy before and after release of obstruction. *Kidney Int* 1972;2:119–130.
129. Buerkert J, Martin D, Head M, et al. Deep nephron function after release of acute unilateral ureteral obstruction in the young rat. *J Clin Invest* 1978;62:1228–1239.
130. Buerkert J, Martin D. Relation of nephron recruitment to detectable filtration and recovery of function after release of ureteral obstruction. *Proc Soc Exp Biol Med* 1983;173:533–540.
131. Provoost AP, Molenaar JC. Renal function during and after a temporary complete unilateral ureter obstruction in rats. *Invest Urol* 1981;18:242–246.

132. Yokoyama M, Yoshioka S, Iwata H, et al. Paradoxical tubular obstruction after release of ureteral obstruction in rat kidney. *J Urol* 1984;132:388–391.
133. Huguenin ME, Thiel GT, Brunner FP, et al. Regeneration du rein apres levee d'une occlusion de l'uretere chez le rat, *Kidney Int* 1974;5:221–232.
134. Tanner GA, Knopp LC. Glomerular blood flow after single nephron obstruction in the rat kidney. *Am J Physiol* 1986; 250:F77–F85.
135. Chevalier RL, Gomez RA, Jones CA. Developmental determinants of recovery after relief of partial ureteral obstruction. *Kidney Int* 1988;33:775–781.
136. Blackshear JL, Wathen RL. Effects of indomethacin on renal blood flow and renin secretory responses to ureteral occlusion in the dog. *Mineral Electrolyte Metab* 1978;1:271–278.
137. Yarger WE, Schocken DD, Harris RH. Obstructive nephropathy in the rat: possible roles for the renin-angiotensin system, prostaglandins, and thromboxanes in postobstructive renal function. *J Clin Invest* 1980;65:400–412.
138. Harris KPG, Schreiner GF, Klahr S. Effect of leukocyte depletion on the function of the postobstructed kidney in the rat. *Kidney Int* 1989;36:210–215.
139. Schnermann J, Traynor T, Pohl H, et al. Vasoconstrictor responses in thromboxane receptor knockout mice: tubuloglomerular feedback and ureteral obstruction. *Acta Physiol Scand* 2000;168:201–207.
140. Yanagisawa H, Morrissey J, Morrison AR, et al. Role of ANG II in eicosanoid production by isolated glomeruli from rats with bilateral ureteral obstruction. *Am J Physiol* 1990;258:F85–F93.
141. Hanss BG, Lewy JE, Vari RC. Alterations in glomerular dynamics in congenital, unilateral hydronephrosis. *Kidney Int* 1994;46:48–57.
142. Kühl PG, Schönig G, Schweer H, et al. Increased renal biosynthesis of prostaglandin E_2 and thromboxane B_2 in human congenital obstructive uropathy. *Pediatr Res* 1990;27:103–107.
143. Yanagisawa H, Morrissey J, Klahr S. Mechanism of enhanced eicosanoid production by isolated glomeruli from rats with bilateral ureteral obstruction. *Am J Physiol* 1991; 261:F248–F255.
144. Yanagisawa H, Morrissey J, Morrison AR, et al. Eicosanoid production by isolated glomeruli of rats with unilateral ureteral obstruction. *Kidney Int* 1990;37:1528–1535.
145. Chevalier RL, Sturgill BC, Jones CE, et al. Morphologic correlates of renal growth arrest in neonatal partial ureteral obstruction. *Pediatr Res* 1987;21:338–346.
146. Chevalier RL, Peach MJ. Hemodynamic effects of enalapril on neonatal chronic partial ureteral obstruction. *Kidney Int* 1985;28:891–898.
147. Carmines PK, Tanner GA. Angiotensin in the hemodynamic response to chronic nephron obstruction. *Am J Physiol* 1983;245:F75–F82.
148. McDougal WS. Pharmacologic preservation of renal mass and function in obstructive uropathy. *J Urol* 1982;128:418–421.
149. Purkerson ML, Blaine EH, Stokes TJ, et al. Role of atrial peptide in the natriuresis and diuresis that follows relief of obstruction in rat. *Am J Physiol* 1989;25:F583–F589.
150. Himmelstein SI, Coffman TM, Yarger WE, et al. Atrial natriuretic peptide-induced changes in renal prostacyclin production in ureteral obstruction. *Am J Physiol* 1990;258:F281–F286.
151. Harris KPG, Purkerson ML, Klahr S. The recovery of renal function in rats after release of unilateral ureteral obstruction: the effects of moderate isotonic saline loading. *Eur J Clin Invest* 1991;21:339–343.
152. Reyes AA, Robertson G, Klahr S. Role of vasopressin in rats with bilateral ureteral obstruction. *Proc Soc Exp Biol Med* 1991;197:49–55.
153. Yarger WE, Newman WJ, Klotman PE. Renal effects of aprotinin after 24 hours of unilateral ureteral obstruction. *Am J Physiol* 1987;253:F1006–F1014.
154. El-Dahr SS, Dipp S. Differential effects of ureteral obstruction on rat kininogen gene family. *J Am Soc Nephrol* 1994;5:102–109.
155. Reyes AA, Martin D, Settle S, et al. EDRF role in renal function and blood pressure of normal rats and rats with obstructive uropathy. *Kidney Int* 1992;41:403–413.
156. Chevalier RL, Thornhill BA, Gomez RA. EDRF modulates renal hemodynamics during unilateral ureteral obstruction in the rat. *Kidney Int* 1992;42:400–406.
157. Hegarty NJ, Young LS, Kirwan CN, et al. Nitric oxide in unilateral ureteral obstruction: effect on regional renal blood flow. *Kidney Int* 2001;59:1059–1065.
158. Morrissey JJ, Ishidoya S, McCracken R, et al. Nitric oxide generation ameliorates the tubulointerstitial fibrosis of obstructive nephropathy. *J Am Soc Nephrol* 1996;7:2202–2212.
159. McDowell KA, Chevalier RL, Thornhill BA, et al. Unilateral ureteral obstruction increases glomerular soluble guanylyl cyclase activity. *J Am Soc Nephrol* 1995;6:1498–1503.
160. Miyajima A, Chen J, Poppas DP, et al. Role of nitric oxide in renal tubular apoptosis of unilateral ureteral obstruction. *Kidney Int* 2001;59:1290–1303.
161. Hochberg D, Johnson CW, Chen J, et al. Interstitial fibrosis of unilateral ureteral obstruction is exacerbated in kidneys of mice lacking the gene for inducible nitric oxide synthase. *Lab Invest* 2000;80:1721–1728.
162. Hammad FT, Wheatley AM, Davis G. Long-term renal effects of unilateral ureteral obstruction and the role of endothelin. *Kidney Int* 2000;58:242–250.
163. Jones DA, George NJR, O'Reilly PH. Postobstructive renal function. *Semin Urol* 1987;5:176–190.
164. Wahlberg J, Stengerg A, Wilson DR, et al. Tubuloglomerular feedback and interstitial pressure in obstructive nephropathy. *Kidney Int* 1984;26:294–302.
165. Boone TB, Allen TD. Unilateral post-obstructive diuresis in the neonate. *J Urol* 1992;147:430–432.
166. Sonnenberg H, Wilson DR. The role of medullary collecting ducts in postobstructive diuresis. *J Clin Invest* 1976;57: 1564–1574.
167. Buttner M, Brown L, Wieland WF, et al. Renal function and (Na+ + K+)-ATPase in chronic unilateral hydronephrosis in dogs. *J Urol* 1986;135:185–190.
168. Brunskill N, Hayes C, Morrissey J, et al. Changes in lipid environment decrease Na,K-ATPase activity in obstructive nephropathy. *Kidney Int* 1991;39:843–849.
169. Wilson DR, Honrath U. Effect of renal denervation, furosemide, and acute saline loading on postobstructive diuresis in the rat. *Can J Physiol Pharmacol* 1981;59:59–64.
170. Hanley MJ, Davidson K. Isolated nephron segments from rabbit models of obstructive nephropathy. *J Clin Invest* 1982; 69:165–174.

171. Frokiaer J, Marples D, Knepper MA, et al. Bilateral ureteral obstruction downregulates expression of vasopressin-sensitive AQP-2 water channel in rat kidney. *Am J Physiol* 1996; 270:F657–F668.
172. Li C, Wang W, Kwon TH, et al. Downregulation of AQP1, -2, and -3 after ureteral obstruction is associated with a long-term urine-concentrating defect. *Am J Physiol* 2001;281:F163–F171.
173. Kekomaki M, Wehle M, Walker RD. The growing rabbit with a solitary, partially-obstructed kidney. Analysis of an experimental model with reference to the renal concentrating ability. *J Urol* 1985;133:870–872.
174. Gade R, Feinfeld DA, Gade MF. Renal microradiography of experimental ureteral obstruction in the rabbit. *J Urol* 1989;142:1619–1623.
175. Solez K, Ponchak S, Buono RA, et al. Inner medullary plasma flow in the kidney with ureteral obstruction. *Am J Physiol* 1976;231:1315–1321.
176. Earley LE. Extreme polyuria in obstructive uropathy: report of a case of "water-losing nephritis" in an infant, with a discussion of polyuria. *New Engl J Med* 1956;255: 600–605.
177. Nguyen HT, Wu HY, Baskin LS, et al. High urinary flow accelerates renal injury in young rats with partial unilateral ureteral obstruction. *J Urol* 2000;163:1904–1907.
178. Batlle DC, Arruda JAL, Kirtzman NA. Hyperkalemic distal renal tubular acidosis associated with obstructive uropathy. *New Engl J Med* 1981;304:373–380.
179. Alon UA, Kodroff MB, Broecker BH, et al. Renal tubular acidosis type 4 in neonatal unilateral kidney diseases. *J Pediatr* 1984;104:855–860.
180. Rodriguez-Soriano J, Vallo A, Oliveros R. Transient pseudohypoaldosteronism secondary to obstructive uropathy in infancy. *J Pediatr* 1983;103:375–380.
181. Marra G, Goj V, Appiani AC, et al. Persistent tubular resistance to aldosterone in infants with congenital hydronephrosis corrected neonatally. *J Pediatr* 1987;110:868–872.
182. Edwards GA, Crumb CK, Suki WN. Renal handling of phosphate following release of ureteral obstruction. *Mineral Electrolyte Metab* 1987;13:377–384.
183. Taki M, Goldsmith DI, Spitzer A. Impact of age on effects of ureteral obstruction on renal function. *Kidney Int* 1983;24:602–609.
184. Hinman F. Renal counterbalance: an experimental and clinical study with reference to the significance of disuse atrophy. *J Urol* 1923;9:289–314.
185. Hayslett JP. Effect of age on compensatory renal growth. *Kidney Int* 1983;23:599–602.
186. Aschinberg LC, Koskimies O, Bernstein J, et al. The influence of age on the response to renal parenchymal loss. *Yale J Biol Med* 1978;51:341–345.
187. Chevalier RL, Thornhill BA, Wolstenholme JT, et al. Unilateral ureteral obstruction in early development alters renal growth: dependence on the duration of obstruction. *J Urol* 1999;161:309–313.
188. Chevalier RL, Kaiser DL. Chronic partial ureteral obstruction in the neonatal guinea pig I: influence of uninephrectomy on growth and hemodynamics. *Pediatr Res* 1984;18:1266–1271.
189. Peters CA. Animal models of fetal renal disease. *Prenat Diagn* 2001;21:917–923.
190. Berman DJ, Maizels M. The role of urinary obstruction in the genesis of renal dysplasia: a model in the chick embryo. *J Urol* 1982;128:1091–1096.
191. Gotoh H, Masuzaki H, Taguri H, et al. Effect of experimentally induced urethral obstruction and surgical decompression in utero on renal development and function in rabbits. *Early Hum Dev* 1998;52:111–123.
192. Liapis H, Barent B, Steinhardt GF. Extracellular matrix in fetal kidney after experimental obstruction. *J Urol* 2001;166:1433–1438.
193. Steinhardt G, Salinas-Madrigal L, Farber R, et al. Experimental ureteral obstruction in the fetal opossum. I. Renal functional assessment. *J Urol* 1990;144:564–566.
194. Steinhardt GF, Liapis H, Phillips B, et al. Insulin-like growth factor improves renal architecture of fetal kidneys with complete ureteral obstruction. *J Urol* 1995;154:690–693.
195. Tanagho EA. Surgically induced partial urinary obstruction in the fetal lamb. *Invest Urol* 1972;10:25–34.
196. Beck AD. The effect of intra-uterine urinary obstruction upon the development of the fetal kidney. *J Urol* 1971;105:784–789.
197. Carr MC, Schlussel RN, Peters CA, et al. Expression of cell growth regulated genes in the fetal kidney: relevance to in utero obstruction. *J Urol* 1995;154:242–246.
198. Gobet R, Park JM, Nguyen HT, et al. Renal renin-angiotensin system dysregulation caused by partial bladder outlet obstruction in fetal sheep. *Kidney Int* 1999;56:1654–1661.
199. Harrison MR, Nakayama DK, Noall R, et al. Correction of congenital hydronephrosis in utero II. Decompression reverses the effects of obstruction on the fetal lung and urinary tract. *J Pediatr Surg* 1982;17:965–974.
200. Glick PL, Harrison MR, Noall RA, et al. Correction of congenital hydronephrosis in utero III: early mid-trimester ureteral obstruction produces renal dysplasia. *J Pediatr Surg* 1983;18:681–687.
201. Gonzales R, Reinberg Y, Burke B, et al. Early bladder outlet obstruction in fetal lambs induces renal dysplasia and the prune-belly syndrome. *J Pediatr Surg* 1990;25:342–345.
202. Glick PL, Harrison MR, Adzick NS, et al. Correction of congenital hydronephrosis in utero IV: in utero decompression prevents renal dysplasia. *J Pediatr Surg* 1984;19:649–657.
203. Edouga D, Hugueny B, Gasser B, et al. Recovery after relief of fetal urinary obstruction: morphological, functional and molecular aspects. *Am J Physiol* 2001;281:F26–F37.
204. Bogaert GA, Gluckman GR, Mevorach RA, et al. Renal preservation despite 35 days of partial bladder obstruction in the fetal lamb. *J Urol* 1995;154:694–699.
205. Nguyen HT, Kogan BA. Renal hemodynamic changes after complete and partial unilateral ureteral obstruction in the fetal lamb. *J Urol* 1998;160:1063–1069.
206. Tarantal AF, Han VKM, Cochrum KC, et al. Fetal rhesus monkey model of obstructive renal dysplasia. *Kidney Int* 2001;59:446–456.
207. Zhang PL, Peters CA, Rosen S. Ureteropelvic junction obstruction: morphological and clinical studies. *Pediatr Nephrol* 2000;14:820–826.
208. Barakat AY, Awazu M, Fleischer AC. Antenatal diagnosis of renal abnormalities: a review of the state of the art. *South Med J* 1989;82:229–234.

209. Coplen DE, Hare JY, Zderic SA, et al. 10-year experience with prenatal intervention for hydronephrosis. *J Urol* 1996;156:1142–1145.
210. Horton CE Jr, Davisson MT, Jacobs JB, et al. Congenital progressive hydronephrosis in mice: a new recessive mutation. *J Urol* 1988;140:1310–1315.
211. Furness PD III, Maizels M, Han SW, et al. Elevated bladder urine concentration of transforming growth factor-β1 correlates with upper urinary tract obstruction in children. *J Urol* 1999;162:1033–1036.
212. Chevalier RL, Thornhill BA, Chang AY. Unilateral ureteral obstruction in neonatal rats leads to renal insufficiency in adulthood. *Kidney Int* 2000;58:1987–1995.
213. Sutaria PM, Ohebshalom M, McCaffrey TA, et al. Transforming growth factor-beta receptor types I and II are expressed in renal tubules and are increased after chronic unilateral ureteral obstruction. *Life Sci* 1998;62:1965–1972.
214. Claesson G, Josephson S, Robertson B. Experimental partial ureteric obstruction in newborn rats. VII. Are the long term effects on renal morphology avoided by release of the obstruction? *J Urol* 1986;136:1330–1334.
215. Claesson G, Josephson S, Robertson B. Renal recovery after release of experimental neonatal ureteric obstruction. *Urol Int* 1987;42:353–359.
216. Josephson S. Experimental obstructive hydronephrosis in newborn rats. III. Long-term effects on renal function. *J Urol* 1983;129:396–400.
217. Claesson G, Josephson S, Robertson B. Experimental partial ureteric obstruction in newborn rats. IV. Do the morphological effects progress continuously? *J Urol* 1983;130:1217–1222.
218. Claesson G, Svensson L, Robertson B, et al. Experimental obstructive hydronephrosis in newborn rats. XI. A one-year follow-up study of renal function and morphology. *J Urol* 1989;142:1602–1607.
219. Stenberg A, Olsen L, Josephson S, et al. Partial ureteric obstruction in weanling rats. I. Long-term effects on the renal morphology. *Scand J Urol Nephrol* 1985;19:139–146.
220. Josephson S, Aperia A, Lannergren K, et al. Partial ureteric obstruction in the pubescent rat. I. Long-term effects on renal function [published erratum appears in *J Urol* 1988;139:432]. *J Urol* 1987;138:414–418.
221. Vaughan ED Jr, Gillenwater JY. Recovery following complete chronic unilateral ureteral occlusion: functional, radiographic and pathologic alterations. *J Urol* 1971;106:27–35.
222. Gonnermann D, Huland H, Schweiker U, et al. Hydronephrotic atrophy after stable mild or severe partial ureteral obstruction: natural history and recovery after relief of obstruction. *J Urol* 1990;143:199–203.
223. Homsy YL, Saad F, Laberge I, et al. Transitional hydronephrosis of the newborn and infant. *J Urol* 1990;144:579–583.
224. Dejter SW Jr, Gibbons MD. The fate of infant kidneys with fetal hydronephrosis but initially normal postnatal sonography. *J Urol* 1989;142:661–662.
225. Peters CA. Urinary tract obstruction in children. *J Urol* 1995;154:1874–1883.
226. Lebowitz RL. Neonatal hydronephrosis: 146 cases. *Radiol Clin North Am* 1977;15:49–59.
227. Flashner SC. Ureteropelvic junction. In: Kelalis PP, King LR, Belman AB, eds. *Clinical pediatric urology*. Philadelphia: Saunders, 1992:693–725.
228. Kelalis PP, Culp OS, Stickler GB, et al. Ureteropelvic obstruction in children: experiences with 109 cases. *J Urol* 1971;106:418–422.
229. Johnston JH, Evans JP, Glassberg KI, et al. Pelvic hydronephrosis in children: a review of 219 personal cases. *J Urol* 1977;117:97–101.
230. Robson WJ, Rudy SM, Johnston JH. Pelviureteric obstruction in infancy. *J Pediatr Surg* 1976;11:57–61.
231. Ureteral structure and ultrastructure. Part II. Congenital ureteropelvic junction obstruction and primary obstructive megaureter. *J Urol* 1976;166:725–730.
232. Notley RG. Electron microscopy of the upper ureter and pelviureteric junction. *Br J Urol* 1968;40:37–52.
233. Johnston JH. The pathogenesis of hydronephrosis in children. *Br J Urol* 1969;41:724–734.
234. Ostling K. The genesis of hydronephrosis, particularly with regard to changes at the ureteropelvic junction. *Acta Scand* 1942;86:1–118.
235. Alcaraz A, Vinaixa F, Tejedo-Mateu A, et al. Obstruction and recanalization of the ureter during embryonic development. *J Urol* 1991;145:410–416.
236. Ruano-Gil D, Coca-Payeras A, Tejedo-Mateu A. Obstruction and normal recanalization of the ureter in the human embryo: its relation to congenital ureteric obstruction. *Eur Urol* 1975;1:287–293.
237. Maizels M, Stephens FD. Valves of the ureters as a cause of primary obstruction of the ureter: anatomic, embryologic and clinical aspects. *J Urol* 1980;123:742–747.
238. Starr NT, Maizels M, Chou P, et al. Microanatomy and morphometry of the hydronephrotic "obstructed" renal pelvis in asymptomatic infants. *J Urol* 1992;148(2 PT 2):519–524.
239. Antonakopoulos GN, Fuggle WJ, Newman J. Idiopathic hydronephrosis. *Arch Pathol Lab Med* 1985;109:1097–1101.
240. Koff SA, Thrall JH. Diagnosis of obstruction in experimental hydroureteronephrosis. *Urology* 1981;17:570–577.
241. Peters CA, Roth JA. Congenital urine flow impairments of the upper urinary tract. In: Gearhart JP, Rink RC, Mouriquand PDE, eds. *Pediatric urology*. Philadelphia: W.B. Saunders, 2001:303–317.
242. Dietl. Nerki wedrujace I ich uwzgnienie. *Przegl Lek (Krakow)* 1864;303–317.
243. Stephens FD. Ureterovascular hydronephrosis and the "aberrant" renal vessels. *J Urol* 1982;128:984–987.
244. Lebowitz RL, Johan BG. The coexistence of ureteropelvic junction obstruction and reflux. *AJR Am J Roentgenol* 1982; 140:231–238.
245. Bernstein GT, Mandell J, Lebowitz RL, et al. Ureteropelvic junction obstruction in the neonate. *J Urol* 1988;140:1216–1221.
246. Hollowell JG, Altman HG, Snyder HM, III, et al. Coexisting ureteropelvic junction obstruction and vesicoureteral reflux: diagnostic and therapeutic implications. *J Urol* 1989; 142:490–493.
247. Koff SA, Campbell KD. The nonoperative management of unilateral neonatal hydronephrosis: natural history of poorly functioning kidneys. *J Urol* 1994;152:593–595.
248. Cartwright PC, Duckett JW, Keating MA, et al. Managing apparent ureteropelvic junction obstruction in the newborn. *J Urol* 1992;148:1224–1228.

249. Brown T, Mandell J, Lebowitz RL. Neonatal hydronephrosis in the era of sonography. *Am J Radiol* 1992;148:959–963.
250. Stephens FD, Smith ED, Hutson JM. *Congenital anomalies of the urinary and genital tracts.* Oxford: Isis Medical Media, 1996.
251. Hoover DL, Duckett JW. Posterior urethral valves, unilateral reflux and renal dysplasia; a syndrome. *J Urol* 1982;128:994–997.
252. Rittenberg MH, Hulbert WC, Snyder HM III, et al. Protective factors in posterior urethral valves. *J Urol* 1988;140:993–996.
253. El-Sherbiny MT, Hafez AT, Shokeir AA. Posterior urethral valves: does young age at diagnosis correlate with poor renal function? *Urology* 2002;60:335–338.
254. Churchillo BM, Krueger RP, Fleisher MH. Complications of posterior urethral valve surgery. *Urol Clin North Am* 1983;10:219–530.
255. Warshaw BL, Hymes LC, Trulock TS, et al. Prognostic features in infants with obstructive uropathy due to posterior urethral valves. *J Urol* 1985;133:240–243.
256. Nakayama DK, Harrison MR, de Lorimier AA. Prognosis of posterior urethral valves presenting at birth. *J Ped Surg* 1986;21:43–45.
257. Parkhouse HF, Barratt TM, Dillon MJ. Long-term outcome of boys with posterior urethral valves. *Br J Urol* 1988;62:59–62.
258. Ebel K. Uroradiology in the fetus and newborn: diagnosis and follow up of congenital obstruction of the urinary tract. *Pediatr Radiol* 1998;28:630–635.
259. Siemens D, Prouse K, MacNiely A. Antenatal hydronephrosis: thresholds of renal pelvic diameter to predict insignificant postnatal pelviectasis. *Tech Urol* 1998;4:198–201.
260. Reddy P, Mandell J. Prenatal diagnosis: therapeutic implications. *Urol Clin North Am* 1998;25:171–180.
261. Shokeir AA, Nijman RJM. Antenatal hydronephrosis: changing concepts in diagnosis and subsequent management. *BJU Int* 2000;85:987–994.
262. Platt JF, Rubin JM, Ellis JH, et al. Duplex Doppler US of the kidney: differentiation of obstructive from nonobstructive dilatation. *Radiology* 1989;171:515–517.
263. Palmer JM, DiSandro M. Diuretic enhanced duplex Doppler sonography in 33 children presenting with hydronephrosis: a study of test sensitivity, specificity and precision. *J Urol* 1995;154:1885–1888.
264. Garcia-Pena BM, Keller MS, Schwartz DS, et al. The ultrasonographic differentiation of obstructive versus nonobstructive hydronephrosis in children: a multivariate scoring system. *J Urol* 1997;158:560–565.
265. Gordon I. Diuretic renography in infants with prenatal unilateral hydronephrosis: an explanation for the controversy about poor drainage. *BJU Int* 2001;87:551–555.
266. Whitaker RH. Methods of assessing obstruction in dilated ureters. *Br J Urol* 1973;45:15.
267. Whitaker RH. The Whitaker test. *Urol Clin North Am* 1979;6:529.
268. Whitaker RH, Buxton-Thomas MS. A comparison of pressure-flow studies and renography in equivocal upper urinary tract obstruction. *J Urol* 1984;131:446.
269. Fung LCT, Churchill BM. Ureteral opening pressure: a novel parameter for the evaluation of pediatric hydronephrosis. *J Urol* 1998;159:1326–1330.
270. Fung LCT, Khoury AE. Urodynamic studies of the upper urinary tract. In: Gearhart JP, Rink RC, Mouriquand PDE, eds. *Pediatric urology.* Philadelphia: W.B. Saunders, 2001:198–224.
271. Fung LCT, Khoury AE, McLorie GA, et al. Evaluation of pediatric hydronephrosis using individualized pressure flow criteria. *J Urol* 1995;154:671–676.
272. Fung LCT, Khoury AE. Pressure decay half-life: a method for characterizing upper urinary tract urine transport. *J Urol* 1996;155:1045–1049.
273. Park J, Bloom D. The pathophysiology of UPJ obstruction: current concepts. *Urol Clin North Am* 1998;25:161–169.
274. Oliveira EA, Diniz JSS, Cabral ACV, et al. Prognostic factors in fetal hydronephrosis: a multivariate analysis. *Pediatr Nephrol* 1999;13:859–864.
275. Oliveira EA, Diniz JSS, Cabral ACV, et al. Predictive factors of fetal urethral obstruction: a multivariate analysis. *Fetal Diagn Ther* 2000;15:180–186.
276. Shimada K, Hosokawa S, Tohda A. Follow up of children after fetal treatment for obstructive uropathy. *Int J Urol* 1998;5:312–316.
277. Harding LJ, Malone PS, Wellesley DG. Antenatal minimal hydronephrosis: is its follow-up an unnecessary cause of concern? *Prenat Diagn* 1999;19:701–705.
278. Austin P, Cain M, Casale A. Prenatal bladder outlet obstruction secondary to ureterocoele. *Urology* 1998;52:1132–1135.
279. Herndon CD, McKenna PH, Kolon TF, et al. A multicenter outcomes analysis of patients with neonatal reflux presenting with prenatal hydronephrosis. *J Urol* 1999;162:1203–1208.
280. Dhillon HK. Prenatally diagnosed hydronephrosis: the Great Ormond Street experience. *Pediatr Radiol* 1998;28:630–635.
281. Koff SA. The prenatal diagnosis of hydronephrosis: when and why not to operate? *Arch Exp Urol* 1998;51:569–574.
282. Koff SA. Postnatal management of antenatal hydronephrosis using an observational approach. *Urology* 2000;55:609–611.
283. Cornford PA, Rickwood AM. Functional results of pyeloplasty in patients with antenatally diagnosed pelviureteric junction obstruction. *Br J Urol* 1998;81:152–155.
284. McAleer IM, Kaplan GW. Renal function before and after pyeloplasty: does it improve? *J Urol* 1999;162:1041–1044.
285. Capolicchio G, Leonard MP, Wong C, et al. Prenatal diagnosis of hydronephrosis: impact on renal function and its recovery after pyeloplasty. *J Urol* 1999;162:1029–1032.
286. Gonzalez R, Schminke C. The prenatal diagnosis of hydronephrosis, when and why to operate? *Arch Exp Urol* 1998; 51:575–579.
287. Hanna MK. Antenatal hydronephrosis and ureteropelvic junction obstruction: the case for early intervention. *Urology* 2000;55:612–615.
288. Takla NV, Hamilton BD, Cartwright PC, et al. Apparent unilateral ureteropelvic junction obstruction in the newborn: expectations for resolution. *J Urol* 1998;160:2175–2178.
289. Subramaniam R, Kouriefs C, Dickson A. Antenatally detected pelviureteric junction obstruction: concerns about conservative management. *Br J Urol Int* 1999;84:335–338.
290. Chertin B, Fridmans A, Knizhnik M, et al. Does early detection of ureteropelvic junction obstruction improve surgical outcome in terms of renal function? *J Urol* 1999;162: 1037–1040.
291. Roth KS, Carter WH Jr, Chan JCM. Obstructive nephropathy in children: long-term progression after relief of posterior urethral valve. *Pediatrics* 2001;107:1004–1010.
292. Holmes N, Harrison MR, Baskin LS. Fetal surgery for posterior urethral valves: long-term postnatal outcomes. *Pediatrics* 2001;108:NIL36–NIL42.

56

BLADDER DYSFUNCTION

DAWN L. McLELLAN
STUART B. BAUER

INTRODUCTION

Physiology of Bladder Function

The function of the bladder is to store urine at low pressure and empty efficiently at a socially acceptable time. This complex process involves integration of activity from the brain, brainstem, spinal cord, detrusor muscle, and external urinary sphincter. The detrusor muscle is composed of relatively large, interlacing smooth muscle fibers in three layers—the outer longitudinal, the middle circular, and the inner longitudinal—that surround the mucosa and submucosa (1). At the level of the bladder neck in males the middle circular layer forms an incomplete ring of the internal (or preprostatic) sphincter mechanism. There is no actual internal sphincter muscle per se, but the smooth muscle arrangement around the bladder neck and proximal urethra act as such. This layer is not prominent in females (1). The external (or voluntary) urinary sphincter in both sexes is composed of smooth and skeletal muscle (2). It is located just distal to the prostate in males and at the midurethra in females.

The innervation of the bladder and sphincter mechanisms is via the autonomic and somatic nervous systems. The somatic input originates from the Onuf nucleus in the anterior horn of the S2 to S4 segments of the spinal cord (3) and travels via the pudendal nerve to the skeletal muscle component of the external urethral sphincter (4). The neurotransmitter acetylcholine provides excitatory stimulation to muscarinic receptors of the external urinary sphincter. In the filling phase, this enables tonic contraction of the external sphincter to keep the bladder outlet closed and aids in the maintenance of continence (2). The primary excitatory input to the bladder that causes a detrusor contraction and a rise in intravesical pressure is the parasympathetic nervous system. The preganglionic parasympathetic input originates at spinal levels S2 to S4 and travels via the pelvic splanchnic nerves (3). The primary neurotransmitter of the parasympathetic system is acetylcholine. Its effect is mediated by the muscarinic receptors of postganglionic nerve fibers distributed primarily in the fundus of the bladder wall (5). The sympathetic nervous system input to the bladder originates from spinal cord levels T10 to L2. Postganglionic sympathetic fibers originate from the paravertebral ganglia as the superior hypogastric plexus, which becomes the right and left hypogastric nerves. The hypogastric nerves blend with the pelvic parasympathetic nerves to form the pelvic plexus (3). Both α and β receptors play a role in the sympathetic input to the bladder, which facilitates bladder storage (6). The β receptors are distributed predominantly over the fundus of the bladder. Release of the neurotransmitter norepinephrine permits relaxation of the detrusor muscle, which allows accommodation of increasing volumes of urine at low pressure. Stimulation of α receptors located almost exclusively at the trigone, bladder outlet, and proximal urethra causes contraction of these smooth muscles (3,6,7), which results in an increase in bladder outlet resistance and thus promotes urine storage and continence.

Coordination of the autonomic and somatic systems to facilitate urine storage and voiding is mediated via the central nervous system. The details of this system are not yet fully understood. It is known that multiple areas of the brain play a role, including the brainstem, hypothalamus, cerebellum, and frontal and parietal lobes of the cerebral cortex (8–10). Within the brainstem, the pontine micturition center plays a crucial role in normal bladder function (5,11).

During bladder filling, sympathetic outflow via the hypogastric nerves promotes relaxation of the majority of bladder muscle bundles through stimulation of β receptors and contraction of the bladder neck mechanism via stimulation of α receptors (12). The guarding reflex causes activation of the striated muscle of the external sphincter (13) through pudendal nerve efferents. This reflex arc is active in response to sudden increases in abdominal pressure (i.e., coughing, Credé maneuver, or Valsalva maneuver) and becomes maximal at bladder capacity, which promotes continence.

Micturition is a reflex initiated by myelinated A-fiber receptors in the mucosa and submucosa of the bladder (14). These free nerve endings act as mechanoreceptors, activated by bladder stretch with low pressure thresholds (≤10 mm Hg). They may also function as chemoreceptors because they are activated by intravesical instillation of noxious agents (15), although unmyelinated C fibers are thought to be the predominant pathway for afferent noxious stimuli (16). The normal micturition reflex elicited by A-fiber afferents is initially lost in cats with a suprasacral transection of the spinal cord. A spinally mediated bladder micturition reflex gradually returns, but it is elicited by C fibers (14).

Bladder stretch activates A-fiber mechanoreceptors in the bladder mucosa. This signal travels to the spinal cord via afferents within the pudendal nerve. Ascending pathways in the lateral spinothalamic tract relay the signal to the pontine micturition center, where it is modulated by descending input from higher, cerebral centers. Descending signals from the pontine micturition center then cause inhibition of the pudendal motor neurons, inhibition of the sympathetic outflow to the bladder, and stimulation of the parasympathetic outflow via the pelvic nerve, which results in a coordinated relaxation of the bladder neck mechanism and external sphincter along with a sustained detrusor contraction leading to low-pressure voiding (12,17).

Development of Urinary Control

A standard pattern is seen for the attainment of urinary and bowel continence. Normally, children achieve nighttime bowel control first, followed by daytime bowel control, then daytime urinary control, and finally nighttime dryness (13). The age at which children attain urinary continence is variable, ranging from 2 to 4 years of age for daytime control (10,18). Eighty-five percent of children have achieved continence at night by age 10 years (13). Cultural differences are known to exist in this achievement and in parental expectations for attainment of developmental milestones (19).

Within an individual there is great variation in the normal voiding pattern with respect to frequency of micturition, volume voided, and postvoid residual urine volume (PVR) (20–22). The infant normally voids approximately once per hour (20,22,23). This frequency gradually decreases with increasing age to 11 voids per 24 hours at age 3 years (23,24). Infants and children are known to empty their bladders almost completely, with minimal PVRs (20,25,26). Bladder capacity is known to increase with age (23,24,26–28). Several formulas have been developed to estimate normal bladder capacity based on age (27,28). For example, for children younger than 2 years of age, the estimated bladder capacity can be calculated by the following equation: $2 \times \text{age (years)} + 2 = \text{capacity (ounces)}$. For children older than 2 years of age, the following equation is used: $\text{age (years)}/2 + 6 = \text{capacity (ounces)}$ (27).

In the past, voiding in the infant was believed to be automatic and uninhibited, a reflex initiated by a specific bladder volume confined to the level of the sacral spinal cord without cortical input. The development of urinary control was thought to be related to maturation of neural pathways (10,18,29). Animal studies have demonstrated the plasticity and maturation of the neural pathways responsible for micturition (30–32). More recent studies of childhood micturition patterns challenge the concept of uninhibited infant voiding unmodified by higher cortical input. Specifically, the demonstration that infants void while awake or during arousal from sleep and never during quiet sleep is evidence of cortical arousal in response to bladder distension (33). It is suggested that the pathways between the peripheral and central nervous systems are well formed at birth, and the development of voluntary control represents a modification of preexisting reflexes (33). Further support is lent to this theory by the demonstration of a higher proportion of fully awake voiding in normal neonates than in premature infants (34). Also supporting this concept is the stepwise decrease in the percentage of interrupted voiding episodes. Interrupted voiding is thought to be a discoordination between the sphincter and detrusor, and is demonstrated in 58% of premature infants (34), 33% of infants 3 months of age, and rarely after 2 years of age (23). The demonstration that voiding pressures in infants are not excessive (23,26,35) and that the bladder wall in normal infants is not thickened (36,37) further substantiates the theory that higher cortical input plays an important role in the voiding reflex of neonates.

Voiding Dysfunction

Voiding dysfunction is an all-encompassing term used to describe abnormalities of the micturition cycle. It may refer to structural or functional causes of abnormal bladder storage and emptying. Normal bladder function requires accommodation by the detrusor of increasing volumes of urine at low pressure with normal sensation, a closed bladder outlet despite increases of abdominal pressure, and the absence of involuntary bladder contractions (38). Therefore, any alteration of bladder compliance or detrusor storage function, innervation of bladder or sphincter mechanisms, or structural changes of the bladder or bladder outlet could result in voiding dysfunction. The symptoms of voiding dysfunction include urgency and urge incontinence, daytime and/or nighttime incontinence, urinary frequency, painful voiding, straining with urination, and urinary tract infection (UTI). The possible causes of voiding dysfunction in children, which will be discussed in detail, are listed in Table 56.1.

In summary, the complex motor and neuronal pathways responsible for micturition are most likely present in infancy but undergo maturation in the early childhood years. Most children attain the ability to voluntarily void by the age of 4 years. However, the age at which continence is achieved, as well as the voiding pattern, varies greatly among individuals and in part is influenced by culture. Over time, the voiding frequency decreases and the bladder capacity increases. The causes and symptoms of voiding dysfunction are diverse. Appropriate evaluation of these disorders will rule out any significant abnormalities that require intervention while minimizing harm from invasive investigations in the pediatric patient.

TABLE 56.1. CAUSES OF DYSFUNCTIONAL VOIDING IN CHILDREN

Neurogenic bladder dysfunction
- Neurospinal dysraphisms
  - Myelodysplasia
  - Lipomeningocele and other spinal dysraphisms
  - Sacral agenesis
  - Associated conditions—imperforate anus
- Central nervous system insults
  - Cerebral palsy
  - Traumatic injuries to the spine

Nonneurogenic bladder dysfunction
- Nonneurogenic neurogenic bladder
- Unstable bladder
- Infrequent voiding syndrome
- Functional bowel disturbances
- Daytime urinary frequency syndrome

EVALUATION OF VOIDING DYSFUNCTION

Some advocate a thorough evaluation of all children with voiding symptoms by means of invasive testing such as cystoscopy and urodynamic and radiographic studies (39,40). However, most accept that a more selective approach is warranted in children who do not have continuous day and night symptoms, anatomic anomalies, neurologic abnormalities, or UTI because of the very low incidence of significant pathology in these patients (41). This selective approach usually includes taking a thorough history, including prenatal, perinatal, and early postnatal information, a physical examination, and urinalysis with culture (42–44). The urine should be checked for abnormal specific gravity and glycosuria to exclude diabetes insipidus and diabetes mellitus, respectively. It is crucial that UTI (often an insidious issue) is excluded as the cause of the voiding dysfunction (45). A history of UTI in a young boy or a girl should be evaluated by a voiding cystourethrogram (VCUG) (males) or nuclear cystography (females) to rule out vesicoureteral reflux (VUR) or another anatomic abnormality (44). Renal ultrasonography should be performed to detect possible congenital causes of obstruction of the urinary tract presenting with UTI. A plain radiograph of the abdomen (kidneys, ureters, and bladder) will reveal evidence of chronic stool retention (46), which indicates a dysfunctional elimination syndrome, and should be obtained when history or symptoms warrant it. Boys with persistent daytime and nighttime wetting with or without UTI or with elevated voiding pressures and hyperreflexia noted on urodynamic studies must have a VCUG to evaluate for posterior urethral valves (47,48).

History and Physical Findings

A complete history should begin with details of the mother's pregnancy and the perinatal period, including insulin-dependent gestational diabetes, prematurity, fetal distress leading to emergency cesarean section, neonatal anoxia, infection, seizures, traumatic birth, birth injury, or respiratory distress requiring pulmonary assistance and/or oxygen administration. Any family history of renal or urologic abnormalities should be elucidated.

The history should be tailored to the age of the patient. For an infant, the number of wet diapers per day and the interval between changes should be detailed. The characteristics of the urinary stream should be noted. Does the infant seem to strain to void or is there constant dribbling of urine? A history of chronic genital dermatitis may also be important for evaluating the possibility of an ectopically placed ureteral orifice. For children of toilet-training age or older, the frequency of voiding and volume voided provide crucial information. A voiding and bowel-emptying diary completed with the assistance of the parents over several days may be the best way to obtain this information. The occurrence of daytime or nighttime incontinence should be detailed with respect to onset, duration, and frequency. Symptoms of urinary frequency or urgency should be documented. Use of a Valsalva or Credé maneuver to void with or without a poor urinary stream may indicate obstruction or a neurologic cause of voiding dysfunction. Postvoid wetting in girls without any nighttime incontinence suggests vaginal trapping of urine during voiding. In females, a normal voiding pattern associated with continuous wetting may indicate the presence of an ectopic ureter that inserts distal to the urethral sphincter. This diagnosis is corroborated by renal ultrasonographic findings of a dilated upper-pole collecting system and a dilated ureter extending behind the bladder beyond the bladder neck. Specific posturing, such as leg crossing, squatting, and Vincent curtsy should be noted (49). Delayed achievement of milestones, impaired fine motor coordination of the upper extremities, poor school performance, or inability to stay focused on activities may be signs of central nervous system dysfunction affecting the lower urinary tract. Hemiatrophy and left-handedness in a family without a history of left-handedness (referred to as pathologic left-handedness) suggests an early perinatal brain injury, which may be associated with voiding dysfunction (50). A history of polyuria or polydipsia is suggestive of undiagnosed diabetes mellitus or insipidus. For patients of all ages, specific questions about the frequency and consistency of bowel movements, fecal soiling, or fecal incontinence should be investigated to elucidate a possible history of constipation or encopresis. UTI or multiple febrile illnesses of unknown cause should be identified. If available, culture documentation of a UTI and means of urine collection (bag vs. catheterization) can provide helpful information. For each UTI, a history of systemic signs or fever should be sought, as this may suggest possible renal parenchymal scarring (5,41,51).

A focused physical examination of the abdomen, back, external genitalia, and lower extremity neurologic system should be performed. Palpation of the abdomen may reveal an enlarged or hydronephrotic kidney, a distended bladder, or evidence of impacted fecal material. The back should be examined for subtle findings suggestive of an occult spinal abnormality, including lipoma, telangiectasia, abnormal pigmentation, spinal dimple, hair patch, gluteal asymmetry, or abnormal gluteal cleft (52). Absence of the upper gluteal cleft suggests sacral agenesis. As well, the presence of the sacrum and completeness of the vertebrae should be confirmed by palpation. In girls, the labia should be separated and the external genitalia examined for separate urethral and vaginal openings, the presence labial adhesions, or epispadias (denoted as a bifid clitoris or patulous urethra). In boys, the urethral meatus should be visualized by gentle retraction of the foreskin to identify its position and appearance. Skin excoriation or genital dermatitis should be noted. The examiner should be alert to signs of sexual abuse. In cases of suspected neurologic dysfunction, the absence or presence of perianal sensation and an anal wink (anocutaneous reflex) should be demonstrated. The bulbocavernosus reflex may be elicited by gently squeezing the glans penis or clitoris while observing a contraction of the anal sphincter (if necessary, this may be accomplished with a digital rectal examination). Assessment of gait, muscle mass, symmetry, and deep tendon reflexes of the lower extremities completes the neurologic examination (45,51).

Worrisome Signs and Symptoms

Certain signs and symptoms should alert the clinician that further investigation is warranted (Table 56.2) (41). Lumbosacral and neurologic abnormalities may be indicative of an occult spinal dysraphism. In this case, further radiographic imaging [spinal ultrasonography for infants younger than 3 months of age and spinal magnetic resonance imaging (MRI) for older children] and urodynamic testing are required. Low specific gravity of the urine could be related to diabetes insipidus. Further investigation for diabetes mellitus should be carried out if glycosuria is detected. As noted earlier, a history of UTI calls for renal ultrasonography and VCUG in males or a radionuclide cystogram in females. Any child with a history of genital pain or discharge should be thoroughly evaluated for possible sexual abuse.

TABLE 56.2. WORRISOME SIGNS AND SYMPTOMS IN EVALUATION OF DYSFUNCTIONAL VOIDING IN CHILDREN

- Signs
  - Lumbosacral spine abnormalities
    - Hairy patch (hypertrichosis)
    - Lipoma
    - Cutaneous abnormalities/dermal vascular malformation (pigmentation, telangiectasia) or dimple
    - Bony irregularities (scoliosis, abnormally appearing gluteal cleft)
  - Reduced anal sphincter tone
  - Lack of lower extremity deep tendon or bulbocavernosus reflex
  - Fixed low urine specific gravity or glycosuria
  - Urinary tract infection
- Symptoms
  - Day and night frequency and wetting
  - Painful urination
  - Rectal pain
  - Penile or vaginal pain or discharge
  - Straining to void

Modified from Koff SA. Evaluation and management of voiding disorders in children. *Urol Clin NA* 1988;15(4):769–775.

Urodynamic Evaluation

Urodynamic studies in children are a time-consuming endeavor and require the patience and experience of a trained pediatric urodynamics nurse. A urodynamic suite tailored to the pediatric patient with toys, videotapes, or other personal security items (e.g., blanket, teddy bear) is beneficial. The importance of patient cooperation cannot be overstated (51). Urodynamic studies may be difficult to interpret when the child is uncooperative.

Noninvasive urodynamic studies do not require catheterization and are easy to perform. Noninvasive studies include urinary flow rate and PVR determination, and an assessment of bladder wall thickness by ultrasonography. More invasive urodynamic studies require catheterization and possibly the placement of perineal electromyographic (EMG) needle electrodes when a neuropathy is considered. These evaluations should be used selectively in those patients who require more thorough investigation.

Children with incontinence, with or without UTI, who have negative findings on physical examination and normal radiographic imaging results are not usually candidates for initial, more invasive studies because they usually respond to empiric therapeutic options such as bladder and bowel retraining and/or anticholinergic medication (51). See Table 56.3.

The most commonly used urodynamic tests are urinary flow rate, cystometrogram (CMG), EMG, and urethral pressure profilometry. The urinary flow rate is the voided volume per unit time, expressed in milliliters per second. This test also provides the volume voided and a flow tracing. The normal flow-tracing voiding pattern is a bell-shaped curve. A Valsalva voider has an intermittent and prolonged curve. Staccato or interrupted voiding is seen in a considerable number of girls with recurrent UTI (53). Nomograms for flow rate and voided volume are available (51).

CMG is a pressure-volume study that characterizes both the filling and voiding phases of bladder function. High intravesical filling pressures and high pressures at urinary leakage (leak point pressure) are associated with upper urinary tract deterioration (54). The CMG can also provide a measurement of bladder compliance, the change in bladder volume divided by the change in bladder pressure, expressed as milliliters per centimeter of water. No standard compliance values are available for children. The filling CMG may also demonstrate involuntary detrusor contractions, or detrusor instability. It is important to fill the bladder slowly with warmed saline to

TABLE 56.3. INDICATIONS FOR URODYNAMIC TESTING IN CHILDREN

Noninvasive
- Nonneurogenic bladder dysfunction (Hinman-Allen syndrome)
- Valve bladder syndrome
- Prune-belly syndrome
- Nocturnal and diurnal enuresis
- Functional voiding dysfunction refractory to standard therapy

Invasive[a]
- Myelodysplasia
- Occult spinal dysraphism
- Sacral agenesis
- Imperforate anus
- VACTERL syndrome association
- Cerebral palsy, attention deficit disorder, or developmental delay
- Spinal cord injury
- Nonneurogenic bladder dysfunction (Hinman-Allen syndrome)
- Valve bladder syndrome
- Prune-belly syndrome

VACTERL, *v*ertebrae, *a*nus, *c*ardiovascular tree, *t*rachea, *e*sophagus, *r*enal system, and *l*imb buds.
[a]In some of these cases noninvasive studies and treatment are attempted first.

avoid inducing bladder contractions (51). Even at these rates compliance measurements may be falsely low when compared to pressures obtained during natural filling (14,55).

EMG is the study of the electrical potentials generated by the depolarization of striated muscle bundles. In urodynamic studies EMG provides information about the degree of denervation of the external urinary sphincter, responses to sacral reflexes, and presence or absence of detrusor-sphincter dyssynergia (51).

Static urethral pressure profilometry measures the passive resistance at a particular point in the urethra at a specific point of bladder stretch. This provides an assessment of bladder outlet resistance. Dynamic urethral pressure profilometry provides the continuous monitoring of a particular point in the urethra as the bladder fills to capacity and then empties (51).

Urodynamic studies can provide useful information in children with voiding dysfunction. One must remember the limitations in performing and interpreting these evaluations of bladder function. These methods are invasive and should be reserved for refractory cases or patients with neurologic or structural abnormalities, with the specific test used to obtain the most valuable information for efficient treatment.

NEUROGENIC CAUSES OF BLADDER DYSFUNCTION IN CHILDREN

Spinal dysraphism, or myelodysplasia, is the most common cause of neurogenic bladder dysfunction in children. The number of children born with myelodysplasia in the United States is approximately 1 per 1000 births (56). The incidence of this disorder is decreasing (57). The reason for the decreasing frequency is unknown, but some speculate that it may be related to elective termination of pregnancy (58) as well as the recommendation that women ingest 400 μg of folic acid daily before becoming pregnant (59). This practice has been shown to reduce the incidence of giving birth to a child with spina bifida by 50% (60). The variations of congenital spinal anomalies classified as spinal dysraphism are listed in Table 56.4 (52). Of the myelodysplastic states, myelomeningocele accounts for more than 85% of cases and usually presents at birth with an obvious open lesion of the back. Lipomeningocele is the second most common type of myelodysplasia. Approximately half of the cases present later in childhood with symptoms of voiding dysfunction and subtle findings on physical examination (61,62). Other causes of neurogenic bladder dysfunction in children include sacral agenesis, imperforate anus, cerebral palsy, and traumatic spinal cord injury.

TABLE 56.4. TYPES OF SPINAL DYSRAPHISM

- Meningocele
- Myelomeningocele
- Myeloschisis
- Spina bifida occulta
- Diastematomyelia
- Diplomyelia
- Tethered conus
- Intraspinal lipoma
- Lipomyelomeningocele
- Dermoid cyst
- Dermal sinus

Myelomeningocele

During embryonic life, the edges of the neural plate proliferate to form the neural folds by 3 weeks of gestation. Starting in the cranial region, these neural folds close in the midline to create a tube that progresses caudally. The lateral ectoderm migrates medially to cover the neural tube, thus separating the neural tissue from the overlying ectodermal surface. This process is complete by the 35th day of gestation (63). The exact etiology of spinal dysraphism is unknown, but a commonly accepted theory is incomplete closure of the neural tube and failure of the mesoderm to encircle the cord and/or ectoderm to cover the underlying tissue (64). The most frequently affected region is the lumbar spine followed by the sacral, thoracic, and cervical areas in descending order of frequency (65,66).

The description of neural tube defects is based on the degree of involvement of the neural elements. *Meningocele* refers to a defect in which the meninges extend beyond the confines of the vertebral canal with no neural elements contained within the sac; *myelomeningocele* refers to a defect that includes neural elements, such as nerve roots or part of the spinal cord, that have protruded along with the meninges; if fatty tissue develops within in the cord structures, it is described as a

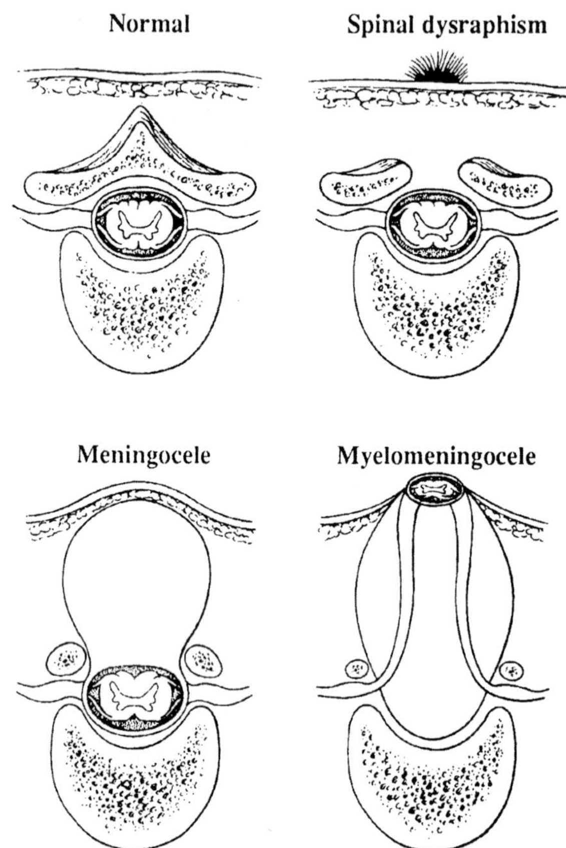

FIGURE 56.1. Defects and locations of neural elements in spinal dysraphism. (From Barrat TM, Avner ED, Harmon W, eds. *Pediatric nephrology*, 3rd ed. Baltimore: Lippincott Williams & Wilkins, 1993, with permission.)

lipomeningocele (Fig. 56.1). It has been demonstrated that neural elements may be abnormal both above and below the site of the bony defect (64). This explains why the level of the bony defect may not always correlate with the type or extent of the neurologic deficit (65,67). The neural elements are usually covered by a thin sac or membrane. Urgent surgical repair and sterile precautions are necessary to prevent progression of neurologic damage and to reduce the risk of infection.

Most children with spinal dysraphism have other associated abnormalities, including orthopedic anomalies and the Arnold-Chiari malformation, a herniation of the cerebellar tonsils through the foramen magnum, which prevents cerebrospinal fluid from entering the subarachnoid space by obstructing the fourth ventricle. Because of the varied defects in these children, a multidisciplinary approach that includes neurosurgical, urologic, and orthopedic assessment and treatment is optimal.

Urologic Evaluation of the Newborn with Myelodysplasia

Initial evaluation of the neonate with myelodysplasia should include a urinalysis, serum creatinine level, and measurement of PVR. Clean intermittent catheterization (CIC) should be initiated if the PVR is greater than 5 mL (approximately one-third of the expected bladder capacity) with spontaneous voiding or following a Credé maneuver. After back closure has been completed, renal ultrasonography and a urodynamic study should be performed. Back closure has been shown to have little effect on detrusor function in neonates (68). It is well known that the neurologic status of patients with myelodysplasia is dynamic, and neonatal urodynamic studies act as an important baseline for future comparisons. The urologic manifestations of the neurologic deficit may improve or worsen over time (67,69,70). The urodynamic studies also guide management and define the risk of neurourologic deterioration (66,71). The bladder capacity of children with myelomeningocele is approximately 25% less than that of age-matched neurologically normal children. Expected bladder capacity for these children may be calculated by the following equation: 24.5 × age (years) + 62 = capacity (mL) (72).

If the renal ultrasonogram is abnormal or if urodynamic studies reveal detrusor sphincter dyssynergia (DSD), a VCUG should be performed to identify possible VUR. If reflux is severe or significant renal parenchymal changes are noted on ultrasonography, a renal scan should be performed to assess renal function and parenchymal damage.

Management of the Neonate with Myelodysplasia

In the past, patients with myelomeningocele were managed expectantly. Therapeutic intervention with sterile (62) or CIC (54) was initiated only when complications such as hydronephrosis or reflux arose. However, up to 50% of the patients managed by self-voiding develop urinary tract deterioration (66,67,70,73,74). Prospective studies have clearly demonstrated that the patients at highest risk of deterioration are those with DSD, high voiding pressure, or high leak point pressure (54,65,71,74–76). Deterioration is most likely to occur within the first 3 years of life (70,76). Early management with CIC and anticholinergic medication for children at high risk has significantly decreased the occurrence of urologic deterioration (74,76).

Because not all children are at risk for deterioration, the primary management and follow-up regimen can be tailored to the initial neonatal urodynamic profile. Three groups may be distinguished on the basis of the urodynamic findings: those with detrusor–external urethral sphincter incoordination (dyssynergy), those with detrusor–external urethral sphincter coordination (synergy), and those with a complete neurologic lesion or no bioelectric activity in the external urethral sphincter (65).

Detrusor sphincter dyssynergy occurs when the external urinary sphincter contracts involuntarily during a detrusor contraction in patients with neurologic lesions of the suprasacral spinal cord (77,78). Because these children are at high risk for urinary tract deterioration and prophylactic therapy has been shown to reduce this risk, CIC should be instituted as standard therapy along with yearly urodynamic studies and renal ultrasonography (76,79). If high bladder filling pressures, high leak point pressure (greater than 40 cm H_2O), or persistent incontinence occurs, anticholinergic medication should be added (74,76,80). If these measures fail to stop progression, urinary tract diversion with cutaneous vesicostomy (81) or bladder augmentation (79) may be required.

Synergy of the voiding reflex is characterized by complete silencing of the external urinary sphincter during a detrusor contraction. Patients with a synergic sphincter are at lower risk of urinary tract deterioration unless they develop dyssynergy (70,71). Therefore, they should undergo annual urodynamic studies and renal ultrasonographic examination to monitor for a change in their neurologic picture. Continence may be improved with timed voiding, CIC, and anticholinergic medication if necessary.

When no bioelectric potentials are detectable in the region of the external urinary sphincter during the voiding cycle or in response to sacral reflex stimulation (including the Credé maneuver), a complete neurologic lesion exists. In this condition the bladder acts as a urinary conduit without any obstruction. These children are at low risk of urinary tract deterioration (74) unless they develop denervation fibrosis of the skeletal muscle component of the external urinary sphincter as evidenced by an increase in residual urine volume or urodynamic study demonstration of an elevated urethral leak point pressure (65). Thus, these children require annual renal ultrasonographic examination and documentation of PVR.

Management of incontinence includes CIC and administration of alpha-agonists to increase bladder neck outlet resistance. If conservative measures fail, surgical options such as artificial urinary sphincter, bladder neck reconstruction, or urinary diversion with a continent catheterizable stoma may be necessary.

Management of Vesicoureteral Reflux

Initial therapy for VUR includes CIC and anticholinergic therapy to establish effective bladder emptying and decrease elevated intravesical pressures (79,82). The indications for surgical repair of VUR in children with myelomeningocele are similar to those in children with primary reflux. They include recurrent UTI despite adequate antibiotic prophylaxis and a routine CIC schedule; development or progression of renal parenchymal damage or scarring, or planned bladder neck reconstruction (83). When combined with CIC, success rates for surgical repair of reflux in neurogenic bladders approaches that of repair in nonneurogenic bladders (84). The Credé maneuver should be avoided in children with reflux who also have an intact sacral reflex arc because they will have a reflexive increase in external urinary sphincter tone when abdominal pressure is increased. This results in inefficient bladder emptying due to increasing urethral resistance, which may cause a worsening in the degree of reflux (85).

Occult Spinal Dysraphisms

Like myelomeningocele, occult spinal dysraphisms have a structural defect of the caudal end of the vertebral canal and spinal cord. However, there is no open vertebral canal. Occult spinal dysraphisms include diastematomyelia, lipoma, dermoid cyst or sinus, aberrant sacral roots, fibrous traction on the conus medullaris, or a tight filum terminale (62). The diagnosis is usually suspected in neonates because of a cutaneous lesion overlying the spine (86). If the dysraphism is not noted in the neonatal period, children usually present between the ages of 2 and 4 with difficulty in toilet training for bladder and/or bowels, or present with urinary tract symptoms around 9 to 13 years of age due to an acceleration in growth during puberty (62,86). These symptoms may include incontinence, UTI, and encopresis or fecal soiling (62,87). Other, less common presenting symptoms include weakness or incoordination of the feet and legs, leg numbness, and back, testicular, or leg pain (63,88). Physical findings include the characteristic cutaneous back lesions listed in Table 56.2, poor anal tone, decreased perianal sensation, high arched foot or feet, leg length discrepancy, abnormal gait, asymmetrical lower leg muscle mass, lower extremity weakness, and altered sensation or deep tendon reflexes of the lower extremities (88,89).

The presenting signs and symptoms of occult dysraphic states are similar to those in patients presenting with tethered spinal cord syndrome, the pathologic fixation of the cord in an abnormal caudal position (87). Patients with a history of prophylactic spinal surgery for repair of a lipomeningocele before 18 months of age have a lower risk of developing secondary tethering of the spinal cord than children who do not have surgery until obvious neurologic abnormalities occur (87,88). The mechanism of neurologic dysfunction is thought to be the result of impaired mitochondrial oxidative metabolism with constant or intermittent cord stretching (90).

Evaluation of suspected occult dysraphic states and tethered spinal cord should include a thorough history taking and physical examination. The diagnosis should be confirmed with spinal ultrasonography in children younger than 3 months of age (91) and with MRI of the spine in children older than 3 months (88,89). A baseline urinalysis, creatinine level, renal ultrasonography, and PVR should be obtained. Urodynamic evaluation is critical, as many of these patients have a normal neurologic examination but a significant neurologic abnormality on urodynamic studies (86,91,92). In fact, up to 40% of children with lipomeningocele may have abnormal urodynamic findings as their sole neurologic deficit (92).

Management of the urinary tract in children with occult dysraphic states and tethered spinal cord is identical to that described earlier for the various urodynamic patterns of myelomeningocele. Early surgical correction of the spinal cord abnormality is associated with a better improvement rate of urinary tract and lower extremity abnormalities than is late repair (61,69,88,91,92).

Sacral Agenesis

Congenital absence of part of one or more of the sacral vertebrae or coccyx is very rare and is referred to as sacral agenesis (93,94). If the lumbar spine is also affected, the term *caudal regression syndrome* is used (94,95). Neurogenic bladder dysfunction will result if the sacral neural segments S2 to S4 are involved (94). As with myelomeningocele, the level of bony abnormality does not predict the level of neurologic abnormality (94,95). The etiology is unknown, but exposure to teratogenic influences is thought to play a role (94). One percent of infants born to diabetic mothers have sacral agenesis, and the incidence of maternal diabetes in children with this anomaly is 12 to 16% (94,96–98).

Approximately half of the cases present in the neonatal period and the remainder are diagnosed at age 4 to 6 years when an evaluation for urinary incontinence is performed (94,99). Presenting signs and symptoms include urinary frequency and urgency, urinary incontinence, recurrent UTI, and constipation (99). Physical examination may reveal flattening of the buttocks, loss of the gluteal cleft, widely spaced buttock dimples, and a palpable sacral defect (98). Perineal sensation is normal in up to 75% of these children (94,97). The bulbocavernosus reflex may or may not be intact (94). Early diagnosis and management help to avoid complications such as renal functional impairment, recurrent UTI, and renal scarring (97,99,100). Associated orthopedic and genitourinary anomalies include club foot or feet, skeletal defects of the tibia and fibula, unilateral renal agenesis, VUR, and renal ectopia (93,94,96,98,99).

The diagnosis is confirmed by anterior-posterior and lateral radiographs of the sacrum, which demonstrate the bony deformity (98,99). Renal ultrasonography or intravenous pyelogram will reveal any associated genitourinary anomalies (97). A VCUG will determine if VUR is present (94). Urodynamic studies show a variable pattern of either an upper motor neuron lesion with hyperreflexia and DSD with an intact sphincter EMG, or detrusor areflexia with extensive denervation in the sphincter (94,97,99).

Management is tailored to the urodynamic profile and includes CIC to achieve complete bladder emptying, antibiotic therapy for infection or reflux, and administration of anticholinergics to improve continence or to help lower abnormally high bladder pressures (94,97,99,100).

Associated Conditions—Imperforate Anus

Ongoing problems with urinary incontinence in some patients with imperforate anus was thought to be related to peripheral nerve injury at the time of the anal pull-through procedure. It was eventually deduced that many of these patients had sacral agenesis or neurospinal dysraphism that resulted in neurogenic bladder dysfunction and incontinence (101). Up to 30% of children with an anorectal malformation have sacral dysplasia (102), and the majority of them have neurogenic bladder and sphincter dysfunction (95). The incidence of sacral agenesis and genitourinary abnormalities, including VUR and DSD, is much greater in those with high lesions of imperforate anus than in those with low lesions (101–103). To determine if sacral agenesis or spinal dysraphism is present, prompt investigation of children with imperforate anus by imaging examination, including plain radiography, ultrasonography, or MRI of the spine, is recommended (88,89,91). A urodynamic study is required if either abnormality is noted. Urodynamic studies may demonstrate a normal voiding pattern, detrusor hyperreflexia or areflexia, and normal or partial denervation of the sphincter with or without DSD (101,104). Urologic management is based on the initial urodynamic profile as described earlier for myelomeningocele.

Central Nervous System Insults

Cerebral Palsy

The incidence of moderate to severe cerebral palsy is estimated to be 1.5 to 2.5 per 1000 live births (105). One-third will report urinary symptoms (106). The most common presenting symptom of voiding dysfunction is daytime urinary incontinence. Patients may be prone to incontinence because of impaired cognitive and communication skills as well as decreased mobility (107). Urgency, urinary frequency, stress incontinence, difficulty initiating voiding, or UTI may also be noted (106–109).

Routine screening of the urinary tract is not warranted in patients with cerebral palsy because fewer than 2% have been demonstrated to have unexpected genitourinary abnormalities by renal ultrasonography (110). If a patient has a history of UTI, however, there is a high likelihood of a structural defect or a significant urodynamic abnormality, such as DSD; therefore, renal ultrasonography and urodynamic studies should be performed (109). Urodynamic studies often show detrusor hyperreflexia and/or a small capacity bladder. An incomplete lesion of the external urinary sphincter may be seen in 10 to 15% of cases, suggesting a spinal cord as well as a central nervous system abnormality. DSD is rare (108,109). Management includes anticholinergic therapy for urgency, incontinence, and hyperreflexia, and CIC for incomplete bladder emptying or DSD (107,109). In children not requiring CIC, the anticholinergic drugs should be administered gingerly with monitoring of residual urine, because these children may develop urinary retention (111).

Traumatic Spinal Cord Injury

Spinal cord injury in the child is a rare event. The incidence of traumatic spinal cord injury is higher in boys than in girls, and the risk of injury increases with age (112,113).

The most likely causes are a sports injury or birth trauma from a high forceps delivery (114). Immediately after the injury, a period of spinal shock exists, the bladder is often areflexic, and the urethral sphincter is nonreactive with normal bioelectric potentials on EMG (115). Initial management of the urinary tract involves placement of an indwelling Foley catheter to maintain bladder emptying until the patient is stable. CIC may then be initiated (116,117). When bladder function returns, there is usually an upper-motor-neuron type of injury with detrusor hyperreflexia and DSD (115). The goals of management are to preserve renal function, achieve continence, and avoid infection and stone formation. Urodynamic studies can help determine which patients are at risk for urinary tract deterioration and should be performed within 2 to 3 months of the initial injury. Follow-up urodynamic studies at 6 to 9 months and again at 2 years after injury help to determine the stability of lower urinary tract function, the need for continued catheterization, and the necessity of further pharmacologic or surgical intervention. Periodic renal ultrasonography to evaluate for hydronephrosis and stone formation is recommended (115).

NONNEUROGENIC CAUSES OF BLADDER DYSFUNCTION IN CHILDREN

As noted previously, the distinction between functional and organic causes of voiding dysfunction can be elucidated by careful history taking and physical examination with special attention to worrisome signs and symptoms (Table 56.2). Children with symptoms of voiding dysfunction will likely fit into one of the following categories of dysfunctional elimination syndromes: the nonneurogenic neurogenic bladder, the unstable bladder, the infrequent voiding syndrome, and functional bowel disturbance. The presence of these dysfunctional elimination syndromes is associated with increased recurrence of UTI, delayed resolution of VUR, and unsuccessful surgical outcome for VUR (118,119). This highlights the importance of diagnosing and treating these syndromes.

Nonneurogenic Neurogenic Bladder (Hinman-Allen Syndrome)

Hinman first described a syndrome that he designated as nonneurogenic neurogenic bladder (120). The disorder was further characterized and described by others and thus has many other names, including Hinman-Allen syndrome (121), occult neuropathic bladder (122), subclinical neurogenic bladder (123), pseudo-obstructed bladder (124), unstable bladder of childhood (125), and occult neurologic bladder (126).

Hinman wrote about a symptom complex of enuresis and daytime wetting associated with UTI, often with upper urinary tract dilatation, as seen in 14 boys in whom no neurologic defects or obstructive lesions could be identified. Incoordination between a detrusor contraction and contraction of the pelvic floor was postulated as a possible cause (127). For the end stage of bladder dysfunction associated with nonneurogenic neurogenic bladder to develop, there must be a failure to inhibit the detrusor reflex and overcompensation by the external sphincter (121). This acquired disorder occurs after toilet training and usually presents before puberty. Symptoms include daytime and nighttime incontinence, fecal retention and soiling, and UTI. Varied degrees of urinary tract changes including renal functional compromise in children with "failure" personalities and domineering parents are noted (122,125,127,128).

Radiologic abnormalities that can be seen include hydronephrosis, a trabeculated bladder with diverticula, a large PVR, VUR, renal parenchymal scarring, and the classic "spinning top urethra" (persistent narrowing of the sphincter area during voiding) (122,124,127,128). Urodynamic study with anal sphincter EMG confirms failure of relaxation or increased external sphincter activity with voiding (125,128). This causes elevated detrusor filling and voiding pressures, which ultimately result in the radiologic changes noted previously.

A multitude of approaches are necessary for successful management of the nonneurogenic neurogenic bladder. Bladder retraining with a timed voiding schedule and double voiding (120,128) are recommended. CIC may be required to achieve adequate bladder emptying (125,129). Biofeedback techniques have been highly successful in modifying learned patterns of bladder sphincter incoordination (130). Some have recommended psychotherapy and hypnosis to assist in the bladder retraining (125). Long-term suppressive antibiotic therapy may be necessary to prevent recurrent UTI (120,131). Management of fecal impaction and constipation plays an important role (120,131). Drug therapy includes anticholinergics to decrease unstable bladder contractions (120,131) and bethanechol chloride to improve bladder contractility; alpha-blockers and diazepam may reduce bladder outflow resistance (125,132).

Unstable Bladder

Children with an unstable bladder have the ability to void normally on command but experience premature detrusor contractions with bladder filling (125). This disorder is thought to arise from a delay in nervous system maturation or a regression in development (10). Therefore, it has also been referred to as "infantile" or "uninhibited" bladder (41). These children often present with symptoms of urgency, urge incontinence, urinary frequency, and enuresis. Characteristic postures such as Vincent curtsy or squatting are often noted by parents (39,41,45,49,125,133). Children with attention deficit disorder (134,135), abnormal neurologic examinations, learning disabilities, or poor fine motor coordination, and left-handed children in a family without left-handedness may present with voiding dysfunction of this type (50).

Urodynamic studies may demonstrate a bladder that is smaller than estimated for the patient's age, a normal voiding pattern, and normal PVR (39,133). Radiographic studies usually do not reveal any abnormalities (125).

Management of the unstable bladder includes a timed voiding schedule with frequent voids (41) and anticholinergic medication to increase the threshold of detrusor filling before an unstable contraction has occurred (41,125,133).

Infrequent Voiding Syndrome

Children with infrequent voiding syndrome tend to delay voiding, eventually developing extremely large bladder capacities (up to 2 standard deviations greater than the mean for their age) with a weak or absent detrusor contraction at capacity (45,125,136). This entity is often referred to as the "lazy bladder syndrome." Patients often complain of urinary leakage, which is due to overflow or stress urinary incontinence (45,125,137). The condition is more common in females and is likely to present after toilet training has been initiated (125,137). Some common presenting signs include infrequent voiding (one to two voids per day), UTIs, a palpable abdominal mass, voiding by straining or Valsalva maneuver, weak urinary stream, constipation, and abdominal pain associated with nausea and vomiting (39,45,125,136–140).

Physical examination may disclose a palpably enlarged bladder. Radiographic studies generally show a normal upper urinary tract (125), an enlarged, smooth-walled bladder (137), and fecal retention. Urodynamic studies confirm incomplete emptying with large PVR, weak flow with voiding by straining, and a weak or absent detrusor contraction at capacity (125,136,137,140). VUR may or may not be present (137).

Management of this disorder is focused on bladder retraining, including double voiding and use of a timed voiding schedule with frequent voids, and improved bowel emptying (45,125,137,138,140). Infection should be treated with an appropriate antibiotic (137,138,140). For those in whom this conservative management fails, CIC may be required to achieve complete bladder emptying (129). Some have suggested the use of alpha-antagonists to relax the bladder outlet and improve bladder emptying (45).

Functional Bowel Disturbances

Constipation usually refers to infrequent hard stools that are difficult and uncomfortable to pass (141,142). A commonly accepted definition is a stool frequency of less than three times a week. Impaired bladder emptying has been demonstrated with constipation and fecal impaction (143). The mechanism by which this occurs is thought to be a physical obstruction of the bladder outlet by the fecal mass in the neighboring rectum (139,144).

Patients present with firm, hard stools that are difficult to pass, infrequent bowel movements, blood-streaked stools from rectal fissures, history of laxative or suppository use, abnormally large-sized bowel movements, or fecal soiling (145). Clinical suspicion can be confirmed and the condition graded by a plain radiograph of the abdomen (46,143).

Constipation and fecal impaction have been noted with multiple urinary tract abnormalities, such as hydronephrosis (139), nonneurogenic neurogenic bladder (122), acute urinary retention (144,146,147), diurnal and nocturnal incontinence (147), and recurrent UTI (141,145,147). Management of constipation without other specific urinary tract therapy has decreased PVRs and hydronephrosis (143,148). Management of constipation had also been shown to significantly reduce the recurrence rate of UTI (145,147) and to eliminate diurnal incontinence in 90% and nocturnal incontinence in 60% of patients (145).

Initial management of severe constipation usually involves digital disimpaction or disimpaction with oral laxatives and enemas (143,147). Dietary modification through increased intake of fiber and water is important (143,145). Scheduled toileting has been very effective (145,147). Continued medical management with daily oral laxatives and lubricants such as mineral oil may be required (143,145). On rare occasions a Malone antegrade continence enema procedure has been performed to provide a means of emptying the colon proximal to the large intestine on a regular basis, with good results reported (149,150). When medication is needed for bladder dysfunction, it is preferable to avoid oxybutynin and instead to use a more bladder-specific (and less constipating) antimuscarinic drug, such as tolterodine (151).

Extraordinary Urinary Frequency

The syndrome of extreme daytime urinary frequency of small volumes has a sudden onset in a previously well, toilet-trained child without evidence of structural urinary tract abnormalities or UTI (152–155). Its cause is unknown, but it has been related to the presence of psychological stresses (152,156). It has been referred to as *pollakiuria* from the Greek *pollakis,* which means "often" (154). Initially, the condition was thought to be quite rare (155); however, it may have been underrecognized, as many large case series now have been reported (152–154,156,157).

This syndrome generally occurs more frequently in boys (154,155). The symptoms are isolated to daytime events for most children. When nocturia does occur, it correlates with an increased incidence of recurrence of symptoms (154,155,157). The age of presentation ranges from 2 to 14 years, with most children developing symptoms between 4 and 6 years of age (153,154,156,157). Generally, there are no other symptoms noted (152). Physical examination is within normal limits (155,156). In some boys, however, signs of urethral meatal stenosis or urethritis may be noted, and the symptom of a thin, fine, forceful, upwardly directed stream can be elicited on querying the child or his parents.

A noninvasive investigation is needed to rule out significant abnormalities. Urinalysis and urine culture results are normal, but these studies should be performed to rule out diabetes mellitus, diabetes insipidus, and UTI (154–156). Renal and bladder ultrasonographic images are also normal (152,153,155,156). Further invasive testing such as urodynamic studies or voiding cystography is not indicated if results of the aforementioned investigations are normal (153,156).

This entity usually resolves spontaneously. Reassurance that the symptoms will resolve between 1 and 3 months from the syndrome's onset is all that is required (152,155,156). Drug therapy, such as administration of anticholinergics, has not improved symptoms (153).

REFERENCES

1. Brooks J. Anatomy of the lower urinary tract and male genitalia. In: Walsh PC, Vaughn ED Jr, Wein AJ, eds. *Campbell's urology*. 7th ed. Vol. 1. Philadelphia: WB Saunders, 1998:89–128.
2. Lapides J, Sweet RB, Lewis LW. Role of striated muscle in urination. *J Urol* 1957;77:247.
3. Hoebeke P, Walle JV. The pharmacology of pediatric incontinence. *Br J Urol Int* 2000;86:581.
4. Tanagho E, Schmidt RA, de Araujo CG. Urinary striated sphincter: what's its nerve supply? *Invest Urol* 1982;20:415.
5. Noto H, Roppolo JR, Steers WD, et al. Excitatory and inhibitory influences on bladder activity elicited by electrical stimulation in the pontine micturition center in the rat. *Brain Res* 1989;492:99.
6. El-Badawi A, Schenk EA. Dual innervation of the mammalian urinary bladder: a histochemical study of the distribution of cholinergic and adrenergic nerves. *Am J Anat* 1966;119:405.
7. Tanagho E. The "internal sphincter": is it under sympathetic control? *Invest Urol* 1969;7:79.
8. Barrington F. The localization of the paths subserving micturition in the spinal cord of the cat. *Brain* 1933;56:126.
9. de Groat W. Anatomy and physiology of the lower urinary tract. *Urol Clin North Am* 1993;20:383.
10. Nash D. The development of micturition control with special reference to enuresis. *Ann R Coll Surg Engl* 1949;5:318.
11. Kruse M, Noto H, Roppolo JR, et al. Pontine control of the urinary bladder and external urethral sphincter in the rat. *Brain Res* 1990;532:182.
12. Steers W. Physiology and pharmacology of the bladder and urethra. In: Walsh PC, Vaughn ED Jr, Wein AJ, eds. *Campbell's urology*. 7th ed. Vol. 1. Philadelphia: WB Saunders, 1998:870–916.
13. Koff S. Enuresis. In: Walsh PC, Vaughn ED Jr, Wein AJ, eds. *Campbell's urology*. 7th ed. Vol. 2. Philadelphia: WB Saunders, 1998:2055–2068.
14. de Groat W, Nedelhaft I, Milne RJ, et al. Organization of the sacral parasympathetic reflex pathways to the urinary bladder and large intestine. *J Auton Nerv Syst* 1981;3:135.
15. Shea V, Cai R, Crepps B, et al. Sensory fibers of the pelvic nerve innervating the rat's urinary bladder. *J Neurophysiol* 2000;84:1924.
16. Sengupta J, Gebhart GF. Mechanosensitive properties of pelvic nerve afferent fibers innervating the urinary bladder of the rat. *J Neurophysiol* 1994;72:2420.
17. Yeates W. Bladder function in normal micturition. In: Kovin I, MacKeith RC, Meadow SR, eds. *Bladder control and enuresis*. London: Spastics International Medical Publications, 1973:28–36.
18. Muellner S. Development of urinary control in children: some aspects of the cause and treatment of primary enuresis. *JAMA* 1960;172:1256.
19. Pachter L, Dworkin PH. Maternal expectations about normal child development in four cultural groups. *Arch Pediatr Adolesc Med* 1997;151:1144.
20. Holmdahl G, Hanson E, Hellstrom AL, et al. Four-hour voiding observation in healthy infants. *J Urol* 1996;156:1809.
21. Mattsson S, Lindstrom S. Diuresis and voiding pattern in healthy school children. *Br J Urol* 1995;76:783.
22. Gladh G, Persson D, Mattsson S, et al. Voiding pattern in healthy newborns. *Neurourol Urodyn* 2000;19:177.
23. Jansson U, Hanson M, Hanson E, et al. Voiding pattern in healthy children 0 to 3 years old: a longitudinal study. *J Urol* 2000;164:2050.
24. Goellner M, Ziegler EE, Fomon SJ. Urination during the first three years of life. *Nephron* 1981;28:174.
25. Roberts D, Rendell B. Postmicturition residual bladder volumes in healthy babies. *Arch Dis Child* 1989;64:825.
26. Wen J, Tong EC. Cystometry in infants and children with no apparent voiding symptoms. *Br J Urol* 1998;81:468.
27. Kaefer M, Zurakowski D, Bauer SB, et al. Estimating normal bladder capacity in children. *J Urol* 1997;158:2261.
28. Berger R, Maizels M, Moran GC, et al. Bladder capacity (ounces) equals age (years) plus 2 predicts normal bladder capacity and aids in diagnosis of abnormal voiding patterns. *J Urol* 1983;129:347.
29. MacKeith R, Meadow R, Turner RK. How children become dry. In: Kovin I, MacKeith RC, Meadow SR, eds. *Bladder control and enuresis*. London: Spastics International Medical Publications, 1973:23–27.
30. Araki I, de Groat WC. Developmental synaptic depression underlying reorganization of visceral reflex pathways in the spinal cord. *J Neurosci* 1997;17:8402.
31. Maggi C, Santicioli P, Meli A. Postnatal development of micturition reflex in rats. *Am J Physiol* 1986;250.
32. Thor K, Blais DP, de Groat WC. Behavioral analysis of the postnatal development of micturition in kittens. *Brain Res Dev Brain Res* 1989;46:137.
33. Yeung C, Godley ML, Ho CKW, et al. Some new insights into bladder function in infancy. *Br J Urol* 1995;76:235.
34. Sillen U, Solsnes E, Hellstrom AL, et al. The voiding pattern of healthy preterm neonates. *J Urol* 2000;163:278.
35. O'Donnell B, O'Connor TP. Bladder function in infants and children. *Br J Urol* 1971;43:25.
36. Yamazaki Y, Yago R, Toma H. Sonographic characteristics of the urinary tract in healthy neonates. *J Urol* 2001;166:1054.
37. Jequier S, Rousseau O. Sonographic measurements of the normal bladder wall in children. *AJR Am J Roentgenol* 1987;149: 563.

38. Wein A. Pharmacology of incontinence. *Urol Clin North Am* 1995;22:557.
39. van Gool J, Vijverberg MAW, de Jong TPVM. Functional daytime incontinence: clinical and urodynamic assessment. *Scand J Urol Nephrol Suppl* 1992;141:58.
40. Webster G, Koefoot RB, Sihelnik S. Urodynamic abnormalities in neurologically normal children with micturition dysfunction. *J Urol* 1984;132:74.
41. Koff S. Evaluation and management of voiding disorders in children. *Urol Clin North Am* 1988;15:769.
42. Parekh D, Pope JC, Adams MC, et al. The use of radiography, urodynamic studies and cystoscopy in the evaluation of voiding dysfunction. *J Urol* 2001;165:215.
43. Cayan S, Doruk E, Bozlu M, et al. Is routine urinary tract investigation necessary for children with monosymptomatic primary nocturnal enuresis? *Urology* 2001;58:598.
44. Williams M, Noe HN, Smith RA. The importance of urinary tract infection in the evaluation of the incontinent child. *J Urol* 1994;151:188.
45. Austin P, Ritchey ML. Dysfunctional voiding. *Pediatr Rev* 2000;21:336.
46. Blethyn A, Jones K, Verrier NR, et al. Radiological assessment of constipation. *Arch Dis Child* 1995;73:532.
47. Bomalaski MD, Anema JG, Coplen DE, et al. Delayed presentation of posterior urethral valves: a not so benign condition. *J Urol* 1999;162:2130.
48. Yamanishi T, Yasuda K, Hamano S, et al. Urethral obstruction in patients with nighttime wetting: urodynamic evaluation and outcome of surgical incision. *Neurourol Urodyn* 2000;19:241.
49. Vincent S. Postural control of urinary incontinence: the curtsy sign. *Lancet* 1966;2:631.
50. Khoshbin S. Pathologic left handedness. In: McLellan D, ed. Boston: 2002.
51. Ewalt D, Bauer SB. Pediatric neurourology. *Urol Clin North Am* 1996;23:501.
52. Drolet B. Cutaneous signs of neural tube dysraphism. *Pediatr Clin North Am* 2000;47:813.
53. Bauer S, Borer JG. Predominant urodynamics parameters in girls with recurrent urinary tract infection. Paper presented at: Annual Meeting of the American Urological Association; 1999; Dallas, TX.
54. McGuire E, Woodside J, Borden T, et al. Prognostic value of urodynamic testing in myelodysplastic patients. *J Urol* 1981; 126:205.
55. Kaefer M, Rosen A, Darbey M, et al. Pressure at residual volume: a useful adjunct to standard fill cystometry. *J Urol* 1997;158:1268.
56. Lary J, Edmonds LD. Prevalence of spina bifida at birth—United States, 1983–1990: a comparison of two surveillance systems. *MMWR Morb Mortal Wkly Rep* 1996;45: 15.
57. Stein S, Feldman JG, Friedlander M, et al. Is myelomeningocele a disappearing disease? *Pediatrics* 1982;69:511.
58. Palomaki GE, Williams JR, Haddow JE. Prenatal screening for open neural-tube defects in Maine. *N Engl J Med* 1999;340: 1049.
59. Desposito FC. Folic acid for the prevention of neural tube defects. Paper presented to: Committee on Genetics, American Academy of Pediatrics; 1999.
60. Laurence K. Double-blind randomized control trial of folate treatment before conception to prevent recurrence of neural tube defects. *BMJ* 1981;282:1509.
61. Khoury A, Hendrick EB, McLorie GA, et al. Occult spinal dysraphism: clinical and urodynamic outcome after division of the filum terminale. *J Urol* 1990;144:426.
62. Mandell J, Bauer SB, Hallett M, et al. Occult spinal dysraphism: a rare but detectable cause of voiding dysfunction. *Urol Clin North Am* 1980;7:349.
63. Anderson F. Occult spinal dysraphism: a series of 73 cases. *Pediatrics* 1975;55:826.
64. Emery J, Lendon RG. The local cord lesion in neurospinal dysraphism (meningomyelocele). *J Pathol* 1973;110:83.
65. Bauer S, Labib KB, Dieppa RA, et al. Urodynamic evaluation of boy with myelodysplasia and incontinence. *Urology* 1977;10:354.
66. Perez L, Khoury J, Webster GD. The value of urodynamic studies in infants less than 1 year old with congenital spinal dysraphism. *J Urol* 1992;148:584.
67. Dator D, Hatchett L, Dyro FM, et al. Urodynamic dysfunction in walking myelodysplastic children. *J Urol* 1992;148:362.
68. Kroovand R, Bell W, Hart LJ, et al. The effect of back closure on detrusor function in neonates with myelomeningocele. *J Urol* 1990;144:423.
69. Lais A, Kasabian NG, Dyro FM, et al. The neurosurgical implications of continuous neurourological surveillance of children with myelodysplasia. *J Urol* 1993;150:1879.
70. Tarcan T, Bauer SB, Olmedo E, et al. Long-term followup of newborns with myelodysplasia and normal urodynamic findings: is followup necessary? *J Urol* 2001;165:564.
71. Bauer S, Hallett M, Khoshbin S, et al. Predictive value of urodynamic evaluation in newborns with myelodysplasia. *JAMA* 1984;252:650.
72. Palmer L, Richards I, Kaplan WE. Age related bladder capacity and bladder capacity growth in children with myelomeningocele. *J Urol* 1997;158:1261.
73. Geraniotis E, Koff SA, Enrile B. The prophylactic use of clean intermittent catheterization in the treatment of infants and young children with myelomeningocele and neurogenic bladder dysfunction. *J Urol* 1988;139:85.
74. Sidi A, Dykstra DD, Gonzalez R. The value of urodynamic testing in the management of neonates with myelodysplasia: a prospective study. *J Urol* 1986;135:90.
75. McLorie G, Perez-Marero R, Csima A, et al. Determinants of hydronephrosis and renal injury in patients with myelomeningocele. *J Urol* 1988;140:1289.
76. Edelstein R, Bauer SB, Kelly MD, et al. The long-term urological response of neonates with myelodysplasia treated proactively with intermittent catheterization and anticholinergic therapy. *J Urol* 1994;154:1500.
77. Blaivas J, Sinha HP, Zayed AH, et al. Detrusor-external sphincter dyssynergia. *J Urol* 1981;125:542.
78. Blaivas J, Sinha HP, Zayed AH, et al. Detrusor-external sphincter dyssynergia: a detailed electromyographic study. *J Urol* 1981;125:545.
79. Hernandez R, Hurwitz RS, Foote JE, et al. Nonsurgical management of the threatened upper urinary tracts and incontinence in children with myelomeningocele. *J Urol* 1994;152:1582.

80. Kasabian N, Bauer SB, Dyro FM, et al. The prophylactic value of clean intermittent catheterization and anticholinergic medication in newborns and infants with myelodysplasia at risk of developing urinary tract deterioration. *Am J Dis Child* 1992;146:840.
81. Mandell J, Bauer SB, Colodny AH, et al. Cutaneous vesicostomy in infancy. *J Urol* 1981;126:92.
82. Kass E, Koff SA, Diokno AC. Fate of vesicoureteral reflux in children with neuropathic bladders managed by intermittent catheterization. *J Urol* 1980;125:63.
83. Bauer S, Colodny AH, Retik AB. The management of vesicoureteral reflux in children with neurogenic bladder. *J Urol* 1976;115:449.
84. Jeffs R, Jonas P, Schillinger JF. Surgical correction of vesicoureteral reflux in children with neurogenic bladder. *J Urol* 1976;115:449.
85. Barbalias G, Klauber GT, Blaivas JG. Critical evaluation of the Credé maneuver: a urodynamic study of 207 patients. *J Urol* 1983;129:720.
86. Keating M, Rink RC, Bauer SB, et al. Neurourological implications of the changing approach in management of occult spinal lesions. *J Urol* 1988;140:1299.
87. Kaplan W, McLone DG, Richards I. The urological manifestations of the tethered spinal cord. *J Urol* 1988;140:1285.
88. Satar N, Bauer SB, Shefner J, et al. The effects of delayed diagnosis and treatment in patients with an occult spinal dysraphism. *J Urol* 1995;154:754.
89. Arikan N, Soygur T, Selcuki M, et al. Role of magnetic resonance imaging in children with voiding dysfunction: retrospective analysis of 81 patients. *Urology* 1999;54:157.
90. Yamada S, Zinke DE, Sanders D. Pathophysiology of "tethered cord syndrome." *J Neurosurg* 1981;54:494.
91. Atala A, Bauer SB, Dyro FM, et al. Bladder functional changes resulting from lipomyelomeningocele repair. *J Urol* 1992;148:592.
92. Foster L, Kogan BA, Cogen PH, et al. Bladder function in patients with lipomyelomeningocele. *J Urol* 1990;143:984.
93. Freedman B. Congenital absence of the sacrum and coccyx: report of a case and review of the literature. *Br J Surg* 1950;37:299.
94. Guzman L, Bauer SB, Hallett M, et al. Evaluation and management of children with sacral agenesis. *Urology* 1983;22:506.
95. Boemers T, van Gool JD, de Jong TPVM, et al. Urodynamic evaluation of children with the caudal regression syndrome (caudal dysplasia sequence). *J Urol* 1994;151:1038.
96. Passarge E, Lenz W. Syndrome of caudal regression in infants of diabetic mothers: observations of further cases. *Pediatrics* 1966;37:672.
97. Koff S, Deridder PA. Patterns of neurogenic bladder dysfunction in sacral agenesis. *J Urol* 1977;118:87.
98. White R, Klauber GT. Sacral agenesis: analysis of 22 cases. *Urol Int* 1976;8:521.
99. Wilmshurst J, Kelly R, Borzyskowski M. Presentation and outcome of sacral agenesis: 20 years' experience. *Dev Med Child Neurol* 1999;41:806.
100. Braren V, Jones WB. Sacral agenesis: diagnosis, treatment, and followup of urological complications. *J Urol* 1979;121:543.
101. Kakizaki H, Nonomura K, Asano Y, et al. Preexisting neurogenic voiding dysfunction in children with imperforate anus: problems in management. *J Urol* 1994;151:1041.
102. Carson J, Barnes PD, Tunell WP, et al. Imperforate anus: the neurologic implication of sacral abnormalities. *J Pediatr Surg* 1984;19:838.
103. Parrott T, Woodard JR. Importance of cystourethrography in neonates with imperforate anus. *Urology* 1979;13:607.
104. Greenfield S, Fera M. Urodynamic evaluation of the patient with an imperforate anus: a prospective study. *J Urol* 1991;146:539.
105. Kuban KC, Leviton A. Cerebral palsy. *N Engl J Med* 1994;330:188.
106. McNeal D, Hawtrey CE, Wolraich ML, et al. Symptomatic neurogenic bladder in a cerebral-palsied population. *Dev Med Child Neurol* 1983;25:612.
107. Reid C, Borzyskowski M. Lower urinary tract dysfunction in cerebral palsy. *Arch Dis Child* 1993;68:739.
108. Mayo M. Lower urinary tract dysfunction in cerebral palsy. *J Urol* 1992;147:419.
109. Decter R, Bauer SB, Khoshbin S, et al. Urodynamic assessment of children with cerebral palsy. *J Urol* 1987;138:1110.
110. Brodak P, Scherz HC, Packer MG, et al. Is urinary tract screening necessary for patients with cerebral palsy? *J Urol* 1994;152:1586.
111. Bauer S. Anticholinergic therapy in children with cerebral palsy. In: McLellan D, ed. Boston: 2002.
112. Anderson JM, Schutt AH. Spinal injury in children: a review of 156 cases seen from 1950 through 1978. *Mayo Clin Proc* 1980;55:499.
113. Pannek J, Diederichs W, Botel U. Urodynamically controlled management of spinal cord injury in children. *Neurourol Urodyn* 1997;16:285.
114. Cass A, Luxenberg M, Johnson CF, et al. Management of the neurogenic bladder in 413 children. *J Urol* 1984;132:521.
115. Bauer S, Koff SA, Jayanthi VR. Voiding dysfunction in children: neurogenic and non-neurogenic. In: Walsh PC, Vaughn ED Jr, Wein AJ, eds. *Campbell's urology*. Philadelphia: Elsevier Science, 2002:2231–2283.
116. Guttmann L, Frankel H. The value of intermittent catheterization in the early management of the traumatic paraplegia and tetraplegia. *Paraplegia* 1966;4:63.
117. Lapides J, Diokno AC, Silber SH, et al. Clean, intermittent self-catheterization in the treatment of urinary tract disease. *J Urol* 1972;107:458.
118. Koff S, Wagner TT, Jayanthi VR. The relationship among dysfunctional elimination syndromes, primary vesicoureteral reflux and urinary tract infections in children. *J Urol* 1998;160:1019.
119. Van Gool J, Hjalmas K, Tamminen-Mobius T, et al. Historical clues to the complex of dysfunctional voiding, urinary tract infection and vesicoureteral reflux. *J Urol* 1992;148.
120. Hinman F. Urinary tract damage in children who wet. *Pediatrics* 1974;54:142.
121. Hinman FJ. Nonneurogenic neurogenic bladder (The Hinman Syndrome)—15 years later. *J Urol* 1986;136:769.
122. Williams D, Hirst G, Doyle D. The occult neuropathic bladder. *J Pediatr Surg* 1974;9:35.
123. Dorfman L, Bailey J, Smith JP. Subclinical neurogenic bladder in children. *J Urol* 1969;101:48.
124. Johnston J, Koff SA, Glassberg KI. The pseudo-obstructed bladder in enuretic children. *Br J Urol* 1978;50:505.
125. Bauer S, Retik AB, Colodny AH, et al. The unstable bladder of childhood. *Urol Clin North Am* 1980;7:321.

126. Martin D, Datta NS, Schweitz B. The occult neurological bladder. *J Urol* 1971;105:733.
127. Hinman F, Baumann FW. Vesical and ureteral damage from voiding dysfunction in boys without neurologic or obstructive disease. *J Urol* 1973;109:7272.
128. Allen T. The non-neurogenic neurogenic bladder. *J Urol* 1976;117:232.
129. Pohl H, Bauer SB, Borer JG, et al. The outcome of voiding dysfunction managed with clean intermittent catheterization in neurologically and anatomically normal children. *Br J Urol Int* 2002;89:923.
130. Coms A, Glassberg AD, Gerdes D, et al. Biofeedback therapy for children with dysfunctional voiding. *Urology* 1998;52:312.
131. Baumann F, Hinman F. The treatment of incontinent boys with non-obstructive disease. *J Urol* 1974;111:114.
132. Austin P, Homsy L, Masel JL, et al. Alpha-adrenergic blockade in children with neuropathic and nonneuropathic voiding dysfunction. *J Urol* 1999;162:1064.
133. Koff S, Lapides J, Piazza DH. Association of urinary tract infection and reflux with uninhibited bladder contractions and voluntary sphincteric obstruction. *J Urol* 1979;122:373.
134. Fergusson DM, Horwood LJ. Nocturnal enuresis and behavioral problems in adolescence: a 15-year longitudinal study. *Pediatrics* 1994;94:662.
135. Kodman-Jones C, Hawkins L, Schulman SL. Behavioral characteristics of children with daytime wetting. *J Urol* 2001;166:2392.
136. Hjalmas K. Urinary incontinence in children: suggestions for definitions and terminology. *Scand J Urol Nephrol Suppl* 1992;141:1.
137. DeLuca F, Swenson O, Fisher JH, et al. The dysfunctional "lazy" bladder syndrome in children. *Arch Dis Child* 1962;37:117.
138. Lapides J, Costello RT. Uninhibited neurogenic bladder: a common cause for recurrent urinary infection in normal women. *J Urol* 1969;101:539.
139. Shopfner C. Urinary tract pathology associated with constipation. *Radiology* 1968;90:865.
140. Lapides J, Diokno AC. Persistence of the infant bladder as a cause for urinary infection in girls. *Trans Am Assoc Genitourin Surg* 1969;61:51.
141. Blethyn A, Jenkins HR, Roberts R, et al. Radiological evidence of constipation in urinary infection. *Arch Dis Child* 1995;73:534.
142. O'Regan S, Schick E, Hamburger B, et al. Constipation associated with vesicoureteral reflux. *Urology* 1986;28:394.
143. Dohil R, Roberts E, Verrier Jones K, et al. Constipation and reversible urinary tract abnormalities. *Arch Dis Child* 1994; 70:56.
144. Gallo D, Presman D. Urinary retention due to fecal impaction in children. *Pediatrics* 1970;45:292.
145. Neumann P, deDomenico IJ, Nogrady MB. Constipation and urinary tract infection. *Pediatrics* 1973;52:241.
146. Baldew I, Van Gelderen HH. Urinary retention without organic cause in children. *Br J Urol* 1983;55:200.
147. Loening-Baucke V. Urinary incontinence and urinary tract infection and their resolution with treatment of chronic constipation of childhood. *Pediatrics* 1997;100:228.
148. Lucanto C, Bauer SB, Hyman PE, et al. Function of hollow viscera in children with constipation and voiding difficulties. *Dig Dis Sci* 2000;45:1274.
149. Sugarman ID, Malone PS, Terry TR, et al. Transversely tubularized ileal segments for the Mitrofanoff or Malone antegrade colonic enema procedures: the Monti principle. *Br J Urol* 1998;81:253.
150. Griffiths DM, Malone PS. The Malone antegrade continence enema. *J Pediatr Surg* 1995;30:68.
151. Chapple CR. Muscarinic receptor antagonists in the treatment of overactive bladder. *Urology* 2000;55:33.
152. Bass L. Pollakiuria, extraordinary daytime urinary frequency: experience in a pediatric practice. *Pediatrics* 1991; 87:735.
153. Koff S, Byard MA. The daytime urinary frequency syndrome of childhood. *J Urol* 1988;140:1280.
154. Waternberg N, Shalev H. Daytime urinary frequency in children. *Clin Pediatr* 1994;33:50.
155. Gupta A, Uppal SS, Salhan RN. Daytime urinary frequency syndrome in childhood. *Indian Pediatr* 1990;27:752.
156. Robson W, Leung AK. Extraordinary urinary frequency syndrome. *Urology* 1993;42:321.
157. Zoubek J, Bloom DA, Sedman AB. Extraordinary urinary frequency. *Pediatrics* 1990;85:1112.

57

UROLITHIASIS

DAWN S. MILLINER

Urolithiasis is increasingly recognized in pediatric patients and is encountered in a variety of clinical settings: the 8-year-old boy with idiopathic hypercalciuria and a single stone, the 14-year-old with cystinuria experiencing her fourth episode of renal colic in the past 6 years, the 10-year-old with inflammatory bowel disease whose two renal stones were recognized incidentally during imaging for evaluation of abdominal pain, the premature infant with asymptomatic nephrocalcinosis and a stone, the 4-year-old with human immunodeficiency virus infection in the emergency room with gross hematuria and abdominal pain after recently starting indinavir medication. All have in common particulate material of mineral origin within the urinary tract, the development of which depends on fundamental physicochemical principles. An understanding of these principles, along with the pathophysiologic states that promote urinary tract calculi, provides the basis for effective clinical management.

MECHANISMS OF STONE FORMATION

Several steps are required for stone formation, beginning with crystallization and followed by crystal growth, aggregation, and adherence of crystals to epithelium. Supersaturation in a specific crystal system is a precondition for solutes to precipitate in the urine and form crystals. Although the concentration of solutes is the principal determinant, supersaturation is dependent on other factors as well, including ionic strength and pH. Promotors and inhibitors present in the urine also play a role in crystallization. Concentrations of mineral solutes, ionic strength, pH, promotors, and inhibitors in the urine vary throughout the day as influenced by fluid intake, dietary constituents, and body metabolism. Urine in healthy individuals is often supersaturated with calcium oxalate, calcium phosphate, or sodium urate. A dynamic process of crystal formation, crystal growth, aggregation, disaggregation, and dissolution of crystals accompanies the diurnal variations in the physicochemical state of the urine. Thus, despite frequent periods of supersaturation, most children do not form urinary tract stones.

Promoters of crystallization are not well characterized but may include urinary macromolecules and lipids (1). Lipids are integral to the organic matrices of mineralized tissues as well as to pathologic calcifications (1). Urinary tract stones are no exception. Khan et al. (1) found that the urine of calcium and uric acid stone formers contained significantly more cholesterol, cholesterol ester, and triglycerides than the urine of healthy controls, with more acidic phospholipids observed in calcium oxalate stone formers only. In addition to reflecting renal cell damage with release of membrane phospholipids into the urine, the lipids appear to promote crystallization of both calcium oxalate and calcium phosphate. Another type of promotion that has received attention is the role played by crystals of one salt in inducing crystallization of another. For example, sodium urate (2–3) or calcium phosphate (4) can act as a nidus for calcium oxalate crystal formation. This circumstance occurs because there is a metastable region between the ion solubility product (below which the urine is undersaturated) and the ion formation product. In this metastable region there is the potential for heterogeneous crystal formation and growth (5). Above the formation product, the solution is unstable and spontaneous homogeneous crystal formation occurs. These principles help to explain the observation that patients with calcium stones are often hyperuricosuric (6).

Inhibitors of crystallization act at the crystal surface, most often interfering at active crystal growth sites (5). Naturally occurring inhibitors of calcium oxalate and calcium phosphate crystal formation in the urine include citrate, pyrophosphate, magnesium, and urinary macromolecules such as glycosaminoglycans, and nephrocalcin. Citrate, phosphate, magnesium, and sulfate also interfere with crystallization by forming soluble complexes with potential crystal ions. These properties can be used to therapeutic advantage in patients with calcium oxalate and calcium phosphate stones (7–8).

From the time filtrate is formed at the glomerulus until the urine reaches the bladder there is an environment of constant flow, so that crystals formed are generally washed out of the urinary tract. For stones to form, the crystals must either aggregate to a size sufficient to obstruct a renal tubule and impair flow (free particle theory) or the crystal must adhere to the renal epithelial cell, the papillary tip, the wall of a calyx, or another location in the urinary tract (fixed particle theory). Adherence is favored by injury to the renal tubular epithelium or the urothelium. Injury may be induced by toxins, by infection, or by crystals themselves. Metabolic factors such as high concentrations of oxalate, which is now recognized to cause direct injury to renal tubular epithelial cells (9), may also play a role. Attention has turned to the interaction of urinary constituents and renal epithelial cells as determinants of crystal formation, crystal structure and growth, and attachment (10–12). Once crystals are relatively stationary in the urinary tract, which permits growth and aggregation, a stone may develop. Stasis of the urinary tract, with or without frank obstruction, is an important contributor. The balance of all of these processes is such that most individuals do not form urinary tract stones. Among children who do form stones, predisposing metabolic factors, infection, and/or urinary stasis are identified in the majority (13).

EPIDEMIOLOGY OF UROLITHIASIS IN CHILDREN AND ADOLESCENTS

Urinary tract calculi have been perceived as uncommon in children and adolescents and account for between 1 in 1000 and 1 in 7600 hospital admissions in this age group in the United States (14–16), a rate that is one-fiftieth to one-seventy-fifth of that reported in adults (13). Because many patients with urolithiasis do not require hospitalization, such data underestimate the incidence and prevalence. There are few population-based studies. That of Johnson et al. found the incidence of urolithiasis in patients older than 10 years to be 109 per 100,000 population per year in men and 36 per 100,000 population per year in women. Patients aged 10 to 19 years accounted for just 3.7% of the total episodes (17).

An explanation for the lower incidence of urolithiasis observed in children is incomplete, but the reason may be related to observations that concentrations of inhibitors of crystal formation and crystal cell attachment such as citrate, magnesium, and certain macromolecules are higher in the urine of children than in that of adults (12,18–19). The ratio of citrate to calcium and magnesium to calcium in the urine is higher in children (18). Miyake et al. (18) noted that nucleation of calcium oxalate crystals was more strongly inhibited in random urine samples from children than from those of adults as determined by measurement of the metastable limit for calcium oxalate. Robertson et al. defined a risk index for calcium oxalate lithiasis and also found this index to be lower in children (20). In another study, Miyake and colleagues (12) found that urinary macromolecules from pediatric patients more strongly inhibited the adhesion of calcium oxalate crystals to renal tubular epithelial cells *in vitro* than did those from adults. This effect may have been potentiated by the higher concentrations of citrate observed in the urine from pediatric patients in the study.

Nonetheless, with appreciation that the presenting symptoms of urolithiasis may be different in children and that improved radiographic techniques are used more liberally than in the past, the diagnosis is now being made more often in pediatric patients. The frequency of occurrence has also been influenced in recent years by factors predisposing premature infants to nephrocalcinosis and urinary tract stones, and advances in medical care that have resulted in the survival through childhood and adolescence of increasing numbers of patients with medical conditions such as cystic fibrosis that are associated with urolithiasis. Finally, an increasing incidence of urolithiasis overall in recent decades has been noted in population-based studies in industrialized countries (21).

Among children and adolescents, boys show a mild preponderance for stone disease overall (17,22–25). Four pediatric series reported a male to female ratio of 1.4:1 to 2.1:1 in the United States, United Kingdom, Brazil, and Armenia (26–29). These ratios contrast with those for symptomatic adult stone formers, among whom males predominate in a ratio of 2:1 to 3:1, and reach a maximum of 4.8:1 from ages 40 to 60 years (21). There are exceptions among certain specific groups, such as young children with developmental anomalies of the urinary tract and associated infection, who tend to be male and younger in age (22,27). It is important to keep in mind that most pediatric series are small and subject to referral bias. The only population-based study showed a ratio of 1.3:1 (17) but did not include children younger than 10 years of age.

CLINICAL FEATURES

Symptoms of renal colic and gross hematuria, pathognomonic of urolithiasis in adults, are seen less reliably in children (22,30). Flank or abdominal pain or hematuria were the initial presenting features in 94% of adolescents and 72% of school-aged children, but in just 56% of children from birth to 5 years of age in one series (Fig. 57.1). In younger children, pain with features of renal colic was the exception, with most reporting or observed to have nonspecific abdominal pain. Indeed, among children up to 5 years of age the diagnosis of urolithiasis was made during investigation of a urinary tract infection or as an incidental radiographic finding during evaluation of other problems in 44% of patients (22).

In North American series, 60 to 78% of urinary tract calculi are found in the kidney at the time of diagnosis (22,26,31). The majority of those found in the ureters, bladder, or urethra have also originated in the kidneys. The bladder appears to be the site of stone formation in fewer

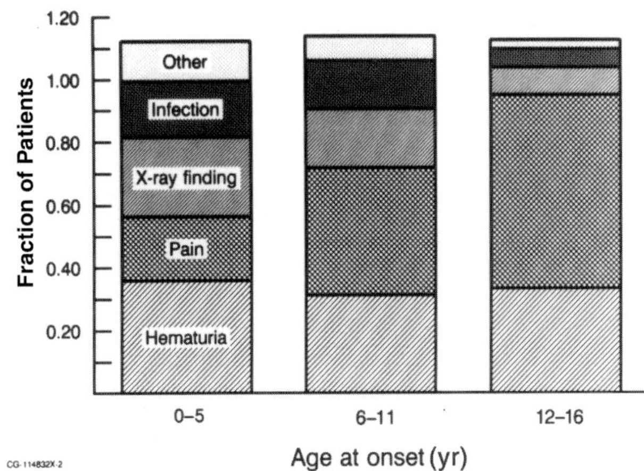

FIGURE 57.1. Clinical features at time of initial presentation of 221 children and adolescents with urolithiasis. (From Milliner DS, Murphy ME. Urolithiasis in pediatric patients. *Mayo Clin Proc* 1993;68:241–248, with permission.)

than 10% of North American children, although in other areas of the world bladder calculi may be seen more often and are often referred to as endemic bladder stones (29,32). Primary bladder stones tend to occur in younger children (21,29). Such stones appear related to dietary factors in developing countries (33,34). A diet with a high content of whole-grain cereals and/or oxalate-rich vegetables together with a low content of calcium, animal protein, and phosphate is believed to be responsible (21,32). The resulting urinary biochemical profile favors precipitation of ammonium acid urate and calcium oxalate, the most frequently occurring constituents of endemic bladder stones (32). Endemic bladder stones of childhood are frequent in several areas of the world, including Thailand, India, Turkey, Syria, Iran, Iraq, Tunisia, Pakistan, Indonesia, and the Sudan (21). There has been a striking decline in such stones in Europe and other developed countries over the last century (21,34). Calculi that form in the bladder in North American children are nearly always associated with bladder malformations or prior surgery such as augmentation cystoplasty and are characterized by infection.

Composition of stones from the upper urinary tract is calcium oxalate in 40 to 60%, calcium phosphate in 15 to 25%, mixed (usually calcium oxalate and calcium phosphate) in 10 to 25%, magnesium ammonium phosphate (struvite) in 17 to 30%, cystine in 6 to 10%, and uric acid in 2 to 10% of stones analyzed in several pediatric series (14,22–24,26,29,35).

CAUSATIVE FACTORS IN UROLITHIASIS

Seventy-five percent of children and adolescents with urolithiasis have identifiable predisposing causes for stone formation (22–24,35). In a compilation of studies that included 492 North American pediatric patients with urolithiasis, Polinsky et al. (13) noted that metabolic causes accounted for approximately 33%, structural urinary tract abnormalities for 32%, and infection for 4% of stones although differences in classification complicated the combining of multiple studies. In most published series, complete metabolic evaluations were not performed for all patients, which likely led to underestimation of the contribution of metabolic factors. This impression is supported by a study in which all patients were screened for metabolic abnormalities (36). In this study, a metabolic cause for stone formation was identified in 25 of 47 patients (53%). In some pediatric reports, especially those from Europe, infection is cited as the cause of urolithiasis in a higher proportion of patients (54% in Polinsky et al.'s combined series of European children) (13,27,29,37). In most series, infants and young children have infection-related stones more frequently than do older children or adolescents (22,27), whereas adolescents account for the majority of those with idiopathic stone disease. No contributing cause for stone formation was identified (idiopathic) in 28% of North American patients and 14% of the European patients in the compilation by Polinsky (13).

It is common to find more than one predisposing factor in a given patient (22). In one study of 221 pediatric patients with urolithiasis, 36% of those with structurally abnormal urinary tracts were also found to have metabolic abnormalities predisposing to stone formation and 39% had chronic infection (22). Among the patients with infection-related stones, 29% also had metabolic abnormalities. Thus the presence of infection, obstruction, or structural anomaly in the urinary tract does not obviate the need for careful metabolic assessment. Among patients with metabolic abnormalities, 21% also had structural anomalies and 10% had chronic infection as additional predisposing factors (22). Because of the high likelihood of identifying causes for stone formation in children and adolescents and in view of the early onset and potential for many years of stone-forming tendency, complete assessment for stone-forming factors is indicated in all children.

Metabolic Factors Predisposing to Stone Formation

High urinary concentrations of calcium, oxalate, uric acid, or cystine resulting from either increased renal excretion or low urine volume results in supersaturation of the urine for the respective crystal systems and thus favors crystal and stone formation. Among naturally occurring inhibitors of stone formation in the urine, citrate, magnesium, and pyrophosphate are the best defined. A number of urinary macromolecules, including glycosaminoglycans, osteopontin, and urinary prothrombin fragment 1, appear to play a role but as yet are not well studied in children and adolescents (38). Identification of the specific predisposing metabolic

TABLE 57.1. METABOLIC ABNORMALITIES ASSOCIATED WITH UROLITHIASIS

	Idiopathic	Secondary	Renal tubule transport disorder or inborn error of metabolism
Hypercalciuria	Inherited Sporadic	Dietary salt excess Dietary calcium excess Vitamin D excess Ketogenic diet Corticosteroids Loop diuretics Immobilization Metabolic acidosis Phosphate depletion Prematurity Prostaglandin E_2 Hypercalcemia Hyperparathyroidism Hyper- or hypothyroidism	Dent's disease RTA Familial hypomagnesemia-hypercalciuria Calcium-sensing receptor mutations
Hyperoxaluria	Mild, associated with idiopathic stone disease	Dietary oxalate excess Enteric hyperoxaluria Parenteral nutrition in premature infants	Primary hyperoxaluria I and II
Cystinuria	—	—	Cystinuria
Hyperuricosuria	Mild, associated with idiopathic stone disease Familial forms	High-protein diet Ketogenic diet High-dose pancreatic enzyme therapy Diabetes Tumor lysis Myeloproliferative, lymphoproliferative disorders SIADH Salicylates Sulfinpyrazone Phenylbutazone	HPRT deficiency, complete (Lesch-Nyhan syndrome) or partial
Hypocitric aciduria	Mild, associated with idiopathic urolithiasis	Metabolic acidosis Ketogenic diet Hypokalemia Bacteriuria	Distal RTA

HPRT, hypoxanthine phosphoribosyltransferase; RTA, renal tubular acidosis; SIADH, syndrome of inappropriate secretion of antidiuretic hormone.

factors (Table 57.1) in each patient is of importance in developing the most effective therapeutic regimen.

Solute Excess

Hypercalciuria as currently defined (greater than 4 mg/kg/day or urinary calcium/creatinine ratio greater than 0.21) is common, occurring in 2.9 to 3.8% of healthy children (39,40), and can predispose to hematuria, dysuria, urinary urgency, and perhaps recurrent urinary tract infections (41–44) as well as to urolithiasis. Hypercalciuria accounts for 30 to 50% of identified metabolic factors in children and adolescents with urolithiasis. Most hypercalciuria is idiopathic, identified as an isolated finding, and may be sporadic or inherited. Inherited forms have been well described, may account for up to 40 to 60% of cases of idiopathic hypercalciuria, and appear to follow an autosomal dominant or codominant pattern (45–48). The gene or genes responsible remain to be identified.

Among children and adults with idiopathic hypercalciuria, two subtypes of the disorder have been described, one related to enhanced gastrointestinal absorption of calcium and the other related to increased renal tubular secretion of calcium (49,50). The former is characterized by hypercalciuria after an oral calcium intake, with normal urine calcium/creatinine ratios in the fasting state. Renal leak hypercalciuria is present in the fasting as well as postprandial state and persists despite dietary calcium restriction. The use of oral calcium loading tests has been advocated to distinguish between these two types (40,49–51), but they often do not allow clear separation among subtypes of hypercalciuria in children (43,52). The inability of this test to distinguish between the two types is in part due to the confounding role of sodium on renal tubular secretion of calcium and the recognition that some children identified as having idiopathic hypercalciuria have sodium-dependent hypercalciuria related to high dietary sodium intake. Other mechanisms of idiopathic hypercalciuria have also been implicated and include renal tubular phosphate leak, increased 1,25-dihydroxyvitamin D synthesis, increased renal prostaglandin E_2 production, and bone resorption (53).

Among children with idiopathic hypercalciuria who did not have urolithiasis at initial diagnosis, the likelihood of developing calculi was 4 to 17% during 1 to 11 years of follow-up in three studies involving a total of 146 patients (42,43,54). The risk of urolithiasis appears to increase with age (44). In addition to playing a role in the development of urolithiasis and urinary tract symptoms, idiopathic hypercalciuria may be associated with reduced bone mass (55,56).

Secondary forms of hypercalciuria are common and occur most often in response to dietary salt excess, long-term use of corticosteroids, and use of loop diuretics such as furosemide. Prolonged immobilization in children or adolescents, excess intake of calcium or vitamin D, and high concentrations of circulating parathyroid hormone all predispose to hypercalciuria. Phosphate depletion causes hypercalciuria mediated by an increase in 1,25-dihydroxyvitamin D synthesis (57). Chronic metabolic acidosis from any cause has the potential to result in hypercalciuria due to bone resorption. In distal renal tubular acidosis (RTA), the deficiency in acid secretion results in significant hypercalciuria. Once the metabolic acidosis is corrected with exogenous administration of base, the hypercalciuria resolves. Hypercalcemia of any cause is likely to result in secondary hypercalciuria.

Rare, inherited forms of hypercalciuria include the X-linked disorders related to mutations of the CLCN5 chloride channel, the gene for which is located on chromosome band Xp11.22. This chloride channel is expressed in the cortical proximal tubule, medullary thick ascending limb of the loop of Henle, and α-intercalated cells of the human nephron (58). Mutations of this channel have now been demonstrated in four conditions previously described as separate clinical entities: X-linked nephrolithiasis with renal failure, Dent's disease, X-linked recessive hypophosphatemic rickets, and low-molecular-weight proteinuria with hypercalciuria and nephrocalcinosis. These conditions have in common hypercalciuria, nephrolithiasis, nephrocalcinosis, renal tubule dysfunction characterized by low-molecular-weight proteinuria and impaired absorption of phosphorus, progressive renal insufficiency, and in some cases rickets (59). The syndromes differ in degree from one another, but it is now established that they are phenotypic variants of a single disease. Although a large number of mutations have been identified, there appears to be no consistent correlation between genotype and phenotype (59). Thus, here all are referred to collectively as Dent's disease (60).

Hypercalciuria in patients with Dent's disease is typically moderate, although it may be as high as 10 mg/kg/day in some children. The reason for the hypercalciuria is not well understood (61). Both fasting hypercalciuria and an exaggerated response to an oral calcium load have been demonstrated in affected patients (62). Parathyroid hormone concentrations are typically below the mean of normal, and 1,25-dihydroxyvitamin D levels are above the mean of normal and are frequently elevated (59). Serum phosphorus level is normal or low. The hypercalciuria may be the result of abnormal regulation of 1α-hydroxylation of vitamin D, perhaps related to generalized proximal renal tubule cell dysfunction (59). Others have suggested that defective CLCN5 channel function resulting in abnormal vesicle acidification may underlie a renal tubular failure to reabsorb low-molecular-weight proteins and calcium (61,63). Notably, both parathyroid hormone and vitamin D–binding protein are normally reabsorbed from luminal fluid and are increased in the urine of ClC-5 "knock-out" mice (61). Hypercalciuria in Dent's disease is responsive to thiazides, which indicates that inactivation of the CLCN5 chloride channel does not impair calcium transport in the distal convoluted tubule (64).

Tubular proteinuria of up to 1 g/day in children is a diagnostic feature of boys affected with Dent's disease (59) and is frequently present in lesser amounts in carrier girls (63). The level of retinol-binding protein is distinctly elevated, and this protein has been shown to be better than β_2-microglobulin or α_1-microglobulin in identifying the tubular proteinuria of Dent's disease (63). Renal tubular dysfunction may be evident as early as the neonatal period; hypophosphatemic rickets may develop in the first years of life; and nephrocalcinosis is often seen in childhood (65). Evidence of other renal tubule dysfunction including aminoaciduria, phosphate or potassium wasting, and glycosuria is observed less consistently. Impaired renal concentrating capacity is often observed in conjunction with nephrocalcinosis or renal insufficiency (59).

Urolithiasis is common in childhood in affected boys, although it is not universal. Occasionally, carrier girls have significant clinical manifestations and may develop nephrolithiasis or renal impairment (66). The most important factor contributing to stone formation appears to be the hypercalciuria. Urine citrate and oxalate excretion rates are typically normal when studied at times of good renal function (59). The hypercalciuria of Dent's disease appears responsive to treatment with thiazide diuretics. However, amiloride was not found to be helpful (59,64).

Other rare, inherited disorders are associated with hypercalciuria, including mutations of the calcium-sensing receptor that lead to hypocalcemia and hypercalciuria (67), and familial hypomagnesemia-hypercalciuria (68).

Hyperoxaluria accounts for 2 to 20% of metabolic factors identified in children and adolescents with urolithiasis (22,69,70). Mild idiopathic hyperoxaluria (ranging from 0.45 to 0.6 mmol/1.73 m^2/24 hr) may be seen and is not infrequently observed in conjunction with mild hypercalciuria in patients with idiopathic stone disease (70,71). The cause of the hyperoxaluria is unknown but has variably been ascribed to metabolic changes that result in increased oxalate production or to enhanced gastrointestinal absorption (71–73). Ten percent to 20% of the oxalate in the urine has traditionally been regarded as derived from dietary sources (74), although some have argued that the contribution of dietary oxalate is higher (75). Marked dietary oxalate excess (particularly if there is concomitant low dietary calcium) (71,75) can lead to hyperoxaluria. Ingestion of starfruit (carambola) has been associated with acute oxalate nephropathy (76). Ethylene glycol, found in antifreeze, is metabolized to oxalate. Ingestion may result in acute renal failure due to oxalate nephropathy.

Under normal conditions, less than 10% of oxalate ingested is absorbed from the gastrointestinal tract (73,77,78). There has been interest in the disposition of fecal oxalate by certain anaerobic bacteria that populate the colon in a significant proportion of healthy individuals. It has been hypothesized that loss of colonization with organisms such as *Oxalobacter formigenes* may result in increased gastrointestinal absorption of oxalate leading to hyperoxaluria (70,79). As of 2003, this interesting hypothesis remains to be convincingly demonstrated.

Increased absorption of oxalate resulting from gastrointestinal disease is termed *enteric hyperoxaluria.* Any abnormality of the intestinal tract that is associated with malabsorption of fat can result in enhanced enteric absorption of oxalate (80). Mechanisms include binding of calcium by fatty acids. This leaves less calcium in the lumen to combine with oxalate, and oxalate is thus absorbed more avidly. In addition, bile salts cause injury to the colonic epithelium, which promotes enhanced oxalate absorption. The degree of hyperoxaluria caused by enteric disease is highly diet dependent and quite variable from mild to severe. Consequences can include not only recurrent urolithiasis but also oxalate nephropathy leading to renal failure. Treatment includes reduction in dietary oxalate, addition of calcium supplements to bind oxalate in the intestinal tract, increased oral fluid intake, a low-fat diet, and in some patients administration of sequestrants of bile acids. If hypocitric aciduria or hypomagnesuria is present, supplementation may be helpful to improve urinary inhibition of calcium oxalate crystal formation.

The primary hyperoxalurias are autosomal recessive inborn errors of metabolism due to deficiency of hepatic alanine:glyoxylate aminotransferase (AGT) (type I) or glyoxylate reductase/hydroxypyruvate reductase (type II) and are associated with moderate to marked elevation of urine oxalate excretion (81,82). Both of these enzymes are important in the metabolic disposition of glyoxylate, a precursor of oxalate found in hepatic cells. The gene encoding AGT is located on chromosome band 2q37.3 (81). A large number of mutations of the gene have been described that lead to a reduction in AGT enzyme activity and/or to a mistargeting of the enzyme from the peroxisome to the mitochondria where it is ineffective in disposition of glyoxylate. A marked increase in the hepatic production of oxalate and variable increases in glycolate result. Excess oxalate must be excreted by the kidney, and the resulting high urinary concentrations lead to supersaturation of the urine with calcium oxalate. The gene responsible for encoding glyoxylate reductase/hydroxypyruvate reductase resides on chromosome 9 (83). Deficiency of enzyme activity leads to hyperoxaluria and hyperglyceric aciduria. Studies in France suggest a prevalence of type I disease of 1.05 per 1 million population (84). Type II is rare, with fewer than 35 cases to date reported in the literature. A small number of children have been reported who have marked hyperoxaluria and clinical features similar to those of type I and II disease, but who have normal hepatic AGT and glyoxylate reductase/hydroxypyruvate reductase activity. Whether these children have an as yet undefined error of hepatic metabolism or whether another mechanism for the hyperoxaluria is responsible remains to be established (70,78,85).

Mean urine oxalate excretion in a comparative study of patients with primary hyperoxaluria was 2.2 mmol/1.73 m^2/24 hr in type I disease and 1.61 mmol/1.73 m^2/24 hr in type II primary hyperoxaluria (86). Due to the degree of hyperoxaluria and the presence of the abnormality from birth, primary hyperoxaluria is characterized by particularly aggressive stone formation. The majority of patients demonstrate urolithiasis and/or nephrocalcinosis during infancy or childhood (Fig. 57.2). Over time, due to repeated stone episodes that may involve obstruction or infection and due to nephrocalcinosis and other effects of oxalate on the renal tubules and

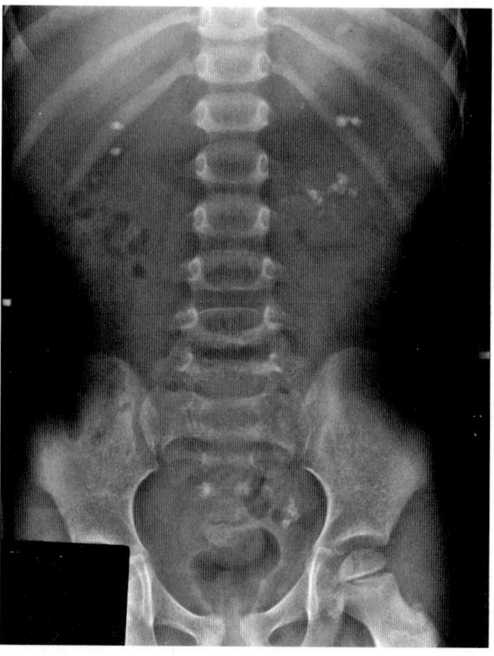

FIGURE 57.2. Multiple calcium oxalate stones in both kidneys of a 5-year-old boy with primary hyperoxaluria type I.

interstitium, renal failure often results. Clinical expression of type I disease is more severe than that of type II (86), with a higher proportion of type I patients progressing to end-stage renal disease at an earlier age. However, there is wide variability of clinical expression in both types, with some patients in renal failure in infancy and others retaining satisfactory renal function until the fourth or fifth decade (87,88). Once the glomerular filtration rate is reduced below 30 mL/min/1.73 m^2, plasma oxalate concentration increases rapidly, with resulting deposition of calcium oxalate in multiple organ systems (oxalosis). If oxalosis cannot be reversed by intensive dialysis and early transplantation, severe morbidity and mortality are the consequence.

Approximately one-third of patients with type I primary hyperoxaluria respond to pharmacologic doses of pyridoxine with a marked reduction in, and in some cases normalization of, oxalate excretion (87,89). Patients with primary hyperoxaluria type I should receive a trial of pyridoxine to assess their response. In all patients with primary hyperoxaluria, intensive efforts to minimize calcium oxalate crystallization and stone formation in the kidneys appear to be helpful in preservation of renal function (87). Neutral phosphate therapy has been shown both to reduce urinary supersaturation of calcium oxalate and to increase urinary inhibitory activity for calcium oxalate crystal formation. Mechanisms include a decrease in total urinary calcium and a decrease in urinary free calcium due to complexing of calcium by phosphate. There is an increase in the urinary concentration of pyrophosphate, an effective inhibitor of calcium oxalate crystal formation, and inhibition is further augmented by the accompanying increase in pH (90). In long-term studies of patients with primary hyperoxaluria, this treatment, along with increased fluid intake, appears beneficial in reducing stone-forming activity and in preserving renal function (87). Citrate therapy has also been advocated (91).

Cystinuria is identified in 2 to 7% of children with metabolic stones (13,22). An inherited defect in the renal tubular reabsorptive transport of cystine and the dibasic amino acids (ornithine, arginine, and lysine) accounts for the high concentrations of cystine in the urine of patients with this disorder. Cystine stones form because cystine excretion rates exceed cystine solubility at usual urine volumes. At a physiologic pH of less than 7, solubility is limited to 1000 μmol/L (240 mg/L) (92). Cystine solubility is enhanced at an alkaline urine pH, so that alkalinization of the urine is an important component of treatment regimens. Even at an optimal urine pH of 7, however, cystine solubility in urine is limited to approximately 1250 μmol/L (300 mg/L) of urine (92). The increased urinary concentrations of the other dibasic amino acids and the accompanying intestinal dibasic amino acid transport defect appear to be without clinical consequence. The prevalence of cystinuria in the general population in the United States and Europe is estimated at 1 in 7000 but varies widely in various parts of the world, ranging from 1 in 2500 in Jews of Libyan origin to 1 in 15,000 in parts of the United States to 1 in 100,000 in Sweden (93,94). The mutant gene appears to be common, with a frequency approaching 1% (93–95).

Three clinical subtypes have been described, based on the level of urinary cystine in obligate heterozygotes (96). Type I accounts for approximately 70% of patients with clinically evident cystinuria and is completely recessive. Patients with type I/I show cystine excretion rates that are generally higher than 1000 μmol/g creatinine by 1 year of age with a mean excretion rate of 4500 μmol/g creatinine (96). Half or more of such patients develop stones within the first decade of life (96). Mutations of the SLC3A1 gene on chromosome arm 2p encoding the rBAT protein important in dibasic amino acid transport have been shown to be responsible (97,98). Types II and III are identified by elevated cystine excretion in obligate heterozygotes (99). Heterozygotes with type II/N have cystine excretion of 400 to 2400 μmol/g creatinine and may form stones. Those with III/N have lower cystine excretion and typically do not develop urolithiasis. Patients with types II/II and III/III have cystine excretion rates similar to that in type I/I. Compound heterozygotes are common. Type I/III patients appear to excrete less cystine and are unlikely to form stones within the first decade of life (96). Other compound heterozygotes have not been as well studied. Mutations of the SLC7A9 gene on chromosome 19 are responsible for types II and III (98,100). With increasing molecular genetic information, some have challenged the traditional classification system (101). Due to the immaturity of renal tubule function during infancy and the complexity of compound heterozygosity, it is difficult definitively to establish the diagnosis of cystinuria before 1 year of age (102).

Patients with homozygous forms of cystinuria have lifelong recurring stone formation (Fig. 57.3). Medical therapy can be highly beneficial. First-line therapy consists of increased

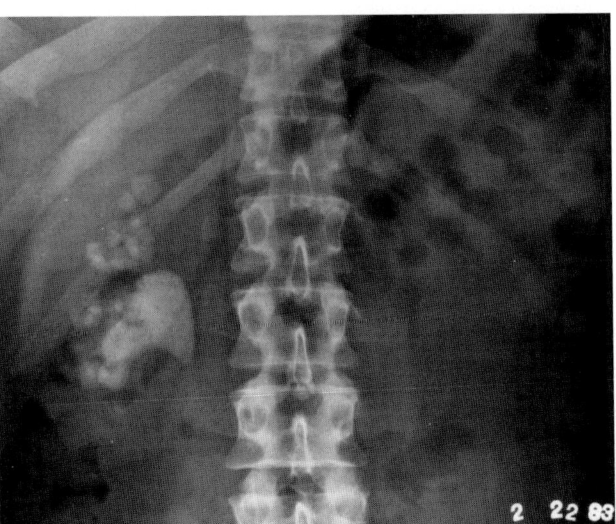

FIGURE 57.3. Staghorn calculus in the right kidney of a patient with cystinuria.

oral fluid intake and a low-salt diet with urinary alkalinization to a pH of 7.0. If formation of cystine stones is not well controlled with these measures, addition of tiopronin (Thiola) or D-penicillamine is recommended. The use of captopril has been advocated but results have been inconclusive (103). Even with optimal medical management, however, urologic procedures are periodically required. With advancing age, elevated serum creatinine concentrations can be encountered in as many as 50% of patients, and a small proportion (approximately 3%) eventually require dialysis (103,104).

Hyperuricosuria is found in 2 to 10% of children and adolescents with metabolic stones. Mild idiopathic hyperuricosuria may be a cause of hematuria (52) and is often found in conjunction with hypercalciuria (22,105). A defect in renal tubular transport of uric acid, due either to reduced proximal tubular reabsorption or to increased secretion, may be found (52,106,107). Idiopathic renal hyperuricosuria is often familial and asymptomatic. Secondary hyperuricosuria may result from diets high in protein or ketogenic diets (108); from medications, including dicumarol, ascorbic acid, probenecid, phenylbutazone, salicylates, and citrate; and from pancreatic extract therapy in patients with cystic fibrosis (52). It can be seen in association with diabetes (109) and the syndrome of inappropriate secretion of antidiuretic hormone (110).

Although uric acid crystals in the urine may contribute to urolithiasis by forming a nidus for calcium oxalate crystallization, uric acid stones are uncommon in childhood. When they occur in children, uric acid stones are generally due to marked overproduction of uric acid such as occurs in tumor lysis syndrome, lymphoproliferative or myeloproliferative disorders, or rare inborn errors of metabolism such as complete (Lesch-Nyhan syndrome) or partial deficiencies of hypoxanthine phosphoribosyltransferase enzyme activity. Urolithiasis occurs in a high proportion of patients with Lesch-Nyhan syndrome and not infrequently develops during the first year of life. Of those with partial hypoxanthine phosphoribosyltransferase deficiency, up to 75% develop uric acid urolithiasis (13). High fluid intake and restriction of dietary purines are recommended. Treatment to achieve urinary alkalinization to a pH of 7.0 will increase solubility, and a trial of allopurinol may be beneficial (80).

Xanthine calculi may occasionally be seen in patients treated with allopurinol for hyperuricemia related to Lesch-Nyhan syndrome or tumor lysis syndrome during chemotherapy (111). Markedly increased urine concentrations of xanthine and hypoxanthine are also seen in patients with a rare autosomal recessive deficiency of xanthine oxidase activity. Xanthine calculi develop in approximately one-third of patients with hereditary xanthinuria (75,112). Urinary tract stone disease in childhood may result from urinary solute excess due to other rare inborn errors of metabolism, including adenine phosphoribosyltransferase deficiency leading to 2,8-dihydroxyadeninuria (113,114), orotic aciduria, and alkaptonuria (115). Treatment with allopurinol is effective in adenine phosphoribosyltransferase deficiency because it blocks production of 2,8-dihydroxyadenine.

Inhibitor Deficiencies

Citrate is a naturally occurring inhibitor of calcium oxalate and calcium phosphate crystallization. Hypocitric aciduria is a frequent finding in a subset of adult patients with idiopathic urolithiasis (80,116). In a study of pediatric patients by Tekin and colleagues, urinary citrate excretion was significantly lower in calcium stone formers than in a control group of healthy children (117). Baggio et al. found lower urinary concentration and excretion rates of citrate in stone-forming children than in control subjects, but the differences did not reach statistical significance (118). Whether or not citrate deficiency is a primary contributing factor to stone formation in a particular patient, increasing a lower citrate concentration to a higher one can be beneficial in minimizing stone-forming activity.

Deficiency of urinary citrate occurs predictably as a result of hypokalemia and systemic or intracellular acidosis. In most such situations, however, the hypocitric aciduria is transient. In distal RTA, hypocitric aciduria appears to be a major contributor to stone formation. The hypocitric aciduria persists until the metabolic acidosis is corrected. The measured urine citrate concentration is predictably reduced in the presence of a urinary tract infection, and measurement should be repeated after antibiotic treatment. Interpretation of urinary citrate concentrations is complicated by relatively few studies of urinary citrate in healthy children of various ages and the fact that citrate is influenced by prandial state, dietary composition, and age.

Pyrophosphate and magnesium in the urine are also known to act as inhibitors of calcium oxalate and calcium phosphate crystal formation. Although both are used for therapeutic benefit, deficiencies of pyrophosphate or magnesium have not been described as a primary cause of urolithiasis.

There has been interest in a variety of urinary macromolecules that appear to inhibit calcium oxalate crystal formation. Those studied include glycosaminoglycans, osteopontin, nephrocalcin, and urinary prothrombin fragment 1, among others. Some researchers have observed relatively lower concentrations of these inhibitors in children who form stones than in the urine of children who do not (119). However, considerable controversy still exists regarding the role of urinary macromolecules in clinical disorders of stone formation (38).

Clinical Conditions Associated with Urolithiasis

A number of clinical conditions are associated with metabolic factors that predispose to stone formation. Distal RTA results in hypocitric aciduria, hypercalciuria, low titratable

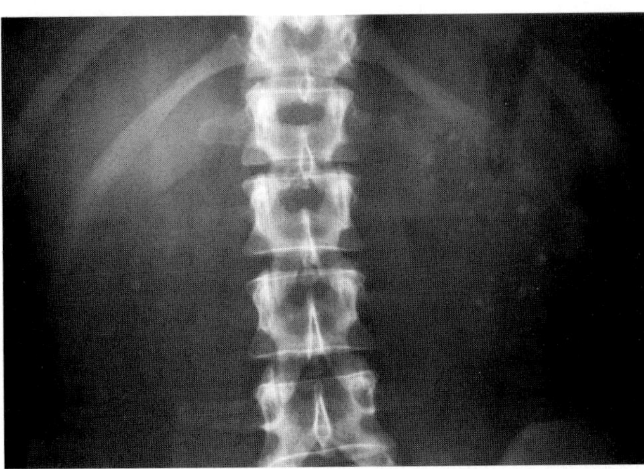

FIGURE 57.4. Small radiopaque stones scattered throughout both kidneys in a patient with distal renal tubular acidosis (RTA). The pattern is characteristic for RTA.

acidity, and high urine pH. Multiple calcifications comprised of calcium phosphate and/or calcium oxalate in the region of the papillary tips of the kidneys are typical and are seen with both incomplete and complete forms of distal RTA (Fig. 57.4). In long-term follow-up of distal RTA in childhood, Caldas et al. (120) found nephrolithiasis and/or nephrocalcinosis in 14 of 28 patients. Nephrocalcinosis tends to occur with increasing age (120). The experience of others suggests that early initiation of alkali therapy may obviate the development of nephrocalcinosis by correcting the hypocitric aciduria and hypercalciuria (121,122). A few patients have been reported among kindreds with RTA that appeared to develop nephrolithiasis and/or nephrocalcinosis due to hypercalciuria without systemic acidosis (123). This and other observations regarding hereditary RTA suggest that the relationships among hypercalciuria, the renal tubule acidification defect, and nephrocalcinosis-urolithiasis are complex (123).

Several autosomal recessive mutations resulting in carbonic anhydrase II deficiency have been described that are accompanied by variable degrees of distal and/or proximal RTA and associated urolithiasis and nephrocalcinosis (124–126). Mutations in the red cell anion exchanger (Band 3, AE1) gene have been confirmed in several families (127), are associated with distal RTA, and usually show autosomal dominant transmission (128). Urolithiasis is a frequent manifestation (127). Secondary distal RTA such as occurs in Wilson's disease and Sjögren's syndrome has also been associated with urolithiasis (129,130). Hypercalciuria and hypocitric aciduria, which increase with age, and distal RTA have been implicated in the nephrolithiasis associated with type 1a glycogen storage disease (131–134). Incomplete distal RTA and urolithiasis have been reported in cerebrotendinous xanthomatosis, an autosomal recessive lipid metabolic disorder (135).

Urolithiasis is not typically associated with proximal RTA (136,137) nor with type IV RTA (138). Although hypercalciuria occurs in proximal RTA, the high associated urinary citrate concentrations may protect against stone formation. In type IV RTA, citrate excretion is reduced, but reduced excretion of calcium appears sufficient to compensate for the reduced urine citrate so that urinary saturation of calcium oxalate remains within normal limits (138). Lower phosphorus and uric acid excretion in patients with type IV RTA may also help prevent stone formation (138).

Medullary sponge kidney is frequently associated with recurrent calcium urolithiasis. Hypercalciuria, hypocitric aciduria, incomplete RTA, and increased urine pH have been variably observed in such patients (139). Nephrolithiasis is seen in 20 to 36% of patients with autosomal dominant polycystic kidney disease, with approximately half of the stones comprised of calcium oxalate and the other half of uric acid (140). The most consistent metabolic abnormality is hypocitric aciduria, with a minority of the patients having hyperuricosuria or hypercalciuria (140,141). Thin basement membrane nephropathy has been associated with hypercalciuria, hyperuricosuria, and resulting nephrolithiasis (142). An increased frequency of urolithiasis and nephrocalcinosis has also been reported in cystinosis (143–146). Children and adults with Wilson's disease may develop urolithiasis. Distal RTA is the most commonly observed factor (129). Some patients, however, demonstrate hypercalciuria and urolithiasis without evidence of RTA (147). Because urolithiasis may be diagnosed before Wilson's disease is clinically evident, any patient with renal stones and unexplained neurologic, bony, or hepatic abnormalities should be screened for Wilson's disease (129). Hypercalciuria and hypocitric aciduria, which increase with age, and distal RTA have been implicated in the nephrolithiasis associated with type 1a glycogen storage disease (131–133).

Inflammatory bowel disease and other diseases of the gastrointestinal tract associated with malabsorption can cause hypocitric aciduria and hypomagnesuria due to loss of bicarbonate and magnesium in the stool, hyperoxaluria from enhanced enteric oxalate absorption, hyperuricosuria due to increased cell turnover, and low urine volume because of diarrhea, which together result in reduced inhibitor activity and high solute concentrations in the urine (148,149).

Calcium oxalate urolithiasis has been reported in 5.2 to 10.4% of young patients with cystic fibrosis (77,150,151), and nephrocalcinosis has been observed in another 6.3% (77). Katz et al. found microscopic nephrocalcinosis at autopsy in 35 of 38 patients (92%) with cystic fibrosis, including 6 patients who were younger than 1 year of age at the time of death (152). Hyperoxaluria appears to be the primary factor (77,150,151,153), although hypocitric aciduria (77,151) and hyperuricosuria (77) have also been observed. Urine calcium has been variably reported as reduced (153), normal (77), or increased (77,151). Crystalluria is commonly seen (150,151). Pancreatic insufficiency with fat malabsorption and resulting enteric hyperoxaluria

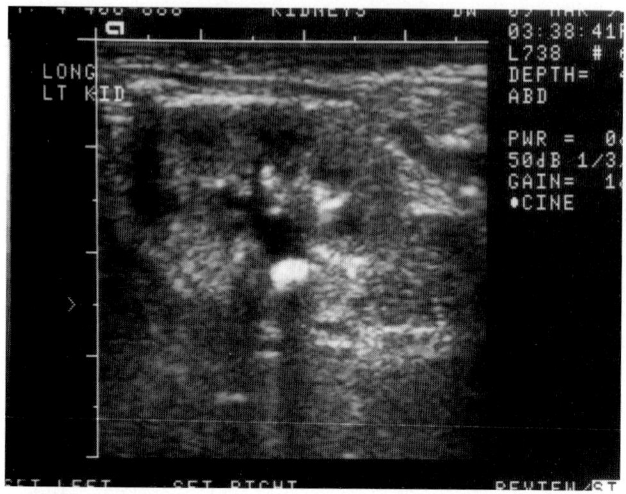

FIGURE 57.5. Ultrasonographic evaluation showing nephrocalcinosis and a shadowing stone in the pelvis of the kidney of a 3-month-old infant born prematurely.

are suggested by the clinical setting, although no correlation could be established between the degree of fat malabsorption and urine oxalate excretion in two studies (151,153). Deficiency of enteric *O. formigenes* due to repeated courses of antibiotics has also been suggested as a risk factor for hyperoxaluria in this patient population (79). Pancreatic enzyme replacement and high-protein diets may contribute to hyperuricosuria. Damage to renal tubules by antibiotic treatment has been implicated by some authors as a contributing cause due to hypercalciuria after a renal phosphate leak (151).

Premature infants have a higher incidence of nephrocalcinosis and nephrolithiasis than healthy term infants (Fig. 57.5). In three prospective studies of infants born at less than 1500 g or less than 32 weeks' gestation, renal calcifications were found to occur in 64%, 16%, and 28% of infants (154–156). The risk of renal calcifications appears higher in smaller infants, those receiving furosemide or postnatal corticosteroids, those undergoing a longer period of mechanical ventilation and parenteral nutrition, white infants, and those with a family history of urolithiasis (156). Metabolic disturbances including hypercalciuria (154), hypophosphatemia and hypercalcemia (both of which can induce hypercalciuria) (157), and hyperoxaluria related to parenteral nutrition (158) have been implicated. Abnormalities of urine composition associated with renal tubule immaturity may play a role. Nephrocalcinosis resolves with time in approximately half of the patients, and new stone formation appears to abate in the majority of patients. However, longer-term studies performed at 4 to 12 years of age in very-low-birth-weight children who had a history of renal calcifications demonstrated hypercalciuria, hypocitric aciduria, and reduced ammonium excretion in response to furosemide in comparison to a control group of children born at term (159). At the time of study 18% of the children still had renal cortical hyperechogenicity and 9% had urolithiasis. Whether the renal tubular abnormalities are the long-term result of renal tubular immaturity at birth, are secondary to renal damage from nephrocalcinosis, or are due to other factors remains to be established.

Nephrocalcinosis is often seen together with urolithiasis and appears to share many of the same metabolic risk factors. In one study of 152 children and adolescents with nephrocalcinosis, idiopathic hypercalciuria was found in 34% and various hereditary renal tubular disorders in 32% (160). A family history of nephrocalcinosis or urolithiasis was noted in 7.2% and 19.1%, respectively (160).

Pharmacologic Agents Implicated in Urolithiasis

Urolithiasis can result from pharmacologic use of a variety of medications. Calculi may result from excretion of concentrations of the medication or a metabolite in the urine that exceed solubility or may occur due to metabolic effects induced by the medication. The protease inhibitor indinavir, used widely in the treatment of human immunodeficiency virus infection, precipitates in the urine as radiolucent crystals and stones; these can cause ureteral obstruction and colic, which are observed in 2 to 28% of patients treated with this agent (161–163). Up to 20% of this parent drug is filtered by the kidney. The drug is poorly soluble at a pH level higher than 5. Distinctive birefringent crystals with plate and starburst structures are observed in 20 to 25% of patients receiving this antiretroviral agent (162,164). The indinavir crystals or small stones may also act as a nidus for calcium oxalate or calcium phosphate, and are also associated with stones of mixed composition that may be radiopaque. There are a number of reports of such effects in children (161,165,166). Due to the radiolucent nature of indinavir stones, they are not visible on noncontrast renal tomography and may be difficult to distinguish from soft tissue by computed tomography (CT) (165). Ultrasonography, intravenous pyelography, or contrast-enhanced CT may be needed to demonstrate indinavir stones and associated ureteral obstruction. Dissolution of stone material may be observed with discontinuation of indinavir, increased fluid intake, and urine acidification (166).

Other medications that can precipitate to form urinary tract stones are ceftriaxone (167,168), sulfonamides, ampicillin, amoxicillin, triamterene, guaifenesin (169), phenazopyridine, and oxypurinol (170). Urinary tract stones are observed only rarely with these agents.

Carbonic anhydrase inhibitors, administered for management of epilepsy and glaucoma among other uses, result in alkaline urine, reduced urine citrate levels, and hypercalciuria (170,171). Agents of this class, including zonisamide, topiramate, and dorzolamide, have been reported to be associated with calcium phosphate and calcium oxalate urolithiasis in children and adolescents (172–174). Commonly used agents such as corticosteroids, calcium supplements, and vitamin D and its analogues are associated with hypercalciuria and can predispose to stone formation. Aminophylline use results in hypercalciuria, alkaline urine, and phosphaturia, countered in part by its diuretic effects (175). Lithium use can induce hypercalcemia and hypercalciuria.

Dietary Considerations

Diets low in animal protein but high in cereals contribute to formation of bladder stones in children (34,176). Large dietary intake of sodium or calcium may induce hypercalciuria. High intake of animal protein predisposes to higher urine uric acid, calcium, and oxalate excretion and reduced urinary citrate and pH, all of which favor calcium oxalate stone formation (21). Frassetto et al. noted that contemporary net acid-producing diets (rich in animal protein and deficient in plant protein and potassium alkali salts) produce a low-grade systemic acidosis in otherwise healthy adults (177). He and others have postulated that the ensuing metabolic changes may, in part, explain the increasing prevalence of urolithiasis in industrialized countries in recent decades (21,177).

Ketogenic diets used for the management of seizures have been reported to be associated with nephrolithiasis in 3 to 10% of children receiving this form of therapy (178). Stones may be comprised of uric acid, calcium phosphate, mixed calcium and uric acid, or ammonium urate (108,178). Urolithiasis appears to be related to ensuing hypercalciuria, hypocitric aciduria, and reduced oral fluid intake (108,178,179). Urine uric acid excretion is normal in most but not all patients (108,178), so that uric acid stone formation appears related primarily to the low volume and acidic pH of the urine. Stone formation has been noted between 7 and 22 months after initiation of the diet (108,178).

Infection as a Lithogenic Factor

Infection of the urinary tract with bacteria producing the enzyme urease leads to hydrolysis of urea with resulting production of ammonium and bicarbonate ions in the urine. In the presence of the increased pH, dissociation of phosphate occurs, with supersaturation of the urine for magnesium ammonium phosphate (struvite) and calcium phosphate apatites, including carbonate apatite (180). Precipitation of stone material follows. A variety of bacterial species produce urease, including *Proteus*, *Staphylococcus*, *Klebsiella*, *Providencia*, *Pseudomonas*, *Enterobacter*, *Ureaplasma urealyticum*, *Corynebacterium urealyticum*, and some anaerobes. Struvite tends to form staghorn calculi that can grow rapidly and are challenging to treat. It is difficult to eradicate infection while stone material remains, because antibiotics do not penetrate well within the interstices of the stone where bacteria reside. Just under half of the patients with infected staghorn calculi can be rendered stone free by extracorporeal shock wave lithotripsy (ESWL) (181), so that combined procedures including percutaneous ultrasonic lithotripsy are often needed (182). Retained stone fragments can serve as a nidus for early recurrence.

Xanthogranulomatous pyelonephritis is a rare but serious infectious process leading to nonfunction of the infected kidney. Obstruction caused by renal calculi has been found in 68% of affected children (183), with approximately half of such calculi being of the staghorn variety (183). Another author reported nephrolithiasis and/or nephrocalcinosis in 71% of such children (184). *Proteus*, *Escherichia coli*, *Klebsiella*, *Pseudomonas*, and *Enterobacter* bacteria (several species of which produce urease) are most often responsible (185). In xanthogranulomatous pyelonephritis, renal stones, obstruction, and infection exacerbate each other. Nephrectomy is required in most circumstances (183–185).

Encrusted pyelitis is another unusual manifestation of infection and mineralization (186). Infection of the kidney with *C. urealyticum*, a urea-splitting organism, leads to encrustation of the wall of the renal pelvis with struvite and associated apatite crystals and proteins (187). Infection with this slow-growing aerobic organism is usually acquired after urologic manipulations of the urinary tract and is most often observed in immunosuppressed patients. Most reports in the literature cite cases in renal allograft recipients (186,188,189). Obstructive uropathy and loss of renal function are common (188,189). The encrustations are tightly adherent to the mucosa and are difficult to dislodge. In addition to prolonged antibiotic therapy, placement of percutaneous nephrostomy tubes for irrigation with acidic Thomas solution (186) or use of acetohydroxamic acid (186,189,190) has been advocated.

Although infection with urease-producing organisms can produce de novo urolithiasis, often the infection exacerbates underlying metabolic factors. With careful evaluation, 20 to 61% of patients with infection-related stones can also be demonstrated to have metabolic factors predisposing to stone formation (22,80,191). Stasis due to urinary tract abnormalities also predisposes to infection, which further illustrates the interaction among infection, metabolic factors, and structural abnormalities of the urinary tract in the genesis of calculi.

Structural Abnormalities of the Urinary Tract

Stasis of urine often accompanies structural abnormalities of the urinary tract, whether congenital or acquired. By compromising the normal continuous flow of urine from the upper urinary tract and interfering with regular and complete emptying of urine from the bladder, stasis promotes crystal retention and stone formation as well as infection. A wide range of structural abnormalities has been associated with urolithiasis, including medullary sponge kidney (139), autosomal dominant polycystic kidney disease, calyceal diverticula (192), ureteropelvic junction obstruction (117,193), horseshoe kidney (194), ureterocele, primary megaureter (31), posterior urethral valves (31), and the bladder extrophy–epispadius complex (195). Medullary sponge kidney is frequently associated with recurrent calcium urolithiasis. In medullary sponge kidney and autosomal dominant polycystic kidney disease, tubular ectasia and cyst formation, respectively, are felt to contribute to stasis of the urine that exacerbates metabolic abnormalities. Patients with myelodysplasia often have impaired bladder emptying, recurrent urinary tract infections, and hypercalciuria from relative immobilization. Partial obstruction can result in renal acidification deficiencies with accompanying hypocitric aciduria. Patients who have undergone enterocystoplasty and urinary diversion using intestinal mucosa are particularly prone to local formation of stones, with 16 to 50% of patients undergoing enterocystoplasty reported to form bladder stones (196–198). The difficulty in eradicating bacteria from the enteral mucosa, stasis, an alkaline urine pH due to infection or to exchange of chloride for bicarbonate across the mucosa, and the presence of mucus in the bladder all favor stone formation (197). Foreign bodies such as sutures or staples, or indwelling stents also can act as a nidus for stone formation.

With the exception of those undergoing enterocystoplasty, however, the overall incidence of stones in children with structurally anomalous, obstructed, or infected urinary tracts is low, on the order of 1 to 5% (199). This suggests that, although these factors are permissive, children who form stones may also have underlying metabolic abnormalities. Hypercalciuria, hyperoxaluria, or hypocitric aciduria have been identified in 66 to 80% of patients with structural abnormalities of the kidneys or ureters who also had urolithiasis and underwent metabolic evaluation (193,200). Tekin and colleagues demonstrated a similar degree of hypocitric aciduria and hyperoxaluria in patients with ureteropelvic junction obstruction and urolithiasis as in those with calcium stone formation but without urinary tract abnormalities. The incidence in both groups was significantly different from that in the control group of healthy children (117). The importance of metabolic abnormalities in patients with stones and urinary tract abnormalities is further suggested by long-term follow-up of a group of pediatric patients with ureteropelvic junction obstruction and renal calculi. Recurrent urolithiasis developed in 68% of the patients despite successful ureteropelvic junction repair. Furthermore, 10 of 19 recurrent stones (53%) formed in the contralateral, uninvolved kidney (193). Accordingly, complete metabolic evaluation is just as important in children with structural abnormalities of the urinary tract or infection-related stones as it is in those without.

DIAGNOSTIC EVALUATION

Recommended initial evaluation of children or adolescents with urolithiasis includes taking medical and diet histories; obtaining family history; performing urinalysis with determination of pH, osmolality, and presence or absence of crystals; and measurement of serum levels of calcium, phosphorus, uric acid, bicarbonate, sodium, potassium, creatinine, alkaline phosphatase, and albumin. An estimate of daily fluid intake is an important aspect of the dietary history, as is an estimate of the daily intake of calcium, sodium, oxalate, and protein. The medical and diet history taking should include an inquiry regarding use of over-the-counter food supplements, vitamins, minerals, or herbal preparations. Analysis of stone composition should always be performed when stone material is available. Urine concentrations and, when possible, excretion rates of solutes should be measured. For infants or young children, older children with developmental delay, or cases in which a reliable timed urine collection cannot be obtained, taking random urine specimens and measuring solute to creatinine ratio can be very useful. Care is advised in interpretation, however, because normal values often vary by age, time of day, and prandial state. Whenever a child is able to cooperate with a timed 24-hour urine collection, this will provide more complete information, including assessment of daily urine volume. Completeness of each collection should be verified with measurement of urine creatinine level. Urine should be analyzed for calcium, oxalate, citrate, uric acid, sodium, cystine, creatinine, and total volume. Metabolic evaluation should be performed while the patient is on his or her usual diet, usual fluid intake, and normal activity level. The studies should not be performed shortly after ESWL or a stone removal procedure and should not be obtained when the child is receiving intravenous fluids. If abnormalities are found, further metabolic evaluation may be indicated.

Normal values for urine analytes are shown in Table 57.2. Solute to creatinine ratios are higher in infancy. After 2 years of age, urine uric acid/creatinine and oxalate/creatinine ratios vary, decreasing by age, but excretion rates are fairly consistent throughout childhood when determined in a timed collection and expressed as milligrams per 1.73 m^2 per 24 hours (201–204). Uric acid can also be expressed as milligrams per deciliter glomerular filtration rate, measured in either a random or timed urine collection (205). Reported normal values for some analytes vary from study to study and vary for oxalate by the measurement method. Because information on normal values is used for diagnosis and treatment, it is helpful to keep in mind that the excretion rate of each of these analytes is a continuous variable and should be regarded as a modifiable risk factor rather than compared to a strictly defined threshold for normal.

Evaluation should include imaging studies of the urinary tract. Stones comprised of calcium oxalate or calcium phosphate are radiodense and are readily seen. Struvite and cystine stones are of intermediate radiodensity. Uric acid, xanthine, 2,8-dihydroxyadenine, and orotic acid stones are radiolucent by conventional radiography but visible by

TABLE 57.2. URINE CHEMISTRY: NORMAL VALUES

Urine constituent	Age	Random	Timed	Comments
Calcium (52,230)	0–6 mo	<0.8 mg/mg creat		Prandial variation
	7–12 mo	<0.6 mg/mg creat		Sodium dependent
	≥2 yr	<0.21 mg/mg creat	<4 mg/kg/24 h	
Oxalate[a] (204,231)	<1 yr	0.15–0.26 mmol/mmol creat		Random urine mmol/mmol highly age dependent
	1 yr to <5 yr	0.11–0.12 mmol/mmol creat		
	5–12 yr	0.006–0.15 mmol/mmol creat	≥2 yr; <0.5 mmol/1.73 m²/24 h	Excretion rate/1.73 m² constant through childhood and adulthood
	>12 yr	0.002–0.083 mmol/mmol creat		
Uric acid (201,205)	Term infant	3.3 mg/dL GFR[b]	<815 mg/1.73 m²/24 h	Excretion rate/1.73 m² from >1 yr age constant through childhood
	>3 yr	<0.53 mg/dL GFR		
Magnesium (13,230)	>2 yr	<0.12 mg/mg creat	<88 mg/1.73 m²/24 h	Excretion rate/1.73 m² constant through childhood
Citrate (232)		>180 mg/g creat (232) >400 mg/g creat (13)		Limited data available for children
Cystine (13,30)		<75 mg/g creat	<60 mg/1.73 m²/24 h	Cystine >250 mg/g creat suggests homozygous cystinuria

creat, creatinine; GFR, glomerular filtration rate.
[a]Oxalate oxidase assay.
[b](mg/dL uric acid) (serum creatinine concentration/urine creatinine concentration).

ultrasonography or unenhanced CT. Ultrasonography is sufficient in many circumstances (206), whereas CT, urography, or intravenous pyelography is required at times, as is voiding cystourethrography. Nimkin and colleagues compared imaging modalities for detection of stones in the pediatric population and reported a sensitivity of 57% for plain films and 77% for ultrasonography compared with stone detection by CT (16). Others have reported better overall sensitivity for ultrasonography (207), but it may fail to detect 30% of small papillary or calyceal stones (208) and may miss ureteral calculi (207). For acute renal colic, noncontrast helical CT scanning is considered the imaging modality of choice, because it is more sensitive and specific for ureteral calculi than all other imaging modalities (209). CT also has the advantage of providing detailed anatomic information (usually without the need for intravenous contrast administration) and improved sensitivity for very small stones or those that are poorly radiopaque (206). Concern has been expressed regarding the degree of radiation exposure from CT (210). With careful attention to radiographic technique, the radiation exposure with CT can be significantly reduced while maintaining good imaging quality (209,211) and may be less than that with other renal imaging techniques such as an intravenous pyelography (212).

Urine culture should be performed for every patient with stones. Colony counts of bacteria in the urine of patients with infected stones may not reach the threshold of 10^5 colony-forming units/mL, so that lower colony counts should be further evaluated. In selected circumstances, such as suspected *Ureaplasma*, *C. urealyticum*, or anaerobic bacterial infection, special culture techniques may be needed.

TREATMENT

Stones causing obstruction or acute renal colic, stones with a high potential for causing acute obstruction (e.g., a large stone in the renal pelvis), and infected stones should be evaluated jointly with a urologist. The majority of stones smaller than 5 mm in diameter will pass spontaneously, even in young children (25). Larger symptomatic stones are likely to require surgical intervention. The range of effective surgical interventions continues to increase, and now even very young patients can often undergo ESWL, ureteroscopic lithotripsy or removal, or percutaneous ultrasonic lithotripsy procedures. Open lithotomy is rarely required. Due to the potential for high-energy shock waves to permanently damage renal tissue, there has been concern regarding possible long-term adverse effects of ESWL on the developing kidney. A careful study of 16 children treated for a single stone found no morphologic changes in the kidneys by ultrasonography after ESWL and no significant changes in serum creatinine level but did document significant posttreatment increases in urinary β_2-microglobulin and enzymuria (213). These changes were considered evidence of proximal renal tubule dysfunction and resolved by 14 days after the procedure. This value can be compared to 7 days for resolution of similar changes in adult patients and may indicate more significant injury in children (213). One study suggested impairment in growth of the kidneys in children after ESWL (214). However, most information involving second-generation or later lithotriptors does not indicate clinically significant renal parenchymal scarring, impaired renal growth, permanent renal function abnormalities, or hypertension in children after ESWL treatment (215). Information is still relatively limited, particularly in children who were under the age of 6 at the time of treatment.

Patients with infected stones who need ESWL, percutaneous ultrasonic lithotripsy, or an open procedure require attentive antibiotic management because bacteria may be released rapidly from stone material on fragmentation during lithotripsy or instrumentation. Struvite stones may be soft and friable, with particular vulnerability to stone fragment retention after ESWL. Any stone fragments remaining may harbor bacteria in the interstices of the fragments, where they are less accessible to antibiotic penetration; this makes eradication of the infection very difficult. In addition, stone fragments provide a nidus for new struvite stone formation, which can occur rapidly. It is for this reason that percutaneous ultrasonic lithotripsy or nephrolithotomy is still sometimes required to assure complete removal of infected stone material.

Stones that are not causing symptoms and are not associated with impending or established obstruction may be managed medically. For all forms of urolithiasis, increased oral fluid intake to maintain a urine volume of greater than 750 mL/day in infants, 1000 mL/day in children under the age of 5, 1500 mL/day to the age of 10, and greater than 2 L/day in preadolescents and adolescents is most helpful to minimize stone growth and recurrent stone formation and is recommended. Increased urine volume has been shown to be significantly associated with a lower risk of stone recurrence in adults with idiopathic stone formation (216). Avoidance of dietary excesses of calcium, oxalate, and sodium is important. However, reduction to less than the recommended daily allowance, particularly of dietary calcium, may be problematic with respect to nutritional adequacy, normal growth, and development. Reduction to the appropriate recommended daily allowance for age for calcium, and no lower, is recommended even in children with known hypercalciuria. Indeed, epidemiologic studies in adults suggest that dietary calcium reduction is associated with an *increased* likelihood of urolithiasis (217), perhaps due to greater absorption of dietary oxalate when less calcium is present in the intestinal tract. Dietary sodium restriction is of particular importance in patients with hypercalciuria and those with cystinuria, because it can reduce the urinary excretion of calcium (54,218) and cystine (219–222), respectively.

Patients with idiopathic urolithiasis who have normal urine chemistry results or mild hypercalciuria only and a single stone may be managed initially with increased fluid intake and dietary modification alone. If metabolic stone-forming activity is not adequately controlled by this approach, addition of potassium citrate therapy—or, for those with hypercalciuria, therapy with a thiazide—is the next step. Treatment of patients with metabolic factors should be directed specifically to the abnormality(ies) found. Suggested initial therapy, and second-line therapy if problems persist despite the initial intervention, are shown in Table 57.3.

TABLE 57.3. SUGGESTED THERAPY FOR UROLITHIASIS CAUSED BY METABOLIC ABNORMALITIES

Metabolic abnormality	Initial treatment	Second-line treatment
Hypercalciuria	Reduction of dietary Na^+ Dietary calcium at RDA Thiazides	Potassium citrate Neutral phosphate
Hyperoxaluria	Adjustment of dietary oxalate Potassium citrate	Neutral phosphate[a] Magnesium Pyridoxine[a]
Hypocitric aciduria	Potassium citrate Bicarbonate	
Hyperuricosuria	Alkalinization	Allopurinol
Cystinuria	Alkalinization Reduction of dietary Na^+	Tiopronin (Thiola) D-penicillamine Captopril

RDA, recommended daily allowance.
[a]Initial therapy in primary hyperoxaluria.

Urolithiasis in children and adolescents, like that in adults, recurs frequently. In one study of 221 children followed for a mean of 59 months (median, 36 months), 67% developed two or more stones during initial evaluation and follow-up (22). Other authors have reported recurrence rates of 20 to 40% with variable follow-up periods (25). Recurrence rates are higher in children with demonstrable metabolic abnormalities (25). Because of the persistence of underlying metabolic abnormalities and known risk of recurrence, long-term follow-up with periodic reassessments of the activity of stone formation is indicated. Evaluation of metabolic stone-forming activity over time, as determined by growth in size of existing stones or formation of new stones, is an important aspect of treatment. The frequency of renal imaging required depends on the type and number of stones and the severity of the metabolic abnormalities detected. In most circumstances and in the absence of symptoms or infection, imaging once yearly or every other year is sufficient. Patients with significant metabolic problems such as primary hyperoxaluria, cystinuria, or marked hypercalciuria, and those with infected stones (which can develop and grow quickly) may require more frequent evaluations. Ultrasonography has the advantage of visualization of radiolucent as well as radiopaque stones, detection of hydronephrosis, and the absence of radiation exposure, and is preferred for most routine follow-up assessments. However, its lack of sensitivity for small stones, the difficulty in comparing the sizes of individual stones over time, its lower sensitivity for visualization of ureteral stones, and the possibility of obstruction in the absence of hydronephrosis will, at times, dictate other imaging modalities. Acute symptoms should prompt reevaluation.

If increase in the size of existing stones or new stone formation occurs despite treatment, a more intensive regimen should be implemented. In patients with active stone formation, additional studies can be helpful in assessing the degree of metabolic stone formation and providing guidance as to the most effective therapies. These may include determination of crystalluria by phase-contrast microscopy, determination of supersaturation of the urine by modelling of various components, measurement of urinary inhibitor activity, evaluation for subtype of hypercalciuria (absorptive, renal leak, sodium dependent), or measurement of enteral absorption of oxalate, among others.

In children of all ages, if compliance with recommendations can be secured, response to treatment is typically excellent, with reduced frequency or elimination of active stone formation. Many metabolic abnormalities, such as idiopathic hypercalciuria, are lifelong, however. Subtle degrees of damage to the renal tubule are suggested by studies showing increased urinary excretion of renal *N*-acetyl-β-glucosaminidase in children with hypercalciuria (223) and in those with urolithiasis (224); a deficiency of distal acidification in children with hypercalciuria and urolithiasis that is not seen in children with hypercalciuria alone (225); and the identification of families in which hypercalciuria appears to be the primary event, with distal RTA developing over the years as an apparent complication of hypercalciuria (123,226). Others have argued that the renal tubule acidification deficiency is primary and that the hypercalciuria and urolithiasis occur secondarily (227). Jaeger and colleagues studied renal tubular function in patients with urolithiasis related to primary hyperparathyroidism, medullary sponge kidneys, hyperuricemia, cystinuria, struvite stone disease, idiopathic hypercalciuria, and normocalciuric idiopathic urolithiasis (219). They found that a significant number of stone formers have dysfunction of the proximal renal tubule, that the abnormalities are found in patients in all of the diagnostic groups, and that the occurrence is related to the presence of stones in the collecting system at the time of study (219). The authors concluded that in nephrolithiasis tubulopathy is the consequence, rather than the cause, of stone disease.

The risk of renal insufficiency has been estimated at 1.7% in idiopathic calcium oxalate urolithiasis (228). In a group of 40 patients with a mean duration of cystinuric stone disease of 26 years, renal insufficiency was found in 70% of patients, although none had reached end-stage renal disease (229). In these patients, stone-preventive treatment appeared effective in preserving renal function (229). Infection-related staghorn stones are associated with end-stage renal disease in 20 to 30% of adult patients with unilateral involvement and a higher percentage of those with bilateral stones (228). Several forms of more severe urolithiasis, such as primary hyperoxaluria, Dent's disease, and 2,8-dihydroxyadeninuria are frequently associated with renal insufficiency or end-stage renal disease.

For these reasons, and despite the excellent response to treatment noted in most children with urolithiasis, long-term nephrologic care is indicated, particularly for those with more complex forms of renal stone disease.

REFERENCES

1. Khan SR, Glenton PA, Backov R, et al. Presence of lipids in urine, crystals and stones: implication for the formation of kidney stones. *Kidney Int* 2002;62:2062–2072.
2. Pak CYC, Arnold LH. Heterogenous nucleation of calcium oxalate by seeds of monosodium urate. *Proc Soc Exp Biol Med* 1975;149:930–932.
3. Fleisch H. Inhibitors and promoters of stone formation. *Kidney Int* 1978;13:361–371.
4. Pak CYC. Potential etiologic role of brushite in the formation of calcium (renal) stones. *J Cryst Growth* 1981;53:202–208.
5. Lingeman JE, Smith LH, Wood JR, et al. Basic considerations of urinary stone formation. In: Moster MB, ed. *Urinary calculi*. Philadelphia: Lea and Febiger, 1989:51–76.
6. Coe FL, Kavalach AG. Hypercalciuria and hyperuricosuria in patients with calcium nephrolithiasis. *N Engl J Med* 1974;291:1344–1350.
7. Burdette DC, Thomas WC, Finlayson B. Urinary supersaturation with calcium oxalate before and during orthophosphate therapy. *J Urol* 1976;115:418–422.
8. Pak CYC, Fuller C, Sakhaee K, et al. Long-term treatment of calcium nephrolithiasis with potassium citrate. *J Urol* 1985;134:11–19.
9. Thamilselvan S, Byer KJ, Hackett RL, et al. Free radical scavengers, catalase and superoxide dismutase provide protection from oxalate-associated injury to LLC-PK1 and MDCK cells. *J Urol* 2000;224–229.
10. Wesson JA, Worcester EM, Wiessner JH, et al. Control of calcium oxalate crystal structure and cell adherence by urinary macromolecules. *Kidney Int* 1998;53:952–957.
11. Lieske JC, Toback FG, Deganello S. Sialic acid–containing glycoproteins on renal cells determine nucleation of calcium oxalate dihydrate crystals. *Kidney Int* 2001;60:1784–1791.
12. Miyake O, Kakimoto K, Tsujihata M, et al. Strong inhibition of crystal-cell attachment by pediatric urinary macromolecules: a close relationship with high urinary citrate secretion. *Urology* 2001;58:493–497.
13. Polinsky MS, Kaiser BA, Baluarte HJ. Urolithiasis in childhood. *Pediatr Clin North Am* 1987;34:683–710.
14. Walther PC, Lamm D, Kaplan GW. Pediatric urolithiasis: a 10-year review. *Pediatrics* 1980;65:1068–1072.
15. Troup CW, Lawnicki CC, Bourne RB, et al. Renal calculus in children. *J Urol* 1972;107:306–307.
16. Nimkin K, Lebowitz RL, Share JC, et al. Urolithiasis in a children's hospital: 1985–1990. *Urol Radiol* 1992;14:139–143.
17. Johnson CM, Wilson DM, O'Fallon WM, et al. Renal stone epidemiology: a 25-year study in Rochester, Minnesota. *Kidney Int* 1979;16:624–631.
18. Miyake O, Yoshimura K, Yoshioka T, et al. High urinary excretion level of citrate and magnesium in children: poten-

tial etiology for the reduced incidence of pediatric urolithiasis. *Urol Res* 1998;26:290–213.
19. Fujisawa M, Morikawa M, Arima S, et al. Analysis of the urinary risk factors of urolithiasis in healthy children [in Japanese]. *J Urol* 1989;80:1187–1194.
20. Robertson WG, Peacock M, Heyburn PJ. Risk factors in calcium stone disease of the urinary tract. *Br J Urol* 1978;50:449–454.
21. Milliner DS. Epidemiology of calcium oxalate urolithiasis in man. In: Kahn S, ed. *Calcium oxalate in biological systems.* Boca Raton, FL: CRC Press, 1995:169–188.
22. Milliner DS, Murphy ME. Urolithiasis in pediatric patients. *Mayo Clin Proc* 1993;68:241–248.
23. Lim DJ, Walker RD III, Ellsworth PI, et al. Treatment of pediatric urolithiasis between 1984 and 1994. *J Urol* 1996; 156:702–705.
24. Choi H, Snyder HM, Duckett JW. Urolithiasis in childhood: current management. *J Pediatr Surg* 1987;22:158–164.
25. Pietrow PK, Pope JC, Adams MC, et al. Clinical outcome of pediatric stone disease. *J Urol* 2002;167:670–673.
26. Gearhart JP, Herzberg GZ, Jeffs RD. Childhood urolithiasis: experiences and advances. *Pediatrics* 1991;87:445–450.
27. Diamond DA. Clinical patterns of paediatric urolithiasis. *Br J Urol* 1991;68:195–198.
28. Perrone HC, dos Santos DR, Santos MV, et al. Urolithiasis in childhood: metabolic evaluation. *Pediatr Nephrol* 1992; 6:54–56.
29. Sarkissian A, Baloyan A, Arikyants N, et al. Pediatric urolithiasis in Armenia: a study of 198 patients observed from 1991 to 1999. *Pediatr Nephrol* 2001;16:728–732.
30. Stapleton FB. Clinical approach to children with urolithiasis. *Semin Nephrol* 1996;16:389–397.
31. Kraus SJ, Lebowitz RL, Royal SA. Renal calculi in children: imaging features that lead to diagnoses: a pictorial essay. *Pediatr Radiol* 1999;29:624–630.
32. Robertson WG. What is the aetiology of urinary calculi? *Pediatr Nephrol* 1996;10:763.
33. Anderson DA. The nutritional significance of primary bladder stones. *Br J Urol* 1962;34:160.
34. Ashworth M. Endemic bladder stones. *BMJ* 1990;301:826–827.
35. Stapleton FB, McKay CP, Noe HN. Urolithiasis in children: the role of hypercalciuria. *Pediatr Ann* 1987;16:980–992.
36. Noe HN, Stapleton FB, Jerkins GR, et al. Clinical experience with pediatric urolithiasis. *J Urol* 1983;129:1166–1168.
37. Basaklar AC, Kale N. Experience with childhood urolithiasis. Report of 196 cases. *Br J Urol* 1991;67:203–205.
38. Ryall RL. Glycosaminoglycans, proteins, and stone formation: adult themes and child's play. *Pediatr Nephrol* 1996;10: 656–666.
39. Moore ES. Hypercalciuria in children. *Contrib Nephrol* 1981; 27:20–32.
40. Kruse K, Kracht U, Kruse U. Reference values for urinary calcium excretion and screening for hypercalciuria in children and adolescents. *Eur J Pediatr* 1984;143:25–31.
41. Vachvanichsanong P, Malagon M, Moore ES. Urinary tract infection in children associated with idiopathic hypercalciuria. *Scand J Urol Nephrol* 2001;35:112–116.
42. Stapleton FB. Idiopathic hypercalciuria: association with isolated hematuria and risk for urolithiasis in children. *Kidney Int* 1990;37:807–811.
43. Garcia CD, Miller LA, Stapleton FB. Natural history of hematuria associated with hypercalciuria in children. *Am J Dis Child* 1991;145:1204–1207.
44. Polito C, La Manna A, Cioce F, et al. Clinical presentation and natural course of idiopathic hypercalciuria in children. *Pediatr Nephrol* 2000;15:211–214.
45. Coe FL, Parks JH, Moore ES. Familial idiopathic hypercalciuria. *N Engl J Med* 1979;300:337–340.
46. Mehes K, Szelid Z. Autosomal dominant inheritance of hypercalciuria. *Eur J Pediatr* 1980;133:239–242.
47. Harangi F, Méhes K. Family investigations in idiopathic hypercalciuria. *Eur J Pediatr* 1993;152:64–68.
48. Goodman JO, Holmes RP, Assimos DG. Genetic factors in calcium oxalate stone disease. *J Urol* 1995;153:301–307.
49. Stapleton FB, Noe HN, Jenkins GR, et al. Urinary excretion of calcium following an oral calcium loading test in healthy children. *Pediatrics* 1982;69:594–597.
50. Hymes LC, Warshaw BL. Idiopathic hypercalciuria: renal and absorptive subtypes in children. *Am J Dis Child* 1984; 138:176–180.
51. Pak CYC, Kaplan R, Bone H, et al. A single test for the diagnosis of absorptive, resorptive, and renal hypercalciuria. *N Engl J Med* 1975;292:497–500.
52. Stapleton FB. Hematuria associated with hypercalciuria and hyperuricosuria: a practical approach. *Pediatr Nephrol* 1994; 8:756–761.
53. Pak CYC. Hypercalciuric calcium nephrolithiasis. In: Resnick M, Pak CYC, eds. *Urolithiasis: a medical and surgical reference.* Philadelphia: WB Saunders, 1990:45–49.
54. Alon US, Berenbom A. Idiopathic hypercalciuria of childhood: 4- to 11-year outcome. *Pediatr Nephrol* 2000;14: 1011–1015.
55. Freundlich M, Haimberg J, Bellorin-Font E, et al. Reduced bone mass in asymptomatic mothers and their children with idiopathic hypercalciuria. *J Am Soc Nephrol* 1997;8:551A.
56. Misael da Silva AM, dos Reis LM, Pereira RC, et al. Bone involvement in idiopathic hypercalciuria. *Clin Nephrol* 2002;57:183–191.
57. Prie D, Ravery V, Boccon-Gibod L, et al. Frequency of renal phosphate leak among patients with calcium nephrolithiasis. *Kidney Int* 2001;60:272–276.
58. Devuyst O, Christie PT, Courtoy PJ, et al. Intra-renal and subcellular distribution of the human chloride channel, CLC-5, reveals a pathophysiological basis for Dent's disease. *Hum Mol Genet* 1999;8:247–257.
59. Scheinman SJ. X-linked hypercalciuric nephrolithiasis: clinical syndromes and chloride channel mutations. *Kidney Int* 1998;53:3–17.
60. Lloyd SE, Gunther W, Pearce SHS, et al. Characterisation of renal chloride channel CLCN5, mutations in hypercalciuric nephrolithiasis (kidney stones) disorders. *Hum Mol Genet* 1997;6:1233–1239.
61. Yu ASL. Role of CIC-5 in the pathogenesis of hypercalciuria: recent insights from transgenic mouse models. *Curr Opin Nephrol Hypertens* 2001;10:415–420.
62. Reinhart SC, Norden AG, Lapsley M, et al. Characterization of carrier females and affected males with X-linked

recessive nephrolithiasis. *J Am Soc Nephrol* 1995;5:1451–1461.

63. Norden AGW, Scheinman SJ, Deschodt-Lanckman MM, et al. Tubular proteinuria defined by a study of Dent's (CLCN5 mutation) and other tubular diseases. *Kidney Int* 2000;57:240–249.
64. Raja KA, Schurman S, D'Mello RG, et al. Responsiveness of hypercalciuria to thiazide in Dent's disease. *J Am Soc Nephrol* 2002;13:2938–2944.
65. Langlois V, Bernard C, Scheinman SJ, et al. Clinical features of X-linked nephrolithiasis in childhood. *Pediatr Nephrol* 1998;12:625–629.
66. Igarashi T, Inatomi J, Ohara T, et al. Clinical and genetic studies of CLCN5 mutations in Japanese families with Dent's disease. *Kidney Int* 2000;58:520–527.
67. Pearce SHS, Williamson C, Kifor O, et al. A familial syndrome of hypocalcemia with hypercalciuria due to mutations in the calcium-sensing receptor. *N Engl J Med* 1996;335:1115–1122.
68. Rodriguez-Soriano J, Vallo A. Pathophysiology of the renal acidification defect present in the syndrome of familial hypomagnesaemia-hypercalciuria. *Pediatr Nephrol* 1994;8:431–435.
69. Bohles H, Brandl U, Schott G, et al. Clinical and chemical factors in kidney calculus formation in childhood. An analysis of 40 patients. *Monatsschr Kinderheilkd* 1984;132:158–162.
70. Neuhaus TJ, Belzer T, Blau N, et al. Urinary oxalate excretion in urolithiasis and nephrocalcinosis. *Arch Dis Child* 2000;82:322–326.
71. Smith LH. Diet and hyperoxaluria in the syndrome of idiopathic calcium oxalate urolithiasis. *Am J Kidney Dis* 1991; 17:370–375.
72. Hatch M. Oxalate status in stone-formers. *Urol Res* 1993; 21:55–59.
73. Hesse A, Schneeberger W, Engfeld S, et al. Intestinal hyperabsorption of oxalate in calcium oxalate stone formers: application of a new test with [$^{13}C_2$] oxalate. *J Am Soc Nephrol* 1999;10:S329–S333.
74. Williams HE, Wandzilak TR. Oxalate synthesis, transport, and the hyperoxaluric syndromes. *J Urol* 1989;141:742–749.
75. Holmes RP, Goodman HO, Assimos DG. Contribution of dietary oxalate to urinary oxalate excretion. *Kidney Int* 2001;59:270–276.
76. Chen CL, Fang HC, Chou KJ, et al. Acute oxalate nephropathy after ingestion of star fruit. *Am J Kidney Dis* 2001;37:418–422.
77. Hoppe B, Hesse A, Bromme S, et al. Urinary excretion substances in patients with cystic fibrosis: risk of urolithiasis? *Pediatr Nephrol* 1998;12:275–279.
78. Monico CG, Ford GC, Persson XMT, et al. Potential mechanisms of marked hyperoxaluria not due to primary hyperoxaluria I or II. *Kidney Int* 2002;62:392–400.
79. Sidhu H, Hoppe B, Hesse A, et al. Absence of *Oxalobacter formigenes* in cystic fibrosis patients: a risk factor for hyperoxaluria. *Lancet* 1998;352:1026–1029.
80. Lingeman JE, Smith LH, Wood JR, et al. Medical evaluation and treatment of the stone patient. In: Moster MB, ed. *Urinary calculi.* Philadelphia: Lea and Febiger, 1989:84–133.
81. Danpure CJ. Primary hyperoxaluria. In: Schriver CR, Beaudet AL, Sly WS, et al., eds. *The metabolic and molecular bases of inherited disease,* 8th ed. New York: McGraw-Hill, 2001:3323–3367.
82. Giafi CF, Rumsby G. Primary hyperoxaluria type 2: enzymology. *J Nephrol* 1998;11:29–31.
83. Cramer SD, Ferree PM, Lin K, et al. The gene encoding hydroxypyruvate reductase (GRHPR) is mutated in patients with primary hyperoxaluria type II. *Hum Mol Genet* 1999;8: 2063–2069.
84. Cochat P, Deloraine A, Rotily M, et al. Epidemiology of primary hyperoxaluria type I. *Nephrol Dial Transplant* 1995; 10:3–7.
85. Van Acker KJ, Eyskens FJ, Espeel MF, et al. Hyperoxaluria with hyperglycoluria not due to alanine:glyoxylate aminotransferase defect: a novel type of primary hyperoxaluria. *Kidney Int* 1996;50:1747–1752.
86. Milliner DS, Wilson DM, Smith LH. Phenotypic expression of primary hyperoxaluria: comparative features of types I and II. *Kidney Int* 2001;59:31–36.
87. Milliner DS, Eickholt JT, Bergstralh E, et al. Primary hyperoxaluria: results of long-term treatment with orthophosphate and pyridoxine. *N Engl J Med* 1994;331:1553–1558.
88. Cochat P, Koch Nogueira PC, Mahmoud MA, et al. Primary hyperoxaluria in infants: medical, ethical, and economic issues. *J Pediatr* 1999;135:746–750.
89. Toussaint C. Pyridoxine-responsive PHI: treatment. *J Nephrol* 1998;11:49–50.
90. Smith LH, Werness PG, Van den Berg CJ, et al. Orthophosphate treatment in calcium urolithiasis. *Scand J Urol Nephrol* 1980;53:253–263.
91. Leumann E, Hoppe B, Neuhaus TJ. Management of primary hyperoxaluria: effect of oral citrate administration. *Pediatr Nephrol* 1993;7:207–211.
92. Dent CE, Senor B. Studies on the treatment of cystinuria. *Br J Urol* 1955;27:317–332.
93. Bruno M, Marangella M. Cystinuria: recent advances in pathophysiology and genetics. *Contrib Nephrol* 1997;122: 173–177.
94. Goodyer P, Boutros M, Rozen R. The molecular basis of cystinuria: an update. *Exp Nephrol* 2000;8:123–127.
95. Scriver CR. Cystinuria. *N Engl J Med* 1986;315:1155–1157.
96. Goodyer P, Saadi I, Ong P, et al. Cystinuria subtype and the risk of nephrolithiasis. *Kidney Int* 1998;54:56–61.
97. Purroy J, Bisceglia L, Calonge MJ, et al. Genomic structure and organization of the human rBAT gene (SLC3A1). *Genomics* 1996;37:249–252.
98. Chesney RW. Mutational analysis of patients with cystinuria detected by a genetic screening network: powerful tools in understanding the several forms of the disorder. *Kidney Int* 1998;54:279–280.
99. Rosenberg LE, Downing SJ, Durant JL, et al. Cystinuria: biochemical evidence for three genetically distinct diseases. *J Clin Invest* 1966;45:365–371.
100. Feliubadalo L, Font M, Purroy J, et al. Non-type I cystinuria caused by mutations in SLC7A9, encoding a subunit ($bo^{,+}AT$) of rBAT. *Nat Genet* 1999;23:52–57.
101. Strologo LD, Pras E, Pontesilli C, et al. Comparison between SLC3A1 and SLC7A9 cystinuria patients and car-

riers: a need for a new classification. *J Am Soc Nephrol* 2002;13:2547–2553.
102. Goodyer PR, Clow C, Reade T, et al. Prospective analysis and classification of patients with cystinuria identified in a newborn screening program. *J Pediatr* 1993;122:568–572.
103. Milliner DS. Cystinuria. In: Smith LH, ed. *Endocrinology and metabolism clinics of North America.* Philadelphia: WB Saunders, 1990:889–907.
104. Jaeger P. Cystinuria. In: Morgan SH, Grunfeld JP, eds. *Inherited disorders of the kidney.* New York: Oxford University Press, 1998:476–486.
105. La Manna A, Polito C, Marte A, et al. Hyperuricosuria in children: clinical presentation and natural history. *Pediatrics* 2001;107:86–90.
106. Baldree LA, Stapleton FD. Uric acid metabolism in children. *Pediatr Clin North Am* 1990;2:391–418.
107. Benjamin D, Sperling O, Weinberger A. Familial hypouricemia due to isolated renal tubular defect. *Nephron* 1977;18: 220–225.
108. Furth SL, Casey JC, Pyzik PL, et al. Risk factors for urolithiasis in children on the ketogenic diet. *Pediatr Nephrol* 2000;15:125–128.
109. Padova J, Pachevsky A, Onesti G. The effect of glucose loads on renal uric acid secretion in diabetic patients. *Metabolism* 1964;28:472–476.
110. Beck LH. Hypouricemia in the syndrome of inappropriate secretion of antidiuretic hormone. *N Engl J Med* 1979;301: 528–530.
111. Greene ML, Fujimoto WY, Seegmiller JE. Urinary xanthine stones: a rare complication of allopurinol therapy. *N Engl J Med* 1969;280:426–427.
112. Carpenter TO, Lebowitz L, Nelson D, et al. Hereditary xanthinuria presenting in infancy with nephrolithiasis. *J Pediatr* 1986;109:307–309.
113. Simmonds HA, Sahota AS, Van Acker KJ. Adenine phosphoribosyltransferase deficiency and 2,8-dihydroxyadenine urolithiasis. In: Scriver CR, ed. *The metabolic and molecular bases of inherited disease,* 7th ed. New York: McGraw-Hill, 1995:1707–1724.
114. Edvardsson V, Palsson R, Olafsson I, et al. Clinical features and genotype of adenine phosphoribosyltransferase deficiency in Iceland. *Am J Kidney Dis* 2001;38:473–480.
115. Zibolen M, Srsnova K, Srsen S. Increased urolithiasis in patients with alkaptonuria in childhood. *Clin Genet* 2000; 58:79–80.
116. Parks JH, Coe FL. A urinary calcium-citrate index for the evaluation of nephrolithiasis. *Kidney Int* 1986;30:85–90.
117. Tekin A, Tekgul S, Atsu N, et al. A study of the etiology of idiopathic calcium urolithiasis in children: hypocitruria is the most important risk factor. *J Urol* 2000;164: 162–165.
118. Baggio B, Gambaro G, Favaro S, et al. Juvenile renal stone disease: a study of urinary promoting and inhibiting factors. *J Urol* 1983;130:1133–1135.
119. Akcay T, Konukolu D, Dincer Y. Urinary glycosaminoglycan excretion in urolithiasis. *Arch Dis Child* 1999;80:271–272.
120. Caldas A, Broyer M, Duchaux M, et al. Primary distal tubular acidosis in childhood: clinical study and long-term follow-up of 28 patients. *J Pediatr* 1992;121:233–241.
121. McSherry E, Pokroy M. The absence of nephrocalcinosis in children with type 1 RTA on high-dose alkali therapy since infancy. *Clin Res* 1978;26:470A.
122. Santos F, Chan JCM. Renal tubular acidosis in children. *Am J Nephrol* 1986;6:289–295.
123. Buckalew VM, Purvis ML, Shulman MG, et al. Hereditary renal tubular acidosis. *Medicine* 1974;53:229–254.
124. Ismail EAR, Saad SA, Sabry MA. Nephrocalcinosis and urolithiasis in carbonic anhydrase II deficiency syndrome. *Eur J Pediatr* 1997;156:957–962.
125. Strisciuglio P, Hu PY, Lim EJ, et al. Clinical and molecular heterogeneity in carbonic anhydrase II deficiency and prenatal diagnosis in an Italian family. *J Pediatr* 1998;132:717–720.
126. Nagai R, Kooh SW, Balfe JW, et al. Renal tubular acidosis and osteopetrosis with carbonic anhydrase II deficiency: pathogenesis of impaired acidification. *Pediatr Nephrol* 1997;11:633–636.
127. Bruce LJ, Unwin RJ, Wrong O, et al. The association between familial distal renal tubular acidosis and mutations in the red cell anion exchanger (band 3, AE1) gene. *Biochem Cell Biol* 1998;76:723–728.
128. Karet FE, Gainza FJ, Gyory AZ, et al. Mutations in the chloride-bicarbonate exchanger gene AE1 cause autosomal dominant but not autosomal recessive distal renal tubular acidosis. *Proc Natl Acad Sci U S A* 1998;95:6337–6342.
129. Wiebers DO, Wilson DM, McLeod RA, et al. Renal stones in Wilson's disease. *Am J Med* 1979;67:249–254.
130. Eriksson P, Denneberg T, Enestrom S, et al. Urolithiasis and distal renal tubular acidosis preceding primary Sjögren's syndrome: a retrospective study 5–53 years after the presentation of urolithiasis. *J Intern Med* 1996;239:483–488.
131. Restaino I, Kaplan BS, Stanley C, et al. Nephrolithiasis, hypocitraturia, and a distal renal tubular acidification defect in type I glycogen storage disease. *J Pediatr* 1992;122:392–396.
132. Chen YT, Coleman RA, Scheinman JI, et al. Renal disease in type 1 glycogen storage disease. *N Engl J Med* 1988;318:7–11.
133. Weinstein DA, Somers MJG, Wolfsdorf JI. Decreased urinary citrate excretion in type 1a glycogen storage disease. *J Pediatr* 2001;138:378–382.
134. Chen YT. Type I glycogen storage disease: kidney involvement, pathogenesis and its treatment. *Pediatr Nephrol* 1991; 5:71–76.
135. Chang WN, Cheng YF. Nephrolithiasis and nephrocalcinosis in cerebrotendinous xanthomatosis: report of three siblings. *Eur Neurol* 1995;35:55–57.
136. Brenner RJ, Spring DB, Sebastian A, et al. Incidence of radiologically evident bone disease, nephrocalcinosis, and nephrolithiasis in various types of renal tubular acidosis. *N Engl J Med* 1982;307:217–221.
137. Rodriguez-Soriano J, Vallo A. Renal tubular acidosis. *Pediatr Nephrol* 1990;4:268–275.
138. Uribarri J, Oh MS, Pak CYC. Renal stone risk factors in patients with type IV renal tubular acidosis. *Am J Kidney Dis* 1994;23:784–787.
139. Osther PJ, Mathiasen H, Hansen AB, et al. Urinary acidification and urinary excretion of calcium and citrate in women with bilateral medullary sponge kidney. *Urol Int* 1994;52:126–130.

140. Torres VE, Erickson SB, Smith LH, et al. The association of nephrolithiasis and autosomal dominant polycystic kidney disease. *Am J Kidney Dis* 1988;11:318–325.
141. Levine E, Grantham JJ. Calcified renal stones and cyst calcifications in autosomal dominant polycystic and kidney disease: clinical and CT study in 84 patients. *Am J Radiol* 1992; 159:77–81.
142. Praga M, Martinez MA, Andres A, et al. Association of thin basement membrane nephropathy with hypercalciuria, hyperuricosuria, and nephrolithiasis. *Kidney Int* 1998;54: 915–920.
143. Black J, Stapleton FB, Roy S, et al. Varied types of urinary calculi in patients with cystinosis without tubular acidosis. *Pediatrics* 1986;78:295–297.
144. Saleem MA, Milford DV, Alton H, et al. Hypercalciuria and ultrasound abnormalities in children with cystinosis. *Pediatr Nephrol* 1995;9:45–47.
145. Van't Hoff WG, Gretz N. The treatment of cystinosis with cysteamine and phosphocysteamine in the United Kingdom and Eire. *Pediatr Nephrol* 1995;9:685–689.
146. Fischbach M, Terzic J, Cavalier A, et al. Renal stones in nephropathic cystinosis treated with phosphocysteamine. *Pediatr Nephrol* 1997;11:787–788.
147. Azizi E, Eshel G, Aladjem M. Hypercalciuria and nephrolithiasis as a presenting sign in Wilson disease. *Eur J Pediatr* 1989;148:548–549.
148. Smith LH, Fromm H, Hofmann AF. Acquired hyperoxaluria, nephrolithiasis, and intestinal disease: description of a syndrome. *N Engl J Med* 1972;286:1371–1375.
149. Smith LH, Werness PG, McCall JT. Enteric hyperoxaluria and other hyperoxaluric states. In: Coe FL, guest ed, Brenner BM, Stein JA, eds. *Contemporary issues in nephrology*, New York: Churchill-Livingstone, 1980:215–238.
150. Chidekel AS, Dolan TF. Cystic fibrosis and calcium oxalate nephrolithiasis. *Yale J Biol Med* 1996;69:317–321.
151. Bohles H, Beggardt B, Beeg T, et al. Antibiotic treatment–induced tubular dysfunction as a risk factor for renal stone formation in cystic fibrosis. *J Pediatr* 2002;140:103–109.
152. Katz SM, Krueger LJ, Falkner B. Microscopic nephrocalcinosis in cystic fibrosis. *N Engl J Med* 1988;319:263–266.
153. Turner MA, Goldwater D, David TJ. Oxalate and calcium excretion in cystic fibrosis. *Arch Dis Child* 2000;83:244–247.
154. Jacinto JS, Modanlou HD, Crade M, et al. Renal calcification incidence in very low birth weight infants. *Pediatrics* 1988;81:31–35.
155. Narendra A, White MP, Rolton HA, et al. Nephrocalcinosis in preterm babies. *Arch Dis Child Fetal Neonatal Ed* 2001; 85:F207–F213.
156. Karlowicz MG, Katz ME, Adelman RD, et al. Nephrocalcinosis in very low birth weight neonates: family history of kidney stones and ethnicity as independent risk factors. *J Pediatr* 1993;122:635–638.
157. Short A, Cooke RWI. The incidence of renal calcification in preterm infants. *Arch Dis Child* 1991;66:412–417.
158. Campfield T, Braden G. Urinary oxalate excretion by very low birth weight infants receiving parenteral nutrition. *Pediatrics* 1989;84:860–863.
159. Monge M, Garcia-Nieto VM, Domenech E, et al. Study of renal metabolic disturbances related to renal lithiasis at school age in very low birth weight children. *Nephron* 1998;79:269–273.
160. Ronnefarth G, Misselwitz J. Nephrocalcinosis in children: a retrospective survey. *Pediatr Nephrol* 2000;14:1016–1021.
161. Noble CB, Klein LT, Staiman VR, et al. Ureteral obstruction secondary to indinavir in the pediatric HIV population. *Pediatr Radiol* 1998;28:627–629.
162. Kopp JB, Miller KD, Mican JM, et al. Crystalluria and urinary tract abnormalities associated with indinavir. *Ann Intern Med* 1997;127:119–125.
163. Saltel E, Angel JB, Futter NG, et al. Increased prevalence and analysis of risk factors for indinavir nephrolithiasis. *J Urol* 2000;164:1895–1897.
164. Gagnon RF, Tecimer SN, Watters AK, et al. Prospective study of urinalysis abnormalities in HIV-positive individuals treated with indinavir. *Am J Kidney Dis* 2000;36:507–515.
165. Zinn HL, Orentlicher RJ, Haller JO, et al. Radiographically occult ureteral calculi in an HIV-positive child undergoing indinavir therapy. *Emerg Radiol* 2000;7:114–116.
166. Van Rossum AM, Dieleman JP, Fraaij PL, et al. Indinavir-associated asymptomatic nephrolithiasis and renal cortex atrophy in two HIV-1 infected children. *AIDS* 2001;15:1745–1747.
167. Cochat P, Cochat N, Jouvenet M, et al. Ceftriaxone-associated nephrolithiasis. *Nephrol Dial Transplant* 1990;5:974–976.
168. De Moor RA, Egberts ACG, Schroder CH. Ceftriaxone-associated nephrolithiasis and biliary pseudolithiasis. *Eur J Pediatr* 1999;158:975–977.
169. Pickens CL, Milliron AR, Russner AL, et al. Abuse of guaifenesin-containing medications generates an excess of a carboxylate salt of beta-(20-methoxyphenoxy)-lactic acid, a guaifenesin metabolite, and results in urolithiasis. *Urology* 1999;54:23–27.
170. Daudon M, Estepa L. Drug induced lithiases. *Presse Med* 1998;11:675–683.
171. Ahlstrand C, Tiselius HG. Urine composition and stone formation during treatment with acetazolamide. *Scand J Urol Nephrol* 1987;21:225–228.
172. Levisohn PM. Safety and tolerability of topiramate in children. *J Child Neurol* 2000;15:S22–S26.
173. Kubota M, Nishi-Nagase M, Sakakihara Y, et al. Zonisamide-induced urinary lithiasis in patients with intractable epilepsy. *Brain Dev* 2000;22:230–233.
174. Carlsen J, Durcan J, Zabriskie N, et al. Nephrolithiasis with dorzolamide. *Arch Ophthalmol* 1999;117:1087–1088.
175. Siwinska A, Gluszek J, Maciejewski J, et al. Intravenous aminophylline increases the degree of saturation of urine with calcium phosphate and struvite. *Int Urol Nephrol* 1997;29:141–146.
176. Valaseri A, Van Reen R. Pediatric bladder stone disease: current status of research. *J Pediatr* 1968;72:546.
177. Frassetto L, Morris RC, Sellmeyer DE, et al. Diet, evolution and aging: the pathophysiologic effects of the post-agricultural inversion of the potassium-to-sodium and base-to-chloride ratios in the human diet. *Eur J Nutr* 2001;40:200–213.
178. Kielb S, Koo HP, Bloom DA, et al. Nephrolithiasis associated with the ketogenic diet. *J Urol* 2000;164:464–466.
179. Herzberg GZ, Fivush BA, Kinsman SL, et al. Urolithiasis associated with the ketogenic diet. *J Pediatr* 1990;117:743–745.

180. Rodman JS. Struvite stones. *Nephron* 1999;81:50–59.
181. Michaels EK, Fowler JE. Extracorporeal shock wave lithotripsy for struvite calculi: prospective study with extended follow-up. *J Urol* 1991;146:728–732.
182. Segura JW. Staghorn calculi. *Urol Clin North Am* 1997;24:71–80.
183. Samuel M, Duffy P, Capps S, et al. Xanthogranulomatous pyelonephritis in childhood. *J Pediatr Surg* 2001;36:598–601.
184. Bingol-Kologlu M, Ciftci AO, Senocak ME, et al. *Eur J Pediatr Surg* 2002;12:42–48.
185. Schulman H, Barki Y, Hertzanu Y, et al. Diffuse xanthogranulomatous pyelonephritis in childhood. *J Clin Ultrasound* 1997;25:207–210.
186. Meria P, Desgrippes A, Fournier R, et al. The conservative management of corynebacterium group D2 encrusted pyelitis. *Br J Urol Int* 1999;84:270–275.
187. Nadler RB, Hoffman TA, McClennan BL, et al. *Corynebacterium urealyticum* (CIC, group D2) associated with staghorn calculus: treatment by percutaneous debulking and chemolysis. *J Endourol* 1996;10:31–34.
188. Aguado JM, Morales JM, Salto E, et al. Encrusted pyelitis and cystitis by *Corynebacterium urealyticum* (CDC group D2): a new and threatening complication following renal transplant. *Transplantation* 1993;56:617–622.
189. Morales JM, Aguado JM, Diaz-Gonzalez R, et al. Alkaline-encrusted pyelitis/cystitis and urinary tract infection due to *Corynebacterium urealyticum:* a new severe complication after renal transplantation. *Transplant Proc* 1992;24:81–82.
190. Soriano F, Ponte C, Santamaria M, et al. Struvite crystal formation by *Corynebacterium* group D2 in human urine and its prevention by acetohydroxamic acid. *Eur Urol* 1987;13:271–273.
191. Verbaeys A, Minnaert H, De Paepe M, et al. Results of urometabolic evaluation in 127 patients with renal calculus disease. *Urology* 1985;25:22–25.
192. Hsu THS, Streem SB. Metabolic abnormalities in patients with caliceal diverticular calculi. *J Urol* 1998;160:1640–1642.
193. Husmann DA, Milliner DS, Segura JW. Ureteropelvic junction obstruction with concurrent renal pelvic calculi in the pediatric patient: a long-term followup. *J Urol* 1995;156:741–743.
194. Glenn JF. Analysis of 51 patients with horseshoe kidney. *N Engl J Med* 1959;261:684–687.
195. Silver RI, Gros DAC, Jeffs RD, et al. Urolithiasis in the exstrophy-epispadias complex. *J Urol* 1997;158:1322–1326.
196. Mathoera RB, Kok DJ, Nijman RJM. Bladder calculi in augmentation cystoplasty in children. *Pediatr Urol* 2000;56:482–487.
197. Khoury AE, Salomon M, Doche R, et al. Stone formation after augmentation cystoplasty: the role of intestinal mucus. *J Urol* 1997;158:1133–1137.
198. Shekarriz B, Upadhyay J, Demirbilek S, et al. Surgical complications of bladder augmentation: comparison between various enterocystoplasties in 133 patients. *Urology* 2000;55:123–128.
199. Wenzl JE, Burke EC, Stickler GB, et al. Nephrolithiasis and nephrocalcinosis in children. *Pediatrics* 1968;41:57–61.
200. Noe HN. Hypercalciuria and pediatric stone recurrences with and without structural abnormalities. *J Urol* 2000;164:1094–1096.
201. Stapleton FB, Linshaw MA, Hassanein K, et al. Uric acid excretion in normal children. *J Pediatr* 1978;92:911–914.
202. Morgenstern BZ, Milliner DS, Murphy ME, et al. Urinary oxalate and glycolate excretion patterns in the first year of life: a longitudinal study. *J Pediatr* 1993;123:248–251.
203. von Schnakenburg C, Byrd DJ, Latta K, et al. Determination of oxalate excretion in spot urines of healthy children by ion chromatography. *Eur J Clin Chem Clin Biochem* 1994;32:27–29.
204. Gibbs DA, Watts RW. The variation of urinary oxalate excretion with age. *J Lab Clin Med* 1969;73:901–908.
205. Stapleton FB, Nash DA. A screening test for hyperuricosuria. *J Pediatr* 1983;102:88–90.
206. Smith SL, Somers JM, Broderick N, et al. The role of the plain radiograph and renal tract ultrasound in the management of children with renal tract calculi. *Clin Radiol* 2000;55:708–710.
207. Diament MJ, Malekzadeh M. Ultrasound and the diagnosis of renal and ureteral calculi. *J Pediatr* 1986;109:980–983.
208. Vrtiska TJ, Hattery RR, King BF, et al. Role of ultrasound in medical management of patients with renal stone disease. *Urol Radiol* 1992;14:131–138.
209. Smergel E, Greenberg SB, Crisci KL, et al. CT urograms in pediatric patients with ureteral calculi: do adult criteria work? *Pediatr Radiol* 2001;31:720–723.
210. Brenner DJ, Elliston C, Hall E, et al. Estimated risks of radiation-induced fatal cancer from pediatric CT. *Am J Radiol* 2001;176:289–296.
211. Donnelly LF, Emery KH, Brody AS, et al. Minimizing radiation dose for pediatric body applications of single detector helical CT: strategies at a large children's hospital. *Am J Radiol* 2001;176:303–306.
212. Rosser CJ, Zagoria R, Dixon R, et al. Is there a learning curve in diagnosing urolithiasis with noncontrast helical computed tomography? *Can Assoc Radiol J* 2000;51:177–181.
213. Villanyi KK, Szekely JG, Farkas LM, et al. Short-term changes in renal function after extracorporeal shock wave lithotripsy in children. *J Urol* 2001;166:222–224.
214. Lifshitz DA, Lingeman JE, Zafar FS, et al. Alterations in predicted growth rate of pediatric kidneys treated with extracorporeal shock wave lithotripsy. *J Endourol* 1998;12:469–475.
215. Brinkman OA, Griehl A, Kuwertz-Broking E, et al. Extracorporeal shock wave lithotripsy in children. *Eur Urol* 2001;39:591–597.
216. Strauss AL, Coe FL, Deutsch L, et al. Factors that predict relapse of calcium nephrolithiasis during treatment. *Am J Med* 1982;72:17–24.
217. Curhan GC, Willett WC, Rimm EB, et al. A prospective study of dietary calcium and other nutrients and the risk of symptomatic kidney stones. *N Engl J Med* 1993;328:833–838.
218. Muldowney FR, Freaney R, Moloney MF. Importance of dietary sodium in the hypercalciuria syndrome. *Kidney Int* 1982;22:292–296.
219. Jaeger P, Portmann L, Saunders L, et al. Anticystinuric effects of glutamine and of dietary sodium restriction. *N Engl J Med* 1986;315:1120–1123.
220. Norman RW, Manette WA. Dietary restriction of sodium as a means of reducing urinary cystine. *J Urol* 1990;143:1193–1195.
221. Peces R, Sanchez L, Gorostidi M, et al. Effects in variation in sodium intake on cystinuria. *Nephron* 1991;57:421–423.

222. Rodriguez LM, Santos F, Malaga S, et al. Effect of a low sodium diet on urinary elimination of cystine in cystinuric children. *Nephron* 1995;71:416–418.
223. Stapleton FB, Chesney RW, Behrmann AT, et al. Increased urinary excretion of renal N-acetyl-β-glucosaminidase in hypercalciuria. *Am J Dis Child* 1985;139:950–952.
224. Balla AA, Salah AM, Abdalmotaal E, et al. N-acetyl-β-D-glucosaminidase excretion in healthy children and in pediatric patients with urolithiasis. *World J Urol* 1998;16:413–416.
225. Bonilla-Felix M, Villegas-Medina O, Vehaskari VM. Renal acidification in children with idiopathic hypercalciuria. *J Pediatr* 1994;124:529–534.
226. Hamed IA, Czerwinski AW, Coats B, et al. Familial absorptive hypercalciuria and renal tubular acidosis. *Am J Med* 1979;67:385–391.
227. Backman U, Danielson BG, Johansson G, et al. Incidence and clinical importance of renal tubular defects in recurrent renal stone formers. *Nephron* 1980;25:96–101.
228. Gambaro G, Favaro S, D'Angelo A. Risk for renal failure in nephrolithiasis. *Am J Kidney Dis* 2001;37:233–243.
229. Lindell A, Denneberg T, Granerus G. Studies on renal function in patients with cystinuria. *Nephron* 1997;77:76–85.
230. Moore ES, Coe FL, McMann BJ, et al. Idiopathic hypercalciuria in children: prevalence and metabolic characteristics. *J Pediatr* 1978;92:906–910.
231. Barratt TM, Kasidas GP, Murdoch I, et al. Urinary oxalate and glycolate excretion and plasma oxalate concentration. *Arch Dis Child* 1991;66:501–503.
232. Norman ME, Feldman NI, Cohn RM, et al. Urinary citrate excretion in the diagnosis of distal renal tubular acidosis. *J Pediatr* 1978;92:394–400.

58

PEDIATRIC RENAL TUMORS

CHRISTOPHER S. COOPER
JACK S. ELDER

WILMS' TUMOR

Incidence

Wilms' tumor is the most common renal malignancy in children and the fourth most common pediatric malignancy (1). Seventy-five percent of Wilms' tumors are seen in children between 1 and 5 years of age, and 90% occur in children younger than 7 years of age; age of peak incidence is 44 months. Boys and girls are almost equally affected by Wilms' tumor (1,2).

Etiology and Pathophysiology

Wilms' tumor is thought to arise from abnormal renal development, with proliferation of metanephric blastema without normal differentiation into tubules and glomeruli. Alterations in genes controlling growth and differentiation have been associated with Wilms' tumor (2).

Nephrogenic rests or nephroblastomatosis may be precursor lesions that have the potential to undergo change and become a Wilms' tumor. A nephrogenic rest consists of a focus of abnormally persistent embryonic kidney cells. Nephrogenic rests occur in 1% of kidneys in newborns but usually regress or differentiate early in childhood. Nephroblastomatosis describes the condition in which multifocal or diffuse nephrogenic rests are present. More than 40% of kidneys from children with Wilms' tumor contain nephrogenic rests, and almost 100% of children with bilateral Wilms' tumors have rests in their kidneys. Children with a Wilms' tumor 1 (*WT-1*) or 2 (*WT-2*) gene mutation have an increased incidence of nephrogenic rests, and a second factor may induce the transformation of these rests into malignancies (3).

Nephrogenic rests can be divided into two categories based on their position relative to the renal lobe. Intralobar nephrogenic rests consist of rests anywhere within the renal lobe, sinus, or pelvicaliceal system. Perilobar nephrogenic rests occur in the lobar periphery. The latter rests probably occur later in development because the renal lobe develops in a centrifugal fashion. Intralobar nephrogenic rests are found in a younger age group, are less common, and are often associated with the WAGR (*W*ilms tumor, *a*niridia, *g*enitourinary malformations, and mental *r*etardation) and Denys-Drash syndromes, which occur in association with *WT-1* mutations (4). Perilobar nephrogenic rests occur more frequently than intralobar nephrogenic rests and are associated with overgrowth syndromes such as hemihypertrophy and the Beckwith-Wiedemann syndromes.

The majority of nephrogenic rests undergo regression and become sclerotic or obsolescent, including those associated with *WT-1* mutations. Some rests grow and become hyperplastic, but even hyperplastic rests may regress. Unfortunately, a dormant, hyperplastic, or regressing rest maintains neoplastic potential, and the microscopic appearance of Wilms' tumor and nephrogenic rests can be indistinguishable. Consequently, the diagnosis of Wilms' tumor depends on the shape and growth characteristics of the lesion. With hyperplasia, a rest tends to maintain its original shape, unlike with a neoplasm, which is often spherical. Serial imaging studies to determine the growth characteristics of a lesion may be required to determine its malignant potential (3).

Multiple genetic mutations have been associated with the development of Wilms' tumor. The *WT-1* gene is located in the 11p13 region and is critical for normal genitourinary development. *WT-1* mutations have been associated with the development of Wilms' tumor as well as Wilms'-associated syndromes such as the Denys-Drash and WAGR syndromes. Mutations in the *WT-1* gene occur in only 6 to 18% of cases of Wilms' tumor (2). Other gene mutations distal to the *WT-1* gene in the 11p15 (*WT-2*) region are associated with Wilms' tumors occurring in the Beckwith-Wiedemann syndrome (5). The putative Wilms' tumor gene at 11p15 has not been identified, and there exist at least 10 imprinted genes at the *WT-2* locus. Several of these genes have been implicated in Wilms' tumorigenesis. Other locations of Wilms' tumor susceptibility genes occur at chromosome arms 16q, 1p, and 7p (2).

Associated Anomalies

Almost 10% of Wilms' tumors occur in children with congenital anomalies and syndromes (2,6). Aniridia consists of hypoplasia of the iris, and the sporadic form occurs in 1 in 50,000 people. The incidence of aniridia in children with Wilms' tumors increases to 1 in 70. The *PAX6* gene is responsible for aniridia and is located next to the WT-1 gene at 11p13. The familial form of aniridia occurring with an isolated *PAX6* mutation and normal WT-1 is not associated with Wilms' tumor, but 1.5% of children with the sporadic form of aniridia develop Wilms' tumor (2,7).

The WAGR syndrome includes Wilms' tumor, aniridia, genitourinary anomalies, and mental retardation. This syndrome is associated with deletion of the *WT-1* gene. Children with the WAGR syndrome generally present before 3 years of age; they also have deformities of the external ear and may have facial or skull dysmorphism (8).

Denys-Drash syndrome occurs as a result of a point mutation in the *WT-1* gene. This mutation results in testicular dysgenesis, male pseudohermaphroditism, and a nephropathy characterized by diffuse mesangial sclerosis. Approximately 90% of these children develop Wilms' tumors. Bilateral nephrectomy and transplantation are indicated in patients with Denys-Drash chromosome due to the progressive nephropathy and high risk of developing Wilms' tumors (90%) in the native kidneys (9).

Hemihypertrophy, in which an asymmetry of the body exists, occurs in 1 in 14,300 people; however, it occurs in 1 in 32 children with Wilms' tumor (2.9%). The tumor may occur on either side. These children have an increased incidence of genitourinary anomalies and other cancers, including adrenal cortical carcinomas and hepatoblastomas.

Children with Beckwith-Wiedemann syndrome have a mutation at chromosome band 11p15. These children develop organomegaly, including enlargement of the adrenal cortex, kidney, liver, pancreas, and gonads. Other associated anomalies in Beckwith-Wiedemann syndrome include omphalocele, hemihypertrophy, microcephaly, ear pits, mental retardation, macroglossia, and hyperinsulinemic hypoglycemia. Neoplasia occurs in one out of ten children with this syndrome and affects the same organs as those with hemihypertrophy, including the liver, adrenal cortex, and kidney (10).

Almost 3% of children with Wilms' tumor have musculoskeletal anomalies. Dermatologic lesions, including hemangiomas, multiple nevi, and café-au-lait spots, occur in 7.9% of children with Wilms' tumors. Genitourinary anomalies, including renal hypoplasia, ectopia, fusions, duplications, cystic disease, hypospadias, cryptorchidism, and pseudohermaphroditism, occur in 4.4% of children with Wilms' tumors (11).

Pathology

Wilms' tumor frequently consists of an encapsulated solitary tumor occurring in any part of the kidney. Necrosis and hemorrhage within the tumor are common. Occasionally the tumor will contain true cysts. The tumor may grow into the renal pelvis and cause obstruction or hematuria (Fig. 58.1). Multiple renal lesions may occur with nephroblastomatosis. Invasion of the renal vein by the tumor occurs in up to 20% of patients. The lymph nodes are frequently enlarged at the time of surgery without metastatic disease, making gross assessment of nodal involvement unreliable.

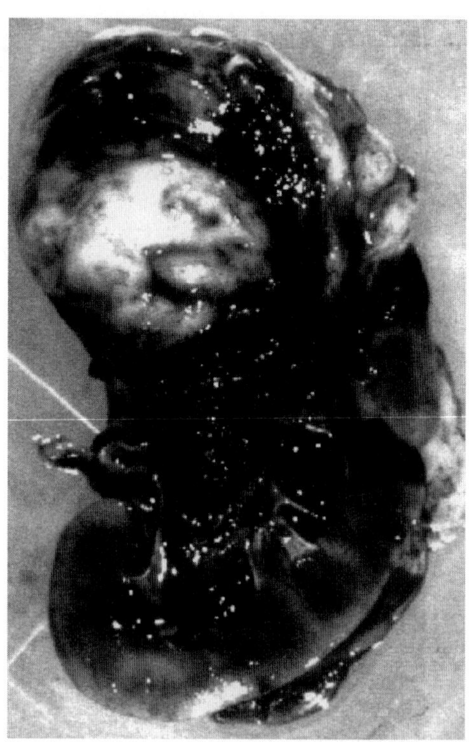

FIGURE 58.1. Gross pathologic view of bivalved kidney demonstrating a superior-pole renal tumor invading the renal pelvis along with thrombus in the renal pelvis and hydronephrosis of the lower pole.

Microscopically, the tumor typically demonstrates a triphasic histologic appearance consisting of blastemal, epithelial, and stromal cells. The "nephrogenic" cells demonstrate a tubuloglomerular pattern against a background of "stromagenic" cells (Fig. 58.2A). The stromal component may differentiate into striated muscle, cartilage, or, rarely, fat or bone. The epithelial component varies from well differentiated, resembling mature tubules, to a very primitive appearance. Most tumors are considered to have "favorable histologic features," which means that they typically demonstrate a favorable response to surgical removal and chemotherapy, with or without radiation therapy.

Some tumors contain anaplasia, which consists of a threefold variation in nuclear size with hyperchromatism and abnormal mitotic figures. The histologic demonstration of anaplasia portends a worse prognosis, is associated with resistance to chemotherapy (Fig. 58.2B), and is termed "unfavorable histologic features." Anaplasia occurs more frequently in older children. Anaplasia is categorized as diffuse

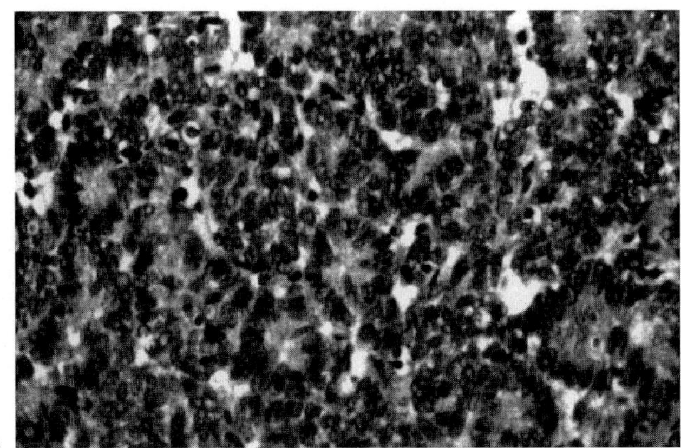
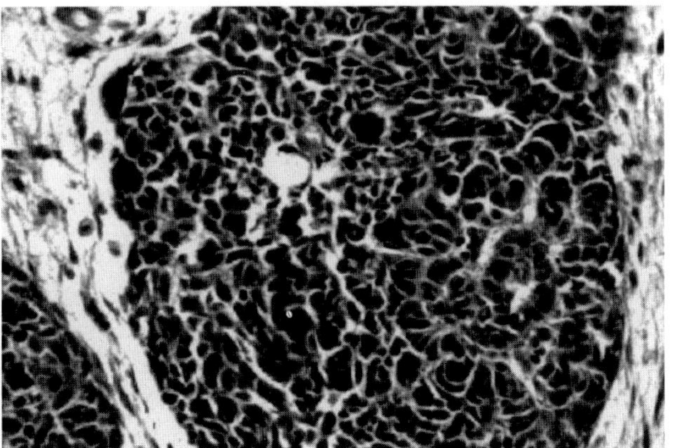

FIGURE 58.2. **A:** Well-differentiated Wilms' tumor with tubular formation (magnification ×150). **B:** Anaplastic Wilms' tumor with evident mitotic activity (magnification ×50). (Images courtesy of Dr. Dale S. Huff.)

or focal. Diffuse anaplasia is diagnosed when anaplastic tissue is present in more than one part of the tumor or at any extrarenal or metastatic site. Diffuse anaplasia conveys a worse prognosis than focal anaplasia, in which sharply localized clusters of anaplastic cells are contained only in the primary tumor. The rhabdoid tumor and clear cell sarcoma of the kidney were once considered forms of Wilms' tumor with poor prognoses but are now considered separate entities (12).

Staging

The staging system used by the National Wilms' Tumor Study Group (NWTSG) is outlined in Table 58.1 (13). The system is based on surgical and pathologic findings and correlates with prognosis.

Presentation

Most children with Wilms' tumor present with an abdominal mass or increasing abdominal girth. Approximately 30% of patients present with abdominal pain, but most children with Wilms' tumor appear well and are asymptomatic. Occasionally, a sudden subcapsular hemorrhage creates pain of acute onset and fever associated with anemia and hypertension. Children with tumor rupture may present with an acute abdomen (14).

Physical examination of the child with Wilms' tumor reveals a firm, nontender, smooth mass that rarely crosses the midline, in contrast with a nodular neuroblastoma, which grows across the midline and presents in an ill-appearing child. Hypertension may occur in up to two-thirds of children with Wilms' tumor and may be secondary to elevated renin levels resulting from renal ischemia caused by the pressure of the tumor. With tumor propagation into the vena cava, a child may develop a varicocele or even congestive heart failure. Physical examination should also assess the presence of any associated anomalies described previously, such as aniridia or hemihypertrophy.

Radiologic Evaluation

Ultrasonography allows the rapid distinction between a renal and nonrenal mass and permits identification of hydronephrosis and multicystic kidney, which also may present as an abdominal mass. Wilms' tumor characteristically demonstrates a solid renal mass with a heterogeneous echo pattern on ultrasonography. Ultrasonographic examination should include assessment of the renal vein and inferior vena cava for tumor thrombus. Excretory urography is used infrequently and demonstrates a mass effect that deforms the calyces.

Magnetic resonance imaging (MRI) accurately evaluates the extent and size of the Wilms' tumor, which frequently gives variable signal intensities (Fig. 58.3). Areas of hemorrhage show increased signal intensity on T1- and T2-weighted pulse sequences. Regions of necrosis demonstrate a decreased signal on T1- but not on T2-weighted pulse sequences (15). MRI is the most accurate study to demon-

TABLE 58.1. NATIONAL WILMS' TUMOR STUDY GROUP STAGING SYSTEM

Stage I:	Tumor within the kidney and completely excised.
Stage II:	Tumor beyond the kidney and completely excised. May have involvement of extrarenal vessels by tumor thrombus or local tumor spillage may have occurred. Includes tumor biopsy.
Stage III:	Residual tumor left within the abdomen; positive lymph nodes, positive surgical margins, peritoneal metastases, diffuse nonconfined tumor spillage.
Stage IV:	Hematogenous metastases (e.g., lung, liver, bone, brain).
Stage V:	Bilateral Wilms' tumor (irrespective of tumor extent/metastases).

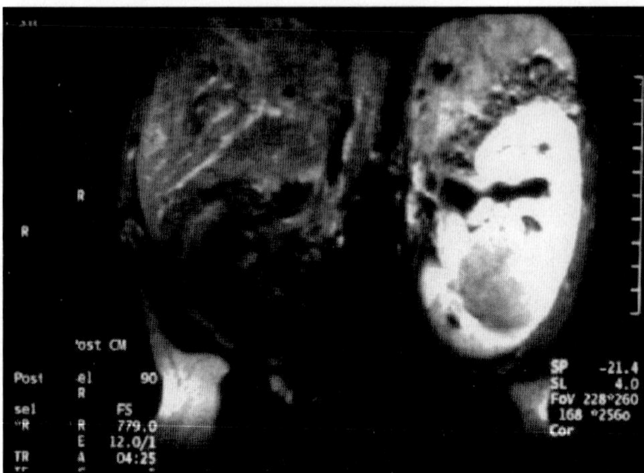

FIGURE 58.3. Magnetic resonance image demonstrating left lower pole Wilms' tumor.

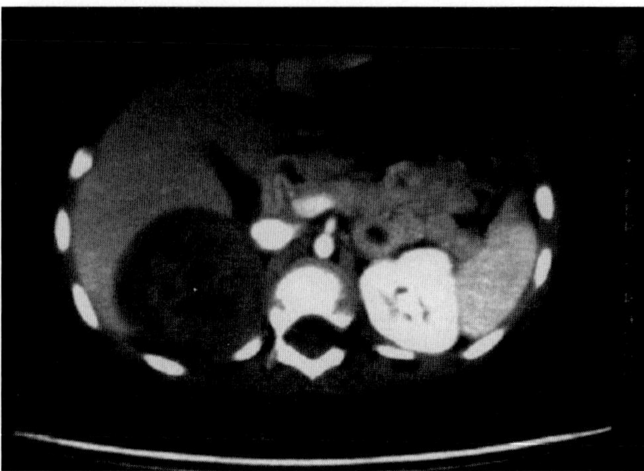

FIGURE 58.4. Computed tomographic scan demonstrating large right-sided Wilms' tumor.

strate tumor extension into the renal vein and inferior vena cava. Computed tomography (CT) with contrast also provides precise anatomic delineation of the renal and retroperitoneal anatomy (Fig. 58.4). Attention must also be directed to the contralateral kidney to assess the presence of lesions and determine contralateral function. Despite the accuracy of these techniques, false-negative results do occur. Consequently, intraoperative contralateral renal exploration is necessary, because bilateral involvement occurs in 10% of cases of Wilms' tumor. Treatment of bilateral Wilms' tumors is different from that for unilateral disease. A chest radiograph should also be obtained to evaluate the lung fields and rule out significant metastatic disease. If the diagnosis of Wilms' tumor is relatively certain, preoperative chest CT may be appropriate (16).

Treatment

Effective treatment of Wilms' tumor relies on the appropriate use of surgery, radiation, and chemotherapy. Refinements in radiation and multiagent chemotherapy have increased survival while minimizing side effects. There have been two multicenter trials of the management of Wilms' tumor in children:

1. National Wilms' Tumor Study (NWTS) (http://www.nwtsg.org) in the United States, in which primary nephrectomy followed by chemotherapy with or without radiotherapy has been used. A total of four cooperative trials have been completed, and children are now being enrolled in NWTS-5. Currently the 4-year survival rate for children with all stages of Wilms' tumor with favorable histologic features exceeds 90% (17).
2. In Europe, cooperative studies by the International Society for Paediatric Oncology (SIOP) (http://www.siop.nl), in which preoperative biopsy with chemotherapy, with or without radiation therapy, followed by tumor removal has been used. The concept is that preoperative therapy reduces the risk of tumor rupture or spill and may allow renal preservation.

Surgical Therapy

The goal of surgical management is removal of the primary tumor. Before the tumor is removed, however, the extent of the tumor is evaluated and the renal vessels, inferior vena cava, liver, and lymph nodes are assessed. Because preoperative imaging misses approximately 7% of bilateral Wilms' tumors, the contralateral kidney should be explored by opening Gerota's fascia and inspecting the entire surface at the time of surgery (18). Biopsy of any suspicious lesion is necessary, because children with bilateral Wilms' tumor are managed with preoperative chemotherapy followed by tumor nephrectomy.

When the kidney can be removed, it is taken along with the adrenal gland if the tumor involves the upper pole. Tumor rupture with diffuse spillage increases the chance of abdominal relapse. Preoperative radiation in addition to chemotherapy decreases this risk. Formal lymph node dissection does not improve survival, although biopsy specimens should be obtained from hilar, paraaortic, iliac, and celiac nodes, because positive lymph node findings portend a worse prognosis and affect postsurgical therapy (5). If the primary tumor involves surrounding organs and cannot be removed safely or if there is inferior vena caval extension above the hepatic vein, preoperative chemotherapy is advised, followed by tumor removal.

Chemotherapy

Actinomycin D, vincristine, and doxorubicin (Adriamycin) have been effective in the treatment of Wilms' tumor. A summary of the current treatment for Wilms' tumor used by NWTSG-V is given in Table 58.2. At present all children in

TABLE 58.2. SUMMARY OF NATIONAL WILMS' TUMOR STUDY GROUP V TREATMENT FOR TUMORS OF STAGES I TO IV AFTER TOTAL NEPHRECTOMY

Stage I or II favorable histologic features, stage I anaplasia: pulse-intensive dactinomycin and vincristine (18 weeks)
Stage III or IV favorable histologic features, stage II–IV focal anaplasia: pulse-intensive dactinomycin, vincristine, doxorubicin (24 weeks), and abdominal radiation based on local tumor stage; stage IV tumors with favorable histologic features: also radiation therapy to both lungs
Stage II–IV diffuse anaplasia: dactinomycin, vincristine, doxorubicin, cyclophosphamide, etoposide, and radiation therapy

NWTSG receive chemotherapy. One NWTSG protocol evaluated the treatment of children younger than 24 months of age who had stage I Wilms' tumor with favorable histologic features, using nephrectomy alone (19). The relapse-free survival rate was marginally inferior to that of children receiving adjuvant chemotherapy, so at this time chemotherapy for all children with Wilms' tumor remains the standard of care. The treatment of bilateral disease (stage V) includes a biopsy followed by preoperative chemotherapy and bilateral partial nephrectomies. When metastatic or recurrent disease is encountered, doxorubicin is routinely given if the patient has received only dactinomycin and vincristine. For those who have already received three-agent chemotherapy, there is no well-established regimen.

Preoperative chemotherapy can be used selectively and is appropriate for inoperable tumors, tumors with vena caval extension above the hepatic vein, or bilateral tumors. SIOP investigators routinely administer preoperative chemotherapy to all patients with the presumptive diagnosis of Wilms' tumor. This approach differs from the NWTSG approach, in which radical nephrectomy is performed before adjuvant chemotherapy (20). The SIOP approach of preoperative chemotherapy may shrink the tumor and produce lower morbidity. It does not influence long-term survival, however, and it may result in down-staging of the tumor with the potential for undertreatment of a tumor that would have been associated with positive lymph node findings. The use of these agents as well as of radiation therapy varies with the tumor stage and histologic findings (5).

Radiation Therapy

The application of radiation therapy in the treatment of Wilms' tumor is shown in Table 58.2. Radiation to the operative site or whole abdomen occurs 1 to 3 days after surgery. The current NWTSG-V protocol recommends 10.8 Gy as the abdominal dose for Wilms' tumor regardless of age (21). Supplemental radiation is directed to regions with residual tumor. In cases of pulmonary metastases radiation is delivered to both lungs regardless of the number or location of metastases. Postoperative brachytherapy has been used in selected children with chemoresistant bilateral Wilms' tumors. The radioactive source is delivered through a catheter left in the tumor bed at the time of surgery (22,23).

Bilateral Wilms' Tumor

Synchronous bilateral Wilms' tumors occur in approximately 6% of children with Wilms' tumor, and metachronous bilateral Wilms' tumors affect another 1%. The mean age of presentation of a child with synchronous bilateral Wilms' tumors is 32 months. These children have more genitourinary anomalies and a higher incidence of hemihypertrophy than those with unilateral Wilms' tumor. The incidence of unfavorable histologic findings is 10%, which is similar to that in children with unilateral disease. Anaplasia is less frequent in children under the age of 2 years with bilateral Wilms' tumors and, accordingly, younger children tend to have a better prognosis.

The overall survival of patients with synchronous bilateral Wilms' tumors with favorable histologic features is 76% at 3 years. In contrast, of children who develop a metachronous bilateral Wilms' tumor, only 39% are disease free 2 years after developing the second Wilms' tumor. The survival rate for children with bilateral Wilms' tumor and anaplasia is severely decreased and ranges from 10% to 26% (22,24,25). The stage of the most advanced lesion, histologic findings, and presence of lymph node metastases are important prognostic indicators in cases of bilateral Wilms' tumors.

Therapy for bilateral Wilms' tumors after diagnosis by radiographic imaging and/or biopsy is chemotherapy and then surgery. The chemoresponsiveness of many large tumors permits a renal-sparing approach with partial nephrectomy or excisional biopsy, and, at times, the larger tumor responds better to chemotherapy than the smaller tumor. In one study, 80% of children treated in this manner retained normal renal function 6 years after treatment (24). Bilateral nephrectomy and renal transplantation are rarely required for children with bilateral Wilms' tumors but may be appropriate for those with anaplasia, given the dismal prognosis and chemoresistance of the tumors (22).

Treatment Complications

A report of surgical complications from NWTSG-IV suggests an incidence of approximately 13% (26). The most frequent surgical complications were bowel obstruction (5.1%), extensive bleeding (1.9%), infection (1.9%), and vascular (1.5%) or splenic (1.1%) injury. Deaths related to surgical complications occurred in 0.5%. Risk factors for surgical complications included tumor extension into the inferior vena cava, tumors larger than 10 cm in diameter, and performance of the procedure by a surgeon not specializing in pediatric urology or pediatric surgery.

There are numerous potential complications of chemotherapy and radiation therapy for Wilms' tumor (Table 58.3).

TABLE 58.3. COMPLICATIONS OF CHEMOTHERAPY AND RADIATION THERAPY FOR WILMS' TUMOR

Bone marrow toxicity—chemotherapy induced
Gastrointestinal toxicity—chemotherapy-induced nausea, vomiting, and diarrhea; radiation-induced enteritis
Hepatic toxicity—induced by chemotherapy (dactinomycin is hepatotoxic) or radiation therapy
Vertebral hypoplasia and scoliosis—radiation induced
Renal toxicity—chemotherapy-induced tubular necrosis or radiation-induced nephritis
Pulmonary toxicity—acute interstitial radiation pneumonitis, reduced lung capacity
Cardiac toxicity—doxorubicin-induced cardiomyopathy, increased when combined with radiation therapy
Gonadal toxicity—ovarian failure after radiation therapy or oligospermia after chemotherapy or radiation therapy
Secondary neoplasms—1.6% of long-term survivors (sarcomas, adenocarcinomas, leukemias); most develop within radiation fields

One of the most common complications is acute hematologic toxicity due to the suppressive effects of chemotherapy on the bone marrow. Chemotherapy also frequently induces an acute gastrointestinal toxicity manifest by nausea, vomiting, and diarrhea. Radiation has the potential to adversely affect any exposed organ and can do so over a long period of time.

There is a low risk of renal failure in patients with a unilateral Wilms' tumor (0.25%) (18). This risk increases with bilateral Wilms' tumor (15% at 5 years). Children treated with nephrectomy and abdominal irradiation are also at increased risk for renal dysfunction. This risk appears to be dose dependent, with dysfunction occurring in over 70% of patients receiving 24 Gy to the remaining kidney and in fewer than 20% of patients receiving 12 Gy (27).

Second malignant neoplasms occur in 1.6% of survivors 15 years after diagnosis. These malignancies are most often leukemias, lymphomas, and skeletal system neoplasms (28). Abdominal irradiation increases the risk of second malignant neoplasms, and doxorubicin potentiates this effect (29). These tumors often arise in the irradiated field and may include sarcomas, adenocarcinomas, bone tumors, and breast and thyroid cancer (27).

Prognosis

Overall survival of patients with Wilms' tumor is almost 90%. Prognosis depends on multiple factors, including the stage and grade of the tumor. The 4-year postnephrectomy survival results from NWTSG-III and NWTSG-IV are listed in Table 58.4 (12,17,30–32). The most important prognostic factor in Wilms' tumor is histologic findings. Approximately 5% of children with Wilms' tumor have anaplasia, and it occurs more frequently in the older child. Children with anaplasia are four times more likely to experience relapse and nine times more likely to die from their disease than children without anaplasia. When

TABLE 58.4. FOUR-YEAR SURVIVAL (%) OF PATIENTS WITH WILMS' TUMOR AFTER NEPHRECTOMY AND CHEMOTHERAPY WITH OR WITHOUT RADIOTHERAPY

	Favorable histologic features		
Stage	RFS[a]	Overall	Unfavorable histologic features
I	94	99	68
II	88	96	55
III	92	96	45
IV	83	90	4

[a]Relapse-free survival.

anaplasia is well circumscribed and focally contained within the primary tumor, it is not considered unfavorable. Focal anaplasia in a stage I Wilms' tumor does not alter the prognosis when the tumor is treated with total nephrectomy and chemotherapy (12).

Hematogenous metastases also worsen the prognosis and are present at diagnosis in 10% to 15% of patients. Metastatic disease to the lungs occurs most often (85%), followed by metastases to the liver, bone, and brain. Metastases to the lymph nodes also predict a worse outcome with increased risk of local recurrence, and thus abdominal radiotherapy is added to chemotherapy. A tumor with renal vascular invasion carries a higher risk of local relapse. When metastatic or recurrent disease occurs, doxorubicin is routinely given if the patient has previously received only dactinomycin and vincristine. For those children already receiving three-agent chemotherapy, there is no well-established regimen.

Follow-Up

Follow-up is directed at detecting recurrence of cancer or the complications of treatment. The abdomen should be palpated and any suspicious findings evaluated with radiologic imaging. For patients with low-stage disease, evaluation of the abdomen with physical examination and of the lungs with a chest radiograph for recurrence may be all that is required, because the most likely site of relapse is in the lungs. In children at risk for abdominal recurrence, such as those with a history of higher-stage disease or contralateral nephrogenic rests, abdominal sonography should be performed every 3 months for at least 4 years. For patients with a history of hematogenous metastasis (brain, lung, liver, and bone), the site of metastasis should be evaluated with imaging every 3 months for the first year, then every 6 months for 2 years, and then yearly until 5 years. Irradiated bone should be monitored for life for any radiation-associated neoplasms. Follow-up for children with Wilms' tumor should include measurement of blood pressure and urinalysis to check for protein and serum creatinine (27).

CLEAR CELL SARCOMA OF THE KIDNEY

Clear cell sarcoma originally was considered to be a variant of Wilms' tumor. The age at diagnosis and the location are the same as for Wilms' tumor. However, unlike Wilms' tumor, clear cell sarcoma is associated with bone and brain metastases. In addition, it is not observed in children with associated congenital anomalies such as aniridia and hemihypertrophy. Treatment includes nephrectomy and systemic chemotherapy with actinomycin D, vincristine, and in many cases doxorubicin. In a review of 351 such tumors, predictors of survival included lower stage, younger age at diagnosis, and absence of tumor necrosis (33). Patients with stage I tumors had a 98% survival rate. In long-term follow-up, 30% of relapses occurred more than 3 years after diagnosis, and in some cases 10 years later (17).

RHABDOID TUMOR OF THE KIDNEY

Rhabdoid tumor is the most aggressive renal tumor in children. This tumor may metastasize to the lungs, abdomen, or liver, as well as the brain. It is also associated with second primary tumors in the brain such as cerebellar medulloblastoma, pineoblastoma, neuroblastoma, and subependymal giant cell astrocytoma. The median age of occurrence is younger than 16 months, and the tumor usually is resistant to chemotherapy (17).

CONGENITAL MESOBLASTIC NEPHROMA

Congenital mesoblastic nephroma (CMN) is a solid renal tumor that is found in neonates and is distinguished from Wilms' tumor in its morphology and relatively benign behavior. This tumor develops in approximately 1 in 500,000 infants and accounts for fewer than 3% of pediatric renal neoplasms. CMN is usually diagnosed at birth or within the first 3 months of life, whereas Wilms' tumor has a peak incidence between 2 and 4 years of age.

The pathogenesis of CMN is controversial. One theory relates to the two-hit concept for Wilms' tumor development; if neoplasia is induced during the early stromagenic phase, a conventional CMN might develop (34). Another theory is that the tumor originates from uninduced nephrogenic mesenchyme (35). Another observation is that trisomy 11 is common in many children with CMN tumors, particularly those with the "cellular" and "mixed" histologic subtypes of CMN (36). It has been proposed that the insulin-like growth factor-II gene, which has been mapped to the short arm of chromosome 11 and is expressed in mesenchymal cells during renal development, may play a key role in the acquisition of the growth properties of neoplasia (36).

Pathology

Three histologic types of CMN have been described: the classic pattern of CMN, the cellular or atypical variant, and a third type, which shows mixed features. A rare cystic variant also has been described.

Classically the involved kidney is enlarged and distorted by the tumor, which ranges from 0.6 to 9.0 cm (Fig. 58.5). The mass has a slightly bulging cut surface that has a whorled, coarsely trabeculated appearance, similar to that of a uterine leiomyoma. Cellular CMNs are softer than the classic type and show areas of hemorrhage, necrosis, and cystic degeneration.

Classic CMN is composed of uniform spindle-shaped cells arranged in interlacing bundles. The cells have pale eosinophilic cytoplasm and ovoid, elongated vesicular nuclei. Foci of extramedullary hematopoiesis are frequently observed. Mitotic activity ranges from zero to one mitotic figure per 10 high-power fields. The cellular variant contains diffuse sheets of closely packed cells with scanty cytoplasm, and thin-walled vascular spaces are scattered throughout. Necrosis and hemorrhage are common. Mitotic activity ranges from 10 to 30 mitotic figures per 10 high-power fields.

Clinical Features

CMN usually presents as an asymptomatic abdominal mass in the newborn or infant, although it has been detected by prenatal sonography (37). Tumors are more common on the left side. Renin-mediated hypertension is common in infants with CMN. Immunochemical studies in removed kidneys indicate that renin production by CMN cells is minimal but is highest in areas of renal cortex entrapped by the tumor (38).

In the majority of cases CMN is a relatively benign lesion, but local invasion, recurrence, and metastasis to

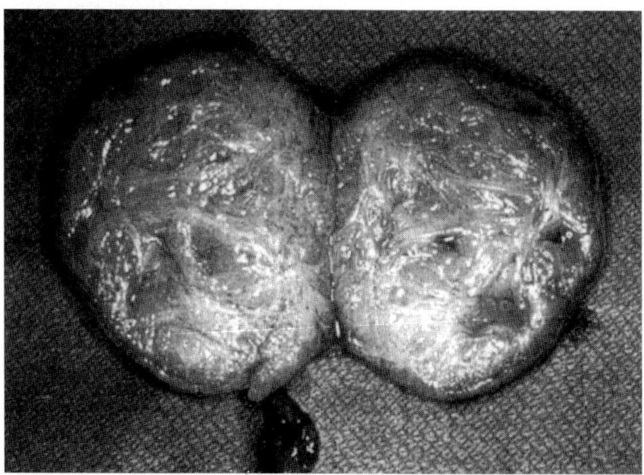

FIGURE 58.5. Gross photograph of infant kidney replaced with congenital mesoblastic nephroma.

the lung and brain can occur. The cellular variant is thought by some to be more likely to exhibit aggressive characteristics. Most infants with aggressive lesions are older than 3 months of age at diagnosis. Consequently, infants older than 3 months of age with a CMN cellular variant or tumor with atypical histologic features should be considered for adjunctive therapy after radical nephrectomy (39).

Diagnosis

In the newborn and infant the abdominal mass is the key to diagnosis, and the tumor usually is confirmed by ultrasonography, which demonstrates a solid mass. Abdominal and chest CT (or MRI) is done to stage the neoplasm preoperatively. MRI of the head should be performed if central nervous system metastases are suspected.

Treatment and Follow-Up

Both the classic and cellular variants of CMN are typically cured by radical nephrectomy. Unlike in Wilms' tumor, bilateral involvement is rare. Adjuvant therapy generally is not required. Recurrent or metastatic tumors may occur, however, usually in the lungs or brain, and close observation of these patients is important.

Congenital Mesoblastic Nephroma and Wilms' Tumor

Several differences exist between CMN and Wilms' tumor:

- CMN usually is diagnosed at birth or within the first 3 months of life, whereas Wilms' tumor has a peak incidence between 2 and 4 years.
- Wilms' tumor is a primitive embryonal neoplasm that is thought to develop from residual metanephric blastemas and histologically mimics different stages of renal development, whereas CMN typically consists of spindle cells that resemble primitive mesenchymal tissue of less definite derivation with few or no neoplastic epithelial cells.
- Clinically, CMN usually is cured by surgery alone, whereas Wilms' tumors require systemic chemotherapy.
- Both CMN and Wilms' tumors arise from primitive renal cells. However, molecular analysis demonstrates significant differences. Wilms' tumor frequently is associated with loss of heterozygosity at chromosome band 11p13 and/or 11p15, but CMN is not. Insulin-like growth factor-II, *N-myc* oncogene, and *WT-1* are highly expressed in Wilms' tumors and fetal kidneys. Insulin-like growth factor-II is detected in CMN, but *N-myc* and *WT-1* are not.
- Bilateral renal involvement is significantly more common in Wilms' tumor.

RENAL ANGIOMYOLIPOMA

Renal angiomyolipoma (AML) is a benign mesenchymal nodule consisting of blood vessels with thickened walls, smooth muscle, and adipose tissue. Between 20% and 40% of AMLs occur in individuals with the tuberous sclerosis complex (TSC) and 40% to 80% of TSC patients develop an AML (40). AML is predominant in females, with a 3:1 or 4:1 female/male ratio. Although AML is common in patients with TSC, distinguishing this tumor from renal cell carcinoma is important (41).

Etiology

TSC is an autosomal dominant condition with genetic locus heterogeneity. Half of patients are mentally retarded, and most have seizures as well as one of the characteristic dermatologic lesions, including adenoma sebaceum (facial angiofibromas), hypopigmented macules (ash leaf patches), and ungual fibromas. Involvement can occur in areas other than the kidney, including cortical tubers, subependymal nodules, retinal astrocytomas, and cardiac rhabdomyomas. Two major gene loci have been identified, including chromosome bands 9q34 (*TSC1*) and 16p13.3 (*TSC2*). These may act as growth suppressor genes in a way analogous to the two-hit model of the traditional tumor suppressor gene in the Knudson hypothesis (42).

Clinical Features

Renal AMLs with tuberous sclerosis are rare in children younger than 5 years of age. They are more common in children between 6 and 10 years of age, and most common in children older than 10 years. There are often tumors of various sizes, and they are usually bilateral. Through screening of tuberous sclerosis patients with ultrasonography or CT, many asymptomatic lesions are being discovered. Symptoms and signs of tumor growth may occur if any of the tumors enlarges significantly.

The vast majority of children with renal AML have some or all of the stigmata of tuberous sclerosis. Among children with renal AML, renal cysts are also common. Cysts that are more than 4 cm in diameter are more likely to cause symptoms such as flank pain, a palpable tender mass, and gross hematuria that require treatment (43–45). Retroperitoneal hemorrhage associated with spontaneous rupture of AML is the most life-threatening presentation of the tumor. The risk of tumor rupture has been attributed to the weak, elastin-poor vascular structures in the tumor.

Pathology

AMLs are vascular tumors consisting of smooth muscle, adipose tissue, and blood vessels with thickened walls. They range in size from small punctate "tubers" to huge masses exceeding 20 cm. The amount of fat in the tumor varies. Microscopic examination shows fat necrosis and collections of xanthoma cells. The

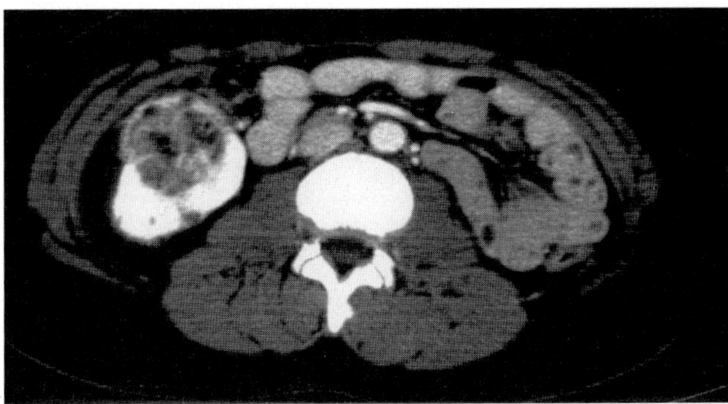

FIGURE 58.6. Computed tomographic scan demonstrating large right lower pole angiomyolipoma (AML) in a teenaged girl with tuberous sclerosis. The patient previously underwent removal of a large aneurysm within an AML in the left kidney.

blood vessels either lack elastic tissue or contain abnormally distributed elastic tissue, which possibly explains their tendency to rupture. In children these tumors are considered benign.

Renal cell carcinoma develops in 1 to 3% of patients with tuberous sclerosis, but these patients are most likely to be young women, not children (46).

Diagnosis

AML is diagnosed most often by sonography or CT. Sonography shows the tumor to be echodense, because of the fatty tissue, and well circumscribed. Similarly, CT establishes the diagnosis if there is a significant amount of fat in the lesion, because the x-ray attenuation of these tumors typically is less than −10 to −15 Hounsfield units. The use of thin cuts on nonenhanced CT scans improves the chances of detecting and measuring these small areas of fat (Fig. 58.6).

On MRI, the fat component has a high signal intensity on unenhanced T1-weighted images and lower intensity on T2-weighted images (47). MRI is particularly useful if sonography and CT scan are inconclusive.

Treatment

The risk of untreated AML includes development of abdominal or flank pain, palpable mass, hemorrhage, hematuria, anemia, and hypertension (43). These tumor complications occur primarily in individuals with tumors larger than 4 cm in diameter. If the lesion is smaller than 4 cm, follow-up with sonography or CT every 6 to 12 months is recommended. Over a period of 4 years, a significant increase in AML size occurred in 39% of males and 100% of females (44). If the lesion is over 4 cm and is growing, or if it is large, selective angiographic embolization or partial nephrectomy may be necessary (41,43,47).

The use of angiographic embolization was reviewed by Nelson and Sanda (45). Various materials have been used for embolization, including absorbable gelatin sponge, absolute alcohol, iodized oil, polyvinyl alcohol particles, and metal coils. Complications were reported in 10% of cases, most commonly abscess formation. Eighty-five percent of the patients experienced a postembolization syndrome of flank pain, fever, leukocytosis, and nausea attributed to inflammatory mediators. Administration of a tapering dose of prednisone over a 2-week period significantly ameliorated these problems (48). After embolization, reduced tumor size is expected. In addition, this form of treatment appears durable for the affected tumor.

Partial nephrectomy is another option for treatment of AML, provided there is significant residual functioning renal tissue (49). In recent years there has been interest in performing this procedure laparoscopically, as well as using cryotherapy, although the latter procedure is experimental.

RENAL CELL CARCINOMA

Older children with solid renal tumors may have a renal cell carcinoma. Radiographically, renal cell carcinoma cannot be distinguished from Wilms' tumor. Although the natural history of renal cell carcinoma appears to be similar in children and adults, it may have a more favorable prognosis in children younger than 10 years of age (50). Adjuvant interferon-alpha therapy may be beneficial also (51).

REFERENCES

1. Miller RW, Young JL Jr, Novakovic B. Childhood cancer. *Cancer* 1995;75:395–405.
2. Dome JS, Coppes MJ. Recent advances in Wilms tumor genetics. *Curr Opin Pediatr* 2002;14:5–11.
3. Beckwith JB. Precursor lesions of Wilms' tumor: clinical and biological implications. *Med Pediatr Oncol* 1993;21:158–168.
4. Ritchey ML. Recent progress in the biology and treatment of Wilms' tumor. *Curr Urol Rep* 2001;2:127–131.
5. Petruzzi MJ, Green DM. Wilms' tumor. *Pediatr Clin North Am* 1997;44:939–952.
6. Pendergrass TW. Congenital anomalies in children with Wilms' tumor: a new survey. *Cancer* 1976;37:403–408.
7. Haicken BN, Miller DR. Simultaneous occurrence of congenital aniridia, hamartoma and Wilms' tumor. *J Pediatr* 1971;78:497–502.
8. Narahara K, Kikkawa K, Kimira S, et al. Regional mapping of catalase and Wilms' tumor—aniridia, genitourinary abnormalities, and mental retardation triad loci to the chromosome segment 11p1305–p1306. *Hum Genet* 1984;66:181–185.
9. Rudin C, Pritchard J, Fernando ON, et al. Renal transplantation in the management of bilateral Wilms' tumor (BWT) and of Denys-Drash syndrome (DDS). *Nephrol Dial Transplant* 1998;13:1506–1510.
10. Sotelo-Avila C, Gonzalez-Crussi F, Fowler JW. Complete and incomplete forms of Beckwith-Wiedemann syndrome: their oncogenic potential. *J Pediatr* 1980;96:47–50.
11. Stay EJ, Vawter G. The relationship between nephroblastoma and neurofibromatosis (Von Recklinghausen's disease). *Cancer* 1977;39:2550–2625.
12. Faria P, Beckwith JB, Mishra K, et al. Focal versus diffuse anaplasia in Wilms tumor—new definitions with prognostic sig-

nificance; a report from the National Wilms Tumor Study Group. *Am J Surg Pathol* 1996;20:909–920.

13. D'Angio GJ, Breslow N, Beckwith JB, et al. Treatment of Wilms' tumor. Results of the Third National Wilms' Tumor Study. *Cancer* 1989;64:349–360.
14. Ramsay NK, Dehner LP, Coccia PF, et al. Acute hemorrhage into Wilms' tumor: a cause of rapidly developing abdominal mass with hypertension, anemia, and fever. *J Pediatr* 1977;91:763–765.
15. Hricak H, Thoeni RF, Carroll PR, et al. Detection and staging of renal neoplasms: a reassessment of MR imaging. *Radiology* 1988;166:643–649.
16. Shamberger RC. Pediatric renal tumors. *Semin Surg Oncol* 1999;16:105–120.
17. Ritchey ML. Pediatric urologic oncology. In: Walsh PC, Retik AB, Vaughan ED Jr, et al., eds. *Campbell's urology*, 8th ed. Philadelphia: WB Saunders, 2002:2419–2507.
18. Ritchey ML, Green DM, Breslow NB, et al. Accuracy of current imaging modalities in the diagnosis of synchronous bilateral Wilms' tumor. A report from the National Wilms' Tumor Study Group. *Cancer* 1995;75:600–604.
19. Green DM, Breslow NE, Beckwith JB, et al. Treatment with nephrectomy only for small, stage I/favorable histology Wilms' tumor: a report from the National Wilms' Tumor Study Group. *J Clin Oncol* 2001;19:3719–3724.
20. Pritchard-Jones K. Controversies and advances in the management of Wilms' tumour. *Arch Dis Child* 2002;87:241–244.
21. Lundin A, Makis RM. Radiotherapy for pediatric genitourinary tumors. *Urol Clin North Am* 2000;27:553–562.
22. Cooper CS, Jaffe WI, Huff DS, et al. The role of renal salvage procedures for bilateral Wilms' tumor: a 15-year review. *J Urol* 2000;163:265–268.
23. Thomas WW Jr, Goldwein JW, D'Angio G. A technique for the use of afterloading 137Cs brachytherapy in renal-sparing irradiation of bilateral Wilms tumor. *Int J Radiat Oncol Biol Phys* 1997;39:1121–1124.
24. Kumar R, Fitzgerald R, Breatnach F. Conservative surgical management of bilateral Wilms tumor: results of the United Kingdom Children's Cancer Study Group. *J Urol* 1998;160:1450–1453.
25. Montgomery BT, Kelalis PP, Blute ML, et al. Extended followup of bilateral Wilms tumor: results of the National Wilms Tumor Study. *J Urol* 1991;146:514–518.
26. Ritchey ML, Shamberger RC, Haase G, et al. Surgical complications after primary nephrectomy for Wilms' tumor: report from the National Wilms' Tumor Study Group. *J Am Coll Surg* 2001;192:63–68.
27. Egeler RM, Wolff JEA, Anderson RA, et al. Long-term complications and post-treatment follow-up of patients with Wilms' tumor. *Semin Urol Oncol* 1999;17:55–61.
28. Cherullo EE, Ross JH, Kay R, et al. Renal neoplasms in adult survivors of childhood Wilms tumor. *J Urol* 2001;165:2013–2017.
29. Breslow NE, Takashima JR, Whitton JA, et al. Second malignant neoplasms following treatment for Wilm's tumor: a report from the National Wilms' Tumor Study Group. *J Clin Oncol* 1995;13:1851–1859.
30. Neville HL, Ritchey ML. Wilms tumor: overview of National Wilms' Tumor Study Group results. *Urol Clin North Am* 2000;27:435–442.
31. Green DM, Breslow NE, Beckwith JB, et al. Comparison between single-dose and divided-dose administration of dactinomycin and doxorubicin for patients with Wilms' tumor: a report from the National Wilms' Tumor Study Group. *J Clin Oncol* 1998;16:237–245.
32. Green DM, Breslow NE, Beckwith JB, et al. Effect of duration of treatment on treatment outcome and cost of treatment for Wilms' tumor: a report from the National Wilms' Tumor Study Group. *J Clin Oncol* 1998;16:3744–3751.
33. Argani P, Perlman EJ, Breslow NE, et al. Clear cell sarcoma of the kidney: a review of 351 cases from the National Wilms Tumor Study Group Pathology Center. *Am J Surg Pathol* 2000;24:4–18.
34. Snyder HM III, Lack EE, Chetty-Baktavizian A, et al. Congenital mesoblastic nephroma: relationship to other renal tumors of infancy. *J Urol* 1981;126:513–516.
35. Nadasdy T, Roth J, Johnson DL, et al. Congenital mesoblastic nephroma: an immunohistochemical and lectin study. *Hum Pathol* 1993;24:413–419.
36. Mascarello JT, Cajulis TR, Krous HF, et al. Presence or absence of trisomy 11 is correlated with histologic subtype of congenital mesoblastic nephroma. *Cancer Genet Cytogenet* 1994;77:50–54.
37. Goldstein I, Shoshani G, Ben-Harus E, et al. Prenatal diagnosis of congenital mesoblastic nephroma. *Ultrasound Obstet Gynecol* 2002;19:209–211.
38. Tsuchida Y, Shimizu K, Hata J, et al. Renin production in congenital mesoblastic nephroma in comparison with that in Wilms' tumor. *Pediatr Pathol* 1993;13:155–164.
39. Heidelberger KP, Ritchey ML, Dauser RC, et al. Congenital mesoblastic nephroma metastatic to the brain. *Cancer* 1993; 72:2499–2502.
40. Kennelly MJ, Grossman HB, Cho KJ. Outcome analysis of 42 cases of renal angiomyolipoma. *J Urol* 1994;152:1988–1991.
41. van Baal JG, Smits NJ, Keeman JN, et al. The evolution of renal angiomyolipomas in patients with tuberous sclerosis. *J Urol* 1994;152:35–38.
42. Green AJ, Johnson PH, Yates JR. The tuberous sclerosis gene on chromosome 9q34 acts as a growth suppressor. *Hum Mol Genet* 1994;3:1833–1834.
43. Steiner MS, Goldman SM, Fishman EK, et al. The natural history of renal angiomyolipoma. *J Urol* 1993;150:1782–1786.
44. Ewalt DH, Sheffield E, Sparagana SP, et al. Renal lesion growth in children with tuberous sclerosis complex. *J Urol* 1998;160:141–145.
45. Nelson CP, Sanda MG. Contemporary diagnosis and management of renal angiomyolipoma. *J Urol* 2002;168:1315–1325.
46. Tello R, Blickman JG, Buonomo C, et al. Meta analysis of the relationship between tuberous sclerosis complex and renal cell carcinoma. *Eur J Radiol* 1998;27:131–138.
47. Vasavada SP, Corrales JG, Elder JS. Renal tumors in children. In: Resnick MI, Older RA, eds. *Diagnosis of genitourinary disease*, 2nd ed. New York: Thieme, 1997:411–424.
48. Bissler JJ, Racadio J, Donnelly LF, et al. Reduction of postembolization syndrome after ablation of renal angiomyolipoma. *Am J Kid Dis* 2002;39:966–971.
49. Fazeli-Matin S, Novick AC. Nephron-sparing surgery for renal angiomyolipoma. *Urology* 1998;52:577–583.
50. Broecker B. Renal cell carcinoma in children. *Urology* 1991;38:54–56.
51. Asanuma H, Nakai H, Takeda M, et al. Renal cell carcinoma in children: experience at a single institution in Japan. *J Urol* 1999;162:1402–1405.

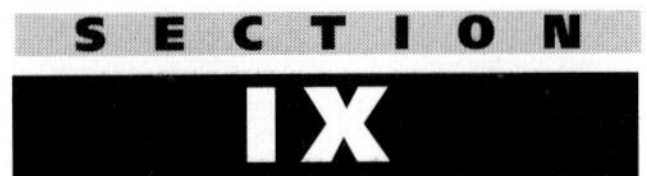

SECTION IX

HYPERTENSION

59

EPIDEMIOLOGY OF HYPERTENSION

JEAN U. BENDER
MELVIN A. BONILLA-FELIX
RONALD J. PORTMAN

Hypertension (HTN) is of immense national importance. Mild to moderate HTN remains one of the major risk factors for the development of atherosclerosis and subsequent cardiovascular disease (CVD) and cerebrovascular disease. The role of the pediatric nephrologist and others caring for children includes not only the management of patients with established high blood pressure (BP) but also the identification of children at risk for HTN and the initiation of preventive measures when indicated. In addition, new evidence suggests that the most prevalent form of HTN in pediatrics is now essential or primary HTN. The prevalence is increasing in concert with the epidemic of childhood obesity. Further, essential HTN during childhood is associated with end-organ damage (EOD) and thus is not benign. The existing definitions of HTN have, by necessity, been epidemiologic in nature. New definitions for both casual and ambulatory measurements must be functional and based on the presence of EOD.

The treatment of HTN has greater beneficial impact on CVD risk than any other intervention. There is renewed interest in the issues surrounding BP measurement. These issues have major impact on the interpretation of important major national and international treatment trials. For example, changes in nocturnal BP when casual BP (CBP) measurements are normal have been correlated with the development of microalbuminuria. Thus, the issues of BP measurement in the assessment of HTN and its treatment require careful scrutiny (1).

This chapter reviews the epidemiology of HTN in childhood, including discussions of the controversial issue of BP measurement; the chronobiology of BP; definitions of HTN; the effects of age, gender, ethnicity, maturation, diet, body mass, and birth weight on BP; genetics of HTN; the course of primary HTN; and the association of BP with EOD.

MEASUREMENT OF BLOOD PRESSURE

Casual Blood Pressure

The proper techniques for the diagnosis and evaluation of HTN in children remain unclear although several decades have passed since the first large-scale normative data became available (2,3). BP is defined as the pressure of the blood within the arteries, maintained by the contraction of the left ventricle, the elasticity of the arterial walls, as well as the viscosity and volume of the blood. Systolic BP (SBP) is defined as the pressure occurring at the moment of ventricular systole, whereas diastolic BP (DBP) is the pressure noted during ventricular diastole, immediately preceding systole. Technical problems exist with all forms of BP measurement. Even the gold standard of intraarterial BP measurement has technical problems and shows variability depending on the chosen artery, catheter positioning within the artery, and the equipment used. The available normative data have been developed using noninvasive techniques. BP measurement by palpation is inaccurate, but because the reappearance of the pulse is an approximation of SBP, it can be used to determine the starting point for an auscultatory measurement. The two major noninvasive CBP techniques are auscultatory and oscillometric. Both present significant technical challenges that are affected by the technology itself, the patient, and the person taking the measurement.

Patient Issues

Patient-related issues are similar for all types of CBP measurement and include the ingestion of stimulants (e.g., caffeine, pseudoephedrine), inclusion of an appropriate resting period, patient position, ambient temperature, and level of anxiety. As outlined in the *Update on the 1987 Task Force Report on High Blood Pressure in Children and Adolescents* (3), the environment should be controlled and the child should rest for 3 to 5 minutes before BP measurements are taken. BP readings are obtained from a child in the seated position (supine for infants) from a fully exposed right arm resting on a supportive surface at heart level with back supported and feet firmly on the floor. One must ensure that the inflatable bladder that encircles the circumference of the arm is wide enough to cover more than 40% of the distance from the acromion to the olecranon and neither obstructs the placement of the stethoscope bell at the antecubital fossa nor interferes with the axilla. Use of a small BP cuff may result in falsely elevated readings; use of too large of a cuff may cause minimally lower readings. Clark et al. (4) described the difficulty in selecting appropriate cuffs from the many available sizes and its critical importance to accurate BP measurement in children with all BP measurement techniques. Incorrect measurement can result in unnecessary investigations, treatment, or follow-up for the misdiagnosis of HTN. Cuff selection is of particular importance in children, who have normal age-dependent variations in body size and BP. One cannot rely on the size listed on the proprietary cuff, for example, "infant" or "child" cuff, as there is tremendous variation between companies in this labeling. Rather, one must measure the arm to select a cuff fulfilling Task Force criteria. Larger BP cuffs are required if upper arm length is used as the primary criterion for cuff selection. In contrast, smaller cuffs are required if 40% of the upper mid-arm circumference is used as a criterion for cuff selection. No single cuff, when used in accordance with current recommendations, yields accurate SBP as well as DBP. How to select a proper cuff size for an accurate measurement of BP remains unresolved, but until better data are available, the Task Force recommendations should be followed.

Technical Issues

Although the proper BP measurement techniques may be debated for years, the critical issue is not comparison of one technique with another but comparison of the readings obtained using any chosen technique with the occurrence of hypertensive EOD.

Auscultation

To obtain a measurement using auscultation, the BP cuff is inflated to approximately 20 mm Hg higher than the pressure necessary to occlude the brachial pulse as determined by palpation; pressure is then released at 2 to 3 mm Hg/sec while the observer identifies Korotkoff sounds over the brachial artery. Too rapid or too slow a rate of deflation results in inaccurate readings, as does parallax when a mercury manometer is used. Two readings should be obtained and averaged at each visit to estimate a child's BP level. Studies from our group show that when three measurements are used, the second of three measurements had the best correlation to the mean of the three, which confirms that 2 measurements are generally sufficient (5).

Identification of appropriate Korotkoff sounds presents an area of difficulty in measuring BP in children. K1 (SBP) is recorded when the first tapping sound is heard as the pressure in the BP cuff is released and is caused by the opening of the artery. K2 is characterized by a constant murmur after the tapping sounds, and K3 occurs as the pressure is further released and the sounds become crisper and more intense. K4 is a low-pitched, muffled sound; K5 is the disappearance of all sounds. In some children, K4 and K5 occur so closely that they are indistinguishable; in others K5 never occurs. By adolescence, however, K5 is easily identified. Despite these difficulties, the American Heart Association and the updated Task Force guidelines (3) have identified K5 as a reliable definition of DBP for children and adolescents of all ages. If K5 is not observed, the DBP can be recorded as K4 if heard. Difficulties in performing auscultatory techniques in smaller children, in developing acceptable definitions of DBP (K4 vs. K5), and in minimizing interobserver variability have led many physicians' offices and clinics to opt for technically easier and more reproducible ways to measure BP.

Despite their status as the gold standard, mercury manometers, when systematically evaluated, show a significant number of problems that may preclude accurate use, even if the observer and patient issues are overcome. In several studies in the United Kingdom, a high prevalence of technical problems (18 to 38%) was noted, such as dirty columns, oxidized mercury, faded column markings, mixing of air in the mercury column, or mercury leakage, which led to inaccurate measurement by 21% of monitors (6–8). In a systematic evaluation of sphygmomanometers, *none* of the 356 instruments tested met all standards, and 86% did not meet safety standards (9). For these reasons, mercury manometers soon are likely to be phased out in Europe and the United States (10) in spite of recommendations by the American Hospital Association and the Seventh Report of the Joint National Committee on Prevention, Detection, Evaluation, and Treatment of High Blood Pressure (JNC VII) to retain their use (6).

The aneroid manometer functions through a system composed of a metal bellows, a mechanical amplifier, springs, and a gauge that displays the pressure in the cuff. Aneroid devices are often felt to be less accurate than mercury columns because of the difficulty in keeping them functional (11,12). Aneroid manometers were evaluated in many of the same studies cited for the assessment of mercury manometers and demonstrated even more inaccuracies.

A trained individual must have good hearing acuity, must be aware of digit preference, and must know the "rules" of the auscultatory method. So prevalent are these technical difficulties that the random zero manometer was developed. With this device, the observer is blinded to the reading until after the measurement has been completed. Although such units are the gold standard for research, they are not readily available on a clinical basis.

If "ideal" auscultation is assumed, how good is the match between BP measured using the Korotkoff sounds and direct measurements of BP? Because they are all measuring some component of BP, the statistical correlations are quite strong. Nevertheless, there can be some remarkable differences between the two. K1 appears on average 3 mm Hg below direct systolic pressures. K5 disappears on average 9 mm Hg above direct diastolic pressure (13). There is still controversy in pediatrics over whether K4 or K5 should be used to assess the "true" diastolic pressure (14). If the data cited here apply to children, K4 would clearly be much higher than true diastole.

Oscillometry

All of these difficulties in measurement, the time required for the measurement in a busy practice, and the interobserver variability led to the development of oscillometric monitors. Development of the first commercial oscillometric device for BP measurement started in the early 1970s and resulted in the Dinamap, an acronym for "device for indirect noninvasive mean arterial pressure" (15). Many oscillometric devices for automated BP measurement have been introduced and new models of the Dinamap updated. With oscillometric devices, cuff inflation and deflation are automated and BP determination is made by a microprocessor using information sent to it from a pressure transducer. A great advantage that makes this technique popular is its ease of use and the elimination of observer bias. The BP cuff automatically inflates on first measurement to a set value determined by algorithm and, with subsequent measurements, inflates to 20 to 35 mm Hg above the previously recorded systolic value. Deflation occurs in a set bleed step such as 4, 8, or 10 mm Hg that varies by device and, in some, can be set at different levels. As the cuff pressure decreases, oscillations of the arterial wall increase in amplitude and reach a maximum when the cuff pressure approaches the mean arterial pressure. With further deflation of the BP cuff, oscillations diminish and eventually stop. The monitor then computes the information and displays heart rate (HR) and mean BP, SBP, and DBP. The precise method of BP determination is complex and uses an algorithm that varies from one device to another. It is unknown whether the device is actually measuring or calculating the displayed values. These algorithms are considered proprietary information and thus are not made public. It is therefore impossible for investigators to verify the accuracy of their underlying physiologic principals. The measurement results of these devices cannot be used interchangeably because of their different algorithms (16). Measurements obtained using both oscillometric and mercury manometers correlated well with intraarterial measurements (17), including those determined with pediatric and neonatal Dinamap models.

What is the agreement between auscultatory and oscillometric measures? In fact, it is not particularly good for many devices. Unfortunately, the most commonly used monitors have been demonstrated to give variable results in multiple studies. This should not be a surprise, because the techniques are not measuring the same "pressure." We have a dilemma facing us. The available normative data from the Task Force are based mostly on auscultatory and mercury technology. The easier-to-use oscillometric technique is now the prevalent technology, but we do not have adequate epidemiologic normative data. Although the techniques measure different "pressures," the definitions of HTN that must be developed are those that are predictive of EOD. Standardized oscillometric monitor certification for use on children, development of new epidemiologic normative data in comparison with EOD, and, finally, careful ongoing calibration of monitors by biotechnicians are needed.

Self-Measurement of Blood Pressure

Measurement of BP outside the clinician's office may provide valuable information for the initial assessment of patients with HTN and for monitoring of the response to treatment (19). Self-measurement of BP (SMBP) has four general advantages: (a) distinguishing sustained HTN from *white-coat HTN* (WCH), (b) assessing response to antihypertensive medication, (c) improving patient adherence to treatment, and (d) potentially reducing costs. There is no universally agreed-upon upper limit of normal home BP, but readings of 135/85 mm Hg or higher in adults should be considered elevated (18). No data are available on pediatric norms for SMBP. SMBP appears to allow improved assessment of BP and its control under pharmacologic therapy. Mercury and aneroid sphygmomanometers are generally not practical for home use. Therefore, validated electronic devices (oscillometric) that have proven to be accurate according to standard testing are recommended for use, along with appropriately sized cuffs. Wrist and finger monitors are inaccurate. Periodically, the accuracy of the patient's device should be checked by comparing its readings with simultaneously recorded auscultatory readings taken with a mercury device. Few of the many self-monitors on the market have passed the criteria of the British Medical Society (20) or the Association for the Advancement of Medical Instrumentation (21). A Task Force of the European Society of Hypertension has suggested new criteria for this assessment (22). A review of available monitors has been published (23).

BPs measured outside of the physician's office tend have lower values. Six studies comparing SMBP and CBP demonstrated a consistently lower BP by SMBP (SBP 5.4 ± 17.7 mm Hg lower and DBP 1.5 ± 6.3 mm Hg lower). Three studies comparing ambulatory BP (ABP) and SBP show similar daytime BP results. Some preliminary studies have examined the prevalence of WCH determined using SMBP and have compared the results to determination of the same diagnosis by ABP, finding similar results (approximately 20% WCH). There were significant methodologic concerns, however, that suggest some problems with this conclusion, such as small sample sizes of heterogeneous populations, variable definitions of HTN by CBP and SMBP, and no reproducible data. Only one study has examined the correlation of SMBP results with clinical events. SMBP showed a marginally better correlation with left ventricular hypertrophy (LVH) than did CBP (SBP: SMPB R = 0.47 vs. CBP R = 0.44; DBP: SMBP R = 0.4 vs. CBP R = 0.37) but no advantage in correlation with microalbuminuria (19).

Better data are available regarding monitoring of the efficacy of antihypertensive therapy using SMBP. Interventions that included SMBP showed improved BP control in 6 of 12 trials (19). SMBP enables monitoring of both BP and BP variation. Along with BP measurements, the time of the measurement and the time and dose of antihypertensive medication should be recorded as specified by the Joint National Committee. In two trials using technology that stored the BP data in a computer, both documented reduced BP from intervention that included this technology. Although the results are inconsistent, there is promise, especially with report-generating monitors, that SMBP can lead to improved BP control.

The reliability and accuracy of the monitors themselves are important; however, another important issue that must be addressed in the use of SMBP is the reliability of the measurement recording. There are several studies performed using a BP device that stores the readings on an internal chip. In the majority of the studies, the devices were given to patients without their knowledge of this capability. The patients were asked to record their BP in a log as usual and then the stored results were compared with the patient-generated log books. Patient reports had mean differences in BP of a least 10 mm Hg for SBP and 5 mm Hg for DBP compared with stored BP readings (24). In another study, 36% of patients underreported and 9% overreported BP readings. Log books also contained phantom readings; conversely, patients failed to report measurements that were taken and stored (25). This type of patient reliability in home monitoring is not unique to BP measurement. Similar findings were observed with the use of glucometers by diabetic patients (26) and in records of metered dose inhaler usage by asthmatic patients (27). Thus, although SMBP has the potential to make an important contribution in BP diagnosis and management, objective recording of the data is strongly advised. SMBP is a useful adjunct to CBP measurement, can be performed by many patients, and is consistent with the goal of self-management.

Ambulatory Blood Pressure Monitoring

The use of ABP monitoring (ABPM) in children has been described in detail by Portman et al. (28). In brief, the ABPM device is attached to the subject's nondominant arm with an appropriately sized BP cuff using Task Force criteria. SBP and DBP levels are measured at 20-minute intervals during the 24-hour period. To avoid subject biofeedback, the monitors can be programmed not to display BP measurements. A bleed step of 8 mm Hg allows accurate readings that are well tolerated by children. These monitors are small and lightweight and have appropriately sized cuffs for use in children of all ages. The keys to successful monitoring are adequate patient instruction, which includes the need to keep the monitor dry, holding the arm motionless during the reading, applying the cuff in the appropriate way, and maintaining an adequate diary and provision of a person to contact about any problems. The diary should include at a minimum the time of going to sleep and the time of waking, including naps or disrupted nighttime sleep, as well as the timing of any medications taken during the period. The monitor's accuracy (within approximately 5 mm Hg) must be validated by comparison with mercury manometry before use. Adequate study is approximately 85% confirmed successful readings. ABPM use is feasible in children, and the measurements obtained using this device correlate well with those obtained using mercury manometry, which conforms to the guidelines proposed by O'Brien et al. (29) for ABPM validation. Monitors using different technologies, including oscillometric, auscultatory, auscultatory with electrocardiogram gating and intraarterial monitors, and Finapres beat-to-beat constant monitoring are available. The authors prefer the oscillometric monitor because it provides fewer nonsense readings in loud environments usually associated with children and is well tolerated. Although standards for monitoring children have yet to be developed, the use of the ABPM in children has great promise for the diagnosis and management of HTN in children.

Chronobiology of Blood Pressure

Biologic functions and processes are organized not only in space, as in physical anatomy, but also in time, as biologic rhythms. These rhythms are endogenous, heritable traits that can be described in specific, quantifiable terms (30). Knowledge of BP rhythms and the factors controlling them is important for the proper diagnosis and treatment of HTN. BP demonstrates a circadian rhythm composed of a daytime (diurnal) period and a nighttime (nocturnal) period. However, the environmental day-night rhythm is superseded by the biologic clock as reflected by the periods of wake and sleep (31). Although a low-amplitude circadian rhythm can be identified, shift workers have BP patterns more closely related to their activity. In addition, BP is the same during a daytime nap as during nighttime sleep. Consequently it is important to classify ABPM data not in terms of day and night, but rather wake and sleep. BP not only follows a circadian rhythm but also varies minute to minute. Thus, the use of a single random BP measurement to characterize circadian BP levels or long-term behavior of a continuous variable is as unrealistic as use of a weekly single measurement of blood glucose level compared to glycosylated hemoglobin (32).

Healthy individuals display a sleep-related fall in BP. Its multifaceted etiology is determined by physical activity, emotional factors, and circadian rhythms in the sympathetic nervous system (SNS), hormone levels, and the cardiovascular system (31). A person whose mean BP falls by 10% from wake to sleep (sleep/wake ratio of <0.9) is termed a *dipper*; an individual whose BP fails to do so is termed a *nondipper*. A person whose BP is higher during sleep periods has a reversed BP rhythm. Reproducibility of "dipper" status on repeated studies remains unclear (33).

TABLE 59.1. THRESHOLDS FOR AMBULATORY BLOOD PRESSURE MEASUREMENTS (mm Hg) IN ADULTS

	95th percentile	Normotension	Hypertension
24 h	132/82	≤130/80	≥135/85
Daytime	138/87	≤135/85	≥140/90
Nighttime	123/74	≤120/70	≥125/75

Note: Thresholds are based on epidemiologic studies of normotensive and hypertensive individuals as well as morbidity and mortality. From Staessen JA et al. *Blood Press Monit* 1999;4:127–36, with permission.

During the active process of sleep (31) there is a progressive fall in BP in the first hour as the stages of sleep progress; BP maximally decreases 15 to 20% after approximately 2 hours of sleep, which coincides with sleep stages 3 and 4. This fall in BP with sleep is accompanied by a decrease in HR and cardiac output. BP tends to rise during REM (rapid-eye-movement) sleep but remains lower than values during wakefulness. BP and HR rapidly increase on awakening in association with activation of the SNS and its receptors. There are normal sleep-related changes in renal function that during pathologic states may contribute to HTN. Renal blood flow and glomerular filtration rate (GFR) fall by approximately 20% in association with a pronounced decrease in urine flow due to an increased tubular reabsorption of water, sodium, and chloride. Plasma catecholamine levels also fall during sleep consistent with diminished SNS activity, whereas plasma renin, aldosterone, and antidiuretic hormone levels steadily rise concomitantly throughout the night. Renin secretion also rises during non-REM sleep and minimally during REM sleep.

Considerable data now define ABPM values in normotensive adults based on EOD (Table 59.1) (34,35). An increasing number of studies in children describe age- and

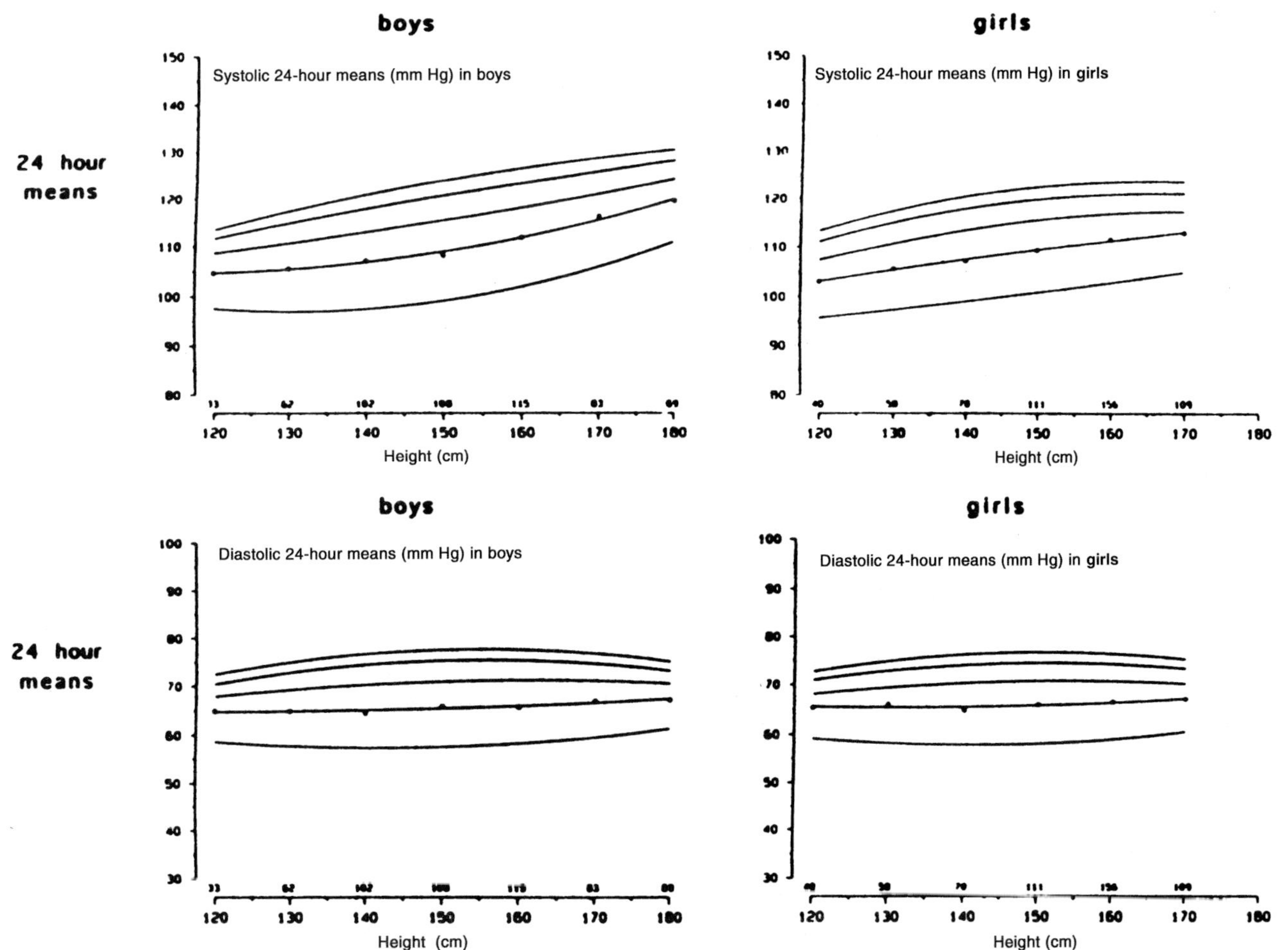

FIGURE 59.1. Twenty-four-hour mean BP values for 1141 children related to height, with systolic blood pressure in the upper two graphs and diastolic in the lower two. Values for boys are on the left side and girls the right. The points show the raw median values for each height group. The lines represent the fitting polynomials for the tenth, fiftieth, ninetieth, and ninety-fifth percentiles. The numbers along the x-axis indicate the number of subjects in each height group. (From Soergel M, Kirschstein M, Busch C. Oscillometric twenty-four-hour ambulatory blood pressure values in healthy children and adolescents: a multicenter trial including 1141 subjects. *J Pediatr* 1997;130:178–184, with permission.)

size-specific normal values for ABP. There have now been several studies in the United States, United Kingdom, Spain, Germany, Italy, and Brazil attempting to establish normal ABPM values for children. However, in none of these studies is the population of sufficient size in each age, size, and ethnic category and the measurements of BP performed with the same techniques and equipment so as to provide true normal data. The International Pediatric Hypertension Association is in the process of combining these studies to develop more generalizable normative data. Future studies examining ABPM will need to incorporate measures of EOD in the definition of HTN. The largest multicenter study, reported by Soergel et al. (36) in central Europe, provides the best available data (Fig. 59.1). The normative data were based on the child's height (115 to 185 cm). Findings show a moderate increase in fiftieth-percentile SBP with increasing height from 103 to 113 mm Hg in girls and from 105 to 120 mm Hg in boys. The fiftieth percentile for DBP was 66 ± 1 mm Hg regardless of gender or height. A new statistical approach to ABPM normalizes data, which permits the use of an SDS score for the purposes of diagnosis (37). Importantly, no statistical technique can really diagnose true HTN, which is the BP that can predict the presence of EOD. The report of the Ambulatory Blood Pressure Monitoring Task Force II (38) stated that, although it is difficult to validate diagnostic reference values based on morbidity and mortality because of low incidence rates in children, functional rather than distribution-based definitions of ambulatory HTN must be developed. This point is critical because most studies of adults and children have shown a better correlation of ABP to EOD than for CBP measures.

DEFINITIONS OF HYPERTENSION

Casual Blood Pressure

HTN is a leading risk factor for CVD, renal disease, and stroke. In addition, it is believed that primary HTN has its roots in childhood. Thus, accurate definition and early identification of HTN risk is imperative but, as yet, not possible. Ideally the definition of HTN would identify individuals at risk for adverse outcomes when BP level exceeds a determined threshold; subjects with BP levels lower than the definition would be at little or no risk for adverse outcomes related to BP. Because no such dividing line exists in the continuum of BP, arbitrary levels (based on CBP) have been established to define persons who are at risk for morbid cardiovascular events and who will benefit from therapy.

The literature for adult patients is replete with studies correlating HTN with various adverse outcomes (39). Information from such studies linking BP elevations to outcomes of mortality, nonfatal myocardial infarction, congestive heart failure, stroke, renal failure, LVH, and advancement of atherosclerosis has been instrumental in guiding expert committees in efforts to reduce the morbidity of HTN. Based on these outcome studies, definitions of HTN have changed, becoming ever lower so that 130/80 is the currently recognized upper limit of normal. In contrast to the situation for adults, BP levels considered to be hypertensive in children have yet to be fully correlated with cardiovascular morbidity and mortality, as they occur infrequently in children. However, convincing evidence has been reported that pediatric HTN is not benign and that many cardiovascular risk factors found in adults begin in childhood. Hypertensive EOD damage is discussed later in the chapter. Although other large studies have been published with somewhat different results, the *Update on the 1987 Task Force Report on High Blood Pressure in Children and Adolescents* (3) is probably the most widely used source of information on BP in children and provides us with statistical definitions of HTN. The Task Force Report is a compilation of data from 10 studies and includes data for more than 60,000 white, African American, and Hispanic children. From these studies, age-specific percentile curves of BP measurements for boys and girls ranging in age from birth to 18 years have been developed with the inclusion of BP tables adjusted for height (Tables 59.2 and 59.3) for children older than 1 year of age. By using these curves, one can compare measured BP levels to age-, gender-, and height-specific norms. To use these tables, a child's BP is measured and the height percentile is calculated using standard growth charts. The measured BP and age-specific height percentile are compared with the values on the gender-specific tables. If the BP is below the ninetieth percentile, the child is normotensive. If the measured BP is between the ninetieth and ninety-fifth percentiles, the patient is considered to have high-normal BP, and observation and consideration of risk factors for HTN are initiated. Measurements higher than the ninety-fifth percentile may indicate a diagnosis of HTN, and repeated measurements are indicated. A new updated Task Force report is expected in the near future that will publish norms based on the latest Centers for Disease Control and Prevention data on height in children as well as more information on oscillometric, ambulatory, and home monitors. No changes in the standards for SBP and DBP for infants younger than 1 year were reported in the 1996 update (3); data for healthy subjects published in the Task Force report of 1987 (40) should be used.

No recommendations on the timing of BP measurement are included in the Task Force recommendations, although repeated measurements over time are encouraged (3). Future Task Force recommendations may include advice such as more information about the 24-hour pattern of BP in children as it becomes available. It is critical to recall that these data are from the *first* measure obtained for each child in each study. It is well recognized, however, that with repeated measurement there is regression to a lower average value. The pediatric definition of HTN, therefore, is arbi-

TABLE 59.2. BLOOD PRESSURE LEVELS FOR THE 90TH AND 95TH PERCENTILES OF BLOOD PRESSURE FOR BOYS AGED 1 TO 17 YEARS BY PERCENTILES OF HEIGHT

		SBP by percentile of height (mm Hg)[b]							DBP by percentile of height (mm Hg)[b]						
Age (yr)	BP percentile[a]	5th	10th	25th	50th	75th	90th	95th	5th	10th	25th	50th	75th	90th	95th
1	90th	94	95	97	98	100	102	102	50	51	52	53	54	54	55
	95th	98	99	101	102	104	106	106	55	55	56	57	58	59	59
2	90th	98	99	100	102	104	105	106	55	55	56	57	58	59	59
	95th	101	102	104	106	108	109	110	59	59	60	61	62	63	63
3	90th	100	101	103	105	107	108	109	59	59	60	61	62	63	63
	95th	104	105	107	109	111	112	113	63	63	64	65	66	67	67
4	90th	102	103	105	107	109	110	111	62	62	63	64	65	66	66
	95th	106	107	109	111	113	114	115	66	67	67	68	69	70	71
5	90th	104	105	106	108	110	112	112	65	65	66	67	68	69	69
	95th	108	109	110	112	114	115	116	69	70	70	71	72	73	74
6	90th	105	106	108	110	111	113	114	67	68	69	70	70	71	72
	95th	109	110	112	114	115	117	117	72	72	73	74	75	76	76
7	90th	106	107	109	111	113	114	115	69	70	71	72	72	73	74
	95th	110	111	113	115	116	118	119	74	74	75	76	77	78	78
8	90th	107	108	110	112	114	115	116	71	71	72	73	74	75	75
	95th	111	112	114	116	118	119	120	75	76	76	77	78	79	80
9	90th	109	110	112	113	115	117	117	72	73	73	74	75	76	77
	95th	113	114	116	117	119	121	121	76	77	78	79	80	80	81
10	90th	110	112	113	115	117	118	119	73	74	74	75	76	77	78
	95th	114	115	117	119	121	122	123	77	78	79	80	80	81	82
11	90th	112	113	115	117	119	120	121	74	74	75	76	77	78	78
	95th	116	117	119	121	123	124	125	78	79	79	80	81	82	83
12	90th	115	116	117	119	121	123	123	75	75	76	77	78	78	79
	95th	119	120	121	123	125	126	127	79	79	80	81	82	83	83
13	90th	117	118	120	122	124	125	126	75	76	76	77	78	79	80
	95th	121	122	124	126	128	129	130	79	80	81	82	83	83	84
14	90th	120	121	123	125	126	128	128	76	76	77	78	79	80	80
	95th	124	125	127	128	130	132	132	80	81	81	82	83	84	85
15	90th	123	124	125	127	129	131	131	77	77	78	79	80	81	81
	95th	127	128	129	131	133	134	135	81	82	83	83	84	85	86
16	90th	125	126	128	130	132	133	134	79	79	80	81	82	82	83
	95th	129	130	132	134	136	137	138	83	83	84	85	86	87	87
17	90th	128	129	131	133	134	136	136	81	81	82	83	84	85	85
	95th	132	133	135	136	138	140	140	85	85	86	87	88	89	89

BP, blood pressure; DBP, diastolic blood pressure; SBP, systolic blood pressure.
[a]BP percentile was determined by a single measurement.
[b]Height percentile was determined by standard growth curves.

trarily higher than the true ninety-fifth percentile for the pediatric population. With repeated measurement, the Task Force (40) and others (41) estimate that only approximately 1% of children and adolescents will ultimately prove to have HTN. However, these estimates of the prevalence of pediatric HTN must be balanced against the observation that the epidemiology of cardiovascular risk factors in children is changing for the worse. In the United States, the prevalence of obesity among children increased from 5 to 11% in national surveys from the 1960s to the 1990s. Current estimates of the prevalence of obesity among school-aged children are even higher. Because the Task Force data were collected primarily in the 1970s and 1980s the current pediatric 95th percentile would almost certainly be higher than in previous decades. More recent studies place the prevalence of HTN much higher than previously reported (42), particularly among ethnic minority adolescents. Sorof et al. (42) reported an estimated prevalence of HTN of 17% after one measurement, comparable to the Task Force data; subsequently the prevalence was reduced to 7% after three measurements were taken. Thus, the current prevalence of pediatric HTN is likely to be greater than the 1% quoted in the Task Force report. One possible explanation for this variance could be that the oscillometric method of BP measurement was used for the Sorof et al. study whereas the auscultatory method was used to collect the data for the Task Force. Oscillometric methods, as noted previously, can yield a higher SBP than auscultatory methods, but even this could not fully explain a sevenfold increase in HTN prevalence. The prevalence of EOD of 47% in a similar group of our patients suggests that the diagnosis is valid. A more likely explanation is the fact that

TABLE 59.3. BLOOD PRESSURE LEVELS FOR THE 90TH AND 95TH PERCENTILES OF BLOOD PRESSURE FOR GIRLS AGED 1 TO 17 YEARS BY PERCENTILES OF HEIGHT

		SBP by percentile of height (mm Hg)[b]							DBP by percentile of height (mm Hg)[b]						
Age (yr)	BP percentile[a]	5th	10th	25th	50th	75th	90th	95th	5th	10th	25th	50th	75th	90th	95th
1	90th	97	98	99	100	102	103	104	53	53	53	54	55	56	56
	95th	101	102	103	104	105	107	107	57	57	57	58	59	60	60
2	90th	99	99	100	102	103	104	105	57	57	58	58	59	60	61
	95th	102	103	104	105	107	108	109	61	61	62	62	63	64	65
3	90th	100	100	102	103	104	105	106	61	61	61	62	63	63	64
	95th	104	104	105	107	108	109	110	65	65	65	66	67	67	68
4	90th	101	102	103	104	106	107	108	63	63	64	65	65	66	67
	95th	105	106	107	108	109	111	111	67	67	68	69	69	70	71
5	90th	103	103	104	106	107	108	109	65	66	66	67	68	68	69
	95th	107	107	108	110	111	112	113	69	70	70	71	72	72	73
6	90th	104	105	106	107	109	110	111	67	67	68	69	69	70	71
	95th	108	109	110	111	112	114	114	71	71	72	73	73	74	75
7	90th	106	107	108	109	110	112	112	69	69	69	70	71	72	72
	95th	110	110	112	113	114	115	116	73	73	73	74	75	76	76
8	90th	108	109	110	111	112	113	114	70	70	71	71	72	73	74
	95th	112	112	113	115	116	117	118	74	74	75	75	76	77	78
9	90th	110	110	112	113	114	115	116	71	72	72	73	74	74	75
	95th	114	114	115	117	118	119	120	75	76	76	77	78	78	79
10	90th	112	112	114	115	116	117	118	73	73	73	74	75	76	76
	95th	116	116	117	119	120	121	122	77	77	77	78	79	80	80
11	90th	114	114	116	117	118	119	120	74	74	75	75	76	77	77
	95th	118	118	119	121	122	123	124	78	78	79	79	80	81	81
12	90th	116	116	118	119	120	121	122	75	75	76	76	77	78	78
	95th	120	120	121	123	124	125	126	79	79	80	80	81	82	82
13	90th	118	118	119	121	122	123	124	76	76	77	78	78	79	80
	95th	121	122	123	125	126	127	128	80	80	81	82	82	83	84
14	90th	119	120	121	122	124	125	126	77	77	78	79	79	80	81
	95th	123	124	125	126	128	129	130	81	81	82	83	83	84	85
15	90th	121	121	122	124	125	126	127	78	78	79	79	80	81	82
	95th	124	125	126	128	129	130	131	82	82	83	83	84	85	86
16	90th	122	122	123	125	126	127	128	79	79	79	80	81	82	82
	95th	125	126	127	128	130	131	132	83	83	83	84	85	86	86
17	90th	122	123	124	125	126	128	128	79	79	79	80	81	82	82
	95th	126	126	127	129	130	131	132	83	83	83	84	85	86	86

BP, blood pressure; DBP, diastolic blood pressure; SBP, systolic blood pressure.
[a]BP percentile was determined by a single reading.
[b]Height percentile was determined by standard growth curves.

45% of the population was either Hispanic or African American and that 38% of the population was overweight or obese. Figure 59.2 shows that the prevalence of HTN increases as body mass index increases (42).

Ambulatory Blood Pressure Monitoring

The interpretation of the ABPM data should be based on the BP levels that are associated with EOD rather than on an epidemiologic definition of HTN. There are numerous studies of adults and now several of the pediatric population demonstrating that various ABPM parameters have an excellent correlation with EOD, whereas correlation with CBP is weaker or absent. As stated in the Sixth Report of the Joint National Committee on Prevention, Detection, Evaluation and Treatment of High Blood Pressure (JNC

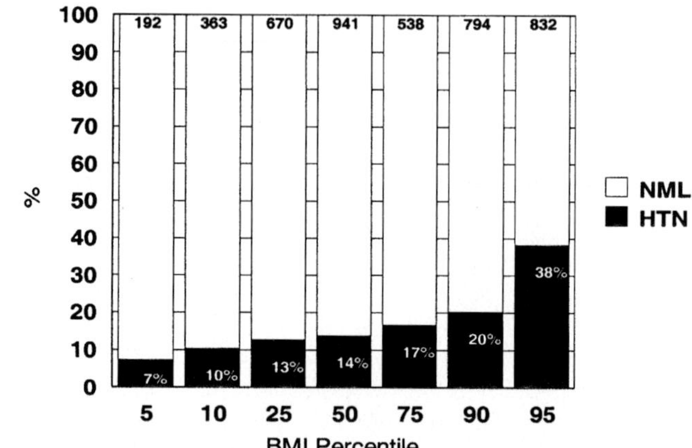

FIGURE 59.2. Hypertension prevalence by body mass index (BMI) percentile. NML, normal; HTN, hypertension.

VI) (18), "Among persons with HTN, an extensive and very consistent body of evidence indicates that ABP correlates more closely than clinic BP with a variety of measures of target organ damage such as left ventricular hypertrophy." The definitions take into account distributions of ABP in normal and hypertensive populations, and validation of diagnostic thresholds in terms of LVH and in terms of morbidity and mortality (Table 59.1) (43). A meta-analysis of 18 studies demonstrated that CBP measurements were higher than 24-hour, wake or sleep ABP measurements (19). ABPM data can be analyzed by a number of different statistical approaches. Which of these is the superior and most clinically applicable is still unanswered. Most observers use the 24-hour mean SBP and DBP and also separate the 24-hour period into day-night or the more appropriate sleep-wake periods (44). Others choose to separate the waking BP periods into 8-hour segments: those of stress such as work or school, those of other activities, and sleep. The first 2 hours of any ABPM may be excluded as an accommodation period during which time BP levels are higher than in the rest of the readings (45).

The BP load for adults is defined as the number of SBP or DBP measurements during the wake period exceeding 135/85 plus the number of BP levels during sleep exceeding 120/75 divided by the total number of measurements during 24 hours times 100 (46,47). For pediatric patients, it is defined as the percentage of total BP measurements exceeding the upper limit of normal for age, size, and time of day. The BP load represents the summation of the peaks of BP and is believed to measure the maximal stress on the heart and other organs. As discussed later, increased BP loads have an excellent correlation with EOD. An advantage of this concept is that BP load can be influenced not only by the mean BP but also by its variability. Thus, a patient with high-amplitude swings in BP can be diagnosed as hypertensive even if the mean BP is near normal. Because the BP load is determined by comparison with age- and size-related normal values, one can compare the BP challenge of diverse patient groups. It is generally accepted that BP loads of 25% or more constitute HTN for a given time period and that BP loads above 40% in adults and 50% in children (48) are strongly associated with EOD. Analysis using BP load data is limited by a ceiling value of 100%. A patient with all BP levels mildly elevated would not be at the same risks as those with more severe BP elevations. A new concept called the BP index (48) can serve as a quantitative assessment of the degree the BP exceeds the upper limit of normal for a given time period. In early studies, it has been demonstrated to have a strong correlation with EOD in children. The index is calculated by dividing the patient's BP by the ninety-fifth percentile. For example, a BP index of 1.2 would be 20% higher than the ninety-fifth percentile for an individual measurement or for a specific time period.

As mentioned previously, mean BP tends to fall by 10 to 20% during sleep periods relative to waking levels. A dipper is a person who has a minimum of a 10% fall in mean BP. Nondippers have been found to have an increased incidence of EOD including LVH, stroke, and cardiovascular events. The status of dipping may be less important than the diagnosis of HTN within the period. A patient with severe HTN may have more than a 10% fall in sleep BP but have significant HTN during sleep. Conversely, 30% of children may not be dippers but may have perfectly normal sleep BP levels. In adults, age, clinic BP, diabetes, duration of sleep, smoking habits, and work activity are the most important determinants in attenuation of the nocturnal BP drop in patients with essential HTN (49). Numerous studies demonstrate very strong association between sleep period HTN and EOD. Conversely, excessive dipping ("super dipping"), especially in the elderly, can be associated with silent cerebrovascular lesions such as lacunar infarcts (50).

These abnormalities observed during the sleep period may occur secondary to a lack of physical and emotional activity, which permits less variability and therefore a heightened sensitivity for the detection of abnormal BP. Alternatively, there are specific changes that occur during sleep that may cause abnormalities not observed during the waking period.

There is a considerable list of conditions associated with sleep-related HTN or nondipper status in adults, including abnormalities of the SNS (diabetes, pheochromocytoma, dysautonomias) and renin system [chronic kidney disease (CKD), end-stage renal disease, renovascular diseases], glucocorticoid therapy or Cushing's syndrome, solid organ transplantation, sleep apnea, and preeclampsia. In particular, a blunted fall in BP appears to be a ubiquitous finding in renal diseases (51). Farmer et al. demonstrated a rise in nondipping prevalence with worsening renal function (Fig. 59.3) (52). Almost 80% of adult patients with sleep apnea syndrome are both obese and hypertensive (53); conversely, 22 to 30% of adult hypertensive patients have sleep apnea. In pediatric patients, a similar phenomena has been observed in, for example, transplant, dialysis, African American, and diabetic patients as well as in those with secondary forms of HTN (48).

The most commonly implicated potential mechanisms of sleep-related HTN in children with CKD are increased activity of the SNS, insulin insensitivity, decreased antidiuretic hormone excretion during sleep, sleep apnea, and, the most often reported, volume overload with decreased sodium excretion. Evidence for the latter also comes from a return to a dipper status when sodium restriction and/or diuretic therapy is instituted (51). Stolarz et al. (33) reviewed the Osahama study and the predictive value of sleep-related HTN with CVD. In that study, a linear and inverse relationship was demonstrated between cardiovascular mortality and the nocturnal decline in BP. Overall, each 5% increment in the systolic or diastolic night-to-day ratio was associated with a 20% rise in the risk of CVD,

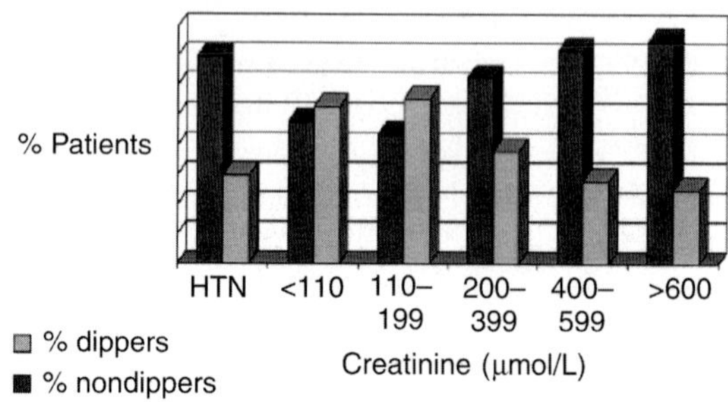

FIGURE 59.3. Blunting of the diurnal blood pressure rhythm of predialysis patients is more severe as renal failure worsens. HTN, hypertension. (From Farmer CKT, Goldsmith DJA, Cox J, et al. An investigation of the effect of advancing uraemia, renal replacement therapy and renal transplantation on blood pressure diurnal variability. *Nephrol Dial Transplant* 1997;12:2301–2307, with permission.)

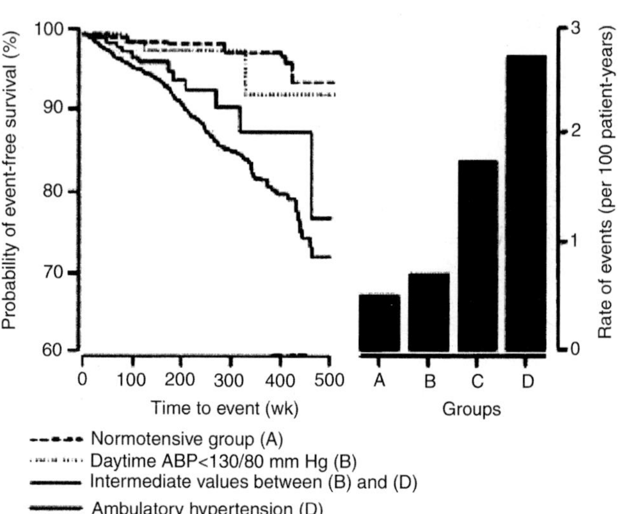

FIGURE 59.4. In the Hypertension and Ambulatory Recording Venetia Study of 942 patients with stage 1 hypertension (HTN), patients with white-coat HTN (WCH) had significantly lower left ventricular mass and microalbuminuria than did patients with established HTN, and there was no difference in end-organ damage between WCH patients and normotensive controls. ABP, ambulatory blood pressure. (From Palatini P, Mormino P, Santonastaso M, et al. Target organ damage in stage 1 hypertensive subjects with white coat and sustained hypertension. Results from the HARVEST study. *Hypertension* 1998;31:57–63, with permission.)

even when 24-hour ABP was within the normotensive range. Patzer (37) published a paper examining the diagnosis of HTN in the sleep period in children with CKD due to renal scarring. The diagnosis of HTN was more specific using ABPM than CBP and it was the nocturnal BP changes that were most specific. New techniques for examining the BP challenge may come from the rate-pressure product (HR BP) × over the 24-hour period. The standard deviation of the BP measurements is considered an excellent measure of variability of BP and has also been considered a separate risk factor for HTN-induced EOD (54).

White-Coat Hypertension

WCH is a conditioned, transient, elevation of BP in a medical setting when the BP is normal at other times. Its reported prevalence as measured by ABPM is 20 to 60% in adults and 28 to 88% in children. The mistaking of WCH for persistent HTN may lead to unnecessary diagnostic studies and medication use. ABP has been most useful in making this diagnosis (55). A meta-analysis by Appel et al. (19) found that the prevalence of WCH was approximately 20% in the population of adults diagnosed as hypertensive by CBP. Too few studies were available to determine the reproducibility of this classification. Under standardized conditions, SMBP is also effective in identifying WCH. There is debate in the literature regarding the question of whether WCH is an intermediate state between normotension and HTN, or a prehypertensive state. The Ambulatory Blood Pressure Monitoring Task Force (56) determined that event-based studies of hypertensive patients have convincingly demonstrated that the risk of CVD is lower in patients with properly defined WCH than in those with higher ABP levels, even after controlling for concomitant risk factors. Based on prognosis in adults, WCH can be defined as a CBP that is persistently 140/90 mm Hg or higher with an average daytime ABP of below 135/85 mm Hg (56). Individuals with WCH were found to have a lower risk of CVD than those with sustained HTN, although the authors concluded that no prospective study adequately compared the risk of those having WCH with that of normotensive patients (55). The finding that patients with WCH have significantly less EOD than those with persistent HTN and the same as control subjects is noted in the Hypertension and Ambulatory Recording Venetia Study (HARVEST) (57) (Fig. 59.4).

We studied 350 pediatric patients younger than 18 years of age with persistently elevated BP who were not taking concurrent antihypertensive medications or other medications that could affect BP levels. Seventy-one patients met these criteria and were studied with ABPM. Over half of these patients (55%) had WCH by ABPM as judged from mean BP; 21% had WCH when a normal BP load was required as well (58). Adult studies suggest that, the higher the JNC VI grade of HTN, the lower the prevalence of WCH. This is also true in children, as seen in Figure 59.5, which shows that the likelihood of diagnosis of WCH is 90% for patients with a BP index of 1.0 (on the 95th percentile) but less than 15% for those with a BP index of 1.2 (20% over the 95th percentile). The prevalence of WCH in patients CKD has not been determined reliably. WCH is more prevalent in patients with milder HTN in both adults and children. Thus, the prevalence of WCH might be lower in patients with CKD.

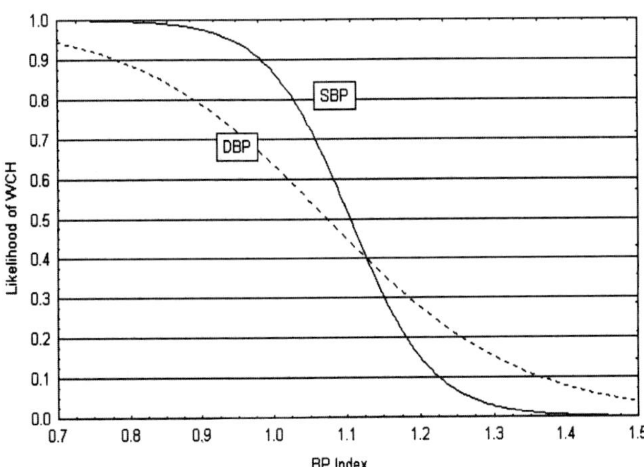

FIGURE 59.5. Blood pressure (BP) index versus probability of white-coat hypertension (WCH). DBP, diastolic blood pressure; SBP, systolic blood pressure.

Ambulatory Blood Pressure Monitoring in Chronic Kidney Disease

The emphasis of this text is pediatric nephrology, and thus the issue of BP in CKD should be carefully examined. Both JNC VI and JNC VII recommend ABPM for specific circumstances, including diagnosis of suspected WCH and evaluation of patients with apparent drug resistance, hypotensive symptoms while taking antihypertensive medications, episodic HTN, and autonomic dysfunction. The Kidney Disease Outcomes and Quality Initiative Hypertension Work Group has suggested that ABPM is valuable in patients with CKD because of the close correlation of the data with EOD and because of the alterations in circadian BP rhythms noted in CKD patients but has stopped short of recommending it for routine use. Authoritative reviews suggest that ABPM has advantages in evaluation of essential HTN (19). ABPM has been widely used for the past decade, but its use has been limited because of the expense of the equipment, the time involved in patient training and data analysis, and, until recently, the lack of consistent insurance reimbursement.

Level of BP and abnormal patterns as measured by ABPM show a high correlation with EOD, such as cardiovascular mortality and events, abnormal LV mass and function, cerebrovascular events, and glomerular and tubular proteinuria, and is capable of identifying abnormal circadian BP rhythms such as nocturnal HTN. ABP is also important in demonstrating the rapid rise in early morning BP that is associated with a high risk for cardiovascular events. There is a growing body of evidence showing that nondipping is associated with a worse prognosis, irrespective of whether nighttime dipping is studied as a continuous or a categorical variable (59). A metaanalysis of 25 studies of the relationship of ABP levels with EOD showed that LV mass was positively associated with ABP (19). In ten studies, at least one dimension of ABP predicted subsequent clinical events prospectively. The metaanalysis agreed that a nondipping or reverse dipping pattern was associated with an increased risk of adverse events. The international conference on ABPM in 2001 agreed that, although the incidence of cardiovascular events has some correlation with CBP, the use of ABPM significantly refined the prediction. In the large Systolic Hypertension in Europe Trial, 24-hour SBP measurements were found to be a significant predictor of cardiovascular risk (60). Some but not all studies have reported an independent and positive relationship between measures of *variability* of daytime and nighttime BP and cardiovascular outcome. Finally, it has been suggested that ABP patterns can be predictive of preeclampsia early in pregnancy and that intervention with aspirin may prove beneficial in prevention (61).

Insufficient evidence exists to conclude that adjusting medications using ABP is superior to adjustment using CBP measurements. The metaanalysis (19) concluded that ABP has not been studied adequately to assess its role in antihypertensive therapy.

The most common circadian rhythm abnormalities seen in CKD patients is sleep-associated HTN and a nondipping BP pattern. Among such patients the prevalence of a nondipping pattern is high (67%) (62–64). These patterns are reproducible, with 67% of CKD patients maintaining their diurnal rhythm and 82% having a predictable pattern on repeated monitorings. The patterns were even more reproducible in transplant and dialysis patients (59). The mechanisms for this pattern have not been carefully elucidated (65). It was also demonstrated that the prevalence of nondipping patterns increases as GFR decreases (Fig. 59.3). Fifty-three percent of CKD patients with a serum creatinine level of 400 mmol/dL had a nondipping pattern; the proportion progressed to 75% for those with a creatinine level of above 600 mmol/dL (66). The nondipping pattern observed in those with type 1 and 2 diabetes (67) has also been related to the presence of microalbuminuria. CKD patients, particularly kidney transplant patients, may have a reversed BP pattern of higher BP during sleep than waking.

Children with CKD have altered patterns of BP that make the diagnosis of HTN in the normal clinic setting difficult. Lingens et al. (68) examined 31 children with CKD of whom 62% were diagnosed as hypertensive by CBP, 38% by home BP measurements, and 26% by ABPM. One-quarter of the patients had abnormal BP rhythms. The primary rhythm abnormality was a blunted sleep-related fall in BP; that is, nondipping status, which was commonly associated with sleep-related HTN. In several studies, isolated sleep-related HTN has been observed with normal wake pressures in unilateral renal dysplasia (69) and in polycystic kidney disease (70). The abnormal patterns increase as GFR declines (71,72). They are also more prevalent in dialysis patients and renal transplant

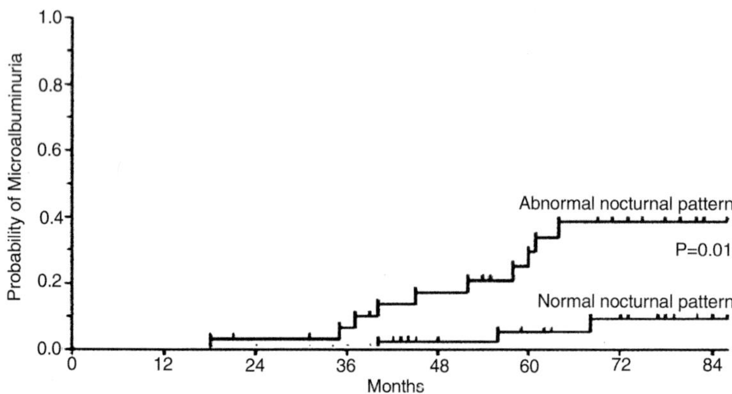

FIGURE 59.6. Followed from the time of enrollment, nocturnal ambulatory blood pressure elevations predated the development of microalbuminuria in patients with type 1 diabetes.

patients (73–75). Up to 78% of transplant patients have been reported to have a nondipping pattern and 24% to have a reversed BP pattern (73). It has been suggested (76) that ABPM can aid in differentiating primary from secondary HTN in children. A combination of daytime DBP load greater than 25% and nocturnal SBP load of greater than 50% was very specific for secondary HTN.

Abnormal ABP patterns have been shown to be related to varying degrees of abnormal protein excretion. Abnormal or nondipping pattern in ABPM measurements is strongly correlated with microalbuminuria and proteinuria, and this correlation is superior to that found with CBP measurement. This has been shown in studies of patients with type 1 diabetes (77,78), type 2 diabetes (67,79), type 1 and type 2 diabetes combined (80–82), and essential HTN (57,83–85). In the few studies examining possible mechanisms, autonomic dysfunction has been implicated (78,82).

Importantly, it has been shown in a landmark article that ABPM can identify individuals at risk for development of CKD. In type 1 diabetes, nocturnal BP elevations determined by ABPM predated the development of microalbuminuria (Fig. 59.6) (77). Identifying individuals at risk for development of microalbuminuria provides an important window of opportunity for primary prevention.

The correlation of EOD with cardiovascular end points is similar in patients with CKD to that reported in hypertensive patients. There are few studies of patients with CKD that examine the relationship of ABP to morbid or mortal events. Three hundred and twenty-five patients with non–insulin-dependent diabetes mellitus (NIDDM) were studied, with ABP circadian rhythm assessed by cosinor analysis (86). After an 8-year follow-up 201 patients had a normal circadian rhythm and 87 a reversed one. Twenty subjects in group 1 (9.9%) had nonfatal (cerebrovascular, cardiovascular, peripheral vascular, or retinal events) or fatal events versus 56 patients (64.4%) in the reversed group. Circadian pattern of BP and age had the greatest effect on adverse events in a Cox proportional hazards model. The same correlation between ABP and measures of LV mass is seen regardless of the cause of CKD: autosomal dominant polycystic kidney disease (87), kidney failure (88,89), glomerulonephritis (90), HTN with albuminuria (91,92) immunoglobulin A nephropathy (93), NIDDM (86), and renal transplantation (64,94). The recurring theme in these articles is positive correlation of LV mass with ABP parameters, most commonly a nondipping pattern or sleep-related HTN. In each of the studies there were either weak or, more commonly, no correlations between CBP and these outcomes. Combining the 24-hour SBP with a measure of dipping, the night to day ratio, was a strong predictor of cardiovascular end points in the Systolic Hypertension in Europe Trial.

Abnormal ABP patterns have been related to more rapid progression of kidney disease. There are five studies that examine the association of ABP with renal disease progression. In 126 patients with immunoglobulin A nephropathy, those who had ambulatory HTN developed higher creatinine values, whereas the normotensive patients, with or without antihypertensive therapy, had stable serum creatinine. Nondippers made up 93% of the hypertensive patients. The normotensive patients who were nondippers also had higher creatinine values than dippers (95). In a 3-year case-control study, 48 patients with CKD were studied: 28 dippers and 20 nondippers (96). Nondippers had a faster decline in GFR (4.4 mL/min/yr) than dippers (3.2 mL/min/yr) and a higher mean protein excretion. In a similar study of diabetic patients, nondippers had a 7.9 mL/min/yr decline compared to 2.9 for nondippers (97). Finally, Nakano et al. (98) examined 257 NIDDM patients with normal circadian rhythms (194 patients) or reversed patterns (63 patients). More patients with a reversed pattern (23.5%) than patients with a normal rhythm (3%) progressed to dialysis (86). Jacobi et al. (99) demonstrated the relationship between creatinine levels 6 months after transplantation and ABP levels.

Due to these abnormal patterns, the correlation between CBP and ABP is poor, as is the relationship of CBP to EOD. A poor correlation (R = 0.61) was found between office BP measurements and ABP measurement in kidney transplant patients (100). Three studies of diabetic patients all showed a significant association between ABP and urinary albumin excretion in cases in which CBP failed to do so. Once again, SBP and nocturnal elevations had the clos-

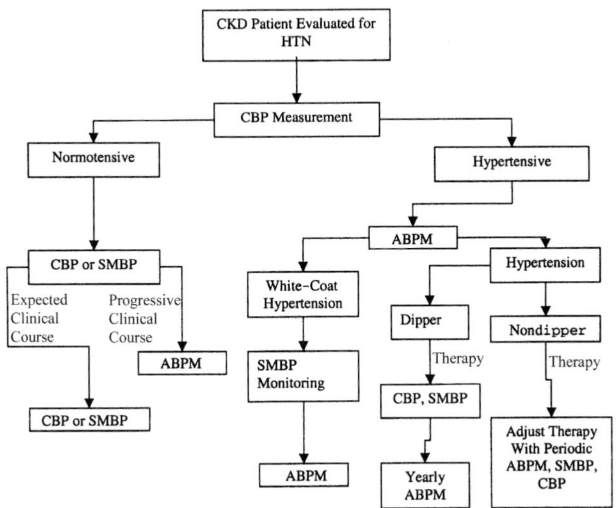

FIGURE 59.7. Proposed paradigm for use of ambulatory blood pressure monitoring in evaluation of hypertension in patients with chronic kidney disease (CKD). ABPM, ambulatory blood pressure monitoring; CBP, casual blood pressure; HTN, hypertension; SMBP, self-measurement of blood pressure.

est correlation to this measure of EOD. In nondiabetic CKD patients, five studies have demonstrated the same finding. McGregor et al. found a nondipping pattern in renal transplant patients. This pattern was associated with LVH, whereas CBP did not show such an association (64). Tucker et al. demonstrated that casual SBP and DBP had a weak correlation of 0.25 to 0.22 with LVH in 16% of his CKD patients, whereas systolic ABP had a correlation of 0.52 and diastolic ABP had a correlation of 0.42. Nocturnal BPs showed an even better correlation (88).

Cardiovascular mortality is rare in pediatric patients, although it is much more common in CKD patients than in the general pediatric population. Thus, determination of more subtle hypertensive damage is critical to an assessment of the effects of HTN or therapy for HTN. ABP correlates better with measures of LVH than does CBP in pediatric CKD patients (101–104). HTN determined by ABPM has also been shown to correlate with evidence of LV dysfunction and increased intimal-medial thickness (105). There have been no long-term studies of the treatment of HTN in children with CKD using ABPM.

The diagnosis of nocturnal HTN could affect the requirement for antihypertensive therapy in CKD patients. The concern in CKD patients who have altered patterns of BP and a nondipping BP pattern is that (a) measuring CBP may not correctly represent BP burden and risk, and (b) confining the definition of WCH to the daytime BP comparison may include patients with sleep-related HTN in the WCH category.

Insufficient evidence exists to determine whether ABPM is a better monitoring tool than CBP for assessing the effect of antihypertensive treatment and outcomes of antihypertensive therapy. LVH was found to be present only when CKD patients were noted to have persistently abnormal ABP, not abnormal CBP. When treatment decisions were made on the basis of CBP, 13% of patients had LVH, compared with none of the patients whose treatment decisions were controlled by ABP criteria (91). A comparison of lisinopril with nisoldipine showed a decrease in microalbuminuria with no differences between albuminuria groups as measured by CBP; however, there were differences between groups in nighttime SBP when measured by ABP (106). A potential paradigm for the integration of various BP measurement technologies in HTN evaluation in CKD patients is presented in Figure 59.7.

PEDIATRIC STUDIES

Epidemiology of Hypertension

Age

BP levels are closely related to growth and maturation (107). Children have lower BP levels than adults, but the levels progressively increase as the child ages. At birth, a term infant has a SBP of close to 70 mm Hg (108). During the first week of life BP increases at a rate of approximately 1 mm Hg/day. After the first week the rise in BP continues at a fairly rapid rate, although slightly slower than in the first week, and then rises more slowly throughout the remainder of the first year of life. DBP begins at approximately 40 mm Hg at birth for a term infant. It also increases during the first week of life but then falls to a nadir at approximately 3 months of age. It then increases in parallel to the SBP throughout the remainder of the first year of life (109). From ages 1 to 13 years, a linear rise in BP is observed. This seems to be the result more of an increase in body size than an increase in age. From childhood to adolescence, SBP rises 1 to 2 mm Hg per year. The rise in DBP is slower (110).

The increase in SBP and DBP during the first year of life occurs at a faster rate in premature infants than in term infants (111). Among groups of premature infants, very-low-birth-weight infants have a more dramatic increase in BP than do larger preterm infants. By approximately 4 months of age, BP levels for both groups of preterm infants are similar to those of term infants.

Gender

Gender plays an important role in BP variability. Not only are there differences in BP levels between the genders, but changes in the pattern of development of BP are also observed from an early age. In girls, SBP rises more rapidly between 6 and 11 years of age than it does from 12 to 17 years of age. In boys, the opposite is seen; a more rapid rise in BP is observed from 12 to 17 years than from 6 to 11 years of age. Although not universal, by the age of 12 to 14 years boys tend to have higher mean BP levels than do girls. These changes probably reflect the gender-specific differences in rates of growth and maturation. Male predominance of higher BP levels lasts until approximately 50 years of age, when women's BP levels once again exceeds men's (109,111,112).

Race

The African American population has an incidence of HTN that is at least twice that among whites for nearly every age- and sex-matched group (113). These racial differences can be observed from childhood (114,115). Not only are CBP levels altered, but the circadian rhythm of BP in African Americans is also different from that in whites, with a blunted nocturnal BP dip (116). Those of African descent living in the Western hemisphere, including African Americans, have BP levels and 24-hour patterns of BP that are different from those of African natives (117,118). This finding suggests that, in addition to genetic factors, the environment plays a key role in BP determination.

HTN in the African American population seems to be sodium mediated. Based on these observations, the potential role of genes encoding for proteins involved in the renin-angiotensin system has been studied in African American populations. Serum levels of angiotensinogen are higher in African American than in white children (119). A higher frequency of a deletion polymorphism in the angiotensin-converting enzyme (ACE) gene has been observed in African Americans with HTN. This suggests a potential role for a salt sensitivity phenotype mediating HTN in blacks (120).

Racial differences in BP levels between African American and white children are not observed until approximately age 12 years. By this age small differences have been reported in some epidemiologic studies. Interestingly, although African American children generally demonstrate higher DBP levels from age 12 years, white children of both genders generally have higher mean SBP levels than do African American children. Some studies report that these differences disappear when socioeconomic status is considered (112). African American adults have a higher incidence of HTN than whites.

Berenson et al. have shown that African American male children have higher supine BP levels than whites and there is little relationship of HR to BP levels or body weight (121). In this same group of children, higher cardiac outputs were demonstrated in white children than in African American children after adjustment for body size. African American children also were noted to have higher peripheral vascular resistance than white children (122). Not surprisingly, BP in African American children was more sensitive to sodium (114,123,124). In addition, greater cardiovascular reactivity has been described in African American children (115,125–127). Higher cardiovascular reactivity to stress, especially in African American patients, may lead to misclassification because of higher office BP measurements. African American children exhibited higher 24-hour mean ABP than white children, and there was a good correlation between BP during stress and mean ABPM results (128).

No dramatic differences in BP levels have been identified among other racial groups. Data from six European studies have been pooled to provide specific percentile values for children in northwest European countries (129). A comparison of the results of this European study to those of the Task Force reveals lower BP means and percentiles in the Task Force results (North American children). The average difference in systolic measurements between the two studies is approximately 6 mm Hg for both genders; the difference in DBP for both genders is approximately 3 mm Hg. The reasons for this difference are unknown but might include methodologic differences as well as actual population differences.

Body Mass

Mechanisms proposed to explain the relationship of obesity and higher BP, none of which has been proven, include increased cardiac output in an arterial tree that is of normal size, expansion of the blood volume, increased sodium intake with increased caloric intake, increased steroid production, and alteration of receptors for pressor substances (130). More recently, leptin has been implicated as a potential factor linking body mass with HTN. Animal and human data suggest that leptin is involved in BP regulation through the leptin receptor (131). Regardless of the cause, weight reduction is associated with a decrease in BP (109,132–137). HTN has been found to be more common in obese children. In a study of 2460 adolescent students (49% Hispanic, 31% African American, 13% white) 17% were found to have HTN after one measurement and 23% were obese (138). Of the HTN students, 88% had isolated systolic HTN. HTN was more prevalent in obese students (33%) than in nonobese students (11%) ($p < .001$). Obese students also had a higher resting HR (85.9 vs. 79.6 beats/min, $p < .001$) consistent with other studies, which suggests a higher activation of the SNS (139). Among those patients studied with ABPM, isolated systolic HTN was found in 51% by CBP and in 62% confirmed by ABPM. BP variability was greater during wake and sleep periods in obese patients ($p < .05$). Sorof and Daniels have reviewed this topic in detail (140).

In addition to weight, height appears to be an independent predictor of BP. Portman et al. (141) and Voors et al. (142) have reported stronger correlation of BP with height than with weight in adolescents. This effect is independent of the level of maturation (143,144). Data suggest that some of the racial differences in BP levels could be explained by differences in body mass index (145). If white and African American populations with low body mass indices are compared, BP levels are higher in blacks. However, at the highest levels of body mass indices, high BP levels and HTN (systolic or diastolic) are more common in whites (146).

Physical Activity

The level of fitness has a significant but variable effect on ABPM profiles, particularly in African American subjects (147). Although exercise is generally promoted to improve overall cardiovascular fitness, its role as an independent factor decreasing BP levels is less clear (132). The effect on BP level may depend on the type of exercise performed. Dynamic (isotonic or aerobic) exercise decreases BP in hypertensive adolescents (148,149) and is generally recommended as part of an overall healthy lifestyle (109,132). In contrast, during static (isometric) exercise, there is a marked increase in DBP due to muscular contraction. The resultant increase in muscle mass leads to an increase in CBP (109,132). Programs emphasizing aerobic forms of exercise can be recommended to improve physical conditioning, whereas those emphasizing isometric exercise should be avoided.

A common area of concern for adolescents and parents of children with HTN is participation in various kinds of sports. Sports that feature dynamic exercise appear to improve overall cardiac fitness; the long-term effect of sports programs that feature static exercise remains less clear. Before embarking in competitive sports and highly static activities, children with cardiac symptomatology should undergo exercise stress testing to identify arrhythmias, ST-segment depression, or excessive BP increases. This may preclude some from participation in sports until clarification of the condition. Patients who have uncontrolled HTN and who have not yet responded to therapy should wait before starting sport activities (149). Once BP is under control, dynamic exercise training should be encouraged for better control of HTN and overall cardiovascular conditioning. Children with controlled HTN should not be restricted from sports participation (149).

Role of Sodium

The relationship between salt intake and BP remains controversial. Although several epidemiologic studies have shown that BP levels are significantly higher in societies with high salt intake, the results from clinical trials involving children and adults have been far less impressive (150–160). It is likely, however, that some people are genetically susceptible to the effects of salt and that at least some of the variability in BP is due to salt intake (161). Salt sensitivity is defined as an elevation in BP during high salt intake. Approximately 50% of patients with essential HTN are salt sensitive (162). Although this phenomenon is more commonly observed in hypertensive subjects, it has been documented in normotensive subjects as well. It is more prevalent among older patients and patients with low plasma renin activity (PRA), or low renin HTN (162).

The BP response to sodium intake seems to be genetically determined. The cross-transplantation experiments of Dahl et al. in 1974 demonstrated that sodium sensitivity was determined largely by the genotype of the donor kidney rather than by that of the recipient (163). Transplantation of a sodium-sensitive kidney to a sodium-resistant rat resulted in sodium sensitivity in the latter, and vice versa. Normotensive first-degree relatives of hypertensive subjects have lower urinary sodium excretion after a saline load than do relatives of nonhypertensive subjects (164). The average U.S. diet contains an overabundance of sodium. Therefore, modest reductions in salt intake may be advisable as a general good health practice for hypertensive patients. However, severe reduction in salt intake may be inappropriate for rapidly growing children and adolescents.

Nephron Number

The idea that HTN is programmed by an adverse environment *in utero* was first proposed by Barker, who reported a strong association between HTN in adult life and retarded growth in fetal life (165,166). The relation between BP and birth weight becomes stronger as the patient ages. At 7 years of age SBP increases by 1.3 mm Hg and DBP by 0.6 mm Hg for each 1-kg decrease in birth weight (167). By age 64 to 71 years, the effect is more marked, with a decrease in SBP of 5.2 mm Hg for every 1-kg increase in birth weight (168). In humans low birth weight, length at birth, and small body in relation to placental size have been related to the development of HTN and coronary heart disease. It has been proposed that undernutrition during fetal life may stimulate an elevation in BP, which is amplified during time and results in HTN in adult life. This suggests that HTN is initiated in fetal life (169). Using ABPM, Lurbe et al. examined 332 children 6 to 16 years of age who were stratified by birth weight tertiles and age. Birth weight was inversely related to daytime SBP and BP load when current height, ponderal index, and age were controlled (170).

Brenner and colleagues have elaborated this hypothesis, suggesting that the relationship between HTN and low birth weight is the result of low nephron number in low-birth-weight infants. This directly relates birth weight to nephron mass at birth and suggests an inverse relationship between nephron number and risk of HTN (171–173). Impaired fetal growth results in a permanent decrease in nephrons. Subsequent accelerated growth leads to excessive metabolic demands for the limited renal mass. Specifically, a decreased ability to handle sodium load results in excessive sodium retention and systemic HTN. In addition, glomerular HTN causes progressive nephron loss and worsening of systemic HTN and renal function (172,173).

TABLE 59.4. GENES RESPONSIBLE FOR SELECTED MONOGENIC VARIANTS OF HYPERTENSION-CAUSING DISORDERS

Syndrome	K+	pH	Renin	Aldo	Specific treatment	Gene loci	Gene
GRA	↓	↑	↓	↑	Spironolactone (amiloride, triamterene)	8q	Chimeric gene (*CYP11B1/CYP11B2*)
Liddle's syndrome	↓	↑	↓	↓	Amiloride, triamterene	16p	β and γ subunit of ENaC
AME	↓	↑	↓	↓	Spironolactone (amiloride, triamterene)	16q	11β-HSD
MR	↓	↑	↓	↓	None, multiple drug therapy	4q	MR
Gordon's syndrome	↑	↓	↓	↓	Hydrochlorothiazide	1q	Unknown
						12p13	WNK1
						17p	WNK4
HBS[a]	N	N	N(↓)	N	None, multiple drug therapy	12p11	Unknown

↑, increase; ↓, decrease; Aldo, aldosterone; AME, apparent mineralocorticoid excess; GRA, glucocorticoid-remediable aldosteronism; HBS, hypertension brachydactyly syndrome; K^+, potassium; MR, mineralocorticold receptor; N, normal.
[a]Contrary to the rest, HBS is not a salt-sensitive condition and is characterized by normal values for the parameters shown.
From Toka HR, Luft FC. Monogenic forms of human hypertension. *Semin Nephrol* 2002;22:81–88, with permission.

This hypothesis seems to be supported in a number of clinical instances. In low-birth-weight infants, for instance, reduced nephron number seems to translate into a more rapid rise in BP than in weight gain and a higher incidence of essential HTN later in life.

GENETICS OF HYPERTENSION

Essential HTN is a complex disease that is influenced by both genetics and the environment. Although Robert Platt believed that BP was inherited in a simple autosomal dominant manner, he was one of the first to recognize the influence of genetics on HTN (174). George Pickering proved this theory wrong and suggested that HTN was caused by multiple genes (174a). Although multiple genes are suspected to cause the variation in BP, no one knows exactly how many genes are involved or how much effect each gene has (175). The heritability of HTN is 30 to 40%, which implies that only 30 to 40% of the interindividual difference in BP is due to genetics (176). Identifying these genes is daunting. One of the challenges is the difficulty in defining the phenotype for HTN. Potential influential genes are discovered usually by genome scans or search for candidate genes. A big advancement in the genetics of HTN is the identification of genes responsible of some of the monogenic variants of HTN (Table 59.4). Understanding the genetics of HTN is beneficial not only in identifying those at risk but also in better predicting the response to treatment and developing new therapies.

Familial Aggregation

Given that HTN is more common and more severe in particular ethnic groups, genes likely play an important role (177). HTN is also known to aggregate in families. Longini et al. studied families from Tecumseh, Michigan, and determined heritabilities of 0.42 and 0.30 for SBP and DBP, respectively (178). Early twin studies have confirmed the heritability of BP variation (179). Adoption studies have also been performed to study the heritability of HTN. Biron et al. performed an adoption study of French-Canadian families. After studying families with adopted children, natural children, and with both adopted and natural children, Annest et al. concluded that 34% of the variability in BP is genetically determined, 11% is due to the environment, and the remaining 55% is due to random factors (176a).

Genome Scans

Identifying the genes influencing BP is a formidable task. Currently, there are three main techniques (180). One way is to perform a genome scan to try to find regions that are similar for patients with HTN. Another method is to look at candidate genes, which are genes whose product is suspected of influencing BP based on its physiologic function. A third method is to identify genes that cause HTN in rare monogenic types of HTN and determining if these genes are altered in essential HTN.

Rice and his colleagues performed a genome scan on patients in the Quebec Family Study. They investigated 206 patients and used 420 polymorphic markers. Although they identified no site with a lod score higher than 3, they did find some peaks on chromosomes 1, 2, 5, 7, 8, and 9 (181). Another design using genome scanning is the study of highly discordant siblings. Krushkal and her group did a genome scan on discordant siblings. She performed a genome scan of 359 polymorphic markers on 427 participants, consisting of 69 discordant sib pairs. Her group identified four regions (on chromosomes 2, 5, 6, and 15) that showed significant results and eight regions that were suggestive. Some of these regions have been identified as containing candidate genes that are known to contribute to BP variation (182). Levy and his group performed a genome scan on 1702 subjects in the Framingham Heart Study and was able to identify a maximum lod score of 4.7 on chromosome 17; interestingly, this chromosome contains the gene responsible for Gordon's syndrome (180). Because HTN is a complex polygenic disorder, genome scans are a difficult way to identify new genes accounting for the variation in BP.

Candidate Genes

Evaluating candidate genes is a popular tool in molecular genetics. Although several genes have been studied, five are most promising at this point. These include angiotensinogen, ACE gene, β_2-adrenergic receptor, α-adducin gene, and G-protein β_3 subunit.

Angiotensinogen Gene

The angiotensinogen gene was the first gene to be associated with high BP (183). Genetic linkage analysis performed on populations from Utah and Paris identified the substitution of methionine by threonine at position 235 to be associated with BP. This 235T variant was associated with higher levels of circulating angiotensinogen and higher BP. Other studies, however, have not been able to replicate these findings. Brand and her colleagues conducted a large European study involving 630 affected sib pairs and were not able to show an association between angiotensinogen levels and the 235T variant (184). A meta-analysis performed by Kunz et al. did find a small association between the 235T variant and HTN (odds ratio 1.2) (185). Therefore, the discrepancy in these studies is most likely due to the fact that, although the angiotensinogen gene does influence BP, its effect is small.

Angiotensin-Converting Enzyme Gene Polymorphism

ACE gene polymorphisms have also been studied for their role in HTN. Although such polymorphism has been associated more with myocardial infarction than with BP, several studies have linked polymorphism to BP in particular groups (186). Busjahn et al. has shown that the D allele is associated with ACE plasma levels and cardiac posterior wall thickness by echocardiography (187). Another study showed a positive association between BP and the ACE gene. Fornage and her group looked at a population from Rochester, Minnesota, and found an association between ACE alleles and variation in DBP for males but not for females (188). O'Donnell et al. also found increased DBP to be associated with the D allele in their male but not in their female subjects (189). Turner et al. determined that the effect of I/D polymorphism on BP was dependent on gender, age, height, and weight (190). Several studies have focused on the influence of genetic differences in the ACE gene in determining the responsiveness to a particular therapy. Jacobsen et al. showed that possessing the deletion polymorphism for the ACE gene resulted in a decrease in response of BP and proteinuria to therapy in diabetic patients (191). Although it exhibits a small effect, the ACE gene is likely to be one of the many genes influencing BP.

β_2-Adrenergic Receptor Gene

Polymorphisms in the β_2-adrenergic receptor gene have been associated with HTN. Kotanko et al. studied 136 hypertensive and 81 normotensive people of African Caribbean descent and detected an association between HTN and a variant in the β_2-adrenergic receptor gene involving a substitution of glycine for arginine at position 16 (192). Busjahn et al. looked at the β_2-adrenergic receptor gene in twins and found that four single nucleotide polymorphisms in the β_2-adrenergic receptor gene were associated with BP levels (193). Bray and her colleagues identified several polymorphisms in the ADRB2 gene that were associated with HTN (194). However, Herrmann et al. conducted a large European study looking at the relation between polymorphisms in the β_2-adrenergic receptor gene and outcome, and did not find an association with HTN or risk for myocardial infarction (195).

α-Adducin Gene

Findings regarding the role of the α-adducin gene in HTN have been conflicting. Glorioso et al. genotyped 490 hypertensive and 176 normotensive people from Sassari, Italy, and 468 hypertensive and 181 normotensive people from Milano, Italy. His group detected an association of the Gly460Trp variant with HTN in the Milano group but not in the Sassari group (196). Province et al. identified an association between the α-adducin gene Gly460Trp variant and HTN in whites but not in African Americans. They genotyped 822 white subjects and 572 African American subjects as part of the HyperGEN study and found an odds ratio of 1.73 [95% confidence interval (CI), 1.17 to 2.54] for whites for the development of HTN. Interestingly, the Gly460Trp variant was actually protective against the development of HTN in African American patients, with an odds ratio of 0.48 (95% CI, 0.25 to 0.90) (197). Bray et al. could not find an association between the α-adducin gene and BP when performing a linkage analysis on sib pairs from Rochester, Minnesota (198). However, Psaty et al. showed that patients possessing the Gly460Trp variant of the α-adducin gene had a decreased risk of myocardial infarction or stroke when their BP was controlled by diuretic therapy versus nondiuretic therapy (odds ratio, 0.49; 95% CI, 0.32 to 0.77) (199).

β_3 Subunit of G Proteins

Siffert et al. identified a polymorphism (C825T) in the β_3 subunit of G proteins that was significantly associated with HTN (200). Turner et al. evaluated the ability of the T allele of the C825T polymorphism from the β_3 subunit of G proteins to predict the response to diuretic therapy. One hundred ninety-seven hypertensive African American adults and 190 hypertensive non-Hispanic whites were genotyped for the β_3 subunit of G proteins. After a 1-month washout period, all participants received hydrochlorothiazide for 4 weeks. The TT patients had the greatest response to the diuretic followed by the TC patients; the CC patients had the smallest response. The investigators predicted that the TT polymorphism accounted for 3.1% and 4.5% of interindividual variation in SBP and DBP response, respectively (201).

Monogenic Hypertension

HTN secondary to specific monogenic mutations, including those causing Liddle's syndrome, glucocorticoid-remediable aldosteronism, and apparent mineralocorticoid excess syndrome (Table 59.4) are described in Chapter 60.

Autosomal Dominant Hypertension with Brachydactyly

Autosomal dominant HTN with brachydactyly is a very rare monogenic hypertensive syndrome that has been identified in only three kindreds, one in northeastern Turkey, one in Canada, and one in the United States (202,203). This syndrome is characterized by severe, salt-insensitive HTN. Although the gene has been mapped to the short arm of chromosome 12, it has not yet been cloned (202,203). Frequently multiple antihypertensive medications are required to control the BP in this disease (204).

TRACKING OF BLOOD PRESSURE

BP tracking refers to the maintenance of one's position in the percentile distribution for BP levels over time. The prevalence of HTN is much higher in adults whose BPs during childhood were in the top quintile. The risk of becoming an hypertensive adult is 3.6 times higher if a child has a SBP in the top quintile and 2.6 times higher if the DBP is in the top quintile. Conversely, almost half of the adults with HTN had elevated BP during childhood (205). If a child has a BP level in the ninetieth percentile, the risk of becoming a hypertensive adult is 2.4 times higher (206). However, although many children and adolescents maintain their BP rank in the population as they mature into adults, there is considerable variability (207,208). It is currently impossible to identify with confidence which children with primary HTN are destined to become hypertensive adults and in whom modification of BP in childhood will alter risks for later coronary artery disease. The correlation seems to be much better in adults; that is, once an adult is identified as hypertensive, he or she will probably remain hypertensive for the remainder of his or her life (132,209).

During the first 6 months of life BP does not track (112). Children followed from birth have low correlation of SBP levels and no correlation of DBP levels by 7 years of age (210). In children beyond the first year of life, tracking correlations range from 0.2 to 0.5 for SBP and from 0.2 to 0.3 for DBP levels (206). These tracking correlations were compiled from several studies and demonstrate that, although some children maintain their rank order for BP over time, others do not track well. Although the predictive value of high BP early in life for future HTN is low, the actual level of a child's BP remains the single best predictor of future BP (211). The variability in the degree of tracking reported by different studies is the result of differences in the analytic methods used and the population studied. The age of the subjects at initial observation, number and spacing of observations longitudinally, and duration of the observation period play an important role. Other factors that might directly affect the BP level could influence the degree of tracking, including body mass, sexual maturation, and family history (208). It has been shown that family history and excessive weight gain in adolescence substantially increase the risk of HTN in adulthood (211).

Improved predictive value can be achieved when serial measurements over time are considered. In the Bogalusa Heart Study, Shear et al. found the predictive value for future hypertensive readings based on a single previous measurement to be only 41.4% for SBP and 34.4% for DBP (212). When three serial measurements over an 8-year period were considered, however, the predictive value of a child's remaining in the upper quartile increased to 68.4% and 62.0% for SBP and DBP, respectively. In addition, when three previous BP measurements were considered, the probability that children could be identified who would not be in the high-BP group in the future was 96.8%. Similarly, Gillman et al. found improved correlation coefficients for both SBP and DBP in children whose BP levels were measured weekly for four visits in each of 4 years (213). In this study, correlation coefficients were 0.69 for SBP levels and 0.54 for DBP levels at the end of the 4-year follow-up. The multiple measurements available with ABPM allow for better predictive values. Twenty-four-hour mean SBP measurements track better than casual SBP readings (214).

END-ORGAN DAMAGE

HTN is associated with an increase in cardiovascular morbidity and mortality in adults. Although cardiovascular mortality is rare in children, those with end-stage renal disease are 1000 times more likely to die of CVD than the general pediatric population (215). The impact of elevated BP alone in children is not as clearly delineated. In contrast to HTN in adults, which is defined by the level of BP associated with an increase in morbidity and mortality, HTN in children is defined by population normative values (3). Studies do show that elevated

BP in children, especially as determined by ABPM, is also associated with EOD. The commonly studied surrogate markers for target organ damage are LVH, carotid intimal-medial wall thickness and radial artery compliance, microalbuminuria, and retinopathy. In adults, the effect of HTN on the central nervous system is evidenced by ischemic stroke, cerebral hemorrhage, and central nerve palsy. Although these events are rare in children, extremely elevated BP can present with seizures (216). Because morbidity and mortality are not usually seen in the pediatric hypertensive patient, it is important to identify surrogate markers for EOD and treat BP aggressively to decrease disease progression in adulthood.

Left Ventricular Hypertrophy

Although many organ systems, such as the brain, eyes, kidney, and blood vessels, are affected by elevated BP, the heart is the most studied of the target organs. LVH is associated with HTN and is an independent predictor of CVD in adults (217–219). Brown et al. showed that, even in the absence of HTN, LVH is a harbinger of coronary heart disease (220). Treating HTN in adults decreases the morbidity and mortality from CVD (221,222). In children there is no clear threshold in LV mass or LV mass index (LVMI) to predict LVH (223–226). Due to the difficulty in defining LVH in children, its prevalence is difficult to predict and has been reported to range from 16 to 51% (102,223,225). In 1981, Laird and Fixler sought to determine the prevalence of LVH in hypertensive children. They evaluated 50 hypertensive and 50 normotensive children. LV mass was indexed by body surface area, and LVH was defined as more than 2 standard deviations above the mean. They identified 16% of hypertensive children and 4% of normotensive children as having LVH (225). Daniels et al. have proposed indexing LV mass by height cubed when controlling for size and gender (227). LVH can then be defined as LV mass greater than either the ninetieth or ninety-fifth percentiles for LVMI. Before this recommendation was made, Daniels et al. indexed LV mass by height when defining LVH. They studied 104 children aged 6 to 23 years and found that 51% were considered to have LVH when LVMI was greater than 90% according to normative values and 38.5% were considered to have LVH when LVMI was greater than 95% (223). Belsha performed ABPM and echocardiography in 33 normotensive and 29 untreated hypertensive children. By defining LVH as LV mass indexed for height cubed, his group identified LVH in 34% of the hypertensive children and none of the normotensive children (102). To control for differences in body size, de Simone and his group recommend indexing LV mass by height to the power of 2.7. Using a 97.5 percentile cutoff of normative values for LV mass divided by height to the power of 2.7, his group detected a fourfold increase in the presence of designated cardiovascular end points in adults (228). The same group documented left atrial enlargement in children with essential HTN. Those with left atrial enlargement had a higher body mass than those without (229).

Many studies show an association between LVMI and BP in children (102,223,224). Burke et al. in the Bogalusha Heart Study examined data for 654 children aged 7 through 22 years who had stable BPs over a 2- to 3-year period and showed that LV wall thickness was correlated with SBP ($R = 0.21$, $p < .001$) (229). Even in normotensive children, there is a correlation of age, body size, and BP to LV mass (226). Treiber and his group evaluated normotensive children with a family history of essential HTN and showed an association of LV mass with SBP but not with DBP (230). Although these studies reveal an association between LV mass and BP in children, they do not provide a threshold in LV mass that predicts LVH.

Elevated BP, as determined by CBP readings and by ABPM, has been found to be positively associated with LVMI in children (102,231). Sorof et al. showed that ABPM was a better predictor of EOD than clinic BP readings (104). His group correlated the findings of ABPM and echocardiography for normotensive and hypertensive children. They found that only systolic parameters and not diastolic parameters were associated with LVMI. In defining LVH, LV mass was indexed by height to the power of 2.7 and defined as the LVMI higher than 51 g/m$^{2.7}$ that corresponds to greater than the ninety-ninth percentile for children. LVMI was significantly greater in the hypertensive groups than in the normotensive groups (41.5 ± 12.0 vs. 32.5 ± 8.1, $p < .001$), even when controlled for age, gender, weight, and height. The LVMI showed highest correlation with ambulatory SBP index, the average 24-hour SBP divided by the pediatric 95th percentile for ambulatory 24-hour SBP ($R = 0.43$, $p = .008$). This correlation was better than the correlation with SBP load ($R = 0.38$, $p = .020$). By assigning ABPM threshold parameters to determine LVH, his group found that, when SBP load is greater than 50% and the SBP index is higher than 1, LVH is present 47% of the time. If neither condition is met, LVH is present only 10% of the time. Therefore, ABPM is a better method to use in determining which children likely have EOD from their elevated BP and need aggressive treatment.

Microalbuminuria

During the mid-1980s the Framingham study reported the association between proteinuria and an increase in morbidity and mortality (232). Since then many studies have concentrated on the early detection of proteinuria by studying microalbuminuria, defined as 30 to 300 mg of albumin/24 hr or 30 to 300 mg of albumin/g creatinine. The Heart Outcomes Prevention Evaluation (HOPE) study of diabetic and nondiabetic adult patients showed that microalbuminuria is an independent risk factor for future cardiovascular events and is probably a signal of vascular damage (233). Treatment with the ACE inhibitor ramipril reduced CVD risk by 26% (233). Other studies have also shown microalbuminuria to be more prevalent in hypertensive patients than in normotensive patients. Jones et al. of the National Health and Nutrition Examination Survey III studied 22,244 people aged 6 years and older to determine the prevalence of microalbuminuria and its association with other diseases such as diabetes and HTN. They identified microalbuminuria in 16% of the hypertensive participants but in only 5.1% of the participants without diabetes, HTN, or CVD (234). However, the sample size for hypertensive children was too small to be reported. The prevalence of persistent microalbuminuria is unknown because the National Health and Nutrition Examination Survey III examined only one urine sample from each participant. Pontremoli et al. evaluated the association between microalbuminuria and early EOD in adults with essential HTN. Although their sample size was small (17 hypertensive participants with microalbuminuria, 16 without microalbuminuria, and 20 controls), they showed that the hypertensive participants with microalbuminuria had significantly higher LVMIs than the hypertensive participants without microalbuminuria and the controls (167 ± 7 g/m^2 vs. 139 ± 9 g/m^2 vs. 118 ± 5 g/m^2, respectively) (235). There are few studies evaluating microalbuminuria in hypertensive children. Belsha and his group looked at 24-hour urinary albumin excretion rates in normotensive and hypertensive adolescents and did not find a difference between the groups (236). Interestingly, normotensive children of hypertensive parents have been shown to have greater amounts of microalbuminuria than the control children who did not have hypertensive parents (3.1 mg/min vs. 2.1 mg/min, p <.05) (237). More studies are needed to determine the role of microalbuminuria in nondiabetic hypertensive children.

Vascular Changes

The vascular system is another "organ" often affected by HTN that has been evaluated in children as evidence of EOD. Two surrogate markers for vessel involvement are a decrease in vascular compliance and an increase in intimal-medial wall thickness of the carotid artery (cIMT). Arnett et al. evaluated arterial compliance by examining radial artery waveforms with an arterial tonometer device (pulse contour analysis). They studied 179 young normotensive adults who had been followed since childhood as part of the Minnesota Children's Blood Pressure Study. Both SBP and DBP were inversely related to large artery compliance (p < .001 and p < .02, respectively). Small artery compliance was inversely related to DBP, but not to SBP (p < .005) (238). Swinford et al. demonstrated markedly decreased compliance in children treated with hemodialysis, with the lowest compliance occurring middialysis (239). Bennett et al. performed studies of middle school children documenting vascular compliance that is lower than that in normal older teens and young adults. Hypertensive children in the screening population were also noted to have decreased compliance compared to normotensive children (240).

Elevated BP is also associated with cIMT. Sass et al. studied 369 men and women aged 10 to 54 years to determine the influence of age, gender, morphologic status, and BP on carotid and femoral intimal-medial wall thickness. They showed that cIMT was not affected by age or gender up to 18 years of age. However, cIMT was correlated with body mass index and BP in children (241). Sorof studied cIMT in hypertensive children. His group determined the prevalence of elevated cIMT to be 28% among hypertensive children with a mean age of 13.9 ± 2.7 years. Those with elevated cIMT also had higher LVMI than did the hypertensive children with normal cIMT (46.8 g/m$^{2.7}$ vs. 31.4 g/m$^{2.7}$, p < .001) (104). Like LVH, radial artery compliance and cIMT can be used to assess the presence of EOD in children.

Retinopathy

There are only a few studies of children showing the association between elevated BP and retinal changes. Daniels and his group evaluated 88 children to determine the prevalence of target organ damage in essential HTN. They identified LVH in 36%, glomerular hyperfiltration in 49%, and retinal vascular changes in 50% of the children (242). Daniels examined retinal photographs in 97 children with essential HTN to determine the presence of arteriolar narrowing, tortuosity, and arteriovenous nicking. Forty-one percent of the children had arteriolar narrowing, 14% had tortuosity, and 8% had arteriovenous nicking; overall, 51% of the children had at least one eye abnormality (243). EOD of the eye can occur in children with HTN.

SUMMARY

The prevalence especially of essential HTN is increasing in children and adolescents parallel to the increase in obesity and the proportion of minorities making up the population in the United States. We anxiously await further population genetic studies that may provide tools to predict which patients will develop HTN. Nonetheless, secondary forms of HTN are also more prevalent in pediatric patients than in adults. The diagnosis of HTN remains an epidemiologic one and is complicated by the continued inability to clarify the optimum method of BP measurement: the more commonly and easily used oscillometry or the more accepted but difficult auscultatory technique. How do we best use these various technologies? Comparison of oscillometric results with standards obtained using auscultatory methods also confuses the diagnosis. ABPM has been well tested in children. The procedure is well tolerated and gives a clearer picture of the BP situation than CBP alone. It is now clear that HTN even during childhood leads to EOD, and ABPM measurements have been documented in children with all forms of HTN to have a superior correlation with EOD. Because the "hard" end points of mortality or cardiovascular events are rarely seen in children, more subtle measures of EOD must be used. There is great hope that new techniques to study the vasculature such as cIMT measurement, vascular profiling, and flow-mediated dilation can identify those patients at risk before damage occurs. Thus future definitions of HTN must take into account the development of EOD damage.

REFERENCES

1. Kurtz TW. False claims of blood pressure-independent protection by blockade of the renin-angiotensin aldosterone system. *Hypertension* 2003;41:193–196.
2. Morgenstern B. Blood pressure, hypertension and ambulatory blood pressure monitoring in children and adolescents. *Am J Hypertens* 2002;15:64S–66S.
3. Update on the 1987 task force report on high blood pressure in children and adolescents: a working group report from the National High Blood Pressure Education Program. *Pediatrics* 1996;98:649–658.
4. Clark JH, Lieh-Lai MW, Sarnaik H, et al. Discrepancies between direct and indirect BP measurement using various recommendations for arm cuff selection. *Pediatrics* 2002;110: 920–923.
5. Sorof JM, Eissa MA, Lai D, et al. Multiple clinic measurements do not improve the relative agreement between clinic and daytime ambulatory BP in children. *Am J Hypertens* 2001;14:235A.
6. Markandu ND, Whitcher F, et al. The mercury sphygmomanometer should be abandoned before it is proscribed. *J Hum Hypertens* 2000;14(1):31–36.
7. Vanasse A, Courteau J. Evaluation of sphygmomanometers used by family physicians practicing outside the hospital environment in Bas-Saint-Laurent [in French]. *Can Fam Physician* 2001;47:281–286.
8. Mion D, Pierin AM. How accurate are sphygmomanometers? *J Hum Hypertens* 1998;12(4):245–248.
9. Knight T, Leech F, et al. Sphygmomanometers in use in general practice: an overlooked aspect of quality in patient care. *J Hum Hypertens* 2001;15(10):681–684.
10. Jones JS, Ramsey W, et al. Accuracy of prehospital sphygmomanometers. *J Emerg Med* 1987;5(1):23–27.
11. Sloan PJ, Zezulka A, et al. Standardized methods for comparison of sphygmomanometers. *J Hypertens* 1984;2(5):547–551.
12. Perloff D, Grim C, et al. Human blood pressure determination by sphygmomanometry. *Circulation* 1993;88(5 Pt 1):2460–2470.
13. McAlister FA, Straus SE. Measurement of blood pressure: an evidence based review. *BMJ* 2001:322:908–911.
14. Alpert BS, Marks L, Cohen M. K5 = diastolic blood pressure [Letter]. *Pediatrics* 1996;98:1002.
15. Ramsey M 3rd. (1991). Blood pressure monitoring: automated oscillometric devices. *J Clin Monit* 7(1):56–67.
16. Kaufmann MA, Pargger H, et al. Oscillometric blood pressure measurements by different devices are not interchangeable. *Anesth Analg* 1996;82(2):377–381.
17. Park MK, Menard SM. Accuracy of blood pressure measurement by the Dinamap monitor in infants and children. *Pediatrics* 1987;79(6):907–914.
18. The Sixth Report of the Joint National Committee on Prevention, Detection, Evaluation and Treatment of High Blood Pressure. National Institutes of Health Publication 98-4080. Bethesda, MD: National Institutes of Health, November 1997.
19. Appel LJ, Robinson KA, Guallar E, et al. Utility of blood pressure monitoring outside of the clinic setting. Evidence Report/Technology Assessment No. 63. AHRQ Publication No. 03-E004. Rockville, MD: US Department of Health and Human Services, Agency for Healthcare Research and Quality, November 2002. Available at http://www.ahrq.gov/clinic/bpmoninv.htm.
20. O'Brien E, Petrie J, Littler WA, et al. The British Hypertension Society protocol for the evaluation of blood pressure measuring devices. *J Hypertens* 1993;11[Suppl 2]:S43–S63.
21. Association for the Advancement of Medical Instrumentation. *American national standard. Electronic or automated sphygmomanometer.* ANSI/AAMI SP 10–1992. Arlington, VA: Association for the Advancement of Medical Instrumentation, 1992.
22. O'Brien E. State of the market for devices for blood pressure measurement. *Blood Press Monit* 2001;6:281–286.
23. O'Brien E, De Gaudemaris R, Bobrie G, et al. Proceedings from a Consensus Conference on Self-Blood Pressure Measurement. Devices and validation. *Blood Press Monit* 2000;5:93–100.
24. Myers MG. Reporting bias in self measurement of blood pressure. *Blood Press Monit* 2001;6:181–183.
25. Mengden T, Hernandez Medina RM, Betran B, et al. Reliability of reporting self-measured BP values by hypertensive patients. *Am J Hypertens* 1998;11:1413–1417.
26. Maaze RS, Shamoom H, Pasmantier R, et al. Reliability of blood glucose monitoring by subjects with diabetes mellitus. *Am J Med* 1984;77:211–217.
27. Gong H, Simmons MS, Clark VA, et al. Metered dose inhaler usage in subjects with asthma: comparison of Nebulizer Chonolog and daily diary recordings. *J Allergy Immunol* 1988;82:5–10.
28. Portman RJ, Yetman RJ, West MS. Efficacy of 24-hour ambulatory blood pressure monitoring in children. *J Pediatr* 1991;118:842–849.
29. O'Brien E, Cox JP, O'Malley K. Ambulatory blood pressure measurements in the evaluation of blood pressure lowering drugs. *J Hypertens* 1989;7:243–247.
30. Smolensky MH, D'Alonzo GE, Portman RJ. Chronobiology and chronotherapeutics: new concepts in cardiovascular medicine. *Am J Osteopath Med (in press).*
31. *Ambulatory monitoring and blood pressure variability.* London: Science Press, 1991:chap 5, 5.1–5.15.
32. Covic A, Goldsmith D. Ambulatory blood pressure monitoring: an essential tool for blood pressure assessment in uraemic patients. *Nephrol Dial Transplant* 2002;17:1737–1741.
33. Stolarz K, Staessen JA, O'Brien ET. Night-time blood pressure: dipping into the future. *J Hypertens* 2002;20:2131–2133.
34. Staessen JA, Bieniaszewski L, O'Brien ET, et al. What is normal blood pressure on ambulatory monitoring? *Nephrol Dial Transplant* 1996;11:241–245.
35. O'Brien E, Staessen J. Normotension and hypertension as defined by 24-hour ambulatory blood pressure monitoring. *Blood Press* 1995;4:266–282.

36. Soergel M, Kirschstein M, Busch C, et al. Oscillometric twenty-four hour ambulatory blood pressure values in healthy children and adolescents: a multicenter trial including 1141 subjects. *J Pediatr* 1997;130:178–184.
37. Patzer L, Seeman T, Luck C, et al. Day- and night-time blood pressure elevation in children with higher grades of renal scarring. *J Pediatr* 2003;142(2):117–122.
38. Staessen JA, Asmar R, De Buyzere M, et al., and participants of the 2001 Consensus Conference on Ambulatory Blood Pressure Monitoring. Task Force II: blood pressure measurement and cardiovascular outcome. *Blood Press Monit* 2001;6:355–370.
39. Laragh JH, Brenner BM. *Hypertension: pathophysiology, diagnosis, and management,* 2nd ed. New York: Raven Press, 1995.
40. Second Task Force on Blood Pressure Control in Children. Report of the Second Task Force on Blood Pressure Control in Children, 1987. *Pediatrics* 1987;79:1–25.
41. Sinaiko AR, Gomez-Marin O, Prineas RJ. Prevalence of "significant" hypertension in junior high school-aged children; the Children and Adolescent Blood Pressure Program. *J Pediatr* 1989;114:664–669.
42. Sorof JM, Poffenbarger T, Franco K, et al. Evaluation of white coat hypertension in children: importance of the definitions of "normal" ambulatory blood pressure and the severity of casual hypertension. *Am J Hypertens* 2001;14:855–860.
43. Staessen JA, O'Brien ET. Development of diagnostic thresholds for automated measurement of blood pressure in adults. *Blood Press Monit* 1999;4:127–136.
44. Pickering TG. How should the diurnal changes of blood pressure be expressed? *Am J Hypertens* 1995;8:681–682.
45. Prasad N, MacFadyn RJ, Ogston S, et al. Elevated blood pressure during the first two hours of ambulatory blood pressure monitoring. *J Hypertens* 1995;13:291–295.
46. White WB, Dey HM, Schulman P. Assessment of the daily blood pressure load as a determinant of cardiac function in patients with mild-to-moderate hypertension. *Am Heart J* 1989;118:782–795.
47. Zachariah PK, Sheps SG, Ilstrup DM, et al. Blood pressure load: a better determinant of blood pressure. *Mayo Clin Proc* 1988;63:94–98.
48. Sorof JM. Prevalence and consequence of systolic hypertension in children. *Am J Hypertens* 2002;15:S57–S60.
49. Schillaci G, Verdecchia P, Borgiono C, et al. Predictors of diurnal blood pressure changes in 2042 subjects with essential hypertension. *J Hypertens* 1996;14:1167–1173.
50. Watanabe N, Imai Y, Nagai K, et al. Nocturnal blood pressure and silent cerebrovascular lesions in elderly Japanese. *Stroke* 1996;27:1319–1327.
51. Covic A, Goldsmith D. Ambulatory blood pressure monitoring: an essential tool for blood pressure assessment in uraemic patients. *Nephrol Dial Transplant* 2002;17:1737–1741.
52. Farmer CK, Goldsmith DJ, Quinn JD, et al. Progression of diabetic nephropathy—is diurnal blood pressure rhythm as important as absolute blood pressure level? *Nephrol Dial Transplant* 1998;13:635–639.
53. Hoffstein V, Chan CK, Slutsky AS. Sleep apnea and systemic hypertension: a causal association review. *Am J Med* 1991;91:190–196.
54. Parati G, Pomidossi G, Albini F, et al. Relationship of 24-hour blood pressure and variability to severity of target organ damage in hypertension. *J Hypertens* 1987;5:93–98.
55. Hoegholm A, Kristensen KS, Bang LE, et al. White coat hypertension and target organ involvement: the impact of different cut-off levels on albuminuria and left ventricular mass and geometry. *J Hum Hypertens* 1998;12:433–439.
56. Staessen JA, Beilin L, Parati G, et al. Task Force IV: clinical use of ambulatory blood pressure monitoring. Participants of the 1999 Consensus Conference on Ambulatory Blood Pressure Monitoring. *Blood Press Monit* 1999;4:319–331.
57. Palatini P, Mormino P, Santonastaso M, et al. Target organ damage in stage 1 hypertensive subjects with white coat and sustained hypertension. Results from the HARVEST study. *Hypertension* 1998;31:57–63.
58. Sorof JM, Portman RJ. White coat hypertension in children with elevated casual blood pressure. *J Pediatr* 2000;137:493–497.
59. Covic A, Goldsmith DJA, Farmer CKT, et al. How reproducible is diurnal blood pressure rhythm in patients with secondary (renal) hypertension? *Rev Med Chir Soc Med Nat Iasi* 1999;103:88–93.
60. Staessen JA, Thijs L, Fargard R, et al., for the Systolic Hypertension in Europe Trial investigators. Predicting cardiovascular risk using conventional vs. ambulatory blood pressure in older patients with systolic hypertension. *JAMA* 1999;282:539–546.
61. Hermida RC, Ayala DE. Prognostic value of office and ambulatory blood pressure measurements in pregnancy. *Hypertension* 2002;40:298–303.
62. Baumgert P, Walger P, Gemen S, et al. Blood pressure elevation during the night in chronic renal failure, hemodialysis and after renal transplantation. *Nephron* 1991;57:293–298.
63. Middeke M, Schrader J. Nocturnal blood pressure in normotensive subjects and those with white coat, primary, and secondary hypertension. *BMJ* 1994;308:630–632.
64. McGregor DO, Olsson C, Lynn KL. Autonomic dysfunction and ambulatory blood pressure in renal transplant recipients. *Transplantation* 2001;71:1277–1281.
65. Cottone S, Panepinto N, Vadala A, et al. Sympathetic overactivity and 24-hour blood pressure pattern in hypertensives with chronic renal failure. *Ren Fail* 1995;17:751–758.
66. Farmer CKT, Goldsmith DJA, Cox J, et al. An investigation of the effect of advancing uraemia, renal replacement therapy and renal transplantation on blood pressure diurnal variability. *Nephrol Dial Transplant* 1997;12:2302–2307.
67. Keller CK, Bergis KH, Fliser D, et al. Renal findings in patients with short term type 2 diabetes. *J Am Soc Nephrol* 1996;7:2627–2645.
68. Lingens N, Freund M, Seeman T, et al. Circadian blood pressure changes in untreated children with kidney disease and conserved renal function. *Acta Paediatr* 1997;86:719–723.
69. Seeman T, John U, Blahova K, et al. Ambulatory blood pressure monitoring in children with unilateral multicystic dysplastic kidney. *Eur J Pediatr* 2001;160:78–83.
70. Seeman T, Sikut M, Konrad M, et al. Blood pressure and renal function in autosomal dominant polycystic kidney disease. *Pediatr Nephrol* 1997;11:592–596.
71. Bald M, Lettgen B, Wingen AM, et al. Twenty-four-hour blood pressure monitoring in children and adolescents after

recovery from hemolytic uremic syndrome. *Clin Nephrol* 1996;46:50–53.

72. Reusz GS, Hobor M, Tulassay T, et al. Twenty-four-hour blood pressure monitoring in health and hypertensive children. *Arch Dis Child* 1994;70:90–94.
73. Sorof JM, Poffenbarger T, Portman R. Abnormal 24-hr blood pressure patterns in children after renal transplantation. *Am J Kidney Dis* 2000;35:681–686.
74. Lingens N, Soergel M, Loirat C, et al. Ambulatory blood pressure monitoring in paediatric patients treated by regular hemodialysis and peritoneal dialysis. *Pediatr Nephrol* 1995;9:167–172.
75. Khan IA, Gajaria M, Stephens D, et al. Ambulatory blood pressure monitoring in children: a large center experience. *Pediatr Nephrol* 2000;14:802–805.
76. Flynn JT. Differentiating between primary and secondary hypertension in children using ambulatory blood pressure monitoring. *Pediatrics* 2002;110:89–93.
77. Lurbe E, Redon J, Kesani A, et al. Increase in nocturnal blood pressure and progression to microalbuminuria in type I diabetes. *N Engl J Med* 2002;347:797–805.
78. Poulsen PL, Ebbehoj E, Hansen KW, et al. Twenty-four-hour blood pressure and autonomic function is related to albumin excretion within the normoalbuminuric range in IDDM patients. *Diabetologia* 1997;40:718–725.
79. Nielsen FS, Gaede P, Vedel P, et al. White coat hypertension in NIDDM patients with and without incipient and overt diabetic nephropathy. *Diabetes Care* 1997;20:859–863.
80. Bauduceau B, Genes N, Chamontin B, et al. Ambulatory blood pressure and urinary albumin excretion in diabetic (non–insulin-dependent and insulin-dependent) hypertensive patients: relationships at baseline and after treatment by the angiotensin converting enzyme inhibitor trandolapril. *Am J Hypertens* 1998;11(9):1065–1073.
81. Garg SK, Chase HP, Icaza G, et al. Twenty-four-hour ambulatory blood pressure and renal disease in young subjects with type I diabetes. *J Diabetes Complications* 1997;11(5):263–267.
82. Chau NP, Bauduceau B, Chanudet X, et al. Ambulatory blood pressure in diabetic subjects. *Am J Hypertens* 1994;7:487–491.
83. Palatini P, Graniero GR, Mormino M, et al., on behalf of the HARVEST study group. Prevalence and clinical correlates of microalbuminuria in stage I hypertension. Results from the Hypertension and Ambulatory Recording Venetia Study (HARVEST Study). *Am J Hypertens* 1996;9:334–341.
84. Hansen HP, Rossing P, Tarnow L, et al. Circadian rhythm of arterial blood pressure and albuminuria in diabetic nephropathy. *Kidney Int* 1996;50:579–585.
85. Martinez MA, Moreno A, Aguirre de Carcer A, et al., on behalf of the MAPA-Madrid Working Group. Frequency and determinants of microalbuminuria in mild hypertension: a primary-care based study. *J Hypertens* 2001:19:319–326.
86. Nakano S, Ogihara M, Tamura C, et al. Reverse circadian blood pressure rhythm independently predicts end stage renal failure in non–insulin dependent diabetes mellitus subjects. *J Diabetes Complications* 1999;13:224–231.
87. Martinez-Vea A, Valero FA, Bardaji A, et al. Left ventricular hypertrophy in hypertensive patients with autosomal dominant polycystic kidney disease: influence of blood pressure and humoral and neurohumeral factors. *Am J Nephrol* 2000;20:193–200.
88. Tucker B, Fabbian F, Giles M, et al. Left ventricular hypertrophy and ambulatory blood pressure monitoring in chronic renal failure. *Nephrol Dial Transplant* 1997;12:724–728.
89. Tucker B, Fabbian F, Giles M, et al. Reduction of left ventricular mass index with blood pressure reduction in chronic renal failure. *Clin Nephrol* 1999;52:377–382.
90. Stefanski A, Schmidt K, Waldherr R, et al. Early increase in blood pressure and diastolic left ventricular malfunction in patients with glomerulonephritis. *Kidney Int* 1996;50:1321–1326.
91. Cuspidi C, Lonati L, Sampieri L, et al. Prevalence of target organ damage in treated hypertensive patients: different impact of clinic and ambulatory blood pressure control. *J Hypertens* 2000;18:803–809.
92. Palatini P, Graniero GR, Canali C, et al. Relationship between albumin excretion rate, ambulatory blood pressure and left ventricular hypertrophy in mild hypertension. *J Hypertens* 1995;13(12 Pt 2):1796–1800.
93. Szelestei T, Kovacs T, Barta J, et al. Circadian blood pressure changes and cardiac abnormalities in IgA nephropathy. *Am J Nephrol* 1999;19:546–551.
94. Covic A, Goldsmith DJA, Georgescu GC, et al. Relationships between blood pressure variability and left ventricular parameters in hemodialysis and renal transplant patients. *Nephrology* 1998;4:87–94.
95. Csiky B, Kovacs T, Wagner L, et al. Ambulatory blood pressure and progression in patients with IgA nephropathy. *Nephrol Dial Transplant* 1999;14:86–90.
96. Timio M, Venanzi S, Lolli S, et al. "Non-dipper" hypertensive patients and progressive renal insufficiency: a 3-year longitudinal study. *Clin Nephrol* 1995;43(6):382–387.
97. Farmer KT, Goldsmith DJA, Quin JD, et al. Progression of diabetic nephropathy—is diurnal blood pressure rhythm as important as absolute blood pressure level? *Nephrol Dial Transplant* 1998;13:635–639.
98. Reference deleted.
99. Jacobi J, Rockstroh J, John S, et al. Prospective analysis of the value of 24-hour ambulatory blood pressure on renal function after kidney transplantation. *Transplantation* 2000;70(5):819–827.
100. Kooman JP, Christiaans M, Boots JMM, et al. A comparison between office and ambulatory blood pressure measurements in renal transplant patients with chronic transplant nephropathy. *Am J Kidney Dis* 2001;37:1170–1176.
101. Calzolari A, Giordano U, Chiara Matteucci M, et al. Hypertension in young patients after renal transplantation, ambulatory blood pressure versus casual blood pressure. *Am J Hypertens* 1998;11:497–501.
102. Belsha CW, Wells TG, McNiece KL, et al. Influence of diurnal BP variations on target organ abnormalities in adolescents with mild essential hypertension. *Am J Hypertens* 1998;11:410–417.
103. Matteucci MC, Giordano U, Calzoni A, et al. Left ventricular hypertrophy, treadmill tests, and 24 hour blood pressure

in pediatric transplant patients. *Kidney Int* 1999;56:1566–1570.
104. Sorof JM, Cardwell G, Franco K, et al. Ambulatory blood pressure and left ventricular mass index in hypertensive children. *Hypertension* 2002;39:903–908.
105. Sorof JM, Alexandrov AV, Cardwell G, et al. Carotid intimal medial thickness and left ventricular hypertrophy in children with elevated blood pressure. *Pediatrics* 2003;111:61–66.
106. Rossing P, Tarnow L, Boelskifte S, et al. Differences between nisoldipine and lisinopril on glomerular filtration rates and albuminuria in hypertensive IDDM patients with diabetic nephropathy during the first year of treatment. *Diabetes* 1997;46:481–487.
107. Katz SH, Heidiger ML, Schall JI, et al. Blood pressure, growth and maturation from childhood through adolescence. Mixed longitudinal analyses of the Philadelphia Blood Pressure Project. *Hypertension* 1980; 2:55–69.
108. Zinner SH, Rosner B, Oh W, et al. Significance of blood pressure in infancy: familial aggregation and predictive effort on late blood pressure. *Hypertension* 1985;7:411–416.
109. Second Task Force on Blood Pressure Control in Children. Report of the Second Task Force on Blood Pressure Control in Children, 1987. *Pediatrics* 1987;79:1–25.
110. Portman RJ, Yetman RJ. Temporal blood pressure patterns in children. *Ann N Y Acad Sci* 1996;783:227–241.
111. Georgieff MK, Mills MM, Gomez-Marin O, et al. Rate of change of blood pressure in premature and full term infants from birth to 4 months. *Pediatr Nephrol* 1996;10:152–154.
112. Szklo M. Epidemiologic patterns of blood pressure in children. *Epidemiol Rev* 1979;1:143–169.
113. Cornoni-Huntley J, Lacroix AZ, Havlik RJ. Race and sex differentials in the impact of hypertension in the United States. The national health and nutrition examination survey I epidemiologic follow-up study. *Arch Intern Med* 1989;149:780–788.
114. Eisner GM. Hypertension: racial differences. *Am J Kidney Dis* 1990;16[Suppl 1]:35–40.
115. Eiber FA, Musanti L, Strong WB, et al. Racial differences in young children's blood pressure: responses in dynamic exercise. *Am J Dis Child* 1989;143:720–723.
116. Harshfield GA, Hwang C, Grim CE. Circadian variation of blood pressure in blacks: influence of age, gender and activity. *J Hum Hypertens* 1990;4:43–47.
117. Grim CE, Robinson M. Blood pressure variation in blacks: genetic factors. *Semin Nephrol* 1996;16:83–93.
118. Grim CE, Wilson TW, Egbunike AC, et al. Nocturnal blood pressure is higher in US born blacks than non-US born blacks. *Circulation* 1990;82:553.
119. Bloem LJ, Manatunga AK, Tweksbur DA, et al. The serum angiotensinogen concentration and variants of the angiotensinogen gene in white and black children. *J Clin Invest* 1995;95:948–953.
120. Duru K, Farrow S, Wang JM, et al. Frequency of a deletion polymorphism in the gene for angiotensin converting enzyme is increased in African-Americans with hypertension. *Am J Hypertens* 1994;7:759–762.
121. Berenson GS, Lawrence M, Soto L. The heart and hypertension in children. *Semin Nephrol* 1989;9:236–246.
122. Soto L, Kikuchi DA, Arcilla RA, et al. Echocardiographic function and blood pressure levels in children and young adults from a biracial population. The Bogolusa Heart Study. *Am J Med Sci* 1989;297:271–279.
123. Luft FC, Rankin LI, Bloch R, et al. Cardiovascular and humoral responses to extremes of sodium intake in normal black and white men. *Circulation* 1979;60:697–706.
124. Falkner B, Kushner H. Interaction of sodium sensitivity and stress in young adults. *Hypertension* 1991;17[Suppl]:I162–I165.
125. Elseed AM, Shinebourne EA, Joseph MC. Assessment of techniques for measurement of blood pressure in infants and children. *Arch Dis Child* 1973;48:932–936.
126. Murphy JK, Alpert BS, Moes DM, et al. Race and cardiovascular reactivity: a neglected relationship. *Hypertension* 1986;8:1075–1083.
127. Murphy JK, Alpert BS, Walker SS, et al. Children's cardiovascular reactivity: stability of racial differences and relation to subsequent blood pressure over a one-year period. *Psychophysiology* 1991;28:447–457.
128. Modesti PA, Pela I, Cecioni I, et al. Changes in blood pressure reactivity and 24-hour blood pressure profile occurring at puberty. *J Vasc Dis* 1994;45:443–450.
129. de Man SA, Andre JL, Bachmann H, et al. Blood pressure in children: pooled findings of six European studies. *J Hypertens* 1991;9:109–114.
130. Dunstan HP. Obesity and hypertension. In: Lauer RM, Shekelle RB, eds. *Childhood prevention of atherosclerosis and hypertension*. New York: Raven Press, 1980:305–312.
131. Rosmond R, Chagnon YC, Holm G, et al. Hypertension in obesity and the leptin receptor gene locus. *J Clin Endocrinol Metab* 2000;85:3126–3131.
132. Final report of the Subcommittee on Nonpharmacological Therapy of the 1984 Joint National Committee on Detection, Evaluation, and Treatment of High Blood Pressure: nonpharmacological approaches to the control of high blood pressure. *Hypertension* 1986;8:444–467.
133. Ingelfinger JR. Nutritional aspects of pediatric hypertension. *Bull N Y Acad Med* 1989;65:1109–1153.
134. Kotchen JM, Holley J, Kotchen TA. Treatment of high blood pressure in the young. *Semin Nephrol* 1989;9:296–303.
135. Reisin ED, Abel R, Modan M, et al. Effect of weight loss without salt restriction on the reduction of blood pressure in overweight hypertensive patients. *N Engl J Med* 1978;298:1–6.
136. Rocchini A, Key J, Bondie D, et al. The effect of weight loss on their sensitivity of blood pressure to sodium in obese adolescence. *N Engl J Med* 1989;321:580–585.
137. Gutin B, Basch C, Shea S, et al. Blood pressure, fitness, and fatness in 5- and 6-year-old children. *JAMA* 1990;264:1123–1127.
138. Sorof JM, Poffenbarger T, Franco K, et al. Isolated systolic hypertension, obesity and hyperkinetic states in children. *J Pediatr* 2002;140:660–666.
139. Julius S. The association of tachycardia with obesity and elevated blood pressure. *J Pediatr* 2002:140:643–645.
140. Sorof JM, Daniels S. Obesity hypertension in children. *Hypertension* 2002;40:441–447.
141. Portman RJ, Lugo-Miro VI, Ikle D, et al. Diagnosis of adolescent hypertension on initial screening by the use of height age. *J Adolesc Health Care* 1990;11:215–222.
142. Voors AW, Webber LS, Frerichs RR, et al. Body height and body mass as determinants of basal blood pressure in chil-

dren: the Bogalusa Heart Study. *Am J Epidemiol* 1977; 106:101–112.
143. Londe S, Johanson A, Kronemer NS, et al. Blood pressure and puberty. *J Pediatr* 1975;87:896–900.
144. Gillum RF, Prineas RJ, Horibe H. Maturation vs. age: assessing blood pressure by height. *JAMA* 1982;74:43–46.
145. Rosner B, Prineas R, Daniels SR, et al. Blood pressure differences between blacks and whites in relation to body size among US children and adolescents. *Am J Epidemiol* 2000;151:1007–1019.
146. Reference deleted.
147. Harshfield GA, Dupaul LM, Alpert BS, et al. Aerobic fitness and the diurnal rhythm of blood pressure in adolescents. *Hypertension* 1990;15:810–814.
148. Hagberg JM, Goldring D, Ehsani AA, et al. Effect of exercise training on the blood pressure and hemodynamic features of hypertensive adolescents. *Am J Cardiol* 1983;52:763–768.
149. Athletic participation by children and adolescents who have systemic hypertension. *Pediatrics* 1997;99:637–638.
150. Kaminer B, Lutz WPW. Blood pressure in bushmen of the Kalahari Desert. *Circulation* 1960;22:289–295.
151. Oliver WJ, Cohen EL, Neel JV. Blood pressure, sodium intake and sodium related hormones in the Yanomamo Indians, a "no-salt" culture. *Circulation* 1975;52:146–151.
152. Dahl LK, Love RM. Evidence of relationship between sodium (chloride) intake and human hypertension. *Arch Intern Med* 1954;94:525–531.
153. Stamler J, Rose G, Elliott P, et al. Findings of the international cooperative INTERSALT study. *Hypertension* 1991;17[Suppl 1]:9–15.
154. Elliott P. Observational studies of salt and blood pressure. *Hypertension* 1991;17[Suppl 1]:3–8.
155. Gillum RF, Elmer PJ, Prineas RJ. Changing sodium intake in children: the Minneapolis children's blood pressure study. *Hypertension* 1981;3:698–703.
156. Whitten CF, Stewart RA. The effect of dietary sodium in infancy on blood pressure and related factors: studies of infants fed salted and unsalted diets for five months at eight months and eight years of age. *Acta Paediatr Scand Suppl* 1980;279:2–17.
157. Miller JZ, Weinberger MH, Daugherty SA, et al. Blood pressure response to dietary sodium restriction in healthy normotensive children. *Am J Clin Nutr* 1988;47:113–119.
158. Cooper R, van Horn L, Liu K, et al. A randomized trial on the effect of decreased dietary sodium intake on blood pressure in adolescents. *J Hypertension* 1984;2:361–366.
159. Simons-Morton DG, Obarzanek E. Diet and blood pressure in children and adolescents. *Pediatr Nephrol* 1997;11:244–249.
160. Law MR, Frost CD, Walt NJ. By how much does dietary salt reduction lower blood pressure? *BMJ* 1991;302:811–823.
161. Campese VM, Karubian F. Renal consequences of salt and hypertension. *Semin Nephrol* 1991;11:561–570.
162. Weinberger MH, Miller JZ, Luft FC, et al. Definitions and characteristics of sodium sensitivity and blood pressure resistance. *Hypertension* 1986;8[Suppl 2]:127–134.
163. Dahl LK, Heine M, Thompson K. Genetic influence of the kidneys on blood pressure: evidence from chronic renal homografts in rats with opposite predispositions to hypertension. *Circ Res* 1974;34:94–101.
164. Grim CE, Miller JZ, Brown PL, et al. Effects of sodium loading and depletion in normotensive first-degree relatives of essential hypertensives. *J Lab Clin Med* 1979;94:764–771.
165. Barker DJ. The fetal origins of adult hypertension. *J Hypertens Suppl* 1992;10:S39–44.
166. Law CM, Barker DJ, Bull AR, et al. Maternal and fetal influences on blood pressure. *Arch Dis Child* 2001;66:1291–1295.
167. Yiu V, Buka S, Zurakowski D, et al. Relationship between birthweight and blood pressure in childhood. *Am J Kidney Dis* 1999;33:253–260.
168. Law CM, de Swiet M, Osmond C, et al. Initiation of hypertension in utero and its implication throughout life. *BMJ* 1993;306:24–27.
169. Barker DJ. The fetal origins of hypertension. *J Hypertens Suppl* 1996;14:S111–S120.
170. Lurbe E, Redon J, Alvarez V, et al. Relationship between birth weight and awake blood pressure in children and adolescents in absence of intrauterine growth retardation. *Am J Hypertens* 1996;9:787–794.
171. Mackenzie HS, Brenner BM. Fewer nephrons at birth: a missing link in the etiology of essential hypertension? *Am J Kidney Dis* 1995;26:91–98.
172. Brenner BM, Garcia DL, Anderson S. Glomeruli and blood pressure. Less of one, more of the other? *Am J Hypertens* 1988;1:335–347.
173. Brenner BM. Congenital oligonephropathy and the etiology of adult hypertension and progressive renal injury. *Am J Kidney Dis* 1994;23:171–175.
174. Platt R. The nature of essential HTN. *Lancet* 1959;55–57.
174a. Pickering GW. The nature of hypertension. *Lancet* 1959; 1027–1028.
175. Corvol P, Persu A, Gimenez-Roqueplo AP, et al. Seven lessons from two candidate genes in human essential hypertension: angiotensinogen and epithelial sodium channel. *Hypertension* 1999;33:1324–1331.
176. Ward R. Familial aggregation and genetic epidemiology of blood pressure. In: Laragh J, Brenner B, eds. *Hypertension: pathophysiology, diagnosis, and management,* 2nd ed. New York: Raven Press, 1997:67–88.
176a. Annest JL, Sing CF, Biron P, et al. Familial aggregation of blood pressure and weight in adoptive families. *Am J Epidemiol* 1997;110:492–503.
177. Crook ED. The genetics of human hypertension. *Semin Nephrol* 2002;22(1):27–34.
178. Longini IMJ, Higgins MW, Hinton PC, et al. Environmental and genetic sources of familial aggregation of blood pressure in Tecumseh, Michigan. *Am J Epidemiol* 1984;120:131–144.
179. Grim CE, Wilson TW, Nicholson GD, et al. Blood pressure in blacks. Twin studies in Barbados. *Hypertension* 1990;15:803–809.
180. Levy D, DeStefano AL, Larson MG, et al. Evidence for a gene influencing blood pressure on chromosome 17. Genome scan linkage results for longitudinal blood pressure phenotypes in subjects from the Framingham heart study. *Hypertension* 2000;36:477–483.
181. Rice T, Rankinen T, Province MA, et al. Genome-wide linkage analysis of systolic and diastolic blood pressure: the Quebec Family Study. *Circulation* 2000;102:1956–1963.

182. Krushkal J, Ferrell R, Mockrin SC, et al. Genome-wide linkage analyses of systolic blood pressure using highly discordant siblings. *Circulation* 1999;99:1407–1410.
183. Jeunemaitre X, Soubrier F, Kotelevtsev YV, et al. Molecular basis of human hypertension: role of angiotensinogen. *Cell* 1992;71:169–180.
184. Brand E, Chatelain N, Keavney B, et al. Evaluation of the angiotensinogen locus in human essential hypertension: a European study. *Hypertension* 1998;31:725–729.
185. Kunz R, Kreutz R, Beige J, et al. Association between the angiotensinogen 235T-variant and essential hypertension in whites: a systematic review and methodological appraisal. *Hypertension* 1997;30:1331–1337.
186. Luft FC. Twins in cardiovascular genetic research. *Hypertension* 2001;37(2 Pt 2):350–356.
187. Busjahn A, Knoblauch H, Knoblauch M, et al. Angiotensin-converting enzyme and angiotensinogen gene polymorphisms, plasma levels, cardiac dimensions. A twin study. *Hypertension* 1997;29:165–170.
188. Fornage M, Amos CI, Kardia S, et al. Variation in the region of the angiotensin-converting enzyme gene influences interindividual differences in blood pressure levels in young white males. *Circulation* 1998;97:1773–1779.
189. O'Donnell CJ, Lindpaintner K, Larson MG, et al. Evidence for association and genetic linkage of the angiotensin-converting enzyme locus with hypertension and blood pressure in men but not women in the Framingham Heart Study. *Circulation* 1998;97:1766–1772.
190. Turner ST, Boerwinkle E, Sing CF. Context-dependent associations of the ACE I/D polymorphism with blood pressure. *Hypertension* 1999;34:773–778.
191. Jacobsen P, Rossing K, Rossing P, et al. Angiotensin converting enzyme gene polymorphism and ACE inhibition in diabetic nephropathy. *Kidney Int* 1998;53:1002–1006.
192. Kotanko P, Binder A, Tasker J, et al. Essential hypertension in African Caribbeans associates with a variant of the $beta_2$-adrenoceptor. *Hypertension* 1997;30:773–776.
193. Busjahn A, Li GH, Faulhaber HD, et al. Beta-2 adrenergic receptor gene variations, blood pressure, and heart size in normal twins. *Hypertension* 2000;35:555–560.
194. Bray MS, Krushkal J, Li L, et al. Positional genomic analysis identifies the beta(2)-adrenergic receptor gene as a susceptibility locus for human hypertension. *Circulation* 2000;101:2877–2882.
195. Herrmann SM, Nicaud V, Tiret L, et al. Polymorphisms of the $beta_2$-adrenoceptor (ADRB2) gene and essential hypertension: the ECTIM and PEGASE studies. *J Hypertens* 2002;20:229–235.
196. Glorioso N, Manunta P, Filigheddu F, et al. The role of alpha-adducin polymorphism in blood pressure and sodium handling regulation may not be excluded by a negative association study. *Hypertension* 1999;34:649–654.
197. Province MA, Arnett DK, Hunt SC, et al. Association between the alpha-adducin gene and hypertension in the HyperGEN Study. *Am J Hypertens* 2000;13:710–718.
198. Bray MS, Li L, Turner ST, et al. Association and linkage analysis of the alpha-adducin gene and blood pressure. *Am J Hypertens* 2000;13(6 Pt 1):699–703.
199. Psaty BM, Smith NL, Heckbert SR, et al. Diuretic therapy, the alpha-adducin gene variant, and the risk of myocardial infarction or stroke in persons with treated hypertension. *JAMA* 2002;287:1680–1689.
200. Siffert W, Rosskopf D, Siffert G, et al. Association of a human G-protein beta3 subunit variant with hypertension. *Nat Genet* 1998;18:45–48.
201. Turner ST, Schwartz GL, Chapman AB, et al. C825T polymorphism of the G protein beta(3)-subunit and antihypertensive response to a thiazide diuretic. *Hypertension* 2001;37:739–743.
202. Schuster H, Wienker TE, Bahring S, et al. Severe autosomal dominant hypertension and brachydactyly in a unique Turkish kindred maps to human chromosome 12. *Nat Genet* 1996;13:98–100.
203. Schuster H, Wienker TF, Toka HR, et al. Autosomal dominant hypertension and brachydactyly in a Turkish kindred resembles essential hypertension. *Hypertension* 1996;28:1085–1092.
204. Toka HR, Luft FC. Monogenic forms of human hypertension. *Semin Nephrol* 2002;22:81–88.
205. Bao W, Threefoot SA, Srinivasan SR, et al. Essential hypertension predicted by tracking of elevated blood pressure from childhood to adulthood: the Bogalusa Heart Study. *Am J Hypertens* 1995;8:657–665.
206. Mahoney LT, Clarke WR, Burns TL, et al. Childhood predictors of high blood pressure. *Am J Hypertens* 1991;4[Suppl]: 608S–610S.
207. Portman RJ, Robson AM. Controversies in pediatric hypertension. In: Tune BM, Mendoza SA, Brenner BM, et al., eds. *Pediatric nephrology*. New York: Churchill Livingstone, 1984:265–296.
208. Nelson MJ, Ragland DR, Syme SL. Longitudinal prediction of adult blood pressure from juvenile blood pressure levels. *Am J Epidemiol* 1992;136:633–645.
209. The Joint National Committee on Detection, Evaluation, and Treatment of High Blood Pressure. The 1980 Report of the Joint National Committee on Detection, Evaluation, and Treatment of High Blood Pressure. *Arch Intern Med* 1980;140:1280–1285.
210. Mahoney LT, Lauer RM. Consistency of blood pressure levels in children. *Semin Nephrol* 1989;9:230–235.
211. Burke V, Beilin LJ, Dunbar D. Tracking of blood pressure in Australian children. *J Hypertens* 2001;19:1185–1192.
212. Shear CL, Burke GL, Freedman DS, et al. Value of childhood blood pressure measurements and family history in predicting future blood pressure status: results from 8 years of follow-up in the Bogalusa Heart Study. *Pediatrics* 1986; 77:862–869.
213. Gillman MW, Rosner B, Evans DA, et al. Use of multiple visits to increase blood pressure tracking correlations in childhood. *Pediatrics* 1991;87:708–711.
214. O'Sullivan JJ, Derrick G, Foxall RJ. Tracking of 24-hour and casual blood pressure: a 1-year follow-up study in adolescents. *J Hypertens* 2000;18:1193–1996.
215. Parekh RS, Carroll CE, Wolfe RA, et al. Cardiovascular mortality in children and young adults with end-stage kidney disease. *J Pediatr* 2002;141:191–197.
216. Proulx F, Lacroix J, Farrell CA, et al. Convulsions and hypertension in children: differentiating cause from effect. *Crit Care Med* 1993;21:1541–1546.
217. Levy D, Garrison RJ, Savage DD, et al. Prognostic implications of echocardiographically determined left ventricular

mass in the Framingham Heart Study. *N Engl J Med* 1990;322:1561–1566.

218. Kannel WB, Gordon T, Offutt D. Left ventricular hypertrophy by electrocardiogram. Prevalence, incidence, and mortality in the Framingham study. *Ann Intern Med* 1969;71:89–105.
219. Kannel WB, Gordon T, Castelli WP, et al. Electrocardiographic left ventricular hypertrophy and risk of coronary heart disease. The Framingham study. *Ann Intern Med* 1970;72:813–822.
220. Brown DW, Giles WH, Croft JB. Left ventricular hypertrophy as a predictor of coronary heart disease mortality and the effect of hypertension. *Am Heart J* 2000;140:848–856.
221. Five-year findings of the Hypertension Detection and Follow-up Program. II. Mortality by race-sex and age. Hypertension Detection and Follow-up Program Cooperative Group. *JAMA* 1979;242:2572–2577.
222. Five-year findings of the Hypertension Detection and Follow-up Program. I. Reduction in mortality of persons with high blood pressure, including mild hypertension. Hypertension Detection and Follow-up Program Cooperative Group. *JAMA* 1979;242:2562–2571.
223. Daniels SD, Meyer RA, Loggie JM. Determinants of cardiac involvement in children and adolescents with essential hypertension. *Circulation* 1990;82:1243–1248.
224. Daniels SR, Kimball TR, Morrison JA, et al. Effect of lean body mass, fat mass, blood pressure, and sexual maturation on left ventricular mass in children and adolescents. Statistical, biological, and clinical significance. *Circulation* 1995;92:3249–3254.
225. Laird WP, Fixler DE. Left ventricular hypertrophy in adolescents with elevated blood pressure: assessment by chest roentgenography, electrocardiography, and echocardiography. *Pediatrics* 1981;67:255–259.
226. Malcolm DD, Burns TL, Mahoney LT, et al. Factors affecting left ventricular mass in childhood: the Muscatine Study. *Pediatrics* 1993;92:703–709.
227. Daniels SR, Kimball TR, Morrison JA, et al. Indexing left ventricular mass to account for differences in body size in children and adolescents without cardiovascular disease. *Am J Cardiol* 1995;76:699–701.
228. de Simone G, Devereux RB, Daniels SR, et al. Effect of growth on variability of left ventricular mass: assessment of allometric signals in adults and children and their capacity to predict cardiovascular risk. *J Am Coll Cardiol* 1995;25: 1056–1062.
229. Daniels SR, Witt SA, Glasock B, et al. Left atrial size in children with hypertension: the influence of obesity, blood pressure and left ventricular mass. *J Pediatr* 2002;141:186–190.
230. Trieber FA, McCaffrey F, Pflieger K, et al. Determinants of left ventricular mass in normotensive children. *Am J Hypertens* 1993;6:505–513.
231. Chamontin B, Amar J, Barthe P, et al. Blood pressure measurements and left ventricular mass in young adults with arterial hypertension screened at high school check-up. *J Hum Hypertens* 1994;8:357–361.
232. Kannel WB, Stampfer MJ, Castelli WP, et al. The prognostic significance of proteinuria: the Framingham study. *Am Heart J* 1984;108:1347–1352.
233. Effects of ramipril on cardiovascular and microvascular outcomes in people with diabetes mellitus: results of the HOPE study and MICRO-HOPE substudy. Heart Outcomes Prevention Evaluation Study Investigators. *Lancet* 2000;355:253–259.
234. Jones CA, Francis ME, Eberhardt MS, et al. Microalbuminuria in the US population: third National Health and Nutrition Examination Survey. *Am J Kidney Dis* 2002;39:445–459.
235. Pontremoli R, Nicolella C, Viazzi F, et al. Microalbuminuria is an early marker of target organ damage in essential hypertension. *Am J Hypertens* 1998;11:430–438.
236. Belsha CW, Wells TG, McNiece KL, et al. Influence of diurnal blood pressure variations on target organ abnormalities in adolescents with mild essential hypertension. *Am J Hypertens* 1998;11:410–417.
237. Grunfeld B, Perelstein E, Simsolo R, et al. Renal functional reserve and microalbuminuria in offspring of hypertensive parents. *Hypertension* 1990;15:257–261.
238. Arnett DK, Glasser SP, McVeigh G, et al. Blood pressure and arterial compliance in young adults: the Minnesota Children's Blood Pressure Study. *Am J Hypertens* 2001;14:200–205.
239. Swinford RD, Sorof JM, Poffenbarger T, et al. Abnormal large and small artery compliance in adolescent hemodialysis patients. Pediatric Academic Societies 2003, Research 2003(abst) *(in press).*
240. Bennett S, Sorof JM, Turner J, et al. Vascular compliance in normal children. Pediatric Academic Societies 2003, Research 2003(abst) *(in press).*
241. Sass C, Herbeth B, Chapet O, et al. Intima-media thickness and diameter of carotid and femoral arteries in children, adolescents and adults from the Stanislas cohort: effect of age, sex, anthropometry and blood pressure. *J Hypertens* 1998;16:1593–1602.
242. Daniels SR, Meyer RA, Strife CF, et al. Distribution of target-organ abnormalities by race and sex in children with essential hypertension. *J Hum Hypertens* 1990;4:103–104.
243. Daniels SR, Lipman MJ, Burke MJ, et al. The prevalence of retinal vascular abnormalities in children and adolescents with essential hypertension. *Am J Ophthalmol* 1991;111: 205–208.

60

PATHOPHYSIOLOGY OF HYPERTENSION

JOSEPH T. FLYNN
ROBERT P. WORONIECKI

Fundamentally, blood pressure is a function of cardiac output and total peripheral resistance. Cardiac output depends on cardiac stroke volume and heart rate. Stroke volume in turn depends on myocontractility and preload. Total peripheral resistance is dependent on vessel elasticity, myocontractility, and afterload. Thus, any factor influencing vessel wall tension or lumen size, extracellular fluid volume, autonomous cardiac rhythm, or cardiac pump function has an impact on blood pressure regulation and thereby can lead to the development of hypertension.

Research has begun to unravel relationships at the cellular and molecular levels that have important effects on blood pressure. The endothelium, intima, vascular smooth muscle, and extracellular matrix interact with each other and with vasomotor, growth, transcriptional, hormonal, and neuronal factors that affect signal transduction, gene transcription, ion transport, tissue remodeling, and cellular response, all in the context of the patient's genetic background.

MECHANISMS OF BLOOD PRESSURE REGULATION

Cardiac Output

Because the mean arterial blood pressure is a function of cardiac output and total peripheral resistance, hypertension is fundamentally a hemodynamic disorder that indicates a disturbance in one of these elements. Cardiac output is a function of stroke volume and heart rate. The preload of cardiac myocytes determines stroke volume, and heart rate is regulated by the sympathetic nervous system (SNS) as well as by the cardiac autonomic pacemaker. The SNS receives homeostatic feedback from baroreceptor-chemoreceptor reflexes and regulates the distribution of cardiac output over the short term. Increased SNS activity is most likely responsible for the mild tachycardia seen in many patients with primary hypertension (1).

Cardiac index (CI) is a function of cardiac output and body surface area. Young patients with mild hypertension have significantly higher cardiac output, CI, and sympathetic nerve burst frequency than age-matched controls (1). In borderline hypertension, CI and heart rate are higher, and calculated total peripheral resistance is normal (2). In nearly all forms of established hypertension, however, total peripheral resistance is increased and cardiac output is reduced. Moreover, in progressive hypertension, a further increase in total peripheral resistance occurs, and cardiac output continues to fall, which indicates reduced vascular compliance (3).

It is clear, however, that not all hypertensive patients start out with a state of increased cardiac output. In some patients, hypertension may develop because of increased total peripheral resistance. In addition, as is discussed later in the chapter, some patients may develop hypertension because of primary renal disease or a genetic defect that increases circulating blood volume through sodium retention.

Total Peripheral Resistance and the Vascular Wall

Because resistance increases as vessel cross-sectional area decreases, total peripheral resistance is mainly a function of small, peripheral resistance vessels. This physical property makes arterioles important regulators of blood pressure. The earliest structural change observed in the arterioles of experimental animals after the onset of hypertension is thickening of the media due to matrix deposition, smooth muscle cell hypertrophy (increase in cell size without division), and hyperplasia (increase in cell number) (4). The medial smooth muscle cells then rearrange themselves to create a smaller lumen without change in cell number or size, a process that has been termed remodeling. Later, a neointima may develop with the appearance of smooth muscle cells inside the internal elastic lamina. There are also local areas of endothelial cell denudation and inflammatory cell infiltration, which can progress to atherosclerotic plaque formation (5). Finally, resorption and loss of blood vessels may occur in the periphery—a process termed *rarefaction*, which has been found in both the early and later stages of hypertension (6).

In larger vessels, the content of elastin and collagen in the media increases and the number of smooth muscle cells decreases (via medial atrophy, necrosis, or apoptosis) (7), which leads to a loss of elasticity and the development of vessel "stiffness." Significant increases in the size and number of vasa vasorum (tiny vessels in the adventitia that supply nutrients and oxygen to the deeper layers of the media) can be observed in larger conduit vessels, which is probably an adaptive process in the sense that the increased smooth muscle cell mass in the hypertensive vessel wall requires more oxygen and nutrients. In summary, the hypertensive vessel wall is generally characterized by increased medial thickness or an increased media/lumen ratio of the resistance arterioles. This structural change is biomechanically adaptive because wall stress is normalized as defined by Laplace's law, but functionally this means that there is greater resistance for a given contractile stimulus (8).

Altered vascular structure in hypertension is also accompanied by functional changes in the cellular components of the vessel wall, specifically decreased relaxation and increased contraction (8). Decreased relaxation has been attributed primarily to endothelial dysfunction, and increased contraction has been attributed to enhanced smooth muscle cell vasoreactivity. Sensitivity to vasoconstrictors may also be increased (6). Decreased relaxation is an effect of impaired endothelial production of vasodilating substances [mainly nitric oxide (NO) and prostacyclin] or increased production of vasoconstricting substances [endothelin, platelet-derived growth factor (PDGF)], or both.

Increased smooth muscle cell responsiveness is caused by alterations in the ability of vasodilating substances to exert their effects, changes in the ability of smooth muscle cells to respond to vasodilators, increased responsiveness to vasoconstrictors because of increased numbers of receptors or an augmented contractile machinery, or all of these. Moreover, vasoconstrictors frequently stimulate smooth muscle cell growth and, conversely, many growth factors have vasoconstrictor activity [e.g., PDGF is a vasoconstrictor (9) and angiotensin II is a potent smooth muscle cell growth factor (10)]. These functional alterations act in concert with the structural changes discussed earlier to perpetuate hypertension, which emphasizes the importance of the vasculature in blood pressure regulation.

Sympathetic Innervation/ Central Nervous System

Renal vessels, tubules, and the juxtaglomerular apparatus are innervated by the renal sympathetic nerves (11). Renal sympathetic nerve activity (RSNA) influences renal hemodynamics, solute and water handling, and hormonal release. Increased RSNA is found in animal models of hypertension and in hypertensive humans (12). SNS activation, as confirmed by increased circulating noradrenaline, muscle sympathetic nerve traffic, and systemic noradrenaline spillover, is almost universally present in essential hypertension (13,14) and has been demonstrated in patients with renovascular hypertension (15). It appears to be particularly pronounced in young and middle-aged patients (14). Renal denervation prevents or alleviates hypertension in virtually all animal models of hypertension.

Increased RSNA constricts the renal vasculature and decreases glomerular filtration rate (GFR) and renal blood flow (16). The hypertensive response to chronic renal adrenergic stimulation is associated with a sustained increase in plasma renin activity and is dependent on an increase in plasma angiotensin II concentration (17). Renin release and increased circulating angiotensin II results in enhanced tubular water and sodium reabsorption throughout the nephron (18). The effect of angiotensin II to raise proximal tubular chloride and water reabsorption is decreased by 75% in animals after experimental renal denervation. Thus, only approximately 25% of the effect of angiotensin II is mediated directly by type 1 angiotensin receptors; the majority of the effect is dependent on intact renal innervation. In experimental renal sympathetic nerve stimulation, angiotensin II enhanced renal venous outflow of norepinephrine, an effect that was blocked by an angiotensin II receptor antagonist (19). This clearly demonstrates the connection between RSNA and angiotensin II, and suggests that angiotensin II exerts a peripheral, presynaptic action on renal sympathetic nerve terminals in renal tubular epithelial cells and vessels to enhance the release of norepinephrine (20).

Studies indicate that angiotensin II also acts centrally on brainstem nuclei that are important in the control of peripheral sympathetic vasomotor tone, for example, the rostral ventrolateral medulla of the hypothalamus (RVLM) (21). Because circulating angiotensin II is not able to cross the blood-brain barrier, it acts on circumventricular organs in which the normal blood-brain barrier is lacking. Those consist of the subfornical organ, the organum vasculosum of the lamina terminalis, the median eminence, and the area postrema (22). Activation of the area postrema by circulating angiotensin II may in turn increase peripheral sympathetic nerve activity via a direct excitatory connection from the area postrema to the RVLM. Experimental microinjection of angiotensin II into the RVLM results in increases in arterial pressure (23) and peripheral sympathetic nerve activity (24), and facilitates arterial baroreflex modulation of RSNA (25). All these effects are blocked by antagonists for angiotensin type 1 (AT1) receptors but not by antagonists for angiotensin type 2 (AT2) receptors (26). Moreover, the RVLM contains angiotensin II immunoreactive nerve terminals, AT1 receptor messenger RNA, and AT1 receptor binding sites (27). These findings suggest that angiotensin peptides of brain origin may have a local paracrine or autocrine action on the RVLM that regulates RSNA and its arterial baroreflex control.

Circadian Rhythm

The circadian rhythm is an intrinsic 24-hour cycle that affects numerous physiologic processes. Vascular tone, total peripheral resistance, heart rate, and blood pressure increase in the early morning hours in both normotensive and hypertensive subjects. This rise corresponds to increased plasma renin activity and a surge in secretion of catecholamines. Blood pressure reaches its peak at approximately 9 a.m. and falls to its lowest level at 3 a.m. A significant rise in blood pressure occurs before awakening. Although environmental factors (especially light-dark cycles) have a significant impact on the circadian variation in blood pressure, some aspects appear to be genetically determined (28). Diurnal variation of blood pressure has been clearly demonstrated in normotensive children (29); in hypertensive children, data suggest that diurnal variation is preserved in children with primary hypertension but is abnormal in those with secondary forms of hypertension (30). (See Chapter 61.)

The central pacemaker in mammals is located in the suprachiasmatic nucleus (SCN) of the brain, which is found in the anterior hypothalamus, immediately above the optic chiasm (31). It receives input about light-dark cycles from the retina via the retinohypothalamic tract and produces several neuropeptides, including vasopressin and vasoactive intestinal peptide (VIP), that appear to have diurnal peaks of expression and release (32). Animal experiments have demonstrated that the SCN is linked to multiple sympathetic pathways that control the cardiovascular system (33). It plays a crucial role in synchronizing the peripheral oscillators that are found in all tissues, including vascular smooth muscle cells and the aorta, and in the execution of rhythmic behavior. The primary mediator of SCN action appears to be melatonin, which is secreted by the pineal gland under control of the SCN (31). Melatonin appears to transmit information about light-dark cycles from the SCN to the peripheral oscillators (28) as well as to other centers in the hypothalamus that regulate cardiovascular activity (33).

Supporting evidence for the role of the SCN and melatonin in blood pressure regulation comes from studies demonstrating that melatonin levels are decreased in hypertensive individuals and that administration of melatonin lowers blood pressure (33). In addition, autopsy studies of patients with primary hypertension have demonstrated that SCN neuronal populations responsible for producing vasopressin and VIP are reduced, which suggests that, in at least some individuals with hypertension, normal function of the intrinsic biologic clock is impaired (34).

Fluid and Electrolyte Balance

The kidneys of an adult with free access to water and salt filter approximately 125 mL/min of plasma containing 140 mEq/L of sodium and 105 mEq/L of chloride. Approximately 100 mEq of sodium and chloride are excreted daily in the urine. The kidneys have the ability to respond to changes in arterial pressure by altering the renal excretion of salt and water; increases in renal perfusion pressure lead to decreases in sodium reabsorption and increases in sodium excretion (pressure natriuresis) (35).

The intrarenal mechanism of pressure natriuresis is related to medullary blood flow, renal interstitial hydrostatic pressure, and renal autocoids (NO, prostaglandins, kinins, and angiotensin II). Increased renal perfusion pressure is associated with increases in renal interstitial hydrostatic pressure and levels of NO, prostaglandin E_2, and kinins, and a decrease in angiotensin II (35–38). Increased blood flow to the renal medulla, which normally receives only 5 to 10% of the total renal blood flow, contributes to washout of the urea gradient. This results in an increase in renal interstitial fluid pressure, which in turn reduces tubular reabsorption of sodium and water; the result is natriuresis and diuresis, which lowers blood pressure (39). Infusion of norepinephrine into the renal medulla results in a pressure natruresis and lowering of arterial blood pressure (40). This depressor response is abolished by chemical medullectomy (41). This finding suggests the presence of an as-yet-to-be-characterized depressor hormone in the renal medulla (42).

Regulation of the number and function of critical renal sodium transporters and channels is another important means by which the kidney controls salt and water balance. Expression of many of these proteins is influenced by aldosterone and other hormones that affect blood pressure (43,44). As discussed later in this chapter, all monogenic forms of human hypertension described thus far can be characterized by alterations in renal ion channels that lead either to increased sodium reabsorption or to decreased excretion. Similarly, in an animal model of essential hypertension, the Dahl salt-sensitive hypertensive rat, AngII/arginine vasopressin receptor dysfunction produces hypertension through increased tubular sodium and fluid reabsorption (45).

Renal Autoregulation

Renal autoregulation, or the kidney's intrinsic ability to maintain constant renal blood flow and GFR despite changes in renal perfusion pressure, serves to protect nephron function. However, major variations in renal perfusion can still influence renal excretory functions, renin release, and arterial blood pressure. Autoregulation occurs in interlobular arteries, side branches of arcuate arteries, and afferent and efferent arterioles. It depends on myogenic mechanisms present in those vessels and is blocked by the smooth muscle relaxant papaverine (46) and by calcium-channel blockade (47). Tubuloglomerular feedback also plays an important but not essential role in autoregulation (48).

Renal autoregulation is reset in animal models of spontaneous hypertension (49). Angiotensin II plays an important role in the resetting of the autoregulation limits (50).

Higher pressures are needed to trigger the vasoconstrictive response in the afferent arteriole (51), but in the intermediate portion of the interlobular artery of the spontaneously hypertensive rat, a lower threshold pressure stimulates a greater myogenic response (52). In the Dahl salt-sensitive hypertensive rat, both the afferent arterioles and the interlobular arteries have reduced myogenic responsiveness to increases in perfusion pressure (53). Studies demonstrating that abnormalities in renal autoregulation are more pronounced in patients with severe hypertension than in those with moderate hypertension (54) suggest that disturbed renal autoregulation can be induced by chronic hypertension. Thus, disturbed renal autoregulation may contribute to the perpetuation of blood pressure elevation in patients with established hypertension.

Renin-Angiotensin System

Renin is secreted from the juxtaglomerular apparatus of the kidney in response to glomerular underperfusion or reduced sodium intake, or in response to stimulation from the SNS. Except for renin, all the components of a local vascular wall renin-angiotensin system appear to be present in normal vessels (55), and their activity is dynamically regulated. In the classic renin-angiotensin system, circulating renal-derived renin cleaves hepatic-derived angiotensinogen to form the decapeptide angiotensin I, which is converted by angiotensin-converting enzyme (ACE) in the lungs to the active component of the renin-angiotensin system, angiotensin II (angiotensin II). ACE exists in plasma, in the interstitium, and within the cell. Tissue ACE is present in all major organs, including the heart, brain, blood vessels, adrenals, kidney, liver, and reproductive organs (56) and is already functional *in utero* (57).

Angiotensin II is a potent vasoconstrictor and thus causes a rise in blood pressure. It also stimulates the release of aldosterone from the zona glomerulosa of the adrenal gland, which results in a further rise in blood pressure from aldosterone-mediated sodium and water retention. In addition, it plays an important physiologic role in the regulation of sympathetic nervous activity (see preceding discussion of the SNS) and the thirst response (58). The effects of angiotensin II are mediated primarily by the plasma membrane receptors AT1 and AT2. Other angiotensin receptors have been described but are not yet fully characterized (59,60).

The AT1 receptor is composed of 359 amino acids and belongs to the seven-membrane-spanning G-protein–coupled receptor family (61,62). In rodents, the AT1 receptor has two functionally distinct subtypes, AT1A and AT1B, with greater than 95% amino acid sequence homology (63). The human AT1 receptor gene has been mapped to chromosome 3 (64). Expression of the AT1 receptor is a subject to negative feedback by angiotensin II (65). AT1 receptor activation stimulates vasoconstriction, vascular cell hypertrophy and hyperplasia, sodium retention, reactive oxygen species generation via induction of nicotinamide adenine dinucleotide phosphate (reduced form) (66), and induction of inflammatory (67), thrombotic (68), and fibrotic processes (69). Some of the pathophysiologic effects of angiotensin II may be mediated through activation of the transcription factor nuclear factor-B (NF-B) (70), which participates in a variety of inflammatory responses (71). Many polymorphisms of the AT1 receptor gene have been identified, but the A1166→C polymorphism has been the most extensively studied. It has been associated with the development of primary hypertension in various populations (72).

The AT2 receptor is a seven-transmembrane-type, G-protein–coupled receptor comprising 363 amino acids. It has low amino acid sequence homology (approximately 34%) with AT1A and AT1B receptors (61,62). The expression of the AT2 receptor is upregulated by sodium depletion (73) and is inhibited by angiotensin II and growth factors such as PDGF and epidermal growth factor (74). Under physiologic conditions, AT2 receptor antagonizes AT1-mediated actions (75) by inhibiting cell growth and by inducing apoptosis and vasodilatation (76,77). Cardiovascular effects of the AT2 receptor appear to be opposite to those of the AT1 receptor (78). Other physiologic effects attributed to the AT2 receptor include modulation of thirst, behavior, and locomotor activity (79). It also has proinflammatory effects, via induction of NF-B (70), and trophic effects leading to vascular (80) and cardiac (81) hypertrophy. The functions of the AT1 and AT2 receptors are summarized and compared in Table 60.1.

Hypertension is associated with remodeling of the left ventricle, alterations in the morphology and mechanical properties of the vasculature, and the development of endothelial dysfunction (82,83). Angiotensin II is capable of mediating these changes, independently of its effect on blood pressure, via its interaction with the AT1 receptor (84). These varied effects of angiotensin II in hypertension provide the physiologic foundation for the use of ACE inhibitors and angiotensin II receptor antagonists in the treatment of patients with hypertension.

TABLE 60.1. COMPARISON OF THE EFFECTS OF ANGIOTENSIN TYPE 1 (AT1) AND ANGIOTENSIN TYPE 2 (AT2) RECEPTORS

AT1	AT2
Vasoconstriction	Vasodilatation
Cell proliferation	Apoptosis
Cell hypertrophy	Growth inhibition
Antinatriuresis	Natriuresis
Superoxide production	Nitric oxide production
Endothelin release	Collagen synthesis
Lipid peroxidation	
Adhesion molecule expression	
Vascular matrix expansion	

Aldosterone

Aldosterone is produced by the mitochondrial enzyme CYP 11B2 (aldosterone synthase) encoded by the *CYP11B2* gene (85). This enzyme is expressed in the zona glomerulosa of the adrenal glands, aorta, endothelial cells and vascular smooth muscle cells, hypothalamus, hippocampus, amygdala, cerebrum, and cerebellum (86,87). Aldosterone and its precursors, 18-hydroxycorticosterone, corticosterone, and deoxycorticosterone, are synthesized from cholesterol. Angiotensin II and III induce aldosterone synthesis. Potassium and adrenocorticotropic hormone (ACTH) stimulate its secretion (88). Atrial natriuretic peptide (ANP) inhibits aldosterone secretion by interfering with extracellular calcium influx (89).

Aldosterone acts via an intracellular, high-affinity type I glucocorticoid receptor. The postreceptor mechanisms of rapid aldosterone action appear to involve protein kinase C, calcium, cyclic adenosine 3',5'-monophosphate and inositol 1,4,5-triphosphate, with downstream effects on a variety of ion pumps and channels (90). Aldosterone induces retention of sodium and potassium excretion. It also activates the SNS by preventing the uptake of norepinephrine by the myocardium and causes baroreceptor dysfunction (91,92) and eventually myocardial and vascular fibrosis (93). The importance of aldosterone in hypertension is highlighted by studies demonstrating that the aldosterone receptor antagonist spironolactone improves endothelial dysfunction, increases NO bioactivity in chronic heart and renal failure, and prevents the development of nephrosclerosis and cerebrovascular lesions (94,95).

Dopamine

Dopamine is an important modulator of systemic blood pressure with direct actions on the heart, arteries, and veins. Dopamine is synthesized in noradrenergic and dopaminergic nerves, and also in nonneural tissues (e.g., kidney, gastrointestinal tract) (96). Dopamine modulates renal epithelial transport, and gastrointestinal sodium uptake (97). It can indirectly modulate blood pressure via release of hormones and humoral agents such as aldosterone, catecholamines, endothelin, prolactin, proopiomelanocortin, renin, and vasopressin (98). Dopamine modulates fluid and sodium intake via "appetite" centers in the brain (99) and, in addition, controls blood pressure by direct action on neuronal cardiovascular centers.

Dopamine increases cardiac output by stimulating myocardial β-adrenergic receptors and plays an important role in modulating vascular smooth muscle tone by a complex series of interactions with various dopamine receptors. Stimulation of D1 and D5 dopamine receptors can cause vasorelaxation, whereas stimulation of D3 receptors produces vasoconstriction. At extremely high concentrations, dopamine produces vasoconstriction by occupation of α_1-adrenergic receptors (100). Dopaminergic blockade is associated with the development of hypertension in rats and potentiates the renal effects of NO inhibition in humans (101).

Moreover, dopamine also regulates the expression of other receptors involved in blood pressure regulation (e.g., endothelin-B, AT1). Both D1- and D2-like receptors downregulate AT1 receptor expression and function (102). Disruption of the D3 receptor gene in mice is associated with renin-dependent hypertension and a decreased ability to excrete an acute saline load (103). Aberrant dopaminergic regulation of aldosterone secretion (via D3 receptors) may be involved in some forms of hyperaldosteronism and hypertension (104,105).

Interindividual variation in systolic blood pressure has been shown in one study to be influenced by the activity of the gene that encodes the type 1A dopamine receptor (106). However, no mutations have been found in the coding region of the D1 receptor in patients with essential hypertension or in genetically hypertensive rats (107). A polymorphism in the noncoding region of the D1 receptor has been reported to be associated with human essential hypertension; however, the mechanism by which this polymorphism induces hypertension remains to be determined (108). Several D2 receptor polymorphisms have been reported, one of which is associated with hypertension (109). It is likely that as molecular genetic and population genetic studies progress, the role of dopamine in the pathogenesis of human hypertension will be further elucidated.

Atrial Natriuretic Peptide

ANP belongs to a family of natriuretic peptides that also includes the B-type and the C-type natriuretic peptides (110). The biologic functions of B-type and C-type natriuretic peptides do not differ from those of ANP. ANP is involved in regulation of salt and water balance and blood pressure homeostasis, and has an antiproliferative effect at the cellular level in the cardiovascular system (111–113). ANP is primarily expressed in cardiac myocytes but is also found in brain, vessels, and kidneys. ANP has potent diuretic, natriuretic, and vasorelaxant effects. In the kidneys, ANP increases GFR through vasodilatation of the afferent arterioles and vasoconstriction of the efferent arterioles (114). Natriuresis occurs by several mechanisms, including inhibition of sodium reabsorption in both the proximal and the distal tubule (115,116) and inhibition of both renin and aldosterone biosynthesis (117,118).

The combined systemic hemodynamic effects of ANP result in reduction of both preload and afterload (119,120). Administration of endogenous ANP results in a significant decrease of blood pressure in humans and in animal models of hypertension by reducing systemic vascular resistance (121,122). The blood pressure–lowering effect of ANP is enhanced in models of renovascular hypertension (123) and in conditions of volume expansion (124). At high plasma levels, ANP decreases heart rate, central venous pressure, and stroke volume (125).

Mutations in the ANP gene have been described in both hypertensive and healthy individuals (126,127). A significant association has been demonstrated between an intronic variant of the ANP gene (HpaII) and salt-sensitive hypertension in African Americans (128). A mutation located within the 5' untranslated region of the ANP gene has been reported to show a marginally significant association with occurrence of hypertension in a Japanese population (129). In a population drawn from the Physicians' Health Study, carriers of a mutation in exon 1 of the ANP gene showed a twofold higher risk of stroke than noncarriers, an effect that was independent from other conventional risk factors such as obesity and diabetes, and occurred in spite of lower blood pressure levels (130). These studies suggest a potentially important role for variants of the ANP gene in the development of hypertension and other cardiovascular disease, although, as with other genetic influences on hypertension (see later), much more research must be done to elucidate exactly how these genetic variants produce blood pressure elevation.

Endothelin-1

Endothelin-1 (ET-1) is an endothelial cell–derived, potent vasoconstrictive peptide containing 21 amino acids (131). Three isopeptides of endothelin (ET-1, ET-2, and ET-3), encoded by separate genes, have been identified (132). Endothelial ET-1 synthesis is activated by vasoactive hormones, growth factors, hypoxia, shear stress, lipoproteins, free radicals, endotoxin, and cyclosporine, and is inhibited by NO, natriuretic peptides, heparin, and prostaglandins (133). Apart from endothelial cells, ET-1 is also produced by the heart, kidney, posterior pituitary, central nervous system, and vascular smooth muscle cells (133). ET-2 is produced in endothelial cells, heart, and kidney (134), but it has not been detected in human plasma. ET-3 is selectively expressed in the endocrine, gastrointestinal, and central nervous system, but not in endothelial cells (135).

ET-1 appears to be primarily a locally acting paracrine substance. Endothelin receptor-binding sites have been identified throughout the body, with the greatest number of receptors in the kidneys and lungs (136). Endothelin signals through two receptor subtypes, ETA and ETB. The ETA receptor is preferentially activated by ET-1 but not by ET-3, whereas the ETB receptor is activated equally by ET-1 and ET-3 (137,138). The vasoconstrictor effects of endothelin are mediated primarily by ETA receptors, but ETB receptors located on vascular smooth muscle also contribute to the vasoconstrictor effects of this peptide (139). ETB receptors located on the endothelium are thought to stimulate release of NO and prostacyclin.

ET-1 closes membrane K^+ channels (140), which prevents efflux of K^+ from the cell and thereby favors depolarization of membrane and contraction of smooth muscle. ET-1 also activates production of prostacyclin and thromboxane A_2 (141). In the kidney, ET-1 contracts afferent and efferent arterioles equally (142) and thus reduces both renal plasma flow and GFR (143,144). It blocks reabsorption of sodium by inhibiting tubular Na^+-K^+–adenosine triphosphatase activity in the proximal tubule and collecting duct (145). ET-1 inhibits release of renin from isolated rat glomeruli (146) but stimulates release of aldosterone from isolated cortical zona glomerulosa cells (147). ET-1 also stimulates production and release of ANP by cultured atrial myocytes (148).

The overall cardiovascular effect of endogenous ET-1 depends on the balance between ETA- and ETB-mediated effects. Activation of vascular smooth muscle ETA receptors causes vasoconstriction and tends to elevate blood pressure, whereas activation of endothelial and renal ETB receptors promotes vasodilatation and natriuresis and tends to decrease blood pressure (149). ETB "knock-out" mice have hypertension secondary to renal retention of sodium, and there is evidence of marked enhancement of vascular expression of ET-1 in salt-sensitive hypertensive rat models (150). ET-1 appears to potentiate sympathetically mediated vasoconstriction only in hypertensive and not in normotensive subjects (151).

Hypertensive patients with normal renal function have concentrations of immunoreactive E-1 similar to those in normotensive patients (152); however, plasma concentrations of ET-1 are raised in patients with accelerated hypertension, and these levels are positively correlated with creatinine clearance (153). Plasma concentrations of ET-1 in patients with chronic renal failure are onefold to twofold greater than normal, whereas values in those undergoing hemodialysis are twofold to fourfold greater than normal (154). In renal transplant patients, production of ET-1 is stimulated by cyclosporine A (155), which also increases the number of renal ET-1 binding sites (156). Tacrolimus also appears to increase secretion of ET-1 *in vitro* (157). These findings suggest that endothelin may be involved in the pathogenesis of calcineurin-induced hypertension.

Genetic variation in ET-1 expression may be involved in the pathogenesis of essential hypertension. African Americans with hypertension have much higher concentrations of immunoreactive endothelin than do whites (158). There is also strong correlation between diastolic blood pressure and polymorphisms of the ET-1 precursor pre–proendothelin-1 between patients with essential hypertension and normotensive controls (159).

Nitric Oxide and Adenosine

Nitric oxide is endothelium-derived gas, synthesized from the amino acid L-arginine by the endothelial isoform of NO synthase (NOS) (160). NO is extremely labile, with a half-life of less than 4 seconds in biologic solutions. It is rapidly oxidized to nitrite and then nitrate by oxygenated hemoglobin before being excreted into the urine (160). Synthesized NO diffuses across the endothelial cell membrane and enters the vascular smooth muscle cells. It activates guanylate cyclase, which leads to production of a second messenger, cyclic guanosine-3',5-monophosphate (cGMP) (160). The cGMP mediates control of vascular tone and platelet function.

NO is a vasodilator, and the balance between NO and various endothelium-derived vasoconstrictors and the SNS maintains physiologic blood vessel tone (161). In addition, NO suppresses platelet aggregation, leukocyte migration, and cellular adhesion to the endothelium. It attenuates vascular smooth muscle cell proliferation and migration, as well as inhibiting activation and expression of certain adhesion molecules, and has an influence on production of superoxide anion.

Endothelium-dependent relaxation is decreased in patients with essential hypertension (162) who have impaired generation of NO (163). Treatment with inhibitors of NO synthesis induces a hypertensive response, whereas L-arginine treatment prevents the development of hypertension in animals prone to this disease (164) and also causes a rapid reduction in systolic and diastolic pressures when infused into healthy humans and patients with essential hypertension (165). Methylated L-arginine derivatives, including NG-NG-dimethylarginine (asymmetric dimethylarginine), an inhibitor of NO synthase, and symmetric dimethylarginine, its inactive isomer, are present in human plasma and urine. These compounds accumulate in the plasma of patients with renal failure (162,166).

Cardiovascular homeostasis is also influenced by neuronal production of NO within the autonomic nervous system. Acting by central and peripheral mechanisms, NO has been shown to have sympathoinhibitory and vagotonic effects. Experiments in hypertensive rats indicate that neuronal NO production is impaired at a number of key central sites concerned with autonomic cardiovascular regulation (167). Because sympathetic overactivity may play a role in the genesis of human hypertension, these experiments suggest that defects in central nervous system neuronal NO production may be an initiating step in this process.

Adenosine is produced from the hydrolysis of adenosine 5'-monophosphate by 5'-nucleotidase (168,169). In the kidney, it regulates GFR, tubuloglomerular feedback, tubular reabsorption, and renin secretion. Adenosine acts via several cell surface receptors that have been designated A1, A2A, A2B, A3, and A4, all of which differentially stimulate or inhibit the production of cyclic adenosine-3',5'-monophosphate. Sites of A1 gene expression include glomeruli, proximal tubule, thick ascending limb of the loop of Henle, juxtaglomerular apparatus, collecting ducts, and microvessels (170). Selective A1 antagonists lead to diuresis and natriuresis and uncouple glomerular filtration and tubular reabsorption (171). A2A and A2B receptors have been described on vascular smooth muscle cells and the endothelium, where they are associated with vasodilatation (171). A2A "knock-out" mice have increased blood pressure and heart rate, and increased platelet aggregation (172).

Other Regulatory Hormones

Thyroid hormone plays an important role in the regulation of blood pressure. Administration of exogenous thyroid hormone results in a decrease in systemic vascular resistance, which in turn results in renin release, activation of the angiotensin–aldosterone axis, increase in renal sodium reabsorption, increase in intravascular volume, and increase in cardiac output and cardiac contractility. Thyroid hormone also stimulates erythropoietin secretion (173). Triiodothyronine (T_3) acts directly on arterioles (vascular smooth muscle cells) and promotes relaxation and vasodilatation by local heat production, and β_2 receptor stimulation (174).

T_3 enters the cell by a specific transporter and forms a complex with nuclear T_3 receptors. This complex binds to thyroid hormone response elements of several genes and regulates their transcription. Genes upregulated by T_3 include those for adrenergic receptors, Na^+-K^+–adenosine triphosphatase, and voltage-gated potassium channels, among others. Genes downregulated by T_3 include those for the Na^+-Ca^{2+} exchanger, adenyl cyclase types V and VI, and the T_3 nuclear receptor. In the short term, T_3 modulates sodium, potassium, and calcium-channel activities in the heart that lead to changes in intracellular calcium and potassium with subsequent increase in inotropy and chronotropy (175). Increased heart rate, widened pulse pressure, and increased cardiac output despite normal or low-serum concentrations of catecholamines is a characteristic feature of patients with hyperthyroidism (176).

Adrenomedullin peptide (ADM), a 52-amino-acid peptide, has been found in the adrenal medulla, cardiac atrium, lung, and kidney. In the kidney, ADM is found in glomeruli, cortical distal tubules, and medullary collecting duct cells (177,178). ADM is also secreted from endothelial cells and vascular smooth muscle cells (179). ADM leads to vasodilatation, natriuresis, diuresis, inhibition of aldosterone production, and enhancement of tumor cell growth (180,181). Increased levels of ADM have been documented in patients with essential hypertension and chronic renal failure (182).

PRIMARY HYPERTENSION

Most hypertension in adults is of unknown cause; therefore, the term *essential hypertension* has been applied as a catch-all diagnosis in individuals in whom an underlying cause for their hypertension cannot be identified. However, because the word *essential* implies that the patient's level of blood pressure is necessary in some way to maintain normal func-

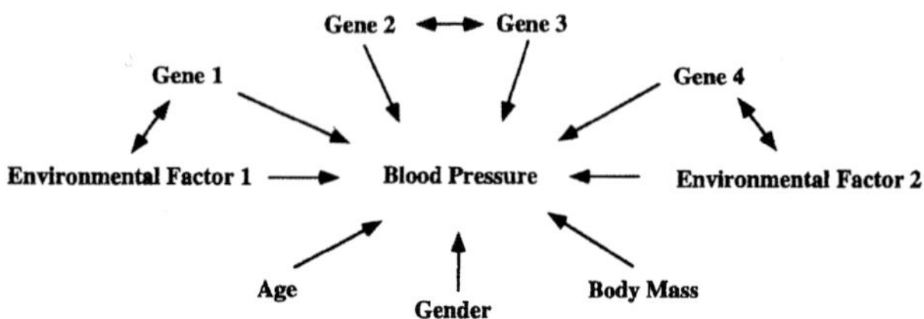

FIGURE 60.1. Multifactorial model of blood pressure determination, demonstrating the potential influence of genes, environmental factors, and demographic factors on blood pressure. The potential interaction of these determining factors is represented by arrows linking different determinants. (From Lifton RP. Genetic determinants of human hypertension. *Proc Natl Acad Sci U S A* 1995;92:8545–8551, copyright 1995, National Academy of Sciences, USA, with permission.)

tion, this term is misleading and should be abandoned in favor of *primary hypertension*. It is likely that, as our unraveling of the human genome progresses and more genetic forms of hypertension are identified (see later), fewer and fewer patients will be diagnosed with primary hypertension; for now, however, primary hypertension remains an important entity and accounts for most human hypertension.

In children, primary hypertension has long been considered an uncommon form of hypertension and accounted for fewer than 25% of cases of childhood hypertension in series from referral centers published through the mid-1990s (183). As studies from less specialized centers and more recent series from referral centers have demonstrated (184,185), however, primary hypertension in children is likely more common than previously thought and is probably also increasing in prevalence, with many children developing hypertension as a manifestation of obesity (see the following discussion), which is also becoming increasingly prevalent in childhood (186).

Primary hypertension is a multifactorial disorder in which elevated blood pressure is caused by different combinations of factors in different individuals (Fig. 60.1). Advances in molecular genetics have caused a great deal of attention to be focused on determining how genetic variation may explain blood pressure elevation in some individuals (187). Although genes are likely to be involved to some extent in nearly every hypertensive individual, however, the genetic contribution to an individual's hypertension may not be as significant as that of other factors, such as body habitus or environment. Although a detailed discussion of every factor possibly involved in the pathogenesis of primary hypertension is beyond the scope of this chapter, some of the more important mechanisms likely to contribute to the development of primary hypertension in children are highlighted.

Genetic Influences on Primary Hypertension

Substantial evidence exists for genetic influence on blood pressure. Twin studies document greater concordance of blood pressures among monozygotic than among dizygotic twins (188), and population studies demonstrate greater similarity of blood pressure within families than between families (189). Studies demonstrating a lack of correlation of blood pressure between parents and their adoptive children would also support the contention that blood pressure is genetically determined (190). Despite intensive efforts over nearly three decades, however, the genetic basis of hypertension has not been fully elucidated thus far.

Studies applying new molecular biologic techniques to the problem of hypertension have focused on identifying candidate genes involved in the pathogenesis of hypertension. To date, however, with the exception of the single-gene forms of hypertension described later in this chapter, most of these studies have failed to demonstrate how the various genetic mutations identified lead to elevated blood pressure. For example, although the studies of Jeunemaitre et al. (191) and Inoue et al. (192) have identified a link between polymorphisms of the angiotensinogen gene and hypertension, and although other studies have shown that angiotensinogen levels are higher in individuals with higher levels of blood pressure (193), how these variations cause hypertension still is not known (187). The same holds true for all of the many other allelic variants identified to date in individuals with primary hypertension.

Studies have demonstrated that, in some people, blood pressure elevation may be not the result of a single mutation but rather the product of multiple genetic variants interacting with each other (194). Similarly, it is probable that the role of some genetic variants in the pathogenesis of primary hypertension may be not to increase blood pressure in and of themselves, but rather to increase the susceptibility of an individual to environmental factors that can elevate blood pressure (195). This would be consistent with the scheme illustrated in Figure 60.1.

Clearly, the delineation of the pathogenesis of primary hypertension from the genetic standpoint is in its early stages. Mapping of the rat genome and the development of new strategies and technologies in molecular genetics, including differential gene expression, expressed sequence tags, and DNA biochips, provide hope that the challenge of elucidating the genetic basis of primary hypertension will be met (196). This in turn should result in improved therapies for the millions of Americans with primary hypertension.

Influence of Birth Weight and Perinatal Factors on Primary Hypertension

The influence of prenatal and postnatal events on future blood pressure has been a topic of great interest to researchers over the past 15 years. Proponents of the "fetal origins" hypothesis maintain that low birth weight is a risk factor for the subsequent development of primary hypertension in adulthood. This hypothesis is based on the findings of large population studies that demonstrate an inverse correlation between birth weight and adult blood pressure (197,198). Proposed explanations for this effect include deficient maternal nutrition (197,199), which possibly leads to acquisition of a reduced number of nephrons *in utero* (200). Other investigators have demonstrated that maternal smoking during pregnancy and bottle-feeding of newborns also may lead to hypertension later in life (201,202), which widens the spectrum of possible influences on later blood pressure from *in utero* factors to postnatal factors as well.

Animal studies have generally supported the epidemiologic evidence cited earlier. Pregnant rats fed low-protein diets bear young that are small at birth and later develop hypertension (203). Maternal diets low in protein result in decreased nephron number as well as suppression of the renin-angiotensin system (204), which leads to elevated blood pressure and reduced GFR. In addition, various pharmacologic manipulations of the fetal milieu also result in changes in fetal renal development that promote the appearance of hypertension after birth (205), which lends further credence to the theory that perinatal events have an important influence on later blood pressure.

Despite the epidemiologic and experimental evidence cited earlier, the effect of perinatal factors on later blood pressure does not appear to be completely straightforward. In contradiction to the studies demonstrating an inverse relationship between birth weight and adult blood pressure, other epidemiologic studies have found that adult blood pressure is more closely related to gestational age at birth (206) or to childhood growth (207) than to birth weight. In addition, studies have shown that twins have lower systolic blood pressures than singletons despite their lower birth weights (208). These challenges to the fetal origins hypothesis not only indicate that further research is needed to determine the effects of prenatal and perinatal factors on future blood pressure but also support the concept illustrated in Figure 60.1 that the development of primary hypertension depends on multiple factors that vary among different individuals.

Activation of the Sympathetic Nervous System in Primary Hypertension

The role of the SNS in blood pressure regulation has been discussed in detail earlier. Many lines of evidence suggest that SNS activation or overactivity is the primary mechanism by which blood pressure elevation is initiated in young individuals with otherwise unexplained primary hypertension. For example, children with primary hypertension have long been known to have higher resting heart rates than normotensive children (209). This has been confirmed by large epidemiologic studies such as the Bogalusa Heart Study, in which resting heart rate was found to correlate with blood pressure (210). Although this characteristic has now been "rediscovered" in obese adolescents with primary hypertension (211), there is a large, established body of literature that links tachycardia not only with elevated blood pressure but also with increased cardiovascular risk in general (212).

Another notable manifestation of SNS activation in hypertensive children is heightened cardiovascular reactivity to stress. Early studies by Falkner demonstrated that hypertensive adolescents had significantly greater increases in heart rate, systolic blood pressure, and diastolic blood pressure during mental stress (performance of difficult arithmetic problems) than did normotensive adolescents (209). Increased cardiovascular reactivity to the cold pressor test has also been shown to predict the subsequent development of hypertension (213). An interaction between genetic factors and SNS activation is suggested by differences in the cardiovascular response to stress in children with different racial backgrounds or family histories of hypertension (214).

Laboratory studies confirm the SNS activation in primary hypertension suggested by the aforementioned clinical and epidemiologic data. Measurement of plasma catecholamine levels demonstrates that both children and young adults with primary hypertension have higher plasma norepinephrine levels than normotensives (13,14). The importance of this as a mechanism in the development of hypertension is highlighted by the fact that elevated catecholamine levels are more commonly found in younger individuals with primary hypertension than in older individuals (14), and also by the fact that such elevations are commonly seen in young individuals with borderline hypertension who later develop more significant blood pressure elevation (215). This phenomenon is also true of the tachycardia described earlier (209). Furthermore, abnormalities in the SNS have recently been demonstrated in normotensive children of hypertensive parents (216), which suggests that SNS activation not only is present in prehypertensives but may also be genetically determined.

Further laboratory evidence for SNS activation in primary hypertension can be found in studies that have demonstrated increased SNS activity by direct recordings of nerve activity. Increased SNS activity has been found in recordings from both peripheral and renal sympathetic nerves in hypertensive individuals (1,217). Taken together, these changes in SNS activity would then lead to the development of hypertension through a rise in cardiac output, with increased peripheral vascular resistance and volume expansion from increased renal sodium and water retention both playing a role. There is also evidence to suggest that the increased circulating levels of catecholamines may be involved in the development of the vascular hypertrophy that is a hallmark of established hypertension (218), which thereby perpetuates increased peripheral resistance. In sum, although it is likely that SNS activation may not be present in later stages of hypertension (2), there is strong evidence that abnormalities of SNS activity are involved in the pathogenesis of primary hypertension, at least in the early phases of blood pressure elevation, which is clearly significant as far as pediatric hypertension is concerned.

White-Coat Hypertension

Individuals with *white-coat hypertension* (WCH) would be considered to have hypertension if the diagnosis were based on casual blood pressure readings obtained in the office setting, but actually have normal blood pressure except for their office readings (219). The diagnosis is best made by ambulatory blood pressure monitoring, a procedure that has become increasingly available in pediatric referral centers over the past several years. WCH is most likely a manifestation of the flight or fight response. Individuals with WCH are typically anxious and demonstrate a mild resting daytime tachycardia (219). Although the role of SNS activation has not been extensively investigated in individuals with WCH, it is a plausible underlying mechanism.

More important, WCH may represent a prehypertensive state, at least in some individuals. Long-term follow-up of adults with WCH has demonstrated a higher left ventricular mass index and greater incidence of cardiovascular events than in normotensive persons (220). This finding suggests that patients with WCH should be followed periodically for the later development of sustained hypertension, probably with serial ambulatory blood pressure monitoring.

Obesity Hypertension

Although a relationship between obesity and the development of hypertension has been recognized for many decades, the exact mechanisms by which obesity causes hypertension remain incompletely understood. In addition, there has been debate over whether obesity hypertension represents a secondary form of hypertension or a variant of primary hypertension. Because many of the mechanisms likely to be operative in individuals with obesity hypertension are similar or even identical to factors already discussed as being present in young individuals with primary hypertension, and given the absence of specific renal or other major organ system diseases in the vast majority of children with obesity hypertension, we have chosen to discuss obesity hypertension in the context of primary hypertension.

The two major hormonal abnormalities in obesity hypertension are hyperinsulinemia, a consequence of peripheral insulin resistance, and hyperleptinemia, a consequence of the increased mass of adipose tissue. It is likely that either insulin or leptin or both is fundamentally involved in the development of hypertension in most, if not all, hypertensive obese individuals.

One of the first investigators to propose that the link between obesity, insulin resistance, and hypertension was SNS activation was Landsberg, who stated "insulin resistance in the obese is a mechanism evolved for limiting further weight gain. Like any compensatory mechanism, however, there is a price to pay. In this situation, that price is the hyperinsulinemia and sympathetic activation which, via effects on the blood vessels, the heart and the kidneys, exerts a pro-hypertensive effect that, in susceptible individuals, causes hypertension" (221). Although the issue of whether the hyperinsulinemia causes the SNS activation or vice versa remains unresolved, most of the experimental evidence supports the presence of SNS activation in obesity hypertension (221,222).

Insulin resistance has been linked to several physiologic mechanisms that can elevate blood pressure. First and foremost among these mechanisms is likely to be an altered renal handling of sodium, which leads to hypertension through an expansion of plasma volume. Insulin increases renal sodium reabsorption, possibly in the distal nephron, although this is not completely certain (223). It is likely that increased activity of renal sympathetic nerves is responsible at least in part for this effect (224). Elevated circulating levels of aldosterone, which have been demonstrated in salt-sensitive obese adolescents, may also be involved (225). Importantly, these effects of hyperinsulinemia on renal sodium handling can be reversed with weight loss (225).

The second major mechanism by which hyperinsulinemia may elevate blood pressure is through effects on vascular structure and function. Although insulin acts as a vasodilator when infused directly into local vascular beds (226), in hypertensive subjects this effect is probably offset by vasoconstriction mediated by increased sympathetic nervous activity (222,226). In addition, impaired vasodilatation in response to insulin infusion has been demonstrated in obese individuals (227). Alternatively, insulin may act to stimulate vascular smooth muscle proliferation in resistance vessels (228), thereby leading to increased peripheral vascular resistance due to vascular medial hypertrophy. In this way, hyperinsulinemia would lead to hypertension by increasing total peripheral resistance.

Leptin is a peptide hormone encoded on chromosome 7 in humans and primarily produced by adipose tissue whose major function seems to be regulation of energy stores. Circulating leptin crosses the blood-brain barrier and binds with receptors in the hypothalamus. In leptin-deficiency states or after weight loss, leptin levels are decreased; this stimulates secretion of neuropeptide Y, which leads to increased food intake and decreased energy expenditure. Conversely, with weight gain, the resulting increase in leptin (caused by the increased mass of adipose tissue) leads to release of melanocyte-stimulating hormone; this hormone in turn binds to and activates the melanocortin-4 receptor, which induces physiologic changes that counteract obesity (229).

In obese hypertensive individuals, leptin levels are elevated and correlate with both blood pressure and heart rate (230). The mechanism by which hyperleptinemia results in hypertension appears to be increased SNS activity. Evidence in support of this hypothesis comes from animal studies, several of which have demonstrated that intraventricular leptin infusions increase RSNA and that intravenous leptin infusions increase blood pressure and heart rate (230,231). However, it is unknown at present whether the same hypothalamic pathways involved in leptin's regulation of energy stores is also involved in the development of hypertension (230). Leptin also has significant intraglomerular effects, including increased synthesis of transforming growth factor β, increased production of type IV collagen by glomerular endothelial cells, and stimulation of type I collagen synthesis by mesangial cells. This, in turn, may lead to glomerular sclerosis via extracellular matrix deposition (232), perhaps contributing to or even accounting for the secondary focal segmental glomerulosclerosis that can be seen in obesity. The role of leptin in the pathogenesis of obesity hypertension has been discovered relatively recently and is likely to be more complex than described here.

Insulin Resistance in Nonobese Hypertensive Individuals

Not all hypertensive individuals with insulin resistance are obese (222,233), which suggests that insulin resistance is a primary mechanism in the development of primary hypertension. Supporting this hypothesis are studies demonstrating a significant inverse relationship between insulin-mediated glucose uptake and blood pressure levels in lean normotensive and borderline hypertensive individuals (234). The mechanisms responsible for the development of elevated blood pressure in lean individuals with insulin resistance are most likely similar to those discussed earlier. What remains unknown at this point is what causes insulin resistance in nonobese hypertensives individuals (222).

Dietary and Environmental Influences on the Development of Primary Hypertension

Numerous dietary constituents have been examined as possible contributors to the development of primary hypertension. Of these, the two that have received the most interest have been sodium and potassium. Population studies of sodium consumption have demonstrated that populations with lower sodium intake have lower blood pressures than those with higher sodium intake (235,236). It is noteworthy that, typically, populations with high sodium intake also demonstrate lower potassium intake (235,237), which suggests a potential pathogenic role for potassium as well. Interventional studies of sodium restriction have generally shown that reducing sodium intake lowers blood pressure in both adults (238) and children (239), whereas the data for potassium supplementation are less clear (239,240). Recently, a diet low in sodium and saturated fats and high in potassium and calcium [the Dietary Approaches to Stop Hypertension (DASH) diet] was shown to be able to substantially lower blood pressure in hypertensive adults (241); this diet has also been advocated as a method of hypertension prevention.

These dietary influences on blood pressure, however, although present when large populations are studied, may not apply to the individual patient (235,242). This is because some hypertensive patients are salt sensitive and others are not. Understanding the mechanisms responsible for salt sensitivity has been a subject of much research (242). What is true is that the mechanisms may vary from individual to individual: in obese hypertensive persons, for example, salt sensitivity is likely related to insulin resistance (see earlier discussion), but in hypertensive individuals with reduced nephron mass, salt sensitivity may simply represent a compensatory mechanism to maintain pressure natriuresis (200). Whatever the mechanism, one cannot ignore the public health implications of dietary sodium restriction: a modest reduction in sodium intake resulting in a 3-mm Hg reduction in systolic blood pressure has been calculated to have significant potential to reduce the incidence of stroke and other cardiovascular disease in the population at large (238).

The other environmental factor felt to play a role in the development of primary hypertension is stress. As noted earlier, stress has been shown to increase blood pressure in experimental settings, most likely through activation of the SNS (209,213,214). At the population level, stress has also been advanced as an explanation for the higher incidence of hypertension among African Americans than among whites (243). An individual's reaction to stress may lead to other changes in the environment that are themselves related to blood pressure (244), such as obesity from increased caloric intake, which would then cause hypertension by the mechanisms discussed earlier.

SECONDARY HYPERTENSION

Mendelian Forms of Blood Pressure Elevation

Molecular genetic studies have now identified mutations in eight genes that affect blood pressure. Common to all of the resulting disorders is altered renal handling of sodium. Mutations that increase renal salt reabsorption raise blood pressure; conversely, those that diminish salt reabsorption lower blood pressure (Fig. 60.2). In this chapter, we focus on the hypertensive syndromes: apparent mineralocorticoid excess (AME), Liddle's syndrome, glucocorticoid-remediable aldosteronism (GRA), and Gordon's syndrome. For a full discussion of the hypotensive syndromes, the reader is referred to the reviews of this topic (196).

The syndrome of *apparent mineralocorticoid excess* is an autosomal recessive disease characterized by early-onset hypertension with hypokalemia and metabolic alkalosis accompanied by suppressed plasma renin activity and the virtual absence of circulating aldosterone. In this disease, steroids other than aldosterone activate the mineralocorti-

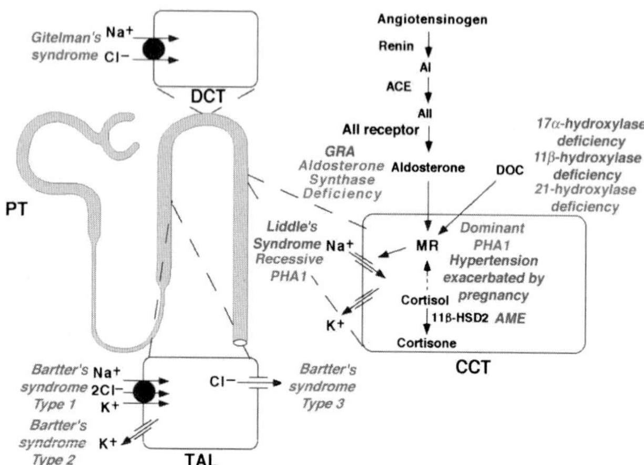

FIGURE 60.2. Single-gene mutations altering blood pressure. A diagram of a nephron, the filtering unit of the kidney, is shown. The molecular pathways mediating NaCl reabsorption in individual renal cells in the thick ascending limb of the loop of Henle (TAL), distal convoluted tubule (DCT), and the cortical collecting tubule (CCT) are indicated, along with the pathway of the renin-angiotensin system, the major regulator of renal salt reabsorption. Inherited diseases affecting these pathways are indicated, with hypertensive disorders in gray and hypotensive disorders in black. 11β-HSD2, 11β-hydroxysteroid dehydrogenase-2; ACE, angiotensin-converting enzyme; AI, angiotensin I; AII, angiotensin II; AME, apparent mineralocorticoid excess; DOC, deoxycorticosterone; GRA, glucocorticoid-remediable aldosteronism; MR, mineralocorticoid receptor; PHA1, pseudohypoaldosteronism type 1; PT, proximal tubule. (From Lifton RP, Ghavari AG, Geller DS. Molecular mechanisms of human hypertension. *Cell* 2001;104:545–556, with permission of Elsevier Science.)

coid receptor (MR). Affected patients have a lack-of-function mutation in the gene encoding the renal isoenzyme of 11β-hydroxysteroid dehydrogenase (11β-HSD), which results in impaired conversion of cortisol to cortisone (245). *In vitro*, cortisol activates MR with potency similar to aldosterone; however, *in vivo* almost all activation of MR is mediated by aldosterone despite its low plasma concentration. The specificity of MR for aldosterone *in vivo* is mediated indirectly by 11β-HSD activity; this "protects" the MR from cortisol by metabolizing it to cortisone, which does not activate the MR (246). In AME, the absence of this enzyme allows cortisol to activate the MR, which results in hypertension mediated by increased sodium retention. Confirmation of the pathogenesis of AME came with the cloning of 11HSD-2; this gene, expressed in the same cells of the nephron that express the epithelial Na^+ channels (ENaC), shows homozygous loss-of-function mutations in AME patients (245).

Liddle's syndrome is an autosomal dominant, low-renin form of hypertension characterized by constitutively elevated renal sodium reabsorption that results from activating mutations in the β or γ subunit of the ENaC. These mutations result in an increase in the number of channels at the cell surface (247). The increased number of channels is due to reduced clearance of ENaC from the cell surface with dramatically longer half-life (248). The clearance of the normal channel from the membrane is dependent on the sequence PPPXY in the cytoplasmic C terminus of both the β and γ ENaC subunits. Loss of this sequence from either subunit in Liddle's syndrome results in prolongation of the cell surface half-life and increased channel numbers, attributable to loss of interaction with WW domain–containing proteins and loss of clearance through clathrin-coated pits. The genetic defect has been localized to a single segment of chromosome 16 that encodes the ENaC subunits. Several different mutations have been described, all of which either cause a frame-shift mutation or introduce premature stop codons (249).

Glucocorticoid-remediable aldosteronism is an autosomal dominant disease characterized by early onset of hypertension with normal or elevated aldosterone levels despite suppressed plasma renin activity (187). GRA is caused by a chimeric gene that results from unequal crossing over of the aldosterone synthase and 11β-hydroxylase genes on chromosome 8. Aldosterone synthase is the rate-limiting enzyme for aldosterone biosynthesis in the adrenal glomerulosa and 11β-hydroxylase is an enzyme involved in cortisol biosynthesis in the adrenal fasciculata whose expression is regulated by ACTH. The resulting chimeric gene is expressed in the adrenal fasciculata and encodes a protein product with aldosterone synthase enzymatic activity whose expression is regulated by ACTH. Consequently, aldosterone synthase activity is ectopically expressed in the adrenal fasciculata under control of ACTH rather than of angiotensin II. Aldosterone secretion becomes linked to cortisol secretion, and maintenance of normal cortisol levels results in constitutive aldosterone secretion, which leads to expanded plasma volume and hypertension (250). The expanded plasma volume suppresses secretion of renin, but this fails to diminish secretion of aldosterone.

The final Mendelian form of hypertension is *Gordon's syndrome*, also known as pseudohypoaldosteronism type II. This is an autosomal dominant disorder characterized by hypertension, increased renal salt reabsorption, and impaired K^+ and H^+ excretion. It has been linked to mutations of genes on chromosome bands 1q31-42 and 17p11-q21 that encode the WNK kinases, a family of serine-threonine kinases (251). These mutations lead to increased expression of WNK1 and WNK4 in the distal nephron. An additional mutation at 12p13 has also been described that produces a similar phenotype (252).

Other Genetic Forms of Hypertension

Hypertension exacerbated in pregnancy by mutations in the MR is an autosomal dominant form of hypertension that is markedly accelerated in pregnancy (253). A systematic screening of patients with early-onset hypertension detected a missense mutation in the ligand-binding domain of the receptor MR S810L. S810L carriers all developed hypertension before age 20, a finding absent in their relatives with wild-type receptors. Steroids lacking 21-hydroxyl groups (progesterone, spironolactone) that normally bind but do not activate MR are all potent agonists of the mutant receptor. Because progesterone levels rise 100-fold during pregnancy, all pregnancies among patients harboring this mutation have been complicated by dramatic acceleration of hypertension associated with complete suppression of the renin-angiotensin system (253).

Hypertension with brachydactyly is characterized by severe hypertension and abnormal skeletal development in the hand and wrist. There are no associated distinguishing biochemical features. This syndrome has been mapped to chromosome band 12p12.2-11.2 (254), but the responsible gene has not yet been identified.

Hypertension in Renal Parenchymal Disease

Hypertension resulting from renal parenchymal disease is multifactorial in origin. Volume expansion secondary to reduced sodium excretion increases cardiac output and activates the renin-angiotensin-aldosterone axis (255). Abnormal activation of the adrenergic system and baroreceptor dysfunction are also present (256). Chronic renal insufficiency leads to accumulation of the NOS inhibitors asymmetric and symmetric dimethylarginine (257) and endothelial dysfunction (258). Decreased production of vasodilators, including kinin and prostaglandins, and increased production of the vasoconstrictor ET-1 are also seen (259). Finally, recombinant human erythropoietin treatment and abnormal parathyroid-calcium homeostasis with elevated intracellular calcium concentrations in the myocardium and platelets is associated with hypertension (260).

Hypertension in Renovascular Disease

In the classic Goldblatt model of hypertension (261), the one-clip one-kidney or two-kidney two-clip model (analogous to renal artery stenosis in a solitary kidney or to bilateral renal artery stenosis in humans), hypertension is sodium and volume dependent. In the one-clip one-kidney or two-kidney two-clip hypertensive model, ACE inhibition has little effect on blood pressure unless the animal has been sodium depleted (262). However, in humans with bilateral renal artery stenosis, both renin and volume factors are involved.

Hypertension in the one-clip two-kidney model (analogous to unilateral renal artery stenosis in humans) is renin dependent (263). Two-kidney one-clip animals also have increased norepinephrine release and SNS activity (264), which implicates the SNS in the development of renovascular hypertension. This has been disputed in animal models (263), but as mentioned previously, studies in humans with renovascular hypertension have clearly demonstrated elevated sympathetic nerve activity (15).

Renal perfusion pressure starts to be affected when renal artery stenosis reaches 50%. The stenosis needs to occlude at least 70% of the lumen, however, before it begins to reduce renal blood flow and raise arterial pressure (265). In the late phase, hypertension persists despite removal of the stenosis or ischemic kidney due to damage to the contralateral kidney (266). In fact, in the one-clip two-kidney model of renovascular hypertension, the vascular, glomerular, and tubulointerstitial damage is greater in the unclipped kidney than in the clipped kidney. The clipped kidney is exposed to elevated angiotensin levels but is protected from hypertension (267). Activation of the renin-angiotensin system also results in an increase in oxidative stress and accelerated atherosclerosis (268).

Hypertension in Acute and Chronic Renal Failure

Acute and severe insult to the kidneys impairs excretion of salt and water, reduces renal blood flow, or both. Dysregulation of salt and water excretion leads to volume expansion, whereas reduction in renal blood flow activates the renin-angiotensin-aldosterone axis. Hypertension in chronic renal failure is primarily volume and salt dependent and results from impaired sodium excretion. Salt plays a crucial role by causing an increase in interchangeable (269) and vascular wall sodium (270), which leads to an expansion in the intravascular volume. The renin-angiotensin system is also stimulated, which in turn produces sodium retention and an increase in total peripheral resistance.

Sympathetic tone increases, as expressed by an increase in plasma noradrenaline, which contributes to increases in total peripheral resistance and cardiac output (256). As discussed previously, ET-1 and ANP are elevated and associated with high blood pressure in chronic renal failure (154,271). Administration of nonsteroidal antiinflammatory drugs in chronic renal failure produces an increase in arterial pressure and a reduction in renal prostaglandins (272), which suggests an important role for prostaglandins in hypertension associated with chronic renal failure. Patients with uremia secondary to impaired renal clearance also have elevated levels of NOS inhibitor (166).

Posttransplantation Hypertension

Hypertension is a common phenomenon after renal transplantation, with up to 70% of pediatric transplantation patients requiring antihypertensive medications in the first month after transplantation (273). The major contributing factors include history of pretransplantation hypertension, persistent native kidney hypertension, the effects of immunosuppressive medications, transplant renal artery stenosis (TRAS), and chronic allograft dysfunction (see Chapter 73).

As can be deduced from the preceding sections, pretransplantation hypertension causes chronic vascular changes that increase peripheral vascular resistance. Although such vascular remodeling can be reversed with effective antihypertensive treatment (274), many patients come to transplantation hypertensive despite therapy, so the same mechanisms that were operative in perpetuating their pretransplantation hypertension will still be at work. In addition, if the patient's native kidneys are still in place, they may continue to release renin (275), thereby further contributing to posttransplantation hypertension.

Immunosuppressive medications, particularly glucocorticoids and calcineurin inhibitors, contribute to posttransplantation hypertension in several ways. Although prednisone may be a significant contributing factor to the development of hypertension in the immediate posttransplantation period, most pediatric immunosuppression protocols try to reduce the dosage of prednisone as far as possible to maximize posttransplantation growth, so that prednisone is a much less important contributing factor later on (275,276). Calcineurin inhibitors affect blood pressure in a variety of ways, including increasing production of the vasoconstrictor endothelin (155,157), decreasing production of vasodilatory substances (276), and activating the SNS (277).

TRAS has been reported to occur in up to 20% of hypertensive pediatric renal transplant recipients (275), although improved surgical techniques have probably decreased its incidence somewhat (276). Causes may include surgical trauma, prolonged ischemia, suturing technique or reactions to suture material, and atheromatous plaques in the donor kidney (276). Elevated renin secretion has been seen in patients with TRAS (278), which suggests that the mechanisms responsible for hypertension in TRAS are similar to those discussed elsewhere in this chapter for renovascular hypertension.

Allograft dysfunction has long been recognized as a significant cause of hypertension in both children and adults with posttransplantation hypertension (275,276). Whether it results from the sequelae of rejection or from calcineurin nephrotoxicity, the primary mechanism of hypertension related to allograft dysfunction appears to be renal sodium retention (276,279). Other mechanisms seen in patients with renal insufficiency of other causes may also be responsible.

Hypertension in Dialysis Patients

Children receiving long-term dialysis have a significant incidence of hypertension: of the children in the North American Pediatric Renal Transplant Cooperative Study dialysis database, 53 to 63% of those receiving hemodialysis and 43 to 56% of those receiving peritoneal dialysis were also receiving antihypertensive medications at the time of the 2002 study annual report (273). The major pathophysiologic mechanism in most dialysis patients seems to be volume overload related to sodium and water retention. This may be more significant in peritoneal dialysis patients than in hemodialysis patients (280). Evidence in favor of fluid overload as the major mechanism can be found in the many studies that demonstrate correction of hypertension after increased fluid removal in both peritoneal dialysis and hemodialysis patients (281,282).

Numerous other factors have been implicated, however, including overactivity of the SNS, activation of the renin-angiotensin system, erythropoietin, parathyroid hormone, and nocturnal hypoxemia (283). Studies have also implicated NO and endothelin in the pathogenesis of dialysis hypertension (283,284). Endothelin and other vasoconstrictive factors have also been shown to be involved in the pathogenesis of erythropoietin-related hypertension (285). Postdialysis hypertension in hemodialysis patients is likely renin mediated and responds to administration of an ACE inhibitor after dialysis (286).

Hypertension in Coarctation of the Aorta

Hypertension associated with aortic coarctation may occur in three clinical settings: before surgical repair, in the immediately postoperative period after surgical repair, and long after surgical repair. Prerepair hypertension is the result of renal hypoperfusion and activation of the renin-angiotensin system. The activity of the SNS may also be increased (287). In the immediately postsurgical period, paradoxical hypertension may be seen, which is probably the result of increased activity of the renin-angiotensin system and the SNS (288).

Despite surgical repair of coarctation, many patients are found to have abnormal blood pressure at rest. Ambulatory blood pressure monitoring is probably superior to casual blood pressure measurement for detection of hypertension in this population (289). Proposed mechanisms for this late or persistent hypertension include altered baroreceptor function, thickening of blood vessels below the site of the coarctation, and elevation of plasma adrenaline and aldosterone levels (290,291). Renal structural changes have also been demonstrated in animal models of coarctation (292). Recoarctation should also be investigated in any patient with the development of late postrepair hypertension.

Hypertension in Vasculitis

Due to the numerous vessels within the renal parenchyma, the kidneys are frequently targeted by systemic vasculitides. Glomerular inflammation, with cellular infiltration, proliferation, and immune complex deposition resulting in nephritis and renal failure, has been well described in systemic lupus erythematosus, microscopic polyarteritis, Wegener's granulomatosis, Schönlein-Henoch purpura, and cryoglobulinemic vasculitis (see Chapters 44 through 46). Takayasu's arteritis, an inflammatory process associated with stenosis and obliteration of the aorta and its primary branches, induces hypertension by mechanisms that are similar to those seen in coarctation of aorta, renovascular hypertension, or ischemic kidney disease as discussed earlier. Necrotizing vasculitides, such as classic polyarteritis nodosa and Kawasaki disease, may lead to hypertension secondary to thrombosis of inflamed major extrarenal and intrarenal arteries with resulting local (intrarenal) renin-angiotensin system activation and infarction of the renal parenchyma (293).

Hypertension in Endocrine Diseases

Adrenocortical Hypertension

Although an excess of exogenous or endogenous glucocorticoids (Cushing syndrome) has long been known to cause hypertension, the exact mechanism or mechanisms that result in blood pressure elevation remain unknown. The hepatic synthesis of angiotensinogen, which stimulates the renin-angiotensin system, is activated, and phospholipase A_2, which releases arachidonic acid from phospholipids and plays an important role in the synthesis of vasodilatory prostaglandins, is inhibited (294). Glucocorticoids also reduce the activity of the depressor kallikrein-kinin system, enhance pressor sensitivity to endogenous vasoconstrictors (epinephrine and angiotensin II) (295,296), and promote sodium influx into vascular smooth muscle cells (297). High levels of cortisol exert mineralocorticoid effects, and in adrenal carcinomas, deoxycorticosterone and aldosterone levels may also be elevated (298).

Hyperaldosteronism may result from either an aldosterone-producing adrenal adenoma or, more commonly, from adrenal hypertrophy (idiopathic hyperaldosteronism). Aldosterone-producing adenoma and idiopathic hyperaldosteronism both produce excess aldosterone secretion and both result in hypertension with similar clinical features: hypokalemia, renal potassium wasting, suppressed plasma renin activity, and increased plasma and urinary levels of aldosterone (299). The blood pressure elevation due to aldosterone excess results from an increase in systemic vascular resistance due to aldosterone-mediated increased plasma sodium concentration, which leads in turn to a rise in the intracellular calcium content. Increase in intracellular calcium results in impaired left ventricular diastolic relaxation (300) and enhanced contractility with reduced vascular compliance (301). The increased aldosterone production in idiopathic hyperaldosteronism reflects increased activity of a rate-limiting mitochondrial cytochrome P-450 isoenzyme, the aldosterone synthase gene CYP 11B2 (302). Polymorphisms of the CYP 11B2 gene determine interindividual variations in aldosterone activity and response to antihypertensive treatment (303,304).

Pheochromocytoma

Pheochromocytomas are catecholamine-secreting tumors of chromaffin cells that may arise from cells of neural crest origin, either in the adrenal glands themselves or in extraadrenal sites. Sustained or paroxysmal hypertension is the most common clinical sign, although it may be less common in children than in adults (305). Although most pheochromocytomas are sporadic, there is a familial predisposition in patients with multiple endocrine neoplasia type 2, von Hippel–Lindau disease, neurofibromatosis type 1, and familial carotid body tumors (306). Pheochromocytoma in multiple endocrine neoplasia type 2 is associated with a germline mutation of the proto-oncogene RET (307) and pheochromocytoma in von Hippel–Lindau disease results from germline mutation of the von Hippel–Lindau gene (308).

Hypertension in pheochromocytoma results from the direct effect of high circulating levels of catecholamines, primarily noradrenaline, adrenaline, and dopamine (305). Some tumors produce the catecholamine precursor L-dopa. Pheochromocytomas also secrete numerous other peptide hormones, among which are renin, VIP, neuropeptide Y, somatostatin, and ET-1. These substances are responsible for many of the nonhypertensive symptoms seen in patients with pheochromocytoma, including flushing, sweating, and diarrhea (305).

Thyroid Disorders

Hypothyroidism produces a reduction in renal blood flow and GFR, as well as decreased cardiac output (309). Compensatory mechanisms, primarily increased peripheral resistance mediated by increased responsiveness to adrenergic stimulation and increased SNS activity (310), lead to diastolic hypertension. Treatment with thyroid hormone corrects the hypertension.

Hyperthyroidism, on the other hand, is associated with activation of the renin-angiotensin-aldosterone axis and increased sodium reabsorption, which leads to expansion of plasma volume (172). There is also β_2-receptor stimulation, which in turn results in vasodilatation, increased cardiac output, and cardiac contractility (173). These physiologic changes result in isolated systolic hypertension (175).

Renin Overproduction

Juxtaglomerular cell tumors of the kidney or ectopic tumors secrete renin and induce hypertension associated with hypokalemia, as well as hyponatremia and other features of renin-angiotensin-aldosterone system activation (311).

Hypertension in Pulmonary Diseases

Hypertension in children with chronic lung disease is most commonly seen in infants with bronchopulmonary dysplasia. Although the pathophysiology of bronchopulmonary dysplasia–associated hypertension is not completely understood, it is likely to be multifactorial in origin. Corticosteroids, especially dexamethasone, when used for prolonged periods elevate blood pressure in such infants, but with withdrawal the hypertension resolves (312). Because the development of hypertension has been correlated with the severity of lung disease, chronic hypoxia may also be an important mechanism (313).

Obstructive sleep apnea, characterized by episodic upper airway obstruction during sleep despite persisting respiratory efforts, leads to asphyxia, hypoxia, hypercapnia, and disruption of sleep architecture. Obstructive sleep apnea is a risk factor for systemic hypertension, myocardial infarction, stroke, and sudden death (314). Acute episodes of hypoxia result in stimulation of peripheral chemoreceptors and increased sympathetic outflow with subsequent activation of the renin-angiotensin system (315). These events lead to cyclic or episodic hypertension that later evolves into sustained hypertension if the sleep apnea remains untreated.

Hypertension in Neurologic Disorders

Systemic hypertension can be seen in a variety of neurologic disorders, including seizures, poliomyelitis, hydrocephalus, head trauma, pseudotumor cerebri (idiopathic intracranial hypertension), Guillain-Barré syndrome, and space-occupying lesions (tumor, bleeding, and abscess). Many of these are associated with increased SNS outflow, which leads to peripheral vasoconstriction and renal sodium retention (see earlier sections).

In Guillain-Barré syndrome, for example, microneurographic studies have demonstrated increased SNS activity in the acute phase of the illness (316). Increased levels of circulating renin and catecholamines have also been reported (317). These abnormalities, and the hypertension, resolve as the neurologic abnormalities subside. Increased sympathetic activity is also seen in patients with spinal cord injury. In familial dysautonomia, hypertension is caused by increased levels of circulating catecholamines and increased responsiveness to circulating catecholamines (318).

Increased intracranial pressure causes systemic hypertension that can be quite labile. The mechanism of hypertension is believed to be the stretching of receptors located under the floor of the fourth ventricle (319). Sympathetic nervous outflow is increased in most patients, and baroreceptor function is disrupted. Circulating levels of catecholamines may be increased. Hemodynamically, hypertension is primarily due to increased total peripheral resistance. In many instances, especially when intracranial pressure is elevated due to trauma, systemic hypertension is an important compensatory mechanism for the maintenance of normal cerebral perfusion (320).

Pregnancy-Induced Hypertension and Preeclampsia

Pregnancy-induced hypertension may affect up to 10% of all first pregnancies in the United States (321). As with many of the forms of hypertension discussed in this chapter, pregnancy-induced hypertension is most likely a multifactorial disorder with many contributing mechanisms. However, because the hypertension associated with preeclampsia develops during pregnancy and remits after delivery, the placenta is thought to play a central role in the disease development. Abnormal cytotrophoblast invasion of spiral arterioles leading to reduced uteroplacental perfusion and ischemia appears to be the initiating event (322).

Placental ischemia results in activation or dysfunction of the maternal vascular endothelium that in turn increases the formation of endothelin and thromboxane, increases vascular sensitivity to angiotensin II, and decreases formation of vasodilators such as NO and prostacyclin (323,324). There is also increased synthesis of inflammatory cytokines such as tumor necrosis factor-α, interleukin-1, and interleukin-6, which is activated by tumor necrosis factor-α (325). Those cytokines, in turn, induce structural and functional alterations in endothelial cells, enhance the formation of endothelin, and reduce acetylcholine-induced vasodilatation (325).

TABLE 60.2. MECHANISMS OF DRUG-INDUCED HYPERTENSION

Drug	Potential mechanism(s) (references)
Caffeine	Vasoconstriction, increased SNS activity, decreased baroreceptor sensitivity (328,329)
Calcineurin inhibitors	SNS activation (277), increased ET-1 secretion (155–157)
Cocaine	Increased heart rate and myocardial oxygen demand, direct vasoconstriction, increased matrix synthesis, glomerular inflammation, and glomerulosclerosis (330)
Erythropoietin	Increased erythrocyte mass, changes in production or sensitivity to endogenous vasopressors, dysregulation of production or responsiveness to endogenous vasodilatory factors, a direct vasopressor effect, arterial remodeling through stimulation of vascular cell growth (285,331)
Ethanol	Abnormal response of blood pressure and plasma renin activity to variations in salt intake (332)
Glucocorticoids	Stimulation of the renin-angiotensin system, inhibition of phospholipase A_2, reduced activity of the kallikrein-kinin system, enhanced pressor sensitivity to endogenous vasoconstrictors, mineralocorticoid effects (295–298)
NSAIDs	Prostaglandin inhibition, decrease glomerular filtration rate, salt and water retention, tubulointerstitial injury (333)
Oral contraceptives	Alteration in sodium balance and the renin-angiotensin-aldosterone system (334,335)
Tobacco	Increased SNS outflow, attenuated endothelium-dependent vasodilatation, increased arterial wall stiffness (336–338)

ET-1, endothelin-1; NSAID, nonsteroidal antiinflammatory drug; SNS, sympathetic nervous system.

Another important mechanism may be defective production of NO. During normal pregnancy, maternal cardiac output and blood volume increase by 40 to 50%, whereas total peripheral resistance and blood pressure tend to decrease. In addition, GFR and renal plasma flow increase 30 to 40%. There is substantial evidence that NO plays an important role in mediating those changes. Plasma and urinary levels of cGMP, the second messenger of NO, increase during pregnancy in rats, and urinary nitrate and nitrite excretion have also been reported to be increased. Chronic NOS inhibition in pregnant rats produces a hypertension associated with peripheral and renal vasoconstriction, proteinuria, intrauterine growth retardation, and increased fetal morbidity, a pattern that closely resembles the symptoms of human pregnancy-induced hypertension (326,327).

Drug-Induced Hypertension

Numerous therapeutic and illicit drugs, as well as various other consumed substances, may influence blood pressure significantly, especially in individuals whose blood pressure regulation is already disturbed. A detailed discussion of the many substances with effects on blood pressure is beyond the scope of this chapter. However, some of the more common mechanisms of blood pressure effects due to drugs are summarized in Table 60.2.

REFERENCES

1. Floras JS, Hara K. Sympathoneural and haemodynamic characteristics of young subjects with mild essential hypertension. *J Hypertens* 1993;11:647–655.
2. Julius S, Pascual AV, Sannerstedt R, et al. Relationship between cardiac output and peripheral resistance in borderline hypertension. *Circulation* 1971;43:382–390.
3. Julius S. Changing role of the autonomic nervous system in human hypertension. *J Hypertens* 1990;8[Suppl 7]:S59–S65.
4. Owens GK. Influence of blood pressure on development of aortic medial smooth muscle hypertrophy in spontaneously hypertensive rats. *Hypertension* 1987;9:178–187.
5. Gibbons GH, Dzau VJ. The emerging concept of vascular remodeling. *N Engl J Med* 1994;330:1431–1438.
6. Vicaut E. Microcirculation and arterial hypertension. *Drugs* 1999;58:1–10.
7. Owens GK, Schwartz SM. Alterations in vascular smooth muscle mass in the spontaneously hypertensive rat. Role of cellular hypertrophy, hyperploidy, and hyperplasia. *Circ Res* 1982;51:280–289.
8. Berk BC. Biology of the vascular wall in hypertension. In: Brenner BM, ed. *Brenner and Rector's the kidney*, 6th ed. Philadelphia: WB Saunders, 2000:1943–1966.
9. Berk BC, Alexander RW, Brock TA, et al. Vasoconstriction: a new activity for platelet-derived growth factor. *Science* 1986;232:87–90.
10. Geisterfer AA, Peach MJ, Owens GK. Angiotensin II induces hypertrophy, not hyperplasia, of cultured rat aortic smooth muscle cells. *Circ Res* 1988;62:749–756.
11. DiBona GF, Kopp UC. Neural control of renal function. *Physiol Rev* 1997;77:75–197.
12. Campese VM, Krol E. Neurogenic factors in renal hypertension. *Curr Hypertens Rep* 2002;4:256–260.
13. McCrory WW, Klein AA, Rosenthal RA. Blood pressure, heart rate, and plasma catecholamines in normal and hypertensive children and their siblings at rest and after standing. *Hypertension* 1982:4:507–513.
14. Goldstein DS, Lake CR, Chernow B, et al. Age-dependence of hypertensive-normotensive differences in plasma norepinephrine. *Hypertension* 1983;5:100–104.
15. Johansson M, Elam M, Rundqvist B, et al. Increased sympathetic nerve activity in renovascular hypertension. *Circulation* 1999;99:2537–2542.
16. Handa RK, Johns EJ. Interaction of the renin-angiotensin system and the renal nerves in the regulation of rat kidney function. *J Physiol* 1985;369:311–321.
17. Reinhart GA, Lohmeier TE, Hord CE Jr. Hypertension induced by chronic renal adrenergic stimulation is angiotensin dependent. *Hypertension* 1995;25:940–949.
18. Hall JE, Brands MW. The renin-angiotensin-aldosterone systems: renal mechanisms and circulatory homeostasis. In: Seldin DW, Giebisch G, eds. *The kidney: physiology and pathophysiology*, 3rd ed. Philadelphia: Lippincott Williams and Wilkins, 2000:1009–1046.
19. Wong PC, Bernard R, Timmermans PB. Effect of blocking angiotensin II receptor subtype on rat sympathetic nerve function. *Hypertension* 1992;19(6 Pt 2):663–667.
20. Boke T, Malik KU. Enhancement by locally generated angiotensin II of release of the adrenergic transmitter in the isolated rat kidney. *J Pharmacol Exp Ther* 1983;226:900–907.
21. DiBona GF. Central sympathoexcitatory actions of angiotensin II: role of type 1 angiotensin II receptors. *J Am Soc Nephrol* 1999;10[Suppl 11]:S90–S94.
22. Ferguson AV, Washburn DL. Angiotensin II: a peptidergic neurotransmitter in central autonomic pathways. *Prog Neurobiol* 1998;54:169–192.
23. Allen AM, Dampney RA, Mendelsohn FA. Angiotensin receptor binding and pressor effects in cat subretrofacial nucleus. *Am J Physiol* 1988;255:H1011–H1017.
24. Sasaki S, Dampney RA. Tonic cardiovascular effects of angiotensin II in the ventrolateral medulla. *Hypertension* 1990;15:274–283.
25. Saigusa T, Iriki M, Arita J. Brain angiotensin II tonically modulates sympathetic baroreflex in rabbit ventrolateral medulla. *Am J Physiol* 1996;271:H1015–H1021.
26. Dampney RA, Fontes MA, Hirooka Y, et al. Role of angiotensin II receptors in the regulation of vasomotor neurons in the ventrolateral medulla. *Clin Exp Pharmacol Physiol* 2002;29:467–472.
27. Song K, Allen AM, Paxinos G, et al. Mapping of angiotensin II receptor subtype heterogeneity in rat brain. *J Comp Neurol* 1992;316:467–484.
28. Portaluppi F, Smolensky MH. Circadian rhythm and environmental determinants of blood pressure regulation in normal and hypertensive conditions. In: White WB, ed.

Blood pressure monitoring in cardiovascular medicine and therapeutics. Totowa, NJ: Humana Press, 2001:79–138.

29. Lurbe E, Thijs L, Redon J, et al. Diurnal blood pressure curve in children and adolescents. *J Hypertens* 1996;14:41–46.
30. Flynn JT. Differentiation between primary and secondary hypertension in children using ambulatory blood pressure monitoring. *Pediatrics* 2002;110:89–93.
31. van Esseveldt LKE, Lehman MN, Boer GJ. The suprachiasmatic nucleus and the circadian time-keeping system revisited. *Brain Res Brain Res Rev* 2000;33:34–77.
32. Neyama T, Krout KE, Van Nguyen X, et al. Suprachiasmatic nucleus: a central autonomic clock. *Nat Neurosci* 1999;2:1051–1053.
33. Sewerynek E. Review: Melatonin and the cardiovascular system. *Neuroendocrinol Lett* 2002;23[Suppl 1]:79–83.
34. Goncharuk VD, vas Heerikhuize J, Dai JP, et al. Neuropeptide changes in the suprachiasmatic nucleus in primary hypertension indicate functional impairment of the biologic clock. *Comp Neurol* 2001;431:320–330.
35. Guyton AC. Kidneys and fluids in pressure regulation. Small volume but large pressure changes. *Hypertension* 1992;19[1 Suppl]:I2–I8.
36. Tornel J, Madrid MI, Garcia-Salom M, et al. Role of kinins in the control of renal papillary blood flow, pressure natriuresis, and arterial pressure. *Circ Res* 2000;86:589–595.
37. Roman RJ, Lianos E. Influence of prostaglandins on papillary blood flow and pressure-natriuretic response. *Hypertension* 1990;15:29–35.
38. Majid DS, Navar LG. Nitric oxide in the control of renal hemodynamics and excretory function. *Am J Hypertens* 2001;14:74S-82S.
39. Cowley AW Jr. Role of the renal medulla in volume and arterial pressure regulation. *Am J Physiol* 1997;273:R1–R15.
40. Correia AG, Madden AC, Bergstrom G, et al. Effects of renal medullary and intravenous norepinephrine on renal antihypertensive function. *Hypertension* 2000;35:965–970.
41. Christy IJ, Woods RL, Courneya CA, et al. Evidence for a renomedullary vasodepressor system in rabbits and dogs. *Hypertension* 1991;18:325–333.
42. Brooks B, Byers LW, Muirhead EE, et al. Purification of class I medullipins from the venous effluent of isolated normal kidneys perfused under high pressure with saline. *Blood Press* 1994;3:407–417.
43. Masilamani S, Kim G-H, Mitchell C, et al. Aldosterone-mediated regulation of ENaC, and subunit proteins in rat kidney. *J Clin Invest* 1999;104:R19–R23.
44. Kim G-H, Masilamani S, Turner R, et al. The thiazide-sensitive Na-Cl cotransporter is an aldosterone-induced protein. *Proc Natl Acad Sci U S A* 1998;95:14552–14557.
45. Ruiz-Opazo N, Lopez LV, Herrera VL. The dual AngII/AVP receptor gene N119S/C163R variant exhibits sodium-induced dysfunction and cosegregates with salt-sensitive hypertension in the Dahl salt-sensitive hypertensive rat model. *Mol Med* 2002;8:24–32.
46. Edwards RM. Segmental effects of norepinephrine and angiotensin II on isolated renal microvessels. *Am J Physiol* 1983;244:F526–F534.
47. Navar LG, Champion WJ, Thomas CE. Effects of calcium channel blockade on renal vascular resistance responses to changes in perfusion pressure and angiotensin-converting enzyme inhibition in dogs. *Circ Res* 1986;58:874–881.
48. Schnermann J, Briggs JP, Weber PC. Tubuloglomerular feedback, prostaglandins, and angiotensin in the autoregulation of glomerular filtration rate. *Kidney Int* 1984;25:53–64.
49. Iversen BM, Sekse I, Ofstad J. Resetting of renal blood flow autoregulation in spontaneously hypertensive rats. *Am J Physiol* 1987;252:F480–F486.
50. Sorensen CM. Role of the renin-angiotensin system in regulation and autoregulation of renal blood flow. *Am J Physiol Regul Integr Comp Physiol* 2000;279:R1017–R1024.
51. Hayashi K, Epstein M, Loutzenhiser R. Pressure-induced vasoconstriction of renal microvessels in normotensive and hypertensive rats. *Circ Res* 1989;65:1475–1484.
52. Hayashi K, Epstein M, Loutzenhiser R. Enhanced myogenic responsiveness of renal interlobular arteries in spontaneously hypertensive rats. *Hypertension* 1992;19:153–160.
53. Takenaka T, Forster H, De Micheli A, et al. Impaired myogenic responsiveness of renal microvessels in Dahl salt-sensitive rats. *Circ Res* 1992;71:471–480.
54. Almeida JB, Saragoca MA, Tavares A, et al. Severe hypertension induces disturbances of renal autoregulation. *Hypertension* 1992;19[2 Suppl]:II279–II283.
55. Muller DN, Luft FC. The renin-angiotensin system in the vessel wall. *Basic Res Cardiol* 1998;93[Suppl 2]:7–14.
56. Hollenberg NK, Fisher ND, Price DA. Pathways for angiotensin II generation in intact human tissue: evidence from comparative pharmacological interruption of the renin system. *Hypertension* 1998;32:387–392.
57. Esther CR, Marino EM, Howard TE. et al. The critical role of tissue angiotensin-converting enzyme as revealed by gene targeting in mice. *J Clin Invest* 1997;99:2375–2385.
58. Steckelings U, Lebrun C, Qadri F, et al. Role of brain angiotensin in cardiovascular regulation. *J Cardiovasc Pharmacol* 1992;19[Suppl 6]:S72–S79.
59. Chaki S, Inagami T. Identification and characterization of a new angiotensin II receptor subtype in differentiated neuro-2A cells. *Biochem Biophys Res Commun* 1992;182:388–394.
60. Swanson GN, Hanesworth JM, Sardinia MF, et al. Discovery of a distinct binding site for angiotensin II (3–8), a putative angiotensin IV receptor. *Regul Pept* 1992;40:409–419.
61. Inagami T, Iwai N, Sasaki K, et al. Cloning, expression and regulation of angiotensin II receptors. *J Hypertens* 1992;10:713–716.
62. Mukoyama M, Nakajima M, Horiuchi M, et al. Expression cloning of type 2 angiotensin II receptor reveals a unique class of seven-transmembrane receptors. *J Biol Chem* 1993; 268:24539–24542.
63. Iwai N, Inagami T. Identification of two subtypes in the rat type I angiotensin II receptor. *FEBS Lett* 1992;298:257–260.
64. Curnow KM, Pascoe L, White PC. Genetic analysis of the human type-1 angiotensin II receptor. *Mol Endocrinol* 1992;6: 1113–1118.
65. Aguilera G, Catt K. Regulation of vascular angiotensin II receptors in the rat during altered sodium intake. *Circ Res* 1981;49:751–758.
66. Rajagopalan S, Kurz S, Munzel T, et al. Angiotensin II-mediated hypertension in the rat increases vascular superoxide production via membrane NADH/NADPH oxidase

activation. Contribution to alterations of vasomotor tone. *J Clin Invest* 1996;97:1916–1923.

67. Muller DN, Dechend R, Mervaala EM, et al. NF-κB inhibition ameliorates angiotensin II-induced inflammatory damage in rats. *Hypertension* 2000;35:193–201.
68. Vaughan DE, Lazos SA, Tong K. Angiotensin II regulates the expression of plasminogen activator inhibitor-1 in cultured endothelial cells. A potential link between the renin-angiotensin system and thrombosis. *J Clin Invest* 1995;95: 995–1001.
69. Nakamura S, Nakamura I, Ma L, et al. Plasminogen activator inhibitor-1 expression is regulated by the angiotensin type 1 receptor in vivo. *Kidney Int* 2000;58:251–259.
70. Ruiz-Ortega M, Lorenzo O, Ruperez M, et al. Angiotensin II activates nuclear transcription factor kappaB through AT(1) and AT(2) in vascular smooth muscle cells: molecular mechanisms. *Circ Res* 2000;86:1266–1272.
71. Barnes PJ, Karin M. Nuclear factor-kappaB: a pivotal transcription factor in chronic inflammatory diseases. *N Engl J Med* 1997;336:1066–1071.
72. Wang WY, Zee RY, Morris BJ. Association of angiotensin II type 1 receptor gene polymorphism with essential hypertension. *Clin Genet* 1997;51:31–34.
73. Ozono R, Wang ZQ, Moore AF, et al. Expression of the subtype 2 angiotensin (AT2) receptor protein in rat kidney. *Hypertension* 1997;30:1238–1246.
74. Ichiki T, Kambayashi Y, Inagami T. Multiple growth factors modulate mRNA expression of angiotensin II type-2 receptor in R3T3 cells. *Circ Res* 1995;77:1070–1076.
75. Ciuffo GM, Alvarez SE, Fuentes LB. Angiotensin II receptors induce tyrosine dephosphorylation in rat fetal membranes. *Regul Pept* 1998;74:129–135.
76. Horiuchi M, Hayashida W, Kambe T, et al. Angiotensin type 2 receptor dephosphorylates Bcl-2 by activating mitogen-activated protein kinase phosphatase-1 and induces apoptosis. *J Biol Chem* 1997;272:19022–19026.
77. Horiuchi M, Lehtonen JY, Daviet L. Signaling mechanism of the AT2 angiotensin II receptor: crosstalk between AT1 and AT2 receptors in cell growth. *Trends Endocrinol Metab* 1999;10:391–396.
78. Matsubara H. Pathophysiological role of angiotensin II type 2 receptor in cardiovascular and renal diseases. *Circ Res* 1998;83:1182–1191.
79. Hein L, Barsh GS, Pratt RE, et al. Behavioural and cardiovascular effects of disrupting the angiotensin II type-2 receptor in mice. *Nature* 1995;377:744–747.
80. Cao Z, Dean R, Wu L, et al. Role of angiotensin receptor subtypes in mesenteric vascular proliferation and hypertrophy. *Hypertension* 1999;34:408–414.
81. Booz GW, Baker KM. Role of type 1 and type 2 angiotensin receptors in angiotensin II-induced cardiomyocyte hypertrophy. *Hypertension* 1996;28:635–640.
82. Heagerty AM. Changes in vascular morphology in essential hypertension. *J Hum Hypertens* 1991;5[Suppl 1]:3–8.
83. Panza JA, Quyyumi AA, Brush JE, et al. Abnormal endothelium-dependent vascular relaxation in patients with essential hypertension. *N Engl J Med* 1990;323:22–27.
84. Griffin SA, Brown WC, MacPherson F, et al. Angiotensin II causes vascular hypertrophy in part by a non-pressor mechanism. *Hypertension* 1991;17:626–635.
85. Curnow KM, Tusie-Luna MT, Pascoe L, et al. The product of the CYP11B2 gene is required for aldosterone biosynthesis in the human adrenal cortex. *Mol Endocrinol* 1991;5:1513–1522.
86. Takeda Y, Yoneda T, Demura M, et al. Cardiac aldosterone production in genetically hypertensive rats. *Hypertension* 2000;36:495–500.
87. MacKenzie SM, Clark CJ, Fraser R, et al. Expression of 11beta-hydroxylase and aldosterone synthase genes in the rat brain. *J Mol Endocrinol* 2000;24(3):321–328.
88. Vinson GP, Laird SM, Whitehouse BJ, et al. The biosynthesis of aldosterone. *J Steroid Biochem Mol Biol* 1991;39:851–858.
89. Chartier L, Schiffrin EL. Role of calcium in effects of atrial natriuretic peptide on aldosterone production in adrenal glomerulosa cells. *Am J Physiol* 1987;252:E485–E491.
90. Funder JW. Non-genomic actions of aldosterone: role in hypertension. *Curr Opin Nephrol Hypertens* 2001;10:227–230.
91. Koenig W, Binner L, Gabrielsen F, et al. Catecholamines and the renin-angiotensin-aldosterone system during treatment with felodipine ER or hydrochlorothiazide in essential hypertension. *J Cardiovasc Pharmacol* 1991;18:349–353.
92. Wang W, McClain JM, Zucker IH. Aldosterone reduces baroreceptor discharge in the dog. *Hypertension* 1992;19:270–277.
93. Lijnen P, Petrov V. Induction of cardiac fibrosis by aldosterone. *J Mol Cell Cardiol* 2000;32:865–879.
94. Rocha R, Chander PN, Khanna K, et al. Mineralocorticoid blockade reduces vascular injury in stroke-prone hypertensive rats. *Hypertension* 1998;31:451–458.
95. Dorrance AM, Osborn HL, Grekin R, et al. Spironolactone reduces cerebral infarct size and EGF-receptor mRNA in stroke-prone rats. *Am J Physiol Regul Integr Comp Physiol.* 2001;281:R944–R950.
96. Bell C, Ferguson M, Petrovic T. Neurochemistry of dopaminergic nerves. In: Bell C, McGrath B, eds. Peripheral actions of dopamine. London: Macmillan, 1988:41–55.
97. Van den Buuse M. Role of the mesolimbic dopamine system in cardiovascular homeostasis. Stimulation of the ventral tegmental area modulates the effect of vasopressin on blood pressure in conscious rats. *Clin Exp Pharmacol Physiol* 1998;25:661–668.
98. Bek MJ, Eisner GM, Felder RA, et al. Dopamine receptors in hypertension. *Mt Sinai J Med* 2001;68:362–369.
99. Zabik JE, Sprague JE, Odio M. Interactive dopaminergic and noradrenergic systems in the regulation of thirst in the rat. *Physiol Behav* 1993;54:29–33.
100. Jose PA, Eisner GM, Felder RA. The renal dopamine receptors in health and hypertension. *Pharmacol Ther* 1998;80:149–182.
101. Montanari A, Tateo E, Fasoli E, et al. Dopamine-2 receptor blockade potentiates the renal effects of nitric oxide inhibition in humans. *Hypertension* 1998;31:277–282.
102. Cheng H-F, Becker BN, Harris RC. Dopamine decreases expression of type-1 angiotensin II receptors in renal proximal tubule. *J Clin Invest* 1996;97:2745–2752.
103. Asico LD, Ladines C, Fuchs S, et al. Disruption of the dopamine D3 receptor gene produces renin-dependent hypertension. *J Clin Invest* 1998;102:493–498.
104. Naruse M, Naruse K, Yoshimoto T, et al. Dopaminergic regulation of aldosterone secretion: its pathophysiologic significance in subsets of primary aldosteronism. *Hypertens Res* 1995;18[Suppl 1]:S59–S64.

105. Williams GH, Gordon MS, Steunkel CA, et al. Dopamine and nonmodulating hypertension. *Am J Hypertens* 1990;3:112S–115S.
106. Krushkal J, Ferrell R, Mockrin SC, et al. Genome-wide linkage analyses of systolic blood pressure using highly discordant siblings. *Circulation* 1999;99:1407–1410.
107. Sanada H, Jose PA, Hazen-Martin D, et al. Dopamine-1 receptor defect in renal proximal tubular cells in essential hypertension. *Hypertension* 1999;33:1036–1042.
108. Sato M, Soma M, Nakayama T, et al. Dopamine D1 receptor gene polymorphism is associated with essential hypertension. *Hypertension* 2000;36:183–186.
109. Thomas GN, Tomlinson B, Critchley JA. Modulation of blood pressure and obesity with the dopamine D2 receptor gene Ta q1 polymorphism. *Hypertension* 2000;36:177–182.
110. Levin ER, Gardner DG, Samson WK. Natriuretic peptides. *N Engl J Med* 1998;339:321–328.
111. Itoh H, Pratt RE, Dzau VJ. Atrial natriuretic polypeptide inhibits hypertrophy of vascular smooth muscle cells. *J Clin Invest* 1990;86:1690–1697.
112. Morishita R, Gibbons GH, Pratt RE, et al. Autocrine and paracrine effects of atrial natriuretic peptide gene transfer on vascular smooth muscle and endothelial cellular growth. *J Clin Invest* 1994;94:824–829.
113. Cao L, Gardner DG. Natriuretic peptides inhibit DNA synthesis in cardiac fibroblasts. *Hypertension* 1995;25:227–234.
114. Maack T, Marion DN, Camargo MJF, et al. Effects of auriculin (atrial natriuretic factor) on blood pressure, renal function, and the renin-aldosterone system in dogs. *Am J Med* 1984;77:1069–1075.
115. Sonnenberg H, Honrath U, Chong CK, et al. Atrial natriuretic factor inhibits sodium transport in medullary collecting duct. *Am J Physiol* 1986;231:1572–1573.
116. Harris PJ, Thomas D, Morgan TO. Atrial natriuretic peptide inhibits angiotensin-stimulated proximal tubular sodium and water reabsorption. *Nature* 1987;326:697–698.
117. Burnett JC Jr, Ganger JP, Opgenorth TS. Effects of synthetic atrial natriuretic factor on renal function and renin release. *Am J Physiol* 1984;247:F863–F866.
118. Aguilera G. Differential effects of atrial natriuretic factor on angiotensin II and adrenocorticotrophin-stimulated aldosterone secretion. *Endocrinology* 1987;120:299–304.
119. Volpe M, Mele AF, Indolfi C, et al. Hemodynamic and hormonal effects of atrial natriuretic factor in patients with essential hypertension. *J Am Coll Cardiol* 1987;10:787–793.
120. Cody RJS, Atlas SA, Laragh JH, et al. Atrial natriuretic factor in normal subjects and heart failure patients: plasma levels and renal, hormonal and hemodynamic responses to peptide infusion. *J Clin Invest* 1986;78:1362–1372.
121. Maack T, Marion DN, Camargo MJF, et al. Effects of auriculin (atrial natriuretic factor) on blood pressure, renal function, and the renin-aldosterone system in dogs. *Am J Med* 1984;77:1069–1075.
122. Hunt PJ, Espiner EA, Nicholls MG, et al. Differing biological effects of equimolar atrial and brain natriuretic peptide infusions in normal man. *J Clin Endocrinol Metab* 1996;81:3871–3876.
123. Volpe M, Odell G, Kleinert HD, et al. Effect of atrial natriuretic factor on blood pressure, renin and aldosterone in Goldblatt hypertension. *Hypertension* 1985;7[Suppl I]:I43–I48.
124. Volpe M, Sosa RE, Muller FB, et al. Differing hemodynamic and hormonal effects of human alpha atrial natriuretic peptide in two models of hypertension. *Am J Physiol* 1986;250:H871–H878.
125. Volpe M, Vecchione F, Cuocolo A, et al. Hemodynamic responses to atrial natriuretic factor in nephrectomized rabbits: attenuation of the circulatory consequences of acute volume expansion. *Circ Res* 1988;63:322–329.
126. Ramasawmy R, Kotea N, Lu CY, et al. A new polymorphic restriction site of the human atrial natriuretic peptide (hANP) gene locus. *Hum Genet* 1993;91:509–510.
127. Ramasawmy R, Kotea N, Lu CY, et al. Investigation of the polymorphic Sca I site by a PCR-based assay at the human atrial natriuretic peptide (hANP) gene locus. *Hum Genet* 1992;90:323–324.
128. Rutledge DR, Sun Y, Ross EA. Polymorphisms within the atrial natriuretic peptide gene in essential hypertension. *J Hypertens* 1995;13:953–955.
129. Kato N, Sugiyama T, Morita H, et al. Genetic analysis of the atrial natriuretic peptide gene in essential hypertension. *Clin Sci* 2000;98:251–258.
130. Rubattu S, Ridker PM, Stampfer JM, et al. The gene encoding atrial natriuretic peptide and the risk of human stroke. *Circulation* 1999;100:1722–1726.
131. Yanagisawa M, Kurihawa H, Kimura S, et al. A novel potent vasoconstrictor peptide produced by vascular endothelial cells. *Nature* 1988;332:411–415.
132. Inoue A, Yanagisawa M, Kimura S, et al. The human endothelin family: three structurally and pharmacologically distinct isopeptides predicted by three separate genes. *Proc Natl Acad Sci U S A* 1989;86:2863–2867.
133. Gray GA. Generation of endothelin. In: Gray GA, Webb DJ, eds. *Molecular biology and pharmacology of the endothelins.* Austin, TX: RG Landes, 1995:13–32.
134. Howard PG, Plumpton C, Davenport AP. Anatomical localisation and pharmacological activity of mature endothelins and their precursors in human vascular tissue. *J Hypertens* 1992;10:1379–1386.
135. Hirata Y. Endothelin peptides. *Curr Opin Nephrol Hypertens* 1996;5:12–15.
136. Ogawa Y, Nakao K, Arai H, et al. Molecular cloning of a non-isopeptide-selective human endothelin receptor. *Biochem Biophys Res Commun* 1991;178:248–255.
137. Arai H, Hori S, Aramori I, et al. Cloning and expression of a cDNA encoding an endothelin receptor. *Nature* 1990;348:730–732.
138. Williams DL, Jones KL, Pettibone DJ, et al. Sarafotoxin S6c: an agonist which distinguishes between endothelin receptor subtypes. *Biochem Biophys Res Commun* 1991;175:556–561.
139. Davenport AP, Maguire JJ. Is endothelin-induced vasoconstriction mediated only by ETA receptors in humans? *Trends Pharmacol Sci* 1994;15:9–11.
140. Miyoshi Y, Nakaya Y, Wakatsuki T. Endothelin blocks ATP-sensitive K^+ channels and depolarises smooth muscle cells of porcine coronary artery. *Circ Res* 1992;70:612–616.
141. Gray GA. Signal transduction mechanisms of the endothelins. In: Gray GA, Webb DJ, eds. *Molecular biology and pharmacology of the endothelins.* Austin, TX: RG Landes, 1995:95–114.
142. Edwards RM, Trizna W, Ohlstein EH. Renal microvascular effects of endothelin. *Am J Physiol* 1990;259:F217–F221.

143. López-Farré A, Montanes I, Millas I, et al. Effect of endothelin on renal function in rats. *Eur J Pharmacol* 1989;163:187–189.
144. King AJ, Brenner BM, Anderson S. Endothelin: a potent renal and systemic vasoconstrictor peptide. *Am J Physiol* 1989;256:F1051–F1058.
145. Zeidel ML, Brady HR, Kone BC, et al. Endothelin, a peptide inhibitor of sodium Na^+-K^+-ATPase, in intact renal tubular endothelial cells. *Am J Physiol* 1989;257:C1101–C1107.
146. Rakugi H, Nakamaru M, Saito H, et al. Endothelin inhibits renin release from isolated rat glomeruli. *Biochem Biophys Res Commun* 1988;155:1244–1247.
147. Cozza EN, Gomez-Sanchez CE, Foecking M, et al. Endothelin binding to cultured calf adrenal zona glomerulosa cells and stimulation of aldosterone secretion. *J Clin Invest* 1989; 84:1032–1035.
148. Fukuda Y, Hirata Y, Yoshimi H, et al. Endothelin is a potent secretagogue for atrial natriuretic peptide in cultured rat atrial myocytes. *Biochem Biophys Res Commun* 1988;155:167–172.
149. Levin N. Endothelins. *N Engl J Med* 1995;333:356–363.
150. Schiffrin EL, Larivière R, Li JS, et al. Enhanced expression of the endothelin-1 gene in blood vessels of DOCA–salt hypertensive rats: correlation with vascular structure. *J Vasc Res* 1996;33:235–248.
151. Haynes WG, Hand M, Johnstone HA, et al. Direct and sympathetically mediated venoconstriction in essential hypertension: enhanced responses to endothelin-1. *J Clin Invest* 1994; 94:1359–1364.
152. Davenport AP, Ashby MJ, Easton P, et al. A sensitive radioimmunoassay measuring endothelin-like immunoreactivity in human plasma: comparison of levels in patients with essential hypertension and normotensive control subjects. *Clin Sci* 1990;78:261–264.
153. Kohno M, Murakawa K-I, Horio T, et al. Plasma immunoreactive endothelin-1 in experimental malignant hypertension. *Hypertension* 1991;18:93–100.
154. Koyama H, Tabata T, Nishzawa Y, et al. Plasma endothelin levels in patients with uraemia. *Lancet* 1989;333:991–992.
155. Bunchman TE, Brookshire CA. Cyclosporine-induced synthesis of endothelin by cultured human endothelial cells. *J Clin Invest* 1991;88:310–314.
156. Nambi P, Pullen M, Contino LC, et al. Upregulation of renal endothelin receptors in rats with cyclosporin A-induced nephrotoxicity. *Eur J Pharmacol* 1990;187:113–116.
157. Moutabarrik A, Ishibashi M, Fukunaga M, et al. FK 506 mechanism of nephrotoxicity: stimulatory effect on endothelin secretion by cultured kidney cells and tubular cell toxicity in vitro. *Transplant Proc* 1991;23:3133–3136.
158. Ergul S, Parish DC, Puett D, et al. Racial differences in plasma endothelin concentrations in individuals with essential hypertension. *Hypertension* 1996;28:652–655.
159. Stevens PA, Brown MJ. Genetic variability of the ET-1 and the ETA receptor genes in essential hypertension. *J Cardiovasc Pharmacol* 1995;26[Suppl 3]:S9–S12.
160. Moncada S, Higgs EA. The L-arginine-nitric oxide pathway. *N Engl J Med* 1993;329:2002–2012.
161. Vallance P, Collier J, Moncada S. Effects of endothelium-derived nitric oxide on peripheral arteriolar tone in man. *Lancet* 1989;2(8670):997–1000.
162. Panza JA, Quyyumi AA, Brush JE Jr, et al. Abnormal endothelium-dependent vascular relaxation in patients with essential hypertension. *N Engl J Med* 1990;323:22–27.
163. Calver A, Collier J, Moncada S, et al. Effect of local intra-arterial NG-monomethyl-L-arginine in patients with hypertension: the nitric oxide dilator mechanism appears abnormal. *J Hypertens* 1992;10:1025–1031.
164. Chen PY, Sanders PW. L-arginine abrogates salt-sensitive hypertension in Dahl/Rapp rats. *J Clin Invest* 1991;88:1559–1567.
165. Nakaki T, Hishikawa K, Suzuki H, et al. L-arginine-induced hypotension. *Lancet* 1990;336:696–696.
166. Vallance P, Leone A, Calver A, et al. Accumulation of an endogenous inhibitor of nitric oxide synthesis in chronic renal failure. *Lancet* 1992;339:572–575.
167. Shibuki K, Okada D. Endogenous nitric oxide release required for long-term synaptic depression in the cerebellum. *Nature* 1991;349:326–328.
168. Spielman WS, Arend LJ. Adenosine receptors and signaling in the kidney. *Hypertension* 1991;17:117–130.
169. Chen Y-F, Li P-L, Zou A-P. Oxidative stress enhances the production and actions of adenosine in the kidney. *Am J Physiol* 2001;281:R1808–R1816.
170. Ledent C, Vaugeois JM, Schiffmann SN, et al. Aggressiveness, hypoalgesia and high blood pressure in mice lacking the adenosine A2a receptor. *Nature* 1997;388:674–678.
171. Dixon AK, Gubitz AK, Sirinathsinghji DJ, et al. Tissue distribution of adenosine receptor mRNAs in the rat. *Br J Pharmacol* 1996;118:1461–1468.
172. Welch WJ. Adenosine A1 receptor antagonists in the kidney: effects in fluid-retaining disorders. *Curr Opin Pharmacol* 2002;2:165–170.
173. Klein I, Levey GS. The cardiovascular system in thyrotoxicosis. In: Braverman LE, Utiger RD, eds. *Werner and Ingbar's the thyroid: a fundamental and clinical text,* 8th ed. Philadelphia: Lippincott Williams and Wilkins, 2000:596–604.
174. Park KW, Dai HB, Ojamaa K, et al. The direct vasomotor effect of thyroid hormones on rat skeletal muscle resistance arteries. *Anesth Analg* 1997;85:734–738.
175. Klein I, Ojamaa K. Thyroid hormone and the cardiovascular system. *N Engl J Med.* 2001;344:501–509.
176. Levey GS, Klein I. Catecholamine-thyroid hormone interactions and the cardiovascular manifestations of hyperthyroidism. *Am J Med* 1990;88:642–646.
177. Kitamura K, Kangawa K, Kawamoto M, et al. Adrenomedullin: a novel hypotensive peptide isolated from human pheochromocytoma. *Biochem Biophys Res Commun* 1993;192:553–560.
178. Ichiki Y, Kitamura K, Kangawa K, et al. Distribution and characterization of immunoreactive adrenomedullin in human tissue and plasma. *FEBS Lett* 1994;338:6–10.
179. Sugo S, Minamino N, Kangawa K, et al. Endothelial cells actively synthesize and secrete adrenomedullin. *Biochem Biophys Res Commun* 1994;201:1160–1166.
180. Miller MJ, Martinez A, Unsworth EJ, et al. Adrenomedullin expression in human tumor cell lines: its potential role as an autocrine growth factor. *J Biol Chem* 1996;271:23345–23351.
181. Shimekake Y, Nagata K, Ohta S, et al. Adrenomedullin stimulates two signal transduction pathways, cAMP accumulation and Ca^{2+} mobilization, in bovine aortic endothelial cells. *J Biol Chem* 1995;270(9):4412–4417.

182. Nishikimi T, Horio T, Kohmoto Y, et al. Molecular forms of plasma and urinary adrenomedullin in normal, essential hypertension and chronic renal failure. *J Hypertens* 2001;19:765–773.
183. Arar MY, Hogg RJ, Arant BS Jr, et al. Etiology of sustained hypertension in children in the southwestern United States. *Pediatr Nephrol* 1994;8:186–189.
184. Wyszynska T, Cichocka E, Wieteska-Klimczak A, et al. A single center experience with 1025 children with hypertension. *Acta Paediatr* 1992;81:244–246.
185. Flynn JT. What's new in pediatric hypertension? *Curr Hypertens Rep* 2001;3:503–510.
186. Troiano RP, Flegal KM. Overweight children and adolescents: description, epidemiology and demographics. *Pediatrics* 1998;101:497–504.
187. Lifton RP. Genetic determinants of human hypertension. *Proc Natl Acad Sci U S A* 1995;92:8545–8551.
188. Feinleib M, Garrison RJ, Fabsitz R, et al. The NHLBI twin study of cardiovascular disease risk factors: methodology and summary of results. *Am J Epidemiol* 1977;106:284–285.
189. Longini IM Jr, Higgins MW, Hinton PC, et al. Environmental and genetic sources of familial aggregation of blood pressure in Tecumseh, Michigan. *Am J Epidemiol* 1984;120:131–144.
190. Mongeau JG. Heredity and blood pressure in humans: an overview. *Pediatr Nephrol* 1987;1:69–75.
191. Jeunemaitre X, Soubrier F, Kotelevtsev YV, et al. Molecular basis of human hypertension: role of angiotensinogen. *Cell* 1992;71:169–180.
192. Inoue I, Nakajima T, Williams CS, et al. A nucleotide substitution in the promoter of human angiotensinogen is associated with essential hypertension and affects basal transcription in vitro. *J Clin Invest* 1997;99:1786–1797.
193. Watt GCM, Harrap SB, Foy CJW, et al. Abnormalities of glucocorticoid metabolism and the renin-angiotensin system: a four-corners approach to the identification of genetic determinants of blood pressure. *J Hypertens* 1992;10:473–482.
194. Williams SM, Addy JH, Phillips III JA, et al. Combinations of variations in multiple genes are associated with hypertension. *Hypertension* 2000;36:2–6.
195. Samani NJ. Molecular genetics of susceptibility to the development of hypertension. *Br Med Bull* 1994;50:260–271.
196. Lifton RP, Gharavi AG, Geller DS. Molecular mechanisms of human hypertension. *Cell* 2001;104:545–556.
197. Law CM, Barker DJP, Bull AR, et al. Maternal and fetal influences on blood pressure. *Arch Dis Child* 1991;66:1291–1295.
198. Zureik M, Bonithon-Kopp C, Lecomte E, et al. Weights at birth and in early infancy, systolic pressure and left ventricular structure in subjects aged 8 to 24 years. *Hypertension* 1996;27(pt 1):339–345.
199. Barker DJP, Gluckman PD, Godfrey KM, et al. Fetal nutrition and cardiovascular disease in adult life. *Lancet* 1993;341:938–941.
200. Mackenzie HS, Lawler EV, Brenner BM. Congenital olionephropathy. The fetal flaw in essential hypertension? *Kidney Int* 1996;55:S30–S34.
201. Beratis NG, Panagoulias D, Varvarigou A. Increased blood pressure in neonates and infants whose mothers smoked during pregnancy. *J Pediatr* 1996;128:806–812.
202. Singhal A, Cole TJ, Lucas A. Early nutrition in preterm infants and later blood pressure: two cohorts after randomized trials. *Lancet* 2001;357:413–419.
203. Langley-Evans SC. Critical differences between two low protein diet protocols in the programming of hypertension in the rat. *Int J Food Sci Nutr* 2000;51:11–17.
204. Woods LL, Ingelfinger JR, Nyengaard JR, et al. Maternal protein restriction suppresses the newborn renin-angiotensin system and programs adult hypertension in rats. *Pediatr Res* 2001;49:460–467.
205. Ingelfinger JR. Perinatal programming, renal development, and adult renal function. *Am J Hypertens* 2002;15:46S-49S.
206. Siewert-Delle A, Ljungman S. The impact of birth weight and gestational age on blood pressure in adult life: a population-based study of 49-year old men. *Am J Hypertens* 1998;11:946–953.
207. Falkner B, Hulman S, Kushner H. Birth weight versus childhood growth as determinants of adult blood pressure. *Hypertension* 1998;31(pt 1):145–150.
208. Williams S, Poulton R. Twins and maternal smoking: ordeals for the fetal origins hypothesis [abridged version]. *BMJ* 1999;318:897–900.
209. Falkner B, Kushner H, Onesti G, et al. Cardiovascular characteristics in adolescents who develop essential hypertension. *Hypertension* 1981;3:521–527.
210. Voors AW, Webber LS, Berenson GS. Resting heart rate and pressure-rate product in a total biracial community: the Bogalusa Heart Study. *Am J Epidemiol* 1982;116:276–286.
211. Sorof JM, Poffenbarger T, Franco K, et al. Isolated systolic hypertension, obesity and hyperkinetic hemodynamic states in children. *J Pediatr* 2002;140:660–666.
212. Palatini P, Julius S. Heart rate and the cardiovascular risk. *J Hypertens* 1997;15:1–15.
213. Menkes MS, Matthews KA, Krantz DS, et al. Cardiovascular reactivity to the cold pressor test as a predictor of hypertension. *Hypertension* 1989;14:524–530.
214. Treiber FA, McCaffrey F, Musante L, et al. Ethnicity, family history of hypertension and patterns of hemodynamic reactivity in boys. *Psychosom Med* 1993;55:70–77.
215. Mauso K, Mikami H, Ogihara T, et al. Sympathetic nerve hyperactivity precedes hyperinsulinemia and blood pressure elevation in a young, nonobese Japanese population. *Am J Hypertens* 1997;10:77–83.
216. Lopes HF, Silva HB, Consolim-Colombo FM, et al. Autonomic abnormalities demonstrable in young normotensive subjects who are children of hypertensive parents. *Brazil J Med Biol Res* 2000;33:51–54.
217. Anderson EA, Sinkey CA, Lawton WJ, et al. Elevated sympathetic nerve activity in borderline hypertensive humans: evidence from direct intraneural recordings. *Hypertension* 1989;14:177–183.
218. Mimura Y, Kobayashi S, Notoya K, et al. Activation by alpha 1-adrenergic agonists of the progression phase in the proliferation of primary cultures of smooth muscle cells in mouse and rat aorta. *Biol Pharm Bull* 1995;18:1373–1376.
219. Koch VH, Furusawa EA, Saito MI, et al. White coat hypertension in adolescents. *Clin Nephrol* 1999;52:297–303.
220. Anwar YA, White WB. Ambulatory monitoring of blood pressure: devices, analysis and clinical utility. In: White WB, ed. *Blood pressure monitoring in cardiovascular medicine and therapeutics*. Totowa, NJ: Humana Press, 2001:57–75.

221. Landsberg L. Insulin-mediated sympathetic stimulation: role in the pathogenesis of obesity-related hypertension (or, how insulin affects blood pressure, and why). *J Hypertens* 2001;19:523–528.
222. Reaven GM, Lithell H, Landsberg L. Hypertension and associated metabolic abnormalities—the role of insulin resistance and the sympathoadrenal system. *N Engl J Med* 1996;334:374–381.
223. Gupta AK, Clark RV, Kirchner KA. Effects of insulin on renal sodium excretion. *Hypertension* 1992;19:I78–I82.
224. Esler M, Rumatir M, Wiesner G, et al. Sympathetic nervous system and insulin resistance: from obesity to diabetes. *Am J Hypertens* 2001;14:304S-309S.
225. Rocchini AP, Key J, Bondie D, et al. The effect of weight loss on the sensitivity of blood pressure to sodium in obese adolescents. *N Engl J Med* 1989;321:580–585.
226. Anderson EA, Hoffman RP, Balon TW, et al. Hyperinsulinemia produces both sympathetic neural activation and vasodilatation in normal humans. *J Clin Invest* 1991;87:2246–2252.
227. Laasko M, Edeelman SV, Brechtel G, et al. Decreased effect of insulin to stimulate skeletal muscle blood flow in obese men. *J Clin Invest* 1990;1844–1852.
228. Bornfeldt KE, Arnqvist HJ, Capron L. In vivo proliferation of rat vascular smooth muscle in relation to diabetes mellitus insulin-like growth factor I and insulin. *Diabetologia* 1992;35:104–108.
229. Ahima RS, Flier JS. Leptin. *Annu Rev Physiol* 2000;62:413–437.
230. Hall JE, Hildebrandt DA, Kuo J. Obesity hypertension: role of leptin and sympathetic nervous system. *Am J Hypertens* 2001;14:103S–115S.
231. Haynes WG, Morgan DA, Walsh SA, et al. Receptor-mediated regional sympathetic nerve activation by leptin. *J Clin Invest* 1997;100:270–278.
232. Wolf G, Chen S, Han DC, et al. Leptin and renal disease. *Am J Kidney Dis* 2002;39:1–11.
233. Ferrannini E, Buzzigoli G, Bonadonna R, et al. Insulin resistance in essential hypertension. *N Engl J Med* 1987;317:350–357.
234. Falkner B, Hulman S, Tannenbaum J, et al. Insulin resistance and blood pressure in young black men. *Hypertension* 1990;16:706–711.
235. Weinberger MH, Miller JZ, Luft FC, et al. Sodium and blood pressure: an overview. In: *Children's blood pressure: report of the 88th Ross Conference on Pediatric Research.* Columbus, OH: Ross Laboratories, 1985:77–85.
236. Law MR, Frost CD, Wald NJ. By how much does dietary salt reduction lower blood pressure? I—Analysis of observational data among populations. *BMJ* 1991;302:811–815.
237. He FJ, MacGregor GA. Potassium intake and blood pressure. *Am J Hypertens* 1999;12:849–851.
238. Cutler JA, Follmann D, Allender PS. Randomized trials of sodium reduction: an overview. *Am J Clin Nutr* 1997;65:643S-651S.
239. Simmons-Morton DG, Obarzanek E. Diet and blood pressure in children and adolescents. *Pediatr Nephrol* 1997;11:244–249.
240. Grimm RH, Neaton JD, Elmer PJ, et al. The influence of oral potassium chloride on blood pressure in hypertensive men on a low-sodium diet. *N Engl J Med* 1990;322:569–574.
241. Appel LJ, Moore TJ, Obarzanek E, et al. A clinical trial of the effects of dietary patterns on blood pressure. *N Engl J Med* 1997;336:1117–1124.
242. Weinberger MH. Salt sensitivity of blood pressure in humans. *Hypertension* 1996;27:481–490.
243. Shapiro D, Goldstein IB, Jammer LD. Effects of cynical hostility, anger out, anxiety and defensiveness on ambulatory blood pressure in black and white college students. *Psychosom Med* 1996;58:354–364.
244. Pickering TG. The effects of environmental and lifestyle factors on blood pressure and the intermediary role of the sympathetic nervous system. *J Hum Hypertens* 1997;11:S9–S18.
245. Mune T, Rogerson FM, Nikkila H, et al. Human hypertension caused by mutations in the kidney isozyme of 11 beta-hydroxysteroid dehydrogenase. *Nat Genet* 1995;10:394–399.
246. Funder JW. Adrenal steroids: new answers, new questions. *Science* 1987;237:236–237.
247. Snyder PM, Price MP, McDonald FJ, et al., Mechanism by which Liddle's syndrome mutations increase activity of a human epithelial Na+ channel. *Cell* 1995;83:969–978.
248. Shimkets RA, Lifton RP, Canessa CM. The activity of the epithelial sodium channel is regulated by clathrin-mediated endocytosis. *J Biol Chem* 1997;272:25537–25541.
249. Hansson JH, Nelson-Williams C, Suzuki H, et al. Hypertension caused by a truncated epithelial sodium channel gamma subunit: genetic heterogeneity of Liddle syndrome. *Nat Genet* 1995;11:76–82.
250. Lifton RP, Dluhy RG, Powers M, et al. Hereditary hypertension caused by chimeric gene duplications and ectopic expression of aldosterone synthase. *Nat Genet* 1992;2:66–74.
251. Wilson FH, Disse-Nicodeme S, Choate KA, et al. Human hypertension caused by mutations in WNK kinases. *Science* 2001;293:1107–1112.
252. Disse-Nicodeme S, Achard JM, Desitter I, et al. A new locus on chromosome 12p13.3 for pseudohypoaldosteronism type II, an autosomal dominant form of hypertension. *Am J Hum Genet* 2000;67:302–310.
253. Geller DS, Farhi A, Pinkerton N, et al. Activating mineralocorticoid receptor mutation in hypertension exacerbated by pregnancy. *Science* 2000;289:119–123.
254. Schuster H, Wienker TF, Toka HR, et al. Autosomal dominant hypertension and brachydactyly in a Turkish kindred resembles essential hypertension. *Hypertension* 1996;28:1085–1092.
255. Alvarez-Lara MA. Blood pressure and body water distribution in chronic renal failure patients. *Nephrol Dial Transplant* 2001;16[Suppl 1]:94–97.
256. Boero R. Sympathetic nervous system and chronic renal failure. *Clin Exp Hypertens* 2001;23:69–75.
257. Fleck C. Serum concentrations of asymmetric (ADMA) and symmetric (SDMA) dimethylarginine in renal failure patients. *Kidney Int Suppl* 2001;78:S14–S18.
258. Morris ST. Impaired endothelial function in isolated human uremic resistance arteries. *Kidney Int* 2001;60:1077–1082.
259. Vajo Z, Moffitt RA, Rarvathala S, et al. Elevated endothelin-1 levels and persistent stage IV hypertension in a non-volume over-loaded anephric patient. *Am J Hypertens* 1996; 9:935–937.

260. van Geet C, van Damme-Loembaerts R, Vanrusselt M, et al. Recombinant human erythropoietin increases blood pressure, platelet aggregability and platelet free calcium mobilization in uremic children: A possible link? *Thromb Haemost* 1990;64:7–10.
261. Goldblatt H, Lynch J, Hanzal RF, et al. Studies on experimental hypertension. I. The production of persistent elevation of systolic blood pressure by means of renal ischemia. *J Exp Med* 1934;59:347–378.
262. Abdi A, Johns EJ. Importance of the renin-angiotensin system in the generation of kidney failure in renovascular hypertension. *J Hypertens* 1996;14:1131–1137.
263. Nystrom HC, Jia J, Johansson M, et al. Neurohormonal influences on maintenance and reversal of two-kidney one-clip renal hypertension. *Acta Physiol Scand* 2002;175:245–251.
264. Nakada T, Kubota Y, Suzuki H, et al. Suppression of sympathetic nervous system attenuates the development of two-kidney, one-clip Goldblatt hypertension. *J Urol* 1996;156: 1480–1484.
265. Imanishi M, Akabane S, Takamiya M, et al. Critical degree of renal artery stenosis that causes hypertension in dogs. *Angiology* 1992;43:833–842.
266. Brown JJ, Cuesta V, Davies DL, et al. Mechanism of renal hypertension. *Lancet* 1976;1:1219–1221.
267. Eng E, Veniant M, Floege J, et al. Renal proliferative and phenotypic changes in rats with two-kidney, one-clip Goldblatt hypertension. *Am J Hypertens* 1994;7:177–185.
268. Higashi Y. Endothelial function and oxidative stress in renovascular hypertension. *N Engl J Med* 2002;346:1954–1962.
269. Kurokawa K. Kidney, salt, and hypertension: how and why. *Kidney Int Suppl* 1996;55:S46–S51.
270. Safar ME, Thuilliez C, Richard V, et al. Pressure-independent contribution of sodium to large artery structure and function in hypertension. *Cardiovasc Res* 2000;46:269–276.
271. Hasegawa K, Matsushita Y, Inoue T, et al. Plasma levels of atrial natriuretic peptide in patients with chronic renal failure. *J Clin Endocrinol Metab* 1986;63:819–822.
272. Bennett WM, Henrich WL, Stoff JS. The renal effects of nonsteroidal anti-inflammatory drugs: summary and recommendations. *Am J Kidney Dis* 1996;28[Suppl 1]:S56–S62.
273. *North American Pediatric Renal Transplant Cooperative Study, 2002 annual report.* Potomac, MD: EMMES Corporation, 2002.
274. Park JB, Schiffrin EL. Effects of antihypertensive therapy on hypertensive vascular disease. *Curr Hypertens Rep* 2000;2:280–288.
275. Broyer M, Guest G, Gagnadoux M-F, et al. Hypertension following renal transplantation in children. *Pediatr Nephrol* 1987;1:16–21.
276. Schwenger V, Zeier M, Ritz E. Hypertension after renal transplantation. *Curr Hypertens Rep* 2001;3:434–439.
277. Scherrer U, Vissing SF, Morgan BJ, et al. Cyclosporine-induced sympathetic activation and hypertension after heart transplantation. *N Engl J Med* 1990;323:693–699.
278. Laskow DA, Curtis JJ. Post-transplant hypertension. *Am J Hypertens* 1990;3:721–725.
279. Luke RG. Pathophysiology and treatment of posttransplant hypertension. *J Am Soc Nephrol* 1991;2:S37–S44.
280. Enia G, Mallamaci F, Benedetto FA, et al. Long-term CAPD patients are volume expanded and display more severe left ventricular hypertrophy than haemodialysis patients. *Nephrol Dial Transplant* 2001;16:1459–1464.
281. Leypoldt JK, Cheung AK, Delmez JA, et al. Relationship between volume status and blood pressure during chronic hemodialysis. *Kidney Int* 2002;61:266–275.
282. Lameire N, Van Biesen W. Importance of blood pressure and volume control in peritoneal dialysis patients. *Perit Dial Int* 2001;21:206–211.
283. Rahman M, Smith MC. Hypertension in hemodialysis patients. *Curr Hypertens Rep* 2001;3:496–502.
284. Erkan E, Devarajan P, Kaskel F. Role of nitric oxide, endothelin-1, and inflammatory cytokines in blood pressure regulation in hemodialysis patients. *Am J Kidney Dis* 2002;40:76–81.
285. Vaziri ND. Cardiovascular effects of erythropoietin and anemia correction. *Curr Opin Nephrol Hypertens*ion 2001;10:633–637.
286. Agarwal R, Lewis R, Davis JL, et al. Lisinopril therapy for hemodialysis hypertension: hemodynamic and endocrine responses. *Am J Kidney Dis* 2001;38:1245–1250.
287. Ross RD, Clapp SK, Gunther S, et al. Augmented norepinephrine and renin output in response to maximal exercise in hypertensive coarctectomy patients. *Am Heart J* 1992;123:1293–1298.
288. Choy M, Rocchini AP, Beekman RH, et al. Paradoxical hypertension after repair of coarctation of the aorta in children: balloon angioplasty versus surgical repair. *Circulation* 1987;75:1186–1191.
289. O'Sullivan JJ, Derrick G, Darnell R. Prevalence of hypertension in children after early repair of coarctation of the aorta: a cohort study using casual and 24 hour blood pressure measurement. *Heart* 2002;88:163–166.
290. Simsolo R, Grunfield B, Gimenez M, et al. Long-term systemic hypertension in children after successful repair of coarctation of the aorta. *Am Heart J* 1988;115:1268–1273.
291. Roegel JC. Vascular and neuroendocrine components in altered blood pressure regulation after surgical repair of coarctation of the aorta. *J Hum Hypertens* 1998;12:517–525.
292. DeBruno MP, Turoni CMJ, Maranon RO, et al. Structural changes in the kidney induced by coarctation hypertension. *Clin Exp Hypertens* 2001;23:501–511.
293. Jennette JC. The pathology of vasculitis involving the kidney. *Am J Kidney Dis* 1994;24:130–141.
294. Gomez-Sanchez CE. Cushing's syndrome and hypertension. *Hypertension* 1986;8:258–264.
295. Mantero F, Boscardo M. Glucocorticoid-dependent hypertension. *J Steroid Biochem Mol Biol* 1992;43:409–413.
296. Sato A, Suzuki H, Murakami M, et al. Glucocorticoid increases angiotensin II type I receptor and its gene expression. *Hypertension* 1994;23:25–30.
297. Kornel L, Manisundaram B, Nelson W. Glucocorticoids regulate Na transport in vascular smooth muscle through the glucocorticoid receptor-mediated mechanism. *Am J Hypertens* 1993;6:736–744.
298. Krakoff L, Nicolis G, Amsel B. Pathogenesis of hypertension in Cushing's syndrome. *Am J Med* 1975;58:216–220.
299. Stewart PM. Mineralocorticoid hypertension. *Lancet* 1999;353:1341–1347.
300. Schlaich MP, Klingbeil A, Hilgers K, et al. Relation between the renin-angiotensin-aldosterone system and left ventricu-

lar structure and function in young normotensive and mildly hypertensive subjects. *Am Heart J* 1999;138:810–817.
301. Duprez DA, De Buyzere ML, Rietzschel ER, et al. Inverse relationship between aldosterone and large artery compliance in chronically treated heart failure patients. *Eur Heart J* 1998;19:1371–1376.
302. Takeda Y, Furukawa K, Inaba S, et al. Genetic analysis of aldosterone synthase in patients with idiopathic hyperaldosteronism. *J Clin Endocrinol Metab* 1999;84:1633–1637.
303. Davies E, Holloway CD, Ingram MC, et al. Aldosterone excretion rate and blood pressure in essential hypertension are related to polymorphic differences in the aldosterone synthase gene CYP11B2. *Hypertension* 1999;33:703–707.
304. Kurland L, Melhus H, Karlsson J, et al. Aldosterone synthase (CYP11B2)-344 C/T polymorphism is related to antihypertensive response: results from the Swedish Irbesartan Left Ventricular Hypertrophy Investigation versus Atenolol (SILVHIA) trial. *Am J Hypertens* 2000;15:389–393.
305. Fonseca V, Bouloux P-M. Phaeochromocyoma and paraganglioma. *Baillières Clin Endocrinol Metab* 1993;7:509–543.
306. Neumann HPH, Berger DP, Sigmund G, et al. Pheochromocytomas, multiple endocrine neoplasia type 2, and Von Hippel–Lindau disease. *N Engl J Med* 1993;329:1531–1538.
307. Mulligan LM, Eng C, Healey CS, et al. Specific mutations of the RET proto-oncogene are related to disease phenotype in MEN 2A and FMTC. *Nat Genet* 1994;6:70–74.
308. Latif F, Duh FM, Gnarra J, et al. von Hippel–Lindau syndrome: cloning and identification of the plasma membrane Ca(++)-transporting ATPase isoform 2 gene that resides in the von Hippel–Lindau gene region. *Cancer Res* 1993;53:861–867.
309. Montenegro J, Gonzalez O, Saracho R, et al. Changes in renal function in primary hypothyroidism. *Am J Kidney Dis* 1996;27:195–198.
310. Fletcher AK, Weetman AP. Hypertension and hypothyroidism. *J Hum Hypertens* 1998;12:79–82.
311. Conn JW, Cohen EL, Lucas CP, et al. Primary reninism: hypertension, hyperreninemia, and secondary aldosteronism due to renin-producing juxtaglomerular cell tumors. *Arch Intern Med* 1972;130:682–696.
312. Smets K, Vanhaesebrouck P. Dexamethasone associated systemic hypertension in low birth weight babies with chronic lung disease. *Eur J Pediatr* 1996;155:573–575.
313. Anderson AH, Warady BA, Daily DK, et al. Systemic hypertension in infants with severe bronchopulmonary dysplasia: associated clinical factors. *Am J Perinatol* 1993;10:190–193.
314. Hla KM, Young TB, Bidwell T, et al. Sleep apnea and hypertension. A population-based study. *Ann Intern Med* 1994;120:382–388.
315. Fletcher EC. Effect of episodic hypoxia on sympathetic activity and blood pressure. *Respir Physiol* 2000;119:189–197.
316. Yamamato K, Sobue G, Iwase S, et al. Skin sympathetic nerve activity in Guillain-Barré syndrome: a microneurographic study. *J Neurol Neurosurg Psychiatry* 1997;63:537–541.
317. Okada T, Hiyoski K, Noto N, et al. A case of Guillain-Barré syndrome accompanied by sympathetic overactivity and hypertensive encephalopathy. *Acta Paediatr* 1996;85:1006–1008.
318. Gitlow SE, Bertani LM, Wilk E, et al. Excretion of catecholamine metabolites by children with familial dysautonomia. *Pediatrics* 1970;46:513–522.
319. Bell GM. Intracranial disorders and hypertension. In: Laragh JH, Brenner BM, eds. *Hypertension: pathophysiology, diagnosis and management*, 2nd ed. New York: Raven Press, 1995:2451–2458.
320. Plets C. Arterial hypertension in neurosurgical emergencies. *Am J Cardiol* 1989;63:40C-42C.
321. Report of the National High Blood Pressure Education Program Working Group on High Blood Pressure in Pregnancy. *Am J Obstet Gynecol* 2000;183:S1–S22.
322. Granger JP, Alexander BT, Bennett WA, et al. Pathophysiology of pregnancy-induced hypertension. *Am J Hypertens* 2001;14:178S-185S.
323. Taylor RN, Varma M, Teng NNH, et al. Women with preeclampsia have higher plasma endothelin levels than women with normal pregnancies. *J Clin Endocrinol Metab* 1990;71:1675–1677.
324. Wang Y, Walsh S, Kay H. Placenta lipid peroxides and thromboxane are increased and prostacyclin is decreased in women with preeclampsia. *Am J Obstet Gynecol* 1992;167:946–949.
325. Conrad KP, Benyo DF. Placental cytokines and the pathogenesis of preeclampsia. *Am J Reprod Immunol* 1997;37:240–249.
326. Yallampalli C, Garfield RE. Inhibition of nitric oxide synthesis in rats during pregnancy produces signs similar to those of preeclampsia. *Am J Obstet Gynecol* 1993;169:1316–1320.
327. Molnar M, Suto T, Toth T, et al. Prolonged blockade of nitric oxide synthesis in gravid rats produces sustained hypertension, proteinuria, thrombocytopenia, and intrauterine growth retardation. *Am J Obstet Gynecol* 1994;170:1458–1466.
328. Pincomb GA, Lovallo WR, Passey RB, et al. Effects of caffeine on vascular resistance, cardiac output and myocardial contractility in young men. *Am J Cardiol* 1985;56:119–122.
329. Evoniuk G, von Borstel RW, Wurtman RJ. Antagonism of the cardiovascular effects of adenosine by caffeine or 8–(p-sulfophenyl)theophylline. *J Pharmacol Exp Ther* 1987;240:428–432.
330. Nzerue CM. Cocaine and the kidney: a synthesis of pathophysiologic and clinical perspectives. *Am J Kidney Dis* 2000;35:783–795.
331. Vaziri ND. Mechanism of erythropoietin-induced hypertension. *Am J Kidney Dis* 1999;33:821–828.
332. Di Gennaro C. Sodium sensitivity of blood pressure in long-term detoxified alcoholics. *Hypertension* 2000;35:869–874.
333. Weir MR. Renal effects of nonselective NSAIDs and coxibs. *Cleve Clin J Med* 2002;69[Suppl 1]:S153–S158.
334. Oelkers W, Schoneshofer M, Blumel A. Effects of progesterone and four synthetic progestogens on sodium balance and the renin-aldosterone system in man. *J Clin Endocrinol Metab* 1974;39:882–890.
335. McAreavey D, Cumming AM, Boddy K, et al. The renin-angiotensin system and total body sodium and potassium in hypertensive women taking oestrogen-progestogen oral contraceptives. *Clin Endocrinol (Oxf)* 1983;18:111–118.
336. Narkiewicz K, van de Borne PJH, Hausberg M, et al. Cigarette smoking increases sympathetic outflow in humans. *Circulation* 1998;98:528–534.
337. Celemajer DS, Adams MR, Charkson P, et al. Passive smoking and impaired endothelium-dependent arterial vasodilatation in healthy young adults. *N Engl J Med* 1996;334:150–154.
338. Liang Y-L, Shiel LM, Teede H, et al. Effects of blood pressure, smoking, and their interaction on carotid artery structure and function. *Hypertension* 2001;37:6–11.

61

EVALUATION OF HYPERTENSION IN CHILDHOOD DISEASES

EILEEN D. BREWER

Evaluation of hypertension in the pediatric age group should be guided by how old the child is at presentation, how severe the hypertension is, and whether the hypertension is sustained or transient. The most common causes of hypertension differ by age group (Table 61.1). Hypertension is more likely to be secondary and sustained in younger age groups, whereas essential hypertension and white-coat hypertension are more likely to be the cause in adolescents (1–3). The current epidemic of childhood obesity has been associated with an increase in the incidence of essential hypertension in adolescence (1,4). Obese children have a threefold higher risk of developing hypertension than nonobese children (4). The increased incidence of essential hypertension in obese adolescents dictates an entirely different evaluation for this group than for younger or nonobese children. Renal disease must be considered in every child with hypertension, because of the prevalence of renovascular and renal parenchymal disorders as a cause of hypertension in any age group. Secondary hypertension from renal disorders is more likely to be severe at presentation than is essential hypertension. Endocrine causes of hypertension are rare, so special diagnostic studies for these disorders should be reserved for those patients whose history, physical examination, and preliminary evaluation indicate that further specific investigation is warranted. This chapter outlines the steps in evaluation of childhood hypertension, starting with the confirmation of the diagnosis of high blood pressure and evaluation of its duration and severity.

CONFIRMATION OF THE DIAGNOSIS OF HYPERTENSION IN CHILDREN AND ADOLESCENTS

Recommended techniques for measuring blood pressure in children are discussed in detail in Chapter 59. A few points are reemphasized here, because confirming the diagnosis of hypertension is the first step in the evaluation. Standards for blood pressure measurement in children and adolescents were revised in 1996 to include assessment of height as well as age and gender to determine normative data for children 1 to 17 years old (1). The new approach minimizes misclassification of children as hypertensive when they are very tall or very short for age. In addition, the fifth Korotkoff sound (point at which the sound disappears) is used to determine diastolic blood pressure in all age groups, even though in some young children no fifth sound can be heard because sounds are still audible at 0 mm Hg. In these children only the systolic measurement can be used to assess hypertension. In infants younger than 1 year of age, the use of systolic blood pressure to define hypertension is recommended, because few data exist for normal diastolic blood pressures (1–2). However, the report of the 1987 Second Task Force on Blood Pressure Control in Children (2) includes standards for both systolic and diastolic blood pressure for awake infants, aged birth to 12 months, based on measurements obtained using either Doppler instruments or sphygmomanometers and the fourth Korotkoff sound (point at which the sound muffles) to determine diastolic blood pressure (2). Blood pressure is lower in sleeping infants, so correction factors of 7 mm Hg for systolic and 5 mm Hg for diastolic blood pressure are recommended when measurements taken during sleep are used to assess for hypertension (2). Standards for adolescents 18 years of age and older are included in those for the adult age group and do not take into account age, gender, or height. In 2003, the Joint National Committee on Prevention, Detection, Evaluation, and Treatment of High Blood Pressure (5) revised adult blood pressure standards. This report set the guidelines for the upper limit of normal blood pressure for all adults, aged 18 years or older, at 120/80 and classified blood pressures between 120/80 and 139/89 as prehypertension.

Tables of normal blood pressure for children and adolescents (1,2) or adults (5) are based on measurements made manually with a sphygmomanometer and auscultation using a stethoscope. Few data are available for normal blood pressures measured with an automatic oscillometric device, such

TABLE 61.1. MOST COMMON CAUSES OF HYPERTENSION BY AGE AT PRESENTATION

Age group	Cause
Newborn	Renal artery thrombosis or embolus (umbilical artery catheter)
	Renal vein thrombosis
	Congenital renal malformations
	Coarctation of aorta
	Renal artery stenosis
	Bronchopulmonary dysplasia
Infancy to 6 yr	Renal parenchymal disease
	Renal artery stenosis
	Coarctation of the aorta
	Medications (corticosteroids, albuterol, pseudoephedrine)
	Endocrine causes
6–10 yr	Renal parenchymal disease
	Renal artery stenosis
	Essential hypertension
	Endocrine causes
Adolescence	Essential hypertension
	White-coat hypertension
	Renal parenchymal disease
	Substance abuse (cocaine, amphetamines, methamphetamines, phencyclidine, methylphenidate, caffeine)
	Endocrine causes

as the Dinamap. Although oscillometric devices are in widespread use in pediatric hospitals in North America, especially for neonates, infants, and toddlers, no established reference standards exist for normal blood pressure in children using these devices (1,6). In practice, values obtained with automatic oscillometric devices are treated as if they were obtained manually and compared with the standard blood pressure tables. In the few studies comparing measurements with oscillometric devices to those with conventional manual sphygmomanometry in children, the blood pressures were not equivalent, and the errors were not systematic for all ages (6–8). In addition, few of the oscillometric devices on the market were actually found to fulfill strict criteria for accuracy (9). Therefore, in instances of borderline or mild hypertension, manual sphygmomanometry should be performed as part of the evaluation to confirm that the diagnosis of hypertension is appropriate.

The conditions under which blood pressure is measured are also important, but sometimes these are not able to be standardized in a busy outpatient clinic or emergency room. The Second Task Force on Blood Pressure Control in Children (1) and the Joint National Committee on Prevention, Detection, Evaluation, and Treatment of High Blood Pressure (5) recommend that blood pressure be measured at least twice in a controlled environment, preferably in the right arm with the cubital fossa at heart level and the patient in a seated position after the patient has rested for 3 to 5 minutes. The bladder of the cuff, not the entire cuff, should be an appropriate size for the patient (1). The bladder width should be approximately 40% of the arm circumference midway between the acromion and olecranon; the length of the bladder should cover 80 to 100% of the circumference of the arm without overlapping. Cuff sizes are not standardized, so determination of the appropriate cuff size should be made according to these guidelines and not according to the name written on the cuff; for example, a small adult cuff might be just the right size for a tall or obese 7-year-old. Measuring blood pressure accurately may be difficult in a severely obese adolescent, unless a large leg cuff is used on the arm. Sometimes, particularly in a small or ill child, blood pressure is most conveniently evaluated using a leg measurement. When the leg blood pressure is abnormal, the value should be compared to values measured in the right arm to be certain of the diagnosis of hypertension. If a patient has coarctation of the aorta, blood pressure may be greatly reduced in the legs and possibly in the left arm, depending on the location of the coarctation, but will still be high in the right arm.

High blood pressure readings may be transient. A blood pressure reading taken in a crying, moving, or anxious child is likely to be high and is not reliable for diagnosing hypertension. Blood pressure measurement should be repeated several times when the child is calm. If blood pressure is not severely high, it should be measured on repeated visits over days to weeks before one diagnoses primary hypertension or embarks on a detailed diagnostic evaluation (1). Blood pressure tends to decrease on subsequent visits as anxiety subsides and the patient becomes more accustomed to the environment and technique of measurement. If white-coat hypertension is suspected after focused detailed history taking and physical examination and minimal screening laboratory tests, ambulatory blood pressure monitoring (ABPM) may be the next step in the evaluation (1,10). ABPM requires a wearable oscillometric blood pressure device, usually placed on the nondominant arm, that automatically measures and records blood pressure at prescribed frequent intervals (e.g., every 20 minutes during awake time and every 30 minutes during sleep) over an entire 24-hour period (10). ABPM allows evaluation of blood pressure throughout the day in the patient's own environment to reduce anxiety-induced elevations in blood pressure. Frequency of hypertension throughout the day (blood pressure load) and changes in the normal circadian pattern of blood pressure are also assessed, which cannot be done by casual blood pressure measurements in the clinic or at home. ABPM is discussed in detail in Chapter 59.

ASSESSMENT OF SEVERITY AND DURATION OF HYPERTENSION

When repeated blood pressure measurements taken under appropriate conditions satisfy the definition of hypertension (1,2,5), the severity of hypertension must be deter-

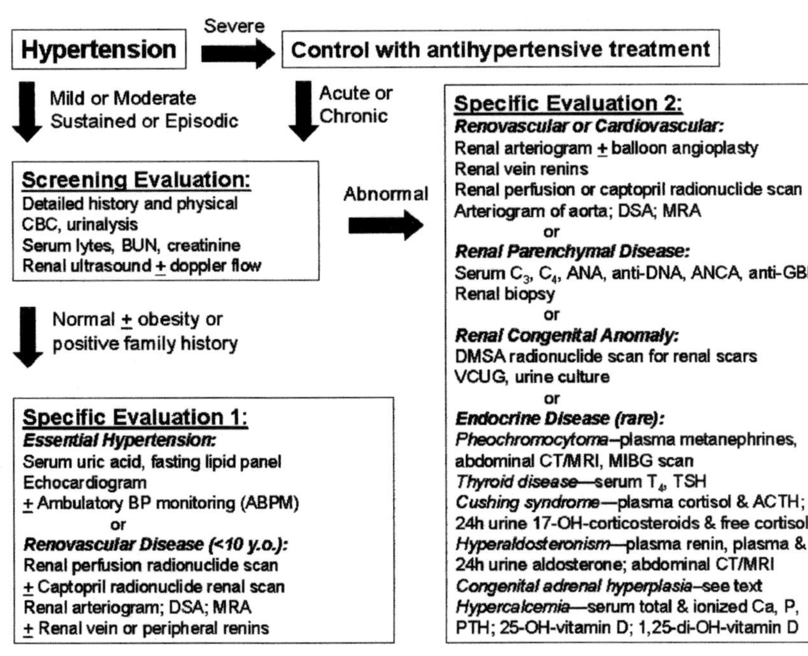

FIGURE 61.1. Algorithm for evaluation of hypertension in children and adolescents. ACTH, adrenocorticotropic hormone; ANA, antinuclear antibody; ANCA, antineutrophil cytoplasmic antibody; anti-DNA, anti–double-stranded DNA antibody; anti-GBM, anti–glomerular basement membrane antibody; BP, blood pressure; BUN, blood urea nitrogen; C_3 and C_4, complements 3 and 4; CBC, complete blood count; CT, computed tomography; DMSA, dimercaptosuccinic acid; DSA, digital subtraction angiography; MIBG, metaiodobenzylguanidine; MRA, magnetic resonance angiography; MRI, magnetic resonance imaging; OH, hydroxy; PTH, parathyroid hormone; T_4, thyroxine; TSH, thyroid-stimulating hormone; VCUG, voiding cystourethrogram; y.o., years old.

mined to direct further evaluation (Fig. 61.1). Guidelines for assessment of the severity of hypertension by age, gender, and height percentile are given in Table 61.2. If hypertension is mild or moderate (intermediate between mild and severe), diagnostic evaluation may continue before treatment is instituted. If hypertension is severe, emergent treatment should be undertaken to reduce the level of hypertension before further diagnostic evaluation (Fig. 61.1). If possible, laboratory tests that might be affected by treatment, such as peripheral plasma renin levels, should be performed before therapy is initiated.

The nature of the hypertension—acute or chronic, transient or sustained, or episodic—helps direct further evaluation. Transient or unsustained hypertension may need only clinical follow-up to be sure it does not recur. Episodic hypertension is best evaluated at the time of an occurrence, because evaluation may be unrevealing between attacks. Acute hypertension is often secondary to other diseases, which may have distinct signs and symptoms that direct specific evaluation at the time of presentation.

Duration of hypertension is first assessed by taking a thorough hypertension-oriented history and performing a physical examination (1,3). Headaches, blurred vision, seizures, chest pain, and frequent epistaxis may be associated with acute onset of hypertension. Episodic symptoms and hypertension are associated with pheochromocytoma or autonomic nervous system dysfunction. A detailed medication history for both prescription and over-the-counter medications, including herbal medicines, may help identify the cause of acute, transient, or episodic hypertension. Recent introduction of medications for which hypertension is a known side effect, like high-dose corticosteroids (11) or albuterol for asthma, large (adult) doses of pseudoephed-

TABLE 61.2. GUIDELINES FOR ASSESSING SEVERITY OF HIGH BLOOD PRESSURE BY AGE, GENDER, AND HEIGHT PERCENTILES

	BP percentile for Ht		
	Mild HBP[a]		Severe HBP[b]
Age group	BP 95% Ht 5%	BP 95% Ht 95%	BP >99% All Ht
Boys			
Newborn	90/—	90/—	>106/—
1–12 mo	98/55	106/59	>115/75
1–3 yr	104/63	113/67	>118/82
4–6 yr	109/72	117/76	>124/84
7–10 yr	114/77	123/82	>130/86
11–13 yr	121/79	130/84	>134/90
14–17 yr	132/85	140/89	>144/92
18 yr or older	No data	140/90[c]	>160/100[c]
Girls			
Newborn	88/—	88/—	>106/—
1–12 mo	101/57	107/60	>115/75
1–3 yr	104/65	110/68	>118/82
4–6 yr	108/71	114/75	>124/84
7–10 yr	116/77	122/80	>130–86
11–13 yr	121/80	128/84	>134/90
14–17 yr	126/83	132/86	>144/92
18 yr or older	No data	>140/90[c]	>160/100[c]

BP, blood pressure; HBP, high blood pressure; Ht, height.
[a]Adapted from Update on the 1987 Task Force report on high blood pressure in children and adolescents: a working group report from the national high blood pressure education program. *Pediatrics* 1996;98:649–658.
[b]Adapted from Report of the Second Task Force on Blood Pressure Control in Children—1987. *Pediatrics* 1987;79:1–25. The fourth Korotkoff sound was used to determine diastolic blood pressure in 1- to 12-month-old infants.
[c]Adapted from Seventh report of the Joint National Committee on Prevention, Detection, Evaluation, and Treatment of High Blood Pressure. *JAMA* 2003;289:2560–2572.

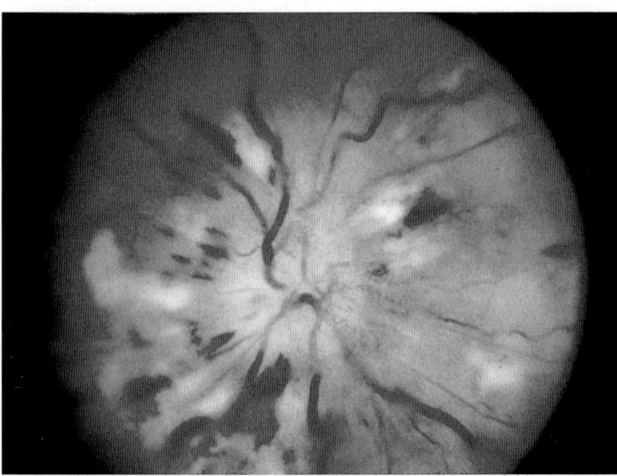

FIGURE 61.2. Severe hypertensive retinopathy in a child with long-standing untreated hypertension showing arteriolar narrowing, hemorrhages and exudates, and papilledema. (See Color Plate 61.2.)

rine for cold symptoms, or phenylephrine eye or nose drops, may be the cause of new-onset but transient hypertension. Adolescents are at risk for substance abuse and should be interviewed in private to maximize the chance of obtaining a history of the use of illicit drugs, tobacco, or high-caffeine or guarana-containing drinks, all of which can cause or contribute to hypertension (1,12,13). Restless sleep, irritability, anorexia, and poor school performance are subtle signs of chronic hypertension and should be specifically elicited in the history. Poor growth may also be a sign of chronic hypertension or underlying chronic renal disease. Obesity with body mass index higher than the 95th percentile for age and gender is often associated with chronic essential hypertension (1,4). The presence of peripheral edema, pleural effusion, rash, or swelling and tenderness of joints suggest acute onset or exacerbation of underlying renal or systemic disease. Retinal changes usually indicate long-standing untreated hypertension and include arteriolar narrowing or tortuosity, arteriovenous nicking, and hemorrhages and exudates (Fig. 61.2).

SCREENING EVALUATION OF HYPERTENSION

Episodic or sustained, acute or chronic hypertension, whether mild or severe, merits further screening and specific detailed evaluation. A convenient algorithm for evaluation of pediatric hypertension in given in Figure 61.1. The direction of further detailed laboratory and radiographic or biopsy evaluation of hypertension should become apparent after taking a detailed personal and family history, performing a careful physical examination, and ordering a few simple laboratory tests.

The personal history taking should include specific questioning regarding the presence of headaches, visual disturbance, nosebleeds, palpitations, episodic rapid pulse, pallor or flushing, joint pains, rash, edema, gross hematuria, excessive weight gain or loss, or decreased height growth. Neonatal history of low birth weight or the use of umbilical artery catheters may provide clues to the diagnosis of essential hypertension in an adolescent (14,15) or hypertension from renal artery thrombosis or emboli in an infant, respectively. Detailed dietary history may reveal excessive intake of sodium or caffeinated beverages, especially soft drinks. Taking a medication history should include specific questions about over-the-counter drugs like pseudoephedrine or herbal preparations like ephedra, St. John's wort, or licorice (16,17), as well as prescription drugs. Adolescents should be questioned in private to obtain a history of substance abuse or the possibility of pregnancy. Identifying a family history of hypertension, heart attacks, or stroke is particularly important for children with essential hypertension. Over 50% of children with essential hypertension have a relative with the same disease (1,2,4,18).

Physical examination may reveal specific signs of genetic disease, such as the elfin facies of Williams syndrome, the café-au-lait spots and small skin neurofibromata of neurofibromatosis type 1, the physical features of Cushing syndrome, or ambiguous genitalia associated with congenital adrenal hyperplasia or Denys-Drash syndrome. Rarely, unilateral facial paralysis (Bell's palsy of the seventh cranial nerve) can be the initial presentation of severe hypertension in a child (19,20). Careful auscultation of the abdomen may reveal a bruit suggestive of renovascular disease, but a bruit is audible only approximately 50% of the time in these patients (21). Femoral pulses may be diminished in patients with coarctation of the aorta or middle aortic syndrome. Determination of height, weight, and body mass index with comparison to percentiles for age and gender should always be included as part of the screening physical examination.

Screening laboratory evaluation should be minimally invasive and cost effective. Screening for rare endocrine causes of hypertension should not be done initially in every pediatric patient with hypertension. Screening studies for all patients should include complete blood count, urinalysis, and levels of serum electrolytes, creatinine, and blood urea nitrogen (BUN) (1–3). In adolescents with suspected essential hypertension for whom there is no suspicion of endocrine abnormalities, measurement of serum electrolytes may not be useful. However, a low potassium concentration with metabolic alkalosis may indicate a rare but treatable disorder, such as primary or secondary hyperaldosteronism or Liddle's syndrome. Elevated serum potassium level in conjunction with metabolic acidosis may suggest chronic renal disease, which is confirmed by the presence of an increased serum creatinine concentration. Creatinine clearance can be estimated from serum creatinine level (Schwartz formula) (22) or measured directly with a 24-hour urine collection. Because renal disease is the most common cause of hypertension in children and the kidney is also a target organ for damage from untreated hypertension, urinalysis is an important screening test. Hematuria and the presence of red cell casts with or without proteinuria suggests glomerular disease. Isolated hematuria also may be associated with dilatation of the urinary tract or trauma. Proteinuria may be seen in nonglomerular conditions such as reflux nephropathy, obstructive uropathy, or interstitial nephritis, as well as glomerular diseases like focal segmental glomerulosclerosis or membranoproliferative glomerulonephritis. Proteinuria alone may be a sign of end-organ damage from hypertension but must be distinguished, especially in adolescents, from orthostatic (postural) proteinuria, which is a benign condition.

A renal ultrasonographic examination is a simple, noninvasive test that is appropriate to perform early in the evaluation of any hypertensive child (3). Although it may not provide much information in the adolescent in whom essential hypertension is strongly suspected, a renal ultrasonogram helps exclude congenital anomalies that have previously gone undetected. The renal ultrasonogram provides information about the size and architecture of each kidney and the lower urinary tract. Abnormal kidneys may be small or asymmetric (renovascular disease, vesicoureteral reflux, or dysplasia); hyperechoic, symmetric, and normal or large (renal parenchymal disease); or large with or without cysts (polycystic kidney disease, multicystic dysplasia). Hydronephrosis and/or hydroureters may be associated with congenital obstructive uropathy or vesicoureteral reflux.

The addition of color-coded Doppler analysis to B-mode ultrasonography is termed *duplex ultrasonography* (23) and provides information about the patency and flow within the main renal vessels to help diagnose renovascular hypertension. Better hardware, software, and transducer technology have improved visualization and evaluation of the more distal segments of the main renal artery (23). During Doppler evaluation care should be taken to scan the entire artery from origin at the aorta to renal hilum to improve sensitivity and accuracy. Obtaining measurements in two views, both anterior and oblique, improves identification of fibromuscular dysplasia in the middle to distal segments of the main renal artery. The limited amount of body fat in many children and the proximity of renal vessels to the skin surface allow the use of high-frequency transducers to improve the technical quality (24). Ultrasonography in obese patients may provide a technical challenge. Color Doppler images can demonstrate global perfusion as well as patency of flow through large renal arteries and veins. Turbulence at a stenotic site alters peak-systolic and end-diastolic blood flow velocities and creates a characteristic pattern of flow detected by the spectral Doppler waveform (Fig. 61.3). The sensitivity of the Doppler flow study is limited for detection of stenosis in accessory renal arteries, intrarenal arteries, or mildly stenotic arteries (24,25). A positive result on a Doppler flow study is helpful in directing further evaluation, but a negative result does not rule out significant renovascular disease.

DIRECTED SPECIFIC EVALUATION OF HYPERTENSION AFTER SCREENING

Specific Evaluation 1

If the screening evaluation described earlier is normal or positive only for obesity or a family history of essential hypertension, detailed evaluation should be directed toward the diagnosis of essential hypertension (Fig. 61.1). Because essential hypertension is largely a diagnosis of exclusion and is less common in young children, renovascular disease must always be ruled out if the child is younger than 10 years of age.

Essential Hypertension

The specific evaluation of essential hypertension is directed primarily at determining the presence of cardiovascular risk factors, such as hyperlipidemia, and assessing any end-organ damage to the heart or kidneys (1). In children elevation of serum uric acid level may help distinguish essential from secondary hypertension. Increased serum uric acid concentrations were noted in children with essential hypertension many decades ago (26) but were largely ignored until reports appeared that serum uric acid level is significantly higher at presentation in children with essential hypertension than in children with secondary hypertension (27). Elevated uric acid levels may play an early pathogenetic role in childhood hypertension by activating cellular pathways that lead to increased renovascular tone, fibrosis, and irreversible arteriolosclerosis (28). ABPM may also help distinguish essential from secondary hypertension, the latter of which is more likely to manifest greater daytime diastolic blood pressure load, greater nocturnal systolic blood pressure load, and blunted nocturnal dipping (29). ABPM is useful to differentiate white-coat hypertension from essential hypertension as well (10).

End-organ damage may already be evident at presentation of essential hypertension in adolescents. An echocardiogram is the best way to screen for left ventricular hypertrophy and also serves as a baseline study for comparison later in the course of therapy (2,30). APBM may also be useful to identify which children may be at greatest risk for developing end-organ damage from hypertension (10,31,32).

Renovascular Disease

Renovascular disease is the cause of hypertension in approximately 10% of children referred for diagnosis (33,34). Children with renovascular hypertension are frequently asymptomatic (35). Hypertension is often severe and may be hard to control with medication before proceeding with spe-

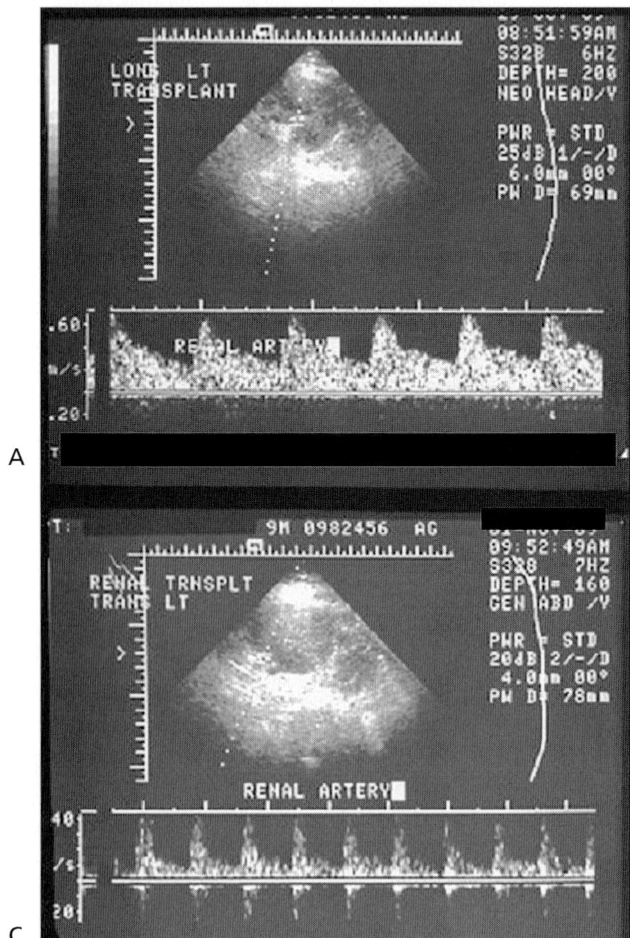

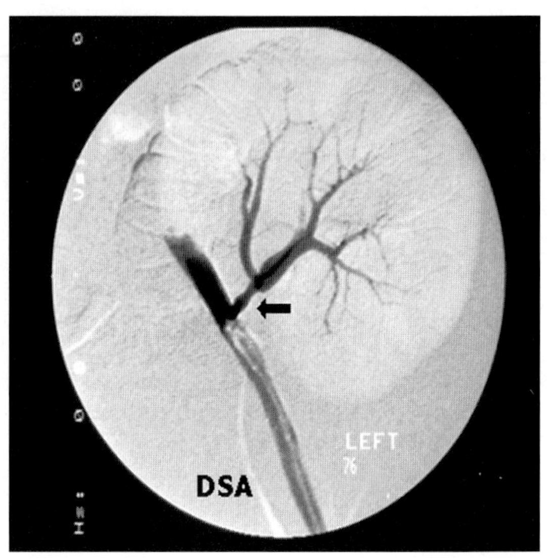

FIGURE 61.3. Renal transplant ultrasound using Doppler flow evaluation in a child. **A:** The high resistive index (0.6) and the turbulent flow pattern suggest transplant renal artery stenosis. **B:** Stenosis was confirmed by digital subtraction angiography (DSA) *(arrow).* **C:** Normalization of the Doppler flow study with resistive index lower (0.4) and no turbulence after successful balloon angioplasty of the stenosis.

cific evaluation (35). An angiotensin-converting enzyme (ACE) inhibitor may provide the best control, but with prolonged use can also lead to loss of function in the affected kidney from reduced arterial flow in an area of severe stenosis (Fig. 61.4). Some patients with bilateral renal artery stenosis may develop acute renal failure at the onset of ACE inhibitor therapy. A child's response to an ACE inhibitor during radionuclide imaging with either diethylenentriaminepenta-acetic acid (DTPA), mercaptoacetyltriglycine (MAG-3), or dimercapto-succinic acid (DMSA) can be used in the evaluation for renal artery stenosis and is often referred to as a captopril renal scan (36–38). Although a captopril renal scan may help lead to a diagnosis, the test is invasive and only moderately sensitive (50 to 70%), especially if disease is bilateral (37,38). Because a renal arteriogram is both diagnostic and potentially therapeutic when coupled with balloon angioplasty, a captopril renal scan may not be a reasonable step in the evaluation of children with a high likelihood of renal artery stenosis at centers with skilled pediatric interventional radiologists.

A renal perfusion scan with DTPA or MAG-3 may be useful to identify segmental areas of hypoperfusion or infarction, especially those associated with an embolus from an umbilical artery catheter used in the neonatal period (39,40). Intravenously administered MAG-3 is initially filtered by the glomerulus, then taken up into the kidney primarily by proximal tubular secretion, so MAG-3 can be used for estimation of tubular function as well as renal plasma flow.

Selective renal arteriography with or without digital subtraction angiography enhancement is the gold standard for diagnosis of renal artery stenosis. In a retrospective review of 15 years' experience with renal arteriography in pediatric hypertensive patients, Shahdadpuri and colleagues (41) showed that renal arteriography had a high positive yield, providing diagnostic findings in 40% of cases when performed for the indication of severe hypertension or inability to control hypertension effectively with one drug. Renal arteriography has the added advantage that therapeutic transluminal balloon angioplasty (42–46) or placement of bridging stents (47) can be performed during the same procedure. Balloon angioplasty may be possible even in small children using balloon catheters designed for coronary artery angioplasty (47). The disadvantage of renal arteriography is that it is invasive, exposes the child to nephrotoxic radiocontrast agents, and usually requires general anesthesia for small or uncooperative children (35). Deep conscious

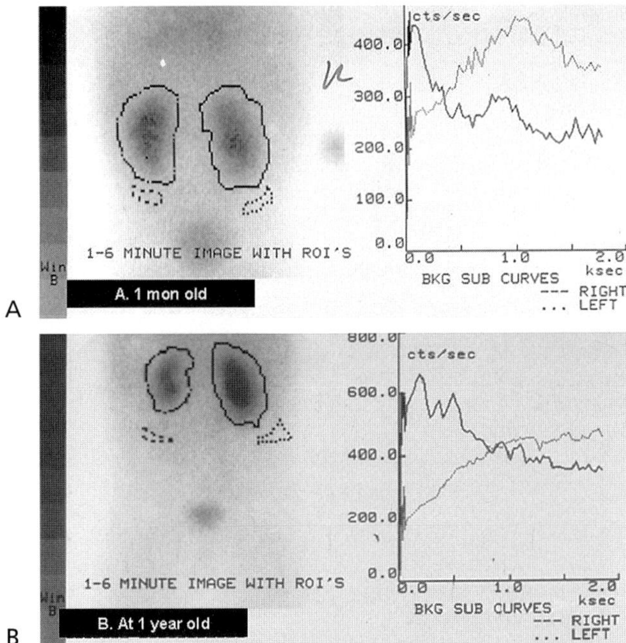

FIGURE 61.4. Sequential technetium 99–diethylenentriamine-penta-acetic acid radionuclide renal scans for an infant with unilateral left renal artery stenosis who was treated medically, because body size was too small to allow transluminal balloon angioplasty. **A:** At diagnosis at 1 month of age; 40% function in left kidney, 60% function in right kidney. **B:** At 1 year of age after 11 months of oral angiotensin-converting enzyme inhibitor therapy for left main renal artery stenosis; 26% function in left kidney, 74% function in right kidney. BKG SUB, background subtraction; cts, counts; ROI, region of interest.

sedation may be effective for cooperative older children and adolescents. If performed by an experienced interventional radiologist, renal arteriography can be performed safely as a 1-day outpatient procedure for most children. The incidence of severe complications, such as intimal tear or injury, renal artery thrombosis, or branch embolus, is very low in experienced hands. Patients must be observed for 4 to 6 hours after the procedure for possible complications. Arterial puncture carries the risk of hematoma formation at the site and vascular compromise to the extremity.

Magnetic resonance angiography (MRA) is emerging as an accurate and sensitive alternative to renal arteriography for evaluation of renovascular disease in adults, especially those with significant renal failure or heart disease (48–50). Unfortunately, published experience of MRA in pediatric hypertensive patients is limited to studies using technology available in the early 1990s, which is now out of date (51). Current three-dimensional (3D) contrast-enhanced MRA technology allows faster scans of higher resolution within a 20- to 30-second breath hold (49). MRA has the advantages of being minimally invasive (requires only a peripheral intravenous line), avoiding ionizing radiation, and using a nonnephrotoxic contrast agent, gadolinium, which provides excellent imaging of the abdominal vasculature. Direct comparison of MRA results with those of conventional angiography shows that MRA has 100% sensitivity and 95 to 98% specificity for detecting greater than 50% renal artery stenosis in adults (48) and children (51). MRA is not yet as good as conventional angiography for delineating the architecture of accessory renal arteries and distal renal artery fibromuscular dysplasia (23,49), but the technology is still evolving. MRA has been a useful evaluation technique at our center for neonates or infants too small to undergo balloon angioplasty and for children and adolescents in whom the indication for invasive renal angiography is not clear-cut.

MRA has a distinct advantage over spiral computerized tomographic renal angiography (CTRA), which can produce excellent images of the renal vasculature but uses ionizing radiation and requires nephrotoxic radiocontrast agents (23,52). Like MRA, CTRA requires only a peripheral intravenous approach and allows 3D visualization with appropriate software (52). A limited computed tomographic (CT) scan of the abdomen may be performed before CTRA to provide additional information about the anatomy of the kidneys, adrenals, and surrounding structures (23). If MRA and conventional renal angiography are not available or possible, spiral CTRA may be a useful alternative (52).

Plasma renin activity measured in samples from peripheral veins or especially from selective renal veins may provide additional useful information for evaluation of renovascular disease (35,53). Selective sampling of renal vein renins may be done conveniently at the time of renal arteriography to provide supporting evidence for unilateral or bilateral disease. The inferior vena cava above and below the renal veins should be sampled at the same time as the renal veins. If the selective renal vein renin concentration is at least 1.5 times greater than the concentration in the contralateral kidney, the result is diagnostic of renin-mediated hypertension from that kidney (35,53). If the contralateral kidney is normal, renal vein renin concentration should actually be decreased due to downregulation of renin production in the normal kidney from increased circulating angiotensin II (54,55). If the ratio between renal vein renin concentration in the contralateral kidney and that in the caudal inferior vena cava is less than 1.3, then renin production is suppressed in the contralateral kidney (53). The combination of results may be useful to determine whether a patient might benefit from or be cured by surgery (53), in the event that angioplasty is only partially successful or not able to be performed.

Peripheral vein renin levels obtained before initiation of antihypertensive therapy may also be useful in evaluation of renovascular hypertension, if they are abnormal (35). Levels must be interpreted within the age-specific normal values for the laboratory performing the test and in light of estimated sodium intake at the time the sample was drawn. Furthermore, the levels may be adversely affected if the blood is not handled properly after the blood draw. The specimen should be drawn into an ethylenediaminetetraacetic acid tube, immediately placed on ice, spun in a

TABLE 61.3. RENOVASCULAR AND CARDIOVASCULAR CAUSES OF HYPERTENSION

Intrinsic renal artery disease
- Fibromuscular dysplasia
- Intimal fibromuscular dysplasia (neurofibromatosis type 1, Williams syndrome)
- Arteritis (Kawasaki, Takayasu, or Moyamoya disease)
- Renal transplant artery stenosis
- Chronic renal allograft nephropathy
- Newborn with umbilical vessel catheters
  - Arterial or venous thrombosis
  - Segmental infarction from embolus
- Renal transplant renal artery or venous thrombosis
- Renal trauma

Extrinsic compression
- Neoplasia
  - Wilms' tumor
  - Neuroblastoma
  - Pheochromocytoma, paraganglioma
  - Neurofibroma
  - Lymphoma
- Perirenal hematoma, trauma
- Retroperitoneal fibrosis
- Congenital fibrous bands

Cardiovascular disease
- Coarctation of aorta
- Middle aortic syndrome (hypoplastic abdominal aorta syndrome)
- Williams syndrome
- Turner syndrome

refrigerated centrifuge, and then kept frozen for later assay. A peripheral renin level that is elevated for age suggests renovascular or renal parenchymal hypertension. A normal level, however, does not exclude significant renovascular hypertension. Low levels of plasma renin in the presence of hypokalemia and elevated plasma and urinary aldosterone levels suggest primary aldosteronism or one of the forms of congenital adrenal hyperplasia as the cause of the hypertension (see the section on endocrine abnormalities later).

Specific Evaluation 2

When the history, physical examination, or screening laboratory evaluation is abnormal, further evaluation should be directed by those results. If the history, physical examination, urinalysis, and other laboratory test results suggest renal artery stenosis or other vascular disease (Table 61.3) or renal parenchymal disease (Table 61.4), evaluation should proceed along the lines outlined in the algorithm presented earlier (Fig. 61.1). If initial screening rules out renal disease but suggests a rare endocrine cause (Table 61.5), evaluation should proceed accordingly (Fig. 61.1).

The need for evaluation for other causes of childhood hypertension, such as neurologic abnormalities, teen pregnancy, drugs, or other illnesses (Table 61.6), should become apparent after a detailed screening history taking and physical examination. The rest of the discussion in

TABLE 61.4. RENAL PARENCHYMAL DISEASES ASSOCIATED WITH HYPERTENSION

Glomerulonephritis
- Acute postinfectious glomerulonephritis
- Immunoglobulin A nephropathy
- Membranoproliferative glomerulonephritis
- Rapidly progressive (crescentic) glomerulonephritis
- Focal segmental glomerulosclerosis

Systemic vasculitis with renal involvement
- Henoch-Schönlein purpura
- Antineutrophil cytoplasmic antibody vasculitis
- Polyarteritis nodosum
- Systemic lupus erythematosus

Hemolytic uremic syndrome

Interstitial nephritis (chronic pyelonephritis)

Hereditary diseases
- Autosomal recessive or dominant polycystic kidney disease
- Medullary cystic disease; juvenile nephronophthisis
- Denys-Drash syndrome
- Sickle cell disease
- Liddle's syndrome

Congenital renal anomalies
- Vesicoureteral reflux
- Obstructive uropathy
- Multicystic dysplastic kidney
- Horseshoe kidney
- Segmental hypoplasia (Ask-Upmark kidney)

TABLE 61.5. ENDOCRINE ABNORMALITIES ASSOCIATED WITH HYPERTENSION

Tumors secreting vasoactive substances (catecholamines, renin)
- Pheochromocytoma, paraganglioma
  - Sporadic or familial (associated with von Hippel–Lindau disease, multiple endocrine neoplasias type 2, neurofibromatosis)
- Neuroblastoma, ganglioneuroblastoma
- Juxtaglomerular cell tumors, Wilms' tumor

Thyroid disorders
- Hyperthyroidism (Graves disease)
- Hypothyroidism

Cushing syndrome
- Adrenocorticotropic hormone (ACTH) dependent
  - Iatrogenic (exogenous glucocorticoid therapy)
  - Adrenocortical tumor (adenoma, carcinoma)
- ACTH independent
  - Iatrogenic (ACTH therapy)
  - Hypothalamic or ectopic corticotropin-releasing hormone–producing tumor
  - Pituitary or ectopic ACTH-producing tumor

Hyperaldosteronism
- Adrenal tumor (adenoma, carcinoma)
- Idiopathic adrenal hyperplasia

Congenital adrenal hyperplasia
- 11β-hydroxylase (P450c11) deficiency
- 17α-hydroxylase (P450c17) deficiency

Hypercalcemia
- Vitamin D intoxication
- Hyperparathyroidism
- Williams syndrome
- Malignancy

P450c11, P450c17, cytochrome P-450 enzymes.

TABLE 61.6. MISCELLANEOUS CAUSES OF HYPERTENSION

Neurologic abnormalities
- Elevated intracranial pressure (associated bradycardia)
- Recent seizure, status epilepticus
- Familial dysautonomia (Riley-Day syndrome)
- Quadriplegia with autonomic nervous system dysfunction
- Femoral nerve traction

Cyclic vomiting syndrome
Polycythemia; recombinant erythropoietin therapy
Anesthetic drugs
- Ketamine
- Naloxone

Drug abuse
- Cocaine
- Amphetamines
- Methamphetamines (e.g., ecstasy)
- Phencyclidine (PCP)
- Methylphenidate

Oral contraceptive use
Teen pregnancy

this chapter is divided into evaluation of hypertension by disease category.

RENOVASCULAR AND CARDIOVASCULAR DISEASE

Renovascular Disease

Multiple types of renovascular abnormalities can lead to hypertension (Table 61.3), but fibromuscular dysplasia is the most common, occurring in approximately 70% of pediatric cases (33,56,57). Most often, the medial layer of the artery is affected, although rarely the intima may be involved, especially in the case of neurofibromatosis type 1 or Williams syndrome (35). Disease may be bilateral or unilateral, but if unilateral, may manifest itself with hypertension from the other kidney at a later date. Multiple stenotic lesions followed by poststenotic aneurysms can resemble a string of beads on a selective angiogram (Fig. 61.5). Branch vessels, as well as peripheral intrarenal vessels, may be involved. Other vessels, including the abdominal aorta, may be stenotic or hypoplastic, especially in association with neurofibromatosis type 1 (Fig. 61.6) or Williams syndrome (58,59). Typically, the lesions of neurofibromatosis are near the origin of the renal arteries (Fig. 61.6), whereas the lesions of fibromuscular dysplasia are often more distal (Fig. 61.7) (33,42). Duplex ultrasonography with color Doppler flow may suggest the diagnosis of these disorders, but renal arteriography is needed for diagnosis and delineation of the extent of the renovascular disease. If the lesion is in the main renal artery and does not involve a long segment of the vessel, transluminal balloon angioplasty may be performed at the same time (Fig. 61.7) (42–44). If the child is too small for

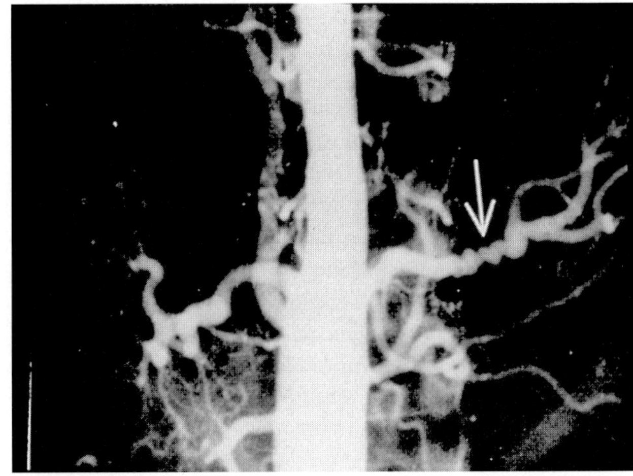

FIGURE 61.5. Renal arteriogram showing typical "string-of-beads" appearance (*arrow*) of fibromuscular dysplasia in the left main renal artery.

balloon angioplasty, hypertension may be controlled with medical therapy, especially ACE inhibitors. Then, a radionuclide renal scan is a useful tool to sequentially evaluate the growth and function of the affected kidney during long-term follow-up (Fig. 61.4).

Duplex ultrasonography with color Doppler is a good screening evaluation test for renal transplant artery stenosis (60,61), which usually occurs at or near the surgical anastomosis (60) (Fig. 61.3). The incidence is as high as 10% in

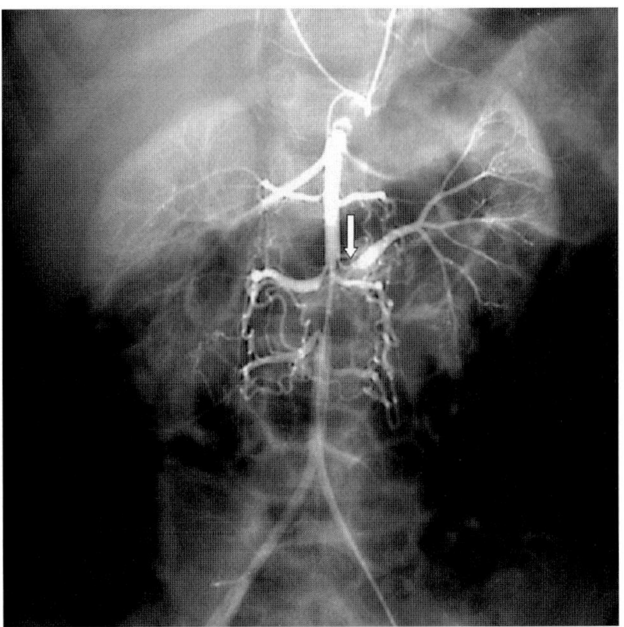

FIGURE 61.6. Abdominal arteriogram in a child with neurofibromatosis type 1 showing long segment tubular stenosis of the aorta with collateral flow as well as severe stenosis of the left main renal artery near its origin (*arrow*). Poststenotic dilatation of the renal artery and delayed uptake of contrast in the left kidney compared to the right are present.

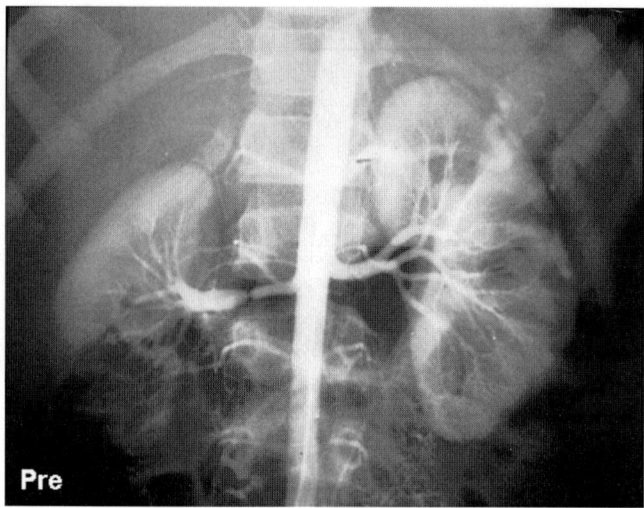

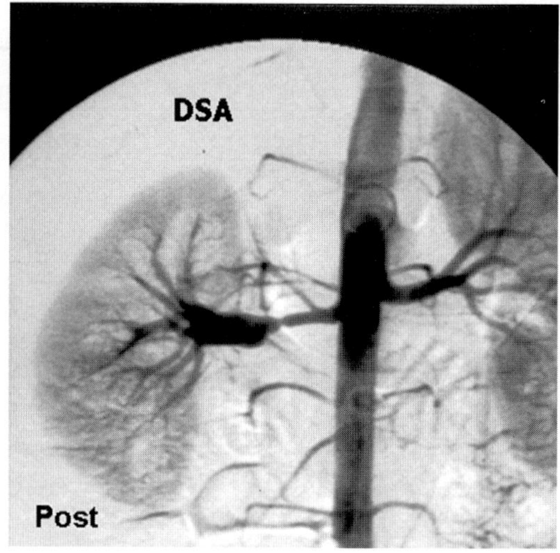

FIGURE 61.7. Renal angiogram for a child showing right main renal artery stenosis from fibromuscular dysplasia pre- and posttransluminal balloon angioplasty. The image after angioplasty shows residual stenosis, but considerable improvement in flow of radiocontrast. DSA, digital subtraction angiography.

children and adults (60,61). Confirmatory arteriography is always necessary (Fig. 61.3), and therapeutic balloon angioplasty may be performed at the same time if indicated. Duplex ultrasonography also may be useful for follow-up to determine continued success or the recurrence of stenosis after balloon angioplasty or surgical intervention (60,61) (Fig. 61.3). MRA may be helpful in equivocal cases (49). However, the presence of metallic surgical clips adjacent to the anastomosis may cause MRA artifacts that mimic stenosis and render the test unreliable.

Mild to severe hypertension is associated with chronic renal allograft nephropathy, the term now used to describe the various processes, including chronic rejection, donor vascular disease, and chronic calcineurin inhibitor nephrotoxicity, that lead to arterial fibrous intimal thickening, interstitial fibrosis, tubular atrophy, and glomerulosclerosis late in the course after renal transplantation (62). The small arteries are affected, so imaging is not useful for diagnosis (60). The diagnosis is made by renal transplant biopsy.

Rarely, hypertension in a child results from extrinsic compression of a renal artery or segment by an extrinsic mass, such as a tumor or traumatic perirenal hematoma. Renal ultrasonography may identify the mass, but MRA technology allows visualization of extensive 3D detail to establish the diagnosis (Fig. 61.8) and direct corrective therapy (49). More than half of patients with Wilms' tumor have concomitant hypertension secondary to either intrarenal vessel compression or renin production by the tumor (63).

Cardiovascular Disease

Coarctation of the aorta accounts for 2% of secondary hypertension in childhood and adolescence but is the underlying disorder in approximately one-third of patients with hypertension seen in the first year of life (64,65). Aortic coarctation may be focal (juxtaductal), diffuse (hypoplastic aortic isthmus), or complete (aortic arch interruption) (66). Screening evaluation of the hypertensive child suggests coarctation when blood pressure is at least 10 mm Hg higher in the right arm or in both arms than in the legs, and the femoral pulses are diminished. A systolic ejection murmur of low intensity may be heard over the base of the heart and precordium and radiates into the left interscapular region. The murmur may be louder over the back. The older child who has developed collateral circulation may have a continuous murmur over large collateral intercostal arteries. When coarctation is suspected on the basis of screening evaluation, the patient should be referred to a pediatric cardiologist for further evaluation.

Echocardiography with color Doppler flow may identify a characteristic wedge-shaped band of tissue to confirm the diagnosis and measure any gradient across the coarcted segment (67–69). The transverse aortic arch also should be imaged to evaluate for hypoplasia. Magnetic resonance imaging (MRI) and MRA are being used increasingly for primary evaluation of thoracic coarctation in children over 4 or 5 years of age or for follow-up after angioplasty or surgical correction (66,70–73). Echocardiography is difficult after surgical repair because of the presence of scar tissue and thorax deformities, which limit the acoustic window. MRI technology, including 3D gadolinium-enhanced MRA, allows excellent visualization of the anatomy of the aorta, estimates the pressure gradient based on peak flow velocity across the stenosis, assesses collateral aortic circulation, and permits a 3D view of the full extent of the aorta (66,71). Conventional angiography still remains the gold standard and allows direct measurement of the pressure gradient across the coarctation, but MRI technology may

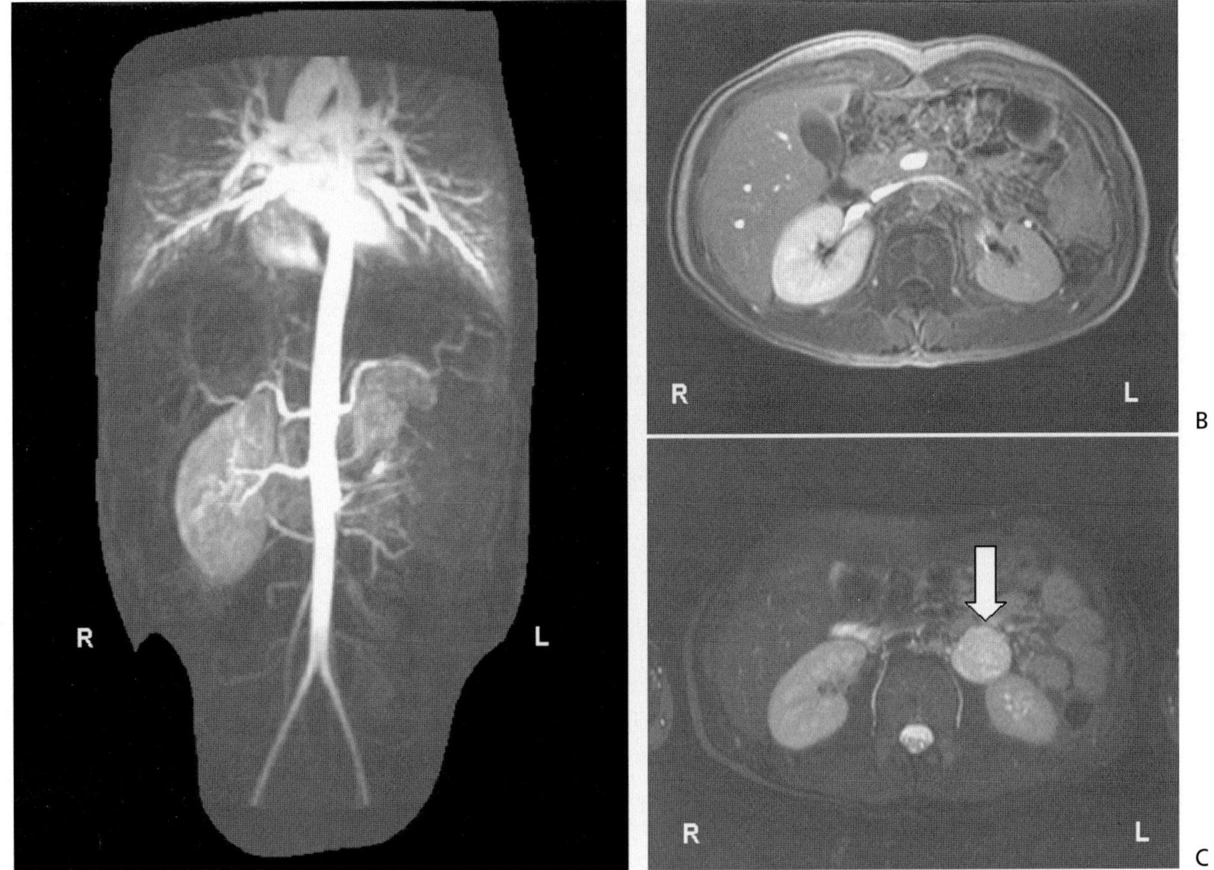

FIGURE 61.8. Images from a three-dimensional gadolinium-enhanced magnetic resonance angiography (MRA) for a teenager with new-onset severe hypertension. MRA shows that each kidney is supplied by two renal arteries **(A)**. The right kidney and left upper pole kidney provide prompt nephrograms, but perfusion of the lower two-thirds of the left kidney is delayed **(A,B)** secondary to compression of the left lower renal artery by a 4-cm paraspinal soft tissue mass (*arrow*) **(C)**.

become an adequate replacement in the near future, especially with new technology (66,72).

Other uncommon forms of cardiovascular disease lead to hypertension in infants and children (Table 61.3). Middle aortic syndrome, a rare entity that may be congenital, acquired from aortitis or vasculitis, or associated with genetic diseases such as neurofibromatosis (Fig. 61.6) or Williams syndrome, may lead to severe life-threatening hypertension as well as lower extremity claudication and mesenteric ischemia (20, 33,74–78). Diagnosis is made by conventional abdominal angiography, which shows tubular stenosis of the aorta and its visceral branches. MRA with gadolinium enhancement may eventually replace angiography in the initial evaluation of middle aortic syndrome, because MRA is much less invasive and gives excellent 3D detail.

Williams syndrome or Turner syndrome should be suspected during screening evaluation because of typical physical findings, including the elfin facies of Williams syndrome and the short stature and webbed neck of Turner syndrome. A variety of cardiovascular abnormalities that can cause hypertension are associated with Williams syndrome, including supravalvular aortic stenosis and thoracic coarctation (58,76,79). Patients with Turner syndrome have a high incidence (20 to 50%) of cardiovascular malformations, including coarctation of the aorta, bicuspid aortic valve, and aortic root dilatation, as well as a high incidence of cardiovascular disease morbidity and mortality as adults (80–83). Hypertension per se may contribute to cardiovascular disease as adults (81–83). ABPM in 75 girls with Turner syndrome revealed abnormal blood pressure circadian rhythm in 50%, suggestive of secondary hypertension (83).

RENAL PARENCHYMAL DISEASE

Most children with secondary hypertension (60 to 80%) have renal parenchymal disease (84,85). A variety of glomerular and a few tubular or interstitial renal disorders may cause hypertension in children and adolescents (Table 61.4). The most common renal parenchymal disorders associated with hypertension are glomerulonephritis and reflux nephropathy (85,86). Further evaluation for renal parenchymal disease is

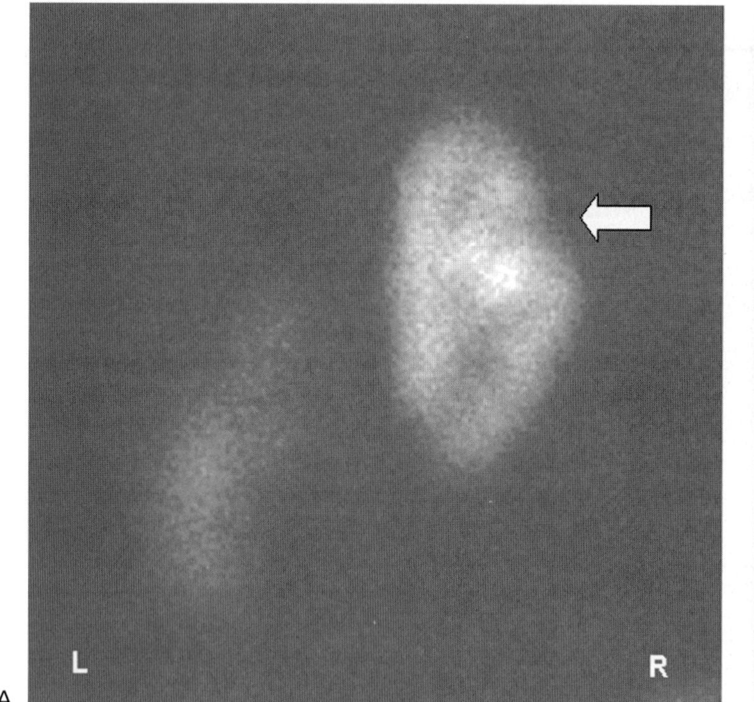

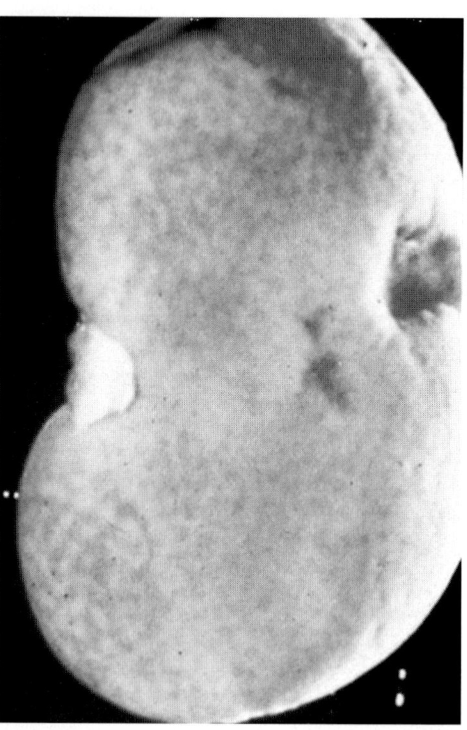

A B

FIGURE 61.9. Dimercaptosuccinic acid (DMSA) radionuclide scan for evaluation of renal scars. **A:** Technetium 99m–DMSA radionuclide scan for a 9-year-old who presented with hypertension and Bell's palsy, showing right upper pole renal scar (*arrow*) and poorly functioning smaller left kidney (relative activity 29%) from vesicoureteral reflux. **B:** Kidney from a different patient showing an upper pole scar from vesicoureteral reflux.

dictated by findings of the screening history and physical examination or abnormal complete blood count, urinalysis, or levels of BUN, serum creatinine, or electrolytes (Fig. 61.1). Hematuria, proteinuria, red blood cell casts on urinalysis, and edema suggest glomerulonephritis. Other systemic signs and symptoms, such as purpuric or malar rash, arthritis, and abdominal pain, are suggestive of systemic vasculitis. Anemia and short stature for age in the presence of elevated BUN and serum creatinine levels are characteristic of chronic renal failure, which can result from most of these diseases. Additional laboratory studies, including serum levels of C3 and C4, anti–glomerular basement membrane antibody, antinuclear antibody, anti–double-stranded DNA, and antineutrophil cytoplasmic antibody, may help make the diagnosis of a specific glomerulonephritis or systemic vasculitis, but a renal biopsy is almost always needed for definitive diagnosis. The diagnosis of hemolytic uremic syndrome may be made clinically, if microangiopathic hemolytic anemia, thrombocytopenia, and uremia are present. These diseases are all discussed in detail in other chapters of this book.

Some hereditary diseases are frequently associated with hypertension. These include autosomal recessive and dominant polycystic kidney disease, medullary cystic disease, juvenile nephronophthisis, Denys-Drash syndrome, and sickle cell disease. Diagnostic evaluation of these disorders is discussed in detail in other chapters of this book. Liddle's syndrome (pseudoaldosteronism) is a familial syndrome characterized by severe hypertension, hypokalemia, metabolic alkalosis, and decreased plasma renin activity and aldosterone levels (87–89). Originally thought to be an endocrine disorder, Liddle's syndrome is known now to result from a primary defect in renal tubular sodium handling that can be suppressed by amiloride therapy with dietary sodium restriction. A mutation in the renal epithelial sodium channel located in the luminal membrane of the collecting duct leads to avid unregulated sodium reabsorption, volume expansion, hypertension, and renal potassium wasting. The gene has been mapped to locus 16p13-p12. The precise mechanism of the abnormal activation of the sodium channel is still under investigation.

Hypertension associated with congenital renal anomalies, especially vesicoureteral reflux, typically presents in late childhood or early adolescence and may be the first sign of disease (19,86). Screening renal ultrasonography may be diagnostic but at least will direct further specific evaluation. Specific evaluation for vesicoureteral reflux should include taking a detailed history to identify undiagnosed fevers or documented urinary tract infections in early childhood and obtaining a voiding cystourethrogram, which can both diagnose and grade reflux. The absence of reflux does not negate the possibility that reflux was present in infancy and early childhood and then spontaneously resolved, but left the child with renal scars and reflux nephropathy. Results of a urinalysis and urine culture should be negative for urinary tract infection before one proceeds with a voiding cystourethro-

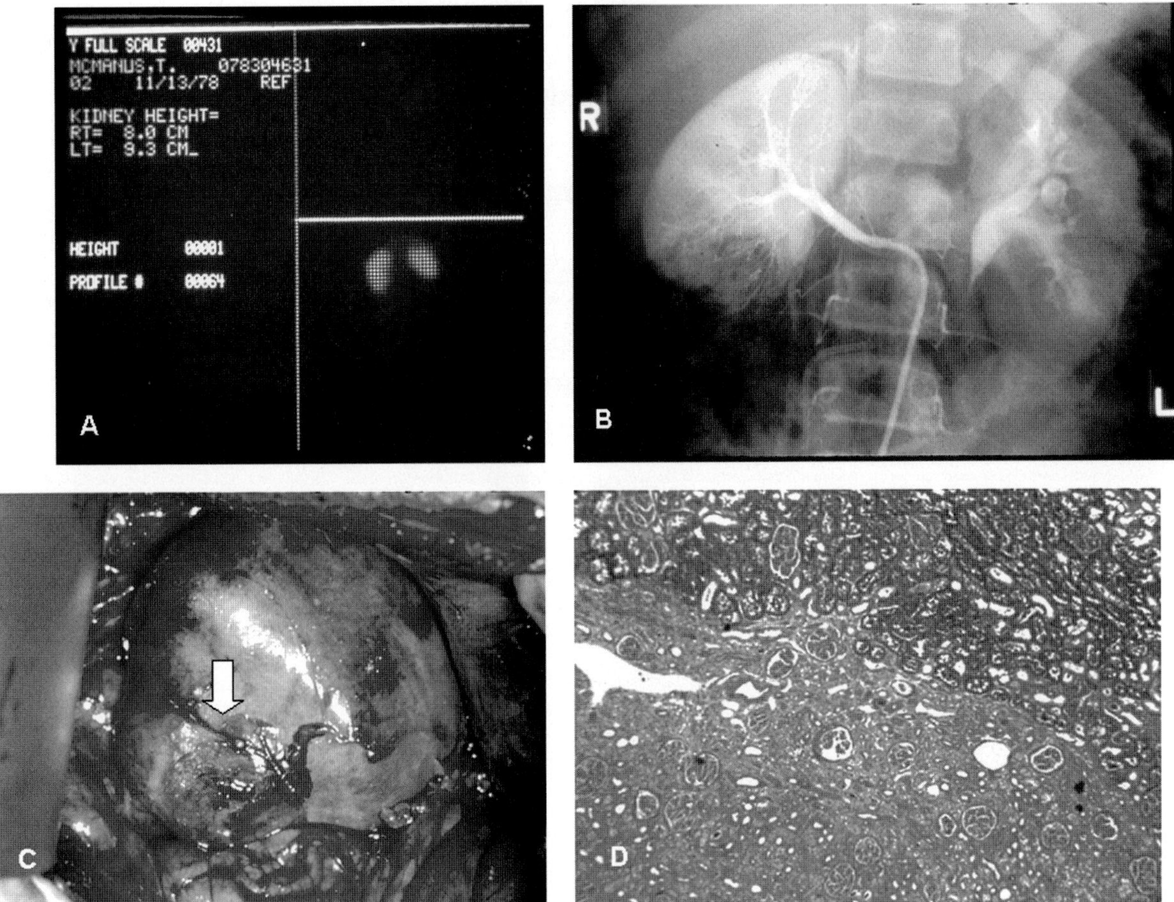

FIGURE 61.10. Ask-Upmark kidney. **A:** Technetium 99–diethylenentriaminepenta-acetic acid (DTPA) radionuclide scan showing right kidney smaller than left. **B:** Selective right renal arteriogram showing no filling of lower pole of right kidney; left kidney with late nephrogram of previous radiocontrast injection. **C:** Intraoperative photograph showing small lower pole of right kidney (*arrow*). **D:** Light microscopy of the junction of the normal portion of the kidney with the hypoplastic lower pole segment (periodic acid–Schiff stain).

gram. Children previously diagnosed with vesicoureteral reflux or other congenital anomalies, such as unilateral multicystic dysplastic kidney found in the neonatal period, may be normotensive at diagnosis and may develop hypertension later in life. Unfortunately, no test is available to predict the risk for developing hypertension, so regular follow-up of blood pressure is recommended (86). To detect the presence of renal scars, a DMSA radionuclide scan is preferred over conventional urography or ultrasonography (90,91). DMSA is filtered and then reabsorbed by the renal tubule to become fixed in the parenchyma, which provides a static image of functional renal tissue (92). Absence of uptake is consistent with a nonfunctioning scar as illustrated by Figure 61.9.

Segmental hypoplasia with atrophy, known as the Ask-Upmark kidney (Fig. 61.10), is a scarred, shrunken segment of the kidney characterized histologically by the presence of colloid-filled tubular microcysts and few or absent glomeruli (93,94). Whether this defect is congenital or the result of injury from vesicoureteral reflux or urinary tract infection is uncertain (94). Partial nephrectomy cures the associated hypertension. Renal arteriography with selective renal vein renin sampling is helpful to identify the exact location and extent of the hypoplastic segment before surgery is undertaken (95).

ENDOCRINE ABNORMALITIES ASSOCIATED WITH HYPERTENSION

Endocrine causes of hypertension in childhood are rare but usually treatable and often curable (96). Specific evaluation should be directed by the suspected disorder (Fig. 61.1). The combination of a good history taking and physical examination, accurate interpretation of screening laboratory data, and sequential ordering of diagnostic tests leads to a diagnosis and is still efficient and cost effective.

Pheochromocytoma

Pheochromocytoma is quite rare in all age groups (96,97) and accounts for fewer than 1% of the cases of secondary

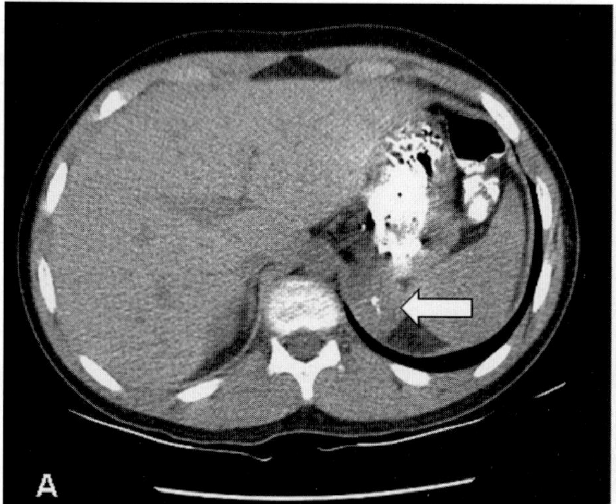

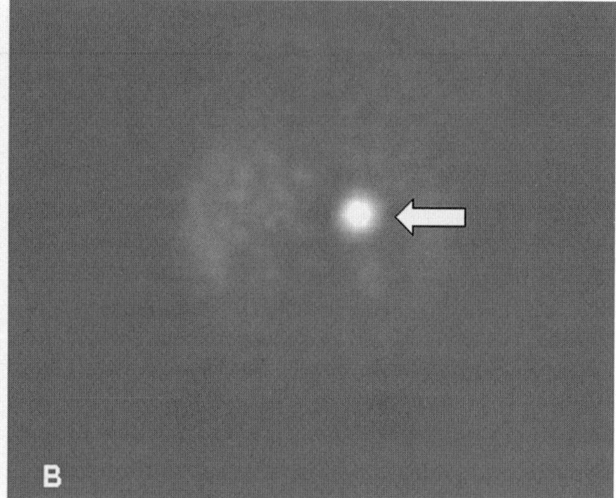

FIGURE 61.11. Diagnostic imaging for pheochromocytoma. **A:** Abdominal computed tomographic scan showing a 3-cm mass with central calcifications (*arrow*) located superior to the left kidney in the left adrenal gland. **B:** Iodine 123 meta-iodobenzyl guanidine (MIBG) scan showing uptake in right adrenal mass (*arrow*).

hypertension in childhood (64). Children are more likely to have multiple tumors, recurrence of tumors, and a positive family history of related tumors (96). Pheochromocytomas are chromaffin cell tumors that arise from the adrenal gland. When they arise in extra-adrenal positions in the autonomic nervous system of the abdomen, thorax, neck, or head, they are more specifically termed *paragangliomas* but are often referred to as extra-adrenal pheochromocytomas (97). Children with pheochromocytomas may present with the classical clinical triad of episodic hypertension, headache, and sweating, but hypertension is sustained approximately 80% of the time in children (96). Other symptoms include pallor, flushing, visual disturbances, abdominal pain, nausea, vomiting, and weight loss. Physical examination may reveal hypertensive retinopathy, features of associated syndromes such as the café-au-lait spots of neurofibromatosis, or rarely an abdominal mass, the palpation of which may lead to an abrupt increase in blood pressure and other symptoms of catecholamine release (96).

Pheochromocytomas in childhood may be sporadic but are familial approximately 30% of the time (96). Advances in genetic mutation analysis have improved identification of familial disease, which allows detection of affected children at an early age, before typical signs and symptoms occur (97). Familial disease is seen mainly in patients with von Hippel–Lindau disease, multiple endocrine neoplasia type 2, neurofibromatosis, or familial carotid body tumors. If pheochromocytoma is the primary manifestation of the family disease, a von Hippel–Lindau gene mutation is the most likely cause, whereas most of the patients with multiple endocrine neoplasia type 2 have medullary thyroid carcinoma.

Pheochromocytoma is a potentially curable cause of severe and sometimes life-threatening bouts of hypertension (96,99), so a thorough evaluation to make the diagnosis is important. Specific evaluation for pheochromocytoma (Fig. 61.1) should start with measurement of plasma metanephrine levels, which are elevated in 80% of patients even when the individuals are asymptomatic (98). Periodic screening with this test can lead to early diagnosis in children with familial disease (97). If the levels are normal, the diagnosis may be excluded. If the levels are only marginally increased, further evaluation with repeated measurement of plasma metanephrines plus plasma catecholamines, or a clonidine or glucagon test should be performed by a clinician experienced with these tests. Plasma concentrations of normetanephrine greater than 2.5 pmol/mL or plasma concentrations of metanephrine greater than 1.4 pmol/mL indicate the presence of pheochromocytoma with 100% specificity and warrant proceeding directly to imaging studies to locate the tumor (97).

The first step in imaging should be a CT or MRI scan of the abdomen (97). CT detects adrenal pheochromocytomas with 93 to 100% sensitivity (Fig. 61.11A) but has only 90% sensitivity for extra-adrenal tumors. MRI has high sensitivity for detecting both. CT and MRI cannot delineate whether a mass is a pheochromocytoma or another adrenal or soft tissue tumor. As an example, the paraspinal tumor depicted by MRA in Figure 61.8 was unexpectedly identified as a paraganglioma histologically after surgical removal. To identify pheochromocytomas preoperatively, the next step should be meta-iodobenzyl guanidine (MIBG) scanning (Fig. 61.11B). MIBG, which localizes in storage granules in adrenergic tissue of neural crest origin, is very specific (95 to 99%) for pheochromocytoma and neuroblastoma in children (100,101). Iodine 123 MIBG offers better imaging quality than iodine 131 MIBG (97). False-negative MIBG results can occur, particularly if tumors are small or in the thorax, neck, or head. Repeated examinations may be necessary to finally localize small tumors. Once localized, the pheochromocytoma may be surgically removed and cures hypertension in 90% of cases (96). Only approximately 10% of childhood pheochromocytomas are malignant (96).

Renin-Producing Tumors

The possibility of a renin-secreting tumor, such as a juxtaglomerular cell tumor (102,103) or Wilms' tumor (63,104), should be entertained in a hypertensive child with hypokalemia, elevated plasma renin activity, and absence of other obvious renal or renovascular disease. For juxtaglomerular cell tumors, abdominal CT or MRI imaging identifies small masses better than does selective renal arteriography, the results of which are normal in approximately 50% of reported cases (103).

Thyroid Disorders

Mild hypertension may be associated with hyperthyroidism from Graves' disease or rarely thyroid adenoma (96). Acquired hypothyroidism in adults is associated with hypertension and is reversible with thyroid replacement therapy in approximately 50% of cases (105). The first step in specific evaluation of thyroid disease is assessment of serum thyroxine and thyroid-stimulating hormone concentration to make the diagnosis of hyperthyroidism or hypothyroidism (Fig. 61.1). Further evaluation is probably best accomplished by referral to a pediatric endocrinologist.

Cushing Syndrome

Exogenous glucocorticoid or adrenocorticotropic hormone (ACTH) therapy, including that used for treatment of asthma, renal disease, rheumatologic disease, neurologic disorders, and cancer or transplantation immunosuppression, is the most common cause of Cushing syndrome and endocrine-associated hypertension in pediatric patients (96). On the other hand, excess endogenous production of glucocorticoids or ACTH from an adrenal or pituitary tumor is unusual in childhood. Obvious physical changes of glucocorticoid excess, including round facies, plethora, truncal obesity, acne, easy bruisability, and abdominal striae, may direct the physician to the diagnosis. If the patient is receiving no glucocorticoid medications, screening by measurement of an 8 a.m. plasma cortisol level, ACTH level, and 24-hour urinary excretion of 17-hydroxycorticosteroids and free cortisol may be appropriate, if referral to a pediatric endocrinologist is not readily available.

Hyperaldosteronism

Hypertension associated with adrenal tumors or idiopathic adrenal hyperplasia is usually mediated by aldosterone or other compounds with mineralocorticoid effects (96). Mineralocorticoid excess leads to salt and water retention, volume expansion, and renal potassium wasting. Hypertension in the presence of hypokalemia and metabolic alkalosis found on screening evaluation should direct the specific evaluation to that for hyperaldosteronism (Fig. 61.1). If plasma renin activity is low, plasma and 24-hour urinary aldosterone levels should be measured. Urinary aldosterone level is elevated in the presence of high plasma aldosterone concentration and decreased in the presence of other compounds with mineralocorticoid effect. Imaging of the adrenal glands with CT or MRI should be the next step for diagnosis and localization of adrenal adenoma or carcinoma in patients with hyperaldosteronism (96).

Congenital Adrenal Hyperplasia

Only two enzyme deficiencies in the cortisol pathway are associated with hypertension, 11β-hydroxylase (96,106) and 17α-hydroxylase (96,107). Deficiency of 11β-hydroxylase is the second most common cause of congenital adrenal hyperplasia but accounts for only approximately 5% of cases (96). Deficiency of 11β-hydroxylase is an autosomal recessive disorder caused by mutations of the CYP11B1 gene located on chromosome band 8q21-q22 (106). An 11β-hydroxylase deficiency results in decreased conversion of 11-deoxycortisol to cortisol and 11-deoxycorticosterone (DOC) to corticosterone, and excess production of androgens from precursors more proximal in the pathway. Decreased cortisol production stimulates secretion of pituitary ACTH, which results in adrenal stimulation and excess production of DOC. DOC has mineralocorticoid effects at high concentration. The excess androgen production results in virilization and ambiguous genitalia in female infants and penile enlargement in males. Hypertension, hypokalemia, and low plasma renin activity are present in most, but not all, affected patients. Referral to a pediatric endocrinologist for more extensive laboratory evaluation is an appropriate next step. Characteristic findings are elevated plasma concentrations of 11-deoxycortisol and DOC and the androgens dehydroepiandrosterone (DHEA) and testosterone, as well as increased urinary excretion of 17-hydroxycorticosteroids, tetrahydro-11-deoxycortisol, and 17-ketosteroids (108). ACTH stimulation testing may be needed to make or confirm the diagnosis, especially in adolescents.

Deficiency of 17α-hydroxylase is very rare, occurring in less than 1% of cases of congenital adrenal hyperplasia (96). The trait is autosomal recessive and caused by mutations in the CYP17 gene on chromosome band 10q24-q25 (107). This enzyme has both 17α-hydroxylase and 17,20-lyase (desmolase) activity (109,110). The enzyme 17α-hydroxylase normally facilitates conversion of progesterone to 17-hydroxyprogesterone and conversion of pregnenolone to

17-hydroxypregnenolone, which lead to the production of cortisol. The enzyme 17,20-lyase is required for the synthesis of androgens and estrogenic C18 steroids. Deficiency of the enzyme limits synthesis of cortisol as well as androgens and estrogens. Unlike patients with 11β-hydroxylase deficiency, patients with 17α-hydroxylase deficiency are not virilized and thus may not be diagnosed before discovery of their hypertension, hypokalemia, and hypogonadism in adolescence. Girls have primary amenorrhea and absent secondary sexual characteristics. Boys usually have complete male pseudohermaphroditism with female external genitalia, a blind vagina, absent uterus, and intraabdominal testes. Laboratory evaluation reveals increased serum progesterone and DOC levels and reduced plasma cortisol, 11-deoxycortisol, DHEA, testosterone, and estradiol concentrations. These cases are very rare and are best evaluated by referral to a pediatric endocrinologist.

Hypercalcemia

Hypercalcemia is well known to cause hypertension as well as polyuria, constipation, abdominal pain, anorexia, and mental status changes. In pediatric cases, the cause is most often vitamin D intoxication, Williams syndrome, or malignancy, and rarely primary hyperparathyroidism (96). Evaluation should include measurement of serum levels of total and ionized calcium, phosphorus, parathyroid hormone, 25-hydroxyvitamin D, and 1,25-dihydroxyvitamin D (Fig. 61.1).

MISCELLANEOUS CAUSES OF HYPERTENSION

Table 61.6 lists a number of miscellaneous causes of hypertension, including some drugs that should be considered in the evaluation of the hypertensive child. In all adolescents or younger children at high risk for drug abuse, a urine drug screen should always be performed as part of the initial evaluation. A few of the other causes of hypertension in children are discussed in more detail here.

Neurologic Abnormalities

A variety of neurologic disorders give rise to hypertension (Table 61.6). In the critically ill child with rising blood pressure and falling heart rate, evolving increased intracranial pressure should always be suspected. The incidence of intracranial pressure is especially high with acute meningitis or encephalitis (111). Children with seizures and status epilepticus may present with hypertension (112). If blood pressure in the postictal period is high but is less than 4 standard deviations above the mean, hypertension is more likely to be transient and seizure induced rather than caused by hypertensive encephalopathy with seizures (112). Disorders of the autonomic nervous system may also lead to hypertension. Familial dysautonomia is the best known of these disorders (113–115). Clinical features include paroxysmal hypertension, swallowing difficulties, speech and motor incoordination, and pain insensitivity. Clinical diagnosis is based on the findings of Ashkenazi Jewish heritage, diminished tear production, lack of an axon flare after intradermal histamine, lack of lingual fungiform papillae, and decreased deep tendon reflexes. The gene for this disorder, IKBKAP, has been isolated and mapped to chromosome band 9q31.

Teen Pregnancy

Pregnant teenagers are at high risk for developing hypertension, which increases their risk for poor outcomes for the baby, including low birth weight, preterm delivery, and congenital malformations (116–118). When hypertension occurs early in gestation, hospitalization with strict supervision and control of blood pressure may be required. Ultrasonographic imaging for evaluation of hypertension is acceptable, but conventional radiographic studies and radioisotopic scans should be avoided because of potential adverse effects on the fetus. ACE inhibitors and angiotensin receptor blockers are teratogenic, and their use in pregnancy is contraindicated (119,120). Pubertal and postpubertal girls with antecedent hypertension should be advised to protect against pregnancy while taking these medications for control of hypertension (120). When preeclampsia or severe hypertension occurs after 36 weeks' gestation, delivery is the therapy of choice. If a teenager with known hypertension becomes pregnant, evaluation should always include serial reassessment of maternal renal function throughout pregnancy.

REFERENCES

1. Update on the 1987 Task Force Report on High Blood Pressure in Children and Adolescents: a working group report from the National High Blood Pressure Education Program. *Pediatrics* 1996;98:649–658.
2. Report of the Second Task Force on Blood Pressure Control in Children—1987. *Pediatrics* 1987;79:1–25.
3. Lieberman E. Pediatric hypertension: clinical perspective. *Mayo Clin Proc* 1994;69:1098–1107.
4. Sorof J, Daniels S. Obesity hypertension in children, a problem of epidemic proportions. *Hypertension* 2002;40:441–447.
5. The seventh report of the Joint National Committee on Prevention, Detection, Evaluation, and Treatment of High Blood Pressure. *JAMA* 2003;289:2560–2572.
6. Butani L, Morgenstern BZ. Are pitfalls of oscillometric blood pressure measurements preventable in children? *Pediatr Nephrol* 2003;18:313–318.
7. Park MD, Menard SW, Yuan C. Comparison of auscultatory and oscillometric blood pressures. *Arch Pediatr Adolesc Med* 2001;155:50–53.

8. Wattigney WA, Webber LS, Lawrence MD, et al. Utility of an automatic instrument for blood pressure measurement in children. The Bogalusa Heart Study. *Am J Hypertens* 1996;9:256–262.
9. O'Brien E, Waeber B, Parati G, et al. Blood pressure measuring devices: recommendations of the European Society of Hypertension. *BMJ* 2001;322:531–536.
10. Sorof J, Portman R. Ambulatory blood pressure monitoring in the pediatric patient. *J Pediatr* 2000;136:578–586.
11. Sanders BP, Portman RJ, Ramey RA, et al. Hypertension during reduction of long-term steroid therapy in young subjects with asthma. *J Allergy Clin Immunol* 1992;89:816–821.
12. Ferdinand KC. Substance abuse and hypertension. *J Clin Hypertens* 2000;2:37–40.
13. Klein-Schwartz W, McGrath J. Poison centers' experience with methylphenidate abuse in preteens and adolescents. *J Am Acad Child Adolesc Psychiatry* 2003;42:288–294.
14. Law CM, Sheill AW, Newsome CA, et al. Fetal, infant, and childhood growth and adult blood pressure: a longitudinal study from birth to 22 years of age. *Circulation* 2002;105:1088–1092.
15. Barker DJ, Osmond C, Goldring J, et al. Growth in utero, blood pressure in childhood and adult life, and mortality from cardiovascular disease. *BMJ* 1989;298:564–567.
16. Ernst E. Cardiovascular adverse effects of herbal medicines: a systematic review of the recent literature. *Can J Cardiol* 2003;19:818–827.
17. Patel S, Robinson R, Burk M. Hypertensive crisis associated with St. John's wort. *Am J Med* 2002;112:507–508.
18. Sorof JM. Systolic hypertension in children: benign or beware? *Pediatr Nephrol* 2001;16:517–525.
19. Siegler RL, Brewer ED, Corneli HM, et al. Hypertension first seen as facial paralysis. *Pediatrics* 1991;87:387–389.
20. Lewis VE, Peat DS, Tizard EJ. Hypertension and facial palsy in middle aortic syndrome. *Arch Dis Child* 2001;85:240–241.
21. Daniels SR, Loggie JM, McEnery Pt, et al. Clinical spectrum of intrinsic renovascular hypertension in children. *Pediatrics* 1987;80:698–704.
22. Schwartz GJ, Brio LP, Spitzer A. The use of plasma creatinine concentration for estimating glomerular filtration rate in infants, children and adolescents. *Pediatr Clin North Am* 1987;34:571–590.
23. Carman TL, Olin JW, Czum J. Noninvasive imaging of the renal arteries. *Urol Clin North Am* 2001;28:815–826.
24. Brun P, Kchouk H, Mouchet B. Value of Doppler ultrasound for the diagnosis of renal artery stenosis in children. *Pediatr Nephrol* 1997;11:27–30.
25. Zierler RE. Is duplex scanning the best screening test for renal artery stenosis? *Semin Vasc Surg* 2001;14:177–185.
26. Prebis JW, Gruskin AB, Polinshy MS, et al. Uric acid in childhood essential hypertension. *J Pediatr* 1981;98:702–707.
27. Feig DI, Johnson RJ. Hyperuricemia in childhood primary hypertension. *Hypertension* 2003 (*in press*).
28. Johnson RJ, Kang DH, Feig D, et al. Is there a pathogenetic role for uric acid in hypertension and cardiovascular and renal disease? *Hypertension* 2003;41:1183–1190.
29. Flynn JT. Differentiation between primary and secondary hypertension in children using ambulatory blood pressure monitoring. *Pediatrics* 2002;110:89–93.
30. Daniels SR, Meyer RA, Loggie JM. Determinants of cardiac involvement in children and adolescents with essential hypertension. *Circulation* 1990;82:1243–1248.
31. Belsha CW, Wells TG, McNiece KL, et al. Influence of diurnal blood pressure variations on target organ abnormalities in adolescents with mild essential hypertension. *Am J Hypertens* 1998;11:410–417.
32. Belsha CW. Ambulatory blood pressure monitoring and hypertensive target-organ damage in children. *Blood Press Monit* 1999;4:161–164.
33. Deal JE, Snell ME, Barratt TM, et al. Renovascular disease in childhood. *J Pediatr* 1992;121:378–384.
34. Sinaiko AR. Childhood hypertension. In: Laragh JH, Brenner BM, eds. *Hypertension: pathophysiology, diagnosis, and management*. New York: Raven Press, 1995:209–225.
35. Ingelfinger J. Renovascular disease in children. *Kidney Int* 1993;43:493–505.
36. Williams CD, Shah V, Uchiyama M. Captopril as an aid to diagnosis in childhood hypertension. *Clin Exp Hypertens* 1986;8:747–781.
37. Van Jaarsveld BC, Krijnen P, Derkz FH, et al. The place of renal scintigraphy in the diagnosis of renal artery stenosis. Fifteen years of clinical experience. *Arch Intern Med* 1997;157:1226–1234.
38. Ng CS, de Bruyn R, Gordon I. The investigation of renovascular hypertension in children: the accuracy of radio-isotopes in detecting renovascular disease. *Nucl Med Commun* 1997;18:1017–1028.
39. Adelman RD. Long-term follow-up of neonatal renovascular hypertension. *Pediatr Nephrol* 1987;1:36–41.
40. Adelman RD, Morrell RE. Coarctation of the abdominal aorta and renal artery stenosis related to an umbilical artery catheter placement in a neonate. *Pediatrics* 2000;106:E36.
41. Shahdadpuri J, Frank R, Gauthier BG, et al. Yield of renal arteriography in the evaluation of pediatric hypertension. *Pediatr Nephrol* 2000;14:816–819.
42. Casalini E, Sfondrin MS, Fassali E. Two-year clinical follow-up of children and adolescents after percutaneous transluminal angioplasty for renovascular hypertension. *Invest Radiol* 1995;30:40–43.
43. Booth C, Preston R, Clark G, et al. Management of renal vascular disease in neurofibromatosis type I and the role of percutaneous transluminal angioplasty. *Nephrol Dial Transplant* 2002;17:1235–1240.
44. Fossali E, Signorini E, Intermite RC, et al. Renovascular disease and hypertension in children with neurofibromatosis. *Pediatr Nephrol* 2000;14:806–810.
45. Tyagi S, Kaul UA, Satsangi DK, et al. Percutaneous transluminal angioplasty for renovascular hypertension in children: initial and long-term results. *Pediatrics* 1997;99:44–49.
46. Hofbeck M, Singer H, Rupprecht T, et al. Successful percutaneous transluminal angioplasty for treatment of renovascular hypertension in a 15-month-old child. *Eur J Pediatr* 1998;157:512–514.
47. Liang CD, Wu CJ, Fang CY, et al. Endovascular stent placement for management of total renal artery occlusion in a child. *J Invasive Cardiol* 2002;14:32–35.
48. Thornton J, O'Callaghan J, Walshe J, et al. Comparison of digital subtraction angiography with gadolinium enhanced magnetic resonance angiography in the diagnosis of renal artery stenosis. *Eur Radiol* 1999;9:930–934.

49. Leung DA, Hagspiel KD, Angle JF, et al. MR angiography of the renal arteries. *Radiol Clin North Am* 2002;40:847–865.
50. Marcos HB, Choyke PL. Magnetic resonance angiography of the kidney. *Semin Nephrol* 2000;20:450–455.
51. Smith HJ, Bakke SJ. MR angiography of in situ and transplanted renal arteries. Early experience using a three-dimensional time-of-flight technique. *Acta Radiol* 1993;34:150–155.
52. Vade A, Agrawal R, Lim-Dunham J, et al. Utility of computed tomographic renal angiogram in the management of childhood hypertension. *Pediatr Nephrol* 2002;17:741–747.
53. Goonasekera CDA, Shah V, Wade AM, et al. The usefulness of renal vein renin studies in hypertensive children: a 25-year experience. *Pediatr Nephrol* 2002;17:943–949.
54. Martinez-Maldonado M. Pathophysiology of renovascular hypertension. *Hypertension* 1991;17:707–719.
55. Pickering TG, Sos TA, James GD. Comparison of renal vein renin activity in hypertensive patients with stenosis of one or both renal arteries. *J Hypertens* 1985;3(suppl 3):S291–293.
56. Fry WJ, Ernst BC, Stanley JC, et al. Renovascular hypertension in the pediatric patient. *Arch Surg* 1973;107:692–698.
57. Makker SP, Moorthy B. Fibromuscular dysplasia of renal arteries. An important cause of renovascular hypertension in children. *J Pediatr* 1979;95:940–945.
58. Ingelfinger JR, Newburger JW. Spectrum of renal anomalies in patients with Williams syndrome. *J Pediatr* 1991;119: 771–773.
59. Pankau R, Partsch CJ, Winter M. Incidence and spectrum of renal abnormalities in Williams-Beuren syndrome. *Am J Med Genet* 1996;63:301–304.
60. Baxter BM. Ultrasound of renal transplantation. *Clin Radiol* 2001;56:802–818.
61. Mutze S, Turk I, Schonberger, et al. Colour-coded duplex sonography in the diagnostic assessment of vascular complications after kidney transplantation in children. *Pediatr Radiol* 1997;27:898–902.
62. Waller JR, Nicholson ML. Molecular mechanisms of renal allograft fibrosis. *Br J Surg* 2001;88:1429–1441.
63. Steinbrecher HA, Malone PS. Wilms tumour and hypertension: incidence and outcome. *Br J Urol* 1995;76:241–243.
64. Londe S. Causes of hypertension in the young. *Pediatr Clin North Am* 1978;25:55–58.
65. Alpert BS, Bain HH, Balfe JW. Role of the renin-angiotensin-aldosterone system in hypertensive children with coarctation of the aorta. *Am J Cardiol* 1979;43:828–831.
66. Soler R, Rodriquez, Requejo I, et al. Magnetic resonance imaging of congenital abnormalities of the thoracic aorta. *Eur Radiol* 1998;540–546.
67. Sanders SP, MacPherson D, Yeager SB. Temporal flow velocity profile in the descending aorta in coarctation. *J Am Coll Cardiol* 1986;7:603–609.
68. Shaddy RE, Snider AR, Silverman NH, et al. Pulsed Doppler findings in patients with coarctation of the aorta. *Circulation* 1986;73:82–88.
69. Lim DS, Ralston MA. Echocardiographic indices of Doppler flow patterns compared with MRI or angiographic measurements to detect significant coarctation of the aorta. *Echocardiography* 2002;19:55–60.
70. Bank ER, Aisen AM, Rocchini AP, et al. Coarctation of the aorta in children undergoing angioplasty: pre-treatment and post-treatment MR imaging. *Radiology* 1987;162:235–240.
71. de Roos A, Roest AA. Evaluation of congenital heart disease by magnetic resonance imaging. *Eur Radiol* 2000;10:2–6.
72. Godart F, Labrot G, Devos P, et al. Coarctation of the aorta: comparison of aortic dimensions between conventional MR imaging, 3D MR angiography, and conventional angiography. *Eur Radiol* 2002;12:2034–2039.
73. Rupprecht T, Nitz W, Wagner M, et al. Determination of the pressure gradient in children with coarctation of the aorta by low-field magnetic resonance imaging. *Pediatr Cardiol* 2002;23:127–131.
74. Sen PK, Kinare SG, Engineer SD, et al. The middle aortic syndrome. *Br Heart J* 1963;25:610–618.
75. Terramani TT, Salim A, Hood DB, et al. Hypoplasia of the descending thoracic and abdominal aorta: a report of two cases and review of the literature. *J Vasc Surg* 2002;36:844–848.
76. Israel G, Krinsky G, Lee V. The "skinny aorta." *Clin Imaging* 2002;26:116–121.
77. Criado E, Izquierdo L, Lujan S. et al. Abdominal aortic coarctation, renovascular hypertension, and neurofibromatosis. *Ann Vasc Surg* 2002;16:363–367.
78. Radford DJ, Pohlner PG. The middle aortic syndrome: an important feature of Williams' syndrome. *Cardiol Young* 2000;10:597–602.
79. Eronen M, Peippo M, Hiippala A, et al. Cardiovascular manifestations in 75 patients with Williams syndrome. *J Med Genet* 2002;39:554–558.
80. Sybert VP. Cardiovascular malformations and complications in Turner syndrome. *Pediatrics* 1998;101:E11.
81. Landin-Wilhelmsen K, Bryman I, Wilhelmsen L. Cardiac malformations and hypertension, but not metabolic risk factors, are common in Turner syndrome. *J Clin Endocrinol Metab* 2001;86:4166–4170.
82. Nathwani NC, Unwin R, Brook CG, et al. Blood pressure and Turner syndrome. *Clin Endocrinol* 2000;52:363–370.
83. Nathwani NC, Unwin R, Brook CG, et al. The influence of renal and cardiovascular abnormalities on blood pressure in Turner syndrome. *Clin Endocrinol* 2000;52:371–377.
84. Dillon MJ. Investigation and management of hypertension in children. A personal perspective. *Pediatr Nephrol* 1987;1:59–68.
85. Arar MY, Hogg RJ, Arant BS, et al. Etiology of sustained hypertension in children in the southwestern United States. *Pediatr Nephrol* 1994;8:186–189.
86. Goonasekera CD, Dillon MJ. Reflux nephropathy and hypertension. *J Hum Hypertens* 1998;12:497–504.
87. Warnock DG. Liddle syndrome: genetics and mechanisms of Na+ channel defects. *Am J Med Sci* 2001;322:302–307.
88. Scheinman SJ, Guay-Woodford LM, Thakker RV, et al. Mechanisms of disease: genetic disorders of renal electrolyte transport. *N Engl J Med* 1999;340:1177–1187.
89. Assadi FK, Kimura RE, Subramanian, et al. Liddle syndrome in a newborn infant. *Pediatr Nephrol* 2002;17:609–611.
90. Gordon I. Indications for 99m technetium dimercapto-succinic acid scan in children. *J Urol* 1987;137:464–467.
91. Stokland E, Hellstrom M, Jakobsson B, et al. Imaging of renal scarring. *Acta Paediatr* 1999;88(suppl):13–21.
92. Peters AM, Jones DH, Evans K, et al. Two routes for 99mTc-DMSA uptake into the renal cortical tubular cell. *Eur J Nucl Med* 1988;14:555–561.

93. Ask-Upmark E, Fagerberg S. Renal arteriography in arterial hypertension. *Acta Med Scand* 1965;178:577–582.
94. Arant BS, Sotelo-Avila C, Bernstein J. Segmental "hypoplasia" of the kidney (Ask-Upmark). *J Pediatr* 1979;95:931–939.
95. Tash JA, Stock JA, Hanna MK. The role of partial nephrectomy in the treatment of pediatric renal hypertension. *J Urol* 2003;169:625–628.
96. Rodd CJ, Sockalosky JJ. Endocrine causes of hypertension in children. *Pediatr Clin North Am* 1993;40:149–164.
97. Pacak K, Linehan WM, Eisenhofer G, et al. Recent advances in genetics, diagnosis, localization, and treatment of pheochromocytoma. *Ann Intern Med* 2001;134:315–329.
98. Eisenhofer G, Lenders JW, Linehan WM, et al. Plasma normetanephrine and metanephrine for detecting pheochromocytoma in von Hippel-Lindau disease and multiple endocrine neoplasia type 2. *N Engl J Med* 1999;340:1872–1879.
99. Reddy VS, O'Neill JA, Holcomb GW, et al. Twenty-five year surgical experience with pheochromocytoma in children. *Am Surg* 2000;66:1085–1091.
100. Leung A, Shapiro B, Hattner R, et al. Specificity of radioiodinated MIBG for neural crest tumors in childhood. *J Nucl Med* 1997;38:1351–1357.
101. Shulkin BL, Shapiro B. Current concepts on the diagnostic use of MIBG in children. *J Nucl Med* 1998;39:679–688.
102. Abbi RK, McVicar M, Teichberg S, et al. Pathologic characterization of a renin-secreting juxtaglomerular cell tumor in a child and review of the pediatric literature. *Pediatr Pathol* 1993;13:443–451.
103. Haab F, Duclos J, Guyenne T, et al. Renin secreting tumors: diagnosis, conservative surgical approach and long-term results. *J Urol* 1995;153:1781–1784.
104. Spahr J, Demers LM, Shochat SJ. Renin producing Wilms' tumor. *J Pediatr Surg* 1981;16:32–34.
105. Dernellis J, Panaretou M. Effects of thyroid replacement therapy on arterial blood pressure in patients with hypertension and hypothyroidism. *Am Heart J* 2002;143:718–724.
106. Cerame BI, New MI. Hormonal hypertension in children: 11beta-hydroxylase deficiency and apparent mineralocorticoid excess. *J Pediatr Endocrinol Metab* 2000;13:1537–1547.
107. Dacou-Voutetakis C, Maniati-Christidi M, Dracopoulou-Vabouli M. Genetic aspects of congenital adrenal hyperplasia. *J Pediatr Endocrinol Metab* 2001;14(suppl 5):1303–1308.
108. White PC, Curnow KM, Pascoe L. Disorders of steroid 11 beta-hydroxylase isoenzymes. *Endocr Rev* 1994;15:421–438.
109. Winter JS, Couch RM, Muller J, et al. Combined 17-hydroxylase and 17,20-desmolase deficiencies. Evidence for synthesis of a defective cytochrome P450c17. *J Clin Endocrinol Metab* 1989;68:309–316.
110. Winter JS. Clinical, biochemical and molecular aspects of 17-hydroxylase deficiency. *Endocr Res* 1991;17:53–62.
111. Rebaud P, Berthier JC, Hartemann E, et al. Intracranial pressure in childhood central nervous system infections. *Intensive Care Med* 1988;14:522–525.
112. Proulx F, Lacroix J, Farrell Ca, et al. Convulsions and hypertension in children: differentiating cause from effect. *Crit Care Med* 1993;21:1541–1546.
113. Axelrod FB. Familial dysautonomia: a 47-year perspective. How technology confirms clinical acumen. *J Pediatr* 1998;132:S2–S5.
114. Axelrod FB, Goldberg JD, Ye X, et al. Survival in familial dysautonomia: impact of early intervention. *J Pediatr* 2002;141:518–523.
115. Fernhoff PM. No pains, many gains. *J Pediatr* 2002;141:470–471.
116. Davis S. Pregnancy in adolescents. *Pediatr Clin North Am* 1989;36:665–680.
117. Murdock NM. Teenage pregnancy. *J Natl Med Assoc* 1998;90:135–136.
118. Gortzak-Uzan L, Hallak M, Press F, et al. Teenage pregnancy: risk factor for adverse perinatal outcome. *J Matern Fetal Med* 2001;10:393–397.
119. Tabacova SA, Kimmel CA. Enalapril: pharmacokinetic/dynamic inferences for comparative developmental toxicity [Review]. *Reprod Toxicol* 2001;15:467–478.
120. Sedman AB, Kershaw DB, Bunchman TE. Recognition and management of angiotensin converting enzyme inhibitor fetopathy. *Pediatr Nephrol* 1999;9:382–385.

62

TREATMENT OF HYPERTENSION

BETH A. VOGT
IRA D. DAVIS

This chapter reviews nonpharmacologic and pharmacologic interventions used to treat hypertension. Therapeutic plans for various causes of hypertension are also discussed.

NONPHARMACOLOGIC TREATMENT OF HYPERTENSION

To the physician, nonpharmacologic therapy of hypertension is appealing. Interventions such as dietary salt restriction, mineral supplementation (potassium, calcium, magnesium), weight loss, exercise, and lifestyle modification (alcohol, cigarettes, stress) are inexpensive, provide health benefits in addition to their blood pressure (BP)–lowering effects, and can delay or prevent the need for antihypertensive medications.

Is there any value in using nonpharmacologic therapies as first-line treatments for mild or moderate hypertension (or as an adjunct to medications in more serious forms of hypertension), when effective, safe, and well-tolerated medications exist? For most children and adolescents, the long-term complications of hypertension have little relevance to their daily life. It is difficult to predict which patients and families will embrace lifestyle modifications necessary for successful nonpharmacologic BP reduction. Currently, the National High Blood Pressure Education Program Task Force report on high blood pressure in children and adolescents recommends the introduction of nonpharmacologic interventions to all children with high-normal BPs (ninety to ninety-fifth percentile for age and height) and those with documented hypertension (1).

Dietary Salt Restriction

There is ample evidence from studies of adults demonstrating that high salt intake adversely affects BP. Observational studies of diet and BP have shown that populations with high dietary salt intake have higher BPs than those with lower salt intake (2,3). In addition, multiple clinical trials have shown that reduced salt intake lowers BP (4–6). It is clear that certain subpopulations, including African Americans; the elderly; and individuals with obesity, diabetes, or renal dysfunction, tend to be more *salt-sensitive* than other populations.

The mechanisms by which excess dietary salt intake may contribute to hypertension are not well understood. One theory suggests that kidneys of hypertensive individuals may have a physiologic defect in their ability to excrete sodium (7). Normally, renal sodium excretion increases when there is an acute increase in BP; in individuals with hypertension, the BP required to excrete a given sodium load is higher and is described as a rightward shift in the pressure-natriuresis curve. The mechanisms leading to this shift in the curve remain uncertain, but may involve (a) a congenital reduction in the number of nephrons limiting sodium filtration (8), (b) genetic alterations in the expression of vasoactive mediators involved in renal sodium handling (9), or (c) a reduction in renal medullary blood flow, leading to local tissue ischemia and sodium retention (10).

Many pediatric intervention studies, in which patients receive a low-salt diet, have failed to demonstrate a diet-specific reduction in BP (11–14). However, several pediatric studies have demonstrated small but measurable reductions in BP (15–17), and a number of interventional trials suggest a beneficial effect of a low-sodium diet in hypertensive adults (4–6).

In the future, research may improve our ability to identify those children and adolescents most likely to benefit from dietary salt restriction. Because dietary salt intake is generally so high in Western countries (average adult intake = 150 mEq Na or 3500 mg Na/day), we currently recommend daily intake of no more than 2400 mg sodium for all children and adolescents with high-normal BP or hypertension (18). Families must be educated that added salt represents only a small proportion of total daily dietary salt intake. Prepared foods, breads, and fast food restaurant items tend to contain large amounts of salt added during food processing. Families should be encouraged to read food package labels, which in the United States and Western Europe contain extensive information about sodium content. Health care providers should provide guidance in interpreting those labels to families interested in reducing sodium intake. Initial consultation and longitudinal follow-up with a qualified dietitian may be particularly beneficial.

Mineral Supplementation

Observational and interventional studies suggest that the adequate mineral content of the diet may be linked to BP variability, in particular salt sensitivity. Therefore, there have been attempts to improve BP control using oral potassium, calcium, and magnesium supplements.

In epidemiologic studies, high dietary potassium intake has been found to be associated with lower BP (19). The mechanisms by which potassium exerts its antihypertensive effects include induction of natriuresis, decreasing urinary calcium excretion, and altering systemic vascular and renal resistance (20). There is evidence of a BP-lowering effect of oral potassium supplementation in adults (21); however, there are no reports to date of a beneficial effect in hypertensive children or adolescents.

Dietary calcium intake has also been found to be inversely related to BP (22). Increased calcium intake may impact BP through a variety of mechanisms, including alteration of vascular smooth muscle tone and cardiac muscle contractility. Dietary calcium supplementation in hypertensive adults yields minimal reductions in BP (23). Although some individuals may benefit more than others, there is currently no way to identify which individuals with hypertension might respond to dietary calcium supplementation. There is no clinical evidence to support dietary calcium supplementation in the pediatric hypertensive patient.

Epidemiologic studies examining dietary magnesium intake (24), as well as the clinical efficacy of magnesium in the treatment of preeclampsia-associated hypertension, suggest that magnesium supplementation may be of benefit in the treatment of chronic hypertension. However, trials of magnesium supplementation have demonstrated minimal (25) or no effect (26) on decreasing BP in adults. There is currently no indication for dietary magnesium supplementation in hypertensive adults or children.

The most compelling evidence supporting a beneficial effect of increased mineral intake comes from the DASH (*D*ietary *A*pproaches to *S*top *H*ypertension) clinical trial (27). In the DASH study, adults consumed a healthy diet that was rich in fruits, vegetables, and low-fat dairy products. The DASH diet provided intake of potassium, calcium, and magnesium at the seventy-fifth percentile of U.S. consumption, while maintaining daily sodium intake at 3 g. In hypertensive adults, the systolic BP was reduced by 11.4 mm Hg and the diastolic BP by 5.5 mm Hg. It is theorized that the increased intake of all three minerals provided by the DASH diet led to an additive effect on BP reduction not previously seen in clinical trials involving supplementation of individual nutrients. On the basis of these data, we recommend that children and adolescents with hypertension consume a healthy diet, rich in fruits, vegetables, and low-fat dairy products similar to the DASH diet, rather than recommending specific nutritional supplements.

Weight Loss

The prevalence of childhood obesity has increased worldwide, particularly in developed nations, as a result of easy access to calorically dense foods and an increasingly sedentary lifestyle (28). Obese children have increased rates of hypertension, as well as other adverse cardiovascular risk factors, including hyperlipidemia and insulin resistance (29).

The mechanisms by which excessive body fat increases BP are complex and likely multifactorial. There is general agreement that obesity-associated hypertension is associated with excessive fluid retention (30), possibly caused by increased sympathetic nervous system activity (31,32), insulin resistance (33), or increased activity of the renin-angiotensin-aldosterone system (34).

Traditionally, obesity has been defined as a weight in excess of 120% of the median weight for a given height or a weight for height greater than the ninetieth percentile on the growth charts from the National Center for Health Statistics. Recently, the body mass index [BMI; weight (kg)/ height $(m)^2$] has been added to the revised 2000 pediatric growth charts and become a useful tool in assessing pediatric obesity (35). A child with a BMI greater than the ninety-fifth percentile for a child of the same age and gender is defined as obese, whereas a child with a BMI greater than the eighty-fifth percentile and less than or equal to the ninety-fifth percentile is considered at risk for obesity.

Reduction of body fat through diet and exercise is an effective way to reduce BP (36–38). Strategies for weight reduction should include counseling regarding the benefits of healthy eating habits and less sedentary lifestyles. In addition, population-based approaches should be initiated, as even small reductions in the percentage of obese patients would significantly lower the incidence of adult cardiovascular disease. In addition, Rocchini (30) has outlined a treatment plan for obese children that recognizes the importance of family participation in an exercise program (Fig. 62.1). The clinician should stress that weight loss is important in obese children, not only to reduce BP, but also to decrease the risk of other obesity-associated complications, including type II diabetes, obstructive sleep apnea, orthopedic complications, cholelithiasis, hepatic steatosis, pseudotumor cerebri, polycystic ovary disease, and psychological consequences, including depression and behavioral problems.

Exercise

There is abundant evidence that regular exercise of mild to moderate intensity lowers BP in both children and adults (39–41). In addition, interventional trials have shown that regular exercise can lead to regression of left ventricular hypertrophy, a

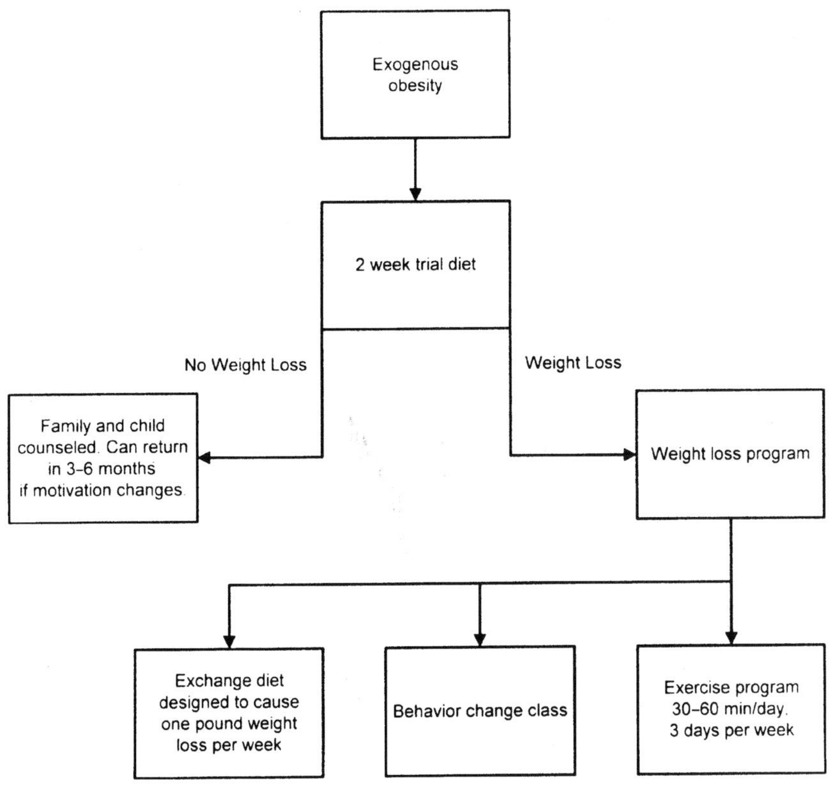

FIGURE 62.1. Suggested treatment plan for obese children. [From Rocchini AP. Adolescent obesity and hypertension. *Pediatr Clin North Am* 1993;40(1):81–92, with permission.]

finding that is recognized as an independent risk factor for cardiovascular disease (42,43). The underlying mechanisms by which exercise reduces BP are not well understood. Exercise may reduce BP by leading to weight loss, but there is general agreement that additional independent mechanisms exist. These mechanisms may include decreased sympathetic tone, decreased insulin resistance, altered baroreceptor responsiveness, increased endorphin production, decreased plasma volume, improved endothelial function, and decreased systemic vascular resistance (44).

Aerobic (dynamic) exercise involves repetitive low resistance movements over a long period of time, usually more than 10 minutes. Aerobic activities include walking, running, swimming, soccer, and basketball. These activities increase cardiac output and mean BP, but they may decrease or only slightly increase diastolic BP and decrease peripheral vascular resistance. Aerobic exercise can be characterized as low intensity [35 to 59% of age-predicted maximal heart rate (PMHR)], moderate intensity (60–79% of PMHR), and high intensity (80% or higher of PMHR). *Anaerobic* (also known as *isometric* or *static*) exercise involves high resistance, low repetition movements over short periods of time (1 to 3 minutes). These activities, which include weight lifting, are characterized by increases in both systolic and diastolic BPs, increased peripheral vascular resistance, and increased cardiac output.

Regular aerobic exercise is strongly recommended as a lifestyle modification for children and adults with hypertension (1,45). Although some studies have shown BP benefits of isometric exercise (46,47), the American College of Sports Medicine does not recommend it as the only form of exercise for hypertensive patients (48).

Clinicians should advise children and adolescents with hypertension or high-normal BP to adopt an active lifestyle with regular aerobic exercise. Unfortunately, in the twenty-first century, physical activity has diminished significantly in children and adolescents, particularly adolescent girls. In all parts of the world, automobiles have replaced walking, and sedentary entertainment exceeds active leisurely pursuits (49). Clinicians should assess the amount of time spent in sedentary leisure activities (television viewing, video games) versus the amount of time spent in organized sports, outdoor play, and physical education classes. Parents should be advised to set time limits for sedentary activities and to schedule a daily time for physical activity. Optimally, all children and adolescents should participate in regular (4 to 5 times/week) activities that involve low to moderate intensity aerobic exercise to maintain optimal cardiovascular health (50).

Media reports of sudden death in competitive athletes have created unwarranted fear in active children and adolescents with hypertension. The largest theoretic risk occurs for those patients with extreme hypertension who choose to participate in weight and power lifting, bodybuilding, and strength training. To date, no episodes of sudden death in children or adolescents during exercise have been attributed to hypertension alone. The American Academy of Pediatrics Committee on Sports Medicine and Fitness recommends that the presence of significant hypertension in the absence of target organ damage or concomitant heart disease should not limit a person's eligibility for competitive athletics (51). Children and adolescents with severe hypertension should be restricted from competitive sports and highly static (isometric) activities until their hypertension is under adequate control and they have no evidence of target organ damage.

Hyperlipidemia

Hyperlipidemia, in particular elevated low-density lipoprotein cholesterol, is recognized as the primary target for risk factor modification in adults to prevent cardiovascular disease (52). Although routine lipid screening is recommended for all adults older than 20 years, routine screening for hyperlipidemia is not recommended in the general pediatric population. The National Cholesterol Education Program of the National Institutes of Health's National Heart, Lung, and Blood Institute National Cholesterol Education Program suggests selective screening of children whose parents or grandparents have a history of atherosclerotic disease or hyperlipidemia, as well as those children with additional risk factors, including hypertension, obesity, and smoking (53).

Because of the combined risks of hyperlipidemia and hypertension, we recommend measurement of fasting lipid profiles in all children and adolescents with hypertension. Initial treatment for children and adolescents found to have lipid abnormalities (hypertriglyceridemia, elevated low-density lipoprotein cholesterol, decreased high-density lipoprotein cholesterol) should include the American Heart Association Step I diet, regular aerobic exercise, and weight loss. Children whose lipid profiles do not improve using this approach should be changed to the American Heart Association Step II diet. Although their use is limited in the pediatric population, lipid-lowering medications may be considered in children refractory to dietary and lifestyle modification, particularly those with familial dyslipidemias or medical conditions that result in altered lipid profiles, such as nephrotic syndrome, end-stage renal disease, or renal transplantation.

Tobacco Use

Cigarette smoking remains a significant problem in adolescents. Sixty-four percent of surveyed U.S. high school students report lifetime smoking (any previous use of cigarettes), 28.5% report current smoking (smoking on 1 or more of the 30 days preceding the survey), and 13.8% report current frequent smoking (smoking on 20 or more of the 30 days preceding the survey) (54). Although these percentages suggest a continued problem with tobacco, the data actually demonstrate a steady decline in tobacco use since 1999, possibly related to national smoking prevention campaigns, increased school-based efforts to prevent tobacco use, and a 70% increase in the retail price of cigarettes between 1997 and 2001. Tobacco use was highest among white adolescents, followed by Hispanic and African American adolescents. The putative causes of adolescent smoking include high levels of stress in individuals with deficient coping resources, peer pressure, and social factors, as well as neurochemical dependence on nicotine (55).

All children and adolescents, particularly those with hypertension, should receive preventative counseling on the health dangers of initiating tobacco use. Hypertensive adolescents who are currently smokers should be strongly urged to discontinue all tobacco use. Smoking cessation programs in adolescents have had varied success in the face of peer pressure, family influences, and social forces but should nevertheless be part of any treatment plan for hypertension.

PHARMACOLOGIC TREATMENT OF HYPERTENSION

Although nonpharmacologic therapies may be effective in reducing BP in children and adolescents with essential hypertension, antihypertensive medications are usually necessary in patients with secondary hypertension or target organ involvement. Pharmacologic therapy is also important in hypertensive patients unwilling to make lifestyle changes. Therapies most likely to be effective are those with simple dosing regimens and minimal side effects.

Pharmacologic treatment of hypertension in children is limited by a lack of controlled clinical trials to assess safety and efficacy, as well as the absence of age-specific pharmacokinetic data for most agents. Many of the reports are limited by retrospective design, small sample size, and absence of a control group. Most pediatric dosing regimens have been simply extrapolated from adult data. As a result, the U.S. Food and Drug Modernization Act of 1997 now grants patent exclusivity to pharmaceutical companies that conducted pediatric safety and efficacy studies. This has led to an increasing number of appropriate pediatric studies (56).

The following sections review the major classes of antihypertensive medications found to be useful in children and adolescents and discusses specific use in hypertensive emergencies, essential hypertension, hypertensive athletes, neonatal hypertension, and chronic kidney disease. Dosing guidelines are based on either specific pediatric data or "best practice" guidelines used by most pediatric nephrologists and cardiologists.

Angiotensin-Converting Enzyme Inhibitors

Angiotensin-converting enzyme (ACE) inhibitors are widely used in the management of both essential and secondary hypertension in pediatric patients. ACE inhibitors prevent the conversion of angiotensin I to angiotensin II (AII), reducing AII-induced vasoconstriction and aldosterone release. In addition, ACE inhibitors indirectly reduce BP by their effects on vasopressin, atrial natriuretic factor, prostaglandins, and sympathetic nervous system activity. Finally, ACE inhibitors inhibit kininase II, which may reduce BP by increasing circulating levels of vasodilatory bradykinins.

Captopril and enalapril were the first ACE inhibitors to be widely used in children (57,58). Because of its relatively short half-life and the ability to carefully titrate dosages by grinding tablets into a powder, captopril is widely used in neonates and in younger children. Dosing every 6 to 8 hours usually results in stable BP control, although some patients may be successfully treated with twice-daily dosing. For older patients, the longer half-life and consequent once- or twice-daily dosing regimens of enalapril favor its use. Pharmacokinetic data have recently been generated for infants and children treated with enalapril (59). The only currently available intravenous ACE inhibitor with established pediatric use is enalaprilat (60). This agent should be used with great caution, as it has been associated with prolonged hypotension and oliguric acute renal failure, particularly in neonates.

Newer ACE inhibitors, formulated primarily to reduce cost, dosing frequency, and side effects, include benazepril, fosinopril, lisinopril, quinapril, and ramipril. Pharmacokinetic and pharmacodynamic studies are currently underway to determine optimal pediatric dosing recommendations for most of these agents. Fixed-dose combinations of ACE inhibitors with diuretics or calcium-channel blockers (CCBs) are now reaching the market. Although these medications may prove to offer improvements over current therapies, there is no pediatric literature to recommend their use at this time. Currently available ACE inhibitors and recommended dosages are listed in Table 62.1.

The side effects of ACE inhibitors in children do not differ from those seen in adults. Renal impairment, hyperkalemia, neutropenia, anemia, dry cough, and angioedema have all been reported in children. Adverse effects on renal function are seen primarily in patients with preexisting renal insufficiency [glomerular filtration rate (GFR) less than 30% of normal], bilateral renal artery stenosis, and renal artery stenosis in a solitary or transplanted kidney. Decreased renal function in patients with the previously mentioned conditions occurs when AII-mediated efferent arteriolar vasoconstriction, necessary for maintenance of glomerular filtration, is reversed by ACE inhibition. The resulting acute renal failure is reversible once ACE inhibitors are discontinued.

Hyperkalemia may be related to medication-induced acute renal failure but may also be seen in patients with relatively normal renal function because of diminished aldosterone levels. Many clinicians periodically measure blood urea nitrogen, creatinine, and electrolytes beginning 1 week after starting ACE inhibitors and after increases in dosage.

TABLE 62.1. SUGGESTED DOSAGES OF ANGIOTENSIN-CONVERTING ENZYME INHIBITORS

Drug	Infant/child	Adult
Benazepril[a]	?	10–80 mg/d PO (QD or ÷BID)
Captopril[b]	1–6 mg/kg/d (÷BID-QID)	12.5–450 mg PO (÷ TID)
Enalapril[c]	0.1–0.5 mg/kg/d (QD or ÷BID)	2.5–40 mg/d PO (QD or ÷BID)
Enalaprilat[d]	5-10 μg/kg/dose IV q8–24h	1.25 mg IV q6h
Fosinopril[e]	?	10–40 mg/d PO (QD or ÷BID)
Lisinopril[f]	?	5–40 mg/d PO (QD)
Quinapril[g]	?	10–80 mg/d PO (QD)
Ramipril[h]	?	1.25–20 mg/d PO (QD or ÷BID)

?, Dosages for these age groups have not been established; ÷, divided.
[a]Available as Lotensin, 5-, 10-, 20-, and 40-mg tablets.
[b]Available as Capoten, 12.5-, 25-, 50-, and 100-mg tablets.
[c]Available as Vasotec or generic enalapril, 2.5-, 5-, 10-, and 20-mg tablets.
[d]Available as 1.25 mg/mL in 1- and 2-mL vials.
[e]Available as Monopril, 10-, 20-, and 40-mg tablets.
[f]Available as Prinivil or Zestril, 2.5-, 5-, 10-, 20-, and 40-mg tablets.
[g]Available as Accupril, 5-, 10-, 20-, and 40-mg tablets.
[h]Available as Altace, 1.25-, 2.5-, 5-, and 10-mg tablets.

Dosage reduction is indicated in the presence of hyperkalemia or a rising serum creatinine. Although hematologic complications are rare and reversible with drug discontinuation, it is prudent to periodically obtain complete blood counts in patients treated with ACE inhibitors.

The inhibition of kininase and accumulation of bradykinin produce several side effects in patients treated with ACE inhibitors. A small but significant number of patients treated with captopril (1 to 5%) report a persistent, nonproductive cough. The incidence of this side effect appears to be less frequent in patients treated with newer ACE inhibitors. The cough is not dose-related and improves when medication is stopped. It is important to ask about cough when monitoring for side effects, because parents and patients may often attribute it to other causes (reactive airway disease, upper respiratory infection). Angioedema and anaphylactoid reactions are less common (0.1%) but serious side effects of ACE inhibitors.

ACE inhibitors are contraindicated during pregnancy. Maternal use of ACE inhibitors during the second and third trimesters of pregnancy has been associated with oligohydramnios, profound fetal hypotension, reversible or irreversible neonatal renal failure, hypocalvaria, and neonatal death (61,62). ACE inhibitors are also contraindicated in patients with bilateral renal artery stenosis, renal artery stenosis in a solitary kidney, and acute renal failure. The need for frequent monitoring of serum creatinine and potassium values also limits their usefulness in patients with chronic renal insufficiency with a GFR of less than 30% of normal.

ACE inhibitors have been shown to have both renoprotective and cardioprotective properties, making them particularly attractive therapeutic agents for patients with chronic hypertension (63–66). The renoprotective properties of ACE inhibitors are most likely due to reduction in AII, which has been implicated as a central effector in the progression of chronic renal injury (63). Several clinical trials have demonstrated that treatment with ACE inhibitors retards the progression of chronic renal disease in both diabetic and nondiabetic nephropathy (64–66). In addition, the HOPE (*H*eart *O*utcomes *P*revention *E*valuation) trial recently demonstrated that treatment with ramipril significantly reduced cardiovascular morbidity and mortality in adult patients with cardiovascular disease (67). These additional beneficial effects of ACE inhibitors add significantly to their value as first-line antihypertensive medications.

TABLE 62.2. SUGGESTED DOSAGES OF ANGIOTENSIN II RECEPTOR ANTAGONISTS

Drug	Infant/child	Adult
Candesartan[a]	?	8–32 mg PO QD
Eprosartan[b]	?	400–800 mg/d PO (QD or ÷BID)
Irbesartan[c]	?	150–300 mg/d PO (QD)
Losartan[d]	?	25–100 mg/d PO (QD or ÷BID)
Telmisartan[e]	?	40–80 mg/d PO (QD)
Valsartan[f]	?	80–320 mg/d PO (QD)

?, Dosages for these age groups have not been established; ÷, divided.
[a]Available as Atacand, 4-, 8-, 16-, and 32-mg tablets.
[b]Available as Teveten, 400- and 600-mg tablets.
[c]Available as Avapro, 75-, 150-, and 300-mg tablets.
[d]Available as Cozaar, 25-, 50-, and 100-mg tablets.
[e]Available as Micardis, 40- and 80-mg tablets.
[f]Available as Diovan, 80-, 160-, and 320-mg tablets.

Angiotensin II Receptor Antagonists

AII receptor antagonists are relatively new agents in the treatment of pediatric hypertension. AII receptor antagonists block the binding of AII to the AT-1 subtype of the AII receptors in blood vessels and other tissues (68). This blockade reduces BP by inhibiting AII-induced vasoconstriction and aldosterone release.

Although AII receptor antagonists are similar to ACE inhibitors in their blockade of AII, there are several major differences that differentiate these two classes of drugs. Because AII receptor antagonists act directly at the AII receptor site, they completely block the effect of AII, including AII formed by ACE-independent pathways such as trypsin, cathepsin, and heart chymase. ACE inhibitors, on the other hand, block only the AII formed by ACE-mediated conversion from angiotensin I. Unlike ACE inhibitors, AII receptor antagonists have minimal effect on bradykinin metabolism. Finally, AII receptor antagonists, but not ACE inhibitors, lead to an exaggerated stimulation of the AT-2 subtype of the AII receptor, which may promote apoptosis and decrease fibrosis (69), possibly reducing renal scarring and cardiac hypertrophy.

Losartan was the first AII receptor antagonist approved for the oral treatment of hypertension in adults and now is increasingly used in the pediatric population (70). Irbesartan, valsartan, candesartan, and telmisartan are additional long-acting AII receptor antagonists that have been approved for the treatment of hypertension and offer the benefit of once-daily dosing (71). Pharmacokinetic and pharmacodynamic studies are currently underway to determine optimal pediatric dosing guidelines for losartan, irbesartan, and valsartan. Currently available AII receptor antagonists and recommended dosages are listed in Table 62.2.

AII receptor antagonists are generally well tolerated, with a favorable side effect profile. Adverse effects on renal function may occur, particularly in patients with preexisting renal insufficiency, bilateral renal artery stenosis, or renal artery stenosis in a solitary or transplant kidney. Hyperkalemia may be related to medication-induced renal insufficiency but also may be seen in patients with normal kidney function as a result of aldosterone inhibition.

Although cough and angioedema occur in patients treated with AII receptor antagonists (72,73), they are observed less frequently than in patients treated with ACE inhibitors. The difference in the frequency of these side effects is most likely due to the difference in effect on bradykinin metabolism between the two drug classes. AII receptor antagonists are contraindicated in pregnancy, as they have been associated with hypocalvaria, oligohydramnios, and fetal death (74).

Several recent large trials have demonstrated that, like ACE inhibitors, AII receptor antagonists exert renoprotective effects in patients with diabetic nephropathy (75–77). In addition, AII receptor antagonists appear to have cardioprotective effects (78–80). The additional renal and cardioprotective effects of AII receptor antagonists make them attractive as therapeutic agents for patients with chronic hypertension and cardiovascular and/or renal disease.

Because AII receptor antagonists and ACE inhibitors suppress the renin-angiotensin system by different mechanisms, they can be used together. Combination has been proven to be safe and more effective at reducing BP (81) and proteinuria (82) than single-drug therapy.

Vasopeptidase Inhibitors

Vasopeptidase inhibitors are a new class of cardiovascular drugs that may become useful in the treatment of pediatric hypertension in the future (83). Vasopeptidase inhibitors simultaneously inhibit ACE and *neutral endopeptidase* (NEP), a metalloproteinase enzyme found principally in the brush-border membrane of renal tubules. The mechanism of action of vasopeptidase inhibitors includes the previously described effects of ACE inhibition, such as reduction in AII-mediated vasoconstriction, reduction in aldosterone synthesis, and increase in circulating bradykinins. In addition, vasopeptidase inhibitors block the effect of NEP, which catalyzes the breakdown of a variety of vasodilatory peptides, including atrial natriuretic peptide, brain natriuretic peptide, C-type natriuretic peptide, adrenomedullin, urodilatin, and bradykinin.

The vasopeptidase inhibitor at the most advanced stage of clinical development is omapatrilat. Several studies have demonstrated favorable antihypertensive effects when compared to lisinopril (84) and amlodipine (85). A large, international, placebo-controlled trial is currently assessing the effects of omapatrilat on survival and cardiovascular outcomes in elderly patients with systolic hypertension (86). Additional vasopeptidase inhibitors under early clinical development include sampatrilat, gemopatrilat, and fasidotrilat.

Flushing, transient facial redness, and dizziness have also been noted in patients treated with omapatrilat. Like ACE inhibitors, omapatrilat has been reported to cause cough and angioneurotic edema, most likely related to its inhibitory effect on bradykinin metabolism. Because ACE inhibition and NEP inhibition both produce increases in bradykinin levels, these side effects potentially may occur more frequently in patients treated with vasopeptidase inhibitors than in patients treated with ACE inhibitors. The full safety profile of vasopeptidase inhibitors remains to be determined with wider clinical development.

Calcium-Channel Blockers

CCBs are among the most commonly used antihypertensive agents in children. CCBs act as direct vasodilators by inhibiting vascular smooth muscle contraction by interfering with cellular calcium influx (87). The relative affinities of the different types of CCBs for different types of contractile tissues (vascular smooth muscle, myocardium) determine their antihypertensive efficacy and their side effect profiles. The three major classes are dihydropyridines (amlodipine, felodipine, isradipine, nicardipine, nifedipine), phenylalkylamines (verapamil), and benzothiazepines (diltiazem). Because of their relative selectivity for arteriolar smooth muscle, the dihydropyridines (particularly amlodipine and nifedipine) are the most widely used CCBs in pediatric hypertension. Because the nondihydropyridines also exert significant effects on cardiac conduction and contractility, their role in pediatric hypertension is not well defined.

One of the primary benefits of CCBs is the availability of long-acting preparations that permit once- or twice-daily administration (88). Although sustained release nifedipine (Procardia XL) was commonly used in the past, its usefulness in smaller children and infants was limited by the ability of the child to swallow the commercially available capsules and tolerate the minimum dosage available. As of 1999, amlodipine became a popular choice, as its long-acting effect is related to the drug's chemical structure rather than a slow-release pill formulation (89,90). Amlodipine tablets may be crushed and/or made into a suspension, extending the drug's usefulness to small children and infants.

TABLE 62.3. SUGGESTED DOSAGES OF CALCIUM CHANNEL BLOCKERS

Drug	Infant/child	Adult
Amlodipine[a]	0.1–0.6 mg/kg/d (÷QD-BID)	2.5–20 mg/d PO (QD)
Diltiazem[b]	1.5–2.0 mg/kg/d (÷TID)	120–360 mg/d PO (QD or ÷BID)
Felodipine[c]	0.1 mg/kg/d (÷QID-BID)	2.5–10 mg PO (QD)
Isradipine[d]	0.05–0.15 mg/kg/dose (TID-QID)	2.5–20 mg/d PO (QD)
Nicardipine[e] (IV)	0.5–5.0 μg/kg/min	5–15 mg/h
Nicardipine[f] (oral)	?	60–120 mg/d PO (BID)
Nifedipine[g] (extended-release)	0.25–3.0 mg/kg/d (QD or ÷BID)	30–120 mg/d PO (QD or ÷BID)
Verapamil[h]	3–8 mg/kg/d (÷TID)	120–480 mg/d PO (QD or ÷BID)

?, Dosages for these age groups have not been established; ÷, divided.
[a]Available as Norvasc, 2.5-, 5.0-, and 10.0-mg tablets.
[b]Available as Cardizem-SR, 60-, 90-, and 120-mg sustained-release capsules (dosed BID), and available as Cardizem-CD, 120-, 180-, 240-, 300-, and 360-mg extended-release capsules (dosed QD).
[c]Available as Plendil, 2.5-, 5.0-, and 10.0-mg extended-release capsules.
[d]Available as Dynacirc, 2.5- and 5.0-mg capsules, which may be made into an extemporaneous suspension stable up to 30 days.
[e]Available as Nicardipine injection, 2.5 mg/mL.
[f]Available as Cardene-SR, 30-, 45-, and 60-mg capsules.
[g]Available as Procardia XL, Adalat-CC, or Nifedipine-ER, 30-, 60-, and 90-mg sustained-release tablets. Also available as Procardia and Adalat, 10- and 20-mg liquid-filled capsules. Liquid may be aspirated from the capsule with a syringe, with a concentration of 10-mg/0.34 mL, although the accuracy of dosing is not consistent. See text for concerns about the use of rapid-acting nifedipine.
[h]Available as Calan-SR, 40-, 80-, and 120-mg capsules.

In contrast to adults, nondihydropyridines (verapamil and diltiazem) are not commonly used for treatment of hypertension in children. Nondihydropyridines are contraindicated in neonates and in patients with left ventricular dysfunction, sick sinus syndrome, second- or third-degree atrioventricular block, and atrial flutter or fibrillation. Currently available CCBs and recommended dosages are listed in Table 62.3.

Nicardipine is the only CCB available in intravenous form and may have an emerging role in the emergency department and intensive care setting for treatment of hypertensive emergencies. Rapid, safe, and effective reductions in BP have been achieved with continuous infusions of 0.5 to 5.0 μg/kg/min in children and neonates, providing an alternative to nitroprusside or intravenous labetalol (91,92).

CCBs are generally well tolerated, with a low incidence of significant side effects. No routine monitoring of blood work is recommended. Headache, flushing, dizziness, and tachycardia may be seen with immediate release CCB formulations as a result of acute vasodilation. Lower extremity edema and erythema may be seen with higher doses of long-acting CCB preparations as a result of a direct effect on local vasculature and not fluid overload. Gingival hyperplasia may occur and may be even more significant when CCBs are administered in conjunction with cyclosporine in transplant patients (93).

In adult patients, short-acting CCBs have been associated with adverse cardiovascular and neurologic sequelae, including myocardial infarction, stroke, and syncope (94). Therefore, their use in the management of acute hypertension in adults has been significantly curtailed. The safety of short-acting CCBs in children is less well defined. Although several surveys and studies suggest that CCBs are safe in the pediatric population (95,96), serious adverse events have been temporally linked to the administration of short-acting nifedipine (97–99). Some clinicians have replaced short-acting nifedipine with isradipine (0.05 to 0.15 mg/kg/dose), which offers a more gradual reduction in BP, theoretically lowering the risk of adverse events associated with abrupt decreases in BP.

CCBs appear to have some immediate and long-term renoprotective properties that have led to widespread use among renal transplant recipients. CCBs decrease mesangial cell proliferation and dilate the afferent arteriole, increasing renal blood flow and GFR. In the long-term, verapamil reduces proteinuria in patients with diabetic nephropathy; however, this beneficial effect does not appear to be uniform among all CCBs.

β-Adrenergic Antagonists

β-Adrenergic antagonists (beta-blockers) were among the first and most widely used antihypertensive medications in children. Several mechanisms for their antihypertensive effect have been proposed, including decreased cardiac output, decreased peripheral vascular resistance, inhibition of renin secretion, decreased circulating plasma volume, and inhibition of central nervous system (CNS) sympathetic activity. The relative importance of each of these mechanisms is unclear and may depend on the specific β-adrenergic agent used.

Characteristics that distinguish one β-adrenergic antagonist from another include differences in cardioselectivity, intrinsic sympathomimetic activity due to partial β-agonist activity, degree of hydrophilicity and lipophilicity, and α-adrenergic antagonism. Use of the prototypic β-adrenergic antagonist, propranolol, is limited by its lack of selectivity for cardiovascular β_1-receptors. Because of propranolol's effects on peripheral β_2-receptors, including bronchoconstriction, impaired glucose tolerance, and altered lipid profiles, drugs with relative cardioselectivity were developed such as atenolol and metoprolol. Intrinsic sympathomimetic activity is another characteristic that is variable among β-adrenergic antagonists. This characteristic may benefit some patients by moderating negative inotropy, bradycardia, peripheral vasoconstriction, and dyslipidemia. Many patients treated with β-adrenergic antagonists experience significant CNS side effects that are minimized by altering the hydrophilicity/lipophilicity of the drug that limits CNS absorption.

Labetalol is a β-adrenergic antagonist with peripheral α-adrenergic antagonism that produces vasodilatation of peripheral vasculature, providing a synergistic antihypertensive effect. Labetalol is not cardioselective and does not have intrinsic sympathomimetic activity. Labetalol can be given safely in children and is an effective agent when administered intravenously for the treatment of hypertensive emergencies (100).

Other cardioselective β-adrenergic antagonists without intrinsic sympathomimetic activity that have been used safely in children include atenolol and metoprolol (101). Esmolol is a short-acting intravenous β-adrenergic antagonist that has been used successfully in children with hypertension after cardiac surgery (102). A randomized double-blind, placebo-controlled trial of the combination drug bisoprolol fumarate, a selective β_1-adrenergic antagonist, and hydrochlorothiazide has recently been shown to have modest effects on lowering BP in hypertensive children precluding its use as a first-line agent (103).

The most common side effects of β-adrenergic antagonists include (a) cardiovascular—bradycardia, fluid retention; (b) CNS—light-headedness, ataxia, dizziness, syncope, sleepiness, irritability, hearing and visual disturbances, vivid dreams/nightmares, weakness, fatigue, depression; (c) gastrointestinal—nausea, diarrhea, cramping, constipation; (d) hematologic—eosinophilia, leukopenia, thrombocytopenia; (e) genitourinary—impotence; and (f) metabolic—delayed recognition of the clinical symptoms of hypoglycemia, blunted recovery from hypoglycemia in insulin-dependent diabetics. β-Adrenergic antagonists that are nonselective or lacking sympathomimetic activity are more likely to result in increased serum triglyceride levels and reduced levels of high-density lipoproteins. β-Adrenergic antagonists are contraindicated in patients with asthma, insulin-dependent diabetes mellitus, Raynaud's phenomenon, congestive heart failure, and atrioventricular conduction disturbances other than first-degree heart block.

No direct comparisons of β-adrenergic antagonists with diuretics, CCBs, or ACE inhibitors as first-line pediatric antihypertensives have been performed. As a result, clinical practice and experience, rather than direct comparison, have relegated β-adrenergic antagonists to second or third choices for the pharmacologic treatment of essential hypertension in children. Nonetheless, β-adrenergic antagonists may be particularly useful when combined with vasodilators that produce reflex tachycardia or in patients for whom ACE inhibitors are contraindicated. Currently available β-adrenergic antagonists and recommended dosages are listed in Table 62.4.

Diuretics

Despite increasing use of ACE inhibitors and CCBs as first-line pediatric antihypertensive medications, diuretics remain

TABLE 62.4. SUGGESTED DOSAGES OF β-ADRENERGIC ANTAGONISTS

Drug	Infant/child	Adult
Atenolol[a]	1–3 mg/kg/d (÷QD, BID)	25–100 mg/d PO (QD or ÷BID)
Bisoprolol[b]	?	2.5–20 mg/d PO (QD)
Labetalol[c]	1–40 mg/kg/d (÷ BID, TID)	200–2400 mg/d PO (÷BID) (usual regimen 400–1200 mg/d)
Metoprolol[d]	?	Short acting: 100–450 mg/d PO (QD or ÷BID) Extended release: 50–400 mg PO (QD)
Nadolol[e]	?	20–320 mg/d PO (QD)
Pindolol[f]	?	10–60 mg/d PO (÷BID, TID)
Propanolol[g]	0.5–8.0 mg/kg/d (÷BID, QID)	80–480 mg/d PO (÷BID)

?, Dosages for these age groups have not been established; ÷, divided.
[a]Available as tablets: 25 mg, 50 mg 100 mg.
[b]Adjust dose in renal failure.
[c]Contains α_1 blocking activity. Available as tablets: 100 mg, 200 mg, 300 mg. Available as suspension: 10 mg/mL.
[d]Available as short-acting tablets: 50 mg, 200 mg. Available as extended release tablets: 47.5 mg, 95 mg, 195 mg.
[e]Adjust dose in renal failure. Available as tablets: 20 mg, 40 mg, 80 mg, 120 mg, 160 mg.
[f]Contains intrinsic sympathomimetic activity. Available as tablets: 5 mg, 10 mg.
[g]Available as short-activity tablets: 10 mg, 20 mg, 40 mg, 60 mg, 80 mg, 90 mg. Available as extended-release tablets: 60 mg, 80 mg, 120 mg, 160 mg. Available as suspension: 20 mg/5 mL, 40 mg/5 mL, and 80 mg/mL.

important adjunctive agents. Diuretics are commonly prescribed because of their long history of safety in children, their low cost, and their effectiveness in most types of pediatric hypertension. They remain the standard by which newer medications are compared.

All diuretics act by blocking solute reabsorption in the nephron, resulting in increased distal delivery of solute, increased urine flow, and ultimately decreased intravascular volume. Some diuretics may also act directly on the peripheral vasculature as vasodilators. The different classes of diuretics are defined by their primary site of action in the nephron (104). Diuretics are secreted by organic acid transporters in the proximal tubule (105). Their secretion may be inhibited in the presence of metabolic acidosis, retained organic anions, or urates.

Quinazolones act by blocking sodium reabsorption in the proximal and distal convoluted tubules. Metolazone, the most commonly used quinazolone, is a long-acting diuretic, which results in the excretion of 5–8% of the filtered sodium load. Although rarely used alone, quinazolones may be used concurrently with diuretics acting at the loop of Henle to increase solute delivery to the distal nephron.

Loop diuretics act primarily in the thick ascending limb of the loop of Henle by binding to the bumetanide-sensitive cotransporter-1 or $Na^+/K^+/2Cl$ cotransporter resulting in the excretion of water, sodium, potassium, chloride, magnesium, calcium, and phosphate. Common loop diuretics include furosemide, bumetanide, and ethacrynic acid. Loop diuretics are potent and effective when rapid diuresis is needed. Unlike thiazides, loop diuretics remain effective in patients with chronic renal insufficiency with GFR between 10 and 30 mL/min. Loop diuretics increase urinary calcium excretion, which may lead to nephrocalcinosis with extended use. Ototoxicity can be seen with higher dosages or when used with other ototoxic agents such as gentamicin. Loop diuretics and thiazides should be used with caution in neonates, because they displace bilirubin from albumin, which increases the risk of hyperbilirubinemia.

Thiazide diuretics, such as chlorothiazide, chlorthalidone, and hydrochlorothiazide, inhibit sodium chloride reabsorption in the distal convoluted tubule by binding to the thiazide-sensitive transporter or Na^+/Cl cotransporter. The safety and effectiveness of thiazides for the treatment of hypertension is well established in the pediatric population. Compared with loop diuretics, thiazides provide a more sustained but less vigorous diuresis. Also, they cause an increase in calcium absorption in the distal nephron, which may lead to hypercalcemia. Thiazide diuretics are relatively ineffective in patients with GFRs less than 30 mL/min.

Potassium-sparing diuretics such as spironolactone, triamterene, and amiloride, inhibit sodium reabsorption in the collecting duct. Spironolactone is a competitive inhibitor of aldosterone, whereas amiloride and triamterene act more directly by inhibiting sodium transport mechanisms. Although these medications have limited antihypertensive effects compared with loop or thiazide diuretics, spironolactone is useful in patients with states of elevated plasma aldosterone such as primary hyperaldosteronism, congestive heart failure, and liver disease, whereas amiloride is valuable in patients with glucocorticoid-remediable hypertension. Potassium-sparing diuretics can also minimize urinary potassium losses and obviate the need for potassium supplementation in patients treated with thiazide or loop diuretics.

SR121463, a selective vasopressin V_2 receptor antagonist, represents a new class of drugs called *aquaretics*, which induce free-water excretion without sodium or potassium urinary excretion (106). This drug has the potential to be therapeutically effective in dilutional causes of hyponatremia such as syndrome of inappropriate antidiuretic hormone, congestive heart failure, liver cirrhosis, and nephrotic syndrome. The potential use of this new class of drugs in patients with hypertension remains to be determined.

Dosages of commonly used diuretics are listed in Table 62.5. Although diuretics are effective, well tolerated, and inexpensive, they have largely been replaced as first-line agents for pediatric hypertension. Potential reasons for the decreasing use of diuretics include the need for monitoring potassium, magnesium, and uric acid levels in patients taking loop and thiazide diuretics; an increased risk of nephrocalcinosis in patients receiving loop diuretics; and adverse

TABLE 62.5. SUGGESTED DOSAGES OF COMMONLY USED DIURETICS

Drug	Infant/child	Adult
Amiloride[a]	?	5–20 mg PO QD
Bumetanide[b]	?	0.5–4.0 mg/d PO (QD or ÷BID)
Chlorothiazide[c]	10–20 mg/kg/d (maximum dose = 375 mg if age <2 yr, 1000 mg if age 2–12 yr)	125–500 mg/d PO (÷BID) (maximum dose, 2000 mg/d)
Furosemide[d]	0.5–4.0 mg/kg/d (QD or ÷BID)	Same as children
Hydrochlorothiazide[e]	1–3 mg/kg/d (÷BID) (maximum dose = 37.5 mg if age <2 yr, 100 mg if age 2–12 yr)	25–200 mg/d PO (QD or ÷BID)
Metolazone[f]	0.2–0.4 mg/kg/d	2.5–20 mg/d PO (QD or ÷BID)
Spironolactone[g]	3.3 mg/kg/d	25–200 mg/d PO (QD or ÷BID)

?, Dosages for these age groups have not been established; ÷, divided.
[a]Available as 5-mg tablets.
[b]Available as tablets: 0.5 mg, 1 mg, and 2 mg.
[c]Available as tablets: 250 mg, 500 mg. Available as oral suspension: 250 mg/5 mL.
[d]Available as tablets: 20 mg, 40 mg, and 80 mg. Available as oral solution: 10 mg/mL.
[e]Available as tablets: 12.5 mg, 25 mg, 50 mg, 100 mg. Available as oral solution: 50 mg/5 mL.
[f]Available as tablets: 2.5 mg, 5 mg, and 10 mg. Available as oral suspension: 0.1 mg/mL.
[g]Available as tablets: 25 mg, 50 mg, and 100 mg. Tablet may be pulverized and administered in oral suspension with cherry syrup.

lipid profiles and hyperglycemia in patients taking thiazide diuretics. However, diuretics remain useful in hypertensive patients with hypervolemia.

Direct Vasodilators

Although direct vasodilators work through different mechanisms, they are discussed together because they are used similarly in hypertensive emergencies or in cases refractory to more commonly used antihypertensives. Their usefulness as first-line medications for treatment of chronic hypertension is limited by their side effects such as headache, palpitations, tachycardia, flushing, fluid and sodium retention, and exacerbation of symptoms in patients with preexisting coronary or cerebrovascular compromise. These side effects are primarily due to nonspecific vasodilation. Concurrent use of β-adrenergic antagonists or diuretics is often effective in reducing these side effects while controlling refractory hypertension in patients treated with vasodilators as first-line antihypertensive agents.

Hydralazine

Although the mechanism of action of hydralazine is not well understood, it affects primarily arteriolar resistance vessels and, to a lesser effect, venous capacitance vessels. Hydralazine has been used extensively in pediatrics, particularly in neonates, because it is available in oral suspension, oral tablets, and intravenous preparations (107,108). Frequent side effects include reflex tachycardia, palpitations, dizziness, headaches, and gastrointestinal discomfort. With long-term use, up to 10% of patients treated with hydralazine may develop a hypersensitivity reaction that resembles systemic lupus erythematosus characterized by fever, arthralgia, splenomegaly, lymphadenopathy, myalgia, chest pain, and edema. These physical findings may be accompanied by the development of antinuclear antibodies and anti–single-stranded DNA antibodies. This syndrome resolves when hydralazine is stopped. As a result of these side effects, hydralazine use is restricted primarily to hypertensive neonates requiring parenteral antihypertensive therapy. Hydralazine is contraindicated in patients with dissecting aortic aneurysm, rheumatic valve disease, cerebrovascular disease, and coronary vascular disease. Pediatric oral dosing of hydralazine is 0.25 to 1 mg/kg per dose two to four times daily up to a maximum dose of 7.5 mg/kg/day or 25 mg per dose. Hydralazine is available as 10-, 25-, 50-, and 100-mg tablets and as a 0.2-mg/mL oral liquid. The intravenous dosage is 0.1 to 0.6 mg/kg per dose every 4 to 6 hours up to a maximum dose of 20 mg in children and 40 mg in adolescents or adults.

Minoxidil

Minoxidil acts on arteriolar resistance vessels to exert a potent antihypertensive effect possibly through inhibition of vascular smooth muscle potassium channels or through modulation of cyclic adenosine monophosphate or guanosine monophosphate–mediated vasodilation. Because of significant side effects, pediatric use usually is limited to hypertensive patients with renal disease who require multiple drugs for BP control (109,110). Fluid and sodium retention is a major problem often leading to congestive heart failure or pericardial effusion. Therefore, patients treated with minoxidil require diuretic therapy, a sodium-restricted diet, and careful attention to fluid balance. In addition, minoxidil therapy is usually associated with tachycardia, which often requires concurrent use of a β-adrenergic antagonist. Other side effects of minoxidil include hirsutism and exacerbation of angina pectoris. Contraindications to the use of minoxidil include pheochromocytoma, congestive heart failure, and recent myocardial infarction. Minoxidil is available as 2.5- and 10.0-mg tablets. Pediatric dosing is 0.2 to 5.0 mg/kg/day given once or twice daily. The maximum dose is 50 mg/day in children and 100 mg/day in adolescents and adults. Therapy is commonly initiated while patients are hospitalized to observe for evidence of congestive heart failure, pericardial effusion, or other evidence of fluid overload.

Nitroprusside

Sodium nitroprusside is a nitric oxide donor that exerts a vasodilatory effect on both venous capacitance and arteriolar resistance vessels. Also, this drug increases renal blood flow with minimal effects on cardiac output. Sodium nitroprusside is administered as a continuous infusion and remains one of the drugs of choice for management of hypertensive emergencies. Because of its immediate onset of action and rapid metabolism, use of nitroprusside requires continuous BP monitoring, preferably with an indwelling arterial catheter. Significant side effects limit the duration of treatment. Prolonged use of nitroprusside results in the production of toxic metabolites, cyanide and thiocyanate, which accumulate in patients with renal and hepatic insufficiency. In patients requiring treatment for longer than 24 hours, concurrent infusion with thiosulfate (10:1 ratio of nitroprusside to thiosulfate) is recommended to eliminate the possibility of cyanide toxicity (111). Clinical signs of cyanide/thiocyanate toxicity include anxiety, headache, dizziness, confusion, jaw stiffness, seizures, metabolic acidosis, and hypoxemia. Other side effects include hypotension, methemoglobinemia, hypothyroidism, tinnitus, visual disturbances, and tachyphylaxis. Nitroprusside is contraindicated in patients with increased intracranial pressure and should be used with caution in patients with coarctation of the aorta. Use of nitroprusside in children is associated with fewer episodes of ischemic events secondary to hypotension compared to bolus injections of diazoxide (112).

Dosing should begin at 0.3 μg/kg/min, and is titrated to a maximum dose of 8 μg/kg/min to achieve the desired BP. Adequate control is usually obtained with a dose of 2 to 4 μg/kg/min. If BP is not adequately controlled at a nitroprusside dose of 8 μg/kg/min, additional medications may be needed such as labetalol, calcium-channel antagonists, or diuretics.

Diazoxide

Diazoxide is a powerful arteriolar vasodilator, although its mechanism of action is not well defined. This drug is available only for parenteral use because of its rapid but unpredictable onset of action. The side effects of diazoxide are similar to other systemic vasodilators. In addition, hyperglycemia, hyperuricemia, nausea, vomiting, constipation, hypertrichosis, skin rash, fever, leukopenia, and thrombocytopenia may occur. Although slow continuous infusion of diazoxide appears to be tolerated as well as nitroprusside (113), diazoxide has been replaced by better-tolerated and safer medications, including intravenous labetalol and nicardipine in the setting of hypertensive emergencies (112). Diazoxide is contraindicated in patients with intracerebral hemorrhage, dissecting aortic aneurysm, acute myocardial infarction, and aortic coarctation. The recommended dosage is 1 to 2 mg/kg per dose via intravenous infusion over 5 to 10 minutes and may be given every 10 to 15 minutes until a response is seen. The maximal daily dose is 10 mg/kg.

Fenoldopam

Fenoldopam mesylate is the first selective peripheral dopamine-1 receptor agonist approved for parenteral use in the treatment of hypertensive emergencies and severe perioperative hypertension (114). This drug is a direct-acting vasodilator that binds to the postsynaptic dopamine-1 receptors in renal, coronary, cerebral, and splanchnic vasculature resulting in dilation of arterial and venous capacitance vessels. Activation of dopamine-1 receptors in the renal vasculature and renal tubular epithelium leads to natriuresis, diuresis, mesangial cell relaxation, and an increase in renal blood flow and GFR.

Due to its poor oral bioavailability, fenoldopam is used exclusively as a parenteral agent to achieve rapid reduction of BP. Peak effects on BP occur within 5 to 15 minutes and steady-state serum levels are achieved by 30 to 60 minutes. In a prospective, randomized, multicenter trial of 153 adults with diastolic BPs exceeding 120 mm Hg, fenoldopam was as effective as sodium nitroprusside in reducing BP (115). A dose-dependent reduction in BP was noted up to 48 hours without evidence of tolerance or rebound on withdrawal. In a study of 107 adults with hypertensive emergencies, fenoldopam was safe and effective in lowering BP using a dose-titration regimen (116). Fenoldopam has also been effective in treating perioperative hypertension, including elevations in BP after coronary bypass surgery. Fenoldopam has been used successfully without significant side effects in four children between the ages 6 weeks and 11 years for treatment of hypertensive emergencies/urgencies and hypertension associated with extracorporeal membrane oxygenation (117). Also, fenoldopam has been used to achieve controlled hypotension intraoperatively (117).

Although fenoldopam has the potential to function as a renal protective agent, no conclusive evidence exists to support this pharmacologic effect (114). Uncontrolled studies with small numbers of patients suggest that fenoldopam may be beneficial in protecting against radiographic contrast nephropathy after percutaneous coronary intervention or angiography and renal dysfunction associated with aortic cross-clamping for repair of aneurysms (118,119).

Adverse effects of fenoldopam include headache, flushing, dizziness, and tachycardia or bradycardia. These effects usually occur within the initial 24 hours of treatment and are self-limited. A more serious adverse effect of fenoldopam is increased intraocular pressure. Therefore, this drug should be used cautiously in patients with glaucoma or high intraocular pressure. Nonspecific T-wave flattening may also be seen. Clinically significant drug interactions have not been reported. Advantages of fenoldopam over nitroprusside include absence of thiocyanate toxicity, lack of degradation on exposure to light, and lack of rebound hypertension after discontinuation.

The recommended initial infusion rate of fenoldopam should be 0.1 μg/kg/min with increments of 0.05 to 0.10 μg/kg/min every 15 to 20 minutes, up to a maximal dose of 5 μg/kg/min. The infusion period should not exceed 48 hours owing to the presence of tolerance beyond this time period. Fenoldopam can be slowly tapered or abruptly discontinued without complications. Oral antihypertensive therapy may be initiated at any time during the fenoldopam infusion.

Central Nervous System Sympathetic Inhibitors

CNS sympathetic inhibitors, such as clonidine, methyldopa, guanabenz, and guanfacine, have been used successfully in children for many years. These drugs inhibit sympathetic tone through stimulation of CNS α_2-adrenergic receptors. Unlike β-adrenergic antagonists and diuretics, these drugs exert favorable cardiovascular effects, including decreased left ventricular mass and stable or improved lipid profiles. In addition, they exert no adverse influence on renal hemodynamics or glucose metabolism. Although these drugs are excellent candidates for the treatment of chronic hypertension, unfavorable side effect profiles have relegated these agents to second or third choices in patients requiring multiple drug regimens. Patients often experience dry mouth, depression, sedation, vivid dreams, nightmares, hallucinations, impotence, decreased libido, or ejaculatory difficulty. A particularly worrisome side effect of these drugs is rebound hypertension, which may precipitate a hypertensive emergency or urgency in patients who suddenly discontinue their use. Because of the concern about rebound hypertension, these drugs should not be administered to patients at high risk for noncompliance, such as adolescents, and should be limited to those patients with a clear understanding of this risk.

Clonidine

Most pediatric experience with clonidine arises from use in children treated with this medication for behavioral problems. It is worth remembering that normotensive children treated with clonidine for behavioral modification may experience rebound hypertension if suddenly withdrawn (120). Patients treated with clonidine may experience transient elevations in liver enzymes, muscle or joint pain, weight gain, and rash, in addition to the previously mentioned side effects of central sympatholytic agents. Clonidine is available in 0.1- and 0.2-mg tablets. The oral dosage is 0.05 to 0.3 mg per dose two to three times daily. Clonidine is also available in transdermal patches, Catapres TTS-1, TTS-2, and TTS-3, which are equivalent to daily doses of 0.1, 0.2, and 0.3 mg, respectively. Patches are changed weekly. Steady-state levels are achieved after 48 to 72 hours of initial placement. Many patients prefer the transdermal patch to the tablets because of administration ease, reduced incidence of rebound hypertension, and fewer side effects due to stable steady-state drug levels. Caution should be exercised in patients with significant hirsutism, such as renal transplant recipients on cyclosporine, or patients with excess sweating due to difficulties in maintaining the patch properly applied to the skin surface.

Methyldopa

Methyldopa is one of the few antihypertensive medications with wide experience and proven safety in pregnancy. Unique side effects include a higher incidence of fluid retention and weight gain than that seen with the other sympatholytics, a less favorable effect on lipid profiles, and development of a positive direct Coombs' reaction in approximately 25% of patients. Five percent of patients who develop this reaction may develop hemolytic anemia or hepatitis that resolves after requiring discontinuation. Although patients may develop positive antinuclear antibodies or rheumatoid factor, overt clinical manifestations of autoimmune disease are uncommon. The pediatric dosage of methyldopa is 5 to 20 mg/kg per dose two to three times daily, and it is available as 125-, 250-, and 500-mg tablets and as a 250-mg/5 mL oral suspension. The use of methyldopa is restricted primarily to hypertension associated with pregnancy.

Guanabenz and Guanfacine

Pediatric experience with guanabenz and guanfacine is limited, and neither has demonstrated side effects that differ from those of the class. Guanabenz appears to have the most favorable effect on lipid profiles. Guanfacine has the longest half-life, often permitting once-daily dosing. No pediatric dosing for these medications has been determined. For older adolescents and adults, guanabenz is available in 4- and 8-mg tablets, and dosing is 4 to 16 mg per dose twice daily. Guanfacine is available as 1- and 2-mg tablets, and usual dosing is 1 to 3 mg per dose as a single daily dose.

Miscellaneous Antihypertensive Medications

Prazosin

Prazosin (along with newer agents terazosin, doxazosin, trimazosin, and indoramin) selectively antagonizes peripheral α_1-adrenergic receptors, resulting in dilation of both arteriolar resistance and venous capacitance vessels. Although these drugs cause less reflex tachycardia, renin release, and catecholamine excretion than direct vasodilators, significant postural hypotension may occur. The safety of peripheral α_1-adrenergic receptor antagonists has recently been questioned after the results of an adult study in which doxazosin was associated with a doubling of the risk for heart failure compared to patients on low-dose chlorthalidone (121). Pediatric experience with this class of drug is limited, and pediatric dosing has not been established. However, prazosin may be most effective when used in combination with ACE inhibitors, CCBs, labetalol, or diuretics when triple-drug therapy is needed for control of refractory hypertension. It is available in 1-, 2-, and 5-mg tablets. The usual adult dosing is 1 to 5 mg three times daily.

Phenoxybenzamine and Phentolamine

Phenoxybenzamine and phentolamine are α-adrenergic antagonists used almost exclusively in the treatment of pheochromocytoma. Phenoxybenzamine, which binds irreversibly to α_1- and α_2-adrenergic receptors, reduces BP and diaphoresis

TABLE 62.6. EFFECTS OF ANTIHYPERTENSIVE AGENTS ON A VARIETY OF PHYSIOLOGIC FACTORS

Factors	Diuretics	Beta-blockers Without ISA	Beta-blockers With ISA	CCBs	ACE inhibitors	Central α-agonists	Alpha-blockers	Direct vasodilators	Alpha-beta-blockers (e.g., labetalol)
Hemodynamic effects of antihypertensive drugs									
Systemic vascular resistance	↔ or ↓	↑	↓	↓	↓	↓	↓	↓	↔ or ↓
Cardiac output	↓	↓	↔ or ↓	↔ or ↑	↑	↔	↔ or ↑	↔ or ↑	↔ or ↓
Left ventricular hypertrophy	↔ or ↓	↓	↑	↓	↓	↓	↔ or ↓	↑	↓
Vascular smooth muscle	↔ or ↑	↔ or ↓	↑	↓	↓	↓	↔ or ↓	↑	↓
Exercise	↔ or ↓	↓	↔ or ↓	↔	↔	↔	↔	↔	↔ or ↓
Intravascular volume	↓	↔ or ↑	↔	↓	↓	↔ or ↓	↔ or ↑	↑	↔ or ↑
Cerebral blood flow	↓	↓	↔	↑	↑	↔ or ↑	↑	↑	↔ or ↓
Heart rate	↑	↑	↔ or ↑	↔ or ↑	↑	↔	↔ or ↑	↑	↔ or ↓
Stroke volume	↓	↓	↔ or ↓	↔ or ↑	↑	↔	↔ or ↑	↑	↔ or ↓
Effects of antihypertensive drugs on coronary heart disease									
Insulin resistance	↑	↑	↑	↔	↓	↔	↓	↔	↔ or ↑
Uric acid	↑	↑	↑	↔	↓	↔	↔	↔	↑
Dyslipidemia	↑	↑	↔	↓	↔	↓	↓	↔	↔
Fibrinogen	↑	?	?	?	?	?	?	?	?
Thrombogenic potential	↑	?	?	↓	?	?	?	?	?
Antiatherogenic potential	No	Yes	?	Yes	Yes	?	?	?	?
Blood viscosity	↑	↔	↔	?	↔	↓	↓	↓	↔
Potassium/magnesium	↓	↔	↔	↔	↔	↔	↔	↔	↔
Glucose intolerance	↑	↑	↑	↔	↓	↔	↓	↔	↑
Effects of antihypertensive drugs on renal function									
Glomerular filtration rate	↓	NC ↓	NC	↑	↑	NC ↑	NC ↑	NC ↑	NC
Renal plasma flow	↓	NC ↓	NC	↑	↑	NC	NC ↑	NC ↑	NC
Renal blood flow	↓	NC ↓	NC ↑	NC ↑	NC ↑	NC ↑	NC ↑	NC ↑	NC ↑
Renal vascular resistance	↑	NC ↑	NC	↓	↓	?	↓	↑	?
Intraglomerular capillary pressure	↑	?	?	NC ↓	↓	?	?	↑	?
Urinary albumin	↑	?	?	NC ↓	↓	?	?	↑	?
Plasma volume	↓	NC	NC	NC ↑	NC ↓	NC ↓	NC ↑	↑	NC ↑
Urinary sodium	↑	NC	NC	↑	↑	NC ↑	NC ↓	↓	NC
Urinary potassium	↑	NC	NC	NC ↑	↓	NC	NC	NC	NC

ACE, angiotensin-converting enzyme; CCBs, calcium-channel blockers; ISA, intrinsic sympathomimetic activity; NC, no change; NC ↑, tends to increase; NC ↓, tends to decrease; ↔, these agents have no effect on this parameter; ↓, decreased by these agents; ↑, increased by these agents; ?, effects of these agents are uncertain or unknown.
From Miller K. Effects of antihypertensive agents on a variety of physiological factors. Pharmacological management of hypertension in paediatric patients: a comprehensive review of the efficacy, safety, and dosage guidelines of the available agents. *Drugs* 1994;48(6):868–887, with permission.

without blockade of β-adrenergic receptors. Phentolamine, which is a competitive antagonist of α_1- and α_2-adrenergic receptors, may be administered parenterally during a pheochromocytoma-associated hypertensive crisis or in the perioperative period during tumor excision. The onset of action is immediate with a duration of action of 30 to 60 minutes. Side effects related to α-blockade include tachycardia, postural hypotension, nasal congestion, fatigue, miosis, gastrointestinal irritation, drowsiness, and inhibition of ejaculation.

Phenoxybenzamine is available as a 10-mg capsule and is used as chronic therapy at an initial dose of 2.5 mg twice daily. Dosage adjustments are made every 4 to 7 days up to a maximum dose of 20 to 25 mg/day in young children and 40 to 100 mg/day in adolescents and adults in two to three divided

TABLE 62.7. POTENTIAL SIDE EFFECTS OF ANTIHYPERTENSIVE DRUGS

Diuretics	β-Adrenergic antagonists	Vasodilators	Central sympatholytics	ACE inhibitors/ AT-II receptor antagonists	CCB
Hypokalemia	Bradycardia	Headache	Sedation	Renal insufficiency	Peripheral edema
Volume depletion	Syncope	Palpitations	Dry mouth	Hyperkalemia	Dizziness
Hypotension	Vision disturbances	Tachycardia	Depression	DO NOT USE in bilateral renal artery stenosis	Light-headedness
Hypomagnesemia	Vivid dreams	Flushing	Vivid dreams	Neutropenia	Headache
Hypercalcemia	Weakness	Fluid/sodium retention	Nightmares	Hypotension	Flushing
Glucose intolerance[a]	Fatigue		Hallucination	Rash	Weakness
Hyperlipidemia[a]	Depression		Rebound hypertension	Dry cough	Transient hypotension
Hyperuricemia	Bronchospasm		Impotence[b]	Bronchospasm	Constipation
Gastric irritation	Impotence[b]			Angioedema	Gingival hyperplasia[c]
Cramping	Hyperlipidemia			Fetopathy	Tachycardia/bradycardia
Impotence[b]					

ACE, angiotensin-converting enzyme; CCB, calcium-channel blocker.
[a]Only with thiazides diuretics.
[b]Patient incidence <2%.
[c]Especially when used with calcineurin inhibitors.

doses. Phentolamine may be administered parenterally at a dose of 0.05 to 0.10 mg/kg per dose up to a maximum of 5 mg 1 to 2 hours before surgery and repeated every 2 to 4 hours as needed.

Combination Antihypertensive Products

A number of fixed-dosage combination products have been designed for the treatment of hypertension. The proposed benefit of such products is the synergistic effect of antihypertensive agents with differing mechanisms of action and the minimization of side effects with the use of lower dosages of different drug classes. Examples of categories of combination drugs include β-adrenergic antagonist-diuretic, ACE-inhibitor–diuretic, AII receptor antagonist-diuretic, diuretic-diuretic, and CCB-ACE inhibitor. Only one study to date has evaluated the pharmacokinetics and efficacy of a combination drug (bisoprolol-hydrochlorothiazide; Ziac) in the pediatric population (103). The use of combination drugs in children and adolescents remains limited at present but may increase over time as pediatricians gain familiarity with these agents.

Comparison of Antihypertensive Medications

In the selection process of an antihypertensive agent, the physician must appraise the physiologic effects on systemic hemody-

TABLE 62.8. COMPARISON OF POTENTIAL FIRST-LINE MEDICATIONS USED IN TREATMENT OF HYPERTENSION

	ACE inhibitors /AR-II B	Calcium-channel blockers	β-Adrenergic antagonists	Diuretics
Lipid metabolism	0	+	–	–
Glucose metabolism	0	0	–	–
Left ventricular hypertrophy	+	+	0	–
Exercise tolerance	0	0	–	0
Electrolytes	0	0	0	–
Glomerular filtration rate	+	+	0/+	–
Renal blood flow	+	+	0/+	–
Proteinuria	+	0/+	0	–
Renoprotective	+	+	0	0
Sedation/depression	0	0	–	0

+, favorable effect; –, unfavorable effect; 0, neutral or unknown effect; ACE, angiotensin-converting enzyme.
Modified from Feld LG, Waz WR. Pharmacologic therapy of hypertension. In: Feld LG, ed. *Hypertension in children*. Boston: Butterworth–Heinemann, 1997:133–178.

TABLE 62.9. CONTRAINDICATIONS TO THE USE OF VARIOUS ANTIHYPERTENSIVE MEDICATIONS

Angiotensin-converting enzyme inhibitors/angiotensin-II receptor blockers
Pregnancy
Bilateral renal artery stenosis (or renal artery stenosis in solitary kidney)
Acute renal failure
Calcium-channel blockers
Left ventricular dysfunction (verapamil and diltiazem)
Sick sinus syndrome, second- or third-degree atrioventricular block (verapamil and diltiazem)
Atrial flutter or atrial fibrillation (verapamil and diltiazem)
Neonates (verapamil and diltiazem)
β-Adrenergic antagonists
Asthma
Insulin-dependent diabetes mellitus
Raynaud's phenomenon
Congestive heart failure
Atrioventricular conduction disturbances (other than first-degree heart block)
Diuretics
Thiazides in neonates with hyperbilirubinemia
Loop diuretics in patients with hypercalciuria/nephrocalcinosis
Potassium-sparing in patients with hyperkalemia, diabetic nephropathy
Direct vasodilators
Hydralazine—coronary artery disease, cerebrovascular disease, mitral valve disease
Minoxidil—pheochromocytoma, congestive heart failure, recent myocardial infarction
Diazoxide—cerebral hemorrhage, dissecting aortic aneurysm, acute myocardial infarction, aortic coarctation
Nitroprusside—coarctation of aorta, increased intracranial pressure
Central sympathetic inhibitors
Clonidine, Guanabenz, Guanfacine—none other than hypersensitivity to drug
Methyldopa—acute/active hepatic disease
Other drugs
Reserpine—mental depression
Prazosin—none other than hypersensitivity to drug

From Feld LG, Waz WR. Pharmacologic therapy of hypertension. In: Feld LG, ed. *Hypertension in children*. Boston: Butterworth–Heinemann, 1997:133–178, with permission.

namics, cardiac and renal function (Table 62.6), potential side effects (Tables 62.7 or 62.8), and cost. Contraindications to the use of various antihypertensive medications is presented in Table 62.9. With attention to these details, the practitioner is able to assess the benefit:risk ratio of any antihypertensive drug.

TREATMENT PLANS FOR SPECIFIC TYPES OF HYPERTENSION

Hypertensive Emergencies

Patients who present with severe hypertension (BP greater than the ninety-ninth percentile for age, height percentile, and gender) or an acute BP elevation require immediate attention if they present with a hypertensive urgency or emergency. A *hypertensive urgency* is a situation in which the possibility exists for progression to a hypertensive emergency requiring a decrease in BP within 12 to 24 hours (112). A hypertensive emergency is defined by elevations in systolic and diastolic BP associated with end-organ injury of the brain, heart, and/or kidneys. Clinical manifestations of hypertensive emergencies include hypertensive encephalopathy, congestive heart failure, pulmonary edema, acute renal failure, stroke, head trauma, myocardial infarction, adrenergic crisis, dissecting aortic aneurysm, or eclampsia. Hypertensive encephalopathy typically presents with a prodrome lasting for at least 12 to 48 hours consisting of headache, altered mental status, visual impairment, seizures, or focal neurologic deficits. The symptoms of hypertensive encephalopathy appear to be a result of disturbances in cerebral autoregulation, which lead to altered cerebral blood flow and perfusion pressure.

An algorithm for treating hypertensive emergencies is shown in Figure 62.2. This algorithm incorporates a 25% reduction in BP during the initial hour after presentation with a hypertensive emergency and recommends not achieving a mean arterial pressure below the ninety-fifth percentile for age and height until 24 to 48 hours after presentation. Excessive reductions in mean arterial pressure must be avoided, because this can lead to diminished cerebral blood flow and syncope that may progress to infarction of the cerebral cortex, brainstem, or retina.

Essential Hypertension

Although hypertensive children younger than 10 years are more likely to have a secondary cause for their hypertension, older children and adolescents most commonly have no identifiable etiology and are considered to have essential hypertension. All children with essential hypertension should be counseled on the nonpharmacologic lifestyle interventions previously described. Antihypertensive therapy in children with essential hypertension should be aimed at reducing BP below the ninetieth percentile and preventing or reversing target organ damage. Figure 62.3 provides a general approach to the treatment of a child with essential hypertension. The choice of antihypertensive drug should take into account the potential for adverse side effects, including hyperlipidemia, electrolyte abnormalities, glucose intolerance, sedation, and behavioral changes (Table 62.7 or 62.8), as well as contraindications of various medications (Table 62.9).

Children without target organ damage and BP between the ninety-fifth and ninety-ninth percentile should be placed on a nonpharmacologic regimen for 3 months before considering the addition of antihypertensive medication. Children with target organ damage and/or severe hypertension (BP greater than ninety-ninth percentile) should receive both nonpharmacologic interventions and antihypertensive medications.

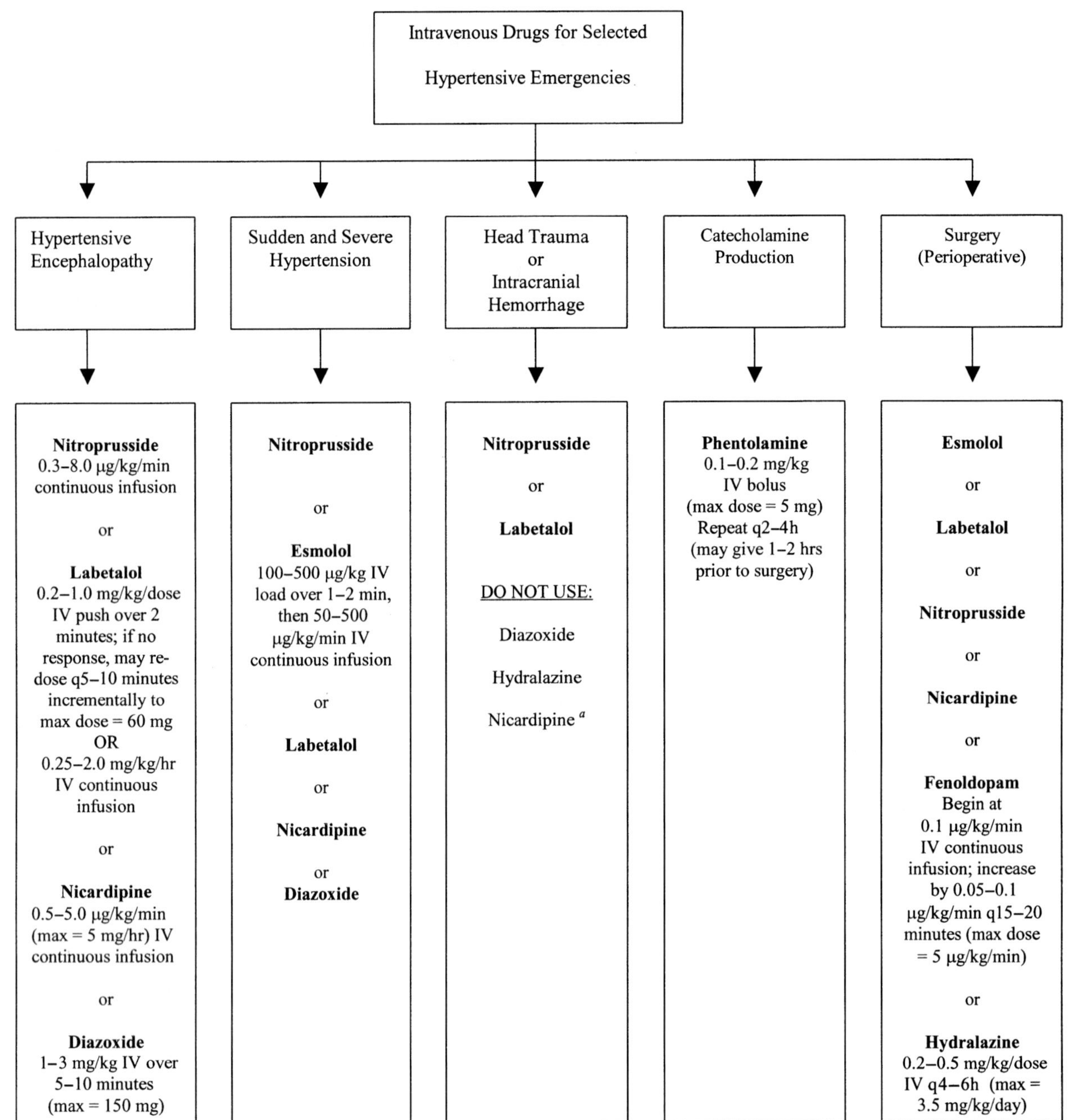

FIGURE 62.2. Suggested treatment options for hypertensive emergencies. [a]Use with extreme caution in children with space-occupying intracranial lesions and severe atelectasis or pneumonia. (Modified from Feld LG, Waz WR. Pharmacologic therapy of hypertension. In: Feld LG, ed. *Hypertension in children*. Boston: Butterworth–Heinemann, 1997:133–178.)

Hypertensive Athlete

Treatment of the hypertensive athlete presents unique issues because of the potential for medication-related side effects. Impairment in athletic performance may result from the use of β-adrenergic antagonists, which reduce cardiac contractility and cardiac output, or diuretics, which reduce intravascular volume. As a result, ACE inhibitors or dihydropyridine CCBs are the preferred agents in hypertensive athletes requiring pharmacologic therapy, because they effectively lower BP without significant adverse effects on cardiac output, cardiac contractility, or intravascular volume that might impair athletic performance (122). Recommendations by the American Academy of Pediatrics Committee on Sports Medicine and Fitness for hypertensive pediatric patients wishing to participate in competitive sports are summarized in Table 62.10 (51).

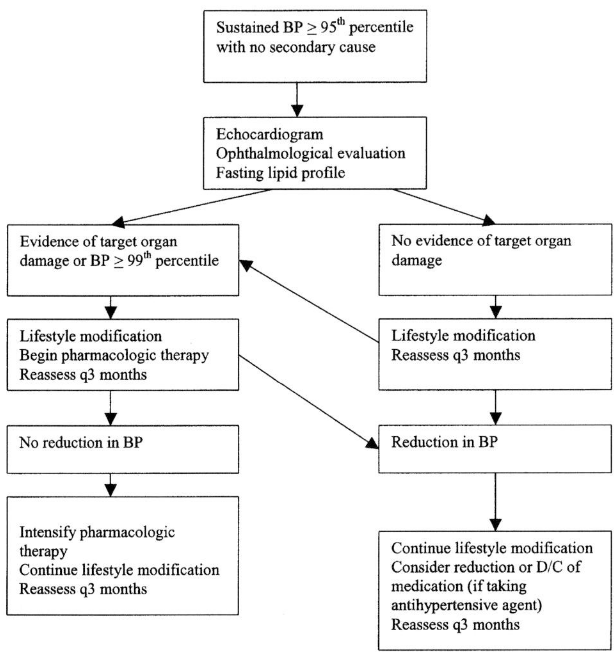

FIGURE 62.3. Suggested treatment of essential hypertension. BP, blood pressure; D/C, discontinue.

Neonatal Hypertension

Hypertension is seen in approximately 2% of term or preterm neonates (123). Premature infants; infants with acute renal failure, respiratory distress, or severe infection; and those with a family history of congenital renal or heart disease are at greatest risk for developing hypertension. Causes of neonatal hypertension are reviewed in Chapter 60. The choice of pharmacologic therapy of neonatal hypertension depends on the underlying cause and severity of the hypertension. Hypertension in some neonates resolves once the underlying cause is properly treated, such as obstructive uropathy, hypervolemia associated with acute renal failure, or coarctation of the aorta. The initial approach to treatment of neonates with hypertension due to thromboembolism from an umbilical artery catheter is catheter removal. Antihypertensive medication may be required for 1 to 2 years in these patients. Medications used in neonatal hypertension are listed in Table 62.11.

TABLE 62.10. RECOMMENDATIONS FOR PARTICIPATION IN COMPETITIVE SPORTS FOR THE HYPERTENSIVE PEDIATRIC PATIENT

1. Patients with mild to moderate hypertension (90th to 99th percentile for age and height; 1996 Task Force) and no evidence of end-organ involvement or other cardiovascular disease can participate in all competitive sports. Blood pressures should be monitored every 2 mo to monitor the impact of participation.
2. Patients with severe hypertension (>99th percentile for age and height; 1996 Task Force) but with no evidence of end-organ involvement or other cardiovascular disease should be restricted, particularly from high-static sports, until blood pressure is controlled. They may then participate as in number 1. For those patients with severe hypertension and evidence of end-organ involvement, the same recommendation may be followed as long as sports participation does not exacerbate the end-organ involvement or place the patient at risk.
3. Patients with hypertension and coexisting cardiovascular disease may require additional restrictions based on the nature of the cardiovascular disease and associated risks.

From American Academy of Pediatrics Committee on Sports Medicine and Fitness. Athletic participation by children and adolescents who have systemic hypertension. *Pediatrics* 1997;99:637–638, with permission.

TABLE 62.11. PHARMACOLOGIC THERAPY OF NEONATAL HYPERTENSION

Angiotensin-converting enzyme inhibitors	
Captopril	0.05–2.0 mg/kg/d PO (÷q6–12h)
Enalaprilat	5–10 μg/kg/dose IV (q8–24h)
Beta-adrenergic antagonists	
Esmolol	100–500 μg/kg IV load over 1–2 min, then 50–500 μg/kg/min IV continuous infusion
Labetalol	1–20 mg/kg/d PO (÷q8–12h) 0.2–1.0 mg/kg/dose IV bolus or 0.25–3.0 mg/kg/h IV continuous infusion
Propranolol	0.5–5.0 mg/kg/d PO (÷q6–12h)
Calcium-channel antagonists	
Amlodipine	0.1–0.6 mg/kg/d PO (÷q12h)
Isradipine	0.05–0.15 mg/kg/dose PO (q6h)
Nifedipine	0.125–0.5 mg/kg/dose PO (÷q6–8h) (max dose = 3 mg/kg/d)
Nicardipine	0.5–3.0 μg/kg/min IV continuous infusion
Diuretics	
Bumetanide	??
Chlorothiazide	20–30 mg/kg/d PO (÷q12h)
Furosemide	0.5–4.0 mg/kg/dose IV/PO (÷q6–8h) (max dose = 4 mg/kg/d)
Hydrochlorothiazide	2–3 mg/kg/day PO (÷q12h)
Vasodilator	
Hydralazine	0.1–0.6 mg/kg/dose IM/IV q4–6h OR 0.75–5.0 μg/kg/min IV continuous infusion
Sodium nitroprusside	0.5–8.0 μg/kg/min IV continuous infusion

÷, divided.

Chronic Kidney Disease

BP control is particularly important in the CKD population, as studies in adult and animal models of kidney disease demonstrate that effective BP control and reduction of proteinuria delay the progression of chronic renal insufficiency (63–66,75–77). Although nonpharmacologic therapies remain a critical component of the therapeutic strategy to properly control BP in patients with CKD, these lifestyle

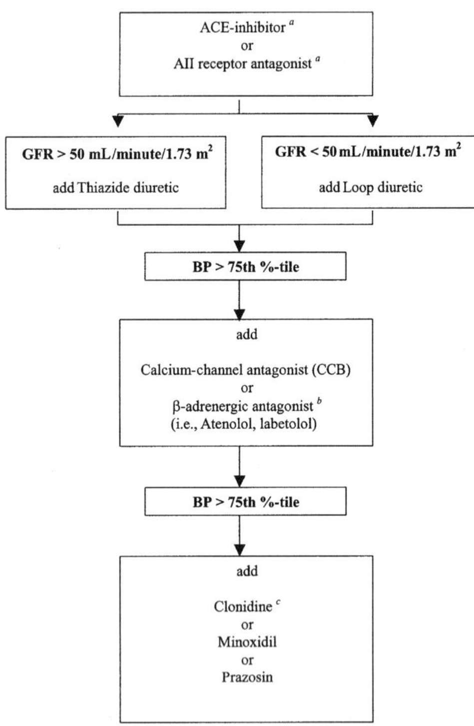

FIGURE 62.4. Suggested pharmacologic approach for treatment of hypertension in chronic kidney disease. Blood pressure (BP) goal should be below the 75th percentile for age, height, and gender. [a]Use with caution in patients with glomerular filtration rate (GFR) <50 mL/min/1.73 m^2 and discontinue if hyperkalemia or acute decrease in GFR. [b]Avoid if patient on β-adrenergic antagonist. [c]May contribute to the development of hyperkalemia. ACE, angiotensin-converting enzyme; CCB, calcium-channel blocker. (Modified from Feld LG, Lieberman E, Mendoza SA, et al. Management of hypertension in the child with chronic renal insufficiency. *J Pediatr* 1996;129:S18.)

modifications are rarely sufficient in achieving BP measurements below the seventy-fifth percentile.

The pharmacologic approach for treating hypertension is different in patients with CKD, compared to those with essential hypertension (124). Guidelines derived from the National Kidney Foundation Hypertension and Diabetes Executive Committees Working Group (125) for treating hypertension in CKD patients are presented in Figure 62.4. Recommended dosage adjustments for antihypertensive agents in children with CKD are outlined in Table 62.12.

The hallmark of therapy in hypertensive CKD patients with a mild impairment in kidney function is blockade of the renin-angiotensin-aldosterone pathway with ACE inhibitors or AII receptor antagonists. Importantly, dose adjustments of antihypertensive medications should not be made more frequently than every 2 to 3 days when maximal dosage effect may occur. Addition of a second antihypertensive agent should not occur until maximum dosage is achieved with the initial drug.

Another important aspect of treating hypertensive CKD patients is sodium restriction and diuretic therapy to reduce the intravascular volume. Mechanisms for loop diuretic resistance in CKD include decreases in loop diuretic basal fractional NaCl reabsorption and proximal tubular secretion. Other factors for loop diuretic resistance include decreased renal clearance and enhanced distal nephron NaCl reabsorption. Strategies to overcome loop diuretic

TABLE 62.12. RECOMMENDED DOSAGE ADJUSTMENTS FOR SELECTED ANTIHYPERTENSIVE DRUGS FOR PATIENTS WITH CHRONIC KIDNEY DISEASE

Drug	Adjustment in CRI	Effect on renin
Diuretics		Increase
Chlorothiazide	Thiazides not effective at GFR <30–40 mL/min/1.73 m^2	
Hydrochlorothiazide		
Furosemide	None	
Bumetanide	Unknown	
Metolazone	Unknown	
β-Adrenergic antagonists		Decrease
Acebutolol	Decrease dose	
Atenolol	Decrease 50% at GFR <50 mL/min/1.73 m^2, give QOD at GFR <10 mL/min/1.73 m^2	
Labetalol	None	
Metoprolol	None	
Propranolol	None	
Vasodilators		Increase
Hydralazine	None	
Minoxidil	None	
Central sympatholytic		Decrease
Clonidine	None	
Angiotensin-converting enzyme inhibitors		Increase
Captopril	Caution with all ACE inhibitors when GFR <50 mL/min/1.73 m^2	
Enalapril		
Lisinopril		
Angiotensin-II receptor antagonists		Increase
Losartan	Caution with all AII receptor blockers when GFR <50 mL/min/1.73 m^2	
Valsartan		
Calcium-channel blockers		None
Nifedipine	May need to limit dose	
Diltiazem	Unknown	
Verapamil	With caution	

AII, angiotensin II; ACE, angiotensin-converting enzyme; CRI, chronic renal insufficiency; GFR, glomerular filtration rate.
Modified from Feld LG, Lieberman E, Mendoza SA, et al. Management of hypertension in the child with chronic renal insufficiency. *J Pediatr* 1996;129:S18.

resistance include maintaining adequate BP and intravascular volume; correction of metabolic acidosis, uremic organic acids, and hyperuricemia; avoiding the use of organic anion medications that compete for the OATs; and addition of thiazides or quinazolones. However, thiazides should be used with caution in patients with mild to moderate renal insufficiency, because they may result in significant reductions of intravascular blood volume leading to hypotension and prerenal azotemia.

REFERENCES

1. National High Blood Pressure Education Program Working Group on Hypertension Control in Children and Adolescents. Update on the 1987 Task Force Report on High Blood Pressure in Children and Adolescents: A Working Group Report from the National High Blood Pressure Education Program. *Pediatrics* 1996;88(4):649–658.
2. Dahl LK. Possible role of salt intake in the development of essential hypertension. In: Cottier P, Bock KD, eds. *Essential hypertension: an international symposium.* Berlin: Springer-Verlag, 1960:53–65.
3. Froment A, Milon H, Gravier C. Relation entre consommation sodee et hypertension arterielle. *Rev Epidemiol Sante Publique* 1979;27:437–454.
4. Cutler JA, Follmann D, Allender PS. Randomized trials of sodium reduction: an overview. *Am J Clin Nutr* 1997;65: 643S–651S.
5. Graudal NA, Galloe AM, Garred P. Effects of sodium restriction on blood pressure, renin, aldosterone, catecholamines, cholesterols, and triglyceride: a meta-analysis. *JAMA* 1998;279:1383–1391.
6. Sacks FM, Svetkey LP, Vollmer WM, et al. Effects on BP of reduced dietary sodium and the Dietary Approaches to Stop Hypertension (DASH) diet. *N Engl J Med* 2001;344:3–10.
7. Johnson RJ, Herrera-Acosta J, Schreiner GF, et al. Subtle acquired renal injury as a mechanism of salt-sensitive hypertension. *N Engl J Med* 2002;346:913–923.
8. Brenner BM, Garcia DL, Anderson S. Glomeruli and blood pressure: less of one, more the other? *Am J Hypertens* 1988; 1:335–347.
9. Lifton R. Molecular genetics of human blood pressure variation. *Science* 1996;272:676–680.
10. Cowley AW, Mattson DL, Lu S, et al. The renal medulla and hypertension. *Hypertension* 1995;25:663–673.
11. Gillum RF, Elmer PJ, Prineas RJ. Changing sodium intake in children: the Minneapolis children's blood pressure study. *Hypertension* 1981;3:698–703.
12. Cooper R, Van Horn L, Liu K, et al. A randomized trial on the effect of decreased dietary sodium intake on blood pressure in adolescents. *J Hypertens* 1984;2:361–366.
13. Grobbee DE, Hofman A, Roelandt JT, et al. Sodium restriction and potassium supplementation in young people with mildly elevated blood pressure. *J Hypertens* 1987;5:115–119.
14. Howe PRC, Cobiac L, Smith RM. Lack of effect of short-term changes in sodium intake on blood pressure in adolescent schoolchildren. *J Hypertens* 1991;9:181–186.
15. Hofman A, Hazebroek A, Valkenburg HA. A randomized trial of sodium intake and blood pressure in newborn infants. *JAMA* 1983;250:370–373.
16. Tucker DT, Smothers M, Lewis C, et al. Effects of decreased dietary salt intake on blood pressure in preschool children. *J Natl Med Assoc* 1983;81:299–302.
17. Miller JZ, Weinberger MH, Daugherty SA, et al. Blood pressure response to dietary sodium restriction in normotensive children. *Am J Clin Nutr* 1988;47:113–119.
18. Krauss RM, Eckel RH, Howard B, et al. AHA Dietary Guidelines. Revision 2000: a statement for healthcare professionals from the Nutrition Committee of the American Heart Association. *Circulation* 2000;102:2284–2299.
19. Rodriguez BL, Labarthe DR, Huang B, et al. Rise of blood pressure with age: new evidence of population differences. *Hypertension* 1994;24:779–785.
20. Coruzzi P, Brambilla L, Brambilla V, et al. Potassium depletion and salt sensitivity in essential hypertension. *J Clin Endocrinol Metab* 2001;86:2857–2862.
21. Whelton PK, He J, Cutler JA, et al. Effects of oral potassium on blood pressure: meta-analysis of randomized controlled clinical trials. *JAMA* 1997;277:1624–1632.
22. Cappuccio FP, Elliott P, Allender PS, et al. Epidemiologic association between dietary calcium intake and blood pressure: a meta-analysis of published data. *Am J Epidemiol* 1995;142:935–945.
23. Allender PS, Cutler JA, Follman D, et al. Dietary calcium and blood pressure: a meta-analysis of randomized clinical trials. *Arch Intern Med* 1996;124:825–831.
24. Harlan WR, Harlac LC. Blood pressure and calcium and magnesium intake. In: Laragh JH, Brenner BM, eds. *Hypertension: pathophysiology, diagnosis, and management,* 2nd ed. New York: Raven Press, 1995:1143–1154.
25. Kawano Y, Matsuoka H, Takishita S, et al. Effects of magnesium supplementation in hypertensive patients: assessment by office, home, and ambulatory blood pressures. *Hypertension* 1998;32:260–265.
26. Yamamoto ME, Applegate WB, Klag MJ, et al. Lack of blood pressure effect with calcium and magnesium supplementation in adults with high-normal blood pressure: results from Phase 1 of the Trials of Hypertension Prevention (TOHP). Trials of Hypertension Prevention (TOHP) Collaborative Research Group. *Ann Epidemiol* 1995;5:96–107.
27. Appel LJ, Moore TJ, Obarzanek E, et al. A clinical trial of the effects of dietary patterns on blood pressure. *N Engl J Med* 1997;336:1117–1124.
28. Ebbeling CB, Pawlak DB, Ludwig DS. Childhood obesity: public health crisis, common sense cure. *Lancet* 2002;473–482.
29. Freedman DS, Dietz WH, Srinivasan SR, et al. The relation of overweight to cardiovascular risk factors among children and adolescents: the Bogalusa Heart Study. *Pediatrics* 1999;103: 1175–1182.
30. Rocchini AP. Obesity hypertension. *Am J Hypertens* 2002; 15:50S–52S.
31. Corry DB, Tuck A. Obesity, hypertension, and sympathetic nervous system activity. *Curr Hypertens Rep* 1999;1:119–126.
32. Masuo K, Mikami H, Itoh M, et al. Sympathetic activity and body mass index contribute to blood pressure levels. *Hypertens Res* 2000;23:303–310.

33. Landsberg L. Hyperinsulinemia: possible role in obesity-induced hypertension. *Hypertension* 1992;19(Suppl I):I61–I66.
34. Tuck MI, Sowers J, Dornfield L, et al. The effect of weight reduction on blood pressure plasma renin activity and plasma aldosterone level in obese patients. *N Engl J Med* 1981;304:930–933.
35. Rosner B, Prineas R, Loggie J, et al. Percentiles for body mass index in US children 5 to 7 years of age. *J Pediatr* 1998;132:211–222.
36. Stevens VJ, Obarzanek E, Cook NR, et al. Long-term weight loss and changes in blood pressure: results of the Trials of Hypertension Prevention, phase II. *Ann Intern Med* 2001;134:1–11.
37. Rocchini AP, Katch V, Anderson J, et al. Blood pressure in obese adolescents: effect of weight loss. *Pediatrics* 1988;82:16–23.
38. Clarke WR, Woolson RF, Lauer RM. Changes in ponderosity and blood pressure in childhood: the Muscatine study. *Am J Epidemiol* 1986;124:195–206.
39. Hansen HS, Froberg K, Hyldebrandt N, et al. A controlled study of eight months of physical training and reduction of blood pressure in children: the Odense schoolchild study. *BMJ* 1991;303:682–685.
40. Alpert BS, Wilmore JH. Physical activity and blood pressure in adolescents. *Pediatr Exercise Sci* 1994;6:361–380.
41. Whelton SP, Chin A, Xin X, et al. Effect of aerobic exercise on blood pressure: a meta-analysis of randomized, controlled trials. *Ann Intern Med* 2002;136:493–503.
42. Hinderliter A, Sherwood A, Gullette ECD, et al. Reduction of left ventricular hypertrophy after exercise and weight loss in overweight patients with mild hypertension. *Arch Intern Med* 2002;162:1333–1339.
43. Kokkinos PF, Narayan P, Colleran JA, et al. Effects of regular exercise on blood pressure and left ventricular hypertrophy in African-American men with severe hypertension. *N Engl J Med* 1995;333:1462–1467.
44. Kokkinos PF, Narayan P, Papademetriou V. Exercise as hypertension therapy. *Cardiol Clin* 2001;19:507–516.
45. The Sixth Report of the Joint National Committee on Prevention, Detection, Evaluation, and Treatment of High Blood Pressure. *Arch Intern Med* 1997;157:2413–2447.
46. Webb DR. Strength training in children and adolescents. *Pediatr Clin North Am* 1990;37:1187–1210.
47. Hagberg JM, Ehsoni AA, Goldring D. Effect of weight training on blood pressure and hemodynamics in hypertensive adolescents. *J Pediatr* 1984;104:147–151.
48. American College of Sports Medicine. Physical activity, physical fitness and hypertension: position stand. *Med Sci Sports Exerc* 1993;25:ix.
49. Kimm SYS, Glynn NW, Kriska AM, et al. Decline in physical activity in black girls and white girls during adolescence. *N Engl J Med* 2002;347:709–715.
50. Williams CL, Hayman LL, Daniels SR, et al. Cardiovascular health in childhood: a statement for health professionals from the Committee on Atherosclerosis, Hypertension, and Obesity in the Young (AHOY) of the Council on Cardiovascular Disease in the Young, American Heart Association. *Circulation* 2002;106:143–160.
51. American Academy of Pediatrics Committee on Sports Medicine and Fitness. Athletic participation by children and adolescents who have systemic hypertension. *Pediatrics* 1997;99:637–638.
52. Executive Summary of the Third Report of the National Cholesterol Education Program (NCEP) Expert Panel on Detection, Evaluation, and Treatment of High Blood Cholesterol in Adults (Adult Treatment Panel III). *JAMA* 2001;285:2486–2509.
53. American Academy of Pediatrics. National Cholesterol Education Program: Report of the Expert Panel on Blood Cholesterol Levels in Children and Adolescents. *Pediatrics* 1992;89(Suppl 3):525–584.
54. Centers for Disease Control and Prevention. Trends in cigarette smoking among high school students—United States, 1991–2001. *MMWR Morb Mortal Wkly Rep* 2002;51:409–412.
55. Pletcher JR, Schwarz DF. Current concepts in adolescent smoking. *Curr Opin Pediatr* 2000;12:444–449.
56. Wolgemuth RL. Realizing the promise of the US Food and Drug Administration Modernization Act. *Clin Ther* 1998;20(Suppl C):C26–C31.
57. Schneeweiss A. Cardiovascular drugs in children. II: angiotensin converting enzyme inhibitors in pediatrics. *Pediatr Cardiol* 1990;11:199–207.
58. O'Dea RF, Mirkin BL, Alward CT, et al. Treatment of neonatal hypertension with captopril. *J Pediatr* 1988;113:403–406.
59. Wells T, Rippley R, Hogg R, et al. The pharmacokinetics of enalapril in children and infants with hypertension. *J Clin Pharmacol* 2001;41:1064–1074.
60. Wells TG, Bunchman TE, Kearns GL. Treatment of neonatal hypertension with enalaprilat. *J Pediatr* 1990;117:664–667.
61. Sedman AB, Kershaw DB, Bunchman TE. Recognition and management of angiotensin converting enzyme inhibitor fetopathy. *Pediatr Nephrol* 1995;9:383–385.
62. Rosenthal T, Oparil S. The effect of antihypertensive drugs on the fetus. *J Hum Hypertens* 2002;16:292–298.
63. Taal MW, Brenner BM. Renoprotective benefits of RAS inhibition: from ACEI to angiotensin II antagonists. *Kidney Int* 2000;57:1803–1817.
64. Lewis EJ, Hunsicker LG, Bain RP, et el. The effect of angiotensin-converting-enzyme inhibition on diabetic nephropathy. *N Engl J Med* 1993;329:1456–1462.
65. The GISEN Group. Randomised placebo-controlled trial of effect of ramipril on decline in glomerular filtration rate and risk of terminal renal failure in proteinuric, non-diabetic nephropathy. *Lancet* 1997;349:1857–1863.
66. Ruggenenti P, Perna A, Gherardi G, et al. Renoprotective properties of ACE-inhibition in non-diabetic nephropathies with non-nephrotic proteinuria. *Lancet* 1999;354:359–364.
67. Yusuf S, Sleight P, Pogue J, et al. Effects of an angiotensin-converting enzyme inhibitor, ramipril, on cardiovascular events in high-risk patients. The Heart Outcomes Prevention Evaluation Study Investigators. *N Engl J Med* 2000;342:145–153.
68. Burnier M, Brunner HR. Angiotensin II receptor antagonists. *Lancet* 2000;355:637–645.
69. Stoll M, Steckelings UM, Paul P, et al. The angiotensin AT2-receptor mediates inhibition of cell proliferation in coronary endothelial cells. *J Clin Invest* 1995; 95:651–657.
70. Conlin PR. Efficacy and safety of angiotensin receptor blockers: a review of losartan in essential hypertension. *Curr Ther Res* 2001;62:79–90.

71. Waeber B. A review of irbesartan in antihypertensive therapy: comparison with other antihypertensive agents. *Curr Ther Res* 2001;62:505–523.
72. Acker G, Greenberg A. Angioedema induced by the angiotensin II blocker losartan. *N Engl J Med* 1995;333:1572.
73. Van Rijnsoever EW, Kwee-Zuiderwijk WJ, Feenstra J. Angioneurotic edema attributed to the use of losartan. *Arch Intern Med* 1998;158:2063–2065.
74. Saji H, Yamanaka M, Hagiwara A, et al. Losartan and fetal toxic effects. *Lancet* 2001;357:363.
75. Brenner BM, Cooper ME, De Zeeuw D, et al. Effects of losartan on renal and cardiovascular outcomes in patients with type 2 diabetes and nephropathy. *N Engl J Med* 2001;345:861–869.
76. Lewis EJ, Hunsicker LG, Clarke WR, et al. Renoprotective effect of the angiotensin-receptor antagonist irbesartan in patients with nephropathy due to type 2 diabetes. *N Engl J Med* 2001;345:851–860.
77. Parving HH, Lehnert H, Brochner-Mortensen J, et al. The effect of irbesartan on the development of diabetic nephropathy in patients with type 2 diabetes. *N Engl J Med* 2001; 345:870–878.
78. Theurmann PA, Kenedi P, Schmidt A, et al. Influence of the angiotensin II antagonist losartan on left ventricular hypertrophy in patients with essential hypertension. *Circulation* 1998;98:2037–2042.
79. Havranek EP, Thomas I, Smith WB, et al. Dose-related beneficial long-term hemodynamic and clinical efficacy of irbesartan in heart failure. *J Am Coll Cardiol* 1999;33:1174–1181.
80. Cohn JN, Tognoni G, for the Valsartan Heart Failure Trial Investigators. A randomized trial of the angiotensin-receptor blocker valsartan in chronic heart failure. *N Engl J Med* 2001;345:1667–1675.
81. Ruilope LM, Aldigier JC, Ponticelli C, et al. Safety of the combination of valsartan and benazepril in patients with chronic renal disease. European Group for the Investigation of Valsartan in Chronic Renal Disease. *J Hypertens* 2000;18:89–95.
82. Russo D, Minutolo R, Pisani A, et al. Coadministration of losartan and enalapril exerts additive antiproteinuria effect in IgA nephropathy. *Am J Kidney Dis* 2001;38:18–25.
83. Weber MA. Vasopeptidase inhibitors. *Lancet* 2001;358:1525–1532.
84. Asmar R, Fredebohm W, Senftleber I, et al. Omapatrilat compared with lisinopril in treatment of hypertension as assessed by ambulatory blood pressure monitoring. *Am J Hypertens* 2000;13:143A.
85. Ruilope LM, Plantini P, Grossman E, et al. Randomized, double-blind comparison of omapatrilat with amlodipine in mild-to-moderate hypertension. *Am J Hypertens* 2000;13(pt 2):134A.
86. Kostis JB, Cobbe S, Johnston C, et al. OPERA Study Group (Omapatrilat in Persons with Enhanced Risk of Atherosclerotic Events). *Am J Hypertens* 2002;15:193–198.
87. Abernethy DR, Schwartz JB. Calcium-antagonist drugs. *N Engl J Med* 1999;314:1447–1457.
88. Flynn JT, Pasko DA. Calcium channel blockers: pharmacology and place in therapy of pediatric hypertension. *Pediatr Nephrol* 2000;15:302–316.
89. Tallian KB, Nahata MC, Turman MA, et al. Efficacy of amlodipine in pediatric patients with hypertension. *Pediatr Nephrol* 1999;13:304–310.
90. Flynn JT, Smoyer WE, Bunchman TE. Treatment of hypertensive children with amlodipine. *Am J Hypertens* 2000; 13:1061–1066.
91. Flynn JT, Mottes TA, Brophy PD, et al. Intravenous nicardipine for treatment of severe hypertension in children. *J Pediatr* 2001;139:38–43.
92. Milou C, Debuche-Benouachkou VD, Semama DS, et al. Intravenous nicardipine as a first-line antihypertensive drug in neonates. *Intensive Care Med* 2000;26:956–958.
93. Miranda J, Brunet L, Roset P, et al. Prevalence and risk of gingival enlargement in patients treated with nifedipine. *J Periodontol* 2001;72:605–611.
94. Grossman E, Messerli FH, Grodzicki T, et al. Should a moratorium be placed on sublingual nifedipine capsules given for hypertensive emergencies and pseudoemergencies? *JAMA* 1996;276:1328–1331.
95. Gauthier B, Trachtman H. Short-acting nifedipine. *Pediatr Nephrol* 1997;11:786–787.
96. Blaszak RT, Savage JA, Ellis EN. The use of short-acting nifedipine in pediatric patients with hypertension. *J Pediatr* 2001;139:34–37.
97. Egger DW, Deming DD, Hamada N, et al. Evaluation of the safety of short-acting nifedipine in children with hypertension. *Pediatr Nephrol* 2002;17:35–40.
98. Leonard MB, Kasner SE, Feldman HI, et al. Adverse neurologic events associated with rebound hypertension after using short-acting nifedipine in childhood hypertension. *Pediatr Emerg Care* 2001;17:435–437.
99. Truttman AC, Zehnder-Schlapback S, Bianchetti MG. A moratorium should be placed on the use of short-acting nifedipine for hypertensive crises. *Pediatr Nephrol* 1998;12:259–261.
100. Bunchman TE, Lynch RE, Wood E. Intravenously administered labetalol for treatment of hypertension in children. *J Pediatr* 1992;120:140–144.
101. Kornbluth A, Frishman WH, Ackerman M. Beta adrenergic blockade in children. *Cardiol Clin North Am* 1987;5:629–649.
102. Wiest DB, Garner SS, Uber WE, et al. Esmolol for the management of pediatric hypertension after cardiac operations. *J Thorac Cardiovasc Surg* 1998;4:890–897.
103. Sorof JM, Cargo P, Graepel J, et al. β-blocker/thiazide combination for treatment of hypertensive children: a randomized double-blind, placebo-controlled trial. *Pediatr Nephrol* 2002;17:345–350.
104. Wells TG. The pharmacology and therapeutics of diuretics in the pediatric patient. *Pediatr Clin North Am* 1990;37:463–504.
105. Sweet DH, Bush KT, Nigam SK. The organic acid transporter family: from physiology to ontogeny and the clinic. *Am J Physiol* 2001;F197–F205.
106. Serradeil-Le GC. An overview of SR121463, a selective non-peptide vasopressin V(2) receptor antagonist. *Cardiovasc Drug Rev* 2001;19:201–2140.
107. Martin GR, Chauvin L, Short BL. Effects of hydralazine on cardiac performance in infants receiving extracorporeal membrane oxygenation. *J Pediatr* 1991;118:944–948.
108. Adelman RD, Merten D, Vogel J, et al. Nonsurgical treatment of renovascular hypertension in the neonate. *Pediatrics* 1978;62:71–76.
109. Puri HC, Maltz HE, Kaiser BA, et al. Severe hypertension in children with renal disease: treatment with minoxidil. *Am J Kidney Dis* 1983;3(1):71–75.

110. Feld LG, Lieberman E, Mendoza SA, et al. Management of hypertension in the child with chronic renal failure. *J Pediatr* 1996;129:S18–S26.
111. Hall VA, Guest JM. Sodium nitroprusside-induced cyanide intoxication and prevention with sodium thiosulfate prophylaxis. *Am J Crit Care* 1992;1:19–25.
112. Fivush B, Neu A, Furth S. Acute hypertensive crises in children: emergencies and urgencies. *Curr Opin Pediatr* 1997;9: 233–236.
113. Thien TA, Huysmans FT, Gerlag PG, et al. Diazoxide infusion in severe hypertension and hypertension crises. *Clin Pharmacol Ther* 1979;35:795–799.
114. Murphy MB, Murray C, Shorten GD. Fenoldopam: a selective peripheral dopamine-receptor agonist for the treatment of severe hypertension. *N Engl J Med* 2001;345:1548–1557.
115. Panacek EA, Bednarczyk EM, Dunbar LM, et al. Randomized, prospective trial of fenoldopam vs sodium nitroprusside in the treatment of acute severe hypertension. *Acad Emerg Med* 1995;2:959–965.
116. Tumlin JA, Dunbar LM, Oparil S, et al. Fenoldopam, a dopamine agonist, for hypertensive emergency: a multicenter randomized trial. *Acad Emerg Med* 2000;7:653–662.
117. Strauser LM, Pruitt RD, Tobias JD. Initial experience with fenoldopam in children. *Am J Ther* 1999;6:283–288.
118. Kini A, Mitre C, Kamran M, et al. Changing trends in incidence and predictors of radiographic contrast nephropathy after percutaneous coronary intervention with use of fenoldopam. *Am J Cardiol* 2002;89:999–1002.
119. Gilbert TB, Hasnain JU, Flinn WR, et al. Fenoldopam infusion associated with preserving renal function after aortic cross-clamping for aneurysm repair. *J Cardiovasc Pharmacol Ther* 2001;6:31–36.
120. Comings DE, Comings BG, Tacket T, et al. The clonidine patch and behavior problems. *J Am Acad Child Adolesc Psychiatry* 1990;29(4):667–668.
121. ALLHAT Collaborative Research Group. Major cardiovascular events in hypertensive patients randomized to doxazosin vs chlorthalidone: the antihypertensive and lipid-lowering treatment to prevent heart attack trial (ALLHAT). *JAMA* 2000;283:1967–1975.
122. Niedfeldt MW. Managing hypertension in athletes and physically active patients. *Am Fam Physician* 2002;66:445–452.
123. Flynn JT. Neonatal hypertension: diagnosis and management. *Pediatr Nephrol* 2000;14:332–341.
124. Feld LG, Lieberman E, Mendoza SA, et al. Management of hypertension in the child with chronic renal failure. *J Pediatr* 1996;129:S18–S26.
125. Bakris GL, Williams M, Dworkin L, et al. Preserving renal function in adults with hypertension and diabetes: a consensus report approach. *Am J Kidney Dis* 1999;36:646–661.

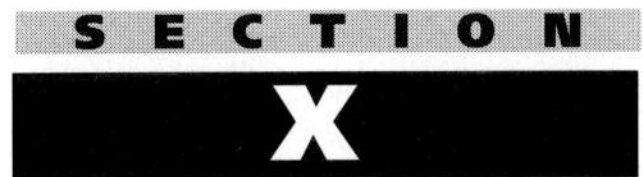

ACUTE RENAL FAILURE

63

PATHOGENESIS OF ACUTE RENAL FAILURE

NORMAN J. SIEGEL
SCOTT K. VAN WHY
PRASAD DEVARAJAN

PATHOPHYSIOLOGIC MECHANISMS

Acute renal failure (ARF) is defined as the sudden loss of renal function that may result from inadequate renal perfusion associated with a decrease in effective circulation, arterial or venous obstruction, renal cell injury, or obstruction to urine flow as occurs in obstructive uropathy (see Chapters 54 and 55). Renal cell injury commonly results from an ischemic or toxic insult that causes acute tubular damage. In this circumstance, the decrease in glomerular filtration rate (GFR), an invariable component of ARF, is a successful adaptive response in that the continued filtration of plasma across the glomerular basement membrane without reabsorption of the filtrate by the renal tubules results in massive losses of salt and water (1). Thus, the decreased GFR associated with ARF prevents severe depletion of extracellular fluid (ECF). This chapter describes the pathophysiology of ARF to provide a contemporary understanding of the cellular and molecular mechanisms that are associated with epithelial cell injury.

PATHOPHYSIOLOGY OF EXPERIMENTAL ACUTE RENAL FAILURE

Initially, studies on the pathophysiology of ARF were descriptive and involved the development of experimental models. Contemporary studies have been concerned with the pathophysiology of cell injury, particularly related to renal tubule function and metabolism. This chapter addresses the cellular, molecular, and metabolic alterations associated with loss and restitution of epithelial cell integrity and functions.

Renal Hemodynamics

Renal vasoconstriction is intense in experimental and clinical ARF (2–4). Because vasoconstriction was considered to be the dominant factor, it was suggested once that the term *vasomotor nephropathy* might be more appropriate than ARF to describe this condition (5). The hypothesis was that an insult to the renal tubular epithelium resulted in release of vasoactive compounds that increased cortical vascular resistance, thereby decreasing renal blood flow (RBF) and perpetuating injury to the tubule. Release of vasoconstrictive compounds diminished GFR by constricting the afferent and efferent arterioles, which led to a diminished urine output, or oliguria (3). Therefore, emphasis has been placed on identifying vasoactive compounds that are stimulated or induced by an ischemic or toxic insult. Candidate systems for vasoconstriction and vascular components of epithelial cell injury include angiotensin, prostaglandins, adenosine, endothelin, and nitric oxide (NO).

Renin-Angiotensin System

The renin-angiotensin system functions in a manner consistent with the renal vasoconstriction hypothesis (3,6). An injury to the more proximal portion of the nephron that impairs reabsorption results in the delivery of more solute and water into the distal nephron. This increased solute load enters the distal nephron and perfuses the macula densa of the juxtaglomerular apparatus, stimulating the intrarenal release of renin with the subsequent generation of angiotensin II, a potent renal vasoconstrictor.

Several findings suggest that this system may have a role in the pathogenesis of ARF:

1. Hyperplasia of the juxtaglomerular apparatus with increased renin granules is reported both in patients and in experimental animals with ARF.
2. Plasma renin activity is increased in patients with ARF.
3. Changing intrarenal renin content modifies the degree of renal functional impairment; for example, animals fed a high-salt diet (which suppresses renin production) before a renal injury have better preservation of

renal function than those fed a low-salt diet (which stimulates renin production).

However, other findings suggest that the renin-angiotensin system does not fully account for the changes in renal hemodynamics associated with ARF. For example, amelioration of the renal injury also follows the induction of a solute diuresis with either mannitol or loop diuretics, neither of which affects intrarenal renin. Furthermore, the degree of renal injury is not affected in animals that have been immunized against renin-angiotensin, treated with angiotensin-converting enzyme inhibitors, or infused with a competitive antagonist to angiotensin II. Therefore, the role of the renin-angiotensin system as the modulator of renal injury in ARF is uncertain.

Prostaglandins

Prostaglandins are potent renal vasodilators. Although inhibition of prostaglandin production is associated with decreased RBF and affects the severity of ARF, the precise role of prostaglandins in the induction and maintenance of acute tubular necrosis is not established (6). However, prostaglandin inhibitors, such as nonsteroidal antiinflammatory drugs, increase the risk for development of ARF and may act to synergize with other insults.

Adenosine

Adenosine, which results from catabolism of adenine nucleotides, is a potent vasoconstrictor of renal vasculature, whereas it is a vasodilator of peripheral vasculature (7). The infusion of methylxanthines, which block adenosine receptors, inhibits the tubuloglomerular feedback mechanism and the decrease in GFR that accompanies reduced tubular absorption, suggesting that adenosine may be involved in the modulation of renal vascular resistance in ARF. In some experimental models, the infusion of methylxanthines has been associated with diminished functional impairment. The proposal that adenosine is an important vasoactive compound after an acute tubule insult is attractive because it would link alterations in cell metabolism with hemodynamic changes.

However, the evidence that adenosine is a major factor in the vasoconstrictive response is inconclusive:

1. Methylxanthines have a variety of effects in addition to the inhibition of adenosine receptors.
2. Although adenosine is produced after the initiation of adenine nucleotide catabolism, it is rapidly catabolized by adenosine deaminase when released into ECF.
3. Intrarenal levels of adenosine diminish very rapidly on the establishment of reflow to the kidney, whereas renal vasoconstriction is continued through the early phases of reperfusion after an ischemic injury.
4. When tissue adenosine levels are increased by inhibition of adenosine deaminase during ischemia, postischemic recovery of renal function is enhanced (8).

Endothelin

Endothelin, a 21-amino-acid peptide, is a very potent renal vasoconstrictor that has other important biologic activities as well (9–11). It contributes to the vasoconstriction that occurs in a number of tissues and organs as a response to hypoxia. Raised endothelin levels in plasma and in both the cortex and medulla of the kidney have been demonstrated in experimental animals after the induction of renal ischemia (9). The postischemic infusion of antiendothelin antibody or endothelin-receptor antagonists provides protection from ischemic injury (9–11). This represents a very early event in the initiation of ARF and may be quite specific for only some types of injuries.

Nitric Oxide

NO is a potent renal vasodilator that is widely distributed in the kidney and is produced by constitutive and inducible synthetases located in endothelial cells and renal tubules (12). Although a specific role for these compounds in cerebral ischemia has been established (13), the effect of either stimulation or inhibition of NO synthetase (NOS) on ischemic or toxic ARF is confusing and, at times, contradictory. The rat kidney was protected from ischemic injury when inducible NOS was targeted with oligodeoxynucleotides, suggesting that NO had a direct cytotoxic effect on renal epithelia (14). A similar cytotoxic effect of NO has been documented in isolated proximal tubule cells subjected to hypoxia (15). Yet, it has been postulated that production of NO after ischemia should help alleviate the vasoconstriction that characterizes ARF, and nonselective NOS inhibition has been shown to result in worsening of renal function and profound vasoconstriction (13). Hence the enigma: Stimulation of NO in the renal vasculature via NOS will modulate vasoconstriction and lessen injury; induction of NO via NOS in renal tubules is cytotoxic (12–14). This complex biologic system may play a role in the pathogenesis of ARF, but the specificity of involvement remains to be determined.

All things considered, renal vasoconstriction is a well-documented factor in initiating ARF, but vasodilation does not consistently result in amelioration of an acute renal insult. Once ARF has been established, the infusion of potent vasodilators such as prostaglandins or dopamine does not lead to sustained improvement in GFR (16,17). The early recovery phase of ARF is associated with an increase in RBF, whereas GFR increases more slowly (18). Although renal hemodynamic factors play an important role in initiating ARF, alterations in renal vascular resistance and renal perfusion may not be the dominant determinants of epithelial cell injury.

Nephronal Factors

The term *nephronal factors* refers to the unique susceptibility of various nephron segments to injury. Best studied, in this regard, are the S_3 segment of the proximal tubule and the medullary thick ascending limb (mTAL). Studies of cellular injury and repair in each of these segments have provided important insights into the pathophysiology of tubule cell injury.

Medullary Thick Ascending Limb

The mTAL is particularly vulnerable to hypoxia because oxygen tension in this, the medullary area, is low, and the mTAL segment has a high rate of oxygen consumption (19). Initial observations that established this relationship were made in isolated kidneys that were perfused with cell-free perfusate. Hypoxic injury to the mTAL progresses rapidly from mitochondrial swelling to nuclear pyknosis and then complete cellular disruption. These lesions in the mTAL are prevented or reversed by increasing oxygen delivery with the addition of red blood cells or hemoglobin to the perfusion media.

The degree of mTAL necrosis also is modified by the workload imposed on this segment. Inhibiting transport by infusing furosemide or ouabain significantly diminishes the degree of injury; increasing the workload has the opposite effect. It has been suggested that lesions in the mTAL may be enhanced because swelling in the S_3 segment of the proximal tubule would decrease venous return from the medullary portion of the kidney by impingement of the swollen S_3 segments on venules.

The relationship of these observations, made largely during *in vitro* studies of the isolated perfused kidney, to the pathogenesis of acute tubular necrosis in humans is controversial. Reducing the inspired oxygen content in experimental animals does not reproduce these lesions *in vivo*, and the experimental models in which the lesions occur *in vivo* are those that combine severe reductions in RBF with the administration of a nephrotoxin. The unique vulnerability of this nephron segment to hypoxia has provided new information concerning important relationships between oxygen supply, workload, and the cellular targets of an ischemic, hypoxic, or anoxic injury (20). In large measure, these pathophysiologic changes may be most pertinent in the synergist effects of agents that would not on their own produce ARF.

Straight Segment of the Proximal Tubule

The straight segment of the proximal tubule (S_3 segment) depends on oxidative phosphorylation for the energy required for its transport functions. It is particularly susceptible to ischemia and to those nephrotoxins that disrupt energy supply or mitochondrial function (6,21). The earliest responses to ischemia are found in the brush border and consist of blebbing and internalization of the luminal membrane. Even mild and short-term (as little as 10 minutes) ischemia can result in sloughing of the brush border and other alterations in the proximal tubule histomorphology. With more prolonged ischemia, these changes progress to a lethal injury of some cells in which the tubule epithelium is denuded from the basement membrane and a sublethal injury characterized by swelling, mitochondrial condensation, and disruption of cellular morphology in other cells. These changes in the S_3 segment result in two important pathophysiologic events.

Intratubular Obstruction and Backleak

Cell and brush-border debris become impacted in the hairpin turn of the loop of Henle and produce obstruction and backleak of tubular fluid in some nephron segments. Intratubular obstruction has been documented by determination of elevated proximal tubular pressure and by histomorphology after ischemic injury (21–23).

A loss of tubular integrity and backleak of tubular fluid have been demonstrated in both experimental animals and patients (21–24). In experimental animals, the microinjection of inulin or horseradish peroxidase into normal nephrons results in the inulin being collected only from that kidney or the staining of horseradish peroxidase only within that tubule lumen. However, microinjection into an injured nephron results in inulin being excreted by the contralateral kidney and the horseradish peroxidase being found in both intratubular and peritubular loci.

In patients with ARF, backleak has been demonstrated by the differential clearance of graded dextrans (24). These observations and an understanding of this mechanism have clinical implications. If inulin, urea, and creatinine leak back into the circulation, the renal clearances of these solutes are no longer suitable for estimating GFR in patients with ARF.

Over the past several years, the cellular and molecular basis for tubule observation and backleak have been documented (25,26). Integrins are proteins that are (a) located on the basal domain of epithelial cells and (b) attach tubules to ligands in the extracellular matrix. After ischemia or adenosine triphosphate (ATP) depletion, these proteins loose their attachment to the extracellular matrix, which allows both injured and viable cells to be liberated from the tubule basement membrane and float into the tubule lumen. In addition, these integrins become displaced from the basal to the luminal domain, which allows individual cells to attach via an arginine-glycine-aspartic acid (RDG sequence) adhesion mechanism (25). This RDG sequence may also promote binding of sloughed tubule cells to Tamm-Horsfall protein, which is produced in the thick ascending limb and distal convoluted tubule and contains an RDG sequence (26). The infusion of RDG peptide abolished the characteristic increase in proximal tubule pressure and substantially improved renal function (27,28).

Cellular and Metabolic Alterations

Reactive Oxygen Molecules

Reactive oxygen molecules have been implicated in a variety of kidney diseases, including reperfusion injury after

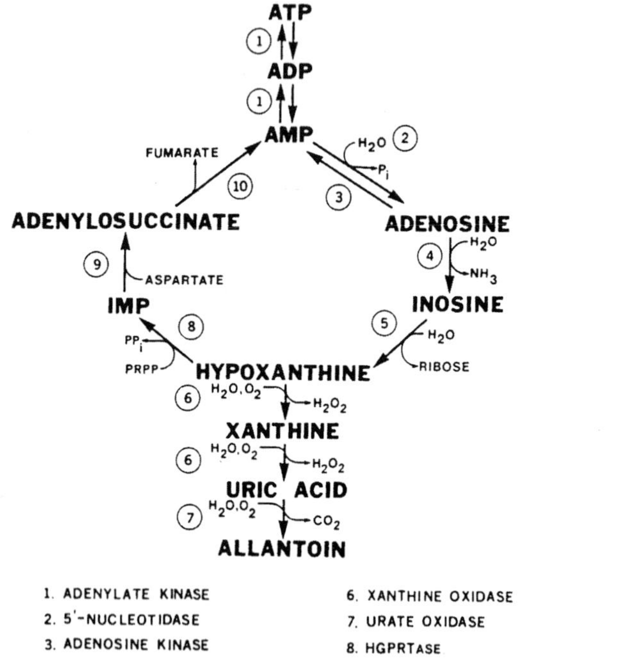

FIGURE 63.1. Schematic of adenosine triphosphate (ATP) metabolism that results from renal ischemia. Adenine nucleotide catabolism proceeds in a clockwise direction.

ischemia (29). The most highly reactive oxygen molecules are free radicals such as hydroxyl radical (OH) or superoxide anion (O_2^-). The very high reactivity and brief existence of these molecules result in injury very close to the site of free radical generation. Other oxygen species such as hydrogen peroxide (H_2O_2) and hypochlorous acid (HOCl), not being free radicals, are less reactive. However, they have longer half-lives than free radicals and in some cases may cross cell membranes to cause injury distant from their site of origin.

Reactive oxygen molecules also are generated during reperfusion of kidneys (29). Ischemia results in a rapid fall in cellular ATP levels with subsequent metabolism of the adenine nucleotides to adenosine, inosine, and hypoxanthine (Fig. 63.1). Ischemia also may cause a conformational change in xanthine dehydrogenase [which uses NAD (nicotinamide adenine dinucleotide) as an electron receptor] to xanthine oxidase, which uses oxygen (30). Once perfusion and oxygen delivery are returned, xanthine oxidase can metabolize hypoxanthine to xanthine and uric acid, generating hydrogen peroxide and superoxide anion (Fig. 63.1). Mitochondria, which produce reactive species through electron transport systems, when damaged by ischemia, may leak the injurious oxygen metabolites. The respiratory burst and myeloperoxidase released from activated polymorphonuclear leukocytes produce superoxide anion, hydrogen peroxide, and hypochlorous acid (29). Prostaglandin metabolism may also provide reactive molecules. Iron can play a significant part by donating electrons to hydrogen peroxide to form the highly damaging hydroxyl radical (31). In this way, iron release may be responsible for the injury resulting in hemoglobin- or myoglobin-induced ARF (32).

Once generated, reactive oxygen molecules damage cellular components and extracellular matrix (33). Many amino acid residues on cellular proteins may be oxidized, resulting in conformational changes with loss of enzymatic activity or loss of the integrity of structural proteins. Membrane lipids and lipoproteins undergo peroxidation by free radicals; these propagate and result in progressive membrane damage. Hydroxyl radicals damage DNA and oxidize matrix proteins. Reactive oxygen metabolites may contribute to ischemia by deleterious interactions with NOSs. Because of the putative effects, a great deal of attention has been paid to determining the role of reactive oxygen molecules in ischemic-reperfusion injury (29,34). The effects of enhancing endogenous antioxidants (superoxide dismutase, glutathione, and catalase) or administering exogenous free radical scavengers have been examined. Despite the large number of studies using these techniques, no final conclusion can be made as to the importance of reactive oxygen species, because strong evidence exists both for and against these compounds having a dominant role.

Adenine Nucleotide Metabolism

Energy depletion and restoration are believed to play a pivotal role in renal cell injury (33). *In vivo*, renal ischemia results in a profound fall in ATP, and, *in vitro*, metabolic inhibition of ATP production is used to induce cellular injury. Within 5 to 10 minutes of renal ischemia, nearly 90% of ATP has been consumed (8). With reperfusion, renal ATP levels recover in a bimodal fashion (Fig. 63.2). In the first few minutes of reper-

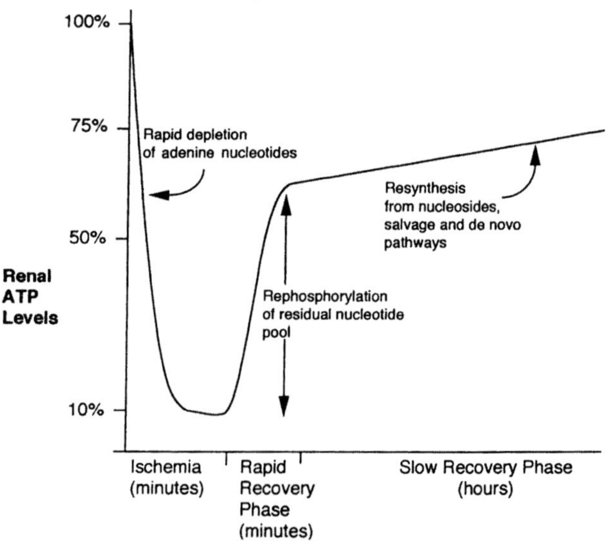

FIGURE 63.2. The course of renal adenosine triphosphate (ATP) depletion and recovery during ischemia and reperfusion. The initial rapid phase of ATP recovery represents phosphorylation of remaining AMP and ADP. Slow recovery phase occurs by resynthesis and phosphorylation of adenine nucleotides.

fusion, there is a rapid, although incomplete, recovery of ATP to 50 to 70% of normal levels, depending on the duration of ischemia (34,35). The longer the interval of ischemia, the smaller the degree of renal ATP recovery during this rapid phase. ATP recovery during this initial phase correlates highly with the total pool of adenine nucleotides (ATP + ADP + AMP) that are present in the kidney at the end of the ischemic interval. The total adenine nucleotide pool, mainly composed of AMP, decreases as the duration of ischemia increases. The catabolism of adenosine by adenosine deaminase results in depletion of the adenine nucleotide pool with extended duration of ischemia (Fig. 63.1). Thus, the predominant means of ATP recovery during the initial period of reoxygenation is through oxidative phosphorylation of the residual cellular nucleotides (AMP and ADP).

After the rapid phase, a second, slow phase of ATP recovery occurs over hours. The ATP recovery rate in this phase also depends on the duration of the preceding ischemia; longer ischemic intervals result in slower recovery rates. The second phase requires resynthesis of ATP from purine nucleotide degradation products and salvage pathways or from precursors provided during reperfusion. A primary role for ATP depletion in the cellular event that leads to epithelial cell injury is supported by several findings:

1. When ATP catabolism is inhibited during ischemia, the structural and functional consequences of renal artery occlusion are significantly ameliorated (18,21,33).
2. Graded reductions in cellular ATP either *in vivo* or *in vitro* determine the severity of cellular disruption (36,37).
3. Augmentation of recovery of ATP during reperfusion substantially enhances recovery of structure and function (33).

Consequently, alterations in adenine nucleotide metabolism are both a consequence and predictor of renal cell injury. In addition, limited cellular ATP sets in motion a sequence of events that lead to disruption of epithelial structure and function: increased intracellular calcium, activation of phospholipases, loss of polarity, and detachments of the cortical cytoskeleton.

Alterations in Intracellular Calcium

Under normal circumstances, ECF calcium concentration exceeds that of intracellular free calcium (Ca_i) by a factor of 10^4. The remarkably low Ca_i is maintained by a variety of mechanisms that exclude calcium from the cell or sequester it within intracellular compartments. Calcium is extruded from cells by plasma membrane Ca^+–adenosine triphosphatase (ATPase) and Na^+-Ca^+ exchanger. Intracellular sequestration is mediated by Ca^+-ATPase in the endoplasmic reticulum and by calcium uptake into mitochondria. A fall in cellular ATP will adversely effect Na^+-K^+-ATPase and Na^+-Ca^+ transporter, which, taken together, would likely result in decreased calcium transport out of cells and a rise in Ca_i. However, a rise in mitochondrial calcium levels after ischemic and toxic cell injury usually occurs after cell injury is lethal because mitochondrial calcium uptake is substantial only when cytosolic levels rise because even damaged mitochondria are able to actively sequester calcium (34). In addition, it has been suggested that release of Ca_i from cellular organelles contributes substantially to the rise in cytosolic Ca.

It is unclear whether high Ca_i levels play a central role in the pathophysiology of cell injury or the intracellular Ca changes are merely secondary to cell death. Increased cell and mitochondrial Ca levels are linked with cell death but are not thought to increase until irreversible changes have occurred (38,39). In light of the many ATP-dependent mechanisms responsible for Ca exclusion from the cytosol, it is surprising that only recently an increase in Ca_i has been documented early in the course of cell injury. After 5 minutes of hypoxia, rat proximal tubules developed a significant rise in Ca_i before evidence of membrane damage and the increase in Ca_i was reversed with reoxygenation (40). An increase in Ca_i could contribute to renal cell injury in several dimensions: increased activity of proteases and phospholipases; calpain activation, which would contribute to degradation of cytoskeleton; and inhibition of mitochondrial oxidative phosphorylation. Nonetheless, controversy remains about the extent to which increased Ca_i contributes to these pathophysiologic mechanisms.

Phospholipids and Phospholipases

The striking morphologic changes that occur in proximal tubules after ischemia, especially brush-border membrane blebbing, and the release of intracellular enzymes such as lactate dehydrogenase suggest that significant membrane alterations may be part of the cellular injury. Changes in intracellular calcium flux have been shown to activate endogenous phospholipase, and some phospholipase may be activated by decreased cellular ATP. Phospholipase activation results in breakdown of membrane phospholipids into products including free fatty acids and lysophospholipids, which may disrupt membranes. The accompanying lack of ATP during ischemia may prevent the synthesis of new phospholipids to replenish membranes. The result is a generalized loss of membrane phospholipids with an accumulation of degradative products that by their detergent activities further disrupt cell membranes and eventually lead to loss of membrane integrity and cell death.

Renal ischemia does indeed result in activation of phospholipase (PLA_2) and a rapid fall in cortical phospholipid levels (41). The detrimental effects of PLA_2 can be offset by unsaturated free fatty acids (42) and suggest that PLA_2 could be cytotoxic by degradation of phospholipids in cell membranes or through accumulation of lysophospholipids (43).

Cell Polarity

Renal tubules are composed of highly specialized cells whose primary function of transport depends on their polar structure (Fig. 63.3). Changes in cell polarity that occur during ARF have important effects on these functions (37). The plasma membrane of proximal tubule cells is divided into apical and basolateral domains by the tight junction that it shares with neighboring cells. The apical membrane, which faces the tubule lumen, differs from the basolateral membrane both in lipid composition and in the types of membrane proteins present. The microvilli of the apical domain are rich in sodium-dependent cotransporters and Na^+-H^+ antiporters, which affect reabsorption of glucose, amino acids, phosphate, and bicarbonate. The sodium gradient across the apical membrane, which drives the resorption of these compounds, is established and maintained by Na^+-K^+-ATPase, located on the basolateral membrane. Plasma membrane polarity is maintained by the tight junctions that prevent lateral diffusion of membrane phospholipids and proteins into the opposite domain. In addition, the cortical cytoskeleton anchors membrane proteins, such as Na^+-K^+-ATPase, in specific domains through an intricate sequence of linked proteins. The actin-based cytoskeleton is a dynamic structure that maintains cellular polarity and mediates a number of processes necessary to sustain both structure and function of renal epithelia (44). Interactions between cytoskeletal proteins and plasma membrane proteins are responsible for functions, including cell adhesion, endocytosis, signal translocation, and ion channels.

Renal ischemia *in vivo* and ATP depletion *in vitro* alter this polarity in that membrane lipids and proteins, which are highly mobile, redistribute between apical and basolateral domains (Fig. 63.3). After as little as 5 minutes of renal ischemia, there is loss, internalization, and blebbing of brush-border membranes and, shortly thereafter, basolateral Na^+-K^+-ATPase migrates to the apical membranes (37). With longer ischemia, the loss of polarity worsens. Proximal tubule tight junction integrity, an obstacle to diffusion of membrane components across domains, is lost. Membrane proteins such as Na^+-K^+-ATPase, which normally are anchored to the actin cortical cytoskeleton, migrate when this attachment is disrupted. The actin cytoskeleton itself plays an important role in both processes because disruption of actin microfilaments results in opening of tight junctions (35,45) and loss of the polar distribution of those proteins that anchor Na^+-K^+-ATPase to the plasma membrane (46). Ankyrin, which links fodrin to Na^+-K^+-ATPase, normally is limited to the basolateral domain. After ischemia, ankyrin migrates along with Na^+-K^+-ATPase to the apical domain. After ATP depletion, spectrin, which normally links actin to ankyrin and Na^+-K^+-ATPase, becomes dissociated and solubilized throughout the cytosol (47). The loss of cellular polarity is a fundamental alteration in renal epithelial injury. These structural changes and the reduction in transepithelial sodium reabsorption that follows ischemia do not return to normal until membrane polarity is reestablished during reflow or ATP repletion.

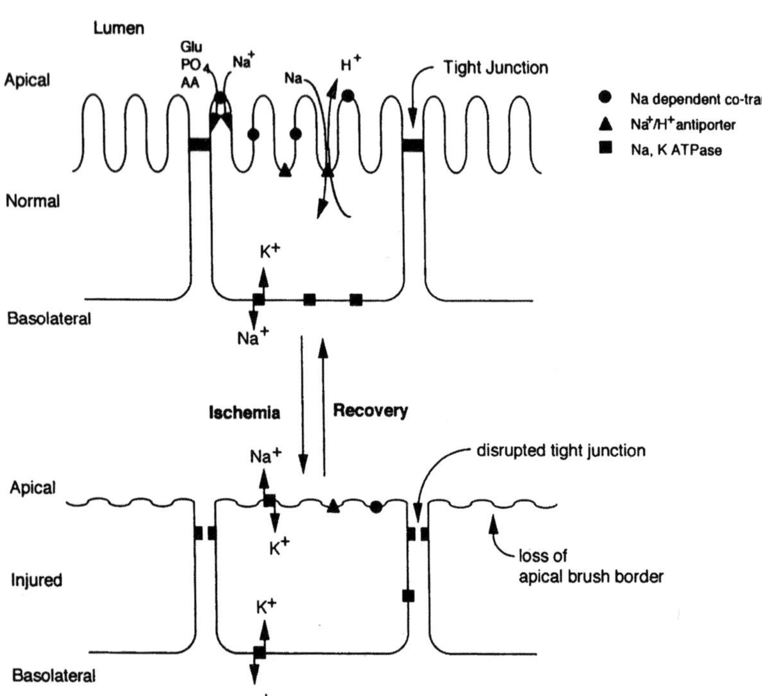

FIGURE 63.3. Disruption of normal proximal tubule cell structure by ischemia includes loss of apical brush border, opening of tight junctions, and depolarization of the plasma membrane. Impairment of transepithelial solute reabsorption coincides with alterations in cell structure. Functional recovery parallels morphologic recovery. ATPase, adenosine triphosphatase.

Apoptosis

In recent years, it has been appreciated that cell death after an ischemic or toxic insult may occur by necrosis or apoptosis—a gene-directed process that results in irrevocable DNA damage (48). The characteristic biochemical marker for apoptosis is endonuclease activation, which has been documented in hypoxic and ischemic tubules (49). In the final analysis, apoptosis is the result of the dynamic interaction of an activator such as tumor necrosis factor and inhibitors such as growth factors. Apoptosis represents an important mechanism of cell death, and its role in ARF is under active investigation (48).

Factors Influencing Recovery

An understanding of factors that may influence the course of recovery from an acute insult offers an opportunity to identify mechanisms that are fundamental to cellular repair and restitution of function.

Adenine Nucleotides and Thyroxine

Because ATP depletion predicts the severity and reversibility of an ischemic injury, altering the recovery of renal ATP is a likely candidate for influencing recovery from injury. Two compounds, ATP-$MgCl_2$ and thyroxine, have been shown to accelerate recovery of renal ATP. In both cases, glomerular and tubular function is improved, cellular structure and polarity are stabilized, and enhanced recovery of renal function is sustained (16,32,35). Although the specific cellular mechanism by which each compound-enhanced ATP recovery is different, the end result is accelerated recovery from an ischemic or toxic insult. Adenine nucleotides–$MgCl_2$ provide essential precursors, particularly adenosine to the sublethally injured cells and stimulate *de novo* purine synthesis (35). Thyroxin stimulates regeneration of ATP by stabilizing the mitochondrial adenine nucleotide transporter (50).

Atrial Natriuretic Factors

Atrial natriuretic factors (ANFs), which, when infused into animals, cause a dramatic increase in salt and water excretion, also increase RBF and GFR through afferent arterial dilation and efferent arterial constriction. As is expected, ANF infusion improves overall renal function in states of volume depletion or high afferent renal artery vascular resistance. ANF is beneficial in toxin-induced renal injury, which may be attributable to its enhancement of RBF and urine flow. Of particular interest are the effects of ANF infusion after renal ischemia. When infused shortly after an interval of renal ischemia, ANF results in rapid and sustained improvement in GFR (51). Renal plasma and urine flow also are increased, as is net tubular reabsorption of sodium. Reports conflict as to whether ANF treatment improves renal histomorphology.

The mechanism of the effects of ANF is not definitively determined but is attributed to its vasodilatory properties, increased RBF, and increased tubular flow rate with concomitant relief of tubular obstruction. Thus, in established ARF, ANF may increase hydraulic pressures in obstructed nephrons sufficiently to dislodge tubule casts downstream, thereby restoring GFR (52). It has also been proposed that ANF ameliorates the ischemic injury through its initial natriuretic effect, reducing tubular reabsorptive work and thus permitting greater energy expenditure for restoring cellular integrity and polarity (51).

Leukocyte-Endothelial Adhesion

In ischemic tissues, leukocytes, particularly neutrophils, are known to adhere to the vascular endothelium and are thought to contribute to tissue injury by release of reactive oxygen species or cytotoxic enzymes (53–55) and may contribute to vascular congestion. Intracellular adhesion molecule I (ICAM-I) on endothelial cells promotes this leukocyte adhesion, and elegant studies have demonstrated that mice deficient in ICAM-I are protected against ischemic injury and that administration of ICAM-I antibody prevents ischemic ARF (54,55).

Calcium-Channel Blockers

Low-extracellular calcium levels ameliorate anoxic injury, whereas high-extracellular calcium levels enhance anoxic injury. Manipulating extracellular calcium levels to potentially ameliorate the course of ARF has obvious clinical limitations. However, calcium-channel blockers, in the setting of ARF, might alter the influx of calcium into injured cells and attenuate further cell damage or prevent cell death. The effects of calcium-channel blockers on the course and recovery from ARF are inconsistent. Specific effects have been seen in some types of injuries (34), particularly cyclosporine-related toxicity, but evidence for ubiquitous effects on basic pathophysiologic mechanisms is lacking.

Heat-Shock Proteins

Heat-shock proteins (HSPs) are a group of highly conserved proteins that are elaborated in cells and respond to injury caused by heat, anoxia, and a number of toxic agents. HSPs are present in nearly every organism studied and appear to be essential to basic cell function and survival by providing routine assistance in intracellular protein handling and trafficking (56). These stress proteins are grouped into families according to size and apparent function. Within each HSP family, certain members are constitutively expressed, and others are expressed only after injury. The pattern of HSP induction varies, depending on species, cell types, and the nature of the agent causing injury.

The loss of cell polarity and disruption of the cytoskeleton are fundamental processes that contribute to

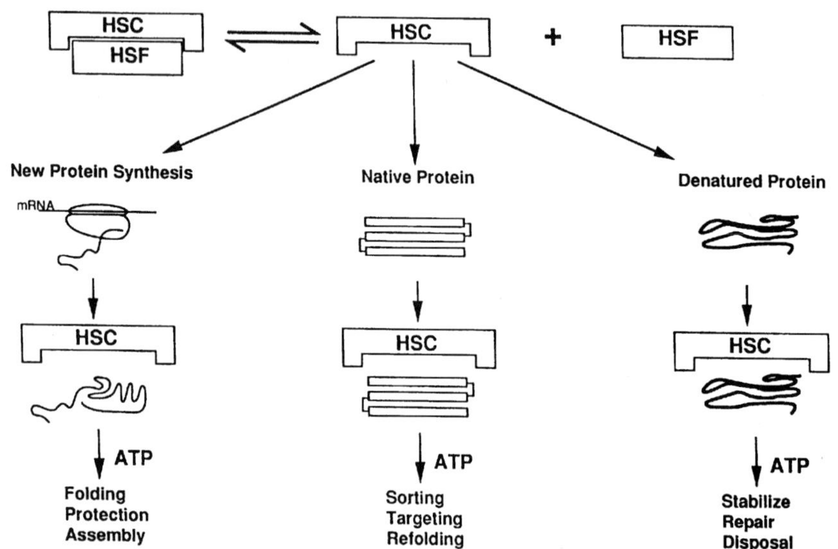

FIGURE 63.4. Known and proposed actions of 70-kDa heat-shock protein (HSP-70) system. Normal cellular protein handling accomplished by heat-shock cognate (HSC; constitutively expressed heat-shock protein). Cellular stress and increased denatured protein increases demand for HSC. Heat-shock factor (HSF; transcription factor for inducible HSP) is reversibly bound to HSC and is released with increased demand for HSC. HSF then initiates transcription of inducible HSP mRNA. ATP, adenosine triphosphate.

the pathogenesis of cellular ARF. Injured tubule cells, which have suffered loss of polarity, appear to regain their polarity through remodeling (37). The recycling of cytoskeletal and plasma membrane proteins is a primary mechanism of cellular repair after ischemia or ATP depletion (47,57).

One family of HSPs that may assist in restitution of cellular polarity and function is the 70-kDa HSP family (HSP-70). Certain members of this family are readily induced by injury and have distinctive cytoprotectant effects different from those of other HSPs. Although first identified by their ability to be induced, most of what is known about HSP-70 activity has been found by studying the constitutively expressed members. HSP-70 proteins provide various functions by their shared ability to unfold peptides and disassemble protein aggregates. These HSPs act as "chaperones" to newly formed proteins, allowing proper folding and preventing "inappropriate" peptide interactions or aggregation. In like manner, HSP-70 members assist in the translocation of proteins across intracellular membranes and assist denatured proteins in refolding or reassembling into normal configuration as part of the process of repair (Fig. 63.4).

When renal ATP levels are reduced below 50% of control values either *in vivo* or *in vitro*, heat-shock transcription factor, the most proximal component of HSP induction, is rapidly activated (36). Newly formed HSP-70/72 mRNA is found within minutes, and its rate of formation peaks within a few hours after a period of ischemia. HSP-72 protein elaboration follows shortly thereafter, accumulates in the first day after the injury, and persists for up to 5 days. HSP-72 is found in membrane protein fractions and among soluble cytoplasmic proteins, suggesting that HSP-72 is interacting with and rescuing diverse proteins (58,59). *In situ* localization of HSP-72 in proximal tubules has a specific pattern of distribution after ischemic injury (59). Within minutes of the relief of ischemia, HSP-72 appears predominantly in the apical domain of proximal tubule cells. This localization coincides with brush-border changes, apical cytoskeletal disruption, and redistribution of basolateral membrane proteins to the apical membrane (see Cell Polarity). During the recovery period, when brush-border morphology is largely restored, HSP-72 migrates away from the apical domain to cytoplasmic and basolateral domains. Thus, the course of induction, elaboration, and localization of HSP-72 coincides with repair of cell morphology, polarity, and function during recovery of the proximal tubule epithelia from ischemic injury. HSP-25, which is able to function as an actin-capping protein, has been shown to be induced after renal ischemia (60). Moreover, this protein moves from a soluble cytosolic distribution to an insoluble actin-associated state rapidly after an ischemic insult. These dynamic interactions of different classes of HSP, each with its specific functions, may be essential to reestablish cellular polarity and integrity.

Growth Factors

Several growth factors are known to bind specific receptors in renal tubules and regulate the proliferative process. After an ischemic insult, the infusion of either epidermal growth factor, hepatocyte growth factor, or insulin-like growth factor I result in (a) improved GFR, (b) diminished morphologic injury, (c) increased thymidine incorporation into tubule DNA, and (d) diminished mortality (61). Insulin-like growth factor I also diminishes loss of body weight associated with ARF in animals. In addition, growth factors may interact with other factors such as thyroxin or ADP to augment recovery from ARF (62–64).

CONCLUSION

Over the past decade, we have begun to unravel and discover the cellular and molecular mechanisms that contribute to the development of and recovery from ARF (65,66). Because ARF is a multifactorial process, it is unlikely that any single mechanism can explain the many dimensions of ARF. The processes described in this chapter and the integration of their effects provides a basis for understanding the complex pathophysiologic events that result in damage to renal epithelial cells and the acute unexpected loss of renal function—ARF.

REFERENCES

1. Thura K. Nephrology: a look into the future. *Kidney Int* 1979;15:1–6.
2. Gaudio KM, Siegel NJ. New approaches to the treatment of acute renal failure. *Pediatr Nephrol* 1987;1:339–347.
3. Gaudio KM, Siegel NJ. Pathogenesis and treatment of acute renal failure. *Pediatr Clin North Am* 1987;34:771–778.
4. Hollenber NK, Epstein M, Rosen SM, et al. Acute oliguric renal failure in man; evidence for preferential renal cortical ischemia. *Medicine* 1968;47:455–474.
5. Oken DE. Acute renal failure (vasomotor nephropathy): micropuncture studies of the pathogenetic mechanisms. *Annu Rev Med* 1975;10:307–319.
6. Stein JH, Lifschitz MD, Barnes LD. Current concepts on the pathophysiology of acute renal failure. *Am J Physiol* 1978;234:F171–F181.
7. Bidani AK, Churchill PC. Aminophylline ameliorates glycerol-induced acute renal failure in rats. *Can J Physiol Pharmacol* 1983;61:567–571.
8. Avison MJ, van Waard A, Stromski ME, et al. Metabolic alterations in the kidney during ischemic acute renal failure. *Semin Nephrol* 1989;9:98–101.
9. Chan L, Chittinandana A, Shapiro JI, et al. Effect of an endothelin-receptor antagonist on ischemic acute renal failure. *Am J Physiol* 1994;266:F135–F138.
10. Kon V, Yoskioka T, Fogo A, et al. Glomerular actions of endothelin in vivo. *J Clin Invest* 1989;83:1762–1767.
11. Kon V, Bodi K. Biologic actions and pathophysiologic significance of endothelin. *Kidney Int* 1991;40:1–12.
12. Peer G, Blum M, Iaina A. Nitric oxide and acute renal failure. *Nephron* 1996;73:375–381.
13. Huang Z, Huang PL, Panahian N, et al. Effects of cerebral ischemia in mice deficient in neuronal nitric oxide synthase. *Science* 1994;265:1883–1885.
14. Noiri E, Peresleni T, Miller F, et al. In vivo targeting of inducible NO synthase with oligodeoxynucleotides protects rat kidney against ischemia. *J Clin Invest* 1996;97:2377–2383.
15. Yu L, Gengaro PE, Niederberger M, et al. Nitric oxide: a mediator in rat tubular hypoxia/reoxygenation injury. *Proc Natl Acad Sci U S A* 1994;91:1691–1695.
16. Gaudio KM, Stromski M, Thulin G, et al. Postischemic hemodynamics and recovery of renal adenosine triphosphate. *Am J Physiol* 1986;20:F603–F609.
17. Paller MS, Anderson RJ. Use of vasoactive agents in the therapy of acute renal failure. In: Brenner BM, Lazarus JM, eds. *Acute renal failure*. Philadelphia: WB Saunders, 1983;723.
18. Finn WF, Chevalier RL. Recovery from postischemic acute renal failure in the rat. *Kidney Int* 1979;16:113–123.
19. Brezis M, Rosen S, Silva P, et al. Renal ischemia: a new perspective (editorial review). *Kidney Int* 1984;26:375–383.
20. Brezis M, Rosen S. Hypoxia of the renal medulla: its implications for disease. *N Engl J Med* 1995;332:647–655.
21. Donohoe JF, Venkatachalam MA, Bernard DB, et al. Tubular leakage and obstruction after renal ischemia: structural-functional correlations. *Kidney Int* 1978;13:208–222.
22. Gaudio KM, Ardito TA, Reilly HF, et al. Accelerated cellular recovery after an ischemic renal injury. *Am J Pathol* 1983;112:338–346.
23. Gaudio KM, Taylor MR, Chaudry IH, et al. Accelerated recovery of single nephron function by the postischemic infusion of ATP-$MgCl_2$. *Kidney Int* 1982;22:13–20.
24. Myers BD, Chui F, Hilberman M, et al. Transtubular leakage of glomerular filtrate in human acute renal failure. *Am J Physiol* 1979;237(4):F319–F325.
25. Gailit J, Colflesh D, Rabiner I, et al. Redistribution and dysfunction of integrins in cultured renal epithelial cells exposed to oxidative stress. *Am J Physiol* 1993;33:F149–F157.
26. Pennica D, Kohr WJ, Kuang WJ, et al. Identification of human uromodulin as the Tamm Horsfall urinary glycoprotein. *Science* 1987;236:83–87.
27. Goligorsky MS, Dibona GF. Pathogenic role of Arg-Gly-Asp recognizing integrins in acute renal failure. *Proc Natl Acad Sci U S A* 1993;90:5700–5704.
28. Noiri E, Gailit J, Sheth D, et al. Cyclic RGD peptides ameliorate ischemic acute renal failure in rats. *Kidney Int* 1994;46: 1050–1058.
29. Andreoli SP. Reactive oxygen molecules, oxidant injury and renal disease. *Pediatr Nephrol* 1991;5:733–742.
30. McKelvey TG, Hollworth ME, Ganger DN, et al. Mechanisms of conversion of xanthine dehydrogenase to xanthine oxidase in ischemic rat liver and kidney. *Am J Physiol* 1988;254:G753–G760.
31. Halliwell B, Gutteridge JMC. Iron and free radical reactions: two aspects of antioxidant protection. *Trends Biochem Sci* 1986;11:372–375.
32. Paller MS. Hemoglobin and myoglobin-induced acute renal failure in rats: role of iron in nephrotoxicity. *Am J Physiol* 1988;255:F539–F544.
33. Siegel NJ, Devarajan P, Van Why SK. Renal cell injury: metabolic and structural alterations. *Pediatr Res* 1994;30:129–136.
34. Weinberg JM. The cell biology of ischemic renal injury. *Kidney Int* 1991;39:476–500.
35. Stromski ME, Cooper K, Thulin G, et al. Chemical and functional correlates of postischemic renal ATP levels. *Proc Natl Acad Sci U S A* 1986;83:6142–6145.
36. Van Why SK, Mann AS, Thulin G, et al. Activation of heat-shock transcription factor by graded reductions in renal ATP, in vivo, in the rat. *J Clin Invest* 1994;94:1518–1523.
37. Molitoris BA. New insights into the cell biology of ischemic acute renal failure. *J Am Soc Nephrol* 1991;1:1263–1270.
38. Arnold PE, Lumlertgul D, Burke TJ, et al. In vitro versus in vivo mitochondrial calcium loading in ischemic acute renal failure. *Am J Physiol* 1985;248:F845–F850.

39. Weinberg JM. Oxygen deprivation-induced injury to isolated rabbit kidney tubules. *J Clin Invest* 1985;76:1193–1208.
40. Kribben A, Wieder ED, Wetzels JF, et al. Evidence for role of cytosolic free calcium in hypoxia-induced proximal tubule injury. *J Clin Invest* 1994;93:1922–1929.
41. Humes HD, Nguyen VD, Cielinski DA. The role of free fatty acids in hypoxia-induced injury to proximal tubules. *Am J Physiol* 1989;256:F688–F696.
42. Zager RA, Burkhart KM, Conrad DS, et al. Phospholipase A2-induced cytoprotection of proximal tubules: potential determinants and specificity for ATP depletion mediated injury. *J Am Soc Nephrol* 1996;7:64–72.
43. Chen Y, Morimoto S, Kitano S, et al. Lysophosphatidylcholine causes calcium influx, enhanced DNA synthesis and cytotoxicity in cultured vascular smooth muscle cells. *Atherosclerosis* 1995;112:69–76.
44. Molitoris BA. Putting the actin cytoskeleton into perspective: pathophysiology of ischemic alterations. *Am J Physiol* 1997;272:F430–F433.
45. Madara JL, Barenberg D, Carlson S. Effects of cytochalasin D on occluding junctions of intestinal absorptive cells: further evidence that the cytoskeleton may influence paracellular permeability and junctional charge selectivity. *J Cell Biol* 1986;102:2125–2136.
46. Kashgarian M, Van Why SK, Hildebrand F, et al. Regulation of expression and polar distribution of Na,K ATPase in renal epithelium during recovery from ischemic injury. In: Kaplan P, Deweer P, eds. *The sodium pump: recent developments*. New York: The Rockefeller University Press, 1991:573–577.
47. Molitoris BA, Dahl R, Hosford M. Cellular ATP depletion induces disruption of the spectrin cytoskeletal network. *Am J Physiol* 1996;271:F790–F798.
48. Liberthal W, Levine JS. Mechanisms of apoptosis and its potential role in renal tubular epithelial cell injury. *Am J Physiol* 1996;271:F477–F488.
49. Squier MKT, Miller ACK, Cohen JJ. Calpain activation in apoptosis. *J Cell Physiol* 1994;159:229–237.
50. Boystun I, Najjar S, Kashgarian M, et al. Postischemic thyroxin stimulates renal mitochondrial adenine nucleotide translocator activity. *Am J Physiol* 1995;268:F651–F656.
51. Nakamoto M, Shapiro JI, Shanley PF, et al. In vitro and in vivo protective effect of atriopeptin III on ischemic acute renal failure. *J Clin Invest* 1987;80:1232–1237.
52. Conger JD, Falk SA, Hammond WS. Atrial natriuretic peptide and dopamine in established acute renal failure in the rat. *Kidney Int* 1991;40:21–28.
53. Marks RM, Todd RF III, Ward PA. Rapid induction of neutrophil-endothelial adhesion by endothelial complement fixation. *Nature* 1989;339:314–317.
54. Kelly KJ, Williams WW, Colvin RB, et al. Intercellular adhesion molecule-I deficient mice are protected against ischemic renal injury. *J Clin Invest* 1996;97:1056–1063.
55. Kelly KJ, Williams WW Jr, Colvin RB, et al. Antibody to intercellular adhesion molecule I protects the kidney against ischemic injury. *Proc Natl Acad Sci U S A* 1994;91:812–816.
56. Nover L, ed. *Heat shock response*. Boca Raton, FL: CRC Press, 1991.
57. Van Why SK, Mann AS, Ardito T, et al. Expression and molecular regulation of Na^+-K^+-ATPase after renal ischemia. *Am J Physiol* 1994;267:F75–F85.
58. Emami A, Schwartz JH, Borkan SC. Transient ischemia or heat stress induces a cytoprotectant protein in rat kidney. *Am J Physiol* 1991;260:F479–F485.
59. Van Why SK, Hildebrandt F, Ardito T, et al. Induction and intracellular localization of HSP-72 after renal ischemia. *Am J Physiol* 1992;32:F769–F775.
60. Aufricht C, Ardito T, Thulin G, et al. Heat-shock protein 25 induction and redistribution during actin reorganization after renal ischemia. *Am J Physiol* 1998;274:F215–F222.
61. Hammerman MR, Miller SB. Therapeutic use of growth factors in renal failure. *J Am Soc Nephrol* 1994;5:1–11.
62. Humes HD, Creslinski DA, Johnson LB, et al. Triiodothyronine enhances renal tubule cell replication by stimulating EGF receptor gene expression. *Am J Physiol* 1992;262:F540–F545.
63. Toback FG. Regeneration after acute tubular necrosis. *Kidney Int* 1992;41:226–246.
64. Fine LG, Hammerman MR, Abboud HE. Evolving role of growth factors in the renal response to acute and chronic disease. *J Am Soc Nephrol* 1992;2:1163–1170.
65. Dagher P, Herget-Rosenthal S, Reuhm S, et al. Newly developed techniques to study and diagnose acute renal failure. *J Am Soc Nephrol* 2003;14:2188–2198.
66. Bonventre J, Weinberg J. Recent advances in the pathophysiology of ischemic acute renal failure. *J Am Soc Nephrol* 2003;14:2199–2210.

64

CLINICAL EVALUATION AND MANAGEMENT

SHARON P. ANDREOLI

DEFINITION

Acute renal failure is characterized by an abrupt increase in the blood concentration of creatinine and nitrogenous waste products, a decrease in the glomerular filtration rate (GFR), and the inability of the kidney to appropriately regulate fluid and electrolyte homeostasis. Increases in the levels of serum creatinine and blood urea nitrogen (BUN) are typical in acute renal failure, but each may be affected by factors other than a decline in the GFR. Because the serum creatinine level is a reflection of muscle mass, children with decreased muscle mass may have substantial decreases in their GFR with minimal to modest changes in the serum creatinine concentration. BUN is affected by multiple factors, including the state of hydration of the child and conditions that increase urea production, such as gastrointestinal bleeding, high protein intake, a hypermetabolic state, or the administration of catabolic medications such as corticosteroids. Each of these states increase the BUN level independently of renal function. In contrast, BUN may be lower than expected in acute renal failure in a child with diminished urea production, such as in severe liver disease, or in a child with protein malnutrition.

Although a decline in urine output is a common clinical manifestation of acute renal failure, some forms of acute renal failure are associated with normal urine output. Children with acute renal failure due to hypoxic-ischemic insults, hemolytic uremic syndrome (HUS), acute glomerulonephritis, rapidly progressive glomerulonephritis, or other causes are more likely to demonstrate oliguria or anuria (urine output <400 to 500 mL/24 hr in older children or urine output <0.5 to 1.0 mL/kg/hr in younger children and infants). Children with acute interstitial nephritis or nephrotoxic renal insults, including aminoglycoside nephrotoxicity and contrast nephropathy, are more likely to have acute renal failure with normal urine output. Several studies have shown that the morbidity and mortality of nonoliguric acute renal failure are substantially lower than those of oliguric renal failure (1–8). Although nonoliguric renal failure is more commonly associated with nephrotoxic insults, studies also suggest that the degree of oliguria or anuria is also related to the severity of the insult, with less severe insults resulting in nonoliguric acute renal failure (3,4).

EPIDEMIOLOGY OF ACUTE RENAL FAILURE

Although the precise incidence and prevalence of acute renal failure in pediatric patients is unknown, studies suggest that the incidence of acute renal failure in hospitalized children may be increasing (5–13). In a large study of adult patients, the incidence of acute renal failure was 209 per 1 million population, and the most common cause of acute renal failure was prerenal in 21% of patients and acute tubular necrosis in 45% of patients (13). Similar epidemiologic studies have not been performed in pediatric patients, but hypoxia-ischemia and nephrotoxicity have been shown to be important causes of acute renal failure in neonates, children, and adolescents (5–7,9). In a study of pediatric patients in a tertiary care center, 227 children received dialysis therapy during an 8-year interval for an overall incidence of 8 per 1 million total population (6). In one study of neonates, the incidence of acute renal failure ranged from 8 to 24% of newborns, and acute renal failure was particularly common in neonates who had undergone cardiac surgery (6–8). Neonates experiencing severe asphyxia had a high incidence of acute renal failure, whereas acute renal failure was less common in neonates with moderate asphyxia and the acute renal failure was nonoliguric, oliguric, and anuric in 60%, 25%, and 15%, respectively (6–8,11).

In addition to environmental risks factors for acute renal failure, some children may also have genetic risks factors for acute renal failure. Polymorphism of the angiotensin-converting enzyme gene or the angiotensin receptor gene with resultant alterations in activity of the renin-angiotensin system might play a role in the development of acute renal failure (14). In a study in neonates, the incidence of angiotensin-converting enzyme I/D allele genotypes or the variants of the angiotensin I receptor gene did not differ in neonates with acute renal failure and neonates without acute renal failure (14). In other studies, polymorphisms of tumor necrosis factor-α, interleukin-1β, interleukin-6, and interleukin-10 genes were investigated in newborns to determine if polymorphisms of these genes would lead to a more intense inflammatory response and predispose newborns to acute renal failure (15). The allelic frequency of the individual genes did not differ between newborns with acute renal failure and those without acute renal failure, but the tumor necrosis factor-α/interleukin-6 AG/GC haplotypes were present in 26% of newborns who developed acute renal failure compared to 6% of newborns who did not develop acute renal failure. The investigators suggested that the combination of these polymorphisms might lead to a greater inflammatory response and the development of acute renal failure in neonates with infection (15). Future studies of the genetic background of the child at risk for acute renal failure due to medication exposure, toxin exposure, ischemic-hypoxic insults, or other insults will likely influence the management of the child at risk for acute renal failure and the management of acute renal failure.

ETIOLOGY OF ACUTE RENAL FAILURE IN CHILDREN

There are many different causes of acute renal failure in neonates, infants, children, and adolescents. Renal failure can be divided into prerenal failure, intrinsic renal disease including vascular insults, and obstructive uropathies (Table 64.1). Some causes of acute renal failure such as cortical necrosis and renal vein thrombosis occur more commonly in neonates, whereas HUS is more common in young children and rapidly progressive glomerulonephritis generally occurs in older children and adolescents. The history, physical examination, laboratory studies, including a urinalysis, and radiographic studies can establish the likely cause(s) of renal failure. In some instances, such as in acute renal failure occurring in hospitalized children, multiple factors are likely to be implicated as the cause of acute renal failure. Tables 64.2 and 64.3 show the clinical, laboratory, and radiographic findings in the more common broad categories of acute renal failure in children.

TABLE 64.1. ETIOLOGY OF ACUTE RENAL FAILURE IN NEONATES, INFANTS, CHILDREN, AND ADOLESCENTS

- **Prerenal failure**
  - **Decreased true intravascular volume**
    - Dehydration
    - Gastrointestinal losses
    - Salt-wasting renal or adrenal disease
    - Central or nephrogenic diabetes insipidus
    - Third-space losses (sepsis, traumatized tissues, nephrotic syndrome)
  - **Decreased effective intravascular volume**
    - Congestive heart failure
    - Pericarditis, cardiac tamponade
- **Intrinsic renal disease**
  - **Acute tubular necrosis**
    - Ischemic-hypoxic insults
    - Drugs
      - Aminoglycosides
      - Intravascular contrast medium
      - Cisplatin
      - Ifosfamide
      - Nonsteroidal antiinflammatory drugs
      - Acetaminophen
    - Toxins
      - Exogenous toxins
        - Ethylene glycol, methanol, bromate, toxic mushrooms
        - Heavy metals
      - Endogenous toxins
        - Myoglobin and hemoglobin
  - **Uric acid nephropathy and tumor lysis syndrome**
  - **Interstitial nephritis**
    - Drug induced—antibiotics, anticonvulsants
    - Idiopathic
  - **Glomerulonephritis**
    - Postinfectious glomerulonephritis
    - Membranoproliferative glomerulonephritis
    - Systemic lupus erythematosus nephritis
    - Nephritis of chronic infection
    - Henoch-Schönlein purpura nephritis
    - Antineutrophil cytoplasmic antibody–positive glomerulonephritis
    - Anti–glomerular basement membrane glomerulonephritis
    - Goodpasture syndrome
    - Idiopathic rapidly progressive glomerulonephritis
  - **Vascular lesions**
    - Hemolytic uremic syndrome (HUS)
      - Vero cytotoxin–producing *Escherichia coli*–associated HUS
      - Drug-induced HUS (mitomycin, birth control pills, quinine)
      - Bone marrow transplant nephropathy
    - Cortical necrosis
    - Renal artery thrombosis
    - Renal venous thrombosis
  - **Infectious causes**
    - Sepsis, with or without disseminated intravascular coagulation
    - Pyelonephritis
- **Obstructive uropathy**
  - **Obstruction in a solitary kidney**
  - **Bilateral ureteral obstruction**
  - **Urethral obstruction**

Prerenal Failure

When a child is at risk for developing acute renal failure, appropriate therapy can prevent or decrease the extent of the injury that leads to acute renal failure. Adequate hydration of the dehydrated child, avoidance of nephrotoxic drugs when possible, and other appropriate measures can minimize or prevent acute deterioration in renal function in children. Specific measures that can help minimize or eliminate acute deterioration in renal function include hydration of the child receiving nephrotoxic drugs such as amphotericin B, cisplatin, and intravascular contrast media as well as avoidance of prostaglandin synthetase inhibitors and angiotensin-converting enzyme inhibitor therapy during volume depletion and renal hypoperfusion (16–26).

TABLE 64.2. EVALUATION OF CAUSES OF ACUTE RENAL FAILURE IN CHILDREN BY SEVERITY OF INSULT

	Prerenal failure	Acute tubular necrosis	Cortical necrosis
Clinical history	Dehydration Vomiting, diarrhea Hemorrhage Diabetes insipidus Third-space losses Congestive heart failure Cardiac tamponade Hepatorenal syndrome	Dehydration, hemorrhage Hypoxia-ischemia Toxins Sepsis Hemoglobinuria Myoglobinuria Nephrotoxic drugs NSAIDs, ACE inhibitors	Hypoxia-ischemia Placental abruption Twin-twin or twin-maternal transfusion Renal artery or vein thrombosis
Urine output	Decreased	Oliguria or nonoliguria	Oliguria
Urinalysis	Normal or minor changes	Granular casts Pigmenturia Epithelial cells Epithelial casts	Gross or microscopic hematuria Proteinuria
Urine osmolality	>400–500 mOsm	<350 mOsm	
Newborn	>350 mOsm	<300 mOsm	
Urine Na	<10 mEq/L	>30–40 mEq/L	
Newborn	<20–30 mEq/L	>30–40 mEq/L	
FE_{Na}	<1%	>2%	
Newborn	<2.5%	>2.5–3.0%	
Laboratory studies	Increased BUN compared to creatinine		Thrombocytopenia Microangiopathy
Imaging studies	US: normal	US: normal or increased echogenicity with loss of corticomedullary differentiation	US: normal or loss of cortomedullary differentiation
	RS normal	RS: normal or slightly decreased blood flow with delayed renal parenchymal accumulation of isotope	RS: poor or no blood flow with no accumulation of isotope

ACE, angiotensin-converting enzyme; BUN, blood urea nitrogen; FE_{Na}, fractional excretion of sodium; NSAID, nonsteroidal antiinflammatory drug; RS, radiographic scan; US, ultrasonographic scan.

TABLE 64.3. EVALUATION OF CAUSES OF ACUTE RENAL FAILURE IN CHILDREN BY TYPE OF INJURY

	Interstitial nephritis	Glomerulonephritis	Hemolytic uremic syndrome	Obstruction
Clinical history	Drug exposure Infection Rash Fever	Previous infection Systemic symptoms Rash Fever	Diarrheal (may be bloody) prodrome	Flank masses Abdominal mass Palpable bladder Posterior urethral valve in newborn
Urine output	Variable Usually nonoliguric	Variable Usually oliguric	Variable Usually oliguric	Variable
Urinalysis	Pyuria WBC casts Eosinophiluria	Gross or microscopic hematuria RBC casts Proteinuria	Hematuria RBC casts Proteinuria	Unremarkable
Urine osmolality	<350 mOsm	>400–500 mOsm	Variable	Variable
Urine Na	>30–40 mEq/L	<10 mEq/L	Variable	Variable
FE_{Na}	>2%	<1%	Variable	Variable
Laboratory studies	Eosinophilia	Positive ANA, ANCA Low C3, C4	Thrombocytopenia Microangiopathic hemolytic anemia	
Imaging studies	US: nephromegaly and increased echogenicity	US: nephromegaly and loss of corticomedullary differentiation	US: normal or loss of corticomedullary differentiation RS: poor flow with decreased function	US: dilated pelvis, ureter, and/or bladder depending on level of obstruction RS: collection of isotope in pelvis, ureter, or bladder depending on level of obstruction

ANA, antinuclear antibodies; ANCA, antineutrophil cytoplasmic antibodies; FE_{Na}, fractional excretion of sodium; RS, radiographic scan; US, ultrasonographic scan.

The prophylactic administration of *N*-acetylcysteine has been shown to dampen the decline in GFR associated with the administration of intravascular contrast agents in adults at risk for contrast nephropathy (23). However, a separate study did not demonstrate such a benefit in adult patients undergoing cardiac angiography (24). Similar studies have not been performed in pediatric patients. The potential hazards and benefits of *N*-acetylcysteine in pediatric patients at risk for contrast nephropathy are unknown, and such studies should be performed.

In prerenal failure, renal function is decreased due to decreased renal perfusion, but the kidney is intrinsically normal. Restoration of renal perfusion results in a prompt return of renal function to normal, whereas the presence of acute tubular necrosis as described later implies that the kidney has suffered intrinsic damage. The evolution of prerenal failure to intrinsic renal failure is not sudden, however, and a number of compensatory mechanisms work together to maintain renal perfusion in the face of adverse renal hemodynamic conditions (16–22). When renal perfusion is compromised, the afferent arteriole relaxes its vascular tone to decrease renal vascular resistance and maintain renal blood flow. Decreased renal perfusion results in increased catecholamine secretion, activation of the renin-angiotensin system, and generation of prostaglandins. During renal hypoperfusion, the intrarenal generation of vasodilatory prostaglandins, including prostacyclin, mediates vasodilatation of the renal microvasculature to maintain renal perfusion (16–18). Administration of aspirin or nonsteroidal antiinflammatory drugs can inhibit this compensatory mechanism and precipitate acute renal insufficiency during renal hypoperfusion. Similarly, when renal perfusion pressure is low, as in renal artery stenosis, the intraglomerular pressure necessary to drive filtration is in part mediated by increased intrarenal generation of angiotensin II to increase efferent arteriolar resistance (19–22). Administration of angiotensin-converting enzyme inhibitors under these conditions can eliminate the pressure gradient needed to drive filtration and precipitate acute renal failure (19–22). It was originally thought that selective cyclooxygenase-2 (COX-2) inhibitors would be renal sparing, but it has been recognized that the selective COX-2 inhibitors can adversely affect renal hemodynamics in a way similar to nonselective COX inhibitors (25). In addition, clinical use of selective COX-2 inhibitors has been associated with acute renal failure (26). Thus, administration of medications that can interfere with compensatory mechanisms to maintain renal perfusion can precipitate acute renal failure in certain clinical circumstances.

Prerenal failure results from renal hypoperfusion due to true volume contraction or from a decreased effective blood volume (1,6–19). True volume contraction results from hemorrhage, dehydration due to gastrointestinal losses, salt-wasting renal or adrenal diseases, central or nephrogenic diabetes insipidus, increased insensible losses such as occur in burns, and disease states associated with third-space losses such as sepsis, nephrotic syndrome, tissue trauma, and capillary leak syndrome. Decreased effective blood volume occurs when the true blood volume is normal or increased but renal perfusion is decreased due to diseases such as congestive heart failure, cardiac tamponade, and hepatorenal syndrome (16–19). Whether prerenal failure is caused by true volume depletion or decreased effective blood volume, correction of the underlying disturbance returns renal function to normal.

Urine osmolality, urine sodium concentration, fractional excretion of sodium, and the renal failure index have all been proposed to help differentiate prerenal failure from vasomotor nephropathy (acute tubular necrosis). This differentiation is based on the concept that the tubules are working appropriately in prerenal failure and are therefore able to conserve salt and water appropriately, whereas in vasomotor nephropathy the tubules have progressed to irreversible injury and are unable to appropriately conserve sodium (1,16,20–22). During prerenal failure, the tubules are able to respond to decreased renal perfusion by appropriately conserving sodium and water so that the urine osmolality is greater than 400 to 500 mOsm/L, the urine sodium level is less than 10 to 20 mEq/L, and the fractional excretion of sodium (FE_{Na}) is less than 1%. FE_{Na} is calculated by the following formula:

$$FE_{Na} = [(U_{Na}/P_{Cr})/(P_{Na}/U_{Cr})] \times 100 \qquad \text{[Eq. 1]}$$

where U_{Na} is urine sodium level, P_{Na} is plasma sodium level, U_{Cr} is urine creatinine level, and P_{Cr} is plasma creatinine level. Because the renal tubules in newborns and premature infants are relatively immature compared to those in older infants and children, the corresponding values suggestive of renal hypoperfusion are a urine osmolality higher than 350 mOsm/L, urine sodium lower than 20 to 30 mEq/L, and an FE_{Na} lower than 2.5% (27–29). When the renal tubules have sustained injury as occurs in acute tubular necrosis, they cannot appropriately conserve sodium and water, so that the urine osmolality is lower than 350 mOsm/L, the urine sodium is higher than 30 to 40 mEq/L, and the FE_{Na} is higher than 2%. However, the use of these values to differentiate prerenal failure from acute tubular necrosis requires that the patient have normal tubular function initially. Although this may be the case in some children, newborns with immature tubules and children with preexisting renal disease, salt-wasting renal adrenal disease, as well as other diseases may have prerenal failure with urinary indices suggestive of acute tubular necrosis. Therefore, it is essential to consider the state of the function of the tubules before the potential onset that might precipitate vasomotor nephropathy and acute tubular necrosis.

In adult patients it has been shown that calculation of the fractional excretion of urea nitrogen (FE_{UN}) is a more sensitive test than FE_{Na} to differentiate prerenal failure from acute tubular necrosis, particularly in patients who have received diuretic therapy (30). FE_{UN} is given by:

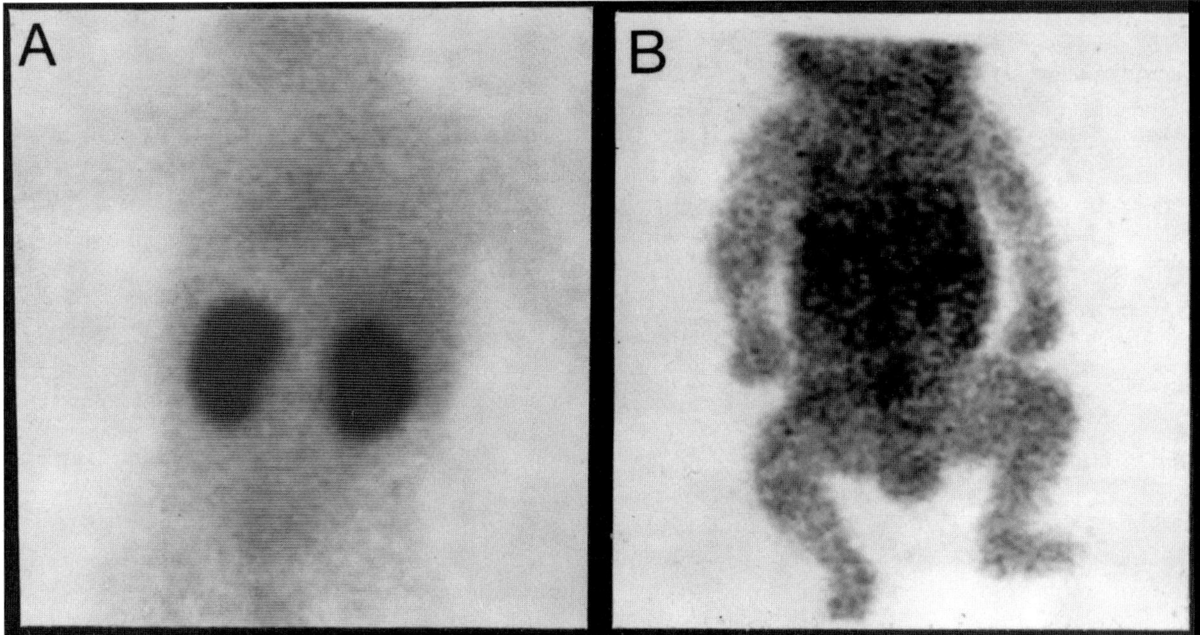

FIGURE 64.1. Mercaptotriglyclglycine renal scan for a 1-year-old with acute tubular necrosis **(A)** and a newborn with cortical necrosis **(B)**. Each scan was made 4 hours after injection of the isotope. **A:** Shows delayed uptake of isotope with parenchymal accumulation of isotope and little or no excretion of isotope into the collecting system. **B:** In contrast, demonstrates no renal parenchymal uptake of isotope.

$$FE_{UN} = [(UUN/U_{Cr})/(BUN/P_{Cr})] \times 100 \quad \text{[Eq. 2]}$$

where UUN is urine urea nitrogen. An FE_{UN} value of less than 35% typically signifies prerenal azotemia and FE_{UN} of more than 50% indicates acute tubular necrosis. FE_{UN} was found to be at least as sensitive and specific an indicator as FE_{Na} in prerenal azotemia, but FE_{UN} did not lose its sensitivity or specificity in differentiation of prerenal failure and acute tubular necrosis when patients had received diuretic therapy (30). Whether FE_{UN} is more sensitive or specific than FE_{Na} in pediatric patients is unknown, and such studies need to be performed to determine if FE_{UN} is a more sensitive measure of tubular function in children.

Intrinsic Renal Disease

Acute Tubular Necrosis

Acute tubular necrosis can evolve from prerenal failure if the insult is severe and sufficient enough to result in vasoconstriction and tubular damage. The pathophysiology of ischemic-hypoxic acute tubular necrosis is thought to be related to early vasoconstriction followed by patchy tubular necrosis. Acute tubular necrosis may also result from toxic injury of tubular epithelial cells caused by drugs, including aminoglycoside antibiotics, cisplatin, ifosfamide, amphotericin B, acetaminophen, and radio-contrast dye, as well as exogenous toxins such as ethylene glycol, methanol, or bromate or endogenous toxins such as myoglobin and hemoglobin (Table 64.1).

Hypoxic-Ischemic Acute Tubular Necrosis

Hypoxic-ischemic acute tubular necrosis evolves from prolonged prerenal failure or severe hypoxic insults. Results of the urinalysis may be unremarkable or may demonstrate low-grade proteinuria and granular casts, and urine indices of tubular function demonstrate an inability to conserve sodium and water as described earlier. The creatinine level typically increases by 0.5 to 1.0 mg/dL/day. Radiographic studies demonstrate kidneys of normal size with loss of corticomedullary differentiation, whereas a radionucleotide renal scan using technetium-99–mercaptotriglyclglycine or technetium-99–diethylenetriaminepenta-acetic acid shows normal or slightly decreased renal blood flow with poor function and delayed accumulation of the radioisotope in the renal parenchyma without excretion of the isotope in the collecting system (Fig. 64.1A).

The prognosis of acute tubular necrosis is good except in cases in which the insult is of sufficient severity to lead to vasculature injury and microthrombi formation with the subsequent development of cortical necrosis. The recovery of the child and the recovery of renal function depend on the underlying events that precipitated the ischemic-hypoxic insults. The mortality and morbidity of acute renal failure is much worse in children and neonates with multiorgan failure, and the child does not succumb to renal failure but rather the child succumbs to renal failure and the associated conditions that precipitated the multiorgan failure (8,11,31–37). In children who recover from acute tubular necrosis, renal function returns to normal, but the length of time before recovery is quite variable. Some children begin to recover renal function within days of the onset of renal failure, whereas recovery may not occur for several weeks in other children. Return of renal function may be accompanied by a diuretic phase with excessive urine output at a time when the tubules have begun to recover from the insult but have not recovered sufficiently to appropriately reabsorb solute and water. When the diuretic phase occurs during recovery, close attention to fluid and electrolyte balance is very important to ensure adequate fluid management so as to promote recovery from acute tubular necrosis and prevent additional renal injury.

Nephrotoxic Acute Renal Failure

Many different drugs and agents may result in nephrotoxic acute renal failure (38,39). Nephrotoxic acute renal failure may result from the administration of a number of different medications as well as the ingestion of poisons or from a nephrotoxic insult from indigenous compounds such as hemoglobin or myoglobin.

Drug-Induced Acute Renal Failure. Medications that are associated with acute renal failure at least in part due to toxic tubular injury include aminoglycoside antibiotics, intravascular contrast media, amphotericin B, chemotherapeutic agents such as ifosfamide and cisplatin, acyclovir, and acetaminophen; other medications have been implicated less commonly (38–49). Aminoglycoside nephrotoxicity usually presents with nonoliguric acute renal failure with a urinalysis showing minimal urinary abnormalities (40). The incidence of aminoglycoside antibiotic nephrotoxicity is related to the dose and duration of the antibiotic therapy as well as the level of renal function before the initiation of aminoglycoside therapy. The cause of aminoglycoside nephrotoxicity is thought to be related to the lysosomal dysfunction of proximal tubules and is reversible once the aminoglycoside antibiotics have been discontinued. After the aminoglycoside is discontinued, however, the serum creatinine level may continue to increase for several days due to ongoing tubular injury from continued high parenchymal levels of the aminoglycoside. Studies have demonstrated that once-daily dosing of aminoglycoside antibiotics is associated with a slightly decreased incidence of nephrotoxicity without compromising efficacy (50,51).

Intravascular contrast media may also precipitate acute renal failure, particularly in patients who are at higher risk for contrast nephropathy, including patients with dehydration, diabetes, or preexisting renal disease and patients with hypergammaglobulinemia (41,42). The incidence of contrast nephropathy can be reduced through the use of nonionic, low-osmolality contrast media (41,42). Use of the iso-osmolar, dimeric nonionic contrast medium iodixanol is associated with an even lower risk of contrast nephropathy (52). The prophylactic administration of *N*-acetylcysteine may decrease the decline in GFR associated with the administration of an intravascular contrast agent in adults at risk for contrast nephropathy (25). Similar studies have not been performed in pediatric patients, and the potential hazards and benefits of *N*-acetylcysteine in pediatric patients at risk for contrast nephropathy are unknown.

Nonsteroidal antiinflammatory drugs may also precipitate acute renal failure by their effect on intrarenal hemodynamics (16–21). Cisplatin, ifosfamide, acyclovir, amphotericin B, and acetaminophen are also nephrotoxic and may precipitate acute renal failure (43–51). Predictors of amphotericin B nephrotoxicity include high daily dosage and concomitant use of cyclosporine (43). The combination of a cephalosporin and acyclovir may be particularly nephrotoxic (49). Several other drugs have also been associated with acute renal failure, but the incidence of acute renal failure with these other drugs is lower.

Exogenous Toxin–Induced Acute Renal Failure. Ingested toxic compounds, either in their native state or after metabolization, may precipitate acute renal failure. The best known of such toxins are ethylene glycol and methanol (53–57). Both ethylene glycol and methanol are not toxic until they are metabolized by alcohol dehydrogenase to organic acids and oxalate for ethylene glycol, and formic acid and formaldehyde for methanol. Once sufficient quantities of the metabolites have been generated, the patient will present with severe metabolic acidosis with a large anion gap. Ethylene glycol intoxication may also be characterized by calcium oxalate crystalluria and hematuria on urinalysis; other laboratory findings may include hypocalcemia. Both ethylene glycol and methanol intoxication can result from the accidental ingestion of antifreeze or transmission fluid or from a suicide attempt in older children. In the past ethylene glycol and methanol intoxication were best treated with an ethanol drip to competitively inhibit ethanol dehydrogenase and decrease the metabolism of ethylene glycol and methanol to their toxic metabolites. In addition, for patients with moderate to severe intoxication as indicated by a substantial metabolic acidosis and/or an initial ethylene glycol or methanol level higher than 50 mg/dL, the patient should be urgently treated with bicarbonate hemodialysis (43–45). This allows removal of ethylene glycol or methanol before it is metabolized to its toxic compounds and treats the acidosis as well. Fomepizole (4-methylpyrazole), an inhibitor of alcohol dehydrogenase, has been shown to be effective in the treatment of ethylene glycol intoxication in adults and pediatric patients (56,57). Fomepizole does not have the adverse effects of ethanol infusion in pediatric patients.

Other compounds that may cause acute renal failure upon ingestion include potassium sodium bromate, which is contained in hair permanent-wave solutions (58,59). Other less common causes of acute renal failure include the ingestion of carbon tetrachloride and heavy metals such as mercury and other compounds (39).

Endogenous Toxin–Induced Acute Renal Failure Including Hemoglobinuria and Myoglobinuria. Hemolysis and rhabdomyolysis from any cause can result in sufficient hemoglobinuria or myoglobinuria to induce tubular injury and precipitate acute renal failure (60–65). Risk factors for acute renal failure during an episode of rhabdomyolysis in children include dehydration, a high serum concentration of myoglobin, the presence of other organ failure, and the presence of the systemic inflammatory response syndrome (61). The mechanisms of injury are complex but may be related to vasoconstriction, precipitation of the pigments in the tubular lumen, and/or heme protein–induced oxidant stress (62–64). If the rhabdomyolysis is a result of tissue injury with substantial third-space fluid losses as occurs in a crush injury, rapid fluid resuscitation can prevent or limit the renal injury (65). Once intravascular volume has been established, diuretic therapy with mannitol or other loop diuretics to promote flow, prevent precipitation of the heme proteins in the tubules, and alkalize the urine to potentially increase the solubility of hemoglobin and myoglobin has been proposed to decrease tubular injury (65). Hyperkalemia, acidosis, and other electrolyte abnormalities may develop rapidly and require prompt therapy.

Uric Acid Nephropathy and Tumor Lysis Syndrome

Acute renal failure may be detected at the time of diagnosis of leukemia or lymphoma due to infiltration of tumor cells in the kidney or due to uric acid nephropathy. Radiographic studies demonstrate either mass lesions in the kidney in the case of lymphoma or diffuse infiltrative disease in the case of leukemia (66–68). Children with acute lymphocytic leukemia and B-cell lymphoma are at the highest risk for uric acid nephropathy and tumor lysis syndrome (68,69). Although the pathogenesis of uric acid nephropathy is complex, an important potential mechanism of injury is the precipitation of uric acid crystals in the tubules to obstruct urine flow or in the renal microvasculature to obstruct renal blood flow (68,69). A more common cause of acute renal failure in leukemia is the development of the tumor lysis syndrome during chemotherapy (68,69). Administration of allopurinol limits the increased excretion of uric acid with chemotherapy, but allopurinol treatment results in a markedly increased excretion of uric acid precursors, including hypoxanthine and xanthine (69). Xanthine is less soluble than uric acid, and precipitation of hypoxanthine and xanthine may play a role in the development of acute renal failure during tumor lysis syndrome. Tumor lysis syndrome results in rapid increases in the levels of serum potassium, BUN, purine metabolite products, and phosphorus with a reciprocal decrease in the serum calcium level as tumor cells are lysed. Acute renal failure due to tumor lysis syndrome is transient, and the patient eventually recovers renal function once tumor lysis is complete. However, frequent hemodialysis or continuous hemofiltration may be necessary to control hyperkalemia and other metabolic abnormalities resulting from the rapid lysis of tumor cells (70–72).

Acute Interstitial Nephritis

Acute interstitial nephritis resulting from a reaction to a drug or idiopathic acute interstitial nephritis may cause acute renal failure. Children with acute interstitial nephritis may have rash, fever, arthralgias, eosinophilia, and pyuria with or without eosinophiluria (73). Uveitis has been reported in several cases of acute interstitial nephritis and is important to recognize, because treatment with topical steroids may be indicated for the uveitis (74). Radiographic studies demonstrate large echogenic kidneys, and a kidney biopsy specimen demonstrates interstitial infiltrate with many eosinophils. The pathogenesis of drug-induced acute interstitial nephritis is thought to be related to a hypersensitivity reaction, with the development of anti–tubular basement membrane antibodies in some cases (73–75). Medications commonly associated with acute interstitial nephritis include methicillin and other penicillin analogues, cimetidine, sulfonamides, rifampin, and nonsteroidal antiinflammatory drugs; other drugs have been associated with acute interstitial nephritis less commonly (73,75). Acute interstitial nephritis associated with nonsteroidal antiinflammatory drugs may also present with high-grade proteinuria and nephrotic syndrome (75). Specific therapy for acute interstitial nephritis includes the withdrawal of the drug implicated in causing the acute interstitial nephritis. In addition, corticosteroids may aid in the resolution of the renal failure.

Rapidly Progressive Glomerulonephritis

Any form of glomerulonephritis at its most severe can present with acute renal failure and rapidly progressive glomerulonephritis. The clinical features include hypertension, edema, hematuria, which is frequently gross, and rapidly rising BUN and creatinine levels. The characteristic pathologic finding in rapidly progressive glomerulonephritis is extensive crescent formation. Some glomerulonephritides, such as postinfectious glomerulonephritis, membranoproliferative glomerulonephritis, Henoch-Schönlein purpura nephritis, and lupus nephritis, present with a rapidly progressive course in a minority of cases. However, other glomerulonephritides, such as antineutrophil cytoplasmic antibody (ANCA)–positive glomerulonephritis, Goodpasture syndrome, and idiopathic rapidly progressive glomerulonephritis, typically present with acute renal failure (76–78). Serologic tests including tests for antinuclear antibodies and ANCA, anti–glomerular basement membrane titers, and complement studies are required to evaluate the cause of the rapidly progressive glomerulonephritis. The presence of active lesions in biopsy specimens is associated with recovery of renal function, and the disorder may be reversible with immunosuppressive therapy (75). Because the treatment depends on the pathologic findings, a biopsy should be performed quite promptly when a child presents with clinical characteristics suggestive of rapidly progressive glomerulonephritis so that specific therapy can be initiated as soon as possible.

Vascular Insults

Large vessel insults such as renal artery thrombosis and renal vein thrombosis present with acute renal failure only if they are bilateral or if they occur in a solitary kidney. Microvascular insults occur in cortical necrosis, in typical (diarrhea positive) and atypical (diarrhea negative) HUS, and in HUS after bone marrow transplantation.

Renal Artery Thrombosis and Renal Venous Thrombosis

Renal artery thrombosis, cortical necrosis, and renal venous thrombosis occur most commonly in newborns and small children. Renal artery thrombosis is strongly associated with an umbilical artery line and a patent ductus arteriosus (79,80). In addition to acute renal failure, children may demonstrate hypertension, gross or microscopic hematuria, thrombocytopenia, and oliguria. In renal artery thrombosis, the initial ultrasonographic image may appear normal or may demonstrate minor abnormalities, whereas a renal scan demonstrates little or no blood flow. In renal vein thrombosis, the ultrasonographic image demonstrates an enlarged, swollen kidney, and the renal scan typically shows decreased blood flow and function. Therapy should be aimed at limiting extension of the clot by removal of the umbilical arterial catheter, and anticoagulant or fibrinolytic therapy can be considered, particularly if the clot is large (79–82).

Cortical Necrosis

Cortical necrosis as a cause of acute renal failure is much more common in young children, particularly in the neonate. Cortical necrosis is associated with hypoxic-ischemic insults due to perinatal anoxia, placental abruption, and twin-twin or twin-maternal transfusions with resultant activation of the coagulation cascade. Children and newborns with cortical necrosis usually have gross or microscopic hematuria and oliguria, and may have hypertension as well (83). In addition to laboratory features of elevated BUN and creatinine levels, thrombocytopenia may also be present due to the microvascular injury. Radiographic features include a normal renal ultrasonogram in the early phase, but in the later phases ultrasonography may show that the kidney has undergone atrophy and has substantially decreased in size. A radionucleotide renal scan shows decreased or no perfusion with delayed or no function (Fig. 64.1B) in contrast to the delayed uptake of the radioisotope that is observed in acute tubular necrosis (Fig. 64.1A). The prognosis of cortical necrosis is much worse than that of acute tubular necrosis. Children with cortical necrosis may have partial recovery or no recovery at all. Typically, children with cortical necrosis will need short- or long-term dialysis therapy, but children who do recover sufficient renal function are at risk for the late development of chronic renal insufficiency and end-stage renal disease.

Hemolytic Uremic Syndrome

HUS is a common cause of intrinsic acute renal failure in children and leads to substantial morbidity and mortality as well as long-term complications that may not become apparent until adulthood (84–110). Typical HUS usually follows a gastrointestinal illness characterized by hemorrhagic colitis associated with infection with vero cytotoxin–producing *Escherichia coli*, of which O157:H7 is the most common serotype. Shiga toxin–producing *E. coli* was first linked to human disease in the early 1980s (89–91). Several well-publicized outbreaks of hemorrhagic colitis and HUS have highlighted the morbidity and mortality of infection with vero cytotoxin–producing *E. coli*. In 1993, an outbreak in the western United States resulted in several cases of severe HUS with substantial extrarenal complications (95). In 1996, over 5000 Japanese schoolchildren were infected with vero cytotoxin–producing *E. coli*. An outbreak in Scotland resulted in 20 deaths. One outbreak in the United States was traced to contaminated apple juice, and several million pounds of contaminated hamburger was recalled by the manufacturers (96,97). In case-control studies, consumption of a beef burger and/or consumption of cold cooked sliced meat was found to be associated with vero cytotoxin–producing *Escherichia coli* O157 infection (98). Although undercooked beef is the most common vector for O157:H7 infection, apple juice, radish sprouts, sausages, and other food sources have been implicated in the spread of vero cytotoxin–producing *E. coli* infections. In the United States and Europe, the O157:H7 serotype is the serotype most commonly implicated in infection with vero cytotoxin–producing organisms, but in other areas of the world non-O157:H7 strains are emerging as important pathogens (99–101). *E. coli* O111:H– caused a large outbreak of hemorrhagic colitis and HUS in Australia, and other serotypes have been associated with hemorrhagic colitis and HUS as well (100,101).

Among persons infected with vero cytotoxin–producing *E. coli*, the percentage of patients who progress to HUS ranges from 5 to 15%. In children under 5 years of age, the rate of progression to hemolytic anemia or HUS is 12.9%, whereas the rate is 6.8 for children aged 5.0 to 9.9 years and 8% for those older than 10 years of age (92). In another separate study, children with a white blood cell count higher than 13,000/mm^3 during the initial 3 days of illness with vero cytotoxin–producing *E. coli* infection had a sevenfold increase in the risk of developing HUS compared to age-matched children with a white blood cell count lower than 13,000/mm^3. The use of antimotility agents was also associated with a higher risk for the development of HUS (102). One study demonstrated that children with hemorrhagic colitis associated with shiga toxin–producing *E. coli* who received antibiotic therapy were much more likely to progress to HUS (103). Environmental or genetic factors that might predispose to the progression of hemorrhagic colitis associated with shiga toxin–producing *E. coli* to HUS are currently unknown. It has been suggested that alterations in the gene for factor H now described in patients with atypical HUS may also be relevant to epidemic diarrhea-positive HUS (93).

At the time the diarrhea is subsiding, the child appears pale and lethargic due to the hemolytic anemia. Irritability is very common, although some children may also develop petechiae due to the thrombocytopenia. Oliguria or anuria occurs in 30 to 50% of children, and 40 to 75% of children will need dialysis therapy. The kidney and gastrointestinal tract are the organs most commonly affected in HUS, but evidence of central nervous system, pancreatic, skeletal, and myocardial involvement may also be present (105–109). Gastrointestinal involvement may lead to rectal prolapse, ischemic colitis, and transmural colonic necrosis requiring surgical intervention. Pancreatic involvement manifested as elevated pancreatic enzyme levels occurs in 10 to 20% of children, whereas glucose intolerance due to pancreatic islet cell involvement occurs in fewer than 10% of children (107). Central nervous system disease may present as seizures, coma, lethargy, and irritability.

Management of HUS requires appropriate attention to fluid and electrolyte balance and nutritional status, and careful attention to the extrarenal complications of HUS. Hemolysis may be brisk and may require frequent transfusions of packed red blood cells (approximately 10 mL/kg given over several hours). Early initiation of dialysis or CVVH (continuous venovenous hemofiltration) may be necessary if the child is oliguric. Because platelet transfusions may add fuel to the fire, platelet transfusions are reserved for patients with active bleeding or for children with severe thrombocytopenia who need to undergo a surgical procedure such as placement of a dialysis catheter or a central line. In general, antibiotic therapy is not indicated, because antibiotic therapy has the theoretical potential to alter the bacterial production of toxin and/or result in the increased release of toxin. Similarly, use of antimotility agents is also not indicated, because they may increase the systemic absorption of toxin due to the slower gastrointestinal transit time. Some studies have demonstrated a harmful effect of antibiotic therapy in hemorrhagic colitis. Children with hemorrhagic colitis associated with shiga toxin–producing *E. coli* who received antibiotic therapy were more likely to develop HUS than were children who did not receive antibiotic therapy (103). Other studies have not demonstrated such an association, and a meta-analysis concluded that administration of antibiotics in people infected with shiga toxin–producing *E. coli* was not associated with the development of HUS (110,111). Although there is no consensus on the benefit versus harm of antibiotic therapy for shiga toxin-producing *E. coli* infection, *in vitro* studies have shown that subinhibitory concentrations of several antimicrobial agents promote and increase the release of vero cytotoxins (112). Plasmapheresis has not been shown to alter the natural history of diarrhea-associated HUS (113).

A diatomaceous silicon diamide compound linked to an oligosaccharide chain (Synsorb Pk) has been developed and has been shown to avidly bind and neutralize shiga toxin. A clinical trial designed to determine if oral administration of Synsorb Pk could decrease the rate of progression of hemorrhagic colitis to HUS or if it could decrease the need for dialysis or the development of extrarenal complications in children who have developed HUS has been completed (114,115). Unfortunately, Synsorb Pk was not found to be beneficial in preventing extrarenal complications nor in decreasing the duration of dialysis in children with new-onset HUS (115). Starfish is a new compound that has been developed and has been shown to bind to shiga toxin 1000 times more efficiently than Synsorb Pk. Starfish is a pentamer that binds shiga toxin and has the potential to be administered intravenously (116).

Atypical HUS is not associated with diarrhea and occurs much less frequently in children. Atypical HUS may be associated with a number of immunologic diseases including systemic lupus erythematosus, with infections such as streptococcal pneumonia, or with the administration of medications such as cyclosporin or birth control pills or chemotherapeutic agents such as mitomycin (94). Acute renal failure may also occur after bone marrow transplantation. The cause is likely to be multifactorial, but a high incidence of microvascular disease resembling HUS has been observed, usually in association with venoocclusive disease (94). Acute renal failure after bone marrow transplantation in children usually has a multifactorial cause and may be associated with long-term renal insufficiency in some children (117). Atypical HUS may lead to end-stage renal disease and can recur in patients with kidney transplants.

SUPPORTIVE THERAPY AND MEDICAL MANAGEMENT

In clinical situations in which renal hypoperfusion and toxic insults are anticipated (such as cardiac surgery, administration of a contrast medium or amphotericin), therapy with fluids, mannitol, diuretics, and dopamine is frequently used to prevent or limit renal injury. Although whether use of these agents helps to prevent or limit renal injury is controversial, increasing urine output makes fluid management easier, aids in maintaining homeostasis of potassium and other electrolytes, and simplifies addressing the nutritional needs of the child. As described earlier, therapy with *N*-acetylcysteine has been shown to significantly decrease the rise in serum creatinine level after the intravascular administration of contrast medium (23). Once intrinsic renal failure has become established, management of the metabolic complications of acute renal failure continues to involve appropriate management of fluid balance, electrolyte status, acid-base balance, and nutrition. Additional renal injury from hypoperfusion or hypoxic-ischemic and nephrotoxic insults that could delay and complicate recovery should be prevented as much as possible.

Vasoactive Agents

The use of "renal-dose" dopamine (0.5 to 5.0 μg/kg/min) to improve renal perfusion after an ischemic insult has become very common in intensive care units. Although dopamine increases renal blood flow by promoting vasodilatation and may improve urine output by promoting natriuresis, there are no definitive studies to demonstrate that low-dose dopamine is effective in decreasing the need for dialysis or improving survival in patients with acute renal failure (118,119). In fact, a placebo-controlled, randomized study of low-dose dopamine therapy in adult patients demonstrated that low-dose dopamine was not beneficial and did not confer clinically significant protection from renal dysfunction (120). When the group receiving dopamine was compared with the placebo group, no difference was found in peak serum creatinine level, the number of patients whose creatinine level exceeded 300 μmol/L, the number of patients who received renal replacement therapy, the duration of intensive care unit stay, the number of hospital days required, or mortality (120). Other studies have demonstrated that renal-dose dopamine is not effective in the treatment of acute renal failure (121,122).

Fenoldopam mesylate is a selective dopamine 1 receptor agonist that has been approved for short-term use in severe hypertension (123). Studies in animals have shown that the effects of fenoldopam on renal hemodynamics may lead to improvement in renal perfusion and carry the potential to preserve renal function. The negative results of studies using low-dose dopamine along with the potential side effects of low- and high-dose dopamine and the nonselective stimulation of dopamine 1 and 2 receptors by dopamine has prompted interest in the use of fenoldopam in the management of acute renal failure. Intravenous fenoldopam increased renal perfusion, urine flow, and excretion of both sodium and potassium in hypoxemic adults (123). Randomized trials are important to determine if selective dopamine agonists are safe and efficacious in acute renal failure.

Anaritide, an atrial natriuretic peptide, increases the GFR by dilating afferent arterioles while constricting efferent arterioles and has been shown to improve GFR, urinary output, and histologic findings in animal models of acute renal failure and in humans with acute renal failure (124). In a randomized clinical trial of anaritide treatment involving over 500 adults with acute renal failure, anaritide did not improve the overall rate of dialysis-free survival (125). However, survival may have been increased in oliguric patients receiving anaritide, whereas survival may have been worse in patients with nonoliguric acute renal failure receiving anaritide. It is hoped that future studies will delineate the clinical conditions under which anaritide may be indicated in the management of acute renal failure.

Diuretic Therapy

Stimulating urine output eases management of acute renal failure, but the conversion of oliguric to nonoliguric acute renal failure has not been shown to alter the course of the disorder (126,127). In theory, diuretic therapy has potential mechanisms to prevent, limit, or improve renal function. Mannitol (0.5 to 1.0 g/kg delivered over several minutes) may increase intratubular urine flow to limit tubular obstruction and may limit cell damage by preventing swelling or by acting as a scavenger of free radicals or reactive oxygen molecules. Furosemide (Lasix) (1 to 5 mg/kg/dose) also increases urine flow rate to decrease intratubular obstruction and inhibits Na^+-K^+–adenosine triphosphatase, which limits oxygen consumption in already damaged tubules with a low oxygen supply. In studies published many years ago, loop diuretic therapy did not alter the need for renal replacement therapy or mortality (127–129).

When mannitol is used in children with acute renal failure, a lack of response to therapy can precipitate congestive heart failure, particularly if the child's intravascular volume is expanded before mannitol infusion. In addition, lack of excretion of mannitol may result in substantial hyperosmolality. Similarly, administration of high doses of furosemide in renal failure has been associated with ototoxicity (127). When diuretic therapy is used in children with acute renal failure, potential risks and benefits need to be considered. When the child is unresponsive to therapy, continued administration of high doses of diuretics is not justified and is unlikely to be beneficial to the child. In patients who do respond to therapy, continuous infusions may be more effective and may be associated with less toxicity than bolus administration (128).

Fluid Balance

Depending on the cause of acute renal failure and the presence or absence of associated symptoms such as vomiting or diarrhea, children with acute renal failure may present with hypovolemia, euvolemia, or fluid overload and pulmonary edema. Patients with salt-wasting renal or adrenal disease, diarrhea, or vomiting may present with fluid deficits that need correction to a euvolemic state, whereas patients with oliguria or anuria more commonly present with hypervolemia and need fluid restriction and/or acute fluid removal to achieve a euvolemic state. Weight, blood pressure, heart rate, skin turgor, and capillary refill are each used to assess the intravascular volume. In children who are intravascularly volume depleted, 10 to 20 mL/kg of normal saline can be infused to reestablish intravascular volume. If urine output does not increase and azotemia does not improve after fluid resuscitation, then central venous pressure monitoring may be necessary to further guide fluid therapy. If the child presents with fluid overload, then fluid restriction and/or fluid removal with dialysis or hemofiltration may be instituted if the child does not respond to diuretic therapy.

Once normal intravascular volume has been reached, euvolemia can be maintained by providing the child with fluid to replace normal water losses from the skin, respiratory tract, and gastrointestinal tract (insensible losses, 400 mL/m^2/24 hr). Excess stool losses such as may occur with diarrhea or excess skin and respiratory tract losses such as may occur with hyperthermia need to be accounted for as well and replaced with the appropriate fluid. Urine losses may also be replaced milliliter for milliliter with the appropriate fluid, which is usually determined by measuring urine electrolytes. Daily weight measurements, blood pressure, accurate fluid input and output records, physical examination, and nutritional needs of the child guide ongoing fluid therapy. Without supplemental enteral or intravenous nutrition, weight loss may be 0.5 to 1.0% of the body weight per day. Children in the diuretic phase of acute tubular necrosis may have substantial fluid and electrolyte losses that require replacement.

Electrolyte and Acid-Base Balance

Mild hyponatremia is very common in acute renal failure and may be due to hyponatremia dehydration, but fluid overload with dilutional hyponatremia is much more common. If the serum sodium level is higher than 120 mEq/L, fluid restriction or water removal by dialytic therapy corrects the serum sodium. However, if the serum sodium level is lower than 120 mEq/L, the child is at higher risk for seizures due to hyponatremia, and correction to a sodium level of approximately 125 mEq/L with hypertonic saline should be considered. The amount of sodium required can by calculated by the following formula:

$$(125 - P_{Na})\ (Wt)\ (0.6) = \text{mEq Na} \qquad \text{[Eq. 3]}$$

where P_{Na} is the current plasma sodium concentration, Wt is the weight in kilograms, and 0.6 is the fraction of the weight that is total body water. The required amount is usually infused over several hours to avoid rapid correction of the serum sodium level. Rapid correction of the serum sodium concentration in adults with chronic hyponatremia has been associated with neurologic injury, particularly central pontine myelinolysis, although the incidence of such injury in children is unknown (130). Restriction of free water further helps to correct hyponatremia.

Because the kidney tightly regulates potassium balance and excretes approximately 90% of dietary potassium intake, hyperkalemia is a common and potentially life-threatening electrolyte abnormality in acute renal failure. Hyperkalemia results from decreased filtration, impaired tubular secretion, altered distribution of potassium by acidosis, which shifts potassium from the intracellular to the extracellular compartment, and release of intracellular potassium due to the associated catabolic state. For each 0.1-unit reduction in arterial pH, the serum potassium level may increase by 0.3 mEq/L. The serum potassium level may be falsely elevated if the technique of the blood draw causes hemolysis or tissue destruction, or if the child has a high white blood cell or platelet count, which can falsely elevate the potassium level (131).

True hyperkalemia results in disturbances of cardiac rhythm by its depolarizing effect on the cardiac conduction pathways. The concentration of serum potassium that results in arrhythmia is dependent on the acid-base balance and the levels of other serum electrolytes. Hypocalcemia, which is common in renal failure, exacerbates the adverse effects of the serum potassium level on cardiac conduction pathways. Tall, peaked T waves are the first manifestation of cardiotoxicity, and prolongation of the PR interval, flattening of P waves, and widening of QRS complexes are later abnormalities. Severe hyperkalemia eventually leads to ventricular tachycardia and fibrillation. Symptoms of hyperkalemia include malaise, nausea, and progressive muscle weakness.

Treatment of hyperkalemia is indicated if cardiac conduction abnormalities are noted or if levels are higher than 6 to 7 mEq/L. Therapy for hyperkalemia is summarized in Table 64.4. Sodium bicarbonate (0.5 to 1.0 mEq/kg/dose) transfers potassium into cells, but, as described later, this therapy may precipitate seizures and tetany if the serum calcium level is low, which results in a decreased ionized calcium level. Intravenous administration of glucose and insulin also transfer potassium from the extracellular to the intracellular compartment (132). Intravenous administration of calcium gluconate increases the threshold potential of the excitable myocardial cells and counteracts the depolarizing effect of the hyperkalemia. Studies in adults have shown that the β-agonist albuterol, given via a nebulizer, can acutely lower the serum potassium level by stimulating intracellular uptake of potassium (133). Each of the aforementioned are temporizing measures and do not remove potassium from the body. Sodium polystyrene sulfonate (Kayexalate) given orally, by nasogastric tube, or by rectum exchanges sodium for potassium in the gastrointestinal tract and results in potassium removal (131,134). Complications of sodium polystyrene sulfonate therapy include possible hypernatremia, sodium retention, and constipation. In addition, sodium polystyrene sulfonate therapy has been associated with intestinal necrosis in adult patients after surgery (135). Depending on the degree of hyperkale-

TABLE 64.4. TREATMENT OF HYPERKALEMIA

Agent	Mechanism	Dose	Onset of effect	Complications
Sodium bicarbonate	Shifts K^+ into cells	1 mEq/kg IV over 10–30 min	15–30 min	Hypernatremia Change in ionized calcium level
Calcium gluconate (10%)	Stabilizes membrane potential	0.5–1.0 mL/kg IV over 5–15 min	Immediate	Bradycardia Arrhythmias Hypercalcemia
Glucose and insulin	Stimulates cellular uptake of K^+	Glucose 0.5 g/kg Insulin 0.1 U/kg IV over 30 min	30–120 min	Hypoglycemia
β-Agonists (albuterol)[a]	Stimulates cellular uptake of K^+	5–10 mg nebulizer (adult dose)	30 min	Tachycardia Hypertension
Sodium polystyrene sulfonate (Kayexalate)	Exchanges Na^+ for K^+ across colonic mucosa	1 g/kg PO or PR in sorbitol	30–60 min	Hypernatremia Constipation

[a]Limited pediatric use.

mia and the need for correction of other metabolic derangements in acute renal failure, hyperkalemia frequently requires the initiation of dialysis or hemofiltration.

Because the kidney excretes net acids generated by diet and intermediary metabolism, acidosis is very common in acute renal failure. As long as the child's central nervous system is intact, respiratory compensation provides partial correction of the acidosis, but if the child is obtunded, respiratory compensation may be compromised, which results in severe acidosis. Severe acidosis can be treated with intravenous or oral sodium bicarbonate, oral sodium citrate solutions, and/or dialysis. When treatment of acidosis is contemplated, it is important to consider the serum ionized calcium level. Under normal circumstances, approximately one-half the total calcium is protein bound; half is free and in the ionized form, and this is what determines the transmembrane potential and electrochemical gradient. Hypocalcemia is common in acute renal failure and acidosis increases the fraction of total calcium in the ionized form. Treatment of acidosis can then shift the ionized calcium to the more normal ratio, decreasing the amount of ionized calcium and precipitating tetany and/or seizures. Thus, base therapy for acidosis should not be considered without knowledge of the total and ionized calcium levels. When base therapy is given, an amount of 0.5 to 1.0 mEq/kg administered over approximately 1 hour is reasonable. Administering sodium bicarbonate generates CO_2 and an intact respiratory system to excrete the excess generated CO_2 is required for bicarbonate therapy to be effective.

Calcium and Phosphate Balance

Because the kidney excretes a large amount of ingested phosphorus, hyperphosphatemia is a very common electrolyte abnormality during acute and chronic renal failure. Hyperphosphatemia should be treated with dietary phosphorus restriction and with oral calcium carbonate or other calcium compounds to bind phosphorus and prevent gastrointestinal absorption of phosphorus (136,137). Sevelamer hydrochloride has been shown to be an effective non–calcium-containing phosphorus binder in chronic renal failure but has not been tested or used in acute renal failure (138). Because most patients with acute renal failure have hypocalcemia, use of calcium-containing phosphate binders provides a source of calcium as well as phosphate-binding capacity. Aluminum-containing compounds should be avoided, because several studies have demonstrated that oral administration of aluminum-containing phosphorus binders results in substantial aluminum absorption and leads to severe aluminum intoxication (139). Dialysis therapy also effectively removes phosphorus, but because phosphorus is a divalent cation, it will cross dialysis membranes less readily than uncharged molecules such as urea or monovalent anions such as potassium.

The cause of hypocalcemia in acute renal failure is multifactorial, and hypocalcemia may result from hyperphosphatemia, inadequate gastrointestinal calcium absorption due to inadequate 1,25-dihydroxyvitamin D production by the kidney, and skeletal resistance to the action of parathyroid hormone. As described earlier, acid-base balance has a profound effect on the ionized calcium level and the interpretation of the calcium level, and therapy must take into consideration the degree of acidosis. If hypocalcemia is severe and/or if bicarbonate therapy is necessary for hyperkalemia, treatment with 10% calcium gluconate (100 mg/kg up to a minimum of 1 g, or 1 mL/kg up to a maximum of 10 mL) should be given over 30 to 60 minutes with continuous electrocardiographic monitoring. Hypocalcemia may also be treated by oral administration of calcium carbonate or other calcium salts.

Medications

When medications are prescribed in acute renal failure, the mechanism of drug elimination and the metabolic pathway of the drug must be considered and adjustments made for renal failure. Many drug adjustment tables are based on the level of renal function (GFR greater than 50 mL/min/1.73 m^2, GFR of 20 to 50 mL/min/1.73 m^2, or GFR less than 20 mL/min/1.73 m^2), and it is important to estimate the child's level of renal function appropriately and to consider the rate of increase in the serum creatinine level rather than the absolute creatinine level. To prevent further insults to the kidney, it is best to avoid nephrotoxic drugs in acute renal failure; however, if potentially nephrotoxic drugs are needed, it is appropriate to use them while monitoring drug levels and potential adverse effects.

Hypertension

Hypertension in acute renal failure is commonly related to volume overload and/or to alterations in vascular tone. If hypertension is related to volume overload, appropriate fluid removal with dialysis or hemofiltration is necessary if the patient has not responded to diuretic therapy. Depending on the degree of blood pressure elevation and the cause of the hypertension, antihypertensive therapy may also be indicated. The choice of antihypertensive therapy depends on the degree of blood pressure elevation, the presence of central nervous system symptoms of hypertension, associated conditions, and the cause of the acute renal failure. For the child who has severe hypertension and/or is encephalopathic, intravenous therapy with sodium nitroprusside (beginning dose, 0.5 to 1.0 μg/kg/min) is indicated with monitoring of the serum levels of thiocyanate, a metabolic product of nitroprusside that is excreted by the kidney. Alternative therapies include intravenous labetalol (0.5 to 3.0 mg/kg/hr), diazoxide (1 to 5 mg/kg/dose), enalaprilat (0.005 to 0.01 mg/kg/day), and nicardipine (1 to 3 μg/kg/min) (140). Intravenous hydralazine or sublingual nifedipine can be used for less severe hypertension. Severe hypotension and tissue ischemia after sublingual administration of nifedipine, which has been observed in adult patients, is distinctly uncommon in pediatric patients (141). Once the blood pressure is controlled, treatment with oral long-acting agents can be initiated.

Nutritional Support

In many instances acute renal failure is associated with marked catabolism, and malnutrition can develop rapidly, leading to delayed recovery from acute renal failure. Prompt and proper nutrition is essential in the management of the child with acute renal failure. Although studies suggesting that proper nutritional support improves the outcome of acute renal failure in children have not been documented, it is reasonable to suppose that the complication rate is reduced and recovery is enhanced by adequate nutrition. If the gastrointestinal tract is intact and functional, enteral feedings with formula (PM60/40 for newborns and infants) should be instituted as soon as possible. In older children, a diet of high-biologic-value protein, low-phosphorus, and low-potassium foods can be used. Dilute formula should be given initially and then feedings can be increased and concentrated to achieve optimal caloric intake. Infants should receive maintenance calories (120 kCal/kg/day) and older children appropriate maintenance calories or higher if needed due to the catabolic state and malnutrition. If enteral feedings are not possible, then hyperalimentation, usually through a central line, with a high concentration of dextrose (25%), lipids (10 to 20%), and protein (1.0 to 2.0 g/kg/day) should be instituted. If the child is oliguric or anuric and sufficient caloric intake cannot be achieved while appropriate fluid balance is maintained, dialysis should be initiated earlier than in the usual case.

Renal Replacement Therapy

The purpose of acute renal replacement therapy is to remove endogenous and exogenous toxins and to maintain fluid, electrolyte, and acid-base balance until renal function returns. Renal replacement therapy may be provided by peritoneal dialysis, intermittent hemodialysis, or continuous renal replacement therapy (CRRT) consisting of hemofiltration with or without a dialysis circuit. CRRT is discussed in detail in Chapter 65 and peritoneal and hemodialysis are discussed in Chapters 70 and 71. It is important to point out that renal replacement therapy for children with acute renal failure has evolved substantially over the past several years (142). The preferential use of CRRT by pediatric nephrologists is increasing, whereas the use of peritoneal dialysis is decreasing except in neonates and small infants (143–145). The choice of a dialytic membrane and daily dialysis in adults with acute renal failure has been shown to affect recovery of renal function and survival substantially (146,147). Although similar studies have not been performed in pediatric patients, these findings should be considered in treating the child with acute renal failure.

Therapy to Decrease Injury and Promote Recovery

Exciting advances in understanding of the cellular and molecular events that precipitate acute renal failure has allowed for the development of strategies to potentially decrease injury and/or promote recovery from acute renal failure. Recovery of renal function after acute tubular necrosis requires a complex and not fully understood set of events that leads to restoration of renal blood flow and regeneration of renal tubular epithelial cells (148). Interesting studies suggest that infusion of RGD peptides prevents renal tubular obstruction and accelerates improvement of renal function after an ischemic injury in an animal model of acute renal failure (149). In other animal studies of acute renal injury, postischemic infusion of growth factors, including insulin-like growth factor-1 (IGF-1), epidermal growth factor, and hepatocyte growth factor, resulted in an accelerated recovery of renal function, less severe histologic alterations, and decreased mortality (150–152). Similar results were seen in nephrotoxic acute renal failure (153). In animal models, administration of melatonin-stimulating hormone, thyroxine, C5a receptor antagonist, selective inhibitors of inducible nitric oxide synthase, statins, and a novel inhibitor of the Na^+/H^+ exchange subtype 3, as well as inhibition of monocyte chemoattractant protein-1 by gene therapy, has been shown to ameliorate acute renal failure (154–161).

Although multiple interventions decrease the severity of acute renal failure and promote recovery in animal models, results of interventional studies in patients with acute renal failure have been disappointing. In a study comparing use of IGF-1 and placebo in adults with acute renal failure, IGF-1 therapy did not accelerate the recovery of renal function and was not associated with differences in dialysis needs or in mortality (162). Thyroxine therapy in adult patients with acute renal failure did not improve scores on a measure of the severity of acute renal failure and was associated with a substantially higher mortality in treated patients due to prolonged suppression of thyroid-stimulating hormone (163). As described earlier, randomized, placebo-controlled trials demonstrated that administration of renal-dose dopamine and atrial natriuretic peptide was ineffective in treating acute renal failure (120,125).

In children in the intensive care unit, the systemic inflammatory response is thought to contribute to renal failure and multiorgan failure by activation of the inflammatory cascade with the participation of cytokines, reactive oxygen species, proteolytic enzymes, and adhesion molecules. Ischemic injury stimulates the activation of neutrophils and the expression of adhesion molecules with resultant tissue injury. Activated neutrophils generate reactive oxygen molecules, including superoxide anion, hydrogen peroxide, hydroxyl radical hypochlorous acid, and peroxynitrate. In addition, activated neutrophils release proteolytic enzymes that can result in substantial tissue injury (62,164,165). Melatonin-stimulating factor has an antiinflammatory activity and has been shown to inhibit ischemic reperfusion injury in mice and rats, even when infused 6 hours after the insult (154). In studies of hypoxic-ischemic acute renal failure in the rat, scavengers of oxidants and free radicals have been shown to decrease renal injury (62,165,166). Infusion of the membrane-permeable scavenger of reactive oxygen molecules resulted in significantly reduced BUN level, creatinine level, and kidney myeloperoxidase activity, and decreased lipid peroxidation in rats undergoing bilateral clamping of the renal pedicle (166). Other studies demonstrate that anti–adhesion molecule therapy markedly decreases ischemic renal injury by preventing adhesion of activated neutrophils to renal cells (167). Potential future therapy to interfere with the inflammatory cascade might modify the severity and/or duration of acute renal failure.

OUTCOME AND PROGNOSIS

The prognosis and recovery of the child with acute renal failure are highly dependent on the underlying cause (31–37). Children who have acute renal failure as a component of multisystem failure have a much higher mortality rate than children with intrinsic renal disease such as HUS, rapidly progressive glomerulonephritis, or acute interstitial nephritis. Factors that are associated with mortality include multiorgan failure, hypotension, need for pressors, hemodynamic instability, and need for mechanical ventilation and dialysis (35–37,168–171). The cause of mortality is nearly always related to associated conditions and not to the renal failure per se. Although the inhospital mortality of patients with acute renal failure is high, studies involving adults have shown that patients who recover from renal failure have a reasonable survival rate and a good quality of life (172). Other factors that affect recovery of renal function and mortality (discussed in detail in the next chapter) include the mode of renal replacement therapy, the type of membrane used in hemodialysis, the use of daily versus alternate-day dialysis, and the dose of dialysis or hemofiltration (146,147,173–175).

Recovery of renal function is also highly dependent on the underlying cause of the acute renal failure. Children with acute interstitial nephritis and acute tubular necrosis typically recover normal renal function and are at low risk for any late complications. In animal models of acute tubular necrosis, however, recovery after a severe ischemic insult resulted in alteration in urinary concentrating ability, diminished capacity to generate a hypertonic medullary interstitium, and tubulointerstitial fibrosis (176). Children who may have suffered substantial loss of nephrons such as may occur in HUS or rapidly progressive glomerulonephritis are at risk for late development of renal failure long after the initial insult. Several studies in animal models and some studies in adults have documented that hyperfiltration of the remnant nephron may eventually lead to progressive glomerulosclerosis of the remaining nephrons (177). Thus, children who have experienced cortical necrosis during the neonatal period and have recovered renal function or children who have experienced an episode of severe Henoch-Schönlein purpura or HUS are clearly at risk for the late development of renal complications. Such children need life-long renal function monitoring, blood pressure monitoring, and urinalysis. Typically, the late development of chronic renal failure first becomes apparent with the appearance of hypertension, proteinuria, and eventually elevated BUN and creatinine levels.

REFERENCES

1. Thadhani R, Pascual M, Bonventre JV. Acute renal failure. *N Engl J Med* 1996;334:1448–1460.
2. Anderson RJ, Linas SL, Berns AS, et al. Nonoliguric acute renal failure. *N Engl J Med* 1977;296:1134–1138.
3. Honda N, Hishida A. Pathophysiology of experimental nonoliguric acute renal failure. *Kidney Int* 1993;43:513–521.
4. Sudo M, Honda N, Hishida A, et al. Renal hemodynamics in oliguric and nonoliguric acute renal failure of rabbits. *Nephron* 1980;25:144–150.

5. Andreoli SP. Acute renal failure. *Curr Opin Pediatr* 2002;17:713–717.
6. Mogal NE, Brocklebank JT, Meadow SR. A review of acute renal failure in children: incidence, etiology and outcome. *Clin Nephrol* 1998;49:91–95.
7. Gouyon JB, Guignard JP. Management of acute renal failure in newborns. *Pediatr Nephrol* 2000;14:1037–1044.
8. Karlowivz MG, Adelman RD. Nonoliguric and oliguric acute renal failure. *Pediatr Nephrol* 1995;9:718–722.
9. Andreoli SP. Renal failure in the newborn unit. In: Polin RA, Yoder MC, Berg FD, eds. *Workbook in practical neonatology*. Philadelphia: W.B. Saunders Company, 2000:322–337.
10. Andreoli SP. Acute and chronic renal failure in children. In: Gearhart JP, Rink RC, Mouriquand PD, eds. *Pediatric urology*. Philadelphia: W.B. Saunders Company, 2001:777–789.
11. Martin-Ancel A, Garcia-Alix A, Gaya F, et al. Multiple organ involvement in perinatal asphyxia. *J Pediatr* 1995;127:786–793.
12. Nolan CR, Anderson RF. Hospital-acquired acute renal failure. *J Am Soc Nephrol* 1998;9:710–718.
13. Liano F, Pascual J. The Madrid Acute Renal Failure Study Group. Epidemiology of acute renal failure: a prospective, multicenter study community-based study. *Kidney Int* 1996;50:811–818.
14. Nobilis A, Kocsis I, Toth-Heyn P, et al. Variance of ACE and AT1 receptor genotype does not influence the risk of neonatal acute renal failure. *Pediatr Nephrol* 2001;16:1063–1066.
15. Treszl A, Toth-Heyn P, Koscic I. Interleukin genetic variants and the risk of renal failure in infants with infection. *Pediatr Nephrol* 2002;17:713–717.
16. Brady HR, Linger GG. Acute renal failure. *Lancet* 1995;346:1533–1540.
17. Schlondorff D. Renal complications of nonsteroidal anti-inflammatory drugs. *Kidney Int* 1993;44:643–653.
18. van Bel F, Guit GL, Schipper J, et al. Indomethacin-induced changes in renal blood flow velocity waveform in premature infants investigated with color Doppler imaging. *J Pediatr* 1991;118:621–626.
19. Badr KF, Ichikawa I. Prerenal failure: a deleterious shift from renal compensation to decompensation. *N Engl J Med* 1988;319:623–628.
20. Hricik DE, Dunn MJ. Angiotensin-converting enzyme inhibitor-induced renal failure: causes, consequences, and diagnostic uses. *J Am Soc Nephrol* 1990;1:845–858.
21. Tack ED, Perlman JM. Renal failure in sick hypertensive premature infants receiving captopril therapy. *J Pediatr* 1988;112:805–810.
22. Wood EG, Bunchman TE, Lynch RE. Captopril-induced reversible acute renal failure in an infant with coarctation of the aorta. *Pediatrics* 1991;88:816–818.
23. Tepel M, van der Giet M, Bashoure TM, et al. Prevention of radiographic-contrast-agent-induced reduction in renal function by acetylcysteine. *N Engl J Med* 2000;20:180–184.
24. Durham JD, Caputo C, Dokko J, et al. AS randomized controlled trial of *N*-acetylcysteine to prevent contrast nephropathy in cardiac angiography. *Kidney Int* 2002;62:2202–2207.
25. Brater DC. Effects of nonsteroidal anti-inflammatory drugs on renal function: focus on cyclooxygenase-2-selective inhibitors. *Am J Med* 1999;107:S65–S71.
26. Perazella MA, Eras J. Are selective COX-2 inhibitors nephrotoxic? *Am J Kidney Dis* 2000;35:937–940.
27. Mathew OP, Jones AS, James E, et al. Neonatal renal failure: usefulness of diagnostic indices. *Pediatrics* 1980;65:57–60.
28. Ellis EN, Arnold WC. Use of urinary indexes in renal failure in the newborn. *Am J Dis Child* 1982;136:615–617.
29. Hodson EM, Kjellstrand CM, Mauer SM. Acute renal failure in infants and children: outcome of 53 patients requiring hemodialysis. *J Pediatr* 1978;93:756–761.
30. Carvounis SP, Nisar S, Guro-Razuman S. Significance of the fractional excretion of urea in the differential diagnosis of acute renal failure. *Kidney Int* 2002;62:2223–2229.
31. Niadet P, Haj-Ibrahim MH, Gagnadous MF, et al. Outcome of children with acute renal failure. *Kidney Int* 1985;S148–S151.
32. Chevalier RL, Campbell F, Brenbridge AN. Prognostic factors in neonatal acute renal failure. *Pediatrics* 1984;74:265–272.
33. Stapleton FB, Jones DP, Green RS. Acute renal failure in neonates: incidence, etiology and outcome. *Pediatr Nephrol* 1987;1:314–320.
34. Bunchman TE, McBryde KD, Motes TE, et al. Pediatric acute renal failure: outcome by modality and disease. *Pediatric Nephrol* 2001;16:1067–1071.
35. Goldstein SL, Currier H, Graf J, et al. Outcome in children receiving continuous venovenous hemofiltration. *Pediatrics* 2001;107:1309–1312.
36. Gallego N, Perez-Caballero C, Estepa R, et al. Prognosis of patients with acute renal failure without cardiomyopathy. *Arch Dis Child* 2001;84:258–260.
37. Goldstein SL. Hemodialysis in the pediatric patient: state of the art. *Adv Ren Replace Ther* 2001;8:173–179.
38. Mendoza SA. Nephrotoxic drugs. *Pediatr Nephrol* 1988;2:466–476.
39. Abuelo JG. Renal failure caused by chemicals, foods, plants, animal venoms, and misuse of drugs. *Arch Intern Med* 1990;150:505–510.
40. Humes HD. Aminoglycoside nephrotoxicity. *Kidney Int* 1988;33:900–911.
41. Barrett BJ. Contrast nephrotoxicity. *J Am Soc Nephrol* 1994;5:125–137.
42. Rudnick MR, Goldfarb S, Wexler L, et al. Nephrotoxicity of ionic and nonionic contrast media in 1196 patients: a randomized trial. *Kidney Int* 1995;47:254–261.
43. Bates DW, Donghui TY, Chertow GM, et al. Correlates of acute renal failure in patients receiving parenteral amphotericin B. *Kidney Int* 2001;60:1452–1459.
44. Skinner R, Pearson ADJ, English MW, et al. Risk factors for ifosfamide nephrotoxicity in children. *Lancet* 1996;348:578–580.
45. Shore R, Greenberg M, Geary D, et al. Iphosphamide-induced nephrotoxicity in children. *Pediatr Nephrol* 1992;6:162–165.
46. Vachvanichsanong P, Patamasucon P, Malagon M, et al. Acute renal failure in a child associated with acyclovir. *Pediatr Nephrol* 1995;9:346–347.
47. Bianchetti MG, Roduit C, Oetliker OH. Acyclovir-induced renal failure: course and risk factors. *Pediatr Nephrol* 1991;5:238–239.
48. Vale JA, Proudfoot AT. Paracetamol (acetaminophen) poisoning. *Lancet* 1995;346:547–552.
49. Vomiero G, Carptenter B, Robb I, et al. Combination of

ceftriaxone and acyclovir—an underestimated nephrotoxic potential? *Pediatr Nephrol* 2002;17:633–637.
50. Hatala R, Dinh T, Cook DJ. Once daily aminoglycoside dosing in immunocompetent adults: a meta-analysis. *Ann Intern Med* 1996;124:717–725.
51. Barza M, Ioannidis JP, Cappelleri JC, et al. Single or multiple doses of aminoglycosides. A meta-analysis. *BMJ* 1996;312:338–345.
52. Aspelin P, Aubry R, Fransson SG, et al. Nephrotoxic effects in high-risk patients undergoing angiography. *New Engl J Med* 2003;348:491–499.
53. Peterson CD, Collins AJ, Himes JM, et al. Ethylene glycol poisoning. Pharmacokinetics during therapy with ethanol and hemodialysis. *N Engl J Med* 1981;304:21–23.
54. Rothman A, Normann SA, Manoguerra AS, et al. Short-term hemodialysis in childhood ethylene glycol poisoning. *J Pediatr* 1986;108:153–155.
55. Jacobsen D, Hewlett TP, Webb R, et al. Ethylene glycol intoxication: evaluation of kinetics and crystalluria. *Am J Med* 1988;84:145–152.
56. Brent J, McMartin K, Phillips S, et al. Fomepizole for the treatment of ethylene glycol poisoning. *N Engl J Med* 1999;340:832–838.
57. Boyer EW, Mejia M, Woolf A, et al. Severe ethylene glycol ingestion treated without hemodialysis. *Pediatrics* 2001; 107:172–174.
58. Warshaw BL, Carter MC. Bromate poisoning from hair permanent preparations. *Pediatrics* 1985;76:975–978.
59. Lichtenberg R, Zeller WP, Gatson R, et al. Bromate poisoning. *J Pediatr* 1989;114:891–894.
60. Kasik JW, Leuschen MP, Bolam DL, et al. Rhabdomyolysis and myoglobinemia in neonates. *Pediatrics* 1985;76:255–258.
61. Watanabe T. Rhabdomyolysis and acute renal failure in children. *Pediatr Nephrol* 2001;16:1072–1075.
62. Andreoli SP. Reactive oxygen molecules, oxidant injury and renal disease. *Pediatr Nephrol* 1991;5:733–742.
63. Zager RA. Rhabdomyolysis and myohemoglobinuric acute renal failure. *Kidney Int* 1996;49:314–326.
64. Zager RA, Burkhart K. Myoglobin toxicity in proximal human kidney cells: roles of Fe, Ca^{2+}, H_2O_2, and terminal mitochondrial electron transport. *Kidney Int* 1997;51:728–738.
65. Vanholder R, Sever MS, Erek E, et al. Rhabdomyolysis. *J Am Soc Nephrol* 2000;11:1553–1561.
66. Mills NE, Goldenberg AS, Liu D, et al. B-cell lymphoma presenting as infiltrative renal disease. *Am J Kidney Dis* 1992;19:181–184.
67. Gilboa N, Lum GM, Urizar RE. Early renal involvement in acute lymphoblastic leukemia and non-Hodgkin's lymphoma in children. *J Urol* 1983;129:364–367.
68. Stapleton FB, Strother DR, Roy S, et al. Acute renal failure at onset of therapy for advanced stage Burkitt lymphoma and B cell acute lymphoblastic lymphoma. *Pediatrics* 1988;82:863–869.
69. Andreoli SP, Clark JH, McGuire WA, et al. Purine excretion during tumor lysis in children with acute lymphocytic leukemia receiving allopurinol: relationship to acute renal failure. *J Pediatr* 1986;109:292–298.
70. Jones DP, Mahmoud H, Chesney RW. Tumor lysis syndrome: pathogenesis and management. *Pediatr Nephrol* 1995;9:206–212.
71. Sakarcan A, Quigley R. Hyperphosphatemia in tumor lysis syndrome: the role of hemodialysis and continuous veno-venous hemofiltration. *Pediatr Nephrol* 1994;8:351–353.
72. Heney D, Essex-Cater A, Brocklebank JT, et al. Continuous arteriovenous hemofiltration in the treatment of tumor lysis syndrome. *Pediatr Nephrol* 1990;4:245–247.
73. Hawkins EP, Berry PL, Silva FG. Acute tubulointerstitial nephritis in children: clinical, morphologic, and lectin studies. *Am J Kidney Dis* 1989;14:466–471.
74. Birnbacher R, Balzar E, Aufricht C, et al. Tubulointerstitial nephritis and uveitis: an immunological disorder? *Pediatr Nephrol* 1995;9:193–195.
75. Michel DM, Kelly CJ. Acute interstitial nephritis. *J Am Soc Nephrol* 1998;10:506–515.
76. Jardim HM, Leake J, Risdon RA, et al. Crescentic glomerulonephritis in children. *Pediatr Nephrol* 1992;6:231–235.
77. Ellis EN, Wood EG, Berry P. Spectrum of disease associated with anti-neutrophil cytoplasmic autoantibodies in pediatric patients. *J Pediatr* 1995;126:40–43.
78. Hauer HA, Bajena UM, van Houwelingen HC. Determinants of outcome in ANCA-associated glomerulonephritis: a prospective clinco-histopathological analysis of 96 patients. *Kidney Int* 2002;62:1732–1742.
79. Payne RM, Martin TC, Bower RJ, et al. Management and follow-up of arterial thrombosis in the neonatal period. *J Pediatr* 1989;114:853–858.
80. Ellis D, Kaye RD, Bontempo FA. Aortic and renal artery thrombosis in a neonate: recovery with thrombolytic therapy. *Pediatr Nephrol* 1997;11:641–644.
81. Chevalier RL. What treatment do you advise for bilateral or unilateral renal thrombosis in the newborn, with or without thrombosis of the inferior vena cava? *Pediatr Nephrol* 1991;5:679.
82. Mocan H, Beattie TJ, Murphy AV. Renal venous thrombosis in infancy: long-term follow-up. *Pediatr Nephrol* 1991;5:45–49.
83. Anand SK, Northway JD, Smith JA. Neonatal renal papillary and cortical necrosis. *Am J Dis Child* 1977;131:773–777.
84. Siegler RL. The hemolytic uremic syndrome. *Pediatr Clin North Am* 1995;421:1505–1529.
85. Siegler RL, Milligan MK, Burningham TH, et al. Long-term outcome and prognostic indicators in the hemolytic-uremic syndrome. *J Pediatr* 1991;118:195–200.
86. Gagnadoux MF, Habib R, Gubler MC, et al. Long-term (15–25 years) outcome of childhood hemolytic-uremic syndrome. *Clin Nephrol* 1996;46:39–41.
87. Moghal NE, Ferreira MAS, Howie AJ, et al. The late histologic finding in diarrhea associated hemolytic uremic syndrome. *J Pediatr* 1998;133:220–223.
88. Spizzirri FD, et al. Childhood hemolytic uremic syndrome in Argentina: long-term follow up and prognostic features. *Pediatr Nephrol* 1997;11:156–160.
89. Repetto HA. Epidemic hemolytic uremic syndrome in children. *Kidney Int* 1997;52:1708–1719.
90. Boyce TG, Swerdlow DL, Griffin PM. *Escherichia coli* O157:H7 and the hemolytic-uremic syndrome. *N Engl J Med* 1995;33:364–368.
91. Su C, Brandt LJ. *Escherichia coli* O157:H7 infection in humans. *Ann Intern Med* 1995;123:698–714.
92. Rowe PC, Orrbine E, Wells GA, et al. Risk of hemolytic uremic syndrome after sporadic *Escherichia coli* O157:H7 infection: results of a Canadian collaborative study. *J Pediatr* 1998;132:777–782.

93. Warwicker P, Goodship TJH, Donne RL, et al. Genetic studies into inherited and sporadic hemolytic syndrome. *Kidney Int* 1998;53:836–844.
94. Kaplan BS, Meyers KE, Schulman SL. The pathogenesis and treatment of the hemolytic uremic syndrome. *J Am Soc Nephrol* 1998;9:1126–1133.
95. Brandt JR, Fouser LS, Watkins SL, et al. *Escherichia coli* O157:H7-associated hemolytic-uremic syndrome after ingestion of contaminated hamburgers. *J Pediatr* 1994;125:519–526.
96. Yamasaki S, Takeda Y. Enterohemorrhagic *Escherichia coli* O157:H7 episode in Japan with a perspective on vero toxins (Shiga-like toxins). *J Toxicol Toxin Rev* 1997;16:229–240.
97. Cody SH, Glynn K, Farrar JA, et al. An outbreak of *Escherichia coli* O157:H7 infection from unpasteurized commercial apple juice. *Ann Intern Med* 1999;130:202–209.
98. Parry SM, Salmon RL, Willshaw GA, et al. Risk factors for and prevention of sporadic infectious with verocytotoxin (Shiga toxin) producing *Escherichia coli* O157. *Lancet* 1998;351:1019–1022.
99. Voss E, Paton AW, Manning PA, et al. Molecular analysis of Shiga toxigenic *Escherichia coli* O111:H– proteins which react with sera from patients with hemolytic uremic syndrome. *Infect Immun* 1998;66:1467–1472.
100. Henning PH, Tham ECB, Martin AA, et al. Hemolytic-uremic syndrome outbreak caused by *Escherichia coli* O111:H–: clinical outcomes. *Med J Aust* 1998;168:552–555.
101. Hashimoto H, Mizukoshi K, Nishi M, et al. Epidemic of gastrointestinal tract infection including hemorrhagic colitis attributing to Shiga toxin 1-producing *Escherichia coli* O118:H2 at a junior high school in Japan. *Pediatrics* 1999;103:E2.
102. Bell BP, Griffin PM, Lozano P, et al. Predictors of hemolytic uremic syndrome in children during a larger outbreak of *Escherichia coli* O157:H7 infections. *Pediatrics* 1997;100:E12.
103. Wong CS, Jelacic S, Habeeb RL, et al. The risk of hemolytic uremic syndrome after antibiotic treatment of *Escherichia coli* O157:H7 infections. *N Engl J Med* 2000;342:1930–1936.
104. Thayu M, Chandler WL, Jelacic S, et al. Cardiac ischemia during hemolytic uremic syndrome. *Pediatr Nephrol* 2003; 18:286–289.
105. Andreoli SP, Bergstein JM. Development of insulin dependent diabetes mellitus during the hemolytic uremic syndrome. *J Pediatr* 1982;100:541–545.
106. Andreoli SP, Bergstein JM. Acute rhabdomyolysis associated with the hemolytic-uremic syndrome. *J Pediatr* 1983;103:78–80.
107. Andreoli SP, Bergstein JM. Exocrine and endocrine pancreatic insufficiency and calcinosis following the hemolytic uremic syndrome. *J Pediatr* 1987;110:816–817.
108. Upadhyaya K, Barwick K, Fishaut M, et al. The importance of nonrenal involvement in hemolytic-uremic syndrome. *Pediatrics* 1980;65:115–120.
109. Andreoli SP III. Pancreatic involvement in the hemolytic uremic syndrome. In: Kaplan BS, Trompeter R, Moak J, eds. *The hemolytic uremic syndrome: thrombotic thrombocytopenia purpura.* New York: Marcel Dekker, Inc., 1992:131–141.
110. Safdar N, Said A, Sangnon RE, et al. Risk of hemolytic uremic syndrome after antibiotic treatment of *Escherichia coli* O157:H7 enteritis: a meta-analysis. *JAMA* 2002;288:996–1001.
111. Molbak K, Mead PS, Griffin PM. Antimicrobial therapy in patients with *Escherichia coli* O157:H7 infection. *JAMA* 2002;288:1014–1016.
112. Grif K, Kierich MP, Karch H, et al. Strain-specific differences in the amount of Shiga toxin released from enterohemorrhagic *Escherichia coli* O157 following exposure to subinhibitory concentrations of antimicrobial agents. *Eur J Clin Microbiol Infect Dis* 1998;17:761–766.
113. Rizzoni G, Claris A, Edefonti A, et al. Plasma infusion for hemolytic uremic syndrome in children: results of a multicenter controlled trial. *J Pediatr* 1988;112:284–290.
114. Armstrong GD, Fodor E, Vanmaele R. Investigation of Shiga-like toxin binding of chemically synthesized oligosaccharide sequences. *J Infect Dis* 1991;164:1160–1167.
115. Trachtman H, Cnaan A, Christen E, et al. Effect of oral Shiga toxin binding agent on diarrhea-related hemolytic uremic syndrome in children: a randomized controlled trial. *JAMA* 2003 (*in press*).
116. Kitov PI, Sadowska JM, George M, et al. Shiga-like toxins are neutralized by tailored multivalent carbohydrate ligands. *Nature* 2000;403:669–672.
117. Kist-van Holthe JE, Goedvolk CA, Brand R, et al. Prospective study of renal insufficiency after bone marrow transplantation. *Pediatr Nephrol* 2002;17:1032–1037.
118. Denton MD, Chertow GM, Brady HR. "Renal-dose" dopamine for the treatment of acute renal failure: scientific rationale, experimental studies and clinical trials. *Kidney Int* 1996;49:4–14.
119. Chertow GM, Sayegh MH, Allgren RL, et al. Is the administration of dopamine associated with adverse or favorable outcomes in acute renal failure? *Am J Med* 1996;101:498–453.
120. Australian and New Zealand Intensive Care Society Clinical Trials Group. Low dose dopamine in patients with early renal dysfunction: a placebo controlled trial. *Lancet* 2000;356:2139–2143.
121. Kellum JA, Decker JM. Use of dopamine in acute renal failure: a meta-analysis. *Crit Care Med* 2001;29:1526–1531.
122. Galley HF. Renal dose dopamine: will the message get through? *Lancet* 2000;356:2112–2113.
123. Murphy MB, Murphy C, Shorten GD. Fenoldopam: a selective peripheral dopamine receptor agonist for the treatment of severe hypertension. *N Engl J Med* 2001;345:1548–1557.
124. Rahman SN, Kim GE, Mathew AS, et al. Effects of atrial natriuretic peptide in clinical acute renal failure. *Kidney Int* 1994;45:1731–1738.
125. Allgren RL, Marbury TC, Rahman SN, et al. Anaritide in acute tubular necrosis. *N Engl J Med* 1997;336:828–834.
126. Lamiere N, Vanholder R. Pathophysiologic features and prevention of human experimental acute tubular necrosis. *J Am Soc Nephrol* 2001;12:S20–S32.
127. Kellum JA. Use of diuretics in the acute care setting. *Kidney Int* 1998;53:67–70.
128. Marti SJ, Danzinger LH. Continuous infusions of loop diuretics in the critically ill. *Crit Care Med* 1994;22:1323–1329.
129. Brown CB, Ogg CS, Cameron JS. High dose furosemide in acute renal failure. *Clin Nephrol* 1981;15:90.
130. Sterns RH, Cappuccio JD, Silver SM, et al. Neurologic sequelae after treatment of severe hyponatremia: a multicenter perspective. *J Am Soc Nephrol* 1994;4:1522–1530.
131. Rodriguez-Soriano J. Potassium homeostasis and its disturbances in children. *Pediatr Nephrol* 1995;9:364–374.

132. Malone TA. Glucose and insulin versus cation-exchange resin for the treatment of hyperkalemia in very low birth weight infants. *J Pediatr* 1991;118:121–123.
133. Allon M, Copkney C. Albuterol and insulin for treatment of hyperkalemia in hemodialysis patients. *Kidney Int* 1990;38:869–872.
134. Bunchman TE, Wood EG, Schenck MH, et al. Pretreatment of formula with sodium polystyrene sulfonate to reduce dietary potassium intake. *Pediatr Nephrol* 1991;5:29–32.
135. Gerstman BB, Kirkman R, Platt R. Intestinal necrosis associated with postoperative orally administered sodium polystyrene sulfonate in sorbitol. *Am J Kidney Dis* 1992;20:159–161.
136. Andreoli SP, Dunson JW, Bergstein JM. Calcium carbonate is an effective phosphorus binder in children with chronic renal failure. *Am J Kidney Dis* 1987;9:206–210.
137. Wallott M, Bonzel KE, Winter A, et al. Calcium acetate versus calcium carbonate as oral phosphate binder in pediatric and adolescent hemodialysis patients. *Pediatr Nephrol* 1996;10:625–630.
138. Amin N. The impact of improved phosphorus control: use of sevelamer hydrochloride in patients with chronic renal failure. *Nephrol Dial Transplant* 2002;17:340–345.
139. Andreoli SP, Bergstein JM, Sherrard DJ. Aluminum intoxication from aluminum-containing phosphate binders in children with azotemia not undergoing dialysis. *N Engl J Med* 1984;310:1079–1084.
140. Adelman RD, Coppi R, Dillon MJ. The emergency management of severe hypertension. *Pediatr Nephrol* 2000;14:422–427.
141. Gauthier B, Trachtman H. Short acting nifedipine. *Pediatr Nephrol* 1997;11:786–787.
142. Belsha CW, Kohaut EC, Warady BA. Dialytic management of childhood acute renal failure: a survey of North American pediatric nephrologists. *Pediatr Nephrol* 1995;9:361–363.
143. Reznik VM, Griswold WR, Peterson BM, et al. Peritoneal dialysis for acute renal failure in children. *Pediatr Nephrol* 1991;5:715–717.
144. Steele BT, Vigneux A, Blatz D, et al. Acute peritoneal dialysis in infants weighing < 1500 g. *J Pediatr* 1987;110:126–129.
145. Mathews DE, West KW, Rescorla FJ, et al. Peritoneal dialysis in the first 60 days of life. *J Pediatr Surg* 1990;25:110–116.
146. Schiffl H, Lang SM, Fischer R. Daily hemodialysis and the outcome of acute renal failure. *N Engl J Med* 2002;346:305–310.
147. Hakim RM, Wingard RL, Parker RA. Effect of the dialysis membrane in the treatment of patients with acute renal failure. *N Engl J Med* 1994;331:1338–1342.
148. Toback FG. Regeneration after acute tubular necrosis. *Kidney Int* 1992;41:226–246.
149. Noiri E, Gailit J, Sheth D, et al. Cyclic RGD peptides ameliorate ischemic acute renal failure. *Kidney Int* 1994;46:1050–1058.
150. Humes HD, Cieslinski DA, Coimbra TM, et al. Epidermal growth factor enhances renal tubule cell regeneration and repair and accelerates the recovery of renal function in post ischemic acute renal failure. *J Clin Invest* 1989;84:1757–1761.
151. Ding H, Kopple JD, Cohen A, et al. Recombinant human insulin-like growth factor-1 accelerates recovery and reduces catabolism in rats with ischemic acute renal failure. *J Clin Invest* 1993;91:2281–2287.
152. Hammerman MR, Miller SB. Therapeutic use of growth factors in renal failure. *J Am Soc Nephrol* 1994;5:1–11.
153. Morin NL, Laurent G, Nonclercq D, et al. Epidermal growth factor accelerates renal tissue repair in a model of gentamycin nephrotoxicity in rats. *Am J Physiol* 1992;263:F806–F811.
154. Chiao H, Kohda Y, McLeroy P, et al. Alpha-melanocyte-stimulating hormone protects against renal injury after ischemia in mice and rats. *J Clin Invest* 1997;99:1165–1172.
155. Andreoli SP, Mallett CP, McAteer JA. Epidermal growth factor accelerated recovery of LLC-PK1 cells following oxidant injury. *In Vitro Cell Devel Biol Anim* 1998;34:824–830.
156. Arumugam TV, Shiels IA, Strachan AJ, et al. A small molecule C5a receptor antagonist protects kidney from ischemia/reperfusion injury. *Kidney Int* 2003;63:134–142.
157. Hropot M, Juretschke HP, Langer KH, et al. S3226, a novel NHE3 inhibitor, attenuates ischemia-induced acute renal failure in rats. *Kidney Int* 2001;60:2283–2289.
158. Chatterjee PK, Patel NSA, Sivarajah A, et al. GW274150, a potent and highly selective inhibitor of iNOS, reduces experimental renal ischemia/reperfusion injury. *Kidney Int* 2003;63:853–865.
159. Gueler F, Rong S, Park JK, et al. Postischemic acute renal failure is reduced by short term statin treatment in a rat model. *J Am Soc Nephrol* 2002;13:2288–2298.
160. Furuichi K, Wada T, Iwata Y, et al. Gene therapy expressing amino terminal truncated monocyte chemoattractant protein-1 prevents renal ischemia-reperfusion injury. *J Am Soc Nephrol* 2003;14:1066–1071.
161. Seigel NJ, Gaudio KM, Katz LA, et al. Beneficial effects of thyroxin on recovery from acute renal failure. *Kidney Int* 1984;25:906–911.
162. Hirschberg RT, Kopple J, Lipsett P, et al. Multicenter clinical trial of recombinant human insulin like growth factor in patients with acute renal failure. *Kidney Int* 1999;55:2423–2432.
163. Acker CG, Singh AR, Flick RP, et al. A trial of thyroxine in acute renal failure. *Kidney Int* 2000;57:293–298.
164. Luster AD. Chemokines: chemotactic cytokines that mediate inflammation. *N Engl J Med* 1998;338:436–445.
165. Heinzelmann M, Mercer-Jones MA, Passmore JC. Neutrophils and renal disease. *Am J Kidney Dis* 1999;34:384–399.
166. Chatterjee PK, Cuzzocrea S, Brown P, et al. Tempol, a membrane permeable radical scavenger, reduces oxidant stress mediated renal dysfunction and injury in the rat kidney. *Kidney Int* 2000;58:658–673.
167. Kelly KJ, Williams WW, Colvin RB, et al. Antibody to intercellular adhesion molecule-1 protects the kidney against ischemic injury. *Proc Natl Acad Sci U S A* 1994;91:812–817.
168. Bunchman TE, Maxvold NJ, Kershaw DB, et al. Continuous venovenous hemodiafiltration in infants and children. *Am J Kidney Dis* 1995;25:17–21.
169. Smoyer WE, McAdams C, Kaplan BS, et al. Determinants of survival in pediatric continuous hemofiltration. *J Am Soc Nephrol* 1995;6:1401–1409.
170. Ellis EN, Pearson D, Belsha CW, et al. Use of pump-assisted hemofiltration in children with acute renal failure. *Pediatr Nephrol* 1997;11:196–200.
171. Maxvold NJ, Smoyer WE, Gardner JJ, et al. Management of acute renal failure in the pediatric patients: hemofiltration versus hemodialysis. *Am J Kidney Dis* 1997;30:S84–S88.

172. Morgera S, Kraft AK, Siebert G, et al. Long-term outcomes in acute renal failure treated with continuous renal replacement therapies. *Am J Kidney Dis* 2002;40:275–279.
173. Phu NH, Hein TT, Mai TH, et al. Hemofiltration and peritoneal dialysis in infection-associated acute renal failure in Vietnam. *N Engl J Med* 2002;347:895–902.
174. Subrtamanian S, Venkataraman R, Kellum JA. Influence of dialysis membranes on outcomes in acute renal failure. *Kidney Int* 2002;62:1819–1823.
175. Bonventre JV. Daily hemodialysis—will treatment each day improve the outcome in patients with acute renal failure? *N Engl J Med* 2002;346:362–464.
176. Basile DP, Donohoe D, Roethe K, et al. Renal ischemic injury results in permanent damage to peritubular capillaries and influences long-term function. *Am J Physiol* 2001;281:F887–F899.
177. Brenner BM, Lawler EV, Mackenzie HS. The hyperfiltration theory: a paradigm shift in nephrology. *Kidney Int* 1996;49:1774–1777.

65

MANAGEMENT OF ACUTE RENAL FAILURE

MARK R. BENFIELD
TIMOTHY E. BUNCHMAN

Acute renal failure (ARF) represents a sudden reduction in kidney function to a level insufficient to adequately filter and excrete solute and water and maintain fluid and electrolyte balance. In spite of many years of clinical recognition, intervention, and research, a precise definition of ARF remains elusive, and commonly used definitions, including oliguria and azotemia, have shortcomings in pediatric practice. Although oliguria is often a presenting finding, this is not invariable, and urine output is a poor indicator of kidney function. ARF is often asymptomatic and noted only on routine screening laboratory evaluation as elevated blood urea nitrogen (BUN) and creatinine (Cr) levels. BUN and Cr are also insensitive markers of kidney function, however. Glomerular filtration rate (GFR) may fall by as much as 50% before serum Cr begins to rise, whereas a large rise in serum Cr may reflect only a small change in GFR in infants and patients with chronic renal insufficiency (1,2). These inaccuracies are further exaggerated in patients with reduced muscle mass, decreased protein intake, or underlying renal anomalies. Early recognition of ARF is important, however, to appropriately treat hypoperfusion, remove nephrotoxic agents or other factors contributing to ARF, and appropriately adjust fluids, electrolytes, and medications (3).

Kidney function is dependent on the adequacy of blood supply to the kidney, the integrity of the renal parenchyma, and the patency of the urinary tract (4). Because of this, the well-established approach to the classification of AFR as prerenal, renal, or postrenal continues to be useful and is employed in this chapter. Although few studies are available to determine the incidence of ARF in pediatric patients, most large studies of adults report the cause of ARF to be prerenal azotemia in 55 to 60% of cases, intrinsic renal parenchymal disease in 35 to 40% [90% of which cases are acute tubular necrosis (ATN)], and secondary to postrenal obstructive disease in fewer than 5% (5). Smaller pediatric studies have similarly demonstrated that hypoxia- and ischemia-induced renal injury is an important cause of ARF in children (6–8).

In developing countries, volume depletion from diarrhea continues to be the most common cause of ARF (9,10). In industrialized countries, however, ARF is more often seen in hospitalized patients with complex conditions who frequently have preexisting kidney disease. ARF is a particularly common complication in critically ill children in intensive care units (ICUs). In the neonatal ICU 3 to 24% of all admissions and as many as 60% of infants with severe asphyxia develop ARF (8,11–13). In adult studies, ARF complicates 5% of hospital admissions and 30% of ICU admissions (14).

In these patients, the causes of ARF are almost always multifactorial, related to underlying diseases and required therapies. Many of these patients have multiple renal insults, none of which alone would be expected to cause ARF. A detailed discussion of the clinical aspects of ARF is found in Chapter 64. This chapter describes in detail the management of ARF, especially in the ICU setting. The following section describes circumstances in which decisions concerning treatment must be made.

CATEGORIES OF ACUTE RENAL FAILURE

Prerenal Causes

Prerenal azotemia is the most common cause of ARF and represents an appropriate physiologic response to renal hypoperfusion (15). During early or mild hypoperfusion states a series of neural and humoral responses are active to maintain renal perfusion and GFR, including increased adrenergic activity, stimulation of the renin-angiotensin-aldosterone system, and the release of antidiuretic hormone. The adrenergic nerves cause diffuse vasoconstriction maintaining systemic blood pressure. However, this leads to increased renal vascular resistance and decreased glomerular blood flow. In response to hypovolemia and hypoperfusion, the renin-angiotensin system is stimulated, which causes increased production of angiotensin II. This has a direct

TABLE 65.1. PATHOGENESIS OF ACUTE RENAL FAILURE: PRERENAL CAUSES

Hypovolemia	
Gastrointestinal losses	Vomiting
	Diarrhea
	Nasogastric drainage
Renal losses	Salt-wasting nephropathy
	Diabetes insipidus
	Adrenal insufficiency
	Diuresis (drug induced or osmotic)
Blood losses	Surgery
	Trauma
	Gastrointestinal bleeding
	Pancreatitis
Insensible losses	Hyperthermia
	Burns
Redistribution	Sepsis
	Nephrotic syndrome
	Heart failure
	Liver failure
	Third-space sequestration

effect on the proximal tubule and, through aldosterone, on the distal tubule, causing reabsorption of salt and water. Furthermore, angiotensin II preferentially increases glomerular efferent arteriolar constriction, which increases the glomerular filtration pressure (15–17). These vasoconstrictive factors are counterbalanced by increased production of prostaglandins and nitric oxide, which stimulate afferent arteriolar vasodilatation (18–20). Cumulatively, these changes may cause an increased filtration fraction and maintain GFR. As the hypoperfusion state worsens, however, these compensatory mechanisms are overwhelmed, which leads to excessive vasoconstriction, decreased glomerular blood flow, and decreased GFR (15,21).

Overall, 60% of cases of ARF are prerenal, usually due to excessive fluid losses from trauma and bleeding or losses from the gastrointestinal system, kidneys, or skin (22,23). Prerenal ARF can complicate any disease process associated with hypovolemia and decreased renal perfusion (Table 65.1). Many of these cases are obvious on initial evaluation and involve overt loss of volume such as through vomiting and diarrhea, or blood loss through surgery or trauma. Other disease states, however, result in reduced effective vascular volume without overt volume loss. These situations include excessive insensible volume loss during hyperthermia or with severe burns, and gastrointestinal losses, as well as redistribution of volume such as seen with sepsis, nephrotic syndrome, heart failure, liver failure, or third-space sequestration.

Infants are particularly susceptible to excessive volume loss. The immature kidney is unable to develop maximally concentrated urine and adequately conserve salt and water, which makes infants particularly vulnerable to dehydration. Furthermore, neonates have a relatively large body surface area compared to body mass, and insensible water loss through the skin during febrile illnesses, while under radiant warmers, and during bilirubin phototherapy can be excessive (24).

Renal losses of salt and water leading to prerenal azotemia are often difficult to recognize. Many of these children have underlying abnormalities causing polyuria, which makes urine output an insensitive tool in assessing kidney function. They also frequently have chronically reduced kidney function, which makes BUN and Cr less useful as diagnostic tools. This form of nonoliguric ARF can be seen in diseases with renal concentrating defects (cystic dysplasia, polycystic kidney diseases, diabetes insipidus) or those with large osmotic loads (hyperglycemia). In many of these illnesses, other laboratory findings of volume contraction, including weight loss, increased BUN, hypernatremia, and increased hematocrit, are clues to the excessive loss of free water (15,25).

In diseases with redistribution of volume, patients often have signs and symptoms of total body volume overload. Because of excessive third-space fluid loss or vasodilatation, however, the effective intravascular volume and renal perfusion are inadequate. In these situations it is important to maintain a high index of suspicion and search carefully for signs and symptoms suggestive of volume contraction and the physiologic responses to inadequate vascular volume. In most cases of prerenal azotemia, careful correction and maintenance of intravascular fluid and perfusion can prevent progression and more profound ARF (ATN).

Renal Causes

When renal causes of ARF are considered, it is useful to classify diseases according to the location of renal injury: vascular, glomerular, tubular, or interstitial (Table 65.2). Large clinical epidemiologic studies involving adults demonstrate that approximately 50% of ARF is due to ischemic ATN, 35% to nephrotoxic injury, and 15% to acute interstitial nephritis or acute glomerulonephritis (14,26–29).

TABLE 65.2. PATHOGENESIS OF ACUTE RENAL FAILURE: RENAL CAUSES

Arterial	Thrombosis
	Arteritis
	Hemolytic uremic syndrome
	Malignant hypertension
Venous	Renal venous thrombosis
Glomerular	Acute glomerulonephritis
Tubular	
Acute tubular necrosis	Ischemia
	Nephrotoxicity
	Pigment nephropathy
Obstructive	Crystal nephropathy
Interstitial	Acute interstitial nephritis
	Pyelonephritis
Congenital anomalies	Hypoplasia and dysplasia
	Polycystic kidney disease
All	Tumor lysis syndrome

The causes of intrinsic renal ARF in pediatrics vary significantly by age. In infancy the most common causes of ARF include (a) hypoxic-ischemic insults secondary to severe gastroenteritis and dehydration, perinatal asphyxia, respiratory distress syndrome, sepsis, necrotizing enterocolitis, and congenital heart disease (8,11,30); (b) nephrotoxic insults from antibiotics (aminoglycosides), antifungal agents (amphotericin B), nonsteroidal antiinflammatory agents given for patent ductus arteriosus, and maternal ingestion of angiotensin-converting enzyme inhibitors; (c) renal vascular obstruction secondary to renal artery and venous thrombosis; and (d) congenital renal anomalies, including obstructive uropathies (posterior urethral valves, bilateral ureteropelvic junction obstruction, ureterocele), hypoplasia and dysplasia syndromes, and autosomal recessive polycystic kidney disease. In the school-aged child glomerular diseases, especially postinfectious glomerulonephritis, and hemolytic uremic syndrome are the most common causes. Finally, trauma and rapidly progressive glomerulonephritis are the most common causes of ARF in adolescent patients.

Vascular

Arterial obstruction is seen almost exclusively during the neonatal period and is most often due to thromboembolic events secondary to the use of umbilical artery catheters. Thromboembolism from umbilical artery catheters most often leads to hypertension; however, with a solitary kidney or massive thromboemboli, ARF can occur (3,31,32). More commonly sepsis, perinatal asphyxia, hypovolemia, shock, maternal diabetes, or polycythemia leads to renal venous thrombosis (RVT) (3,33–37). Outside of the neonatal period RVT is also seen in children with severe dehydration or with hypercoagulable states associated with nephrotic syndrome, systemic lupus erythematosus, antiphospholipid syndrome, and congenital deficiencies in proteins of the coagulation cascade, including protein C, protein S, antithrombin III, plasminogen, factor V Leiden mutation, prothrombin variant, methylenetetrahydrofolate reductase variant, and increased lipoprotein(a) (14,38–43). RVT typically presents with enlarged kidneys, gross hematuria, thrombocytopenia, hypertension, decreased urine output, and increasing BUN and Cr levels (3,44,45). Anatomically, venous thrombosis usually involves the entire venous system, and thrombectomy is rarely indicated or possible. Controversy exists as to the usefulness of anticoagulation or thrombolytic therapy. Multiple single-center reports describe the use of heparin, streptokinase, urokinase, and tissue plasminogen activator (34,36,46–48). Although some reports suggest recovery of renal function, others have noted significant incidence of bleeding complications and significant renal atrophy on long-term follow-up (46). Clearly, different approaches would be used and different outcomes expected for patients with RVT secondary to congenital absence of coagulation factors and for those with severely altered blood flow secondary to sepsis and shock. Nevertheless, recovery has been reported and is likely because of patchy venous thrombosis and/or associated ATN. It is certainly possible that anticoagulation may prevent progression of existing thrombosis to uninvolved parenchyma or to the contralateral kidney; however, carefully controlled multicenter studies are needed to answer these questions.

Other diseases lead to direct injury of renal vasculature that leads to ischemia-hypoxia and ARF. Hemolytic uremic syndrome is a largely reversible disorder usually initiated by verotoxin-producing organisms (especially *Escherichia coli* O157:H7) causing endothelial damage, hemorrhagic colitis, microangiopathic hemolytic anemia, thrombocytopenia, and renal failure. The care for hemolytic uremic syndrome continues to be supportive and frequently involves early dialysis to prevent fluid and electrolyte imbalance and allow transfusions of red blood cells and adequate nutritional support.

Malignant hypertension is a clinical diagnosis defined as severely elevated blood pressure with signs or symptoms of acute target organ damage (central nervous, cardiovascular, renal systems) (49). The primary pathophysiology involves blood pressure elevation beyond the level at which local autoregulation can control blood flow to tissues. This is usually associated with frank inflammation, arteritis, and ischemia, and in the case of the kidneys has been described to cause ARF. These patients often present with hematuria and worsening kidney function. In cases of ARF, recovery of renal function is quite variable and may take a prolonged period of time (49–56).

Glomerular

Acute glomerulonephritis as a cause of ARF is seldom subtle. These patients often have findings that include edema, hypertension, and active urinary sediment which help guide the diagnosis to this category. Acute glomerulonephritis is rare in infants and toddlers. In school-aged children, postinfectious glomerulonephritis continues to be the most common acute glomerulonephritis and is often associated with mild to moderate ARF. However, almost any of the glomerulonephritides of childhood can present with a rapidly progressive course and ARF. Patients with ARF secondary to acute glomerulonephritis require prompt evaluation, and diagnosis with renal biopsy is important to guide definitive therapies.

Tubular

Although prerenal azotemia and ischemic ATN are discussed as separate entities, they represent a spectrum of disease, and all of the diseases in Table 65.1 can be associated with either prerenal azotemia or ischemic ATN. In each of the diseases described earlier, unless renal perfusion is restored or nephrotoxic agents withdrawn, prerenal azotemia often progresses to

TABLE 65.3. ACUTE RENAL FAILURE: NEPHROTOXIC AGENTS

Hyperoncotic state	Dextran
	Mannitol
Prerenal state	Diuretics
	Interleukins
	Angiotensin-converting enzyme inhibitors
	Antihypertensives
Tubular toxicity	
Direct toxicity	Aminoglycosides
	Cisplatin
	Vancomycin
	Foscarnet
	Pentamidine
	Radiocontrast agents
	Amphotericin B
	Heavy metals
Tubular swelling	Intravenous immune globulin
	Dextran
	Maltose
	Sucrose
	Mannitol
Endothelial injury	Cyclosporine
	Tacrolimus
	Mitomycin C
	Cocaine
	Estrogen
	Quinine
Altered vascular reactivity	
Afferent arteriolar constriction	Nonsteroidal antiinflammatory drugs
	Radiocontrast agents
	Amphotericin B
Efferent arteriolar dilatation	Angiotensin-converting enzyme inhibitors
	Angiotensin II receptor antagonists
Crystalluria	Sulfonamides
	Methotrexate
	Acyclovir
	Triamterene
	Ethylene glycol
	Protease inhibitors
Glomerulopathy	Gold
	Penicillamine
	Nonsteroidal antiinflammatory drugs
Interstitial nephritis	Multiple agents
Pigmenturia	Multiple agents

Adapted from Nolan CR, Anderson RJ. Hospital-acquired acute renal failure. *J Am Soc Nephrol* 1998;9:710–718.

the intrinsic renal disease of ischemic-nephrotoxic ATN. Nephrotoxic agents are important causes of ARF. The number of nephrotoxins is large, and the mechanisms by which they contribute to ARF are diverse (Table 65.3) (57–59).

Pigment nephropathy is caused by the sudden release of large quantities of heme proteins, especially hemoglobin from breakdown of red blood cells and myoglobin from breakdown of muscle cells, into the blood (60–62). Pigment nephropathies are seen clinically in the setting of rhabdomyolysis secondary to trauma, crush injury, heat stroke, sepsis, or underlying myopathy and during episodes of rapid hemolysis.

Although hemoglobin and myoglobin are not toxic, the heme proteins associated with their breakdown have multiple toxicities. The renal damage caused by pigment nephropathy has three distinct mechanisms: (a) renal vasoconstriction, (b) direct heme protein–induced tubular cell toxicity, and (c) intraluminal cast formation. Renal vasoconstriction is likely the prominent mechanism, and the reduced renal blood flow and urine production accentuate the other mechanisms of injury. Rhabdomyolysis is invariably associated with rapid movement of fluid from the vascular space into injured muscles, which causes severe contraction of the extracellular fluid volume. Without aggressive volume resuscitation, this causes ischemic ATN. The heme proteins are rapidly filtered in the glomerulus, and in the renal tubule produce reactive oxygen metabolites that are directly toxic to the tubules and are scavengers of nitrous oxide, which causes unopposed renal medullary vasoconstriction (60,63–66). In an acidic environment myoglobin and hemoglobin also dissociate to ferrihemate, which is directly toxic to the renal tubule. Finally, tubular pigment can precipitate, which causes tubular obstruction (63,67). This precipitation of heme proteins is also enhanced in an acid environment (60,68,69).

Pigment nephropathy is usually diagnosed by noting obvious precipitating events in the history and by urine that gives positive dipstick results for hemoglobin but has minimal cellular elements on microscopic examination. Confirmatory tests include evaluation of serum creatine phosphokinase levels. Treatment includes expansion of the vascular volume to assure adequate renal blood flow, forced diuresis and alkalinization of urine to reduce the production of reactive oxygen metabolites and ferrihemate, and maximization of urine flow to reduce the precipitation of heme proteins.

In contrast-induced nephropathy, ARF is produced predominantly by acute vasoconstriction and ATN (70,71) and is best minimized by assuring adequate hydration before exposure. The use of newer nonionic contrast materials and alternate imaging techniques (e.g., magnetic resonance imaging) and contrast materials has not reduced the incidence of contrast-induced nephropathy (26,72–74).

Other causes of intrinsic renal disease leading to ARF include direct toxicities of drugs and other substances. These include aminoglycoside antibiotics, cisplatin, cyclosporine, tacrolimus, mannitol, amphotericin B, methotrexate, foscarnet, pentamidine, organic solvents, heavy metals, cocaine, intravenous immunoglobulin, and radiocontrast agents. Amphotericin B has been clearly described as causing distal tubular damage leading to decreased urinary concentrating capacity, distal renal tubular acidosis, potassium wasting, and magnesium wasting. Amphotericin B nephrotoxicity can best be minimized by assuring adequate hydration and renal perfusion. Liposomal preparations of amphotericin B have been associated with less nephrotoxicity.

Interstitial Disease

A long list of medications has been associated with acute interstitial nephritis. Many of these are considered to be very safe and are in broad usage. Acute interstitial nephritis is discussed in detail elsewhere. Although these drugs are often associated with peripheral and urinary eosinophilia, a high index of suspicion is necessary to accurately diagnose this disorder.

Postrenal Causes

Obstructive uropathy is one of the most common causes of renal failure in pediatrics. Obstruction of the urinary tract is an uncommon cause of ARF. However, patients with chronic obstructive uropathies and urinary concentrating defects are at significantly increased risk of renal failure associated with prerenal hypoxic-ischemic insults and nephrotoxic agents. Proper diagnosis of urinary obstruction is obviously necessary to provide appropriate treatment.

ASSESSMENT OF THE PATIENT WITH ACUTE RENAL FAILURE

In most patients with ARF, the causes of renal disease are evident from the history and physical examination. Historical findings of surgery or trauma associated with large blood loss, sepsis or other cause of unstable blood pressure and generalized hypoperfusion, excessive vomiting and diarrhea, burns, and so on, would quickly suggest a renal hypoperfusion state and either prerenal azotemia or ischemic ATN. In the hospitalized patient this is further enhanced by review of hospital records for serially determined fluid balance, weight, and urine output to assess volume status as well as for drug exposures and other procedures or interventions that may contribute to azotemia. ARF often has a multifactorial cause, however. In many patients, no single instigating event can be identified; a combination of chronic disease, relative hypoperfusion, and nephrotoxic medications cause decreased kidney function.

The physical examination also gives many clues to the cause of ARF. Findings suggestive of hypovolemia, including tachycardia, orthostatic blood pressure changes, dry mucous membranes, and decreased skin turgor, would support the diagnosis of prerenal azotemia. Patients with nephrotic syndrome, heart failure, liver failure, and other diseases with decreased effective intravascular volume often have obvious physical findings of the primary organ dysfunction. On the other hand, patients with inflammatory diseases of the kidney have evidence for volume overload, including edema and hypertension.

Prerenal ARF is often associated with oliguria, elevated BUN and Cr levels, and other metabolic derangements. By definition, however, renal parenchymal integrity is maintained, and recovery is complete when perfusion is restored. The diagnosis of prerenal ARF is made by identifying the normal systemic responses to hypovolemia and the normal renal tubular responses to hypoperfusion. These include history and physical examination findings of volume contraction, including increased thirst, dry mucous membranes, decreased skin turgor, and tachycardia. The normal renal tubular response to hypoperfusion is seen with decreased urine flow, increased urinary concentration, and decreased urinary excretion of sodium. Several urine tests have been developed to help demonstrate these tubular responses (Table 65.4).

Although evaluation of BUN and Cr is important in making the diagnosis of ARF, and electrolyte analysis is helpful in determining complications related to ARF, urinary sediment and indices are perhaps the most important factors in determining the cause of ARF. Urine specific gravity begins to give clues related to effective vascular volume and renal blood flow. Significant hematuria and proteinuria are suggestive of a glomerulonephritis. Urine dipstick test results positive for blood with no cells on

TABLE 65.4. LABORATORY EVALUATIONS OF ACUTE RENAL FAILURE

Test	Prerenal	Intrinsic renal	Postrenal
BUN/Cr ratio	>20	10–20	10–20
Urine specific gravity	>1.020	~1.010	<1.010
Urine osmolality	>350	~300	~300
Urine sodium	<20	>30	>40
FE_{Na}[a]	<1%	>2%	>3%
Urine Cr/plasma Cr	>40	<20	<20
Urine microscopy	Normal	ATN: dark granular casts, renal epithelial cells/casts	Normal
	Hyaline casts	GN: RBCs, RBC casts, WBCs, proteinuria AIN: urine eosinophilia, WBCs, hyaline casts	Hyaline casts

AIN, acute interstitial nephritis; ATN, acute tubular necrosis; BUN, blood urea nitrogen; Cr, creatinine; FE_{Na}, fractional excretion of sodium; GN, glomerulonephritis; RBC, red blood cell; WBC, white blood cell.
[a]Falsely low FE_{Na} seen with acute GN, radiocontrast-induced nephropathy, rhabdomyolysis.
From Albright RC Jr. Acute renal failure: a practical update. *Mayo Clin Proc* 2001;76:67–74, with permission.

microscopic examination of the urine is highly suggestive of myoglobin or hemoglobin in the urine and pigment nephropathy. Urine indices are designed to assess renal tubular function and are useful in differentiating prerenal from intrinsic renal causes of ARF (75,76). A particularly useful test is the fractional excretion of sodium (FE_{Na}):

$$FE_{Na} = (P_{Na}/U_{Na})/(P_{Cr}/U_{Cr})$$

where P_{Na} and P_{Cr} are the plasma levels of sodium and creatinine, and U_{Na} and U_{Cr} are the urine levels of sodium and creatinine, respectively.

Multiple studies have demonstrated that an FE_{Na} of less than 1% is seen with prerenal azotemia and a value higher than 2% is seen in intrinsic renal causes of ARF. However, it is important to note that several causes of intrinsic renal ARF are associated with a falsely low FE_{Na}, including some acute glomerulonephritides, contrast-induced nephropathy, and rhabdomyolysis. Also the FE_{Na} is difficult to interpret in the presence of medications that alter Na reabsorption, such as diuretics.

TREATMENT OF THE PATIENT WITH ACUTE RENAL FAILURE

Nondialytic Therapy

Although dialysis remains the only proven complete treatment for ARF, many other treatment regimens have been used to prevent or treat ARF. Many clinical trials of pharmaceutical agents have been conducted, but none of these has demonstrated convincing results. To date the only effective nondialytic treatment of ARF entails restoration of adequate renal blood flow, avoidance of nephrotoxic medications or those that interfere with renal compensatory mechanisms, and assurance that renal perfusion has been maximized before exposure to nephrotoxic agents.

A long-followed medical approach to management of patients at risk for ARF has been the use of "renal-dose dopamine" (1 to 3 μg/kg/min). Although this approach has been associated with increased urine output, the effect is short lived (1 to 3 days), and existing data demonstrate no effect on survival or delay in the need for dialysis (6,26,77–82).

Similarly, diuretics have also been used in patients with oliguric ARF. Diuretics occasionally improve urine flow and thus may provide enough urine output to allow medications and nutrition to be provided safely. Furthermore, the increased urine flow may decrease the concentration of toxins such as myoglobin or hemoglobin in the renal tubules. The increased urine flow does not reflect improved GFR, however, and has not been demonstrated to prevent or ameliorate ATN (26,83–87). In fact, diuresis may worsen ARF in prerenal azotemia and radiocontrast-induced ARF, as well as ARF after cardiac surgery (26,88,89).

Mannitol is an osmotic diuretic that has also been used to treat a variety of diseases with high risk of ARF (26,90). Although mannitol may be beneficial in organ preservation solutions and when given extremely early after a crush injury to produce diuresis, it has not been shown to be useful in prevention or treatment of ARF.

Hyperkalemia is a common life-threatening complication of ARF. Until removal of potassium is possible, other methods are often needed to shift potassium from the intravascular to intracellular space. Infusions of calcium (10 mg/kg elemental calcium as calcium chloride or calcium gluconate) have been demonstrated to stabilize cell membranes and decrease the risk of cardiac arrhythmias but do not change the serum potassium concentration. Intravenous glucose and insulin (0.25 U regular insulin per gram of glucose) have been demonstrated to cause a shift of potassium from the extracellular to the intracellular space. The β-agonists have also been demonstrated to lower serum potassium acutely and can be administered by inhalation in situations in which intravenous access is not available (91,92). Enteric exchange resins (sodium polystyrene sulfonate, or Kayexalate, 1 g/kg body weight, repeated up to hourly) effectively remove potassium from the body. However, this removal may be slow and inconsistent, and administration may be difficult, especially if multiple treatments are necessary. Although parenteral bicarbonate therapy (1 mEq/kg body weight) has been widely used to alkalinize the blood and drive intracellular shifting of potassium, multiple studies have demonstrated that bicarbonate therapy has little to no effect on potassium levels in the long term (93).

Acidosis related to enhanced metabolic rate and inflammation frequently occurs in ARF and complicates its management. In this setting, removal of the acid load can be accomplished only by some method of dialysis. Buffering by administration of an oral or parenteral bicarbonate may provide temporary improvement, but its use is often limited because of the concomitant provision of sodium.

Other solutes such as sodium phosphorus or uric acid accumulate in the blood of patients with ARF. Attention should be paid to avoiding the compounding of those abnormalities in the conservative management of ARF. If the concentrations of these substances reach critical levels, treatment by some form of dialysis is indicated.

Adequate nutrition is a critically important component of the treatment of ARF, especially in the ICU setting. Provision of nutrition may be very difficult when oliguria is present. Nutrition should not be compromised, however, and the need for its provision may itself be an indication for initiation of dialysis.

Dialytic Therapy

Because of the complex metabolic abnormalities associated with ARF, dialysis is often the treatment of choice to quickly restore fluid and electrolyte balance. There are currently three dialysis modalities in common use for ARF: peritoneal dialysis (PD), hemodialysis (HD), and continuous renal replacement therapy (CRRT). The choice of dialysis modality is best made in keeping with the local standard of care and is based on a number of considerations (94). The first consideration is experience with the modality. It would be inappropriate to introduce a new or unfamiliar form of dialysis therapy during the care of an acutely ill patient with a complex condition. The second consideration is access. If the peritoneal membrane is disrupted or scarred, PD is impossible. If sufficient vascular access cannot be attained, HD cannot be attempted. The third consideration is hemodynamic stability of the patient. Patients who are hemodynamically unstable often will not tolerate the rapid fluid shifts associated with intermittent HD as opposed to more continuous modalities such as PD or CRRT. The fourth consideration is the goal of the dialysis. When the goal is fluid removal, any of these modalities works effectively. When solute clearance is critical, however, HD is the most efficient method and is often preferred over other modalities to obtain the maximum solute clearance in the least amount of time (95). Optimum care of the child with ARF is best achieved by assuring access to multiple forms of treatment.

Other chapters in this book describe the technical details of PD and HD, and their application in the child with ARF is very similar to their use in children with end-stage renal disease. This chapter focuses on CRRT as a treatment for ARF in the ICU.

Types of Continuous Renal Replacement Therapy

CRRT is a term coined to describe a continuous mode of dialysis at the bedside. Historically this included PD or hemofiltration (HF), but now the term is used almost interchangeably with HF. Continuous HF can be accomplished via either arteriovenous or venovenous access. The major difference between the two is that arteriovenous HF uses an arterial access and arterial blood pressure to pump blood through the circuit, whereas venovenous HF uses a pump to circulate blood through the extracorporeal system. Studies have shown that arteriovenous HF is associated with inadequate solute clearance, more serious vascular complications, and a more frequent need to change to other modalities compared with venovenous HF (96). As a result, arteriovenous HF has largely fallen from use. Therefore the major focus of this discussion is on venovenous HF.

Venovenous HF can be accomplished by three methods. These include continuous venovenous HF (CVVH), CVVH with dialysis (CVVHD), and continuous venovenous hemodiafiltration (CVVHDF). The major difference between CVVH and CVVHDF is that convective solute removal is used in CVVH whereas solute is removed by diffusion in CVVHDF.

Continuous Venovenous Hemofiltration

CVVH combines ultrafiltration with convective clearance. An ultrafiltrate of blood passes through a membrane and is replaced with either a prefilter or a postfilter sterile infusion of an isotonic solution. Based on the principles of convective clearance, solute is removed in the ultrafiltrate and replaced with a solution free of this solute. Over time the remaining solute is diluted. Both small and mid-sized molecules are convectively cleared based on their concentration in the blood, the rate of ultrafiltration, and the molecule's sieving coefficient. The sieving coefficient is related to the molecular weight, the charge of the HF membrane, and the protein binding of the solute. Convection is effective but is not as efficient as diffusion.

Continuous Venovenous Hemofiltration with Dialysis

CVVHD is achieved by perfusing the space on the opposite side of the membrane from the patient's blood with a dialysate solution. As with HD, this permits diffusion of solutes across the membrane driven by a concentration gradient. The components of the dialysate must be physiologic. The transfer of solute across the membrane is again related to the sieving coefficient of the solute as well as the charge and pH of the membrane and the concentration gradient across the membrane. Low-molecular-weight compounds have a sieving coefficient approaching 1.0, and transfer is similar with convective or diffusive clearance. For compounds of middle and higher molecular weight, the sieving coefficient becomes less than 1.0, and better transfer is achieved by convective therapies. Work by Maxvold et al. has compared the mass transfer of urea in CVVH to that in CVVHD (97). In the former, clearance is related to the ultrafiltration rate, whereas in the latter, the dialysate flow rate is generally rate limiting.

Continuous Venovenous Hemodiafiltration

CVVHDF methods include a combination of both convective and diffusive solute removal. During CVVHDF, prefilter or postfilter infusion of replacement fluid is combined with high ultrafiltration rates to achieve convection, and a dialysis fluid is used to achieve diffusion. This combination of diffusive and convective clearance may improve clearance over that using either method alone. However, the data have not shown a practical increase in solute clearance sufficient to compensate for the increased complexity of the procedure.

Ultrafiltration

Ultrafiltration in a setting of CRRT is based on the concept of net fluid removal. As opposed to PD, in which ultrafiltration is controlled by osmolar fluid shifts, the ultrafiltration in CRRT is achieved by a transmembrane pressure. Ultrafiltration can be increased either by increasing the venous return pressure or by creating a higher vacuum ("negative pressure") across the membrane on the ultrafiltrate side. The newer generation of CRRT devices controls ultrafiltration by computer software and is accurate to 1 to 2%.

Equipment

Historically, in the late 1980s and early 1990s all equipment related to HF was adapted from previously existing blood pumps, intravenous pumps, and/or HD machines. Adapted devices were easy to use at the bedside but lacked technical safeguards such as air leak detectors, blood warmers, and ultrafiltration controllers. These adapted devices allowed for the early provision of CRRT at the bedside but also increased the work of the nursing staff and also increased the potential for errors associated with temperature control and ultrafiltration (98,99).

Newer equipment has taken the historical benefits of adapted devices at bedside and added a warming device for replacement or dialysate fluid, very accurate ultrafiltration control devices, and appropriate failure detectors. These additional three components have made CRRT much safer. These devices incorporate computer modules that allow for continuous readout of several parameters. In North America, these modern devices include the B. Braun Diapact System, the Gambro Prisma system, the Aquarius system (Edwards LifeScience, Missisagua, Ontario), and the Baxter BM-25 and, in the near future, Accura systems (Baxter, McGaw Park, IL); also available is the CRRT option for the model 2008H and 2008K HD machines by Fresenius. Outside North America, HF machines include the Hygieia Plus (Kimal, Middlesex, UK), EQUASmart (Medica, Medolla, Italy), and Rand Performer (Italy). All of these devices provide variable blood flow rates from 10 to 300 mL/min, variable dialysate flow rates from 0 to 3 L/hr, variable replacement flow rates from 0 to 5 L/hr, variable ultrafiltration rates including accurate ultrafiltration controllers with a range of ±1 to 2%, and accurate temperature control. In addition, all these devices have air leak detectors as well as blood-side pressure monitors.

The B. Braun, Edwards Life Sciences, Baxter, and Fresenius devices allow the user to choose a dialysis membrane. The membrane can be any of the commercially available membranes. The Gambro Prisma system has a cassette system that enhances the ease of administration and commencement of CRRT but requires the operator to use the specific membrane associated with their cassette.

Membranes

The membranes used for CRRT are similar to those used for HD. They vary in the components of the membranes, sieving coefficient, and surface area. The two major types of membranes for HF are composed of polysulfone or acrylonitrile. Both have the advantages that they are slightly negatively charged, they have a fairly high sieving coefficient that allows for adequate ultrafiltration and solute clearance either by convective or by diffusive techniques, and they are considered "biocompatible." Table 65.5 lists the various membranes available.

The acrylonitrile (AN69) membrane has a unique property that is problematic in acidotic patients. When the acidic plasma interacts with the membrane, bradykinin production ensues. When infused back into the patient, these activated bradykinins can cause an anaphylactic-like response. This response is accentuated in patients who are small or who require blood priming during the onset of HF. Blood bank blood has a pH between 6.2 and 6.4, a very high concentration of potassium, and a very low concentration of calcium. There have been several reports of anaphylaxis in patients during blood priming with the AN69 membrane. This is easily prevented by dialyzing the blood for a period of time to bring the pH close to 7.6 and the potassium and calcium to physiologic levels. Alternatively, a bypass maneuver may be used (100).

TABLE 65.5. PEDIATRIC CIRCUIT VOLUMES AND HEMOFILTER PROPERTIES

Patient weight (kg)	Hemofilter	Material and surface area	Priming volume (mL)	Arterial/venous line volume
<10	Amicon Minifilter Plus	Polysulfone	15	3 mL/3 mL
		0.07 m^2		TCV = 21 mL
>10	Renaflo II HF	Polysulfone		7 mL/7 mL
	400	0.3 m^2	28	TCV = 42 mL
	700	0.7 m^2	53	TCV = 67 mL
	1200	1.25 m^2	83	TCV = 97 mL
>10	Hospal (Lyon, France) Multiflow 60	Acrylonitrile and sodium methallyl sulfonate copolymer	48	6.5 mL/13.8 mL
		0.6 m^2		TCV = 67.3 mL
>10	Asahi PAN	Polyacrylonitrile		
	0.3	0.3 m^2	33	
	0.6	0.6 m^2	63	
	1.0	1.0 m^2	87	

TCV, total circuit volume.
Note: Venovenous hemofiltration requires larger circuit volume depending on the pumps used. For the nonadapted systems, such as the Prisma, the filter is the Multiflow 60, and the circuit volume is fixed at around 100 mL.

Tubing

Tubing for CRRT is available from several companies. Presently the Edwards LifeScience Aquarius and the Baxter Accura devices are in production. Edwards systems with the Aquarius now has pediatric tubing, whereas the Baxter Accura system does not. The Fresenius HD machine that can be adapted for CRRT can use all HD tubing, including neonatal, pediatric, and adult tubing. Gambro (Prisma system) is in the process of developing a system that is 50% smaller. The B. Braun device has both pediatric and adult tubing that allows for various sizes of membranes. The current Baxter BM-25 has both low- and high-volume tubing.

Historically, many nephrologists have been told that if one has more than 10% of blood volume in an extracorporeal device, blood priming is necessary to maintain hemodynamic stability. This approach is probably inappropriate, because one is taking a process used for an outpatient stable population with chronic disease and applying it to an inpatient unstable population. Therefore, blood priming should no longer be based on the extracorporeal blood volume but on a combination of the extracorporeal blood volume and the hemodynamic stability of the patient. Except with the AN69 membrane, blood priming should be considered necessary for any patient with hemodynamic instability at the time of onset of need for HF.

Access

Access for CRRT can be achieved with either a cuffed or a noncuffed catheter. In most settings a noncuffed catheter is used for acute treatment. Table 65.6 provides a list of vascular catheters for CRRT. The noncuffed catheter can be placed in the internal jugular (IJ), subclavian, or femoral space. Many nephrologists would prefer to avoid the use of subclavian catheters in patients who may develop end-stage renal disease and whose subsequent treatment is complicated by subclavian stenosis. The advantage of the IJ catheter is that it is not compromised by the patient's motion and appears to give adequate blood flow with minimal resistance or recirculation. The disadvantage of the IJ catheter is the increased risk of both pneumothorax and hemothorax at the time of placement. The advantage of a femoral catheter is that it is associated with less risk at the time of placement than is a subclavian or IJ catheter. The disadvantages of the femoral line includes a theoretical increased risk of infection and the possibility that movement during therapy may affect blood flow or cause intermittent inhibition of blood flow.

Solutions

The U.S. Food and Drug Administration (FDA) considers anything that is placed in the vascular space to be a drug. The FDA has yet to approve any specific solution as a replacement fluid in CVVH. Therefore, many programs are using either saline or lactated Ringer solution as the standard replacement fluid. Furthermore, many programs are having the pharmacy make solutions to meet the needs of each specific patient. The FDA Modernization Act of 1997 (http://www.fda.gov/opacom/backgrounders/modact.htm) does allow for local judgment in using a device (i.e., a dialysis solution) as a drug (replacement) if it is safer than other options. Therefore, many programs use dialysis solutions as replacement fluids for CRRT.

Dialysis solutions are not considered drugs but are considered devices that have been approved by the FDA. Two solutions are available for dialysis in the United States. These are the Baxter (lactate-based) hemofiltration solution and Dialysis Solutions (Richmond Hills, Ontario, Canada) Normocarb (bicarbonate-based) solutions. In Canada, Hemosol L0 and B0 (Hospal, Lyon, France) are also available.

Lactate-based and bicarbonate-based solutions are available for CRRT. If bicarbonate is placed directly into plastic bags, over a short period of time the bicarbonate will leach out as CO_2 and the solution will lose its buffering capacity. Lactate has been used because it is stable in these solutions.

When these solutions are used, lactate is delivered to the patient. The use of lactate solutions can be associated with rising lactate levels in patients, and it can be difficult to discriminate whether this level is related to endogenous lactate resulting from conditions such as bowel ischemia or low cardiac output, or is due to the lactate in the solution. One could discriminate between these two by determining

TABLE 65.6. SUGGESTED SIZE AND SELECTION OF HEMOFILTRATION VASCULAR ACCESS DEVICES FOR PEDIATRIC PATIENTS

Patient weight	Catheter size and source	Site of insertion
Neonate	Single-lumen 18, 16, 14 gauge (Cook)	Femoral artery or vein
	Single-lumen 5.0 French (Medcomp)	Femoral artery or vein, or umbilical vein
	Dual-lumen 7.0 French (Cook, Medcomp)	Internal/external jugular, subclavian, or femoral vein
3–6 kg	Dual-lumen 7.0 French (Cook, Medcomp)	Internal/external jugular, subclavian, or femoral vein
	Triple-lumen 7.0 French (Medcomp, Arrow)	Internal/external jugular, subclavian, or femoral vein
6–30 kg	Dual-lumen 8.0 French (Kendall, Arrow)	Internal/external jugular, subclavian, or femoral vein
>25 kg	Dual-lumen 9.0 French (Medcomp)	Internal/external jugular, subclavian, or femoral vein
>40 kg	Triple-lumen 12.5 French (Arrow, Kendall)	Internal/external jugular, subclavian, or femoral vein

whether the lactate is the L or the D form. To make that determination, however, frequently requires a protracted time, and this limits its usefulness.

The development of a Normocarb concentrate stored in a glass bottle permits the fresh preparation of a physiologic bicarbonate-based solution for dialysate or replacement. Comparison data have shown that not only is bicarbonate solution more physiologic but its use is also correlated with improved outcome, fewer instances of hemodynamic instability, lower vasopressor requirements, and less frequent requirement for bicarbonate replacement. These data reinforce that lactate solutions should not be used in CRRT (101).

Anticoagulation

At least three options are available for anticoagulation in CRRT. The first approach is to use none; the second is to use heparin; and the third is to use citrate.

The use of no anticoagulation during CRRT has been shown repeatedly to decrease the duration of each circuit. No anticoagulation is typically used in a patient with disseminated intravascular coagulation who has a low platelet count and abnormal coagulation test results. Many of these patients, however, have a paradoxical hypercoagulability that requires some anticoagulation to prevent clotting in the system. Furthermore, many of these patients are being given continuous fresh frozen plasma replacement and platelet infusions that will correct the underlying anticoagulation problem.

Historically, many programs have used heparin. Heparin is infused in the system prefilter and is used to anticoagulate the system. Heparin's anticoagulation effect is assessed by measuring postfilter partial thromboplastin time or activated clotting time.

When heparin is used as an anticoagulant, the target is an activated clotting time between 180 and 220 seconds or a partial thromboplastin time between 1.5 and 2 times normal (98). A significant disadvantage of heparin usage is that it is associated with systemic anticoagulation of the patient. Furthermore, heparin use can be associated with heparin-induced thrombocytopenia, which further increases the risk of bleeding. In many patients with multiorgan system failure who require CRRT, systemic heparinization may be an additional risk factor.

Citrate anticoagulation is carried out by infusing citrate into the system postpatient and prefilter. Citrate then binds to the plasma calcium. Because coagulation is a calcium-dependent process, the patient is partially anticoagulated. To avoid citrate toxicity and systemic hypocalcemia, calcium must be infused into the patient separately from the dialysis system. Therefore, two processes must be monitored when citrate anticoagulation is used. The first is infusion of the citrate into the system to maintain the ionized calcium level in the extracorporeal system at between 0.25 and 0.4 mmol/L. The second is infusion of calcium back into the patient to maintain the patient's ionized calcium level at between 1.1 and 1.3 mmol/L (102,103).

The use of citrate anticoagulation may cause citrate toxicity or a metabolic alkalosis. Citrate toxicity occurs when the delivery rate of citrate exceeds the clearance rate. The clearance rate of citrate is related to both the clearance of the dialysis membrane and hepatic metabolism. One millimole of citrate is converted to 3 mmol of bicarbonate by the liver. Therefore, one sign of excessive citrate exposure is metabolic alkalosis (102).

The second sign of citrate excess is the "citrate gap." The citrate gap is seen when there is a rise in total calcium with a drop in ionized calcium. The citrate gap can be easily corrected by stopping the citrate delivery for 20 minutes to 2 hours and restarting the citrate at 70% of the previous rate.

Metabolic alkalosis can easily be corrected by decreasing the citrate exposure, by increasing the clearance of citrate by dialysis, or by infusing an acidic solution back into the patient. Many programs use citrate anticoagulation with a bicarbonate-based solution such as Normocarb and the result will be metabolic alkalosis. The pH of normal saline is 5 to 5.4; therefore, the use of replacement fluid of normal saline can easily correct this metabolic alkalosis.

Nutrition

CRRT provides continuous ultrafiltration, thus permitting a continuous delivery of nutrition. This continuous treatment, however, inevitably results in some loss of nutrients through the clearance of CRRT. A prospective crossover study by Maxvold et al. demonstrated that a standard CVVH or CVVHD prescription with a delivery of 1.5 g/kg/day of protein results in clearance of approximately 20% of amino acids by CRRT (97). If not accounted for, this could result in a negative nitrogen balance. Furthermore, many of the parenteral formulas are lacking in glutamine, which is also cleared by CRRT. Therefore a negative glutamine balance could place the patient at risk of impaired protein synthesis, which is controlled in part by glutamine. A more recent study by Bellomo et al. demonstrated that a delivery rate of 2.5 g/kg/day in adults with multiorgan system failure was only partially successful in restoring nitrogen balance (104).

Thus many pediatric programs provide delivery of 2 to 3 g/kg/day of protein and adjust to a target BUN level of 40 to 50 mg/dL.

Drug Clearance

The proper dosing of medications is based on the balance between the rate of administration of the drug, the dose of the drug, the metabolism of the drug, and the CRRT clearance of the drug. Understanding the factors that affect mass transfer helps the clinician determine a reasonable estimate of medication losses (105).

1. Convective transfer through CVVH yields a greater proportional solute clearance of middle- and larger-sized molecules than the diffusive transfer through CVVHD.
2. Protein binding affects clearance, with greater binding resulting in less transfer.
3. The molecular weight of the solute affects clearance. Large molecules pass through the membranes less readily than smaller ones.
4. The type of membrane and the charge of the membrane affect adherence of the particle to the membrane as well as the permeability of the membrane.

Therefore, when the renewal of medications is determined, all of the aforementioned need to be considered. For a septic child on CRRT, many err on the side of putting the child at risk for overtreatment instead of undertreatment.

Complications of Continuous Renal Replacement Therapy

The complications of CRRT include overanticoagulation associated with heparin use, citrate toxicity, citrate hypocalcemia, as well as metabolic alkalosis associated with citrate use. All these complications are easily identifiable and correctable.

Excessive ultrafiltration can occur in patients on CRRT. This happened more commonly with older systems when intravenous pumps were used as a way to inhibit ultrafiltration rates. These pumps may have been useful to measure ultrafiltration but have been found to have up to a 30% error rate in control of ultrafiltration. The newer devices allow for accurate ultrafiltration within a 1 to 2% error rate (97). Temperature control instability can be seen in patients treated with CRRT. This needs to be monitored closely, especially in small children.

Initiation of Continuous Renal Replacement Therapy

No prospective data exist to determine the optimal point at which to begin CRRT. Ronco et al. showed that, in adults on CRRT, increasing doses of replacement fluid statistically improved outcome. Patients given prescriptions of both 35 and 45 mL/kg/hr showed better survival rates than those receiving 25 mL/kg/hr. Furthermore, they showed that there was a statistical improvement in survival when patients were placed on CRRT by the time BUN had risen to 80 mg/dL as opposed to higher levels. These results suggest that early intervention based on solute clearance may improve outcome (106).

Goldstein et al. showed that the amount of fluid overload at the time of commencing CRRT affected outcome in a series of children receiving CRRT. Survivors had an average fluid overload of 16%, whereas nonsurvivors had an average of 32% (107). These data suggest that early intervention from an ultrafiltration perspective also affects survival.

Outcome

ARF continues to be a devastating complication and is associated with a high risk of mortality. Simple ARF without other underlying illness has been reported to have a 7 to 23% mortality rate. When it is associated with other diseases in the ICU setting, the mortality rate for patients with ARF is 50 to 80% (26,27,108–116). Although it is difficult to determine the role of ARF as opposed to that of other comorbid diseases, these numbers illustrate the serious nature of this complication.

REFERENCES

1. Doolan PD, Alpen EL, Theil GB. A clinical appraisal of the plasma concentration and endogenous clearance of creatinine. *Am J Med* 1962;32:65.
2. Bennet WM, Porter GA. Endogenous creatinine clearance as a clinical measure of glomerular filtration rate. *BMJ* 1971;4:84.
3. Stewart CL, Barnett R. Acute renal failure in infants, children, and adults. *Crit Care Med* 1997;13:575–590.
4. Barratt TM. Acute renal failure. In: Holliday MA, Barratt TM, Vernier RL, eds. *Pediatric nephrology*. Baltimore: Williams & Wilkins, 1987:766–772.
5. Brady HR, Brenner BM, Clarkson MR, et al. Acute renal failure. In: Brenner BM, Levine SA, eds. *Brenner & Rector's the kidney*. Philadelphia: W.B. Saunders, Co., 2000:1201–1246.
6. Andreoli AP. Acute renal failure. *Curr Opin Pediatr* 2002; 14:183–188.
7. Moghal NE, Brocklebank JT, Meadow SR. A review of acute renal failure in children: incidence, etiology and outcome. *Clin Nephrol* 1998;49:91–95.
8. Karlowicz MG, Adelman RD. Nonoliguric and oliguric acute renal failure in asphyxiated term neonates. *Pediatr Nephrol* 1995;9:718–722.
9. Airede A, Bello M, Weerasinghe HD. Acute renal failure in the newborn: incidence and outcome. *J Paediatr Child Health* 1997;33:246–249.
10. Kandoth PW, Agarwal GJ, Dharnidharka VR. Acute renal failure in children requiring dialysis therapy. *Indian Pediatr* 1994;31:305–309.
11. Karlowicz MG, Adelman RD. Acute renal failure in the neonate. *Clin Perinatol* 1992;19:139–158.
12. Gouyon JB, Guignard JP. Management of acute renal failure in newborns. *Pediatr Nephrol* 2000;14:1037–1044.
13. Chan JC, Williams DM, Roth KS. Kidney failure in infants and children. *Pediatr Rev* 2002;23:47–60.
14. Hou SH, Bushinsky DA, Wish JB, et al. Hospital-acquired renal insufficiency: a prospective study. *Am J Med* 1983; 74:243–248.
15. Blantz RC. Pathophysiology of pre-renal azotemia. *Kidney Int* 1998;53:512–523.

16. Steiner RW, Tucker BJ, Blantz RC. Glomerular hemodynamics in rats with chronic sodium depletion: effect of saralasin. *J Clin Invest* 1979:503–512.
17. Tucker BJ, Blantz RC. Mechanism of altered glomerular hemodynamics during chronic sodium depletion. *Am J Physiol* 1983:F11–F18.
18. Dzau VJ, Packer M, Lilly LS, et al. Prostaglandins in severe congestive heart failure: relation to activation of the renin-angiotensin system and hyponatremia. *N Engl J Med* 1984; 310:347–352.
19. De Nicola L, Blantz RC, Gabbai FB. Nitric oxide and angiotensin II. Glomerular and tubular interaction in the rat. *J Clin Invest* 1992;89:1248–1256.
20. Baylis C, Brenner BM. Modulation by prostaglandin synthesis inhibitors of the action of exogenous angiotensin II on glomerular ultrafiltration in the rat. *Circ Res* 1978;43:889–898.
21. Badr KF, Ichikawa I. Prerenal failure: a deleterious shift from renal compensation to decompensation. *N Engl J Med* 1988;319:623–629.
22. Albright RC Jr. Acute renal failure: a practical update. *Mayo Clin Proc* 2001;76:67–74.
23. Liano F, Pascual J. Epidemiology of acute renal failure: a prospective, multi-center, community-based study. Madrid Acute Renal Failure Study Group (MARFS) *Kidney Int* 1996;50:811–818.
24. Drukker A, Guignard JP. Renal aspects of the term and preterm infant: a selective update. *Curr Opin Pediatr* 2002;14:175–182.
25. Miller PD, Krebs RA, Neal BJ, et al. Polyuric pre-renal failure. *Arch Intern Med* 1980;140:907–909.
26. Star RA. Treatment of acute renal failure. *Kidney Int* 1998;54:1817–1831.
27. Thadhani R, Pascual M, Bonventre JV. Acute renal failure. *N Engl J Med* 1996;334:1448–1460.
28. Rasmussen HH, Ibels LS. Acute renal failure. Multivariate analysis of causes and risk factors. *Am J Med* 1982;73:211–218.
29. Nash K, Hafeez A, Hou SH. Hospital acquired renal insufficiency. *Am J Kidney Dis* 2002;39:930–936.
30. Coulthard MG, Vernon B. Managing acute renal failure in very low birthweight infants. *Arch Dis Child Fetal Neonatal Ed* 1995;73:F187–F192.
31. Bauer SB, Feldman SM, Gelis SS, et al. Neonatal hypertension: a complication of umbilical artery catheterization. *N Engl J Med* 1975;293:1032–1033.
32. Adelman RD. The hypertensive neonate. *Clin Perinatol* 1988;15:567–583.
33. Lin GJ, Yang PH, Wang ML. Neonatal renal venous thrombosis—a case report describing serial sonographic changes. *Pediatr Nephrol* 1994;8:589–591.
34. Schmidt B, Andrew M. Neonatal thrombosis: report of a prospective Canadian and international registry. *Pediatrics* 1995;96:939–943.
35. Avery ME, Oppenheimer EH, Gordon HH. Renal-vein thrombosis in infants of diabetic mothers. *N Engl J Med* 1957;256:1134–1138.
36. Nuss R, Hays T, Manco-Johnson M. Efficacy and safety of heparin anticoagulation for neonatal renal vein thrombosis. *Am Journal Pediatr Hematol Oncol* 1994;16:127–131.
37. Katzman GH. Thrombosis and thromboembolism in an infant of a diabetic mother. *J Perinatol* 1989;9:137–140.
38. Cohen AH, Wang H, Bider WA, et al. Acute renal failure due to acute tubular necrosis in lupus nephritis. *Proc Am Soc Nephrol* 1982;15:26A.
39. Munchow N, Kosch A, Schobess R, et al. Role of genetic prothrombotic risk factors in childhood caval vein thrombosis. *Eur J Pediatr* 1999;158:S109–S112.
40. Sutor AH, Uhl M. Diagnosis of thromboembolic disease during infancy and childhood. *Semin Thromb Hemost* 1997;23:237–246.
41. Schobess R, Junker R, Auberger K, et al. Factor V G1691A and prothrombin G20210A in childhood spontaneous venous thrombosis—evidence of an age-dependent thrombotic onset in carriers of factor V G1691A and prothrombin G20210A mutation. *Eur J Pediatr* 1999;158:S105–S108.
42. Llach F. Hypercoagulability, renal vein thrombosis, and other thrombotic complications of nephrotic syndrome. *Kidney Int* 1985;28:429.
43. Llach F, Papper S, Massry SG. The clinical spectrum of renal vein thrombosis: acute and chronic. *Am J Med* 1980;69:819.
44. Keidan I, Lotan D, Gazit G, et al. Early neonatal renal venous thrombosis: long-term outcome. *Acta Paediatr* 1994;83:1225–1227.
45. Pinto E, Guignard JP. Renal masses in the newborn. *Biol Neonate* 1995;68:175–184.
46. Zigman A, Yazbeck S, Emil S, et al. Renal vein thrombosis: a 10-year review. *J Pediatr Surg* 2000;35:1540–1542.
47. Weinschenk N, Pelidis M, Fiascone J. Combination thrombolytic and anticoagulant therapy for bilateral renal vein thrombosis in a premature infant. *Am J Perinatol* 2001; 18:293–297.
48. Markowitz GS, Brignol F, Burns ER, et al. Renal vein thrombosis treated with thrombolytic therapy: case report and brief review. *Am J Kidney Dis* 1995;25:801–806.
49. McRae RP Jr, Liebson PR. Hypertensive crisis. *Med Clin North Am* 1986;70:749–767.
50. Adelman RD, Russo J. Malignant hypertension: recovery of renal function after treatment with antihypertensive medications and hemodialysis. *J Pediatr* 1981;98:766–768.
51. Bakir A, Dunea G. Accelerated and malignant hypertension: experience from a large American inner city hospital. *Int J Artif Organs* 1989;12:675–676.
52. Barcenas CG, Eigenbrodt E, Long DL, et al. Recovery from malignant hypertension with anuria after prolonged hemodialysis. *South Med J* 1976;69:1230–1233.
53. Cordingley FT, Jones NF, Wing AJ, et al. Reversible renal failure in malignant hypertension. *Clin Nephrol* 1980;14:98–103.
54. Isles CG, McLay A, Jones JM. Recovery in malignant hypertension presenting as acute renal failure. *Q JM* 1984;53:439–452.
55. Yaqoob M, McClelland P, Ahmad R. Delayed recovery of renal function in patients with acute renal failure due to accelerated hypertension. *Postgrad Med J* 1991;67:829–832.
56. Nicholson GD. Long-term survival after recovery from malignant nephrosclerosis. *Am J Hypertens* 1988;1:73–75.
57. Nolan CR, Anderson RJ. Hospital-acquired acute renal failure. *J Am Soc Nephrol* 1998;9:710–718.
58. Choudhury D, Ahmed Z. Drug-induced nephrotoxicity. *Med Clin North Am* 1997;81:705–717.
59. Cayco AV, Perazella MA, Harplett JP. Renal insufficiency after intravenous immune globulin therapy: a report of two

cases and analysis of literature. *J Am Soc Nephrol* 1997;8: 1788–1794.

60. Visweswaran P, Guntupalli J. Environmental emergencies. *Crit Care Clin* 1999;15:415–428.
61. Vanholder R, Sever MS, Erek E, et al. Disease of the month. *J Am Soc Nephrol* 2000:11.
62. Holt SG, Moore KP. Pathogenesis and treatment of renal dysfunction in rhabdomyolysis. *Intensive Care Med* 2001; 27:803–811.
63. Weldon BC, Monk TG. The patient at risk for acute renal failure. Recognition, prevention, and preoperative optimization. *Anesthesiol Clin North Am* 2000;18:705–717.
64. Baxter. Acute renal insufficiency complicating trauma and surgery. In: Shires GT, ed. *Principles of trauma care.* New York: McGraw-Hill, 1985:502.
65. Fridovich I. The biology of oxygen radicles: the superoxide radicle is an agent of oxygen toxicity. *Science* 1978;201: 875–880.
66. Lampert MB, Weiss SJ. The chlorinating potential of the human monocyte. *Blood* 1983;62:645–651.
67. Dubrow A, Flamenbaum W. Acute renal failure associated with myoglobinuria and hemoglobinuria. *Acute Renal Failure* 1988;2:279–293.
68. Zager RA, Cotran RS, Hoyer JR. Pathological localization of Tamm-Horsfall protein in interstitial deposits in renal disease. *Lab Invest* 1878;38:52–57.
69. Pollak UE, Arbel C. The distribution of Tamm-Horsfall mucoprotein (uromucoid) in the human nephron. *Nephron* 1969;6:667–672.
70. Bakris GL, Burnett JC. A role of calcium in radiocontrast-induced reductions in renal hemodynamics. *Kidney Int* 1985;27:465–468.
71. Russo D, Minutolo R, Cianciaruso B, et al. Early effects of contrast media on renal hemodynamics and tubular function in chronic renal failure. *J Am Soc Nephrol* 1994;6: 1451–1458.
72. Berns AS. Nephrotoxicity of contrast media. *Kidney Int* 1989;36:730–740.
73. Solomon R. Contrast–medium-induced acute renal failure. *Kidney Int* 1998;53:230–242.
74. Lasser EC, Lyon SG, Berry CC. Reports on contrast media reactions: analysis of data from reports to the U.S. Food and Drug Administration. *Radiology* 1997;203:605–610.
75. Musch W, Thimpont J, Vandervelde D, et al. Combined fractional excretion of sodium and urea better predicts response to saline in hyponatremia than do usual clinical and biochemical parameters. *Am J Med* 1995;99:348–355.
76. Tapia-Rombo CA, Velasquez-Jones L, Fernandez-Celis JM, et al. Usefulness of fractional excretion of sodium in critically ill pre-term newborns. *Arch Med Res* 1997;28:253–257.
77. Bellomo R, Chapman M, Finfer S, et al. Low-dose dopamine in patients with early renal dysfunction: a placebo controlled randomized trial. Australian and New Zealand Intensive Care Society (ANZICS). *Lancet* 2000;356:2139–2143.
78. Galley. Renal-dose dopamine: will the message now get through? *Lancet* 2000;356:2112–2113.
79. Ichai C, Passeron C, Carles M, et al. Prolonged low-dose dopamine infusion induces a transient improvement in renal function in hemodynamically stable, critically ill patients: a single-blind, prospective, controlled study. *Crit Care Med* 2000;28:1329–1335.
80. Chertow GM, Sayegh MH, Allgren RL, et al. Is the administration of dopamine associated with adverse or favorable outcomes in acute renal failure? *Am J Med* 1996;101:49–53.
81. Denton MD, Chertow GM, Brady HR. "Renal-dose" dopamine for the treatment of acute renal failure: scientific rationale, experimental studies and clinical trials. *Kidney Int* 1996;49:4–14.
82. Kellum JA, Decker JM. Use of dopamine in acute renal failure: a meta-analysis. *Crit Care Med* 2001;29:1526–1531.
83. Conger. Interventions in clinical acute renal failure: What are the data? *Am J Kidney Dis* 1995;26:565–576.
84. Kellum. Use of diuretics in the acute care setting. *Kidney Int* 1995;53:S67–S70.
85. Fink. Are diuretics useful in the treatment or prevention of acute renal failure? *South Med J* 1982;75.
86. Lieberthal W, LN. Treatment of acute tubular necrosis. *Semin Nephrol* 1990:10.
87. Shilliday IR, Quinn KJ, Allison ME. Loop diuretics in the management of acute renal failure: a prospective, double-blind, placebo-controlled, randomized study. *Nephrol Dial Transplant* 1997;12:2592–2596.
88. Solomon R, Werner C, Mann D, et al. Effects of saline, mannitol, and furosemide to prevent acute decreases in renal function induced by radiocontrast agents. *N Engl J Med* 1994;331:1416–1420.
89. Lassnigg A, Donner E, Grubhofer G, et al. Lack of renoprotective effects of dopamine and furosemide during cardiac surgery. *J Am Soc Nephrol* 2000;11:97–104.
90. Better OS, Rubinstein I, Winaver JM, et al. Mannitol therapy revisited. *Kidney Int* 1997;52:886–894.
91. Kemper MJ, Harps E, Muller-Wiefel DE. Hyperkalemia: therapeutic options in acute and chronic renal failure. *Clin Nephrol* 1996;46:67–69.
92. Singh BS, Sadiq HF, Noguchi A, et al. Efficacy of albuterol inhalation in treatment of hyperkalemia in premature neonates. *J Pediatr* 2002;141:16–20.
93. Bulumberg A, Weidmann P, Perrari P. Effect of prolonged bicarbonate administration on plasma potassium in terminal renal failure. *Kidney Int* 1992;41:369–374.
94. Lowrie L. Renal replacement therapies in pediatric multiorgan dysfunction syndrome. *Pediatr Nephrol* 2000;14:6–12.
95. Chadha V, Warady BA, Blowey DL, et al. Tenckhoff catheters prove superior to cook catheters in pediatric acute peritoneal dialysis. *Am J Kidney Dis* 2000;35:1111–1116.
96. Bunchman TE, Maxvold NJ, Kershaw DB, et al. Continuous venovenous hemodiafiltration in infants and children. *Am J Kidney Dis* 1995;25:17–21.
97. Maxvold NJ, Smoyer WE, Custer JR, et al. Amino acid loss and nitrogen balance in critically ill children with acute renal failure: a prospective comparison between classic hemofiltration and hemofiltration with dialysis. *Crit Care Med* 2000;28:1161–1165.
98. Bunchman TE, McBryde KD, Mottes TE, et al. Pediatric acute renal failure: outcome by modality and disease. *Pediatr Nephrol* 2001;16:1067–1071.
99. Jenkins R, Harrison H, Chen B, et al. Accuracy of intravenous infusion pumps in continuous renal replacement therapies. *Trans Am Soc Artif Intern Organs* 1992;38:808.

100. Brophy PD, Mottes TA, Kudelka TL, et al. AN-69 membrane reactions are pH-dependent and preventable. *Am J Kidney Dis* 2001;38:173–178.
101. Barenbrock M, Hausberg M, Matzkies F. Effects of bicarbonate and lactate buffered replacement fluids on cardiovascular outcome in CVVH patients. *Kidney Int* 2000;58: 1751–1757.
102. Bunchman TE, Maxvold NJ, Barnett J, et al. Pediatric hemofiltration: Normocarb® dialysate solution with citrate anticoagulation. *Pediatr Nephrol* 2002;17:150–154.
103. Chadha V, Garg U, Warady BA. Citrate clearance in children receiving continuous venovenous renal replacement therapy. *Pediatr Nephrol* 2002;17:819–824.
104. Bellomo R, Tan H, Bhonagiori S, et al. High protein intake during continuous hemodiafiltration: impact on amino acids and nitrogen balance. *Int J Artif Organs* 2002;25:263–268.
105. Schetz M, Ferdinade P, Van den Berghe G, et al. Pharmacokinetics of continuous renal replacement therapy. *Intensive Care Med* 1995;21:612–620.
106. Ronco C, Bellomo R, Homel P, et al. Effects of different doses in continuous venovenous haemofiltration on outcomes of acute renal failure: a prospective randomized trial. *Lancet* 2000;356:26–30.
107. Goldstein S, Currier H, Graf J, et al. Outcome in children receiving continuous venovenous hemofiltration. *Pediatrics* 2001;107:1309–1312.
108. Liano F, Junco E, Pascual J, et al. The spectrum of acute renal failure in the intensive care unit compared with that seen in other settings. *Kidney Int* 1998;53:S16–S24.
109. Briglia A, Paganini EP. Acute renal failure in the intensive care unit. Therapy overview, patient risk stratification, complications of renal replacement, and special circumstances. *Clin Chest Med* 1999;20(2):347-366.
110. Mehta R. Acute renal failure in the intensive care unit: a tale of two eras. *Mayo Clin Proc* 1996;71:117.
111. Yagi N, Paganini EP. Acute dialysis and acute renal replacement: the emergence of new technology involving the nephrologist in the intensive care setting. *Semin Nephrol* 1997;17:306.
112. Chertow GM, Christiansen CL, Cook EF, et al. Preoperative renal risk satisfaction. *Circulation* 1997;95:878–884.
113. Paganini EP, Tapolyai M, Goormastic M, et al. Establishing a dialysis therapy patient outcome link in intensive care unit acute dialysis for patients with acute renal failure. *Am J Kidney Dis* 1996;28:S81–S89.
114. Chertow GM, Christiansen CL, Cleary PD, et al. Prognostic stratification in critically ill patients with acute renal failure requiring dialysis. *Arch Intern Med* 1995;155:1505–1511.
115. Kierdorf HP, Sieberth HG, Heintz B, et al. Continuous renal replacement therapies versus intermittent hemodialysis in acute renal failure: What do we know? *Am J Kidney Dis* 1995;28:S90.
116. Lewis JL, Chertow GM, Paganini EP, et al. A multicenter survey of patient characteristics, practice patterns and outcomes in critically ill patients with acute renal failure. *J Am Soc Nephrol* 1997;8:142a.

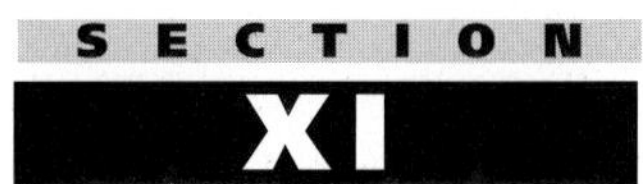

CHRONIC RENAL FAILURE

66

PATHOPHYSIOLOGY OF PROGRESSIVE RENAL DISEASE

AGNES B. FOGO
VALENTINA KON

Progressive renal disease occurs in all age groups. The incidence of chronic renal insufficiency among children younger than 16 years varies between 1.5 and 3.0 per million. Congenital structural anomalies, including reflux, obstruction, hypoplasia, and dysplasia are the principal underlying causes of end-stage renal disease, particularly in the very young child. Older children also develop end-stage renal disease from glomerulopathies, including focal segmental glomerulosclerosis (FSGS), hemolytic uremic syndrome, immune complex diseases, and hereditary nephropathies, such as Alport's disease (1) (Fig. 66.1). Although diabetic nephropathy does not result in chronic renal insufficiency in childhood, most patients with diabetes who develop end-stage renal disease in their 20s and 30s are those whose diabetes presented during childhood. This period between onset of disease during childhood and later development of diabetic nephropathy in adolescence or adulthood is an example of an opportunity for the physician to apply new therapeutic strategies outlined in this chapter, which may affect ultimate development of what has become the number one cause of end-stage renal disease in adults.

The remarkably similar histologic appearance of chronic renal diseases regardless of the primary insult suggests a common final pathway, with variations dependent on unique disease-specific factors and individual susceptibility. The alterations and adaptations in nephrons remaining after the initial insult are thought ultimately to cause scarring and further nephron loss, thus perpetuating a vicious cycle that results in the end-stage kidney. However, individual genetic variations and disease-specific mechanisms contribute to variability in progression and response to therapy (2). Possible mechanisms of progressive renal damage include, but are not limited to, hemodynamic factors, shear stress, growth factors, cell-specific damage, and metabolic factors such as a diabetic milieu and hyperlipidemia. The balance of cell growth versus cell death and the balance of matrix accumulation versus degradation determine whether injury results in healing with remodeling and resolution of damage or ongoing sclerosis (Fig. 66.2).

EXPERIMENTAL EVIDENCE

Systemic and Glomerular Hypertension

Systemic hypertension often accompanies renal disease. It results from and contributes to progression of renal damage. Hypertension accelerates progression of chronic renal disease in humans, as discussed later. Systemic blood pressure not only can affect the glomerulus by transmission of pressures but also may affect other determinants of progressive injury. In addition, intrarenal factors related to the unique aspects of kidney structure and function may be important. The glomerulus has both an afferent and an efferent arteriole, which permits modulation of perfusion and pressure within the glomerular capillary bed differentially from systemic blood pressure. Therefore, attention has been focused on the potential impact of local (i.e., glomerular) hemodynamic changes in structural glomerular injury.

Numerous studies in the last decade have examined the remnant kidney or renal-ablation model of progression in the rat. The ablation model was initially described nearly 100 years ago (3). In this model, removal of a large portion of renal mass results in progressive hyperperfusion, hyperfiltration, and sclerosis in a heterogeneous pattern (i.e., focal and segmental glomerulosclerosis) (4–6). Kidney weight increases, and tubular and glomerular growth occur. The structural changes after loss of nephrons include hyperplasia and hypertrophy. So-called glomerular hypertrophy represents both cellular hypertrophy (increase in cell size) and hyperplasia (increase in cell number). Age and the extent of renal ablation affect the relative contributions of hypertrophy and hyperplasia. Although new nephrons do not form after term birth, hyperplasia is more prominent in the young and is greater after extensive nephron loss (7–9). The postulated intermediary factors for progressive glomer-

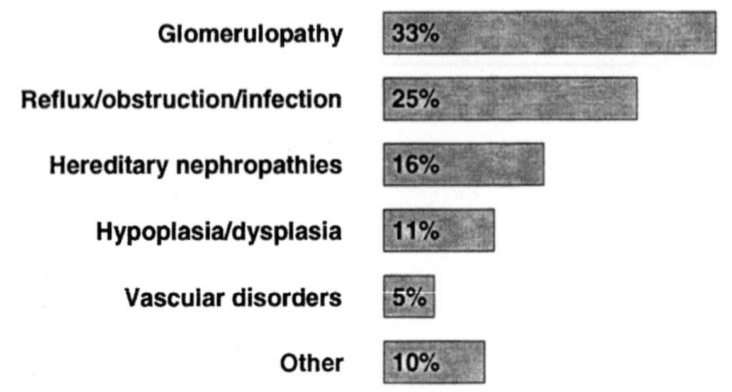

FIGURE 66.1. Causes of end-stage renal disease in combined series of 4136 children. Glomerulopathy includes immune complex diseases and focal segmental glomerulosclerosis. Hereditary disorders include cystinosis, oxalosis, and Alport's disease. Vascular diseases include hemolytic uremic syndrome, hypertensive nephrosclerosis, arteritis, renal vein thrombosis, and diabetes. (Data from Foreman JW, Chan JCM. Chronic renal failure in infants and children. *J Pediatr* 1988;113:793–800.)

ulosclerosis have also been investigated in other models in which nephrons are not removed and the initial injury is more diffuse. Thus, both the puromycin aminonucleoside and Adriamycin models of renal disease show initial proteinuria and epithelial cell damage similar to human minimal-change disease, followed by progressive focal and segmental glomerulosclerosis.

The initial observations that single nephron function was increased after renal ablation led to further studies (3) and the hypothesis that hyperfiltration was injurious (6). It was postulated that this maladaptive change after removal of nephrons results in the ongoing loss of glomeruli, and, thus, a cycle of hyperfiltration and glomerulosclerosis is perpetuated (10). Manipulations of hyperfiltration by feeding a low-protein diet or by giving angiotensin I–converting enzyme inhibitors (ACEIs), lipid-lowering agents, or heparin were effective in ameliorating glomerular sclerosis. However, in some studies, glomerular sclerosis was decreased without altering glomerular hyperfiltration (11). In addition, experimental maneuvers that actually increased glomerular hyperperfusion (such as thromboxane synthase inhibitors or exercise training) not only did not accelerate progression but also actually slowed the process. Finally, glomerular sclerosis was noted to occur even in the absence of intervening hyperperfusion (9,12).

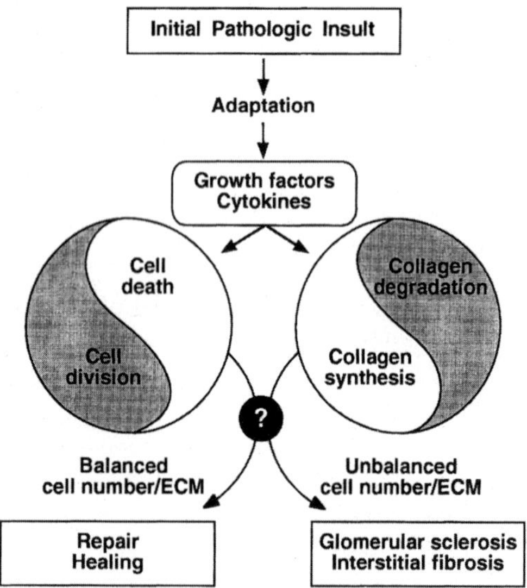

FIGURE 66.2. Postulated mechanisms for progressive sclerosis in chronic renal disease. Glomerulosclerosis results from the net effects of growth promoters and inhibitors on cell growth and matrix accumulation. The balance of cell proliferation versus apoptosis and matrix production versus degradation determines whether scarring or healing ensues in response to injury. ECM, extracellular matrix. (From Neilson EG, Couser WG, eds. *Immunologic renal disease*. Philadelphia: Lippincott–Raven, 1997, with permission.)

The absence of a tight link between hyperperfusion and glomerular sclerosis shifted focus from hyperperfusion/hyperfiltration to glomerular hypertension, another element of the increased glomerular stress that follows renal ablation. Glomerular hypertension is typical in many models of chronic renal failure. Maneuvers that increase glomerular capillary pressure, such as therapy with erythropoietin, glucocorticoids, or high-protein diet, accelerated glomerulosclerosis. Maneuvers that induce systemic and/or glomerular hypertension, such as uninephrectomy, superimposed on other forms of renal disease, including nephrotoxic serum nephritis, immune complex nephritis, or diabetic nephropathy, worsen both functional and structural deterioration (9,12).

There appears to be better correlation between increased glomerular pressure and glomerulosclerosis than hyperfiltration/hyperperfusion and sclerosis. Mechanisms by which increased pressure might promote sclerosis include altered mechanical and/or shear stress. Mesangial cells in culture subjected to pulsatile mechanical stretch/relaxation cycles changed production of cytokines that affect matrix production and proliferation of glomerular cells and altered type and amount of matrix production (13). Many maneuvers that had been used to ameliorate matrix accumulation and, thus, glomerulosclerosis *in vivo* also affected glomerular pressures. Decreased glomerular pressure, in response to dietary protein restriction (14) or antihypertensive drugs (9,12,15,16), is associated with slower progression. As discussed later, these maneuvers also have other effects. Of special interest are the findings of protection against glomerulosclerosis with ACEIs (17). This has been attributed to the unique actions of ACEIs to decrease glomerular capillary pressure by preferential dilation of the efferent arteriole (1). ACEIs also act as kininase inhibitors and activate bradykinin. Bradykinin is postulated to be the mediator effecting vasodilatation of the efferent arteriole by ACEIs (18). Newer antihypertensive drugs that inhibit the renin-angiotensin system include angiotensin II (Ang II) type 1 receptor antagonists (RAs). They do not have kininase activity and therefore do not alter bradykinin activity. Because both of these modes of inhibition of the renin-angiotensin system are effective in protecting against glomerulosclerosis, the specific effect of ACEI to decrease efferent arteriolar resistance does not appear to be critical for amelioration of glomerulosclerosis. Rather, inhibition of Ang II actions per se is postulated to be involved in the effect of these drugs (17). Ang II also affects mesangial and vascular smooth muscle cell growth and matrix production (see later).

After loss of nephrons, whether removed surgically or damaged by disease, the remaining glomerular tufts enlarge. One study in rats examined the heterogeneous changes in function in individual nephrons after renal ablation. Glomerular filtration and pressure were assessed repeatedly by micropuncture in the same nephrons over a 6-week period. When the single-nephron glomerular filtration rate (GFR) and glomerular capillary pressure were correlated with the degree of sclerosis in the same glomerulus, no correlation was found between the levels of these hemodynamic parameters and the degree of sclerosis. Thus, the nephrons with the greatest hyperfiltration or highest glomerular capillary pressure did not show the most severe sclerosis at the end of the study, indicating that glomerular hypertension or hyperperfusion per se did not directly account for the glomerular damage (19). Similar conclusions were reached based on experiments in another nonhypertensive model, the puromycin aminonucleoside nephropathy, in which ACEIs also were effective in slowing glomerulosclerosis (9).

Further along these lines are observations of disorders characterized by glomerular hypertension, which do not develop sclerosis (15,20). For example, in the diabetic nephropathy model in the rat, although glomerular capillary hypertension is typically seen, only mild mesangial expansion results rather than overt glomerulosclerosis (12). In another study, hyperfiltration was induced either by renal ablation or by diversion of urine into the peritoneal cavity. Similar degrees of glomerular hyperperfusion, hyperfiltration, and hypertension developed in both ureter-diverted and renal-ablation groups. Glomeruli of the ureter-diverted rats did not hypertrophy, whereas those of the renal-ablation rats did. Significant glomerulosclerosis developed only in the renal-ablation group (20). Overall, these findings indicate that glomerulosclerosis can develop without glomerular hypertension, and glomerulosclerosis can be ameliorated without altering glomerular hemodynamics. These results suggest that glomerular hyperfiltration, hyperperfusion, or glomerular hypertension alone do not fully explain the development of glomerular hypertrophy or sclerosis.

On the other hand, it has been postulated that individual factors such as glomerular hypertrophy and glomerular pressures interact to produce heightened injury by affecting factors such as wall tension. Increased wall tension, resulting from a combination of increased pressures and increased size of the glomerular capillary as predicted by Laplace's law, has been proposed as a mechanism for progressive glomerulosclerosis (21,22). However, in several animal models, glomerular enlargement occurs through lengthening and/or branching of the capillaries rather than by increased capillary diameter (23–25). In children with reflux nephropathy, glomerular growth resulted from increased capillary branching and not increased capillary diameter (26). These observations cast doubt on whether increased wall tension actually occurs, at least in such settings of glomerular growth. Other synergistic contributions proposed to be deleterious include systemic blood pressure, which may modulate glomerular injury either by direct transmission of altered shear stress and pressures or by altering the elaboration of vasoactive substances that affect the microcirculation (9).

Growth Factors

After initial loss of nephrons, growth promoters are increased and act on remaining glomeruli. Glomerular sclerosis is often closely associated with glomerular hypertrophy in a variety of animal and human diseases (9). Stimuli that induce glomerular hypertrophy often accelerate glomerular sclerosis, which has focused research on possible roles of these growth factors in progression of renal disease (Fig. 66.3). In the remnant kidney in rats, structural lesions

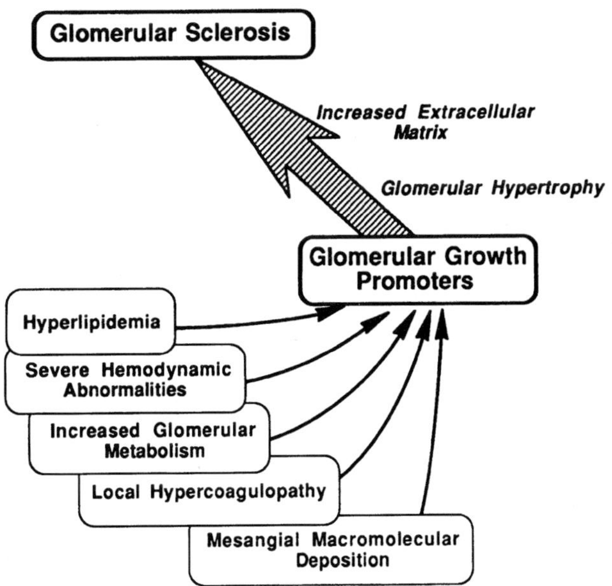

FIGURE 66.3. Speculation on relationship between glomerular growth promoters and other potentially pathogenic intermediary mechanisms for glomerular sclerosis. Currently available experimental observations in renal and nonrenal tissues suggest the possibility that these other mechanisms may interact with glomerular growth promoters, which have the capacity to induce both glomerular hypertrophy and mesangial matrix accumulation, leading to the typical glomerular sclerotic lesion. (From Fogo A, Ichikawa I. Role of glomerular growth promoters in progression of renal disease. In: Andreucci VE, Fine LG, eds. *International yearbook of nephrology*. Boston: Kluwer Academic Publishers, 1991:21–45, with permission.)

develop that closely resemble human FSGS. Like those seen in humans, these changes occur initially in the deep juxtamedullary glomeruli (7,27). In young animals in which maturational growth is occurring, injury after renal ablation is more severe than in adults (8,28). Detailed analysis of the distribution of this glomerular injury revealed more focal and severe glomerulosclerosis in the deep (vs. the superficial) glomeruli in the young rats. Hemodynamic factors did not differ between the two age groups. Although after renal ablation more glomerular enlargement occurred in the young rat than in the adult rat, glomerular enlargement occurred proportionally in both superficial and deep nephron populations. The more severe injury of the deep glomeruli in the young immature rat was, therefore, postulated to be related to factors unique to the young growing kidney, which is characterized by centripetal growth and differentiation. The mechanisms that promote hyperplasia rather than hypertrophy in the accentuated growth and wound healing in response to nephron loss may also promote scarring (28).

Uninephrectomy, a stimulus for hypertrophy, also accelerates glomerular sclerosis in other models (e.g., experimental glomerulonephritis, minimal-change disease, focal sclerosis, and diabetic nephropathy) (9,12). Excess growth hormone, whether endogenously produced (i.e., transgenic mice) (29) or exogenous (30,31), is associated with marked glomerular hypertrophy and accelerated glomerulosclerosis. Even in normal young rats, recombinant human growth hormone (rhGH) caused glomerular hypertrophy and severe sclerosis (31). Although these normal rats did not develop uremia over the course of observation, these findings raise important issues for the treatment of children with rhGH, as discussed in Growth Hormone.

Although hypertrophic stimuli accelerate glomerular sclerosis, the converse is also true: Decreasing the hypertrophic response is associated with decreased glomerular sclerosis. Dwarf rats with a defect in growth hormone are resistant to the development of glomerulosclerosis after renal ablation (30). A rat strain characterized by a larger number of small glomeruli and a minimal hypertrophic response to loss of nephrons, the PVGc strain, has proved resistant to the development of glomerulosclerosis after the removal of one kidney (9). Interventions that ameliorate glomerulosclerosis have a similar effect on glomerular hypertrophy. Treatment with low-protein diets ameliorates sclerosis; however, it may be effective only when the diet is low enough in calories to inhibit growth (32). Antihypertensive drugs also inhibit both glomerular growth and glomerulosclerosis.

In vivo and *in vitro* evidence suggests that many cytokines can promote glomerular cell growth and enhance extracellular matrix release, thus promoting sclerosis as well as growth. Numerous growth factors affect renal growth and scarring. Several growth factors appear to play key roles in progression of glomerular and tubulointerstitial scarring. These factors and their roles may differ at the various stages of injury. Altered gene expressions in pathophysiologic settings implicate factors, including the following: platelet-derived growth factor (PDGF), transforming growth factor β (TGFβ), TGFα, insulin-like growth factor-1 (IGF-1), growth hormone, epidermal growth factor, interleukin-1 (IL-1) and -6, tumor necrosis factor-α (TNF-α), Ang II, basic fibroblast growth factor (basic FGF), and endothelin (9,33,34). A recent study showed that inhibition of a specific growth factor, either TGFβ or PDGF, could decrease mesangial matrix expansion in the anti-Thy1 model (35,36). Conversely, animals transgenic for TGFβ develop progressive renal disease (37). The biologic actions of TGFβ are complex, and depend not only on cell state, but on presence of decorin, which binds and modifies its activity (38). Further study is necessary to determine the specific role each of these factors plays at varying stages of glomerular injury.

The contribution of Ang II is particularly relevant because it can be inhibited by currently clinically available agents, and extensive clinical evidence shows the efficacy of Ang inhibition on progression of renal disease. The mechanisms by which Ang II affects growth and matrix include both direct and indirect effects via induction of other growth factors, including basic FGF, PDGF, and TGFβ, and modulation of fibrinolysis/proteolysis (9,38). The effects of Ang to induce plasminogen activator inhibitor-1 (PAI-1) provide a link of the renin-angiotensin system to thrombosis (39,40). Importantly, PAI-1 inhibits proteolysis as well as fibrinolysis. Recent studies have also shown linkage of injury and increased PAI-1 expression *in vivo* in a model of radiation-induced endothelial injury with thrombosis followed by glomerulosclerosis. Inhibition of Ang II or aldosterone, either by ACEI or Ang type 1 (AT1) RA, or with the aldosterone RA spironolactone, prevented PAI-1 upregulation and injury (41,42).

Recent studies have examined whether Ang II and aldosterone induce PAI-1 expression and subsequent fibrosis independent of TGFβ activation (43). These studies examined the effect of Ang II and aldosterone on tubulointerstitial fibrosis induced by unilateral ureteral obstruction (UUO) in $\alpha_v\beta_6$ knock-out mice, in which the local activation of TGFβ is impaired. The integrin $\alpha_v\beta_6$ serves as a ligand for latency-associated peptide (LAP) and is expressed in epithelia in lung, skin, and kidney (44). TGFβ circulates bound to LAP and is locally activated when LAP binds to $\alpha_v\beta_6$ and TGFβ is cleaved. Consistent with prior studies indicating that $\alpha_v\beta_6$ mice are protected against bleomycin-induced pulmonary fibrosis (44), the knock-out animals demonstrated attenuated PAI-1 expression, collagen I and III expression, and markedly decreased renal fibrosis after UUO compared to wild-type animals, even though macrophage infiltration was not altered in the $\alpha_v\beta_6$ mice (43). However, treatment with Ang II, aldosterone, or both increased PAI-1 expression and rendered the animals equally susceptible to UUO-induced fibrosis as the wild-type animals. This study suggests that Ang II or aldosterone can induce PAI-1 expression and fibrosis through a TGFβ-independent pathway (43).

Ang II has additional effects on the vascular system, promoting migration of endothelial and vascular smooth muscle cells and hypertrophy and hyperplasia of smooth muscle cells and mesangial cells (9,45). Ang II is present in monocytes, which may thus serve as yet another source of Ang II in immune-mediated glomerular injuries (46). Local transfection to the carotid artery of ACE resulted in increased DNA synthesis and medial hypertrophy, associated with local Ang II generation without systemic changes (47). Glomerular transfection *in vivo* with angiotensinogen or renin similarly induced activation of mesangial cells and increased matrix (48). Recent data implicate the Ang type 2 receptor in growth inhibition and apoptosis in vascular injury and remodeling as well as in development (49–51). Pharmacologic inhibition or absence of the AT2 receptor in null mutant mice, with resulting deficient apoptosis after injury, leads to increased fibrosis in models of kidney and heart fibrosis (52,53). Apoptosis may serve as a healing mechanism, eliminating injured cells with minimal stimulation of immune/inflammatory mechanisms and cytokines. However, disproportionate apoptosis of cells that cannot regenerate may have deleterious consequences. Indeed, combined therapy with AT1 and AT2 RAs was more effective than monotherapy in amelioration of progression in the remnant kidney model (54). In contrast, mechanisms of regression of existing injury are distinct, with recent data suggesting a particular advantage of maintaining activity of the AT2 receptor to achieve optimal remodeling (55). Furthermore, the AT2 receptor tonically inhibits ACE activity, which may dampen Ang II generation (56). Thus, AT2 receptor-transduced Ang actions may counter some of AT1-mediated effects and has potential implications for effects of ACEI versus newly available AT1 RAs in various disease settings. The net effect of Ang II thus depends on the balance of AT1- and AT2-mediated effects, as well as induction of proliferative growth factors, such as PDGF and basic FGF, and matrix modulators, such as PAI-1, versus TGF-β1, which promotes matrix synthesis and inhibits or promotes cellular proliferation depending on conditions.

Combined ACEI and AT1 RA treatment thus could have theoretic advantage, allowing further blockade of Ang II actions while maintaining preferential local availability of the AT2 receptor. However, in the remnant kidney model, combined ACEI+AT1RA therapy did not result in added benefit on glomerulosclerosis when compared to single-drug therapy with similar blood pressure control (57). However, in the rat transgenic for renin (mREN-2) 27, combination therapy was more effective than monotherapy in reducing blood pressure and in limiting end-organ injury (58). Combination of AT1RA and ACEI in small clinical studies in normotensive patients with either immunoglobulin A (IgA) nephropathy or diabetic nephropathy resulted in more profound decrease in proteinuria than treatment with either drug alone, not attributable to effects on systemic blood pressure (59,60). In a large study of hypertensive patients with diabetic nephropathy and microalbuminuria, combined therapy resulted in greater blood pressure and albuminuria reduction than either drug alone (61). Combination therapy appears to be safe, and may even have additional antifibrotic effects versus monotherapy by decreasing urinary TGFβ independent of blood pressure or proteinuria effects (62). In this connection, patients receiving ACEI long term still have measurable ACE in plasma, and, in an experimental rat model, even suprapharmacologic doses of ACE inhibition did not achieve complete suppression of the local RAS (63). It is possible that non-ACE–dependent Ang II generation by chymotrypsin-sensitive generating enzyme occurs in humans. New directions under investigation include development of renin antagonists that could obviate these effects.

Further study is necessary to determine the specific role of each of the many potential growth factors that can affect matrix accumulation at varying stages of glomerular injury. Increased release of growth factors may be triggered by local increase in shear stress or hydraulic pressures or by insults that include, but are not limited to, increased glomerular metabolism, heightened reactive oxygen species, altered lipid metabolism, mesangial deposition of macromolecules, and abnormal hemostasis (Fig. 66.3) (9,12,64,65).

Glomerular Cells in Progression

The endothelial cells interact with other cells and affect both growth-promoting and growth-inhibiting factors. Some of the factors upregulated after endothelial injury, such as plasminogen activators and inhibitors and collagenases, not only affect coagulation and thrombosis but also have been linked to matrix remodeling. Thus, scarring may be a late sequela of endothelial cell injury. Endothelial cells release cytokines that affect vascular tone and express adhesion molecules for circulating cells. Normally, endothelial cells inhibit smooth muscle cell migration and proliferation. When injured, they release growth factors that promote proliferation and matrix, lipoproteins, and cholesterol accumulation (66). Endothelial cells produce numerous cytokines that modulate mesangial cell growth (e.g., endothelin, PDGF, and endothelial-derived relaxing factor); some endothelial-derived factors act in synergy with heparin-like substances. For example, endothelin, a powerful vasoconstrictor, results in hyperplasia, hypertrophy, and increased matrix in mesangial cells in culture; it also enhances PDGF release, another key factor augmenting these processes (67).

Recent studies have pointed to a primary importance in progressive renal disease of endothelial cells in an extraglomerular site, namely in the peritubular capillary. Decreased peritubular capillary density, possibly modulated by decreased vascular endothelial derived growth factor or other angiogenic factors, has been proposed as a mechanism in various progressive renal diseases (68). Future studies may demonstrate whether these interstitial microvascular lesions are causal or consequential in the development of interstitial injury.

Glomerular visceral epithelial cells are the primary targets in many glomerular diseases, including FSGS and the experimental models of Adriamycin and puromycin aminonucleoside-induced nephropathies. Specific antigens of these cells (e.g., megalin) are targets in immune-mediated glomerulonephritis (69,70). The glomerular visceral epithelial cells are pivotal for maintenance of normal permselectivity and are a source of matrix in both physiologic and pathophysiologic settings. In contrast to the ability of mesangial and endothelial cells to regenerate after injury, the glomerular visceral epithelial cell is growth challenged. This limited proliferation in the mature glomerular visceral epithelial cell is accompanied by high expression of a cyclin-dependent kinase inhibitor, p27kip1 (71). This cyclin-dependent kinase inhibitor seems to be a rate-limiting step for the growth response of the visceral epithelial cell. Either too much or too little proliferation of the visceral epithelial cell in response to genetic manipulation of p27kip1 is postulated to be detrimental (72). Inadequate growth of the visceral epithelial cell is postulated to give rise to areas of dehiscence and insudation of plasma proteins, which progress to adhesions and sclerosis (73). Another cyclin-dependent kinase inhibitor, p21, appears necessary for development of injury after 5/6 nephrectomy in mice, pointing to the crucial importance of cell growth responses in determining response to injury (74).

Glomerular visceral epithelial cells normally produce an endogenous heparin-like substance that inhibits mesangial cell growth; thus, injury may decrease this growth inhibitory effect and allow increased mesangial growth. Glomerular visceral epithelial cells are the main renal source of vascular endothelial growth factor, an endothelial cell–specific mitogen that plays a key role in both physiologic and pathologic angiogenesis and vascular permeability (75). Epithelial cell integrins are key modulators of cell interactions and cell-matrix binding, and antibodies to β_1 integrins or epithelial slit pores caused proteinuria acutely (76,77). Decreased α_3 and α_5 integrins are seen localized to areas of sclerosis (78). Together, these structural changes may underlie the foot process fusion and altered cell-cell and cell-matrix interactions.

New studies of the molecular biology of the podocyte and identification of genes mutated in rare familial forms of nephrotic syndrome or FSGS, such as nephrin, α-actinin-4, and podocin, have given important new insights into mechanisms of progressive glomerulosclerosis. The gene mutated in congenital nephrotic syndrome, nephrin (*NPHS1*), is localized to chromosome region 19q13 (79). Nephrin localizes to the slit diaphragm over the podocyte and is tightly associated with CD2-associated protein (CD2AP). Nephrin functions as a zona occludens–type junction protein and, along with CD2AP, provides a crucial role in receptor patterning and cytoskeletal polarity. Mice engineered to be deficient in CD2AP develop congenital nephrotic syndrome, similar to congenital nephrotic syndrome of Finnish type (80). Additional important genes interacting with this complex have been identified in rare cases of familial FSGS. Autosomal dominant FSGS is caused by mutation in α-actinin-4, also localized to chromosome 19q13 (81). This is hypothesized to cause altered actin cytoskeleton interaction, causing FSGS through a gain-of-function mechanism, and contrasting the loss-of-function mechanism implicated for disease caused by the nephrin mutation (81). Patients with α-actinin-4 mutation progress to end stage by age 30 years, with rare recurrence in a transplant. Podocin, another podocyte-specific gene (*NPHS2*), is mutated in autosomal recessive FSGS that has an early onset in childhood with rapid progression to end stage (82). Podocin is an integral stomatin protein family member and interacts with the CD2AP-nephrin complex, indicating that podocin could serve in the structural organization of the slit diaphragm.

An additional interesting connection to progressive renal disease has been discovered from new insights in the nail-patella syndrome. This is caused by a mutation in the *LMX1B* gene, which codes a LIM-homeodomain transcription factor. The knock-out mouse for this gene has abnormal podocytes lacking typical slit diaphragms, and also has greatly reduced CD2AP and podocin, indicating a primary dependency of slit diaphragm development on *LMX1B* gene expression (83). Recently, an overlap in the *NPHS1*/*NPHS2* mutation spectrum has been detected, modifying the phenotype of congenital nephrotic syndrome of Finnish type to congenital FSGS when mutations in both are inherited. These findings further point to key functional interrelationships between *NPHS1* and *NPHS2* (84). Currently, investigators are examining whether acquired FSGS also may involve alteration in expression of some of these key podocyte genes. Indeed, occasional patients with nonfamilial forms of FSGS have been found to have podocin mutations (85).

Acquired disruption of some of these complexly interacting podocyte molecules has been demonstrated in experimental models and in human proteinuric diseases. Thus, in puromycin aminonucleoside nephropathy, a model of FSGS, nephrin localization, and organization were altered (86). Similar decreases in nephrin were observed in hypertensive diabetic rat models with significant proteinuria (87). The recently developed *NPHS1*-mutated mouse, generated by gene trapping, shows severe glomerulosclerosis and proteinuria and diffuse effacement of foot processes. The few remaining interpodocyte junctions lacked slit diaphragms, implicating that nephrin is essential for the integrity of both the foot processes and slit diaphragms (88). New molecular technologies targeting specific podocyte genes using podocyte-specific promoters exist and will elucidate the pathogenesis of FSGS (89). Treatments that ameliorated these experimental models preserved glomerular nephrin expression, providing further support for a key causal role for slit diaphragm and nephrin preservation in nephrotic syndrome (90). Of interest, the Na+/H+ exchanger regulator factor 2 (Nherf2) also functions in maintenance of the foot processes by linking the podocyte protein podocalixin to the cytoskeleton. In the puromycin aminonucleoside nephropathy model of FSGS, this complex is disrupted, and leads to the dramatic loss of foot processes and nephrotic syndrome (91).

Recent observations underscore the importance of the interactions between the podocyte and the underlying basement membrane. Dystroglycan is an integral component of the glomerular basement membrane. Decreased dystroglycan staining was observed in patients with minimal change disease (92). Dystroglycan expression was maintained in the nonsclerotic segments in FSGS, suggesting that minimal change disease and FSGS are indeed different disease processes and not merely different stages of one disease.

Because sclerosis ultimately is comprised of obliterated capillary loops and excess matrix, the mesangial cell also contributes to glomerular sclerosis (34). The mesangial cells share many characteristics with vascular smooth muscle cells; they contract and proliferate in response to numerous vasoactive substances, such as Ang II, and growth factors/cytokines, such as IGF-1 and TNF-α (9). After initial injury, the activated mesangial cell changes phenotype, expressing fibroblast-like myosin (93). These changes may alter their susceptibility to injury. Ang II induces mesangial cell hypertrophy, increases matrix production from mesangial cells *in vitro*, and induces the smooth muscle cell *c-fos* oncogene (34). TGFβ, a cytokine released from a variety of cells, increases both collagen and proteoglycan production by mesangial cells and, depending on the cell-cycle stage, acts synergistically with other growth factors (9,38). Many growth factors initially may be released from infiltrating macrophages, platelets, or resident glomerular cells (i.e., endothelial and epithelial cells). Macrophage influx is associated with PDGF production; prevention of this influx, by dietary or other maneuvers, decreases subsequent injury (94). PDGF is increased in several models of glomerulosclerosis (67). Mesangial cells in culture release both IL-1 and a PDGF-like factor, suggesting that both autocrine and paracrine regulation of mesangial cell proliferation occur.

Therapy and Growth Factors

An important role for growth factors in glomerulosclerosis is underscored by the observation that therapies that reduce sclerosis may do so through antiproliferative effects. Antihypertensive therapies, in addition to altering blood pressure, have effects on growth. Results with ACEIs are of particular interest in view of the potent effects Ang II has on renal hemodynamics and mesangial cell growth. Treatment with ACEIs markedly attenuates glomerular hypertrophy, ameliorates glomerulosclerosis in the renal ablation model (16), and decreases glomerulosclerosis, even in a nonhypertensive model (puromycin aminonucleoside nephropathy) (9). Furthermore, ACEIs attenuate hypertrophy of nonrenal blood vessels independently of their vasodilating effects in animals with hypertension (17). Similar effects on vascular lesions and glomerulosclerosis were seen with AT1 RAs (17). Other antihypertensives, including combination therapy (with vasodilators and diuretics) and calcium channel blockers, have shown varying efficacy. Combination therapy in large doses ameliorated both glomerulosclerosis and glomerular hypertrophy without affecting glomerular pressures (16). In spontaneously hypertensive rats after uninephrectomy, both nifedipine and enalapril prevented glomerular sclerosis and decreased glomerular hypertension and renal hypertrophy. Nifedipine decreased glomerular hypertrophy and sclerosis in desoxycorticosterone acetate–salt hypertension and the renal ablation model without normalizing glomerular pressure. Verapamil, another calcium-channel blocker, has shown differing effects: In the renal ablation model, renal injury was worsened, whereas, in another study, doses insufficient to decrease blood pressure showed protection (12).

Dietary Factors

A high-protein diet accelerates progression of renal disease in rats regardless of the primary injury. Conversely, protection with low-protein diets has been observed in the renal ablation model, Adriamycin nephropathy, nephrotoxic serum nephritis, and in the nonclipped kidney of Goldblatt hypertensive rats (95,96). The studies are difficult to assess, because altering dietary protein also results in change in other dietary components. Postulated dietary mediators of progressive renal disease include calcium, salt, phosphate, and fat. Reduction in caloric intake per se may be pivotal in the protection against progressive injury (32). A low-protein diet slows progression in the nonhypertensive puromycin aminonucleoside nephropathy model; when combined with ACEI, sclerosis was even reversed. A high-protein diet that accelerates progression augments gene expression of the renin-angiotensin system both in normal rats and in those with renal ablation; this provides a potential basis for the augmented effects of the combined ACEI and low-protein therapy. Among other mechanisms postulated for the effect of low-protein diets are altered T-cell function, decreases in macrophage influx, calcium-phosphate precipitation–induced tubular injury, proteinuria, and oxygen radicals (97).

Other dietary manipulations shown to affect glomerulosclerosis include salt. A low-salt diet decreased systemic blood pressure and attenuated glomerular hypertrophy and sclerosis in the remnant kidney model. Stimulation of glomerular growth by androgens did not affect intraglomerular pressures but increased sclerosis (94). A high-salt diet increased glomerular volume, sclerosis, and proteinuria in the ablation model without affecting arterial or intraglomerular pressures (21). Thus, in addition to its well-known effect on blood pressure, salt restriction affects glomerular growth.

A further caveat in extrapolating from these studies is to consider the differences in the experimental models and human renal disease (97). The renal ablation model in the rat is characterized by marked compensatory growth as well as ongoing maturational growth. Rats continue to have renal, especially glomerular, growth during most of their life span; human glomerular growth is complete when body growth is completed. Therefore, the effects of restricted diets that affect both maturational and pathophysiologic growth processes may be more extreme in rats than they are in humans.

Lipids and Hyperlipidemia

Lipids are important in modulating glomerular sclerosis in rats; analogous studies in humans are incomplete (64,98). Hypercholesterolemia per se appears to have little effect on glomerular injury in humans or in animal modes. However, glomerular injury was increased in experimental models of kidney disease when excess cholesterol was added to diets of rats with preexisting glomerular disease, ablation nephropathy, or hypertension. Histologic evidence of abnormal renal lipid accumulation has long been noted (9). Glomerular disease has been reported in the rare familial disease, lecithin cholesterol acyltransferase deficiency, and with excess apolipoprotein E. However, renal disease is not typical in the more common forms of primary hyperlipidemias. Patients with minimal-change disease or membranous glomerulonephritis, characterized by hyperlipidemia as part of their nephrotic syndrome, usually do not develop glomerular scarring. Evidence of the effects of manipulation of lipids is currently limited to animal studies (64).

Lipoprotein levels are also modulated by severe proteinuria. Proteinuria itself has been proposed to be injurious by affecting glomerular mesangial and epithelial cells or by cast formation with subsequent tubular epithelial damage and interstitial inflammation (99). When glomerular disease is accompanied by severe proteinuria, the prognosis is worse. Whether proteinuria is merely a marker of injury or a contributor to progressive injury has been debated.

Glomerulosclerosis shares several features with atherosclerosis: Both are affected by macrophages, PDGF, and lipids. Macrophage accumulation resulting from high cholesterol levels has been postulated to be a key early step for glomerulosclerosis. These cells are potential sources of numerous cytokines and eicosanoids that affect the glomerulus (64,98). Support for this hypothesis is seen with the protective effects of maneuvers that decrease macrophage influx (100). In a rat model of UUO, administration of ACEI ameliorated interstitial monocyte/macrophage infiltration and decreased fibrosis (101). However, macrophages may also play a beneficial role in scarring. The specific role of the macrophage AT1a receptor in renal fibrosis was examined in studies of bone marrow transplantation in wild-type mice with UUO mice reconstituted with either wild-type macrophages or macrophages devoid of the AT1a receptor. There was more severe interstitial fibrosis in mice with the AT1a-deficient macrophages even though fewer infiltrating macrophages were observed, suggesting that the macrophage AT1a receptor functions to protect the kidney from fibrogenesis (102).

Interesting new data have pointed to the importance of the tubulointerstitial lesion in progression. Elegant morphometric studies of human diabetic nephropathy show that the earliest changes in the interstitium are due to an increase in total interstitial cell volume (which may represent increased cell size and/or number), preceding the accumulation of interstitial collagen (103). This is in stark contrast to the diabetic mesangial lesion in which the expanded mesangial area is largely due to increased matrix accumulation rather than hypercellularity. Further understanding of the nature of these interstitial cells, which do not appear to be accounted for by infiltrating lymphocytes and/or macrophages, will shed additional light onto an important pathogenetic mechanism in progressive diabetic nephropathy. These cells could possibly represent interstitial myofibroblasts, postulated to play a key role in interstitial fibrosis. These activated interstitial cells are a major source of collagen synthesis, and increased expression of α-smooth muscle actin, a marker of myofibroblasts, predicts progressive renal dysfunction both in human and experimental renal disease. The source of myofibroblasts is a topic of controversy. Bone marrow–derived or potential renal stem cells may give rise not only to interstitial cells but also to regenerating parenchymal cells (104).

Epithelial-mesenchymal transformation is another possible mechanism for generation of interstitial myofibroblasts (105). This seamless plasticity of cells changing from epithelial to mesenchymal phenotypes exists during early development. Data indicate that epithelial-mesenchymal transformation may also occur in the adult after injury. Injured tubular epithelial cells can change phenotype both *in vivo* and *in vitro*, with *de novo* expression of a fibroblast-specific protein (FSP1) and possibly migrate into the interstitium as myofibroblasts. The components of the surrounding matrix regulate this process.

Obesity and Renal Scarring

Obesity in adult and pediatric populations is increasing at an epidemic proportion in the United States and other industrialized countries. The prevalence of obesity in childhood and adolescence ranges from 12 to 40% of the population (106). Obesity has been shown to be a precursor to various disorders, including hypertension, type II diabetes mellitus, lipid abnormalities, obstructive sleep apnea, and orthopedic problems. Recently, obesity has also been recognized to lead to glomerulosclerosis. Glomerular hypertrophy is a common feature in obesity-associated FSGS and may be implicated in its genesis. Other additional mechanisms contributing to sclerosis have been suggested, including hyperlipidemia, hyperfiltration, glomerular hypertension, reactive oxygen species, and abnormal growth factor environment (107). In particular, hyperinsulinemia may contribute to the genesis of the glomerulomegaly (106). The pediatric patients reported in a study of obesity-linked FSGS were all African American, nephrotic, and had rapid deterioration in renal function, a finding that contrasts a large review of obesity-related glomerulopathy in adults, in which patients were more often white, had less than nephrotic range proteinuria, and had slow progression (108,109). Renal biopsies revealed some features suggestive of a contribution of diabetic injury, including glomerulomegaly, mesangial matrix expansion, and glomerular basement membrane thickening, in addition to the segmental sclerosis. Of note, weight reduction dramatically reduced proteinuria in some of these patients. Approaches with combined therapies are now being investigated. Experimental studies suggest that inhibition of the renin angiotensin system and HMG Co-A reductase inhibitor (so-called statins) have further beneficial effects in a severe experimental nephropathy model (110).

Obese patients are particularly at risk for developing glomerulopathy in the setting of additional injuries. Thus, among patients undergoing unilateral nephrectomy, approximately one-fourth had significant proteinuria. More than one-half of these patients also had renal insufficiency associated with a significantly higher body mass index (BMI) compared to those with preserved renal function (111). The adverse effect of obesity in addition to other risk factors has also been shown in a transplant setting, in which renal transplant recipients with elevated BMI showed inferior patient survival compared to patients with lower BMI. This elevated BMI was also associated with worse graft survival independent of patient survival (112).

Recent studies have examined the possible role of leptin in obesity. Leptin is the product of the *ob* gene and is produced by adipose tissue. Its concentration in plasma is related to the total amount of body fat. Administration of leptin to mice with a genetic defect in its production, the ob/ob mice, increases energy expenditure, reduces food intake, and causes loss of body weight, mediated through the leptin receptor localized in the hypothalamus. Leptin may also have direct tissue effects. Some patients with obesity have high circulating leptin levels. *In vitro* and *in vivo* studies support a moderate effect of leptin to promote growth and profibrogenic mechanisms, such as increased TGFβ and collagen type IV expression (113).

Thrombosis/Fibrinolysis

Altered hemostasis is postulated to be another mechanism for progressive renal disease. Several anticoagulant agents and platelet inhibitors ameliorate glomerulosclerosis *in vivo* and affect the proliferation of glomerular cells in culture. Heparin is of particular interest, because epithelial cells produce a heparin-like substance that inhibits mesangial cells. Fractions of heparin, both with and without anticoagulant activity, when added to cell cultures decrease glomerulosclerosis and suppress mesangial cell growth and matrix production. Thromboxane is another vasoactive substance that affects coagulation and renal injury. Antagonism of thromboxane's actions is protective in several forms of progressive renal disease (9). Mechanisms may relate to prevention of microthrombi, a finding seen with severe injury, or prevention of platelet and monocyte activation with ensuing release of cytokines.

The plasmin-plasminogen activator system is comprised of the plasminogen activators and their inhibitors, which together modulate the production of plasmin. Plasmin, which is generated from the inactive precursor plasminogen by the action of plasminogen activators, is not only the primary effector of fibrinolysis but also a major contributor to the degradation of matrix glycoproteins and vascular remodeling (39,114). PAI-1 modulates plasminogen activation, and thereby fibrinolytic activity, by inhibiting tissue-type plasminogen activator and urokinase-type plasminogen activator. Increased PAI-1 levels have been identified in atherosclerosis, in some patients with myocardial infarction, in diabetics, and in animal models of glomerulosclerosis (39,41,115). A PAI-1 polymorphism (4G vs. 5G) has been associated with increased risk for cardiovascular complications in diabetics (39). Interestingly, Ang, in addition to its established effects on vasoconstriction and as a growth factor, increases PAI-1 expression, and aldosterone enhances this effect (40,42). Thus, Ang inhibition has the potential to modulate thrombotic/fibrinolytic and remodeling mechanisms (114–116) (see Growth Factors).

CLINICAL FACTORS THAT INFLUENCE PROGRESSION

Severity of Initial Renal Damage

The renal parenchyma in two normal kidneys has more than adequate reserve. Loss of even one-half of the total renal parenchyma (uninephrectomy) results in prompt compensation by the remaining tissue. Within 2 to 3 months, the remaining kidney increases in size by one-half, and the GFR is within 10 to 20% of the prenephrectomy level and therefore adequate to maintain metabolic function of a normal individual. While these compensatory responses return renal mass and GFR toward normal values, the compensatory response places the kidney at increased risk for progressive renal damage. For example, adults who have lost one kidney because of trauma or individuals who donate a kidney for transplantation have a slightly higher incidence of hypertension and more proteinuria than the normal population. Similarly, individuals with unilateral renal agenesis are at greater risk for progressive renal damage (117,118). Thus, the loss of even 50% of renal parenchyma does expose the remaining nephron population to a small but clinically significant risk for renal damage. Greater nephron loss brings greater risk for progressive renal damage. The reason for this deterioration likely relates to limited renal reserve and increased risk of progressive structural damage from superimposed injury from infection, dehydration, drugs, and toxins that activate or promote mechanisms outlined in the preceding sections. The extent of initial nephron loss necessary for initiating progression, while unclear, probably exceeds 75% of renal mass. A study of 14 patients undergoing up to 7/8 nephrectomy for removal of tumor showed mild to severe proteinuria in most. Renal biopsies in four who had lost the most renal mass showed focal segmental or global glomerulosclerosis (119). Most renal disease in humans that leads to chronic renal failure is diffuse; the remaining nephrons have great heterogeneity in function. Whereas some nephrons are severely affected, others have enhanced function. However, if the removal/destruction of renal parenchyma is extensive, this apparent initial compensation may subsequently result in a progressive downward course.

Removal of one kidney in children (e.g., due to Wilms' tumor) has somewhat more ominous consequences than loss of nephrons in adults: Renal growth was most marked in those who had surgery at a younger age, and this increased kidney growth was associated with microalbuminuria, which developed in 11 of 34 patients (120). Likewise, in patients with unilateral renal agenesis there is significantly increased risk for proteinuria (in 19%), hypertension (47%) and renal insufficiency (13%), with death due to renal disease in 6 of 157 patients in a large series (121). These findings suggest that the number of remnant nephrons in the congenital solitary kidney may, in fact, be decreased (i.e., hypogenesis), thereby representing a more severe form of reduction in nephron population than surgical unilateral nephrectomy. The possibility that the remnant glomeruli of congenital solitary kidney are under greater hypertrophic stress is indeed supported by quantitative morphometric studies. The volume of each glomerulus in solitary kidneys was found to be 5 to 6 times normal, a value close to that found in oligomeganephronia, an extreme condition of decreased nephron number (see Nature of Insult and Host Factors) (122).

Nature of Insult and Host Factors

The initial renal injury may be limited or it may affect all nephrons; it may be a one-time episode, continuous, or recurrent (Fig. 66.4). A single episode affecting a limited number of nephrons, as occurs with pyelonephritis, usually does not have long-term consequences. Multiple episodes that damage many nephrons lead to progression and renal failure. Diseases that are diffuse, such as poststreptococcal glomerulonephritis, usually do not damage glomerular structure severely enough to cause progressive injury and sclerosis. However, injury that is diffuse and either prolonged or recurrent, such as occurs in diabetes, lupus nephritis, or membranoproliferative glomerulonephritis, increases the risk of irreversible damage and progressive renal injury. Delay in therapy prolongs the initial injury and potentially increases both the initial and subsequent renal damage.

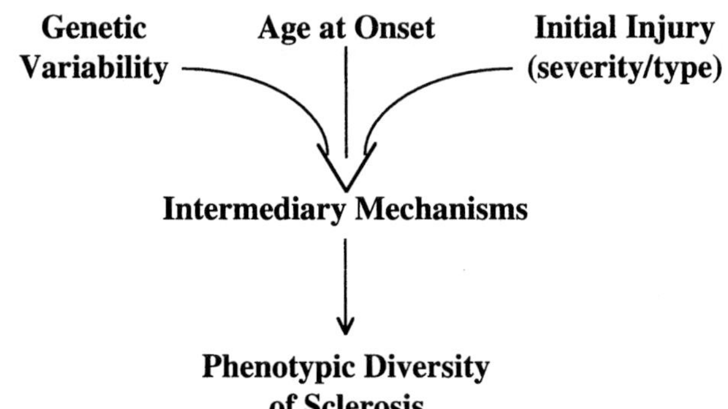

FIGURE 66.4. Diversity of morphologic appearance of sclerosis reflects specific contributions of an individual's genetic make-up, type and severity of the initial injury, and the patient's age at disease onset. These factors activate diverse intermediary mechanisms that determine the course of renal damage.

Individual patients also vary in their susceptibility to particular injuries (Fig. 66.4). For example, individual differences in susceptibility to renal damage have been described in patients with urinary tract infections; the uroepithelium in some patients binds bacteria more avidly than in others (see Chapter 53). Heightened inflammatory response to immunologic or infectious injury leads to enhanced leukocyte infiltration and greater release of free radicals, which also damage renal parenchyma. (See also Chapter 29.) Individual differences in host response may contribute to the great variability in the degree of renal injury in patients with hemolytic uremic syndrome. A recent study suggests that weakened or absent PI antigen expression on red blood cells increases risk for hemolytic uremic syndrome and for more severe involvement (123).

Predisposition of certain populations to the pathophysiologic factors outlined in the preceding section also varies. Glomerular size is greater in African Americans than in whites (124). The Pima Indians, who have a high incidence of diabetic nephropathy, also have larger glomeruli, even before development of renal disease (125). The increased risk of development of end-stage renal disease does not only reflect increased incidence of renal disease in these populations but also reflects the course of progression for given diseases. Thus, even when controlled for blood pressure levels, the risk of end-stage renal disease associated with hypertension is greater in African Americans than whites. Microalbuminuria is also more prevalent in African

American versus white hypertensive patients even at similar age, BMI, degree or duration of hypertension, or antihypertensive treatment (126). Hypertension and moderate renal insufficiency are associated with extensive global glomerulosclerosis in the African American patients, far greater than reported in other populations (127). The phenotype of this global glomerulosclerosis differs in African Americans versus whites, with more of the solidified type (i.e., replacement of the glomerular tuft by collagen) in the former and the usual obsolescent type (i.e., collagenous material filling in Bowman's space with a globally sclerosed glomerulus) prevalent in whites. These findings suggest possible different mechanisms of glomerular scarring associated with hypertension in these two populations (128). Of note, the African American Study of Kidney Disease trial demonstrated that ACEI was a superior treatment to preserve GFR in African Americans with moderate renal insufficiency and hypertension, although multiple additional antihypertensive drugs and higher doses were necessary to achieve target blood pressure goals (129).

It is possible that factors that underlie kidney development and glomerular number/size also contribute to the increased susceptibility of African Americans to develop end-stage renal disease. The course of lupus nephritis in a prospective, randomized National Institutes of Health trial was more severe in African Americans than whites, with more extensive crescent formation and interstitial fibrosis and greater likelihood of end-stage renal disease in the former population (130). Even the manifestations of human immunodeficiency virus (HIV) infection in the kidney differ markedly in the two populations: HIV-associated renal disease in African Americans is typically an aggressive FSGS, contrasting HIV-positive whites with renal disease who more frequently have immune-complex–mediated glomerulonephritides (131). These observations underscore the importance of genetic factors in response to injuries.

Impact of Genetics

The extent or virulence of a given disease varies among individuals. Even when patients are stricken with a given disease, the risk of progressive organ damage varies greatly (Fig. 66.4). Only a portion of patients with diabetes mellitus, IgA nephropathy, or postinfectious glomerulonephritis develop progressive glomerulosclerosis. Thus, a patient's genetic burden impacts assessment of organ damage due to increased variability of the disease process and also influences the choice and efficacy of therapeutic interventions.

Occurrence of renal diseases has been linked to genotype. In African-Americans, HLA-DR3 was consistently associated with end-stage renal disease due to hypertension, diabetic nephropathy due to insulin-dependent diabetes mellitus, or membranous glomerulonephritis. Excess HLA-D3 was present in whites with end-stage renal disease when end-stage renal disease was caused by insulin-dependent diabetes mellitus, lupus, or membranous glomerulonephritis, although no association was found with end-stage renal disease due to hypertension, IgA nephropathy, or FSGS. The possibility that the HLA class II association is due to linkage disequilibrium with the HLA class III TNF locus is currently being investigated, owing to the close physical proximity of these two genes on chromosome 6 (132). Taken together, differences in genetic make-up among different racial groups appear to influence the occurrence of renal disease.

Genetic background also modulates susceptibility in experimental models. The hypertrophic response, or lack thereof, and subsequent development of sclerosis are dependent on the genetic background, suggesting that complex genetic traits modulate the response of glomerular cells to pathogenic stimuli. Mice with reduced nephron number due to a radiation-induced mutation that results in approximately 50% nephron reduction in association with oligosyndactyly ($Os^{+/+}$) developed severe glomerular enlargement and sclerosis when this abnormality occurred on the sclerosis-prone ROP genetic background but not in the sclerosis-resistant C57BL6/J strain (133). Glomerular hypertrophy was proportional to reduction of nephron mass in the former strain. In contrast, a threshold for glomerular size was observed in the C57BL6/J mice.

Susceptibility may be influenced by renin gene polymorphisms. Some mouse strains (e.g., C57BL6/J) have one gene (*Ren-1^c*), whereas other strains (e.g., 129) have two (*Ren-1^d* and *Ren-2*) (134). The *Ren-1* genes govern expression of renin in the kidney in the juxtaglomerular apparatuses, whereas the *Ren-2* gene controls submaxillary gland renin expression and has very low renal expression. Mice with two renin genes (i.e., 129 strain) have tenfold higher plasma renin activity, angiotensin-dependent hypertension, and increased blood pressure and cardiac and renal hypertrophic responses to salt compared to one renin gene mice (i.e., C57BL6/J). Renin gene status, thus, could have a major effect on susceptibility to injuries where the renin angiotensin aldosterone system plays a role (134).

There is also accumulating evidence that genes in humans modulate the course and rate of organ damage. Polymorphisms in several genes within the RAS system, including ACE, angiotensinogen, and the angiotensin type 1 receptor, have been linked with cardiovascular and renal disorders, including diabetic nephropathy, IgA nephropathy, and uropathies (135–139). Polymorphisms of all three genes were evaluated in patients with IgA nephropathy as well as in diabetics (135,136,140,141). The ACE DD genotype frequency was increased in the patients who ultimately experienced progressive decline in renal function during follow-up compared to those whose function remained stable over the same time. Notably, exclusion of patients with known risk factors for progression, such as hypertension and significant proteinuria, strengthened the association of the DD genotype and progression of renal dysfunction in IgA nephropathy (140). Although environmental and other genetic factors may contribute, similar ACE polymorphism distributions in progressive IgA nephropathy in genetically distinct and geographically remote populations point to a significant functional role for the deletion allele of the ACE polymorphism (139,141).

Intron 16 encompassing the ACE I/D segment has a repeated sequence, comprising the terminal bases of one end of the "insert" and flanking the opposite end. This arrangement suggests a possible origin of the D allele. During meiosis, one of these two repeats could align with the complement of the other, thus producing a "loop-out" of the intervening fragment. This structure implies that the mutational event may actually occur by a deletion rather than insertion (140). Interestingly, in normal as well as diabetic whites, those with the II genotype have the lowest serum ACE levels, DD subjects have the highest, and those with the ID genotype have intermediate levels, supporting that the D allele contributes to the activation of ACE (142). This suggests that the "insert" may contain a silencer element, the absence of which activates the ACE gene. A functional relevance of this genetic variant is supported by the observation that normotensive men with the DD genotype had increased systemic pressor responsiveness to infusion of Ang I when compared with II genotype (143). Moreover, the plasma Ang II levels were also higher across the dose range of angiotensin I infusion, implying increased generation of Ang II in the DD individuals. It is interesting that in a recent large-scale study of diabetics, in addition to ACE polymorphism, an angiotensinogen gene polymorphism also predicted occurrence of nephropathy and progression of renal dysfunction. The angiotensinogen polymorphism modulates circulating angiotensinogen levels and, together with ACE I/D phenotype, affects constitutive levels of Ang II and, therefore, renal parenchymal damage and response to Ang inhibition. Thus, it appears that these polymorphic loci likely directly affect renal disease and are not just markers for another gene variant which more directly contributes to progression. Polymorphisms of TGFβ are also implicated in hypertension and progressive fibrosis. The Arg 25 polymorphism may be increased in African Americans, who also may have greater elevation of circulating TGFβ when they reach end-stage renal disease, compared to whites (144).

Congenital Disease/Nephron Number

Several factors contribute to the importance of age at time of injury as a variable affecting progression (Fig. 66.4). First, duration of the disease process before diagnosis and institution of therapy may be prolonged. Also, underlying developmental/structural abnormalities amplify the destructive process because of the decreased number of nephrons in these congenital abnormalities. In addition, these disorders reflect abnormal organization of the nephron, which may predispose it to subsequent injury.

There is clinical and experimental evidence that loss of nephrons early in life leads to a more active growth response that is followed by a greater tendency to glomerulosclerosis later on (117,118). Children with agenesis of one kidney show exaggerated glomerular hypertrophy and glomerulosclerosis relative to individuals who have a nephrectomy later in life. In the child, increased metabolic load associated with growth may augment these risks for injury. Focal and segmental glomerulosclerosis is particularly pronounced and often commences in the deep nephrons, which develop first and attain larger glomerular size. These changes are postulated to relate to the environment of the young host, including growth factors that, when overstimulated, may promote scarring. In a three-dimensional study of the distribution of lesions in idiopathic FSGS, children showed a predominance of peripheral, small lesions, in contrast to adults, who showed frequent lesions with a hilar component. The location of sclerosis (i.e., hilar vs. peripheral) and the extent of involvement may have impact on the course and response to therapy (145). Of interest, children with FSGS may have a good response to intensive treatment with IV methylprednisolone and oral alkylating agents (146).

Recently, variations in nephron endowment at birth, not related to prematurity, have been recognized. Experimental models have demonstrated that various intrauterine insults, such as gentamicin exposure, hyperglycemia, corticosteroids, and vitamin A deficiency can result in decreased nephron number (147–149). Decreased nephron number has been postulated to occur secondary to low term birth weight, defined as less than 2500 g. Lower nephron number may increase risk of renal disease and may be one of the mechanisms whereby individuals with low birth weight have increased incidence of progressive renal disease in adulthood (150). These fewer nephrons are postulated to be under greater hemodynamic stress, thus contributing to progressive sclerosis. Of interest, glomerular size in normal African Americans is larger than in whites and could possibly reflect smaller nephron number (124). This finding could contribute to the increased incidence of end-stage renal disease in African Americans compared to whiteswhites. Mechanisms other than hemodynamic stress, which could underlie these differences in normal glomerular populations and also relate to increased incidence of end-stage renal disease, include functional polymorphisms of genes that are involved both in renal and glomerular development and contribute to amplified scarring mechanisms, such as the renin-angiotensin system (151).

Glomerular Growth and Glomerulosclerosis

Abnormal glomerular growth and glomerulosclerosis are associated in many diseases (151). The most extreme glomerulomegaly described in humans is that seen in oligomeganephronia. This congenital renal disease is characterized by a decreased number of nephrons, each of which is markedly enlarged, and an increase in FSGS (152). In diabetic nephropathy, the number of functioning nephrons is normal at the early stage, but the glomeruli enlarge and hyperfunction from the onset of diabetes (153,154). The severity of glomerular sclerosis correlates with the degree of glomerular growth. Mean glomerular size and mesangial volumes are smaller in diabetic patients after pancreas and renal transplantation than in control renal transplant patients (155).

In patients with FSGS, the processes linked to glomerular growth appear to be primary and not secondary to nephron loss (Fig. 66.3) (i.e., glomerular growth precedes nephron dropout due to sclerosis). Kidney biopsies from patients with FSGS or minimal-change disease were compared with tissue from patients with no renal disease. Both adults and children with FSGS had substantially larger glomeruli than age-matched normal individuals or those with minimal-change nephrotic syndrome (156). Children with apparent minimal-change disease who in repeat biopsies progressed to overt FSGS had enlarged glomeruli in their initial biopsies, compared with glomeruli of age-matched normal controls. Patients with minimal-change disease who continued with typical benign clinical courses and who, on repeat biopsies (performed in two-thirds) continued with minimal-change disease, had normal-sized glomeruli on the initial biopsy. In patients aged 1 to 5 years with minimal-change disease, initial glomerular size was equal to or less than that of autopsy control. These patients continued to have a benign clinical course. In contrast, all those with an initial glomerular size more than 1.5 times the average size of normal glomeruli developed FSGS. Thus, this cutoff level of glomerular size was a highly sensitive and specific predictor of those patients who develop FSGS among those with an initial diagnosis of apparent minimal-change disease. Increased glomerular size also predicted subsequent glomerular sclerosis in the setting of recurrent FSGS in the transplant kidney. Thus, children who did not develop FSGS in their transplants did not show increased glomerular size in the initial months after transplantation. In contrast, children who developed recurrent FSGS had marked abnormal glomerular growth, which preceded overt manifestation of FSGS (157). The linkage of growth with glomerular sclerosis has been noted in patients with reflux nephropathy and those with sickle cell glomerulopathy, obesity, HIV nephropathy, and a remnant kidney resulting from removal of more than one kidney (9,119). Glomerular enlargement could therefore be a marker in the early phase of disease—before overt sclerosis is detectable—for aberrant growth factor expression ultimately leading to scarring of the kidney. Molecular detection of these early processes could potentially be an even earlier, more sensitive marker of progression.

CLINICAL IMPLICATIONS/INTERVENTION

Treatments Associated with Progression

Treatments directed to some of the complications of renal failure may accelerate progression. We describe one example: growth hormone. Other factors, such as calcium and vitamin D, also affect progression.

Growth Hormone

rhGH has been used to stimulate growth in children who are growth retarded owing to renal failure and also as treatment of short stature after renal transplantation where its effects have been impressive (158). However, experimental evidence and clinical experience have raised questions about whether treatment may accelerate progression in compromised kidneys and, in rats, injure even normal kidneys. rhGH given to rats with renal ablation accelerated progression of glomerulosclerosis. Normal young rats treated chronically with hGH developed glomerulosclerosis (31). Although renal function in the latter group was not affected, the severity of the lesions indicated that functional potential had been compromised. In one clinical report, eight children who were post–renal transplant and growth retarded were given hGH for 6 to 21 months. In four of these patients, creatinine clearances decreased, one sufficient to cause the physician to stop treatment (159). Recent study of children with renal transplants showed, although renal function was not compromised, there was more proximal tubule atrophy in patients receiving hGH than in transplanted patients without hGH treatment (160). Increased urinary albumin excretion rate was observed in children with short stature who received hGH even without underlying renal disease (161). These studies hint that treatment of short stature, whether accompanying renal failure or not, may be a double-edged sword. There is somatic growth. However, because hGH can enhance B- and T-lymphocyte function, development of cytotoxic T cells, and natural killer cell activity, there is the possibility of increased acute and chronic rejection (162–164). The proinflammatory properties of hGH can also accelerate sclerosis (164). The study further suggests that the destructive process takes root and progresses, even when at the onset of growth hormone treatment renal damage is not profound or there is no initial renal damage. A recent study showed that rhGH in transplanted children did result in increased somatic growth. There was not an observed increase in acute rejection, although, of note, immunosuppression was such that 2 of the 68 patients developed posttransplant lymphoproliferative disease, and one developed Hodgkin's lymphoma. Furthermore, two of the rhGH-treated patients had graft loss due to chronic allograft nephropathy, compared to one graft loss due to noncompliance in the control group (165).

Treatment Used to Slow Progression

Intervention strategies aimed at slowing progression include early detection of patients with primary diseases, diet modification, antihypertensive drugs, and therapy aimed at forestalling diabetic nephropathy.

Early Detection and Treatment

Identification of those with renal disease is important in initiating treatment to slow progression. Sonography of fetuses during gestation identifies those with urologic abnormalities. Preschool screening of urine for abnormalities has been disappointing in detecting urinary tract infections and glomerular disease. Programs now are directed at identifying children with urinary tract infections and/or urinary tract abnormalities in the first 1 to 2 years of life, when treatment will have more impact (see also Chapter 53). If effective, these measures would detect children with urinary tract abnormalities, who currently constitute the largest population of children developing chronic renal failure (Fig. 66.1). Microalbuminuria, most commonly used to detect early diabetic nephropathy, may prove to be a useful indicator of renal damage in reflux nephropathy and hypertension (166,167). Although some patients with ureteral reflux/obstruction corrected before the age of 1 year still progress to end-stage renal disease, early detection and treatment are likely beneficial (168). Probability of progressive renal damage relates to the extent of the original damage, associated abnormalities, superimposed infections or nephrotoxic antibiotics, and compensatory changes that are discussed in this chapter.

Potential Regression of Sclerosis

Glomerulosclerosis is an ongoing, dynamic process. Various diseases show heterogeneous appearance of glomerulosclerosis. Thus, nodular, collapsing, cellular, hilar, peripheral, or "tip" (i.e., at the tubular pole) patterns of sclerosis have been postulated to have etiologic and also prognostic significance and may also reflect distinct mechanisms of sclerosis (169) (Fig. 66.4). Glomeruli also show heterogeneous injury at a given time in an individual patient. Heterogeneity in glomerulosclerosis was examined in humans with FSGS. This relationship, as well as the response to therapy, was assessed in animals with progressive renal failure after 5/6 nephrectomy. Morphologic analyses of the size and degree of sclerosis of individual glomeruli were done by three-dimensional methods (16,169). A biphasic relationship between glomerular hypertrophy and sclerosis was noted. There was a strong positive correlation between these two indices in glomeruli with early sclerosis, whereas the correlation was negative in glomeruli with advanced sclerosis (Fig. 66.5). This biphasic pattern was maintained after treatment with antihypertensives in the rat; the effectiveness of treatment appeared to depend on the stage of glomeruli along the pathway to sclerosis. Rats with remnant kidneys treated with an ACEI after injury were established and showed continued progression in the glomeruli that were already severely sclerotic. In contrast, glomeruli with only moderate degrees of sclerosis at the onset of treatment were protected by treatment.

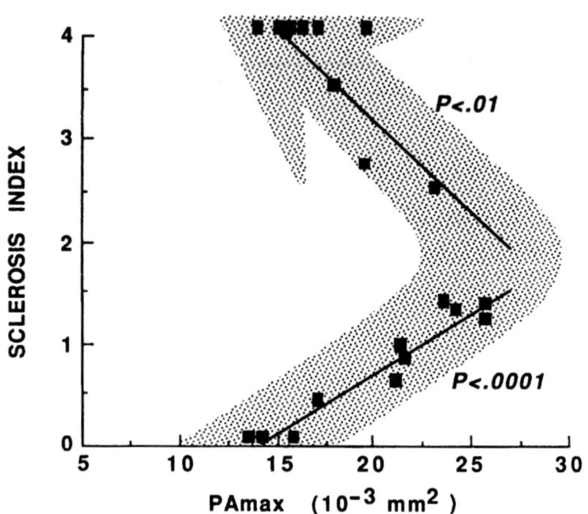

FIGURE 66.5. Relationship of glomerular hypertrophy and sclerosis in individual glomeruli within one kidney at 12 weeks after 5/6 nephrectomy. When sclerosis index (0–4 scale by serial section) and maximum planar area (PAmax) were evaluated for each of 22 glomeruli in a single remnant rat kidney 12 weeks after subtotal nephrectomy, a significant correlation with a biphasic pattern was found between these parameters. Thus, there was a negative correlation for the glomeruli with advanced sclerosis and a positive correlation for the glomeruli with early-stage sclerosis, pointing to a potential linkage between the pathogenesis of glomerular hypertrophy and sclerosis. (From Fogo A, Ichikawa I. Evidence for the central role of glomerular growth promoters in the development of sclerosis. *Semin Nephrol* 1989;9:329–342, with permission.)

Regression of injury can be accomplished. A shift in the balance of synthesis/degradation must occur to accomplish regression of sclerosis. Most challenging is the remodeling of obliterated capillary lumina (Table 66.1). Injured cells have to be replenished, repaired, or deleted to regenerate or restore capillary loops that may affect filtration. The following obstacles have to be overcome: (a) the net loss of endothelial cells, which must regenerate; (b) the variable increase in mesangial cells before the sclerotic acellular lesion develops, and mesangial cells must regrow; and (c) the limited growth capacity of the visceral epithelial cell. New glomeruli cannot be generated after term birth in humans, so regeneration of open loops has to occur by new capillary loop growth within injured glomeruli, with reabsorption of the sclerosed segments within that glomerulus. Regression could thus be mediated by new growth of capillaries, which take the place of the sclerosed, reabsorbed segments. Evidence in humans and animals indicate that glomerular growth with injury may indeed be achieved by lengthening or branching of the capillary loops (23–26). Consideration of the biologic potential of each of these processes in the glomerulus indicates that remodeling and regression of glomerulosclerosis indeed is theoretically possible. Emerging data show that this can actually be accomplished in practice as well.

TABLE 66.1. POTENTIAL MECHANISMS OF REGRESSION VS. PROGRESSION OF GLOMERULOSCLEROSIS

Factors favoring regression	Factors favoring progression
Proteases expressed in glomerulus (e.g., MMP-2, MMP-9, t-PA, u-PA)	Protease inhibitors expressed in glomerulus (e.g., TIMP-1, TIMP-2, PAI-1) Resistance to proteolysis (e.g., glycation, cross-linking)
Factors decreasing ECM synthesis (e.g., ACEI, AT1RA)	Growth factors causing increased ECM synthesis (e.g., angiotensin, TGF-β)
Growth factors stimulating cell regeneration (e.g., VEGF)	Growth factors causing apoptosis Limited growth potential of the podocyte
New capillary growth within the glomerulus (capillary lengthening/branching)	No glomerulogenesis after birth

ACEI, angiotensin I–converting enzyme inhibitor; ECM, extracellular matrix; MMP, matrix metalloproteinase; PAI, plasminogen activator inhibitor; TGF, transforming growth factor; TIMP, tissue inhibitor of metalloproteinase; t-PA, tissue-type plasminogen activator; u-PA, urokinase-type plasminogen activator; VEGF, vascular endothelial growth factor.

In contrast to the extensive investigation of factors promoting matrix synthesis, modulators of increased matrix degradation, which could allow resolution, have not been well characterized. Several proteases and protease inhibitors are expressed in the glomerulus, indicating that modulation of matrix can occur (114,115). Recent evidence has added PAI-1 to this array of matrix modulators in the kidney. PAI-1 inhibits not only fibrinolysis but also proteolysis by inhibiting activation of plasminogen activators. PAI-1 has been linked to sclerosis, and regression of sclerosis is tightly linked to its downregulation (114–116).

Higher doses of an ACEI or AT1RA (having the same hemodynamic effects) resulted in regression of existing glomerulosclerosis, linked to decreased extracellular matrix synthesis with decreased TGFβ, and increased extracellular matrix degradation, linked to marked decrease of PAI-1 (115). In a study of rats with puromycin aminonucleoside nephropathy that were treated with combined therapy—low-protein diet and an ACEI—this potential to decrease established glomerulosclerosis also was demonstrated (170). These findings emphasize that early aggressive treatment is important not only in limiting initial injury but also in controlling progression. The application of these conclusions has been investigated in diabetic patients with normal renal function and no overt proteinuria. The results show that early aggressive therapy with an ACEI given to diabetics with normal blood pressure and GFR maintained GFR and decreased proteinuria (171,172). Either ACEI or AT1RA was also effective in slowing progression in hypertensive patients with established diabetic nephropathy (173–175). Cure of diabetes by pancreas transplant in patients with moderate diabetic nephropathy resulted in regression of existing glomerulosclerosis and tubulointerstitial fibrosis over a 10-year period (176). Regression of existing lesions also occurred in relatively early IgA nephropathy in response to high-dose corticosteroids and tonsillectomy (177).

Dietary Protein

A relationship between diet and progressive loss of renal function has long been recognized. The potentially nephrotoxic factors in the diet include protein, carbohydrate, lipid, calcium, phosphorus, and sodium. Among these, low-protein diets have been studied most for several reasons:

1. Low-protein diets alleviate uremic symptoms.
2. Compared with other dietary constituents, dietary protein intake and output can be monitored. Protein restriction preserves renal function and morphology in several rat models of chronic renal failure (96).

Protein restriction has several effects that may ameliorate the pathophysiologic processes leading to progressive renal failure. These include reduction in glomerular perfusion and pressure and decrease in glomerular hypertrophy. Protein restriction also decreases serum lipid levels, reduces immune cell activation, and alters cellular growth factors. The recently published data of the Modification of Diet in Renal Disease study did not demonstrate the expected dramatic effects of protein restriction on progression, perhaps not surprising in view of the diverse underlying conditions in the populations studied (178). The resistance to therapy in some diseases, such as polycystic kidney disease, also underscores the heterogeneous mechanisms in different renal diseases. Furthermore, protein restriction has side effects that include malnutrition, which is emerging as an important contributor to morbidity and mortality of patients with end-stage renal disease. Overall, the current sentiment in treating children with progressive renal disease is to not restrict the diet other than to limit protein and phosphorus to recommended daily allowance levels.

Antihypertensive Treatment

Long-term clinical evidence clearly demonstrates the benefit of reducing blood pressure in patients with hypertension with or without renal disease. Untoward clinical events occur not only in the relatively few individuals with severe disease, but also affect the large number of patients with only mild hypertension. This recognition has led to changes in both the definition of hypertension and treatment recommendations. The Joint National Committee on the Detection, Evaluation, and Treatment of High Blood Pressure has, for the first time since the original report in 1977, reclassified normal diastolic blood pressure as less than 85 mm Hg (179). The report also emphasizes the importance of systolic blood pressure as a predictor of adverse events, in that normal systolic blood pressure is now taken to be less than 130 mm Hg. In parallel, clinical practice has evolved from treating only markedly high blood pressures to intervening when pressures are only modestly elevated. In diabetics, decreased systemic blood pressure below normal levels may benefit progression (171) by decreasing systemic and/or glomerular pressures, as well as modulating specific endothelial-derived factors. Control of blood pressure, however, does not necessarily prevent progression nor does its presence predict inevitable dire consequences. Other factors, such as genetic predisposition and race, may modulate the effects of systemic blood pressure on progression.

Independent of effects on systemic blood pressure, antihypertensive treatment preserves glomerular function and structure through its effects at specific sites within the renal circulation, as well as its nonhemodynamic effects (12,22,180,181). Among the various antihypertensives, ACEIs appear to be most consistent in arresting glomerular destruction in animals (115,180,182). This effect has been ascribed to the intrarenal effects of ACEIs that decrease glomerular pressure. However, the benefits of inhibiting the renin-angiotensin system go beyond systemic or glomerular antihypertensive effects. In this regard, protection similar to that with ACEIs is seen with AT1RA. Furthermore, greater benefit on scarring was observed with higher doses of ACEIs or AT1RAs, although systemic and local glomerular pressures were not further altered. Finally, contrasting potentially adverse effects on glucose and lipid metabolism ascribed to other antihypertensive treatment, notably hydrochlorothiazide, ACEIs may have beneficial effects on potential mediators of the pathophysiologic processes. Therapies that inhibit the renin angiotensin system appear particularly effective in both human and animal models (181). However, the efficacy in humans has been assessed only by GFR and not by long-term effects on structural lesions. These studies have shown benefit of ACEI over other antihypertensive treatments in both normotensive diabetics and in patients with nondiabetic progressive renal disease (173,182,183).

Another class of antihypertensive vasodilators that is being studied is the calcium antagonists. The results on renal function and histology in animal models are mixed. Several animal models, including diabetes, renal ablation, and several forms of hypertension, showed protection (22,184), but this was not a uniform finding. Calcium-channel blockers appear to have particularly beneficial effects in preserving renal allograft function. The mechanisms for this preservation include decreased vasoconstriction (primarily by dilating the afferent arteriole); augmenting immunosuppression, either directly or by increasing cyclosporine levels; and antiproliferative effects (184). The complementary mechanisms of actions of ACEI and calcium-channel blockers suggest synergistic benefit with combined therapy by decreasing both Ang II and downstream calcium-mediated effector mechanisms linked to vascular injury (185).

In addition to antihypertensive treatment being applied to a variety of renal diseases, new therapies are aimed at affecting progression in specific disorders. Diabetic nephropathy develops in approximately 40% of diabetics. On average, 17 years after diagnosis of juvenile-onset diabetes, diabetic nephropathy manifests as proteinuria followed by declining renal function within a few years. The dire consequences of diabetic nephropathy and the long preclinical phase before it becomes overt have targeted this entity for intense investigation for therapeutic maneuvers, including control of systemic blood pressure, low-protein diets, strict glucose control, and inhibitors of advanced glycation end products (186). Pancreas transplantation has become more successful in diabetic patients, and early studies indicate that restoring normal insulin control does decrease and even regress structural renal injury (155,176). Future efforts may be directed toward not only altering secondary, intermediary mechanisms of sclerosis but also the cure of the initial disease (e.g., with islet cell transplant in diabetes mellitus).

ASSESSMENT OF EFFICACY OF INTERVENTIONS

To assess which new therapies are most effective, we need to evaluate critically their effects on renal function and structure. The most commonly used indicators of renal function are GFR and proteinuria. Proteinuria has commonly been used as an indicator for progressive renal injury, and a change in proteinuria in response to treatment has been viewed as a beneficial effect of therapy. However, proteinuria is determined by several factors. Thus, proteinuria may reflect an underlying structural injury and disruption in the integrity of the permeability barrier. Proteinuria may also reflect abnormal glomerular hemodynamics in structurally, relatively intact glomeruli. In this regard, high glomerular pressure alters the sieving properties of the glomerular capillary bed. Glomerular hypertension can increase the relative number of large pores postulated to be the sole channel for macromolecular (i.e., protein) transport to the urinary space. Decreased protein excretion does not necessarily reflect improvement in progression of renal disease. This is particularly relevant for interpretation of data from short-term studies in which lessened proteinuria accompanies a decrease in GFR in response to antihypertensive therapy. In these studies, the mechanisms underlying decreased proteinuria include lower glomerular pressure (187). In particular, ACEI, by augmenting bradykinin, decreases efferent arteriolar resistance and, thus, decreases GFR and proteinuria acutely via these reversible hemodynamic effects (18). These ACEI effects make interpretation of clinical trials more challenging, as this decrease in GFR acutely masks anticipated benefit on sclerosing mechanisms, which ultimately result in preserved GFR over a longer time course.

The biopsy is frequently used as a diagnostic tool in nephrology. Based on new insights into pathogenesis, this technique may be used as a prognosticator as well. The renal biopsy may allow us to gauge long-term responses to therapy. Future evaluation may include more sophisticated techniques, such as morphometry, to assess glomerular size or degree of tubulointerstitial injury, *in situ* hybridization, or PCR of specific areas by laser capture microdissection to examine specific abnormal gene expression and its alteration by therapy (188).

Finally, due to the limitations of prospective randomized, controlled studies to address issues such as the proposed pathogenetic mechanisms outlined in this chapter, metaanalysis has been applied to cumulatively study results of clinical trials (189). Although there may be potential bias from selection and heterogeneity of studies, this method may yield answers to some key questions. This approach has been applied to the many studies of effects of antihypertensive treatment on the kidney in diabetes (182).

ACKNOWLEDGMENT

This work was supported in part by National Institutes of Health grants DK44757 (ABF, VK), DK39261 (ABF), and DK 56942 (ABF).

REFERENCES

1. Foreman JW, Chan JC. Chronic renal failure in infants and children. *J Pediatr* 1988;113:793–800.
2. Jungers P, Hannedouche T, Itakura Y, et al. Progression rate to end-stage renal failure in non-diabetic kidney diseases: a multivariate analysis of determinant factors. *Nephrol Dial Transplant* 1995;10:1353–1360.
3. Olson JL, Heptinstall RH. Nonimmunologic mechanisms of glomerular injury. *Lab Invest* 1988;59:564–578.
4. Morrison AB, Howard RM. The functional capacity of hypertrophied nephrons: effect of partial nephrectomy on the clearance of inulin and PAH in the rat. *J Exp Med* 1966;123:829–844.
5. Shimamura T, Morrison AB. A progressive glomerulosclerosis occurring in partial five-sixths nephrectomized rats. *Am J Pathol* 1975;79:95–106.
6. Hostetter TH, Olson JL, Rennke HG, et al. Hyperfiltration in remnant nephrons: a potentially adverse response to renal ablation. *Am J Physiol* 1981;241:F85–F93.
7. Aschinberg LC, Koskimies O, Bernstein J, et al. The influence of age on the response to renal parenchymal loss. *Yale J Bio Med* 1978;51:341–345.
8. O'Donnell MP, Kasiske BL, Raij L, et al. Age is a determinant of the glomerular morphologic and functional responses to chronic nephron loss. *J Lab Clin Med* 1985;106:308–313.
9. Fogo A, Ichikawa I. Glomerular growth promoter—the common channel to glomerular sclerosis. In: Mitch WE, ed. *Contemporary issues in nephrology: the progressive nature of renal disease*, 2nd ed. New York: Churchill Livingstone, 1992:23–54.
10. Brenner BM, Meyer TW, Hostetter TH. Dietary protein intake and the progressive nature of kidney disease: the role of hemodynamically mediated glomerular injury in the pathogenesis of progressive glomerular sclerosis in aging, renal ablation, and intrinsic renal disease. *N Engl J Med* 1982;307:652–659.
11. Nath KA, Kren SM, Hostetter TH. Dietary protein restriction in established renal injury in the rat. Selective role of glomerular capillary pressure in progressive glomerular dysfunction. *J Clin Invest* 1986;78:1199–1205.
12. Neuringer JR, Anderson S, Brenner BM. The role of systemic and intraglomerular hypertension. In: Mitch WE, ed. *The progressive nature of renal disease*, 2nd ed. New York: Churchill Livingstone, 1992:1–21.
13. Harris RC, Haralson MA, Badr KF. Continuous stretch-relaxation in culture alters mesangial cell morphology, growth characteristics, and metabolic activity. *Lab Invest* 1992;66:548–554.
14. Hostetter TH, Meyer TW, Rennke HG, et al. Chronic effects of dietary protein in the rat with intact and reduced renal mass. *Kidney Int* 1986;30:509–517.
15. Anderson S, Meyer TW, Rennke HG, et al. Control of glomerular hypertension limits glomerular injury in rats with reduced renal mass. *J Clin Invest* 1985;76:612–619.
16. Yoshida Y, Fogo A, Ichikawa I. Effects of anti-hypertensive drugs on glomerular morphology. A close linkage between their anti-hypertrophic and anti-sclerotic action on remnant glomeruli. *Kidney Int* 1989;36:626–635.
17. Kakinuma Y, Kawamura T, Bills T, et al. Blood-pressure independent effect of angiotensin inhibition on vascular lesions of chronic renal failure. *Kidney Int* 1992;42:46–55.
18. Kon V, Fogo A, Ichikawa I. Bradykinin causes selective efferent arteriolar dilatation during angiotensin I converting enzyme inhibition. *Kidney Int* 1993;44:545–550.
19. Yoshida Y, Fogo A, Shiraga H, et al. Serial micropuncture analysis of single nephron function in the rat model of subtotal renal ablation. *Kidney Int* 1988;33:855–867.
20. Yoshida Y, Fogo A, Ichikawa I. Glomerular hemodynamic changes vs. hypertrophy in experimental glomerular sclerosis. *Kidney Int* 1989;35:654–660.
21. Daniels BS, Hostetter TH. Adverse effects of growth in the glomerular microcirculation. *Am J Physiol* 1990;258:F1409–F1416.
22. Dworkin LD. Effects of calcium antagonists on glomerular hemodynamics and structure in experimental hypertension. *Am J Kidney Dis* 1991;17:89–93.
23. Nyengaard JR. Number and dimensions of rat glomerular capillaries in normal development and after nephrectomy. *Kidney Int* 1993;43:1049–1057.
24. Marcussen N, Nyengaard JR, Christensen S. Compensatory growth of glomeruli is accomplished by an increased number of glomerular capillaries. *Lab Invest* 1994;70:868–874.
25. Nyengaard JR, Rasch R. The impact of experimental diabetes mellitus in rats on glomerular capillary number and sizes. *Diabetologia* 1993;36:189–194.
26. Akaoka K, White RHR, Raafat F. Glomerular morphometry in childhood reflux nephropathy, emphasizing the capillary changes. *Kidney Int* 1995;47:1108–1114.

27. Rich AR. A hitherto undescribed vulnerability of the juxtamedullary glomeruli in lipoid nephrosis. *Bull Johns Hopkins Hosp* 1957;100:173–175.
28. Ikoma M, Yoshioka T, Ichikawa I, et al. Mechanism of the unique susceptibility of deep cortical glomeruli of maturing kidneys to severe focal glomerular sclerosis. *Pediatr Res* 1990;28:270–276.
29. Doi T, Striker LJ, Gibson CC, et al. Glomerular lesions in mice transgenic for growth hormone and insulinlike growth factor-I. I. Relationship between increased glomerular size and mesangial sclerosis. *Am J Pathol* 1990;137:541–552.
30. El Nahas AM, Bassett AH, Cope GH, et al. Role of growth hormone in the development of experimental renal scarring. *Kidney Int* 1991;40:29–34.
31. Allen DB, Fogo A, El-Hayek R, et al. Effects of prolonged growth hormone administration in rats with chronic renal insufficiency. *Pediatr Res* 1992;31:406–410.
32. Tapp DC, Wortham WG, Addison JF, et al. Food restriction retards body growth and renal pathology in remnant kidneys regardless of protein intake. *Lab Invest* 1989;60:184–195.
33. Fine LG, Hammerman MR, Abboud HE. Evolving role of growth factors in the renal response to acute and chronic disease. *J Am Soc Nephrol* 1992;2:1163–1170.
34. Kashgarian M, Sterzel RB. The pathobiology of the mesangium. *Kidney Int* 1992;41:524–529.
35. Johnson RJ, Raines EW, Floege J, et al. Inhibition of mesangial cell proliferation and matrix expansion in glomerulonephritis in the rat by antibody to platelet-derived growth factor. *J Exp Med* 1992;175:1413–1416.
36. Border WA, Okuda S, Languino LR, et al. Suppression of experimental glomerulonephritis by antiserum against transforming growth factor beta 1. *Nature* 1990;346:371–374.
37. Kopp JB, Factor VM, Mozes M, et al. Transgenic mice with increased levels of TGF-β1 develop progressive renal disease. *Lab Invest* 1996;74:991–1003.
38. Ketteler M, Noble NA, Border WA. Transforming growth factor-β and angiotensin II: The missing link from glomerular hyperfiltration to glomerulosclerosis? *Annu Rev Physiol* 1995;57:279–295.
39. Brown NJ, Vaughan DE. The renin-angiotensin and fibrinolytic systems. *Trends Cardiovasc Med* 1996;6:239–243.
40. Kerins DM, Hao Q, Vaughan DE. Angiotensin induction of PAI-1 expression in endothelial cells is mediated by the hexapeptide angiotensin IV. *J Clin Invest* 1995;96:2515–2520.
41. Oikawa T, Freeman M, Lo W, et al. Modulation of plasminogen activator inhibitor-1 (PAI-1) in vivo: a new mechanism for the anti-fibrotic effect of renin-angiotensin inhibition. *Kidney Int* 1997;51:164–172.
42. Brown NJ, Kim KS, Chen YQ, et al. Synergistic effect of adrenal steroids and angiotensin II on plasminogen activator inhibitor-1 expression. *J Clin Endocrinol Metab* 2000;85:336–344.
43. Ma LJ, Yang H, Gaspert, et al. Transforming growth factor (TGF)-β dependent and independent pathways of induction of tubulointerstitial fibrosis in β6-/- mice. *Am J Pathol (in press).*
44. Munger JS, Huang X, Kawakatsu H, et al. The integrin alpha v beta 6 binds and activates latent TGF beta 1: a mechanism for regulating pulmonary inflammation and fibrosis. *Cell* 1999;96:319–328.
45. Orth SR, Weinreich T, Bönisch S, et al. Angiotensin II induces hypertrophy and hyperplasia in adult human mesangial cells. *Exp Nephrol* 1995;3:23–33.
46. Kitazono T, Padgett RC, Armstrong ML, et al. Evidence that angiotensin II is present in human monocytes. *Circulation* 1995;91:1129–1134.
47. Morishita R, Gibbons GH, Ellison KE, et al. Evidence for direct local effect of angiotensin in vascular hypertrophy: in vivo gene transfer of angiotensin converting enzyme. *J Clin Invest* 1994;94:978–984.
48. Arai M, Wada A, Isaka Y, et al. In vivo transfection of genes for renin and angiotensinogen into the glomerular cells induced phenotypic change of the mesangial cells and glomerular sclerosis. *Biochem Biophys Res Commun* 1995;206: 525–532.
49. Kakuchi J, Ichiki T, Kiyama S, et al. Developmental expression of renal angiotensin II receptor genes in the mouse. *Kidney Int* 1995;47:140–147.
50. Yamada T, Horiuchi T, Dzau VJ. Angiotensin II type 2 receptor mediates programmed cell death. *Proc Natl Acad Sci U S A* 1996;93:156–160.
51. Stoll M, Steckelings M, Paul M, et al. The angiotensin AT2-receptor mediates inhibition of cell proliferation in coronary endothelial cells. *J Clin Invest* 1995;95:651–657.
52. Ma LJ, Nishimura H, Fogo A, et al. Accelerated fibrosis and collagen deposition develop in the renal interstitium of angiotensin type 2 receptor null mutant mice during ureteral obstruction. *Kidney Int* 1998;53:937–944.
53. Ohkubo N, Matsubara H, Nozawa Y, et al. Angiotensin type 2 receptors are reexpressed by cardiac fibroblasts from failing myopathic hamster hearts and inhibit cell growth and fibrillar collagen metabolism. *Circulation* 1997;96:3954–3962.
54. Cao Z, Bonnet F, Candido R, et al. Angiotensin type 2 receptor antagonism confers renal protection in a rat model of progressive renal injury. *J Am Soc Nephrol* 2002;13:1773–1787.
55. Ma LJ, Nakamura S, Nakamura I, et al. High dose angiotensin II type 1 receptor antagonist and angiotensin converting enzyme inhibitor in regression of glomerulosclerosis [abstract]. *J Am Soc Nephrol* 2002;13:342A.
56. Hunley TE, Tamura M, Stoneking BJ, et al. The angiotensin type II receptor tonically inhibits angiotensin-converting enzyme in AT2 null mutant mice. *Kidney Int* 2000;57:570–577.
57. Ots M, Mackenzie HS, Troy JL, et al. Effects of combination therapy with enalapril and losartan on the rate of progression of renal injury in rats with 5/6 renal mass ablation. *J Am Soc Nephrol* 1998;9:224–230.
58. Richer C, Bruneval P, Menard J, et al. Additive effects of enalapril and losartan in (mREN-2) 27 transgenic rats. *Hypertension* 1998;31:692–698.
59. Russo D, Pisani A, Balletta MM, et al. Additive antiproteinuric effect of converting enzyme inhibition and losartan in normotensive patients with IgA nephropathy. *Am J Kidney Dis* 1999;33:851–856.
60. Hebert LA, Falkenhain ME, Nahman NS Jr, et al. Combination ACE inhibitor and angiotensin II receptor antagonist therapy in diabetic nephropathy. *Am J Nephrol* 1999;19:1–6.
61. Mogensen CE, Neldam S, Tikkanen I, et al. Randomised controlled trial of dual blockade of renin-angiotensin system in patients with hypertension, microalbuminuria, and non-

insulin dependent diabetes: the candesartan and lisinopril microalbuminuria (CALM) study. *BMJ* 2000;321(7274): 1440–1444.
62. Taal MW, Brenner BM. Combination ACEI and ARB therapy: additional benefit in renoprotection? *Curr Opin Nephrol Hypertens* 2002;11:377–381.
63. Nishiyama A, Seth DM, Navar LG. Renal interstitial fluid concentrations of angiotensins I and II in anesthetized rats. *Hypertension* 2002;39:129–134.
64. Keane WF, Mulcahy WS, Kasiske BL, et al. Hyperlipidemia and progressive renal disease. *Kidney Int* 1991;39(suppl 31): S41–S48.
65. Klahr S, Schreiner G, Ichikawa I. The progression of renal disease. *N Engl J Med* 1988;318:1657–1666.
66. Gerritsen ME, Bloor CM. Endothelial cell gene expression in response to injury. *FASEB J* 1993;7:523–532.
67. Floege J, Alpers CE, Burns MW, et al. Glomerular cells, extracellular matrix accumulation, and the development of glomerulosclerosis in the remnant kidney model. *Lab Invest* 1992;66:485–497.
68. Kang DH, Kanellis J, Hugo C, et al. Role of the microvascular endothelium in progressive renal disease. *J Am Soc Nephrol* 2002;13:806–816.
69. Bruijn JA, de Heer E. Adhesion molecules in renal disease. *Lab Invest* 1995;72:387–394.
70. Farquhar MG, Kerjaschki D, Lundstrom M, et al. gp330 and RAP: the Heyman nephritis antigenic complex. *Ann N Y Acad Sci* 1994;737:96–113.
71. Combs HL, Shankland SJ, Setzer SV, et al. Expression of the cyclin kinase inhibitor, p27kip1, in developing and mature human kidney. *Kidney Int* 1998;53:892–896.
72. Shankland SJ. Cell cycle regulatory proteins in glomerular disease. *Kidney Int* 1999;56:1208–1215.
73. Kriz W, Gretz N, Lemley KV. Progression of glomerular diseases: Is the podocyte the culprit? *Kidney Int* 1998;54:687–697.
74. Megyesi J, Price PM, Tamayo E, et al. The lack of a functional p21(WAF1/CIP1) gene ameliorates progression to chronic renal failure. *Proc Natl Acad Sci U S A* 1999;96:10830–10835.
75. Aiello LP, Avery RL, Arrigg PG, et al. Vascular endothelial growth factor in ocular fluid of patients with diabetic retinopathy and other retinal disorders. *N Engl J Med* 1994;331:1480–1487.
76. Adler S, Chen X. Anti-Fx1A antibody recognizes a b1-integrin on glomerular epithelial cell and inhibits adhesion and cell growth. *Am J Physiol* 1992;31:F770–F776.
77. Salant DJ. The structural biology of glomerular epithelial cells in proteinuric diseases. *Curr Opin Nephrol Hypertens* 1994;3:569–574.
78. Kemeny E, Mihatsch MJ, Durmuller U, et al. Podocytes loose their adhesive phenotype in focal segmental glomerulosclerosis. *Clin Nephrol* 1995;43:71–83.
79. Ruotsalainen V, Ljungberg P, Wartiovaara J, et al. Nephrin is specifically located at the slit diaphragm of glomerular podocytes. *Proc Natl Acad Sci U S A* 1999;96:7962–7967.
80. Shih NY, Li J, Karpitskii V, et al. Congenital nephrotic syndrome in mice lacking CD2-associated protein. *Science* 1999;286:312–315.
81. Kaplan JM, Kim SH, North KN, et al. Mutations in ACTN4, encoding alpha-actinin-4, cause familial focal segmental glomerulosclerosis. *Nat Genet* 2000;24:251–256.
82. Boute N, Gribouval O, Roselli S, et al. NPHS2, encoding the glomerular protein podocin, is mutated in autosomal recessive steroid-resistant nephrotic syndrome. *Nat Genet* 2000;24:349–354.
83. Miner JH, Morello R, Andrews KL, et al. Transcriptional induction of slit diaphragm genes by Lmx1b is required in podocyte differentiation. *J Clin Invest* 2002;109:1065–1072.
84. Koziell A, Grech V, Hussain S, et al. Genotype/phenotype correlations of NPHS1 and NPHS2 mutations in nephrotic syndrome advocate a functional inter-relationship in glomerular filtration. *Hum Mol Genet* 2002;11:379–388.
85. Karle SM, Uetz B, Ronner V, et al. Novel mutations in NPHS2 detected in both familial and sporadic steroid-resistant nephrotic syndrome. *J Am Soc Nephrol* 2002;13:388–393.
86. Kawachi H, Koike H, Kurihara H, et al. Cloning of rat nephrin: expression in developing glomeruli and in proteinuric states. *Kidney Int* 2000;57:1949–1961.
87. Forbes JM, Bonnet F, Russo LM, et al. Modulation of nephrin in the diabetic kidney: association with systemic hypertension and increasing albuminuria. *J Hypertens* 2002;20:985–992.
88. Rantanen M, Palmen T, Patari A, et al. Nephrin TRAP mice lack slit diaphragms and show fibrotic glomeruli and cystic tubular lesions. *J Am Soc Nephrol* 2002;13:1586–1594.
89. Eremina V, Wong MA, Cui S, et al. Glomerular-specific gene excision in vivo. *J Am Soc Nephrol* 2002;13:788–793.
90. Benigni A, Tomasoni S, Gagliardini E, et al. Blocking angiotensin II synthesis/activity preserves glomerular nephrin in rats with severe nephrosis. *J Am Soc Nephrol* 2001;12:941–948.
91. Takeda T, McQuistan T, Orlando RA, et al. Loss of glomerular foot processes is associated with uncoupling of podocalyxin from the actin cytoskeleton. *J Clin Invest* 2001;108:289–301.
92. Regele HM, Fillipovic E, Langer B, et al. Glomerular expression of dystroglycans is reduced in minimal change nephrosis but not in focal segmental glomerulosclerosis. *J Am Soc Nephrol* 2000;11:403–412.
93. Johnson RJ, Floege J, Yoshimura A, et al. The activated mesangial cell: a glomerular "myofibroblast"? *J Am Soc Nephrol* 1992;2(suppl 2):S190–S197.
94. van Goor H, Fidler V, Weening JJ, et al. Determinants of focal and segmental glomerulosclerosis in the rat after renal ablation. Evidence for involvement of macrophages and lipids. *Lab Invest* 1991;64:754–765.
95. Klahr S, Levey AS, Beck GJ, et al. The effects of dietary protein restriction and blood-pressure control on the progression of chronic renal disease. *N Engl J Med* 1994;330:877–884.
96. Mitch WE. Dietary protein restriction in chronic renal failure: nutritional efficacy, compliance, and progression of renal insufficiency. *J Am Soc Nephrol* 1991;2:823–831.
97. Lax DS, Benstein JA, Tolbert E, et al. Effects of salt restriction on renal growth and glomerular injury in rats with remnant kidneys. *Kidney Int* 1992;41:1527–1534.
98. Oda H, Keane WF. Recent advances in statins and the kidney. *Kidney Int* 1999;71(suppl):S2–S5.
99. Remuzzi G, Bertani T. Is glomerulosclerosis a consequence of altered glomerular permeability to macromolecules? *Kidney Int* 1990;38:384–394.
100. Kipari T, Hughes J. Macrophage-mediated renal cell death. *Kidney Int* 2002;61:760–761.

101. Ishidoya S, Morrissey J, McCracken R, et al. Angiotensin II receptor antagonist ameliorates renal tubulointerstitial fibrosis caused by unilateral ureteral obstruction. *Kidney Int* 1995;47:1285–1294.
102. Nishida M, Fujinaka H, Matsusaka T, et al. Absence of angiotensin II type 1 receptor in bone marrow-derived cells is detrimental in the evaluation of renal fibrosis. *J Clin Invest* 2002;110:1859–1868.
103. Katz A, Caramori ML, Sisson-Ross S, et al. An increase in the cell component of the cortical interstitium antedates interstitial fibrosis in type 1 diabetic patients. *Kidney Int* 2002;61:2058–2066.
104. Al-Awqati Q, Oliver JA. Stem cells in the kidney. *Kidney Int* 2002;61:387–395.
105. Okada H, Inoue T, Suzuki H, et al. Epithelial-mesenchymal transformation of renal tubular epithelial cells in vitro and in vivo. *Nephrol Dial Transplant* 2000;6(15 suppl):44–46.
106. Robinson TN, Dietz WH. *Rudolph's pediatrics*. Stamford, CT: Appleton & Lange, 1996:156–159.
107. Adelman RD. Obesity and renal disease. *Curr Opin Nephrol Hypertens* 2002;11:331–335.
108. Adelman RD, Restaino IG, Alon US, et al. Proteinuria and focal segmental glomerulosclerosis in severely obese adolescents. *J Pediatr* 2001;138:481–485.
109. Kambham N, Markowitz GS, Valeri AM, et al. Obesity-related glomerulopathy: an emerging epidemic. *Kidney Int* 2001;59:1498–1509.
110. Zoja C, Corna D, Rottoli D, et al. Effect of combining ACE inhibitor and statin in severe experimental nephropathy. *Kidney Int* 2002;61:1635–1645.
111. Praga M, Hernandez E, Herrero JC, et al. Influence of obesity on the appearance of proteinuria and renal insufficiency after unilateral nephrectomy. *Kidney Int* 2000;58:2111–2118.
112. Meier-Kriesche HU, Arndorfer JA, Kaplan B. The impact of body mass index on renal transplant outcomes: a significant independent risk factor for graft failure and patient death. *Transplantation* 2002;73:70–74.
113. Wolf G, Chen S, Han DC, et al. Leptin and renal disease. *Am J Kidney Dis* 2002;39:1–11.
114. Fogo AB. The role of angiotensin II and plasminogen activator inhibitor-1 in progressive glomerulosclerosis. *Am J Kidney Dis* 2000;35:179–188.
115. Fogo A. Progression and potential regression of glomerulosclerosis. Nephrology forum. *Kidney Int* 2001;59:804–819.
116. Brown NJ, Vaughan DE, Fogo AB. The renin-angiotensin-aldosterone system and fibrinolysis in progressive renal disease. *Semin Nephrol* 2002;22(5):399–406.
117. Kiprov DD, Colvin RB, McCluskey RT. Focal and segmental glomerulosclerosis and proteinuria associated with unilateral renal agenesis. *Lab Invest* 1982;46:275–281.
118. Wikstad I, Celsi G, Larsson L, et al. Kidney function in adults born with unilateral renal agenesis or nephrectomized in childhood. *Pediatr Nephrol* 1988;2:177–182.
119. Novick AC, Gephardt G, Guz B, et al. Long-term follow-up after partial removal of a solitary kidney. *N Engl J Med* 1991;325:1058–1062.
120. Di Tullio MT, Casale F, Indolfi P, et al. Compensatory hypertrophy and progressive renal damage in children nephrectomized for Wilms' tumor. *Med Pediatr Oncol* 1996;26:325–328.
121. Argueso L, Ritchey ML, Boyle ET Jr, et al. Prognosis of patients with unilateral renal agenesis. *Pediatr Nephrol* 1992;6:412–416.
122. Bhathena DB, Julian BA, McMorrow RG, et al. Focal sclerosis of hypertrophied glomeruli in solitary functioning kidneys of humans. *Am J Kidney Dis* 1985;5:226–232.
123. Taylor CM, Milford DV, Rose PE, et al. The expression of blood group P1 in post-enteropathic haemolytic uraemic syndrome. *Pediatr Nephrol* 1990;4:59–61.
124. Pesce C, Schmidt K, Fogo A, et al. Glomerular size and the incidence of renal disease in African Americans and Caucasians. *J Nephrol* 1994;7:355–358.
125. Fogo A, Breyer JA, Smith MC, et al. Accuracy of the diagnosis of hypertensive nephrosclerosis in African Americans—a report from the African American Study of Kidney Disease (AASK) trial. *Kidney Int* 1997;51:244–252.
126. Schmidt K, Pesce C, Liu Q, et al. Large glomerular size in Pima Indians. Lack of change with diabetic nephropathy. *J Am Soc Nephrol* 1992;3:229–235.
127. Summerson JH, Bell RA, Konen JC. Racial differences in the prevalence of microalbuminuria in hypertension. *Am J Kidney Dis* 1995;26:577–579.
128. Marcantoni C, Ma LJ, Federspiel C, et al. Hypertensive nephrosclerosis in African-Americans vs Caucasians. *Kidney Int* 2002;62:172–180.
129. Agodoa LY, Appel L, Bakris GL, et al. Effect of ramipril vs amlodipine on renal outcomes in hypertensive nephrosclerosis: a randomized controlled trial. African American Study of Kidney Disease and Hypertension (AASK) Study Group. *JAMA* 2001;285:2719–2728.
130. Austin HA, Boumpas DT, Vaughan EM, et al. High-risk features of lupus nephritis: importance of race and clinical and histological factors in 166 patients. *Nephrol Dial Transplant* 1995;10:1620–1628.
131. Casanova S, Mazzucco G, Barbiano di Belgiojoso G, et al. Pattern of glomerular involvement in human immunodeficiency virus-infected patients: an Italian study. *Am J Kidney Dis* 1995;26:446–453.
132. Freedman BI, Bowden DW. The role of genetic factors in the development of end-stage renal disease. *Curr Opin Nephrol Hypertens* 1995;4:230–234.
133. Esposito C, He CJ, Striker GE, et al. Nature and severity of the glomerular response to nephron reduction is strain-dependent in mice. *Am J Pathol* 1999;54:891–897.
134. Wang Q, Hummler E, Nussberger J, et al. Blood pressure, cardiac, and renal responses to salt and deoxycorticosterone acetate in mice: role of renin genes. *J Am Soc Nephrol* 2002;13:1509–1516.
135. Yoshida H, Kuriyama S, Atsumi Y, et al. Angiotensin-I converting enzyme gene polymorphism in non-insulin dependent diabetes mellitus: risk for progression to chronic renal failure and mortality. *Kidney Int* 1996;50:657–664.
136. Marre M, Jeunemaitre X, Gallois Y, et al. Contribution of genetic polymorphism in the renin-angiotensin system to the development of renal complications in insulin-dependent diabetes. *J Clin Invest* 1997;99:1585–1595.
137. Brock JW III, Hunley TE, Adams MC, et al. Role of the renin-angiotensin system in disorders of the urinary tract. *J Urol* 1998;160:1812–819.
138. Cambien F, Poirier O, Lecerf L, et al. Deletion polymorphism in the gene for angiotensin-converting enzyme is a

potent risk factor for myocardial infarction. *Nature* 1992; 359:641–644.

139. Yoshida H, Kon V, Ichikawa I. Polymorphisms of the renin-angiotensin system genes in progressive renal diseases. *Kidney Int* 1996;50:732–744.
140. Hunley TE, Julian BA, Phillips JA III, et al. Angiotensin converting enzyme gene polymorphism: potential silencer motif and impact on progression in IgA nephropathy. *Kidney Int* 1996;49:571–577.
141. Yoshida H, Mitarai T, Kawamura T, et al. Role of the deletion polymorphism of the angiotensin converting enzyme gene in the progression and therapeutic responsiveness of IgA nephropathy. *J Clin Invest* 1995;96:2162–2169.
142. Rigat B, Hubert C, Alhenc-Gelas F, et al. An insertion/deletion polymorphism in the angiotensin I-converting enzyme gene accounting for half the variance of serum levels. *J Clin Invest* 1990;86:1343–1346.
143. Ueda S, Elliott HL, Morton JJ, et al. Enhanced pressor response to angiotensin I in normotensive men with the deletion genotype (DD) for angiotensin-converting enzyme. *Hypertension* 1995;25:1266–1269.
144. August P, Leventhal B, Suthanthiran M. Hypertension-induced organ damage in African Americans: transforming growth factor-beta(1) excess as a mechanism for increased prevalence. *Curr Hypertens Rep* 2000;2:184–191.
145. Fogo A, Glick AD, Horn SL, et al. Is focal segmental glomerulosclerosis really focal? Distribution of lesions in adults and children. *Kidney Int* 1995;47:1690–1696.
146. Tune BM, Kirpekar R, Sibley RK, et al. Intravenous methylprednisolone and oral alkylating agent therapy of prednisone-resistant pediatric focal segmental glomerulosclerosis: a long-term follow-up. *Clin Nephrol* 1995;43:84–88.
147. Schwedler SB, Gilbert T, Moreau E, et al. Nephrotoxin exposure in utero reduces glomerular number in sclerosis-prone but not sclerosis-resistant mice. *Kidney Int* 1999;56:1683–1690.
148. Lelievre-Pegorier M, Vilar J, Ferrier ML, et al. Mild vitamin A deficiency leads to inborn nephron deficit in the rat. *Kidney Int* 1998;54:1455–1462.
149. Lelievre-Pegorier M, Merlet-Benichou C. The number of nephrons in the mammalian kidney: environmental influences play a determining role. *Exp Nephrol* 2000;8:63–65.
150. Garrett PJ, Bass PS, Sandeman DD. Barker, Brenner, and babies—early environment and renal disease in adulthood. *J Pathol* 1994;173:299–300.
151. Fogo AB. Glomerular hypertension, abnormal glomerular growth and progression of renal diseases. *Kidney Int* 2000; 57(Suppl 75):S15–S21.
152. Elfenbein IB, Baluarte HJ, Gruskin AB. Renal hypoplasia with oligomeganephronia. *Arch Pathol* 1974;97:143–149.
153. Østerby R, Parving HH, Nyberg G, et al. A strong correlation between glomerular filtration rate and filtration surface in diabetic nephropathy. *Diabetologia* 1988;31:265–270.
154. Mauer SM, Steffes MW, Ellis EN, et al. Structural-functional relationships in diabetic nephropathy. *J Clin Invest* 1984;74:1143–1155.
155. Bilous RW, Mauer SM, Sutherland DER, et al. The effects of pancreas transplantation on the glomerular structure of renal allografts in patients with insulin-dependent diabetes. *N Engl J Med* 1989;321:80–85.
156. Fogo A, Hawkins EP, Berry PL, et al. Glomerular hypertrophy in minimal change disease predicts subsequent progression to focal glomerular sclerosis. *Kidney Int* 1990;38:115–123.
157. Fogo A, Hawkins EP, Verani R, et al. Focal segmental glomerulosclerosis (FGS) in renal transplants is associated with marked glomerular hypertrophy [abstract]. *J Am Soc Nephrol* 1991;2:797.
158. Fine RN. Growth hormone and the kidney: the use of recombinant human growth hormone (rhGH) in growth-retarded children with chronic renal insufficiency. *J Am Soc Nephrol* 1991;1:1136–1145.
159. Jabs K, Van Dop C, Harmon WE. Growth hormone treatment of growth failure among children with renal transplant. *Kidney Int* 1993;43:S71–S75.
160. Laine J, Krogerus L, Sarna S, et al. Recombinant human growth hormone treatment. *Transplantation* 1996;61:898–903.
161. Sasaki H, Takeda N, Kawamura I, et al. Urinary albumin excretion in short children treated with recombinant human growth hormone. *Clin Nephrol* 1996;46:6–9.
162. Chavers BM, Doherty L, Nevins TE, et al. Effects of growth hormone on kidney function in pediatric transplant recipients. *Pediatr Nephrol* 1995;9:176–181.
163. Tyler G, Berg U, Reinholt F. Acute renal graft rejection after treatment with human growth hormone. *Lancet* 1990;336: 1455–1456.
164. Kelley KW. The role of growth hormone in modulation of the immune response. *Ann N Y Acad Sci* 1990;594:95–103.
165. Fine RN, Stablein D, Cohen AH, et al. Recombinant human growth hormone post-renal transplantation in children: a randomized controlled study of the NAPRTCS. *Kidney Int* 2002;62:688–696.
166. Karlén J, Linné T, Wikstad I, et al. Incidence of microalbuminuria in children with pyelonephritic scarring. *Pediatr Nephrol* 1996;10:705–708.
167. Cerasola G, Cottone S, Mule G, et al. Microalbuminuria, renal dysfunction and cardiovascular complication in essential hypertension. *J Hypertens* 1996;14:915–920.
168. Warshaw BL, Edelbrock HH, Ettenger RB, et al. Progression to end-stage renal disease in children with obstructive uropathy. *J Pediatr* 1982;100:183–187.
169. Fogo A, Ichikawa I. Focal segmental glomerulosclerosis—a view and review. *Pediatr Nephrol* 1996;10:374–391.
170. Marinides GN, Groggel GC, Cohen AH, et al. Enalapril and low protein reverse chronic puromycin aminonucleoside nephropathy. *Kidney Int* 1990;37:749–757.
171. Marre M, LeBlanc H, Suarez L, et al. Converting enzyme inhibition and kidney function in normotensive diabetic patients with persistent microalbuminuria. *BMJ* 1987;294: 1448–1452.
172. Mathiesen ER, Hommel E, Giese J, et al. Efficacy of captopril in postponing nephropathy in normotensive insulin dependent diabetic patients with microalbuminuria. *BMJ* 1991;303:81–87.
173. Lewis EJ, Hunsicker LG, Bain RP, et al. The effect of angiotensin-converting-enzyme inhibition on diabetic nephropathy. *N Engl J Med* 1993;330:1456–1462.
174. Brenner BM, Cooper ME, de Zeeuw D, et al. Effects of losartan on renal and cardiovascular outcomes in patients

with type 2 diabetes and nephropathy. *N Engl J Med* 2001;345:861–869.

175. Lewis EJ, Hunsicker LG, Clarke WR, et al. Renoprotective effect of the angiotensin-receptor antagonist irbesartan in patients with nephropathy due to type 2 diabetes. *N Engl J Med* 2001;345:851–860.
176. Fioretto P, Steffes MW, Sutherland DE, et al. Reversal of lesions of diabetic nephropathy after pancreas transplantation. *N Engl J Med* 1998;339:69–75.
177. Hotta O, Furuta T, Chiba S, et al. Regression of IgA nephropathy: a repeat biopsy study. *Am J Kidney Dis* 2002;39: 493–502.
178. Levey A, Gassman JJ, Hall PM, et al. Assessing the progression of renal disease in clinical studies: effects of duration of follow-up and regression to the mean. *J Am Soc Nephrol* 1991;1:1087–1094.
179. Gifford RWJ. The fifth report of the Joint National Committee on detection, evaluation, and treatment of high blood pressure. *Arch Intern Med* 1993;153:154–187.
180. Keane WF, Anderson S, Aurell M, et al. Angiotensin converting enzyme inhibitors and progressive renal insufficiency. Current experience and future directions. *Ann Intern Med* 1989;111:503–516.
181. Fogo A, Kon V. Treatment of hypertension. *Semin Nephrol* 1996;16:555–566.
182. Kasiske BL, Kalil RSN, Ma JZ, et al. The effect of blood pressure treatment on the kidney in diabetes: a meta-regression analysis. *Ann Intern Med* 1993;118:129–138.
183. Maschio G, Alberti D, Janin G, et al. Effect of the angiotensin-converting-enzyme inhibitor benazepril on the progression of chronic renal insufficiency. *N Engl J Med* 1996;334:939–945.
184. Bakris GL. The effects of calcium antagonists on renal hemodynamics, urinary protein excretion, and glomerular morphology in diabetic states. *J Am Soc Nephrol* 1991;2:S21–S29.
185. Lüscher TF, Wenzel RR, Moreau P, et al. Vascular protective effects of ACE inhibitors and calcium antagonists: theoretical basis for a combination therapy in hypertension and other cardiovascular diseases. *Cardiovasc Drugs Ther* 1995;9:509–523.
186. Vlassara H. Advanced glycosylation in nephropathy of diabetes and aging. *Adv Nephrol Necker Hosp* 1996;25:303–315.
187. Meyer TW, Morelli E, Loon N, et al. Converting enzyme inhibition and glomerular size selectivity in diabetic nephropathy. *J Am Soc Nephrol* 1990;1:S64–S68.
188. Kretzler M, Cohen CD, Doran P, et al. Repuncturing the renal biopsy: strategies for molecular diagnosis in nephrology. *J Am Soc Nephrol* 2002;13:1961–1972.
189. Kassirer JP. Clinical trials and meta-analysis. What do they do for us? *N Engl J Med* 1992;327:273–274.

67

CONSERVATIVE MANAGEMENT OF CHRONIC RENAL INSUFFICIENCY

RICHARD N. FINE
DILYS A. WHYTE
IVY I. BOYDSTUN

Chronic renal insufficiency (CRI) causes substantial morbidity in virtually every major organ system of the body. Many of these complications can be controlled through diet and medications, a regimen generally termed *conservative management.* This chapter describes these therapies in detail. Moreover, CRI inevitably progresses to end-stage renal disease (ESRD), which is, by definition, a degree of renal insufficiency that requires either dialysis or renal transplantation to sustain life. Because chronic dialysis therapy replaces only some of the ultrafiltration and clearance functions of the native kidneys, the same therapies used during conservative management of CRI must be continued or enhanced during chronic dialysis therapy. Any changes in these treatments required by either peritoneal dialysis or hemodialysis are addressed in the chapters covering these specific treatments. Because renal transplantation restores normal renal function, these conservative measures can generally be discontinued at the time of the procedure, although some of the consequences of long-standing CRI must be addressed after the procedure.

GROWTH RETARDATION IN CHRONIC RENAL INSUFFICIENCY

Etiology of Growth Retardation

Growth retardation is one of the most onerous complications of CRI. The initial use of the therapeutic modalities of dialysis and transplantation was successful in extending the lives of children afflicted with ESRD, but neither treatment was completely successful in restoring normal growth.

The cause of the growth retardation has been considered to be multifactorial. Age at onset of CRI and primary renal disease are clearly correlates of the severity of growth retardation. Metabolic acidosis, inadequate nutritional (caloric) intake, anemia, and renal osteodystrophy are each identified as sufficient contributing factors. However, individual correction of each of these factors was found to be insufficient to restore normal growth rates. More recently, perturbations of the growth hormone (GH)–insulin-like growth factor (IGF) axis have been shown to be preeminent in altering normal growth patterns in children with CRI, and treatments for these abnormalities have been far more successful.

Although an unequivocal precise defect that impairs linear growth in association with reduced renal function has not been described, the following abnormalities have been identified: (a) reduction in the number of hepatic GH receptors with a concomitant reduction in circulating levels of GH-binding protein; (b) increase in the levels of various IGF-binding proteins, especially IGF-binding protein 3; and (c) reduction in "free" IGF levels. The latter presumably stimulates the epiphyseal growth plate and thus produces increments in linear height.

The classical data of Betts and McGrath (1) published more than a quarter century ago demonstrated that suboptimal growth associated with CRI was apparent during the initial 2 years of life and at the time of puberty. Accelerated growth velocity is normally present during these two time periods, with impairment adversely affecting stature. More recent data from the North American Pediatric Transplant Cooperative Study (NAPRTCS) CRI registry indicate that with current management practices accelerated growth in infants and young children with CRI is possible, but maximization of the pubertal growth spurt remains a challenge (Fig. 67.1).

Even when dialysis is initiated, growth retardation persists, and growth velocity may decrease compared to that occurring in CRI. Because peritoneal dialysis is the modality of choice for infants and young children, and hemodialysis is primarily used for adolescents, it is difficult to determine currently if either modality offers any advantage regarding increments in growth velocity.

Accelerated growth after renal transplantation occurs primarily in infants and preschool-aged children, with

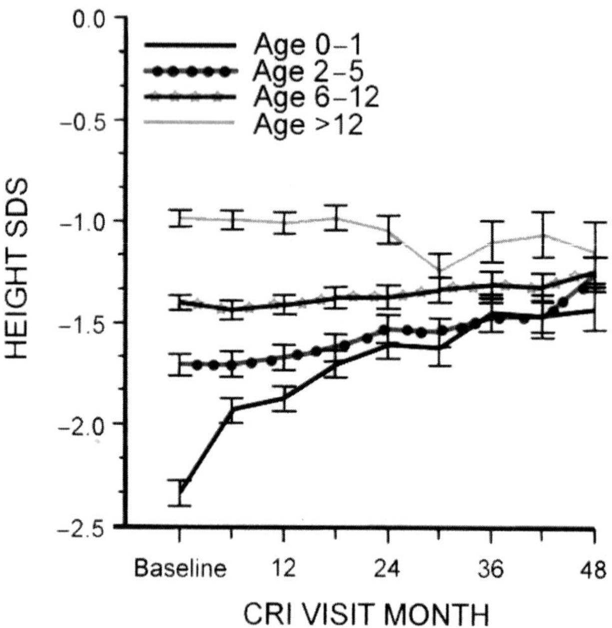

FIGURE 67.1. Change in height standard deviation score (SDS) of patients enrolled in the North American Pediatric Transplant Cooperative Study chronic renal insufficiency (CRI) registry. No improvement during puberty is demonstrated in patients who were older than 12 years of age at enrollment.

school-aged children and adolescents either maintaining normal growth velocity for age or demonstrating a worsening of standard deviation score (SDS). This pattern has not changed for more than a decade despite changes in the immunosuppressive regimens and improvement in patient and graft survival rates as shown by NAPRTCS data.

There are limited data detailing the precise variation in pubertal growth associated with CRI. Schaefer et al. (2) detailed the most extensive study, which demonstrated a reduction in the pubertal height gain in both boys and girls compared to unaffected adolescents. The length of the pubertal growth spurt was also shortened. Most children with CRI do not reach final adult height until after they have developed ESRD and have undergone successful transplantation. Data from NAPRTCS indicate that the mean Z score of 1075 individuals who were at least 19 years of age was –1.51; however, 25% had scores of –2.4 or worse, and 10% had scores higher than –3.4. Although there has been significant improvement in final adult height during the past decade, most of these children do not reach their genetic potential in final height. Importantly, much of the improvement has been related to treatment during CRI rather than growth after transplantation.

Management of Growth Retardation

Optimal management of growth retardation would entail prevention throughout the course of CRI. Because the maximum growth velocity occurs during infancy, a strategy directed toward this patient population has evolved. In addition to assiduous attention to correcting any fluid and electrolyte imbalances and concomitant acidosis, assurance of optimal caloric (nutritional) intake with supplemental nasogastric or gastrostomy tube feeding is necessary. Control of secondary hyperparathyroidism is obtained through close attention to the prevention of hypophosphatemia or hyperphosphatemia and judicious use of hydroxylated vitamin D and calcium supplementation. This regimen has been associated with normal growth patterns in young infants with CRI. For children with ESRD, there are limited data about the effects of the dialysis regimen on growth. Tom et al. (3) demonstrated an improvement in growth velocity associated with increments in hemodialysis Kt/V.

Suboptimal growth after renal transplantation has been attributed primarily to graft dysfunction, which leads to a reduction in glomerular filtration rate (GFR), and the deleterious impact of corticosteroids on growth. Data on steroid withdrawal (4) and steroid avoidance (5) after transplantation are encouraging. Improvements in SDS are not currently realized after transplantation in school-aged children and adolescents, however, and it is likely that the height centile at transplantation will be the final adult height centile. In this regard, it is encouraging that between 1987 and 2001 the mean SDS of children at the time of transplantation markedly improved (Fig. 67.2), presumably because of changes in treatment practices. This may be reflected in improvement in final adult height in this patient population in the future.

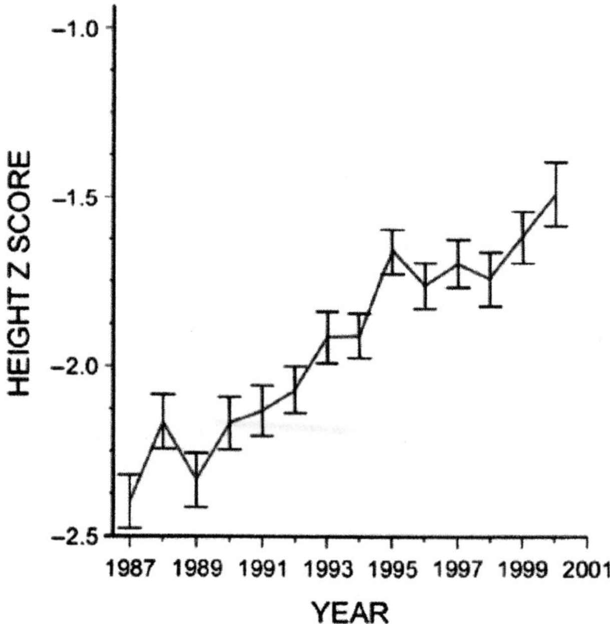

FIGURE 67.2. Height Z scores at the time of transplantation over a 15-year period from 1987 to 2001, demonstrating that height of recipients at the time of transplantation has steadily improved during this time interval.

Recombinant Human Growth Hormone

After the initial report of the safety and efficacy of recombinant human GH (rhGH) in treating children with CRI (6), a randomized, double-blind, placebo-controlled study was undertaken to obtain U.S. Food and Drug Administration (FDA) approval of the use of rhGH to improve the growth velocity of growth-retarded children with CRI and those undergoing dialysis (7). After 2 years there was a significant difference in the change in Z score between the rhGH-treated children and an untreated control group (Fig. 67.3). This led the FDA to approve the use of rhGH in this patient population. The indication for the use of rhGH in children with CRI is the presence of growth retardation (SDS more negative than –2.00) in children with irreversible renal insufficiency (GFR less than 75 mL/min/1.73 m^2). No provocative testing for GH levels is required before initiation of rhGH treatment. The dosage of rhGH that has been recommended is 0.05 mg/kg/day, 7 days per week, subcutaneously. A newer depot formulation of rhGH is likely effective, but precise recommendations for the dose and frequency are not yet available.

Before rhGH therapy is initiated, it is imperative to correct acidosis and any fluid electrolyte abnormalities, assure optimal caloric intake, and minimize the coexistence of renal osteodystrophy. Suppression of excessive secondary hyperparathyroidism [parathyroid hormone (PTH) level more than three times the normal value] is advantageous because either the response to rhGH will be suboptimal in the presence of secondary hyperparathyroidism or rhGH will accentuate the deformities of osteodystrophy. Care must be taken, however, to simultaneously prevent adynamic bone disease.

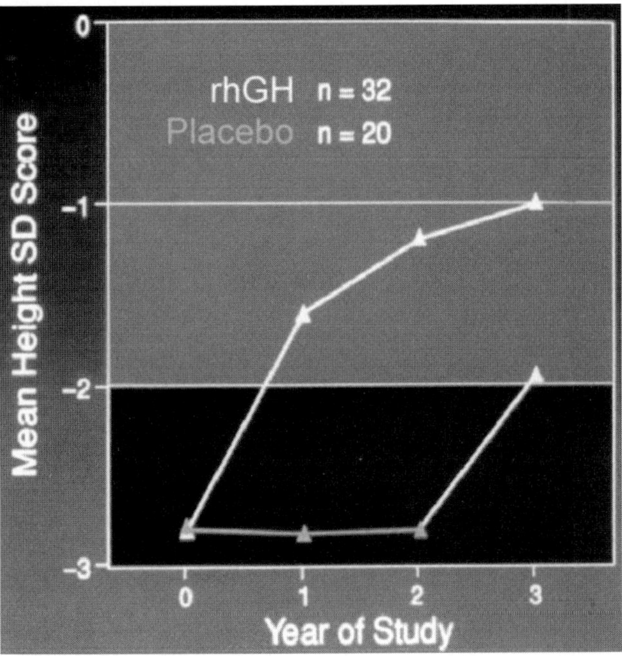

FIGURE 67.3. Change in height standard deviation (SD) score during a 2-year period of treatment with recombinant human growth hormone (rhGH) or placebo. Marked improvement in height SD score is demonstrated in the rhGH-treated group, whereas no improvement is seen in the placebo-treated group. The white line indicates patients receiving rhGH and the gray line indicates patients receiving a placebo. Those in the latter group received rhGH after 2 years.

Because of the potential adverse events of intracranial hypertension, avascular necrosis, and slipped capital femoral epiphysis associated with rhGH treatment, it is recommended that an ophthalmologic consultation and hip radiographs be obtained before initiating rhGH treatment.

During the first year of life, growth is minimally dependent on GH; therefore, limited data are available on the use of rhGH in infants younger than 2 years of age. Data from a multicenter study, however, have demonstrated the efficacy and safety of its use in infants as young as 6 months of age at initiation of therapy (8). Likewise, rhGH has been effective in adolescents at stages III and IV of puberty (9).

A dilemma that has not been resolved unequivocally is the approach to the child who reaches target height (fiftieth percentile for midparental height) after initiation of rhGH treatment. Because occasionally the child will track along the fiftieth percentile after discontinuation of rhGH, a pause of treatment has been recommended in this circumstance. Immediate resumption is indicated, however, if a significant reduction in growth velocity results.

Growth of children with CRI after long-term treatment with rhGH has demonstrated continued improvement in SDS (10). Although the greatest magnitude of increase in SDS occurs in the first and second year of rhGH treatment, continued positive change in SDS can be demonstrated for at least 5 years of treatment.

Numerous adverse events have been attributed to rhGH treatment in children with GH deficiency. Although isolated cases of some adverse events have been reported in children with CRI treated with rhGH, an NAPRTCS report noted no increased incidence of intracranial hypertension, aseptic necrosis, slipped capital femoral epiphyses, and malignancy compared with an untreated control population (11).

Early reports of the use of rhGH in an ESRD population had suggested the efficacy of its use in children undergoing peritoneal dialysis. However, a European report indicated that the effectiveness of rhGH therapy was suboptimal in children undergoing dialysis (12). Nevertheless, a multicenter study in France demonstrated that the short-term efficacy of rhGH therapy in children undergoing hemodialysis was comparable to that achieved in CRI patients (13).

As indicated previously, growth is frequently suboptimal after transplantation, especially in school-aged children and adolescents. Isolated reports and four controlled studies (14–17) (Table 67.1) have demonstrated the efficacy and safety of rhGH treatment of children after transplantation. The major concern that rhGH would either precipitate acute rejection episodes or accelerate the course of chronic

TABLE 67.1. RESULTS OF RECOMBINANT HUMAN GROWTH HORMONE (RHGH) TREATMENT IN PEDIATRIC RENAL ALLOGRAFT RECIPIENTS

		Growth (cm/yr)		
Study	No. of patients	rhGH	Control	*p* Value
Hokken-Koelega et al. (14)	5	3.9[a]	1.0	<.0001
	6	5.3	1.5	
Maxwell and Rees (15)	15[b]	8.1	3.7	<.0005
	7[c]	10.1	3.9	
Guest et al. (16)	90	7.7	4.6	<.0001
Fine et al. (17)	67	9.0	4.2	<.0001

[a]Per 6 months.
[b]Prepubertal.
[c]Pubertal.

rejection has not been substantiated in any of the controlled studies. However, rhGH is not yet currently approved by the FDA for use in renal transplant recipients with growth retardation.

DEVELOPMENTAL ABNORMALITIES ASSOCIATED WITH CHRONIC RENAL INSUFFICIENCY

Although the adverse impact of uremia on the functioning of the nervous system has been appreciated in the past, it is only more recently that the magnitude of the problem in children has been described. Baluarte and coworkers described a distinct syndrome in six children, aged 26 months to 10 years, with congenital renal disorders that was characterized by myoclonus, dysarthria, seizures, dementia, and coma (18). The syndrome was evident when there was significant renal functional impairment (GFR less than or equal to 5 to 10 mL/min/1.73 m^2) and was irreversible, despite dialysis and successful transplantation. Bale and colleagues noted similar neurologic abnormalities of seizures and intellectual impairment in three children with congenital renal abnormalities (19). The findings were observed initially when the GFR was 15 to 25 mL/min/1.73 m^2. Aluminum intoxication was implicated by Baluarte et al. (18); however, the cerebrospinal fluid aluminum concentration was measured in one child by Bale et al. (19) and was found to be normal.

The magnitude of the problem was emphasized in the report of Rotundo et al. (20), who undertook a retrospective analysis of 23 children with chronic renal failure diagnosed before 1 year of age. Of the 23 children, 20 had progressive encephalopathy characterized by developmental delay (19), microcephaly (15), hypotonia (13), seizures (13), and dyskinesia (11). A specific cause was not identified; however, four patients developed central nervous system symptoms before receiving any oral aluminum therapy, and all patients had symptoms before initiation of dialysis. All of these patients had associated significant growth impairment, and 15 of the 20 patients with progressive encephalopathy had progressive reduction in head size.

The relationship between the onset of CRI during the first year of life and subsequent developmental delay was emphasized in the report of McGraw and Haka-Ikse (21), who studied 12 boys with onset of chronic renal failure at less than 1 month of age. Developmental testing at 13 to 54 months of age in 10 of the 12 patients revealed the following: normal development in 2 of 10 (20%), developmental quotient (DQ) of 60 to 80 in 3 of 10 (30%), DQ of 40 to 60 in 4 of 10 (40%), and DQ of less than 40 in 1 of 10 (10%). Serial head circumference measurements were less than 2 standard deviations below the mean in 9 of 12 patients, and 9 of 12 patients had a history of seizures. Linear growth retardation was present in eight patients (67%). A progressive neurologic disorder occurred in one patient who did not remit after successful transplantation.

These reports implicate an adverse impact of uremia on the developing brain, because all patients had evidence of renal functional impairment during the first year of life. An additional etiologic possibility is the toxic effect of aluminum on the developing brain. All of the patients described in the report of McGraw and Haka-Ikse (21) had received aluminum-containing phosphate binders; only 4 of the 20 patients reported by Rotundo et al. (20) had not received aluminum-containing compounds.

A report by Freundlich et al. (22) described elevated aluminum levels in the brains of two infants with chronic renal failure who died in the first year of life without receiving aluminum-containing phosphate binders and implicated the infants' formula as the source of the high aluminum levels in the brain. The latter finding suggests that aluminum toxicity may be the cause of the neurologic manifestations in infants with chronic renal failure who did not receive aluminum-containing phosphate binders. Although an unequivocal relationship between neurologic impairment and aluminum toxicity does not exist, it would be prudent to avoid aluminum-containing compounds in infants with CRI and to use other phosphate-binding agents (23). Bale et al. (19) and Rotundo et al. (20) suggested that earlier initiation of dialysis and/or transplantation should be considered in infants with congenital renal abnormalities to avoid these neurologic sequelae.

A more recent follow-up report to that of McGraw and Haka-Ikse (21) from the same institution (24) was considerably less pessimistic regarding neurologic development of infants with chronic renal failure. Thirty-three children in whom chronic renal failure was detected in the first year of life were tested for neurologic function on two occasions approximately 2 years apart. Aluminum usage was exceptional, and assiduous attempts were made to optimize caloric intake. Initially, 11 of 33 children had a DQ of less than 80; 10 of 11 children were mildly delayed, and 1 child was moderately delayed in development. When last evaluated, 10 of 33 children had a DQ of less than 80; 8 of 10 children were mildly delayed, and 2 of 10 children were moderately delayed. The latter two patients had experienced cerebrovascular accidents. This incidence of developmental delay (±30%) was much lower than the 60 to 85% previously reported (25).

Additional experience continues to provide a more optimistic outlook for infants with CRI and ESRD. In 1999 Warady et al. (26) reviewed the outcome of 34 infants who began dialysis before 3 months of age. Calcium carbonate was the only phosphate binder used, and 27 of 28 infants who survived longer than 1 year received supplemental nasogastric tube feeding. At 1 year of age, the 28 patients had a mean head circumference SDS of –0.96 ± 1.2. The mental developmental score of 22 patients (79%) fell in the average range, whereas only 1 child (4%) was significantly delayed. Of 19 children retested at 4 years of age or older, 15 (79%) performed in the average range and 1 (5%) performed in the impaired rage. Of 16 patients 5 years of age or older, 15 (94%) attended school full time and in age-appropriate classrooms. Twenty-four patients received their initial kidney transplant at a mean age of 2.1 ± 0.8 years. This experience provides evidence that the combination of aggressive nutrition, elimination of aluminum as a phosphate binder, and appropriate provision of dialysis and transplantation all contribute to a favorable developmental outcome in children who have ESRD in early infancy.

This optimism regarding the neurologic development of infants with CRI and ESRD was substantiated by the report of Qvist et al. (27). These authors evaluated 33 children who received an initial renal allograft at less than 5 years of age. Twenty-nine of the patients (88%) had Finnish-type congenital nephrotic syndrome, and the mean age at initial transplant was 2.4 ± 1.1 years with a mean duration of dialysis of 1.3 ± 1.2 years. It is apparent that this group of patients would be at high risk for neurodevelopmental abnormalities. At a mean age of 8 years at follow-up, 26 of the children (79%) attended regular school and 76% had normal motor performance. Risk factors for abnormal neurodevelopment were an increased number of hypertensive crises ($p = .002$) and seizures ($p = .03$) during dialysis and not serum aluminum levels or number of septic episodes. The authors concluded that, in a previously lethal disease, the overall neurodevelopmental outcome of infants with ESRD is now reassuring.

Further evidence that current clinical practice results in acceptable neurologic development of infants with CRI and ESRD was provided by Ledermann et al. (28), who treated 20 infants (mean age, 0.34 years) with long-term dialysis and subsequent renal transplantation. Head circumference SDS improved from –1.9 at initiation of peritoneal dialysis to –0.9 at 1 year of age ($p = .015$). Fourteen of the 16 survivors (88%) achieved normal developmental milestones or attended mainstream schools.

The current clinical practice of avoiding any additional aluminum intake in infants, optimizing nutritional intake with supplemental feeding, preventing the emergence of secondary hyperparathyroidism, and avoiding hypertensive crisis should optimize neurologic development in infants with CRI and ESRD.

Limited data are available that have addressed the concern that cognitive functioning in children may be impaired during dialysis and/or renal transplantation. Brouhard et al. (29) undertook an elegant study to compare cognitive function in 62 patients with ESRD with that of their sibling controls. The controls were chosen so as to neutralize the impact of ethnicity and economic status. The average intelligence quotient rank of the patients was significantly lower than that of their siblings, and the patients tended to score lower on achievement tests than did their siblings. Increased dialysis time predicted lower scores on achievement tests. The authors concluded that factors related to ESRD are the risk factor for lower intelligence quotient and academic achievement. These data suggest that optimizing cognitive development requires limitation of the time that children experience ESRD.

The current approach to the infant with chronic renal failure includes careful surveillance of growth and head circumference with the intent to initiate dialysis once growth deviates from the normal curve. Developmental testing in infants is not sufficiently precise to warrant therapeutic intervention only on the basis of deviant test results. Abnormalities of growth and head circumference may be more precise indicators of the adverse effects of uremia. Whether the earlier initiation of ESRD care in these infants might prevent the development of the neurologic sequelae of uremia has not been completely proven. Nonetheless, this issue should be carefully considered when making clinical decisions about individual infants.

There are no definitive answers to the two other philosophical issues regarding management of the mentally challenged child with CRI. Observation of children with mild to moderate degrees of mental retardation has indicated that they do not respond as well to the imposed constraints of ESRD care as do children with normal intellectual capacity (30). The family of a mentally retarded child should be given a dispassionate assessment of the various therapeutic options. If the family decides against ESRD care, it is imperative that the health care team provide continued psychological, emotional, and medical support. Abandonment of the child and family after the decision not to embark on ESRD care could lead the family to question the wisdom of their decision.

Also, if the child presents with a history of long-standing chronic renal failure that had its onset in infancy and the child is mentally retarded, it is appropriate to assume that the child's intellectual impairment is not related to a sudden decline in renal function. It is important, however, to detail the premorbid mental capacity of the child with a sudden onset of ESRD who appears to be functioning at a subnormal level. The uremic milieu depresses cognitive function and the reality of ESRD produces psychological depression, both of which may be reversed by successful renal transplantation. A detailed analysis of the child's intellectual functioning in the premorbid state is vital before the family is counseled regarding the potential therapeutic options.

CARDIOVASCULAR ABNORMALITIES ASSOCIATED WITH CHRONIC RENAL INSUFFICIENCY

Cardiovascular disease is the leading cause of mortality in adults with ESRD, accounting for almost 50% of all deaths (31). Mortality related to cardiovascular disease is 10 to 20 times higher in adult patients with ESRD than in the general population (32). In adults with ESRD the two major risk factors for cardiovascular disease mortality are atherosclerotic coronary artery disease (CAD) and left ventricular hypertrophy (LVH) (33).

Mortality in children with CRI and ESRD is substantially lower than that reported in adult patients. Of 5039 children with CRI enrolled in the NAPRTCS CRI registry between 1994 and 2001, only 50 (2.7%) died. Of the 2361 children enrolled in the NAPRTCS dialysis registry since 1992, whose first reported course appears to be the first ever without a history of renal transplantation, the 3-year patient survival rate was 86.8 ± 1.5% (standard error). Of the 436 deaths, cardiopulmonary reasons were cited in 92 (21.1%). Patient survival among 7247 index transplant patients enrolled in NAPRTCS since 1987 (3704 given living donor organs and 2964 cadaveric organs) was 94.0 ± 0.4% at 5 years. There were 329 deaths (5.5%), with cardiopulmonary death cited in 55 (15.1%) (34).

The 1999 U.S. Renal Data System report indicated that 33% of deaths in children with ESRD were related to cardiovascular causes (35). Similarly, data on European pediatric patients who died while receiving renal replacement therapy between 1987 and 1990 indicated a cardiovascular cause of death in 51% of those on dialysis and 37% of those who had undergone transplantation (36).

Therefore, although mortality in children with CRI and ESRD does not approach the magnitude observed in adult patients, cardiovascular events are a significant cause of death. Little is known about the development of cardiovascular disease in children and adolescents with CRI and ESRD. Moreover, current treatment modalities are extending longevity into adulthood, and the factors responsible for subsequent development of clinical cardiovascular disease may be prevalent in childhood and adolescence.

In 1976 Pennisi et al. (37) noted a significant prevalence of fasting hypertriglyceridemia and hypercholesterolemia in 35 pediatric renal allograft recipients and 15 children and adolescents undergoing maintenance hemodialysis. Autopsy material from 12 children who had undergone maintenance hemodialysis and/or renal transplantation was compared to that from age-matched controls. An increased collagenous content of the intima that was possibly an early indication of CAD was noted more frequently in the patients with ESRD than in the control subjects ($p < .0006$). More recently, Goodman et al. (38) used electron beam computed tomography to screen for coronary artery calcification in 39 patients with ESRD undergoing dialysis who were 7 to 30 years of age (mean of 19 ± 7 years). None of the patients younger than 20 years of age had evidence of coronary artery calcification; however, 14 of 16 patients 20 to 30 years of age did have such evidence. These data emphasize that the factors responsible for the development of cardiovascular disease may have their origins in childhood and adolescence in those with CRI and ESRD. Scharer et al. (39) reviewed cardiac function and structure in children with CRI. The authors delineated the hemodynamic, vascular, humoral, metabolic, and toxic factors influencing cardiac function and structure in patients with CRI. Most of the available information was from studies of adult patients. Limited data were available regarding LVH and hypertension.

Morris et al. (40) in 1994 noted a reduction in left ventricular mass (LVM) in seven children undergoing dialysis after correction of anemia with recombinant human erythropoietin (rHuEpo). After transplantation this group was compared with a group who did not require rHuEpo during dialysis to determine the impact of correction of the uremic milieu on cardiovascular function. Because limited improvement was seen in the latter group after transplantation, the authors concluded that anemia had an important influence on cardiovascular function in ESRD.

In 1996 Johnstone et al. (41) described left ventricular abnormalities in 32 children, adolescents, and young adults with CRI, 10 undergoing chronic peritoneal dialysis, and 30 who had received renal transplants. The results were compared with data for 60 controls. Using echocardiographic measurement of LVM, the authors noted an increase compared to controls in 22% of the CRI group, 30% of the peritoneal dialysis group, and 63% of the transplant group. An important correlation between serum creatinine level and LVH was noted in the CRI group, which indicates that progressive uremia may correlate with increasing LVM. The incidence and severity of the LVH in the transplant group, which was not correlated with the presence of hypertension, indicates the potential for cardiovascular disease with longevity in children with ESRD.

More recently, Matteucci et al. (42) performed echocardiography, 24-hour ambulatory blood pressure monitoring (ABPM), and treadmill testing in 28 pediatric allograft recipients. LVH was found in 82% of the recipients; however, only 43% (10 of 23) of those with LVH were hypertensive by 24-hour ABPM. Unfortunately, serial evaluations were not undertaken to determine the impact of prior LVH on the posttransplantation abnormalities.

Factors prevalent during the course of CRI may affect the incidence of cardiovascular disease in pediatric patients with ESRD. Mitsnefes et al. (43) in 2000 retrospectively evaluated echocardiographic findings in 64 dialysis patients 20 months to 22 years of age. LVH was present in 75%, including 85% of those on hemodialysis and 68% of those on peritoneal dialysis. The duration of CRI before initiation of dialysis was significantly related to the severity of the LVH. The relationship between hypertension and LVH has been validated in adults, and LVH has been identified as one of the indicators of end-organ damage in children with hypertension (44). Data delineating the incidence of hypertension in children with CRI and the relationship to the development of LVH are limited.

NAPRTCS does not collect data on specific blood pressure readings; however, the latest report of NAPRTCS indicated that 37% of patients with CRI were receiving antihypertensive medications at enrollment. A special analysis of NAPRTCS data encompassing 5251 renal allograft recipients indicated that hypertension persists during the course of ESRD care (45). At 5 years after transplantation, 58% of recipients were receiving antihypertension medications.

If a precise relationship between the incidence and prevalence of hypertension and the relationship to the development of LVH in pediatric patients with CRI and ESRD is to be ascertained, more precise serial measurements of blood pressure must be obtained. The use of 24-hour ABPM has received limited attention. Sorof (46) used 24-hour ABPM in pediatric ESRD patients and noted a reclassification of more than one-third of the patients when 24-hour ABPM results were compared with casual blood pressure recordings. The author correlated 24-hour ABPM findings with a 20% incidence of LVH in transplant recipients. Similarly, Koch et al. (47) demonstrated that casual recordings were not representative of blood pressure measurements assessed by 24-hour ABPM in children undergoing dialysis. End-organ damage was also noted in patients judged normotensive by casual readings.

Because of the relationship between hyperlipidemia and CAD in the general population (48) and because CAD contributes to the 10 to 20 times greater incidence of cardiovascular mortality in adults with ESRD (32), it is important to delineate the incidence and prevalence of hyperlipidemia in pediatric patients. Querfeld (49) reviewed the problem of hyperlipidemia in children with CRI. Initial reports suggested that children with CRI have mild hypertriglyceridemia and slightly elevated serum cholesterol levels (50,51). With reduction in the GFR (10 to 20 mL/min/1.73 m^2), a decrease in high-density lipoprotein cholesterol was noted. Evaluation of 68 pediatric patients at initiation of dialysis noted that 90% had hypertriglyceridemia and 69% had hypercholesterolemia (52). Subsequently, Querfeld et al. (53) noted that 8 of 20 children (40%) with CRI had elevated lipoprotein(a) levels.

More recently, Silverstein et al. (54) analyzed the risk factors for hyperlipidemia in long-term pediatric renal allograft recipients. Of 62 pediatric recipients surviving with a functioning graft for a mean of 6.7 ± 3.1 years, more than 50% had hypercholesterolemia; 45% had high low-density lipoprotein levels and 9% had low levels of high-density lipoprotein. A prominent risk factor for posttransplantation hyperlipidemia was pretransplantation hyperlipidemia, which indicates the importance of identification and management of hyperlipidemia in children during the course of CRI. No data are available on the optimal therapeutic approach to management of hyperlipidemia in children with CRI.

Hyperhomocysteinemia has been identified as a risk factor for CAD in adult patients with CRI and ESRD (55). Limited data are available addressing this issue in a pediatric population. Schroder et al. (56) measured plasma homocysteine levels in 21 children with ESRD undergoing dialysis and compared the results with those for 234 healthy controls. The median level was 9.1 mol/L in the control population and 20 mol/L in the ESRD population. Four weeks of treatment with folic acid reduced the plasma homocysteine concentration to 12 mol/L in the patients undergoing dialysis. The potential contribution of elevated homocysteine levels to CAD in a pediatric population with CRI and ESRD remains to be identified, and an optimal approach to lowering the plasma homocysteine level requires delineation.

A consensus conference on the prevention of posttransplantation cardiovascular disease noted that "little information is available regarding long-term cardiac morbidity and mortality in pediatric solid organ recipients" (57). The following risk factors were identified: (a) pretransplantation cardiovascular disease, (b) hypertension, (c) hyperlipidemia, (d) obesity and sedentary lifestyle, (e) diabetes mellitus, and (f) hypertriglyceridemia. Guidelines were provided to manage these risk factors; however, the authors acknowledge that "further research is required to develop definitive guidelines."

One of the potential reasons for the incidence of cardiovascular morbidity and mortality in children with CRI and ESRD is the development of arrhythmias consequent to the prolongation of corrected QT interval (QTc). Prolonged QTc has been proposed as a cause of sudden infant death syndrome (58). It has also been described with electrolyte abnormalities such as hypokalemia (59) and hypocalcemia (60) and as a side effect of some medications (61).

Limited data are available delineating the incidence of prolonged QTc in children with CRI and ESRD. Bosch et al. (62) have noted a high incidence of prolonged QTc in a limited number of children with CRI and ESRD using Holter monitoring. No data are available, however, correlating serial electrocardiographic evidence of prolonged QTc, echocardiographic findings, and electrolyte abnormalities in a pediatric population with CRI and ESRD.

In summary, acute cardiovascular events lead to significant morbidity and mortality in pediatric patients with CRI and ESRD. Risk factors for the development of long-term cardiovascular disease in children with CRI and

ESRD are evident in childhood and adolescence. Limited data are available to identify these putative factors precisely so that potential therapeutic approaches could be initiated to limited long-term consequences of cardiovascular disease in a population of patients with anticipated increasing longevity. In the meantime, blood pressure, anemia, and lipid levels should be carefully controlled, and appropriate diet and exercise should be maintained in children with CRI and ESRD.

ANEMIA IN CHRONIC RENAL INSUFFICIENCY

Definition

Anemia is defined as a reduction in the red blood cell volume or hemoglobin concentration below the range of values occurring in healthy persons (63). Anemia should be addressed in patients with chronic renal disease when hemoglobin levels decline to 80% of the mean level defined for healthy subgroups (64). Generally, a significant reduction in hemoglobin concentrations develops in patients with CRI when the GFR declines below 35 mL/min/1.73 m^2 (65). Based on morbidity, mortality, and quality-of-life data, the Dialysis Outcomes Quality Initiative guidelines recommend a target range of 33 to 36% for hematocrit and 11 to 12 g/dL for hemoglobin for patients with CRI (66).

Impact of Anemia

Before the availability of rHuEpo, transfusions were required in almost all pediatric patients with ESRD. These transfusions were associated with the development of total body iron overload as well as increased exposure to HLA antigens and infectious agents. It now appears that the development of anemia, and not the accumulation of ill-defined uremic toxins, was responsible for many of the symptoms seen in CRI and ESRD. Appetite, physical activity, libido, school attendance in children, and in, some studies, performance on intelligence quotient testing are all improved after the correction of anemia using rHuEpo. Because children with CRI have complex conditions that contribute to morbidity, the impact of anemia may best be assessed by improvements that occur with correction of hemoglobin concentrations. It has been proposed that anemia contributes to impaired cognitive function, exercise intolerance, growth retardation, and school absences. Studies of adult and pediatric patients have shown improved memory, concentration, and speed of information processing in cognitive evaluations, improved cardiac function, improved exercise performance, and decreased mortality after partial correction of anemia (67,68). In anemic children without kidney disease, investigators have demonstrated elevations in heart rate with physical activity (69), blunted cardiovascular response to exercise, and decreased peak exercise duration (70) compared to nonanemic age-matched control children. Growth impairment has been documented in children with anemia due to sickle cell disease and thalassemia, with improved growth in thalassemia patients on hypertransfusion protocols (71,72). Studies of children with anemia secondary to kidney disease have involved mostly children with ESRD, and have found improved exercise capacity with correction of hematocrit from 21.7 to 33.4% (73). Objective improvement in exercise tolerance and subjective improvement in physical performance, general health, and school attendance was reported by Morris et al. (74) for this population. The effects of correction of anemia on growth and nutritional status in children with CRI were reviewed by Jabs (75). Although most patients reported subjective improvements in appetite and food, correction of mean hematocrit from 21 to 31% did not improve weight gain, anthropometric measures, or SDS height scores in any age group. In children who had had multiple transfusions, the levels of previously formed panel-reactive antibodies and cytotoxic antibodies to a T-cell panel decreased after the initiation of rHuEpo treatment and the cessation of transfusions (76,77). A lower level of preformed antibodies may allow this group of children to be transplanted more readily. Montini et al. evaluated brainstem auditory evoked responses and peripheral nerve conduction velocity at baseline and during rHuEpo treatment (78). At baseline, five of nine children evaluated had abnormal auditory evoked responses, and in four of them the responses normalized after the hematocrit increased. In contrast, there was no improvement in peripheral nerve conduction velocity. An additional benefit of rHuEpo treatment is a decrease in uremic coagulopathy. The bleeding time as measured by the Ivy method improved significantly during rHuEpo treatment (78,79). The improved bleeding time and platelet aggregation (79) may decrease uremic bleeding, including gastrointestinal blood loss.

Causes of Anemia

Anemia in children with CRI may be secondary to inadequate erythropoiesis due to insufficient production of erythropoietin by diseased kidneys (80) or to iron deficiency (81). Children with CRI are at increased risk for development of iron deficiency for several reasons. There is often decreased appetite with progressive disease or poor iron intake due to dietary restrictions. In addition, only a small percentage of ingested iron is actually absorbed by the gut, and the amount is further decreased by medications, including phosphate binders, prescribed to be taken with meals. In addition to poor intake, the annual iron loss via the gastrointestinal tract has been estimated to be 0.9 g/1.73 m^2 in predialysis pediatric patients (82). Not only is red cell production inadequate, but red cell survival is shortened (83), and often iatrogenic blood loss as well as occult gastrointestinal bleeding occur. Contributing factors that inhibit effective erythropoiesis include infection, severe hyperparathyroidism (84), and coexisting acute and chronic inflammation (85).

After successful renal transplantation, anemia may be present in a significant number of patients, with reports indicating that from 12 to 39% of kidney transplant patients have persistent anemia (86,87). Data concerning anemia in pediatric kidney transplant recipients are unavailable. In patients with renal insufficiency of the allograft, inadequate production of erythropoietin may play a role. Iron deficiency may be present at the time of transplantation or may develop over the subsequent months (88). Special consideration must be given to the potential effects of immunosuppressive agents in the development of chronic as well as acute anemia. Azathioprine and mycophenolate mofetil may cause anemia associated with leukopenia and thrombocytopenia (89) but may also exert a selective erythroid toxicity (90). Children younger than 6 years of age treated with mycophenolate mofetil were more likely to develop anemia and other side effects of this drug than were older children (91). Microangiopathic hemolytic anemia may be caused by cyclosporine (92), tacrolimus (93), or OKT3 (muromonab-CD3) (94), often in association with hypertension, thrombocytopenia, and acute renal failure. This process may be reversed by withdrawal of the drug and treatment of the hypertension (89). Minor ABO incompatibility between recipient and donor may also result in hemolytic anemia in as many as 14 to 20% of cases (95). Clinically, hemolysis may begin 3 to 22 days after transplantation, with spontaneous remission occurring after 7 to 10 days, and patients treated with cyclosporine may be at increased risk (96). Other drugs used in the posttransplantation period may also be implicated, especially angiotensin-converting enzyme (ACE) inhibitors, which may cause a fall in hematocrit of 10% or more that is reversible with discontinuation of the drug (97). Kidney transplant patients with anemia must also be evaluated for gastrointestinal blood loss, occult infection, chronic inflammation, and vitamin B_{12} deficiency.

Evaluation of Anemia

Careful evaluation of anemia is warranted to assure effective therapy for its correction. A complete blood count with red cell indices, hemoglobin concentration and hematocrit, and reticulocyte count, and a review of the smear provide initial information and a baseline. Stool should be tested for occult blood, and coexisting conditions such as hyperparathyroidism or systemic inflammatory disease should be considered. Parameters for assessment of iron status include serum iron level and total iron-binding capacity. Transferrin saturation (TSAT) can be calculated by multiplying the serum iron value by 100 and dividing by the total iron-binding capacity. Serum iron level and TSAT measure the iron immediately available for hemoglobin synthesis, with a target for TSAT of above 20%. TSAT values lower than 20% indicate the need for iron replacement therapy. Serum ferritin levels reflect total body iron stores, but because ferritin is also an acute-phase reactant, results may be affected by systemic inflammation. Ferritin target values in the absence of significant inflammation are higher than 100 ng/mL (98). Adequate iron stores and TSAT with a low reticulocyte count may reflect inadequate erythropoietin production. In patients who do not respond to adequate iron and erythropoietin therapy, folic acid and vitamin B_{12} levels should be checked. Drugs that suppress bone marrow function must also be considered, including ACE inhibitors, antibiotics, and immunosuppressive agents. Elevated PTH levels may also diminish the efficacy of erythropoietin (99,100).

Treatment of Anemia

Laboratory evidence of iron deficiency begins with decreases in serum ferritin levels, followed by a fall in serum iron and increase in total iron-binding capacity. These findings are accompanied by a fall in the calculated TSAT. If iron deficiency persists, hypochromia and microcytic anemia develop. Effective therapy with iron results in reticulocytosis by 72 hours, which peaks by 5 to 7 days. Increased hemoglobin concentrations are detectable by 4 to 30 days, with repletion of stores after 1 to 3 months of continuous effective supplementation (101).

Oral iron therapy should target delivery of 2 to 3 mg/kg/day of elemental iron in two to three divided doses. Iron is best absorbed without food and is recommended to be taken 1 to 2 hours after meals, which would also avoid interference in absorption by phosphate binders. Side effects include gastric irritation, constipation, and diarrhea. For patients with ongoing blood loss or inability to tolerate or absorb adequate iron via the oral route, parenteral iron therapy should be considered. Especially after the initiation of hemodialysis, in which significant additive blood loss occurs with each treatment, even well-tolerated oral supplementation is often inadequate to maintain iron stores. Parenteral iron supplements are currently available as iron dextran, iron gluconate, and iron sucrose. Use of iron dextran requires administration of a test dose due to risk of allergic or anaphylactic reaction, which is less likely with iron gluconate. Iron sucrose preparations have been used in Europe and Japan and are under review by the FDA for use in the United States. Protocols for parenteral iron therapy are available in the literature (98).

Erythropoietin use is almost universal in children with advanced CRI. NAPRTCS reports showed that 96% of children were receiving erythropoietin at the time of initiation of chronic dialysis, which resulted in an increase of hematocrits to a median of 31% at 6-month follow-up (102). Erythropoietin can be administered either intravenously, subcutaneously, or intraperitoneally. The subcutaneous route is the most common method of administration for children with CRI and for those receiving chronic peritoneal dialysis (103). Subcutaneous injections of erythropoietin are generally given once or twice per week. This method of administration leads to a prolonged half-life and a decrease in the total weekly dose (104). Reported total initial weekly doses have ranged between 30 and 300 U/kg, whereas maintenance dosages varied between 60 and 600 U/kg/wk (105). Most pediatric patients respond to between 100 and 200 IU/kg/wk (106–110). The large dosage variation appears to be related to several factors: the target hematocrit; ongoing blood loss (either gastrointestinal or via dialysis) (82); patient age, with younger children requiring higher dosages than older individuals (105,109); presence of infection or inflammation (110); and, in some studies, hyperparathyroidism (99,100,111). The best predictor of response to erythropoietin appears to be the patient's iron status.

The intravenous route is generally reserved for children receiving chronic hemodialysis. Although the subcutaneous route is more cost effective, amelioration of the discomfort associated with that method of administration is generally used to justify intravenous administration in those with a hemodialysis access site. The initial dose should be sufficient to eliminate the need for transfusions while increasing the hematocrit slowly enough to allow adjustments in volume status and antihypertensive medications to maintain a normal blood pressure. A reasonable starting dose is 40 to 60 U/kg administered intravenously at each hemodialysis treatment three times a week (98). The dose of rHuEpo required to maintain the hematocrit in the target range varies with patient age. Children younger than 5 years of age frequently require higher weekly doses than older children and adults (greater than 300 U/kg vs. 80 to 120 U/kg) (109,112). In one multicenter European trial of rHuEpo in hemodialysis patients 2 to 21 years of age, the median weekly maintenance rHuEpo dose varied from 136 U/kg in those over 15 years to 321 U/kg in children younger than 5 years of age (109). Similar results have been found in a multicenter U.S. trial (112).

Intraperitoneal administration was developed for peritoneal dialysis patients and was found to be most effective if the agent was instilled in small volume into a "dry" peritoneal cavity where absorption could be maximized (113). Subsequent studies have shown that approximately 7% of the medication may be adsorbed onto plastic components of the dialysis delivery system (114). Although some studies have shown that erythropoietin can be administered effectively via the intraperitoneal route to patients receiving chronic peritoneal dialysis (115), there is concern about the side effects of this method and its cost effectiveness (115–117).

A longer-lasting formulation of an erythropoiesis-stimulating drug, darbepoietin alpha, has been studied and its pharmacokinetic profile seems to be similar in adults and children (118). This formulation has a terminal half-life two to four times longer than that of the traditional formulation, which permits less frequent dosing. Long-term studies designed to determine optimal administration in children are ongoing.

ELECTROLYTE DISORDERS IN CHRONIC RENAL INSUFFICIENCY

With advancing CRI, the total number of remaining functional nephrons is reduced, which requires the residual nephrons to compensate by increasing their fractional excretion of solutes to maintain homeostasis (119). Fluid and electrolyte balance is generally well maintained until 75% of function is lost, due to compensatory mechanisms that develop as nephron mass declines. Limitations to this adaptation are related to the magnitude and time frame for adjustment in filtered load. Gradual changes are met by appropriate adjustments in fractional excretion. Sudden changes in volume status or solute load may result in loss of homeostasis, because already compensating nephrons cannot respond instantaneously (120). In addition, the degree of adaptation to nephron loss depends on the substance that must be handled by the kidney. No adaptive mechanism exists for clearance of urea and creatinine; hence, the serum concentration increases almost inversely with the fall in GFR. For other substances, such as phosphate and hydrogen ion, there is significant adaptation by residual nephrons, which maintain serum concentrations at normal physiologic values until only approximately 25% of function remains. Adaptation for sodium and potassium handling is relatively complete until GFR falls to very low levels (121,122).

Water Balance

Depending on the cause of CRI, patients may have a fixed volume of urine output. There may be difficulty in excreting an acute water load due to loss of filtration or renal injury, which results in defects of normal diluting mechanisms. Conversely, and perhaps more commonly in children, a significant concentrating defect may be present, as seen in patients with sickle cell nephropathy, juvenile nephronophthisis, or obstructive uropathy. Even with a very low GFR, the kidneys filter 14 L of plasma per day, which can lead to a large urine volume if water reabsorption mechanisms cannot respond appropriately to concentrate urine. In addition, there remains an obligate urine output volume necessary to excrete the daily filtered load. Some patients maintain fairly steady fluid balance even in advanced insufficiency, in part due to an intact thirst mechanism if the child is old enough and has free access to water. Difficulties arise when these children are challenged by an acute dehydrating illness such as gastroenteritis or poor intake from pharyngitis, or when they are stressed iatrogenically by being restricted to nothing by mouth before a procedure, or conversely, suffer fluid overload from injudicious use of intravenous fluids.

In CRI, defective urinary concentrating ability may be the result of one or more impaired mechanisms, including tubular resistance to antidiuretic hormone. Vasopressin-resistant hyposthenuria in patients with CRI caused by primary tubular or interstitial disorders has been characterized by Holliday et al. (122). As CRI progresses, there develops an increased osmotic diuresis per residual nephron as fractional excretion of solutes rises to compensate for a decreased number of functional units. This adaptation results in continual osmotic diuresis and hyposthenuria (123). There may be structural anatomic derangement of renal tubules and medullary vasculature impairing the development of hypertonic interstitium, necessary for appropriate concentrating ability (123,124). Conversely, the functional defect affecting water and solute clearance in CRI in response to a fluid challenge is characterized by impairment in the ability to increase urinary volume after water loading. This is in part due to a decreased ability to dilute urine due to a fixed ratio of free water clearance to GFR (123).

Sodium Balance

Sodium balance is generally maintained in CRI by a progressive increase in the fractional excretion of sodium by remaining nephrons (125). This increase in sodium excretion is due to decreased sodium reabsorption by both the proximal and distal tubules in CRI (126) but is poorly understood. Water diuresis leads to increased sodium excretion because of a limited capacity of the distal nephron to reduce tubular fluid sodium concentration; therefore sodium excretion becomes dependent on urine flow rate (127). Children with polyuria may thus have difficulty conserving sodium and develop a salt-wasting state that requires careful supplementation. Clinically, hyponatremia may develop acutely due to a significant free water load or gradually due to depletion from chronic urinary losses. Use of diuretics, antihypertensive agents, and prostaglandin synthesis inhibitors alters sodium handling in normal and diseased kidneys. Urinary tract obstruction or infection may result in tubular hyporesponsiveness to aldosterone, described in infants with hyperkalemia and hyponatremia (128). One further concern regarding sodium balance involves removal of significant amounts of NaCl by peritoneal dialysis, especially in infants, which results in a clinically significant NaCl deficit (123).

Conversely, hypernatremia may be seen from an excess exogenous sodium load. Fractional excretion of sodium cannot exceed 20 to 30% of the filtered load in normal or diseased kidneys (129). If remaining nephrons have already reached maximal sodium excretion capacity, no further compensation can take place with further increases in sodium load. If some reserve remains, nephrons require time to increase sodium excretion and reestablish sodium balance.

Potassium Balance

Potassium handling in healthy and diseased kidneys involves reabsorption of almost all the filtered load by the proximal tubule and loop of Henle, with distal nephron secretion determining potassium excretion in the urine (130,131). Up to 90% of daily dietary potassium intake is secreted by the kidneys in normal individuals. As CRI progresses, potassium homeostasis is maintained by increasing distal tubular potassium secretion by remaining nephrons (132,133). With significant loss of kidney function, increased potassium secretion occurs through the colon (134–137), with as much as 35% of dietary potassium excreted in the stool (135). Aldosterone stimulates increasing sodium-potassium exchange in both the distal tubule (138,139) and colonic mucosa (140,141).

Hyperkalemia may result from increased dietary load that exceeds the ability of the compensatory mechanisms to maintain homeostasis. Certain drugs may lead to significant elevations in serum potassium through, for example, competitive inhibition of aldosterone by spironolactone, inhibition of distal potassium secretion by triamterene or amiloride, or decrease in remaining glomerular filtration by ACE inhibitors (142). ACE inhibitors may also cause transient pseudohypoaldosteronism, which contributes to their hyperkalemic effects (143). Repair of obstructive uropathy in infants may result in a similar phenomenon (144,145). Acute metabolic acidosis may create life-threatening hyperkalemia by moving intracellular potassium to the extracellular compartment in patients who maintain a fragile balance while well. Some patients with CRI secondary to diabetes mellitus or interstitial nephritis have been determined to have low plasma renin and aldosterone levels, which lead to hyperkalemia in excess of that usually associated with their level of renal failure (146,147). In children with CRI, the renin-aldosterone axis and potassium handling were studied by Rodriguez-Soriano and colleagues, who found hyperkalemia in 13% of 23 children studied. These hyperkalemic children had low aldosterone levels and plasma renin activity, without overt salt wasting (148). CRI patients with sickle cell disease, lupus nephritis, or a kidney transplant may develop hyperkalemia due to diminished distal tubular secretory capacity (149). Chronic obstructive uropathy may lead to tubular resistance to aldosterone (150), which puts these patients at particular risk for hyperkalemia and salt wasting.

Hypokalemia may be present in patients with tubular defects involving potassium loss, such as renal tubular acidosis or Fanconi syndrome. These patients may require potassium supplementation, although careful monitoring and adjustments must be made as renal function declines. Iatrogenic hypokalemia may also develop through the use of diuretics, especially in patients with poor nutritional status.

Acid-Base Balance

Impairment of mechanisms responsible for normal acid-base balance in CRI include abnormal reabsorption of filtered bicarbonate, reduction in renal ammonia synthesis, decreased excretion of titratable acid, and decreased acidification of tubular luminal fluid by the distal nephron (130,151). When GFR declines below 50% of normal, systemic metabolic acidosis becomes a significant clinical feature (152). Bicarbonate reabsorption per unit GFR is reduced in humans with CRI (130) and is further reduced by hyperkalemia, increased extracellular fluid volume, and hyperparathyroidism (153–155). Declining reabsorption of bicarbonate is clinically important in that it limits the effectiveness of base therapy to correct acidosis (155). Other patients with CRI due to tubular defects may have bicarbonate wasting, which is seen in proximal forms of renal tubular acidosis.

Although net ammonia production per remaining proximal tubule has been demonstrated to increase in response to nephron loss (156,157), as CRI progresses the compensation becomes inadequate and absolute ammonia excretion declines (158). Structural abnormalities may also lead to disruption of the tubulomedullary ammonium concentration gradient, decreasing ammonium trapping, which results in ammonium excretion (158,159). Excretion of titratable acid and distal urinary acidification generally remain well preserved as CRI progresses (142) but may also be decreased in advanced disease. The titratable acid excretion remains relatively normal primarily through increased excretion of phosphate per remaining nephron (160). Eventually, fractional excretion of phosphate cannot increase further, so that total urinary titratable acid excretion diminishes (120).

Therapy for acid-base disturbances involves correction of acidosis through oral base therapy, because persistent acidosis may adversely influence growth. A serum bicarbonate level of 20 to 22 mEq/L should be maintained, and sudden increases in endogenous hydrogen ion production through catabolic states, volume depletion, and phosphate deficiency should be avoided (123).

Renal Osteodystrophy

The kidney plays a major role in mineral homeostasis. Calcium, phosphorus, and magnesium balance are maintained via the kidney. The substances 1,25-dihydroxyvitamin D_3 and 24,25-dihydroxyvitamin D_3 are synthesized within the kidney, and PTH is degraded and cleared by the kidney. Hence, it is easy to see how renal failure can affect bone development and maintenance. In chronic renal failure, secondary hyperparathyroidism develops because of several factors. There is resistance to the calcemic action of PTH, low calcitriol levels, hyperphosphatemia, and downregulation of PTH bone cell receptors (161,162). High-low bone turnover and histologic as well as radiologic changes are the resultant features of renal osteodystrophy. The goal is to initiate a therapeutic intervention before endosteal resorption leads to osteitis fibrosa and fractures.

Secondary hyperparathyroidism can be controlled in several ways. The two most important mechanisms are adequate hydroxylated vitamin D replenishment and correction of hyperphosphatemia and hypocalcemia. Synthesis of 1,25-dihydroxyvitamin D_3 from 25-dihydroxyvitamin D_3 is stimulated by hypocalcemia, PTH, and decreased dietary intake of phosphate. Without sufficient 1,25-dihydroxy vitamin D_3, intestinal absorption of calcium is reduced, which causes hypocalcemia. Hypocalcemia then allows for increased PTH formation (163–165). Initial studies were performed on patients undergoing regular dialysis treatment, and it was noted that intravenous administration of calcitriol suppressed PTH secretion (166,167). Subsequent studies demonstrated that both intravenous and oral calcitriol administration reduced PTH secretion. The available forms of vitamin D are dihydrotachysterol, 25-hydroxyvitamin D_3 (calcifediol), 1 α-hydroxyvitamin D_3, and 1,25-dihydroxyvitamin D_3 (calcitriol), all of which have been shown to reduce PTH secretion.

The role of hyperphosphatemia in the development of secondary hyperparathyroidism has been demonstrated in several studies (167,168). Prevention of hyperphosphatemia can be achieved with the use of phosphate binders such as calcium carbonate, calcium acetate, and noncalcium binders (Renagel). The use of calcium-containing binders helps to increase calcium levels and thus suppresses PTH secretion. Aluminum-based binders should be avoided in the pediatric age group, especially in infants, because of the increased possibility of aluminum toxicity in renal failure (169,170). Restriction of dietary phosphorus also decreases hyperphosphatemia as well as PTH secretion (171).

Another mechanism to control secondary hyperparathyroidism is the use of calcimimetic drugs to decrease the secretion of PTH. These drugs stimulate the calcium-sensing receptors in the parathyroid glands, making them more sensitive to extracellular calcium. Initial studies of therapy with these medications indicated that plasma levels of intact PTH were decreased in uremic patients (172,173), and further investigations into their benefits are in progress.

Parathyroidectomy should be considered in patients when levels of intact PTH are more than five to seven times the upper limit of normal in the presence of hypercalcemia after assiduous medical management has failed. Coexistent abnormal radiologic findings and metastatic calcification provide additional indications (174).

Serum alkaline phosphatase activity has been demonstrated to correlate with histologic features of osteitis fibrosa (165,175). Monitoring the activity of this bone isoenzyme may be more specific in the management of patients with renal osteodystrophy; however, patients receiving rhGH may also have an increase in alkaline phosphatase unrelated to bone disease (175,176).

PROTEIN RESTRICTION IN PREVENTION OF PROGRESSION OF CHRONIC RENAL INSUFFICIENCY IN CHILDREN

Reduction in dietary protein has been associated with delayed progression of CRI (177,178) as a result of a decrease in one or more of the following: uremia (179), metabolic acidosis, hypertension, hyperkalemia, or renal osteodystrophy (179,180). Restriction in protein intake leads to a reduction in levels of metabolites that may be detrimental to the kidney, such as phosphates, sulfates, sodium, and potassium. Definitive correlation between protein restriction and progression of CRI in humans has not been clearly established, however. Initial animal studies demonstrated that a high-protein diet was associated with an increased incidence of interstitial damage and hypertension as well as a higher mortality rate (180,181). The pathogenesis was thought to involve hyperfiltration that led to increased glomerular pressure and ultimately to glomerular sclerosis (182). The baboon model, however, did not show this association (183). Human studies in which protein intake was restricted to a level of 0.6 to 1.1 g/kg/day produced variable results (184,185).

The pathophysiology of fasting involves breakdown of stored proteins into amino acids, which are required for (hepatic) gluconeogenesis (186). Feeding induces anabolism and thus suppression of protein degradation. This occurs with or without stimulation of protein synthesis (187). As a result of this response, lean body mass is preserved and nitrogen balance is maintained (188,189). Protein restriction leads to decreased amino acid oxidation and use of essential amino acids, which thereby produces suppression of protein degradation and synthesis. In CRI, protein restriction thus theoretically would reduce the amount of protein byproducts. In addition, acidosis, a factor leading to growth impairment, would also be diminished (190).

Restriction of dietary protein in childhood raises concern for impaired growth in comparison with that of older children and adults, because growing children require a higher protein intake (191). Growth factors such as IGF-1 are necessary for normal bone growth (192). Both animal and human studies implicate IGF-1 in mediation of hyperfiltration and glomerular hypertrophy (193). In children, restricted protein intake has been found to be associated with decreased IGF-1 levels (194). However, further studies are necessary to determine the effect of IGF-1 on CRI progression.

The Modification of Diet in Renal Disease study in adults demonstrated that consumption of low-protein diets of approximately 0.6 g/kg/day was not associated with any physical changes such as changes in midarm circumference or body weight (185). None of the patients enrolled in this study appeared to have suffered malnutrition. However, analysis of the data on protein restriction revealed minimal benefit in reducing the rate of progression of renal disease (195). The European Study Group for Nutritional Treatment of Chronic Renal Failure in Childhood found that consumption of a low-protein diet with a protein level of 0.8 to 1.1 g/kg/day did not have a deleterious effect on height in children with CRI; however, no correlation between protein restriction and progression of CRI was established (196). Studies have demonstrated that the use of low-protein diets supplemented with ketoacids slowed progression to renal failure (197). These supplements increase the energy intake, which is required in renal failure. Limited data are available on the efficacy of this approach in children.

Proteinuria has been implicated in the causal pathway of renal failure (198). Studies have shown that the progression of CRI centers on impaired glomerular permselectivity to plasma macromolecules, such as proteins (199), which is thought to be due to long-standing glomerular hypertension. High glomerular capillary pressure may increase the radii of pores within the glomerular basement membrane, which leads to excessive ultrafiltration of plasma proteins in the proximal tubule lumen. Furthermore, this alteration may be partially mediated by angiotensin II, and the proteins may be potentially nephrotoxic (200), giving rise to the inflammatory component leading to CRI progression. In addition, upregulation of various genes that encode proinflammatory and vasoactive molecules occurs as a result of protein reabsorption. Inflammatory mediators such as endothelin-1 (201,202), as well as cytokines such as RANTES (*r*egulated upon *a*ctivation, *n*ormal *T* cell *e*xpressed and *s*ecreted) and MCP-1 (monocyte chemotactic protein-1), have all been shown to be produced in response to this protein reabsorption (203,204). These factors may play a significant role in the pathogenesis of renal scarring (205). In addition to the aforementioned processes, telomere shortening has now been proposed as another cause of deterioration in renal function. At a crucial point in cell division, if the telomere is too short, cell senescence and finally apoptosis will result (206).

ACE inhibitors are useful therapeutic agents in the reduction of proteinuria associated with progression of CRI (207). This therapeutic effect of ACE inhibitors was initially observed in patients with renal disease secondary to scleroderma and later was demonstrated in animal models (208–210). The animal studies suggested that the antiproteinuric effect of ACE inhibitors may be due to reduced glomerular hydraulic pressure resulting from a decrease in one or more of the following factors: postglomerular arteriolar resistance, GFR, and filtration fraction (211). Angiotensin II, however, may produce an increase in glomerular capillary hydraulic pressure via vasoconstriction of the afferent arterioles. These data demonstrate that the mechanism by which ACE inhibitors reduce proteinuria is a decrease in glomerular capillary hydraulic pressure. Remuzzi et al. showed that ACE inhibitors also improved glomerular basement permselectivity (212).

In clinical practice, it is difficult to separate proteinuria and hypertension as two distinct risk factors for progression of CRI. Early studies attempted to evaluate this concept in diabetic patients with CRI. In these clinical trials, diabetic patients treated with captopril were found to have a decreased incidence of CRI, independent of blood pressure changes (213). Later studies examining the use of enalapril in non–insulin-dependent diabetes mellitus demonstrated stabilization of renal function as well as proteinuria (214,215). Furthermore, the Ramipril Efficacy in Nephropathy trial demonstrated a correlation between improved renal function and reduction in proteinuria in nondiabetic adult patients with nephropathy (216).

The European Study Group for Nutritional Treatment of Chronic Renal Failure in Childhood analyzed the nutritional status of children in the mid-1990s and concluded that proteinuria and hypertension were independent predictors of progression of renal disease (196). This study showed that children with decreased protein excretion had a slower progression to CRI. In addition, lower blood pressure was associated with a better creatinine clearance.

In addition to the ACE inhibitors, angiotensin II receptor antagonists (ARAs) are another class of antihypertensive agents. The mechanism of action involves the renin-angiotensin system, as with the ACE inhibitors. Specifically, the ARAs block the angiotensin II type 1 receptor, which leads to a reduction in blood pressure. Unlike the ACE inhibitors, the ARAs do not typically accentuate kinin activity or enhance prostaglandin synthesis (217). Therefore, ARAs appear to have an antiproliferative effect.

ARAs are currently considered to be an additional class of agents useful in reduction of proteinuria. Lafayette and colleagues (218) were among the first to demonstrate ARAs to be effective in reducing the progression of renal injury in rats with a five-sixths nephrectomy. This study demonstrated that both the ACE inhibitors, enalapril, and the ARA losartan decreased proteinuria as well as blood pressure. Other studies demonstrated that candesartan, another ARA, prevented the development of proteinuria (219). ARAs also are being used in combination with ACE inhibitors to maximize the antiproteinuric effect produced by the administration of each agent (220).

Therefore, currently the control of hypertension, the reduction in the magnitude of proteinuria using ACE inhibitors and/or ARAs, and the potential minimization of hyperfiltration by ACE inhibitors and ARAs are used to modulate the progression of CRI in children. These treatments are widely used despite the lack of controlled studies demonstrating efficacy in this patient population.

HEALTH MAINTENANCE AND IMMUNIZATIONS IN CHRONIC RENAL INSUFFICIENCY

Children who have chronic diseases are seen frequently in medical facilities, and general health issues are sometimes overlooked. It is essential that primary care providers continue to monitor these children for routine health maintenance and preventive medicine issues. Similarly, these children should be encouraged to participate in educational, social, and athletic activities appropriate for age, developmental level, and physical capabilities.

The provision of routine immunizations to children with CRI and ESRD has been shown to be safe and generally effective, even after renal transplantation. Thus, as much as possible, these immunizations should be provided at routine intervals, in a strategy that permits the best opportunity for adequate response (221,222). Immunizations that are routinely administered to children include diphtheria and tetanus toxoids and pertussis vaccine, measles-mumps-rubella vaccine, varicella vaccine, *Haemophilus influenzae* type b vaccine, and hepatitis B virus vaccine. Children with chronic diseases often receive influenza and pneumococcal vaccines. In some cases, booster immunizations are necessary. Antibody responses of children with CRI and ESRD to several currently recommended vaccines have been variable (223–226). Possible explanations for the reduced protection include lower seroconversion rate due to immunocompromise related to chronic disease or to the concomitant use of immunosuppressive medications, lower peak antibody titers, and a more rapid decline of antibody levels as a consequence of diminished production or loss of immunoglobulins in urine or in peritoneal dialysate (227–231).

Diphtheria-pertussis-tetanus vaccine is routinely administered to infants and diphtheria-tetanus boosters are given throughout life. Some concerns have been raised about their immunostimulatory effects after transplantation. However, a study of 42 children with renal transplants demonstrated safety and a protective response in 95% (237). Interestingly, a study of 71 hemodialysis patients with an unknown previous immunization history revealed only a 38% protective conversion rate after a single diphtheria-tetanus immunization, which suggests a worse response on dialysis than after transplantation (234). Thus, not only should immunization be ensured before transplantation, but protective antibody levels should be ascertained frequently.

Varicella vaccine has been available in Europe for over 15 years but has only more recently been made available in the United States. Varicella is a potentially fatal infection in immunosuppressed individuals (238). Pretransplantation vaccination of children is successful in preventing or mitigating the disease (239). Pretransplantation vaccination is generally successful and cost effective (236,240). Even posttransplantation vaccination seems to be safe and reasonably effective (241).

Hepatitis B vaccination of patients who have CRI or are receiving dialysis is frequently less successful than that of normal individuals, and increased vaccine administration, change of route of administration, or the use of adjuvant immunomodulating therapy have been suggested (224, 225,232).

The most commonly administered form of the pneumococcal vaccine contains 23 antigens from pneumococcal serotypes. The vaccine is generally given only once, when the patient reaches at least 2 years of age. However, revaccination should be considered for children younger than 10 years of age who are at risk for severe pneumococcal disease, such as those with CRI, particularly those receiving chronic peritoneal dialysis. Revaccination should also be considered in older children maintained on chronic peritoneal dialysis for more than 6 years. Administration to children with CRI or those on dialysis is successful in the majority of cases, but protection seems to decline rapidly (233), and failures have been reported (235). Provision after kidney transplantation seems to be at least safe (233,242).

Influenza vaccine has been recommended for children with chronic renal disease, including those who have CRI and those who have undergone transplantation (221,222, 243). The vaccine is generally given annually in the fall, and young children may need repeated doses.

In general, therefore, children with CRI should receive routine immunizations. Even live virus vaccines appear to be safe after transplantation, and no increased incidence of rejection has been reported after immunostimulation due to the immunization. Vigilance with regard to sustained protection is important in these children.

REFERENCES

1. Betts PR, Magrath G. Growth patterns and dietary intake of children with chronic renal insufficiency. *BMJ* 1974;2:189–193.
2. Schaefer F, Seidel C, Binding A, et al. Pubertal growth in chronic renal failure. *Pediatr Res* 1990;28:5–10.
3. Tom A, McCauley L, Bell L, et al. Growth during maintenance hemodialysis: impact of enhanced nutrition and clearance. *J Pediatr* 1999;134(4):464–471.
4. Ellis D. Growth and renal function after steroid-free tacrolimus-based immunosuppression in children with renal transplants. *Pediatr Nephrol* 2000;14:689–694.
5. Sarwal MM, Yorgin PD, Alexander S, et al. Promising early outcomes with a novel, complete steroid avoidance immunosuppression protocol in pediatric renal transplantation. *Transplantation* 2001;72:13–21.
6. Koch VH, Pippe BM, Nelson PA, et al. Accelerated growth after recombinant human growth hormone treatment of children with chronic renal failure. *J Pediatr* 1989;115:365–371.
7. Fine RN, Kohaut EC, Brown D, et al. Growth in children with chronic renal failure: report of a multicenter randomized double-blind placebo-controlled study. *J Pediatr* 1994;124:374–382.
8. Fine RN, Attie KM, Kuntze J, et al. The Genetech Collaborative Study Group. Recombinant human growth hormone in infants and young children with chronic renal insufficiency. *Pediatr Nephrol* 1995;9:451–457.
9. Hokken-Koelega AC, Stjnen T, De Ridder MA, et al. Growth hormone treatment in growth-retarded adolescents after renal transplant. *Lancet* 1994;343:1313–1317.
10. Fine RN, Kohaut E, Brown D, et al. Long-term treatment of growth retarded children with chronic renal insufficiency, with recombinant human growth hormone. *Kidney Int* 1996;49:781–785.
11. Fine RN, Ho M, Tejani A, et al. Adverse events with rhGH treatment of CRI and ESRD patients. *J Pediatr* 2003;142:539–545.
12. Wuhl E, Haffner D, Schaefer F, et al. The German Study Group for Growth Hormone Treatment in Children with Chronic Renal Failure. Short children on dialysis treatment respond less to growth hormone than patients with chronic renal failure prior to dialysis. *Pediatr Nephrol* 1996;10:294–298.
13. Berard E, Crosnier H, Six-Beneton A, et al. Recombinant human growth hormone treatment of children on hemodialysis. *Pediatr Nephrol* 1998;12:304–310.
14. Hokken-Koelega A, Stijnen T, De Jong R, et al. A placebo-controlled, double blind trial of growth hormone treatment in prepubertal children after renal transplant. *Kidney Int* 1996;49:S128–S134.
15. Maxwell H, Rees L. Randomized controlled trial of recombinant human growth hormone in prepubertal and pubertal renal transplant recipients. *Arch Dis Child* 1998;79:481–487.
16. Guest G, Berard E, Crosnier H, et al. Effects of growth hormone in short children after renal transplantation. *Pediatr Nephrol* 1998;12:437–446.
17. Fine RN, Stablein D, Cohen AH, et al. Recombinant human growth hormone post-renal transplantation in children: a randomized controlled study of the NAPRTCS. *Kidney Int* 2002;62:688–696.
18. Baluarte HJ, Gruskin AB, Hiner LB, et al. Encephalopathy in children with chronic renal failure. *Proc Clin Dial Transplant Forum* 1977;7:95.
19. Bale JF Jr, Siegler RL, Bray P, et al. Encephalopathy in young children with moderate chronic renal failure. *Am J Dis Child* 1980;134:581.
20. Rotundo A, Nevins TE, Lipton M, et al. Progressive encephalopathy in children with chronic renal insufficiency in infancy. *Kidney Int* 1982;21:486.
21. McGraw ME, Haka-Ikse K. Neurologic-developmental sequelae of chronic renal failure in infancy. *J Pediatr* 1985;106:579.
22. Freundlich M, Zilleruelo G, Arbitol C, et al. Infant formula as a cause of aluminum toxicity in neonatal uraemia. *Lancet* 1985;2:527.
23. Salusky IB, Coburn JW, Foley J, et al. Effects of oral calcium carbonate on control of serum phosphorus and changes in plasma aluminum levels after discontinuation of aluminum-containing gels in children receiving dialysis. *J Pediatr* 1986;108:767.
24. Geary DF, Haka-Ikse K. Neurodevelopmental progress of young children with chronic renal disease. *Pediatrics* 1989;84:68.
25. Polinsky MS, Kaiser BA, Stover JB, et al. Neurologic development of children with severe chronic renal failure from infancy. *Pediatr Nephrol* 1987;1:157.
26. Warady BA, Belden B, Kohaut E, et al. Neurodevelopmental outcome of children initiating peritoneal dialysis in early infancy. *Pediatr Nephrol* 1999;13:759–765.
27. Qvist E, Pihko H, Fagerudd P, et al. Neurodevelopmental outcome in high-risk patients after renal transplantation in early childhood. *Pediatr Transplant* 2002;6:53–62.

28. Ledermann SE, Scanes ME, Fernando ON, et al. Long-term outcome of peritoneal dialysis in infants. *J Pediatr* 2000;136:24–29.
29. Brouhard BH, Donaldson LA, Lawry KW, et al. Cognitive functioning in children on dialysis and post-transplantation. *Pediatr Transplant* 2000;4:261–267.
30. Francis VR, Fine RN, Korsch BM, et al. Physiologic and social adjustment to external hemodialysis and renal homotransplantation in 42 children. *Proc Eur Dial Transplant Assoc* 7:366.
31. The USRDS 1998 annual report causes of death. *Am J Kidney Dis* 1998;32(suppl 1):S81–S88.
32. Foley RN, Parfrey PS, Sarnak MJ, et al. Clinical epidemiology of cardiovascular disease in chronic renal disease. *Am J Kidney Dis* 1998;32(suppl 3):S112–S119.
33. Levy D, Garrison RJ, Savage DD, et al. Prognostic implications of echocardiographically determined left ventricular mass in the Framingham heart study. *N Engl J Med* 1990;322:1561–1566.
34. Seikaly M, Ho PL, Emmett L, et al. The 12th annual report of the North American Pediatric Renal Transplant Cooperative Study: renal transplantation from 1987 through 1998. *Pediatric Transplant* 2001;5:215–231.
35. The USRDS 1998 annual report. Pediatric end-stage renal disease. *Am J Kidney Dis* 1998;32(suppl 1):S98–S108.
36. Ehrich JMH, Loirat C, Brunner FP, et al. Report on management of renal failure in children in Europe XXII, 1991. *Nephrol Dial Transplant* 1992;7(suppl 2):36–42.
37. Pennisi AJ, Heuser ET, Mickey MR, et al. Hyperlipidemia in pediatric hemodialysis and renal transplant patients: associated with coronary artery disease. *Am J Dis Child* 1976;130:957–961.
38. Goodman WG, Goldin J, Kuizon BD, et al. Coronary-artery calcification in young adults with end-stage renal disease who are undergoing dialysis. *N Engl J Med* 2000;342:1478–1483.
39. Scharer K, Schmidt KG, Soergel M, et al. Cardiac function and structure in patients with chronic renal failure. *Pediatr Nephrol* 1999;13:951–965.
40. Morris KP, Skinner JR, Hunter S, et al. Cardiovascular abnormalities in end stage renal failure: the effect of anaemia or uraemia? *Arch Dis Child* 1994;71:119–122.
41. Johnstone LM, Jones CL, Grigg LE, et al. Left ventricular abnormalities in children, adolescents, and young adults with renal disease. *Kidney Int* 1996;50:998–1006.
42. Matteucci MC, Giordano U, Calzolari A, et al. Left ventricular hypertrophy, treadmill tests, and 24-hour blood pressure in pediatric transplant patients. *Kidney Int* 1999;56:1566–1570.
43. Mitsnefes MM, Daniels SR, Schwartz SM, et al. Severe left ventricular hypertrophy in pediatric dialysis: prevalence and predictors. *Pediatr Nephrol* 2000;14:898–902.
44. Bostom AD, Brown RS Jr, Chavers BM, et al. Prevention of post-transplant cardiovascular disease—report and recommendations of an ad hoc group. *Am J Transplant* 2002;2:491–500.
45. Sorof JM, Sullivan EK, Tejani A, et al. Antihypertensive medication and renal allograft failure: a North American Pediatric Renal Transplant Cooperative Study report. *J Am Soc Nephrol* 1999;10:1324–1330.
46. Sorof JM. Ambulatory blood pressure monitoring in pediatric end-stage renal disease: chronic dialysis and transplantation. *Blood Press Monit* 1999;4:171–174.
47. Koch VH, Furusawa EA, Ignes E, et al. Ambulatory blood pressure monitoring of chronically dialyzed pediatric patients. *Blood Press Monit* 1999;4:213–216.
48. Foley RN, Parfrey PS, Sarnak MJ, et al. Clinical epidemiology of cardiovascular disease in chronic renal disease. *Am J Kidney Dis* 1998;32(suppl 3):S112–S119.
49. Querfeld U. Disturbances of lipid metabolism in children with chronic renal failure. *Pediatr Nephrol* 1993;7:749–757.
50. Berger M, James GP, Davis ER, et al. Hyperlipidemia in uremic children: response to peritoneal dialysis and hemodialysis. *Clin Nephrol* 1978;9:19–24.
51. Papadopoulou ZL, Sandler P, Tina LU, et al. Hyperlipidemia in children with chronic renal insufficiency. *Pediatr Res* 1981;15:887–891.
52. Querfeld U, Salusky IB, Nelson P, et al. Hyperlipidemia in pediatric patients undergoing peritoneal dialysis. *Pediatr Nephrol* 1998;2:447–452.
53. Querfeld U, Lang M, Friedrich JB, et al. Lipoprotein (a) serum levels and apolipoprotein (a) phenotypes in children with chronic renal disease. *Pediatr Res* 1993;34:772–776.
54. Silverstein DM, Palmer J, Polinsky MS, et al. Risk factors for hyperlipidemia in long-term pediatric renal transplant recipients. *Pediatr Nephrol* 2000;14:105–110.
55. Dennis VW, Robinson K. Homocysteinemia and vascular disease in end-stage renal disease. *Kidney Int* 1996;50:S11–S17.
56. Schroder CH, de Boer AW, Giesen A, et al. Treatment of hyperhomocystinemia in children on dialysis by folic acid. *Pediatr Nephrol* 1999;13:583–585.
57. Bostom AD, Brown RS, Chavers BM, et al. Prevention of post-transplant cardiovascular disease-report and recommendations of an ad hoc group. *Am J Transplant* 2002;2:491–500.
58. Jervell A, Lange-Nielsen F. Congenital deaf-mutism, functional heart diseases, with prolongation of the QT interval and sudden death. *Am Heart J* 1957;54:598.
59. Williams MJ, Hammond-Tooke GD, Restieaux NJ, et al. Hypokalemic periodic paralysis with cardiac arrhythmia and prolonged QT interval. *Aust N Z J Med* 1995;25:549.
60. Huang TC, Cecchin FC, Mahoney P, et al. Corrected QT interval (QTc) prolongation and syncope associated with pseudohypoparathyroidism and hypocalcemia. *J Pediatr* 2000;136:404–407.
61. Brandriss MW, Richardson WS, Barold SS, et al. Erythromycin-induced QT prolongation and polymorphic ventricular tachycardia (torsades de pointes): case report and review. *Clin Infect Dis* 1994;18:995–998.
62. Bosch A, Ulmer HE, Keller HE, et al. Electrocardiographic monitoring in children with chronic renal failure. *Pediatr Nephrol* 1999;4:140–144.
63. Schwartz E. The anemias. In: Behrman RE, Kliegman RM, Jenson HB, eds. *Nelson textbook of pediatrics*, 16th ed. Philadelphia: W.B. Saunders Company, 2000:1461.
64. National Kidney Foundation, Kidney Disease Outcomes Quality Initiative. Clinical practice guidelines for anemia of chronic kidney disease, 2000:21.
65. McGonigle RJS, Boineau FG, Beckman B, et al. Erythropoietin and inhibitors of in vitro erythropoiesis in the development of anemia in children with renal disease. *J Lab Clin Med* 1985;105:449–458.
66. National Kidney Foundation, Kidney Disease Outcomes Quality Initiative. Clinical practice guidelines for anemia of chronic kidney disease, 2000:27–32.

67. Temple RM, Deary IJ, Winney RJ, et al. Recombinant erythropoietin improves cognitive function in patients maintained on chronic ambulatory peritoneal dialysis. *Nephrol Dial Transplant* 1995;10:1733–1783.
68. Yorgin PD, Belson A, Al-Uzri AY, et al. The clinical efficacy of higher hematocrit levels in children with chronic renal insufficiency and those undergoing dialysis. *Semin Nephrol* 2001;21(5):451–462.
69. Nelson M, Bakaliou F, Trivedi A, et al. Iron-deficiency anemia and physical performance in adolescent girls from different ethnic backgrounds. *Br J Nutr* 1994;72:427–433.
70. Kapoor RK, Kumar A, Chandra M, et al. Cardiovascular responses to treadmill testing in anemia. *Indian Pediatr* 1997;34:607–612.
71. Kramer MS, Rooks Y, Washington L, et al. Pre- and postnatal growth and development in children with sickle cell anemia. *J Pediatr* 1980;96:857–860.
72. Kattamis C, Touliatos N, Haidas S, et al. Growth of children with thalassemia and effect of different transfusion regimens. *Arch Dis Child* 1970;45:502–505.
73. Martin GR, Ongkingo JR, Turner ME, et al. Recombinant erythropoietin (Epogen) improves cardiac exercise performance in children with end-stage renal disease. *Pediatr Nephrol* 1993;7:276–280.
74. Morris KP, Sharp J, Watson S, et al. Non-cardiac benefits of human recombinant erythropoietin in end-stage renal failure and anemia. *Arch Dis Child* 1993;69:580–586.
75. Jabs K. The effects of recombinant human erythropoietin on growth and nutrition status. *Pediatr Nephrol* 1996;10:324–327.
76. Rigden SP, Montini G, Morris M, et al. Recombinant human erythropoietin therapy in children maintained by haemodialysis. *Pediatr Nephrol* 1990;4:618–622.
77. Grimm PC, Sinai-Trieman L, Sekiya NM, et al. Effects of recombinant human erythropoietin on HLA sensitization and cell mediated immunity. *Kidney Int* 1990;38:12–18.
78. Montini G, Zacchello G, Baraldi E, et al. Benefits and risks of anemia correction with recombinant human erythropoietin in children maintained by hemodialysis. *J Pediatr* 1990;117:556–560.
79. Fabris F, Cordiano I, Randi ML, et al. Effect of human recombinant erythropoietin on bleeding time, platelet number and function in children with end-stage renal disease maintained by haemodialysis. *Pediatr Nephrol* 1991;5:225–228.
80. Eschbach JW. The anemia of chronic renal failure: pathophysiology and the effects of recombinant erythropoietin. *Kidney Int* 1989;35:134–148.
81. Parker PA, Izard MW, Maher JF, et al. Therapy of iron deficiency anemia in patients on maintenance dialysis. *Nephron* 1979;23:181–186.
82. Muller-Wiefel DE, Sinn H, Gilli G, et al. Hemolysis and blood loss in children with chronic renal failure. *Clin Nephrol* 1990;8:481–486.
83. Eschbach JW, Funk DD, Adamson J, et al. Erythropoiesis in patients with renal failure undergoing chronic dialysis. *N Engl J Med* 1967;276:653–658.
84. Potasman I, Better OS. The role of secondary hyperparathyroidism in the anemia of chronic renal failure. *Nephron* 1983;33:229–231.
85. Adamson JW, Eschbach JW. Management of the anemia of chronic renal failure with recombinant erythropoietin. *Q JM* 1989;73:1093–1101.
86. Miles AM, Markell MS, Daskalakis P, et al. Anemia following renal transplantation: erythropoietin response and iron deficiency. *Clin Transplant* 1997;11(4):313–315.
87. Lorenz M, Kletzmayr J, Perschl A, et al. Anemia and iron deficiencies among long-term renal transplant recipients. *J Am Soc Nephrol* 1992;13(3):794–797.
88. Moore LW, Smith SO, Winsett RP, et al. Factors affecting erythropoietin production and correction of anemia in kidney transplant recipients. *Clin Transplant* 1994;8(4):358–364.
89. Aroldi A. Musculoskeletal, ocular and hematological complications. In: Kahan BD, Ponticelli C, eds. *Principles and practice of renal transplantation.* Martin Dunitz Ltd, 2000;711–714.
90. McGrath BP, Ibels LS, Raik E, et al. Erythroid toxicity of azathioprine: macrocytosis and selective marrow hypoplasia. *QJM* 1975;44(173):57–63.
91. Bunchman T, Navarro M, Broyer M, et al. The use of mycophenolate mofetil suspension in pediatric renal allograft recipients. *Pediatr Nephrol* 2001;16(12):978–984.
92. Nizze H, Mihatsch MJ, Zollinger HU, et al. Cyclosporine-associated nephropathy in patients with heart and bone marrow transplants. *Clin Nephrol* 1988;30(5):248–260.
93. Trimarchi HM, Troung LD, Brennan S, et al. FK 506-associated thrombotic microangiopathy: report of two cases and review of the literature. *Transplantation* 1999;67(4):539–543.
94. Doutrelepont JM, Abramowicz D, Florquin S, et al. Early recurrence of hemolytic uremic syndrome in a renal transplant patient during prophylactic OKT3 therapy. *Transplantation* 1992;53(6):1378–1383.
95. Povlsen JV, Rasmussen A, Hansen HE, et al. Acquired haemolytic anemia due to isohemagglutinins of donor origin following ABO-minor incompatible kidney transplantation. *Nephrol Dial Transplant* 1990;5(2):148–151.
96. Ramsey G. Red cell antibodies arising from solid organ transplants. *Transfusion* 1991;31:76–86.
97. Vlahakos DV, Canzanello VJ, Madaio MP, et al. Enalapril-associated anemia in renal transplant recipients treated for hypertension. *Am J Kidney Dis* 1991;17(2):199–205.
98. NKF-DOQI clinical practice guidelines for the treatment of anemia of chronic renal failure. National Kidney Foundation-Dialysis Outcomes Quality Initiative. *Am J Kidney Dis* 1997;30(4 suppl 3):S194–S240.
99. Seeherunvong W, Rubio L, Abitbol CL, et al. Identification of poor responders to erythropoietin among children undergoing hemodialysis. *J Pediatr* 2001;138:710–714.
100. Van Damme-Lombaerts R, Herman J. Erythropoietin treatment in children with renal failure. *Pediatr Nephrol* 1999;13:148–152.
101. Schwartz E. The anemias. In: Behrman RE, Kliegman RM, Jenson HB, eds. *Nelson textbook of pediatrics*, 16th ed. Philadelphia: W.B. Saunders Company, 2000;1470–1472.
102. Neu AM, Ho PL, McDonald RA, et al. Chronic dialysis in children and adolescents. The 2001 NAPRTCS annual report. *Pediatr Nephrol* 2002;17:656–663.
103. Warady BA, Hébert D, Sullivan EK, et al. Renal transplantation, chronic dialysis, and chronic renal insufficiency in

children and adolescents. The 1995 annual report of the North American Pediatric Renal Transplant Cooperative Study. *Pediatr Nephrol* 1997;11:49–64.

104. Levin N, Lazarus J, Nissenson A. The National Cooperative rHu Erythropoietin Study Group. National Cooperative rHu Erythropoietin Study in patients with chronic renal failure—an interim report. *Am J Kidney Dis* 1993;22(suppl 1):3–12.
105. Jabs K, Harmon W. Recombinant human erythropoietin therapy in children on dialysis. *Adv Ren Replace Ther* 1996;3:24–36.
106. Navarro M, Alonso A, Avilla J, et al. Anemia of chronic renal failure: treatment with erythropoietin. *Child Nephrol Urol* 1991;11:146–151.
107. Ongkingco J, Ruley E, Turner M. Use of low-dose erythropoietin in end-stage renal disease: experience in children receiving continuous cyclic peritoneal dialysis. *Am J Kidney Dis* 1991;18:446–450.
108. Brant JR, et al. Safety and efficacy of erythropoietin in children with chronic renal failure *Pediatr Nephrol* 1999;13:143–147.
109. Scigalla P. Effect of recombinant human erythropoietin treatment on renal anemia and body growth of children with end-stage renal disease. In: Gurland H, Moran J, Samtleben W, et al., eds. *Erythropoietin in renal and non-renal anemias*. Basel: Karger, 1991:201–211.
110. Hymes L, SM H, Clowers B. Impaired response to recombinant human erythropoietin therapy in children with peritonitis. *Dial Transplant* 1994;23:462–463.
111. McGonigle R, Wallin J, Husserl F, et al. Potential role of parathyroid hormone as an inhibitor of erythropoiesis in the anaemia of renal failure. *J Lab Clin Med* 1984;104:1016–1026.
112. Jabs K, Alexander S, McCabe D, et al. Primary results from the U.S. multicenter pediatric recombinant erythropoietin study. *J Am Soc Nephrol* 1994;5:456.
113. Reddingius R, Schröder C, Koster A, et al. Pharmacokinetics of recombinant erythropoietin in children treated with continuous peritoneal dialysis. *Eur J Pediatr* 1994;153:850–854.
114. Schroder CH, Swinkels LM, Reddingius RE, et al. Adsorption of erythropoietin and growth hormone to peritoneal dialysis bags and tubing. *Perit Dial Int* 2001;21:90–92.
115. Kausz AT, Watkins SL, Hansen C, et al. Intraperitoneal erythropoietin in children on peritoneal dialysis: a study of pharmacokinetics and efficacy. *Am J Kidney Dis* 1999;34: 651–656.
116. Montini G, Zacchello G, Perfumo F, et al. Pharmacokinetics and hematologic response to subcutaneous administration of recombinant human erythropoietin in children undergoing long-term peritoneal dialysis: a multicenter study. *J Pediatr* 1993;122:297–302.
117. Ateshkadi A, Johnson CA, Oxton LL, et al. Pharmacokinetics of intraperitoneal, intravenous, and subcutaneous recombinant human erythropoietin in patients on continuous ambulatory peritoneal dialysis. *Am J Kidney Dis* 1993;21:635–642.
118. Lerner G, Kale AS, Warady BA, et al. Pharmacokinetics of darbepoetin alfa in pediatric patients with chronic kidney disease. *Pediatr Nephrol* 2002;17:933–937.
119. Bricker NS, Fine LG, Kaplan M, et al. "Magnification phenomenon" in chronic renal disease. *N Engl J Med* 1978;299:1287–1293.
120. Morrison G, Murray TG. Electrolyte, acid base and fluid homeostasis in chronic renal failure. *Med Clin North Am* 1981;65:429–447.
121. Mackenzie HS, Taal MW, Luyckx VA, et al. Adaptation to nephron loss. In: Brenner BM, ed. *Brenner & Rector's the kidney*. Philadelphia: W.B. Saunders Company, 2000:1901–1942.
122. Holliday MA, Egan TJ, Morris RC Jr, et al. Pitressin-resistant hyposthenuria in chronic renal disease. *Am J Med* 1967;42:378–387.
123. Rodriguez-Soriano J, Arant BS, Brodehl J, et al. Fluid and electrolyte imbalances in children with chronic renal failure. *Am J Kidney Dis* 1986;7:268–274.
124. Fine LG, Salehmoghaddam S. Water homeostasis in acute and chronic renal failure. *Semin Nephrol* 1984;4:289–294.
125. Bricker NS, Shapiro MS, Levine MM, et al. Physiology and pathology of electrolyte metabolism in chronic renal disease. In: Seldin DW, Giebish G, eds. *The kidney: physiology and pathophysiology*. New York: Raven, 1985:1837–1862.
126. Hayslett JP, Kashgarian M, Epstein SH, et al. Mechanism of change in the excretion of sodium per nephron when renal mass is reduced. *J Clin Invest* 1969;48:1002–1006.
127. Coleman AJ, Arias M, Carter NW, et al. The mechanism of salt wastage in chronic renal disease. *J Clin Invest* 1966;45:1116–1125.
128. Rodriguez-Soriano J, Vallo A, Oliveros R, et al. Transient pseudohypoaldosteronism secondary to obstructive uropathy in infancy. *J Pediatr* 1983;103:375–380.
129. Kleeman CR, Oken R, Heller RJ, et al. The renal regulation of sodium and potassium in patients with chronic renal failure (CRF) and the effect of diuretics on excretion of these ions. *Ann N Y Acad Sci* 1966;139:520–539.
130. Hayslett JP. Functional adaptation to reduction in renal mass. *Physiol Rev* 1979;59:137–164.
131. Bengele HH, Evan A, McNamara ER, et al. Tubular sites of potassium regulation in the normal and uninephrectomized rat. *Am J Physiol* 1978;234:F146–F153.
132. Giebisch G. Some reflections on the mechanism of renal tubular transport of potassium. *Yale J Biol Med* 1975;48:315–366.
133. Schon DA, Silva P, Hayslett JP, et al. Mechanism of potassium excretion in renal insufficiency. *Am J Physiol* 1974; 227:1323–1330.
134. Bastl C, Hayslett JP, Binder HJ, et al. Increased large intestinal secretion of potassium in renal insufficiency. *Kidney Interact* 1977;12:8–16.
135. Hayes CP, McLeod MI, Robinson R, et al. An extra-renal mechanism for the maintenance of potassium balance in severe CRF. *Trans Assoc Am Physicians* 1967;80:207–216.
136. Van Ypersele C. Potassium homeostasis in renal failure. *Kidney Int* 1977;11:491–504.
137. Fine LG, Yanagowa N, Schultze RG, et al. Functional profile of the isolated uremic nephron. Potassium adaptation in the rabbit cortical collecting duct. *J Clin Invest* 1979; 64:1033–1043.
138. Schrier RW, Regal EM. Influence of aldosterone on sodium, water, and potassium metabolism in chronic renal disease. *Kidney Int* 1972;1:156–168.
139. Hays CP, McLeod MF, Robinson RR, et al. An extrarenal mechanism for the maintenance of potassium balance in

severe chronic renal failure. *Trans Assoc Am Physicians* 1967;80:207–216.

140. Berl T, Katz FH, Henrich WL, et al. Role of aldosterone in the control of sodium excretion in patients with advanced chronic renal disease. *Kidney Int* 1978;14:228–235.
141. Bia MJ, DeFronzo R. Extrarenal potassium homeostasis. *Am J Physiol* 1981;240:F257–F268.
142. Chan L, Alfrey AC. Chronic renal failure: manifestations and pathogenesis. In: Schrier RW, ed. *Renal and electrolyte disorders*. Philadelphia: Lippincott-Raven, 1997:507–543.
143. Wassner SJ. Conservative management of chronic renal insufficiency. In: Holliday MA, Barratt TM, Avner ED, eds. *Pediatric nephrology*, 3rd ed. Baltimore: Williams & Wilkins, 1994;1314–1338.
144. Klahr S, Harris K, Purkerson ML, et al. Effects of obstruction on renal functions. *Pediatr Nephrol* 1988;3:34–42.
145. Rodriguez-Soriano J, Vallo A, Oliveros R, et al. Transient pseudohypoaldosteronism secondary to obstructive uropathy in infancy. *J Pediatr* 1983;103:375–380.
146. Schambelan M, Stockist JR, Biglieri EG, et al. Isolated hypoaldosteronism in adults: a renin-deficiency syndrome. *N Engl J Med* 1972;287:573–578.
147. Schambelan M, Sebastian A, Biglieri EG, et al. Prevalence, pathogenesis, and functional significance of aldosterone deficiency in hyperkalemic patients with chronic renal insufficiency. *Kidney Int* 1980;17:89–101.
148. Rodriguez-Soriano J, Vallo A, Sanjuro P, et al. Hyporeninemic hypoaldosteronism in children with chronic renal failure. *J Pediatr* 1986;109:476–482.
149. Battle DC, Arruda JAL, Kurtzman NA, et al. Hyperkalemic distal tubular acidosis associated with obstruction. *N Engl J Med* 1981;304:373–379.
150. Windmer B, Gerhardt RE, Harrington JT, et al. Serum electrolyte and acid-base composition. The influence of graded degrees of chronic renal failure. *Arch Intern Med* 1979;139:1099–1102.
151. Arruda JA. Acidosis of renal failure. *Semin Nephrol* 1981;1:275–280.
152. Muldowney FP, Donohoe JF, Carrol DV, et al. Parathyroid acidosis in uremia. *QJM* 1972;41:321–342.
153. Purkerson ML, Lubowitz H, White RW, et al. On the influence of extracellular fluid volume expansion on bicarbonate reabsorption in the rat. *J Clin Invest* 1969;48:1754–1760.
154. Sastrasinh S, Tanen RL. Effect of plasma potassium on renal NH3 production. *Am J Physiol* 1983;244:F383–F391.
155. Narins RG. The renal acidoses. In: Brener BM, Stein JH, eds. *Contemporary issues in nephrology: acid-base and potassium homeostasis*. New York: Churchill Livingstone, 1978; 30–64.
156. Schoolwerth AC, Sandler RS, Hoffman PM, et al. Effects of nephron reduction and dietary protein content on renal ammoniagenesis in the rat. *Kidney Int* 1975;7:397–404.
157. Klahr S, Schwab SJ, Stokes TJ, et al. Metabolic adaptations of the nephron in renal disease. *Kidney Int* 1986;29:80–89.
158. Buerkert J, Martin D, Trigg D, et al. Effect of reduced renal mass on ammonia handling and net acid formation by the superficial and juxtamedullary nephron of the rat. Evidence for re-entrapment rather than decreased production of ammonium in the acidosis of uremia. *J Clin Invest* 1983;71: 1661–1675.
159. Finkelstein FO, Hayslett JP. Role of medullary structures in the functional adaptation of renal insufficiency. *Kidney Int* 1974;6:419–425.
160. Gonick HC, Kleeman CR, Rubini MD et al. Functional impairment in chronic renal disease. II. Studies of acid excretion. *Nephron* 1969;6:28–49.
161. Feinfeld DA, Sherwood LM. Parathyroid hormone and 1,25(OH)2 D3 in chronic renal failure. *Kidney Int* 1988;33:1049–1058.
162. Felsenfeld AJ, Llach F. Parathyroid gland function in chronic renal failure. *Kidney Int* 1993;43:771–789.
163. Cheung AK, Manolagas SC, Catherwood BD, et al. Determinants of serum levels in renal disease. *Kidney Int* 1983;24:104.
164. Chesney RW, Hamstra AJ, Mazees RB, et al. Circulating vitamin D metabolite concentrations in childhood diseases. *Kidney Int* 1982;21:65.
165. Salusky IB. Bone and mineral metabolism in childhood end-stage renal disease. *Pediatr Clin North Am* 1995;42:1531–1547.
166. Slatopolsky E, Weerts C, Thielan J, et al. Marked suppression of secondary hyperparathyroidism by the intravenous administration of 1,25 dihydroxycholecalciferol in uremic patients. *J Clin Invest* 1984;74:2136–2143.
167. Rodriguez M, Felsenfeld AJ, Williams C, et al. The effect of long-term intravenous calcitriol administration on parathyroid function in hemodialysis patients. *J Am Soc Nephrol* 1991;2:1014–1020.
168. Slatopolsky E, Caglar S, Pennell JP, et al. On the pathogenesis of hyperparathyroidism in chronic experimental renal insufficiency in the dog. *J Clin Invest* 1971;50:492.
169. Salusky IB, Colburn JW, Paunier L, et al. Role of aluminum hydroxide in raising serum aluminum levels in children undergoing continuous ambulatory peritoneal dialysis. *J Pediatr* 1984;105:717.
170. Griswold WR, Reznik V, Mendoza SA, et al. Accumulation of aluminum in a nondialyzed uremic child receiving aluminum hydroxide. *Pediatrics* 1983;71:56.
171. Combe C, Aparicio M. Phosphorus and protein restriction and parathyroid function in chronic renal failure. *Kidney Int* 46:1381–1386.
172. Strewler GJ. Hormones and disorders of mineral metabolism. *Endocrinol Metab Clin North Am* 2002;29:9–11.
173. Gowen J. Antagonizing the parathyroid calcium receptor stimulates parathyroid hormone secretion and bone formation in osteopenic rats. *J Clin Invest* 105:1595–1604.
174. Hottelart C, Bako G, Oprisiu R, et al. Renal osteodystrophy: in treatment before dialysis. *Nephrologie* 2000;21:275–282.
175. Pierides AM, Skillen AW, Ellis HA, et al. Serum alkaline phosphatase in azotemic and hemodialysis osteodystrophy. A study of isoenzyme patterns, their correlation with bone histology and their changes in response to treatment with 1alpha(OH) D3 and 1,25(OH)2D3. *J Lab Clin Med* 1979;93:899.
176. Salusky IB, Goodman WG. Growth hormone and calcitriol as modifiers of bone formation in renal osteodystrophy. *Kidney Int* 1995;48:657.
177. Rosman JB, Sluiter WJ, Donker AJM, et al. Dietary protein in chronic renal failure. *Lancet* 1985;1:465–466.
178. Hostetter TH, Meyer TW, Rennke HG, et al. Chronic effects of dietary protein in the rat with intact and reduced renal mass. *Kidney Int* 1986;30:509–517.

179. Greiber S, Mitch WE. Catabolism in uremia: metabolic acidosis and activation of specific pathways. *Contrib Nephrol* 1992;982–927.
180. Maroni BJ, Mitch WE. Role of nutrition in prevention of the progression of renal disease. *Annu Rev Nutr* 1997;17: 435–455.
181. Brenner BM, Meyer TW, Hostetter TH, et al. Dietary protein intake and the progressive nature of kidney disease: the role of hemodynamically mediated glomerular sclerosis in aging, renal ablation, and intrinsic renal disease. *N Engl J Med* 1982;307:652–659.
182. Hostetter TH, Olson JL, Rennke HG, et al. Hyperfiltration in remnant nephrons: a potentially adverse response to renal ablation. *Am J Physiol* 1981;241:F85–F93.
183. Bourgoignie JJ, Gavellas G, Sabnis SG, et al. Effect of protein diets on the renal function of baboons (*Papio hamadryas*) with remnant kidneys: a 5 year follow-up. *Am J Kidney Dis* 1994;23:199–204.
184. Cianciaruso B, Bellizzi V, Capuano A, et al. Short-term effects of low protein-normal sodium diet on renal function in chronic renal failure. *Kidney Int* 45:852–860.
185. Kopple JD, Levey AS, Greene T, et al. Effect of dietary protein restriction on nutritional status in Modification of Diet in Renal Disease (MDRD) Study. *Kidney Int* 1997;52:778–791.
186. Mitch WE. Mechanisms causing loss of lean body mass in kidney disease. *Am J Clin Nutr* 1998;67:359–366.
187. Felig P. Amino acid metabolism in man. *Annu Rev Biochem* 1975;44:935–955.
188. McNurlan MA, Garlick PJ. Influence of nutrient intake on protein turnover. *Diabetes Metab Rev* 1989;5:165–189.
189. Quevedo MR, Price GM, Halliday D, et al. Nitrogen homeostasis in man: diurnal changes in nitrogen excretion, leucine oxidation and whole body leucine kinetics during a reduction from a high to a moderate protein intake. *Clin Sci* 1994;86:185–193.
190. Kleinkecht C, Maniar S, Zhou X, et al. Acidosis prevents growth hormone-induced growth in experimental uremia. *Pediatr Nephrol* 1996;10:256–260.
191. Committee on dietary allowances recommended dietary allowances. Washington, DC: National Academy of Science, 1989.
192. Wang J, Zhou J, Bondy CA. Igf1 promotes longitudinal bone growth by insulin-like actions augmenting chondrocyte hypertrophy. *FASEB J* 1999;13:1985–1990.
193. Fine LG. The role of hypertrophy of renal tissue. *Kidney Int* 1987;32:S2–S8.
194. Underwood LE. Special considerations in the design of trials involving children. *J Nutr* 1999;129:1251–1258.
195. Mitch WE. Dietary therapy in uremia: the impact on nutrition and progressive renal failure. *Kidney Int* 2000;57:S38–S43.
196. Wingren AM, Fabian-Bach C, Schaefer F, et al. Randomized multicenter study of a low-protein diet on the progression of chronic renal failure in children. *Lancet* 1997;349: 1117–1123.
197. Walser M, Hill S, Ward L, et al. Progression of chronic renal failure on substituting a ketoacid supplement for an amino acid supplement. *J Am Soc Nephrol* 1992;2:1178–1185.
198. Remuzzi G, Ruggenenti P, Benigni A, et al. Understanding the nature of renal disease progression. *Kidney Int* 1997;51:2–15.
199. Yoshioka T, Rennke HG, Salant DJ, et al. Role of abnormally high transmural pressure in the permselectivity defect of glomerular capillary wall: a study in early passive Heymann nephritis. *Circ Res* 1987;61:531–538.
200. Bohrer MP, Deen WM, Robertson CR, et al. Mechanism of angiotensin II induced proteinuria in the rat. *Am J Physiol* 1977;233:F13–F21.
201. Zoja C, Morigi M, Figliuzzi M, et al. Proximal tubular cell synthesis and secretion of endothelin-1 on challenge with albumin and other proteins. *Am J Kidney Dis* 1995;26:834–941.
202. Perico N, Remuzzi G. Vascular endothelin in glomerular injury. *Kidney Int* 1993;43:S76–S80.
203. Zoja C, Bonadelli R, Colleoni S, et al. Protein overload stimulates RANTES production by proximal tubular cells depending on NF-kappa B activation. *Kidney Int* 1998;53:1608–1615.
204. Wang Y, Chen J, Chen L, et al. Induction of monocyte chemoattractant protein-1 in proximal tubule cells by urinary protein. *J Am Soc Nephrol* 1997;8:1537–1545.
205. Pisoni R, Ruggenent P, Remuzzi G, et al. Renoprotective therapy in patients with nondiabetic nephropathies. *Drugs* 2001;61:733–745.
206. Ding GH, Reddy K, Kapasi AA, et al. Angiotensin II induces apoptosis in rat glomerular epithelial cells. *Am J Physiol Renal Physiol* 2002;283:F173–F180.
207. Hollenberg NK, Raij L. Angiotensin-converting enzyme-inhibition and renal protection: an assessment of implications for therapy. *Arch Intern Med* 1993;153:2426–2435.
208. Lopez-Ovejero JA, Saal SDF, D'Angelo, et al. Reversal of vascular and renal crises of scleroderma by oral angiotensin-converting enzyme blockade. *N Engl J Med* 1979;300:1417–1419.
209. Thurn RH, Alexander JC. Captopril in the treatment of scleroderma renal crisis. *Arch Intern Med* 1984;144:733–735.
210. Dworkin LD, Grosser M, Feiner HD, et al. Renal vascular effects of antihypertensive therapy in uninephrectomized SHR. *Kidney Int* 1989;35:790–798.
211. de Jong PE, Anderson S, Dezeeuw D, et al. Glomerular preload and afterload reduction as a tool to lower urinary protein leakage: Will such treatments also help to improve renal function outcome? *J Am Soc Nephrol* 1993;3:1333–1341.
212. Remuzzi A, Perticucci E, Ruggenenti P, et al. Angiotensin converting enzyme inhibition improves glomerular size selectivity in IgA nephropathy. *Kidney Int* 1991;39:1267–1273.
213. Lewis EJ, Hunsicker LG, Bain RP, et al. The effect of angiotensin-converting enzyme inhibition on diabetic nephropathy. *N Engl J Med* 1993;329:1456–1462.
214. Ravid M, Savin H, Jutrin I, et al. Long term stabilizing effect of angiotensin-converting enzyme inhibition on plasma creatinine and on proteinuria in normotensive type II diabetic patients. *Ann Intern Med* 1993;118:577–581.
215. Ravid M, Lang R, Rachmani R, et al. Long-term renoprotective effect of angiotensin-converting enzyme inhibition on non-insulin dependent diabetes mellitus. A 7-year follow-up study. *Arch Intern Med* 1996;156:286–289.
216. The Gisen Group. Randomized placebo-control trial of ramipril on decline in glomerular filtration rate and risk of terminal renal failure in proteinuric, non-diabetic nephropathy. *Lancet* 1997;349:1857–1863.
217. Goldberg MR, Bradstreet TE, McWilliams, et al. Biochemical effects of losartan, a nonpeptide angiotensin II receptor

antagonist, on the renin-angiotensin-aldosterone system in hypertensive patients. *Hypertension* 1995;25:37–46.

218. Lafayette RA, Mayer G, Park SK, et al. Angiotensin II receptor blockade limits glomerular injury in rats with reduced renal mass. *J Clin Invest* 1992;9:766–771.
219. Mackenzie HS, Troy JL, Rennke HG, et al. TVC 116 prevents progressive renal injury in rats with extensive renal mass ablation. *J Hypertens* 1994;12:S11–S16.
220. Russo D, Pisani A, Balletta MM, et al. Additive antiproteinuric effect of converting enzyme inhibitor and losartan in normotensive patients with IgA nephropathy. *Am J Kidney Dis* 1999;33:851–856.
221. American Academy of Pediatrics. *2003 red book: report on the Committee on Infectious Diseases*, 24th ed. Elk Grove Village, IL: American Academy of Pediatrics, 1997:21–23, 69–81.
222. Fivush BA, Furth SL, Neu AM. Immunizations in children on PD: current guidelines and recommendations. *Adv Perit Dial* 1995;11:270–273.
223. Johnson DW, Fleming SJ. The use of vaccines in renal failure. *Clin Pharmacokinet* 1992;22:434–436.
224. Moxey-Mims MM, Preston K, Fivush BA, et al. Heptavax-B in pediatric dialysis patients: effect of systemic lupus erythematosus. *Pediatr Nephrol* 1990;4:171–173.
225. Watkins SL, Hoss RJ, Alexander SR, et al. Response to recombinant hepatitis B vaccine (Recombivax HB) in children with chronic renal failure. *J Am Soc Nephrol* 1994;5:344.
226. Neu AM, Lederman H, Warady B, et al. Humoral immunity in infants on CPD. *J Am Soc Nephrol* 1994;5:467.
227. Fivush BA, Case B, May MW, et al. Hypogammaglobulinemia in children undergoing continuous ambulatory peritoneal dialysis. *Pediatr Nephrol* 1989;3:186–188.
228. Fivush BA, Case B, Warady BA, et al. Defective antibody response to *Haemophilus influenzae* type b immunization in children receiving peritoneal dialysis. *Pediatr Nephrol* 1993;7:548–550.
229. Neu AM, Lederman H, Warady B, et al. Immunization with conjugated haemophilus influenza vaccine in infants on CPD. *J Am Soc Nephrol* 1994;5:467.
230. Schulman SL, Deforest A, Kaiser BA, et al. Response to measles-mumps-rubella vaccine in children on dialysis. *Pediatr Nephrol* 1992;6:179–181.
231. Hisano S, Miyazaki C, Hatae K, et al. Immune status of children on continuous ambulatory peritoneal dialysis. *Pediatr Nephrol* 1992;6:179–181.
232. Jilkova E, Jilek D, Bitterova Z, et al. [Hepatitis B vaccination in patients with chronic renal failure]. *Epidemiol Mikrobiol Imunol* 1997;46:135–139.
233. Fuchshuber A, Kuhnemund O, Keuth B, et al. Pneumococcal vaccine in children and young adults with chronic renal disease. *Nephrol Dial Transplant* 1996;11:468–473.
234. Kruger S, Seyfarth M, Sack K, et al. Defective immune response to tetanus toxoid in hemodialysis patients and its association with diphtheria vaccination. *Vaccine* 1999;17:1145–1150.
235. Laube GF, Berger C, Goetschel P, et al. Immunization in children with chronic renal failure. *Pediatr Nephrol* 2002;17:638–642.
236. Webb NJ, Fitzpatrick MM, Hughes DA, et al. Immunisation against varicella in end stage and pre-end stage renal failure. Trans-Pennine Paediatric Nephrology Study Group. *Arch Dis Child* 2000;82:141–143.
237. Enke BU, Bokenkamp A, Offner G, et al. Response to diphtheria and tetanus booster vaccination in pediatric renal transplant recipients. *Transplantation* 1997;64:237–241.
238. Lynfield R, Herrin JT, Rubin RH. Varicella in pediatric renal transplant recipients. *Pediatrics* 1992;90:216–220.
239. Broyer M, Tete MJ, Guest G, et al. Varicella and zoster in children after kidney transplantation: long-term results of vaccination. *Pediatrics* 1997;99:35–39.
240. Olson AD, Shope TC, Flynn JT. Pretransplant varicella vaccination is cost-effective in pediatric renal transplantation. *Pediatr Transplant* 2001;5:44–50.
241. Zamora I, Simon JM, Da Silva ME, et al. Attenuated varicella virus vaccine in children with renal transplants. *Pediatr Nephrol* 1994;8:190–192.
242. Kazancioglu R, Sever MS, Yuksel-Onel D, et al. Immunization of renal transplant recipients with pneumococcal polysaccharide vaccine. *Clin Transplant* 2000;14:61–65.
243. Kasiske BL, Vazquez MA, Harmon WE, et al. Recommendations for the outpatient surveillance of renal transplant recipients. American Society of Transplantation. *J Am Soc Nephrol* 2000;11:S1–S86.

68

ENDOCRINE AND GROWTH DISORDERS IN CHRONIC RENAL FAILURE

FRANZ SCHAEFER

ENDOCRINE DISORDERS IN CHRONIC RENAL FAILURE

Pathophysiologic Mechanisms

Uremia interferes with metabolism and regulation of hormones by various mechanisms. Disturbed endocrine function may arise either from inappropriate circulating hormone *concentrations* or from altered hormone *action* at the target tissue level. Both conditions may be present in the uremic state.

Increased Plasma Hormone Concentrations

Renal catabolism accounts for one-third to two-thirds of the metabolic clearance rates of various polypeptide hormones (1). Most polypeptide hormones are almost freely filtered in the glomerulus, followed by either intratubular degradation (brush-border peptidases) or intracellular degradation (cytosolic or lysosomal) in tubular cells. Moreover, certain hormones are subject to receptor-mediated uptake across the basolateral tubular cell membrane. Hence, any reduction of renal mass results in a decrease in the metabolic clearance of most peptide hormones (Fig. 68.1). If catabolic mechanisms differ for different isoforms or subunits of a hormone, an imbalance of these constituents may arise, altering the relation between biologically active and inactive hormone fragments (see later). In addition to renal clearance, *extrarenal hormone elimination* may also be reduced in renal failure. For example, degradation of insulin in skeletal muscle tissue is diminished (2), and hepatic catabolism of biologically active parathyroid hormone (PTH) is reduced in uremia (3). Finally, *hypersecretion* of various hormones or hormone-binding proteins occurs in renal failure, either as an appropriate response to secretory stimuli (e.g., PTH) or without an apparent homeostatic signal (e.g., prolactin).

Decreased Plasma Hormone Concentrations

The reduction in functional renal mass is assumed to be the main cause for decreased levels of hormones produced by the *kidney* (erythropoietin; 1,25-dihydroxyvitamin D_3). In addition, the uremic milieu may suppress the production of these hormones by alterations of the internal milieu. For example, intracellular phosphate accumulation may inhibit 1α-hydroxylase even before the reduction of renal mass becomes quantitatively important. Levels of *extrarenal hormones* may be decreased when the hormone-producing gland is the final effector organ of a complex hormonal axis (e.g., testis–testosterone, ovary–estradiol). In these cases, insufficient production of hormones may result either from direct toxic damage to the endocrine gland, from insufficient stimulatory input from the superior part of the hormonal axis, or from hyporesponsiveness of the gland.

Disorders of Hormone Action

Disturbed Activation of Prohormones

Concentrations of certain prohormones are elevated in chronic renal failure (CRF), for example, pro–insulin-like growth factor IA, a precursor of insulin-like growth factor-1 (IGF-1), which is not detectable in normal serum (4), and proinsulin, which is not converted appropriately to insulin or C-peptide in patients with end-stage renal disease (ESRD) (5). Peripheral conversion of thyroxine (T_4) to tissue-active triiodothyronine (T_3) is impaired (6). Some prohormones may block hormone action by competitively inhibiting receptor binding at the tissue level.

Multimolecular Forms of Variable Bioactivity

Some polypeptide hormones circulate in plasma in multiple isoforms characterized by varying composition of their carbohydrate side chains. In CRF, altered glycosylation and sialization (7) may shift the isohormone spectrum toward less bioactive forms [e.g., luteinizing hormone (LH) (8)]. This may be due to alterations of posttranslational processing or to differences in the renal clearance of individual isoforms.

Hormone Binding to Plasma Proteins

Excessive concentrations of several IGF-binding proteins are found in CRF (9,10). Binding proteins can compete for

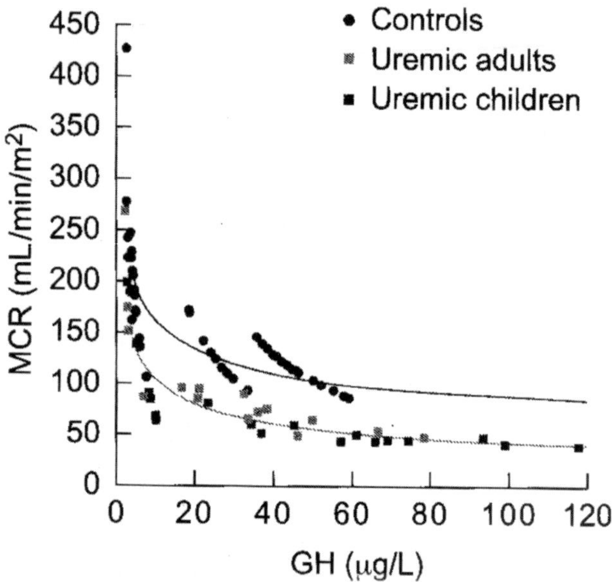

FIGURE 68.1. Total metabolic clearance rate (MCR) as a function of steady-state plasma growth hormone (GH) concentrations in controls and patients with chronic renal failure (CRF). MCR is reduced in children and adults with CRF at any prevailing plasma GH level. (From Haffner D, Schaefer F, Girard J, et al. Metabolic clearance of recombinant human growth hormone in health and chronic renal failure. *J Clin Invest* 1994;93:1163–1171, with permission.)

the hormone with target organ receptors, and this explains in part the reduced somatomedin bioactivity in the presence of normal total serum IGF. Abnormal concentrations of other polypeptide binding proteins may similarly be related to abnormal hormone action in uremia.

Alterations of Target Tissue Sensitivity

Diminished target organ responsiveness is observed in various endocrine systems in uremia. Mechanisms for altered target tissue sensitivity include reduced cellular receptor activation due to the diminished receptor abundance, the presence of inhibitory substances, the accumulation of molecules inhibiting hormone-receptor interaction (e.g., IGF-1), and structural changes of either the hormone or its receptor (9). Moreover, defects of hormone-receptor complex–dependent intracellular signaling may occur. Such postreceptor events seem to play a key role in the pathogenesis of insulin (11) and growth hormone (GH) (12) resistance in uremia.

Gonadotropic Hormone Axis

Clinical Findings

The onset of puberty is usually delayed in adolescents with CRF. At least 50% of adolescents with ESRD enter puberty beyond the normal age range (13) and achieve the pubertal milestones beyond the normal age range (14–16). Late puberty is observed both in children on dialysis and after renal transplantation. In the Cooperative Study for Pubertal Development in CRF, the onset of puberty was delayed by 2 to 2.5 years on average (17). The start of genital maturation (Tanner stage G2) was delayed by 1.8 years in uremic boys and 2.5 years in boys undergoing transplantation. Full genital maturation was achieved with a delay of 2.2 and 3.2 years, respectively. Thus, once started, puberty appears to proceed at a normal rate. However, in individual patients, particularly those on long-term dialysis, pubertal maturation may arrest for years. Almost half of the girls treated by dialysis or renal transplantation fail to menstruate before the upper normal age limit of 15 years. Menarche tends to occur even later in girls undergoing transplantation than in girls on dialysis (14).

Unlike the development of secondary sexual characteristics, which is delayed but not permanently halted in CRF, reproductive function may be permanently impaired. In autopsy studies of boys with CRF, germ cell depletion in the testicular tubules has been described (18). These changes do not appear reversible after renal transplantation (19). Persistently reduced sperm counts were observed in 10 of 12 young adults who successfully underwent transplantation who had suffered from ESRD during childhood (19). Erectile dysfunction, decreased libido, and decreased fertility are primarily organic in nature and are due to uremia as well as to other comorbid conditions, fatigue, and psychosocial factors (20). The frequency of conception is decreased in women with chronic renal insufficiency, and pregnancy is very uncommon in adolescents with ESRD. The percentage of surviving infants ranges from 70 to 100% in women with CRF on conservative treatment or after renal transplantation (19) and from 50 to 80% in women on dialysis (21–23). Intrauterine growth retardation is frequent, and the birth weight is reduced by nearly 1 kg (16,20,21).

Gonadal Hormones

In adults with CRF plasma concentrations of *testosterone* (T) are usually low or low normal (24), due to reduced synthesis and, perhaps, increased metabolic clearance rate (25,26). In prepubertal children with predialytic renal failure, low total and free T and dihydrotestosterone (DHT) plasma concentrations have been reported (27). However, because the adrenal cortex is the major site of androgen production before puberty and the levels of specific adrenal androgens are also low in children with CRF (28), low prepubertal plasma androgen levels do not provide evidence for gonadal damage before puberty (29,30). In pubertal patients, normal or slightly subnormal plasma T concentrations are observed (31–33). In late puberty, however, DHT concentrations are significantly lower in children with CRF than in healthy children or those who have undergone transplantation (F.S., unpublished observation). Impaired conversion of T to DHT due to decreased 5α-reductase activity has been suggested (34,35). Because this metabolite is responsible for many tissue actions of the andro-

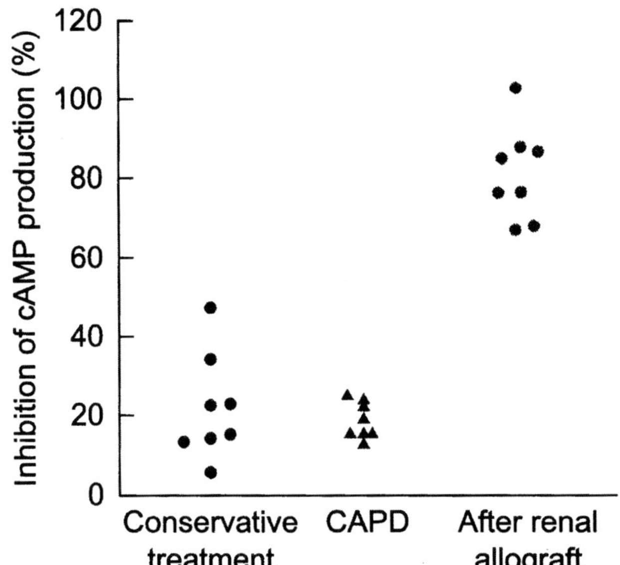

FIGURE 68.2. Evidence for circulating luteinizing hormone (LH) inhibitor in sera of boys with chronic renal failure. Inhibition is suppressed in presence of serum of patients on conservative treatment or continuous ambulatory peritoneal dialysis (CAPD). Human chorionic gonadotropin (HCG)–induced production of cyclic adenosine monophosphate (cAMP) by cell line expressing human LH/HCG receptor is suppressed by a fraction containing 30- to 60-kDa proteins (data not shown). [Adapted with permission from Dunkel L, Raivio T, Laine J, et al. Circulating luteinizing hormone receptor inhibitor(s) in boys with chronic renal failure. *Kidney Int* 1997;51:777–784.]

gens, reduced conversion of T to DHT may explain the frequently sparse development of secondary sexual characteristics in boys with advanced renal failure.

The testicular response to supraphysiologic stimulation by human chorionic gonadotropin is impaired in adult men (24) as well as in prepubertal and pubertal boys with CRF. Testicular insufficiency is most prominent in boys on hemodialysis (31). Leydig cell resistance is caused by a cyclic adenosine monophosphate (cAMP)–dependent mechanism (36). The presence of an endogenous LH inhibitor in uremic serum has been demonstrated (37) (Fig. 68.2). The disorder is reversible after renal transplantation (31).

The physiologic age-related decrease of sex hormone–binding globulin is conserved in prepubertal children on dialysis (32); however, at a given age sex hormone–binding globulin concentrations are higher and the unbound T fraction is lower than in normal children. The increase of sex hormone–binding globulin may be due to accumulation in end-stage renal failure; a normal fraction of free T has been reported in prepubertal children on conservative treatment (27).

The plasma concentration of *inhibin*, a polypeptide produced by the Sertoli and granulosa cells, is elevated in peripubertal boys with CRF (38).

Estradiol plasma concentrations in the low-normal range are observed in women with CRF (39). In pubertal girls with CRF, estradiol plasma levels are normal or low when related to pubertal stage (40,41). An inverse correlation between serum creatinine levels and estradiol concentrations was found in patients with predialytic CRF. Longitudinal analysis revealed an insufficient increase in estradiol during puberty in those patients whose renal function deteriorated, whereas after renal transplantation, even after several years of dialysis, estradiol concentrations increased (41).

Gonadotropins

Plasma LH levels are high normal or elevated in adult men, women, and prepubertal and pubertal boys and girls with CRF (8,24,27,39,40,42); follicle-stimulating hormone (FSH) concentrations are also usually elevated in both adults and children with CRF. After transplantation, LH levels usually return to normal, whereas plasma FSH frequently remains elevated.

The combination of elevated gonadotropins and decreased or low-normal gonadal hormone levels has been taken as evidence for a state of compensated hypergonadotropic hypogonadism (27,43). However, the degree of hypergonadotropism in CRF is usually inadequate for the prevailing degree of hypogonadism, which suggests an additional defect of hypophyseal gonadotropin secretion.

An alteration at the pituitary level is suggested by the blunted increase of plasma LH and FSH after stimulation by a bolus of exogenous gonadotropin-releasing hormone (GnRH) in men, women, boys, and girls with CRF (24,27,40). These abnormalities appear even more marked when the diminished metabolic clearance of gonadotropins is taken into account (44). The gonadotropin response to GnRH is normalized after successful transplantation (40).

LH is released from the pituitary gland in episodic (pulsatile) bursts occurring every 90 to 120 minutes. The plasma LH concentration peaks reflect intermittent secretion of hypothalamic GnRH into the hypophyseal-portal bloodstream (45). Hence, the analysis of plasma LH pulses gives indirect information about the functional state of the hypothalamic GnRH "pacemaker." A differentiation of the secretion and elimination components underlying the fluctuating plasma LH concentration patterns by means of deconvolution methodology (46) revealed that the elevation of basal plasma LH concentrations is entirely due to the diminished renal metabolic clearance of the hormone (44) both in humans (47) and in rats (48). Plasma half-life of LH is inversely correlated with GFR (47). In contrast, actual pituitary LH secretion rates are decreased in CRF; pubertal dialysis patients secrete 3 times less immunoreactive LH and 2.5 times less bioactive LH in episodic nocturnal peaks than normal adolescents (47). This abnormality, which has been reproduced in experimental uremia (49), gives strong evidence for a dysregulation of the gonadotropic axis at the hypothalamopituitary level. After transplantation, a regular pattern of LH pulses is reestablished (8,50). Because the onset of puberty is heralded by the emergence of a nocturnal pattern of pulsatile LH secre-

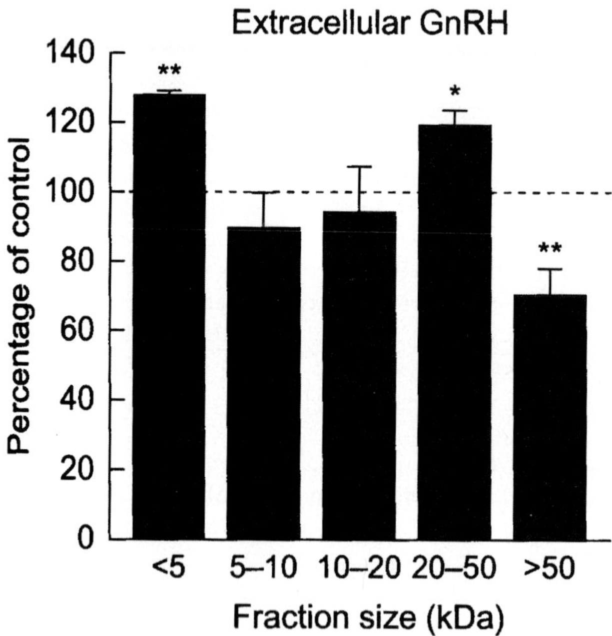

FIGURE 68.3. Selective inhibition of gonadotropin-releasing hormone (GnRH) secretion from cultured neurons of a hypothalamic cell line by incubation with a high-molecular-weight fraction of uremic serum. GnRH supernatant concentrations observed with serum fractions from control animals were defined as 100%. *, *p* <.05; **, *p* <.01. (Adapted from Daschner M, Philippin B, Nguyen T, et al. Circulating inhibitor of gonadotropin releasing hormone secretion from hypothalamic neurons in uremia. *Kidney Int* 2002;62:1582–1590.)

tion, the observed disturbance of pulsatile LH secretion suggests that the delayed pubertal development in CRF is caused by a primary hypothalamic defect. Experimental evidence confirms that the subnormal pituitary gonadotropin secretion is caused by diminished release of GnRH into the hypophyseal portal circulation (48,51). In cultured GnRH-producing neurons an inhibition of GnRH release was observed on addition of a high-molecular-weight fraction of uremic serum. Further investigation suggested that the inhibitor is a hydrophilic protein suppressing GnRH exocytosis but not synthesis (52) (Fig. 68.3). Moreover, with the use of *in vivo* intracerebral microdialysis in experimentally uremic rats, we observed an increased tone of the neuroinhibitory amino acid γ-aminobutyric acid in the extracellular fluid of the hypothalamic medial preoptic area, the region where the GnRH neurons reside (53). Hence, the accumulation of γ-aminobutyric acid in the central nervous system may be another mechanism of downregulation of the gonadotropic hormone axis in uremia.

In summary, clinical and experimental evidence indicates that the neuroendocrine control of pulsatile LH secretion is altered in CRF. Although overt hypogonadotropism is masked by a simultaneous reduction of metabolic clearance rates, the deficient physiologic pulsatile GnRH-LH signal may be the key abnormality underlying the delayed onset of puberty in chronic renal disease. The observed disorders of LH secretion and metabolism appear to be reversible after successful renal transplantation.

Not only is there quantitative insufficiency of the hypothalamopituitary unit, but the biologic *quality* of the circulating gonadotropins is also altered in uremia. LH bioactivity, measured by the potency of a plasma sample in inducing testosterone secretion in a Leydig cell culture, depends on the degree of glycosylation and sialization of this glycoprotein hormone (54). During normal puberty, the relative bioactivity of LH gradually increases (55). In pubertal (56,57) and adult patients (50) on dialysis, the ratio of bioactive to immunoreactive plasma LH is reduced, which suggests that the spectrum of circulating LH molecules is shifted toward bioinactive forms (8,47,50,58). This may be attributed to altered glycosylation of plasma proteins in uremia (7). The physiologic increase in hormone bioactivity during puberty is absent in dialysis patients (57). The inhibitor of LH action circulating in the serum of uremic boys may represent an accumulating LH fragment (37) (Fig. 68.2). After successful renal transplantation, LH biopotency tends to normalize.

Prolactin

Prolactin is a proteohormone secreted by the pituitary that is involved in the hormonal regulation of lactation. Its function in nonpuerperal women, in men, and in children is not clear. However, prolactin attenuates gonadotropin release. Plasma prolactin levels are elevated in men (59) and, more markedly, in women and pubertal girls (40,59) with CRF. Uremic hyperprolactinemia appears to result from both decreased metabolic clearance rate and increased production of the hormone (60). Hyperprolactinemia may play a role in the pathogenesis of uremic hypogonadism, because elevated prolactin levels exert a suppressive effect on the GnRH-LH pulse generator (61). The physiologic sleep-related nocturnal prolactin surge is absent (62), and the circadian rhythm of secretion is deranged (63). Prolactin secretion in CRF patients is insensitive to stimulation by thyrotropin-releasing hormone (TRH) (64), chlorpromazine, metoclopramide, arginine, or insulin-induced hypoglycemia (65). Neither L-dopa nor dopamine is effective in suppressing prolactin secretion (65); however, hyperprolactinemia may be corrected by long-term treatment with dopaminergic agonists (66,67). Uremic hyperprolactinemia may be related to other complications of CRF such as vitamin D deficiency and renal anemia. Administration of 1,25-dihydroxyvitamin D_3 (68) and erythropoietin (69) leads to a partial normalization of plasma prolactin levels.

In conclusion, various physiologic studies and pharmacologic tests reveal a partial disintegration of the gonadotropic hormone axis at the hypothalamopituitary level, in addition to alterations of gonadal function. The analysis of hormone secretory patterns has confirmed that the central nervous dysregulation is not restricted to the functional reserve capacity of the reproductive hormone system but affects physiologic spontaneous hormone secretion. The reversibility of the observed changes after successful renal transplantation gives further evidence that regulatory mechanisms, rather than toxic end-organ damage, affect gonadal function in uremia. It remains to be shown to what extent the apparent dysregulation of hormone secretion represents a "physiologic" adaptation to an adverse metabolic environment.

Growth Hormone–Insulin-Like Growth Factor Axis

During normal childhood, the somatotrophic hormone axis plays a key role in the regulation of body growth. In addition, GH is part of a complex system of counterregulatory hormones maintaining the homeostasis of carbohydrate metabolism.

Growth Hormone

Serum Concentrations and Kinetics

Fasting GH concentrations are variably elevated in uremic children and adults depending on the extent of renal failure (70,71). The kidney is a major site of GH degradation (72). In patients with end-stage renal failure, the metabolic clearance rate of GH is reduced by approximately 50% (73,74) (Fig. 68.1). Deconvolution analyses of GH plasma concentration profiles revealed that the increase in plasma GH concentrations is due mainly to an increased plasma half-life of the hormone; the actual pituitary GH secretion rate varied among patients and across studies. GH secretion rate was high normal in prepubertal children with ESRD and increased in adult patients on hemodialysis, possibly as a result of attenuated bioactive IGF-1 feedback of the hypothalamopituitary unit (75,76). In pubertal patients with advanced CRF, reduced GH secretion rates were observed, which indicated an altered sensitivity of the somatotropic hormone axis to the stimulatory effect of sex steroids during this stage of development (77). The variability of plasma GH levels in CRF may be due in part to associated conditions such as acidosis and malnutrition, which independently affect GH secretion. Metabolic acidosis suppresses GH release in both rodents and humans (78).

Neuroendocrine Control of Growth Hormone Release

Dysregulation of GH secretion may be related to abnormalities of central neuroendocrine control mechanisms. Evidence for this is provided by several hypothalamopituitary function tests. The GH response to intravenous administration of GH-releasing hormone is augmented and prolonged in children (79). Exogenous TRH, which does not affect GH release in healthy subjects, markedly enhances GH secretion in subjects with renal failure (70,80). Also, CRF patients respond to acute hyperglycemia with a paradoxical increase of GH secretion (70,81). Stimulation tests such as arginine infusion and insulin-induced hypoglycemia lead to a sustained, exaggerated increase of GH (70,82,83). However, the altered metabolic clearance rates of GH as well as of the provocative agents in renal failure (84) make a meaningful clinical interpretation of such tests virtually impossible.

Growth Hormone Receptor Signaling and Tissue Action

Growth failure despite elevated circulating GH concentrations suggests a state of GH resistance in children with CRF. Indeed, GH-induced hepatic IGF-1 synthesis is markedly reduced in rats with CRF (12,85). This GH insensitivity may in part be due to deficient GH receptor expression, although this is controversial. Reduced hepatic GH receptor messenger RNA (mRNA) and receptor binding has been reported in some but not all studies carried out with animals (12,85–88). These discrepancies may be related to the effect of reduced nutritional intake. Indeed, controlling for the anorexia of chronic uremia by pair-feeding control animals abolished the difference in GH receptor protein expression and binding to liver plasma membranes seen when ad lib feeding controls and uremic animals are compared (12,87), although receptor mRNA levels remained subnormal (12). On the other hand, reduced GH receptor protein expression was observed in the growth cartilage of rats with CRF even though nutritional intake was controlled (89). In humans serum levels of GH-binding protein, putatively reflecting hepatic GH receptor status, were found to be decreased in some studies but normal in others (74,90–93).

Another mechanism accounting for the resistance to GH in uremia is provided by a marked *postreceptor* GH signaling defect observed in livers of chronically uremic rats (12). Despite unaltered GH receptor protein levels, phosphorylation of the GH receptor–associated tyrosine kinase janus kinase 2 (JAK2) was diminished by 75% (Fig. 68.4). This resulted in a similar suppression of GH-JAK2–dependent phosphorylation of specific downstream signaling molecules, namely, signal transducer and activator of transcription 1 (STAT1), 3 (STAT3), and 5 (STAT5). This defect was possibly caused by upregulation of two intracellular JAK2 inhibitors, suppressors of cytokine signaling 2 (SOCS2) and 3 (SOCS3). Because these regulatory proteins are induced by inflammatory cytokines, it may be postulated that GH resistance in uremia is caused by a microinflammatory state.

Insulin-Like Growth Factors

Because most metabolic effects of GH are mediated by IGF-1, GH insensitivity in uremia may also be due to IGF resistance. Indeed, numerous studies in the rat as well as in humans have clearly documented marked IGF-1 resistance in CRF (94–97).

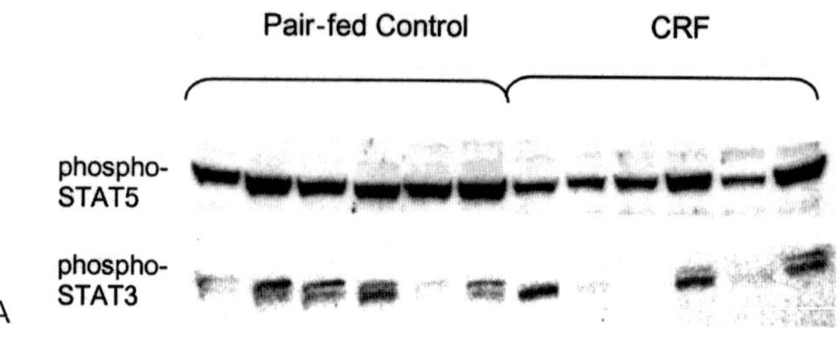

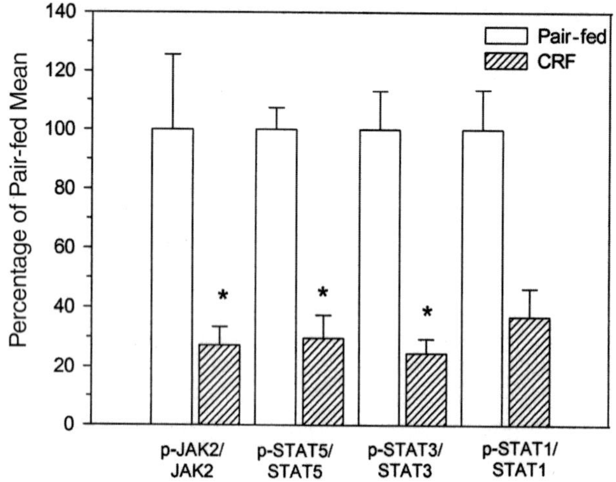

FIGURE 68.4. Impaired postreceptor growth hormone signaling in rats with experimental uremia. **A:** Deficient nuclear accumulation of tyrosine-phosphorylated signal transducer and activator of transcription 5 (STAT5) and 3 (STAT3) protein in livers of rats with chronic renal failure (CRF) compared to pair-fed controls. **B:** Increased messenger RNA abundance of suppressor of cytokine signaling 2 (SOCS2) in rats with CRF treated with recombinant growth hormone. SOCS2 inhibits STAT phosphorylation by binding to tyrosine kinase janus kinase 2 (JAK2). p-JAK2, phosphorylated janus kinase 2; p-STAT1, p-STAT3, p-STAT5, phosphorylated signal transducer and activator of transcription 1, 3, and 5. (From Schaefer F, Chen Y, Tsao T, et al. Impaired JAK-STAT signal transduction contributes to growth hormone resistance in chronic uremia. *J Clin Invest* 2001;108:467–475, with permission.)

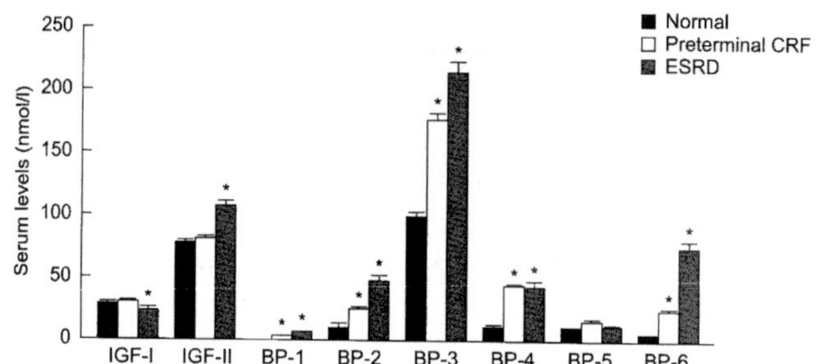

FIGURE 68.5. Molar concentrations of insulin-like growth factors (IGFs) and IGF-binding proteins (BPs) in children with pre–end-stage chronic renal failure (CRF) and children with end-stage renal disease (ESRD) on dialysis compared with age-matched healthy children. [From Ulinski T, Mohan S, Kiepe D, et al. Serum insulin-like growth factor binding protein (IGFBP)-4 and IGFBP-5 in children with chronic renal failure: relationship to growth and glomerular filtration rate. *Pediatr Nephrol* 2000;14:589–597, with permission.]

Insulin-Like Growth Factor Serum Concentrations

The effect of GH on longitudinal growth is partially mediated by stimulation of the production of somatomedins, the two most important of which are the IGF-1 and IGF-2. Serum IGF-1 and IGF-2 levels in children with preterminal CRF are in the normal range, whereas in ESRD mean age-related serum IGF-1 levels are slightly decreased and IGF-2 levels are moderately elevated (98). Hence, total immunoreactive IGF levels in CRF serum are normal. In contrast, IGF *bioactivity* is markedly reduced. Similarly, the level of free IGF-1 is reduced by 50% in relation to the degree of renal dysfunction (99). This is one of the key abnormalities of the GH-IGF axis in children with CRF.

Insulin-Like Growth Factor Plasma Binding and Tissue Action

The discrepancy between low somatomedin activity by bioassay and normal or elevated IGF by radioimmunoassay or radioreceptor assay suggests the presence of circulating somatomedin inhibitors in uremia. An early study indicated the presence of a low-molecular-weight IGF inhibitor (approximately 1 kDa), but its molecular structure has not been characterized further (100).

The most likely explanation for the inhibition of somatomedin action in uremia has emerged from the identification of six IGF-binding proteins (IGFBP1 to IGFBP6). IGFBP3 appears to be the most abundant in humans, constituting more than 95% of total circulating IGFBP. In children with CRF, the serum concentrations of IGFBP1, IGFBP2, IGFBP4, and IGFBP6 are increased in a manner inversely related to GFR (9,10,98,101–104) (Fig. 68.5). Ligand blotting shows that the elevation of radioimmunoassayable IGFBP3 is due to an increase in low-molecular-weight forms mainly in the range of 14 to 19 kDa, whereas intact IGFBP3 (38 to 41 kDa) is markedly reduced (105,106). IGFBP1, IGFBP2, and IGFBP6 inhibit somatomedin bioactivity *in vitro* (107). Somatomedin bioactivity in uremic serum can be returned to normal by removing unsaturated IGFBP (108). Experimental evidence suggests that the increase of IGFBP1 and IGFBP2 is due not only to reduced renal metabolic clearance but also to increased hepatic synthesis (109). An important question is whether the imbalance between normal total IGF and the excess of unsaturated IGFBPs contributes to growth failure in children with CRF. Serum levels of IGFBP1, IGFBP2, and IGFBP4 correlate inversely with standardized height in children with CRF (98,104,110). Although it is tempting to speculate that these IGFBPs could contribute to growth failure in these children, proving causality is difficult because IGFBP levels and height standard deviation score (SDS) are all correlated with GFR.

Apart from the increased plasma IGF-1–binding capacity, a postreceptor IGF-1 signaling defect may also contribute to IGF-1 resistance in CRF. In uremic rats the effect of IGF-1 and various IGF-1 analogues on protein turnover was suppressed (94). The observation that the inhibitory effect of IGF-1 and its analogues were affected to a similar degree indicates that the resistance arises because of a defect at a cellular level and not because of changes in IGFBP levels. Deficient autophosphorylation of the IGF-1 receptor in skeletal muscle of uremic rats has been reported (94) but was not confirmed in a later study (111).

Growth Hormone–Insulin-Like Growth Factor-1 Homeostasis in Chronic Renal Failure

The pattern of elevated GH, normal total IGF, and markedly elevated IGFBP plasma concentrations in uremia has interesting implications with respect to the estimated IGF production rate. In a functioning homeostatic system, the diminished free IGF-1 levels would be expected to stimulate IGF production to restore the steady state between bound and unbound hormone at a higher level. In uremia, however, total IGF concentrations are normal rather than increased. Kinetic modeling suggests that the metabolic half-life of IGFs is markedly elevated, and the IGF production rate is decreased 10- to 100-fold in uremia (112). Taken together, the markedly deficient IGF-1 synthesis and the modest elevation of plasma GH levels, which is due mainly to impaired metabolic clearance, in the presence of increased IGF-binding capacity strongly support the notion of a multilevel homeostatic failure of the GH–IGF-1 system in uremia. Pituitary GH secretion is insufficiently feedback-stimulated by reduced free IGF-1 levels, and marked tissue GH resistance prevents an increase in total IGF-1 levels in the presence of elevated GH levels.

Glucocorticoids and the Growth Hormone–Insulin-Like Growth Factor-1 Hormone Axis

After renal transplantation, the use of glucocorticoids for immunosuppression interferes with the GH–IGF-1 axis on various levels. Endogenous GH secretion is reduced in pediatric renal allograft recipients, mainly by a reduction of amplitudes of the GH secretory bursts (33,113). The physiologic increase of GH burst amplitudes during puberty is blunted, and the normal correlation between sex steroid plasma levels and GH secretion rate is absent (33). GH release after insulin-induced hypoglycemia is inadequate (113). The insufficiency of spontaneous and stimulated GH secretion in patients after transplantation is most likely explained by a glucocorticoid-induced enhancement of hypothalamic somatostatin release (114). On the target tissue level, glucocorticoids suppress GH receptor and IGF-1 gene transcription (115,116). Nevertheless, basal IGF-1 plasma levels in renal transplant recipients are in the normal range (117–119). This discrepancy between clinical and experimental findings suggests that glucocorticoids alter translation, synthesis, and/or secretion of IGF-1 in such a way that the IGF-1 mRNA redundancy no longer reflects IGF-1 protein synthesis. Whereas circulating immunoreactive IGF-1 concentrations are not consistently reduced, IGF bioactivity is markedly diminished in patients on glucocorticoid treatment (117,120). This may be due to the induction of IGF inhibitors of 12 to 20 kDa molecular weight and/or to increased serum IGFBP3 levels (117,120). Moreover, increased IGFBP2 concentrations are found in patients with Cushing syndrome (121). IGFBP2 may be another functional IGF-1 inhibitor in patients receiving long-term glucocorticoid treatment.

Glucocorticoids also interfere with chondrocyte growth and enchondral bone formation in various ways. They inhibit sulfate incorporation into cartilage matrix as well as mineralization and formation of new bone (122). In cultured epiphyseal chondrocytes, dexamethasone decreases DNA synthesis and cell proliferation, GH receptor expression, and paracrine IGF-1 secretion (123).

Thyroid Hormone Axis

Clinical Findings

The thyroid hormone axis plays an important role in the regulation of tissue metabolism. Throughout childhood, thyroid hormone is involved in growth and skeletal maturation, stimulating both cartilage proliferation and epiphyseal differentiation.

The prevalence of goiter is increased in patients with ESRD (124,125). The prevalence of hypothyroidism ranges between 0 and 9.5% (124). Whereas primary hypothyroidism is observed 2.5 times more frequently in dialysis patients than in patients with other chronic nonrenal diseases, the prevalence of hyperthyroidism is not different (124). In children, the prevalence of hypothyroidism may be higher due to the greater proportion of patients treated for cystinosis and nephrotic syndrome. In cystinotic patients, deposition of cystine crystals in the thyroid can lead to destruction of the gland and frank hypothyroidism (126). Children with severe nephrotic syndrome, particularly those with the congenital form (127), may become hypothyroidal due to the renal loss of thyroid hormone–binding globulin (TBG).

Because some manifestations of hypothyroidism, such as hypothermia, pallor, and dry skin, also occur in uremia, the exclusion of the diagnosis of hypothyroidism on clinical grounds may be difficult in a uremic child. Therefore, exploration of the hormonal status of a patient is essential for the recognition of an accompanying thyroidal disorder.

Thyroid Hormones

Inorganic iodine is physiologically excreted by the kidney, and plasma inorganic iodine levels increase as kidney function decreases (128).

The plasma levels of total T_4 (thyroxine) and T_3 (triiodothyronine) are decreased in patients with CRF (129). Significant depression of T_4 and T_3 levels usually occurs once the GFR falls below 50%. Thyroid hormone *production rates* are normal in patients with CRF (130,131). Metabolic clearance rates of the hormones may (132) or may not (131) be increased. Due to impaired peripheral deiodination of T_4 to T_3 (6,132), there is a more distinct suppression of T_3 than of T_4 levels. In ESRD, diminished T_4 levels are found in one-third of patients and diminished T_3 levels in 50% of patients (125,133–136), including children (137). Concentrations of reverse T_3 (rT_3), the inactive metabolite of T_4 in plasma, are low (138) or normal (136). Production and metabolic clearance rates of rT_3 are normal (130), but extravascular binding of rT_3 is increased (131).

The more pronounced decrease of plasma T_3 than of T_4 levels in CRF resembles the thyroid hormone pattern observed in other states of chronic nonthyroidal diseases (sick euthyroid or low T_3 syndrome). However, whereas in the sick euthyroid syndrome rT_3 levels are elevated as a result of impaired peripheral conversion of T_4 to T_3, rT_3 levels are in the low-normal range in CRF. This constellation has been explained by a redistribution of rT_3 into extravascular compartments in uremia (131).

Binding Proteins

Circulating thyroid hormones are bound to TBG, albumin, and prealbumin. TBG levels usually are normal in hemodialysis patients (133,139); they are frequently low in patients on continuous ambulatory peritoneal dialysis (CAPD), who lose thyroid hormone–binding proteins via the dialysate (139,140). Patients with severe nephrotic syndrome may have markedly low TBG plasma levels due to urinary protein loss. Only the unbound (free) T_4 (fT_4) and T_3 (fT_3) fractions are biologically active. Plasma levels of fT_4 and fT_3 as measured by radioimmunoassay are low (141), and dissociation constants for specific T_4 and T_3 binding are normal (142).

Thyroid-Stimulating Hormone

Despite low plasma total and free T_4 and T_3 levels, thyroid-stimulating hormone (TSH) concentrations are usually normal in adults (133,141) and children with CRF (137). Normal TSH in the face of low fT_3 and fT_4 points to altered regulation of the hypothalamopituitary–thyroid axis. Experimental evidence suggests that the sensitivity of the thyrotroph to feedback inhibition is increased in uremia. In addition, TRH administration causes a blunted, delayed rise of plasma TSH (6,80,142). The duration of the TSH response is prolonged due to decreased metabolic clearance and increased half-lives of both TRH and TSH (84,143). Although basal iodine uptake is low (133), thyroid responsiveness to stimulation by TSH is normal (144).

The most convincing evidence for a primary hypothalamic defect comes from studies on the temporal organization of TSH release. The physiologic nocturnal TSH surge is frequently blunted in children and adults with ESRD (137,145), and the pattern of pulsatile TSH secretion is altered toward low-amplitude, high-frequency pulses (145).

In summary, CRF is associated with a resetting of the central thyrostat toward lower levels of circulating thyroid hormones. The lacking upregulation of spontaneous TSH secretion despite low thyroid hormone levels either may indicate a failure of the thyrotroph to respond to the physiologic stimulus of low thyroid hormone concentrations or may be interpreted as a "physiologic" downregulation resulting from a reduced *demand* for thyroid hormone in the specific state of metabolism caused by uremia.

Children with nephropathic cystinosis are exceptional in that, even in advanced renal failure, they exhibit an exaggerated TSH response to TRH stimulation. This reflects primary hypothyroidism due to destruction of the thyroid gland by deposition of cystine crystals (126). TSH level may also be elevated in children with severe nephrotic syndrome (127), which reflects a hypothyroid state due to renal loss of TBG-bound thyroid hormones.

Thyroid Hormone Action

Clinically, patients with CRF usually appear euthyroid. Measurements of basal metabolic rate and rough clinical indices yield normal results (134,146). Normal TSH concentrations suggest that euthyroidism is also present in pituitary thyrotrophs. In experimental uremia an upregulation of T_3 receptor expression, possibly as a compensatory mechanism to low circulating levels of T_3, and normal expression of T_3-dependent hepatic proteins have been observed (147,148). Although endogenous hormone action appears efficient, CRF patients show a marked resistance against exogenous thyroid hormone administration with regard to thermogenesis. Oxygen uptake is neither stimulated by administration of T_3 nor suppressed by its antagonist sodium ipodate (149) (Fig. 68.6). In contrast to normal subjects, in CRF patients T_3 supplementation results in exaggerated protein degradation and a negative nitrogen balance (138,150,151), similar to that observed in patients with chronic illness or malnutri-

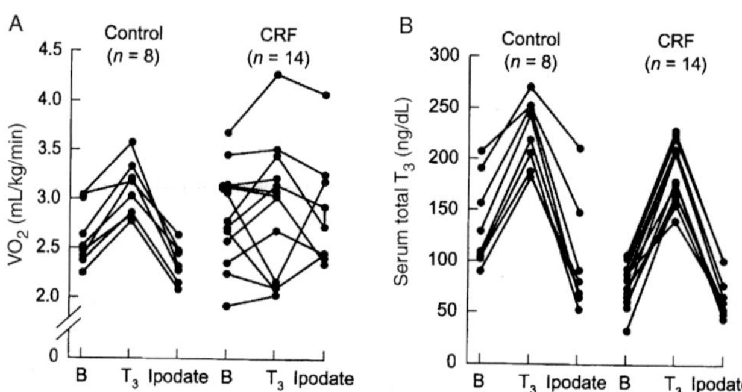

FIGURE 68.6. Failure of thyroxin administration to stimulate, and of thyroid suppression to reduce, oxygen consumption (VO_2) **(A)** despite adequate changes in plasma triiodothyronine (T_3) levels **(B)** in patients with chronic renal insufficiency (CRF). B, baseline level. (From Lim VS, Zavala DC, Flanigan MJ, et al. Blunted peripheral tissue responsiveness to thyroid hormone in uremic patients. *Kidney Int* 1987;31:808–814, with permission.)

tion (152). Hence, the low T_3 syndrome of uremia may in part be interpreted as a physiologic adaptation to conserve energy in an adverse metabolic environment, and supplementary thyroid hormone treatment might be not only useless but even harmful.

Diagnosis and Clinical Management of Thyroid Disorders in Chronic Renal Failure

In a uremic patient, hypothyroidism should be diagnosed only if total and free T_4 levels are distinctly low, the TBG concentrations are normal, and basal TSH levels are elevated (>20 μU/mL). A normal plasma TSH level is probably a valid indicator of tissue euthyroidism. Treatment with thyroid hormones should be limited to patients with clinical hypothyroidism and elevated plasma TSH levels. The increased risk for induction of tissue catabolism by thyroid hormone treatment needs to be recognized.

In hemodialysis patients heparin may interfere with the thyroid hormone status. Heparin competes with T_4 at intra- and extravascular binding sites, and thus increases total and free T_4 serum levels for at least 24 hours after dialysis (153). Therefore, strict standardization of the timing of investigations relative to dialysis is essential. Other substances, for example, high-dose frusemide, can cause similar artifacts (154).

Patients with CRF who undergo repeated radiologic investigations with iodinated contrast agents may be at increased risk of developing iodine-induced hyperthyroidism because of reduced iodine clearance.

Adrenal Hormone Axis

Clinical Findings

Dysfunction of the pituitary-adrenal axis may be difficult to diagnose in patients with CRF. Uremia shares certain clinical signs and symptoms with Cushing syndrome, such as osteopenia, proximal muscle weakness with atrophy, glucose intolerance, negative nitrogen balance, and hypertension (155); therefore, Cushing syndrome may easily be missed if it occurs concomitantly with renal failure. Similarly, adrenal insufficiency may present with symptoms that are not uncommon in renal failure, for example, hypotension, weakness, and hyperkalemia. To confirm or reject the diagnoses of Cushing syndrome or adrenal failure, the clinician must rely on the evaluation of the patient's hormonal status under basal and stimulated conditions.

Cortisol

Cortisol is conjugated in the liver to water-soluble metabolites, which are predominantly excreted by the kidney and accumulate in renal failure. Although normal morning fasting cortisol levels are found in the majority of adult and pediatric patients with CRF (156–159), 24-hour integrated mean total and free cortisol concentrations are consistently elevated (160). Basal hypercortisolism is particularly prevalent in patients on hemodialysis (159). The diurnal rhythm and the pulsatile mode of cortisol secretion is conserved in renal failure; however, the half-life of the endogenous secretory peaks is prolonged (156,160,161). In hemodialysis patients, the secretory activity is shifted toward the dialysis hours, whereas a normal pattern is observed on days off dialysis (160).

Stimulation of the zona fasciculata with exogenous adrenocorticotropic hormone (ACTH) in uremic patients yields a normal cortisol response, irrespective of whether supraphysiologic (159,162,163) or low doses of ACTH are used (163). Zona glomerulosa steroids (aldosterone, 18-hydroxycorticosterone) are stimulated normally in CAPD (163) but not in hemodialysis patients (164). Transient hyporesponsiveness to ACTH is observed in the majority of patients who returned to dialysis after transplant failure (165).

Adrenal Androgens

Adrenarche marks an important milestone in endocrine maturation. Adrenarche occurs approximately 2 years before the initiation of puberty and is independent of it. Low plasma levels of dehydroepiandrosterone and dehydroepiandrosterone sulfate, the marker hormones of the zona reticularis, are observed in adult men as well as in pre- and midpubertal boys on hemodialysis, whereas normal levels are found in patients on conservative treatment (30,166,167). Conversely, levels of androstenedione, an adrenal androgen produced by the ACTH-dependent zona fasciculata, are elevated in patients on conservative treatment, and normal or elevated in hemodialysis patients (30,159). A similar elevation of androstenedione level is observed in girls with CRF (41). In renal allograft recipients, glucocorticoid treatment invariably lowers adrenal androgen production to almost undetectable levels (29,30,159).

Adrenocorticotropic Hormone

Basal ACTH levels are normal (159) or elevated (157,162) in patients with CRF. The functional status of pituitary corticotrophs in uremia is still under discussion. ACTH secretion is not suppressible by standard oral doses of dexamethasone (162,168). Oral absorption of dexamethasone is reduced in uremia (156), however, and suppression of ACTH can be achieved at higher doses (156,160). After intravenous administration of dexamethasone, only incomplete suppression of plasma cortisol levels is observed; however, the metabolic clearance of dexamethasone is possibly increased in uremia (156,169). The responsiveness of the corticotroph to stimulation by metapyrone may (162) or may not (156) be reduced in uremia. The ACTH release after administration of corticotropin-releasing hormone occurs early but is blunted (157). In normal subjects acute hypoglycemia elicits a counterregulatory stimulation of the corticotropin-releasing hormone–ACTH–cortisol axis. In patients with CRF this stress reaction is markedly suppressed. The increase of ACTH and cortisol after insulin-induced hypoglycemia is blunted in patients on hemodialysis (156), which provides further evidence of a disordered hypothalamopituitary regulation of the corticotropic axis in uremia.

Diagnosis and Management of Pituitary-Adrenal Disorders

The most frequent circumstance in which a pediatric nephrologist encounters adrenocortical failure is on discontinuation of glucocorticoids in patients returning to dialysis after transplant failure. Also, accidental adrenectomy can occur during nephrectomy, particularly in young infants, and adrenal hemorrhage leading to functional disorders is not uncommon in the perinatal period, in children with coagulation disorders, and as a side effect of therapeutic anticoagulation. Also, adrenal insufficiency is occasionally seen as a complication of amyloidosis that also compromises renal function, as typically seen in patients with severe chronic vasculitis or familial Mediterranean fever. Demonstration of low cortisol levels and insufficient cortisol response to ACTH is required to confirm the diagnosis.

In transplant recipients adrenal responsiveness is suppressed by steroid treatment (165). This poses the risk of acute adrenal insufficiency during severe stress, for example, surgical procedures or abrupt steroid withdrawal.

The diagnosis of Cushing syndrome in a patient with CRF requires the finding of elevated plasma cortisol levels, measured by a radioimmunoassay in extracted serum. Although a single measurement of cortisol may be misleading, loss of diurnal rhythm (24-hour cortisol profile) is a characteristic of Cushing syndrome not seen in uremia-related adrenal dysfunction. Failure of high-dose dexamethasone given orally (0.11 mg/kg) or intravenously (0.03 mg/kg) to suppress ACTH and cortisol levels is confirmatory evidence.

Hormones Involved in Carbohydrate Metabolism

Glucose intolerance is a common feature of CRF. The introduction of the euglycemic and hyperglycemic clamp techniques has been important in understanding insulin and glucose metabolism in patients with CRF (170). In the euglycemic insulin clamp technique, a given level of insulinemia is maintained and blood glucose is kept constant by infusing glucose at a continuously adjusted rate. Thus, the infusion rate equals tissue glucose uptake and metabolism. This allows quantitation of tissue sensitivity to insulin. In the hyperglycemic clamp technique, blood glucose levels are acutely raised by a priming infusion of glucose and then maintained constant at approximately twice the fasting level by a variable glucose infusion. Under these steady-state conditions, the glucose infusion rate is a measure of glucose uptake and metabolism by all cells of the body. The early plasma insulin response is an index of beta cell responsiveness to the hyperglycemic stimulus, whereas the late insulin response is a measure of peripheral tissue sensitivity to insulin.

Insulin Secretion

Fasting serum insulin levels are usually normal or slightly elevated in patients with CRF. In contrast, serum levels of proinsulin and C-peptide are elevated. This discrepancy is explained by differences in the relative contribution of the kidney to the metabolic clearance rates of these peptides (171). Nevertheless, insulin half-life is increased two- to threefold in CRF. When this is taken into account, a relative insulin hyposecretion is present under fasting conditions in CRF patients (172).

In hyperglycemic clamp studies, the early insulin response, an indicator of the pancreatic beta-cell sensitivity to glucose, is variable: Decreased (173), delayed (174), normal (175), and even increased (176,177) responses have been reported. A decreased initial insulin release in response to high glucose concentrations is found in isolated pancreatic islets of uremic rats (178). The late insulin response is invariably increased in uremic patients, which indicates tissue resistance to insulin, and improves with dialysis (179).

Insulin is physiologically secreted in frequent (every 8 minutes), low-amplitude oscillations that are superimposed on slow, high-amplitude secretory pulsations (every 75 minutes). Unlike in other states of insulin resistance, a characteristic slowing of both rhythms as well as hyperrhythmicity and exaggerated width and amplitude of the low-frequency insulin pulses in response to meals was observed in patients with CRF, which points to a specific abnormality in the neuroendocrine regulation of insulin secretion (172).

The variable beta-cell response may explain why only some patients develop overt glucose intolerance despite constant peripheral insulin resistance. Glucose intolerance becomes manifest only when the beta-cell insulin response to glucose is so impaired that it can no longer increase and overcome peripheral insulin resistance (81).

Some evidence suggests a role for PTH in the deranged beta-cell function of CRF. In children with CRF and severe secondary hyperparathyroidism, glucose intolerance resolves after parathyroidectomy through an improvement of the pancreatic insulin secretory capacity, whereas insulin insensitivity persists (180,181). High PTH levels, with or without uremia, impair insulin secretion by a cAMP-independent mechanism (182). Chronic hyperparathyroidism might enhance calcium entry into the pancreatic islets, which results in an accumulation of calcium that impairs insulin release. This hypothesis is supported by the prevention of glucose intolerance and the normalization of islet insulin secretion in uremic rats treated with the calcium channel blocker verapamil (183).

Tissue Resistance to Insulin

Euglycemic insulin clamp studies in adults (184) and children (185) with preterminal renal failure unanimously show marked decreases in tissue sensitivity to insulin, glucose uptake, and metabolic clearance of insulin. After 10 weeks of dialysis treatment all indices are markedly improved. The two major sites of carbohydrate metabolism are the liver and the muscle tissue. Impaired insulin action may be characterized by diminished splanchnic glucose extraction, increased hepatic gluconeogenesis, decreased peripheral glucose uptake, or a combination of these. Most studies of uremic patients report normal basal and insulin- or glucose-suppressed hepatic glucose output (11,184,186). However, these observations may be valid only for supraphysiologic insulin concentrations. When endogenous insulin secretion is blocked by somatostatin and insulin infused in physiologic doses, suppression of hepatic gluconeogenesis is incomplete in uremic patients (187). Moreover, isotope studies suggest reduced glucose oxidation to CO_2 and increased glucose recycling (186). In contrast to these subtle changes of hepatic glucose turnover, glucose metabolism in the peripheral tissue is markedly impaired (184,188,189). Hence, the major site of resistance to insulin-mediated glucose uptake in uremia is the peripheral tissue, mainly skeletal muscle.

In principle, insulin resistance may be due to changes at the membrane receptor level, the postreceptor level, or a combination of these. Studies of adipocytes, monocytes, hepatocytes, and human muscle tissue showed normal or even elevated density and binding affinities of the insulin receptor and normal receptor-mediated transmembranous hexose transport (11,190–194). In uremic patients, glucose disposal was subnormal even after suppression of endogenous insulin secretion by somatostatin (195). This observation suggests that the stimulation of glucose uptake by insulin is unchanged, but insulin-independent glucose uptake is impaired. Thus, receptor expression and binding are normal or even increased, possibly as a result of homeostatic upregulation in response to insulin resistance, and the stimulation of glucose uptake by insulin is intact.

Insulin membrane receptors are expressed in abundance, and maximal hormone action occurs when only 10% of receptors are occupied. Consequently, insulin resistance at the receptor level can be overcome by high insulin concentrations, whereas a postreceptor defect cannot. Glucose uptake evaluated by the euglycemic clamp technique remains severely reduced in uremic patients even at the highest dose of insulin (11) (Fig. 68.7). This observation is

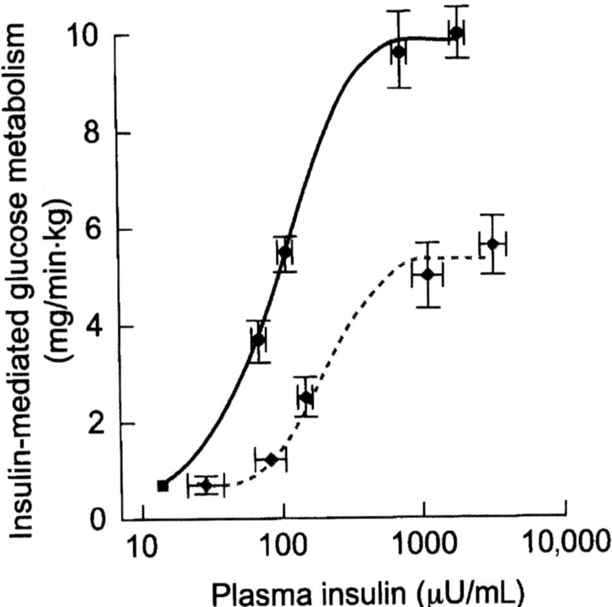

FIGURE 68.7. Dose-response relationship between the plasma insulin concentration and insulin-mediated glucose metabolism in patients with chronic renal failure (*dashed line*) and control subjects (*solid line*). Diminished maximal insulin-mediated glucose metabolism suggests insulin resistance by postreceptor defect. (From Smith D, Defronzo RA. Insulin resistance in uremia mediated by post binding defects. *Kidney Int* 1982;22:54–62, with permission.)

The exact step in the sequence of insulin-induced signaling events that accounts for the postreceptor defect is not yet known. In human muscle tissue, insulin-receptor kinase activity is normal (194). Insulin stimulates glycogen synthesis and glycolysis by increasing the activity of glycogen synthase, phosphofructokinase, pyruvate kinase, and pyruvate dehydrogenase. Glycogen levels are normal and maximal glycogen synthase activity is even elevated in muscle tissue of uremic patients (194), whereas phosphofructokinase activity is diminished (196). On the other hand, basal and stimulated lactate formation is normal or even increased in erythrocytes of uremic patients, which suggests no impairment of glycolysis in this tissue (191). Kalhan et al. demonstrated diminished glucose oxidation and increased recycling of glucose carbon in uremic patients, which suggests impaired glucose metabolism via the Krebs cycle (186).

Etiology of Insulin Resistance

Glucose intolerance in patients with CRF is partially corrected by dialysis (179,197). This observation suggests the presence of one or more dialyzable factors in uremic serum that compromise the biological actions of insulin. Apart from dialysis, glucose metabolism is also improved by consumption of low-protein diets in children (198) and adults (199) with CRF. It was hypothesized that low protein intake reduces the synthesis of a peptide inhibiting insulin action. Several peptides possibly interfering with glucose metabolism in uremia have been isolated (200–202). Evidence suggests that 1,25-dihydroxyvitamin D_3 deficiency may play a role in the pathogenesis of insulin resistance in uremia (203). Furthermore, insulin resistance improves in adolescents on dialysis after correction of anemia and amelioration of iron overload by recombinant erythropoietin therapy (204).

Glucagon

Glucagon plasma levels are markedly increased in uremia. This increase is in part due to cross reactivity with the bioinactive 9-kDa proglucagon molecule (205). The biologically active 3.5-kDa glucagon moiety is increased threefold. This increase is entirely due to decreased metabolic clearance; secretion is normal (206). Glucagon exerts its hyperglycemic action primarily by stimulating hepatic gluconeogenesis. Patients with CRF exhibit reduced endogenous glucose output after a glucagon challenge (187). Diminished glucagon binding with unchanged binding affinity by hepatic membranes was demonstrated in chronically uremic rats (207). Normal basal but diminished stimulated adenylate cyclase activity was found. These results may be explained by receptor downregulation in response to chronic glucagon excess, because healthy rats treated with exogenous glucagon exhibit similar changes.

Carbohydrate Metabolism during Peritoneal Dialysis

Long-term peritoneal dialysis is characterized by continuous glucose absorption from the peritoneal fluid, which amounts to 2 to 3 g/kg/day in children on an average peritoneal dialysis regimen. In view of the known glucose intolerance of uremia, this has raised some concern. Basal glucose and insulin levels are normal or increased in CAPD patients (174,208,209). A transient increase of plasma glucose and insulin levels occurs during a CAPD cycle, which is correlated with the glucose content of the peritoneal dialysis fluid (208). The area under the curve after an oral glucose load is higher in uremic patients on CAPD than in nondialyzed and hemodialyzed patients (191). Conflicting results have been reported with respect to the effect of CAPD on glucose tolerance and glucoregulatory hormones (190,209). Peripheral insulin sensitivity improves after initiation of CAPD (210); the improvement is significantly better with peritoneal dialysis than with hemodialysis treatment (197). Insulin-binding affinity and receptor numbers decrease on adipocytes of CAPD patients within the first 3 months of CAPD treatment, but no change in insulin sensitivity is observed as assessed by the effect of insulin on glucose uptake and lipogenesis (190).

The presently available information indicates that glucose intolerance is not exaggerated in patients on CAPD. Insulin resistance tends to improve after initiation of peritoneal dialysis, even more so than in newly hemodialyzed patients. This may be explained by removal of circulating inhibitors of insulin action. The observed decrease of membrane insulin-binding capacity *in vitro* (190) may reflect receptor downregulation due to chronic hyperinsulinemia. Whether the chronic hyperinsulinemia in CAPD patients has deleterious long-term effects is as yet unknown.

GROWTH AND DEVELOPMENTAL DISORDERS IN CHRONIC RENAL FAILURE

Impact of Developmental Stage on Growth in Chronic Renal Failure

The regulatory mechanisms of statural growth during childhood differ at the successive stages of development. During the first 2 years of life, growth is driven mainly by nutritional factors, particularly the intake of energy and protein. In later childhood, growth appears to depend mainly on the somatotropic hormone axis, with nutrition exerting a more permissive influence. In puberty, the growth process is dominated by the gonadotropic hormone axis, which stimulates and finally terminates body growth by direct action on the growth cartilage and by modulation of the somatotropic hormone axis. In view of these differences in growth regulation, the description of growth in renal disorders deserves to be separated for the periods of infancy, mid-childhood, and puberty.

The first 2 years of life are the most dynamic period of growth. Some 30% of total postnatal statural growth normally is achieved during this period. Any disturbance of growth in infancy has a greater impact on growth potential than disturbance at later stages of development. Spontaneous growth in children with congenital CRF is characterized by a rapidly increasing height deficit during the first 2 years of life, followed by a rather percentile-parallel growth pattern in the mid-childhood years. In the late prepubertal period, height velocity again decreases disproportionately, resulting in a further deviation from the normal percentiles. A late pubertal growth spurt of diminished amplitude eventually results in an irreversible loss of growth potential, which leads to a stunted adult height.

Infancy

Untreated CRF during early infancy is usually associated with severe growth retardation (211–214). The mean loss in relative height in untreated patients is as high as 0.6 standard deviation (SD) per month during the first year of life. A detailed analysis of the early infantile growth pattern observed in children with congenital CRF by means of the infancy-childhood-puberty model revealed that the infancy growth phase, starting in intrauterine life and vanishing during the second year of life, is affected in 50% of patients

(215). Height SDS was already reduced at birth, decreased further during the first 3 postnatal months, behaved normally between the third and ninth months, and again decreased between the tenth and twelfth months of life. The intrauterine period, the first 3 postnatal months, and the period preceding the first birthday each contributed by approximately one-third to the overall reduction in height SDS observed in infants with congenital CRF. The observed intrauterine growth retardation raises the question of whether the prenatal accumulation of certain circulating substances not cleared by the placenta in children with severe renal hypoplasia may compromise fetal growth. Conversely, intrauterine malnutrition could be the primary cause not only of fetal growth retardation but also of abnormal renal morphogenesis, if it is present in the early stages of pregnancy. In early postnatal life, anorexia, water and electrolyte imbalances due to uremia, recurrent vomiting, catabolic responses to infections, metabolic acidosis, and secondary hyperparathyroidism are the main factors compromising growth. If appropriate management is instituted early enough, severe stunting can usually be prevented. Forced enteral feeding using nasogastric tubes, gastrostomies, and even fundoplication as required appears essential to prevent or reverse malnutrition (216,217). Under optimal conditions it is possible to keep infants with CRF within 1 to 2 SD below the mean height for age (217,218).

After a transient stabilization of growth rates, a variable further loss in relative height is commonly seen between 9 and 18 months of age. According to the infancy-childhood-puberty model, this period reflects the transition from the infancy growth phase to the childhood growth phase. An irregular onset or maintenance of the childhood growth component was observed in 60% of patients and resulted in a further decrease in mean standardized height of 0.7 SDS (215). The reasons for this secondary deterioration of growth in infancy, which may occur despite adequate nutritional and medical supplementation, are poorly understood.

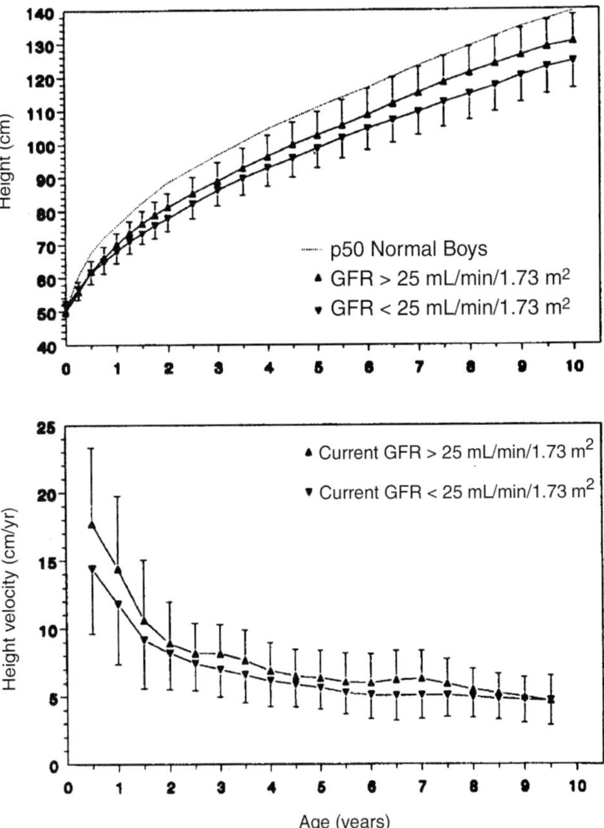

FIGURE 68.8. Glomerular filtration rate (GFR)–dependent growth pattern in children with chronic renal failure due to hypoplastic and dysplastic renal disorders. Approximately 100 children per age interval were evaluated. Mean ±1 standard deviation of height is shown for children with average GFR less than and greater than 25 mL/min/1.73 m^2. p50, fiftieth percentile. (Adapted from Schaefer F, Wingen AM, Hennicke M, et al. Growth charts for prepubertal children with chronic renal failure due to congenital renal disorders. European Study Group for Nutritional Treatment of Chronic Renal Failure in Childhood. *Pediatr Nephrol* 1996;10:288–293.)

Mid-Childhood

After the period of rapid infantile growth, height velocity slows down to an almost constant increment per year. During this period endocrine mechanisms regulate growth.

In mid-childhood, patients with hypoplastic renal diseases usually grow in keeping with the percentile attained around the end of infancy (219). Patients who develop CRF after the second year of life exhibit a loss of relative height early in the course of disease and follow the growth percentile reached after stabilization of the disease process. The degree of renal dysfunction is the principal determinant of the variability in growth during this period. Spontaneous mid-childhood growth tends to be subnormal when GFR is below 25 mL/min/1.73 m^2 (212,219–221) (Fig. 68.8). Mid-childhood growth rates are consistently correlated with GFR, although only 10 to 15% of the variability in growth is actually accounted for by this parameter (219). The degree of anemia, metabolic acidosis, and malnutrition contributes only marginally to annual growth rates.

The more or less percentile-parallel growth of uremic children in mid-childhood has been interpreted as a "normal" growth pattern that could be expected after a loss of growth potential in early infancy. Such readjustment of the growth channel is seen in children with cardiac diseases after surgery or in children with adrenal insufficiency overtreated in infancy (222). However, the observation that complete catchup growth, although not common, does occur in children in whom renal function is normalized by successful renal transplantation, and that glucocorticoid treatment can be withdrawn (223), suggests that catchup growth is continuously suppressed in the uremic milieu. The percentile-parallel growth pattern during this period may therefore reflect a net balance between the growth-suppressive effect of uremia and the organism's inherent tendency for catchup growth.

Puberty

The height gain achieved during the pubertal growth spurt is usually reduced (17,118,224,225). In a longitudinal analysis of the growth curves of 29 adolescents with various degrees of CRF, the growth spurt started with an average delay of 2.5 years (17). The degree of the delay was correlated with the duration of CRF. Although a distinct acceleration of growth occurred during puberty, the total pubertal height gain was reduced in both sexes to approximately 50% of that of healthy late-maturing children. This reduction was due to a marked suppression of the late prespurt height velocity, a subnormal peak height velocity, and a shortening of the pubertal growth period by 1 year in boys and 1.5 years in girls. Notably, the prolonged prepubertal growth phase, which resulted from the delayed onset of the pubertal growth spurt, permitted the patients to grow up to an almost normal immediately prespurt height (–1 SDS in boys, +0.1 SDS in girls). Subsequently, relative height was gradually lost during the pubertal growth spurt, so that patients ended up with an average relative height of –2.9 SDS in boys and –2.3 SDS in girls. This pattern of pubertal growth was confirmed in a control group of ESRD patients followed in the late 1990s who were not treated with rGH (226).

In prepubertal children with long-standing renal failure, bone maturation is invariably retarded (227–230). In dialysis patients, skeletal maturation is increasingly retarded before the start of puberty and then accelerates dramatically. This observation and the fact that uremic boys respond to exogenous application of testosterone esters by an exaggerated increase in skeletal maturation (230) suggest that the sensitivity of the growth plate to sex steroids is at least conserved. Because proliferation (i.e., growth) cannot keep pace with differentiation (i.e., bone maturation), growth potential may irreversibly be lost during puberty in uremia.

In contrast, in many transplant patients, an apparent standstill of bone maturation is observed, even when the patient is growing and puberty is progressing. This phenomenon is thought to be related to direct interference of corticosteroids with the differentiation of the growth plate. Despite the delayed bone maturation, late growth is usually not observed (17,231,232). In fact, the successive stages of the pubertal growth spurt seem to occur at increasingly earlier bone ages than would be assumed in a normal population (17).

Final Height

A crucial question in the rehabilitation of children with chronic renal disease is the degree to which final height is compromised. Of the patients with childhood-onset ESRD in the European Dialysis and Transplant Association Registry, 50% achieved adult heights below the third percentile. Children who underwent continued dialysis until adulthood reached a lower mean final height than children who received a renal transplant (231,233–238). Final height appears to be more severely compromised in boys than in girls, which reflects the higher incidence of congenital nephropathies in boys. Final height is most compromised in patients with severe congenital renal disorders, among which nephropathic cystinosis leads to the most obvious growth retardation (239). However, patients with acquired glomerular diseases usually exhibit a very marked loss in height SDS in the early course of the disease, which results in the need for growth-promoting treatment in a large proportion of this patient group as well.

Impact of Underlying Renal Disease on Statural Growth

Hypoplastic and Dysplastic Nephropathies

Congenital renal hypoplasia or dysplasia, with or without urinary tract obstruction, is the most common cause of ESRD during the first 5 years of life. Renal dysplasia is characterized by tubular dysfunction with electrolyte losses and polyuria, and a gradual decline of GFR. The time to ESRD is highly variable and depends on the degree of hypoplasia and tubular dysfunction, and the incidence of infections. Growth failure usually develops during the first year of life. Thereafter, growth rates remain more or less stable and are usually sufficient to keep the patient's height parallel to the centiles. In the care of these patients, it is important to compensate for tubular electrolyte losses and acidosis. Pharmacologic renoprotective therapy with renin-angiotensin system antagonists may slow the progression of renal failure and thereby have a positive long-term impact on statural growth.

Glomerulopathies

Progressive glomerular injury may appear as acute or chronic glomerulonephritis, or as nephrotic disease. Growth rates decline in patients with progressive glomerulonephritis as glomerular function deteriorates. Growth velocity is affected even in mild renal insufficiency (220). In patients with nephrotic syndrome, proteinuria per se impairs growth, both in congenital nephrosis and resistant nephrotic syndrome that appears later in childhood (240,241). The dosage and duration of glucocorticoid treatment in nephrotic syndrome and the evolution of renal function are predominant factors affecting growth. Prolonged high-dose corticosteroid administration suppresses growth rates (241–244). Although partial catchup growth occurs after steroid withdrawal, final height is correlated with the cumulative glucocorticoid dose (241). Congenital nephrotic syndrome usually is associated with severe stunting during the first months of life while

GFR still is in the normal range but massive edema and proteinuria are present. Growth failure in these infants may be secondary to edema, recurrent infections, endocrine alterations due to losses of peptide and protein-bound hormones, and protein-calorie malnutrition. Bilateral nephrectomy, which replaces proteinuria, edema, and cachexia by ESRD, may be associated with improved growth (245).

Tubular and Interstitial Nephropathies

Primary *tubular dysfunctions* and *interstitial disorders* may lead to severe growth impairment even in the absence of chronic renal insufficiency. Patients with either proximal or distal renal tubular acidosis may present with growth failure during the first years of life (246,247). Growth impairment may be due to tissue catabolism, volume depletion, electrolyte disorders, and/or malnutrition. Catchup growth is observed after correction of *acidosis* with alkaline therapy in distal renal tubular acidosis (246,248). Growth retardation occurs in approximately 50% of patients with nephrogenic *diabetes insipidus*; hypernatremia, volume contraction, and malnutrition interfere with growth. Maintenance of water balance and treatment with indomethacin are associated with catchup growth (249). Bartter's syndrome and related disorders with chronic *potassium depletion* usually are characterized by a failure to thrive (250). Experimental potassium deficiency leads to growth failure characterized by both reduced endogenous GH secretion and complete resistance to exogenous GH (251,252). In patients with hyper–prostaglandin E syndrome, indomethacin medication leads to partial catchup growth (253). In view of the various isolated tubular deficiencies that can cause growth impairment, it is conceivable that children with complex disorders of proximal and distal tubular function, such as idiopathic *Fanconi syndrome* (254,255) or hereditary *fructose intolerance,* may develop severe growth failure. In these cases, only partial catchup growth is possible even with rigorous electrolyte supplementation (246,248,250,253). Severe growth failure may also develop in children with systemic diseases such as *cystinosis* or *oxalosis* that involve not only the kidneys but also other organs. In patients with cystinosis, growth failure is usually the first clinical symptom of tubular dysfunction, which generally develops around 6 to 18 months of age. Growth failure occurs even with optimal substitution of tubular losses, however, due to the generalized deposition of cystine crystals, which results in local growth plate and hypothalamopituitary dysfunction and hypothyroidism. In a survey by the EDTA only 13 of 106 cystinotic patients on renal replacement therapy who were between 8 and 21 years of age had a height above the third percentile (256). The introduction of cystine-depleting agents has offered new prospects for children with cystinosis. Treatment with cysteamine or phosphocysteamine appears to slow the rate of deterioration of GFR and to improve growth rates (257–259). Recombinant GH is effective in stimulating growth independently of renal function and cysteamine treatment (239).

In patients with chronic or recurrent interstitial disease, a minor degree of growth retardation may develop. Persistent or recurrent *urinary tract infections* may cause growth impairment by tubular dysfunction, the catabolic effect of chronic disease, and/or progressive renal insufficiency. Growth rates may increase after medical and/or surgical intervention (260–262). In patients with vesicoureteric reflux, moderate growth retardation has been demonstrated in cases of bilateral disease and significant renal scarring (263). Whereas previous reports noted a growth spurt after successful antireflux surgery (261,262), multiple regression analysis encompassing 54 patients with obstructive urinary tract malformations suggested a positive relationship between the increase in relative height and the duration of antibiotic treatment, but no independent effect of surgical intervention (264). Severe growth failure was observed in patients with posterior urethral valves; it was most marked in patients with severe symptoms diagnosed early (265).

Etiology of Growth Failure in Chronic Renal Failure

The pathogenesis of impaired growth in CRF is complex and only partially understood. Although a particular cause can occasionally be found, a combination of several factors is generally responsible for growth impairment. Furthermore, the patient's age; the type, duration, and severity of renal disease; the treatment modality; and the patient's social environment all play important roles.

One of the cardinal abnormalities associated with CRF is a *loss of appetite*. Adequate energy intake is required for anabolism and growth. Energy intake is inversely related to the degree of renal failure (266) and is correlated with growth rates if it is lower than 80% of the recommended dietary allowance (267). However, further augmentation of energy intake above this level results in obesity rather than in a further stimulation of growth (267,268). Energy malnutrition is particularly prevalent in uremic infants during the first year of life, when metabolic rate is high in relation to body mass. Height SDS is correlated with body cell mass and serum transferrin or albumin levels in infants, which emphasizes the importance of malnutrition in growth failure in this age group (211,269,270). In later childhood, spontaneous food intake is usually low for the patient's age but normal when adjusted for body mass (271,272). Thus, it is difficult to differentiate whether low energy intake is the cause or the consequence of impaired growth. The same is true for the body protein content of children with CRF and short stature, which generally is adequate for height but not for age (273).

At any given protein intake, the conversion of dietary protein to body protein is less efficient in uremic animals than in pair-fed controls (274). Resistance to the anabolic effects of insulin and IGF-1 and increased protein breakdown by activation of proteolytic pathways may contribute to poor growth. In contrast to deficient calorie intake, protein malnutrition is infrequently seen in children with CRF (271,272). In a prospective study that deliberately limited protein intake to the safe levels set by the World Health Organization (e.g., 0.8 to 1.1 g/kg/day) but ensured adequate calorie intake, no impairment of weight gain and length gain was seen over 3 years (275).

Disturbances of Water and Electrolyte Metabolism

Many congenital renal diseases that slowly progress toward CRF lead to a loss of electrolytes and a reduced ability of the kidney to concentrate urine. In particular, sodium chloride is lost in patients with obstructive uropathies and renal hypoplasia, and potassium is lost in patients with tubular damage, particularly those with nephropathic cystinosis. Polyuria, an expression of the reduced ability of the kidney to concentrate the urine, is seen in Fanconi syndrome and nephronophthisis, but also in hypoplastic kidney disease.

It is not possible to independently assess the extent to which disturbances in water and electrolyte metabolism contribute to growth retardation in individual patients with CRF. The probability of these factors' being significant, however, has been shown by analogous clinical and animal studies. In rats, sodium deficiency leads to a decrease in protein synthesis and growth, which is only partially reversible by sodium repletion (276,277). Part of the effects usually attributed to sodium deficiency are actually caused by concomitant depletion of chloride; selective removal of chloride from a sodium-replete diet causes growth retardation and diminished muscle protein synthesis (278).

Metabolic Acidosis

Metabolic acidosis is inevitably observed in CRF if a 50% reduction in normal GFR is noted, due to the kidney's reduced ability to excrete ammonia. The acidosis is aggravated by nutritional protein and acid load, catabolism, and altered electrolyte balance. Metabolic acidosis is associated with increased glucocorticoid production and increased protein degradation by the activation of branched-chain ketoacid catabolism and the ubiquitin-proteasome pathway (279–281). In young children with CRF, the degree of protein wasting is tightly correlated with serum bicarbonate levels (282). Moreover, metabolic acidosis has profound suppressive effects on the somatotropic hormone axis by downregulating GH secretion (78), GH receptor and IGF-1 gene expression (283), and serum IGF-1 levels (284). Hence acidosis per se causes a state of GH insensitivity.

Anemia

Children with CRF develop increasing anemia as a result of erythropoietin deficiency. It is not certain if or to what extent chronic anemia leads to growth impairment. Children with chronic anemia (e.g., thalassemia major) show retardation of growth and development. When these patients are treated with high-frequency transfusion regimens to keep hematocrits close to the normal range, growth rates may improve (285). Theoretically, anemia may interfere with growth via various mechanisms such as poor appetite, intercurrent infections, cardiac complications, and poor oxygenation of the cartilage cells in the growth plate. The introduction of recombinant erythropoietin for the treatment of renal anemia has offered the opportunity to study whether changes in growth are induced by compensation for renal anemia. Whereas short-term stimulatory effects of erythropoietin were observed in single patients (286), no persistent growth improvement was seen in prospective trials (287). Likewise, blood transfusion and erythropoietin treatment of uremic rats did not result in improved growth (288).

Renal Osteodystrophy

Although gross skeletal deformities can contribute to the retardation of a child's growth, the appearance of renal osteodystrophy is not inevitably paralleled by alterations in epiphyseal growth of the long bones. Severe metaphyseal skeletal changes are often detected radiologically in patients with relatively good growth rates. In such cases, osteopathy is unmasked by rapid growth. Growth is arrested completely only when secondary hyperparathyroidism results in severe destruction of the metaphyseal bone architecture.

Whereas treatment with vitamin D and 1,25-dihydroxyvitamin D_3 improves growth in uremic rats (289), an equivalent therapeutic success has not been achieved in children with CRF. Treatment with 5000 to 10,000 IU vitamin D_3 per day did not affect growth in children on dialysis (290). An early optimistic report involving four patients receiving 1,25-dihydroxyvitamin D_3 (291) could not be validated in the long term (292).

The extent to which secondary hyperparathyroidism contributes to growth impairment is unclear. PTH is an anabolic hormone and an intrinsic growth factor, stimulating mitosis in osteoprogenitor cells and growth plate chondrocytes and upregulating the vitamin D receptor (293,294). Intermittent PTH administration stimulates the skeletal growth of normal and uremic rats (295). However, resistance to the effect of PTH is observed in uremia, characterized by reduced cAMP production in growth plate chondrocytes (293). A low bone turnover state induced by relatively low PTH levels may contribute to growth impairment (296). At the other end of the spectrum, excessive secretion of PTH can lead to the destruction of growth plate architecture (297), epiphyseal displacement (298), and metaphyseal fractures (299).

Hormonal Factors

The multiple alterations of endocrine systems associated with CRF have been described earlier. Of particular relevance for statural growth is the complex state of GH and IGF-1 resistance, which results in an impaired promotion of endochondral and appositional growth by IGF-1.

Impact of Treatment on Growth in Chronic Renal Failure

General Aspects

Adequate *nutritional intake* is the most important prerequisite for early infantile growth. Growth rates in this period are correlated with energy intake (267). Consequently, forced feeding via nasogastric tube, gastrostomy, or even fundoplication is an essential component in the management of infantile CRF (216,217,300). In later childhood, adequate nutrition is a permissive factor for growth; however, catchup growth cannot be obtained by dietary manipulations alone. *Metabolic acidosis* should be treated systematically, and *water and electrolyte losses* must be consequently compensated (218,301,302). Prevention of renal osteodystrophy by *vitamin D* treatment is a further precondition for optimal growth rates. Except in the period of infancy, however, none of the aforementioned therapeutic procedures has been demonstrated to induce catchup growth in short children with CRF.

The initiation of *dialysis* usually does not improve growth in uremic children. Several large studies found mean annual losses of 0.4 to 0.8 SD standardized height (303–305). This is conceivable if the hypothesis is correct that uremic growth failure inhibition is caused mainly by the accumulation of IGFBPs, which are not removed by standard hemodialysis. On the other hand, a single-center study reported improved growth, with an annual height gain of 0.3 SD, under intensified hemodialysis achieving a Kt/V of 2.0 by almost 15 hours of dialysis per week (306).

As with standard hemodialysis, catchup growth is not commonly observed in children on *peritoneal dialysis*. Whereas early experience suggested continued significant losses of standardized height with treatment by CAPD or continuous cyclical peritoneal dialysis (214,307–309), more recent studies suggest percentile-parallel growth patterns or slight losses of less than 0.5 SD per year (310,311). Residual renal function is a more important predictor of growth in patients on peritoneal dialysis than is dialytic clearance (311). In addition, a high peritoneal transporter state, a known morbidity and mortality risk factor in adults, predicted poor growth (−0.5 SD/yr) in a prospective study of 51 children followed for 18 months (310). It is currently believed that, apart from causing increased dialytic protein losses, the high transporter status may be an indicator of microinflammation, a putative cause of GH resistance in uremia (see earlier). In fact, growth failure may represent the pediatric equivalent of the malnutrition-inflammation-atherosclerosis syndrome of adult ESRD patients (312,313). Adverse clinical outcomes including a two- to threefold elevated risk of death have been associated with growth failure in children on dialysis (314,315).

Only successful *renal transplantation* is able to restore the conditions for normal growth compromised by the uremic state. Growth rates after transplantation vary widely, however, from further deterioration of height SDS to complete catchup growth (118,224,316–324). In an analysis of the North American Pediatric Renal Transplant Cooperative Study, the mean effect of transplantation before puberty on adult height was 0.0 SDS (325), which confirms that the relative height achieved at the time of transplantation is the most important predictor of final height (322,323). Whereas pubertal patients tend to lose relative height after transplantation (326), a potential for posttransplantation catchup growth exists in patients younger than 6 years of age (321,324,327,328) (Fig. 68.9). Infant allograft recipients typically exhibit excellent spontaneous growth rates, with a relative height gain of 1.5 SD within 2 to 7 years (316,324,329). Apart from the inverse relationship with age, the degree of growth retardation positively predicts posttransplantation growth rate (321,323,324,328,330). Furthermore, posttransplantation growth critically depends on graft function (236,321,323–325,328–330). A marked deceleration in posttransplantation growth is observed when GFR is below 60 mL/min/1.73 m^2, and in the French experience catchup growth occurred only in children with a GFR above this value (225).

The daily dose as well as the cumulative dose of corticosteroids seems to be inversely related to the posttransplantation growth rate (17,331,332). The hope that the prednisolone derivative deflazacort would interfere less with catchup growth

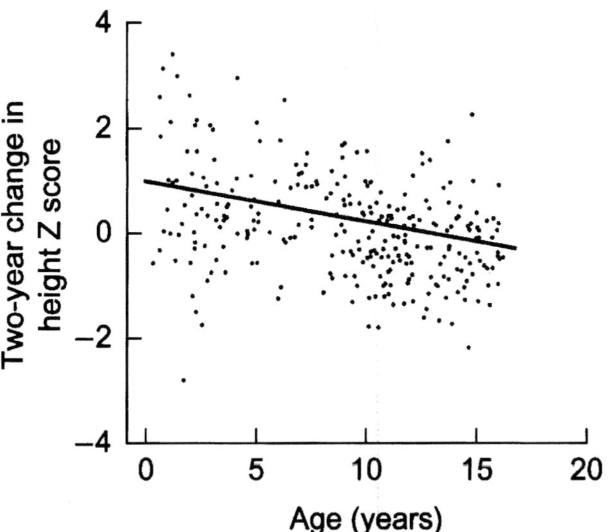

FIGURE 68.9. Change in standardized height during the first 2 years after transplantation. Improvement in mean height Z score is limited to children of preschool age. (From Tejani A, Fine RN, Alexander S, et al. Factors predictive of sustained growth in children after renal transplantation. The North American Pediatric Renal Transplant Cooperative Study. *J Pediatr* 1993;122:397–402, with permission.)

at equivalent immunosuppressive biopotency has not been substantiated so far (333,334). Alternate-day corticosteroid administration has been demonstrated in a controlled, randomized trial to improve growth by 0.25 to 0.5 SD of height per year (318,335). The most impressive catchup growth has been observed in patients in whom steroids could be completely withdrawn (223,317,336–338). In these patients, an improvement of 0.6 to 0.8 SD during the first posttransplantation year was observed. Ellis et al. found a cumulative height increment of 1.5 SD within 3 years in children younger than 5 years of age given tacrolimus monotherapy and apparent catchup growth even in pubertal patients (337). The results of steroid withdrawal studies should be interpreted with caution because usually only patients with low risk for rejection and good allograft function were included. Nevertheless, several potent new immunosuppressive agents have been developed that may allow the option to completely withdraw or even primarily avoid steroid use in pediatric renal transplantation cases (338,339). The risk of rejection and loss of renal function by steroid withdrawal, historically rated as 40 to 50% (317,340,341), may have diminished considerably with the new immunosuppressive protocols, but this awaits confirmation in prospective trials. Hence, alternate-day steroid administration should be standard, and complete cessation should be considered after transplantation in short children with good renal function who do not exhibit spontaneous catchup growth.

Treatment of Renal Growth Failure with Recombinant Growth Hormone

The GH resistance observed in uremia and during glucocorticoid treatment and the experimental proof that GH resistance can be overcome by supraphysiologic doses of exogenous GH (342) have provided a rationale for treating children with CRF and those undergoing renal transplantation with rGH. Administration of rGH raises IGF-1 production to a greater degree than it raises IGFBP concentrations and thereby increases the availability of free IGF-1 at the tissue level (93) (Fig. 68.10).

Use of Recombinant Growth Hormone in Prepubertal Children

In prepubertal children with predialytic CRF numerous studies, including two double-blind placebo-controlled trials, demonstrated that rGH induces a nearly twofold increase in height velocity during the first treatment year, with a diminishing but still significant effect on growth rate during the second year (343–350). Although the maximal height increment occurs in the first three treatment years, standardized height continues to increase slightly during extended treatment. After 5 or 6 years of rGH administration, mean height SDS had increased from –2.6 at baseline to –0.7 in a North American study (349), from –3.4 to –1.9 in German children (348), and from –3 to –0.5 in Dutch patients (350). The remarkable prepubertal growth acceleration was not associated with a disproportionate advancement of bone age, which resulted in a remarkable increase in predicted adult height at the end of the prepubertal phase (348). Prepubertal children on *dialysis* respond less well to rGH than children with CRF on conservative treatment (348,351). In the German multicenter study, 13 prepubertal dialysis patients gained only 0.8 SDS in height on average during the first two treatment years, compared to an increment of 1.3 SDS in 41 CRF patients (348) (Fig. 68.11). These results were confirmed in a large cohort of French children on hemodialysis, who had only a 0.5-SDS height gain during the first treatment year, with continued small annual increments for up to 5 years (352). Children on long-term peritoneal dialysis do not respond differently to rGH than do hemodialysis patients (353). In prepubertal children with *nephropathic cystinosis*, GH administration increased height by 0.8 SDS during the first year and by 1.7 SDS within five treatment years (354). In *prepubertal renal allograft patients*, in whom alternate-day corticosteroid treatment does not induce catchup growth and discontinuation of corticosteroid medication is not considered an option for safety reasons, a therapeutic trial with GH may be considered. Several studies have demonstrated a growth-promoting effect of GH in prepubertal children with renal allografts over average treatment periods of 1 to 3 years (119,355–360). Treatment efficacy was slightly inferior to that observed in CRF patients on conservative treatment, with mean cumulative height gains of 1 to 1.5 SD during the first 3 years.

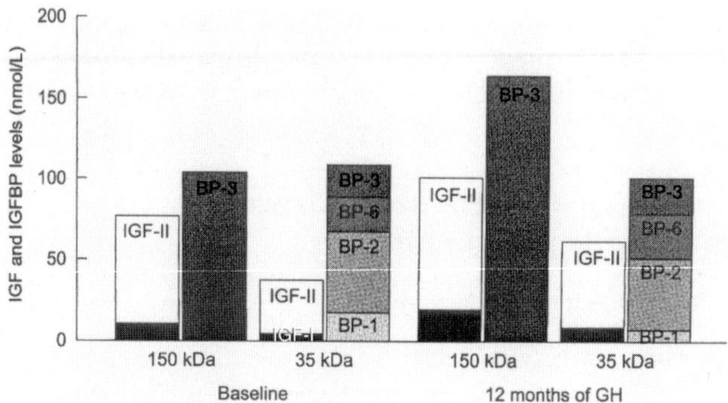

FIGURE 68.10. Balance between insulin-like growth factor–binding proteins (IGFBPs) and IGFs in serum of children with chronic renal failure before (baseline) and after 12 months of treatment with recombinant growth hormone (GH). Recombinant GH increases the IGF/IGFBP ratio in the 35-kDa complex. BP, binding protein. (Adapted from Powell DR, Durham SK, Liu F, et al. The insulin-like growth factor axis and growth in children with chronic renal failure: a report of the Southwest Pediatric Nephrology Study Group. *J Clin Endocrinol Metab* 1998;83:1654–1661.)

Recombinant Growth Hormone Use in Puberty

A systematic analysis of rGH treatment efficacy in pubertal children is difficult due to methodologic problems (361).

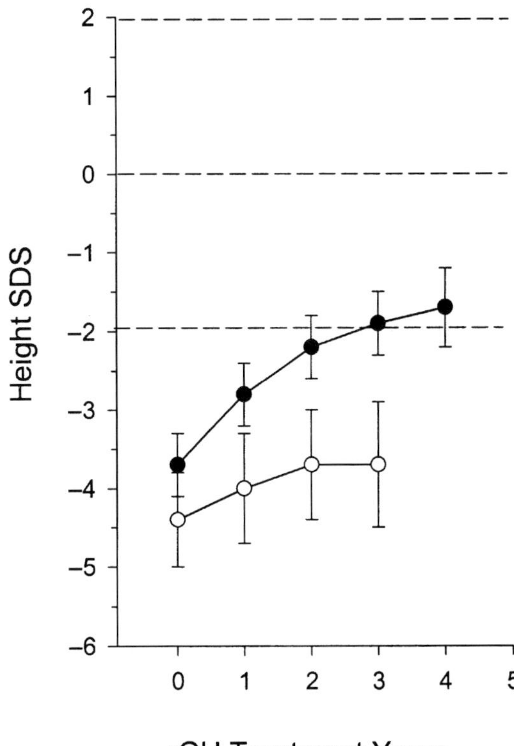

FIGURE 68.11. Superior efficacy of recombinant growth hormone (rGH) treatment in children with pre–end-stage chronic renal failure (•, n = 19) compared to children on dialysis (o, n = 6). SDS, standard deviation score. (Adapted from Haffner D, Wühl E, Schaefer F, et al. Factors predictive of the short- and long-term efficacy of growth hormone treatment in prepubertal children with chronic renal failure. German Study Group for Growth Hormone Treatment in Children with Chronic Renal Failure. *J Am Soc Nephrol* 1998;9:1899–1907.)

These include delayed puberty with a lack of appropriate growth reference data, potential effects of rGH on the onset and duration of the pubertal growth spurt, and frequent changes in treatment modalities with variable relative efficacy of rGH. In addition, rGH administration is usually discontinued at the time of transplantation but is sometimes reinstituted if the growth rate remains low, which introduces large variability in the duration of rGH treatment during puberty. Hence, only controlled long-term observations, ideally recording total pubertal height gain in treated and untreated patients with comparable distributions of treatment modalities, permit a meaningful analysis of rGH efficacy in puberty.

Haffner et al. followed 38 children with CRF in whom rGH administration was initiated at a prepubertal age and continued until they reached adult height (226) (Figs. 68.12 and 68.13). Because rGH was stopped at the time of transplantation, the patients received GH during 50% of the pubertal observation time. Fifty children, matched for age and degree of CRF, who did not receive rGH because they still had normal height served as controls. The children receiving rGH showed sustained catchup growth, whereas the control children developed progressive growth failure (Fig. 68.12). Dissection of the prepubertal and pubertal growth phases disclosed that the additional height gain relative to the control group was limited almost entirely to the prepubertal period, whereas pubertal height gain was insignificantly greater in the rGH-treated patients than in the controls (Fig. 68.13). The apparent inefficacy of rGH administration in puberty may be explained in part by the incomplete continuation of treatment, as is suggested by a positive correlation of the fractional duration of rGH therapy with total pubertal height gain. In fact, Hokken-Koelega et al. demonstrated that allograft recipients may respond very well to rGH even in late puberty (346), with an almost threefold greater 2-year height gain compared to untreated historical controls (362).

In neither the German children nor the Dutch cohort (350) was an advanced onset of puberty observed, although a subtle acceleration of bone maturation and a slight shortening of the pubertal growth spurt was noted by Haffner et al. (226).

Adult Height after Recombinant Growth Hormone Treatment

Fifteen years after the start of the first therapeutic trials with rGH, final height outcome data are beginning to

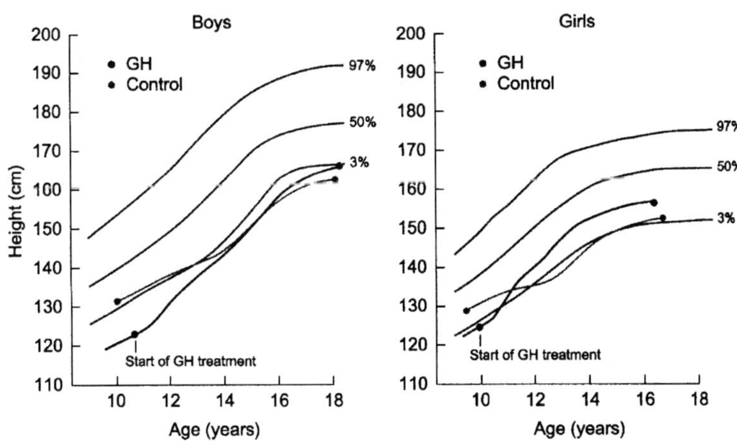

FIGURE 68.12. Favorable effect of long-term treatment with recombinant growth hormone (GH) on final adult height in children with chronic renal failure (CRF). Synchronized mean growth curves during GH treatment for 38 children (32 boys and 6 girls) with CRF are compared with those for 50 control children with CRF not treated with GH. Normal values are indicated by the third, fiftieth, and ninety-seventh percentiles. The circles indicate the time of the first observation (the start of GH treatment in the treated children) and the end of the pubertal growth spurt. (From Haffner D, Schaefer F, Nissel R, et al. Effect of growth hormone treatment on adult height of children with chronic renal failure. *N Engl J Med* 2000;343:923–930, with permission.)

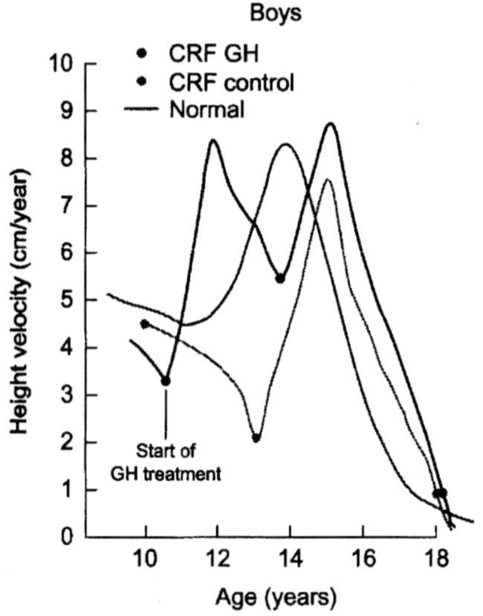

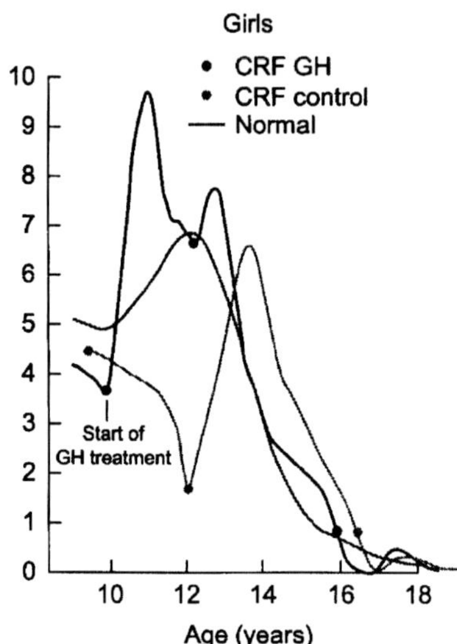

FIGURE 68.13. Synchronized mean height velocity curves during growth hormone (GH) treatment for the same children as shown in Figure 68.12. The circles indicate the time of the first observation (the start of GH treatment in the treated children), the time of minimal prespurt height velocity, and the end of the pubertal growth spurt. CRF, chronic renal failure. (From Haffner D, Schaefer F, Nissel R, et al. Effect of growth hormone treatment on adult height of children with chronic renal failure. *N Engl J Med* 2000;343:923–930, with permission.)

emerge, which will permit assessment of the ultimate efficacy of rGH therapy. In the German multicenter study, the mean adult height of 38 children who received rGH for a mean of 5.3 years was –1.6 SDS, with two-thirds of patients ending up at a height above the third percentile (226). The patients ultimately gained 1.4 SD compared to their standardized height at baseline. Conversely, mean height SDS decreased in the untreated control group from –1.5 to –2.1 SDS at attainment of adult height (Fig. 68.13). Figures in the same range were reported from several other trials (Table 68.1). Of course, the variability in final height outcomes is large. Cumulative height gain appears to be positively affected by the height deficit at the start of rGH treatment and the total duration of rGH administration (226), and negatively affected by the cumulative time spent on dialysis. Height gain was positively associated with the initial target height deficit and the duration of rGH therapy, and was negatively associated with the

TABLE 68.1. SYNOPSIS OF STUDIES REPORTING ADULT HEIGHT DATA AFTER RECOMBINANT GROWTH HORMONE (RGH) TREATMENT OF GROWTH FAILURE DUE TO CHRONIC RENAL FAILURE (CRF)

Study	No. of patients studied	CRF treatment modalities	Age at start of rGH (yr)	Pubertal status at start of rGH	Duration of follow-up (yr)	Duration of rGH (yr)	Initial height SDS	Final height SDS	Change in height SDS
Netherlands (350)	4	Cons Rx/dialysis	<11.0	Prepubertal	>5.0	>5.0	n.i.	–0.2[a]	n.i.
Germany (393)	12	Cons Rx/dialysis	11.9	Prepubertal	n.i.	5.0	n.i.	n.i.	+1.0
United Kingdom (363)	2	Cons Rx	9.9[a]	Prepubertal	10.0[a]	0.4[a]	–2.2[a]	–1.1[a]	+1.1[a]
	5	Transplant	11.9	Prepubertal	>6.0	2.9	–3.3	–3.0	+0.3
	6	Transplant	15.6	Pubertal	>5.0	1.4	–3.4	–2.5	+0.9
North America	9	Cons Rx	n.i.	n.i.	3.2	<3.2	–3.0	–2.2	+0.7
(394)	22	Dialysis	n.i.	n.i.	4.1	<4.1	–3.6	–3.2	+0.4
	72	Transplant	n.i.	n.i.	3.7	<3.7	–3.0	–2.5	+0.5
Germany (226)	38	47% cons Rx, 24% dialysis, 29% post-transplant[b]	10.4	Prepubertal	7.6	5.3	–3.1	–1.6	+1.4
Belgium (359)	17	Transplant	n.i.	n.i.	n.i.	3.4	–3.0	–1.8	+1.2
Netherlands (357)	18	Transplant	15.5	Pubertal	n.i.	n.i.	n.i.	n.i.	Total height gain 19 cm

Cons Rx, conservative treatment; n.i., no information given; SDS, standard deviation score.
Note: Mean values are given for age, time period, and SDS values unless indicated otherwise.
[a]Median.
[b]Percent patient years spent in each treatment category.

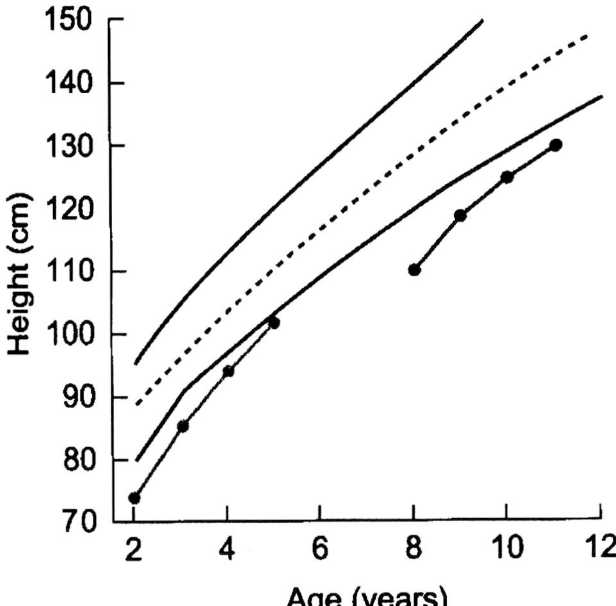

FIGURE 68.14. Age-dependent relative efficacy of growth hormone (GH) treatment exemplified by individual growth curves predicted for two patients aged 2 and 8 years, started on GH at a basal height standard deviation score (SDS) of −3.5 and a height velocity SDS of −2.0. The reference lines indicate the third, fiftieth, and ninety-seventh percentiles of the healthy population. Growth is accelerated over baseline height velocity in both patients by 4.5 cm in the first treatment year, 1.9 cm in the second, and 1.0 cm in the third (empirical means observed in patients on conservative treatment followed for 3 years). The younger child reaches the third percentile within 3 years, whereas the older child does not. (From Haffner D, Wühl E, Schaefer F, et al. Factors predictive of the short- and long-term efficacy of growth hormone treatment in prepubertal children with chronic renal failure. German Study Group for Growth Hormone Treatment in Children with Chronic Renal Failure. *J Am Soc Nephrol* 1998;9:1899–1907, with permission.)

percentage of the observation period spent on dialysis (226,350). The relative height attained at the time of transplantation seems to be maintained to final height; neither spontaneous catchup growth nor catchdown growth after discontinuation of GH seems to be common (363,364).

Strategies to Optimize Growth by Recombinant Growth Hormone Treatment

The response to rGH is influenced positively by the residual GFR, target height, initial target height deficit, and duration of GH treatment, and is influenced negatively by the age at the start of treatment (361). A curvilinear dose-response relationship appears to exist. Although a dosage of 4 IU/m^2/day was more efficient than 2 IU/m^2/day in a double-blind trial (365), no further improvement of the growth response was observed with 8 IU/m^2/day, at least in a pubertal cohort (362). Daily dosing is more efficacious than three administrations per week (366). Discontinuation of GH treatment results in loss of height SDS in 75% of children with CRF on conservative treatment (367), whereas catchdown growth seems to be uncommon when rGH is discontinued due to renal transplantation (363).

Because the absolute growth response to rGH (in centimeters of height gain per year) is independent of age but the reference range increases with age (348), rGH treatment should be started as early as possible in the course of renal disease (Fig. 68.14). A fixed daily dose of 4 IU/m^2 (= 12 mg/m^2) should be used. Treatment should not be stopped if the annual gain of height SDS diminishes after the third treatment year to avoid the risk of catchdown growth. Treatment should also be continued when the patient becomes dialysis dependent. If rGH therapy is initiated in a small child already on dialysis, transplantation should not be postponed for the sake of approved rGH treatment, because the efficacy of rGH therapy in dialysis patients is limited and short lasting. Treatment should be stopped at the time of renal transplantation to observe the spontaneous evolution of growth. If no growth or insufficient catchup growth occurs within 12 months, glucocorticoid withdrawal is the first option. If this is unsuccessful, rGH reinstitution should be considered. Treatment decisions should be made without delay to preserve growth potential. The question of rGH continuation through puberty is still controversial. The pubertal growth spurt occurs independent of concomitant rGH treatment, which renders any judgment about treatment efficacy exceedingly difficult. Controlled prospective study results are not available. Hence, the decision to continue or restart rGH therapy in puberty must be made on an individual basis, with consideration of the degree of growth retardation, the residual growth potential, and the expected therapeutic compliance of the adolescent.

Whether a low growth rate (height velocity below the twenty-fifth percentile over several years) should also be a treatment indication in a child whose relative height is still in the normal range remains uncertain. Such preventive therapy might prove to be more effective in increasing adult height than initiation of treatment when short stature is already established. This treatment strategy appears justified if a growth arrest is noted that is not explained by nonendocrine factors. It is also an issue of current consideration whether in patients with imminent or early puberty skeletal maturation should be delayed by pharmacologic intervention with GnRH analogues or aromatase inhibitors to prolong the prepubertal growth phase to facilitate GH treatment.

Adverse Effects of Growth Hormone Treatment

Given its remarkable efficacy, GH treatment causes surprisingly few side effects in children with CRF.

Concern was raised initially that prolonged GH treatment might provoke *diabetes mellitus*, because patients with CRF already show impaired glucose tolerance due to peripheral insulin resistance (see earlier). Notwithstanding this concern, oral glucose tolerance remained unaltered in children with CRF and in those undergoing transplantation who were treated with GH for up to 5 years (368). Insulin secretion increased during the first treatment year, however, and remained elevated thereafter. This increase was most pronounced in transplant recipients. The long-term consequences of increased insulin secretion are uncertain. Theoretically it may contribute to atherosclerosis or induce diabetes mellitus by exhaustion of pancreatic beta cells. Although not a single case of irreversible diabetes mellitus has been observed in children with CRF (369,370), a report of increased incidence of type 2 diabetes mellitus in nonrenal children undergoing GH therapy requires prospective surveillance (371).

Epiphyseal slipping (372,373) and femoral head necrosis (374) have been reported as rare events during treatment with rGH. Whether these complications were caused or intensified by rGH is unclear, because both complications are noted with increased incidence in children with CRF who do not receive GH treatment (297,299). An aggravation of secondary *hyperparathyroidism* has been reported rarely (375,376). This seems not to be due to direct stimulation of the parathyroid gland by GH, but to represent an indirect effect of small decreases of ionized calcium as a consequence of GH-stimulated bone apposition or an increase in serum phosphate concentration secondary to improved appetite. Furthermore, preexisting renal osteodystrophy may be unmasked by an increased growth rate and may become radiographically apparent (377).

Concern has also been raised that GH may cause glomerular hyperfiltration and accelerated deterioration of *renal function*. However, the physiologic acute increase in GFR induced by GH in healthy subjects is obliterated in patients with CRF (378). Long-term observations of up to 8 years showed no acceleration of renal failure progression in predialytic patients with CRF due to cystinosis (354) or other renal disorders (226,348,350), or in renal allograft recipients (226).

Because GH is an immunomodulatory substance (379), *allograft rejection* might be triggered by rGH administration in patients after transplantation. However, several controlled trials provided evidence that an increased risk of rejection is limited to high-risk patients with more than one acute rejection episode before the start of GH treatment (358,360,380,381).

Contrary to previous concerns (382), an extended survey of thousands of patients failed to disclose any significant relationship between GH treatment and *malignancy* (383–385). A review of adverse events in 583 patients with CRF and ESRD treated with GH revealed one solid tumor and one B-cell lymphoma among patients undergoing peritoneal dialysis and one lymphoma in a transplant recipient (386). Reports of renal cell carcinoma in two patients who had received GH occurring 9 and 11 years after transplantation, a case of leukemia in an 18-year-old GH-treated patient with a failing transplant (383), and a report of premalignant tubuloepithelial changes in a pediatric renal allograft (387) raise the suspicion that tumor risk may be selectively increased by GH in posttransplantation children receiving long-term immunosuppression.

GH induces an IGF-1–mediated increase in distal tubular sodium reabsorption and upregulates the renin-angiotensin system (388,389). As a consequence, a transient, usually mild *retention of sodium and water* occurs during the first few days of treatment. In this context, *benign intracranial hypertension* has been reported as a rare adverse effect of GH treatment in patients with various underlying diseases. In CRF, the risk for this complication is increased tenfold (390,391). One survey noted signs or symptoms of intracranial hypertension in 15 out of 1670 patients with renal disease receiving rGH (0.9%) (392). All but two patients were symptomatic; the symptoms generally abated when GH therapy was discontinued, but two patients had persistent blindness. At least four of these patients experienced recurrence of intracranial hypertension after reinitiation of GH therapy. Intracranial hypertension manifested within a median of 13 weeks of treatment. We therefore recommend performing a baseline funduscopy and gradually increasing the dose from 50 to 100% of the maintenance dose within 4 weeks. Because hypertension and fluid overload may be predisposing factors, the state of hydration should be well controlled at the start of treatment. Headache, vomiting, and other clinical signs of increased intracranial hypertension mandate careful clinical investigation, including funduscopy. The risk-benefit ratio should be evaluated carefully when considering reinitiation of rGH treatment after reversal of symptoms.

REFERENCES

1. Emmanouel DS, Lindheimer MD, Katz AI. Pathogenesis of endocrine abnormalities in uremia. *Endocr Rev* 1980;1:28–44.
2. Rabkin R, Unterhalter SA, Duckworth WC. Effect of prolonged uremia on insulin metabolism by isolated liver and muscle. *Kidney Int* 1979;16:433–439.
3. Hruska KA, Korkor A, Martin K, et al. Peripheral metabolism of intact parathyroid hormone. *J Clin Invest* 1981; 67:885–892.
4. Powell DR, Lee PDK, Chang D, et al. Antiserum developed for the E peptide region of insulin-like growth factor IA prohormone recognizes a serum protein by both immunoblot and radioimmunoassay. *J Clin Endocrinol Metab* 1987; 65:868–875.
5. Zilker TR, Rebel C, Kopp KF, et al. Kinetics of biosynthetic human proinsulin in patients with terminal renal insufficiency. *Horm Metab Res* 1988;18(suppl):43–48.
6. Lim VS, Fang VS, Katz AI, et al. Thyroid dysfunction in chronic renal failure. *J Clin Invest* 1977;60:522–534.
7. Kishore BK, Arakawa M, Geiyo F. Altered glycosylation and sialisation of serum proteins and lipid bound sialic acids in chronic renal failure. *Postgrad Med J* 1983;59:551–555.

8. Schaefer F, Seidel C, Mitchell R, et al. Pulsatile immunoreactive and bioactive luteinizing hormone secretion in pubertal patients with chronic renal failure. *Pediatr Nephrol* 1991;5:566–571.
9. Blum WF, Ranke MB, Kietzmann K, et al. Excess of IGF-binding proteins in chronic renal failure: evidence for relative GH resistance and inhibition of somatomedin activity. In: Drop SLS, Hintz RL, eds. *Insulin-like growth factor binding proteins.* Amsterdam: Elsevier Science Publishers, 1989:93–99.
10. Lee PD, Hintz RL, Sperry JB, et al. IGF binding proteins in growth-retarded children with chronic renal failure. *Pediatr Res* 1989;26:308–315.
11. Smith D, Defronzo RA. Insulin resistance in uremia mediated by postbinding defects. *Kidney Int* 1982;22:54–62.
12. Schaefer F, Chen Y, Tsao T, et al. Impaired JAK-STAT signal transduction contributes to growth hormone resistance in chronic uremia. *J Clin Invest* 2001;108:467–475.
13. Schärer K, Chantler C, Brunner FP, et al. Combined report on regular dialysis and transplantation of children in Europe, 1975. *Proc Eur Dial Transplant Assoc* 1976;13:3–103.
14. Rizzoni G, Broyer M, Brunner FP, et al. Combined report on regular hemodialysis and transplantation in Europe, 1985. *Proc EDTA* 1986;23:55–83.
15. Schärer K. Study on pubertal development in chronic renal failure. Growth and development of children with chronic renal failure. *Acta Paediatr Scand* 1990;366(suppl):90–92.
16. Ehrich JHH, Rizzoni G, Brunner FP, et al. Combined report on regular dialysis and transplantation in Europe, 1989. *Nephrol Dial Transplant* 1991;6(suppl):37–47.
17. Schaefer F, Seidel C, Binding A, et al. Pubertal growth in chronic renal failure. *Pediatr Res* 1990;28:5–10.
18. Burke BA, Lindgren B, Wick M, et al. Testicular germ cell loss in children with renal failure. *Pediatr Pathol* 1989;9:433–444.
19. Schaefer F, Walther U, Ruder H, et al. Reduced spermaturia in adolescent and young adult patients after renal transplantation. *Nephrol Dial Transplant* 1991;6:840.
20. Palmer BF. Sexual dysfunction in uremia. *J Am Soc Nephrol* 1999;10:1381–1388.
21. Hou S. Pregnancy in chronic renal insufficiency and end-stage renal disease. *Am J Kidney Dis* 1999;33(2):235–252.
22. Chan WS, Okun N, Kjellstrand CM. Pregnancy in chronic dialysis: a review and analysis of the literature. *Int J Artif Organs* 1998;21(5):259–268.
23. Nakabayashi M, Adachi T, Itoh S, et al. Perinatal and infant outcome of pregnant patients undergoing chronic hemodialysis. *Nephron* 1999;82(1):27–31.
24. Handelsman DJ. Hypothalamic-pituitary gonadal dysfunction in renal failure, dialysis and renal transplantation. *Endocr Rev* 1985;6:151–182.
25. Corvol B, Bertagna X, Bedrossian J. Increased steroid metabolic clearance rate in anephric patients. *Acta Endocrinol (Copenh)* 1974;75:756–761.
26. Stewart-Bentley M, Gans D, Horton R. Regulation of gonadal function in uremia. *Metabolism* 1974;23:1065–1072.
27. Oertel PJ, Lichtwald K, Häfner S, et al. Hypothalamo-pituitary-gonadal axis in children with chronic renal failure. *Kidney Int* 1983;24:34–39.
28. Forest MG. Physiological changes in circulating androgens. In: *Androgens in childhood. Pediatric and adolescent endocrinology.* Vol 19. Basel: Karger, 1989:104–129.
29. Ferraris J, Saenger P, Levine L, et al. Delayed puberty in males with chronic renal failure. *Kidney Int* 1980;18:344–350.
30. Schärer K, et al. Adrenal androgens in plasma of boys with chronic renal failure. Cooperative Study Group on Pubertal Development in Chronic Renal Failure. *Pediatr Nephrol* 1992;6:C179.
31. Schärer K, Broyer M, Vecsei P, et al. Damage to testicular function in chronic renal failure of children. *Proc Eur Dial Transplant Assoc* 1980;17:725–729.
32. Belgorosky A, Ferraris JR, Ramirez JA, et al. Serum sex hormone-binding globulin and serum nonsex hormone-binding globulin-bound testosterone fractions in prepubertal boys with chronic renal failure. *J Clin Endocrinol Metab* 1991;73:107–110.
33. Schaefer F, et al. Pulsatile growth hormone secretion in peripubertal patients with chronic renal failure. Cooperative Study Group on Pubertal Development in Chronic Renal Failure. *J Pediatr* 1991;119:568–577.
34. Gupta D, Bundschu HD. Testosterone and its binding in the plasma of male subjects with chronic renal failure. *Clin Chim Acta* 1972;36:479–486.
35. Van Kammen E, Thijssen JHH, Schwarz F. Sex hormones in male patients with chronic renal failure. I. The production of testosterone and androstendione. *Clin Endocrinol* 1978;8:7–12.
36. Kreusser W, Spiegelberg U, Sis J, et al. Hypergonadotroper Hypogonadismus bei Niereninsuffizienz—eine Folge gestörter cAMP-Bildung. *Verh Dtsch Ges Inn Med* 1978;84:1446–1448.
37. Dunkel L, Raivio T, Laine J, et al. Circulating luteinizing hormone receptor inhibitor(s) in boys with chronic renal failure. *Kidney Int* 1997;51:777–784.
38. Mitchell R, Schaefer F, Morris ID, et al. Elevated serum immunoreactive inhibin levels in pubertal boys with chronic renal failure. *Clin Endocrinol* 1993;39:27–33.
39. Lim VS, Henriquez C, Sievertsen G, et al. Ovarian function in chronic renal failure: evidence suggesting hypothalamic anovulation. *Ann Intern Med* 1980;93:21–27.
40. Ferraris JR, Domene HM, Escobar ME, et al. Hormonal profile in pubertal females with chronic renal failure: before and under haemodialysis and after renal transplantation. *Acta Endocrinol (Copenh)* 1987;115:289–296.
41. Schärer K, Schaefer F, Trott M, et al. Pubertal development in children with chronic renal failure. In: Schärer K, ed. *Growth and endocrine changes in children and adolescents with chronic renal failure. Pediatric and adolescent endocrinology.* Vol 20. Basel: Karger, 1989:151–168.
42. Swamy AP, Woolf PD, Cestero RVM. Hypothalamic-pituitary-ovarian axis in uremic women. *J Lab Clin Med* 1979;93:1066–1072.
43. Blackman MR, Weintraub BD, Kourides IA, et al. Discordant elevation of the common alpha-subunit of the glycoprotein hormones compared to β-subunits in serum of uremic patients. *J Clin Endocrinol Metab* 1981;53:39–48.
44. Holdsworth S, Atkins RC, de Kretser DM. The pituitary-testicular axis in men with chronic renal failure. *N Engl J Med* 1977;296:1245–1249.
45. Corley KP, Valk TW, Kelch RP, et al. Estimation of GnRH pulse amplitude during pubertal development. *Pediatr Res* 1981;15:157–162.

46. Veldhuis JD, Carlson ML, Johnson ML. The pituitary gland secretes in bursts: appraising the nature of glandular secretory impulses by simultaneous multiple-parameter deconvolution of plasma hormone concentrations. *Proc Natl Acad Sci U S A* 1987;84:7686–7690.
47. Schaefer F, Veldhuis JD, Robertson WR, et al. Immunoreactive and bioactive luteinizing hormone in pubertal patients with chronic renal failure. Cooperative Study Group on Pubertal Development in Chronic Renal Failure. *Kidney Int* 1994;45:1465–1476.
48. Schaefer F, Daschner M, Veldhuis JD, et al. In vivo alterations in the gonadotropin-releasing hormone pulse generator and the secretion and clearance of luteinizing hormone in the castrate uremic rat. *Neuroendocrinology* 1994;59:285–296.
49. Dong Q, Handelsman DJ. Regulation of pulsatile luteinizing hormone secretion in experimental uremia. *Endocrinology* 1991;128:1218–1222.
50. Talbot JA, Rodger RSC, Robertson WR. Pulsatile bioactive luteinising hormone secretion in men with chronic renal failure and following renal transplantation. *Nephron* 1990;56:66–72.
51. Wibullaksanakul S, Handelsman DJ. Regulation of hypothalamic gonadotropin-releasing hormone secretion in experimental uremia: in vitro studies. *Neuroendocrinology* 1991;54:353–358.
52. Daschner M, Philippin B, Nguyen T, et al. Circulating inhibitor of gonadotropin releasing hormone secretion from hypothalamic neurons in uremia. *Kidney Int* 2002;62:1582–1590.
53. Schaefer F, Vogel M, Kerkhoff G, et al. Experimental uremia affects hypothalamic amino acid neurotransmitter milieu. *J Am Soc Nephrol* 2001;12:1218–1227.
54. Robertson WR, Lambert A, Loveridge N. The role of modern bioassays in clinical endocrinology. *Clin Endocrinol (Oxf)* 1987;27:259–278.
55. Celani MF, Montanini V, Baraghini GF, et al. Biological and immunological profiles of serum luteinizing hormone (LH) during male sexual maturation. *Acta Med Auxol* 1983;15:195–204.
56. Schaefer F, Mitchell R, Schärer K, et al. Gonadotrophin secretion in pubertal children on dialysis or after renal transplantation. *J Endocrinol* 1989;121(suppl):230.
57. Giusti M, Perfumo F, Verrina E, et al. Biological activity of luteinizing hormone in uremic children: spontaneous nocturnal secretion and changes after administration of exogenous pulsatile luteinizing hormone releasing hormone. *Pediatr Nephrol* 1991;5:559–565.
58. Mitchell R, Bauerfeld C, Schaefer F, et al. Less acidic forms of luteinizing hormone are associated with lower testosterone secretion in men on hemodialysis treatment. *Clin Endocrinol* 1994;41:65–73.
59. Gomez F, de la Cueva R, Wauters JP, et al. Endocrine abnormalities in patients undergoing long-term hemodialysis—the role of prolactin. *Am J Med* 1980;68:522–530.
60. Sievertsen GD, Lim VS, Nakawatase C, et al. Metabolic clearance and secretion rates of human prolactin in normal subjects and in patients with chronic renal failure rate. *J Clin Endocrinol Metab* 1980;50:846–852.
61. Winters SJ, Troen P. Altered pulsatile secretion of luteinising hormone in hypogonadal men with hyperprolactinemia. *Clin Endocrinol* 1984;21:257–263.
62. Schmitz O. Absence of diurnal plasma prolactin rhythm in diabetic and non-diabetic uremic patients. *Acta Endocrinol (Copenh)* 1984;105:173–178.
63. Biasioli S, Mazzali A, Foroni R, et al. Chronobiological variations of prolactin (PRL) in chronic renal failure (CRF). *Clin Nephrol* 1988;30:86–92.
64. Czernichow P, Dauzet MC, Broyer M, et al. Abnormal TSH, PRL and GH response to TSH releasing factor in chronic renal failure. *J Clin Endocrinol Metab* 1976;43:630–637.
65. Ramirez G, O'Neill WM, Bloomer HA. Abnormalities in the regulation of prolactin in patients with chronic renal failure. *J Clin Endocrinol Metab* 1977;45:658–661.
66. Bommer J, Ritz E, del Pozo E, et al. Improved sexual function in male haemodialysis patients on bromocriptine. *Lancet* 1979;2:496–497.
67. Ruilope L, Garcia-Robles R, Paya C, et al. Influence of lisuride, a dopaminergic agonist, on the sexual function of male patients with chronic renal failure. *Am J Kidney Dis* 1985;5:182–185.
68. Verbeelen D, Vanhaelst L, van Steirteghem AC, et al. Effect of 1,25-dihydroxyvitamin D3 on plasma prolactin in patients with renal failure on regular dialysis treatment. *J Endocrinol Invest* 1983;6:359–362.
69. Schaefer RM, Kokot F, Kuerner B, et al. Normalization of serum prolactin levels in hemodialysis patients on recombinant human erythropoietin. *Int J Artif Organs* 1989;12:445–449.
70. Ramirez G, O'Neill WM, Bloomer A, et al. Abnormalities in the regulation of growth hormone in chronic renal failure. *Arch Intern Med* 1978;138:267–271.
71. Davidson MB, Fisher MB, Dabir-Vaziri N, et al. Effect of protein intake and dialysis on the abnormal growth hormone, glucose, and insulin homeostasis in uremia. *Metabolism* 1976;25:455–464.
72. Johnson V, Maack T. Renal extraction, filtration, absorption, and catabolism of growth hormone. *Am J Physiol* 1977;233:F185–F196.
73. Haffner D, Schaefer F, Girard J, et al. Metabolic clearance of recombinant human growth hormone in health and chronic renal failure. *J Clin Invest* 1994;93:1163–1171.
74. Schaefer F, Baumann G, Haffner D, et al. Multifactorial control of the elimination kinetics of unbound (free) growth hormone (GH) in the human: regulation by age, adiposity, renal function, and steady state concentrations of GH in plasma. *J Clin Endocrinol Metab* 1996;81:22–31.
75. Tönshoff B, Veldhuis JD, Heinrich U, et al. Deconvolution analysis of spontaneous nocturnal growth hormone secretion in prepubertal children with chronic renal failure. *Pediatr Res* 1995;37:86–93.
76. Veldhuis JD, Iranmanesh A, Wilkowski MJ, et al. Neuroendocrine alterations in the somatotropic and lactotropic axes in uremic men. *Eur J Endocrinol* 1994;131:489–498.
77. Schaefer F, Veldhuis J, Stanhope R, et al. Alterations in growth hormone secretion and clearance in peripubertal boys with chronic renal failure and after renal transplantation. *J Clin Endocrinol Metab* 1994;78:1298–1306.
78. Challa A, Krieg RJ Jr, Thabet MA, et al. Metabolic acidosis inhibits growth hormone secretion in rats: mechanism of growth retardation. *Am J Physiol* 1993;265:E547–E553.
79. Bessarione D, Perfumo F, Giusti M, et al. Growth hormone response to growth hormone-releasing hormone in normal

and uraemic children: comparison with hypoglycemia following insulin administration. *Acta Endocrinol (Copenh)* 1987;114:5–11.
80. Giordano C, De Santo NG, Carella C, et al. TSH response to TRH in hemodialysis and CAPD patients. *Int J Artif Organs* 1984;7:7–10.
81. Alvestrand A, Mujagic M, Wajngot A, et al. Glucose intolerance in uremic patients: the relative contributions of impaired beta-cell function and insulin resistance. *Clin Nephrol* 1989;31:175–183.
82. Marumo F, Sakai T, Sato S. Response of insulin, glucagon and growth hormone to arginine infusion in patients with chronic renal failure. *Nephron* 1979;24:81–84.
83. Rodger RSC, Dewar JH, Turner SJ, et al. Anterior pituitary dysfunction in patients with chronic renal failure treated by hemodialysis or continuous ambulatory peritoneal dialysis. *Nephron* 1986;43:169–172.
84. Duntas L, Wolf CF, Keck FS, et al. Thyrotropin-releasing hormone: pharmacokinetic and pharmacodynamic properties in chronic renal failure. *Clin Nephrol* 1992;38:214–218.
85. Chan W, Valerie KC, Chan JCM. Expression of insulin-like growth factor-1 in uremic rats: growth hormone resistance and nutritional intake. *Kidney Int* 1993;43:790–795.
86. Tönshoff B, Eden S, Weiser E, et al. Reduced hepatic growth hormone (GH) receptor gene expression and increase in plasma GH binding protein in experimental uremia. *Kidney Int* 1994;45:1085–1092.
87. Villares SM, Goujon L, Maniar S, et al. Reduced food intake is the main cause of low growth hormone receptor expression in uremic rats. *Mol Cell Endocrinol* 1994;106: 51–56.
88. Martínez V, Balbín M, Ordónez FA, et al. Hepatic expression of growth hormone receptor/binding protein and insulin-like growth factor I genes in uremic rats. Influence of nutritional deficit. *Growth Horm IGF Res* 1999;9:61–68.
89. Edmondson SR, Baker NL, Oh J, et al. Growth hormone receptor abundance in tibial growth plates of uremic rats: GH/IGF-I treatment. *Kidney Int* 2000;58:62–70.
90. Baumann G, Shaw MA, Amburn K. Regulation of plasma growth hormone-binding proteins in health and disease. *Metabolism* 1989;38:683–689.
91. Postel-Vinay MC, Tar A, Crosnier H, et al. Plasma growth-hormone binding is low in uremic children. *Pediatr Nephrol* 1991;5:545–547.
92. Tönshoff B, Cronin MJ, Reichert M. Reduced concentration of serum growth hormone (GH)-binding protein in children with chronic renal failure: correlation with GH insensitivity. *J Clin Endocrinol Metab* 1997;82:1007–1013.
93. Powell DR, Liu F, Baker BK, et al. Modulation of growth factors by growth hormone in children with chronic renal failure. The Southwest Pediatric Nephrology Study Group. *Kidney Int* 1997;51:1970–1979.
94. Ding H, Gao XL, Hirschberg R, et al. Impaired actions of insulin-like growth factor 1 on protein synthesis and degradation in skeletal muscle of rats with chronic renal failure. Evidence for a postreceptor defect. *J Clin Invest* 1996;97: 1064–1075.
95. Phillips LS, Kopple JD. Circulating somatomedin activity and sulfate levels in adults with normal and impaired kidney function. *Metabolism* 1981;30:1091–1095.
96. Fouque D. Insulin-like growth factor 1 resistance in chronic renal failure. *Miner Electrolyte Metab* 1995;22:133–137.
97. Fouque D, Peng SC, Kopple JD. Impaired metabolic response to recombinant insulin-like growth factor-1 in dialysis patients. *Kidney Int* 1995;47:876–883.
98. Tönshoff B, Blum WF, Wingen AM, et al. Serum insulin-like growth factors (IGFs) and IGF binding proteins 1, 2 and 3 in children with chronic renal failure: relationship to height and glomerular filtration rate. *J Clin Endocrinol Metab* 1995;80:2684–2691.
99. Frystyk J, Ivarsen P, Skjaerbaek C, et al. Serum-free insulin-like growth factor I correlates with clearance in patients with chronic renal failure. *Kidney Int* 1999;56:2076–2084.
100. Phillips LS, Fusco AC, Unterman TG, et al. Somatomedin inhibitor in uremia. *J Clin Endocrinol Metab* 1984;59:764–772.
101. Powell DR, Liu F, Baker B, et al. Insulin-like growth factor-binding protein-6 levels are elevated in serum of children with chronic renal failure: a report of the Southwest Pediatric Nephrology Study Group. *J Clin Endocrinol Metab* 1997;82:2978–2984.
102. Powell DR, Durham SK, Brewer ED, et al. Effects of chronic renal failure and growth hormone on serum levels of insulin-like growth factor-binding protein-4 (IGFBP-4) and IGFBP-5 in children: a report of the Southwest Pediatric Nephrology Study Group. *J Clin Endocrinol Metab* 1999;84:596–601.
103. Powell DR, Liu F, Baker BK, et al. Effect of chronic renal failure and growth hormone therapy on the insulin-like growth factors and their binding proteins. *Pediatr Nephrol* 2000;14:579–583.
104. Ulinski T, Mohan S, Kiepe D, et al. Serum insulin-like growth factor binding protein (IGFBP)-4 and IGFBP-5 in children with chronic renal failure: relationship to growth and glomerular filtration rate. *Pediatr Nephrol* 2000;14: 589–597.
105. Liu F, Powell DR, Hintz RL. Characterization of insulin-like growth factor-binding proteins in human serum from patients with chronic renal failure. *J Clin Endocrinol Metab* 1989;70:620–628.
106. Lee DY, Park SK, Yorgin PD, et al. Alteration in insulin-like growth factor-binding proteins (IGFBPs) and IGFBP-3 protease activity in serum and urine from acute and chronic renal failure. *J Clin Endocrinol Metab* 1994;79:1376–1382.
107. Kiepe D, Ulinski T, Powell DR, et al. Differential effects of IGFBP-1, -2, -3, and -6 on cultured growth plate chondrocytes. *Kidney Int* 2002;62:1591–1600.
108. Blum WF, Ranke MB, Kietzmann K, et al. GH resistance and inhibition of somatomedin activity by excess of insulin-like growth factor binding protein in uremia. *Pediatr Nephrol* 1991;5:539–544.
109. Tönshoff B, Powell DR, Zhao D, et al. Decreased hepatic insulin-like growth factor (IGF)-I and increased IGF binding protein-1 and -2 gene expression in experimental uremia. *Endocrinology* 1997;138:938–946.
110. Powell D, Liu F, Baker B, et al. Modulation of growth factors by growth hormone in children with chronic renal failure. *Kidney Int* 1997;51:1970–1979.
111. Tsao T, Fervenza FC, Friedlaender M, et al. Effect of prolonged uremia on insulin-like growth factor-I receptor auto-

phosphorylation and tyrosine kinase activity in kidney and muscle. *Exp Nephrol* 2002;10:285–292.

112. Blum WF. Insulin-like growth factors (IGF) and IGF-binding proteins in chronic renal failure: evidence for reduced secretion of IGF. *Acta Paed Scand* 1991;379(suppl):24–31.
113. Pennisi AJ, Costin G, Phillips LS, et al. Somatomedin and growth hormone studies. *Am J Dis Child* 1979;133:950–954.
114. Wehrenberg WB, Janowski BA, Piering AW. Glucocorticoids: potent inhibitors and stimulators of growth hormone secretion. *Endocrinology* 1990;126:3200–3203.
115. Luo J, Murphy LJ. Dexamethasone inhibits growth hormone induction of insulin-like growth factor-I (IGF-I) messenger ribonucleic acid (mRNA) in hypophysectomized rats and reduces IGF-I mRNA abundance in the intact rat. *Endocrinology* 1989;125:165–171.
116. Gabrielsson BG, Carmignac DF, Flavell DM, et al. Steroid regulation of growth hormone (GH) receptor and GH binding protein messenger ribonucleic acids in the rat. *Endocrinology* 1995;133:2445–2452.
117. Tönshoff B, et al. Children with renal allografts. Efficacy and safety of growth hormone treatment in short children with renal allografts: three year experience. *Kidney Int* 1993;44:199–207.
118. Rees L, Greene SA, Adlard P, et al. Growth and endocrine function after renal transplantation. *Arch Dis Child* 1988; 63:1326–1332.
119. van Dop C, Jabs KL, Donohue PA, et al. Accelerated growth rates in children treated with growth hormone after renal transplantation. *J Pediatr* 1992;120:244–250.
120. Unterman TG, Phillips LS. Glucocorticoid effects on somatomedins and somatomedin inhibitors. *J Clin Endocrinol Metab* 1985;61:618–626.
121. Bang P, Degerblad M, Thoren M. Insulin like growth factor (IGF) I and II and IGF binding protein (IGFBP) 1, 2 and 3 in serum from patients with Cushing's syndrome. *Acta Endocrinol* 1993;128:397–404.
122. Silbermann M, Maor G. Mechanisms of glucocorticoid-induced growth retardation: impairment of cartilage mineralization. *Acta Anatomica* 1978;101:140–149.
123. Jux C, Leiber K, Hügel U, et al. Dexamethasone inhibits growth hormone (GH)-stimulated growth by suppression of local insulin-like growth factor (IGF)-I production and expression of GH- and IGF-I receptor in cultured rat chondrocytes. *Endocrinology* 1998;139:3296–3305.
124. Kaptein EM, Quion-Verde H, Chooljian CJ, et al. The thyroid in end-stage renal disease. *Medicine (Baltimore)* 1988;67:187–197.
125. Hegedus L, Andersen JR, Poulsen LR, et al. Thyroid gland volume and serum concentrations of thyroid hormones in chronic renal failure. *Nephron* 1985;40:171–174.
126. Burke JR, El-Bishti MM, Maisey MN, et al. Hypothyroidism in children with cystinosis. *Arch Dis Child* 1978;53:947–951.
127. McLean RH, Kennedy TL, Psoulpour M, et al. Hypothyroidism in the congenital nephrotic syndrome. *J Pediatr* 1982;101:72–75.
128. Koutras DA, Marketos SG, Rigopoulos GA, et al. Iodine metabolism in chronic renal insufficiency. *Nephron* 1972;9:55–65.
129. Schaefer F, Ritz E. Endocrine disorders in chronic renal failure. In: Cameron JS, Davison AM, Grünfeld JP, et al., eds. *Oxford textbook of clinical nephrology*. Oxford: Oxford University Press, 1992:1317–1329.
130. Kaptein EM, Feinstein EI, Nicoloff JT, et al. Serum reverse triiodothyronine and thyroxine kinetics in patients with chronic renal failure. *J Clin Endocrinol Metab* 1983;57:181–189.
131. Kaptein EM, Kaptein JS, Chang EI, et al. Thyroxine transfer and distribution in critical nonthyroidal illnesses, chronic renal failure, and chronic ethanol abuse. *J Clin Endocrinol Metab* 1987;65:606–616.
132. Faber J, Heaf J, Kirkegaard C, et al. Simultaneous turnover studies of thyroxine, 3,5,3'- and 3,3',5'-triiodothyronine, 3,5-, 3,3', and 3',5'-diiodothyronine, and 3'-monoiodothyronine in chronic renal failure. *J Clin Endocrinol Metab* 1983;56:211–217.
133. Ramirez G, Jubiz W, Gutch CF, et al. Thyroid abnormalities in renal failure. A study of 53 patients on chronic hemodialysis. *Ann Intern Med* 1973;79:500–504.
134. Spector DA, Davis PJ, Helderman H, et al. Thyroid function and metabolic state in chronic renal failure. *Ann Intern Med* 1976;85:724–730.
135. Kosowicz J, Malczewska B, Czekalski S. Serum reverse triiodothyronine (3,3',5'-L-triiodothyronine) in chronic renal failure. *Nephron* 1980;26:85–89.
136. De-Marchi S, Cecchin E, Villalta D, et al. Serum reverse T3 assay for predicting glucose intolerance in uremic patients on dialysis therapy. *Clin Nephrol* 1987;27:189–198.
137. Pasqualini T, Zantleifer D, Balzaretti M, et al. Evidence of hypothalamic-pituitary thyroid abnormalities in children with end-stage renal disease. *J Pediatr* 1991;118:873–878.
138. Verger MF, Verger C, Hatt-Magnien D, et al. Relationship between thyroid hormones and nutrition in chronic failure. *Nephron* 1987;45:211–215.
139. Pagliacci MC, Pelicci G, Grignani F, et al. Thyroid function tests in patients undergoing maintenance dialysis: characterization of the "low-T4 syndrome" in subjects on regular hemodialysis and continuous ambulatory peritoneal dialysis. *Nephron* 1987;46:225–230.
140. Robey C, Shreedhar K, Batuman V. Effects of chronic peritoneal dialysis on thyroid function tests. *Am J Kidney Dis* 1989;13:99–103.
141. Hardy MJ, Ragbeer SS, Nascimento L. Pituitary-thyroid function in chronic renal failure assessed by a highly sensitive thyrotropin assay. *J Clin Endocrinol Metab* 1988;66:233–236.
142. Beckett GJ, Henderson CJ, Elwes R, et al. Thyroid status in patients with chronic renal failure. *Clin Nephrol* 1983;19:172–178.
143. Davis FB, Spector DA, Davis PJ, et al. Comparison of pituitary-thyroid function in patients with end-stage renal disease and in age- and sex-matched controls. *Kidney Int* 1982;21:362–364.
144. Silverberg DS, Ulan RA, Fawcett DM, et al. Effects of chronic hemodialysis on thyroid function in chronic renal failure. *Can Med Assoc J* 1973;189:282–286.
145. Wheatley T, Clark PMS, Clark JDA, et al. Abnormalities of thyrotrophin (TSH) evening rise and pulsatile release in the hemodialysis patients: evidence for hypothalamic-pituitary changes in chronic renal failure. *Clin Endocrinol* 1989;31:39–50.
146. Holliday MA, Chantler C. Metabolic and nutritional factors in children with renal insufficiency. *Kidney Int* 1978; 14:306–312.

147. Williams GR, Franklyn JA, Neuberger JM, et al. Thyroid hormone receptor expression in the "sick euthyroid" syndrome. *Lancet* 1989;2:1477–1481.
148. Kinlaw WB, Schwartz HL, Mariash CN, et al. Hepatic messenger ribonucleic acid activity profiles in experimental azotemia in the rat. *J Clin Invest* 1984;74:1934–1941.
149. Lim VS, Zavala DC, Flanigan MJ, et al. Blunted peripheral tissue responsiveness to thyroid hormone in uremic patients. *Kidney Int* 1987;31:808–814.
150. Lim VS, Flanigan MJ, Zavala DC, et al. Protective adaptation of low serum triiodothyronine in patients with chronic renal failure. *Kidney Int* 1985;28:541–549.
151. Lim VS. Thyroid function in patients with chronic renal failure. *Am J Kidney Dis* 2001;38:S80–S84.
152. Spaulding SW, Chopra IJ, Sherwin RS, et al. Effect of caloric restriction and dietary composition on serum T3 and reverse T3 in man. *J Clin Endocrinol Metab* 1976;42:197–200.
153. van Leusen R, Meinders AE. Cyclical changes in serum thyroid hormone concentrations related to hemodialysis: movement of hormone into and out of the extravascular space as a possible mechanism. *Clin Nephrol* 1982;18:193–199.
154. Liewendahl K, Tikanoja S, Mahonen H, et al. Concentrations of iodothyronines in serum of patients with chronic renal failure and other nonthyroidal illnesses: role of free fatty acids. *Clin Chem* 1987;33:1382–1386.
155. Sharp NA, Devlin JT, Rimmer JM. Renal failure obfuscates the diagnosis of Cushing's disease. *JAMA* 1986;256:2564–2565.
156. Ramirez G, Gomez-Sanchez C, Meikle WA, et al. Evaluation of the hypothalamic hypophyseal adrenal axis in patients receiving long-term hemodialysis. *Arch Intern Med* 1982;142:1448–1452.
157. Luger A, Lang I, Kovarik J, et al. Abnormalities in the hypothalamic-pituitary-adrenocortical axis in patients with chronic renal failure. *Am J Kidney Dis* 1987;9:51–54.
158. Betts PR, Hose PM, Morris R. Serum cortisol concentrations in children with chronic renal insufficiency. *Arch Dis Child* 1975;50:245–247.
159. Ferraris JR, Ramirez JA, Goldberg V, et al. Glucocorticoids and adrenal androgens in children with end-stage renal disease. *Acta Endocrinol (Copenh)* 1991;124:245–250.
160. Wallace EZ, Rosman P, Toshav N, et al. Pituitary-adrenocortical function in chronic renal failure: studies of episodic secretion of cortisol and dexamethasone suppressibility. *J Clin Endocrinol Metab* 1980;50:46–51.
161. Cooke CR, Whelton PK, Moore MA, et al. Dissociation of the diurnal variation of aldosterone and cortisol in anephric patients. *Kidney Int* 1979;15:669–675.
162. McDonald WJ, Golper TA, Mass RD, et al. Adrenocorticotropin-cortisol axis abnormalities in hemodialysis patients. *J Clin Endocrinol Metab* 1979;48:92–95.
163. Zager PG, Spalding CT, Frey HJ, et al. Low dose adrenocorticotropin infusion in continuous ambulatory peritoneal dialysis patients. *J Clin Endocrinol Metab* 1985;61:1205–1210.
164. Williams GH, Bailey GL, Hampers CL. Studies on the metabolism of aldosterone in chronic renal failure and anephric man. *Kidney Int* 1973;4:280–288.
165. Rodger RSC, Watson MJ, Sellars L, et al. Hypothalamic-pituitary-adrenocortical suppression and recovery in renal transplant patients returning to maintenance dialysis. *QJM* 1986;61:1039–1046.
166. van Coevorden A, Stolear JC, Dhaene M, et al. Effect of chronic oral testosterone undecanoate administration on the pituitary-testicular axis of hemodialyzed male patients. *Clin Nephrol* 1986;26:48–54.
167. Mastrogiacomo I, de Besi L, Zucchetta P, et al. Male hypogonadism of uremic patients on hemodialysis. *Arch Androl* 1988;20:171–175.
168. Rosman PM, Farag A, Peckham R, et al. Pituitary-adrenocortical function in chronic renal failure: blunted suppression and early escape of plasma cortisol levels after intravenous dexamethasone. *J Clin Endocrinol Metab* 1982;54:528–533.
169. Kawai S, Ichikawa Y, Homma M. Differences in metabolic properties among cortisol, prednisolone, and dexamethasone in liver and renal diseases: accelerated metabolism of dexamethasone in renal failure. *J Clin Endocrinol Metab* 1985;60:848–854.
170. Defronzo RA, Tobin J, Andres R. The glucose clamp technique. A method or the quantification of beta cell sensitivity to glucose and of tissue sensitivity to insulin. *Am J Physiol* 1979;237:E214–E223.
171. Katz AI, Rubenstein AH. Metabolism of proinsulin, insulin, and C-peptide in the rat. *J Clin Invest* 1973;52:1113–1121.
172. Feneberg R, Sparber M, Veldhuis JD, et al. Altered temporal organization of plasma insulin oscillations in chronic renal failure. *J Clin Endocrinol Metab* 2002;87:1965–1973.
173. Hampers CL, Soeldner JS, Doak PB, et al. Effect of chronic renal failure and hemodialysis on carbohydrate metabolism. *J Clin Invest* 1966;45:1719–1731.
174. Smith WG, Hanning I, Johnston DG, et al. Pancreatic beta-cell function in CAPD. *Nephrol Dial Transplant* 1988;3:448–452.
175. Lowrie EG, Soeldner JS, Hamoers CL, et al. Glucose metabolism and insulin secretion in uremic, prediabetic, and normal subjects. *J Lab Clin Med* 1976;76:603.
176. Spitz IM, Rubinstein AH, Behrson I, et al. Carbohydrate metabolism in renal disease. *QJM* 1970;39:201–226.
177. Schmitz O. Effects of physiologic and supraphysiologic hyperglycemia on early and late-phase insulin secretion in chronically dialyzed uremic patients. *Acta Endocrinol (Copenh)* 1989;121:251–258.
178. Nakamura Y, Yoshida T, Kajiyama S, et al. Insulin release from column-perifused isolated islets of uremic rats. *Nephron* 1985;40:467–469.
179. Defronzo RA, Tobin JD, Rowe JW, et al. Glucose intolerance in uremia. *J Clin Invest* 1978;62:425–435.
180. Mak RH, Bettinelli A, Turner C, et al. The influence of hyperparathyroidism on glucose metabolism in uremia. *J Clin Endocrinol Metab* 1985;60:229–233.
181. Mak RHK, Turner C, Haycock GB, et al. Secondary hyperparathyroidism and glucose intolerance in children with uremia. *Kidney Int* 1983;24:S128–S133.
182. Fadda GZ, Akmal M, Premdas FH, et al. Insulin release from pancreatic islets: effects of CRF and excess PTH. *Kidney Int* 1988;33:1066–1072.
183. Fadda GZ, Akmal M, Soliman AR, et al. Correction of glucose intolerance and the impaired insulin release of chronic renal failure by verapamil. *Kidney Int* 1989;36:773–779.

184. Defronzo RA, Alvestrand A. Glucose intolerance in uremia: site and mechanism. *Am J Clin Nutr* 1980;33:1438–1445.
185. Mak RH, Haycock GB, Chantler C. Glucose intolerance in children with chronic renal failure. *Kidney Int* 1983;24:S22–S26.
186. Kalhan SC, Ricanati ES, Tserng KY, et al. Glucose turnover in chronic uremia: increased recycling with diminished oxidation of glucose. *Metabolism* 1983;32:1155–1162.
187. Schmitz O. Peripheral and hepatic resistance to insulin and hepatic resistance to glucagon in uraemic subjects. *Acta Endocrinol (Copenh)* 1988;118:125–134.
188. Westervelt FB, Schreiner GE. The carbohydrate intolerance of uremic patients. *Ann Intern Med* 1962;57:266–275.
189. Deferrari G, Garibotto G, Robaudo C, et al. Glucose interorgan exchange in chronic renal failure. *Kidney Int* 1983;24: S115–S120.
190. Taylor R, Heaton A, Hetherington CS, et al. Adipocyte insulin binding and insulin action in chronic renal failure before and during continuous ambulatory peritoneal dialysis. *Metabolism* 1986;35:430–435.
191. Weisinger JR, Contreras NE, Cajias J, et al. Insulin binding and glycolytic activity in erythrocytes from dialyzed and nondialyzed uremic patients. *Nephron* 1988;48:190–196.
192. Pedersen O, Schmitz O, Hjøllund E, et al. Postbinding defects of insulin action in human adipocytes from uremic patients. *Kidney Int* 1985;27:780–784.
193. Maloff BL, McCaleb M, Lockwood DH. Cellular basis of insulin resistance in chronic uremia. *Am J Physiol* 1983;245: E178–E184.
194. Bak JF, Schmitz O, Sorensen SS, et al. Activity of insulin receptor kinase and glycogen synthase in skeletal muscle from patients with chronic renal failure. *Acta Endocrinol (Copenh)* 1989;121:744–750.
195. Schmitz O, Arnfred J, Orskov L, et al. Influence of hyperglycemia on glucose uptake and hepatic glucose production in non-dialyzed uremic patients. *Clin Nephrol* 1988;30:27–34.
196. Guarnieri G, Toigo G, de Marchi S, et al. Muscle hexokinase and phosphofructokinase activity in chronically uremic patients. In: Giordano C, Friedman EA, eds. *Uremia*. Milano: Wichtig, 1981:278.
197. Mak RH. Insulin resistance in uremia: effect of dialysis modality. *Pediatr Res* 1996;40:304–308.
198. Mak RH, Turner C, Thompson T, et al. The effect of a low protein diet with amino acid/keto acid supplements on glucose metabolism in children with uremia. *J Clin Endocrinol Metab* 1986;63:985–989.
199. Gin H, Aparicio M, Potaux L, et al. Low protein and low phosphorus diet in patients with chronic renal failure: influence on glucose tolerance and tissue insulin sensitivity. *Metabolism* 1987;36:1080–1085.
200. Hörl WH, Haag-Weber M, Georgopoulos A, et al. The physicochemical characterization of a novel polypeptide present in uremic serum that inhibits the biological activity of polymorphonuclear cells. *Proc Natl Acad Sci U S A* 1990;87:6353–6357.
201. Dzúrik R, Hupková V, Cernacek P, et al. The isolation of an inhibitor of glucose utilization from the serum of uraemic subjects. *Clin Chim Acta* 1973;46:77–83.
202. McCaleb ML, Wish JB, Lockwood DH. Insulin resistance in chronic renal failure. *Endocr Res* 1985;11:113–125.
203. Mak RHK, Chang S, Xie WW. 1,25 Dihydroxycholecalciferol reverses inulin resistance and hypertension in the uremic rat. *Pediatr Res* 1991;29:346A.
204. Mak RH. Effect of recombinant human erythropoietin on insulin, amino acid, and lipid metabolism in uremia. *J Pediatr* 1996;129:97–104.
205. Jaspan JB, Rubenstein AH. Circulating glucagon. Plasma profiles and metabolism in health and disease. *Diabetes* 1977;26:887–902.
206. Sherwin RS, Bastl C, Finkelstein FO, et al. Influence of uremia and hemodialysis on the turnover and metabolic effects of glucagon. *J Clin Invest* 1976;57:722–731.
207. Dighe RR, Rojas FJ, Birnbaumer L, et al. Glucagon-stimulable adenylyl cyclase in rat liver. Effects of chronic uremia and intermittent glucagon administration. *J Clin Invest* 1984;73:1004–1012.
208. Heaton A, Johnston DG, Burrin JM, et al. Carbohydrate and lipid metabolism during continuous ambulatory dialysis (CAPD): the effect of a single dialysis cycle. *Clin Sci* 1983;65:539–545.
209. Lindholm B, Karlander SG. Glucose tolerance in patients undergoing continuous ambulatory peritoneal dialysis. *Acta Med Scand* 1986;220:477–483.
210. Heaton A, Taylor R, Johnston DG, et al. Hepatic and peripheral insulin action in chronic renal failure before and during continuous ambulatory peritoneal dialysis. *Clin Sci* 1989;77:383–388.
211. Jones RWA, Rigden SP, Barratt TM, et al. The effects of chronic renal failure in infancy on growth, nutritional status and body composition. *Pediatr Res* 1982;16:784–791.
212. Kleinknecht C, Broyer M, Huot D, et al. Growth and development of nondialyzed children with chronic renal failure. *Kidney Int* 1983;24:40–47.
213. Rizzoni G, Basso T, Setari M. Growth in children with chronic renal failure on conservative treatment. *Kidney Int* 1984;26:52–58.
214. Warady BA, Kriley MA, Lovell H, et al. Growth and development of infants with end-stage renal disease receiving long-term peritoneal dialysis. *J Pediatr* 1988;112:714–719.
215. Karlberg J, Schaefer F, Hennicke M, et al. Early age-dependent growth impairment in chronic renal failure. European Study Group for Nutritional Treatment of Chronic Renal Failure in Childhood. *Pediatr Nephrol* 1996;10:283–287.
216. Ramage IJ, Geary DF, Harvey E, et al. Efficacy of gastrostomy feeding in infants and older children receiving chronic peritoneal dialysis. *Perit Dial Int* 1999;19:231–236.
217. Kari JA, Gonzalez C, Lederman SE, et al. Outcome and growth of infants with severe chronic renal failure. *Kidney Int* 2000;57:1681–1687.
218. Van Dyck M, Bilem N, Proesmans W. Conservative treatment for chronic renal failure from birth: a 3-year follow-up study. *Pediatr Nephrol* 1999;13:865–869.
219. Schaefer F, Wingen AM, Hennicke M, et al. Growth charts for prepubertal children with chronic renal failure due to congenital renal disorders. European Study Group for Nutritional Treatment of Chronic Renal Failure in Childhood. *Pediatr Nephrol* 1996;10:288–293.
220. Hodson EM, Shaw PF, Evans RA, et al. Growth retardation and renal osteodystrophy in children with chronic renal failure. *J Pediatr* 1983;103:735–740.

221. Polito C, Greco L, Totino SF, et al. Statural growth of children with chronic renal failure on conservative treatment. *Acta Paediatr Scand* 1987;76:97–102.
222. Rappaport R, Bouthreuil E, Marti-Henneberg C, et al. Linear growth rate, bone maturation and growth hormone secretion in prepubertal children with congenital adrenal hyperplasia. *Acta Paediatr Scand* 1973;62:513–519.
223. Klare B, Strom TM, Hahn H, et al. Remarkable long-term prognosis and excellent growth in kidney-transplant children under cyclosporine monotherapy. *Transplant Proc* 1991;23: 1013–1017.
224. Offner G, Hoyer PF, Jüppner H, et al. Somatic growth after kidney transplantation. *Am J Dis Child* 1987;141:541–546.
225. Broyer M, Guest G. Growth after kidney transplantation—a single centre experience. In: Schärer K, ed. *Growth and endocrine changes in children and adolescents with chronic renal failure. Pediatric and adolescent endocrinology*. Vol 20. Basel: Karger, 1989:36–45.
226. Haffner D, Schaefer F, Nissel R, et al. Effect of growth hormone treatment on adult height of children with chronic renal failure. *N Engl J Med* 2000;343:923–930.
227. Schärer K. Growth and development of children with chronic renal failure. Cooperative Study Group on Pubertal Development in Chronic Renal Failure. *Acta Paediatr Scand* 1990;366(suppl):90–92.
228. Betts PR, White RHR. Growth potential and skeletal maturity in children with chronic renal insufficiency. *Nephron* 1976;16:325–332.
229. Cundall DB, Brocklebank JT, Buckler JMH. Which bone age in chronic renal insufficiency and end-stage renal disease? *Pediatr Nephrol* 1988;2:200–204.
230. van Steenbergen MW, Wit JM, Donckerwolcke RA. Testosterone esters advance skeletal maturation more than growth in short boys with chronic renal failure and delayed puberty. *Eur J Pediatr* 1991;150:676–780.
231. van Diemen-Steenvoorde R, Donckerwolcke RA, Brackel H, et al. Growth and sexual maturation in children after kidney transplantation. *J Pediatr* 1987;110:351–356.
232. Grushkin CM, Fine RN. Growth in children following renal transplantation. *Am J Dis Child* 1973;125:514–516.
233. Rizzoni G, Broyer M, Brunner FP, et al. Combined Report on Regular Hemodialysis and Transplantation in Europe, 1985. *Proc EDTA* 1986;23:55–83.
234. Chantler C, Broyer M, Donckerwolcke RA, et al. Growth and rehabilitation of long-term survivors of treatment for end-stage renal failure in childhood. *Proc Eur Dial Transplant Assoc* 1981;18:329–339.
235. Gilli G, Mehls O, Schärer K. Final height of children with chronic renal failure. *Proc Eur Dial Transplant Assoc* 1984;21: 830–836.
236. Fennell RS III, Love JT, Carter RL, et al. Statistical analysis of statural growth following kidney transplantation. *Eur J Pediatr* 1986;145:377–379.
237. Schaefer F, Gilli G, Schärer K. Pubertal growth and final height in chronic renal failure. In: Schärer K, ed. *Growth and endocrine changes in children and adolescents with chronic renal failure. Pediatric and adolescent endocrinology*. Vol 20. Basel: Karger, 1989:59–69.
238. Hokken-Koelega AC, Van Zaal MA, van Bergen W, et al. Final height and its predictive factors after renal transplantation in childhood. *Pediatr Res* 1994;36:323–328.
239. Wühl E, Haffner D, Offner G, et al. Long-term treatment with growth hormone in short children with nephropathic cystinosis. *J Pediatr* 2001;138:880–887.
240. Polito C, la Manna A, Olivieri AN, et al. Proteinuria and statural growth. *Child Urol Nephrol* 1988;9:286–289.
241. Schärer K, Essigmann HC, Schaefer F. Body growth of children with steroid-resistant nephrotic syndrome. *Pediatr Nephrol* 1999;13:828–834.
242. Lam CN, Arneil GC. Long-term dwarfing effects of corticosteroid treatment for childhood nephrosis. *Arch Dis Child* 1968;43:589–594.
243. Foote KD, Brocklebank JT, Meadow SR. Height attainment in children with steroid-responsive nephrotic syndrome. *Lancet* 1985;2:917–919.
244. Rees L, Greene SA, Adlard P, et al. Growth and endocrine function in steroid sensitive nephrotic syndrome. *Arch Dis Child* 1988;63:484–490.
245. Holtta TM, Ronnholm KA, Jalanko H, et al. Peritoneal dialysis in children under 5 years of age. *Perit Dial Int* 1997;17:573–580.
246. Nash MA, Torrado AD, Greifer I, et al. Renal tubular acidosis in infants and children. *J Pediatr* 1972;80:738–748.
247. Tsuru N, Chan JCM. Growth failure in children with metabolic alkalosis and with metabolic acidosis. *Nephron* 1987;45: 182–185.
248. Morris RC, Sebastian AC. Renal tubular acidosis and Fanconi syndrome. In: Stanbury JB, Wyngaarden JB, Frederickson DS, eds. *The metabolic basis of inherited disease*, 3rd ed. New York: McGraw-Hill, 1983:1808.
249. Niaudet P, Dechaux M, Trivin C. Nephrogenic diabetes insipidus. Clinical and pathophysiological aspects. *Adv Nephrol* 1983;13:247–260.
250. Simopoulos AP. Growth characteristics in patients with Bartter's syndrome. *Nephron* 1979;23:130–135.
251. Taymans JM, Wintmolders C, Riele TE, et al. Detailed localization of regulator of g protein signaling 2 messenger ribonucleic acid and protein in the rat brain. *Neuroscience* 2002;114:39–53.
252. Bergwitz C, Abou-Samra AB, Hesch RD, et al. Rapid desensitisation of parathyroid hormone dependent adenylate cyclase in perifused human osteosarcoma cells (SaOS-2). *Biochim Biophys Acta* 1994;1222:447–156.
253. Seidel C, Timmermanns G, Seyberth H, et al. Body growth in hyperprostaglandin E syndrome (HPGS) treated by indomethacine. *Pediatr Nephrol* 1992;6:C108.
254. Haffner D, Weinfurth A, Seidel C, et al. Body growth in primary de Toni-Debre-Fanconi syndrome. *Pediatr Nephrol* 1997;11:40–45.
255. Haffner D, Weinfurth A, Manz F, et al. Long-term outcome of paediatric patients with hereditary tubular disorders. *Nephron* 1999;83:250–260.
256. Ehrich JHH. Combined report on regular dialysis and transplantation in Europe part III: renal replacement therapy in children. Presentation at the XXIX Congress of European Renal Association—The European Dialysis and Transplant Association; June 28 –July 1, 1992; Paris.
257. da Silva VA, Zurbrügg RP, Lavanchy P, et al. Long-term

treatment of infantile nephropathic cystinosis with cysteamine. *N Engl J Med* 1985;313:1460–1463.
258. Gahl WA, Reed GF, Thoene JG, et al. Cysteamine therapy for children with nephropathic cystinosis. *N Engl J Med* 1987;316:971–977.
259. van't Hoff WG, Gretz N. The treatment of cystinosis with cysteamine and phosphocysteamine in the United Kingdom and Eire. *Pediatr Nephrol* 1995;9:685–689.
260. Smellie JM, Preece MA, Paton AM. Normal somatic growth in children receiving low-dose prophylactic co-trimoxazole. *Eur J Pediatr* 1983;140:301–304.
261. Merrell RW, Mowad JJ. Increased physical growth after successful antireflux operation. *J Urol* 1979;122:523–527.
262. Sutton R, Atwell JD. Physical growth velocity during conservative treatment and following subsequent surgical treatment for primary vesicoureteric reflux. *Br J Urol* 1989;63: 245–250.
263. Polito C, la Manna A, Capacchione A, et al. Height and weight in children with vesicoureteral reflux and renal scarring. *Pediatr Nephrol* 1996;10:564–567.
264. Seidel C, Schaefer F, Schärer K. Body growth in urinary tract malformation. *Pediatr Nephrol* 1993;7:151–155.
265. Drozdz D, Drozdz M, Gretz N, et al. Progression to end-stage renal disease in children with posterior urethral valves. *Pediatr Nephrol* 1998;12:630–636.
266. Norman LJ, Coleman JE, Macdonald IA, et al. Nutrition and growth in relation to severity of renal disease in children. *Pediatr Nephrol* 2000;15:259–265.
267. Arnold WC, Danford D, Holliday MA. Effects of calorie supplementation on growth in uremia. *Kidney Int* 1983; 24:205–209.
268. Betts PR, Magrath G, White RHR. Role of dietary energy supplementation in growth of children with chronic renal insufficiency. *BMJ* 1977;1:416–418.
269. Lucas LM, Kumar KL, Smith DL. Gynecomastia: a worrisome problem for the patient. *Postgrad Med* 1987;82:73–81.
270. Jones RWA, Dalton RN, Turner C, et al. Oral essential amino acid and ketoacid supplements in children with chronic renal failure. *Kidney Int* 1983;24:95–103.
271. Orejas G, Santos F, Malaga S, et al. Nutritional status of children with moderate chronic renal failure. *Pediatr Nephrol* 1995;9:52–56.
272. Foreman JW, Abitbol CL, Trachtman H, et al. Nutritional intake in children with renal insufficiency: a report of the Growth Failure in Children with Renal Diseases Study. *J Am Coll Nutr* 1996;15:579–585.
273. Baur LA, Knight JF, Crawford BA, et al. Total body nitrogen in children with chronic renal failure and short stature. *Eur J Clin Nutr* 1994;48:433–441.
274. Mehls O, Ritz E, Gilli G, et al. Nitrogen metabolism and growth in experimental uremia. *Int J Pediatr Nephrol* 1980; 1:34–41.
275. Wingen AM, Fabian-Bach C, Schaefer F, et al. Randomised multicentre study of a low-protein diet on the progression of chronic renal failure in children. European Study Group of Nutritional Treatment of Chronic Renal Failure in Childhood. *Lancet* 1997;349:1117–1123.
276. Wassner SJ. Altered growth and protein turnover in rats fed sodium-deficient diets. *Pediatr Res* 1989;26:608–613.
277. Wassner SJ. The effect of sodium repletion on growth and protein turnover in sodium-depleted rats. *Pediatr Nephrol* 1991;5:501–504.
278. Heinly MM, Wassner SJ. The effect of isolated chloride depletion on growth and protein turnover in young rats. *Pediatr Nephrol* 1994;8:555–560.
279. May RC, Kelly RA, Mitch WE. Metabolic acidosis stimulates protein degradation in rat muscle by a glucocorticoid-dependent mechanism. *J Clin Invest* 1986;77:614–621.
280. May RC, Hara Y, Kelly RA, et al. Branched-chain amino acid metabolism in rat muscle: abnormal regulation in acidosis. *Am J Physiol* 1987;252:E712–E718.
281. Bailey JL, Wang X, England BK, et al. The acidosis of chronic renal failure activates muscle proteolysis in rats by augmenting transcription of genes encoding proteins of the ATP-dependent ubiquitin-proteasome pathway. *J Clin Invest* 1996;97:1447–1453.
282. Boirie Y, Broyer M, Gagnadoux MF, et al. Alterations of protein metabolism by metabolic acidosis in children with chronic renal failure. *Kidney Int* 2000;58:236–241.
283. Challa A, Chan W, Krieg RJ Jr, et al. Effect of metabolic acidosis on the expression of insulin-like growth factor and growth hormone receptor. *Kidney Int* 1993;44:1224–1227.
284. Brüngger M, Hulter HN, Krapf R. Effect of chronic metabolic acidosis on the growth hormone/IGF1 endocrine axis: new cause of growth hormone insensitivity in humans. *Kidney Int* 1997;51:216–221.
285. Kattamis CA, Kattamis AC. Management of thalassemias: growth and development, hormone substitution, vitamin supplementation, and vaccination. *Semin Hematol* 1995;32:269–279.
286. Seidel C, Schaefer F, Walther U, et al. The application of knemometry in renal disease: preliminary observations. *Pediatr Nephrol* 1991;5:467–471.
287. Schaefer F, André JL, Krug C, et al. Growth and skeletal maturation in dialysed children treated with recombinant human erythropoietin (rhEPO)—a multicenter study. *Pediatr Nephrol* 1991;5:C61.
288. Huth MD. Structured abstracts for papers reporting clinical trials. *Ann Intern Med* 1987;106:626–627.
289. Mehls O, Ritz E, Gilli G, et al. Effect of vitamin D on growth in experimental uremia. *Am J Clin Nutr* 1978;31:1927–1931.
290. Mehls O, Ritz E, Gilli G, et al. Role of hormonal disturbances in uremic growth failure. *Contrib Nephrol* 1986;50: 119–129.
291. Chesney RW, Moorthy AV, Eisman JA, et al. Increased growth after long-term oral 1-alpha-25-vitamin D3 in childhood renal osteodystrophy. *N Engl J Med* 1978;298:238–242.
292. Chesney RW, Moorthy AV, Eisman JA, et al. Influence of oral 1,25-vitamin D in childhood renal osteodystrophy. *Contrib Nephrol* 1980;18:55–71.
293. Kreusser W, Weinkauf R, Mehls O, et al. Effect of parathyroid hormone, calcitonin and growth hormone on cAMP content of growth cartilage in experimental uremia. *Eur J Clin Invest* 1982;12:337–343.
294. Klaus G, von Eichel B, May T, et al. Synergistic effects of parathyroid hormone and 1,25-dihydroxyvitamin D3 on proliferation and vitamin D receptor expression of rat growth cartilage cells. *Endocrinology* 1994;135:1307–1315.

295. Schmitt CP, Hessing S, Oh J, et al. Intermittent administration of parathyroid hormone (1-37) improves growth and bone mineral density in uremic rats. *Kidney Int* 2000;57:1484–1492.
296. Kuizon BD, Goodman WG, Jüppner H, et al. Diminished linear growth during intermittent calcitriol therapy in children undergoing CCPD. *Kidney Int* 1998;53:205–211.
297. Krempien B, Mehls O, Ritz E. Morphological studies on pathogenesis of epiphyseal slipping in uremic children. *Virchows Arch A Pathol Anat Histol* 1974;362:129–143.
298. Mehls O, Ritz E, Krempien B, et al. Slipped epiphyses in renal osteodystrophy. *Arch Dis Child* 1975;50:545–554.
299. Mehls O, Ritz E, Oppermann HC, et al. Femoral head necrosis in uremic children without steroid treatment or transplantation. *J Pediatr* 1981;6:926–929.
300. Strife CF, Quinlan M, Mears K, et al. Improved growth of three uremic children by nocturnal nasogastric feedings. *Am J Dis Child* 1986;140:438–443.
301. Rodriguez-Soriano J, Arant BS, Brodehl J, et al. Fluid and electrolyte imbalances in children with chronic renal failure. *Am J Kidney Dis* 1986;7:268–269.
302. Parekh RS, Flynn JT, Smoyer WE, et al. Improved growth in young children with severe chronic renal insufficiency who use specified nutritional therapy. *J Am Soc Nephrol* 2001;12:2418–2426.
303. Trachtman H, Hackney P, Tejani A. Pediatric hemodialysis: a decade's (1974-1984) perspective. *Kidney Int* 1986;30:S15–S22.
304. Fennell RS III, Orak JK, Hudson T, et al. Growth in children with various therapies for end-stage renal disease. *Am J Dis Child* 1984;138:28–31.
305. Chantler C, Donckerwolcke RA, Brunner FP, et al. Combined Report on Regular Dialysis and Transplantation of Children in Europe, 1976. In: Vereerstraeten P, Hawkins JB, eds. *Dialysis transplantation nephrology. European Dialysis and Transplant Association.* Vol 14. Tunbridge Wells: Pitman Medical Publications, 1977.
306. Tom A, McCauley L, Bell L, et al. Growth during maintenance hemodialysis: impact of enhanced nutrition and clearance. *J Pediatr* 1999;134:464–471.
307. Potter DE, Luis ES, Wipfler JE, et al. Comparison of continuous ambulatory peritoneal dialysis and hemodialysis in children. *Kidney Int* 1986;30:S11–S14.
308. von Lilien T, Gilli G, Salusky IB. Growth in children undergoing continuous ambulatory or cycling peritoneal dialysis. In: Schärer K, ed. *Pediatric and adolescent endocrinology*. Vol 20. Basel: Karger, 1989:27–35.
309. Fine RN, Mehls O. CAPD/CCPD in children: four years' experience. *Kidney Int* 1986;30:S7–S10.
310. Schaefer F, Klaus G, Mehls O, et al. Peritoneal transport properties and dialysis dose affect growth and nutritional status in children on chronic peritoneal dialysis. *J Am Soc Nephrol* 1999;10:1786–1792.
311. Chadha V, Blowey DL, Warady BA. Is growth a valid outcome measure of dialysis clearance in children undergoing peritoneal dialysis? *Perit Dial Int* 2001;21:S179–S184.
312. Heaf J. High transport and malnutrition-inflammation-atherosclerosis (MIA) syndrome. *Perit Dial Int* 2003;23:109–110.
313. Stenvinkel P, Alvestrand A. Inflammation in end-stage renal disease: sources, consequences, and therapy. *Semin Dial* 2002;15:329–337.
314. Furth SL, Stablein D, Fine RN, et al. Adverse clinical outcomes associated with short stature at dialysis initiation: a report of the North American Pediatric Renal Transplant Cooperative Study. *Pediatrics* 2002;109:909–913.
315. Furth SL, Hwang W, Yang C, et al. Growth failure, risk of hospitalization and death for children with end-stage renal disease. *Pediatr Nephrol* 2002;17:450–455.
316. Ingelfinger JR, Grupe WE, Harmon WE, et al. Growth acceleration following renal transplantation in children less than 7 years of age. *Pediatrics* 1981;68:255–259.
317. Reisman L, Lieberman KV, Burrows L, et al. Follow-up of cyclosporine-treated pediatric renal allograft recipients after cessation of prednisone. *Transplantation* 1990;49:76–80.
318. Broyer M, Guest G, Gagnadoux MF. Growth rate in children receiving alternate-day corticosteroid treatment after kidney transplantation. *J Pediatr* 1992;120:721–725.
319. Kaiser BA, Polinsky MS, Palmer JA, et al. Growth after conversion to alternate-day corticosteroids in children with renal transplants: a single-center study. *Pediatr Nephrol* 1994;8:320–325.
320. Hokken-Koelega AC, Van Zaal MA, de Ridder MA, et al. Growth after renal transplantation in prepubertal children: impact of various treatment modalities. *Pediatr Res* 1994;35:367–371.
321. Fine RN. Growth post-renal transplantation in children: lessons from the North American Pediatric Renal Transplant Cooperative Study (NAPRTCS). *Pediatr Transplant* 1997;1:85–89.
322. Rodriguez-Soriano J, Vallo A, Quintela MJ, et al. Predictors of final adult height after renal transplantation during childhood: a single-center study. *Nephron* 2000;86:266–273.
323. Ninik A, McTaggart SL, Gulati S, et al. Factors influencing growth and final height after renal transplantation. *Pediatr Transplant* 2002;6:219–223.
324. Qvist E, Marttinen E, Rönnhom K, et al. Growth after renal transplantation in infancy or early childhood. *Pediatr Nephrol* 2002;17:438–443.
325. Fine RN, Ho M, Tejani A. The contribution of renal transplantation to final adult height: a report of the North American Pediatric Renal Transplant Cooperative Study (NAPRTCS). *Pediatr Nephrol* 2001;16:951–956.
326. Tejani A, Cortes L, Sullivan EK. A longitudinal study of the natural history of growth post-transplantation. *Kidney Int Suppl* 1996;53:103–108.
327. Pennisi AJ, Costin G, Phillips LS, et al. Linear growth in long-term renal allograft recipients. *Clin Nephrol* 1977;8:415–421.
328. Englund MS, Tyden G, Wikstad I, et al. Growth impairment at renal transplantation—a determinant of growth and final height. *Pediatr Transplant* 2003;7:192–199.
329. So SKS, Chang PN, Najaran JS, et al. Growth and development in infants after renal transplantation. *J Pediatr* 1987;110:343–350.
330. Tejani A, Fine R, Alexander S, et al. Factors predictive of sustained growth in children after renal transplantation. The North American Pediatric Renal Transplant Cooperative Study. *J Pediatr* 1993;122:397–402.
331. DeShazo CV, Simmons RL, Berstein SM, et al. Results of renal transplantation in 100 children. *Surgery* 1974;76:461–463.

332. Sarna S, Hoppu K, Neuvonen PJ, et al. Methylprednisolone exposure, rather than dose, predicts adrenal suppression and growth inhibition in children with liver and renal transplantation. *J Clin Endocrinol Metab* 1997;82:75–77.
333. Ferraris JR, Pasqalini T, Legal S, et al. Effect of deflazacort versus methylprednisolone on growth, body composition, lipid profile, and bone mass after renal transplantation. The Deflazacort Study Group. *Pediatr Nephrol* 2000;14:682–688.
334. Schärer K, Feneberg R, Klaus G, et al. Experience with deflazacort in children and adolescents after renal transplantation. *Pediatr Nephrol* 2000;14:457–463.
335. Jabs K, Sullivan EK, Avner ED, et al. Alternate-day steroid dosing improves growth without affecting graft survival or long-term graft function. A report of the North American Pediatric Renal Transplant Cooperative Study. *Transplantation* 1996;61:31–36.
336. Chao SM, Jones CL, Powell HR, et al. Triple immunosuppression with subsequent prednisolone withdrawal: 6 years' experience in paediatric renal allograft recipients. *Pediatr Nephrol* 1994;8:26–29.
337. Ellis D. Growth and renal function after steroid-free tacrolimus-based immunosuppression in children with renal transplants. *Pediatr Nephrol* 2000;14:689–694.
338. Motoyoma O, Hasagawa A, Ohara T, et al. A prospective trial of steroid cessation after renal transplantation in pediatric patients treated with cyclosporine and mizoribine. *Pediatr Transplant* 1997;1:29–36.
339. Chakrabarti P, Wong HY, Scantlebury VP, et al. Outcome after steroid withdrawal in pediatric renal transplant patients receiving tacrolimus-based immunosuppression. *Transplantation* 2000;5:760–764.
340. Ingulli E, Sharma V, Singh A, et al. Steroid withdrawal, rejection and the mixed lymphocyte reaction in children after renal transplantation. *Kidney Int* 1993;43(suppl):S36–S39.
341. Klaus G, Jeck N, Konrad M, et al. Risk of steroid withdrawal in pediatric renal transplant patients with suspected steroid toxicity. *Clin Nephrol* 2001;56:S37–S42.
342. Mehls O, Ritz E, Hunziker EB, et al. Improvement of growth and food utilization by human recombinant growth hormone in uremia. *Kidney Int* 1988;33:45–52.
343. Koch VH, Lippe BM, Nelson PA, et al. Accelerated growth after recombinant human growth hormone treatment of children with chronic renal failure. *J Pediatr* 1989;115:365–371.
344. Rees L, Rigden SPA, Ward G, et al. Treatment of short stature in renal disease with recombinant human growth hormone. *Arch Dis Child* 1990;65:856–860.
345. Tönshoff B, Dietz M, Haffner D, et al. Effects of two years growth hormone treatment in short children with renal disease. *Acta Paediatr Scand* 1991;379(suppl):33.
346. Hokken-Koelega AC, Stijnen T, de Muinck-Keizer-Schrama SM, et al. Placebo controlled, double blind, cross-over trials of growth hormone treatment in prepubertal children with chronic renal failure. *Lancet* 1991;338:585–590.
347. Fine RN, Kohaut EC, Brown D, et al. Growth after recombinant human growth hormone treatment in children with chronic renal failure. Genentech Cooperative Study Group. *J Pediatr* 1993;124:374–382.
348. Haffner D, Wühl E, Schaefer F, et al. Factors predictive of the short- and long-term efficacy of growth hormone treatment in prepubertal children with chronic renal failure. German Study Group for Growth Hormone Treatment in Children with Chronic Renal Failure. *J Am Soc Nephrol* 1998;9:1899–1907.
349. Fine RN, Kohaut E, Brown D, et al. Long-term treatment of growth retarded children with chronic renal insufficiency, with recombinant human growth hormone. *Kidney Int* 1996;49:781–785.
350. Hokken-Koelega A, Mulder P, De Jong R, et al. Long-term effects of growth hormone treatment on growth and puberty in patients with chronic renal insufficiency. *Pediatr Nephrol* 2000;14:701–706.
351. Wühl E, Haffner D, Nissel R, et al. Short dialyzed children respond less to growth hormone than patients prior to dialysis. German Study Group for Growth Hormone Treatment in Chronic Renal Failure. *Pediatr Nephrol* 1996;10:294–298.
352. Berard E, Crosnier H, Six-Beneton A, et al. Recombinant human growth hormone treatment of children on hemodialysis. French Society of Pediatric Nephrology. *Pediatr Nephrol* 1998;12:304–310.
353. Schaefer F, Wühl E, Haffner D, et al. Stimulation of growth hormone in children undergoing peritoneal or hemodialysis treatment. *Adv Perit Dial* 1994;10:321–326.
354. Wühl E, Haffner D, Gretz N, et al. Treatment with recombinant human growth hormone in short children with nephropathic cystinosis: no evidence for increased deterioration rate of renal function. *Pediatr Res* 1998;43:484–488.
355. Johannson G, et al. Treatment with Genotropin in short children with chronic renal failure, either before active replacement therapy or with functioning renal transplants. An interim report on five European studies. *Acta Paediatr Scand* 1990;370(suppl):36–42.
356. Fine RN, Yadin O, Nelson PA, et al. Recombinant human growth hormone treatment of children following renal transplantation. *Pediatr Nephrol* 1991;5:147–151.
357. Hokken-Koelega AC, Stijnen T, de Jong RC, et al. A placebo-controlled, double-blind trial of growth hormone treatment in prepubertal children after renal transplant. *Kidney Int* 1996;53(suppl):S128–S134.
358. Guest G, Berard E, Crosnier H, et al. Effects of growth hormone in short children after renal transplantation. *Pediatr Nephrol* 1998;12:437–446.
359. Janssen F, Van Damme-Lombaerts R, Van Dyck M, et al. Impact of growth hormone treatment on a Belgian population of short children with renal allografts. *Pediatr Transplant* 1997;1:190–196.
360. Fine RN, Stablein D, Cohen AH, et al. Recombinant human growth hormone post-renal transplantation in children: a randomized controlled study of the NAPRTCS. *Kidney Int* 2002;62:688–696.
361. Haffner D, Wühl E, Tönshoff B, et al. Growth hormone treatment in short children: 5-year experience. German Study Group for Growth Hormone Treatment in Chronic Renal Failure. *Nephrol Dial Transplant* 1994;9:960–961.
362. Hokken-Koelega AC, Stijnen T, de Ridder MA, et al. Growth hormone treatment in growth-retarded adolescents after renal transplant. *Lancet* 1994;343:1313–1317.
363. Rees L, Ward G, Rigden SPA. Growth over 10 years follow-

ing a 1-year trial of growth hormone therapy. *Pediatr Nephrol* 2000;14:309–314.
364. Fine RN, Sullivan EK, Kuntze J, et al. The impact of recombinant human growth hormone treatment during chronic renal insufficiency on renal transplant recipients. *J Pediatr* 2000;136: 376–382.
365. Hokken-Koelega AC, Stijnen T, de Jong MC, et al. Double blind trial comparing the effects of two doses of growth hormone in prepubertal patients with chronic renal insufficiency. *J Clin Endocrinol Metab* 1994;79:1185–1190.
366. Fine RN, et al. Recombinant human growth hormone (rhGH) treatment in children with chronic renal failure (CRF): long-term (one to three years) outcome. *Pediatr Nephrol* 1991;5: 477–481.
367. Fine RN, Brown DF, Kuntze J, et al. Growth after discontinuation of recombinant human growth hormone therapy in children with chronic renal failure. *J Pediatr* 1996;129: 883–891.
368. Haffner D, Nissel R, Wühl E, et al. Metabolic effects of long-term growth hormone treatment in prepubertal children with chronic renal failure and after kidney transplantation. *Pediatr Res* 1997;43:209–215.
369. Filler G, Franke D, Amendt P, et al. Reversible diabetes mellitus during growth hormone therapy in chronic renal failure. *Pediatr Nephrol* 1998;12:405–407.
370. Stefanidis CP, Papathanassiou A, Michelis K, et al. Diabetes mellitus after therapy with recombinant human growth hormone. *Br J Clin Pract* 1996;85(suppl):66–67.
371. Cutfield WS, Wilton P, Bennmarker H, et al. Incidence of diabetes mellitus and impaired glucose tolerance in children and adolescents receiving growth hormone treatment. *Lancet* 2000;355:610–613.
372. Mehls O, Broyer M. Growth response to recombinant human growth hormone in short prepubertal children with chronic renal failure with or without dialysis. European/ Australian Study Group. *Acta Paediatr* 1994;399(suppl):81.
373. Watkins SL. Is severe renal osteodystrophy a contraindication for recombinant human growth hormone treatment? *Pediatr Nephrol* 1996;10:351.
374. Boechat M, Winters W, Hogg R, et al. Avascular necrosis of the femoral head in children with chronic renal disease. *Radiology* 2001;218:411–413.
375. Kaufman D. Growth hormone and renal osteodystrophy: a case report. *Pediatr Nephrol* 1998;12:157–159.
376. Picca S, Cappa M, Rizzoni G. Hyperparathyroidism during growth hormone treatment: a role for puberty? *Pediatr Nephrol* 2000;14:56–58.
377. Mehls O, Salusky IB. Recent advances and controversies in childhood renal osteodystrophy. *Pediatr Nephrol* 1987;1:212–223.
378. Haffner D, Zacharewicz S, Mehls O, et al. The acute effect of growth hormone on GFR is obliterated in chronic renal failure. *Clin Nephrol* 1989;32:266–269.
379. Auernhammer CJ, Strasburger CJ. Effects of growth hormone and insulin-like growth factor I on the immune system. *Eur J Endocrinol* 1995;133:635–645.
380. Hokken-Koelega ACS, Stijnen T, de Jong RC, et al. A placebo-controlled double-blind trial of growth hormone treatment in prepubertal children with renal allografts. *Kidney Int* 1996;49(suppl):S128–S134.
381. Maxwell H, Rees L. Randomised controlled trial of recombinant human growth hormone in prepubertal and pubertal renal transplant recipients. British Association for Paediatric Nephrology. *Arch Dis Child* 1998;79:481–487.
382. Stahnke N, Zeisel HJ. Growth hormone therapy and leukaemia. *Eur J Pediatr* 1989;148:591–596.
383. Tyden G, Wernersson A, Sandberg J, et al. Development of renal cell carcinoma in living donor kidney grafts. *Transplantation* 2000;70:1650–1656.
384. Boose AR, Pieters R, Delemarre-Van de Waal HA, et al. Growth hormone therapy and leukemia. *Tijdschr Kindergeneeskd* 1992:1.
385. Furlanetto R. Guidelines of the use of growth hormone in children with short stature. A report by the Drug and Therapeutics Committee of the Lawson Wilkins Pediatric Endocrine Society. *J Pediatr* 1995;127:857.
386. Cochat P, Six-Beneton A. Adverse effects of recombinant human growth hormone in renal patients. Proceedings: 3rd Novo Nordisk Workshop on CRI, 1997:19–23.
387. Janssen F, Van Damme-Lombaerts R, Van Dyck M, et al. Impact of growth hormone treatment on a Belgian population of short children with renal allografts. *Pediatr Transplant* 1997;1:190–196.
388. Lampit M, Nave T, Hochberg Z. Water and sodium retention during short-term administration of growth hormone to short normal children. *Horm Res* 1998;50: 83–88.
389. Hanukoglu A, Belutserkovsky O, Phillip M. Growth hormone activates renin-aldosterone system in children with idiopathic short stature and in a pseudohypoaldosteronism patient with a mutation in epithelial sodium channel alpha subunit. *J Steroid Biochem Mol Biol* 2001; 77:49–57.
390. Malozowski S, Tanner LA, Wysowski D, et al. Growth hormone, insulin-like growth factor I and benign intracranial hypertension. *N Engl J Med* 1993;329:665–666.
391. Wingenfeld P, Schmidt B, Hoppe B, et al. Acute glaucoma and intracranial hypertension in a child on long-term peritoneal dialysis treated with growth hormone. *Pediatr Nephrol* 1995;9:742–745.
392. Koller EA, Stadel BV, Malozowski SN. Papilledema in 15 renally compromised patients treated with growth hormone. *Pediatr Nephrol* 1997;11:451–454.
393. Mehls O, Berg U, Broyer M, et al. Chronic renal failure and growth hormone treatment: review of the literature and experience in KIGS. In: Ranke MB, Wilton P, eds. *Growth hormone therapy in K–10 years experience.* Heidelberg: Barth, 1999:327–340.
394. Fine RN, Sullivan EK, Tejani A. The impact of recombinant human growth hormone treatment on final adult height. *Pediatr Nephrol* 2000;14:679–681.

69

RENAL OSTEODYSTROPHY

BEATRIZ D. KUIZON
ISIDRO B. SALUSKY

The association between renal failure and bone disease in children was described more than a century ago. The kidney plays a major role in bone and mineral homeostasis: It regulates calcium, phosphorus, and magnesium metabolism; participates in the catabolism of parathyroid hormone (PTH); excretes aluminum and β_2-microglobulin; and, more importantly, synthesizes calcitriol or 1,25-dihydroxyvitamin D_3, the most potent and active vitamin D metabolite, through the action of the 1α-hydroxylase enzyme. As such, renal bone disease is a common consequence of chronic renal insufficiency (CRI) and may lead to growth retardation and osseous deformities if left untreated during the critical years of skeletal growth and development. As the longevity of children with CRI increases because of advances in medical management, dialysis, and renal transplantation, the prevention and treatment of renal osteodystrophy should remain a major component in the overall management of these children.

Renal osteodystrophy encompasses a spectrum of high- to low-turnover skeletal lesions, and the impact of various therapies may change the histologic pattern. Because renal osteodystrophy changes with progression of CRI, reference is made to the stages of CRI, which are based on the measured or estimated glomerular filtration rate (GFR), as recommended by the National Kidney Foundation Kidney Disease Outcomes Quality Initiative (K/DOQI) (Table 69.1). This chapter summarizes the major aspects of the pathogenesis, clinical manifestations, histologic features, and therapeutic interventions currently used in the management of renal osteodystrophy in children. The clinical and histologic features of bone diseases after successful kidney transplantation are also provided.

PATHOGENESIS OF RENAL BONE DISEASE

High-Turnover Bone Lesions (Bone Lesions Associated with Secondary Hyperparathyroidism)

Several factors contribute to the development of secondary hyperparathyroidism in most patients with end-stage renal disease (ESRD). These factors include phosphate retention, hypocalcemia, impaired renal calcitriol synthesis, alterations in PTH secretion, skeletal resistance to the calcemic actions of PTH, and alterations in the calcium-sensing receptor (CaR). The severity of secondary hyperparathyroidism varies considerably depending on the cause, duration, and rate of progression of renal disease. Some patients with mild CRI may have elevated serum PTH levels and bone histologic patterns characteristic of secondary hyperparathyroidism (1). If left untreated, the severity of secondary hyperparathyroidism worsens with the progressive decline in renal function. Indeed, the majority of patients demonstrate bone histologic abnormalities when the GFR decreases to less than 50 ml/min and serum PTH levels inversely correlate with the GFR (1–3). Serum PTH levels remain significantly elevated with accompanying enlargement of the parathyroid glands, leading to overt hyperparathyroid bone disease and adverse effects on other tissues. Therefore, the major objective in the treatment of these patients is to prevent or reverse the effects of excess PTH secretion on the skeleton and nonskeletal organs.

Phosphorus Retention

Normal serum phosphorus levels are usually maintained in patients with mild to moderate CRI by increasing urinary phosphate excretion. However, hyperphosphatemia develops when the GFR declines to 25 to 30% of normal (4,5). Hyperphosphatemia promotes the secretion of PTH indirectly by lowering serum calcium levels and by reducing calcitriol synthesis through inhibition of the enzyme 1α-hydroxylase, which is responsible for conversion of 25-hydroxyvitamin D to the active metabolite 1,25-dihydroxyvitamin D_3. Indeed, dietary phosphorus restriction has been shown to ameliorate the development of secondary hyperparathyroidism in uremic dogs and completely abolish parathyroid cell proliferation in nephrectomized rats (6–9). In children and adults with moderate renal failure, dietary phosphorus restriction has likewise suppressed serum PTH levels and increased serum calcitriol levels (10) (Fig. 69.1).

TABLE 69.1. STAGES OF CHRONIC RENAL INSUFFICIENCY

Stage	Description	GFR (mL/min/1.73 m²)
1	Kidney damage with normal or increased GFR	>90
2	Kidney damage with mild decreased GFR	60–89
3	Moderate decreased GFR	30–59
4	Severe decreased GFR	15–29
5	Kidney failure	<15 or dialysis

GFR, glomerular filtration rate.

In addition, the direct effects of phosphorus on parathyroid gland function were demonstrated in uremic animals that developed increased serum PTH levels and parathyroid gland hyperplasia independent of changes in serum calcium or calcitriol levels during phosphorus supplementation (11,12). This effect of phosphorus appeared to involve posttranscriptional mechanisms because pre-pro-PTH mRNA levels were not increased in the animals given a high phosphorus diet (11). Conversely, when animals with established secondary hyperparathyroidism were then given dietary phosphorus restriction, serum phosphorus and PTH levels normalized, but the parathyroid glands remained hyperplastic, and no evidence of apoptosis was found (13). Moreover, no difference in PTH synthesis, parathyroid gland cytosolic PTH, or the parathyroid gland secretory response to calcium was demonstrated, suggesting alterations in PTH exocytosis (13). It is not yet known whether there is a specific receptor for phosphorus, but a specific parathyroid cell sodium-dependent phosphate co-transporter (PiT-1) has been demonstrated (14). Because PiT-1 mRNA levels are upregulated by vitamin D and phosphorus restriction, this co-transporter may mediate the actions of phosphate and vitamin D on PTH secretion (14).

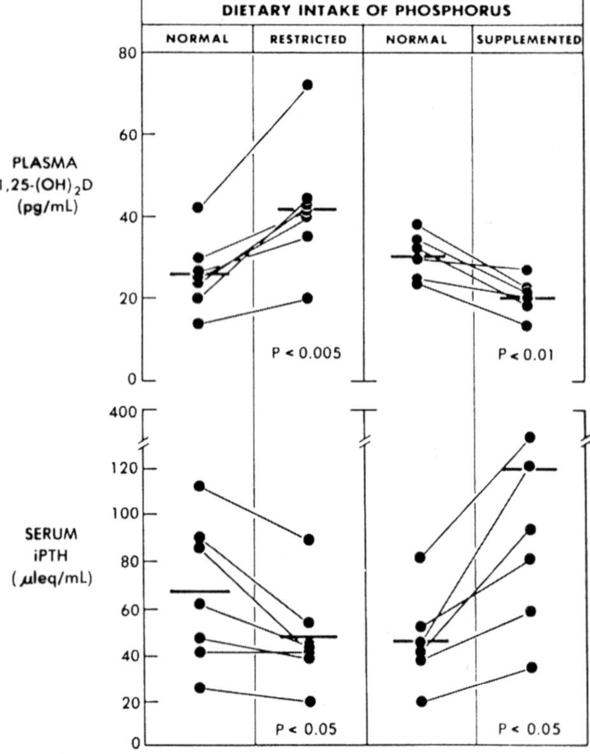

FIGURE 69.1. Effects of dietary phosphorus restriction on plasma levels of parathyroid hormone (PTH) and children in moderate renal failure. iPTH, intact PTH. (From Portale AA, Booth BE, Halloran BP, et al. Effect of dietary phosphorus on circulating concentrations of 1,25-dihydroxyvitamin D and immunoreactive parathyroid hormone in children with moderate renal insufficiency. *J Clin Invest* 1984;73:1580–1589, with permission.)

Hyperphosphatemia has also been implicated in pathogenesis of parathyroid gland hyperplasia in renal failure. Phosphorus supplementation increases parathyroid cell proliferation, whereas phosphorus restriction inhibits this process in animal models of renal failure (8,15). There is limited information, however, regarding the mechanism by which phosphorus stimulates parathyroid cell proliferation in renal failure. Recently, Dusso et al. demonstrated the potential role of cyclin/cyclin-dependent kinase (Cdk) inhibitor p21 and transforming growth factor α (TGFα) in mediating the effects of phosphorus on parathyroid cell proliferation in uremia (16). These investigators demonstrated that phosphorus restriction may prevent parathyroid hyperplasia in early renal failure by stimulating p21. In contrast, parathyroid hyperplasia induced by phosphorus supplementation is mediated by upregulating parathyroid TGFα expression (16).

Alterations in Vitamin D Metabolism

The proximal tubule is the primary site of calcitriol synthesis, in which the conversion of 25-hydroxyvitamin D_3 (predominant form in the blood) to 1,25-dihydroxyvitamin D_3 occurs through the action of the rate-limiting enzyme 1α-hydroxylase (17,18). The gene encoding 1α-hydroxylase has been cloned from rat, mouse, and human tissues, and mutations in the gene result in vitamin D–dependent rickets, type 1 (19–21). The activity of this enzyme is modulated by PTH, calcium, phosphorus, insulin-like growth factor-1 (IGF-1), and other factors. The activity of this enzyme is also dependent on the availability of 25-hydroxyvitamin D_3, which is bound to its plasma carrier; vitamin D–binding protein, filtered through the glomerulus; and, more recently, has been shown to require reabsorption by megalin, an endocytic receptor located in the proximal tubule (22,23). With progressive impairment in renal function, a significant reduction in calcitriol synthesis occurs, leading to subnormal blood levels (Fig. 69.2) (24–26). The decline in calcitriol production may be compensated in part by reduced metabolic clearance of calcitriol in CRI (27,28). The factors responsible for this change have not been determined, but inhibition of the normal pathways of calcitriol degradation by substances retained in uremic plasma may contribute to this problem (29).

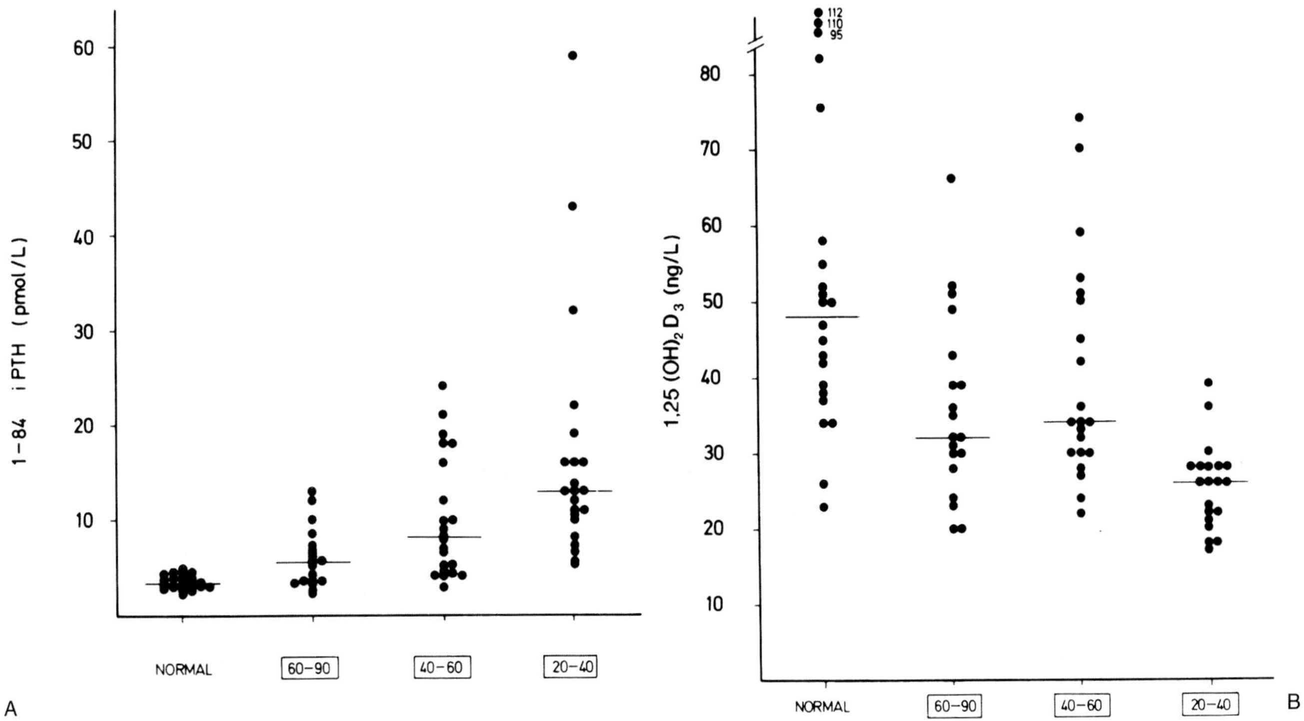

FIGURE 69.2. Changes in serum PTH (IRMA) **(A)** and calcitriol **(B)** levels in patients with different degrees of chronic renal insufficiency. iPTH, intact PTH. (From Reichel H, Deibart B, Schmidt-Gayk H, et al. Calcium metabolism in early chronic renal failure: implications for the pathogenesis of hyperparathyroidism. *Nephrol Dial Transplant* 1991;6:162–169, with permission.)

Low levels of calcitriol impair the absorption of calcium, causing hypocalcemia and hypocalciuria, which are characteristic of patients with CRI. In addition, calcitriol deficiency contributes to alterations in parathyroid gland function and parathyroid gland hyperplasia. Calcitriol inhibits pre-pro-PTH gene transcription through the negative vitamin D response elements in the PTH gene both *in vitro* in bovine parathyroid cells and *in vivo* in rats (30,31). Moreover, calcitriol regulates PTH synthesis via the vitamin D receptor (VDR). By increasing VDR gene expression in the parathyroid gland, calcitriol enhances the feedback inhibition of PTH gene transcription, particularly, because renal failure is associated with reduced binding of VDR to the osteocalcin VDR element and because parathyroid glands of animals and humans with secondary hyperparathyroidism have diminished VDR expression (32–35).

Vitamin D is also one of the major factors involved in the regulation of parathyroid cell proliferation in renal failure, but the mechanism is poorly understood (36–38). Vitamin D has been shown to inhibit parathyroid gland hyperplasia by upregulating Cdk inhibitor p21 expression and decreasing parathyroid TGFα expression in animal models of renal failure (39). Furthermore, because vitamin D exerts potent antiproliferative effects, calcitriol deficiency and diminished VDR expression in parathyroid tissues may contribute to the pathogenesis of parathyroid hyperplasia. Another mechanism may involve the CaR, the expression of which is reduced in hyperplastic parathyroid tissues obtained from patients with renal secondary hyperparathyroidism (40). Vitamin D has been shown to modify CaR expression in parathyroid tissue (41). Indeed, vitamin D–deficient animals had decreased parathyroid CaR mRNA expression, and vitamin D therapy resulted in a dose-dependent increase in CaR mRNA levels (41).

Whereas these studies have demonstrated the inhibitory effects of vitamin D on PTH release and parathyroid cell proliferation in renal failure, recent studies in mice with null mutations of the VDR suggest that vitamin D actions are not necessary to inhibit the development of parathyroid gland hyperplasia. These animals had hypocalcemia, markedly elevated serum PTH levels, parathyroid gland hyperplasia, and histologic evidence of rickets (42). When these animals were given dietary calcium and phosphorus supplementation to normalize serum calcium and phosphorus levels, the development of rickets was prevented despite the absence of VDR (43,44). However, the significance of these findings in secondary hyperparathyroidism remains uncertain.

Abnormalities in Parathyroid Gland Function

Hyperplasia of the parathyroid glands and alterations in the regulation of PTH release are generally considered the two major determinants of excess PTH secretion in CRI. *In vitro* studies of parathyroid tissues and parathyroid cells, the application of molecular biology techniques, and *in vivo* clinical assessments each provide insight into the regulation of PTH secretion in normal and pathologic conditions, and they have substantially increased our understanding of the role of certain factors as key modifiers of parathyroid gland function in CRI.

Results from early *in vitro* studies of dispersed parathyroid cells indicated that the set point for calcium-regulated PTH release was greater than normal in cells obtained from patients with primary hyperparathyroidism, whereas less significant increases in set point were found in parathyroid cells obtained from patients with secondary hyperparathyroidism (45,46). These *in vitro* observations using the four-parameter model provide the basis for the concept that the set point for calcium-regulated PTH release is greater than normal not only in primary hyperparathyroidism but also in secondary hyperparathyroidism due to CRI. Thus, the sigmoidal curve depicting the relationship between ionized calcium levels and PTH secretion is shifted to the right, and higher *in vitro* concentrations of calcium are required to achieve equivalent reductions in PTH release in parathyroid cells from adenomatous or hyperplastic parathyroid glands (45,46).

Over the last decade, dynamic tests of parathyroid gland function have been widely used to examine the regulation of PTH release by calcium in patients with CRI. However, differences in either experimental methods and/or mathematic modeling of PTH secretion have, in part, contributed to inconsistencies in the results of *in vivo* assessments of parathyroid gland function. Indeed, initial studies demonstrated abnormalities of set point in patients undergoing hemodialysis with different types of renal osteodystrophy and after calcitriol therapy (47–49). However, using the four-parameter model originally described by Brown et al., we found no difference in set point between normal subjects and dialysis patients with mild and moderate secondary hyperparathyroidism or those with adynamic renal osteodystrophy (45,50–53). The set point for calcium-regulated PTH release was higher than normal only in patients with ESRD and advanced secondary hyperparathyroidism before parathyroidectomy (Fig. 69.3) (54). Such observations are in accord with *in vitro* data on dispersed parathyroid cells analyzed using the same four-parameter method.

A shortcoming of *in vivo* dynamic testing of parathyroid gland function as currently applied is the inability to correct for variations in the size of the parathyroid glands. Such methodologic considerations may account for the disparity between *in vivo* findings in patients with secondary hyperparathyroidism, in whom basal serum PTH varies widely, and those of *in vitro* studies using defined numbers of cells obtained from hyperplastic parathyroid tissues; they also serve as a reminder of the limitation of *in vivo* models for studying the physiology of PTH secretion (48,50,52,53,55).

Because of the controversy about the various methods for evaluating parathyroid gland function *in vivo* in patients with CRI, alternative approaches to examining PTH secretion in

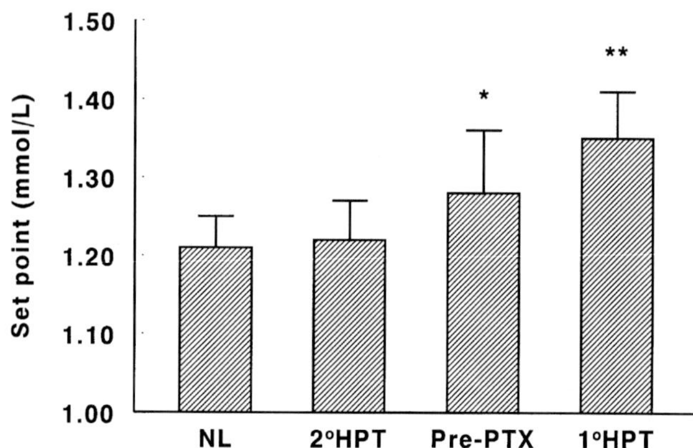

FIGURE 69.3. Set point values for calcium-regulated parathyroid hormone release in volunteers with normal renal function (NL), dialysis patients with mild or moderate secondary hyperparathyroidism (2°HPT), dialysis patients with severe secondary hyperparathyroidism before parathyroidectomy (pre-PTX), and patients with primary hyperparathyroidism (1°HPT).

CRI are of considerable interest (56–58). In this regard, intravenous infusions of calcium have been used to assess parathyroid gland function in other clinical disorders, such as familial hypocalciuric hypercalcemia (FHH) and primary hyperparathyroidism (59); therefore, this technique has been used to compare the responses among patients with various types of renal osteodystrophy. The responses to calcium infusion suggest that the inhibitory effect of calcium on PTH release *in vivo* did not differ between adynamic renal osteodystrophy and secondary hyperparathyroidism (53). The results of that study suggest that differences in functional parathyroid gland mass rather than alterations in calcium sensing by the parathyroid glands are the major determinants of the prevailing serum PTH level in patients with renal osteodystrophy. Assessment in patients with secondary hyperparathyroidism undergoing regular hemodialysis reached similar conclusions (60). Although the histologic type of tissue hyperplasia, variations in VDR expression, and monoclonal expansion of subpopulations of parathyroid cells may contribute, variations in the degree of parathyroid gland hyperplasia are likely to account not only for the marked difference in basal serum PTH levels between adynamic renal osteodystrophy and secondary hyperparathyroidism but also for the moderate but persistent elevations in serum PTH values commonly seen in patients with adynamic renal osteodystrophy.

Alterations in the Calcium-Sensing Receptor

The homeostasis of extracellular calcium concentration is maintained by the rapid actions of PTH and the ability of bone, intestine, and kidney to respond to changes in circulating levels of PTH and 1,25-dihydroxyvitamin D. The CaR cloned by Brown et al., which has been localized in the kidney, parathyroid gland, brain, and gastrointestinal tract and other tissues, plays an important role in calcium-regulated

PTH secretion by detecting minute changes in extracellular calcium ion concentration and activating other G protein–coupled receptors (61,62). In the parathyroid glands, the CaR allows for precise regulation of the extracellular ionized calcium concentration. Changes in CaR expression may play a role in the alterations of the set point for calcium-regulated PTH secretion described in patients with primary and advanced secondary hyperparathyroidism (63).

Mutations of the CaR gene have been demonstrated in patients with benign FHH, autosomal dominant hypocalcemia, and neonatal severe hyperparathyroidism (64,65). Although no mutations of the CaR have been demonstrated in the parathyroid glands of patients with primary and secondary hyperparathyroidism, a significant reduction in the immunoreactivity of the CaR has been shown in adenomas and hyperplastic glands (40,66). Moreover, Gogusev et al. describe downregulation of the CaR in the nodular areas of the parathyroid glands obtained from patients with uremic hyperparathyroidism (63). It is unclear whether phosphorus or calcitriol plays a role in the regulation of the CaR. Several investigators have shown that phosphorus, calcium, and calcitriol did not affect CaR mRNA expression when administered in the uremic and vitamin D–deficient rat (67,68). In contrast, Brown et al. describe upregulation of the CaR expression in the kidney and parathyroid gland of the vitamin D–deficient rats that were treated with calcitriol (41) and moderate changes in serum-ionized calcium did not affect CaR expression.

The localization of the CaR protein in the parathyroid glands has led to development of novel therapeutic agents for the management of hyperparathyroid states. Calcimimetic compounds decrease the threshold for calcium-mediated activation of the CaR and reduce PTH secretion from parathyroid cells. Clinical trials have demonstrated their efficacy in lowering PTH levels in patients with primary hyperparathyroidism and in adult dialysis patients with secondary hyperparathyroidism (69–71) (*vide infra*).

Skeletal Resistance to Parathyroid Hormone

Rapid mobilization of calcium and phosphorus from the skeleton occurs in the presence of PTH. In patients with moderate to severe CRI, however, this rapid response to intravenous infusion of PTH is greatly diminished (72). Moreover, delayed recovery after hypocalcemic stimulation was shown in patients with early renal failure and in uremic dogs despite marked elevation of PTH levels (73). Although the precise mechanisms by which skeletal resistance to PTH affects the calcemic response in patients with renal failure are unclear, unspecified uremic toxins, hyperphosphatemia, and alterations in vitamin D metabolism have been implicated. Additional mechanisms may involve the PTH/PTH-related protein receptor; diminished PTH/PTHrP receptor mRNA expression has been demonstrated in the kidney and growth plate of uremic rats and in the osteoblasts of patients with ESRD (74–76). The potential role of molecular markers localized in skeletal tissues of patients with CRI may provide more information on the pathogenesis of this abnormality. Also, calcitriol administration has been shown to partially restore the calcemic response to PTH in patients with moderate CRI and in experimental animals (77).

Low-Turnover Bone Lesions (Adynamic Bone and Osteomalacia)

In children with CRI, osteomalacia may result from inadequate dietary intake of calcium, phosphorus, or vitamin D, particularly during rapid growth, when the skeletal demand for these nutrients is high. In young children with tubulointerstitial disease, renal calcitriol production may decline at an early stage of renal failure and may contribute to the development of osteomalacia. In the 1980s, osteomalacia and adynamic bone lesions associated with aluminum toxicity were prevalent (78–80); the main sources were aluminum-containing phosphate-binding agents and contaminated dialysate solutions. Aluminum-related bone disease has become much less common with the greater use of calcium-containing phosphate-binding agents and avoidance of other sources of aluminum loading.

Over the last decade, the occurrence of adynamic renal osteodystrophy without aluminum deposition has increased in adult patients undergoing hemodialysis or peritoneal dialysis and in those immediately before commencing dialysis therapy (81,82). Although the prevalence of adynamic lesions of bone has remained less than 20% in children and adolescents with ESRD who were treated with daily doses of calcitriol, adynamic bone developed in 33% of patients who were given high intermittent calcitriol therapy for control of secondary hyperparathyroidism (82).

Adynamic renal osteodystrophy is characterized by decreased osteoblastic activity and rates of bone formation. Serum PTH and alkaline phosphatase levels are often low to normal, suggesting a relative state of hypoparathyroidism (83). Often, patients develop hypercalcemic episodes, reflecting the skeleton's inability to incorporate an increased calcium load (84). Disorders that are associated with longstanding or irreversible reductions in osteoblastic activity and bone formation include age-related or postmenopausal osteoporosis, steroid-induced osteoporosis, idiopathic or surgically induced hypoparathyroidism, and diabetes mellitus. Reversible causes of adynamic renal osteodystrophy include lesions that develop after subtotal parathyroidectomy in patients with ESRD, prolonged treatment with calcium-containing phosphate-binding medications, use of high dialysate calcium concentration, aggressive vitamin D therapy and aluminum toxicity (85).

CLINICAL MANIFESTATIONS

Renal osteodystrophy in children presents with nonspecific signs and symptoms and often goes unnoticed. Clinically, patients may restrain physical activity, making early diagnosis difficult, and radiographic changes may not reflect the severity of bone disease. Careful and detailed physical examination must be performed in the evaluation of these patients.

Growth Retardation

A substantial proportion of children with CRI have significant growth impairment. Based on the North American Pediatric Renal Transplant Cooperative Study (NAPRTCS), the mean height standard deviation scores (SDSs) were 1.64 below the appropriate age- and gender-adjusted height levels at the start of dialysis in more than 3000 patients studied; of these, males and younger patients were more growth impaired (86). At time of transplant, the mean height SDS was −1.91 in more than 6600 patients studied, with greater height deficits in males, younger patients, and in those with previous renal transplants.

Multiple factors may be responsible for growth retardation in children with CRI, including persistent metabolic acidosis, calcitriol deficiency and renal osteodystrophy, inadequate protein and caloric intake, and disturbances in certain growth factors. Acidosis has been linked to delayed linear growth in patients with renal tubular acidosis and normal renal function, and correction of metabolic acidosis often leads to acceleration in growth velocity (87). Acidotic rats have been found to have decreased growth hormone (GH) secretion, serum IGF-1, and hepatic IGF-1 mRNA expression. Moreover, metabolic acidosis has been shown to inhibit the effects of GH in rats with normal and decreased renal function (88–90). In the growth plate, incubation of murine mandibular condyles in acidic medium diminished the expressions of the GH receptor, IGF-1 receptor, and IGF-1 (both with and without GH treatment) and upregulated the expressions of IGF-binding proteins (IGFBPs) 2 and 4, which are negative modulators of IGF-1 (91). However, the role of metabolic acidosis in renal failure remains to be determined.

Calcitriol deficiency has also been thought to contribute to growth retardation and bone disease in children with CRI. Indeed, treatment with daily doses of calcitriol, or 1,25-dihydroxyvitamin D_3, has been reported to improve linear growth in small numbers of children with stable CRI and in those receiving regular dialysis (92–94). Such findings provide the rationale for the routine administration of calcitriol to nearly all children with CRI. However, enhanced growth velocity was not demonstrated on long-term follow-up (94) and further studies have not shown that calcitriol consistently improves linear growth in children with CRI (95–97).

Secondary hyperparathyroidism remains prevalent in children with advanced renal disease, and osteitis fibrosa continues to be the most common skeletal lesion of renal osteodystrophy in those undergoing regular dialysis despite regular treatment with daily doses of oral calcitriol (78,98). Large intermittent doses of calcitriol have thus been used to treat secondary hyperparathyroidism (82,99–102). This approach has been shown to significantly reduce bone formation and suppress osteoblastic activity in both adults and children (77,101). However, diminished linear growth has been reported in prepubertal children with secondary hyperparathyroidism who developed adynamic renal osteodystrophy after treatment with large intermittent doses of calcitriol (103). It is not known whether impaired growth resulted from a direct inhibitory effect of either high doses or intermittent dosing of calcitriol on chondrocyte activity or whether it was a consequence of oversuppression of PTH (103). In a recent study, linear growth and PTH suppression did not differ during daily or twice-weekly administration of similar doses of calcitriol in prepubertal patients with CRI. Nonetheless, a direct correlation between growth velocity and PTH levels was found, suggesting that PTH levels may act as an additional modulator of growth (104).

Although the mechanisms responsible for the inhibitory actions of calcitriol on epiphyseal growth plate cartilage remain poorly understood, it is well-known that calcitriol, or 1,25-dihydroxyvitamin D, exerts dose-dependent inhibitory effects on cell proliferation *in vitro* both in chondrocytes and in osteoblast-like cells, and neither GH nor IGF-1 can overcome these inhibitory effects (36–38). In addition, recent studies demonstrate that vitamin D sterols increase expressions of a number of IGFBPs (IGFBP-2, -3, -4, -5), which may indirectly suppress proliferation by sequestering IGF-1 and/or may exert IGF-1–independent antiproliferative effects through its own receptors (105–108). IGFBPs may also inhibit IGF-1R signaling, block the cell cycle in the G1/G0 phase, or promote apoptosis (109,110).

GH resistance has been described as one of the factors responsible for impaired linear growth in renal failure. Poor growth develops despite normal or increased serum GH levels due to enhanced pituitary GH secretion and decreased renal clearance of GH (111,112). There is limited information, however, regarding the underlying molecular mechanisms for GH insensitivity in CRI. Animals with renal failure have been found to have diminished expressions of the hepatic GH receptor and IGF-1 mRNA and postreceptor defects in GH-mediated signal transduction in the liver (113,114). Moreover, reductions in serum GH-binding protein levels (derived from the extracellular domain of the GH receptor) have been described in children and adults with CRI (115). In addition, increased synthesis and reduced clearance of IGFBP-1, -2, -4, and -6 and low-molecular-weight fragments of IGFBP-3 are found in uremic serum, and levels of IGFBP-1, -2, and -4 inversely correlate with height (116–118). These excess IGFBPs, which have high affinity for IGF-1, may decrease the bioavailability of IGF-1 and may also exert direct, IGF receptor–independent actions on cell proliferation via their own receptors (107,108). As such, improved growth velocity during recombinant human GH (rhGH) therapy has been ascribed to increased bioavailability of IGF-1 to target tissues because GH stimulates each component of the 150-kDa serum ternary complex (acid-labile subunit, IGFBP-3, IGF-1, and IGF-2) and reduces serum IGFBP-1 level. However, children who are undergoing regular dialysis respond less well to rhGH therapy than children with less severe CRI. The mechanisms for the differences in response to GH therapy remain to be determined, but the potential interaction between calcitriol and rhGH in the growth plate cartilage should be considered.

Bone Pain

In the early course of renal osteodystrophy, bone pain is nonspecific and difficult to distinguish from common aches and pains. Pain is more often present in patients with low-turnover bone lesions associated with aluminum toxicity. A great variability in clinical presentation occurs among patients. As the disease progresses, the pain localizes to the lower back and to weight-bearing joints, including hips, knees, and ankles. Symptoms worsen with pressure and changes in posture. Limping requires prompt and thorough evaluation in a previously ambulatory child with secondary hyperparathyroidism because of the increased prevalence of fracture and slipped epiphysis in this population (119).

Slipped Epiphyses

Slipped epiphyses are one of the most severe and physically incapacitating manifestations of bone disease in children with CRI. In preschool children, the upper and lower femoral epiphyses are often affected, whereas, in older children, the upper femur and the radial/ulnar epiphyses are involved. Other epiphyses that can be affected include the distal radius and metacarpal and metatarsal heads (119). In one report, slipped epiphyses were found in 10 of 33 children with newly diagnosed CRI and in 1 of 82 of those who are undergoing dialysis therapy (119). Clinical presentation may include limping, waddling gait, limitation of the range of motion, and inability to ambulate. Mehls et al. demonstrated that children with epiphysiolysis have severe osteitis fibrosa with high serum PTH levels and marked endosteal fibrosis; a dense fibrous tissue may be present between the growth plate cartilage and the adjacent metaphysis, where the plane of slippage may occur (120). The diagnosis is usually established by roentgenograms. Total joint replacement is often required when the proximal femur is involved.

Skeletal Deformities

Bone deformities may be one of the major manifestations of renal osteodystrophy in children with long-term untreated CRI. The pattern of bone deformities varies with the child's age. Bowing may affect both the upper and lower extremities (Fig. 69.4). Patients younger than 4 years will have skeletal abnormalities similar to those due to vitamin D–deficient rickets, which include rachitic rosary; metaphyseal widening, leading to wrist and ankle enlargement; craniotabes; and frontal bossing (121). Because of the rapid increase in growth velocity in children younger than 10 years, bone deformities in the long bones, particularly in the lower extremities, are much more evident. Radiographic changes similar to Blount disease are commonly seen, although these changes occur in the lateral aspect of the proximal tibial metaphysis and epiphysis. Cor-

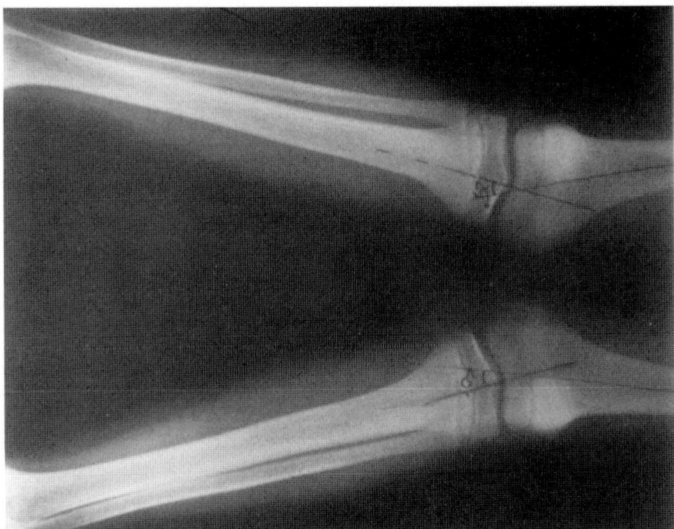

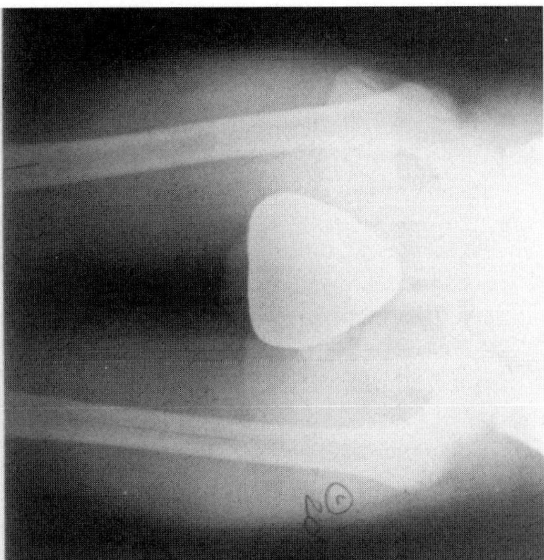

FIGURE 69.4. Roentgenographic evidence of genu valgum in a 14-year-old boy with secondary hyperparathyroidism.

rective orthopedic surgeries may be required in some patients despite calcitriol therapy. Patients may also present with ulnar deviation, pes varus, pseudo-clubbing, and dental abnormalities.

Muscle Weakness

Myopathy in children with CRI may present in a progressive manner. Initially, patients may complain of nonspecific aches and pains, which can progress to inability to perform activities of daily living. Gait disturbances may be seen with the characteristic waddling gait, which resembles the proximal muscle weakness seen in patients with nutritional vitamin D deficiency (122,123). An underrecognized but significant consequence of myopathy in children is the restriction of physical activity, which impairs the quality of life and social development. Progressive and debilitating myopathy that develops in association with severe bone pain is a common manifestation of aluminum-related bone disease. The mechanism for the development of proximal myopathy in children is not well understood, although contributing factors include secondary hyperparathyroidism, phosphate depletion, aluminum bone disease, and disorders of vitamin D metabolism (124,125).

The diagnosis of proximal myopathy is usually made from a complete history and physical examination, because no specific tests are available. Electromyographic studies do not show specific findings, and serum levels of various muscle enzymes such as creatine phosphokinase, aldolase, and transaminases are usually within normal limits. No specific treatment is available, although an improvement in muscle strength in both proximal and distal muscles has been shown after treatment with vitamin D (126). Improvement in symptoms during vitamin D therapy may be due, in part, to the presence of VDRs in skeletal muscle (127). Subtotal parathyroidectomy also results in clinical improvement.

Extraskeletal Calcification

Soft tissue calcifications are more commonly seen in adults with CRI but they also occur in children with ESRD (128). Autopsy data from 120 children who had undergone dialysis or renal transplantation identified soft tissue calcifications in 60%, and the most commonly affected sites were blood vessels, lung, kidney, myocardium, coronary arteries, central nervous system, and gastric mucosa (128). Calcification was associated with multiple factors such as treatment with vitamin D, peak calcium-phosphorus product, age at onset of CRI, and male gender. Of these, vitamin D sterols, particularly calcitriol, had the strongest correlation with calcification. Consistent with data in adults with CRI, such results suggest a potential role of altered mineral metabolism in extraskeletal calcification.

There are three types of soft tissue calcification: visceral, tumoral or periarticular, and vascular. Deposition of calcium and phosphorus in the conjunctiva results in inflammation often called the *red-eye syndrome*, which has been described in approximately 10% of dialyzed patients. Calcifications in the cornea are demonstrated by slit-lamp examination and they can result in band keratopathy. Pulmonary calcifications may lead to restrictive lung disease, which may progress despite optimal dialysis therapy (Fig. 69.5). Often, parathyroidectomy and renal transplantation are the best therapeutic options (129). Calcific periarthritis is characterized by episodes of acute inflammation in and around small joints, with periarticular warmth and erythema. Radiographic findings demonstrate small effusions within the joint and calcifications in adjacent periarticular tissues.

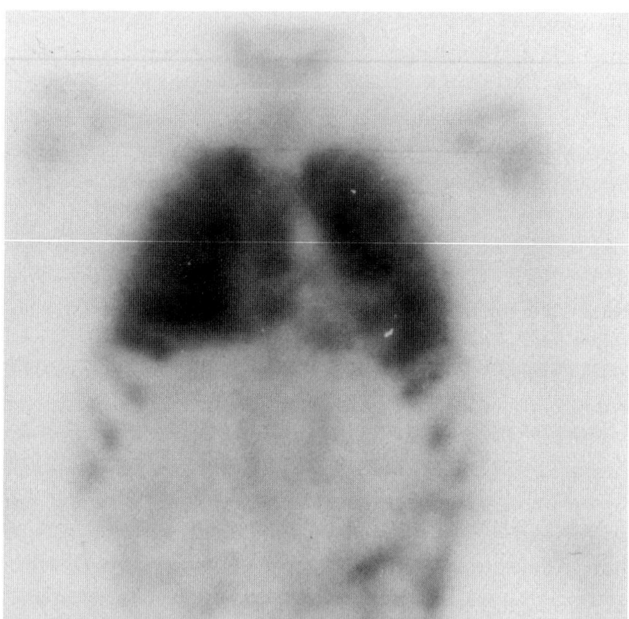

FIGURE 69.5. Diffuse bilateral lung calcifications diagnosed by scintigraphy with technetium-labeled diphosphonate in a 17-year-old girl with severe secondary hyperparathyroidism.

Cardiac calcifications, particularly in the mitral valve and aortic valve, occur in more than 50% of adult patients who have been on chronic dialysis therapy, and these findings were even more common in the presence of hypertension (130,131). Vascular calcification in renal failure occurs in the media, where it is more common (Mönckeberg's sclerosis), and in the intima, where it is usually associated with atherosclerosis. Schwarz et al. have recently shown that patients with CRI have heavily calcified plaques compared to subjects with intact renal function who have fibroatheromatous plaques (132). Vascular calcifications may contribute to the exceedingly high mortality rate in CRI. In addition, it may complicate the establishment of vascular access for hemodialysis (133), and the rigid wall may make blood pressure and pulse determinations more difficult and may also be falsely elevated.

Cardiac calcifications involving valves and coronary vessels can be assessed using the high-resolution electron beam com-

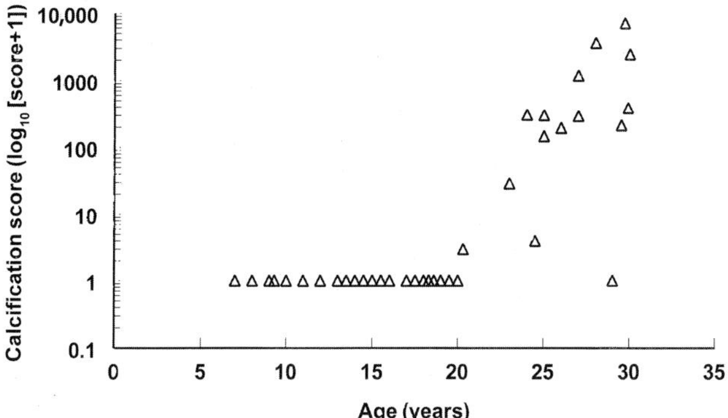

FIGURE 69.6. Coronary artery calcification scores assessed by electron beam computed tomography according to age in children and young adults undergoing dialysis. (From Goodman WG, Goldin J, Kuizon BD, et al. Coronary artery calcification in young adults with end-stage renal disease who are undergoing dialysis. *N Engl J Med* 2000;342:1478–1483, with permission.)

puted tomography (EBCT), whereas vascular calcifications in the extremities are best demonstrated in the lateral radiographs of the ankles or anteroposterior views of the hands and feet (134). For subjects with normal renal function, reports indicate that coronary calcification measured by EBCT corresponds to the extent and severity of lesions detected by angiography. Using this technique in adult patients with ESRD, markedly elevated calcification scores were found compared to subjects of the same age with normal renal function, and the scores in these patients increased after 1 year (130). Likewise, positive EBCT scans were found in young adult patients who had started dialysis in childhood (135–137) (Fig. 69.6), and calcification scores doubled after less than 2 years of follow-up (135) (Fig. 69.7). Factors associated with positive EBCT scans include older age, longer treatment with dialysis, increased calcium-phosphorus ion product (135,137), higher intake of calcium-containing phosphate-binders (135), hyperparathyroidism (137), microinflammation (137), and hyperhomocystinemia (137). These findings underscore the role of disturbances in mineral metabolism in the development and progression of coronary artery calcification in patients with ESRD, and they may contribute to the markedly high mortality rate from cardiovascular disease in these patients (138).

Although vascular calcification has been thought to develop from passive tissue deposition of calcium in the past, recent data indicate that it is an active and regulated process similar to bone ossification. Several studies have demonstrated the expression of factors normally involved in skeletal metabolism in both intimal and medial calcification. In fact, PTH-related peptide and the PTH/PTHrP receptor, bone morphogenetic protein-2, and osteocalcin and osteopontin expressions were localized within human intimal atherosclerotic lesions (139–143). In medial calcification, Shanahan et al. reported diminished expressions of constitutively inhibitory proteins such as matrix Gla protein, osteonectin, osteoprotegerin, and aggrecan by vascular smooth muscle cells and increased expressions of alkaline phosphatase, bone sialoprotein, bone Gla protein, and collagen in association with transcription factors that control the expression of these genes (144–146). When the vascular smooth muscle cells obtained from vessels with medial calcification were examined, features that were characteristic of osteoblasts were found, and they were able to calcify *in vitro* (146).

Likewise, the expressions of osteopontin, bone sialoprotein, alkaline phosphatase and type I collagen have been reported in calcified vessels obtained from adult patients with ESRD (147). Greater expressions of Cbfa1, a transcription factor for osteoblast differentiation, and osteopontin were demonstrated in calcified vessels than in normal vessels. Furthermore, uremic serum upregulated the expression of Cbfa1 and osteopontin in bovine smooth muscle cells *in vitro* (148). Overall, these results emphasize the role of abnormalities in bone and min-

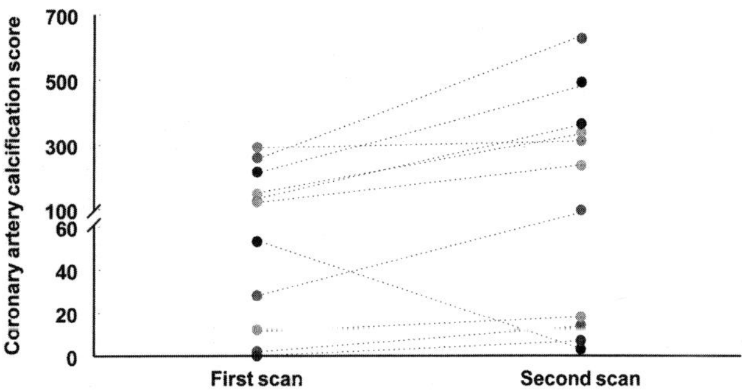

FIGURE 69.7. Coronary calcification scores in ten patients with positive scores on initial scan and in two patients whose scans became positive after less than 2-year follow-up. Calcification scores nearly doubled in nine of the ten patients who had an initial positive scan. (From Goodman WG, Goldin J, Kuizon BD, et al. Coronary artery calcification in young adults with end-stage renal disease who are undergoing dialysis. *N Engl J Med* 2000;342:1478–1483, with permission.)

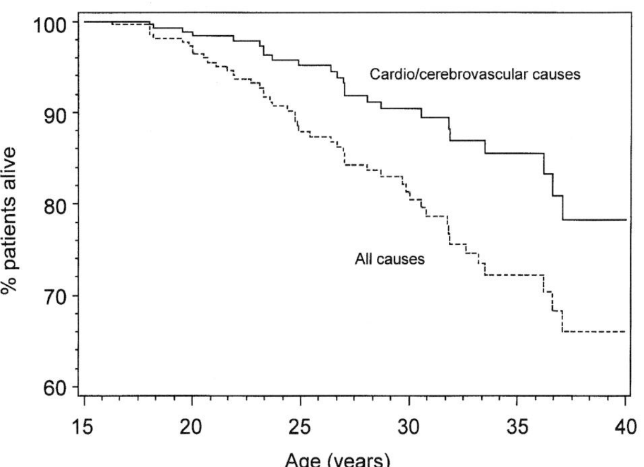

FIGURE 69.8. Follow-up of young adults with childhood-onset chronic renal insufficiency showed that one-half of the patients died from a cardiovascular or cerebrovascular event. (From Oh J, Wunsch R, Turzer M, et al. Advanced coronary and carotid arteriopathy in young adults with childhood-onset chronic renal failure. *Circulation* 2002;106:100–105, with permission.)

eral metabolism in vascular calcification in the context of CRI. Thus, it is critical that therapeutic measures for the prevention of such complications in the growing child are taken into consideration, particularly because cardiovascular disease is the leading cause of death in children and adults with ESRD, and the mortality rate is markedly higher than in the general population (137,138,149) (Fig. 69.8).

DIAGNOSTIC EVALUATIONS

Biochemical Determinations

Calcium

Serum calcium levels are usually low in patients with moderate or advanced CRI. Hypocalcemia often resolves during treatment with calcium-containing phosphate binders, vitamin D, and with initiation of dialysis. The concentration of calcium in most dialysis solutions is 2.5 mEq/L; this concentration is generally adequate to maintain serum calcium within acceptable limits.

Recurrent or persistent hypercalcemia in patients with CRI is not common. Possible etiologies include severe secondary hyperparathyroidism, aluminum-related bone disease, adynamic bone, vitamin D sterols, use of large amounts of calcium-containing phosphate-binding agents, and prolonged immobilization (46,97,150–152). Malignancy and extrarenal production of calcitriol in disorders such as sarcoidosis or tuberculosis result in hypercalcemia, but these conditions are uncommon in the pediatric age group. Patients with adynamic bone lesion without evidence of aluminum toxicity are prone to develop hypercalcemic episodes, which are related to the skeleton's inability to incorporate an acute calcium load (84).

Phosphorus

Serum phosphorus levels are often maintained within normal limits in early CRI. However, when the GFR falls below 30 mL/min/1.73 m^2 (stage 4 CRI), phosphorus excretion decreases and leads to hyperphosphatemia (4). Hyperphosphatemia is a common problem in patients with more advanced CRI, and measures to maintain serum phosphorus levels within age-appropriate levels and calcium phosphorus product lower than 55 mg^2/dL^2 must be initiated to prevent the development and progression of secondary hyperparathyroidism and vascular calcifications. Indeed, disturbances in mineral metabolism (hyperphosphatemia, hypercalcemia, increased calcium phosphorus product) and vitamin D therapy have been associated with vascular calcification. Although extraskeletal and vascular calcification are well-recognized consequences of CRI in adult dialysis patients and were regarded as rare in the pediatric population, more recent studies demonstrate evidence of vascular calcifications in young adult dialysis patients who had started dialysis in childhood (135,137). Moreover, elevations in levels of serum phosphorus and calcium-phosphorus product have been demonstrated to be independent risk factors for mortality in adult patients treated with dialysis (153).

The normal range for serum phosphorus levels is age-adjusted. Values are higher in infants and decline to adult values by late adolescence. During the first 3 months of life, values range from 4.8 to 7.4 mg/dL (mean, 6.2 mg/dL); levels decrease to 4.5 to 5.8 mg/dL (mean, 5.0 mg/dL) at age 1 to 2 years, and 3.5 to 5.5 mg/dL (mean, 4.4 mg/dL) during childhood (154).

Alkaline Phosphatase

Serum total alkaline phosphatase is a biochemical marker of osteoblastic activity. Values generally correspond to the histologic severity of osteitis fibrosa, and serial measurements may be helpful in the follow-up of children with renal osteodystrophy. During intermittent calcitriol therapy, serum alkaline phosphatase levels have been found to be good predictors of adynamic renal osteodystrophy (103). Indeed, serum alkaline phosphatase levels often decrease below baseline in patients with bone biopsy–proven secondary hyperparathyroidism, and such changes correspond to marked reductions in bone formation documented by bone biopsy. In addition, changes in Z-scores for height during intermittent calcitriol therapy correlate with serum alkaline phosphatase levels, although a similar relationship is not observed during daily calcitriol therapy (103). Bone-specific alkaline phosphatase may be useful in predicting the histologic lesion of renal osteodystrophy. Values below 27 U/L have been used to exclude high-turnover bone lesions.

Parathyroid Hormone

Accurate measurements of the concentration of PTH in serum or plasma are essential for the proper assessment of renal osteodystrophy (81,155–158). Indeed, determinations of PTH levels are used as surrogates for bone histology, which remains the most reliable method to establish the diagnosis of renal osteodystrophy (78,159,160).

Serum PTH levels are usually elevated in patients with moderate and severe CRI (10,161). Previous assays measuring the epitopes located in the midregion or carboxy-terminal portions of the PTH molecule resulted in high values because of inactive fragments that are retained in renal failure (155). Andress et al. demonstrated that the amino terminal, which cross-reacts with the intact PTH molecule, may be a better predictor of osteitis fibrosa than the inactive carboxyterminal/midregion PTH fragments (162). The first clinically useful two-site immunometric PTH assay (PTH-IMA) used two antibodies directed against amino- and carboxyl-terminal epitopes, respectively, and was, therefore, predicted to measure only full length PTH(1-84) (163).

Over the last decade, this first-generation PTH-IMA (1st PTH-IMA) proved to be a reasonably reliable predictor of the different subtypes of renal osteodystrophy, and it performed well in assessing the therapeutic response to active vitamin D sterols in patients with renal failure (81,157,158). Serum PTH levels greater than 200 pg/mL were 95% sensitive and 86% specific for identifying those with high-turnover bone lesions from secondary hyperparathyroidism in patients treated with dialysis (157). In contrast, in adult patients with stable stage 3 CRI (GFR, 30 to 59 mL/min/1.73 m^2), serum PTH levels between 100 and 150 pg/mL were associated with bone biopsy findings consistent with osteitis fibrosa (2). On the other hand, serum PTH levels less than 200 pg/mL were 100% sensitive but only 79% specific for diagnosing patients with adynamic bone lesion; specificity was increased when serum calcium greater than 10 mg/dL was included in patients treated with dialysis. In dialysis patients receiving intermittent calcitriol therapy, however, serum PTH levels were not as predictive; the levels remained elevated despite a significant decline in bone formation rate (82). This disparity between histologic and biochemical findings suggests that intermittent calcitriol administration can reduce bone formation in patients with secondary hyperparathyroidism, at least in part, by a mechanism that is independent of vitamin D–induced reductions in serum PTH levels (82).

On the other hand, recent observations highlight important shortcomings of this and other PTH-IMAs (164,165). In particular, a series of studies by D'Amour and colleagues (164–166) demonstrated that 1st PTH-IMAs detect not only the intact hormone, but also additional PTH fragments truncated at the amino-terminus [ntPTH(1-84)]. Indeed, most of the detection antibodies, which are usually directed against epitopes within the amino-terminus of the hormone, detect not only PTH(1-84) but also one or several ntPTH(1-84) fragments, some of which co-elute from reverse-phase high-performance liquid chromatography column with synthetic PTH(7-84) (165). In contrast, a more recently developed second-generation PTH-IMA (2nd PTH-IMA) using a detection antibody raised against the first four amino-terminal amino acids of human PTH recognizes only PTH(1-84) and possibly PTH fragments that are truncated at the carboxyl-terminus but not PTH(7-84) (Fig. 69.9) (167–169). Consistent with this assessment, human PTH(1-34) but not human PTH(2-34) or other amino-terminally truncated fragments of human PTH(1-34) cross-reacted with the detection antibody (167–169). 1st PTH-IMAs, thus, overestimate the true concentration of PTH(1-84) in serum or plasma both in patients with ESRD and in those with normal renal function (166,167,169–172) (Fig. 69.10).

Recent *in vitro* and *in vivo* experimental data also indicate that one or more amino-terminally truncated PTH(1-84) fragments antagonize the calcemic actions of

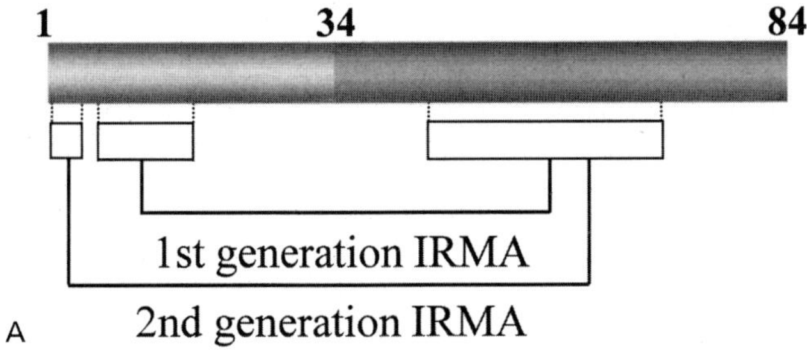

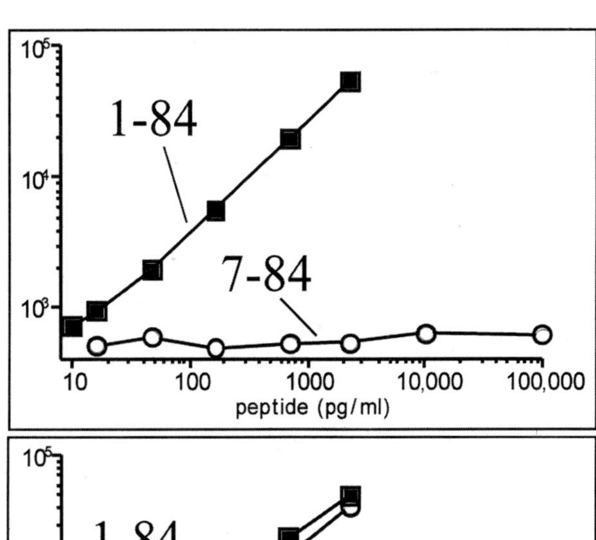

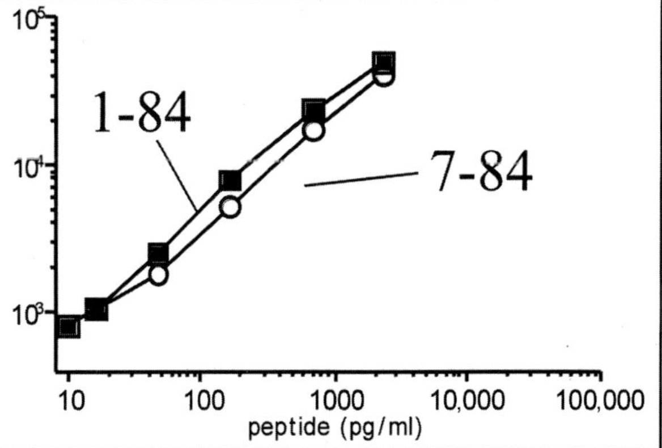

FIGURE 69.9. A: The first generation immunoradiometric assay (IRMA) uses an antibody directed against the 13-34 region of the parathyroid hormone (PTH) molecule, whereas the second generation IRMA uses an antibody against an initial epitope within the amino terminus (residues 1-3). Both assays use antibodies against epitopes within the 39-84 region of the PTH molecule. (From Salusky IB, Goodman WG, Kuizon BD, et al. Similar predictive value of bone turnover using first- and second-generation immunometric PTH assays in pediatric patients treated with peritoneal dialysis. *Kidney Int* 2003;63:1801–1808, with permission.) **B:** The first generation IRMA assay (*top*) had similar cross-reactivity for PTH(1-84) and PTH(7-84), whereas the second generation IRMA assay (*bottom*) detected only PTH(1-84) and possibly PTH fragments that are truncated at the carboxyl-terminus but not PTH(7-84) even at markedly high concentrations. (From Jon MR, Goodman WG, Gao P, et al. A novel immunoradiometric assay detects full-length human PTH but not amino-terminally truncated fragments: implications for PTH measurements in renal failure. *J Clin Endoc Metab* 1999;84:4287–4290, with permission.)

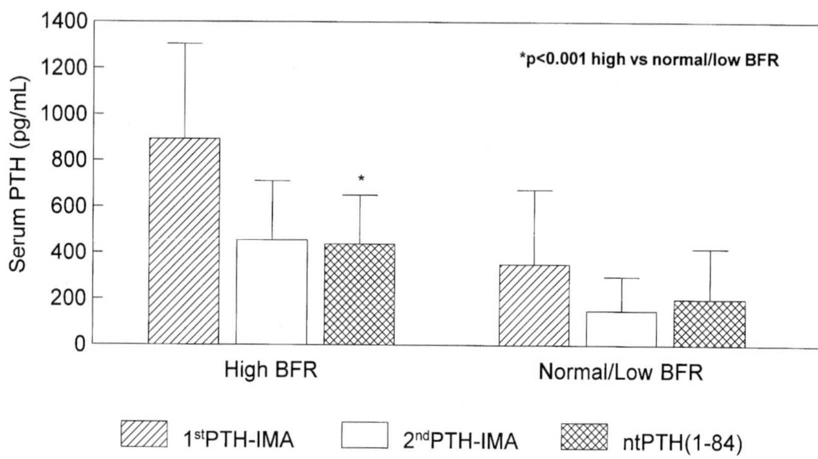

FIGURE 69.10. Serum parathyroid hormone (PTH) levels measured using the first (*hatched bars*) and second (*open bars*) generation immunometric assays (IMA) in patients with high and normal or low bone formation rates (BFR). First generation IMAs also detect additional PTH fragments truncated at the amino-terminus [ntPTH(1-84)].

PTH(1-84) and diminish bone cell activity and may, thereby, modulate bone metabolism. These actions are possibly mediated through a receptor distinct from the type I PTH/PTHrP receptor (168,173). Such findings suggest that amino-truncated PTH(1-84) fragments may contribute to the skeletal PTH resistance that occurs in patients with renal failure (168,173). It, therefore, appears plausible that an independent assessment of PTH(1-84) and amino-truncated PTH(1-84) fragments may have better value for diagnosis of the different subtypes of renal osteodystrophy than each parameter alone. Indeed, it has been suggested that estimates of the ratio between PTH(1-84) and amino-truncated PTH(1-84) fragments more accurately predicts bone remodeling and turnover in patients with ESRD (170). On the other hand, two reports in adult and pediatric patients treated with dialysis failed to confirm such findings (172,174).

Taking into consideration the crucial role of serum PTH concentrations in the diagnosis and treatment of renal osteodystrophy, 2nd PTH-IMA may provide important new insights into the physiology of parathyroid gland function. However, current findings demonstrated that measurements of PTH using either 1st or 2nd PTH-IMAs provided similar accuracy for predicting bone turnover in pediatric patients undergoing maintenance peritoneal dialysis (Fig. 69.11) (172,174). Therefore, the current recommendations for indications of therapy with active vitamin D sterols should be based on the relationship between indices of bone formation and PTH levels determined by first-generation immunometric assays. The following are the target values of PTH in patients' varying stages of CRI:

Stage 3 CRI (GFR, 30 to 59 mL/min/1.73 m^2): 6 to 65 pg/mL

Stage 4 CRI (GFR, 15 to 29 mL/min/1.73 m^2): 100 to 200 pg/mL

Stage 5 CRI (GFR, less than 15 mL/min/1.73 m^2 or dialysis): 150 to 300 pg/mL

Further studies are needed to establish the value of the new generation of PTH assays for assessing bone disease in renal failure and during therapy with vitamin D and to address

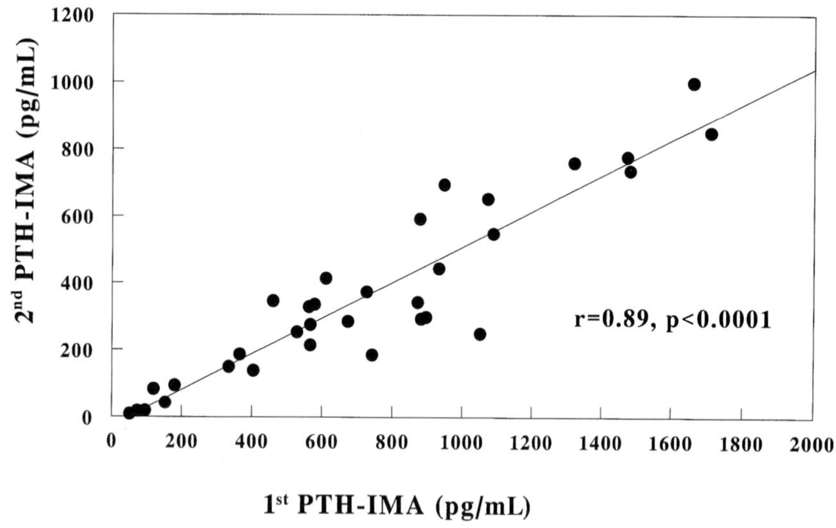

FIGURE 69.11. Relationship between parathyroid hormone (PTH) levels measured using the first generation immunometric PTH assay (1st PTH-IMA) and the second generation immunometric PTH assay (2nd PTH-IMA). (From Salusky IB, Goodman WG, Kuizon BD, et al. Similar predictive value of bone turnover using first- and second-generation immunometric PTH assays in pediatric patients treated with peritoneal dialysis. *Kidney Int* 2003;63:1801–1808, with permission.)

the need for higher PTH levels determined by either assay for preventing the development of adynamic osteodystrophy and its consequences on the growing skeleton (175).

Aluminum

Plasma aluminum levels are useful in the monitoring of patients who are undergoing chronic dialysis therapy and receiving aluminum-containing phosphate-binding agents for prolonged periods. Plasma aluminum values measured using electrothermal atomic absorption spectrometry are often accurate and reproducible. Although plasma aluminum levels reflect more recent exposure, the levels do not reflect aluminum deposits accurately. The presence of aluminum deposits in the bone and liver do not correlate with the plasma levels (176). Aluminum toxicity occurs in dialysis patients or CRI patients with GFR less than 30 mL/min/1.73 m^2 because aluminum that is absorbed from the gut or enters the body from the dialysate or other parenteral route is not excreted or is inadequately excreted by the diseased kidney. The accumulation occurs in various tissues, including bone, brain, parathyroid glands, and other organs. Such accumulation can produce toxicity with several distinct syndromes depending on the rate and magnitude of the aluminum loading. The first to be described was dialysis encephalopathy, as well as fracturing dialysis osteomalacia and microcytic anemia.

A deferoxamine (DFO) test should be performed if the plasma aluminum levels are between 60 and 200 µg/L or if clinical signs and symptoms of aluminum toxicity are present or before parathyroid surgery if the patient has had aluminum exposure. The DFO infusion test is performed by infusing 5 mg/kg of DFO during the last hour of the dialysis session. Serum aluminum should be measured before DFO infusion and, 2 days later, before the next dialysis session (177). The test is considered positive if the increment of serum aluminum is greater than 50 µg/L. The presence of aluminum bone disease can be predicted by a rise in serum aluminum of 50 µg/L, combined with a plasma PTH (1st PTH-IMA) of less than 150 pg/mL. However, the gold standard for the diagnosis of aluminum bone disease is a bone biopsy showing increased aluminum staining of the bone surface (greater than 15 to 25%) and histologic evidence of adynamic bone or osteomalacia. A DFO test should not be performed if the serum levels of aluminum are more than 200 µg/L to avoid DFO-induced neurotoxicity.

Radiographic Features

The primary radiographic feature of children with secondary hyperparathyroidism is evidence of increased bone resorption, which is usually located in the subperiosteal or endosteal surfaces of cortical bone within cortical regions. The extent of bone resorption correlates with serum PTH levels (162,178). Subperiosteal resorption may occur at the distal ends of the clavicles, ischial and pubis surfaces, sacroiliac joints, junction of the metaphysis and diaphysis of long bone, and in the phalanges (Fig. 69.12) (179,180). A diffuse ground-glass appearance, generalized mottling, focal radiolucencies, and sclerotic areas may be evident in the skull (181). Metaphyseal changes, called *growth zone lesions* or *rickets-like lesions*, are best demonstrated in hand radiographs (182). Although subperiosteal erosions are a hallmark of secondary hyperparathyroidism, these lesions can also be seen in patients with aluminum-related bone disease, which may represent unhealed lesions from a previous state of secondary hyperparathyroidism (183). To enhance the sensitivity of hand radiographs, the use of fine-grain films and magnification by hand lens has been recommended (180).

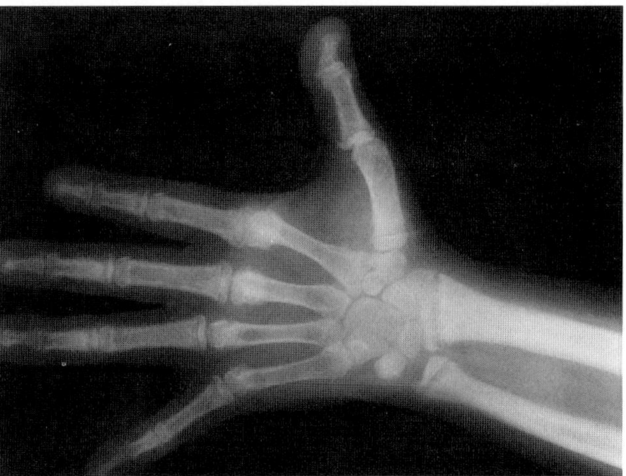

FIGURE 69.12. Subperiosteal erosions of the midphalanges in a patient with severe secondary hyperparathyroidism.

The radiographic features of osteomalacia are less evident, particularly in older children and adolescents. In young children, widening of the epiphyseal growth plate and other deformities of the growth plate cartilage are evident, whereas pseudofractures and looser zones, which appear as straight, wide radiolucent bands within the cortex, may be the only findings in older children and adults. The radiographic density of bone on conventional skeletal radiographs is reduced in many patients with renal osteodystrophy, but osteosclerotic changes or localized increases in bone density are a prominent finding in children with chronic renal failure.

Bone Scintigraphy

Bone scans using the technetium-99–labeled diphosphonate are helpful in estimating the severity of bone disease and differentiating between high-turnover lesions of osteitis fibrosa and low-turnover lesions of osteomalacia (184). Uptake is usually diffuse and symmetric in patients with severe secondary hyperparathyroidism, whereas patients with osteomalacia exhibit a more diffuse and less intense uptake (184). Extraskeletal calcifications may also be demonstrated using the bone scan in various organ systems, such as the lungs and heart (185).

Bone Biopsy

Iliac crest bone biopsy provides valuable diagnostic information in children with renal osteodystrophy (186). The procedure is safe and well tolerated in children and is done in an outpatient setting (78). Bone biopsy provides information about the histologic appearance and dynamics of bone formation and mineralization. For bone labeling, tetracycline is administered at 15 mg/kg/day in two to three doses for 2 days, 14 days apart. For children younger than 8 years, tetracycline dosage is usually kept below 10 mg/kg/day to avoid toxicity. Histochemical staining procedures demonstrate the deposition of abnormal components within bone such as iron, aluminum, and oxalate (78,187). Indications for bone biopsy include investigation of persistent hypercalcemia before parathyroidectomy with and without vitamin D therapy, unexplained hypercalcemia associated with PTH levels between 200 and 500 pg/mL, assessment of skeletal response to certain therapeutic modalities, and diagnosis of aluminum bone disease.

Osteitis fibrosa is one of the most common histologic lesions in children with chronic renal failure (78,186). Histologically, large numbers of osteoclasts are present, with a proportional increase in bone resorption (Table 69.2). Fibrous tissue often accumulates within the bony trabeculae, and, in severe cases, fibrous tissue deposition occurs in the marrow space (Fig. 69.13). The development of severe osteitis fibrosa may worsen the anemia of CRI by displacing erythroid precursors from the marrow space.

In uncomplicated osteitis fibrosa, bone formation rates are elevated to approximately two to three times normal (78,186); this is coupled with a marked increase in osteoblastic number and activity (188). Peritrabecular fibrosis is absent in mild lesions of secondary hyperparathyroidism. Nevertheless, activity of both osteoclasts and osteoblasts is increased, and the rate of bone formation is greater than normal (78,186). Tetracycline-based measurements of bone formation are valuable in differentiating this less severe lesion of secondary hyperparathyroidism from the low-turnover disorders (78,186).

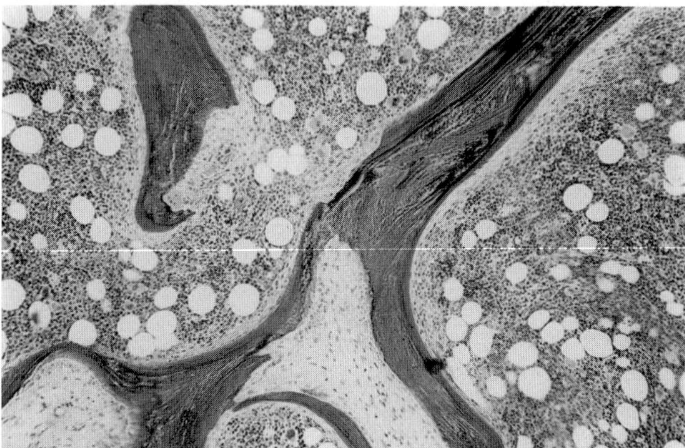

FIGURE 69.13. Histologic lesion of osteitis fibrosa characterized by increased resorptive surface on mineralized bone by osteoclasts and fibrosis.

Osteomalacia is the most striking histologic feature of low-turnover bone disease. Excess osteoid or unmineralized bone collagen accumulates because of a defect in skeletal mineralization (189). Osteoid seams are thickened, with a multilaminated or lamellar appearance. Osteoblastic activity is usually reduced, and the rate of bone formation often cannot be measured because of absence of tetracycline uptake into bone. In patients with suspected aluminum-related bone disease, histochemical staining provides useful information. In these cases, the severity of histochemical changes of osteomalacia corresponds with the amount of surface-stainable aluminum in the cancellous bone (190).

Adynamic or aplastic bone is characterized by the presence of normal to reduced osteoid formation, absence of fibrosis, and diminished numbers of osteoblasts and osteoclasts; bone formation rate is characteristically absent to subnormal (78,186,191) (Table 69.3). The absence of osteoid accumulation differentiates it from osteomalacia (Fig.

TABLE 69.2. HIGH-TURNOVER LESIONS OF RENAL OSTEODYSTROPHY

	Mild lesion	Osteitis fibrosa
Bone formation		
Osteoblast number	High	Very high
Osteoid volume	Normal-high	Normal-high
Osteoid seam width	Normal	Normal-high
Bone formation rate	High	Very high
Bone resorption		
Osteoclast number	High	Very high
Resorption perimeter	High	Very high
Fibrosis	Absent	Present

TABLE 69.3. LOW-TURNOVER LESIONS OF RENAL OSTEODYSTROPHY

	Adynamic	Osteomalacia
Bone formation		
Osteoblast number	Low	Low
Osteoid volume	Normal-low	High
Osteoid seam width	Normal-low	High
Bone formation rate	Low	Low
Bone resorption		
Osteoclast number	Low	Normal-low
Resorption perimeter	Low	Low-normal
Fibrosis	Absent	Absent

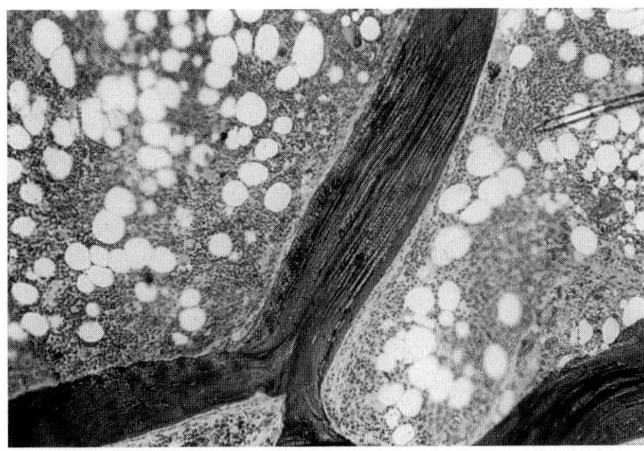

FIGURE 69.14. Histologic lesion of adynamic bone characterized by diminished amount of osteoid formation, osteoblasts and osteoclasts, and markedly reduced tetracycline uptake.

69.14). In the past decade, aluminum deposits in the bone were evident in patients with adynamic bone; however, currently, an increasing proportion of patients have been reported to have adynamic bone lesions without aluminum deposition (78,192).

Occasionally, patients may exhibit mixed lesion of renal osteodystrophy, which is characterized by histologic changes of both osteitis fibrosa and osteomalacia (159). These patients often have high serum PTH levels and histologic manifestations of impaired bone formation and mineralization. Mixed lesions are seen with high-turnover bone disease in patients who are developing aluminum toxicity or in patients with low-turnover aluminum-related bone disease during DFO therapy (193). In these cases, mixed lesion represents a transitional stage between high-turnover and low-turnover bone disease.

TREATMENT

Particular attention must be made to the bone and mineral metabolism of children with CRI to minimize complications in the growing skeleton and to prevent extraskeletal, particularly, vascular calcifications.

Dietary Manipulation

Evaluation of dietary intake and growth must be performed at regular intervals to maximize the growth potential of children with CRI. Nutritional requirements are based on the recommended dietary allowances for energy and protein. Nutritional supplements, which may be given orally or through a nasogastric or gastrostomy tube, are recommended when recommended dietary allowances for energy and protein are not achieved by dietary intake alone or when there is impaired linear growth and/or weight gain.

The dietary reference intake (DRI) for phosphorus for the different age groups is based on the report from the Food and Nutrition Board (Table 69.4) (194). Based on this report, the average phosphorus intake of children in the United States is higher than the DRI and is approximately 1500 to 2000 mg/day, of which 60 to 70% is absorbed. Phosphorus is present in nearly all foods and its highest concentration is in meat and dairy products. Dietary phosphorus intake is frequently restricted to 600 to 1200 mg/day when serum phosphorus levels exceed age-appropriate normal levels and to keep the calcium phosphorus product less than 55 mg^2/mL^2 (177). Similar restrictions are recommended for patients with serum PTH levels that are higher than the target range according to the stage of CRI. In dialysis patients, phosphorus removal by peritoneal dialysis (240 to 440 mg/day) or hemodialysis (600 mg during a 4-hour session) is inadequate to maintain target phosphorus levels (195,196); therefore, dietary phosphorus restriction is usually required. More frequent hemodialysis, however, such as nocturnal hemodialysis, which is performed 6 to 7 nights per week for 8 to 10 hours during sleep at home, has been shown to remove twice as much phosphate per week than conventional hemodialysis (197). As such, adult patients undergoing nocturnal hemodialysis do not require phosphate binders, are able to ingest higher dietary phosphate and protein intake, and some require phosphorus supplementation in the dialysate (197,198). However, this dialytic modality has not been performed in pediatric dialysis patients.

TABLE 69.4. DIETARY REFERENCE INTAKE FOR PHOSPHORUS

Age (yr)	Dietary reference intake (mg/d)	Tolerable upper intake (mg/d)
0–0.5	100	Not determined
0.6–1.0	275	Not determined
1–3	460	3000
4–8	500	3000
9–18	1250	4000

Although dietary phosphorus restriction is recommended in the majority of patients with more advanced CRI, long-term compliance to such restrictions is difficult because of protein requirements for growth and the unpalatability of low phosphate diets. Accordingly, the use of phosphate-binding agents becomes an integral component of the treatment of these children. Serum phosphorus levels should be measured at least every 3 months after starting the phosphorus-restricted diet to prevent hypophosphatemia, particularly in those who are also given large doses of phosphate-binding agents. Infants are particularly at risk for hypophosphatemia because of the use of low phosphorus-containing formulas, aggressive use of phosphate binders, increased phosphate removal by peritoneal dialysis probably due to higher surface area, and possibly nutritional repletion (199). Patients with severe and persistent hypophosphatemia have been reported to develop

TABLE 69.5. DIETARY REFERENCE INTAKE FOR CALCIUM

Age (yr)	Dietary reference intake (mg/d)	Tolerable upper intake (mg/d)
0–0.5	210	420
0.6–1.0	270	520
1–3	500	1000
4–8	800	1600
9–18	1300	2500

bone disease such as osteomalacia and rickets, proximal myopathy, rhabdomyolysis, and congestive heart failure (199,200). The use of calcitriol may also complicate the management of hyperphosphatemia because it enhances intestinal phosphorus absorption; in these cases, higher dosages of phosphate binding agents are required (201).

The DRI for calcium for the different age groups is shown in Table 69.5 (194). Calcium intake to meet the DRI and regular exercise are strongly recommended throughout childhood and adolescence to increase peak bone mass, and thereby reduce fracture rates and prevent osteoporosis later in life. In patients with CRI stages 1 to 4, the recommended calcium intake is based on the DRI for age (177). The main source of calcium is milk and dairy products, although various foods such orange juice and cereals are fortified with calcium. Calcium supplementation is recommended when the DRI is not met by dietary intake. In patients with CRI stage 5 or those undergoing dialysis, calcium intake from both diet and calcium containing phosphate binders should be limited to no more than 2500 mg/day (Table 69.5) (177).

Phosphate-Binding Agents

Phosphate-binding agents are recommended in patients with hyperphosphatemia despite dietary phosphorus restriction. They form poorly soluble complexes with phosphorus in the intestinal tract, thereby decreasing phosphorus absorption. Calcium-containing phosphate binders are widely used as the initial agent for the management of hyperphosphatemia. They also provide an additional source of calcium. Several calcium-containing salts, such as calcium carbonate, calcium acetate, and calcium citrate are commercially available. Schaefer et al. found similar effectiveness in controlling serum phosphorus levels using calcium carbonate or calcium acetate, but calcium acetate has been shown to bind twice more phosphorus using equivalent doses in adult studies (202). Calcium citrate is not recommended in patients with CRI who are also receiving aluminum-containing phosphate binders, because citrate increases intestinal aluminum absorption (203).

Overall, calcium carbonate is the calcium salt that is largely prescribed, and its effectiveness in reducing serum phosphorus levels has been reported in adult and pediatric patients (152,204). In addition, calcium carbonate therapy alone decreased serum intact PTH levels in adult patients with secondary hyperparathyroidism (205,206). The dose of calcium-based phosphate binders varies widely among children and should be adjusted to maintain normal calcium levels and age-appropriate serum phosphorus levels. Calcium salts should be given immediately after meals if they are used as phosphate binders and they should be given between meals if used for hypocalcemia. Hypercalcemia is a major complication associated with the long-term use of high doses of calcium-based phosphate-binding agents, particularly in patients treated with vitamin D or those with adynamic bone lesion (207,208). Hypercalcemia usually resolves with lowering the dose of vitamin D and calcium-based binders. Vitamin D should be given at bedtime in patients treated with calcium-based binders to decrease intestinal calcium absorption. In patients with CRI stage 5 or those undergoing dialysis, calcium intake from both diet and calcium-containing phosphate binders should be limited to no more than 2500 mg/day (177).

Over the last few years, the use of calcium-containing binders has been linked with the development of vascular calcifications in adult and pediatric patients treated with maintenance dialysis (135). Furthermore, there is substantial evidence that abnormalities in mineral metabolism, hypercalcemia, hyperphosphatemia, and elevated calcium-phosphorus ion product are associated with the development of soft tissue and vascular calcifications (128,135,137,209). Thus, intake of calcium from calcium-containing phosphate binders as well as the use of active vitamin D sterols have been implicated in the process of vascular calcifications, and they may play a role in the development of accelerated cardiovascular disease that occurs in adult patients treated with dialysis (128,135). Although the mortality rate is low in children with ESRD, current evidence indicates that vascular calcifications are present in young adults treated with dialysis or renal transplantation with childhood-onset renal disease (135–137). Thus, in dialysis patients, it is recommended that the amount of elemental calcium from these compounds and from diet should not exceed 2500 mg/day (177).

Alternative phosphate binders have thus been developed because of the risks of hypercalcemia and vascular calcification associated with the use of calcium salts and because of toxicity from long-term ingestion of aluminum-containing phosphate binders. Sevelamer hydrochloride (Renagel), a calcium- and aluminum-free hydrogel of cross-linked poly(allylamine-hydrochloride), has been reported to lower serum phosphorus, calcium-phosphorus ion product, and intact PTH without inducing hypercalcemia in adult and pediatric patients with ESRD (210–213). Serum total cholesterol and low-density lipoprotein cholesterol levels also decreased, whereas high-density lipoprotein increased during sevelamer treatment (212), and these effects may offer additional benefits in reducing cardiovascular complications in patients with ESRD. More importantly, the process of vascular calcification was halted during treatment with sevelamer hydrochloride when compared to calcium-containing binders in adult patients treated with hemodialysis (214). Sevelamer may be used as the primary agent, particularly in patients who are prone to develop hypercalcemia and in those requiring large doses of vitamin D, but further studies are warranted to evaluate the long-term effects of this new therapy on bone disease in children with renal failure.

Additional phosphate binders include magnesium, iron, and lanthanum compounds. Magnesium carbonate reduces serum phosphorus levels, but, because of the risk of developing hypermagnesemia in patients treated with dialysis, a dialysate with lower magnesium content is recommended (215). Diarrhea can also develop if large doses of magnesium carbonate are used, therefore limiting its use as a single agent. Iron compounds, such as stabilized polynuclear iron hydroxide and ferric polymaltose complex, are novel phosphate binders that are effective in short-term studies in adults with CRI (216,217). Another new agent, lanthanum chloride hydrate, decreased intestinal phosphate absorption in experimental studies and in a clinical trial (218,219). Because it is a heavy metal, however, studies to address its potential for long-term complications should be considered.

Aluminum-containing gels are effective phosphate-binding agents that were primarily used before the 1980s. The development of bone disease, encephalopathy, and bone disease associated with long-term administration, however, led to the restriction of its use to patients with hypercalcemia or increased calcium phosphorus product, because both conditions worsen with calcium salts. Plasma aluminum levels in children correlate well with the quantity of aluminum-containing phosphate-binding agents (220). Thus, guidelines for maximum safe dosages of aluminum hydroxide have been proposed: 30 mg/kg/day for children and 2000 to 3000 mg/day for adults (80,221). Despite the recommended dosages, aluminum accumulation still occurs, as seen by a rise in plasma aluminum level after DFO infusion and by histologic evidence of aluminum deposits in the bone (222). The lowest possible dose must be used for a limited period of approximately 4 to 6 weeks, and plasma aluminum levels should be followed closely. The simultaneous use of aluminum-containing agents and citrate must be avoided to prevent toxic accumulation of aluminum, because citrate enhances aluminum absorption by altering tight junctions in the intestinal epithelium (203). Citrate-containing medications that are usually used in patients with CRI include calcium citrate, Alka-Seltzer, Shohl's solution, sodium citrate (Bicitra/Polycitra), and even citrus fruits.

Vitamin D Therapy

One of the goals in the management of secondary hyperparathyroidism with vitamin D is to inhibit PTH release through its direct effects on pre-pro-PTH gene transcription and the VDR or indirectly through hypocalcemia. In pediatric patients with CRI, additional benefit was reported on promoting linear growth during treatment with daily doses of calcitriol (92,93). Several vitamin D sterols are currently available, and clinical trials have demonstrated their efficacy in lowering PTH levels. In the United States, calcitriol is frequently prescribed, whereas 1α-hydroxyvitamin D is commonly administered in Europe and Japan.

In patients with CRI stage 3 (GFR, 30 to 59 mL/min/1.73 m^2), vitamin D therapy is indicated when PTH levels measured by 1st PTH-IMA are above 65 pg/mL; in those with stage 4 CRI (GFR, 15 to 29 mL/min/1.73 m^2), when values are above 100 pg/mL; and in patients undergoing dialysis (stage 5 CRI), therapy is indicated when PTH levels exceed 300 pg/mL (177). Before starting treatment with vitamin D, however, it is important to ensure that serum phosphorus levels are within the normal range for age. Calcitriol or alfacalcidol may be started at a daily dose of 0.25 to 0.5 μg, and the dose is gradually titrated in 0.25- to 0.5-μg increments to achieve 1st PTH-IMA levels within the normal range. Dosage regimens have generally ranged from 0.25 to 1.0 μg/day. Serum levels of calcium, phosphorus, and 1st PTH-IMA should be monitored monthly for the first 3 months after start of vitamin D therapy. Hypercalcemia is the most common side effect, but it is often reversible by withholding or reducing the dose. Although initial studies have demonstrated a more rapid deterioration in renal function during vitamin D therapy, subsequent studies have shown no adverse effects on progression of renal failure (223–225).

In patients with CRI stage 5 or those requiring regular dialysis, vitamin D therapy is recommended when 1st PTH-IMA levels exceed 300 pg/mL despite maintaining serum phosphorus within age-appropriate levels (177). Daily calcitriol or alfacalcidol therapy may be initiated at a dose of 0.25 to 0.5 μg, and the dose is gradually increased in 0.25- to 0.5-μg increments to achieve first PTH-IMA levels between 150 and 300 pg/mL. Intermittent doses may be considered when serum PTH levels are greater than 500 to 600 pg/mL. The initial dose is 0.5 to 1.0 μg three times per week administered by the oral or intravenous route. The intraperitoneal route of calcitriol administration is currently not approved by the U.S. Food and Drug Administration. The use of a dialysate calcium concentration of 2.5 μg/L is recommended for patients treated with either hemodialysis or peritoneal dialysis. Decreasing the dialysate calcium concentration may allow higher doses of calcitriol to be given. Long-term treatment with high pulse doses of calcitriol should be undertaken with caution in prepubertal children with secondary hyperparathyroidism. Suppressing PTH levels below 200 pg/mL should be avoided because of the risk for growth retardation in those who develop adynamic renal osteodystrophy (103). Findings by Schmitt et al. in 2003 in children with CRI before dialysis support this initial observation (104). Additional studies are needed to define the optimal PTH levels during calcitriol treatment that would support normal rates of bone formation and linear growth in pediatric patients with renal osteodystrophy.

Control of secondary hyperparathyroidism should be considered before initiation of rhGH in children with CRI. It is recommended that serum phosphorus levels are less than 1.5 times the upper limit for age and 1st PTH-IMA levels less than 1.5 times the upper target values for the CRI stage before starting rhGH (177). It is expected that therapy with rhGH will increase serum PTH levels during the initial first months of therapy; therefore, monthly PTH should be monitored more frequently during that period. Therapy with rhGH should be temporarily discontinued if PTH levels exceed three times the upper target value for the CRI stage despite at least 3 months of vitamin D therapy and restarted once values are below 1.5 times the upper target value for the CRI stage (177). In addition, it is important to maximize the control of serum phosphorus levels.

New vitamin D compounds that retain the suppressive effects on PTH but induce less hypercalcemia and hyperphosphatemia are being evaluated. However, studies that compare the biochemical and histologic responses of these new compounds with standard therapy (calcitriol or alfacalcidol) are not yet available. 22-Oxacalcitriol inhibits PTH mRNA expression *in vitro* and *in vivo*, and it prevents the reduction in VDR in the parathyroid glands of rats with renal failure (226). Short-term treatment with OCT lowered serum PTH levels and bone formation rates without inducing hypercalcemia in experimental animals with either normal or reduced renal function (227). Long-term administration, however, resulted in hypercalcemia and hyperphosphatemia in uremic dogs (228). Moreover, although OCT diminished abnormal woven osteoid, lamellar osteoid, and fibrosis, it did not decrease bone formation rates on repeat biopsy (228). In early clinical trials, OCT controlled secondary hyperparathyroidism, but hypercalcemia prevented further increases in dose for one-half of the subjects (229,230). Although controlled studies are needed, preliminary findings involving a small number of patients do not support an advantage of OCT over calcitriol.

Another new vitamin analog is 1α(OH)-vitamin D_2 (1αD_2, doxercalciferol), which is equipotent to 1, α(OH)-vitamin D_3 in intestinal calcium absorption and bone calcium mobilization in vitamin D–deficient rats, but it requires larger doses than 1αD_3 to induce hypercalcemia and toxicity in normal rodents (231). Initial clinical trials demonstrated suppression of PTH levels during treatment with daily or intermittent oral doses of 1αD_2 (starting dose 4 μg/day or 4 μg thrice weekly) in 24 adult hemodialysis patients with moderate to severe secondary hyperparathyroidism. Serum calcium levels increased moderately, from 8.8 ± 0.18 to 9.5 ± 0.21 (p <.001), and treatment had to be stopped only once for hypercalcemia (232). In a subsequent multicenter trial involving 80 adults undergoing hemodialysis, treatment with larger intermittent oral doses of 1αD_2 (10 μg thrice weekly) effectively decreased serum PTH levels with minimal hypercalcemia and hyperphosphatemia (233). While these results are encouraging, studies that compare this compound to either calcitriol or 1αD_3 are needed. Doxercalciferol has recently been approved for treatment of secondary hyperparathyroidism in the United States.

Another vitamin D analog, 19-nor-1α,25$(OH)_2D_2$ (paricalcitol), was initially reported to reduce PTH secretion without changing the concentrations of plasma ionized calcium or plasma phosphorus in rats with renal failure (234). In addition, parathyroidectomized rats fed either a low-calcium or a low-phosphate diet had less increments in plasma calcium or phosphorus levels during treatment with paricalcitol than with similar doses of calcitriol (235). Results of double-blind, placebo-controlled, randomized clinical trials demonstrate the efficacy of paricalcitol in suppressing PTH, and these were associated with increases in final mean serum calcium levels compared to baseline values, although levels were still within normal range (236,237). In a comparative study of intravenous paricalcitol versus calcitriol, paricalcitol reduced PTH levels more rapidly with fewer episodes of hyperphosphatemia, but with no differences in serum calcium levels between the groups (238). Similarly, comparison studies against standard treatment regimens and trials using this agent in pediatric patients have yet to be done.

CALCIMIMETIC COMPOUNDS

Calcimimetic compounds are allosteric activators of the CaR in the parathyroid gland, kidney, and other tissues. They lower the set point for activation of the CaR by calcium, thereby decreasing PTH secretion from parathyroid cells. Thus, they offer a novel approach for the treatment of secondary hyperparathyroidism in patients with CRI, because they inhibit PTH secretion without resulting in hypercalcemia and/or hyperphosphatemia. First-generation calcimimetic compounds, which are based on a phenylalkylamine structure as typified by R-568, have been reported to reduce PTH secretion and parathyroid gland proliferation and ameliorate histologic evidence of osteitis fibrosa in animal models of secondary hyperparathyroidism (239–241). Inhibition of PTH release has likewise been shown after a single dose of NPSR-568 in patients with primary hyperparathyroidism and after two consecutive daily doses of the drug in adult dialysis patients with mild secondary hyperparathyroidism (242,243). In a subsequent study, administration of R-568 for 15 days lowered serum PTH levels in adult dialysis patients with moderate to severe secondary hyperparathyroidism (70).

Second-generation calcimimetic agents, such as AMG 073, were developed because of the low bioavailability of the first-generation compounds. In an 18-week double-blind, randomized, placebo-controlled, dose titration study, AMG 073 decreased PTH levels in adult hemodialysis patients with secondary hyperparathyroidism (69,244). PTH levels declined by 26%, and calcium phosphorus product decreased by 12% in AMG 073–treated patients compared to the placebo group. There were no major side effects noted. Thus, these short-term trials have consistently shown the efficacy of calcimimetic agents in suppressing PTH secretion in patients with primary hyperparathyroidism and in those with varying degrees of secondary hyperparathyroidism due to CRI. Calcimimetic agents may be advantageous for patients who are refractory to calcitriol or in whom calcitriol treatment is limited by hypercalcemia and/or hyperphosphatemia. Although these studies have all been conducted in adult patients, there is concern for its use in pediatric patients because the CaR expression has also been localized to chondrocytes in the growth plate cartilage (245).

PARATHYROIDECTOMY

Parathyroid gland hyperplasia, which is characterized by serum PTH elevations and osteitis fibrosa on bone biopsy, is a result of poorly controlled secondary hyperparathyroidism. Calcitriol resistance may develop in the presence of an enlarged nodular hyperplastic parathyroid gland because of the decrease in the number of VDRs and the presence of monoclonal proliferation in the nodular areas (35,246). When vitamin D therapy fails to correct the signs of secondary hyperparathyroidism, parathyroidectomy must be considered. Urgent indications for parathyroidectomy include persistent or recurrent hypercalcemia (particularly when associated with intractable pruritus not responding to intensive dialysis), progressive extraskeletal calcifications, bone pain, multiple and recurrent fractures, and the appearance of calciphylaxis (128).

Before the 1980s, the development of hypercalcemia in patients receiving little or no vitamin D suggested that aluminum-related bone disease may have been present. Currently, hypercalcemia is more commonly due to administration of high doses of vitamin D and calcium-containing compounds. A substantial proportion of patients develop adynamic/aplastic bone lesions not related to aluminum deposition. Parathyroidectomy may be indicated for persistent hypercalcemia in patients with PTH levels of 200 to 500 pg/mL (247).

Hypocalcemia may develop after parathyroidectomy in patients with severe secondary hyperparathyroidism. This condition, called *hungry bone syndrome*, is caused by a high rate of skeletal calcium uptake, which may continue for some time after serum PTH levels are lowered by parathyroidectomy. Serum calcium decreases 24 to 36 hours after surgery; daily doses of calcitriol at 0.5 to 1.0 μg/day for 2 to 6 days before surgery can be administered to prevent hypocalcemic episodes. Once the serum calcium declines below 8.5 mg/dL, calcium gluconate infusion should be started to provide 100 to 150 mg of elemental calcium per hour for the first 4 to 6 hours and infusion rate adjusted according to serum calcium measurements. Hypophosphatemia may develop concurrently, but supplemental phosphorus is not given because it may aggravate hypocalcemia unless the serum level is below 2.0 mg/dL. Ideally, serum phosphorus levels should be maintained between 3.5 and 4.5 mg/dL to avoid further reductions in serum calcium levels.

BONE DISEASE AFTER SUCCESSFUL KIDNEY TRANSPLANTATION

Successful kidney transplantation corrects many of the metabolic abnormalities associated with the development of renal osteodystrophy, but despite a well-functioning graft, osteopenia, growth failure, spontaneous fractures, and avascular necrosis remain prevalent in adult and pediatric kidney recipients (248–254). Significant bone loss has been described by several investigators to occur as early as 3 to 6 months after kidney transplantation (253,254). Several factors have been implicated in the development of bone disease after transplantation; these include persistent secondary hyperparathyroidism, prolonged immobilization, and, most important, use of immunosuppressive agents, which are required to maintain graft function.

Bone loss has been attributed largely to prolonged and often high-dose corticosteroid use. Corticosteroids have been demonstrated to directly and indirectly affect skeletal metabolism by decreasing intestinal calcium absorption, enhancing urinary calcium excretion, inhibiting osteoblastic activity, decreasing bone formation, and significantly increasing osteoclastic activity and bone resorption (255–258). Likewise, cyclosporine has been reported to increase both bone formation and bone resorption and reduce cancellous bone volume in the rat (259,260); similar findings have been described in adult renal transplant recipients (261). In contrast, Bryer et al. demonstrated in rat studies that azathioprine does not have a significant impact on skeletal remodeling (262). The role of other immunosuppressive agents, such as mycophenolate mofetil, as potential modifiers of bone formation and bone resorption has not been evaluated.

After successful kidney transplantation, growth may be accelerated by an improvement in kidney function, but several investigators have shown that catch-up growth may not be observed even in children who undergo transplantation very early in life (263). Moreover, height deceleration occurs in approximately 75% of patients who undergo transplantation before the age of 15 years (264). The use of alternate-day steroids and a better SDS for height at the time of transplant may serve as better predictors of the final height attained (263–265); rhGH has been used in children with significant height deficit after kidney transplantation. A substantial increase in linear growth has been reported within the first year of rhGH therapy, but the magnitude of growth response may decline thereafter (266).

In the adult kidney recipients, Julian et al. reported that histologic changes associated with secondary hyperparathyroidism resolved 6 months after kidney transplantation (254). However, an imbalance of bone remodeling still occurred, because the mineral apposition rate was markedly reduced, and these changes were accompanied by substantial reductions in bone mass as determined by dual-energy x-ray absorptiometry (254). Moreover, Velasquez-Forero et al. described findings of adynamic bone lesion in 12 of 16 adult kidney recipients 7 years after kidney transplantation despite moderately elevated serum PTH levels (267). A recent report describes the spectrum of bone disease in 47 pediatric kidney recipients with stable graft function: 67% had histologic features of normal bone formation, 10% had adynamic bone lesion, and 23% had bone lesions characteristic of secondary hyperparathyroidism (268). Although there was restoration of normal bone formation in the majority of patients, a number of these patients exhibited increases in osteoid perimeter and eroded bone perimeter when compared with reference values obtained from children and adolescents with normal renal function. These findings may reflect a component of persistent secondary hyperparathyroidism because serum PTH levels remained elevated in some patients, or perhaps they were related to cyclosporine therapy (268). The factors responsible for the persistent increase in osteoid formation and resorption surface despite normalization of kidney function and the role of multiple immunosuppressive agents required to maintain the allograft remain to be determined.

REFERENCES

1. Malluche HH, Ritz E, Lange HP, et al. Bone histology in incipient and advanced renal failure. *Kidney Int* 1976;9:355–362.
2. Hamdy NA, Kanis JA, Beneton MNC, et al. Effect of alfacalcidol on natural course of renal bone disease in mild to moderate renal failure. *BMJ* 1995;310:358–363.
3. Norman ME, Mazur AT, Borden S, et al. Early diagnosis of juvenile renal osteodystrophy. *J Pediatr* 1980;97:226–232.
4. Goldman R, Bassett SH. Phosphorus excretion in renal failure. *J Clin Invest* 1954;33:1623–1628.
5. Coburn JW, Popovtzer M, Massry SG, et al. The physiochemical state and renal handling of divalent ions in chronic renal failure. *Arch Intern Med* 1969;124:302–311.
6. Rutherford WE, Bordier P, Marie P, et al. Phosphate control and 25-hydroxycholecalciferol administration in preventing experimental renal osteodystrophy in the dog. *J Clin Invest* 1977;60:332–334.
7. Slatopolsky E, Caglar S, Gradowska L, et al. On the prevention of secondary hyperparathyroidism in experimental chronic renal disease using "proportional reduction" of dietary phosphorus intake. *Kidney Int* 1972;2:147–151.
8. Naveh-Many T, Rahamimov R, Livni N, et al. Parathyroid cell proliferation in normal and chronic renal failure rats. The effects of calcium, phosphate, and vitamin D. *J Clin Invest* 1995;96:1786–1793.
9. Lopez-Hilker S, Dusso A, Rapp N, et al. Phosphorus restriction reverses hyperparathyroidism in uremia independent of changes in calcium and calcitriol. *Am J Physiol* 1990;259:F432–F437.
10. Portale AA, Booth BE, Halloran BP, et al. Effect of dietary phosphorus on circulating concentrations of 1,25-dihydroxyvitamin D and immunoreactive parathyroid hormone in children with moderate renal insufficiency. *J Clin Invest* 1984;73:1580–1589.
11. Slatopolsky E, Finch J, Denda M, et al. Phosphorus restriction prevents parathyroid gland growth. High phosphorus directly stimulates PTH secretion *in vitro*. *J Clin Invest* 1996;97:2534–2540.
12. Denda M, Finch J, Slatopolsky E. Phosphorus accelerates the development of parathyroid hyperplasia and secondary hyperparathyroidism in rats with renal failure. *Am J Kidney Dis* 1996;28:596–602.
13. Takahashi F, Denda M, Finch JL, et al. Hyperplasia of the parathyroid gland without secondary hyperparathyroidism. *Kidney Int* 2002;61:1332–1338.
14. Tatsumi S, Segawa H, Morita K, et al. Molecular cloning and hormonal regulation of PiT-1, a sodium-dependent phosphate cotransporter from rat parathyroid glands. *Endocrinology* 1998;139:1692–1699.
15. Yi H, Fukagawa M, Yamato H, et al. Prevention of enhanced parathyroid hormone secretion, synthesis and hyperplasia by mild dietary phosphorus restriction in early chronic renal failure in rats: possible direct role of phosphorus. *Nephron* 1995;70:242–248.
16. Dusso AS, Pavlopoulos T, Naumovich L, et al. p21(WAF1) and transforming growth factor-alpha mediate dietary phosphate regulation of parathyroid cell growth. *Kidney Int* 2001;59:855–865.
17. Fraser DR, Kodicek E. Unique biosynthesis by kidney of a biologically active vitamin D metabolite. *Nature* 1970;228:764.
18. Gray R, Boyle I, DeLuca HF. Vitamin D metabolism: The role of kidney tissue. *Science* 1971;172:1232–1234.
19. Shinki T, Shimada H, Wakino S, et al. Cloning and expression of rat 25-hydroxyvitamin D3-1alpha-hydroxylase cDNA. *Proc Natl Acad Sci U S A* 1997;94:12920–12925.
20. Kitanaka S, Takeyama K, Murayama A, et al. Inactivating mutations in the 25-hydroxyvitamin D3 1alpha-hydroxylase gene in patients with pseudovitamin D-deficiency rickets. *N Engl J Med* 1998;338:653–661.
21. Yoshida T, Monkawa T, Tenenhouse HS, et al. Two novel 1alpha-hydroxylase mutations in French-Canadians with vitamin D dependency rickets type I1. *Kidney Int* 1998;54:1437–1443.
22. Nykjaer A, Dragun D, Walther D, et al. An endocytic pathway essential for renal uptake and activation of the steroid 25-(OH) vitamin D3. *Cell* 1999;96:507–515.
23. Leheste JR, Melsen F, Wellner M, et al. Hypocalcemia and osteopathy in mice with kidney-specific megalin gene defect. *FASEB J* 2003;17:247–249.
24. Portale AA, Boothe BE, Tsai HC, et al. Reduced plasma concentration of 1,25-dihydroxy-vitamin D in children with moderate renal insufficiency. *Kidney Int* 1982;21:627–632.
25. Wilson L, Felsenfeld A, Drezner MK, et al. Altered divalent ion metabolism in early renal failure: role of 1,25(OH)2D. *Kidney Int* 1985;27:565–573.

26. Reichel H, Deibart B, Schmidt-Gayk H, et al. Calcium metabolism in early chronic renal failure: implications for the pathogenesis of hyperparathyroidism. *Nephrol Dial Transplant* 1991;6:162–169.
27. Hsu CH, Patel S, Young EW, et al. Production and degradation of calcitriol in renal failure rats. *Am J Physiol* 1987; 253:F1015–F1019.
28. Hsu CH, Patel S, Buchsbaum BL. Calcitriol metabolism in patients with chronic renal failure. *Am J Kidney Dis* 1991;171: 185–190.
29. Patel SR, Ke HQ, Hsu CH. Effect of vitamin D metabolites on calcitriol degradative enzymes in renal failure. *Kidney Int* 1994;45:509–514.
30. Silver J, Russell J, Sherwood LM. Regulation by vitamin D metabolites of messenger ribonucleic acid for preproparathyroid hormone in isolated bovine parathyroid cells. *Proc Natl Acad Sci U S A* 1985;82:4270–4273.
31. Silver J, Naveh-Many T, Mayer H, et al. Regulation by vitamin D metabolites of parathyroid hormone gene transcription *in vivo* in the rat. *J Clin Invest* 1986;78:1296–1301.
32. Naveh-Many T, Marx R, Keshet E, et al. Regulation of 1,25-dihydroxyvitamin D3 receptor gene expression by 1,25-dihydroxyvitamin D3 in the parathyroid in vivo. *J Clin Invest* 1990;86:1968–1975.
33. Brown AJ, Zhong M, Finch J, et al. The roles of calcium and 1,25-dihydroxyvitamin D3 in the regulation of vitamin D receptor expression by rat parathyroid glands. *Endocrinology* 1995;136:1419–1425.
34. Patel SR, Ke HQ, Vanholder R, et al. Inhibition of calcitriol receptor binding to vitamin D response elements by uremic toxins. *J Clin Invest* 1995;96:50–59.
35. Fukuda N, Tanaka H, Tominaga Y, et al. Decreased 1,25-dihydroxyvitamin D3 receptor density is associated with a more severe form of parathyroid hyperplasia in chronic uremic patients. *J Clin Invest* 1993;92:1436–1443.
36. Saggese G, Federico G, Cinquanta L. *In vitro* effects of growth hormone and other hormones on chondrocytes and osteoblast-like cells. *Acta Paediatr* 1993;391(suppl):54–59.
37. Scharla SH, Strong DD, Mohan S, et al. 1,25-dihydroxyvitamin D3 differentially regulates the production of insulin-like growth factor-I (IGF-I) and IGF-binding protein-4 in mouse osteoblasts. *Endocrinology* 1991;129:3139–3146.
38. Akiyama H, Hiraki Y, Shigeno C, et al. 1a,25-Dihydroxyvitamin D3 inhibits cell growth and chondrogenesis of a clonal mouse EC cell line, ATDC5. *J Bone Miner Res* 1996;11:22–28.
39. Cozzolino M, Lu Y, Finch J, et al. p21WAF1 and TGF-alpha mediate parathyroid growth arrest by vitamin D and high calcium. *Kidney Int* 2001;60:2109–2117.
40. Kifor O, Moore FD Jr, Wang P, et al. Reduced immunostaining for the extracellular Ca2+-sensing receptor in primary and uremic secondary hyperparathyroidism. *J Clin Endocrinol Metab* 1996;81:1598–1606.
41. Brown AJ, Zhong M, Finch J, et al. Rat calcium-sensing receptor is regulated by vitamin D but not by calcium. *Am J Physiol* 1996;270:F454–F460.
42. Li YC, Pirro AE, Amling M, et al. Targeted ablation of the vitamin D receptor: an animal model of vitamin D-dependent rickets type II with alopecia. *Proc Natl Acad Sci U S A* 1997;94:9831–9835.
43. Amling M, Priemel M, Holzmann T, et al. Rescue of the skeletal phenotype of vitamin D receptor-ablated mice in the setting of normal mineral ion homeostasis: formal histomorphometric and biomechanical analyses. *Endocrinology* 1999;140:4982–4987.
44. Li YC, Amling M, Pirro AE, et al. Normalization of mineral ion homeostasis by dietary means prevents hyperparathyroidism, rickets, and osteomalacia, but not alopecia in vitamin D receptor-ablated mice. *Endocrinology* 1998;139: 4391–4396.
45. Brown EM. Four-parameter model of the sigmoidal relationship between parathyroid hormone release and extracellular calcium concentration in normal and abnormal parathyroid tissue. *J Clin Endocrinol Metab* 1983;56:572–581.
46. Brown EM, Wilson RE, Eastmen RC, et al. Abnormal regulation of parathyroid hormone release by calcium in secondary hyperparathyroidism due to chronic renal failure. *J Clin Endocrinol Metab* 1982;54:172–179.
47. Felsenfeld AJ, Rodriguez M, Dunlay R, et al. A comparison of parathyroid-gland function in haemodialysis patients with different forms of renal osteodystrophy. *Nephrol Dial Transplant* 1991;6:244–251.
48. Dunlay R, Rodriguez M, Felsenfeld AJ, et al. Direct inhibitory effect of calcitriol on parathyroid function (sigmoidal curve) in dialysis. *Kidney Int* 1989;36:1093–1098.
49. Delmez JA, Tindira C, Grooms P, et al. Parathyroid hormone suppression by intravenous 1,25-dihydroxyvitamin D. A role for increased sensitivity to calcium. *J Clin Invest* 1989;83:1349–1355.
50. Ramirez JA, Goodman WG, Gornbein J, et al. Direct *in vivo* comparison of calcium-regulated parathyroid hormone secretion in normal volunteers and patients with secondary hyperparathyroidism. *J Clin Endocrinol Metab* 1993;76:1489–1494.
51. Goodman WG, Belin T, Gales B, et al. Calcium-regulated parathyroid hormone release in patients with mild or advanced secondary hyperparathyroidism. *Kidney Int* 1995;48:1553–1558.
52. Goodman WG, Veldhuis JD, Belin TR, et al. Suppressive effect of calcium on parathyroid hormone release in adynamic renal osteodystrophy and secondary hyperparathyroidism. *Kidney Int* 1997;51:1590–1595.
53. Sanchez CP, Goodman WG, Ramirez JA, et al. Calcium-regulated parathyroid hormone secretion in adynamic renal osteodystrophy. *Kidney Int* 1995;48:838–843.
54. Goodman WG, Veldhuis JD, Belin TR, et al. Calcium-sensing by parathyroid glands in secondary hyperparathyroidism. *J Clin Endocrinol Metab* 1998;83:2765–2772.
55. Ouseph R, Leiser JD, Moe SM. Calcitriol and the parathyroid hormone-ionized calcium curve: a comparison of methodologic approaches. *J Am Soc Nephrol* 1996;7:497–505.
56. Felsenfeld AJ, Llach F. Parathyroid gland function in chronic renal failure. *Kidney Int* 1993;43:771–789.
57. Giangrande A, Castiglioni A, Solbiati L, et al. Chemical parathyroidectomy for recurrence of secondary hyperparathyroidism. *Am J Kidney Dis* 1994;24:421–426.
58. McCarron DA, Muther RS, Lenfesty B, et al. Parathyroid function in persistent hyperparathyroidism: relationship to gland size. *Kidney Int* 1982;22:662–670.
59. Khosla S, Ebelling PR, Firek AF, et al. Calcium infusion suggests a "set point" abnormality of parathyroid gland function in familial benign hypercalcemia and more com-

plex disturbances in primary hyperparathyroidism. *J Clin Endocrinol Metab* 1993;76:715–720.
60. Indridason OS, Heath H III, Khosla S, et al. Non-suppressible parathyroid hormone secretion is related to gland size in uremic secondary hyperparathyroidism. *Kidney Int* 1996;50:1663–1671.
61. Brown EM, Gamba G, Riccardi D, et al. Cloning and characterization of an extracellular Ca(2+)-sensing receptor from bovine parathyroid. *Nature* 1993;366:575–580.
62. Brown EM, Hebert SC. Calcium-receptor-regulated parathyroid and renal function. *Bone* 1997;20:303–309.
63. Gogusev J, Duchambon P, Hory B, et al. Depressed expression of calcium receptor in parathyroid gland tissue of patients with hyperparathyroidism. *Kidney Int* 1997;51:328–336.
64. Pollak MR, Seidman CE, Brown EM. Three inherited disorders of calcium sensing. *Medicine (Baltimore)* 1996;75:115–123.
65. Baron J, Winer KK, Yanovski JA, et al. Mutations in the Ca(2+)-sensing receptor gene cause autosomal dominant and sporadic hypoparathyroidism. *Hum Mol Genet* 1996;5:601–606.
66. Hosokawa Y, Pollak MR, Brown EM, et al. Mutational analysis of the extracellular Ca(2+)-sensing receptor gene in human parathyroid tumors. *J Clin Endocrinol Metab* 1995;80:3107–3110.
67. Rogers KV, Dunn CK, Conklin RL, et al. Calcium receptor messenger ribonucleic acid levels in the parathyroid glands and kidney of vitamin D-deficient rats are not regulated by plasma calcium or 1,25-dihydroxyvitamin D3. *Endocrinology* 1995;136:499–504.
68. Hernandez A, Torres A, Concepcion MT, et al. Parathyroid gland calcium receptor gene expression is not regulated by increased dietary phosphorus in normal and renal failure rats. *Nephrol Dial Transplant* 1996;11(suppl 3):11–14.
69. Goodman WG, Hladik GA, Turner SA, et al. The calcimimetic agent AMG 073 lowers plasma parathyroid hormone levels in hemodialysis patients with secondary hyperparathyroidism. *J Am Soc Nephrol* 2002;13:1017–1024.
70. Goodman WG, Frazao JM, Goodkin DA, et al. A calcimimetic agent lowers plasma parathyroid hormone levels in patients with secondary hyperparathyroidism. *Kidney Int* 2000;58:436–445.
71. Collins MT, Skarulis MC, Bilezikian JP, et al. Treatment of hypercalcemia secondary to parathyroid carcinoma with a novel calcimimetic agent. *J Clin Endocrinol Metab* 1998;83:1080–1083.
72. Massry SG, Coburn JW, Lee DBN, et al. Skeletal resistance to parathyroid hormone in renal failure. *Ann Intern Med* 1973;78:357–364.
73. Galceran T, Martin KJ, Morrissey JJ, et al. The role of 1,25(OH)2 D3 on the pathogenesis of skeletal resistance to parathyroid hormone in chronic renal failure. *Kidney Int* 1987;32:801–807.
74. Ureña P, Ferreira A, Morieux C, et al. PTH/PTHrP receptor mRNA is downregulated in epiphyseal cartilage growth plate of uraemic rats. *Nephrol Dial Transplant* 1996;11:2008–2016.
75. Moore P, Gokal RG, Freemont AJ, et al. Downregulation of osteoblast PTH receptor (PTH-R) mRNA expression in end-stage renal failure. *J Pathol* 1997;181(suppl):12A.
76. Sanchez CP, Salusky IB, Kuizon BD, et al. Growth of long bones in renal failure: roles of hyperparathyroidism, growth hormone and calcitriol. *Kidney Int* 1998;54:1879–1887.
77. Massry SG, Stein R, Garty J, et al. Skeletal resistance to the calcemic action of parathyroid hormone in uremia: role of 1,25(OH)2D3. *Kidney Int* 1976;9:467–474.
78. Salusky IB, Coburn JW, Brill J, et al. Bone disease in pediatric patients undergoing dialysis with CAPD or CCPD. *Kidney Int* 1988;33:975–982.
79. Andreoli SP, Bergstein JM, Sherrard DJ. Aluminum intoxication from aluminum-containing phosphate binders in children with azotemia not undergoing dialysis. *N Engl J Med* 1984;310:1079–1084.
80. Sedman AB, Miller NL, Warady BA, et al. Aluminum loading in children with chronic renal failure. *Kidney Int* 1984;26:201–204.
81. Sherrard DJ, Hercz G, Pei Y, et al. The spectrum of bone disease in end-stage renal failure—an evolving disorder. *Kidney Int* 1993;43:436–442.
82. Goodman WG, Ramirez JA, Belin TR, et al. Development of adynamic bone in patients with secondary hyperparathyroidism after intermittent calcitriol therapy. *Kidney Int* 1994;46:1160–1166.
83. Hercz G, Pei Y, Greenwood C, et al. Aplastic osteodystrophy without aluminum: the role of "suppressed" parathyroid function. *Kidney Int* 1993;44:860–866.
84. Kurz P, Monier-Faugere MC, Bognar B, et al. Evidence for abnormal calcium homeostasis in patients with adynamic bone disease. *Kidney Int* 1994;46:855–861.
85. Cohen-Solal ME, Sebert JL, Boudailliez B, et al. Non-aluminic bone disease in non-dialyzed uremic patients: A new type of osteopathy due to overtreatment? *Bone* 1992;13:1–5.
86. Neu AM, Ho PL, McDonald RA, et al. Chronic dialysis in children and adolescents. The 2001 NAPRTCS annual report. *Pediatr Nephrol* 2002;17:656–663.
87. Nash MA, Torrado AD, Greifer I, et al. Renal tubular acidosis in infants and children. *J Pediatr* 1972;80:747–748.
88. Challa A, Chan W, Krieg RJ Jr, et al. Effect of metabolic acidosis on the express of insulin-like growth factor and growth hormone receptor. *Kidney Int* 1993;44:1224–1227.
89. Maniar S, Kleinknecht C, Zhou X, et al. Growth hormone action is blunted by acidosis in experimental uremia on acid load. *Clin Nephrol* 1996;46:72–76.
90. Challa A, Krieg RJ Jr, Thabet MA, et al. Metabolic acidosis inhibits growth hormone secretion in rats: mechanism of growth retardation. *Am J Physiol* 1993;265:E547–E553.
91. Green J, Maor G. Effect of metabolic acidosis on the growth hormone/IGF-I endocrine axis in skeletal growth centers. *Kidney Int* 2000;57:2258–2267.
92. Chesney RW, Moorthy AV, Eisman JA, et al. Increased growth after long-term oral 1,25-vitamin D3 in childhood renal osteodystrophy. *N Engl J Med* 1978;298:238–242.
93. Langman CB, Mazur AT, Baron R, et al. 25-Hydroxyvitamin D3 (calcifediol) therapy of juvenile renal osteodystrophy: beneficial effect on linear growth velocity. *J Pediatr* 1982;100:815–820.
94. Chan JC, Kodroff MB, Landwehr DM. Effects of 1,25-dihydroxyvitamin-D3 on renal function, mineral balance, and growth in children with severe chronic renal failure. *Pediatrics* 1981;68:559–571.

95. Chan JCM, McEnery PT, Chinchilli VM, et al. A prospective, double-blind study of growth failure in children with chronic renal insufficiency and the effectiveness of treatment with calcitriol versus dihydrotachysterol. *J Pediatr* 1994;124:520–528.
96. Hodson EM, Evans RA, Dunstan CR, et al. Treatment of childhood renal osteodystrophy with calcitriol or ergocalciferol. *Clin Nephrol* 1985;24:192–200.
97. Salusky IB, Fine RN, Kangarloo H, et al. "High-dose" calcitriol for control of renal osteodystrophy in children on CAPD. *Kidney Int* 1987;32:89–95.
98. Goodman WG, Salusky IB. Evolution of secondary hyperparathyroidism during daily oral calcitriol therapy in pediatric renal osteodystrophy. *Contrib Nephrol* 1991;90:189–195.
99. Slatopolsky E, Weerts C, Thielan J, et al. Marked suppression of secondary hyperparathyroidism by intravenous administration of 1,25-dihydroxycholecalciferol in uremic patients. *J Clin Invest* 1984;74:2136–2143.
100. Andress DL, Norris KC, Coburn JW, et al. Intravenous calcitriol in the treatment of refractory osteitis fibrosa of chronic renal failure. *N Engl J Med* 1989;321:274–279.
101. Martin KJ, Bullal HS, Domoto DT, et al. Pulse oral calcitriol for the treatment of hyperparathyroidism in patients on continuous ambulatory peritoneal dialysis: preliminary observations. *Am J Kidney Dis* 1992;19:540–545.
102. Klaus G, Mehls O, Hinderer J, et al. Is intermittent oral calcitriol safe and effective in renal secondary hyperparathyroidism? *Lancet* 1991;337:800–801.
103. Kuizon BD, Goodman WG, Jüppner H, et al. Diminished linear growth during treatment with intermittent calcitriol and dialysis in children with chronic renal failure. *Kidney Int* 1998;53:205–211.
104. Schmitt CP, Ardissino G, Testa S, et al. Growth in children with chronic renal failure on intermittent versus daily calcitriol. *Pediatr Nephrol* 2003;18:440–444.
105. Colston KW, Perks CM, Xie SP, et al. Growth inhibition of both MCF-7 and Hs578T human breast cancer cell lines by vitamin D analogues is associated with increased expression of insulin-like growth factor binding protein-3. *J Mol Endocrinol* 1998;20:157–162.
106. Nickerson T, Huynh H. Vitamin D analogue EB1089-induced prostate regression is associated with increased gene expression of insulin-like growth factor binding proteins. *J Endocrinol* 1999;160:223–229.
107. Miyakoshi N, Richman C, Kasukawa Y, et al. Evidence that IGF-binding protein-5 functions as a growth factor. *J Clin Invest* 2001;107:73–81.
108. Richman C, Baylink DJ, Lang K, et al. Recombinant human insulin-like growth factor-binding protein-5 stimulates bone formation parameters in vitro and in vivo. *Endocrinology* 1999;140:4699–4705.
109. Longobardi L, Torello M, Buckway C, et al. A novel insulin-like growth factor (IGF)-independent role for IGF binding protein-3 in mesenchymal chondroprogenitor cell apoptosis. *Endocrinology* 2003;144:1695–1702.
110. Collard TJ, Guy M, Butt AJ, et al. Transcriptional upregulation of the insulin-like growth factor binding protein IGFBP-3 by sodium butyrate increases IGF-independent apoptosis in human colonic adenoma-derived epithelial cells. *Carcinogenesis* 2003;24:393–401.
111. Samaan NA, Freeman RM. Growth hormone levels in severe renal failure. *Metabolism* 1970;19:102–113.
112. Tonshoff B, Veldhuis JD, Heinrich U, et al. Deconvolution analysis of spontaneous nocturnal growth hormone secretion in prepubertal children with preterminal chronic renal failure and with end-stage renal disease. *Pediatr Res* 1995;37:86–93.
113. Tonshoff B, Eden S, Weiser E, et al. Reduced hepatic growth hormone (GH) receptor gene expression and increased plasma GH binding protein in experimental uremia. *Kidney Int* 1994;45:1085–1092.
114. Schaefer F, Chen Y, Tsao T, et al. Impaired JAK-STAT signal transduction contributes to growth hormone resistance in chronic uremia. *J Clin Invest* 2001;108:467–475.
115. Tonshoff B, Cronin MJ, Reichert M, et al. Reduced concentration of serum growth hormone (GH)-binding protein in children with chronic renal failure: correlation with GH insensitivity. *J Clin Endocrinol Metab* 1997;82:1007–1013.
116. Powell DR. Effects of renal failure on the growth hormone-insulin-like growth factor axis. *J Pediatr* 1997;131:S13–S16.
117. Tonshoff B, Blum WF, Mehls O. Derangements of the somatotropic hormone axis in chronic renal failure. *Kidney Int* 1997;58(suppl):S106–S113.
118. Powell D, Liu F, Baker BK, et al. Modulation of growth factors by growth hormone in children with chronic renal failure. *Kidney Int* 1997;51:1970–1979.
119. Kirkwood JR, Ozonoff MB, Steinbach HL. Epiphyseal displacement after metaphyseal fracture in renal osteodystrophy. *AJR Am J Roentgenol* 1972;115:547–554.
120. Mehls O, Ritz E, Krempien B, et al. Slipped epiphyses in renal osteodystrophy. *Arch Dis Child* 1975;50:545.
121. Mehls O. Renal osteodystrophy in children: etiology and clinical aspects. In: Fine RN, Gruskin AB, eds. *Endstage renal disease in children.* Philadelphia: W.B. Saunders, 1984: 227–250.
122. Schott GD, Wills MR. Muscle weakness in osteomalacia. *Lancet* 1976;1:626–629.
123. Smith R, Stern G. Myopathy, osteomalacia and hyperparathyroidism. *Brain* 1967;90:593–602.
124. Mallette LE, Patten BM, Engel WK. Neuromuscular disease in secondary hyperparathyroidism. *Ann Intern Med* 1975;82: 474–483.
125. Birge SJ. Vitamin-D, muscle and phosphate homeostasis. *Miner Electrolyte Metab* 1978;1:57.
126. Henderson RG, Russell RGG, Ledingham JGG, et al. Effects of 1,25-dihydroxycholecalciferol on calcium absorption, muscle weakness, and bone disease in chronic renal failure. *Lancet* 1974;1:379–384.
127. Bischoff HA, Borchers M, Gudat F, et al. In situ detection of 1,25-dihydroxyvitamin D3 receptor in human skeletal muscle tissue. *Histochem J* 2001;33:19–24.
128. Milliner DS, Zinsmeister AR, Lieberman E, et al. Soft tissue calcification in pediatric patients with end stage renal disease. *Kidney Int* 1990;38:931–936.
129. Conger JD, Hammond WS, Alfrey AC, et al. Pulmonary calcification in chronic dialysis patients. Clinical and pathologic studies. *Ann Intern Med* 1975;83:330–336.
130. Braun J, Oldendorf M, Moshage W, et al. Electron beam computed tomography in the evaluation of cardiac calcifications in chronic dialysis patients. *Am J Kidney Dis* 1996;27: 394–401.
131. Kuzela DC, Huffer WE, Conger JD, et al. Soft tissue calcifica-

tion in chronic dialysis patients. *Am J Clin Pathol* 1977;86: 403–424.
132. Schwarz U, Buzello M, Ritz E, et al. Morphology of coronary atherosclerotic lesions in patients with end-stage renal failure. *Nephrol Dial Transplant* 2000;15:218–223.
133. Gipstein RM, Coburn JW, Adams JA, et al. Calciphylaxis in man: a syndrome of tissue necrosis and vascular calcification in 11 patients with chronic renal failure. *Arch Intern Med* 1976;136:1273–1280.
134. Meema HE, Oreopoulos DG, DeVeber GA. Arterial calcification in severe chronic renal disease and their relationship to dialysis treatment, renal transplant and parathyroidectomy. *Radiology* 1976;121:315–321.
135. Goodman WG, Goldin J, Kuizon BD, et al. Coronary artery calcification in young adults with end-stage renal disease who are undergoing dialysis. *N Engl J Med* 2000;342:1478–1483.
136. Eifinger F, Wahn F, Querfeld U, et al. Coronary artery calcifications in children and young adults treated with renal replacement therapy. *Nephrol Dial Transplant* 2001;15:1892–1894.
137. Oh J, Wunsch R, Turzer M, et al. Advanced coronary and carotid arteriopathy in young adults with childhood-onset chronic renal failure. *Circulation* 2002;106:100–105.
138. Foley RN, Parfrey PS, Sarnak MJ. Clinical epidemiology of cardiovascular disease in chronic renal disease. *Am J Kidney Dis* 1998;32:S112–S119.
139. Bostrom K, Watson KE, Horn S, et al. Bone morphogenetic protein expression in human atherosclerotic lesions. *J Clin Invest* 1993;91:1800–1809.
140. Giachelli CM, Bae N, Almeida M, et al. Osteopontin is elevated during neointima formation in rat arteries and is a novel component of human atherosclerotic plaques. *J Clin Invest* 1993;92:1686–1696.
141. Fitzpatrick LA, Severson A, Edwards WD, et al. Diffuse calcification in human coronary arteries. Association of osteopontin with atherosclerosis. *J Clin Invest* 1994;94:1597–1604.
142. Ozeki S, Ohtsuru A, Seto S, et al. Evidence that implicates the parathyroid hormone-related peptide in vascular stenosis. Increased gene expression in the intima of injured carotid arteries and human restenotic coronary lesions. *Arterioscler Thromb Vasc Biol* 1996;16:565–575.
143. Levy RJ, Gundberg C, Scheinman R. The identification of the vitamin K-dependent bone protein osteocalcin as one of the gamma-carboxyglutamic acid containing proteins present in calcified atherosclerotic plaque and mineralized heart valves. *Atherosclerosis* 1983;46:49–56.
144. Shanahan CM, Proudfoot D, Tyson K, et al. Expression of mineralisation-regulating proteins in association with human vascular calcification. *Z Kardiol* 2000;89:63–68.
145. Tyson KL, Reynolds JL, McNair R, et al. Osteo/chondrocytic transcription factors and their target genes exhibit distinct patterns of expression in human arterial calcification. *Arterioscler Thromb Vasc Biol* 2003;23:489–494.
146. Shanahan CM, Cary NR, Salisbury JR, et al. Medial localization of mineralization-regulating proteins in association with Mönckeberg's sclerosis: evidence for smooth muscle cell-mediated vascular calcification. *Circulation* 1999;100:2168–2176.
147. Reslerova M, Moe SM. Vascular calcification in dialysis patients: pathogenesis and consequences. *Am J Kidney Dis* 2003;41:S96–S99.
148. Moe SM, Duan D, Doehle BP, et al. Uremia induces the osteoblast differentiation factor Cbfa1 in human blood vessels. *Kidney Int* 2003;63:1003–1111.
149. Chavers BM, Li S, Collins AJ, et al. Cardiovascular disease in pediatric chronic dialysis patients. *Kidney Int* 2002;62:648–653.
150. Brown EM. Set point for calcium: its role in normal and abnormal secretion. In: Cohn DV, Talmage RV, Matthews JL, eds. *Hormonal control of calcium metabolism*. Amsterdam: Excerpta Medica, 1981:35.
151. Coburn JW, Nebeker HG, Hercz G, et al. Role of aluminum accumulation in the pathogenesis of renal osteodystrophy. In: Robinson RR, ed. *Nephrology*. Vol 2. New York: Springer-Verlag, 1984:1383–1395.
152. Salusky IB, Coburn JW, Foley J, et al. Effects of oral calcium carbonate on control of serum phosphorus and changes in plasma aluminum levels after discontinuation of aluminum-containing gels in children receiving dialysis. *J Pediatr* 1986;108:767–770.
153. Block GA, Hulbert-Shearon TE, Levin NW, et al. Association of serum phosphorus and calcium x phosphorus product with mortality risk in chronic hemodialysis patients: a national study. *Am J Kidney Dis* 1998;31:607–617.
154. Portale AA. Calcium and Phosphorus. In: Barratt T, Avner E, Harmon W, eds. *Pediatric nephrology*, 4 ed. Baltimore: Lippincott Williams & Wilkins, 1999:191–213.
155. Cohen-Solal ME, Sebert JL, Boudailliez B, et al. Comparison of intact, midregion, and carboxy-terminal assays of parathyroid hormone for the diagnosis of bone disease in hemodialyzed patients. *J Clin Endocrinol Metab* 1991;73:516–524.
156. Quarles LD, Lobaugh B, Murphy G. Intact parathyroid hormone overestimates the presence and severity of parathyroid-mediated osseous abnormalities in uremia. *J Clin Endocrinol Metab* 1992;75:145–150.
157. Salusky IB, Ramirez JA, Oppenheim WL, et al. Biochemical markers of renal osteodystrophy in pediatric patients undergoing CAPD/CCPD. *Kidney Int* 1994;45:253–258.
158. Mathias RS, Salusky IB, Harmon WH, et al. Renal bone disease in pediatric patients and young adults treated by hemodialysis in a childrens hospital. *J Am Soc Nephrol* 1993;12:1938–1946.
159. Sherrard DJ, Baylink DJ, Wergedal JE, et al. Quantitative histological studies on the pathogenesis of uremic bone disease. *J Clin Endocrinol Metab* 1974;39:119–135.
160. Malluche HH, Monier-Faugere MC. The role of bone biopsy in the management of patients with renal osteodystrophy. *J Am Soc Nephrol* 1994;4:1631–1642.
161. Llach F, Massry SG. On the mechanism of secondary hyperparathyroidism in moderate renal insufficiency. *J Clin Endocrinol Metab* 1985;61:601–606.
162. Andress DL, Endres DB, Maloney NA, et al. Comparison of parathyroid hormone assays with bone histomorphometry in renal osteodystrophy. *J Clin Endocrinol Metab* 1986;63:1163–1169.
163. Nussbaum SR, Zahradnik RJ, Lavigne JR, et al. Highly sensitive two-site immunoradiometric assay of parathyrin, and its clinical utility in evaluating patients with hypercalcemia. *Clin Chem* 1987;33:1364–1367.
164. Brossard JH, Cloutier M, Roy L, et al. Accumulation of a non-(1-84) molecular form of parathyroid hormone (PTH) detected by intact PTH assay in renal failure: importance in

the interpretation of PTH values. *J Clin Endocrinol Metab* 1996;81:3923–3929.

165. Lepage R, Roy L, Brossard JH, et al. A non-(1-84) circulating parathyroid hormone (PTH) fragment interferes significantly with intact PTH commercial assay measurements in uremic samples. *Clin Chem* 1998;44:805–809.
166. Brossard JH, Yamamoto LN, D'Amour P. Parathyroid hormone metabolites in renal failure: bioactivity and clinical implications. *Semin Dial* 2002;15:196–201.
167. John MR, Goodman WG, Gao P, et al. A novel immunoradiometric assay detects full-length human PTH but not amino-terminally truncated fragments: implications for PTH measurements in renal failure. *J Clin Endocrinol Metab* 1999;84: 4287–4290.
168. Slatopolsky E, Finch J, Clay P, et al. A novel mechanism for skeletal resistance in uremia. *Kidney Int* 2000;58:753–761.
169. Gao P, Scheibel S, D'Amour P, et al. Development of a novel immunoradiometric assay exclusively for biologically active whole parathyroid hormone 1-84: implications for improvement of accurate assessment of parathyroid function. *J Bone Miner Res* 2001;16:605–614.
170. Monier-Faugere MC, Geng Z, Mawad H, et al. Improved assessment of bone turnover by the PTH-(1-84)/large C-PTH fragments ratio in ESRD patients. *Kidney Int* 2001;60:1460–1468.
171. Salomon R, Charbit M, Gagnadoux MF, et al. High serum levels of a non-(1-84) parathyroid hormone (PTH) fragment in pediatric haemodialysis patients. *Pediatr Nephrol* 2001;16:1011–1014.
172. Salusky IB, Goodman WG, Kuizon BD, et al. Similar predictive value of bone turnover using first- and second-generation immunometric PTH assays in pediatric patients treated with peritoneal dialysis. *Kidney Int* 2003;63:1801–1808.
173. Nguyen-Yamamoto L, Rousseau L, Brossard JH, et al. Synthetic carboxyl-terminal fragments of parathyroid hormone (PTH) decrease ionized calcium concentration in rats by acting on a receptor different from the PTH/PTH-related peptide receptor. *Endocrinology* 2001;142:1386–1392.
174. Coen G, Bonucci E, Ballanti P, et al. PTH 1-84 and PTH "7-84" in the noninvasive diagnosis of renal bone disease. *Am J Kidney Dis* 2002;40:348–354.
175. Salusky IB, Goodman WG. Adynamic renal osteodystrophy: Is there a problem? *J Am Soc Nephrol* 2001;12:1978–1985.
176. Alfrey AC. Aluminum metabolism. *Kidney Int* 1986;29(suppl 18):S8–S11.
177. Pediatric bone metabolism and disease in chronic kidney disease. TBA 2003.
178. Ritz E, Prager P, Krempien B, et al. Skeletal x-ray findings and bone histology in patients on hemodialysis. *Kidney Int* 1978;13:316–323.
179. Dent CE, Hodson CJ. Radiological changes associated with certain metabolic bone diseases. *Br J Radiol* 1954;27:605–608.
180. Meema HE, Rabinovich S, Meema S, et al. Improved radiological diagnosis of azotemic osteodystrophy. *Radiology* 1972; 102:1–10.
181. Parfitt AM. Clinical and radiographic manifestations of renal osteodystrophy. In: David DS, ed. *Calcium metabolism in renal failure and nephrolithiasis.* New York: John Wiley & Sons, 1977:150–190.
182. Mehls O, Krempien B, Ritz E, et al. Renal osteodystrophy in children on maintenance hemodialysis. *Proc Eur Dial Transplant Assoc* 1973;10:197–201.
183. Parfitt AM, Massry SG, Winfield AC. Osteopenia and fractures occurring during maintenance hemodialysis: a "new" form of renal osteodystrophy. *Clin Orthop* 1972;87:287–302.
184. Olgaard K, Heerfordt, Madsen S. Scintigraphic skeletal changes in uremic patients on regular hemodialysis. *Nephron* 1976;17:325–334.
185. Wright RS, Mehls O, Ritz E, et al. Musculoskeletal manifestation of chronic renal failure, dialysis and transplantation. In: Bacon P, Hadler N, eds. *Renal manifestations in rheumatic disease.* London: Butterworth Publishers, 1982:352.
186. Sherrard DJ, Ott SM, Maloney NA, et al. Uremic osteodystrophy: classification, cause and treatment. In: Frame B, Potts J, eds. *Clinical disorders of bone and mineral metabolism.* Amsterdam: Excerpta Medica, 1983:254–259.
187. Maloney NA, Ott SM, Alfrey AC, et al. Histological quantitation of aluminum in iliac bone from patients with renal failure. *J Lab Clin Med* 1982;99:206–216.
188. Serrano S, Mariposo ML, Torres A, et al. Osteoblastic proliferation in bone biopsies from patients with end-stage chronic renal failure. *J Bone Miner Res* 1997;12:191–199.
189. Blumenthal NC, Posner AS. *In vitro* model of aluminum-induced osteomalacia: inhibition of hydroxyapatite formation and growth. *Calcif Tissue Int* 1984;36:439–441.
190. Hodsman AB, Sherrard DJ, Alfrey AC, et al. Bone aluminum and histomorphometric features of renal osteodystrophy. *J Clin Endocrinol Metab* 1982;54:539–546.
191. Andress DL, Maloney NA, Endres DB, et al. Aluminum-associated bone disease in chronic renal failure: high prevalence in a long-term dialysis population. *J Bone Miner Res* 1986;1:391–398.
192. Parisien M, Charhon SA, Arlot M, et al. Evidence for a toxic effect of aluminum on osteoblasts: a histomorphometric study in hemodialysis patients with aplastic bone disease. *J Bone Miner Res* 1988;3:259–267.
193. U.S. Renal Data System. USRDS 1994 annual data report. Bethesda, MD: The National Institute of Health, National Institute of Diabetes and Digestive and Kidney Diseases, 1994:43–54.
194. Institute of Medicine, Food and Nutrition Board. Dietary reference intakes for calcium, phosphorus, magnesium, vitamin D, and fluoride. Washington: National Academy Press, 1997.
195. Blumenkrantz MJ, Kopple JD, Moran JK, et al. Metabolic balance studies and dietary protein requirements in patients undergoing continuous ambulatory peritoneal dialysis. *Kidney Int* 1982;21:862–867.
196. Albertini B, Miller JH, Gardner PW, et al. High-flux hemodiafiltration: under six hours/week treatment. *Trans Am Soc Artif Intern Organs* 1984;28:302–307.
197. Pierratos A, Ouwendyk M, Francoeur R, et al. Nocturnal hemodialysis: three-year experience. *J Am Soc Nephrol* 1998;9:859–868.
198. Mucsi I, Hercz G, Uldall R. Control of serum phosphorus without any phosphate binders in patients treated with nocturnal hemodialysis. *Kidney Int* 1998;53:1399–1404.
199. Roodhooft AM, Van Hoeck KJ, Van Acker KJ. Hypophosphatemia in infants on continuous ambulatory peritoneal dialysis. *Clin Nephrol* 1990;34:131–135.

200. Tejeda A, Saffarian N, Uday K, et al. Hypophosphatemia in end stage renal disease. *Nephron* 1996;73:674–678.
201. Brickman AS, Coburn JW, Massry SG, et al. 1,25-Dihydroxyvitamin D3 in normal man and patients with renal failure. *Ann Intern Med* 1974;80:161–168.
202. Schaefer K, Sheer J, Asmus G, et al. The treatment of uremic hyperphosphatemia with calcium acetate and calcium carbonate: a comparative study. *Nephrol Dial Transplant* 1991;6:171–175.
203. Coburn JW, Mischel MG, Goodman WG, et al. Calcium citrate markedly enhances aluminum absorption from aluminum hydroxide. *Am J Kidney Dis* 1991;17:708–711.
204. Alon U, Davidai G, Bentur L, et al. Oral calcium carbonate as phosphate-binder in infants and children with chronic renal failure. *Miner Electrolyte Metab* 1986;12:320–325.
205. Tsukamoto Y, Moriya R, Nagaba Y, et al. Effect of administering calcium carbonate to treat secondary hyperparathyroidism in nondialyzed patients with chronic renal failure. *Am J Kidney Dis* 1995;25:879–886.
206. Indridason OS, Quarles LD. Comparison of treatments for mild secondary hyperparathyroidism in hemodialysis patients. *Kidney Int* 2000;57:282–292.
207. Slatopolsky E, Weerts C, Lopez-Hilker S, et al. Calcium carbonate is an effective phosphate binder in patients with chronic renal failure undergoing dialysis. *N Engl J Med* 1986;315:157–161.
208. Fournier A, Moriniere PH, Sebert JL, et al. Calcium carbonate, an aluminum-free agent for control of hyperphosphatemia, hypocalcemia and hyperparathyroidism in uremia. *Kidney Int* 1986;29:S115–S119.
209. Ibels LS, Alfrey AC, Huffer WE, et al. Arterial calcification and pathology in uremic patients undergoing dialysis. *Am J Med* 1979;66:790–796.
210. Slatopolsky EA, Burke SK, Dillon MA. RenaGel, a nonabsorbed calcium- and aluminum-free phosphate binder, lowers serum phosphorus and parathyroid hormone. The RenaGel Study Group. *Kidney Int* 1999;55:299–307.
211. Bleyer AJ, Burke SK, Dillon M, et al. A comparison of the calcium-free phosphate binder sevelamer hydrochloride with calcium acetate in the treatment of hyperphosphatemia in hemodialysis patients. *Am J Kidney Dis* 1999;33:694–701.
212. Chertow GM, Burke SK, Dillon MA, et al. Long-term effects of sevelamer hydrochloride on the calcium x phosphate product and lipid profile of haemodialysis patients. *Nephrol Dial Transplant* 1999;14:2709–2714.
213. Mahdavi H, Kuizon BD, Gales B, et al. Sevelamer hydrochloride: an effective phosphate binder in children treated with dialysis. *Pediatr Nephrol* 2003.
214. Chertow GM, Burke SK, Raggi P. Sevelamer attenuates the progression of coronary and aortic calcification in hemodialysis patients. *Kidney Int* 2002;62:245–252.
215. Parsons V, Baldwin D, Moniz C, et al. Successful control of hyperparathyroidism in patients on continuous ambulatory peritoneal dialysis using magnesium carbonate and calcium carbonate as phosphate binders. *Nephron* 1993;63:379–383.
216. Hergesell O, Ritz E. Phosphate binders on iron basis: A new perspective? *Kidney Int* 1999;73(suppl):S42–S45.
217. Chang JM, Hwang SJ, Tsai JC, et al. Effect of ferric polymaltose complex as a phosphate binder in haemodialysis patients. *Nephrol Dial Transplant* 1999;14:1045–1047.
218. Graff L, Burnel D. A possible non-aluminum oral phosphate binder? A comparative study on dietary phosphorus absorption. *Res Commun Mol Pathol Pharmacol* 1995;89:373–388.
219. Nelson R. Novel phosphate binder is effective in patients on haemodialysis. *Lancet* 2002;360:1483.
220. Salusky IB, Coburn JW, Paunier L, et al. Role of aluminum hydroxide in raising serum aluminum levels in children undergoing continuous ambulatory peritoneal dialysis. *J Pediatr* 1984;105:717–720.
221. Winney RJ, Cowie JF, Robson JS. The role of plasma aluminum in the detection and prevention of aluminum toxicity. *Kidney Int* 1986;29(suppl 18):S91–S95.
222. Salusky IB, Foley J, Nelson P, et al. Aluminum accumulation during treatment with aluminum hydroxide and dialysis in children and young adults with chronic renal disease. *N Engl J Med* 1991;324:527–531.
223. Eke FU, Winterborn MH. Effect of low dose 1α-hydroxycholecalciferol on glomerular filtration rate in moderate renal failure. *Arch Dis Child* 1984;58:810–813.
224. Christiansen C, Rodbro P, Christensen MS, et al. Is 1,25-dihydroxy-cholecalciferol harmful to renal function in patients with chronic renal failure? *Clin Endocrinol (Oxf)* 1981;15:229–236.
225. Tougaard L, Sorensen E, Brochner-Mortensen J, et al. Controlled trial of 1a-hydroxycholecalciferol in chronic renal failure. *Lancet* 1976;1:1044–1047.
226. Denda M, Finch J, Brown AJ, et al. 1,25-Dihydroxyvitamin D3 and 22-oxacalcitriol prevent the decrease in vitamin D receptor content in the parathyroid glands of uremic rats. *Kidney Int* 1996;50:34–39.
227. Hirata M, Katsumata K, Masaki T, et al. 22-Oxacalcitriol ameliorates high-turnover bone and marked osteitis fibrosa in rats with slowly progressive nephritis. *Kidney Int* 1999;56:2040–2047.
228. Monier-Faugere MC, Geng Z, Friedler RM, et al. 22-Oxacalcitriol suppresses secondary hyperparathyroidism without inducing low bone turnover in dogs with renal failure. *Kidney Int* 1999;55:821–832.
229. Kurokawa K, Akizawa T, Suzuki M, et al. Effect of 22-oxacalcitriol on hyperparathyroidism of dialysis patients: results of preliminary study. *Nephrol Dial Transplant* 1996;11:121–124.
230. Tsukamoto Y, Hanaoka M, Matsuo T, et al. Effect of 22-oxacalcitriol on bone histology of hemodialyzed patients with severe secondary hyperparathyroidism. *Am J Kidney Dis* 2000;35:458–464.
231. Sjöden G, Smith C, Lindgren JU, et al. 1α-Hydroxyvitamin D2 is less toxic than 1a-hydroxyvitamin D3 in the rat. *Proc Soc Exp Biol Med* 1985;178:432–436.
232. Tan AU Jr, Levine BS, Mazess RB, et al. Effective suppression of parathyroid hormone by 1 alpha-hydroxy-vitamin D2 in hemodialysis patients with moderate to severe secondary hyperparathyroidism. *Kidney Int* 1997;51:317–323.
233. Frazao J, Chesney RW, Coburn JW. Intermittent oral 1alpha-hydroxyvitamin D2 is effective and safe for the suppression of secondary hyperparathyroidism in haemodialysis patients. 1alphaD2 Study Group. *Nephrol Dial Transplant* 1998;13(suppl 3):68–72.
234. Slatopolsky E, Finch J, Ritter C, et al. A new analog of calcitriol, 19-nor-1,25-$(OH)_2D_2$, suppresses parathyroid hormone secretion in uremic rats in the absence of hypercalcemia. *Am J Kidney Dis* 1995;26:852–860.

235. Finch JL, Brown AJ, Slatopolsky E. Differential effects of 1,25-dihydroxy-vitamin D3 and 19-nor-1,25-dihydroxy-vitamin D2 on calcium and phosphorus resorption in bone. *J Am Soc Nephrol* 1999;10:980–985.
236. Martin KJ, Gonzalez EA, Gellens M, et al. 19-Nor-1-α-25-dihydroxyvitamin D2 (paricalcitol) safely and effectively reduces the levels of intact parathyroid hormone in patients on hemodialysis. *J Am Soc Nephrol* 1998;9:1427–1432.
237. Llach F, Keshav G, Goldblat MV, et al. Suppression of parathyroid hormone secretion in hemodialysis patients by a novel vitamin D analogue: 19-nor-1,25-dihydroxyvitamin D2. *Am J Kidney Dis* 1998;32:S48–S54.
238. Sprague SM, Lerma E, McCormmick D, et al. Suppression of parathyroid hormone secretion in hemodialysis patients: comparison of paricalcitol with calcitriol. *Am J Kidney Dis* 2001;38:S51–S56.
239. Wada M, Furuya Y, Sakiyama J, et al. The calcimimetic compound NPS R-568 suppresses parathyroid cell proliferation in rats with renal insufficiency. Control of parathyroid cell growth via a calcium receptor. *J Clin Invest* 1997;100: 2977–2983.
240. Wada M, Nagano N, Furuya Y, et al. Calcimimetic NPS R-568 prevents parathyroid hyperplasia in rats with severe secondary hyperparathyroidism. *Kidney Int* 2000;57:50–58.
241. Wada M, Ishii H, Furuya Y, et al. NPS R-568 halts or reverses osteitis fibrosa in uremic rats. *Kidney Int* 1998;53:448–453.
242. Silverberg SJ, Bone HG III, Marriott TB, et al. Short-term inhibition of parathyroid hormone secretion by a calcium-receptor agonist in patients with primary hyperparathyroidism. *N Engl J Med* 1997;337:1506–1510.
243. Antonsen JE, Sherrard DJ, Andress DL. A calcimimetic agent acutely suppresses parathyroid hormone levels in patients with chronic renal failure. Rapid communication. *Kidney Int* 1998;53:223–227.
244. Lindberg JS, Moe SM, Goodman WG, et al. The calcimimetic AMG 073 reduces parathyroid hormone and calcium x phosphorus in secondary hyperparathyroidism. *Kidney Int* 2003;63:248–254.
245. Chang W, Tu C, Chen TH, et al. Expression and signal transduction of calcium-sensing receptors in cartilage and bone. *Endocrinology* 1999;140:5883–5893.
246. Arnold A, Brown MF, Ureña P, et al. Monoclonality of parathyroid tumors in chronic renal failure and in primary parathyroid hyperplasia. *J Clin Invest* 1995;95:2047–2053.
247. Ott SM, Maloney NA, Coburn JW, et al. The prevalence of bone aluminum deposition in renal osteodystrophy and its relation to the response to calcitriol therapy. *N Engl J Med* 1982;307:709–713.
248. Offner G, Aschendorff C, Brodehl J. Growth after renal transplantation: an update. *Pediatr Nephrol* 1991;5:472–476.
249. Potter DE, Genant HK, Salvatierra O Jr. Avascular necrosis of bone after renal transplantation. *Am J Dis Child* 1978;132:1125–1129.
250. Van Damme-Lombaerts R, Pirson Y, Squifflet JP, et al. The avascular necrosis of bone after renal transplantation in children. *Transplant Proc* 1985;17:184–186.
251. Feber J, Cochat P, Braillon P, et al. Bone mineral density after renal transplantation. *J Pediatr* 1994;125:870–875.
252. Chesney RW, Rose PG, Mazess RB. Persistence of diminished bone mineral content following renal transplantation in childhood. *Pediatrics* 1984;73:459–466.
253. Grotz WH, Mundinger FA, Gugel B, et al. Bone mineral density after kidney transplantation. A cross-sectional study in 190 graft recipients up to 20 years after transplantation. *Transplantation* 1995;59:982–986.
254. Julian BA, Laskow DA, Dubovsky J, et al. Rapid loss of vertebral mineral density after renal transplantation. *N Engl J Med* 1991;325:544–550.
255. Allen DB, Goldberg BD. Stimulation of collagen synthesis and linear growth by growth hormone in glucocorticoid-treated children. *Pediatrics* 1992;89:416–421.
256. Root AW, Bongiovanni AM, Eberlein WR. Studies of the secretion and metabolic effects of human growth hormone in children with glucocorticoid-induced growth retardation. *J Pediatr* 1969;75:826–832.
257. Ortoft G, Oxlund H. Qualitative alternations of cortical bone in female rats after long-term administration of growth hormone and glucocorticoid. *Bone* 1996;18:581–590.
258. Wehrenberg WB, Janowski BA, Piering AW, et al. Glucocorticoids: potent inhibitors and stimulators of growth hormone secretion. *Endocrinology* 1990;126:3200–3203.
259. Aubia J, Masramon J, Serrano S, et al. Bone histology in renal transplant patients receiving cyclosporin. *Lancet* 1988;2:1048–1049.
260. Movsowitz C, Epstein S, Fallon M, et al. Cyclosporin-A *in vivo* produces severe osteopenia in the rat: effect of dose and duration of administration. *Endocrinology* 1988;123:2571–2577.
261. del Pozo E, Lippuner K, Ruch W, et al. Different effects of cyclosporin A on bone remodeling in young and adult rats. *Bone* 1995;16:271S–275S.
262. Bryer HP, Isserow JA, Armstrong EC, et al. Azathioprine alone is bone sparing and does not alter cyclosporin A-induced osteopenia in the rat. *J Bone Miner Res* 1995;10: 132–138.
263. Warady BA, Hebert D, Sullivan EK, et al. Renal transplantation, chronic dialysis, and chronic renal insufficiency in children and adolescents. The 1995 annual report of the North American Pediatric Renal Transplant Cooperative Study. *Pediatr Nephrol* 1997;11:49–64.
264. Hokken-Koelega AC, van Zaal MA, van Bergen W, et al. Final height and its predictive factors after renal transplantation in childhood. *Pediatr Res* 1994;36:323–328.
265. Hokken-Koelega AC, de Muinck Keizer-Schrama SM, Drop SL. Effects of alternate-date or daily prednisone treatment on GH and cortisol levels in growth-retarded children after renal transplantation. *J Pediatr Endocrinol* 1994;7:119–125.
266. Fine RN, Yadin O, Nelson PA, et al. Recombinant human growth hormone treatment of children following renal transplantation. *Pediatr Nephrol* 1991;5:147–151.
267. Velasquez-Forero F, Mondragon A, Herrero B, et al. Adynamic bone lesion in renal transplant recipients with normal renal function. *Nephrol Dial Transplant* 1996;11:38–64.
268. Sanchez CP, Salusky IB, Kuizon BD, et al. Bone disease in children and adolescents undergoing successful renal transplantation. *Kidney Int* 1998;53:1358–1364.

70

PERITONEAL DIALYSIS

BRADLEY A. WARADY
BRUCE Z. MORGENSTERN
STEVEN R. ALEXANDER

Pediatric nephrologists have long recognized the importance of peritoneal dialysis (PD) as a renal replacement therapy (RRT) for children. PD was first used to treat children with acute renal failure more than 50 years ago and to treat children with end-stage renal disease (ESRD) more than 30 years ago (1,2). Recent developments have dramatically increased reliance on PD as a maintenance RRT for children with ESRD. As more pediatric nephrologists have become directly involved in the management of children receiving maintenance PD, our understanding of the technique and its pediatric applications has increased substantially.

This chapter reviews current approaches to the clinical applications of PD in pediatric patients. However, entire textbooks have been published on the subject of PD (3,4), as have extensive monographs focused on various aspects of the use of this therapy in children (5,6). Although every effort has been made in this chapter to summarize accurately current knowledge specific to this field, no attempt has been made to do so completely; interested readers are encouraged to consult source materials cited throughout this chapter for more details. In addition, topics such as growth, osteodystrophy, and anemia, which are pertinent to all pediatric patients with ESRD irrespective of dialysis modality, are discussed in other chapters of this book.

NOTES ON THE HERITAGE OF PEDIATRIC PERITONEAL DIALYSIS

The peritoneal cavity has been used in the treatment of serious illness in children for at least 80 years. In 1918, Blackfan and Maxcy described the successful use of intraperitoneal injections of saline solution in dehydrated infants (7), a method that is still used today in rural areas of some developing countries. The first reports of the use of PD to treat children with renal failure were published by Bloxsum and Powell in 1948 and by Swan and Gordon in 1949 (1,8). These papers appeared when the worldwide reported clinical experience with PD was less than 100 patients (9). As detailed by Swan and Gordon (8), the technique allowed large volumes of dialysate to flow continuously by gravity from 20-L carboys through a rigid metal catheter that had been surgically implanted into the upper abdomen. Dialysate was constantly drained from the peritoneal cavity by water suction through an identical catheter implanted in the pelvis. This technique today is termed *continuous peritoneal lavage*, and, in some ways, it foretold the current emphasis on continuous as opposed to intermittent PD (IPD) therapies.

Swan and Gordon maintained fluid balance in their young patients by adjusting the dialysate dextrose content between 2 and 4 g/100 mL, as is generally done today. Excellent solute removal was achieved with an average dialysate delivery of 33 L daily. Dialysate temperature was regulated by adjusting the number of illuminated 60-watt incandescent light bulbs in a box placed over the dialysate inflow path. Although two of the three children treated for acute renal failure by Swan and Gordon survived after 9 and 12 days of continuous peritoneal lavage, this technique did not attract much interest among physicians treating children with renal failure during this period because it was more than a decade before the use of PD in children was again reported. During the 1950s, the development of disposable nylon catheters and commercially prepared dialysis solutions made PD a practical short-term treatment for acute renal failure (10). Successful adaptation of the technique, known then and now as *acute IPD*, for use in infants and children with acute renal failure was first reported in 1961 by Segar et al. (11) and in 1962 by Etteldorf et al. (12).

Although successful in treating acute renal failure, PD did not appear to be useful in the treatment of children with ESRD. Early acute IPD techniques required reinsertion of the dialysis catheter for each treatment (2), making prolonged use in small patients essentially impossible. The development of a "permanent" peritoneal catheter, first proposed by Palmer et al. (13,14) and later perfected by Tenckhoff and Schecter (15), made long-term IPD an accessible form of RRT for pediatric ESRD patients. When Boen et al. (16) and then Tenckhoff et al. (17) devised an automated dialysate delivery system that could be used in the home, long-term IPD became a practical and potentially desirable alternative to long-term hemodialysis (HD) for children with ESRD.

A new era in the history of PD as a treatment for children with ESRD was heralded by the description in 1976 by Popovich et al. of a "novel portable/wearable equilibrium dialysis technique" that is now called continuous ambulatory PD (CAPD) (18). Pediatric nephrologists were quick to recognize the potential advantages CAPD offered to their young patients, perhaps because PD was familiar to those who regularly treated children with acute renal failure. Advantages over HD of special importance to children included near steady-state biochemical control, no disequilibrium syndrome, greatly reduced dietary restrictions and fluid limits, and freedom from repeated dialysis needle punctures. CAPD also allowed children of all ages to receive dialysis in the home and thus to have more normal childhoods. Importantly, CAPD made possible the routine treatment of very young infants with ESRD, thereby extending the option of RRT to an entire patient population previously considered too young to be suitable for chronic treatment.

CAPD was first used in a child in 1978 in Toronto (19,20). Since 1975, CAPD and its many modifications [which together can be called *continuous PD* (CPD)] have become the dialysis treatment modalities most commonly prescribed for children with ESRD throughout much of the world (21). Because CPD is now so important to pediatric dialysis programs, much of the information presented is devoted to a review of current CPD practices that are, in many instances, based on the results of clinical investigative efforts conducted since 1999.

PERITONEAL MEMBRANE ANATOMY AND PHYSIOLOGY IN CHILDREN

Peritoneal Ultrastructure

The peritoneum is a serous membrane composed of thin layers of loose connective tissue covered by a sheet of mesothelium. It is a "living membrane" considered to have two principal parts: the parietal peritoneum lining the inner surface of the abdominal and pelvic walls (including the diaphragm) and the visceral peritoneum, which covers the intraperitoneal organs, forms the visceral mesentery and omentum, and connects loops of bowel (22). The peritoneal cavity ordinarily contains only small amounts of fluid.

The arterial blood supply to the parietal peritoneum comes from the vasculature of adjacent structures; the visceral peritoneum receives arterial blood from the celiac and superior and inferior mesenteric arteries. Almost all venous blood from both visceral and parietal peritoneum is drained ultimately to the portal vein. The portion of the peritoneal capillary bed that actually participates in solute and fluid exchange during PD is unknown and is the subject of some controversy. Studies in the rat have suggested that most of the small vessels capable of exchange are located in the reflections of peritoneum over loops of bowel (23), whereas other experimental data in eviscerated rats demonstrated that the visceral peritoneum is not necessary for fluid and solute exchange (24,25). The peritoneum has an active lymphatic system, which is comprised of specialized structures located on the undersurface of the diaphragm (the lacunae). Drainage via these subdiaphragmatic lacunae ultimately reaches the right lymphatic duct and, to a lesser extent, the thoracic duct.

Peritoneal Surface Area

The precise overall size of the peritoneal membrane relative to the body size of the child is uncertain. Clearly, the peritoneal membrane grows along with a growing child. This then raises the question of whether the membrane bears some constant relationship to body size, either for weight, height, or surface area. Clinical and experimental data (26) suggest that throughout life the membrane is proportional more to body surface area (BSA) than body weight.

There are few actual measures of the peritoneum that have been published. Originally estimated to equal BSA (27), it is clear that the size of the membrane that actually participates in exchange is significantly smaller than that (28,29). The total membrane size is likely less relevant than the total membrane pore area or, more precisely, the membrane pore area of that part of the peritoneum which is engaged in exchanges. There are limited data available on this topic in children, and that which is available has been derived from kinetic modeling of transperitoneal exchanges. It has been estimated from three-pore models of transperitoneal solute and solvent movement that the total pore area with respect to the diffusion distance (A_0/Δ_x) is between 1.53 and 2.40 m^2/cm of diffusion distance/1.73 m^2 (30,31). Further data using the same model and both lactate-based and bicarbonate-based dialysate found a steady-state A_0/Δ_x of 2.65 ± 0.98 $m^2/cm/1.73m^2$. To demonstrate the varying nature of a living membrane, the A_0/Δ_x at 30 minutes into the exchange was much higher than the steady-state value, 4.27 ± 1.37 $m^2/cm/1.73$ m^2 using bicarbonate-based buffer and 4.56 ± 1.20 $m^2/cm/1.73$ m^2 with lactate-based fluid (32). The mechanisms underlying the vasodilation that is presumed to be the etiology of this finding have not yet been elucidated.

Peritoneum as a Dialyzing Membrane

The peritoneal exchange process is the sum of two simultaneous and interrelated transport mechanisms: diffusion and convection. *Diffusion* refers to the movement of solute down a concentration gradient, whereas *convection* refers to movement of solutes that are "transported" in a fluid flux, the magnitude of which is determined by the ultrafiltration rate (33). As noted, it is the functional and not the anatomic peritoneal surface area that is important in peritoneal exchange.

Diffusion and convection are clinically linked processes under most circumstances, since the most commonly used agent to generate a gradient to drive the fluid flux that is necessary for convection is glucose. Glucose acts osmotically, and the osmotic forces serve to draw water from the vascular space into the peritoneal cavity. Glucose, however, is a small molecule and is subject to the diffusive process, because intraperitoneal glucose concentrations at the start of an exchange are much greater than blood glucose concentrations.

The living nature of the peritoneum and the interdependence between the processes of diffusion and convection make the scientific study of transperitoneal exchange quite complex and difficult. Several theories have been developed to model the movement of water and solute across the peritoneal membrane, each progressively more complex but each, in turn, more accurate. The development of CAPD in the mid-1970s was also accompanied by the development of a distributed pore model. Recently, a more comprehensive model has been developed that is known as the three-pore model. As one would expect from the name, the model postulates three types of pores:

1. Ultra-small transcellular water pores or channels, which comprise perhaps 1 to 2% of the total pore area, yet account for 40% of water flow, and are driven by osmotic forces.
2. Small pores, which are 4 to 6 nm in diameter and comprise 90% of total pore area. These pores are subject to both concentration gradients (diffusive forces) and osmotic gradients (convective forces).
3. Large pores, which are greater than 40 nm in diameter and comprise the remaining 5 to 7% of total pore area. These pores allow larger molecules, such as albumin, to leave capillaries, probably driven by hydrostatic forces within the capillary bed.

Although water moves through all three pores, only the small and large pores allow convective solute transfer (34). The three-pore model has been applied to PD studies in infants and children (30,31).

Diffusive Transport

In the absence of an osmotic gradient between blood and dialysate, the rate of diffusive transfer of a solute is directly related to the product of the concentration gradient of the solute across the peritoneal membrane and the mass transfer area coefficient (MTAC) of that solute. The solute concentration gradient is dynamic during an exchange and decreases exponentially for small solutes. For larger solutes, diffusion is so slow that the loss of the gradient is essentially linear. The MTAC is equal to the theoretic maximum clearance the membrane allows for a given solute—at the point when the dialysate concentration is zero—and is the product of the permeability of the peritoneum and the effective surface area. MTAC is a parameter that, as a physiologic principle, is independent of dialysis mechanics (i.e., exchange volume, dialysate dextrose concentration) (33). The MTAC, as applied to current three-pore models of transperitoneal solute and water flux, is equal to the product of the free diffusion coefficient for the solute, the fractional area available for diffusion (which is a percent of the area of the unrestricted pores), and the term A_0/Δ_x, which was described in Peritoneal Surface Area (35). There are no simple methods for determining MTACs. Precise estimates require rigorously performed PD exchanges and computer solutions of complex equations. There are some formulas that allow reasonable estimates of MTAC (36).

A few studies have measured MTAC values in pediatric patients; some have been calculated based on the mathematic model of peritoneal membrane transport devised by Popovich et al. (37); some by the simpler formulas, often from data obtained during a peritoneal equilibration test (PET) test (see later); and still others using the three-pore models. In an early study, Morgenstern et al. found MTAC values for urea, creatinine, uric acid, and glucose in eight children, 1.5 to 18.0 years of age, to be similar to adult reference values (38). Geary et al. determined MTAC values in 28 pediatric patients and provided evidence to suggest that solute transport capacity varies with age and does not approach adult values until later childhood (39).

Warady et al. determined the MTACs for urea, creatinine, glucose, and potassium in 95 children ranging in ages from less than 1 to 20 years of age who were evaluated in a standardized manner with the test exchange volume scaled to BSA (i.e., 1100 mL/m^2) (36). When MTAC was scaled for BSA, using analysis of variance, there were only differences by age for the MTAC for glucose and potassium (the younger children having a higher value). However, by quadratic regression analysis, there was greater transport capacity in the youngest patients (those younger than 3 years) for these two solutes and creatinine. This enhanced transport is likely the result of differences in either permeability or effective surface area (36). MTAC has also been determined in children undergoing PD studies based on the three-pore model. The values for children, when scaled for BSA, are similar to those of adults (40).

Diffusive transfer, as noted earlier, is dependent on the MTAC and the transmembrane concentration gradient, which diminishes during exchanges. The rate of diminishment is influenced by factors such as cycle frequency and dialysate volume. The impact of dialysate volume is felt to rest on the principle of geometry of diffusion (41), which simply states that the larger the dialysate volume, the longer the transperitoneal concentration gradient will persist to drive diffusion. In children, this principle has been a confounding variable in many studies of PD, because the studies have often been performed with fill volumes that were not scaled properly to body size (currently accepted to be scaling to BSA).

This issue has been particularly apparent in studies of PD in infants, who have a greater ratio of BSA to weight than do older children and adults. Therefore, a 40-mL/kg body weight exchange in an infant represents a smaller volume/m^2 BSA than a 40-mL/kg exchange does in an adult. This relatively smaller volume results in more rapid equilibration of solute and the inaccurate perception of enhanced membrane transport capacity (26,42). The importance of scaling fill volume to BSA has been verified by Kohaut et al. (26), Schaefer et al. (43), de Boer et al. (44), and Warady et al. (45) in association with the Pediatric Peritoneal Dialysis Study Consortium (PPDSC).

The concentration gradient and hence diffusive transport is also impacted by the presence of residual peritoneal volume from previous exchanges. Residual volume can be substantial in children (36,46). Small solutes in the residual fluid will likely have equilibrated with serum; this will lead to a time "zero" solute concentration that is much greater than zero, despite the fact that the instilled dialysate concentration of a solute was zero. This will limit fluid flux and solute transport.

Convective Mass Transfer and Ultrafiltration

The removal of fluid during a PD exchange reflects the interaction of many factors: the hydraulic permeability of the peritoneal membrane, the permeability of the peritoneum to the osmotically active solutes on either side of the membrane, the absorption of fluid into peritoneal tissue, and lymphatic absorption. These latter phenomena serve to counteract transperitoneal ultrafiltration. Convective mass transfer, which is dependent on fluid removal, is not thought to participate to a great degree in the mass transfer of small solutes, whereas large solutes are removed almost exclusively by convection (33). Pyle has estimated that the contribution of convection to urea transport in a 4-hour CAPD exchange with 4.25% glucose is 12%; for inulin, 45%; and for total protein, 86% (47).

Although early reports and much clinical experience suggested that adequate ultrafiltration was more difficult to achieve in infants and young children, subsequent studies have failed to confirm these differences. As mentioned previously, proper scaling of the exchange volume is an important determinant of the rate of dissipation of the osmotic gradient that determines ultrafiltration. Other aspects of solute flux and convection have been far more difficult to solve, and these difficulties reconciling theory with clinical findings have been critical in the development of the three-pore model of fluid and solute transfer (48). The third pore has been postulated to be composed of water-only channels, a theory supported by the finding of aquaporin-1 channels in the peritoneum (49).

Peritoneal Fluid and Lymphatic Absorption

During PD, fluid is lost continuously from the peritoneal cavity both directly into the tissues surrounding the peritoneal cavity and via lymphatic vessels. Fluid absorption out of the peritoneal cavity remains poorly understood (48). Initially, flow through lymphatic vessels was believed to be the dominant pathway (50). Most recently, fluid absorption is believed to move primarily directly into the tissues surrounding the peritoneal cavity (51). Lymphatic absorption is only thought to account for 20% of fluid reabsorption (52). The limited data on lymphatic absorption in children are conflicting (53,54).

Fluid absorption rates can be determined when a PD exchange is modeled using the three-pore model. It is believed to be driven by intraperitoneal hydraulic pressure (51) and may be explained by the movement of dialysate into interstices in the peritoneal cavity, which allow for water absorption at the same time that ultrafiltration is occurring in the portion of the peritoneum where the bulk of the fluid remains (48). There are limited data available on fluid absorption using the three-pore model in children. In one study, the absorption rate increased with body size in absolute terms but decreased when normalized to body size. The decrease was slight when scaled to BSA but marked when scaled to body weight (30).

Principles of the Peritoneal Equilibration Test

The PET was developed by Twardowski et al. as a simple means of characterizing solute transport rates across the peritoneum that could have direct clinical applications (55). The construction of reference curves based on the kinetics of solute equilibration between dialysate and plasma (D:P ratio) after a 2-L exchange volume made possible the categorization of adult patients into those with high, high-average, low-average, and low peritoneal membrane solute transport rates and served as the basis for dialysis prescription (see later).

Twardowski's adult PET reference curves have not enjoyed widespread application in the pediatric PD population for two reasons. First, there has been the widely acknowledged but unproven perception that the solute transport function of the pediatric peritoneal membrane is different from that of the adult (56,57). The second reason is the uniform 2-L test exchange volume that is provided to all study patients, regardless of their size, in the Twardowski scheme. Obviously, this approach does not allow for modification of the exchange volume to reflect differences in body size (e.g., pediatric patient, small adult, large adult) and has contributed to the limited usefulness of this approach in children.

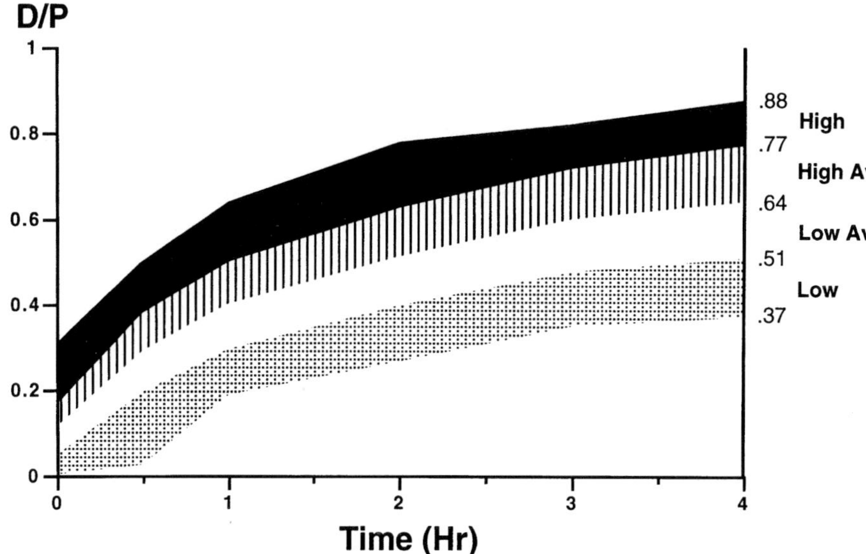

FIGURE 70.1. Peritoneal equilibration test results for creatinine. Shaded areas represent high, high-average, and low transport rates. The white band represents the low-average transport rate. The four categories are bordered by the maximal, mean +1 SD, mean, mean −1 SD, and minimal values for the population. D/P, dialysate:plasma ratio. (From Warady BA, Alexander SR, Hossli S, et al. Peritoneal membrane transport function in children receiving long-term dialysis. *J Am Soc Nephrol* 1996;7:2385–2391, with permission.)

Application of a standardized PET procedure for children has resulted from an appreciation of the previously mentioned age-independent relationship between BSA and peritoneal membrane surface area and the recommended use of an exchange volume scaled to BSA whenever one conducts studies of peritoneal transport kinetics (26,36,44,58,59). In the largest pediatric study to date, the PPDSC evaluated 95 children using a test exchange volume of 1100 mL/m^2 BSA to develop reference kinetic data (e.g., D:P and D:Do ratios), which can be used to categorize an individual pediatric patient's peritoneal membrane solute transport capacity (Figs. 70.1 and 70.2) (36). Similar reference data have been generated from pediatric studies in Europe with a test exchange volume of 1000 mL/m^2 BSA (59).

Because the transport capacity of a patient's peritoneal membrane is such an important factor to consider when determining the dialysis prescription, a PET evaluation should be conducted soon after the initiation of dialysis (60,61). However, there is evidence that a PET performed within the first week after initiation of PD may yield higher transport results than a PET performed several weeks later (62). Accordingly, whereas it may be most convenient to perform the initial PET at the conclusion of PD training, the results after 1 month of PD may more accurately reflect peritoneal transport properties (62,63). The PET evaluation should be repeated when knowledge of the patient's current membrane transport capacity is necessary for determination of the patient's PD prescription, especially when

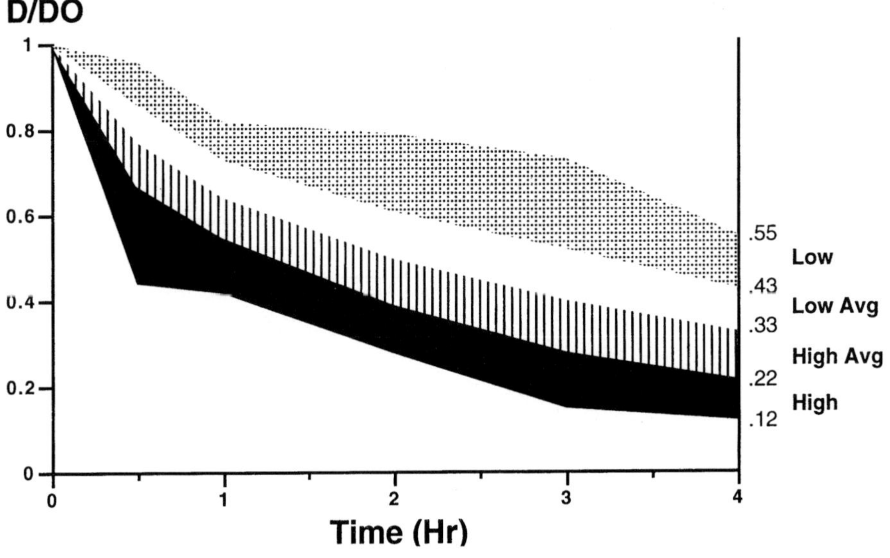

FIGURE 70.2. Peritoneal equilibration test results for glucose. Shaded areas represent high, high-average, and low transport rates. The white band represents the low-average transport rate. The four categories are bordered by the maximal, mean +1 SD, mean, mean −1 SD, and minimal values for the population. D/DO, dialysate glucose:initial dialysate glucose concentration ratio. (From Warady BA, Alexander SR, Hossli S, et al. Peritoneal membrane transport function in children receiving long-term dialysis. *J Am Soc Nephrol* 1996;7:2385–2391, with permission.)

clinical events have occurred (e.g., repeated peritonitis) that may have altered transport characteristics. In addition, knowledge of a patient's transport capacity may have a profound impact on their overall care because of the important relationships that exist between transport status and patient outcome in children and adults (64–67).

Proper evaluation of the data obtained requires that dialysate creatinine values be corrected for glucose interference because falsely elevated creatinine values may result when creatinine is measured by the Jaffe method (55). In addition, measured plasma solute concentrations must be divided by 0.9 to account for their presence in plasma water only and not in whole plasma. Failure to do so has resulted in solute D:P ratios greater than unity (68).

In summary, the contributions of diffusion and convection to peritoneal membrane kinetics in children have been characterized by the careful performance of standardized assessments of peritoneal membrane transport capacity. The uniform use of BSA as the scaling factor for the peritoneal exchange volume used in these evaluations has been particularly important. The accurate use of such assessments on a clinical basis (e.g., PET evaluation) requires the same attention to detail.

PERITONEAL DIALYSIS FOR ACUTE RENAL FAILURE

Indications and Contraindications

The conservative management of acute renal failure in infants and children requires meticulous attention to every detail of fluid and electrolyte balance. In these small patients, relatively minor errors can have grave consequences. However, several factors at work in pediatric patients tend to defeat even the most carefully conceived conservative management plans. Children have higher metabolic rates and thus can generate harmful solutes more rapidly. It is difficult to meet relatively greater dietary energy requirements in the oliguric child while abiding by stringent limitations on allowable fluid intake. Children with acute renal failure typically are profoundly catabolic, resulting in accumulation of potentially harmful amounts of potassium, phosphate, and other solutes at surprisingly rapid rates. Consequently, RRT tends to be used sooner and more often in pediatric patients with acute renal failure, especially neonates and young children (69,70). Widely accepted clinical indications for RRT in children with acute renal failure are covered in the Section X. Acute Renal Failure.

Traditionally, the convenience, simplicity, and relative safety of PD have allowed the nephrologist to begin dialysis in the child as soon as it is needed, without undue alarm over possible complications associated with the procedure itself. Two factors may make PD more suitable than HD for critically ill pediatric patients: ready access to the peritoneum (vs. typically more difficult vascular access) and better tolerance of PD by hemodynamically unstable children. The recent development of continuous hemofiltration techniques for children has provided a third option for treatment of the most critically ill pediatric patients (71–74). Although continuous hemofiltration does require vascular access similar to HD, it appears to be well tolerated by hemodynamically unstable children, especially those with cardiac failure in whom peritoneal perfusion is often poor, thereby interfering with the effectiveness of PD. Clear indications for one RRT over the others in the individual child with acute renal failure are rarely present, and often the experience of the treating center weighs most heavily in the choice of RRT modality (75,76).

Contraindications to acute PD are few. Absolute contraindications all relate to the lack of an adequate peritoneal cavity. Neonates with omphalocele, diaphragmatic hernia, or gastroschisis cannot be treated with PD. Recent abdominal surgery is not an absolute contraindication to PD as long as there are no draining abdominal wounds. However, such patients can often be treated more effectively with continuous venovenous hemofiltration or with HD if hemodynamically stable. Children with vesicostomies and other urinary diversions, polycystic kidneys, colostomies, gastrostomies, prune belly syndrome, and recent bowel surgery have been successfully treated with PD (77–79). PD has also been used routinely to treat acute renal failure related to allograft dysfunction after renal transplantation, as long as the allograft has been placed in an extraperitoneal location.

Technical Considerations

Catheters: Temporary versus Permanent

As with long-term PD, a reliable catheter is mandatory for successful therapy. The choice between a percutaneously placed temporary catheter and a "permanent" catheter placed surgically under direct vision is usually somewhat arbitrary, reflecting local practice. An increased incidence of peritonitis historically has been associated with the use of temporary catheters for longer than 72 hours (80), although a longer period of peritonitis-free use has also been documented (81).

Surgical placement of the same catheter that would be used for long-term PD has the advantage of assurance of good immediate function. The use of fibrin glue at the site of catheter entry into the peritoneum also may facilitate prompt catheter use without dialysate leakage (82). This advantage must be weighed in the patient against the risks and delays associated with a surgical procedure requiring general anesthesia in the operating room. Anesthesiologists are often reluctant to administer anesthesia to a child with the metabolic derangements of acute renal failure, despite the fact that those very metabolic derangements (e.g., hyperkalemia, acidemia, fluid overload) dictate the need for a PD catheter and thus an operative procedure. It may be

TABLE 70.1. PERITONEAL DIALYSIS SOLUTION CONTAINING BICARBONATE[a]

Component	mL	Na^+ (mEq)	Cl^- (mEq)	Mg^{2+} (mEq)	SO^{2-}_4 (mEq)	HCO_3^- (mEq)	Hydrous dextrose (g)
NaCl (0.45%)	896	69	69	—	—	—	—
NaCl (2.5 mEq/mL)	12	30	30	—	—	—	—
$NaHCO_3$ (1.0 mEq/mL)	40	40	—	—	—	40	—
$MgSO_4$ (10%)	1.8	—	—	1.5	1.5	—	—
$D_{50}W$	50	—	—	—	1.5	—	25
Total	999.8	139	99	1.5	3	40	25

[a]Calculated osmolality = 423 mOsm/kg H_2O.
Modified from Nash MA, Russo JC. Neonatal lactic acidosis and renal failure: the role of peritoneal dialysis. *J Pediatr* 1977;91:101–105.

more reasonable to initially place a percutaneous PD catheter under local anesthesia in patients who are to receive PD and who are considered to be at high risk for general anesthesia for any reason and then proceed to surgical catheter placement after the child is stable, and it is clear that more than 3 to 5 days of dialysis will be needed. For unstable infants in intensive care units, surgical catheter placement at the bedside using local anesthesia is readily accomplished in many pediatric centers (83,84).

Temporary catheters inserted percutaneously at the bedside have been used for decades. The classic nylon stylet-type catheter (Trocath, McGaw, Irvine, CA) has been replaced in most pediatric centers by a soft polyurethane or Teflon catheter that is placed over a guide wire using the Seldinger technique and a peel-away sheath (Cook Critical Care, Bloomington, IN). A similar technique has been developed for bedside placement of the same silastic Tenckhoff catheter that is used in chronic PD (85). Although percutaneously placed catheters rarely leak, poor dialysate drainage due to omental wrapping during outflow can be a common problem that is best remedied by replacement with a surgically placed catheter (86,87).

Dialysate

Dialysate is available from several manufacturers in standard hydrous dextrose concentrations of 1.5, 2.5, and 4.25%. Acute dialysis often is begun with 2.5% dextrose solution to obtain better ultrafiltration at the outset, when fluid overload often is a problem. Higher dextrose concentrations can be used but increase the risk of hyperglycemia and hypernatremia in small infants.

The usual electrolyte composition of commercially available dialysate is sodium, 132 mEq/L; chloride, 102 mEq/L; lactate, 35 mEq/L; magnesium, 1.5 mEq/L; and calcium, 3.5 mEq/L. Lower calcium (2.5 mEq/L) and magnesium (0.5 mEq/L) concentrations are readily available. Some critically ill infants do not tolerate the lactate that is absorbed from standard dialysate (88). These babies are often hypoxic and hypotensive, with an ongoing metabolic acidosis that is primarily due to accumulation of lactic acid. Additional lactate absorbed from the dialysate only worsens the situation. Such infants may do better if they are treated from the outset with a dialysate that has been specially formulated to contain bicarbonate instead of lactate. One approach to such a prescription is shown in Table 70.1. Note that calcium should be given by an alternate route when bicarbonate-based dialysate is used; typically, calcium may be provided as part of the total parenteral nutrition solutions in such critically ill infants. The recent development of pH-neutral, bicarbonate-buffered dialysis solutions designed for use in children with ESRD offers another possible approach to PD in the acidic infant that has yet to be tested in the acute renal failure setting (32).

Newly available (outside the United States) CPD solutions that contain a bicarbonate/lactate mixture, amino acids, or glucose polymers (89–91) may provide additional treatment options to meet the specific needs of selected patients with acute renal failure. A recent review from the European Paediatric Peritoneal Dialysis Working Group summarizes available information on the use of these new solutions in children receiving CPD (92).

Dialysate must always be warmed to body temperature before infusion into the child. Whereas adults may complain of discomfort during the inflow of unwarmed dialysate, small infants commonly respond to cool dialysate with a sudden fall in blood pressure. To avoid this problem, either blood transfusion warming devices placed in the dialysate inflow circuit or the heating device on an automated cycler can be used to warm the dialysate bags.

Acute Peritoneal Dialysis Equipment

A simple manual exchange method using a three-way stopcock, several intravenous line extension tubes, one or two in-line volumetric infusion chambers (Buretrol, Baxter Healthcare Corp., Deerfield, IL), and a urinary drainage bag can be easily prepared in an emergency for use in infants requiring only small exchange volumes. A closed infant dialysis administration set is also commercially available (Gesco Dialy-Nate Set, Gesco, San Antonio, TX) and adds the advantage of an in-line warming coil for infused dialysate. When the exchange volume exceeds 100 mL, an automated cycler can be used in most patients. Recent advances in cycler technology have allowed the use of exchange volumes as low as 50 mL (93).

Acute Peritoneal Dialysis Prescription

The PD prescription must specify dialysate composition, exchange volume, inflow, dwell, and drain times of each exchange and the number of exchanges to be performed in 24 hours. During the initial 24 hours after catheter placement, the exchange volume is kept low, no more than 500 mL/m^2 (i.e., 10 to 20 mL/kg) to reduce the risk of dialysate leakage. Over the ensuing 5 to 10 days, the exchange volume is increased gradually to reach a maximum of 1100 mL/m^2 (i.e., 35 to 45 mL/kg). Respiratory embarrassment and hydrothorax have been reported with the use of exchange volumes approaching 50 mL/kg (94–96).

Initial stabilization on PD often requires several days of continuous short exchanges (e.g., 30 to 60 minutes each) to remove accumulated solutes and excess fluid. This period corresponds to a traditional acute IPD regimen. Once the patient is stabilized, dialysis may be continued indefinitely. By gradually increasing exchange volumes toward 1100 mL/m^2 while either extending dwell periods (as in CAPD and continuous cycling PD) or introducing time off dialysis (as in nightly IPD), a typical maintenance CPD regimen may be reached in a few days. Familiarity with CPD as a treatment for ESRD has led to the popularity of standard CPD regimens in the treatment of acute renal failure. Although there have been no systematic studies of this approach to the acute PD prescription, the advantages of near steady-state biochemical and fluid control achievable with CPD are compelling, especially in infants and small children whose cardiovascular and nutritional status is often precarious. Finally, there is no need to periodically suspend CPD to see whether renal function will return; in the euvolemic child, renal function improves at its own pace, regardless of the presence or absence of CPD.

Complications of Acute Peritoneal Dialysis

Peritonitis

Peritonitis is a common complication of both acute and chronic PD that is discussed later.

Bleeding

Blood-tinged dialysate that clears after a few exchanges is frequently seen at dialysis initiation and is due to localized bleeding from the catheter insertion wound. Heparin should be added to bloody dialysate (250 to 500 U/L) to prevent catheter obstruction by small blood clots. Of much greater concern is bleeding from a laceration or perforation of a major organ or large vessel, as can be rarely seen with percutaneously placed catheters. The use of abdominal ultrasound guidance at the time of bedside catheter placement reduces the risk of serious catheter trauma and should be used routinely or whenever abdominal distention clouds the findings on physical examination.

The severity of intraperitoneal bleeding can be difficult to judge from the color of drained dialysate; as little as a few mL of blood will give a blood-tinged appearance to a relatively large volume of dialysate. When in doubt, a hematocrit can be obtained on the effluent.

Bladder Perforation

Perforation of the bladder can occur when the bladder is not completely emptied immediately before percutaneous catheter placement. Infants (in whom the normal bladder position frequently rises above the pelvis) and children with neuropathic or obstructed bladders are at particular risk. Bladder perforation may not be detectable until dialysis commences, when the sudden appearance of a suprapubic mass, polyuria, gross hematuria, and glycosuria make the diagnosis obvious. Careful catheter drainage of the bladder before dialysis catheter insertion and the use of abdominal/pelvic ultrasound to guide percutaneous catheter placement help prevent this complication.

Pain

After the catheter insertion wound has healed, PD should be a painless procedure. The presence of pain on inflow can be due to peritonitis, dialysate that is not at body temperature, local reaction to the low pH of commercial dialysate, local irritation from rapid dialysate inflow when straight catheters are used, omental or adhesion trapping of the catheter tip, and excessive distention of the abdomen. Rectal or suprapubic pain is usually due to migration or faulty placement of the catheter tip too deep in the pelvis between the bladder and the rectum. Shoulder pain is due to air under the diaphragm. Outflow pain can be seen early in the course of dialysis when the peritoneal cavity is drained too completely.

Investigation of painful dialysis should include abdominal radiographs (flat plate and cross-table lateral views) that provide a three-dimensional picture of catheter location. Constipation is a frequent contributing factor to both poor catheter drainage and painful dialysis. The use of laxatives and increased physical activity can sometimes relocate a poorly placed, painful catheter, but most often surgical repositioning, either open or laparoscopically, is required. The temporary addition of a low concentration of sodium bicarbonate to the dialysate often results in the resolution of pain that is secondary to the low dialysate pH (97).

Dialysate Leakage

Leakage most often occurs during the first few days of dialysis and can occur when initial exchange volumes are too large, when the catheter is frequently manipulated (as in too aggressive exit site care), or when traction of any type is placed on the catheter, as can occur during weighing or repositioning of the patient. Leakage is less likely when use of a new catheter can be delayed for 24 hours.

Temporary suspension of dialysis may be necessary. When this is not an option, the replacement of a percutaneous catheter over a guide wire with a larger catheter can be effective.

Poor Dialysate Flow

Reduced dialysate drainage is most often due to omental trapping of the catheter. Typically, dialysate inflow is adequate, but poor outflow leads to abdominal distention and fluid overload. Constipation, intraperitoneal adhesions, fibrin, blood clots, catheter migration or faulty position, tubing kinks, and running the dialysate directly into the drainage bag are additional considerations. Drainage will occasionally improve with simple flushing of the catheter using heparinized saline or dialysate. The instillation of a solution containing a fibrinolytic agent such as urokinase or tissue plasminogen activator may be helpful (98,99).

Hyponatremia/Hypernatremia

Hyponatremia is frequently seen in infants receiving nutrition based on human breast milk or standard formulas that are low in sodium (100). Both the removal of relatively large amounts of sodium in the ultrafiltrate that is in electrolyte equilibrium with serum and ongoing urinary sodium losses contribute to overall negative sodium balance. Aggressive oral or intravenous sodium supplementation is necessary to prevent symptomatic hyponatremia, which can present as the sudden onset of seizures.

Hypernatremia may occur as a consequence of peritoneal membrane sodium sieving during vigorous ultrafiltration with hypertonic dialysate (101). Additional free water may correct the hypernatremia but will make overall fluid removal goals more difficult to achieve.

Hypokalemia/Hyperkalemia

Hypokalemia can develop early in the course of acute dialysis, especially when high concentrations of dextrose are used in the dialysate and in parenteral nutrition solutions. Addition of potassium chloride to the dialysate at concentrations of 3 to 4 mEq/L should be undertaken when the serum potassium concentration falls below 4 mEq/L. The use of higher dialysate potassium concentrations (up to 20 mEq/L) has been reported but should be avoided in all but the most urgent situations; the intraperitoneal administration of nonphysiologic concentrations of potassium can be painful and may be damaging to the peritoneum (102).

Life-threatening hyperkalemia should not be treated with acute PD except as a last resort when no other RRT is available. Although potassium quickly equilibrates between serum and dialysate during an exchange, overall mass transfer of potassium is slow and inefficient. Acute HD remains the treatment of choice for severe hyperkalemia.

Respiratory Distress

Increased intraperitoneal pressure due to excessive or retained dialysate can cause dyspnea, hypoxemia, and respiratory failure, especially in small infants whose respiratory status is often fragile in the setting of acute renal failure and multiple organ system dysfunction. Hydrothorax due to a diaphragmatic hernia or eventration of the diaphragm (103) must also be ruled out. Thoracentesis can be used to establish the diagnosis of a diaphragmatic defect by demonstrating the high dextrose content of aspirated fluid. The addition of the dye methylene blue to the dialysate before thoracentesis can cause chemical peritonitis and is no longer recommended (104). In difficult cases, isotope scanning may be helpful (105).

Hypotension

Critically ill infants and small children may experience fluctuations in blood pressure as a consequence of the PD exchange procedure. Dialysate that is infused at room temperature can produce acute hypotension. Rapid infusion of dialysate can sometimes cause blood pressure to fall during aggressive ultrafiltration. A more frequent observation is hypotension during dialysate drain cycles. Both of the latter situations are usually the result of marginal hypovolemia and can be remedied by intravascular volume expansion.

Chyloperitoneum

Chylous ascites occurs when major intraperitoneal lymphatic drainage channels are interrupted and the patient ingests a fatty meal. Thus, chyloperitoneum will not occur until the patient with acute renal failure has begun oral feeds. Although the complication is rare, it can occur spontaneously in neonates (106) and has been reported in association with catheter insertion (107). The presence of cloudy, almost milky dialysate in the absence of any indication of peritonitis suggests the diagnosis; a dialysate triglyceride level that exceeds the plasma triglyceride level can confirm it, as can lipoprotein electrophoresis analysis of drained dialysate (108). A diet containing only medium chain triglycerides may allow continuation of PD (106).

PERITONEAL DIALYSIS FOR END-STAGE RENAL DISEASE

Indications for End-Stage Renal Disease Therapy

The indication for initiating dialysis therapy in children with ESRD depends on a combination of the biochemical and clinical characteristics of the child. When possible, dialysis should be initiated early enough to prevent the development of malnutrition and/or any significant uremic symptomatology. Although there is no definite level of blood urea nitrogen or serum creatinine concentration that mandates dialysis initiation, in most cases, dialysis should be started when the residual creatinine clearance has declined to a value between 9 and 14 mL/min per 1.73 m^2 or the weekly renal Kt/V_{urea} falls below 2.0 (63).

Selection of Peritoneal Dialysis or Hemodialysis for Children with End-Stage Renal Disease

It is not surprising that CPD is the most commonly used dialysis modality in specialized pediatric dialysis centers (109). Because CPD proceeds over prolonged periods (i.e., 24 hours per day for CAPD or continuous cycling PD; 8 to 12 hours for nightly IPD), body fluid composition and volume change slowly, resulting in a near steady state (110). The disequilibrium syndrome does not occur in children receiving CPD. Almost all children receiving CPD may be encouraged to eat an essentially unlimited diet, relatively high in protein, and with generous allowances for fluid and sodium. The relative simplicity and safety of CPD allow performance at home in all but the most exceptional circumstances, thereby returning the child with ESRD to regular school attendance (109) and facilitating family vacations and other normal childhood activities. CPD avoids the many difficulties associated with the maintenance of vascular access in children and eliminates the need for regular dialysis needle punctures.

It must be remembered, however, that there have been no randomized comparative studies of CPD and HD in children. Pediatric dialysis programs that once focused almost entirely on CPD have recognized that the availability of a chronic HD program designed for pediatric patients is of equal importance to the provision of optimum care for children with ESRD (111). Recent advances in HD techniques and equipment have made chronic HD an attractive alternative to CPD in many centers. Whenever possible, patients and families must be given the opportunity to participate fully in the selection of the chronic dialysis modality that is best suited to their individual needs and lifestyle.

Use of Continuous Peritoneal Dialysis for Children with End-Stage Renal Disease

Dramatic growth in the use of CPD as a maintenance dialysis treatment for children occurred throughout the world during the 15 years after its introduction to pediatric dialysis in 1978 (21). By 1993, ESRD patient registry reports showed that CPD was the most commonly prescribed long-term dialysis modality for children younger than 15 years in the United States, Canada, Australia, New Zealand, United Kingdom, former West Germany, Israel, Netherlands, and a few other countries (109,112).

Data on more recent CPD use in North American children have been compiled by the North American Pediatric Renal Transplant Cooperative Study (NAPRTCS). The NAPRTCS collects data on pediatric dialysis from more than 152 pediatric dialysis centers located in the United States, Canada, Mexico, and Costa Rica. Between 1992 and 2001, the NAPRTCS enrolled 4139 pediatric dialysis patients ages 1 day to 20 years (113). Of these, 2971 (65.4%) were receiving CPD. Although the majority of patients in all age groups were receiving CPD, the preference for CPD over HD was most pronounced among younger patients. Eighty-seven percent of infants and young children 0 to 5 years of age were receiving CPD, compared to 67% of children 6 to 12 years and 54% of patients older than 12 years.

It must be remembered that participation in the NAPRTCS is restricted to specialized pediatric dialysis centers staffed by pediatric nephrologists, a fact that may influence such observations as dialysis modality choice. Recent studies by Furth et al. have shown that older children treated in nonpediatric units are more likely to receive maintenance HD than CPD (114).

Patient Selection

CPD can be attempted in any child whose peritoneal cavity is intact and will admit a sufficient volume of dialysate. Experience has shown that CPD can be used successfully in children with the following conditions: polycystic kidney disease (usually after unilateral or bilateral nephrectomy), vesicostomy, cutaneous ureterostomy, colostomy, prune belly syndrome, bilateral Wilms' tumor, recent abdominal surgery (if no draining wounds are present), ventriculoperitoneal shunt, and concurrent immunosuppressive therapy (77,79,115–117). Patient age, gender, primary renal disease, and renal transplant status have no apparent influence on CPD outcome.

CPD is the clear treatment of choice for infants (113,118,119). Before the introduction of CPD, some pediatric dialysis programs did not accept infants for treatment. It is now widely recognized that CPD can be an effective maintenance RRT in babies who develop ESRD as early as the first few days or weeks of life (120). Despite these successes, mortality rates among infants on CPD are higher than in all other age groups. The NAPRTCS has shown that 1-year mortality risk for infants is more than three times greater than that for older age groups (121). Recent studies have suggested that the presence of extrarenal organ system injury and oligoanuria are the major contributing mortality risk factors for patients receiving CPD during the first 2 years of life (122,123).

Finally, a treating facility that provides CPD to children also should be able to provide the necessary multidisciplinary services required by the child and family. Successful CPD for children is a team effort. The team consists of CPD nurse specialists, nephrologists, urologists, general surgeons, renal dietitians, renal social workers, child psychologists, child psychiatrists, child development specialists, child life therapists, speech pathologists, and chaplains, all of whom are pediatric specialists. Children require a great investment of time and resources from the CPD team, and the effort that is involved is often several orders of magnitude greater than that required to care for the typical adult CPD patient (111).

Permanent Peritoneal Catheters for CPD

A reliable peritoneal catheter is the cornerstone of successful CPD, well worth the attention and effort required to "perfect" the procedure in each center that proposes to treat children with long-term PD. There are multiple types of PD catheters presently available, with a variety of configurations. In general, most long-term PD catheters are constructed of soft material, such as silicone rubber or polyurethane. The catheters can be thought of as having two separate regions: the intraperitoneal portion and the extraperitoneal portion. The intraperitoneal portion contains holes or slots to allow passage of peritoneal fluid. The shape of the intraperitoneal portion typically is straight or curled, the latter configuration often associated with less patient pain with dialysate inflow and a decreased predisposition to omental wrapping of the catheter. The most common catheters with these characteristics used by pediatric patients have been the straight and curled Tenckhoff catheters. The extraperitoneal portion of each of these catheters has one or two Dacron cuffs to prevent fluid leaks and bacterial migration and to fix the catheter's position. The shape of this portion of the catheter is variable and may be straight or have a preformed angle (e.g., swan neck or pail handle) to help create a downward-directed catheter exit site.

In general, it is believed that infants and young children with vesicostomies, ureterostomies, or colostomies require placement of the catheter exit site as far from the stoma as possible to prevent contamination and infection. Placement of the exit site on the chest wall has successfully limited the number of infections in such high-risk situations in a small number of children and adults (124–126). The primary reason for catheter revision is catheter malfunction, often caused by omental wrapping of the catheter (109). However, the decision to perform an omentectomy in conjunction with catheter placement is not universal (127). Catheter occlusion by fibrin may also occur but can usually be successfully relieved by the installation of fibrinolytic agents into the catheter (98,99).

In a 1995 report from the 18 centers of the PPDSC, most preferred a curled Tenckhoff catheter (88%), with fewer centers using a catheter with a straight intraperitoneal segment (127). The most common extraperitoneal design consisted of a straight tunnel with a single cuff (69%). Fewer centers used dual-cuff catheters with angled extraperitoneal regions. In most of the centers, the peritoneal catheter was placed by a surgeon, and in 53% of the centers, an omentectomy was performed. Finally, the exit site was directed downward in 69% of the centers, and 25% of centers indicated an upward exit site. Although no correlation between catheter characteristics and infection rate was provided, this small experience confirmed the significant variation in PD catheter choice and implantation strategies.

Daschner et al. have reported on the laparoscopic placement of 25 two-cuff Tenckhoff catheters in 22 pediatric patients (128). Postoperative leakage occurred in only two patients, and the procedure facilitated the performance of adhesionolysis and inguinal hernia repair at the time of catheter placement.

In the most recent report of the NAPRTCS, catheter characteristics were reported from 2971 independent courses of CPD accumulated from 1992–2001 (113). As was shown in previous reports, the annualized peritonitis rate decreased with increasing age and was best in association with Tenckhoff catheters with straight intraperitoneal segments, double cuffs, swan-neck tunnels, and downward pointed exit sites (109,121,129). In addition, time to first peritonitis episode was longer for catheters with two cuffs compared to one, with swan-neck tunnels compared to straight tunnels, and with downward exit sites compared to lateral exit sites or exit sites directed upward. These results confirm findings from the adult PD population (130).

Peritoneal Dialysis Prescription

In general, the PD prescription for children has evolved empirically from guidelines that adapted adult CAPD for pediatric patients. A CAPD regimen of four to five exchanges per day with an exchange volume of 900 to 1100 mL/m^2 BSA (35 to 45 mL/kg) of 2.5% dextrose dialysis solution has routinely yielded net ultrafiltration volumes of up to 1100 mL/m^2 per day. Using similar exchange volumes, the greatest percentage of children receiving CPD receive cycler dialysis with a regimen consisting of 6 to 10 exchanges over 8 to 10 hours per night.

The current goal of achieving dialysis adequacy in the most cost-effective manner has highlighted the need to be cognizant of a patient's BSA, peritoneal membrane solute transport capacity, and residual renal function when designing the dialysis prescription (36,61,131,132). In most patients (except for the rapid transporter), the most effective way to increase solute clearance is to initially increase the exchange volume followed by an increase in dialysis duration by prolonging the dwell time. Ideally, the prescription for all children should include an exchange volume of 1100 to 1400 mL/m^2 BSA, as tolerated by the patient. Measurement of the intraperitoneal pressure generated by escalating exchange volumes can be useful in determining the optimum dialysis prescription (133–135). In the case of the rapid transporter, an increase in the number of exchanges and a reduction of the dwell time per cycle can result in improved solute clearance.

As mentioned, the categorization of a patient's peritoneal membrane transport capacity can best be determined by the performance of a PET and comparison of the individual patient data to reference values (36). In turn, this information makes it possible to optimize the dialysis prescription in terms of dwell time. Recognizing that it is often impractical to consider the provision of a dialysis prescription based solely on kinetic data without reference to social constraints (e.g., school attendance, working parent), the use of the results of a PET evaluation can be particularly helpful in determining a cost-effective approach to PD modality selection (e.g., high transporter–cycling PD; high-average to low-average transporter CAPD or cycling PD ± additional daytime exchange). Often, this can be most easily achieved with the use of one of several computer-modeling programs that have been validated in pediatric patients and that can provide accurate estimates of solute clearance (30,136,137). It must be emphasized that in pediatrics, as well as in adults, predicted values are only estimates and do not substitute for actual measurements of solute clearance (see Peritoneal Dialysis Adequacy).

The residual renal function, a characteristic that appears to be better preserved by PD versus HD, is calculated as the average of urea and creatinine clearance and assumes greatest importance in the patient who does not attain target clearances with dialysis alone (63,138). Whereas the contribution of residual renal function toward a target goal may be significant early in the course of dialysis, a progressive loss of residual renal function usually occurs and mandates an associated enhancement of the dialysis prescription if target clearances are to be maintained (139–141).

Peritoneal Dialysis Adequacy

Until recently, most studies with adult PD patients in which clinical outcome parameters (e.g., frequency of hospitalization, patient mortality) have been monitored have characterized dialysis adequacy in terms of small solute clearance as a total (residual renal + PD) weekly Kt/V_{urea} greater than or equal to 2.0 and a total weekly creatinine clearance greater than or equal to 60 L/1.73 m^2 for the patient receiving CAPD (63). Minor differences in the recommendations exist for the cycler dialysis patient. Over the past several years, however, two publications have provided data that challenge current recommendations and require consideration. An analysis of data generated in the Canada-USA study by Churchill et al. has revealed superior patient and technique survival in the adult CAPD population with low/low average transport capacity and lower total creatinine clearance values compared to those patients who are high transporters (66). This has resulted in a change of the target creatinine clearance recommendation to 50 L/1.73 m^2/wk for this subset of patients in the guidelines of the National Kidney Foundation-Kidney Disease Outcomes Quality Initiative (NKF-K/DOQI) and the Canadian Society of Nephrology (63,142). In the ADEMEX study, adult CAPD patients were prospectively randomized to their routine CPD prescription versus a prescription targeted to a creatinine clearance of 60 L/1.73 m^2/wk. This study found no improvement in patient survival when the peritoneal clearance of small solutes was increased to the adequacy targets recommended by K/DOQI (143). However, deaths attributable to uremia and inadequate fluid removal were higher in the control population. Not unexpectedly, this experience has prompted a further reassessment of PD adequacy criteria in adults.

Current clinical experience supports the use of similar (or greater) target clearances for children. Reports by Höltta et al., McCauley et al., and Chadha et al. have all presented data suggestive of a correlation between patient outcome and solute clearance (144–147). The experience of Chadha et al. was also significant for demonstrating the influence that residual renal function has on patient outcome and the apparent contradiction of the presumed equivalence of PD and native solute clearance (147). The contribution of residual renal function is most apparent with respect to total creatinine clearance, as well as middle molecule clearance (148).

Can the solute clearance targets be achieved by children on CPD without introducing a prescription that has a significant negative impact on their quality of life? Whereas data by van der Voort et al. (149) suggests otherwise, the clinical experiences of Höltta et al. and Chadha and Warady provide good evidence that if the dialysis exchange volume is maximized and if the frequency of the exchanges is individualized and adjusted according to the peritoneal membrane transport characteristics, it should be possible to achieve the current K/DOQI clearance targets, at least for Kt/V_{urea}, in most children receiving CPD (144,150).

The ability to accurately estimate a patient's total body water (or V) is integral to the determination of Kt/V_{urea} as an adequacy measure. The K/DOQI guidelines have recommended the use of the gender-specific formulas of Mellits-Cheek for total body water assessment, despite the fact that the formulas were derived from studies of healthy children (151). Recently, more accurate estimates of V have at last become feasible after the analysis of additional body water data in the literature and after study of pediatric dialysis patients by bioelectrical impedance analysis as well as with the use of D_2O or H_2O^{18} (152–155). It is noteworthy, however, that there are few data to support the preference of one solute clearance measure (Kt/V_{urea} vs. creatinine clearance) over another and that discrepancies in the results may occur in as many as 20% of patients. This has prompted the recommendation that the evaluation of adequacy be based on the results of both clearance measures and an ongoing assessment of the patient's clinical condition (156,157). If there is discordance in achieving these targets, it has been suggested that the Kt/V_{urea} be the immediate determinant of adequacy because it directly reflects protein metabolism and is less affected by extreme variations in residual renal function (63).

Implicit in the approach to achieve and maintain dialysis adequacy is the need to repeatedly measure total solute clearance. Ideally, 24-hour collections of urine and dialysate fluid should be obtained three times per year or when there have been significant changes in the patient's clinical status that may influence dialysis performance (e.g., severe or repeated peritonitis).

In summary, current knowledge supports the clinical use of a target total weekly Kt/V_{urea} of greater than or equal to

2.0 and a total weekly creatinine clearance of greater than or equal to 60 L/1.73 m^2 to achieve dialysis adequacy in most children receiving CAPD (63). Patients receiving cycling PD likely require slightly greater clearances, and low transporters may do well with lower clearances if the pediatric experience is comparable to that of the adults. The continued accumulation of patient outcome data is critical to the ongoing assessment of these criteria.

Nutritional Management of Children Receiving Continuous Peritoneal Dialysis

The achievement of normal growth is uncommon among children treated with CPD, despite access to an essentially unlimited diet (158,159). Compared with normal healthy children, pediatric patients receiving CPD have significantly lower energy intake, as well as diminished height, weight, triceps skinfold thickness, and mid-arm muscle circumference (160). Hypoalbuminemia, hypertriglyceridemia, and hypercholesterolemia are commonly seen (161). Current guidelines from the National Kidney Foundation's K/DOQI program suggest the need to provide an energy intake of at least 100% of the recommended daily allowance (RDA) for children of the same gender and chronologic age (162). High-calorie formulas are often helpful to meet these requirements, particularly in infants who may require supplemental tube feeding by the nasogastric or gastrostomy routes (163–165). The K/DOQI guidelines recommend that supplemental nutritional support be considered when a child does not have a normal height velocity or is failing to consume the RDA for energy and/or protein, the latter problem often magnified by protein losses into dialysate (166,167). Supplementation by the oral route is preferred followed by enteral tube feeding (162).

The potential need for sodium, potassium, and phosphorus supplementation requires special attention. Young infants may have significant sodium loss in dialysate, as well as from their native kidneys as a result of underlying obstructive uropathy. Hypophosphatemia is especially common in association with the use of low phosphorus infant formulas (168). Either hyperkalemia or hypokalemia can also result from a combination of dialysate losses and dietary intake.

The nutritional status of every pediatric patient must be repeatedly and regularly evaluated to be certain that individual patient needs are constantly met. According to K/DOQI guidelines, the most valid measures of protein and energy nutrition status in children treated with maintenance dialysis include a dietary interview/diary, the serum albumin, the child's height or length, the estimated dry weight, the weight-for-height index, anthropometric measures (mid-arm circumference, muscle circumference or area, and skinfold thickness), head circumference for children younger than 3 years, and the standard deviation score (or Z score) for height (162).

Little prospective evidence is available to support supplementing water-soluble vitamins above the RDA or the dietary reference intakes for age (162,169,170). Supplements of the fat-soluble vitamins A, E, and K should be avoided, because elevated levels of vitamin A have been reported in children receiving CPD (171).

Peritonitis

The single most common complication that occurs in children maintained on CPD is peritonitis (121,172–176). Unfortunately, present data make it clear that children have a significantly greater rate of peritonitis than adults, with a substantial number of children experiencing an episode of peritonitis during their first year of CPD treatment. Reductions in observed peritonitis rates have been reported in both adults and children in association with treatment of *Staphylococcus aureus* nasal carriage; use of a two-cuff catheter, as well as with recent technical developments such as newer disconnect systems; and the flush-before-fill technique (172,176–181). The important contribution of prolonged dialysis training has also been demonstrated (182).

Recent evaluation of the NAPRTCS database has revealed a total of 2965 reported episodes of peritonitis in 3621 years of follow-up, resulting in an annualized peritonitis rate of 0.82 or one infection every 14.7 patient months (113). The rate of peritonitis was highest in the youngest patients (0 to 1 years of age) who had an annualized peritonitis rate of 1.02 or 1 infection every 11.8 months versus an annualized rate of 0.75 or 1 episode every 16.1 patient months in children more than 12 years of age. In this same report, gram-positive infections comprised slightly more than 50% of the episodes of peritonitis and gram-negative infections slightly more than 20%. Fungal peritonitis represented 2.3% of peritonitis episodes.

The current approach to the treatment of peritonitis relies primarily on the intraperitoneal administration of antibiotics. A key development has been the recent publication of the *Consensus Guidelines for the Treatment of Peritonitis in Pediatric Patients Receiving Peritoneal Dialysis* by an international committee of physicians and nurses under the auspices of the International Society of Peritoneal Dialysis (180). This set of 15 guidelines includes recommendations for empiric antibiotic therapy, treatment of gram-positive, gram-negative, and fungal peritonitis, and indications for catheter removal and replacement (Figs. 70.3, 70.4, and 70.5). The concern that has arisen regarding the development of vancomycin-resistant organisms and the vestibular, renal, and audiologic complications of aminoglycosides has influenced the content of several of the recommendations (183–185). An international registry is currently accumulating data regarding the application of these guidelines into clinical care.

Finally, sclerosing encapsulating peritonitis is a rare but extremely serious clinical entity characterized by the presence of continuous, intermittent, or recurrent bowel obstruction associated with gross thickening of the perito-

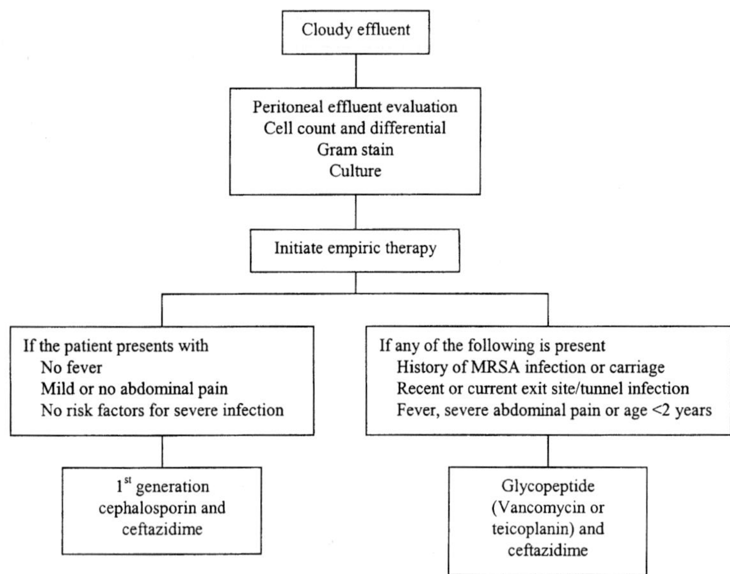

FIGURE 70.3. Treatment algorithm for empiric therapy of peritonitis. MRSA, methicillin-resistant *Staphylococcus aureus*. (From Warady BA, Schaefer F, Alexander S, et al. Consensus guidelines for the treatment of peritonitis in pediatric patients receiving peritoneal dialysis. *Perit Dial Int* 2000;20:610–624, with permission.)

neum (186). Although primarily diagnosed in adults, it may also occur in children, typically those who have received CPD for more than 5 years (187,188). The presence of peritoneal calcifications on abdominal computed tomography scan in association with ultrafiltration failure is highly suggestive of the diagnosis and may be an indication to discontinue CPD.

TREATMENT OUTCOME

Functional Integrity of the Peritoneal Membrane

The stability of the peritoneum as a dialyzing membrane is of particular interest because of the potential for the long-term need for CPD. Infection would seem to be a likely contributor to decreased long-term membrane function, but the data are conflicting. In a retrospective study in children, it has been reported that peritonitis caused by *Pseudomonas aeruginosa* or alpha streptococcal organisms was an independent predictor of membrane failure, defined as the severe loss of ultrafiltration capacity (189). When two other groups of children were assessed by means of solute D:P ratios derived during the performance of a PET conducted without standardized study mechanics, either no change over time or a deterioration was demonstrated (190,191). The peritonitis history of the cohort of children studied to develop the pediatric PET curves was reanalyzed and revealed higher MTAC for glucose and creatinine in those who had previous episodes of peritonitis (36,192). Similarly, in the one pediatric prospective evaluation of the peritoneal membrane as assessed by PET testing over a mean of 20 months between studies, there were no changes in MTAC for glucose or creatinine over time. However, in

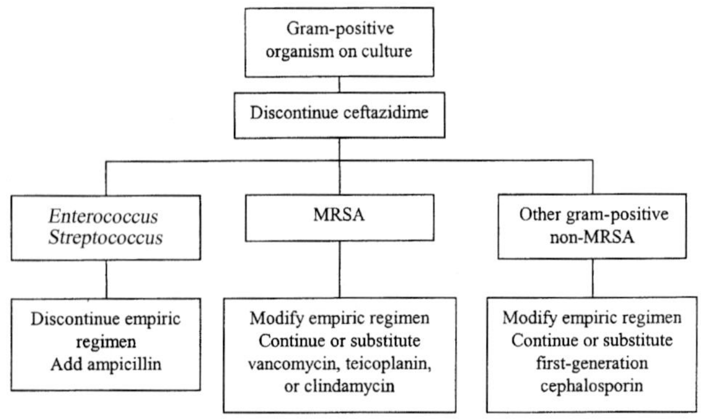

FIGURE 70.4. Treatment algorithm for gram-positive peritonitis. MRSA, methicillin-resistant *Staphylococcus aureus*. (From Warady BA, Schaefer F, Alexander S, et al. Consensus guidelines for the treatment of peritonitis in pediatric patients receiving peritoneal dialysis. *Perit Dial Int* 2000;20:610–624, with permission.)

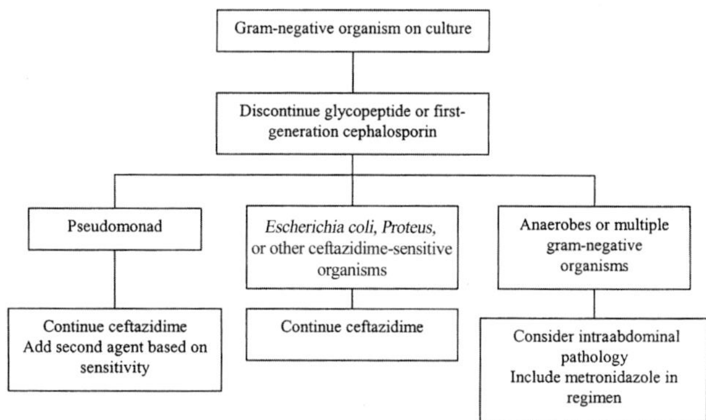

FIGURE 70.5. Treatment algorithm for gram-negative peritonitis. (From Warady BA, Schaefer F, Alexander S, et al. Consensus guidelines for the treatment of peritonitis in pediatric patients receiving peritoneal dialysis. *Perit Dial Int* 2000;20:610–624, with permission.)

the children with a history of peritonitis, the MTAC values increased (193). Finally, in one of the few studies evaluating peritoneal biopsy material from children, a reduced density of mesothelial microvilli presumably related to the duration of PD treatment and the presence of peritonitis was documented, as was fibrosis of the peritoneal membrane (194). However, the latter did not correlate with the frequency of peritonitis or the duration of PD therapy.

Quality-of-Life Issues

Health-related quality of life refers to the measure of a patient's functioning, well-being, and general health perception in each of three domains: physical, psychological, and social (195). In turn, a patient's quality of life is an important indicator of the effectiveness of the medical therapy he or she receives (196). Several characteristics of CPD permit an improved quality of life for many children and their families as reflected in one report in which older children who experienced both therapies preferred CPD over HD (197). The ability to attend school every day may be one of the most beneficial features of CPD for children. Data from the NAPRTCS showed that among patients maintained on PD, 77% were attending school full-time and 15% part-time or at home (113). Comparable values for the HD population were 46 and 36%, respectively. Very few restrictions to physical activities are necessary. However, children receiving CPD should avoid tackle football, wrestling, and some gymnastic exercises involving appliances (e.g., uneven parallel bars). Swimming is permitted, although attention must be paid to securing the catheter while in the water, and only chlorine-treated swimming pools (rather than lakes or rivers) are recommended. This philosophy also facilitates the ability of these children to participate in summer camping experiences that are commonly coordinated by dialysis team personnel (198). Nevertheless, data suggesting a decline in the quality of life over time for adult patients on CPD mandate the performance of formal investigations of quality of life in pediatric CPD patients to better evaluate this critical aspect of patient care (196,197,199).

Termination of Continuous Peritoneal Dialysis

Data on termination of CPD therapy are available from the NAPRTCS Registry (113). Of the 472 children who terminated CPD for reasons other than transplant, 45% of the children changed dialysis modality because of excessive infection. Patient/family choice and access failure were the reasons for modality change in 8% and 7%, respectively. In a single center study, Gulati et al. found the likelihood of technique failure to be increased in PD patients with hypoalbuminemia 1 month after dialysis initiation (200).

Patient Mortality

In the most recent annual report of NAPRTCS, an overall mortality rate of 8.5% was noted for the pediatric CPD population (113). An assessment related to age revealed a mortality rate of 14.9% for patients younger than 5 years at dialysis initiation, which was significantly greater than the mortality rate of 5.7% and 4.5% for patients in the 6 to 12 and older than 13 years age groups. The mortality rate for patients 0 to 1 years and 2 to 5 years was 18.9% and 8.3% with 1- and 3-year postinitiation mortality rates of 15.3% and 32.5% for the youngest patients, and 5.8% and 13.7% for the 2- to 5-year age group. These data confirm the high-risk status of the infant and young child with ESRD and are similar to data collected from children in Italy and Japan (112,201). The primary reported causes of death for all PD patients were infection (27.9%) and cardiopulmonary disease (20.9%). The primary causes of death for patients 0 to 5 years of age were the same with infection accounting for 27.1% of deaths and cardiopulmonary disease 19.8%. Although the specific reasons for the higher death rates seen in infants receiving CPD have not been well delineated, recent work has suggested that the presence of extrarenal disease, particularly pulmonary disease/hypoplasia and oliguria or anuria, are important risk factors (122,123).

REFERENCES

1. Bloxsum A, Powell N. The treatment of acute temporary dysfunction of the kidneys by peritoneal irrigation. *Pediatrics* 1948;1:52–57.
2. Feldman W, Baliah T, Drummond KN. Intermittent peritoneal dialysis in the management of chronic renal failure in children. *Am J Dis Child* 1968;116:30–36.
3. Gokal R, Khanna R, Krediet R, et al., eds. *The textbook of peritoneal dialysis*, 2nd ed. Boston: Kluwer Academic Publishers, 2000.
4. Khanna R, Nolph KD, Oreopoulos DG, eds. *The essentials of peritoneal dialysis*. Dordrecht: Kluwer Academic Publishers, 1993.
5. Fine RN, ed. *Chronic ambulatory peritoneal dialysis (CAPD) and chronic cycling peritoneal dialysis (CCPD) in children*. Boston: Martinus Nijhoff, 1987.
6. Fine RN, Alexander SR, Warady BA, eds. *Chronic ambulatory peritoneal dialysis (CAPD) and chronic cycling peritoneal dialysis (CCPD) in children*, 2nd ed. Boston: Kluwer Academic Publishers, 1998.
7. Blackfan KD, Maxcy KF. The intraperitoneal injection of saline solution. *Am J Dis Child* 1918;15:19–28.
8. Swan H, Gordon HH. Peritoneal lavage in the treatment of anuria in children. *Pediatrics* 1949;4:586–595.
9. Odel HM, Ferris DO, Power MH. Peritoneal lavage as an effective means of extra-renal excretion. *Am J Med* 1959;170:917–924.
10. Maxwell MH, Rockney RB, Kleeman CR, et al. Peritoneal dialysis: I. technique and applications. *JAMA* 1959;917–924.

11. Segar WE, Gibson RK, Rhamy R. Peritoneal dialysis in infants and small children. *Pediatrics* 1961;27:603–613.
12. Etteldorf JN, Dobbins WT, Sweeney MJ, et al. Intermittent peritoneal dialysis in the management of acute renal failure in children. *J Pediatr* 1962;60:327–339.
13. Palmer RA, Quinton WE, Gray JF, et al. Prolonged peritoneal dialysis for chronic renal failure. *Lancet* 1964;1:700–702.
14. Palmer RA, Newell JE, Gray JF, et al. Treatment of chronic renal failure by prolonged peritoneal dialysis. *N Engl J Med* 1966;274:248–254.
15. Tenckhoff H, Schecter H. A bacteriologically safe peritoneal access device. *Trans Am Soc Artif Intern Organs* 1966;14:181–186.
16. Boen ST, Mion CM, Curtis FK, et al. Periodic peritoneal dialysis using the repeated puncture technique and an automated cycling machine. *Trans Am Soc Artif Intern Organs* 1964;10:409–414.
17. Tenckhoff H, Meston B, Shilipetar G. A simplified automatic peritoneal dialysis system. *Trans Am Soc Artif Intern Organs* 1972;18:436–440.
18. Popovich RP, Moncrief JW, Decherd JW, et al. The definition of a novel wearable/portable equilibrium peritoneal dialysis technique. *Trans Am Soc Artif Intern Organs* 1976;5:64.
19. Oreopoulos DG, Katirtzoglou A, Arbus G, et al. Dialysis and transplantation in young children [Letter]. *BMJ* 1979;1:1628–1629.
20. Balfe JW, Irwin MA. Continuous ambulatory peritoneal dialysis in children. In: Legrain M, ed. *Continuous ambulatory peritoneal dialysis*. Amsterdam: Excerpta Medica, 1980.
21. Alexander SR, Honda M. Continuous peritoneal dialysis for children: a decade of worldwide growth and development. *Kidney Int* 1993;43:S65–S74.
22. Twardowski ZJ. Physiology of peritoneal dialysis. In: Nissenson AR, Fine RN, Gentile DE, eds. *Clinical dialysis*. Norwalk: Appleton & Lange, 1990.
23. Miller FN, Nolph KD, Joshua JG. The osmolality component of peritoneal dialysis solutions. In: Legrain M, ed. *Continuous ambulatory peritoneal dialysis*. Amsterdam: Excerpta Medica, 1980.
24. Fox SD, Leypoldt JK, Henderson LW. Visceral peritoneum is not essential for solute transport during peritoneal dialysis. *Kidney Int* 1991;40:612–620.
25. Alon U, Bar-Maor JA, Bar-Joseph G. Effective peritoneal dialysis in an infant with extensive resection of the small intestine. *Am J Nephrol* 1988;8:65–67.
26. Kohaut EC, Waldo FB, Benfield MR. The effect of changes in dialysate volume on glucose and urea equilibration. *Perit Dial Int* 1994;14:236–239.
27. Wegner G. Chirurgische Bemerkungen umlautuber die peritoneal Humlautohle, mit besonder Berucksichtigung der Ovariotomie. *Arch Klin Chir* 1887;20:51.
28. Chagnac A, Herskovitz P, Weinstein T, et al. The peritoneal membrane in peritoneal dialysis patients: estimation of its functional surface area by applying stereological methods to computerized tomography scans. *J Am Soc Nephrol* 1999;10:342–346.
29. Flessner MF, Lofthouse J, Zakaria ER. Improving contact area between the peritoneum and intraperitoneal therapeutic solutions. *J Am Soc Nephrol* 2001;12:807–813.
30. Schaefer F, Haraldsson B, Haas S, et al. Estimation of peritoneal mass transport by three-pore model in children. *Kidney Int* 1998;54:1372–1379.
31. Fischbach M, Haraldsson B. Dynamic changes of the total pore area available for peritoneal exchange in children. *J Am Soc Nephrol* 2001;12:1524–1529.
32. Schmitt CP, Haraldsson B, Doetschmann R, et al. Effects of pH-neutral, bicarbonate-buffered dialysis fluid on peritoneal transport kinetics in children. *Kidney Int* 2002;61:1527–1536.
33. Rippe B, Stelin G. Simulations of peritoneal transport during CAPD. Application of two-pore formalism. *Kidney Int* 1989;35:1234–1244.
34. Flessner MF. The peritoneal dialysis system: importance of each component. *Perit Dial Int* 1997;17:S91–S97.
35. Haraldsson B. Assessing the peritoneal dialysis capacities of individual patients. *Kidney Int* 1995;47:1187–1198.
36. Warady BA, Alexander SR, Hossli S, et al. Peritoneal membrane transport function in children receiving long-term dialysis. *J Am Soc Nephrol* 1996;7:2385–2391.
37. Popovich RP, Pyle WK, Rosenthal DA, et al. Kinetics of peritoneal dialysis in children. In: Moncrief JW, Popovich RP, eds. *CAPD update*. New York: Masson, 1981.
38. Morgenstern BZ, Pyle WK, Gruskin AB, et al. Convective characteristics of pediatric peritoneal dialysis. *Perit Dial Bull* 1984;4:S155–S158.
39. Geary DF, Harvey EA, Balfe JW. Mass transfer area coefficients in children. *Perit Dial Int* 1994;14:30–33.
40. Bouts AH, Davin JC, Groothoff JW, et al. Standard peritoneal permeability analysis in children. *J Am Soc Nephrol* 2000;11:943–950.
41. Morgenstern BZ. Equilibration testing: close, but not quite right. *Pediatr Nephrol* 1993;7:290–291.
42. Mendley SR, Majkowski NL. Peritoneal equilibration test results are different in infants, children, and adults. *J Am Soc Nephrol* 1995;6:1309–1312.
43. Schaefer F, Haas S, Mehls O. Analysis of peritoneal transport characteristic by peritoneal dialysis capacity (PDC) test in children. *Perit Dial Int* 1996;16:S11.
44. de Boer AW, van Schaijk TC, Willems HL, et al. The necessity of adjusting dialysate volume to body surface area in pediatric peritoneal equilibration tests. *Perit Dial Int* 1997;17:199–202.
45. Warady BA, Alexander S, Hossli S, et al. The relationship between intraperitoneal volume and solute transport in pediatric patients. *J Am Soc Nephrol* 1995;5:1935–1939.
46. Fukuda M, Kawamura K, Okawa T, et al. The peritoneal equilibration test variables in pediatric CAPD patients. *Acta Paediatr Jpn* 1994;36:57–61.
47. Pyle WK. *Mass transfer in peritoneal dialysis* [dissertation]. Austin: University of Texas, 1981.
48. Leypoldt JK. Solute transport across the peritoneal membrane. *J Am Soc Nephrol* 2002;13:S84–S91.
49. Krediet RT. The physiology of peritoneal solute transport and ultrafiltration. In: Gokal R, Khanna R, Krediet RT, et al., eds. *Textbook of peritoneal dialysis*. Dordrecht: Kluwer Academic Publishers, 2000.
50. Mactier RA, Khanna R, Twardowski ZJ, et al. Contribution of lymphatic absorption to loss of ultrafiltration and solute clearances in continuous ambulatory peritoneal dialysis. *J Clin Invest* 1987;80:1311–1316.

51. Flessner MF. Transport kinetics during peritoneal dialysis. In: Leypoldt JK, Austin RG, eds. *The artificial kidney: physiological modeling and tissue engineering.* Landes, 1999.
52. Rippe G. Is lymphatic absorption important for ultrafiltration? *Perit Dial Int* 1995;15:203–204.
53. Mactier RA, Khanna R, Moore H, et al. Kinetics of peritoneal dialysis in children: role of lymphatics. *Kidney Int* 1988;34:82–88.
54. Schroder CH, Reddingius R, van Dreumel JA, et al. Transcapillary ultrafiltration and lymphatic absorption during childhood continuous ambulatory peritoneal dialysis. *Nephrol Dial Transplant* 1991;6:571–573.
55. Twardowski ZJ, Nolph KD, Khanna R, et al. Peritoneal equilibration test. *Perit Dial Bull* 1987;7:378–383.
56. Putiloff PV. Materials for the study of the laws of growth of the human body in relation to the surface areas of different systems: the trial on Russian subjects of planigraphic anatomy as a means for exact anthropometry; one of the problems of anthropology. Report of Dr. P.V. Putiloff at the meeting of the Siberian Branch of the Russian Geographic Society, 1884.
57. Kohaut EC, Alexander SR. Ultrafiltration in the young patient on CAPD. In: Moncrief JW, Popovich RP, eds. *CAPD update.* New York: Masson, 1981.
58. Sliman GA, Klee KM, Gall-Holden B, et al. Peritoneal equilibration test curves and adequacy of dialysis in children on automated peritoneal dialysis. *Am J Kidney Dis* 1994;24:813–818.
59. Schaefer F, Lagenbeck D, Heckert KH, et al. Evaluation of peritoneal solute transfer by the peritoneal equilibration test in children. *Adv Perit Dial* 1992;8:410–415.
60. Warady BA. The peritoneal equilibration test (PET) in pediatrics. *Contemp Dial Nephrol* 1994:21–41.
61. Blake P, Burkart JM, Churchill DN, et al. Recommended clinical practices for maximizing peritoneal dialysis clearances. *Perit Dial Int* 1996;16:448–456.
62. Rocco MV, Jordan JR, Burkart JM. Changes in peritoneal transport during the first month of peritoneal dialysis. *Perit Dial Int* 1995;15:12–17.
63. NKF-K/DOQI. *Clinical practice guidelines for peritoneal dialysis adequacy.* New York: National Kidney Foundation, 2001.
64. Schaefer F, Günter K, Mehls O, et al. Peritoneal transport properties and dialysis dose affect growth and nutritional status in children on chronic peritoneal dialysis. *J Am Soc Nephrol* 1999;10:1786–1792.
65. Fried L. Higher membrane permeability predicts poorer patient survival. *Perit Dial Int* 1997;17:387–388.
66. Churchill DN, Thorpe KE, Nolph KD, et al. Increased peritoneal membrane transport is associated with decreased patient and technique survival for continuous peritoneal dialysis patients. The Canada-USA (CANUSA) Peritoneal Dialysis Study Group. *J Am Soc Nephrol* 1998;9:1285–1292.
67. Kagan A, Bar-Khayim Y. Role of peritoneal loss of albumin in the hypoalbuminemia of continuous ambulatory peritoneal dialysis patients: relationship to peritoneal transport of solutes. *Nephron* 1995;71:314–320.
68. Waniewski J, Heimburger D, Werynski A, et al. Aqueous solute concentrations and evaluation of mass transport coefficients in peritoneal dialysis. *Nephrol Dial Transplant* 1992;7:50–56.
69. Parekh RS, Bunchman TE. Dialysis support in the pediatric intensive care unit. *Adv Ren Replace Ther* 1996;3:326–336.
70. Renzik VM, Randolph G, Collins CM, et al. Cost analysis of dialysis modalities for pediatric acute renal failure. *Perit Dial Int* 1993;13:311–313.
71. Belsha CW, Kohaut EC, Warady BA. Dialytic management of childhood acute renal failure: a survey of North American pediatric nephrologist. *Pediatr Nephrol* 1995;9:361–363.
72. Warady BA, Bunchman TE. Dialysis therapy for children with acute renal failure: survey results. *Pediatr Nephrol* 2000;15:11–13.
73. Ronco C, Parenzan L. Acute renal failure in infancy: treatment by continuous renal replacement therapy. *Intensive Care Med* 1995;21:490–499.
74. Bunchman TE, Donckerwolcke RA. Continous arterial-venous diahemofiltration and continuous veno-venous diahemofiltration in infants and children. *Pediatr Nephrol* 1994;8:96–102.
75. Bunchman TE, McBryde KD, Mottes TE, et al. Pediatric acute renal failure: outcome by modality and disease. *Pediatr Nephrol* 2001;16:1067–1071.
76. Goldstein SL, Currier H, Graf JM, et al. Outcome in children receiving continuous hemofiltration. *Pediatrics* 2001;107:1309–1312.
77. Alexander SR. Pediatric CAPD update. *Perit Dial Bull* 1983;(suppl 3):S15–S22.
78. Flynn JT. Choice of dialysis modality for management of pediatric acute renal failure. *Pediatr Nephrol* 2002;17:61–69.
79. Alexander SR, Lubischer JT. Continuous ambulatory peritoneal dialysis in pediatrics: 3 years' experience at one center. *Nefrologia* 1982;11:53–62.
80. Day RE, White RHR. Peritoneal dialysis in children: review of 8 years' experience. *Arch Dis Child* 1977;52:56–61.
81. Bunchman TE. Acute peritoneal dialysis access in infant renal failure. *Perit Dial Int* 1996;16:S509–S511.
82. Sojo E, Bisigniano L, Falke G, et al. Is fibrin glue (FG) useful in preventing dialysate leakage (DL) in children on CAPD? Preliminary results of a prospective randomized study. *Perit Dial Int* 1997;17:S89.
83. Leumann EP, Knecht B, Dangel P, et al. Peritoneal dialysis in newborns: technical improvements. In: Bulla M, ed. *Renal insufficiency in children.* New York: Springer-Verlag, 1982.
84. Borzotta A, Harrison HL, Groff DB. Technique of peritoneal dialysis cannulation in neonates. *Surg Gynecol Obstet* 1983;157:73–74.
85. Reznik VM, Griswold WR, Peterson BM, et al. Peritoneal dialysis for acute renal failure. *Pediatr Nephrol* 1991;5:715–717.
86. Lewis MA, Nycyk JA. Practical peritoneal dialysis—the Tenckhoff catheter in acute renal failure. *Pediatr Nephrol* 1992;6:470–475.
87. Chadha V, Warady BA, Blowey DL. Tenckhoff catheters prove superior to Cook catheters in pediatric acute peritoneal dialysis. *Am J Kidney Dis* 2000;35:1111–1116.
88. Nash MA, Russo JC. Neonatal lactic acidosis and renal failure: the role of peritoneal dialysis. *J Pediatr* 1977;91:101–105.

89. Tranaeus A. A long-term study of bicarbonate/lactate-based peritoneal dialysis solution—clinical benefits. *Perit Dial Int* 2000;20:516–523.
90. de Boer AW, Schroder CH, van Vliet R, et al. Clinical experience with icodextrin in children: ultrafiltration profiles and metabolism. *Pediatr Nephrol* 2000;15:21–24.
91. Canepa A, Verrina E, Perfumo F, et al. Value of intra-peritoneal amino acids in children treated with chronic peritoneal dialysis. *Perit Dial Int* 1999;19:S435–S440.
92. Schroder CH. European Paediatric Peritoneal Dialysis Working Group. The choice of dialysis solutions in pediatric chronic peritoneal dialysis: guidelines of an ad hoc European committee. *Perit Dial Int* 2001;21:568–574.
93. Warady BA, Lane J, Mentser M, et al. Use of HomeChoice automated peritoneal dialysis cycler with low fill volume drain logic in pediatric patients with peritoneal dialysis fill volumes less than 1000 mL. *Perit Dial Int* 2002;22(suppl 1):S76.
94. Lorentz WB. Acute hydrothorax during peritoneal dialysis. *J Pediatr* 1979;94:417–419.
95. Rose GM, Conley SB. Unilateral hydrothorax in small children on chronic continuous peritoneal dialysis. *Pediatr Nephrol* 1989;3:89–91.
96. Kawaguchi AL, Dunn JC, Fonkalsrud EW. Management of peritoneal dialysis-induced hydrothorax in children. *Am Surg* 1996;62:820–824.
97. Bunchman TE, Ballal SH. Treatment of inflow pain by pH adjustment of dialysate in peritoneal dialysis. *Perit Dial Int* 1991;11:179–180.
98. Stadermann MB, Rusthoven E, van de Kar NC, et al. Local fibrinolytic therapy with urokinase for peritoneal dialysis catheter obstruction in children. *Perit Dial Int* 2002;22:84–86.
99. Shea M, Hmiel SP, Beck AM. Use of tissue plasminogen activator for thrombolysis in occluded peritoneal dialysis catheters in children. *Adv Perit Dial* 2001;17:249–252.
100. Paulsen WD, Bock GH, Nelson AP, et al. Hyponatremia in the very young chronic peritoneal dialysis patient. *Am J Kidney Dis* 1989;14:196–199.
101. Ahearn DJ, Nolph KD. Controlled sodium removal with peritoneal dialysis. *Trans Am Soc Artif Intern Organs* 1972;18:423–428.
102. Spital A, Sterns R. Potassium supplementation via dialysate in continuous ambulatory peritoneal dialysis. *Am J Kidney Dis* 1985;6:173–176.
103. Bjerki HS, Adkins ES, Foglia RP. Surgical correction of hydrothorax from diaphragmatic eventration in children on peritoneal dialysis. *Surgery* 1991;109:550–554.
104. Macia M, Gallego E, Garcia-Cobaleda I, et al. Methylene blue as a cause of chemical peritonitis in a patient on peritoneal dialysis. *Clin Nephrol* 1995;43:136.
105. Mestas D, Wauquier JP, Escande G, et al. Diagnosis of hydrothorax complicating CAPD and demonstration of successful therapy by scintigraphy [Letter]. *Pediatr Dial Int* 1991;11:283–285.
106. Melnick JZ, McCarty CM, Hunchik MP, et al. Chylous ascites complicating neonatal peritoneal dialysis. *Pediatr Nephrol* 1995;9:753–755.
107. Pomeranz A, Reichenberg Y, Schurr D, et al. Chyloperitoneum: a rare complication of peritoneal dialysis. *Perit Dial Bull* 1984;4:114–117.
108. Porter J, Wang WH, Oliveria DB. Chylous ascites and CAPD. *Nephrol Dial Transplant* 1991;6:659–661.
109. Warady BA, Hebert D, Sullivan EK, et al. Renal transplantation, chronic dialysis, and chronic renal insufficiency in children and adolescents. The 1995 annual report of the North American pediatric renal transplant cooperative study. *Pediatr Nephrol* 1997;11:49–64.
110. Baum M, Powell D, Calvin S, et al. Continuous ambulatory peritoneal dialysis in children: comparison with hemodialysis. *N Engl J Med* 1982;307:1537–1542.
111. Warady BA, Alexander SR, Watkins SL, et al. Optimal care of the pediatric end-stage renal disease patient on dialysis. *Am J Kidney Dis* 1999;33:567–583.
112. Honda M, Iitaka K, Kawaguchi H, et al. The Japanese national registry data on pediatric CAPD patients: a ten-year experience. A report of the Study Group of Pediatric PD Conference. *Perit Dial Int* 1996;16:269–275.
113. Neu AM, Ho PL, McDonald RA, et al. Chronic dialysis in children and adolescents. The 2001 NAPRTCS annual report. *Pediatr Nephrol* 2002;17:656–663.
114. Furth SL, Powe NR, Hwang W, et al. Does greater pediatric experience influence treatment choices in chronic disease management? Dialysis modality choice for children with ESRD. *Arch Pediatr Adolesc Med* 1997;151:545–550.
115. Balfe JW, Vigneaux A, Williamson J, et al. The use of CAPD in the treatment of children with end-stage renal disease. *Perit Dial Bull* 1981;1:35–38.
116. Fine RN, Salusky IB, Ettenger RB. The therapeutic approach to the infant, child, and adolescent with end-stage renal disease. *Pediatr Clin North Am* 1987;34:789–801.
117. Evans ED, Greenbaum LA, Ettenger RB. Principles of renal replacement therapy in children. *Pediatr Clin North Am* 1995;42:1579–1602.
118. Warady BA, Bunchman TE. An update on peritoneal dialysis and hemodialysis in the pediatric population. *Curr Opin Pediatr* 1996;8:135–140.
119. Neu AM, Warady BA. Dialysis and renal transplantation in infants with irreversible renal failure. *Adv Ren Replace Ther* 1996;3:48–59.
120. Warady BA, Belden B, Kohaut E. Neurodevelopmental outcome of children initiating peritoneal dialysis in early infancy. *Pediatr Nephrol* 1999;13:759–765.
121. Warady BA, Sullivan EK, Alexander SR. Lessons from the peritoneal dialysis patient database: a report of the North American pediatric renal transplant cooperative study. *Kidney Int* 1996;49:S68–S71.
122. Ellis EN, Pearson D, Champion B, et al. Outcome of infants on chronic peritoneal dialysis. *Adv Perit Dial* 1995;11:266–269.
123. Wood EG, Hand M, Briscoe DM, et al. Risk factors for mortality in infants and young children on dialysis: a report of the North American Pediatric Renal Transplant Cooperative Study (NAPRTCS). *Am J Kidney Dis* 2001;37:573–579.
124. Sieniawska M, Roszkowska-Blaim M, Warchol S. Preliminary results with the swan neck presternal catheter for CAPD in children. *Adv Perit Dial* 1993;9:321–324.
125. Twardowski ZJ, Prowant BF, Pickett B, et al. Four-year experience with swan neck presternal peritoneal dialysis catheter. *Am J Kidney Dis* 1996;27:99–105.

126. Chadha V, Jones LL, Ramirez ZD, et al. Chest wall peritoneal dialysis catheter placement in infants with a colostomy. *Adv Perit Dial* 2000;16:318–320.
127. Neu AM, Kohaut EC, Warady BA. Current approach to peritoneal access in North American children: a report of the pediatric peritoneal dialysis study consortium. *Adv Perit Dial* 1995;11:289–292.
128. Daschner M, Gfrörer S, Zachariou Z, et al. Laparoscopic Tenckhoff catheter implantation in children. *Perit Dial Int* 2002;22:22–26.
129. Lerner GR, Warady BA, Sullivan EK, et al. Chronic dialysis in children and adolescents. The 1996 annual report of the North American Pediatric Renal Transplant Cooperative Study. *Pediatr Nephrol* 1999;13:404–417.
130. Golper TA, Brier ME, Bunke M, et al. Risk factors for peritonitis in long-term peritoneal dialysis: the Network 9 peritonitis and catheter survival studies. *Am J Kidney Dis* 1996;28:428–436.
131. Burkart JM, Schreiber M, Korbet SM, et al. Solute clearance approach to adequacy of peritoneal dialysis. *Perit Dial Int* 1996;16:457–470.
132. Rocco MV. Body surface area limitations in achieving adequate therapy in peritoneal dialysis patients. *Perit Dial Int* 1996;16:617–622.
133. Fischbach M, Terzic J, Becmeur F, et al. Relationship between intraperitoneal hydrostatic pressure and dialysate volume in children on PD. *Adv Perit Dial* 1996;12:330–334.
134. Fischbach M, Terzic J, Menouer S, et al. Impact of fill volume changes on peritoneal dialysis tolerance and effectiveness in children. *Adv Perit Dial* 2000;16:321–323.
135. Fischbach M, Terzic J, Menouer S, et al. Optimal volume prescription for children on peritoneal dialysis. *Perit Dial Int* 2000;20:603–606.
136. Warady BA, Watkins SL, Fivush BA, et al. Validation of PD Adequest 2.0 for pediatric dialysis patients. *Pediatr Nephrol* 2001;16:205–211.
137. Verrina E, Amici G, Perfumo F, et al. The use of the PD Adequest mathematical model in pediatric patients on chronic peritoneal dialysis. *Perit Dial Int* 1998;18:322–328.
138. Fischbach M, Terzic J, Menouer S, et al. Effects of automated peritoneal dialysis on residual daily urinary volume in children. *Adv Perit Dial* 2001;17:269–273.
139. Ferber J, Scherer K, Schaefer F, et al. Residual renal function in children on haemodialysis and peritoneal dialysis therapy. *Pediatr Nephrol* 1994;8:579–583.
140. Canada-USA (CANUSA) Peritoneal Dialysis Study Group. Adequacy of dialysis and nutrition in continuous peritoneal dialysis: association with clinical outcomes. *J Am Soc Nephrol* 1996;7:198–207.
141. Lures R, Perlmutter J, Holley JL, et al. Loss of residual renal function in patients on peritoneal dialysis. *Adv Perit Dial* 1993;9:165–168.
142. Churchill DN, Blake PG, Jindal KK, et al. Clinical practice guideline for initiation of dialysis. *J Am Soc Nephrol* 1999;10:S289–S291.
143. Paniagua R, Amato D, Vonesch E, et al. Effects of increased peritoneal clearances on mortality rates in peritoneal dialysis: ADEMEX, a prospective, randomized, controlled trial. *J Am Soc Nephrol* 2002;13:1307–1320.
144. Höltta T, Rönnholm K, Jalanko H, et al. Clinical outcome of pediatric patients on peritoneal dialysis under adequacy control. *Pediatr Nephrol* 2000;14:889–897.
145. McCauley L, Champoux S, Parvex P, et al. Enhanced growth in children on peritoneal dialysis (PD): dialysis dose, nutrition, and metabolic control. *Perit Dial Int* 2000; 20(suppl 1):S89.
146. Champoux S, McCauley L, Sharma A, et al. Enhanced response to growth hormone in children on peritoneal dialysis. *Perit Dial Int* 2001;21(suppl 1):S86.
147. Chadha V, Blowey DL, Warady BA. Is growth a valid outcome measure of dialysis clearance in children undergoing peritoneal dialysis? *Perit Dial Int* 2001;21:S179–S184.
148. Montini G, Amici G, Milan S, et al. Middle molecule and small protein removal in children on peritoneal dialysis. *Kidney Int* 2002;61:1153–1159.
149. van der Voort JH, Harvey EA, Braj B, et al. Can the DOQI guidelines be met by peritoneal dialysis alone in pediatric patients? *Pediatr Nephrol* 2000;14:717–719.
150. Chadha V, Warady BA. What are the clinical correlates of adequate peritoneal dialysis? *Semin Nephrol* 2001;21:480–489.
151. Mellits ED, Cheek DB. The assessment of body water and fatness from infancy to adulthood. *Monogr Soc Res Child Dev* 1970;35:12–26.
152. Morgenstern B, Sreekumaran NK, Lerner G, et al. Impact of total body water errors on Kt/V estimates in children on peritoneal dialysis. *Adv Perit Dial* 2001;17:260–263.
153. Wühl E, Fusch CH, Schäarer K, et al. Assessment of total body water error in paediatric patients on dialysis. *Nephrol Dial Transplant* 1996;11:75–80.
154. Morgenstern B, Warady BA. Estimating total body water in children based upon height and weight: a reevaluation of the formulas of Mellits and Cheek. *J Am Soc Nephrol* 2002;13:1884–1888.
155. Morgenstern BZ, Mahoney DW, Wuehl E, et al. Total body water (TBW) in children on peritoneal dialysis. *J Am Soc Nephrol* 2002;13:2A.
156. Chen HH, Shetty A, Afthentopoulos IE, et al. Discrepancy between weekly Kt/V and weekly creatinine clearance in patients on CAPD. *Adv Perit Dial* 1995;11:83–87.
157. Twardowski ZJ. Relationship between creatinine clearance and Kt/V in peritoneal dialysis: a response to the defense of the DOQI document. *Perit Dial Int* 1999;19:199–203.
158. Canepa A, Perfumo F, Carrea A, et al. Nutritional status in children receiving chronic peritoneal dialysis. *Perit Dial Int* 1996;16:S526–S531.
159. Salusky IB. Nutritional management of pediatric patients on chronic dialysis. In: Nissenson AR, Fine RN, Gentile DE, eds. *Clinical dialysis.* Norwalk: Appleton & Lange, 1995.
160. Coleman JE, Edefonti A, Watson AR, et al. Guidelines by an ad hoc European committee on the assessment of growth and nutrition status in children on chronic peritoneal dialysis. *Pediatr Dial Int* [serial online] 2002;22.
161. Scolnik D, Balfe JW. Initial hypoalbuminemia and hyperlipidemia persist during chronic peritoneal dialysis in children. *Perit Dial Int* 1993;13:136–139.
162. K/DOQI, National Kidney Foundation. Clinical practice guidelines for nutrition in chronic renal failure: II. Pediatric guidelines. *Am J Kidney Dis* 2000;35:S105–S136.

163. Warady BA, Weis L, Johnson L. Nasogastric tube feeding in infants on peritoneal dialysis. *Perit Dial Int* 1996;16:S521–S525.
164. Coleman JE, Watson AR. Gastrostomy buttons: the optimal route for nutritional support in children with chronic renal failure. *J Ren Nutr* 1992;3:21–26.
165. Geary DF, Chait PG. Tube feeding in infants on peritoneal dialysis. *Perit Dial Int* 1996;16:S517–S520.
166. Quan A, Baum M. Protein losses in children on continuous cycler peritoneal dialysis. *Pediatr Nephrol* 1996;10:728–731.
167. Brem AS, Lambert C, Hill C, et al. Prevalence of protein malnutrition in children maintained on peritoneal dialysis. *Pediatr Nephrol* 2002;17:527–530.
168. Roodhooft AM, Van Hoeck KJ, Van Acker KJ. Hypophosphatemia in infants on continuous ambulatory peritoneal dialysis. *Clin Nephrol* 1990;34:131–135.
169. Kriley M, Warady BA. Vitamin status of pediatric patients receiving long-term peritoneal dialysis. *Am J Clin Nutr* 1991;531:1476–1479.
170. Warady BA, Kriley M, Alon U, et al. Vitamin status of infants receiving long-term peritoneal dialysis. *Pediatr Nephrol* 1994;8:354–356.
171. Parrott KA, Stockberger R, Alexander SR, et al. Plasma vitamin A levels in children on CAPD. *Perit Dial Bull* 1987;7:90–92.
172. Verrina E, Honda M, Warady BA, et al. Prevention of peritonitis in children on peritoneal dialysis. *Perit Dial Int* 2000;20:625–630.
173. Warady BA, Campoy SF, Gross SP, et al. Peritonitis with continuous ambulatory peritoneal dialysis and continuous cycling peritoneal dialysis. *J Pediatr* 1984;105:726–730.
174. Watson AR, Vigneaux A, Bonnatyne RM, et al. Peritonitis during continuous ambulatory peritoneal dialysis in children. *Can Med Assoc J* 1986;134:1019–1022.
175. Levy M, Balfe JW. Optimal approach to the prevention and treatment of peritonitis in children undergoing continuous ambulatory and continuous cycling peritoneal dialysis. *Semin Dial* 1994;7:442–449.
176. Harvey E, Secker D, Braj B, et al. The team approach to the management of children on chronic peritoneal dialysis. *Adv Ren Replace Ther* 1996;3:3–13.
177. Watkins S, Warady BA, Ogrinc F, et al. Impact of flush-before-fill methodology on peritonitis rates in patients receiving automated peritoneal dialysis. *J Am Soc Nephrol* 1998;9:716A.
178. Kingwatanakul P, Warady BA. *Staphylococcus aureus* nasal carriage in children receiving long-term peritoneal dialysis. *Adv Perit Dial* 1997;13:280–283.
179. Oh J, Von Baum H, Klaus G, et al. Nasal carriage of *staphylococcus aureus* in families of children on peritoneal dialysis. *Adv Perit Dial* 2000;16:324–327.
180. Warady BA, Schaefer F, Alexander S, et al. Consensus guidelines for the treatment of peritonitis in pediatric patients receiving peritoneal dialysis. *Perit Dial Int* 2000;20:610–624.
181. Oh J, Baum M, Wühl E, et al. Nasal mupirocin prophylaxis reduces the incidence of PD-related *S. aureus* infections in children: results of a double-blind, placebo-controlled multicenter trial. *Perit Dial Int* 2002;22(suppl 1):S74.
182. Holloway M, Mujais S, Kandert M, et al. Pediatric peritoneal dialysis training: characteristics and impact on peritonitis rates. *Perit Dial Int* 2001;21:401–404.
183. Troidle L, Kliger AS, Gorban-Brennan N, et al. Nine episodes of CPD-associated peritonitis with vancomycin-resistant enterococci. *Kidney Int* 1996;50:1368–1372.
184. Warady BA, Reed L, Murphy G, et al. Aminoglycoside ototoxicity in pediatric patients receiving long-term peritoneal dialysis. *Pediatr Nephrol* 1993;7:178–181.
185. Von Baum H, Schehl J, Geiss HK, et al. Prevalence of vancomycin-resistant enterococci among children with end-stage renal failure. *Clin Infect Dis* 1999;29:912–916.
186. Warady BA. Sclerosing encapsulating peritonitis: What approach should be taken with children? *Perit Dial Int* 2000;20:390–391.
187. Araki Y, Hataya H, Tanaka Y, et al. Long-term peritoneal dialysis is a risk factor of sclerosing encapsulating peritonitis for children. *Perit Dial Int* 2000;20:445–451.
188. Hoshii S, Honda M, Itami N, et al. Sclerosing encapsulating peritonitis in pediatric dialysis patients. *Pediatr Nephrol* 2000;14:275–279.
189. Andreoli SP, Langefeld CD, Stadler S, et al. Risks of peritoneal membrane failure in children undergoing long-term peritoneal dialysis. *Pediatr Nephrol* 1993;7:543–547.
190. Schroder CH, van Dreumel MJ, Reddingius R, et al. Peritoneal transport kinetics of glucose, urea, and creatinine during infancy and childhood. *Perit Dial Int* 1991;12:322–325.
191. Nishi A, Ito Y, Amamoto Y, et al. Longitudinal changes in peritoneal equilibration test with or without peritonitis in children. *Pediatr Nephrol* 1995;9:562–565.
192. Andreoli SP, Leiser J, Warady BA, et al. Adverse effect of peritonitis on peritoneal membrane function in children on dialysis. *Pediatr Nephrol* 1999;13:1–6.
193. Warady BA, Fivush BA, Andreoli SP, et al. Longitudinal evaluation of transport kinetics in children receiving peritoneal dialysis. *Pediatr Nephrol* 1999;13:571–576.
194. Schneble F, Bonzel KE, Waldheer R, et al. Peritoneal morphology in children treated by continuous ambulatory peritoneal dialysis. *Pediatr Nephrol* 1992;6:542–546.
195. Valderrabano F, Jofre R, Lopez-Gomez M. Quality of life in end-stage renal disease patients. *Am J Kidney Dis* 2001;38:443–464.
196. Bakewell AB, Higgins RM, Edmunds ME. Quality of life in peritoneal dialysis patients: decline over time and association with clinical outcomes. *Kidney Int* 2002;61:239–248.
197. Furth SL, Gerson AC, Neu AM, et al. The impact of dialysis and transplantation on children. *Adv Ren Replace Ther* 2001;8:206–213.
198. Warady BA. Therapeutic camping for children with end-stage renal disease. *Pediatr Nephrol* 1994;8:387–390.
199. Gerson A, Fivush BA, Kaskel F, et al. Functional outcome in adolescents with renal failure: assessing a generic health status questionnaire. *Perit Dial Int* 2001;21:S89.
200. Gulati S, Stephens D, Balfe JA, et al. Children with hypoalbuminemia on continuous peritoneal dialysis are at risk for technique failure. *Kidney Int* 2001;59:2361–2367.
201. Verrina E, Zacchello G, Perfumo F, et al. Clinical experience in the treatment of infants with chronic peritoneal dialysis. *Adv Perit Dial* 1995;11:281–284.

71

HEMODIALYSIS

STUART L. GOLDSTEIN
KATHY JABS

Hemodialysis is a procedure that uses extracorporeal perfusion to clear accumulated solutes or toxins from the blood by diffusion and convection across a semipermeable membrane. End-stage renal disease (ESRD) and acute renal failure are uncommon disease states in children. As a result, technologic advances and professional expertise specific for pediatric patients with renal failure have often developed relatively slowly. The hemodialysis procedure has become increasingly sophisticated, however, and many of the theoretical and technological advances studied previously in adult patients have been applied to children receiving hemodialysis. Provision of optimal pediatric hemodialysis requires a specialized and integrated health care team to manage the medical, nursing, nutrition, development, and psychosocial aspects of care for the pediatric patient with ESRD. In addition, neonates, children, and adolescents with acute renal failure often require short-term dialysis treatment until adequate renal function is restored. This chapter reviews the fundamental principles of hemodialysis and provides practical information regarding the provision of hemodialysis to children with acute and chronic renal failure.

INCIDENCE AND ETIOLOGY OF END-STAGE RENAL DISEASE

The incidence rate of ESRD in the United States is 11 to 14 per 1 million for individuals under 20 years of age and has remained relatively stable over the past 30 years. In 1999, 5935 children in the United States carried the diagnosis of ESRD; 939 of them received hemodialysis as long-term renal replacement therapy (1). The number of neonates and infants receiving acute and chronic hemodialysis has steadily increased over the past decade as a result of improved pediatric dialysis nursing expertise and the availability of pediatric- and neonatal-sized catheters and blood tubing that minimize the blood volume of the extracorporeal circuit (2–4). The success of renal transplantation in young children has further stimulated programs to develop satisfactory dialysis treatment facilities to prepare these infants optimally for transplantation (4).

PHYSIOLOGY OF HEMODIALYSIS

The goal of the hemodialysis treatment is to remove prescribed quantities of solutes and fluid that have accumulated between dialysis sessions. Solute removal (clearance) and fluid removal (ultrafiltration) are accomplished via blood perfusion of an extracorporeal filter membrane across which runs a countercurrent balanced electrolyte solution.

Solute clearance during hemodialysis occurs by two physiologic mechanisms: diffusion and convection. Diffusion refers to solute migration across a semipermeable membrane. The factors governing the rate of transfer are membrane permeability (i.e., the number and size of the pores in the membrane), solute size and charge, membrane surface area, and magnitude of the concentration gradient across the membrane. Solute transfer rates are inversely proportional to particle size—smaller particles diffuse more rapidly than larger particles. On the other hand, solute transfer rates are directly proportional to membrane surface area and concentration gradient, both of which can be manipulated by prescription to improve clearance.

Convection refers to the phenomenon of solute movement (or solute drag) across the membrane independent of concentration gradient. The main determinant of solute drag is the osmotic gradient achieved by the amount of plasma water pushed across the membrane (ultrafiltrate). The amount of convective transfer of a particular solute is proportional to both the amount of ultrafiltrate achieved during the treatment and the sieving properties of particular dialyzers. A sieving coefficient for each solute-dialyzer pair reflects the interaction between the size and charge of the solute, and the pore number and pore size of the dialyzer.

Because the extracorporeal circuit is in contact with only the intravascular component of the extracellular space, clearance of solute by dialysis and fluid removal via ultrafiltration do not occur simultaneously through the various

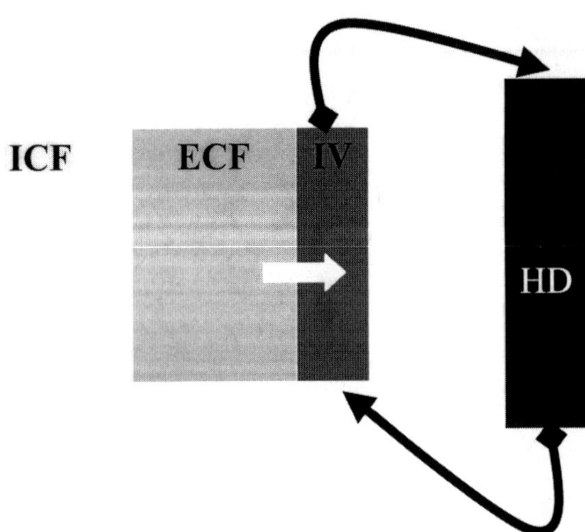

FIGURE 71.1. This extracorporeal circuit model demonstrates that the dialysis circuit has access only to the intravascular (IV) space. As a result, both solute and fluid removal occur initially from the IV space. Removal from the interstitial and intracellular spaces occurs after fluid and solutes move down dialysis-induced hydrostatic and concentration gradients, respectively. ECF, extracellular fluid; HD, hemodialysis; ICF, intracellular fluid.

body compartments. Before the initiation of dialysis, accumulated solutes are distributed across patient total body water, which is comprised of the intracellular and extracellular spaces. Solute clearance and fluid removal occur instantaneously from the extracorporeal circuit in the dialyzer space. Fluid in the extravascular space must move down the concentration and hydrostatic gradients created during the dialysis treatment into the intravascular space before being processed in the extracorporeal circuit (Fig. 71.1). The extravascular to intravascular transfer rates have important practical effects on the quantification of solute removal and tolerable ultrafiltration rates. These effects are discussed later in the chapter.

HEMODIALYSIS TREATMENT AND EQUIPMENT

Hemodialysis Circuit

The hemodialysis circuit is comprised of the patient's blood compartment access in the form of an arteriovenous fistula (AVF) or arteriovenous graft (AVG) or a venous catheter, polyethylene tubing through which the patient's blood travels to and from the dialyzer, and the dialyzer itself. Blood tubing is produced in a variety of sizes and should be matched to patient size to allow for optimal blood flow while minimizing the volume of the extracorporeal circuit, which is the sum of the blood tubing volume and hollow fiber dialyzer volume. To prevent excessive repeated blood loss in the circuit and hemodynamic instability, the extracorporeal circuit should not exceed 10% of the patient's calculated blood volume. Neonatal lines with a volume of 40 mL are available for use in children who weigh less than 15 kg. A wide variety of dialyzers with different blood volumes are available from various manufacturers that can be matched to pediatric patient sizes.

To prevent hypovolemia during initiation of a dialysis treatment, the circuit should be primed with either saline or colloid. For some infants, for whom even the smallest blood tubing-dialyzer volumes exceed 10% of patient blood volume, the circuit should be primed with colloid (5% albumin or packed red blood cells diluted with albumin to a measured hematocrit of 35%) instead of crystalloid. Weekly serum hematocrit values should be obtained to monitor for anemia resulting from excessive blood loss in the hemodialysis circuit for infants of less than 10 kg maintained on chronic hemodialysis. Special considerations for infants receiving chronic hemodialysis are discussed at the end of the chapter.

A primary determinant of the amount of solute clearance during the hemodialysis treatment is the blood pump flow rate (Q_b, in milliliters per minute) through the dialyzer. A calibrated roller pump housed in the hemodialysis machine drives extracorporeal blood from the patient access through the blood tubing to the dialyzer and then back to the patient access. The Q_b should be prescribed to provide safe and optimal clearance of solute. Use of a maximum Q_b of less than 400 mL/min/1.73 m^2 of patient body surface area minimizes the risk of cardiovascular compromise.

Ultrafiltration is achieved via creation of a hydrostatic pressure gradient across the dialyzer membrane (transmembrane pressure or TMP). Newer dialysis machines equipped with volumetric control automatically establish the necessary TMP to provide the ultrafiltration volume prescribed over the duration of the treatment. Volumetric control machines can provide ultrafiltration volumes within 10 to 100 mL of prescribed volumes and have eliminated the need for dialysis staff to calculate and create the appropriate TMP.

Hemodialyzer

Current dialyzers are manufactured with a hollow fiber design to minimize blood volume and provide reliable and predictable solute clearance and ultrafiltration coefficients. Advancements in dialyzer manufacturing processes have led to improvements in clearance efficiency and biocompatibility.

Dialyzer clearance is a function of the dialyzer surface area and its clearance characteristic (K_oA, in milliliters per minute) for a particular solute (5), the blood flow rate (Q_b, in milliliters per minute), and the countercurrent dialysate flow rate (Q_d, in milliliters per minute). To enhance diffusion and prevent saturation of dialysate with solute, the prescribed Q_d should exceed the Q_b by at least 50%. In fact, *in vitro* and *in vivo* studies have shown that increasing Q_d has a significant affect on urea clearance and may further improve clearance in patients with sufficient Q_b and dialysis times and add very little to the cost of the procedure (6). The clearance rate for a particular solute is generally inversely proportional to the molecular size of the solute. Most modern dialyzers permit clearance of solutes up to a molecular weight of 5000 to 10,000 daltons.

Figure 71.2 depicts different relative clearance characteristics for dialyzers with a different K_oA at various blood pump flow rates. This figure demonstrates that clearance is equivalent for both dialyzers at low blood flow rates, because equilibration of solute occurs between the blood space and dialysate space within the dialyzer at low flow rates. The figure also illustrates the nonlinear association between blood flow rates and dialyzer clearance (K_d), because at higher blood flow rates, diffusion and convection are maximized at a point at which blood travels rapidly through the dialyzer and back to the patient. The differences between the two dialyzers are the blood flow rate at which the maximum clearance is achieved and the maximum clearance that can be achieved.

The ultrafiltration coefficient of the dialyzer is determined by the charge of the dialyzer surface area and the size of the pores through which solutes traverse from the blood space to the dialysate space. The ultrafiltration coefficient should be sufficient to allow for the prescribed volume of fluid removal during the 3- to 4-hour hemodialysis treatment. Hemodialysis machines with volumetric control have been a major advancement to prevent excessive fluid removal by ultrafiltration in smaller children receiving hemodialysis.

Activation of proinflammatory cytokines, leukocytes, and other mediators can occur when blood comes into contact with an inorganic surface. Although few pediatric data currently exist, numerous studies in adults have suggested that repeated exposure to certain dialysis membranes may result in prolonged immune system activation, protein catabolism, and alteration of host proteins, which may have long-term adverse clinical consequences (7–14). For instance, proinflammatory cytokine induction by dialysis membrane exposure has been posited to lead to glycosylation of β_2-microglobulin. The advanced glycosylation end-products are thought to contribute to dialysis-associated amyloid deposition in soft tissues (15,16). Furthermore, inflammation may be a contributory factor for development of the coronary artery calcifications often observed in adult patients receiving chronic hemodialysis, which in turn are thought to contribute to the increased cardiovascular mortality rates seen in young adult patients with ESRD (17).

Newer-generation dialysis membranes constructed from materials such as polysulfone and polymethylmethacrylate cause less proinflammatory cytokine activation than older generation membranes made from cellulose or cuprophane (18,19). There are no data available on changes in outcomes with polysulfone or polymethylmethacrylate membranes, although the incidence of anaphylactoid, complement-mediated immediate membrane reactions is far lower with biocompatible membranes.

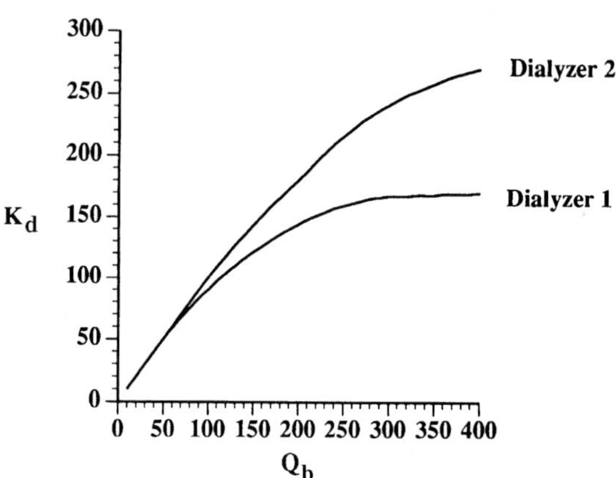

FIGURE 71.2. The relationship between blood flow (Q_b) and dialyzer clearance (K_d) for two different dialyzers. Dialyzer 2 has a K_oA value (clearance characteristic) twice as large as that of dialyzer 1.

Water Treatment System

The hemodialysis water treatment system must remove all potentially hazardous substances from source water before distribution to the unit's dialysis machines. Source water is usually derived from a municipal water supply. Although standards for hemodialysis water treatment vary from state to state, compliance with minimum standards and components outlined by the Association for the Advancement of Medical Instrumentation is required for all systems operating in the United States (20).

The components of hemodialysis water treatment systems and their basic functions are listed in Table 71.1. Critical components include sediment filters to remove particulates, softener tanks to remove calcium and magne-

TABLE 71.1. COMPONENTS AND FUNCTIONS OF A HEMODIALYSIS WATER TREATMENT SYSTEM

Component	Function
Backflow preventer	Prevents reverse flow of water through the valve
Temperature blending valve	Maintains constant water temperature of 25°C
Multimedia filter	Filters out particulates 10–20 μm or larger
Softener and exchange filter	Removes water hardness (calcium and magnesium) in exchange for sodium
Carbon tank (two needed)	Removes chlorine and chloramines: 6 min EBCT for chlorine, 10 min EBCT for chloramine
Prefilter	Filters out particulates 3–5 μm in size
Reverse osmosis membrane	Removes 96–99% of incoming particles >200 molecular weight, endotoxins, viruses, and bacteria
Deionization tank	Removes charged ions from water
Ultraviolet light	Kills or alters DNA of bacteria as water passes through lamp

EBCT, empty bed contact time.

sium, ultrafilters to remove bacteria and endotoxins, carbon tanks to remove chlorine and chloramines, and ultraviolet irradiators to destroy bacteria. The heart of the water treatment system is the reverse osmosis membrane, which removes 99% of bacteria and 95% of charged ions.

Once the source water has been treated and rendered safe for dialysis, it is delivered to the unit and each patient station by means of distribution piping. Bacterial overgrowth and the resultant establishment of biofilm is a constant hazard for all water treatment systems. Measures that help prevent bacterial overgrowth include use of nonporous tubing, minimization of dead ends and bends in the distribution loop, and generation of high water flow rates of greater than 3 ft/sec to create turbulent flow and thereby prevent bacterial attachment. Regular monitoring for bacterial contamination of dialysis water from various segments of the treatment system and at each patient station is crucial to assure the safety of hemodialysis. In addition, regular periodic disinfection of the water treatment system is warranted.

Data demonstrate that dialysis water levels of endotoxin below levels that produce pyrogenic reactions (and below the limits set by Association for the Advancement of Medical Instrumentation standards) may still cause chronic inflammation in some patients. Ultrapure water, similar to that used for pharmaceutical injection and semiconductor manufacturing, leads to a decrease in cytokine-mediated inflammation when used for dialysis fluid (21) but is extremely expensive to produce.

The electrolytic composition of dialysis water is critical to ensure safe diffusive treatment. Standard dialysis baths contain sodium (140 mEq/L), potassium (2 to 3 mEq/L), chloride (100 to 102 mEq/L), bicarbonate (40 mEq/L), magnesium (1.5 to 2.0 mEq/L), calcium (ionized concentration 1.5 to 3.0 mEq/L), and glucose (100 mg/dL). Bicarbonate is preferred to acetate for acid buffering, because the use of acetate has been associated with hypotension in dialysis patients (22,23). Current dialysis machines can alter the sodium concentration during the course of the treatment. Use of sodium-modeling programs, which deliver higher sodium concentrations earlier in the treatment followed by lower concentrations later in the treatment, has been shown to decrease both intra- and interdialytic patient symptoms (24–26).

VASCULAR ACCESS

Adequate provision of hemodialysis depends on a properly functioning vascular access. Current hemodialysis access options are divided into two categories: permanent access in the form of an AVF or AVG and semipermanent access in the form of catheters with a subcutaneous cuff for long-term dialysis or without a cuff for short-term hemodialysis.

Permanent vascular access of an AVF or AVG can function for many years and is preferred over indwelling catheters in children and adults. However, the majority of children receiving hemodialysis in the United States are still dialyzed via a catheter (27). Reasons for high catheter prevalence rates include lack of local surgical experience in permanent access creation in smaller patients, anticipation of a short dialysis course before transplantation, or dialysis unit philosophy to decrease painful procedures (i.e., repeated needle sticks for children with AVFs or AVGs).

AVFs are created by connection of a patient's native artery to vein. The most common sites for AVFs are the wrist (radiocephalic or Brescia-Cimino fistula) and the antecubital fossa (brachial artery to cephalic vein). If possible, the wrist location is preferable for the first access to preserve more proximal vessels for future access placement [National Kidney Foundation Kidney-Dialysis Outcomes Quality Initiative (NKF-KDOQI) recommendation] (28). The arterial to venous connection results in a communication between the high-pressure arterial system and the low-pressure venous system. Before initial use, the venous portion of the AVF must be allowed to "mature" or expand to produce a size large enough for safe needle placement. Maturation time depends on patient size and AVF location but should be a minimum of 4 weeks and preferably 3 to 4 months (28). Some AVFs in smaller children require 4 to 6 months to mature (29). Thus, to allow for ample maturation time and avoid the use of temporary venous catheters, AVF placement should occur in advance of the patient's immediate need for dialysis if possible. Current guidelines recommend placement of an AVF or AVG when patient glomerular filtration rate (as measured by creatinine clearance) is less than 25 mL/min/1.73 m^2 (28).

AVGs are composed of prosthetic polytetrafluoroethylene (Gore-Tex) tubing connecting a patient's artery to vein. The advantages of AVGs over AVFs include increased options for site placement (thigh, forearm, and upper arm) and configuration (straight and looped). In addition, AVGs are technically easier to construct and do not require maturation times as prolonged as those for AVFs. AVGs should not be used within 4 weeks of placement to allow the luminal portion to become lined with endothelium (28).

AVF complications include development of venous collaterals, arterial inflow stenosis with resultant poststenotic dilatation, and aneurysm formation caused by repeated needle puncture in the same site. Furthermore, patients with very high flow rates of greater than 2000 mL/min may be at risk for hypoxia from extracardiac shunting or ischemia of the limb distal to the AVF anastomosis. A thorough physical examination should be performed before AVF placement to ensure that the limb receives good blood flow from an artery other than the vessel planned for arterial anastomosis.

Thrombosis of permanent access sites is a significant cause of morbidity for the hemodialysis patient population (30). In many instances, thrombosis results from decreased access flow caused by a stenosis of the access venous outflow tract (31,32).

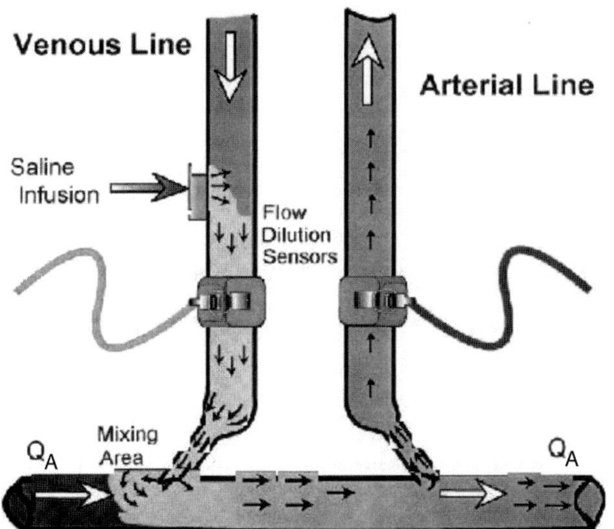

FIGURE 71.3. Ultrasound dilution monitor configuration. The patient's dialysis lines are temporally reversed to create recirculation. A 20-mL saline bolus is injected upstream of the first sensor. The saline enters the patient access site, and most of the bolus goes into the patient circulation. In the presence of venous stenosis, more saline returns to the dialysis circuit and is detected by the second sensor. Both sensors are connected to a computer, which interprets the data and calculates the flow by the Fick equation. Q_A, access flow. (Courtesy of Transonic Systems, Inc., Ithaca, New York.)

Substantial clinical research has been performed over the past decade to devise methods to assess for vascular access outflow stenosis in adult patients receiving hemodialysis, but many methods have significant drawbacks that preclude routine use (33–38). Ultrasound dilution (UD) is a practical, noninvasive, and reliable indicator of vascular access flow and has been used effectively to identify venous stenosis in adult patients receiving hemodialysis (39–43). The technique employs two reusable sensors, one attached to the venous and one to the arterial line while the patient is receiving hemodialysis. During the first hour of a hemodialysis treatment, the hemodialysis lines are temporarily reversed (to create temporary recirculation) and a 20-mL bolus of saline is then injected quickly into the venous line proximal to the venous sensor. The sensors are attached to a computer that interprets the changes in Doppler velocity within each line as the hematocrit changes in relation to dialyzer blood flow (Fig. 71.3).

When the access flow (Q_A, in milliliters per minute) reported by the UD monitor is corrected for patient size (Q_{Acorr}, in milliliters per minute per 1.73 m^2), a Q_{Acorr} lower than 650 mL/min/1.73 m^2 is extremely sensitive and specific for predicting AVG and AVF stenosis in pediatric patients receiving hemodialysis (44). Furthermore, when patients with a Q_{Acorr} lower than 650 mL/min/1.73 m^2 were referred for venography and balloon dilatation angioplasty within 48 hours of UD measurement, a 90% reduction in vascular access thrombosis rate was observed (45). This reduction in thrombosis rate was associated with decreased patient hospitalization and a 40% reduction in unit cost per patient for vascular access management.

TABLE 71.2. CUFFED HEMODIALYSIS CATHETER AND PATIENT SIZE GUIDELINE

Patient size (kg)	Catheter options
<20	8 French dual lumen
20–25	7 French twin Tesio
25–40	10 French dual lumen
	10 French Ash split
	10 French twin Tesio
>40	10 French twin Tesio
	11.5 or 12.5 French dual lumen

Other noninvasive venoarterial flow measurements include ionic dialysance and transcutaneous access flow, but neither has been studied in a pediatric hemodialysis patient population (46,47).

Long-term survival of AVGs and AVFs has recently been evaluated for pediatric patients (48). One-, 3-, and 5-year pediatric AVF survival rates are 90, 60, and 40%, respectively. One-, 3-, and 5-year pediatric AVG survival rates are 90, 50, and 40%, respectively. The data demonstrated that, although 5-year AVG and AVF survival rates are not significantly different, AVGs do exhibit higher thrombosis and surgical intervention rates.

Although the method is not preferred for hemodialysis vascular access, lack of local surgical expertise and small patient size have rendered semipermanent access in the form of cuffed catheters crucial for provision of hemodialysis to children. Current catheter configurations can be divided into three types: dual-lumen catheters with both lumens fixed to each other for the entire length of the catheter, dual-lumen catheters that have split the venous and arterial lumens of the distal portion of the catheter to allow for free tip movement within the vein (Ash split catheter), and twin separate single-lumen catheter systems that can be inserted into the same vein with different exit sites or in different veins altogether (Tesio catheter system). Table 71.2 lists some of the available cuffed hemodialysis catheter options and provides a guideline for matching catheter size and type with patient size.

Hemodialysis catheter tip placement in the right atrium allows for the blood flows required to provide adequate dialysis; catheter tips that rest in the superior vena cava may be at risk for collapse against the vessel wall. In considering sites for placement of temporary or cuffed catheters, the risk of central venous stenosis should be considered. A central venous stenosis may increase venous pressure and result in poor flow or thrombosis of the AVF or AVG. The right internal jugular site is associated with venous thrombosis less frequently than subclavian sites. It is also preferable to place the catheter on the contralateral side to a planned AVF or AVG (28). A chest radiograph should be obtained before the first use of a catheter to ensure proper catheter placement and absence of pneumothorax or hemothorax.

To prevent catheter thrombosis, packing with concentrated heparin (1000 U/mL for children smaller than 40 kg, 2000 U/mL for children larger than 40 kg) is recommended. Even with heparin packing, catheter thrombosis remains a significant problem that can preclude the delivery of adequate dialysis. Initial studies of the use of trisodium citrate to lock hemodialysis catheters demonstrated significant reduction in thrombosis rates in adult patients, but cases of inadvertent infusion of citrate into the bloodstream and resultant patient hemorrhage lead to the discontinuation of approval for citrate catheter locking.

Treatment of catheter thrombosis is currently limited to the instillation of tissue plasminogen activator into the catheter (1 to 2 mg/mL for 2 hours) and intraluminal brushing to dislodge the clot. The presence of intra- and extraluminal fibrin sheaths can be diagnosed reliably only by injecting venous contrast through the catheter. Pharmacologic treatment of fibrin sheaths around catheters has been unrewarding. Some centers currently strip fibrin sheaths from catheters using wire-guided scrapers that are inserted into the patient's femoral vein and advanced to the catheter tip under fluoroscopic imaging.

A few pediatric studies have assessed the survival rates and complications for pediatric hemodialysis catheters (49–51). The most common complications observed include infection (either tunnel infection or line sepsis), kinking of the catheter, and thrombosis. Gram-positive organisms, especially *Staphylococcus* species, are the most common causative organisms in hemodialysis catheter infections. Because hemodialysis is a life-sustaining procedure and cannot be interrupted, many centers attempt to treat hemodialysis catheter infections with antibiotics alone and do not immediately remove the catheter. Catheter removal should be performed when patients are repeatedly symptomatic from shedding of bacteria in the bloodstream during the dialysis treatment, as manifested by high fever, rigors, chills, and/or hypotension, or when the infection cannot be eradicated. In addition, catheter removal will likely be necessary in patients with fungal line infections, which are very difficult to eradicate with antimicrobials alone.

Pediatric studies demonstrate a median survival of 204 to 280 days for a dual-lumen hemodialysis catheter (49–51). In a single-center comparison, pediatric Tesio catheters exhibited significantly longer survival and provided adequate hemodialysis more reliably than dual-lumen catheters of similar size (50).

TARGET DRY WEIGHT AND ULTRAFILTRATION PRACTICE

For many reasons, accurate determination of patient target weight is a challenging task when treating hemodialysis patients. Symptoms of hypovolemia may be difficult to assess, as the behavior of small children receiving dialysis is often hard to interpret. Although overly rapid acute fluid removal may cause temporary intravascular volume depletion and patient cramping, hypotension, dizziness, and/or nausea, some young children are not able to verbalize their symptoms to dialysis personnel or may act distressed because of anxiety or fear unrelated to true physical discomfort. Month-to-month target weight assessment is difficult in children due to widely ranging ratios of total body water to body mass that vary with age. Furthermore, children are growing and have variable appetites, so that real weight loss and weight gain may occur more frequently than in adults.

Nonetheless, accurate determination of pediatric target weight is critical, because an underestimation of dry weight can lead to hypovolemia with acute symptoms noted earlier and to enhanced postdialysis thirst that results in immediate posttreatment overdrinking and increased interdialytic fluid gain. Continual overestimation of target weight can lead to chronic volume overload with resultant hypertension, pulmonary edema, congestive heart failure, and left ventricular hypertrophy. Ultrafiltration-associated symptoms may occur with an appropriately determined dry weight, especially in patients with large interdialytic weight gains. These symptoms are the result of intravascular volume depletion while awaiting refilling from the extravascular space. Approaches to minimize ultrafiltration-associated symptoms include sequential ultrafiltration and dialysis (or isolated ultrafiltration at the start of a treatment), sodium modeling, and noninvasive monitoring (NIVM) of hematocrit.

Sodium Modeling

Sodium modeling is a machine-programmed algorithm that varies the dialysate sodium concentration during the treatment. Most modeling programs use hyperosmolar dialysate sodium concentrations at the beginning of treatment and then decrease sodium concentration, either by linear, logarithmic, or stepwise algorithms, throughout the remainder of the treatment. The increase in sodium concentration caused by sodium diffusion into the serum at the beginning of the treatment is designed to offset the decrease in serum osmolarity resulting from urea removal during dialysis. A return to normal sodium concentrations at the end of the treatment decreases the interdialytic thirst that would result from dialysis against a constantly high sodium level. Sodium modeling has been shown to be effective in decreasing both intradialytic and interdialytic symptoms in adolescent and adult patients receiving hemodialysis (25,56). Similarly, isolated ultrafiltration at the start of dialysis maintains the osmolality of the intravascular space by removing solutes only by convection and helps with refill of the intravascular space during ultrafiltration.

Noninvasive Monitoring

Because red cell volume remains constant during dialysis, changes in hematocrit are inversely proportional to changes in intravascular volume. Continuous optical methods of NIVM of hematocrit take advantage of this relationship to demonstrate a real-time association between fluctuating hematocrit and intravascular volume during the hemodialysis treatment.

Optical methods of NIVM to continuously monitor changes in intravascular volume can help decrease symptomatology during a dialysis treatment (52–54). For example, if fluid removal is too rapid as detected by a rapidly increasing hematocrit and steep declining slope on the NIVM monitor, the ultrafiltration rate can be decreased before hypovolemic symptoms occur. If fluid removal is too slow as suggested by a stable hematocrit and a flat slope on the NIVM monitor, then the ultrafiltration rate may be increased safely to achieve the patient's actual target weight.

The use of NIVM has been studied in pediatric patients receiving hemodialysis (55,56). Rates of ultrafiltration-associated events (defined as hypotension, headache, or cramping that required a nursing intervention such as administration of a saline bolus, placement in the Trendelenburg position, or a slowing or stopping of ultrafiltration) were lower when NIVM was performed, especially among patients weighing less than 35 kg. The decrease in symptom event rates with NIVM occurred without a sacrifice in target weight achievement. When NIVM was performed, symptom events occurred in the first 90 minutes of treatment only with a blood volume change of greater than 8% per hour as registered on the NIVM monitor. Seventy-one percent of events occurring after 60 minutes of treatment initiation were associated with a blood volume change greater than 4% per hour. These treatment time and event observations have been used to model ultrafiltration rates to optimize fluid removal during dialysis, lessen the need for antihypertensive medications, and minimize intra- and interdialytic patient symptoms (57). The model prescribes half of the total treatment ultrafiltration volume to be removed in the first 90 minutes of treatment with a maximum of a total 12% blood volume change as registered on the NIVM monitor. The remainder of the ultrafiltration volume is then removed during the final hours of treatment.

DIALYSIS PRESCRIPTION

Initiation of Hemodialysis

The first few hemodialysis treatments may be associated with large transcellular osmolar shifts if the pretreatment blood urea nitrogen (BUN) levels are very high, with resultant disequilibrium syndrome, cerebral edema, and seizures. Maneuvers aimed at limiting large osmolar shifts include infusion of mannitol (0.5 g/kg over 1 hour starting 30 minutes into the treatment) or limiting the amount of clearance until the pretreatment BUN is lower than 100 mg/dL. The amount of urea reduction can be prescribed using the following equation:

$$-\ln (C_t/C_0) = Kt/V \qquad \text{[Eq. 1]}$$

where C_t is the BUN concentration after t minutes of dialysis, C_0 is the time 0 or prehemodialysis BUN concentration, K is the urea clearance of the dialyzer (in milliliters per minute) at the blood flow prescribed, t is the duration of dialysis in minutes, and V is the patient urea distribution volume (total body water). The initial estimate of V is 600 mL/kg body weight. To prevent dialysis disequilibrium, one can prescribe a 30% urea reduction for the first treatment as depicted in the following example.

Hemodialysis is being initiated for a 13-year-old 50-kg girl with focal segmental glomerulosclerosis. A dialyzer with a surface area of 1.3 m^2 and a K of 210 mL/min at a Q_b of 200 mL/min is chosen. Her estimated V is 50 kg × 600 mL/kg, or 30,000 mL. To determine the duration of dialysis needed to effect an approximate 30% urea reduction, the equation is solved as follows:

$$-\ln (70/100) = 210 \text{ mL/min} \times t/30{,}000 \text{ mL or}$$

$$0.35 = 210 \text{ mL/min} \times t/30{,}000 \text{ mL}$$

$$t = 0.35 \times 30{,}000 \text{ mL}/210 \text{ mL/min or}$$

$$t = 51 \text{ min}$$

A pretreatment and posttreatment BUN level should be measured for the first treatment. Using the measured C_t and C_0 from the first treatment, one can solve for V and obtain a more accurate estimate of the patient's total body water. The new V can be used to prescribe an approximate 50% clearance for the second treatment, and this iterative process can be repeated to prescribe an approximate 70% urea clearance for the next few treatments. Once a prescription is found that maintains the pretreatment BUN at a relatively consistent value below 100 mg/dL, the adequacy of the patient's dialysis can then be evaluated more formally.

Hemodialysis Adequacy

The concept of hemodialysis adequacy is derived from the mechanistic analysis of the National Cooperative Dialysis Study (NCDS) published in 1985 (58). A main result inferred from the NCDS was a higher probability of "patient failure" (i.e., patient death or hospitalization) in adult patients who received lower doses of hemodialysis and/or had worse nutrition. The definition of hemodialysis adequacy that should ensue from the NCDS result is the minimum amount of urea clearance and nutritional intake to prevent these failure outcomes (59–61).

Figure 71.4 graphically depicts the serum concentration changes of urea, or any readily dialyzable solute, during and between dialysis treatments. The total mass of urea removed during the treatment is based on the fractional reduction of urea during the hemodialysis treatment. The interdialytic accumulation of urea reflects the amount of protein catabolized during the time between dialysis treatments (62). In a steady state, this protein catabolic rate (in grams per day) is indicative of the amount of protein ingested by the patient and hence is a marker of nutritional status (63–69).

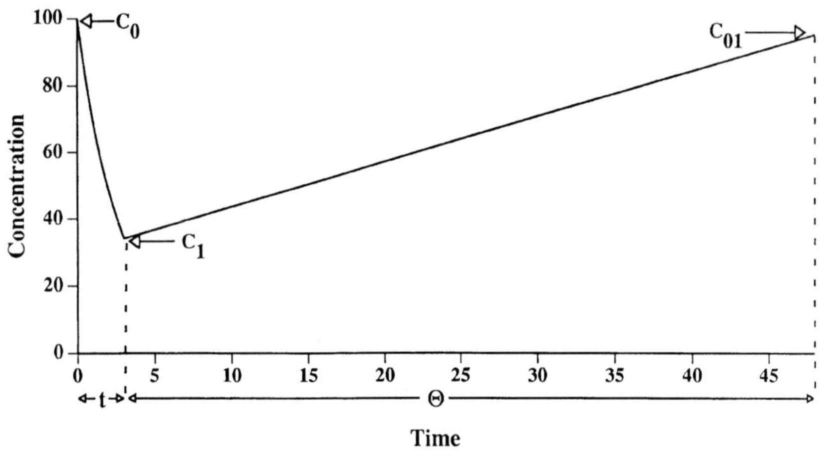

FIGURE 71.4. Changes in concentration of a readily dialyzed solute during (t; hours) and between (Θ; hours) hemodialysis treatments. C_0 depicts solute concentration at the beginning of dialysis. C_1 depicts the concentration of solute at the end of dialysis. The concentration fall during dialysis is depicted in a first-order fashion. Between treatments, the solute concentration increases in a zero-order fashion until it reaches the predialysis concentration, C_{01}.

Most studies of hemodialysis adequacy since the NCDS analysis have focused on refinement of Kt/V measurement and determination of the potential effect of the dose of hemodialysis on adult patient outcome. Decreasing all-cause mortality in adult hemodialysis patients has been correlated with progressively increasing Kt/V levels up to 1.3 (59). Current NKF-DOQI recommendations on dialysis adequacy in adult hemodialysis patients call for a minimum Kt/V of 1.2 (70). Although routine measurement of urea clearance by Kt/V has been reported for children receiving hemodialysis, there are no data on the association between delivered dialysis dose and outcomes for pediatric patients (71–78). Until such data are available, it is reasonable to provide children with at least a single-pool Kt/V of 1.2.

Formal urea kinetic modeling (UKM) solves two differential equations to yield the two variables of patient urea distribution volume (V_d, total body water in milliliters) and urea generation rate (G, in milligrams per minute). Treatment data needed for calculation of V_d are pretreatment and posttreatment BUN levels, the dialyzer urea clearance at a particular blood flow rate (K, in milliliters per minute), the hemodialysis treatment duration (t, in minutes), and the patient's pretreatment and posttreatment weight (in kilograms). Normalized urea clearance during hemodialysis can then be expressed by the unitless term Kt/V. Normalized protein catabolic rate (NPCR, in grams of protein per kilogram per day) is calculated from the urea generation rate (G) using the modified Borah equation (62).

The superiority of formal UKM over other methods for hemodialysis adequacy measurement resides in the ability of UKM to provide a unique solution for urea clearance by Kt/V and nutritional status by NPCR. Although formal UKM is recognized as the gold standard for hemodialysis adequacy measurement, evaluation of simpler surrogate methods to approximate Kt/V has been an active area of investigation. The natural logarithm formula of Daugirdas has been recognized and endorsed as the only valid alternative to formal UKM for Kt/V calculation in adults (28,78):

$$Kt/V = -\ln (C_1/C_0 - 0.008 \times t) + (4 - 3.5 \times C_1/C_0) \times UF/W \quad \text{[Eq. 2]}$$

where C_0 is predialysis BUN (in milligrams per deciliter), C_1 is postdialysis BUN (in milligrams per deciliter), t is session duration (in hours), UF is ultrafiltration volume (in kilograms), and W is postdialysis weight (in kilograms). The accuracy of the Daugridas natural logarithm formula lies in its accounting for dialysis treatment duration and urea removed by ultrafiltration.

The natural logarithm formula has been shown to be a reliable and practical alternative to formal UKM for estimation of Kt/V in a large group of pediatric patients receiving hemodialysis (71,79,80) and has been validated in comparison with formal UKM in children. In this same study, NPCR was also accurately and reliably estimated using a urea generation rate derived from the difference between the posttreatment and pretreatment BUN levels:

$$estG\ (mg/min) = [(C_2 \times V_2) - (C_1 \times V_1)]/t \quad \text{[Eq. 3]}$$

where C_1 is postdialysis BUN (in milligrams per deciliter), C_2 is predialysis BUN (in milligrams per deciliter), V_1 is postdialysis total body water (in deciliters; V_1 = 5.8 dL/kg × postdialysis weight in kilograms), V_2 is predialysis total body water (in deciliters; V_2 = 5.8 dL/kg × predialysis weight in kilograms), and t is time (in minutes) from the end of the dialysis treatment to the beginning of the following treatment. Then, estNPCR was calculated using the modified Borah equation:

$$estNPCR = 5.43 \times estG/V_1 + 0.17 \quad \text{[Eq. 4]}$$

where V_1 is total body water (in liters) postdialysis (0.58 × weight in kilograms).

Single-Pool versus Double-Pool Kt/V

Kt/V calculation is based on sampling of pretreatment and posttreatment BUN level. In adults and children, the posthe-

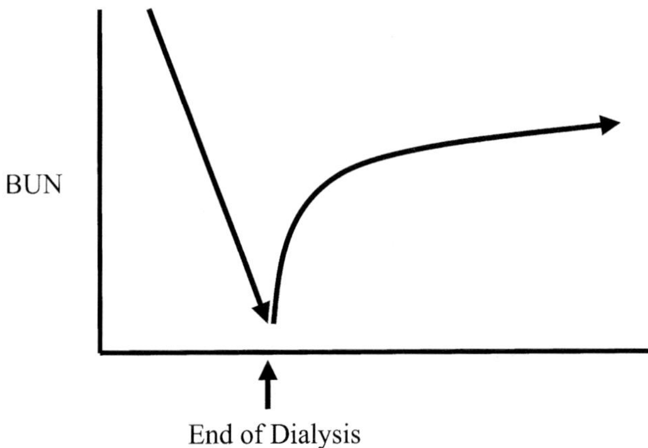

FIGURE 71.5. Depiction of urea rebound after a hemodialysis treatment. Blood urea nitrogen (BUN) moves from the extravascular space to the intravascular space by first-order kinetics until it reaches equilibration, a process that occurs over 30 to 60 minutes.

modialysis BUN concentration rises in a logarithmic fashion until equilibration occurs 30 to 60 minutes after a hemodialysis treatment (73,81,82). This rise in BUN concentration has been termed *urea rebound* (Fig. 71.5). As the BUN rises with equilibration after hemodialysis, the resultant calculation of Kt/V yields lower values. Urea rebound includes the early phenomena of access and cardiopulmonary recirculation, that is, the flow of the most recently dialyzed blood through urea-rich tissues and the later process of transcellular movement of urea after the cessation of dialysis.

Calculation of Kt/V by single-pool kinetics (spKt/V) using the immediate, 30-second postdialysis BUN ($BUN_{30\ sec}$) sample does not take urea rebound into account and leads to overestimation of the true urea mass removed during dialysis. Calculation of Kt/V by double-pool kinetics (eqKt/V) is based on a postdialysis BUN level actually determined through blood draw or estimated after the completion of urea rebound. Numerous studies of both children and adults have demonstrated that urea rebound ranges from 7.6 to 24.0% and accounts for a 12.3 to 16.8% difference between spKt/V and eqKt/V values (72–76). Despite inaccuracies, single-pool kinetic assessment has remained in use at some centers as a matter of convenience.

Because it is impractical to wait 1 hour after a treatment to obtain an equilibrated BUN (eqBUN) level for calculation of eqKt/V, several formulas have been devised to estimate eqKt/V by applying a cofactor to spKt/V and relying solely on a pretreatment and 30-second posttreatment BUN level (74,83–85). Because urea rebound is primarily characterized by a first-order logarithmic, concentration-dependent movement of urea from intracellular fluid to extracellular fluid, a more recent method (73) for estimating eqBUN extrapolates the rise in BUN from 30 seconds to 15 minutes after treatment (ΔBUN). Because urea rebound is 69% complete at 15 minutes after dialysis (72), eqBUN can be estimated (estBUN) using the following formula:

$$estBUN = [(BUN_{15\ min} - BUN_{30\ sec})/0.69] + BUN_{30\ sec} \quad \text{[Eq. 5]}$$

The difference between eqKt/V using a measured eqBUN and estimated eqKt/V using the estBUN by logarithmic extrapolation was less using this approach than with other published eqKt/V estimation methods (83–85).

The important relationship between nutritional status and outcome for patients with ESRD prompted the NKF-KDOQI to create guidelines to assess for and treat malnutrition in both children and adults with ESRD. The pediatric NKF-DOQI guidelines recommend measurement of serum albumin level, height or length, dry weight, midarm circumference, skinfold thickness, fronto-occipital circumference, and height Z score to monitor nutritional status and intensive enteral nutrition administration to treat protein energy malnutrition (86). Data also show that prealbumin is a more sensitive measure of current nutritional status. Although these measures may be important to monitor for and treat protein energy malnutrition, they may not be sufficient in all cases. Many adult outcome studies use NPCR as an independent marker of nutritional status. NPCR is derived from the interdialytic rise in BUN levels and has been shown to correlate with nutritional status in adult patients receiving hemodialysis (65–67). Minimal investigation into the validity of NPCR has been carried out since the early 1980s and demonstrated a positive correlation between dietary protein intake and NPCR (67,68). These studies suggested that positive nitrogen balance, which is essential for growth, could be achieved with moderate protein intake and without an increase in dialysis requirements. Research is now showing NPCR to be more sensitive and specific than serum albumin as a marker for nutritional status in pediatric hemodialysis patients (69,87).

Provision of adequate nutrition is essential to the delivery of optimal dialysis. Research has correlated increased protein administration and urea clearance with improved growth in well-nourished children undergoing hemodialysis (77). Intradialytic parenteral nutrition has been used effectively to treat severe protein energy malnutrition in children receiving hemodialysis (69,88). Intradialytic parenteral nutrition is comprised of dextrose (70%) and amino acids (15%) and is delivered during the dialysis treatment to provide 1.3 g/kg of protein.

Medications for Patients Receiving Hemodialysis

The physiology and treatment for ESRD-related anemia, renal osteodystrophy, and growth failure are discussed elsewhere in Chapter 67. Just as advances have been made in hemodialysis techniques, ongoing advances are being realized in the development of intravenous forms of medications for treatment of complications of ESRD. As a result of these advances, recombinant erythropoietin (rHuEpo) rather than red cell transfusion is administered during dialysis. Although higher rHuEpo doses may be required to correct anemia when given intravenously than when administered subcutaneously (89,90), ease of administration continues to make the intravenous route the preferred one in most pediatric dialysis units. Oral iron supplementation is rarely sufficient to maintain the iron stores, so treatment with intravenous iron complexes (iron dextran, ferric gluconate, iron sucrose) is necessary for optimum erythropoiesis (91–94). Investigation into maintenance intravenous iron dosing demonstrates decreased rHuEPO requirements with such dosing in both children and adult patients receiving hemodialysis (95–97). Intravenous forms of the vitamin D analogues calcitriol and paricalcitol are currently available to treat the secondary hyperparathyroidism associated with renal failure (98,99); pediatric dosing and efficacy trials are under way in the United States. Increased use of intravenous medications has led to increased nursing responsibilities during the hemodialysis treatment.

Acute Hemodialysis Considerations

The epidemiology and pathophysiology of acute renal failure are discussed in the Acute Renal Failure section. Acute hemodialysis requires the same type of equipment discussed earlier. Most acute dialysis access occurs via a temporary, uncuffed dual-lumen catheter placed in the femoral, internal jugular, or subclavian vein. Infants often require dialysis via two separate single-lumen venous catheters, for example, via umbilical vessels, because dual-lumen catheters may not be of appropriate size for their smaller vessel diameters. Many patients with acute renal failure are too ill to be transported to a chronic hemodialysis unit, so water treatment is accomplished using commercially available portable reverse osmosis machines. Many medications, including antimicrobials, anticonvulsants, sedatives, and chemotherapeutic agents, are removed by hemodialysis. Therefore, additional doses of these medications may be required during or after the hemodialysis treatment to maintain therapeutic serum concentrations. Patients who require two or more pressors to maintain normotension may be too unstable for intermittent hemodialysis and attendant intermittent ultrafiltration and might be treated more appropriately with continuous renal replacement therapy (100–102).

Acute hemodialysis is also indicated in certain clinical situations that are not accompanied by renal failure, such as tumor lysis syndrome in patients with newly diagnosed leukemia or lymphoma, and hyperammonemia in patients with inborn errors of metabolism and drug intoxications. In such clinical cases, close attention to and supplementation of the patient's serum phosphorus and potassium are required, because protracted hemodialysis can rapidly lead to hypophosphatemia and hypokalemia in a patient with normal renal function. Hemodialysis is indicated for the elimination of a toxin if there is a potential clinical benefit to the patient of removing the toxin more quickly than the endogenous clearance rate, if a significant amount of the toxin can be removed, and if there is a clear relationship between the blood levels of an agent and toxic effects. Toxins that can be successfully removed by dialysis are distributed in body water, have low molecular weights, and are not bound to plasma or tissue proteins.

HEMODIALYSIS FOR INFANTS

Although all pediatric hemodialysis requires specialized nursing and medical expertise, hemodialysis for neonates is an especially complicated procedure. As noted previously, neonatal-sized blood tubing is available to minimize the blood volume of the extracorporeal circuit. The neonatal tubing is one-fourth the diameter of standard tubing, so the blood pump speed must be quadrupled to deliver the same blood volume per minute (e.g., an apparent Q_b of 160 mL/min on the dialysis machine yields an actual blood flow of 40 mL/min through the dialyzer when neonatal tubing is used). Even with smaller neonatal tubing, the extracorporeal volume is usually greater than 10% of the patient's blood volume, so the circuit should be primed with packed red blood cells mixed to a concentration of 35%.

Current volumetric hemodialysis machines produce an ultrafiltration accuracy of 50 to 100 mL, which is acceptable for most pediatric patients but is not tolerable for neonates. Digital scales, which are accurate to within 10 g, can be placed under an infant warmer and help guide ultrafiltration during a neonatal hemodialysis treatment.

OPTIMAL PEDIATRIC HEMODIALYSIS

Evaluation and refinement of methods and technologies addressed in this chapter have been important steps toward establishing an evidence-based standard of optimal care for children receiving hemodialysis. Optimal pediatric hemodialysis care requires not only attention to these specific medical and nursing areas but also provision of adequate psychosocial, educational, and dietary support to patients and their families. Child-life specialists lend critical expertise to provide developmentally appropriate evaluation and assistance for pediatric patients with ESRD, who undergo many surgical procedures and are faced with the never-ending cycle of dialysis and renal transplantation. ESRD-trained social work personnel are essential to assess the psychosocial development of children with ESRD and to assist families with the complex socioeconomic challenges and barriers associated with ESRD. Dieticians expert in the nutritional requirements and restrictions imposed by ESRD are vital to develop palatable menus for children with ESRD and to monitor a multitude of nutritional status markers, including weight, growth, body mass index, NPCR, mid-arm circumference, triceps skinfold thickness, and results of bioimpedance analysis.

Furthermore, relevant short-term and long-term outcome measures for children with ESRD are lacking. Although standard outcome measures used for adult patients, such as death and hospitalization rates, are important outcome measures for children, they are clearly insufficient. In addition, factors to assess adult health-related quality of life (HRQOL), including work status and sexual function, are not generally appropriate for a pediatric population. Other factors including growth, exercise capacity, school attendance and performance, self-reliance, and functional development are crucial components for assessing the HRQOL for a pediatric patient with ESRD. Currently, no HRQOL measurement tool exists that is specific for a pediatric patient with ESRD. In addition, few data exist to describe the physical functioning capabilities and limitations for children with ESRD, and the data that are available do not follow children longitudinally over extended periods and are not linked with an assessment of HRQOL (103–106).

Most research into the HRQOL of pediatric ESRD patients occurred a number of years ago (106–112). These studies demonstrate that, although pediatric patients with ESRD certainly have some developmental and psychosocial issues similar to those of children with other chronic illnesses, they also have challenges specifically related to ESRD. Obstacles common to most chronically ill children include physical changes related to illness, the need to take many medications and undergo medical treatment, and time away from school and peers, which can lead to perceived differences and isolation. Children with ESRD have additional challenges such as maintaining a restricted dietary and fluid regimen, chronic dependence on medical equipment to sustain life, very obvious physical changes associated with transplantation, and the knowledge that they will live their whole lives with the recurrent cycle of dialysis and transplantation. To date, no follow-up from these studies has been published.

Both the acute and chronic effects of hemodialysis on short-term and long-term outcomes must be assessed. Potential areas for investigation include evaluation of the effects of different ultrafiltration modeling algorithms on postdialysis thirst, fatigue, interdialytic weight gain, exercise capacity, and patient attitude toward dialysis. In addition, establishing pediatric vascular access monitoring standards with UD or other noninvasive techniques will likely prolong vascular access survival rates and decrease patient morbidity and hospitalization. Such studies can only help to optimize patient physical and psychological well-being.

MULTICENTER END-STAGE RENAL DISEASE REGISTRIES

Although long-term prospective interventional outcome studies must be multicenter in design and will likely follow patients from hemodialysis through transplantation, current descriptive multicenter pediatric registries have been crucial to outline the state of pediatric ESRD-associated care.

Continued advances in acute and chronic hemodialysis treatment in children require accurate data on treatments and their outcomes in children. Improvements in hemodialysis techniques over the last 20 years have come from lessons learned in adults, results of single-center trials or surveys, and registry studies. The number of pediatric patients in even the largest pediatric centers is not large or diverse enough to provide sufficient data to optimally advance the practice of hemodialysis in children. Multiple national or multinational ESRD-related registries have been established in the last several decades, including the European Dialysis and Transplantation Association–European Renal Association (EDTA-ERA) registry, the United States Renal Data Renal Data System (USRDS), the Canadian Organ Replacement Register (CORR), the Registry of the Japanese Society for Dialysis Therapy, and the Australia and New Zealand Dialysis and Transplant Registry (ANZ DATA) (113). Center participation in all the registries is voluntary with the exception of the USRDS. Few of the registries have a focus or special analysis of pediatric patients. Detailed description of these registries is beyond the scope of this text; however, an overview of selected registries with significant pediatric components follows.

The EDTA-ERA registry, the oldest and largest of the registries of renal replacement therapy, has collected data since 1964. It currently covers 670 million people in 36 countries in Europe and the Mediterranean coastal region and is funded by the European Renal Association, some participating countries, industry, and educational grants. Participation varies by country with 50 to 90% of patients included in the database (114,115). In 1970 a survey of the members of the European Society of Pediatric Nephrology found a death rate from chronic renal failure of 0.75 per 1 million total population. Although that figure was thought to be an underestimate, the decision was made to develop a separate registry for "pediatric cases" within the EDTA (115). Pediatric patients are defined as those younger than 15 years at the start of renal replacement therapy. In 1971 there were 296 children registered; this increased to a total of 8850 by 1990 with an overall rate of 4.6 children per 1 million child population. Survey materials include questionnaires sent to centers about current practices as well as individual patient questionnaires. There are yearly dialysis and transplant reports providing a snapshot of the characteristics and status of patients with ESRD. There have also been special studies examining topics such as oxalosis, focal segmental glomerulosclerosis, and rehabilitation in adults who received renal replacement therapy as children. These studies are conducted through occasional mini-questionnaires. Information is also collected on the number of children cared for in "pediatric centers," defined by the presence of a pediatrician, a dietitian, a social worker, a child psychologist, school facilities, a children's ward, and a combined dialysis and transplantation program. In 1989, 77% of children were treated in pediatric centers (113).

The USRDS was established in 1988 with research funds from the National Institutes of Health with the following goals: to characterize patients receiving dialysis in the United States; to report trends in incidence, modalities, and outcomes over time; and to identify opportunities for more focused special studies (116). Data have been collected from Medicare-approved ESRD facilities since 1972 and include information on dialysis and transplantation. All patients whose treatment is paid for by the U.S. government are included in the United States, so the database includes approximately 94% of patients receiving dialysis in the United States. Data are transmitted through 18 regional ESRD networks to the Centers for Medicare and Medicaid Services (CMS; formerly the Health Care Financing Administration) and then to the National Institutes of Health. The data are analyzed by a coordinating center, currently at the Minneapolis Medical Research Foundation. Annual data reports are available at the USRDS web site, and individual investigators can download portions. Investigators can submit special data requests (117).

Subanalyses of pediatric dialysis and transplant patients, defined as those younger than 20 years of age, are performed using information in the USRDS database. In the 1997 to 1999 cohort, the ESRD incidence rates ranged from 7.0 per 1 million population for children 5 to 9 years of age to 26.5 per 1 million population for those 15 to 19 years of age (118). The data reported here have been supplied by the USRDS. The interpretation and reporting of these data are the responsibility of the authors and in no way should be viewed as an official policy or interpretation of the U.S. government.

In addition to the USRDS database analyses, CMS currently funds the ESRD Clinical Performance Measures Project based on periodic data collection involving a random sample of adult dialysis patients. Since 2000, a supplemental project has collected demographic data and information on dialysis adequacy, vascular access, management of anemia, and serum albumin levels on all in-center hemodialysis patients 12 to 18 years of age. The 2000 project included 433 patients. Seventy-nine percent of these had a mean calculated delivered Kt/V of more than 1.2; 41% had a catheter for vascular access; 55% had a mean hemoglobin level of more than 11 g/dL; and 83% had a serum albumin level within the normal range (119).

The North American Pediatric Renal Transplant Cooperative Study (NAPRTCS) is a voluntary registry that includes children and adolescents younger than 21 years of age at the initiation of dialysis or transplantation who receive care at 130 pediatric dialysis centers in the United States, Canada, Mexico, and Costa Rica. NAPRTCS is unique among the registries described in this section in that it includes only pediatric patients. Investigators organized NAPRTCS, and the registry portion of this study is funded by grants from industry. The registry was organized in 1987 to study renal transplantation in children and adolescents; it was expanded in 1992 to include pediatric hemodialysis and peritoneal dialysis patients at participating NAPRTCS centers, and in 1994 also included children with chronic renal insufficiency who did not yet require renal replacement therapy. Data-gathering forms soliciting information on patient demographics, treatment characteristics (e.g., dialysis access type, erythropoietin and growth hormone treatment), school attendance, and adverse effects are collected at enrollment, at 30 days, and then every 6 months. A clinical coordinating center and data-coordinating center organize data collection and analyses. Annual reports are generated and circulated to the participating investigators and are available on the World Wide Web (http://www.naprtcs.org). Registry reports describing trends in treatment and outcomes are periodically published. The 1996 annual report summarized data collected from 1992 to 1996 on 2208 patients in whom 2787 courses of dialysis were carried out (27). The 2002 annual report listed 4886 children in the dialysis registry, 2184 of whom had had at least one course of hemodialysis. In addition, periodic special studies (in which additional data are collected) or special analyses (in which additional analyses of existing data are carried out) are performed. Special analyses or studies may be requested by participating center investigators. A special studies committee reviews such requests, and the performance of these studies is based on scientific merit, the amount of additional time that will be required by the center investigators and coordinators, and the cost. In some cases, investigators must solicit additional funding to perform special studies or analyses. The NAPRTCS organization has also performed prospective clinical trials, funded principally by the National Institutes of Health.

The strength of these registries lies in the numbers of patients included and their descriptions of patients, treatments, and outcomes in a defined region during a specific time period. In theory, the existence of multiple registries should allow comparisons of different patient populations and treatment practices. The registries also share the weakness of including centers that dialyze varying numbers of patients and have varying personnel responsible for data collection, which may affect the patient population and the nature of the data collected. These registries describe children with ESRD and the outcomes of their treatment in hopes of improving patient care. However, they can only generate and not test specific hypotheses. Therefore, there is room for a more selective multicenter study of pediatric hemodialysis to address the unanswered questions in the care of children requiring acute and chronic hemodialysis.

A multicenter prospective pediatric continuous renal replacement therapy registry has been established with the purpose of identifying optimal continuous renal replacement therapy intervention strategies and rapidly testing new devices and medications for the treatment of critically ill children with acute renal failure.

REFERENCES

1. US Renal Data System. Excerpts from the USRDS 2001 annual data report. *Am J Kidney Dis* 2001;38:S1–S248.
2. Knight F, Gorynski L, Bentson M. Hemodialysis of the infant or small child with chronic renal failure. *ANNA J* 1990;20:315–323.
3. Bunchman T. Chronic dialysis in the infant less than 1 year of age. *Pediatr Nephrol* 1995;9:S18–S22.
4. Neu AM, Warady BA. Dialysis and renal transplantation in infants with irreversible renal failure. *Adv Ren Replace Ther* 1996;3:48–59.
5. Gotch FA, Autian J, Colton CK, et al. *The evaluation of hemodialyzers.* Washington, DC: DHEW Publ. No. NIH-73-103, 1973.
6. Hauk M, Kuhlmann MK, Riegel W, et al. In vivo effects of dialysate flow rate on Kt/V in maintenance hemodialysis patients. *Am J Kidney Dis* 2000;35:105–111.
7. Horl WH. Hemodialysis membranes. Interleukins, biocompatibility, and middle molecules. *J Am Soc Nephrol* 2002;13(suppl 1):S62–S71.
8. Kim PK, Deutschman CS. Inflammatory responses and mediators. *Surg Clin North Am* 2000;80:885–894.
9. Dinarello CA. Pro-inflammatory cytokines. *Chest* 2000; 118:503–508.
10. Brivet FG, Emilie D, Galanaud. Pro- and anti-inflammatory cytokines during acute severe pancreatitis: an early and sustained response, although unpredictable of death. *Crit Care Med* 1999;27:749–755.
11. Gloor B, Uhl W, Tcholakov O, et al. Hydrocortisone treatment of early SIRS in acute experimental pancreatitis. *Dig Dis Sci* 2001;456:2154–2161.
12. Herbelin A, Nguyen AT, Zingraff J, et al. Influence of uremia and hemodialysis on circulating interleukin-1 and tumor necrosis alpha. *Kidney Int* 1990;37:116–125.
13. Latscha B. Elevated circulating levels of interleukin-6 in patients with chronic renal failure. *Kidney Int* 1991;39:954–960.
14. Zwolinska D, Medynska A, Szprynger K, et al. Serum concentration of IL-2, IL-6, TNF-alpha and their soluble receptors in children on maintenance hemodialysis. *Nephron* 2000;86:441–446.
15. Sebekova K, Podracka L, Heidland A, et al. Enhanced plasma levels of advanced glycation end products (AGE) and pro-inflammatory cytokines in children/adolescents with chronic renal insufficiency and after renal replacement therapy by dialysis and transplantation—are they interrelated? *Clin Nephrol* 2001;56:S21–S26.
16. Danesh F, Ho LT. Dialysis-related amyloidosis: history and clinical manifestations. *Semin Dial* 2001;14:80–85.
17. Wang AYM, Woo J, Wang M, et al. Association of inflammation and malnutrition with cardiac valve calcification in continuous ambulatory peritoneal dialysis patients. *J Am Soc Nephrol* 2001;12:1927–1936.
18. Memoli B, Marzano L, Bisesti V, et al. Hemodialysis-related lymphomononuclear release of interleukin-12 in patients with end-stage renal disease. *J Am Soc Nephrol* 1999;10: 2171–2176.
19. Memoli B, Postiglione L, Cianciaruso B, et al. Role of different dialysis membranes in the release of interleukin-6-soluble receptor in uremic patients. *Kidney Int* 2000;58: 417–424.
20. Association for the Advancement of Medical Instrumentation. Water treatment equipment for hemodialysis applications. RD 62, 2001.
21. Baz M, Durand C, Ragon A, et al. Using ultrapure water in hemodialysis delays carpal tunnel syndrome. *Int J Artif Organs* 1991;14:681–685.
22. Ruder MA, Alpert MA, Van Stone J, et al. Comparative effects of acetate and bicarbonate hemodialysis on left ventricular function. *Kidney Int* 1985;27:768–773.
23. Leenen FH, Buda AJ, Smith DL, et al. Hemodynamic changes during acetate and bicarbonate hemodialysis. *Artif Organs* 1984;8:411–417.
24. Dheenan S, Henrich WL. Preventing dialysis hypotension: a comparison of usual protective maneuvers. *Kidney Int* 2001;59:1175–1181.
25. Sadowski RH, Allred EN, Jabs K. Sodium modeling ameliorates intradialytic and interdialytic symptoms in young hemodialysis patients. *J Am Soc Nephrol* 1993;4:1192–1198.
26. Sang GL, Kovithavongs C, Ulan R, et al. Sodium ramping in hemodialysis: a study of beneficial and adverse effects. *Am J Kidney Dis* 1997;29:669–677.
27. Lerner GR, Warady BA, Sullivan EK, et al. Chronic dialysis in children and adolescents. The 1996 annual report of the North American Pediatric Renal Transplant Cooperative Study. *Pediatr Nephrol* 1999;13:404–417.
28. NKF-K/DOQI. Clinical practice guidelines for vascular access: update 2000. *Am J Kidney Dis* 2001;37(suppl 1):S137–S181.
29. Bourquelot P, Cussenot O, Corbi P, et al. Microsurgical creation and follow-up of arteriovenous fistulae for chronic haemodialysis in children. *Pediatr Nephrol* 1990;4:156–159.
30. Excerpts from the United States Renal Data System 1999 annual data report. *Am J Kid Dis* 1999;34(suppl 1):S1–S176.
31. Swedberg SH, Brown BG, Sigley R, et al. Intimal fibromuscular hyperplasia at the venous anastomosis of PTFE grafts in hemodialysis patients. Clinical, immunocytochemical, light and electron microscopic assessment. *Circulation* 1989;80:1726–1736.
32. Kanterman RY, Vesely TM, Pilgram TK, et al. Dialysis access grafts: anatomic location of venous stenosis and results of angioplasty. *Radiology* 1995;195:135–139.
33. Albers FJ. Causes of hemodialysis access failure. *Adv Ren Replace Ther* 1994;1:107–118.
34. Dousset V, Grenier N, Douws C, et al. Hemodialysis grafts: color Doppler flow imaging correlated with digital subtraction angiography and functional status. *Radiology* 1991;181:89–94.
35. May RE, Himmelfarb J, Yenicesu M, et al. Predictive measures of vascular access thrombosis: a prospective study. *Kidney Int* 1997;52:1656–1662.
36. Oudenhoven LF, Pattynama PM, de Roos A, et al. Magnetic resonance, a new method for measuring blood flow in hemodialysis fistulae. *Kidney Int* 1997;45:884–889.
37. Schwab SJ, Raymond JR, Saeed M, et al. Prevention of hemodialysis fistula thrombosis. Early detection of venous stenoses. *Kidney Int* 1989;36:707–711.

38. Cinat ME, Hopkins J, Wilson SE. A prospective evaluation of PTFE graft patency and surveillance techniques in hemodialysis access. *Ann Vasc Surg* 1999;13:191–198.
39. Krivitski NM. Theory and validation of access flow measurement by dilution technique during hemodialysis. *Kidney Int* 1995;48:244–250.
40. Neyra NR, Ikizler TA, May RE, et al. Change in access blood flow over time predicts VAT. *Kidney Int* 1999;54:1714–1719.
41. May RE, Himmelfarb J, Yenicesu M, et al. Predictive measures of VAT: a prospective study. *Kidney Int* 1997;52:1656–1662.
42. Schwab SJ, Oliver MJ, Suhocki P, et al. Hemodialysis arteriovenous access: detection of stenosis and response to treatment by vascular access blood flow. *Kidney Int* 2001;59:358–362.
43. McCarley P, Wingard RL, Shyr Y, et al. Vascular access blood flow monitoring reduces access morbidity and costs. *Kidney Int* 2001;60:1164–1172.
44. Goldstein SL, Allsteadt A. Ultrasound dilution evaluation of pediatric hemodialysis vascular access. *Kidney Int* 2001;59:2357–2360.
45. Goldstein SL, Allsteadt A, Smith CM, et al. Ultrasound dilution monitoring of pediatric hemodialysis vascular access: effects of a proactive monitoring program on thrombosis rates. *Kid Int* 2002; 62:272–275
46. Mercadal L, Hamani A, Bene B, et al. Determination of access blood flow from ionic dialysance: theory and validation. *Kidney Int* 1999;56:1560–1565.
47. Steuer RR, Miller DR, Zhang S, et al. Noninvasive transcutaneous determination of access blood flow rate. *Kidney Int* 2001;60:284–391.
48. Sheth RD, Brandt ML, Brewer ED, et al. Permanent hemodialysis vascular access survival in children and adolescents with ESRD. *Kidney Int* (*in press*).
49. Goldstein SL, Macierowski CT, Jabs K. Hemodialysis catheter survival and complications in children and adolescents. *Pediatr Nephrol* 1997;11:74–77.
50. Sheth RD, Kale AS, Brewer ED, et al. Successful use of Tesio catheters in pediatric patients receiving chronic hemodialysis. *Am J Kidney Dis* 2001;38:553–559.
51. Sharma A, Zilleruelo G, Abitbol C, et al. Survival and complications of cuffed catheters in children on chronic hemodialysis. *Pediatr Nephrol* 1997;13:245–248.
52. Steuer RR, Leypoldt JK, Cheung AK, et al. Hematocrit is an indicator of blood volume and a predictor of intradialytic morbid events. *ASAIO J* 1994;40:M691–M696.
53. Swartz RD, Somermeyer MG, Hsu CH. Preservation of plasma volume during hemodialysis depends on the dialysate osmolality. *Am J Nephrol* 1982;2:189–194.
54. Steuer RR, Leypoldt JK, Cheung AK, et al. Reducing symptoms during hemodialysis by continuously monitoring the hematocrit. *Am J Kidney Dis* 1996;27:525–532.
55. Jain SR, Smith L, Brewer ED, et al. Non-invasive intravascular monitoring in the pediatric hemodialysis population. *Ped Nephrol* 2001;16:15–18.
56. Dheenan S, Henrich WL. Preventing dialysis hypotension: a comparison of usual protective maneuvers. *Kidney Int* 2001;59:1175–1181.
57. Michael M, Brewer ED, Goldstein SL. Non-invasive monitoring of hematocrit (NIVM) optimizes achievement of target weight (wt) without increasing intra- or interdialytic symptoms (sx) in children and adolescents receiving hemodialysis (HD). *J Am Soc Nephrol* 2001;12:398(abst).
58. Gotch FA, Sargent JA. A mechanistic analysis of the National Cooperative Dialysis Study (NCDS). *Kidney Int* 1985;28:526–534.
59. Held PJ, Port FK, Wolfe RA, et al. The dose of hemodialysis and patient mortality. *Kidney Int* 1996;50:550–556.
60. Bloembergen WE, Stannard DC, Port FK, et al. Relationship of dose of hemodialysis and cause-specific mortality. *Kidney Int* 1996;50:557–565.
61. Hakim RM, Breyer J, Ismail N, et al. Effects of dose of dialysis on morbidity and mortality. *Am J Kid Dis* 1994;23:661–669.
62. Borah MF, Schoenfeld PY, Gotch FA, et al. Nitrogen balance during intermittent dialysis therapy of uremia. *Kidney Int* 1978;14:491–500.
63. Combe C, Chauveau P, Laville M, et al. Influence of nutritional factors and hemodialysis adequacy on the survival of 1,610 French patients. *Am J Kidney Dis* 2001;37(1 suppl 2):S81–S88.
64. Cappy CS, Jablonka J, Schroeder ET. The effects of exercise during hemodialysis on physical performance and nutrition assessment. *J Ren Nutr* 1999;9:63–70.
65. Sobh MA, Sheashaa H, Tantawy AE, et al. Study of effect of optimization of dialysis and protein intake on neuromuscular function in patients under maintenance hemodialysis treatment. *Am J Nephrol* 1998;18:399–403.
66. Maggiore Q, Nigrelli S, Ciccarelli C, et al. Nutritional and prognostic correlates of bioimpedance indexes in hemodialysis patients. *Kidney Int* 1996;50:2103–2108.
67. Grupe WE, Harmon WE, Spinozzi NS. Protein and energy requirements in children receiving chronic hemodialysis. *Kidney Int* 1983;15(suppl 1):S6–S10.
68. Harmon WE, Spinozzi NS, Sargent JR, et al. Determination of protein catabolic rate (PCR) in children on hemodialysis by urea kinetic modeling. *Pediatr Res* 1979;13:513.
69. Goldstein SL, Baronette SD, Vital-Gambrell T, et al. nPCR assessment and IDPN treatment of malnutrition in pediatric hemodialysis patients. *Pediatr Nephrol* 2002:(*in press*).
70. NKF-K/DOQI. Clinical practice guidelines for hemodialysis adequacy: update 2000. *Am J Kidney Dis* 2001;37(1 suppl 1):S7–S64.
71. Goldstein SL, Sorof JM, Brewer ED. Natural logarithmic estimates of Kt/V in the pediatric hemodialysis population. *Am J Kidney Dis* 1999;33:518–522.
72. Goldstein SL, Sorof JM, Brewer ED. Evaluation and prediction of urea rebound and equilibrated Kt/V in the pediatric hemodialysis population. *Am J Kidney Dis* 1999;34:49–54.
73. Goldstein SL, Brewer ED. Logarithmic extrapolation of a 15-minute postdialysis BUN to predict equilibrated BUN and calculate double-pool Kt/V in the pediatric hemodialysis population. *Am J Kidney Dis* 2000;36:98–104.
74. Marsenic OD, Pavlicic D, Peco-Antic A, et al. Prediction of equilibrated urea in children on chronic hemodialysis. *ASAIO J* 2000;46:283–287.
75. Sharma A, Espinosa P, Bell L, et al. Multicompartment urea kinetics in well-dialyzed children. *Kidney Int* 2000;58:2138–2146.
76. Evans JH, Smye SW, Brocklebank JT. Mathematical modelling of haemodialysis in children. *Pediatr Nephrol* 1992; 6:349–353.

77. Tom A, McCauley L, Bell L, et al. Growth during maintenance hemodialysis: impact of enhanced nutrition and clearance. *J Pediatr* 1999;134:464–471.
78. Brem AS, Lambert C, Hill C, et al. Outcome data on pediatric dialysis patients from the end-stage renal disease clinical indicators project. *Am J Kidney Dis* 2000;36:310–317
79. Daugirdas JT. Second generation logarithmic estimates of single-pool variable volume Kt/V: an analysis of error. *J Am Soc Nephrol* 1993;4:1205–1213.
80. Goldstein SL. Pediatric hemodialysis—state of the art. *Adv Ren Replace Ther* 2001;8:173–179.
81. Pedrini LA, Zereik S, Rasmy S. Causes, kinetics and clinical implications of post-hemodialysis urea rebound. *Kidney Int* 1988;34:817–824.
82. Daugirdas JT, Schneditz D. Overestimation of hemodialysis dose depends on dialysis efficiency by regional blood flow but not by conventional two pool urea kinetic analysis. *ASAIO J* 1995;41:M719–M724.
83. Daugirdas JT, Depner TA, Gotch FA, et al. Comparison of methods to predict equilibrated Kt/V in the HEMO Pilot Study. *Kidney Int* 1997;52:1395–1405.
84. Tattersall J, DeTakats D, Chamney P, et al. The post-hemodialysis rebound: predicting and quantifying its effect on Kt/V. *Kidney Int* 1996;50:2094–2102.
85. Maduell F, Garcia-Valdecasas J, Garcia H, et al. Validation of different methods to calculate Kt/V considering postdialysis rebound. *Nephrol Dial Transplant* 1997;12:1928–1933.
86. Clinical practice guidelines for nutrition in chronic renal failure. *Am J Kidney Dis* 2000;35(suppl 2):S105–S136
87. Goldstein SL, Brewer ED. Low nPCR is an earlier marker than low serum albumin (Alb) for impending weight loss and potential malnutrition in pediatric hemodialysis (HD) patients (Pts). *J Am Soc Nephrol* 2001;12:448(abst).
88. Krause I, Shamir R, Davidovits M, et al. Intradialytic parenteral nutrition in malnourished children treated with hemodialysis. *J Ren Nutr* 2002;12:55–59
89. Paganini EP, Eschbach JW, Lazarus JM, et al. Intravenous versus subcutaneous dosing of epoetin alfa in hemodialysis patients. *Am J Kidney Dis* 1995;26:331–340
90. Ashai NI, Paganini EP, Wilson JM. Intravenous versus subcutaneous dosing of epoetin: a review of the literature. *Am J Kidney Dis* 1993;22(2 suppl 1):23–31.
91. Fishbane S, Wagner J. Sodium ferric gluconate complex in the treatment of iron deficiency for patients on dialysis. *Am J Kidney Dis* 2001;37:879–883.
92. Fishbane S, Lynn RI. The efficacy of iron dextran for the treatment of iron deficiency in hemodialysis patients. *Clin Nephrol* 1995;44:238–240.
93. Chandler G, Harchowal J, Macdougall IC. Intravenous iron sucrose: establishing a safe dose. *Am J Kidney Dis* 2001;38:988–991.
94. Faich G, Strobos J. Sodium ferric gluconate complex in sucrose: safer intravenous iron therapy than iron dextrans. *Am J Kidney Dis* 1999;33:464–470.
95. Greenbaum LA, Pan CG, Caley C, et al. Intravenous iron dextran and erythropoietin use in pediatric hemodialysis patients. *Pediatr Nephrol* 2000;14:908–911.
96. Morgan HE, Gautam M, Geary DF. Maintenance intravenous iron therapy in pediatric hemodialysis patients. *Pediatr Nephrol* 2001;16:779–783.
97. Besarab A, Amin N, Ahsan M, et al. Optimization of epoetin therapy with intravenous iron therapy in hemodialysis patients. *J Am Soc Nephrol* 2000;11:530–558.
98. Sprague SM, Lerma E, McCormmick D, et al. Suppression of parathyroid hormone secretion in hemodialysis patients: comparison of paricalcitol with calcitriol. *Am J Kidney Dis* 2001;38(suppl 5):S51–S56.
99. Andress DL. Intravenous versus oral vitamin D therapy in dialysis patients: What is the question? *Am J Kidney Dis* 2001;38(suppl 5):S41–S44.
100. Maxvold NJ, Smoyer WE, Gardner JJ, et al. Management of acute renal failure in the pediatric patient: hemofiltration versus hemodialysis. *Am J Kidney Dis* 1997;30(suppl 4):S84–S88.
101. Smoyer WE, McAdams C, Kaplan BS, et al. Determinants of survival in pediatric continuous hemofiltration. *J Am Soc Nephrol* 1995;6:1401–1409.
102. Goldstein SL, Currier H, Graf JM, et al. Outcome in children receiving continuous veno-venous hemofiltration. *Pediatrics* 2001;107:1309–1312.
103. Warady BA, Sabath RJ, Smith, et al. Recombinant human erythropoietin therapy in pediatric patients receiving long-term peritoneal dialysis. *Pediatr Nephrol* 1991;5:718–723.
104. Martin GR, Ongkingo JR, Turner, et al. Recombinant erythropoietin improves cardiac exercise performance in children with end-stage renal disease. *Pediatr Nephrol* 1993;7:276–280.
105. Giordano U, Calzolari A, Matteucci et al. Exercise tolerance and blood pressure response to exercise testing in children and adolescents after renal transplantation. *Pediatr Cardiol* 1998;19:471–473.
106. Krull F, Schulze-Neick I, Hatopp A, et al. Exercise capacity and blood pressure response in children and adolescents after renal transplantation. *Acta Paediatr* 1994;83:1296–1302.
107. Brownbridge G, Fielding DM. Psychosocial adjustment and adherence to dialysis treatment regimes. *Pediatr Nephrol* 1994;8:744–749.
108. Fukunishi I, Honda M. School adjustment of children with end-stage renal disease. *Pediatr Nephrol* 1995;9:553–557.
109. Garralda ME, Jameson RA, Reynolds JM, et al. Psychiatric adjustment in children with chronic renal failure. *J Child Psychol Psychiatry* 1988;29:79–90.
110. Brownbridge G, Fielding DM. Psychosocial adjustment to end-stage renal failure: comparing haemodialysis, continuous ambulatory peritoneal dialysis and transplantation. *Pediatr Nephrol* 1991;5:612–616.
111. Rosenkranz J, Bonzel KE, Bulla M, et al. Psychosocial adaptation of children and adolescents with chronic renal failure. *Pediatr Nephrol* 1992;6:459–463.
112. Frauman AC, Gilman CM, Carlson JR. Rehabilitation and social and adaptive development of young renal transplant recipients. *ANNA J* 1996;23:467–471.
113. D'Amico G. Comparability of the different registries on renal replacement therapy. *Am J Kidney Dis* 1995;25:113–118.
114. Mallick NP, Jones E, Selwood N. The European (European Dialysis and Transplantation Association-European Renal Association) Registry. *Am J Kidney Dis* 1995;25:176–187.
115. Broyer M, Chantler C, Donckerwolcke R, et al. The paediatric registry of the European Dialysis and Transplant Asso-

ciation: 20 years' experience. *Pediatr Nephrol* 1993;7:758–768.

116. Agodoa LY, Eggers PW. Renal replacement therapy in the United States: data from the United States Renal Data System. *Am J Kidney Dis* 1995;25:119–133.
117. United States Renal Data System. *Researcher's guide to the USRDS database.* Bethesda, MD: National Institutes of Health, National Institute of Diabetes and Digestive and Kidney Diseases, 2002.
118. U.S. Renal Data System. *USRDS 2001 annual data report: atlas of end-stage renal disease in the United States.* Bethesda, MD: National Institutes of Health, National Institute of Diabetes and Digestive and Kidney Diseases, 2001.
119. A study of pediatric (>12<18 years old) in-center hemodialysis patients: results for the 2000 End Stage Renal Disease Clinical Performance Measures Project. The Health Care Financing Administration, January 2001.

72

TRANSPLANTATION IMMUNOBIOLOGY

ALAN M. KRENSKY
CAROL CLAYBERGER

A basic understanding of the cellular and molecular basis of organ transplant acceptance and rejection helps in diagnosing and treating rejection more readily and prolonging allograft survival. Although much is already understood about the basic processes involved, the mechanisms of discrimination of self from nonself are complex. This chapter reviews current knowledge of the immunobiology of transplantation; another chapter discusses the current status of clinical renal transplantation.

MAJOR HISTOCOMPATIBILITY COMPLEX

A major function of the immune system is the discrimination of self from nonself. Although this system almost assuredly arose to allow the individual to keep out foreign infectious invaders, the same basic mechanisms are responsible for the cascade of events that result in organ transplant rejection. T lymphocytes recognize antigen as proteolyzed fragments (peptides) bound to major histocompatibility complex (MHC) molecules (1–3). MHC molecules, called HLA for human leukocyte antigens in the human, are polymorphic, and most individuals differ in their expression of these cell-surface antigens. When lymphocytes from one individual interact with cells from an unrelated individual, the lymphocytes recognize antigens on the unrelated tissue as nonself and are activated (called the *alloresponse*). These cells proliferate in numbers and differentiate to activate effector arms of the immune system (Fig. 72.1) (4–8). The major histocompatibility antigens responsible for these events are encoded by a cluster of genes on human chromosome 6 (Fig. 72.2) (9,10). These genes encode proteins of three distinct structural and functional groups, designated HLA class I, class II, and class III. The HLA class I antigens are constitutively expressed by most cells and tissues. They are composed of a 44,000-d polymorphic heavy chain associated with an invariant 12,000-d light chain, β_2-microglobulin (encoded on chromosome 15). These class I antigens can be subdivided based on genetic clustering and sequence homologies into families designated HLA-A, HLA-B, and HLA-C. Although HLA class I typing arose from microcytotoxicity assays using antisera, these reactivity patterns correlate well with the sequence information that has been obtained (11). The most common HLA class I type is HLA-A2, as originally identified by typing antisera. Subsequent serotyping, biochemical analysis, and sequence information shows that there is microheterogeneity within HLA molecules, which gives rise to subtypes within particular HLA families. For instance, there are currently 31 recognized subtypes for HLA-A2 and 16 for HLA-B27 (12,13). It is certain that the number of subtypes, based on sequence microheterogeneity, will continue to grow and that HLA types will prove to be even more complex than previously thought. Although the HLA-C antigens are structurally very similar to the HLA-A and HLA-B antigens, they are less polymorphic and do not elicit as strong an allogeneic response (antigenic response between individuals of the same species) as the HLA-A and HLA-B antigens.

The function of HLA class I molecules is to present peptide antigens to a subpopulation of T lymphocytes that perform specific functions, including HLA-restricted cytotoxicity and suppression (see later). The crystal structure of HLA-A2 revealed a groove on its external surface that allows a peptide to bind and in turn be "presented" to the immune system (Fig. 72.3) (14,15). Subsequent crystallographic studies showed that these peptides fit into anchoring pockets along the groove, which determines which peptides can fit into a particular HLA molecule and thereby be presented to the immune system (16). HLA class I molecules bind peptide antigens within the endoplasmic reticulum, which biases the peptides bound to those derived from intracellular (or endogenous) antigens (17,18).

HLA class II molecules are structurally and functionally distinct. They are constitutively expressed by a relatively small number of cell types—B lymphocytes, macrophages, monocytes, and follicular dendritic cells—but they can be induced by interferon and other agents on several other cell types, including T lymphocytes, endothelial cells, renal tubular cells, and pancreatic islet cells. HLA class II molecules are composed of a 44,000-d heavy chain associated

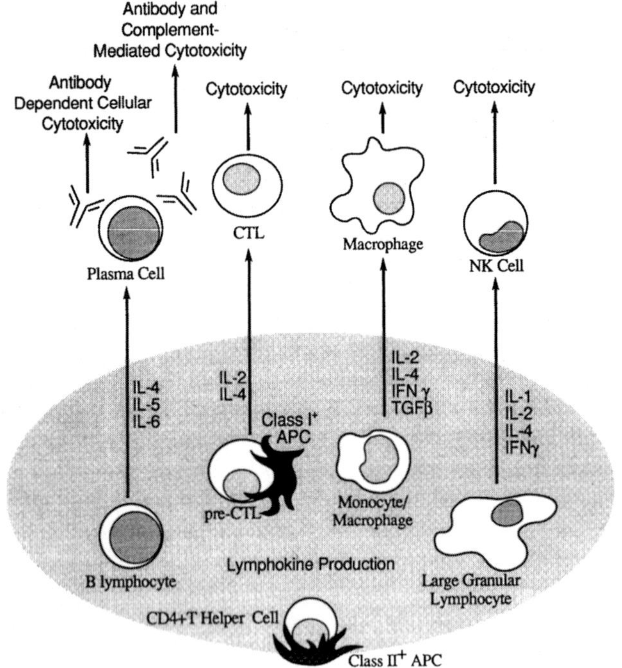

FIGURE 72.1. Cellular basis of transplant rejection. CD4+ T helper lymphocytes recognize HLA class II antigens expressed on allograft cells and release lymphokines, which in association with foreign antigens, activate the effector arms of the immune system. APC, antigen-presenting cell; CTL, cytotoxic T lymphocyte; IL, interleukin; IFN, interferon; NK cell, natural killer cell; TGF, transforming growth factor. (Adapted from Krensky AM. Molecular basis of transplant rejection and acceptance. *Pediatr Nephrol* 1991;5:422–427.)

with a 39,000-d light chain. Although both chains are polymorphic, most of the allelic polymorphism resides in the aminoterminal domains (α_1 and β_1), which correlates well with the key role these external parts are known to play in antigen presentation and T cell recognition (19). HLA class II molecules are divided into three subgroups: HLA-DR, HLA-DP, and HLA-DQ. These molecules bind peptides in compartments of the endocytic pathway and, therefore, generally present exogenously supplied antigens (17,18). HLA class II molecules present antigen to helper T lymphocytes, which, in response, proliferate, amplify, and coordinate the immune response. HLA-DR antigens are the strongest inducers of the proliferative response to nonself. The specialized functions of HLA-DP and HLA-DQ antigens are less clear, although there is some evidence that HLA-DQ may be involved in tolerance induction (20) (see later).

HLA class III molecules are structurally and functionally more diverse (21). Included in this region are the genes for several proteins of the complement cascade, including C4, C2, and factor B (Bf). Although these molecules are important components of the effector arm of the immune response, they do not appear to be relevant to proximal events in transplant rejection.

Subsequent work uncovered non–class II genes in the class II region (22). Although several of these genes have no obvious relevance to the immune system, others are part of the antigen-processing machinery for HLA class I molecules. Two genes (*t*ransporter *a*ssociated with antigen *p*rocessing 1, or TAP 1 [RING 4], and TAP 2 [RING 11]) encode peptide transporters (23,24), whereas closely linked genes (large multifunctional protease 2, or LMP 2 [RING 12], and LMP 7 [RING 10]) encode components of a large cytoplasmic organelle, the proteasome, which generates peptide fragments (25,26). A current model (Fig. 72.4) suggests that intact antigen binds to the proteasome, which then degrades the protein into peptide fragments (27). These peptides in turn are pumped by the peptide transporters across the membrane of the endoplasmic reticulum, where newly synthesized HLA class I molecules, peptides, and β_2-microglobulin associate to form the HLA molecules, which are then routed to the cell surface.

Minor Transplantation Antigens

Rejection episodes documented between HLA-identical siblings support studies in experimental animals that indicate that there are minor transplantation antigens (28,29).

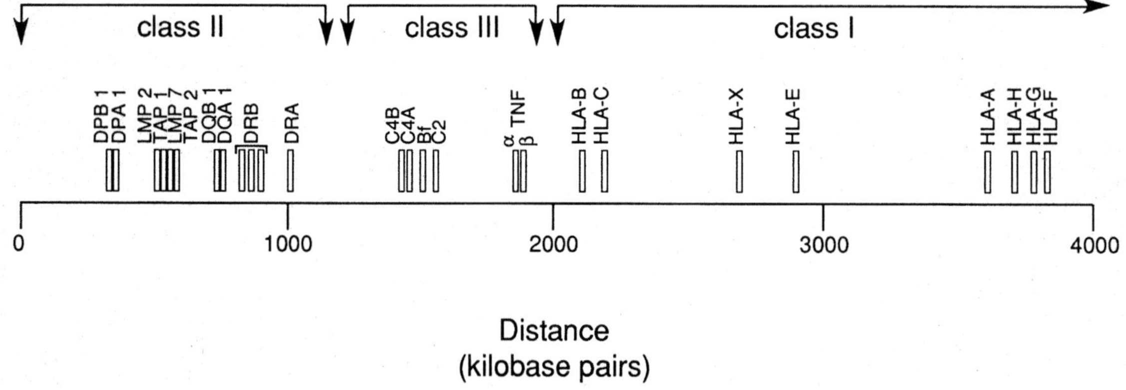

FIGURE 72.2. Map of the human major histocompatibility complex.

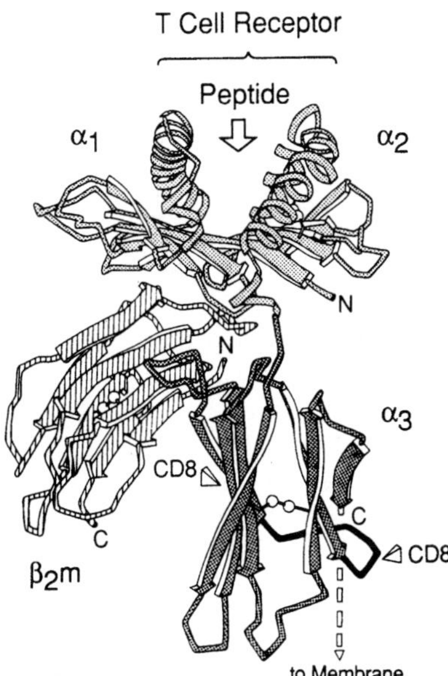

FIGURE 72.3. Structure of HLA-A2. The α_1 and α_2 domains (*dotted*) form the peptide-binding site, with the groove in which the peptide binds and the face with which the T-cell receptor is thought to interact indicated at the top. β_2-Microglobulin (*hatched*) and α_3 (*heavily shaded*) are immunoglobulin-like domains adjacent to the cell membrane. The diagram does not show the membrane anchor and cytoplasmic domains, which are at the carboxy end of the α_3 domain. N and C denote the amino and carboxy ends, respectively. The putative CD8 binding region is indicated in black. (Adapted from Bjorkman PJ, Saper MA, Samraoui B, et al. Structure of the human class I histocompatibility antigen, HLA-A2. *Nature* 1987;329:506–512; and Krensky AM, Weiss A, Crabtree G, et al. T-lymphocyte-antigen interactions in transplant rejection. *N Engl J Med* 1990;322:510–517.)

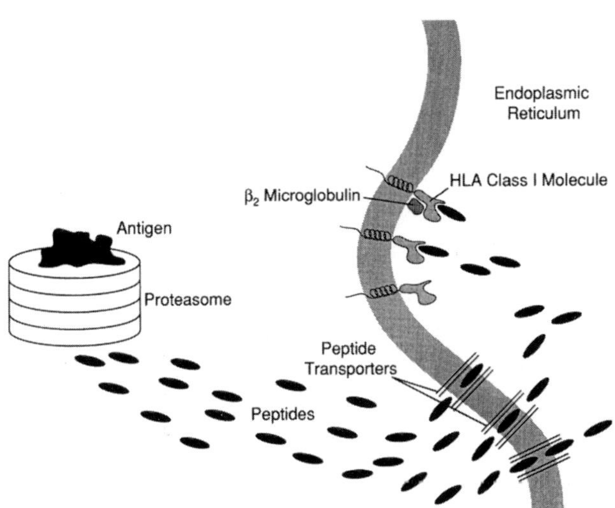

FIGURE 72.4. Antigen-processing machinery. It is postulated that antigens are proteolyzed into peptide fragments in proteasomes located in the cytosol. Peptides enter the endoplasmic reticulum via specialized transporters and associate with HLA class I molecules. β_2-Microglobulin associates with the peptide–HLA heavy chain complex, and mature HLA molecules are routed to the cell surface. (Adapted from Parham P. Transporters of delight. *Nature* 1990;348:674–675; and Robertson M. Proteasomes in the pathway. *Nature* 1991;353:300–301.)

Numerous minor systems, all with limited polymorphism, have been identified in mice and can result in vigorous rejection between HLA-identical individuals. Because minor histocompatibility antigens are recognized as peptides in association with HLA molecules, rather than as intact antigens, it proved difficult to raise antibodies against them. The generation of T-cell clones and elution of peptides from HLA molecules, however, has allowed the molecular characterization of at least some of these antigens (30,31). Peptides derived from self-proteins that vary among members of the same species function as minor histocompatibility antigens. Examples include mitochondrial proteins and gender-associated antigens (e.g., H-Y) (30,31). The large number of single-nucleotide polymorphisms identified in humans suggests the theoretical opportunity for a very large number of minor histocompatibility mismatches.

ALLOGENEIC RESPONSE

Molecular Basis of the Alloresponse

The immune response between genetically unrelated individuals of the same species, designated the alloresponse, is largely due to the proliferative response induced by HLA class II molecules and cytolytic response directed at HLA class I molecules (4,7). The process by which HLA differences lead to graft rejection is a variation on the normal function of these molecules as described earlier, although the precise role of HLA-associated peptide in the alloresponse remains incompletely defined (4,32).

The allogeneic response is stronger than the T-cell response against nominal antigens, such as viruses. There are at least 100-fold more peripheral T lymphocytes primed to react to nonself HLA than there are T lymphocytes capable of recognizing self HLA plus a particular antigen, such as influenza. The explanation for this probably lies in the natural high affinity of T-cell receptors for HLA antigens. T cells must go through the thymus before they appear in the periphery. It is in the thymus that T cells with appropriate self-reactivity are selected (educated to self). T cells with too high an affinity for self HLA are deleted (negative selection), whereas those with "proper" affinity are selected (positive selection) (Fig. 72.5) (33,34). T cells with too low an affinity die due to a lack of positive selection. Because T cells do not know in advance what the particular self HLA polymorphism will be, the T-cell repertoire must cover the entire spectrum of HLA types. In organ transplantation across an HLA barrier, T cells that escaped negative selection in the thymus may now (in the periphery) encounter donor HLA antigens for which they have very high affinity. This natural affinity of T-cell receptors for HLA molecules may in part account for the magnitude of the allogeneic response. An alternative explanation is that there is "molecular mimicry" between HLA-plus-peptide combinations such that nonself HLA plus X is recognized as self HLA plus Y (35).

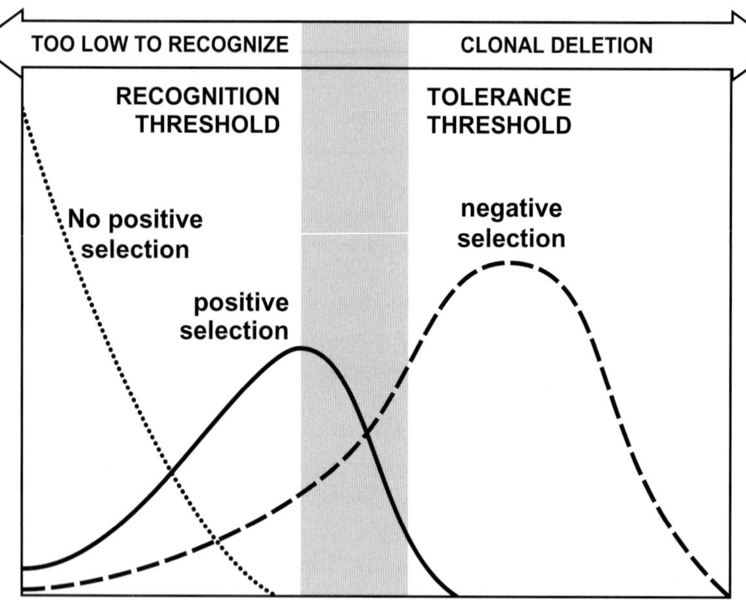

FIGURE 72.5. Positive and negative selection. T lymphocytes are selected in the thymus for proper affinity to self HLA. T cells with too low an affinity for self are not positively selected; T cells with too high an affinity for self are deleted by negative selection. Only T cells with receptors with "proper" affinity for self are positively selected and emerge from the thymus. TCR, T-cell receptor. (From Krensky AM. Immunologic tolerance. *Pediatr Nephrol* 2001;16:675–679, with permission.)

There remains the question of the precise molecular nature of the alloantigen. Is the strong allogeneic response directed at the HLA molecule devoid of peptide, with a particular peptide, or with any peptide? Rammensee and his colleagues shed light on this important question (36,37). Anchoring pockets in the HLA molecule restrict the peptides that can fit into a given HLA molecule. HLA-A2, for instance, tends to bind peptides with a leucine or methionine at position 2 and a valine or leucine at position 9 (36). HLA-B27, on the other hand, contains peptides that have an arginine at position 2 and an arginine or lysine at position 9 (38). Thus, HLA molecules have a restricted pattern of peptides that they are capable of binding. In some cases, it appears that the T cell recognizes these anchor positions in the context of the HLA molecule, whereas in other instances one particular peptide or perhaps an empty molecule may be recognized (32,35–39). Thus, the robustness of the allogeneic response depends not only on the natural affinity of T-cell receptors for HLA molecules but also on the variety of different T cell–peptide–HLA interactions that can result in allorecognition.

Cellular Basis of the Immune Response

The immune response in general, and allogeneic response in particular, are orchestrated by T helper cells, which recognize HLA class II antigens (Fig. 72.1) (4,40,41). A T lymphocyte has on its surface a clonally restricted T-cell receptor (42,43). These T-cell receptors structurally resemble immunoglobulin molecules with variable, constant, and joining regions. The variable and joining regions determine antigen specificity and account for the specificity encoded in the T-cell repertoire. In addition, T cells express other invariant cell-surface molecules that are associated with the antigen-specific T-cell receptor. These include the CD3 complex (42,44) and the CD4 and CD8 molecules (45) (Fig. 72.6). The CD3 complex consists of three invariant dimers, CD3 ε-γ, ε-δ, and ζ-ζ, that transduce signals from

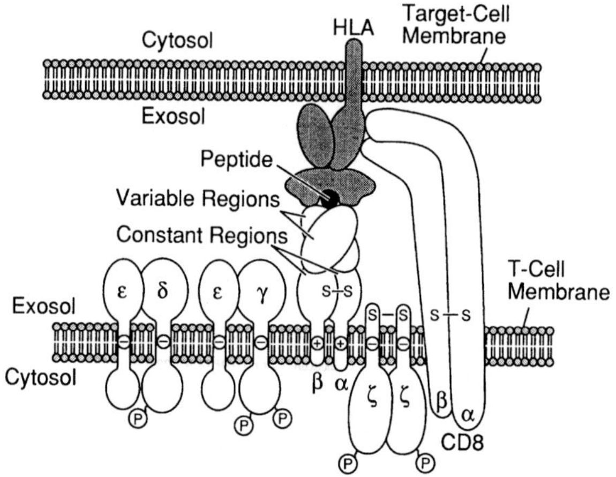

FIGURE 72.6. The T-cell receptor complex. The T-cell receptor α and β chains are linked by disulfide bonds to form a heterodimer that recognizes peptides associated with HLA molecules on the target cell membrane. CD3 polypeptides form invariant dimers that are thought to function in signal transduction. The CD8 molecule transiently associates with the T-cell receptor complex and recognizes invariant sequences of the HLA class I α_3 domain. P, phosphorylation sites. (Adapted from Krensky AM, Weiss A, Crabtree G, et al. T-lymphocyte-antigen interactions in transplant rejection. *N Engl J Med* 1990;322: 510–517.)

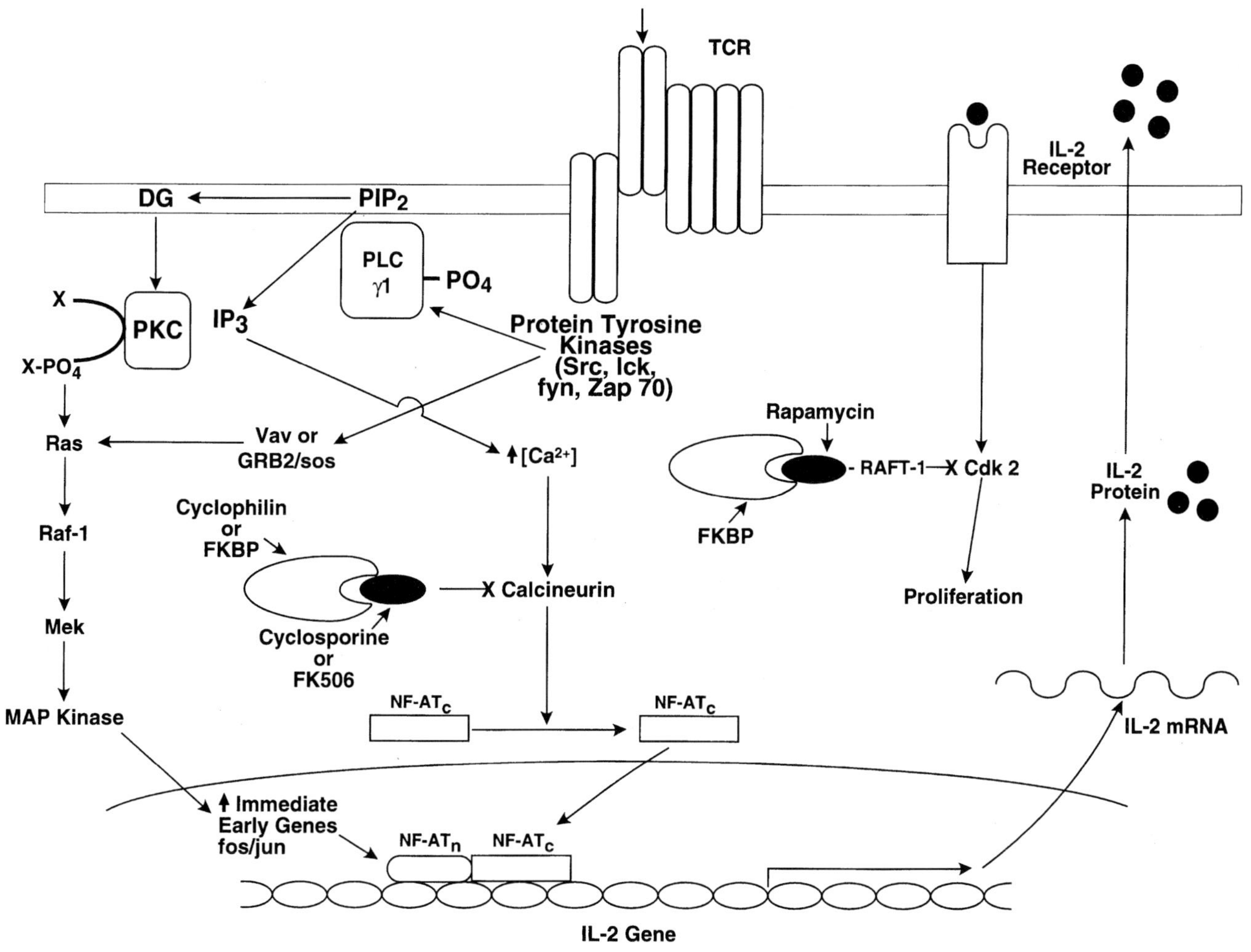

FIGURE 72.7. Cytoplasmic and nuclear events in T-cell activation. Triggering of the T-cell receptor (TCR) complex by specific antigen activates phospholipase C (PLC), tyrosine kinase, protein kinase C (PKC), and calcium ion flux. Through as yet undefined pathways, these cell surface biochemical events induce the transcription of activation-associated genes in the T-cell nucleus. For details, see references 4, 48, and 49. DG, diacylglycerol; FK506, tacrolimus; FKBP, FK506-binding protein; IL, interleukin; IP_3, inositol 1,4,5-triphosphate; MAP, mitogen-activated protein; mRNA, messenger RNA; $NF\text{-}AT_c$ and $NF\text{-}AT_n$, cytoplasmic component and nuclear component, respectively, of nuclear factor of T-cell activation; PIP_2, phosphatidylinositol 4,5-biphosphate. (From Clayberger C, Krensky AM. Mechanisms of allograft rejection. In Neilson EG, Couser WG, eds. *Immunologic renal diseases*, 2nd ed. Philadelphia: Lippincott Williams & Wilkins, 2001:321–346, with permission.)

the antigen-specific T-cell receptor into the cell (see later) (42,46). The CD4 and CD8 molecules, on the other hand, function as "co-receptors" in antigen recognition (45,47). Most mature peripheral blood lymphocytes express either CD4 or CD8. CD4 binds and recognizes HLA class II molecules, whereas CD8 interacts with HLA class I. Therefore, most helper T lymphocytes, which tend to recognize HLA class II molecules, are CD4+; most cytotoxic T lymphocytes recognize HLA class I antigens and express CD8.

Thus, when specific T-cell receptors on CD4+ helper T lymphocytes of a transplant recipient encounter foreign HLA-DR antigens on a transplanted organ, the helper T lymphocytes are triggered (4,48,49). Signals are sent from the T-cell receptor complex into the T cell (46,48). Several pathways are activated, including the flux of calcium across the T-lymphocyte membrane, a phosphatidylinositol signaling pathway, protein kinase C, and tyrosine kinases (Fig. 72.7) (46,48). The connections between these biochemical events near the cell surface and the ensuing functional events have become increasingly clear. The cytoplasmic domains of the T-cell receptor invariant chains contain a common motif that couples these proteins to intracellular protein kinases. *Src* family members, *lck* and *fyn*, interact with these antigen recognition activation motifs, which results in the phosphorylation of the motifs and recruitment of ZAP70 kinase to the membrane receptor complex. Both CD4 and CD8 bind *lck* through a common cysteine-containing motif, bringing *lck* into proximity of the T-cell receptor complex

TABLE 72.1. LYMPHOKINES

Name	Biologic activities
IL-1	Activates resting T cells, stimulates lymphokine synthesis, activates macrophages and endothelial cells, has multiple other effects
IL-2	T-cell growth factor; induces lymphokine synthesis, activates cytotoxic T cells
IL-3	Multicolony-stimulating factor, mast cell growth factor; shows histamine release activity
IL-4	B- and T-cell growth factor; induces HLA-DR; enhances cytotoxic T-cell activity, immunoglobulin isotype regulation (induces IgE), mast cell growth factor
IL-5	B-cell growth and differentiation factor; enhances IL-2–mediated killer cell induction, eosinophil colony-stimulating factor
IL-6	B-cell growth factor; myeloid growth factor; T-cell costimulatory activity; induces HLA class I expression, immunoglobulin secretion, and hepatic acute-phase proteins
IL-7	B- and T-cell growth factor (stromal cell factor)
IL-8	Neutrophil chemotactic and activating factor
IL-9	T-cell, mast cell, erythroid (hematopoietic) growth factor
IL-10	Cytokine synthesis inhibitory factor, B-cell–derived T-cell growth factor, mast cell growth factor; increases MHC class II expression
IL-11	Megakaryocyte stimulatory factor
IL-12	NK (natural killer) cell stimulatory factor
IL-13	B-cell growth and differentiation factor; inhibits macrophage inflammatory cytokine production
IL-15	T-cell growth factor; IL-2–like in action
GM-CSF	Granulocyte, eosinophil, and macrophage colony formation, histamine release activity
IFN-γ	Induces MHC and other cell surface antigen expression; activates macrophages and endothelial cells; antiviral
TNF-α	"Cachectin," direct cytotoxin for tumors; induces acute-phase responses, induces lymphokines, stimulates macrophages and endothelial cells, mediates inflammation
TNF-β	"Lymphotoxin"; induces MHC expression, B-cell growth factor, antiviral; activates endothelial cells, granulocytes, and osteoclasts

GM-CSF, granulocyte-macrophage colony-stimulating factor; IFN, interferon; IgE, immunoglobulin E; IL, interleukin; MHC, major histocompatibility complex; TNF, tumor necrosis factor.

and perhaps stabilizing the interaction. The role of interacting nonenzymatic proteins as the structural core of T-cell receptor signaling has been elucidated (49). Scaffolds, adaptors, and linkers, including linkers of activated T cells (LAT), SH2 (*src* homology 2)–containing leukocyte-specific protein of 76 kDa (SLP-76), and SLP-76–associated phosphoprotein of 130 kDa (SLP-130), are thought to coordinate signaling pathways by performing anchoring, targeting, and kinetic thresholding functions (49).

In a related but separate pathway, tyrosine phosphorylation of *vav* activates the *ras* signal transduction pathway. The oncogene *ras*, a guanosine triphosphate–binding protein with guanosine triphosphatase activity, interacts directly with Raf-1, a serine-threonine kinase, which regulates a cascade of kinases, including Mek and MAP (mitogen-activated protein) kinase. These events lead to the binding of c-fos and c-jun transcription factors to the interleukin (IL)-2 promoter. With the nuclear factor of activated T lymphocytes (NF-AT), these factors lead to the transcription of new genes, such as IL-2, in T lymphocytes (50). Immune cells are triggered to make soluble mediators (cytokines or, when made by leukocytes, ILs), which in turn trigger specific effector arms of the immune system (Fig. 72.1) (48,50). For example, activated helper T lymphocytes make IL-2, a potent inducer of lymphocyte proliferation, as well as upregulate IL-2 receptors on their surfaces. These cells then induce themselves to proliferate and differentiate (autocrine stimulation) as numerous other well-characterized factors are elaborated by the helper T lymphocytes (Table 72.1) (51–53). These include interferon-gamma, which induces both the de novo and increased expression of HLA class II antigens, which in turn amplify the stimulation, as well as families of chemoattractants, growth and differentiation factors, and lytic effector molecules (51–53) (see later).

When a $CD8^+$ precytolytic T lymphocyte recognizes an HLA class I molecule and receives stimulation by growth factors, including IL-2, IL-4, and IL-5 from nearby helper T lymphocytes, it too proliferates and differentiates (54). These cells in turn are capable of damaging and eventually killing target cells by at least two processes (Fig. 72.8) (55–57). In one process, cytolytic T lymphocytes release granules that contain perforin, granzymes, and granulysin. Perforin is a complement C9–like molecule that makes pores in target cells, which results in osmotic lysis within minutes (55). Granzymes are serine esterase molecules that enter through the pores and rapidly induce the disintegration of target cell DNA and cell death (56). Granulysin is a member of the saposin-like family of proteins and induces apoptosis via caspase-dependent and caspase-independent mechanisms (57). The second process results in apoptotic cell death after interaction of cell surface molecules Fas and Fas ligand. Fas is a transmembrane 48,000-d glycoprotein that shares homology with tumor necrosis factor (TNF)-α. Cross-linking Fas by antibody or binding to its natural ligand (Fas ligand) induces cell death characterized by DNA fragmentation (58).

Some of the factors produced by the $CD4^+$ helper T lymphocytes (IL-4, IL-5, and IL-6) induce resting B cells, which express cell surface immunoglobulin specific for donor antigens, to proliferate and differentiate (59,60). Fully differentiated B cells become plasma cells and make large amounts of specific antibody. Antibody in turn binds target tissues, leading to direct destruction by binding complement or directing cell-mediated cytotoxicity by K cells (61) (Fig. 72.1).

Natural killer (NK) cells, macrophages, eosinophils, and granulocytes also respond to factors made by helper T lym-

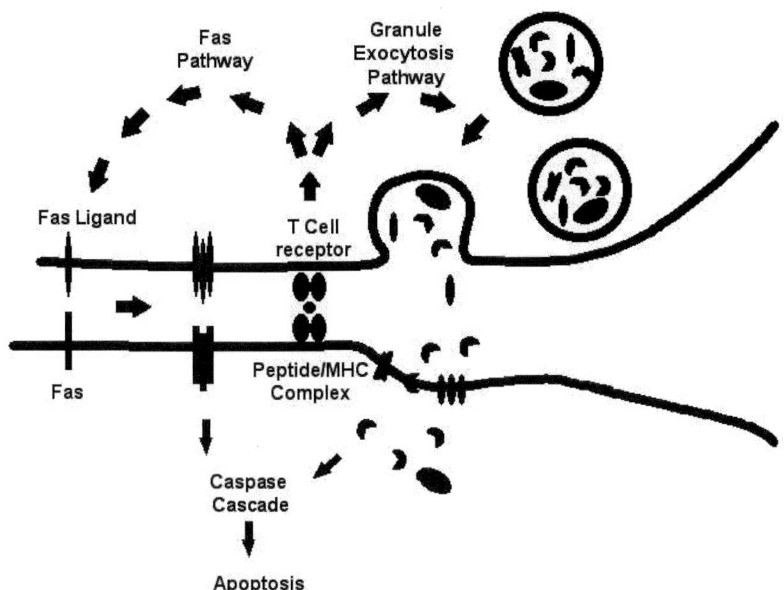

FIGURE 72.8. Mechanisms of cytotoxic T lymphocyte–mediated cytolysis. Granules containing perforin and granzymes mediate a secretory pathway for target cell lysis. A nonsecretory pathway involves the interaction of Fas (CD95) on target cells with Fas ligand on cytotoxic T lymphocytes. MHC, major histocompatibility complex.

phocytes and contribute to graft dysfunction and rejection (50–53).

TRANSPLANT REJECTION

The cellular and molecular events described earlier account for only some of the well-characterized pathologic and clinical patterns of rejection (62,63). The rejection process is more complex than the classical patterns of (a) hyperacute rejection associated with preformed antibodies (Fig. 72.9A,B) and (b) acute/subacute to chronic rejection associated with cellular infiltrates (Fig. 72.9C–E). Increasingly, chronic forms of rejection associated with vascular and interstitial changes (Fig. 72.9F) have been appreciated (64). These may result from the elaboration of cytokines and other factors that are still poorly understood. Both immunologic and nonimmunologic factors contribute to chronic allograft rejection (65).

Hyperacute rejection is characterized by immediate and massive damage to the allograft (66). Preexisting antibodies to ABO, HLA, and other polymorphic antigens bind the allograft endothelium and activate complement. The result is fibrinoid necrosis of the vessel walls, platelet and fibrin thrombus formation, mononuclear and polymorphonuclear cell infiltration, and ischemic necrosis within minutes to hours. Although the cause of sensitization (pregnancy, transfusion, previous transplants) is not always apparent, routine crossmatching has virtually eliminated this fulminant type of rejection.

The histologic hallmark of acute/subacute rejection is the infiltration of the graft with T cells and injury to parenchymal cells (67). Macrophages, NK cells, and granulocytes are also variably present. Foreign HLA class II antigens in the graft are recognized by circulating immune cells. This antigen-presenting function may be performed by "professional" antigen-presenting cells, resident macrophages, dendritic cells, or passenger leukocytes. There is now considerable evidence, however, that B cells (and even endothelial and epithelial cells), once induced to express HLA class II antigens, can perform this function, which triggers $CD4^+$ helper T lymphocytes and activates the cascade of events described earlier (Fig. 72.1) (68).

Almost immediately after triggering, T cells upregulate the expression of several cell surface receptors that are important in cell adhesion and intracellular signaling (Table 72.2) (69–75). As these molecules are expressed or increased in expression, cells begin to adhere to the vascular endothelium (margination) (Fig. 72.10). After a brief period of "rolling" (weak attachment), they adhere firmly and eventually invade the endothelium and enter the renal parenchyma (76). Like immune cells, endothelial and parenchymal cells regulate expression of various cell surface receptors on activation or injury (74). Vascular endothelial cells downregulate certain receptors and upregulate others. These new molecules serve as ligands for the receptors newly expressed on T lymphocytes (Table 72.2), and these new adhesive interactions control immune cell adhesion to the vessel wall and entry into the graft tissue (76,77). New receptors, many of which are members of the integrin family of cell surface α-β heterodimers (Table 72.3), are expressed on T cells and bind to extracellular matrix components, thereby regulating immune cell movement through the tissues (75–81).

Chemoattractant cytokines (chemokines) are pivotal in attracting immune cells into the allograft (Fig. 72.10) (82). Stressed tissues in the allograft release proinflammatory cytokines, such as IL-1 and TNF-α, which in turn activate parenchymal cells to release chemokines that bind to glycosaminoglycans on the vessel wall and serve as signposts to attract immune cells. Immune cells bind to the vascular

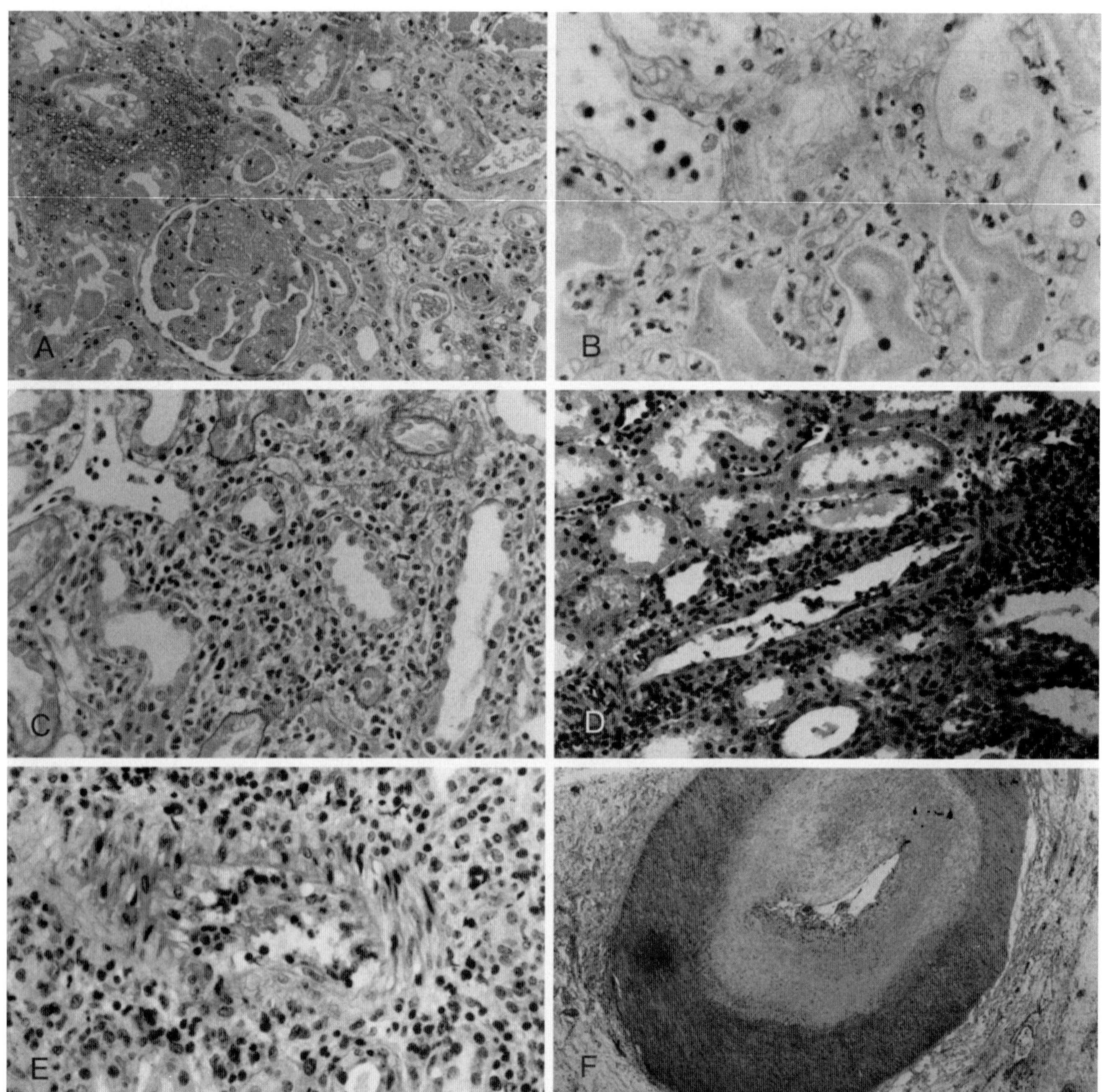

FIGURE 72.9. Pathology of transplant rejection. **A:** Hyperacute rejection with edema of stroma, focal hemorrhage, thrombus formation, polymorphonuclear cell infiltration, and mesangiolysis. **B:** Hyperacute rejection 1 hour later, with tubular and epithelial cell necrosis and increased polymorphonuclear cell infiltration. **C:** Acute cellular rejection with inflammatory cell infiltration. **D:** Acute cellular rejection with "endotheliitis," inflammatory cells permeating the vascular intima. **E:** Acute cellular rejection with vessel wall infiltration. **F:** Chronic rejection with dense intimal fibrosis. (Courtesy Dr. Robert Colvin, Massachusetts General Hospital, Boston, Massachusetts.)

endothelium by haptotaxis and enter the tissue along a chemotactic gradient. Once T cells reach the site of antigen-specific triggering, they release additional chemokines, most notably RANTES (regulated upon activation, normal T cell expressed and secreted), which is expressed late (3 to 5 days) after T-cell activation and prolongs the process in time and space. The regulation of these events is complex and, until recently, it was difficult to dissect the relative roles of the numerous chemokines present, because many chemokines and G-protein–associated chemokine receptors appeared redundant. Studies using "knock-out" mice, however, have begun to shed light on the relative roles, and specific inhibitors show dramatic therapeutic activity in preclinical animal models (83).

TABLE 72.2. RECEPTOR-LIGAND PAIRS IN THE INTERACTION BETWEEN T LYMPHOCYTES AND TARGETS

Receptor	Counterreceptor (ligand)	Reference
T-cell receptor	HLA and peptide	42
CD4	MHC class II	45
CD8	MHC class I	45
CD11a, 18 (LFA-1)	CD54 (ICAM-1), ICAM-2	70
CD43	CD54 (ICAM-1)	71
CD2 (LFA-2)	CD58 (LFA-3)	70
CD5	CD72	72
CD44 (Hermes)	Glycan bearing addressin	73
Leu 8 (Mel 14)	Glycan bearing addressin	74
ELAM-1	Glycan sialylated Lewis X antigen	74
VCAM-1	VLA-4	74

ELAM, endothelial-leukocyte adhesion molecule; ICAM, intercellular adhesion molecule; LFA, lymphocyte funtion-associated antigen; MHC, major histocompatibility complex; VCAM, vascular cell adhesion molecule; VLA, very late antigen.

TABLE 72.3. EXTRACELLULAR MATRIX RECEPTORS ON LYMPHOCYTES

Name	Structure		Putative ligand(s)
Integrins			
	alpha	*beta*	
VLA-1	CD49a	CD29	Collagen, laminin
VLA-2	CD49b	CD29	Collagen, laminin
VLA-3	CD49c	CD29	Collagen, laminin, fibronectin
VLA-4	CD49d	CD29	Fibronectin
VLA-5	CD49e	CD29	Fibronectin
VLA-6	CD49f	CD29	Laminin
	CD51	CD61	Fibronectin, vitronectin, fibrinogen
Others			
CD26	Dipeptidyl peptidase		Fibronectin, collagen
CD44	Cartilage link protein		Hyaluronic acid
CD73	Ectoenzyme 5' nucleotidase		Fibronectin, laminin

VLA, very late antigen.

As described earlier, $CD4^+$ helper T lymphocytes orchestrate the further recruitment, activation, and functional differentiation of a variety of effector cells. They produce IL-2 and IL-4, which induce the proliferation and differentiation of T cells. Interferon-gamma, TNF-β, and IL-6 cause increased expression of HLA molecules. IL-4, IL-5, and IL-6 activate B cells, which in turn differentiate and divide. Some cytokines, including IL-1, TNF-α, and TNF-β, can directly cause cell damage. These events result in increased inflammatory infiltrate and upregulation of HLA expression. Extracellular matrix is damaged and destroyed by inflammatory proteases, and debris is phagocytosed by macrophages and granulocytes (84,85). Fibroblasts undergo morphologic changes and begin to produce large amounts of collagen, fibronectin, and proteoglycans; these are organized into new extracellular matrix, which results in scar formation (86). These highly regulated events are designed to maintain the structural integrity of the organ despite considerable parenchymal injury, but invariably, if not halted, they result in progressive loss of graft function.

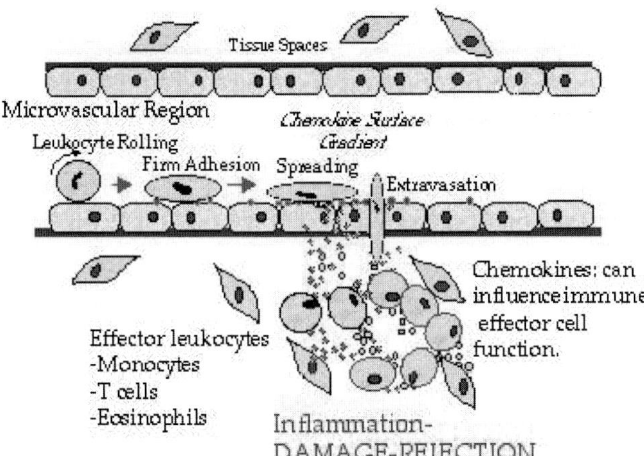

FIGURE 72.10. Chemokine gradients facilitate recruitment of inflammatory cells from peripheral circulation into sites of inflammation. This multistep process is central to the generation of inflammatory infiltrate in kidney transplant rejection. (From Nelson PJ, Krensky AM. Chemokines and allograft rejection; narrowing the list of suspects. *Transplantation* 2001;72:1195–1197, with permission.)

The major problem associated with kidney transplantation is long-term graft loss, and this is usually due to an incompletely understood constellation of pathophysiologic events that have been collectively called chronic rejection or chronic allograft nephropathy (CAN). It is accepted that this entity is the end result of both immune-mediated and non–immune-mediated events (87), including elements of chronic rejection, chronic calcineurin inhibitor nephrotoxicity, and renal lesions resulting from multiple insults related to transplantation. Despite improvements in immunosuppression and a decrease in the incidence of acute rejection, the incidence of late graft loss due to CAN has remained essentially unchanged over the last decade. Clinically, CAN is defined as progressive and persistent renal allograft functional impairment not attributable to known entities such as recurrence of primary renal disease, vascular complications, overt drug toxicity, or acute rejection. The process is marked by a gradual rise in serum creatinine levels 90 days or more after renal transplantation and is accompanied by pathologic findings, including (a) fibrous intimal thickening that results in renal vessel occlusion and ischemic transplant glomerulopathy, (b) tubular atrophy, (c) interstitial fibrosis, and (d) mononuclear cell infiltration (88). Retransplantation is the only available therapy.

The pathogenesis and molecular events leading to CAN remain poorly characterized. Evidence to support the presence of underlying immune triggers to the development of CAN are the following: There is a correlation between the development of CAN and (a) the incidence of acute rejection (more than two acute rejections have been associated with a 12-fold increase in the incidence of chronic rejection), (b) the degree of HLA disparity, (c) the recipient's pretransplant sensitization state as reflected by panel-reactive antibody, and (d) a history of underimmunosuppression as reflected by low drug levels of immunosuppressives (88–90). In the absence of obvious immune-mediated injury, however, CAN sometimes still develops. There is an association between development of CAN and preexisting hypertension, hyperlipidemia, obesity, smoking, donor age, organ ischemia time, delayed graft function, cytomegalovirus infection, and bacterial infection (91–93).

Although it was originally believed that CAN was not impacted by current immunosuppressive protocols, more recent analyses of adult renal transplant cases indicates that long-term outcomes are improving, which suggests that better early immunosuppression and decreased acute rejection episodes do somewhat protect from CAN (94). Administration of mycophenolate mofetil (MMF) decreased the relative risk of chronic allograft failure by 27% (risk ratio, 0.73; p <.001) and improved censored graft survival (85.6% vs. 81.9% at 4 years) (95). In other studies, patients who experienced gradual loss of renal function while taking cyclosporine A, prednisone, and azathioprine therapy were transferred to alternate protocols in which azathioprine was replaced with MMF (96) or the dose of cyclosporine A was reduced in combination with MMF replacement of azathioprine (97). In both studies, there was a beneficial effect of replacing azathioprine with MMF, but reduction of cyclosporine A alone appears to slow the rate of renal deterioration (98).

IMMUNOPHARMACOLOGY OF GRAFT REJECTION

Although most of the drugs approved for use in organ transplantation have been developed as a result of drug screening and optimization by pharmaceutical companies, elucidation of the cellular and molecular events underlying the allogeneic response allows a better understanding of the mechanisms of action of existing therapies and potentially helps in the design of new immunotherapies.

Drug Therapy

General Approach to Organ Transplant Therapy

Organ transplant therapy is organized around five general principles:

1. Careful patient preparation and tissue matching are performed.
2. A multitiered approach is taken to immunosuppression, much like combination therapy in cancer chemotherapy. Several agents are used simultaneously, each directed at a different molecular target. Because the various immunotherapies described later inhibit rejection at different points, combination therapies can provide additive or even synergistic immunosuppression without added toxicity (99,100). In addition, when therapies are combined, dosages can be decreased and toxicities further reduced.
3. Greater immunosuppression is required for promotion of early engraftment and/or treatment of established rejection than for maintenance. Therefore, more intensive induction and tapering maintenance therapies are used.
4. Careful evaluation of each episode of transplant dysfunction is required to clarify whether the cause is rejection, drug toxicity, infection, or some combination of these.
5. Drugs are reduced or withdrawn when toxicity exceeds the therapeutic benefit.

Current protocols often involve three or four different drugs in combination. Future protocols will undoubtedly use combinations of therapies to further alleviate the various side effects associated with current approaches.

Adrenocortical Steroids

Corticosteroids were the first drugs to prove efficacious for reversal of acute rejection. Steroids are currently used at moderate dosages for prevention of rejection and at high dosages for treatment of acute rejection (101). Steroids lyse and possibly redistribute lymphocytes, causing a rapid, transient decrease in peripheral blood lymphocyte counts. Longer term effects are due to the binding of either glucocorticoid receptors or glucocorticoid-induced proteins to DNA in the vicinity of response elements that regulate the transcription of numerous genes (Fig. 72.11) (102,103). Glucocorticoid-receptor complexes increase inhibitor of κB expression,

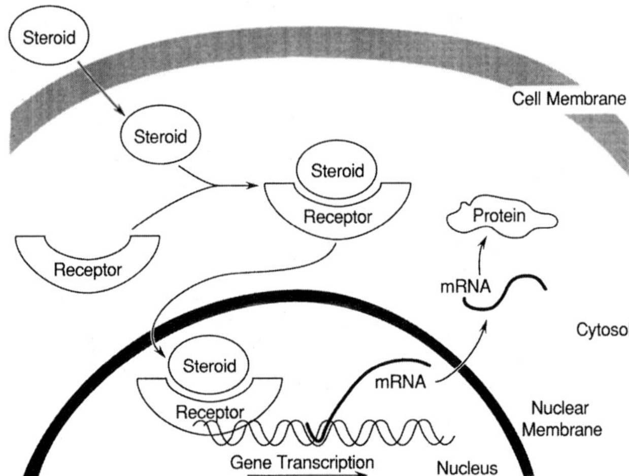

FIGURE 72.11. Mechanism of action of steroids. Glucocorticoids bind receptors in the cytosol and are transported to the cell nucleus. These receptors and/or glucocorticoid-induced proteins bind to DNA in the vicinity of response elements that regulate the transcription of numerous genes. mRNA, messenger RNA.

decrease nuclear factor-κB levels, and cause apoptosis of activated T cells (104). Of great significance is downregulation of important proinflammatory cytokines, such as IL-1 and IL-6, which are important factors in macrophage activation of T cells (51–53,105). T cells, in turn, are inhibited from producing IL-2 and proliferating. Neutrophils and monocytes display poor chemotaxis and decreased lysosomal enzyme release (106). Thus, steroids have broad immunosuppressive and antiinflammatory effects on T cells, monocytes, and neutrophils. Steroids have little effect, however, on humoral immunity (107). Because there are numerous responsive tissues and genes, steroids have multiple side effects, including growth retardation, avascular necrosis of bone, osteopenia, increased risk of infection, poor wound healing, cataract development, hyperglycemia, and hypertension. For these reasons, steroid-sparing and now even steroid-avoidance protocols are being evaluated (108,109).

Calcineurin Inhibitors

The most effective immunosuppressive drugs in routine clinical use are the calcineurin inhibitors cyclosporine and tacrolimus, drugs that target intracellular signaling pathways downstream of T-cell receptor triggering (110). Although these two drugs are structurally unrelated and bind to different (but related) molecular targets, their general mechanisms of action are similar (Fig. 72.12).

Cyclosporine

The discovery of cyclosporine and its application to organ transplantation was an important milestone (111). It improved graft survival for kidneys and made other types of organ transplantations a clinical reality. Cyclosporine, an 11-amino-acid cyclic peptide of fungal origin, is highly immunosuppressive (112). Importantly, cyclosporine appears to be highly specific for helper T lymphocytes, while having little if any effect on other arms of the immune response (113). Cyclosporine inhibits transcription of IL-2 and other lymphokines (114). Because it acts early in T-cell activation, it has broad secondary effects on other cell types dependent on T-cell products, as well as late functions of T cells. Cyclosporine inhibits the DNA-binding activity of several proteins involved in regulation of early T-cell activation genes. Cyclophilin, a cyclosporine-binding protein, is identical to a peptidylprolyl *cis-trans* isomerase, which is required for the proper folding of many proteins (115). When it was discovered that another potent drug, tacrolimus (FK506), inhibits a similar isomerase (designated FKBP for FK506-binding protein), it was suggested that this was the mode of action of these most potent immunosuppressives (116). Subsequent data, however, demonstrate that the mechanism of action is more complex. The isomerase activity may not be involved; rather, it may be the proline-binding tendency of the various cyclophilins that is relevant.

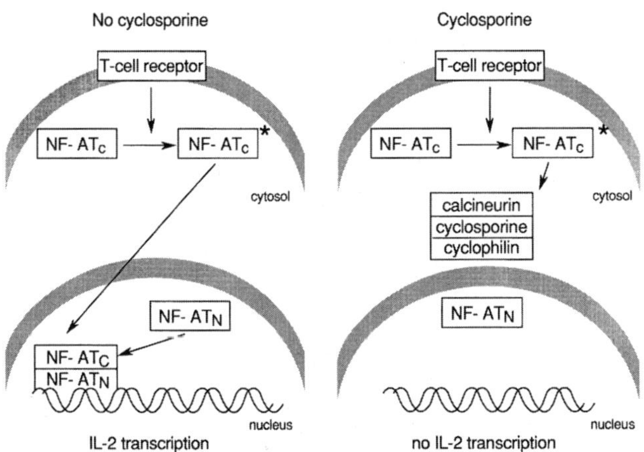

FIGURE 72.12. Mechanism of action of cyclosporine. In the presence of cyclosporine, a cytoplasmic component of the nuclear factor of T-cell activation (NF-AT_c) is unable to gain access to the nucleus. As a result, the nuclear component of NF-AT (NF-AT_N) is unable to bind DNA, and there is no interleukin-2 (IL-2) gene transcription (117). *, activated.

A current model is shown in Figure 72.12 (117). The inhibitory drug–immunophilin complex blocks transcription regulated by a T-cell–specific activation factor, NF-AT (nuclear factor of activated T cells). NF-AT is composed of at least two subunits; one is widely expressed and localized in the nucleus, whereas the other is T-cell specific and is found in the cytoplasm of resting T cells. These subunits must associate for transcription of early T-cell–activation genes, including IL-2 and other cytokines, to occur. Cyclosporine or FK506 binds to its particular intracytoplasmic immunophilin (cyclophilin or FKBP), and, in turn, this complex binds a phosphatase, calcineurin, which is required for translocation of the cytoplasmic portion of NF-AT to the nucleus (118). If the NF-AT cytoplasmic component is not translocated to the nucleus, it cannot bind to the enhancers-promoters of IL-2 and other early activation genes, thus preventing T-cell activation and helper T-cell function.

When little or no IL-2 is secreted, T cells do not proliferate and the immune response is not amplified, interferon-gamma is not secreted, HLA class II antigens are not induced, and macrophages are not further activated. Although such helper functions are potently inhibited, cyclosporine therapy appears to spare or even support suppressor T cells (119). Cyclosporine also increases expression of transforming growth factor β (TGF-β), a potent inhibitor of IL-2–stimulated T-cell proliferation and generation of cytotoxic T lymphocytes (120). Although cyclosporine is remarkably nontoxic to other hematopoietic lineages, its use is limited by its marked nephrotoxicity (121). The precise mechanism of nephrotoxicity is unknown, but it is clear that cyclosporine interferes with intrarenal blood flow (122) and that certain cyclosporine-binding proteins are expressed in high amounts by kidney cells (123). Other side effects of cyclosporine include hyperkalemia, hypertension, hepatotoxicity, hirsutism, and gingival hyperplasia.

Tacrolimus

Tacrolimus (FK506) is a macrolide that blocks T-cell activation by mechanisms similar to those of cyclosporine. Tacrolimus binds to binding proteins (FKBP). This complex, in turn, binds calcineurin and interrupts NF-AT translocation to the nucleus and IL-2 production (Fig. 72.12). Tacrolimus is more potent than cyclosporine on a molecular-weight basis (124) but appears to have similar limiting side effects, particularly nephrotoxicity (125). Other side effects include neurotoxicity (tremor, headache, motor disturbances, and seizures), gastrointestinal complaints, impaired glucose tolerance, and hypertension. Tacrolimus has slowly gained market share with cyclosporine over the past several years, largely due to ease of use and some differences in toxicity.

Antiproliferative and Antimetabolic Drugs

Sirolimus

Like tacrolimus, sirolimus is a macrolide that binds FKBP, but it does not block the transcription of cytokine genes. Rather, it inhibits signal transduction mediated by IL-2 and other growth factors, thereby blocking cell cycle progression from G_1 to S phase (126). One or more cellular proteins, mammalian target(s) of rapamycin (mTOR), bind the rapamycin-FKBP complex (127). These proteins have sequence homology to the catalytic domain of the P-110 subunit of phosphatidylinositol 3 kinase. Sirolimus and tacrolimus are pharmacologic antagonists, whereas cyclosporine and sirolimus may act synergistically. In addition, sirolimus blocks the transcription of a molecule required for cell cycle progression, PCNA (proliferating cell nuclear antigen) (128). In animal models, sirolimus inhibits both transplant rejection and autoimmune disease, as well as chronic vascular disease associated with rejection (129). Sirolimus causes diabetes in rats, but not in primates, and is reported to be less nephrotoxic than cyclosporine. Severe gastrointestinal and testicular toxicities described in animals (130) do not yet appear limiting for use in humans. The major limiting toxicity in humans is dose-dependent increase in serum lipid levels (131). Although sirolimus is not nephrotoxic on its own, in combination with cyclosporine, it carries an increased incidence of nephrotoxicity compared to the use of cyclosporine with azathioprine or placebo. Anemia, leukopenia, thrombocytopenia, hypokalemia, hyperkalemia, fever, and gastrointestinal complaints have also been associated with sirolimus use.

Azathioprine

Azathioprine (Imuran) was first introduced as an immunosuppressive agent in 1961 and continues to prove useful for the prevention of organ transplant rejection (132). It is a thiopurine, the *S*-imidazolyl derivative of 6-mercaptopurine, and is metabolized *in vivo* to 6-thioinosinic acid and other 6-mercaptopurine derivatives that become incorporated into DNA, inhibiting purine synthesis and metabolism, hindering RNA and DNA synthesis, and blocking gene replication and cell proliferation (133). It is a powerful inhibitor of primary responses but does not block secondary responses and therefore is not useful for treatment of ongoing rejection (134). Early withdrawal of azathioprine increases the likelihood of rejection, whereas late withdrawal has less effect (135). Azathioprine inhibits most T-cell functions, including the mixed lymphocyte response, cytotoxic T lymphocytes, suppressor phenomena, NK cells, and antibody-dependent cellular cytotoxicity (136–138). In addition, it inhibits primary antibody synthesis and decreases circulating granulocytes and mononuclear cells. Its major side effect is bone marrow suppression, with leukopenia and (less frequently) thrombocytopenia or anemia. Other important side effects include increased susceptibility to viral infection (especially varicella or herpes simplex), hepatotoxicity, alopecia, and increased risk of neoplasia.

Mycophenolate Mofetil

MMF (CellCept) is the 2-morpholinoethyl ester of mycophenolic acid (139). Mycophenolic acid, like azathioprine, inhibits nucleotide biosynthesis (140). It is a selective, noncompetitive, and reversible inhibitor of inosine monophosphate dehydrogenase, an important enzyme in the de novo pathway of guanine nucleotide synthesis (141). B and T cells are highly dependent on this pathway for proliferation, in contrast to other cell types that use salvage pathways. Mycophenolic acid, therefore, selectively inhibits lymphocyte proliferation and other functions, including antibody formation, cell adhesion, and migration (142). This drug is more potent and efficacious than azathioprine and reduces the incidence of acute rejection in combination therapy (143). In rodent models, it prolongs allograft and xenograft survival, reverses advanced rejection, prevents graft vascular disease, and induces alloantigen unresponsiveness (142). Its use, however, is limited by gastrointestinal and hematologic side effects, including diarrhea, constipation, nausea, vomiting, leukopenia, anemia, thrombocytopenia, and hypochromic anemia (144). There is also an increased incidence of some infections, especially cytomegalovirus-associated sepsis.

New Drugs

Although the rate of development of new drugs (corticosteroids, azathioprine, and cyclosporine) was relatively slow from 1950 to 1990, the profound success of cyclosporine provided additional impetus for pharmaceutical companies to develop new immunosuppressives. Several are currently in clinical trials and may become available for use. For the most part, however, these new drugs are merely variations on those previously developed. In general, they fall into the same families and have similar mechanisms of action. One drug with an apparently novel mechanism of action is FTY720. This drug has been shown to prolong allograft survival in a variety of preclinical models and is being evaluated in several clinical trials (145). It is reported to alter lymphocyte recirculation and homing after modulation of chemokine G-protein–coupled receptors (146,147). Other drugs affecting chemokine function have shown promising results in preclinical models and may soon be evaluated clinically (83).

The relative efficacies, mechanisms of action, pharmacokinetics, and toxicities of these new drugs are currently being assessed. Preliminary results with all of these drugs are encouraging, and at least some will probably come into general use. There is hope that they may prove more efficacious than current drugs, but the potential for steroid-sparing, additive combinatorial effects and decreased myelotoxicities (azathioprine) and nephrotoxicities (cyclosporine and tacrolimus) make these new drugs potentially important. Perhaps the most exciting of the new drugs are those capable of inducing and maintaining immunologic tolerance (see later).

Antibody Therapy

Both polyclonal and monoclonal antibodies against lymphocyte cell-surface antigens are widely used for prevention and treatment of organ transplant rejection.

Polyclonal Immune Globulins

Purified gamma globulin fractions from polyclonal antisera generated by immunizing horses or rabbits with lymphocytes [antilymphocyte globulin (ALG)] or thymocytes [antithymocyte globulin (ATG)] are useful for preventing and/or treating acute allograft rejection (148,149). These preparations contain a heterogeneous group of antibodies that eliminate circulating T cells by several mechanisms, including clearance of lymphocytes by the reticuloendothelial system, blocking of lymphocyte function by binding to important T-cell surface receptors, antibody-dependent cellular cytotoxicity, and classical antibody- and complement-mediated lympholysis (148–150). In addition, some reports suggest that these sera expand suppressor cell populations *in vivo* (151). Because each polyclonal immune globulin preparation varies in its constituent antibodies, variable and sometimes unpredictable efficacy and side effects are seen across batches. The lack of standardization has hampered assessment of various polyclonal antisera, but in general, they are highly efficacious for induction immunosuppression and treatment of acute rejection in combination with other drugs (152–154). A course of ALG is often used in patients with delayed graft function to allow withdrawal of nephrotoxic calcineurin inhibitors and thereby aid in recovery from ischemic reperfusion injury. Side effects vary among different preparations but include thrombocytopenia, granulocytopenia, serum sickness, and glomerulonephritis. Local pain, fever, urticaria, and hypotension are generally controlled by steroids and other premedications. Increased susceptibility to infection, particularly viral infections, has also been described.

Monoclonal Antibodies

Many of the problems associated with the lack of standardization of the polyclonal antisera were overcome with the advent of monoclonal antibodies. Kohler and Milstein described methodologies to generate essentially unlimited amounts of antibodies of a single specificity (Fig. 72.13) (155). Mice are immunized with human T lymphocytes, and the murine spleen cells are harvested and fused with a suitable B-cell myeloma that has been selected for the inability to grow in a medium supplemented with hypoxanthine, aminopterin, and thymidine (HAT). Only B-cell

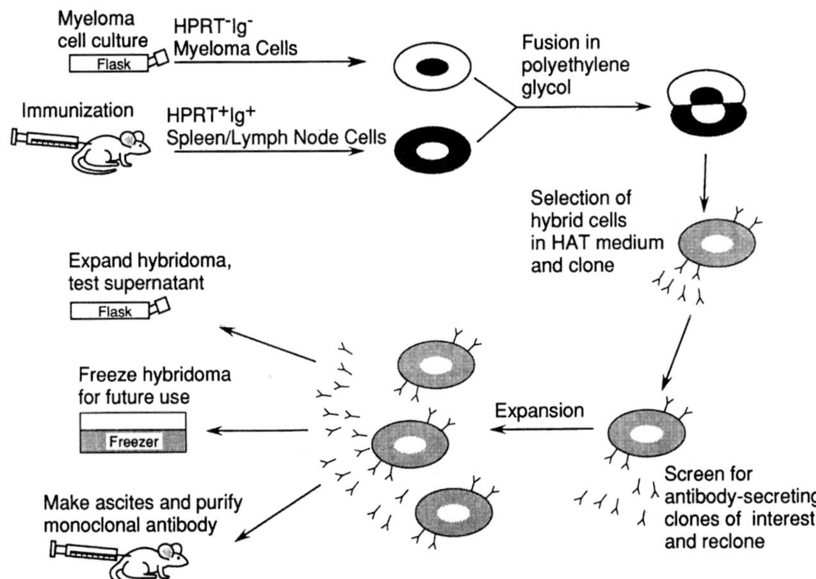

FIGURE 72.13. Generation of monoclonal antibodies. Mice are immunized, and spleen or lymph node B cells are harvested and fused with a suitable B-cell myeloma that has been selected for the inability to grow in a medium supplemented with hypoxanthine, aminopterin, and thymidine (HAT). Only B-cell myeloma cells that fuse with mouse B cells can survive in a HAT-supplemented medium. After these hybridomas have expanded, those of interest are identified and cloned. Monoclonal antibodies can be used directly as culture supernatants or purified from supernatants or ascites fluid from mice injected intraperitoneally with the hybridoma. HPRT, hypoxanthinephospho-ribosyltransferase; Ig, immunoglobulin (155).

TABLE 72.4. SELECTED MONOCLONAL ANTIBODIES AT LEAST PARTIALLY EFFECTIVE AS IMMUNOTHERAPY FOR TRANSPLANT REJECTION

Target antigen	Reference
CD3	160
CD4	162
CD6 (T12)	163
CD8	164
CD11a, CD18 (LFA-1)	165
CD25 (IL-2 receptor)	166
CD45	168
CDw52 (Campath-1M)	169
CD54 (ICAM-1)	170

ICAM-1, intercellular adhesion molecule-1; IL-2, interleukin-2; LFA-1, leukocyte factor antigen-1.

myeloma cells that have fused with splenic B cells can survive in a HAT-supplemented medium. Once these hybridomas have expanded, those of interest can be identified and cloned. Many T-cell–specific and more broadly expressed antigens have been identified and characterized using such monoclonal antibodies, and many of these have been tested therapeutically (Table 72.4) (156–170). The two major groups of monoclonal antibodies used clinically are against the CD3 antigen and the IL-2 receptor.

OKT3

OKT3 was the first U. S. Food and Drug Administration–approved monoclonal antibody available for therapeutic use in transplantation in the United States (171,172). OKT3 antibody binds the 20,000-d δ chain of the CD3 complex. This antibody is a potent inhibitor of virtually every T-cell function. When the antibody binds to the T-cell receptor complex, this all-important recognition complex is shed from the cell surface and/or is internalized. Many $CD3^+$ cells are destroyed (T-cell depletion). As a result, the T lymphocytes are unable to recognize the offending (allo)antigen, and the rejection process is blocked. Although OKT3 therapy is highly efficacious for reversing acute rejection (173), its use is limited by the propensity of the recipient to develop antiimmunoglobulin responses to the mouse portions of the antibody (174,175). Chimeric or "humanized" antibodies containing largely human sequences (176,177) still elicit antibody responses to the antigen-specific portions of the immunoglobulin molecule (antiidiotypic responses) (178) but in general are better tolerated. The major side effects associated with OKT3 therapy include fever, shaking chills, nausea, vomiting, diarrhea, headache, anorexia, weakness, and a capillary leak syndrome (179). This constellation of symptoms is thought to be due to T-cell activation and cytokine release induced by the OKT3 antibody. In general, this syndrome can be controlled with prednisone (180). In addition, treatment with "nonmitogenic" anti-OKT3 is less frequently associated with such side effects. In any case, a decrease in the incidence of acute rejection episodes as a result of the use of mycophenolic acid, anti–IL-2 receptor monoclonal antibodies, and other therapies has resulted in decreased use of anti-OKT3 in general.

Anti–Interleukin-2 Receptor Antibodies

Monoclonal antibodies recognizing other T-cell surface molecules have been evaluated for use in transplantation but only anti–IL-2 receptor antibodies have gained general use. Daclizumab (Zenapax), a humanized murine complementarity-determining region/human immunoglobulin G1 chimeric monoclonal antibody, and basiliximab (Simulect), a murine-human chimeric antibody, have been produced by recombinant DNA technology (181). Both antibodies bind to the α subunit (CD25) of the IL-2 receptor present on activated, but not resting, T lymphocytes. They block IL-2–mediated T-cell activation. Both are used for prophylaxis against acute rejection as part of combination (induction) therapy (182).

Nonpharmacologic Immunosuppression

Nonpharmacologic immunosuppression can be provided in several forms. Plasmapheresis to remove antibodies has been attempted for acute vascular rejection, but this approach does not appear to be generally effective for treatment of acute rejection episodes (183,184). Splenectomy is controversial and is rarely performed. Although the immunosuppressive effects of pretransplantation splenectomy are clear, the risk of overwhelming infection outweighs the potential benefit (185). Irradiation is an effective immunosuppressive therapy (186). Although total-body irradiation was originally abandoned because of the high risk of infection, studies suggest that it may be a useful adjuvant, especially in the development of immunologic tolerance (187) or as rescue therapy for intractable rejection (188). Lastly, retrospective and prospective studies showed that blood transfusions were once beneficial for graft survival (189,190). The effect has diminished or disappeared in the cyclosporine era (191), however, and donor-specific or other transfusion protocols are seldom used today. Although the mechanism of the blood transfusion effect remains unknown, evidence suggests that donor cells, even blood cells, may be effective tolerogens for the induction of specific immunologic unresponsiveness (192) and may be useful in inducing tolerance.

TOLERANCE

Immunosuppression is predicated on blocking the immune response and is therefore associated with multiple unwanted side effects, including the occurrence of opportunistic infections and secondary tumors. It would be preferable to work with the immune response rather than against it. Immunologic tolerance, then, defined as the active state of antigen-specific immune unresponsiveness, is the ultimate goal of transplant biologists.

Mechanisms

An individual who encounters a new antigen must constantly discriminate self from nonself, destroying harmful invaders while leaving self tissues unharmed. Owen first showed that immune responsiveness was an active process when he noted that freemartins, bovine twins who shared a common placenta, became hematologic chimeras and did not recognize their sibling's blood cells as foreign (193). This experiment of nature led Burnet to hypothesize that there was a critical period in development when the fetus learned to discriminate self from nonself and developed tolerance to self (194). Medawar and his colleagues showed that freemartins could in fact accept skin grafts from each other but would reject grafts from third parties and that similar "neonatal tolerance" would develop in mice that received allogeneic skin transplants (195). In fact, mice injected with foreign cells in the neonatal period maintained lifelong tolerance of the foreign-donor transplant antigens but still rejected third-party grafts. These seminal observations, which showed that the immune response could be manipulated to lose reactivity with a transplanted organ, laid the foundation for modern transplantation immunobiology.

There are several theories to explain immunologic tolerance. In clonal deletion, all of the T cells capable of recognizing a particular antigen are deleted from the T-cell repertoire. For example, mice expressing a certain HLA class II molecule (I-E) delete all T cells expressing a particular T-cell receptor variable region (V β 17) (34). This type of tolerance is induced while thymocytes are maturing in the thymus. Experiments in which tissues (glomeruli, pancreatic islets, or spleen cells) injected directly into the thymus induce transplant tolerance may work by inducing clonal deletion of recipient T cells capable of recognizing the injected cells (196,197).

Although T-cell deletion during ontogeny leads to immune tolerance, T cells that have exited the thymus can also be deleted. In the periphery, mature T cells can undergo apoptosis by two distinct pathways: activation-induced cell death (AICD) and passive cell death. AICD occurs in repetitively stimulated T cells and acts to limit the extent of the immune response. AICD is largely mediated through Fas and other members of the TNF receptor family and appears to require IL-2. Once activated, T cells upregulate expression of Fas and Fas ligand, and when these cells are brought together, as would occur on an antigen-presenting cell, the interaction of Fas and Fas ligand results in apoptosis. Interestingly, certain tissues such as testis and the anterior chamber of the eye are characterized by a state of immune privilege. These tissues constitutively express Fas ligand, which triggers apoptosis in invading Fas^+ T cells (198). Thus, these tissues are not rejected on transplantation into HLA-mismatched recipients. Passive cell death occurs when activated T cells are deprived of growth factors, perhaps due to the action of regulatory T cells. In addition, phagocytosis of apoptotic cells by macrophages often leads to production of IL-10 and TGF-β (199), which contribute to the development of tolerance (200).

Studies have shown that, once induced, tolerance can be "infectious"; that is, T cells from a tolerant animal can transfer tolerance to another animal. This observation led Gershon and Kondo to hypothesize that there were cells (which they called suppressor T cells) actively involved in dampening the immune response (201). Therapies such as cyclosporine (202), ATG (203), and total lymphoid irradiation (204) may induce suppressor cells. Moreover, it now appears that long-term maintenance of peripheral tolerance depends on self-perpetuating immunoregulatory mechanisms that actively inhibit alloreactive T cells. $CD4^+$ regulatory T cells, first identified in 1990 (205,206), are now recognized as critical effectors in both the control of autoimmunity (207–209) and the maintenance of peripheral tolerance (210,211). The mechanisms by which CD4 regulatory T cells exert their effects remain controversial, however. Regulatory T cells inhibit production of IL-2 by the responding T cells (212,213). Suppression of T-cell proliferation by regulatory T cells appears to involve secretion of antiinflammatory cytokines such as IL-10 (214) and TGF-β (215), whereas in other cases suppression requires direct cell contact, possibly through cell-surface molecules such as cytotoxic T lymphocyte A4 (CTLA4) (216) or TGF-β (217).

Tolerance can occur during T-cell selection (central tolerance) or after T cells have moved into the blood and lymphoid organs (peripheral tolerance). Anergy is an important mechanism by which mature T cells are rendered tolerant. The interaction of the T-cell receptor with specific antigen in the context of self HLA activates the T cell only if a second signal is also provided (Fig. 72.14) (218,219). Thus, a T cell that does not receive the second signal will not be activated, proliferate, or differentiate into an effector T cell. Furthermore, these cells become anergic; that is, for a prolonged period of time, they will not respond to the appropriate antigenic stimulus even in the presence of the second signal. Addition of exogenous IL-2 can sometimes overcome this anergy, and, therefore, triggering the IL-2 receptor is one means of providing a second signal. Clinically, anergy appears to be inducible with soluble antigens, through either donor-specific transfusions (220) or soluble HLA molecules that seem to be released in liver transplantation (221). Provision of such first signals (tolerogens) without an accompanying second signal may be a potent and general means of inducing tolerance.

Several observations suggest that there may be different ways to provide a second signal. One of the best-defined pathways involves the interaction of the T-cell surface mol-

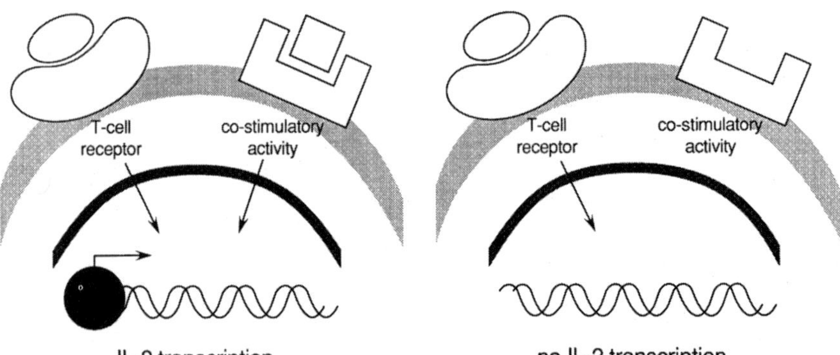

FIGURE 72.14. Two signals for T-cell activation. T cells require two signals to be activated to make interleukin-2 (IL-2) and proliferate. If the T-cell receptor complex is engaged without simultaneous provision of a second signal, the T cell is anergic, does not secrete IL-2, and does not proliferate (218,219).

ecule, CD28, with its ligands, B7-1 (CD80) and B7-2 (CD86), expressed on antigen-presenting cells (Fig. 72.15) (222,223). In humans, CD28 is constitutively expressed on 95% of resting CD4$^+$ cells and 50% of resting CD8$^+$ peripheral blood T cells. Its expression increases after T-cell activation. It has been known for some time that monoclonal antibodies to CD28 could activate T cells (222); in addition, B7 molecules are natural ligands capable of sending this intracellular signal (223). CD28 triggering activates a response element present in the promoter of the IL-2 gene, triggering IL-2 expression (224). CTLA4, another molecule highly homologous to CD28 but restricted in expression to activated T lymphocytes, is capable of binding B7 with even higher affinity (225). The signaling consequences of CTLA4 binding are quite different, however. CTLA4 "knock-out" mice die within 4 weeks of birth from uncontrolled activation and accumulation of T lymphocytes (226). This definitive experiment complements earlier studies that suggested that CTLA4 engagement sends a negative signal into the T cell, turning off activation. In contrast, CD28 "knock-out" mice lack a positive second signal, and T-cell responses are diminished (227). Thus, a pair of related ligands (B7-1 and B7-2) interact with a pair of T-cell surface receptors (CD28 and CTLA4) to dynamically control T-cell activation and deactivation. A soluble, recombinant form of CTA4, called CTLA4Ig, binds with high avidity to both B7 molecules, inhibits T-cell–dependent antibody responses, prolongs transplant survival, slows autoimmune disease progression, and induces long-term donor-specific tolerance (228,229). Additional novel molecules, identified by mutation of CTLA4Ig, appear more potent and selective in their binding to the B7-1 ligand (230). Although blocking second-signal pathways appears to be an attractive alternative to providing tolerogen, there may be several different ways to provide the second signal, and many approaches may prove clinically useful. Nevertheless, ongoing studies of CD28-B7 and other receptor-ligand pairs will provide new insights into the mechanism of T-cell activation and, reciprocally, anergy.

Therapeutic Approaches

Based on preclinical studies in rodents and nonhuman primates, therapeutic approaches for induction and maintenance of immunologic tolerance are being evaluated clinically. These include donor cell chimerism, costimulatory blockade, immune deviation, and soluble HLA molecules.

Donor Cell Chimerism

Chimerism refers to persistence of donor cells in the peripheral blood of the recipient (231). This can be "macro" or "micro" depending on the percentage of donor cells circulating in the periphery. Both forms have been associated with long-term graft acceptance in both animal models and human patients (232). It is unclear whether these cells survive because of tolerance or whether they are responsible for induction and/or maintenance of tolerance. In general, approaches aimed at obliteration of the immune response with immunosuppressive agents is followed by provision of tolerogen as blood, bone marrow, or stem cells. Sachs, Sykes, Cosimi, and their colleagues reported the first deliberate induction of mixed lymphohematopoietic chimerism after a nonmyeloablative preparative regimen to treat hematologic malignancy and to provide tolerance for a kidney transplant (233).

Costimulatory Blockade

Costimulatory blockade is predicated on the two-signal model described earlier. Reagents that block costimulation, including anti-CD28, CD80, CD86, CD40, and CD40L,

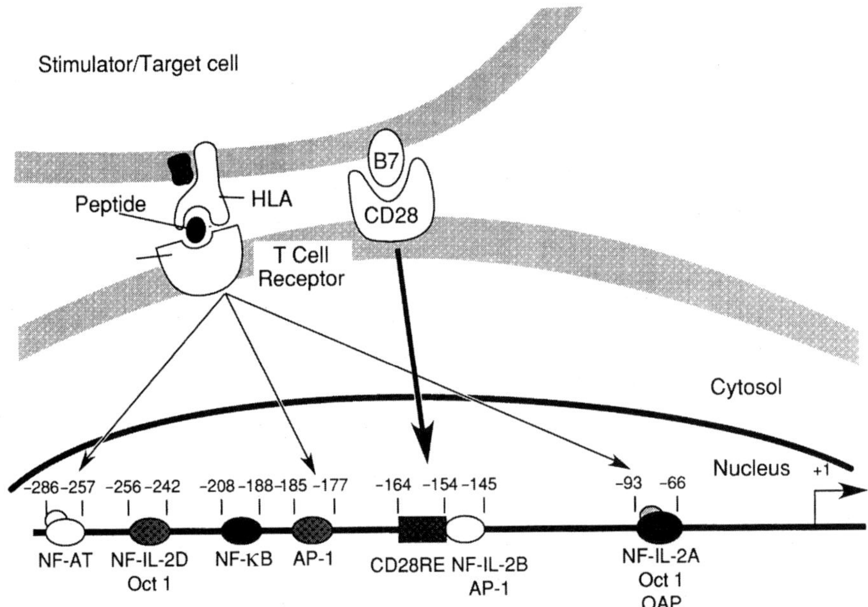

FIGURE 72.15. CD28 second-signal pathway. Activation of the CD28 molecule by engagement with its ligand, B7, sends signals to a CD28 response element (CD28RE) present in the interleukin-2 (IL-2) gene promoter-enhancer, which results in transcription (224). NF-AT, nuclear factor of activated T lymphocytes; NF-IL-2B, nuclear factor of interleukin-2B; NF-IL-2D, nuclear factor of interleukin-2D; NF-κB, nuclear factor-κB; OAP, octamer binding protein.

as well as the chimeric molecule CTLA4Ig, are therapeutic in a variety of preclinical models and are beginning to be evaluated in clinical trials for immune-mediated diseases. Early studies appear to be limited by unexpected side effects.

Immune Deviation

Immune deviation is based on the concept that the helper T response involves two competing arms (234): the Th1 subset of helper T cells produces IL-2 and interferon-gamma, regulates cell-mediated immunity, and is associated with rejection. The Th2 subset produces IL-4, IL-10, and IL-13, and is associated with humoral immunity and tolerance. Immune deviation, switching from a Th1 to a Th2 phenotype, has been associated with tolerance in a number of model systems, although it is possible to have transplant rejection without IL-2 and transplant tolerance without IL-4 (235). The balance of such responses is dependent on the cytokine milieu, antigen-presenting cells, the strength of the T-cell receptor signal, and the array of costimulatory molecules expressed. The use of monoclonal antibodies against CD3 and other approaches can produce immune deviation experimentally and are being evaluated clinically.

Soluble HLA Molecules

HLA molecules function in antigen presentation to T cells and NK cells but also can inhibit immune responses in soluble form (236). Synthetic peptides composed of HLA amino acid sequences have unexpected regulatory effects *in vitro* and *in vivo* (237). They are antiproliferative, block cell cycle progression, and induce anergy and apoptosis. Such reagents have been evaluated clinically (238) and may explain the transfusion effects associated with prolonged graft survival in the precyclosporine era (239).

XENOTRANSPLANTATION

As the demand for organs for transplantation increases, alternatives to both organs from living related individuals and cadaveric organs must be sought. One alternative is transplantation of organs from another species, such as other primates or pigs (240–242). Although successful xenotransplantation of primate kidney was accomplished several decades ago (243), most now would avoid using nonhuman primates because the number of organs these species might provide is few and because use of these animals as a source of organs carries the risk of fatal zoonotic disease. On the other hand, nonprimates such as pigs have as one advantage the fact that they can be genetically engineered. The xenoresponse triggers a different set of immune responses than the alloresponse. The first major immunologic hurdle to xenotransplantation is hyperacute rejection. As in allotransplantation, this process is characterized pathologically by interstitial hemorrhage and thrombosis, and the transplanted organ is destroyed within minutes. In pig to primate transplantation, however, this process is almost exclusively attributable to the binding of xenoreactive antibodies and activation of complement on blood vessels in the donor organ. Surprisingly, most xenoreactive antibodies recognize only one structure, Galα1-3gal (244,245), a saccharide expressed by lower mammals but not by humans, apes, or Old World monkeys. A variety of methods have been developed to overcome recognition of this sugar moiety. Specific depletion by solid-phase immunoabsorption (246), blocking by polymerized saccharides or peptide mimotopes (247), and reduction or elimination of expression of the antigen via genetic engineering (248) have prevented (or, in the case of reduction of antigen expression, promise to prevent) hyperacute rejection. The role of complement has similarly been moderated by the administration of complement inhibitors (249) or expression by genetic engineering of cell-associated complement-regulatory proteins, such as decay-accelerating factor (CD55) and membrane inhibitor of reactive lysis (CD59) (250,251). These approaches also have successfully bypassed hyperacute rejection in a variety of models.

The second immunologic hurdle is acute vascular rejection. Endothelial swelling, focal ischemia, inflammation, and diffuse intravascular coagulation may begin within 24 hours of transplantation, but weeks may pass before the graft is destroyed. This form of rejection also appears to be mediated by xenoreactive antibodies and complement, but cellular components, including NK cells, also may be involved. Of particular interest, depletion of antidonor antibodies from the graft recipient results in a state of "accommodation," whereby enduring graft survival ensues even if antidonor antibodies later return to the circulation (252). The mechanism of accommodation is still unclear. Even if these vascular assaults are inhibited, it is possible that cell-mediated responses involving xenoantigen-associated peptides presented in the context of recipient antigen-presenting cells will provide yet another barrier. Perhaps current approaches aimed at immunosuppression or tolerance induction in the alloresponse will also prove useful in this regard. Even if all of these immunologic barriers are overcome, however, additional problems, such as potential zoonoses (infections passed from animals to humans) and animal rights issues, may prove limiting.

CONCLUSION

Clinical organ transplantation is at a crossroad. Progress in tissue typing, clinical care, and immunosuppression has made renal transplantation a safe and reliable therapy. Nevertheless, opportunistic infection, the increased potential for neoplasm, and poorly understood chronic vascular rejection persist. Therefore, although new and better immunosuppressive therapies should and will continue to be sought, the ultimate goal for clinical transplantation remains the attainment of specific unresponsiveness, immunologic tolerance. Although such tolerance can be routinely attained in animal models (253,254) and is occasionally reported in patients (187,255), we still do not understand how to reproducibly obtain this most desired outcome. Current experimental protocols are aimed at a three-step process: (a) obliterating the normal immune response with irradiation, immunosuppressive drugs, and/or antibody treatment (ATG or OKT3) followed by (b) providing donor-specific antigen (tolerogen) as blood or bone marrow transfusion (256–258), and (c) allowing the immune response to return, now recognizing nonself as self. Such protocols suggest that future approaches to transplantation using organs from living related donors and organs from cadavers will diverge. For transplantation of organs from living related donors, antigen-specific treatments involving pretransplant irradiation and donor-specific tolerogens (transfusions, thymic injections, etc.) may in fact provide immunologic tolerance. Transplantation of cadaveric organs, on the other hand, does not allow sufficient time pretransplantation for such therapies. Without tremendous progress in longer-term tissue preservation, more classical approaches with better donor selection and more potent but less toxic immunosuppression may be the future. Although tolerance-induction protocols are still experimental, there is every reason to expect that we will someday be able to harness the immune response to provide normal protection from foreign invaders while still accepting the transplanted organ as self. When this is possible, transplantation will be a true cure for kidney failure.

REFERENCES

1. Zinkernagel RM, Doherty PC. Restriction of in vitro T cell mediated cytotoxicity in lymphocytic choriomeningitis within a syngeneic or semiallogeneic system. *Nature* 1974;248:701–702.
2. Shimonkevitz R, Kappler J, Marrack P, et al. Antigen recognition by H-2 restricted T cells. I. Cell-free antigen processing. *J Exp Med* 1983;158:303–316.
3. Babbitt BP, Allen PM, Matsueda G, et al. Binding of immunogenic peptides to Ia histocompatibility molecules. *Nature* 1985;317:359–361.
4. Krensky AM, Weiss A, Crabtree G, et al. T-lymphocyte-antigen interactions in transplant rejection. *N Engl J Med* 1990;322:510–517.
5. Tax WJ, Koene RA. Effector mechanisms in renal allograft rejection. *Nephrol Dial Transplant* 1995;10:1569–1571.
6. Krensky AM, Clayberger C. The HLA-T cell interaction in transplant rejection. *Graft* 1998;4:135–141.
7. Hernandez-Fuentes MP, Baker RJ, Lechler RI. The alloresponse. *Rev Immunogenet* 1999;1:282–296.
8. Krensky AM. Molecular biology of transplantation. *Nephron* 2000;86:260–265.
9. Margulies DH. The major histocompatibility complex. In: Paul WE, ed. *Fundamental immunology*, 4th ed. Philadelphia: Lippincott-Raven, 1999:263–286.
10. Krensky AM, Clayberger C. Structure of HLA molecules and immunosuppressive effects of HLA derived peptides. *Int Rev Immunol* 1996;13:173–185.
11. Zemmour J, Parham P. HLA class I nucleotide sequences, 1991. *Immunobiology* 1991;182:347–367.
12. Bodmer JG, Marsh SGE, Albert E, et al. Nomenclature for factors of the HLA system, 1995. *Tissue Antigens* 1995;46:1–18.
13. Marsh SGE, Parham P, Barber LD. *The HLA facts book*. San Diego: Academic Press, 2000.

14. Bjorkman PJ, Saper MA, Samraoui B, et al. Structure of the human class I histocompatibility antigen, HLA-A2. *Nature* 1987;329:506–512.
15. Bjorkman PJ, Saper MA, Samraoui B, et al. The foreign antigen binding site and T-cell recognition regions of class I histocompatibility antigens. *Nature* 1987;329:512–518.
16. Madden DR, Gorga JC, Strominger JL, et al. The structure of HLA-B27 reveals nonamer self-peptides bound in an extended conformation. *Nature* 1991;353:321–325.
17. Allen PM. Antigen processing at the molecular level. *Immunol Today* 1987;8:270–273.
18. Morrison LA, Lukacher AE, Braciale VL, et al. Differences in antigen presentation to MHC class I and class II restricted influenza virus-specific cytotoxic T lymphocyte clones. *J Exp Med* 1986;163:903–921.
19. Brown JH, Jardetzky T, Saper MA, et al. A hypothetical model of the foreign antigen binding site of class II histocompatibility molecules. *Nature* 1988;332:845–850.
20. Streilein JW, Socarras S, Powell TJ. Influence of I-E expression on induction of neonatal tolerance. *Eur J Immunol* 1991;21:261–266.
21. Campbell RD, Dunham I, Sargent CA. Molecular mapping of the HLA-linked complement genes and the RCA linkage group. *Exp Clin Immunogenet* 1988;5:81–98.
22. Trowsdale J, Ragoussis J, Campbell RD. Map of the human MHC. *Immunol Today* 1991;12:443–446.
23. Trowsdale J, Hanson I, Mockridge I, et al. Sequences encoded in the class II region of the MHC related to the "ABC" superfamily of transporters. *Nature* 1990;348:741–744.
24. Spies T, Bresnahan M, Bahram S, et al. A gene in the human major histocompatibility complex class II region controlling the class I antigen presentation pathway. *Nature* 1990;348:744–747.
25. Robertson M. Proteasomes in the pathway. *Nature* 1991;353:300–301.
26. Glynne R, Powis SH, Beck S, et al. A proteasome-related gene between the two ABC transporter loci in the class II region of the human MHC. *Nature* 1991;353:357–360.
27. Parham P. Transporters of delight. *Nature* 1990;348:674–675.
28. Goulmy E, Pool J, van Lochem E, et al. The role of human minor histocompatibility antigens in graft failure: a minireview. *Eye* 1995;9:180–184.
29. Lindahl KF. Minor histocompatibility antigens. *Trends Genet* 1991;7:219–224.
30. den Haan JM, Sherman NE, Blokland E, et al. Identification of a graft versus host disease-associated human minor histocompatibility antigen. *Science* 1995;268:1476–1480.
31. Simpson E, Chandler P, Goulmy E. Separation of the genetic loci for the H-Y antigen and testis determination on the Y chromosome. *Nature* 1987;326:876–878.
32. Krensky AM, Clayberger C. The nature of allorecognition. *Curr Opin Nephrol Hypertens* 1993;2:898–903.
33. von Boehmer H, Teh HS, Kisielow P. The thymus selects the useful, neglects the useless, and destroys the harmful. *Immunol Today* 1989;10:57–61.
34. Kappler JW, Roehm N, Marrack P. T cell tolerance by clonal elimination in the thymus. *Cell* 1987;49:273–280.
35. Batchelor JR, Kaminski E, Lombardi G, et al. Individual variation in alloresponsiveness and the molecular basis of allorecognition. *Hum Immunol* 1990;28:96–103.
36. Falk K, Rotzschke O, Stevanovic S, et al. Allele specific motifs revealed by sequencing of self peptides eluted from MHC molecules. *Nature* 1991;351:290–295.
37. Rotzcchke O, Falk K. Naturally-occurring peptide antigens derived from the MHC class I restricted processing pathway. *Immunol Today* 1991;12:447–455.
38. Jardetzky TS, Lane WS, Robinson RA, et al. Identification of self peptides bound to purified HLA-B27. *Nature* 1991;353:326–329.
39. Buxton SE, Benjamin RJ, Clayberger C, et al. Anchoring pockets in HLA class I molecules: analysis of the conserved B ("45") pocket of HLA-B27. *J Exp Med* 1992;175:809–820.
40. Tilney NL. Renal transplantation. *Curr Prob Surg* 1989;26:601–669.
41. Muluk SC, Clerici M, Via CS, et al. Correlation of in vitro CD4+ T helper cell function with clinical graft status in immunosuppressed kidney transplant recipients. *Transplantation* 1991;52:284–291.
42. Davis MM, Bjorkman PJ. T cell receptor genes and T cell recognition. *Nature* 1988;344:395–402.
43. Allison JP, Lanier LL. Structure, function and serology of the T-cells antigen receptor complex. *Annu Rev Immunol* 1987;5:503–540.
44. Clevers H, Alarcon B, Wileman T, et al. The T-cell receptor/CD3 complex: a dynamic protein ensemble. *Annu Rev Immunol* 1988;6:629–662.
45. Parnes JR. Molecular biology and function of CD4 and CD8. *Adv Immunol* 1989;44:265–312.
46. Cantrell D. T cell antigen receptor signal transduction pathways. *Annu Rev Immunol* 1996;14:259–274.
47. Salter RD, Benjamin RJ, Wesley PK, et al. A binding site for the T cell receptor co-receptor, CD8, on the alpha 3 domain of HLA-A2. *Nature* 1990;345:41–46.
48. Clayberger C, Krensky AM. Mechanisms of allograft rejection. In: Neilson EG, Couser WG, eds. *Immunologic renal diseases*, 2nd ed. Philadelphia: Lippincott Williams & Wilkins, 2001:321–346.
49. Burack WR, Cheng AM, Shaw AS. Scaffolds, adaptors and linkers of TCR signaling: theory and practice. *Curr Opin Immunol* 2002;14:312–316.
50. Ullman KS, Northrup JP, Verweij CL, et al. Transmission of signals from the T lymphocyte antigen receptor to the genes responsible for cell proliferation and immune function: the missing link. *Annu Rev Immunol* 1990;8:421–452.
51. O'Garra A, Umland S, DeFranco T, et al. "B cell factors" are pleiotropic. *Immunol Today* 1988;9:45–54.
52. O'Garra A. Interleukins and the immune system. *Lancet* 1989;1:943–947, 1003–1005.
53. Liles WC, Van Voorhis WC. Nomenclature and biologic significance of cytokines involved in inflammation and the host immune response [review]. *J Infect Dis* 1995;172:1573–1580.
54. Mescher MF. Molecular interactions in the activation of effector and precursor cytotoxic T lymphocytes. *Immunol Rev* 1995;146:177–210.
55. Liu CC, Persechini PM, Young JD. Perforin and lymphocyte-mediated cytolysis. *Immunol Rev* 1995;146:145–175.
56. Smyth MJ, Trapiani JA. Granzymes: exogenous proteinases that induce target cell apoptosis. *Immunol Today* 1995;16:202–206.

57. Kumar J, Okada S, Clayberger C, et al. Granulysin: a novel antimicrobial. *Exp Opin Invest Drugs* 2001;10:321–330.
58. Kagi D, Vignaux F, Ledermann B, et al. Fas and perforin pathways as major mechanisms of T-cell mediated cytotoxicity. *Science* 1994;265:528–531.
59. IL4 and 5: biology and genetics. *Immunol Rev* 1988;102:1–212.
60. Wong GG, Clark SC. Multiple actions of interleukin 6 within a cytokine network. *Immunol Today* 1988;9:137–139.
61. Trinchieri G. Biology of natural killer cells. *Adv Immunol* 1989;47:187–376.
62. Colvin RB. Renal allografts. In: Colvin RB, Bahn AK, McCluskey RT, eds. *Diagnostic immunopathology*. New York: Raven Press, 1988:151–197.
63. Rao KV. Mechanism, pathophysiology, diagnosis, and management of renal transplant rejection. *Med Clin North Am* 1990;74:1039–1057.
64. Koskinen P, Lemstrom K, Hayry P. Chronic rejection. *Curr Opin Nephrol Hypertens* 1996;5:269–272.
65. Kreis HA, Ponticelli C. Causes of late renal allograft loss; chronic allograft dysfunction, death, and other factors. *Transplantation* 2001;71:SS5–SS9.
66. Kissmeyer-Nielsen F, Olsen S, Peterson VP, et al. Hyperacute rejection of kidney allografts associated with pre-existing humoral antibodies against donor cells. *Lancet* 1966;2:662–665.
67. Guettier C, Nochy D, Hinglais N, et al. Distinct phenotypic composition of diffuse interstitial and perivascular infiltrates in renal allografts: a morphometric analysis of cellular infiltration under conventional immunosuppressive therapy and under cyclosporine A. *Clin Nephrol* 1988;30:97–105.
68. Larsen CP, Austyn JM, Morris PJ. The role of graft derived dendritic leukocytes in the rejection of vascularized organ allografts. Recent findings on the migration and function of dendritic leukocytes after transplantation. *Ann Surg* 1990;212:308–317.
69. Krensky AM, Clayberger C. Diagnostic and therapeutic implications of T cell surface antigens. *Transplantation* 1985;39:339–348.
70. Springer TA. Adhesion receptors of the immune system. *Nature* 1990;346:425–434.
71. Rosenstein Y, Park JK, Hahn WC, et al. CD43, a molecule defective in Wiskott-Aldrich syndrome, binds ICAM-1. *Nature* 1991;354:233–235.
72. Van de Velde H, von Hoegen I, Luo W, et al. The B cell surface protein CD72/Lyb-2 is the ligand for CD5. *Nature* 1991;351:662–665.
73. Dianzani U, Malavasi F. Lymphocyte adhesion to endothelium. *Crit Rev Immunol* 1995;15:167–200.
74. Pober JS, Cotran RS. Immunologic interactions of T lymphocytes with vascular endothelium. *Adv Immunol* 1991;50:261–302.
75. Springer TA, Dustin ML, Kishimoto TK, et al. The lymphocyte function associated LFA-1, CD2, and LFA-3 molecules: cell adhesion receptors of the immune system. *Annu Rev Immunol* 1987;5:223–252.
76. Dustin ML, Springer TA. Role of lymphocyte adhesion receptors in transient interactions and cell locomotion. *Annu Rev Immunol* 1991;9:27–66.
77. Larson RS, Springer TA. Structure and function of leukocyte integrins. *Immunol Rev* 1990;114:181–217.
78. Kuncio GS, Neilson EG, Haverty T. Mechanisms of tubulointerstitial fibrosis. *Kidney Int* 1991;39:550–556.
79. Shimizu Y, Shaw S. Lymphocyte interactions with the extracellular matrix. *FASEB J* 1991;5:2292–2299.
80. deSousa M, Tilney NL, Kupiec-Weglinski JW. Recognition of self within self: specific lymphocyte positioning and the extracellular matrix. *Immunol Today* 1991;12:262–266.
81. Hemler ME. VLA proteins in the integrin family: structures, functions, and their role on leukocytes. *Annu Rev Immunol* 1990;8:365–400.
82. Nelson PJ, Krensky AM. Chemokines, chemokine receptors, and allograft rejection. *Immunity* 2001;14:377–386.
83. Nelson PJ, Krensky AM. Chemokines and allograft rejection; narrowing the list of suspects. *Transplantation* 2001;72:1195–1197.
84. Root RK. Leukocyte adhesion proteins: their role in neutrophil function. *Trans Am Clin Climatol Assoc* 1989;101:207–226.
85. Nacy CA, Meltzer MS. T-cell mediated activation of macrophages. *Curr Opin Immunol* 1991;3:330–335.
86. Kovacs EJ. Fibrogenic cytokines: the role of immune mediators in the development of scar tissue. *Immunol Today* 1991;12:17–23.
87. Halloran PF, Melk A, Barth C. Rethinking chronic allograft nephropathy: the concept of accelerated senescence. *J Am Soc Nephrol* 1999;10:167–181.
88. Grimm PC, Nickerson P, Gough J, et al. Quantitation of allograft fibrosis and chronic allograft nephropathy. *Pediatr Transplant* 1999;3:257–270.
89. Tullius SG, Tilney NL. Both alloantigen-dependent and -independent factors influence chronic allograft rejection. *Transplantation* 1995;59:313–318.
90. Paul LC. Chronic renal transplant loss. *Kidney Int* 1995; 47:1491–1499.
91. Toyoda M, Carlos JB, Galera OA, et al. Correlation of cytomegalovirus DNA levels with response to antiviral therapy in cardiac and renal allograft recipients. *Transplantation* 1997;63:957–963.
92. Tuazon TV, Schneeberger EE, Bhan AK, et al. Mononuclear cells in acute allograft glomerulopathy. *Am J Pathol* 1987;129:119–132.
93. Heemann U, Azuma H, Schmid C, et al. Effects of mycophenolic acid mofetil on acute rejection of kidney allografts in rats. *Clin Nephrol* 1996;45:355–357.
94. Nickerson P, Jeffery J, Gough J, et al. Effect of increasing baseline immunosuppression on the prevalence of clinical and subclinical rejection: a pilot study. *J Am Soc Nephrol* 1999;10:1801–1805.
95. Ojo AO, Meier-Kriesche HU, Hanson JA, et al. Mycophenolate mofetil reduces late renal allograft loss independent of acute rejection. *Transplantation* 2000;69:2405–2409.
96. Di Maria L, Bertoni E, Rosati A, et al. Mycophenolate mofetil (MMF) in the treatment of chronic renal rejection. *Clin Nephrol* 2000;53:33–34.
97. Pascual M, Williams WW, Cosimi AB, et al. Chronic renal allograft dysfunction: a role for mycophenolate mofetil? *Transplantation* 2000;69:1749–1750.
98. Weir MR, Ward MT, Blahut SA, et al. Long-term impact of discontinued or reduced calcineurin inhibitor in patients with chronic allograft nephropathy. *Kidney Int* 2001;59:1567–1573.
99. Hong JC, Kahan BD. Immunosuppressive agents in organ

transplantation: past, present, and future. *Semin Nephrol* 2000;20:108–125.
100. Hirose R, Vincenti F. Review of transplantation—1999. *Clin Transpl* 1999;295–315.
101. Rugstad HE. Antiinflammatory and immunoregulatory effects of glucocorticoids: mode of action. *Scand J Rheumatol* 1988;76S:257–264.
102. Wahli W, Martinez E. Superfamily of steroid nuclear receptors: positive and negative regulators of gene expression. *FASEB J* 1991;5:2243–2249.
103. Beato M. Gene regulation by steroid hormones. *Cell* 1989;56:335–344.
104. Auphan N, DiDonato JA, Rosette C, et al. Immunosuppression by glucocorticoids: inhibition of NF-kappa B activity through induction of I kappa B synthesis. *Science* 1995;270:286–290.
105. Balow JE, Hunninghake GW, Fauci AS. Corticosteroids in human lymphocyte mediated cytotoxic reactions. *Transplantation* 1977;23:322–328.
106. Goldstein IM. Effects of steroids on lysosomes. *Transplant Proc* 1975;7:21–24.
107. Stevens C, Lempert N, Freed BM. The effects of immunosuppressive agents on in vitro production of human immunoglobulins. *Transplantation* 1991;51:1240–1244.
108. Hricik DE. Steroid withdrawal in renal transplant recipients: pro point of view. *Transplant Proc* 1998;30:1380–1382.
109. Sarwal MM, Yorgin PD, Alexander S, et al. Promising early outcomes with a novel, complete steroid avoidance immunosuppression protocol in pediatric renal transplantation. *Transplantation* 2001;72:13–21.
110. Hemenway CS, Heitman J. Calcineurin. Structure, function, and inhibition. *Cell Biochem Biophys* 1999;30:115–151.
111. Morris PJ. Cyclosporine A. Overview. *Transplantation* 1981;32:349–354.
112. Borel JF. Comparative study of in vitro and in vivo drug effects on cell mediated cytotoxicity. *Immunology* 1976;31:631–641.
113. Borel JF, Feurer C, Gubler HU, et al. The biologic effects of cyclosporin A: a new antilymphocytic agent. *Agents Actions* 1976;6:468–475.
114. Faulds D, Goa KL, Benfield P. Cyclosporin. A review of its pharmacodynamic and pharmacokinetic properties, and therapeutic use in immunoregulatory disorders. *Drugs* 1993;45:953–1040.
115. Schreiber SL. Chemistry and biology of immunophilins and their immunosuppressive ligands. *Science* 1991;251:283–287.
116. Harding WM, Galat A, Uehling DE, et al. A receptor for the immunosuppressant FK506 is a cis-trans peptidyl-prolyl isomerase. *Nature* 1989;341:758–760.
117. Schreiber SL, Crabtree GR. The mechanism of action of cyclosporin A and FK506. *Immunol Today* 1992;13:136–142.
118. Liu J, Farmer JD, Lane WS, et al. Calcineurin is a common target of cyclophilin-cyclosporin A and FKBP-FK506 complexes. *Cell* 1991;66:807–815.
119. Kupiec-Weglinski JW, Filho MA, Strom TB, et al. Sparing of suppressor cells: a critical action of cyclosporine. *Transplantation* 1984;38:97–101.
120. Khanna A, Li B, Stenzel KH, et al. Regulation of new DNA synthesis in mammalian cells by cyclosporine. Demonstration of a transforming growth factor beta-dependent mechanism of inhibition of cell growth. *Transplantation* 1994;57:577–582.
121. Humes HD, Coffman T, Halderman H, et al. Cyclosporine nephrotoxicity: a workshop to discuss mechanisms, diagnosis, and treatment. *Transplant Proc* 1988;20S:833–840.
122. Youngelman DF, Kahng KU, Rosen BD, et al. Effects of chronic cyclosporine administration on renal blood flow and intrarenal blood flow distribution. *Transplantation* 1991;51:503–509.
123. Friedman J, Weissman I. Two cytoplasmic candidates for immunophilin action are revealed by affinity for a new cyclophilin: one in the presence and one in the absence of CsA. *Cell* 1991;66:799–806.
124. Peters DH, Fitton A, Plosker GL, et al. Tacrolimus. A review of its pharmacology, and therapeutic potential in hepatic and renal transplantation. *Drugs* 1993;46:746–794.
125. Fung JJ, Starzl TE. FK506 in solid organ transplantation. *Ther Drug Monit* 1995;17:592–595.
126. Kahan BD. Sirolimus: a comprehensive review. *Expert Opin Pharmacother* 2001;2:1903–1917.
127. Brunn GJ, Williams J, Sabers C, et al. Direct inhibition of the signaling functions of the mammalian target of rapamycin by the phosphoinositide 3-kinase inhibitors, wortmannin and LY294002. *EMBO J* 1996;15:5256–5267.
128. Feuerstein N, Huang D, Prystowsky MB. Rapamycin selectively blocks interleukin-2-induced proliferating cell nuclear antigen gene expression in T lymphocytes. Evidence for inhibition of CREB/ATF binding activities. *J Biol Chem* 1995;270:9454–9458.
129. Sehgal SN. Rapamune (sirolimus, rapamycin): an overview and mechanism of action. *Ther Drug Monit* 1995;17:660–665.
130. Saunders RN, Metcalfe MS, Nicholson ML. Rapamycin in transplantation: a review of the evidence. *Kidney Int* 2001;53:3–16.
131. Murgia MG, Jordan S, Kahan BD. The side effect profile of sirolimus: a phase I study in quiescent cyclosporine-prednisone-treated renal transplant patients. *Kidney Int* 1996;49:209–216.
132. Murray JE, Merrill JP, Harrison JH, et al. Prolonged survival of human kidney homografts by immunosuppressive drug therapy. *N Engl J Med* 1963;268:1315–1323.
133. Elion GB. Biochemistry and pharmacology of purine analogues. *Fed Proc* 1967;26:898–904.
134. Strom TB. Immunosuppressive agents in renal transplantation. *Kidney Int* 1984;26:353–365.
135. Haesslein HC, Pierce JC, Lee HM, et al. Leukopenia and azathioprine management in renal homotransplantation. *Surgery* 1972;71:598–604.
136. Dimitriu A, Fauci AS. Differential sensitivity of human lymphocyte subpopulations to azathioprine. *Transplant Proc* 1979;11:878–881.
137. Prince HE, Ettenger RB, Dorey FJ, et al. Azathioprine suppression of natural killer cell activity and antibody dependent cellular cytotoxicity in renal transplant recipients. *Transplant Proc* 1984;16:1475–1477.
138. Galanaud P, Crevon MC, Duclos, et al. New data on the effect of azathioprine at the cellular level. *Adv Nephrol Necker Hosp* 1980;6:371–382.
139. Allison AC, Eugui EM. Mycophenolate mofetil and its mechanism of action. *Immunopharmacology* 2000;47:85–118.
140. Ransom JT. Mechanism of action of mycophenolate mofetil. *Ther Drug Monit* 1995; 17:681–684.

141. Natsumeda Y, Carr SF. Human type I and II IMP dehydrogenases as drug targets. *Ann N Y Acad Sci* 1993;696:88–93.
142. Fulton B, Markham A. Mycophenolate mofetil. A review of its pharmacodynamic and pharmacokinetic properties and clinical efficacy in renal transplantation. *Drugs* 1996;51:278–298.
143. Halloran P, Mathew T, Tomlanovich S, et al. Mycophenolate mofetil in renal allograft recipients: a pooled efficacy analysis of three randomized, double-blind, clinical studies in prevention of rejection. The International Mycophenolate Mofetil Renal Transplant Study Groups. *Transplantation* 1997;63:39–47.
144. Pirsch JD, Sollinger HW. Mycophenolate mofetil—clinical and experimental experience. *Ther Drug Monit* 1996;18: 357–361.
145. Budde K, Schmouder RL, Brunkhorst R, et al. First human trial of FTY720, a novel immunomodulator, in stable renal transplant patients. *J Am Soc Nephrol* 2002;13:1073–1083.
146. Chen S, Bacon KB, Garcia G, et al. FTY720, a novel transplantation drug, modulates lymphocyte migratory responses to chemokines. *Transplant Proc* 2001;33:3057–3063.
147. Li H, Meno-Tetang GM, Chiba K, et al. Pharmacokinetics and cell trafficking dynamics of 2-amino-2-[2-(4-octylphenyl)ethyl]propane-1,3-diol hydrochloride (FTY720) in cynomolgus monkeys after single oral and intravenous doses. *J Pharmacol Exp Ther* 2002;301:519–526.
148. Mannick JA, Davis RC, Cooperband SR, et al. Clinical use of rabbit antihuman lymphocyte globulin in cadaver-kidney transplantation. *N Engl J Med* 1982;284:1109–1115.
149. Uittenbogaart CH, Robinson BJ, Malekzadeh MH, et al. The use of antilymphocyte globulin (dose by rosette protocol) in pediatric renal allograft recipients. *Transplantation* 1979;28:291–293.
150. Bonnefoy-Berard N, Vincent C, Revillard JP. Antibodies against functional leukocyte surface molecules in polyclonal antilymphocyte and antithymocyte globulins. *Transplantation* 1991;51:669–673.
151. Mjornsteadt L, Olansson M, Lindholm L, et al. Mechanisms maintaining transplantation tolerance in antilymphocyte globulin treated rats. *Transplantation* 1987;44:669–673.
152. Filo RS, Smith EJ, Leapman SB. Therapy of acute cadaveric renal allograft rejection with adjunctive antithymocyte globulin. *Transplantation* 1980;30:445–449.
153. Hardy MA, Nowygrod R, Elberg A, et al. Use of ATG in treatment of steroid resistant rejection. *Transplantation* 1980;29:162–164.
154. Szczech LA, Feldman HI. Effect of anti-lymphocyte antibody induction therapy on renal allograft survival. *Transplant Proc* 1999;31:9S–11S.
155. Kohler G, Milstein C. Continuous cultures of fused cells secreting antibody of predefined specificity. *Nature* 1975; 256:495–497.
156. Cosimi AB, Colvin RB, Burton RC, et al. Use of monoclonal antibodies to T cell subsets for immunological monitoring and treatment in recipients of renal allografts. *N Engl J Med* 1981;305:308–314.
157. Waldmann H. Manipulation of T-cell responses with monoclonal antibodies. *Annu Rev Immunol* 1989;7:404–444.
158. Chatenoud L, Bach JF. Selective immunosuppression with anti-T cell monoclonal antibodies. *Clin Nephrol* 1992; 38(suppl 1):S53–S60.
159. Cobbold SP, Adams E, Marshall SE, et al. Mechanisms of peripheral tolerance and suppression induced by monoclonal antibodies to CD4 and CD8. *Immunol Rev* 1996;149:5–33.
160. Chatenoud L, Bach JF. Monoclonal antibodies to CD3 as immunosuppressants. *Semin Immunol* 1990;2:437–447.
161. Leone MR, Barry JM, Alexander SR, et al. Monoclonal antibody OKT3 therapy in pediatric kidney transplant recipients. *J Pediatr* 1990;116:S86–S91.
162. Sablinski T, Hancock WW, Tilney NL, et al. CD4 monoclonal antibodies in organ transplantation—a review of progress. *Transplantation* 1991;52:579–589.
163. Milford EL, Carpenter CB, Kirkman RL, et al. Anti-T12 monoclonal antibody therapy of acute renal allograft rejection. *Transplant Proc* 1987;19:1910.
164. Wee SL, Colvin RB, Phenlan JM, et al. Fc receptor for mouse IgG1 (Fc gamma RII) and antibody mediated cell clearance in patients treated with Leu 2a antibody. *Transplantation* 1989;48:1012–1017.
165. Hourmant M, Bedrossian J, Durand D, et al. A randomized multicenter trial comparing leukocyte function-associated antigen-1 monoclonal antibody with rabbit antithymocyte globulin as induction treatment in first kidney transplantations. *Transplantation* 1996;62:1565–1170.
166. Vincenti F, Lantz M, Birnbaum J, et al. A phase I trial of humanized anti-interleukin 2 receptor antibody in renal transplantation. *Transplantation* 1997;63:33–38.
167. van Gelder T, Zietse R, Mulder AH, et al. A double-blind, placebo-controlled study of monoclonal anti-interleukin-2 receptor antibody (BT563) administration to prevent acute rejection after kidney transplantation. *Transplantation* 1995;60:248–252.
168. Lazarovits AI, Poppema S, Zhang Z, et al. Prevention and reversal of renal allograft rejection by antibody against CD45RB. *Nature* 1996;380:717–720.
169. Friend PJ, Hale G, Waldmann H, et al. Campath-1M—prophylactic use after kidney transplantation. A randomized controlled clinical trial. *Transplantation* 1989;48:248–253.
170. Zeng Y, Gage A, Montag A, et al. Inhibition of transplant rejection by pretreatment of xenogeneic pancreatic islet cells with anti-ICAM-1 antibodies. *Transplantation* 1994;58: 681–689.
171. Norman DJ, Leone MR. The role of OKT3 in clinical transplantation. *Pediatr Nephrol* 1991;5:130–136.
172. Hooks MA, Wade CS, Millikan WJ Jr. Muromonab CD3: a review of its pharmacology, pharmacokinetics, and clinical use in transplantation. *Pharmacotherapy* 1991;11:26–37.
173. Ortho Multicenter Transplant Study Group. A randomized clinical trial of Orthoclone OKT3 monoclonal antibody for acute rejection of cadaveric renal transplants. *N Engl J Med* 1985;313:337–342.
174. Muromonab CD3: a reappraisal of its pharmacology and use as prophylaxis of solid organ transplant rejection. *Drugs* 1996;51:865–894.
175. Shield CF III, Norman DJ, Marlett P, et al. Comparison of antimouse and antihorse antibody production during the treatment of allograft rejection with OKT3 or antilymphocyte globulin. *Nephron* 1987;46:48–51.
176. Riechman L, Clark M, Waldmann H, et al. Reshaping human antibodies for therapy. *Nature* 1988;332:323–327.
177. Winter G, Milstein C. Man-made antibodies. *Nature* 1991;349:293–299.

178. Isaacs JD. The antiglobulin response to therapeutic antibodies. *Semin Immunol* 1990;2:449–456.
179. Cosimi AB. OKT3: first dose safety and success. *Nephron* 1987;46:12–18.
180. Thistlethwaite JR Jr, Stuart JK, Mayes JT, et al. Complications and monitoring of OKT3 therapy. *Am J Kidney Dis* 1988;11:112–119.
181. Wiseman LR, Faulds D. Daclizumab: a review of its use in the prevention of acute rejection in renal transplant recipients. *Drugs* 1999;58:1029–1042.
182. Cibrik DM, Kaplan B, Meier-Kriesche HU. Role of anti-interleukin-2 receptor antibodies in kidney transplantation. *BioDrugs* 2001;15:655–666.
183. Naik RB, Ashlin R, Wilson C, et al. The role of plasmapheresis in renal transplantation. *Clin Nephrol* 1979;11: 245–250.
184. Frasca GM, Martella D, Vangelista A, et al. Ten years experience with plasma exchange in renal transplantation. *Int J Artif Organs* 1991;14:51–55.
185. Fryd DS, Sutherland DER, Simmons RL, et al. Results of a prospective randomized study on the effect of splenectomy versus no splenectomy in renal transplant patients. *Transplant Proc* 1881;13:48–56.
186. Pilepich MV, Dicard GA, Breaux SR, et al. Renal graft irradiation in acute rejection. *Transplantation* 1983;35:208–211.
187. Saper V, Chow D, Engelman ED, et al. Clinical and immunologic studies of cadaveric renal transplant recipients given total lymphoid irradiation and maintained on low dose prednisone. *Transplantation* 1988;45:540–546.
188. Myburgh JA. Total lymphoid irradiation in transplantation. *Transplant Proc* 1988;20S:118–121.
189. Opelz G, Terasaki PI. Improvement of kidney graft survival with increased numbers of blood transfusions. *N Engl J Med* 1978;299:799–803.
190. Carpenter CB. Blood transfusion effects in kidney transplantation. *Yale J Biol Med* 1990;63:435–443.
191. Potter DE, Portale AA, Melzer JS, et al. Are blood transfusions beneficial in the cyclosporine era? *Pediatr Nephrol* 1991;5:168–172.
192. de Waal LP, van Twuyver E. Blood transfusion and allograft survival: Is mixed chimerism the solution for tolerance induction in clinical transplantation? *Crit Rev Immunol* 1991;10:417–425.
193. Owen RD. Immunogenetic consequences of vascular anastomosis between bovine twins. *Science* 1945;102:400–401.
194. Burnet FM. *Clonal selection theory of acquired immunity.* Cambridge: Cambridge University Press, 1959.
195. Billingham RE, Brent L, Medawar PB. Actively acquired tolerance of foreign cells. *Nature* 1953;172:603–606.
196. Remuzzi G, Rossini M, Imberti O, et al. Kidney graft survival in rates without immunosuppressants after intrathymic glomerular transplantation. *Lancet* 1991;337:750–752.
197. Perico N, Rossini M, Imbert O, et al. Thymus mediated immune tolerance to renal allografts is donor but not tissue specific. *J Am Soc Nephrol* 1991;2:1063–1071.
198. Griffith TS, Brunner T, Fletcher SM, et al. Fas ligand-induced apoptosis as a mechanism of immune privilege. *Science* 1995;270:1189–1192.
199. Chen JJ, Sun Y, Nabel GJ. Regulation of the proinflammatory effects of Fas ligand (CD95L). *Science* 1998;282:1714–1717.
200. Sauter B, Albert ML, Francisco L, et al. Consequences of cell death: exposure to necrotic tumor cells, but not primary tissue cells or apoptotic cells, induces the maturation of immunostimulatory dendritic cells. *J Exp Med* 2000;191: 423–34.
201. Gershon RK, Kondo K. Infectious immunological tolerance. *Immunology* 1971;21:903–914.
202. Nisco SJ, Hissink RJ, Vriens PW, et al. In vivo studies of the maintenance of peripheral transplant tolerance after cyclosporine. Radiosensitive antigen-specific suppressor cells mediate lasting graft protection against primed effector cells. *Transplantation* 1995;59:1444–1452.
203. Fukuzaki T, Hancock WW, Monaco AP, et al. Indefinite survival of skin allografts in adult thymectomized, antilymphocyte serum-treated mice given bone marrow and thymus grafts of donor origin: tolerance induction by donor bone marrow and thymus. *Transplantation* 1998;65:1036–1043.
204. Strober S. Total lymphoid irradiation: basic and clinical studies in transplantation immunity. *Prog Clin Biol Res* 1986;224:251–262.
205. Hall BM, Pearce NW, Gurley KE, et al. Specific unresponsiveness in rats with prolonged cardiac allograft survival after treatment with cyclosporine. III. Further characterization of the CD4+ suppressor cell and its mechanisms of action. *J Exp Med* 1990;171:141–157.
206. Sakaguchi S, Sakaguchi N. Thymus and autoimmunity: capacity of the normal thymus to produce pathogenic self-reactive T cells and conditions required for their induction of autoimmune disease. *J Exp Med* 1990;172:537–545.
207. Takahashi T, Tagami T, Yamazaki S, et al. Immunologic self-tolerance maintained by CD25(+)CD4(+) regulatory T cells constitutively expressing cytotoxic T lymphocyte antigen associated antigen 4. *J Exp Med* 2000;192:303–310.
208. Suri-Payer E, Amar AZ, Thornton AM, et al. CD4+CD25+ T cells inhibit both the induction and effector function of autoreactive T cells and represent a unique lineage of immunoregulatory cells. *J Immunol* 1998;160:1212–1218.
209. Salomon B, Lenschow DJ, Rhee L, et al. B7/CD28 costimulation is essential for the homeostasis of the CD4+CD25+ immunoregulatory T cells that control autoimmune diabetes. *Immunity* 2000;12:431–40.
210. Hara M, Kingsley CI, Niimi N, et al. IL-10 is required for regulatory T cells to mediate tolerance to alloantigens in vivo. *J Immunol* 2001;166:37:89–96.
211. Taylor PA, Noelle RJ, Blazar BR. CD4(+)CD25(+) immune regulatory cells are required for induction of tolerance to alloantigen via costimulatory blockade. *J Exp Med* 2001;193:1311–1318.
212. Thornton AM, Shevach EM. Suppressor effector function of CD4+CD25+ immunoregulatory T cells is antigen nonspecific. *J Immunol* 2000;164:183–190.
213. Powrie F, Carlino J, Leach MW, et al. A critical role for transforming growth factor-beta but not interleukin 4 in the suppression of T helper type 1 mediated colitis by CD45RB(low) CD4+ T cells. *J Exp Med* 1996;183:2669–2674.

214. Groux H, O'Garra A, Bigler M, et al. A CD4+ T cell subset inhibits antigen specific T cell responses and prevents colitis. *Nature* 1997;389:737–742.
215. Weiner HL. Induction and mechanism of action of transforming growth factor-beta-secreting Th3 regulatory cells. *Immunol Rev* 2001;182:207–214.
216. Read S, Malmstrom V, Powrie F. Cytotoxic T lymphocyte associated antigen 5 plays an essential role in the function of CD25(+)CD4(+) regulatory cells that control intestinal inflammation. *J Exp Med* 2000;192:295–302.
217. Nakamura K, Kitani A, Strober W. Cell contact-dependent immunosuppression by CD4(+)CD25(+) regulatory T cells is mediated by cell surface bound transforming growth factor beta. *J Exp Med* 2001;194:629–644.
218. Schwartz RH. Acquisition of immunologic self tolerance. *Cell* 1989;57:1073–1081.
219. Schwartz RH. A cell culture model for T lymphocyte clonal anergy. *Science* 1990;248:1349–1356.
220. Opelz G, Vanrenterghem Y, Kirste G, et al. Prospective evaluation of pretransplant blood transfusions in cadaver kidney recipients. *Transplantation* 1997;63:964–967.
221. Davies HF, Pollard SG, Calne RY. Tolerogenic and immunosuppressive properties of liver grafts in animals and man. *Transplant Proc* 1991;23:2248–2249.
222. Lenschow DJ, Walunas TL, Bluestone JA. CD28/B7 system of T cell costimulation. *Annu Rev Immunol* 1996;14:233–258.
223. Bluestone JA. Costimulation and its role in organ transplantation. *Clin Transplant* 1996;10:104–109.
224. Fraser JD, Irving BA, Crabtree GR, et al. Regulation of interleukin-2 gene enhancer activity by the T-cell accessory molecule CD28. *Science* 1991;251:313–316.
225. Linsley PS, Brady W, Urnes M, et al. CTLA4 is a second receptor for the B cell activation antigen B7. *J Exp Med* 1991;174:561–569.
226. Tivol EA, Borriello F, Schweitzer AN, et al. Loss of CTLA-4 leads to massive lymphoproliferation and fatal multiorgan tissue destruction, revealing a critical negative regulatory role of CTLA-4. *Immunity* 1995;3:541–547.
227. Shahinian A, Pfeffer K, Lee KP, et al. Differential T cell costimulatory requirements in CD28-deficient mice. *Science* 1993;261:609–612.
228. Lin H, Wei RQ, Gordon D, et al. Review of CTLA4Ig use for allograft immunosuppression. *Transplant Proc* 1994;26: 3200–3201.
229. Judge TA, Tang A, Turka LA. Immunosuppression through blockade of CD28:B7-mediated costimulatory signals. *Immunol Res* 1996;15:38–49.
230. Greene JL, Leytze GM, Emswiler J, et al. Covalent dimerization of CD28/CTLA-4 and oligomerization of CD80/CD86 regulate T cell costimulatory interactions. *J Biol Chem* 1996;271:26762–26771.
231. Starzl TE, Demetris AJ, Murase N, et al. Donor cell chimerism permitted by immunosuppressive drugs: a new view of organ transplantation. *Immunol Today* 1993;14:326–332.
232. Sykes M, Sachs DH. Mixed chimerism. *Philos Trans R Soc Lond B Biol Sci* 2001;356:707–726.
233. Spitzer TR, Delmonico F, Tolkoff-Rubin N, et al. Combined histocompatibility leukocyte-antigen matched donor bone marrow and renal transplantation for multiple myeloma with end-stage renal disease: the induction of allograft tolerance through mixed lymphohematopoietic chimerism. *Transplantation* 1999;68:480–484.
234. Rocken M, Shevach EM. Immune deviation—the third dimension of nondeletional T cell tolerance. *Immunol Rev* 1996;149:175–194.
235. Strom TB, Roy-Chaudhury P, Manfro R, et al. The Th1/Th2 paradigm and the allograft response. *Curr Opin Immunol* 1996;8:688–693
236. Krensky AM. The HLA system, antigen processing and presentation. *Kidney Int* 1997;51:S2–S7.
237. Murphy B, Krensky AM. HLA derived peptides as novel immunomodulatory therapeutics. *J Am Soc Nephrol* 1999;10:1346–1355.
238. Giral M, Cuturi MC, Nguyen JM, et al. Decreased cytotoxic activity of natural killer cells in kidney allograft recipients treated with human HLA-derived peptide. *Transplantation* 1997;63:1004–1011.
239. Barber WH, Mankin JA, Laskow DA, et al. Long-term results of a controlled prospective study with transfusion of donor-specific bone marrow in 57 cadaveric renal allograft recipients. *Transplantation* 1991;51:70–75.
240. Cascalho M, Platt JL. Xenotransplantation and other means of organ replacement. *Nature Rev Immunol* 2001;1:154–160.
241. Cozzi E, White DJ. Xenotransplantation. *Curr Opin Nephrol Hypertens* 1996;5:514–518.
242. Platt JL. Xenotransplantation; recent progress and current perspectives. *Curr Opin Immunol* 1996;8:721–728.
243. Starzl TE, Marchioro TL, Peters GN, et al. Renal heterotransplantation from baboon to man: experience with 6 cases. *Transplantation* 1964;2:752–776.
244. Good AH, Cooper DKC, Malcolm AJ, et al. Identification of the carbohydrate structures that bind human anti-porcine antibodies: implications for discordant xenografting in humans. *Transplant Proc* 1992;24:559–562.
245. Collins BH, Cotterell AH, McCurry KR, et al. Hyperacute rejection of cardiac xenografts between primate species: evidence to support the significance of the alpha-galactosyl determinant. *J Immunol* 1995;154:5500–5510.
246. Sachs DH, Sablinski T. Tolerance across discordant xenogeneic barriers. *Xenotransplantation* 1995;2:234-239.
247. Kooyman DL, Parker WR, McClellan SB, et al. Identification and characterization of a galactosyl peptide mimetic. *Transplantation* 1996;61:851–855.
248. Sharma A, Okabe JF, Birch P, et al. Reduction in the level of Gal(alpha 1,3) Gal in transgenic mice and pigs by the expression of an alpha(1,2) fucosyltransferase. *Proc Natl Acad Sci U S A* 1996;93:7190–7195.
249. Leventhal JR, Dalmasso AP, Cromwell JW, et al. Prolongation of cardiac xenograft survival by depletion of complement. *Transplantation* 1993;55:857–866.
250. Platt JL, Vercellotti GM, Dalmasso AP, et al. Transplantation of discordant xenografts: a review of progress. *Immunol Today* 1990;11:450–456.
251. Dalmasso AP, Vercellotti GM, Platt JL, et al. Inhibition of complement-mediated endothelial cell cytotoxicity by decay accelerating factor: potential for prevention of xenograft hyperacute rejection. *Transplantation* 1991;52:530–533.

252. Parker W, Saadi S, Lin SS, et al. Transplantation of discordant xenografts: a challenge revisited. *Immunol Today* 1996;17:373–378.
253. Hall BM, Gurley K, Dorsch SE. Specific unresponsiveness in rats with prolonged allograft survival is dependent upon the graft and suppressor T cells. *Transplant Proc* 1986;19:495–496.
254. Roser BJ, Dorsch S. The cellular basis of transplantation tolerance in the rat. *Immunol Rev* 1979;46:46–54.
255. Chow D, Saper V, Strober S. Renal transplant patients treated with total lymphoid irradiation show specific unresponsiveness to donor antigens in the mixed lymphocyte reaction (MLR). *J Immunol* 1987;138:3746–3750.
256. Monaco AP. Future trends in transplantation in the 1990s: prospects for the induction of clinical tolerance. *Transplant Proc* 1991;23:67–72.
257. Krensky AM. Immunologic tolerance. *Pediatr Nephrol* 2001;16:675–679.
258. Brennan DC, Mohanakumar T, Flye MW. Donor-specific transfusion and donor bone marrow infusion in renal transplantation tolerance: a review of efficacy and mechanisms. *Am J Kidney Dis* 1995;26:701–715.

73

PEDIATRIC RENAL TRANSPLANTATION

WILLIAM E. HARMON

INTRODUCTION

Role of Transplantation

Chronic dialysis and renal transplantation are both satisfactory treatments for end-stage renal disease (ESRD). The majority of adults with ESRD are receiving dialysis rather than undergoing renal transplantation, although the number seeking renal transplantation is continuing to rise substantially (1). There is a survival advantage of transplantation for virtually all candidates. Unfortunately, the lack of suitable donors has limited the number of people who can receive transplants. Renal transplantation was recognized as the better form of treatment for children with ESRD some two decades ago (2). Both peritoneal dialysis, delivered as continuous ambulatory peritoneal dialysis or continuous cyclical peritoneal dialysis, and hemodialysis lead to a deceleration of growth. Data from the dialysis component of the North American Pediatric Renal Transplant Cooperative Study (NAPRTCS) registry (3) showed that the overall height deficit of –1.8 standard deviation units at initiation of dialysis became more negative, reaching a value of –2.16 standard deviation units at 24 months. In addition, children do not tolerate being dependent on dialysis, and maintenance dialysis induces loss of self-esteem and emotional maladjustment (4). Cognitive achievement test scores may diminish with prolonged time on dialysis (5). In contrast, the mobility and freedom from dietary restrictions afforded by a functioning renal transplant enable children to live nearly normal lives despite complex immunosuppressive regimens. Although renal transplantation has resulted in normal growth for all children, dramatic short-term improvements in height can be seen in many, and final adult height is improving after transplantation (6–9). Most importantly, successful transplantation permits the child to attend school and to develop normally. School function test scores improve dramatically after transplantation (10,11). Importantly, young children now have the best long-term outcomes of all age groups among transplant recipients, which confirms the usefulness of transplantation in this age group (12). For all of these reasons, successful renal transplantation remains the primary goal for children with ESRD.

Incidence and Frequency of Transplantation

NAPRTCS has registered approximately 500 pediatric kidney transplantations each year since its inception in 1987, which account for 75% of all those performed in North America, and that number has remained relatively constant over the time span. In 2002, there were approximately 14,700 kidney transplants performed in the United States, which suggests that pediatric patients comprise approximately 5% of all transplant recipients. Although the number of pediatric transplants performed each year has not varied by more than 10%, the donor origin has undergone substantial changes. Data of the Scientific Registry of Transplant Recipients show that living kidney donation has expanded substantially, and the number of living donors (LDs) exceeded the number of cadaveric donors (CADs) for the first time in 2001 (1). Living donations now account for 43% of all kidney transplants in the United States. In 1987, only 40% of all transplants performed in children were from an LD source; by 1991, the figure had risen to 53%, and since 1998 LDs have accounted for over 60% of all pediatric renal transplants (Table 73.1) (13). Parents comprise 82% of LDs. Mothers comprise the majority of parent donors; fathers account for 46%. There is no outcome advantage to donation from one parent versus the other with the possible exception that infants younger than 1 year of age seem to experience fewer rejections if the mother is the donor (14,15). Due to the fact that children most often have siblings who are too young to donate (younger than 18 years), the NAPRTCS registry has recorded only 305 transplants between siblings. Of these, 150 grafts were from donors younger than 21 years of age. A review of the NAPRTCS registry data identified only 12 LDs under 18 years of age, of which 11 involved transplants between siblings and one a transplant from parent to child. It is quite clear that most programs are very reluctant to use young donors (16,17). However, a review of United Network of Organ Sharing (UNOS) data revealed that, of approximately 40,000 LDs in the United States between 1987 and 2000, 60 were donors younger than 18 years of age (18). Twenty-four of the recipients were children and 36 were adults; only seven of the transplantations were

TABLE 73.1. CHARACTERISTICS OF PEDIATRIC KIDNEY DONORS AND RECIPIENTS

	1987	1989	1991	1993	1995	1997	1999	2001
Living donors (%)	43	46	51	51	52	55	58	63
Recipients younger than 6 yr (%)	25	23	22	23	15	18	17	17
Cadaveric donors younger than 10 yr (%)	35	33	19	16	15	10	10	10

Adapted from Seikaly M, Ho PL, Emmett L, et al. The 12th annual report of the North American Pediatric Renal Transplant Cooperative Study: renal transplantation from 1987 through 1998. *Pediatr Transplant* 2001;5:215–231.

between identical twins. There has been a substantial interest in organ donation by living unrelated individuals in the adult transplant literature because the outcome of the grafts has been shown to be better than that using cadaver source kidneys (19). NAPRTCS identified 123 transplantations involving living unrelated donors between 1987 and 2001. A preliminary analysis of the first 38 recipients of grafts from living unrelated donors showed that 23 (61%) were male, 30 (79%) were white, 8 were younger than 6 years of age, and 20 were older than 12 years of age (20). This was the primary transplant for 29 of the 38 recipients. Of the 38 donors, 22 were nonbiological parents, and family friends were the donors in 10 of the cases.

The majority of cadaveric kidneys used in children are recovered from adult donors. In the 1980s there was a tendency to preferentially place kidneys recovered from infants into infant recipients, which led to disastrous consequences for patient and graft survival (21). As a result of widespread dissemination of these data (22,23), there has been a marked change in this practice (Table 73.1). From 1987 through 1990, the percentage of CADs older than 10 years of age ranged from 59 to 68%. From 1991 through 1994, these percentages ranged from 78 to 88%. Before 1991, children younger than 2 years of age comprised 3.2% of CADs. In 1991, no pediatric recipient received a kidney from a CAD under 2 years of age; and in 1995 and 1996, there were no such kidneys used in children (24). Between 1991 and 2002, fewer than 1% (23 of 2464) of CADs for children were younger than 2 years of age (13). This change in allocation of kidneys from young donors led to improvement in graft survival (21). Some specialized pediatric programs have reported good results with young donors (25), but many programs reserve grafts from very young donors for en bloc transplantation into older recipients (26).

Primary Diagnosis

Because of the large NAPRTCS database, it is now possible to determine the percentages of each disease category leading to ESRD by age at transplantation as well as by gender and race. ESRD in children is generally due to congenital or inherited diseases. When 7651 transplantations were reviewed, the most common congenital diagnoses were found to be obstructive uropathy and aplastic-hypoplastic-dysplastic kidneys, each representing approximately 16% of cases (13) (Table 73.2). Among glomerular disorders, focal segmental glomerulosclerosis (FSGS) is the most common; 873 children received a renal transplant for FSGS between 1987 and 2002. The primary diagnosis also varies with the race of the recipient. Overall in the NAPRTCS registry, white children account for 62% of all recipients; however, white children account for less than 50% of the children undergoing transplantation for FSGS. The data regarding the role of FSGS as a cause of ESRD can be better appreciated by observations from the dialysis section of the registry, in which the two most common diagnoses are FSGS and aplastic-dysplastic kidneys, each accounting for 14% of cases. White children make up only 34% of 733 children with FSGS on dialysis, with African American and Hispanic children accounting for 62% of these patients. Twenty-four percent of African American children on dialysis and 30% of those older than 12 years of age have FSGS. Table 73.2 shows the primary diagnoses by gender and race of 7651 children who have received a transplant as recorded by NAPRTCS since 1987, as well as the percentage of biopsy-proven diagnoses. It is important to observe that confirmation of the primary diagnosis by biopsy was made in 94% of patients with FSGS, 93% of those with systemic immunologic diseases, and 90% of patients with congenital nephrotic syndrome. The information regarding primary diagnosis becomes critical in predicting graft survival as well as recurrence of the original disease, as discussed later.

Age at Transplantation

Kidney transplantation in infants younger than 6 months of age or below a weight of 6 kg is exceptional. From 1987 to 2002, NAPRTCS recorded 81 transplantations performed in children younger than 12 months (13). Of these, 5 transplantations were performed in children between 3 and 5 months, 21 were performed in children between 6 and 8 months, and 55 were performed in children between 9 and 11 months of age. Only 12 infants have been reported to have undergone transplantation since 1996. In general, the number of kidney transplantations performed in infants and young children seems to be declining (Table 73.1). Because infants and adolescents have different risk factors for both patient and graft survival, children have been grouped into five age categories: 0 to 1 year, 2 to 5 years, 6 to 12 years, 13 to 17 years, and 18 to 21 years of age. It had been suggested that children 0 to 5 years of age

TABLE 73.2. GENDER AND RACE DISTRIBUTION OF PEDIATRIC KIDNEY TRANSPLANT PATIENTS BY PRIMARY DIAGNOSIS

	N	%	% Male	% White	% Biopsied
Total	7651		60	62	56
Diagnosis					
Obstructive uropathy	1237	16	86	66	32
Aplasic-hypoplastic-dysplastic kidney	1222	16	62	65	28
Focal segmental glomerulosclerosis	873	11	58	48	94
Reflux nephropathy	397	5	45	74	33
Chronic glomerulonephritis	279	4	42	47	75
Polycystic disease	213	3	52	75	56
Medullary cystic disease	212	3	50	83	66
Hemolytic uremic syndrome	206	3	56	80	53
Prune-belly syndrome	201	3	99	61	38
Congenital nephrotic syndrome	192	3	51	66	90
Familial nephritis	177	2	82	58	72
Cystinosis	162	2	50	90	44
Idiopathic crescentic glomerulonephritis	151	2	35	53	95
Membranoproliferative glomerulonephritis type 1	150	2	46	55	97
Pyelonephritis, interstitial nephritis	146	2	47	71	75
Systemic lupus erythematosus nephritis	124	2	19	27	96
Renal infarct	119	2	49	78	37
Henoch-Schönlein nephritis	101	1	41	67	85
Berger (immunoglobulin A) nephritis	100	1	57	63	93
Membranoproliferative glomerulonephritis type 2	68	1	50	76	96
Wilms' tumor	43	1	49	79	91
Drash syndrome	43	1	63	65	93
Oxalosis	43	1	58	81	74
Wegener's granulomatosis	42	1	40	79	93
Membranous nephropathy	36	1	61	56	97
Other systemic immunologic disease	30	0.4	13	53	93
Sickle cell nephropathy	14	0.2	57	0	71
Diabetic glomerulonephritis	8	0.1	25	38	62
Other	596	8	54	63	65
Unknown	466	6	51	31	30

Adapted from Seikaly M, Ho PL, Emmett L, et al. The 12th annual report of the North American Pediatric Renal Transplant Cooperative Study: renal transplantation from 1987 through 1998. *Pediatr Transplant* 2001;5:215–231.

were at higher risk for graft failure (27,28). In 1987, 25% of all pediatric transplantations were performed in children 0 to 5 years of age (29), whereas in 1995, the same age group accounted for 15%, and in 1995 the figure was 17% (24). Currently the proportion is 17% (13). Whether the decreased number of transplantations in this group is due to an awareness of the vulnerability of these children or to improvements in dialysis has not been established. It is important to note that excellent results have been obtained in very young patients at some centers (30,31). The concept that the immune response is heightened in young recipients is currently controversial (32–34). Thus, the unique problems associated with transplantation in young recipients may be related to infections, technical issues, and differences in immunosuppressive drug pharmacokinetics (14,35–38) rather than immune response. Reports of outstanding long-term graft survival rates in these young children seem to indicate that their specific problems can be overcome successfully (12).

Indications for Transplantation

Because of the shortage of donors for kidney transplantation, the evaluation of potential recipients and the indications for transplantation have been reviewed (39,40). Virtually all children reaching ESRD are considered to be candidates for renal transplantation. In some settings, the definition of ESRD is related to the need for chronic dialysis to sustain life. Currently in the United States, dialysis is rarely indicated in adults until the creatinine level has exceeded 8 mg/dL. The definition of dialysis dependency is inadequate in pediatrics, however, because a significant number of children receive a preemptive kidney transplant without ever having been on dialysis (41). In a review of

7053 primary kidney transplantations in children from 1987 through 2002, NAPRTCS noted that 1713 (24%) of the patients had never received maintenance dialysis (13). In the past, growth failure was considered one indication for transplantation, but the success of recombinant human growth hormone therapy in overcoming this complication of chronic renal insufficiency (CRI) in children (8,42) has virtually eliminated growth failure as an absolute indication. A very disturbing result from an analysis of UNOS data was that African Americans in the United States are less likely to be wait-listed for transplantation at any time after their first dialysis treatment than are whites (43). The point at which a child with CRI should be considered for renal transplantation remains controversial.

Preemptive Transplantation

Because preemptive transplantation is an important treatment modality for children, NAPRTCS conducted a special study to determine the frequency and outcome of this approach (41) and has updated it in the annual reports (13). From 1987 through 1992, 26% of the patients were registered as having had preemptive transplantation. The study compared data for those recipients who had been on maintenance dialysis and for patients who had had no previous dialysis. Of 2213 primary transplantations during that time period, 1150 grafts (52%) were from an LD source, whereas in the preemptive group 70% were recipients of an LD kidney. More recently, of 7053 primary transplantations, 1713 (24%) were preemptive. Preemptive transplantation was more common in those receiving LD grafts (33%) than in those given CAD grafts (13%), and was more common in males (27%) than in females (20%). The rate of preemptive transplantation varied among age groups and was 20%, 24%, 28%, 27%, and 20% for the 0- to 1-year, 2- to 5-year, 6- to 12-year, 13- to 17-year, and 18- to 20-year age groups, respectively. It also varied by race, with whites, African Americans, Hispanics, and "other" races showing rates of 30%, 14%, 16%, and 16%, respectively. As noted earlier, African Americans were also less likely than whites to be wait-listed after initiation of dialysis (43). One objection to preemptive transplantation has been that, if the patient did not undergo the rigors of prior dialysis, compliance with the immunosuppressive regimen might be poor. To determine whether this hypothesis was correct, graft survival was compared for the two groups and was determined not to be different at 1 or 4 years (41). When causes for graft loss were analyzed, the preemptive group did not have a higher incidence due to noncompliance. NAPRTCS also surveyed the motives for preemptive transplantation and determined that the primary reasons were parents' desire to avoid dialysis (34%) and the nephrologist's recommendation (18%). Desire for improved growth was considered a contributory factor for 50% of patients (41).

Contraindications to Transplantation

There are few absolute contraindications to transplantation. The concern of further immunosuppressing an already compromised host makes positivity for human immunodeficiency virus (HIV) in children a relative contraindication. Many children who develop HIV nephropathy succumb to the systemic ravages of the virus, either before or very shortly after reaching ESRD status (44). However, marked advances in the treatment of HIV-positive patients, especially treatment with protease inhibitors and other antiretroviral agents, makes consideration of kidney transplantation more likely (45,46). Ironically, initial results from a few centers suggest that HIV-positive patients with reasonable CD4 cell counts may have more problems with rejection than with infection after transplantation.

Another relative contraindication is a preexisting malignancy. The NAPRTCS dialysis registry contains 70 children with Wilms' tumor or Denys-Drash syndrome (47). Thirteen of these did not receive a transplant because of metastatic disease and all 13 died. The transplant registry lists 86 children who have these diagnoses and who have received a kidney transplant, and no recurrences of malignancy have been reported in any of them. The outcome of those who received transplants was similar to that in recipients without Wilms' tumor or Denys-Drash syndrome. Children with already existing metastatic disease are generally not considered transplant candidates, however. Also, children with devastating neurologic dysfunction may not be suitable transplant candidates, but the wishes of the parents, as well as the potential for long-term rehabilitation, must be considered in these circumstances. Potential for recurrence of the original renal disease is of major concern but generally has not precluded at least an initial transplant. Oxalosis, which once was considered an absolute contraindication due to a high incidence of recurrence, can be treated successfully with combined liver and kidney transplantation (48,49), although the complication rate remains high (31,50,51).

PRETRANSPLANTATION PREPARATION

Recipient Preparation

Before a child can undergo transplantation, the problems caused by CRI must be addressed and remedied if possible. In those cases in which ESRD is due to urologic abnormalities, corrective reconstructive surgery should be undertaken, especially to the lower urinary tract, before transplantation. Two of the major consequences of CRI are anemia and growth retardation, which should both be addressed before transplantation. A report of final height in pediatric renal transplant recipients suggests that the current improvement in final adult height after transplantation is related more to improvement of height deficits before transplantation than to any net gains achieved after transplantation (8,9). Uremia also leads to wasting and undernutrition in the child, and this can compromise the success of the procedure. For example, prophylactic native nephrectomy and reversal of protein wasting and malnutrition improve the outcome of transplantation in children with congenital nephrotic syndrome (52–54). Careful preparation is particularly important in children undergoing preemptive transplantation. Although there are descriptions of evaluation of the adult transplant recipient (39,40), there are no similar published reports for pediatric patients. Nonetheless, Table 73.3 details typical preparation used before surgery for pediatric recipients.

Urologic Evaluation

Children with the diagnoses described in Table 73.4 require a thorough urologic evaluation before transplantation. In the NAPRTCS report, 1878 of 7651 pediatric transplant recipients (25%) were identified as having lower urinary tract abnormalities (13). For all such patients, a history of voiding pattern before development of renal failure is most helpful. Preliminary investigations consist of measurement of urinary flow rate and ultrasonographic estimation of the postmicturition urine volume. Urinary flow rate should be at least 15 mL/sec (55), and the residual volume should be less than 30 mL. Further investigations would include urethrocystoscopy in patients suspected of a urethral stricture, and a voiding cystometrogram is essential for complete assessment of bladder function (56). This provides information about bladder capacity, pressure rise, and the efficiency of voiding. Still more information can be obtained by combining the urodynamic studies with radioisotope imaging. Routine voiding cystourethrography is not indicated in older patients without lower urinary tract symptoms (57).

A bladder with a very small capacity may not be adequate for a functioning transplant. Occasionally a small-capacity bladder may be seen in patients with prolonged oliguria or anuria. If the bladder is distensible and the bladder wall compliant, however, such a bladder may be used safely in kidney transplantation. Other criteria for a useable bladder are an end-filling pressure lower than 30 cm H_2O and a good flow rate. In patients with a poor flow rate, if urethral and bladder outlet obstruction are ruled out, the problem may be due to detrusor malfunction (55). When a bladder fails to empty completely, infection and obstruction are potential complications that may shorten graft survival. Intermittent, clean self-catheterization, which is widely used in urologic practice, can be safely used after transplantation in patients in whom the primary abnormality is inefficient, uncoordinated detrusor function.

Most pediatric patients have a urinary bladder that will adapt to the new kidney. Although the bladder may not appear to have the capacity, especially in patients on long-term dialysis before transplantation, it will most often distend with usage (48). However, in patients with a truly low capacity or high pressure, bladder augmentation may be necessary before transplantation (58–60). Augmentation cystoplasty consists of adding bowel or gastric wall to the bladder. In substitution cystoplasty, most of the bladder is excised and replaced with bowel. The use of gastric remnants for augmentation has been popular; however, such remnants do tend to cause excessive loss of acid in the urine, which leads to discomfort and metabolic alkalosis. Attempts to reconstruct bladders with bioengineered material are ongoing. There are promising reports of bioengineered bladder material, although these have not yet been tried in transplant recipients (61,62). In those patients in whom augmentation has been performed before transplantation, long-term antibiotic therapy and intermittent catheterization may have to be used to prevent urine stasis and infection. In a very small subset of patients whose bladder is

TABLE 73.3. STANDARD PREPARATION OF PEDIATRIC RENAL TRANSPLANT CANDIDATES

History and physical examination
Laboratory tests
- Hematology (CBC, platelets, differential)
- Coagulation (PT, PTT, TT)
- Chemistry (serum electrolytes, BUN, creatinine, liver function, lipid profile, Ca, PO_4, PTH)
- Urine volume, culture, and urinalysis
- Blood bank/immunology (ABO blood type, HLA type, histocompatibility testing, anti-HLA antibody screening, hepatitis profile, HIV screening)
- Virology (CMV, EBV, MMR titers)

Radiography (VCUG[a], CXR, bone age)
Consults
- Dentist
- Social worker
- Nutritionist

Vaccines
- DPT/polio, MMR, HIB, HBV
- *Pneumococcus*
- Varicella (Varivax)

PPD

BUN, blood urea nitrogen; CBC, complete blood count; CMV, cytomegalovirus; CXR, chest radiograph; DPT, diphtheria-pertussis-tetanus; EBV, Epstein-Barr virus; HBV, hepatitis B virus; HIB, *Haemophilus influenzae* type B; HIV, human immunodeficiency virus; HLA, human leukocyte antigen; MMR, measles-mumps-rubella; PPD, purified protein derivative (of tuberculin); PT, prothrombin time; PTH, parathyroid hormone; PTT, partial thromboplastin time; TT, thrombin time; VCUG, voiding cystourethrogram.
[a]For selected recipients.

TABLE 73.4. POSSIBLE LOWER URINARY TRACT ABNORMALITIES OF PEDIATRIC RENAL TRANSPLANT RECIPIENTS

Bladder exstrophy
Neuropathic bladder (meningomyelocele, spinal cord trauma, neurologic disease)
Posterior urethral valves
Prune-belly syndrome
Vesicoureteral reflux

unusable and in whom augmentation is unsuccessful, some form of urinary diversion may be necessary (48).

Pretransplantation Blood Transfusions

In the precyclosporine era blood transfusions were shown to have a beneficial effect on graft outcome (63), but their effect subsequently diminished (64) and they are currently rarely used. The early beneficial effect of pretransplant transfusions in children was similar to that seen in adults. In the past, donor-specific transfusions were also given to children. Early results from such studies suggested better graft survival; however, more prolonged follow-up with improved immunosuppression showed diminished benefit (65), and the use of donor-specific transfusions has now been largely abandoned in pediatric renal transplantation. However, two reports of the beneficial effects of deliberate pretransplant transfusions have renewed interest in their use (66,67). Because of the theoretical advantages of pretransplant tolerance induction by antigen presentation, their possible use remains intriguing (68).

The role of random pretransplantation transfusions in improving graft survival remains unclear. In 1992, NAPRTCS, in a study of 1667 transplants of which 57% were of CAD origin, did not observe any beneficial or detrimental effect of pretransplantation blood transfusions (29). Subsequently, however, a deleterious effect of pretransplantation transfusion became apparent. For LD source transplants, the use of five or more prior transfusions was associated with graft loss with a relative risk (RR) of 1.8 (22). By 1995, the use of prior transfusions was found to be a risk factor for CAD source transplants as well, and the use of five or more transfusions was associated with graft loss with an RR of 1.3 (3). The 1996 NAPRTCS report, which analyzed 4714 transplants, showed that the use of more than five transfusions was associated with graft loss with an RR of 1.7 for LD grafts and 1.3 for CAD grafts (24). An NAPRTCS special analysis indicated that multiple transfusions have a deleterious effect on graft survival, but fewer than five transfusions may be associated with a decreased incidence of acute rejection episodes (69). Sixty-five percent of pediatric LD renal transplant recipients and 56% of CAD recipients now receive no random transfusions before transplantation, and donor-specific transfusion is rarely performed (13). Pretransplantation blood transfusions would be of only historical interest except for a renewed interest related to tolerance induction and the reports mentioned earlier (66,67). Whether they will be used in the future for this indication is unknown.

Effect of the Age of the Cadaver Donor

For many years there was a tendency to use kidneys recovered from infants and young children for transplantation into young recipients (21). Early studies showed that 25% of all cadaver transplants used in children were recovered from children under 10 years of age (29). A special NAPRTCS study (70) demonstrated that the preferential placement of small kidneys into infants and very young children had disastrous consequences for graft survival, and this was subsequently confirmed by a larger study (71). As a result, CAD allocation policies for pediatric recipients were changed, which led to improved outcome (21). More recent information shows that this practice has now undergone substantial change (13). Since 1991, fewer than 1% of cadaver kidneys for pediatric recipients have come from donors younger than 2 years of age. During the same time, the percentage of kidneys recovered from donors over the age of 10 years increased from 78% to 88%. Importantly, the kidneys from young donors have not been discarded but have been used for transplantation into adult recipients via the en bloc technique (26,71,72). Single centers have reported better success with grafts from young donors, using carefully controlled protocols (25). Advanced donor age is also associated with diminished long-term graft survival (73,74), and likely should be avoided for young recipients (70,75,76).

HLA Matching Results in Children

For CAD transplants the NAPRTCS registry data indicate that a 2-DR mismatch graft has a relative hazard (RH) of first rejection of 1.27 and an RH of graft failure of 1.21 (p = .002) compared to a 0-DR mismatch (13). These outcomes are consistent with the relationship between histocompatability matching and graft outcome in adults (77,78). Unfortunately, because children have waiting-time preference in the CAD waiting list in the United States, HLA matching is poorer for them than for adults (12). Because most LDs of renal transplants for children are parents, these transplants are mismatched at one haplotype.

ABO Blood Type in Children

NAPRTCS has recorded 27 confirmed kidney transplants across ABO blood group compatibility barriers. Of these, most are O recipients of grafts from A donors. An NAPRTCS special study of 11 of these patients concluded that the procedure could be successful if performed under carefully controlled conditions (79). Evaluation of recipient isohemagglutinin levels may be helpful to identify suitable donor-recipient pairs. A more recent strategy for ABO mismatching entails "donor swaps," either with a complimentary donor-recipient pair or with a recipient on a CAD waiting list (80,81).

TRANSPLANTATION PROCEDURE

Technical Issues in Transplantation

The operative technique for transplantation differs depending on the weight of the child. For small children of less than 15 kg, the transplantation is frequently performed through a

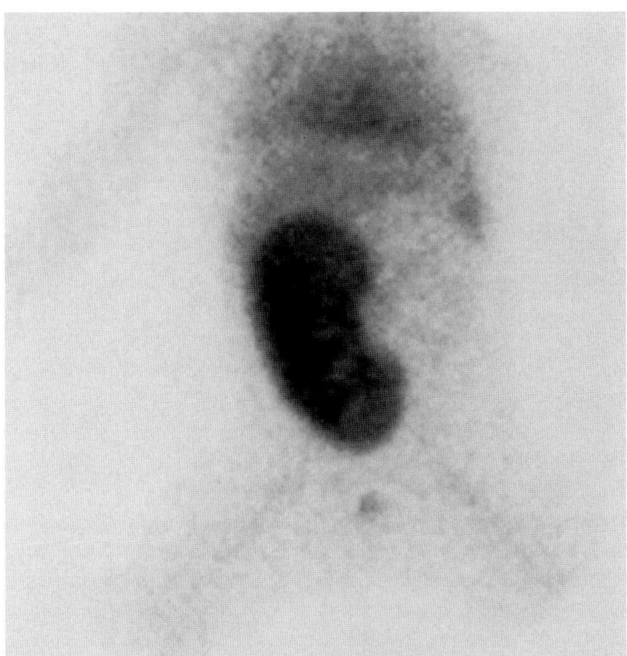

FIGURE 73.1. Technetium 99m–mercaptoacetyltriglycerine radionuclide renal scan for a 9-month-old infant who received a living-donor renal transplant from his father. The graft is intraperitoneal and occupies most of the right side of the peritoneal space. Note the relative sizes of the graft and the heart.

midline incision, and the larger vessels are used for anastomosis with the donor kidney (48). After reflection of the cecum and the right colon, the anterior wall of the aorta and the inferior vena cava are exposed and dissected (82). The aorta is mobilized from above the inferior mesenteric artery to the external iliac artery on the right side. After the lumbar branches are ligated and divided, the iliac arteries and the inferior mesenteric are encircled. Next the inferior vena cava is mobilized from the left renal vein to the iliac veins. After the lumbar veins are ligated, the iliac veins are encircled. The donor renal vein is anastomosed to the recipient vena cava using an end-to-side technique (83). The donor renal artery is then anastomosed to the recipient aorta in an end-to-side fashion. Careful attention must be paid to the recipient hemodynamic response on clamping and unclamping of the major vessels, and it is desirable to maintain a central venous pressure of 15 to 18 cm H_2O before unclamping (48,82). The filling of the transplanted kidney may be slow due to the fact that a large adult kidney takes up a significant portion of the normal pediatric blood volume. Hemodynamic studies suggest that the cardiac output of infants must double to perfuse the adult donor kidney adequately (84). Thus, volume replacement is critical (Fig. 73.1). The ureteral anastomosis is done by implanting the donor's ureter into the recipient's bladder using either a Leadbetter-Politano procedure or a modification of it. Many surgeons now prefer a nonrefluxing extravesical rather than transvesical approach for ureteroneocystostomy because it is faster, a separate cystotomy is not required, and less ureteral length is necessary, which thus assures adequate distal ureteral blood supply (85–87).

The transplantation technique used in children with a body weight greater than 15 kg is similar to that used in adults. Whereas the transperitoneal approach is necessary in younger children, in older children the procedure is extraperitoneal, with the renal vein anastomosed to the common iliac or the external iliac vein (82). The arterial anastomosis can be to either the common iliac or internal iliac artery. The ureterovesicular anastomosis is done using the techniques described earlier.

Evaluation of Graft Dysfunction

At the completion of the vascular anastomosis and release of the vascular clamps, immediate function of the transplanted kidney is demonstrated by the production of urine. Various causes may prevent initial function, however, and evaluation of immediate nonfunction and the differential diagnosis of this condition is a critical component of the transplant physician's role.

Acute Tubular Necrosis

Acute tubular necrosis (ATN) represents the most frequent cause of immediate graft nonfunction. Data from the NAPRTCS 1996 annual report showed that ATN was observed in 5% of LD and 19% of CAD transplants (24). Because the NAPRTCS definition for ATN is stringent, requiring dialysis in the first posttransplant week, these figures probably underrepresent the actual incidence of ATN. The risk of early ATN in LD kidneys is related to factors such as prior transplantations and use of more than five transfusions. Similarly, the risk factors of ATN in CAD kidneys include prolonged cold ischemia, absence of prophylactic antibody therapy, and the use of more than five blood transfusions. The diagnosis is confirmed in most cases by radionuclide scan (Fig. 73.2). If recovery of graft function is delayed, however, a transplant biopsy may be necessary, because other diagnostic tests cannot distinguish between ATN and rejection (88,89). Importantly, early acute rejection can mimic ATN or coexist with it. The presence of ATN does not auger well for the transplant, particularly those of cadaveric source, because graft failure and death are more common among patients with ATN (50). The NAPRTCS data showed that 71% of CAD grafts without ATN were functioning at 4 years compared to only 51% of those with ATN (90).

Graft Thrombosis

Graft thrombosis is an almost unique complication of pediatric transplantation. Although usually a major cause of immediate graft nonfunction, it can be seen later on in the course and has been recorded to occur as late as 15 days after transplantation after initial engraftment and function. Graft thrombosis has been the third most common cause of graft failure in pediatric renal transplantation (13), and the rate

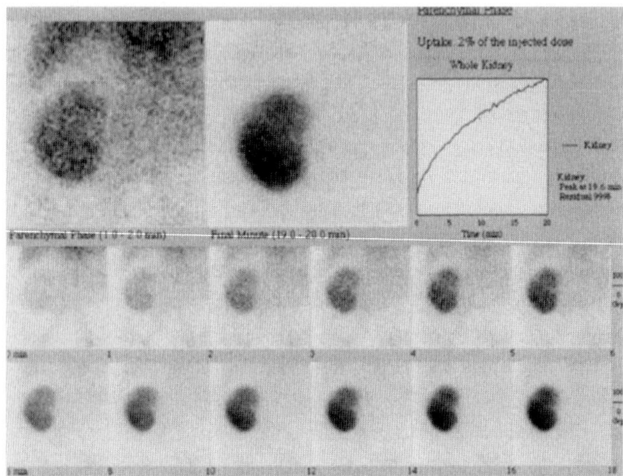

FIGURE 73.2. Technetium 99m–mercaptoacetyltriglycerine radionuclide renal scan of a cadaveric-donor renal transplant in a 15-year-old boy performed on the first postoperative day. The cold ischemia time exceeded 24 hours, and the recipient experienced oliguric acute tubular necrosis. Note the good perfusion, followed by little excretion and washout of the tracer from the graft.

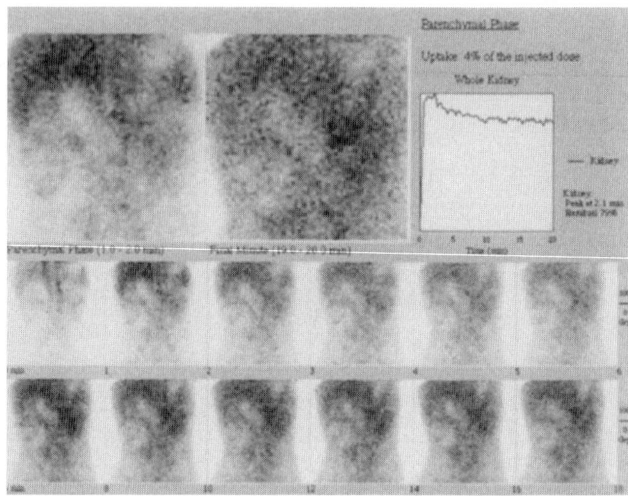

FIGURE 73.3. Technetium 99m–mercaptoacetyltriglycerine radionuclide renal scan for a 6-year-old girl with focal segmental glomerulosclerosis who received a living-donor renal transplant, taken 16 hours postoperatively. Note the photopenic area in the right abdomen, which indicates thrombosis of the graft with no perfusion.

may rise further if acute rejection rates continue to fall (91). The critical nature of this complication can be appreciated from the fact that it accounts for 11% of graft failures in index transplantations and 13% in repeat transplantations in the NAPRTCS registry. A dreaded event, this condition is irreversible in most cases and necessitates removal of the graft. Graft thrombosis should be suspected in cases in which there has been immediate function followed by the development of oliguria or anuria. The diagnosis is established by a radionuclide scan using diethylenetriaminepenta-acetic acid (DTPA) or mercaptoacetyltriglycerine (MAG-3) (92), which reveals a photopenic defect with no uptake by the transplanted kidney (Fig. 73.3).

Because the outcome of graft thrombosis is uniformly dismal, numerous studies have been conducted in an attempt to understand and anticipate this complication. The etiology of graft thrombosis is multifactorial, but it is more commonly seen in young recipients (93). In a special study of 2060 LD and 2334 CAD kidney transplants (94), NAPRTCS showed that a history of prior transplantation increases the risk, whereas increasing recipient age has a protective effect for LD kidneys. The prophylactic use of antilymphocyte antibody also decreases the risk, and this may be particularly true for the monoclonal interleukin-2 (IL-2) receptor antibodies (91). For CAD kidneys, a cold ischemia time longer than 24 hours increases the risk of thrombosis. The use of antibody induction therapy, the use of donors older than 5 years of age, and increasing recipient age were factors that decreased the risk of thrombosis. A heightened thrombotic state has also been implicated (92,95,96). One study showed that centers that performed fewer infant transplantations had higher rates of graft thrombosis (97), and another suggested that pretransplantation use of peritoneal dialysis increased the risk of thrombosis (98,99). Some centers routinely administer anticoagulants to pediatric recipients at high risk of graft thrombosis, but no clinical studies of their effectiveness have been performed and their use is not without complications (100). The incidence of graft thrombosis has not changed over the past 15 years (13); however, a preliminary report suggests that a new approach to induction therapy may have led to a decrease (91).

Obstruction and Urinary Leak

An uncommon but correctable cause of immediate graft dysfunction is obstruction of the urinary flow, which presents as decreasing urine output and the development of hydronephrosis. An ultrasonographic or radionuclide scan with a furosemide washout enables the clinician to establish this diagnosis. Obstruction can be due to kinking of the ureter, to edema or blockage of the implantation site of the ureter, or to development of a lymphocele. A more ominous cause of immediate nonfunction is the rare case of urinary leak due to disintegration of the distal ureter or rupture of the bladder. This condition is extremely painful due to the extravasation of urine into the pelvis or peritoneal cavity, and its presence is established by radionuclide scan (Fig. 73.4). The appearance of the tracer in the peritoneal cavity or in the scrotal, vulval, or inguinal area clinches the diagnosis. Immediate surgical correction is necessary.

Induction Therapy

T-Cell Antibodies

Prophylactic therapy with anti–T-cell antibody has been used for quite some time to improve graft survival (101). The

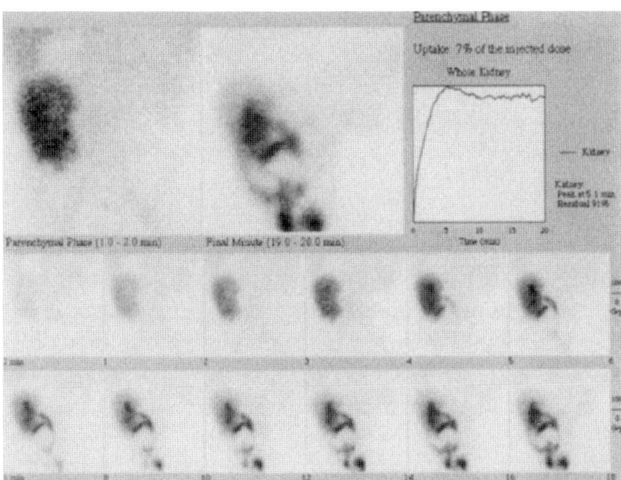

FIGURE 73.4. Technetium 99m–mercaptoacetyltriglycerine radionuclide renal scan for an 8-year-old girl who received a cadaveric renal transplant, taken 12 hours postoperatively. Note the good perfusion of the graft and the rapid concentration and excretion from the kidney. Tracer, however, rapidly accumulates in the right lower quadrant, outside of the bladder. Investigation demonstrated a traumatic bladder rupture.

rationale for this practice is to preempt the development of the first rejection, which is injurious to long-term graft survival. Retrospective data from NAPRTCS does show a beneficial effect. In a review of data for LD transplants, 5-year graft survival was 81% in 1041 patients who received T-cell antibody therapy compared to 75% in 1399 patients who did not receive this therapy. Similar figures for CAD kidneys were 66% in 1423 T-cell antibody–treated patients, compared to 56% in 1034 patients who did not receive T-cell antibody therapy (24). A major problem with these analyses is that several different types of T-cell antibodies were used. In the early years a polyclonal antibody was used, the most common form of which was prepared from horse serum and designated as MALG (Minnesota antilymphocyte globulin) (101). A monoclonal antibody directed at subsets of T-cells, called OKT3, was subsequently used (102).

Two polyclonal antibodies currently available are Atgam (Upjohn) and Thymoglobulin (Sangstat). Atgam, due to the sclerosing nature of the preparation, is given intravenously through a central catheter for 10 to 15 days. The dosage used is 15 mg/kg, and calcineurin inhibitors are generally withheld during the administration of the antibody. Thymoglobulin is provided through a peripheral vein at 1.5 to 2.0 mg/kg/dose. A report suggests daily monitoring of $CD3^+$ subsets to guide therapy: the daily dose is given only when the $CD3^+$ count exceeds 20 cells/mm^3 (103). Thymoglobulin therapy has been studied in small groups of pediatric renal transplant recipients and was found to be effective (104). Comparison in the efficacy of removal of circulating T cells suggested that Thymoglobulin may have some advantage over Atgam (105), but no comparisons of clinical outcomes have been performed. The monoclonal antibody OKT3 is administered as a bolus injection into a peripheral vein daily for 10 to 14 days at a dose of 5 mg for older children and 2.5 mg for children weighing less than 30 kg. Calcineurin inhibitors are also withheld during the use of OKT3. The major problems with these induction therapies include the "first-dose reaction" (106,107), neurologic difficulties (108), and the potential for the development of superimposed infections, such as cytomegalovirus (CMV) or Epstein-Barr virus (EBV) disease. Although retrospective analysis of pediatric kidney transplantation continues to show a clear benefit to the use of prophylactic induction antibody therapy (13), a prospective randomized trial of OKT3 induction showed no clear advantage (109). Currently, fewer than 10% of pediatric renal transplant recipients receive an anti–T-cell antibody for induction therapy (13).

Interleukin-2 Receptor Antibodies

There are two high-affinity chimeric or humanized antibodies that act on the inducible α-chain of the IL-2 receptor on the surface of the activated lymphocyte: basiliximab (Simulect, Novartis) and Daclizumab (Zenapax, Roche). Basiliximab is generally given as a two-dose regimen (generally 10 mg for children weighing less than 40 kg and 20 mg for those weighing more than 40 kg) on days 0 and 4 after transplantation (110). A pharmacologic study showed that basiliximab clearance in children is reduced by approximately half compared with that in adults and is independent of age, weight, or body surface area (111). One study has noted that pediatric recipients receiving basiliximab may have significantly elevated levels of cyclosporine and may require reduced dosages to avoid toxicity (112). Daclizumab is generally given in a dose of 1 mg/kg intravenously on the day of transplantation and every 14 days thereafter for a total of 5 doses (113). Higher doses may be required for saturation of IL-2 receptors in younger children (6). Both antibodies are generally well tolerated without substantial side effects. The use of both antibodies has been studied extensively in children and both have been shown to be safe and effective (6,110,112,114–116). The precise mechanism of action of the antibodies is not known but is presumed to be saturation of the IL-2 receptor and subsequent competitive antagonism of IL-2–dependent proliferation. A novel 6-month dosing schedule of Daclizumab has been reported as part of a steroid-avoidance pilot study program and appears to be well tolerated (6). There are no studies comparing the two antibodies. Up to 65% of pediatric renal transplant recipients are now receiving an IL-2 receptor antibody as induction therapy (13).

Other Induction Therapies

If T-cell antibody is not chosen for induction therapy, one of the calcineurin inhibitors may be used instead. Currently there are two such drugs, cyclosporine and tacrolimus, which have similar mechanisms but act at different sites to inhibit calcineurin. The major complication of this type of induction, particularly if it is given intravenously, is delayed graft function (117,118). The data in the twelfth annual NAPRTCS report show that approximately 35% of children receive no induction antibody therapy (13).

Maintenance Immunosuppression

Cyclosporine

Cyclosporine was first used in renal transplantation by Calne et al. in 1978 (119). The initial experience was followed by controlled trials in the United States, Canada, and Europe, all of which showed a significant improvement in graft survival over that with existing therapies. The drug was licensed in the United States in 1983 and has been used in all types of solid organ transplantation for over 20 years. There have been no controlled trials in children, but over the years of use a large body of information regarding its dosing and side effects has accumulated (13).

Induction Dosage

For induction purposes cyclosporine is given intravenously at a dosage of 165 mg/m^2 daily for children under 6 years of age and 4.5 mg/kg daily in children over 6 years. The dosage for younger children is calculated in square meter format because they metabolize the drug differently. The drug is preferably given in a continuous infusion over a 24-hour period starting intraoperatively. If practicality precludes a continuous infusion, the drug should be administered in three divided doses daily but over as long an interval as possible. If possible, induction therapy using intravenous cyclosporine should be continued for only 48 hours and then converted to oral cyclosporine therapy. The recommended starting oral dosage for children younger than 6 years of age is 500 mg/m^2 daily, administered in three divided doses; for children older than 6 years, it is 15 mg/kg daily, administered in two divided doses. These dosages are higher than those prescribed for adults because experience over the last 10 years has determined that the drug is metabolized more rapidly in children (120). A calcium-channel blocker is typically given with cyclosporine to reduce toxicity (121).

Maintenance Dosage

Because of the drug's irregular absorption and inherent nephrotoxicity, dosage adjustments of cyclosporine are constantly necessary (122). Data from NAPRTCS show that at 1 year after transplantation the mean cyclosporine dose can vary from 5.6 mg/kg to 8 mg/kg (24). It has also been demonstrated that higher maintenance dosages are associated with diminished chronic graft rejection (120). Among cadaveric kidney recipients the rate of rejection was 16% in those receiving doses higher than 8 mg/kg at 1 year after transplantation, compared with 24% in those receiving less than 6 mg/kg daily (123). The difficulty of maintaining constant dosing has led to several methods of measuring cyclosporine blood levels (118). Either high-pressure liquid chromatography or fluorescence polarization immunoassay techniques are used. Drug adequacy is considered to be a range of 100 to 200 ng/mL high-pressure liquid chromatography whole-blood trough level or 200 to 450 ng/mL radioimmunoassay whole-blood levels for patients more than 3 months after transplantation. Higher levels are necessary in the first 3 months. Newer data suggest that measuring the level 2 hours after the dose is received may allow more accurate dosing, assessment of the true area under the curve, and avoidance of toxicity (124–126).

Side Effects

Treatment with cyclosporine is associated with nephrotoxicity, hypertension, and hepatotoxicity. A major concern in children is hypertrichosis and facial dysmorphism (127). Hyperkalemia is common in patients taking cyclosporine (128) and also responds to dosage reduction. The mechanism is possibly related to diminished tubular excretion. Renal handling of uric acid is also altered, which leads to hyperuricemia (129). Hypomagnesemia is also observed as a result of altered tubular function (130). Tremors, convulsions, and paresthesias have been recorded in patients taking cyclosporine (131). These side effects may be multidrug induced rather than resulting from cyclosporine alone; however, they are often seen with high blood levels of the drug. Both hypertension and hyperlipidemia are observed in patients taking cyclosporine. A worrisome side effect in children is gingival hypertrophy (132), seen more often with higher dosages and in the presence of poor dental hygiene (133). NAPRTCS registry data published in 2001 showed that slightly fewer than 50% of renal transplant recipients were currently receiving cyclosporine as initial immunosuppression (13).

Tacrolimus

Tacrolimus (Prograf, Fujisawa) was introduced as an immunosuppressant for kidney transplantation in the mid-1990s (134–136). NAPRTCS data show that slightly fewer than 50% of children are being maintained on tacrolimus at 31 days after transplantation (13).

Dosage

One method of initiation of tacrolimus therapy is to provide 0.1 mg/kg/24 hr as a continuous infusion, with a switch to oral therapy within 2 to 3 days. However, because of the good absorption of the oral preparation and the concern about nephrotoxicity, many programs begin treatment by mouth or nasogastric tube very early posttransplantation. Initial oral dosages should not exceed 0.15 mg/kg twice daily and should be reduced to 0.1 mg/kg as a maintenance dose. Blood monitoring is necessary as with cyclosporine, and target whole-blood trough levels, measured by enzyme-linked immunosorbent assay, should be maintained between 5 and 20 ng/mL. Diarrhea, which is common, particularly in infants, may lead to increased tacrolimus levels (137).

Side Effects

Because tacrolimus has a similar mechanism of action, virtually all of the side effects of cyclosporine therapy are also seen with tacrolimus therapy (135). The nephrotoxic effect is similar (138). The hypertrichosis and dysmorphic features noted with cyclosporine are not seen with tacrolimus (139). Neurologic side effects are common and may be seen more frequently than with cyclosporine (140,141). A concern for the use of tacrolimus in pediatric renal transplantation was the development of posttransplantation diabetes mellitus, because in an early Japanese report one-third of patients developed hyperglycemia requiring insulin therapy (142). This has also been reported from other single centers (143,144). The mechanism may be related to a diminished insulin secretion in association with the insulin resistance associated with steroid use (145). The incidence of posttransplantation lymphoproliferative disorder (PTLD) was much higher with the use of tacrolimus than with the use of other immunosuppressants during early experience (136,146). However, a more recent retrospective analysis showed that the use of tacrolimus was not a risk factor for development of PTLD, likely due to the lower dosages currently used (147).

Choice of Calcineurin Inhibitor

Calcineurin inhibitors have been mainstays of immunosuppression in pediatric transplantation for the past decade and likely account for the continuing improvement in graft survival rates (12,148,149). The choice between drugs has often been based on a center preference. An open-label randomized trial of the two drugs with steroids and azathioprine was completed (150). Tacrolimus-treated patients had a lower rate of acute rejection (37%) than cyclosporine-treated patients (59%), although both rates were higher than current standards (13) and not all episodes were biopsy proven. One-year graft survival rates were similar, although the glomerular filtration rate was higher in the tacrolimus-treated group. Rates of hypomagnesemia, diarrhea, and posttransplantation diabetes mellitus were higher in the tacrolimus group, and rates of hypertrichosis and gum hyperplasia were higher in the cyclosporine group. In a retrospective analysis of NAPRTCS data on therapy with the two drugs given with mycophenolate mofetil (MMF) and steroids (139), there was no difference in early rejection rate (29%), risk of rejection, or risk of graft loss. At 2 years, graft survival was no different with the two agents (tacrolimus, 91%; cyclosporine, 95%). Tacrolimus-treated patients were less likely to require antihypertensive medication and had higher glomerular filtration rates at 2 years.

Azathioprine

For pediatric patients azathioprine is given at a dosage of 1 to 2 mg/kg/day. Patients taking higher dosages should be closely monitored for myelosuppression. In the early years of transplantation azathioprine was routinely used in all transplant recipients; when cyclosporine became available it was still widely used as an adjunct drug. In 1989 and 1990, 80% of pediatric patients in the NAPRTCS registry were receiving azathioprine, but as familiarity with MMF has increased, the use of azathioprine has diminished substantially, and it is currently given to fewer than 10% of patients (13).

Mycophenolate Mofetil

As of 1996, the NAPRTCS registry noted that only 6.5% of patients were being maintained on MMF (24), but the figures published in 2001 show that it is used in approximately two-thirds of pediatric kidney transplant recipients (13). Results concerning its advantages over azathioprine have been mixed (151–154). A well-controlled study, however, concluded that it was safe and effective for use in pediatric renal transplant recipients (155). A major difficulty in widespread use of the drug in children has been gastrointestinal disturbance, especially in young children (156). Both nausea and vomiting are common, but in some patients the drug has to be withdrawn due to intolerable diarrhea. An advantage of MMF over azathioprine is that the drug is less likely to induce leukopenia. The current recommended dosage of MMF for pediatric patients is 1200 mg/m^2/day, divided into two, three, or four doses (157). It is likely that therapeutic monitoring should be used, but clear standards are not yet available to guide treatment (158–163).

Corticosteroids

The NAPRTCS reports show that 96% of children with a functioning graft are maintained on prednisone (24). The numerous mechanisms of action of steroids lead to side effects and toxicities. The important concern in children is growth retardation. Studies have shown that dosages in excess of 8.5 mg/day impair normal growth (164). Other side effects include increased susceptibility to infection, impaired wound healing, aseptic necrosis of the bone, cataracts, glucose intolerance, hypertension, cushingoid facies, and acne (165). The preparations commonly used are prednisolone, its 11-keto metabolite prednisone, and methylprednisolone. Although the half-lives of these preparations are very short, they can be administered once daily because their effect on inhibition of lymphocyte production persists for 24 hours (166). The dosage is usually high in the period immediately after transplantation, approximately 2 mg/kg/day, with a gradual reduction to 0.2 to 0.3 mg/kg/day within a 6-month to 1-year period. Because of the multiple side effects of maintenance steroid therapy, attempts have been made to withdraw steroids altogether and have been reported in both adult and pediatric kidney transplantation cases (167). Unfortunately, the majority of these attempts have failed because of the development of acute rejection episodes (168–170). The use of alternate-day steroid therapy, which appears to reduce the growth-inhibiting effect without unduly increasing rejection episodes (171,172), seems reasonable, but only a minority of pediatric renal transplant recipients are receiving steroids in that manner (13). Several ongoing studies are investigating the use of steroid avoidance or steroid withdrawal protocols, and it is likely that steroids will not be used for immunosuppression in the future.

Rapamycin

Rapamycin (sirolimus; Rapamune, Wyeth) is the newest immunosuppressive agent used for kidney transplantation. It is the product of a fungus that was discovered on Easter Island (Rapa Nui) in 1969. It was first investigated for antifungal properties, and its immunosuppressant characteristics were first discovered in 1988. The agent was approved by the Food and Drug Administration in 1999. A similar compound that may be an analogue, SDZ-RAD, is currently undergoing clinical trials. Rapamycin is classified as a TOR inhibitor. TOR is a cytosolic enzyme that regulates differentiation and proliferation of lymphocytes. TOR is then activated as a result of the cascade of reactions in lymphocytes caused by the proliferation of cytokines and initiates production of messenger RNAs that trigger cell-cycle progression from G_1 to S phase. The TOR inhibitors bind to the immunophilin FKBP12 and inhibit the actions of TOR (173–178). TOR inhibitors may be particularly important in long-term immunosuppression because they stimulate T-cell apoptosis. TOR inhibitors also inhibit mesenchymal proliferation, which may prove to be important in graft vascular disease (179,180). Also, because the mechanism of action of rapamycin is different from that of other currently available immunosuppressants, it can be used in combination with all of them. Rapamycin has been found to be effective in combination with calcineurin inhibitors (181–185), in a calcineurin-inhibitor–sparing protocol (186), and in a steroid-free protocol (187). The role of rapamycin or SDZ-RAD therapy in pediatric transplantation is actively being studied (36,188,189).

Dosage

Rapamycin is available as an oral preparation, either as a solid or a liquid. Rapamycin was shown to have a prolonged half-life in adults that allowed once-daily dosing in adults (183–185). However, pharmacokinetic studies in children have demonstrated a much shorter half-life, as short as 12 hours (36,190). Thus, children may require twice-per-day schedules to maintain therapeutic levels. Retrospective analysis of early trials of rapamycin have suggested a relationship between blood levels and risk of rejection (191). Current suggestions for therapeutic levels remain speculative and range between 25 ng/mL in the early posttransplantation period without use of calcineurin inhibitors (36,186) to 5 to 10 ng/mL later in the course of transplantation.

Side Effects

The major side effects of rapamycin are hyperlipidemia, thrombocytopenia and leukopenia, and possibly delayed wound healing (183). The former complications can respond to the use of lipid-lowering drugs or dosage reduction. The latter complication may require suspension of the drug until the wound heals completely.

Maintenance Immunosuppression Combinations

Most pediatric renal transplant recipients are treated with triple immunosuppressive agents (13). When the number of drugs was limited, the number of possible combinations was small. However, there are at least 20 possible combinations of the six drugs now available, and when the induction antibodies are added, there are over 60 possible reported protocols (192). No "best" protocol for children has been established, although most clinical trials are currently directed at eliminating either steroids or calcineurin inhibitors or both. Currently most children are receiving prednisone, MMF, and cyclosporine or tacrolimus after kidney transplantation (13).

There are many possible targets for immunosuppression strategies for children (193). One promising new protocol of steroid avoidance has been reported (6). This approach consists of 6 months of administration of anti–IL-2 receptor antibody, tacrolimus, and MMF. Short-term patient and graft survival rates have been excellent, and growth rates have been very good. Major complications have included bone-marrow suppression and nephrotoxicity. Other protocols currently under investigation include calcineurin inhibitor avoidance or withdrawal and costimulation blockade with the eventual goal of avoiding both corticosteroids and calcineurin inhibitors.

ALLOGRAFT REJECTION

In the absence of tolerance the renal allograft is destined for loss by some form of rejection. Rejections are classified as hyperacute (occurring immediately on grafting), accelerated acute (occurring within the first week after transplantation), acute (generally occurring within the first year of transplantation), late acute (occurring after the first year), and chronic, for which the time sequence is difficult to establish because it may occur as early as 3 months but generally occurs years later in the course of the transplant.

Hyperacute Rejection

Hyperacute rejection is the result of specific recurrent anti-donor antibodies against HLA, ABO, or other antigens

(194). Irreversible rapid destruction of the graft occurs. Histologically there is glomerular thrombosis, fibrinoid necrosis, and polymorphonuclear leukocyte infiltration. In the early years of transplantation, when the HLA matching techniques were not well developed, hyperacute rejection was more common. In most centers, it occurs very rarely. The latest data from NAPRTCS show the incidence of hyperacute rejection to be less than 0.25% (17 cases) over the last 15 years (13). The only treatment is surgical removal of the allograft.

Acute Rejection

Information regarding the incidence and outcome of acute rejection in pediatric renal transplantation is available from the NAPRTCS data. Because NAPRTCS receives data from multiple sites that use many different diagnostic and treatment protocols, the definition of a rejection episode is based on the patient's having received antirejection therapy, although biopsy confirmation is becoming more common. In a review of 8777 rejection episodes over a 15-year study, there were, on average, 0.89 rejection episodes for each LD transplant and 1.23 for each CAD transplant. A remarkable decrease in the incidence of acute rejection has occurred since 1987 (Table 73.5). In a study of two cohorts of pediatric renal transplant recipients (1469 in 1987 to 1989; 1189 in 1997 to 1999), the rejection ratios dropped from 1.6 per patient to 0.7 per patient (195). Sixty percent of the latter group was rejection free compared to 29% of the former group, and 1-year graft survival was 94% compared to 80%. Historically, over half of patients experienced a rejection in the first weeks after transplantation; now the majority experience a rejection-free first year. Risk factors for CAD transplants include the absence of prophylactic T-cell antibody therapy, donor age younger than 5 years, black race, and no DR matches. Risk factors for LD source transplants are the absence of T-cell antibody, one or two DR mismatches, black race, and presence of ATN. In an earlier study NAPRTCS noted that, when data were reviewed by age groupings, rejection ratios, time to first rejection, and mean number of rejection episodes were no different across age groups; however, as the initial rejection episode, recipients younger than 6 years of age had significantly increased irreversible rejections leading to graft loss (23). Data are conflicting regarding whether infants and small children have a "heightened" immune response and an increased incidence of acute rejection episodes. Indirect evidence suggested a more vigorous immune response, especially in infants (27). Also, data from the UNOS registry demonstrated a higher rate of acute rejections in young children after both LD and CAD transplantation, although adolescents were noted to have a higher rate of late acute rejections (14). On the other hand, data from surveillance transplant biopsy specimens suggest equivalent rejection responses in all groups (33). Data from one large pediatric transplant program demonstrated that infants have a lower rate of acute rejection than older children (35). A report of the Scientific Registry of Transplant Recipients demonstrated that infants and young children now have the best outcomes of all age groups (12). Thus, either the proposed heightened immune response has been overcome by improved immunosuppression or the previously poor outcomes were related to other factors.

TABLE 73.5. TWELVE-MONTH PROBABILITY OF FIRST REJECTION BY TRANSPLANT YEAR

	Living donor		Cadaveric donor	
Transplant year	%	SE	%	SE
1987–1990	54.2	1.7	69.2	1.4
1991–1994	45.2	1.5	60.8	1.6
1995–1998	34.0	1.4	41.0	1.7
1999–2002	27.2	1.8	31.2	2.5

SE, standard error.
Adapted from Seikaly M, Ho PL, Emmett L, et al. The 12th annual report of the North American Pediatric Renal Transplant Cooperative Study: renal transplantation from 1987 through 1998. *Pediatr Transplant* 2001;5:215–231.

Diagnosis of Acute Rejection

Rejection is suspected when there is decreasing urinary outflow and a rising serum creatinine level. In the past, classical signs of acute rejection included fever and graft tenderness. With the use of calcineurin inhibitors and prophylactic antibody therapy, however, these signs are rarely seen; thus early evidence of graft dysfunction, even without other signs, should initiate concern. The differential diagnosis consists of ureteral obstruction, renal vascular compromise from stenosis, urinary leak, and an infectious process. When rejection is suspected, a urinalysis and urine culture should be performed to assess the possibility of infection. The urinalysis is also helpful if it suggests intragraft inflammation or immune response as evidenced by proteinuria and the presence of leukocytes and other cells in the sediment. Blood or urinary cytokine analysis may also be useful for diagnosing rejection (196,197), and examination of the sediment may be useful in detecting other reasons for graft dysfunction. Ultrasonography is performed to rule out anatomical obstruction. Obstruction can be the result of perirenal fluid collection, a large lymphocele, hematoma, or, rarely, an abscess. The ultrasonographic scan can also provide information about intragraft blood flow and pressure (88). A radionuclide renal scan using a tracer such as MAG-3 is a very helpful tool in establishing some diagnoses (Figs. 73.2 to 73.4) (198). Rejection is suggested by rapid uptake of the tracer by the kidney but a delayed excretion. Unfortunately, radionuclide scans cannot distinguish among various causes of intragraft dysfunction, such as rejection, cyclosporine toxicity, and ATN.

Thus, a definitive diagnosis of rejection requires a transplant biopsy.

Renal Transplant Biopsy

The renal transplant biopsy procedure is very easy and safe when conscious sedation and ultrasonographic guidance are used. Data evaluating over 150 pediatric renal transplant biopsy specimens, including some in intraperitoneal kidneys and many performed during the first week after transplantation, have demonstrated a very low risk (89). A major factor in reducing postbiopsy bleeding is the use of an automated biopsy "gun" with a small (18-gauge) needle rather than the standard (15-gauge) needle.

A good biopsy core includes glomeruli, tubules, interstitial tissue, and vessels. Obtaining such a sample is facilitated if a dissecting microscope is used at the time of the procedure to identify glomeruli and tubules in the specimen. In acute rejection glomerular changes are restricted to increased prominence of the mesangial stalk. However, it is the presence of tubular changes that is significant in early acute rejection, and tubulitis is considered the hallmark. Semiquantitative analysis and grading of acute rejection biopsy findings is done using the Banff criteria (199). Grade I is the presence of focal interstitial lymphocytic infiltrate with mild tubulitis and normal vessels. In Grade II there is extensive interstitial infiltrate with tubulitis and vacuolation in arterial vessels, whereas Grade III shows extensive interstitial infiltration with tubulitis and lymphocytic infiltration of arterial walls with occasional fibrinoid change.

Treatment of Acute Rejection

Standard treatment for an episode of acute rejection is intravenous methylprednisolone in a single daily dose of 20 to 25 mg/kg (maximum dose: 0.5 to 1.0 g) for 3 consecutive days. Most grade I and grade II rejections respond to steroid therapy. Steroid-resistant rejection episodes are treated with T-cell antibody, either the monoclonal OKT3 or the polyclonal antithymocyte globulin (Atgam or Thymoglobulin). OKT3 is administered in a dose of 2.5 mg for children with a body weight of 30 kg and 5 mg for children over 30 kg for 10 to 14 days. Atgam is given in a dose of 15 mg/kg through a central venous catheter for 10 to 14 days, depending on the white cell and platelet counts, as it frequently depletes all formed elements in the blood system. It is advisable to maintain the white cell count above 2000/mm^3 and the platelet count above 20,000/mm^3. Thymoglobulin is given in a dose of 1.5 to 2.0 mg/kg for a total of 10 to 14 days. It may be advisable to monitor levels of CD3$^+$ cells during treatment and to restrict dosing only to days when the count is higher than 20 cells/mm^3 (103). All antibody therapies have several side effects. Of concern are the first-dose symptoms of OKT3 due to cytokine release (106,107). These are clinically observed as fever with chills and, rarely, as pulmonary edema. Defervescents, such as acetaminophen, should be given every 4 hours, and the administration of the antibody should be preceded by a bolus dose of 500 mg of methylprednisolone 1 hour before administration. Respiratory compromise, in the form of extravasation of fluid into the pulmonary capillary bed, is seen only in patients with fluid overload. Dialytic fluid removal should be considered before the administration of OKT3 in patients whose body weight exceeds 5% of their baseline. Precaution against a potential anaphylactic reaction to polyclonal antibodies consists of administration of 500 mg of methylprednisolone with the infusion of the antibody and administration of an antihistamine, such as diphenhydramine (Benadryl), one-half hour before drug administration.

Reversibility of Acute Rejection

NAPRTCS data demonstrate that among LD kidneys 55% of rejection episodes are completely reversed, 40% are partially reversed, and 5% end in graft failure. Similar figures for CAD kidneys are 48%, 45%, and 7%, respectively (24). When data are stratified by age, young transplant recipients are found to more frequently experience irreversible rejection episodes. Ten percent of acute rejections among infants receiving an LD kidney end in graft failure, compared to 4% for older children. For CAD kidneys the rate of graft failure in infants is 15%, compared to 7% for older children. Not only is rejection frequency decreasing, but complete rejection reversal in pediatric LD recipients seems to be increasing in more recent age cohorts (13). Molecular or genomic characterization of rejection biopsy specimens may be helpful in describing different types of acute rejection (196,197,200–202).

Rescue Therapy

In those patients in whom neither steroids nor antibody therapy successfully reverses a rejection episode, conversion to an alternative calcineurin inhibitor or to other immunosuppressants appears to be warranted. There have been no controlled studies to document reversal of rejection with conversion to tacrolimus; however, anecdotal reports do suggest that in some cases conversion helps stabilize graft function (135,136,170).

Chronic Rejection

The gradation from acute to chronic rejection is gradual; however, many biopsy specimens show features of both, and some characteristic vascular changes of chronic rejection may be seen as early as 10 days after transplantation (203). The clinical picture is that of gradually declining renal function together with varying degrees of proteinuria and hypertension. An ongoing controversy exists as to whether the changes seen in chronic rejection are immune mediated, ischemic in nature, or nonimmunologic injury due to hyperfiltration (204,205). Data for children have shown clearly that acute rejection is a predictor of chronic rejection (148). In a study of 1699 patients receiving LD grafts and 1795 receiving CAD grafts, NAPRTCS noted that acute rejection was an RR factor for chronic rejection (RR = 3.1), and multiple acute rejections increased the RR to 4.3. Late acute rejections are also clinical correlates of chronic rejection (206). Even if acute rejection is the most critical element in the genesis of chronic rejection, other immune mechanisms may mediate its progression. One possible explantation would be that, in patients who go on to develop chronic rejection, the immune mediators of acute rejection, such as granzyme B, perforin, and Fas ligand, are expressed in a more robust fashion and the responses are quantitatively different from the responses of an acute rejection that does not lead to chronic rejection. Alternatively, the immune mediators of chronic rejection may be qualitatively different from those associated with an acute episode. For example, the multifunctional cytokine transforming growth factor β1, which has fibrogenic properties, is present in biopsy tissue of patients with chronic rejection (207). Identification of the mechanism of initiation or progression of chronic rejection is vital to any attempts to control it.

Treatment of symptoms is currently the only available method of dealing with chronic rejection. Hypertension should be controlled, and the proteinuria may occasionally respond to angiotensin-converting enzyme inhibitors; however renal function will continue to decline. In children, chronic rejection produces an additional burden, because decreased renal function results in deceleration of growth (208,209). It is in this context that prevention of chronic rejection by early aggressive therapy in patients who have had an episode of acute rejection may be rewarding. Because currently available immunosuppressive medications have been unsuccessful in preventing or slowing the progression of chronic rejection, the use of immunosuppressive agents other than those currently approved may be reasonable.

GRAFT SURVIVAL

Pediatric renal centers reporting graft survival show varying results. Because the number of patients at any one center is small, such data cannot represent the pediatric transplant population at large. Furthermore, multiple factors affect graft survival, such as donor and recipient age, histocompatibility matching, recipient race, and so forth. Thus, graft survival rates cannot be described accurately without classification of the important variables. To obtain a proper population mix representing gender, age, and racial diversity, the NAPRTCS annual reports have been used (13).

A total of 2201 graft failures occurred in 8399 transplantations (26%). Of index transplantations, 1924 of 7651 (23%) failed, whereas 277 of 748 subsequent transplantations (37%) experienced graft failure. Among patients whose grafts failed, 1648 (75%) were returned to dialysis and 132 (6%) underwent retransplantation at the time of failure. Table 73.6 provides the distribution of

TABLE 73.6. CAUSES OF GRAFT FAILURE

	Index graft failures		Subsequent graft failures		All graft failures	
	N	%	N	%	N	%
Total	1924	100	227	100	2201	100
Death with functioning graft	183	9.5	21	7.6	204	9.3
Primary nonfunction	48	2.5	4	1.4	52	2.4
Vascular thrombosis	206	11.0	36	13.0	242	11.0
Other technical problems	29	1.5	4	1.4	33	1.5
Hyperacute rejection, less than 24 h	13	0.7	4	1.4	17	0.8
Accelerated acute rejection, 2–7 d	32	1.7	8	2.9	40	1.8
Acute rejection	267	14.0	36	13.0	303	14.0
Chronic rejection	628	33.0	93	34.0	721	33.0
Recurrence of original disease	121	6.3	25	9.0	146	6.6
Renal artery stenosis	15	0.8	—	—	15	0.7
Bacterial or viral infection	39	2.0	40	1.4	43	2.0
Cyclosporine toxicity	10	0.5	—	—	10	0.5
De novo disease	6	0.3	2	0.7	8	0.4
Patient discontinuation of medication	93	4.8	8	2.9	101	4.6
Malignancy	27	1.4	101	4.6	28	1.3
Other or unknown	99	5.1	16	5.8	115	5.2

Adapted from Seikaly M, Ho PL, Emmett L, et al. The 12th annual report of the North American Pediatric Renal Transplant Cooperative Study: renal transplantation from 1987 through 1998. *Pediatr Transplant* 2001;5:215–231.

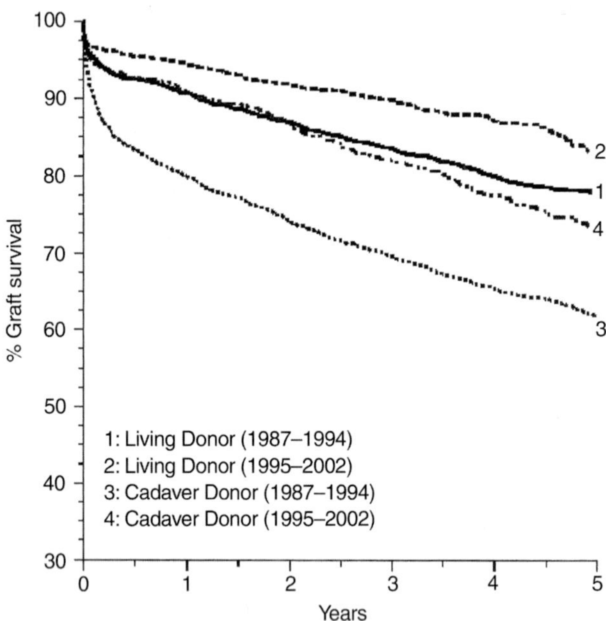

FIGURE 73.5. Five-year actuarial graft survival in children receiving transplants from living and cadaveric donors. (Adapted from Seikaly M, Ho PL, Emmett L, et al. The 12th annual report of the North American Pediatric Renal Transplant Cooperative Study: renal transplantation from 1987 through 1998. *Pediatr Transplant* 2001;5:215–231.)

causes of graft failure. With increased length of follow-up, chronic rejection continues to increase in importance. It is now the most common cause of graft failure. Overall, 47% of graft failures are caused by rejection, with chronic rejection accounting for 33% and acute rejection accounting for 14%. Recurrence of original disease as a cause of graft failure was observed 146 times (FSGS, 66; membranoproliferative glomerulonephritis type 2, 13; oxalosis, 10; hemolytic uremic syndrome, 16; chronic glomerulonephritis, 6; other disorders, 35). Vascular thrombosis remains a major cause of failure, and 327 graft failures were attributed to primary nonfunction, vascular thrombosis, or miscellaneous technical causes. These data show that such problems occur in 3.8% of pediatric transplantations (93–95,97–99,210).

Overall 5-year graft survival curves by donor source are shown in Figure 73.5. Current graft survival rates for index transplants at 1, 3, and 5 years are 95%, 90%, and 83%, respectively, for LD kidneys and 91%, 82%, and 73%, respectively, for CAD kidneys. These values are substantially better than previous results (Table 73.7). Table 73.8 shows RHs for graft failure associated with selected transplant characteristics for both LD and CAD kidneys. Five-year graft survival rates by selected variables for LD grafts are shown in Figure 73.6 and for CAD grafts are shown in Figure 73.7. An important trend toward improved graft survival in pediatric LD and CAD renal transplantation has been reported (12,123), and data published in 2001 and 2003 are shown in Figures 73.8 and 73.9.

TABLE 73.7. PERCENTAGE GRAFT SURVIVAL BY SOURCE AND EUROPEAN RENAL ASSOCIATION

	Years after transplantation		
	1 (%)	3 (%)	5 (%)
Living donor			
1995–2001	94.5	90.0	83.1
1987–1994	90.1	83.5	77.8
Cadaveric donor			
1995–2001	90.8	81.9	73.4
1987–1994	79.9	69.6	61.8

Adapted from Seikaly M, Ho PL, Emmett L, et al. The 12th annual report of the North American Pediatric Renal Transplant Cooperative Study: renal transplantation from 1987 through 1998. *Pediatr Transplant* 2001;5:215–231.

Registry-based graft survival data can be used to establish risk factors. RRs of graft failure are derived using Cox proportional hazards regression models. For LD kidneys the risk factors for graft failure include black race (RH = 1.88), receipt of more than five prior transfusions (RH = 1.41), and absence of HLA-B matches (RH = 1.39) (Table 73.8). Lack of receipt of induction antibody therapy is also a risk factor (RH = 1.13) as is transplant era (RH = 0.95) (13). A similar risk factor analysis for CAD kidneys has been reported (13,24,211), and data from the twelfth annual report of NAPRTCS are presented in Table 73.8. The risk factors are similar to those seen with LD grafts, with additional hazards such as young age of recipient (RH = 1.80), young age of donor, and prolonged cold ischemia time (RH = 1.20). Some factors that increase the RR of cadaveric graft failure in children, such as recipient age, are

TABLE 73.8. RELATIVE HAZARD (RH) ANALYSIS FOR GRAFT FAILURE IN MULTIVARIATE PROPORTIONAL HAZARDS MODEL

	Living donor		Cadaveric donor	
	RH	*p* Value	RH	*p* Value
Young recipient age (<2 years)	1.02	NS	1.80	<.0001
Prior transplant	1.30	NS	1.41	<.0001
No induction antibody therapy	1.13	.0090	1.14	.0430
More than five transfusions in lifetime	1.41	.0003	1.32	<.0001
No HLA-B matches	1.39	.0180	1.19	.0067
No HLA-DR matches	1.09	NS	1.21	.0022
Black race	1.88	<.0001	1.55	<.0001
Prior dialysis	1.20	.0240	1.29	.0130
Graft cold storage time >24 h	—	—	1.20	.0060
Transplant year	0.95	<.0001	0.93	<.0001

Adapted from Seikaly M, Ho PL, Emmett L, et al. The 12th annual report of the North American Pediatric Renal Transplant Cooperative Study: renal transplantation from 1987 through 1998. *Pediatr Transplant* 2001;5:215–231.

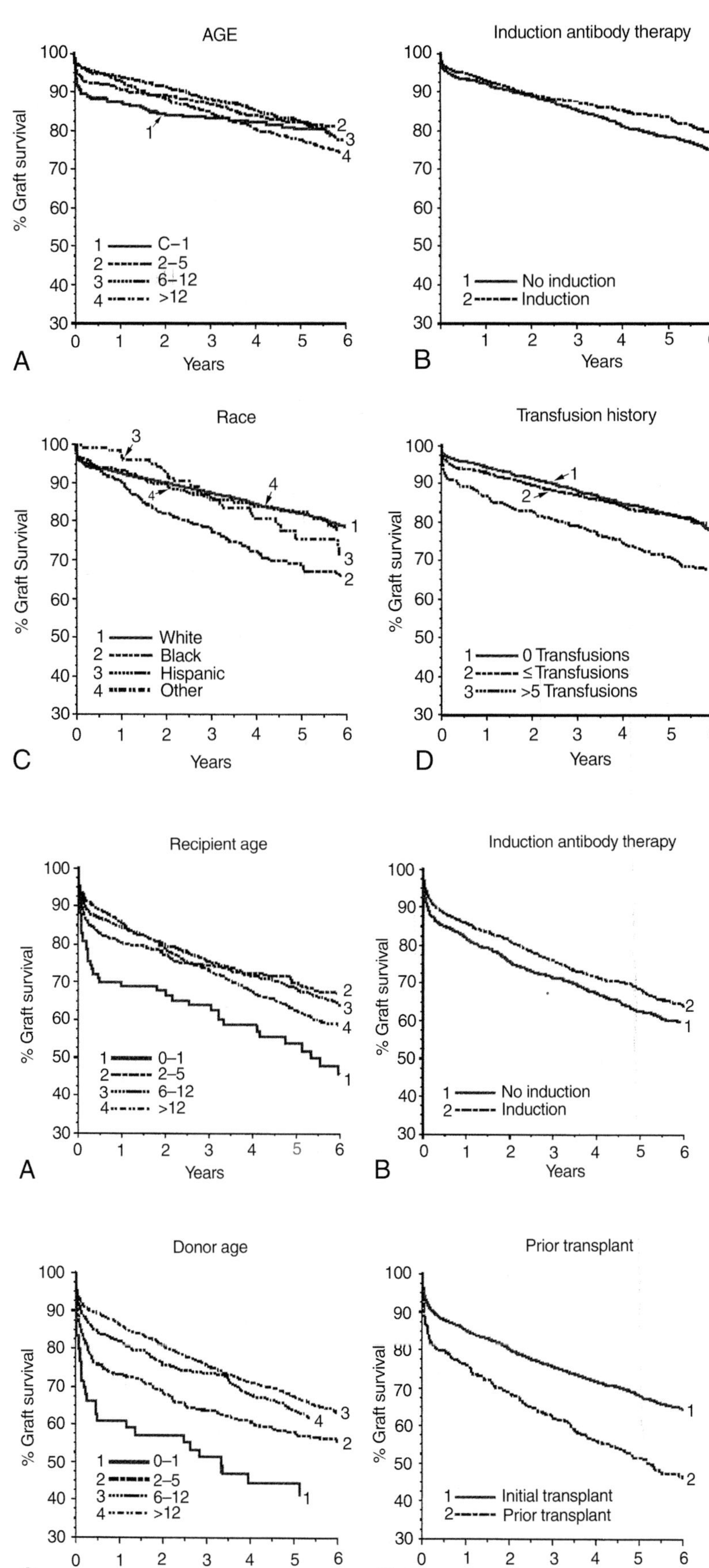

FIGURE 73.6. Five-year actuarial graft survival after living-donor renal transplantation in children by recipient age **(A)**, use of antibody induction therapy **(B)**, race **(C)**, and number of pretransplantation blood transfusions **(D)**. (Adapted from Seikaly M, Ho PL, Emmett L, et al. The 12th annual report of the North American Pediatric Renal Transplant Cooperative Study: renal transplantation from 1987 through 1998. *Pediatr Transplant* 2001;5:215–231.)

FIGURE 73.7. Five-year actuarial graft survival after cadaveric-donor renal transplantation in children by recipient age **(A)**, use of antibody induction therapy **(B)**, donor age **(C)**, and prior transplant history **(D)**. (Adapted from Seikaly M, Ho PL, Emmett L, et al. The 12th annual report of the North American Pediatric Renal Transplant Cooperative Study: renal transplantation from 1987 through 1998. *Pediatr Transplant* 2001;5:215–231.)

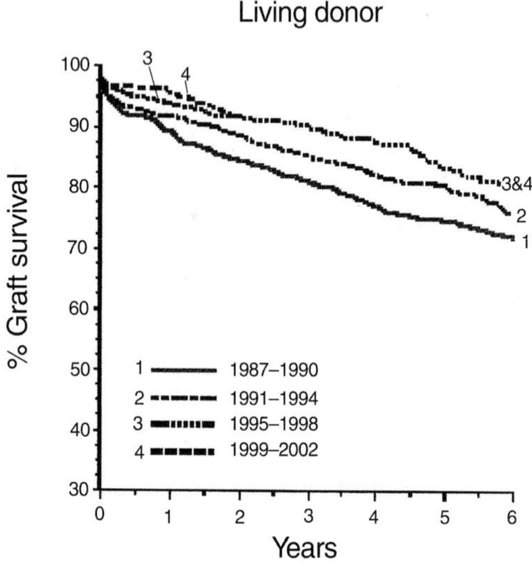

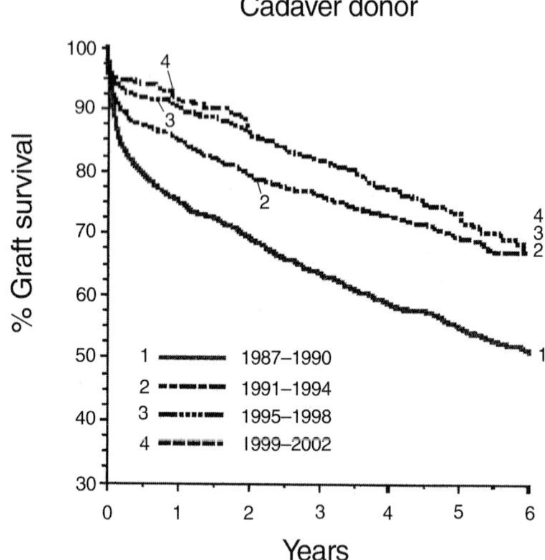

FIGURE 73.8. Actuarial survival of grafts from living and cadaveric donors by year of renal transplantation. (Adapted from Seikaly M, Ho PL, Emmett L, et al. The 12th annual report of the North American Pediatric Renal Transplant Cooperative Study: renal transplantation from 1987 through 1998. *Pediatr Transplant* 2001;5:215–231.)

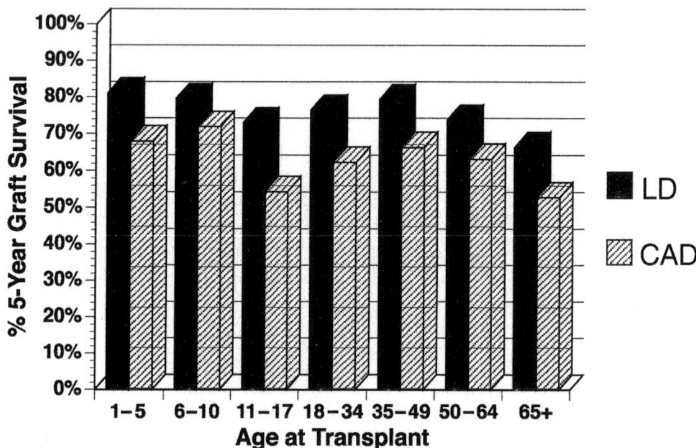

FIGURE 73.9. Five-year actuarial survival of living-donor (LD) and cadaveric (CAD) grafts in children and adults undergoing renal transplantation by recipient age. Young children currently have the best long-term outcomes of all age groups. [Adapted from Colombani PM, Dunn SP, Harmon WE, et al. Pediatric transplantation. *Am J Transplant* 2003;3(Suppl 4):53–63.]

integral to pediatrics. Other factors, such as recipient race, the degree of HLA matching, and prior transplantation, cannot be easily altered. Improvement in cadaveric allograft survival rates can be achieved, however, by judicious choice of donors, appropriate pretransplantation management, changes of induction therapy, and optimization of immunosuppressive therapy (23).

Another measure of long-term graft function is the calculation of graft half-life. An analysis of 8922 pediatric and 78,418 adult renal transplant cases demonstrated superior long-term graft function in young pediatric recipients (14). Infants (aged 0 to 2 years) had worse 1-year graft survival rates (71%) than children 3 to 12 years (83%), adolescents 13 to 21 years (85%), and adults (86%). However, among all grafts that survived at least 1 year, those in infants had the longest projected half-life (18 years), exceeding that of grafts in children (11 years), adolescents (7 years), and adults (11 years). A similar analysis of UNOS data showed that grafts in young recipients who received adult donor kidneys and had immediate graft function had projected half-lives of longer than 25 years, even better than that in adult recipients of grafts from HLA-identical adult donors (212).

The primary disease causing ESRD can have an effect on graft survival. Children with oxalosis used to have poor outcomes, so that this diagnosis was considered a contraindication to transplantation. However, improvements in outcome related to combined liver-kidney transplantation have been encouraging (31,49–51). Similarly, infants with congenital nephrotic syndrome often had very poor outcomes (50,213), but strategies designed to reduce the risk of thrombosis and improve nutrition before transplantation have led to marked improvements (52–54,96). FSGS can be a devastating disease that recurs very quickly after renal transplantation, sometimes as early as the first day after transplantation (213–217). Although recurrence is no more frequent in LD transplants than in CAD transplants, the graft survival advantage of LD transplantation is lost for children with FSGS (218). Little is known about the pathophysiology of the disorder or the cause of recurrence (219,220). There are several proposed approaches to preventing or treating recurrence, most involving enhanced immunosuppression with plasmapheresis (217,221–226). Lupus nephritis surprisingly does not recur after renal transplantation to any great extent. Patients with lupus have outcomes similar to those of other patients (227,228), except for a slight increase in mortality (228), an increase in incidence of recurrent rejections, and a slight tendency to graft failure in those patients receiving CAD grafts after peritoneal dialysis (227). Children with sickle cell disease and ESRD can receive kidney transplants successfully

(229), as can those with Down syndrome (230,231). Hemolytic uremic syndrome has been variably described as likely to recur or not (213,232). When the etiologic factors are distinguished, data show that epidemic shiga toxin–associated hemolytic syndrome is unlikely to recur after renal transplantation (233,234), whereas atypical or familial hemolytic uremic syndrome may recur with devastating and irreversible consequences (234).

GROWTH AFTER TRANSPLANTATION

A major feature distinguishing pediatric from adult recipients is the need for statural growth and maturation. The growth failure commonly observed in children at the time of transplantation is multifactorial; however, the most important cause is the reduced response to endogenous growth hormone (42), which is related to several mechanisms. Growth failure often begins insidiously early in the course of CRI. In an NAPRTCS analysis of data for 1768 children with CRI (glomerular filtration rate less than 75 mL/min/m^2), over one-third had a height deficit of more than 2 standard deviation scores. It has been amply demonstrated that CRI beginning in infancy leads to permanent reduction in growth potential (235). Growth retardation continues in children who are on a dialysis regime, whether the mode of dialysis is peritoneal dialysis or hemodialysis. For several years it has been suggested that a functioning transplant would enable the child to achieve catchup growth (7). Unfortunately, long-term data from registry studies have revealed a more disappointing outcome.

NAPRTCS data show that the mean height deficit at the time of transplantation is –1.88. Males (–1.92) and younger recipients have greater height deficits at the time of transplantation (13). Younger children can show catchup growth (7) with complete inversion of Z-score up to 0.60 at 2 years in those younger than 5 years of age at the time of transplantation. Older children may grow at a normal rate but rarely show catchup growth. The Z-score for 19-year-olds is –1.5. Final adult height for children with ESRD is improving, but all of the improvements seem to be related to the gains achieved during treatment for CRI rather than after transplantation (8).

These studies on long-term growth after transplantation are disappointing; however, they do focus on mechanisms that prevent growth despite a milieu with normal renal function. Studies at individual centers have adopted a variety of techniques, such as discontinuation of prednisone (236,237), alternate-day steroid therapy (171,172,238), steroid avoidance (6), or the use of recombinant human growth hormone (239). It has been known for several years that use of steroids for immunosuppression inhibits growth (167). It has also been demonstrated that steroids affect growth hormone secretion (208,240–242). Measurements of pulsatile and pharmacologically stimulated hormone release reveal that steroids play an inhibitory role (167,243). Conversion of children to alternate-day steroid therapy has resulted in improvement in growth (171,172); however, the best catchup growth is seen in patients from whom steroids are completely withdrawn (6,136,168). Numerous uncontrolled studies have shown that steroids can be withdrawn from children after transplantation (6,136,244); however, acute rejection tends to occur shortly afterward in many of these patients (169), with marked detrimental long-term effects. An alternative method of attaining catchup growth after transplantation is the use of growth hormone. Recombinant human growth hormone is not approved for use in children after transplantation; however, numerous uncontrolled studies have shown its ability to accelerate growth in this setting (245). Several possible complications of the use of recombinant human growth hormone after transplantation have been identified (245–248), but a controlled trial demonstrated that it could be used safely and effectively (249).

MORBIDITY

Hospitalization

The median duration of hospitalization at the time of transplantation cited in the twelfth annual NAPRTCS report was 13 days, with longer stays required for young patients and for recipients of CAD transplants (13). The mean hospital stay fell by approximately 8 days between 1987 and 2001. Most children require rehospitalization at least once after the initial discharge after renal transplantation. Fifty percent of LD graft recipients and 62% of CAD graft recipients are hospitalized during the first 6 months after transplantation. The hospitalization rate falls with increasing time after transplantation, but 16% require at least one hospital stay in the fourth posttransplant year (24). The most common reason for hospitalization used to be for treatment of rejection. However, an analysis of recent data indicates that treatment of viral and bacterial infections is now the most common reason for hospitalization (250). The most common bacterial infection in children 5 years of age or younger is *Clostridium difficile* diarrhea; in those older than 5 years, it is urinary tract infection (UTI) (35). CMV infection appears to be the most common viral infection in older children. Treatment for hypertension is the cause for hospitalization in 5 to 8% of recipients in the first 6 months after transplantation; the rate falls to approximately 1% 5 years after transplantation (24).

Posttransplantation Lymphoproliferative Disease and Malignancy

Although PTLD has been reported as a complication of pediatric organ transplantation for many years (251), the number of published reports seems to be increasing (252).

It is not clear whether this indicates that the incidence of this potentially lethal complication of immunosuppression is increasing or that it is just more readily recognized. If the incidence is increasing, it may be the unfortunate consequence of "improved" immunosuppression (146). A review of UNOS data indicates that the incidence of PTLD after pediatric renal transplantation is clearly increasing, and age younger than 18 years, white race, and male gender are significant risk factors (253). The current incidence of PTLD is 1 to 2% of all pediatric renal transplant patients.

PTLD often presents within lymph nodes, but it can be extranodal, frequently occurring within the gastrointestinal tract (254), proximate to or within the graft (255), or distant from it (256). Presentation of PTLD within the central nervous system is often devastating and rapidly fatal. PTLD is generally thought to emanate from an EBV infection (254,257,258). Thus, the pretransplantation EBV status of the donor and recipient may be an important determinant of the disease and may explain why the disease is more common in children than in adults (259,260). In several reports, the incidence rate of PTLD for EBV-seronegative recipients was many times higher than that for EBV-seropositive recipients (261,262), and in others, the source was the donor in most of the cases (263). Concomitant primary infection with CMV may increase the risk of PTLD fivefold (261). The intensity of immunosuppression may also predispose the child to PTLD (264). Treatment with antilymphocyte antibodies, such as OKT3, as either induction or antirejection therapy, may increase the risk of developing PTLD substantially (261,262,265). Although PTLD has been reported after both cyclosporine and tacrolimus treatment, the experience of programs that have used both drugs has suggested that the incidence is higher in tacrolimus-treated recipients (146,259,266). However, a registry report indicated that neither MMF treatment nor tacrolimus therapy was an independent risk factor for PTLD; rather, the overall intensity of immunosuppression was most important (147).

The diagnosis of PTLD has generally been made on the basis of characteristic pathologic findings, and the diagnosis cannot be made without biopsy material. Advances in detection of EBV DNA (267–271) and in the outgrowth of transformed lymphocytes (272,273) have permitted early detection of patients at high risk of developing PTLD. Surveillance of blood and prospective adjustment of immunosuppression has been proposed, but there are no universally accepted standards in this area (274). Similar test results have been used also to guide treatment (267), but their absolute value for this function is not established.

The mainstay of treatment of PTLD is the reduction or discontinuation of immunosuppressive therapy (263,275,276). Of interest, in many of these cases, the graft is not rejected despite the marked lowering or discontinuation of immunosuppressive medications. Interferon-alpha and intravenous gamma globulin (277,278), ganciclovir (279), and even chemotherapy have been suggested, but their efficacy has been variable. In high-risk patients prophylaxis may be useful (280). Treatment with the monoclonal antibody rituximab has shown promising results (281–285).

Other Infections

Immunosuppression renders the recipient susceptible to numerous viral and bacterial infections. Infections account for the majority of complications after transplantation in children and are the principal cause of morbidity. Most centers use prophylactic therapy against the more common infections seen in the context of a renal transplantation.

Cytomegalovirus Infection

CMV is an extremely important cause of infectious complications affecting transplant recipients. Unlike the situation in nonimmunocompromised individuals, CMV infection in renal allograft recipients more often causes serious symptoms. CMV presents as a primary infection in seronegative patients; in seropositive patients the infection is secondary due to reactivation of the patient's own latent virus. Clinically the two types cannot be distinguished, although the former is generally more severe. Because of the high risk to the patient and renal allograft, prophylactic therapy is indicated for all seronegative patients who receive a seropositive kidney, and for all patients who receive induction therapy with a T-cell antibody. Prophylaxis can be carried out either with specific antiviral therapy or with high-titer CMV immunoglobulin, or both. The incidence of virologically confirmed CMV-associated syndromes was reduced from 60% in control subjects to 21% in recipients of CMV immunoglobulin. CMV immunoglobulin is generally given in the first 4 months after transplantation. Both acyclovir (286) and ganciclovir (287) have been shown to be effective as prophylactic therapy; however, the latter should replace the former since the introduction of an oral preparation, which has been shown to be highly efficacious (288,289). The dosage of oral ganciclovir is 500 to 700 mg/m^2 every 8 hours (290). There have been no controlled trials comparing CMV immunoglobulin to ganciclovir, so the relative merits of and indications for the two preparations are unknown, although the former seems to ameliorate the severity of CMV disease whereas the latter decreases the frequency.

Pneumocystis carinii *Pneumonia*

Because of their defective cellular immunity, transplant patients are susceptible to respiratory infection by opportunistic organisms that are not of concern to normal children. Pneumonia is a common cause of morbidity in children with a renal allograft, and *Pneumocystis carinii* is the most important cause. *P. carinii* pneumonia occurs in approximately 3% of all renal transplant recipients (291). *Pneumocystis* produces a diffuse pneumonia in which shortness of breath and hypoxemia are salient features. If it is diagnosed quickly, it can be treated effectively; however, delay can be fatal, and hence prophylaxis is standard therapy in most centers. The risk is highest in the first year, and trimethoprim-sulfamethoxazole (Bactrim), in a dosage of 10 mg/kg three times per week, should be given during the period of highest risk.

Varicella

Chickenpox is one of the constant worries of both the transplant physician and the patient's family, because exposure in the pediatric age range is extremely high (35). The rash in an immunocompromised patient may become confluent, bullous, and hemorrhagic. If the disease becomes systemic, the fatality rate can be high (292). Treatment of varicella in immunocompromised children generally consists of intravenous administration of acyclovir at least until all lesions are crusted (291,293). Prophylaxis, consisting of the administration of varicella-zoster immunoglobulin, is carried out routinely in all transplanted seronegative children on exposure (291). The administration of varicella vaccine (Varivax) before transplantation substantially reduces the frequency and severity of the disease after transplantation (294). The use of varicella vaccine after transplantation has been reported in only a small series (295).

Urinary Tract Infection

UTIs are extremely common during the first 3 months after transplantation and may be seen in as many as 50% of patients (35,296). Beyond the first 3 months, episodes of asymptomatic bacteriuria appear more common. During the first 3 months, however, UTIs may be a common source of bacteremia (297). Chemoprophylaxis through the administration of trimethoprim-sulfamethoxazole as described for *P. carinii* infection should be provided in the first month for all patients and may be continued up to 1 year in patients whose original disease was urologic in origin.

Polyoma Virus Infection

Polyoma BK virus infection may be an increasingly important cause of graft dysfunction and graft loss after renal transplantation (298), but there has been little information about its frequency or severity in children. In one retrospective analysis of 100 pediatric renal transplant patients, BK virus was detected in the urine of 26 patients and in the blood of 5 (299). Those with viremia had elevated serum creatinine levels and evidence of interstitial nephritis in graft biopsy specimens. Screening of susceptible patients by urine analysis for BK messenger RNA has been proposed (300).

Hypertension

The incidence of hypertension after transplantation is demonstrated in an NAPRTCS investigation in which 70% of patients required antihypertensive medications at 1 month after transplantation; the incidence decreased to 59% at 24 months (301). Hypertension is detected more commonly if ambulatory blood pressure monitoring methods are used (302,303). Hypertension after transplantation is primarily related to the side effects of drug therapy. The two most widely used immunosuppressive agents—calcineurin inhibitors and prednisone—both exacerbate preexisting hypertension. Hypertension has been correlated with multiple complications of transplantation, including reduced graft survival and cardiovascular complications (304–307).

With dosage reduction of prednisone and calcineurin inhibitors, hypertension can be managed in almost all patients, although multiple drug regimens may be necessary in some patients. An effective and safe drug to use is a calcium-channel blocker such as nifedipine, which also reduces cyclosporine toxicity (121,308). Another drug particularly favored for adolescent patients due to concerns of noncompliance is clonidine, which is available in a transdermal patch. Clonidine may induce drowsiness, and sudden withdrawal tends to produce rebound hypertension. In patients who complain of palpitations due to drug-induced reflux tachycardia, prazosin is more effective because it induces the least amount of tachycardia. Minoxidil, an acute vasodilator, should be used only in cases of severe hypertension and for only a limited time because it causes hirsutism. Care must be exercised to restrict the use of angiotensin-converting enzyme inhibitors, because converting enzyme inhibition in a single kidney model leads to reduction in glomerular filtration (309,310).

Hyperlipidemia

Steroids, calcineurin inhibitors, and rapamycin induce hyperlipidemia. A fall in serum cholesterol levels on conversion from cyclosporine to azathioprine has been demonstrated (311). The mechanism by which calcineurin inhibitors might increase plasma cholesterol is unclarified. The drugs are highly lipophilic, and up to 80% is transported in plasma by binding to lipoproteins, particularly low-density lipoprotein (LDL). It is conceivable that the binding to LDL cholesterol results in impaired clearance of LDL from the circulation via cell surface receptors (312). Posttransplantation hyperlipidemia in adults has an adverse effect on cardiovascular morbidity (313,314). NAPRTCS reviewed data for posttransplantation patients maintained under a rigid common protocol of immunosuppression and observed that at 1 year after transplantation they did exhibit significantly higher levels of plasma cholesterol and very low density lipoprotein cholesterol than healthy controls; however, the elevated cholesterol levels (mean of 213 mg/dL) were not high enough to require the use of lipid-lowering agents (315). In patients with higher serum lipid levels (cholesterol level of 250 mg/dL or higher), 3-hydroxy-3-methylglutaryl coenzyme A reductase inhibitors are particularly effective in reducing total cholesterol levels

(316,317). The use of rapamycin may increase the need for lipid-lowering agents in the future.

Posttransplantation Diabetes Mellitus

Hyperglycemia and posttransplantation diabetes mellitus in children may be increasing in frequency (144). Corticosteroid use leads to peripheral insulin insensitivity and hyperglycemia that is relatively insensitive to exogenous insulin. Steroid withdrawal has led to improvements in this condition (318). An NAPRTCS investigation described an overall incidence of less than 3% among pediatric renal transplant recipients, with African Americans at higher risk (319). Tacrolimus use was identified as a significant risk factor, a finding confirmed by other reports, some of which showed incidence rates exceeding 50% (135,142–144,320). Tacrolimus may diminish insulin secretion (145). Treatment may be aided by reducing the dosage of or eliminating corticosteroids or calcineurin inhibitors (318,321).

Noncompliance with Therapeutic Regimen

Noncompliance with the therapeutic regimen is often cited as a cause of long-term graft loss in pediatric renal transplant recipients, especially adolescents. A major reason for noncompliance is thought to be the alteration in appearance that accompanies the use of immunosuppressive medications, including the cushingoid facies and growth retardation related to long-term daily corticosteroid administration and the hirsutism and gingival hypertrophy associated with cyclosporine use. However, the true incidence of noncompliance is unknown. Noncompliance rates of 22% (322), 43% (323), and as high as 64% in adolescents (324) have been reported. Some factors, such as young age, adolescence, poor socioeconomic status, and family stress, have been associated with increased levels of noncompliance (322,324–326). Importantly, however, health care workers are not able to identify a significant proportion of noncompliant patients (327). Treatments such as educational programs (323) and family-based therapy (328) have been proposed, but these types of programs have not been universally successful in changing motivation.

LONG-TERM OUTCOME

Rehabilitation

Organ transplantation typically results in dramatic improvement of all aspects of physical, emotional, and social functioning. Importantly, cognitive skills improve after successful renal transplantation (11), which suggests stabilization of neurophysiologic functioning. Scores on health-related quality-of-life measures are generally good, especially in older children and adolescents, although all ages report some problems with usual activities (329). Interestingly, the perceived emotional status of the children was actually better than that of controls, especially during and after adolescence (329).

Long-term survival is generally excellent (330), and measures of quality of life have demonstrated excellent rehabilitation in long-term survivors (331,332). More than 90% have rated their health as good or excellent, and most did not feel that their health condition interfered with normal functioning. Most of them were full-time students or were employed. The majority were below normal in height and up to one-third were dissatisfied with their body appearance. In one report, only a small minority of long-term survivors were married (333), but in another, 50% were married and half of those had children (332).

Mortality

Infection is generally the major cause of death, particularly in the first years after transplantation (13). Other major causes include cancer and malignancy, cardiopulmonary disorders, and dialysis-related complications. The best patient survival results are found in older pediatric recipients and in recipients of LD transplants (50). Risk factors for excess mortality include young recipient age, graft dysfunction (ATN) at 30 days after transplantation, and certain underlying renal diseases (oxalosis, congenital nephrotic syndrome, Denys-Drash syndrome) (50). Mortality after 10 years posttransplantation seems to be related primarily to cardiovascular causes (330), which may be linked to the hyperlipidemia and hypertension associated with chronic immunosuppression. The mortality rate of children, except for the very youngest, is very low and is generally better than that found in adults.

REFERENCES

1. Gaston RS, Alveranga DY, Becker BN, et al. Kidney and pancreas transplantation. *Am J Transplant* 2003;3(suppl 4):64–77.
2. Fine RN. Renal transplantation for children—the only realistic choice. *Kidney Int* 1985;17(suppl):S15–S17.
3. Warady BA, Hebert D, Sullivan EK, et al. Renal transplantation, chronic dialysis, and chronic renal insufficiency in children and adolescents. The 1995 annual report of the North American Pediatric Renal Transplant Cooperative Study. *Pediatr Nephrol* 1997;11:49–64.
4. Trachtman H, Hackney P, Tejani A. Pediatric hemodialysis: a decade's (1974–1984) perspective. *Kidney Int* 1986;19(suppl): S15–S22.
5. Brouhard BH, Donaldson LA, Lawry KW, et al. Cognitive functioning in children on dialysis and post-transplantation. *Pediatr Transplant* 2000;4:261–267.
6. Sarwal MM, Yorgin PD, Alexander S, et al. Promising early outcomes with a novel, complete steroid avoidance immunosuppression protocol in pediatric renal transplantation. *Transplantation* 2001;72:13–21.
7. Ingelfinger JR, Grupe WE, Harmon WE, et al. Growth acceleration following renal transplantation in children less than 7 years of age. *Pediatrics* 1981;68:255–259.

8. Fine RN, Ho M, Tejani A. The contribution of renal transplantation to final adult height: a report of the North American Pediatric Renal Transplant Cooperative Study (NAPRTCS). *Pediatr Nephrol* 2001;16:951–956.
9. Fine RN. Growth following solid-organ transplantation. *Pediatr Transplant* 2002;6:47–52.
10. Mendley SR, Zelko FA. Improvement in specific aspects of neurocognitive performance in children after renal transplantation. *Kidney Int* 1999;56:318–323.
11. Fennell EB, Fennell RS, Mings E, et al. The effects of various modes of therapy for end stage renal disease on cognitive performance in a pediatric population—a preliminary report. *Int J Pediatr Nephrol* 1986;7:107–112.
12. Colombani PM, Dunn SP, Harmon WE, et al. Pediatric transplantation. *Am J Transplant* 2003;3(suppl 4):53–63.
13. Seikaly M, Ho PL, Emmett L, et al. The 12th annual report of the North American Pediatric Renal Transplant Cooperative Study: renal transplantation from 1987 through 1998 (updated at www.naprtcs.org). *Pediatr Transplant* 2001;5:215–231.
14. Cecka JM, Gjertson DW, Terasaki PI. Pediatric renal transplantation: a review of the UNOS data. *Pediatr Transplant* 1997;1:55–64.
15. Neu AM, Stablein DM, Zachary A, et al. Effect of parental donor sex on rejection in pediatric renal transplantation: a report of the North American Pediatric Renal Transplant Cooperative Study. *Pediatr Transplant* 1998;2:309–312.
16. Spital A. Should children ever donate kidneys? Views of U.S. transplant centers. *Transplantation* 1997;64:232–236.
17. Price DP. Minors as living donors: ethics and law. *Transplant Proc* 1996;28:3607–3608.
18. Delmonico FL, Harmon WE. The use of a minor as a live kidney donor. *Am J Transplant* 2002;2:333–336.
19. Terasaki PI, Cecka JM, Gjertson DW, et al. High survival rates of kidney transplants from spousal and living unrelated donors. *N Engl J Med* 1995;333:333–336.
20. Al-Uzri A, Sullivan EK, Fine RN, et al. Living-unrelated renal transplantation in children: a report of the North American Pediatric Renal Transplant Cooperative Study. *Pediatr Transplant* 1998 (*in press*).
21. Davies DB, Breen TJ, Guo T, et al. Waiting times to pediatric transplantation: an assessment of the August 1990 change in renal allocation policy. *Transplant Proc* 1994;26:30–31.
22. McEnery PT, Alexander SR, Sullivan K, et al. Renal transplantation in children and adolescents: the 1992 annual report of the North American Pediatric Renal Transplant Cooperative Study. *Pediatr Nephrol* 1993;7:711–720.
23. Tejani A, Stablein D, Alexander S, et al. Analysis of rejection outcomes and implications—a report of the North American Pediatric Renal Transplant Cooperative Study. *Transplantation* 1995;59:500–504.
24. Feld LG, Stablein D, Fivush B, et al. Renal transplantation in children from 1987–1996: the 1996 annual report of the North American Pediatric Renal Transplant Cooperative Study. *Pediatr Transplant* 1997;1:146–162.
25. Filler G, Lindeke A, Bohme K, et al. Renal transplantation from donors aged <6 years into children yields equal graft survival when compared to older donors. *Pediatr Transplant* 1997;1:119–123.
26. Hiramoto JS, Freise CE, Randall HR, et al. Successful long-term outcomes using pediatric en bloc kidneys for transplantation. *Am J Transplant* 2002;2:337–342.
27. Ettenger RB, Blifeld C, Prince H, et al. The pediatric nephrologist's dilemma: growth after renal transplantation and its interaction with age as a possible immunologic variable. *J Pediatr* 1987;111:1022–1025.
28. Ettenger R, Marik J, Rosenthal JT. Sequential therapy in pediatric cadaveric renal transplantation: a critical analysis. *J Am Soc Nephrol* 1992;2:S304–S311.
29. McEnery PT, Stablein DM, Arbus G, et al. Renal transplantation in children. A report of the North American Pediatric Renal Transplant Cooperative Study. *N Engl J Med* 1992;326:1727–1732.
30. Briscoe DM, Kim MS, Lillehei C, et al. Outcome of renal transplantation in children less than two years of age. *Kidney Int* 1992;42:657–662.
31. Najarian JS, Frey DJ, Matas AJ, et al. Renal transplantation in infants. *Ann Surg* 1990;212:353–365.
32. Ingulli E, Matas AJ, Nevins TE, et al. Impact of age on renal graft survival in children after the first rejection episode. *Pediatr Nephrol* 1996;10:474–478.
33. Strehlau J, Sharma VK, Pavalakis M, et al. Do children have a heightened immune response to acute allograft rejection? A preliminary comparative study of intragraft gene transcripts of immune activation markers in adult and pediatric graft rejection. The 16th annual meeting of the American Society of Transplant Physicians, Chicago, 1997(abst).
34. Scomik JC, Cecka M. Clinical parameters of immune responsiveness in children and African American transplant patients. The 16th annual meeting of the American Society of Transplant Physicians, Chicago, 1997(abst).
35. Chavers BM, Gillingham KJ, Matas AJ. Complications by age in primary pediatric renal transplant recipients. *Pediatr Nephrol* 1997;11:399–403.
36. Schachter AD, Meyers KE, Spaneas LD, et al. Short sirolimus half-life in pediatric renal transplant recipients on a calcineurin inhibitor-free protocol. *Pediatr Transplant* 2003 (*in press*).
37. Lemire J, Capparelli EV, Benador N, et al. Neoral pharmacokinetics in Latino and Caucasian pediatric renal transplant recipients. *Pediatr Nephrol* 2001;16:311–314.
38. Hoppu K, Koskimies O, Holmberg C, et al. Pharmacokinetically determined cyclosporine dosage in young children. *Pediatr Nephrol* 1991;5:1–4.
39. Ramos EL, Kasiske BL, Alexander SR, et al. The evaluation of candidates for renal transplantation. The current practice of U.S. transplant centers. *Transplantation* 1994;57:490–497.
40. Kasiske BL, Ramos EL, Gaston RS, et al. The evaluation of renal transplant candidates: clinical practice guidelines. Patient Care and Education Committee of the American Society of Transplant Physicians [Review]. *J Am Soc Nephrol* 1995;6:1–34.
41. Fine RN, Tejani A, Sullivan EK. Pre-emptive renal transplantation in children: report of the North American Pediatric Renal Transplant Cooperative Study (NAPRTCS). *Clin Transplant* 1994;8:474–478.
42. Fine RN, Kohaut EC, Brown D, et al. Growth after recombinant human growth hormone treatment in children with chronic renal failure: report of a multicenter randomized double-blind placebo-controlled study. Genentech Cooperative Study Group. *J Pediatr* 1994;124:374–382.

43. Furth SL, Garg PP, Neu AM, et al. Racial differences in access to the kidney transplant waiting list for children and adolescents with end-stage renal disease. *Pediatrics* 2000;106:756–761.
44. Ingulli E, Tejani A, Fikrig S, et al. Nephrotic syndrome associated with acquired immunodeficiency syndrome in children. *J Pediatr* 1991;119:710–716.
45. Roland ME, Stock PG. Review of solid-organ transplantation in HIV-infected patients. *Transplantation* 2003;75:425–429.
46. Kuo PC, Stock PG. Transplantation in the HIV+ patient. *Am J Transplant* 2001;1:13–17.
47. Kist-van Holthe JE, Ho PL, Harmon WE, et al. Outcome of children after renal transplantation for Wilms' tumor and Drash syndrome: a report of the North American Pediatric Renal Transplant Cooperative Study. *Am J Transplant* 2003;3:154.
48. Salvatierra O, Tanney D, Mak R, et al. Pediatric renal transplantation and its challenges. *Transplant Rev* 1997;11:51–69.
49. Gagnadoux MF, Lacaille F, Niaudet P, et al. Long term results of liver-kidney transplantation in children with primary hyperoxaluria. *Pediatr Nephrol* 2001;16:946–950.
50. Tejani A, Sullivan EK, Alexander S, et al. Posttransplant deaths and factors that influence the mortality rate in North American children. *Transplantation* 1994;57:547–553.
51. Ellis SR, Hulton SA, McKiernan PJ, et al. Combined liver-kidney transplantation for primary hyperoxaluria type 1 in young children. *Nephrol Dial Transplant* 2001;16:348–354.
52. Kim MS, Primack W, Harmon WE. Congenital nephrotic syndrome: preemptive bilateral nephrectomy and dialysis before renal transplantation. *J Am Soc Nephrol* 1992;3:260–263.
53. Fasola CG, Gillingham KJ, Troppmann C, et al. Kidney transplant or retransplant can effectively treat congenital nephrotic syndrome: a single-center experience. *Transplant Proc* 1994;26:9.
54. Holmberg C, Jalanko H, Koskimies O, et al. Renal transplantation in small children with congenital nephrotic syndrome of the Finnish type. *Transplant Proc* 1991;23:1378–1379.
55. Rudge CJ. Transplantation and the abnormal bladder. In: Morris PJ, ed. *Kidney transplantation: principles and practice.* Philadelphia: W.B. Saunders, 1994:138–148.
56. Lopez Pereira P, Jaureguizar E, Martinez Urrutia MJ, et al. Does treatment of bladder dysfunction prior to renal transplant improve outcome in patients with posterior urethral valves? *Pediatr Transplant* 2000;4:118–122.
57. Ramirez SP, Lebowitz RL, Harmon WE, et al. Predictors for abnormal voiding cystourethrography in pediatric patients undergoing renal transplant evaluation. *Pediatr Transplant* 2001;5:99–104.
58. Koo HP, Bunchman TE, Flynn JT, et al. Renal transplantation in children with severe lower urinary tract dysfunction. *J Urol* 1999;161:240–245.
59. Power RE, O'Malley KJ, Khan MS, et al. Renal transplantation in patients with an augmentation cystoplasty. *BJU Int* 2000;86:28–31.
60. Nahas WC, Mazzucchi E, Arap MA, et al. Augmentation cystoplasty in renal transplantation: a good and safe option—experience with 25 cases. *Urology* 2002;60:770–774.
61. Atala A. Bladder regeneration by tissue engineering. *BJU Int* 2001;88:765–770.
62. Atala A. Future trends in bladder reconstructive surgery. *Semin Pediatr Surg* 2002;11:134–142.
63. Opelz G, Sengar DP, Mickey MR, et al. Effect of blood transfusions on subsequent kidney transplants. *Transplant Proc* 1973;5:253–259.
64. Opelz G. Improved kidney graft survival in nontransfused recipients. *Transplant Proc* 1987;19:149–152.
65. Potter DE, Portale AA, Melzer JS, et al. Are blood transfusions beneficial in the cyclosporine era? *Pediatr Nephrol* 1991;5:168–172.
66. Niaudet P, Dudley J, Charbit M, et al. Pretransplant blood transfusions with cyclosporine in pediatric renal transplantation. *Pediatr Nephrol* 2000;14:451–456.
67. Otsuka M, Yuzawa K, Takada Y, et al. Long-term results of donor-specific blood transfusion with cyclosporine in living related kidney transplantation. *Nephron* 2001;88:144–148.
68. Fedoseyeva EV, Tam RC, Popov IA, et al. Induction of T cell responses to a self-antigen following allotransplantation. *Transplantation* 1996;61:679–683.
69. Chavers BM, Sullivan EK, Tejani A, et al. Pre-transplant blood transfusion and renal allograft outcome: a report of the North American Pediatric Renal Transplant Cooperative Study. *Pediatr Transplant* 1997;1:22–28.
70. Harmon WE, Alexander SR, Tejani A, et al. The effect of donor age on graft survival in pediatric cadaver renal transplant recipients—a report of the North American Pediatric Renal Transplant Cooperative Study. *Transplantation* 1992;54:232–237.
71. Bresnahan BA, McBride MA, Cherikh WS, et al. Risk factors for renal allograft survival from pediatric cadaver donors: an analysis of united network for organ sharing data. *Transplantation* 2001;72:256–261.
72. Ruff T, Reddy KS, Johnston TD, et al. Transplantation of pediatric en bloc cadaver kidneys into adult recipients: a single-center experience. *Am Surg* 2002;68:857–859.
73. Takemoto S, Terasaki PI. Donor age and recipient age. *Clin Transpl* 1988:345–356.
74. Terasaki PI, Gjertson DW, Cecka JM, et al. Significance of the donor age effect on kidney transplants. *Clin Transplant* 1997;11:366–372.
75. Tejani AH, Stablein DM, Sullivan EK, et al. The impact of donor source, recipient age, pre-operative immunotherapy and induction therapy on early and late acute rejections in children: a report of the North American Pediatric Renal Transplant Cooperative Study (NAPRTCS). *Pediatr Transplant* 1998;2:318–324.
76. Toma H, Tanabe K, Tokumoto T, et al. Time-dependent risk factors influencing the long-term outcome in living renal allografts: donor age is a crucial risk factor for long-term graft survival more than 5 years after transplantation. *Transplantation* 2001;72:940–947.
77. Cho YW, Cecka JM, Terasaki PI. HLA matching effect: better survival rates and graft quality. *Clin Transplant* 1994:435–449.
78. Terasaki PI, Cho Y, Takemoto S, et al. Twenty-year follow-up on the effect of HLA matching on kidney transplant survival and prediction of future twenty-year survival. *Transplant Proc* 1996;28:1144–1145.
79. Osorio AV, Sullivan EK, Alexander SR, et al. ABO-mismatched renal transplantation in children: a report of the

North American Pediatric Renal Transplant Cooperative Study (NAPRTCS) and the Midwest Organ Bank (MOB). *Pediatr Transplant* 1998;2:26–29.
80. Ross LF, Rubin DT, Siegler M, et al. Ethics of a paired-kidney-exchange program. *N Engl J Med* 1997;336:1752–1755.
81. Delmonico FL, Morrissey PE, Lipkowitz GS, et al. Donor kidney exchange for incompatible donors. *Am J Transplant* 2003;3(suppl 5):550.
82. Jones JW, Matas AJ, Najarian JS. Surgical technique. In: Tejani AH, Fine RN, eds. *Pediatric renal transplantation.* New York: Wiley-Liss, 1994:187–200.
83. Lee HM. Surgical techniques of renal transplantation. In: Morris PJ, ed. *Kidney transplantation: principles and practice.* Philadelphia: W.B. Saunders, 1994:127–137.
84. Salvatierra O, Singh T, Shifrin R, et al. Transplantation of adult-sized kidneys into infants induces major blood flow changes. *Transplantation* 1998 (*in press*).
85. French CG, Acott PD, Crocker JF, et al. Extravesical ureteroneocystostomy with and without internalized ureteric stents in pediatric renal transplantation. *Pediatr Transplant* 2001;5:21–26.
86. Zaontz MR, Maizels M, Sugar EC, et al. Detrusorrhaphy: extravesical ureteral advancement to correct vesicoureteral reflux in children. *J Urol* 1987;138:947–949.
87. Wacksman J, Gilbert A, Sheldon CA. Results of the renewed extravesical reimplant for surgical correction of vesicoureteral reflux. *J Urol* 1992;148:359–361.
88. Briscoe DM, Hoffer FA, Tu N, et al. Duplex Doppler examination of renal allografts in children: correlation between renal blood flow and clinical findings. *Pediatr Radiol* 1993;23:365–368.
89. Benfield MR, Herrin J, Feld L, et al. Safety of kidney biopsy in pediatric transplantation: a report of the Controlled Clinical Trials in Pediatric Transplantation Trial of Induction Therapy Study Group. *Transplantation* 1999;67:544–547.
90. Tejani A, Sullivan EK, Alexander SR, et al. Predictive factors for acute tubular necrosis (ATN) and its impact on renal graft survival in children. The 16th annual meeting of the American Society of Transplant Physicians, Chicago, 1997(abst).
91. Smith JM, McDonald RA, Stablein D, et al. The impact of interleukin-2 receptor antibodies on renal allograft thrombosis: an analysis of the North American Pediatric Renal Transplant Cooperative Study. *Am J Transplant* 2003;3(suppl 5):166.
92. Balachandra S, Tejani A. Recurrent vascular thrombosis in an adolescent transplant recipient [Review]. *J Am Soc Nephrol* 1997;8:1477–1481.
93. Harmon WE, Stablein D, Alexander SR, et al. Graft thrombosis in pediatric renal transplant recipients. A report of the North American Pediatric Renal Transplant Cooperative Study. *Transplantation* 1991;51:406–412.
94. Singh A, Stablein D, Tejani A. Risk factors for vascular thrombosis in pediatric renal transplantation: a special report of the North American Pediatric Renal Transplant Cooperative Study. *Transplantation* 1997;63:1263–1267.
95. Wheeler MA, Taylor CM, Williams M, et al. Factor V Leiden: a risk factor for renal vein thrombosis in renal transplantation. *Pediatr Nephrol* 2000;14:525–526.
96. Kim MS, Stablein D, Harmon WE. Renal transplantation in children with congenital nephrotic syndrome: a report of the North American Pediatric Renal Transplant Cooperative Study (NAPRTCS). *Pediatr Transplant* 1998;2:305–308.
97. Schurman SJ, Stablein DM, Perlman SA, et al. Center volume effects in pediatric renal transplantation. A report of the North American Pediatric Renal Transplant Cooperative Study. *Pediatr Nephrol* 1999;13:373–378.
98. Vats AN, Donaldson L, Fine RN, et al. Pretransplant dialysis status and outcome of renal transplantation in North American children: a NAPRTCS Study. North American Pediatric Renal Transplant Cooperative Study. *Transplantation* 2000;69:1414–1419.
99. McDonald RA, Smith JM, Stablein D, et al. Pretransplant peritoneal dialysis and graft thrombosis following pediatric kidney transplantation: a NAPRTCS report. *Pediatr Transplant* 2003;7:204–208.
100. Lundin C, Bersztel A, Wahlberg J, et al. Low molecular weight heparin prophylaxis increases the incidence of lymphocele after kidney transplantation. *Ups J Med Sci* 2002; 107:9–15.
101. Simmons RL, Canafax DM, Fryd DS, et al. New immunosuppressive drug combinations for mismatched related and cadaveric renal transplantation. *Transplant Proc* 1986;18:76–81.
102. Norman DJ. Mechanisms of action and overview of OKT3 [Review]. *Ther Drug Monit* 1995;17:615–620.
103. Peddi VR, Bryant M, Roy-Chaudhury P, et al. Safety, efficacy, and cost analysis of thymoglobulin induction therapy with intermittent dosing based on CD3+ lymphocyte counts in kidney and kidney-pancreas transplant recipients. *Transplantation* 2002;73:1514–1518.
104. Ault BH, Honaker MR, Osama Gaber A, et al. Short-term outcomes of thymoglobulin induction in pediatric renal transplant recipients. *Pediatr Nephrol* 2002;17:815–818.
105. Brophy PD, Thomas SE, McBryde KD, et al. Comparison of polyclonal induction agents in pediatric renal transplantation. *Pediatr Transplant* 2001;5:174–178.
106. Norman DJ, Chatenoud L, Cohen D, et al. Consensus statement regarding OKT3-induced cytokine-release syndrome and human antimouse antibodies [Review]. *Transplant Proc* 1993;25:89–92.
107. Robinson ST, Barry JM, Norman DJ. The hemodynamic effects of intraoperative injection of muromonab CD3. *Transplantation* 1993;56:356–358.
108. Shihab FS, Barry JM, Norman DJ. Encephalopathy following the use of OKT3 in renal allograft transplantation. *Transplant Proc* 1993;25:31–34.
109. Tejani A, Harmon W, Benfield MR. A randomized, prospective, multicenter trial of T-cell antibody induction therapy in pediatric renal transplantation. *Transplantation* 2000; 69:S111(abst).
110. Offner G, Broyer M, Niaudet P, et al. A multicenter, open-label, pharmacokinetic/pharmacodynamic safety, and tolerability study of basiliximab (Simulect) in pediatric de novo renal transplant recipients. *Transplantation* 2002;74:961–966.
111. Kovarik JM, Offner G, Broyer M, et al. A rational dosing algorithm for basiliximab (Simulect) in pediatric renal transplantation based on pharmacokinetic-dynamic evaluations. *Transplantation* 2002;74:966–971.
112. Strehlau J, Pape L, Offner G, et al. Interleukin-2 receptor antibody-induced alterations of ciclosporin dose require-

ments in paediatric transplant recipients. *Lancet* 2000;356: 1327–1328.
113. Ciancio G, Burke GW, Suzart K, et al. Daclizumab induction, tacrolimus, mycophenolate mofetil and steroids as an immunosuppression regimen for primary kidney transplant recipients. *Transplantation* 2002;73:1100–1106.
114. Swiatecka-Urban A, Garcia C, Feuerstein D, et al. Basiliximab induction improves the outcome of renal transplants in children and adolescents. *Pediatr Nephrol* 2001;16:693–696.
115. Vester U, Kranz B, Testa G, et al. Efficacy and tolerability of interleukin-2 receptor blockade with basiliximab in pediatric renal transplant recipients. *Pediatr Transplant* 2001;5:297–301.
116. Zamora I, Berbel O, Simon J, et al. [Anti-CD25 monoclonal antibody against polyclonal antibodies in pediatric renal transplantation]. *Nefrologia* 2002;22:66–70.
117. Jablonski P, Harrison C, Howden B, et al. Cyclosporine and the ischemic rat kidney. *Transplantation* 1986;41:147–151.
118. Kahan BD. Cyclosporine [Review]. *N Engl J Med* 1989;321: 1725–1738.
119. Calne RY, Rolles K, White DJ, et al. Cyclosporin A initially as the only immunosuppressant in 34 recipients of cadaveric organs: 32 kidneys, 2 pancreases, and 2 livers. *Lancet* 1979;2: 1033–1036.
120. Harmon WE, Sullivan EK. Cyclosporine dosing and its relationship to outcome in pediatric renal transplantation. *Kidney Int* 1993;43(suppl):S50–S55.
121. Suthanthiran M, Haschemeyer RH, Riggio RR, et al. Excellent outcome with a calcium channel blocker-supplemented immunosuppressive regimen in cadaveric renal transplantation. A potential strategy to avoid antibody induction protocols. *Transplantation* 1993;55:1008–1013.
122. Tejani A, Sullivan EK. Higher maintenance cyclosporine dose decreases the risk of graft failure in North American children: a report of the North American Pediatric Renal Transplant Cooperative Study. *J Am Soc Nephrol* 1996;7:550–555.
123. Tejani A, Sullivan EK, Fine RN, et al. Steady improvement in renal allograft survival among North American children: a five year appraisal by the North American Pediatric Renal Transplant Cooperative Study. *Kidney Int* 1995;48:551–553.
124. David-Neto E, Araujo LP, Feres Alves C, et al. A strategy to calculate cyclosporin A area under the time-concentration curve in pediatric renal transplantation. *Pediatr Transplant* 2002;6:313–318.
125. Belitsky P, Dunn S, Johnston A, et al. Impact of absorption profiling on efficacy and safety of cyclosporin therapy in transplant recipients. *Clin Pharmacokinet* 2000;39:117–125.
126. Dunn SP. Neoral monitoring 2 hours post-dose and the pediatric transplant patient. *Pediatr Transplant* 2003;7:25–30.
127. Crocker JF, Dempsey T, Schenk ME, et al. Cyclosporin A toxicity in children. *Transplant Rev* 1993;7:72.
128. Foley RJ, Hamner RW, Weinman EJ. Serum potassium concentrations in cyclosporine- and azathioprine-treated renal transplant patients. *Nephron* 1985;40:280–285.
129. Chapman JR, Griffiths D, Harding NG, et al. Reversibility of cyclosporin nephrotoxicity after three months' treatment. *Lancet* 1985;1:128–130.
130. Allen RD, Hunnisett AG, Morris PJ. Cyclosporin and magnesium [Letter]. *Lancet* 1985;1:1283–1284.
131. Beaman M, Parvin S, Veitch PS, et al. Convulsions associated with cyclosporin A in renal transplant recipients. *BMJ* 1985;290:139–140.
132. Thomas DW, Baboolal K, Subramanian N, et al. Cyclosporin A-induced gingival overgrowth is unrelated to allograft function in renal transplant recipients. *J Clin Periodontol* 2001;28:706–709.
133. Seymour RA, Jacobs DJ. Cyclosporin and the gingival tissues [Review]. *J Clin Periodontol* 1992;19:1–11.
134. Shapiro R, Jordan ML, Scantlebury VP, et al. The superiority of tacrolimus in renal transplant recipients—the Pittsburgh experience [Review]. *Clin Transplant* 1995:199–205.
135. McKee M, Segev D, Wise B, et al. Initial experience with FK506 (tacrolimus) in pediatric renal transplant recipients. *J Pediatr Surg* 1997;32:688–690.
136. Ellis D. Clinical use of tacrolimus (FK-506) in infants and children with renal transplants [Review]. *Pediatr Nephrol* 1995;9:487–494.
137. Eades SK, Boineau FG, Christensen ML. Increased tacrolimus levels in a pediatric renal transplant patient attributed to chronic diarrhea. *Pediatr Transplant* 2000;4:63–66.
138. Shapiro R, Jordan M, Fung J, et al. Kidney transplantation under FK 506 immunosuppression. *Transplant Proc* 1991;23: 920–923.
139. Neu AM, Ho PL, Fine RN, et al. Tacrolimus vs. cyclosporine A as primary immunosuppression in pediatric renal transplantation: a NAPRTCS study. *Pediatr Transplant* 2003;7:217–222.
140. Eidelman BH, Abu-Elmagd K, Wilson J, et al. Neurologic complications of FK 506. *Transplant Proc* 1991;23:3175–3178.
141. Neu AM, Furth SL, Case BW, et al. Evaluation of neurotoxicity in pediatric renal transplant recipients treated with tacrolimus (FK506). *Clin Transplant* 1997;11:412–414.
142. Japanese FK506 Study Group. Morphological characteristics of renal allografts showing renal dysfunction under FK506 therapy: is graft biopsy available to reveal the morphological findings corresponding with FK506 nephropathy? *Transplant Proc* 1993;25:624.
143. Furth S, Neu A, Colombani P, et al. Diabetes as a complication of tacrolimus (FK506) in pediatric renal transplant patients. *Pediatr Nephrol* 1996;10:64–66.
144. Greenspan LC, Gitelman SE, Leung MA, et al. Increased incidence in post-transplant diabetes mellitus in children: a case-control analysis. *Pediatr Nephrol* 2002;17:1–5.
145. Filler G, Neuschulz I, Vollmer I, et al. Tacrolimus reversibly reduces insulin secretion in paediatric renal transplant recipients. *Nephrol Dial Transplant* 2000;15:867–871.
146. Ciancio G, Siquijor AP, Burke GW, et al. Post-transplant lymphoproliferative disease in kidney transplant patients in the new immunosuppressive era. *Clin Transplant* 1997;11:243–249.
147. Dharnidharka VR, Ho PL, Stablein DM, et al. Mycophenolate, tacrolimus and post-transplant lymphoproliferative disorder: a report of the North American Pediatric Renal Transplant Cooperative Study. *Pediatr Transplant* 2002;6:396–399.
148. Tejani A, Ho PL, Emmett L, et al. Reduction in acute rejections decreases chronic rejection graft failure in children: a report of the North American Pediatric Renal Transplant Cooperative Study (NAPRTCS). *Am J Transplant* 2002;2: 142–147.

149. Tejani A, Stablein DM, Donaldson L, et al. Steady improvement in short-term graft survival of pediatric renal transplants: the NAPRTCS experience. *Clin Transplant* 1999:95–110.
150. Trompeter R, Filler G, Webb NJ, et al. Randomized trial of tacrolimus versus cyclosporin microemulsion in renal transplantation. *Pediatr Nephrol* 2002;17:141–149.
151. Benfield MR, Symons JM, Bynon S, et al. Mycophenolate mofetil in pediatric renal transplantation. *Pediatr Transplant* 1999;3:33–37.
152. Butani L, Palmer J, Baluarte HJ, et al. Adverse effects of mycophenolate mofetil in pediatric renal transplant recipients with presumed chronic rejection. *Transplantation* 1999;68:83–86.
153. Jungraithmayr T, Staskewitz A, Kirste G, et al. Pediatric renal transplantation with mycophenolate mofetil-based immunosuppression without induction: results after three years. *Transplantation* 2003;75:454–461.
154. Filler G, Gellermann J, Zimmering M, et al. Effect of adding mycophenolate mofetil in paediatric renal transplant recipients with chronical cyclosporine nephrotoxicity. *Transplant Int* 2000;13:201–206.
155. Staskewitz A, Kirste G, Tonshoff B, et al. Mycophenolate mofetil in pediatric renal transplantation without induction therapy: results after 12 months of treatment. German Pediatric Renal Transplantation Study Group. *Transplantation* 2001;71:638–644.
156. Bunchman T, Navarro M, Broyer M, et al. The use of mycophenolate mofetil suspension in pediatric renal allograft recipients. *Pediatr Nephrol* 2001;16:978–984.
157. Ettenger R, Cohen A, Nast C, et al. Mycophenolate mofetil as maintenance immunosuppression in pediatric renal transplantation. *Transplant Proc* 1997;29:340–341.
158. Oellerich M, Shipkova M, Schutz E, et al. Pharmacokinetic and metabolic investigations of mycophenolic acid in pediatric patients after renal transplantation: implications for therapeutic drug monitoring. German Study Group on Mycophenolate Mofetil Therapy in Pediatric Renal Transplant Recipients [Erratum in: *Ther Drug Monit* 2000;22(4):500]. *Ther Drug Monit* 2000;22:20–26.
159. Filler G, Feber J, Lepage N, et al. Universal approach to pharmacokinetic monitoring of immunosuppressive agents in children. *Pediatr Transplant* 2002;6:411–418.
160. Shipkova M, Armstrong VW, Weber L, et al. Pharmacokinetics and protein adduct formation of the pharmacologically active acyl glucuronide metabolite of mycophenolic acid in pediatric renal transplant recipients. *Ther Drug Monit* 2002;24:390–399.
161. Weber LT, Schutz E, Lamersdorf T, et al. Therapeutic drug monitoring of total and free mycophenolic acid (MPA) and limited sampling strategy for determination of MPA-AUC in paediatric renal transplant recipients. The German Study Group on Mycophenolate Mofetil (MMF) Therapy. *Nephrol Dial Transplant* 1999;14:34–35.
162. Weber LT, Schutz E, Lamersdorf T, et al. Pharmacokinetics of mycophenolic acid (MPA) and free MPA in paediatric renal transplant recipients—a multicentre study. The German Study Group on Mycophenolate Mofetil (MMF) Therapy. *Nephrol Dial Transplant* 1999;14:33–34.
163. Weber LT, Shipkova M, Armstrong VW, et al. The pharmacokinetic-pharmacodynamic relationship for total and free mycophenolic acid in pediatric renal transplant recipients: a report of the German study group on mycophenolate mofetil therapy. *J Am Soc Nephrol* 2002;13:759–768.
164. Potter D, Belzer FO, Rames L, et al. The treatment of chronic uremia in childhood. I. Transplantation. *Pediatrics* 1970;45:432–443.
165. Baqi N, Tejani A. Maintenance immunosuppression regimens. In: Tejani AH, Fine RN, eds. *Pediatric renal transplantation.* New York: Wiley-Liss, 1994:201–210.
166. Danovitch GB. *Handbook of kidney transplantation.* Boston: Little, Brown and Company, 1996.
167. Ingulli E, Tejani A. Steroid withdrawal after renal transplantation. In: Tejani AH, Fine RN, eds. *Pediatric renal transplantation.* New York: Wiley-Liss, 1994:221–238.
168. Ingulli E, Sharma V, Singh A, et al. Steroid withdrawal, rejection and the mixed lymphocyte reaction in children after renal transplantation. *Kidney Int* 1993;43(suppl):S36–S39.
169. Reisman L, Lieberman KV, Burrows L, et al. Follow-up of cyclosporine-treated pediatric renal allograft recipients after cessation of prednisone. *Transplantation* 1990;49:76–80.
170. Hymes LC, Warshaw BL. Tacrolimus rescue therapy for children with acute renal transplant rejection. *Pediatr Nephrol* 2001;16:990–992.
171. Broyer M, Guest G, Gagnadoux MF. Growth rate in children receiving alternate-day corticosteroid treatment after kidney transplantation. *J Pediatr* 1992;120:721–725.
172. Jabs K, Sullivan EK, Avner ED, et al. Alternate-day steroid dosing improves growth without adversely affecting graft survival or long-term graft function. A report of the North American Pediatric Renal Transplant Cooperative Study. *Transplantation* 1996;61:31–36.
173. Sehgal SN, Molnar-Kimber K, Ocain TD, et al. Rapamycin: a novel immunosuppressive macrolide [Review]. *Med Res Rev* 1994;14:1–22.
174. Kim HS, Raskova J, Degiannis D, et al. Effects of cyclosporine and rapamycin on immunoglobulin production by preactivated human B cells. *Clin Exp Immunol* 1994;96:508–512.
175. Ferraresso M, Tian L, Ghobrial R, et al. Rapamycin inhibits production of cytotoxic but not noncytotoxic antibodies and preferentially activates T helper 2 cells that mediate long-term survival of heart allografts in rats. *J Immunol* 1994;153:3307–3318.
176. Aagaard-Tillery KM, Jelinek DF. Inhibition of human B lymphocyte cell cycle progression and differentiation by rapamycin. *Cell Immunol* 1994;156:493–507.
177. Dumont FJ, Staruch MJ, Koprak SL, et al. Distinct mechanisms of suppression of murine T cell activation by the related macrolides FK-506 and rapamycin. *J Immunol* 1990;144:251–258.
178. Wood MA, Bierer BE. Rapamycin: biological and therapeutic effects, binding by immunophilins and molecular targets of action. *Perspect Drug Discov Des* 1994;2:163–184.
179. Marx SO, Jayaraman T, Go LO, et al. Rapamycin-FKBP inhibits cell cycle regulators of proliferation in vascular smooth muscle cells. *Circ Res* 1995;76:412–417.
180. Cao W, Mohacsi P, Shorthouse R, et al. Effects of rapamycin on growth factor-stimulated vascular smooth muscle cell DNA synthesis. Inhibition of basic fibroblast growth factor and platelet-derived growth factor action and antagonism of rapamycin by FK506. *Transplantation* 1995;59:390–395.

181. El-Sabrout R, Weiss R, Butt F, et al. Rejection-free protocol using sirolimus-tacrolimus combination for pediatric renal transplant recipients. *Transplant Proc* 2002;34:1942–1943.
182. Montgomery SP, Mog SR, Xu H, et al. Efficacy and toxicity of a protocol using sirolimus, tacrolimus and daclizumab in a nonhuman primate renal allotransplant model. *Am J Transplant* 2002;2:381–385.
183. Kahan BD, Camardo JS. Rapamycin: clinical results and future opportunities. *Transplantation* 2001;72:1181–1193.
184. Kahan BD, Julian BA, Pescovitz MD, et al. Sirolimus reduces the incidence of acute rejection episodes despite lower cyclosporine doses in Caucasian recipients of mismatched primary renal allografts: a phase II trial. Rapamune Study Group. *Transplantation* 1999;68:1526–1532.
185. Kahan BD, Podbielski J, Napoli KL, et al. Immunosuppressive effects and safety of a sirolimus/cyclosporine combination regimen for renal transplantation. *Transplantation* 1998;66:1040–1046.
186. Kreis H, Cisterne JM, Land W, et al. Sirolimus in association with mycophenolate mofetil induction for the prevention of acute graft rejection in renal allograft recipients. *Transplantation* 2000;69:1252–1260.
187. Mital D, Podlasek W, Jensik SC. Sirolimus-based steroid-free maintenance immunosuppression. *Transplant Proc* 2002;34: 1709–1710.
188. Vester U, Kranz B, Wehr S, et al. Everolimus (Certican) in combination with Neoral in pediatric renal transplant recipients: interim analysis after 3 months. *Transplant Proc* 2002;34:2209–2210.
189. Van Damme-Lombaerts R, Webb NA, Hoyer PF, et al. Single-dose pharmacokinetics and tolerability of everolimus in stable pediatric renal transplant patients. *Pediatr Transplant* 2002;6:147–152.
190. Sindhi R, Webber S, Goyal R, et al. Pharmacodynamics of sirolimus in transplanted children receiving tacrolimus. *Transplant Proc* 2002;34:1960.
191. MacDonald A, Scarola J, Burke JT, et al. Clinical pharmacokinetics and therapeutic drug monitoring of sirolimus. *Clin Ther* 2000;22:B101–B121.
192. Harmon WE, Stablein DM, Sayegh MH. Trends in immunosuppression strategies in pediatric kidney transplantation. *Am J Transplant* 2003;3(suppl 5):285.
193. Sho M, Samsonov DV, Briscoe DM. Immunologic targets for currently available immunosuppressive agents: what is the optimal approach for children? *Semin Nephrol* 2001;21:508–520.
194. Tilney NL. Early course of a patient. In: Morris PJ, ed. *Kidney transplantation: principles and practice*. Philadelphia: W.B. Saunders, 1988:278–283.
195. McDonald R, Ho PL, Stablein DM, et al. Rejection profile of recent pediatric renal transplant recipients compared with historical controls: a report of the North American Pediatric Renal Transplant Cooperative Study (NAPRTCS). *Am J Transplant* 2001;1:55–60.
196. Dadhania D, Muthukumar T, Ding R, et al. Molecular signatures of urinary cells distinguish acute rejection of renal allografts from urinary tract infection. *Transplantation* 2003;75:1752–1754.
197. Strehlau J, Pavlakis M, Lipman M, et al. Quantitative detection of immune activation transcripts as a diagnostic tool in kidney transplantation. *Proc Natl Acad Sci U S A* 1997;94: 695–700.
198. Treves ST, Majd M, Kuruc A, et al. Kidneys. In: Treves WT, ed. *Pediatric nuclear medicine.* New York: Springer-Verlag, 1995:339–399.
199. Solez K, Axelsen RA, Benediktsson H, et al. International standardization of criteria for the histologic diagnosis of renal allograft rejection: the Banff working classification of kidney transplant pathology. *Kidney Int* 1993;44:411–422.
200. Ding R, Li B, Muthukumar T, et al. CD103 mRNA levels in urinary cells predict acute rejection of renal allografts. *Transplantation* 2003;75:1307–1312.
201. Li B, Hartono C, Ding R, et al. Noninvasive diagnosis of renal-allograft rejection by measurement of messenger RNA for perforin and granzyme B in urine. *N Engl J Med* 2001;344:947–954.
202. Sarwal M, Chua MS, Kambham N, et al. Molecular heterogeneity in acute renal allograft rejection identified by DNA microarray profiling. *N Engl J Med* 2003;349:125–138.
203. Dunnill MS. Histopathology of renal allograft rejection. In: Morris PJ, ed. *Kidney transplantation: principles and practice.* Philadelphia: WB Saunders, 1994:266–285.
204. Feehally J, Harris KP, Bennett SE, et al. Is chronic renal transplant rejection a non-immunological phenomenon? *Lancet* 1986;2:486–488.
205. Tilney NL, Guttmann RD. Effects of initial ischemia/reperfusion injury on the transplanted kidney [Review]. *Transplantation* 1997;64:945–947.
206. Tejani A, Cortes L, Stablein D. Clinical correlates of chronic rejection in pediatric renal transplantation. A report of the North American Pediatric Renal Transplant Cooperative Study. *Transplantation* 1996;61:1054–1058.
207. Sharma VK, Bologa RM, Xu GP, et al. Intragraft TGF beta 1 mRNA: a correlate of interstitial fibrosis and chronic allograft nephropathy. *Kidney Int* 1996;49:1297–1303.
208. Jabs KL, Van Dop C, Harmon WE. Endocrinologic evaluation of children who grow poorly following renal transplantation. *Transplantation* 1990;49:71–76.
209. Harmon WE, Jabs K. Factors affecting growth after renal transplantation [Review]. *J Am Soc Nephrol* 1992;2:S295–S303.
210. van Lieburg AF, de Jong MC, Hoitsma AJ, et al. Renal transplant thrombosis in children. *J Pediatr Surg* 1995;30:615–619.
211. Tejani A, Fine RN. Cadaver renal transplantation in children. Incidence, immunosuppression, outcome, and risk factors [Review]. *Clin Pediatr* 1993;32:194–202.
212. Sarwal MM, Cecka JM, Millan MT, et al. Adult-size kidneys without acute tubular necrosis provide exceedingly superior long-term graft outcomes for infants and small children: a single center and UNOS analysis. United Network for Organ Sharing. *Transplantation* 2000;70:1728–1736.
213. Kashtan CE, McEnery PT, Tejani A, et al. Renal allograft survival according to primary diagnosis: a report of the North American Pediatric Renal Transplant Cooperative Study. *Pediatr Nephrol* 1995;9:679–684.
214. Tejani A, Stablein DH. Recurrence of focal segmental glomerulosclerosis posttransplantation: a special report of the North American Pediatric Renal Transplant Cooperative Study. *J Am Soc Nephrol* 1992;2:S258–S263.
215. Baum MA, Ho M, Stablein D, et al. North American Pediatric Renal Transplant Cooperative Study. Outcome of renal

transplantation in adolescents with focal segmental glomerulosclerosis. *Pediatr Transplant* 2002;6:488–492.
216. Benfield MR, McDonald R, Sullivan EK, et al. The 1997 annual renal transplantation in children report of the North American Pediatric Renal Transplant Cooperative Study (NAPRTCS). *Pediatr Transplant* 1999;3:152–167.
217. Schachter AD, Harmon WE. Single-center analysis of early recurrence of nephrotic syndrome following renal transplantation in children. *Pediatr Transplant* 2001;5:406–409.
218. Baum MA, Stablein DM, Panzarino VM, et al. Loss of living donor renal allograft survival advantage in children with focal segmental glomerulosclerosis. *Kidney Int* 2001;59:328–333.
219. Schachter AD, Strehlau J, Zurakowski D, et al. Increased nuclear factor-kappaB and angiotensinogen gene expression in posttransplant recurrent focal segmental glomerulosclerosis. *Transplantation* 2000;70:1107–1110.
220. Sharma M, Sharma R, McCarthy ET, et al. "The FSGS factor": enrichment and in vivo effect of activity from focal segmental glomerulosclerosis plasma. *J Am Soc Nephrol* 1999;10: 552–561.
221. Belson A, Yorgin PD, Al-Uzri AY, et al. Long-term plasmapheresis and protein A column treatment of recurrent FSGS. *Pediatr Nephrol* 2001;16:985–989.
222. Dall'Amico R, Ghiggeri G, Carraro M, et al. Prediction and treatment of recurrent focal segmental glomerulosclerosis after renal transplantation in children. *Am J Kidney Dis* 1999;34:1048–1055.
223. Greenstein SM, Delrio M, Ong E, et al. Plasmapheresis treatment for recurrent focal sclerosis in pediatric renal allografts. *Pediatr Nephrol* 2000;14:1061–1065.
224. Ohta T, Kawaguchi H, Hattori M, et al. Effect of pre- and postoperative plasmapheresis on posttransplant recurrence of focal segmental glomerulosclerosis in children. *Transplantation* 2001;71:628–633.
225. Raafat R, Travis LB, Kalia A, et al. Role of transplant induction therapy on recurrence rate of focal segmental glomerulosclerosis. *Pediatr Nephrol* 2000;14:189–194.
226. Cochat P. Is there a need for a multicenter study to determine the optimal approach to recurrent nephrotic syndrome following renal transplantation? *Pediatr Transplant* 2001;5:394–397.
227. Bartosh SM, Fine RN, Sullivan EK. Outcome after transplantation of young patients with systemic lupus erythematosus: a report of the North American Pediatric Renal Transplant Cooperative Study. *Transplantation* 2001;72:973–978.
228. Gipson DS, Ferris ME, Dooley MA, et al. Renal transplantation in children with lupus nephritis. *Am J Kidney Dis* 2003;41:455–463.
229. Warady BA, Sullivan EK. Renal transplantation in children with sickle cell disease: a report of the North American Pediatric Renal Transplant Cooperative Study (NAPRTCS). *Pediatr Transplant* 1998;2:130–133.
230. Edvardsson VO, Kaiser BA, Polinsky MS, et al. Successful living-related renal transplantation in an adolescent with Down syndrome. *Pediatr Nephrol* 1995;9:398–399.
231. Baqi N, Tejani A, Sullivan EK. Renal transplantation in Down syndrome: a report of the North American Pediatric Renal Transplant Cooperative Study. *Pediatr Transplant* 1998;2:211–215.
232. Broyer M, Selwood N, Brunner F. Recurrence of primary renal disease on kidney graft: a European pediatric experience. *J Am Soc Nephrol* 1992;2:S255–S257.
233. Ferraris JR, Ramirez JA, Ruiz S, et al. Shiga toxin-associated hemolytic uremic syndrome: absence of recurrence after renal transplantation. *Pediatr Nephrol* 2002;17:809–814.
234. Quan A, Sullivan EK, Alexander SR. Recurrence of hemolytic uremic syndrome after renal transplantation in children: a report of the North American Pediatric Renal Transplant Cooperative Study. *Transplantation* 2001;72:742–745.
235. Betts PR, Magrath G. Growth pattern and dietary intake of children with chronic renal insufficiency. *BMJ* 1974;2:189–193.
236. Tejani A, Ingulli E. Growth in children post-transplantation and methods to optimize post-transplant growth. *Clin Transplant* 1991;5:214–218.
237. Shapiro R, Scantlebury VP, Jordan ML, et al. Pediatric renal transplantation under tacrolimus-based immunosuppression. *Transplantation* 1999;67:299–303.
238. McEnery PT, Gonzalez LL, Martin LW, et al. Growth and development of children with renal transplants. Use of alternate-day steroid therapy. *J Pediatr* 1973;83:806–814.
239. Johansson G, Sietnieks A, Janssens F, et al. Recombinant human growth hormone treatment in short children with chronic renal disease, before transplantation or with functioning renal transplants: an interim report on five European studies. *Acta Paediatr Scand* 1990;370(suppl):36–42.
240. Kaufmann S, Jones KL, Wehrenberg WB, et al. Inhibition by prednisone of growth hormone (GH) response to GH-releasing hormone in normal men. *J Clin Endocrinol Metab* 1988;67:1258–1261.
241. Rees L, Greene SA, Adlard P, et al. Growth and endocrine function after renal transplantation. *Arch Dis Child* 1988;63:1326–1332.
242. Wehrenberg WB, Janowski BA, Piering AW, et al. Glucocorticoids: potent inhibitors and stimulators of growth hormone secretion. *Endocrinology* 1990;126:3200–3203.
243. Schaefer F, Hamill G, Stanhope R, et al. Pulsatile growth hormone secretion in peripubertal patients with chronic renal failure. Cooperative Study Group on Pubertal Development in Chronic Renal Failure. *J Pediatr* 1991;119:568–577.
244. Ghio L, Tarantino A, Edefonti A, et al. Advantages of cyclosporine as sole immunosuppressive agent in children with transplanted kidneys. *Transplantation* 1992;54:834–838.
245. Ingulli E, Tejani A. An analytical review of growth hormone studies in children after renal transplantation [Review]. *Pediatr Nephrol* 1995;9:S61–S65.
246. Broyer M. Results and side-effects of treating children with growth hormone after kidney transplantation—a preliminary report. Pharmacia & Upjohn Study Group. *Acta Paediatr* 1996;417(suppl):76–79.
247. Jabs K, Van Dop C, Harmon WE. Growth hormone treatment of growth failure among children with renal transplants. *Kidney Int* 1993;43(suppl):S71–S75.
248. Chavers BM, Doherty L, Nevins TE, et al. Effects of growth hormone on kidney function in pediatric transplant recipients [Review]. *Pediatr Nephrol* 1995;9:176–181.
249. Fine RN, Stablein D, Cohen AH, et al. Recombinant human growth hormone post-renal transplantation in children: a randomized controlled study of the NAPRTCS. *Kidney Int* 2002;62:688–696.

250. Dharnidharka V, Stablein D, Harmon W. Risk of hospitalization due to infection now exceeds risk due to acute rejection at early and late time points in pediatric renal transplantation. *Am J Transplant* 2003;3(suppl 5):319.
251. Hanto DW, Frizzera G, Purtilo DT, et al. Clinical spectrum of lymphoproliferative disorders in renal transplant recipients and evidence for the role of Epstein-Barr virus. *Cancer Res* 1981;41:4253–4261.
252. Nocera A, Ghio L, Dall'Amico R, et al. De novo cancers in paediatric renal transplant recipients: a multicentre analysis within the North Italy Transplant programme (NITp), Italy. *Eur J Cancer* 2000;36:80–86.
253. Dharnidharka VR, Tejani AH, Ho PL, et al. Post-transplant lymphoproliferative disorder in the United States: young Caucasian males are at highest risk. *Am J Transplant* 2002;2:993–998.
254. Chang H, Wu JD, Cheng KK, et al. Epstein-Barr virus-associated lymphoproliferative disorders in oral cavity after heart transplantation: report of a case. *J Formos Med Assoc* 1994;93:332–336.
255. Renoult E, Aymard B, Gregoire MJ, et al. Epstein-Barr virus lymphoproliferative disease of donor origin after kidney transplantation: a case report. *Am J Kidney Dis* 1995;26:84–87.
256. Gonthier DM, Hartman G, Holley JL. Posttransplant lymphoproliferative disorder presenting as an isolated skin lesion. *Am J Kidney Dis* 1992;19:600–603.
257. Cen H, Williams PA, McWilliams HP, et al. Evidence for restricted Epstein-Barr virus latent gene expression and anti-EBNA antibody response in solid organ transplant recipients with posttransplant lymphoproliferative disorders. *Blood* 1993;81:1393–1403.
258. Delecluse HJ, Kremmer E, Rouault JP, et al. The expression of Epstein-Barr virus latent proteins is related to the pathological features of post-transplant lymphoproliferative disorders. *Am J Pathol* 1995;146:1113–1120.
259. Cox KL, Lawrence-Miyasaki LS, Garcia-Kennedy R, et al. An increased incidence of Epstein-Barr virus infection and lymphoproliferative disorder in young children on FK506 after liver transplantation. *Transplantation* 1995;59:524–529.
260. Andrews W, Sommerauer J, Roden J, et al. 10 years of pediatric liver transplantation. *J Pediatr Surg* 1996;31:619–624.
261. Walker RC, Marshall WF, Strickler JG, et al. Pretransplantation assessment of the risk of lymphoproliferative disorder. *Clin Infect Dis* 1995;20:1346–1353.
262. Cockfield SM, Preiksaitis JK, Jewell LD, et al. Post-transplant lymphoproliferative disorder in renal allograft recipients. Clinical experience and risk factor analysis in a single center. *Transplantation* 1993;56:88–96.
263. Sokal EM, Caragiozoglou T, Lamy M, et al. Epstein-Barr virus serology and Epstein-Barr virus-associated lymphoproliferative disorders in pediatric liver transplant recipients. *Transplantation* 1993;56:1394–1398.
264. Srivastava T, Zwick DL, Rothberg PG, et al. Posttransplant lymphoproliferative disorder in pediatric renal transplantation. *Pediatr Nephrol* 1999;13:748–754.
265. Swinnen LJ, Costanzo-Nordin MR, Fisher SG, et al. Increased incidence of lymphoproliferative disorder after immunosuppression with the monoclonal antibody OKT3 in cardiac-transplant recipients. *N Engl J Med* 1990;323:1723–1728.
266. Ellis D, Shapiro R, Jordan ML, et al. Comparison of FK-506 and cyclosporine regimens in pediatric renal transplantation. *Pediatr Nephrol* 1994;8:193–200.
267. Kenagy DN, Schlesinger Y, Weck K, et al. Epstein-Barr virus DNA in peripheral blood leukocytes of patients with posttransplant lymphoproliferative disease. *Transplantation* 1995;60:547–554.
268. Campe H, Jaeger G, Abou-Ajram C, et al. Serial detection of Epstein-Barr virus DNA in sera and peripheral blood leukocyte samples of pediatric renal allograft recipients with persistent mononucleosis-like symptoms defines patients at risk to develop post-transplant lymphoproliferative disease. *Pediatr Transplant* 2003;7:46–52.
269. Gupta M, Filler G, Kovesi T, et al. Quantitative tissue polymerase chain reaction for Epstein-Barr virus in pediatric solid organ recipients. *Am J Kidney Dis* 2003;41:212–219.
270. Jabs WJ, Hennig H, Kittel M, et al. Normalized quantification by real-time PCR of Epstein-Barr virus load in patients at risk for posttransplant lymphoproliferative disorders. *J Clin Microbiol* 2001;39:564–569.
271. Wagner HJ, Wessel M, Jabs W, et al. Patients at risk for development of posttransplant lymphoproliferative disorder: plasma versus peripheral blood mononuclear cells as material for quantification of Epstein-Barr viral load by using real-time quantitative polymerase chain reaction. *Transplantation* 2001;72:1012–1019.
272. Rooney CM, Loftin SK, Holladay MS, et al. Early identification of Epstein-Barr virus-associated post-transplantation lymphoproliferative disease. *Br J Haematol* 1995;89:98–103.
273. Falco DA, Nepomuceno RR, Krams SM, et al. Identification of Epstein-Barr virus-specific CD8+ T lymphocytes in the circulation of pediatric transplant recipients. *Transplantation* 2002;74:501–510.
274. Shroff R, Trompeter R, Cubitt D, et al. Epstein-Barr virus monitoring in paediatric renal transplant recipients. *Pediatr Nephrol* 2002;17:770–775.
275. Harris KM, Schwartz ML, Slasky BS, et al. Posttransplantation cyclosporine-induced lymphoproliferative disorders: clinical and radiologic manifestations. *Radiology* 1987;162:697–700.
276. Chen JM, Barr ML, Chadburn A, et al. Management of lymphoproliferative disorders after cardiac transplantation. *Ann Thorac Surg* 1993;56:527–538.
277. Taguchi Y, Purtilo DT, Okano M. The effect of intravenous immunoglobulin and interferon-alpha on Epstein-Barr virus-induced lymphoproliferative disorder in a liver transplant recipient. *Transplantation* 1994;57:1813–1815.
278. Shapiro RS, Chauvenet A, McGuire W, et al. Treatment of B-cell lymphoproliferative disorders with interferon alfa and intravenous gamma globulin [Letter]. *N Engl J Med* 1988; 318:1334.
279. Pirsch JD, Stratta RJ, Sollinger HW, et al. Treatment of severe Epstein-Barr virus-induced lymphoproliferative syndrome with ganciclovir: two cases after solid organ transplantation. *Am J Med* 1989;86:241–244.
280. Davis CL, Harrison KL, McVicar JP, et al. Antiviral prophylaxis and the Epstein Barr virus-related post-transplant lymphoproliferative disorder. *Clin Transplant* 1995;9:53–59.
281. Herman J, Vandenberghe P, van den Heuvel I, et al. Successful treatment with rituximab of lymphoproliferative disorder in a child after cardiac transplantation. *J Heart Lung Transplant* 2002;21:1304–1309.

282. Berney T, Delis S, Kato T, et al. Successful treatment of posttransplant lymphoproliferative disease with prolonged rituximab treatment in intestinal transplant recipients. *Transplantation* 2002;74:1000–1006.
283. McGhee W, Mazariegos GV, Sindhi R, et al. Rituximab in the treatment of pediatric small bowel transplant patients with posttransplant lymphoproliferative disorder unresponsive to standard treatment. *Transplant Proc* 2002;34:955–956.
284. Serinet MO, Jacquemin E, Habes D, et al. Anti-CD20 monoclonal antibody (rituximab) treatment for Epstein-Barr virus-associated, B-cell lymphoproliferative disease in pediatric liver transplant recipients. *J Pediatr Gastroenterol Nutr* 2002;34:389–393.
285. Dotti G, Rambaldi A, Fiocchi R, et al. Anti-CD20 antibody (rituximab) administration in patients with late occurring lymphomas after solid organ transplant. *Haematologica* 2001;86:618–623.
286. Balfour H, Jr., Chace BA, Stapleton JT, et al. A randomized, placebo-controlled trial of oral acyclovir for the prevention of cytomegalovirus disease in recipients of renal allografts. *N Engl J Med* 1989;320:1381–1387.
287. Schmidt GM, Horak DA, Niland JC, et al. A randomized, controlled trial of prophylactic ganciclovir for cytomegalovirus pulmonary infection in recipients of allogeneic bone marrow transplants. The City of Hope-Stanford-Syntex CMV Study Group. *N Engl J Med* 1991;324:1005–1011.
288. Ahsan N, Holman MJ, Yang HC. Efficacy of oral ganciclovir in prevention of cytomegalovirus infection in post-kidney transplant patients. *Clin Transplant* 1997;11:633–639.
289. Brennan DC, Garlock KA, Singer GG, et al. Prophylactic oral ganciclovir compared with deferred therapy for control of cytomegalovirus in renal transplant recipients. *Transplantation* 1997;64:1843–1846.
290. Pescovitz MD, Brook B, Jindal RM, et al. Oral ganciclovir in pediatric transplant recipients: a pharmacokinetic study. *Clin Transplant* 1997;11:613–617.
291. Harmon WE. Opportunistic infections in children following renal transplantation [Review]. *Pediatr Nephrol* 1991;5:118–125.
292. Lynfield R, Herrin JT, Rubin RH. Varicella in pediatric renal transplant recipients. *Pediatrics* 1992;90:216–220.
293. Kashtan CE, Cook M, Chavers BM, et al. Outcome of chickenpox in 66 pediatric renal transplant recipients. *J Pediatr* 1997;131:874–877.
294. Broyer M, Tete MJ, Guest G, et al. Varicella and zoster in children after kidney transplantation: long-term results of vaccination. *Pediatrics* 1997;99:35–39.
295. Zamora I, Simon JM, Da Silva ME, et al. Attenuated varicella virus vaccine in children with renal transplants. *Pediatr Nephrol* 1994;8:190–192.
296. Prat V, Horcickova M, Matousovic K, et al. Urinary tract infection in renal transplant patients. *Infection* 1985;13:207–210.
297. Peterson PK, Ferguson R, Fryd DS, et al. Infectious diseases in hospitalized renal transplant recipients: a prospective study of a complex and evolving problem. *Medicine* 1982;61:360–372.
298. Drachenberg CB, Beskow CO, Cangro CB, et al. Human polyoma virus in renal allograft biopsies: morphological findings and correlation with urine cytology. *Hum Pathol* 1999;30:970–977.
299. Ginevri F, De Santis R, Comoli P, et al. Polyomavirus BK infection in pediatric kidney-allograft recipients: a single-center analysis of incidence, risk factors, and novel therapeutic approaches. *Transplantation* 2003;75:1266–1270.
300. Ding R, Medeiros M, Dadhania D, et al. Noninvasive diagnosis of BK virus nephritis by measurement of messenger RNA for BK virus VP1 in urine. *Transplantation* 2002;74:987–994.
301. Baluarte HJ, Gruskin AB, Ingelfinger JR, et al. Analysis of hypertension in children post renal transplantation—a report of the North American Pediatric Renal Transplant Cooperative Study (NAPRTCS). *Pediatr Nephrol* 1994;8:570–573.
302. Morgan H, Khan I, Hashmi A, et al. Ambulatory blood pressure monitoring after renal transplantation in children. *Pediatr Nephrol* 2001;16:843–847.
303. Sorof JM, Poffenbarger T, Portman R. Abnormal 24-hour blood pressure patterns in children after renal transplantation. *Am J Kidney Dis* 2000;35:681–686.
304. Wigger M, Druckler E, Muscheites J, et al. Course of glomerular filtration rate after renal transplantation and the influence of hypertension. *Clin Nephrol* 2001;56:S30–S34.
305. Mitsnefes MM, Schwartz SM, Daniels SR, et al. Changes in left ventricular mass index in children and adolescents after renal transplantation. *Pediatr Transplant* 2001;5:279–284.
306. Mitsnefes MM, Omoloja A, McEnery PT. Short-term pediatric renal transplant survival: blood pressure and allograft function. *Pediatr Transplant* 2001;5:160–165.
307. Lilien MR, Stroes ES, Op't Roodt J, et al. Vascular function in children after renal transplantation. *Am J Kidney Dis* 2003;41:684–691.
308. Shin GT, Cheigh JS, Riggio RR, et al. Effect of nifedipine on renal allograft function and survival beyond one year. *Clin Nephrol* 1997;47:33–36.
309. Cohen LS, Friedman EA. Losartan-induced azotemia in a diabetic recipient of a kidney transplant [Letter]. *N Engl J Med* 1996;334:1271–1272.
310. Grekas D, Dioudis C, Kalevrosoglou I, et al. Renal hemodynamics in hypertensive renal allograft recipients: effects of calcium antagonists and ACE inhibitors. *Kidney Int* 1996;55 (suppl):S97–S100.
311. Harris KP, Russell GI, Parvin SD, et al. Alterations in lipid and carbohydrate metabolism attributable to cyclosporin A in renal transplant recipients. *BMJ* 1986;292:16.
312. Raine AE. Cardiovascular complications after renal transplantation. In: Morris PJ, ed. *Kidney transplantation: principles and practice*. Philadelphia: WB Saunders, 1994:339–355.
313. Vathsala A, Weinberg RB, Schoenberg L, et al. Lipid abnormalities in cyclosporine-prednisone-treated renal transplant recipients. *Transplantation* 1989;48:37–43.
314. Drueke TB, Abdulmassih Z, Lacour B, et al. Atherosclerosis and lipid disorders after renal transplantation [Review]. *Kidney Int* 1991;31(suppl):S24–S28.
315. Singh A, Tejani C, Benfield M, et al. Natural history of lipid abnormalities in children post-transplantation. The 16th annual meeting of the American Society of Transplant Physicians, Chicago, 1997(abst).
316. Grundy SM. HMG-CoA reductase inhibitors for treatment of hypercholesterolemia [Review]. *N Engl J Med* 1988;319:24–33.
317. Silverstein DM. Indications and outcome of treatment of hyperlipidemia in pediatric allograft recipients. *Pediatr Transplant* 2003;7:7–10.

318. Hricik DE, Bartucci MR, Moir EJ, et al. Effects of steroid withdrawal on posttransplant diabetes mellitus in cyclosporine-treated renal transplant recipients. *Transplantation* 1991; 51:374–377.
319. Al-Uzri A, Stablein DM, A Cohn R. Posttransplant diabetes mellitus in pediatric renal transplant recipients: a report of the North American Pediatric Renal Transplant Cooperative Study (NAPRTCS). *Transplantation* 2001;72: 1020–1024.
320. Ferraresso M, Ghio L, Edefonti A, et al. Conversion from cyclosporine to tacrolimus in pediatric kidney transplant recipients. *Pediatr Nephrol* 2002;17:664–667.
321. Butani L, Makker SP. Conversion from tacrolimus to Neoral for postrenal transplant diabetes. *Pediatr Nephrol* 2000;15: 176–178.
322. Meyers KE, Weiland H, Thomson PD. Paediatric renal transplantation non-compliance. *Pediatr Nephrol* 1995;9: 189–192.
323. Beck DE, Fennell RS, Yost RL, et al. Evaluation of an educational program on compliance with medication regimens in pediatric patients with renal transplants. *J Pediatr* 1980;96: 1094–1097.
324. Ettenger RB, Rosenthal JT, Marik JL, et al. Improved cadaveric renal transplant outcome in children. *Pediatr Nephrol* 1991;5:137–142.
325. Foulkes LM, Boggs SR, Fennell RS, et al. Social support, family variables, and compliance in renal transplant children. *Pediatr Nephrol* 1993;7:185–188.
326. Bell F. Post-renal transplant compliance. *Journal Child Health Care* 2000;4:5–9.
327. Blowey DL, Hebert D, Arbus GS, et al. Compliance with cyclosporine in adolescent renal transplant recipients. *Pediatr Nephrol* 1997;11:547–551.
328. Fennell RS, Foulkes LM, Boggs SR. Family-based program to promote medication compliance in renal transplant children. *Transplant Proc* 1994;26:102–103.
329. Apajasalo M, Rautonen J, Sintonen H, et al. Health-related quality of life after organ transplantation in childhood. *Pediatr Transplant* 1997;1:130–137.
330. Kim MS, Jabs K, Harmon WE. Long-term patient survival in a pediatric renal transplantation program. *Transplantation* 1991;51:413–416.
331. Morel P, Almond PS, Matas AJ, et al. Long-term quality of life after kidney transplantation in childhood. *Transplantation* 1991;52:47–53.
332. Potter DE, Najarian J, Belzer F, et al. Long-term results of renal transplantation in children. *Kidney Int* 1991;40:752–756.
333. Ehrich JH, Rizzoni G, Broyer M, et al. Rehabilitation of young adults during renal replacement therapy in Europe. 2. Schooling, employment, and social situation. *Nephrol Dial Transplant* 1992;7:579–586.

74

ETHICAL CONSIDERATIONS

MICHEL J. C. BROYER

Many ethical considerations arise in the clinical practice of pediatric nephrology. Issues range from the appropriate use of modern-day molecular genetic technology in renal diagnostics to choice of therapies in children with retracting symptoms and/or progressive renal failure.

PRINCIPLES

Medical ethics is based on three well-established principles. *First,* the benevolence/nonmalevolence interpretation of the *primum non nocere* principle of the Hippocratic corpus must be used. This states that, in any given case, treatment must confer net benefit over harm, a calculation that is not always readily apparent. *Second,* the principle of autonomy mandates appropriate informed consent. This requires that not only the parents but also the child as much as possible have accurate information, knowledge of possible alternatives, and general understanding, and that their comprehension be confirmed. *Third,* the principle of justice must be constantly applied. This means that equal access to optimal levels of care must be available—abrogation of the rights of some to satisfy the needs of others cannot be condoned.

In addition to following these principles, one also must take into account the impact of cultural, religious, and legal factors that may affect medical decisions. The application of these principles is far from straightforward in most clinical settings. In many cases, the answer to an ethical question may be controversial, with well-developed and contrary positions effectively presented.

From a global perspective, it is obvious that ethics must take into account international conventions and existing national laws. Fundamental is the United Nations Convention for the Rights of Children, which reinforces the human dignity of children and seeks respect for children by endorsing the principle of nondiscrimination and always working in the best interest of the child with his or her participation (1).

ETHICS AND CLINICAL RESEARCH

Research involving human subjects must follow strict rules that originated with the Nuremberg Code and the Declaration of Helsinki. Regularly revised guidelines have been adopted and issued by the World Health Organization. In many countries, national laws define the investigator's obligations in clinical research. Besides these regulations, research on humans must also take into account a series of ethical principles well summarized by Beauchamp and Childress in 1979 (2): First, acknowledge the dignity and the autonomy of individuals with special protection for potentially vulnerable populations such as children. Second, ascertain that the risks always be justified by the expected benefits of the research. Third, research should not involve persons from groups that are unlikely to benefit from subsequent applications of the research. These principles carry strong moral imperatives. Difficult ethical dilemmas may arise when they conflict, which appropriately result in the abandonment of the proposed project.

In the United States, the protection of human subjects is defined in the Code of Federal Regulations (3), and the protocol for any federally sponsored research project involving human subjects must first be submitted to the Office for Human Subject Research, which determines if an Institutional Review Board review is required. The protocol is then submitted to the Institutional Review Board, which approves, disapproves, or requests modifications. A similar process is followed in other countries. In France, for example, a law was enacted in 1988 (4) requiring that all research projects involving human subjects be approved by the Committee for the Protection of Persons Submitted to Biomedical Research. Children, in particular, are protected from research not yielding a direct benefit. Such research is permitted only if the following three conditions are met: (a) there is no foreseeable serious risk to subjects, (b) results are potentially useful specifically for children, and (c) the information yielded could not readily be obtained by other means. In addition, any indemnity is forbidden. The informed consent of the parents (and the child, if possible) is required. In the United Kingdom, the active informed consent of those older than 16 years of age is mandatory.

In conclusion, before any research project involving children is contemplated, the appropriate answers must be given to five questions well formulated by Alderson (5):

1. Are children likely to suffer any harm as a result of the research in the form of emotional distress or intrusion?
2. Do the benefits of the research clearly outweigh these possible risks?
3. Who will benefit from the research: children or only the researchers?
4. Are children given the proper information about the research?
5. Are children offered the opportunity to refuse to participate or to answer particular questions?

ETHICS AND GENETICS TESTING

The application of functional genomics to kidney diseases creates controversies in the assessment of information provided to patients and possible interventions. This is a particularly complex area that has been extensively reviewed (6). National regulations have been developed concerning genetic testing. The intent behind these regulations is to respect the privacy of any tested individual and to limit the practice of testing in children to special situations. Informed consent is mandatory, because results may have serious impact on the individual, especially when asymptomatic disease with possible severe clinical evolution and the risk of transmission to descendants is identified. With regard to children, because no therapies may be available to prevent the development or progression of disease, it may be argued that the negative impact of a "genetic diagnosis" is serious enough to warrant limiting genetic testing to situations in which the child or the child's family may derive a direct benefit from immediate curative or preventive measures. In France, for example, genetic testing of children is legally forbidden if this latter criterion is not fulfilled. It is still debatable, however, whether yearly renal investigation throughout childhood and adolescence is preferable to genetic testing in individuals at risk for an inherited disease such as nephronophthisis. Another important point to emphasize is that the results of genetic tests must not be delivered directly to the patient by a testing laboratory. It is mandatory that a knowledgeable physician provide and interpret test results as part of the physician-patient relationship. In addition, any patient may accept or refuse to know the results; the subject has the right not to know, a consequence of respecting the patient's autonomy. Results concerning other members of the family are protected by medical confidentiality, and test results must be given to each individual separately.

In the area of genetic renal diseases, it is best that a multidisciplinary team (i.e., pediatrician, genetic counselor, geneticist, social worker, mental health professional) be involved with pediatric patients and their families.

CLINICAL EXAMPLES: ETHICAL DILEMMAS

Antenatally Detected Abnormalities of the Urinary Tract

Routine fetal sonography is able to detect important renal abnormalities such as kidney agenesis, cystic or dysplastic kidneys, or obstructive uropathy (7). Kidney morphology and the volume of amniotic fluid may be assessed. Studies of the composition of amniotic fluid may provide additional information, but further studies are needed to determine the true value of such assessment. Communication with parents requires the constant participation of the several specialists involved: radiologist, obstetrician, and pediatric nephrologist. In the case of urinary obstruction *in utero,* intervention has been extremely disappointing to date. New data concerning the prevention of neonatal death (due to pulmonary hypoplasia) by amniotic fluid infusion deserve comment. In the case of severe oligoaminos, ethical rationale would consider the risk of fetal intervention justified in view of the 93% mortality rate, acknowledging, of coarse, the futility of such an intervention should exclusion criteria exist, such as chromosomal abnormalities, renal agenesia, or presumed irreversible renal damage (8). This may be particularly true if exclusion criteria such as chromosomal abnormalities, renal agenesi, or presumed irreversible renal damage are met. In these cases, after full information is disclosed, parents may opt for pregnancy termination when legally allowed. Others have argued that the present possibilities of neonatal dialysis and early transplantation may not warrant these exclusions. As is noted later in this chapter, this raises ethical questions regarding renal replacement therapy (RRT) in neonates.

Amnioinfusion with saline or, preferably, lactated Ringer solution to prevent or limit lung hypoplasia, a consequence of oligohydramnios (9), is an extreme approach that seems effective in limiting lung hypoplasia and the development of Potter syndrome. It does not modify the renal disease. Amnioinfusion, an experimental therapy, is performed only with the fully informed consent of the parents in a decision made together with the obstetrician, perinatologists, and pediatric nephrologist.

Renal Insufficiency in Premature Babies

Renal insufficiency is not uncommon in the very-low-birth-weight premature infant. Peritoneal dialysis is best adapted to this situation given the very large ratio of peritoneal surface area to body weight, but in some cases such infants have been treated with hemodialysis or hemofiltration. The ideal case to treat is the very-low-birth-weight infant with acute reversible renal insufficiency without structural renal abnormalities secondary to toxic or ischemic vasomotor nephropathy. An association with other major renal parenchymal damage or multiorgan abnormalities clearly represents a contraindication for intervention in most pediatric nephrology centers worldwide. In a review, Coulthard and Vernon (10) reported survival of 13 infants out of 21 with a birth weight lower than 1 kg, and of 2 infants out of 4 with a birth weight between 1.0 and 1.5 kg.

Such expensive and labor- and resource-intensive therapy raises serious ethical issues: Is it considered unacceptable overtreating, or, if treatment is withheld, is it nonassistance to an endangered individual? As stated by Coulthard, the choice is between certain death and a slight chance of survival, and for many, death will occur at a later date. Is such treatment an act of cruelty for families whose hopes have been raised only to be dashed, or alternatively is it a welcome opportunity to relate, bringing greater meaning to a life, albeit for a brief period? In such cases, the principles of benevolence and nonmalevolence can support either treatment option. In any specific case, the actual course of action is determined only with the active involvement of parents and all members of the health care delivery team, with constant and consistent communication.

ETHICAL PROBLEMS IN THE TREATMENT OF END-STAGE RENAL DISEASE IN CHILDREN

Treatment by dialysis was first selectively applied to adult patients in the mid-1960s. It was difficult at the time even to imagine that children could be treated using this modality. The prospect of performing kidney transplantation with some success and the dramatic technical progress in vascular access and dialysis modalities changed this attitude, and in the 1970s specialized centers started to accept children into dialysis and transplant programs. At the time, this approach was criticized by certain pediatricians, mental health professionals, and others, who considered it unethical to submit children to such difficult treatments. Nevertheless, from that time onward, desperate parents almost always chose to save their children through dialysis, even though the long-term effects (complications, long-term survival, quality of life) were still unknown. With advances in therapy, it is now clear that most if not all children reaching end-stage renal failure may benefit from RRT as routine treatment. Such therapy, although expensive and labor intensive, is usually compatible with survival and a satisfactory quality of life, as measured by a variety of methodologies. Indeed, if parents actively refused such intervention in the United States, they would immediately be subject to acute investigation for possible child endangerment.

End-Stage Renal Disease in Newborns and Infants

End-stage renal disease (ESRD) in newborns still presents a series of ethical challenges. Two possibilities clinically lead to different courses of action: bilateral renal agenesis and kidney malfunction in the presence of renal parenchyma. In the first case, the decision is usually made not to initiate RRT, but this is not uniform and is discussed later. In the second instance, dialysis may be contemplated when it is believed that renal damage may be reversible; this dialysis should be initiated only with the informed consent of the parents and should continue only long enough for the diagnosis and prognosis to be established.

Newborns with Renal Agenesis or Irreversibly Damaged Kidneys

In the case of newborns with renal agenesis or irreversibly damaged kidneys, there are two possibilities: either withholding all treatment or using an aggressive approach and initiating dialysis. This is always a difficult scenario for both the parents and the medical-nursing team. The decision is made only after the parents have been fully informed. It must be clearly stated to the parents that, although dialysis and/or transplant treatment can be applied to children with some success, their use is much more difficult in an infant (11) and involves serious treatment and frequent hospitalizations during critical stages of development. Treatment is far more intensive than that for older children. In addition, success is not guaranteed, and almost all studies of this age group report significant morbidity and mortality. Long-term home therapy can be challenging for even the more motivated and intensively trained family members, who become "amateur intensivists" in the home. The consequences of this workload are serious. One of the two parents must dedicate himself or herself full time to this occupation. Family life is disrupted, and the impact on siblings, although significant, remains poorly studied. Overall, the quality of life of an infant on dialysis is far from normal due to the connection to the dialysis machine and all the necessary care. In addition to dialysis, patients also need an aggressive approach to nutrition, which usually necessitates tube or gastrostomy feeding. The overall objective is to perform kidney transplantation after 12 to 18 months of dialysis when the infant has reached at least 12 kg of real body weight. There are centers that perform kidney transplantation in very young patients with good results (12), but it must be noted that these single-center results have not been obtained in larger multicenter studies worldwide. Another concern, besides mortality, is the question of long-term quality of life, particularly neurocognitive development (13). Resource allocation becomes a major issue in countries with limited overall medical resources and health care delivery systems. Several reports have been more encouraging (14–17). A study by Warady and colleagues (16) reports the 5-year outcomes of 34 infants who were started on dialysis before 3 months of age: 6 died within the first year, 28 survived, 24 have received grafts, and only 1 had delayed psychomotor development. In this series, of the 16 who were older than 5 years of age, 15 had normal intellectual development and were at age-appropriate schooling levels. A study by Ledermann (17) reports on a series of 20 children starting dialysis within the first year of life (mean = 3.5 months) with a follow-up of 1 to 5 years. Of the 16 survivors in this series, 14 had normal psychomotor and neurocognitive development. The importance of comorbidity is nevertheless stressed: there were a number of peritoneal dialysis catheter replacements, and more than one peritonitis episode in 30% of cases. Nevertheless, the height, weight, and head circumference were not more than 1 standard deviation below the mean normal values. All these publications, however encouraging, deal with a limited number of infants treated in the first days of life and cannot be used as a compelling argument.

Attitudes of Pediatricians to the Management of End-Stage Renal Disease in Newborns and Infants

Several surveys have addressed the attitudes of pediatricians to the management of ESRD in newborns and infants. A multicenter study involving 217 pediatric nephrology centers in eight different countries was published in 1998 (18); by definition, these centers had the capacity to offer dialysis treatment to at least some infants aged 1 to 12 months. The survey asked whether the nephrologists offered RRT to any or all infants with ESRD, and, if parents refused RRT for otherwise normal children with ESRD, whether this was ever acceptable to the nephrologist. Ninety-three percent of the centers stated that they offered dialysis to some infants younger than 1 month of age; 41% offered it to all infants of this age, but 53% offered it to all children 1 to 12 months of age. The opinion of pediatric nephrologists as to the parents' right to refuse RRT for their children was varied: 50% of physicians thought that this refusal was ethically acceptable for infants younger than 1 month of age, but only 25% held this opinion in the case of infants 1 to 12 months of age. For 19% of physicians, this refusal was never acceptable for infants younger than 1 month of age, and for 38%, it was not acceptable for infants 1 to 12 months of age. Among factors influencing the decision to withhold RRT were the presence of coexistent multiorgan defects, the anticipation of morbidity for the child, the family's right to decide, and the medical staff's right to decide. Economic constraints were not an important factor; neither was the socioeconomic status of the family. There were no clear differences in the attitudes of pediatric nephrologists in different countries except for opinions concerning the right of the parents to refuse RRT, which was much less accepted in Italy and in Japan than in other countries such as Germany, the United Kingdom, and the United States.

In an additional study of 37 level 3 university neonatal units, 34 units answered a questionnaire on the attitudes concerning newborns with ESRD or preterminal ESRD who needed RRT within months or a few years (19). With regard to newborns with ESRD, 23 of 34 units refused any form of RRT, 3 were in favor, and 8 gave no opinion. In the case of newborns with preterminal ESRD, 18 accepted the idea of RRT, 3 refused it, and 13 gave no opinion. Those that did not give an opinion pointed out that the decision rested on several elements and that each case deserved an individual decision.

End-Stage Renal Disease in Children Older Than 12 Months

As mentioned earlier, for over 20 years children with ESRD have regularly received RRT in specialized centers. However, children under 5 years of age have not always been accepted into such programs. Data of the European Dialysis and Transplantation Association registry (20) reveal a progressive increase in the youngest groups of patients receiving RRT: the proportion of new patients under 2 years of age increased from 0.6 to 9.5%, and the proportion of those 2 to 5 years old increased from 4.7 to 14% from the period 1968–1973 to the period 1986–1991. In other words, in most European countries, RRT for children became progressively acceptable as a routine treatment during the 1980s. Despite this, however, initiation of dialysis in children still provokes ethical controversy. The Spanish Society of Pediatric Nephrology conducted a survey in 1998 (21) with the purpose of defining the criteria for starting RRT in children with ESRD. According to this study, 90% of pediatric nephrologists concluded that some patients ought not to receive RRT and that the main criteria for withholding this treatment were a prognosis of a short life and serious physical or neurologic defects. Fauriel et al. (22) studied via "semidirected" interviews the attitude of French pediatric nephrologists toward the decision of withholding or withdrawal of RRT. Of 20 physicians, 19 answered that withholding RRT was sometimes necessary and only 1 was absolutely against the idea. The reasons given for withholding treatment were poor quality of life, protection of the family, and avoidance of "unbearable treatment."

One of the few publications that report the withholding of RRT in children with ESRD deals with a series of patients with primary hyperoxaluria (23). In this study of 78 cases in 24 countries on three continents, 65 patients reached ESRD, and RRT was withheld from 40% for one or more reasons. The reasons were economic and organizational in 10 cases, "ethical" in 17 cases, and based on parental decision in 16 cases. Most of these children were younger than 1 year of age, and ESRD developed before the time that liver transplantation was generally advised for this indication.

Withholding or Withdrawal of Life-Sustaining Therapy: The Decision-Making Process

In the process leading to a decision to withhold or withdraw a life-saving treatment, Steinberg (24) recognized three major factors: (a) relevant medical facts, such as diagnosis, the various therapeutic options available, the potential complications, and the spectrum of short- and long-term prognosis; (b) the parent-physician relationship, with stress on the importance of an atmosphere of trust; and (c) general sociocultural, ethical, legal, and religious principles, for which consulting experts in these fields is also important. Besides these obvious factors, a number of other issues must be considered.

Quality of Life

The concept of quality of life has replaced the concept of "life at any cost." However, the definition of unacceptable quality of life is difficult to establish (25). An adult individual, even a mature adolescent, may be able to judge that his or her own quality of life is unacceptable, at least to some extent. The case of newborns unable to express themselves is challenging. In this instance, professionals and parents must have reached an agreement that the quality of life of the infant is unacceptable and without future promise. Admittedly, this assessment is subjective and could be biased. Errors are possible with regard to the diagnosis, the prognosis, the possible benefit of a treatment or its adverse effects, the complications of the disease, and the level of suffering of the child and his or her family. Because there is no precise benchmark beyond which quality of life becomes unacceptable, it is possible to imagine slippery slopes toward decisions that would be clearly unethical. Here, mention may be made of the Dutch legislation (26) permitting euthanasia and possibly leading to more or less acceptable decisions.

Parents' Role

The parents are generally in the best position to determine what is in their child's best interest. It is also the parents who bear the consequences of any decisions, more than any professional. Centralizing all decision making exclusively with the parents may lead to problems, however. Parents may sometimes make a decision that is not in the best interest of the child. In addition, an objective decision is sometimes difficult to make in the emotional context of the birth of a child with a severe medical problem. The postpartum period is often accompanied by a decreased ability to make decisions and a transitory deficit of cognitive function (27). Parents may wish to continue a treatment that has been judged as futile by the medical staff (28).

Patient's Rights, When They Apply to an Opinion Expressed by a Minor

The patient's wish may be considered only if formed by a mature adolescent who is judged to be intellectually capable. When dealing with adolescents, it is important to bear in mind the characteristics of their age: the need for privacy, independence, mobility, schooling, and the company of their peers (29). The request to withdraw from dialysis is considered ethically and legally acceptable when expressed by adults (30). Consequently, there is no formal reason to dismiss *a priori* such a request from a young patient who perceives his or her future as hopeless with no possibility of improvement. Nevertheless, caution must be exercised regarding the idea of competency. Competency should include a basic understanding of the disease and of the different treatment options, the possible hope of a transplantation, and so on. Maturity, which is acquired with age, is an important part of the decision-making capacity, permitting a value judgment on the world and the surrounding social environment so that one can situate oneself despite the handicap. In fact, maturity and competence are extremely variable at any given age. The irreversibility of the decision justifies physicians' hesitation in accepting an adolescent's request for treatment withdrawal. There is first the evaluation of the cognitive ability to give informed consent, which may have been distorted by social and familial history or by psychological trauma leading to behavior regression. Thus a 14-year-old adolescent may refuse treatment irrationally, and the physician must analyze the situation and make the necessary decision, including an eventual appeal to a psychiatrist. There are cases, however, such as one reported many years ago (31), in which a treatment deemed intolerable may be stopped at the request of an adolescent.

In the case of a minor exhibiting his or her wish to die by refusing dialysis without medical reasons, one must carefully review all information on the different modes of dialysis and the possibility and result of transplantation. It is useful to organize meetings with other adolescents in a similar situation who are being treated by dialysis or who have a functioning graft. The strategy must also be based on allowing some freedom and proposing a trial period with one of the modes of dialysis chosen by the patient; this may permit the patient to gain control of the situation and at the same time may constitute an opening toward treatment acceptance.

Professionals

Professionals have a central role in the decision process. They provide the information that is the basis for a patient's decision. It must be remembered that there are different attitudes regarding withholding treatment (32,33). One must bear in mind the obligation to be as objective as possible, to avoid lies of omission, and to provide the essential elements to permit ethical decisions to be made.

Ethics Committee

The multidisciplinary composition of ethics committees may be useful in difficult cases or those that involve conflict. Such committees are composed not only of experts in the medical field but also of psychologists, social workers, jurists, religious representatives, philosophers, and lay members of the community. Such a committee may be capable of furnishing reasonable advice and may be able to harmonize various views. Existing national advisory ethics committees may also be useful, as was the case in France, where a study examined the problems raised by intensive care of newborns with borderline medical status (34). Responsibility, discernment, and humanity were the key concepts in this report and should guide decisions on whether to withhold or withdraw a life-sustaining treatment, with the role of the parents being central in the decision process.

Legal Field

The legal field is rather complex because of differences in laws among countries. An important body of court decisions is available in the United States, developed to protect the lives of disabled children, for whom one might abandon treatment. The Baby Doe amendment (35) makes it an obligation to administer medical treatment needed by the child with the parents' agreement in all situations except the following: (a) the child is in irreversible coma; (b) treatment merely prolongs dying, does not correct all of the infant's life-threatening anomalies, and is useless in ensuring the infant's survival; and (c) such treatment would be futile in the infant and its pursuit would be inhumane.

To what extent this amendment applies to a newborn with ESRD is worth discussion, because it could be argued that an infant treated by dialysis may suffer not only from the treatment itself but also from its complications, which may render such treatment inhumane. As a matter of fact, dialysis for ESRD in newborns is one of these ambiguous situations in which contradictory points of view may be held. The decision to initiate such treatment remains controversial (35). In Europe there has been no court decision on the subject. Basic medical principles dictate that the physician is obliged to prescribe the treatment needed by the patient or, in cases without any hope, to apply palliative care. In addition, although the legal regulations generally define euthanasia as a crime, they also define as a criminal offense the exposure of a person to a risk of death. It is important to note that courts are not involved in these decisions in countries such as France or Australia (36), because, although a tribunal gives an *a priori* guarantee of objectivity, judges are less sensitive and more remote than health professionals, the latter of whom are closely connected emotionally with the treatment. In Holland, although the law defines situations allowing euthanasia, the withholding of medical treatment for a non-medical reason (e.g., social, economic, or based on quality of life) is illegal; to perform a futile medical act is also illegal.

Economic Factors

Economic factors are not usually considered a determinant among the reasons to withhold or withdraw treatment for children in developed countries. They were considered unimportant in the study of Geary (18) and are completely absent in the Spanish survey (21). Nevertheless, it remains true that use of a dialysis program in newborns and infants is associated with a number of days of hospitalization, requires more nurses and physicians for a nonguaranteed result, and is associated with a death rate that may be as high as 20 to 30%. This cost is at present covered by many government programs in the Western world but presents severe problems in other countries. In some areas, allocation of resources must be based on priorities (37). It may be argued that in poor countries priority must be given to preventive and therapeutic measures that offer a basic level of health care to large numbers of individuals at low cost and that expensive treatments which benefit only a small number of the population cannot even be considered.

Development of Recommendations Concerning Withholding or Withdrawal of Renal Replacement Therapy

General Case

In recent years, the question of withholding or withdrawing life-support treatment has been discussed largely in neonatology, with the elaboration of a regulated approach, following a consensus, as in the United Kingdom or France.

In the United Kingdom, the recommendations of the Royal College of Paediatrics and Child Health lists five situations justifying withholding or withdrawing treatment (38): (a) brain death, (b) irreversible vegetative state, (c) the no-chance situation, in which treatment will merely delay death and will offer no significant relief from the suffering caused by the disease, (d) the no-purpose situation, in which treatment may be life saving but will leave the child with a degree of mental or physical impairment so great that the quality of life for the child is without hope of improvement, and (e) the unbearable situation, in which additional treatment may only cause further suffering.

Along with these recommendations, some other considerations were noted: first, expert palliative care must be provided when curative treatment is withheld; and, second, good communication with the parents is needed at the time of the decision to withhold treatment. It is also necessary to provide appropriate measures for the parents after the death of their child. A survey of the application of these recommendations (39) showed their soundness.

In France, neonatologists have developed principles concerning withholding or withdrawing treatment in the newborn, simultaneously with the Comité Consultatif National d'Ethique (National Consulting Committee on Ethics) (33). The consensual document published by the Federation of French Neonatologists (40) mainly insisted on the need for an organized process with several steps. The first is discussion of the case, with the participation of medical and nursing staff and other experts, which may lead to a conclusion. The second step is to inform the parents, with the notion (extremely strong in France) that parents must not be left alone to make a decision and that their agreement to a possible decision to end life by withholding or withdrawing treatment must be obtained over time and with the attempt to avoid a situation in which the parents are obliged to bear the weight of this decision. Third is the final decision taken in a measured way by experienced professionals, with the whole staff participating in or being informed of the decision.

Specific Case of End-Stage Renal Disease in Children

Recommendations for starting dialysis in children with ESRD were elaborated by the Spanish Society of Pediatric Nephrology (41). In what follows, articles dealing with withholding or withdrawal are given in italics.

1. All pediatric patients receiving dialysis must meet the following criteria:
   - The patient must be diagnosed with ESRD.
   - Informed consent must be given by the parents or the legal guardian.
   - The patient must have real possibilities for kidney transplantation.
   - There must be a reasonable expectation that the patient will enjoy an acceptable quality of life during dialysis therapy and after kidney transplantation.
   - The patient and the parent(s) or guardian(s) must demonstrate a willingness to participate in and cooperate with the dialysis procedure and follow medical advice.
2. Patients with irreversible diseases that make survival extremely unlikely will not be considered as candidates for dialysis.
3. Those patients meeting the criteria stated in guideline 1 will not be refused dialysis treatment for economic, social, or psychological reasons, nor will age, sex, race, or physical handicap be taken into consideration.
4. Dialysis treatment will not be withdrawn against the wishes of the parent(s) or guardian(s).
5. The cessation of dialysis will be considered if results are not satisfactory or it is certain that results will not improve. A decision to stop treatment must always be made with the agreement of the responsible physician, the patient, and the parenr(s) or guardian(s).

Recommendations for withholding or withdrawing dialysis have been published for adult patients (42); these recommendations are not appropriate for children. Except for newborns with isolated renal failure, it is always in cases where ESRD is associated with other serious medical problems (e.g., malignant disease at the last stage, severe neurologic disease) that the issue is raised. It is not possible to foresee all the situations in which the question of whether to perform RRT will arise. As was proposed by the Royal College of Paediatrics and Child Health and the Federation of French Neonatologists, it would be reasonable that such a decision follow a stepwise process, with the best interests of the child kept in mind. This process might be summarized as follows:

1. Gather all elements of the medical history and discuss the details with the different relevant experts, especially neurologists, to determine as precisely as possible the life prognosis, as well as the functional prognosis, with consideration of the quality of life in the short and long term and acknowledgment that some subjectivity may enter into the discussion. In this analysis, the participation of the nursing staff is necessary. The conclusion must be noted in the medical file.
2. Discuss the severity of the case with the family and obtain their agreement for withholding or withdrawal of treatment. This is sometimes possible only after several meetings involving other professionals such as the family's general practitioner or a religious representative.
3. In case of disagreement or conflict, propose that a second opinion be obtained from another group or physician in the same specialty.
4. The advice of an ethical committee may be useful at this stage.
5. If the parents continue to ask that treatment be continued against the physician's recommendation, the problem is difficult, and there is no rule that can prevail absolutely. Some physicians stick to their decisions and are ready to stop a treatment considered to be unethical; others believe they should follow the parents' request, even if it opposes their own feelings.
6. Special cases:
   a. Adolescent requesting withdrawal from dialysis: This request is to be considered in context and cannot be accepted unless the conditions of intellectual competence, possession of appropriate information, and maturity are present.
   b. Newborn in ESRD: This case is controversial, and the process described earlier can be applied only in a situation involving trained medical and nursing staff and availability of the necessary medical equipment. It could be useful to show the parents other babies receiving dialysis and also to have them meet other parents who have been faced with a similar situation and are willing to discuss their experience.

In conclusion, pediatric nephrologists are sometimes faced with the question of withholding or withdrawing dialysis in children with ESRD in special situations. It is always a difficult decision, given that opposing positions (43,44) may be put forward. This is another example of a common dilemma of medical ethics in which there are no ready-made answers.

SOME ETHICAL ISSUES IN PEDIATRIC KIDNEY TRANSPLANTATION

Among a number of ethical questions related to kidney transplantation, several issues have been selected for discussion in this chapter: indications and contraindications for transplantation, informed consent, the priority of children on the waiting list, the living donor approach, and the use of commercial donors.

Appropriateness of Contraindications

Rereading the textbooks written in the 1980s and 1990s, one finds that contraindication to transplantation in children was considered justified in cases involving disabilities, some diseases such as oxalosis, or infection with human immunodeficiency virus (HIV).

Today, most of these contraindications are disappearing. Disabilities per se are not an ethically acceptable reason for denying access to transplantation. For example, a number of trisomic patients have successfully received grafts (45). The prognosis of primary oxaluria, previously associated with a constant recurrence in the graft and severe associated extrarenal pathology due to oxalate accumulation, has been completely changed by combined liver-kidney transplantation. HIV infection, aggravated by the effects of immunosuppressors and, in any case, having a poor prognosis, today may be treated effectively by means of triple antiviral therapy and thus is no longer an absolute contraindication (46).

In fact, when a possible contraindication to kidney transplantation in a child is discussed, the individual case deserves to be examined in depth from an ethical point of view. The answer should be given after considering the three basic principles of medical ethics: Do the benefits expected from transplantation clearly outweigh the negative effects? Do the parents and, if possible, the patient still agree after full information has been provided? Is distributive justice contradicted? A reasonable balance must be achieved between protecting the health of the patient and not wasting valuable organs. Today, there probably remains only a very small number of cases for which a contraindication persists—those patients with a short life expectancy or those with very severe brain damage, for example.

Pediatric Priority

Pediatricians have worked in many countries to obtain priority for children on transplantation waiting lists. This has been the case in France since 1997 (47).

From an ethical point of view, some are opposed to granting any kind of priority because it would breach one of the basic principles concerning distributive justice. There is a valid reason for violating this principle, however: childhood is a very special time in the life of human beings during which education and socialization are developmentally necessary for the individual to reach an acceptable adult level. Only a successful transplantation allows completion of these developmental tasks; long periods on dialysis have been associated with the irreversible loss of both education and socialization (48).

Informed Consent

For at least two decades it has been clear that kidney transplantation is the best therapeutic modality for children with ESRD. Nevertheless, the decision to perform this treatment cannot be made without the informed consent of the parents and the child, depending on his or her age. The main potential complications, including the risk of death, must be described, even if they occur relatively rarely these days, and the need for medical follow-up and for indefinite immunosuppressive treatment must be made clear. Provision of a written document that summarizes the oral information is part of good practice. The information given to the child should of course be adapted to his or her level of understanding. Refusal of transplantation, especially by an adolescent, must be respected until the time that he or she may be more willing to accept it, such as after further information is provided or the individual experiences dialysis. Consent during adolescence is especially mandatory, because compliance with the medical treatment is crucial.

Living Donor

First, one must remember that to take a kidney from a healthy individual breaches the basic principle of Hippocratic medicine, the *primum non nocere*. To do so is possible only when the benefits to the recipient are considered to outweigh the harm to the donor. Consequently, physicians must always keep this balance in mind before making such a decision. For this purpose, a strict protocol must be applied. In the process of live donor transplantation, the initial information given by the physicians is of major importance because it greatly influences the individual who receives it. So that complete autonomy is respected, the initial information must be neutral and must not present the use of a live donor as the best approach when a cadaver program is also available. The recommendations of working groups, such as the consensus statement of the National Kidney Foundation and the American Society of Transplantation (49), are useful and stress the fact that the live donor must be competent, must be willing to donate free of any form of coercion, must be medically and psychologically suitable, and must be fully informed of the risks to himself or herself and the risks and benefits to the recipient, as well as of the available treatment alternatives. It is the physician's duty to verify the correct understanding of the information, especially when the family is from another country and does not speak the same language as the medical staff. It is also important to double-check the consent using a multidisciplinary approach involving the nurses, psychologist, and so on. If a risk factor for the donor is identified at the time of evaluation, the risk-benefit balance must be carefully considered, with the idea that it is better not to take any supplementary risk involving a donor. This point of view is challenged by some "ethicists," who claim that donor autonomy must be respected nonetheless and that physicians may only act as the service providers. From an ethical point of view, if the risk—even a seemingly suicidal one—taken by the donor might still be considered ethically legitimate in the aim of alleviating the suffering of another, it remains that the intervention can only be accomplished at the hands of the doctor who must obey his or her own moral principles, as well as the professional code of ethics, which states that one can not be the instrument of injury to others.

Nonrelated Living Donor

Recently, a new donor category has emerged, especially in the United States: the altruistic donor (50). The altruistic donor decides to give a kidney to an unknown individual without expecting any reward. He or she may be considered a kind of holy person, and from an ethical point of view there may be no opposition to such a decision. The real issue lies in the certainty of this decision. An in-depth psychosocial evaluation is needed before such donors are used. Very few donors were ultimately retained in the first such series (50). Altruistic organ donation for a child raises the problem of hidden commerce, which it is never completely possible to exclude.

Commercial Donor

Commercial organ donation is universally banned by the Transplant Society, the European Dialysis and Transplant Association, the World Health Organization, and the Council of Europe, and is illegal under national laws almost everywhere because it is ethically unacceptable. Unfortunately, however, commerce in human kidneys exists in several countries and is actively (though on a limited basis) taking place in Europe. Most worrying is the fact that some self-defined ethicists as well as some physicians have recently defended this commerce. Their arguments hold that the principle that "the body cannot be sold" is obsolete because the world is ruled by the marketplace. They respond to the argument that such donors are compelled by abject misery by proposing to let people be free. To the argument that such a practice will benefit mainly the rich, they respond that this is also true for other areas of medical activity and could be solved by creating a central agency. To the risk of hidden viral contaminations, they propose multiplication of screening procedures. And to the suggestion that commercial organ donation may evolve into a criminal activity, they reply that that is the work of the police. It appears easy to supply a reply to all these arguments. Then why is the commerce in organs unethical? Because converting human beings into products will undermine the fundamental values requisite both for respect of others and for self-esteem. In addition, the organ trade is likely to take unfair advantage of poor people and poor countries, and will do nothing to solve the problem of poverty. It will alter the attitude of society toward medical professionals, with the development of suspicion and loss of respect (51). Thus, we must remember that the ends (*of increasing kidney transplantation*) do not justify the means (*for obtaining organs*).

CONCLUSION

Although ethical considerations are a part of any medical act, the most significant questions deal with the treatment of ESRD in children. Even if technically feasible, dialysis may not be appropriate, and transplantation may create more harm than benefits. There is no definitive answer to ethical dilemmas, which require multidisciplinary teamwork with the participation of the parents and the child. The best interests of the child must always be the primary consideration.

ACKNOWLEDGMENT

I am indebted to Louise Taylor, who revised the language of the manuscript.

REFERENCES

1. Convention for the Rights of the Child UNICEF (2000) [Web site]. Available at: http://www.unicef.org/crc/convention.htm.
2. Beauchamp T, Childress J. *Principles of biomedical ethics.* New York: Oxford University Press, 1979.
3. Code of Federal Regulations (2002) [Web site]. Available at: http://ohsr.od.nih.gov/info/ainfo_1.php3.
4. *Guide pratique. Loi du 20 décembre 1988 modifiée sur la protection des personnes qui se prêtent aux recherches biomédicales.* Paris: Doin, 1995.
5. Alderson P. *Listening to children: children, ethics and social research.* London: Barnados, 1995.
6. Kielstein R, Sass HM. Genetics: ethical issues in kidney disease. In: Levinsky N, ed. *Ethics and the kidney.* London: Oxford University Press, 2001:167–182.
7. Colodny AH. Antenatal diagnosis and management of urinary abnormalities. *Pediatr Clin North Am* 1987;34:1365–1381.
8. Freedman AL, Johnson MP, Gonzalez R. Fetal therapy for obstructive uropathy: Past present...future? *Pediatr Nephrol* 2000;14:167–176.
9. Cameron T, Lupton PA, Farquarson D, et al. Amnioinfusion in renal agenesis. *Obstet Gynecol* 1994;83:872–876.
10. Coulthard MG, Vernon B. Managing acute renal failure in very low birth weight infants. *Arch Dis Child Fetal Neonatal Ed* 1995;73:F187–F192.

11. Bunchman TE. The ethics of infant dialysis. *Perit Dial Int* 1996;16(suppl 1):S505–S508.
12. Najarian JS, Almond PS, Mauer M, et al. Renal transplantation in the first year of life, the treatment of choice for infants with end stage renal disease. *J Am Soc Nephrol* 1992;2:S228–S233.
13. Currier C. Ethical issues in the neonatal patient with end stage renal disease. *J Perinat Neonatal Nurs* 1994;8:74–78.
14. Honda M, Kamiyama Y, Kawamura K, et al. Growth, development and nutritional status in Japanese children under 2 years on continuous ambulatory peritoneal dialysis. *Pediatr Nephrol* 1995;9:543–548.
15. Becker N, Brandt JR, Sutherland TA, et al. Improved outcome of young children on lately automated peritoneal dialysis. *Pediatr Nephrol* 1997;11:676–679.
16. Warady BA, Belden et Kohaut E. Neurodevelopmental outcome of children initiating peritoneal dialysis in early infancy. *Pediatr Nephrol* 1999;13:759–765.
17. Ledermann SE, Scanes ME, Fernando EN, et al. Long term outcome of peritoneal dialysis in infants. *J Pediatr* 2000;136:24–29.
18. Geary DF. Attitude of pediatric nephrologists to management of end stage renal disease in infant. *J Pediatr* 1998;133:154–156.
19. Burguet A, Abraham-Lerat L, Cholley F, et al. Insuffisance rénale chronique terminale et pré-terminale du nouveau-né dans les services de réanimation français: enquête de la Société de néphrologie pédiatrique auprès du Groupe francophone de réanimation et d'urgences pédiatriques. *Arch Pediatr* 2002:9(sous presse).
20. Loirat C, Ehrich JH, Geerlings W, et al. Report on management of renal failure in children in Europe XXIII, 1992. *Nephrol Dial Transplant* 1994;9(suppl 1).26–40.
21. Riano I , Malaga S. Encuesta sobre criterios de inclusion en programas de dialisis y trasplante de ninos en situacion de insufisciencia renal terminal. *An Esp Pediatr* 1998;48:33–38.
22. Fauriel I, Moutel G, François I, et al. Modes of decision making concerning the withholding or withdrawal of potential life-sustaining treatments in paediatric nephrology a multicentre study in French-speaking countries. *Arch Pediatr Adolesc* 2003.
23. Cochat P, Koch-Nogueira PC, Mamhoud A, et al. Primary hyperoxaluria in infants: medical, ethical and economical issues. *J Pediatr* 1999;135:746–750.
24. Steinberg A. Decision making and the role of surrogacy in withdrawing or withholding of therapy in neonate. *Clin Perinatol* 1998;25:779–790.
25. Kodadek MP. Cessation of treatment decision for infants: the role of quality of life. *Nursingconnections* 1996;9:40–47.
26. Orlowski JP, Smith ML, Van Zwienen J. Pediatric euthanasia. *Am J Dis Child* 1992;146:1440–1446.
27. Eidelman AI, Hoffmann NW, Kaitz M. Cognitive deficits in women after childbirth. *Obstet Gynecol* 1993;81:764–767.
28. Clarke CM. Do parents or surrogates have the right to demand treatment deemed futile? An analysis of the case of baby L. *J Adv Nurs* 2000;32:757–763.
29. Doyal L, Henning B. Stopping treatment for end stage renal failure: the right of children and adolescents. *Pediatr Nephrol* 1994;8:768–771.
30. Neu S, Kjelstrand CM. An empirical study of withdrawal of life supporting treatment. *N Engl J Med* 1986;314:14–20.
31. Schowalter JE, Ferholt JB, Mann NM. The adolescent patient's decision to die. *Pediatrics* 1973;51:97–103.
32. Randolph AG, Zollo MB, Wigton RS, et al. Factors explaining variability among caregivers in the intent to restrict life support interventions in a pediatric intensive care unit. *Crit Care Med* 1997;25:435–439.
33. Kachaner J. Cardiopathies néonatales intraitables: une controverse. *Arch Pediatr* 2002;9(suppl 1):49S–54S.
34. Comité Consultatif National d'Ethique Rapport N° 65: Réflexions éthiques autour de la réanimation néonatale. Paris septembre 2000. Available at: http://www.ccne-ethique.org.
35. Cohen C. Ethical legal considerations in the case of infants with end stage renal disease whose parents elect conservative therapy. An American perspective. *Pediatr Nephrol* 1987; 1:466–471.
36. Ward C, Myers NA. Babies born with major disabilities: the medical legal interface. *Pediatr Surg Int* 1999;15:310–319.
37. Saieh-Andonie. The management of end stage renal diseases in under developed countries: a moral and economic problem. *Pediatr Nephrol* 1990;4:199–201.
38. Royal College of Pediatrics and Child Health. *Withholding or withdrawing life saving treatment in children. Framework for practice.* London: RCP CH, 1997.
39. Tournai AE. Withdrawal of medical treatment in children. *West J Med* 2000;173:407–411.
40. Ropert JC. Les dilemmes éthiques des décisions de fin de vie en période périnatale. *Arch Pediatr* 2002;9(suppl 1):43S–48S.
41. Riano I, Malaga S, Callis L, et al. Towards guidelines for dialysis in children with end stage renal diseases. *Pediatr Nephrol* 2000:15:157–162.
42. Galla JH. Clinical practice guidelines on shared decision making in the appropriate initiation of and withdrawal from dialysis. *J Am Soc Nephrol* 2000;11:1340–1342.
43. Currier H. Dialysis in the newborn with chronic renal insufficiency: ethical considerations. *ANNA J* 1998;25:74–76.
44. Bunchman T. Infant dialysis: the future is now. *J Pediatr* 2000;136:1–2.
45. Baqi N, Tejani A, Sullivan EK. Renal transplantation in Down syndrome: a report of the North American Pediatric Renal Transplant Study. *Pediatr Transplant* 1998;3:211–215.
46. Kuo PC, Stock PG. Transplantation in the HIV+ patient. *Am J Transplant* 2001;1:13–17.
47. Loirat L, Chalem Y, Golmard JL. Organ allocation in pediatric transplantation in France. *Pediatr Nephrol* 2001;16:964–970.
48. Fior S, Broyer M, Guest G, et al. Devenir social professionnel et familial des patients traités depuis l'enfance par dialyse et/ou transplantation rénale. *Arch Pediatr* 1996;3(suppl 1):138S–140S.
49. Consensus statement on the live organ donor (NKF and American Societies of Transplantation). *JAMA* 2000;284: 2919–2926.
50. Matas AJ, Garvey CA, Jacob CL, et al. Non-directed donation of kidneys from living donors. *N Engl J Med* 2000;343:433–436.
51. Phadke K, Anandh U. Why is the commerce of organs unethical? *Pediatr Nephrol* 2002;17:309–311.

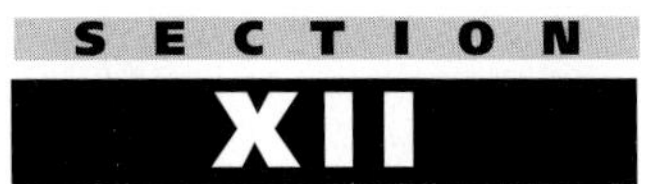

SECTION XII

PEDIATRIC NEPHROLOGY AROUND THE WORLD

75A

OVERVIEW

MATTHIAS BRANDIS
IRA GREIFER

The subspecialty of pediatric nephrology has developed within the last 40 to 50 years. Sophisticated diagnostic and therapeutic standards have been achieved for the care of children with congenital or acquired renal diseases. The technical equipment developed for adults has been adapted to children.

A series of reports entitled "Nephrology around the World" was first presented in the second edition of this book to draw attention to the variation in the clinical spectrum of renal disease in children in various parts of the world, with particular emphasis on differences from the pattern seen in Europe and North America (1). Cameron, reviewing the historical, social, and geographic factors affecting the pattern of renal disease in children, used the challenging phrase "pediatric nephrology in an unjust world" to describe the fact that most contemporary pediatric nephrology arose from and was relevant to only a minority of the world's children (2). The situation has hardly changed since that time. The only difference is that more and more pediatricians around the world have become interested in this field of patient care and clinical research (3,4). There has been an impressive change in the distribution of competence and knowledge within the recent past. The increase in activities on the South American continent, which has its own regional society (the Latin American Association of Pediatric Nephrology) (4), the productive and efficient organization of the Asian Society of Pediatric Nephrology with steadily rising numbers of participants at the various congresses in that region, and last but not least the establishment of an African Society of Pediatric Nephrology (AFSPN), which has already organized its second congress, are undoubtedly signs of an increasing conscience about the care of children with kidney disease. These signs of increasing interest and motivation on the part of young pediatricians in the field of nephrology are prompted by the sincere desire to provide better care for children with renal disease and to achieve this goal by initiating better and more adequate training.

Many of the old problems remain. The proper management of renal disease in children is expensive, particularly the provision of renal replacement therapy for end-stage renal disease. Poor countries are doubly deprived: not only is their gross national product low, but also a smaller fraction of it is made available for health care (5). Nevertheless a concern about renal disease in children has developed in all regional societies and working groups. The newest regional society of the International Pediatric Nephrology Association (IPNA), the AFSPN, is trying slowly to reach pediatricians with interest in this subspecialty within the African continent, despite the existence of a wide variety of ethnic and economic issues. The huge distances and differences in social, economic, and political problems between South African and North African countries, and the quite different structures within Central Africa are only some of the tremendous problems that exist, even independent of the difficult economical questions. Notwithstanding these obvious issues, there is an increasing conscience and willingness to launch better care for children. Different incidences and epidemiologic characteristics of diseases in developing and tropical countries than in developed countries reinforce the interest of the field of nephrology in the pathogenesis and outcome of similar diseases in various parts of the world. One can conclude that, in spite of the economic differences and difficult political situations, the pediatric nephrology societies have an increasing professional interest in studying the clinical and pathologic differences in kidney diseases in various parts of the world (6–10).

To address the prevailing problem of economic limitations to the distribution of equitable diagnostic and high-quality therapeutic services in all parts of the world, the community of pediatric nephrologists has a growing conviction that they must help to increase the knowledge of basic care for children with renal disease (11). Sophisticated research or introduction of technical procedures, which for the near future is not achievable, is not on the main worldwide agenda.

Children have a right to treatment every bit as sophisticated and to resources just as well developed as those available to adults; yet in countries in transition to new demographic and economic patterns, children still have difficulty competing with adults for limited resources, as the reports from Latin America (see Chapter 75F) and Africa (see Chapter 75E) clearly show.

The modern structure of the specialty can be traced to the formation of the International Study of Kidney Disease in Children (ISKDC) in the second half of the 1960s (12,13). Such multicenter studies are of value not only for the power that they bring to the resolution of a clinical problem by virtue of the large numbers of cases available for study, but also for the professional relationships, understanding, and standards that they foster. This study was naturally followed by the formation of several regional pediatric nephrology societies and by the IPNA, which held its first congress in Paris in 1971. In this section the different regional societies are represented to outline the specific geographic, ethnic, and socioeconomic aspects of pediatric renal disease around the world.

The European Society for Pediatric Nephrology (see Chapter 75B) and the American Society of Pediatric Nephrology (see Chapter 75D) have the longest tradition. Both are associated with registries that maintain a database of children on renal replacement programs: the registry of the European Dialysis and Transplantation Association and European Renal Association, and the registry of the North American Pediatric Renal Transplant Cooperative Study (14,15), which in particular developed the best resource of actual data not only on transplantation but on other renal diseases as well. There is no other registry in the world of comparable quality.

The European Society for Pediatric Nephrology is addressing the issues that arise from the harmonization of standards within the European Community with particular focus on the adaptation of the countries in Eastern Europe. Special training courses have been implemented within the Eastern European community in Russia, Rumania, and the Baltic states. This program has been received with enthusiasm by local pediatric nephrologists.

The American Society of Pediatric Nephrology has taken the lead in defining the requirements for pediatric nephrologists in developed countries (16).

The Japanese Society for Pediatric Nephrology is the oldest and largest of the regional pediatric nephrology societies (see Chapter 75C). A unique feature of pediatric nephrology in Japan is that children are screened annually by urinalysis in a nationwide program (17). This screening has provided invaluable epidemiologic information and the opportunity to set up clinical trials involving children in the early stages of disease.

Asia accounts for 57% of the world's population and an even higher proportion of its children because of that region's demographic characteristics. The Asian Pediatric Nephrology Association has developed into a well-recognized society with yearly conferences that are well received. Educational courses have been introduced to extend competence into areas in which there is less access to financial and technical resources. Because of this, generous space has been allocated to this region in this section of the book (see Chapter 75H). The Asian Pediatric Nephrology Association and the Latin American Association of Pediatric Nephrology (see Chapter 75F) are principally concerned with the problems of delivering health care to children with renal disease in countries in transition to new demographic and economic structures.

The Australasian Pediatric Nephrology Association is a well-organized, smaller regional society that took responsibility for organizing the IPNA congress in 2004 (see Chapter 75G).

The youngest society, the AFSPN, had its first congress in Cairo, Egypt, in 2000 and its second congress in 2002 in Nigeria with participants primarily from Nigeria but also from South Africa and Egypt (see Chapter 75E).

The IPNA provides a coordinating framework for the regional associations. In April 2002, it had a membership of more than 1600. It promotes the specialty of pediatric nephrology by holding a triennial international congress (next scheduled for Adelaide, Australia in the fall of 2004), supporting other meetings and teaching ventures, and publishing the journal *Pediatric Nephrology.*

REFERENCES

1. Nephrology around the world. In: Holliday MA, Barratt TM, Vernier RL, eds. *Pediatric nephrology*, 2nd ed. Baltimore: Williams & Wilkins, 1987:348–367.
2. Cameron JS. Historical, social, and geographical factors: paediatric nephrology in an unjust world. In: Holliday MA, Barratt TM, Vernier RL, eds. *Pediatric nephrology*, 2nd ed. Baltimore: Williams & Wilkins, 1987:341–347.
3. Gruenberg J, Nogueira A. Paediatric nephrology in poor countries: an educational and cultural outlook. *Pediatr Nephrol* 1995;9:541.
4. Grunberg J, Kummann E, Srivaszava RN, et al. Paediatric nephrology in countries with limited resources. *Pediatr Nephrol* 1994;8:522–524.
5. Chantler C. Pediatric nephrology on the threshold of European integration. *Pediatr Nephrol* 1991;5:428–432.
6. van Buuren AS, Bates WD, Muller N. Nephrotic syndrome in Namibian children. *S Afr Med J* 1999;89:1088–1091.
7. Okoro BA, Okafor HU, Nnolis LK. Childhood nephrotic syndrome in Enugu, Nigeria. *West Afr J Med* 2000;19:137–141.
8. Asinobi AO, Gbadegesin RA, Adeyemo AA, et al. The predominance of membranoproliferative glomerulonephritis in childhood nephrotic syndrome in Ibadan, Nigeria. *West Afr J Med* 1999;18:203–206.
9. Kadiri S, Arije A, Salako BL. Traditional herbal preparations and acute renal failure in South-West Niger. *Trop Doct* 1999;29:244–246.
10. Gbadoe AD, Atakouma DY, Napo-Koura G, et al. Primary nephrotic syndrome in the black African child. *Arch Pediatr* 1999;6:985–989
11. Gruenberg J. Appropriate training in paediatric nephrology for developing countries. *Pediatr Nephrol* 1990;4:290–295.

12. Abramowicz M, Barnett HL, Edelmann CM, et al. Controlled trial of azathioprine in children with nephrotic syndrome. A report of the International Study of Kidney Disease in Children. *Lancet* 1970;2:959–961.
13. Churg J, Habib R, White RHR. Pathology of the nephrotic syndrome in children. Report of the International Study of Kidney Disease in Children. *Lancet* 1970;1:1299–1302.
14. Broyer M, Chantler C, Donckerwolcke R, et al. The paediatric registry of the European Dialysis and Transplant Association: 20 years' experience. *Pediatr Nephrol* 1993;7:758–768.
15. Seikaly M, Ho PL, Emmett L, et al. The report of the North American Pediatric Renal Transplant Cooperative Study: renal transplantation from 1987 to 1998. *Pediatr Transplant* 2001;5:215–231.
16. Stapleton FB, Andreoli S, Ettenger R, et al. Future workforce for pediatric nephrology: an analysis of the nephrology workforce and training requirements by the American Society of Pediatric Nephrology. *J Am Soc Nephrol* 1997;8:S5–S8.
17. Iitaka K. Japan: screening problems. In: Holliday MA, Barratt TM, Avner ED, eds. *Pediatric nephrology*, 3rd ed. Baltimore: Williams & Wilkins, 1994:1434–1435.

75B

EUROPE

JOCHEN H. H. EHRICH
ANITA AMINA ELGENDI

OUTLINE

Among European countries there are major differences in the type and quality of medical care given to children. With regard to pediatric renal care, until now only incomplete data have been available on national organization and provision of health care for children with kidney diseases. The European Society for Pediatric Nephrology (ESPN) suggests that the need to improve the availability of pediatric renal care throughout Europe, especially Eastern Europe, is great. Differences throughout Europe concerning pediatric renal care are related to factors such as population size, geographical and political situation, primary pediatric care patterns, and the economic situation. In 1998, the number of pediatric nephrologists per million child population (pmcp) was related to the different European pediatric care systems. Generally, the general practitioner care system had significantly fewer pediatricians involved in renal care than the pediatric or the combined care system. The difference in access to renal replacement therapy (RRT) is related to the different health insurance systems (public, mixed, and private): Although the syllabus for training in pediatric nephrology is defined by the ESPN, the definition of a pediatric nephrologist is different in Eastern European countries than in Western European countries. In Eastern Europe dialysis and transplantation care for children is not always undertaken by pediatric nephrologists.

Europe, at the end of the twentieth century, had far from equal access to RRT for children. In times of financial constraint, national priorities in pediatric care need to be identified and programs agreed upon. The goal of equal access to RRT for children throughout Europe remains a challenge in the early twenty-first century.

INTRODUCTION

The vision of "health for all" (HFA) was born during the World Health Assembly in 1977 and launched at the Alma-Ata Conference in 1978. HFA, adopted by the world community in May 1998, aimed to realize a vision of providing maximal health care for all by setting out global priorities and targets for the first two decades of the twenty-first century. The regional HFA policy for the European region of the World Health Organization (http://www.who.org) in Copenhagen had recognized 21 European targets in 1999 and concluded that this is a vision that could be realized. With the theoretical approach of these targets borne in mind, Europe needs "clearly focused and committed action and strong leadership" to transform the vision of HFA into a practical and sustainable reality (1). At the beginning of the twenty-first century, the reality was far from "health for all" in Europe. Approximately 800 million people live in the European region in more than 40 countries. Europe contains both highly developed, rich countries and economically challenged countries. Some countries are still struggling with the consequences of the democratic, social, and economic transition that began in the early 1990s. During this time the average life expectancy of people in the European region actually declined for the first time since the Second World War. This was due largely to a deterioration in health care systems in the newly independent states and some Central and Eastern European countries, with an actual life-span variation of up to 15 years. According to the human development report of 1997 issued by the United Nations Development Program, poverty-level income has spread from a small part of the population of these countries to approximately one-third, with 120 million people living below the poverty line of US$4 per day (1). The situation in Europe, therefore, reflects the global situation of widening gaps between countries and within societies (2).

SYSTEMS OF PEDIATRIC CARE IN EUROPE

At the end of the last century there were at least three different systems in Europe offering general pediatric care, defined according to the proportion of the country's children aged younger than 15 years and seen primarily either by pediatricians or by family physicians or general practitioners (3):

1. The pediatric system (12 of 34 countries): more than 75% of children were under the care of pediatricians, with 1 pediatrician per 600 to 1250 children, mostly in Eastern European countries.
2. The combined system (16 of 34 countries): both pediatricians and general practitioners offered primary care to almost equal numbers of children (50 ± 25%), with 1 pediatrician per 1250 to 2500 children, mostly in Central Europe.
3. The general practitioner system (6 of 34 countries): more than 75% of children were under the care of family physicians or general practitioners, with 1 pediatrician per 2500 to 7500 children, exclusively in Western European countries.

HISTORY OF PEDIATRIC RENAL CARE IN EUROPE

The ESPN is the representative body for pediatric nephrology in Europe and is recognized by the Confederation of European Specialists in Paediatrics. The ESPN was founded in 1967, and by the year 2000 had 398 registered members from 35 different countries. The aims of the ESPN include (a) the continuous updating of recommendations for the training of pediatric nephrologists, (b) the development of international standards for all pediatric nephrology centers, and (c) the development of guidelines for quality assessment of clinical care of children with renal disease and for collaborative research in pediatric nephrology. The ESPN is committed to support training courses in Eastern and Central Europe on a yearly basis. Furthermore, training grants for young pediatric nephrologists from Eastern Europe are available from the ESPN, which include coverage of expenses for a 2-month training course at an established pediatric nephrology center in Europe. Travel grants to congresses are also awarded annually by the ESPN. In addition, the ESPN is creating a basis for international cooperation in nationally controlled trials and published a handbook on pediatric nephrology in 2002.

Since 1965, the European Dialysis and Transplantation Association (EDTA) has gathered data on RRT in children and adults with end-stage renal failure. In 1995 there were more than 2000 centers in 36 European and Mediterranean countries reporting to the EDTA registry. Approximately 150 of these centers were pediatric nephrology centers (4,5). Until 1998, data were supplied on a voluntary basis through three types of questionnaire: (a) those gathering data from each center practicing RRT, (b) those obtaining data on each patient on RRT (pediatric questionnaire for patients younger than 15 years), and (c) specific mini-questionnaires generated by working groups on particular topics (6). In 1998, 70% of 40 European countries reported on their patients to either a national or international registry, or both, on RRT. The percentage of countries not reporting to any registry was higher in Eastern European countries, with only 50% of countries reporting as opposed to 100% of European Union countries. In 1998, it became evident that the EDTA registry could not continue without major changes because it faced a number of unresolved problems, including incomplete data collection, inadequate management of its database, and financial pressures (7). A new EDTA office was set up in Amsterdam and is based in a university department with access to advice on computing and epidemiology. From now on, only a small set of core data will be collected from national registries, which thus increases the possibility of complete data collection and decreases the burden on contributors. Specific questions will be analyzed through mini-questionnaires.

PEDIATRIC NEPHROLOGISTS IN EUROPE

The Union of National European Paediatric Societies and Associations and the ESPN studied pediatric renal care management in Europe with the help of a questionnaire directed to the presidents of national pediatric nephrology societies. In 1998 there were 842 pediatric nephrologists working in 42 European countries with a median of 9 pediatric nephrologists per country (range, 0 to 150). The median number of pediatric nephrologists pmcp was 4.9, ranging from 0 to 15. The median number of children per pediatric nephrologist was 168,480, ranging from 67,130 to 878,940, excluding five European countries with no pediatric nephrologists at all. The situation in pediatric nephrology varied depending on the pediatric primary care system; for example, fewer nephrologists were reported from countries with a combined system or a general practitioner care system than from countries with a pediatric care system.

In addition, there were a total of 1087 general pediatricians with a part-time interest in pediatric nephrology in Europe in 1998. Eastern European countries with a mean number of 16.7 general pediatricians with a part-time interest pmcp had the highest number of those specialists, and countries with a pediatric care system had significantly more than those with a general practitioner care system. There were approximately 170,000 pediatricians in Europe in 1998, and the proportion of pediatric nephrologists among all pediatricians ranged from 1 in 60 to 1 in 200.

The extent to which the staffing of pediatric nephrology units has affected access to and/or quality of pediatric renal care remains unclear. Hörl et al. (8) found differences in the renal care given to adults depending on their different health insurance systems. Public systems (national health service financed through taxes) had fewer doctors involved in treating end-stage renal disease (ESRD) than health insurance systems (personally financed), as well as lower acceptance rates for RRT, lower prevalence of patients on dialysis, and a higher proportion of patients undergoing transplantation. Eighty percent of countries with a general practitioner care system are countries with a national health service system, and parallels were found concerning the number of doctors involved in pediatric renal care. Chantler (9) stated in 1991 that in many instances there is no shortage of doctors, nurses, and hospital beds but there is a need to change the administrative and academic structures and to introduce appropriate technology.

Boesken et al. (10) described a fragmentation of nephrology services in some Eastern European countries. There were three types of specialists practicing nephrology in countries of the former Soviet Union: (a) "therapeutists" (nephrologists treating general nephrology problems), (b) dialysis specialists (often surgeons), and (c) transplant surgeons. Renal biopsies were often performed by urologists. The training to become a pediatric nephrologist in these countries starts in medical school. There are three different types of medical schools: adult, pediatric, and dental. Two to 3 years of postgraduate surgical, medical, or pediatric training normally follow graduation from medical school, and after this only a 4- to 6-month course in nephrology is sufficient to qualify as a pediatric nephrologist. These significant differences lead to the conclusion that most pediatric nephrologists in Eastern European countries would not be considered as such in European Union countries, and therefore the high number of "pediatric nephrologists" in Eastern countries may be based on different definitions of this specialty. In these countries no real subdivision of pediatrics has taken place; rather, pediatric subspecialties have arisen in other disciplines such as surgery (10). The extent of fragmentation is not the same in all Eastern European countries, however, and some countries have changed their organization of medical care (3). The integration process of a "European house" will need time to train pediatricians and to take the necessary organizational steps. The importance of pursuing this goal is strengthened when one considers that the decision-making processes for promoting a better economic and/or medical rationale are seldom in the hands of health care professionals. Although training recommendations do their part in contributing to better care, they are largely developed following the recommendations of national medical organizations.

The goal of achieving specialized pediatric nephrology centers (defined as a center offering general pediatric nephrology, dialysis, and transplantation) and determining how many centers per country to establish is difficult to define and differs according to geographical, social, and financial factors. In 1990 a median of 1.4 centers pmcp provided 24-hour service with a median of four pediatric nephrologists per center (5). It appears that there are enough pediatric nephrologists in most Western, Central, and Eastern European countries to meet the demands of comprehensive renal care. However, an unlimited exchange of pediatric nephrologists across borders is possible only within the European Union.

AVAILABILITY OF RENAL REPLACEMENT THERAPY

In recent years the incidence of ESRD has been evaluated by the EDTA registry based on the number of patients accepted into dialysis-transplantation programs. Therefore, these figures underestimate the incidence of children with ESRD because they exclude those children who are not treated due to technical reasons, lack of facilities, or health or social policies in countries with limited resources. In Western European countries the incidence of chronic renal failure has remained stable in children, whereas the prevalence has increased steadily as a consequence of improved RRT and prolonged survival of children on RRT (5). The mean number of new pediatric patients pmcp reported in countries with large child populations such as France, Germany, Spain, and Italy was 2.3 in 1973, 5.6 in 1988, and 4.2 in 1991. In countries with a smaller child population such as Belgium, the Netherlands, Finland, Norway, and Sweden, the mean number of new pediatric patients pmcp was 3.3 in 1973, 8 in 1988, and 6.6 in 1991. Thus, despite wide variations in countries and over time, the number of children younger than 15 years of age who need RRT each year is at least 4 to 6 pmcp and may reach 9 pmcp or more. Data for the former Soviet Union were not available for many years, even after the end of the Cold War. Rutkowski et al. (11) on behalf of the Central and Eastern European Advisory Board on Chronic Renal Failure published the first reliable data in 1998; however, there were no separate pediatric data. In 1995 it was estimated that only 3% of all children with ESRD received appropriate treatment in countries of the former Soviet Union (10). With regard to the availability of pediatric RRT in European countries, data show that 92% of all European countries offered pediatric dialysis for acute renal failure, 90% offered pediatric dialysis for chronic renal failure, and 55% offered pediatric transplantation. The availability of pediatric transplantation was associated significantly with the size of the child population and with the gross national product. Only 30% of Eastern European countries offered pediatric transplantation as opposed to 87% of European Union countries. The fact that, according to available data, approximately 90% of European countries provide pediatric dialysis for chronic renal failure but only 55% provide pediatric renal transplantation indicates inadequate care, as does the association of availability of renal transplantation with the GNP, when one considers the clinical and financial long-term superiority of renal transplantation (12). Some of those Eastern countries that did not offer renal transplantation for children at all did offer transplantation for adults (11). These findings unfortunately reinforce the fact that in numerous developing countries, long-term dialysis and transplantation have been developed for adults but are still unavailable for children. In 1995 in Rumania, for example, only 20% of children younger than 15 years of age with ESRD were treated with RRT, whereas 60% of those in the 25- to 44-year age group were treated (13). Efforts must be undertaken to ensure that children receive equal access to RRT, not only in different European countries but also in the different social groups within a given country.

The discussion of factors contributing to the mode of selection between peritoneal dialysis and hemodialysis in RRT is long-standing. In pediatric patients an expansion of peritoneal dialysis as an effective treatment modality has been increasingly recognized in Europe (14). In European countries, the distribution of the use of peritoneal dialysis as treatment varies significantly (14) despite the absence of major medical differences between the two types of techniques. Nissenson et al. (15) found the cost and reimbursement rate to be the most important factors influencing choice of treatment. In countries with fixed annual health care allocations to hospitals or regions, use of peritoneal dialysis was high, which reflects its lower cost. Vecchi et al. (16) found cost and reimbursement patterns to be similar in the majority of countries and attributed differences in treatment selection to differences in microeconomics of the provider. Hemodialysis is a treatment with high fixed costs (personnel and structure); peritoneal dialysis is a treatment with low fixed costs but high variable costs (supplies) and low need for investments. Differences in microeconomics are one reason why peritoneal dialysis is not only more expensive in most Eastern European countries than in Western European countries but also more expensive than hemodialysis in Eastern European countries. As with most new pharmaceutical products, all necessary supplies, including lines, bags, fluids, connectors, and so on, must be imported from Western countries (10).

COSTS OF PEDIATRIC NEPHROLOGIC CARE

Data on the costs of RRT in Europe are scanty; they mainly evaluate adult services and fail to link outcome with cost and resource use. RRT is known to be more expensive in children than in adults, due to various factors such as the need for psychosocial care and growth therapy, and feeding problems. The total costs for all pediatric patients, however, are much less due to the lower incidence and prevalence of ESRD in children than in adults. Neuhaus et al. (12) evaluated the costs of RRT in children younger than 5 years of age, including costs for erythropoietin, growth hormone, vaccinations, psychosocial support, travel expenses for diagnosis, treatment, and rehabilitation, and costs of nursing support at home. They found the overall costs of medical treatment before initiation of RRT to be similar to the annual costs after successful renal transplantation [30,000 Swiss francs (SFr) per patient per year]. The highest costs were incurred in the year of transplantation (130,000 SFr per patient per year), followed by dialysis therapy (93,000 SFr). After all, renal transplantation remains the treatment of choice for children with ESRD, not only with regard to survival and quality of life but also with regard to long-term costs.

An effective program for the development and improvement of RRT was implemented in Poland and provides an example of successful enhancement of RRT through targeted health policies. Improvement of RRT in Poland took place due to the enormous effort of the nephrology community, which resulted in a better appreciation of the problem by the authorities on various levels. Their program was prepared by the National Committee for the Promotion of Nephrology and was accepted by the Ministry of Health and the parliamentary health commission. Each year a budget is allocated by the Ministry of Health to cover the expenses of the program. Central purchasing was organized and a major portion of dialysis equipment was purchased in this way and distributed according to patient load. In addition, a new law on transplantation has been passed by the Polish parliament (17).

COOPERATION AMONG EUROPEAN PEDIATRIC NEPHROLOGISTS

"If inequities are to be lessened and the security and cohesion of Europe to be maintained, a much stronger collective effort must be made by Member States to increase their volume, effectiveness and coordination of support to countries in most need in the Region. Receiving countries for their part should give very high priority to the formulation of HFA policies and make health and development plans" (1). According to our data, the cooperation rate among individual European pediatric nephrologists was reported to be high; however, this is not without difficulties. Access to telephone, fax, E-mail, and the Internet is more difficult in developing countries than in developed countries, and there are more obstacles, such as language barriers (i.e., insufficient knowledge of English) and the lack of a history of cooperation in Eastern Europe due to former political policies. Collaboration between national pediatric societies has many facets, and many challenges will need to be met in the global European context. Participation in international meetings is another area of scientific cooperation. Travel grants for scientists with limited financial resources are provided by the ESPN to allow large groups of junior doctors to attend meetings. Because the attendance of a junior doctor at a congress often depends on the acceptance of an abstract, the ESPN studied the acceptance rate of abstracts for the ESPN congress in 1997 in Greece. In actual fact, the acceptance rate varied according to country. For example, Eastern European countries had an acceptance rate of 30 to 45%, whereas 75 to 85% of all abstracts from Western European countries were accepted (C. Stefanidis, *personal communication*). These differences underline the need for collaborative, multinational research activities. Our analysis also showed that not only the total number of ESPN members per country but also the proportion of membership among pediatric nephrologists was lower in Eastern European than in European Union countries.

Efforts have to be made by the ESPN to implement training courses on a regular basis. Very successful courses were held in Russia, Georgia, and Lithuania. Furthermore, training grants were offered to young pediatric nephrologists in Eastern Europe that covered the expenses for a 2-month training course at an established pediatric nephrology center in Europe.

Another important challenge for the European pediatric nephrology community and others is to effectively meet the needs of emergency situations such as natural catastrophes, epidemics, and armed conflicts (18). Major disasters create emergencies that often require rapid and large-scale foreign aid for the affected country. By their very nature, disasters and complex human emergencies constitute an international concern and provoke responses at an international level. During the 1990s the European region has experienced armed conflicts in ten member states, and earthquakes in Armenia in 1988 and in Turkey in 1999. Responding to this situation, hundreds of organizations and many donor countries have been involved in emergency assistance, often in a very uncoordinated way. The desperate need for a coordinated and multilateral organized approach through a European pediatric nephrology task force is apparent. In the postemergency phase, "action for health" can be used as an effective entry point to strengthen national health concerns and to promote solidarity and social cohesion (18,19).

REFERENCES

1. WHO, Health 21. The health for all policy framework for the WHO European region, 1999.
2. Walt G. Globalisation of international health. *Lancet* 1998; 351:434–437.
3. Katz M, Rubino A, Collier J, et al. Demography of pediatric primary care in Europe: delivery of care and training. *Pediatrics* 2002;109(5):788–796.
4. Mallick NP, Jones E, Selwood N. The European (European Dialysis and Transplantation Association-European Renal Association) Registry. *Am J Kidney Dis* 1995;25:176–187.
5. Loirat C, Ehrich JHH, Geerling W, et al. Report on management of renal failure in children in Europe, XIII, 1992. *Nephrol Dial Transplant* 1994;1(suppl):26–40.
6. Wing AJ, Brunner FP. Twenty-three years of dialysis and transplantation in Europe: experiences of the EDTA Registry. *Am J Kidney Dis* 1989;14:341–346.
7. Mehls O, Rigden S, Ehrich JHH, et al. Report on management of renal failure in Europe, XXV, 1994. The child-adult interface. *Nephrol Dial Transplant* 1996;11(suppl 1):22–36.
8. Hörl WH, Alvaro F, Williams PF. Healthcare systems and end stage renal disease (ESRD) therapies, an international review: access to ESRD treatments. *Nephrol Dial Transplant* 1999;14(suppl 6):10–14.
9. Chantler C. Paediatric nephrology on the threshold of European Integration. *Pediatr Nephrol* 1991;5:428–432.
10. Boesken WH, Ahmed KEY, Méry JP, et al. Observations on renal replacement services in Russia, Belarus and Lithuania. *Nephrol Dial Transplant* 1995;10:2013–2016.
11. Rutkowski B. Changing pattern of end-stage renal disease in central and eastern Europe. *Nephrol Dial Transplant* 2000; 15:156–160.
12. Neuhaus TJ, Goetschel P, Leumann E. Small patients—big costs: economic aspects of medical treatment of children with early onset of chronic renal failure. *Praxis* 1998;87: 1593–1599.
13. Ursea N, Mircescu G, Constantinovici N, et al. Nephrology and renal replacement therapy in Romania. *Nephrol Dial Transplant* 1997;4:684–690.
14. Rizzoni G, Broyer M, Ehrich JHH, et al. The use of continuous peritoneal dialysis in Europe for the treatment of children with end-stage renal failure: data from the EDTA Registry. *Nephrol Dial Transplant* 1990;5:985–990.
15. Nissenson AR, Prichard SS, Cheng IKP, et al. Non-medical factors that impact on ESRD modality selection. *Kidney Int* 1993;43(suppl 40):120–127.
16. Vecchi AF, Dratwa M, Wiedemann ME. Healthcare systems and end-stage renal disease (ESRD) therapies—an international review: costs and reimbursement/funding of ESRD therapies. *Nephrol Dial Transplant* 1999;14(suppl 6):31–41.
17. Rutkowski B, Puka J, Lao M, et al. Renal replacement therapy in an era of socioeconomic changes—report from the Polish registry. *Nephrol Dial Transplant* 1997;12:1105–1108.
18. Leumann E, Bernhardt JP, Babloyan A, et al. From dialysis to basic paediatric nephrology: an unorthodox project applied in Yerevan, Armenia. *Pediatr Nephrol* 1994;8:252–255.
19. Sukru Sever M, Erek E. Sincere thanks of Turkish nephrologists to their European friends. *Nephrol Dial Transplant* 2000;15:1478–1480.

75C

JAPAN

KOICHI NAKANISHI
MASATAKA HONDA
NORISHIGE YOSHIKAWA

SCHOOL URINARY SCREENING PROGRAM

One of the unique features of pediatric nephrology in Japan is that children are screened annually by urinalysis in a nationwide program (1), which has provided invaluable epidemiologic information and the opportunity for setting up clinical trials involving individuals in the early stages of disease. Urine screening of elementary and junior high school students in Japan has been mandated by the School Health Law since 1974. One of the major purposes of this program is the detection of glomerulonephritis to allow early therapeutic intervention.

First-voided early morning urine has been tested on an annual basis for each student. Urine samples are collected at home, with participants instructed to empty the bladder on the preceding night and collect a midstream sample on first urination the following morning. The first-voided early morning urine specimen is examined by a simple dipstick method for the detection of proteinuria and hematuria. If a urine test result is positive (±30 mg/dL or more), a second test is performed in the same manner. A repeat urinalysis is performed 2 weeks later if the initial collection occurred at the time of menstruation (the first examination). Individuals with hematuria ±30 mg/dL or more and/or proteinuria ±30 mg/dL or more are referred to family doctors for the second examination. If needed, blood investigations are performed. Those with persistent hematuria + or more and/or persistent proteinuria +15–30 mg/dL or more in the second examination are referred to nephrologists for special follow-up (the third examination).

Table 75C.1 summarizes the findings of the first urine examination in the city of Kobe in 1998. The first urinalysis revealed that elementary school children (aged 6 to 11 years) had proteinuria, hematuria, or both abnormalities at prevalences of 0.17%, 0.30%, and 0.06%, respectively. The corresponding prevalences among junior high school students (aged 12 to 14 years) were 0.69%, 0.57%, and 0.25%, respectively. The prevalence rates of hematuria and proteinuria were higher in girls than in boys, and higher in junior high school children than in elementary school children as shown in Table 75C.1.

In the second examination, 34 elementary school students (0.04%) and 43 junior high school students (0.09%) showed positive findings.

The school urinary screening program allows the establishment of clinical trials involving individuals in the early stages of disease. As a consequence of this program, in more than half of the patients with immunoglobulin A (IgA) nephropathy, the most prevalent glomerular disease among Japanese children, this disease is detected at an early stage by routine urinalysis (2). The disorder has been detected in 31% of renal biopsy specimens obtained in Japanese hospitals since 1981. IgA nephropathy is the leading cause of chronic renal disease and end-stage renal failure in Japan. The occurrence of end-stage renal failure in adult patients (3) and long-term studies assessing the prognosis in children have challenged earlier views that the condition represents a benign disorder (2). The long-term follow-up of 241 Japanese children indicated that 5% of patients had developed chronic renal failure by 5 years from the onset of the disease, 6% by 10 years, and 11% by 15 years. Thus, IgA nephropathy presents a therapeutic challenge in both adults and children. Because of the variable rate of progression to renal failure and because of the probable multifactorial pathogenesis of the disease, the effectiveness of treatment can be properly evaluated only by means of a controlled trial.

The controlled trial of the Japanese Pediatric IgA Nephropathy Treatment Study Group demonstrated that treatment with prednisolone, azathioprine, heparin-warfarin, and dipyridamole for 2 years early in the course of disease prevents immunologic renal injury and progression of the disease in children with severe IgA nephropathy (4). In this study, 82% of the patients presented with microscopic hematuria and/or asymptomatic proteinuria. This high figure presumably reflects the high detection rate of the school screening program, which revealed a high prevalence of asymptomatic urinary abnormalities, rather than regional variation in the expression of IgA nephropathy. Renal biopsy specimens are

TABLE 75C.1. FINDINGS OF THE FIRST URINE EXAMINATION IN THE CITY OF KOBE IN 1998

Age (yr)		No. students	No. examined (%)	Total no. cases with positive test results (%)	Proteinuria: No. with positive results (%)	Hematuria: No. with positive results (%)	Proteinuria and hematuria: No. with positive results (%)
6–11	Male	44,018	43,825 (99.6)	141 (0.32)	44 (0.10)	81 (0.18)	16 (0.04)
	Female	41,230	41,031 (99.5)	311 (0.75)	103 (0.25)	173 (0.42)	35 (0.08)
	Total	85,248	84,856 (99.5)	452 (0.53)	147 (0.17)	254 (0.30)	51 (0.06)
12–14	Male	23,723	23,120 (97.5)	231 (0.97)	156 (0.66)	50 (0.21)	25 (0.11)
	Female	22,007	21,538 (97.9)	459 (2.09)	161 (0.73)	210 (0.95)	88 (0.40)
	Total	45,730	44,658 (97.7)	690 (1.51)	317 (0.69)	260 (0.57)	113 (0.25)

usually obtained from children with microscopic or macroscopic hematuria and persistent proteinuria.

The long-term effects of the combination therapy on the rate of progression to chronic renal failure was examined. The treated group of children with IgA nephropathy showing diffuse mesangial proliferation (combination therapy group; N = 40) was compared with a historical control group of untreated children with IgA nephropathy showing diffuse mesangial proliferation (control group; N = 48). Renal survival was significantly better in the combination therapy group than in the control group (100% vs. 77% at the twelfth year after initial biopsy).

To determine whether similar results could be obtained with prednisolone alone, the effects of prednisolone treatment were compared with those of treatment with prednisolone, azathioprine, warfarin, and dipyridamole in 78 children with newly diagnosed IgA nephropathy showing diffuse mesangial proliferation. The patients were randomly assigned to receive either prednisolone alone or prednisolone, azathioprine, warfarin, and dipyridamole for 2 years. This study demonstrated that treatment of children with severe IgA nephropathy with prednisolone alone for 2 years early in the course of disease reduces urinary protein excretion and serum IgA concentration but does not prevent increase of sclerosed glomeruli and progression of the disease.

A controlled trial is in progress to compare the effects of a combination of prednisolone, mizoribine, warfarin, and dipyridamole with those of prednisolone and mizoribine alone in children with severe IgA nephropathy.

NATIONAL REGISTRY DATA FOR CHILDREN UNDERGOING PERITONEAL DIALYSIS

The Japanese Pediatric Peritoneal Dialysis Study Group has collected data on pediatric patients younger than 16 years of age from the National Registry of Chronic Peritoneal Dialysis (5,6). In Japan, 84% of the children with all types of end-stage renal disease were introduced to peritoneal dialysis (PD) as the first treatment modality (0 to 4 years, 90%; 5 to 9 years, 84%; 10 to 14 years, 80%).

The database records the patient number, age, outcome, cause of death, reason for terminating PD therapy, type of PD therapy, occurrence of peritonitis, and catheter survival. From 1981 to the end of 1999, data accrued on 931 patients. Of these 931 patients, 83 patients (8.9%) were younger than 1 year of age and 308 patients (33.1%) were younger than 6 years of age. The duration of PD for these patients was 5 years or longer for 257 patients (27.6%); the number of long-term PD patients increased from 11% in 1991 (5). The number of patients on automated PD increased to 78% in 1999 from 9% in 1991.

The outcome of the total patient population of 931 as of the end of 1999 is as follows: 221 patients (23.7%) were being successfully treated with PD, 99 patients (10.6%) died, 328 patients (35.2%) received a kidney transplant, and 169 (18.2%) were transferred to hemodialysis (HD). The patient survival rate was 92% at 3 years and 87% at 5 years. The technique survival rate (percentage who remained on PD) was 84% at 3 years and 72% at 5 years. Survival rates were compared for 354 patients who began PD before 1990 and 577 patients who began PD after 1990 (Table 75C.2). Although patient survival rate was significantly worse (p <.0001) in children younger than 6 years old, technique survival rate showed no significant change. Two major causes of death were infection and cardiovascular disorders. Before 1990, 20 of 62 deaths (32%) were due to infection. Subsequently 8 of 36 deaths (22%) have been due to infection. Cardiovascular deaths increased from 33% to 44% during the same period. Of the 169 patients who were transferred

TABLE 75C.2. PATIENT AND TECHNIQUE SURVIVAL RATE IN CHILDREN ON PERITONEAL DIALYSIS BEFORE AND AFTER 1990

		No. patients	Survival rate (%) 1 yr	3 yr	5 yr	7 yr
Patient[a]	Before 1990	354	96	88	82	78
	1990 and after	577	97	93	91	89
Technique[b]	Before 1990	354	92	78	64	55
	1990 and after	577	96	88	78	70

[a] p <.02 by generalized Wilcoxon method. Patient survival rate for children before 1990 versus that for children in 1990 and after.
[b] p = .01 by generalized Wilcoxon method. Technique survival rate for children before 1990 versus that for children in 1990 and after.

from PD to HD, 76 patients (45%) were transferred because of peritonitis and 38 patients (22%) were transferred because of ultrafiltration failure. The number of patients who transfer to HD due to ultrafiltration failure has increased, and encapsulating peritoneal sclerosis has been identified as a long-term side effect of PD (7). The rate of peritonitis was one episode over 31 patient months (0.39/year). Both the number of patients with peritonitis and the peritonitis rate were worse in children younger than 6 years of age (0.47/year) than in older children (0.36/year). Double-cuff swan-neck catheters showed significantly better survival and an improved peritonitis-free rate compared to other catheters.

REFERENCES

1. Iitaka K. Japan: screening problems. In: Holliday MA, Barratt TM, Avner ED, eds. *Pediatric nephrology*, 3rd ed. Baltimore: Williams & Wilkins, 1994:1434–1435.
2. Yoshikawa N, Tanaka R, Iijima K. Pathophysiology and treatment of IgA nephropathy in children. *Pediatr Nephrol* 2001;16:446–457.
3. Emacipator SN, Gallo GR, Lamm ME. IgA nephropathy: perspective on pathogenesis and classification. *Clin Nephrol* 1985;24:161–179.
4. Yoshikawa N, Ito H, Sakai T, et al. A controlled trial of combined therapy for newly diagnosed severe childhood IgA nephropathy. The Japanese Pediatric IgA Nephropathy Treatment Study Group. *J Am Soc Nephrol* 1999;10:101–109.
5. Honda M, Iitaka K, Kawaguchi H, et al. The Japanese national registry data on pediatric CAPD patients: a ten-year experience. A report of The Study Group of Pediatric PD Conference. *Peri Dial Int* 1996;16:269–275.
6. Honda M. The 1997 report of the Japanese national registry data on pediatric peritoneal dialysis patients. *Peri Dial Int* 1999;19:473–478.
7. Hoshii S, Honda M, Itami N, et al. Sclerosing encapsulating peritonitis in pediatric peritoneal dialysis patients. *Pediatr Nephrol* 2000;14:275–279.

75D

NORTH AMERICA

SHARON P. ANDREOLI

Pediatric nephrologists in North America are a diverse and active group of academic pediatric nephrologists and practitioners, pediatric department chairmen, medical school deans, and physicians employed in the pharmaceutical or biotechnology industry. Pediatric nephrologists are clinicians, basic scientists, clinical and translational researchers, and advocates for pediatric patients with renal disease. Whatever the primary activity of North American pediatric nephrologists, each is likely to participate in at least some capacity as a clinician, teacher, researcher, and mentor to future pediatric nephrologists.

AMERICAN SOCIETY OF PEDIATRIC NEPHROLOGY

The American Society of Pediatric Nephrology (ASPN; http://www.aspneph.com) was established in 1969 to promote optimal care for children with renal disease and to disseminate advances in the clinical practice and basic science of pediatric nephrology. A major goal of the ASPN has been to organize an annual national scientific meeting at which pediatric nephrologists and other health care professionals have the opportunity to meet and learn about new advancements in the care of children with renal disease. In 2002, the ASPN initiated a formal partnership with the Pediatric Academic Societies. Since that time, the ASPN annual meeting has been held jointly with that of the Pediatric Academic Societies in a convocation forum at which advances in the clinical and basic science of pediatric nephrology have been presented in the overall context of pediatric academics for trainees, pediatric nephrologists, and pediatric subspecialty colleagues in many disciplines.

A major focus of the ASPN is to promote clinical and basic scientific research in pediatric nephrology and to support training of physicians and allied health care professionals who will provide clinical care to children with kidney disease. In the late 1990s, the ASPN urged the National Institute of Diabetes and Digestive and Kidney Diseases of the National Institutes of Health to develop and implement plans to address the special research needs of children with kidney disease. The National Institute of Diabetes and Digestive and Kidney Diseases and the ASPN formed a task force of pediatric nephrologists experienced in basic, clinical, and translational research that analyzed the research needs in pediatric nephrology. The task force produced a report that focused on genetics and developmental diseases, acute renal failure, immune-related renal diseases, chronic renal failure, and pediatric transplantation (1) This report has served as a blueprint for the implementation of a number of specific basic research institutes and national multicenter clinical trials for renal transplantation, treatment of focal segmental glomerulosclerosis, and identification of risk factors for progression of chronic kidney disease in childhood.

A major goal of the ASPN is to support training of pediatricians to care for children with kidney disease. As in many pediatric subspecialties in the United States, the number of pediatric nephrology fellows currently in training is inadequate to fill current and projected personnel needs. The ASPN, in association the other major nephrology societies, commissioned an analysis to determine the number of pediatric nephrologists necessary to meet the clinical needs of children with kidney disease by the year 2010 (2). In addition to documenting a major personnel shortage, the workforce survey identified two major differences between the practice of pediatric nephrology and internal medicine nephrology. First, clinical care of children and adolescents with end-stage renal disease (ESRD) requires a greater time commitment than care of adults with ESRD as a direct result of greater disease acuteness and changing maturational and developmental needs of chronically ill children. Second, the vast majority of pediatric nephrologists are members of full-time academic faculties or maintain significant affiliations with academic medical centers. Their mission includes teaching and other academic activities in addition to patient care. These differences must be taken into account in assessing future workforce needs in pediatric nephrology (3).

The distribution of pediatric nephrologists in North America is quite diverse. According to ASPN data detailing the number of ASPN members in each state, a few states such as Alaska and Montana have no pediatric nephrologists, whereas California has 50 and New York has 57 pedi-

TABLE 75D.1. NUMBER OF PEDIATRIC NEPHROLOGISTS PER CAPITA IN SELECTED STATES BASED ON THE MOST RECENT DATA OF THE U.S. CENSUS AND AMERICAN SOCIETY OF PEDIATRIC NEPHROLOGY

East	
Massachusetts	1 per 318,965
New York	1 per 333,532
New Hampshire	1 per 1,259,181
Pennsylvania	1 per 616,692
South	
Alabama	1 per 1,116,089
Florida	1 per 819,825
Tennessee	1 per 382,668
Virginia	1 per 598,977
Midwest	
Kansas	1 per 1,347,320
Missouri	1 per 351,856
Minnesota	1 per 414,357
Ohio	1 per 454,954
Mountain	
Colorado	1 per 1,104,428
Texas	1 per 561,184
West	
California	1 per 710,022
Nevada	1 per 702,024
Oregon	1 per 578,811
Washington	1 per 460,613
Canada	1 per 1,852,095
Puerto Rico	1 per 678,412

atric nephrologists (active members, emeritus members, and fellow members). Rough per capita data demonstrate state-by-state and regional variability (Table 75D.1).

The ASPN promotes the provision of quality care to children with kidney disease and assists ASPN membership in fostering sound fiscal clinical programs. The Clinical Affairs Committee of the ASPN serves as a liaison with other organizations that have the responsibility of developing clinical practice guidelines and educational and clinical care materials for physicians and families of children with renal disease. Over the past several years, the Clinical Affairs Committee of the ASPN has participated in a review of clinical practice guidelines produced by the Kidney/Dialysis Outcome Quality Initiative (see later) and reviewed fact sheets for the National Institutes of Health and other organizations.

The Public Policy Committee of the ASPN advocates for public policies and programs that promote the interests of children with kidney disease and the educational and research mission of the society. This committee is quite active in representing the interests of the ASPN, patients, and their families in coalition with similar organizations before the U.S. Congress and federal agencies. The Public Policy Committee gathers, analyzes, and disseminates information pertinent to it members and provides advice in the development and evaluation of the ASPN formal positions, initiatives, and responses pertaining to public policy. The research committee and the Public Policy Committee work together in the development and promotion of research policies.

NORTH AMERICAN PEDIATRIC RENAL TRANSPLANT COOPERATIVE STUDY AND SOUTHWEST PEDIATRIC NEPHROLOGY STUDY GROUP

The North American Pediatric Renal Transplant Cooperative Study (NAPRTCS) is a research effort organized in 1987 to obtain data on all pediatric renal transplant recipients in North America (4) (http://spitfire.emmes.com/study/ped). Scientific objectives included capture of information about current practice and trends in immunosuppressive therapy with an ultimate goal of improving care of pediatric renal allograft recipients. In 1992, the study was expanded to include pediatric dialysis patients and in 1994 the registry was further expanded to include pediatric patients with chronic renal failure (estimated glomerular filtration rate of less than 75 mL/min/1.73 m^2 as calculated by the Schwartz formula). The goal is to register and follow more than 80% of the children receiving renal allografts in the United States and Canada and to study the clinical course and natural history of patients with renal dysfunction as they progress to ESRD. At the time of data closure for the 2001 annual report, nearly 12,000 patients had been registered in various arms of NAPTRCS. In addition to the registry components of NAPTRCS, randomized prospective clinical trials were initiated by NAPTRCS in the mid-1990s using a study of OKT3 (muromonab-CD3) induction therapy in children and adolescents undergoing renal transplant. Clinical trials to investigate the use of growth hormone in dialysis patients and in children and adolescents are currently underway. Finally, NAPTRCS is currently carrying out studies to evaluate sirolimus therapy in children and adolescents who have undergone transplantation and experience acute or chronic rejection.

The Southwest Pediatric Nephrology Study Group (SPNSG) was formed in 1980 to develop multicenter collaborative studies of renal diseases in newborns, children, and adolescents (http://www.spnsg.org). Over the past several years, the SPNSG has carried out randomized clinical trials of therapy for immunoglobulin A nephropathy, including a comparison of treatment with placebo, fish oil, and alternate-day prednisone. This study is completed and data analysis is underway. The SPNSG has initiated a second study of immunoglobulin A nephropathy using mycophenolate. NAPTRCS and the SPNSG are each participating in the multicenter trial of therapy for focal segmental glomerulosclerosis.

UNITED STATES RENAL DATA SYSTEM

Since 1988, the United States Renal Data System has produced an annual report on ESRD including a report of pediatric ESRD. This report provides valuable information on the demographics, epidemiology, modes of therapy, morbidity, and mortality in pediatric patients with ESRD.

The 2001 United States Renal Data System Annual Report demonstrated that the incidence rates of ESRD in children rose 2 to 3% over the prior decade and revealed unexplained geographical variability in the development of ESRD (5). Overall, congenital and hereditary renal disease and glomerulonephritis are the most common causes of renal failure. However, the age, gender, and racial background of the child are directly related to the cause of renal failure. Glomerulonephritis is the most common primary diagnosis in African American, Native American, and Asian pediatric patients, whereas cystic, hereditary, and congenital disease occurs most often in young white and Native American patients. Interestingly, Asian children are almost twice as likely as children of other races to have a primary diagnosis of glomerulonephritis/vasculitis. Hospitalizations for children with ESRD are directly related to age, and infection is the most important cause of complications requiring hospitalization. Survival rates also differ by age and modality of therapy. For example, by 5 years after the start of ESRD, 69% of children whose end stage began between birth and 4 years of age are still alive on dialysis, compared with 82% of children in other age groups.

KIDNEY DISEASE OUTCOMES QUALITY INITIATIVE GUIDELINES

The Dialysis Quality Initiative Guidelines published in 1997 by the National Kidney Foundation represented the first comprehensive effort to give evidence-based guidance to decrease variations in dialysis practices in the United States. A goal of the Dialysis Quality Initiative Guidelines was to develop concrete plans that could have a measurable impact on improving the quality of life for dialysis patients. The initial guidelines addressed adequacy of hemodialysis, adequacy of peritoneal dialysis, management of vascular access, and management of anemia. Although these guidelines were focused on patients with ESRD, the update of these guidelines was extended to cover patients with chronic renal failure before initiation of renal replacement therapy. This new initiative is known as the Kidney Disease Outcomes Quality Initiative (K/DOQI) (6). Although comprehensive guidelines were targeted to adult patients, specific issues related to pediatric patients are addressed in most of the guidelines.

Several guidelines have covered important aspects of the care of pediatric patients. Pediatric K/DOQI guidelines addressing nutritional issues including evaluation of protein-energy nutritional status, management of acid-base status, energy and protein intake for children treated with dialysis, and vitamin and mineral requirements were published in 2000 (7). A classification of stages of renal disease in adult and pediatric patients was published in 2002 (8). Specific goals of these guidelines have included the definition and classification of chronic kidney disease irrespective of the underlying cause, the evaluation of laboratory measurement and clinical assessment of kidney disease, the association of the stratification of the level of kidney function with complications of chronic kidney disease, and the risk for loss of kidney function with the development of cardiovascular disease. Guidelines under various stages of development include management of dyslipidemias, management of bone disease, and blood pressure management in chronic kidney disease. Each of these guidelines will address problems specific to pediatric patients with renal diseases. Detailed guidelines published to date are available on the National Kidney Foundation web site at http://www.kidney.org.

REFERENCES

1. Research needs in pediatric kidney disease: 2000 and beyond. Pediatric Nephrology Task Force Meeting. Bethesda, MD: National Institute of Diabetes and Digestive and Kidney Diseases, 1999. Available at: http://www.niddk.nih.gov. Accessed August 2003.
2. Ad Hoc Committee on Nephrology Manpower Needs. The Ad Hoc Committee report on estimating workforce and training requirements for nephrologists through the year 2010. *J Am Soc Nephrol* 1997;8(suppl 9):1–32.
3. Stapleton FB, Andreoli S, Ettenger R, et al. Future workforce needs for pediatric nephrology: an analysis of the nephrology workforce and training requirement by the Workforce Committee of the American Society of Pediatric Nephrology. *J Am Soc Nephrol* 1997;8:S5–S8.
4. North American Pediatric Renal Transplant Cooperative Study: 2001 annual report.
5. Pediatric end stage renal disease. United States Renal Data System's 2001 annual report 2001;38(suppl):S107–S116.
6. K/DOQI clinical practice guidelines: update 2001. *Am J Kidney Dis* 2001;37:S5–S6.
7. K/DOQI clinical practice guidelines for nutrition in chronic renal failure. *Am J Kidney Dis* 2000;35:S105–S136.
8. K/DOQI clinical practice guidelines for chronic kidney disease: evaluation, classification, and stratification. *Am J Kidney Dis* 2002;38:S1–S130.

75E

AFRICA

BAHIA HASSAN MOUSTAFA
FELICIA EKE
RAJENDRA BHIMMA

Many children with kidney disease in Africa do not receive proper medical care. Pediatric nephrologists are lacking in many African countries, and even when they are available, their numbers are far below that required for the child population in their areas. In Egypt there is one pediatric nephrologist per 500,000 child population, in Nigeria there is one per 10 million, and in South Africa there is one per 1.5 million. Therefore, pediatricians and general practitioners commonly treat these children (1). In the last two decades pediatric nephrology units have developed throughout the continent. They are concentrated mainly (a) in the northern region in Egypt, Tunisia, Algeria, Libya, and Morocco; (b) in the eastern region in Kenya, Sudan, and Ethiopia; (c) in the western region in Nigeria; and (d) in the southern region in South Africa. Most of these units provide primary and secondary renal care. Some provide tertiary care (i.e., limited dialysis), and very few provide quaternary care (i.e., comprehensive dialysis and transplantation). In the northern region of Africa dialysis and transplantation programs are well developed; however, they are run by internist nephrologists in many areas because of the high ratio of internist to pediatric nephrologists. In Egypt, efficient pediatric nephrology units are university-related units. There are approximately 12 university pediatric nephrology units. They act as regional centers for upper and lower Egypt and provide training and treatment. Over the last 2 years the Ministry of Health has established a number of pediatric hemodialysis units in national hospitals. Medical insurance covers the costs for patients treated in university or national hospital units. Transplantation for children is provided mainly by adult nephrologists. This situation is slowly changing as more pediatric nephrologists are being trained.

In the east, only Kenya has organized renal services including peritoneal dialysis, hemodialysis, and renal transplantation. In the western and central zones, Nigeria is the largest and richest country. There are seven pediatric nephrologists serving a child population of approximately 80 million, among whom 7.5 children per million per year are expected to develop end-stage renal failure. There are 12 adult hemodialysis units of variable quality and reliability. There are no transplantation centers and no pediatric hemodialysis units, but peritoneal dialysis is available for children with acute renal failure (ARF). Continous ambulatory peritoneal dialysis (CAPD) is not undertaken because of poor socioeconomic and hygienic conditions. Children with chronic renal failure (CRF) whose parents can afford the costs travel to Western countries for dialysis and transplantation. In South Africa, in spite of the deficiency of trained pediatric nephrologists in relation to child population, there are several centers that provide secondary levels of renal care, and most have facilities and expertise for peritoneal dialysis. Care for children with end-stage renal disease who need dialysis and transplantation is centralized in three major centers: Cape Town, Johannesburg, and Durban. In Durban, renal replacement therapy is limited to older children, but with the commissioning of the Inkosi Albert Luthuli Central Hospital, tertiary and quaternary renal care will be offered to all age groups. The policy of the country is to centralize quaternary care to limited designated sites for the entire country, whereas provision of various levels of renal replacement therapy will remain regionalized within a handful of cities.

The profile of renal diseases prevalent in Africa is unique with respect to etiology and clinical presentation. Endemic infections are a major cause of many renal diseases. The low socioeconomic status in many areas, lack of clean water supply, poor sanitation and irrigation systems, and overcrowded housing promote endemic infections such as schistosomiasis, malaria, tuberculosis, hepatitis, and infection with *Streptococcus*, *Salmonella*, *Shigella*, *Filaria,* and human immunodeficiency virus (HIV). The second major category contributing to the unique pattern of renal diseases in Africa includes the overuse of drugs, use of herbal and traditional medicines, toxins from bites, and local environmental pollutants. Obviously the dry environment and tropical climate with inadequate water supply leads to a high incidence of nephrolithiasis in the population.

African children demonstrate unique clinical presentations for various renal diseases. Infection and malnutrition

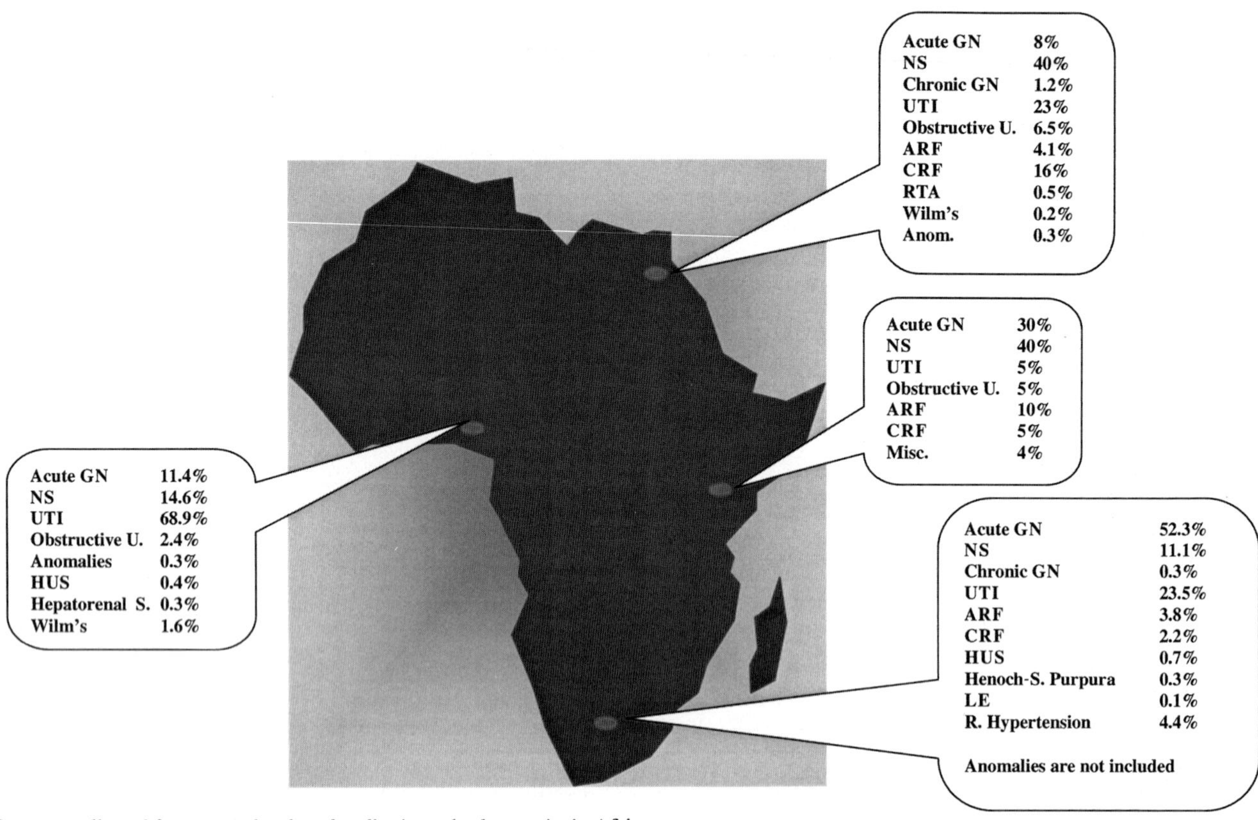

Data are collected from most developed pediatric nephrology units in Africa:

- **Cairo University Children's Hospital, Egypt**
- **Kenyata National Hospital Nairobi, Kenya**
- **King Edward VIII Hospital Durban, South Africa**
- **University of Port Harcourt Teaching Hospital, Nigeria**

FIGURE 75E.1. Renal disorders in northern, eastern, western, and southern Africa. Anom., anomalies; ARF, acute renal failure; CRF, chronic renal failure; GN, glomerulonephritis; Henoch-S. Purpura, Henoch-Schönlein purpura; Hepatorenal S., hepatorenal syndrome; HUS, hemolytic uremic syndrome; LE, lupus erythematosus; Misc., miscellaneous; NS, nephrotic syndrome; R., renal; RTA, renal tubular acidosis; U., uropathy; UTI, urinary tract infection.

commonly complicate the picture of the renal disorder. Infection either may be the primary cause of the kidney disease or may be acquired during treatment. The higher mortality and morbidity observed in these children can be attributed in large extent to late diagnosis and late referral to specialized units. Moreover, the poor intradialytic care children receive in some units because of limited resources or insufficient staff explains poor quality of life compared to that of similarly treated children in developed countries. The most prevalent renal disorders in Africa include nephrotic syndrome (NS), urinary tract infections (UTIs), and ARF and CRF (Fig. 75E.1).

NEPHROTIC SYNDROME

NS is the most common childhood renal disorder in Africa. It accounts for 14.6% of renal disorders in eastern Nigeria (2), 40% in Sudan (3), and 40% in Egypt (4). It has a very diverse profile in the black continent. In northern regions it resembles that in Western countries to a great extent; minimal change NS (MCNS) constitutes the major cause with a prevalence of 88% in Egypt (4), 85% in Libya (5), and 37% in Sudan (3). In Tunisia (6), however, it is not considered the most common pattern. In Egypt, children with nil disease show an excellent response to steroids and a satisfactory outcome. Children experiencing frequent relapse and steroid-dependent children constitute 42% and 36% of children with MCNS in the Cairo unit (4) and 21% and 15% in the Mansoura unit (7), respectively. In most patients, relapse rate correlates with compliance with the steroid therapy regimen. Infection is the main complication commonly reported. Pneumonia, subcutaneous abscesses, UTIs, peritonitis, and septicemia show prevalences of 35%, 22%, 28%, 5%, and 2%, respectively. Hypovolemic shock after infectious diarrhea was reported in 5% of nephrotic children. Intravascular thrombosis was reported in 2%. The death rate in this study was 2% (4). Among other pathologic types of NS in Egypt, a high prevalence of focal segmental glomerulosclerosis (FSGS) was seen during the 1980s in the Cairo unit (4). Later data from the same unit in the 1990s showed an almost equal prevalence of mesangial proliferative glomerulonephritis (MPGN) (22.7%) and FSGS (21.3%) (8). Subsequently MPGN (34.3%) was prevalent through the next 10 years when data for 394 nephrotic children undergoing renal biopsy were analyzed. Secondary forms of NS are less common in northern Africa than in other parts of the continent. An incidence of 6.6% was reported in Egypt (7). A postinfection pattern is the most common, with schistosomal nephropathy endemic in the north in the Nile delta in Egypt, Ethiopia, and Sudan. The causative parasite is *Schistosoma haematobium* in East, West, and Central Africa as well as the Nile delta. *Schistosoma mansoni* is endemic in the Nile valley, and the western and southern regions of Africa. Such patterns correlate with prevalence of the snail host and poor hygiene. Infected children present with hematuria, glomerulonephritis, NS, or renal failure. Hepatosplenomegaly with the presence of bilharzial ova in urine or stools commonly point to the diagnosis. Patients demonstrate unselective proteinuria, marked reduction in total serum levels of proteins with a characteristic high gamma globulin fraction, normal serum cholesterol level, normal to low serum complement profile, low urine osmolality, and normal to low glomerular filtration rate (GFR). Many such patients are chronic *Salmonella* carriers with intermittent bacteruria, especially those with refractory anemia and persistent fever. Urinary tract imaging may reveal bladder calcification and/or obstructive uropathies and vesicoureteral reflux (VUR); renal biopsy results revealed diffuse MPGN (38%), FSGS (20%), membranous nephropathy (12%), focal MPGN (7%), or mesangiocapillary glomerulonephritis (18%) (9). Different immune mechanisms have been implicated in the pathogenesis of these lesions (10). Current statistics have shown a marked decline in the prevalence of schistosomal nephropathy in many African countries, mainly the Nile delta of Egypt. This has been attributed to aggressive use of chemotherapy among schoolchildren and extensive snail eradication. Trials for manufacture of a new protective vaccine are promising (11).

Hepatitis B is increasingly more prevalent as a cause of NS in northern Africa, with a 44% incidence among secondary forms of NS reported in Egypt (12). Hepatitis C was less commonly reported in the same region (13). Tuberculosis and filariasis are now less prevalent in the northern region. Lupus erythematosus nephropathy is found in 8% of nephrotic children undergoing biopsy (4) in Egypt. Sickle cell nephropathy is rare in North Africa, although the disease is not rare. Ochratoxins and aflatoxins, which are common constituents in foodstuffs in Africa, were detected in urine, serum, and kidney biopsy specimens of children with NS or renal failure in Tunisia and Egypt (14). Cadmium and aluminum, which are common environmental pollutants in Africa, were recorded as toxic causes for NS in Africa.

In West and Central Africa the profile of NS is unlike that in the Western world. Idiopathic NS is not common. When it affects black children it is often associated with a high rate of steroid nonresponse. This is true in Togo, West Africa (15), western Nigeria (16), northern Nigeria (17), Uganda (18), and Zaire (19). In Port Harcourt (20) and Yaoude, Cameroon (21), however, steroid responsiveness is not uncommon. Infections play a major role in the pathogenesis of NS in West and Central Africa. Quartan malarial nephropathy, first described in Ibadan, western Nigeria, is detected in up to 81% of renal biopsy specimens in children (16). Quartan malarial nephropathy is predominantly associated with *Plasmodium malariae* and also with *Plasmodium falciparum* infection (17). Typically there is focal and segmental glomerulonephritis with thickening of capillary walls but without endothelial cell proliferation. Finding of *P. malariae* or *P. falciparum* antigen in the glomeruli by immunofluorescence is diagnostic. In eastern Nigeria, MCNS is the most common pathologic diagnosis in cases undergoing biopsy (21). Other infections reported in West and Central Africa include hepatitis B with membranous nephropathy (22). NS often complicates poststreptococcal glomerulonephritis in this region. Schistosomiasis, filariasis, and leprosy are also recorded.

In eastern Nigeria, sickle cell nephropathy is common and sickle cell anemia is common with a heterozygous carrier rate of 25%. FSGS and renal papillary necrosis are explained by endothelial damage caused by occlusion by sickled cells and microinfarcts. There are numerous cases of unexplained renal pathology, with NS possibly caused by toxins found in herbal remedies or environmental contamination.

In South Africa, the etiology of NS has undergone considerable change after 1995 as compared to earlier records (Table 75E.1). During the 1970s and 1980s, the pattern in Indian and white children was similar to that seen in the

TABLE 75E.1. HISTOLOGIC PATTERN OF NEPHROTIC SYNDROME BEFORE AND AFTER 1995 IN DURBAN, SOUTH AFRICA

Histologic findings	1976–1994	1995–2000
Minimal change disease	95	11
Focal segmental glomerulosclerosis	41	43
Membranous nephropathy	44	6
Membranous nephropathy (hepatitis B associated)	63	24
Diffuse mesangial proliferative glomerulonephritis	26	1
Focal mesangial proliferative glomerulonephritis	13	2
Mesangiocapillary glomerulonephritis	4	1
Total	286	88

Western world (23). Those of mixed race had a similar histologic pattern of disease but a less gratifying response to steroid therapy. In all of these racial groups, minimal change disease, the presence of which strongly correlated with steroid responsiveness, was the most common lesion. NS among black children in South Africa is characterized by a paucity of minimal change disease, steroid resistance, and a less satisfactory outcome and unidentifiable causative agents in many (24,25). During these two decades the most common histopathologic form of NS seen among black children in the coastal regions was membranous nephropathy, whereas that seen in regions such as Johannesburg was FSGS (26). Membranous nephropathy accounted for 40% of all cases of NS in black children; it was associated with chronic hepatitis B virus carriage in over 86% of cases and showed a strong male predominance (27,28). Minimal change disease accounted for 14 to 25% of all cases of NS; it was less common in coastal regions such as Durban (24,27). Over the last decade there has been a substantial change in the pattern of NS in coastal regions of South Africa. FSGS has increased among Indian and black children, accounting for 50% of all cases of NS in children. More than 95% of these patients are steroid unresponsive. Black patients tend to have more aggressive disease with progression to end-stage disease over a short of period of time (29). The introduction of hepatitis B vaccine in April 1995 had a major impact on the incidence of hepatitis B virus–associated NS. In Durban, the number of new cases remained steady up to 1999 with a marked decline thereafter (30). Other secondary causes of NS in South Africa include congenital syphilis, cytomegalovirus infection, and poststreptococcal glomerulonephritis. Schistosomal nephropathy and malarial nephropathy are rare in South Africa. The HIV infection and acquired immunodeficiency syndrome that have overwhelmed Sub-Saharan Africa over the last decade have had little reported impact on the pattern of NS seen in children. There have been no reports on HIV-associated nephropathies in children in South Africa to date.

URINARY TRACT INFECTIONS

UTIs are common in Africa, in both rural and urban areas and among neonates, preschool children, and school-aged children. UTIs show a prevalence of 22% in symptomatic children in Cairo, Egypt. Asymptomatic bacteruria has a recorded incidence of 4.2% in girls and 2.8% in boys among schoolchildren in urban Egypt (31) and 11% in girls and 3.6% in boys in rural Egypt (32). In Central and West Africa, UTIs have an incidence from 8.2 to 72% in symptomatic children (33) and of 48% in an asymptomatic rural community (34). In Cape Town, approximately 1000 cases of UTI are seen yearly. In fact, because of the nonspecific complaints in neonates and young children, many cases are missed, especially in rural areas. The microbiology of UTIs in Africa is consistent over the continent (35). In the northern region of Egypt, the recorded causative organism is *Escherichia coli* in 70% of cases, *Proteus* in 10%, *Klebsiella* in 5%, and *Pseudomonas* in 5% (36). Schistosomiasis is considered a common predisposing factor for UTI in Egypt (36), Senegal (37), and Cameroon (38). Stones, developmental anomalies of the urinary tract, and VUR are also common structural changes that favor infection in Egypt, with prevalences of 2.5%, 12%, and 17%, respectively (36). VUR is rare in West and Central Africa whereas posterior urethral valves and meatal and urethral strictures are reported to have an incidence of 29.3% among children with UTIs (35). In South Africa, local predisposing factors include malnutrition, congenital anomalies, immunodeficiency states, and VUR. The latter is rare in black children but common in whites (39,40). Adhikari (40) reported 2 Indian children with VUR out of 26 children with anomalies, and 7 cases of PUV out of 14 with obstructive uropathies. Renal growth and GFR are commonly affected in African children with UTI because of late diagnosis and referral, as well as patient noncompliance with treatment. Impaired renal growth was reported in 36% of cases referred to the Cairo University unit, whereas low GFR was reported in 5% of the same patients (36). *E. coli* strains resistant to amoxicillin and co-trimoxazole were reported in Africa with 88% and 86% resistance to these drugs, respectively, in Cape Town.

ACUTE RENAL FAILURE

ARF has unique epidemiology in African children. Infection is the major cause. Bacterial infections commonly reported include streptococcosis, cholera, salmonellosis, shigellosis, leptospirosis, tetanus, and diphtheria. Viral infections include HIV infection, hepatitis B, hepatitis C, hepatitis A, and cytomegalovirus infection. Common parasitic infections are malaria and schistosomiasis. Among all pathogen-related causes, diarrheal diseases, schistosomiasis, and malaria remain the most common. Infection precipitates ARF through immune mechanisms and alteration of kidney hemodynamics (41). Toxins present after snakebites, scorpion stings, or other insect stings, or after ingestion of herbal medicines or overuse of drugs are also unique causes of ARF in Africa. Table 75E.2 summarizes causes of ARF in Egypt (42), Nigeria (43), and South Africa. Septicemia, gastroenteritis, and hemolytic uremic syndrome (HUS) are common causes in the three regions. Epidemic forms of ARF after use of native herbal medicines and holy water were reported in Nigeria (44). In South Africa, an epidemic of *Shigella* dysentery type 1 occurred in 1994 to 1996 in Sub-Saharan Africa, starting in Burudi and progressing to the Cape (45). One hundred fifty-nine cases of HUS occurred in black children after this bloody diarrhea. Among 81 cases of post-*Shigella*-induced HUS in Durban, complications included ARF in 90.1%,

TABLE 75E.2. CAUSES OF ACUTE AND CHRONIC RENAL FAILURE IN SELECTED LOCATIONS IN AFRICA

	Egypt (%)	Nigeria (%)	Cape Town (%)	Durban blacks (%)
Acute renal failure				
Septicemia and urinary obstruction	21	16	24.1	—
Gastroenteritis	27	34	7.4	—
Poststreptococcal glomerulonephritis	29	—		—
Lupus erythematosus	12		—	—
Hemolytic uremic syndrome	6	11	9.3	—
Nephrotoxins	3	—		—
Unknown	2	5	—	—
Acute glomerulonephritis	—	12		—
Malaria	—	10	—	—
Birth asphyxiation	—	12	—	—
Postcardiac surgery	—	—	16.7	—
Myocarditis	—	—	11.1	—
Rapidly progressive glomerulonephritis	—	—	9.3	—
Necrotizing enterocolitis	—	—	7.4	—
Kwashiorkor	—	—	7.4	—
Leukemia	—	—	7.4	—
Chronic renal failure				
Reflux nephropathy	15	—	—	—
Glomerulonephritis	26	72	—	45
Unknown	28	14	—	—
Urinary obstruction	31	7	—	—
Pyelonephritis	—	7	—	—
Focal segmental glomerulonephritis	—	—	—	25
Anomalies	—	—	—	26
Other causes	—	—	—	4

encephalopathy in 37%, convulsions in 14.8%, hemiplegia in 2.3%, intestinal perforation in 9.9%, protein-losing enteropathy in 32.1%, toxic megacolon in 4.9%, rectal prolapse in 6.2%, hepatitis in 13.6%, myocarditis in 6.2%, disseminated intravascular coagulation in 21%, CRF in 32.1%, impaired renal function in 9.9%, ESRD in 1.2%, and death in 17.3% (46). During the last 2 years *E. coli*–induced HUS, especially coexistent with HIV infection, has been reported in Cape Town.

CHRONIC RENAL FAILURE

The pattern of CRF in African children is unique with respect to its etiology, clinical presentation, and management. Causes of CRF in Egypt (47), Nigeria (2), and South Africa are summarized in Table 75E.2. It is evident that obstructive uropathies and reflux nephropathy are prevalent causes in Egypt, whereas glomerulonephritis is common in Nigeria and South Africa. Late referral of cases explains the preponderance of unknown diagnoses among Egyptian children who already have atrophic kidneys at their first visit to a pediatric nephrology unit.

Signs of CRF in African children are aggravated by three distinct elements: infection (whether causing CRF or acquired during dialysis), malnutrition (especially deficiencies of iron, vitamin D, and trace elements), and late diagnosis and poor management (which aggravate anemia, growth retardation, and bone disabilities).

DIALYSIS AND TRANSPLANTATION

Acute peritoneal dialysis is the most common type of dialysis in Africa and is more readily available than acute hemodialysis. Chronic intermittent peritoneal dialysis is the most common technique used in CRF cases in developing countries in Africa. The use of continuous cycling peritoneal dialysis is less common. In developed areas such as Cape Town in South Africa, however, use of CAPD is predominant. Efficiency of dialysis varies among pediatric nephrology centers in Africa. It depends on availability of funds as well as trained staff. African children on regular dialysis demonstrate lack of compliance with the regimen because of psychosocial and economic factors, and most of them experience poor quality of life. Factors that contribute to their poor outcome include deficient dialysis, undernutrition, infection, and lack of appropriate interdialytic care due to nonavailability of erythropoietin, iron, active vitamin D, and growth hormone (1).

Although renal transplantation is more cost effective than dialysis, it is not available in most African countries.

Reported centers are concentrated in the northern region and in South Africa. Ethical and religious factors in each country determine whether cadaveric or living donor grafts are used. In South Africa, cadaver organ–based programs are widely used, whereas in Egypt, only living related donor–based programs are permitted. Morbidity and mortality of patients undergoing renal transplantation are higher in Africa than in developed countries.

Most African countries lack national kidney foundations as well as medical insurance systems. Therefore, funding for ESRD therapy remains a significant handicap for most African countries. Prevention of ESRD is the best strategy when approaching the problem of CRF in Africa. Simple measures include health education to combat unhygienic habits and use of traditional remedies, many of which are nephrotoxic. Additional measures include infection control through antischistosomal and antimalarial campaigns and obligatory vaccination against tuberculosis and hepatitis. Screening for renal diseases among schoolchildren might identify patients early in the disease course and maximize appropriate intervention.

The development of the African Pediatric Nephrology Association (AFPNA) in 1999 with its affiliation to the International Pediatric Nephrology Association carries new prospects for upgrading the practice of pediatric nephrology in Africa. Training programs supported by the IPNA to increase the number of trained pediatric nephrologists are now planned to cover northern, central, and southern regions of Africa. Shortage of specialists and trained staff as well as restricted financial resources remain a major handicap in many areas. Development of regional pediatric nephrology societies such as the Egyptian Society of Pediatric Nephrology and the South African transplantation and pediatric nephrology groups as well as improved education offer promise for dramatic improvements in pediatric nephrology care in Africa over the next decade.

ACKNOWLEDGMENTS

The authors would like to thank Prof. M. Adhikari (Durban) and Dr. M. McCulloch and Dr. P. Sinclair (Red Cross Children's Hospital, Cape Town) for providing valuable data from their centers. The authors also offer special thanks to colleagues in different pediatric nephrology units throughout the continent for their assistance in data collection and collation.

REFERENCES

1. Moustafa B. Mapping of pediatric nephrology in Africa. 1st Congress for African Pediatric Nephrology Association (A.F.P.N.A.), February, 2000:P9.
2. Eke FU, Eke NN. Renal disorders in children: a Nigerian study. *Pediatr Nephrol* 1994;8:383–386.
3. Musa AR, Veress B, Kordofani AM, et al. Pattern of the nephrotic syndrome in Sudan. *Ann Trop Med Parasitol* 1980;74:37–44.
4. Moustafa B, El Zawahry K, El Kolally S. Epidemiological profile of nephrotic syndrome in Egypt. *Gaz Egypt Paediatr Assoc* 1984;32:39–45.
5. El Zouki AY, Amin F, Jaiswal OP. Primary nephrotic syndrome in Arab children. *Arch Dis Child* 1984;59:253–255.
6. Maiz HB, Moussa FB, Abderrahim E, et al. N.S. in childhood, study of 381 cases. The 25th annual meeting of the European society of Pediatric Nephrology. *Pediatr Nephrol* 1991;5:C26(abst).
7. Sarhan AA, Baker AM, Hammad AM, et al. Pattern of NS in P.N. unit Mansoura University, Egypt in the last 5 years. The 33rd annual meeting of the European Society of Pediatric Nephrology. *Pediatr Nephrol* 1999;13:C61(abst).
8. Moustafa B, Zahran M, Francis M, et al. Pathological profile of glomerulopathies among Egyptian children. *JAC* 1996;7(1):25–46.
9. Moustafa B. Schistosomal nephropathy. Egyptian experience. 1st Congress of A.F.P.N.A., Cairo, February, 2000:P9.
10. Barsoom R. Schistosomal glomerulopathies. *Kidney Int* 1993;44:1.
11. Alsherbiny MM. New schistosomal vaccine. WHO/TDR program supported by the Schistosomiasis Vaccine Development Project (SVDP). *A.F.P.N.A. Newsletter* September, 2001.
12. Farid F, Moselhy S, Rafik, M, et al. Hepatitis B virus related glomerulopathies in Egyptian children. 1997;18(2):437–448.
13. Moselhy S, Gaffar A, Hememy N. Hepatitis C associated glomerulopathies in Egyptian children. *New Egypt J Med* 1997;17(3):267–274.
14. Saadi MG, Abdallah S, Fadel F, et al. Prevalence of okra toxin OT among Egyptian children and adults with different renal diseases. *Med J Cairo Univ* 1996;64(2):497–506.
15. Gbadoe AD, Atakouma DY, Napo-Koura G, et al. Primary nephrotic syndrome in the black African child. *Arch Pediatr* 1999;6:985–989.
16. Hendrickse RG, Adeniyi A, Edington GM, et al. Quartan malarial nephrotic syndrome. Collaborative clinicopathological study in Nigerian children. *Lancet* 1972;1:1143–1149.
17. Abdurrahma MB. The role of infectious agents in the etiology and pathogenesis of childhood nephrotic syndrome in Africa. *J Infect* 1983;8:100–109.
18. Odiit A, Tindyebwa D. Selective protein index and clinical features of childhood nephrotic syndrome in Kampala. *East Afr Med J* 1997;74:207–209.
19. Pakasa M, Mangani N, Dikassa L. Focal and segmental glomerulosclerosis in nephrotic syndrome: a new profile of adult nephrotic syndrome in Zaire. *Mod Pathol* 1993;6:125–128.
20. Eke, FU. Nephrotic syndrome in Port Harcourt—clinical presentation and response to steroids. *Nig J Paediatr* 1990;17:59–63.
21. Mbakop A, Youmbissi TJ, Gonsu JD, et al. [Renal puncture biopsy in nephrotic syndrome in Cameroonian children, adolescents, and adults: histopathologic profile according to age]. *Arch Anat Cytol Pathol* 1990;38:104–107.
22. Seggie J, Nathoo K, Davies PG. Association of hepatitis B (HBs) antigenaemia and membranous glomerulonephritis in Zimbabwean children. *Nephron* 1984;38:115–119.

23. Bhimma R, Coovadia HM, Adhikari M. Nephrotic syndrome in South African children: changing perspectives over 20 years (1976–1995). *Pediatr Nephrol* 1997;11:429–434.
24. Adhikar M, Coovadia HM, Morel-Margoer L. Absence of true minimal change nephrotic syndrome in African children in South Africa. *J Trop Med Hyg* 1993;88:223–228.
25. Coovadia HM, Adhikari M, Morel-Maroger L. Clinicopathological features of the nephrotic syndrome in South African children. *QJM* 1979;48:77–91.
26. Thomson PD. Glomerulonephritis in children: a South African perspective. *Specialist Medicine* 2000:21–32.
27. Bhimma R, Coovadia HM, Adhikari M. Hepatitis B virus—associated nephropathy in black South African children. *Pediatr Nephrol* 1998;12:479–484.
28. Gilbert DR, Wiggelinkhulzen J. The clinical courses of Hepatitis B virus nephropathy. *Pediatr Nephrol* 1994;8:11–14.
29. Adhikari M, Bhimma R, Coovadia HM. Focal segmental glomerulosclerosis in children from KwaZulu/Natal, South Africa. *Clin Nephrol* 2001;55(1):16–24.
30. Kew MC. Progress towards the comprehensive control of hepatitis B in Africa: a view from South Africa. *Gut* 1996; 38(suppl 2):S31–S36.
31. Moustafa B. UTIs in Egyptian children. 19th Congress of Egyptian Society of Nephrology and Transplantation, Gona, Egypt, 2000:P27.
32. El-Gamal SA, Saleh LH. Asymptomatic bacteriuria in school children in a rural area, Egypt. *J Egypt Public Health Assoc* 1991;66:113–121.
33. Anoukoun T, Agbodjan-Djossou O, Atakouma YD, et al. [Epidemiologic and etiologic features of urinary infections in children at the pediatrics service of the CHU-Campus de Lome (Togo)]. *Ann Urol* 2001;35:178–184.
34. Azubike CN, Nwamadu OJ, Oji RU, et al. Prevalence of urinary tract infection among school children in a Nigerian rural community. *West Afr J Med* 1994;13:48–52.
35. Eke FU, Eke N. Urinary tract infection in Nigerian children. *Nephron* 1995;70:132.
36. Moustafa B, Soliman N, Kamalo M, et al. Profile of UTI in Cairo University PN unit through last 8 years. *J Egypt Soc Pediatr Nephrol Transplant* (*in press*).
37. Verle P, Stelma F, Desreumaux P, et al. Preliminary study of urinary schistosomiasis in a village in the delta of the Senegal river basin, Senegal. *Trans R Soc Trop Med Hyg* 1994:88.
38. Cunin P, Griffet A, Poste B, et al. Epidemic Schistosoma mansoni in a known S. Haematobium area. *Trans R Soc Trop Med Hyg* 2000;94:657–660.
39. Reed RP, Wegerhoff FO. Urinary tract infection in malnourished rural African children. *Ann Trop Paediatr* 1995;15:21–26.
40. Jeena PM, Coovadia HM, Adhikari M. Bacteriuria in children attending a primary health care clinic: a prospective study of catheter stream urine samples. *Ann Trop Paediatr* 1996;16:293–398.
41. Quezado ZMN, Natanson C. Systemic haemodynamic abnormalities and vasopressor therapy in sepsis and septic shock. *Am J Kidney Dis* 1992;20:214.
42. Moustafa B, Baha El-Din H, Shoman M. Acute renal failure among Egyptian children. Causes and outcome. XXI International Congress of Pediatrics, Cairo, Egypt, September 10–15, 1995:P526.
43. Eke FU. Acute renal failure as seen in Port Harcourt over fifteen years. 12th Congress of the International Pediatric Nephrology Assoc, 2001:55.
44. AdelekunTA, Ekwere TR, Akinsola A. The pattern of acute toxic nephropathy in Ife, Nigeria. *West Afr J Med* 1999;18: 60–63.
45. Bhimma R, Rollins N, Coovadia HM, et al. Post dysenteric hemolytic-uraemic syndrome in children during an epidemic of shigella dysentery in Kwazulu/Natal. *Centr Afr J Med* 1997;43:152–158.
46. Bhimma R, Nigel CR, Coovadia HM, et al. Post-dysenteric hemolytic uremic syndrome in children during an epidemic of shigella dysentery in Kwazulu/Natal Ped. *Nephrol* 1997; 11:560–564.
47. Safouh H, El Hetw M. Chronic renal failure in Egyptian children. XXI International Congress of Pediatrics, Cairo, Egypt, September 10 to 15, 1995:P658.

75F

LATIN AMERICA

RAMON ALFONSO EXENI

DEMOGRAPHY

Latin America comprises nations in North, Central, and South America in which the prevailing languages derive from Latin. It encompasses an extensive territory with significant cultural and socioeconomic differences and sharp contrasts. Aboriginal inhabitants live in extremely poor conditions in some regions, and considerable social imbalances characterize urban areas. However, some noteworthy features, such as hospitality, tolerance, and respect for ethnic differences, have arisen from the fusion between the ancient indigenous cultures and the European colonization.

LATIN AMERICAN ASSOCIATION OF PEDIATRIC NEPHROLOGY

The Latin American Association of Pediatric Nephrology (ALANEPE) was created in Buenos Aires, Argentina, in a meeting held by the Sociedad Argentina de Pediatría [Argentine Society of Pediatrics] on November 27, 1981, by 48 founding members. The objective of ALANEPE was to promote knowledge and science in pediatric nephrology and to improve the care of Latin American children with kidney diseases.

ALANEPE is divided in three regions:

- Region 1: Mexico, Guatemala, El Salvador, Costa Rica, Nicaragua, Honduras, Panama, Caribbean islands, Cuba, Dominican Republic, Puerto Rico
- Region 2: Venezuela, Colombia, Ecuador, Peru, Bolivia
- Region 3: Chile, Argentina, Brazil, Paraguay, Uruguay

These regions comprise a population of approximately 457 million (Table 75F.1).

In 2001, the publication of ALANEPE's official journal, *Archivos latinoamericanos de nefrología pediátrica* [Latin American Archives of Pediatric Nephrology], was initiated. This is a teaching journal with reviews, recommendations, practical nephrology items, news, and reports of societal activities. This publication has increased interest in the specialty on the part of pediatricians and has served as continuing medical education for pediatric nephrologists. Like the triennial ALANEPE congress, it is a symbol of ALANEPE's commitment to its mission.

PEDIATRIC NEPHROLOGY DEVELOPMENT IN LATIN AMERICA

The field of pediatric nephrology in Latin America had the privilege of having two figures that greatly fostered its development in two geographically separated regions. In 1954, Dr. Gustavo Gordillo created one of the first departments of pediatric nephrology in the world in the Children's Hospital of Mexico. Dr. Carlos Gianantonio, in Argentina, championed the specialty in the south. Due to the extremely high incidence of hemolytic uremic syndrome (HUS) in Argentina, Dr. Gianantonio dedicated extraordinary effort to understanding the basic pathophysiology, clinical course, and management of this disease. The influence of these two leaders of the field promoted the creation of pediatric nephrology centers in both countries, which then spread throughout Latin America. Their nephrology departments turned into educational centers for nephrologists from all the regions of the continent. Dr. Renee Habib (France) and Dr. Juan Rodríguez Soriano (Spain) have also promoted and influenced the development of pediatric nephrology in Latin America.

ALANEPE has grown from 48 to 540 members, and the emergence of pediatric nephrology in Latin America is well documented through analysis of the number of Latin American abstracts submitted to the last four congresses of the International Pediatric Nephrology Association (Table 75F.2) and the Latin American papers published in *Pediatric Nephrology*, the official journal of this organization, over the past 15 years (1987 to 2002) (Fig. 75F.1; Table 75F.3).

SPECIFIC AREAS OF CLINICAL AND RESEARCH INTEREST: HEMOLYTIC UREMIC SYNDROME

The world's highest incidence of HUS (see Chapter 47) is reported in Argentina, with 22 cases per 100,000 children younger than 5 years of age. In this country, approximately

TABLE 75F.1. LATIN AMERICA POPULATION (× 1000 INHABITANTS) (1)

Argentina	34,293	Bolivia	7896	Brazil	160,737	Chile	14,161
Colombia	26,200	Costa Rica	3419	Cuba	10,938	Dominican Republic	7948
Ecuador	10,891	El Salvador	5870	Guatemala	11,000	Honduras	5460
Mexico	93,986	Nicaragua	4206	Panama	2681	Paraguay	5358
Peru	24,087	Puerto Rico	3691	Uruguay	3223	Venezuela	21,005

400 new cases are reported annually. Nearly all of them are secondary to infections caused by verotoxin-producing *Escherichia coli* O157:H7. After Gasser's description in 1955, Dr. Carlos Gianantonio and colleagues published a seminal study of 64 cases in 1964 (2). Gianantonio's greatest achievement was the implementation of peritoneal dialysis in these children, which reduced acute mortality from 50% to 5%.

The Nephrology Committee of the Argentine Society of Pediatrics registered 7570 HUS patients in 11 centers in Argentina between 1965 and 2001. In that period, mortality varied between 2 and 5.6% during the acute phase. There were no significant differences between the sexes. Mean patient age of 11 months in 1990 increased to 18 months in 2001. Cases have been observed throughout the year, with a greater incidence between November and March (summertime). These cases underestimate actual disease incidences, because they reflect data only from public hospitals. A considerable number of children go to private centers and were not included in this report.

The high incidence of HUS in Argentina is related to the high rate of ingestion of bovine meat and its early introduction in young children's diets. Several centers in Argentina have participated in collaborative studies using Synsorb, and many are involved in a multicenter study using therapy with monoclonal antibodies. Table 75F.4 summarizes 30 years' experience in the treatment of HUS in two major reference centers: Ricardo Gutiérrez Children's Hospital in Buenos Aires and San Justo Children's Hospital in a Buenos Aires suburb. It was at the Ricardo Gutiérrez Children's Hospital where Dr. Gianantonio performed his research on this disease.

TABLE 75F.2. ORIGIN OF ABSTRACTS SUBMITTED TO THE LAST FOUR INTERNATIONAL CONGRESSES OF THE INTERNATIONAL PEDIATRIC NEPHROLOGY ASSOCIATION

	Congress			
	Jerusalem (Israel), 1992	Santiago (Chile), 1995	London (United Kingdom), 1998	Seattle (United States), 2001
Total number of abstracts	420	465	582	590
Number (%) of Latin American abstracts	22 (5.23)	89 (19.13)	56 (9.6)	61 (10.3)
Countries				
Argentina	5	38	14	10
Brazil	13	22	24	35
Colombia	1	—	—	1
Chile	1	18	7	8
Mexico	1	1	2	1
Uruguay	1	1	—	—
Venezuela	1	9	9	6

COLLABORATIVE STUDIES

National Collaborative Studies

Venezuela

The Pediatric Nephrology Chapter of the Venezuelan Society of Pediatrics and the Venezuelan Society of Nephrology reported epidemiologic data on renal disorders in children of that country (4). Information was obtained from 14 centers for the period January through December 1998. A total of 3624 patients were evaluated either through a first outpatient consultation or at a first hospital admission.

The patients were grouped into the following categories: (a) urinary tract infections (32%), with detection of abnormalities of the urinary tract in 25%; (b) metabolic disorders (28%), mainly idiopathic hypercalciuria and hyperuricosuria; and (c) glomerulonephritis (9.5%). The remaining 30% included children with urolithiasis (7%), nephritic syndrome (4.5%), primary hematuria (4.2%), acute renal failure (2.8%, with 43% of cases secondary to acute dehydration, 15% due to birth asphyxia, 14% due to secondary septicemia, and 23% due to multiple factors), chronic renal failure

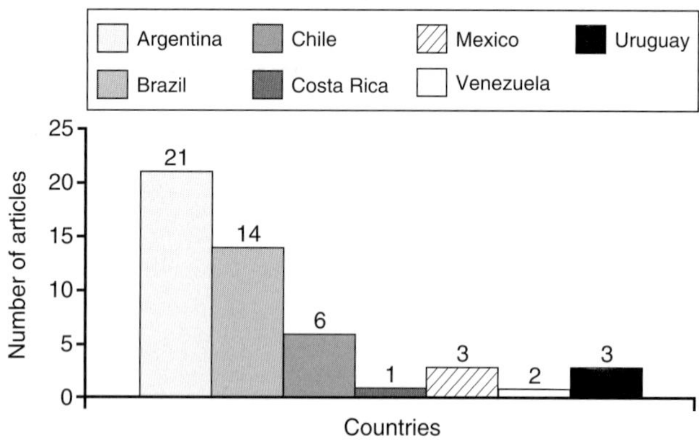

FIGURE 75F.1. Number of Latin American articles published in *Pediatric Nephrology* from 1987 to 2002.

TABLE 75F.3. TOPICS OF THE ARTICLES PUBLISHED BY LATIN AMERICAN PEDIATRIC NEPHROLOGISTS IN *PEDIATRIC NEPHROLOGY*

Topic	No.
Acid-base balance and electrolytic disturbances	2
Acute renal failure	1
Chronic renal failure	1
Glomerulopathies	1
Hemolytic uremic syndrome	11
Hypertension	2
Kidney transplantation	5
Neonatal disorders	2
Nephrolithiasis and hypercalciurias	5
Nephrologic policies and social issues	5
Nephrotic syndrome	6
Peritoneal dialysis	1
Tubulopathies	1
Urinary tract infections and uropathies	6

(CRF) (1.6%; secondary to glomerulopathies, predominantly focal glomerulosclerosis, structural abnormalities of the urinary tract, hereditary disorders, and renal hypoplasia and dysplasia), and miscellaneous diseases (4.8%).

Chile: Chronic Peritoneal Dialysis in Chile—A Multicenter Study

Dr. Angela Delucchi coordinated a multicenter study of continuous ambulatory peritoneal dialysis (CAPD) in five Chilean centers: Luís Calvo Mackenna Hospital, Roberto del Río Hospital, Guillermo Grant Benavente Hospital, Exequiel González Cortés Hospital, and School of Public Health—University of Chile, Santiago, Concepción. (5) One hundred and twenty-nine children younger than 18 years of age were evaluated; 97 of them, with at least 6 months of follow-up, were included in the analysis. Causes of disease were renal hypoplasia or dysplasia (26%), glomerulopathies (17%), reflux nephropathy (15%), obstructive uropathy (15%), vascular diseases (15 %), and other disorders (12%). Serum calcium levels increased from 8.9 mg/dL to 9.3 mg/dL after CAPD (p <.05). Parathyroid hormone and alkaline phosphatase levels were correlated significantly (p <.0004). Mean Z score for height and age was –2.2 ± 1.6. A progressive but not significant impairment of Z score height was found; growth failure was lower in children who started peritoneal dialysis at a younger age.

This study demonstrates that the use of CAPD has progressively increased in Chile in recent years. An increase in the number of children starting CAPD at a younger age was also observed. Hematologic and biochemical parameters improved on CAPD. Poor growth rate was related to a longer mean duration of dialysis. Dialysis doses were inversely related to age.

Staphylococcus aureus accounted for the majority of episodes of peritonitis, and the incidence of this complication was 0.67 episodes per patient per year, a rate similar to that reported in the literature. The mean weekly urea K_t/v was 2.9 ± 1.9.

TABLE 75F.4. HEMOLYTIC UREMIC SYNDROME: RICARDO GUTIÉRREZ CHILDREN'S HOSPITAL (BUENOS AIRES) AND SAN JUSTO CHILDREN'S HOSPITAL (BUENOS AIRES PROVINCE), 1970–2000

Acute manifestations	
Prodromes	
Diarrhea: mucous-bloody	1249 (96%)
No diarrhea	53 (4%)
Upper respiratory infection	130 (10%)
Hematologic manifestations	
Hemolytic anemia	1302 (100%)
Thrombocytopenia	1302 (100%)
Leukocytosis	218 (67%)
Acute renal failure	100%
Anuria fewer than 7 days	660 (50.69%)
Anuria more than 7 days	312 (23.97%
No anuria	298 (22.89%)
Anuria without diuresis recovery	32 (2.45%)
Hypertension	348 (33%)
Major neurologic manifestations	260 (20%)
Mortality	35 (2.6%)
Long-term follow-up (3)	
No. patients: 152	
Mean follow-up: 10.3 years (range, 5–27 years)	
Functional status:	
Group A: 107 (70%)—normal renal function without proteinuria or hypertension	
Group B: 21 (13.8%)—normal renal function, proteinuria ± hypertension	
Group C: 19 (2.6%)—decreased glomerular filtration rate, proteinuria ± hypertension	
Group D: 5 (5.3%)—end-stage renal disease	

Argentina: National Register of Chronic Renal Disease, Dialysis, and Transplantation

In 1996, Argentina initiated a centralized registry of pediatric patients with end-stage CRF undergoing conservative management, dialysis, and transplantation (6). The coordinator of this national register is Dr. Irene Grimoldi. The 1996 results, which were based on data from 14 centers, were the following.

One hundred and thirty-five patients were registered; 62 (45.9%) were being managed conservatively; 51 (37.8%) were receiving dialysis; and 22 (16.3%) received kidney transplantations. The following were reported as primary renal diseases: glomerulopathies (27.4%), obstructive uropathy (17.7%), reflux nephropathy (16.3%), HUS (10.3%), aplasia-dysplasia-hypoplasia (8.8%), and other (19.5%). Of 51 patients on dialysis, 41.2% received peritoneal dialysis and 58.8% hemodialysis. In the group that was being managed conservatively, the mean age was 8.8 years, whereas for transplantation patients the mean age was 12.3 years. Among transplantation patients, 72.7% received an organ from a living donor and 27.3% from a cadaveric donor.

Mexico: Experience of Ten Years of Kidney Transplantation in Mexican Children

A study reported on 240 children undergoing kidney transplantation between November 1989 and June 1999 who were admitted to the Service of Nephrology, Urology, and Transplantation at the Pediatric Hospital of Children's Hospital, Department of Nephrology, Occident National Medical Center, from Social Security Medical Institute, in Guadalajara, Jalisco, Mexico (7).

One hundred and thirty-six (56%) were boys and 104 (44%) were girls. Mean age was 11 years (range, 3 to 16). The causes of the renal disorders included glomerulopathies in 59 (25%), obstructive uropathy in 31 (13%), hereditary diseases in 15 (6%), interstitial nephritis in 10 (4%), and unspecified disorders in 125 (52%). Seventy-five percent were receiving CAPD and 25% were on hemodialysis when they underwent transplantation. Ninety-five percent of transplant organ were from living donors (75% from parents, 15% from siblings). One hundred and thirteen (47%) had blood group O, 106 (44%) had blood group A, 16 had blood group B (6%), and 5 (3%) had blood group AB. With regard to HLA, 26 (11%) were identical, 209 (87%) shared one haplotype, and 5 (2%) had different antigens in all their loci. At the end of 1999, 216 (85%) had normal renal function.

International Latin American Collaborative Studies

Epidemiology of Nephrolithiasis in Childhood

The study on the epidemiology of nephrolithiasis (see Chapter 57) was coordinated by Dr. H. Perrone, and 13 centers in Latin America participated (8). Eight hundred and seventy children were recruited; 552 (63%) were boys and 318 (37%) were girls. The age at which the disease was detected ranged from 2 months to 17 years. Only 4% of the subjects were asymptomatic. The initial symptoms reported most frequently were hematuria in 337 (39%) patients, abdominal and/or lumbar pain in 235 (27%), and hematuria associated with pain in 147 (17%). Additional findings were dysuria in 71 (8%), recurrent urinary tract infections in 146 (17%), and elimination of calculi in 28 (3%). Kidney malformations were found in 78 (8.9%).

Epidemiologic Aspects of Chronic Renal Failure in Latin American Countries

Dr. Nelson Orta coordinated a study on the epidemiology of CRF study (9). Its most relevant conclusions are presented in the following paragraphs.

The incidence of CRF shows a wide variability that ranges between 2.8 and 15.8 new cases per 1 million inhabitants (Table 75F.5).

The causes of CRF are glomerulopathies in 36%, obstructive uropathies and reflux nephropathy in 31%, systemic diseases in 9%, and other disorders in 15%. The histopathologic entity most frequently associated with CRF is focal segmental sclerosis. At present, HUS is an important cause of CRF—but not the most frequent one—in Argentina.

TABLE 75F.5. ANNUAL INCIDENCE OF CHRONIC RENAL DISEASES IN LATIN AMERICAN COUNTRIES

Country	Incidence (patients per 1 million inhabitants)
Argentina	15.8
Brazil	6.5
Colombia	2.8
Mexico	3.5
Uruguay	4.4
Venezuela	12.6

Data from Orta Sibu N. Epidemiological aspects of chronic renal failure in Latin American countries. *Rev Venez Pediatr* 1999;62[Suppl 2]:83.

Antibodies against Streptococcal Zymogen in the Sera of Patients with Acute Glomerulonephritis—A Multicenter Study

One hundred and fifty-three patients with poststreptococcal acute glomerulonephritis from Argentina, Chile, and Venezuela were studied (10); 140 were male and 49 were female. The source of infection was the skin in 84 patients, the throat in 44, and unknown in the remaining 14. Furthermore, 23 patients with streptococcal infections without glomerulonephritis and 93 healthy controls were also studied.

Antizymogen and antiproteinase titers were determined. The conclusion was that antizymogen antibody titer is the best available marker for streptococcal infections associated with glomerulonephritis.

ORGANIZATION AND RESOURCES

The nephrologic care of children in Latin America varies; countries range from those having medical systems that provide care to all patients who need dialysis procedures to others offering no possibilities to provide dialysis or transplantation to children with end-stage CRF. Even in countries in which hemodialysis, CAPD, and kidney transplantation programs are available, such services are markedly hampered by economic problems. Health authorities appropriately give priority to prevention and treatment of common diseases, and it is difficult to obtain funds for children with chronic renal disease—a small number of patients in need of expensive resources. This is worsened by the current state of devaluation of Latin American currencies, because the relative cost of the materials for treatment of end-stage renal disease, all of which are of foreign origin, constantly increases. To determine the situation in each of these countries, we sent a questionnaire that was answered by nephrologists skilled in these procedures. The assessment was begun in January 2002. Argentina, Brazil, Venezuela, Chile, and Mexico have well-structured programs. CAPD and hemodialysis programs, as well as kidney transplantation programs, have an adequate infrastructure. Uruguay has adequate hemodialysis programs and was a pioneer in CAPD. The program of transplantation in public

TABLE 75F.6. ORGANIZATION OF PEDIATRIC NEPHROLOGY IN LATIN AMERICAN COUNTRIES

	Yes	No
National society of pediatric nephrology	11	3
National certification in pediatric nephrology	8	6
Pediatric chronic renal replacement therapy (CRRT) facilities	12	2
Legislation on/regulation of CRRT	11	3
Equity in access to CRRT for pediatric population	8	6

Data from Grunberg J, Verocay C. Pediatric nephrology around the world. In: Barrat M, Avner E, Harmon B, eds. *Pediatric nephrology,* 4th ed. Baltimore: Lippincott Williams & Wilkins, 1999:1368–1370.

hospitals is in its initial phase. Cuba and Costa Rica have adequate programs of hemodialysis and transplantation. CAPD is not used. Other countries, such as Paraguay, Ecuador, and Colombia, are developing new programs for hemodialysis, CAPD, and renal transplantation. We do not have information about national programs in the other countries. Table 75F.6 shows some aspects of the organization of pediatric nephrology services in Latin American countries (11).

MEDICAL EDUCATION SYSTEMS

Pediatric nephrology residency programs exist in Argentina, Brazil, Chile, Mexico, Costa Rica, and Venezuela. Besides the residency in public hospitals, Argentina has developed a postgraduate training program in pediatric nephrology at Buenos Aires University. Currently there are three centers for this postgraduate education: Ricardo Gutiérrez Children's Hospital in Buenos Aires, and Alejandro Posadas National Hospital and San Justo Children's Hospital, both in Buenos Aires Province.

TABLE 75F.7. NUMBER OF PEDIATRIC NEPHROLOGISTS AND POPULATION YOUNGER THAN 14 YEARS

Country	No. pediatric nephrologists	Population younger than 14 yr (thousands)
Argentina	93	104
Brazil	100	518
Bolivia	3	1069
Colombia	14	825
Costa Rica	3	393
Cuba	38	68
Chile	20	216
Dominican Republic	4	717
Guatemala	3	1582
Mexico	70	482
Paraguay	4	485
Peru	11	769
Venezuela	50	148
Uruguay	15	51

Data from Grunberg J. Pediatric nephrology workforce in Latin America. *Pediatr Nephrol* 1998;12(9):796–798.

The number of pediatric nephrologists varies by country. Table 75F.7 presents such data in the context of the number of children younger than 14 years in each country (12).

In conclusion, there is a great discrepancy in the quality of care available in the different Latin American countries, and many challenges remain. However, dramatic improvement has been made in the care of children with renal disease over the past decade in this area of the world.

ACKNOWLEDGMENTS

The author gratefully acknowledge the questionnaires sent by Dr. Carlos Saieh (Chile), Dr. Michelle López (Venezuela), Dr. Digna Espinosa (Cuba), Dr. Reyner Loza (Peru), Dr. Noemia Perlí Goldraich (Brazil), Dr. Gustavo Gordillo Paniagua (México), Dr. Jorge de la Cruz (Colombia), Dr. Jannetthe Salguero Aparicio (Bolivia), Dr. Cristina Mayado (Uruguay), Dr. Osvaldo Freire Valencia (Ecuador), Dr. Leticia Florentín de Merech (Paraguay), Dr. Mabel Sandoval Díaz (Nicaragua), and Dr. Gilbert Madrigal Campos (Costa Rica).

REFERENCES

1. Challu A, Martinez Maldonado M. Latin American nephrology: present and future concerns. *Kidney Int* 1997;52:583–588.
2. Gianantonio C, Vitaco M, Mendilaharzu F, et al. Hemolytic uremic syndrome. *J Pediatr* 1964;64:478–491.
3. Exeni R, Grimoldi I, Amore A, et al. Hemolytic uremic syndrome: our experience in 283 cases. *Pediatr Nephrol* 1998;12 (7):C179.
4. Orta-Sibu N, Lopez M, Moriyon J, et al. Renal diseases in Venezuela, South America. *Pediatr Nephrol* 2002(*in press*).
5. Delucchi A, Bidegain A, Contreras A, et al. Chronic peritoneal dialysis in Pediatrics. Chilean experience. *Pediatr Nephrol* 2001;16(8):401.
6. Grimoldi I, Bibiloni N, Caletti M, et al. Registro Nacional de Enfermedad Renal Cronica, Diálisis y Trasplante. *Arch Venez Pediatr* 1999;62(suppl 2):155.
7. Ojeda Duran S, Ochoa Ponce C, Ortiz Lopez H, et al. Experiencia de 10 años de trasplante renal en niños en el Occidente de México. *Arch Venez Pediatr* 1999;62(suppl 2):179.
8. Perrone Cattini H. Epidemiology of nephrolithiasis. *Pediatr Nephrol* 1998;12:10(suppl 3):C46.
9. Orta Sibu N. Epidemiological aspects of chronic renal failure in Latin American countries. *Rev Venez Pediatr* 1999;62(suppl 2):83.
10. Parra GR, Iturbe B, Batsford S, et al. Antibody to streptococcal zymogen in the serum of patients with glomerulonephritis. A multicentric study. *Kidney Int* 1998;54(2):509–517.
11. Grunberg J, Verocay C. Pediatric nephrology around the world. In: Barrat M, Avner E, Harmon B, eds. *Pediatric nephrology,* 4th ed. Baltimore: Lippincott Williams & Wilkins, 1999:1368–1370.
12. Grunberg J. Pediatric nephrology workforce in Latin America. *Pediatr Nephrol* 1998;12(9):796–798.

75G

AUSTRALIA AND NEW ZEALAND

JOHN R. BURKE
WILLIAM WONG

DEMOGRAPHY

Australia and New Zealand have well-established health services giving outcomes comparable to those seen in Europe and North America. Both countries are well served by pediatric nephrologists—25 for the 23 million population of Australia, and 3 for the 4 million population of New Zealand. In Australia, most of the population lives close to the coast, and pediatric nephrology units are confined to five cities that provide outreach services for the appropriate states. In New Zealand, pediatric nephrology is concentrated in the largest center, Auckland, a city of 1.1 million. The service is staffed by two pediatric nephrologists who provide outreach services to other cities in the country and undertake the majority of the end-stage renal failure (ESRF) management. Significant improvement is required in both pediatric and adult health care in New Guinea, however, and for the indigenous people of Australia (Aborigines) and New Zealand (Maoris).

EPIDEMIOLOGY

New Guinea

New Guinea has a population of 4 million, and most people live in remote areas with limited access to a regional hospital. In Papua New Guinea, children die at a rate 20 times higher than Australian children. The mortality rate for children under 5 years of age is 120 per 1000 live births. The major causes of child mortality are streptococcal pneumonia, malnutrition, measles, meningitis, and neonatal sepsis. Less than one-third of women give birth with the assistance of a skilled health worker.

There are no facilities for chronic dialysis or transplantation for adult or pediatric patients, and no adult or pediatric nephrologist resides in New Guinea. A few patients, accompanied by a donor, are sent to Australia for live related donor organ transplantation at considerable cost to their families. There is no health insurance except for employees of some large companies. The process of obtaining informed consent from the kidney donor is often difficult, and follow-up is inadequate because of the high expense of the immunosuppressive drugs, which must be paid by the families, and the lack of a local nephrology service. Nephrologic disorders seen by local doctors include poststreptococcal glomerulonephritis related to impetigo, urinary tract infections, and nephrotic syndrome that is often steroid resistant. Hemolytic uremic syndrome (HUS) is uncommon. Diagnostic capabilities outside major centers are limited to dipstick testing and urine microscopy. Immunologic services and biopsy facilities are generally not available.

Major improvements in health delivery depend on the return of the village health worker, particularly in the New Guinea highlands and Bougainville; restoration and funding of rural vaccination programs; improvement in maternal education; and economic development (1). Regular teaching and surgical specialty team visits by Australian and New Zealand specialists are coordinated through various organizations, including the International Nephrology Association.

Australian Aborigines

ESRF is a significant problem among adult Australian Aborigines (2). In the Northern Territory, the prevalence is 1 per 3000 of the total Aboriginal population, which is 10 times higher than in the non-Aboriginal population. These patients are more likely to be young adult women and to have renal pathology showing glomerulomegaly and non–immunoglobulin A mesangiocapillary glomerulonephritis. Contributing factors may include genetics, low birth weight, infections, smoking, alcoholism, and type 2 diabetes.

Epidemiologic screening for renal disease in both children and adults has commenced in some Aboriginal communities. People with a history of poststreptococcal glomerulonephritis in childhood have a risk of overt albuminuria more than six times that of those without such a history (3). Skin infections occur in up to 70% of Aboriginal children, with the major pathogens being group A streptococci (4). On Tiwi Island, approximately 10% of children have microalbuminuria by the midteenage years. In some communities angiotensin-converting enzyme inhibitors are prescribed for people who have albuminuria, but controlled studies are not available.

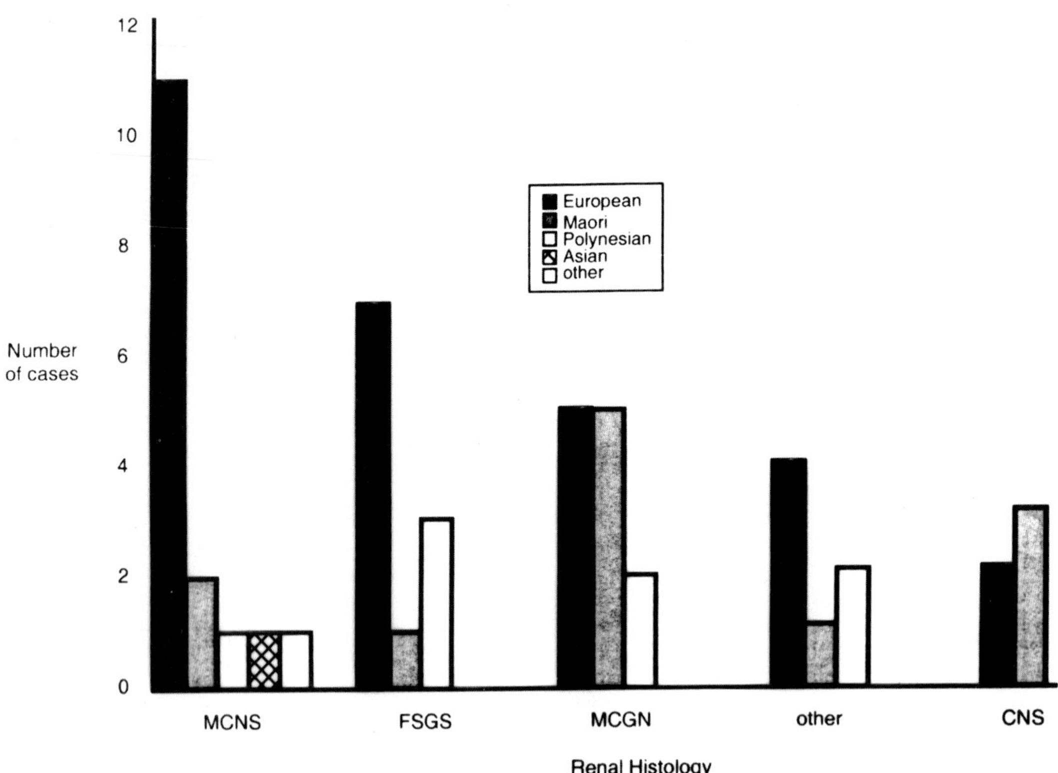

FIGURE 75G.1. Glomerular histologic findings in childhood nephrotic syndrome in New Zealand. CNS, congential nephrotic syndrome; FSGS, focal segmental glomerulosclerosis; MCGN, mesangiocapillary glomerulonephritis; MCNS, minimal change nephrotic syndrome.

Increased incidence of urate urolithiasis is seen in young Aboriginal children, particularly those living in arid zones (5,6). Development of these stones has been attributed to consumption of a high-cereal, high-protein diet and dehydration. However, some cases occur in breast-fed children younger than 6 months of age, and the disorder is seen occasionally in urban communities. No evidence of a defect in the urate pathway has been identified. These stones tend not to recur and are not a contributing cause of renal failure.

New Zealand Maoris and Polynesians

The incidence of glomerulonephritis in adult Maoris and Pacific Islanders is higher than that in New Zealanders of European descent (7). Histologic analysis in this group shows an increased incidence of mesangiocapillary glomerulonephritis, postinfectious glomerulonephritis, and focal segmental glomerulosclerosis. Among patients with childhood nephrotic syndrome, Maori children are more likely to have mesangiocapillary glomerulonephritis followed by minimal change disease, whereas white and Pacific Island children tend to have minimal change disease followed by focal segmental glomerulosclerosis (Fig. 75G.1). It is also of interest that lupus nephritis occurs predominantly in Maori and Pacific Island children with very few whites represented (8). A prospective national surveillance study currently in progress will provide a more accurate picture of nephrotic syndrome in New Zealand.

RENAL FAILURE

Hemolytic Uremic Syndrome

In Australia and New Zealand HUS is usually a sporadic disorder. In Australia between 1994 and 1998, 98 cases

TABLE 75G.1. PATIENTS' AGE AND TREATMENT ON DECEMBER 31, 2000

		Age group				
Country	**Treatment**	**0–5 yr**	**5–10 yr**	**10–15 yr**	**15–19 yr**	**Total**
Australia	Hemodialysis	0	2	5	29	36
	Peritoneal dialysis	9	10	6	19	44
	Transplantation	11	36	56	87	193
	Total	20	51	67	135	273
New Zealand	Hemodialysis	1	0	1	9	11
	Peritoneal dialysis	0	3	3	7	13
	Transplantation	3	6	14	14	37
	Total	4	9	18	30	61

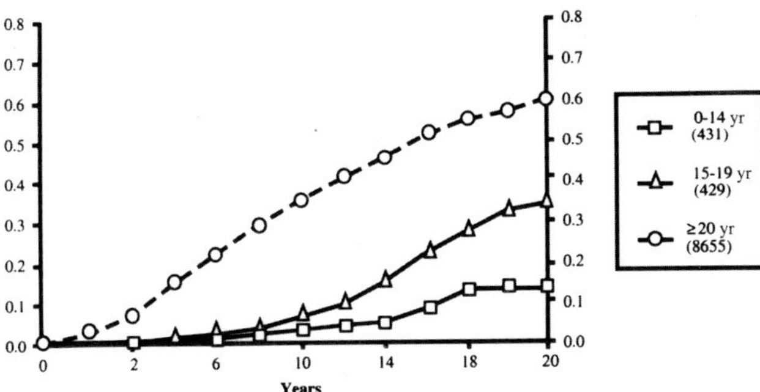

FIGURE 75G.2. Risk of skin cancer, by age group, in all transplantation patients with surviving grafts (from both cadaveric donors and living related donors).

TABLE 75G.2. SKIN CANCER IN PEDIATRIC RENAL TRANSPLANTATION PATIENTS

		Median age (range)		
Type of skin cancer	No. cases	At first treatment for renal disease	At transplantation	At cancer diagnosis
Squamous cell carcinoma	22	12.6 (7.8–14.8)	13.3 (8.2–16.7)	28.3 (18.4–45.0)
Basal cell carcinoma	12	12.1 (9.1–14.7)	13.3 (9.8–15.1)	27.8 (14.7–41.3)
Merkel cell tumor	1	14.8	15.2	29.5
Total	35	12.5 (7.8–14.8)	13.3 (8.2–16.7)	28.4 (14.7–45.0)

were identified. Eighty-four were associated with diarrhea (64 cases sporadic, 20 constituting an outbreak), and 14 were atypical. Shiga toxin–producing *Escherichia coli* O111:H- was the most common isolate in sporadic HUS and caused the outbreak. Shiga toxin–producing *Escherichia coli* O157:H7 was not isolated in any case (9). Of five children with T activation caused by pneumococcal pneumonia, all had a complete recovery of renal function (10). The New Zealand Paediatric Society Surveillance Unit study, currently into its fifth year, showed that the most common serotype was *E. coli* O157 and that more than 90% of cases occurred in the North Island.

Chronic Renal Failure

The incidence of ESRF in Australia and New Zealand is 5 to 6 per million population aged 0 to 15 years. In the adolescent age group, the incidence is 13 per million population aged 15 to 18 years (11). Table 75G.1 shows the number of children and adolescents (up to 20 years of age) who commenced treatment for ESRF from 1995 to 2000. The trend in the last 5 years is hospital-based peritoneal dialysis for small children (0 to 4 years) and hospital-based hemodialysis for adolescents. Preemptive renal transplantation occurred in 20% of children.

Australian and New Zealand adult transplant patients have a high incidence of skin cancers relating to the hot climate (12). Figure 75G.2 shows the incidence of skin cancer in different transplant age groups. The risk over 20 years is 10% in children, 30% in adolescents, and 60% in adults. In children the median interval between transplantation and diagnosis of the first skin cancer lesion (basal cell carcinoma or squamous cell carcinoma) is approximately 15 years (Table 75G.2).

The management of adolescent transplant patients continues to encounter difficulties. Analysis by era shows an improvement in graft survival for the 0- to 14-year age group but not the 15- to 19-year age group (Fig. 75G.3). This is most likely related to poor compliance with the medication regimen. Overall patient survival between 1990 and 2000 for the 0- to 19-year age group was 93%.

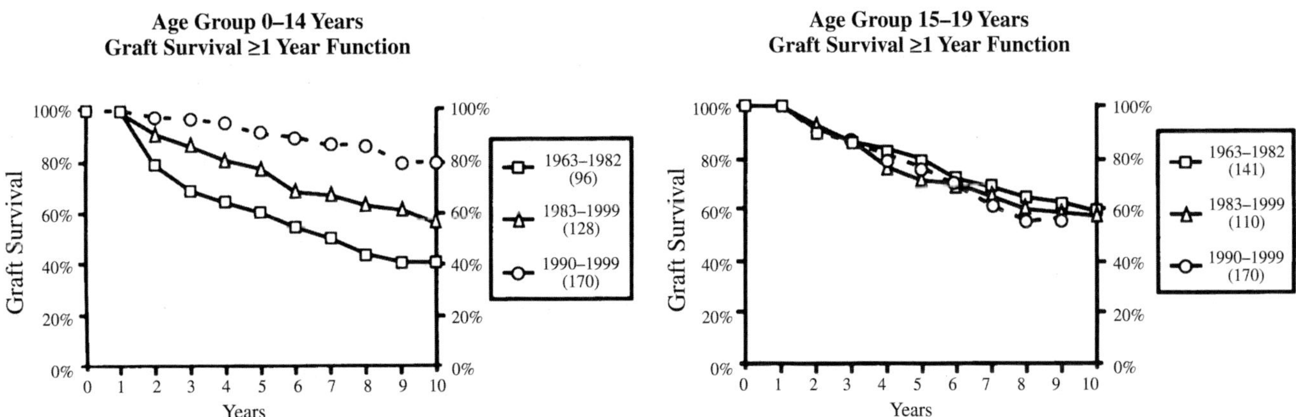

FIGURE 75G.3. Graft survival in Australian pediatric and adolescent transplant recipients by era.

REFERENCES

1. Duke T. Decline in child health in rural Papua New Guinea. *Lancet* 1999;354:1291–1294.
2. Spencer JL, Silva DT, Snelling P, et al. An epidemic of renal failure among Australian Aborigines. *Med J Aust* 1998;168:537–541.
3. White AV, Hoy WE, McCreadie DA. Childhood post-streptococcal glomerulonephritis as a risk factor for chronic renal failure in later life. *Med J Aust* 2001;174: 492–496.
4. Currie BJ, Carapetis JR. Skin infections and infestations in Aboriginal communities in Northern Australia. *Australas J Dermatol* 2000;41:139–143.
5. Williams WM, Nicholas JJ, Nungurrayi PB, et al. Pediatric urolithiasis in a remote Australian Aboriginal community. *J Paediatr Child Health* 1996;32:344–346.
6. Thambi Dorai CR, Dewan PA, Boucaut HA, et al. Urolithiasis in Australian Aboriginal children. *Aust N Z J Surg* 1994;64:99–101.
7. Bailey RR, Hannan SF, Neale TJ, et al. The New Zealand Glomerulonephritis Study: introductory report. *Clin Nephrol* 1989;5:239–246.
8. Simpson AK, Wong W, Morris MC. Paediatric nephrotic syndrome in Auckland, New Zealand. *J Paediatr Child Health* 1998;34:360–362.
9. Elliott EJ, Robins-Browne RM, O'Laughlin EV, et al. Nationwide study of haemolytic uraemic syndrome; clinical, microbiological, and epidemiological features. *Arch Dis Child* 2001;85:125–131.
10. McTaggart SJ, Burke JR. Streptococcus pneumonia-induced haemolytic uraemic syndrome. *J Paediatr Child Health* 1998; 34:192–195.
11. Russ GR. 24th Report of Australia and New Zealand dialysis and transplantation registry, 2001.
12. Disney A. 23rd Report of Australia and New Zealand dialysis and transplantation registry, 2000.

75H

ASIA

CARMELO A. ALFILER
HUI-KIM YAP
MAN-CHUN CHIU

OVERVIEW

The United Nations Population Fund reported that 60% of the world's population of 6.1 billion at the end of 2001 resided in Asia (1). The majority of Asia's people are from developing countries with large populations, which results in major problems in education and health care. This chapter describes the current status of pediatric nephrology in the member countries of the Asian Pediatric Nephrology Association (the report for Japan is in Chapter 78C).

Since the last update (2), there has been a marked increase in the number of postresidency fellowship programs across the region, which has contributed to improvement in care of children with kidney diseases. Better diagnostic and therapeutic facilities in many Asian medical centers have increased the chances of survival and quality of life. The widespread use of oral rehydration solutions has caused a significant decrease in the incidence of acute renal failure due to gastroenteritis-related dehydration. Mass urinary screening programs have been conducted among apparently healthy schoolchildren to help identify kidney and urinary tract abnormalities that can be managed early, in the hope of preventing and retarding progression to chronic renal failure.

EAST ASIA

China

China has more than 1 billion people, of whom nearly one-third are children. In 1979, pediatric nephrologists in China formed a cooperative study group, which led to the establishment of the Chinese Society of Pediatric Nephrology in 1986. In recent years, its membership has reached more than 250. Several projects have been undertaken, including standardization of the clinical classification of glomerular diseases (1979), nationwide investigation of kidney diseases in hospitals (1982, 1992), nationwide urinary screening (1986), and cooperative study of renal biopsy specimens (1995). In 2000, new clinical guidelines on the diagnosis and management of nephrotic syndrome and other glomerular diseases, based on current practice in China, were formulated by the Chinese Association of Pediatrics and replaced the previous guidelines established in 1982 (3).

In a 1982 survey of 105 hospitals in 20 provinces, acute glomerulonephritis was common, accounting for 54% of renal cases requiring hospital admission (4). Its incidence appears to have declined, as a similar survey done in 1992 showed that such cases constituted only 37% of renal admissions. Acute glomerulonephritis was usually preceded by upper respiratory tract infections in the north and by skin infections in the south. In the 1982 survey, renal diseases requiring hospital admission were nephrotic syndrome (21%), urinary tract infection (8%), and Henoch-Schönlein nephritis (5%). Hepatitis B virus infection was commonly associated with membranous nephropathy, which occurred in 144 of 204 cases.

Renal involvement was commonly seen in Chinese children with systemic lupus erythematosus and commonly affected those in their teens (5). In a review encompassing 105 children with lupus nephritis, the clinical types were nephrotic syndrome (45%), nephritic syndrome (34%), rapidly progressive nephritis (9%), chronic nephritis (2%), and mild proteinuria (10%). Treatment agents included prednisone and cyclophosphamide. Methylprednisolone and cyclophosphamide pulse therapy were used to treat severe cases (6).

A nationwide urinary screening for proteinuria and hematuria was performed in 2- to 14-year-old children in 1986 (7). Of 224,291 children screened, 0.85% were found to have urinary abnormalities, which included asymptomatic hematuria, nephritis, urinary tract infection, asymptomatic bacteriuria, urinary stones, hydronephrosis, and urinary malformations. Urinary abnormalities were more common in girls than in boys (0.85% vs. 0.62%).

In an analysis of the causes of acute renal failure prevalent 10 to 20 years ago (8), acute nephritis was found in 40% of cases; the other causes were progressive glomerulonephritis, infection, septicemia, and congenital renal malformations.

The average mortality was 38%. Peritoneal dialysis is the main modality of dialysis for acute renal failure in many hospitals, but hemodialysis is carried out in a few centers. No data are available on chronic dialysis in children, and few children have undergone renal transplantation.

Hong Kong

Hong Kong has a population of 6.73 million of which 1.55 million (23%) are 0 to 19 years of age. Children with renal diseases are cared for in most major acute-care hospitals. Since 1999, a pediatric renal center for dialysis and transplantation has been in operation, in which children with chronic renal failure are offered treatment in a centralized end-stage renal disease program (9).

The Hong Kong Pediatric Nephrology Society was formed in the 1980s to bring together pediatricians working on pediatric renal diseases to promote nephrology work in children. Several surveillances and a renal registry have been set up for hospital patients. The number of new cases per year of nephrotic syndrome, lupus nephritis, cystic kidney diseases, and hereditary tubular disorders were 57, 10, 12, and 2, respectively (10). An average of seven new cases per year of chronic renal failure with glomerular filtration rates lower than 25 mL/min/1.73 m^2 were seen in children under 15 years old. A collaborative study on primary nocturnal enuresis involving 100 children was carried out; results showed that combined use of an enuresis alarm and desmopressin was most effective and yielded a lower relapse rate.

The incidence of end-stage renal disease in children younger than 15 years of age was estimated to be 4 per million children in the early 1990s (10). More recently, however, the incidence for those younger than 20 years of age was 34 per million adjusted population (11). The incidence for those between 11 and 20 years of age was six times that of children 10 years old or younger. The common causes of end-stage renal failure were chronic glomerulonephritis (26%), chronic pyelonephritis (18%), hypoplastic or dysplastic kidneys (18%), and hereditary or familial diseases (9%); no cases due to cystinosis or hemolytic uremic syndrome were reported (10).

Chronic ambulatory peritoneal dialysis was started in the 1980s, and since 1996, automated peritoneal dialysis has been provided to nearly all children on peritoneal dialysis. In a review encompassing 24 children on automated peritoneal dialysis, a very low peritonitis rate of 1 in 87.5 patient-months was recorded (9). Chronic hemodialysis was offered to older children or those deemed clinically unsuitable for peritoneal dialysis. In a review involving 12 patients on chronic hemodialysis, no major complications were encountered, and establishment of suitable vascular access remained the main obstacle to overcome in small children (9).

Renal transplantation in children has been available since the late 1980s, and in a review conducted in the mid-1990s involving seven children, all grafts were functioning after a follow-up period of 37.9 months, with a mean serum creatinine level of 134 μmol/L (12). In a review of outcomes for 20 transplanted grafts, 1- and 3-year actuarial graft survival rates were 92.3% and 83.1% for cadaveric donor grafts, and 100% and 100% for living donor grafts, respectively (13). The longest graft survival was more than 10 years.

A comprehensive renal registry including both adults and children with end-stage renal disease has been set up in Hong Kong. The 2002 data showed that, of children younger than 10 years of age, four were on peritoneal dialysis, one was on hemodialysis, and three had undergone transplantation. Among adolescents 11 to 20 years of age, 15 were on peritoneal dialysis, 9 were on hemodialysis, and 27 had received transplants (11).

Korea

South Korea had 47,343,000 inhabitants in 2001, and 28.5% were younger than 19 years of age (14). The Korean Society of Pediatric Nephrology, established in October 1994, has over 70 members. There are 45 universities and general hospitals capable of performing renal diagnosis and therapy in Korea. Ten university hospitals have dialysis and transplantation centers for children and offer postresidency fellowship programs in pediatric nephrology.

At the Department of Pediatrics, Seoul National University Children's Hospital, one of the tertiary referral hospitals in Korea, children with renal disease comprised 5.8% of total inpatients in 1999. Urinary tract infection (29%), nephrotic syndrome (22%), and chronic renal failure (17%) were the leading causes of admissions among renal patients (15).

In a review of more than 1400 renal biopsy specimens performed at two tertiary referral centers (16,17), the most frequent pathologic findings were minimal change lesion (26% and 25%), immunoglobulin A (IgA) nephropathy (15% and 10%), focal segmental glomerulosclerosis (14% and 9%), and Henoch-Schönlein nephritis (7% and 14%).

In 2000, a nationwide survey of childhood chronic renal failure was performed by the Korean Society of Pediatric Nephrology (18). The incidence of chronic renal failure was 3.68 per 1 million child population per year and the male to female ratio was 1.73:1. Reflux nephropathy (16%), focal segmental glomerulosclerosis (11%), and renal hypoplasia or dysplasia (9%) were the leading causes of chronic renal failure. The initial mode of renal replacement therapy for end-stage renal disease patients was hemodialysis in 42% of cases, peritoneal dialysis in 35% of cases, and renal transplantation in 23% of cases.

Taiwan

Taiwan is an island of more than 22 million people of whom 6.4 million are between 1 and 19 years of age. A biannual mass urinary screening of elementary and junior high school students has been in operation since 1990. The first morning urine is tested for pH, protein, occult blood, and glucose. Children whose test results are positive undergo repeat testing 10 to 15 days later, with the addition of sulfosalicylic acid and urine sediment examination. Results from the screening of 2.6 million children showed that 0.10 to 0.35% had proteinuria and 0.07 to 0.21% had hematuria (19). A third examination involves procurement of a blood sample by a public health nurse, which is subsequently tested for 11 substances, including total protein, albumin, globulin, blood urea nitrogen, creatinine, antistreptolysin O, complement C3, cholesterol, hepatitis B surface antigen, IgA, and glucose. The children are classified into grades A to E after analysis of the results. Those in grades D and E are referred to a hospital for further investigation.

In an epidemiologic study of 132,686 schoolchildren screened by renal ultrasonography, 0.5% were found to have renal abnormalities, including hydronephrosis (0.19%), unilateral renal agenesis (0.08%), unilateral small kidneys (0.10%), renal cystic disorders (0.07%), and ectopic kidney (0.02%) (20). Fifty children underwent surgical correction of the abnormality.

Eighty children are registered for chronic ambulatory peritoneal dialysis or automated peritoneal dialysis, and 152 children younger than age 18 are registered for hemodialysis. Dialysis is performed in ten centers throughout Taiwan. Those undergoing chronic ambulatory peritoneal dialysis have peritonitis rates of one episode per 36 patient-months. The first pediatric kidney transplant program was started in Taipei in 1985. To date, 44 children have undergone transplantation, and currently four centers perform pediatric transplantation. More than 90% of transplants were cadaveric organs. Thirty-four patients had prolonged graft function, eight had graft failure, and two died. Common complications in transplantation patients with long-term survival were osteoporosis and cataracts. Although short stature was of great concern, physical and psychosocial rehabilitation has been successful.

SOUTHEAST ASIA

Indonesia

In Indonesia, a country of at least 200 million people in which approximately 30%, or 70 million, are younger than 15 years of age, there are 11 centers for renal diagnosis and therapy; 9 offer dialysis and only 2 perform renal transplantation. One of these centers offers postresidency fellowship training in pediatric nephrology.

Seven university hospitals throughout Indonesia undertook a collaborative retrospective-prospective study from 1984 to 1988 to investigate the spectrum of renal diseases among hospitalized children (21). Of the 104,457 patients admitted to the hospitals over this period, 2892 (3%) had some kidney or urinary tract complaint. The most common kidney diseases encountered were nephrotic syndrome (35%), acute glomerulonephritis (26%), and urinary tract infections (23%). The study showed that the profile of renal diseases was uniform throughout the country and that no noticeable changes in incidences of disease occurred during the 5-year period.

Between 1991 and 1995, data from the general hospital in Jakarta showed that 688 (or 6.2%) of 11,162 children hospitalized were admitted for renal diseases (22). This was almost double the number of children hospitalized for the same reason between 1984 and 1988, that is, 489 (or 3.3%) of 14,480 children (23). Nephrotic syndrome was still the most frequent cause of renal disease, found in 41.4% of all cases. It was also the main cause of end-stage renal disease (47%), followed by chronic glomerulonephritis (8.8%) and urinary tract infection and/or malformations (44%) (22). In addition, a collaborative study of eight child health departments in teaching hospitals between 1997 and 2001 reported 276 cases of acute glomerulonephritis, mainly poststreptococcal in cause. There were 139 boys (50.4%) and 137 girls (49.6%), aged between 2.5 and 14.5 years, of whom the majority (77.1%) were older than 6 years (24).

Urinary incontinence has been increasingly reported. Between 1989 and 2001, 20 cases were seen in Jakarta, composed of ten boys and ten girls. Seven cases were due to spinal dysraphism, three cases of osteolytic lesion in the vertebrae were due to malignancy, six patients had non-neurogenic bladder, and four had anatomical abnormalities. Eleven out of the 20 children (55%) developed chronic renal failure (25).

Among the causes of acute renal failure in older children, jengkol bean intoxication or poisoning is still the most prominent cause, responsible for 20 out of 64 casees (31%) of children hospitalized with acute renal failure in the general hospital in Jakarta between 1984 and 1993 (26). Jengkol bean is widely consumed in Indonesia, especially in rural areas. The pathophysiologic mechanisms of acute renal failure include obstruction of the renal tubules by jengkolic acid crystals, as well as a direct toxic effect on the tubular cells.

Tuberculosis is one of the most common complications in children with nephrotic syndrome. A cross-sectional study of 100 children with nephrotic syndrome revealed that 15% had tuberculosis. The majority of cases (80%) occurred in children with frequently relapsing and steroid-dependent nephrotic syndrome (27).

Malaysia

Malaysia has a total population of 23,795,300, of whom 10,293,000 (43.26%) are in the 0- to 19-year age group. There are currently eight pediatric nephrologists in the country. Dialysis facilities for children with end-stage renal failure are available in four centers, and pediatric renal transplantation is offered in one center. The 2001 report of the Malaysian Dialysis and Transplant Registry indicated that the dialysis provision rate for children aged 0 to 14 years was 4 per 1 million child population (28), with more than 70 children on dialysis. More than 90% of children on dialysis were on chronic ambulatory peritoneal dialysis. Only two children were on automated peritoneal dialysis. Dialysis treatment for children is subsidized by the Ministry of Health.

More than 90 children younger than 18 years of age have undergone transplantation since the inception of the program in 1986; 90% of donors were living related relatives. The patient and graft survival rates have been comparable to those in other countries.

Singapore

Singapore has a child population (younger than the age of 15 years) of 769,182. Over the last two decades, the pattern of renal diseases in Singapore children has changed drastically. Previously poststreptococcal acute glomerulonephritis was the most common type of glomerulonephritis seen (29). Over the last decade, idiopathic nephrotic syndrome has taken on increasing prominence as a cause of morbidity in children. In a retrospective study of 91 children with steroid-responsive nephrotic syndrome, 61.5% subsequently developed steroid dependency (30). The median age at onset was 3.1 years, and there was no correlation between increasing age at onset and steroid dependency as reported in other studies (31). The incidence of hematuria at presentation of nephrotic syndrome was 31.1%, but this did not correlate with development of steroid dependency. On the other hand, a prolonged duration of treatment before achieving remission was shown to be a significant predictor of steroid dependency (30). In fact, 76.3% of patients who had not achieved remission by day 9 subsequently became steroid dependent, whereas all patients who were still proteinuric at day 21 developed steroid dependency. Of the nephrotic children with steroid resistant disease, almost half had focal segmental glomerulosclerosis, whereas 42% had minimal change disease. Over a period of 10 years, 57.7% of children with focal segmental glomerulosclerosis had progressed to end-stage renal failure. Nonresponse to cyclosporine therapy was a significant predictor of progression to renal failure (32).

Singapore has seen a change in the pattern and modalities of treatment of acute renal failure in children. In an 18-year study of children requiring acute dialysis, it was found that 91% of children underwent dialysis for acute renal failure, whereas the remaining 9% had metabolic disorders (33). The main causes of acute renal failure in this cohort were acute tubular necrosis (62.2%), hepatorenal syndrome (15.1%), acute glomerulonephritis (4.5%), hemolytic uremic syndrome (7.6%), and obstructive uropathy (1.5%). Approximately one-fourth of children undergoing dialysis for acute renal failure were treated in the first 15 years of the study when acute peritoneal dialysis was the sole modality of dialysis, whereas 75% of them were treated in the last 3 years, when continuous hemodiafiltration was used more frequently in the critical care setting. Despite the implementation of continuous hemodiafiltration for acute dialysis, the mortality rose from 63.9% in the first 15 years to 72.4% over the last 3 years of the study. This increase in mortality was probably related to the changes in patient selection profile because more critically ill children with multiorgan dysfunction syndrome underwent dialysis. Previously, many of these children would have been deemed "undialyzable," especially those with intra-abdominal pathology such as necrotizing enterocolitis and postabdominal surgery, because the sole modality of dialysis was peritoneal dialysis.

The chronic dialysis and transplantation program was first started in 1988 (34). With an annual incidence of end-stage renal failure of 5 to 6 per 1 million children younger than 15 years of age, a total of 46 children have required chronic dialysis, almost half of whom have undergone transplantation. The main causes of end-stage renal failure are chronic glomerulonephritis (43%), renal dysplasia and hypoplasia (27%), and reflux nephropathy (11%). The main modality of chronic dialysis was night intermittent peritoneal dialysis. Although infections remain a major cause of morbidity, the peritonitis rate of 1 case per 17 patient-months was comparable with that in many centers in Europe and North America. Cardiovascular disease has been identified as one of the major causes of morbidity in adults and children on long-term dialysis. Approximately 35% of the children in the chronic dialysis program had evidence of left ventricular hypertrophy, as measured by a left ventricular mass index of greater than 51 $g/m^{2.7}$. This was shown to correlate significantly with the degree of anemia as measured by the hematocrit in these children.

Pediatric renal transplantation was first performed in Singapore in 1989. Since then, 24 children have received transplants, of whom 67% were given allografts from living related donors. The 5-year allograft survival rate for cadaveric transplants was 58%, whereas the 5- and 10-year allograft survival rates for transplants from living related donors were 92% and 76%, respectively. Viral infections, especially cytomegalovirus infection, occurred in 33% of transplant recipients. Noncompliance with the immunosuppressive treatment regimen was a major problem in 29% of patients.

Screening programs aimed at detecting renal disease and hypertension at an early stage have been initiated in several countries, with the goal of instituting effective interventions to prevent progression to chronic renal failure. In Singapore, a pilot program was launched in 1999 to screen for urinary abnormalities and hypertension in a cohort of 12-year-old schoolchildren (35). Approximately 2000 schoolchildren, or

93.7% of the target population, participated in this program. The prevalence of abnormalities in the target population was high, with hypertension in 13% (predominantly systolic hypertension of 8.4%), proteinuria in 2%, and hematuria in 8%. Increasing weight was found to be a significant predictor for hypertension, which emphasizes the importance of weight control as a potential effective adjunctive strategy for the management of hypertension. On the other hand, low body weight was found to be a significant risk factor for proteinuria in this multiethnic population (36).

Thailand

Thailand has a population of 62 million, of whom 24% are younger than 15 years of age. Common renal problems in children include acute poststreptococcal glomerulonephritis, primary nephrotic syndrome, lupus nephritis, urinary tract anomalies, and infection and urolithiasis. More than 90% of children with primary nephrotic syndrome responded well to corticosteroid therapy (37). Results of renal biopsies performed in selected cases (those with steroid-resistant disease, frequent relapse, and steroid-dependent disease) showed mild mesangial proliferative glomerulonephritis with mesangial immunoglobulin M deposits in 60 to 70%, followed in frequency by focal segmental glomerulosclerosis. Children with immunoglobulin M nephropathy tended to relapse when treated with corticosteroids; however, they were as responsive to oral cyclophosphamide therapy as patients with minimal change disease (38).

Lupus nephritis was the most common secondary cause of glomerulonephritis in Thai children. Diffuse proliferative glomerulonephritis (World Health Organization class IV) was the most common histopathologic finding, identified in more than 50% of the biopsy specimens (39). The prognosis of severe lupus nephritis has improved greatly with the use of intravenous pulse cyclophosphamide therapy (40). IgA nephropathy, as in adults in Thailand, was not a common cause of primary glomerulonephritis in children—only 5% of the biopsy specimens showed mesangial IgA deposits.

Acute renal failure from diarrheal dehydration has been decreasing due to the widespread home use of oral rehydration solution. Hemolytic uremic syndrome as a cause of acute renal failure is rarely seen in Thai children. In the past, bladder calculi were an important problem in the northeast region. With the improvement in nutrition, the prevalence of bladder stones has also been declining. Hence the pattern of childhood renal diseases in Thailand has changed in recent years in association with overall improvement in the socioeconomic climate and health care practices.

Philippines

As of July 2001, the total population of the Philippines was 82,841,518 (41). In 1994, the Pediatric Nephrology Society of the Philippines (PNSP) was established. Its mission is the continuing education of pediatricians-trainees, community service, advocacy for children with kidney disease, and research. Currently, the PNSP has 40 certified members. Four accredited centers offer postresidency fellowships in pediatric nephrology.

Ninety-one hospitals in the country with accredited residency training programs offer facilities for diagnosis and treatment of renal disease; 48 of these are located in metropolitan Manila. There are 138 hospital centers for both hemodialysis and peritoneal dialysis, 49 in metropolitan Manila and 89 in other regions. The majority of kidney transplantations are performed in metropolitan Manila hospitals, with the National Kidney and Transplant Institute performing 71% of procedures (42).

Since 1991, kidney disease has consistently ranked among the top ten causes of mortality in the government's registry of diseases. For every 100,000 population in 1998, nephritis and nephrotic syndrome accounted for 10.2 cases or 2.1% of total deaths (43). From January to December 1998, urinary tract infection was the eighth leading cause of morbidity as reported by Philippine Pediatric Society–accredited hospitals nationwide (44). In a 6-year review, the PNSP reported a total of 5861 admissions in four accredited tertiary medical centers with fellowship programs in pediatric nephrology; of these admissions, 1533 patients (26%) had postinfectious acute glomerulonephritis, 1302 (22%) had idiopathic nephrotic syndrome, 812 (14%) were in renal failure for various causes, 335 (6%) had secondary chronic glomerulonephritis, 204 (3.5%) had bladder dysfunction, 188 (3%) had congenital or inherited renal disease, 113 (2%) had IgA nephropathy, 80 (1.5%) had urolithiasis, 79 (1.4%) had tumors, and 415 (7%) had miscellaneous disorders such as hypertension and renal tubular disease (45). The spectrum of renal and urinary tract disease has not changed since the last census. It is interesting to note, however, that the number of reported renal tubular disorders has been increasing through the years and that the incidence of acute renal failure due to leptospirosis has remained high.

The Philippines has one of the highest numbers of kidney transplantations in Asia. From 1983 to 2000, 1829 transplantations were performed at the National Kidney and Transplant Institute, 69 of which were in pediatric patients aged 5 to 18 years of age (3.78%). There were 66 first and 3 second transplantations, mostly with grafts from live donors. The most common cause of end-stage renal disease was chronic glomerulonephritis, representing 88% of cases (R. M. Rosete-Liquete, "Profile of pediatric renal transplant patients in the Philippines," *unpublished data*, 2002).

In June 1993, the Department of Health, in cooperation with many governmental and nongovernmental agencies, launched the Philippine Preventive Nephrology Project, a mass urinary screening program for apparently healthy public elementary schoolchildren in grades 1 to 6. In 1999, at the end of the project, 5,758,241 of the targeted 9,800,000 children enrolled in the 1994–1995 school year were tested; 24% of them showed at least one urinary abnormality by dipstick testing. After two formal urinalyses in 361,965 children, the prevalence rate of urine abnormality was 165 per 10,000 cases. Among 19,947 pupils who completed initial and subsequent diagnostic investigations, the following kidney problems were identified, with prevalence rates expressed per 10,000 cases: pyuria, 104; urinary tract infection, 23; benign hematuria, 17; glomerulonephritis, 10; asymptomatic proteinuria, 7; nephrotic syndrome 0.5; and others, 2 (46). The Philippine Preventive Nephrology Project is now known as the Renal Disease Control Program.

SOUTH ASIA

Bangladesh

Bangladesh is the eighth most populous country in the world, with approximately 133 million inhabitants recorded in 2001. Of these, 40% are younger than 15 years of age (41).

A Division of Pediatric Nephrology was established at the Institute of Child Health in the capital city of Dhaka. A masters-level subspecialty program has been started for pediatric nephrology and a Kidney Institute for both adult and pediatric disease has been established.

The pattern of renal disorders and the socioeconomic constraints are similar to those in India (see later). Postdysenteric hemolytic uremic syndrome is a common cause of acute renal failure. A large outbreak of acute renal failure occurred in Bangladesh in 1995 secondary to ingestion of ethylene glycol–contaminated liquid paracetamol preparations. That epidemic was associated with a high mortality rate (47).

India

India had more than 1 billion people in 2001. Children between the ages of 0 and 19 years comprise 46.5% of the population (48). A network of state-managed health centers, and district and referral hospitals has been in place for more than 50 years. The resources available at these centers are often limited, and a large proportion of the population obtains medical care through a parallel private sector.

A nucleus of pediatric nephrology was established in New Delhi in 1969. The growth of the specialty received a further impetus when the Indian Academy of Pediatrics created specialty chapters and instituted training fellowships. The Indian Pediatric Nephrology Group has 210 members, who are pediatricians trained in nephrology. Most of them are located in departments of pediatrics of medical schools and major hospitals. The Indian Pediatric Nephrology Group provides short-term training fellowships in the specialty. A 1-year postresidency fellowship has been started in Bangalore. Consensus recommendations on the management of idiopathic nephrotic syndrome, urinary tract infections, and antenatally detected hydronephrosis have been formulated by the group (49–51).

Idiopathic nephrotic syndrome is a common problem, although its exact incidence is unknown. The clinicopathologic features and response to therapy are similar to those reported in the developed countries (52). The incidence of serious infections, which complicate the course of the illness, is higher (53). The use of medications like cyclosporin is limited by economic factors. Levamisole has been found effective and is widely used as a steroid-sparing agent for patients with frequent relapses and steroid dependence (54).

The incidence of poststreptococcal glomerulonephritis was high during the 1970s but has gradually declined. Acute renal failure caused by severe hypovolemia from acute gastroenteritis has also decreased due to the widespread use of oral rehydration therapy (55). Acute intravascular hemolysis in individuals with glucose-6-phosphate dehydrogenase deficiency, snakebite in coastal regions and rural areas, and *Plasmodium falciparum* malaria are important causes of acute renal failure in children. A large increase in the number of patients with hemolytic uremic syndrome occurred during the latter part of the 1970s, and hemolytic uremic syndrome was the most common cause of acute renal failure until the early 1990s (56). Clinical and epidemiologic evidence led to the conclusion that most of these cases were associated with *Shigella*-caused dysentery. Over the last 5 to 7 years, the incidence of hemolytic uremic syndrome has declined. Infection caused by verotoxin-producing *Escherichia coli* appears to be rare in the Indian subcontinent. Perinatal asphyxia, septicemia, and injudicious use of aminoglycoside drugs are important etiologic factors in acute renal failure in the newborn period. Peritoneal dialysis is the most commonly used dialysis modality for patients with acute renal failure.

The incidence of hepatitis B nephropathy is very low, although the carrier rate of hepatitis B surface antigen is approximately 3%. IgA nephropathy is also uncommon in children in India. The incidence of familial and genetic disorders, collagen vascular diseases, and renal tubular disorders appears to be similar to that in the United States and Europe. Takayasu's disease (idiopathic aortoarteritis) is an important cause of hypertension in children (57).

The chief causes of chronic renal failure include obstructive uropathy, reflux nephropathy, and chronic glomerulonephritis. Provision of renal replacement therapy is constrained by socioeconomic factors. Facilities for chronic hemodialysis and renal transplantation are available at six pediatric nephrology centers in the country. The use of continuous ambulatory peritoneal dialysis is limited due to its cost and the necessity to import consumable supplies. Although a Human Organ Transplantation Act came into force in 1994, the cadaveric transplant program is not well developed. Neither the state nor insurance companies subsidize the costs of therapy, which are high, particularly in relation to per capita gross national product.

Pakistan

The total population of Pakistan in 2001 was estimated to be 152 million. Of this, the pediatric population younger than 18 years of age is 73.6 million (48.37%) (58). Pakistan has a large rural population (65%) that is served by inadequate medical facilities. Larger cities with university hospitals have well-equipped centers.

In 1997, the Pakistan Pediatric Nephrology Group was formed under the umbrella of the Pakistan Pediatric Association. It has approximately 50 members, including pediatricians with special interest in nephrology. The group provides training in pediatric nephrology to family physicians, undergraduate medical students, and postgraduate students in fellowships in pediatrics. A formal fellowship program in pediatric nephrology has not been developed to date.

In one study, nephrotic syndrome was found to be the most common renal disease (59). Response to steroid therapy and clinical presentation in nephrotic syndrome are found to be similar to those in Europe and the United States. Seroprevalence of hepatitis B virus is high in Pakistan, but its association with nephrotic syndrome has not been demonstrated (60). Poststreptococcal acute glomerulonephritis has shown a decline compared to the level in previous studies, whereas congenital renal anomalies and renal calculi have been recognized more frequently (59). Vesicoureteric reflux and posterior urethral valves are the two most common structural abnormalities and account for 60% of the congenital anomalies.

Urolithiasis is the third most common cause of renal morbidity, particularly in southern parts of the country. The province of Sindh has the highest prevalence of stone disease in the world (61). The high prevalence may be due to multiple factors, such as hot and humid climate with inadequate fluid intake, consumption of a mainly cereal-based diet due to poverty, and recurrent diarrhea in malnourished children. There may also be a genetic predisposition.

Urolithiasis was found to be the most common cause of acute and chronic renal failure (59). Urolithiasis was also responsible for end-stage renal failure in 20% of 75 children who underwent renal transplantation (62).

There are approximately 15 centers in the country that provide peritoneal dialysis and appropriate investigations to manage children with renal problems, although hemodialysis services are limited to 5 centres. The majority of kidney transplants in the pediatric age group are performed at the Sindh Institute of Urology and Transplantation in Karachi. To date the institute has performed 100 transplantations, all with organs from living related donors. The province of Punjab has two centers in the private sector performing kidney transplantation.

REFERENCES

1. United Nations Population Fund (UNFPA): World population. US Department of State's Office of International Information Programme [Web site]. Available at: http://www.usinfo.state.gov.
2. Alfiler CA, Srivastava RN, Chiu MC. Pediatric nephrology around the world: Asia. In: Barratt TM, Avner ED, Harmon WE, eds. *Pediatric nephrology*. Baltimore: Lippincott Williams & Wilkins, 1999:1357–1362.
3. The Chinese Society of Pediatric Nephrology. Clinical classification, diagnosis and treatment of glomerular diseases in children. *Chinese Pediatr J* 2000;39:746–749.
4. National Paediatrc Nephrology Study Group. Survey on paediatric nephrology diseases. *Chinese Pediatr J* 1986;24:69–72.
5. Ziang XY. 6th Asian Congress of Pediatric Nephrology. Symposium on Lupus nephritis. Manila, 1996.
6. Pediatric Nephrology Group of Chinese Pediatric Society. Renal biopsy findings in Chinese children: a national cooperative study on 2315 cases. *Chinese Pediatr J* 1996;34:319–323.
7. Pediatric Nephrology Group. Survey on pediatric urogenital diseases—national 21 provinces urinary screening results. *Chinese Pediatr J* 1989;27:344–346.
8. Pediatric Nephrology Group. An analysis of medical pediatric urogenital diseases hospital admissions. *Chinese Pediatr J* 1988;26:102–103.
9. Chiu MC, Tse KC, Lai WM. Dialysis and transplantation in children. *H K J Paediatr* 2002:7.
10. Chiu MC. The problems of childhood chronic renal failure in Hong Kong. *H K J Paediatr* 1993;10:9–13.
11. Renal Registry, Hong Kong Hospital Authority.
12. Chiu W, Wong SN, Chan TM, et al. Paediatric renal transplantation—a single center experience. *J Paediatr Child Health* 1997;suppl:S71.
13. Tse KC, Chiu MC, Lai WM, et al. 10 years experience of paediatric kidney transplantation at a paediatric nephrology center. *H K J Paediatr* 2002;7:173–178.
14. Ministry of Health and Welfare, Republic of Korea. Main Health and Social Welfare Indices, 2002.
15. Seoul National University Hospital. Annual report, 1999.
16. Department of Pediatrics, Seoul National University Children's Hospital. Data not published.
17. Choi IJ, Jeong HJ, Han DS, et al. An analysis of 4514 cases of renal biopsy in Korea. *Yonsei Med J* 2001;42:247–254.
18. Kim KS. The Korean Society of Pediatric Nephrology. Chronic renal failure in children: a nationwide survey in Korea. *Korean J Pediatr Nephrol* 2000;4:92–101.
19. Lin CY. 4th Asian Congress of Pediatric Nephrology, 1993.
20. Sheih CP, Liu MB, Hung CS, et al. Renal abnormalities in school children.
21. Kosnadi L. Studi kolaboratif pola penyakit ginjal anak di Indonesia. 4th National Pediatric Nephrology Symposium, 1989(abst).
22. Alatas H, Pardede SO, Tambunan T, et al. Pola penyakit ginjal dan saluran kemih pada anak di FKUI-RSCM Jakarta (abst). 10th National Congress of Pediatrics, 1996.
23. Tambunan T, Wila Wirya IGN, Alatas H. Spectrum of chronic failure in children in Cipto Mangunkusumo Hospital, Jakarta. *Pediatr Indones* 1990;30:227–232.
24. Albar H, Rauf S. Acute glomerulonephritis in children in Indonesia. A preliminary report of a multi-center study. 12th National Congress of Child Health and 11th ASEAN Pediatric Federation Congress, 2002(abst).

25. Tambunan T. Urinary incontinence in children in Cipto Mangunkusumo Hospital, Jakarta. *Pediatr Indones* 2001;41:171–174.
26. Alatas H. Acute renal failure due to jengkol intoxication in children in Jakarta. *Pediatr Indones* 1989;31:663–671.
27. Tambunan T, Dewanti A, Madiyono B, et al. Pulmonary tuberculosis in childhood nephrotic syndrome (a cross sectional study). *Pediatr Indones* 2001;41:106–110.
28. Lim TO, Lim YN. 8th Report of the Malaysian Dialysis and Transplant Registry, 2001.
29. Yap HK, Chia KS, Murugasu B, et al. Acute glomerulonephritis—changing patterns in Singapore children. *Pediatr Nephrol* 1990;4:482–484.
30. Yap HK, Han EJ, Heng CK, et al. Risk factors for steroid dependency in children with idiopathic nephrotic syndrome. *Pediatr Nephrol* 2001;16:1049–1052.
31. Kabuki N, Okugawa T, Hayakawa H, et al. Influence of age at onset on the outcome of steroid-sensitive nephrotic syndrome. *Pediatr Nephrol* 1998;12:467–470.
32. Yap HK, Gong WK, Foong PP, et al. Predictors of poor outcome to therapy in children with focal segmental glomerulosclerosis. *Pediatr Nephrol* 2001;16:C113(abst).
33. Gong WK, Tan TH, Murugasu B, et al. 18 Years experience in pediatric acute dialysis: analysis of predictors of outcome. *Pediatr Nephrol* 2001;16:212–215.
34. Yap HK. Renal replacement therapy in children: viable options in Singapore. *J Singapore Pediatr Soc* 1992;34:156–160.
35. Yap HK, Ramirez SPB, Chan T, et al. A pilot screening program for hematuria, proteinuria and hypertension in Singapore school children. *Pediatr Nephrol* 2001;16:C34(abst).
36. Ramirez SP, Hsu SI, McClellan W. Low body weight is a risk factor for proteinuria in multiracial Southeast Asian pediatric population. *Am J Kidney Dis* 2001;38:1045–1054.
37. Kashemsant C, Sritubtim W, Tapaneya-Olarn W, et al. The primary nephrotic syndrome in children at Ramathibodi hospital: clinical and clinicopathological study. *J Med Assoc Thai* 1989;72(suppl 1):18–25.
38. Tapaneya-Olarn W. 6th Asian Congress of Pediatric Nephrology, Manila, 1996(abst).
39. Tapaneya-Olarn W, Tapaneya-Olarn C, Boonpucknavig V, et al. Lupus nephritis in children at Ramathibodi hospital. *Ramathibodi Med J* 1989;12:203–207.
40. Tangnararatchakit K, Tapaneya-Olarn C, Tapaneya-Olarn W. The efficacy of intravenous pulse cyclophosphamide in the treatment of severe lupus nephritis in children. *J Med Assoc Thai* 1999;82(suppl 1):S104–S110.
41. Countries of the World 2001 [Web site]. Available at: http://www.ncbuy.com/reference/couintry/th-intro.html. Accessed August 2003.
42. Department of Health Renal Disease Control Program (REDCOP). Philippine Society of Nephrology Renal Disease Registry Report, 2001.
43. Philippine Health Statistics, 1998.
44. Philippine Pediatric Society Registry of Childhood Diseases Update, January–December 1998.
45. Pediatric Nephrology Society of the Philippines Research Study Group Report, 1995–2000.
46. Department of Health Renal Disease Control Program (REDCOP). Philippine Preventive Nephrology Project, 1994–1999.
47. Hanif M, Mobarak MR, Ronan A, et al. Fatal renal failure caused by diethylene glycol in paracetamol elixir—the Bangladesh epidemic. *BMJ* 1995;311:88–91.
48. International Institute for Population Studies (IIPS) and ORC Macro. National Family Health Survey (NFHS-2), 1998-99: India. Mumbai: IIPS, 2000.
49. Indian Pediatric Nephrology Group. Consensus statement on management of steroid sensitive nephrotic syndrome. *Indian Pediatr* 2001;38:975–986.
50. Indian Pediatric Nephrology Group. Consensus statement on management of urinary tract infections. *Indian Pediatr* 2001;38:1106–1115.
51. Consensus statement on management of antenatally detected hydronephrosis. *Indian Pediatr* 2001;38:1244–1251.
52. Srivastava RN, Bagga A. Nephrotic syndrome. In: *Pediatric nephrology*, 3rd ed. New Delhi: Jaypee Brothers, 2001.
53. Gulati S, Kher V, Gupta A, et al. Spectrum of infections in Indian children with nephrotic syndrome. *Pediatr Nephrol* 1995;9:431–434.
54. Bagga A, Sharma A, Srivastava RN. Levamisole therapy in corticosteroid-dependent nephrotic syndrome. *Pediatr Nephrol* 1997;11:415–417.
55. Srivastava RN, Bagga A, Moudgil A. Acute renal failure in north Indian children. *Indian J Med Res* 1990;92:404–408.
56. Srivastava RN, Moudgil A, Bagga A, et al. Hemolytic uremic syndrome in children in northern India. *Pediatr Nephrol* 1991;5:284–288.
57. Hari P, Bagga A, Srivastava RN. Sustained hypertension in children. *Indian Pediatr* 2000;37:268–274.
58. The state of the world's children. 2001 UNICEF.statis.table 1:78–81.
59. Ramzan A, Jamro S, Lakhani B. Nephrotic syndrome in Pakistani children: clinical profile and response to steroid therapy. *Pak Pediatr J* 1995;19:141–145.
60. Ramzan A, Moorani KH. Pattern of renal diseases in children. *J Surg Pakistan* 2001;6:4–12.
61. Colin BA. The epidemiology, formation, composition and medical management of idiopathic stone disease. *Curr Opin Urol* 1993;3:316–322.
62. Rizvi SAH, Naqvi SAA, Hussain Z, et al. Living-related pediatric renal transplants: a single-center experience from a developing country. *Pediatr Transplant* 2002;6:101–110.

INDEX

Note: Page numbers followed by *f* refer to figures; page numbers followed by *t* refer to tables.

F

H

M

O

Q

R

S

T

U

V

W

X

Y

Z